StudentConsult.com

Log on now to access content beyond the print book

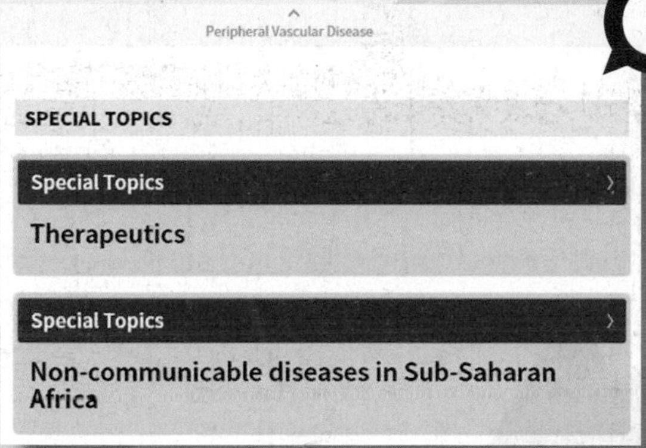
Peripheral Vascular Disease
SPECIAL TOPICS
Special Topics
Therapeutics
Special Topics
Non-communicable diseases in Sub-Saharan Africa

- Special Topics: more drug information, and specific diseases and situations worldwide.

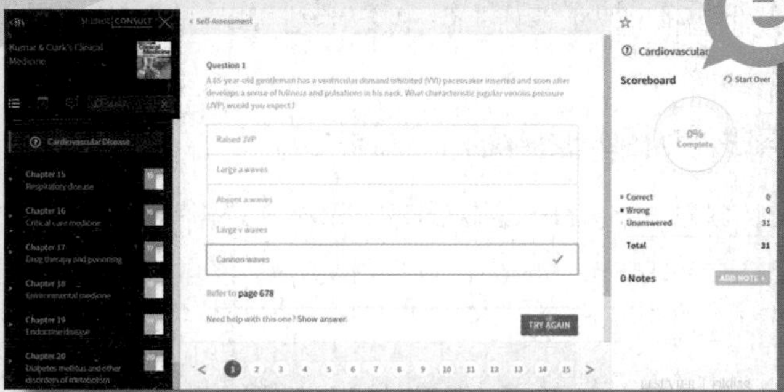

- Self-Assessment: interactive and scored, with feedback.

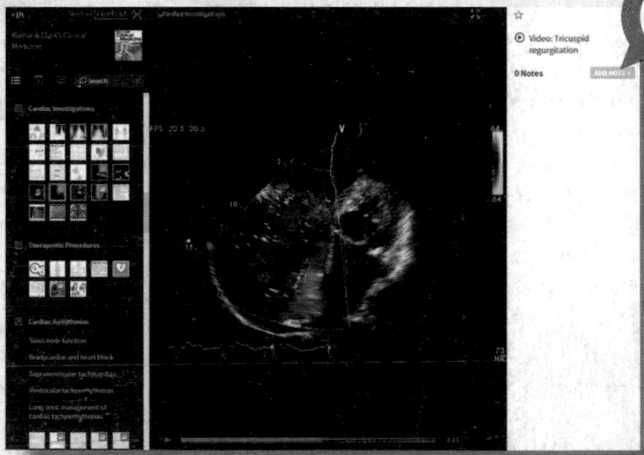

- Videos and Audio: accessible at relevant places in the text, as well as gathered together in a resources chapter to view/listen to what you're most interested in.

- Many more images, to show you, not just tell you.

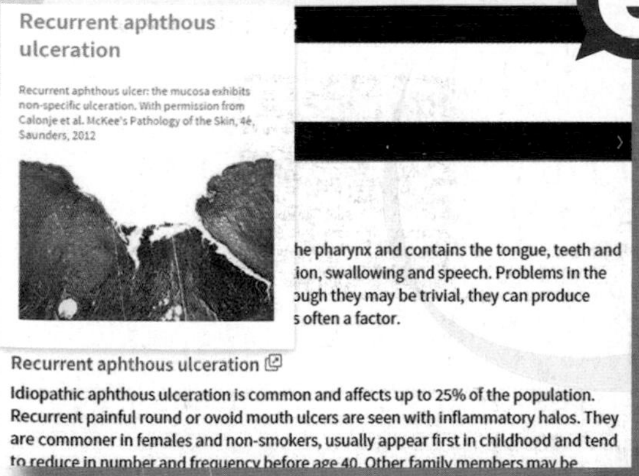
Recurrent aphthous ulceration
Recurrent aphthous ulcer: the mucosa exhibits non-specific ulceration. With permission from Calonje et al. McKee's Pathology of the Skin, 4e, Saunders, 2012
Recurrent aphthous ulceration
Idiopathic aphthous ulceration is common and affects up to 25% of the population. Recurrent painful round or ovoid mouth ulcers are seen with inflammatory halos. They are commoner in females and non-smokers, usually appear first in childhood and tend

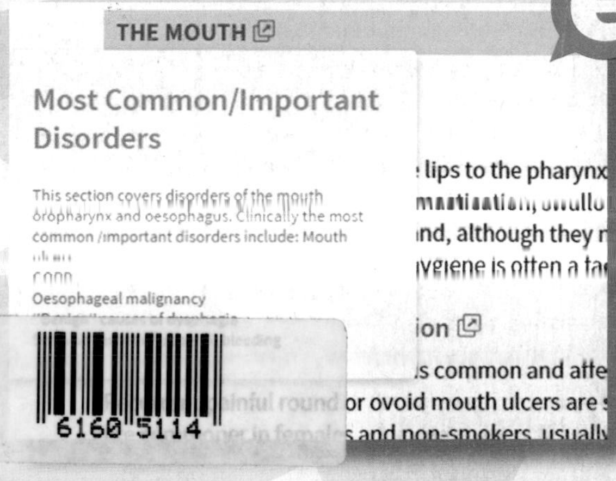
THE MOUTH
Most Common/Important Disorders
Oesophageal malignancy

- Tips, summaries and more from trainees, registrars and young consultants, who know what you need to know.

ELSEVIER

Ninth Edition 2017
Eighth Edition 2012
Seventh Edition 2009
Sixth Edition 2005
Fifth Edition 2002
Fourth Edition 1998
Third Edition 1994
Second Edition 1990
First Edition 1987

Notices

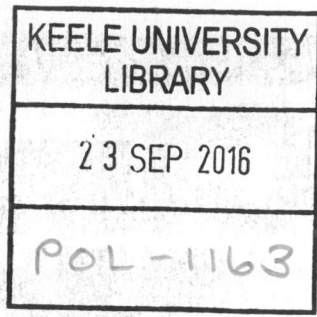

Knowledge and best practice in this field are constantly changing. As new research and experience broaden our understanding, changes in research methods, professional practices, or medical treatment may become necessary.

Practitioners and researchers must always rely on their own experience and knowledge in evaluating and using any information, methods, compounds, or experiments described herein. In using such information or methods they should be mindful of their own safety and the safety of others, including parties for whom they have a professional responsibility.

With respect to any drug or pharmaceutical products identifi ed, readers are advised to check the most current information provided (i) on procedures featured or (ii) by the manufacturer of each product to be administered, to verify the recommended dose or formula, the method and duration of administration, and contraindications. It is the responsibility of practitioners, relying on their own experience and knowledge of their patients, to make diagnoses, to determine dosages and the best treatment for each individual patient, and to take all appropriate safety precautions.

To the fullest extent of the law, neither the Publisher nor the authors, contributors, or editors, assume any liability for any injury and/or damage to persons or property as a matter of products liability, negligence or otherwise, or from any use or operation of any methods, products, instructions, or ideas contained in the material herein.

The Publisher

ISBN 978-0-7020-6601-6
International ISBN 978-0-7020-6599-6
eBook ISBN 978-0-7020-6600-9
Inkling ISBN 978-0-7020-6598-9

For Elsevier
Senior Content Strategist: Pauline Graham
Senior Content Development Specialist: Ailsa Laing
e-Product Content Development Specialist: Kim Benson
Project Manager: Anne Collett
Designer/Design Direction: Christian Bilbow
Illustration Manager: Amy Faith Naylor
Illustrators: Bruce Hogarth, Richard Morris, Ethan Danielson

Printed in The Netherlands

Last digit is the print number: 9 8 7 6 5 4 3 2 1

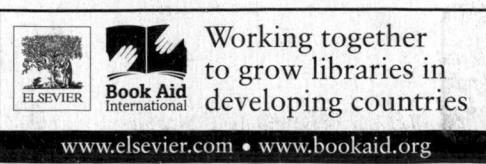

KUMAR & CLARK'S

Clinical Medicine

Ninth Edition

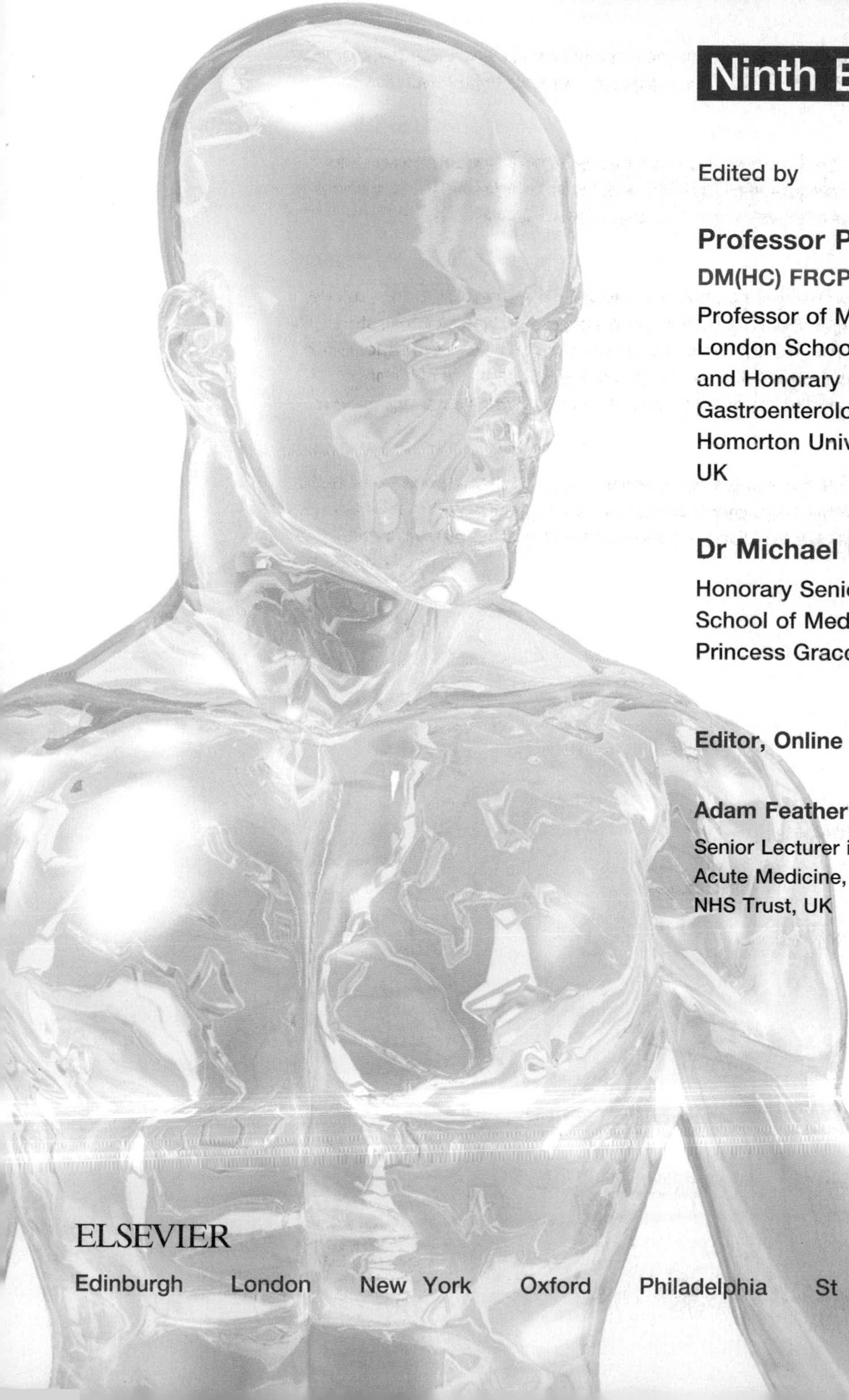

Edited by

Professor Parveen Kumar CBE BSc MD DM(HC) FRCP(L&E) FRCPath
Professor of Medicine and Education, Barts and The London School of Medicine and Dentistry, QMUL, and Honorary Consultant Physician and Gastroenterologist, Barts Health NHS Trust and Homerton University Hospital NHS Foundation Trust, UK

Dr Michael Clark MD FRCP
Honorary Senior Lecturer, Barts and The London School of Medicine and Dentistry, QMUL, and Princess Grace Hospital, UK

Editor, Online Content

Adam Feather FRCP FAcadMEd
Senior Lecturer in Medical Education and Clinical Lead in Acute Medicine, The Royal London Hospital, Barts Health NHS Trust, UK

ELSEVIER

Edinburgh London New York Oxford Philadelphia St Louis Sydney Toronto 2017

Acknowledgements

We would like to thank our many colleagues who have helped in the preparation of this edition by giving us useful advice, helping us to collect photographs and images and reading the manuscripts. A book of this size cannot be accomplished without the help and advice of many. In particular, we would like to acknowledge Peter Garrard, Monica Wolhuter and Susannah Leaver.

We are delighted to welcome several new contributors to this edition and we would like to thank the authors who have stepped down from the book after many years of commitment and loyalty:

- Caroline Byrne (Molecular biology)
- John Camm (Cardiology)
- Charles Clarke (Environmental medicine)
- Meredydd Harries (Special senses)
- Trevor Howlett (Endocrinology)
- Andrew Lister (Oncology)
- James Wainscoat (Haematology)
- David Watson (Critical care)

John Camm and Charles Clarke had been with us since the first edition! We were extremely saddened by the death of Andrew Burroughs (Liver Disease), who was a highly valued colleague and author.

We are very grateful to our specialist registrars, junior trainees and medical students across the world for their input and feedback.

Over the course of several editions, we have made many new friends and colleagues across the world. Our international travels give us much insight into the practice of medicine in different countries. We would like to thank the many colleagues who have escorted us through their hospitals and medical schools. We are extremely grateful to our International Advisory Board members who provide very helpful advice about their regions and contribute articles to the e-book. In particular we would like to thank Professor Janaka de Silva and Professor Senaka Rajapake for their advice, expertise and careful editing of these online contributions.

We are extremely grateful for the support of our publisher, Elsevier, whose staff has maintained a long-term commitment and loyalty to the book. Pauline Graham, our commissioning editor, has now taken us through many editions and has been a constant support. Ailsa Laing, our development editor, has managed the day-to-day work on this edition with great patience and endless good humour. We would also very much like to acknowledge the production team: Anne Collett (production), Christian Bilbow (design), and Kim Benson (development editor for all the electronic content accompanying this book) who have all worked hard to create this extremely high-quality edition. We are also grateful for the meticulous work of the copy editor, Wendy Lee, and proofreader, Glenys Norquay. There are so many other people behind the scenes who have contributed in many ways, and we thank them all for their loyalty and hard work.

Finally, we would like to thank Jillian Linton for secretarial help and the Princess Grace Hospital, London for administrative assistance.

Contents

See your e-book for key learning points, clinical tips, drug tips, extra tables, extra images, interactive Figures, audio, videos, learning challenges, case studies, MCQs and Special Topics from the International Advisory Board.

Online Special Topics

From the International Advisory Board

Contents

e See your e-book for key learning points, clinical tips, drug tips, extra tables, extra images, interactive Figures, audio, videos, learning challenges, case studies, MCQs and Special Topics from the International Advisory Board.

Online Special Topics

From the International Advisory Board

Contributors

Jane Anderson BSc PhD MBBS FRCP
Consultant Physician and Director, Centre for the Study of Sexual Health and HIV, Homerton University Hospital NHS Foundation Trust; Professor, Institute of Cell and Molecular Science, Barts and The London School of Medicine and Dentistry, QMUL, UK
Sexually transmitted infections and human immunodeficiency virus

John V Anderson MD MA MBBS FRCP
Consultant Physician, Homerton University Hospital NHS Foundation Trust and Barts Health NHS Trust, London, UK
Diabetes mellitus
Lipid and metabolic disorders

Neil Ashman PhD FRCP
Consultant Nephrologist and Clinical Director, Department of Renal Medicine and Transplantation, Barts Health NHS Trust, London, UK
Kidney and urinary tract disease

Gavin Barlow MBChB DTM&H MD FRCP
Consultant Physician in Infectious Diseases/General Medicine, Hull and East Yorkshire Hospitals NHS Trust; Clinical Associate, Centre for Immunology and Infection, University of York, UK
Infectious diseases and tropical medicine

Sara Booth MD FRCP
Macmillan Consultant in Palliative Medicine, Clinical Director of Palliative Care, Palliative Care Service, Addenbrooke's Hospital, Cambridge University Hospitals NHS Foundation Trust, UK
Palliative medicine and symptom control

Julius Bourke MBBS MRCPsych
Clinical Lecturer, Centre for Psychiatry, Wolfson Institute of Preventive Medicine, Barts and The London School of Medicine and Dentistry, QMUL, UK
Psychological medicine

Deborah Bowman PhD
Senior Lecturer in Medical Ethics and Law, Division of Population Health Sciences and Education, St George's, University of London, UK
Ethics, law and communication

Sally M Bradberry BSc MD FRCP FAACT FEAPCCT
Deputy Director, National Poisons Information Service (Birmingham Unit) and Director, West Midlands Poisons Unit, City Hospital, UK
Poisoning

Matthew S Buckland MSc PhD FRCP FRCPath FHEA
Consultant in Clinical Immunology, Royal London Hospital, Barts Health NHS Trust, UK
The immune system and disease

Nicholas H Bunce BSc MBBS MD
Consultant Cardiologist, St George's Healthcare NHS Trust, London, UK
Cardiovascular disease

Rachel Buxton-Thomas MBBS MRCP
Consultant Respiratory Physician, Brighton and Sussex University Hospitals, UK
Respiratory disease

Richard Conway MD
Rheumatology Specialist Registrar, Department of Rheumatology, Galway University Hospitals, Ireland
Bone disease

Annie Cushing PhD FDSRCS(Eng) BDS(Hons)
Reader in Clinical Communication Skills, Institute of Health Sciences Education, Barts and The London School of Medicine and Dentistry, QMUL, UK
Ethics, law and communication

Sarah R Doffman MB ChB FRCP
Consultant Respiratory Physician, Brighton and Sussex University Hospitals NHS Trust, Royal Sussex County Hospital, UK
Respiratory disease

Marinos Elia BSc(Hons) MD FRCP
Professor of Clinical Nutrition and Metabolism, Institute of Human Nutrition, University of Southampton, UK
Nutrition

Gail E Eva PhD
Research Fellow, Department of Brain Repair and Rehabilitation, Institute of Neurology, University College London, UK
Palliative medicine and symptom control

Graham Foster BA FRCP PhD
Professor of Hepatology, Barts and The London School of Medicine and Dentistry, QMUL; Consultant, Barts Health NHS Trust, UK
Liver disease

Anthony J Frew MA MD FRCP
Professor of Allergy and Respiratory Medicine, Brighton and Sussex Medical School; Chief Physician, Brighton and Sussex University Hospitals NHS Trust, UK
Respiratory disease

Edwin AM Gale MBBChir FRCP
Professor of Diabetic Medicine, University of Bristol, UK
Diabetes mellitus
Lipid and metabolic disorders

Christopher J Gallagher MBChB PhD FRCP
Consultant Medical Oncologist, St Bartholomew's Hospital, Barts Health NHS Trust, London, UK
Malignant disease

Ian Giles BSc MBBS MRCP PhD
Reader in Rheumatology, Centre for Rheumatology, Department of Medicine, University College London, UK
Rheumatic disease

Helena Gleeson MBBS MRCP(UK) MD
Consultant in Endocrinology, Department of Endocrinology, Queen Elizabeth Hospital, Birmingham, UK
Endocrine disease

Robin D Hamilton MBBS DM FRCOphth
Consultant Ophthalmologist, Moorfields Eye Hospital, London, UK
Ear, nose and throat and eye disease

Charles J Hinds FRCP FRCA
Professor of Intensive Care Medicine, William Harvey Research Institute, Barts and The London School of Medicine and Dentistry, QMUL, and Barts Health NHS Trust, UK
Critical care medicine

Katharine Hurt MBBS MRCP
Consultant Respiratory Physician, Brighton and Sussex University Hospitals, UK
Respiratory disease

William L Irving MA PhD MBBChir MRCP FRCPath
Professor of Virology, University of Nottingham, UK
Infectious diseases and tropical medicine

Paul Jarman MA MBBS(Hons) PhD
Consultant Neurologist, National Hospital for Neurology and Neurosurgery, London, UK
Neurological disease

Miriam J Johnson MD FRCP MRCGP MBChB(Hons)
Senior Lecturer in Palliative Medicine, Hull York Medical School, UK
Palliative medicine and symptom control

David P Kelsell PhD
Professor of Human Molecular Genetics, Centre for Cutaneous Research, Blizard Institute of Cell and Molecular Sciences, Barts and The London School of Medicine and Dentistry, QMUL, UK
Molecular cell biology and human genetics

Louise Langmead MRCP MD
Consultant Gastroenterologist, Royal London Hospital, Barts Health NHS Trust, UK
Gastrointestinal disease

Susan A Lanham-New BA MSc PhD RNutr FAfN FSB
Professor of Nutrition, Head of Department of Nutritional Sciences, School of Biosciences and Medicine, University of Surrey, Guildford, UK
Nutrition

Miles J Levy MD FRCP
Consultant Physician and Endocrinologist, Leicester Royal Infirmary, University Hospitals of Leicester NHS Trust, UK
Endocrine disease

James Lindsay MA PhD BMBCh MRCP
Consultant Gastroenterologist, Barts Health NHS Trust, Royal London Hospital, UK
Gastrointestinal disease

Kenneth J Linton PhD
Professor of Protein Biochemistry, Centre for Cutaneous Research, Blizard Institute of Cell and Molecular Sciences, Barts and The London School of Medicine and Dentistry, QMUL, UK
Molecular cell biology and human genetics

Kieran McCafferty MA MBBChir MRCP MD(res)
Consultant Nephrologist, Department of Nephrology, Barts Health NHS Trust; Senior Lecturer, Department of Nephrology, Barts and The London School of Medicine and Dentistry, QMUL, UK
Water, electrolytes and acid–base balance

Adam Mead MD PhD MRCP FRCPath
Associate Professor of Haematology, Weatherall Institute of Molecular Medicine, University of Oxford, UK
Haematological disease

Nishchay Mehta BSc MBBS MRCS DOHNS
Specialist Registrar in Otorhinolaryngology, University College London Hospital, UK
Ear, nose and throat and eye disease

Peter J Moss MBChB MD FRCP DTMH
Consultant in Infectious Diseases, Department of Infection and Tropical Medicine, and Director of Infection Prevention and Control, and Deputy Medical Director, Hull and East Yorkshire Hospitals NHS Trust, UK
Infectious diseases and tropical medicine

Edward WS Mullins PhD MRCOG
Editor, *Chief Medical Officer's Annual Report*, NW London Obstetrics and Gynaecology Training Programme, UK
Women's Health

Michael F Murphy MD FRCP FRCPath
Professor of Blood Transfusion Medicine, University of Oxford; Consultant Haematologist, NHS Blood and Transplant and Department of Haematology, Oxford Radcliffe Hospitals NHS Trust, UK
Haematological disease

Catherine Nelson-Piercy MA FRCP FRCOG
Professor of Obstetric Medicine, Women's Health Academic Centre, St Thomas' Hospital; Consultant Obstetric Physician, Guy's and St Thomas' NHS Foundation Trust, London, UK
Women's health

Alastair O'Brien MBBS BSc MRCP PhD
Clinical Senior Lecturer, Division of Medicine, University College London, UK
Liver disease

Michael J O'Dwyer MBBS FFARCSI FCICM PhD
Senior Lecturer in Intensive Care Medicine, Barts and The London School of Medicine and Dentistry, QMUL, UK
Critical care medicine

Donncha O'Gradaigh MB PhD FFSEM MRCPI
Consultant Rheumatologist, Department of Rheumatology, Waterford Regional Hospital, Ireland
Bone disease

David G Paige MA MBBS FRCP
Consultant Dermatologist, Barts Health NHS Trust, London, UK
Skin disease

K John Pasi PhD MBChB FRCP FRCPath FRCPCH
Professor of Haemostasis and Thrombosis, Centre for Haematology, Institute of Cell and Molecular Science, Barts and The London School of Medicine and Dentistry, QMUL, UK
Haematological disease

Mark Peakman MBBS BSc MSc PhD FRCPath
Professor of Clinical Immunology, King's College London School of Medicine, UK
The immune system and disease

Rupert M Pearse MD
Senior Lecturer, Barts and The London School of Medicine and Dentistry, QMUL; Consultant in Intensive Care Medicine, Barts Health NHS Trust, UK
Critical care medicine

Sir Munir Pirmohamed MBChB(Hons) PhD FRCP FRCP(Edin) FMedSci
David Weatherall Chair of Medicine and NHS Chair of Pharmacogenetics, Head of Department of Molecular and Clinical Pharmacology, Wolfson Centre for Personalised Medicine, Institute of Translational Medicine, University of Liverpool, UK
Clinical pharmacology

Sean L Preston BSc(Hons) PhD MBBS MRCP
Consultant Gastroenterologist, Barts Health NHS Trust, Royal London Hospital, UK
Gastrointestinal disease

Anisur Rahman MA PhD BMBCh FRCP
Professor of Rheumatology, University College London, UK
Rheumatic disease

Sir Michael Rawlins MD FRCP FMedSci
Chair of the Medicines and Healthcare Products Regulatory Agency; Chairman of UK Biobank, UK
Clinical pharmacology

Robin Ray MBBS MA(Oxon) MRCP PhD
Consultant in Heart failure and Cardiac Imaging, St George's University Hospitals NHS Foundation Trust, London, UK

Lesley Regan MD DSC FRCOG FACOG
Professor of Obstetrics and Gynaecology, Imperial College at St Mary's Hospital, London, UK
Women's health

Babulal Sethia BSc MBBS FRCS
Consultant Congenital Heart Surgeon, Royal Brompton Hospital; President and Lead for Global Health, Royal Society of Medicine, London, UK
Global health

Jonathan Shamash MBChB MD FRCP
Consultant Medical Oncologist, Barts Health NHS Trust, London, UK
Malignant disease

Matthew Smith MA MD MRCP FRCPath
Consultant Haemato-Oncologist, Barts Health NHS Trust, London, UK
Malignant disease

J Allister Vale MD FRCP FRCP(Edin) FRCP(Glasg) FFOM FAACT FBTS FBPhS FEAPCCT Hon FRCPS(Glasg)
Director, National Poisons Information Service (Birmingham Unit), City Hospital, UK
Poisoning

Francis Vaz MBBS BSc(Hons) FRCS(ORL-HNS)
Consultant Ear, Nose and Throat/Head and Neck Surgeon, Department of ENT/Head and Neck Surgery, University College London Hospital, UK
Ear, nose and throat and eye disease

Christopher Wadsworth MBBS PhD MRCP
Consultant Gastroenterologist and Hepato-Pancreato-Biliary Physician, Hammersmith Hospital, Imperial College Healthcare NHS Trust, London, UK
Biliary tract and pancreatic disease

Sarah H Wakelin BSc MBBS FRCP
Consultant Dermatologist, Imperial College Healthcare NHS Trust, London, UK
Skin disease

David Westaby MA(Cantab) FRCP
Consultant Physician and Gastroenterologist, Director of Endoscopic Service, Lead for Hepatobiliary Medicine, Imperial College Healthcare NHS Trust, Hammersmith Hospital, London, UK
Biliary tract and pancreatic disease

Peter D White MD FRCP FRCPsych
Professor of Psychological Medicine, Centre for Psychiatry, Wolfson Institute of Preventive Medicine, Barts and The London School of Medicine and Dentistry, QMUL, UK
Psychological medicine

Janet D Wilson MBChB FRCP
Consultant in Genitourinary Medicine and HIV, Centre for Sexual Health, Leeds Teaching Hospitals NHS Trust, UK
Sexually transmitted infections and human immunodeficiency virus

M Magdi Yaqoob MD FRCP
Professor of Nephrology, William Harvey Research Institute, Barts and The London School of Medicine and Dentistry, QMUL; Consultant, Department of Renal Medicine and Transplantation, Barts Health NHS Trust, UK
Kidney and urinary tract disease
Water, electrolytes and acid–base balance

Online contributors

Jahangir Ahmed MA MRCS DoHNS PGCMed PhD
Specialist Registrar in Otolaryngology, North Thames Deanery, London, UK

Neil Chauhan MBBS MRCP FRCPath PGCert
Consultant Haematologist, Homerton University Hospital NHS Foundation Trust, London, UK

Subathira Dakshina BSc(Hons) MBChB MRCP DipGUM DFSRH
Specialist Registrar in Genitourinary Medicine and HIV, Barts Health NHS Trust, London, UK

Adam Feather FRCP FAcadMEd
Senior Lecturer in Medical Education and Clinical Lead in Acute Medicine, The Royal London Hospital, Barts Health NHS Trust, UK

Jessica Gale MBChB MRCP
Dermatology Registrar, The Royal London Hospital, UK

Khalid Ghufoor MBBS BSC FRCS(CSiG) FRCS(ORL-HNS)
ENT Head and Neck Consultant Surgeon, Head of Department, The Royal London and St Bartholomew's Hospital and The Royal National Throat Nose and Ear Hospital, University College London Hospital, UK

Matthew D Gillam BMBCh MA(Oxon)
Specialist Trainee in Ophthalmology, Department of Ophthalmology, Royal London Hospital, UK

Rebecca J Gorrigan BSc MBChB(Hons) MRCP
Diabetes & Endocrinology Registrar, Royal London Hospital, UK

Salman Haider BSc(Hons) MRCP
Specialty Registrar in Neurology, London Deanery, UK

Sibylle Herzig van Wees PhD (c) MSc BSc
Teaching Fellow in Global Health, King's Centre for Global Health, King's College London, UK

Noor Jawad BSc MBBS PhD MRCP
Consultant Gastroenterologist, Barts Health NHS Trust, London, UK

Vikas Kapil MA MBBS MRCP PhD
Consultant, Barts Heart Centre, Barts Health NHS Trust, London, UK

Charleen Lia MD MRCOG
Senior Clinical Fellow in Obstetrics and Gynaecology, Addenbrooke's Hospital, Cambridge, UK

Deirdre Ashling Lillis BA(Cantab) MBBS MRCP(UK)
Acute Medicine Registrar, King George Hospital, Essex, UK

Angela McGilloway BMedSci MBBS MRCPsych MRes
ST5 Psychiatry Trainee, East London NHS Foundation Trust, UK

Rebecca Marcus BSc MBChB MRCP DTMH DipGU DFSRH
Specialist Registrar, Genitourinary and HIV Medicine, Barts Health NHS Trust, London, UK

Anjali Mullick MBBCh MA
Medical Director and Consultant in Palliative Medicine, St Peter's Hospice, Bristol, UK

Angela Pakozdi MD PhD
Specialist Registrar in Rheumatology, Department of Rheumatology, Barts Health NHS Trust, London, UK

Rishma Pau MBChB BSc MRCP(UK)
Specialty Registrar in Palliative Medicine, St Joseph's Hospice, London, UK

Sarah JL Payne MRCP PhD
Senior Clinical Fellow in Medical Oncology, Guy's and St Thomas' NHS Trust, London, UK

Jessica Potter MBBCh BA(Hons)
Clinical Lecturer, Centre for Primary Care and Public Health, Blizard Institute, QMUL, London, UK

Christopher Primus MBBS(DICP) BSc(Hons) MRCP(London)
Cardiology Registrar, Barts Heart Centre, Barts Health NHS Trust, London, UK

David Randall MA MRCP
Specialty Registrar, Renal Medicine, Department of Renal Medicine and Transplantation, Royal London Hospital, Barts Health NHS Trust, UK

M Ashwin Reddy MA MBBChir MD FRCOphth
Consultant Ophthalmologist, Department of Ophthalmology, Royal London Hospital, and Department of Paediatrics, Moorfields Eye Hospital, UK

Lesley Robson BSc PhD
Head of Year 1 and 2 MBBS, Reader in Musculoskeletal Medicine, Institute of Health Science Education, Barts and The London School of Medicine and Dentistry, QMUL, UK

Meera Shah MBChB BSc(Hons) MRCP (UK)
Specialist Registrar in Gastroenterology and Hepatology, The Royal London Hospital, Barts Health NHS Trust, UK

Johannes de Vos BSc MD FRCPath
Consultant Haematologist, Haematology Department, Royal Surrey County Hospital, Guildford, UK

SPECIAL ADVISOR

Vikas Kapil MA MBBS MRCP PhD
Consultant, Barts Heart Centre, Barts Health NHS Trust, London, UK

International Advisory Board

Preface to the Ninth Edition

Clinical Medicine is now approaching its 30th anniversary. It was first published in 1987 and is now firmly established as a companion to all medical students, young doctors and healthcare professionals. The book has been described as the 'gold standard' guide to clinical medicine and, with an excellent author team, we have striven to keep to these high standards.

There are several innovations in this edition. We have added two new chapters: Women's health and Global health. Women's health has been added to include women's disorders as well as those occurring in pregnancy. Global health has now entered the curricula in many medical schools in acknowledgement that inequalities and inadequacies of healthcare worldwide need to be vigorously tackled to improve the health of all people.

Infections travel fast across continents, as we have seen with the emergence of Ebola and Zika virus epidemics. To allow for fuller discussion of diseases posing particular problems in specific parts of the world, further short Special Topics have been written for the e-book by expert members of our International Advisory Board.

It is a difficult task to be both a comprehensive reference book and also be learner-friendly. However, we have taken much advice from our readers and sought to address this challenge in two main ways. In the print book we have redistributed information in several chapters to break down the content and facilitate learner engagement. Larger chapters have been sub-divided. We have added diagrammatic overviews to all the appropriate systems-based chapters; headings have been put into colour to define whether the text relates to management, disease or basic science. In the e-book that accompanies your print copy, we have appointed a team of registrars, under the editorship of Adam Feather, to take on the task of providing online key learning outcomes, clinical tips, drug tips, videos, audio, extra images, and self-assessment to help learners of all levels to get what they need from the content. Keep checking your e-book to be advised of further developments, as we are also working to provide 'scaled' versions of the text online (which allow the reader to 'zoom' in or out for different levels of detail).

We very much hope you will enjoy reading this edition and find the information easily accessible for learning. Thank you all for your suggestions, which are always welcome.

Parveen Kumar and Mike Clark

HOW TO USE THIS BOOK

The **First Section** contains general topics for the overall practice of medicine, and the Second Section contains the basic sciences. Essentially these contain communication skills, general topics such as pharmacology, poisoning and global health, and the fundamental basics of science. These chapters can be read alone but can also be used as a reference for other chapters where a basic mechanism has been discussed.

The **Third Section** contains clinical chapters with the medical specialities for easy accessibility and to aid the day-to-day practice of medicine.

Chapter format

Each clinical chapter has its own anatomy, physiology and pathology for understanding the presentation of the problems of that speciality. This is followed, where appropriate, by clinical symptoms and signs in general. For the appropriate systems chapters a diagrammatic overview of the anatomy and physiology has been provided.

Individual diseases have an introduction, followed by pathogenesis, aetiology, clinical features, investigations, management and prognosis. These have colour codes to make them easy to follow:

Conditions-related headings (e.g. 'pernicious anaemia')
Disease-specific headings (e.g. 'investigations')
Anatomy/physiology headings (e.g. 'structure')

Boxes

Boxes have been classified by the type of information they provide and have the following symbols:

- Pearls and Tips
- Table
- Emergency
- Information
- Differential diagnosis
- Frailty
- Practical

Emergency Boxes are in red

E-Book enhancements

Click on icons throughout the e-Book to popup the added clinical and drug tips, images, key learning outcomes, videos, audio, extra images, and self-assessment, etc. Click on selected figures to open interactive versions.

Prescribing

We have used the recommended International Non-proprietary Names (rINNs) for all drugs. In some diseases where a particular formulation of a drug is required, the proprietary name is used. Drugs have been spelled by their international names, e.g. bendroflumethazide and not bendrofluazide, and amfetamine and not amphetamine. For adrenaline and noradrenaline, we have added epinephrine and norepinephrine in brackets as these names are often used in emergency guidelines across the world.

Dosages have been given where appropriate but we recommend that all readers check with their national formularies for the exact dosages. We would strongly recommend that this is done every time you use a drug which is unfamiliar to you and not part of your daily practice.

Units of measurements

We have used the International System of Units (SI units) throughout the book. On occasion, if there is a possibility for confusion, we have also used non-SI-units and given a conversion factor.

Evidence based medicine

This is embedded within the book and not singled out as we feel it is a part of one's learning and the way we should practise medicine.

Also in the Kumar & Clark family:

- *Kumar & Clark's Medical Management and Therapeutics*
- Ballinger: *Essentials of Kumar & Clark's Clinical Medicine*
- Kumar & Clark: *Cases in Clinical Medicine*
- Henry & Thompson: *Clinical Surgery*
- O'Reilly et al.: *Essentials of Obstetrics and Gynaecology 2E*
- Thalange et al.: *Essentials of Paediatrics 2E*
- Franklin et al.: *Essentials of Clinical Surgery 2E*

1 Ethics, law and communication

Deborah Bowman, Annie Cushing

See your e-book for MCQs and situational judgement tests.

ETHICS AND THE LAW

ETHICS

The practice of medicine is inherently moral:

- Biomedical expertise and clinical science have to be applied by and to people.
- Medical decisions are underpinned by values and principles.
- Potential courses of action will have implications that are often uncertain.
- Technological advancements sometimes have unintended or unforeseen consequences.

The profession has to agree on its collective purpose, aims and standards. People are much more than a collection of symptoms and signs – they have preferences, priorities, fears and hopes. Doctors too are much more than interpreters of symptoms and signs – they also have preferences, priorities, fears and hopes. Ethics is part of practice; it is a practical pursuit.

The study of the moral dimension of medicine is known as ***medical ethics*** in the UK and ***bioethics*** internationally. Becoming, and practising as, a doctor require an awareness of, and reflection on, one's ethical attitudes. All of us have personal values and moral intuitions. In the field of ethics, a necessary part of learning is to become aware of the assumptions on which these personal values are based, to reflect on them critically, and to listen and respond to challenging or opposing beliefs.

Ethics is commonly characterized as the consideration of big moral questions that preoccupy the media. Questions about cloning, stem cells and euthanasia are what many immediately think of when the words 'medical ethics' are used. However, ethics pervades all of medicine. The daily and routine workload is rife with ethical questions and dilemmas; introductions to patients, dignity on the wards, the use of resources in clinic, the choice of antibiotic and the medical report for a third party are as central to ethics as the issues that pervade the popular representation of this area.

The study and practice of ethics incorporate knowledge, cognitive skills such as reasoning, critique and logical analysis, and clinical skills. Abstract ethical understanding has to be integrated with other clinical knowledge and applied thoughtfully and appropriately in practice.

Ethical practice: sources, resources and approaches

Engaging with an ethical issue in clinical practice depends on:

- discerning the relevant moral question(s)
- looking at the relevant ethical theories and/or tools
- identifying applicable guidance (e.g. from a professional body)
- integrating the ethical analysis with an accurate account of the law (both national and international).

Personal views must be taken into account, but other perspectives should be acknowledged and supported by reasoning, and located in an accurate understanding of the current law and relevant professional guidance.

Ethical theories and frameworks

Key ethical theories are summarized in ***Box 1.1***.

Many doctors find that ethical frameworks and tools that focus on the application of ethical theory to clinical problems are useful. Perhaps the best known is the 'Four Principles' approach, in which the principles are:

1. ***Autonomy***: allowing 'self-rule', i.e. letting patients make their own choices and decide what happens to them
2. ***Beneficence***: doing good, i.e. acting in a patient's best interests
3. ***Non-maleficence***: avoiding harm
4. ***Justice***: treating people equitably and fairly.

Box 1.1 Key ethical theories

- ***Deontology***: a universally applicable rule or duty-based approach to morality, e.g. a deontologist would argue that one should always tell the truth, irrespective of the consequences.
- ***Consequentialism***: an approach that argues that morality is located in consequences. Such an approach will focus on likely risks and benefits.
- ***Virtue ethics***: an approach in which particular traits or behaviours are identified as desirable.
- ***Rights theory***: an assessment of morality with reference to the justified claims of others. Rights are either 'natural' and arise from being human, or legal and therefore enforceable in court. Positive rights impose a duty on another to act, whilst negative rights prohibit interference by others.
- ***Narrative ethics***: an approach that argues that morality is embedded in the stories shared between patient and clinician, and allows for multiple perspectives.

For some, a consistent process that incorporates the best of each theoretical approach is helpful. So, whatever the ethical question, one should:

- summarize the problem and state the moral dilemma(s)
- identify the assumptions being made or to be made
- analyse with reference to ethical principles, consequences, professional guidance and the law
- acknowledge other approaches and state the preferred approach with explanation.

People respond differently to ethical theories and approaches. Do not be afraid to experiment with ways of thinking about ethics. It is worthwhile understanding other ethical approaches, even in broad terms, as it helps in understanding how others might approach the same ethical problem, especially given the increasingly global context in which healthcare is delivered.

PROFESSIONAL GUIDANCE AND CODES OF PRACTICE

As well as ethical theories and frameworks, there are codes of practice and professional guidelines. For example, in the UK, the standards set out by the General Medical Council (GMC) are the basis on which doctors are regulated within the UK; if a doctor falls below the expectations of the GMC, disciplinary procedures may follow, irrespective of the harm caused or whether legal action ensues. In other countries, similar professional bodies exist to license doctors and regulate healthcare. All clinicians should be aware of the regulatory framework and professional standards in the country within which they are practising.

Increasingly, ethical practice and professionalism are considered significant from the earliest days of medical study and training. In the UK, attention has turned to the standards expected of medical students. For example, in the UK, all medical schools are required to have 'Fitness to Practise' procedures. Students should be aware of their professional obligations from the earliest days of their admission to a medical degree. All medical schools are effectively vouching for a student's suitability for provisional registration at graduation. Medical students commonly work with patients from the earliest days of their training and are privileged in the access they have to vulnerable people, confidential information and sensitive situations. As such, medical schools have particular responsibilities to ensure that students behave professionally and are fit to study, and eventually to practise, medicine.

The Hippocratic Oath, although well known, is outdated and something of an ethical curiosity, with the result that it is rarely, if ever, sworn. The symbolic value of taking an oath remains, however, and many medical schools expect students to make a formal commitment to maintain ethical standards.

Further reading

General Medical Council. *Good Medical Practice*. London: GMC; 2012.
General Medical Council. *Medical Students: Professional Values and Fitness to Practise*. London: GMC; 2009.
General Medical Council. *The 21st Century Doctor: Understanding the Doctors of Tomorrow*. London: GMC; 2010.

THE LAW

As it pertains to medicine, the law establishes boundaries for what is deemed to be acceptable professional practice. The law that applies to medicine is both national and international: for example, the European Convention on Human Rights ***(Box 1.2)***. Within the UK, along with other jurisdictions, both statutes and common law apply to the practice of medicine ***(Box 1.3)***.

The majority of cases involving healthcare arise in the civil system. Occasionally, a medical case is subject to criminal law: for example, when a patient dies in circumstances that could constitute manslaughter.

Box 1.2 European Convention on Human Rights: substantive rights that apply to evaluating good medical practice

- Right to life (Article 2)
- Prohibition of torture, inhuman or degrading treatment or punishment (Article 3)
- Prohibition of slavery and forced labour (Article 4)
- Right to liberty and security (Article 5)
- Right to a fair trial (Article 6)
- No punishment without law (Article 7)
- Right to respect for private and family life (Article 8)
- Freedom of thought, conscience and religion (Article 9)
- Freedom of expression (Article 10)
- Right to marry (Article 12)
- Prohibition of discrimination (Article 14)

Box 1.3 Statutes and common law

Statutes

- Primary legislation made by the state, e.g. Acts of Parliament in the UK, such as the Mental Capacity Act 2005
- Secondary (or delegated) legislation: supplementary law made by an authority given the power to do so by the primary legislation
- Implementation (or statutory) guidance, e.g. the Mental Health Act Code of Practice

Common law

- Judicial decisions made in cases: these establish precedents that are then applied to future cases
- Precedent: whether a decision constitutes a precedent depends on which court made the decision – higher-level courts have authority over lower-level courts

RESPECT FOR AUTONOMY: CAPACITY AND CONSENT

Capacity

Capacity is at the heart of ethical decision-making because it is the gateway to self-determination ***(Box 1.4)***. People are able to make choices only if they have capacity. The assessment of capacity is a significant undertaking; a patient's freedom to choose depends on it. If a person lacks capacity, it is meaningless to seek consent. In the UK, the Mental Capacity Act 2005 sets out the criteria for assessing whether a person has the capacity to make a decision (see Ch. 22, p. 930).

Box 1.4 Principles of self-determination[a]

- Every adult has the right to make his/her own decisions and to be assumed to have capacity unless proved otherwise.
- Everyone should be encouraged and enabled to make his/her own decisions, or to participate as fully as possible in decision-making.
- Individuals have the right to make eccentric or unwise decisions.
- Proxy decisions should consider best interests, prioritizing what the patient would have wanted, and should be the 'least restrictive of basic rights and freedoms'.

[a]Principles underlying the Mental Capacity Act 2005 (England and Wales), which applies to patients over the age of 16 years.

Assessment of capacity is not a one-off judgement. Capacity can fluctuate and assessments of capacity should be regularly reviewed. Capacity should be understood as task-oriented. People may have capacity to make some choices but not others, and capacity is not automatically precluded by specific diagnoses or impairments. The way in which a doctor communicates can enhance or diminish a patient's capacity, as can pain, fatigue and the environment.

Consent

Consent is integral to ethical and lawful practice. To act without, or in opposition to, a patient's expressed, valid consent is, in many jurisdictions, to commit an assault or battery. Obtaining informed consent fosters choice and gives meaning to autonomy. Valid consent is:

- given by a patient who has capacity to make a choice about his or her care
- voluntary, i.e. free from undue pressure, coercion or persuasion
- sufficiently informed
- continuing, i.e. patients should know that they can change their mind at any time.

The basis of informed consent

Those seeking consent for a particular procedure must be competent in the knowledge of how the procedure is performed and its problems. Whilst it is common and good practice for written information to be provided to patients, the existence of written material and a consent form does not remove the responsibility to talk to the patient. The information given to a patient should be that which a 'reasonable person' would require whilst being alert to the particular priorities and concerns of individuals. Information shared should:

- cover risks and benefits
- explain possible consequences of treatment and non-treatment
- explain options
- disclose uncertainty; this should be as much part of the discussion as sharing what is well understood.

Patients should be encouraged to ask questions and express their concerns and preferences. Since it is the health and lives of patients that are potentially at risk, the moral focus of such disclosure should be on what is acceptable to patients rather than to the professionals.

Consent in educational settings

Much medical education and training takes place in the clinical environment. Future doctors have to learn new skills and apply their knowledge to real patients. However, patients must be given a choice as to whether they wish to participate in educational activities. The principles of seeking consent for education are identical to those applied to clinical situations.

Advance decisions

Advance decisions (sometimes colloquially described as 'living wills') enable people to express their wishes about future treatment or interventions. The decisions are made in anticipation of a time when a person ceases to have capacity. Different countries have differing approaches to advance decision-making and it is necessary to be aware of the relevant law in the area in which one is practising. Within the UK, advance decisions are governed by legislation; for example, the Mental Capacity Act 2005 applies in England and Wales. The criteria for a legally valid advanced decision are that it is:

- made by someone with capacity
- made voluntarily
- based on appropriate information
- specific and applicable to the situation in which it is being considered.

In practice, it is often the requirement of specificity that is most difficult for patients to fulfil because of the inevitable uncertainty surrounding future illness and potential treatments or interventions. There is one issue that, for many, goes to the heart of an ethical objection to advance decision-making: namely, the difficulty in anticipating the future and how one is likely to feel about that future.

Scope

An advance decision can be made to refuse treatment and to express preferences, but cannot be used to demand treatment. In general, no patient has the right to demand or request treatment that is not clinically indicated. Therefore it would be inconsistent to allow patients to include in their advance decisions requests for specific treatments, procedures or interventions. An advance decision cannot be used to refuse basic care, such as maintaining hygiene.

Format

Advance decisions are made orally or in writing. However, advance decisions on the withdrawal or withholding of life-sustaining treatment must be in written form and witnessed, and the decision should state explicitly that it is intended to apply even to life-saving situations. The more informal and non-specific the advance decision is, the more likely it is to be challenged or disregarded as being invalid. If working in a country where advance decisions are recognized, clinicians should make reasonable attempts to establish whether there is a valid advance decision in place; the presumption is to save life where there is ambiguity about either the existence or the content of an advance decision. Advance decisions should be periodically reviewed and amendments, revocations or additions are possible, provided that the person concerned still has capacity.

Ethical and practical rationale

The ethical rationale for the acceptance of advance decisions is usually said to be respect for patient autonomy and it represents the extension of the right to make choices about healthcare in the future. True respect for autonomy and the freedom to choose necessarily involves allowing people to make choices that others might consider misguided. Some suggest that giving patients the opportunity to express their concerns, preferences and reservations about the future management of their health fosters trust and effective relationships with clinicians. However, it could also be argued that none of us will ever have the capacity to make decisions about our future care because the person we become when ill is qualitatively different from the person we are when we are healthy.

Lasting power of attorney

Many countries allow for the appointment of a proxy, or for a third party, to make substituted judgements for people lacking capacity. In England and Wales, consent or refusal can be expressed by someone who has been granted a lasting power of attorney (LPA). Once a person's lack of capacity has been registered with the Public Guardian and the LPA granted, the person holding the power of attorney is charged with representing a patient's best interests. Therefore, it is imperative to establish whether there is a valid LPA in respect of an incapacitous patient and to adhere to the wishes of the person acting as attorney. The only circumstances in which clinicians need not follow the LPA is where the attorney appears not to be acting in the patient's best interests. In such situations, the case should be referred to the Court of Protection. Like advance decisions, the ethical rationale for the existence of LPAs is that prospective autonomy is desirable and facilitates informed care, rather than second-guessing patient preferences.

Best interests of patients who lack capacity

Where an adult lacks capacity to give consent, and there is no valid advance decision or power of attorney in place, clinicians are obliged to act in the patient's best interests. This encompasses more than an individual's best *medical* interests. In practice, the determination of best interests is likely to involve a number of people: for example, members of the healthcare team, professionals with whom the patient had a longer-term relationship, and relatives and carers.

In England and Wales, an Independent Mental Capacity Advocacy Service provides advocates for patients who lack capacity and have no family or friends to represent their interests. 'Third parties' in such a situation, including Independent Mental Capacity Advocates, are not making decisions; rather, they are being asked to give an informed sense of the patient and his or her likely preferences. In some jurisdictions – for example, in North America – clinical ethicists play an advocacy role and seek to represent the patient's best interests.

Provision or cessation of life-sustaining treatment

A common situation requiring determination of a patient's best interests is the provision of life-sustaining treatment, often at the end of life, for a patient who lacks capacity and has neither an advance decision nor an advocate to speak for them. It is considered acceptable not to use medical means to prolong the lives of patients where:

- based on good evidence, the team believes that further treatment will not save life
- the patient is already imminently and irreversibly close to death
- the patient is so permanently or irreversibly brain-damaged that he or she will always be incapable of any future self-directed activity or intentional social interaction.

Moral and religious beliefs vary widely and, in general, decisions not to provide or continue life-sustaining treatment should always be made with as much consensus as possible amongst both the clinical team and those close to the patient. Where there is unresolvable conflict between those involved in decision-making, a court should be consulted. In emergencies in the UK, judges are always available in the relevant court.

Where clinicians decide not to prolong the lives of imminently dying and/or extremely brain-damaged patients, the legal rationale is that they are acting in the patient's best interests and seeking to minimize suffering rather than intending to kill, which would constitute murder. In ethical terms, the significance of intention, along with the moral status of acts and omissions, is integral to debates about assisted dying and euthanasia.

Assisted dying

Currently, in many countries, there is no provision for lawful assisted dying. For example, physician-assisted suicide, active euthanasia and suicide pacts are all illegal in the UK. In contrast, some jurisdictions, including the Netherlands, Switzerland, Belgium and certain states in the USA, permit assisted dying. However, even where assisted dying is not lawful, withholding and withdrawing treatment is usually acceptable in strictly defined circumstances, where the intention of the clinician is to minimize suffering, not to cause death. Similarly, the doctrine of double effect may apply. It enables clinicians to prescribe medication that has as its principal aim the reduction of suffering by providing analgesic relief but which is acknowledged to have side-effects such as the depression of respiratory effort (e.g. opiates). Such prescribing is justifiable on the basis that the intention is benign and the side-effects, whilst foreseen, are not intended to be the primary aim of treatment. End-of-life care pathways, which provide for such approaches where necessary, are discussed in Chapter 3.

Although assisted dying is unlawful in the UK, the Director of Public Prosecutions (DPP) has issued guidance on how prosecution decisions are made in response to a request from the courts, following an action brought by Debbie Purdy. Thus, there are now guidelines that indicate what circumstances are likely to weigh either in favour of, or against, a prosecution. Nevertheless, the law itself is unchanged by the DPP's guidance; for a clinician to act to end a patient's life remains a criminal offence.

Mental health and consent

The vast majority of people being treated for psychiatric illness have capacity to make choices about healthcare. However, there are some circumstances in which mental illness compromises an individual's capacity to make his or her own decisions. In such circumstances, many countries have specific legislation that enables people to be treated without consent on the basis that they pose a risk to themselves and/or to others.

People who have, or are suspected of having, a mental disorder may be detained for assessment and treatment in England and Wales under the Mental Health Act 2007 (which amended the 1983 statute). There is one definition of a mental disorder for the purposes of the law. The Mental Health Act 2007 defines a mental disorder as 'any disorder or disability of the mind'. Addiction to drugs and alcohol is excluded from the definition. Appropriate medical treatment should be available to those who are admitted under the Mental Health Act. In addition to assessment and treatment in hospital, the legislation provides for Supervised Community Treatment Orders, which consist of supervised community treatment after a period of detention in hospital. The law is tightly defined with multiple checks and limitations that are essential, given the ethical implications of detaining and treating someone against his or her will.

Even in situations in which it is lawful to give a detained patient psychiatric treatment compulsorily, efforts should be made to obtain consent if possible. For concurrent physical illness, capacity should be assessed in the usual way. If the patient does have capacity, consent should be obtained for treatment of the physical illness. If a patient lacks capacity because of the severity of a psychiatric illness, treatment for physical illness should be given on the basis of best interests or with reference to a proxy or advance decision, if applicable. If treatment can be postponed without seriously compromising the patient's interests, consent should be sought when the patient once more has capacity.

Consent and children

Where a child does not have the capacity to make decisions about his or her own medical care, treatment will usually depend upon obtaining proxy consent. In the UK, consent is sought on behalf of the child from someone with 'parental responsibility'. In the absence of someone with parental responsibility – for example, in emergencies, where treatment is required urgently – clinicians proceed on the basis of the child's best interests.

Sometimes parents and doctors disagree about the care of a child who is too young to make his or her own decisions. Here, both national and European case law demonstrates that the courts are prepared to override parental beliefs if they are perceived to compromise the child's best interests. However, the courts have also emphasized that a child's best *medical* interests are not necessarily the same as a child's best *overall* interests. Whenever the presenting patient is a child, clinicians are dealing with a family unit. Sharing decisions, and paying attention to the needs of the child as a member of a family, are the most effective and ethical ways of practising.

As children grow up, the question of whether a child has capacity to make his or her own decisions is based on principles derived from a case called *Gillick v. West Norfolk and Wisbech Area Health Authority*, which determined that a child can make a choice about his or her health where:

- the patient, although under 16, can understand medical information sufficiently
- the doctor cannot persuade the patient to inform, or give permission for the doctor to inform, his or her parents
- a minor is seeking contraception, in cases where the patient is very likely to have sexual intercourse with or without adequate contraception
- the patient's mental or physical health (or both) is likely to suffer if treatment is not provided
- it is in the patient's best interests for the doctor to treat without parental consent.

The *Gillick* case recognized that children differ in their abilities to make decisions and established that function, not age, is the prime consideration when considering whether a child can give consent. Situations should be approached on a case-by-case basis, taking into account the individual child's level of understanding of a particular treatment. It is possible (and perhaps likely) that a child may be considered to have capacity to consent to one treatment but not another. Even where a child does not have capacity to make his or her own decision, clinicians should respect the child's dignity by discussing the proposed treatment, even if the consent of the parents also has to be obtained.

In the UK, once a child reaches the age of 16, the Mental Capacity Act 2005 states that he or she should be treated as an adult, except for the purposes of advance decision-making and appointing a lasting power of attorney.

Further reading

British Medical Association. *Assisted Suicide: Guidance for Doctors in England, Wales and Northern Ireland*. London: BMA; 2010.
British Medical Association. *Children and Young People: Toolkit*. London: BMA; 2010.
British Medical Association. *The Mental Capacity Act 2005 – Guidance for Health Professionals*. London: BMA; 2009.
General Medical Council. *0–18 Years: Guidance for All Doctors*. London: GMC; 2007.
General Medical Council. *Consent: Patients and Doctors Making Decisions Together*. London: GMC; 2008.
General Medical Council. *Treatment and Care Towards the End of Life*. London: GMC; 2010.
Heath I. Opt in not out: why is patient's consent presumed for cardiopulmonary resuscitation? *BMJ* 2011; 343:5251.
IMCA. *Making Decisions: The Independent Mental Capacity Advocate (IMCA) Service*. London: Department of Health; 2009.
UK House of Lords. R (Purdy) v Director of Public Prosecutions (2009) UKHL 45; http://www.publications.parliament.uk/pa/ld200809/ldjudgmt/jd090730/rvpurd-1.htm.

CONFIDENTIALITY

Confidentiality is essential to therapeutic relationships. If clinicians violate the privacy of their patients, they risk causing harm, disrespect autonomy, undermine trust, and call the medical profession into disrepute. The diminution of trust is a significant ethical challenge, with potentially serious consequences for both the patient and the clinical team. Within the UK, confidentiality is protected by common and statutory law. Some jurisdictions make legal provision for privacy. Doctors who breach the confidentiality of patients may face severe professional and legal sanctions. For example, in some jurisdictions, breaching a patient's confidentiality is a statutory offence.

Respecting confidentiality in practice

Patients should understand that information about them will be shared with other clinicians and healthcare workers involved in their treatment. Usually, by giving consent for investigations or treatment, patients are deemed to give their implied consent for information to be shared within the clinical team. Very rarely, patients might object to information being shared, even within a team. In such situations, the advice is that the patient's wish should be respected, unless it compromises treatment. In almost all clinical circumstances, therefore, the confidentiality of patients must be respected. Unfortunately, confidentiality can be easily breached inadvertently. For example, clinical conversations take place in lifts, corridors and cafés. Even on wards, confidentiality is routinely compromised by the proximity of beds and the visibility of whiteboards containing medical information. Students and doctors should be alert to the incidental opportunities for breaches of confidentiality and seek to minimize their role in unwittingly revealing sensitive information.

When confidentiality must or may be breached

The duty of confidence is not absolute. Sometimes, the law requires that clinicians must reveal private information about patients to others, even if they wish it were otherwise ***(Box 1.5)***. There are also circumstances in which a doctor has the discretion to share confidential information within defined terms. Such circumstances

Box 1.5 Examples of circumstances in which a doctor is required to share confidential information

- Notifiable diseases, which, by virtue of public health legislation, must be notified to the relevant consultant in communicable disease control
- Court orders
- Road traffic accidents that lead to requests from the police
- Actual or suspected terrorist activity

highlight the ethical tension between the rights of individuals and the public interest.

Aside from legal obligations, there are three broad categories of qualifications that exist in respect of the duty of confidentiality, namely:

1. The patient has given consent.
2. It is in the patient's best interests to share the information but it is impracticable or unreasonable to seek consent.
3. It is in the public interest.

These three categories are useful as a framework within which to think about the extent of the duty of confidentiality and they also require considerable ethical discretion in practice, particularly in relation to situations where sharing confidential information might be considered to be in the 'public interest'. In England and Wales, there is legal guidance on what constitutes sufficient 'public interest' to justify sharing confidential information, which is derived from the case of *W v. Egdell*. In that case, the Court of Appeal held that only the 'most compelling circumstances' could justify a doctor acting contrary to the patient's perceived interest in the absence of consent. The court stated that it would be in the public interest to share confidential information where:

- there is a real and serious risk of harm
- the risk is of physical harm
- there is a risk to an identifiable individual or individuals.

Consent should be sought wherever possible, and disclosure on the basis of the 'public interest' should be a last resort. Each case must be weighed on its own individual merits and a clinician who chooses to disclose confidential information on the ground of 'public interest' must be prepared to justify his or her decision. Even where disclosure is justified, confidential information must be shared only with those who need to know.

If there is a perceived risk to the public interest, does a doctor have a duty to warn? In some jurisdictions there is a duty to warn, but in England and Wales there is no professional duty to warn others of potential risk. The judgement of *W v. Egdell* provides a justification for breaches of confidence in the public interest but it does not impose an obligation on clinicians to warn third parties about potential risks posed by their patients.

Further reading

British Medical Association. *Confidentiality and Disclosure of Health Information: Toolkit*. London: BMA; 2009.
General Medical Council. *Confidentiality: Protecting and Providing Information*. London: GMC; 2009; www.gmc-uk.org.

RESOURCE ALLOCATION

Resources should be considered broadly to encompass all aspects of clinical care, i.e. they include time, knowledge, skills and space, as well as treatment. In circumstances of scarcity, waste and inefficiency of any resource are of ethical concern.

Access to healthcare is considered to be a fundamental right and has been captured in international law since it was included in the Universal Declaration of Human Rights. However, resources are scarce and the question of how to allocate limited resources is a perennial ethical question. Within the UK, the courts have made it clear that they will not force National Health Service (NHS) Trusts to provide treatments that are beyond their means. Nevertheless, the courts also demand that decisions about resources must be made on reasonable grounds.

Fairness

Both ethically and legally, prejudice or favouritism is unacceptable. Methods for allocating resources should be fair and just. In practice, this means that scarce resources should be allocated to patients on the basis of their comparative need and the time at which they sought treatment. It is respect on the part of clinicians for these principles of equality – equal need and equal chance – that fosters fairness and justice in the delivery of healthcare. For example, a well-run Accident and Emergency Department will draw on the principles of equality of need and chance to:

- decide who to treat first and how
- offer treatment that has been shown to deliver optimal results for minimal expense
- use triage to determine which patients are most in need and ensure that they are seen first, the queue (or waiting list) being based on need and time of presentation.

People should not be denied potentially beneficial treatments on the basis of their lifestyles. Such decisions are almost always prejudicial. For example, why single out smokers or the obese for blame, as opposed to those who engage in dangerous sports? Patients are not equal in their abilities to lead healthy lives and to make wise healthcare choices.

Education, information, economic worth, confidence and support are all variables that contribute to, and socially determine, health and wellbeing. As such, to regard all people as equal competitors and to reward those who, in many ways, are already better off is unjust and unfair.

Global perspectives

Increasingly, resource allocation is being considered from an international or global perspective. Beyond the boundaries of the NHS and the borders of the UK, moral questions about the availability of, and access to, effective healthcare are rightly attracting the attention of ethicists and clinicians. Anyone who is training for, or working in, medicine in the 21st century should consider fundamental moral questions about resource allocation, in particular those being raised by issues such as:

- the role and work of pharmaceutical companies
- the mobility of trained clinicians
- the preoccupation of funded and commercial biomedical research with diseases that are prevalent in developed countries
- notions of rights to health and life
- the status of those seeking asylum
- persistent inequalities in health.

Further reading

British Medical Association. *The Right to Health: Toolkit*. London: BMA; 2007.
General Medical Council. *Good Medical Practice*. London: GMC; 2012; paras 84–88.
Newdick C. *Who Should We Treat? Rights, Rationing and Resources in the NHS*. Oxford: Oxford University Press; 2005.

PROFESSIONAL COMPETENCE AND MISTAKES

Doctors have a duty to work to an acceptable professional standard. There are essentially three sources that inform what it means to be a 'competent' doctor, namely:

1. the law
2. professional guidance from bodies such as the GMC
3. policy.

In practice, there is frequently overlap and interaction between the categories: for example, a doctor may be both a defendant in a negligence action and the subject of fitness to practise procedures. Professional bodies are established by, and work within, a legal framework and, in order to implement policy, legislation is required and interpretative case law will often follow.

Standards and the law

In most countries, the law provides the statutory framework within which the medical profession is regulated. For example, in the UK, it is the function of the GMC to maintain the register of medical practitioners, provide ethical guidance, guide and quality-assure medical education and training, and conduct fitness to practise procedures. Therefore it is the GMC that defines standards of professional practice and has responsibility for investigation when a doctor's standard of practice is questioned.

Clinicians have a responsibility not only to reflect on their own practice, but also to be aware of and, if necessary, respond to the practice of colleagues, even in the absence of formal 'line management' responsibilities. In England and Wales, for example, the Public Interest Disclosure Act 1998 provides statutory protection for those who express formal concern about a colleague's performance, provided the expression of concern:

- constitutes a 'qualifying disclosure'
- is expressed using appropriate procedures, *and*
- is made in good faith.

Clinical negligence

Negligence is a civil claim where damage or loss has arisen as a result of an alleged breach of professional duty, such that the standard of care was not, on the balance of probabilities, that which could be reasonably expected.

Of the components of negligence, duty is the simplest to establish: all doctors have a duty of care to their patients (although the extent of that duty in emergencies and social situations is uncertain and contested in relation to civil law). Whether a doctor has discharged his or her professional duty adequately is determined by expert opinion about the standards that might reasonably be expected and his or her conduct in relation to those standards. If doctors have acted in a way that is consistent with a reasonable body of their peers and their actions or omissions withstand logical analysis, they are likely to meet the expected standards of care. Lack of experience is not taken into account in legal determinations of negligence.

The most common reason for a negligence action to fail is causation, which is notoriously difficult to prove in clinical negligence claims. For example, the alleged harm may have occurred against the background of a complex medical condition or course of treatment, making it difficult to establish the actual cause.

Clinical negligence remains relatively rare and undue fear of litigation can lead to defensive and poor practice. All doctors make errors and these do not necessarily constitute negligence or indicate incompetence. Inherent in the definition of incompetence is time, i.e. on-going review of a doctor's practice to see whether there are patterns of error or repeated failure to learn from error. Regulatory bodies and medical defence organizations recommend that doctors should be honest and apologetic about their mistakes, remembering that to do so is not necessarily an admission of negligence (see p. 14). Such honesty and humility, aside from its inherent moral value, have been shown to reduce the prospect of patient complaints or litigation.

Professional bodies

Professional bodies have diverse but often overlapping roles in developing, defining and revising standards for doctors. The principal publications in which the GMC sets out standards and obligations relating to competence and performance, are *Duties of a Doctor* and *Good Medical Practice*.

Policy

There have been an exponential number of policy reforms that have shaped the ways in which the medical competence and accountability agendas have evolved. One of the most notable is the increase in the number of organizations concerned broadly with 'quality' and performance. The increased scrutiny of doctors' competence has found further policy translation in the development of appraisal schemes and the revalidation process. There have been other policy initiatives that adopt the rhetoric of 'quality', such as increased use of clinical and administrative targets, private finance initiatives, and the development of specialist screening facilities and treatment centres.

The issue of professional accountability in medicine is a hot topic. The law, professional guidance and policy documentation provide a starting point for clinicians. Complaints and possible litigation are often brought by patients who feel aggrieved for reasons that may be unconnected with the clinical care that they have received. When patients are asked about their decisions to complain or to sue doctors, it is common for poor communication, insensitivity, administrative errors and lack of responsiveness to be cited as motivation (see p. 14). There is less to fear than doctors sometimes believe. The courts and professional bodies are concerned neither with best practice, nor with unfeasibly high standards of care. What is expected is that doctors behave in a way that accords with the practice of a reasonable doctor – and the reasonable doctor is not perfect. As long as clinicians adhere to some basic principles, it is possible to practise *defensible* rather than *defensive* medicine. It should be reassuring that complaints and litigation are avoidable, simply by developing and maintaining good standards of communication, organization and administration – and good habits begin in medical school. In particular, effective communication is a potent weapon in preventing complaints and, ultimately, encounters with the legal and regulatory systems.

Further reading

Buchan, A. *Buchan and Lewis: Clinical Negligence*, 7th edn. London: Bloomsbury Professional; 2012.

General Medical Council. *Acting as an Expert Witness*. London: GMC; 2008.

General Medical Council. *Duties of a Doctor Registered with the GMC*. London: GMC; http://www.gmc-uk.org/guidance/ethical_guidance/7162.asp.

COMMUNICATION

COMMUNICATION IN HEALTHCARE

Good communication in healthcare is fundamental to achieving optimal patient care, safety and health outcomes. The aim of every healthcare professional is to provide evidence-based, ethically sound and patient-centred care. This depends on a consulting style that fosters trust and demonstrates flexibility, openness, partnership, and collaboration with the patient.

Doctors work in multiprofessional teams and modern healthcare is more effective, more complex and more hazardous. Successful team communication is therefore vital.

What is patient-centred communication?

Patient-centred communication involves reaching a common ground about the illness, its treatment, and the roles that the clinician and the patient will assume ***(Fig. 1.1)***. A good history is the key to diagnosis. Both the biomedical facts of the patient's illness and the patient's ideas, concerns, expectations and feelings are needed in order to discover what is the matter with the patient and what matters to the patient. This information is essential for accurate diagnosis and for gaining the patient's confidence, trust and involvement in appropriate management.

The historical approach of 'doctor knows best' with patients' views not being considered is very outdated; this is not just societal but is driven by evidence about improved health outcome.

- Patients increasingly expect information and want their views taken into account in deciding treatment. This does not mean clinicians totally abdicate power. Patients want their doctors' expert opinions and may still prefer to leave matters to the clinician.
- Many health problems are long-term conditions and patients have to become expert to manage their conditions and reduce risks from lifestyle habits in a partnership approach to care.
- Patients expect humanity and empathy from their doctors, as well as competence. Clinicians can usually offer practical help with patients' concerns and expectations but, if not, they can always listen supportively.

Patient-centred communication requires a good balance between:

- clinicians asking all the questions needed to include or exclude diagnoses
- patients being asked to express their thoughts, ideas, concerns and expectations
- clinicians explaining and advising in ways patients can understand so that they can be involved in decisions about their care.

What are the effects of communication?

Enormous benefits accrue from good communication ***(Box 1.6)***. Patients' problems are identified more accurately and efficiently, expectations for care are agreed, and patients and clinicians experience greater satisfaction. Poor communication results in missed problems and concerns, strained relationships, complaints and litigation.

Diagnostic accuracy

Clinicians commonly interrupt patients after an average of 24 seconds, whether or not a patient has finished explaining the problem. A golden rule involves listening for 1 minute before interrupting. Clinicians are failing if a serious point is raised only as the patient is preparing to leave. One study found that, in 50% of visits, patients and doctors disagreed on the main presenting problem.

Health outcomes

Physical, emotional and functional health is improved by good communication. Conversely, the main predictive factor for patients

Box 1.6 Benefits of good communication

- Diagnostic accuracy
- Physical health outcomes (blood pressure, diabetes, asthma, pain)
- Emotional health and functioning
- Patient adherence
- Patient and clinician satisfaction
- Improved time management and costs
- Patient safety
- Reduced litigation

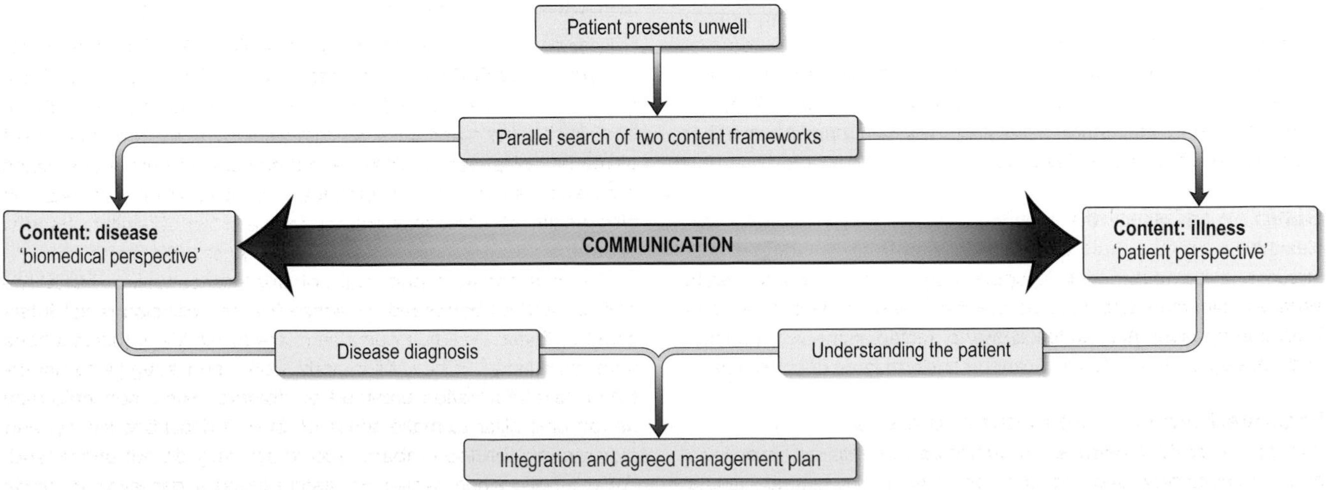

Figure 1.1 The patient-centred clinical interview. *(Adapted from Levenstein JH. In: Stewart M, Roter D, eds.* Communicating with Medical Patients. *Thousand Oaks, CA: Sage; 1989.)*

Box 1.7 Factors that improve adherence to clinical advice

Clinician
- Listens to and understands the patient
- Uses an appropriate tone of voice
- Elicits all of the patient's health concerns

Patient
- Is comfortable asking questions
- Feels sufficient time is spent with the clinician

(From Stewart M, Brown JB, Boon H et al. Evidence on patient communication. Cancer Prevention and Control *1999; 3(i): 25–30, with permission.)*

Box 1.8 Behaviours influencing litigation

Patients are less likely to sue when clinicians:
- Orientate patients, e.g. 'We are going to do this first and then go on to that'
- Use facilitative comments, e.g. 'Uh huh, I see'
- Use active listening
- Check understanding
- Ask patients their opinions
- Use humour and laughter appropriately
- Conduct slightly longer visits (18 versus 15 min)

developing depression on learning of the diagnosis of cancer is the way bad news is broken.

Adherence to treatment

Some 45% of patients are not following treatment advice properly. There is a 19% higher risk of non-adherence where physicians communicate poorly. Errors in use of medications are costly and risk patient safety. Patients may not understand or remember what they were told, while others actively decide not to follow advice and commonly do not tell their doctors. Research shows that clinicians rarely check patients' understanding or views, yet these affect adherence ***(Box 1.7)***.

Patient satisfaction and dissatisfaction

Satisfaction is largely a result of patients knowing they are:
- getting the best medical care
- being treated humanely as individuals and not as items on a conveyer belt.

Satisfaction affects psychological wellbeing and adherence to treatment, both of which have a knock-on effect on clinical outcomes. It also reduces patient complaints and litigation ***(Box 1.8)***. Some 70% of lawsuits are a result of poor communication rather than failures of biomedical practice.

Clinician satisfaction

Healthcare professionals have a very high rate of occupational stress and burnout, which is costly both to them and to health services. Notwithstanding pressure from staffing shortages and inadequate resources, it is the quality of relationships with patients and colleagues that affects clinician satisfaction and happiness.

Improved time management and costs

Integrating ***patient-centred communication*** into all interviews actually saves time and reduces non-essential investigations and referrals, which waste resources. Hospital visits, admissions, length of stay and mortality rate are reduced where clinicians used a

Box 1.9 Common barriers and difficulties in communication

Clinician factors
- Lack of knowledge of:
  - Role of psychosocial issues
  - Skills of communication
- Attitude:
  - Authoritarian manner and negative attitude to shared care
  - Unwillingness to examine own communication skills
- Skills:
  - Distancing to avoid difficult topics
  - Use of jargon
  - Lack of empathy

Shared factors
- Different first language
- Lack of privacy
- Lack of time
- Different cultural backgrounds
- Computers

Patient factors
- Anxiety
- Feeling powerless
- Reticence to disclose concerns
- Misconceptions
- Low health literacy
- Forgetfulness
- Hearing/visual and speech impairment

Box 1.10 Strategies that doctors use to distance themselves from patients' worries

Patient says: 'I have this headache and I'm worried …'
- ***Selective attention to cues***: 'What is the pain like?'
- ***Normalizing***: 'It's normal to worry. Where is the pain?'
- ***Premature reassurance***: 'Don't worry. I'm sure you'll be fine'
- ***False reassurance***: 'Everything is OK'
- ***Switching topic***: 'Forget that. Tell me about …'
- ***Passing the buck***: 'Nurse will tell you about that'
- ***Jollying along***: 'Come on now, look on the bright side'
- ***Physical avoidance***: Passing the bedside without stopping

(From Maguire P. Communication Skills for Doctors. *London: Arnold; 2000, with permission.)*

biopsychosocial approach to managing people with medically unexplained symptoms (25–50% of primary care visits are for medically inexplicable complaints). Patients given the latest evidence on treatment options commonly choose more conservative management with no adverse effects on health outcomes. This has potential for considerable savings in health budgets.

Barriers and difficulties in communication

Communication is not straightforward ***(Box 1.9)***. Time constraints can prevent both doctors and patients from feeling that they have each other's attention and that they fully understand the problem from each other's perspective. Under-estimation of the influence of psychosocial issues on illness and their costs to healthcare means clinicians may resort to avoidance strategies when they fear the discussion will unleash emotions that are too difficult to handle, upset the patient or take too much time ***(Box 1.10)***.

Patients, for their part, will not disclose concerns if they are anxious and embarrassed, or sense that the clinician is not interested or thinks that their complaints are trivial. Many patients have poor knowledge of how their body works and struggle to understand new information provided by doctors. Some concepts may be too unfamiliar to make sense of, even if described simply, and patients may be too embarrassed to say they do not understand. For example, when explaining fasting blood sugar levels to newly diagnosed diabetics it was found that many did not realize that there is sugar in their blood.

Clinicians are human and are often rushed and stressed. They work against the clock and in fallible systems. However, as professionals, it is they, together with healthcare managers, who bear the responsibility for dealing with these difficulties and problems, not the patient.

Further reading

Coulter A. Do patients want a choice and does it work? *BMJ* 2010 Oct 14; 341:c4989. doi: 10.1136/bmj.c4989.

Royal College of Psychiatrists. Guidance for health professionals on medically unexplained symptoms (MUS); 2011; http://www.rcpsych.ac.uk.

THE MEDICAL INTERVIEW

Structure and skills for effective interviewing

Clinicians conduct some 200 000 medical interviews during their careers. Flexibility is key because each patient is different and a framework helps clinicians use time productively. The example below applies to a first consultation and may vary slightly in a follow-up appointment or emergency visit.

There are seven essential steps in the medical interview.

1. Building a relationship

Because patients are frequently anxious and may feel unwell, introductions and first impressions are critical to create rapport and trust. Without this, effective communication is impossible. Well-organized arrangements for appointments, reception and punctuality put patients at ease. Clinicians' non-verbal messages, body language, voice tone and unspoken attitudes have a huge impact on the emotional atmosphere of the interview. Seating arrangements, eye contact, facial expression and tone of voice should all convey friendliness, interest and respect.

2. Opening the discussion

The aim is to obtain all the patients' concerns, remembering that they commonly have at least three. Ask 'What problems have brought you to see me today?'

Listen attentively without interrupting. Ask 'And is there something else?' to screen for other problems before exploring the history in detail.

Only when all concerns are identified can the agenda be prioritized, balancing the patients' main concerns with the clinician's medical priorities.

3. Gathering information

The components of a complete history are shown in ***Box 1.11***.

Listening skills

Attentive listening is essential. Ask patients to tell the story of the problem in their own words from when it first started up to the present. Patients will recognize that clinicians are listening if the clinicians look at them and not the notes or computer. Occasional nods encourage the patient to continue. Avoid interrupting before the patient has finished talking.

Questioning styles

The way a clinician asks questions determines whether the patient speaks freely or just gives one-word or brief answers ***(Box 1.12)***. Start with open questions ('What problems have brought you in today?') and move to screening ('Is there anything else?'), focused ('Can you tell me more about the pain?') and closed questions ('Where is the pain?'). Open methods allow clinicians to listen and to generate their problem-solving approach. Closed questions are necessary to check specific symptoms, but if used too early, they may lead to inaccuracies by missing patients' problems.

Leading questions that imply the expected answer ('You've given up drinking, haven't you?') risk inaccurate responses, as patients may just say yes rather than disagree.

4. Understanding the patient

Finding out the patient's thoughts is an essential step towards holistic care and achieving common ground.

Ideas, concerns and expectations (ICE)

Patients seek help because of their own ideas or concerns about their condition. If these are not heard, they may think the clinician

Box 1.11 Components of a medical interview

- Nature of the key problems
- Date and time of onset
- Development over time
- Precipitating factors
- Help given to date
- Impact of the problem on the patient's life
- Availability of support
- Patient's **i**deas, **c**oncerns and **e**xpectations (ICE)
- Screening question

Box 1.12 Questioning style

Closed questioning style

Dr: 'You say chest pain. Where is the pain?' (*closed Q*)
Pt: 'Just here.' (pointing to sternum)
Dr: 'And is it a sharp or dull pain?' (*closed Q*)
Pt: 'Quite sharp.'
Dr: 'Does it go anywhere else?' (*closed Q*)
Pt: 'No, just there.'
Dr: 'And you don't smoke now, do you?' (*leading Q*)
Pt: 'Well ... just the occasional one.'

Open questioning style

Dr: 'Can you tell me about the pain you've been having?' (*open/focused Q*)
Pt: 'Well, it's been getting worse over the past few weeks and waking me up at night. It's just here (points to sternum), very sharp and I get a burning and bad acid taste in the back of my throat. I try to burp to clear it. I've taken antacids, which help a little, but I'm a bit worried about it. I'm losing sleep and I've got a busy workload, so that's a worry too.'
Dr: 'I see. So it's bothering you quite a lot. Anything else you've noticed?' (*empathic statement, open screening Q*)
Pt: 'I get it more after I've had a few drinks. I have been drinking and smoking a bit more recently. Actually, I've been getting lots of headaches too, which I've just taken ibuprofen for.'
Dr: 'You say you're worried. Is there anything in particular that concerns you?' (*picks up on patient's cue and uses reflecting Q*)
Pt: 'I wondered if it might be an ulcer.'
Dr: 'I see. So this sharp pain under your breastbone, with some acid reflux for several weeks, is worse at night and aggravated by drinking and smoking but not relieved by antacids. You're busy at work, getting headaches, drinking and smoking a bit more and not sleeping well. You're concerned this could be an ulcer.' (*summarizing*)
Pt: 'Yes, a friend had problems like this.'
Dr: 'I can appreciate why you might be thinking that, then.' (*validation*)
Pt: 'Yes, and he had to have a "scope" so I wondered whether I would need one?'(*expectation*)
Dr: 'Well, let me explain first what I think this might be and then what I would recommend next ... ' (*signposting*)

has not got things right and then not follow the advice. Moreover, any misconceptions will go uncorrected. A patient's views can emerge if the clinician listens carefully and picks up on cues. If these views are not forthcoming, it is necessary to ask specific questions, for example:

- 'What were you worried this might be?'
- 'Are there any particular concerns you have about ...?'
- 'Was there anything you were hoping we might do about this?'

The example in ***Box 1.12*** shows how, if the clinician listens, information that may be biomedically relevant emerges and the patient's views are revealed.

Non-verbal communication

In adult conversation, some 5% of meaning derives from words, 35% from tone of voice and 60% from body language and non-verbal communication. When there is a mismatch between words and tone, the non-verbal communication elements hold the truer meaning. Patients who are anxious, uneasy, puzzled or confused are more likely to communicate this through expression and/or restless activity – for example, of the feet and hands – than to tell the clinician outright. The observant clinician can pick up on this: 'You seem uneasy about what I have said ... ', thus inviting the patient to share their concerns. Doctors' non-verbal behaviour is also important. Voice tone, if harsh or uncaring, can even increase the risk of being sued.

Empathizing

Empathy has been described as 'imagination for others'. It is different from sympathy (feeling sorry for the patient), which rarely helps. Empathy is a key skill in building the patient–clinician relationship and is highly therapeutic. The starting point is attentive listening and observing patients to try to understand their predicament. This understanding then needs to be conveyed back in a supportive way. Whilst empathy is about trying to understand, the phrase 'I understand' may be met with 'how could you?' It is usually more helpful to reflect back using some of the patient's own words and ideas. For example: 'It sounds like ...' (patient heard); 'I can see you are upset' (patient seen); 'I realize that this is a shock' (acknowledgement); 'Most people in your circumstances would feel angry' (accepting the patient).

Empathy can be developed with practice but it has to be genuine and cannot be counterfeited by a repertoire of routine mannerisms.

5. Sharing information

Tailoring information to what patients want to know and the level of detail they prefer helps understanding. Most patients, irrespective of socioeconomic group, want to know 'is this problem serious and how will it affect me; what can be done about it; and what is causing it?' Research shows they cannot take in explanations about cause if they are still worrying about the first two concerns.

- Information must be not only related to the biomedical facts, but also tailored to patients' ideas and concerns.
- With adaptations for age, 70–80% of even the most unfamiliar, complex or alarming information can be understood and recalled if explained well ***(Box 1.13)***.

6. Reaching agreement on management

Once the situation is understood, the clinician and patient need to agree on the best course for possible investigations and treatments.

Box 1.13 Giving information: the 3E model: explore, explain, explore

Explore

- ***Ask***. Ask what the patient already knows or thinks is wrong. This allows you to confirm, correct or add new information.

Explain

- ***Chunk and check***. Give information in chunks that are easy to assimilate, one thing at a time. Check after each chunk that the patient is understanding.
- ***Signpost***. 'I'll explain first of all ...'; 'Can I move on now to explain treatment options ...?'
- ***Link***. Explain the cause and effect of the condition in the context of the patient's symptoms, e.g. 'The reason you are experiencing ... is because ...'
- ***Plain language***. Use clear, concise language; 'translate' any unavoidable medical terms and write them down.
- ***Aid recall***. Make use of simple diagrams and leaflets; recommend websites and support organizations.

Explore

- ***'Teach back'***. Use the universal precaution of always asking patients to recap to check you have explained it clearly enough.

Negotiating – enlisting the patient's collaboration

The clinician's opinion should be given and the patient's views sought. Check whether the patient wants to be involved or to leave decisions to the clinician. Partnership requires:

- a frank exchange of information
- the negotiation of options
- active involvement in decisions.

Summarizing

This allows information to be added and misunderstandings corrected. Summarizing is a feature of shared decision-making.

7. Providing closure

A final summary and an outline of next steps indicate the closing stage of the interview. Plans are confirmed for follow-up and for informing other healthcare professionals involved in the patient's care.

Some clinicians close the interview by asking whether the consultation has been useful, before saying goodbye.

Clinical records

All medical interviews should be well documented. Good records are the responsibility of everyone in the healthcare team ***(Box 1.14)***, as is maintenance of confidentiality. They are vital in providing best care, reducing error and ensuring patient safety.

In many countries, patients have the right to see their records, which provide essential information when a complaint or claim for negligence is made. They are also valuable as part of audit to improve standards of healthcare.

Electronic patient records are increasingly replacing written ones. They include more information, overcome problems of legibility and reduce prescription error by 66% compared to handwritten ones. With adequate data protection, they offer immense potential for unifying record systems and allowing access across the healthcare team in primary, secondary and tertiary care sectors. Increasingly, patients will have access and even be contributors to their records.

Box 1.14 Essentials of record-keeping

What records should include
- Relevant clinical and psychosocial information – history and examination
- Relevant findings, both positive and negative
- Diagnosis, including uncertainties
- Investigations arranged
- Test results
- Correspondence, including e-mails and text messages
- Decisions made
- Information given to patients
- Consent
- Drugs or other treatments prescribed
- Follow-up and referrals

Criteria for good records[a,b]
- Clear, accurate, legible and contemporaneous
- Dated and signed with printed name
- Written in pen (if not electronic)
- Written first hand
- Original – never altered (using a signed, dated additional note alongside any mistake)
- Kept secure

[a]*GMC* Good Medical Practice *2012.* [b]*MPS* Guide to Medical Records *2010; http://www.medicalprotection.org/uk/booklets/medical-records.*

Box 1.15 'ATTEND': a mnemonic for patient–physician communication using the electronic medical record

Acquaint yourself with the medical record
- Acquaint yourself with the patient's record beforehand, allowing for less review 'screen time' while in the patient's presence

Take a minute
- Start the visit technology-free, giving the patient and his/her concerns your full attention

Triangulate placement of computer, patient, clinician
- Arrange the room so that it allows you to look at both the screen and the patient, and the patient to look at you and the screen

Engage, explain, educate
- Engage the patient in your use of the computer as a tool during the visit
- Explain what you are doing in both entering data and looking for information on the computer (signposting)
- Educate the patient by letting him/her see what you are seeing on the screen, especially graphs, images

No more screen
- When discussing sensitive issues, completely disengage from the screen (look at the patient, turn away from the screen, take your hands off the keys)

Describe the discharge/Don't forget to log out
- Be explicit about what orders you are entering in the computer at the end of the visit and what the patient should expect (e.g. scheduling, tests)

(Rosenbaum M, Jansen KL, Shen W, Skelly K, Wilbur J. University of Iowa Carver College of Medicine, 2014. Personal communication.)

The computer can, however, act as a considerable barrier to communication and guidelines exist for best practice when using one ***(Box 1.15)***.

Further reading

Robertson K, updated by Cushing A. *Communication Skills*. BMJ Learning Online; 2014; http://www.learning.bmj.com.
Roter DL, Frankel RM, Hall JA et al. The expression of emotion through nonverbal behaviour in medical visits. *J Gen Intern Med* 2006; 21:S28–34.
Royal College of Physicians. *A Clinician's Guide to Record Standards*; 2009; http://www.rcplondon.ac.uk.

Box 1.16 SBAR: a structure for team communication

S – Situation
- My name is …
- I am the junior doctor on ward …
- I am calling about Mr …, under consultant …
- The reason I am calling is …

B – Background
- The patient was admitted on … for …
- The significant medical history …
- Brief summary: medications, laboratory results, diagnostic tests, procedures

A – Assessment
- Summarize relevant information gathered on examination of the patient, charts and results
- Vital signs: heart rate, respiratory rate, oxygen saturation, blood pressure, temperature; assessment of alertness, voice, pain, unresponsiveness (AVPU)
- Early warning or similar score
- What has changed
- Interpretation of this

R – Recommendation (examples)
- I think the patient may need …
- I need your advice on how to proceed …
- I think the patient needs urgent review in the next (timeframe) …

Silverman J, Kurtz Z, Draper J. The Calgary–Cambridge guide: a guide to the medical interview. In: *Skills for Communicating with Patients*, 3rd edn. Abingdon: Radcliffe Medical Press; 2013; http://www.skillscascade.com.

TEAM COMMUNICATION

Modern healthcare is complex and patients are looked after by multiple healthcare professionals working in shifts. Effective team communication is absolutely essential and this is never more vital than when people are busy or a patient is critically ill. Contexts for team communication include ward handovers, requests for help, acceptance of referrals and communication in the operating theatre. Prior to an operation, all clinical staff take a 'time out' and go through a final checklist. This consists of staff introductions, check of the patients' details, site and side of surgery, and a rundown of the drugs being used. Lessons from industries such as aviation show how to reduce errors caused by poor communication.

Problems arise when information is not transmitted, is misunderstood or is not recorded. Communication styles vary. Some people are indirect and more elaborate in their speech, whilst others come straight to the point, leaving out detail and their own rationale. Each type can feel irritated, offended or puzzled by the other and most complaints in teams relate to communication. Handover between teams is helped when everyone adopts a clear system.

Frameworks such as **SBAR** (**S**ituation–**B**ackground–**A**ssessment–**R**ecommendation) use standardized prompt questions in four sections to ensure team members share concise and focused information at the correct level of detail ***(Box 1.16)***. This increases patient safety.

Hierarchies make it harder for people to speak up. This can be dangerous if, for example, a nurse or junior doctor feels unable to point out an error, offer information or ask a question. Hinting and hoping is not good communication. Team leaders who 'flatten' the hierarchy by knowing and using people's names, routinely have briefings and debriefings, do not let their own self-image override doing the right thing, and positively encourage colleagues to speak up, reduce the number of adverse events. Teamwork requires collaboration, open sharing of ideas and a readiness to discuss weaknesses and errors.

Communication on discharge is just as essential and primary care physicians need sufficient information, including details of medication, to continue care safely.

Further reading

British Medical Association. *Safe Handover: Safe Patients. Guidance on Clinical Handover for Clinicians and Managers*. London: BMA; 2009; http://www.bma.org.uk.

Royal College of Physicians. *Ward Rounds in Medicine*. London: RCP; 2012; https://www.rcplondon.ac.uk.

World Health Organization. *The WHO Surgical Safety Checklist*; 2009; http://www.who.int.

BREAKING BAD NEWS

Bad news is any information that is likely to alter a patient's view of the future drastically. The way news is broken has an immediate and long-term effect. When it is skilfully performed, the patient and family are enabled to understand, cope and make the best of even very bad circumstances. These interviews are difficult because biomedical measures may be of little or no help, and patients are upset and can react unpredictably. The clinician may also feel upset, more so if there is an element of medical mishap. The two most difficult things that clinicians report are how to be honest with the patient whilst not destroying hope, and how to deal with the patient's emotions.

Withholding information from patients or telling only the family is a thing of the past and becoming so even in parts of the world where traditionally disclosure did not occur. Although truth can hurt, deceit hurts more. It erodes trust and deprives patients of the information they need to make choices. Most people now express the wish to be told the truth and the evidence is that patients:

- usually know more than anyone realizes and may imagine things worse than they are
- appreciate clear information about even the worst news and want the opportunity to talk openly and ask questions, rather than join in a charade of deception
- differ in how much they can take in at a time.

A framework: the S–P–I–K–E–S strategy

Having a framework helps clinicians to present bad news in a factual, unhurried, balanced and empathic fashion whilst responding to each patient. Prepare the key points you want the patient to understand about the diagnosis, implications and prognosis, what can be done and the next steps.

S - Setting

- See the patient as soon as the current information has been gathered.
- Ask not to be disturbed and hand bleeps to colleagues.
- If possible, patients should have someone with them.
- Choose a quiet place; seat and introduce everyone.
- Indicate your status, the extent of your responsibility towards the patient and the time available.

P - Perception

Ask before telling. Find out what has happened since the last appointment and what has been explained or construed so far. This stage helps gauge the patient's perception but should not be too drawn out.

I - Invitation

- Indicate you have the results and ask if the patient wants you to explain.
- Assess how much the patient would like to know.
- If patients do not want details, offer to answer any questions they may have later or to talk to a relative or friend.

K - Knowledge

If the patient wishes to know:

- Give a warning to help the patient prepare: 'I'm afraid it looks more serious than we hoped.'
- Then give the details.
- At this point, WAIT: allow the patient to think, and only continue when the patient gives some lead to follow. This pause may be long – commonly, a matter of minutes – but it helps patients take in the situation. They may shut down and be unable to hear anything further until their thoughts settle down.
- Give direct information, in small chunks. Avoid technical terms. Check understanding frequently – 'Is this making sense so far?' – before moving on. Watch for signs the patient can take no more.
- Invite questions.
- Emphasize which things – for example, pain and other symptoms – are fixable and which others are not.
- Be prepared for the question: 'How long have I got?' Avoid providing a figure to an individual, which is bound to be inaccurate. Common faults are to be overly optimistic. Some patients wish to know survival rates for their condition. Tell them as much as is appropriate. Stress the importance of ensuring that their quality of life is made as good as possible from day to day.
- Provide some positive information and hope, tempered with realism.

E - Empathy

Responding to the patient's emotions is about the human side of medical care and also helps patients to take in and adjust to difficult information. A range of emotions are experienced in seriously and terminally ill patients ***(Box 1.17)***.

- Be prepared for the patient to have disorderly emotional responses of some kind. Acknowledge them and wait for them to settle before continuing.
- Crying can be a release for some patients. Allow time rather than rushing in to stop the crying.
- Learn to judge which patients wish to be touched and which do not. You can always reach out and touch their chair.
- Keep pausing to allow patients to think and frame their questions.
- Watch for shutdown; stop the interview if necessary and arrange to resume later.

Box 1.17 Emotional responses to serious illness

- Despair
- Denial
- Anger
- Bargaining
- Depression
- Acceptance

S – Strategy and summary

Patients who have a clear plan for the next and future steps are likely to feel less anxious and uncertain. The clinician must ensure that:

- the patient has understood what has been discussed because, at times of emotion, misconceptions can take root
- crucial information is written down to take away
- the patient knows how to contact the appropriate team member and thus has a safety net in place, and when the next appointment is (preferably soon), who it is with and its purpose
- family members are invited to meet clinicians as the patient wishes and further sources of information are provided
- everyone is bid goodbye, starting with the patient.

Follow-up

Bad news is a process and not a one-off. Patients may well not remember everything from the last visit and recapping is necessary. Always start by asking what they have understood so far. It is extremely distressing for patients to hear conflicting things from different clinicians. Keep colleagues informed and document accurately what was said to a patient and what the patient's wishes are.

The move from active treatment to palliative care is particularly difficult. Patients will want to know what happens next: for example, 'Will I be in pain?', 'Can I stay at home?' and 'How long do I have?' Give clear answers with acknowledgement of any uncertainty. The priorities in patient care now are relief of symptoms, quality of life and enabling the patient to settle family matters or unfinished business.

The clinician's role is to mediate between the patient, other medical staff and the patient's relatives whilst continuing to be an empathic and caring doctor.

Further reading

Baile WF, Lenzi R, Kudelka AP et al. SPIKES – a six-step protocol for delivering bad news: application to the patient with cancer. *Oncologist* 2000; 5:302–311.

Chaturvedi SK. Truth telling and communication skills. *Indian J Psychiatry* 2009; 51:227.

Cheng SY, Hu WY, Liu WJ. Good death study of elderly patients with terminal cancer in Taiwan. *Palliat Medic* 2008; 22:626–632.

Clayton JM, Hancock K, Parker S et al. Sustaining hope when communicating with terminally ill patients and their families: a systematic review. *Psychooncology* 2008; 17:641–659.

WHEN THINGS GO WRONG

When things go wrong, as inevitably they do at some time, even in the best of medical care, it is distressing for all concerned. Doctors need to communicate honestly and clearly to minimize distress and act immediately to put matters right, if that is possible. The consultation that occurs after an adverse experience is crucial in influencing any decision to sue.

Being open is recognized as good practice internationally. Doctors should offer an apology and explain fully and promptly what has happened, and the likely short-term and long-term effects of any harm. Reluctance to say 'sorry' comes from a fear that it is an admission of fault, which later implies liability, but guidelines from official bodies emphasize that this is not so. As well as being morally right, an honest approach decreases the trauma felt by patients and relatives following an adverse event and is more likely to lead to forgiveness. Examples of an open approach in the USA, Australia and Singapore have actually reduced the costs of complaints.

Having a clear framework also helps to reduce clinicians' stress and develop their professional reputation for handling difficult situations properly.

Box 1.18 Responding to complaints

- Remember the complainant is still a patient, to whom there is a duty of care
- Listen and express regret for distress
- Acknowledge when things have gone wrong – be objective, not resentful or defensive
- Apologize for actual or perceived shortcomings
- Provide easily understood information or explanations
- Offer appropriate redress
- Explain how things will improve
- Leave medical records strictly unaltered

Complaints

Much of the enormous increase in complaints and medical lawsuits is related to failures in communication. Whilst avoidance and defensiveness are common human responses, professionals must deal with dissatisfaction and complaints as soon as they happen, to save problems escalating and becoming major traumas for all concerned.

The majority of complaints come from the exasperation of patients who:

- feel deserted and devalued by their clinician
- have not been able to obtain clear information
- feel that they are owed an apology
- are concerned that other patients will go through what they have.

Many complaints are resolved satisfactorily once these points are dealt with promptly and appropriately ***(Box 1.18)***.

These interactions are very difficult for everyone and training is recommended to help all healthcare professionals. Clinicians should work in a professional culture that regards complaints as a valuable source of feedback, which deserves to be noted, collected and used constructively to improve services.

Lawsuits

Lawsuits, the extreme form of complaint, are commonly rooted in poor communication or miscommunication, aggravated by a sense of grievance. Clinicians with authoritarian paternalistic styles are more likely to be sued. Some 17% of patients affected by medical injury in the UK want financial compensation or disciplinary action. Any clinician faced with a lawsuit must seek specialist advice.

CULTURE AND COMMUNICATION

Whilst doctors strive to treat all patients equally, those from minority cultures receive poorer healthcare irrespective of socioeconomic status and even when they speak the same language as the clinician. They experience fewer expressions of empathy, shorter consultations and less inclusion in shared decision-making. They also tend to say less in consultations.

Clinicians commonly express anxiety and uncertainty about how to respond to cultural diversity, how to use advocates (interpreters) and how to avoid causing offence.

Beliefs

We all take our culture for granted but it can profoundly affect ideas about symptoms, causes of illness, and appropriate behaviour and treatment.

Beliefs influence when a patient seeks medical assistance, what patients and doctors expect of the consultation, and how they communicate. In some cultures, for example, it is very difficult for a woman to see a male doctor. Sometimes, family members may think it is their duty to talk for the patient whilst the doctor will expect to talk directly with the patient. Sensitive topics may be more difficult but avoidance could jeopardize care. It helps to apologize if offence is inadvertently caused and explain why such questions are required. Clinicians vary too. Those from traditional cultures may have a more paternalistic style than some patients want.

Language

Patients sometimes bring a family member or friend to interpret. The latter may not understand medical questions and may be censoring sensitive matters or expressing their own views rather than the patient's. Confidentiality cannot be guaranteed and patients may feel restricted in what they can say. On the other hand, patients may want a trusted family member to translate. Children should not be used to interpret.

Ideally, a trained interpreter should be used. Ask for the correct pronunciation of a patient's name and about any cultural differences in body language. Arrange seating to see both the patient and the advocate but always look and speak directly to the patient. Speak in short phrases, avoid jargon and find out the patient's ideas, concerns and expectations. Watch for non-verbal communication and check that the patient understands.

Clinicians sometimes worry that interpreters are editing, when long exchanges are followed by only a short summary back to them. It helps to ask interpreters to translate exactly what has been said. The interpreter can stand outside the curtain during examination. Always thank the interpreter at the end. If professional interpreters are not available, use telephone language lines. Advocates are people from the patient's culture who not only translate but also can explain beliefs and concerns that are relevant in the patient's culture. They also help patients to understand the workings of the healthcare system.

Non-verbal communication

Awareness of cultural taboos – for example, handshaking, eye contact, personal space and sensitive subjects – can help in maintaining dignity and respect.

Paraverbal communication varies across cultures. We infer things from tone of voice, stress on words and phrases, silence, pace, and politeness conventions that are used. Some cultures are more open, direct and assertive than others. Some languages do not differentiate gender in common nouns and pronouns, so 'he' and 'she' may be used interchangeably. It is hardly surprising that misunderstandings occur and it can be much harder to create a rapport. It is worth remembering that smiling is a universal expression of kindness and warmth.

Patients may be more or less traditional, so check out assumptions.

Box 1.19 Communicating with people who are deaf or hard of hearing

- Ask if they need to lip-read when you are speaking
- Position yourself on the better hearing side
- Smile and use eye contact
- Face the light
- Do not cover your face or mouth
- Use plain language
- Speak clearly but not too slowly
- Do not shout
- If stuck, write it down
- Check for understanding
- Never say 'Forget it'!

(RNID: http://www.rnid.org.uk/information_resources/factsheets.)

PATIENTS WHO HAVE IMPAIRED FACULTIES FOR COMMUNICATION

All healthcare professionals need patience, ingenuity and willingness to learn to be able to communicate effectively with patients who have impaired communication faculties.

Impaired hearing

Some 55% of people over 60 are deaf or hard of hearing. Patients may be accompanied by a signer but less than 1% of hearing-impaired people sign. Many hard of hearing people lip-read and some common sense tips are listed in **Box 1.19**. Clinicians who mumble, speak fast or have strong accents have a responsibility to make particular efforts to be understood.

Conversation aids may be available or patients may be asked how best to communicate with them.

Impaired vision

Patients who have visual impairment can miss non-verbal cues in communication. It may sound obvious, but it helps to make more conscious efforts to use the patients' names so they know they are being spoken to. Clinicians should avoid sudden touch, explain what they are about to do, and say what they are doing as they go along. Large-print information sheets should be available, with audio recordings, Braille and Moon versions for blind people (http://www.rnib.org.uk).

PATIENTS WHO HAVE LIMITED UNDERSTANDING OR SPEECH

Aphasia is a communication disorder following strokes. Even though hearing and thought processes are unaffected, patients find it hard to understand, or they know what they want to say but cannot find the words; they are literally 'lost for words'. This also affects their ability to write, gesture, draw or mime their thoughts.

Patients may have a strength in one area – for example, understanding – with a weakness in another other area – for example, expression – or vice versa.

It helps to find a quiet place without distractions, to make eye contact and attract the person's attention. Speak slowly and clearly, use simple phrases and leave plenty of time between sentences to allow for extra processing time. Make it obvious when changing the subject.

Closed questions requiring 'yes' or 'no' answers are easier. Write down key words or headings to which both the patient and the clinician can refer. This helps because the auditory memory needed to 'hold on to' the spoken word taxes the patient's language system. Use pictures and have pen and paper to hand if the patient can use them.

Much can be learnt from carers or watching speech and language therapists. Visit: http://www.ukconnect.org.

Further reading

Cooper LA, Roter DL et al. The associations of clinicians' implicit attitudes about race with medical visit communication and patient ratings of interpersonal care. *Am J Public Health* 2012; 102:979–987.

Kai J. Enhancing consultations with interpreters: learning more about how. *Brit J Gen Pract* 2013; 63:66–67.

National Patient Safety Agency. *Being Open: Communicating Patient Safety Incidents with Patients, Their Families and Carers*; 2009; available at www.nrls.npsa.nhs.uk.

Parliamentary and Health Service Ombudsman. *Principles of Good Complaint Handling*. London: HMSO; 2009.

World Health Organization. *Patient Safety: Curriculum Guide for Medical Schools*. Topic 8. Engaging with patients and carers. Geneva: WHO; 2009; pp. 183–199.

INFLUENCES ON COMMUNICATION

The internet

The internet has revolutionized ready access to information, and in 2010 some 65% of the UK population surfed the net with medical queries. Research on its impact on the doctor–patient relationship is emerging. People report feeling more able to ask informed questions and having less fear of the unknown. Most doctors support internet use in enhancing consultations and especially post diagnosis, when it helps patients understand and manage their illness.

Directing patients to trustworthy, reputable internet sites is helpful.

Decision aids

Weighing up treatment benefits and risks where both may be substantial but not guaranteed is very hard for patients. Decision aids that are evidence-based, are written in non-technical language and often include visual representations help people digest complex statistical information. They are reliable and from independent sources. Formats include web applications, DVDs, computer programs, leaflets and structured counselling. They are growing in number and are listed on the Cochrane register (see 'Significant websites').

Studies show these resources do not increase patients' anxiety and their use results in a 21–44% reduction in choice of invasive surgical options over more conservative treatments without adverse effects on health.

TRAINING IN COMMUNICATION SKILLS

This chapter has covered principles and practical advice on communication in healthcare. There is clear evidence that communication ability is not just innate; it is a professional skill that can be improved and used in everyday practice. The need for clinicians to update their skills continually is recognized as working patterns in healthcare, societal expectations and technological advances change. However, skills cannot be learned entirely from books; the opportunity to practise and receive constructive feedback on performance is essential.

Further reading

Coulter A, Collins A. *Making Shared Decision-making a Reality. No Decision About Me Without Me*. London: King's Fund; 2011.

O'Connor AM, Stacey D, Entwhistle V et al. Decision aids for people facing health treatment or screening decisions (Cochrane Review). Chichester: Cochrane Library; 2008; issue 2.

Pletneva N, Cruchet S, Simonet MA et al. *Results of the 10th HON Survey on Health and Medical Internet Use*. Geneva: Health on the Net Foundation; 2010; http://www.HON.ch.

Significant websites

http://www.bma.org.uk/ethics *British Medical Association ethics*
http://www.each.eu/ *European Association for Communication in Healthcare*
http://www.gmc-uk.org/ *General Medical Council*
http://www.hkma.org/eindex.htm *Hong Kong Medical Association*
http://ima-india.org *Indian Medical Association*
http://www.ohri.ca/decisionaid *Patient decision aids*
http://www.pickereurope.org *Picker Institute Europe*

Reliable internet information for patients

http://www.HON.ch
http://www.nationalvoices.org.uk
http://www.nhs.uk

2 Clinical pharmacology

Michael Rawlins, Munir Pirmohamed

See your e-book for key learning points, clinical tips, drug tips, learning challenges, case studies and MCQs.

INTRODUCTION

Prescribing is a key skill required by all doctors, at least at some stage in their careers. This chapter provides an introduction to the principles of rational therapeutics. The 1984 'Nairobi Declaration' emphasized that prescribing should be to the *right patient* with the *right drug* at the *right dose*, and at an *affordable cost*. Thus, the prescription of a medicine needs to take into account the potential benefits and harms of that medicine, and ensure that every step is taken to maximize the benefit: harm ratio. The key principles of prescribing are described in ***Box 2.1***.

WHY DO PATIENTS NEED DRUGS?

There are many reasons for prescribing drugs to patients. These are as follows:

Disease treatment

A reliable diagnosis is crucial before starting treatment, which may either cure or, more often, control a disease process. An accurate diagnosis ensures that a patient is not exposed, unnecessarily, to the hazards or costs of a particular intervention. However, a prior diagnosis may not be possible in every circumstance; for example, in infection, the initiation of 'blind' antimicrobial therapy is justified when delay would expose a patient to hazard or discomfort.

The choice of the drug often depends on clinical factors (such as age, concomitant disease and concurrent therapy), pharmaceutical factors (the availability of other medicines and relative cost-effectiveness) and, increasingly, individual (host) factors. For instance, trastuzumab is only of value in women with breast cancer whose malignant cells express the HER2 epidermal growth factor receptor. Tailoring or targeting treatment, dependent on the use of biomarkers (e.g. genetic polymorphisms or gene expression pattern), is increasingly being used. This promising approach has become known as 'personalized medicine'.

Symptom relief

Drugs are frequently used in the relief of symptoms: for example, in the treatment of severe pain, constipation or pruritus. The issue here is to monitor the patient so that the effectiveness of symptom relief can be judged and, if it is inadequate, either the dose or drug can be altered. Ensure that the drug is stopped when no longer indicated. Doctors are good at starting drugs but very bad at stopping them!

Prevention

Medicines are also given to otherwise healthy individuals. In such circumstances, there must be a very clear imperative to ensure that the benefits to the individual outweigh the harm. Examples include:

- immunization against serious microbial infections (e.g. influenza vaccination)
- the reduction of individual risk factors to prevent later disease (e.g. the use of antihypertensive or lipid-lowering agents to reduce the chances of ischaemic heart disease and stroke)
- oral contraceptives in sexually active women wishing to avoid pregnancy.

THE CHOICE OF DRUG

Selecting the right drug involves three elements:

- the drug's clinical efficacy for the proposed use
- the balance between the drug's efficacy and safety
- patient preference.

The most common approach to assessing a drug's efficacy is the randomized controlled trial (RCT), although other approaches (see p. 28) can be informative. The demonstration of absolute efficacy (against placebo) may, itself, be insufficient. Where there is more than one treatment for the same indication, these should be compared with one another, taking account of the magnitude of their benefits, their individual adverse reaction profiles, and their costs. There are also ethical concerns to the use of placebos; these

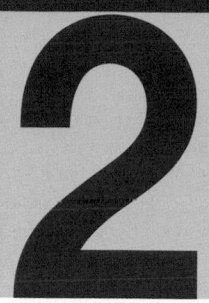

Box 2.1 Key principles of prescribing

- ***Be clear about the reasons for prescribing.*** Obtain an accurate diagnosis and have clear aims of what the benefits will be from prescribing the drug.
- ***Obtain an accurate drug history.*** Patients should be asked about their current medications, over-the-counter herbal medicines, and illicit drug usage. A past history of intolerances, including true allergic reactions, is also required.
- ***Obtain an accurate history of other factors that might affect the benefit : harm ratio of drugs.*** Take note of liver and renal impairment, age, whether patient is pregnant or breast-feeding, and co-morbidities.
- ***Establish what the patient expects from the drug, and deal with any concerns.*** Provide good information for the patient and answer any questions clearly.
- ***Select the most clinically effective, cost-effective and safe medicine for the patient, based on an assessment of the individual.*** Optimize the benefit : harm balance by choosing the right dose and frequency, and the right drug, in the the best formulation, route of administration and duration of treatment. Prescribe within the licence of the medicine, except when no alternative is available.
- ***Adhere to guidelines and local and national formularies.*** Based on the needs of the individual patient, use the most reliable information to identify the medicine most suited to the patient.
- ***Write prescriptions legibly using the correct documents, or prescribe electronically, depending on availability.*** Take care to avoid medication errors.
- ***Monitor the patient for both efficacy and safety after starting the drug.*** This is essential to optimize dose, identify adverse reactions, and determine when to stop the medicine. Report adverse reactions using spontaneous reporting schemes, if appropriate.
- ***Communicate clearly with other healthcare professionals and patients about the reasons for prescribing decisions.*** Communication is essential to optimize the benefit : harm ratio of drugs, particularly when there are multiple prescribers for a single patient.
- ***Prescribe within your competencies.*** Prescribing should be within the limits of your knowledge and experience. Do not be afraid to ask for advice, and ensure that complex prescriptions are checked (e.g. when calculating doses).

(Adapted from British Pharmacological Society; http://www.bps.ac.uk/SpringboardWebApp/userfiles/bps/file/Clinical/BPSPrescribingStatement03Feb2010.pdf.)

should only be used when there are no other effective treatments, when withholding drugs poses no serious risk of harm, and when there are methodological reasons (but where there is no risk of harm from withholding treatment).

Direct comparisons of one treatment versus another are particularly useful but are often unavailable. In such cases, indirect techniques can be used. For example, none of the novel oral anticoagulants (dabigatran, rivaroxaban, apixaban and edoxaban) has been tested against the others, but comparative effectiveness can be modelled using indirect comparison of the individual RCTs in which each drug was compared with warfarin.

Patients' own preferences should be discussed to enable them to be equal partners in decision-making about whether, and how, they wish to be treated. Moreover, a full understanding of the reasons for considering treatment, the likely benefits and the possible adverse reactions has repeatedly been shown to improve 'concordance' with treatment regimens.

Further reading

Millum J, Grady C. The ethics of placebo-controlled trials: methodological justifications. *Contemp Clin Trials* 2013; 36:510–514.
Skjoth F, Larsen TB, Rasmussen LH. Indirect comparison studies – are they useful? Insights from the novel oral anticoagulants for stroke prevention in atrial fibrillation. *Thromb Haemost* 2012; 108:405–406.

THE DOSE

The dose administered to the patient is crucial in determining both efficacy and safety of medicines. Appropriate drug dosages will usually have been determined from the results of so-called '***dose-ranging***' studies during the original development programme.

In some cases, drug doses are ***fixed,*** with all patients being given the same dose; for example, levonorgestrel for emergency contraception. However, these situations are unusual. For example, although the majority of patients are given 75 mg per day of aspirin, doses of up to 300 mg per day have been used for the secondary prevention of myocardial infarction.

More commonly, doses are ***titrated***. For many drugs, there are wide inter-individual variations in response. As a consequence, whilst a particular dose may, in one person, lack any therapeutic effect, the same dose in another may cause serious toxicity. Prescribers should start at a low dose and titrate to the most effective dose, which should, in all cases, determine the lowest effective dose. This is necessary because of the inter-individual variability in the dose–response curve, whereby there is an increase in response with an increase in dose, until a plateau effect is reached ***(Fig. 2.1)***.

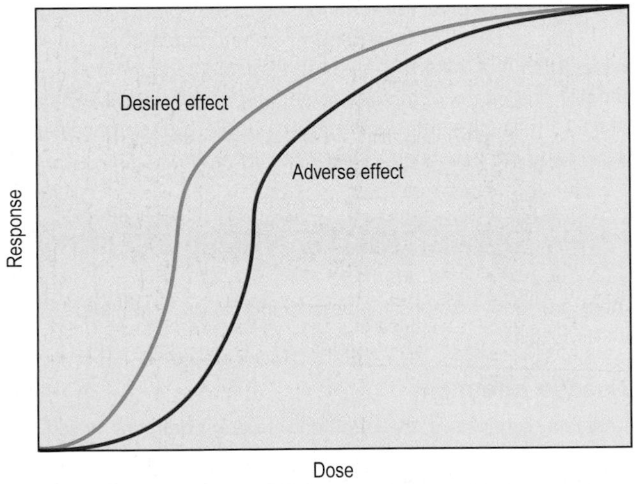

Figure 2.1 Dose–response curve, showing the variable response of the same dose in different patients.

The reasons for this ***variability in response*** can be divided into two broad areas:

- ***Pharmacokinetic*** factors, where the dose administered does not necessarily equate with systemic or tissue drug concentrations: that is, exposure. This may be due to differences in the rates of drug absorption, metabolism and/or excretion.
- ***Pharmacodynamic*** factors, where there are differences in the sensitivity of the drug target that generally fall into the categories of receptors, enzymes, ion channels, transporters, DNA or transcription factors.

Box 2.2 Routes of drug administration

Route	Description	Example
Buccal	Rapid absorption, avoids first-pass metabolism	Midazolam for status epilepticus
Epidural	Used for analgesia	Epidural anaesthetic for pain relief during labour
Inhaled	Achieves high concentrations at site of disease with limited systemic absorption	Salbutamol for acute asthma relief
Intramuscular	Easier than intravenous route but absorption is less predictable	Adrenaline (epinephrine) in anaphylaxis
Intranasal	Often used for local delivery	Intranasal corticosteroids in allergic conditions
Intrathecal	Used to achieve high local levels	Methotrexate in acute lymphoblastic leukaemia
Intravenous	100% of dose enters systemic circulation but invasive and inconvenient	Intravenous teicoplanin for treatment of invasive MRSA infections
Oral	Most common route, convenient, but subject to first-pass metabolism for certain drugs	Ramipril for hypertension
Subcutaneous	Good absorption, can be self-administered	Insulin for diabetes
Sublingual	Rapid absorption, avoids first-pass metabolism	GTN for acute relief of angina chest pain
Topical	Used for local application of cutaneous or joint diseases	Corticosteroids for eczema
Transdermal	Absorption through the skin via a patch	Nicotine replacement therapy for smoking cessation

GTN, glyceryl trinitrate; MRSA, meticillin-resistant *Staphylococcus aureus*

Box 2.3 Key pharmacokinetic parameters

- ***Area under the curve***: A plasma concentration time curve and a measure of the actual body exposure to a drug after administration of a dose of the drug; expressed in mg/L x h.
- ***Bioavailability***: The fraction or proportion of a drug that enters the systemic circulation. Thus, while intravenous formulations have 100% bioavailability, administration via other routes will have <100% bioavailability.
- ***Clearance***: Volume of plasma cleared of the drug per unit time.
- ***C_{max}***: Peak plasma concentration after drug administration.
- ***Concentration***: Amount of drug in a given volume. Even when the dose is similar, concentrations (and thus exposure) will vary between individuals.
- ***Dose***: Amount of drug administered. This may be micrograms, milligrams or grams. Occasionally, drugs are administered per body weight or body surface area.
- ***Elimination half-life***: The time required for the drug concentration to reach half its original value.
- ***T_{max}***: Time to reach C_{max}.
- ***V_d***: Volume of distribution – the apparent volume in which a drug is distributed. Drugs with low V_d are predominantly in the circulation, while drugs with a high V_d have diffused into the peripheral tissue compartment.

PHARMACOKINETICS

Pharmacokinetics is the study of ***what the body does to a drug***. This can be divided into four different processes: absorption, distribution, metabolism and excretion.

Absorption

Drugs can be administered by various different routes ***(Box 2.2)*** but oral administration is the most common. The main determinants of a drug's plasma concentration after oral administration are its bioavailability (Box 2.3) and its rate of systemic clearance (by hepatic metabolism or renal excretion). A drug's oral bioavailability depends on the extent to which it is:

- *Destroyed in the gastrointestinal tract*, especially by gastric acid.
- *Unable to cross the gastrointestinal epithelium*. Drugs can cross either by passive diffusion or by active uptake by transporters that are abundant in the gut epithelial barrier. Such transporters can be either influx transporters (pumping drugs from the gut lumen into the cell, such as the PEPT1 transporter for the absorption of penicillins) or efflux transporters (pumping drugs from cells back into the gut lumen, such as the P-glycoprotein that can limit the absorption of many drugs).
- *Metabolized by the liver* before reaching the systemic circulation (so-called pre-systemic or 'first-pass' metabolism). First-pass metabolism can be avoided by the intravascular, intramuscular or sublingual routes.

Distribution

This is the process by which drugs are distributed from the bloodstream to organs and cells. Most drugs will circulate in the bloodstream bound to plasma proteins, most commonly albumin. Free drug, which is the active drug, is usually in dynamic equilibrium with protein-bound drug, with the latter being released as the free drug concentration decreases.

Metabolism

Metabolism takes place in many different organs, the liver being the most common site. The function of metabolism is to convert lipid-soluble drugs to water-soluble drugs that can then be excreted by the kidneys. Metabolism usually inactivates a drug, but in some cases, it can convert a prodrug into an active drug (e.g. enalapril to enalaprilat), or lead to the formation of toxic metabolites (e.g. the formation of N-acetyl-para-benzoquinoneimine in paracetamol overdose). Drug metabolism occurs in two stages:

- ***Phase I*** is the modification of a drug, by oxidation, reduction or hydrolysis. Of these, oxidation is the most frequent route and is largely undertaken by a family of isoenzymes known as the cytochrome P450 system. Inhibition or induction of cytochrome P450 isoenzymes is a major cause of drug interactions (see p. 24).
- ***Phase II*** involves conjugation with glucuronate, sulphate, acetate or other substances to render the drug more water-soluble and therefore able to be excreted in the urine.

Excretion

Excretion of drugs and their metabolites occurs most commonly via the kidneys, although faeces, breath and sweat represent other routes of excretion. In the kidney, free drug is filtered through the glomerulus and excreted in the urine as long as it is water-soluble. Lipid-soluble drugs are usually reabsorbed in the renal tubules. Some drugs, such as benzylpenicillin, are actively excreted by cells in the proximal convoluted tubule. Renal impairment reduces the elimination of water-soluble drugs, and thus reduction of the maintenance dose must be undertaken to avoid toxicity.

PHARMACODYNAMICS

Pharmacodynamics is the study of ***what the drug does to the body***. Pharmacodynamic sources of variation in drug action can be due to changes in the expression of the drug target, their affinity or their selectivity. This can be caused by genetic factors (see p. 25) and also by disease. For example, in renal impairment, pharmacodynamic factors determine the sensitivity to a drug.

Pharmacodynamic tests can be used in clinical practice to target therapy or to avoid undue sensitivity. Examples include the following:

- Expression of oestrogen and HER2 receptors in women with breast cancer are used as markers of responsiveness to anti-oestrogens and trastuzumab (respectively).
- The *V600E BRAF* somatic gene mutation in patients with malignant melanoma is used to determine whether vemurafenib will be effective (see p. 25).
- Pseudocholinesterase (also known as butyrylcholinesterase) inactivates the neuromuscular blocking agent suxamethonium. Patients with mutations in the pseudocholinesterase gene can develop prolonged paralysis after the administration of suxamethonium.

Pharmacodynamic sources of variation in drug response have not been as well studied as pharmacokinetic factors. The prospect for 'personalized prescribing' will be enhanced when the interplay between pharmacokinetics and pharmacodynamics is better understood, which will then permit drug selection and dosing to become much more precise.

Further reading

Mcleod HL. Cancer pharmacogenomics: early promise, but concerted effort needed. *Science* 2013; 339:1563–1566.

AFFORDABILITY AND COST-EFFECTIVENESS

All healthcare systems try to provide their populations with the highest standards of care within the resources they have at their disposal. The money countries spend on healthcare, however, varies widely ***(Fig. 2.2)***. The differences between countries' expenditure on healthcare are almost entirely determined by their wealth, as reflected in per capita gross domestic product (GDP), with richer countries spending more on healthcare than poorer ones. Consequently, an intervention that might be affordable in the USA, Norway or Sweden is not necessarily affordable in China, India or Indonesia. Increasing use is therefore being made of formal analyses of costs and benefits, by both developed and, to a lesser extent, lower- to middle-income countries, to help decide on healthcare priorities.

There are a number of different approaches to the economic evaluation of healthcare interventions but the main one is known as 'cost–utility analysis'. The main features are as follows:

- The costs are reflected in the price of the product, together with additional sums associated with its administration (including extra costs of any associated hospital care, and additional investigations, for the care of patients with adverse drug reactions). Any savings that may accrue from the use of an intervention are also included in the calculation.
- The benefits are assessed from the increase in quality of life (sometimes known as the ***gain in health utility***) as a result of using an intervention, in comparison with alternative forms of treatment (which, in the absence of an active comparator, may be '***best supportive care***'). The utility gain is expressed on a scale of 0 (dead) to 1 (perfect health). This utility gain is then multiplied by the number of years for which it is 'enjoyed', to provide the ***quality-adjusted life years (QALY)*** gained.
- The ***incremental cost-effectiveness ratio (ICER)*** is estimated by dividing the total net costs (which includes any savings) by the QALY gained. In England, ICERs of an intervention costing less than £20 000 per QALY gained are likely to be regarded as cost-effective; as the ICER rises, so does the likelihood of the intervention being rejected for use in the National Health Service on grounds of cost-ineffectiveness.

The virtue of cost–utility analysis, in the evaluation of both new and established products, is that it allows comparisons to be

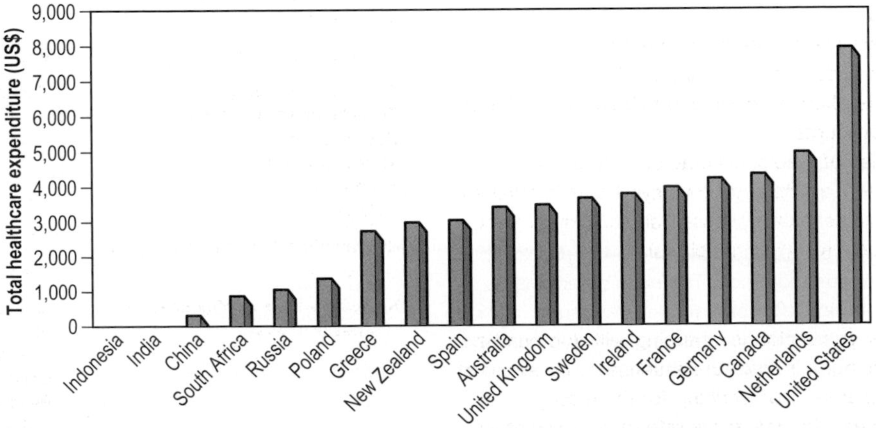

Figure 2.2 Total healthcare expenditure (US$) in various countries, as US$ per head of the population (data for 2009).

Box 2.4 Incremental cost-effectiveness ratios (ICERs), expressed as £ per quality-adjusted life years (QALY) gained, for selected pharmaceutical products

Product	Indication	Comparator	Most plausible ICER[a]
Alimtuzumab	Relapsing–remitting multiple sclerosis	Glatiramer acetate	26 000
Alteplase	Acute ischaemic stoke (0–4.5 h post onset)	Best supportive care	4500
Apixaban	Prevention of stroke and systemic embolism in atrial fibrillation	Warfarin	13 000
Dabigatran	Prevention of stoke and systemic embolism in atrial fibrillation	Warfarin	18 000
Imatinib	Chronic myeloid leukaemia (chronic phase)	Interferon-alpha	26 000
Rituximab	Chronic lymphatic leukaemia (first-line)	Fludarabine + cyclophosphamide	22 500
Rivaroxaban	Prevention of stroke and systemic embolism in atrial fibrillation	Warfarin	18 800
Trastuzumab	Early-stage breast cancer (after surgery and chemotherapy)	Best supportive care	18 000

[a]Based on estimates published by the National Institute for Health and Care Excellence (NICE).

made between differing treatments for differing conditions. Examples of the ICERs of some of the interventions examined by the National Institute for Health and Care Excellence (NICE) are shown in ***Box 2.4***.

PRESCRIBING IN SPECIAL POPULATIONS

Neonates, infants, children and adolescents

The use of drugs in young people poses special problems. Extrapolating from adult dosage regimens, merely adjusting for weight, leads to excessive (and potentially toxic) doses because:

- the rates of hepatic metabolism and renal excretion of drugs are reduced in neonates and infants
- premature babies have approximately 1% of their body weight as fat (compared with 20% in adults), leading to a marked increase in plasma drug levels of fat-soluble drugs.

There are other difficulties in prescribing for children:

- Many treatments have never been subject to formal trials in either children or adolescents and their benefits and risks have not, therefore, been appropriately assessed in these age groups. In order to redress this, regulatory agencies, such as the European Medicines Agency, now require manufacturers to provide Paediatric Investigation Plans if a new drug is licensed for adults only.
- For many drugs, there are no paediatric preparations or formulations. Instead, adult products are used.
- Precise oral dosing is often impossible in babies, who spit out unpleasant-tasting products!
- Adverse effect profiles of medicines may be different in children compared with adults (e.g. Reye syndrome in children given aspirin, suicidal ideas in depressed adolescents treated with selective serotonin reuptake inhibitors).

The elderly

The demography of our population is changing with the numbers of elderly people increasing. It is therefore essential to be aware of the potential issues that arise in prescribing for the elderly:

- Renal function declines with age at the rate of approximately 1 mL/min after the age of 40 years. Extrapolation of drug dosages, from those appropriate in younger adults, may therefore lead to toxic plasma levels in older patients.
- Changes in drug distribution due to changes in body composition, and the preferential distribution of the cardiac output to the brain, may also predispose to toxicity.
- Co-morbidity, often associated with polypharmacy, leads to increased opportunities for disease–drug and drug–drug interactions.
- Concordance with treatment regimens diminishes as the number of prescribed drugs increases, and is especially poor in the face of cognitive impairment.
- Exaggerated pharmacodynamic effects of drugs acting on the central nervous, cardiovascular and gastrointestinal systems are common.

Examples of common problems encountered in the use of drugs amongst older people are shown in ***Box 2.5***.

Box 2.5 Common adverse reactions to drugs in the elderly

Drug or drug class	Effect
Beta-blockers (including eye drops) **Digoxin**	Bradycardia
Nitrates **α-Adrenoceptor-blockers** **Loop diuretics**	Postural hypotension
Diuretics (thiazides)	Glucose intolerance, gout
Antimuscarinic drugs **Tricyclic antidepressants** **Neuroleptics** **Anticonvulsants** **Hypnotics** **Opioids**	Confusion, cognitive dysfunction
Bisphosphonates (mainly alendronic acid)	Oesophageal ulceration and stricture formation
Non-steroidal anti-inflammatory drugs (NSAIDs)	Gastric erosions Small bowel and colonic lesions (less frequently than gastric) Upper gastrointestinal bleeding Perforated peptic ulcer Salt and water retention Renal impairment

Box 2.6 Some human teratogens

Drug or drug class	Effect
ACE inhibitors/antagonists	Oligohydramnios
Retinoids, e.g. isotretinoin	Multiple abnormalities
Carbimazole	Neonatal hypothyroidism Abnormalities of bone growth
Fluconazole	Fallot's tetralogy
Antiepileptics: carbamazepine, lamotrigine, phenytoin, valproate	Cleft palate, facial abnormalities, neural tube defect Neural tube defects, neurodevelopmental delay
NSAIDs	Delayed closure of the ductus arteriosus
Cytotoxic drugs	Most are presumed teratogens
Lithium	Ebstein's anomaly
Misoprostol	Moebius syndrome (rare neurological condition)
Thalidomide (and possibly lenalidomide)	Phocomelia

Note: All drugs should be avoided in pregnancy unless benefit clearly outweighs the risk.

Pregnant women

Clinicians should be extremely cautious about prescribing drugs to pregnant women and only essential treatments should be given. When a known teratogen is needed during pregnancy (e.g. an anticonvulsant drug or lithium), the potential adverse effects should be discussed with the parents, preferably before conception. Teratogens are best known for causing structural malformations: for example, congenital heart disease. However, teratogens can also lead to neurodevelopmental problems without any obvious structural damage. For example, exposure to sodium valproate *in utero* can lead to developmental neurotoxicity, which is manifested as cognitive and behavioural problems. Some known human teratogens are shown in ***Box 2.6***.

Breast-feeding women

Although most drugs can be detected in breast milk, the quantity is generally small. This is because, for most drugs, the concentration in milk is in equilibrium with plasma water (i.e. the non-protein-bound fraction). A few drugs (e.g. aspirin, carbimazole, methotrexate) may, however, cause harm to the infant if ingested in breast milk. The relevant drug literature should be consulted when prescribing for nursing mothers.

MONITORING DRUG THERAPY

The combination of pharmacokinetic and pharmacodynamic causes of variability makes monitoring of the effects of treatment essential. Three approaches are used.

Pre-treatment dose selection

In patients who have known, or suspected, impaired renal function, it is usually possible to predict dose requirements from their estimated glomerular filtration rate (eGFR), usually based on serum creatinine levels. If treatment needs to be started before the eGFR is available, in patients who have very advanced renal impairment or if renal function is fluctuating, then treatment can be started with conventional doses but the prescriber should be prepared to make dose adjustments within 24 hours.

Box 2.7 Drugs for which therapeutic drug monitoring is used

Drug	Therapeutic plasma concentration range	Toxic level	Optimum post-dose sampling time (h)
Carbamazepine	20–50 µmol/L	>50 µmol/L	>8
Ciclosporin	50–200 µg/L	>200 µg/L	Pre-dose
Digoxin	1.3–2.6 nmol/L	>2.6 nmol/L	>8
Gentamicin	Trough <2 mg/L	>14 mg/L	Pre-dose
	Peak 5–10 mg/L	>12 mg/L	>1
Lithium	0.6–1.0 mmol/L	>1.5 mmol/L	>10
Phenytoin	40–80 µmol/L	>80 µmol/L	>10
Theophylline	55–110 µmol/L	>110 µmol/L	>4
Vancomycin	15–20 mg/L	–	Pre-dose

Measuring plasma drug concentrations

For a few drugs, dosages can be effectively monitored by reference to their plasma concentrations ***(Box 2.7)***. This technique is only useful, however, if both of the following criteria are fulfilled:

- There is a reliable and available drug assay.
- Plasma concentrations correlate well with both therapeutic efficacy and toxicity.

Measuring drug effects

For many drugs, dosage adjustments are made in line with patients' responses. Monitoring can involve dose titration against a therapeutic end-point or a toxic effect. Objective measures (such as monitoring antihypertensive therapy by measuring blood pressure, or cytotoxic therapy with serial white blood cell counts) are most helpful, but subjective ones are necessary in many instances (as with antipsychotic therapy in people with schizophrenia).

ADVERSE DRUG REACTIONS

Adverse drug reactions (ADRs), defined as 'the unwanted effects of drugs occurring under normal conditions of use', are a significant cause of morbidity and mortality. The burden of ADRs on hospitals is huge in both adults and children ***(Box 2.8)***. ADRs also account for about 2.5% of emergency room visits, and about 1 in 4 patients in primary care will have an adverse reaction, but fortunately these are mild in most cases. Unwanted effects of drugs are 5–6 times more likely in the elderly than in young adults, and the risk of an ADR rises sharply with the number of drugs administered. ADRs are also more common in women than in men.

Classification

Two types of ADR are recognized.

Type A (augmented) reactions (Box 2.9)

These:

- are qualitatively normal, but quantitatively abnormal, manifestations of a drug's pharmacological or toxicological properties

Box 2.8 Burden of adverse drug reactions (ADRs) in hospitals

Study	Setting	Number of patients studied	Frequency of ADRs
Adults			
Davies et al[a]	Patients in hospital	3695	14.7%
Children			
Gallagher et al[b]	Patients requiring hospital admission	8345	2.9%
Thiesen et al[c]	Inpatients	16601	17.7%

[a]Davies EC, Green CF, Taylor S et al. Adverse drug reactions in hospital in-patients: a prospective analysis of 3695 patient episodes. *PLoS One* 2009; 4:e4439.
[b]Gallagher RM, Mason JR, Bird KA et al. Adverse drug reactions causing admission to a paediatric hospital. *PLoS One* 2012; 7:e50127.
[c]Thiesen S, Conroy EJ, Bellis JR et al. Incidence, characteristics and risk factors of adverse drug reactions in hospitalized children – a prospective observational cohort study of 6,601 admissions. *BMC Medicine* 2013; 11:237.

- are predictable from its known pharmacological or toxicological actions
- generally show a clear dose–response relationship
- are usually common
- are only occasionally serious.

Whilst some reactions, such as hypotension with angiotensin-converting enzyme (ACE) inhibitors, may occur after a single dose, others may develop only after months (pulmonary fibrosis with amiodarone) or years (second malignancies with anticancer drugs).

Type B (idiosyncratic) reactions (see Box 2.9)

These have no resemblance to the recognized pharmacological or toxicological effects of the drug. They:

- are qualitatively abnormal responses to the drug
- are unpredictable from its known pharmacological or toxicological actions
- show a dose–response relationship that is complex and not easily discernible
- are usually rare
- are often serious.

Box 2.9 Examples of adverse drug reactions

Type of reaction and drug (or drug class)	Adverse reaction
Type A (augmented)	
ACE inhibitors, e.g. ramipril	Hypotension Chronic cough
Angiotensin receptor antagonists, e.g. losartan	Hypotension
Anticoagulants, e.g. warfarin	Gastrointestinal bleeding Intracerebral haemorrhage
Antipsychotics, e.g. haloperidol	Acute dystonia/dyskinesia Parkinsonian symptoms Tardive dyskinesia
Cytotoxic agents, e.g. 5-fluorouracil	Bone marrow dyscrasias Cancer
Diuretics, e.g. furosemide	Dehydration, renal impairment
Glucocorticosteroids, e.g. prednisolone	Hypoadrenalism Osteoporosis
Insulin	Hypoglycaemia
Tricyclic antidepressants, e.g. amitriptyline	Dry mouth
Type B (idiosyncratic)	
Benzylpenicillin Radiological contrast media	Anaphylaxis
Broad-spectrum penicillins. e.g. co-amoxiclav	Maculopapular rash
Carbamazepine Lamotrigine Phenytoin Sulphonamides	Toxic epidermal necrolysis Stevens–Johnson syndrome
Carbamazepine Diclofenac Isoniazid Phenytoin Rifampicin	Hepatotoxicity
Isotretinoin SSRIs[a], e.g. fluoxetine	Depression Suicidal ideation

ACE, angiotensin-converting enzyme; SSRIs, selective serotonin reuptake inhibitors.
[a]In children and adolescents.

Diagnosis

All ADRs mimic some naturally occurring disease, and the distinction between an iatrogenic aetiology and an event unrelated to the drug is often difficult. The patient should be asked not only about prescription drugs but also about over-the-counter medicines, herbal medicines and illicit drugs. Although some effects are obviously iatrogenic (e.g. acute anaphylaxis occurring a few minutes after intravenous penicillin), many are less so.

Causality assessment of a suspected ADR can be difficult, particularly in patients on multiple drugs. The following simple rules (remembered by the mnemonic TREND) can help in assessing causality:

- ***Temporal relationship***. The time interval between the administration of a drug and the suspected adverse reaction should be appropriate. Acute anaphylaxis usually occurs within a few minutes of administration, whilst aplastic anaemia will only become apparent after a few weeks (because of the lifespan of erythrocytes). Drug-induced malignancy, however, will take years to develop.
- ***Rechallenge***. Re-institution of the suspected drug, to see if the event recurs, is often regarded as an absolute diagnostic test. This is, in many instances, correct but there are two caveats. First, it is rarely justifiable to subject a patient to further hazard. Second, some ADRs develop because of particular circumstances, which may not necessarily be replicated on rechallenge (e.g. hypoglycaemia with an antidiabetic agent).
- ***Exclusion of other causes***. An ADR is a diagnosis of exclusion, and other causes should be excluded by taking a careful clinical history and undertaking relevant investigations. For example, in drug-induced liver injury, it may be necessary to exclude viral, autoimmune and metabolic causes by blood tests, and cholelithiasis by ultrasound. In a few instances, the diagnosis of an adverse reaction can be inferred from the plasma concentration (see ***Box 2.7***).
- ***Nature and novelty of the reaction***. Many ADRs have been reported before, which can help in assessing causality. Some conditions (e.g. angio-oedema or toxic epidermal necrolysis)

are so typically iatrogenic that an ADR is very likely. Where an event is a manifestation of the known pharmacological property of the drug, it can be recognized as a type A ADR (e.g. hypotension with an antihypertensive agent, or hypoglycaemia with an antidiabetic drug).

- ***Dechallenge***. Failure of remission when the drug is withdrawn (i.e. 'dechallenge') is unlikely to be an ADR. The diagnostic reliability of dechallenge is not, however, absolute; if the ADR has caused irreversible organ damage (e.g. malignancy), then dechallenge will result in a false-negative response.

Management

As a general rule, type A reactions can usually be managed by a reduction in dosage, whilst type B reactions almost invariably require the drug to be withdrawn (and never re-instituted). Most ADRs resolve spontaneously when the drug is withdrawn, but specific therapy is sometimes required for ADRs such as bleeding with warfarin (vitamin K), acute dystonias (benztropine) or acute anaphylaxis (see Emergency ***Box 8.24***). Desensitization is sometimes carried out for immune-mediated reactions but this should be done by a specialist with appropriate resuscitation facilities.

When a patient suffers an ADR, this should be reported to the regulatory agency: for example, through the UK's ***yellow card reporting*** scheme to the Medicines Healthcare Products Regulatory Agency. The criteria for reporting vary across the world but, in general, all ADRs to new drugs should be reported, while only the serious ADRs to established drugs (i.e. those that have been on the market for more than 2 years) should be reported.

Further reading

Pirmohamed M. Anticipating, investigating and managing the adverse effects of drugs. *Clin Med* 2005; 5:23–26.

DRUG INTERACTIONS

Drugs can interact with each other (drug–drug interactions; DDIs), with food (drug–food interactions) and with herbal medicines (drug–herbal interactions) ***(Box 2.10)***. These interactions, in general, can be either pharmacokinetic (affecting the processes of absorption, distribution, metabolism and excretion), pharmacodynamic (synergistic or antagonistic) or mixed. Approximately 1% of all ADRs that lead to hospital admission are due to DDIs. A major risk factor for DDIs is polypharmacy, which is becoming more common because of the co-morbidities associated with an ageing population. About 57% of patients above the age of 65 years are on more than five drugs, with 12% being on more than ten drugs. The use of multiple drugs in a patient is necessary in some cases, but regular review of medicines is essential in order to optimize doses and stop those drugs that are no longer required. Prescribing additional drugs in a patient already on medicines should only be done after a careful history, if it is clinically indicated, and with adjustment of dose through regular monitoring (clinical and/or laboratory, as appropriate).

Food–drug interactions are also becoming increasingly recognized. A common example is grapefruit juice and drugs metabolized

Box 2.10 Some examples of drug interactions

Implicated drug(s)	Affected drug(s)	Mechanism	Clinical effect
Pharmacokinetic: absorption			
Colestyramine	Digoxin	Binding of colestyramine to digoxin	Reduced digoxin plasma concentration and reduced efficacy
Pharmacokinetic: enzyme induction			
Carbamazepine Phenytoin Phenobarbital Rifampicin St John's Wort	Oral contraceptive Warfarin Ciclosporin	CYP3A4 induction CYP2C9 induction CYP3A4 and P-glycoprotein induction	Contraceptive failure Thrombosis Allograft rejection
Pharmacokinetic: enzyme inhibition			
Amiodarone	Warfarin	CYP2C9 inhibition	Haemorrhage
Cimetidine	Warfarin	CYP2C9 inhibition	Haemorrhage
Ciprofloxacin	Theophylline	CYP1A2 inhibition	Arrhythmias
Grapefruit juice	Simvastatin	CYP3A4 inhibition	Myopathy
Itraconazole	Verapamil	CYP3A4 inhibition	Bradycardia
Ritonavir	Fluticasone	CYP3A4 inhibition	Cushing syndrome
Pharmacokinetic: excretion			
Naproxen	Methotrexate	Inhibition of methotrexate excretion	Methotrexate toxicity
Bendroflumethiazide	Lithium	Inhibition of lithium excretion	Lithium toxicity
Pharmacodynamic: synergistic interaction			
Verapamil	Atenolol	Atrioventricular node block	Bradycardia, heart block
Ramipril	Spironolactone	Reduced excretion of potassium	Hyperkalaemia
Pharmacodynamic: antagonistic interaction			
Salbutamol	Atenolol	Opposing effects at the β_2-receptor	Lack of bronchodilatation
Furosemide	Digoxin	Hypokalaemia	Digoxin toxicity

by CYP3A4 (e.g. simvastatin – see ***Box 2.10***, verapamil and tacrolimus, to name a few). Grapefruit juice inhibits CYP3A4 in the intestinal wall, increasing the bioavailability of these drugs and resulting in higher exposure, and toxicity.

Herbal medicines are taken by almost 20% of the population but rarely asked about when a patient's clinical history is taken. Many different herbal–drug interactions have been described, the best recognized of which is with St John's Wort (SJW), which is an inducer of P450 enzymes and drug transporters such as P-glycoprotein. SJW can lead to increased drug metabolism, reduction in drug concentration, and failure of therapeutic effect. An example is interaction with immunosuppressants such as prednisolone and ciclosporin, where the use of SJW has led to allograft rejection.

Further reading

Bailey DG, Dresser G, Arnold JM. Grapefruit–medication interactions: forbidden fruit or avoidable consequences? *CMAJ* 2013; 185:309–316.

Magro L, Moretti U, Leone R. Epidemiology and characteristics of adverse drug reactions caused by drug–drug interactions. *Expert Opin Drug Saf* 2012; 11:83–94.

INTER-INDIVIDUAL VARIABILITY IN DRUG RESPONSE

Patients vary in the way they respond to drugs, in terms of both efficacy and safety. In some circumstances, this may be due to clinical and environmental factors. Age, body weight, renal and hepatic function, concomitant drugs, co-morbidities, diet, smoking and alcohol are all known to affect the pharmacokinetics and sometimes the pharmacodynamics of drugs. Genetic factors affecting both the pharmacokinetics and pharmacodynamics of drugs also play a role in determining how individuals respond to drugs.

Genetic causes of altered pharmacokinetics

Both pre-systemic hepatic metabolism and the rate of systemic hepatic clearance may vary markedly between healthy individuals. Variability in the genes that encode drug-metabolizing enzymes ***(Box 2.11)*** is a major determinant of the inter-individual differences in the therapeutic and adverse responses to drug treatment. Genetic polymorphisms can affect both phase I and phase II drug-metabolizing enzymes.

Box 2.11 Genetic polymorphisms affecting drug response

Organ or system involved	Associated gene/ allele	Drug/drug response phenotype	Pharmacokinetic/ pharmacodynamic
Blood			
Red blood cells	*G6PD*	Primaquine and others	Pharmacodynamic
	*TPMT*2*	Azathioprine/6MP-induced neutropenia	Pharmacokinetic
Neutrophils	*UGT1A1*28*	Irinotecan-induced neutropenia	Pharmacokinetic
Platelets	*CYP2C19*2*	Stent thrombosis	Pharmacokinetic
Coagulation	*CYP2C9*2, *3, VKORC1*	Warfarin dose requirement	Mixed
Brain and peripheral nervous system			
CNS depression	*CYP2D6*N*	Codeine-related sedation and respiratory depression	Pharmacokinetic
Anaesthesia	Butyrylcholinesterase	Prolonged apnoea	Pharmacokinetic
Peripheral nerves	*NAT-2*	Isoniazid-induced peripheral neuropathy	Pharmacokinetic
Drug hypersensitivity and liver injury			
	*HLA-B*57:01*	Abacavir hypersensitivity	Pharmacodynamic
	*HLA-B*15:02*	Carbamazepine-induced Stevens–Johnson syndrome (in some Asian groups)	Pharmacodynamic
	*HLA-A*31:01*	Carbamazepine-induced hypersensitivity in Caucasians and Japanese	Pharmacodynamic
	*HLA-B*58:01*	Allopurinol-induced serious cutaneous reactions	Pharmacodynamic
	*HLA-B*57:01*	Flucloxacillin hepatotoxicity	Pharmacodynamic
Malignancy			
Breast cancer	*CYP2D6*	Response to tamoxifen	Pharmacokinetic
Chronic myeloid leukaemia	*BCR-ABL*	Imatinib and other tyrosine kinase inhibitors	Pharmacokinetic
Colon cancer	*KRAS*	Cetuximab efficacy	Pharmacokinetic
Gastrointestinal stromal tumours	*c-kit*	Imatinib efficacy	Pharmacokinetic
Lung cancer	*EGFR*	Gefitinib efficacy	Pharmacokinetic
	EML4-ALK	Crizotinib efficacy	Pharmacokinetic
Malignant melanoma	*BRAF V600E*	Vemurafenib efficacy	Pharmacodynamic
Muscle			
General anaesthetics	Ryanodine receptor	Malignant hyperthermia	Pharmacodynamic
Statins	*SLCO1B1*	Myopathy/rhabdomyolysis	Pharmacokinetic

(Adapted from Pirmohamed M. Pharmacogenetics: past, present and future. *Drug Discov Today* 2011; 16:852–861.)

Approximately 25% of all medicines currently in use are substrates for CYP2D6. The frequencies of the variant alleles show racial variation and a small proportion of individuals may have three or more copies of the active gene. The phenotypic consequences of the defective CYP2D6 include the increased risk of toxicity with those antidepressants or antipsychotics that undergo metabolism by this pathway. Additionally, reduced conversion of a prodrug to the active metabolite may also compromise efficacy in some patients; for example, poor metabolizers of CYP2D6 may be at increased risk of breast cancer relapse with tamoxifen. Conversely, in individuals with multiple copies of the active gene (ultra-rapid metabolizers), there are extremely rapid rates of metabolism and therapeutic failure at conventional doses. Ultra-rapid metabolizers may also be at increased risk of toxicity with the conversion of prodrugs to active metabolites; this has been shown with codeine, which is metabolized to morphine and has caused respiratory depression, particularly in children.

Warfarin is predominantly metabolized by CYP2C9. In most populations, between 2% and 10% are homozygous for an allele that results in low enzyme activity. Such individuals will therefore metabolize warfarin more slowly, leading to higher plasma levels, a greater risk of bleeding, and a requirement for lower doses if the international normalized ratio (INR) is to be maintained within the therapeutic range. When combined with the genetic polymorphisms in the vitamin K epoxide reductase complex (*VKORC1*) genes (a pharmacodynamic variation), and age and body mass index (BMI), over 50% of the variation in individual daily dose requirement can be predicted. Pre-prescription genotyping for *CYP2C9* and *VKORC1* has been shown to improve anticoagulation control.

Individual differences in the activity of thiopurine methyltransferase (TPMT), a phase II enzyme, are used to determine the appropriate doses of mercaptopurine and azathioprine. Testing for TMPT activity is therefore undertaken routinely in children undergoing treatment for acute lymphatic leukaemia and people with Crohn's disease. Slow acetylators (deficient in N-acetyltransferase type 2) have an increased risk of hepatotoxicity with isoniazid, while individuals with deficient *UGT1A1* activity are at increased risk of toxicity from irinotecan.

Genetic causes of altered pharmacodynamics

Genetic variation also affects pharmacodynamic targets, which can, in turn, lead to variation in both the efficacy and the safety of drugs. For example, variation in the β_2-adrenoceptor gene can affect response to salbutamol (albuterol). Glucose-6-phosphate dehydrogenase deficiency, the most common enzyme deficiency in the world, can predispose patients to acute red cell haemolysis with certain drugs such as primaquine, dapsone, sulphonamides and rasburicase. The biggest clinical advances in this area have occurred in two therapeutic areas:

- ***Cancer***. Sequencing of the cancer genome has identified novel driver mutations. This has led to the development of targeted therapies, which have been remarkably successful in the treatment of some malignancies, even when they are at an advanced stage (e.g. melanoma, see p. 20).
- ***Drug safety***. Some immune-mediated reactions involving the skin and liver can now be predicted by genotyping for certain human leucocyte antigen (HLA) polymorphisms. For example, pre-prescription genotyping for *HLA-B*57:01* has been shown to be clinically effective and cost-effective in preventing hypersensitivity to the anti-human immunodeficiency virus (HIV) drug abacavir. Similarly, *HLA-B*15:02* predisposed patients from South-east Asia to Stevens–Johnson syndrome with carbamazepine.

Future perspective

As we learn more about the human genome, and the fact that many drugs undergo metabolism via many pathways and act on a number of targets, most of which show polymorphic expression, it may be possible in the future to utilize this information to personalize drug therapy to improve both efficacy and safety of drugs. This represents one component of the drive towards personalized medicine.

Further reading

Pirmohamed M. The applications of pharmacogenetics to prescribing: what is currently known? *Clin Med* 2009; 9:493–495.

Pirmohamed M, Burnside G, Eriksson N et al. A randomized trial of genotype-guided dosing of warfarin. *N Engl J Med* 2013; 369:2294–2303.

Wang L, McLeod JL, Weinshilboum RM. Genomics and drug response. *N Engl J Med* 2011; 364:1144–1153.

Woodcock J, Lesko LJ. Pharmacogenetics – tailoring treatment for outliers. *N Engl J Med* 2009; 360:811–813.

EVIDENCE-BASED MEDICINE

Clinical practice should, as far as possible, be based on formal evidence of benefit rather than theoretical speculation, anecdote or authoritative pronouncements.

One of the main applications of evidence-based medicine has been in therapeutics. Treatments should only be introduced into routine clinical care if they have been demonstrated to be effective in appropriate studies. Three approaches are used:

1. randomized controlled trials
2. controlled observational trials
3. uncontrolled observational studies.

Randomized controlled trials (RCTs)

In this type of study, patients with a particular condition are allocated – at random – to one of two (and sometimes more) treatments. At the end of the study, the outcomes in the groups are compared. The purpose of the RCT is to minimize bias and confounding. In order to minimize patient bias, the participants themselves are generally unaware of their treatment allocations (a 'single-blind' trial); and in order to reduce doctor bias, treatment allocations are also withheld from the investigators (a 'double-blind' trial). To recruit sufficient numbers of patients, and to examine the effects of treatment in different settings, it is often necessary to conduct the trial at several locations (a 'multicentre' trial).

RCTs may be designed to assess whether one treatment is better than another (a 'superiority' trial), or whether one treatment is similar to another (an 'equivalence' trial). There are a number of other variants, including crossover trials, cluster randomized controlled trials, inferiority trials and futility trials (see 'Further reading').

Assessing randomized controlled trials

In assessing the relevance and reliability of an RCT, a number of features in its design and analysis need to be taken into account.

Randomization

The method of randomization should be robust and, in particular, the investigator should be unaware of which treatment a patient entering a trial will receive. This avoids selection bias.

Maintaining blindness

Ideally, in RCTs, neither the investigator nor the patient should be aware of the treatment allocations until the end of the study. This, though, is not always possible. Adverse drug reactions, for example, may make it obvious which treatment a patient has been given. Nevertheless, maintaining 'blindness' is necessary where the outcome is subjective (e.g. relief of pain, alleviation of depression) if bias is to be avoided.

Were the treatment groups comparable?

The key questions to ask are:

- Were the patients in each group similar in their 'baseline' characteristics?
- Were they, for example, of similar age, with similar severity and duration of illness?
- If not, are the differences likely to influence the results?
- Has the statistical analysis (using analysis of co-variance or Cox's proportional hazards model – see below) tried to adjust for them?

Box 2.12 shows some of the baseline characteristics of a trial comparing prednisolone with placebo in the treatment of Bell's palsy.

Box 2.12 Summary of a multicentre randomized placebo-controlled trial of prednisolone (25 mg twice daily, for 10 days) in the treatment of Bell's palsy

	Placebo (*n* = 245)		Prednisolone (*n* = 251)	
	n	*(%)*	*n*	*(%)*
Baseline characteristics				
Gender				
Male	118	48.2	135	53.8
Female	127	51.8	116	46.2
Age (years) (mean±SD)	44.9±16.6		43.2±16.2	
Score on House–Brackmann scale[a] (mean±SD)	3.8±1.3		3.5±1.2	
Time between onset of symptoms and start of treatment				
Within 24 h	147	60.0	120	47.8
>24 to <48 h	64	26.1	95	37.8
>48 to <72 h	18	7.3	25	10.0
Unknown (but <72 h)	16	6.5	11	4.4
Results at 3 and 12 months				
Grade 1 on House–Brackmann scale[a]				
At 3 months[b]	152/239	63.1	205/247	83.0
At 12 months[b]	200/245	81.6	237/251	94.4

SD, standard deviation.
[a]The House Brackmann scale scores facial nerve function from 1=normal to 6=complete paralysis. [b]$p<0.001$.
(From Sullivan FM, Swan IRC, Donnan PT et al. Early treatment with prednisolone or acyclovir in Bell's palsy. *N Engl J Med* 2007; 357:1598–1607, with permission.)

Outcomes

There are two ways to analyse the outcomes of an RCT:

- Per protocol analysis: this includes only those who completed the study.
- Intention-to-treat analysis: this includes all patients from the time of randomization.

Ideally, there should be no difference in the results of these two types of analysis but, in reality, the results of a per protocol analysis are usually more advantageous to a treatment than an intention-to-treat analysis. The reason is that the intention-to-treat analysis will take account of patients who have withdrawn from the trial because of adverse reactions. It is therefore a much more robust approach. The results of the intention-to-treat analysis, in the trial of prednisolone in Bell's palsy, are shown in ***Box 2.12***. The trial results indicate, with a high probability, that treatment of Bell's palsy with prednisolone will increase the chances of a full recovery of facial nerve function.

Are the results generalizable?

Were the patients enrolled into the study a reasonable reflection of those likely to be treated in routine clinical practice? Or were they a selected population that excluded significant patient groups (such as the elderly)? If the latter is true, view the results with caution.

Analysis of a superiority trial

The analysis of a superiority trial is based on the premise – the 'null hypothesis' – that there is no difference between the treatments. The null hypothesis is rejected if the probability of the observed result occurring by chance, the p value, is less than 1 in 20 (i.e. $p<0.05$). There are three caveats, though:

- Any difference may still be due to chance; and it is often better to await the results of at least two independent studies before adopting a new treatment.
- A trial may show no 'statistically significant' difference, when one in fact exists, because too few patients have been included. In other words, the trial lacked sufficient 'power'. The 'power' of a study (the number of patients needed in each treatment group to detect a pre-defined difference) should have been defined at the outset. If the study was under-powered, the results of the study should be interpreted with extreme care.
- A statistically significant difference may not necessarily be clinically relevant. Scrutiny of the magnitude of the effect, and its 95% confidence intervals (CI), is a far better guide than the p value.

Effect size. The results of the well-designed trial in ***Box 2.12*** show, very convincingly, that the treatment of Bell's palsy with prednisolone increases the chances of complete recovery of facial nerve function, at 12 months, from 81.6% to 94.4%. This is a far more convincing description of the benefits of treatment than the p value.

Number needed to treat (NNT). Another expression of the benefit of a treatment can be derived from the NNT. This is an estimate of the numbers of patients who need to be treated with a drug to achieve one positive result. In the study shown in ***Box 2.12***, the NNT to enable one patient with Bell's palsy to regain normal facial nerve function, after prednisolone treatment, is 8.

Analysis of an equivalence trial

The aim of an equivalence trial is to determine whether two (or possibly more) treatments produce similar benefits. During the design of such trials, it is necessary to decide what difference is unimportant from a clinical perspective and then to calculate the number of patients needed in order to have an 80% or 90% chance of showing this. In equivalence trials, such power calculations show that the number of patients required is invariably greater than those needed for superiority trials. In equivalence studies, the comparator itself must, of course, already have been shown to be effective.

Meta-analysis

It is possible to summate the results of all the controlled trials that have been performed in the treatment of a particular condition so as to refine the estimate of effectiveness. This technique minimizes random error in the assessment of the effect size of a treatment because more patients are included than could be accommodated in any single trial. A meta-analysis should be performed (and interpreted) because of the heterogeneity of the individual studies used in it. Meta-analyses are most often based on the results of the summary statistics reported in the original reports. Occasionally (but more often in the past few years), meta-analyses use the data from the individual patients involved in the original studies. This technique is time-consuming and requires the original triallists to agree to providing the necessary data.

Controlled observational trials

Three types of observational study have been used to test the clinical effectiveness of therapeutic interventions:

- historical controlled trials
- case–control studies
- before-and-after studies.

Historical controlled trials

Despite the value of the prospective RCT, there are many treatments that have never been subjected to this technique; their efficacy, however, is unquestioned. Examples include insulin in the treatment of diabetic ketoacidosis, thyroxine for hypothyroidism, vitamin B_{12} in pernicious anaemia and defibrillation for ventricular fibrillation. In a historical controlled trial, the outcome in patients treated with the study drug is compared to that of previously untreated people with the same disease. Treatments can be accepted into routine use on the basis of favourable comparisons with historical controls when the following criteria are met:

- There should be a biologically plausible basis for the observed benefits.
- There should be no appropriate treatment that could be reasonably used as a control.
- The condition should have a known and predictable natural history.
- The treatment should not be expected to have adverse effects that would compromise its potential benefits.
- There should be a reasonable expectation that the magnitude of the therapeutic effects of treatment will be large enough to make the interpretation of its benefits unambiguous.

Case–control studies

This type of study design compares people with a particular condition (the 'cases') with those without (the 'controls'). The approach has been used predominantly to identify epidemiological 'risk factors' for specific conditions such as lung cancer (smoking) or sudden infant death syndrome (lying prone), as well as in the evaluation of potential ADRs (such as deep venous thrombosis with oral contraceptives).

Box 2.13 Estimation of odds ratio

	Cases	Controls
Risk factor present	a	c
Risk factor absent	b	d

The odds ratio (OR) = (a ÷ b) / (c ÷ d)

A case–control design allows an estimation of the odds ratio (OR), which is the ratio of the probability of an event occurring to the probability of the event not occurring ***(Box 2.13)***. An OR that is significantly greater than unity indicates a statistical association that may be causal. The ORs for deep venous thrombosis and the current use of oral contraceptives varies from 2 to 4 (depending on the preparation); this indicates that the risk of developing a deep venous thrombosis on oral contraceptives is between 2 and 4 times greater than the background rate.

In some studies, the OR for a particular observation has been found to be significantly less than unity, suggesting 'protection' from the condition under study. Some studies of women with myocardial infarction indicated protection in those using hormone-replacement therapies but it has subsequently been shown that the result was due to bias. On the other hand, case–control studies have consistently shown that aspirin and other non-steroidal anti-inflammatory drugs (NSAIDs) are associated with a reduced risk of colon cancer. This seems to be a causal effect.

Case–control studies claiming to demonstrate the efficacy of a drug need to be interpreted with great care; the possibility of bias and confounding is substantial, as in the studies of hormone-replacement therapy and myocardial infarction. Confirmation from one or more RCT is usually essential.

Before-and-after studies

It has sometimes been inferred that observed improvements seen in patients before, and after, the use of a particular treatment is evidence of efficacy. Such an approach is fraught with difficulties; the combination of a placebo effect, as well as regression to the mean, is likely to negate most studies using this type of design. Nevertheless, there are some circumstances where genuine efficacy can be confidently concluded with such designs: the benefits of hip replacement and cataract surgery are good examples. Such instances can be regarded as special examples of the use of implicit historical controls.

Uncontrolled observational studies

Uncontrolled case series cannot provide primary evidence for efficacy, unless they are undertaken in circumstances that are virtually those of historical controlled trials. Case series can, however, sometimes be of value in demonstrating the generalizability of the results of RCTs.

Evaluation of new drugs

New drugs are subjected to a vigorous programme of pre-clinical and clinical testing before they are licensed for general use ***(Box 2.14)***. At the time new products are licensed there can be confidence in their efficacy for their agreed indications. Conclusions about their safety must, at this point, be provisional, which is why emphasis is placed on post-marketing.

Box 2.14 Evaluation of new drugs

Phase I: Healthy human subjects (usually men)
- First use in humans
- Evaluation of safety and toxicity
- Pharmacokinetic assessment
- Sometimes pharmacodynamic assessment
- Approximately 100 subjects

Phase II: First assessment in patients
- Safety and toxicity evaluated
- Dose range identified
- Pharmacokinetic and pharmacodynamic monitoring
- Approximately 500 subjects

Phase III: Use in wider patient population
- Efficacy main objective
- Safety and toxicity also carefully monitored
- Often multicentre trials
- Approximately 2000 patients involved

Phase IV: Post-marketing surveillance
- All patients prescribed drug monitored
- Efficacy, safety and toxicity measured
- Quantification of unusual drug adverse effects
- Yellow Card and spontaneous reports of adverse reactions
- Often very large numbers of patients observed

STATISTICAL ANALYSES

The relevance of statistics is not confined to those who undertake research but extends to anyone who wants to understand the relevance of research studies to their clinical practice.

The average

Clinical studies may describe, quantitatively, the value of a particular variable (e.g. height, weight, blood pressure, haemoglobin) in a sample from a defined population. The 'average' value (or 'central tendency', in statistical language) can be expressed as the mean, median or mode, depending on the circumstances ***(Fig. 2.3)***.

- The ***mean*** is the average of a distribution of values that are grouped symmetrically around the central tendency.
- The ***median*** is the middle value of a sample. It is used, particularly, where the values in a sample are asymmetrically distributed around the central tendency.
- The ***mode*** is the interval in a frequency distribution of values that contains more values than any other.

In a symmetrically distributed population, the mean, median and mode are the same. The average value of a sample, on its own, is of only modest interest. Of equal (and often greater) relevance is the confidence we can place on the sample average as truly reflecting the average value of the population from which it has been drawn. This is most often expressed as a **confidence interval**, which describes the probability of a sample mean being a certain distance from the population mean. If, for example, the mean systolic blood pressure of 100 undergraduates is 124 mmHg, with a 95% confidence interval of ±15 mmHg, we can be confident that if we replicated the study 100 times, the value of the mean would be within the range 109–139 mmHg on 95 occasions. It is intuitively obvious that the larger the sample, the smaller will be the size of the confidence interval.

Correlation

In clinical studies, two or more independent variables may be measured in the same individuals in a sample population (e.g. weight and blood pressure). The degree of correlation between the two can be investigated by calculating the correlation coefficient (often abbreviated to 'r').

The **correlation coefficient** measures the degree of association between the two variables and may range from 1 to –1:

- If r=1, there is complete and direct concordance between the two variables.
- If r=–1, there is complete but inverse concordance.
- If r=0, there is no concordance.

Statistical tables are available to inform investigators as to the probability that r is due to chance. As in other areas of statistics, if the probability is less than 1 in 20 ($p < 0.05$), then by custom and practice it is regarded as statistically significant. There are, however, two caveats:

- The 1 in 20 rule is a convention and does not exclude the possibility that a presumed association is due to chance.

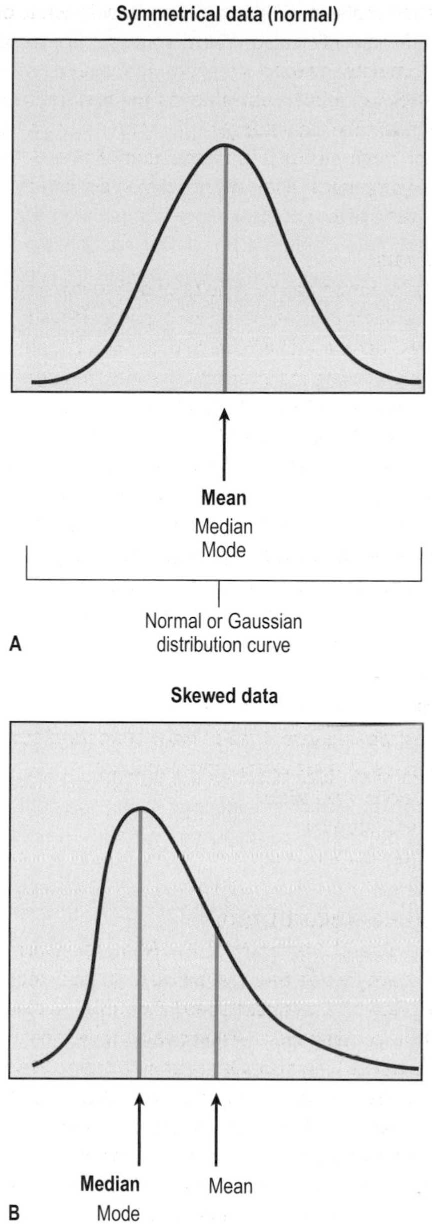

Figure 2.3 Averages. In symmetrical data, the mean, mode and median are the same.

- The fact that there is an association between two variables does not necessarily mean that it is causal. For example, a correlation between blood pressure and weight, with $r=0.75$ and $p < 0.05$, does not mean that weight has a direct effect on blood pressure (or vice versa).

Correlation analyses can become complicated. The simplest (least squares regression analysis) presumes a straight-line relationship between the two variables. More complicated techniques can be used to estimate r where a non-linear relationship is presumed (or assumed); where the distributions deviate from normal; where the scales of one or both variables are intervals or ranks; or where a correlation between three or more variables is sought.

Survival analyses

In studies where individuals are observed over a long(ish) period of time, and in which it is unreasonable (or erroneous) to assume that event rates are constant, the technique of survival analysis is used. This is most commonly reported as the **hazard ratio (HR)** with its 95% confidence interval. The HR is the probability that, if an event in question has not already occurred, it will happen in the next (short) time interval.

Continuous outcomes

Studies such as that in ***Box 2.12*** may report outcomes using one or more continuous scales. In this study of the effects of prednisolone in the treatment of Bell's palsy, the House–Brackmann measure of facial nerve function was used as the outcome measure. Conventional tests of statistical significance using Student's t-test, for example, can be calculated to assess whether the null hypothesis can be rejected.

Number needed to treat (NNT)

As discussed earlier, the NNT is an estimate of the number of patients that need to be treated for one to benefit compared to no treatment. If the probabilities of the end-points with the active drug and no treatment (i.e. placebo) are respectively p_{active} and $p_{\text{no treatment}}$, then the NNT can be calculated thus:

$$\text{NNT} = 1/(p_{\text{active}} - p_{\text{no treatment}})$$

An analogous measure – the **number needed to harm (NNH)** – is the number of patients that need to be treated with a drug to cause one patient to be subject to a specific harm.

Other statistical techniques

Statisticians have developed a range of sophisticated methods to handle a wide variety of biomedical problems. Unless an investigator is supremely (and usually unwisely) confident, it is sensible to seek professional advice in analysing numerical data that look complicated. In doing so, it is invariably wiser to do so at the time the study is being designed rather than after the results have been generated!

Further reading

Jadad AR, Enkin MW. *Randomized Controlled Trials: Questions, Answers and Musings*, 2nd edn. London: Blackwell; 2007.
Matthews JN. *Introduction to Randomized Controlled Trials*, 2nd edn. London: Chapman & Hall; 2006.
Morris S, Devlin N, Parkin D. *Economic Analysis in Health Care*. Chichester: John Wiley & Sons; 2007.
Rawlins MD. *Therapeutic Evidence and Decision-Making*. London: Hodder; 2011.

INFORMATION SOURCES

Pharmacotherapy moves at a very rapid pace and it is impossible for anyone to keep up with contemporary advances. Reliable prescribing advice can be found in:

- The *Summary of Product Characteristics (SmPCs)* produced by manufacturers and vetted by drug regulatory authorities (for the UK, these are the Medicines and Healthcare Products Regulatory Agency and the European Medicines Agency).
- The relevant national formulary. Many countries have their own formularies: for example, the UK has the *British National Formulary* (BNF), produced jointly by the British Medical Association and the Royal Pharmaceutical Society.
- Guidance produced by national health technology agencies such as the UK's National Institute for Health and Care Excellence (NICE).
- Advice on the management of individual conditions, available in the form of clinical guidelines (systematically developed statements to assist practitioner and patient decisions about appropriate healthcare for specific clinical circumstances). Some of these are published by national medical societies. In the UK, NICE is the main developer of clinical guidelines.

Patient information leaflets are supplied with all prescribed medication.

Significant websites

http://www.nice.org.uk *National Institute for Clinical Excellence (NICE) clinical guidelines*
http://www.sign.ac.uk/ *Scottish Intercollegiate Guidelines Network (SIGN) clinical guidelines*
http://www.guideline.gov *National Guideline Clearinghouse clinical guidelines in the USA*

3 Palliative medicine and symptom control

Miriam J Johnson, Gail E Eva, Sara Booth

See your e-book for key learning points, clinical tips, drug tips, extra tables, case studies and MCQs.

INTRODUCTION AND GENERAL ASPECTS

Palliative care is the active total care of patients who have advanced, progressive, life-shortening disease. It should be based on needs and not diagnosis, and is required in non-malignant diseases as well as in cancer ***(Box 3.1)***.

The ***goal*** of palliative care is to achieve the best possible quality of life for patients and their carers by:

- managing physical, psychological, social and spiritual problems so as to provide excellent symptom control
- enabling patients to be cared for and to die in the place of their choice
- enabling the acceptance of death as a normal process when life-prolonging treatments no longer improve or maintain quality of life
- providing the opportunity to say goodbye and bring closure.

Who provides palliative care?

A hallmark of palliative care is the multiprofessional team, as single professionals cannot provide the breadth of necessary expertise. The emotional demands of working in this area require team support to enable balanced, compassionate and professional care.

All healthcare providers should have basic palliative care skills and access to a specialist palliative care (SPC) team. They should be aware of the services that the local SPC teams can offer and recognize when referral is appropriate. A problem-based approach to disease management will ensure that patients and carers obtain access to appropriate support services, including SPC, and will avoid an either/or approach ('either curative treatment or palliative care').

Good communication between members of the healthcare team, and between patient and carer, underpins the successful management of advanced disease and end-of-life care. Effective liaison between the hospital, primary care and hospice is also essential.

When should palliative care needs be assessed – problems rather than prognosis?

Early assessment of needs, with SPC referral if required, is crucial to achieving the best outcome for rehabilitation and for maintaining or improving quality of life for both patient and carer. Palliative care is most effective when it is included as part of routine care as soon as possible after diagnosis, alongside disease-specific therapy, such as radio/chemotherapy for cancer or cardiac medication for heart failure. Early referral links palliative care with quality-of-life improvements; positive associations increase the likelihood that patients and families continue to use palliative care services when they need them over the course of the illness. In cancer, there is good evidence that integrating palliative care and anti-tumour treatment soon after diagnosis reduces long-term distress and increases survival in selected cases.

If palliative care is seen only as relevant to the end-of-life phase, patients who have non-malignant disease are denied expert help for complex symptoms. Timely management of physical and psychosocial issues earlier in the course of disease prevents intractable problems later ***(Box 3.2)***.

What are the patient's needs and what is the patient's understanding?

The causes of a patient's symptoms are often multifactorial, and a holistic assessment is central for optimum management. Assessment of the patient's understanding of the disease, understanding their future wishes and acknowledging their concerns, will help the team plan and implement effective support. Patients will have differing needs for information, and will deal with 'bad news' in different ways. A sensitive approach, respecting individual requirements, is crucial.

How can patients use palliative care services?

Changes in the provision of SPC services have been forced by the increase in the number of patients who survive malignant disease, as well as recognition of the needs of patients who have

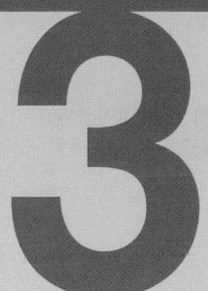

Box 3.1 Key components of a modern palliative care service

- Management based on *needs*, not diagnosis: the symptom burden of non-malignant disease often equals that of cancer
- Care that is independent of the patient's location and that helps patients to remain at home if possible, avoiding unwanted admissions to hospital
- Rehabilitation for people with advanced disease
- Support for carers
- Bereavement care for people with pathological grief problems
- Telephone advice for other clinicians; dissemination of palliative care knowledge
- Teaching for clinicians, from undergraduate level to postgraduate life-long learning

Box 3.2 Problems arising when specialist palliative care (SPC) is delayed until the end of life

- There is insufficient time to achieve good symptom control by combining non-pharmacological and pharmacological components
- SPC services are deemed less acceptable by patient and family, being associated with 'dying' or 'giving up' or 'giving in' to illness
- Psychological distress and physical symptoms become intractable and contribute to complex grief
- It becomes too late to adopt a rehabilitative approach or teach/use non-pharmacological interventions that need a degree of training and patient motivation (e.g. cognitive behavioural approaches, mindfulness meditation, attendance at day therapy)

non-malignant disease. Many patients will use SPC services for a limited period (weeks to months) for complex problems to be addressed, and then are discharged. They have the opportunity for re-referral if help is required later.

Further reading

Parilch RB, Kirch RA, Smith TJ et al. Early specialty palliative care. *N Engl J Med* 2013; 369:2347–2351.
Zimmermann C, Swami N, Krzyzanowska M et al. Early palliative care for patients with advanced cancer: a cluster-randomised controlled trial. *Lancet* 2014; 383:1721–1730.

SYMPTOM CONTROL

Good palliative care integrates the control of symptoms with appropriate non-pharmacological approaches, such as anxiety management and rehabilitation (see p. 36).

Pain

Pain (see also pp. 818–820) is a feared symptom in cancer. At least two-thirds of people with cancer suffer significant pain. Pain has a number of causes, and not all pains respond equally well to opioid analgesics ***(Fig. 3.1)***. The pain is related to the tumour either directly (e.g. pressure on a nerve) or indirectly (e.g. due to weight loss or pressure ulcers). It may result from a co-morbidity such as arthritis. Emotional and spiritual distress may be expressed as physical pain (termed 'opioid irrelevant pain') or will exacerbate physical pain.

The term 'total pain' encompasses a variety of influences that contribute to pain:

- ***Biological***: the cancer itself, cancer therapy (drugs, surgery, radiotherapy).

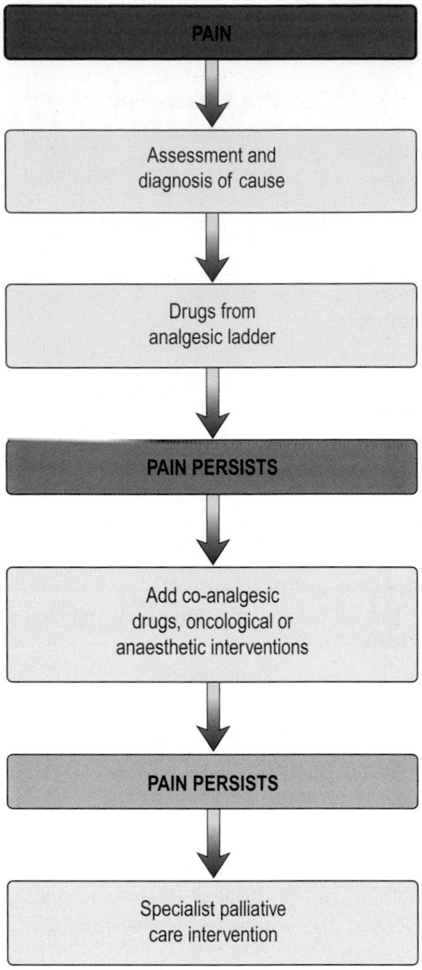

Figure 3.1 Management of cancer pain.

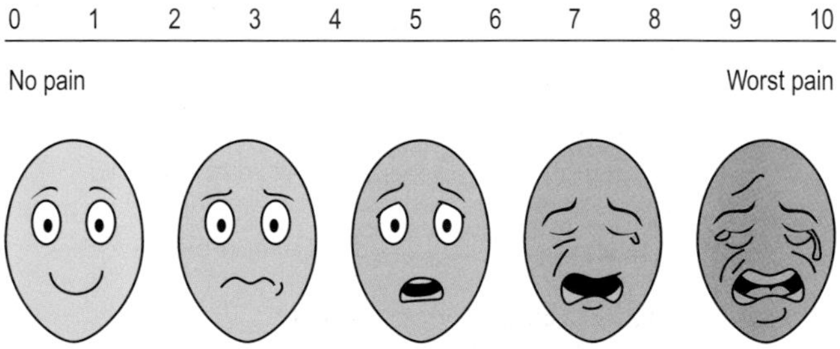

Figure 3.2 Visual analogue scale for pain assessment. A verbal rating scale can also be used: none, mild, moderate, severe.

- ***Social***: family distress, loss of independence, financial problems from job loss.
- ***Psychological***: fear of dying, of pain, or of being in hospital; anger at dying or at the process of diagnosis and delays. Depression can stem from all of the above.
- ***Spiritual***: fear of death, questions about life's meaning, guilt.

A visual analogue scale for pain can be used ***(Fig. 3.2)***.

The WHO analgesic ladder

Most cancer pain can be managed with oral or commonly used transdermal preparations. The World Health Organization (WHO) cancer pain relief ladder guides the choice of analgesic according to pain ***severity*** ***(Fig. 3.3, Box 3.3)***.

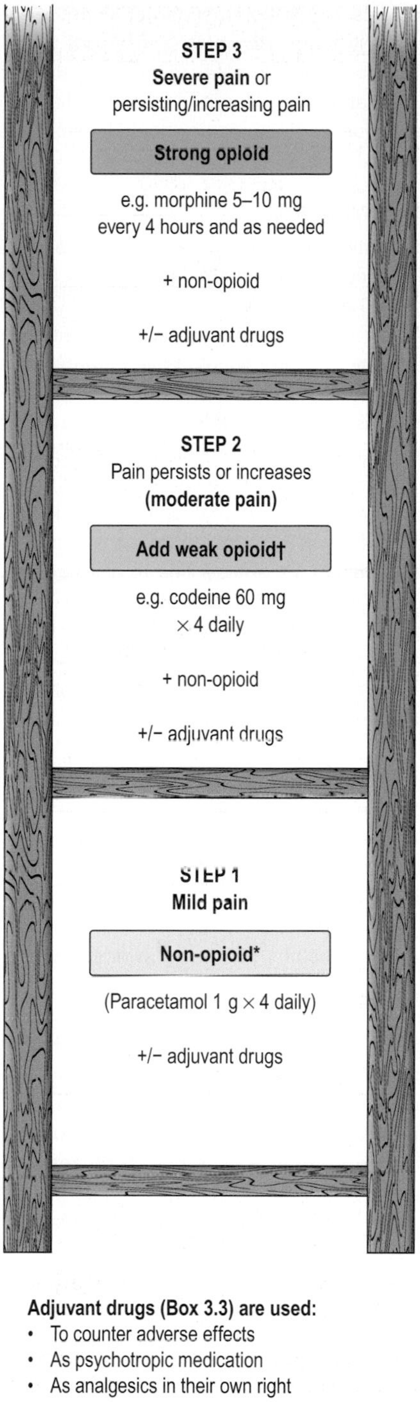

STEP 3
Severe pain or persisting/increasing pain
Strong opioid
e.g. morphine 5–10 mg every 4 hours and as needed
+ non-opioid
+/− adjuvant drugs
STEP 2
Pain persists or increases (moderate pain)
Add weak opioid†
e.g. codeine 60 mg × 4 daily
+ non-opioid
+/− adjuvant drugs
STEP 1
Mild pain
Non-opioid*
(Paracetamol 1 g × 4 daily)
+/− adjuvant drugs
Adjuvant drugs (Box 3.3) are used:
• To counter adverse effects
• As psychotropic medication
• As analgesics in their own right

Figure 3.3 WHO analgesic ladder for cancer and other chronic pain. Step 2 can be omitted, going to morphine immediately. Adjuvant drugs are listed in ***Box 3.3***. *Opioids include all drugs with an action similar to that of morphine, i.e. binding to endogenous opioid receptors. †Continue non-steroidal anti-inflammatory drug (NSAID)/paracetamol regularly when opioid started.

If *regular* use of optimum dosing (e.g. paracetamol 1 g×4 daily for step 1) does not control the pain, then an analgesic from the next step of the ladder is prescribed. As pain has different physical aetiologies, an adjuvant analgesic may be needed in addition: for example, the tricyclic antidepressant amitriptyline for neuropathic pain (see ***Box 3.3***).

Box 3.3 Commonly used adjuvant analgesics

Drugs	Indication
Non-steroidal anti-inflammatory drugs (NSAIDs), e.g. naproxen	Bone pain, inflammatory pain
Anticonvulsants, e.g. gabapentin (600–2400 mg daily) or pregabalin (150 mg at start, increasing up to 600 mg daily)	Neuropathic pain
Tricyclic antidepressants, e.g. amitriptyline (10–75 mg daily)	Neuropathic pain
Bisphosphonates, e.g. disodium pamidronate, zoledronic acid	Metastatic bone disease
Dexamethasone	Neuropathic pain, inflammatory pain (e.g. liver capsule pain), headache from cerebral oedema due to brain tumour

Strong opioid drugs

Dose titration and route

Morphine is the drug of choice and, in most circumstances, should be given regularly by mouth. The dose should be tailored to the individual's needs by allowing 'as required' doses; morphine does not have a 'ceiling' effect. If a patient has needed further doses in addition to the regular daily dose, then the amount in the additional doses can be added to the following day's regular dose until the daily requirement becomes stable: a process called 'titration'. When the stable daily dose requirement has been established, the morphine can be changed to a sustained-release preparation. For example:

20 mg morphine elixir 4-hourly
=120 mg morphine per day
=60 mg twice daily of a 12-hour preparation *or*
=120 mg daily of a 24-hour preparation.

The starting dose of morphine is usually 5–10 mg every 4 hours, depending on patient size, renal function and whether a weak opioid is already being given.

If there is significant renal dysfunction, morphine should be used in low doses and should not be given in continuous dose regimens (e.g. by subcutaneous infusions) because of the risk of metabolite accumulation (it is renally excreted). In renal impairment, an alternative opioid (e.g. fentanyl) can be given transdermally (e.g. 72-hour self-adhesive patches) or by subcutaneous infusion.

N.B. A word of caution about opioid transdermal patches: serum levels do not change quickly with transdermal patches, and they are also cumbersome to titrate in patients with escalating or unstable pain. They should be kept at a stable dose, and a more dose-responsive preparation used to gain pain control.

If a patient is unable to take oral medication due to weakness, swallowing difficulties, or nausea and vomiting, the opioid should be given parenterally. For cancer patients who are likely to need continuous analgesia, continuous subcutaneous infusion is the preferred route.

Both doctors and patients may have erroneous beliefs, such as the fear of addiction, which mean that adequate doses of opioids are not prescribed or taken. However, iatrogenic addiction is very rare, with the risk being <0.01%; the adverse effects and morbidity from uncontrolled pain are much higher.

Side-effects

The most common side-effects are:

- ***Nausea and vomiting***. These can usually be managed or prevented with antiemetics (such as metoclopramide). Some antiemetic solutions for injection can be combined with an opioid for continuous subcutaneous infusion, e.g. haloperidol or metoclopramide; always check compatibility data.
- ***Constipation***. This is common and should be anticipated with administration of a combination of stool softener (e.g. macrogols) and stimulants, either separately or in one preparation. Naltrexone is a peripherally acting opioid receptor antagonist that is used if response to other laxatives is poor.

If side-effects are intractable, a change of opioid is often helpful.

Toxicity

Confusion, persistent and undue drowsiness, myoclonus, nightmares and hallucinations indicate opioid toxicity. This may follow rapid dose escalation and responds to dose reduction and slower retitration. It may indicate pain that is poorly responsive to opioids and the need for adjuvant analgesics.

Antipsychotics such as haloperidol may help settle the patient's distress whilst waiting for resolution of toxicity. Some patients will tolerate an alternative opioid such as oxycodone better, or an alternative route such as subcutaneous injection.

Adjuvant analgesics

The most commonly used adjuvant analgesics are described in ***Box 3.3***. Other treatments, such as radio/chemotherapy, anaesthetic or neurosurgical interventions, acupuncture and transcutaneous electrical nerve stimulation (TENS), may be useful in selected patients.

Regular review is necessary to achieve optimal pain control, including regular assessment to distinguish pain severity from pain distress.

Further reading

Quigley C. Opioids in people with cancer-related pain. *Clin Evid (Online)* 2008; http://www.ncbi.nlm.nih.gov/pmc/articles/PMC2907984/.

SIGN. *Control of Pain in Adults with Cancer*. Publication No. 106. Edinburgh: SIGN; 2008; http://www.sign.ac.uk/pdf/SIGN106.pdf.

Gastrointestinal symptoms

Anorexia, weight loss, malaise and weakness

These result from the cancer-cachexia syndrome of advanced disease and carry a poor prognosis. Although attention to nutrition is necessary, the syndrome is mediated through chronic stimulation of the acute phase response, and tumour-secreted substances (e.g. lipid mobilizing factor and proteolysis-inducing factor). Thus, calorie–protein support alone gives limited benefit; parenteral feeding has been shown to make no difference to patient survival or quality of life.

Management is supportive unless the patient is fit enough for and responds to anti-tumour drugs. Specific therapies such as eicosapentaenoic acid (EPA), fish oil, cyclo-oxygenase (COX) inhibition with non-steroidal anti-inflammatory drugs (NSAIDs) and antioxidant treatments are used.

Advice from a dietician is helpful. Some patients benefit from a trial of a food supplement that contains EPA and antioxidants. Megestrol may help appetite but weight gain is usually caused by fluid or fat. The drug is also thrombogenic and is of little benefit and should therefore not be used.

Corticosteroids were recommended as appetite stimulants and are still commonly used. However, the weight gained is usually caused by fluid, and muscle catabolism is accelerated leading to a proximal myopathy. Any benefit in appetite stimulation tends to be short-lived. Thus, corticosteroids should be limited to short-term use only.

Nausea and vomiting

Nausea and vomiting are common, and often due to use of opioids without antiemetics such as haloperidol 1.5 mg×1–2 daily or metoclopramide 10–20 mg×3 daily.

When nausea and vomiting are associated with:

- ***Chemotherapy***. Patients should have an antiemetic, starting with metoclopramide or domperidone, but if the risk of nausea and vomiting is high, give a specific 5-hydroxytryptamine$_3$ (5-HT$_3$) antagonist, e.g. ondansetron 8 mg orally or by slow i.v. injection.
- ***Chemical causes*** e.g. hypercalcaemia. Haloperidol 1.5–3 mg daily is the first choice. Metoclopramide is also a prokinetic and therefore useful for emesis due to gastric stasis or constipation. Cyclizine 50 mg×3 daily is also used.
- ***Any cause of vomiting***. It may be necessary to start antiemetic therapy parenterally by continuous subcutaneous infusion to gain control. If the patient has gastrointestinal obstruction, this route may need to be continued.

Gastric distension

Gastric distension due to pressure on the stomach by the tumour (squashed stomach syndrome) is treated with a prokinetic: for example, domperidone 10 mg×3 daily.

Bowel obstruction

Metoclopramide is helpful but to be avoided in complete bowel obstruction, where an antispasmodic such as hyoscine butylbromide is preferred. A dose of 60–120 mg/24 hours s.c. is usually recommended, but much higher doses (300–480 mg) may be needed as parenteral hyoscine butylbromide can be rapidly inactivated in humans.

Octreotide (a somatostatin analogue) is commonly used in bowel obstruction to try to reduce gut secretions and the volume of vomitus, but a recent randomized controlled trial failed to show any benefit over placebo. ***Ranitidine*** may have a role in reducing gastric secretions.

Physical measures, such as a defunctioning colostomy or a venting gastrostomy, may be helpful. Occasionally, a lower bowel obstruction is resolved with insertion of a stent, or transrectal resection of tumour in selected individuals. Steroids shorten the length of episodes of obstruction, if resolution is possible.

In ***advanced disease***, patients should be encouraged to drink and take small amounts of soft diet as they wish. With good mouth care, the sensation of thirst is often avoidable, thus sometimes preventing the need for parenteral fluids unless otherwise indicated.

Further reading

Clark K, Lam L, Currow D. Reducing gastric secretions – a role for histamine 2 antagonists or proton pump inhibitors in malignant bowel obstruction? *Support Care Cancer* 2009; 17:1463–1468.

Currow D et al. A randomized double blind placebo controlled trial of infusional subcutaneous octreotide in the management of malignant bowel obstruction in people with advanced cancer. Abstract OA25. *Palliat Med* 2012; 26:403.

Currow DC, Quinn S, Agar M et al. Double-blind, placebo-controlled, randomized trial of octreotide in malignant bowel obstruction. *J Pain Symptom Manage* 2015; 49:814–821.

van der Meij BS, Langius JA, Smit EF et al. Oral nutritional supplements containing (n-3) polyunsaturated fatty acids affect the nutritional status of patients with stage III non-small cell lung cancer during multimodality treatment. *J Nutr* 2010; 140:1774–1780.

Respiratory symptoms

Breathlessness

Breathlessness remains one of the most distressing and common symptoms in palliative care, causing the patient serious discomfort. It is highly distressing for carers to witness. Full assessment and active treatment of all reversible conditions, such as drainage of pleural effusions, or optimization of treatment of heart failure or chronic pulmonary disease is mandatory. In advanced cancer, breathlessness is often multifactorial in origin and many of the contributory factors are irreversible (e.g. cachexia), so a 'complex intervention' combining a number of different treatment strategies has the greatest impact. Aspects of breathlessness management are summarized in ***Box 3.4***. Intractable severe breathlessness in a patient who is dying may require sedation in order to provide comfort but more invasive interventions are usually avoided. Non-invasive ventilation (NIV) has been shown to alleviate distressing dyspnoea and is also associated with a reduced opioid requirement; this may be helpful in selected patients.

Box 3.4 Key points for successful management of breathlessness

- ***Start treatment early***. Patients who are likely to develop breathlessness should learn non pharmacological approaches early in the disease course, before breathlessness has become severe.
- ***Involve the carer in the treatment strategy***. Watching breathlessness episodes and being unable to help is a terrifying experience (and promotes the panic–anxiety cycle); if patients and carers develop a joint ritual for crises, chronic anxiety can be reduced.
- ***Ensure management is rehabilitative*** (see p. 36). This increases physical fitness, hope and self-efficacy, and may enable patient and carer to achieve goals that once seemed impossible.
- ***Integrate psychological, physical and social interventions***. These are important, as with all palliative care.

Breathlessness with panic and anxiety

Patients often experience a panic–breathlessness cycle and fear dying during an acute episode of breathlessness. This is unlikely in chronic disease, unless there is an acute complication, and reassurance will help. The perception of breathlessness is mediated by the central nervous system and can be modulated by thoughts and feelings about the sensation. Education about breathlessness and exploration of psychological precipitators or maintainers can reduce its impact.

Measures to alleviate breathlessness

Non-pharmacological approaches, such as using a hand-held fan, pacing or prioritizing activities to maximize activity within limitations, breathing training and anxiety management, are helpful, along with a tailored exercise programme ***(Box 3.5)***. There is no evidence to suggest that oxygen therapy reduces the sensation of breathlessness in advanced disease more than just cool airflow. A hand-held fan should be used before oxygen, unless the latter is indicated by significant hypoxaemia or disease management. Opioids, used orally or parenterally, can palliate breathlessness. If panic/anxiety is significant, a quick-acting benzodiazepine such as lorazepam (used sublingually for rapid absorption) is useful.

Cough

Persistent unproductive cough can be helped by the antitussive effect of opioids (e.g. morphine). Excessive respiratory secretions can be treated with hyoscine hydrobromide 400–600 µg every

Box 3.5 Key non-pharmacological interventions for breathlessness

Intervention	Putative mechanism of action	Most useful
Hand-held fan	Cools area served by second and third branches of trigeminal nerve Reduces temperature of air flowing over nasal receptors, altering signal to brainstem respiratory complex and so changing respiratory pattern	For reducing length of episodes of SOB on exertion or at rest For giving patient and carer confidence by having an intervention they can use
Exercise	Stops spiral of disability developing Changes muscle structure: less lactic acid produced	In patients who are still quite mobile In patients who have not developed onset of SOB, lessening/deferring symptoms by reducing deconditioning
Anxiety reduction, e.g. CBT (needs skilled clinician to administer) or simple relaxation therapy	Works on central perception of breathlessness, reducing impact Interrupts panic–anxiety cycle	In people with higher levels of anxiety at baseline (i.e. when first seen) In patients willing to persevere with learning a new skill
Carer support	Reduces carer anxiety and distress, which are part of 'total' anxiety–panic cycle	Where carer is isolated, under extra pressures (e.g. looking after elderly parent, going through divorce)
Breathing retraining	Improves mechanical effectiveness of respiratory system	For chronic advanced respiratory disease and in those with anxiety-related breathlessness
Pacing (finding a balance between activity and rest, and prioritizing daily activities)	Avoids over-exertion, which can lead to exhaustion, inactivity and subsequent deconditioning	In patients who are able and willing to modify daily routines
Neuromuscular electrical stimulation	Increases muscle bulk, simulating effect of exercise	In patients who: live alone are unable to attend a rehabilitation group have a short prognosis have co-morbidities that prevent exercise

CBT, cognitive behavioural therapy; SOB, shortness of breath (breathlessness).

4–8 hours but does give a dry mouth. Glycopyrronium is also useful by subcutaneous infusion of 0.6–1.2 mg in 24 hours.

Further reading

Nava S, Ferrer M, Esquinas A et al. Palliative use of non-invasive ventilation in end-of-life patients with solid tumours: a randomised feasibility trial. *Lancet Oncol* 2013; 14:219–227.
Parshall MB, Schwartzstein RM, Adams L et al. An official American Thoracic Society statement: update on the mechanisms, assessment, and management of dyspnea. *Am J Respir Crit Care Med* 2012; 185:435–452.
http://www.cuh.org.uk/breathlessness *More on interventions for breathlessness.*

Other physical symptoms

People with cancer may develop other physical symptoms caused by the tumour directly (e.g. hemiplegia due to brain secondaries) or indirectly (e.g. bleeding or venous thromboembolism due to disturbances in coagulation). Symptoms may also result from treatment, such as lymphoedema following treatment for breast or vulval cancer, or heart failure secondary to anthracycline or trastuzumab therapy. The principles of holistic assessment, reversal of reversible factors and appropriate involvement of the multiprofessional team should be applied.

Lymphoedema

The pain and disabling swelling associated with lymphoedema can be alleviated through complete decongestive therapy (CDT), a treatment that employs a massage-like technique and comprises manual lymphatic drainage, compression bandaging and gentle exercise. Diuretics should not be used. Referral to a specialist lymphoedema therapist or nurse is useful.

Fatigue

Fatigue is a significant and debilitating problem for palliative patients. It has physical, cognitive and affective components; unlike normal tiredness, it is not relieved by usual sleep or rest. An assessment for reversible contributory factors, such as anaemia, hypokalaemia or over-sedation due to poorly optimized medication, should be undertaken. Management strategies are:

- ***non-pharmacological***: relaxation, sleep hygiene, resting 'pro-actively' rather than collapsing when exhausted, and planning, pacing and prioritizing daily activities
- ***pharmacological***: low-dose methylphenidate (central nervous system stimulant), or short-term corticosteroids used in conjunction with the SPC team, may help.

Loss of function, disability and rehabilitation

Some of the most pressing concerns include increasing physical frailty, loss of independence, and perceived burden on others. Evidence suggests that functional problems are not routinely assessed, and not as well managed as pain and other symptoms. Rehabilitation can:

- contribute to patients' quality of life by providing strategies for managing declining physical function and fatigue, and by offering resources that might make life easier for patients and carers (e.g. equipment or a wheelchair)
- support patients' adaptation to disability, helping them to increase social participation and find fulfilment in everyday living
- minimize carer stress and distress.

A referral to physiotherapy or occupational therapy is helpful for patients whose ability to carry out daily activities is compromised by illness or its treatment. However, it must be remembered that effective rehabilitation is a team effort and is not solely the domain of nursing and allied health professionals. Doctors also have a major role to play in attending to functional problems and fatigue; they should not see these as inevitable, unavoidable and insoluble.

There is a need to take into account changing performance status as well as changes in goals and priorities. It can be helpful to identify short-term, achievable goals and focus on these. Most patients wish to remain at home for as long as possible and to die at home, given adequate support. Patients' community rehabilitation needs should not be neglected.

Psychosocial issues

Depression is a common feature of life-limiting and disabling illness, and is often missed or dismissed as 'understandable'. However, it may well respond to the usual antidepressant drugs and/or to non-pharmacological measures such as cognitive behavioural therapy, increased social support (e.g. day therapy) and support for family relationships. Such interventions can make a big difference to the patient's quality of life and ability to cope with the situation.

Further reading

Hudson PL, Remedios C, Thomas K. A systematic review of psychosocial interventions for family carers of palliative care patients. *BMC Palliat Care* 2010; 9:17.

EXTENDING PALLIATIVE CARE TO PEOPLE WITH NON-MALIGNANT DISEASE

The principles of palliative care can be applied throughout medical practice so that all patients, irrespective of care setting (home, hospital or hospice), receive appropriate care from the staff looking after them and have access to SPC services for complex issues. Some principles are outlined in ***Box 3.6.*** Patients who have chronic non-malignant disease, such as organ failures (heart, lung and kidney), degenerative neurological disease and human immunodeficiency virus (HIV) infection:

- have a similar or greater symptom burden than people with cancer
- may live longer with these difficulties
- benefit from a palliative care approach with access to SPC for complex problems.

There may be a less clear end-stage of disease but the principles of symptom control are the same: holistic assessment, reversal of reversible factors and multiprofessional support.

Box 3.6 Key points in palliative care

- Patients should always be involved in decisions about their care.
- Quality of life is increased when treatment goals are clearly understood by everyone, including patient and carer.
- The multidisciplinary team provide a high standard of care but there must be realism and honesty about what can be achieved.
- End-of-life care is often delivered in hospices or the home.
- Care at home should be encouraged for as long as possible, even if the patient's preferred place of death is elsewhere.
- Discussions about end-of-life care planning are best held outside times of crisis, with clinicians with whom the patient has a good relationship. Discussions must be recorded and made known to everyone involved in the patient's care.

Box 3.7 Differences between palliative care for people with malignant and non-malignant diseases

Cancer	Non-malignant disease
Standard treatment regimens, even in advanced disease	Advanced disease often needs bespoke pharmacological interventions, which may interact with palliative drugs. Close teamwork is essential to avoid adversely affecting outcomes, e.g. in use of opioids and many other drugs
Relatively new diagnosis (weeks to months)	Usually many years of illness with loss of social networks, employment and practical support
Sudden death is rare (although it can happen, e.g. pulmonary embolus, neutropenic sepsis)	Sudden death is relatively frequent as a result of cardiovascular/diabetic complications (e.g. in chronic kidney disease)
Cancer and associated problems are the main morbidities	Co-morbidities due to disease or treatment often cause most problems and shape end-of-life care
Prognosis is usually predictable	Prognosis difficult to determine: patients with many 'near-death experiences' and admissions can recover
Support from SPC services is often started early in the disease course	Main support may be from a medical unit, e.g. dialysis unit
Standard hospice services (e.g. day therapy) often suit treatment patterns well	Standard hospice service may not be offered (clinician ignorance) or may not be feasible (e.g. for dialysis patient attending hospital 3 days a week)

Patients who have non-malignant disease may have very close relationships with their usual team, and an integrated approach is essential to allow optimization of disease-directed medication as well as palliation. People with non-malignant disease may live for years with a difficult illness and so their palliative care needs to differ in some respects from that of cancer patients ***(Box 3.7)***. However, symptom management is largely transferable, with some exceptions and extra complexities as outlined below.

Throughout the course of the illness, careful open discussion of possible future options is essential. Early discussion of difficult choices is as helpful for patients who have non-malignant disease as it is for those with cancer, and these discussions are ideally held when the patient is relatively well and outside an acute episode. Discussions delayed until the crisis of acute admission may lead to acceptance of an invasive treatment that is later regretted by the patient.

Heart failure

There are special considerations with respect to cardiac medication in advanced disease:

- ***Drugs*** that are commonly used in palliative care but usually contraindicated in heart failure, such as amitriptyline and NSAIDs, may be appropriate when the patient is dying.
- ***Sudden death*** is more common than in patients who have malignancy and a patient may have an implanted defibrillator in place. If present, these devices should be reprogrammed to pacemaker mode in advanced disease because they have not been shown to improve survival in severe heart failure and it will be distressing for patient, carer and staff if the defibrillator discharges as the patient is dying.
- ***Peripheral oedema*** can become a major problem and more resistant to diuretic therapy; careful balancing of medication regimens is therefore required. Ultimately, symptom relief is prioritized over renal function.
- ***Medications*** should be rationalized to reduce polypharmacy, e.g. ceasing drugs prescribed to reduce long-term secondary risk (e.g. statins) and continuing drugs that help symptom control (including angiotensin-converting enzyme inhibitors, which benefit symptoms as well as survival). Beta-blockers may have to be stopped if the patient can no longer maintain non-symptomatic hypotension.

Regarding statins, a recent randomized trial of withdrawal versus continuation of statin in those thought to be in the last year of life showed no detrimental effect on quality of life with withdrawal.

Chronic respiratory disease

Chronic obstructive pulmonary disease (COPD)

COPD is the most common chronic respiratory disease. Patients may live increasingly restricted lives for years, rather than the months or weeks that are common once someone with cancer becomes breathless. Patients usually reach late middle age or old age before becoming very disabled, and an elderly spouse often has to carry significant physical burdens.

Because of the risk of dependency, falls and memory problems, non-pharmacological approaches to anxiety are more appropriate than benzodiazepines (see ***Box 3.5***). Short-acting benzodiazepines should be reserved for severe panic episodes.

Palliative care breathlessness services can be very helpful for those unable to comply with pulmonary rehabilitation. Emergency admissions to hospital for non-medical reasons are often due to anxiety and the support offered by community palliative care services working with respiratory teams can help prevent these.

Other chronic respiratory diseases

Other chronic respiratory illnesses that often require palliative care include:

- ***Idiopathic pulmonary fibrosis***. This has a trajectory similar to that of cancer, with rapidly developing breathlessness and cough. The breathlessness of idiopathic pulmonary fibrosis is particularly frightening but may respond well to opioids; early access to hospice services is particularly relevant to help with symptom control and anxiety.
- ***Cystic fibrosis***. Patients are teenagers or young adults who usually have known their respiratory team all their lives. An integrated team involving SPC clinicians ensures good symptom control and provides useful support when difficult decisions have to be made about treatments (e.g. lung transplant), as well as offering psychosocial care to the family.
- ***Primary pulmonary hypertension***. Patients are often young and treated far from home in specialist centres. They require symptom control in close consultation with the medical team, and it is essential for any dependent children to receive the care they need.

Ventilatory support (see pp. 1163–1167)

For many patients who have respiratory failure, non-invasive ventilation (NIV) has superseded the use of intermittent positive pressure ventilation (IPPV) on intensive therapy units. However, there are patients who are likely to need IPPV during admission for an acute exacerbation. For some of this group, life has become burdensome, rendering the net benefit for this procedure less or negligible. These patients should be put in contact with hospice services when they are relatively stable (not during acute exacerbations), anticipating an alternative place of admission in the event of subsequent deteriorating health.

Opioid titration in non-malignant respiratory disease

In non-malignant respiratory disease, opioid titration may need to follow a different pattern from that used in malignant disease, in which many patients are already on opioids for pain control before they develop breathlessness. Some clinicians recommend a cautious approach for these chronically breathless patients who have non-malignant disease, but the evidence indicates that those with adequate renal function may safely be started on 5–10 mg modified release morphine, given appropriate monitoring. Constipation can be a problem (see p. 34) but recently naloxegol (a pegylated derivative of the μ-opioid receptor antagonist naloxone) has been shown to be helpful without reducing the analgesic effect of opioids.

Further reading

Boland J, Martin J, Wells AU et al. Palliative care for people with non-malignant lung disease: summary of current evidence and future direction. *Palliat Med* 2013; 27:811–816.

http://www.medpagetoday.com/MeetingCoverage/ASCO/46070 *Stopping statins in terminal illness.*

Renal disease

All care for patients who have end-stage chronic kidney disease (CKD) is directed towards maintenance or improvement of renal function. Prescribing is complicated, particularly if patients are receiving dialysis. Care must be taken not to cause renal damage inadvertently with potentially renotoxic medication, and close liaison with the renal team is mandatory.

In patients who have CKD, co-morbidities such as cardiovascular disease, diabetes or osteoporosis may cause greater problems than the renal disease. Those with a fluctuant course of symptoms, such as the 25–33% who have coexisting cardiac disease, bear disproportionately greater physical and psychological burdens.

Patients who are on dialysis

Patients attend three times per week (and receive social support from this). Thus additional attendance at a hospice day therapy service may be too tiring. If further support from SPC services is needed, then outpatient clinics, community support (for patient and/or carer) or even admission may be more suitable.

Withdrawal of dialysis

Withdrawal of dialysis is necessary if the effort of attendance becomes too great when there is little improvement in quality of life and the impact of other co-morbidities becomes intrusive.

If there is no residual renal function, survival after withdrawal of dialysis is likely to be a few days at most. In contrast, patients who have some residual function (usually those who have had dialysis for only a few weeks or months) may live for months or even a year after withdrawal. Patients and carers need to understand these differences in order to make informed choices.

Patients who are not on dialysis

Maximizing and preserving remaining renal function are critical considerations in deciding which medications can or should be prescribed:

- Medication that accelerates loss of renal function may markedly reduce survival in patients who can live on very little remaining renal function.
- The renal impact of both dose and drug choice must be taken into account. For example, morphine and diamorphine metabolites accumulate in end-stage renal dysfunction; thus strong opioids such as alfentanil or fentanyl should be used instead.

Close liaison with the medical team is essential for drug prescribing.

Further reading

Kane PM, Vinen K, Murtagh FE. Palliative care for advanced renal disease: a summary of the evidence and future direction. *Palliat Med* 2013; 27:817–821.

Neurological disease

People who suffer from chronic degenerative neurological diseases have a considerable burden of palliative care needs, including:

- difficulties in swallowing (e.g. in motor neurone disease)
- loss of mental capacity – the ability to understand, weigh up, come to a decision and communicate that decision.

Ideally, discussions regarding the patient's wishes should take place in advance, if the patient is able to do this, so that these can be supported.

Motor neurone disease

Motor neurone disease is usually rapidly progressive, often requiring hospice support. Percutaneous endoscopic gastrostomy (see p. 213) feeding may be required. In addition, if ventilatory failure develops, nocturnal NIV may be offered. Patients and their carers need to understand:

- why this treatment has been offered (to prevent hypercarbia and morning headache and confusion)
- when this treatment will be withdrawn (when it is no longer helping to maintain or improve quality of life in the face of advancing disease).

Patients need to be given a clear understanding of what alternative symptom control will be offered at withdrawal.

Multiple sclerosis

Pain is often prominent in multiple sclerosis because of muscle spasm; patients may become too disabled to attend outpatient clinics and then receive very little surveillance. Hospice day therapy service, rehabilitation and support for the family can make a huge impact on quality of life.

Dementia

Dementia-related palliative care needs arise in the context of neurological conditions that:

- tend to occur in older people (Alzheimer's disease and multi-infarct dementia)
- also affect younger people (e.g. Parkinson's disease, multiple sclerosis, Huntington's disease).

It is often difficult to ascertain whether these patients are in pain. An assessment tool that assesses behavioural response to pain, such as the Abbey and Doloplus, which uses vocalization (e.g. groaning), facial expression (e.g. frowning), change in body language (fidgeting, rocking), behaviour change (e.g. confusion, refusing to eat) and physical changes, can be useful.

Dementia poses special problems with respect to inpatient palliative care. For example, in the UK, many hospice inpatient units will not accept mobile patients who have dementia because the patient's safety cannot be guaranteed. However, they will care for those at the end of life with other SPC needs – for example, a distressed young family – or pain, and will often support other services by providing advice on symptom control.

Further reading

Richfield EW, Jones EJ, Alty JE. Palliative care for Parkinson's disease: a summary of the evidence and future directions. *Palliat Med* 2013; 27:805–883.

PALLIATIVE CARE OF THE FRAIL ELDERLY

People worldwide are living longer as diseases, both communicable and non-communicable, are better managed. However, the palliative care needs of older patients often go unrecognized and are therefore under-treated. The physiological effects of ageing itself are compounded by co-morbidity, polypharmacy and unhealthy lifestyles. These factors lead to a higher mortality than expected, a heavy symptom burden and shortened life expectancy, compared to those who remain in good health at the same advanced age. Recognition of and attention to the care of these patients can improve outcomes by encouraging carers to produce individual care plans for the elderly frail.

Frailty is an emerging syndrome in the elderly. It has many definitions but can be thought of as a state of extreme vulnerability with 'a progressive physiological decline in multiple organ systems'. This leads to a marked loss of function, loss of physiological reserve and an increased vulnerability to disease and death. There are a number of physiological changes that are associated with normal ageing ***(Box 3.8)***, as well as the cumulative impact of chosen or imposed 'unhealthy' ways of life and chronic pre-existing diseases. The proportion of detrimental changes that can be prevented or ameliorated by different behaviour earlier in life, or by supporting people to maintain healthy habits into older age, is debatable. ***Box 3.9*** shows the 'five ways to wellbeing', which, if practised with other public health teaching on moderate alcohol intake, maintenance of a healthy weight and rejection of smoking, would help to preserve health and activity as life advances.

Box 3.8 Normal physiological changes with ageing that show great inter-individual variation

Physiological change	Result	Possible changes in behaviour and outcomes	Comments
Reduction in activity of immune system	Greater susceptibility to infection	Greater incidence of and rapid, severe deterioration with relatively minor infections, e.g. urinary tract infection	Sudden confusion/deterioration in elderly person commonly caused by infection Vaccination (e.g. against influenza) of importance in prevention
Changes in HPA axis function	Altered circadian rhythm	Need for less sleep, with early wakening Neural cell impairment and compensatory gliosis at many levels of HPA axis	Particularly evident in hypothalamus/hippocampus and limbic system, leading to reduced memory
Possible cognitive decline	Difficulty managing complex medication regimens, understanding illness and consequences	Forgetfulness, difficulty in working out complex problems	Some authorities suggest that cognitive decline largely results from modern lifestyle and illnesses rather than being an inevitable part of ageing Admission to hospital can uncover/exacerbate cognitive impairment
Reduction in balance and coordination	Falls more common, which can lead to catastrophic global deterioration, e.g. need for sheltered care or complications of immobility leading to death	Fear of going out, particularly in winter or after dark, which in turn can exacerbate social isolation, poor nutrition, lack of sunlight and deconditioning	Can be detected on physical examination in modalities of vibration sense, balance in central nervous system
Reduction in body's ability to maintain homeostasis, e.g. stable body temperature	Higher incidence of hypothermia in winter and heat stroke in summer	Increased mortality in this group during periods of extreme heat or cold	Prevention by urging behavioural change (e.g. use of heating) or staying indoors in heat or cold
Reduction in muscle mass	Reduced ability to be mobile (which may become entrenched into spiral of disability)	Can exacerbate isolation and loneliness through fear of going out in case unable to complete activity	What proportion of muscle loss can be prevented by greater exercise is uncertain but it is clear that exercise is beneficial
Deterioration in five senses	Difficulty taking part in or achieving some activities of daily living and participating fully in social life	Loss of confidence, reduction in social life	Macular degeneration, and other changes in sight related to associated morbidity (e.g. diabetes) Age-related hearing loss multifactorial (mostly related to changes in middle ear)
Reduced metabolic rate	Prolonged half-life of drugs	May lead to effective overdosage, or increase in adverse effects of some drugs	E.g. prolonged half-life of sedatives can lead to falls and confusion

HPA axis, hypothalamic–pituitary–adrenal axis.

Box 3.9 Five ways to wellbeing (New Economics Foundation)

Connect with people
- Help the older person to find ways to be in contact with other people to avoid social isolation and loneliness. *Evidence shows that we need both depth and breadth in our relationships for optimum health at any age.*

Be active
- Encourage physical activity that is enjoyable. Incorporate exercise into daily routines as much as possible. A slow walk to the toilet is better than a commode by the bedside. *Exercise facilitates the achievement of the other ways to wellbeing and increases the likelihood of successful self-care, as well as being of key importance for maintaining and improving the health of cardiovascular and musculoskeletal systems.*

Take notice
- Facilitate the older person's interest in current affairs and local news, as well as their immediate surroundings. *Meditation and/or relaxation techniques to manage anxiety are of value at any age and help people to live in the present moment rather than being disabled by past fears and worries or anxiety about the future. They can be taught in hospital by occupational therapists/physiotherapists, psychologists and some specialist nurses and physicians, and education can be maintained on discharge by community resources.*

Keep learning
- Encourage the older person to try something new. *There is accumulating evidence that continuing to learn new skills or maintain learning in established interests is good for mental health, possibly slows cognitive decline and helps with symptom control (distraction).*

Give
- Doing things for others is rewarding. Encourage the older person to see themselves as worthwhile, valuable contributors in their own communities, however small that might be. *Evidence shows that altruism is good for mental health and the palliative care literature demonstrates that even the very ill welcome opportunities to be involved in work that helps others.*

Adapted from http://www.neweconomics.org/projects/entry/five-ways-to-well-being.

Frailty, however, implies vulnerability to a loss of function in many areas. There are a number of scoring indices for frailty. The Fried Frailty Score assesses:
- ***slowness in walking***
- ***exhaustion***
- ***weakness*** (decreased hand grip strength)
- ***physical inactivity*** (low energy expenditure)
- ***weight loss*** (body mass index <18.5 or >5% weight loss in the last year).

A score of 3 or more defines frailty, although slow walking, low physical activity and weight loss, as well as cognitive impairment, were independently associated with disability and a poorer prognosis.

Assessment of the frail elderly person presenting in a medical setting

The frail elderly person may present acutely to medical services in a number of different ways. It is essential for there to be an individual focus on improving and/or maintaining the current quality of life. As there is a high mortality in this group, all care of the frail elderly person can be considered 'palliative'. A central tenet of palliative care is to assess the presence and severity of symptoms and to elicit the patient's priorities for future management. This will identify frail adults. Thus acute hospital admissions provide an opportunity to begin discussions with patients and their families about their preferences for future care. Treatment should be offered on the basis of individual need and potential for benefit for that individual, rather than chronological age. The aims of assessment and management are to:
- identify and treat reversible causes of decline
- detect and control troublesome symptoms and form individualized treatment plans
- screen for weight loss, pain, dyspnoea, falls, depression and insomnia
- assess severity of frailty and identify those with worse prognostic indicators (see above)
- communicate to the patient and the family the prognostic implications of frailty, its likely course, and available support.

Context of the consultation

Care with regard to the setting and conduct of the consultation is necessary to enable individuals to tell their story and make their wishes clear. Assessment may need to be phased to obtain all the necessary information and should involve the multidisciplinary team, as medical and social care needs can often not be differentiated; one is only possible when the other is implemented effectively.

The following are questions to ask:
- ***Is the individual frail elderly person being treated in a dignified way?*** Are they being called by their title and surname, and not a diminutive? Are people shouting at them or belittling them? Are they dressed, covered up, sitting comfortably and/or adequately supported if in bed?
- ***Does the patient have problems with hearing or sight?*** Do they have particular communication needs, e.g. a quiet side room to avoid background noise, help with their hearing aid (is it in? is it working?), assistance finding their glasses.
- ***Do they need help with information to support their use of drug treatment or understanding of their illness?***
- ***Have they come from home or somewhere else?*** Does this setting suit them or is it now part of the problem (see ***Box 3.8***)?

A full assessment of mental capacity is necessary. In those who are unable to provide their own full history, details should be sought from other sources of information such as:
- those looking after them in their nursing or residential home
- their primary care team
- their relatives who support them to live independently/with whom they live.

Ensure that you know whom to contact for advice if you have any doubts about the individual's ability to make informed decisions for themselves. Always take advice from a senior clinician if you have doubts.

Management of the frail elderly person

Following the comprehensive assessment, an early priority is to reverse what is reversible; rehabilitation should be provided, again tailored to the individual's potential for improvement or adaptation.
- ***Treat symptoms***. Investigation and treatment of known medical problems should be appropriate for the individual ***(Box 3.10)***. Investigation and management of any new disease will follow the general principles as for other age groups but remembering that the frail elderly will have a high mortality in the year after admission.

Box 3.10 Care of the frail elderly person: an example

Mrs Jones is found to have a urinary tract infection, which responds well to oral antibiotics. An assessment demonstrates that her hearing aid needs changing and that her sight might be improved by anti-vascular epithelial growth factor injections for her macular degeneration. She no longer requires metformin and her statin is stopped, as it is no longer providing her with benefit. Rehabilitation with more mobility aids is enabling her to transfer from bed to chair and so get up during the day. She is found to have an abdominal mass but declines investigation of it beyond the CT scan. However, she does report that the mass is painful and she is referred to the hospital palliative care team. Her pain is easily controlled on a small regular dose of oral opioid and a community palliative care nurse specialist follows her up with primary care in her nursing home, where she dies 3 months later, without further admission.

- ***Discuss the future sensitively***. Discussions about wishes for future care are complex with anyone who has life-threatening disease. They may not see themselves that way and assumptions should not be made about what frail elderly individuals want or how they view their health status. They may not feel that they are particularly ill or even that they have a poor prognosis, despite having reached a great age. General medical management needs to be integrated with symptom control. The SPC team should be contacted for advice or involved with management when there are difficulties with this or with complex discussions with the individual or their family.
- ***Review the drug chart***. One feature of frailty is that patients are often taking large numbers of drugs, some of which may be causing disabling adverse effects without any immediate benefit for that individual's quality of life. Reviewing every drug with the patient may be very helpful in lessening symptom burden and may help reduce confusion and sedation.

In summary, palliative care should be available to everyone on the basis of need. It is frequently not offered to the frail elderly and symptoms are known to be both under-detected and under-treated in this group. Ensure this does not happen when you are caring for a frail elderly person. Contact the palliative care team for advice, even if referral for transfer of care is not necessary.

Further reading

Iliffe S, Swift CG. Assessment and prevention of falls in older people – concise guidance. *Clin Med* 2014; 14:658–662.
Moorhouse P, Rockwood K. Frailty and its quantitative clinical evaluation. *J R Coll Physicians Edinb* 2012; 42:333–340.
Pal LM, Manning L. Palliative care for frail older people. *Clin Med* 2014; 14:292–295.
Rodriguez-Mañas L, Fried LP. Frailty in the clinical scenario. *Lancet* 2015; 385:E7.
Song X, Mitnitski A, Rockwood K. Prevalence and 10-year outcomes of frailty in older adults in relation to deficit accumulation. *J Am Geriatr Soc* 2010; 58:681–687.
Wou F, Conroy S. The frailty syndrome. *Medicine* 2013; 41:13–15.
https://www.youtube.com/watch?v=MTcopj6dYWQ *Dignity in care.*

CARE OF THE DYING

Most people express a wish to die in their own homes, provided their symptoms are controlled and their carers are supported. However, patients die in any setting and so all healthcare professionals should be proficient in end-of-life care.

Reports of inadequate hospital care have led to the development of integrated pathways of care for the dying. Pathways act as prompts of care, including psychological, social, spiritual and carer concerns in those who are diagnosed as dying. The latter is a decision reached by a multiprofessional team through careful assessment of the patient and exclusion of reversible causes of deterioration.

Box 3.11 Stages in the Liverpool Care Pathway – an end-of-life tool

- Recognition of the dying phase
- Initial assessment (which includes the patient's and carers' understanding and psychological state)
- Ongoing assessment and monitoring
- Care of the carers after the patient's death

Do not attempt resuscitation (DNAR) orders

- The resuscitation status of every patient should be discussed by senior doctors at the time of admission and the decision documented in the notes.
- Many hospitals have specific DNAR forms. Deciding a person's resuscitation status is a careful balance of risk versus benefit. The patient's co-morbidities and pre-morbid quality of life should be taken into account.
- The patient and family should be involved in this discussion, and the medical reasoning behind the decision explained. If the patient requests that cardiopulmonary resuscitation is not performed in the event of cardiopulmonary arrest, those wishes should be respected.

Remember that a decision not to resuscitate a patient is not the same as the decision to withhold other treatment. A patient who is not for resuscitation may still be eligible for antibiotics, fluids, endoscopy and even surgery. Management should remain positive, allowing the patient to die free of distress and with dignity.

Care of the dying tools

The Liverpool Care Pathway (LCP; ***Box 3.11***) has come in for a great deal of criticism. It is a four-stage end-of-life tool designed to transfer the standard of hospice care of the dying into the hospital (see ***Box 3.10***). Now adapted for any setting, it was the most commonly used pathway for care of the dying in the UK and is still in use in several other countries.

The LCP has provision for departures from the 'prompts of care' – for example, discontinuation of intravenous antibiotics or parenteral fluids – if a clinical need can be demonstrated. The patient is reviewed regularly (at least daily). Occasionally, the patient improves whilst on the pathway and can be returned to usual care if this is deemed more appropriate by the clinical team. For those who do not improve, the LCP prompts advanced prescription of medication to ease the symptoms most likely to arise in the dying phase (pain, breathlessness, nausea, agitation and excess respiratory secretions) to allow timely action.

Engagement with family and carers is vital, and it should not be assumed that they will recognize or understand the signs of imminent death. The LCP has supportive information leaflets that carers should find useful.

UK national hospital audits have assessed and monitored the level of care documented against the standards set in the LCP. However, following some well-publicized errors of implementation of the tool in the UK in 2013–2014, and in the face of a lack of randomized controlled trial evidence to support its use, the LCP was withdrawn and replaced by individual care plans outlined by the Leadership Alliance for the Care of Dying People. Since then, a cluster randomized trial of the LCP in cancer patients has reported no significant difference in overall quality of care, but did show improvements in coordination of care, treatment with dignity, family self-efficacy, and respect and information and decision-making.

Further reading

Costantini M, Romoli V, Leo SD et al. Liverpool Care Pathway for patients with cancer in hospital: a cluster randomised trial. *Lancet* 2014; 383:226–237.

General Medical Council. *Treatment and Care Towards the End of Life: Good Practice in Decision Making*. London: GMC; 2010.

Hawkes N. Doctors need more training in care of the dying. *BMJ* 2015; 351:h4792.

Heath I. Role of fear in over-diagnosis and over-treatment – an essay by Iona Heath. *BMJ* 2014; 349:g6123.

Kelley AS, Morrison RS. Palliative care for the seriously ill. *N Engl J Med* 2015; 373:747–755

Leadership Alliance for the Care of Dying People. *One Chance to Get it Right: Improving People's Experience of Care in the Last Few Days or Hours of Life*; 2014; https://www.gov.uk.

Lyons D. The confused patient in the acute hospital: legal and ethical challenges for clinicians in Scotland. *J R Coll Physicians Edinb* 2013; 43:61–67.

Marie Curie Palliative Care Institute Liverpool (MCPCIL) in collaboration with the Clinical Standards Department of the Royal College of Physicians (RCP). *National Care of the Dying Audit – Hospitals (NCDAH) Round 2, 2008–9*. Supported by the Marie Curie Cancer Care and the Department of Health End of Life Care Programme. London: MCPCIL/RCP; 2009.

http://www.legislation.gov.uk/ukpga/2005/9/contents *Mental Capacity Act 2005*.

NICE. *Care of dying adults in the last days of life*. NICE guidelines [NG31]; 2015. https://www.nice.org.uk/guidance/ng31

Bibliography

British National Formulary. *Guidance on Prescribing: Prescribing in Palliative Care. British National Formulary*. London: BMJ Group and RPS Publishing. http://www.bnf.org

Goldstein NE, Fischberg D. Update in palliative medicine. *Ann Intern Med* 2008; 148:135–140.

Twycross R, Wilcock A, Howard P. *Palliative Care Formulary*, 5th edn. Nottingham: palliativedrugs.com; 2014.

Significant websites

http://www.cancerresearchuk.org *UK charity*
http://www.cuh.org.uk *Breathlessness information*
http://www.macmillan.org.uk *UK patient organization*
http://www.palliativedrugs.com *Palliative drugs information*
http://uk.sagepub.com/en-gb/eur/journal/palliative-medicine *Palliative medicine*

4 Global health

Babulal Sethia, Parveen Kumar

See your e-book for key learning points, clinical tips and learning challenges.

INTRODUCTION

The discipline of 'global health' evolved from 'international health', which focused historically on the study and management of infectious tropical diseases.

There is no universally agreed definition of 'global health' (GH). It is 'an area of study, research and practice that places a priority on improving health and achieving equity in health for all people worldwide'. It recognizes that health is determined by problems, issues and concerns that transcend national boundaries, and looks at the healthcare needs of people across the world as well as in individual nations. Such needs are seen in high-, as well as low- and middle-income countries (LMICs), but may be particularly acute, for example, during or after conflicts of war, with the consequences of population displacement or of direct trauma, including rape. Effective delivery of GH needs inevitably requires multidisciplinary collaboration between healthcare workers, politicians, economists and scientists in pursuit of both individual wellbeing and population-based prevention and care. Examples of successful interventions include campaigns for the provision of vaccines by the Global Alliance for Vaccines and Immunization (GAVI), and initiatives to reduce the economic exploitation of child labour. On the infection front, the African Programme for Onchocerciasis control has used the safe drug, ivermectin, which, as a single dose given annually, has transformed the lives of millions. Another example is the use of praziquantel for the eradication of schistosomiasis (bilharzia), one of the most common but neglected tropical diseases, initiated by the Schistosomiasis Control Programme and funded by many organizations.

The scale of the problem worldwide

Data published by the World Health Organization (WHO) in 2012 show that although life expectancy had increased by 6 years since 1990 (mean 70 years in males, range 62–70 years), several unacceptable facts remain true:

- Around 6.6 million children under the age of 5 years die each year.
- Preterm birth (before 37 weeks' gestation) accounts for >1 million deaths per year.
- Each day, 800 women die due to complications of pregnancy and childbirth.
- Cardiovascular diseases are the leading cause of death globally.
- Some 70% of deaths from the human immunodeficiency virus/acquired immunodeficiency syndrome (HIV/AIDS) occur in sub-Saharan Africa.
- Mental health disorders, such as depression, are amongst the 20 leading causes of disability worldwide.
- Tobacco kills nearly 6 million people each year (and is predicted to kill 8 million per year by 2030).
- Almost 1 in 10 people has diabetes.
- Nearly 1.24 million people die from road traffic accidents every year.

Further reading

HM Government. *Health is Global: UK Government Strategy 2008-2013.* London: Department of Health; 2008

Koplan JP, Bond TC, Merson MH et al. Towards a common definition of global health. *Lancet* 2009; 373:1993–1995.

MILLENNIUM DEVELOPMENT GOALS

At the Millennium Summit in September 2000, world leaders from 189 countries adopted a series of time-bound goals, to be achieved by 2015. Twenty-one targets were enshrined within the eight Millennium Development Goals (MDGs). These goals are listed in ***Figure 4.1***.

The goals provided a focus for a major increase in GH investment from all countries, particularly for disease-specific entities (MDG 6: HIV/AIDS, malaria). However, critics have noted that much of the early financial investment for these commitments was used to defray existing debt in low- and middle-income countries (LMICs), whilst progress in the achievement of the targets by 2015 was very uneven. Furthermore, it has been suggested that failures in achievement of MDG targets was inevitably promoted by a lack of local participation in their original development (MDGs 1, 2 and 7). A significant deficiency in the MDGs was a failure to mention agriculture specifically, an essential component of the challenge to eradicate extreme hunger and poverty posed in MDG 1.

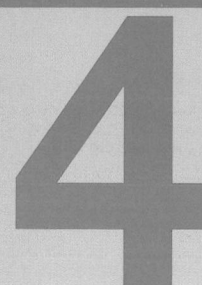

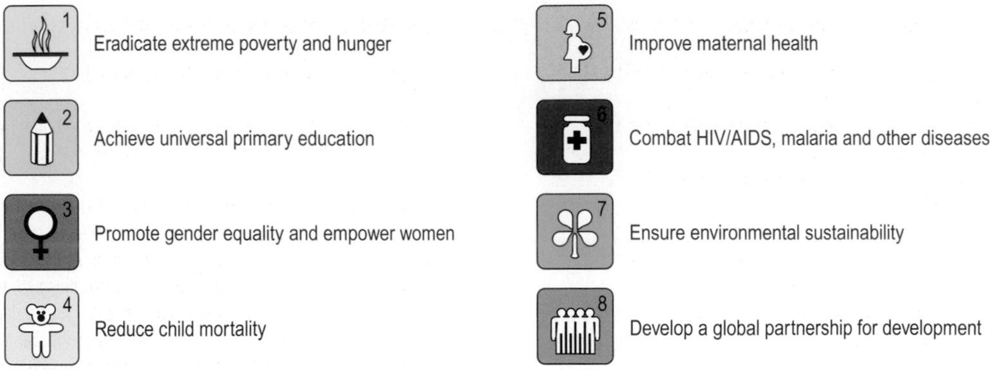

1
Eradicate extreme poverty and hunger
2
Achieve universal primary education
3
Promote gender equality and empower women
4
Reduce child mortality
5
Improve maternal health
6
Combat HIV/AIDS, malaria and other diseases
7
Ensure environmental sustainability
8
Develop a global partnership for development

Figure 4.1 Millennium development goals.

Box 4.1 Achievement of millennium development goals (MDGs): key facts

- Globally, the number of deaths of children under 5 years of age fell from 12.6 million in 1990 to 6.6 million in 2012
- In developing countries, the percentage of underweight children under 5 years old dropped from 25% in 1990 to 15% in 2012
- Births attended by a skilled health worker have increased globally, but still fewer than 50% of births are attended in the WHO African region
- Globally, new HIV infections declined by 33% between 2001 and 2012
- Existing cases of tuberculosis are declining, along with deaths among HIV-negative tuberculosis cases
- In 2010, the world met the United Nations MDG target on access to safe drinking water, as measured by the proxy indicator of access to improved drinking-water sources, but more needs to be done to achieve the sanitation target

(Adapted from WHO Factsheet No. 290, updated May 2015.)

Notwithstanding a variety of criticisms, much progress in achieving parts of the MDGs was reported by 2014, as noted in the update issued by the WHO in 2014 ***(Box 4.1)***.

The new set of goals, targets and indicators issued by the UN states are called ***Sustainable Development Goals*** **(SDGs)**, to be achieved by 2030. These demonstrate a wide-ranging and more integrated approach between the agreed goals, especially with regard to those that succeed MDGs 1, 2 and 7. There are 17 proposed goals incorporating 169 targets. They are worthy aims but may turn out to be unrealistic, as they cover a vast area for improvement ***(Box 4.2)***. Health is only explicitly mentioned in one target (Goal 3) and this emphasizes the fact that the concept of health is inextricably linked to the other major players like politics, economics and agriculture. Goal 3 has been expanded to be more explicit and includes nine targets and four additional targets that were missing from the MDGs. They now include non-communicable diseases, mental ill health, road accident injuries and universal health coverage ***(Box 4.3)***. The UN Secretary General, Ban Ki-moon, has offered conceptual guidance, suggesting six essential overarching SDG elements: 'dignity, prosperity, justice, partnership, planet, people'.

Box 4.2 Sustainable Development Goals: the 17 proposed aims

1. End poverty in all its forms everywhere
2. End hunger, achieve food security and improved nutrition, and promote sustainable agriculture
3. Ensure healthy lives and promote wellbeing for all at all ages
4. Ensure inclusive and equitable quality education and promote life-long learning opportunities for all
5. Achieve gender equality and empower all women and girls. A target example: eliminating violence against women
6. Ensure availability and sustainable management of water and sanitation for all
7. Ensure access to affordable, reliable, sustainable and modern energy for all
8. Promote sustained, inclusive and sustainable economic growth, full and productive employment, and decent work for all
9. Build resilient infrastructure, promote inclusive and sustainable industrialization, and foster innovation
10. Reduce inequality within and amongst countries
11. Make cities and human settlements inclusive, safe, resilient and sustainable
12. Ensure sustainable consumption and production patterns
13. Take urgent action to combat climate change and its impacts
14. Conserve and sustainably use the oceans, seas and marine resources for sustainable development
15. Protect, restore and promote sustainable use of terrestrial ecosystems, sustainably manage forests, combat desertification and halt and reverse land degradation, and halt biodiversity loss
16. Promote peaceful and inclusive societies for sustainable development, provide access to justice for all and build effective, accountable and inclusive institutions at all levels
17. Strengthen the means of implementation and revitalize the global partnership for sustainable development

For the 169 targets enshrined within the goals, see http://www.un.org/sustainabledevelopment/.

GLOBAL BURDEN OF DISEASE

In 2006, 90% of GH funds were spent in high-income countries that carried only 10% of the disease burden ***(Fig. 4.2)***. Clearly, the world faces many health challenges that are difficult to prioritize.

The Global Burden of Disease (GBD) Study 2010 provides critical data for guiding prevention and other interventions. This study is a worldwide collaboration across 302 institutions and has retrospectively reassessed the data from 1990, 2005 and 2010 using the same methodology, thus enabling accurate comparisons of health trends. This gives an understanding of the present and future health priorities for the global community and for individual countries. It was made possible by the introduction of a new metric in 2010, which gave a single measure to quantify the burden of diseases, injuries and risk factors. This **disability-adjusted life year (DALY)** metric allowed the comparison of burden across diseases, both

Box 4.3 The nine main targets and four additional targets (3.a–d) of the Sustainable Development Goal for health (GOAL 3)

3.1. By 2030, reduce the global maternal mortality ratio to less than 70 per 100 000 live births
3.2. By 2030, end preventable deaths of newborns and children under 5 years of age, with all countries aiming to reduce neonatal mortality to at least as low as 12 per 1000 live births and under-5 mortality to at least as low as 25 per 1000 live births
3.3. By 2030, end the epidemics of AIDS, tuberculosis, malaria and neglected tropical diseases, and combat hepatitis, water-borne diseases and other communicable diseases
3.4. By 2030, reduce by a third premature mortality from non-communicable diseases through prevention and treatment, and promote mental health and wellbeing
3.5. Strengthen the prevention and treatment of substance abuse, including narcotic drug abuse and harmful use of alcohol
3.6. By 2020, halve the number of global deaths and injuries from road traffic accidents
3.7. By 2030, ensure universal access to sexual and reproductive healthcare services, including family planning, information, and education, and the integration of reproductive health into national strategies and programmes
3.8. Achieve universal health coverage, including financial risk protection, access to quality essential healthcare services, and access to safe, effective, quality and affordable essential medicines and vaccines for all
3.9. By 2030, substantially reduce the number of deaths and illnesses from hazardous chemicals and air, water, and soil pollution and contamination
3.a. Strengthen the implementation of the WHO Framework Convention on Tobacco Control in all countries, as appropriate
3.b. Support the research and development of vaccines and medicines for the communicable and non-communicable diseases that primarily affect developing countries, provide access to affordable essential medicines and vaccines in accordance with the Doha Declaration on the TRIPS Agreement and Public Health, which affirms the right of developing countries to use to the full the provisions in the TRIPS Agreement regarding flexibilities to protect public health, and, in particular, provide access to medicines for all
3.c. Substantially increase health financing and the recruitment, development, training and retention of the health workforce in developing countries, especially in the least developed countries and small island developing states
3.d. Strengthen the capacity of all countries, in particular developing countries, for early warning, risk reduction and management of national and global health risks

TRIPS, Trade-Related Aspects of Intellectual Property Rights.
(From Maurice J. Special report: UN set to change the world with new development goals. Lancet *2015; 386:1121–1124, with permission.)*

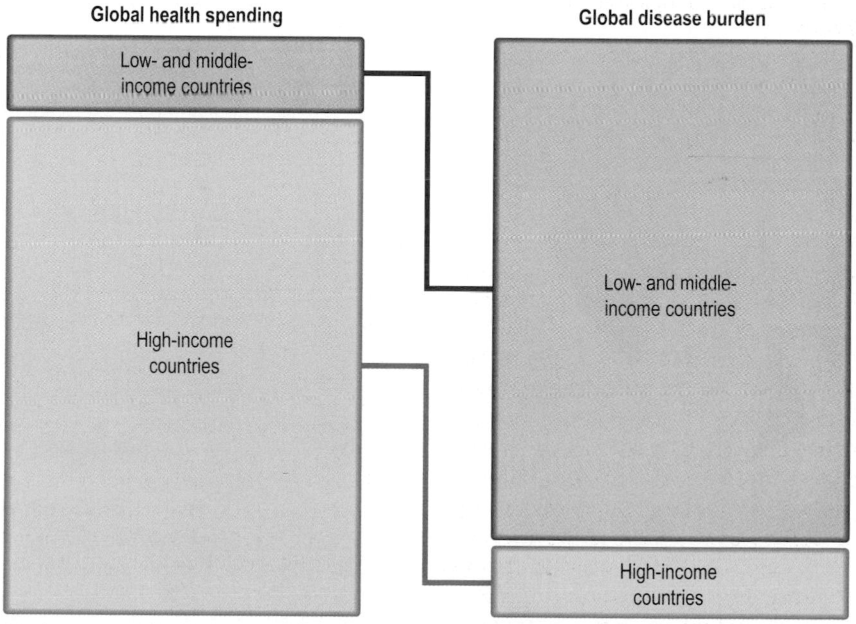

Figure 4.2 Mismatch between health spending and resources. *(From Gottet P, Schieber G.* Health Financing Revisited: A Practitioner's Guide. *Washington: World Bank; 2006.)*

untreated and treated, mortality, morbidity, disability, injuries and risk factors. DALYs measure health gaps, as opposed to health expectancies. They are derived from the calculation of the years of life lost due to early death (YLL) and years lived with disability (YLD).

$$DALY = YLL + YLD$$

Unfortunately, this GBD equation has some deficiencies and limitations. It does not, for example, address rapid transitions in GH, such as demographic changes, changes in causes of death, and changes in causes of disability. DALYs do not identify the transitional demographic changes of increases in population number, and of population age. A change in DALYs, whilst a potentially useful indicator of health outcomes, must therefore be interpreted with care. Both a decrease and an increase in DALYs may reflect improved outcomes. A decrease in DALYs for maternal and neonatal deaths can be accounted for by better education, nutrition or obstetric facilities. However, an increase in DALYs is seen when an ageing population requires treatment for chronic ill health, despite a reduction in mortality.

Further reading

Murray CJL, Lopez AD. Measuring the global burden of disease. *N Engl J Med* 2013; 369:448–457.

POVERTY

More than 3 billion people, nearly half of the world population, live in poverty (defined as living on less than US$2.50 per day), and more than 1.3 billion individuals receive less than US$1.25 per day (extreme poverty). Some 1 billion children worldwide live in poverty.

In 'The Future We Want', the outcome document of the 2012 Rio+20 Conference on the Sustainable Development Agenda, the need to accord the highest priority to poverty eradication was agreed. The 2016 SDGs (see ***Box 4.2***) include five goals (SDGs 1, 2, 12, 13 and 15) relating to this ambition.

Poverty, hunger, agriculture and climate change

These issues are inextricably interdependent. Food production is compromised when agricultural land is directed towards alternative uses, such as industrial development. On the other hand, 25% of food is wasted in LMICs by crop deterioration due to deficiencies in transport and storage. The UK and US together waste approximately US$81 billion of food each year.

In 2009, the UCL–Lancet Commission on 'Managing the Health Effects of Climate Change' called climate change 'the biggest global health threat of the 21st century'. Changes in climate pose major threats to human health, either directly (heatwaves, floods, droughts), or indirectly (agricultural losses, mass migration). For example, a 1° rise in mean temperature in India would result in the loss of 7 million tons of wheat ***(Fig. 4.3)***. By limiting the use of fossil fuels and reducing carbon emissions, it is possible to avoid a potentially catastrophic rise in global temperature ***(Fig. 4.4)***. Urgent action is essential if the gains in GH and development of the last 50 years are to be maintained.

Pain and suffering, especially in LMICs, is often caused by the catastrophic expenditure associated with chronic illness and disease. Every year, as many as 150 million people face financial catastrophe as a result of having to pay for health care.

Further reading

Watts N, Adger WN, Agnolucci P et al. Health and climate change: policy responses to protect public health. *Lancet* 2015; 386:1861–1914.

Xu K, Evans DB, Carrin G et al. *Designing Health Financing Systems to Reduce Catastrophic Health Expenditure.* WHO 2005; http://www.who.int/health_financing/.

http://www.grida.no/publications/ *The Environmental Food Crisis.*

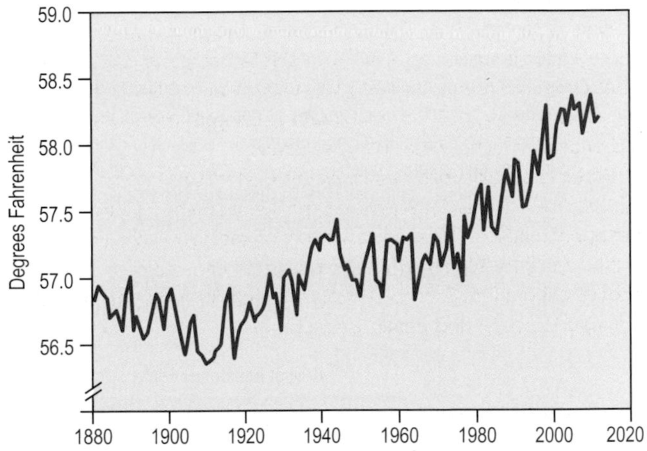

Figure 4.4 Rise in average global temperatures 1880–2012.

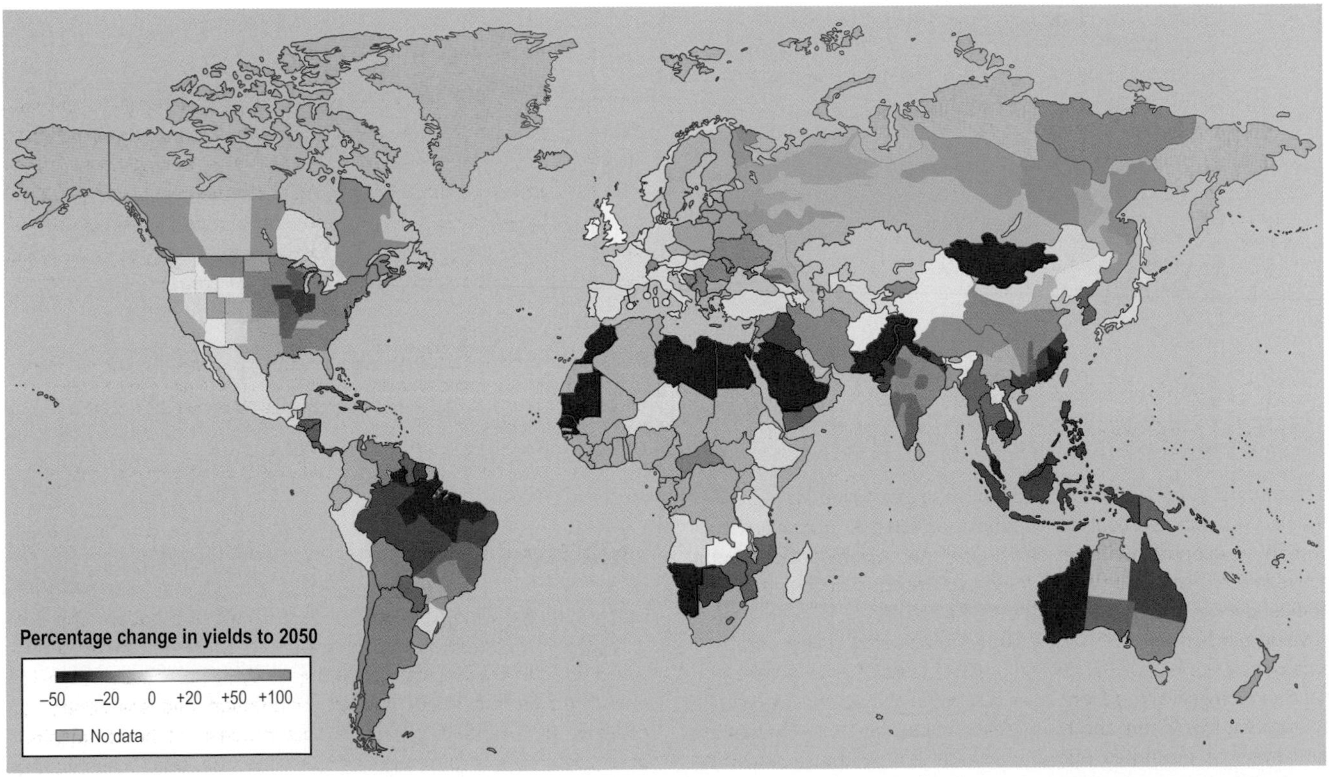

Figure 4.3 Climate change and modelled cereal grain yields to 2050. A rise in global temperature will make currently 'hot' countries (red) hotter, decreasing their grain yield. Alternatively, current cold countries (green) will get warmer with an increased yield of grain. *(From UN Development Programme 2009.)*

WATER AND SANITATION

Poor water, sanitation and hygiene are major causes of early mortality, particularly in children. In 2010, 11% of the world population lacked access to clean water supplies. WHO/UNICEF defined an improved water supply as 'one that, by nature of its construction or through active intervention, is protected from outside contamination, in particular from contamination with faecal matter'. The statement also stipulated that each person should have access to at least 20 L of water per day from a source within 1 km of the user's dwelling.

The target to halve the proportion of people without sustainable access to safe drinking water and basic sanitation by 2015 (MDG 7) was not met.

One in five people still defecates in the open, and 13% live where water is collected from unprotected sources. Some of the other consequences of inadequate sanitation are listed in ***Box 4.4***. It is clear that most of the mortality resulting from poor sanitation and unsafe drinking water is preventable.

Water is usually collected by women, often from distant sources; this can be a hazardous journey, as the women are unprotected and open to abuse. A secondary effect of improved access to water is that the time saved in collecting water can now be spent on income generation, food production, education and activities that can lead to social and health benefits.

Box 4.4 Sanitation

- 2.5 billion people lack adequate sanitation
- Open defecation results in the death of >750 000 children under 5 years of age annually
- 80% of diseases in LMICs are caused by poor sanitation/unsafe water
- More than 7 out of 10 people without improved sanitation were rural inhabitants (2006)
- Every $1 spent on sanitation brings a $5.5 return by keeping people healthy and productive
- Improvement in sanitation could save 1.5 million children each year.

LMICs, low- and middle-income countries.

(Data from: 1. United Nations Department of Public Information. The Future We Want: Water and Sanitation. Rio +20 United Nations Conference on Sustainable Development*; 2012. 2. UN-Water.* Sanitation. *Factsheet; 2014. From http://www.unwater.org. 3. Sanitation Drive* Factsheet 1, Sanitation for All: Making the right a reality*; 2015. From http://www.sanitationdrive2015.org.)*

ORGANIZATIONS AND THE GLOBAL HEALTH AGENDA

International support for GH initiatives may be directed at disease-specific projects (vertical care models) or allied to national health system development. Some of the vast number of organizations active in these areas are listed in ***Box 4.5***. The contributions of these bodies overlap considerably but cover the key areas for health development and infrastructural support, including the response to emergency situations (war and natural disasters). The areas encompass service delivery, patient care, education and training, research, equipment, medicines and human resources. Investment in healthcare systems promotes public health benefit by the provision of vaccination, hygiene and sanitation, as well as major infrastructural projects including technology and communications, such as building roads.

Box 4.5 Some organizations involved in global aid

International organizations
- World Health Organization (WHO)
- Global Fund to fight AIDS, Tuberculosis and Malaria
- Joint United Nations Programme on HIV/AIDS (UNAIDS)
- World Bank
- Department for International Development (DFID; UK)
- President's Emergency Plan for AIDS Relief (PEPFAR; USA)
- Global Alliance for Vaccines and Immunization (GAVI)

Scientific and educational organizations
- Mainly disease-specific, e.g. microbiology, diabetes, infectious diseases
- Consortium of Universities for Global Health (CUGH)
- Global Health through Education, Training and Service (GHETS)

Advocacy and policy organizations
- Centre for Strategic and International Studies (CSIS)
- Global Health Policy Centre
- Global Alliance for Chronic Diseases (GACD)
- Global Health Council
- Global Health Technologies Coalition (GHTC)
- The Earth Institute (Columbia University)
- Kaiser Family Foundation (KFF)
- US Global Health Policy
- Tropical Health and Education Trust (THET)

Foundations
- Bill and Melinda Gates Foundation
- Wellcome Trust
- UN Foundation (UNF)
- Accordia Global Health Foundation

Other non-governmental organizations
- Save the Children
- United Nations International Children's Emergency Fund (UNICEF)
- Red Cross
- Oxfam
- International Rescue Committee (IRC)
- Médecins sans Frontières (MSF)

Empowering the local population to help themselves by delivering local appropriate education is of paramount importance. Global Health through Education Training and Service (GHETS) is an American non-governmental, non-profit organization that works with a network of medical and nursing schools to increase the number of locally trained, primary healthcare workers. These schools build community-based clinics in rural and urban areas.

Further reading

http://gapminder.org *Gapminder: global trends, and health and wealth of nations.*
http://www.ghets.org *Global Health through Education, Training and Service.*
http://www.globalfamilydoctor.com *Rural Medical Education Guidebook (WONCA): free online book for family doctors.*
http://www.thet.org *Tropical Health and Education Trust.*
http://worldmapper.org *Worldmapper: countries resized according to topic.*

EDUCATION

Education has a major impact on the health of a nation. There is evidence to suggest that the more years spent in schooling, the better the health outcomes. Literacy and, in particular, health literacy can have a major impact on nutrition and the control of disease: for example, by the simple process of hand washing. Education helps to promote healthier lifestyles, both by improving nutrition and development, and by reducing the risks associated with infectious diseases. As a result, unemployment falls whilst family and community wellbeing is improved.

Women have a crucial role in the welfare of their families and the development of a country's good health. Traditionally, women have a lower social status in societies where they are suppressed. Nevertheless, it is they who have the dominant impact on the health of the family and the wellbeing of children. They shoulder all the demands of child care, and of care of the elderly and the sick, as well as all household responsibilities.

Approximately 25% of girls in 'developing countries' become mothers before the age of 18. These pregnancies have a high rate of deaths from complications of pregnancy and childbirth. The cost to a country's economy of adolescent pregnancy, as a share of gross domestic product, can be as high as 30%. The education and welfare of women should be major issues in any developing society, as they reduce poverty and aid a country's development.

Further reading

Chaaban J, Cunningham W. *World Bank Policy Research Working Paper 5753: Measuring the Economic Gain of Investing in Girls: the Girls Effect Dividend.* World Bank 2011; http://papers.ssrn.com/.

United Nations Population Fund. *State of World Population 2014*. New York: UN; 2014.

MATERNAL HEALTH AND CHILD HEALTH

Maternal health (see also Ch. 29)

Women remain disadvantaged in many parts of the world. Every second, 380 women become pregnant, 190 women face unplanned or unwanted pregnancy (e.g. from rape), 110 women experience a pregnancy-related complication, 40 women have an unsafe abortion, and 1 woman dies from a pregnancy-related complication. These stark data support the arguments for women to control their own health and fertility.

Of major concern, 303 000 women die in childbirth every year and 80% of these deaths are avoidable (WHO). Maternal mortality figures are more than 100 times greater in low-income countries (LICs) compared to higher-income countries (HICs). The risk of dying in pregnancy varies from 1 : 8 in Mali, compared to 1 : 17 400 in Sweden. The major medical causes of death are haemorrhage, hypertensive disease of pregnancy and infections. Haemorrhage can be intra- or pre-partum, when the most common cause is placental abruption, or postpartum, when the uterus fails to contract, causing fatal haemorrhage. Hypertensive disease can be complicated by pre-eclampsia (see p. 1303). Infections can be caused, for example, by bacteria, HIV, malaria and syphilis. Obstructed labour is another potentially fatal complication and can be due to the fibrosis caused by female genital mutilation (FGM), traditionally practised in some countries.

As most maternal and neonatal deaths occur around delivery, the need for basic and emergency care around the time of labour and delivery is paramount. The presence of a skilled birth attendant has been shown to reduce both maternal and neonatal mortality in many LMICs.

Child health

Globally, the under 5 years mortality rate has fallen mainly due to the prevention of pneumonia, diarrhoea and malaria by organizations and governments working together. Nevertheless, over 50% of these deaths could have been prevented by access to simple and affordable interventions. Most of these deaths are caused by pre-term complications, birth asphyxia, diarrhoea, pneumonia and malaria. Almost half are linked to malnutrition. These children die from common, otherwise non-fatal, childhood ailments. Deaths in children under 5 years of age are mainly concentrated in Southern Asia and in sub-Saharan Africa, where children are 15 times more likely to die compared with children in developed regions. In the rest of the world, mortality figures dropped from 32% (1990) to 18% (2013; WHO).

Vaccination

The World Health Assembly produced a framework to prevent millions of deaths by more equitable access to vaccines, and adopted a 'Decade of Vaccines Global Vaccine Action Plan 2011–2020'. GAVI plays a critical role in this area by financing and facilitating delivery of vaccine platforms. By 2013, it had immunized 440 million additional children and prevented 6 million future deaths.

Child labour

The global number of children engaged in child labour declined by one-third between 2000 and 2012 (246 million dropping to 168 million). More than half (85 million) are engaged in hazardous work. Agriculture remains the most important sector utilizing child labour (98 million).

Child nutrition

Improving child nutrition remains a global imperative. According to data from UNICEF (2013), stunting affects 165 million children under 5 years of age. This problem can be mitigated by interventions during maternal pregnancy and before the child is 2 years old.

Further reading

Bustreo F, Okwo-Bele JM, Kamara L. World Health Organization perspectives on the contribution of the Global Alliance for Vaccines and Immunization on reducing child mortality. *Arch Dis Child* 2015; 100:S34–S37.

Diallo Y, Etienne A, Mehran F and International Programme on the Elimination of Child Labour. *Global Child Labour Trends 2008 to 2012*. Geneva: International Labour Organization; 2013.

International Programme on the Elimination of Child Labour. *Marking Progress Against Child Labour: Global Estimates and Trends 2000–2012*. Geneva: International Labour Organization; 2013.

United Nations Children's Fund (UNICEF). *Improving Child Nutrition: the Achievable Imperative for Global Progress*. New York: UNICEF; 2013.

MENTAL HEALTH

Mental health (including psychological and neurological problems) constitutes 13% of the Global Burden of Disease (GBD). This exceeds the figures for cardiovascular disease and cancer.

Depression represents a major clinical challenge with 350 million patients worldwide. It is the third commonest contributor to GBD. Alcohol and illicit drug misuse account for >5% of the global mental health burden. Additionally, it is estimated that suicide will account for 1.5 million deaths each year by 2020, with a further 15–30 million people attempting suicide.

Globally, the incidence of dementia is accelerating and 7.7 million new cases occur each year. This increased burden disproportionately affects low- and middle-income countries, where resources are few. All of this represents a major worldwide financial burden.

Further reading

Collins PY, Patel V, Joestl SS et al. Grand challenges in global mental health. *Nature* 2011; 475:27–30.

Saxena S, Wortmann M, Prince M et al. *Dementia: a Public Health Priority*. Geneva: WHO; 2012.

ACCIDENTS AND TRAUMA

We are currently in the midst of a global trauma epidemic. It is estimated that 5.8 million people die each year as a result of injury and trauma. At least 2 million of these deaths are potentially avoidable.

Injuries are a significant and increasing cause of mortality and morbidity; more than 90% of injury-related deaths occur in LMICs.

Around 5 billion people do not have access to safe, affordable surgical and anaesthesia care when needed, particularly in LMICs. Many of those who do access care risk personal financial ruin. The WHO estimates that, by 2030, trauma from road traffic accidents will be the third most common cause worldwide of both mortality and disability (as measured in DALYs).

The *Guidelines for Essential Trauma Care* (WHO 2004) have established a core list of 11 essential trauma care services ***(Box 4.6)***. The implementation of these recommendations has been hampered by deficiencies in planning and infrastructure that need to be addressed by national governments.

Further reading

Mock C, Joshipura M, Lormand J et al. Strengthening trauma systems globally: the Essential Trauma Care Project. *J Trauma* 2005; 59:1243–1246.
Sakran J, Greer SE, Werlin E et al. Care of the injured worldwide: trauma still the neglected disease of modern society. *Scand J Trauma Resusc Emerg Med* 2012; 20:64.

Box 4.6 International guidelines for essential trauma care ('rights of the injured')

- Obstructed airways cleared and maintained
- Impaired breathing supported until the injured person is self-ventilating
- Pneumothorax and haemothorax promptly relieved
- Bleeding stopped promptly
- Shock recognized and treated with intravenous fluid replacement
- Traumatic brain injury treated with timely decompression of space-occupying lesions
- Intestinal and other abdominal injuries promptly addressed
- Disabling extremity injuries corrected
- Unstable spinal cord injuries managed appropriately with early immobilization
- Appropriate rehabilitative services available
- Medications for the above and for pain control readily available

(Adapted from Mock C, Joshipura M, Goosen J, Maier R. Overview of the Essential Trauma Care Project. World J Surg 2006; 30:919–929.)

CONFLICT AND CATASTROPHE

Recent years have seen a number of natural disasters; examples include earthquakes in Haiti (2010) and Nepal (2015), the Sri Lanka tsunami (2004), and typhoon Haiyan in the Philippines (2013). Conflicts also persist in Syria, South Sudan, the Ukraine and numerous other parts of the world. Effective global action following these unexpected events is frequently compromised by deficiencies in the disaster response, including the provision of inappropriate resources and inexperienced personnel. Many such deficiencies can be rectified by appropriate training in disaster response. Other elements of an effective international response must address long-term restructuring issues. Following conflict, regulation of the trade in armaments is critical.

Conflicts and catastrophes severely disrupt healthcare provision, especially for women and children. The use of rape as a weapon of war magnifies this tragedy. Furthermore, disruption to education, together with the physical sequelae of conflict, leads to increased long-term societal healthcare burdens, especially in the field of mental health.

ECONOMICS AND POLITICS IN GLOBAL HEALTH

Funding for initiatives in the GH development of LMICs (also known as Development Assistance for Health, DAH) has, historically, originated from multiple sources (see Box 4.5). Whilst these initiatives may have been beneficial for some specific diseases like malaria (see pp. 297–301), tuberculosis (pp. 1106–1113) and HIV/AIDs (pp. 331–355), health systems development has frequently lagged behind such high-profile schemes. The consequences of this were seen in the slow response of the WHO and others to the 2014 outbreak of Ebola in Africa.

Improvements in healthcare result in economic growth. For example, a 10% reduction of malaria in endemic areas is associated with a 0.3% increase in GDP. Treatment of HIV-positive patients with anti-retroviral drugs results in net economic benefit through increased productivity and a reduction in medical care treatment costs. A failure to invest in health and health systems is a threat to future global prosperity, particularly in poor countries. As an example, surgery is currently a neglected component of health systems and it is estimated that 5 billion people currently lack access to safe, affordable surgical and anaesthesia care when needed. The cumulative loss of economic productivity between 2015 and 2030, in the absence of a significant scaling up of global surgical services, is estimated at US$12.3 trillion.

Political decisions regarding investment in healthcare and health systems also need to focus on infrastructure, including food and agriculture, the environment and human rights issues, especially the rights of women. In essence, the pursuit of 'pro-poor' policies that place the poor at the centre of development policy is essential for future global prosperity.

Further reading

Figuera J, McKee M. *Health Systems, Health, Wealth and Societal Well-being.* Maidenhead: McGraw Hill/Open University Press; 2012.
Meara JG, Leather AJM, Hagander L et al. and the Lancet Commission on Global Surgery. Global surgery 2030; evidence and solutions for achieving health, welfare, and economic development. *Lancet* 2015; 386:569–624.
Resch S, Korenromp E, Stover J et al. Economic returns to investment in AIDS treatment in low and middle income countries. *PLoS ONE* 2011; 6:e25310.

SOCIAL DETERMINANTS OF HEALTH

The drivers of health inequities reside in the social, economic and political environments. The WHO (2008) defined the social determinants of health as 'the conditions in which people are born, grow, live, work, and age. These circumstances are shaped by the distribution of money, power and resources at global, national and local levels.' The social gradient of health follows the socioeconomic pattern from the top to the bottom. In general, the lower the individual is within their socioeconomic position, the worse their health; this is seen globally in HICs, as well as LMICs. The socioeconomic status of a person is their social position in society and this is determined by their education, income and occupation.

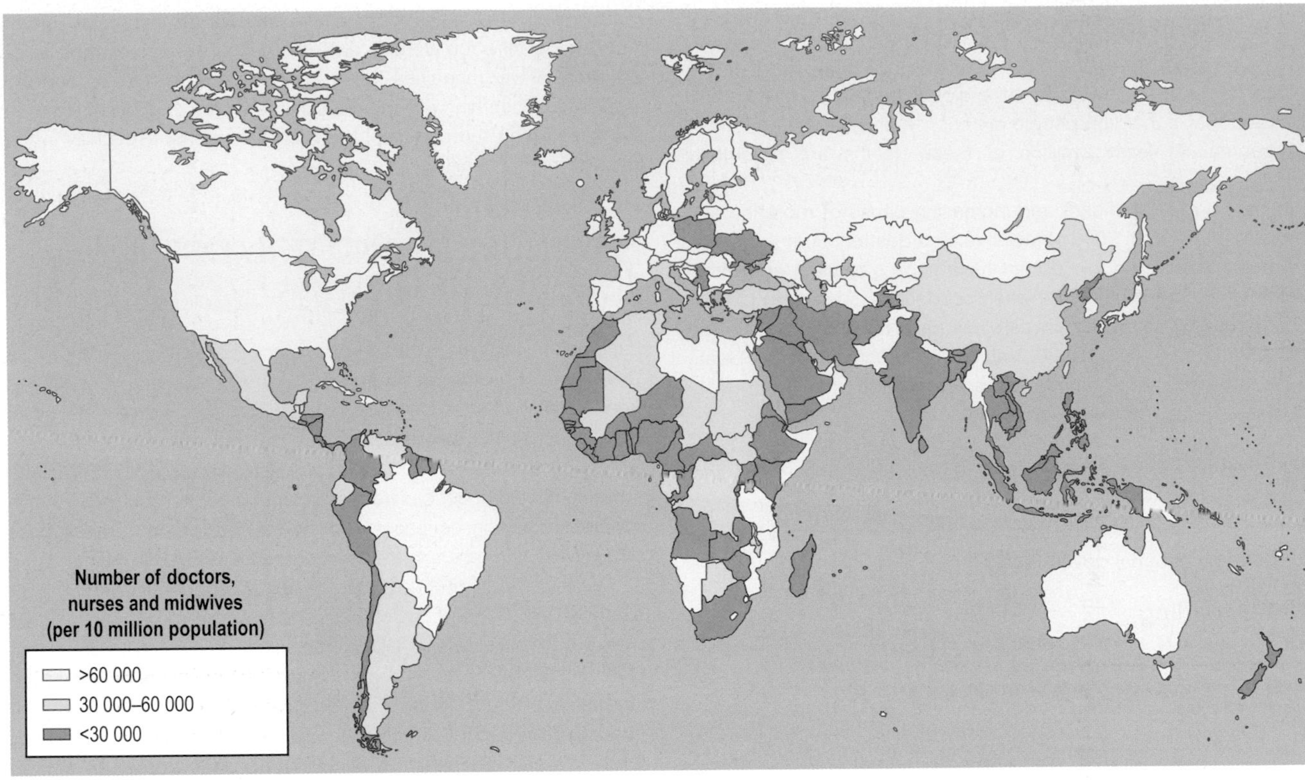

Figure 4.5 Worldwide shortage of healthcare workers. There are 57 countries with a critical shortage of 2.4 million health service providers (doctors, nurses and midwives). Africa has 25% of the world's healthcare burden and 1.3% of the providers. *(From Crisp N, Cheng L. Global supply of health professionals.* N Engl J Med *2014; 370:950–957 [Figure 1], with permission.)*

There is now clear evidence to justify national policies that aim to reduce health inequity and the health divide across all countries. It has also been suggested that reduction in health inequities should become one of the main criteria used to assess the effectiveness of health systems and governments as a whole.

Further reading

Marmot M, Allen J, Bell R et al and World Health Organization. European review of social determinants of health and health divide. *Lancet* 2012; 38:1011–1029.

HUMAN RIGHTS AND THE VALUE OF ENGAGEMENT IN GLOBAL HEALTH

The Universal Declaration of Human Rights (1948), whilst not legally binding, serves as a 'common standard for all peoples and all nations'. It has given rise to two new legally binding covenants: the International Covenant on Civil and Political Rights and the International Covenant on Economic, Social and Cultural Rights.

The WHO is a specialized agency of the United Nations with a remit for international public health. Its constitution enshrines 'the highest attainable standard of health' as a fundamental right of every human being. The right to health contains four elements: availability (of programmes of public health), accessibility (of health facilities and services in a non-discriminating fashion), acceptability (ethical and cultural requirements), and good-quality care.

There is a worldwide shortage of healthcare workers from all disciplines ***(Fig. 4.5)***. Engagement in GH challenges helps to promote patterns of behaviour that benefit healthcare workers, as well as the recipients of their endeavours. Altruistic behaviours, team-working and appreciation of cultural diversity are but a few benefits of participation in GH challenges.

Medical electives

Both medical students and doctors may undertake periods of time visiting and working in unfamiliar environments, often in other countries. This is mutually beneficial to all participants, provided that a culture of shared learning is embraced. All such visits should have clear objectives and measurable educational outcomes. Pre-departure preparation should include consideration of culture, ethical challenges and security issues. All visitors must work within their approved competencies and comply with national guidance on good medical practice. It is essential for the appropriate processes for bipartite support and supervision to be secure.

Maximum benefit is achieved when there is a mutual commitment to long-term partnership. This type of experience promotes personal altruistic behaviours.

Further reading

http://www.ohchr.org/ *International Bill of Human Rights.*
http://www.un.org/ *Universal Declaration of Human Rights.*

Bibliography

Crisp N. *Turning the World Upside Down. The Search for Global Health in the 21st Century*. London: Royal Society of Medicine Press; 2010.
Global Burden of Disease Study 2013 Collaboration. Global, regional, and national incidence, prevalence, and years lived with disability for 301 acute and chronic diseases and injuries in 188 countries, 1990–2013: a systematic analysis for the Global Burden of Disease Study 2013. *Lancet* 2015; 386:743–800.
Marmot M. *The Health Gap. The Challenge of an Unequal World*. London: Bloomsbury Publishing; 2015.

5 Environmental medicine

Michael L Clark

See your e-book for key learning points, clinical tips, learning challenges, MCQs and Special Topics from the International Advisory Board.

DISEASE AND THE ENVIRONMENT

The incidence and prevalence of disease and causes of death within a community are a reflection of interrelated factors:

- ***Genetic predisposition.***
- ***Nutrition, poverty and affluence*** (see p. 183), some countries having a grossly uneven distribution between rich and poor. This leads to chronic disease such as diabetes and obesity mainly in the cities, with malnutrition and infectious disease in the rural areas.
- ***Purity of water sources*** and ***sanitation facilities*** (see p. 47).
- ***Atmospheric pollution.***
- ***Environmental disasters and accidents.***
- ***Background ionizing radiation*** and man-made radiation exposure, deliberate or accidental.
- ***Environmental temperature.***
- ***Patterns of infective disease*** (see p. 222).
- ***Political forces*** determining levels of healthcare, preventative strategies and effects of war on civilian populations (see p. 49).

Some of these environmental effects have been clearly documented within the last decade: for example, the massive civilian mortality and morbidity during the Afghan war, previous Iraq wars and current military action in the Middle East. Loss of life and disease prevalence following the 2006 tsunami, the earthquakes in Szechuan (2008) and Haiti (2010), and cyclone Nargis in the Irawaddy delta have been huge. Aspects related to ***global health*** are discussed in more detail in Chapter 4.

Flooding caused by El Nino in East Africa resulted not only in an increase in breeding sites for mosquito vectors but also in a major outbreak of Rift Valley fever due to the enforced close proximity of cattle and humans.

Tobacco use (active and passive), obesity (see pp. 206–212) and excess alcohol consumption also play a significant role in disease. Physical inactivity has an effect on mortality that is equivalent to tobacco use or obesity. Worldwide health programmes have been established in most countries to reduce these effects.

Further reading

Van Rooyen MS. Medical complications associated with earthquakes. *Lancet* 2012; 379:748–757.

ENVIRONMENTAL TEMPERATURE

Climate change is an unquestionable phenomenon due mainly to increased carbon dioxide production and changes in our habitat.

The effect of environmental temperature (T_{Env}) is paramount in infective diseases; increases as small as 1°C cause major changes in disease vectors. Patterns of infective disease are likely to change radically within the next 20 years. Climate effects are already becoming apparent, such as:

- changes in the patterns of malaria in South-east Asia
- the occurrence of dengue fever in southern Italy
- outbreaks of cholera, and seasonal variation in diarrhoea and vomiting.

Research into the effect of climate change on the changing patterns of infective diseases will point to potential ways in which national and international efforts can be targeted.

HEAT INJURY

Body core temperature (T_{Core}) is maintained at 37°C by the thermoregulator centre in the hypothalamus, which integrates information from skin temperature sensors with core temperatures from receptors in the brain and in the walls of large blood vessels.

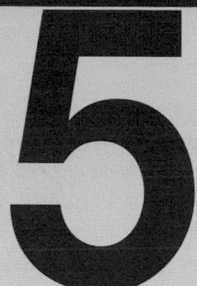

Heat is produced by cellular metabolism and is dissipated through the skin by both vasodilatation and sweating, and in expired air via the alveoli. When the environmental temperature (T_{Env}) is >32.5°C, profuse sweating occurs.

Sweat evaporation is the principal mechanism for controlling T_{Core} following exercise or in response to an increase in T_{Env}.

Heat acclimatization takes place over several weeks. The sweat volume increases and the sweat salt content falls. Increased evaporation of sweat reduces T_{Core}.

Heat cramps

Painful muscle cramps, usually in the legs, often occur in fit people when they exercise excessively, especially in hot weather. Cramps are probably due to low extracellular sodium caused by excess intake of water over salt. They can be prevented by increasing dietary salt. They respond to combined salt and water replacement, and in the acute stage to stretching and muscle massage. T_{Core} remains normal.

Heat exhaustion

At any environmental temperature (especially with T_{Env} of >25°C), and with a high humidity, strenuous exercise in clothing that inhibits sweating, such as a wetsuit or military uniform, can cause an elevation in T_{Core} in less than 15 minutes. Weakness/exhaustion, cramps, dizziness and syncope, with T_{Core} >37°C, define heat exhaustion. Elevation of T_{Core} is more critical than water and sodium loss. Heat exhaustion may progress to heat stroke, a serious emergency (see below).

Management

Reduce (T_{Env}) if possible and cool the patient with sponging and fans. Give O_2 by mask. Other causes of high T_{Core}, such as malaria, should be ruled out if appropriate.

Oral rehydration with *both* salt and water (25 g of salt per 5 L of water/day) is given in the first instance, with adequate replacement thereafter. In severe heat exhaustion, intravenous fluids are needed; 0.9% saline is given. Monitor serum sodium and correct secondary potassium loss.

Heat stroke

Heat stroke is an acute life-threatening situation in which T_{Core} rises >41°C. There is headache, nausea, vomiting and weakness, progressing to confusion, coma and death. The skin *feels* intensely hot to the touch. Sweating is often absent but not invariably so.

Heat stroke can develop in unacclimatized people in hot, humid, windless conditions, even without exercise. Sweating may be limited by prickly heat (plugging or rupture of the sweat ducts, leading to a pruritic, papular, erythematous rash).

Excessive exercise in inappropriate clothing, such as exercising on land in a wetsuit, can lead to heat injury in temperate climates. Diabetes, alcohol and drugs, such as antimuscarinics, diuretics and phenothiazines, can contribute. Heat stroke can lead to a fall in cardiac output, lactic acidosis and intravascular coagulation.

Prevention

Acclimatization, fluids, avoidance of inappropriate clothing and common sense are required.

Management

- Apply standard life support measures (ABCDE).
- Reduce T_{Env} if possible.
- Arrange cold water immersion if facilities are available. Otherwise, cool the patient with sponging, icepacks or fanning.
- Give O_2 by mask.
- Move the patient to a medical facility. Manage in intensive care: monitor cardiac output and respiration; measure biochemistry, clotting and muscle enzymes.
- Give fluids intravenously so the intravascular volume remains normal.

Prompt treatment is essential and can be curative, even with a T_{Core} of >41°C. Morbidity and mortality are directly related to the duration of the high T_{Core}.

Complications are hypovolaemia, intravascular coagulation, cerebral oedema, rhabdomyolysis, and renal and hepatic failure.

Malignant hyperpyrexia

See page 889.

Further reading

Hajat S, O'Connor M, Kosatsky T. Health effects of hot weather: from awareness of risk factors to effective health protection. *Lancet* 2010; 375:856–863.

COLD INJURY

Cold injury may be divided into hypothermia, which is whole-body cooling, and peripheral cold injury ***(Box 5.1)***.

Hypothermia

Hypothermia occurs in many settings.

At home. Hypothermia can occur when T_{Env} is <8°C, if there is poor heating, inadequate clothing and poor nutrition. Depressant drugs, such as hypnotics, as well as alcohol, hypothyroidism or intercurrent illness also contribute. Hypothermia is commonly seen in the poor, frail and elderly. The elderly have a diminished ability to sense cold and also have little insulating fat.

Neonates and infants become hypothermic rapidly because of a relatively large surface area in proportion to subcutaneous fat.

Outdoors on land. Hypothermia is a prominent cause of death in climbers, skiers and polar travellers, and in wartime. Wet, cold conditions with wind chill, physical exhaustion, injuries and inadequate clothing are contributory. Babies and children are at risk because they cannot take action to warm themselves.

Cold water immersion. Dangerous hypothermia can develop following immersion for more than 30 min to 1 hour in water temperatures of 15–20°C. In T_{Water} <12°C, limbs rapidly become numb and weak. Recovery takes place gradually, over several hours following rescue.

Clinical features

Mild hypothermia (T_{Core} <32°C) causes shivering and initially intense discomfort. However, the hypothermic subject, though alert, may not act appropriately to rewarming: for example, by huddling, wearing extra clothing or exercising. As the T_{Core} falls below 32°C,

Box 5.1 Cold injury

- ***Hypothermia*** is defined as a core temperature of <32°C
- ***Peripheral cold injury*** includes:
  - ***Frostbite:*** the local cold injury that follows freezing of tissue
  - ***Non-freezing cold injury:*** the damage – usually to feet – following prolonged exposure to a T_{Env} between 0° and 5°C, usually in damp conditions

severe hypothermia causes impaired judgement – including lack of awareness of cold – and drowsiness and coma. Death follows, usually from ventricular fibrillation.

Diagnosis

Diagnosis is straightforward, if a low-reading thermometer is available. If not, rapid clinical assessment is reliable. Someone who *feels* icy to the touch – abdomen, groin, axillae – is *probably* substantially hypothermic. If the person is clammy, uncooperative or sleepy, T_{Core} is almost certainly <32°C.

Sequelae

Pulse rate and systemic blood pressure fall. Cardiac output and cerebral blood flow are low in hypothermia and can fall further if the upright position is maintained or the thorax restrained by a harness, or by hauling during evacuation. This is why helicopter and lifeboat winch rescues are often carried out with a stretcher rather than a chest harness.

Respiration becomes shallow and slow. Muscle stiffness develops; tendon reflexes become sluggish, then absent. As coma ensues, pupillary and other brainstem reflexes are lost; pupils are fixed and may be dilated in severe hypothermia. Metabolic changes are variable, with either metabolic acidosis or alkalosis. Arterial PO_2 may appear normal: that is, falsely high.

There is shift of the oxygen dissociation curve (see p. 90) to the left because of the reduction in temperature of haemoglobin. Thus, if an arterial blood sample from a hypothermic patient is analysed at 37°C, the PO_2 will be falsely high. Within the range 37–33°C, this factor is around 7% per degree centigrade. Many blood gas machines also calculate the arterial saturation; this too will be falsely high. When a patient is monitored using a pulse oximeter, the level of arterial oxygen saturation (S_aO_2) will, however, be correct, but if S_aO_2 is then converted by calculation to P_aO_2, a downward correction must be applied – simply due to hypothermia.

Bradycardia with 'J' waves (above the isoelectric line at the junction of the QRS complex and ST segment; ***Fig. 5.1***) are pathognomonic of hypothermia. Prolongation of PR and QT intervals and the QRS complex also occurs. Ventricular dysrhythmia (tachycardia/fibrillation) or asystole is the usual cause of death.

Management

- Maintain the patient horizontal or slightly head-down.
- Rewarm gradually.

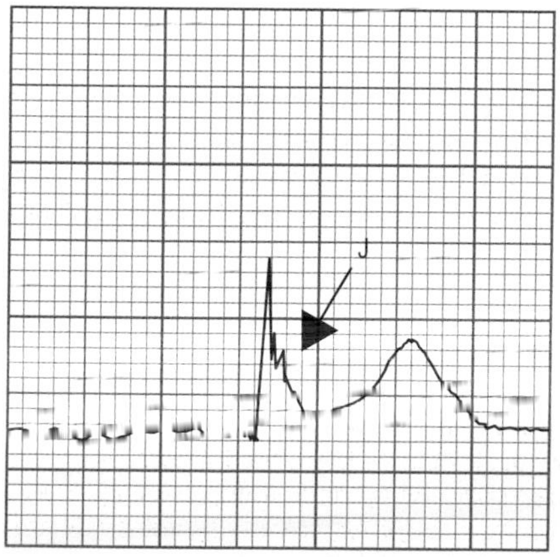

Figure 5.1 Electrocardiogram showing J waves in hypothermia.

- Correct metabolic abnormalities.
- Anticipate and treat dysrhythmias.
- Check for hypothyroidism (see pp. 1202–1204).

If the patient is awake, with a core temperature of >32°C, place in a warm room, use a foil wrap and give warm fluids orally. Outdoors, add extra dry clothing, huddle together and use a warmed sleeping bag. Rewarming may take several hours. Avoid alcohol: this adds to confusion, boosts confidence factitiously, causes peripheral vasodilatation and further heat loss, and can precipitate hypoglycaemia.

Severe hypothermia

In severe hypothermia, people look dead. Always exclude hypothermia before diagnosing brainstem death (see p. 1172). Warm gradually, aiming at a 1°C/hour increase in T_{Core}. Direct mild surface heat from an electric blanket can be helpful. Treat any underlying condition promptly, such as sepsis. Monitor all vital functions. Correct dysrhythmias. Check for sedative drugs.

Give warm intravenous fluids slowly. Correct metabolic abnormalities. Hypothyroidism, if present, should be treated with liothyronine. Various methods of artificial rewarming exist: inhaled warm humidified air, gastric or peritoneal lavage, and haemodialysis. These are rarely used. Hypothermia is frequently lethal when T_{Core} falls below 30°C. Survival with full recovery has, however, been recorded with a T_{Core} of <16°C.

Prevention

Hypothermia in the field can often be prevented by forethought and action. For the elderly, improved home heating and insulation, central heating in bedrooms and electric blankets are helpful in cold spells. This can be expensive and unaffordable for some people, so supplemental finance is required.

Peripheral cold injury

Frostbite

Ice crystals form within skin and superficial tissues when the temperature of the tissue (T_{Tissue}) falls to –3°C: T_{Env} generally must be below –6°C. Wind chill is frequently a factor. Typically, fingers, toes, nose and ears become frostbitten.

Frostbitten tissue is pale, greyish and initially doughy to the touch. Later, tissue freezes hard, looking like meat from a freezer. Frostbite can easily occur when working or exercising in low temperatures and typically develops without the patient's knowledge. Below a T_{Env} of 5°C, hands or feet that have lost their feeling are at risk of cold injury.

Management

Transport the patient – or if this is impossible, make them walk, even on frostbitten feet – to a place of safety before commencing warming. Warm the frozen part by immersion in hand-hot water at 39–42°C, if feasible. Assess hypothermia. Continue warming until obvious thawing occurs; this can be painful. Vasodilator drugs have no part in management. Blisters form in a few days and, depending on the depth of frostbite, a blackened shell – the ***carapace*** – develops as blisters regress or burst. Dry, non-adherent dressings and aseptic precautions are essential, though hard to achieve. Frostbitten tissues are anaesthetic and at risk from further trauma and infection. Recovery takes place over many weeks and may be incomplete. Surgery may be needed, but should be avoided in the early stages.

Chilblains

These are small, purplish itchy inflammatory lesions, occurring on toes and fingers. They occur in cold, wet conditions. They are more common in women and heal in 7–14 days. Prevention is by keeping warm and wearing gloves and warm footwear.

Non-freezing cold injury

Non-freezing cold injury (NFCI, trench foot) describes tissue damage following prolonged exposure, usually for several hours or more, at T_{Env} around or slightly above freezing, but without frostbite. Wet socks and boots are the usual cause. There is severe vasoconstriction, and blotchiness of the lower limbs, with pain and oedema on rewarming. Recovery usually follows over several weeks. There may be a prolonged late susceptibility to cold. NFCI is a prominent cause of morbidity in troops operating in low temperatures and is a subsequent cause of litigation.

Prevention of frostbite and NFCI is largely by education and common sense: avoid damp feet and wet boots. Always carry spare dry socks, gloves and headgear.

Further reading

Sheridan RL, Goldstein MA, Stoddard FJ Jr et al. Case records of the Massachusetts General Hospital. Case 41-2009. A 16-year-old boy with hypothermia and frostbite. *N Engl J Med* 2009; 361:2654–2662.
Wira CR, Becker JU, Martin G et al. Anti-arrhythmic and vasopressor medications for the treatment of ventricular fibrillation in severe hypothermia. *Resuscitation* 2008; 78:21–29.
http://www.hypothermia.org *Hypothermia prevention, recognition and treatment.*

HIGH ALTITUDE

The partial pressure of atmospheric oxygen – and hence alveolar and arterial oxygen – falls in a near-linear relationship as barometric pressure drops with increasing altitude ***(Fig. 5.2)***.

Commercial aircraft are pressurized to around 24 000 m (lowering the oxygen saturation by 3–4%). This trivial reduction is not noticed by healthy individuals. Air travel is discussed on page 61.

On land, below 3000 m there are few clinical effects. The resulting hypoxaemia causes breathlessness only in those with severe cardiorespiratory disease. Above 3000–3500 m, hypoxia causes a spectrum of related syndromes that affect high-altitude visitors, principally climbers, trekkers, skiers and troops ***(Box 5.2)***, especially when they exercise. These conditions occur largely during acclimatization, a process that takes several weeks; once completed, this can enable humans to live – permanently, if necessary – up to about 5600 m. At greater heights, although people can survive for days or weeks, deterioration due to chronic hypoxia is inevitable.

The world's highest railway runs to Lhasa in Tibet, reaching altitudes of over 5000 m. Emergency oxygen is provided in the carriages. Roads at similar altitudes in Central Asia are used extensively but since road passengers do not exercise, serious altitude-related illnesses are unusual. Climbing the world's highest summits is just possible without supplementary oxygen, though it is often used on peaks above 7500 m. At the summit of Mount Everest (8848 m), the barometric pressure is 34 kPa (253 mmHg). An acclimatized mountaineer has an alveolar PO_2 of 4.0–4.7 kPa (30–35 mmHg) – near humans' absolute physiological limit. In 2007, arterial blood samples from acclimatized doctors on Everest at altitude 8400 m, breathing air, showed an average PO_2 of 24.6 mmHg (3.3 kPa).

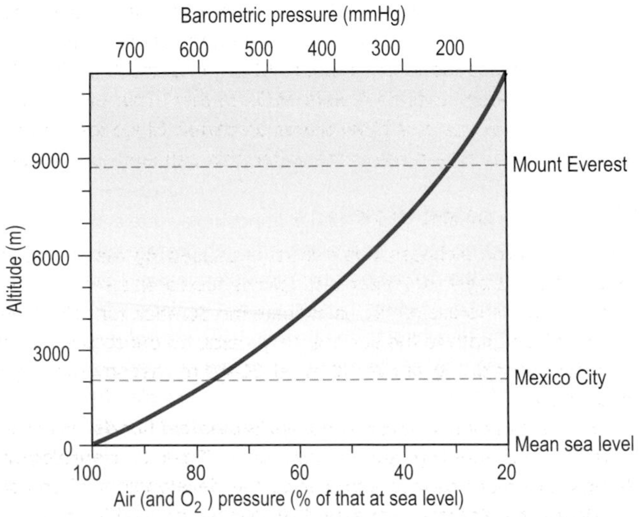

Figure 5.2 The decrease in oxygen and barometric pressure with increasing altitude.

Acute mountain sickness

Acute mountain sickness (AMS) describes malaise, nausea, headache and lassitude that affect the majority of people for a few days, above 3500 m. Following arrival at this altitude, there is usually a latent interval of 6–36 hours before symptoms begin. Treatment is rest, with analgesics if necessary. Recovery is usually spontaneous over several days.

Prophylactic treatment with acetazolamide, a carbonic anhydrase inhibitor and respiratory stimulant, is of some value in preventing AMS. Acclimatizing – that is, ascending gradually – provides better and more natural prophylaxis.

In the minority, more serious sequelae – high-altitude pulmonary oedema and high-altitude cerebral oedema – develop.

High-altitude pulmonary oedema

Predisposing factors include youth, rapidity of ascent, heavy exertion and severe AMS. Breathlessness, occasionally with frothy blood-stained sputum, indicates established oedema. Unless treated rapidly, this leads to cardiorespiratory failure and death. Milder forms are common. Breathlessness at rest should raise the suspicion of pulmonary oedema.

High-altitude cerebral oedema

Cerebral oedema is the result of an abrupt increase in cerebral blood flow that occurs even at modest altitudes of 3500–4000 m. It is unusual below 4500 m, and occurs typically in the first 2 weeks, during acclimatization. Cerebral oedema can also develop suddenly in well-acclimatized climbers above 7000 m. Headache is followed

Box 5.2 Conditions caused by sustained hypoxia

Condition	Incidence (%)	Usual altitude (m)
Acute mountain sickness	70	3500–4000
Acute pulmonary oedema	2	4000
Acute cerebral oedema	1	4500
Retinal haemorrhage	50	5000
Deterioration	100	≥6000
Chronic mountain sickness	Rare	3500–4000

by drowsiness, ataxia and papilloedema, with coma and death if brain oedema progresses.

Management

Any but the milder forms of AMS require urgent treatment. Oxygen should be given by mask if available, and descent should take place as quickly as possible. Nifedipine reduces pulmonary hypertension and is used in pulmonary oedema. Dexamethasone is effective in reducing brain oedema. Portable pressure bags inflated by a foot pump are widely used; the patient is enclosed in the bag.

Retinal haemorrhage

Small flame haemorrhages within the retinal nerve fibre layer are common above 5000 m and usually symptomless. Rarely, a haemorrhage will cover the macula, causing painless loss of central vision. Recovery is usual.

Deterioration

Prolonged residence between 6000 and 7000 m leads to weight loss, anorexia and listlessness after several weeks. Above 7500 m, the effects of deterioration become apparent over several days, although it is possible to survive for a week or more at altitudes near 8000 m without supplementary oxygen.

Chronic mountain sickness

Chronic mountain sickness occurs in long-term residents at high altitudes, usually after several decades, and is seen in the Andes and in Central Asia.

Headache, polycythaemia, lassitude, cyanosis, finger clubbing, congested cheeks and ear lobes, and right ventricular enlargement develop. Chronic mountain sickness is gradually progressive.

Coronary artery disease and hypertension are rare in high-altitude native populations.

Further reading

Grocott MP, Martin DS, Levett DZ et al. Arterial blood gases and oxygen content in climbers on Mount Everest. *N Engl J Med* 2009; 360:140–149.

Imray CH, Grocott MP, Wilson MH et al. Extreme, expedition and wilderness medicine. *Lancet* 2015; 386:2520–2525.

Wilson MH, Habig K, Wright C et al. Pre-hospital emergency medicine. *Lancet* 2015; 386:2526–2534.

http://www.thebmc.co.uk *Union Internationale des Associations d'Alpinisme (UIAA) Mountain Medicine Data Centre leaflets, available from British Mountaineering Council, 177–179 Burton Road, Manchester M20 2BB, UK.*

http://www.wms.org *Wilderness Medical Society Information, PO Box 2463, Indianapolis, Indiana 462206, USA.*

DIVING

Free diving by breath-holding is possible to around 5 m, or with practice to greater depths. Air can be supplied to divers by various methods.

A ***snorkel*** provides air to a depth of about 0.5 m; inspiratory effort is the limiting factor. At depths >0.5 m – that is, with a longer snorkel tube, forced negative-pressure ventilation can cause pulmonary capillary damage with haemorrhagic alveolar oedema.

Scuba divers – recreational sports diving descending to 30 m – carry bottled compressed air or a nitrogen–oxygen mixture.

Commercial divers who work at great depths breathe helium–oxygen or nitrogen–oxygen mixtures, delivered by hose from the surface.

Ambient pressures at various depths are shown in ***Box 5.3***.

Box 5.3 Depth and pressure

Water depth (m)	Pressure	
	Atmospheres	*mmHg*
0	1	760
10	2	1520
50	6	4560
90	10	7600

Problems during descent

Middle ear barotrauma (squeeze) is common and is due to an inability to equalize pressure in the middle ear; Eustachian tube blockage is the usual cause. Pain and hearing loss occur, sometimes with tympanic membrane rupture and acute vertigo.

Sinus squeeze is intense local pain due to blockage of the nasal and paranasal sinus ostia.

Management is by holding the nostrils closed and swallowing, or similar manœuvres, as well as use of decongestants. Diving with a respiratory or sinus infection should be avoided.

Oxygen narcosis

Pure oxygen is not used for diving because of oxygen toxicity. Lung atelectasis, endothelial cell damage and pulmonary oedema occur when alveolar oxygen pressure exceeds 1.5 atmospheres, at depths of around 5 m. At around 10 m, the central nervous system (CNS) becomes affected: apprehension, nausea and sweating are followed by muscle twitching and generalized convulsions.

Nitrogen narcosis

When compressed air is breathed below 30 m, the narcotic effects of nitrogen begin to impair brain function. Poor judgement is hazardous; this also occurs with nitrogen–oxygen mixtures in recreational diving. Nitrogen narcosis is avoided by replacing air with helium–oxygen mixtures, enabling descent to 700 m. At these extreme depths, the direct effect of pressure on neurones can cause tremor, hemiparesis and cognitive impairment.

Problems during and following ascent

Free divers who breath-hold often hyperventilate deliberately prior to plunging in. This drives off CO_2, reducing the stimulus to inspire. During the subsequent breath-hold, P_aCO_2 rises and P_aO_2 falls. On surfacing, decompression lowers P_aO_2 further. This can lead to syncope, known as a ***shallow water blackout***. Since loss of consciousness can take place in the water, this can lead to fatalities.

Decompression sickness

Decompression sickness (the bends) is caused by the release of bubbles of nitrogen or helium and follows too rapid a return to the surface. Decompression tables indicate the duration for safe return from a given depth to the surface. In general, no decompression is necessary for diving above 30 m; at 30–60 m, decompression is necessary.

Bends can be mild (***type 1, non-neurological bends***), with skin irritation and mottling and/or joint pain. ***Type 2, neurological bends***, are more serious and involve the development of cortical blindness, hemiparesis, sensory disturbances or cord lesions.

If bubbles form in pulmonary vessels, divers experience retrosternal discomfort, breathlessness and cough, known as ***the***

chokes. These develop within minutes or hours of a dive. Decompression problems do not only occur immediately on reaching the surface; they may take some hours to become apparent. Over the subsequent 24 hours, further ascent, such as air travel, can occasionally provoke the bends.

Other problems during ascent include paranasal sinus pain and nosebleeds – medically minor but dramatic, with excruciating pain and a mask full of bloody fluid. Toothache can be caused by gas bubbles within rotten fillings.

Management

All but the mildest forms of decompression sickness, such as skin mottling alone, require recompression in a pressure chamber, following strict guidelines. Recovery is usual. A long-term problem is aseptic necrosis of the hip due to nitrogen bubbles causing infarction. Focal neurological damage may persist, but complaints of fatigue and poor concentration are issues compounded by litigation that commonly follows diving accidents. Objective, evidence-based assessments are essential.

Lung rupture, pneumothorax and surgical emphysema

These emergencies occur when divers breath-hold during emergency ascents after gas supplies become exhausted. There is dyspnoea, cough and haemoptysis. Pneumothorax and surgical emphysema resolve with 100% oxygen. Air embolism can also occur and is treated with recompression.

Further reading

Brubakk A, Neuman TS. *Bennett and Elliott's Physiology and Medicine of Diving*, 5th edn. London: WB Saunders; 2002.
Edmonds C, Thomas B, McKewzie B et al. *Diving Medicine for Scuba Divers*; 2012; available at http://www.divingmedicine.info.
Lynch JH, Bove AA. Diving medicine: a review of current evidence. *J Am Board Fam Med* 2009; 22:399–407.
http://www.diversalertnetwork.org/ *Divers Alert Network (DAN).*
http://www.divingmedicine.info/ *Diving Medicine for Scuba Divers.*

DROWNING

Drowning is defined as a process resulting in primary respiratory impairment from submersion or immersion in a liquid medium. Terms such as 'near-drowning and 'wet drowning' should not be used.

Drowning is a common cause of accidental death worldwide. In the UK, some 40% of drownings occur in children under 5 years of age. Drowning can also follow a seizure or a myocardial infarct. Exhaustion, alcohol, drugs and hypothermia all contribute to deaths following submersion.

Fresh or seawater aspiration destroys pulmonary surfactant, leading to alveolar collapse, ventilation/perfusion mismatch and hypoxaemia. Aspiration of hypertonic seawater (5% NaCl) pulls additional fluid into the alveoli with further ventilation/perfusion mismatch. In practice, there is little difference between saltwater and freshwater aspiration. In both, severe hypoxaemia develops rapidly. Severe metabolic acidosis develops in the majority of survivors.

Management and prognosis

Clearance of the airway and ventilation are the major requirements for submerged people, and bystanders should start resuscitation immediately once the person is stable on land. Rescue breaths and chest compression come before the initiation of standard cardiopulmonary resuscitation as used in cardiac arrest (see pp. 956–959). Patients have survived for up to 30 minutes under water without suffering brain damage – and sometimes for longer periods if T_{Water} is near 10°C. Survival is probably related to the protective role of the ***diving reflex***; submersion causes bradycardia and vasoconstriction. Oxygen consumption is also decreased by hypothermia.

Resuscitation should always be attempted, even with absent pulse and fixed dilated pupils. Patients frequently make a dramatic recovery. All survivors should be admitted to hospital for intensive monitoring, as acute respiratory distress syndrome (ARDS) can develop during the subsequent 48 hours.

Recovery is frequently complete if consciousness is regained within several minutes of commencing resuscitation but poor if a patient remains stuporose or in coma at 30 minutes.

Prevention

This includes making sure that all people can swim, particularly young children. Any water can be dangerous, and swimming should only be undertaken in supervised areas.

Further reading

Szpilman D, Bierens JJ, Handley AJ et al. Drowning. *N Engl J Med* 2012; 366:2102–2110.
Vanden Hoek TL, Morrison LJ, Shuster M et al. Part 12: Cardiac arrest in special situations: 2010 American Heart Association Guidelines for Cardiopulmonary Resuscitation and Emergency Cardiovascular Care. *Circulation* 2010; 122:S829.

AIR POLLUTION

Epidemiology

Air pollution is one of the biggest problems facing the world currently. It has become a public health emergency as it leads to chronic diseases and exacerbates respiratory, cardiac and other medical problems. According to the United Nations, air pollution is the cause of 3.7 million premature deaths per year, most of which are from heart attacks and strokes. Annually, pollution is the cause of 1.4 million deaths in China, 645 000 in India and 110 000 in Pakistan, and figures are rising. It is also the single largest environmental risk in Europe, causing 430 000 premature deaths. It has been estimated that air pollution kills more people in a year than malaria and HIV combined and about ten times more deaths than road accidents in some countries. Atmospheric air pollution, due to the burning of coal for energy and heat, has been a feature of urban living in developed countries for at least two centuries. It consists of black smoke and sulphur dioxide (SO_2) and, from combustion of hydrocarbon fuels in motor vehicles, nitrogen oxides (NO and NO_2), diesel particulates, polyaromatic hydrocarbons and ozone, a secondary pollutant generated by photochemical reactions in the atmosphere. Levels of NO_2 can be high in poorly ventilated kitchens and living rooms where gas is used for cooking and in fires.

Particulate matter consists of coarse particles (10–2.5 μm in aerodynamic diameter), produced by construction work and farming, and fine particles (<2.5 μm) generated from burning fossil fuels. Fine particulates ($PM_{2.5}$) remain airborne for long periods and are carried into rural areas. Several respiratory and cardiac problems are exacerbated by these very small particles.

The World Health Organization (WHO) global air-quality guidelines suggest 24-hour values of <25 μg/m^3 for $PM_{2.5}$ for the short term and 10 μg/m^3 in the long term. In Europe, 70% of the particulates present in urban air result from the combustion of diesel fuel, providing a background concentration of 3–5 μg/m^3. The WHO

Box 5.4 Air pollutants and their health effects

Pollutant	Average concentration	Poor air quality	Susceptible individuals	Mechanisms of health effects
Sulphur dioxide (SO_2)	5–15 ppb	>125 ppb	Asthmatics	Bronchoconstriction through neurogenic mechanism
Ozone (O_3)	10–30 ppb	>90 ppb	All affected, particularly during exercise	Restrictive lung defect Airway inflammation Enhanced response to allergen
Nitrogen dioxide (NO_2)	25–40 ppb	>100 ppb	Allergic individuals	Airway inflammation Enhanced response to allergen
Particulate matter				
PM_{10}	25–30 μg/m³	>65 μg/m³	Elderly Allergic individuals	Airway and alveolar inflammation Enhanced selective production of the allergy antibody (IgE)
$PM_{2.5}$	3–5 μg/m³	>10 μg/m³	Those with cardiac and respiratory disease	Airway inflammation

ppb, parts per billion.

estimates that air pollution causes 800 000 premature deaths worldwide every year.

Deaths from respiratory and cardiovascular disease occur mainly in older populations; air pollution mainly causes bronchitis in children. Pollution from motor vehicles has been linked to increased hospital admissions, reduced lung function in children and younger adults, and an increase in lung cancer (polyaromatic hydrocarbons). Although it has been proposed that air pollution may cause asthma and other allergic diseases, there is no current evidence for this ***(Box 5.4)***. However, air pollution does adversely affect lung development in teenage children, while both NO_2 and ozone enhance the nasal and lung airway responses to inhaled allergen in people with established allergic disease.

Management

When air quality is poor, asthmatics are advised to avoid exercising outdoors and to increase their anti-inflammatory medication (i.e. inhaled corticosteroids). Short- and long-term measures are required to reduce air pollution, particularly diesel particulates (which are predicted to increase as more diesel engines are used). Such measures include increased motor engine efficiency, catalytic converters, diesel particulate traps and decreased reliance on cars and trucks.

Further reading

Editorial. Short-lived climate pollutants: a focus for hot air. *Lancet* 2015; 386:1707.

Beelen R, Raaschou-Nielsen O, Stafoggia M et al. Effects of long-term exposure to air pollution on natural-cause mortality: an analysis of 22 European cohorts within the multicentre ESCAPE project. *Lancet* 2014; 383:785–795.

IONIZING RADIATION

Ionizing radiation is either penetrating (X-rays, γ-rays or neutrons) or non-penetrating (α- or β-particles). Penetrating radiation affects the skin and deeper tissues, while non-penetrating radiation affects the skin alone. All radiation effects depend on the type of radiation, the distribution of dose and the dose rate.

Dosage is measured in ***joules per kilogram*** (J/kg): 1 J/kg = 1 gray (1 Gy) = 100 rads.

Radioactivity is measured in ***becquerels*** (Bq); 1 Bq is defined as the activity of a quantity of radioactive material in which one nucleus decays per second; 3.7×10^{10} Bq = 1 ***curie*** (Ci), the older, non-SI unit.

Box 5.5 Systemic radiation effects

Acute effects
- Haemopoietic syndrome
- Gastrointestinal syndrome
- CNS syndrome
- Radiation dermatitis

Delayed effects
- Infertility
- Teratogenesis
- Cataract
- Neoplasia:
  - Acute myeloid leukaemia
  - Thyroid
  - Salivary glands Skin
  - Others

Radiation differs in the density of ionization it causes. Therefore, a dose-equivalent called a ***sievert*** (Sv) is used. This is the absorbed dose weighted for the damaging effect of the radiation. The annual background radiation is approximately 2.5 mSv. A chest X-ray delivers 0.02 mSv, and CT of the abdomen/pelvis about 10 mSv (see Box 17.5). A cumulative risk of cancer following repeated imaging procedures has been established and X-ray exposures should be reduced if possible.

Excessive exposure to ionizing radiation follows accidents in industry, nuclear power plants and hospitals, and deliberate nuclear explosions designed to eliminate populations – and exceptionally, by poisoning, with polonium, for example.

Mild acute radiation sickness

Nausea, vomiting and malaise follow doses of approximately 1 Gy. Lymphopenia occurs within several days, followed 2–3 weeks later by a fall in all white cells and platelets.

Acute radiation sickness

Many systems are affected; the extent depends on the dose of radiation ***(Box 5.5)***

Haemopoietic syndrome

Absorption of 2–10 Gy is followed by transient vomiting in some individuals, followed by a period of improvement. Lymphocytes are particularly sensitive to radiation damage; severe lymphopenia develops over several days. A decrease in granulocytes and platelets follows 2–3 weeks later, since no new cells are formed in the

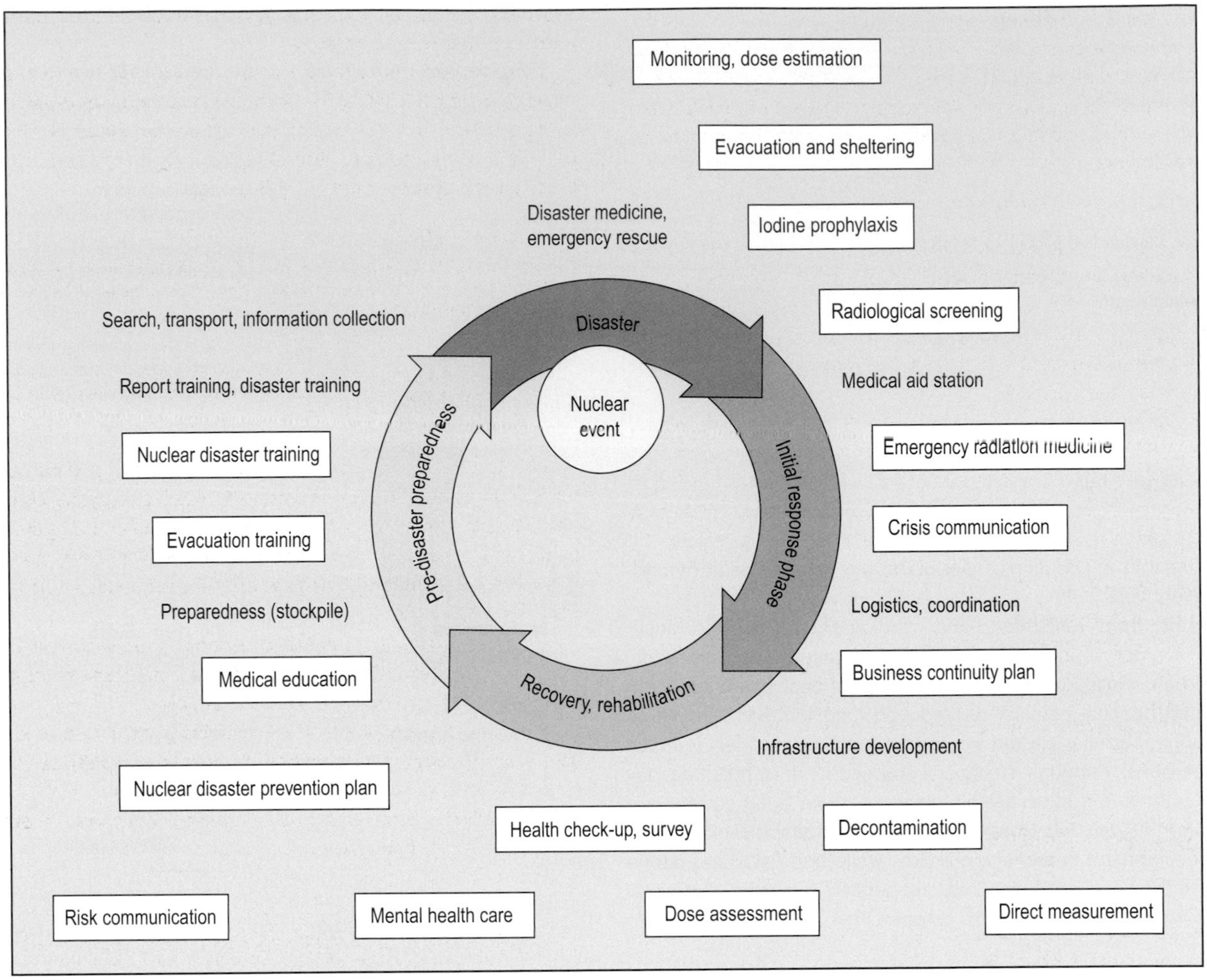

Figure 5.3 General disaster and nuclear disaster cycle. The measures shown in boxes refer to a programme specifically for a nuclear disaster. Those not in boxes are measures required for any large-scale disaster. *(From Ohtsuru A, Tanigawa K, Kumagai A et al. Nuclear disasters and health: lessons learned, challenges, and proposals. Lancet 2015; 386:489–499, with permission.)*

marrow. Thrombocytopenia develops with bleeding and frequent overwhelming infections; there is a high mortality.

Gastrointestinal syndrome

Doses >6 Gy cause vomiting several hours after exposure. This then stops, only to recur some 4 days later, accompanied by diarrhoea. The villous lining of the intestine becomes denuded. Intractable bloody diarrhoea follows, with dehydration, secondary infection and sometimes death.

CNS syndrome

Exposures of >30 Gy are followed rapidly by nausea, vomiting, disorientation and coma. Death due to cerebral oedema can follow, usually within 36 hours.

Radiation dermatitis

Skin erythema, purpura, blistering and secondary infection occur. Total loss of body hair is a bad prognostic sign and usually follows an exposure of >5 Gy.

Late effects of radiation exposure

Survivors of the nuclear bombing of Hiroshima and Nagasaki in 1945 provided data on long-term radiation effects. Risks of acute myeloid leukaemia and cancer, particularly of skin, thyroid and salivary glands, increase. Infertility, teratogenesis and cataract are also late sequelae, developing years after exposure.

Major nuclear power plant accidents

Two high-level nuclear accidents have occurred: the first in 1986 in Chernobyl in the Ukraine (part of the Soviet Union at the time), and the second in 2011 in Fukushima in Japan.

In Chernobyl, 30 people died in the first 3 months due to radiation and other factors. The majority of the people in the area received only a very low dose of radiation and only cancer of the thyroid has been found as a long-term consequence.

In the Fukushima disaster, which occurred following an earthquake that generated tsunamis along the east coast of Japan, radiation release was 10–30% of that released in Chernobyl. There were no immediate deaths due to radiation and the long-term effect of radiation is thought likely to be small.

The major problems caused by both disasters relate to psychological and social effects, as a result of the populations' evacuation and removal from their homes for years following the accidents, as well as a general concern about the effects of radiation on themselves and their children.

Figure 5.3 shows the measures needed in a nuclear disaster.

Therapeutic radiation

The sequelae of therapeutic radiation – early, early-delayed and late-delayed radiation effects – are discussed on page 604. Focusing techniques are used to target radiation towards the field being treated, so that radiosensitive structures, such as the ovaries, are protected by shielding.

Management

Acute radiation sickness is an emergency. Absorption of the initial radiation dose can be reduced by removing contaminated clothing.

Management is largely supportive: prevention and treatment of infection, haemorrhage and fluid loss. Harvesting of blood products is sometimes carried out.

Accidental ingestion of, or exposure to, bone-seeking radioisotopes (e.g. ^{90}strontium and ^{137}caesium) is treated with chelating agents, such as EDTA and massive doses of oral calcium. Radioiodine contamination should be treated immediately with potassium iodide to block radio-iodine absorption by the thyroid.

Further reading

Christodouleas JP, Forrest RD, Ainsley CG et al. Short-term and long-term health risks of nuclear-power-plant accidents. *N Engl J Med* 2011; 364:2334–2341.

Clancey G, Chhem R. Hiroshima, Nagasaki and Fukushima. *Lancet* 2015; 386:405–406.

Ohtsuru A, Tanigawa K et al. A nuclear shadow from Hiroshima and Nagasaki to Fukushima. *Lancet* 2015; 386:403.

ELECTRIC SHOCK

Electric shock can produce:

- ***Pain and psychological sequelae***. The common domestic electric shock is typically painful, but rarely fatal or followed by serious sequelae. Nevertheless, it is an unpleasant and intensely frightening experience. A brief, immediate jerking episode can occur, which is not an epileptic seizure. There is usually no lasting neurological, cardiac or skin damage.
- ***More serious effects***. These are distinctly rare following accidents in the home or in industry, but claims by survivors following industrial accidents are frequently made.
- ***Cardiac, neurological and muscle damage***. Ventricular fibrillation, muscular contraction and spinal cord damage *can* follow a major shock.
- ***Electrical burns***. These are commonly restricted to the skin. Muscle necrosis and spinal cord damage can also occur.
- ***Electrocution***. This means death following ventricular fibrillation, either accidentally, or deliberately as a method of execution. In the USA, at executions, an initial voltage of >2000 volts was applied for some 15 s in the electric chair, causing loss of consciousness and ventricular fibrillation, before the voltage was lowered. The T_{Core} during the execution process would sometimes reach >50°C, leading to severe damage to internal organs.

LIGHTNING STRIKE

Cloud-to-ground lightning originating in thunderstorms. Human tissues are directly damaged by the high-voltage DC current of >10 million volts that lasts only for a few milliseconds. The result is cardiac arrest due to asystole.

Fern-shaped burns are seen on the skin. The victim's clothes explode off the body and the person is pulseless, not breathing and in coma. The only chance of survival at this stage is bystander cardiopulmonary resuscitation. The mortality is high and those who survive are left with variable CNS damage.

Further reading

Davis C, Engeln A, Johnson E et al. Wilderness Medical Society practice guidelines for the prevention and treatment of lightning injuries. *Wilderness Environ Med* 2012; 23:260.

SMOKE

Smoke is air containing toxic and/or irritant gases and carbon particles, coated with organic acids, aldehydes and synthetic materials. Carbon monoxide, sulphur dioxide, sulphuric and hydrochloric acids, and other toxins may also be present. The highly toxic polyvinyl chloride is no longer used in household goods. Air pollution is discussed on page 56.

On smoke inhalation, patients become breathless and tachypnoeic immediately. Choking and stridor may require intubation. Pulmonary oedema and hypoxia can be fatal.

Breathing through a wet towel or clothing is the best emergency treatment. Remove the victim from the scene as rapidly as possible. Give oxygen and arrange ITU support.

Prevention. Smoke alarms, regularly checked, should be installed in every household.

NOISE

Sound ***intensity*** is expressed as the square of ***sound pressure***. The ***bel*** is the ratio equivalent to a 10-fold increase in sound intensity; a ***decibel*** (dB) is one-tenth of a bel. Sound is made up of a number of frequencies ranging from 30 Hz to 20 kHz, most being between 1 and 4 kHz. In practice, a scale known as ***A-weighted sound*** is used; sound levels are reported as dB(A). A hazardous sound source is defined as one with an overall sound pressure of >90 dB(A).

Repeated, prolonged exposure to loud noise, particularly between 2 and 6 kHz, causes first temporary and later permanent hearing loss, by physically destroying hair cells in the organ of Corti and, eventually, auditory neurones. Noise-induced hearing loss is a common occupational problem, not only in industry and the armed forces, but also in the home (drills and sanders), in sport (motor racing) and in entertainment (musicians, DJs and their audiences).

Serious noise-induced hearing loss is almost wholly preventable by personal protection (ear muffs, ear plugs). Little can be offered once hearing loss has become established.

Other effects of noise

Noise is intensely irritating, increasing or producing anxiety and anger. Excessive, repetitive noise is used in torture. Excess noise possibly affects child development and reading skills.

Further reading

Basner M, Babisch W, Davis A et al. Auditory and non-auditory effects of noise on health. *Lancet* 2014; 383:1325–1322.

BIOTERRORISM/BIOWARFARE

Interest in biological warfare and bioterrorism intensified during the 1991 Iraq war and later, following the destruction of the Twin Towers in New York in 2001. The potential of bacteria as weapons is illustrated by a suggestion that several kilograms of anthrax spores might kill as many people as a Hiroshima-sized nuclear weapon.

Potential pathogens

The US Centers for Disease Control and Prevention in Atlanta, Georgia, have developed a classification of potential biological agents ***(Box 5.6)***.

Smallpox

Smallpox is a highly infectious disease with a mortality of >30%. There is no proven therapy but there is an effective vaccine. Universal vaccination was stopped in the early 1970s; the vast majority of the world's population is now unprotected against the variola virus (see p. 251). The potential exists for a worldwide epidemic of smallpox, possibly initiated by a bioterrorist act.

Smallpox has an incubation period of around 12 days, allowing any initial source of infection to go undetected until the rash ***(Fig. 5.4)***, similar to that of chickenpox, develops on the second or third day of the illness. Infection is transmitted by the airborne route; the patient becomes infectious to others 12–24 hours before the rash appears, thus allowing a potential infected volunteer to pass infection to others before being recognized as suffering from smallpox.

Box 5.6 Critical biological agents

Category	Pathogens
A. Very infectious and/or readily disseminated organisms: high mortality with a major impact on public health	Smallpox, anthrax, botulism, plague, tularaemia, viruses
B. Moderately easy to disseminate organisms: moderate morbidity and mortality	Q fever, brucellosis, glanders, food-/water-borne pathogens, influenza
C. Emerging and possible genetically engineered pathogens	Viral haemorrhagic fevers, encephalitis viruses, drug-resistant tuberculosis

(Adapted from Khan AS, Morse S, Lillibridge S. Public health preparedness for biological terrorism in the USA. *Lancet* 2000; 356:1179–1182, with permission.)

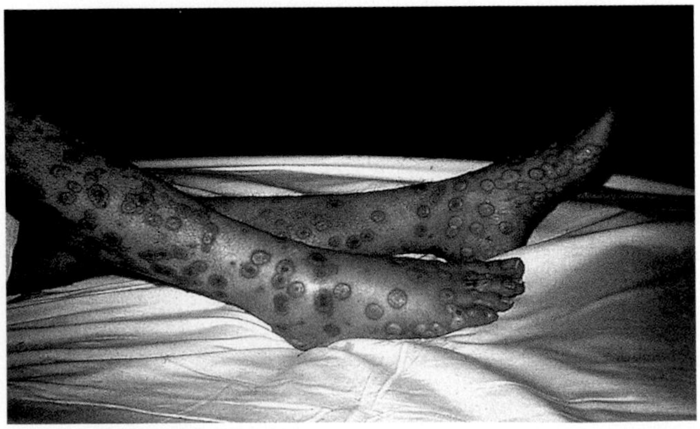

Figure 5.4 Smallpox rash.

If vaccines were to be administered widely to those potentially infected within 3 days of contact, an epidemic might well be prevented. Smallpox virus is stored in two secure laboratories: in Russia and in the USA. Supplies of vaccine are potentially available worldwide.

Anthrax

In late 2001, anthrax organisms (see p. 287) were sent through the US mail and infected 22 individuals. Of these, 11 developed pulmonary anthrax, 5 of whom died; 11 suffered from cutaneous anthrax.

A simulated anthrax attack postulated release of anthrax powder from a truck passing a sports stadium with 74 000 spectators; 16 000 were estimated to have become infected, with a death rate of 25%. In Russia, following accidental release of anthrax from a bioweapons factory, the death rate was substantial in those nearby, especially downwind.

Botulism

The toxin produced by *Clostridium botulinum* is one of the most potent poisons known (see p. 280).

As a bioweapon, botulinum toxin could be transmitted in food or by air: for example, from a crop-spraying light aircraft. The toxin is inactivated by chlorine in domestic water supplies. There is no vaccine available.

Plague

Plague (see p. 291) could potentially be used as a bioweapon either by airborne dissemination or by transmission by infected rats. Immunization is of limited value.

Other potential infective agents are listed in ***Box 5.6***.

Emergency planning

Many countries have plans to deal with bioterrorist attacks. These include training of healthcare staff and police. Such plans indicate the governments' awareness of the possibility of these threats. Stockpiling of vaccines, antibiotics and protective clothing is essential.

Further reading

Adaja AA, Toner A, Inglesby TV. Clinical management of potential bioterrorism-related conditions. *New Engl J Med* 2015; 372:954–962.

Berkelman RL, Hartley DM. Syndromic surveillance and bioterrorism-related epidemics. *Emerg Infect Dis* 2003; 10:1197–1204.

TRAVEL

Motion sickness

This common problem is caused by repetitive stimulation of the labyrinth. Motion sickness occurs frequently at sea and in cars (especially in children), but also with less usual forms of transport such as camels or elephants. Nowadays, motion sickness is rare during commercial flights, but it is a problem during space travel and on airships – one reason why the airship industry has not flourished.

Nausea, sweating, dizziness, vertigo and profuse vomiting occur, accompanied by an irresistible desire to stop moving. Prostration and intense incapacitating malaise can develop: for example, in seasickness.

Prophylactic antihistamines, vestibular sedatives (hyoscine or cinnarizine) and stem ginger are of some value.

Air travel

The incidence of deep venous thrombosis and pulmonary embolism is slightly greater in sedentary passengers on long-haul flights than in a similar population at sea level. Dehydration and alcohol probably contribute. Prophylactic aspirin is not recommended but moving the legs regularly and walking around the cabin every hour may be beneficial.

Commercial aircraft cabins are pressurized (see p. 54). Patients with respiratory disease, particularly chronic obstructive pulmonary disease, may well require oxygen therapy. They should seek advice from their airline.

All patients must be sure to take tablets and other therapy with them in the cabin in case they are required during the flight. Always consult the airline if there is any concern regarding health issues.

Inflight medical emergencies

Half of inflight emergencies are attended by doctors. The main problems are syncope, chest symptoms (cough and pain) and gastrointestinal symptoms. Most patients are managed successfully but approximately 25% require hospitalization on arrival at their destination.

Jet-lag

Jet-lag (circadian dyschronism) is the well-known phenomenon that follows travelling through time-zones, particularly from west to east. Intense insomnia, fatigue, poor concentration, irritability and loss of appetite are common. Headaches may occur. Symptoms last several days.

Mechanisms relate to the hypothalamic body clock within the suprachiasmatic nuclei. The clock is regulated by various *Zeitgebers* (time-givers), such as light and melatonin.

Management of jet lag includes its acceptance as a phenomenon causing poor performance – and thus waiting for 3–5 days to recover, drinking plenty of fluid and avoiding alcohol. Various hypnotics can help insomnia but their value is disputed. Oral melatonin is widely used to reduce jet-lag but is not available on prescription in the UK. Melatonin probably hastens resetting of the body clock.

Further reading

Peterson DC, Mortongill C, Guyetta FX et al. Outcomes of medical emergencies on commercial aircraft flights. *New Engl J Med* 2013; 368:2075–2083.
Sack R. Jet lag. *N Engl J Med* 2010; 362:440–447.
Silverman D, Gendeau M. Medical issues associated with commercial flights. *Lancet* 2009; 373:2067–2077.
Waterhouse J, Reilly T, Atkinson G. Jetlag: trends and coping strategies. *Lancet* 2007; 369:1117–1129.

BUILDING-RELATED ILLNESSES

Non-specific building-related illness

Multi-storey buildings typically have a controlled environment, often with automated heating and air-conditioning, and no ready access to external ventilation. More than half the adult workforce in developed countries works in such buildings.

Headache, fatigue and difficulty concentrating, sometimes in epidemics, are the main complaints but these have become less frequent. Psychological factors are thought to play a substantial role. Temperature, humidity, dust, volatile organic compounds, such as paints and solvents, and even low-level carbon monoxide toxicity have all been blamed, none with any scientific foundation.

Specific building-related illness

Legionnaires' disease (see p. 1105) can follow contamination of air-conditioning systems.

Humidifier fever (see p. 1117) is also due to contaminated systems, probably by fungi, bacteria and protozoa. Many common viruses are potentially transmissible in an enclosed environment, such as the common cold, influenza and, rarely, pulmonary tuberculosis. Allergic disorders, like rhinitis, asthma and dermatitis, also occur following exposure to indoor allergens such as dust mites and plants. Office equipment – for example, fumes from photocopiers – has also been implicated. Passive smoking (see p. 1075) is no longer an issue in Europe and North America, following legislation against smoking.

6 Poisoning

J Allister Vale, Sally M Bradberry

See your e-book for key learning points, clinical tips, drug tips, extra tables, learning challenges, MCQs and Special Topics from the International Advisory Board.

INTRODUCTION

In developed countries, poisoning is responsible for approximately 10% of acute hospital medical presentations and 1% of admissions. In such cases, poisoning is usually by self-administration of prescribed and over-the-counter medicines, or illicit drugs.

- ***Poisoning in children*** aged <6 months is most commonly iatrogenic, e.g. with paracetamol. Children between 8 months and 5 years of age may ingest poisons accidentally (due to inappropriate storage of drugs such as digoxin or quinine, and drugs of misuse purchased or prescribed for a parent or carer). Drugs may also be administered deliberately to cause harm (abuse by proxy).
- ***Self-poisoning in adults*** is commonly a 'cry for help'. Those involved are most often females <35 years in good physical health. They take an overdose in circumstances where they are likely to be found or in the presence of others. In the over-55s, there is a preponderance of men who are suffering from a depressive illness or are in poor physical health.
- ***Occupational poisoning*** due to dermal or inhalational exposure to chemicals is more common in the developing world.
- Poisoning may be ***iatrogenic***, e.g. digoxin toxicity.
- The ***type of agent*** taken in overdose is heavily influenced by availability and culture. In the UK, paracetamol poisoning is responsible for approximately one-third of all admissions, whereas in Sri Lanka, for example, the agents ingested are more often pesticides (e.g. organophosphorus insecticides) or plants (e.g. oleander), and in South India, copper sulphate is a problem. In addition, ingestion of heating fuels (e.g. petroleum distillates), antimalarials, antituberculous drugs and traditional medicine is reported frequently in the developing world. Poisoning from snake venoms is also a problem in rural areas.

A third of patients admitted with an overdose in the UK state that they are unaware of the toxic effects of the substance involved; the majority take whichever drug is easily available at home (***Box 6.1***, p. 66). Studies reveal that:

- Acute overdoses often involve more than one agent; alcohol is the most commonly implicated second agent.
- There is often a poor correlation between the drug history and the toxicological analytical findings. Therefore, a patient's statement about the type and amount of drug ingested cannot always be relied on.

The majority of patients do not require intensive medical management, as they ingest relatively non-toxic agents. All patients require a sympathetic and caring approach, with a psychiatric and social assessment. Fatalities in the UK are due predominantly to antidepressants, paracetamol, analgesic combinations containing paracetamol and an opioid, heroin, methadone or cocaine.

CLINICAL APPROACH TO THE POISONED PATIENT

History

More than 80% of adults are conscious on arrival at hospital and the diagnosis of self-poisoning can usually be made from the history (***Box 6.2***, p. 66). In any patient with an altered level of consciousness, acute poisoning must always be considered in the differential diagnosis.

Examination

On arrival at hospital, the patient must be assessed urgently (***Box 6.3***, p. 66). The 'cluster of features' on presentation may be distinctive and diagnostic. For example, sinus tachycardia, fixed dilated pupils, exaggerated tendon reflexes, extensor plantar responses and coma suggest tricyclic antidepressant poisoning (see ***Box 6.4***).

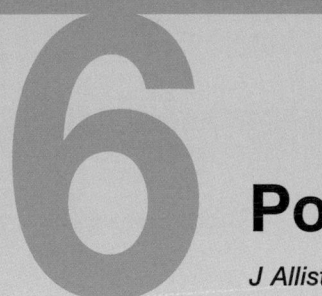

CLINICAL EXAMINATION

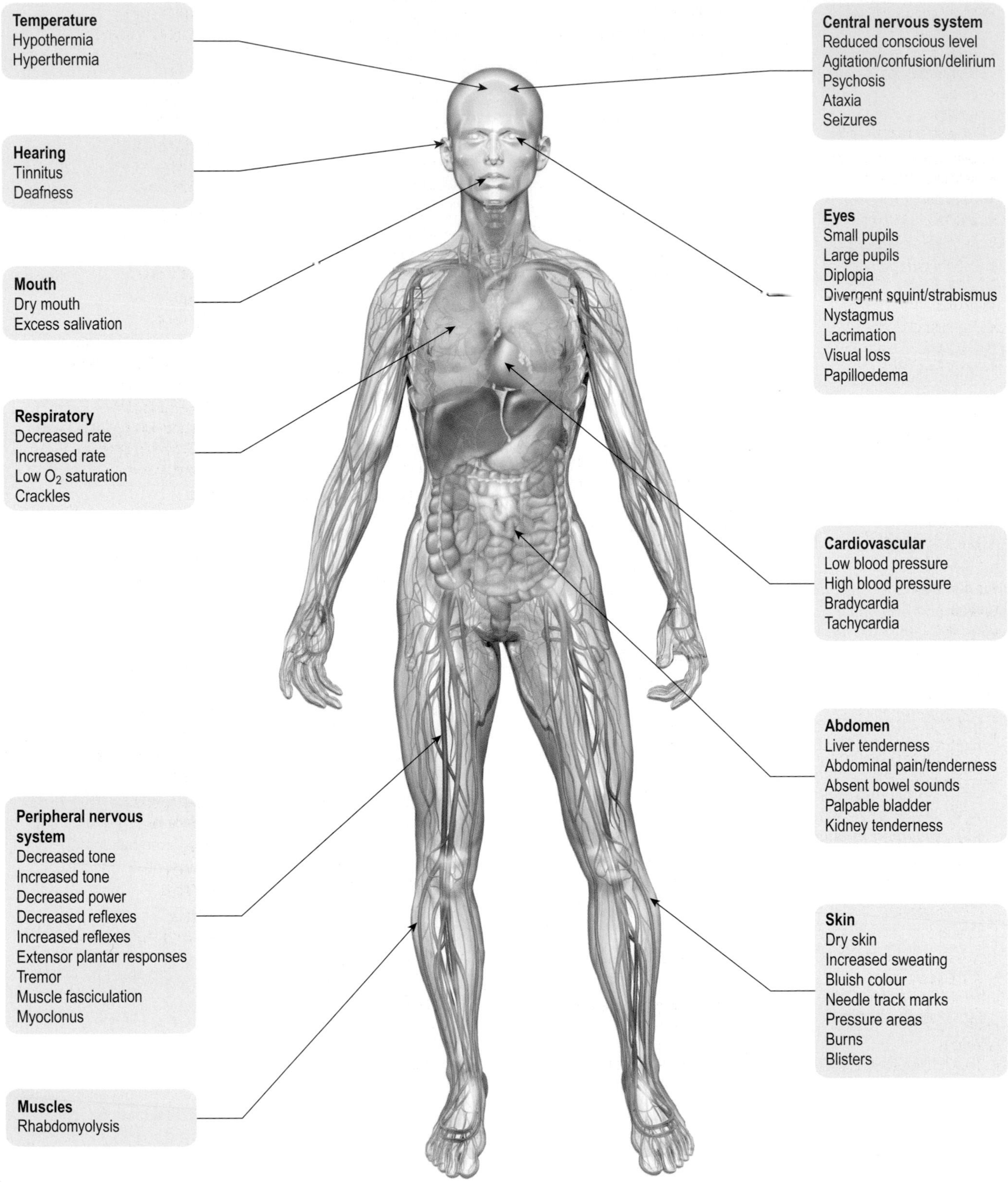
Temperature
Hypothermia
Hyperthermia
Hearing
Tinnitus
Deafness
Mouth
Dry mouth
Excess salivation
Respiratory
Decreased rate
Increased rate
Low O_2 saturation
Crackles
Peripheral nervous system
Decreased tone
Increased tone
Decreased power
Decreased reflexes
Increased reflexes
Extensor plantar responses
Tremor
Muscle fasciculation
Myoclonus
Muscles
Rhabdomyolysis
Central nervous system
Reduced conscious level
Agitation/confusion/delirium
Psychosis
Ataxia
Seizures
Eyes
Small pupils
Large pupils
Diplopia
Divergent squint/strabismus
Nystagmus
Lacrimation
Visual loss
Papilloedema
Cardiovascular
Low blood pressure
High blood pressure
Bradycardia
Tachycardia
Abdomen
Liver tenderness
Abdominal pain/tenderness
Absent bowel sounds
Palpable bladder
Kidney tenderness
Skin
Dry skin
Increased sweating
Bluish colour
Needle track marks
Pressure areas
Burns
Blisters

SOME POISON-SPECIFIC CLINICAL FEATURES

Central nervous system

Reduced conscious level
- Anticonvulsants
- Antimuscarinic drugs
- Benzodiazepines
- Ethanol
- Opiates
- Tricyclic antidepressants

Agitation/confusion/delirium
- Antimuscarinic drugs
- Cannabis
- Ethanol
- Novel psychoactive substances
- Other drugs of misuse

Psychosis
- Antimuscarinic drugs
- Cannabis
- Novel psychoactive substances

Ataxia
- Carbamazepine
- Ethanol
- Tricyclic antidepressants

Seizures
- Carbamazepine
- Mefenamic acid
- Tramadol

Peripheral nervous system

Decreased tone
- Benzodiazepines
- Ethanol

Increased tone
- Antimuscarinic drugs
- Antipsychotic drugs
- Tricyclic antidepressants

Decreased power
- Barium salts
- Nerve agents
- Organophosphorus insecticides

Decreased reflexes
- Benzodiazepines
- Ethanol

Increased reflexes
- Antipsychotic drugs
- Tricyclic antidepressants

Extensor plantar responses
- Tricyclic antidepressants

Tremor
- Lithium
- Mercury and mercury salts
- Nerve agents
- Organophosphorus insecticides

Muscle fasciculation
- Nerve agents
- Organophosphorus insecticides

Myoclonus
- Baclofen

Temperature

Hypothermia
- Central nervous system depressant drugs
- Environmental exposure

Hyperthermia
- Cocaine
- Ecstasy and other amfetamines
- Salicylates
- Selective serotonin reuptake inhibitors (SSRIs)

Muscles

Rhabdomyolysis
- Cocaine
- Drugs causing coma
- Drugs causing seizures
- Ecstasy

Respiratory system

Decreased respiratory rate
- Benzodiazepines
- Opioids

Increased respiratory rate
- Salicylates

Low O_2 saturations
- Benzodiazepines
- Opiates

Crackles
- Aspiration of gastric contents
- Non-cardiogenic pulmonary oedema (heroin, inhaled irritant chemicals)
- Pulmonary oedema (cardiotoxic drugs)

Cardiovascular system

Low blood pressure
- Beta-blockers
- Calcium-channel blockers
- Tricyclic antidepressants
- Antimalarials

High blood pressure
- Adrenoceptor agonists
- Cocaine
- Amfetamines

Bradycardia
- Beta-blockers
- Calcium-channel blockers
- Digoxin

Tachycardia
- Stimulant drugs
- Vasodilators

Abdomen

Liver tenderness
- Paracetamol

Abdominal pain/tenderness
- Antimuscarinic drugs
- Body stuffers
- Corrosives
- Non-steroidal anti-inflammatory drugs (NSAIDs)

Absent bowel sounds (ileus)
- Antimuscarinic drugs
- Colchicine

Palpable bladder
- Antimuscarinic drugs

Kidney tenderness
- Paracetamol

Eyes

Small pupils
- Nerve agents
- Opioids
- Organophosphorus insecticides

Large pupils
- Amfetamines and other stimulants
- Cocaine
- Tricyclic antidepressants
- Antimuscarinic drugs

Diplopia
- Tricyclic antidepressants

Divergent squint/strabismus
- Tricyclic antidepressants

Nystagmus
- Carbamazepine
- Ethanol
- Phenytoin

Lacrimation
- Nerve agents
- Organophosphorus insecticides

Visual loss
- Methanol
- Quinine

Papilloedema
- Carbon monoxide
- Methanol

Hearing

Tinnitus/deafness
- Quinine
- Salicylates

Mouth

Dry mouth
- Antimuscarinic drugs
- Tricyclic antidepressants
- Carbamazepine

Excess salivation
- Nerve agents
- Organophosphorus insecticides

Skin

Dry skin
- Antimuscarinic drugs

Increased sweating
- Nerve agents
- Organophosphorus insecticides
- Salicylates

Bluish colour
- Cyanosis (e.g. opiates)
- Methaemoglobinaemia (e.g. dapsone)

Needle track marks
- Heroin

Pressure areas
- Sedative drugs

Burns
- Acids
- Alkalis

Blisters
- Drugs causing coma

Box 6.1 Prevention of self-poisoning

Patients usually take what is readily available at home.
- Only small amounts of drugs should be sold
- Foil-wrapped drugs are less likely to be taken in overdose
- Drugs should always be kept in a safe place
- Drugs and liquids should be kept in their original containers
- Child-resistant drug containers should be used
- Care should be taken in prescribing all drugs
- Prescriptions for any susceptible patient (e.g. the depressed) must be monitored carefully
- Household products should be labelled and kept safely away from children

Box 6.2 History-taking in poisoning (record in notes)

- Obtain history (if possible) from patient, relatives, friends, paramedics, witnesses
- Seek evidence of overdose
- Establish whether suicide note was left
- Ascertain what drugs/poisons were taken
- Establish time/route taken
- Ask about additional drugs, e.g. alcohol
- Seek details from GP, e.g. prescribed medicines
- Assess suicide risk
- Assess capacity to make decisions
- Record a general history – past history, allergies, family history, social history

Box 6.3 Quick examination guide for the poisoned patient

1. A B C D E (see p. 826)
2. Level of consciousness (Glasgow Coma Scale; see p. 825)
3. Ventilation – pulse oximetry
4. Blood pressure and pulse rate
5. Pupil size and reaction to light
6. Temperature
7. Head injury complicating poisonings
8. If patient is unconscious, check cough and gag reflex

Some physical signs help to identify the poison – see ***Box 6.4***

Box 6.4 Common feature clusters in acute poisoning

Feature clusters	Poisons
Coma, hypertonia, hyper-reflexia, extensor plantar responses, myoclonus, strabismus, mydriasis, sinus tachycardia	Tricyclic antidepressants; less commonly, antihistamines, orphenadrine
Coma, hypotonia, hyporeflexia, plantar responses (flexor or non-elicitable), hypotension	Barbiturates, benzodiazepine and alcohol combinations, tricyclic antidepressants
Coma, miosis, reduced respiratory rate	Opioid analgesics
Nausea, vomiting, tinnitus, deafness, sweating, hyperventilation, vasodilatation, tachycardia	Salicylates
Hyperthermia, tachycardia, delirium, agitation, mydriasis	Ecstasy (MDMA) or other amfetamines, cathinones, cocaine
Miosis, hypersalivation, rhinorrhoea, bronchorrhoea	Organophosphorus and carbamate insecticides, nerve agents

Box 6.5 Management strategy in acute poisoning

Immediate decisions
- Supportive treatment
- Is an antidote appropriate? (see ***Box 6.6***)
- Is it appropriate to try to reduce poison absorption?
- Is it appropriate to perform toxicological investigations?
- Is it appropriate to try to enhance elimination?

Practical points – contact with poison

Eyes
- Remove contact lenses
- Wash eyes with 0.9% saline or water for about 15 min
- Assess corneal damage (if necessary) with slit lamp and fluorescein stain

Skin
- Remove clothing
- Wash thoroughly with soap and water if, e.g., chemical exposure

PRINCIPLES OF MANAGEMENT OF POISONING

Most people with self-poisoning require only general care and support of the vital systems (***Box 6.5***). However, for a few poisons, additional therapy is required.

Care of the unconscious patient

(See also pp. 826–829.) In all cases, the patient should be nursed in the lateral position with the lower leg straight and the upper leg flexed; in this position, the risk of aspiration is reduced. A clear passage for air should be ensured by the removal of any obstructing object, vomit or dentures, and by head tilt and chin lift or jaw thrust. Nursing care of the mouth and pressure areas should be instituted. Immediate catheterization of the bladder is usually unnecessary, as it can be emptied by gentle suprapubic pressure. Insertion of a venous cannula is usual, but administration of intravenous fluids is unnecessary unless the patient has been unconscious for more than 12 hours, is dehydrated or is hypotensive.

Ventilatory support

If respiratory depression is present, as determined by pulse oximetry or preferably by arterial blood gas analysis, an oropharyngeal airway should be inserted and supplemental oxygen should be administered. Pulse oximetry alone will not detect hypercapnia. Loss of the cough or gag reflex is the prime indication for intubation. The gag reflex can be assessed by positioning the patient on one side and making him or her gag using a suction tube. In many severely poisoned patients, the reflexes are depressed sufficiently to allow intubation without the use of sedatives or relaxants. The complications of endotracheal tubes are discussed on pages 1163–1164. If ventilation remains inadequate after intubation, as shown by hypoxaemia and hypercapnia, intermittent positive-pressure ventilation (IPPV) should be instituted.

Cardiovascular support

Although hypotension (systolic blood pressure <80 mmHg) is a recognized feature of acute poisoning, the classic features of shock – tachycardia and pale, cold skin – are observed only rarely.

Hypotension and shock may be caused by:

- ***a direct cardio-depressant action*** of the poison (e.g. beta-blockers, calcium-channel blockers, tricyclic antidepressants)

- ***vasodilatation and venous pooling*** in the lower limbs (e.g. angiotensin-converting enzyme (ACE) inhibitors, phenothiazines)
- ***a decrease in circulating blood volume*** because of gastrointestinal losses (e.g. profuse vomiting from salicylate poisoning), increased insensible losses (e.g. salicylate poisoning), increased renal losses (e.g. poisoning due to diuretics) and increased capillary permeability.

Hypotension may be exacerbated by coexisting hypoxia, acidosis and dysrhythmias. In people with marked hypotension, volume expansion with crystalloids should be used. Urine output (aiming for 35–50 mL/h) is a useful guide to the adequacy of the circulation. If a patient fails to respond to the above measures, more intensive therapy is required. In such individuals, it is helpful to initiate central venous pressure monitoring to confirm that adequate volume replacement has been administered. Volume replacement and the use of inotropes are discussed on page 1148. All patients with cardiogenic shock should have electrocardiographic (ECG) monitoring.

Systemic hypertension can be caused by a few drugs taken in overdose. If this is mild and associated with agitation, treatment with a benzodiazepine may suffice. In more severe cases – for example, severe cocaine or amfetamine poisoning – there may be a risk of arterial rupture, particularly intracranially. To prevent this, intravenous nitrates such as glyceryl trinitrate are given, starting at a dose of 1–2 mg/h, gradually increasing the dose to a maximum of 12 mg/h until blood pressure is controlled. Calcium antagonists, such as verapamil 240–480 mg daily in divided doses, are an alternative second-line therapy. Sodium nitroprusside 0.5–1.5 μg/kg/min (to a maximum of 8 μg/kg/min) is an option for patients with increased blood pressure when there is no evidence of cardiac ischaemia, but caution is required as it may cause a rapid fall in blood pressure.

Arrhythmias can occur, such as tachyarrhythmias following ingestion of a tricyclic antidepressant or theophylline, or brady-arrhythmias with digoxin poisoning. Known arrhythmogenic factors, such as hypoxia, acidosis and hypokalaemia, should be corrected.

Other problems

Hypothermia

A rectal temperature <35°C is a recognized complication of poisoning, especially in older patients or those who are comatose. The patient should be covered with a 'space blanket' and, if necessary, given intravenous and intragastric fluids at normal body temperature. The administration of heated (37°C), humidified oxygen delivered by face mask is also useful.

Hyperthermia

Body temperature can rarely increase to being potentially fatal after poisoning with central nervous stimulants such as cocaine and amfetamines, including ecstasy (MDMA). Muscle tone is often increased and convulsions and rhabdomyolysis are common. Cooling measures, sedation with diazepam and, in severe cases, dantrolene (a skeletal muscle relaxant) 1 mg/kg body weight i.v. should be given.

Skin blisters

Skin blisters may be found in poisoned patients who are, or have been, unconscious and do not move. Such lesions are not diagnostic of specific poisons but are sufficiently common in poisoned patients (and sufficiently uncommon in patients unconscious from other causes) to be of diagnostic value.

Rhabdomyolysis

Rhabdomyolysis can occur from pressure necrosis in drug-induced coma, or it may complicate poisoning in the absence of coma, such as in ecstasy (MDMA) abuse. People with rhabdomyolysis are at risk of developing, firstly, acute kidney injury from myoglobinaemia, particularly if they are hypovolaemic and have an acidosis; and, secondly, wrist or ankle drop from the development of a compartment syndrome (see p. 662).

Convulsions

These may occur in poisoning from many drugs, including tricyclic antidepressants, mefenamic acid and opioids. Usually seizures are short-lived but, if they are prolonged, diazepam 10–20 mg i.v. or lorazepam 4 mg i.v. should be administered. Persistent fits must be controlled rapidly to prevent severe hypoxia, brain damage and laryngeal trauma. If diazepam or lorazepam in repeated dose is ineffective, second-line treatments include intravenous phenytoin (loading dose 20 mg/kg at not more than 50 mg/min) or intravenous phenobarbital sodium (10 mg/kg at not more than 100 mg/min). Phenytoin is contraindicated in cases of poisoning with sodium channel-blocking drugs (such as tricyclic antidepressants) and is relatively contraindicated in all cases of poisoning with cardiotoxic drugs.

Stress ulceration and bleeding

Intravenous omeprazole or ranitidine should be given to prevent stress ulceration of the stomach in the elderly and patients with a previous history of ulceration.

Body 'packers' and body 'stuffers'

Body 'packers' (sometimes called 'mules' or 'swallowers') are those who swallow a substantial number of packages containing illicit drugs for the purpose of smuggling. Heroin used to be the drug of choice but this has been superseded by cocaine. Although each package contains a potentially lethal amount of drug, packets are now usually machine-manufactured using a material that does not leak. Body packers may ingest up to 100–200 packages.

Body 'stuffers' swallow a small number of packages containing an illicit drug, usually heroin, cocaine, cannabis or an amfetamine, in an unplanned attempt to conceal evidence when on the verge of being arrested. These drugs are usually either unpackaged or poorly packaged and, as a consequence, leakage may occur over the ensuing 3–6 hours and cause significant symptoms. Some also hide illicit drug packages in their rectum or vagina with the same intent (these are sometimes known as ***body 'pushers'***).

The ***role of imaging*** is usually confined to body packers; imaging has little role in the care of body stuffers or pushers. Ultrasound is of similar accuracy to abdominal X-ray in locating packages but is less accurate than computed tomography (CT). A urine screen for drugs of misuse should be performed. A screen that is positive for one or more drugs of misuse suggests that either the patient has used the drug in the previous few days, or at least one packet is leaking. A negative screen strongly suggests that no packet is leaking. Screens should be repeated daily, or immediately if the patient develops features of intoxication, to confirm the diagnosis.

Management. Packages can be removed most expeditiously in body stuffers by employing whole-bowel irrigation (see p. 68). In the past, early surgery was advocated in body packers. However, with the development of improved packaging, a more conservative approach using whole-bowel irrigation can now be adopted, with which there is a complication rate of <5%. Immediate surgery is indicated if acute intestinal obstruction develops, or when packets

Box 6.6 Antidotes of value in poisoning

Poison	Antidotes
Aluminium	Desferrioxamine
Arsenic	DMSA, dimercaprol
Benzodiazepines	Flumazenil
β-adrenoceptor-blocking drugs	Atropine, glucagon
Calcium-channel blockers	Atropine
Carbamate insecticides	Atropine
Carbon monoxide	Oxygen
Copper	D-penicillamine, Unithiol (DMPS)
Cyanide	Oxygen, dicobalt edetate, hydroxocobalamin, sodium nitrite, sodium thiosulphate
Diethylene glycol	Fomepizole, ethanol
Digoxin and digitoxin	Digoxin-specific antibody fragments
Ethylene glycol	Fomepizole, ethanol
Hydrogen sulphide	Oxygen
Iron salts	Desferrioxamine
Lead (inorganic)	Succimer (DMSA), sodium calcium edetate
Methaemoglobinaemia	Methylthioninium chloride (methylene blue)
Methanol	Fomepizole, ethanol
Mercury (inorganic)	Unithiol (DMPS)
Nerve agents	Atropine, HI-6, obidoxime, pralidoxime
Oleander	Digoxin-specific antibody fragments
Opioids	Naloxone
Organophosphorus insecticides	Atropine, HI-6, obidoxime, pralidoxime
Paracetamol	Acetylcysteine
Thallium	Berlin (Prussian) blue
Warfarin and similar anticoagulants	Phytomenadione (vitamin K)

DMPS, dimercaptopropanesulphonate; DMSA, dimercaptosuccinic acid.

can be seen radiologically and there is clinical or analytical evidence to suggest leakage, particularly if the drug involved is cocaine.

Packets in the vagina can usually be removed manually.

Specific management of the poisoned patient

Antidotes

Specific antidotes are available for a small number of poisons only ***(Box 6.6)***.

Antidotes may exert a beneficial effect by:

- ***forming an inert complex*** with the poison (e.g. desferrioxamine, D-penicillamine, dicobalt edetate, digoxin-specific antibody fragments, dimercaprol, HI-6, hydroxocobalamin, obidoxime, pralidoxime, protamine, Prussian (Berlin) blue, sodium calcium edetate, succimer (dimercaptosuccinic acid; DMSA), Unithiol (dimercaptopropanesulphonate; DMPS))
- ***accelerating detoxification*** of the poison (e.g. acetylcysteine, sodium thiosulphate)
- ***reducing the rate of conversion*** of the poison to a more toxic compound (e.g. ethanol, fomepizole)
- ***competing with the poison*** for essential receptor sites (e.g. oxygen, naloxone, phytomenadione)
- ***blocking essential receptors*** through which the toxic effects are mediated (e.g. atropine)
- ***bypassing the effect*** of the poison (e.g. oxygen, glucagon).

Gut decontamination

While it appears logical to assume that removal of unabsorbed drug from the gastrointestinal tract will be beneficial (gut decontamination), the efficacy of gastric lavage and syrup of ipecacuanha (to induce vomiting) remains unproven and efforts to remove small amounts of non-toxic drugs are clinically not worthwhile or appropriate.

Gastric lavage should only be performed if a patient has ingested a potentially life-threatening amount of a poison, e.g. iron, and the procedure can be undertaken within 60 minutes of ingestion. Intubation is required if airway protective reflexes are lost. Lavage is contraindicated if a hydrocarbon with high aspiration potential or a corrosive substance has been ingested.

Syrup of ipecacuanha to induce vomiting should *not* be used, as the amount of drug recovered is highly variable and diminishes with time; there is no evidence that it improves the outcome of poisoned patients.

Single-dose activated charcoal is able to adsorb a wide variety of compounds. Exceptions are strong acids and alkalis, ethanol, ethylene glycol, iron, lithium, mercury and methanol. In studies in volunteers given 50 g activated charcoal, the mean reduction in absorption was 40%, 16% and 21%, at 60 min, 120 min and 180 min, respectively, after ingestion. Based on these studies, activated charcoal should be given to those who have ingested a potentially toxic amount of a poison (known to be adsorbed by charcoal). There are insufficient data to support or exclude its use after 1 hour. There is no evidence that administration of activated charcoal improves clinical outcome.

Cathartics have no role in the management of the poisoned patient.

Whole-bowel irrigation requires the insertion of a nasogastric tube into the stomach and the introduction of polyethylene glycol electrolyte solution 1500–2000 mL/h in an adult, which is continued until the rectal effluent is clear. Whole-bowel irrigation may be used for potentially toxic ingestions of sustained-release or enteric-coated drugs, or to remove illicit drug packets.

Increasing poison elimination

***Multiple-dose activated charcoal* (MDAC)** involves the repeated administration of oral activated charcoal to increase elimination of a drug that has already been absorbed. Most absorbed drugs re-enter the gut from the villi capillaries by passive diffusion (a few by an active process) if the concentration in the gut is lower than that in the blood (this is called the entero-enteric circulation). Some drugs are also secreted in the bile (enterohepatic circulation). Activated charcoal will bind any drug that is in the gut lumen, so keeping the concentration in the gut low and favouring further diffusion from blood to gut lumen.

Elimination of drugs with a small volume of distribution (<1 L/kg), low p*K*a (which maximizes transport across membranes), low binding affinity and prolonged elimination half-life following overdose is particularly likely to be enhanced by MDAC. MDAC also improves total body clearance of the drug when endogenous processes are compromised by liver and/or renal failure.

Although MDAC has been shown to increase drug elimination significantly, it has not reduced morbidity and mortality in controlled studies. At present, MDAC should be used only in patients who have ingested a life-threatening amount of carbamazepine, dapsone, phenobarbital, quinine or theophylline.

In *adults*, charcoal should be administered in an initial ***dose*** of 50–100 g and then at a rate of not less than 12.5 g/h, preferably via a nasogastric tube; usually, 200 g is sufficient. If the patient has ingested a drug that induces protracted vomiting (e.g. theophylline), intravenous ondansetron 4–8 mg is an effective antiemetic and thus enables MDAC administration.

Urine alkalinization enhances elimination of salicylate, phenobarbital and chlorophenoxy herbicides (e.g. 2,4-dichlorophenoxyacetic acid) by mechanisms that are not clearly understood. Urine alkalinization is not recommended as first-line therapy for poisoning with phenobarbital, as MDAC is superior. A substantial diuresis is required in addition to urine alkalinization to achieve clinically relevant elimination of chlorophenoxy herbicides.

Urine alkalinization is a metabolically invasive procedure requiring frequent biochemical monitoring and medical and nursing expertise. Before urine alkalinization is commenced, plasma volume depletion, electrolytes (administration of sodium bicarbonate exacerbates pre-existing hypokalaemia) and metabolic abnormalities should be corrected. Sufficient bicarbonate is administered to ensure that the pH of the urine, which is measured by narrow-range indicator paper or a pH meter, is >7.5 and preferably close to 8.5. In one study, sodium bicarbonate 225 mmol was the mean amount required initially. This is most conveniently administered as 225 mL of an 8.4% solution (1 mmol bicarbonate/mL) i.v. over 1 hour.

Haemodialysis and haemodiafiltration are of little value in patients poisoned with drugs that have large volumes of distribution (e.g. tricyclic antidepressants) because the plasma contains only a small proportion of the total amount of drug in the body. These methods are indicated in patients with severe clinical features and high plasma concentrations of ethanol, ethylene glycol, isopropanol, lithium, methanol and salicylate: that is, drugs with small volumes of distribution.

Lipid emulsion therapy involves the intravenous administration of 20% Intralipid® (fractionated soya oil) 1.5 mL/kg, followed by 0.25–0.5 mL/kg/min for 30–60 min to an initial maximum of 500 mL. Use of lipid emulsion as an antidote for severe poisoning with highly lipid-soluble drugs is based on experience of its efficacy in local anaesthetic poisoning. It is believed to increase the intravascular lipid phase, so creating a 'lipid sink' to reduce the amount of active drug in plasma. Other proposed mechanisms of benefit include increasing myocardial fatty acid energy substrate and improving the function of cell membrane-bound ion channels (particularly Ca^{2+} and Na^{+}). The role of Intralipid® in the management of poisoning with highly lipid-soluble drugs is not well defined but case reports suggest some benefit in life-threatening cardiotoxicity that is resistant to other measures.

Investigations

Box 6.7 sets out investigations that may be helpful in poisoned patients. On admission, or at an appropriate time post overdose, a timed blood sample should be taken if it is suspected that aspirin, digoxin, ethylene glycol, iron, lithium, methanol paracetamol, paraquat, quinine or theophylline has been ingested ***(Box 6.8)***. The determination of the concentrations of these drugs will be valuable in management. Drug screens on blood and urine are occasionally indicated in severely poisoned patients in whom the cause of coma is unknown. A poison information service will advise.

Some routine investigations ***(Box 6.9)*** are of value in the differential diagnosis of coma or the detection of poison-induced hypokalaemia, hyperkalaemia, hypoglycaemia, hyperglycaemia, hepatic or renal failure or metabolic acidosis ***Box 6.10***. Measurement of carboxyhaemoglobin, methaemoglobin and cholinesterase activities are of assistance in the diagnosis and management of cases of poisoning due to carbon monoxide, methaemoglobin-inducing

i Box 6.7 Investigations that may be helpful in poisoned patients

- Urea, electrolytes, creatinine, estimated glomerular filtration rate
- Creatine kinase activity
- Acid–base assessment (arterial gas, unless no concern regarding ventilation; see p. 66)
- Blood for specific poisons (see p. 69)
- Electrocardiography (see p. 70)
- Urine saved (plain tube) for possible drug screen
- Radiology (see p. 70)

i Box 6.8 Laboratory analysis for toxins

- Carbon monoxide (carboxyhaemoglobin)
- Ethanol (when monitoring treatment in glycol and methanol poisoning
- Ethylene glycol
- Iron
- Lithium
- Methanol
- Paracetamol
- Salicylate
- Theophylline

i Box 6.9 Relevant non-toxicological investigations with examples

Investigation	Situation
Serum sodium	Hyponatraemia in Ecstasy (MDMA) poisoning
Serum potassium	Hypokalaemia in theophylline poisoning Hyperkalaemia in digoxin poisoning
Plasma creatinine concentration	Estimated glomerular filtration rate (eGFR) in acute kidney injury in ethylene and diethylene glycol poisoning
Acid–base disturbances	Including metabolic acidosis (see ***Box 6.10***)
Blood glucose concentration	Hypoglycaemia in insulin poisoning Hyperglycaemia in salicylate poisoning
Serum calcium concentration	Hypocalcaemia in ethylene glycol poisoning
Liver function (prothrombin time)	In paracetamol poisoning
Carboxyhaemoglobin concentration	In carbon monoxide poisoning
Methaemoglobinaemia	In nitrite poisoning
Cholinesterase activities	Organophosphorus insecticide and nerve agent poisoning
ECG	Wide QRS in tricyclic antidepressant poisoning (see p. 71)
X-ray	Including identification of complications

i Box 6.10 Some poisons that induce metabolic acidosis

- Carbon monoxide
- Cyanide
- Diethylene glycol
- Ethanol
- Ethylene glycol
- Iron
- Isoniazid
- Metformin
- Methanol
- Paracetamol
- Salicylates
- Tricyclic antidepressants

agents such as nitrites, and organophosphorus insecticides, respectively.

ECG

Routine ECG is of limited diagnostic value, but continuous ECG monitoring should be undertaken in those ingesting potentially cardiotoxic drugs; for example, sinus tachycardia with prolongation of the PR and QRS intervals in an unconscious patient suggests tricyclic antidepressant overdose. QT interval prolongation is an adverse effect of several drugs (e.g. quetiapine and quinine).

Radiology

Routine radiology is of little diagnostic value. It can confirm ingestion of metallic objects (e.g. coins, button batteries) or injection of globules of metallic mercury. Some enteric-coated or sustained-release drugs or ingested packets of illicit substances may be seen on plain abdominal X-rays. Radiology can confirm complications of poisoning, such as aspiration pneumonia, non-cardiogenic pulmonary oedema (salicylates) and acute respiratory distress syndrome (ARDS).

Further reading

Barceloux D, McGuigan M, Hartigan-Go K et al. Position paper: cathartics. *Clin Toxicol* 2004; 42:243–253.
Benson BE, Hoppu K, Troutman WG et al. Position paper update: gastric lavage for gastrointestinal decontamination. *Clin Toxicol* 2013; 51:140–146.
Thanacoody R, Bedry R, Caravati EM. Position paper update: ipecac syrup for gastrointestinal decontamination. *Clin Toxicol* 2013; 51:134–139.
Thanacoody R, Caravati EM, Troutman WG et al. Position paper update: whole bowel irrigation for gastrointestinal decontamination of overdose patients. *Clin Toxicol* 2015; 53:5–12.

SPECIFIC POISONS

Drugs and other chemicals

- *All patients must be reviewed by senior medical staff.*
- *All should have relevant blood tests and monitoring when appropriate.*
- The general principles of management of self-poisoning outlined above will always need to be applied.

In this section, only the specific treatment regimens are outlined. The physical signs of the effects of individual drugs are shown on p. 65.

Amfetamines, including Ecstasy (MDMA)

The medicinal product is the dextro-isomer, dexamfetamine. The *N*-methylated derivative, metamfetamine (the crystalline form of this salt is known as 'crystal meth' or 'ice'), and 3,4-methylenedioxymetamfetamine (MDMA), commonly known as Ecstasy, are misused worldwide.

Amfetamines are central nervous system (CNS) and cardiovascular stimulants. These effects are mediated by increasing synaptic concentrations of adrenaline (epinephrine) and dopamine.

Clinical features

Amfetamines cause euphoria, extrovert behaviour, a lack of desire to eat or sleep, tremor, dilated pupils, tachycardia and hypertension. More severe intoxication is associated with agitation, paranoid delusions, hallucinations and violent behaviour. Convulsions, rhabdomyolysis, hyperthermia and cardiac arrhythmias may develop in severe poisoning. Rarely, intracerebral and subarachnoid haemorrhage may occur and can be fatal.

Ecstasy poisoning is characterized by agitation, tachycardia, hypertension, widely dilated pupils, trismus and sweating. In more severe cases, hyperthermia, disseminated intravascular coagulation, rhabdomyolysis, acute kidney injury and hyponatraemia (secondary to inappropriate antidiuretic hormone secretion) predominate.

Management

Agitation is controlled by diazepam 10–20 mg i.v. or haloperidol 5 mg i.m. The peripheral sympathomimetic actions of amfetamines can be antagonized by β-adrenoceptor-blocking drugs. If hyperthermia is present, dantrolene 1 mg/kg body weight i.v. should be considered (see 'Hyperthermia' on p. 67).

Anticonvulsants

Clinical features

The clinical features of poisoning with anticonvulsant drugs are summarized in ***Box 6.11***.

Management

Elimination of carbamazepine can be significantly increased by multiple-dose activated charcoal.

Box 6.11 Clinical features of poisoning with anticonvulsant drugs

Anticonvulsant drug	Clinical features of poisoning
Carbamazepine and oxcarbazepine (a prodrug of carbamazepine)	Dry mouth, coma, convulsions, ataxia, incoordination, hallucinations (particularly in the recovery phase) Ocular: nystagmus, dilated pupils (common), divergent strabismus, complete external ophthalmoplegia (rare)
Phenytoin	Nausea, vomiting, headache, tremor, cerebellar ataxia, nystagmus, loss of consciousness (rare)
Sodium valproate	Most frequent: drowsiness, impairment of consciousness, respiratory depression Uncommon complications: liver damage, hyper-ammonaemia, metabolic acidosis Very severe poisoning: myoclonic jerks, seizures, cerebral oedema
Gabapentin and pregabalin	Lethargy, ataxia, slurred speech, gastrointestinal symptoms
Lamotrigine	Lethargy, coma, ataxia, nystagmus, seizures, cardiac conduction abnormalities
Levetiracetam	Lethargy, coma, respiratory depression
Tiagabine	Lethargy, facial grimacing, nystagmus, posturing, agitation, coma, hallucinations, seizures
Topiramate	Lethargy, ataxia, nystagmus, myoclonus, coma, seizures, metabolic acidosis (secondary to carbonic anhydrase inhibition)

If hepatotoxicity and encephalopathy develop in severe valproate poisoning, early intravenous supplementation with L-carnitine will reduce the formation of ammonia and other toxic metabolites of valproic acid. Haemodialysis increases the elimination of valproate and should be instituted if severe hyper-ammonaemia and electrolyte and acid–base disturbances occur.

Antidepressants: tricyclics and selective serotonin reuptake inhibitors

Tricyclic antidepressants block the reuptake of monoamines (e.g. norepinephrine (noradrenaline) and serotonin) into peripheral and intracerebral neurones, thereby increasing the concentration of these neurotransmitters in these areas (see ***Fig. 22.3***). They also have antimuscarinic actions and class 1 antiarrhythmic (quinidine-like) sodium-channel-blocking activity.

Selective serotonin reuptake inhibitors (SSRIs) (e.g. citalopram, escitalopram, fluoxetine, fluvoxamine, paroxetine and sertraline) lack the antimuscarinic and sodium-channel-blocking actions of tricyclic antidepressants.

Clinical features

Tricyclic antidepressants. Mild poisoning commonly causes drowsiness, sinus tachycardia, dry mouth, dilated pupils, urinary retention (all antimuscarinic effects), and increased reflexes and extensor plantar responses. Severe intoxication leads to coma, convulsions, and occasionally divergent strabismus. Plantar, oculocephalic and oculovestibular reflexes may be abolished temporarily. An ECG will often show a wide QRS interval and there is a reasonable correlation between the width of the QRS complex and the severity of poisoning. Life-threatening arrhythmias may ensue. Metabolic acidosis and cardiorespiratory depression are observed in severe cases.

SSRIs. Even in large overdoses, SSRIs appear to be relatively safe unless potentiated by ethanol. Most patients will show no signs of toxicity but drowsiness, nausea, diarrhoea and sinus tachycardia have been reported. Rarely, junctional bradycardia, seizures and hypertension have been encountered and influenza-like symptoms may develop.

The serotonin syndrome occasionally occurs (see p. 910).

Management

The majority of patients recover with supportive therapy alone (adequate oxygenation, control of convulsions and correction of acidosis), although a small percentage who ingest a tricyclic will require assisted ventilation for 24–48 hours. The onset of supraventricular tachycardia and ventricular tachycardia should be treated with sodium bicarbonate (8.4%) 50 mmol i.v. over 20 min, even if there is no acidosis present; a second bolus may be required.

Antidiabetic drugs

Insulin (if injected but not if ingested) and ***sulphonylureas*** cause hypoglycaemia. This is not seen with ***metformin***, since its mode of action is to increase glucose utilization, but lactic acidosis is a potentially serious complication of metformin poisoning.

Clinical features

Features of severe hypoglycaemia include drowsiness, coma, convulsions, depressed limb reflexes, extensor plantar responses and cerebral oedema. Hypokalaemia also occurs. Cranial (neurogenic) diabetes insipidus and persistent vegetative states are possible long-term complications if hypoglycaemia is prolonged.

Management

The blood or plasma glucose concentration should be measured urgently and intravenous glucose given, if necessary. Glucagon produces only a slight rise in blood glucose, although it can reduce the amount of glucose required (see p. 1258).

Severe insulin poisoning. A continuous infusion of 10–20% glucose (with K^+ 10–20 mmol/L) is required, together with carbohydrate-rich meals, though there may be difficulty in maintaining normoglycaemia.

Sulphonylurea poisoning. The administration of glucose increases already high circulating insulin concentrations. Octreotide (50 µg i.v.), which inhibits insulin release, should be given as well as glucose.

Antimalarials

Clinical features

Chloroquine. Hypotension is often the first clinical manifestation of chloroquine poisoning. It may progress to acute heart failure, pulmonary oedema and cardiac arrest. Agitation, acute psychosis, convulsions and coma may ensue. Hypokalaemia is common and is due to chloroquine-induced potassium-channel blockade. Bradyarrhythmias and tachyarrhythmias are common, and ECG conduction abnormalities are similar to those seen in quinine poisoning.

Quinine. Cinchonism (tinnitus, deafness, vertigo, nausea, headache and diarrhoea) is common. In more severe poisoning, convulsions, hypotension, pulmonary oedema and cardiorespiratory arrest are seen (due to ventricular arrhythmias that are often preceded by ECG conduction abnormalities, particularly QT prolongation). Quinine cardiotoxicity is due to sodium-channel blockade. Patients may also develop ocular features, including blindness, which can be permanent.

Primaquine. The main concern is primaquine's propensity to cause methaemoglobinaemia and haemolytic anaemia.

Management

Multiple-dose oral activated charcoal increases quinine and probably chloroquine clearance. Hypokalaemia should be corrected. Sodium bicarbonate 50–100 mmol i.v. is given if the ECG shows QRS prolongation but it will exacerbate hypokalaemia, which should be corrected first. Mechanical ventilation, the administration of an inotrope (see pp. 1158–1160) and high doses of diazepam (1 mg/kg as a loading dose and 0.25–0.4 mg/kg per hour maintenance) may reduce the mortality in severe chloroquine poisoning. Overdrive pacing may be required if torsades de pointes (see p. 975) occurs in quinine poisoning and does not respond to magnesium sulphate infusion (see p. 975). If clinically significant methaemoglobinaemia (generally above 30%) develops in primaquine poisoning, methylthioninium (methylene blue) 1–2 mg/kg body weight should be administered.

Arsenic

Arsenic poisoning worldwide is commonly caused by contamination of the ground water by inorganic arsenates, particularly in Asia. Occasionally, arsenic is found in Chinese and Indian traditional remedies.

Clinical features

Acute ingestion causes abdominal pain, vomiting and diarrhoea. Hypovolaemic shock and acute tubular necrosis occur in severe cases.

Chronic exposure to lower doses produces gastrointestinal effects, accompanied by skin changes (hyperkeratosis of palms and soles, 'raindrop' pattern of hyperpigmentation and alopecia), neurological features (headache, sensorimotor neuropathy), abnormal liver biochemistry (non-cirrhotic portal hypertension is recognized), peripheral vascular arteriosclerosis and haematological abnormalities (pancytopenia).

Management

The identification of, and removal from, the source of exposure to arsenic is vital. Chelation therapy with oral DMSA 30 mg/kg per day or DMPS 30 mg/kg per day i.v. may be indicated.

Benzodiazepines

Benzodiazepines are commonly taken in overdose but rarely produce severe poisoning, except in the elderly or those with chronic respiratory disease.

Clinical features

Benzodiazepines produce drowsiness, ataxia, dysarthria and nystagmus. Coma and respiratory depression develop in severe intoxication.

Management

If respiratory depression is present in patients who have severe benzodiazepine poisoning, flumazenil 0.5–1.0 mg i.v. is given in an adult and this dose often needs repeating. Flumazenil use often avoids the need for assisted ventilation. It is relatively contraindicated in patients with mixed proconvulsant (e.g. tricyclic antidepressants)/benzodiazepine poisoning and those with a history of epilepsy because it may cause convulsions.

Beta-adrenoceptor-blocking drugs

Clinical features

In mild poisoning, sinus bradycardia is the only feature, but if a substantial amount has been ingested, coma, convulsions and hypotension develop. Less commonly, delirium, hallucinations and cardiac arrest supervene. Bronchospasm and hypoglycaemia are rare complications.

Management

Glucagon 50–150 μg/kg (typically 5–10 mg in an adult), followed by an infusion of 5–10 mg/h, is the most effective agent. It acts by bypassing the blocked beta-receptor, thus activating adenyl cyclase and promoting formation of cyclic adenosine monophosphate (cAMP) from adenosine triphosphate (ATP); cAMP, in turn, exerts a direct beta-stimulant effect on the heart. Atropine 0.6–1.2 mg i.v. can be used to treat bradycardia but is usually less effective. High-dose insulin (initial intravenous bolus of 1.0 IU/kg, followed by 0.5–2.0 IU/kg/h) with hypertonic glucose to avoid hypoglycaemia, has been shown to improve myocardial contractility and systemic perfusion.

Calcium-channel blockers

Calcium-channel blockers all act by blocking voltage-gated calcium channels. Dihydropyridines (e.g. amlodipine, felodipine, nifedipine) are predominantly peripheral vasodilators, while verapamil (a phenylalkylamine) and diltiazem (a benzothiazepine) also have significant cardiac effects. Poisoning, particularly with verapamil and diltiazem, causes heart block and hypotension; in severe poisoning, there is a substantial fatality rate. When a sustained-release preparation has been ingested, the onset of severe features is delayed, sometimes for more than 12 hours. Overdose with even small amounts can have profound effects.

Clinical features

Hypotension occurs due to peripheral vasodilatation, myocardial depression and conduction block. The ECG may progress from sinus bradycardia through first, then higher, degrees of block, to asystole. Cardiac and non-cardiac pulmonary oedema may ensue in severely poisoned patients. Other features include nausea, vomiting, seizures and a lactic acidosis.

Management

Intravenous atropine 0.6–1.2 mg, repeated as required, should be given for bradycardia and heart block. The initial dose can be repeated every 3–5 min, but if there is no response in pulse rate or blood pressure after three such doses, it is unlikely that further boluses will be helpful. The response to atropine is sometimes improved following intravenous 10% calcium chloride, 5–10 mL (at 1–2 mL/min). If there is an initial response to calcium, a continuous infusion is warranted; this is given as 10% calcium chloride, 1–10 mL/h.

Cardiac pacing has a role if there is evidence of atrioventricular conduction delay but failure to capture occurs.

Treat hypotension initially with intravenous crystalloid. If significant hypotension persists despite volume replacement, administer glucagon, which activates myosin kinase independent of calcium. Give glucagon 5–10 mg (150 μg/kg) i.v. as a slow bolus and repeat, if necessary. If there is a favourable response in blood pressure, an infusion of 5–10 mg/h can be commenced.

Insulin–glucose euglycaemia has been shown to improve myocardial contractility and systemic perfusion, and should be considered in cases of resistant hypotension. Insulin is given as a bolus dose of 1 U/kg, followed by an infusion of 1–10 U/kg per hour with 10% glucose and frequent monitoring of blood glucose and potassium.

Cannabis (marijuana) and cannabinoids

Cannabis is usually smoked but may be ingested as a 'cake', made into a tea or injected intravenously. The major psychoactive constituent is δ-11-tetrahydrocannabinol (THC). THC possesses activity at the benzodiazepine, opioid and cannabinoid receptors.

A number of synthetic cannabinoids have been developed recently and are sold as herbal incense or 'spice'. Typically, these are considerably more potent than THC.

Clinical features

Initially, there is euphoria, followed by distorted and heightened images, colours and sounds, altered tactile sensations and sinus tachycardia. Visual and auditory hallucinations and acute psychosis are particularly likely to occur after substantial ingestion in naive cannabis users. Intravenous injection leads to watery diarrhoea, tachycardia, hypotension and arthralgia.

Heavy users suffer impairment of memory and attention, and poor academic performance. There is an increased risk of anxiety and depression. Regular users are at risk of dependence. Cannabis use results in an overall increase in the relative risk for later schizophrenia and psychotic episodes (see p. 924). Cannabis smoke is probably carcinogenic.

Management

Reassurance is usually the only treatment required, although sedation with intravenous diazepam 10–20 mg i.v. in an adult or haloperidol 2–5 mg i.m./oral in an adult is sometimes required. Hypotension requires intravenous fluids.

Carbamate insecticides

Carbamate insecticides inhibit acetylcholinesterase but the duration of this inhibition is comparatively short-lived in comparison with organophosphorus insecticides (see p. 79), since the carbamate–enzyme complex tends to dissociate spontaneously.

Clinical features

Although carbamate insecticide poisoning is generally less severe than organophosphorus insecticide poisoning, acute poisoning with a carbamate can be severe and fatal. Cholinergic symptoms usually develop within a few minutes. In the most severe cases, muscle twitching, profound weakness, profuse sweating, incontinence, mental confusion and progressive cardiac and respiratory failure ensue. In less severe cases, cholinergic symptoms are usually evident within 2 hours and typically resolve within 24 hours. Seizures are relatively uncommon, since carbamate penetration into the CNS is limited.

Management

Mild cases require no specific treatment other than the removal of soiled clothing. Atropine 2 mg i.v. should be given every 3–5 min if necessary to reduce increased secretions, rhinorrhoea and bronchorrhoea. If this measure fails, the patient should be intubated and mechanical ventilation instituted. Since carbamates have a shorter duration of action than organophosphorus insecticides, pralidoxime should be used only rarely in carbamate poisoning. If intoxication is life-threatening, give pralidoxime chloride 30 mg/kg body weight i.v. over 5–10 min, followed by an infusion of 8–10 mg/kg per hour.

Carbon monoxide

The most common source of carbon monoxide is an improperly maintained and poorly ventilated heating system. In addition, inhalation of methylene chloride (found in paint strippers) may also lead to carbon monoxide poisoning, as methylene chloride is metabolized *in vivo* to carbon monoxide. Carbon monoxide has a greater affinity for haemoglobin and forms carboxyhaemoglobin (COHb), thereby reducing the oxygen-carrying capacity. The affinity of the remaining haem groups for oxygen is increased. This shifts the oxyhaemoglobin dissociation curve to the left, impairing liberation of oxygen to the cells and leading to tissue hypoxia. In addition, carbon monoxide also inhibits cytochrome oxidase a_3.

Clinical features

Symptoms of mild to moderate exposure to carbon monoxide may be mistaken for a viral illness.

- A peak COHb concentration of <10% is not normally associated with symptoms
- A peak COHb concentration of 10–30% usually causes headache and mild exertional dyspnoea.
- Higher concentrations of COHb are associated with coma, convulsions and cardiorespiratory arrest. Metabolic acidosis, myocardial ischaemia, hypertonia, extensor plantar responses, retinal haemorrhages and papilloedema also occur.

Neuropsychiatric features may develop after apparent recovery from carbon monoxide exposure.

Management

In addition to removing the patient from carbon monoxide exposure, high-flow oxygen should be administered using a tightly fitting face mask (see p. 1166). Endotracheal intubation and mechanical ventilation are required in those who are unconscious. Several controlled studies of hyperbaric oxygen have been published but none has shown long-term clinical benefit.

Cathinones

Cathinone (khat) is a naturally occurring stimulant derived from the plant *Catha edulis*. The drug is released during prolonged chewing of plant leaves. An increasing number of synthetic cathinone derivatives are available, the best-known of which is mephedrone (4-methyl methcathinone). While typically sold as 'plant foods' or 'bath salts', these 'legal highs' are purchased for their recreational abuse potential. Synthetic cathinones may be taken by mouth, nasal insufflation or injection.

Clinical features

Cathinones can cause euphoria, extrovert behaviour, a lack of desire to eat or sleep, tremor, dilated pupils, tachycardia and hypertension. More severe intoxication is associated with marked agitation, paranoid delusions, and hallucinations. Convulsions, rhabdomyolysis, hyperthermia and cardiac arrhythmias may develop in severe poisoning.

Management

Agitation is controlled by diazepam 10–20 mg i.v. or haloperidol 5 mg i.m. The peripheral sympathomimetic actions can be antagonized by β-adrenoceptor-blocking drugs. If hyperthermia persists despite sedation and cooling measures, expert advice should be sought and dantrolene 1 mg/kg body weight i.v. should be given.

Cocaine

Cocaine hydrochloride ('street' cocaine, 'coke') is a water-soluble powder or granule that can be taken orally, intravenously or intranasally ('snorting'). 'Freebase' or 'crack' cocaine comprises crystals of relatively pure cocaine without the hydrochloride moiety and is obtained in rocks (150 mg of cocaine). It is more suitable for smoking in a pipe or mixed with tobacco; it can also be heated on foil and the vapour inhaled (approximately 35 mg of drug per 'line' or a 'rail'). The effects of cocaine are experienced almost immediately after intravenous administration or smoking, about 10 min following intranasal administration and 45–90 min after oral ingestion. The effects start to resolve in about 20 min but may last up to 90 min. In severe poisoning, death occurs in minutes but survival beyond 3 hours is not usually fatal.

Cocaine blocks the reuptake of biogenic amines:

- Inhibition of dopamine reuptake is responsible for the psychomotor agitation that commonly accompanies cocaine use.
- Blockade of noradrenaline (norepinephrine) reuptake produces tachycardia.
- Inhibition of serotonin reuptake induces hallucinations.
- CNS arousal is enhanced by potentiating the effects of excitatory amino acids.
- Cocaine is a powerful local anaesthetic and vasoconstrictor.

Clinical features

After initial euphoria, cocaine produces agitation, tachycardia, hypertension, sweating, hallucinations, convulsions, metabolic acidosis, hyperthermia, rhabdomyolysis and ventricular arrhythmias. Dissection of the aorta, myocarditis, myocardial infarction, dilated cardiomyopathy, subarachnoid haemorrhage, and cerebral haemorrhage or infarction may occur. If a young person presents with a stroke or myocardial infarction, cocaine poisoning, because of its vasoconstrictor effect, is a possible cause.

Management

- Diazepam 10–20 mg i.v. is used to control agitation and convulsions.
- Active external cooling should be employed for hyperthermia.
- Hypertension and tachycardia usually respond to sedation and cooling. If hypertension persists, give glyceryl trinitrate starting at 1–2 mg/h and gradually increase the dose (maximum 12 mg/h) until the blood pressure is controlled.
- Calcium-channel blockers, such as nifedipine, verapamil or diltiazem, are an alternative second-line therapy. The use of beta-blockers is controversial.
- Early use of a benzodiazepine is often effective in relieving cocaine-associated non-cardiac chest pain.
- Myocardial ischaemia/infarction should be treated conventionally.

Copper sulphate

Copper sulphate is used in fungicides, algicides, electroplating, dyes, inks, disinfectants and wood preservatives.

Clinical features

Ingestion causes vomiting, abdominal pain, diarrhoea, headache, dizziness and a metallic taste. Gastrointestinal haemorrhage, intravascular haemolysis, methaemoglobinaemia, rhabdomyolysis, coma, convulsions and hepatorenal failure may ensue and fatalities have occurred. Body secretions may be blue/green.

Management

Treatment is supportive with replenishment of lost fluids/blood. Blood copper concentrations correlate with the severity of poisoning; a copper concentration of >8 mg/L is indicative of severe poisoning. Early endoscopy (or CT scan with contrast if endoscopy is not possible) is recommended if corrosive damage is suspected. Methaemoglobinaemia of >30% should be treated with intravenous methylthionium chloride 2 mg/kg. Renal failure may require extracorporeal support.

Corrosive agents

Strong acids and alkalis cause chemical burns. Inorganic acids such as hydrochloric and sulphuric acid are generally more toxic than organic acids such as acetic acid. Hydrofluoric acid is considered separately (see p. 76). Some household products, such as water-sterilizing tablets, are strong alkalis. Following corrosive ingestion, the vital aspects of management are early (within 24 h) assessment of the severity of injury (ideally with endoscopy, or alternatively with CT imaging) and prompt surgical intervention to remove necrotic tissue, if indicated.

Cyanide

Cyanide and its derivatives are used widely in industry. Hydrogen cyanide is also released during the thermal decomposition of polyurethane foams, such as that in mattresses. Cyanide reversibly inhibits cytochrome oxidase a_3, so that cellular respiration ceases.

Clinical features

Inhalation of hydrogen cyanide produces symptoms within seconds and death within minutes. By contrast, the ingestion of a cyanide salt may not produce features for 1 hour. After exposure, initial symptoms are non-specific and include a feeling of constriction in the chest and dyspnoea. Coma, convulsions and metabolic acidosis may then supervene.

Management

Oxygen should be administered and, if it is available, dicobalt edetate 300 mg should be administered intravenously; the dose is repeated in severe cases. Dicobalt edetate (and the free cobalt contained in the preparation) complexes free cyanide. An alternative but expensive antidote is hydroxocobalamin 5 g i.v., which enhances endogenous cyanide detoxification; a second dose may be required in severe cases. If these two antidotes are not available, sodium thiosulphate 12.5 g i.v., which acts by enhancing endogenous detoxification, and sodium nitrite 300 mg i.v. should be administered. Sodium nitrite produces methaemoglobinaemia; methaemoglobin combines with cyanide to form cyanmethaemoglobin.

Digoxin

Toxicity occurring during chronic administration is common, though acute poisoning is infrequent. Oleander poisoning (see p. 84) produces similar features.

Clinical features

These include nausea, vomiting, dizziness, anorexia and drowsiness. Rarely, confusion, visual disturbances and hallucinations occur. Sinus bradycardia is often marked and may be followed by supraventricular arrhythmias with or without heart block, ventricular premature beats and ventricular tachycardia. Hyperkalaemia occurs due to inhibition of the sodium–potassium activated ATPase pump.

Management

- Atropine 1.2–2.4 mg i.v. is given to reduce sinus bradycardia, atrioventricular block and sinoatrial standstill.
- Digoxin-specific antibody fragments (digoxin-Fab) should be given intravenously for significant hyperkalaemia, marked arrhythmias (usually severe bradycardia compromising the cardiac output) and asystole. In both acute and chronic poisoning, only half the estimated dose required for full neutralization (calculated from amount of drug taken or serum digoxin concentration) need be given initially; a further dose is given if clinically indicated.

Ethanol

Ethanol is commonly ingested in beverages and deliberately with other substances in overdose. It is also present in many cosmetic and antiseptic preparations. Following absorption, ethanol is oxidized to acetaldehyde and then to acetate. Ethanol is a CNS depressant and the features of ethanol intoxication are generally related to blood concentrations ***(Box 6.12)***.

Clinical features

In children in particular, severe hypoglycaemia may accompany alcohol intoxication due to inhibition of gluconeogenesis. Hypoglycaemia is also observed in those who are malnourished or who have fasted in the previous 24 hours. In severe cases of intoxication, coma and hypothermia are often present, and lactic acidosis, ketoacidosis and acute kidney injury have been reported.

Management

As ethanol-induced hypoglycaemia is not responsive to glucagon, glucose 10–20% i.v. should be infused at a rate determined by the blood sugar. Haemodialysis should be considered if the blood ethanol concentration exceeds 7500 mg/L and if a severe metabolic acidosis (see p. 1150) is present, which has not been corrected by fluids and intravenous bicarbonate.

Ethylene and diethylene glycol

Ethylene and diethylene glycol are found in a variety of common household products, including antifreeze, windshield washer fluid, brake fluid and lubricants. The features observed in poisoning with these agents are due to metabolites predominantly, not the parent chemical. Ethylene glycol ***(Fig. 6.1)*** is metabolized to glycolate, the cause of the acidosis. A small proportion of glyoxylate is metabolized to oxalate. Calcium ions chelate oxalate to form insoluble calcium oxalate, which is responsible for renal toxicity. Diethylene glycol is metabolized to 2-hydroxyethoxyacetate ***(Fig. 6.2)***, which is the cause of metabolic acidosis, and diglycolic acid (the cause of kidney injury).

Clinical features

Initially, the features of ethylene glycol poisoning are similar to those of ethanol intoxication (though there is no ethanol on the breath). Coma and convulsions follow and a variety of neurological abnormalities, including nystagmus and ophthalmoplegias, are seen. Severe metabolic acidosis, hypocalcaemia and acute kidney injury are well-recognized complications.

In diethylene glycol poisoning, nausea and vomiting, headache, abdominal pain, coma, seizures, metabolic acidosis and acute kidney injury commonly occur. Pancreatitis and hepatitis, together with cranial neuropathies and demyelinating peripheral neuropathy, are also seen.

Box 6.12 Clinical features of ethanol poisoning

Blood (ethanol) mg/L	mmol/L	Clinical features
500–1500	11.0–32.5	Emotional lability Mild impairment of coordination
1500–3000	32.5–65.0	Visual impairment Incoordination Slowed reaction time Slurred speech
3000–5000	65.0–108.5	Marked incoordination Blurred or double vision Stupor Occasionally, hypoglycaemia, hypothermia and convulsions
>5000	>108.5	Depressed reflexes Respiratory depression Hypotension Hypothermia Death (from respiratory or circulatory failure, or from aspiration)

Management

If the patient presents early after ingestion, the priority is to inhibit metabolism using either intravenous fomepizole or ethanol; the former does not require monitoring of blood concentrations.

- ***Fomepizole*** 15 mg/kg body weight should be administered, followed by four 12-hourly doses of 10 mg/kg, then 15 mg/kg every 12 h until glycol concentrations are not detectable. Following a substantial ingestion, haemodialysis or haemodiafiltration should be employed to remove the glycol and metabolites. If dialysis is used, the frequency of fomepizole dosing should be increased to 4-hourly because fomepizole is dialysable.
- ***Ethanol*** Alternatively, a loading dose of ethanol 50 g can be administered, followed by an intravenous infusion of ethanol 10–12 g/h to produce blood ethanol concentrations of 500–1000 mg/L (11–22 mmol/L). The infusion is continued until the glycol is no longer detectable in the blood. If haemodialysis is employed, the rate of ethanol administration will need to be increased to 17–22 g/h, as ethanol is dialysable.

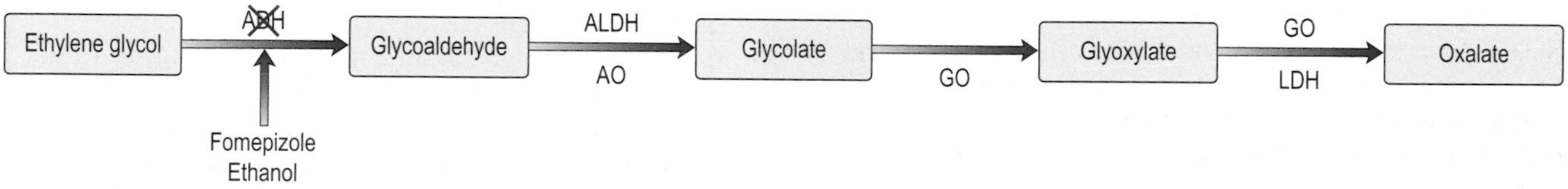

Figure 6.1 The metabolism of ethylene glycol. Fomepizole and ethanol inhibit ADH. ADH, alcohol dehydrogenase; ALDH, aldehyde dehydrogenase; AO, aldehyde oxidase; GO, glycolate oxidase; LDH, lactate dehydrogenase.

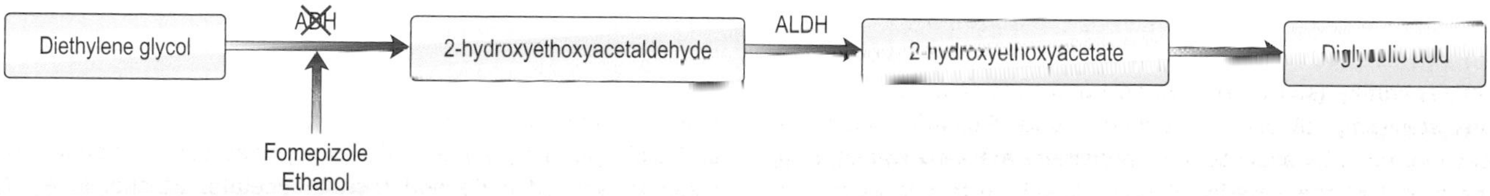

Figure 6.2 The metabolism of diethylene glycol. Fomepizole and ethanol inhibit ADH. ADH, alcohol dehydrogenase; ALDH, aldehyde dehydrogenase.

Supportive measures to combat shock, hypocalcaemia and metabolic acidosis should be instituted.

Gamma-hydroxybutyric acid

Gamma-hydroxybutyric acid (GHB) occurs naturally in mammalian brain, where it is derived metabolically from gamma-aminobutyric acid (GABA). GHB, as well as gamma-butyrolactone (another sedative agent with psychedelic effects), is a major recreational drug for body building, weight loss and production of a 'high'. Street names include 'cherry meth' and 'liquid X'. They are taken as a colourless liquid dissolved in water.

Clinical features

Poisoning is characterized by aggressive behaviour, ataxia, amnesia, vomiting, drowsiness, bradycardia, respiratory depression and apnoea, seizures and coma, which characteristically is short-lived.

Management

In a patient who is breathing spontaneously, the management of GHB poisoning is primarily supportive, with oxygen supplementation and the administration of atropine for persistent bradycardia, as necessary. Those who are severely poisoned will require mechanical ventilation, although recovery is usually complete within 6–8 hours.

Household products

The agents most commonly involved are bleach, cosmetics, toiletries, detergents, disinfectants, and petroleum distillates such as paraffin and white spirit. Ingestion of household products is usually accidental and is most common among children less than 5 years of age.

Clinical features

If ingestion is accidental, features very rarely occur, except in the case of petroleum distillates where aspiration is a recognized complication because of their low surface tension. Powder detergents, sterilizing tablets, denture cleaning tablets and industrial bleaches (which contain high concentrations of sodium hypochlorite) are corrosive to the mouth and pharynx if ingested. Nail polish and nail polish remover contain acetone, which may produce a coma if ingested in substantial quantities. Inhalation by small children of substantial quantities of talcum powder has occasionally given rise to severe pulmonary oedema and death.

Hydrofluoric acid and hydrogen fluoride

Hydrofluoric acid, a solution of hydrogen fluoride in water, is a colourless, fuming liquid that is widely used in industry. It is particularly dangerous because of its unique ability among acids to penetrate tissue.

Clinical features

Dermal exposure to hydrofluoric acid results in rapid liquefactive necrosis and erosion of bone. If more than 1% of the body surface area is contaminated with a 50% or higher solution of hydrofluoric acid, there is a high risk of hypocalcaemia from the formation of calcium fluoride. This may lead to cardiac conduction disturbances, notably QT interval prolongation and an increased risk of ventricular arrhythmias, particularly torsades de pointes (see p. 975).

Ingestion of hydrofluoric acid causes severe corrosive injury to the gastrointestinal tract.

Inhalation of hydrogen fluoride causes irritation of the eyes and nose, with sore throat, cough, chest tightness, headache, ataxia and confusion. Dyspnoea and stridor due to laryngeal oedema may follow, depending on the concentration of hydrogen fluoride. Haemorrhagic pulmonary oedema with increasing breathlessness, wheeze, hypoxia and cyanosis may take up to 36 hours to develop.

Management

- ***Dermal exposure***. Immediate irrigation of the skin with copious volumes of water is the priority, followed by the prompt application of calcium gluconate gel to reduce pain and limit skin damage.
- ***Ingestion***. This is a medical emergency with the need for immediate assessment for surgery after endoscopy or CT.
- ***Inhalation***. If the patient has clinical features of bronchospasm after inhalation, then treat conventionally with nebulized bronchodilators and steroids. Treat pulmonary oedema and/or ARDS (see pp. 1168–1169) with continuous positive airway pressure (CPAP), or in severe cases with intermittent positive pressure ventilation (IPPV).

Iron

Unless more than 60 mg of elemental iron per kg of body weight is ingested (a ferrous sulfate tablet contains 60 mg of iron), features are unlikely to develop. As a result, poisoning is seldom severe but deaths still occur. Iron salts have a direct corrosive effect on the upper gastrointestinal tract.

Clinical features

The initial features are characterized by nausea, vomiting (the vomit may be grey or black in colour), abdominal pain and diarrhoea. Severely poisoned patients develop haematemesis, hypotension, coma and shock at an early stage. Usually, however, most patients suffer only mild gastrointestinal symptoms. A small minority deteriorate 12–48 hours after ingestion and develop shock, metabolic acidosis, acute tubular necrosis and hepatocellular necrosis. Rarely, up to 6 weeks after ingestion, intestinal strictures occur due to corrosive damage. The serum iron concentration should be measured some 4 hours after ingestion; if the concentration exceeds the predicted normal iron-binding capacity (usually >5 mg/L; 90 μmol/L), free iron is circulating and treatment with desferrioxamine is required.

Management

The majority of patients ingesting iron do not require desferrioxamine therapy. If a patient develops coma or shock, desferrioxamine should be given without delay in a dose of 15 mg/kg per hour i.v. (the total amount of infusion usually not to exceed 80 mg/kg in 24 h). If the recommended rate of administration is continued for several days, adverse effects, including pulmonary oedema and ARDS (see pp. 1167–1169), have been reported.

Isopropanol

Isopropanol is found in aftershave lotions, disinfectants and window-cleaning solutions, and is used as a sterilizing agent and 'rubbing' alcohol. It is usually ingested, but inhalation and topical exposure have led to poisoning. Isopropanol is oxidized to acetone by hepatic alcohol dehydrogenase.

Clinical features

Coma, which may be prolonged, and respiratory depression are the major sequelae of substantial exposure. Other features following ingestion include haemorrhagic gastritis, haematemesis, acetone on the breath, hypotension, hypothermia, sinus tachycardia, frequent premature ventricular beats, renal tubular necrosis, acute myopathy and haemolytic anaemia. Ataxia, headache, dizziness, drowsiness, stupor, hallucinations, areflexia and muscle weakness may occur.

Hypoglycaemia or hyperglycaemia, haemolysis, ketonuria, renal tubular acidosis, hepatic dysfunction and rhabdomyolysis have been reported. Prolonged skin contact and inhalation may also result in systemic features.

Management

The mainstay of treatment is supportive care. In addition, since isopropanol has a small volume of distribution (0.6–0.7 L/kg) and is responsible together with its metabolite, acetone, for toxicity, there is a role for haemodialysis in the management of severely poisoned patients.

Lead

Exposure to lead occurs occupationally, children may eat lead-painted items in their homes (pica), and the use of lead-containing cosmetics or 'drugs' has also resulted in poisoning.

Clinical features

Mild intoxication may result in no more than lethargy and occasional abdominal discomfort, though abdominal pain, vomiting, constipation and encephalopathy (seizures, delirium, coma) may develop in more severe cases. Encephalopathy is more common in children than in adults but is rare in the developed world. Typically, though very rarely, lead poisoning results in foot drop attributable to peripheral motor neuropathy.

Anaemia (normally normochromic normocytic) occurs due both to inhibition by lead of several enzymes involved in haem synthesis, and to haemolysis. The latter results from damage to the red cell membrane by aggregates of RNA that accumulate owing to inhibition by lead of pyrimidine-5-nucleotidase, causing characteristic 'basophilic stippling' of erythrocytes.

Management

The social and occupational dimensions of lead poisoning must be recognized. Simply giving patients chelation therapy and then returning them to a contaminated environment is of no value.

The decision to use chelation therapy is based not only on the blood lead concentration but also on the presence of symptoms. Parenteral sodium calcium edetate 75 mg/kg per day or oral succimer (DMSA) 30 mg/kg per day is of similar efficacy. At least 5 days' treatment is usually required. As chelation of zinc may occur with sodium calcium edetate, serum zinc concentrations should be checked.

Lithium

Lithium toxicity is usually the result of therapeutic dosing (chronic toxicity) rather than deliberate self poisoning (acute toxicity). However, single large doses are occasionally ingested by individuals on long-term treatment with the drug (acute-on-therapeutic toxicity). The target therapeutic plasma lithium concentration range is narrow (0.8–1.2 mmol/L).

Clinical features

Features of intoxication include diarrhoea and vomiting, tremor, malaise, thirst, polyuria and, in more serious cases, impairment of consciousness, hypertonia and convulsions; irreversible neurological damage may occur. Measurement of the serum lithium concentration confirms the diagnosis. Acute massive overdose may produce concentrations of 5 mmol/L (34.7 mg/L) without causing toxic features, whereas chronic toxicity may be associated with neurological features at plasma concentrations as low as 1.5 mmol/L (6.9 mg/L).

Management

Since lithium is eliminated unchanged via the kidneys, diuresis with sodium chloride 0.9% is effective in increasing clearance. Haemodialysis is far superior and is used if neurological features are present and/or if renal function is impaired. It is employed particularly in cases of chronic toxicity.

Lysergic acid diethylamide

Clinical features

Lysergic acid diethylamide (LSD) is a potent synthetic hallucinogen. When ingested, usually on impregnated absorbent paper, effects appear within 30 minutes and last 8–12 hours. Visual disturbances are common and may be associated with life-threatening behaviour. Dilated pupils, tachycardia and hypertension are usually present. Psychosis may last several days and subsequent 'flashbacks' are common.

Management

Treatment is supportive, with reassurance and benzodiazepines if required. Antipsychotics are best avoided, as they may lower the seizure threshold.

Mercury

Mercury is the only metal that is liquid at room temperature. It exists in three oxidation states (elemental/metallic Hg^0, mercurous Hg_2^{2+} and mercuric Hg^{2+}) and can form inorganic (e.g. mercuric chloride) and organic (e.g. methylmercury) compounds. Metallic mercury is very volatile; when spilled, it has a large surface area so that high atmospheric concentrations may be produced in enclosed spaces, particularly when environmental temperatures are high. Thus, great care should be taken in clearing up a spillage. If ingested, metallic mercury will usually be eliminated per rectum, though small amounts may settle in the appendix and remain there for years. Mercury salts are well absorbed following ingestion, as is mercury vapour following inhalation.

Clinical features

Acute inhalation of mercury vapour causes headache, nausea, cough, chest pain and, occasionally, a chemical pneumonitis. Proteinuria and nephrotic syndrome are observed rarely.

Ingestion of inorganic or organic mercury compounds causes an irritant gastroenteritis. Mercurous (Hg_2^{2+}) compounds are less corrosive and less toxic than mercuric (Hg^{2+}) salts.

Systemic accumulation of mercury from any source and by any route of exposure leads to characteristic neurological features, including a fine tremor, lethargy, memory loss, insomnia, personality changes and ataxia. Peripheral nerve damage has also been observed, as has renal tubular damage.

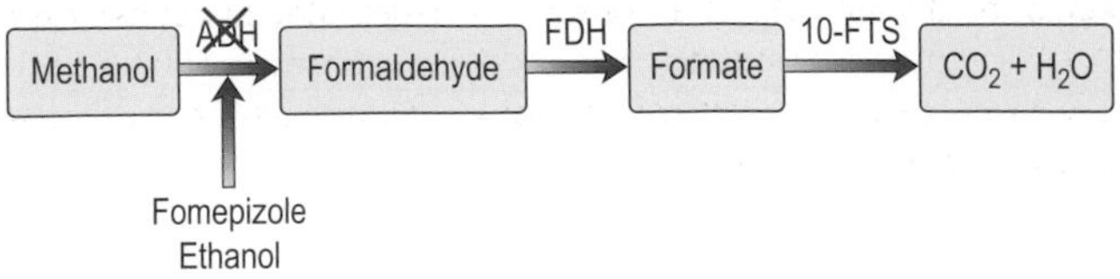

Figure 6.3 The metabolism of methanol. Fomepizole and ethanol inhibit ADH. ADH, alcohol dehydrogenase; FDH, formaldehyde dehydrogenase; 10-FTS, 10-formyl tetrahydrofolate synthetase.

Management

Unithiol (DMPS) is the antidote of choice and is given in a dose of 30 mg/kg i.v. per day. At least 5 days' treatment is usually required.

Methanol

Methanol is used widely as a solvent and is found in antifreeze solutions. Methanol is metabolized to formaldehyde and formate ***(Fig. 6.3)***. The concentration of formate increases greatly and is accompanied by accumulation of hydrogen ions, leading to metabolic acidosis.

Clinical features

Methanol causes inebriation and drowsiness. After a latent period, coma supervenes. Blurred vision and diminished visual acuity occur due to formate accumulation. The presence of dilated pupils that are unreactive to light suggests that permanent blindness is likely to ensue. A severe metabolic acidosis may develop and be accompanied by hyperglycaemia and a raised serum amylase activity. A blood methanol concentration of 500 mg/L (15.6 mmol/L) confirms severe poisoning. The mortality correlates well with the severity and duration of metabolic acidosis. Survivors may show permanent neurological sequelae, including parkinsonian-like signs as well as blindness.

Management

Treatment is similar to that of ethylene glycol poisoning (see pp. 75–76) with the addition of folinic acid 30 mg i.v. 6-hourly for 48 h, which accelerates formate metabolism, thereby reducing ocular toxicity.

Neuroleptics and atypical neuroleptics

Neuroleptic (antipsychotic) drugs are thought to act predominantly by blockade of dopamine D_2 receptors. The ***first-generation neuroleptics*** include the phenothiazines (chlorpromazine), the butyrophenones (benperidol, haloperidol) and the substituted benzamides (sulpiride). More ***selective second-generation (or 'atypical') antipsychotics*** include amisulpride, aripiprazole, clozapine, olanzapine, quetiapine and risperidone.

Clinical features

These include impaired consciousness, hypotension, respiratory depression, hypothermia or hyperthermia, antimuscarinic effects such as tachycardia, dry mouth and blurred vision, occasionally seizures, rhabdomyolysis, cardiac arrhythmias (both atrial and ventricular) and ARDS. Extrapyramidal effects, including acute dystonic reactions, occur but are not dose-related. Most 'atypical' antipsychotics have less profound sedative actions than the older neuroleptics. QT interval prolongation and subsequent ventricular arrhythmias (including torsades de pointes) have occurred following overdose with the atypical neuroleptics. Unpredictable fluctuations in conscious level, with variations between agitation and marked somnolence, have been particularly associated with olanzapine overdose.

Management

Procyclidine 5–10 mg i.v. in an adult is occasionally required for the treatment of dyskinesia and oculogyric crisis. After acidosis has been corrected with sodium bicarbonate, the preferred treatment for arrhythmias caused by antipsychotic drugs (usually torsades de pointes) is intravenous magnesium (see p. 1005) or cardiac pacing (p. 960).

Nerve agents

Nerve agents are related chemically to organophosphorus insecticides (see below) and have a similar mechanism of toxicity but a much higher mammalian acute toxicity, particularly via the dermal route. In addition to inhibition of acetylcholinesterase, a chemical reaction known as 'aging' also occurs rapidly and more completely than in the case of insecticides. This makes the enzyme resistant to spontaneous reactivation or treatment with oximes (pralidoxime, obidoxime or HI-6).

Two classes of nerve agent are recognized: G agents (named after Gerhard Schrader, who synthesized the first agents) and V agents (V allegedly standing for venomous). G agents include tabun, sarin, soman and cyclosarin. The V agents, e.g. VX, were introduced later. The G agents are both dermal and respiratory hazards, whereas the V agents, unless aerosolized, are contact poisons.

Agents used in bioterrorism are described on page 60.

Clinical features

Systemic features include increased salivation, rhinorrhoea, bronchorrhoea, miosis (which is characteristic) and eye pain, abdominal pain, nausea, vomiting and diarrhoea, involuntary micturition and defecation, muscle weakness and fasciculation, tremor, restlessness, ataxia and convulsions. Bradycardia, tachycardia and hypotension occur, depending on whether muscarinic or nicotinic effects predominate. Death occurs from respiratory failure within minutes but mild or moderately exposed individuals usually recover completely. Diagnosis is confirmed by measuring the erythrocyte cholinesterase activity.

Management

The administration of atropine 2 mg i.v., repeated every 3–5 min as necessary, to patients presenting with rhinorrhoea and bronchorrhoea may be life-saving. In addition, an oxime should be given to all those requiring atropine as soon as possible after exposure before 'aging' has occurred: for example, pralidoxime chloride 30 mg/kg i.v., followed by an infusion of pralidoxime chloride 8–10 mg/kg per hour. Alternatively, boluses of pralidoxime chloride 30 mg/kg may be given 4- to 6-hourly. Intravenous diazepam 10–20 mg, repeated as required, is useful in controlling apprehension, agitation, fasciculation and convulsions.

Non-steroidal anti-inflammatory drugs

Self-poisoning with non-steroidal anti-inflammatory drugs (NSAIDs) has increased, particularly now that ibuprofen is available without prescription, over the counter, in many countries.

Clinical features and management

In most cases, minor gastrointestinal disturbance is the only feature but, in more severe cases, coma, convulsions and acute kidney injury have occurred. Transient renal impairment is common after ibuprofen overdose. Poisoning with mefenamic acid commonly results in convulsions, though these are usually short-lived.

Treatment is symptomatic and supportive.

Opiates and opioids

Clinical features

Cardinal signs of opiate poisoning are pinpoint pupils, reduced respiratory rate and coma. Hypothermia, hypoglycaemia and convulsions are occasionally observed in severe cases. Non-cardiogenic pulmonary oedema has been reported in severe heroin overdose.

Management

Naloxone 1.2–2.0 mg i.v. will reverse severe respiratory depression and coma, at least partially. In severe poisoning, larger initial doses or repeat doses will be required. The duration of action of naloxone is often less than the drug taken in overdose: for example, methadone, which has a very long half-life. For this reason, an infusion of naloxone is often required. Non-cardiogenic pulmonary oedema should be treated with mechanical ventilation.

Organophosphorus insecticides

Organophosphorus (OP) insecticides are used widely throughout the world and are a common cause of poisoning, leading to thousands of deaths annually in the developing world. Intoxication may follow ingestion, inhalation or dermal absorption. OP insecticides inhibit acetylcholinesterase, causing accumulation of acetylcholine at central and peripheral cholinergic nerve endings, including neuromuscular junctions. Many OP insecticides require biotransformation before becoming active and so the features of intoxication may be delayed.

Clinical features

Poisoning is characterized by anxiety and restlessness, which is typically followed by nausea, vomiting, abdominal colic, diarrhoea (particularly if exposure is by ingestion), tenesmus, sweating, hypersalivation and chest tightness. Respiratory failure will ensue in severe cases and is exacerbated by the development of bronchorrhoea and pulmonary oedema. Miosis is characteristic. Muscle fasciculation and flaccid paresis of limb muscles, and, occasionally, paralysis of extraocular muscles are observed. Coma and convulsions occur in severe poisoning.

Diagnosis is confirmed by measuring the erythrocyte acetylcholinesterase activity; plasma cholinesterase activity is less specific but may also be depressed.

The ***intermediate syndrome*** usually becomes established 1–4 days after exposure, when the symptoms and signs of the acute cholinergic syndrome are no longer obvious. The characteristic features of the syndrome are weakness of the muscles of respiration (diaphragm, intercostal muscles and accessory muscles, including neck muscles) and of proximal limb muscles. Accompanying features often include weakness of muscles innervated by some cranial nerves.

Delayed polyneuropathy is a rare complication of acute exposure to some OP insecticides not marketed in most countries. It presents with glove and stocking paraesthesiae some 1–4 weeks after exposure, followed by an ascending motor polyneuropathy in many cases. It is initiated by phosphorylation, and subsequent aging, of at least 70% of an esterase – neuropathy target esterase (NTE) – in peripheral nerves. Most mild cases improve with time but severe cases can be left with an upper motor neurone syndrome and permanent disability.

Management

Mild cases require no specific treatment other than the removal of soiled clothing. Atropine 2 mg i.v. should be given every 3–5 min if necessary, to reduce increased secretions, rhinorrhoea and bronchorrhoea.

Symptomatic patients should also be given an oxime (pralidoxime, obidoxime) to reactivate inhibited acetylcholinesterase: for example, pralidoxime chloride 30 mg/kg by slow intravenous injection, followed by an infusion of pralidoxime chloride 8–10 mg/kg per hour. There is no specific treatment for the intermediate syndrome apart from supportive care, including prolonged ventilation, though a prospective trial suggested that early treatment with oximes could reduce the likelihood of the syndrome developing. Most patients recover in 2–3 weeks.

Paracetamol (acetaminophen)

In ***therapeutic doses***, paracetamol is conjugated with glucuronide and sulphate. A small amount of paracetamol is metabolized by mixed-function oxidase enzymes to form a highly reactive toxic compound (*N*-acetyl-*p*-benzoquinoneimine, NAPQI), which is then immediately conjugated with glutathione and subsequently excreted as cysteine and mercapturic conjugates.

In ***overdose***, large amounts of paracetamol are metabolized by oxidation because of saturation of the sulphate conjugation pathway. Liver glutathione stores become depleted so that the liver is unable to deactivate NAPQI. Paracetamol-induced kidney injury probably results from a mechanism similar to that responsible for hepatotoxicity.

Clinical features

Following the ingestion of an overdose of paracetamol, patients usually remain asymptomatic for the first 24 hours or, at the most, develop anorexia, nausea and vomiting. Liver damage is not usually detectable by routine liver function tests until at least 18 hours after ingestion of the drug. Liver damage usually reaches a peak, as assessed by measurement of alanine transferase (ALT) activity and prothrombin time (INR), at 72–96 hours after ingestion. Without treatment, a small percentage of patients will develop fulminant hepatic failure. Acute kidney injury due to acute tubular necrosis occurs in 25% of patients who have severe hepatic damage and in a few without evidence of serious disturbance of liver function.

Management

Acetylcysteine is an effective protective agent, provided that it is administered within 8–10 hours of ingestion of the overdose. It acts by replenishing cellular glutathione stores, though it may also repair oxidation damage caused by NAPQI. The treatment regimen is shown in ***Box 6.13***.

Box 6.13 Regimen for acetylcysteine

- Acetylcysteine 150 mg/kg in 200 mL 5% glucose over 60 min, then 50 mg/kg in 500 mL of 5% glucose over the next 4 h and then 100 mg/kg in 1000 mL of 5% glucose over the ensuing 16 h
- Total dose 300 mg/kg over 21 h

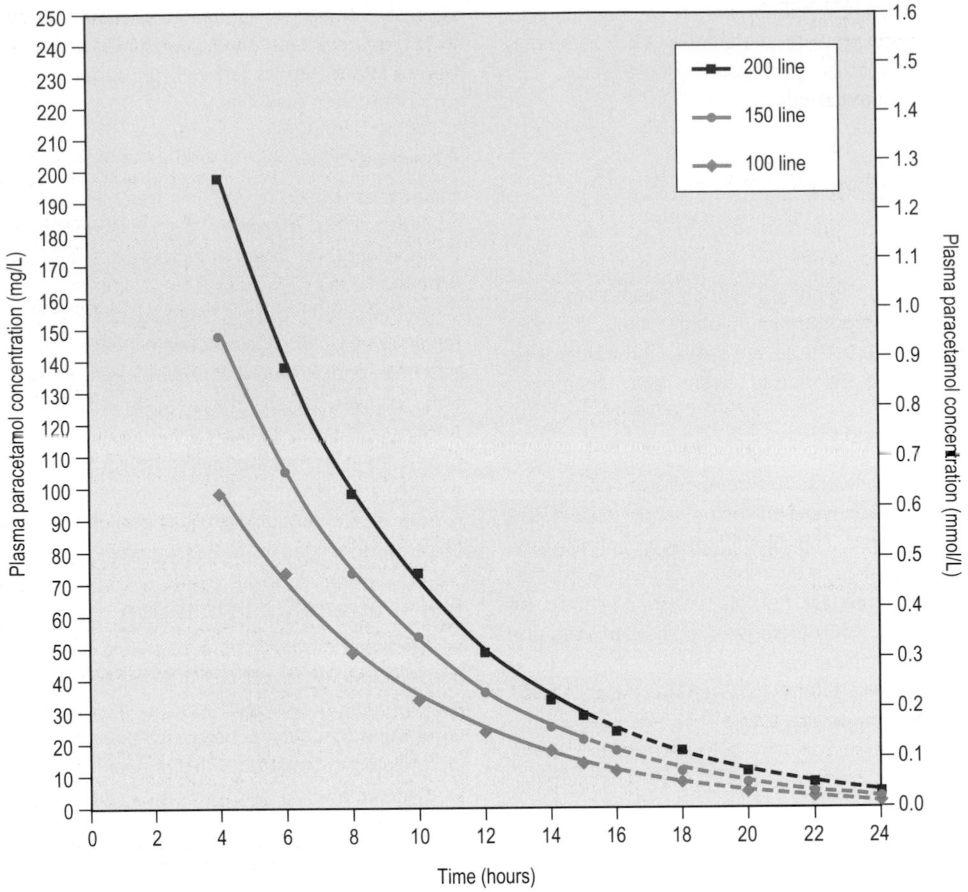

Figure 6.4 Nomogram for treatment of paracetamol poisoning. Note that the treatment lines are uncertain if the patient presents 15 hours or more after ingestion, or has taken a modified-release preparation of paracetamol. Although these lines are often extended to 24 hours (dotted lines), the concentrations are not based on clinical trial data.

There are now two main approaches to treatment worldwide. In the UK, following a decision by the Medicines and Healthcare products Regulatory Agency (MHRA) in 2012 to abandon a detailed risk assessment in the decision to treat, it is deemed that patients with concentrations above a 'treatment line' starting at 100 mg/L 4 hours after ingestion ***(Fig. 6.4)*** should be given treatment with acetylcysteine. In most other countries, a parallel line starting at 150 mg/L 4 hours after ingestion is used, though some still follow the original treatment line starting at 200 mg/L 4 hours after ingestion. The treatment lines ***(Fig. 6.4)*** are uncertain if the patient presents 15 hours or more after ingestion, or has taken a modified-release preparation of paracetamol. Although these lines are often extended to 24 hours (dotted lines), the concentrations are not based on clinical trial data.

Patients who ingest multiple overdoses or take repeated therapeutic excess are at greater risk of liver damage, and decisions to treat are generally based on the dose ingested. In the UK, treatment with acetylcysteine is given if more than 75 mg/kg has been ingested in 24 hours.

Up to 15% of patients treated with intravenous acetylcysteine develop a rash, angio-oedema, hypotension and bronchospasm. These reactions, which are related to the initial bolus, are seldom serious and discontinuing the infusion is usually all that is required. In more severe cases, chlorphenamine 10–20 mg i.v. in an adult should be given.

If liver or renal failure ensues, this should be treated conventionally, though there is evidence that a continuing infusion of acetylcysteine (continue 16-h infusion until recovery) will improve the morbidity and mortality. Liver transplantation has been performed successfully in patients who have paracetamol-induced acute hepatic failure (see p. 463).

Phosphides

Aluminium and zinc phosphides are used as rodenticides and insecticides. They react with moisture in the air (and the gastrointestinal tract) to produce phosphine, the active pesticide. Acute poisoning with these compounds may be direct, due to ingestion of the salts, or indirect, from accidental inhalation of phosphine generated during their approved use.

Clinical features

Ingestion causes vomiting, epigastric pain, peripheral circulatory failure, severe metabolic acidosis, acute kidney injury and disseminated intravascular coagulation, in addition to the features induced by phosphine.

Exposure to phosphine causes lacrimation, rhinorrhoea, cough, breathlessness, chest tightness, dizziness, diplopia, headache, nausea, drowsiness, intention tremor and ataxia. Acute pulmonary oedema, hypertension, cardiac arrhythmias, convulsions and jaundice have been described in severe cases.

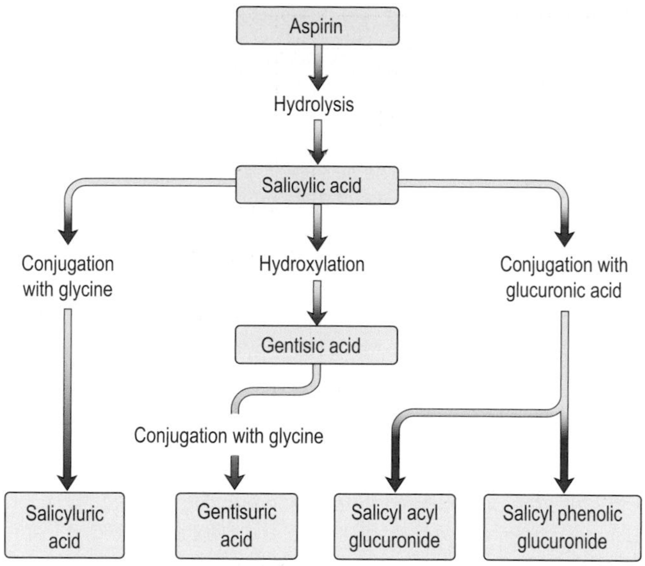

Figure 6.5 **The metabolism of aspirin.**

Management

Treatment is symptomatic and supportive. Gastric lavage should not be used, as it can speed up the rate of disintegration of the product ingested and increase toxicity. Activated charcoal may bind metal phosphides. The mortality is high, despite supportive care.

Salicylates

Aspirin is metabolized to salicylic acid (salicylate) by esterases present in many tissues, especially the liver, and subsequently to salicyluric acid and salicyl phenolic glucuronide ***(Fig. 6.5)***; these two pathways become saturated, with the consequence that the renal excretion of salicylic acid increases after overdose; this excretion pathway is extremely sensitive to changes in urinary pH.

Clinical features

Salicylates stimulate the respiratory centre, increase the depth and rate of respiration, and induce a respiratory alkalosis. Compensatory mechanisms, including renal excretion of bicarbonate and potassium, result in a metabolic acidosis. Salicylates also interfere with carbohydrate, fat and protein metabolism, and disrupt oxidative phosphorylation, producing increased concentrations of lactate, pyruvate and ketone bodies, all of which contribute to the acidosis.

Thus, tachypnoea, sweating, vomiting, epigastric pain, tinnitus and deafness develop. Respiratory alkalosis and metabolic acidosis supervene and a mixed acid–base disturbance is commonly observed. Rarely, in severe poisoning, non-cardiogenic pulmonary oedema, coma and convulsions ensue.

The severity of salicylate toxicity is dose-related.

Management

Fluid and electrolyte replacement is required and special attention should be paid to potassium supplementation. Severe metabolic acidosis requires at least partial correction, with the administration of sodium bicarbonate intravenously. Mild cases of salicylate poisoning are managed with parenteral fluid and electrolyte replacement only. Patients whose plasma salicylate concentrations are in excess of 500 mg/L (3.6 mmol/L) should receive urine alkalinization (see p. 69). Haemodialysis is the treatment of choice for severely poisoned patients (plasma salicylate concentration >700 mg/L; >5.1 mmol/L), particularly those with coma and metabolic acidosis.

Further reading

Barceloux DG, Bond GR, Krenzelok EP et al. American Academy of Clinical Toxicology practice guidelines on the treatment of methanol poisoning. *Clin Toxicol* 2002; 40:415–446.
Bodmer M, Liechti ME, Enzler F et al. Acute cocaine-related health problems in patients presenting to an urban emergency department in Switzerland: a case series. *BMC Res Notes* 2014; 7:173.
Bradberry S. Lithium. *Medicine* 2016; 44:180–181.
Bradberry S, Sheehan T, Vale A. Use of oral dimercaptosuccinic acid (succimer; DMSA) in adult patients with inorganic lead poisoning. *QJM* 2009; 102:721–732.
Bradberry SM, Thanacoody HK, Watt BE et al. Management of the cardiovascular complications of tricyclic antidepressant poisoning: role of sodium bicarbonate. *Toxicol Rev* 2005; 24:195–204.
Bradberry SM, Vale JA. Poisoning due to metals, and their salts: mercury and mercury salts. In: Bateman DN, Jefferson RD, Thomas SHL et al (eds). *Oxford Desk Reference: Toxicology*. Oxford: Oxford University Press; 2014; pp. 279–282.
Brent J. Fomepizole for ethylene glycol and methanol poisoning. *N Engl J Med* 2009; 360:2216–2223.
Buckley NA, Juurlink DN, Isbister G et al. Hyperbaric oxygen for carbon monoxide poisoning. *Cochrane Database of Syst Rev (Online)* 2011; 4:CD002041.
Chan BSH, Buckley NA. Digoxin-specific antibody fragments in the treatment of digoxin toxicity. *Clin Toxicol* 2014; 52:824–836.
Chiew AL, Buckley NA. Carbon monoxide poisoning in the 21st century. *Crit Care (London)* 2014; 18:221.
Dawson A, Buckley N. Digoxin. *Medicine* 2016; 44;158–159
Dear JW, Bateman DN. Iron. *Medicine* 2016; 44:173–174.
Dines AM, Wood DM, Galicia M et al and Euro-DEN Research Group. Presentations to the emergency department following cannabis use – a multi-centre case series from ten European countries. *J Med Toxicol* 2015; 11:415–421.
Engebretsen KM, Kaczmarek KM, Morgan J et al. High-dose insulin therapy in beta-blocker and calcium channel-blocker poisoning. *Clin Toxicol* 2011; 49:277–283.
Ghannoum M, Laliberté M, Nolin TD et al. Extracorporeal treatment for valproic acid poisoning: systematic review and recommendations from the EXTRIP workgroup. *Clin Toxicol* 2015; 53:454–465.
Glatstein M, Scolnik D, Bentur Y. Octreotide for the treatment of sulfonylurea poisoning. *Clin Toxicol* 2012; 50:795–804.
Hill SL, Thomas SHL. Drugs of abuse. *Medicine* 2016; 44:160–169.
Isbister GK, Bowe SJ, Dawson A et al. Relative toxicity of selective serotonin reuptake inhibitors (SSRIs) in overdose. *Clin Toxicol* 2004; 42:277–285.
Lheureux PE, Hantson P. Carnitine in the treatment of valproic acid-induced toxicity. *Clin Toxicol* 2009; 47:101–111.
Marrs TC, Rice P, Vale JA. The role of oximes in the treatment of nerve agent poisoning in civilian casualties. *Toxicol Rev* 2006; 25:297–323.
Proudfoot AT. Aluminium and zinc phosphide poisoning. *Clin Toxicol* 2009; 47:89–100.
Schep LJ, Slaughter RJ, Beasley DM. The clinical toxicology of metamfetamine. *Clin Toxicol* 2010; 48:675–694.
Schep LJ, Slaughter RJ, Temple WA et al. Diethylene glycol poisoning. *Clin Toxicol* 2009; 47:525–535.
Slaughter RJ, Mason RW, Beasley DMG et al. Isopropanol poisoning. *Clin Toxicol* 2014; 52:470–478.
St-Onge M, Dubé P-A, Gosselin S et al. Treatment for calcium channel blocker poisoning: a systematic review. *Clin Toxicol* 2014; 52:926–944.
Thanacoody HK, Thomas SH. Tricyclic antidepressant poisoning: cardiovascular toxicity. *Toxicol Rev* 2005; 24:205–214.
Thanacoody R. Quinine and chloroquine. *Medicine* 2016; 44:197–198.
Whyte I, Buckley N, Dawson A. Calcium channel blockers. *Medicine* 2016; 44:148–150.
Vale A. Alcohols and glycols. *Medicine* 2016; 44:128–132.
Vale A, Lotti M. Organophosphorus and carbamate insecticide poisoning. *Handb Clin Neurol* 2015; 131:149–168.

Marine animals

Amnesic shellfish (domoic acid) poisoning

The syndrome should be known more accurately as domoic acid poisoning because amnesia is not always present. In one outbreak, the first symptoms were experienced between 15 minutes and 38 hours after mussel consumption. There are now legal limits on the domoic acid concentrations allowed in mussels.

Clinical features and management

The most common symptoms are nausea, vomiting, abdominal cramps, headache, diarrhoea and short-term memory loss. Axonal sensory motor neuropathy, seizures, coma and death have also been reported. Treatment is symptomatic and supportive.

Diarrhoeic shellfish (okadaic) poisoning

Okadaic poisoning occurs worldwide, often after eating bivalve molluscs such as mussels and scallops. Okadaic acid is produced by dinoflagellates belonging to the genera *Dinophysis* spp. It inhibits the activity of the protein phosphatases 1 and 2a. As a result, increased phosphorylation of intestinal transport proteins, with increased permeability to solutes, leads to diarrhoea.

Clinical features and management

The predominant symptoms are diarrhoea, nausea, vomiting and abdominal pain. Symptoms tend to occur between 30 minutes and a few hours after shellfish consumption, with patients recovering within 2–3 days. Treatment is symptomatic and supportive.

Neurotoxic shellfish (brevetoxin) poisoning

Neurotoxic shellfish poisoning is caused by brevetoxins produced by the dinoflagellate *Gymnodinium breve*. Brevetoxins open voltage-gated sodium ion channels in cell walls and enhance the inward flow of sodium ions into the cell.

Clinical features and management

The symptoms of neurotoxic shellfish poisoning occur within 30 minutes to 3 hours and last a few days; they include nausea, vomiting, diarrhoea, chills, sweats, reversal of temperature sensation, hypotension, arrhythmias, numbness, tingling, paraesthesiae of the lips, face and extremities, cramps, bronchoconstriction, paralysis, seizures and coma. Treatment is symptomatic and supportive.

Paralytic shellfish (saxitoxin) poisoning

This is caused by bivalve molluscs being contaminated with neurotoxins, including saxitoxin, produced by toxic dinoflagellates on which the molluscs graze. Saxitoxin blocks voltage-gated sodium channels in nerve and muscle cell membranes, thereby blocking nerve signal transmission.

Clinical features and management

Symptoms develop within 30 minutes. The illness is characterized by paraesthesiae of the mouth, lips, face and extremities, and is often accompanied by nausea, vomiting and diarrhoea. In more severe cases, dystonia, dysphagia, muscle weakness, paralysis, ataxia and respiratory depression occur. In one outbreak involving 187 cases, there were 26 deaths. Treatment is symptomatic and supportive.

Ciguatera fish poisoning

Over 400 fish species have been reported as ciguatoxic (*cigua* is Spanish for poisonous snail), though barracuda, red snapper, amberjack and grouper are most commonly implicated. Ciguatera fish contain ciguatoxin, maitotoxin and scaritoxin, which are lipid-soluble, heat-stable compounds that are derived from dinoflagellates such as *Gambierdiscus toxicus*. Ciguatoxin opens voltage-sensitive sodium channels at the neuromuscular junction and maitotoxin opens calcium channels of the cell plasma membrane.

Clinical features and management

The onset of symptoms occurs from a few minutes to 30 hours after ingestion of toxic fish. Typically, features appear between 1 and 6 hours, and include abdominal cramps, nausea, vomiting and watery diarrhoea. In some cases, numbness and paraesthesiae of the lips, tongue and throat occur. Other features described include malaise, dry mouth, metallic taste, myalgia, arthralgia, blurred vision, photophobia and transient blindness. In more severe cases, hypotension, cranial nerve palsies and respiratory paralysis have been reported. Treatment is symptomatic and supportive. Recovery takes from 48 hours to 1 week in the mild form, and from 1 to several weeks in the severe form. The mortality in severe cases may be as high as 12%.

Scombroid fish poisoning

This is due to the action of bacteria such as *Proteus morgani* and *Klebsiella pneumoniae* in the decomposing flesh of fish such as tuna, mackerel, mahi-mahi, bonito and skipjack stored at insufficiently low temperatures. The spoiled fish can contain excessively high concentrations of histamine (muscle histidine is broken down by the bacteria to histamine), though the precise role of histamine in the pathogenesis of the clinical syndrome is uncertain.

Clinical features and management

Clinically, the mean incubation period is 30 minutes. The illness is characterized by flushing, headache, sweating, dizziness, burning of the mouth and throat, abdominal cramps, nausea, vomiting and diarrhoea; it is usually short-lived, the mean duration being 4 hours. Treatment is symptomatic and supportive. Antihistamines may alleviate the symptoms.

Stings from marine animals

Several species of fish have venomous spines in their fins. These include the weaver fish, short-spine cottus, spiny dogfish and stingray. Bathers and fishermen may be stung if they tread on or handle these species. The immediate result of a sting is intense local pain, swelling, bruising, blistering, necrosis and, if the poisoned spine is not removed, chronic sepsis (although this is uncommon). Occasionally, systemic symptoms, including vomiting, diarrhoea, hypotension and tachycardia, occur. Treatment by immersing the affected part in hot water may relieve local symptoms, as this denatures the thermolabile toxin.

Jellyfish stings

Most of the jellyfish found in North European coastal waters are non-toxic, as their stings cannot penetrate human skin. A notable exception is the 'Portuguese man-o'-war' (*Physalia physalis*), whose sting contains a toxic peptide, phospholipase A, and a histamine-liberating factor. Toxic jellyfish are found more frequently in Australia and some, notably the box jellyfish, *Carukia barnesi*, cause the Irukandji syndrome (see below).

Clinical features and management

Local pain occurs, followed by myalgia, nausea, griping abdominal pain, dyspnoea and even death. The cluster of severe systemic symptoms that constitute the Irukandji syndrome occur some 30 minutes after the jellyfish sting. The symptoms include severe low back pain, excruciating muscle cramps in all four limbs, abdomen and chest, sweating, anxiety, restlessness, nausea, vomiting, headache, palpitations, life-threatening hypertension and cardiogenic pulmonary oedema.

Adhesive tape may be used to remove any tentacles still adherent to the bather. Local application of 5% acetic acid is said to prevent stinging cells adherent to the skin discharging. Local analgesia and antihistamine creams provide symptomatic relief. Other features should be treated symptomatically and supportively.

Further reading

Clark RF, Girard RH, Rao D et al. Stingray envenomation: a retrospective review of clinical presentation and treatment in 119 cases. *J Emerg Med* 2007; 33:33–37.

Li L, McGee RG, Isbister G et al. Interventions for the symptoms and signs resulting from jellyfish stings. *Cochrane Database Syst Rev* 2013; 12:CD009688.

Venomous animals

Insect stings and bites

Insect stings from wasps and bees, and bites from ants produce pain and swelling at the puncture site. Following the sting or bite, patients should be observed for 2 hours for any signs of evolving urticaria, pruritus, bronchospasm or oropharyngeal oedema. The onset of anaphylaxis requires urgent treatment (see pp. 143–144).

Scorpions

Scorpion stings are a serious problem in North Africa, the Middle East and the Americas. Scorpion venoms stimulate the release of acetylcholine and catecholamines, causing both cholinergic and adrenergic symptoms.

Clinical features and management

Severe pain occurs immediately at the site of puncture, followed by swelling. Signs of systemic involvement, which may be delayed for 24 hours, include vomiting, sweating, piloerection, abdominal colic and diarrhoea. In some cases, depending on the species, cardiogenic shock, respiratory depression and pulmonary oedema may develop.

Local infiltration with anaesthetic or a ring block will usually alleviate local pain, though systemic analgesia may be required. Specific antivenom, if available, should be administered as soon as possible.

Spiders

The black widow spider (*Latrodectus mactans*) is found in North America, the tropics and, occasionally, in Mediterranean countries.

Clinical features and management

The bite quickly becomes painful, and generalized muscle pain, sweating, headache and shock may occur. No systemic treatment is required except in cases of severe systemic toxicity, when specific antivenom should be given, if this is available.

Venomous snakes

Approximately 15% of the 3000 species of snake found worldwide are considered to be dangerous to humans. Snake bite is common in some tropical countries; rural areas of West Africa, South-east Asia, the Indian subcontinent, New Guinea and the Amazon region are particularly affected. Bites by venomous snakes cause more than 100000 deaths and many permanent sequelae each year (some 46000 people are killed each year in India alone).

There are three main groups of venomous snakes, representing some 200 species, which have in their upper jaws a pair of enlarged teeth (fangs) that inject venom into the tissues of their victim. These are:

- *Viperidae* (with two subgroups: Viperinae – European adders and Russell's vipers; and Crotalinae – American rattlesnakes, moccasins, lance-headed vipers and Asian pit vipers)
- *Elapidae* (African and Asian cobras, Asian kraits, African mambas, American coral snakes, Australian and New Guinean venomous snakes, including the death adder – *Acanthophis antarcticus* – and sea snakes)
- *Hydrophiidae* (sea snakes).

In addition, some members of the family *Colubridae* are mildly venomous (mongoose snake).

Clinical features

The main effects of envenoming are:

- local swelling, bruising, blistering, regional lymph node enlargement and necrosis
- anti-haemostatic defects: consumption coagulopathy and spontaneous systemic bleeding from gums, nose, skin, gut, genitourinary tract and intracranial haemorrhage
- shock (hypotension) and myocardial damage
- descending paralysis: progressing from ptosis and external ophthalmoplegia to bulbar, respiratory muscle and total flaccid paralysis
- generalized rhabdomyolysis with myoglobinuria
- intravascular haemolysis
- acute kidney injury.

Viperidae (Viperinae and Crotalinae)

Russell's viper causes most of the snake-bite mortality in India, Pakistan and Myanmar. There is local swelling at the site of the bite ***(Fig. 6.6)***, which may become massive. Local tissue necrosis may occur. Evidence of systemic involvement (***envenomation***) occurs within 30 minutes, including vomiting, shock and hypotension. Haemorrhage due to incoagulable blood can be fatal. Envenomation by European adders (*Vipera berus*) is rarely fatal.

Elapidae

There is not usually any swelling at the site of the bite, except with Asian cobras and African spitting cobras; in these cases, the bite is painful and is followed by local tissue necrosis. Vomiting occurs first, followed by shock and then neurological symptoms and muscle weakness, with paralysis of the respiratory muscles in severe cases. Cardiac muscle can be involved.

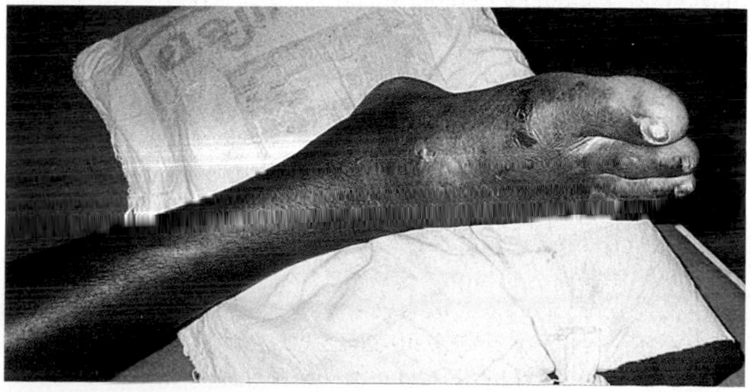

Figure 6.6 Snake bite showing swelling at the site.

Hydrophiidae

Envenomation produces muscle involvement, myalgia and myoglobinuria, which can lead to acute kidney injury. Cardiac and respiratory paralysis may occur.

Management

Following a snake bite, all efforts should be made to transport the patient quickly to a hospital or dispensary. Traditional methods should be discouraged, as they are often ineffective and may harm the patient. Arterial tourniquets should *not* be used, and incision or excision of the bite area should *not* be performed.

As a first aid measure, a firm pressure bandage should be placed over the bite and the limb immobilized, as this may delay the spread of the venom. Local wounds often require little treatment. If necrosis is present, antibiotics should be given. Skin grafting may be required later. Anti-tetanus prophylaxis must be given. The type of snake should be identified, if possible.

In about 50% of cases, no venom has been injected by the bite but, nevertheless, careful observation for 12–24 hours is necessary in case envenomation develops. General supportive measures should be carried out, as necessary. These include intravenous fluids with volume expanders for hypotension and diazepam for anxiety. Treatment of acute respiratory, cardiac and kidney injury is instituted as necessary.

Antivenoms are not generally indicated unless envenomation is present, as they can cause severe allergic reactions. Antivenoms can rapidly neutralize venom, but only if an amount in excess of the amount of venom is given. Large quantities of antivenom may be required; as antivenoms cannot reverse the effects of the venom, they must be given early to minimize some of the local effects and may prevent necrosis at the site of the bite. Antivenoms should be administered intravenously by slow infusion, the same dose being given to children and adults.

Allergic reactions are frequent, and adrenaline (epinephrine) 1 in 1000 solution should be available. In severe cases, the antivenom infusion should be continued even if an allergic reaction occurs, with subcutaneous injections of adrenaline being given as necessary. Some forms of neurotoxicity, such as those induced by the death adder, respond to anticholinesterase therapy with neostigmine and atropine.

Further reading

Warrell DA. Snake bite. *Lancet* 2010; 375:77–88.
Warrell DA. Venomous animals. *Medicine* 2016; 44:120–124.

Plants

Life-threatening poisoning from plant ingestion is rare, though many plants contain potentially toxic substances. These include antimuscarinic agents, calcium oxalate crystals, cardiogenic glycosides, pro-convulsants, cyanogenic compounds, mitotic inhibitors, nicotine-like alkaloids, alkylating agent precursors, sodium channel activators and toxic proteins (toxalbumins). While many plants contain gastrointestinal toxins, these rarely give rise to life-threatening sequelae. In contrast, other botanical poisons may cause specific organ damage, and death may occur from only small ingestions of yew (genus: *Taxus*), oleander (*Thevetia peruviana* and *Nerium oleander*) and cowbane (*Cicuta*).

Atropa belladonna

Atropa belladonna (deadly nightshade) contains hyoscyamine and atropine. It causes antimuscarinic effects – a dry mouth, nausea and vomiting – leading to blurred vision, hallucinations, confusion and hyperpyrexia.

Cicuta species

Cicuta spp. (water hemlock) and the related genus *Oenanthe* contain cicutoxin, a potent CNS stimulant that produces violent seizure activity. The CNS effects of cicutoxin are similar to those of picrotoxin, a known inhibitor of GABA. Severe gastrointestinal symptoms, diaphoresis, salivation and skeletal muscle stimulation may precede the seizure activity.

Conium maculatum

Conium maculatum (poison hemlock) contains a variety of volatile piperidine alkaloids, which have a toxic activity similar to that of nicotine. Large doses produce non-polarizing neuromuscular blockade, which may result in respiratory depression and death.

Datura stramonium

Datura stramonium (jimsonweed) and other *Datura* spp. contain L-hyoscyamine and atropine. These alkaloids are potent antagonists of acetylcholine at muscarinic receptors and produce the anticholinergic syndrome. While morbidity is significant, fatalities are rare and are the consequence of hyperthermia, seizures and/or arrhythmias.

Digitalis purpurea, *Nerium oleander*, *Thevetia peruviana* (yellow oleander)

Ingestion of *Digitalis purpurea* or the common (*Nerium oleander*) or yellow (*Thevetia peruviana*) oleander can produce a syndrome similar to digoxin poisoning (see p. 74). A randomized controlled trial has shown that digoxin-specific antibody fragments can rapidly and safely reverse yellow oleander-induced arrhythmias, restore sinus rhythm, and rapidly reverse bradycardia and hyperkalaemia. The administration of multiple doses of activated charcoal is used but the effect on survival is debated.

Further reading

Bradberry S, Vale A. Plants. *Medicine* 2016; 44:113–115.

Mushrooms

Poisoning due to mushrooms is usually accidental, though ingestion of hallucinogenic ('magic') mushrooms is invariably intentional.

Cytotoxic mushrooms

Cytotoxic mushroom poisoning is caused by amatoxins and orellanin. Amatoxins are found in *Amanita phalloides*, *A. virosa* and *A. verna*, and in some *Galerina* and *Lepiota* spp. Amatoxins inhibit transcription from DNA to mRNA by the blockade of nuclear RNA polymerase II; this results in impaired protein synthesis and cell death.

Clinical features and management

Intense watery diarrhoea starts 8–24 hours after ingestion and persists for 24 hours or longer. Patients often become severely dehydrated. Signs of liver damage appear during the second day and hepatic failure may ensue. Impaired kidney function is often seen both because of fluid loss and as a result of direct kidney injury. In all patients, fluid, electrolyte and acid–base disturbances should be corrected and renal and hepatic function supported. The value of silibinin and benzylpenicillin is not proven. Occasionally, liver transplantation is necessary.

Gyromitrin poisoning

Gyromitrin is found in *Gyromitra* spp., including in particular the false morel (*Gyromitra esculenta*) and *Cudonia circinans*. Gyromitrin decomposes in the stomach, to form hydrazines that inhibit pyridoxine kinase and thus produce functional pyridoxine deficiency. GABA deficiency ensues since pyridoxine is an essential co-factor in GABA synthesis. Seizures may result. Hydrazines also cause haemolysis, methaemoglobin formation and hepatorenal toxicity.

Clinical features and management

Vapours from the mushrooms are irritating to the eyes and respiratory tract. Gastrointestinal symptoms appear 5–8 hours after exposure. Vertigo, sweating, diplopia, headache, dysarthria, incoordination, ataxia and seizures may follow. Symptomatic and supportive care is required. Pyridoxine 25 mg/kg as an infusion over 30 min should be given if severe CNS toxicity develops; repeat doses may be required.

Hallucinogenic mushroom poisoning

Psilocybin produces pharmacological effects similar to those of LSD (see p. 77) and is found in *Psilocybe* and *Panaeolus* spp.

Clinical features and management

Symptoms occur within 20–60 min. Effects include altered time and space sense, depersonalization, hallucinations, derealization and euphoria. Symptoms are usually maximal within 2 hours and disappear within 4–6 hours, though ‘flashbacks’ may recur after weeks or months. Anxiety and agitation should be treated with diazepam, 10–20 mg i.v., repeated as necessary.

Isoxazole poisoning

Isoxazoles (e.g. ibotenic acid, muscimol, muscazone) occur in *Amanita muscaria* and *A. pantherina*, and act as GABA agonists.

Clinical features and management

Nausea, vomiting, inebriation, euphoria, confusion, anxiety, visual disturbances and hallucinations occur often within 30 minutes. Drowsiness is common and a coma-like state may ensue. Severe agitation and violent behaviour are seen occasionally. Other features include myoclonic jerks, muscle fasciculation, and seizures. Symptomatic and supportive care should be given as necessary. Diazepam 10–20 mg i.v., repeated as required, should be administered for anxiety, agitation and seizures.

Neurotoxic mushroom poisoning

Muscarine is found in, for example, *Inocybe* spp., *Clitocybe* spp. and *Mycena pura*. Muscarine stimulates cholinergic receptors in the autonomic nervous system.

Clinical features and management

Diarrhoea, abdominal pain, diaphoresis, salivation, lacrimation, miosis, bronchorrhoea, bronchospasm, bradycardia and hypotension occur. Atropine 0.6–2 mg i.v. should be given to manage the cholinergic syndrome.

Orellanin poisoning

Orellanin is a potent nephrotoxin found in, for example, *Cortinarius orellanus* and *C. speciosissimus*. A metabolite of orellanin inhibits protein synthesis in the kidneys.

Clinical features and management

Symptoms are typically delayed for 2–4 days. Some patients suffer a mild gastrointestinal disturbance before developing signs of renal impairment, headache, fatigue, intense thirst, chills, myalgia and abdominal, lumbar and flank pain. Transient polyuria with proteinuria, haematuria and, characteristically, leucocyturia is followed by oliguria and then anuria. Renal function may recover only partially; chronic kidney disease is reported in about 10–40% of cases. Management involves careful monitoring and haemodialysis/haemofiltration if renal failure supervenes. Renal transplantation may be required.

Significant websites

http://www.toxbase.co.uk *Toxbase – database of the UK National Poisons Information Service*
http://www.toxinz.com *Database of the New Zealand Poisons Centre*
http://www.toxnet.nlm.nih.gov *US National Library of Medicine's Toxnet*
http://www.who.int/gho/phe/chemical_safety/poisons_centres/en/ *Contact details of all poisons centres worldwide*
http://www.wikitox.org *Home of the Clinical Toxicology Teaching Resource Project*

7

Molecular cell biology and human genetics

David P Kelsell, Kenneth J Linton

See your e-book for key learning points, clinical tips, interactive Figures and MCQs.

CELL BIOLOGY

Cells consist of cytoplasm enclosed within a lipid sheath (the plasma membrane). The cytoplasm contains a variety of organelles (subcellular compartments enclosed within their own membranes) in a mixture of salts and organic compounds (the cytosol). These are held within an adaptive internal scaffold (the cytoskeleton) that radiates from the nucleus outwards to the cell surface ***(Fig. 7.1)***. Many cells have special functions and their size, shape and behaviour adapt to meet their physiological roles. Cells can be organized into tissues and organs in which the individual component cells are in contact and able to send and receive messages, both directly and indirectly. Coordinated cellular responses can be achieved through systemic signalling – for example, via steroid or protein signalling molecules (hormones or cytokines), or near-acting, short-lived cyclic lipids (eicosanoids).

CELL STRUCTURE

Cellular membranes

Lipid bilayers

Lipid bilayers separate the cell contents from the external environment and compartmentalize distinct cellular activities into organelles. The membranes comprise a large variety of glycerophospholipids and sphingolipids, which usually have two hydrophobic acyl chains, linked via glycerol or serine to polar hydrophilic head groups ***(Fig. 7.2)***. Their cylindrical shape and their amphiphilic nature, with a 'water-loving' head and a 'water-hating' tail, mean that, in aqueous solution, membrane lipids self-associate into a tail-to-tail bilayer, with their hydrophobic chains separated from the aqueous phase by their polar head groups.

Plasma membrane and organelle lipids

Plasma membrane and organelle (except that surrounding the endoplasmic reticulum) lipids are organized asymmetrically in the bilayer, with the outer leaflet of the plasma membrane enriched in phosphatidylcholine (PC) and sphingolipids, whereas the inner leaflet is enriched in phosphatidylserine (PS), phosphatidylinositol (PI) and phosphatidylethanolamine (PE). This arrangement is required for barrier function and also normal physiology. For example, PC is extracted from the outer leaflet of the canalicular membrane of hepatocytes to form the lipid/bile-salt micelles of bile. The appearance of PS in the outer leaflet of the membrane is an early step in the apoptotic pathway and signals to macrophages to clear the dying cell, while PI and PE, once cleaved by phospholipase, each produce two signalling molecules as second messengers (see p. 96), diacylglycerol and the polar head group. Cholesterol is also an essential component of the plasma membrane and

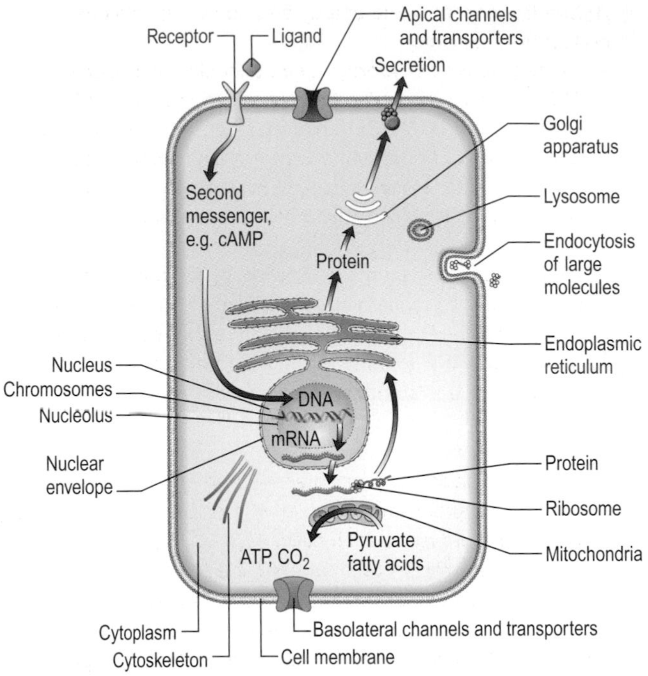

Figure 7.1 Diagrammatic representation of the cell. The major organelles and receptor activation, intracellular messengers, protein formation and secretion, endocytosis of large molecules and production of adenosine triphosphate (ATP) are shown. cAMP, cyclic adenosine monophosphate.

cannot be substituted by plant sterols, which have a subtly different shape. For this reason, the liver secretes plant sterols back into the gut. Membrane lipids are also exploited by pathogens. For example, the sphingolipid GM1-ganglioside is the receptor for cholera toxin (see pp. 288–289).

Membrane proteins

Cells can absorb gases or small hydrophobic compounds directly across the plasma membrane by passive diffusion, but membrane proteins are required to take up hydrophilic nutrients or secrete hydrophilic products, to mediate cell–cell communication and to respond to endocrine, paracrine and cytokine signals. Membrane proteins can be integral to the membrane (i.e. their protein chain traverses the membrane one or multiple times) or they can be anchored to the membrane by an acyl chain ***(Fig. 7.2)***.

The major classes are membrane channel proteins, transporters and receptors.

Membrane channel proteins *(Fig. 7.3)*

Membrane proteins that form solute channels through the membrane only work downhill and only to equilibrium. Solute moves down its electrochemical gradient, a combined force of the electric potential and the solute concentration gradient across the membrane. The bulk flow can be very high, the opening and closing of the channel can be regulated, and they can be selective for specific solutes. For example, the cystic fibrosis transmembrane regulator (CFTR; see ***Fig. 7.26***), the protein whose malfunction causes cystic fibrosis, is a chloride channel found on the apical surface of epithelial cells. CFTR functions to regulate the fluidity of the extra-epithelial mucous layer. When the channel opens in the gut and lung, millions of negatively charged chloride ions typically flow out of the cell down their electrochemical gradient. This induces positively

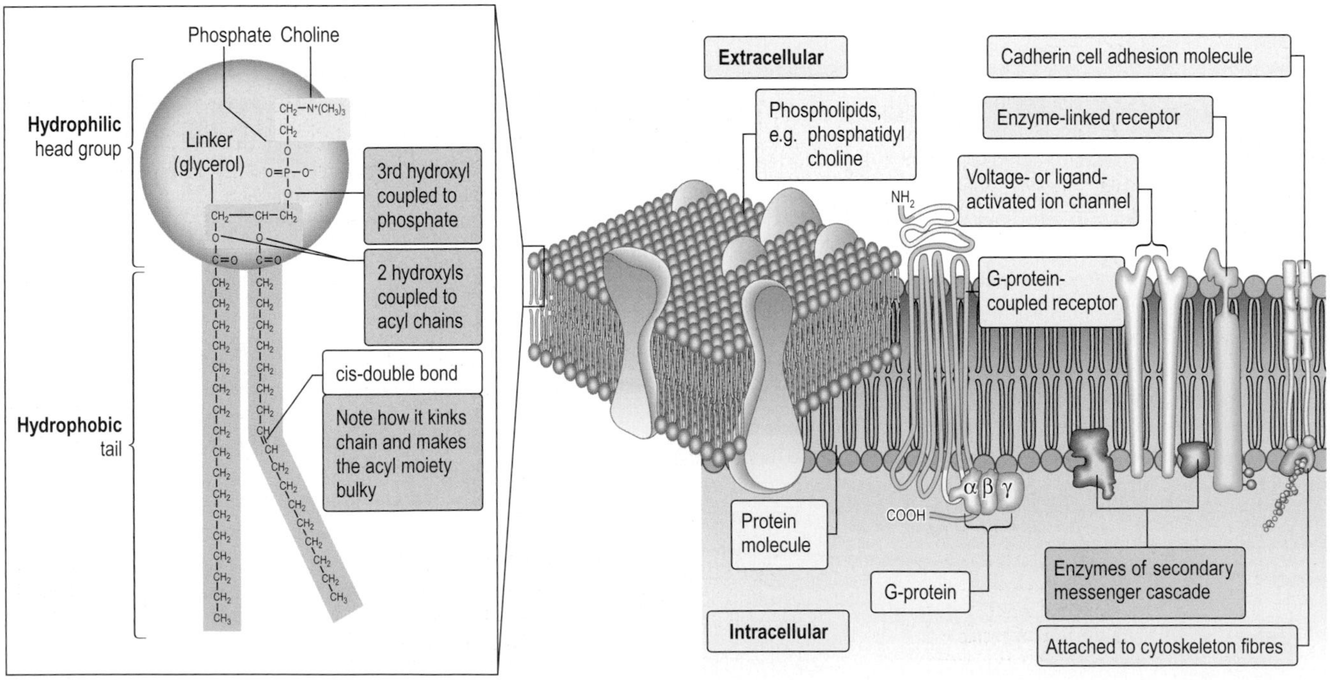

A B

Figure 7.2 Composition and structure of the plasma membrane. A. Membrane lipid phosphatidyl-choline structure. The phospholipid structure is expanded to show its detail. **B.** Cell membrane showing lipid structures and a selection of integral proteins such as receptors, G-proteins, channels, secondary messenger enzyme complexes and cell adhesion molecules.

charged sodium ions to flow between the cells of the epithelium (via a paracellular pathway) to balance the electrical charge. Water follows the efflux of sodium chloride by osmosis, thus maintaining the fluidity of the mucus.

Transporters

In contrast to channels, transporters ***(Fig. 7.3)*** have a low capacity and work by binding solute on one side of the membrane; this induces a conformational change that exposes the solute binding site on the other side of the membrane for release.

- ***Passive transporters*** work without an energy source and can only transport downhill to equilibrium.

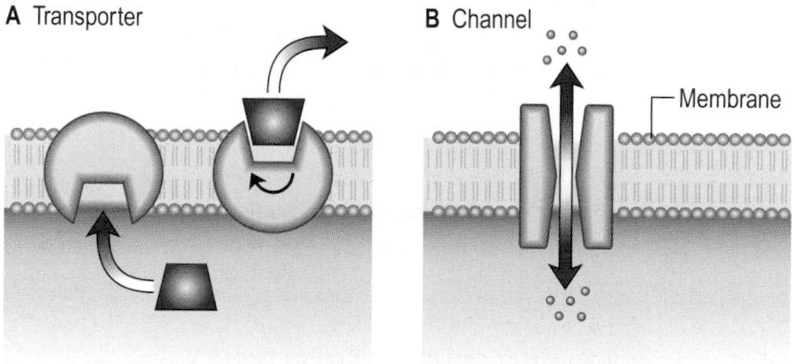

Figure 7.3 **The difference between a transporter and a channel. A.** Transporters expose specific solute binding sites alternately on different sides of the membrane. They can function uphill if coupled to an energy source (active transport) or be downhill only (facilitated diffusion). They are low-capacity. **B.** Channels form a continuous pore through the membrane. They can be regulated and selective, and only work downhill; bulk flow is high.

- ***Active transporters*** use energy and can work uphill to concentrate a solute.
  - *Primary active transporters* use adenosine triphosphate (ATP) hydrolysis to drive the translocation cycle. ATP binding cassette (ABC) transporters are a major class of primary-active transporters whose malfunction causes dozens of human diseases, including a spectrum of liver, eye and skin diseases, bleeding disorders and adrenoleukodystrophy.
  - *Secondary-active pumps* are driven by ion gradients, which are themselves made and maintained by primary-active pumps; thus primary and secondary active pumps often work in concert, as illustrated for the transcellular uptake of glucose across the intestinal epithelium.

Receptors

There are three major receptor categories: receptors that mediate endocytosis, anchorage receptors (e.g. integrins; see p. 94) and signalling receptors (see 'Cell signalling', p. 96).

There are two forms of receptor-mediated endocytosis:

- ***Phagocytosis***. Specialized phagocytic cells such as macrophages and neutrophils can engulf, or phagocytose approximately 20% of their surface in pursuit of large particles such as bacteria or apoptotic cells for digestion and recycling. Phagocytosis is only triggered when specific cell surface receptors – such as the macrophage Fc receptor – are occupied by their ligand.
- ***Pinocytosis***. Pinocytosis is phagocytosis on a small scale and occurs continually in all cells. Smaller molecular complexes, such as low-density lipoprotein (LDL) ***(Fig. 7.4a)***, are internalized during pinocytosis via clathrin-coated pits. The LDL receptor

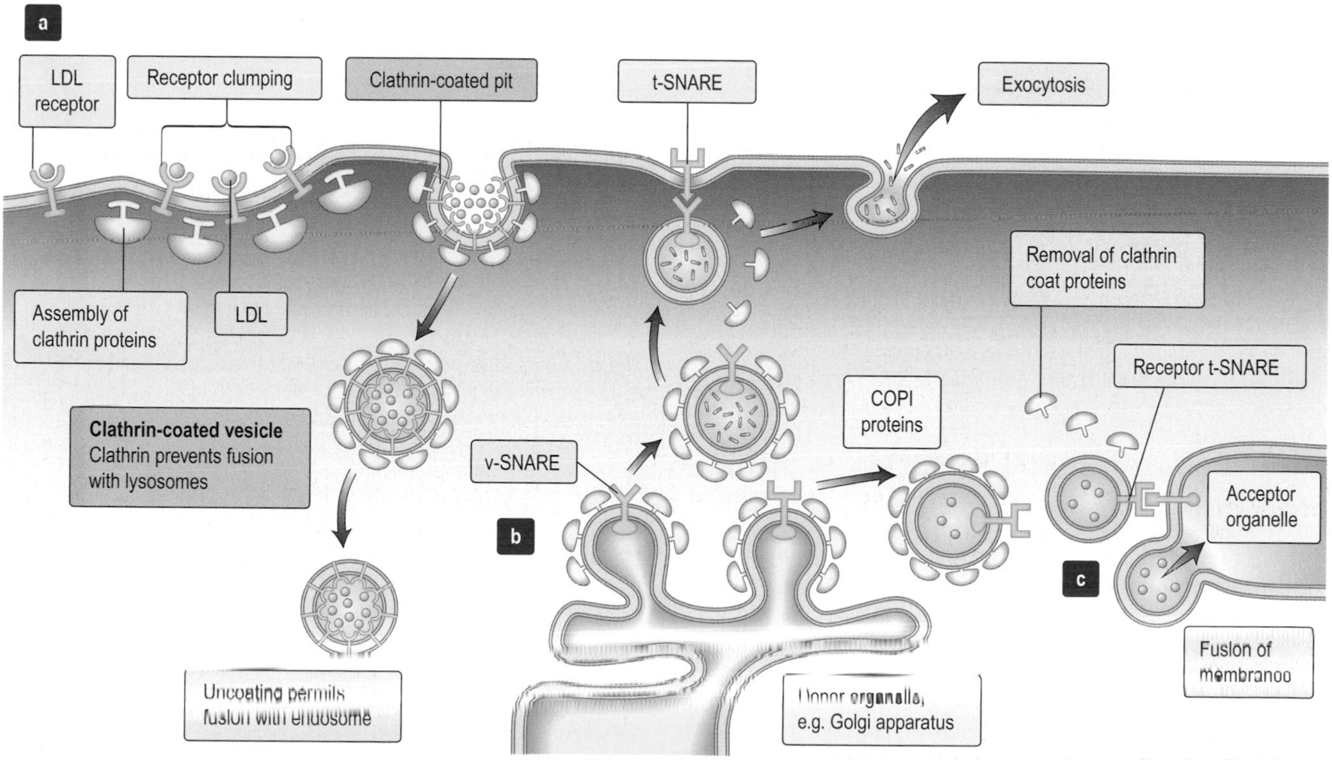

Figure 7.4 **Intracellular transport. (a)** Receptor-mediated endocytosis or pinocytosis. **(b)** Trafficking of vesicles containing synthesized proteins to the cell surface (e.g. hormones). **(c)** Traffic between organelles is also mediated by v- and t-SNARE-containing organelles. COPI, coat protein; LDL, low-density lipoprotein; t-SNARE, target-specific SNARE; v-SNARE, vesicle-specific SNARE. SNARE is an acronym for **S**oluble (**N**-ethylmaleimide-sensitive factor) **A**ttachment **RE**ceptors that mediate vesicle fusion.

has a large extracellular domain that binds circulating LDL. This induces a conformational change in the intracellular domain, which allows it to bind clathrin from the cytosol. Clathrin bends the membrane to form a pit that pinches inwards to become an intracellular clathrin-coated vesicle. Loss of the clathrin coat can allow fusion with other intracellular organelles or vesicles (e.g. with lysosomes to catabolize the cargo), or the coat can be retained during transcellular transport. Defects in each step of pinocytosis can lead to disease. For example, hypercholesterolaemia (see pp. 1280–1282) can result from mutation to the LDL receptor's extracellular domain that prevents LDL binding, but the most common LDL receptor mutation results in loss of the intracellular domain and prevents recruitment of clathrin.

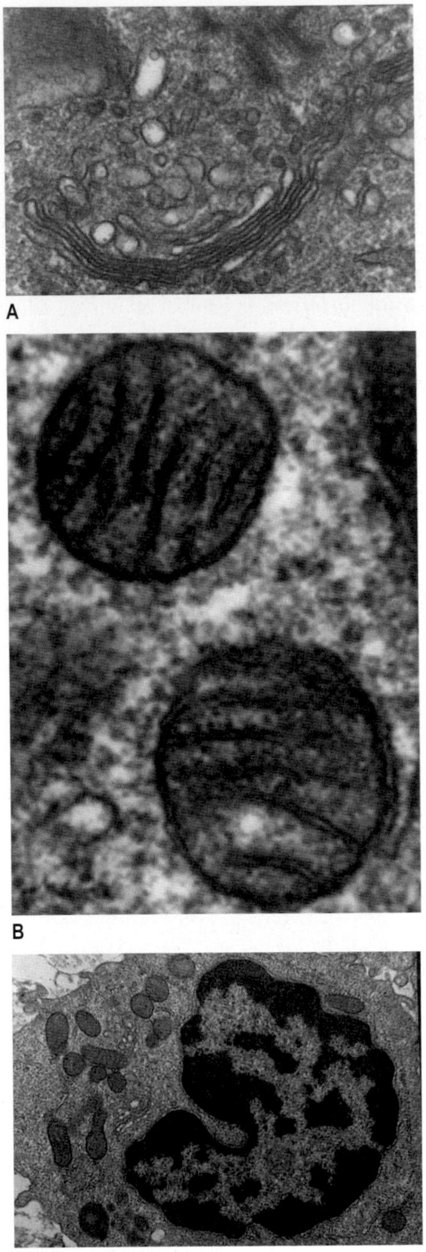

Figure 7.5 **Cell organelles. A.** Golgi apparatus. **B.** Mitochondria. **C.** Nucleus showing dark regions of heterochromatin and lighter euchromatin. *(Courtesy of Louisa Howard, Dartmouth EM Facility.)*

Organelles

Cytoplasmic organelles

Endoplasmic reticulum

Endoplasmic reticulum (ER) is an array of interconnecting tubules or flattened sacs (cisternae) that is contiguous with the outer nuclear membrane (see ***Fig. 7.1***). There are three types of ER:

- ***Rough ER*** carries ribosomes on its cytosolic surface, which synthesize secreted or membrane proteins.
- ***Smooth ER*** is where lipids and sterols are synthesized, and where steroids and drugs are metabolized. It is also a store of calcium that can be released into the cytosol via channel proteins for signalling.
- ***Sarcoplasmic reticulum*** is a form of ER found in muscle, where calcium release on excitation is necessary for muscle contraction (see ***Fig. 23.3***).

Golgi apparatus *(Fig. 7.5A)*

The Golgi apparatus has flattened cisternae similar to those of the ER but arranged in a stack (see ***Fig. 7.1***). Vesicles that bud from the ER with cargo destined for secretion, for the plasma membrane or for other organelles, fuse with the Golgi stack. The proteins, lipids and sterols synthesized in the ER are exported to the Golgi apparatus to complete maturation (for example, the final stages of membrane protein glycosylation occurs here). The mature products are then sorted into vesicles that bud from the Golgi for transport to their final destination (see ***Fig. 7.4b and c***). Golgin proteins control the morphology of the Golgi and vesicle trafficking. Achondrogenesis type 1A is caused by mutation of golgin GMAP-210, which disrupts the Golgi architecture, particularly in bone cells.

Lysosomes

Lysosomes mature from vesicles that bud from the Golgi. They contain digestive enzymes such as lipases, proteases, nucleases and amylases that work in an acidic environment. The membrane of the lysosome therefore includes a proton ATPase pump to acidify the lumen of the organelle. Lysosomes fuse with phagocytotic vesicles (endosomes) to digest their contents ***(Fig. 7.6)***. This is crucial to the function of macrophages and polymorphs (neutrophils and eosinophils) in killing and digesting infective agents, in tissue remodelling during development, and osteoclast remodelling of bone. Not surprisingly, many metabolic disorders result from impaired lysosomal function (see pp. 1287–1288).

Peroxisomes

Peroxisomes contain enzymes for the catabolism of long-chain fatty acids and other organic substrates like bile acids and D-amino acids. Hydrogen peroxide (H_2O_2), a by-product of these reactions, is a highly reactive oxidizing agent, so peroxisomes also contain catalase to detoxify the peroxide. Catalase can reduce H_2O_2 to water while oxidizing harmful phenols and alcohols, thus beginning their detoxification. Peroxisome dysfunction can lead to rare metabolic disorders such as leukodystrophies and rhizomelic dwarfism.

Mitochondria *(Fig. 7.5B)*

Mitochondria are the engines of the cell, providing energy in the form of ATP. They can be small, discrete and few in number in cells with low energy demand, or large and abundant in cells with a high energy

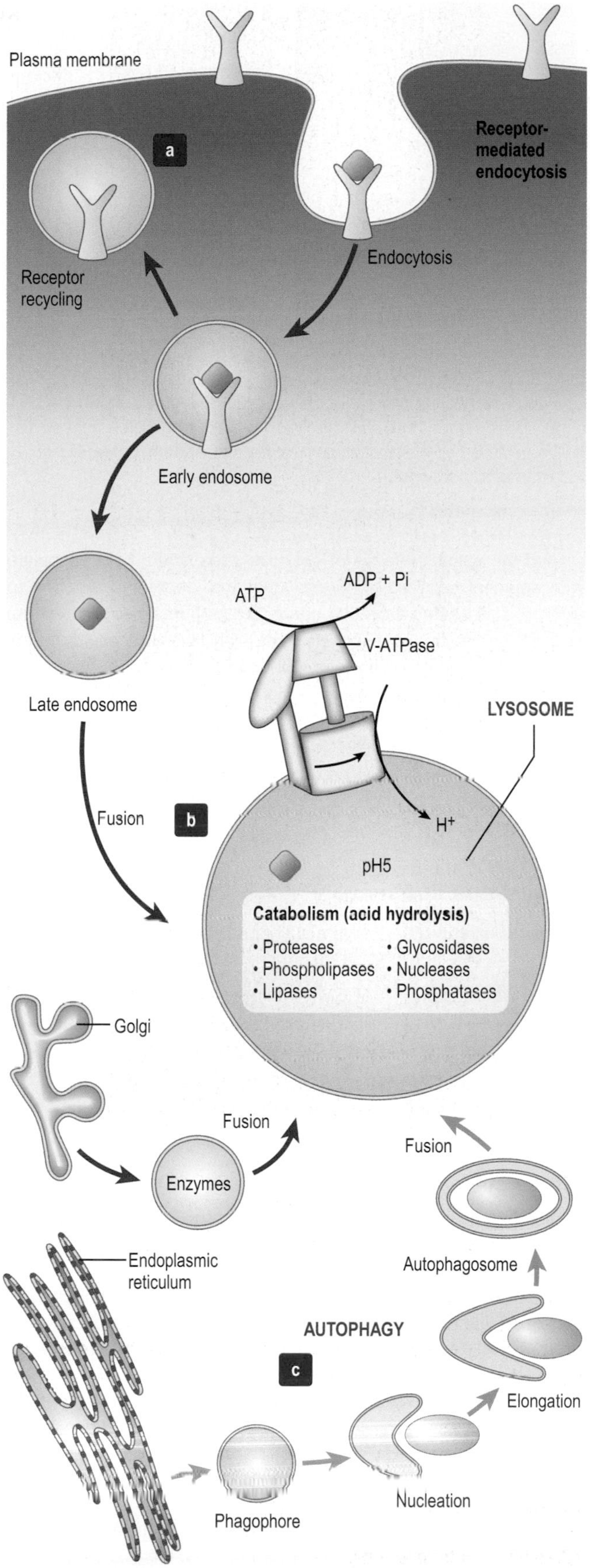

Figure 7.6 A cell showing the action of lysosomes in catabolizing engulfed nutrients and recycling cellular contents. (a) Nutrients taken up by receptor-mediated endocytosis are internalized into vesicles called endosomes. As these mature, the lumen is acidified, causing the receptor to release its cargo. The receptor is trafficked back to the plasma membrane but the cargo may be catabolized by acid hydrolysis in the lysosome **(b)** in which the lumen is acidified by the vacuolaradenosine triphosphatase (V-ATPase). Lysosomes are also involved in autophagy **(c)**. Vesicles (phagophores) bud from the ER and nucleate to engulf cellular components (cytosol and organelles) in an autophagosome. The autophagosome, which has an unusual double membrane, fuses with lysosomes to degrade and recycle the engulfed contents. ADP, adenosine diphosphate; Pi, phosphate.

demand like hepatocytes or muscle cells. The mitochondrion has its own genome encoding 13 proteins. The other proteins (approximately 1000) required for mitochondrial function are encoded by the nuclear genome and imported into the mitochondrion. The mitochondrion has a double membrane surrounding a central matrix. The central matrix contains the enzymes for the Krebs cycle, which accepts the products of sugar and fatty acid catabolism and uses them to produce co-factors that donate their electrons into the electron transport chain of the inner membrane (see pp. 103–104). The inner membrane is highly folded into cristae to increase its effective surface area. The protein complexes of the electron transport chain accept and donate electrons in redox reactions, releasing energy to efflux protons (H^+) into the inter-membrane space. ATP synthase, another integral membrane protein, uses this H^+ electrochemical gradient to drive formation of ATP. Mitochondria have many additional functions, including roles in apoptosis (see p. 105) and supply of substrates for biosynthesis. Mitochondria are also necessary for the synthesis of porphyrin, deficiency of which causes a range of diseases collectively called porphyrias (see pp. 1289–1291).

Nucleus

The most prominent cellular organelle, the nucleus ***(Fig. 7.5C)***, has a double membrane (the outer membrane is continuous with the ER) enclosing the human genome. The double membrane contains nuclear pores, through which gene regulatory proteins, transcription factors and ribonucleic acid (RNA) that has been transcribed from the deoxyribonucleic acid (DNA) are transported. The nuclear matrix is highly organized. Microscopically dense regions of heterochromatin represent highly compacted chromosomal DNA, which tends to be transcriptionally repressed. Lighter regions of euchromatin contain extended chromosomes, which tend to be transcriptionally active. The most prominent nuclear compartment, the nucleolus, is where ribosomal RNA (rRNA) is synthesized and ribosomal subunits are assembled.

Further reading

Artenstein AW, Opal SM. Proprotein convertases in health and disease. *N Engl J Med* 2011; 365:2507–2518.

Linton KJ, Holland IB. *The ABC Transporters of Human Physiology and Disease*. New Jersey: World Scientific; 2011.

Lowe M. Structural organization of the Golgi apparatus. *Curr Opin Cell Biol* 2011; [illegible]

http://www.cytochemistry.net/cell-biology/ *Further explanation and additional images of cells and organelles.*

The cytoskeleton

A complex network of structural proteins regulates the shape, strength and movement of the cell, and the traffic of internal

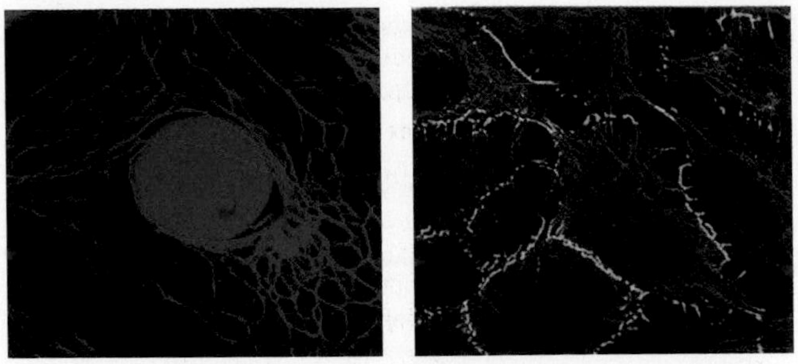
A B

Figure 7.7 Cytoskeleton of epithelial cells. **A.** Keratin red, nuclei stained in blue. **B.** Keratin filaments (in red) and a desmosomal plaque component desmoplakin in green. *(From Moll R, Divo M, Langbein L. The human keratins: biology and pathology.* Histochemistry and Cell Biology *2008; 129:705–733, with permission.)*

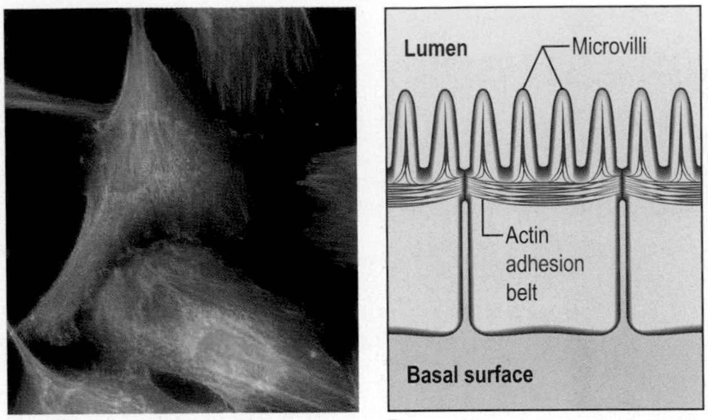

A B

Figure 7.8 Cell cytoskeleton. **A.** Actin microfilament network in an epithelial cell. Actin is orange, nuclei are blue, and green shows the endoplasmic reticulum. **B.** Microfilament (actin) cytoskeleton adhesion belt in polarized epithelial cells. *(**A**, Courtesy of Carolyn Byrne, Queen Mary University of London.)*

organelles and vesicles. The major components are microtubules, intermediate filaments and microfilaments.

Microtubules

Microtubules (20–25 nm diameter) are polymers of α- and β-tubulin. These tubular structures resist bending and stretching, and are polar with plus and minus ends. Their minus ends are anchored in the microtubule organizing centre (MTOC), a complex of centrioles, γ-tubulin and other proteins, with their plus ends extending into the cell. At their plus ends, repeated cycles of assembly and disassembly permit rapid changes in length. Microtubules form a 'highway', transporting organelles and vesicles through the cytoplasm. The two major microtubule-associated motor proteins (kinesin and dynein) allow movement of cargo towards the plus and minus ends, respectively. During cell division, the MTOC forms the mitotic spindle (see p. 101). Drugs that disrupt microtubule assembly (e.g. colchicine and vinca alkaloids) or stabilize microtubules (taxanes) preferentially kill dividing cells by preventing mitosis.

Intermediate filaments

Intermediate filaments (approximately 10 nm) form a network around the nucleus extending to the periphery of the cell. They make cell-to-cell contacts with adjacent cells via desmosomes, and with basement matrix via hemidesmosomes (***Fig. 7.7***; see also ***Fig. 31.34***). Their function is structural integrity; they are prominent in cellular tissues under stress and their disruption in genetic disease can cause structural defects or cell collapse. More than 40 different types of proteins polymerize to form intermediate filaments specific to particular cell types. For example, keratin intermediate fibres are found only in epithelial cells whilst vimentin is in mesothelial (fibroblastic) cells. Lamin intermediate filaments form the nuclear membrane skeleton in most cells.

Microfilaments

Microfilaments (3–6 nm) are polymers of actin, one of the most abundant proteins in all cells. The actin microfilament network ***(Fig. 7.8)*** controls cell shape, prevents cellular deformation, and is involved in cell–cell and cell–matrix adhesion, in cell movements such as crawling and cytokinesis (cell division), and in intracellular vesicle transport. Bundles of actin filaments form the structural core of cellular protrusions such as microvilli, lamellipodia and filopodia (see below). Actin microfilament bundles within the cell can associate with myosin II to form contractile stress fibres, similar to muscle sarcomeres. Stress fibres are often found as circumferential belts around the apical surfaces of epithelial cells where cells associate with adjacent cells via adherens junctions, permitting reaction to external stresses as a cellular sheet. Stress fibres also form where actin interacts via accessory proteins with the extracellular matrix at sites of focal adhesion (see ***Fig. 7.11c***). This occurs when cells move and is prominent during inflammation, wound healing and metastasis. During cytokinesis, actin–myosin II bundles form the contractile ring separating dividing cells. Like microtubules, microfilaments are polar, so can be used to transport secretory vesicles, endosomes and mitochondria, powered by motor proteins, including myosin I and V.

Cell shape and motility

The cytoskeleton determines cell shape and surface structures.

Microvilli

The apical surface of some epithelial cells is covered in tiny microvilli (approximately 1 µm long), forming a brush border of thousands of small, finger-like projections of the plasma membrane that increase the surface area for uptake or efflux ***(Fig. 7.9)***. At their core are 20–30 cross-linked actin microfilaments.

Motile cilia

Motile cilia are also fine, finger-like protrusions but these are longer (approximately 10–20 µm long) ***(Fig. 7.9)***. At their core is an axoneme, a bundle of nine cross-linked tubulin microtubule doublets surrounding a central pair. The action of the motor domain dynein serves to bend the cilium. Neighbouring cilia tend to beat in unison, generating waves of motion that move fluid over the cell surface in the gut and airways (see ***Fig. 24.9***), and also in the fallopian tubes.

Non-motile or primary cilia

Most cells also have a single ***primary cilium***. These cilia have a variant axoneme with no central pair of microtubules and, while they have dynein, they are non-motile (the dynein is used to traffic cargo along the axoneme). Rich in receptor proteins, the primary cilia are used for signalling during development and in the adult. Other related non-motile cilia are found in specialized cells: for example, in the photoreceptors of the retina, the sensory neurones of the

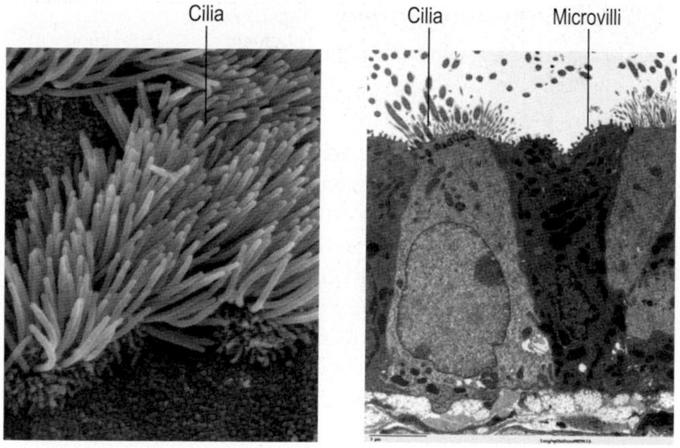

A B

Figure 7.9 Cilia and microvilli in trachea. A. Scanning electron microscope image of longer cilia-bearing cells with adjacent microvilli-bearing cells. **B.** Transmission electron microscope image of section A. *(Courtesy of Louisa Howard, Dartmouth EM Facility.)*

olfactory system, and the sensory hair cells of the cochlea. A range of human ***ciliopathies (Fig. 7.10)*** has been described, with pleiotropic symptoms depending on which cilia are affected. These include polycystic kidney disease, Bardet–Biedl syndrome, Joubert syndrome and Ellis–van Creveld syndrome.

Flagella

The single flagellum – for example, that found on sperm – is structurally related to cilia but is longer (approximately 40 μm) and has a whip-like motion.

Cell motility

Cell motility is essential during development and in the adult: for example, when macrophages migrate to sites of infection, keratinocytes migrate to close wounds, osteoclasts and osteoblasts tunnel into and remodel bone, and fibroblasts migrate to sites of injury to repair the extracellular matrix. Most cell motility in the adult human takes the form of cell crawling, which is dependent on remodelling of the actin cytoskeleton. How the actin cytoskeleton is remodelled determines the mode of migration:

- ***Filopodia***. Actin remodelled essentially in one dimension produces a long filament, pushing the leading edge of the plasma membrane forwards as spikes, similar to long, thin villi.
- ***Lamellipodia***. If remodelled in two dimensions, a network of cross-linked actin microfilaments forms a broad, flat skirt or lamellipodium.
- ***Pseudopodia***. These are more three-dimensional projections, as the actin cytoskeleton is remodelled into a gel-like lattice.

Movement

A similar mechanism involving the coordinated remodelling of the cytoskeleton and the formation and release of cell adhesive proteins underlies all three modes of migration. Essentially, actin is polymerized at the leading edge, extending the plasma membrane forwards. New adhesions are formed with the substratum (to other cells and/or extracellular matrix) at the leading edge to provide purchase. Release of attachments and depolymerization of the actin filaments at the trailing edge allow the cell to move forwards. Myosin and myosin motor proteins may also be involved at the trailing edge, providing the tractive force to pull the cell body forwards. The complex coordination of these processes is controlled by signalling pathways involving members of the Rho protein family of guanosine triphosphatases (GTPases). Key signalling targets are the WASp family of proteins, which stimulate actin polymerization. The significance of cell motility in humans is illustrated by mutation of the WASp expressed in blood cell lineages, which causes Wiskott–Aldrich syndrome (see p. 140), and is characterized by severe immunodeficiency and thrombocytopenia (platelet deficiency).

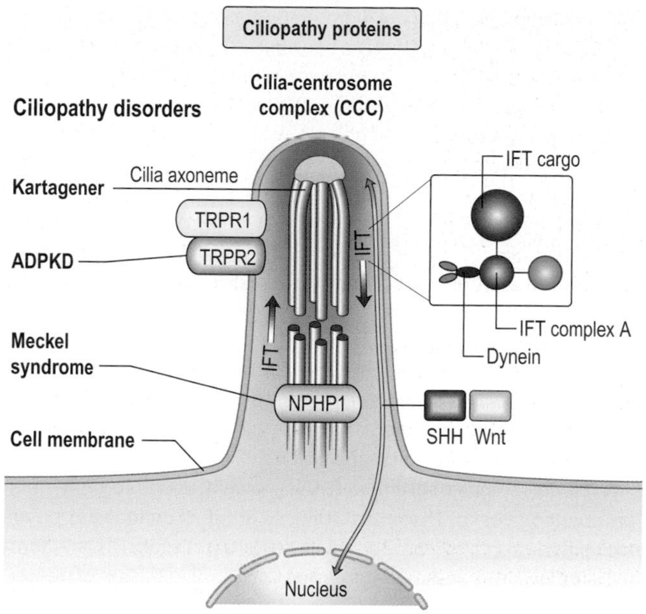

Figure 7.10 Structure of a cilium showing ciliopathy proteins and intraflagellar transport (IFT). Some single-gene ciliopathies are shown, along with their gene products, situated in the cilia–centrosome complex (CCC). Receptors on cilia receive external cell signals that are processed via sonic hedgehog (SHH) and Wnt pathways. The gene mutation can act during morphogenesis (e.g. Meckel syndrome) or during tissue maintenance and repair, leading to degenerative disorders. The IFT system transports axoneme and membrane compounds in raft macromolecular particles (IFT cargo and complex). Retrograde transport occurs via cytoplasmic dynein. ADPKD, autosomal dominant polycystic kidney disease; NPHP1, nephronophthisis type 1; TRPR1 and 2, polycystin 1 and 2. *(Adapted from Hildebrandt F, Benzing T, Katsanis N. Ciliopathies.* New England Journal of Medicine *2011; 364:1533–1543.)*

Further reading

Hildebrandt F, Benzing T, Katsanis N. Ciliopathies. *N Engl J Med* 2011; 364:1533–1543.

THE CELL AND ITS ENVIRONMENT

Most cells differentiate or specialize to perform particular functions within tissues where they interact with the extracellular matrix (ECM) or other cells. The major tissue types are epithelia, connective tissue, muscle and neural tissue.

- ***Epithelial tissues*** comprise layers of cells held tightly together by intercellular junctions and are usually separated from underlying tissue by specialized ECM called the basal lamina. Epithelia cover surfaces (e.g. epidermis, tongue surface) and line passageways (airways, digestive tract, blood vessels), providing protection and regulating absorption and secretion.
- ***Connective tissues*** support other tissues and give organs shape. Connective tissue is a non-rigid matrix of fibres such

as collagen, in which cells are embedded (primarily fibroblasts that secrete the matrix but also other cell types, depending on the type of tissue). Matrix such as bone will include osteoblasts and osteoclasts; cartilage will include chondrocytes and chondroblasts, which reshape and remodel the connective tissue.

Extracellular matrix

The ECM is the gel matrix outside the cell, usually secreted by fibroblasts. ECM determines tissue properties; for example, in bone it is calcified, in tendons it is tough and rope-like, and in neural tissue it is almost absent. However, ECM is more than just a support matrix. It affects cell shape, migration, cell–cell communication and signalling, proliferation and survival.

The gel or ground substance of the ECM is made from polysaccharides (glycosaminoglycans, GAGs), usually bound to proteins to form proteoglycans. These are a diverse group of molecules conferring different matrix properties in different tissues. They form hydrated gels that resist compression yet permit diffusion of metabolites and signalling molecules.

- ***Hyaluronan***, a very large hydrated GAG, is secreted into the joint space in synovial joints (see p. 647), which it lubricates and which helps reduce compressive forces.
- ***Aggrecan***, a very large proteoglycan, forms part of the articular cartilage of joints (see p. 647) and also contributes to compression resistance.
- ***Decorin*** is a much smaller proteoglycan from the loose connective tissue of skin and has structural and signalling functions (through binding and regulating growth factor activity).

Fibrous proteins of ECM include collagens and tropoelastin, which polymerize into collagen and elastin fibres, and fibronectin, which is insoluble in many tissues but soluble in plasma. Collagen provides tensile strength, while elastin confers elasticity. The widely distributed fibronectin adheres to both cells and ECM, thus positioning cells within the ECM. Collagens, the most abundant proteins in the body, are also widespread and play structural roles in skin and bone, where collagen defects and disorders often manifest. Elastin fibres, abundant in arteries, lung and skin, have a fibrillin sheath (fibrillin mutations underlie Marfan syndrome; see pp. 1028–1029). The ECM can be degraded and remodelled by proteins of the matrix metalloproteinase (MMP) family. These are needed for angiogenesis and morphogenesis, and are also involved in the pathophysiology of cancer, cirrhosis and arthritis.

Basal lamina or basement membrane (lamina propria) is a specialized form of ECM, which separates cells from underlying tissue and plays a supportive, anchoring and protective role. Basal lamina can also act as molecular filters (e.g. glomerular filtration barrier; see ***Fig. 20.2***) and mediate signalling between adjacent tissues (e.g. epidermal–dermal signalling in skin). Type IV collagen, heparan sulphate proteoglycan, laminin and nidogen are key basal lamina proteins. Inherited abnormalities in these proteins cause skin blistering diseases (see ***Fig. 31.34***). Breach of the basal lamina by invading cancer cells is a key stage in progression of epithelial carcinoma *in situ* to a malignant carcinoma.

Cell–cell adhesion

Cells need to interact directly for barrier function, tissue strength and communication. This is mediated by several types of protein that form junctions between cells.

Cell–cell adhesion proteins *(Fig. 7.11a)*

Cells adhere to each other through multiprotein junctions and also individual transmembrane proteins.

Immunoglobulin-like cell adhesion molecules

Immunoglobulin-like cell adhesion molecules (iCAMs or CAMs) ***(Fig. 7.11a)*** are structurally related to antibodies. The neural cell adhesion molecule (N-CAM) is found predominantly in the nervous system, where it mediates homophilic (like–like) adhesion. When bound to an identical molecule on another cell, N-CAM can also associate laterally with a fibroblast growth factor receptor and stimulate its tyrosine kinase activity to induce neurite growth, thus triggering cellular responses by indirect activation of the recipient.

Selectins

Unlike most adhesion molecules, which bind to other proteins, the selectins interact with carbohydrate ligands or ***mucin complexes*** on leucocytes and endothelial cells (vascular and haematological systems).

- ***Leucocyte-selectin*** (CD62L) mediates the homing of lymphocytes to lymph nodes.
- ***Endothelial-selectin*** (CD62E) is expressed after activation by inflammatory cytokines; the small basal amount of E-selectin in many vascular beds appears to be necessary for the migration of leucocytes.
- ***Platelet-selectin*** (CD62P) is stored in the alpha granules of platelets and the Weibel–Palade bodies of endothelial cells, but it moves rapidly to the plasma membrane upon cell stimulation.

All three selectins play a part in leucocyte rolling (see ***Fig. 8.9***).

Integrins

Integrins are membrane glycoproteins with α and β subunits that exist as active and inactive forms. The amino acid sequence arginine–glycine–aspartic acid (RGD) is a potent recognition system for integrin binding.

Focal adhesion junctions between adjacent cells

See ***Figure 7.11b.***

Tight junctions (zonula occludens)

These are mediated by the claudin and occluden integral membrane proteins that hold cells together. They form at the top (apical) side of epithelial cells in intestine, skin and kidney, and in endothelial cells of blood vessels ***(Fig. 7.11)*** to provide a regulated barrier to the movement of ions and solutes between cells (paracellular flow). Tight junctions also confer polarity to cells by acting as a barrier between the apical and the basolateral membranes, preventing diffusion of membrane lipids and proteins. Twenty-four ***claudins*** are differentially expressed in different cell types to regulate paracellular transport. For example, changes in claudin expression in the kidney nephron correlate with permeability changes. Mutations in claudin 16 (previously named parcellin-1) and 19, expressed in the thick ascending limb of the loop of Henle in the kidney, cause an inherited renal disorder, familial hypomagnesaemia with hypercalciuria and nephrocalcinosis (FHHNC; see p. 169).

Gap junctions

Gap junctions ***(Fig. 7.11)*** allow low-molecular-weight substances to pass directly between cells, permitting metabolic and electric

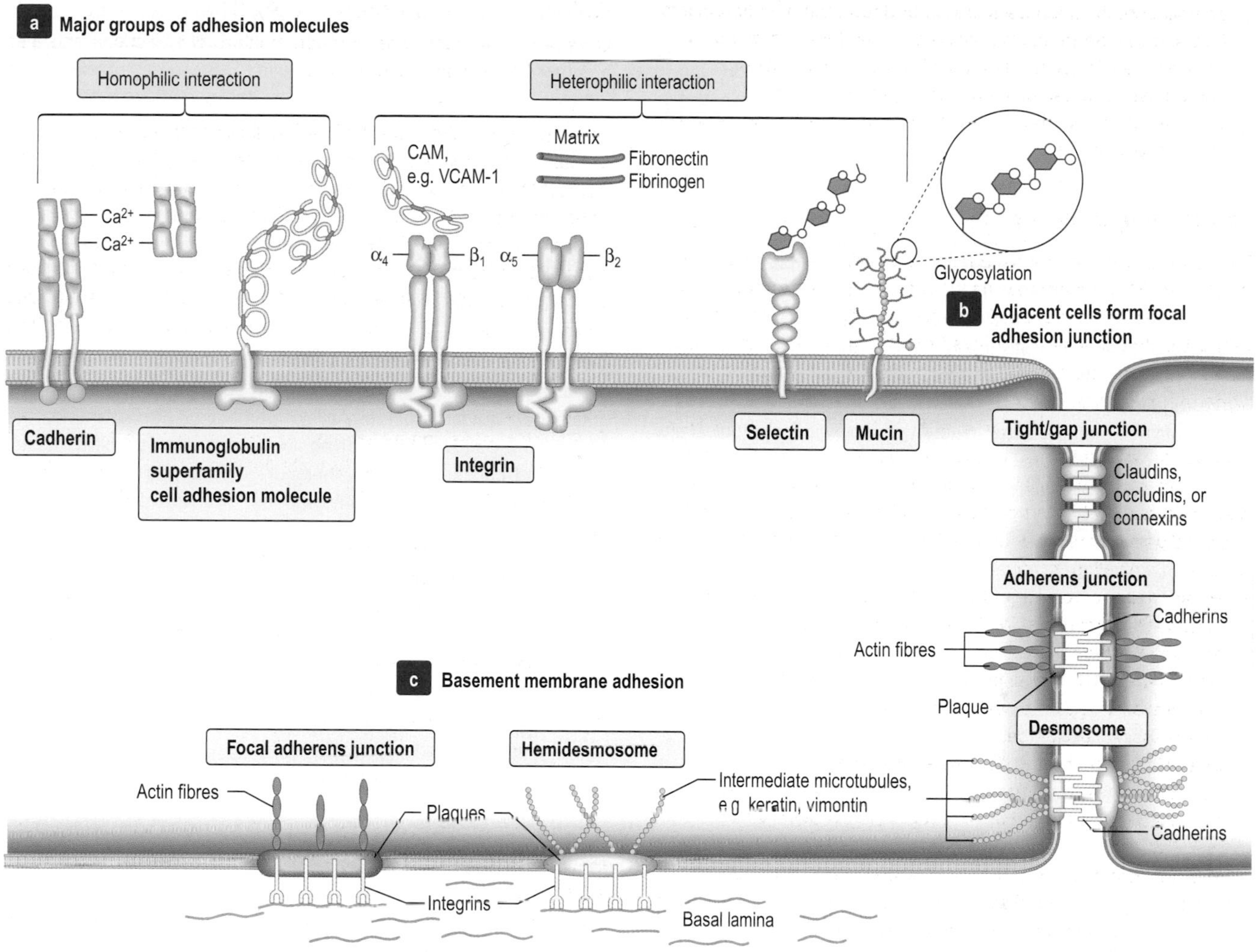

Figure 7.11 Cell adhesion molecules and cellular junctions. (a) Major groups of adhesion molecules. **(b)** Adjacent cells form focal adhesion junctions. **(c)** Basement membrane adhesion.

coupling (e.g. in cardiomyocytes). Protein channels made of six ***connexin*** proteins (as well as ***claudins*** and ***occludens***) are aligned between adjacent cells and allow the passage of solutes of up to 1000 kDa (e.g. amino acids, sugars, ions, chemical messengers). The channels are regulated by many factors such as intracellular Ca^{2+}, pH and voltage. Gap junctions form in almost all interacting cells but connexin family members are differentially expressed. Connexin mutations underlie many inherited disorders, such as the X-linked form of Charcot–Marie–Tooth disease (*GJB1*; see p. 886) and are also a major cause of genetic hearing loss (*GJB2*).

Adherens junctions

Adherens junctions are multiprotein intercellular adhesive structures prominent in epithelial tissues such as the ***fascia adherens*** in cardiac muscle ***(Fig. 7.11b)***. They attach principally to actin microfilaments inside the cell with the aid of multiple additional proteins, and also attach and stabilize microtubules. At the apical sides of epithelial cells, a prominent type of adherens junction, the ***zonula adherens***, attaches to the circumferential actin stress fibres. Transmembrane proteins of the cadherin family provide the adhesion through homotypic interaction of their extracellular domains. Downregulation of cadherins is a feature of cancer progression in many cells.

Desmosomes (macula adherens)

Desmosomes provide strong attachment between cells and are prominent in tissues subject to stress, such as skin and cardiac muscle (see ***Fig. 7.7***, ***Fig. 7.11b*** and ***Fig. 31.1***). Like adherens junctions, they are multiprotein complexes, where adhesion is provided by transmembrane cadherin proteins, desmogleins and desmocollins. However, within the cell, desmosomes interact principally with intermediate filaments rather than microfilaments and microtubules. Germline mutations in genes encoding desmosomal associated proteins are a cause of cardiomyopathy with or without cutaneous features and in ***pemphigus vulgaris*** and ***pemphigus foliaceus*** (see pp. 1368–1369)

Basement membrane adhesion

Cells adhere ***(Fig. 7.11c)*** to non-basal lamina ECM via secreted proteins such as fibronectin and collagen, and to basal lamina proteins via focal adhesion and hemidesmosome multiprotein complexes (e.g. keratin or vimentin). Here, ***integrins*** replace cadherins as the key surface adhesive proteins. Integrins are transmembrane sensors or receptors, which change shape upon binding to ECM. Inside the cell, integrins interact with the cytoskeleton and a complex array of over 150 proteins that influence intracellular signalling pathways affecting proliferation, survival, shape, mobility and gene expression.

- ***Outside-in signalling***. This forms the basis for anoikis or apoptotic death, such as occurs in cancer cells that inappropriately lose cell–substratum adhesion.
- ***Inside-out signalling***. Intracellular changes can also cause integrins to switch from an inactive to an adhesive conformation. This 'inside-out' signalling occurs when platelet integrins glycoprotein IIb-IIIa (GPIIb-IIa) are activated to bind fibrinogen at sites of vessel injury, resulting in platelet aggregation (see p. 565 and ***Fig. 16.39***).

Defective integrins are associated with many immunological and clotting disorders such as Bernard–Soulier syndrome and Glanzmann's thrombasthenia (see ***Box 16.31***).

Further reading

De Matteis MA, Luini A. Mendelian disorders of membrane trafficking. *N Engl J Med* 2011; 365:927–928.
Jean C, Gravelle P, Fournie JJ et al. Influence of stress on extracellular matrix and integrin biology. *Oncogene* 2011; 30:2697–2706.
Thomason HA, Scothern A, McHarg S et al. Desmosomes: adhesive strength and signalling in health and disease. *Biochem J* 2010; 429:419–433.

CELLULAR MECHANISMS

Cell signalling

Signalling or communication between cells is often via extracellular molecules or ligands, which can be proteins (e.g. hormones, growth factors), small molecules (e.g. lipid-soluble steroid hormones such as oestrogen and testosterone) or dissolved gases such as nitric oxide. The signal is usually received by membrane protein receptors, although some signals, such as steroid hormones, enter the target cell, where they interact with intracellular receptors ***(Fig. 7.12)***. Some signalling, especially in the immune system, relies on cell–cell contact, where the signalling molecule (ligand) and receptor are on adjacent cells.

Receptors

Receptors transduce signals across the membrane to an intracellular pathway or second messengers to change cell behaviour, often ultimately affecting gene expression ***(Figs 7.12*** and ***7.13)***. The membrane-bound receptors fall into three main groups based on downstream signalling pathways:

- ***Ion channel-linked receptors*** (voltage- or ligand-activated ion channels; see ***Fig. 7.3***). At synaptic junctions between neurones (see ***Fig. 21.1***), these receptors open in response to neurotransmitters such as glutamate, adrenaline (epinephrine) or acetylcholine to cause a rapid depolarization of the membrane.
- ***G-protein-linked receptors***, such as the odorant and light (opsin) family of receptors. These belong to a large family of seven-pass transmembrane proteins (see ***Figs 7.2*** and ***7.12***). On activation by ligand, G-protein-linked receptors bind a GTP-binding protein (G-protein), which activates adjacent enzyme complexes or ion channels (***Figs 7.12*** and ***21.1***). The adjacent enzyme can be adenylcyclase (see below).
- ***Enzyme-linked receptors*** (***Figs 7.2*** and ***7.12***) typically have an extracellular ligand-binding domain, a single transmembrane-spanning region, and a cytoplasmic domain that has intrinsic enzyme activity or which will bind and activate other membrane-bound or cytoplasmic enzyme complexes. This group of receptors is highly variable but many have kinase activity or associate with kinases, which act by phosphorylating substrate proteins, usually on a tyrosine (e.g. the platelet-derived growth factor (PDGF) receptor) or a serine/threonine (e.g. the transforming growth factor-beta (TGF-β) receptor).

Signal transduction

Signal transduction from the receptor to the site of action in the cell is mediated by small signalling molecules called second messengers, or by signalling proteins ***(Fig. 7.12)***. Changes in activity of signalling proteins by acquired mutation occur in cancer, and many anticancer drugs target signalling pathways. For example, the ***Hedgehog*** pathway is involved in human development, tissue repair and cancer ***(Fig. 7.13)***. Inhibitors of this pathway are being developed for therapeutic interventions. The ***Wnt*** pathway is also involved in bone formation (see p. 708).

Second messengers

These include cyclic adenosine monophosphate (cAMP) and membrane lipid-derived inositol triphosphate (IP_3) and diacylglycerol ***(Fig. 7.12)***. These molecules diffuse from the receptor to bind and change the activity of downstream proteins propagating the signal. Cyclic-AMP triggers a protein signalling cascade by activating a cAMP-dependent protein kinase. Diacylglycerol activates protein kinase C while IP_3 mobilizes calcium from intracellular stores (e.g. from the ER; see ***Fig. 23.9***).

G-proteins

G-proteins or GTP-binding proteins are signalling proteins that switch between an active state when GTP is bound and an inactive state when bound to guanosine diphosphate (GDP). The best-known members are the Ras superfamily, comprising Ras, Rho, Rab, Arf and Ran families. Activation of Ras members by somatic mutation is found in approximately 33% of human cancers. Ras members are often activated downstream of tyrosine kinase receptors, and they transmit signals by activating a cascade of protein kinases, including mitogen-activated protein (MAP) kinase ***(Fig. 7.12)***. Ras signalling molecules have roles in many cellular activities, including regulation of the cell cycle, intracellular transport, and apoptosis.

Kinase and phosphatase signalling proteins

These are enzymes that respectively phosphorylate or dephosphorylate residues on proteins to alter their activity. Phosphorylation cascades transduce and amplify signals from the membrane receptor to the site of action in the cell. The tyrosine kinase receptors phosphorylate each other after ligand binding causes the receptor to dimerize (see ***Fig. 7.12***). The membrane-bound and cytosolic targets of these activated receptor complexes are most commonly the Ras family members, or protein kinase C, which often transduce signals through the MAP kinase cascade, or which phosphorylate the inhibitor of kappa B (IκB), causing it to release its DNA-binding protein, nuclear factor kappa B (NFκB). For example, activated Ras binds and activates the kinase Raf, the first of a set of three MAP kinases that transmit signals by successive phosphorylation of target proteins that ultimately effect transcription ***(Fig. 7.12)***. The receptors for cytokines, such as interleukins, interferons, growth hormone and erythropoietin, transduce signals through the Janus

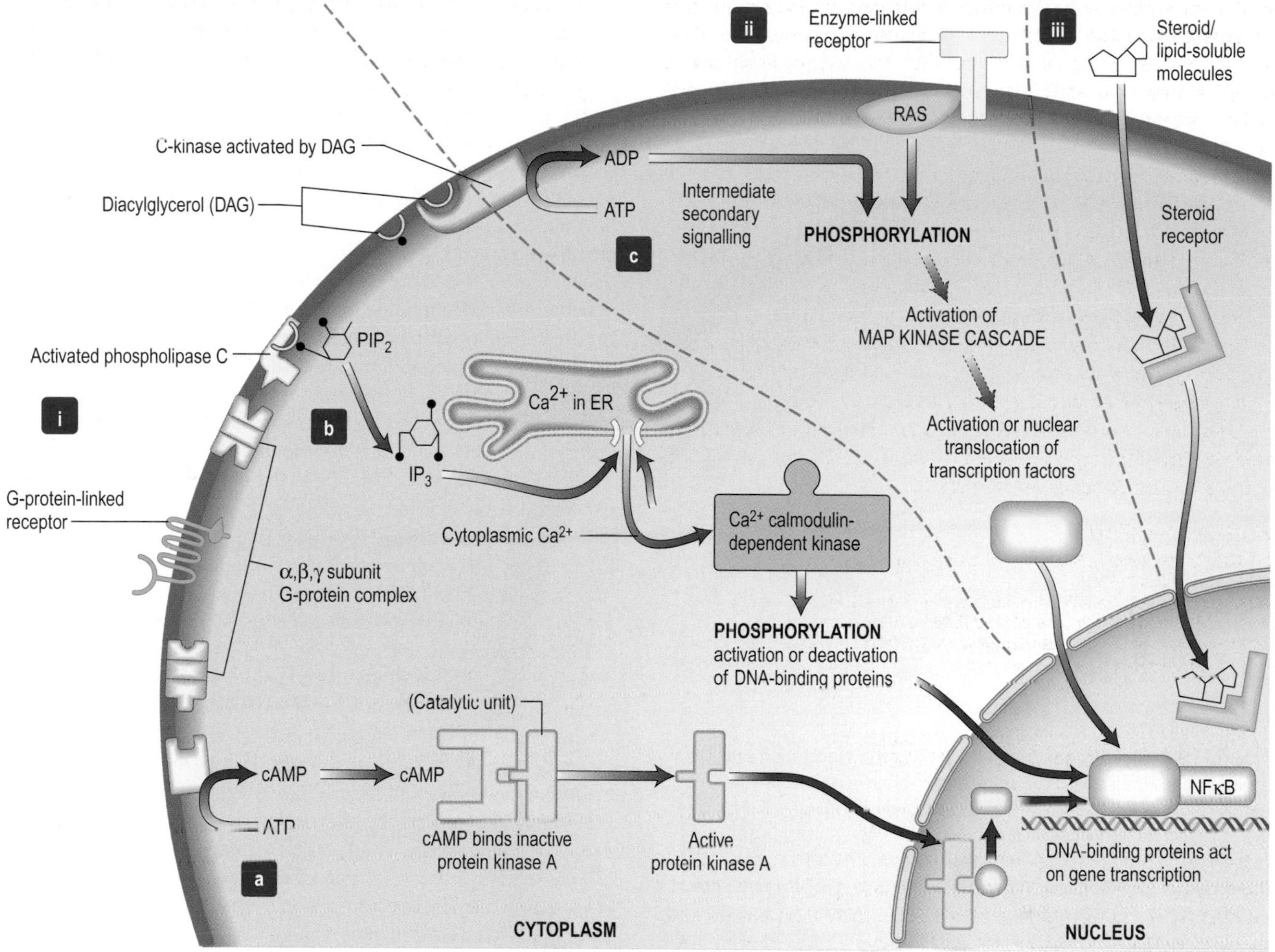

Figure 7.12 **Cell signalling.** **(i)** *G-protein receptor binds ligand (e.g. hormone) and activates G-protein complex.* The G-protein complex can activate three different secondary messengers: **(a)** cAMP generation; **(b)** inositol 1,4,5-trisphosphate (IP_3) and release of Ca^{2+}; **(c)** diacylglycerol (DAG) activation of C-kinase and subsequent protein phosphorylation.
(ii) *Enzyme-linked receptors often dimerize upon ligand binding.* Intracellular domains cross-phosphorylate and link to the phosphorylation cascades such as the mitogen-activated protein (MAP) kinase cascade, via molecules such as Ras.
(iii) *Lipid-soluble molecules, e.g. steroids, pass through the cell membrane and bind to cytoplasmic receptors*, which enter the nucleus and bind directly to DNA.
ADP, adenosine diphosphate; ATP, adenosine triphosphate; cAMP, cyclic adenosine monophosphate; ER, endoplasmic reticulum; NFκB, nuclear factor kappa B; PIP2, phosphatidylinositol 4,5-bisphosphate.

kinase–signal transducer and activator of transcription (JAK-STAT) pathways. Cytokine binding to the receptor activates the associated JAK, which phosphorylates its STAT. The phosphorylated STATs dimerize and translocate to the nucleus to alter gene expression. Kinases and phosphatases are frequently mutated in cancers or underlie developmental conditions. Somatic mutations in *B-Raf* occur in approximately 60% of malignant melanomas (usually the mutation V600E) and are common in other cancers (see pp. 1373–1374). Mutations in the Ras-MAPK signal transduction pathway are the cause of Noonan syndrome.

Further reading

Alberts B, Johnson A, Lewis J et al. *Molecular Biology of the Cell*, 6th edn. New York: Garland Science; 2014.
Briscoe J, Therond PP. The mechanisms of Hedgehog signalling and its roles in development and disease. *Nat Rev Mol Cell Biol* 2013; 14:416–429.
Flaherty KT, Infante JR, Daud A et al. Combined BRAF and MEK inhibition in melanoma with BRAF V600 mutations. *N Engl J Med* 2012; 367:1694–1703.
O'Shea JJ, Holland MD, Staudt LM. JAKs and STATs in immunity, immunodeficiency, and cancer. *N Engl J Med* 2013; 368:161–170.
Roberts AE, Allanson JE, Tartaglia M et al. Noonan syndrome. *Lancet* 2013; 381:333–342.
http://www.biochemj.org/ *Cell signalling information*

Nuclear control

DNA and RNA structure

Hereditary information is contained in the sequence of the building blocks of double-stranded deoxyribonucleic acid (DNA) ***(Fig. 7.14)***. Each strand of DNA is made up of a deoxyribose-phosphate backbone and a series of purine (adenine (A) and guanine (G)) and pyrimidine (thymine (T) and cytosine (C)) bases; because of the way the sugar–phosphate backbone is chemically coupled, each strand has a polarity, with a phosphate at one end (the 5′ end) and a hydroxyl at the other (the 3′ end). The two strands of DNA are held together by hydrogen bonds between the bases. A can only pair with T, and G can only pair with C; therefore each strand is the antiparallel complement of the other ***(Fig. 7.14A)***. This is key to DNA

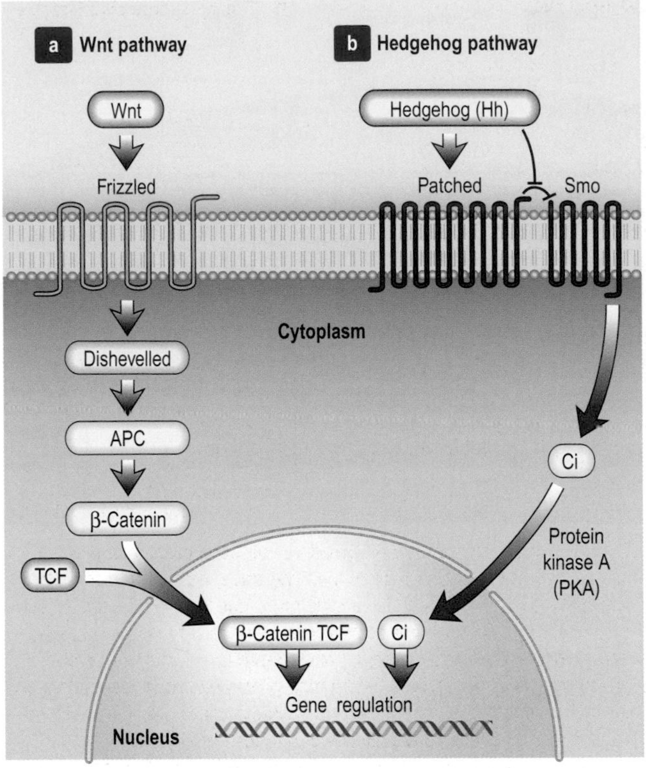

Figure 7.13 Signal transduction showing the Hedgehog and Wnt signalling pathway. (a) ***Wnt signalling*** *has three pathways*: the canonical (β-catenin), Wnt/Ca^{2+} and planar cell polarity pathways. Wnt binds to the Frizzled protein, and then Dishevelled activity via other pathways inhibits phosphorylation of β-catenin. This alters gene transcription. (b) ***Hedgehog ligand (Hh)*** *binds to a 12-transmembrane protein receptor Patched* (Ptc). This acts as an inhibitor of smoothened (Smo), another transmembrane protein related to the Frizzled family of Wnt receptors. In the presence of Hh, the inhibitory effects of Ptc on Smo are removed and Smo is phosphorylated by protein kinase A and other kinases. This prevents cleavage of cubitus interruptus, a zinc finger protein (Ci), which enters the nucleus, inducing the transcription of Hh target genes.
APC, adenomatous polyposis coli protein; TCF, T-cell factor.

replication because each strand can be used as a template to synthesize the other.

The two strands twist to form a double helix with a major and a minor groove, and the large stretches of helical DNA are coiled around histone proteins to form nucleosomes ***(Fig. 7.14C)***. They can be condensed further into the chromosomes that can be visualized by light microscopy at metaphase (see below, and ***Figs 7.14*** and ***7.23***).

To express the information in the genome, cells transcribe the code into the single-stranded ribonucleic acid (RNA). RNA is similar to DNA in that it comprises four bases – A, G and C but with uracil (U) instead of T – and a sugar–phosphate backbone with ribose instead of deoxyribose. Several types of RNA are made by the cell. Messenger RNA (mRNA) codes for proteins that are translated on ribosomes. Ribosomal RNA (rRNA) is a key catalytic component of the ribosome, and amino acids are delivered to the nascent peptide chain on transfer RNA (tRNA) molecules. There are also a variety of RNAs that regulate gene expression or RNA processing. These include microRNA (miRNA) and small interfering RNA (siRNA) (see p. 99) that typically bind to a subset of mRNAs and inhibit their translation and/or initiate their degradation (siRNA only initiates degradation). Other non-coding RNAs are involved in X-inactivation and telomere maintenance or RNA splicing and maturation.

DNA transcription

A gene is usually 20–40 kilobases of DNA (but the muscle protein dystrophin is 2.4 Mb long) that contains the code for a polypeptide sequence. Three adjacent nucleotides (a codon) specify a particular amino acid, such as AGA for arginine. There are only 20 common amino acids, but 64 possible codon combinations make up the genetic code. This redundancy means that most amino acids are encoded by more than one triplet, and additional codons are used to signal initiation or termination of polypeptide-chain synthesis.

RNA is transcribed from the DNA template by an enzyme complex of more than 100 proteins, including RNA polymerase, transcription factors and enhancer proteins. Promoter regions upstream of the gene dictate the start point and direction of transcription. The complex binds to the promoter region, the nucleosomes are remodelled to allow access, and a DNA helicase unwinds the double helix. RNA, like DNA, is synthesized in the 5′ to 3′ direction as ribonucleotides are added to the growing 3′ end of a nascent transcript. RNA polymerase does this by base-pairing the ribonucleotides to the DNA template strand it is reading in the 3′ to 5′ direction. Messenger RNA is modified as it is synthesized ***(Fig. 7.15)***. It is capped at the 5′ end with a modified guanine that is required for efficient processing of the mRNA and translation. The 3′ end of the mRNA is modified with up to 200 A nucleotides by the enzyme poly-A polymerase. This 3′ poly-A tail is essential for nuclear export (through the nuclear pores), stability and efficient translation into protein by the ribosome. Human protein coding sequences (exons) are interrupted by intervening sequences that are non-coding (introns) at multiple positions ***(Fig. 7.15)***. These are spliced from the nascent message in the nucleus by an RNA/protein complex called a spliceosome. Differential splicing can cause exons to be spliced alongside their intervening introns. This contributes significantly to the complexity of the human transcriptome, as proteins translated from these messages lack particular domains and therefore have different activity.

Control of gene expression

The genome of all cells in the body encodes the same genetic information, yet different cell types express very different subsets of proteins. Gene expression is controlled at many steps from transcription to protein degradation. However, for many genes, transcription is the key point of regulation. This is controlled primarily by proteins, which bind to short sequences within the promoter regions that either repress or activate transcription, or to more distant sequences where proteins bind to enhance expression. These transcription factors and enhancers are often the end-points of signalling pathways that transduce extracellular signals to change gene expression (see ***Fig. 7.12***).

This level of regulation often involves the translocation of an activated factor from the cytoplasm to the nucleus. In the nucleus, these DNA binding proteins recognize the shape and position of hydrogen bond acceptor and donor groups within the major and minor grooves of the double helix (i.e. the double helix does not need to unwind). There are several classes of DNA binding protein that differ in the protein structural motif that allows them to interact with the double helix. These primarily include ***helix-turn-helix***, ***zinc finger*** and ***leucine zipper*** motifs, although protein ***loops*** and ***β-sheets*** are used by some proteins. More permanent control of gene expression patterns can be achieved epigenetically.

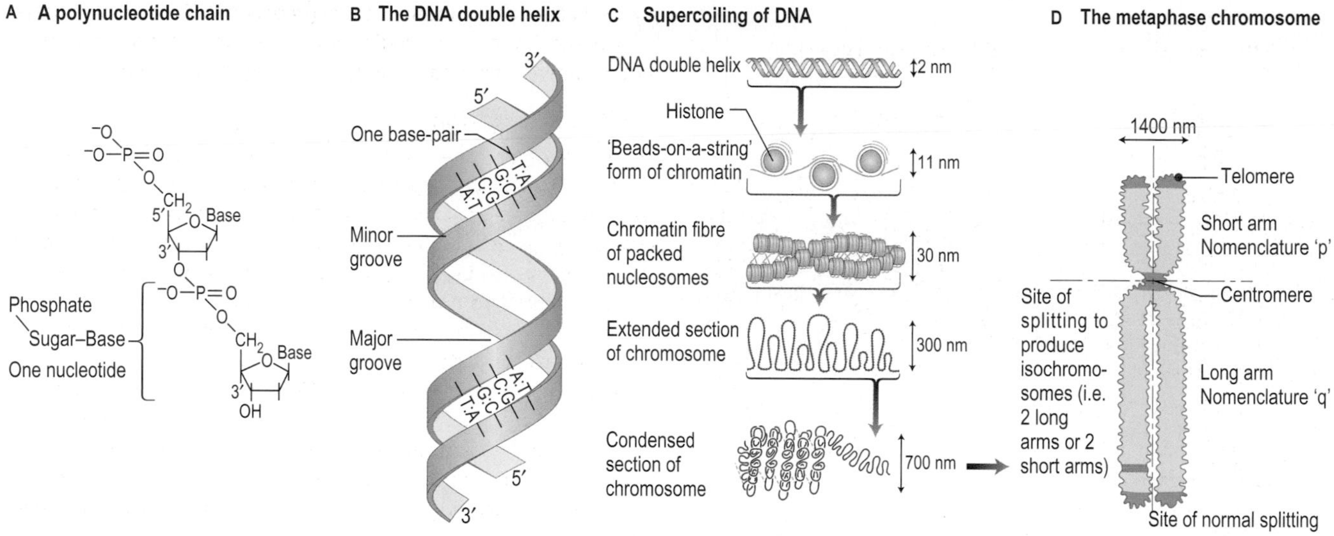

Figure 7.14 DNA and its relationship to human chromosomes. A. Individual nucleotides form a ***polymer*** linked via the deoxyribose sugars to form a single-strand DNA (ssDNA). The 5′ carbon of the sugar is covalently joined to phosphate. The 3′ carbon links the phosphate on the 5′ carbon of the ribose of the next nucleotide, forming the sugar–phosphate backbone of the nucleic acid. The 5′ to 3′ linkage gives orientation to a sequence of DNA. **B. *Double-stranded DNA.*** The two strands of DNA are held together by hydrogen bonds between the bases. T pairs with A, and G with C. The orientation of the complementary ssDNA is thus complementary and antiparallel. The helical three-dimensional structure has major and minor grooves, and a complete turn of the helix contains 12 base-pairs. The grooves are structurally important: DNA-binding proteins predominantly interact with the major grooves. **C. *Supercoiling of DNA.*** The large helical DNA is coiled into nucleosomes by winding around nuclear proteins (histones), and further condensed by coiling and supercoiling into the chromosomes that are visible at metaphase. **D. *At the end of the metaphase**, DNA replication* results in a twin chromosome joined at the centromere. Chromosomes are assigned a number or X or Y, plus short arm (p) or long arm (q). The region or subregion is defined by the transverse light and dark bands observed when staining with Giemsa (hence G-banding) or quinacrine, and numbered from the centromere outwards. ***Chromosome constitution=chromosome number+sex chromosomes+abnormality***; e.g. 46XX=normal female; 47XX+21=Down syndrome (trisomy 21); 46XYt (2;19) (p21; p12) – male with a normal number of chromosomes but a translocation between chromosome 2 and 19 with breakages at short-arm bands 21 and 12 of the respective chromosomes.

The term '***epigenetics***' is used to explain changes in gene expression that do not involve changes in the underlying DNA sequence. Despite not altering the decoding sequence, the effects of epigenetic changes are stable over rounds of cell division, and sometimes between generations. A number of systems initiate and sustain these changes:

- ***Modifications to DNA's surface structure***, but not its base pair sequence – DNA methylation resulting in cytosine being converted to 5-methyl cytosine. This occurs mainly in sites where a cytosine molecule is next to a guanidine nucleotide, a CpG site. When CpG islands (groups of CpG sites) in the promoter region are methylated, gene expression is repressed.
- ***Modification of chromatin proteins*** (in particular, acetylation of histones), which will not only support DNA but bind it so tightly as to regulate gene expression. At the extreme, such binding can permanently prevent the DNA sequences being exposed to, let alone acted on by, gene transcription (DNA-binding) proteins.

Most of the genome is transcribed but only a minority of transcripts encode proteins (see 'Human genetics', p. 106). The non-coding RNAs (ncRNAs) include a group that regulate gene expression (see 'DNA and RNA structure', pp. 97–98). miRNAs and siRNAs are short ncRNAs (19–29 base-pairs (bp)) that together regulate expression of approximately 30% of genes by degradation of transcripts or repression of protein synthesis. A growing range of additional regulatory ncRNA classes are being identified, many of which control gene expression by epigenetic mechanisms.

Epigenetic modification is also 'heritable', meaning that a dividing liver cell, for example, can give rise to two daughter cells with the same epigenetic signals, such that they express the appropriate transcriptome for a liver cell. Epigenetic change forms the basis of genomic imprinting (see p. 115).

Epigenetic change in gene expression also occurs in cancer. An example is DNA methylation repressing tumour suppressor genes. Targeted therapy is already playing a big role in the control of malignant disease

Further reading

Rivera CM, Ren B. Mapping human epigenomes. *Cell* 2013; 155:39–55.
Zhou H, Hu H, Lai M. Non-coding RNAs and their epigenetic regulatory mechanisms. *Biol Cell* 2010; 102:645–655.

The cell cycle and mitosis

The cell duplication cycle has four phases – G1, S, G2 and mitosis ***(Fig. 7.16)*** – and takes about 20–24 hours to complete for a rapidly dividing adult cell. G1, S and G2 are collectively known as interphase, during which the cell doubles in mass (the two gap phases are for growth) and duplicates its 46 chromosomes (S phase). ***Mitosis*** describes, in four subphases (prophase, metaphase, anaphase and telophase; ***Fig. 7.17***), the process of chromosome separation and nuclear division before cytokinesis (division of the cytoplasm into two daughter cells).

Synthesis phase: DNA replication

DNA synthesis by a multi-enzyme complex is initiated simultaneously at multiple replication forks in the genome. The key components of the replication machinery are DNA helicase, DNA primase, DNA polymerase and single-stranded DNA binding proteins.

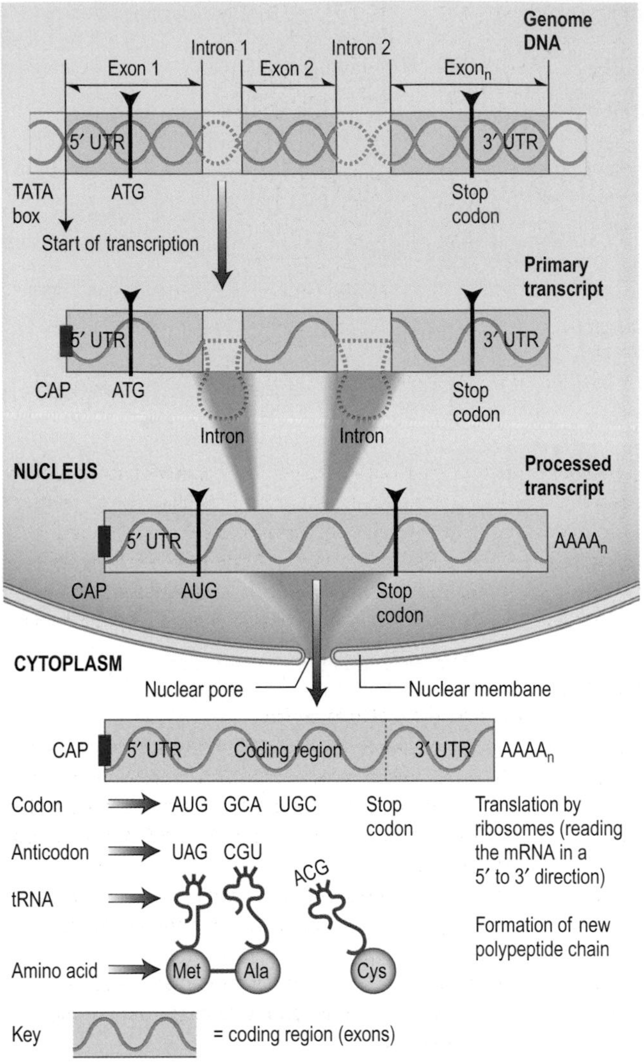

Figure 7.15 **Transcription and translation (DNA to RNA to protein).** **RNA polymerase** transcribes an RNA copy of the DNA gene sequence. The **transcript** is capped at the 5′ end by the addition of an inverted guanine residue, which is then methylated to form 7-methylguanosine. At the 3′ end, the sequence AAUAAA is recognized by endonuclease, and the transcript cleaved 20 base-pairs further downstream. **Poly-A polymerase** then adds adenosine residues to the 3′ end, forming a poly-A tail (polyadenylation). The **introns** are then spliced to produce the mature messenger RNA (mRNA), which is trafficked to the cytosol via nuclear pores. **Ribosomal subunits** assemble on the 5′ end of the mRNA to translate the message into protein for which transfer RNAs (tRNAs) deliver the amino acid building blocks.

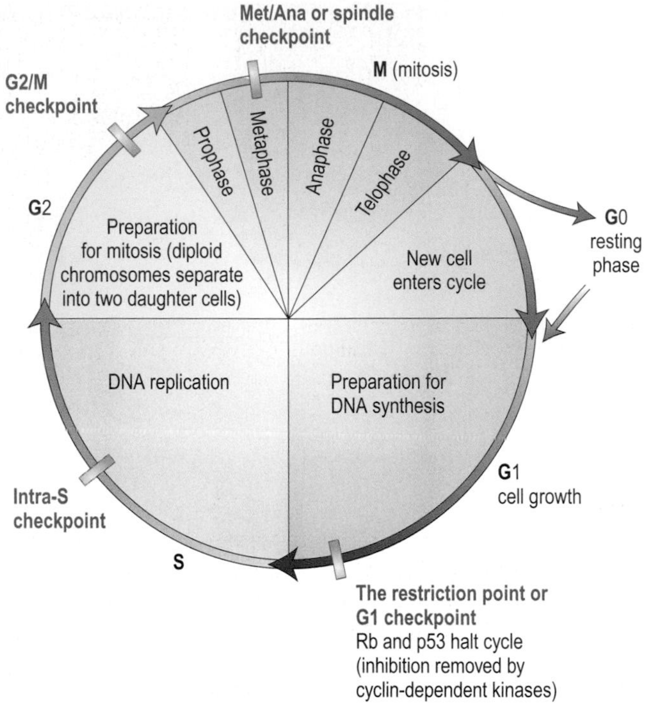

Figure 7.16 **The cell cycle.** Cells are stimulated to leave non-cycle **G0** to enter G1 phase by growth factors. **During G1**, transcription of the DNA synthesis molecules occurs. Rb is a 'checkpoint' (inhibition molecule) between G1 and S phases and must be removed for the cycle to continue. This is achieved by the action of the cyclin-dependent kinase produced during G1. During the **S phase**, any DNA defects will be detected and p53 will halt the cycle (see p. 119). Following DNA synthesis (S phase), cells enter **G2**, a preparation phase for cell division. Mitosis takes place in the **M phase**. The new daughter cells can now either enter **G0** and differentiate into specialized cells, or re-enter the cell cycle.

DNA helicase

DNA helicase hydrolyses ATP to unwind the double helix and expose each strand as a template for replication. The two strands are antiparallel, and DNA can only be extended by addition of nucleotide triphosphates to the hydroxyl of the 3′ end of the growing chain. For the leading template strand, the replication fork moves in a 3′ to 5′ direction along the template, meaning that the newly synthesized strand is synthesized in a 5′ to 3′ direction. At the same replication fork, the antiparallel strand is being exposed in a 5′ to 3′ direction and therefore requires a distinct priming process.

DNA primase

DNA primase synthesizes a short (approximately 10 nucleotide) RNA molecule annealed to the DNA template, which acts as a primer for DNA polymerase.

DNA polymerase

DNA polymerase extends the primer by adding nucleotides to the 3′ end. For the leading template strand, the RNA primer is only required to initiate synthesis once and polymerization continues just behind the replication fork. For the antiparallel strand, DNA primase synthesizes RNA primers at approximately every 200 nucleotides to prime DNA synthesis in the opposite direction to the movement of the replication fork. To allow for this, the synthesis against this template is delayed and so it is called the lagging strand and requires more of the strand to be exposed for DNA primase and DNA polymerase to engage.

Single-stranded DNA binding proteins

These are required to bind to the exposed single-stranded DNA and stabilize it. DNA polymerase extends the RNA primer to cover the 200 nucleotides between each RNA primer on the lagging strand. These RNA/DNA hybrids are called ***Okazaki fragments***.

- *RNAase H* removes the RNA primer from the preceding Okazaki fragment; DNA polymerase extends the new strand over the gap.
- *DNA ligase* joins the two DNA fragments together.

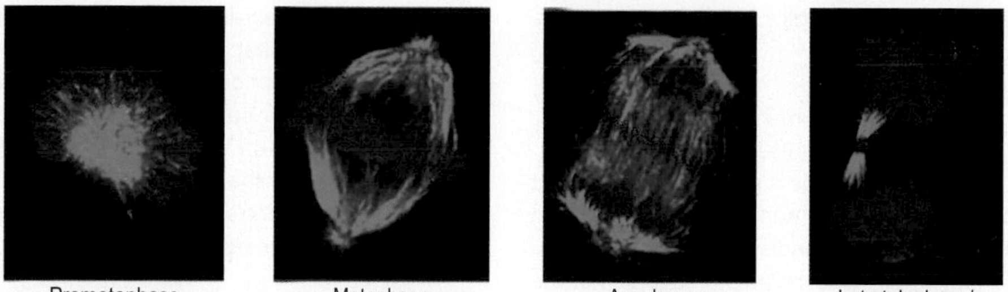

Figure 7.17 Phases of mitosis. DNA is in blue and the microtubules of the cytoskeleton and mitotic spindle are in green. The red marker CENP-V labels kinetochores in prometaphase and metaphase, the mid-zone in anaphase and the mid-body in cytokinesis. *(Courtesy of Tadeu AM, Ribeiro S, Johnston J et al. CENP-V is required for centromere organization, chromosome alignment and cytokinesis.* EMBO Journal *2008; 27:2510–2522.)*

The phases of mitosis

Prophase

The two sister chromatids (the replicated chromosomes held together by proteins called cohesins) condense in the nucleus. The two centrosomes, between which the microtubules of the mitotic spindle will form, move apart in the cytoplasm. At the end of prophase (sometimes known as prometaphase), the nuclear membrane breaks down and the spindle microtubules attach to the kinetochore protein complex bound to the sister chromatids.

Metaphase

The chromosomes are aligned on a central plane with the two centrosomes at opposite poles. The sister chromatids are attached to microtubules from different centrosomes via the kinetochore.

Anaphase

The cohesins break down and the sister chromatids are pulled in opposite directions as the microtubules shorten towards their respective spindle poles.

Telophase

Each set of daughter chromosomes is held at a spindle pole and the nuclear envelope reforms around the genome of each new daughter cell.

Cytokinesis

Binary fission of the cytoplasm begins in telophase, before the completion of mitosis, with the appearance of a ring of actin and myosin filaments around the equator of the cell. Cytokinesis is completed as the ring contracts to create a cleavage furrow and separate the two daughter cells.

Control of the cell cycle and checkpoints

Cells can exit the cell cycle and become quiescent. Indeed, most terminally differentiated adult cells are in a phase termed G0, in which the cycling machinery is switched off. In some cell types, the switch is irreversible (e.g. in neurones), but others, like hepatocytes, retain the ability to re-enter the cell cycle and proliferate. This gives the liver a significant ability to regenerate following damage.

Cyclin-dependent kinases (Cdks), Retinoblastoma protein (Rb) and p53

Progression through the cell cycle is tightly controlled and punctuated by three key checkpoints when the cell interprets environmental and cellular signals to determine whether it is appropriate or safe to proceed ***(Fig. 7.16)***. The switches that allow progression beyond these checkpoints are a family of small protein complexes called cyclin-dependent kinases (Cdks) that phosphorylate serines or threonines in key target proteins at each stage. It is the regulatory cyclin subunit of the Cdks that oscillates during the cell cycle (the actual kinase subunit may be present throughout but only activated by the transient expression of its cognate cyclin).

Checkpoints

Restriction point (G1 checkpoint)

The restriction point works to ensure that the cell cycle does not progress into S-phase unless growth conditions are favourable and the genomic DNA is undamaged. The cyclin-Cdk complexes active early in S-phase are denoted S-Cdk (cyclin A with Cdk1 or Cdk2).

S-Cdks have two roles:

- to phosphorylate their target proteins to initiate helix unwinding of the DNA at origins of replication, allowing the replication complex to begin DNA synthesis
- to prevent re-initiation at the same origin during the same cell cycle (because it would be deleterious to copy parts of the genome more than once).

S-Cdks are themselves subject to regulation by G1-Cdk (cyclin D1–3 with Cdk4 or Cdk5) and G1/S-Cdk (cyclin E with Cdk2), both of which can stimulate cyclin A synthesis. Two major cancer pathways converge on this checkpoint via the cyclin-Cdks:

- ***G1-Cdk*** responds positively to mitogenic (pro-growth) environmental signals like platelet-derived growth factor (PDGF) or epidermal growth factor (EGF). Activated G1-Cdk phosphorylates and inactivates the retinoblastoma protein (Rb), which releases the transcription factor E2F to stimulate G1/S-Cdk and S-Cdk synthesis that is necessary for progression.
- ***G1/S-Cdk and S-Cdk*** also respond to DNA damage via the p53 pathway. On DNA damage, the transcription factor p53 is phosphorylated and stimulates transcription of the *p21* gene. p21 protein is an inhibitor of both G1/S-Cdk and S-Cdk. Both Rb and p53 are regulators of the restriction point. Loss of function of either disables aspects of the negative control pathways. *Rb* and *p53* are commonly mutated in cancer and both are therefore considered 'tumour suppressor genes' (see p. 115).

G2/M checkpoint

The G2/M checkpoint prevents entry into mitosis in the presence of DNA damage or non-replicated DNA. M-Cdk (cyclin B with Cdk1) accumulates towards the end of G2 but is inactive. Activation of M-Cdk is complex and includes dephosphorylation of M-Cdk by the phosphatase Cdc25. Activated M-Cdk has three roles at the G2/M checkpoint:

- to initiate chromosome condensation
- to promote breakdown of the nuclear membrane
- to initiate assembly of the mitotic spindle.

To achieve this, M-Cdk phosphorylates a number of proteins at this checkpoint. The phosphorylation of condensin is required to coil the DNA and initiate chromosome condensation; phosphorylation of nuclear pore and lamina proteins initiates breakdown of the nuclear membrane; and phosphorylation of microtubule-associated proteins and catastrophe factors are both required for assembly of the mitotic spindle. DNA damage and the presence of non-replicated DNA negatively regulate M-Cdk and prevent entry into mitosis. The kinases that phosphorylate p53 in response to DNA damage and block progression through the restriction point can also phosphorylate and inhibit Cdc25, inactivating M-Cdk. Thus DNA damage also blocks cell cycle progression at this checkpoint.

Met/Ana checkpoint

The metaphase to anaphase checkpoint is regulated by protein degradation. The anaphase-promoting complex APC/C, which is activated by Cdc20, is a ubiquitin ligase that transfers a small protein, ubiquitin, to other proteins, marking them for degradation. The primary targets are securin, and the S- and M-cyclins of the cyclin-Cdks present at the start of mitosis.

Securin is an inhibitor of a protease called 'separase', which, on release, digests the cohesin that holds the two sister chromatids together, allowing them to be pulled apart by the mitotic spindle. APC/C activity is tightly controlled but the complete mechanism remains obscure. It includes a negative feedback loop involving M-Cdk, which phosphorylates APC/C and increases its affinity for Cdc20. Thus M-Cdk induces its own inactivation by activating the ligase that ensures degradation of its own cyclin. APC/C is also negatively regulated via an unknown pathway by kinetochores that remain unattached to the mitotic spindle; thus chromatid separation is inhibited until all 46 duplicated chromosomes are on the spindle.

Protein synthesis and secretion

Protein translation

The mature mRNA is transported through the nuclear pore into the cytoplasm for translation into protein by ribosomes (see ***Fig. 7.15***).

- The two subunits of ribosomes (the 40S and 60S) are formed in the nucleolus from multiple proteins and several rRNAs, before transport to the cytoplasm.
- In the cytoplasm, the two subunits interact on an mRNA molecule, usually via ribosome binding sites encoded in the untranslated 5′ region of the message. The mRNA is then pulled through the ribosome until a translation initiation codon is encountered (usually an AUG coding for methionine).
- As the mRNA is pulled through the ribosome in the 5′ to 3′ direction, codons 3′ to the AUG are recognized by complementary sequences, or anticodons, in tRNA molecules that dock on the ribosome.
- Each tRNA molecule carries an amino acid specific to the anticodon. The amino acids are transferred from tRNA molecules and sequentially linked to the carboxy-terminus of the growing polypeptide by the peptidyl transferase activity of the ribosome.
- The poly-A tail of the mRNA is not translated (3′ untranslated region) and is preceded by a translational stop codon: UAA, UAG or UGA.

Translation of secreted or integral membrane proteins is different. Typically, the first few amino acids of the amino terminus of the nascent polypeptide exit the ribosome and are recognized by a signal recognition particle (SRP) that stops translation until the complex is docked on to the ER via the SRP receptor. Translation then continues and the protein is translocated into or through the ER membrane via the Sec61 translocation complex as it is being synthesized (***co-translational transport***).

Protein structure

The amino acid sequence of a polypeptide chain (its ***primary structure***) ultimately determines its shape. The weak bonds (hydrogen bonds, electrostatic and van der Waals interactions) formed between the side-chains of the different amino acids and/or the peptide backbone provide the ***secondary structure*** (α-helices, β-strands, loops). These are in turn folded into a three-dimensional, ***tertiary structure*** to provide functional protein domains of 40–350 amino acids. The modular nature of domains allows their functionality to be combined in protein complexes of different proteins. This final level of organization is the ***quaternary structure***.

The folding of polypeptides into fully functional proteins is facilitated by an assortment of molecular chaperones, e.g. heat shock proteins (HSP), which bind to partially folded polypeptides and prevent the formation of inappropriate bonds.

Lipid synthesis

Fatty acids, molecules with a hydrocarbon chain of 4–28 carbons, are central to cellular life and human metabolism. They form the hydrophobic moiety of membrane lipids (see p. 87); they are precursors for short-lived, near-acting lipid paracrines such as leukotrienes and prostaglandins; and they are energy stores, particularly in the form of triglycerides.

Fatty acids as an energy store

Long-chain fatty acids can be incorporated into triglycerides, which are relatively inert, lipophilic compounds that can be stored as fat droplets in cells (particularly adipocytes). When blood glucose is low, these triglycerides are hydrolysed, secreted into the bloodstream as free fatty acids, and distributed as an energy source for the cells of the body. In the recipient cell, fatty acids are metabolized in the mitochondrion to produce acetyl-CoA for the Krebs cycle (see pp. 103–104). This is a particularly efficient storage system as, gram for gram, triglyceride produces six times the amount of energy than glycogen and occupies less volume in the cell.

Essential fatty acids

Unsaturated fatty acids (UFAs) have carbon–carbon double bonds that are introduced by desaturase enzymes by removal of the hydrogens. The remaining hydrogens on either side of the double bond can be on the same side of the chain (*cis*) or on opposite sides (*trans*). The acyl chain of *cis* UFAs is kinked, which influences the packing of membrane lipids and the function of the membrane barrier. Humans have desaturases that can introduce some double bonds but lack a desaturase required to make linoleic acid or alpha-linolenic acid. These fatty acids have double bonds 6 and 3 carbons from their respective omega ends (the methyl end of the chain). Omega-6 and omega-3 UFAs are essential fatty acids that must be obtained from the diet (see pp. 186–187). They are precursors of arachidonic acid and eicosapentaenoic acid, respectively, from which cyclo-oxygenase 1 and 2 (COX-1 and 2) (see ***Fig. 24.30***) produce the paracrines that play roles in inflammation, pain, fever and airway constriction.

Intracellular trafficking, exocytosis (secretion) and endocytosis

The molecular composition, the lipids and proteins of each type of organelle membrane, is different and distinct from that of the plasma membrane, yet there is a continuous flux of material between many of the different compartments. Much of this flow is via vesicles that carry cargo and bud from one compartment to fuse with another. The process is regulated by an array of lipids and membrane proteins (coat proteins, adaptors, signalling molecules and fusion proteins).

- ***Budding*** of vesicles involves recruitment of coat proteins and adaptors to the membrane. Thus, a receptor, on binding to its ligand, may stimulate a kinase to phosphorylate phosphatidylinositol, or activate a small GTPase like Arf or Sarl, increasing their affinities for a coat protein or adaptor. The coat protein (clathrin at the plasma membrane, COPI at the Golgi, and COPII in the ER) forms a mesh around the developing vesicle (see ***Fig. 7.4***). Fully-formed vesicles normally shed their coat (often triggered by GTP hydrolysis by the GTPase), leaving the adaptor/receptor/lipid combination to identify the vesicle.
- ***Targeting and trafficking*** are mediated by a different family of GTPases (Rab proteins) that recognize the combination of vesicle surface markers and target them appropriately. Once activated by GTP, the Rab proteins are lipid-anchored to the vesicle, where they engage with a diverse pool of Rab effectors. These can be motor proteins that traffic the vesicle along the microfilament and microtubule fibres of the cytoskeleton, or tethering proteins on the target membrane.
- ***Fusion*** is accomplished by membrane-fusion SNARES (see ***Fig. 7.4***). The v-SNARE protein on the vesicle (often associated with the Rab effector) interacts with the t-SNARE on the target membrane to facilitate fusion of the two compartments (distinct combinations of v-SNARE and t-SNARE specify particular pathways).

Vesicles that fuse with the plasma membrane replenish membrane lipids and proteins, and also release cargo extracellularly (exocytosis; see ***Fig. 7.4***). Clathrin-coated vesicles are also used to recycle protein from the plasma membrane, and import extracellular cargo to internal compartments called ***endosomes*** in a process called ***endocytosis***. From endosomes, the receptors may be recycled back to the membrane, while the cargo is sent for degradation in the lysosome.

Pinocytosis and ***phagocytosis*** (see p. 89) are forms of endocytosis. Endocytosis can also occur via plasma membrane microdomains or lipid rafts called caveolae, which pinch in to form uncoated vesicles that fuse with endosomes. Endocytosed vesicles can also be transported across the cell in a process called transcytosis. For example, cargo can be endocytosed at the apical surface of an epithelial cell and exocytosed across the basolateral membrane.

Energy production

As food is catabolized, cells temporarily store the energy released in carrier molecules. These include reduced nicotinamide adenine dinucleotide (***NADH***) and reduced nicotinamide adenine dinucleotide phosphate (***NADPH***), which release energy as they are oxidized to NAD^+ and $NADP^+$. The molar ratio of NAD^+ to NADH is typically high in a cell because NAD^+ is used as an oxidizing agent in catabolic pathways. In contrast, the molar ratio of $NADP^+$ to NADPH is typically low because NAPH is used as a reducing agent in anabolic reactions. The most versatile carrier is adenosine triphosphate (***ATP***). ATP can be hydrolysed to ADP and phosphate (Pi) and the release of energy used to power less favourable reactions.

Lipids and polysaccharides provide most energy in a human diet, although protein can also be used. Enzymes secreted into the gut break down these polymers to their respective building blocks of fatty acids and sugars, which are absorbed by the apical membrane of the gut epithelium (the transporters involved in the transcellular transport of glucose across the enterocyte are described in ***Fig. 13.30***). Fatty acids and sugars are catabolized by the cell to produce an array of activated carrier molecules.

Glycolysis

The six-carbon glucose is primarily catabolized in ten steps by enzymes of the glycolytic pathway (see ***Fig. 16.22***) to produce two three-carbon molecules of the carboxylic acid, pyruvate. Glycolysis occurs in the cytosol and the first three steps actually consume energy (2×ATP), but the remaining steps generate 4×ATP and 2×NADH, giving a net return of 2×ATP and 2×NADH.

Pyruvate is central to metabolism. It can be catabolized as fuel for the Krebs cycle and oxidative phosphorylation. It can regulate the cellular redox state by dehydration to lactate and regeneration of NADH. It can be a precursor for anabolism of fuels (glucose, glycogen and fatty acids), or amino acids via conversion to alanine. The fate of pyruvate depends on the environmental conditions and needs of the cell.

Under anaerobic conditions (e.g. in skeletal muscle following prolonged exercise), NAD^+ must be regenerated (because it is needed as an oxidizing reagent in the catabolism of glucose), and pyruvate is *red*uced to lactate as NADH is *ox*idized to NAD^+ in a 'redox' reaction catalysed by lactate dehydrogenase. This allows the muscle to continue to catabolize glucose to generate ATP under conditions in which metabolic oxygen is limiting. The lactate is secreted into the bloodstream and is ultimately metabolized by the liver back into glucose by gluconeogenesis, consuming 6×ATP in the process. This cycle of anaerobic respiration that produces lactate in muscle, which is released into the bloodstream to be taken up by the liver for reconversion to glucose, is known as the ***Cori cycle*** (see ***Fig. 14.3***).

Krebs cycle

Under aerobic conditions, the fate of pyruvate is different. It is transported into the mitochondrion, where it is decarboxylated to acetyl-CoA and NADH, with CO_2 released as a waste product. The acetyl-CoA formed from pyruvate (or from catabolism of amino acids or β-oxidation of fatty acids) enters the ***Krebs cycle*** in the matrix of the mitochondrion, where it is condensed with the four-carbon oxaloacetate to form the six-carbon citric acid. Citric acid has three carboxylate groups, providing the alternative names for the Krebs cycle (*the citric acid or tricarboxylic acid cycle*). In eight reactions, the Krebs cycle oxidizes two of the six carbons of citric acid to 2×CO_2, regenerates oxaloacetate to enter the next cycle, and in the process, provides enough energy to produce 1×GTP, 3×NADH and 1×reduced flavin adenine dinucleotide ($FADH_2$, a carrier of electrons much like NADH). The latter two products feed their electrons into the electron transport chain, where they are used to make ATP from ADP and Pi, a process known as ***oxidative phosphorylation***.

In addition to energy production, glycolysis and the Krebs cycle provide precursors for the anabolism of amino acids, cholesterol, fatty acids, nucleotides, amino sugars and lipids.

Oxidative phosphorylation

The activated carriers NADH and $FADH_2$ carry high-energy electrons as hydride (a proton H^+ and two electrons), which are donated to complexes of the electron transport chain, in the process regenerating NAD^+ and FAD as oxidizing agents for continued oxidative metabolism. The electrons are passed down the series of inner membrane proteins of the mitochondrion, moving to a lower-energy state at each step until they are finally transferred to oxygen to produce water (hence the requirement for molecular oxygen). The energy released by the electrons is used to efflux protons (H^+) into the inter-membrane space, setting up an H^+ electrochemical gradient, which the ATP synthase (or F_0F_1 ATPase), another integral membrane protein, uses to drive the formation of ATP from ADP and Pi. Oxidative phosphorylation produces the bulk of the cellular ATP. A single molecule of glucose is able to produce a net yield of approximately 30×ATP. Only two of these come from glycolysis directly.

Cellular degradation and death

Cell dynamics

Cell components are continually being formed and degraded. Most of the degradation steps involve ATP-dependent multi-enzyme complexes. Old cellular proteins are identified and modified by 'ubiquitin', a small 8.5 kDa protein present in all living cells. 'Ubiquitination' can deactivate a protein and trigger its internalization from the membrane (both of which are reversible), or it can target the protein for degradation by the lysosome or proteosome (a large proteolytic multi-enzyme complex). Failure to remove dysfunctional or misfolded proteins can result in the development of chronic debilitating disorders. For example, Alzheimer's and frontotemporal dementias are associated with the accumulation of proteins that are resistant to ubiquitin-mediated proteolysis. Similar proteolytic-resistant ubiquitinated proteins give rise to the inclusion bodies found in myositis and myopathies. This resistance can be due to point mutation in the target protein itself (e.g. mutant *p53* in cancer; see p. 119) or can result from an external factor that alters the conformation of the normal protein to create a proteolytic-resistant shape, as in the prion protein of variant Creutzfeldt–Jakob disease (vCJD). Other conditions include von Hippel–Lindau syndrome (see p. 791) and Liddle syndrome (see p. 166).

Free radicals

A free radical is any atom or molecule that contains one or more unpaired electrons, making it more reactive than the native species. The major free radical species produced in the human body are the hydroxyl radical (OH), the superoxide radical (O_2^-) and nitric oxide (NO).

Free radicals are implicated in a large number of human diseases. The hydroxyl radical is by far the most reactive species but the others can generate more reactive species as breakdown products. When a free radical reacts with a non-radical, a chain reaction ensues, which results in direct tissue damage by membrane lipid peroxidation. Furthermore, hydroxyl radicals can cause genetic mutations by attacking purines and pyrimidines. Superoxide dismutase (SOD) converts superoxide to hydrogen peroxide and is thus an inherent protective antioxidant mechanism. Patients with dominant familial forms of amyotrophic lateral sclerosis (motor neurone disease; see pp. 879–880) have mutations in the gene for Cu-Zn SOD-1 catalase. Glutathione peroxidases are enzymes that remove hydrogen peroxide generated by SOD in the cell cytosol and mitochondria.

Free radical scavengers bind reactive oxygen species. Alpha-tocopherol, urate, ascorbate and glutathione remove free radicals non-catalytically by direct interaction. Severe deficiency of α-tocopherol (vitamin E deficiency) causes neurodegeneration. There is some evidence that cardiovascular disease and cancer can be prevented by a diet rich in substances that diminish oxidative damage (see p. 201). The principal dietary antioxidants are vitamin E, vitamin C, β-carotene and flavonoids.

Heat shock proteins

The heat shock response is a highly conserved and ancient response to tissue stress (chemical and physical) that is mediated by activation of specific genes, leading to the production of specific heat shock proteins (HSPs). The diverse functions of HSPs include the transport of proteins in and out of specific cell organelles, acting as molecular chaperones (the catalysis of protein folding and unfolding) and the degradation of proteins (often by ubiquitination pathways). As well as heat, cytotoxic chemicals and free radicals can trigger HSP expression. The unifying feature, which leads to the activation of HSPs, is the accumulation of damaged intracellular protein. Tumours have an abnormal thermotolerance, which is the basis for the observation of the enhanced cytotoxic effect of chemotherapeutic agents in hyperthermic subjects. HSPs are expressed in a wide range of human cancers and are implicated in tumour cell proliferation, differentiation, invasion, metastasis, cell death and immune response.

Autophagy

Cells continually recycle material. For example, cellular proteins are degraded by the proteasome (see p. 104), and mRNA can be de-tailed and degraded by the exosome or decapping complex. Cells respond to stresses like starvation by degrading much of their cytoplasmic contents in order to recycle components and survive.

Cells achieve this by autophagy, during which everything from sugars, lipids, protein aggregates, ribosomal particles and organelles are enclosed in a double membrane (a vesicle that forms a cup shape and extends around the material to be degraded; see ***Fig. 7.6***). The new autophagosome then fuses with a lysosome to degrade the contents by acid hydrolysis. Autophagic induction is complex and still not completely understood, but it has roles in tumour growth and elimination of intracellular microorganisms and toxic misfolded proteins, such as those that give rise to neurodegenerative disorders. Autophagy can suppress apoptotic cell death induced by chemotherapy, while excessive autophagy in response to starvation can lead to autophagic cell death.

Necrotic cell death

In necrotic cell death, external factors (e.g. hypoxia, chemical toxins, injury) damage the cell irreversibly. Necrotic cell death is associated with ischaemia and stroke, cardiac failure, neurodegeneration and pathogen infection, and occurs in the centre of tumours deprived of a blood supply. Characteristically, there is an influx of water and ions, after which the cell and its organelles swell and rupture. Lysosomal proteases released into the cytosol cause widespread degradation. There is a rise in cytosolic calcium, increased reactive oxygen species production, intracellular acidification and ATP depletion. Necrosis is regulated and is sometimes referred to as necroptosis; the cellular processes and activated pathways are still being investigated. Necrotic cell lysis induces acute inflammatory responses owing to the release of lysosomal enzymes into the extracellular environment.

Apoptotic cell death

Most terminally differentiated cells can no longer replicate and eventually die by apoptosis, a type of programmed cell death. Apoptosis occurs through the deliberate activation of cellular pathways, which causes cell suicide. In contrast to necrosis, apoptosis is orderly. Cells are destroyed and their remains phagocytosed by adjacent cells and macrophages without inducing inflammation. Apoptosis is essential for many life processes, including tissue maintenance in the adult, tissue formation in embryogenesis, and normal metabolic processes such as the autodestruction of thickened endometrium leading to menstruation in a non-conception cycle. Cells that have accumulated irreparable DNA damage from toxins or ultraviolet radiation also trigger apoptosis via p53 to prevent replication of mutations or progression to cancer. Many chemotherapy and radiotherapy regimens work by triggering apoptotic pathways in the tumour cell.

Apoptosis has characteristic features:

- shrinkage of the cell and its nucleus
- chromatin aggregation into membrane-bound vesicles called apoptotic bodies
- cell 'blebs' (which are intact membrane vesicles) and exposure of phosphatidylserine on the cell surface
- absence of inflammatory response.

Apoptosis requires proteases called caspases, whose action is very tightly regulated. Caspases not only destroy cell organelles, but also cleave nuclear lamin, causing collapse of the nuclear envelope, and activate, through cleavage, nucleases that degrade DNA. Caspase activation can be achieved by:

- signals from outside the cell (the ***extrinsic apoptotic pathway*** or the ***death receptor pathway***)
- internal signals, such as DNA damage (the ***intrinsic apoptotic pathway*** or the ***mitochondrial pathway***) ***(Fig. 7.18)***.

Extrinsic pathway

The extrinsic pathway is required for tissue remodelling and induction of immune self-tolerance. Cells ubiquitously express a member of the tumour necrosis factor (TNF) death receptor family, such as Fas, on their cell surface. Ligand binding (e.g. by Fas ligand expressed on lymphocytes) causes assembly of a death-inducing signalling complex that produces a cascade of caspase activation. The extrinsic pathway can be amplified by induction of the intrinsic pathway.

Intrinsic pathway

In the intrinsic pathway, increased mitochondrial permeability releases pro-apoptotic proteins like cytochrome C. Cellular stresses, such as growth factor withdrawal, p53-dependent cell cycle arrest, DNA damage and intracellular reactive oxygen species accumulation, induce expression of pro-apoptotic Bcl-2 proteins, Bax and Bak. These enter the outer mitochondrial membrane, forming pores that release cytochrome C, which forms a complex (the apoptosome) with other proteins. The apoptosome activates a caspase cascade.

Further reading

Choi AMK, Ryter SW, Levine B. Autophagy in human health and disease. *N Engl J Med* 2013; 368:651–662.

Hotchkiss RS, Strasser A, McDunn JE et al. Cell death. *N Engl J Med* 2009; 361:1570–1583.

Linkermann A, Green DR. Necroptosis. *N Engl J Med* 2014; 370:455–465.

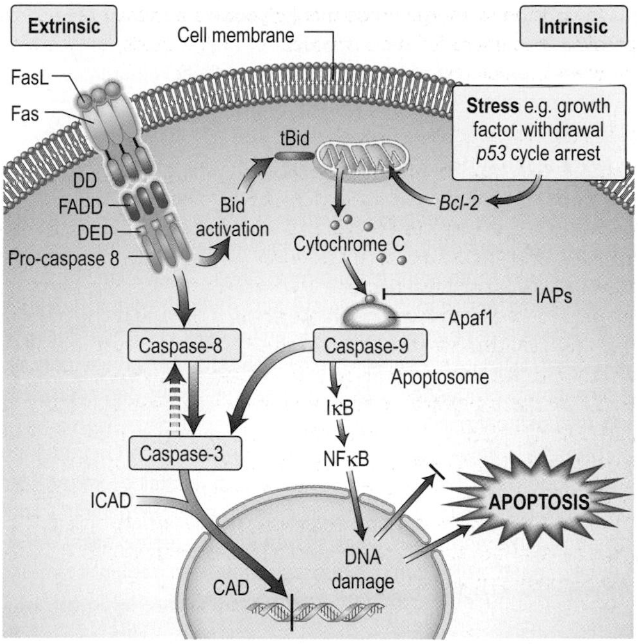

Figure 7.18 **Extrinsic and intrinsic apoptotic signalling network.** The ***Fas protein and Fas ligand (FasL)*** are two proteins that interact to activate an apoptotic pathway. Fas and FasL are both members of the tumour necrosis factor (TNF) family; Fas is part of the transmembrane receptor family and FasL is part of the membrane-associated cytokine family. When the ***homotrimer of FasL binds to Fas***, it causes Fas to trimerize and brings together the ***death domains (DD)*** on the cytoplasmic tails of the protein. The ***adaptor protein***, ***FADD*** (Fas-associating protein with death domain), binds to these ***activated death*** domains and they bind to pro-caspase 8 through a set of ***death effector domains (DED)***. When ***pro-caspase 8s*** are brought together, they transactivate and cleave themselves to release caspase 8, a protease that cleaves protein chains after aspartic acid residues. ***Caspase 8*** then cleaves and activates other caspases, which eventually leads to activation of caspase 3. ***Caspase 3*** cleaves ICAD, the inhibitor of caspase activated DNase (CAD), which frees CAD to enter the nucleus and cleave DNA. Although caspase 3 is the pivotal execution caspase for apoptosis, the processes can be initiated by intrinsic signalling, which always involves mitochondrial release of cytochrome C and activation of caspase 9. The release of ***cytochrome C*** and ***mitochondrial inhibitor of IAPs*** is mediated via Bcl-2 family proteins (including Bax and Bak), forming pores in the mitochondrial membrane. Interestingly, the extrinsic apoptotic signal is aided and amplified by activation of tBid, which recruits Bcl-2 family members and hence also activates the intrinsic pathway. Apaf1, apoptotic protease activating factor 1; Bid, family member of Bcl-2 protein; IAPs, inhibitor of apoptosis proteins; IκB, inhibitor of kappa B; NFκB, nuclear factor kappa B.

STEM CELLS

Following fertilization, the newly formed fertilized cell (the zygote) and those following the first few divisions are totipotent, meaning that they can differentiate into any cell type in the adult body. At the blastula stage of embryonic development, these cells undergo a primary differentiation event to become either the trophectoderm or the inner cell mass (ICM). The trophectoderm gives rise to the fetal cells of the placenta, while the ICM cells are pluripotent and give rise to all other cell types of the body (except those of the placenta); they are more commonly called embryonic stem (ES) cells. Stem cells have two properties:

- ***self-renewal***: the ability to divide indefinitely without differentiating
- ***pluripotency*** or ***totipotency***: the capability to differentiate, given the appropriate signals, into any cell type (except fetal placental cells).

As they begin to differentiate, their ability to self-renew and their potency are reduced but adult progenitor cells (sometimes erroneously referred to as stem cells) remain; these have a limited ability to self-renew and can differentiate into multiple related lineages (multipotent, like haemopoietic 'progenitor cells') or single lineages (unipotent, like muscle satellite cells). The body uses these partially differentiated progenitor cells to replace or repair damaged cells and tissues continually.

Stem cells have great therapeutic potential and can be obtained from blood from the umbilical cord, which contains embryo-like stem cells (which are not as primitive as ES cells but can differentiate into many more cells types than adult progenitor cells). Alternatively, adult cells can be reprogrammed to regain stem-like properties (induced pluripotent stem cells, IPSC).

Cancer 'stem cells'

Only a very small proportion (<1%) of the individual cells from a cancer can form a cancer in a recipient immunodeficient mouse. These cells equate with the population that exclude the fluorescent drug Hoechst 33342 due to presence of a primary active (ABC) drug transporter on their cell surface. They have the characteristics of adult progenitor cells. The high relapse rate of many cancers may well be due to the persistence of these cancer 'stem cells', and new therapies are required to target these in the initial treatment regimen.

Further reading

Ben-David U, Benvenisty N. The tumorigenicity of human embryonic and induced pluripotent stem cells. *Nat Rev Cancer* 2011; 11(4):268–277.
Clevers H. The cancer stem cell: premises, promises and challenges. *Nat Med* 2011; 17:313–319.
Forraz N, McGuckin CP. The umbilical cord: a rich and ethical stem cell source to advance regenerative medicine. *Cell Prolif* 2011; 44(Suppl 1):60–69.
Rice CM, Kemp K, Wilkins A et al. Cell therapy for multiple sclerosis: an evolving concept with implications for other neurodegenerative diseases. *Lancet* 2013; 382:1204–1213.
Wu SM, Hochedlinger K. Harnessing the potential of induced pluripotent stem cells for regenerative medicine. *Nat Cell Biol* 2011; 13:497–505.

HUMAN GENETICS

In 2003, the Human Genome Project was completed, with all 3.2×10^9 bp of DNA sequenced. Over 99% of the DNA sequence is identical between individuals, but still millions of different base-pair variations occur (variants that occur at a frequency >1% are called polymorphisms; pathological polymorphisms are called mutations; single nucleotide polymorphisms are called SNPs, pronounced 'snips'). In addition, the genome contains segmental, duplication-rich regions, where the number of duplications varies between people. These are called copy number variations (CNVs). These variations underlie most human differences, and confer genetic disease and susceptibility to many common diseases. To understand this variation, the 1000 Genomes Project was undertaken and completed in 2015. It involved the sequencing of many genomes from people of Asian, West African and European ancestry. This has now been extended and over 90 000 exomes (protein coding regions of the genome) have been sequenced via the Exome Aggregation Consortium (ExAC).

Genomic DNA encodes approximately 21 000 genes. However, these protein-encoding genes (the exome) comprise only about 1.5% of the human genome. About 90% of the remaining genome is not 'junk' DNA but can be transcribed to form RNA molecules, which are not translated into protein (non-coding RNA, ncRNA). Some of these RNAs have known regulatory roles including microRNAs that can repress gene expression. The remaining DNA also contains evolutionarily conserved non-coding regions, some with known enhancer functions, moderately repeated elements (transposons) with probable viral origin, and microsatellites consisting of short, simple sequence (1–6 nucleotide) repeats. About 10% of the genome is highly repetitive or 'satellite' DNA, consisting of long arrays of tandem repeats. The function of non-protein coding DNA is being intensively investigated, for example, within the ENCODE (Encyclopedia of DNA Elements) project.

Further reading

ENCODE Project Consortium. Identification and analysis of functional elements in 1% of the human genome by the ENCODE pilot project. *Nature* 2007; 447:799–816.
Lander ES. Initial impact of the sequencing of the human genome. *Nature* 2011; 470:187–197.
Nagano T, Fraser P. No-nonsense functions for long noncoding RNAs. *Cell* 2011; 145:178–181.
Zhou H, Hu H, Lai M. Non-coding RNAs and their epigenetic regulatory mechanisms. *Biol Cell* 2010; 102:645–655.
http://genome.wellcome.ac.uk/
http://genome.ucsc.edu/ENCODE/
http://exac.broadinstitute.org/

TOOLS FOR HUMAN GENETIC ANALYSIS

The polymerase chain reaction (PCR)

This technique revolutionized genetic research because minute amounts of DNA – for example, from buccal cell scrapings, blood spots or single embryonic cells – can be amplified over a million times within a few hours. The DNA is amplified between two short (generally 17–25 bases) single-stranded DNA fragments ('oligonucleotide primers') that are complementary to the sequences on different strands at each end of the DNA of interest ***(Fig. 7.19)***.

Hybridization arrays

A fundamental property of DNA is that when two strands are separated – for example, by heating – they will always re-associate and stick together again because of their complementary base sequences. Therefore, the presence or position of a particular gene can be identified using a gene 'probe' consisting of DNA or RNA, with a base sequence that is complementary to that of the sequence of interest. A DNA probe is thus a piece of single-stranded DNA that can locate and bind to its complementary sequence. Hybridization is utilized in array-based platforms, where thousands and thousands of probes can be analysed in one experiment to investigate global gene expression, large-scale genotyping, gene methylation status and/or to seek chromosomal aberrations, including small chromosomal deletion/insertion events or copy number changes ***(Fig. 7.20)***.

DNA sequencing

A chemical process known as dideoxy-sequencing, or Sanger sequencing (after its inventor), allows identification of the exact nucleotide sequence of a piece of DNA. As in PCR, an oligonucleotide primer is annealed adjacent to the region of interest. This primer acts as the starting point for a DNA polymerase to build a new DNA chain that is complementary to the sequence under investigation. Chain extension can be prematurely interrupted when a dideoxynucleotide becomes incorporated (because it lacks the necessary 3′-hydroxyl group). As the dideoxynucleotides are present at a low concentration, not all the chains in a reaction tube will incorporate a dideoxynucleotide in the same place; so the tubes contain sequences of different lengths but which all terminate with a particular dideoxynucleotide. Each base dideoxynucleotide (G, C, T, A) has a different fluorochrome attached, and thus each termination base can be identified by its fluorescent colour. As each strand can be separated efficiently by capillary electrophoresis according to its size/length, simply monitoring the fluorescence as the reaction products elute from the capillary will give the gene sequence ***(Fig. 7.21)***.

Sequencing technology has developed dramatically to the extent that it is now cost-effective and quick to sequence an individual's whole genome in one experiment. This has massive implications in disease gene discovery but also can raise serious ethical considerations. There are a number of different platforms to perform this high-throughput sequencing (or 'next generation sequencing') and new faster and cheaper ones are being developed. For under £500 (2016 price), it is possible to sequence all the coding genes in an individual's human genome (termed the 'exome') to catalogue

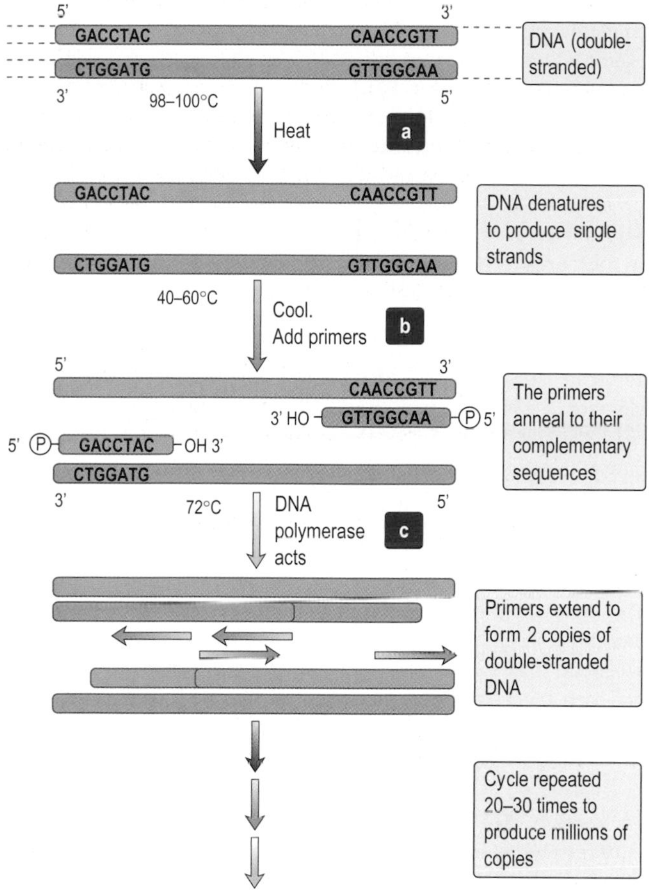

Figure 7.19 Polymerase chain reaction. The technique is based on thermal cycling and has three basic steps. **(a)** The double-stranded genomic DNA is heat-denatured into single-stranded DNA. **(b)** The sample is cooled to favour annealing of the primers to their target DNA. **(c)** A thermostable DNA polymerase extends the primers over the target DNA. After one cycle, there are two copies of double-stranded DNA, after two cycles there are four copies, and so on.

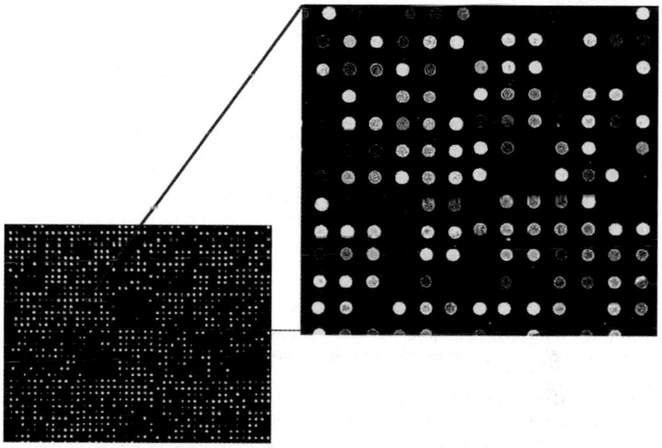

Figure 7.20 Expression microarray. Example of part of a gene chip with hundreds of DNA sequences in microspots. The enlarged area shows the colour coding of no expression (black), over-expression (red), under-expression (green) and equal expression (yellow) of detected mRNA in two related samples.

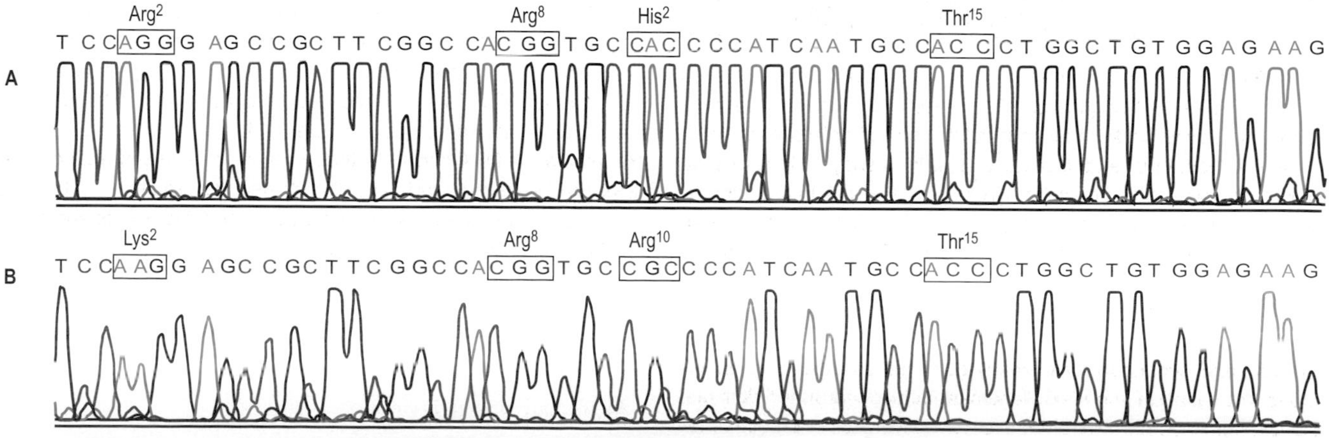

Figure 7.21 Gene sequencing: sequence profiles. A. Part of the normal luteinizing hormone beta chain gene. **B.** A polymorphic variant. The base changes and consequential alterations in amino acid residues are indicated.

all possible disease-associated and non-disease-associated variants in every human gene. As well as sequencing genomic DNA, the technology can be used to sequence RNA (termed RNAseq) to assess gene expression levels accurately, in addition to determining all splice variations and allelic copy number. This can also be used to assess the effect of epigenetic modifications on gene expression.

Identification of gene function

Following sequencing of the genome, the challenge is to understand the function of the protein-coding genes. Most tools rely on the comparison of a cell or animal's phenotype in the presence or absence of the gene in question. Each tool has different merits and faults.

Cell culture

Human cells can be grown in culture flasks in the laboratory and their behaviour (growth rate, morphology, motility, gene expression profile and biochemistry) characterized. A specific gene can then be introduced in a small plasmid (a circle of DNA from which the gene of interest can be expressed) or incorporated into a virus, and the change in cell behaviour assessed to provide an indication of gene function. Alternatively, if the cell line in question already expresses the gene of interest, its expression can be knocked down by RNA interference.

RNA interference (RNAi)

RNAi takes advantage of the cellular machinery that allows microRNAs encoded by the genome to regulate the expression of many genes at the level of messenger RNA stability and translation (see 'Control of gene expression', pp. 98–99). This phenomenon has been exploited in the laboratory to study the function of a gene of interest or, on a much larger scale, the function of each gene in the genome. In such an RNAi screen, a small interfering (si) RNA specific for each gene in the genome is introduced into cells grown *in vitro,* in effect knocking down expression of each gene in approximately 20 000 separate experiments. The phenotype of the cells in each experiment is then monitored to test the effect of loss of gene expression.

Animal models

The effect of a gene at organism level can also be tested by mis-expression/over-expression or knockout of a particular gene in a model animal. Nematode worms (*Caenorhabditis*), fruit flies (*Drosophila*), zebrafish and rodents have all been genetically engineered to identify the function of a gene of interest. Knockout models of the higher organisms can be particularly helpful for medical research to provide a model of disease for exploration of therapeutic intervention. Large-scale mutagenesis programmes are knocking out every gene or regulatory element in the mouse genome. However, it should be noted that the physiology of rodents and humans can differ.

Genetic polymorphisms and linkage studies

Techniques have been developed to identify and quantitate genetic polymorphisms such as single nucleotide polymorphisms (SNPs; see p. 106), microsatellites and copy number variants (CNVs). For example, SNPs consist usually of two nucleotides at a particular site and vary between populations and ethnic groups. They must occur in at least 1% of the population to be a SNP. SNPs can be in coding or non-coding regions of the genes or be between genes, and thus may not change the amino acid sequence of the protein.

Linkage disequilibrium

Polymorphisms that are closer together are more likely to have alleles that move together in a block than those further apart. This phenomenon is called 'linkage disequilibrium' and enables, for example, one SNP variant (tag SNP) in this block to act as a marker for the presence of other SNP variants. Linkage analysis has provided many breakthroughs in mapping the positions of genes that cause genetic diseases, such as the gene for cystic fibrosis, which was found to be tightly linked to a marker on chromosome 7.

The International Hapmap Project

As SNPs close together are inherited in blocks (haplotypes), tag SNPs for each haplotype block are typed and can then be correlated with a specific phenotype. An International Hapmap Project was developed. The Wellcome Trust Case Control Consortium was set up to analyse thousands of DNA samples from patients with different diseases in which there is thought to be a genetic component. Utilizing the Hapmap data and high-density SNP hybridization arrays, genetic risk-associated sequence variants have been found in many diseases and traits, including diabetes, cancer, hypertension, Crohn's disease, height and metabolism.

The 'lod score'

The likelihood of recombination between the marker under study and the disease allele must be taken into account. This degree of likelihood is known as the 'lod score' (the logarithm of the odds) and is a measure of the statistical significance of the observed co-segregation of the marker and the disease gene, compared with what would be expected by chance alone.

- Positive lod scores make linkage more likely.
- Negative lod scores make linkage less likely.

By convention, a lod score of +3 is taken to be definite evidence of linkage because this indicates 1000:1 odds that the co-segregation of the DNA marker and the disease did not occur by chance alone.

Genome databases

Information arising from human genome sequencing is publicly available, providing biological information on every gene in the human genome. Information on any gene describing its protein product, function, tissue specific expression, disease association and sequence variation/mutation can all be easily obtained by searching and manipulating computer-based databases.

Further reading

Biesecker LG, Green RC. Diagnostic clinical genome and exome sequencing. *N Engl J Med* 2014; 370:2418–2425.
http://www.ensembl.org/index.html *Ensembl*
http://genome.ucsc.edu *UCSC Genome Bioinformatics*
http://www.ncbi.nlm.nih.gov *National Center for Biotechnology Information*
http://www.ncbi.nlm.nih.gov/omim *Online Mendelian Inheritance in Man, for information on gene products and their disease association*

THE BIOLOGY OF CHROMOSOMES

Human chromosomes

The nucleus of each diploid cell contains 6×10^9 bp of DNA in long molecules called *chromosomes* (see ***Fig. 7.14***). Chromosomes are massive structures containing one linear molecule of DNA that is wound around histone proteins into small units called nucleosomes, and these are further wound to make up the structure of the chromosome itself.

Diploid human cells have 46 chromosomes, 23 inherited from each parent; thus there are 23 'homologous' pairs of chromosomes (22 pairs of '***autosomes***' and two '***sex chromosomes***'). The sex chromosomes, called X and Y, are not homologous but are different in size and shape. Males have an X and a Y chromosome; females have two X chromosomes. (Primary male sexual characteristics are determined by the *SRY* gene – sex-determining region, Y chromosome.)

The chromosomes are classified according to their size and shape, the largest being chromosome 1. The constriction in the chromosome is the ***centromere***, which can be in the middle of the chromosome (metacentric) or at one extreme end (acrocentric). The centromere divides the chromosome into a short arm and a long arm, referred to as the ***p arm*** and the ***q arm***, respectively ***(Fig. 7.14D)***.

Chromosomes can be stained when they are in the metaphase stage of the cell cycle and are very condensed. The stain gives a different pattern of light and dark ***bands*** that is diagnostic for each chromosome. Each band is given a number, and gene-mapping techniques allow genes to be positioned within a band within an arm of a chromosome. For example, the *CFTR* gene (in which a defect gives rise to cystic fibrosis) maps to 7q21: that is, on chromosome 7 in the long arm in band 21.

During cell division (mitosis), each chromosome divides into two so that each daughter nucleus has the same number of chromosomes as its parent cell. During gametogenesis, however, the number of chromosomes is halved by meiosis, so that, after conception, the number of chromosomes remains the same and is not doubled. In the female, each ovum contains one or other X chromosome, but in the male, the sperm bears either an X or a Y chromosome.

Chromosomes can only be seen easily in actively dividing cells. Typically, lymphocytes from the peripheral blood are stimulated to divide and are processed to allow the chromosomes to be examined. Cells from other tissues can also be used for chromosomal analysis: for example, amniotic fluid, placental cells from chorionic villus sampling, bone marrow and skin ***(Box 7.1)***.

The X chromosome and inactivation

Although females have two X chromosomes (XX), they do not have two doses of X-linked genes (compared with just one dose for a male XY) because of the phenomenon of X inactivation or ***Lyonization*** (after its discoverer, Dr Mary Lyon). In this process, one of the two X chromosomes in the cells of females is epigenetically (see p. 99) silenced through the action of a regulatory ncRNA, so the cell has only one dose of the X-linked genes. Inactivation is random and can affect either X chromosome.

Telomeres and immortality

The ends of chromosomes, telomeres (see ***Fig. 7.14D***, p. 99), do not contain genes but many repeats of a hexameric sequence, TTAGGG. Replication of linear chromosomes starts at coding sites (origins of replication) within the main body of chromosomes and not at the two extreme ends. The extreme ends are therefore susceptible to single-stranded DNA degradation back to double-stranded DNA. Thus, cellular ageing can be measured as a genetic consequence of multiple rounds of replication, with consequential telomere shortening. This leads to chromosome instability and cell death.

Box 7.1 Indications for chromosomal analysis

Chromosome studies may be indicated in the following circumstances:

Antenatal
- Pregnancies in women over 35 years
- Positive maternal serum screening test for aneuploid pregnancy
- Ultrasound features consistent with an aneuploid fetus
- Severe fetal growth retardation
- Sexing of fetus in X-linked disorders

In the neonate
- Congenital malformations
- Suspicion of trisomy or monosomy
- Ambiguous genitalia

In the adolescent
- Primary amenorrhoea or failure of pubertal development
- Growth retardation

In the adult
- Screening of parents of a child with a chromosomal abnormality for further genetic counselling
- Infertility or recurrent miscarriages
- Learning difficulties
- Certain malignant disorders (e.g. leukaemias and Wilms' tumour)

Stem cells have longer telomeres than their terminally differentiated daughters. However, germ cells replicate without shortening of their telomeres. This is because they express an enzyme called telomerase, which protects against telomere shortening by acting as a template primer at the extreme ends of the chromosomes. Most somatic cells (unlike germ and embryonic cells) switch off the activity of telomerase after birth and die as a result of apoptosis. Many cancer cells, however, reactivate telomerase, contributing to their immortality. Conversely, cells from patients with progeria (premature ageing syndrome) have extremely short telomeres. Transient expression of telomerase in various stem and daughter cells is part of their normal biology.

The mitochondrial chromosome

In addition to the 23 pairs of chromosomes in the nucleus of every diploid cell, the mitochondria in the cytoplasm of the cell also have their own genome. The mitochondrial chromosome is a circular DNA (mtDNA) molecule of approximately 16 500 bp, and every base-pair makes up part of the coding sequence. These genes principally encode proteins or RNA molecules involved in mitochondrial function. These proteins are components of the mitochondrial respiratory chain involved in oxidative phosphorylation, producing ATP. They also have a critical role in apoptotic cell death. Every cell contains several hundred mitochondria, and therefore several hundred mitochondrial chromosomes. Virtually all mitochondria are inherited from the mother, as the sperm head contains no (or very few) mitochondria. Disorders mapped to the mitochondrial chromosome are shown in ***Figure 7.22*** and discussed on pages 111–112.

GENETIC DISORDERS

The spectrum of inherited or congenital genetic disorders can be classified as the chromosomal disorders, including mitochondrial chromosome disorders, the Mendelian and sex-linked single-gene disorders, a variety of non-Mendelian disorders, and the multifactorial and polygenic disorders (***Boxes 7.2*** and ***7.3***). All are a result of a

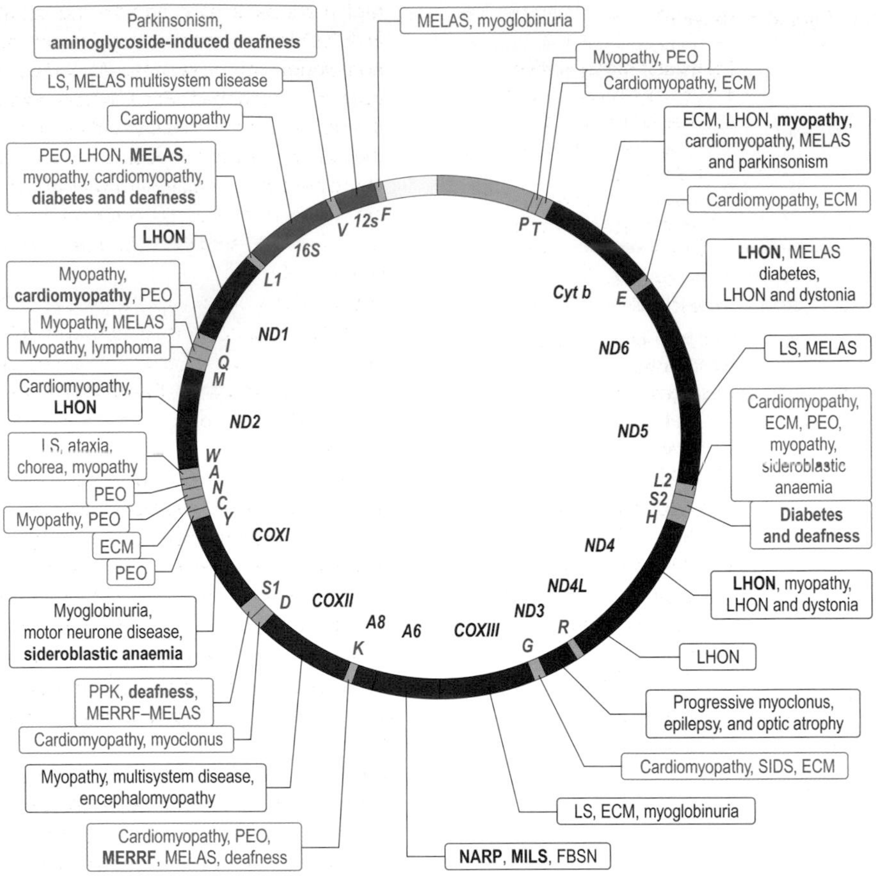

Figure 7.22 Mitochondrial chromosome abnormalities. Disorders that are frequently or prominently associated with mutations in a particular gene are shown in **bold.** Diseases due to mutations that impair mitochondrial protein synthesis are shown in **blue.** Diseases due to mutations in protein-coding genes are shown in **red.** ECM, encephalomyopathy; FBSN, familial bilateral striatal necrosis; LHON, Leber's hereditary optic neuropathy; LS, Leigh syndrome; MELAS, mitochondrial encephalomyopathy, lactic acidosis and stroke-like episodes; MERRF, myoclonic epilepsy with ragged-red fibres; MILS, maternally inherited Leigh syndrome; NARP, neuropathy, ataxia and retinitis pigmentosa; PEO, progressive external ophthalmoplegia; PPK, palmoplantar keratoderma; SIDS, sudden infant death syndrome.

mutation in the genetic code. This may be a change of a single base-pair of a gene, resulting in functional change in the product protein (e.g. thalassaemia) or gross rearrangement of the gene within a genome (e.g. chronic myeloid leukaemia). These mutations can be congenital (inherited at birth) or somatic (arising during a person's life).

Chromosomal disorders

Chromosomal abnormalities are much more common than is generally appreciated. Over half of spontaneous abortions have chromosomal abnormalities, compared with only 4–6 abnormalities per 1000 live births. Specific chromosomal abnormalities can lead to well-recognized and severe clinical syndromes, although autosomal aneuploidy (a differing from the normal diploid number) is usually more severe than the sex-chromosome aneuploidies. Abnormalities may occur in either the number or the structure of the chromosomes.

Abnormal chromosome numbers

If a chromosome or chromatids fail to separate ('non-disjunction') in either meiosis or mitosis, one daughter cell will receive two copies of that chromosome and one daughter cell will receive no copies of the chromosome. If this non-disjunction occurs during meiosis, it can lead to an ovum or sperm having:

- *either* ***an extra chromosome***, so resulting in a fetus that is 'trisomic' and has three instead of two copies of the chromosome
- *or* ***no chromosome***, so the fetus is 'monosomic' and has one instead of two copies of the chromosome.

Non-disjunction can occur with autosomes or sex chromosomes. However, only individuals with trisomy 13, 18 and 21 survive to birth, and most children with trisomy 13 and trisomy 18 die in early childhood. ***Trisomy 21*** (***Down syndrome***) is observed with a frequency of 1 in 650 live births, regardless of geography or ethnic background. This should be reduced with widespread screening (see p. 116). Full ***autosomal monosomies*** are extremely rare and very deleterious. ***Sex-chromosome trisomies*** (e.g. Klinefelter syndrome, XXY) are relatively common. The ***sex-chromosome monosomy*** in which the individual has an X chromosome only and no second X or Y chromosome (i.e. X0) is known as ***Turner's syndrome*** and is estimated to occur in 1 in 2500 live-born girls.

Occasionally, non-disjunction can occur during mitosis shortly after two gametes have fused. It will then result in the formation of two cell lines, each with a different chromosome complement; the person is termed a 'mosaic' individual.

Box 7.2 Prevalence of genetic disease[a]

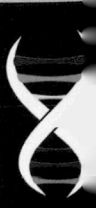

Genetic disease
- 0.5% of all newborns have a chromosomal abnormality
- 7% of all stillborns have a chromosomal abnormality
- 20–30% of all infant deaths are due to genetic disorders
- 11% of paediatric hospital admissions are for children with genetic disorders
- 12% of adult hospital admissions are for genetic causes
- 15% of all cancers have an inherited susceptibility
- 10% of chronic diseases of the adult population (heart, diabetes, arthritis) have a significant genetic component

Congenital malformation
- 3–5% of all births result in congenital malformations
- 30–50% of post-neonatal deaths are due to congenital malformations
- 18% of paediatric hospital admissions are for children with congenital malformations

European incidences per 1000 births

Single-gene disorders: 10
Dominant: 7.0
Recessive: 1.66
X-linked: 1.33

Chromosomal disorders: 3.5
Autosomes: 1.69
Sex chromosomes: 1.80

Congenital malformations: 31
Genetically determined: 0.6
Multifactorial: 30
Non-genetic: ~0.4

[a]*Although individual genetic diseases are rare, regional variation is enormous; the incidence of Down syndrome varies from 1/1000 to 1/100 worldwide. Single-gene diseases collectively comprise over 15 500 recognized genetic disorders. The global prevalence of all single-gene diseases at birth is approximately 10/1000.*

Box 7.3 Genetic disorders

Mendelian
- Inherited or new mutation
- Mutant allele or pair of mutant alleles at single locus
- Clear pattern of inheritance (autosomal or sex-linked) dominant or recessive
- High risk to relatives

Chromosomal
- Loss, gain or abnormal rearrangement of one or more of 46 chromosomes in diploid cells
- No clear pattern of inheritance
- Low risk to relatives

Multifactorial
- Common
- Interaction between genes and environmental factors
- Low risk to relatives

Mitochondrial
- Due to mutations in mitochondrial genome
- Transmitted through maternal line
- Different pattern of inheritance from Mendelian disorders

Somatic cell
- Mutations in somatic cells
- Somatic event is not inherited
- Often give rise to tumours

Very rarely, the entire chromosome set will be present in more than two copies, so the individual may be triploid rather than diploid and have a chromosome number of 69. Triploidy and tetraploidy (four sets) result in spontaneous abortion.

Abnormal chromosome structures

As well as abnormal numbers of chromosomes, chromosomes can have abnormal structures, and the disruption to the DNA and gene sequences may give rise to a genetic disease.

- ***Deletions*** of a portion of a chromosome may give rise to a disease syndrome if two copies of the genes in the deleted region are necessary, and the individual will not be normal with just the one normal copy remaining on the non-deleted homologous chromosome. Many deletion syndromes have been well described. For example, ***Prader–Willi syndrome*** is the result of cytogenetic events resulting in deletion of part of the long arm of chromosome 15; ***Wilms' tumour*** is characterized by deletion of part of the short arm of chromosome 11; and microdeletions in the long arm of chromosome 22 give rise to ***DiGeorge syndrome*** (see p. 140)
- ***Duplications*** occur when a portion of the chromosome is present on the chromosome in two copies, so the genes in that chromosome portion are present in an extra dose. A form of neuropathy, ***Charcot–Marie–Tooth disease*** (see p. 886), is due to a small duplication of a region of chromosome 17.
- ***Inversions*** involve an end-to-end reversal of a segment within a chromosome: for example, 'abcdefgh' becomes 'abcfedgh', as in ***haemophilia*** (see pp. 571–573).
- ***Translocations*** occur if two chromosome regions join together, when they would not do so normally. Chromosome translocations in somatic cells may be associated with tumorigenesis (see p. 607 and ***Fig. 17.21***).

Translocations can be very complex, involving more than two chromosomes, but most are simple and fall into one of two categories:

- ***Reciprocal translocations*** occur when any two non-homologous chromosomes break simultaneously and rejoin, swapping ends. In this case, the cell still has 46 chromosomes but two of them are rearranged. Someone with a balanced translocation is likely to be normal (unless a translocation breakpoint interrupts a gene); however, at meiosis, when the chromosomes separate into different daughter cells, the translocated chromosomes will enter the gametes and any resulting fetus may inherit one abnormal chromosome and have an unbalanced translocation, with physical manifestations.
- ***Robertsonian translocations*** occur when two acrocentric chromosomes join and the short arm is lost, leaving only 45 chromosomes. This translocation is balanced, as no genetic material is lost and the individual is healthy. However, any offspring have a risk of inheriting an unbalanced arrangement. This risk depends on which acrocentric chromosome is involved. The 14/21 Robertsonian translocation is clinically relevant. A woman with this karyotype has a 1 in 8 risk of having a baby with Down syndrome (a male carrier has a 1 in 50 risk). However, they have a 50% risk of producing a carrier like themselves; hence the necessity for genetic family studies. Relatives should be alerted to the increased risk of Down syndrome in their offspring, and should have their chromosomes checked.

Box 7.4 shows some of the syndromes resulting from chromosomal abnormalities.

Mitochondrial chromosome disorders

The mitochondrial chromosome (see ***Fig. 7.11***) carries its genetic information in a very compact form; for example, there are no introns in the genes. Therefore, any mutation has a high chance of having an effect. However, as every cell contains hundreds of mitochondria, a single altered mitochondrial genome will not be noticed. As mitochondria divide, there is a statistical likelihood that there will

Box 7.4 Chromosomal abnormalities: examples of a few syndromes

Syndrome	Chromosome karyotype	Incidence and risks	Clinical features	Mortality
Autosomal abnormalities				
Trisomy 21 (Down syndrome)	47, +21 (95%) Mosaicism Translocation 5%	1:650 (overall) (risk with a 20- to 29-year-old mother 1:1000; >45-year-old mother 1:30)	Flat face, slanting eyes, epicanthic folds, small ears, simian crease, short and stubby fingers, hypotonia, variable learning difficulties, congenital heart disease (up to 50%)	High in first year, but many survive to adulthood
Trisomy 13 (Patau syndrome)	47, +13	1:5000	Low-set ears, cleft lip and palate, polydactyly, micro-ophthalmia, learning difficulties	Rarely survive for more than a few weeks
Trisomy 18 (Edwards syndrome)	47, +18	1:3000	Low-set ears, micrognathia, rocker-bottom feet, learning difficulties	Rarely survive for more than a few weeks
Sex-chromosome abnormalities				
Fragile X syndrome	46, XX, fra (X) 46, XY, fra (X)	1:2000	Most common inherited cause of learning difficulties, predominantly in male Macro-orchidism	
Female				
Turner's syndrome	45, XO	1:2500	Infantilism, primary amenorrhoea, short stature, webbed neck, cubitus valgus, normal IQ	
Triple X syndrome	47, 000	1:1000	No distinctive somatic features, learning difficulties	
Others	48, 000X 49, 000XX	Rare	Amenorrhoea, infertility, learning difficulties	
Male				
Klinefelter syndrome	47, XXY (or XXYY)	1:1000 (more in sons of older mothers)	Decreased crown–pubis:pubis–heel ratio, eunuchoid, testicular atrophy, infertility, gynaecomastia, learning difficulties (20%; related to number of X chromosomes)	
Double Y syndrome	47, XYY	1:800	Tall, fertile, minor mental and psychiatric illness, high incidence in tall criminals	
Others	48, 000Y 49, 000XY		Learning difficulties, testicular atrophy	

be more mutated mitochondria and, at some point, this will give rise to a mitochondrial disease.

Most mitochondrial diseases are myopathies and neuropathies with a maternal pattern of inheritance. Other abnormalities include retinal degeneration, diabetes mellitus and hearing loss. Many syndromes have been described.

Myopathies include chronic progressive external ophthalmoplegia (CPEO); encephalomyopathies include myoclonic epilepsy with ragged-red fibres (MERRF) and mitochondrial encephalomyopathy, lactic acidosis and stroke-like episodes (MELAS) (see p. 892).

Kearns–Sayre syndrome includes ophthalmoplegia, heart block, cerebellar ataxia, deafness and mental deficiency due to long deletions and rearrangements.

Leber's hereditary optic neuropathy (LHON) is the most common cause of blindness in young men, with bilateral loss of central vision and cardiac arrhythmias, and is an example of a mitochondrial disease caused by a point mutation in one gene.

Multisystem disorders include ***Pearson syndrome*** (sideroblastic anaemia, pancytopenia, exocrine pancreatic failure, subtotal villous atrophy, diabetes mellitus and renal tubular dysfunction). In some families, hearing loss is the only symptom, and one of the mitochondrial genes implicated may predispose patients to aminoglycoside cytotoxicity.

Analysis of chromosome disorders

The cell cycle can be arrested at mitosis with colchicine and, following staining, the chromosomes with their characteristic banding can be seen and any abnormalities identified ***(Fig. 7.23)***. This is an automated process with computer scanning software searching for metaphase spreads and then automatic binning of each chromosome to allow easy scoring of chromosome number and banding patterns. Another approach utilizes genome-wide array-based platforms (comparative genomic hybridization (CGH) or chromosomal microarray analysis (CMA)) to identify changes in chromosome copy number and can identify very small interstitial deletions and insertions (<1 Mb in size).

Large region-specific probes are labelled with fluorescently tagged nucleotides and used to allow rapid identification of metaphase chromosomes. This approach allows easy identification of

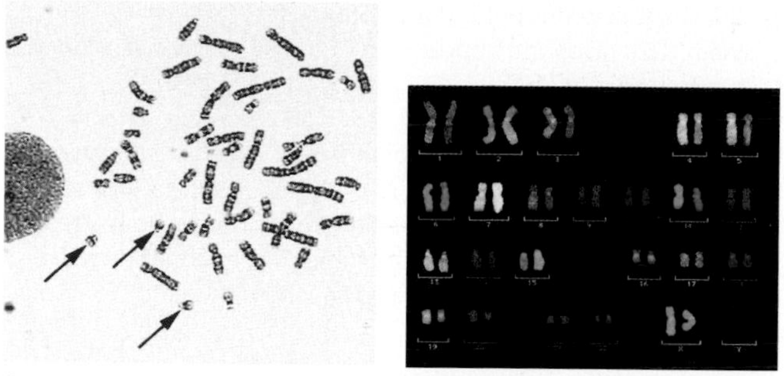
A B

Figure 7.23 Karyotyping. A. G-banded spread of metaphase chromosomes, showing trisomy 21 (arrowed), Down syndrome. **B.** Whole-chromosome painting probes labelled with different fluorochromes or fluorochrome combinations on 24-colour or multiplex fluorescence *in situ* hybridization (mFISH) analysis is based on a DNA probe kit. Digital image analysis software analyses the colour information and identifies the chromosomal origin of each individual pixel within the image. Inter-chromosomal rearrangements will show up as colour changes within the aberrant chromosome. *(Courtesy of D. Lillington, Medical Oncology Unit, St Bartholomew's Hospital.)*

Figure 7.24 Fluorescence *in situ* hybridization (FISH). Two-coloured FISH using a red paint for the *ABL* gene on chromosome 9 and a green paint for the *BCR* gene on chromosome 22 in the anaphase cell nucleus. Where a translocation has occurred, the two genes become juxtaposed on the Philadelphia chromosome and a hybrid yellow fluorescence can be seen only in the affected cell nucleus on the right. *(Courtesy of D. Lillington, Medical Oncology Unit, St Bartholomew's Hospital.)*

chromosomal translocations ***(Fig. 7.24)***. Whole genome sequencing is becoming a common method for identifying deletions, insertions and translocation breakpoints.

Further reading

Archer SL. Mitochondrial dynamics – mitochondrial fission and fusion in human diseases. *N Engl J Med* 2013; 369:2236–2251.

Park CB, Larsson N-G. Mitochondrial DNA mutations in disease and aging. *J Cell Biol* 2011; 193:809–818.

Gene defects

Mendelian and sex-linked single-gene disorders are the result of mutations in coding sequences and their control elements. These mutations can have various effects on the expression of the gene, as explained below, but all cause a dysfunction of the protein product.

Mutations

Although DNA replication is a very accurate process, occasionally mistakes occur and produce changes or mutations. These changes can also occur because of other factors such as radiation, ultraviolet light or chemicals. Mutations in gene sequences or in the sequences that regulate gene expression (transcription and translation) may alter the amino acid sequence in the protein encoded by that gene. In some cases, protein function will be maintained; in other cases, it will change or cease, perhaps producing a clinical disorder. Many different types of mutation occur.

Point mutation

This is the simplest type of change and involves the substitution of one nucleotide for another, so changing the codon in a coding sequence and leading to an amino acid substitution (non-synonymous). For example, **in sickle cell disease**, a mutation within the globin gene changes one codon from GAG to GTG so that, instead of glutamic acid, valine is incorporated into the polypeptide chain, which radically alters its properties. However, substitutions may have no effect on the function or stability of the proteins produced, as several codons code for the same amino acid (synonymous).

Insertion or deletion

Insertion or deletion of one or more bases is a more serious change, particularly if the inserted or deleted DNA is not a multiple of three bases, as this will cause the following sequence to be out of frame.

Splicing mutations

If the DNA sequences that direct the splicing of introns from mRNA are mutated, then abnormal splicing may occur. In this case, the processed mRNA that is translated into protein by the ribosomes may carry intron sequences or miss exons, so altering amino acid composition.

Nonsense mutations

A nonsense mutation is a point mutation in a sequence of DNA that results in a premature stop codon.

Single-gene disease

Monogenetic disorders involving single genes can be inherited as dominant, recessive or sex-linked characteristics. Although classically divided into autosomal dominant, recessive or X-linked disorders, many syndromes show multiple forms of inheritance pattern. For example, in **Ehlers–Danlos syndrome**, we find autosomal dominant, recessive and X-linked inheritance. In addition, there is a spectrum between autosomal recessive and autosomal dominance, in that having just one defective allele gives a mild form of the disease (semi-dominant), while having both alleles with the mutation results in a more severe form of the syndrome. In some cases, such as **factor V Leiden disease**, the boundary between dominant and recessive forms is very blurred.

Some monogenetic disorders show a racial or geographical prevalence. For example, **thalassaemia** (see pp. 535–538) is seen mainly in Greeks, South-east Asians and Italians; **porphyria variegata** in the South African white population; and **Tay–Sachs disease** (see p. 1287) in Ashkenazi Jewish people. Thus, although the prevalence of some single-gene diseases is very low worldwide, it is much higher in specific populations.

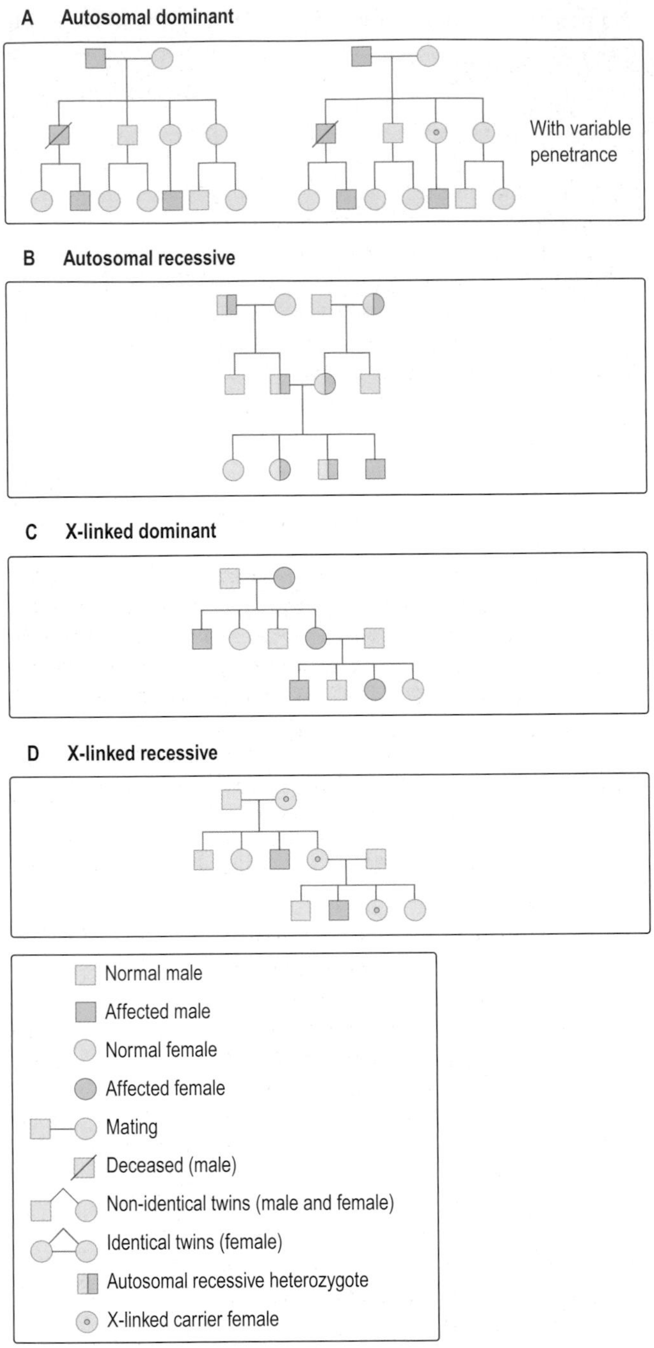

Figure 7.25 Modes of inheritance of simple gene disorders. A key to the standard pedigree symbols is also shown.

Autosomal dominant disorders

Each diploid cell contains two copies of all the autosomes. An autosomal dominant disorder ***(Fig. 7.25A)*** occurs when one of the two copies has a mutation and the protein produced by the normal form of the gene cannot compensate. In this case, a heterozygous individual who has two different forms (or alleles) of the same gene will manifest the disease. The offspring of heterozygotes have a 50% chance of inheriting the chromosome carrying the disease allele, and therefore also of having the disease. However, estimation of risk to offspring for counselling families can be difficult because of three factors:

- Some disorders have a great variability in their manifestation. 'Incomplete penetrance' may occur if patients have a dominant disorder but it does not manifest itself clinically in them. This gives the appearance of the gene having 'skipped' a generation.
- Dominant traits are extremely variable in severity (variable expression) and a mildly affected parent may have a severely affected child.
- New cases in a previously unaffected family may be the result of a new mutation. In this case, the risk of a further affected child is negligible. Most cases of achondroplasia, for example, are due to new mutations.

Autosomal recessive disorders

These disorders ***(Fig. 7.25B)*** manifest themselves only when an individual is homozygous or a compound heterozygote for the disease allele: that is, both chromosomes carry the same gene mutation (homozygous) or two different mutations in the same gene (compound heterozygote). The parents are unaffected carriers (heterozygous for the disease allele). If carriers marry, the offspring have a 1 in 4 chance of carrying both mutant copies of the gene and being affected, a 1 in 2 chance of being a carrier, and a 1 in 4 chance of being genetically normal. Consanguinity increases the risk.

Sex-linked disorders

Genes carried on the X chromosome are said to be 'X-linked', and can be dominant or recessive in the same way as autosomal genes (***Fig. 7.25C and D***).

X-linked dominant disorders

These are rare. Females who are heterozygous for the mutant gene and males who have one copy of the mutant gene on their single X chromosome will manifest the disease. Half the male or female offspring of an affected mother and all the female offspring of an affected man will have the disease. Affected males tend to have the disease more severely than the heterozygous female.

X-linked recessive disorders

These disorders present in males and present only in homozygous females (usually rare). X-linked recessive diseases are transmitted by healthy female carriers or affected males if they survive to reproduce. An example of an X-linked recessive disorder is **haemophilia A** (see pp. 571–573), which is caused by a mutation in the X-linked gene for factor VIII. It has been shown that in 50% of cases there is an intrachromosomal rearrangement (inversion) of the tip of the long arm of the X chromosome (one breakpoint being within intron 22 of the factor VIII gene).

Of the offspring from a carrier female and a normal male:

- 50% of the girls will be carriers, as they inherit a mutant allele from their mother and the normal allele from their father; the other 50% of the girls inherit two normal alleles and are themselves normal
- 50% of the boys will have haemophilia, as they inherit the mutant allele from their mother (and the Y chromosome from their father); the other 50% of the boys will be normal, as they inherit the normal allele from their mother (and the Y chromosome from their father).

The male offspring of a male with haemophilia and a normal female will not have the disease, as they do not inherit his X chromosome. However, all the female offspring will be carriers, as they all inherit his X chromosome.

Box 7.5 Examples of trinucleotide repeat genetic disorders			
Syndrome inheritance pattern	**Disease prevalence**	**Gene, product, location and disorder**	**Genetic test detection rate (%)**
Friedreich's ataxia – AR	2–4/100 000	*FRDA* (frataxin) 9q13 – GAA trinucleotide repeat expansion disorder in intron 1 of *FRDA*	96
Fragile X syndrome – X-linked	16–25/100 000	*FMR1* (fragile X mental retardation 1 protein) Xq27.3 – CGG trinucleotide repeat expansion and methylation changes in the 5′ untranslated region of *FMR1* exon 1	99
Huntington's disease – AD	3–15/100 000	*HD* (Huntingtin protein) 4p16.3 – CAG trinucleotide repeat expansion within the translated protein, giving rise to long tracts of repeat glutamine residues in *HD*	98
Myotonic dystrophy – AD	1/20 000	*DMPK* (myotonin–protein kinase) 19q13.2–13.3 – CTG trinucleotide repeat expansion in the 3′ untranslated region of the *DMPK* gene (dystrophia myotonica 1, DM1). Less common form – expanded. CCTG repeat in zinc finger protein 9 (*ZNF9*) gene (DM2)	100

AD, autosomal dominant; AR, autosomal recessive.

Other single-gene disorders

These are disorders that may be due to mutations in single genes but which do not manifest as simple monogenic disorders. They can arise from a variety of mechanisms, including the following:

Triplet repeat mutations

In the gene responsible for myotonic dystrophy (see p. 891), the mutated allele was found to have an expanded 3′UTR region in which three nucleotides, CTG, were repeated up to about 200 times. In families with myotonic dystrophy, people with the late-onset form of the disease had 20–40 copies of the repeat, but their children and grandchildren who presented with the disease from birth had vast increases in the number of repeats, up to 2000 copies. It is thought that some mechanism during meiosis causes this 'triplet repeat expansion' so that the offspring inherit an increased number of triplets. The number of triplets affects mRNA and protein function ***(Box 7.5)***. See also page 116 for the phenomenon of 'anticipation'.

Mitochondrial disease

As discussed on pages 111–112, various mitochondrial gene mutations can give rise to complex disease syndromes with incomplete penetrance maternal inheritance (see ***Fig. 7.22***).

Imprinting

It is known that normal humans need a diploid number of chromosomes of 46. However, the maternal and paternal contributions can be different. The mechanism that regulates the differential expression of two alleles of the same gene is termed ***genetic imprinting***.

Imprinting is relevant to human genetic disease because different phenotypes may result, depending on whether the mutant chromosome is maternally or paternally inherited. A deletion of part of the long arm of chromosome 15 (15q11-q13) will give rise to the ***Prader–Willi syndrome*** (PWS), if it is paternally inherited. A deletion of a similar region of the chromosome gives rise to ***Angelman syndrome*** (AS) if it is maternally inherited. The affected gene has been identified as ubiquitin (*UBE3A*).

Complex traits: multifactorial and polygenic inheritance

Characteristics resulting from a combination of genetic and environmental factors are said to be multifactorial; those involving multiple genes are said to be polygenic. There has been an explosion of genetic discovery about these complex traits with the development of high-throughput genome-wide SNP arrays, which has allowed cost-effective and unbiased screening of large case–control cohorts (in excess of 1000 cases). This has permitted unequivocal identification of SNPs associated with a variety of traits and diseases. For example, over 30 SNPs in immune-related gene loci have been associated with coeliac disease, with over half also associated with other immune-mediated or inflammatory diseases. This indicates that there are many low-risk genetic risk factors associated with complex traits, and common pathways are implicated in different diseases.

Most human diseases, such as heart disease, diabetes and common mental disorders, are multifactorial traits ***(Box 7.6)***.

Box 7.6 Examples of disorders that may have a polygenic inheritance		
Disorder	**Frequency (%)**	**Heritability (%)[a]**
Hypertension	5	62
Asthma	4	80
Schizophrenia	1	85
Congenital heart disease	0.5	35
Neural tube defects	0.5	60
Congenital pyloric stenosis	0.3	75
Ankylosing spondylitis	0.2	70
Cleft palate	0.1	76

[a]Percentage of the total variation of a trait that can be attributed to genetic factors.

Further reading

De Matteis MA, Luini A. Mendelian disorders of membrane trafficking. *N Engl J Med* 2011; 365:927–938.

Manolio TA. Genomewide association studies and assessment of the risk of disease. *N Engl J Med* 2010; 363:166–176.

http://www.genetests.org *Information on autosomal single-gene disorders*

http://www.genome.gov/gwastudies/ *A Catalogue of published Genome-wide Association studies*

http://www.ncbi.nlm.nih.gov/omim *Information on autosomal single-gene disorders*

POPULATION GENETICS

The genetic constitution of a population depends on many factors. The ***Hardy–Weinberg equilibrium*** is a concept, based on a mathematical equation, that describes the outcome of random mating within populations. It states that 'in the absence of mutation, non-random mating, selection and genetic drift, the genetic constitution of the population remains the same from one generation to the next'.

This genetic principle has clinical significance in terms of the number of abnormal genes in the total gene pool of a population. The Hardy–Weinberg equation states that:

$$p^2 + 2pq + q^2 = 1$$

where p is the frequency of the normal gene in the population, q is the frequency of the abnormal gene, p^2 is the frequency of the normal homozygote, q^2 is the frequency of the affected abnormal homozygote, $2pq$ is the carrier frequency, and $p+q=1$

Example: The equation can be used, for example, to find the frequency of heterozygous carriers in cystic fibrosis. The incidence of cystic fibrosis is 1 in 2000 live births. Thus $q^2=1/2000$, and therefore $q=1/44$. Since $p=1-q$, then $p=43/44$. The carrier frequency is represented by $2pq$, which in this case is 1/22. Thus 1 in 22 individuals in the whole population is a heterozygous carrier for cystic fibrosis.

Further reading

Rotimi CN, Jorde LB. Ancestry and disease in the age of genomic medicine. *N Engl J Med* 2010; 363:1551–1558.

CLINICAL GENETICS AND GENETIC COUNSELLING

Genetic disorders pose considerable health and economic problems because often there is no effective therapy. In any pregnancy, the risk of a serious developmental abnormality is approximately 1 in 50 pregnancies; approximately 15% of paediatric inpatients have a multifactorial disorder with a predominantly genetic element. In addition, 50% of clinical genetics referrals are adults with late-onset disease, including neurological, endocrine, gastrointestinal or cancer.

People with a history of a congenital abnormality in a member of their family often seek advice as to why it happened and about the risks of producing further abnormal offspring. Interviews must be conducted with great sensitivity and psychological insight, as parents may feel a sense of guilt and blame themselves for the abnormality in their child.

Genetic counselling should have the following aims:

- ***Obtaining a full history***. The pregnancy history, drug and alcohol ingestion during pregnancy, and maternal illnesses (e.g. diabetes) should be detailed.
- ***Establishing an accurate diagnosis***. Examination of the child may help in diagnosing a genetically abnormal child with characteristic features (e.g. trisomy 21) or ascertaining whether a genetically normal fetus was damaged *in utero*.
- ***Drawing a family tree***. This is essential. Questions should be asked about abortions, stillbirths, deaths, marriages, consanguinity, and medical history of family members. Diagnoses may need verification from other hospital reports.
- ***Estimating the risk of a future pregnancy being affected or carrying a disorder***. Estimation of risk should be based on the pattern of inheritance. Mendelian disorders (see p. 113) carry a high risk; chromosomal abnormalities other than translocations typically carry a low risk. Empirical risks may be obtained from population or family studies.
- ***Information giving***. Information on prognosis and management should be supplied, with adequate time allowed for it to be discussed openly and freely, and repeated as necessary.
- ***Continued support and follow-up***. Explanation should be provided of the implications for other siblings and family members.
- ***Genetic screening***. This includes prenatal diagnosis or pre-implantation genetic diagnosis (*in vitro* fertilization followed by testing of embryos before implantation) if requested, carrier detection and data storage in genetic registers. A large number of molecular genetic tests are available.
- ***The near future?*** With the development of cheap, high-throughput sequencing, couples could be tested for all genetic variations in their genome (termed 'exome' sequencing for all coding genes, or whole-genome sequencing for all coding *and* non-coding genomic DNA), prior to starting a family, to assess whether they are carriers of recessive mutations in the same disease-associated gene. This information could then be used in prenatal diagnosis.

Genetic counselling should be non-directive, with the couple making their own decisions on the basis of an accurate presentation of the facts and risks in a way they can understand.

Genetic anticipation

It has been noted that successive generations of people with, for example, dystrophia myotonica or Huntington's chorea, present earlier and with progressively worse symptoms. This 'anticipation' is due to unstable mutations occurring within the disease gene. Trinucleotide repeats, such as CTG (dystrophia myotonica) and CAG (Huntington's chorea), expand within the disease gene with each generation, and somatic expansion with cellular replication is also observed. This type of genetic mutation can occur within the translated region or untranslated (and presumably regulatory) regions of the target genes. This genetic distinction has been used to subclassify a number of genetic diseases that have now been shown to be caused by trinucleotide repeat expansion and display phenotypic 'anticipation' (see ***Box 7.5***).

Prenatal diagnosis for chromosomal disorders

This should be offered to *all* pregnant women. Practice and uptake vary in different maternity units, with some offering screening only to high-risk mothers. The risks of Down syndrome increase disproportionately and rapidly for children born to mothers older than 35 years. Infants born to mothers with a history or family history of other conditions due to chromosomal abnormalities may be at increased risk.

Personal choice

There should be a detailed discussion with all mothers as to the possible consequences of each screening test before they are offered it. In particular, they should have an understanding of the failure rates, the detection rates, and the false positive and the false negative rates of each test so that they can properly exercise choice.

Investigations

The choice of investigation depends on gestational age:

7–11 weeks (vaginal ultrasound)

Ultrasound is used to confirm viability, fetal number and gestation by crown–rump measurement.

11–13 weeks and 6 days (combined test)

The combined test comprises:

- ultrasound for nuchal translucency measurement (normal fold <6 mm) to attempt to detect major chromosomal abnormalities (e.g. trisomies and Turner syndrome)
- testing of maternal serum for pregnancy-associated plasma protein-A (PAPP-A from the syncytial trophoblast) and β-human chorionic gonadotrophin for trisomy 21.

All serum marker measurements are corrected for gestational ages, a multiple of the mean (MOM) value for the appropriate week of gestation. If abnormalities are detected, it is necessary to continue to discuss whether further investigation is desired or not. Chorionic villus sampling (CVS) at 11–13 weeks under ultrasound control to sample the placental site, or amniocentesis at 15 weeks to sample amniotic fluid and obtain the fetal cells necessary for cytogenetic testing, is the next option.

The combined test is more accurate than the triple test alone at 16 weeks (see below).

14–20 weeks (serum triple or quadruple test)

A serum triple or quadruple test is done if the pregnancy is too advanced for the earlier tests or if the combined test was not offered.

The triple test for chromosomal abnormalities consists of testing maternal serum for:

- α-fetoprotein (low)
- unconjugated oestradiol (low)
- human chorionic gonadotrophin (high) for Down syndrome and for neural tube defects.

The α-fetoprotein is high for neural tube defects.

The quadruple test also measures inhibin A – high in Down syndrome.

14–22 weeks

Ultrasound detects structural abnormalities (e.g. neural tube defects; the gestation period for detection depends on severity). The best time to detect congenital heart defects is 18–22 weeks.

Reported detection rates for all congenital defects vary: for example, from 14–61% for hypoplastic ventricle to 97–100% for anencephaly.

In time, some of these tests are likely to be superseded by salvage of fetal cells from the maternal blood or cervical secretions, or by retrieval of maternal plasma cell free fetal DNA. Other conditions, such as myotonic dystrophy and Huntington's chorea, may be detected from fetal circulating nucleic acids.

Further reading

Feero WG, Guttmacher AE, Collins FS. Genomic medicine – an updated primer. *N Engl J Med* 2010; 362:2001–2011.

Joann Bodurtha J, Strauss JF. Genomics and perinatal care. *N Engl J Med* 2012; 366:64–73.

National Institute for Health and Care Excellence. *NICE Clinical Guideline 62: Antenatal Care.* NICE 2016; https://www.nice.org.uk/guidance/cg62.

http://www.geneclinics.org *Information on molecular genetic tests*

GENOMIC MEDICINE

Gene therapy

Some genetic disorders, such as ***phenylketonuria*** or ***haemophilia***, can be managed by diet or replacement therapy, but most have no effective treatment. One approach to managing inherited genetic disease entails placing a normal copy of a gene into the cells of a patient who has a defective copy of the gene; this is termed gene therapy.

There are many technical problems to overcome in gene therapy, particularly in finding delivery systems to introduce DNA into a mammalian cell. Very careful control and supervision of gene manipulation will be necessary because of its potential hazards and the ethical issues.

Two major factors are involved in gene therapy:

- the introduction of the functional gene sequence into target cells
- the expression and permanent integration of the transfected gene into the host cell genome.

Cystic fibrosis

CFTR, the cystic fibrosis transmembrane regulator (see also p. 1088), is an unusual ABC transporter in that it does not function as a primary active transporter but as a ligand-gated chloride channel ***(Fig. 7.26)***. The common CF mutation is a 3 bp deletion in exon 10 that results in the removal of a codon specifying phenylalanine (F508del). In this mutation, the CFTR protein is misfolded, thereby causing ineffective biosynthesis and consequently disrupting the delivery of the protein to the cell surface. In the mutation G551 D-CFTR, glycine in position 551 is replaced by aspartate; the CFTR channel reaches the cell surface but fails to open. This has introduced a new era of treatment. VX-770, a potentiating agent that can be given orally, has been developed. It increases the fraction of time for which the phosphorylated G551 D-CFTR channel is open, allowing bicarbonate and chloride flow across the membrane. Early clinical results are encouraging.

There are also over 1000 different mutations of the *CFTR* gene, many of which map to the ATP-binding domains. Two other routes

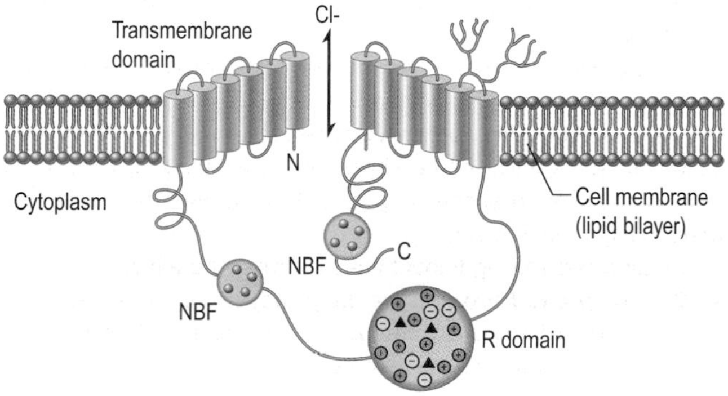

Figure 7.26 **Model of cystic fibrosis transmembrane regulator (CFTR).** This is an integral membrane glycoprotein, consisting of two repeated elements. The cylindrical structures represent six membrane-spanning helices in each half of the molecule. The **nucleotide-binding folds (NBFs)** are in the cytoplasm. The **regulatory (R)** domain links the two halves and contains charged individual amino acids and protein kinase phosphorylation sites (black triangles). **N** and **C** are the amino and carboxy termini of the protein, respectively. The branched structure top right represents potential glycosylation sites.

of gene therapy have been tried, placing the wild-type *CFTR* complementary DNA (cDNA) either into an adenovirus vector to allow infection of human cells, or into a plasmid (an engineered circle of DNA) that is then encapsulated into a liposome to allow transfection of human cells. The latter can be conveyed via an aerosol spray to the lung, where the liposome fuses with the cell membrane to deliver the *CFTR* cDNA into the cell. However, neither of these methods is a treatment option yet. An alternative method is to suppress premature termination codons and thus permit translation to continue; topical nasal gentamicin (an aminoglycoside antibiotic) has been shown to result in the expression of functional *CFTR* channels.

Adenosine deaminase (ADA) deficiency

Successful gene therapy for this rare immunodeficiency disease has entailed introducing a normal human *ADA* gene into the patient's lymphocytes to reconstitute the function of the cellular and humoral immune system in severe combined immunodeficiency (SCID).

Pharmacogenomics

This is the study of individual SNPs that determine drug behaviour to explain why some patients give a variable response to the particular drug. The potential of pharmacogenomic approaches is usually related to single-gene traits that affect drug metabolism: for example, SNPs in the gene encoding thiopurine-*S*-methyltransferase (TPMT), which metabolizes immunosuppressant drugs (e.g. azathioprine). Patient-specific therapies based on their genetic profile will lead to the development of drugs (or drug combinations).

Stem cell therapy

Stem cell therapy has the potential to change the treatment of human disease radically (see pp. 105–106). A number of adult stem cell therapies already exist, particularly bone marrow transplants. It is currently anticipated that technologies derived from stem cell research can be used to treat a wider variety of diseases in which replacement of destroyed specialist tissues is required, such as in Parkinson's disease, spinal cord injuries and muscle damage.

Ethical considerations

Ethical considerations must be taken into account in any discussion of clinical genetics. For example, prenatal diagnosis with the option of termination may be unacceptable on moral or religious grounds. With diseases for which there is no cure and currently no treatment (e.g. Huntington's chorea), genetic tests can accurately predict which family members will be affected; however, many people would rather not have this information. One very serious outcome of the new genetic information is that disease susceptibility may be predictable – for example, in Alzheimer's disease – so the medical insurance companies can decline to issue policies for individuals at high risk. Society has not decided who should have access to an individual's genetic information and to what extent privacy should be preserved.

Further reading

Dietz HC. New therapeutic approaches to Mendelian disorders. *N Engl J Med* 2010; 363:852–863.
McDermott U, Downing JR, Stratton MR. Genomics and the continuum of cancer care. *N Engl J Med* 2011; 364:340–350.
Wang L, McLeod HL, Weinshilboum RM. Genomics and drug response. *N Engl J Med* 2011; 364:1144–1153.
Welsh MJ. Targeting the basic deficit in cystic fibrosis. *N Engl J Med* 2010; 263:2056–2057.

THE GENETIC BASIS OF CANCER

Cancers are genetic diseases and involve changes to the normal function of cellular genes. However, multiple genes interact during oncogenesis and an almost stepwise progression of defects leads from an over-proliferation of a particular cell to the breakdown of control mechanisms such as ***apoptosis (programmed cell death)***. This would be triggered if a cell were to attempt to survive in an organ other than its tissue of origin. For the vast majority of cancer cases (especially those in older people), the multiple genetic changes that occur are somatic. For some cancers, however (where the cancer normally occurs at an earlier age), a dominant inherited single-gene defect can give rise to an almost Mendelian trend with lifetime risks of nearly 90%.

Autosomal dominant inheritance

The following are examples of cancer syndromes (see ***Box 17.2***, p. 588) that exhibit dominant inheritance:

- ***Retinoblastoma***. This is an eye tumour found in young children. It occurs in both hereditary (40%) and non-hereditary (60%) forms. In the hereditary form, there is a germline mutation in the retinoblastoma gene (*RB1*) and people are also at risk for developing other tumours, particularly osteosarcoma.
- ***Breast and ovarian cancer***. Two major genes have been identified – *BRCA1* and *BRCA2*. A strong family history along with germline mutation of these genes accounts for most cases of familial breast cancer and over half of familial ovarian cancers. BRCA1 and 2 proteins bind to the DNA repair enzyme Rad51 to make it functional in repairing DNA breaks. Mutations in the *BRCA* genes will lead to accumulation of unrepaired mutations in tumour suppressor genes and crucial oncogenes.
- ***Neurofibromatosis***. Inactivation of the *NF1* gene will lead to constitutive activation of Ras proteins.
- ***Multiple endocrine adenomatosis syndromes*** (see pp. 1239–1240). Multiple endocrine neoplasia type 1 is associated with the *MEN1* gene, and type 2 (*MEN2*) is associated with mutations in the *RET* proto-oncogene on chromosome 10; as such, these diseases are the exception to all the other syndromes that involve tumour suppressor genes.

Autosomal recessive inheritance

Some relatively rare autosomal recessive diseases associated with abnormalities of DNA repair predispose to the development of cancer:

- ***Xeroderma pigmentosum***. There is an inability to repair DNA damage caused by ultraviolet light and by some chemicals, leading to a high incidence of skin cancer.
- ***Ataxia telangiectasia***. Mutation results in an increased sensitivity to ionizing radiation and an increased incidence of lymphoid tumours.
- ***Bloom syndrome and Fanconi's anaemia***. An increased susceptibility to lymphoid malignancy is seen.

Oncogenes

The genes coding for growth factors, growth factor receptors, secondary messengers or even DNA-binding proteins would act as promoters of abnormal cell growth if mutated. This concept was verified when viruses were found to carry genes that, when integrated into the host cell, promoted oncogenesis. These were

Box 7.7 Examples of acquired/somatic mutations and proto-oncogenes

Point mutation
- *K-RAS*: Colorectal and pancreatic cancer
- *B-RAF*: Melanoma, thyroid
- *ALK*: Lung cancer

DNA amplification
- *MYC*: Neuroblastoma
- *HER2*-neu: Breast cancer

Chromosome translocation
- *BCR/ABL*: Chronic myeloid leukaemia, acute lymphoblastic leukaemia
- *PML/RARA*: Acute promyelocytic leukaemia
- *BCL2/IGH*: Follicular lymphoma
- *IGH/CCND1*: Mantle cell lymphoma
- *MYC/IgH*: Burkitt's lymphoma

originally termed viral or 'v-oncogenes'; later, their normal cellular counterparts, c-oncogenes, were found. Thus, oncogenes encode proteins that are known to participate in the regulation of normal cellular proliferation: for example, *erb-A* on chromosome 17q11-q12 encodes for the thyroid hormone receptor.

Activation of oncogenes

Non-activated oncogenes, which are functioning normally, have been referred to as 'proto-oncogenes' ***(Box 7.7)***. Their transformation to oncogenes can occur by three routes: mutation, chromosomal translocation and viral stimulation.

Mutation

Carcinogens, such as those found in cigarette smoke, ionizing radiation and ultraviolet light, can cause point mutations in genomic DNA encoding tumour suppressor genes or oncogenes.

Chromosomal translocation

If an error occurs during cell division and two chromosomes translocate, so that a portion swaps over, the translocation breakpoint may occur in the middle of two genes. If this happens, then the end of one gene is translocated on to the beginning of another gene, giving rise to a 'fusion gene'. Therefore, sequences of one part of the fusion gene are inappropriately expressed because they are under the control of the other part of the gene.

An example of such a fusion gene (the Philadelphia chromosome) occurs in ***chronic myeloid leukaemia*** (see pp. 612–613). Similarly in ***Burkitt's lymphoma*** (see p. 623), a translocation causes the regulatory segment of the *myc* oncogene to be replaced by a regulatory segment of an unrelated immunoglobulin.

Viral stimulation

When viral RNA is transcribed by reverse transcriptase into viral cDNA and in turn is spliced into the cellular DNA, the viral DNA may integrate within an oncogene and activate it. Alternatively, the virus may pick up cellular oncogene DNA and incorporate it into its own viral genome. Subsequent infection of another host cell might result in expression of this viral oncogene. For example, the Rous sarcoma virus of chickens was found to induce cancer because it carried the *ras* oncogene.

After the initial activation event, other changes occur within the DNA. A striking example of this is amplification of gene sequences, which can affect the *myc* gene, for example. Instead of the normal two copies of a gene, multiple copies of the gene appear either within the chromosomes (these can be seen on stained chromosomes as homogeneously staining regions) or as extrachromosomal particles (double minutes). *N-myc* sequences are amplified in neuroblastomas, as are *N-myc* or *L-myc* in some lung small-cell carcinomas.

Tumour suppressor genes

These genes restrict undue cell proliferation (in contrast to oncogenes), and induce the repair or self-destruction (apoptosis) of cells containing damaged DNA. Therefore, mutations in these genes, which disable their function, lead to uncontrolled cell growth in cells with active oncogenes. An example is the germline mutations in genes found in non-polyposis colorectal cancer, which are responsible for repairing DNA mismatches (see p. 422).

The ***RB gene*** was the first tumour suppressor gene to be described (see p. 588). In the familial variety, the first mutation is inherited and, by chance, a second somatic mutation occurs with the formation of a tumour. In the sporadic variety, by chance, both mutations occur in both of the *RB* genes in a single cell.

Since the finding of *RB*, other tumour suppressor genes have been described, including the ***gene p53***. Mutations in *p53* have been found in almost all human tumours, including sporadic colorectal carcinomas, carcinomas of breast and lung, brain tumours, osteosarcomas and leukaemias. The protein encoded by *p53* is a cellular 53 kDa nuclear phosphoprotein that plays a role in DNA repair and synthesis, in the control of the cell cycle, cell differentiation and programmed cell death – apoptosis. p53 is a DNA-binding protein that activates many gene expression pathways but it is normally only short-lived. In many tumours, mutations that disable *p53* function also prevent its cellular catabolism. Although in some cancers there is a loss of *p53* from both chromosomes, in most cancers (particularly colorectal carcinomas; see ***Fig. 17.2***) such long-lived mutant *p53* alleles can disrupt the normal alleles' protein. As a DNA-binding protein, p53 is likely to act as a tetramer.

Thus, a mutation in a single copy of the gene can promote tumour formation because a hetero-tetramer of mutated and normal p53 subunits would still be dysfunctional. p53 and RB are involved in normal regulation of the cell cycle. Other cancer-associated genes are also intimately involved in control of the cell cycle (see ***Fig. 7.16***).

Further reading

Dawson MA, Kouzarides A, Huntly BJP. Targeting epigenetic readers in cancer. *N Engl J Med* 2012; 367:647–657.

Dhanak D, Jackson P. Development and classes of epigenetic drugs for cancer. *Biochem Biophys Res Commun* 2014; 455:58–69.

Hoeijmakers JH. DNA damage, aging, and cancer. *N Engl J Med* 2009; 361:1475–1485.

Khanna A. DNA Damage in cancer therapeutics: a boon or a curse? *Cancer Res* 2015; 75:2133–8.

Bibliography

Alberts B, Johnson A, Lewis J et al. *Molecular Biology of the Cell*, 5th edn. New York: Garland Science; 2007.

Lodish H, Berk A, Kaiser CA et al. *Molecular Cell Biology*, 6th edn. New York: WH Freeman; 2007.

Significant websites

http://www.ncbi.nlm.nih.gov/omim *McKusick's Online Mendelian Inheritance in Man (OMIM)*

8 The immune system and disease

Mark Peakman, Matthew S Buckland

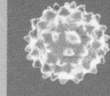

See your e-book for key learning points, clinical tips, drug tips, interactive Figures and MCQs.

ANATOMY AND PRINCIPLES OF THE IMMUNE SYSTEM

Immunity can be defined as protection from infection, whether bacterial, viral, fungal or due to multicellular parasites. The immune system is composed of cells and molecules organized into specialized tissues ***(Fig. 8.1)***.

The ***primary lymphoid organs*** (thymus and bone marrow) are where the cells originate. Cells and molecules of the immune system circulate in the blood; immune responses do not take place there but are at the site of infection (typically the mucosa or skin). They are then propagated and refined in the ***secondary lymphoid organs*** (e.g. lymph nodes). Following resolution of the infection, immunological memory specific for the pathogen is generated and resides in cells (lymphocytes) in the spleen and lymph nodes, as well as being widely secreted in a molecular form (antibodies). Secondary lymphoid organs also include adenoids, tonsils, spleen, Peyer's patches in the small intestine, lymphoids (cervical, axillary, inguinal) and thoracic duct.

Cells involved in immune responses: origin and function

All immune cells derive from pluripotent stem cells generated in the bone marrow. They have diverse functions ***(Box 8.1)***. ***T lymphocytes*** undergo 'education' in the thymus to avoid self-recognition, and populate the peripheral lymphoid tissue, where B lymphocytes also reside. Both sets of lymphocytes undergo activation in the peripheral tissue, to become mature effector cells. ***B lymphocytes*** may further differentiate into antibody-secreting plasma cells. Lymphoid tissue is frequently found at mucosal surfaces in non-encapsulated patches, termed ***mucosa-associated lymphoid tissue*** (MALT).

The immune system

Cells and molecules involved in immune responses are classified into innate and adaptive systems:

- ***The innate immune system*** is inborn and operates throughout life (pp. 123–128).
- ***The adaptive immune system*** changes in response to the pathogens it encounters (pp. 128–132).

There are also non-immunological barriers that are involved in host protection, and lowering of these may allow a pathogen to gain a foothold ***(Box 8.2)***.

The immune system is immensely powerful, in terms of its ability to inflame, damage and kill, and it has a capacity to recognize a myriad of molecular patterns in the microbial world. However, immune responses are not always beneficial. They can give rise to a range of autoimmune and inflammatory diseases, known as ***immunopathologies***. Conversely, the immune system may fail, giving rise to immune deficiency states. These conditions are grouped under the umbrella of clinical immunology.

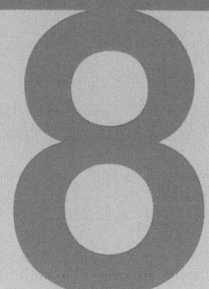

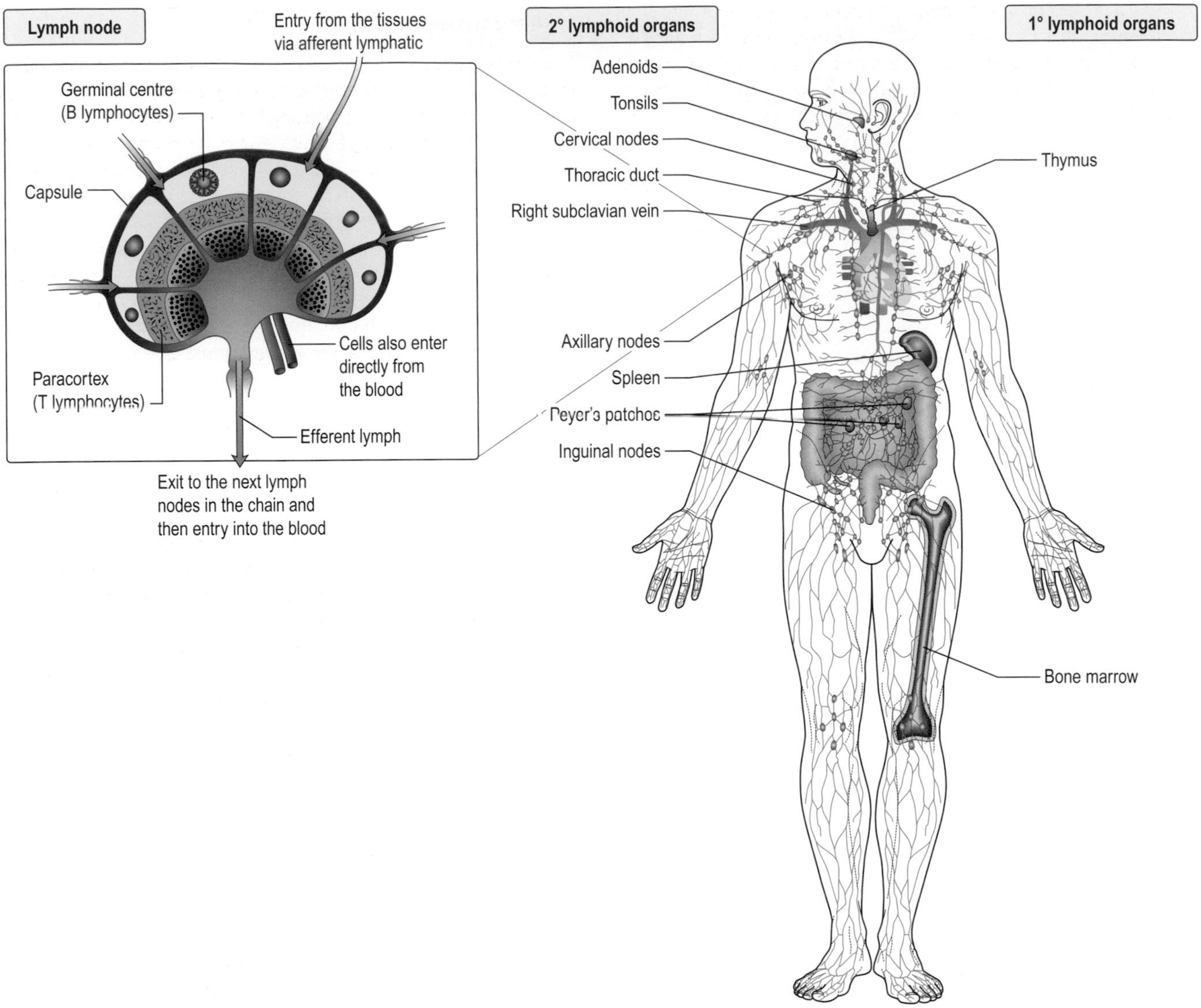

Figure 8.1 Lymph node. Lymphocytes are generated as precursors in the bone marrow and differentiate into T (thymus) or B (bone marrow) lymphocytes in the primary lymphoid tissue. Once differentiated, 98% of lymphocytes reside in the secondary lymphoid tissue where the adaptive immune response takes place.

Box 8.1 Main cells involved in the immune response: functions and origin

Category	Cells	Main functions	Origin	Special features
Myeloid	Neutrophils	Immunity to bacteria and fungi	Bone marrow	Major first-line defence against pathogens
	Eosinophils, mast cells and basophils	Immunity to parasites	Bone marrow	Role in allergy
	Monocytes and macrophages	Immunity to bacteria, fungi, parasites	Bone marrow	Specialized phagocytes; cytokine secretion
Lymphoid	Dendritic cells	Antigen presentation to T lymphocytes	Bone marrow	Key role in activating T lymphocytes
	B lymphocytes	Antibody production	Bone marrow	Have specific receptor for antigen (called 'antibody'). Mature into plasma cells that are 'antibody factories'
	T lymphocytes	Orchestration of immune response against bacteria, fungi, parasites and viruses	Precursors come from bone marrow and undergo selection process in the thymus to avoid self-reactivity	Have specific receptor for antigen (called T cell receptor). Two major subsets: CD4 ('helper' and 'regulatory') and CD8 ('cytotoxic')

A major feature of the immune system is the complexity of its surface-bound, intracellular and soluble mediators. In particular, it is necessary to be aware of the clusters of differentiation (CD) classification ***(Box 8.3)*** and the functions of cytokines and chemokines. The CD classification is the ultimate way of defining a cell.

Cytokines

These are small polypeptides released by a cell in order to change the function of the same or another cell. These chemical messengers are found in many organ systems, but especially the immune system. Cytokines have become markers in the investigation of disease pathogenesis; they are also therapeutic agents in their own right, and the targets of therapeutic agents (see pp. 146–147). The key features of a cytokine are:

- ***pleiotropy***: has different effects on different cells
- ***autocrine function***: modulates the cell secreting it
- ***paracrine function***: modulates adjacent cells
- ***endocrine effects***: modulates cells and organs at remote sites
- ***synergistic activity***: acts in concert with other cytokines to achieve effects greater than the summation of their individual actions.

The main immune cytokines are the ***interferons*** (IFNs) and the ***interleukins*** (ILs). The IFNs are limited to a few major types (α, β and γ), whereas there are 38 interleukins.

Chemokines

The defining feature of chemokines is their function as chemotactic molecules: that is, they attract cells along a gradient of low to high chemical concentration, particularly from the blood into the tissues, and tissues into lymphatics. They also have the ability to activate immune cells. All chemokines have a similar structure relating to the configuration of cysteine residues, which gives rise to four families ***(Box 8.4)***.

Cell-surface receptors for chemokines are denoted by 'R'. CCR5 is a co-receptor for human immunodeficiency virus (HIV; see pp. 333–334) and drugs to block this and other chemokine receptors are under active development to combat inflammation and cancer (by promoting migration of immune cells into tumours).

INNATE IMMUNE SYSTEM

Innate immunity provides immediate, first-line host defence. The key features of this system (as well as the adaptive system, p. 128) are shown in ***Box 8.5***. It is present at birth and remains operative at comparable intensity into old age. Innate immunity is mediated by a variety of cells and molecules ***(Box 8.6)***. Activation of innate immune responses is mediated through interaction between the:

- pathogen side, comprising a relatively limited array of molecules (pathogen-associated molecular patterns, PAMPs)
- host side, a limited portfolio of receptors (pattern recognition receptors, PRRs).

Box 8.2 Non-immunological host defence mechanisms

Normal barriers	Events that may compromise barrier function
Physical barriers	
Skin and mucous membranes	Trauma, burns, i.v. cannulae
Cough reflex	Suppression, e.g. by opiates, neurological disease
Mucosal function	Ciliary paralysis (e.g. smoking) Increased mucus production (e.g. asthma) Abnormally viscid secretions (e.g. cystic fibrosis) Decreased secretions (e.g. sicca syndrome)
Urine flow	Stasis (e.g. prostatic hypertrophy)
Chemical barriers	High gastric pH (gastric acid secretion inhibitors)
Resistance to pathogens provided by commensal skin and gut organisms	Changes in flora (e.g. broad-spectrum antibiotics)

Box 8.3 The CD classification

- Immune cells are distinguished by the surface receptors and proteins that they express in order to mediate their particular range of immunological functions, e.g. cell–cell signalling, cell activation.
- The surfaces are covered with such proteins and indicate the cell lineage or differentiation pathway. The discovery of monoclonal antibodies (proteins tailor-made to bind to a specific target) made this feasible.
- Surface molecules defining the origin and function of selected groups of cells are known as clusters of differentiation (CD). Over 360 CD numbers exist.
- A clinical example is the number of peripheral blood lymphocytes expressing CD4 ('the CD4 count'), which is used to monitor human immunodeficiency virus (HIV) infection (see p. 339)

An updated listing is available at: http://www.hcdm.org/.

Box 8.4 Features of chemokine mediators and receptors

Chemokine family	Structure	Receptor family	Pathological or therapeutic target
CXC	Two cysteines (C) separated by any other amino acid residue (X)	CXCR	CXCR4 – co-receptor for late HIV infection
CC	Two cysteines next to each other	CCR	CCR5 – co-receptor for early HIV infection and blocked by 'entry inhibitors'
C	One cysteine	CR	XCR1 – target of Kaposi's sarcoma human virus protein
CX3C	Two cysteines separated by any three amino acids	CX3CR	Possible survival factor in myeloma

R, receptor.

Box 8.5 Features of the innate and adaptive immune responses

Innate	Adaptive
No memory: quality and intensity of response invariant	Memory: response adapts with each exposure
Recognition of limited number of non-varying, generic molecular patterns on, or made by, pathogens	Recognition of vast array of specific antigens[a] on, or made by, pathogens
Pattern recognition mediated by a limited array of receptors	Antigen recognition mediated by a vast array of antigen-specific receptors
Response immediate on first encounter	Response on first encounter takes 1–2 weeks; on second encounter, 3–7 days

[a]Antigen is a molecular structure (protein, peptide, lipid, carbohydrate) that generates an immune response.

Box 8.6 Soluble components of innate immunity

Molecules	Name (examples)	Function	Provide immunity against
Complement	Cascade of >40 proteins	Lyse bacteria; opsonize[a] bacteria; promote inflammation; recruit and activate immune cells	Bacteria, viruses
Collectins	Mannose-binding lectin	Binds bacteria; activates complement	Bacteria
Pentraxins	C-reactive protein[b]	Opsonize bacteria	Bacteria
Enzymes	Lysozyme	Present in secretions; cleaves bacterial cell wall	Bacteria

[a]Opsonize = coat bacteria to enhance phagocytosis by granulocytes and monocytes/macrophages.
[b]C-reactive protein (CRP) is an acute phase protein. Blood level rises 10–100-fold within hours of the start of an infective or inflammatory process, making it extremely useful in monitoring infective or inflammatory diseases, and their response to treatment.

Activation of certain cells in the innate immune system leads to activation of the ***adaptive immune response*** (see p. 128).

The ***dendritic cell*** is especially involved in this process, and forms a bridge between innate and adaptive systems.

Complement

Complement proteins are produced in the liver and circulate in an inactive form. When triggered, complement molecules become enzymatically active and trigger several molecules of the next stage in a series. This ***complement cascade*** is initiated via three distinct pathways: alternative, classical and mannose-binding lectin ***(Fig. 8.2)***. Each pathway culminates in the cleavage of C3 and C5. Cleavage of C3 has a number of biological consequences; breakdown of C5 achieves the same and, in addition, provides the triggering stimulus to the final common ('membrane attack') pathway, which provides most of the biological activity ***(Fig. 8.2)***.

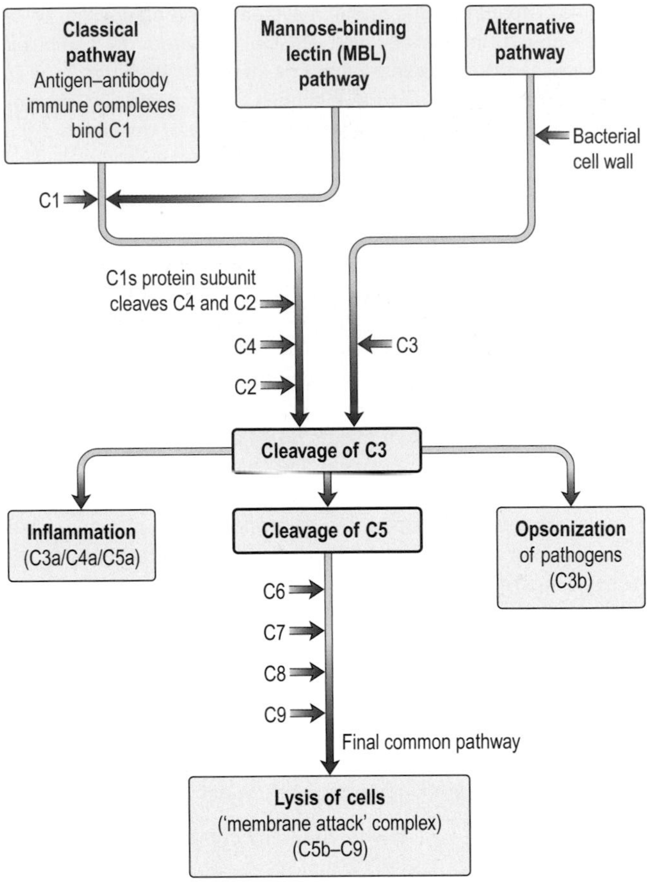

Figure 8.2 The complement pathways and their effector functions.

The main functions of complement activation are to:

- promote inflammation (e.g. through the actions of the anaphylatoxins C3a, C4a and C5a)
- recruit cells (e.g. through chemoattractants)
- kill targeted cells, such as bacteria
- solubilize antigen–antibody ('immune') complexes and remove them from the circulation.

During an immune response, removal of immune complexes protects unaffected tissues from the deposition of these large, insoluble composites, which could result in unwanted inflammation. Failure of this protective mechanism can result in immunopathology: for example, in the joints, kidney and eye.

Neutrophils

Neutrophils (see pp. 562–563) phagocytose and kill microorganisms by releasing antimicrobial compounds (e.g. defensins). They are derived from the bone marrow, which can produce between 10^{11} (healthy state) and 10^{12} (during infection) new cells per day. In health, neutrophils are rarely seen in the tissues.

Neutrophil phagocytosis is activated by interaction with bacteria, either directly or after bacteria have been coated (opsonized) to make them more ingestible ***(Fig. 8.3)***. The contents of neutrophil granules are released both intracellularly (predominantly azurophilic granules) and extracellularly (specific granules) following fusion with the plasma membrane. Approximately 100 different molecules in neutrophil granules ***(Box 8.7)*** kill and digest microorganisms, for example:

- ***Myeloperoxidase and cytochrome b_{558}*** are key components of major oxygen-dependent bactericidal systems.

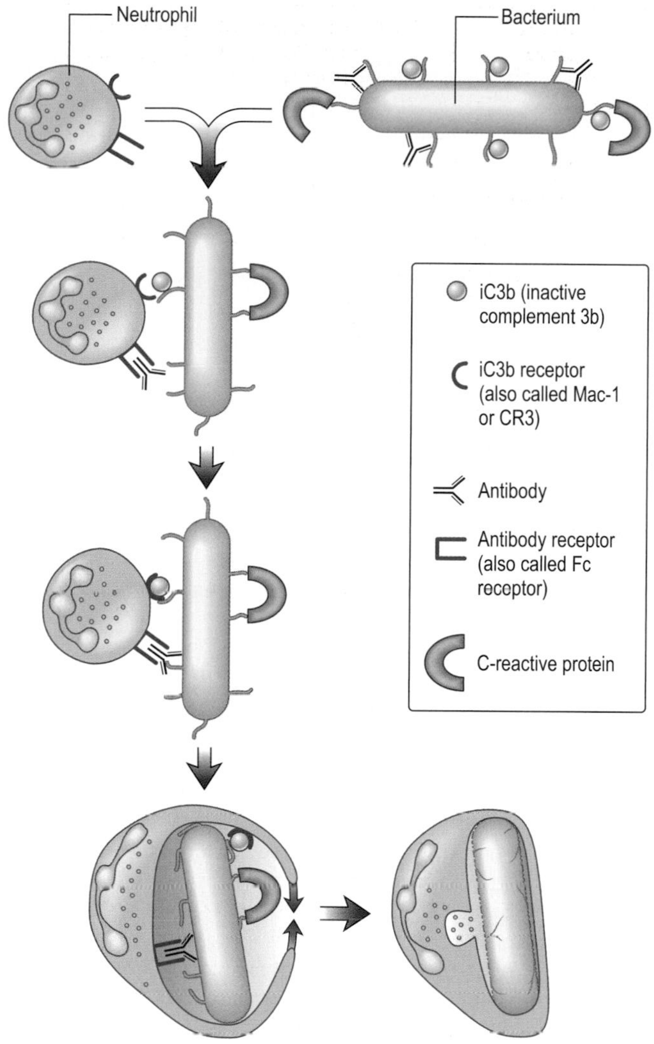

Figure 8.3 **Opsonization.** Bacteria are coated with a variety of soluble factors from the innate immune system (opsonins), which enhance phagocytosis. This leads to engulfment of the bacteria into phagosomes and fusion with granules to release antibacterial agents.

Box 8.7 Contents and function of key neutrophil granules

Function	Primary or azurophilic granules	Secondary or specific granules
Antibacterial	Lysozyme Defensins Myeloperoxidase (MPO) Proteinase-3 Elastase Cathepsins Bactericidal/permeability inducing protein (BPI)	Respiratory burst components (e.g. cytochrome b_{558}) producing reactive oxygen metabolites, such as hydrogen peroxide, hydroxyl radicals and singlet oxygen Lysozyme Lactoferrin
Cell movement		Collagenase CD11b/CD18 (adhesion molecule) *N*-formyl-methionyl-leucylphenylalanine receptor (FMLP-R)

- ***Cathepsins, proteinase-3 and elastase*** are deadly to Gram-positive and Gram-negative organisms, as well as some *Candida* species.
- ***Defensins*** are naturally occurring cysteine-rich antibacterial and antifungal polypeptides (29–35 amino acids).
- ***Collagenase and elastase*** break down fibrous structures in the extracellular matrix, facilitating progress of the neutrophil through the tissues.

Granule release is initiated by the products of bacterial cell walls, certain complement proteins, leukotrienes (LTB_4) and chemokines (e.g. CXCL8), and cytokines such as tumour necrosis factor-alpha (TNF-α).

Eosinophils

Eosinophils release pro-inflammatory mediators to provide immunity against parasites. In contrast to neutrophils, several hundred times more eosinophils are present in the tissues than in the blood, particularly at epithelial surfaces, where they survive for several weeks. The main role of eosinophils is protection against multicellular parasites such as worms (helminths). This is achieved by the release of pro-inflammatory mediators, which are toxic, cationic proteins. In populations and societies in which such parasites are rare, eosinophils contribute mainly to allergic disease, particularly asthma (see p. 1094). Eosinophils have two types of granules:

- ***Specific granules*** (95%) contain the cationic proteins, of which there are four main types: ***major basic protein (MBP), eosinophil cationic protein (ECP)*** and ***eosinophil neurotoxin***, which are all potently toxic to helminths, and ***eosinophil peroxidase***, similar to neutrophil myeloperoxidase.
- ***Primary granules*** (5%) synthesize and release ***leukotrienes*** C_4 ***and*** D_4 and ***platelet-activating factor*** (PAF), which alter airway smooth muscle and vasculature (see p. 1095).

Eosinophils are activated and recruited by a variety of mediators via specific surface receptors, including complement factors and LTB_4. In addition, the chemokines eotaxin-1 (CCL11) and eotaxin-2 (CCL24) are highly selective in eosinophil recruitment. There are surface receptors for the cytokines IL-3 and IL-5, which promote the development and differentiation of eosinophils.

Mast cells and basophils

Mast cells release pro-inflammatory and vasoactive mediators, and have a role in allergy. Mast cells and basophils share features in common, especially in containing:

- histamine-containing granules
- high-affinity receptors for immunoglobulin E (IgE, an antibody type that is involved in allergic disease; see pp. 142–144).

Mast cells are found in tissues (especially skin and mucosae) and basophils in the blood. Both mast cells and basophils release pro-inflammatory mediators, which are either pre-formed or synthesized *de novo* ***(Box 8.8)***.

Histamine is a low-molecular-weight amine (111 Da) with a blood half-life of less than 5 minutes; it constitutes 10% of the mast cell's weight. When injected into the skin, histamine induces the typical 'weal and flare' or 'triple' response: reddening (erythema) due to increased blood flow, swelling (weal) due to increased vascular permeability, and distal vascular changes (flare) due to effects on local axons.

The ***complement-derived anaphylatoxins*** C3a, C4a and C5a activate basophils and mast cells, as does IgE. The mast cell also has a role in the early response to bacteria through release of TNF-α, in cell recruitment to inflammatory sites such as arthritic joints,

Box 8.8 Mast cell and basophil mediators

Mediators	Effects
Pre-formed	
Histamine	Vasodilatation Vascular permeability ↑ Smooth muscle contraction in airways
Proteases	Digestion of basement membrane causes ↑vascular permeability and aids migration
Proteoglycans (e.g. heparan)	Anticoagulant activity
Synthesized *de novo*	
Platelet-activating factor (PAF)	Vasodilatation
LTB_4, LTC_4, LTD_4	Neutrophil and eosinophil activation and chemoattraction Vascular permeability ↑ Bronchoconstriction
Prostaglandins (mainly PGD_2)	Vascular permeability ↑ Bronchoconstriction Vasodilatation

in promotion of tumour growth by enhancing neovascularization and in allograft tolerance.

Monocytes and macrophages

Monocytes (in blood) and macrophages (in tissue) ingest and kill bacteria, release pro-inflammatory molecules, present antigen to T lymphocytes, and are necessary in immunity to intracellular pathogens such as mycobacteria.

Cells of the monocyte/macrophage lineage are highly sophisticated phagocytes. ***Monocytes*** are the blood form of a cell that spends a few days in the circulation before entering into the tissues to differentiate into ***macrophages***, and possibly some types of dendritic cells.

Blood monocytes

Blood monocytes can be divided into subsets according to expression of CD14 (a receptor for lipopolysaccharide, a bacterial cell wall component) and CD16 (a receptor for IgG antibodies). *In vitro*, monocytes have the potential to differentiate into myeloid dendritic cells (after culture with IL-4 and granulocyte-monocyte colony stimulating factor, GM-CSF) and into macrophages, which may exist in specialized forms (e.g. alveolar and gut macrophages and osteoclasts).

Tissue macrophages

A key role of tissue macrophages is the maintenance of tissue homeostasis, through clearance of cellular debris, especially following infection or inflammation. They are responsive to a range of pro-inflammatory stimuli, using their pattern recognition receptors (PRRs) to recognize pathogen-associated molecular patterns (PAMPs). Once activated, they engulf and kill microorganisms, especially bacteria and fungi. In doing so, they release a range of pro-inflammatory cytokines and have the capacity to present fragments of the microorganisms to T lymphocytes (see below) in a process called ***antigen presentation***. Evidence suggests that evolutionarily conserved molecular patterns in mitochondria (organelles that originally were derived from bacteria) can also activate monocytes. These damage-associated molecular patterns (DAMPs) could play a major role in the systemic inflammatory response that follows extensive tissue damage (e.g. following ischaemic injury).

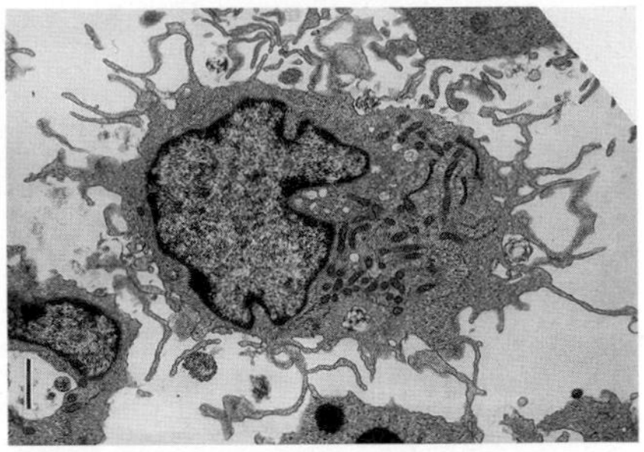

Figure 8.4 Mature dendritic cell. The cell ingests pathogens, migrates to lymph nodes and presents pathogen-derived antigen to T lymphocytes to enable adaptive immunity.

It has been observed that some PAMPs induce the cytoplasmic assembly of large oligomeric structures of PRRs termed ***inflammasomes***. There are numerous examples: members of the Nod-like receptor (NLR) family can be activated by stimuli such as viruses, bacterial toxins and, interestingly, crystallized endogenous molecules, including urate. Inflammasomes have potent effects in activating caspases, leading to processing and secretion of pro-inflammatory cytokines such as IL-1β and IL-18.

Macrophages have pro-inflammatory and microbicidal capabilities similar to those of neutrophils. Under activation conditions, antigen presentation (see p. 135) is enhanced and a range of cytokines secreted, notably TNF-α, IL-1 and IFN-γ. These are necessary for the removal of certain pathogens that live within mononuclear phagocytes (e.g. mycobacteria). Macrophages and related cells may also undergo a process termed ***autophagy*** (see p. 104). This self-cannibalization is a critical property of many cell types under starvation conditions, but is used by the immune system to destroy intracellular pathogens such as *Mycobacterium tuberculosis*, which otherwise persist within cells and block normal antibacterial processes. Autophagy is also a means of enhancing antigen presentation pathways. Dysregulation of the autophagic pathway has been associated with a number of diseases including cancer, inflammatory disease and infections.

Tissue macrophages involved in chronic inflammatory foci may undergo terminal differentiation into multinucleated giant cells, typically found at the site of the granulomata characteristic of tuberculosis and sarcoidosis (see pp. 1118–1120).

Dendritic cells

The major function of dendritic cells (DCs) is activation of naive T lymphocytes to initiate adaptive immune responses (see p. 127); they are the only cells capable of this. The definition of a dendritic cell is one that has:

- dendritic morphology ***(Fig. 8.4)***
- machinery for sensing pathogens
- the ability to process and present antigens to CD4 and CD8 T lymphocytes, coupled with the ability to activate these T lymphocytes from a naive state
- the ability to dictate the T lymphocyte's future function and differentiation.

This is a powerful cell type that functions as a critical bridge between the innate and adaptive immune systems.

Types of dendritic cell

The major types are the ***myeloid DC*** (***mDC***), the ***plasmacytoid DC*** (***pDC***) and a variety of specialized DCs found in tissues that resemble mDCs (e.g. the Langerhans cell in the skin; see ***Fig. 31.1***).

Box 8.9 Molecules on dendritic cells

	Myeloid DC		Plasmacytoid DC	
	Immature	*Mature*	*Immature*	*Mature*
CD1c	+	++	–	–
CD123 (IL-3 receptor)	–	–	+	++
Molecules involved in co-stimulation of T lymphocytes (CD80, CD86)	+	+++	+	+++
HLA class I and II molecules for antigen presentation to T lymphocytes	+	+++	+	+++

Box 8.10 Toll-like receptors (TLR)

Pattern recognition receptor (PRR)	Pathogen-associated molecular pattern (PAMP)	Pathogen	PRR expressed by
TLR2	Peptidoglycan	Gram-positive bacteria	mDC
TLR3	Double-stranded RNA	Viruses	mDC
TLR4	Lipopolysaccharide	Gram-negative bacteria	mDC
TLR7	Single-stranded RNA	Viruses	pDC
TLR9	Double-stranded DNA	Viruses	pDC

mDC, myeloid dendritic cell; pDC, plasmacytoid dendritic cell.

DCs have several distinctive cell surface molecules, some of which have pathogen-sensing activity (e.g. the antigen uptake receptor DEC205 on mDCs) whilst others are involved in interaction with T lymphocytes ***(Box 8.9)***. Immature mDCs and pDCs are present in the blood, but at very low levels (<0.5% of lymphocyte/monocyte cells).

Pathogen sensing is a key component of the function of immature DCs, as well as monocytes/macrophages, and is achieved through expression of a limited array of specialized PRR molecules capable of binding to structures common to pathogens, aided by long cell dendrites and pinocytosis (constant ingestion of soluble material).

PRRs include:

- ***Mannose-binding lectin***, which initiates complement activity, inducing opsonization (see p. 124).
- ***Signalling receptors***, such as the PRR known as toll-like receptor 4 (TLR4), which binds lipopolysaccharide, a molecular pattern found in the cell walls of many Gram-negative bacteria ***(Box 8.10)***. Other TLRs bind double-stranded and single-stranded RNA from viruses and other non-self antigens. Innate immunity critically depends on toll-like receptor signalling. These receptors act through a key adaptor molecule, myeloid differentiation factor 88 (MyD88), to regulate the activity of nuclear factor kappa B (NF-κB) pathways. Some anti-inflammatory pathways (such as transforming growth factor-beta, TGF-β) specifically inhibit MyD88 to limit immune-mediated damage.
- ***Endocytic pattern recognition receptors***, which act by enhancing antigen presentation on macrophages, by recognizing microorganisms with mannose-rich carbohydrates on their surface, or by binding to bacterial cell walls and scavenging [illegible] from the circulation. All lead to ***phagocytosis***.
- ***TREM-1*** (triggering receptor expressed on myeloid cells), a cell surface receptor, which, when bound to its ligand, triggers secretion of pro-inflammatory cytokines. It is upregulated by bacterial lipopolysaccharides but not in non-infective disorders. Interestingly, rare variants in the gene encoding the related protein TREM-2 confer a significant risk of Alzheimer's disease, implying a role for immune cells in preventing the buildup of amyloid plaque (see p. 878).

The key principle at play here is that the immune system has devised a means of identifying most types of invading microorganisms by using a limited number of PRRs recognizing common molecular patterns, or PAMPs. This recognition event has been termed a 'danger signal'; it alerts the immune system to the presence of a pathogen. Sensing danger is a key role of the DC and a key first step towards activation of the adaptive immune system.

Dendritic cells and T cell activation

In a sequence of events that spans 1–2 days, immature DCs are activated by PAMPs or DAMPs in the tissues binding to a PRR on DCs. The immature pDC is a small, rounded cell that develops dendrites upon activation and secretes enormous quantities of IFN-α, a potent antiviral and pro-inflammatory cytokine. On activation, the DC migrates to the local lymph node with the engulfed pathogen. During migration, the DC matures, changing its shape, gene and molecular profile and function within a matter of hours to take on a mature form, with altered functions ***(Box 8.11, Fig. 8.5)***, in particular upregulating machinery required to activate T lymphocytes. Once in the lymph node, the mature DC interacts with naive T lymphocytes (antigen presentation), resulting in two key outcomes:

1. activation of T cells with the ability to recognize peptide fragments (termed epitopes) of the pathogen
2. polarization of the T cell towards a functional phenotype (see below) that is tailored to the particular pathogen.

The mature DC provides three major signals to naive T cells ***(Fig. 8.5)***:

- ***signal 1***=presentation of peptide fragments from the pathogen bound to surface human leucocyte antigen (HLA) molecules
- ***signal 2***=co-stimulation through CD80 and CD86 interacting with CD28 on T cells
- ***signal 3***=secretion of cytokines, notably IL-12.

Natural killer cells

Natural killer (NK) cells are described on page 132.

Further reading

Chola MK, Ryrer SW, Levine B. Autophagy in human health and disease. *N Engl J Med* 2013; 368:651–662.
Collin M, McGovern N, Haniffa M. Human dendritic cell subsets. *Immunology* 2013; 140:22–30.
Manfredi AA, Rovere-Querini P. The mitochondrion – a Trojan horse that kicks off inflammation? *N Engl J Med* 2010; 362:2132–2133.
Netea M, van der Pleer JW. Immunodeficiency and genetic defects of pattern recognition receptors. *N Engl J Med* 2011; 364:60–70.
Reis E, Sousa C. Innate regulation of adaptive immunity. *Eur J Clin Invest* 2010; 41:907–916.
http://www.copewithcytokines.de/ *Cytokine listings, functions of cytokines and chemokines, and related drugs in development*

Box 8.11 Myeloid dendritic cell (mDC) maturation

Immature mDC	Mature mDC
Is highly pinocytotic	Ceases pinocytosis
Has low-level expression of molecules required for T lymphocyte activation	Upregulates CD80, CD86 and HLA molecules
Has low-level expression of machinery required to process and present microbial antigens	Begins to process microbial antigens (break down into small peptides) in readiness to present them to T lymphocytes (using HLA molecules)
Is generally localized and sedentary	Begins active migration to local lymph node
Minimally secretes cytokines	Actively secretes cytokines in readiness to stimulate T lymphocytes, in particular IL-12

CD, cluster of differentiation; HLA, human leucocyte antigen; IL-12, interleukin 12.

ADAPTIVE IMMUNE SYSTEM

The information gained by DCs that interact with a pathogen is passed on, in the form of signals 1–3 (see ***Fig. 8.5b***). These activate T lymphocytes in the adaptive immune system, which recognize the same pathogen. T lymphocytes may be involved in pathogen removal directly (e.g. by killing) or indirectly (e.g. by recruiting B lymphocytes to make specific antibody). Lymphocytes orchestrate immune responses via cell-to-cell interactions and cytokine release.

Antigen receptors on T and B lymphocytes

One of the key features of the adaptive immune system is specificity for antigen. For example, if you are immunized against the measles virus, you do not have immunity to hepatitis B, and vice versa. Specificity is conferred by two types of receptor: the T cell receptor (TCR) on T lymphocytes and an equivalent on B lymphocytes, the BCR. BCRs are also termed surface immunoglobulin (sIg) and differ from TCRs in also being secreted in large quantities by end-stage B lymphocytes (plasma cells) as soluble immunoglobulins, also known as antibodies.

To maintain protection against the multiplicity of pathogens in our environment, each of us generates great diversity amongst TCRs and antibodies. This is achieved through a mechanism shared by both TCR and antibody, in which distinct families of genes are encoded in the germline, each family (called constant, variable, diversity and joining) contributing a sequence to part of the receptor. Recombination between randomly selected members of each family ensures diversity in the end product. Recombination frequently involves base deletions and additions, adding to the diversity. In the case of antibodies, the result is a potential capacity of more than 10^{14} different antibody molecules; for TCRs, it may be as high as 10^{18}.

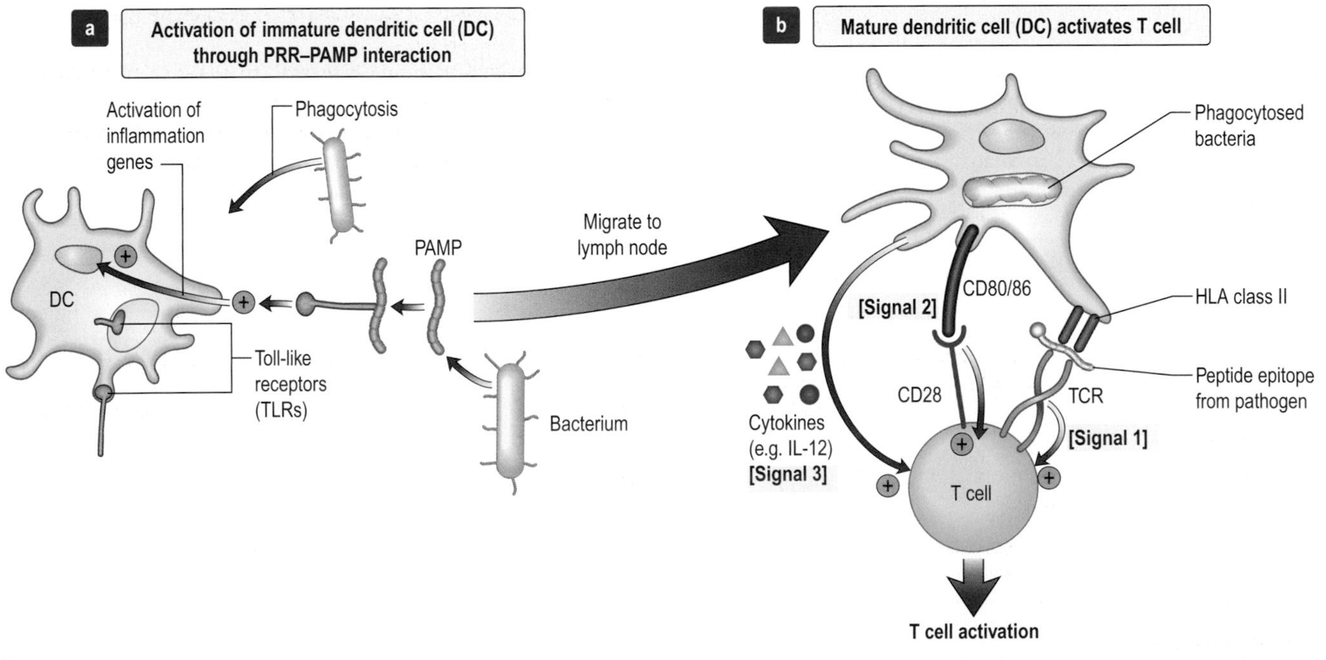

Figure 8.5 Dendritic cell activation of T lymphocytes. (a) Immature dendritic cells (DCs) in the tissues are activated by pathogens through pathogen-associated molecular pattern–pattern recognition receptor (PAMP–PRR) interaction. **(b)** Multiple rapid changes in gene expression lead to migration to the lymph node as the DC takes on the mature phenotype. During migration, there is synthesis of the machinery required for activation of T lymphocytes, shown here in response to **signals 1–3**. CD, cluster of differentiation; HLA, human leucocyte antigen; IL-12, interleukin 12; TCR, T cell receptor.

Immunoglobulins

In structural terms, antibodies have four chains: two identical heavy and two identical light chains ***(Fig. 8.6)***. Each chain contains both highly variable *and* essentially constant regions. The variable parts of the heavy and light chains pair to form the potentially diverse part of the antibody molecule that binds antigen. The constant region of the heavy chain dictates the function of the antibody, and belongs to one of the classes M, G1–4, A1–2, D and E, giving rise to antibodies called IgM, IgG1–4, IgA1–2, IgD and IgE. The characteristics of these different isotypes are shown in ***Box 8.12***.

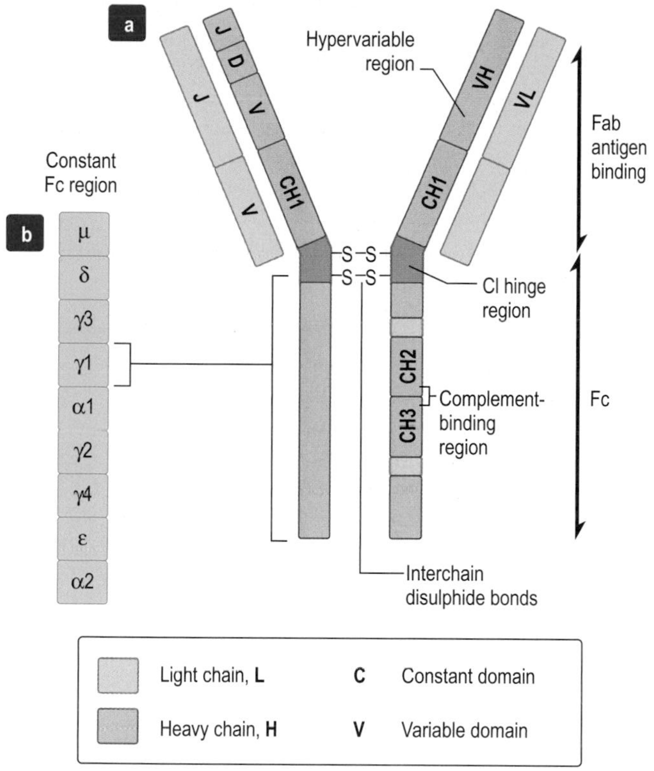

Figure 8.6 **Immunoglobulin structure. (a)** Basic subunit consisting of two heavy and two light chains. **(b)** Genes on the Fab and Fc regions of an immunoglobulin. The chain is made up of a V (variable) gene, which is translocated to the J (joining) chain. The VJ segment is then spliced to the C (constant) gene. Heavy chains have an additional D (diversity) segment, which forms the VDJ segment that bears the antigen-binding site determinants.

Antibody production

Essential points about antibody production are as follows:

- IgM is the first isotype to be made in a primary immune response and thus measurement of pathogen-specific IgM is a useful diagnostic test for recent infection.
- IgG dominates in the second exposure to antigen.
- IgG and IgM are the most efficient complement activators when bound to antigen in an immune complex.
- IgG antibodies cross the placenta, and can carry both immunity and disease to the unborn fetus.
- IgA antibodies are present in secretions (tears, saliva, gastrointestinal tract) to give protection to the mucosae.
- As it matures, and under the instruction of T lymphocytes, a B lymphocyte may change the class (class switching), but never the specificity, of the antibody it makes.
- As B lymphocytes mature and are stimulated to undergo further division, minor changes in antibody gene sequence can take place (somatic mutation), potentially allowing antibodies with higher affinity to arise and be selected for the effector response (affinity maturation).

Antibody function

Essential points about antibody function are as follows:

- In host defence, antibodies target, neutralize and remove infectious organisms and toxins from the circulation and tissues, often through recruitment of innate host effector mechanisms such as complement, phagocytes and mast cells (by binding to specific surface receptors on these cells).
- In clinical medicine, specific anti-pathogen antibody levels are used in diagnosing/monitoring infectious disease, and may also be administered as serum pools to provide host protection passively.
- Antibodies can be raised in animals to generate monoclonal antibodies, which are commonly used in diagnostic immunology tests and increasingly employed as therapeutics (e.g. to target cancer cells), often after 'humanization' (see below).

Box 8.12 Characteristics of the immunoglobulins

	IgG	IgM	IgA	IgE	IgD
Description	Dominant class of antibody	Produced first in immune response	Found in mucous membrane secretions	Responsible for symptoms of allergy: used in defence against nematode parasites	Found almost solely on B lymphocyte surface membranes
Heavy chain	γ	μ	α	ε	δ
Mean adult serum levels (g/L)	IgG (total) = 8–16 G1 = 6.5 G2 = 2.5 G3 = 0.7 G4 = 0.3	0.5–2	IgA (total) = 1.4–4 A1 = 1.5 A2 = 0.2	17–450 ng/mL	0–0.4
Half-life (days)	21	10	6	2	3
Complement fixation					
Classical	++	+++	+	–	–
Alternative	–	–	–	–	–
Binding to mast cells	–	–	–	+	–
Crosses placenta	+	–	–	–	–

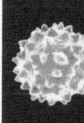

T cell receptor genes and receptor diversity

The genomic organization of T cell receptor (TCR) genes and principles of generation of receptor diversity are similar to those of immunoglobulin genes. The TCR exists as a heterodimer, with a similar overall structure to the antibody molecule. There are two TCR types:

- α and β chains (αβ TCR; expressed on all CD4 T lymphocytes and approximately 90% of CD8 T lymphocytes; play a role in adaptive immune responses)
- γ and δ chains (γδ TCR; fewer in number, mainly on intraepithelial lymphocytes; involved in epithelial defence).

The chains of each type of TCR are divided into variable and constant domains, each domain being encoded by separate gene pools. Like the B lymphocyte producing a single clone of immunoglobulin molecules, the T lymphocyte expresses only one form of TCR once the genes have been rearranged. Unlike antibodies, TCRs do not undergo somatic hypermutation and are not secreted.

T lymphocyte development and activation

T lymphocytes are generated from precursors in the bone marrow, which migrate to the thymus ***(Fig. 8.7)***. Only 1% of the cells that enter the thymus will leave it as naive T lymphocytes to populate the lymph nodes. This process (termed thymic selection) leads to a cohort of cells ***(Box 8.13)*** with:

- functionally rearranged genes allowing surface expression of a receptor for antigen (the TCR) alongside the CD3 accessory molecule involved in transducing the antigen-specific signal
- selection of a co-receptor, either CD4 or CD8, to stabilize the interaction between TCR and peptide-HLA:
  - CD4 T cell responses require presentation of peptide antigens by *self* HLA class II molecules
  - CD8 T cell responses require presentation of peptide antigens by *self* HLA class I molecules
- a reduced or absent tendency of the selected TCR to recognize self antigens (thus avoiding autoimmunity).

Thus, during thymic education, most TCRs are rejected for further use (negative selection), either because they are unable to bind self HLA molecules, or because they bind with too strong an affinity, which would run the risk of self-reactivity and autoimmune disease. The chosen TCRs (positive selection) have low/intermediate affinity for self HLA molecules. During post-thymic activation of T lymphocytes in the lymph node, TCR interaction with HLA has to be bolstered by additional signals (co-stimulation) provided by dendritic cells. This ensures that T lymphocytes are activated only when the checkpoint of DC maturation has been passed, which will happen only in the presence of pathogens.

Co-stimulation of T cells is a competitive process, ensuring that when the activation requirements of T cells have been reduced and the original stimulus (e.g. infection) has been dealt with, the immune response can be switched off. The competition may be provided by alternative ligands for the same molecule with an opposing action. For example, CTLA-4 competes with CD80 and CD86 for CD28, and provides a negative signal, reducing T cell activation. Alternatively, different pairs of molecules, such as programmed cell death protein-1 (PD-1) and its ligand (PD-L1), may be expressed and trigger cell deactivation or death. These pathways can be exploited in therapies for inflammatory diseases: for example, blocking the interaction between CD80/86 and CD28 (via a drug called abatacept) is a highly successful treatment for rheumatoid arthritis. Co-stimulation is also at the centre of a revolution in cancer immunotherapy. Monoclonal antibodies (see pp. 146–147), designed to promote co-stimulation and prevent deactivation, are having dramatic effects on several solid tumours such as melanoma and renal cell carcinoma.

Most naive T lymphocytes are resident in the lymph nodes or spleen, whilst 2% are present in the blood, representing a recirculating pool. Naive T lymphocytes are activated for the first time in the lymph node by antigens presented to their TCRs as short peptides bound to major histocompatibility complex (MHC) molecules on the surface of DCs (see ***Fig. 8.5***). Provision of signals

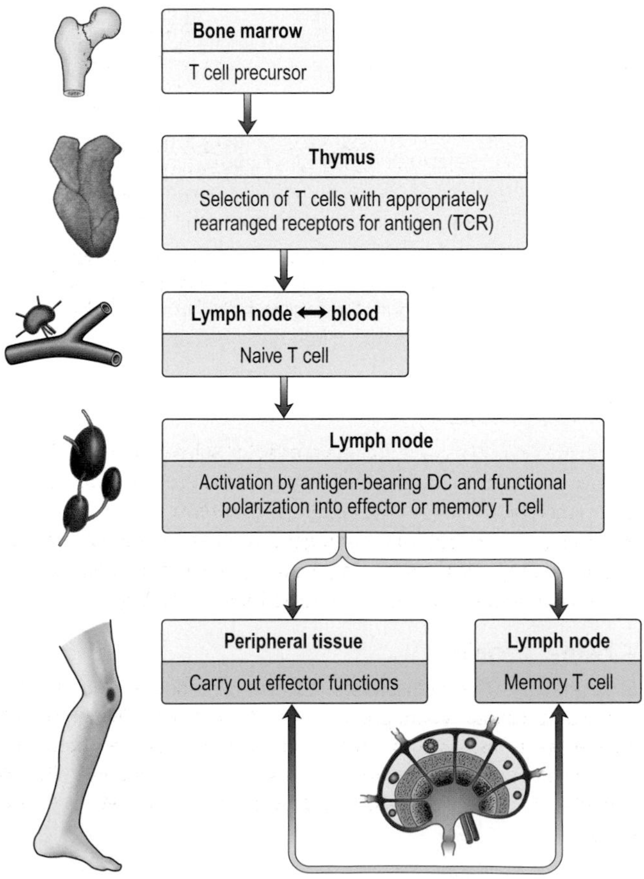

Figure 8.7 Development of T lymphocytes in the thymus and life cycle in the secondary lymphoid tissue. DC, dendritic cell; TCR, T cell receptor.

Box 8.13 Identification of T lymphocytes

T cell population	Marker	Typical percentages in blood	Additional information
T lymphocytes	T cell receptor CD3	100% of T cells (70% of lymphocytes)	All T cells are thymus-derived
Helper T lymphocytes (Th)	CD4	66% of T cells	Th interact with antigen presented by MHC class II molecules
Cytotoxic T lymphocytes (CTL)	CD8	33% of T cells	CTL interact with antigen presented by MHC class I molecules

MHC, major histocompatibility complex.

Box 8.14 Identification of CD4 T lymphocyte subsets by function

T cell type	Main cytokines causing polarization	Main cytokines produced	Functions	Major role in physiological immune response
T helper 1 (Th1) cells	IL-12	IFN-γ, IL-2, TNF-α	Pro-inflammatory	Organize killing of bacteria, fungi and viruses; activate macrophages to kill intracellular bacteria; instruct cytotoxic T cell responses
T helper 2 (Th2) cells	IL-4	IL-4, IL-5, IL-13	Pro-inflammatory	Organize killing of parasites by recruiting eosinophils; promote antibody responses, especially switching to IgE
T helper 17 (Th 17) cells	IL-6, IL-23, TGF-β	IL-17	Pro-inflammatory	Not yet fully defined; capable of recruiting cells and damaging targets; may be more resistant to Treg than Th1/Th2 cells
Regulatory T cells (Treg)	IL-10, TGF-β	IL-10, TGF-β	Regulatory	Regulation of inflammation

IFN-γ, interferon-gamma; IgE, immunoglobulin E; IL, interleukin; TGF-β, transforming growth factor beta; TNF-α, tumour necrosis factor alpha.

1–3 (see p. 127) sets off an intracellular cascade of signalling molecule activation, leading to induction of gene transcription in T lymphocytes.

Nuclear factor kappa B (NF-κB) is a pivotal transcription factor in chronic inflammatory diseases and malignancy (see ***Fig. 7.12***). It is found in the cytoplasm bound to an inhibitor, IκB, which prevents it from entering the nucleus. It is released from IκB on stimulation of the cell and passes into the nucleus, where it binds to promoter regions of target genes involved in inflammation. It is stimulated by, for example, cytokines, protein C activators and viruses. The outcome is T lymphocyte activation, cell division and functional polarization, which is the acquired ability to promote a selected type of adaptive immune response. These processes take several days to achieve. The best-described polarities of T cell responses ***(Box 8.14)*** are:

- $CD4^+$ pro-inflammatory T lymphocytes; T helper 1 (Th1), Th2 and Th17
- $CD8^+$ cytotoxic T lymphocytes (CTLs) ***(Box 8.15)***
- $CD4^+$ regulatory responses (Treg).

Through cell division, a proportion of the T lymphocytes that are activated in response to a pathogen undertake these effector or regulatory functions, whilst a proportion is assigned to a memory pool. Once established, effector and memory T lymphocytes have lesser requirements for subsequent activation, which can be mediated by monocytes, macrophages and B lymphocytes.

CD4 T lymphocyte functions

As the pivotal cell in immune responses, the CD4 T lymphocyte influences most aspects of immunity, either through the release of cytokines, or via direct cell–cell interaction, a process often termed 'licensing'. Licensing critically involves the pairing of CD40 on the antigen presenting cell and CD40 ligand (CD154) on the CD4 T lymphocyte; defects in this process result in antibody deficiency (see below).

Major functions of CD4 T lymphocytes are:

- ***licensing of DCs*** during antigen presentation to activate CD8 T lymphocytes and generate cytotoxic cells
- ***licensing of B lymphocytes*** to initiate and mature antibody responses, leading to class switching, affinity maturation of antibodies, and generation of plasma cells or memory cells
- ***secretion of cytokines*** responsible for growth and differentiation of a range of cell types, especially other T lymphocytes, macrophages and eosinophils
- ***regulation of immune reactions***.

Box 8.15 Major T lymphocyte subsets

Name	Major marker	Cytokines	Major features
Th1	CD4	IFN-γ, TNF-α	Are main subset of effector CD4 T lymphocytes Protect from intracellular pathogens
Th2	CD4	IL-4, IL-5, IL-13	Protect from extracellular pathogens such as parasites Play role in allergic disease
Th17	CD4	IL-17	Protect from fungi Play role in autoimmune inflammatory diseases
CTL	CD8	IFN-γ, TNF-α	Kill target cells via recognition of HLA class I+peptide Protect from viruses

CD, cluster of differentiation; CTL, cytotoxic T lymphocytes; HLA, human leucocyte antigen; IFN-γ, interferon-gamma; IgE, immunoglobulin E; IL, interleukin; TGF-β, transforming growth factor beta; Th, T helper; TNF-α, tumour necrosis factor alpha.

T helper 1 cells

T helper 1 cells (Th1) are the main effector subtype of CD4 T lymphocytes. In physiology, they drive activation of monocytes/macrophages and CTLs. In pathology, they have a key role in protection against intracellular pathogens such as viruses and mycobacteria. Th1 cells are recognized by their secretion of the pro-inflammatory cytokines IFN-γ and TNF-α ***(Box 8.15)***.

T helper 2 cells

In physiology, Th2 cells drive antibody responses, especially IgE, and also promote eosinophil granulocyte functions. In pathology, they have a key role in protection from extracellular parasites (helminths) and also in the immune responses that underlie allergic disease. Th2 cells are recognized by secretion of IL-4, IL-5 and IL-13.

T helper 17 cells

In physiology, Th17 cells drive inflammatory responses, especially via recruitment of neutrophil granulocytes. In pathology, they are necessary for protection from fungal infections, and are increasingly recognized as having a role in chronic inflammatory diseases such as multiple sclerosis, rheumatoid arthritis and inflammatory bowel disease. They are recognized by secretion of IL-17.

Regulatory T lymphocytes

The generation of B and T lymphocytes provides a potentially vast array of rearranged antigen receptors. Although there are selection processes to remove lymphocytes with 'dangerous' avidity for 'self', these are not foolproof and the potential for autoreactivity remains. The fact that there is no self-destruction in the vast majority of people implies that the norm is a state of immunological self-tolerance: the controlled inability to respond to self. Several mechanisms operate to maintain this state, including CD4 T lymphocytes that respond to antigenic stimulation by suppressing ongoing immune responses. At least two different types of regulatory T lymphocytes (Treg) are recognized:

- ***$CD4^{+}$ $CD25^{hi}$ Tregs***. These express high levels of CD25, the receptor for IL-2; regulate other T lymphocytes by cell–cell contact, and also secrete the immune-suppressive cytokines IL-10 and TGF-β; and can be generated in the thymus or post-thymically in the periphery. Their key feature is high expression of the transcription factor Foxp3.
- ***Tr1 Tregs***. These are generated naturally or induced (e.g. by repeated antigen injection); they regulate through production of IL-10.

Evidence that Tregs are clinically relevant is given by the example of immune deficiency states in which they are defective. For example, genetic defects in the Foxp3 gene give rise to IPEX (*i*mmune dysregulation, *p*olyendocrinopathy, *e*nteropathy, *X*-linked syndrome). Patients with this rare syndrome have defective Tregs and develop a range of conditions soon after birth, including organ-specific autoimmune disease such as type 1 diabetes. Much research effort is directed at harnessing this natural regulatory potential, for example to control organ graft rejection and autoimmune disease.

CD8 T lymphocyte functions

Cytotoxic CD8 T lymphocytes (CTLs) are involved in defence against viruses. CTLs kill virus-infected cells following recognition of viral peptide-HLA class I complexes. CTLs must be activated first in the lymph node by a DC cross-presenting the *same* viral peptide, and licensed by a CD4 T lymphocyte recognizing viral peptide-HLA class II complexes. The same defence mechanism may also apply in tumour surveillance. This is a checkpoint that ensures that CTL responses, which have great destructive power, are only activated against a target for which there is also a CD4 T cell response. CTLs kill via three mechanisms:

- cytotoxic granule proteins (cytolysins such as perforin, granzyme B)
- toxic cytokines (e.g. IFN-γ, TNF-α)
- death-inducing surface molecules (e.g. Fas ligand binds Fas on target cells mediating apoptosis via caspase activation; see ***Fig. 7.18***).

Natural killer cells

Natural killer (NK) cells are bone marrow-derived, present in the blood and lymph nodes, and represent 5–10% of lymphoid cells. The name reflects two features. Unlike B and T lymphocytes, NK cells are able to:

Box 8.16 Examples of natural killer (NK) cell receptors

Receptors on NK cells	Ligand
Inhibitory	
KIR2DL1	HLA-C molecules
KIR3DL1	HLA-B molecules
KIRDL2	HLA-A molecules
NKG2A	HLA-E molecules
Activating	
CD16 (low-affinity receptor for IgG)	IgG
NKG2D	MHC class I chain related gene A (MICA)
KIR2DS1	HLA-C

HLA, human leucocyte antigen; KIR, killer cell immunoglobulin-like receptor; MHC, major histocompatibility complex.

- Mediate their effector function *spontaneously* (i.e. *killing* of target cells through release of perforin, a pore-forming protein) in the absence of previous known sensitization to that target.
- Achieve this with a very limited repertoire of germline-encoded receptors that do not undergo somatic recombination.

Despite their close resemblance to T and B lymphocytes in morphology, the lack of requirement for sensitization and the absence of gene rearrangement to derive receptors for target cells mean that NK cells are also categorized as a part of the innate immune system. For identification purposes, the main surface molecules associated with NK cells are CD16 (see below) and CD56 (note that NK cells are CD3- and TCR-negative).

The role of NK cells is to kill 'abnormal' host cells, typically cells that are virus-infected, or tumour cells. Killing is achieved in similar ways to CTLs. NK cells also secrete copious amounts of IFN-γ and TNF-α, through which they can mediate cytotoxic effects and activate other components of the innate and adaptive immune system. To become activated, NK cells integrate the signal from a potential target cell through a series of receptor–ligand pairings ***(Box 8.16)***. These pairings provide activating and inhibitory signals, and it is the overall balance of these that determines the outcome for the NK cell. The balance can be abnormal on a virus-infected or tumour cell, which might have altered expression of HLA molecules, for example, that mark them out for NK cytotoxicity.

In addition, through CD16, which is the low-affinity receptor for IgG (FcgRIIIA), NK cells can kill IgG-coated target cells in a process termed antibody-dependent cellular cytotoxicity (ADCC).

Further reading

Campbell KS, Hasegawa J. Natural killer cell biology: an update and future directions. *J Allergy Clin Immunol* 2013; 132:536–44.
Esensten JH, Wofsy D, Bluestone JA. Regulatory T cells as therapeutic targets in rheumatoid arthritis. *Nat Rev Rheumatol* 2009; 5:560–5.
Gaffen SL. Recent advances in the IL-17 cytokine family. *Curr Opin Immunol* 2011; 23:613–619.
Long EO, Kim HS, Liu D et al. Controlling natural killer cell responses: integration of signals for activation and inhibition. *Ann Rev Immunol* 2013; 31:227–258.
Sakaguchi S, Miyara M, Costantino CM et al. FOXP3+ regulatory T cells in the human immune system. Nat Rev Immunol 2010; 10:490–500.
Schmitt N, Ueno H. Regulation of human helper T cell subset differentiation by cytokines. *Curr Opin Immunol* 2015; 34:130–136.
Wolchok JD, Kluger H, Callahan MK et al. Nivolumab plus ipilimumab in advanced melanoma *New Engl J Med* 2013; 369:122–123.
http://www.biology.arizona.edu/immunology/ *Antibody resources for educators and researchers*

CELL MIGRATION

Immune cells are mobile. They can migrate into the lymph node to participate in an evolving immune response (e.g. a pathogen-loaded DC from the skin, or a recirculating naive T lymphocyte), or can migrate from the lymph node, via the blood, to the site of a specific infection in the tissues. Such migration takes place along blood and lymphatic vessels, and is a highly regulated process.

To take the example of a DC migrating into the lymph node from the tissues via the lymphatics ***(Fig. 8.8)***, this is highly dependent upon expression of the chemokine receptor CCR7 by the migrating cell and of its ligand (CCL21) by the target tissue. Likewise, circulating naive lymphocytes are CCR7^{+} and migrate with ease into the lymph nodes from the blood or via tissue recirculation. In addition, naive lymphocytes express L-selectin, which binds a glycoprotein cell adhesion molecule (GlyCAM-1) found on the high endothelial venules of lymph nodes. This system can be upregulated in an inflamed lymph node, leading to an influx of naive lymphocytes and the typical symptom of a swollen node.

Migration into inflamed tissue requires that:

- an affected organ or tissue signals that there is a focus of injury/infection *and*
- responding immune cells bind and adhere specifically to that tissue.

This process is highly organized and has a similar basis for all immune cells, involving three basic steps: rolling, adhesion and trans-migration. Each of these is dependent on specialized adhesion molecules, as shown in ***Figure 8.9***.

The expression of these molecules (e.g. LFA-1) is upregulated on T lymphocytes after activation in the lymph node. ICAM-1 expression on tissue endothelium is sensitive to numerous pro-inflammatory molecules and allows immune cells to be guided from the blood into the tissues. Once there, cells move along a gradient

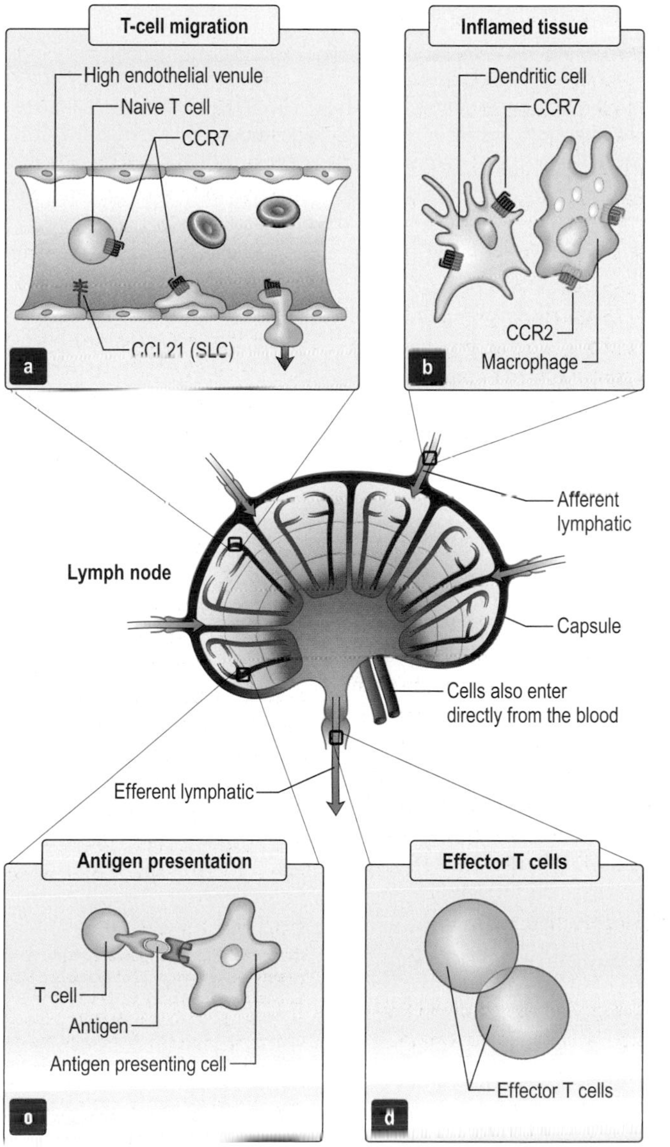

Figure 8.8 Migration of an immune cell through a lymph node.
(a) T lymphocytes migrate through endothelial venules, which express the chemokine CCL21 (secondary lymphoid tissue chemokine, or SLC).
(b) Dendritic cells (expressing CCR7) and macrophages (expressing CCR2) enter lymph nodes via afferent lymphatics and localize in the paracortex.
(c) Antigen presentation (see also Figs 8.12 and 8.13) results in activation of T lymphocytes. **(d) Effector T lymphocytes** leave lymph node via efferent lymphatics.

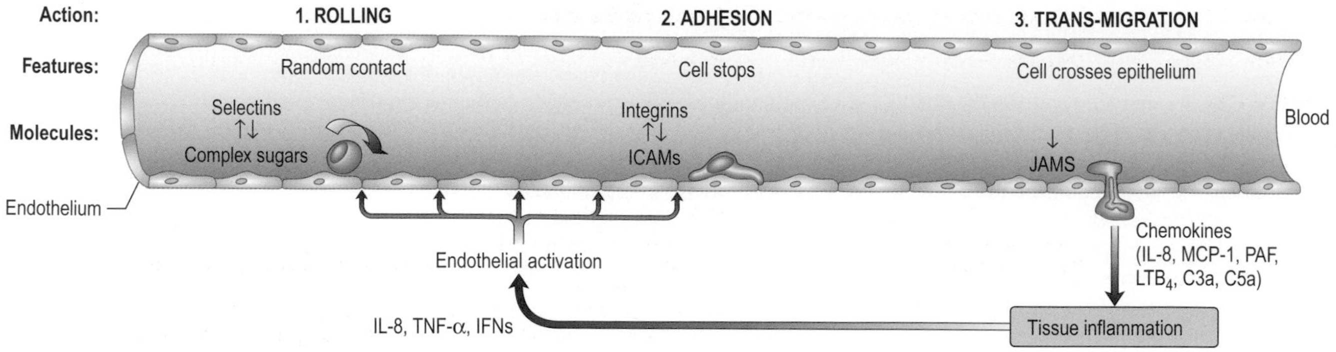

Figure 8.9 Neutrophil migration. Neutrophils arrive at the site of the inflammation, attracted by various chemoattractants.
(1) They ***roll*** along the blood vessel wall through interaction between L-selectin, on their surface, binding to a carbohydrate structure (e.g. sialyl-Lewis^X) on the endothelium. E-selectin on the endothelium mediates a similar effect. P-, E- and L-selectin (*p*latelet, *e*ndothelium and *l*eucocyte, respectively) are named after the predominant cell type that expresses them and bind to carbohydrate moieties such as sialyl-Lewis^X (CD15s) on immune cells, inducing them to slow and roll along the vessel lumen.
(2) ***Firm adhesion*** is then mediated via interaction between integrins on the neutrophil and intercellular and vascular cell adhesion molecules (ICAM-1 and VCAM-1) on the endothelium. The best-known integrin is the heterodimer of CD11a/CD18 (leucocyte function associated antigen-1 – LFA-1), which binds ICAM-1.
(3) ***Trans-migration*** (diapedesis) then occurs: this is a complex process that involves platelet-endothelial cell adhesion molecule-1 (PECAM-1) and junctional adhesion molecules (JAMs).
Following trans-migration (diapedesis), mediators such as interleukin-8 (IL-8), macrophage-chemotactive factor and tumour necrosis factor alpha (TNF-α) attract and activate the neutrophil to the infected tissue, where it phagocytoses and destroys the C3b-coated bacteria.
IFNs, interferons; LTB_4, leukotriene B_4; MCP-1, monocyte chemoattractant protein-1 (CCL2); PAF, platelet-activating factor.

of increasing concentration of mediators such as chemokines in the process of chemotaxis.

HLA MOLECULES AND ANTIGEN PRESENTATION

On the short arm of chromosome 6 is a collection of genes termed the major histocompatibility complex (MHC; known as the human leucocyte antigens, or HLA, in humans), which plays a critical role in immune function. MHC genes code for proteins expressed on the surface of a variety of cell types that are involved in antigen recognition by T lymphocytes. The T lymphocyte receptor for antigen recognizes its ligand as a short antigenic peptide embedded within a physical groove at the extremity of the HLA molecule ***(Fig. 8.10)***.

The HLA genes are particularly interesting for clinicians and biologists. First, differences in HLA molecules between individuals are responsible for tissue and organ graft rejection (hence the name 'histo'(*tissue*)-compatibility). Second, possession of certain HLA genes is linked to susceptibility to particular diseases ***(Box 8.17)***.

The human major histocompatibility complex

The human MHC comprises three major classes (I, II and III) of genes involved in the immune response ***(Fig. 8.11)***.

HLA classes

Classical HLA class I genes

Classical HLA class I genes (also termed Ia) are designated *HLA-A*, *HLA-B* and *HLA-C*. Each encodes a class I α chain, which combines with a β chain to form the class I HLA molecule (see ***Fig. 8.10***). While there are several types of α chain, there is only one type of β chain, β_2 microglobulin. The HLA class I molecule has the role of

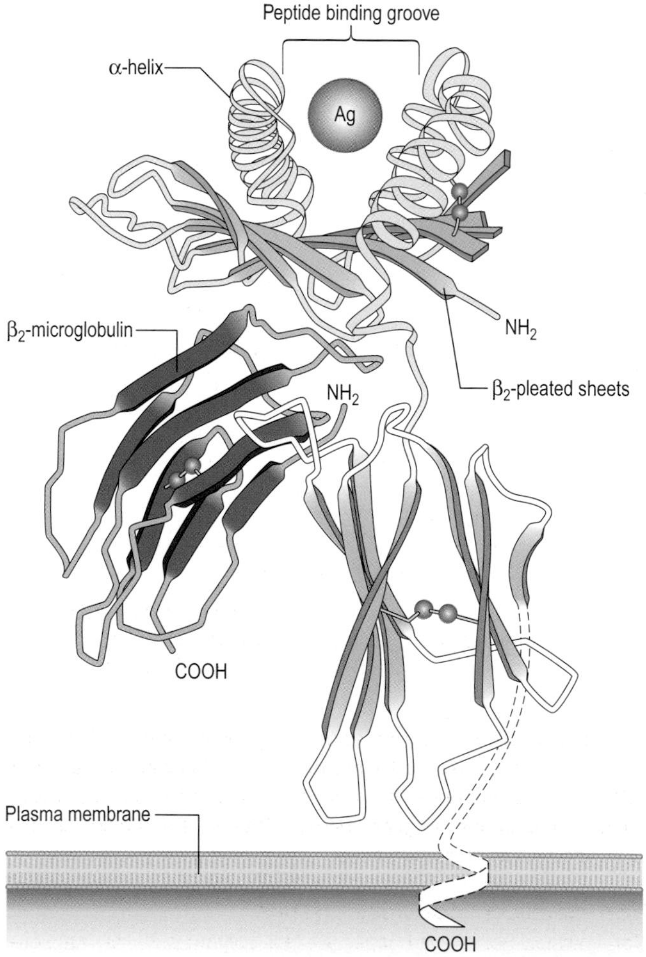

Figure 8.10 Structure of human leucocyte antigen (HLA) class I molecule. The peptide binding groove that is used to present antigen (Ag) to T lymphocytes.

Box 8.17 HLA associations with immune-mediated and infectious diseases

Disease process	Disease	HLA type
Autoimmunity	Type 1 diabetes	Class II: *DQA1*03:01/DQB1*03:02* (susceptibility) *DQA1*05:01/DQB1*02:01* (susceptibility) *DQA1*01:02/DQB1*06.02* (protection) Class I: *HLA-A*24, HLA-B*18, HLA-B*39*
	Multiple sclerosis	*HLA-DRB1*15:01* (susceptibility)
	Myasthenia gravis	*HLA-A*01, -B*08* and *–DRB1*03* extended haplotype (susceptibility) predominates in younger females *HLA-B*07-DRB1*15* (susceptibility) predominates in older males *HLA-DRB1*16, HLA-DRB1*14, HLA-DQB1*05* (susceptibility) for MUSK variant myasthenia
	Behçet syndrome	*HLA-B*51:01* (susceptibility)
	Rheumatoid arthritis	*HLA-DRB1*0404* (susceptibility)
	Autoimmune hepatitis	*HLA-DRB1*03,- DRB1*04* (susceptibility)
	Goodpasture syndrome (anti-glomerular basement membrane disease)	*HLA-DRB1*15:01* (susceptibility)
	Pemphigus vulgaris	*HLA-DRB1*04:02, -DQB1*05:03* (susceptibility)
Inflammatory	Coeliac disease	*HLA-DQA1*05:01/DQB1*02:01* (susceptibility)
	Ankylosing spondylitis	*HLA-B*27* (susceptibility)
	Psoriasis Idiopathic membranous nephropathy	*HLA-Cw*06:02* (susceptibility) *HLA-DQA1* (susceptibility)
Infectious	Human immunodeficiency virus infection	*HLA-B*27, HLA-B*51, HLA-B*57* (associated with slow progression of disease) *HLA-B*35* (associated with rapid progression)
Other	Narcolepsy	*HLA-DQA1*01:02, -DQB1*06:02* (susceptibility) *HLA-DQB1*03:01* (worsens) *HLA-DQB1*05:01, -DQB1*06:01* (protect)

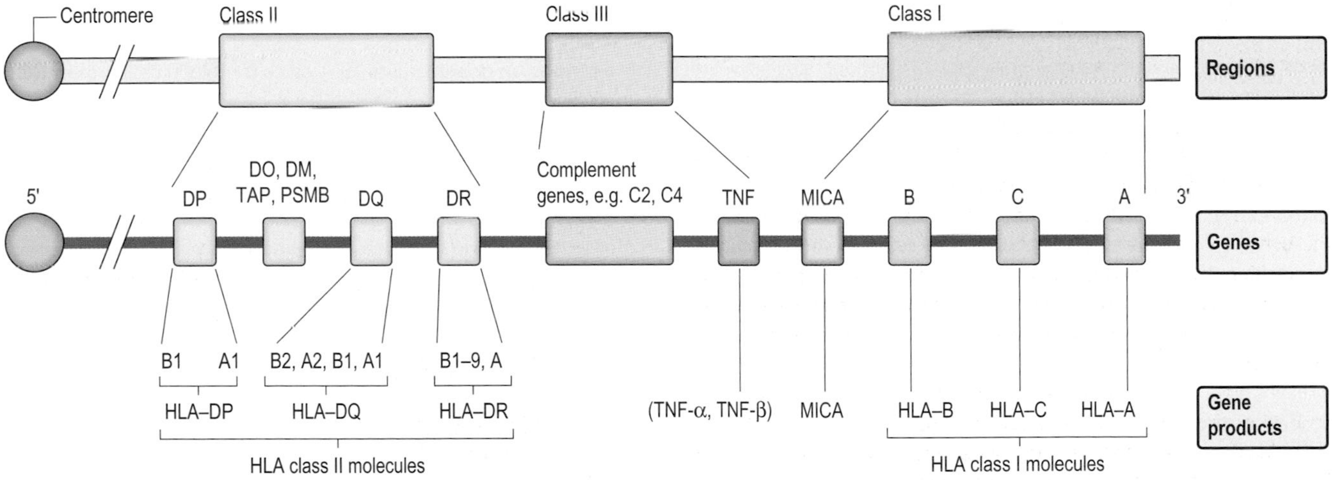

Figure 8.11 The HLA system in humans. On chromosome 6 are three major HLA regions (classes I–III) including genes that encode the HLA class I and II molecules, complement genes, the cytokine tumour necrosis factor (TNF) and other genes involved in antigen presentation (HLA-DO, HLA-DM; transporter associated with processing, TAP; proteasome subunit beta, PSMB; and the non-classical HLA class Ic molecule, MICA).

presenting short (8–10 amino acids) antigenic peptides to the T cell receptor on the subset of T lymphocytes that bear the co-receptor CD8. As an example of HLA polymorphism, there are nearly 200 allelic forms at the *A* gene locus. Class I HLA molecules are expressed on all nucleated cells.

Non-classical HLA class I genes

Non-classical HLA class I genes are less polymorphic, have a more restricted expression on specialized cell types, and present a restricted type of peptide or none at all. These are the *HLA-E*, *F* and *G* (Ib genes) and MHC class I-related (MIC, or class Ic) genes, *A* and *B*. The products of these genes are predominantly found on epithelial cells, signal cellular stress and interact with lymphoid cells, especially natural killer cells (see p. 132).

HLA class II genes

The class II genes have three major subregions: *DP*, *DQ* and *DR*. In these subregions are genes encoding *A* and *B* genes that combine to form dimeric αβ molecules that present short (12–15 amino acid) peptides to T lymphocytes that bear the CD4 co-receptor. Class II HLA genes (apart from *DRA*) are highly polymorphic. Other genes in this region encode proteins with key roles in antigen presentation

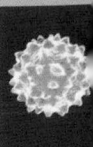

(e.g. TAP, HLA-DM, HLA-DO, proteasome subunits; see below). Class II HLA genes are expressed on a restricted cohort of cells that go by the general term of antigen presenting cells (APCs; DCs, monocyte/macrophages, B lymphocytes).

HLA class III genes

HLA class III genes encode proteins that can regulate/modify immune responses, e.g. tumour necrosis factor (TNF), heat shock protein (HSP) and complement protein (C2, C4).

HLA genotypes and the range of their protein products

HLA genotype is denoted first by the letters that designate the locus (e.g. *HLA-A*, *HLA-DR*, *HLA-DQ*). For class I alleles, this is followed by an asterisk and then a 2- to 4-digit number defining the allelic variant at that locus, often called the HLA type (e.g. *HLA-A*02* is the 02 variant of the *HLA-A* gene). The class II nomenclature is the same, except that both *A* and *B* genes are named (although HLA-DR molecules only require the name of the *B* gene because the *A* gene is the same in all of us).

Some general principles apply to the HLA genes and their protein products:

- The presence of multiple genes on each chromosome, and the fact that both maternal and paternal genes are co-dominantly expressed, allow considerable breadth in the number of HLA molecules that an individual expresses.
- The existence of polymorphisms at each locus provides great breadth in the number of HLA molecules expressed at a population level. The polymorphic forms of HLA molecules differ predominantly in the peptide-binding groove (see ***Fig. 8.10***).

Overall, then, each human can bind a range of peptide epitopes from pathogens to enhance individual protection; similarly, the population has an even greater range of protection, to ensure population survival.

Antigen presentation

HLA molecules bind short peptide fragments that are processed ('chopped up') from larger proteins (antigens) derived from pathogens. The peptide–HLA complex is presented on antigen presenting cells (APCs) for recognition by T cell receptors (TCRs) on T lymphocytes. There are three major routes to antigen processing and presentation:

- ***The endogenous route (Fig. 8.12)*** is a property of all nucleated cells; the internal milieu is sampled to generate peptide–HLA class I complexes for display ('presentation') on the cell surface. In a healthy cell, the peptides are derived from self proteins in the cytoplasm ***(Fig. 8.12)*** and are ignored by the immune system. In a virus-infected cell, viral proteins are processed and presented. The resulting viral peptide–HLA class I complex is presented to CD8 T lymphocytes that have cytotoxic (killer) function. In an immune response against a virus infection, CD8 T lymphocytes recognizing viral peptide–HLA complexes on the surface of an infected cell will kill it as a means to limit and eradicate infection.
- ***The exogenous route (Fig. 8.13)*** is a property of APCs; the external milieu is sampled. Antigens are internalized, either in the process of phagocytosis of a pathogen, through pinocytosis, or through specialized surface receptors (e.g. for antigen/antibody/complement complexes). The antigen is broken down by a combination of low pH and proteolytic enzymes for 'loading' into HLA class II molecules. At the APC surface, the pathogen peptide–HLA class II complex is presented to, and able to interact with, CD4 T lymphocytes. Presentation by DCs can initiate an adaptive immune response by activating a naive, pathogen-specific CD4 T lymphocyte. Presentation by monocyte/macrophages and B lymphocytes can maintain and enhance this response by activating effector and memory pathogen-specific CD4 T lymphocytes.
- ***Cross-presentation*** refers to the ability of some APCs (mainly DCs) to internalize exogenous antigens and process them through the endogenous route (see ***Fig. 8.12***). This is an essential component in the activation of CD8 cytotoxic T cell responses against a virus.

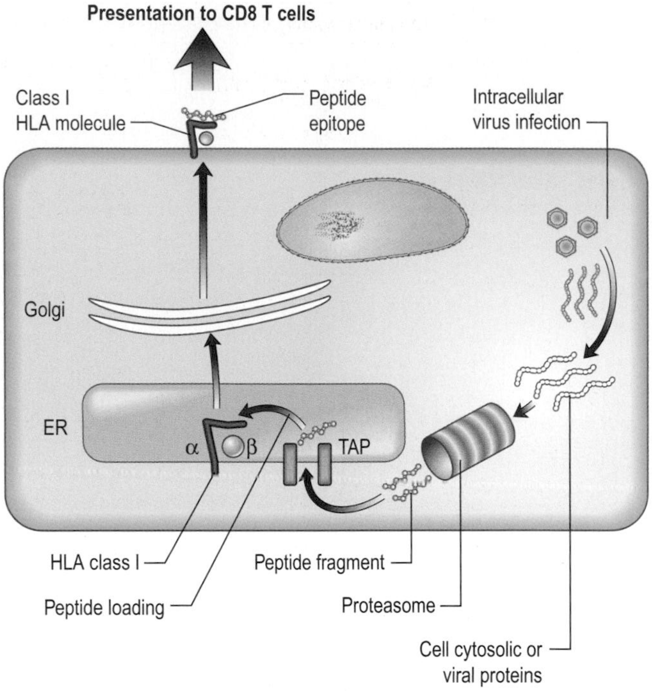

Figure 8.12 **The *endogenous route* of antigen presentation.** Antigen is presented to CD8 T lymphocytes. Cytosolic proteins derived from self (resting cells) or viruses (virus-infected cells) are broken down by the proteasome (a sort of 'protein recycler') into fragments 2–25 amino acids long. Some of these are taken into the endoplasmic reticulum (ER) by a transporter (TAP), trimmed, and loaded into empty HLA class I molecules. These are exported to the surface membrane for presentation to CD8 T lymphocytes.

Further reading

http://hla.alleles.org/ *Information on the human MHC.*

Lázaro S, Gamarra D, Del Val M. Proteolytic enzymes involved in MHC class I antigen processing: a guerrilla army that partners with the proteasome. *Mol Immunol.* 2015; 68:72–76.

Sadegh-Nasseri S, Kim A. Exogenous antigens bind MHC class II first, and are processed by cathepsins later. *Mol Immunol.* 2015; 68:81–84.

THE IMMUNE SYSTEM IN CONCERT

Acute inflammation: events and symptoms

This is the early and rapid host response to tissue injury. To take a bacterial infection as the classic example:

- Local expansion of pathogen numbers leads to direct activation of complement in the tissues, with ensuing degranulation of mast cells.

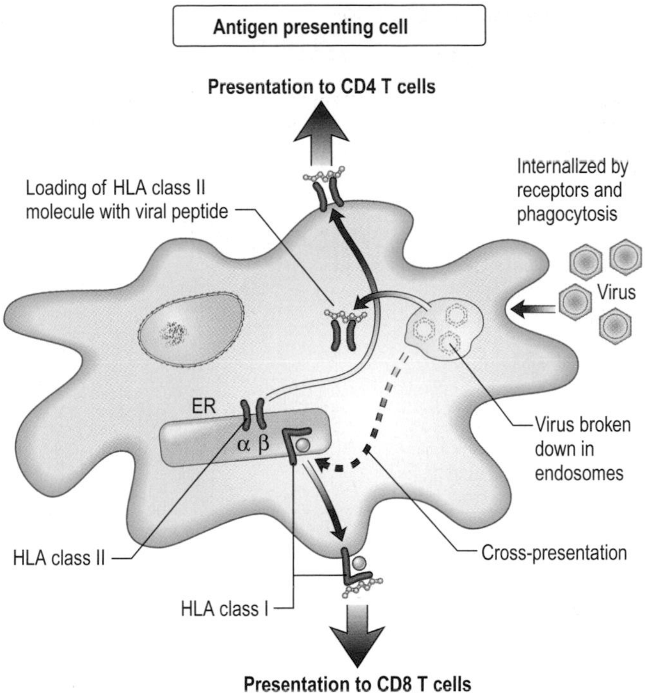

Figure 8.13 The *exogenous route* of antigen presentation and cross-presentation. External material (e.g. virus particles) is taken into an antigen presenting cell and broken down into specialized compartments by a combination of low pH and proteolysis. Peptides are then loaded into HLA class II molecules for presentation to CD4 T lymphocytes. Material may also be transferred across the cell so that it is loaded on to HLA class I molecules for presentation to CD8 T lymphocytes. This process of cross-presentation is restricted to specialized antigen presenting cells such as dendritic cells.

- Inflammatory mediators (from mast cells and complement) change the blood flow and attract and activate granulocytes (neutrophils).
- Concomitantly, there are the local symptoms of heat, pain, swelling and redness, and perhaps more systemic symptoms such as fever due to the effect of circulating cytokines (IL-1, IL-6, TNF-α) on the hypothalamus. Indeed, gene mutations that lead to excessive actions of IL-1 (e.g. mutation of the *IL1RN* gene, which encodes a natural IL-1 antagonist) give rise to rare disease with just these symptoms, as well as bone erosion and skin rashes, which are treatable with IL-1 blockade using soluble IL-1 receptor antagonist (anakinra) or monoclonal anti-IL-1β antibody.
- Systemically active mediators (especially IL-6) also initiate the production of C-reactive protein (CRP) in the liver.
- Bacterial lysis follows through the actions of complement and neutrophils, leading to formation of fluid in the tissue space containing dead and dying bacteria and host granulocytes ('pus').
- At the site of pathogen entry, there is often relative tissue hypoxia. The low oxygen tension has the effect of amplifying the responses of innate immune cells and suppressing the response of adaptive immune cells. This is probably an effective means of preventing excessive immune activation, which can result in collateral damage ***(Fig. 8.14)***.
- The inflammation may become organized and walled off through local fibrin deposition to protect the host.
- Antigens from the pathogen travel via the lymphatics (which may become visible as red tracks in the superficial tissues – lymphangitis) in soluble form or are carried by DCs to establish an adaptive immune response, which, at the first host–pathogen encounter, takes approximately 7–14 days. DCs are activated via the PRR–PAMP system (see ***Fig. 8.5***).
- The adaptive immune response leads to activation of pathogen-specific T lymphocytes and of B lymphocytes, and production of pathogen-specific antibody, initially of the IgM class and of low–moderate affinity, and subsequently of the IgG class (or IgA if the infection is mucosal) and of high affinity.
- Resolution of the infection is aided by the scavenging activity of tissue macrophages.

Chronic inflammation: events and symptoms

Inflammation arising in response to immunological insults that cannot be resolved in days/weeks gives rise to chronic inflammation. Examples include infectious agents (viruses that cause chronic infections such as hepatitis B and C, or intracellular bacteria such as mycobacteria) and environmental toxins (such as asbestos and silicon). At the intracellular level, key processes of inflammasome generation (see p. 126) and autophagy (see p. 104) serve to enhance the chronic inflammatory process. Chronic inflammation is also a hallmark of some forms of allergic disease, autoimmune disease and organ graft rejection.

Mycobacterial disease

The common feature of these pathological processes is that the inciting stimulus is not easy to remove. For example, some viruses and mycobacteria remain hidden intracellularly. In many ways, the pathology that results is thus inadvertent; the immune system is caught between the repercussions of not dealing with the infection/insult and the tissue damage that is caused by chronic activation of lymphoid and mononuclear cells.

- ***Mycobacterium leprae.*** In *Mycobacterium leprae* infection (leprosy; see p. 285) this is well demonstrated. With the same infecting organism, two very different forms of disease are seen: lepromatous or tuberculous. In the tuberculous form, there is a good immune response to chronic infection but the immune response causes nerve damage and numb patches of skin. In the lepromatous form, Th1 responses are less pronounced and infection is widespread but there is less nerve damage.

  In both of these forms of mycobacterial disease, the chronic inflammation may lead to permanent organ damage or impaired vascular function, and can be fatal. If the inciting stimulus is removed, inflammation resolves. With leprosy, this is achieved with antibiotics. However, inflammation can return rapidly (24–48 hours) on re-exposure. This rapid recall response is the basis for patch testing to identify the cause of contact dermatitis, another form of chronic inflammation, and also for the Mantoux (skin) or the interferon gamma release (IGRA) blood test of tuberculosis immunity.

  The main immunological event is the presence of a pro-inflammatory focus comprising T and B lymphocytes and APCs, especially macrophages. If antigen persists, inflammation becomes chronic and the macrophages in the lesion fuse to form giant cells and epithelioid cells. Both Th1 and Th2 reactivity is recognized but specific syndromes may be polarized towards one or the other (e.g. chronic

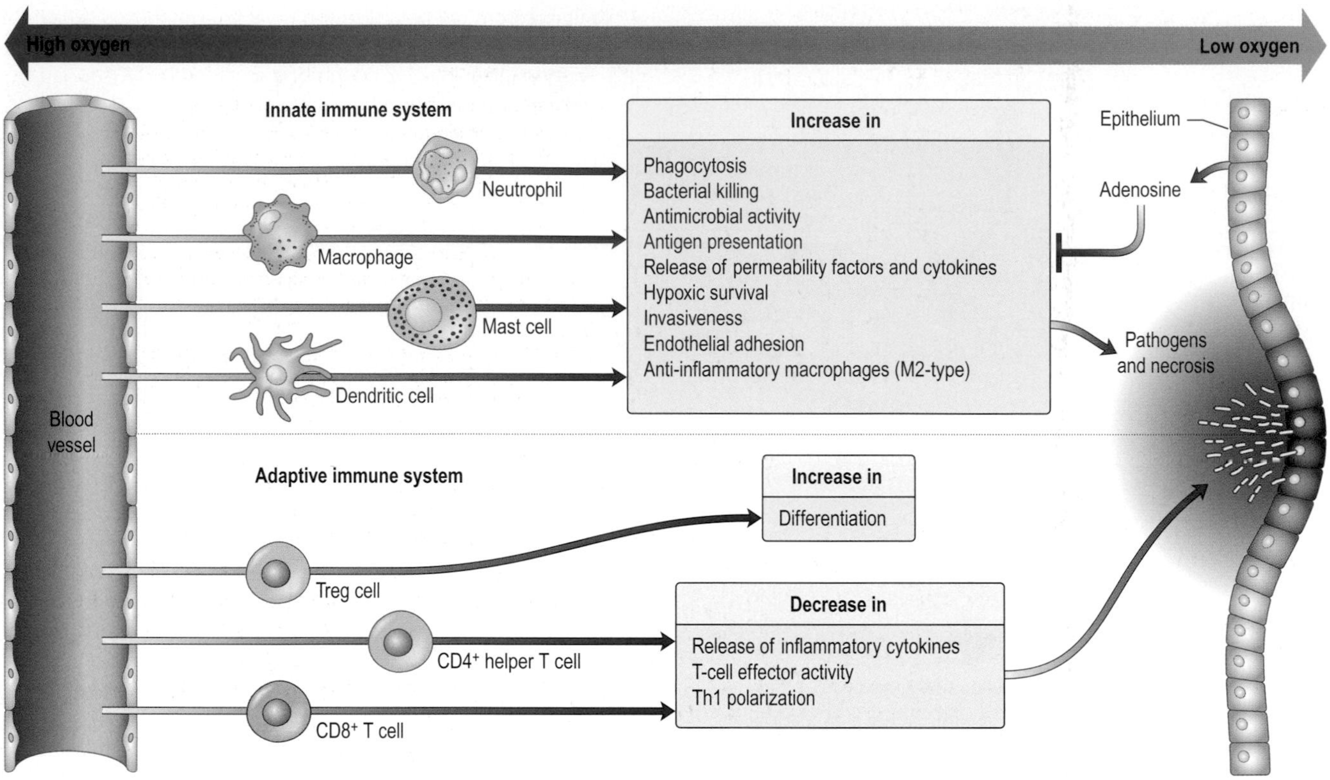

Figure 8.14 Hypoxia and inflammation. At the site of pathogen invasion and necrosis, the oxygen tension is low. Hypoxia acts upon the inflammatory process by amplifying innate immune cell responses and dampening down the adaptive response. Overall, this benefits the host by avoiding an excessive, uncontrolled immune response.

mycobacterial or viral infection initiates Th1 responses, chronic allergic inflammation Th2).

When the inflammation is sufficiently chronic, it may take on the appearance of organized lymphoid tissue resembling a lymph node germinal centre (e.g. in the joints in rheumatoid arthritis; see pp. 672–674). There is massive cytokine production by T lymphocytes and APCs, which contributes to local tissue damage. Granulomata, which 'wall off' the inciting stimulus, may also arise and result in fibrosis and calcification. Symptoms typically relate to the site of the inflammation and the type of pathology, but there may also be systemic effects such as fever and weight loss.

- ***Crohn's disease.*** Chronic inflammation is a hallmark of several immune-mediated and autoimmune diseases but it is often unclear what kick-starts or maintains the inflammatory process. Large-scale studies that identify the genetic basis for these disorders (genome-wide association studies, GWAS) are beginning to provide some clues. A good example is Crohn's disease (CD). Several of the polymorphisms associated with CD reside in genes known to be involved in inflammasome induction, such as *NOD2*. Cytokine regulation has also emerged as a critical disease pathway in GWAS studies on CD: most notably, *IL-23R* (the IL-23 receptor gene), which influences Th17 cell differentiation. Clues like these point to patients with CD having impaired ability to control or terminate inflammasome activity, as well as a predisposition to make polarized pro-inflammatory cytokine responses. This information can now be exploited to devise novel therapeutic approaches, such as monoclonal antibodies that target the key cytokines.

Further reading

Eltzschig HK, Carmeliet P. Hypoxia and inflammation. *N Engl J Med* 2011; 364:656–665.

LABORATORY INVESTIGATIONS OF THE IMMUNE SYSTEM

In the clinical immunology laboratory, proteins and cells can be measured to ascertain the status of the immune system. The results may indicate an undiagnosed inflammatory or infectious disease (e.g. through high CRP level); a state of immune deficiency (e.g. low concentration of IgG); or a state of immune pathology (e.g. the presence of autoantibodies or allergen-specific IgE).

Examples of the more common tests and their interpretation are shown in ***Box 8.18***.

CLINICAL IMMUNODEFICIENCY

Secondary (acquired) versus primary immunodeficiency

Most forms of immunodeficiency are secondary to infection (mainly HIV) or therapy (e.g. corticosteroids, anti-TNF-α monoclonal antibody therapy, cytotoxic anticancer drugs, bone marrow ablation pre-transplant). Examples of other secondary immunodeficiencies are:

- ***Acquired neutropenias***, which are common (e.g. due to myelosuppression by disease or drugs, or the increased rate

Box 8.18 Examining the immune system in the clinical immunology laboratory

	Measurement	Interpretation
Proteins	C-reactive protein	Raised levels indicate infection or inflammation
	Total immunoglobulins	Low levels indicate antibody deficiency, usually a result of underlying disease or primary immunodeficiency. High levels, e.g. ↑ IgM, are seen in acute viral infection (e.g. hepatitis A)
	IgG subclasses	Specific reductions in IgG subclasses (1–4) may indicate immune deficiency. High levels of IgG4 are observed in IgG4 disease
	Complement level and function	Low levels indicate consumption of complement in immune complex disease or primary complement deficiency, which can be confirmed with testing of the alternate or classical pathway function
	IgE	Raised levels are seen in allergy; allergen-specific IgE is useful to pinpoint the inciting stimulus (e.g. pollen, grass), component allergens may be useful in assessing anaphylaxis risk or cross-reactivity between allergens
Cells	Neutrophils	High levels are seen in bacterial infection; low levels in secondary immune deficiency
	Eosinophils	High levels are seen in allergic or parasitic disease
	CD4 T lymphocytes	Low levels are seen in HIV infection
Function	Neutrophil respiratory burst	Absent in immune deficiency chronic granulomatous disease
	T lymphocyte proliferation	Abnormally low in primary T cell immune deficiency disease
Autoantibodies (see also ***Box 8.25*** and ***Box 18.37***)	Rheumatoid factor, anti-citrullinated peptide antibodies (ACPA)	Rheumatoid arthritis
	Double-stranded DNA autoantibodies	Systemic lupus erythematosus
	Acetylcholine receptor antibodies	Myasthenia gravis
	Anti-neutrophil cytoplasmic antibodies (ANCA)	Vasculitis
	Mitochondrial	Primary biliary cholangitis

of destruction in hypersplenism or autoimmune neutropenia) and carry a high risk of infection once the neutrophil count falls below 0.5×10^9/L.

- ***Acquired reductions in levels of immunoglobulins*** (hypogammaglobulinaemia), which are seen in patients with myeloma and chronic lymphocytic leukaemia or lymphoma.
- ***Impairment of defence against capsulated bacteria***, especially pneumococcus, following splenectomy; such patients should receive pneumococcal, meningococcal and Hib vaccinations as a matter of course (see ***Box 16.20***).

Primary immunodeficiency is rare and arises at birth as the congenital effect of a developmental defect or as a result of genetic abnormalities ***(Box 8.19)***. Gene defects may not become manifest until later in infancy or childhood, and some forms of immunodeficiency typically present in adolescence or adulthood.

Clinical features of immunodeficiency

The infections associated with immunodeficiency have several typical features:

- They are often chronic, severe or recurrent.
- They resolve only partially with antibiotic therapy or return soon after cessation of therapy.
- The organisms involved are often unusual ('opportunistic' or 'atypical').

The pattern of infection, in terms of the type of organism involved, is indicative ***(Box 8.20)***:

- ***'Opportunistic' organisms*** are of low virulence but become invasive in immunodeficient states, e.g. atypical mycobacteria, *Pneumocystis jiroveci, Staphylococcus epidermidis*.
- ***Phagocyte defects*** cause deep skin infections, abscesses and osteomyelitis, for example.
- ***Defective antibody*** producers experience infections with pyogenic ('pus-forming') bacteria.

Box 8.19 Classification of immunodeficiencies and the main diseases in each category[a]

Immune component	Examples of diseases
T lymphocyte deficiency	DiGeorge syndrome Acquired immunodeficiency syndrome (AIDS)/human immunodeficiency virus (HIV) infection T cell activation defects (e.g. CD3γ chain mutation) X-linked hyper-IgM syndrome (XHIM; CD40L deficiency)
B lymphocyte deficiency	X-linked agammaglobulinaemia (XLA) Common variable immunodeficiency (CVID) Selective IgA deficiency (IgAD)
Combined T and B cell defects	Severe combined immunodeficiency (SCID) (e.g. due to defects in common γ chain receptor for IL-2, 4, 7, 9, 15)
T cell–APC interactions	IFN-γ receptor deficiency IL-12 deficiency and IL-12 receptor deficiency
Neutrophil defects	Chronic granulomatous disease (CGD) Leucocyte adhesion deficiency (LAD)
Deficiency of complement components	Classical pathway Alternative pathway Common pathway Regulatory proteins Mannose binding lectin

[a]Apart from AIDS, all diseases shown here are primary immunodeficiencies.

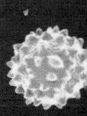

Box 8.20 Immune defects and associated infections

Neutropenia and defective neutrophil function
- *Staphylococcus aureus*
- *Staphylococcus epidermidis*
- *Escherichia coli*
- *Klebsiella pneumoniae*
- *Proteus mirabilis*
- *Pseudomonas aeruginosa*
- *Serratia marcescens*
- *Bacteroides* spp.
- *Aspergillus fumigatus*
- *Candida* spp. (systemic)

Opsonin defects (antibody/complement deficiency)
- *Pneumococcus*
- *Haemophilus influenzae*
- *Meningococcus*
- *Streptococcus* spp. (capsulated)

Antibody deficiency only
- *Campylobacter* spp.
- *Mycoplasma* spp.
- *Ureaplasma* spp.
- Echovirus
- *Pseudomonas* spp.

Complement lytic pathway defects (C5–9)
- Meningococcus
- Gonococcus (disseminated)

Defect in T cell or T cell–APC responses
- *Listeria monocytogenes*
- *Legionella pneumophilae*
- *Salmonella* spp. (non-*typhi*)
- *Nocardia asteroides*
- *Mycobacterium tuberculosis*
- Atypical mycobacteria, especially *M. avium-intracellulare*
- *Candida* spp. (mucocutaneous)
- *Cryptococcus neoformans*
- *Histoplasma capsulatum*
- *Pneumocystis jiroveci*
- *Toxoplasma gondii*
- Herpes simplex
- Herpes zoster
- Cytomegalovirus
- Epstein–Barr virus

- ***T lymphocyte deficiency*** causes infection with fungi, protozoa and intracellular microorganisms.
- ***Congenital deficiencies*** of antibody production are not revealed for several months after birth, due to the 28-day half-life of maternal IgG.

The family history may reveal unexplained sibling death, the fact that only males of the family are affected (X-linked), or consanguinity; each of these makes a primary genetic syndrome more likely. Graft-versus-host disease (GVHD) may arise as a complication of primary or secondary T lymphocyte immunodeficiency. For GVHD to arise, there must be impaired T lymphocyte function in the recipient and the transfer of immunocompetent T lymphocytes from an HLA non-identical donor (see below). GVHD usually arises from therapeutic interventions such as transfusions or transplantation.

Primary immunodeficiency

T lymphocyte deficiency

DiGeorge syndrome

This is due to T lymphocyte deficiency. The third and fourth pharyngeal arches, which normally give rise to the parathyroid glands, aortic arch and the thymus, fail to develop. DiGeorge syndrome arises in 1–5 per 100 000 of the population and presents at birth with dysmorphic facies, hypoparathyroidism and cardiac defects, followed by infections (fungi, protozoa) in later months.

This combination of *c*ardiac abnormalities**,** *a*bnormal facies, *t*hymic dysfunction, *c*left deformities, *h*ypocalcaemia/ hypoparathyroidism and mutations on chromosome *22* is remembered by the acronym CATCH-22. The lack of a location for T lymphocyte development – that is, the thymus – means that affected children have reduced/absent T lymphocyte number and proliferation responses. Apart from calcium supplementation, correction of cardiac abnormalities and prophylactic antibiotics, cure has been reported with thymic transplantation using fetal tissue or stem cell transplant (SCT) from HLA identical siblings.

Other T lymphocyte deficiencies

Other T lymphocyte deficiencies caused by single-gene defects have been characterized and typically present from the age of 3 months with candidal infections of the mouth and skin, protracted diarrhoea, fever and failure to thrive. Examples include deficiency of CD3 itself; defects in signal transduction pathways; and deficiency of IL-2. These disorders are similar in presentation and management to the combined (T and B lymphocyte) immune deficiencies.

T and B lymphocyte deficiency

Severe combined immunodeficiencies

Severe combined immunodeficiencies (SCID) are a heterogeneous group of rare (1–2 live births per 100 000), genetically determined disorders resulting from impaired T, NK and B lymphocyte immunity. The most common form of SCID is an X-linked defect in the IL-2 receptor γ chain, interfering with the function of not just IL-2 but also IL-4, IL-7, IL-9 and IL-15, which share this component in their receptors. Clinical features are similar to those of pure T lymphocyte deficiency and, in the blood, T and NK cells are lacking whilst B lymphocyte numbers may be normal. The most successful treatment for all forms of SCID is SCT, preferably from HLA-identical donors such as siblings. For a few disorders such as γ chain SCID, gene therapy is possible if no appropriate HLA-matched donor can be found.

Hyper-IgM syndrome

This is a mixed deficiency, which may not be diagnosed until later in life. It results from an X-linked defect in the gene encoding CD40 ligand (CD40L, also called CD154). Signalling between CD40 on B lymphocytes and CD40L on T lymphocytes is necessary for the generation of class-switched B lymphocytes bearing high-affinity immunoglobulin, as well as for the maturation of the T cell response. In CD40L deficiency, B lymphocytes are to class switch, producing only IgM. Levels of other types of immunoglobulin IgG and IgA are absent/low and there are mild defects in T cell function.

Opportunistic infections occur: for example, with *Pneumocystis, Cryptosporidium*, *Candida*, *Cryptococcus* and herpes viral infections.

Wiskott–Aldrich syndrome

This is an X-linked defect (at Xp11–23) in a gene involved in signal transduction and cytoskeletal function with associated eczema and thrombocytopenia; a mainly cell-mediated defect with falling immunoglobulins is seen, and autoimmune manifestations and lymphoreticular malignancy may develop. Activating mutations in the same gene have been described that cause severe congenital neutropenia, highlighting the key role of Wiskott–Aldrich serine protease (WASP) in immune regulation.

Ataxia telangiectasia

Patients with this disease have defective DNA repair mechanisms and have cell-mediated defects with low IgA and IgG_2; lymphoid malignancy is again common and a shortened life expectancy often results from the neurological disease.

X-linked lymphoproliferative disease (Epstein–Barr virus)-associated immunodeficiency (Duncan syndrome)

Apparently normal but genetically predisposed (usually X-linked) individuals develop overwhelming Epstein–Barr virus (EBV) infection, polyclonal EBV-driven lymphoproliferation, combined immunodeficiency, aplastic anaemia and lymphoid malignancy. EBV appears to act as a trigger for the expression of a hitherto silent immunodeficiency. Two genetically distinct forms (X-linked lymphoproliferative disease 1 and 2, XLP1 and XLP2) are described, which have defects in the *SH2D1A* and *XIAP* gene, respectively.

B lymphocyte deficiency

X-linked agammaglobulinaemia

X-linked agammaglobulinaemia (XLA) presents soon after maternal IgG protection falls, with recurrent infections of the upper and lower respiratory tract involving pyogenic organisms, enteritis and malabsorption. Morbidity and mortality are high if the condition is untreated, mainly due to chronic lung disease and central nervous system infections with enteroviruses. IgG levels are usually much less than 2.0 g/L (a 1–2-year-old child will usually have an IgG level of 3.5–14 g/L) and all five classes of immunoglobulins are affected, with total levels of less than 2.5 g/L (typically >4 g/L at age 1–2 years). B lymphocyte development is arrested at the pre-B stage, and B lymphocytes are absent in the blood. The cause is a loss-of-function mutation on chromosome Xq22 that affects the gene for a tyrosine kinase involved in cell activation and maturation.

Treatment

Treatment is with replacement immunoglobulins (intravenous or subcutaneous, IVIg or SCIg) to a level that controls infections. Trough IgG concentrations should remain well within normal limits (i.e. >5–6 g/L). Prognosis has improved in recent years as more patients survive into adulthood, but chronic lung disease and lymphomas are life-threatening complications.

Selective IgA deficiency

Selective IgA deficiency (IgAD; serum IgA <0.05 g/L), with normal levels of IgG and IgM, is found in approximately 1/600 Northern Europeans, making it the most common primary immunodeficiency, although the underlying defect is unknown. Most individuals are asymptomatic but patients may present at any age with recurrent infections caused by pyogenic organisms and affecting mucosal sites.

Treatment

When required, this comprises antibiotics. Some IgAD patients produce anti-IgA antibodies of the IgG and IgE classes. Infusion of exogenous IgA (e.g. during a blood transfusion) could therefore result in anaphylaxis. Thus IgAD patients should be screened for anti-IgA antibodies if there is a history of transfusion reaction, and transfused if necessary with washed red cells, blood from an IgAD donor or stored aliquots of their own blood.

Common variable immunodeficiency

Common variable immunodeficiency (CVID) is a heterogeneous disease affecting 1/50 000 and arising during late childhood and early adulthood, with IgG levels <0.5 g/L. It is the most common profound immune deficiency. Presentation with recurrent upper and lower respiratory tract infections is typical and may progress to chronic bronchiectatic lung disease, malabsorption and diarrhoea. There may be additional features of T lymphocyte deficiency, and autoimmunity and granulomatous disease are found in up to 15% of cases. Genetic defects underlying the condition have revealed mutations in multiple genes including *ICOSLG* (ligand for inducible co-stimulator) on activated T lymphocytes in some cases. In most patients, the underlying defect is not known and IVIg or subcutaneous Ig (SCIg) and antibiotics are the treatments of choice.

Defects in antigen presenting cell function

A series of rare genetic defects have been uncovered in which APCs demonstrate an inability to mount protective responses to intracellular bacteria, particularly low-virulence mycobacteria and salmonella. The axis affected is the interplay between CD4 T lymphocytes and APCs that drives Th1 responses, and therefore in turn activates mononuclear cells such as macrophages to kill and eradicate intracellular pathogens. Defective genes so far identified include those encoding a component chain of IL-12; a component chain of the IL-12 receptor; and IFN-γ receptor chains 1 or 2 or the intracellular signalling pathway (STAT 1).

Neutrophil defects

Chronic granulomatous disease

Chronic granulomatous disease (CGD) is a rare (1/250 000) immunodeficiency due to a defect in neutrophil killing and characterized by deep-seated infections. The functional defect is an inability to generate antibacterial metabolites through the respiratory burst (see **Box 8.7**). Typical onset is at toddler age. Neutrophil numbers are normal or increased. A simple respiratory burst test of neutrophil function is diagnostic. The inability to clear infection and frustrated apoptosis adequately by dysfunctional neutrophils leads to granulomatous inflammation.

Treatment

Treatment of infections and prophylactic antibiotic and antifungal therapy are required. Immunotherapy with interferons may have a role in patients with intractable infections, and in some cases SCT is necessary.

Leucocyte adhesion deficiency

Leucocyte adhesion deficiency (LAD) results from defects in integrins (see p. 94). Numerous underlying defects in the genes encoding one of the component chains, *CD18*, have been described in LAD-1. LAD-1 has an autosomal recessive inheritance presenting almost immediately after birth, with delayed umbilical cord separation. In later life, there is a characteristic failure to lose primary dentition and severe gingivitis. Recurrent infections similar to those in chronic granulomatous disease appear during the first decade of life. Blood neutrophil levels are high but cells are absent from the sites of infection, which require aggressive antimicrobial and antifungal treatment, and SCT for cure.

Hyper-IgE syndrome (Job syndrome)

This is an autosomal dominant (occasionally sporadic) immune disorder with high serum IgE levels, dermatitis, boils, pneumonias with cyst formation, and bone and dental abnormalities. Mutations in *STAT3* and *DOCK8* have been found.

Schwachman–Diamond syndrome

This can resemble cystic fibrosis clinically, with exocrine pancreatic insufficiency and pyogenic infections. A mild neutropenia is associated with a defect of neutrophil migration.

Chédiak–Higashi syndrome

This is a rare, recessive disorder due to a mutation in the lysosomal trafficking regulator gene (*LYST*) on chromosome 1q42–45. There are defects in neutrophil function with defective phagolysosome fusion, and large lysosome vesicles are seen in phagocytes. Patients have recurrent infections, neutropenia, anaemia and hepatomegaly. As with Schwachman–Diamond syndrome, tissue infiltration with histiocytes is usually seen, including bone marrow, and Chédiak–Higashi syndrome is one of several genetic causes of primary haemophagocytic lymphohistiocytosis (HLH). Similar genetic abnormalities in melanocytes cause partial oculocutaneous albinism.

Complement deficiency

The consequences of deficiency of complement proteins can be predicted from their functions (see ***Fig. 8.2***):

- Failures in innate response components (e.g. the alternative pathway) lead to impaired non-specific immunity with an increase in bacterial infections.
- Genetically determined low levels of mannose-binding lectin (MBL) are associated with a number of inflammatory and infectious diseases.
- Failure of the classical pathway results in a tendency towards infection and also towards diseases in which immune complex deposition causes inflammation, such as systemic lupus erythematosus (SLE; e.g. C1 and C4 deficiency), vasculitis and glomerulonephritis.

An unexpected finding is that neisserial infections (e.g. meningitis due to *N. meningitidis*) are often encountered in patients with complement defects of the membrane attack complex (C6–9).

Complement regulatory proteins

Deficiency of C1 inhibitor (***C1 esterase deficiency***; see also pp. 1356–1357) is relatively rare. Since this enzyme is involved in regulation of several plasma enzyme systems (e.g. the kinin system) and is continuously consumed, a single parental chromosome defect resulting in 50% of normal production barely copes with the demand and fails under stress (hence has an autosomal dominant effect). As a result, uncontrolled activation of complement and the kinins may occur, leading to oedema of the deep tissues affecting the face, trunk, viscera and airway, explaining the alternative name of hereditary angio-oedema (HAE). Treatment is with C1 inhibitor concentrate or a selective bradykinin-2 receptor antagonist (icatibant). Steroids and antihistamines are not useful in this form of angio-oedema. A rarer acquired form (AAE) may be seen in lymphoproliferative disease or complicating autoimmunity. The treatment is largely as for HAE.

Further reading

Craig TI, Aygören-Pürsün E, Bork K et al. WAO guideline for the management of hereditary angioedema. *World Allergy Organ J* 2012; 5:182–199.
Wood P, Stanworth S, Burton J et al. Recognition, clinical diagnosis and management of patients with primary antibody deficiencies: a systematic review. *Clin Exper Immunol* 2007; 149:410–423.

TYPE I (IMMEDIATE) HYPERSENSITIVITY AND ALLERGIC DISEASE

Normally, host defence can cope with potentially harmful cells and molecules. Under some circumstances, a harmless molecule can initiate an immune response that can lead to tissue damage and death. Such exaggerated, inappropriate responses are termed hypersensitivity reactions or allergic disease.

In ***allergic hypersensitivity***, the binding of an antigen to specific IgE bound to its high-affinity receptor on a mast cell surface results in massive and rapid cell degranulation and the inflammatory response outlined on page 125. The antigens involved are typically inert molecules present in the environment (these are termed allergens; see pp. 1091–1092).

Box 8.21 Mediators involved in the allergic response

Pre-formed mediators	Newly formed mediators (membrane-derived)
• Histamine and serotonin: – Bronchoconstriction – Increased vascular permeability • Neutrophil chemotactic factor (NCF) and eosinophil chemotactic factor (ECF): – Induction of inflammatory cell infiltration	• Leukotriene (LT) B_4: – Chemoattractant • LTC_4, LTD_4, LTE_4 (slow-reacting substance of anaphylaxis, SRS-A): – Sustained bronchoconstriction and oedema • Prostaglandins and thromboxanes: – Platelet-activating factor (PAF) Prolonged airway hyperactivity

The immediate effects of allergen exposure are often very florid (***early phase response***). Allergic disorders also have a second phase, occurring a few hours after exposure and lasting up to several days. These '***late phase responses***' (LPRs) are mediated by Th2 cells recognizing peptide epitopes of the allergen. Recruitment of eosinophils is often a prominent feature.

From a pathological and therapeutic viewpoint, the LPR gives rise to chronic inflammation, which is difficult to control. In ***asthma***, the LPR causes prolonged wheezing, which can be fatal. Immediate hypersensitivity is usually responsive to antihistamines but the LPR is not, requiring powerful immune modulators such as corticosteroids.

In immunopathological terms, in the LPR:

- Neutrophils and eosinophils are prominent in the first 6–18 hours and may persist for 2–3 days.
- Th2 cells accumulate around small blood vessels and persist for 1–2 days.
- Mediators responsible for the cellular infiltrate include platelet-activating factor and leukotrienes ***(Box 8.21)***.
- Th2 cytokines IL-4 and IL-5 and chemokines such as eotaxin act as growth and activation stimuli for eosinophils, which are capable of extensive tissue damage. Th2 cytokines are also responsible for the class switch of Ig production towards IgE, maintaining the cycle of immediate and late responses.

What makes an allergen so powerful?

Several allergens are proteolytic enzymes, allowing them to cross skin and mucosal barriers. They are often contained within small, aerodynamic particles (e.g. pollen grains) that gain access to nasal and bronchial mucosa.

Why do some people react and others not?

The tendency to develop allergic responses (known as atopy) shows strong heritability. Between 20% and 30% of the UK population is atopic and two, one or no atopic parents pass on the atopic trait to their children with a risk of 75%, 50% and 15%, respectively. In developing nations, the tendency to allergy is estimated at one-tenth of the rate in industrialized countries. Amongst the predisposing genes are those encoding the β chain of the high-affinity receptor for IgE and IL-4, both strongly associated with Th2 pathways. The presence of Th2 cells recognizing allergens is the pathological hallmark of allergy.

What environmental factors are involved?

Early exposure to allergens (even *in utero*) may be a factor in developing atopy. Over-zealous attention to cleanliness (the hygiene hypothesis) in developed societies (use of antibiotics, reduced exposure to pathogens that might favour a Th1-like environment) may favour a reduction in Treg activity. This environmental factor is shown by the rapid increase of allergy in the eastern part of Germany following reunification in 1990.

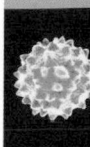

In clinical terms, approximately two-thirds of atopic individuals (who can be identified as those with circulating allergen-specific IgE) have ***clinical allergic disease*** (equating to 15–20% of the UK population). Allergy accounts for up to one-third of school absences because of chronic illness. Allergic disorders include allergic rhinitis (hay fever), allergic eczema, bee and wasp venom allergy, some forms of food allergy, urticaria and angio-oedema.

Diagnosis. Diagnosis of allergic disease is usually made on the history and backed up by skin-prick testing (insertion of a tiny quantity of allergen under the skin and measurement of the size of the weal) and/or measurement of serum allergen-specific IgE. Mast cell tryptase serum levels peak 1–2 hours after an event, remaining high for 24 hours.

Treatment. Avoidance is the first line of therapy. Other measures are as follows:

- ***Antihistamines*** are effective for many immediate hypersensitivity reactions (but have no role in the treatment of asthma).
- ***Corticosteroids*** have several well-identified modifying actions in the allergic process: production of prostaglandin and leukotriene mediators is suppressed, inflammatory cell recruitment and migration are inhibited, and vasoconstriction leads to reduced cell and fluid leakage from the vasculature.
- ***Cysteinyl leukotriene receptor antagonists*** (***LTRAs***) inhibit leukotrienes (LTs) by blocking the type I receptor (e.g. montelukast, used in asthma, particularly the aspirin-induced type).
- ***Omalizumab*** is a monoclonal antibody that binds IgE. It is used in severe asthma (see p. 1099) that cannot be controlled with a corticosteroid plus a long-acting β_2 agonist. Treatment must be initiated in a specialist centre where staff have experience of treating severe, persistent asthma.
- ***Desensitization*** (***allergen immunotherapy***) can be used. It works on the principle that allergy can be prevented by inoculation if the allergen is given in a controlled way. Desensitization is indicated for disorders in which the hypersensitivity is IgE-mediated: for example, life-threatening allergy to insect stings, drug allergy and allergic rhinitis. An induction course of subcutaneous injections of increasing doses of the allergen extract, given once every 1–2 weeks, is followed by maintenance injections monthly for 2–3 years. A systematic review of 51 published randomized, placebo-controlled clinical trials, enrolling a total of nearly 3000 participants, showed a low risk of adverse events with consistent clinical benefit. From an immunological viewpoint, desensitization seems capable of modifying the allergic response at several levels ***(Box 8.22)***. Sublingual allergen immunotherapy (using grass pollen extract tablets of Phl p 5 from timothy grass; see p. 1077) is used in hay fever that has not responded to anti-allergic drugs (the first dose is given under medical supervision).

Anaphylaxis

Anaphylaxis is a serious allergic reaction that is rapid in onset and may cause death. It arises as an acute, generalized IgE-mediated immune reaction involving specific antigen, mast cells and basophils. The reaction requires priming by the allergen, followed by re-exposure. To provoke anaphylaxis, the allergen must be systemically absorbed, after either ingestion or parenteral injection. A range of allergens that provoke anaphylaxis has been identified ***(Box 8.23)***.

Box 8.22 Mechanism of action of desensitization for allergy

Probable mechanism	Effect
IgG blocking antibodies	During repeated exposure to desensitizing allergen, IgG class antibodies develop (especially IgG4 subclass); these compete with the pathogenic IgE for allergen binding and/or prevent IgE–allergen complexes binding to mast cell high-affinity IgE receptors
Regulation	Exposure to repeated desensitizing allergen induces Treg cells, which recognize allergen but invoke regulatory immune responses, dampening down migration, infiltration and inflammation
Immune deviation	A shift away from Th2- to Th1-producing CD4 cells results in the generation of cytokines (e.g. IFN-γ) that are inhibitory to IgE production

Box 8.23 Sources of allergens known to provoke anaphylaxis

Foods
- Nuts: peanuts (protein-arachis hypogaea Ara h 2), Brazil, cashew
- Shellfish: shrimp (allergen Met e 1), lobster
- Dairy products
- Egg
- More rarely: citrus fruits, mango, strawberry, tomato

Venoms
- Wasps, bees, yellow-jackets, hornets

Medications
- Antisera (tetanus, diphtheria), dextran, latex, some antibiotics

Anaphylaxis is rare, and the symptom/sign constellation ranges from widespread urticaria to cardiovascular collapse, laryngeal oedema, airway obstruction and respiratory arrest leading to death:

- Fatal reactions to penicillin occur once every 7.5 million injections.
- Between 1 in 250 and 1 in 125 individuals have severe reactions to bee and wasp stings, and a death takes place every 6.5 million stings, with 60–80 deaths per year in North America and 5–10 in the UK.

Central to the pathogenesis of anaphylaxis is the activation of mast cells and basophils, with systemic release of some mediators and generation of others. The initial symptoms may appear innocuous: tingling, warmth and itchiness. The ensuing effects on the vasculature give vasodilatation and oedema. The consequence of these may be no more than a generalized flush, with urticaria and angio-oedema. More serious sequelae are hypotension, bronchospasm, laryngeal oedema and cardiac arrhythmia or infarction. Death may occur within minutes.

Serum platelet-activating factor (PAF) levels correlate directly with the severity of anaphylaxis, whereas PAF acetylhydrolase (the enzyme that inactivates PAF) correlates inversely and is significantly lower in peanut-sensitive patients with fatal anaphylactic reactions.

Management

Early recognition and treatment are essential ***(Box 8.24)***.

The best treatment is prevention. Avoidance of triggering foods, particularly nuts and shellfish, may require almost obsessive

Box 8.24 Treatment of acute anaphylaxis

Clinical features
- Bronchospasm
- Facial and laryngeal oedema
- Hypotension
- Nausea, vomiting and diarrhoea

Management
- ABCDE (airway, breathing, circulation, disability, exposure)
- Position the patient lying flat with feet raised
- Ensure the airway is free
- Give oxygen
- Monitor blood pressure
- Establish venous access
- Administer 0.5 mg *intramuscular* adrenaline (epinephrine) 0.5 mL of 1 : 1000 adrenaline, i.e. 1 mg/mL, and repeat after 5 min if shock persists. (Dose reduced for children or adults on beta-blockers)
- Administer intravenous antihistamine (e.g. 10–20 mg chlorphenamine) slowly
- Administer 100 mg intravenous hydrocortisone.
  - If hypotension persists, give 1–2 L of intravenous fluid
  - If hypoxia is severe, assisted ventilation may be required
  - Take blood for tryptase levels (aids diagnosis)

self-discipline. Patient education is necessary and many are instructed in the self-administration of adrenaline (epinephrine) and carry pre-loaded syringes. Desensitization has a well-established place in the management of this disorder, particularly if exposure is unavoidable or unpredictable, as in insect stings. In peanut allergy (see p. 216), it has been shown that early introduction of peanuts in children modulates the response in later life.

Further reading

Serhan CN, Chiang N, Dalli J, Levy BD. Lipid mediators in the resolution of inflammation. *Cold Spring Harb Perspect Biol.* 2014; 7:a016311.
http://www.allergen.org/allergen.aspx *Allergen nomenclature*

AUTOIMMUNE DISEASE

Autoimmunity is when the immune response turns against self, i.e. recognizes 'self' antigens. The vast array of possible T cell receptors (TCRs) and antibodies that can be generated by the host make it highly probable that at least a small proportion can recognize self (i.e. are autoreactive). Moreover, a degree of autoreactivity is physiological – the TCR is designed to interact both with the peptide epitope in the HLA molecule binding groove *and* with the HLA molecule itself.

The critical event in the development of autoimmune disease is when T and B lymphocytes bearing these receptors for 'self' become activated. The following are the major checkpoints that the immune system has in place to prevent this:

1. removal of TCRs with very strong affinity for 'self' in the thymus
2. the presence of naturally arising regulatory T lymphocytes (Tregs)
3. the requirement for a danger signal to license dendritic cells to activate CD4 T lymphocytes.

Autoimmune diseases affect 5% of the population at some stage of their life.

Failure of checkpoint 1, thymic education

During thymic education, TCRs with dangerously high affinity for self are deleted. It has become apparent that this process relies upon the thymic expression of self antigens. Situations that compromise the expression of a self protein would be expected to favour the development of autoimmunity. Indeed, in a rare group of patients who develop multiple autoimmune disorders affecting the adrenal and parathyroid glands (autoimmune polyglandular syndrome type 1; see p. 1239), there is a defect in the autoimmune regulator (*AIRE*) gene, which controls thymic expression of a host of self genes. When the gene malfunctions, there is reduced expression of self proteins in the thymus and autoimmune disease is a consequence.

Failure of checkpoint 2, regulatory T lymphocytes

An example of Treg failure is the defect in the gene encoding Foxp3, a critical transcription factor in Tregs (see p. 132), which leads to IPEX (see p. 132). IPEX is very rare but it serves to indicate how Treg defects can lead to autoimmune disease. Laboratory studies in this area are revealing subtle Treg defects in several autoimmune diseases (e.g. type I diabetes, multiple sclerosis, rheumatoid arthritis). The role of FoxP3 in regulating peripheral immune responses highlights the control of immune expansion and regulation of immunological 'space'. Another component of this process is the contraction of an immune response once the infection has been dealt with. Autoimmune lymphoproliferative syndrome (ALPS) is a disorder with defects in either Fas, its ligand (FasL or CD95) or the associated intracellular signalling pathway. Individuals develop multiple cytopenias, organ-specific autoimmunity, and lymphoproliferation that may mimic lymphoma. The common problem is the inability to 'switch off' activated T cells. Treatment is with haemopoietic stem cell transplantation if the disorder is severe. Many patients with multiple cytopenias, including Evans syndrome (autoimmune thrombocytopenia and haemolytic anaemia), are revealed to have ALPS defects when appropriately tested.

Failure of checkpoint 3, CD4 T lymphocyte activation against an autoantigen (or its mimic)

For an autoimmune disease to develop, there must be presentation of autoantigens to a naive, potentially autoreactive CD4 T lymphocyte by activated DCs. This could happen in one of two ways:

- Tissue damage due to infection leads to both the release of hidden self antigens and the provision of sufficient danger signals to activate DCs, which in turn activate autoreactive CD4 T lymphocytes, as well as the pathogen-specific ones. This is often termed 'bystander activation'.
- A pathogen mimics a self antigen. In the process of making an entirely appropriate immune response against the pathogen, T or B lymphocytes are generated that also have the capacity to recognize self. This is termed molecular mimicry.

It is unlikely that, for the common autoimmune diseases ***(Box 8.25)***, there is a 'single checkpoint' explanation. Rather, it is likely that multiple subtle defects, at various checkpoints, are at play.

Mechanisms of tissue damage in autoimmune disease

Figure 8.15 illustrates potential mechanisms of immune damage in autoimmune disease.

Tissue damage via chronic inflammation

In a number of autoimmune diseases (e.g. type 1 diabetes, multiple sclerosis), autoreactive T lymphocytes are likely to be the main drivers of disease and tissue damage. Th1 cells, CTLs and Th17 cells induce chronic inflammation and release cytokines that recruit other effector cells (macrophages) or are directly toxic (e.g.

insulin-producing β-cells are susceptible to the combined effects of IL-1β, IFN-γ and IL-17 in type 1 diabetes).

IgG4 disease

IgG4 disease is a fibro-inflammatory condition with the formation of swellings at multiple sites infiltrated with IgG4-producing plasma cells and a tendency to high circulating levels of IgG4. Unlike many autoimmune disorders, IgG4-related disease is driven by Th2 T cells in association with high numbers of $FoxP3^+$ T cells. The first recognized form of this disorder was autoimmune pancreatitis, but lesions in the biliary tree, salivary glands, periorbital tissues, kidneys, lungs, lymph nodes, meninges, aorta, breast, prostate, thyroid, pericardium and skin are recognized ***(Box 8.26)***. The current hypothesis is that Th2 cells drive the activation of macrophages and myofibroblasts, leading to fibrosis and IgG4 plasma cell proliferation.

Box 8.25 Some autoimmune diseases and their autoantigens

Disease	Antigens
Addison disease	21 α-hydroxylase
Goodpasture syndrome	Alpha-3 chain of type IV collagen
Granulomatosis with polyangiitis	Neutrophil proteinase 3
Graves' thyroiditis	Thyroid-stimulating hormone receptor
Hashimoto's thyroiditis	Thyroid peroxidase, thyroglobulin
Multiple sclerosis	Myelin basic protein Myelin oligodendrocyte glycoprotein
Myasthenia gravis	Acetylcholine receptor, muscle-specific kinase (MuSK)
Pemphigus vulgaris	Desmoglein-3
Pernicious anaemia	H^+/K^+-ATPase, intrinsic factor
Polymyositis/dermatomyositis	Transfer RNA synthases (e.g. Jo-1, PL7, PL12)
Primary biliary cholangitis	Pyruvate dehydrogenase complex
Rheumatoid arthritis	Citrullinated cyclic peptide, IgM
Scleroderma	Topoisomerase
Sjögren syndrome	Ro/La ribonuclear proteins
Systemic lupus erythematosus	Sm/RNP, Ro/La (SS-A/SS-B), histone and native double-stranded DNA
Type 1 diabetes	Pro-insulin, glutamic acid decarboxylase, IA-2, ZNT8
Vitiligo	Pigment cell antigens

Tissue damage via autoantibodies

Examples of damage through direct binding to a target cell or structure, with recruitment of complement and other destructive processes, include:

- ***myasthenia gravis*** (autoantibodies against the acetylcholine receptor cause damage to the neuromuscular junction)
- ***autoimmune haemolytic anaemia*** (autoantibody targets red blood cell autoantigens, leading to lysis)
- ***Goodpasture syndrome*** (anti-glomerular basement membrane autoantibodies damage glomerular integrity).

Autoantibodies can also bind their antigen in the circulation to form immune complexes. When these are deposited in the tissues, complement- and cell-mediated immune reactions are initiated. Immune complexes preferentially deposit in sites such as the kidney glomerulus, leading to chronic kidney disease. This is a feature of SLE, in which the autoantigen within the immune complexes is DNA.

Autoantibody binding may act by binding to surface receptors. In Graves' thyroiditis, for example, the anti-thyroid stimulating hormone receptor antibody stimulates follicular cells to produce thyroid hormones, leading to hyperthyroidism.

Common autoimmune diseases

There are now over 80 diseases classified as autoimmune. The autoimmune origin of some of these diseases is very clear-cut but that is not so for others, and both major and minor factors must be defined.

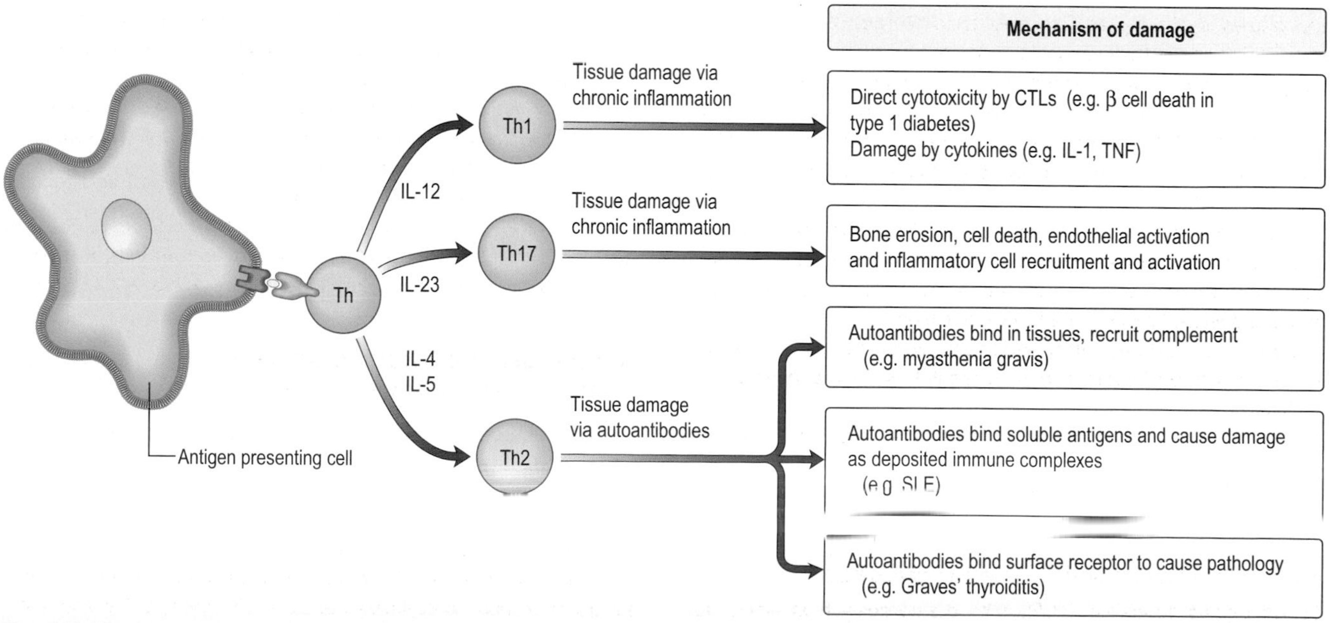

Figure 8.15 Potential mechanisms of immune damage in autoimmune disease. CTL, cytotoxic T lymphocyte; IL, interleukin; SLE, systemic lupus erythematosus; Th, helper T lymphocyte; TNF, tumour necrosis factor.

Major criteria

- There is evidence of autoreactivity (e.g. activated or memory autoreactive T lymphocytes or autoantibodies).
- A clinical response to immune suppression can be demonstrated.
- Passive transfer of the putative immune effector (e.g. autoreactive T lymphocyte or autoantibody) causes the disease (this is the hardest criterion to satisfy in humans but is the most stringent).

Minor criteria

- An animal model exists that resembles the human condition, and in which there is a similar loss of immunological tolerance to self.
- There is evidence that, in the animal model, passive transfer of the putative immune effectors reproduces the disease in a naive animal.
- There is an HLA association (a frequent indicator that a disease is autoimmune).

Box 8.26 IgG4-related disease

Condition	Affected organ or tissue
Chronic stenotic sialadenitis	Submandibular glands
Eosinophilic angiocentric fibrosis	Orbits, upper respiratory tract
Fibrosing mediastinitis	Mediastinum
Hypertrophic pachymeningitis	Dura mater
Idiopathic hypocomplementaemic tubulointerstitial nephritis with extensive tubulointerstitial deposits	Kidney
Inflammatory aortic aneurysm	Aorta
Inflammatory pseudotumour	Orbits, lungs, kidneys and other organs
Mikulicz syndrome	Salivary and lacrimal glands
Multifocal fibrosclerosis	Orbits, thyroid gland, retroperitoneum, mediastinum, and other tissues and organs
Periaortitis and periarteritis	Aorta and large blood vessels
Retroperitoneal fibrosis (Ormond disease)	Retroperitoneum
Riedel's thyroiditis	Thyroid
Sclerosing mesenteritis	Mesentery
Sclerosing pancreatitis	Pancreas

(After Mahajan VS, Mattoo H, Deshpande V, Pillai SS, Stone JH. IgG4-related disease. *Ann Rev Pathology* 2014; 9:315–347.)

Further reading

Cho JH, Gregerson PK. Genomics and the multifactorial nature of human autoimmune disease. *N Engl J Med* 2011; 365:1621–1623.
Goodnow C. Multistep pathogenesis of autoimmune disease. *Cell* 2007; 130:25–35.
Kamisawa T, Zen Y, Pillai S, Stone JH. IgG4-related disease. *Lancet* 2015;385:1460–1470.

ORGAN REJECTION IN CLINICAL TRANSPLANTATION

The outcome of an allograft (i.e. a graft between genetically non-identical members of the same species) in the absence of adequate immunosuppressive therapy is ***immunological rejection***. Histological analysis of rejected organs shows a range of immunological processes in action ***(Box 8.27)***. With modern tissue-matching approaches, hyperacute rejection is rare and acute rejection can usually be prevented or treated with immunosuppression. The process of chronic rejection typically takes place over several years and is the main reason for organ graft failure.

The antigens recognized in acute and chronic graft responses are donor HLA molecules (alloantigens):

- In acute rejection, it is thought that the predominant response is against intact HLA molecules (***direct allorecognition***) and is mediated by $CD4^+$ and $CD8^+$ T lymphocytes.
- As the rejection process becomes more chronic, peptides from donor HLA molecules are processed and presented to T lymphocytes by host HLA molecules (***indirect allorecognition***).

IMMUNE-BASED THERAPIES

Manipulating the immune response in a therapeutic setting has seen many successes, as evidenced by the control of organ rejection in clinical transplantation through targeted immunosuppression ***(Box 8.27)***. Monoclonal antibodies offer the opportunity to neutralize the unwanted effects of cytokines, or to direct immune responses, drugs, toxins or irradiation against a specific target, whether it be a tumour cell or an immune cell involved in a damaging autoimmune response. Natural antiviral mediators, such as the interferons, are already in the clinic as therapies for chronic viral infection, amongst other things.

Monoclonal antibody therapy (targeted therapy)

The combined power of monoclonal antibody (MAb) and recombinant DNA technology has led to a series of 'designer' drugs, which have been engineered so that they:

- are exquisitely targeted
- have optimal effector function

Box 8.27 Classification of rejection

Description	Timing of response	Immunological mechanism	Management
Hyperacute	Minutes to hours	Pre-formed antibodies (e.g. anti-blood group, anti-HLA)	Prevention with typing to avoid mismatch, or depleting antibodies for 'high risk' transplants
Accelerated acute	1–5 days	T lymphocytes	Combinations of immune suppression used prophylactically and as required, e.g. corticosteroids, ciclosporin, tacrolimus, sirolimus, polyclonal antibodies (e.g. against all T lymphocytes) and monoclonal antibodies (e.g. against activated T lymphocytes expressing CD25)
Acute	7–14 days onwards	T lymphocytes	
Chronic	Months to years	Antibodies, complement, endothelial cell changes	Chronic oral immunosuppression

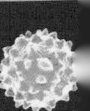

- do not carry antigenic segments that may incite a neutralizing response in the host.

In general, this has meant a process of 'humanizing' antibodies of mouse origin and selecting an appropriate effector function. For example, a MAb designed to remove a subpopulation of lymphocytes from the patient should have good complement-fixing ability or bind well to receptors on phagocytes, whereas a MAb designed to 'modulate' a cell without depletion should have these functions removed. An example of the latter is an anti-CD3 MAb that has modified Fc regions and is designed to downregulate functionally, but not deplete, T lymphocytes. Many examples of MAbs in current use are described in individual chapters. Therapeutic MAbs are potent modifiers of essential components of immune responses and therefore carry both predictable and unpredictable risks. For example, anti-TNF therapies increase the risk of invasive viral and mycobacterial infection. The new inhibitors of integrins, such as natalizumab, have been associated with JC virus reactivation in patients, leading to progressive multifocal leukoencephalopathy (PML). Since integrins are essential for the migration of T cells into tissues, the blockade prevents egress into inflammatory sites, but also reduces immune surveillance of infection. Emerging therapies require an increasing vigilance for side-effects and appropriate counselling of patients.

Immunosuppressive drugs

- ***Glucocorticosteroids*** (cortisone, hydrocortisone, prednisone and prednisolone) are the most commonly used steroids and have a variety of effects on immune function, including:
  - potent effects on monocyte production of the pro-inflammatory cytokines IL-1 and TNF-α
  - blockade of T lymphocyte production of IL-2 and IFN-γ
  - reduced activation and migration of a range of innate and adaptive immune cells.
- ***Ciclosporin, tacrolimus and rapamycin*** (sirolimus) have similar effects on T lymphocyte function. Ciclosporin and tacrolimus are calcineurin inhibitors and inhibit Ca^{2+}-dependent second messenger signals in T lymphocytes following activation via TCRs. By contrast, sirolimus achieves a similar effect but acts at the level of post-activation events in the nucleus.
- ***Purine analogues*** such as azathioprine are also frequently used as anti-inflammatory drugs in conjunction with steroids and act by inhibiting DNA synthesis in dividing adaptive immune cells. Similar in mode of action, but more powerful, is mycophenolate mofetil (MMF).
- ***Alkylating agents*** that interfere with DNA synthesis, such as cyclophosphamide, are also used for immunosuppression.
- ***Kinase inhibitors*** have profoundly improved the treatment of some malignancies with previously very poor outcomes. Tyrosine kinases (TYK) are ubiquitous regulators of cell activation, promoting cell division and proliferation in response to growth factors and cytokines. Inhibition of the signalling pathways can lead to immune suppression. In immune cells, the relevant kinases include the Janus kinases (JAK) that signal through the STAT pathway. Inherited mutations in JAK-STAT pathway molecules can lead to immunodeficiency or, if the mutation causes constant (constitutive) activation, can cause uncontrolled cell division independent of growth factors: that is, cancer. Specific inhibitors of TYK have been developed for a range of cancers and as T and B cell immune suppressants.

Cytokines and anticytokines

Cytokines are pleiotropic agents with powerful pro-inflammatory and immunosuppressive effects, and are attractive targets for therapies that inhibit or enhance their function. TNF-α targeting agents (cytokine modulators) have been tested in rheumatoid arthritis, as has the recombinant IL-1 receptor antagonist anakinra, although with much less success. None the less, the good safety profile of anakinra has prompted its use in other diseases, and a beneficial effect has been shown in type 2 diabetes, which may have an innate inflammatory component. IL-2 and its receptor (CD25) are also obvious candidates for immune therapies. Interferons are successfully used to boost pro-inflammatory immunity in chronic virus infection.

Restoring tolerance in autoimmune diseases and allergy

One of the goals for immune-based therapies for autoimmune disease is not simply to achieve immunosuppression, but also to restore immunological tolerance against the relevant autoantigens. In animal models, an effective means of achieving this is to administer the autoantigen itself, or key peptide epitopes from it. This is known as antigen-specific or peptide immunotherapy and is under trial in several autoimmune diseases, where it appears to induce Tregs. The diseases that have the most advanced clinical data are in the field of allergy. For example, administration of cocktails of peptides of the cat allergen Fel d 1 has led to a reduction in detectable skin-prick responses and improved clinical scores.

Intravenous Immunoglobulin

Intravenous immunoglobulin (IVIg) is a preparation of polyspecific IgG chemically purified from the plasma of large numbers (>20 000) of healthy donors. IVIg is used as a replacement therapy in patients with primary and secondary antibody deficiencies. However, when used for inflammatory conditions, there is also a therapeutic benefit, although randomized placebo-controlled studies are few. In the USA, IVIg is only recommended for a small number of diseases in addition to antibody deficiency. These include: immune-mediated thrombocytopenia, Kawasaki syndrome, chronic inflammatory demyelinating polyneuropathy and post-transfusion purpura.

The mechanism of action is not known, but may include:

- blockade of Fc receptors to prevent pathogenic antibodies binding to phagocytes
- inhibition of autoantibody synthesis by B lymphocytes
- modulation of dendritic cell function
- inhibition of complement activation
- inhibition of specific cytokines
- induction of T cell regulation.

Further reading

Bluestone JA. Interleukin-mediated immunotherapy. *N Engl J Med* 2011; 365:2129–2139.

Gelfand EW. Intravenous immunoglobulin in autoimmune and inflammatory diseases. *N Engl J Med* 2012; 367:2015–2025.

Lachmann HJ, Kone-Paut I, Kuemmerle-Deschner JB et al. Use of canakinumab in the cryopyrin-associated periodic syndrome. *N Engl J Med* 2009; 360:2416–2425.

[illegible] Applying synthetic lethality for selective targeting of cancer. *N Engl J Med* 2014; 371:1725–1735.

O'Shea JJ, Holland SM, Staudt LM. JAKs and STATs in immunity, immunodeficiency and cancer. *N Engl J Med* 2013; 368:161–170.

9 Water, electrolytes and acid–base balance

M Magdi Yaqoob, Kieran McCafferty

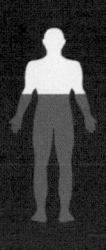

See your e-book for key learning points, clinical tips, extra tables, extra images, interactive Figures and MCQs.

WATER AND ELECTROLYTES

DISTRIBUTION AND COMPOSITION OF BODY WATER

In normal, healthy people, the total body water constitutes 50–60% of lean body weight in men and 45–50% in women. In a healthy 70 kg male, total body water is approximately 42 L. This is contained in three major compartments:

- intracellular fluid (28 L, about 35% of lean body weight)
- extracellular – the interstitial fluid that bathes the cells (9.4 L, about 12%)
- plasma (also extracellular) (4.6 L, about 4–5%).

In addition, small amounts of water are contained in bone, dense connective tissue and epithelial secretions, such as the digestive secretions and cerebrospinal fluid (CSF).

The intracellular and interstitial fluids are separated by the cell membrane; the interstitial fluid and plasma are separated by the capillary wall ***(Fig. 9.1)***. In the absence of solute, water molecules move randomly and in equal numbers in either direction across a semi-permeable membrane. However, if solutes are added to one side of the membrane, the intermolecular cohesive forces reduce the activity of the water molecules. As a result, water tends to stay in the solute-containing compartment because there is less free diffusion across the membrane. This ability to hold water in the compartment can be measured as the osmotic pressure.

Osmotic pressure

Osmotic pressure is the primary determinant of the distribution of water among the three major compartments. The concentrations of the major solutes in the compartments differ, each having one solute that is primarily limited to that compartment and therefore determines its osmotic pressure:

- The intracellular fluid contains mainly potassium (K^+) (most of the cell Mg^{2+} is bound and osmotically inactive).
- In the extracellular compartment, Na^+ salts predominate in the ***interstitial fluid***, and proteins in the plasma.

Regulation of the plasma volume is somewhat more complicated because of the tendency of the plasma proteins to hold water in the vascular space by an oncotic effect that is partly counterbalanced by the hydrostatic pressure in the capillaries that is generated by cardiac contraction ***(Fig. 9.1)***. The composition of intracellular and extracellular fluids is shown in ***Box 9.1***.

Osmotically active solutes cannot freely leave their compartment. The capillary wall, for example, is relatively impermeable to plasma proteins, and the cell membrane is 'impermeable' to Na^+ and K^+ because the Na^+/K^+-adenosine triphosphatase (ATPase) pump largely restricts Na^+ to the extracellular fluid and K^+ to the intracellular fluid. By contrast, Na^+ freely crosses the capillary wall and achieves similar concentrations in the interstitium and plasma; as a result, it does not contribute to fluid distribution between these compartments. Similarly, urea crosses both the capillary wall and the cell membrane, and is osmotically inactive. Thus, the retention of urea in renal failure does not alter the distribution of the total body water.

To conclude, body Na^+ stores are the primary determinant of the extracellular fluid volume. Thus, the extracellular volume – and therefore tissue perfusion – are maintained by appropriate alterations in Na^+ excretion. For example, if Na^+ intake is increased, the extra Na^+ will initially be added to the extracellular fluid. The associated increase in extracellular osmolality will cause water to move out of the cells, leading to extracellular volume expansion. Balance is restored by excretion of the excess Na^+ in the urine.

Distribution of different types of replacement fluids

Figure 9.2 shows the relative effects on the compartments of the addition of identical volumes of water, saline and colloid solutions. Thus, 1 L of water given intravenously as 5% glucose (which is rapidly metabolized to energy, water and carbon dioxide) is distributed equally into all compartments, whereas the same amount of 0.9% saline remains in the extracellular compartment. The latter is thus the correct treatment for extracellular water depletion – sodium

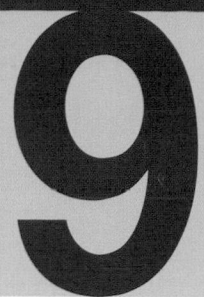

Box 9.1 Electrolyte composition of intracellular and extracellular fluids (mmol/L)

	Plasma	Interstitial fluid	Intracellular fluid
Na^+	142	144	10
K^+	4	4	160
Ca^{2+}	2.5	2.5	1.5
Mg^{2+}	1.0	0.5	13
Cl^-	102	114	2
HCO_3^-	26	30	8
PO_4^{2-}	1.0	1.0	57
SO_4^{2-}	0.5	0.5	10
Organic acid	3	4	3
Protein	16	0	55

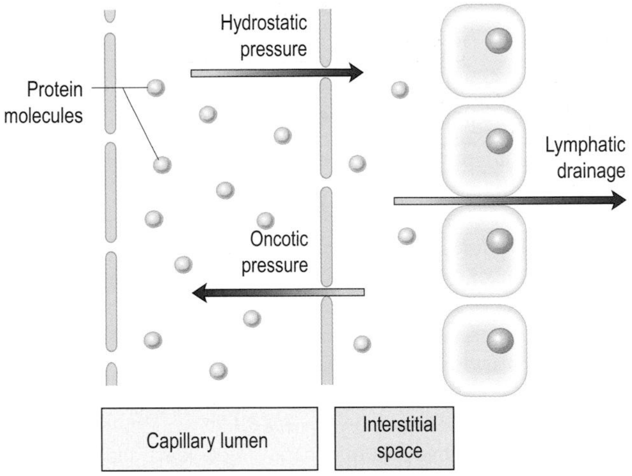

Figure 9.1 Distribution of water between the vascular and extravascular (interstitial) spaces. This is determined by the equilibrium between hydrostatic pressure, which tends to force fluid out of the capillaries, and oncotic pressure, which acts to retain fluid within the vessel. The net flow of fluid outwards is balanced by 'suction' of fluid into the lymphatics, which returns it to the bloodstream. Similar principles govern the volume of the peritoneal and pleural spaces.

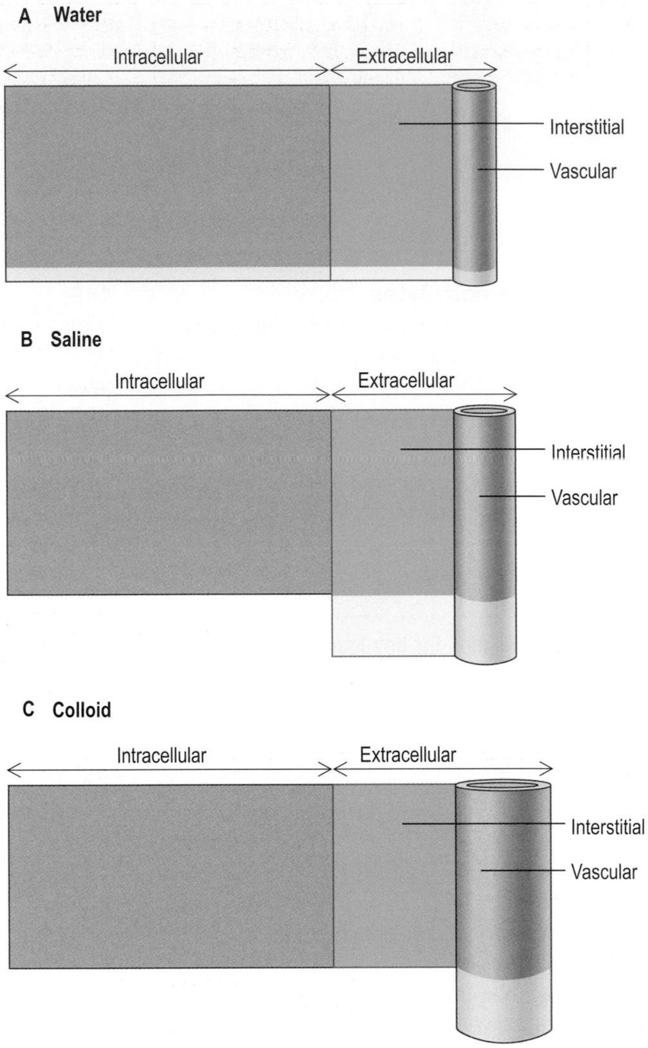

Figure 9.2 Relative effects of the addition of 1 L of (A) water, (B) saline 0.9% and (C) a colloid solution.

keeping the water in this compartment. The addition of 1 L of colloid with its high oncotic pressure stays in the vascular compartment and was a treatment for hypovolaemia, but 0.9% saline is now used.

Regulation of extracellular volume *(Fig. 9.3)*

The extracellular volume is determined by the sodium concentration. The regulation of extracellular volume is dependent upon a tight control of sodium balance, which is exerted by normal kidneys. Renal Na^+ excretion varies directly with the effective circulating volume. In a 70 kg man, plasma fluid constitutes one-third of extracellular volume (4.6 L); of this, 85% (3.9 L) lies in the venous side and only 15% (0.7 L) resides in the arterial circulation.

The fullness of the arterial vascular compartment (***effective arterial blood volume***, EABV) is the primary determinant of renal sodium and water excretion: that is, the ***effective circulatory volume*** for the purposes of body fluid homeostasis.

The fullness of the arterial compartment depends upon a relationship between cardiac output and peripheral arterial resistance. Thus, diminished EABV is initiated by a fall in cardiac output or a fall in peripheral arterial resistance (an increase in the holding capacity of the arterial vascular tree). When the EABV is expanded, the urinary Na^+ excretion is increased and can exceed 100 mmol/L. By contrast, the urine can be rendered virtually free of Na^+ in the presence of EABV depletion and normal renal function.

These changes in Na^+ excretion can result from alterations both in the filtered load, determined primarily by the glomerular filtration rate (GFR), and in tubular reabsorption, which is affected by multiple factors. In general, it is changes in tubular reabsorption that constitute the main adaptive response to fluctuations in the effective circulating volume. How this occurs can be appreciated from ***Box 9.2*** and ***Figure 9.4***, and from ***Figure 20.3*** (see p. 725), which depicts the sites and determinants of segmental Na^+ reabsorption. Although the loop of Henle and distal tubules make a major overall contribution to net Na^+ handling, transport in these segments primarily varies with the amount of Na^+ delivered; that is, reabsorption is flow-dependent. In comparison, the neurohumoral regulation of Na^+ reabsorption according to body needs occurs primarily in the proximal tubules and collecting ducts. The diseases associated with malfunction of each section of the tubule are shown in ***Box 9.3***.

Neurohumoral regulation of extracellular volume

This is mediated by volume receptors that sense changes in the EABV rather than alterations in the sodium concentration. These receptors are distributed in both the renal and cardiovascular tissues.

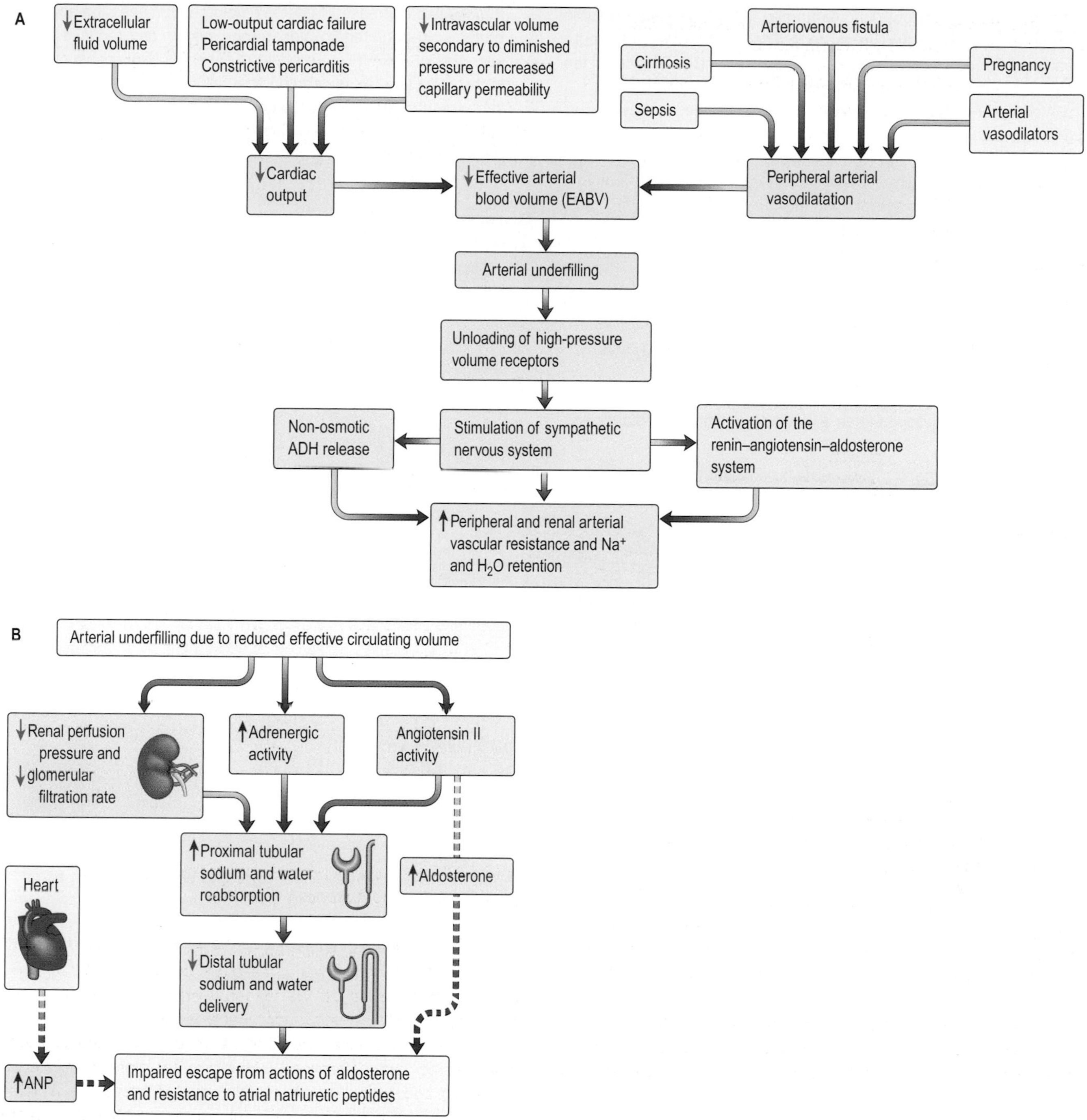

Figure 9.3 **Regulation of extracellular volume. A.** Sequence of events in which a decrease in cardiac output or peripheral arterial dilatation initiates renal sodium and water retention. **B.** Mechanism of impaired escape from the actions of aldosterone and resistance to atrial natriuretic peptides (ANP). ADH, antidiuretic hormone. *(Modified with permission from Schrier RW.* Renal and Electrolyte Disorders, *7th edn. Philadelphia: Lippincott Williams & Wilkins, 2010.)*

- ***Intrarenal receptors***. Receptors in the walls of the afferent glomerular arterioles respond, via the juxtaglomerular apparatus, to changes in renal perfusion, and control the activity of the renin–angiotensin–aldosterone system (see pp. 727–728). In addition, sodium concentration in the distal tubule and sympathetic nerve activity alter renin release from the juxtaglomerular cells. Prostaglandins I_2 and E_2 are also generated within the kidney in response to angiotensin II, acting to maintain glomerular filtration rate and sodium and water excretion, and modulating the sodium-retaining effect of this hormone.
- ***Extrarenal receptors***. These are located in the vascular tree in the left atrium and major thoracic veins, and in the carotid sinus body and aortic arch. These volume receptors respond to a slight reduction in effective circulating volume and this results in increased sympathetic nerve activity and a rise in catecholamines. In addition, volume receptors in the cardiac atria control the release of a powerful natriuretic hormone – atrial natriuretic peptide (ANP) – from granules located in the atrial walls (see p. 983).

High-pressure arterial receptors (carotid, aortic arch, juxtaglomerular apparatus) predominate over low-pressure volume receptors in volume control in mammals. The low-pressure volume receptors are distributed in thoracic tissues (cardiac atria, right ventricle, thoracic veins, pulmonary vessels) and their role in the volume regulatory system is marginal.

Aldosterone and possibly ANP are responsible for day-to-day variations in Na^+ excretion, through their respective ability to augment and diminish Na^+ reabsorption in the collecting ducts.

- A ***salt load***, for example, leads to an increase in the effective circulatory and extracellular volume, raising both renal perfusion pressure, and atrial and arterial filling pressure. The increase in the renal perfusion pressure reduces the secretion of renin, and subsequently that of angiotensin II and aldosterone (see ***Fig. 20.6***), whereas the rise in atrial and arterial filling pressure increases the release of ANP. These factors combine to reduce Na^+ reabsorption in the collecting duct, thereby promoting excretion of excess Na^+.
- By contrast, in patients on a ***low Na^+*** intake or in those who become volume-depleted as a result of vomiting and diarrhoea, the ensuing decrease in effective volume enhances the activity of the renin–angiotensin–aldosterone system and reduces the secretion of ANP. The net effect is enhanced Na^+ reabsorption in the collecting ducts, leading to a fall in Na^+ excretion. This increases the extracellular volume towards normal.

With ***more marked hypovolaemia***, a decrease in GFR leads to an increase in proximal and thin ascending limb Na^+ reabsorption,

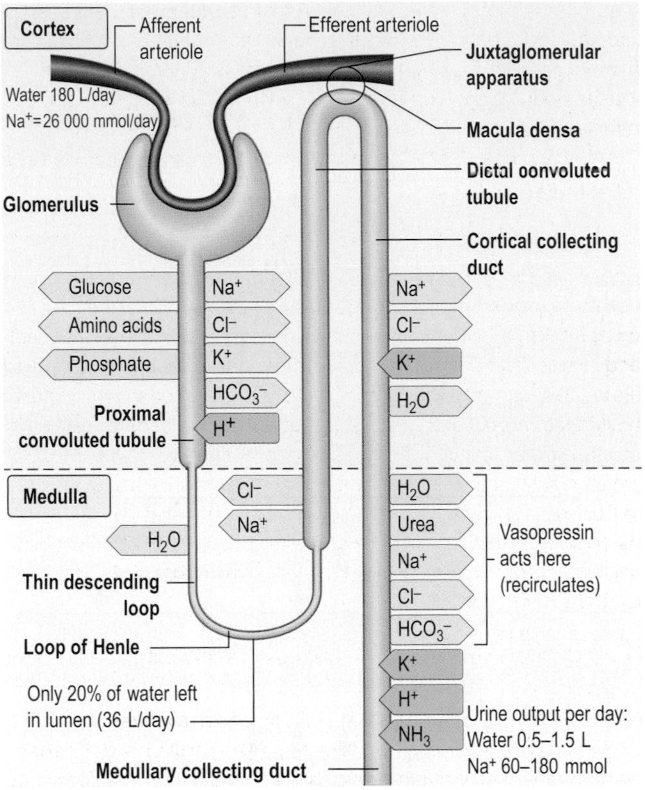

Figure 9.4 The nephron – electrolyte and water exchange. Some 180 L of water and 26000 mmol of sodium/day enter the nephrons via the afferent arterioles to the kidneys. Removal or addition of electrolytes results in the excretion of approximately 1 L of water and 60–180 mmol of sodium/day.

Box 9.2 Mechanisms of sodium transport in the various nephron segments

	Filtered Na reabsorbed (%)	Major mechanisms of luminal Na^+ entry	Major factors regulating transport
Proximal tubule	60–70	Na^+–H^+ exchange and co-transport of Na^+ with glucose, phosphate and other organic solutes	Angiotensin II Noradrenaline (norepinephrine)
Loop of Henle	20–25	Na^+–K^+–$2Cl^-$ co-transport	Flow Pressure natriuresis mediated by nitric oxide
Distal tubule	5	Na^+–Cl^- co-transport	Flow
Collecting ducts	4	Na^+ channels	Aldosterone Atrial natriuretic peptide

Box 9.3 Major functions of each section of the tubule and associated diseases

Site	Function	Diseases associated with this section of nephron
Proximal convoluted tubule (PCT)	**Early PCT:** Solute reabsorption: glucose, amino acids, bicarbonate, phosphate, low-molecular-weight proteins **Late PCT:** Urate secretion/absorption Straight PCT secretion of drugs (loop and thiazide diuretics) and drug metabolites	Fanconi syndrome: failure to reabsorb solutes and low-molecular-weight proteins. Leads to glycosuria, phosphaturia, aminoaciduria and low-molecular-weight proteinuria. May be caused by drugs, myeloma, Wilson's disease and rare genetic diseases Type 2 renal tubular acidosis (see p. 178)
Loop of Henle	Site of counter-current multiplier, which sets up loop, enabling control of final urine concentration	Bartter syndrome (see p. 166)
Distal convoluted tubule	Involvement in sodium and chloride transport, and calcium and magnesium reabsorption	Gitelman syndrome (see p. 166) Gordon syndrome (see p. 167)
Collecting ducts	Na^+ and water reabsorption Secretion of potassium Secretion of bicarbonate or H^+	Liddle syndrome (see p. 166) Pseudohypoaldosteronism type 1 (see p. 167) Nephrogenic diabetes insipidus: resistance to actions of vasopressin. Leads to large volume of dilute urine with polyuria/polydipsia Syndrome of inappropriate antidiuretic hormone secretion (SIADH; see pp. 1234–1235) Type 1 renal tubular acidosis (see p. 178)

which contributes to Na^+ retention. This is brought about by enhanced sympathetic activity acting directly on the kidneys and indirectly by stimulating the secretion of renin/angiotensin II (see **Fig. 9.3B**) and non-osmotic release of antidiuretic hormone (ADH), also called vasopressin. The pressure natriuresis phenomenon may be the final defence against changes in the effective circulating volume. Marked persistent hypovolaemia leads to systemic hypotension and increased salt and water absorption in the proximal tubules and ascending limb of Henle. This process is partly mediated by changes in renal interstitial hydrostatic pressure and local prostaglandin and nitric oxide production. Recurrent episodes of hypovolaemia may, over time, lead to chronic kidney disease (CKD, Mesoamerican nephropathy). This condition is seen in young to middle-aged male agricultural workers along the Pacific coast in Central America, where strenuous work in high temperatures is thought to be a cause.

Volume regulation in oedematous conditions

Sodium and water are retained despite increased extracellular volume in oedematous conditions such as cardiac failure, hepatic cirrhosis and hypoalbuminaemia. Here the principal mediator of salt and water retention is the concept of arterial underfilling due to either reduced cardiac output or diminished peripheral arterial resistance. Arterial underfilling in these settings leads to reduction of pressure or stretch (i.e. 'unloading' of arterial volume receptors), which results in activation of the sympathetic nervous system, activation of the renin–angiotensin–aldosterone system and non-osmotic release of ADH. These neurohumoral mediators promote salt and water retention in the face of increased extracellular volume (see **Fig. 9.3A**).

Mechanism of impaired escape from actions of aldosterone and resistance to ANP

Not only is the activity of the renin–angiotensin–aldosterone system increased in oedematous conditions such as cardiac failure, hepatic cirrhosis and hypoalbuminaemia, but also the action of aldosterone is more persistent than in normal subjects and patients with primary hyperaldosteronism (Conn syndrome), who have increased aldosterone secretion (see p. 1230).

In normal subjects, high doses of mineralocorticoids initially increase renal sodium retention so that the extracellular volume is increased by 1.5–2 L. However, renal sodium retention then ceases, sodium balance is re-established, and there is no detectable oedema. This escape from mineralocorticoid-mediated sodium retention explains why oedema is not a characteristic feature of primary hyperaldosteronism. The escape is dependent on an increase in delivery of sodium to the site of action of aldosterone in the collecting ducts. The increased distal sodium delivery is achieved by high extracellular volume-mediated arterial overfilling. This suppresses sympathetic activity and angiotensin II generation, and increases cardiac release of ANP with resultant increase in renal perfusion pressure and GFR. The net result of these events is reduced sodium absorption in the proximal tubules and increased distal sodium delivery, which overwhelms the sodium-retaining actions of aldosterone.

In patients with the above oedematous conditions, such as heart failure, escape from the sodium-retaining actions of aldosterone does *not* occur and therefore they continue to retain sodium in response to aldosterone. Accordingly, they have substantial natriuresis when given spironolactone, which blocks mineralocorticoid receptors. Alpha-adrenergic stimulation and elevated angiotensin II increase sodium transport in the proximal tubule, and reduced renal perfusion and GFR further increase sodium absorption from the proximal tubules by presenting less sodium and water in the tubular fluid. Sodium delivery to the distal portion of the nephron, and thus the collecting duct, is reduced. Similarly, increased cardiac ANP release in these conditions requires optimum sodium concentration at the site of its action in the collecting duct for its desired natriuretic effects. Decreased sodium delivery to the collecting duct is therefore the most likely explanation for the persistent aldosterone-mediated sodium retention, absence of escape phenomenon and resistance to natriuretic peptides in these patients (see **Fig. 9.3B**).

Regulation of water excretion

Body water homeostasis is affected by thirst and the urine-concentrating and diluting functions of the kidney. These, in turn, are controlled by intracellular osmoreceptors, principally in the hypothalamus, to some extent by volume receptors in capacitance vessels close to the heart, and via the renin–angiotensin system. Of these, the major and best-understood control is via osmoreceptors. Changes in the plasma Na^+ concentration and osmolality are sensed by osmoreceptors that influence both thirst and the release of ADH (vasopressin) from the supraoptic and paraventricular nuclei of the anterior hypothalamus.

ADH plays a central role in urinary concentration by increasing the water permeability of the normally impermeable cortical and medullary collecting ducts. There are three major G-protein coupled receptors for vasopressin (ADH):

- V_{1A} found in vascular smooth muscle cells: activation induces vasoconstriction.
- V_{1B} in the anterior pituitary and throughout the brain: this mediates the effect of ADH on the pituitary, leading to ACTH release.
- V_2 receptors in the principal cells of the kidney distal convoluting tubule and collecting ducts: these mediate the ADH response.

The ability of ADH to increase the urine osmolality is related indirectly to transport in the ascending limb of the loop of Henle, which reabsorbs NaCl without water. This process, which is the primary step in the counter-current mechanism, has two effects: it makes the tubular fluid dilute and the medullary interstitium concentrated. In the absence of ADH, little water is reabsorbed in the collecting ducts, and a dilute urine is excreted. By contrast, the presence of ADH promotes water reabsorption in the collecting ducts down the favourable osmotic gradient between the tubular fluid and the more concentrated interstitium. As a result, there is an increase in urine osmolality and a decrease in urine volume.

The cortical collecting duct has two cell types (see also p. 724) with very different functions:

- ***Principal cells*** (about 65%) have sodium and potassium channels in the apical membrane and, as in all sodium-reabsorbing cells, Na^+/K^+-ATPase pumps in the basolateral membrane.
- ***Intercalated cells***, in comparison, do not transport NaCl (since they have a lower level of Na^+/K^+-ATPase activity) but play a role in hydrogen and bicarbonate handling and in potassium reabsorption in states of potassium depletion.

The ADH-induced increase in collecting duct water permeability occurs primarily in the principal cells. ADH acts on V_2 (vasopressin) receptors located on the basolateral surface of principal cells, resulting in the activation of adenyl cyclase. This leads to protein kinase activation and to pre-formed cytoplasmic vesicles that contain unique water channels (called aquaporins) moving to and then being inserted into the luminal membrane. Four renal aquaporins have

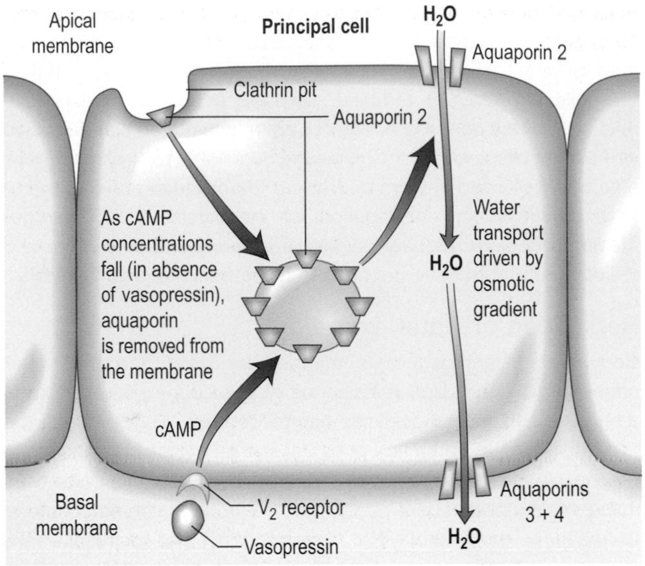

Figure 9.5 Aquaporin-mediated water transport in the renal collecting duct. Stimulation of the vasopressin 2 receptor causes cyclic adenosine monophosphate (cAMP)-mediated insertion of the aquaporin into the apical membrane, allowing water transport down the osmotic gradient. *(Adapted from Connolly DL, Shanahan CM, Weissberg PL. Water channels in health and disease.* Lancet *1996; 347:211, with permission from Elsevier.)*

been well characterized and are localized in different areas of the cells of the collecting duct. The water channels span the luminal membrane and permit water movement into the cells down a favourable osmotic gradient ***(Fig. 9.5)***. This water is then rapidly returned to the systemic circulation across the basolateral membrane. When the ADH effect has worn off, the water channels aggregate within clathrin-coated pits, from which they are removed from the luminal membrane by endocytosis and returned to the cytoplasm. A defect in any step in this pathway, such as in attachment of ADH to its receptor or the function of the water channel, can cause resistance to the action of ADH and an increase in urine output. This disorder is called ***nephrogenic diabetes insipidus***.

Plasma osmolality

In addition to influencing the rate of water excretion, ADH plays a central role in osmoregulation because its release is directly affected by the plasma osmolality. At a plasma osmolality of <275 mosmol/kg, which usually represents a plasma Na^+ concentration of <135–137 mmol/L, there is essentially no circulating ADH. As the plasma osmolality rises above this threshold, however, the secretion of ADH increases progressively.

Two simple examples will illustrate the basic mechanisms of osmoregulation, which is so efficient that the plasma Na^+ concentration is normally maintained within 1–2% of its baseline value.

1. ***Ingestion of a water load*** leads to an initial reduction in the plasma osmolality, thereby diminishing the release of ADH. The ensuing reduction in water reabsorption in the collecting ducts allows the excess water to be excreted in a dilute urine.
2. ***Water loss*** resulting from sweating is followed by, in sequence, a rise in both plasma osmolality and ADH secretion, enhanced water reabsorption, and the appropriate excretion of a small volume of concentrated urine. This renal effect of ADH minimizes further water loss but does not replace the existing water deficit. Thus, optimal osmoregulation requires an increase in water intake, which is mediated by a concurrent stimulation of thirst. The importance of thirst can also be illustrated by studies in patients with central diabetes insipidus, who are deficient in ADH. These patients often complain of marked polyuria, which is caused by the decline in water reabsorption in the collecting ducts. However, they do not typically become hypernatraemic because urinary water loss is offset by the thirst mechanism.

Osmoregulation versus volume regulation

A common misconception is that regulation of the plasma Na^+ concentration is closely correlated with the regulation of Na^+ excretion. It is, however, related to volume regulation, which has different sensors and effectors (volume receptors) from those involved in water balance and osmoregulation (osmoreceptors).

The roles of these two pathways should be considered separately when evaluating patients.

- A ***water load*** is rapidly excreted (in 4–6 h) by inhibition of ADH release so that there is little or no water reabsorption in the collecting ducts. This process is normally so efficient that volume regulation is not affected and there is no change in ANP release or in the activity of the renin–angiotensin–aldosterone system. Thus, a dilute urine is excreted and there is little alteration in the excretion of Na^+.
- ***0.9% saline*** administration, by contrast, causes an increase in volume but no change in plasma osmolality. In this setting, ANP secretion is increased, aldosterone secretion is reduced and ADH secretion does not change. The net effect is the appropriate excretion of the excess Na^+ in a relatively iso-osmotic urine.

In some cases, both volume and osmolality are altered and both pathways are activated. For example, if a person with normal renal function eats salted crisps and peanuts without drinking any water, the excess Na^+ will increase the plasma osmolality, leading to osmotic water movement out of the cells and increased extracellular volume. The rise in osmolality will stimulate both ADH release and thirst (the main reason why many restaurants and bars supply free salted foods), whereas the hypervolaemia will enhance the secretion of ANP and suppress that of aldosterone. The net effect is increased excretion of Na^+ without water.

This principle of separate volume and osmoregulatory pathways is also evident in the ***syndrome of inappropriate antidiuretic hormone secretion*** (***SIADH***). Patients with SIADH (see pp. 1234–1235) have impaired water excretion and hyponatraemia (dilutional) caused by the persistent presence of ADH. However, the release of ANP and aldosterone is not impaired and, thus, Na^+ handling remains intact. These findings have implications for the correction of the hyponatraemia in this setting, which initially requires restriction of water intake.

ADH is also secreted by non-osmotic stimuli such as stress (e.g. surgery, trauma), markedly reduced effective circulatory volume (e.g. cardiac failure, hepatic cirrhosis), psychiatric disturbance and nausea, irrespective of plasma osmolality. This is mediated by the effects of sympathetic overactivity on supraoptic and paraventricular nuclei. In addition to water retention, ADH release in these conditions promotes vasoconstriction owing to the activation of V_{1A} (vasopressin) receptors distributed in the vascular smooth muscle cells.

Regulation of cell volume

Most cells respond to swelling or shrinkage by activating specific metabolic or membrane-transport processes that return cell volume to its normal resting state. Within minutes of exposure to hypotonic solutions and resulting cell swelling, a common feature of many cells is the increase in plasma membrane potassium and chloride conductance. Although extrusion of intracellular potassium certainly contributes to a regulatory volume decrease, the role of chloride efflux itself is modest, given the relatively low intracellular chloride concentration. Other intracellular osmolytes, such as taurine and other amino acids, are transported out of the cell to achieve a regulatory volume decrease. By contrast, these regulatory mechanisms are operative in reverse to protect cell volume under hypertonic conditions, as is the case in the renal medulla. The tubular cells at the tip of renal papillae, which are constantly exposed to a hypertonic extracellular milieu, maintain their cell volume on a long-term basis by actively taking up smaller molecules, such as betaine, taurine and myoinositol, and by synthesizing more sorbitol and glycerophosphocholine.

Increased extracellular volume

Increased extracellular volume occurs in numerous disease states. The physical signs depend on the distribution of excess volume and on whether the increase is local or systemic. According to Starling principles, distribution depends on:

- venous tone, which determines the capacitance of the blood compartment and thus hydrostatic pressure
- capillary permeability
- oncotic pressure – mainly dependent on serum albumin
- lymphatic drainage.

Depending on these factors, fluid accumulation may result in expansion of interstitial volume, blood volume or both.

Clinical features

Peripheral oedema is caused by expansion of the extracellular volume by at least 2 L (15%). The ankles are normally the first part of the body to be affected, although they may be spared in patients with lipodermatosclerosis (where the skin is tethered and cannot expand to accommodate the oedema). Oedema may be noted in the face, particularly in the morning. In a patient in bed, oedema may accumulate in the sacral area. Expansion of the interstitial volume also causes pulmonary oedema, pleural effusion, pericardial effusion and ascites. Expansion of the blood volume (overload) causes a raised jugular venous pressure, cardiomegaly, added heart sounds and basal crackles, as well as a raised arterial blood pressure.

Aetiology

Extracellular volume expansion is due to sodium chloride retention. Increased oral salt intake does not normally cause volume expansion because of rapid homeostatic mechanisms that increase salt excretion. However, a rapid intravenous infusion of a large volume of saline will cause volume expansion. Most causes of extracellular volume expansion are associated with renal sodium chloride retention.

Heart failure

Reduction in cardiac output and the consequent fall in effective circulatory volume and arterial filling lead to activation of the renin–angiotensin–aldosterone system, non-osmotic release of ADH, and increased activity of the renal sympathetic nerves via volume receptors and baroreceptors (see ***Fig. 9.3B***). Sympathetic overdrive also indirectly augments ADH and renin–angiotensin–aldosterone response in these conditions. The cumulative effect of these mediators results in increased peripheral and renal arteriolar resistance and water and sodium retention. These factors lead to extracellular volume expansion and increased venous pressure, causing oedema formation.

Hepatic cirrhosis

The mechanism is complex but involves peripheral vasodilatation, due to increased nitric oxide generation, resulting in reduced EABV and arterial filling. This leads to an activation of a chain of events common also to other conditions with marked peripheral vasodilatation and heart failure (see ***Fig. 9.3***). The cumulative effect results in increased peripheral and renal resistance, water and sodium retention, and oedema formation.

Nephrotic syndrome

Interstitial oedema is a common clinical finding with hypoalbuminaemia, particularly in the nephrotic syndrome. Expansion of the interstitial compartment is secondary to the accumulation of sodium in the extracellular compartment. This is due to an imbalance between oral (or parenteral) sodium intake and urinary sodium loss, as well as alterations of fluid transfer across capillary walls. The intrarenal site of sodium retention is the cortical collecting duct (CCD), where Na^+/K^+-ATPase expression and activity are increased threefold along the basolateral surface (see ***Fig. 9.4***). In addition, amiloride-sensitive epithelial sodium channel activity is also increased in the CCD. The renal sodium retention should normally be counterbalanced by increased secretion of sodium in the inner medullary collecting duct, brought about by the release of ANP. This regulatory pathway is altered in patients with nephrotic syndrome by enhanced ***kidney-specific*** catabolism of cyclic guanosine monophosphate (cGMP, the second messenger for ANP) following phosphodiesterase activation.

Oedema generation was classically attributed to the decrease in plasma oncotic pressure and the subsequent increase in the transcapillary oncotic gradient. However, the oncotic pressure and transcapillary oncotic gradient remain unchanged and the transcapillary hydrostatic pressure gradient is not altered.

The mechanism for oedema seen in nephrotic syndrome is increased capillary hydraulic conductivity (a measure of permeability). This is determined by intercellular macromolecular complexes between the endothelial cells consisting of tight junctions (made of occludins, claudins and zonula occludens (ZO) proteins) and adherens junctions (made of cadherin, catenins and actin cytoskeleton). Elevated tumour necrosis factor alpha (TNF-α) levels in nephrotic syndrome activate protein kinase C, which changes phosphorylation of occludin and capillary permeability. In addition, increased circulating ANP can increase capillary hydraulic conductivity by altering the permeability of intercellular junctional complexes. Furthermore, reduction in effective circulatory volume and the consequent fall in cardiac output and arterial filling can lead to a chain of events, as in cardiac failure and cirrhosis (see above and ***Fig. 9.3***). These factors result in extracellular volume expansion and oedema formation.

Sodium retention

A decreased GFR decreases the renal capacity to excrete sodium. This may be acute, as in the acute nephritic syndrome (see p. 740), or may occur as part of the presentation of chronic kidney disease (CKD). In end-stage renal failure, extracellular volume is controlled by the balance between salt intake and its removal by dialysis.

Numerous drugs cause renal sodium retention, particularly in patients whose renal function is already impaired:

- ***Oestrogens*** cause mild sodium retention, due to a weak aldosterone-like effect. This is the reason for weight gain in the premenstrual phase.

- ***Mineralocorticoids and liquorice*** (the latter potentiates the sodium-retaining action of cortisol) have aldosterone-like actions.
- ***Non-steroidal anti-inflammatory drugs (NSAIDs)*** cause sodium retention in the presence of activation of the renin–angiotensin–aldosterone system by heart failure, in cirrhosis and in renal artery stenosis.
- ***Thiazolidinediones (TZDs***; see p. 1253) are widely used to treat type 2 diabetes. Their mechanism of action is attributed to binding and activation of the peroxisome proliferator-activated receptor gamma (PPAR-γ) system. PPARs are nuclear transcription factors, essential to the control of energy metabolism, which are modulated via binding with tissue-specific fatty acid metabolites. Of the three PPAR isoforms, γ has been extensively studied and is expressed at high levels in adipose and liver tissues, macrophages, pancreatic β cells and principal cells of the collecting duct. These drugs have been associated with salt and water retention and are contraindicated in patients with heart failure. TZD-induced oedema (like insulin) is also due to upregulation of epithelial Na transporter channel (ENaC) but by different pathways. Diuretics of choice for TZD-induced oedema are amiloride and triamterene.

Substantial amounts of sodium and water may accumulate in the body without clinically obvious oedema or evidence of raised venous pressure. In particular, several litres may accumulate in the pleural space or as ascites; these spaces are then referred to as 'third spaces'. Bone may also act as a 'sink' for sodium and water.

Other causes of oedema

- Initiation of insulin treatment for type 1 diabetes and refeeding after malnutrition are both associated with the development of transient oedema. The mechanism is complex but involves upregulation of ENaC in the principal cell of the collecting duct. This transporter is amiloride-sensitive, which makes amiloride or triamterene the diuretic of choice in insulin-induced oedema.
- Oedema may result from increased capillary pressure owing to relaxation of pre-capillary arterioles. The best example is the peripheral oedema caused by dihydropyridine calcium-channel blockers such as nifedipine, which affects up to 10% of the patients. Oedema is usually resolved by stopping the offending drug.
- Oedema is also caused by raised interstitial oncotic pressure as a result of increased capillary permeability to proteins. This can occur as part of a rare complement-deficiency syndrome; with therapeutic use of interleukin 2 in cancer chemotherapy; or in ovarian hyperstimulation syndrome (see p. 1222).

Idiopathic oedema of women

This, by definition, occurs in women without heart failure, hypoalbuminaemia, and renal or endocrine disease. Oedema is intermittent and often worse in the premenstrual phase. The condition remits after the menopause. Patients complain of swelling of the face, hands, breasts and thighs, and a feeling of being bloated. Sodium retention during the day and increased sodium excretion during recumbency are characteristic; an abnormal fall in plasma volume on standing, caused by increased capillary permeability to proteins, may be the cause of this. The oedema may respond to diuretics but returns when they are stopped. A similar syndrome of diuretic-dependent sodium retention can be caused by abuse of diuretics – for instance, as part of an attempt to lose weight – but not all women with idiopathic oedema admit to having taken diuretics, and the syndrome was described before diuretics were introduced for clinical use, so the cause remains unclear.

Local increase in oedema

This does not reflect disturbances of extracellular volume control *per se* but can cause clinical confusion. Examples are ankle oedema due to venous damage following thrombosis or surgery, ankle or leg oedema due to immobility, oedema of the arm due to subclavian thrombosis, and facial oedema due to superior vena caval obstruction.

Management

The underlying cause should be treated where possible. Heart failure, for example, should be treated and offending drugs such as NSAIDs withdrawn.

Sodium restriction has only a limited role but is useful in patients who are resistant to diuretics. Sodium intake can easily be reduced to approximately 100 mmol (2 g) daily; reductions below this are often difficult to achieve without affecting the palatability of food.

Manœuvres that increase venous return (e.g. strict bed rest or water immersion) stimulate salt and water excretion by effects on cardiac output and ANP release, but they are seldom of practical value.

The mainstay of treatment is the use of ***diuretic agents***, which increase sodium, chloride and water excretion in the kidney ***(Box 9.4)***. These agents act by interfering with membrane ion pumps that are present on numerous cell types; they mostly achieve specificity for the kidney by being secreted into the proximal tubule, resulting in much higher concentrations in the tubular fluid than in other parts of the body.

Clinical use of diuretics

Loop diuretics

These potent diuretics are useful in the treatment of any cause of systemic extracellular volume overload. They stimulate excretion of both sodium chloride and water by blocking the sodium-potassium-2-chloride (NKCC2) channel in the thick ascending limb of Henle ***(Fig. 9.6)*** and are useful in stimulating water excretion in states of relative water overload. They also act by causing increased venous capacitance, resulting in rapid clinical improvement in patients with left ventricular failure, preceding the diuresis. Unwanted effects include:

- urate retention, causing gout
- hypokalaemia
- hypomagnesaemia
- decreased glucose tolerance
- allergic tubulointerstitial nephritis and other allergic reactions
- myalgia – especially with high-dose bumetanide
- ototoxicity (due to an action on sodium pump activity in the inner ear) – particularly with furosemide
- interference with excretion of lithium, resulting in toxicity.

There is little to choose between the drugs in this class. Bumetanide has a better oral bioavailability than furosemide, particularly in patients with severe peripheral oedema, and has more beneficial effects than furosemide on venous capacitance in left ventricular failure.

Thiazide diuretics

Thiazide diuretics (see p. 985) are less potent than loop diuretics. They act by blocking a sodium chloride channel in the ***distal convoluted tubule*** (Gitelman syndrome; see p. 166) ***(Fig. 9.7)***. They

Box 9.4 Types and clinical uses of diuretics

Class	Major action	Examples	Clinical uses	Potency
Loop diuretics	↓ Na^+-Cl^--K^+ co-transport in thick ascending limb of loop of Henle	Furosemide Bumetanide Torasemide	Volume overload (CCF, nephrotic syndrome, CKD) ?Acute kidney injury SIADH	+++
Thiazide and related diuretics	↓ Na^+-Cl co-transport in early distal convoluted tubule	Bendroflumethiazide Chlortalidone Metolazone Indapamide	Hypertension Volume overload (CCF) Hypercalciuria	++
Potassium-sparing diuretics	↓ Na^+ reabsorption (in exchange for K^+) in collecting duct (principal cells)	Aldosterone antagonists, e.g. spironolactone, eplerenone Others: amiloride, triamterene	Hyperaldosteronism (primary and secondary) Bartter syndrome Heart failure Cirrhosis with fluid overload Prevention of K^+ deficiency in combination with loop or thiazide	+
Carbonic anhydrase inhibitors	↓ Na^+ HCO_3^- reabsorption in proximal collecting duct ↓ Aqueous humour formation	Acetazolamide	Metabolic alkalosis Glaucoma	±
Vasopressin/ADH receptor blockers (aquaretics)	Block V_2 receptor in collecting ducts producing free water diuresis	Lixivaptan Tolvaptan Satavaptan I.v. conivaptan (also blocks V_{1A})	Heart failure, cirrhosis, SIADH	+

CCF, congestive cardiac failure; CKD, chronic kidney disease; SIADH, syndrome of inappropriate antidiuretic hormone secretion.

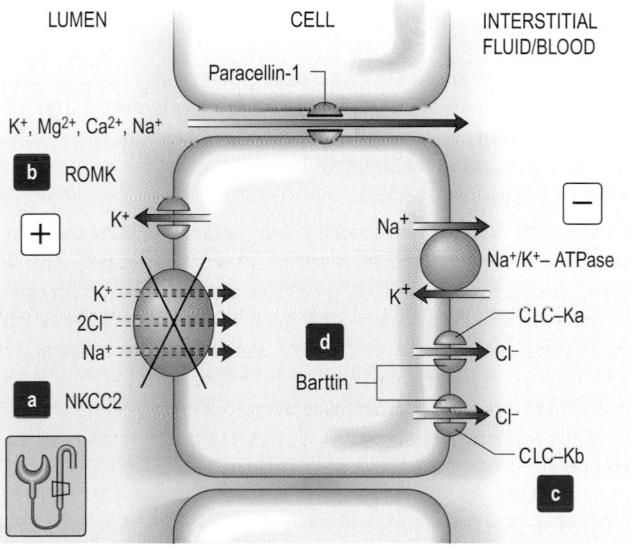

Figure 9.6 Transport mechanisms in the thick ascending limb of the loop of Henle. Sodium chloride is reabsorbed in the thick ascending limb by the bumetanide-sensitive sodium–potassium-2–chloride co-transporter (NKCC2). The electroneutral transporter is driven by the low intracellular sodium and chloride concentrations generated by the Na^+/K^+-ATPase and the kidney-specific basolateral chloride channel (CLC-Kb). The availability of luminal potassium is rate-limiting for NKCC2, and recycling of potassium through the ATP-regulated potassium channel (renal outer medulla K^+ channel, ROMK) ensures the efficient functioning of the NKCC2 and generates a lumen-positive transepithelial potential. Calcium and magnesium, along with potassium and sodium, are also absorbed paracellularly in the thick ascending loop. ***Bartter syndrome:*** loss of function mutations for the different types of syndrome. **(a)** NKCC2 (type I). **(b)** ROMK (type II). **(c)** CLC-Kb (type III). **(d)** Barttin (type IV). In addition, type V may be caused by a gain of function mutation of the calcium-sensing receptor (not shown).

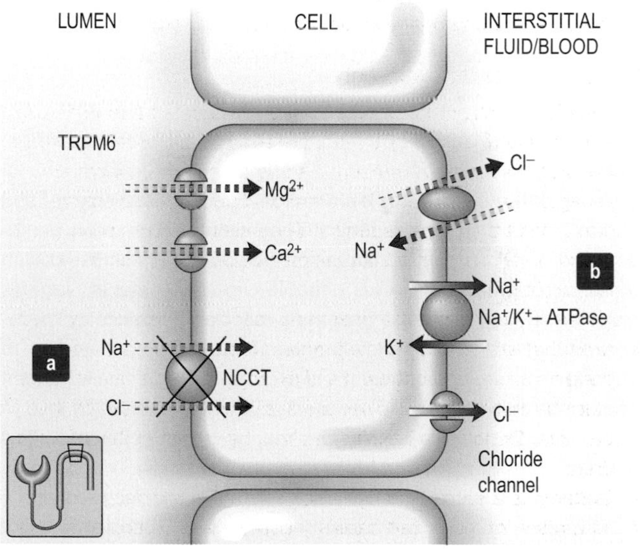

Figure 9.7 Transport mechanisms in the distal convoluted tubule. **(a)** Sodium chloride is usually reabsorbed by the apical *thiazide-sensitive* sodium–chloride co-transporter (**NCCT**) in the distal convoluted tubule. **(b)** The electroneutral transporter is driven by the low intracellular sodium and chloride concentrations generated by the Na^+/K^+-ATPase, and an undefined basolateral chloride channel. In this nephron segment, there is an apical calcium channel and a basolateral sodium-coupled exchanger. The mechanisms for the transport of magnesium are similar to those for calcium. **TRPM6** is a member of the transient receptor potential family. Mutation of NCCT leads to decreased reabsorption of sodium chloride and increased absorption of calcium (***Gitelman syndrome***). Overactivity of NCCT leads to *Gordon syndrome* (see pp. 167–168).

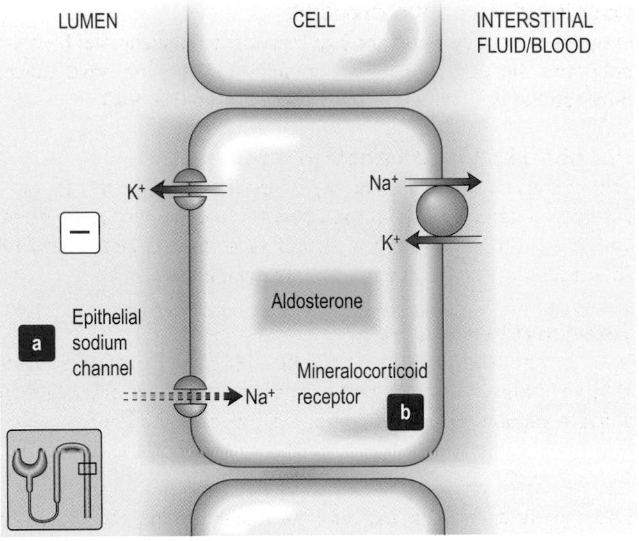

Figure 9.8 Aldosterone-regulated transport in the cortical collecting ducts. Under normal conditions, the ***epithelial sodium channel*** is the rate-limiting barrier for the normal entry of sodium from the lumen into the cell. The resulting lumen-negative transepithelial voltage (indicated by the minus sign) drives potassium secretion from the principal cells and proton secretion from the α-intercalated cells (see ***Fig. 9.12***). **(a)** Site of action of amiloride and triamterene and mutation of epithelial sodium channel gene (***Liddle syndrome***) produces reabsorption of sodium and increased secretion of potassium (not shown). **(b)** Site of action of aldosterone antagonists. Mutation of the gene encoding mineralocorticoid receptor leads to salt wasting and decreased secretion of potassium.

cause relatively more urate retention, glucose intolerance and hypokalaemia than loop diuretics. They interfere with water excretion and may cause hyponatraemia, particularly if combined with amiloride or triamterene. This effect is clinically useful in diabetes insipidus. Thiazides reduce peripheral vascular resistance by mechanisms that are not completely understood but do not appear to depend on their diuretic action, and are widely used in the treatment of essential hypertension. They are also used extensively in mild to moderate cardiac failure. Thiazides reduce calcium excretion. This effect is useful in patients with idiopathic hypercalciuria but may cause hypercalcaemia. Numerous agents are available, with varying half-lives but little else to choose between them. Metolazone is not dependent for its action on glomerular filtration, and therefore retains its potency in renal impairment.

Potassium-sparing diuretics

Potassium-sparing diuretics (see ***Fig. 9.8***) are of two types:

- ***Aldosterone antagonists***, which compete with aldosterone in the collecting ducts and reduce sodium absorption, e.g. spironolactone and eplerenone (which has a shorter half-life). Spironolactone is used in patients with heart failure because it significantly reduces the mortality in these individuals by antagonizing the fibrotic effect of aldosterone on the heart. Eplerenone is devoid of antiandrogenic or antiprogesterone properties.
- ***Amiloride and triamterene***, which inhibit sodium uptake by blocking epithelial sodium channels in the collecting duct and reduce renal potassium excretion by reducing lumen-negative transepithelial voltage. They are mainly used as potassium-sparing agents with thiazide or loop diuretics.

Carbonic anhydrase inhibitors

These are relatively weak diuretics and are seldom used, except in the treatment of glaucoma. They cause metabolic acidosis and hypokalaemia.

Aquaretics (vasopressin or antidiuretic hormone antagonists)

Vasopressin V_2 receptor antagonists are very useful agents in the treatment of conditions associated with elevated levels of vasopressin, such as heart failure, cirrhosis and SIADH (see p. 1235). Non-peptide vasopressin V_2 receptor antagonists are efficacious in producing free water diuresis in humans. Studies in patients with heart failure and cirrhosis suggest that such agents will allow normalization of serum osmolality with less water restriction (see p. 164).

Resistance to diuretics

Resistance may occur as a result of:

- poor bioavailability
- reduced GFR, which may be due to decreased circulating volume despite oedema (e.g. nephrotic syndrome, cirrhosis with ascites) or intrinsic renal disease
- activation of sodium-retaining mechanisms, particularly aldosterone.

Intravenous administration of diuretics may establish a diuresis. ***High doses*** of loop diuretics are required to achieve adequate concentrations in the tubule if GFR is depressed. However, the daily dose of furosemide must be limited to a maximum of 2 g for an adult because of ototoxicity. Intravenous albumin solutions restore plasma oncotic pressure temporarily in the nephrotic syndrome and allow mobilization of oedema but do not increase the natriuretic effect of loop diuretics.

Combinations of various classes of diuretics are extremely helpful in patients with resistant oedema. A loop diuretic plus a thiazide inhibit two major sites of sodium reabsorption; this effect may be further potentiated by addition of a potassium-sparing agent. Metolazone in combination with a loop diuretic is particularly useful in refractory congestive cardiac failure because its action is less dependent on glomerular filtration. However, this potent combination can cause severe electrolyte imbalance. Both aminophylline and dopamine increase renal blood flow and may be useful in refractory cardiogenic sodium retention. In addition, theophyllines, by inhibiting phosphodiesterase activity in the inner medullary collecting duct, prolong the action of cGMP (a second messenger of ANP).

Effects on renal function

All diuretics may increase plasma urea concentrations by increasing urea reabsorption in the medulla. Thiazides may also promote protein breakdown. In certain situations, diuretics also decrease GFR:

- Excessive diuresis causes volume depletion and pre-renal failure.
- Diuretics can cause allergic tubulointerstitial nephritis.
- Thiazides may directly cause a drop in GFR; the mechanism is complex and not fully understood.

Further reading

Berl T. Vasopressin antagonists. *N Engl J Med* 2015; 372:2207–2216.
Dorrance AM. Interfering with mineralocorticoid receptor activation: the past, present, and future. *F1000PrimeRep* 2014; 6:61.

Godin M, Bouchard J, Mehta RL. Fluid balance in patients with acute kidney injury: emerging concepts. *Nephron Clin Pract* 2013; 123:238–245.
Knepper MA, Kwon T-H, Nielson S. Molecular physiology of water balance. *N Engl J Med* **2015; 372:1349–1358.**
Walsh S, Unwin RJ. Renal tubular disorders. *Clin Med* 2012; 12:476–479.

Decreased extracellular volume

Deficiency of sodium and water causes shrinkage both of the interstitial space and of the blood volume, and may have profound effects on organ function.

Clinical features

Symptoms

Thirst, muscle cramps, nausea and vomiting, and postural dizziness occur. Severe depletion of circulating volume causes hypotension and impairs cerebral perfusion, causing confusion and eventual coma.

Signs

Signs can be divided into those due to loss of interstitial fluid and those due to loss of circulating volume.

- ***Loss of interstitial fluid*** leads to loss of skin elasticity ('turgor') – the rapidity with which the skin recoils to normal after being pinched. Skin turgor decreases with age, particularly at the peripheries. The turgor over the anterior triangle of the neck or on the forehead is a very useful sign in all ages.
- ***Loss of circulating volume*** leads to decreased pressure in the venous and (if severe) arterial compartments. Loss of up to 1 L of extracellular fluid in an adult may be compensated for by venoconstriction and may cause no physical signs.

  Loss of more than this amount causes the following:

Postural hypotension

Normally, the blood pressure rises if a subject stands up, as a result of increased venous return due to venoconstriction (this maintains cerebral perfusion). Loss of extracellular fluid (underfill) prevents this and causes a fall in blood pressure. This is one of the earliest and most reliable signs of volume depletion, as long as the other causes of postural hypotension are excluded ***(Box 9.5)***.

Box 9.5 Postural hypotension: some causes of a fall in blood pressure from lying to standing

Decreased circulating volume (hypovolaemia)

Autonomic failure
- Diabetes mellitus
- Systemic amyloidosis
- Shy–Drager syndrome
- Parkinson's disease
- Ageing

Interference with autonomic function by drugs
- Tricyclic antidepressants

Interference with peripheral vasoconstriction by drugs
- Nitrates
- Calcium-channel blockers
- α-Adrenoceptor-blocking drugs

Prolonged bed rest (cardiovascular deconditioning)

Low jugular venous pressure

In hypovolaemic patients, the jugular venous pulsation can be seen only with the patient lying completely flat, or even head down, because the right atrial pressure is lower than 5 cmH_2O.

Peripheral venoconstriction

This causes cold skin with empty peripheral veins, which are difficult to cannulate just when the patient needs intravenous therapy the most! This sign is often absent in sepsis, where peripheral vasodilatation contributes to effective hypovolaemia.

Tachycardia

This is not always a reliable sign. Beta-blockers and other antiarrhythmics may prevent tachycardia, and hypovolaemia may activate vagal mechanisms and actually cause bradycardia.

Aetiology

Salt and water may be lost from the kidneys, the gastrointestinal tract or the skin. Examples are given in ***Box 9.6***.

In addition, there are a number of situations where signs of volume depletion occur despite a normal or increased body content of sodium and water:

- Septicaemia causes vasodilatation of both arterioles and veins, resulting in greatly increased capacitance of the vascular space. In addition, increased capillary permeability to plasma proteins leads to loss of fluid from the vascular space to the interstitium.
- Diuretic treatment of heart failure or nephrotic syndrome may lead to rapid reduction in plasma volume. Mobilization of oedema may take much longer.
- There may be inappropriate diuretic treatment of oedema (e.g. when the cause is local rather than systemic).

Investigations

Blood tests are, in general, not helpful in the assessment of extracellular volume. Plasma urea may be raised owing to increased urea reabsorption and, later, to pre-renal failure (when the creatinine rises as well), but this is very non-specific. Urinary sodium is low if the kidneys are functioning normally, but is misleading if the cause of the volume depletion involves the kidneys (e.g. diuretics, intrinsic renal disease). Urine osmolality is high in volume depletion (owing to increased water reabsorption) but may also often mislead.

Assessment of volume status is shown in ***Box 9.7***.

Management

The overriding principle is to replace what is missing.

Box 9.6 Causes of extracellular volume depletion (hypovolaemia)

Haemorrhage
- External
- Concealed, e.g. leaking aortic aneurysm

Burns

Gastrointestinal losses
- Vomiting
- Diarrhoea
- Ileostomy losses
- Ileus

Renal losses
- Diuretic use
- Impaired tubular sodium conservation
- Reflux nephropathy
- Papillary necrosis
  - Analgesic nephropathy
  - Diabetes mellitus

Sickle cell disease

Haemorrhage

The rational treatment of acute haemorrhage is the infusion of a combination of red cells and a plasma substitute or (if unavailable) whole blood. (Chronic anaemia causes salt and water retention rather than volume depletion by a mechanism common to conditions with peripheral vasodilatation.)

Loss of plasma

Loss of plasma, as occurs in burns or severe peritonitis, should be treated with human plasma or a plasma substitute (see pp. 1157–1158).

Loss of water and electrolytes

Loss of water and electrolytes, as occurs with vomiting, diarrhoea or excessive renal losses, should be treated by replacement of the loss. If possible, this should be with oral water and sodium salts. These are available as slow sodium (600 mg, approximately 10 mmol each of Na^+ and Cl^- per tablet), the usual dose of which is 6–12 tablets/day with 2–3 L of water. They are used in mild or chronic salt and water depletion, such as that associated with renal salt wasting.

Sodium bicarbonate (500 mg, 6 mmol each of Na^+ and HCO_3^- per tablet) is given in doses of 6–12 tablets/day with 2–3 L of water. This is used in milder chronic sodium depletion with acidosis (e.g. CKD, post-obstructive renal failure, renal tubular acidosis). Sodium bicarbonate is less effective than sodium chloride in causing positive sodium balance. Oral rehydration solutions are described in ***Box 11.32***.

Intravenous fluids

These are sometimes required (***Box 9.8***). Rapid infusion (e.g. 1000 mL per hour or even faster) of 0.9% Na Cl is necessary if there is hypotension and evidence of impaired organ perfusion (e.g. oliguria, confusion). Repeated clinical assessments are vital in this situation, usually complemented by frequent measurements of central venous pressure (see p. 1146 for the management of shock). Severe hypovolaemia induces venoconstriction, which maintains venous return; over-rapid correction does not give time for this to reverse, resulting in signs of circulatory overload (e.g. pulmonary oedema), even if a total body extracellular fluid deficit remains. In less severe extracellular fluid depletion (such as in a patient with postural hypotension complicating acute tubular necrosis), the fluid should be replaced at a rate of 1000 mL every 4–6 h, again with repeated clinical assessment. If all that is required is avoidance of fluid depletion during surgery, 1–2 L can be given over 24 h, remembering that surgery is a stimulus to sodium and water retention and that over-replacement may be as dangerous as under-replacement. Regular monitoring by fluid balance charts, body weight and plasma biochemistry is mandatory.

Box 9.7 Assessment of volume status

Best achieved by simple clinical observations, which you should carry out yourself. Check:

- Jugular venous pressure
- Central venous pressure: both basal and after intravenous fluid challenge (see pp. 1146–1147)
- Postural changes in blood pressure
- Chest X-ray
- Serial weights of the patient
- Urine output measurements at regular intervals

Loss of water alone

This causes extracellular volume depletion only in severe cases because the loss is spread evenly among all the compartments of body water. In the rare situations where there is a true deficiency of water alone, as in diabetes insipidus or in a patient who is unable to drink (e.g. after surgery), the correct treatment is to give water.

If intravenous treatment is required, water is given as 5% glucose with K^+ because pure water would lead to osmotic lysis of blood cells.

Further reading

Braam B, Joles JA, Danishwar AH et al. Cardiorenal syndrome–current understanding and future perspectives. *Nat Rev Nephrol* 2014; 10:48–55.

Damkjær M, Isaksson GL, Stubbe J et al. Renal renin secretion as regulator of body fluid homeostasis. *Pflugers Arch* 2013; 465:153–165.

Moritz ML, Ayus JC. Maintenance intravenous fluids in acutely ill patients. *N Engl J Med* 2015; 373:1350–1360.

DISORDERS OF SODIUM CONCENTRATION

These are best thought of as disorders of body water content. As discussed above, sodium content is regulated by volume receptors; water content is adjusted to maintain, in health, a normal osmolality and (in the absence of abnormal osmotically active solutes) a

Box 9.8 Intravenous fluids in general use for fluid and electrolyte disturbances

I.v. fluid	Na^+ (mmol/L)	K^+ (mmol/L)	HCO_3^- (mmol/L)	Cl^- (mmol/L)	Indication[a]
Normal plasma values	**142**	**4.5**	**26**	**103**	
Sodium chloride 0.9%	150	–	–	150	1
Sodium chloride 0.18% + glucose 4%	30	–	–	30	2
Glucose 5% + potassium chloride 0.3%	–	40	–	40	3
Sodium bicarbonate 1.26%	150	–	150	–	4
Hartmann's[b]	131	5	29 (as lactate)	111	4,5

[a]1. Volume expansion in hypovolaemic patients. Rarely, to maintain fluid balance when there are large losses of sodium. The sodium (150 mmol/L) is higher than in plasma and hypernatraemia can result. It is often necessary to add KCl 20–40 mmol/L.
2. Maintenance of fluid balance in normovolaemic, normonatraemic patients.
3. To replace water. Can be given with or without potassium chloride. May be alternated with 0.9% saline as an alternative to (2).
4. For volume expansion in hypovolaemic, acidotic patients, alternating with (1). Occasionally, for maintenance of fluid balance combined with (2) in salt-wasting, acidotic patients.
5. For volume expansion in hypovolaemic patients. May be better than 0.9% saline for patients with sepsis and relative hypovolaemia.

[b]Hartmann's solution also contains 2 mmol/L of calcium.

normal sodium concentration. Disturbances of sodium concentration are caused by disturbances of water balance.

Hyponatraemia

Hyponatraemia (Na <135 mmol/L) is the most common biochemical abnormality in hospitalized patients, with up to 35% of inpatients developing hyponatraemia during their stay. The causes depend on the associated changes in extracellular volume:

- hyponatraemia with hypovolaemia ***(Box 9.9)***
- hyponatraemia with euvolaemia ***(Box 9.10)***
- hyponatraemia with hypervolaemia ***(Box 9.11)***.

Rarely, hyponatraemia may be a 'pseudo-hyponatraemia'. This occurs in hyperlipidaemia (either high cholesterol or high triglyceride) or hyperproteinaemia where there is a spuriously low measured sodium concentration, the sodium being confined to the aqueous phase but having its concentration expressed in terms of the total volume of plasma. In this situation, plasma osmolality is normal and therefore treatment of 'hyponatraemia' is unnecessary. Note that artefactual 'hyponatraemia', caused by taking blood from the limb into which fluid of low sodium concentration is being infused, should be excluded.

Box 9.9 Causes of hyponatraemia with decreased extracellular volume (hypovolaemia)

Extrarenal (urinary sodium <20 mmol/L)
- Vomiting
- Diarrhoea
- Haemorrhage
- Burns
- Pancreatitis

Kidney (urinary sodium >20 mmol/L)
- Osmotic diuresis (e.g. hyperglycaemia, severe uraemia)
- Diuretics
- Adrenocortical insufficiency
- Tubulointerstitial renal disease
- Unilateral renal artery stenosis
- Recovery phase of acute tubular necrosis

Box 9.10 Causes of hyponatraemia with normal extracellular volume (euvolaemia)

Abnormal antidiuretic hormone (ADH) release
- Vagal neuropathy (failure of inhibition of ADH release)
- Deficiency of adrenocorticotrophic hormone (ACTH) or glucocorticoids (Addison's disease)
- Hypothyroidism
- Severe potassium depletion

Syndrome of inappropriate antidiuretic hormone secretion (SIADH)
- See ***Box 26.46***

Psychiatric illness
- 'Psychogenic polydipsia'
- Non-osmotic ADH release?
- Antidepressant therapy

Increased sensitivity to ADH
- Chlorpropamide
- Tolbutamide

ADH-like substances
- Oxytocin
- Desmopressin

Unmeasured osmotically active substances stimulating osmotic ADH release
- Glucose
- Chronic alcohol misuse
- Mannitol
- Sick-cell syndrome (leakage of intracellular ions)

Hyponatraemia with hypovolaemia

This is due to salt loss in excess of water loss; the causes are listed in ***Box 9.9***. In this situation, ADH secretion is initially suppressed (via the hypothalamic osmoreceptors) but, as fluid volume is lost, volume receptors override the osmoreceptors and stimulate both thirst and the release of ADH. This is an attempt by the body to defend circulating volume at the expense of osmolality.

With extrarenal losses and normal kidneys, the urinary excretion of sodium falls in response to the volume depletion, as does water excretion, leading to concentrated urine containing <10 mmol/L of sodium. However, in salt-wasting kidney disease, renal compensation cannot occur and the only physiological protection is increased water intake in response to thirst.

Clinical features

With sodium depletion, the clinical picture is usually dominated by features of volume depletion (see p. 159). The diagnosis is usually obvious where there is a history of gut losses, diabetes mellitus or diuretic abuse. Examination of the patient is often more helpful than the biochemical investigations, which include plasma and urine electrolytes and osmolality.

Box 9.12 shows the potential daily losses of water and electrolytes from the gut. Losses due to renal or adrenocortical disease may be less easily identified but a urinary sodium concentration of >20 mmol/L, in the presence of clinically evident volume depletion, suggests a renal loss.

Management

This is directed at the primary cause whenever possible.

In a healthy patient:

- Give oral electrolyte–glucose mixtures (see pp. 288–289).
- Increase salt intake with slow sodium 60–80 mmol/day.

In a patient with vomiting or severe volume depletion:

- Give intravenous fluid with potassium supplements, i.e. 1.5–2 L 5% glucose (with 20 mmol K^+) and 1 L 0.9% saline over 24 h *plus* measurable losses.
- Correction of acid–base abnormalities is usually not required.

Hyponatraemia with euvolaemia

Hyponatraemia with euvolaemia (see ***Box 9.10***) results from an intake of water in excess of the kidney's ability to excrete it (dilutional hyponatraemia); there is no change in body sodium content but the plasma osmolality is low.

- With normal kidney function, dilution hyponatraemia is uncommon even if a patient drinks approximately 1 L per hour.
- The most common iatrogenic cause is over-generous infusion of 5% glucose into postoperative patients; in this situation, it

Box 9.11 Causes of hyponatraemia with increased extracellular volume (hypervolaemia)

- Heart failure
- Liver failure
- Oliguric kidney injury
- Hypoalbuminaemia

Box 9.12 Average concentrations and potential daily losses of water and electrolytes from the gut

	Na^+ (mmol/L)	K^+ (mmol/L)	Cl^- (mmol/L)	Volume (mL in 24 h)
Stomach	50	10	110	2500
Small intestine				
Recent ileostomy	120	5	110	1500
Adapted ileostomy	50	4	25	500
Bile	140	5	105	500
Pancreatic juice	140	5	60	2000
Diarrhoea	130	10–30	95	1000–2000+

is exacerbated by an increased ADH secretion in response to stress.
- Postoperative hyponatraemia is a common clinical problem (almost 1% of patients) with *symptomatic* hyponatraemia occurring in 20% of these patients.
- Marathon runners who drink excess water can become hyponatraemic. Even so-called 'isotonic sports drinks' can lead to hyponatraemia, as they contain little sodium, their osmolality being made up with carbohydrates, which are metabolized into energy and water.
- Premenopausal females are at most risk for developing hyponatraemic encephalopathy postoperatively, with postoperative ADH values in young females being 40 times higher than in young males.

To prevent hyponatraemia, avoid using hypotonic fluids postoperatively and administer 0.9% saline unless clinically contraindicated. The serum sodium should be measured daily in any patient receiving continuous parenteral fluid.

Some degree of hyponatraemia is usual in acute oliguric kidney injury, while in CKD it is most often due to ill-given advice to 'push' fluids.

Clinical features

Dilutional hyponatraemia

Symptoms of dilutional hyponatraemia are common when hyponatraemia develops *acutely* (<48 h, often postoperatively). Overt neurological symptoms rarely occur until the serum sodium is less than 125 mmol/L and are more usually associated with values around 115 mmol/L or lower, particularly when *chronic*. In elderly patients, however, even mild hyponatraemia with a serum sodium of 130–135 mmol/L has been associated with increased falls risk and subtle changes in cognition. They are due to the movement of water into brain cells in response to the fall in extracellular osmolality.

Hyponatraemic encephalopathy

Symptoms and signs include headache, confusion and restlessness leading to drowsiness, myoclonic jerks, generalized convulsions and eventually coma. Magnetic resonance imaging (MRI) of the brain may reveal cerebral oedema but, in the context of electrolyte abnormalities and neurological symptoms, can help to make a confirmatory diagnosis.

Risk factors for developing hyponatraemic encephalopathy

The brain's adaptation to hyponatraemia initially involves extrusion of blood and CSF, as well as sodium, potassium and organic osmolytes, in order to decrease brain osmolality. Various factors can interfere with successful adaptation. These factors, rather than the absolute change in serum sodium, predict whether a patient will suffer hyponatraemic encephalopathy.
- ***Children*** under 16 years are at increased risk due to their relatively large brain-to-intracranial volume ratio compared with adults.
- ***Premenopausal women*** are more likely to develop encephalopathy than postmenopausal females and males because of inhibitory effects of sex hormones and the effects of vasopressin on cerebral circulation, resulting in vasoconstriction and hypoperfusion of the brain.
- ***Hypoxaemia*** is a major risk factor for hyponatraemic encephalopathy. Patients with hyponatraemia who develop hypoxia, due to either non-cardiac pulmonary oedema or hypercapnic respiratory failure, have a high risk of mortality. Hypoxia is the strongest predictor of mortality in patients with symptomatic hyponatraemia.

Investigations

The cause of hyponatraemia with apparently normal extracellular volume requires investigation:
- *Plasma and urine electrolytes and osmolalities*. The plasma concentrations of sodium, chloride and urea are low, giving a low osmolality. The urine sodium concentration is usually high and the urine osmolality is typically higher than the plasma osmolality. However, maximal dilution (<50 mosmol/kg) is not always present.
- *Further investigations*. These are needed to exclude Addison's disease, hypothyroidism, syndrome of inappropriate ADH secretion (SIADH) and water retention induced by drugs, e.g. chlorpropamide.

Potassium depletion and magnesium depletion potentiate ADH release and are causes of diuretic-associated hyponatraemia.

SIADH is often over-diagnosed. Some causes are associated with a lower set-point for ADH release, rather than completely autonomous ADH release; an example is chronic alcohol use.

Management *(Box 9.13)*

The underlying cause should be corrected where possible.
- ***Most patients***. Most cases are simply managed by restriction of water intake (to 1000 or even 500 mL/day) with review of diuretic therapy. Magnesium and potassium deficiency must be corrected. In mild sodium deficiency, 0.9% saline given slowly (1 L over 12 h) is sufficient.
- ***Acute onset with symptoms***. The most common cause of acute hyponatraemia in adults is postoperative iatrogenic hyponatraemia. Excessive water intake associated with

Box 9.13 Key points in the management of hyponatraemia

- Always treat the underlying cause
- What is the volume status of the patient?
  - If hypovolaemic: rehydrate with 0.9% saline
  - If euvolaemic (SIADH): restrict fluid to 500–700 mL/day
  - If hypervolaemic (chronic kidney disease/heart failure): restrict fluid and salt
- Does the patient have symptomatic hyponatraemia (seizures/coma)?
  - Yes: involve critical care input early; 3% saline 1 mL/kg over 1 h
- Is the hyponatraemia acute or chronic?
  - If acute: more likely to develop symptomatic hyponatraemia
  - If chronic: increased risk of osmotic demyelination due to rapid correction
  - If unsure: give 3% saline very slowly
- Check sodium levels frequently: may need to check Na every 1–2 h
- Correction must not exceed 10 mmol in first 24 h and 18 mmol in 48 h

psychosis, marathon running and use of Ecstasy (a recreational drug) are other causes. All are acute medical emergencies and should be treated aggressively and immediately. In patients who demonstrate severe neurological signs, such as fits, coma or cerebral oedema, ***hypertonic saline*** (3%, 513 mmol/L) should be used. It must be given very slowly (not more than 70 mmol/h), the aim being to increase the serum sodium by 4–6 mmol/L in the first 4 hours, but the absolute change should not exceed 15–20 mmol/L over 48 hours. In general, the plasma sodium should not be corrected to >125–130 mmol/L. Assuming that total body water comprises 50% of total body weight, 1 mL/kg of 3% sodium chloride will raise the plasma sodium by 1 mmol/L.

- ***Symptomatic hyponatraemia in patients with intracranial pathology***. This should be managed aggressively and immediately with 3% saline, as for acute hyponatraemia.
- ***Chronic/asymptomatic hyponatraemia***. If hyponatraemia has developed slowly, as it does in the majority of patients, the brain will have adapted by decreasing intracellular osmolality and the hyponatraemia can be corrected slowly.

However, clinically, it can be difficult to know how long the hyponatraemia has been present for and 3% hypertonic saline may still be required.

Osmotic demyelination syndrome

Avoiding osmotic demyelination syndrome

A rapid rise in extracellular osmolality, particularly if there is an 'overshoot' to high serum sodium and osmolality, will result in the osmotic demyelination syndrome (ODS), formerly known as central pontine demyelination, which is a devastating neurological complication. Plasma sodium concentration in patients with hyponatraemia should not rise by more than 8 mmol/L per day. The rate of rise of plasma sodium should be even lower in patients at higher risk for ODS: for example, those with alcohol excess, cirrhosis, malnutrition or hypokalaemia. Other factors predisposing to demyelination are pre-existing hypoxaemia and central nervous system radiation (see above). ODS is diagnosed by the appearance of characteristic hypointense lesions on T_1-weighted images and hyperintense lesions on T_2 weighted images on MRI; these can take 2 weeks or more to appear.

The pathophysiology of ODS is not fully understood. The most plausible explanation is that the brain loses organic osmolytes very quickly in order to adapt to hyponatraemia so that osmolarity is similar between the intracellular and extracellular compartments. However, neurones reclaim organic osmolytes slowly in the phase of rapid correction of hyponatraemia, resulting in a hypo-osmolar intracellular compartment and shrinkage of cerebral vascular endothelial cells. Consequently, the blood–brain barrier is functionally impaired, allowing lymphocytes, complement and cytokines to enter the brain, damage oligodendrocytes, activate microglial cells and cause demyelination.

The most crucial issue in the treatment of hyponatraemia is to ***prevent rapid correction***. A rapid rise in plasma sodium is almost always due to a water diuresis, which happens when vasopressin (ADH) action stops suddenly: for example, with volume repletion in patients with intravascular volume depletion, cortisol replacement in patients with Addison's disease, or resolution of non-osmotic stimuli for vasopressin release such as nausea or pain. Sometimes, however, chronic hyponatraemia can develop in the absence of vasopressin excess. Even in these cases, water diuresis due to ***increased distal delivery of filtrate*** is the main cause of rapid rise in plasma sodium.

In the absence of vasopressin, it is *generally assumed* that the total urine volume is equal to the volume of filtrate delivered to the distal nephron, which is the GFR minus the volume reabsorbed in the proximal convoluted tubule. Approximately 80% of the GFR is reabsorbed in proximal convoluted tubule under normal circumstance (and increases even more in the presence of intravascular volume depletion). However, *in real life*, water excretion will be less than the volume of distal delivery of filtrate, even in the absence of vasopressin, because a significant degree of water is reabsorbed in the inner medullary collecting duct through its residual water permeability, prompted by a very high osmotic force in the interstitium (see ***Fig. 20.3***).

Even a modest water diuresis in the elderly with reduced muscle mass is large enough to cause a rapid rise in plasma sodium. Moreover, there is a higher risk for ODS if hypokalaemia is present. In such cases, if plasma sodium rises too quickly due to anticipated water diuresis, administration of desmopressin to stop the water diuresis is beneficial. If plasma sodium rises regardless, then lowering plasma sodium to the maximum limit of correction (<8 mmol/L per day) with the administration of 5% glucose solution is the best strategy.

Reversible hyponatraemia culminating in hypernatraemia

In many patients, the cause of water retention is reversible (e.g. hypovolaemia, thiazide diuretics). On correction of the cause, vasopressin levels fall and plasma sodium rises by up to 2 mmol/L per hour as a result of excretion of dilute urine. This excessive water diuresis should be anticipated and prevented by use of desmopressin.

Patients who are chronically hyponatraemic with concomitant hypokalaemia are especially susceptible to overcorrection. Plasma sodium is a function of the ratio of exchangeable body sodium plus potassium to total body water, so potassium administration increases sodium concentration. For example, a mildly symptomatic hyponatraemic patient with a plasma sodium of <120 mmol/L and potassium of <2 mmol/L can potentially develop ODS as a result of overcorrection of hyponatraemia simply as a direct result of replacing the large potassium deficit.

Antidiuretic hormone antagonists (vasopressin antagonists)

Vasopressin V_2 receptor antagonists (see p. 158), which produce a free water diuresis, are being used in clinical trials for the treatment of hyponatraemic encephalopathy. Three oral agents, lixivaptan, tolvaptan and satavaptan, are selective for the V_2 (antidiuretic) receptor, while conivaptan blocks both V_{1A} and V_2 receptors.

These agents produce a selective water diuresis without affecting sodium and potassium excretion; they raise the plasma sodium concentration in patients with hyponatraemia caused by SIADH, heart failure and cirrhosis.

The efficacy of oral tolvaptan in ambulatory patients has been demonstrated in individuals with hyponatraemia (mean plasma sodium 129 mmol/L) caused by SIADH, heart failure or cirrhosis who had a sustained rise in plasma sodium to 136 mmol/L for 4 weeks. Tolvaptan is now approved for use in patients with euvolaemic hyponatraemia and those with SIADH. In addition, intravenous conivaptan is available and is also approved for the treatment of euvolaemic hyponatraemia (i.e. SIADH) in some countries. The approved dosing for conivaptan is a 20 mg bolus followed by continuous infusion of 20 mg over 1–4 days. The continuous infusion increases the risk of phlebitis, which requires the use of large veins and change of infusion site every 24 hours.

Hyponatraemia with hypervolaemia

The common causes of hyponatraemia due to water excess are shown in ***Box 9.11***. In all these conditions, there is usually an element of reduced GFR with avid reabsorption of sodium and chloride in the proximal tubule. This leads to reduced delivery of chloride to the 'diluting' ascending limb of the loop of Henle and a reduced ability to generate 'free water', with a consequent inability to excrete dilute urine. This is commonly compounded by the administration of diuretics that block chloride reabsorption and interfere with the dilution of filtrate either in the loop of Henle (loop diuretics) or distally (thiazides).

Syndrome of inappropriate ADH secretion

This is described on pages 1234–1235. There is inappropriate secretion of ADH, causing water retention and hyponatraemia.

Hypernatraemia

This is much rarer than hyponatraemia and nearly always indicates a water deficit. Causes are listed in ***Box 9.14***.

? Box 9.14 Causes of hypernatraemia

Antidiuretic hormone (ADH) deficiency
- Pituitary diabetes insipidus (see pp. 1233–1234)

Iatrogenic
- Administration of hypertonic sodium solutions
- Administration of drugs with a high sodium content (e.g. piperacillin)
- Use of 8.4% sodium bicarbonate after cardiac arrest

Insensitivity to ADH (nephrogenic diabetes insipidus)
- Lithium
- Tetracyclines
- Amphotericin B
- Acute tubular necrosis
- Osmotic diuresis
- Total parenteral nutrition
- Hyperosmolar hyperglycaemic state (see p. 1264)

Plus
- Deficient water intake: impaired thirst or consciousness
- Excessive water loss through skin or lungs

Hypernatraemia is always associated with increased plasma osmolality, which is a potent stimulus to thirst. None of the factors listed in ***Box 9.14*** causes hypernatraemia unless thirst sensation is abnormal or access to water limited. For instance, a patient with diabetes insipidus will maintain a normal serum sodium concentration by maintaining a high water intake until an intercurrent illness prevents this. Thirst is frequently deficient in elderly people, making them more prone to water depletion. Hypernatraemia may occur in the presence of normal, reduced or expanded extracellular volume, and does not necessarily imply that total body sodium is increased.

Clinical features

Symptoms of hypernatraemia are non-specific. Nausea, vomiting, fever and confusion may occur. A history of longstanding polyuria, polydipsia and thirst suggests diabetes insipidus. Assessment of extracellular volume status guides resuscitation. Mental state should be assessed. Convulsions occur in severe hypernatraemia.

Investigations

Simultaneous urine and plasma osmolality and sodium should be measured. Plasma osmolality is high in hypernatraemia. Passage of urine with an osmolality lower than that of plasma in this situation is clearly abnormal and indicates diabetes insipidus. In pituitary diabetes insipidus, urine osmolality will increase after administration of desmopressin; the drug (a vasopressin analogue) has no effect in nephrogenic diabetes insipidus (see p. 1234). If urine osmolality is high, this suggests either an osmotic diuresis due to an unmeasured solute (e.g. in parenteral feeding) or excessive extrarenal loss of water (e.g. heat stroke).

Management

Treatment is that of the underlying cause. For example:
- In ADH deficiency, replace ADH in the form of desmopressin, a stable non-pressor analogue of ADH.
- Remember to withdraw nephrotoxic drugs where possible and replace water either orally or, if necessary, intravenously.

In ***severe*** (>170 mmol/L) hypernatraemia, 0.9% saline (150 mmol/L) should be used initially. Avoid too rapid a drop in serum sodium concentration; the aim is correction over 48 hours, as over-rapid correction may lead to cerebral oedema.

In ***less severe*** (e.g. >150 mmol/L) hypernatraemia, the treatment is 5% glucose or 0.45% saline; the latter is obviously preferable in hyperosmolar diabetic coma. Very large volumes – 5 L/day or more – may need to be given in diabetes insipidus.

If there is clinical evidence of volume depletion (see p. 159), this implies that there is a sodium deficit as well as a water deficit. Treatment of this is discussed on page 160.

Further reading

Combs S, Berl T. Dysnatremias in patients with kidney disease. *Am J Kidney Dis* 2014; 63:294–303.

King JD, Rosner MH. Osmotic demyelination syndrome. *Am J Med Sci* 2010; 339:561–567.

Nemerovski C, Hutchinson DJ. Treatment of hypervolemic or euvolemic hyponatremia associated with heart failure, cirrhosis, or the syndrome of inappropriate antidiuretic hormone with tolvaptan: a clinical review. *Clin Ther* 2010; 32:1015–1032.

Rozen-Zvi B, Yahav D, Gheorghiade M et al. Vasopressin receptor antagonists for the treatment of hyponatremia: systematic review and meta-analysis. *Am J Kidney Dis* 2010; 56:325–337.

Spasovski G, Vanholst R, Allolio B et al. Clinical practice guidelines on diagnosis and treatment of hyponatraemia. *Eur J Endocrinol* 2014; 170: G1–47.

Sterns RH. Disorders of plasma sodium – causes, consequences and correction. *N Engl J Med* 2015; 372:55–65.

Verbalis JG, Goldsmith SR, Greenberg A et al. Diagnosis, evaluation, and treatment of hyponatremia: expert panel recommendations. *Am J Med* 2013; 126(10 Suppl 1):S1–42.

DISORDERS OF POTASSIUM CONCENTRATION

Regulation of serum potassium concentration

The World Health Organization (WHO) recommends a dietary intake of 90 mmol/day to reduce blood pressure; most people have a dietary intake of between 80 and 150 mmol daily, depending upon fruit and vegetable intake. Most of the body's potassium (3500 mmol in an adult) is intracellular. Serum potassium levels are controlled by:

- uptake of K^+ into cells
- renal excretion
- extrarenal losses (e.g. gastrointestinal).

Uptake of potassium into cells is governed by the activity of the Na^+/K^+-ATPase in the cell membrane and by H^+ concentration.

Uptake is ***stimulated*** by:

- insulin
- β-adrenergic stimulation
- theophyllines.

Uptake is ***decreased*** by:

- α-adrenergic stimulation
- acidosis – K^+ exchanged for H^+ across cell membranes
- cell damage or cell death – resulting in massive K^+ release.

The ***kidney*** plays the pivotal role in the maintenance of potassium balance by varying its secretion with changes in dietary intake. Over 90% of the filtered potassium is reabsorbed in the proximal tubule and the loop of Henle and only <10% of the filtered load is delivered to the early distal tubule. Potassium absorption in the proximal tubule is entirely passive and follows that of sodium and water, while its reabsorption in the thick ascending limb of the loop of Henle is mediated by the sodium–potassium-2-chloride co-transporter. However, potassium is secreted by the principal cells in the cortical and outer medullary collecting tubule. Secretion in these segments is very tightly regulated in health and can be varied according to individual needs; it is responsible for most of urinary potassium excretion.

Renal excretion of potassium is increased by aldosterone, which stimulates K^+ and H^+ secretion in exchange for Na^+ in the principal cells of the collecting duct ***(Fig. 9.8)***. Because H^+ and K^+ are interchangeable in the exchange mechanism, acidosis decreases and alkalosis increases the secretion of K^+. Aldosterone secretion is stimulated by hyperkalaemia and increased angiotensin II levels, as well as by some drugs, and this acts to protect the body against hyperkalaemia and against extracellular volume depletion. The body adapts to dietary deficiency of potassium by reducing aldosterone secretion. However, because aldosterone is also influenced by volume status, conservation of potassium is relatively inefficient, and significant potassium depletion may therefore result from prolonged dietary deficiency.

A number of drugs affect K^+ homeostasis by affecting aldosterone release (e.g. heparin, NSAIDs) or by directly affecting renal potassium handling (e.g. diuretics).

Other endogenous proteins and metabolites also affect potassium homeostasis. Klotho, an anti-ageing protein expressed in the distal tubule (and other organs), increases potassium excretion. CD63, a tetra-spanning protein, inhibits its excretion. Moreover, protein kinase A- and C-mediated phosphorylation inhibits conductance of K^+ channels in the principal cells of the collecting duct but the cytochrome P450-epoxygenase-mediated metabolite of arachidonic acid (11–12-epoxyeicosatrienoic acid) activates these channels and plays a role in overall potassium homeostasis.

Normally, only about 10% of daily potassium intake is excreted in the gastrointestinal tract. Vomit contains around 5–10 mmol/L of K^+, but prolonged vomiting causes hypokalaemia by inducing sodium depletion, stimulating aldosterone, which increases renal potassium excretion. Potassium is secreted by the colon, and diarrhoea contains 10–30 mmol/L of K^+; profuse diarrhoea can therefore induce marked hypokalaemia. Colorectal villous adenomas may rarely produce profuse diarrhoea and K^+ loss.

Hypokalaemia

Aetiology

Common causes

The most common causes of chronic hypokalaemia are diuretic treatment (particularly thiazides) and hyperaldosteronism. Acute hypokalaemia is often caused by intravenous fluids without potassium and redistribution into cells, particularly in the case of diabetic ketoacidosis (see pp. 1261–1264), where the use of fluids without potassium combined with insulin treatment can cause a rapid fall in the serum potassium. The common causes are shown in ***Box 9.15***.

Rare causes

These rare causes are discussed in detail because they show the mechanisms of how diuretics can affect the kidney.

Box 9.15 Causes of hypokalaemia

Increased renal excretion
(Urinary K^+ >20 mmol/day)
- Diuretics:
  - Thiazides
  - Loop diuretics

Increased aldosterone secretion
- Liver failure
- Heart failure
- Nephrotic syndrome
- Cushing syndrome
- Conn syndrome
- ACTH-producing tumours

Exogenous mineralocorticoid
- Corticosteroids
- Liquorice (potentiates renal actions of cortisol)

Renal disease
- Renal tubular acidosis types 1 and 2
- Renal tubular damage (diuretic phase)
- Acute leukaemia
- Nephrotoxicity:
  - Amphotericin
  - Aminoglycosides
  - Cytotoxic drugs
- Release of urinary tract obstruction
- Bartter syndrome
- Liddle syndrome
- Gitelman syndrome

Reduced intake of K+
- Intravenous fluids without K^+
- Dietary deficiency

Redistribution into cells
- β-Adrenergic stimulation
- Acute myocardial infarction
- Beta-agonists, e.g. fenoterol, salbutamol
- Insulin treatment, e.g. treatment of diabetic ketoacidosis
- Correction of megaloblastic anaemia, e.g. B_{12} deficiency
- Alkalosis
- Hypokalaemic periodic paralysis

Gastrointestinal losses
(Urinary K^+ <20 mmol/day)
- Vomiting
- Severe diarrhoea
- Purgative abuse
- Villous adenoma
- Ileostomy or ureterosigmoidostomy
- Fistulae
- Ileus/intestinal obstruction

Bartter syndrome

Bartter syndrome (clinically similar to the effects of treatment with loop diuretics) consists of metabolic alkalosis, hypokalaemia, hypercalciuria, occasionally hypomagnesaemia (see p. 170), normal blood pressure, and an elevated plasma renin and aldosterone. The primary defect in this disorder is an impairment in sodium and chloride reabsorption in the thick ascending limb of the loop of Henle (see ***Fig. 9.6***). Mutation in the genes encoding either the sodium–potassium-2–chloride co-transporter (NKCC2), the ATP-regulated renal outer medullary potassium channel (ROMK) or kidney-specific basolateral chloride channels (CLC-Kb) – Bartter syndrome types I, II and III, respectively – causes loss of function of these channels, with consequent impairment of sodium and chloride reabsorption. There is also an increased intrarenal production of prostaglandin E_2 (PGE_2), which is secondary to sodium and volume depletion, hypokalaemia and the consequent neurohumoral response rather than a primary defect. PGE_2 causes vasodilatation and may explain why the blood pressure remains normal.

Barttin, a β-subunit for CLC-Ka and CLC-Kb chloride channels, is encoded by the *BSND* (Bartter syndrome with sensorineural deafness) gene. Loss-of-function mutations cause type IV Bartter syndrome, which is associated with sensorineural deafness and renal failure. Barttin co-localizes with a subunit of the chloride channel in basolateral membranes of the renal tubule and inner ear epithelium. It appears to mediate chloride exit in the *t*hick *a*scending *l*imb (TAL) of the loop of Henle and chloride recycling in potassium-secreting strial marginal cells in the inner ear. A very rare variant of type IV is a disorder with an impairment of both chloride channels (CLC-Ka and CLC-Kb), producing the same phenotypic defects.

A gain-of-function mutation of the calcium-sensing receptor (CaSR), which leads to autosomal dominant hypocalcaemia, has also been recognized in Bartter syndrome. In the kidney, the CaSR is expressed mainly in the basolateral membrane of cortical TAL. Activation of CaSR by high calcium or magnesium or by gain-of-function mutation triggers intracellular signalling, including release of arachidonic acid and inhibition of adenylate cyclase. Both actions result in inhibition of ROMK activity, which in turn leads to reduction in the lumen-positive electrical potential and transcellular absorption of calcium. This effect of CaSR explains why patients with mutations in this receptor may present with hypocalcaemia, hypercalciuria and renal wasting of NaCl, resulting in a Bartter-like syndrome.

In summary, these defects in sodium chloride transport initiate the following sequence, which is almost identical to that seen with chronic ingestion of a loop diuretic: the initial salt loss leads to mild volume depletion, resulting in activation of the renin–angiotensin–aldosterone system; the combination of hyperaldosteronism and increased distal flow (owing to the reabsorptive defect) enhances potassium and hydrogen secretion at the secretory sites in the collecting tubules, leading to hypokalaemia and metabolic alkalosis.

Diagnostic pointers include high urinary potassium and chloride despite low serum values, as well as increased plasma renin. (N.B. In primary aldosteronism, renin levels are low.) Hyperplasia of the juxtaglomerular apparatus is seen on renal biopsy (careful exclusion of diuretic abuse is necessary). Hypercalciuria is a common feature but magnesium wasting, though rare, also occurs.

Treatment is with combinations of potassium supplements, amiloride and indometacin.

Gitelman syndrome

Gitelman syndrome (similar to the effects of treatment with thiazide diuretics) is a phenotype variant of Bartter syndrome characterized by hypokalaemia, metabolic alkalosis, hypocalciuria, hypomagnesaemia, normal blood pressure, and elevated plasma renin and aldosterone. There are striking similarities between Gitelman syndrome and the biochemical abnormalities induced by chronic thiazide diuretic administration. Thiazides act in the distal convoluted tubule to inhibit the function of the apical sodium–chloride co-transporter (NCCT) (see ***Fig. 9.7***). Analysis of the gene encoding the NCCT has identified loss-of-function mutations in Gitelman syndrome.

As in Bartter syndrome, defective NCCT function leads to increased solute delivery to the collecting duct, with resultant solute wasting, volume contraction and an aldosterone-mediated increase in potassium and hydrogen secretion. Unlike in Bartter syndrome, the degree of volume depletion and hypokalaemia is not sufficient to stimulate PGE_2 production. Impaired function of NCCT is predicted to cause hypocalciuria, as does thiazide administration. Impaired sodium reabsorption across the apical membrane, coupled with continued intracellular chloride efflux across the basolateral membrane, causes the cell to become hyperpolarized. This in turn stimulates calcium reabsorption via apical, voltage-activated calcium channels. Decreased intracellular sodium also facilitates calcium efflux via the basolateral sodium–calcium exchanger. The mechanism for urinary magnesium losses is described on pages 169–170.

Treatment consists of potassium and magnesium supplementation ($MgCl_2$) and a potassium-sparing diuretic. Volume resuscitation is usually not necessary, because patients are not dehydrated. Elevated PGE_2 does not occur (see above) and, therefore, NSAIDs are not indicated in this disorder.

Liddle syndrome

This is characterized by potassium wasting, hypokalaemia and alkalosis, but is associated with low renin and aldosterone production, and high blood pressure. There is a mutation in the gene encoding for the amiloride-sensitive epithelial sodium channel in the distal tubule/collecting duct. This leads to constitutive activation of the epithelial sodium channel, resulting in excessive sodium reabsorption with coupled potassium and hydrogen secretion. Unregulated sodium reabsorption across the collecting tubule causes volume expansion, inhibition of renin and aldosterone secretion, and development of low-renin hypertension (see ***Fig. 9.8***).

Therapy consists of sodium restriction, along with amiloride or triamterene administration. Both are potassium-sparing diuretics that directly close the sodium channels. The mineralocorticoid antagonist spironolactone is ineffective, since the increase in sodium-channel activity is not mediated by aldosterone.

Hypokalaemic periodic paralysis

This condition may be precipitated by carbohydrate intake, suggesting that insulin-mediated potassium influx into cells may be responsible. This syndrome also occurs in association with hyperthyroidism (thyrotoxic periodic paralysis; see p. 889), which occurs in Asians.

Clinical features

Hypokalaemia is usually asymptomatic but severe hypokalaemia (<2.5 mmol) causes muscle weakness. Potassium depletion may also cause symptomatic hyponatraemia (see p. 162).

Hypokalaemia is associated with an increased frequency of atrial and ventricular ectopic beats. This association may not always be causal because adrenergic activation (for instance, after myocardial infarction) results in both hypokalaemia and increased cardiac irritability. Hypokalaemia in patients without cardiac disease is unlikely to lead to serious arrhythmias.

Box 9.16 Treatment of hypokalaemia

Cause	Treatment
Dietary deficiency	Increase intake of fresh fruit/vegetables or oral potassium supplements (20–40 mmol daily). (Potassium supplements can cause gastrointestinal irritation)
Hyperaldosteronism, e.g. cirrhosis, thiazide therapy	Spironolactone/eplerenone. Co-prescription of a potassium-sparing diuretic with a similar onset and duration of action
Intravenous fluid replacement	Add 20 mmol of K^+/L of fluid with monitoring

Hypokalaemia seriously increases the risk of digoxin toxicity by increasing binding of digoxin to cardiac cells, potentiating its action and decreasing its clearance.

Chronic hypokalaemia is associated with interstitial renal disease but the pathogenesis is not completely understood.

Management

The underlying cause should be identified and treated where possible. ***Box 9.16*** shows some examples.

Acute hypokalaemia may correct spontaneously. In most cases, withdrawal of oral diuretics or purgatives, accompanied by the oral administration of potassium supplements in the form of slow-release potassium or effervescent potassium, is all that is required. Intravenous potassium replacement is needed only in conditions such as cardiac arrhythmias, muscle weakness or severe diabetic ketoacidosis. When intravenous therapy is used in the presence of poor renal function, replacement rates <2 mmol per hour should only be used, with hourly monitoring of serum potassium and electrocardiogram changes. Ampoules of potassium should be thoroughly mixed in 0.9% saline; do not use a glucose solution, as this would make hypokalaemia worse.

The treatment of adrenal disorders is described on page 1199.

Failure to correct hypokalaemia may be due to concurrent hypomagnesaemia. Serum magnesium should be measured and any deficiency corrected.

Hyperkalaemia

Aetiology

Common causes

Acute self-limiting hyperkalaemia occurs normally after vigorous exercise and is of no pathological significance. Hyperkalaemia in all other situations is due either to increased release from cells or to failure of excretion ***(Box 9.17)***. The most common causes are renal impairment and drug interference with potassium excretion. The combination of angiotensin-converting enzyme (ACE) inhibitors with potassium-sparing diuretics or NSAIDs is particularly dangerous.

Rare causes

Hyporeninaemic hypoaldosteronism

This is also known as type 4 renal tubular acidosis (see p. 177). Hyperkalaemia occurs because of acidosis and hypoaldosteronism.

Pseudohypoaldosteronism type 1 (autosomal recessive and dominant types)

This is a disease of infancy, apparently due to resistance to the action of aldosterone. It is characterized by hyperkalaemia and evidence of sodium wasting (hyponatraemia, extracellular volume depletion). Autosomal recessive forms result from loss of function because of mutations in the gene for epithelial sodium-channel activity (the opposite to Liddle syndrome). Pseudohypoaldosteronism type 1 involves multiple organ systems and is especially marked in the neonatal period. With aggressive salt replacement and control of hyperkalaemia, these children can survive and the disorder appears to become less severe with age. The autosomal dominant type is due to mutations affecting the mineralocorticoid receptor (see ***Fig. 9.8***). These patients present with salt wasting and hyperkalaemia but do not have other organ-system involvement.

Box 9.17 Causes of hyperkalaemia

Decreased excretion
- Acute kidney injury[a]
- Drugs:[a]
  - Amiloride
  - Triamterene
  - Spironolactone/eplerenone
  - ACE inhibitors/ACE blockers
  - NSAIDs
- Ciclosporin treatment
- Heparin treatment
- Aldosterone deficiency
- Hyporeninaemic hypoaldosteronism (RTA type 4)
- Addison's disease
- Acidosis[a]
- Gordon syndrome

Increased release from cells
(Decreased Na^+/K^+-ATPase activity)
- Acidosis
- Diabetic ketoacidosis
- Rhabdomyolysis/tissue damage
- Tumour lysis
- Succinylcholine (amplified by muscle denervation)
- Digoxin poisoning
- Vigorous exercise (α-adrenergic; transient)

Increased extraneous load
- Potassium chloride
- Salt substitutes
- Transfusion of stored blood[a]

Spurious
- Increased *in vitro* release from abnormal cells
- Leukaemia
- Infectious mononucleosis
- Thrombocytosis
- Familial pseudohyperkalaemia, e.g. haemolysis in syringe
- Increased release from muscles
- Vigorous fist clenching during phlebotomy

[a]Common causes.
ACE, angiotensin-converting enzyme; NSAIDs, non-steroidal anti-inflammatory drugs; RTA, renal tubular acidosis.

Hyperkalaemic periodic paralysis

Hyperkalaemic periodic paralysis (see p. 891) is precipitated by exercise, and is caused by an autosomal dominant mutation of the skeletal muscle sodium-channel gene.

Gordon syndrome (familial hyperkalaemic hypertension, pseudohypoaldosteronism type 2)

This appears to be a mirror image of Gitelman syndrome (see p. 166), in which primary renal retention of sodium causes hypertension, volume expansion, low renin/aldosterone, hyperkalaemia and metabolic acidosis. There is also an increased sensitivity of sodium reabsorption to thiazide diuretics, suggesting that the thiazide-sensitive sodium–chloride co-transporter (NCCT) is involved (see ***Fig 9.7***). Genetic analyses, however, have excluded abnormalities in NCCT. The involvement of two loci on chromosomes 1 and 12 and further genetic heterogeneity have also been found. These genes

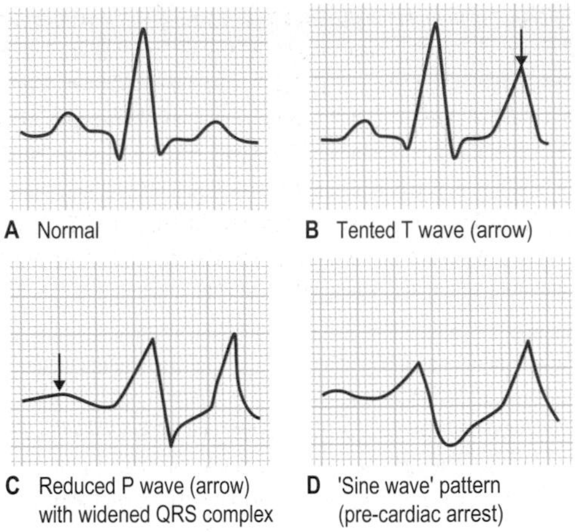

Figure 9.9 Progressive ECG changes with increasing hyperkalaemia.

do not correspond to ionic transporters but to unexpected proteins, WNK (*w*ith *no* lysine *k*inase) 1 and WNK 4, which are two closely related members of a novel serine–threonine kinase family. WNK 4 normally inhibits NCCT by preventing its membrane translocation from the cytoplasm. Loss-of-function mutation in *WNK 4* results in escape of NCCT from normal inhibition and its overactivity, as seen from the patient's phenotype. WNK 1 is an inhibitor of WNK 4 and, in some patients with Gordon syndrome, gain-of-function mutation in *WNK 1* results in functional deficiency of WNK 4 and overactivity of NCCT.

Suxamethonium and other depolarizing muscle relaxants

These cause release of potassium from cells. Induction of muscle paralysis during general anaesthesia may result in a rise of plasma potassium of up to 1 mmol/L. This is not usually a problem unless there is pre-existing hyperkalaemia.

Clinical features

Serum potassium of >7.0 mmol/L is a medical emergency and is associated with ECG changes ***(Fig. 9.9)***. Severe hyperkalaemia may be asymptomatic and may predispose to sudden death from asystolic cardiac arrest. Muscle weakness is often the only symptom, unless (as is commonly the case) the hyperkalaemia is associated with metabolic acidosis, causing Kussmaul respiration. Hyperkalaemia causes depolarization of cell membranes, leading to decreased cardiac excitability, hypotension, bradycardia and eventual asystole.

Management

Treatment for severe hyperkalaemia requires both urgent measures to save lives and maintenance therapy to keep potassium down, as summarized in ***Box 9.18***. The cause of the hyperkalaemia should be found and treated.

High potassium levels are cardiotoxic, as they inactivate sodium channels. Divalent cations, e.g. calcium, restore the voltage dependability of the channels. ***Calcium ions*** protect the cell membranes from the effects of hyperkalaemia but do not alter the potassium concentration.

Supraphysiological intravenous insulin (20 units) drives potassium into the cell and lowers plasma potassium by 1 mmol in 60 min, but must be accompanied by intravenous glucose to avoid hypoglycaemia. Regular measurements of blood glucose for at least 6 h after use of insulin should be performed and extra glucose must be available for immediate use. The use of glucose alone in non-diabetic patients, to stimulate endogenous insulin release, does not produce the high levels of insulin required and therefore is not recommended.

Intravenous or nebulized salbutamol (10–20 mg) has not yet found widespread acceptance and may cause disturbing muscle tremors at the doses required.

Correction of acidosis with hypertonic (8.4%) sodium bicarbonate causes volume expansion due to the high sodium concentration, and should only be used in emergency situations; 1.26% is used with severe acidosis (pH <6.9). Gastric aspiration will remove potassium and leads to alkalosis.

Ion-exchange resins (polystyrene sulphonate resins) are used as maintenance therapy to keep potassium down after emergency treatment. They make use of the ion fluxes that occur in the gut to remove potassium from the body and are the only way, short of dialysis, of removing potassium from the body. They may cause fluid overload (resonium contains Na^+) or hypercalcaemia (calcium resonium). Resins do not appear to enhance the excretion of potassium significantly, beyond the effect of diarrhoea induced by osmotic or secretory cathartics. Two new binders (patiromer and zirconium) selectively bind potassium in the gut. They may be more potent than traditional polystyrene sulphonate resins.

In general, all of these measures are simply ways of buying time either to correct the underlying disorder or to arrange removal of potassium by dialysis, which is the definitive treatment for hyperkalaemia in renal failure.

Box 9.18 Correction of severe hyperkalaemia

Stop all potassium supplements and drugs reducing urinary excretion of potassium.

Immediate
- ECG monitor and i.v. access

Protect myocardium
- 10 mL of 10% calcium gluconate i.v. over 5 min
- Effect is temporary but dose can be repeated after 15 min

Drive K^+ into cells
- Insulin 10 units + 50 mL of 50% glucose i.v. over 10–15 min, followed by regular checks of blood glucose and plasma K^+
- Repeat as necessary:
  - and/or correction of severe acidosis (pH <6.9) – infuse $NaHCO_3$ (1.26%)
  - and/or salbutamol 0.5 mg in 100 mL of 5% glucose over 15 min (rarely used)

Later

Deplete body K^+ (to decrease plasma K^+ over the next 24 h)
- Polystyrene sulphonate resins:
  - 15 g orally up to three times daily with laxatives
  - 30 g rectally followed 9 h later by an enema
- Haemodialysis or peritoneal dialysis if the above fails

Further reading

Bubien JK. Epithelial Na^+ channel (ENaC), hormones, and hypertension. *J Biol Chem* 2010; 285:23527–23531.

Furgeson SB, Linas S. Mechanisms of type I and type II pseudohypoaldosteronism. *J Am Soc Nephrol* 2010; 21:1842–1845.

Glover M, O'Shaughnessy KM. SPAK and WNK kinases: a new target for blood pressure treatment? *Curr Opin Nephrol Hypertens* 2011; 20:16–22.

Gumz M, Rabinowitz L, Wingo CS. An interpreted view of potassium homeostasis. *N Engl J Med* 2015; 373:60–72.

Packham DK, Rasmussen HS, Lavin PT et al. Zirconium cyclosilicate in hyperkalaemia. *N Engl J Med* 2015; 372: 222–231.

Wang WH, Yue P, Sun P et al. Regulation and function of potassium channels in aldosterone-sensitive distal nephron. *Curr Opin Nephrol Hypertens* 2010; 19:463–470.

DISORDERS OF MAGNESIUM CONCENTRATION

Magnesium (Mg^{2+}) plays a pivotal role in many biological processes such as enzymatic reactions, gene transcription, bone remodelling and neuromuscular stability. Approximately 99% of the Mg^{2+} in the body is in the intracellular compartment, mainly in bone (approximately 85%) and in muscle and soft tissues (approximately 14%). The other 1% is in the extracellular fluid.

Plasma magnesium levels are normally maintained within the range 0.7–1.1 mmol/L (1.4–2.2 mEq/L). The average daily magnesium intake is 15 mmol, which is absorbed mainly in the small intestine and, to a lesser extent, in the colon. In the healthy adult, there is no net gain or loss of magnesium from bone, so that balance is achieved by the urinary excretion of the net magnesium absorbed. The kidney reabsorbs between approximately 95% and 98% of the filtered Mg^{2+} and plays a major role in maintaining plasma Mg^{2+} concentrations within the normal range.

Control and renal handling of magnesium

Cortical thick ascending limb of Henle

Approximately 30% of Mg^{2+} is bound to plasma proteins but the remaining fraction is freely filterable. The major site of magnesium transport is the cortical thick ascending limb (cTAL) of the loop of Henle, where 65–70% of the filtered load is reabsorbed, with only 10–20% being reabsorbed in the proximal tubule (see ***Fig. 9.6***). This transport is passive, paracellular and carried out by tight junction proteins (paracellin-1 and claudins). This process is driven by the lumen-positive electrochemical gradient, characteristic of this segment. This voltage gradient is created by the apical disproportionate net transport of two Cl^- to one Na^+ (by the bumetanide-sensitive sodium–potassium-2–chloride transporter) and the secretion of K^+ (via the ROMK) (see ***Fig. 9.6***). Loss-of-function mutations in these key reabsorptive processes lead to hypomagnesaemia as part of the distinctive clinical syndromes described below.

Bartter syndrome

Hypomagnesaemia is rare in Bartter syndrome (see p. 166). This is because the transepithelial voltage, which is responsible for magnesium reabsorption, is preserved and any additional filtered magnesium will be offset by a compensatory increase in absorption in the distal convoluted tubule.

Familial hypomagnesaemia, hypercalciuria and nephrocalcinosis

Familial hypomagnesaemia, hypercalciuria and nephrocalcinosis (FHHNC) is characterized by excessive renal magnesium and calcium wasting; the main defect lies in cTAL. Ten different mutations have been identified in a novel gene that encodes for paracellin-1 and claudins 16/19 complex, in the tight junction proteins (see p. 94).

Individuals develop bilateral nephrocalcinosis and progressive CKD. Patients also have elevated parathyroid hormone levels, which precedes any reduction in GFR. A substantial proportion of patients show incomplete distal renal tubular acidosis, hypocitraturia and hyperuricaemia. Extrarenal involvement, such as myopia, nystagmus and chorioretinitis, has been reported.

Distal convoluted tubule

The reabsorption rate in the distal convoluted tubule (DCT) – 10% – is much lower than in the cTAL, but it defines the final urinary excretion, as there is no significant reabsorption in the collecting duct; 3–5% of filtered magnesium is finally excreted in the urine. Magnesium reabsorption in the DCT is transcellular and active (see ***Fig. 9.7***). The DCT has a slight lumen-negative voltage of approximately −5 mV. The luminal Mg^{2+} concentration in the DCT ranges between 0.2 and 0.7 mmol/L, whereas the intracellular concentration of Mg^{2+} is estimated to be maintained at around 0.2–1.0 mmol/L. Therefore the voltage difference across the apical membrane plays a key role in Mg^{2+} transport within the DCT.

Magnesiotropic proteins

These include the following:

- ***TRPM6***, the *t*ransient *r*eceptor *p*otential channel *m*elastatin member 6, is an Mg^{2+}-permeable channel that is also expressed in the luminal membrane of the intestinal epithelium. Inactivating mutations of TRPM6 (a rare autosomal recessive disease) thus cause a combination of impaired gut absorption of Mg^{2+} and renal wasting known as ***hypomagnesaemia with secondary hypocalcaemia*** (HSH). Clinically, patients have disturbed neuromuscular excitability, muscle spasms, tetany and generalized convulsions. Severe hypomagnesaemia (0.1–0.4 mmol/L) is seen due to impaired intestinal Mg^{2+} absorption and renal reabsorption.
- ***The pro-epidermal growth factor (EGF)*** resides on the basolateral surface of the DCT cells. It markedly stimulates the activity of TRPM6. Loss-of-function mutation results in an autosomal recessive form of ***isolated renal hypomagnesaemia*** (IRH). IRH presents with hypomagnesaemia (0.53–0.66 mmol/L) and an inappropriately high fractional excretion of Mg^{2+} with epileptic seizures and moderate mental retardation. In contrast to HSH, Ca^{2+} handling is not affected in IRH patients. Cancer therapies that inhibit EGF also cause hypomagnesaemia by the above mechanism.
- ***Thiazide-sensitive Na^+–Cl^+ co-transporter in the DCT*** plays a role in sodium and chloride absorption and maintenance of lumen-negative voltage. Loss-of-function mutation in this co-transporter results in ***Gitelman syndrome*** (see p. 166 and ***Fig. 9.7***). Hypomagnesaemia is likely to be due to a reduced abundance of TRPM6. The observed hypocalciuria is caused by an increased proximal tubular reabsorption, a process that occurs in response to the mild volume depletion.
- ***The γ-subunit of the Na^+/K^+-ATPase*** on the basolateral aspect of the DCT plays a pivotal role in the sodium and chloride absorption and maintenance of lumen-negative voltage (a key requirement for magnesium absorption) in this segment of the nephron. A loss-of-function mutation in the *FXYD2* gene (transcription factor for the gamma chain of Na^+/K^+-ATPase) causes ***isolated dominant hypomagnesaemia***. The affected individuals present with renal Mg^{2+} wasting, accompanied by hypocalciuria.
- ***The HNF1b gene*** encodes a transcription factor linked to the regulation of the *FXYD2* gene. Defects in the *HNF1b* gene have been implicated in genetic defects of β-cell function (see ***Box 27.4***). Interestingly, almost half of the carriers of a mutation in the *HNF1b* gene display hypomagnesaemia (<0.65 mmol/L) due to renal wasting of Mg^{2+}. As in patients with *FXYD2* mutations, hypocalciuria is present.
- ***ATP-sensitive inward rectifier potassium channel 10 (Kir4.1)*** is present on the basolateral surface of the DCT. It allows K^+ ions to recycle across the basolateral membrane, thereby maintaining an adequate supply of K^+ to sustain the

high Na^+/K^+-ATPase activity observed in this segment. Loss of its function has been linked to the hypomagnesaemic (EAST) syndrome, in which the impaired electrogenic Na^+/K^+-ATPase transport causes depolarization of the apical membrane and reduces inward transport of Mg^{2+} via TRPM6. Patients have epilepsy, ataxia, sensorineural deafness (Kir 4.1 is present in the inner ear), and tubulopathy (of a Gitelman-like phenotype).

Hypomagnesaemia

In addition to the familial causes described above, hypomagnesaemia most often develops as a result of deficient intake, defective gut absorption, or excessive gut or urinary loss **(Box 9.19)**. It can also occur with acute pancreatitis, possibly owing to the formation of magnesium soaps in the areas of fat necrosis and drug treatment with aminoglycosides and cisplatinum compounds. The serum magnesium is usually <0.7 mmol/L (1.4 mEq/L). Due to the severe effects of hypomagnesaemia, routine measurements of serum Mg^{2+} should be conducted in the critically ill, as well as in patients who are exposed to drugs and other conditions associated with Mg^{2+} deficiency.

Clinical features

Symptoms and signs (indicating a deficit of 0.5–1 mmol/kg) include irritability, tremor, ataxia, carpopedal spasm, hyper-reflexia, confusional and hallucinatory states, and epileptiform convulsions. An ECG may show a prolonged QT interval, broad flattened T waves and occasional shortening of the ST segment.

Management

This involves the withdrawal of precipitating agents such as diuretics or purgatives. If symptomatic (or with hypocalcaemia), give a parenteral infusion of 50 mmol of magnesium chloride in 1 L of 5% glucose or other isotonic fluid over 12–24 h. This should be repeated daily and continued for 2 days after normal plasma levels have been achieved.

Box 9.19 Causes of hypomagnesaemia

Decreased magnesium absorption
- Malabsorption (severe)
- Malnutrition
- Alcohol excess
- Hypomagnesaemia with secondary hypocalcaemia (see p. 1239)

Increased renal excretion
- Drugs:
  - Loop diuretics
  - Thiazide diuretics
  - Digoxin
  - Proton pump inhibitors
- Diabetic ketoacidosis
- Hyperaldosteronism
- SIADH
- Alcohol excess
- Hypercalciuria
- 1,25-(OH)-vitamin D_3 deficiency
- Drug toxicity:
  - Amphotericin
  - Aminoglycosides
  - Cisplatin
  - Ciclosporin

Gut losses
- Prolonged nasogastric suction
- Excessive purgation
- Gastrointestinal/biliary fistulae
- Severe diarrhoea

Inherited tubular wasting
- Bartter syndrome
- Familial hypomagnesaemia, hypercalciuria and nephrocalcinosis
- Isolated dominant hypomagnesaemia
- Gitelman syndrome (see p. 166)
- Isolated recessive hypomagnesaemia
- Hypomagnesaemia with secondary hypocalcaemia (HSH)
- EAST syndrome

Miscellaneous
- Acute pancreatitis

EAST, epilepsy, ataxia, sensorineural deafness and tubulopathy; SIADH, syndrome of inappropriate antidiuretic hormone secretion.

Relationship between hypomagnesaemia and plasma calcium

Calcium deficiency usually, but not always, develops with hypomagnesaemia. Hypomagnesaemia can be further subdivided into three main groups:

- ***Hypercalciuria*** with hypomagnesaemia. This occurs from defects in Mg^{2+} absorption in cTAL, such as in several forms of Bartter syndrome, loop diuretic administration and FHHNC.
- ***Normocalciuria***. This includes autosomal dominant hypomagnesaemia due to mutations in Kv1.1, and IRH due to mutations in the *EGF* gene.
- ***Hypocalciuria with hypomagnesaemia***. This is a hallmark feature of thiazide diuretic use and Gitelman syndrome, and has also been reported in the EAST syndrome, due to mutations in *NCC* and *Kir4.1*, respectively. Genetic defects of β-cell function and isolated dominant hypomagnesaemia (IDH) caused by mutations in *HNF1b* (see p. 169) and *FXYD2* also lead to hypomagnesaemia with accompanying hypocalciuria.

Relationship between hypomagnesaemia and plasma potassium

Magnesium depletion can lead to refractory hypokalaemia. The intracellular magnesium blocks secretory K^+ currents through ROMK channels; therefore, magnesium depletion promotes K^+ loss. Furthermore, this magnesium-mediated inhibition of K^+ secretion increases as extracellular K^+ decreases, which appropriately reduces K^+ loss in the presence of K^+ deficiency. Close monitoring, with potassium supplements if necessary, is required in patients presenting with primary symptomatic low plasma magnesium levels.

Hypermagnesaemia

This primarily occurs in patients with acute or chronic kidney disease given magnesium-containing laxatives or antacids. It can also be induced by magnesium-containing enemas. Mild hypermagnesaemia may occur in patients with adrenal insufficiency. Causes are given in **Box 9.20**.

Clinical features

Symptoms and signs relate to neurological and cardiovascular depression, and include weakness with hyporeflexia proceeding to narcosis, respiratory paralysis and cardiac conduction defects. Symptoms usually develop when the plasma magnesium level exceeds 2 mmol/L (4 mEq/L).

Management

Treatment requires withdrawal of any magnesium therapy. An intravenous injection of 10 mL of calcium gluconate 10% (2.25 mmol

Box 9.20 Causes of hypermagnesaemia

- Impaired renal excretion:
  - Chronic kidney disease
  - Acute kidney injury
- Increased magnesium intake:
  - Purgatives, e.g. magnesium sulphate
  - Antacids, e.g. magnesium trisilicate
- Haemodialysis with high $[Mg^{2+}]$ dialysate

calcium) is given to antagonize the effects of hypermagnesaemia, along with glucose and insulin (as for hyperkalaemia; see p. 168) to lower the plasma magnesium level. Dialysis may be required in patients with severe kidney disease.

Further reading

Ayuk J, Gittoes NJ. Contemporary view of the clinical relevance of magnesium homeostasis. *Ann Clin Biochem* 2014; 51(Pt 2):179–188.

San-Cristobal P, Dimke H, Hoenderop JG et al. Novel molecular pathways in renal Mg2+ transport: a guided tour along the nephron. *Curr Opin Nephrol Hypertens* 2010; 19:456–462.

Yang L, Frindt G, Palmer LG. Magnesium modulates ROMK channel-mediated potassium secretion. *J Am Soc Nephrol* 2010; 21:2109–2116.

DISORDERS OF PHOSPHATE CONCENTRATION

Phosphate forms an essential part of most biochemical systems. The regulation of plasma phosphate level is both direct and closely linked to calcium.

About 85% of all body phosphorus is within bone, plasma phosphate normally ranging from 0.80 to 1.15 mmol/L (2.5–3.6 mg/dL) and accounts for only 1% of the total body phosphate. However, plasma phosphate levels correlate in most circumstances with total body sodium. Phosphate reabsorption from the glomerular filtrate occurs entirely and actively in the renal proximal tubule and is hormonally regulated. It is decreased by parathyroid hormone (PTH), mediated by a cyclic adenosine monophosphate (cAMP)-dependent mechanism; thus primary hyperparathyroidism is associated with low plasma levels of serum phosphate. Other factors that are known to control phosphate reabsorption in the proximal tubule are 1,25-dihydroxyvitamin D_3, sodium delivery to the proximal tubule, serum concentrations of calcium, bicarbonate, carbon dioxide tension, glucose, alanine, serotonin, dopamine and sympathetic activity.

Osteoblast-secreted phosphaturic factors (phosphatonins), such as fibroblast growth factor 23 (FGF23), matrix extracellular phosphoglycoprotein (MEPG) and frizzled-related protein 4 (FRP-4), play a role in phosphate homeostasis. FGF23 is the most extensively investigated phosphatonin. It binds to its receptor, FGFR1, in the kidney and causes phosphaturia; it also regulates vitamin D by inactivation of 1α-hydroxylase (CYP27B1) and upregulation of 24 hydroxylase (CYP24A1) enzymes, with the net result of low 1,25-vitamin D synthesis. Serum FGF23 is also the earliest marker of abnormal phosphate handling in CKD patients, occurring before changes in serum phosphate, calcium or PTH ***(Fig. 9.10)***. Moreover, FGF23 requires Klotho (see p. 165) to act as a co-receptor with FGFR1 for its activity. Loss-of-function mutation in either FGF23 or Klotho results in a similar phenotype of shortened lifespan, premature ageing (see p. 109) and hyperphosphataemia, and, as expected from the mode of action, increases 1,25 vitamin D levels. Klotho can also inhibit phosphate absorption directly in the absence of FGF23 or PTH.

Phosphate absorption is an active process carried out by a family of sodium–phosphate co-transporters (NPT) in the gut and kidneys. NPT2a and NPT2c are expressed in the brush border of the renal proximal tubule whilst NPT2b is expressed in lungs and intestine. NPT2a plays a central role in the renal reabsorption of phosphate but essentially requires a companion protein called sodium hydrogen exchanger regulatory factor 1 (NHERF1) for membrane sorting. Intestinal absorption is carried out by NPT2b but its mutation does not cause any alteration in serum phosphate due to compensation by the renal expression of NPT2a and possibly NPT2c. Under normal circumstances, plasma phosphate levels are kept constant; for example, after a phosphate-rich meal, the bone releases FGF23, which inhibits NPT2a and causes phosphate excretion. Moreover, phosphate in the plasma causes the release of PTH, either directly or indirectly by lowering ionized calcium. PTH also inhibits NPT2a, NPT2C and NHERF1, resulting in phosphaturia ***(Fig. 9.10)***. These two principal mechanisms keep plasma phosphate levels within normal limits on a daily basis.

Hypophosphataemia

Significant hypophosphataemia (<0.4 mmol/L or <1.25 mg/dL) occurs in a number of clinical situations, owing to redistribution into cells, renal losses or decreased intake ***(Box 9.21)***.

Clinical features include:

- muscle weakness, e.g. diaphragmatic weakness, decreased cardiac contractility, skeletal muscle rhabdomyolysis
- a left shift in the oxyhaemoglobin dissociation curve (reduced 2,3-bisphosphoglycerate, 2,3-BPG) and rarely haemolysis
- confusion, hallucinations and convulsions.

Mild hypophosphataemia often resolves without specific treatment. However, diaphragmatic weakness may be severe in acute hypophosphataemia, and may impede the weaning of a patient from a ventilator. Interestingly, chronic hypophosphataemia (in X-linked hypophosphataemia) is associated with normal muscle power.

Aetiology

Primary hyperparathyroidism is a common cause of hypophosphataemia. Very rarely, gain-of-function mutations of the PTH1 receptor cause hypophosphataemia and Jansen's metaphyseal chondrodysplasia due to constitutive activation of PTH signalling, even in the presence of low or absent circulating PTH levels.

Hypophosphataemia can be part of osteomalacia and rickets due to vitamin D deficiency, either dietary (globally, the most

? Box 9.21 Causes of hypophosphataemia

Redistribution
- Respiratory alkalosis
- Treatment of diabetic ketoacidosis (insulin drives phosphate into cells)
- Refeeding (particularly with carbohydrate) after fasting or starvation
- After parathyroidectomy (hungry bone disease)

Decreased intake/absorption
- Diet
- Malabsorption
- Vomiting
- Gut phosphate binders, e.g. sevelamer
- Vitamin D deficiency
- Alcohol withdrawal

Renal losses
- Hyperparathyroidism
- Renal tubular defects
- Diuretics
- Tenofovir treatment

Hypophosphataemic rickets
- Vitamin D-dependent rickets types I and II
- Tumour-induced
- Autosomal dominant and recessive
- X-linked dominant
- Dent's disease

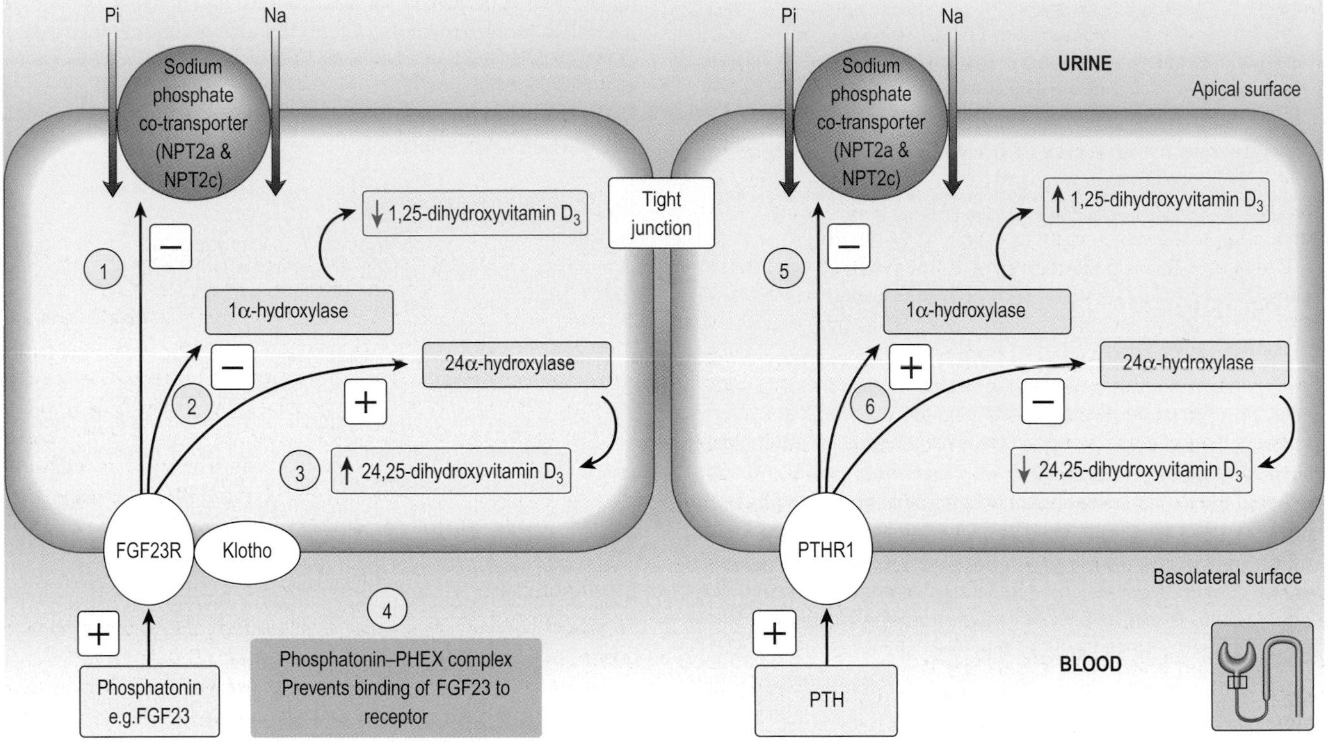

Figure 9.10 ***PHEX*** **and PTH regulation of phosphate transport and vitamin D metabolism in the proximal tubule.**
(1) **Fibroblast growth factor 23 (FGF23)** inhibits the sodium–phosphate co-transporter (NPT2a, c), causing phosphaturia.
(2) **Binding of FGF23 to the FGFR1–Klotho complex** leads to lower levels of the active form of vitamin D (1,25-vitamin D) by inhibiting 1α-hydroxylase.
(3) It also increases levels of inactive **vitamin D** (24,25-vitamin D) by stimulating 24α-hydroxylase.
(4) ***PHEX*** (**phosphate-regulating gene with homologies to endopeptidase on the X chromosome**) acts as a competitive inhibitor, binding FGF23 and blocking its action.
(5) **Parathyroid hormone (PTH)** also inhibits NPT2a, which leads to phosphaturia.
(6) **PTH has opposite effects on vitamin D metabolism** compared with FGF23 by stimulating 1α-hydroxylase and inhibiting 24α-hydroxylase.

common cause) or genetic, and is usually accompanied by hypocalcaemia (calcipenic) and secondary hyperparathyroidism.

Vitamin D-dependent rickets type I

Also known as ***pseudo-vitamin D-deficient rickets***, this is caused by 1α-hydroxylase deficiency due to inactivating mutations in its gene. This condition manifests clinically in the first year of life with severe hypocalcaemia, often complicated by tetany, moderate hypophosphataemia and enamel hypoplasia. The characteristic biochemical findings are normal serum levels of 25-hydroxyvitamin D, low values of 1,25-dihydroxyvitamin D and, usually, relatively high PTH levels. The treatment of choice is replacement therapy with calcitriol.

Vitamin D-dependent rickets type II

This is a form of vitamin D resistance and is known as ***hereditary vitamin D-resistant rickets***. It is an autosomal recessive disorder and is usually caused by loss-of-function mutations in the gene encoding the vitamin D receptor. The clinical manifestations vary widely, depending upon the type of mutation within the vitamin D receptor and the amount of residual vitamin D receptor activity. Affected children usually develop rickets within the first 2 years of life, with alopecia in two-thirds of cases, which is due to lack of vitamin D receptor action within keratinocytes. The treatment involves a therapeutic trial of calcitriol and calcium supplementation. Long-term infusion of calcium into a central vein is a possible alternative for severely resistant patients. Oral calcium therapy may be sufficient once radiographic healing has been observed.

Decreased renal reabsorption of phosphate

Excessive phosphatonins (FGF23)

This condition also occurs in patients with ***tumour-induced osteomalacia*** (TIO), ***X-linked dominant hypophosphataemic rickets*** (XLR) and ***autosomal dominant hypophosphataemic rickets*** (ADHR). These syndromes have similar biochemical and osseous phenotypes. Patients have osteomalacia or rickets, reduced tubular phosphate reabsorption, hypophosphataemia, normal or low serum calcium, normal PTH and PTH-related protein concentrations, and normal or low 1,25-dihydroxyvitamin D_3. Urinary cAMP levels are generally in the normal range.

In ***TIO***, there is excessive production of phosphaturic agents (which are normally produced by osteoblasts and function as hormones by acting on kidneys and regulating phosphate absorption and vitamin D activation): for example, FGF23, MEPG and FRP-4. These are resistant to degradation by *PHEX* (phosphate-regulating gene with homologies to endopeptidases on the X chromosome). The result is excess inhibition of the sodium–phosphate co-transporter in the proximal tubule and phosphaturia.

In ***ADHR***, FGF23 is mutated so that it is resistant to PHEX proteolysis. In XLR, mutations in PHEX prevent binding to FGF23 and FRP-4, resulting in a net relative excess of phosphatonins.

Normal adaptive increases in 1,25-dihydroxyvitamin D_3 synthesis in response to low phosphate levels do not occur in TIO, ADHR and XLR, aggravating phosphaturia ***(Fig. 9.10)***.

Autosomal recessive hypophosphataemia with high FGF23 levels has been described in patients with mutations in the gene encoding dentin matrix protein 1 (*DMP1*), which is a transcription factor produced by odontoblasts, osteoblasts and osteocytes. It is also secreted and can modulate the formation of mineralized matrix.

Reduced NPT2a/NHERF1 activity

Mutations in NPT2a (sodium–phosphate co-transporter 2a) and NHERF1 (sodium hydrogen regulator factor 1) have been identified in patients with low phosphate levels and a reduced ratio of the maximum tubular reabsorption of phosphate (TmP) normalized for GFR (TmP/GFR ratio). Heterozygous loss-of-function mutation in NPT2a and NHERF1 in patients is characterized by hypophosphataemia, low TmP/GFR and normal PTH. Carriers of these mutations do not have hypercalcaemia, which means these mutations do not affect the action of PTH on bones.

Dent's disease

Dent's disease is the generally accepted name for a group of hereditary tubular disorders, including X-linked recessive nephrolithiasis with chronic renal disease, X-linked recessive hypophosphataemic rickets, and idiopathic low-molecular-weight proteinuria. It is characterized by low-molecular-weight proteinuria, hypercalciuria, hyperphosphaturia, nephrocalcinosis, kidney stones and eventual renal failure, with some patients developing rickets or osteomalacia.

Dent's disease is caused, in 60% of cases, by loss-of-function mutation of a proximal tubular endosomal chloride channel, CLC5. Mutations in OCRL1 occur in 15% of cases. This chloride channel, along with the proton pump, is essential for acidification of proximal tubular endosomes. The process is linked with normal endocytosis, degradation and recycling of absorbed proteins, vitamins and hormones. Defective endosomal acidification (owing to the mutated *CLC5* gene) results in impaired endosomal degradation and recycling of endocytosed hormones such as PTH with the clinical phenotype of hyperparathyroidism. Moreover, the receptors (megalin and cubilin) for reabsorption of low-molecular-weight proteins and albumin in the proximal tubules are decreased in Dent's disease. This explains the low-molecular-weight proteinuria and excessive urinary leaks of cytokines, hormones and chemokines. This urinary profile is associated with progressive renal fibrosis and more rapid decline in renal function.

Box 9.22 Causes of hyperphosphataemia

- Acute kidney injury
- Chronic kidney disease
- Phosphate-containing enemas
- Hyperparathyroidism/pseudohyperparathyroidism
- Tumour lysis
- Rhabdomyolysis
- Familial tumoral calcinosis

Diagnosis

Patients with hypophosphataemia should have their urinary fractional excretion of phosphate measured. A value of <0.7 mmol/L indicates renal phosphate wasting. If PTH levels are high, then the patient is very likely to have hyperparathyroidism, either primary or secondary to vitamin D deficiency (acquired or genetic) or Dent's disease. If PTH levels are low, then the only possibility is gain-of-function mutation in PTH1R. If PTH levels are normal, then assess FGF23 levels. High FGF23 serum levels will indicate possible mutated genes in FGF23/Klotho, PHEX and DMP1. Normal FGF23 and PTH levels point to mutations in NPT2a, NPT2c and NHERF1.

Management

Oral phosphate supplementation and calcitriol (1,25-dihydroxyvitamin D) administration is required if there is vitamin D deficiency.

Treatment of ***acute hypophosphataemia*** is with intravenous phosphate at a maximum rate of 9 mmol every 12 hours. Repeated measurements of calcium and phosphate are required, as over-rapid administration of phosphate may lead to severe hypocalcaemia, particularly in the presence of alkalosis. ***Chronic hypophosphataemia*** can be corrected with oral effervescent sodium phosphate.

Hyperphosphataemia

Hyperphosphataemia is common in patients with CKD (see p. 779 and ***Box 9.22***). Hyperphosphataemia is usually asymptomatic but may result in precipitation of calcium phosphate, particularly in the presence of a normal or raised calcium level or of alkalosis. Uraemic itching may be caused by a raised calcium phosphate product. Prolonged hyperphosphataemia causes hyperparathyroidism and periarticular and vascular calcification.

Familial tumoral calcinosis is characterized by calcifications of muscles, skin, eyelids and vessels, as well as hyperostosis. Absence of glycosylation of FGF23 makes it unstable and more sensitive to proteolysis. This results in its deficiency and hyperphosphataemia due to increased renal phosphate reabsorption through increased NPT2a activity.

Usually, no treatment is required for acute hyperphosphataemia, as the causes are self-limiting. Treatment of chronic hyperphosphataemia is with gut phosphate binders and dialysis (see p. 780).

Further reading

Markadieu N, Bindels RJ, Hoenderop JG. The renal connecting tubule: resolved and unresolved issues in Ca(2+) transport. *Intl J Biochem Cell Biol* 2011; 43:1–4.

Nanes MS. Phosphate wasting and fibroblast growth factor 23. *Curr Opin Endocrinol Diabetes Obes* 2013; 20:523–531.

Scialla JJ, Wolf M. Roles of phosphate and fibroblast growth factor 23 in cardiovascular disease. *Nat Rev Nephrol* 2014; 10:268–278.

Tiosano D, Hochberg Z. Hypophosphatemia: the common denominator of all rickets. *J Bone Miner Metab* 2009; 27:392–401.

Wagner CA, Rubio-Aliaga I, Biber J et al. Genetic diseases of renal phosphate handing. *Nephrol Dial Transplant* 2014; 29(Suppl 4):iv45–54.

ACID–BASE DISORDERS

The concentration of hydrogen ions in both extracellular and intracellular compartments is extremely tightly controlled, and very small changes lead to major cell dysfunction. The blood pH is tightly regulated and is normally maintained at between 7.38 and 7.42. Any deviation from this range indicates a change in the hydrogen ion concentration $[H^+]$ because blood pH is the negative logarithm of $[H^+]$ ***(Box 9.23)***. The $[H^+]$ at a physiological blood pH of 7.40 is 40 nmol/L. An increase in the $[H^+]$ (a fall in pH) is termed acidaemia. A decrease in $[H^+]$ (a rise in the blood pH) is termed alkalaemia. The disorders that cause these changes in the blood pH are acidosis and alkalosis, respectively.

Normal acid–base physiology

The normal adult diet contains 70–100 mmol of acid (H^+). Throughout the body there are buffers that minimize any changes in blood pH that these ingested hydrogen ions might cause. Such buffers include intracellular proteins (e.g. haemoglobin) and tissue components (e.g. the calcium carbonate and calcium phosphate in bone), as well as the bicarbonate–carbonic acid buffer pair generated by the hydration of carbon dioxide. This buffer pair is clinically most relevant, in part because its contribution can be measured and because alterations in this buffer pair reveal changes in all other buffer systems. Bicarbonate ions $[HCO_3^-]$ and carbonic acid (H_2CO_3) exist in equilibrium; and in the presence of carbonic anhydrase, carbonic acid dissociates to carbon dioxide and water, as expressed in the following equation:

$$H^+HCO_3^- \rightleftarrows H_2CO_2 \xrightleftharpoons{\text{carbonic anhydrase}} CO_2 + H_2O.$$

The addition of hydrogen ions drives the reaction to the right, decreasing the plasma bicarbonate concentration $[HCO_3^-]$ and increasing the arterial carbon dioxide pressure (P_aCO_2). As shown in the following **Henderson–Hasselbalch equation**, a fall in the plasma $[HCO_3^-]$ increases $[H^+]$ and thus lowers blood pH:

$$[H^+] = 181 \times P_aCO_2[HCO_3^-]$$

where $[H^+]$ is expressed in nmol/L, P_aCO_2 in kilopascals, $[HCO_3^-]$ in mmol/L and 181 is the dissociation coefficient of carbonic acid. Alternatively the equation can be expressed as:

$$pH = pK + \log[HCO_3^-]/[H_2CO_3]$$

where pK=6.1. Thus, the bicarbonate used in the buffering process must be regenerated to maintain normal acid–base balance.

Although the acidaemia stimulates an increase in ventilation, which blunts this change in pH, increased ventilation does not regenerate the bicarbonate used in the buffering process. Consequently, the kidney must excrete hydrogen ions to return the plasma $[HCO_3^-]$ to normal. Maintenance of a normal plasma $[HCO_3^-]$ under physiological conditions depends not only on daily regeneration of bicarbonate but also on reabsorption of all bicarbonate filtered across the glomerular capillaries.

Box 9.23 Relationship between [H+] and pH

pH	$[H^+]$ (nmol/L)
6.9	126
7.0	100
7.1	79
7.2	63
7.3	50
7.4	40
7.5	32
7.6	25

Renal reabsorption of bicarbonate

The plasma $[HCO_3^-]$ is normally maintained at approximately 25 mmol/L. In individuals with a normal GFR (120 mL/min), about 4500 mmol of bicarbonate is filtered each day. If this filtered bicarbonate were not reabsorbed, the plasma $[HCO_3^-]$ would fall, along with blood pH. Thus, maintenance of normal plasma $[HCO_3^-]$ requires that essentially all of the bicarbonate in the glomerular filtrate be reabsorbed ***(Fig. 9.11)***.

The proximal convoluted tubule reclaims 85–90% of filtered bicarbonate; by contrast, the distal nephron reclaims very little. This difference is caused by the greater quantity of luminal (brush border) carbonic anhydrase in the proximal tubule than in the distal nephron. As a result of these quantitative differences, bicarbonate that escapes reabsorption in the proximal tubule is excreted in the urine.

Proximal tubular bicarbonate reabsorption is catalysed by the Na^+/K^+-ATPase pump located in the basolateral cell membrane. By exchanging peritubular potassium ions for intracellular sodium ions, the pump keeps the intracellular sodium concentration low, allowing sodium ions to enter the cell by moving down the sodium concentration gradient from the tubule lumen to the cell interior. Hydrogen ions are transported in the opposite direction (at the Na^+–H^+ antiporter), thereby maintaining electroneutrality. Before bicarbonate enters the proximal tubule, it combines with secreted

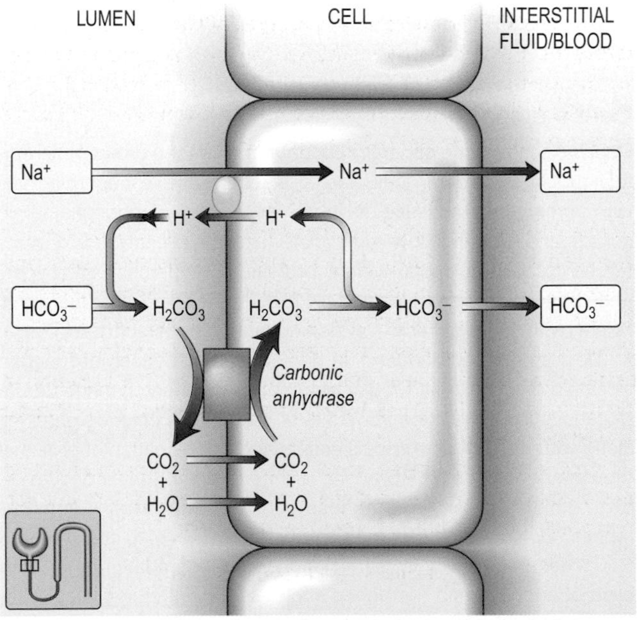

Figure 9.11 Resorption of sodium bicarbonate in the renal (mainly proximal) tubule. Bicarbonate is reclaimed by the secretion of H^+ in exchange for Na^+ into the tubule. This results in the formation of H_2CO_3, which is then broken down to CO_2. This is reabsorbed and converted back to H_2CO_3, which now dissociates into H^+ and HCO_3^-. The net result is reabsorption of Na^+ and HCO_3^-. This process is dependent on carbonic anhydrase within the cells and on the luminal surface of the tubular cell.

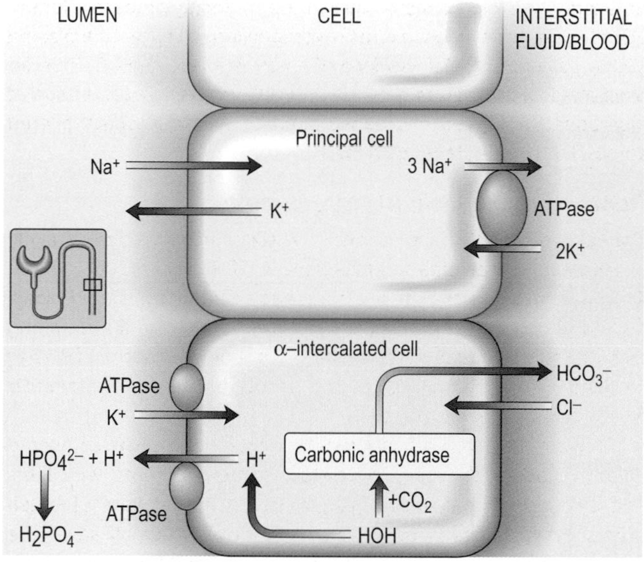

Figure 9.12 Renal excretion of H^+. H^+ excretion is indirectly controlled by aldosterone in the cortical collecting ducts. Aldosterone enhances sodium absorption and potassium excretion by opening sodium channels and enhancing the activity of the Na^+/K^+-ATPase in the principal cell. These actions set up an electrochemical gradient favouring H^+ excretion. Aldosterone also facilitates H^+ excretion by stimulating H^+-ATPase in the intercalated cell.

hydrogen ions, forming carbonic acid. In the presence of luminal carbonic anhydrase (CA-IV), carbonic acid rapidly dissociates into carbon dioxide and water, which can then rapidly enter the proximal tubular cell. In the cell, carbon dioxide is hydrated by cytosolic carbonic anhydrase (CA-II), ultimately forming bicarbonate, which is then transported down an electrical gradient from the cell interior, across the membrane into the peritubular fluid, and into the blood. In this process, each hydrogen ion secreted into the proximal tubule lumen is reabsorbed and can be resecreted; there is no net loss of hydrogen ions or net gain of bicarbonate ions.

Renal excretion of [H^+] *(Fig. 9.12)*

More acid is secreted into the proximal tubule (up to 4500 nmol of hydrogen ions each day) than in any other nephron segment. However, the hydrogen ions secreted into the proximal tubule are almost completely reabsorbed with bicarbonate; consequently, proximal tubular hydrogen ion secretion does not contribute significantly to hydrogen ion elimination from the body. The excretion of the daily acid load requires hydrogen ion secretion in more distal nephron segments.

Most dietary hydrogen ions come from sulphur-containing amino acids that are metabolized to sulphuric acid (H_2SO_4), which then reacts with sodium bicarbonate as follows:

$$H_2SO_4 + 2NaHCO_3 \rightarrow Na_2SO_4 + 2CO_2 + 2H_2O.$$

Excess sulphate is excreted in the urine, whereas excess hydrogen ions are buffered by bicarbonate and lower the plasma [HCO_3^-]. This fall in plasma [HCO_3^-] leads to a slight decrease in the blood pH, although a smaller decrease in the blood pH than would have occurred if buffer were unavailable. The subsequent excretion of hydrogen ions takes place primarily in the collecting duct and results in the regeneration of 1 mmol of bicarbonate for every mmol of hydrogen ions excreted in the urine.

The **collecting duct** has three types of cells:

- The ***principal cell*** with an aldosterone-sensitive Na^+ absorption site. These cells reabsorb Na^+ and H_2O and secrete K^+ under the influence of aldosterone.
- The ***α-intercalated cell***, which possesses the proton pump for the active secretion of hydrogen ions in exchange for reabsorption of K^+ ions. Aldosterone increases H^+ ion secretion.
- The ***β-intercalated cells*** are mirror images of α-intercalated cells. Here the H^+-ATPase pump is located in the basolateral rather than the apical membrane, whereby H^+ ions are secreted into the peritubular capillary. The HCO_3^- ions, on the other hand, are secreted into the tubular lumen by an anion exchanger in the apical membrane. The identity of this transporter is uncertain, however, as it does not appear to represent the same Cl^--HCO_3^- exchanger that is present in the basolateral membrane of the H^+-secreting intercalated cells.

Secretion of hydrogen ions from the cortical collecting duct is indirectly linked to sodium reabsorption.

- Aldosterone has several facilitating effects on hydrogen ion secretion. Aldosterone opens sodium channels in the luminal membrane of the ***principal cell*** and increases Na^+/K^+-ATPase activity. The subsequent movement of cationic sodium into the principal cell creates a negative charge within the tubule lumen. Potassium ions from the principal cells and hydrogen ions from the α-intercalated cells move out from the cells down the electrochemical gradient and into the lumen.
- Aldosterone also stimulates directly the H^+-ATPase in the α-intercalated cell, further enhancing hydrogen ion secretion. The H^+ to be secreted arises from the reassociation of H_2O and CO_2 in the presence of carbonic anhydrase; thus, a bicarbonate molecule is regenerated each time an H^+ is eliminated in the urine.

When hydrogen ions are secreted into the lumen of the collecting tubule, a tiny, but physiologically critical, fraction of these excess hydrogen ions remains in solution. Here, they increase the urinary [H^+] and lower urinary pH below 4.0. Nevertheless, below this urine pH, inhibition of proton-secreting pumps, such as H^+-ATPase, severely restricts kidney secretion of more hydrogen ions. Consequently, secretion of hydrogen ions depends on the presence of buffers in the urine that maintain the urine pH at a level higher than 4.0.

In the presence of alkali excess, the homeostatic needs are reversed. Although the kidney can excrete excess alkaline load by reducing reabsorption of filtered bicarbonate in the proximal and distal tubule, the collecting ducts also contribute by secreting bicarbonate brought about by switching to β-intercalated cells. This switch enables kidneys to secrete bicarbonate and conserve H^+ ions.

Buffer systems in acid excretion

Two buffer systems are involved in acid excretion: the titratable acids, such as phosphate, and the ammonia system. Each system is responsible for excreting about half of the daily acid load of 50–100 mmol under physiological conditions *(Fig. 9.12)*.

Titratable acid

A titratable acid is a filtered buffer substance having a conjugate anion that can be titrated within the pH range occurring physiologically in the urine. Phosphoric acid (pK_a 6.8) is the usual titratable urinary buffer. Hydrogen ions bind to the conjugate anions of the titratable acids and are excreted in the urine. For each hydrogen

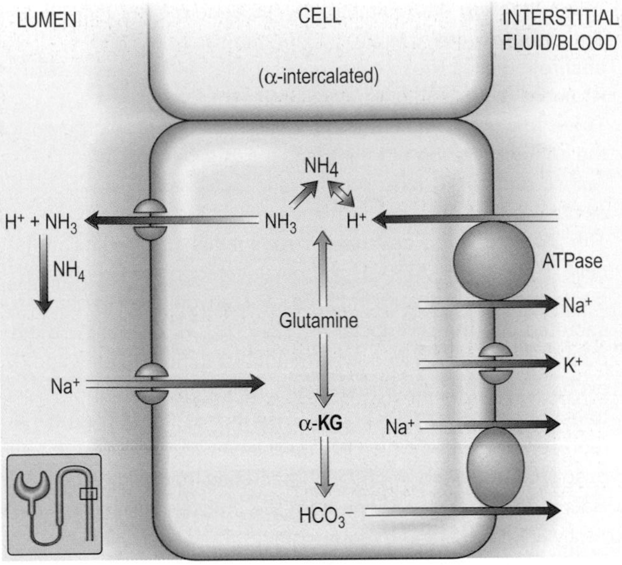

Figure 9.13 The ammonia buffering system in the kidney. All ammonia used to buffer H^+ in the collecting duct is synthesized in the proximal convoluted tubule, and glutamine is the main source of this ammonia. As glutamine is metabolized, α-ketoglutarate (α-KG) is formed, which ultimately breaks down to bicarbonate that is then secreted into the peritubular fluid at an Na^+-HCO_3^- co-transporter.

ion excreted in this form, a bicarbonate ion is regenerated within the cell and returned to the blood ***(Fig. 9.12)***.

Ammonium (NH_4^+)

In the setting of metabolic acidosis, titratable acids cannot increase significantly because the availability of titratable acid is fixed by the plasma concentration of the buffer and by the GFR. The ammonia buffer system, by contrast, can increase several hundred-fold when necessary. Consequently, impaired renal excretion of hydrogen ions is always associated with a defect in ammonium excretion ***(Fig. 9.13)***.

All ammonia used to buffer urinary hydrogen ions in the collecting tubule is synthesized in the proximal convoluted tubule. Glutamine is the primary source of ammonia. It undergoes deamination catalysed by glutaminase, resulting in α-ketoglutaric acid ***(Fig. 9.13)*** and ammonia. Once formed, ammonia can diffuse into the proximal tubule lumen and become acidified, forming ammonium. Once in the proximal tubule lumen, ammonium flows along the tubule to the thick ascending limb of the loop of Henle. Here, it is transported out of the tubule into the medullary interstitium. Ammonium then dissociates to ammonia, leading to a high interstitial ammonia concentration. The notion that ammonia diffuses down its concentration gradient into the lumen of the collecting tubule has been challenged by the discovery of rhesus (Rh)-associated glycoproteins acting as ammonia transport proteins, also called RhCG/Rhcg, which are expressed in the basolateral and apical surfaces of the DCT, inner medullary collecting duct and type α intercalated cells. These proteins play a fundamental role in renal ammonia excretion under both basal and acidotic states. Once secreted, NH_3 reacts with the hydrogen ions secreted by the collecting tubular cells to form ammonium. Because ammonium (NH_4) is not lipid-soluble, it is trapped in the lumen and excreted in the urine as ammonium chloride. Two conditions predominantly promote ammonia synthesis by the proximal tubular cell: systemic acidosis and hypokalaemia.

Box 9.24 Changes in arterial blood gases

	pH	P_aCO_2	HCO_3^-
Respiratory acidosis	N or ↓	↑↑	↑ (compensated)
Respiratory alkalosis	N or ↑	↓↓	↓ (slight)
Metabolic acidosis	N or ↓	↓	↓↓
Metabolic alkalosis	N or ↑	↑ (slight)	↑↑

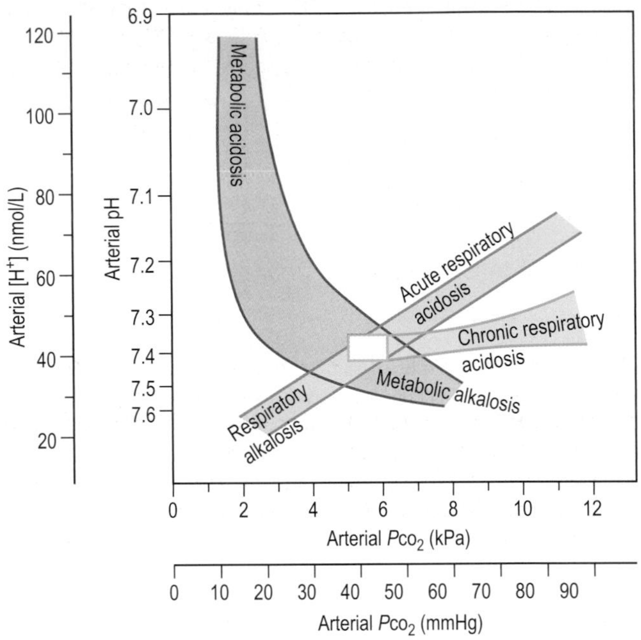

Figure 9.14 The Flenley acid–base nomogram. This was derived from a large number of observations in patients with 'pure' respiratory or metabolic disturbances. The bands show the 95% confidence limits representing the individual varieties of acid–base disturbance. The central white box shows the approximate limits of arterial pH and PCO_2 in normal individuals.

Aetiology of acid–base disturbance

Acid–base disturbance may be caused by:

- abnormal CO_2 removal in the lungs ('respiratory' acidosis and alkalosis)
- abnormalities in the regulation of bicarbonate and other buffers in the blood ('metabolic' acidosis and alkalosis).

Both may, and usually do, coexist. For instance, metabolic acidosis causes hyperventilation (via medullary chemoreceptors, see p. 1061), leading to increased removal of CO_2 in the lungs and partial compensation for the acidosis. Conversely, respiratory acidosis is accompanied by renal bicarbonate retention, which could be mistaken for primary metabolic alkalosis. The situation is even more complex if a patient has both respiratory disease and a metabolic disturbance.

Diagnosis

Clinical history and examination usually point to the correct diagnosis. ***Box 9.24*** shows the typical blood changes, but in complicated patients the acid–base nomogram ***(Fig. 9.14)*** is invaluable. The $[H^+]$ and P_aCO_2 are measured in arterial blood (for precautions), as well as the bicarbonate. If the values from a patient lie in one of the bands in the diagram, it is likely that only one abnormality is present.

If the $[H^+]$ is high (pH low) but the P_aCO_2 is normal, the intercept lies between two bands: the patient has respiratory dysfunction, leading to failure of CO_2 elimination, but this is partly compensated for by metabolic acidosis, stimulating respiration and CO_2 removal (this is the most common 'combined' abnormality in practice).

Respiratory acidosis and alkalosis

Respiratory acidosis

This is caused by retention of CO_2, commonly seen in chronic obstructive pulmonary disease (COPD). The P_aCO_2 and $[H^+]$ rise. Renal retention of bicarbonate may partly compensate, returning the $[H^+]$ towards normal (see p. 1150).

Respiratory alkalosis

Increased removal of CO_2 is caused by hyperventilation, so there is a fall in P_aCO_2 and $[H^+]$ (see p. 1150).

Metabolic acidosis and alkalosis

Metabolic acidosis

This is due to the accumulation of any acid other than carbonic acid, and there is a primary decrease in the plasma $[HCO_3^-]$. Several disorders can lead to metabolic acidosis: acid administration, acid generation (e.g. lactic acidosis during shock or cardiac arrest), impaired acid excretion by the kidneys, or bicarbonate losses from the gastrointestinal tract or kidneys. Calculation of the plasma anion gap is extremely useful in narrowing this differential diagnosis.

The anion gap

The first step is to identify whether the acidosis is due to retention of H^+Cl^- or to another acid. This is achieved by calculation of the anion gap.

- The normal cations present in plasma are Na^+, K^+, Ca^{2+}, Mg^{2+}.
- The normal anions present in plasma are Cl^-, HCO_3^-, negative charges present on albumin, phosphate, sulphate, lactate and other organic acids.
- The sums of the positive and negative charges are equal.
- Measurement of plasma $[Na^+]$, $[K^+]$, $[Cl^-]$ and $[HCO_3^-]$ is usually easily available.

As there are more unmeasured anions than cations, the ***normal anion gap*** is 12–16 mmol/L, although calculations with more sensitive methods place this at 3–9 mmol/L. Albumin normally makes up the largest portion of these unmeasured anions. As a result, a fall in the plasma albumin concentration from the normal value of about 40 g/L to 20 g/L may reduce the anion gap by as much as 6 mmol/L because each 1 g/L of albumin has a negative charge of 0.2–0.28 mmol/L.

Metabolic acidosis with a normal anion gap

If the anion gap is normal in the presence of acidosis, this suggests that H^+Cl^- is being retained or that $Na^+HCO_3^-$ is being lost. Causes of a normal-anion-gap acidosis are given in ***Box 9.25***. In these conditions, plasma bicarbonate decreases and is replaced by chloride to maintain electroneutrality. Consequently, these disorders are sometimes referred to collectively as hyperchloraemic acidoses.

Renal tubular acidosis

The term 'renal tubular acidosis' (RTA) refers to systemic acidosis caused by impairment of the ability of the renal tubules to maintain acid–base balance. This group of disorders is uncommon and only rarely a cause of significant clinical disease.

Box 9.25 Causes of metabolic acidosis with a normal anion gap

Increased gastrointestinal bicarbonate loss
- Diarrhoea
- Ileostomy
- Ureterosigmoidostomy

Increased renal bicarbonate loss
- Acetazolamide therapy
- Proximal (type 2) renal tubular acidosis
- Hyperparathyroidism
- Tubular damage, e.g. drugs, heavy metals, paraproteins

Decreased renal hydrogen ion excretion
- Distal (type 1) renal tubular acidosis
- Type 4 renal tubular acidosis (aldosterone deficiency)

Increased HCl production
- Ammonium chloride ingestion
- Increased catabolism of lysine, arginine

Box 9.26 Features of type 4 renal tubular acidosis (hyporeninaemic hypoaldosteronism)

- Hyperkalaemia (in the absence of drugs known to cause hyperkalaemia)
- Low plasma bicarbonate and hyperchloraemia
- Normal adrenocorticotrophic hormone (ACTH) stimulation test (see p. 1182)
- Low basal 24 h urinary aldosterone
- Subnormal response of plasma renin and plasma aldosterone to stimulation: samples taken over 2 h supine and again after 40 mg furosemide (80 mg if creatinine >120 μmol/L) and 4 h upright posture
- Correction of hyperkalaemia by fludrocortisone 0.1 mg daily

Type 4 renal tubular acidosis

This results from a deficiency or unresponsiveness to aldosterone and, as such, type 4 RTA is also called 'hyporeninaemic hypoaldosteronism'. This is the most common form of RTA. The cardinal features are hyperkalaemia and acidosis occurring in a patient with mild CKD, usually caused by tubulointerstitial disease (e.g. reflux nephropathy) or diabetes. Hyperkalaemia maintains the acidosis through impairment of ammonia production in the proximal tubule leading to a reduction in net acid excretion. Gordon syndrome (see pp. 167–168) shares biochemical abnormalities but differs in having normal GFR and hypertension. Plasma renin and aldosterone are found to be low, even after measures that would normally stimulate their secretion. Features of type 4 RTA are shown in ***Box 9.26***. An identical syndrome is caused by chronic ingestion of NSAIDs, which impair renin and aldosterone secretion. In the presence of acidosis, urine pH may be low. Treatment is with fludrocortisone, sodium bicarbonate, diuretics or ion exchange resins to remove potassium, or a combination of these. Resolution of hyperkalaemia may correct the metabolic acidosis through increased ammonium excretion. Dietary potassium restriction alone is ineffective.

Type 3 renal tubular acidosis

This condition is vanishingly rare, and represents a combination of type 1 and type 2 RTA. Inherited type 3 RTA is caused by mutations resulting in carbonic anhydrase type II deficiency, which is characterized by osteopetrosis, RTA of mixed type, cerebral calcification and mental retardation.

Box 9.27 Causes of type 1 distal renal tubular acidosis

Primary
- Idiopathic
- Genetic
- Marfan syndrome
- Ehlers–Danlos syndrome
- Sickle cell anaemia

Nephrocalcinosis
- Chronic hypercalcaemia
- Medullary sponge kidney

Hypergammaglobulinaemic states
- Amyloidosis[a]
- Cryoglobulinaemia
- Chronic liver disease

Drugs and toxins
- Amphotericin B
- Lithium carbonate
- NSAIDs

[a]*May also cause proximal renal tubular acidosis.*

Box 9.28 Diagnosis of renal tubular acidosis

Plasma HCO_3^- <21 mmol/L, urine pH >5.3 = renal tubular acidosis.

Distal RTA: defect in dietary acid excretion. Urine pH always >5.5

Proximal RTA: defect in bicarbonate reabsorption. Urine pH variable

Bicarbonate infusion test

To differentiate between proximal and distal RTA, perform the bicarbonate infusion test:
- Use a bicarbonate infusion (0.5–1 mmol/kg per hour) to raise serum bicarbonate to 18–20 mmol/L.
- If urine pH rises to >7.5 and the fractional excretion of bicarbonate (Fe HCO_3)[a] rises to >15%, then the defect is bicarbonate reabsorption and diagnosis is proximal RTA.
- If there is little change in urine pH and fractional excretion of bicarbonate remains low, the diagnosis is distal RTA.

Acid load test

If plasma HCO_3^- is >21 mmol/L but there is suspicion of partial renal tubular acidosis (e.g. nephrocalcinosis-associated diseases), an acid load test is required:
- Give 100 mg/kg ammonium chloride by mouth.
- Check urine pH hourly and plasma HCO_3^- at 3 h.
- Plasma HCO_3^- should drop below 21 mmol/L unless the patient vomits (in which case the test should be repeated with an antiemetic).
- If urine pH remains >5.3 despite a plasma HCO_3^- of 21 mmol/L, the diagnosis is confirmed.

[a]*Fe HCO_3 = (urine bicarbonate × serum creatinine)/(serum bicarbonate/urine creatinine) × 100.*

Type 2 ('proximal') renal tubular acidosis

This is very rare in adult practice. It is caused by failure of sodium bicarbonate reabsorption in the proximal tubule. The cardinal features are acidosis, hypokalaemia, an inability to lower the urine pH below 5.5 despite systemic acidosis, and the appearance of bicarbonate in the urine despite a subnormal plasma bicarbonate. This disorder normally occurs as part of a generalized tubular defect, together with other features such as glycosuria and amino-aciduria. Inherited forms of isolated type 2 RTA are described as both autosomal dominant and recessive patterns of inheritance, where putative mutations are in the Na^+–H^+ antiporter in the apical membrane and Na^+–HCO_3^- co-transporter in the basolateral membrane of proximal tubular cells, respectively (see ***Fig. 9.11***). Treatment is with sodium bicarbonate; massive doses may be required to overcome the renal 'leak'.

Type 1 ('distal') renal tubular acidosis

This is due to a failure of H^+ excretion in the distal tubule ***(Box 9.27)***. It consists of:
- acidosis
- hypokalaemia (few exceptions)
- inability to lower the urine pH below 5.3 despite systemic acidosis
- low urinary ammonium production.

These features may be present only in the face of increased acid production; hence the need for an acid load test in diagnosis ***(Box 9.28)***. Other features include:
- low urinary citrate (owing to increased citrate absorption in the proximal tubule, where it can be converted to bicarbonate)
- hypercalciuria.

These abnormalities result in osteomalacia, renal stone formation and recurrent urinary infections:
- ***Osteomalacia*** is caused by buffering of H^+ by Ca^{2+} in bone, resulting in depletion of calcium from bone.
- ***Renal stone formation*** is caused by hypercalciuria, hypocitraturia (citrate inhibits calcium phosphate precipitation) and alkaline urine (which favours precipitation of calcium phosphate).
- ***Recurrent urinary infections*** are caused by renal stones.

Both autosomal dominant and recessive inheritance patterns have been reported in primary distal RTA. In autosomal recessive distal RTA, a substantial proportion of patients have sensorineural deafness, and this is associated with a loss-of-function mutation in the H^+-ATPase at the apical surface of intercalated cells.

Treatment is with sodium bicarbonate, potassium supplements and citrate. Thiazide diuretics are useful because they cause volume contraction and increased proximal sodium bicarbonate reabsorption.

Urinary anion gap

Another useful tool in the evaluation of metabolic acidosis with a normal anion gap is the urinary anion gap:

$$\text{URINARY ANION GAP} = \{\text{urinary }[Na^+] + \text{urinary }[K^+]\} - \text{urinary }[Cl^-].$$

This calculation can be used to distinguish the normal-anion-gap acidosis caused by diarrhoea (or other gastrointestinal alkali loss) from that caused by distal RTA. In both disorders, the plasma $[K^+]$ is characteristically low. In patients with RTA, urinary pH is always greater than 5.3.

Although excretion of urinary hydrogen ions in the patient with diarrhoea should acidify the urine, hypokalaemia leads to enhanced ammonia synthesis by the proximal tubular cells. Despite acidaemia, the excess urinary buffer increases the urine pH to a value above 5.3 in some patients with diarrhoea.

Whenever urinary acid is excreted as ammonium chloride, the increase in urinary chloride excretion decreases the urinary anion gap. Thus, the urinary anion gap should be negative in the patient with diarrhoea, regardless of the urine pH. On the other hand, although hypokalaemia may result in enhanced proximal tubular ammonia synthesis in distal RTA, the inability to secrete hydrogen ions into the collecting duct in this condition limits ammonium chloride formation and excretion; thus, the urinary anion gap is positive in distal RTA.

Metabolic acidosis with a high anion gap

If the anion gap is increased, there is an unmeasured anion present in increased quantities. This is either one of the acids normally present in small but unmeasured quantities, such as lactate, or an exogenous acid. Causes of a high-anion-gap acidosis are given below and in ***Box 9.29***.

Box 9.29 Causes of metabolic acidosis with an increased anion gap: think GOLD MARK

- **G**lycols (ethylene and propylene): ingestions (see pp. 75–76)
- **O**xoproline (pyroglutamic acid): chronic paracetamol ingestion
- **L**-lactate: type A and type B
- **D**-Lactate: small bowel bacterial overgrowth
- **M**ethanol: acute ingestion (see p. 78)
- **A**spirin: salicylate overdose (see p. 81)
- **R**enal failure: accumulation of organic acids
- **K**etoacidosis: diabetic, starvation, alcohol

(From Mehta AN, Emmett JB, Emmett M. GOLD MARK: an anion gap mnemonic for the 21st century. Lancet *2008; 372(9642): 892.)*

Chronic kidney disease

Chronic acidosis is most often caused by chronic kidney disease (CKD), in which there is a failure to excrete fixed acid. Up to 40 mmol of hydrogen ions may accumulate daily. These are buffered by bone, in exchange for calcium. Chronic acidosis is therefore a major risk factor for renal osteodystrophy and hypercalciuria.

Chronic acidosis has also been shown to be a risk factor for muscle wasting in renal failure, and may also contribute to the inexorable progression of some types of renal disease.

Kidney disease causes acidosis in several ways:

- Reduction in the number of functioning nephrons decreases the capacity to excrete ammonia and H^+ in the urine.
- Tubular disease may cause bicarbonate wasting.

Acidosis is a particular feature of those types of CKD in which the tubules are particularly affected, such as reflux nephropathy and chronic obstructive uropathy.

Uraemic acidosis should be corrected because of the effects on growth, muscle turnover and bones. Oral sodium bicarbonate 2–3 mmol/kg daily is usually enough to maintain serum bicarbonate above 20 mmol/L but may contribute to sodium overload. Calcium carbonate improves acidosis and also acts as a phosphate binder and calcium supplement, and is commonly used. Acidosis in end-stage kidney disease is usually fully corrected by adequate dialysis.

Lactic acidosis

Increased lactic acid production occurs when cellular respiration is abnormal, because of either a lack of oxygen in the tissues (**'type A'**) or a metabolic abnormality, such as that induced by drugs such as metformin (**'type B'**). The most common cause in clinical practice is type A lactic acidosis, occurring in septic or cardiogenic shock (see p. 1154). Significant acidosis can occur despite a normal blood pressure and P_aCO_2, owing to splanchnic and peripheral vasoconstriction. Acidosis worsens cardiac function and vasoconstriction further, contributing to a downward spiral and fulminant production of lactic acid.

Raised serum D-lactate occurs with fermentation of glucose by abnormal bowel flora in the short gut syndrome.

Ketoacidosis (see pp. 1261–1264)

There is a high-anion-gap acidosis due to the accumulation of acetoacetic and hydroxybutyric acids, owing to increased production and some reduced peripheral utilization in diabetic ketoacidosis. Ketoacidosis without hypoglycaemia occurs in starvation and after alcohol overdose.

Mixed metabolic acidosis

Both types of acidosis may coexist. For instance, cholera would be expected to cause a normal-anion-gap acidosis owing to massive gastrointestinal losses of bicarbonate, but the anion gap is often increased owing to renal failure and lactic acidosis as a result of hypovolaemia.

To help ascertain if there is an additional normal-anion-gap acidosis as well as, for example, a ketoacidosis, the delta anion gap can be calculated. This is the difference between the upper reference value of the anion gap and the calculated anion gap. This value should equal the fall in the bicarbonate concentration from the lower limit of normal. If the bicarbonate is significantly ***lower*** than predicted (>5 mmol/L), then an additional normal-anion-gap ***acidosis*** must be present. Similarly, if the bicarbonate is >5 mmol/L ***higher*** than expected, an additional normal-anion-gap ***alkalosis*** must be present.

Clinical features of acidosis

Clinically, the most obvious effect is stimulation of respiration, leading to the clinical sign of 'air hunger', or Kussmaul respiration. Interestingly, patients with profound hyperventilation may not complain of breathlessness, although in others it may be a presenting complaint.

Acidosis increases delivery of oxygen to the tissues by shifting the oxyhaemoglobin dissociation curve to the right, but it also leads to inhibition of 2,3-BPG production, which returns the curve towards normal (see ***Fig. 25.2***). Cardiovascular dysfunction is common in acidotic patients, although it is often difficult to dissociate the numerous possible causes of this. Acidosis is negatively inotropic. Severe acidosis also causes venoconstriction, resulting in redistribution of blood from the peripheries to the central circulation, and increased systemic venous pressure, which may worsen pulmonary oedema caused by myocardial depression. Arteriolar vasodilatation also occurs, further contributing to hypotension.

Cerebral dysfunction is variable. Severe acidosis is often associated with confusion and fits, but numerous other possible causes are usually present.

As mentioned earlier, acidosis stimulates potassium loss from cells, which may lead to potassium deficiency if renal function is normal, or to hyperkalaemia if renal potassium excretion is impaired.

General treatment of acidosis

Treatment should be aimed at correcting the primary cause. In lactic acidosis caused by poor tissue perfusion ('type A'), treatment should be aimed at maximizing oxygen delivery to the tissues by protecting the airway, and improving breathing and circulation. This usually requires inotropic agents, mechanical ventilation and invasive monitoring. In 'type B' lactic acidosis, treatment is directed at the underlying disorder – for example:

- insulin in diabetic ketoacidosis
- treatment of methanol and ethylene glycol poisoning with ethanol
- removal of salicylate by dialysis.

The question of whether severe acidosis should be treated with bicarbonate is extremely controversial:

- Rapid correction of acidosis may result in tetany and fits owing to a rapid decrease in ionized calcium.
- Administration of sodium bicarbonate (8.4%) provides 1 mmol/mL of sodium, which may lead to extracellular volume expansion, exacerbating pulmonary oedema.
- Bicarbonate therapy increases CO_2 production and will therefore correct acidosis only if ventilation can be increased to remove the added CO_2 load.

- The increased amounts of CO_2 generated may diffuse more readily into cells than bicarbonate, worsening intracellular acidosis.

Administration of sodium bicarbonate (50 mmol, as 50 mL of 8.4% sodium bicarbonate i.v.) is still occasionally given during cardiac arrest and is often necessary before arrhythmias can be corrected. Correction of hyperkalaemia associated with acidosis is also of undoubted benefit. In other situations, there is no clinical evidence to show that correction of acidosis improves outcome, but it is standard practice to administer sodium bicarbonate when $[H^+]$ is above 126 nmol/L (pH <6.9), using intravenous 1.26% (150 mmol/L) bicarbonate infused over 2–3 h with electrolyte and pH monitoring. Intravenous sodium lactate should never be given.

Metabolic alkalosis

Metabolic alkalosis is common, comprising half of all the acid–base disorders in hospitalized patients. This observation should not be surprising since vomiting, the use of diuretics, and nasogastric suction are common among hospitalized patients. The mortality associated with metabolic alkalosis is substantial; the mortality rate is 45% in patients with an arterial pH of 7.55 and 80% when the pH is over 7.65. Although this relationship is not necessarily causal, severe alkalosis should be viewed with concern.

Classification and definitions

Metabolic alkalosis has been classified on the basis of underlying pathophysiology ***(Box 9.30)***:

- ***chloride depletion***, the most common cause, which can be corrected without potassium repletion
- ***potassium depletion***, usually with mineralocorticoid excess
- ***metabolic alkalosis***, due to both potassium and chloride depletion.

Box 9.30 Causes of metabolic alkalosis

Chloride depletion
- Gastric losses: vomiting, mechanical drainage, bulimia
- Chloruretic diuretics, e.g. bumetanide, furosemide, chlorothiazide, metolazone
- Diarrhoeal states: villous adenoma, congenital chloridorrhoea
- Cystic fibrosis (high sweat chloride)

Potassium depletion/mineralocorticoid excess
- Primary aldosteronism
- Secondary aldosteronism
- Apparent mineralocorticoid excess:
  - Primary deoxycorticosterone excess: 11α- and 17α-hydroxylase deficiencies
  - Drugs: liquorice (glycyrrhizic acid) as a confection or flavouring, carbenoxolone
  - Liddle syndrome
  - Bartter and Gitelman syndromes and their variants
  - Laxative abuse, clay ingestion

Hypercalcaemic states
- Hypercalcaemia of malignancy
- Acute or chronic milk–alkali syndrome

Others
- Amoxicillin or penicillin therapy
- Bicarbonate ingestion: massive or smaller ingestion with kidney disease
- Recovery from starvation
- Hypoalbuminaemia

Chloride may be lost from the gut, kidney or skin. The loss of gastric fluid rich in acid results in alkalosis because bicarbonate generated during the production of gastric acid returns to the circulation. In Zollinger–Ellison syndrome (see p. 512) or gastric outflow obstruction, these losses can be massive. Although sodium and potassium loss in the gastric juice is variable, the obligate urinary loss of these cations is intensified by bicarbonaturia, which occurs during disequilibrium.

Chloruretic agents all directly produce loss of chloride, sodium and fluid in the urine. These losses in turn promote metabolic alkalosis by several mechanisms:

- Diuretic-induced increases in sodium delivery to the distal nephron enhance potassium and hydrogen ion secretion.
- Extracellular volume contraction stimulates renin and aldosterone secretion, which blunts sodium losses but accelerates potassium and hydrogen ion secretion.
- Potassium depletion augments bicarbonate reabsorption in the proximal tubule and stimulates ammonia production, which in turn will increase urinary net acid excretion.

Urinary losses of chloride exceed those for sodium and are associated with alkalosis, even when potassium depletion is prevented. The cessation of events that generate alkalosis is not necessarily accompanied by resolution of the alkalosis. A widely accepted hypothesis for the maintenance of alkalosis is chloride depletion rather than volume depletion. Although normal functioning of the proximal tubule is essential for bicarbonate absorption, the collecting duct appears to be the major nephron site for altered electrolyte and proton transport in both maintenance and recovery from metabolic alkalosis. During maintenance, the α-intercalated cells in the cortical collecting duct do not secrete bicarbonate because insufficient chloride is available for bicarbonate exchange. When chloride is administered and luminal or cellular chloride concentration increases, bicarbonate is promptly excreted and alkalosis is corrected.

Metabolic alkalosis in ***hypokalaemia*** is generated primarily by an increased intracellular shift of hydrogen ion, causing intracellular acidosis. Potassium depletion is also associated with enhanced ammonia production and increased obligate net acid excretion. This is the corollary to the acidosis seen with hyperkalaemia in type 4 RTA. Infusion of potassium alone can correct systemic alkalosis and intracellular acidosis as cells exchange extracellular potassium for intracellular hydrogen, which can then buffer extracellular bicarbonate.

Milk–alkali syndrome in which both bicarbonate and calcium are ingested, produces alkalosis by vomiting, calcium-induced bicarbonate absorption and reduced GFR. Cationic antibiotics in high doses can cause alkalosis by obligatory bicarbonate loss in the urine.

Clinical features

The symptoms of metabolic alkalosis *per se* are difficult to separate from those of chloride, volume or potassium depletion. Tetany (see ***Box 26.50***), apathy, confusion, drowsiness, cardiac arrhythmias and neuromuscular irritability are common when alkalosis is severe. The oxyhaemoglobin dissociation curve is shifted to the left. Respiration may be depressed.

Management

Chloride-responsive metabolic alkalosis

Although replacement of the chloride deficit is essential in chloride depletion states, selection of the accompanying cation – sodium, potassium or proton – is dependent on the assessment of extracellular fluid volume status (see p. 159), the presence or absence of associated potassium depletion, and the degree and reversibility of any depression of GFR. If kidney function is normal, bicarbonate and base equivalents will be excreted with sodium or potassium, and metabolic alkalosis will be rapidly corrected as chloride is made available.

If chloride and extracellular depletion coexist, then isotonic saline solution is appropriate therapy.

In the clinical setting of fluid overload, saline is contraindicated. In such situations, intravenous hydrochloride acid or ammonium chloride can be given. If GFR is adequate, acetazolamide, which causes bicarbonate diuresis by inhibiting carbonic anhydrase, can also be used. When the kidney is incapable of responding to chloride repletion, dialysis is necessary.

Chloride-resistant metabolic alkalosis

Metabolic alkalosis due to potassium depletion is managed by correction of the underlying cause (see 'Hypokalaemia', pp. 165–167). Mild to moderate alkalosis requires oral potassium chloride administration. However, the presence of a cardiac arrhythmia or generalized weakness requires intravenous potassium chloride.

Further reading

Berend K, de Vries AP, Gans RO. Physiological approach to assessment of acid–base disturbances. *N Engl J Med* 2014; 371:1434–1445.
Kraut JA, Madias NE. Lactic acidosis. *N Engl J Med* 2015; 372:1078–1079.
Seifter JL. Integration of acid–base and electrolyte disorders. *N Engl J Med* 2014; 371:1821–1831.
Weiner ID, Verlander JW. Ammonia transport in the kidney by Rhesus glycoproteins. *Am J Physiol Renal Physiol* 2014; 306:F1107–1120.

Bibliography

Burns GP. Arterial blood gases made easy. *Clin Med* 2014; 14:66–68.
Greenlee MM, Lynch IJ, Gumz ML et al. The renal H,K-ATPases. *Curr Opin Nephrol Hypertens* 2010; 19:478–482.
Kaplan LJ, Kellum JA. Fluids, pH, ions and electrolytes. *Curr Opin Crit Care* 2010; 16:323–331.
Karet FE. Disorders of water and acid–base homeostasis. *Nephron Physiol* 2011; 118:28–34.
Kraut JA, Madias NE. Lactic acidosis. *New Engl J Med* 2014; 371:2309–2319.
Seifter JL. Integration of acid–base and electrolyte disorders. *N Engl J Med* 2014; 371:1821–1831.
Sterns RH. Disorders of fluids and electrolytes. *N Engl J Med* 2015; 372:55–65.

10 Nutrition

Marinos Elia, Susan A Lanham-New

See your e-book for key learning points, clinical tips, learning challenges, extra tables, interactive Figures, MCQs and Special Topics from the International Advisory Board.

INTRODUCTION

The interface between normal and abnormal nutrition can be difficult to define. There is no universally accepted definition of malnutrition, but a reasonable definition is as follows: 'Malnutrition is a state of nutrition in which a deficiency, excess or imbalance of energy, protein and other nutrients causes measurable adverse effects on tissue/body form (body shape, size and composition) and function, and on clinical outcome.'

In developing countries, the lack of food and poor usage of the available food, often in association with ongoing inflammatory processes, result in what has traditionally been called protein–energy malnutrition (PEM). However, nutrient deficiencies often accompany PEM and they may contribute to its development. Worldwide, in 2011, 165 million children under 5 years of age were affected by stunting, and at least 52 million by wasting. Obesity has also been a growing problem in developing countries and the combination of stunting with obesity has been increasing. In developed countries, excess food is available, and overweight and obesity are the most common nutritional problems. However, under-nutrition (often referred to as 'malnutrition') continues to remain a major clinical and public health problem worldwide.

Diet and disease are inter-related in many ways:

- ***Excess energy intake contributes to a number of diseases***, including ischaemic heart disease and diabetes, particularly when high in animal (saturated) fat content.
- ***There is a relationship between food intake and cancer***, as found in many epidemiological studies. An excess of energy-rich foods (i.e. those containing fat and sugar), often combined with physical inactivity, plays a role in the development of certain cancers, while diets high in vegetables and fruits reduce the risk of most epithelial cancers. Numerous carcinogens, intentional additions (e.g. nitrates for preserving foods) or accidental contaminants (e.g. moulds producing aflatoxin and fungi) may also be involved in the development of cancer.
- ***The proportion of processed foods eaten may affect the development of disease***. Some processed convenience foods have a high sugar and fat content and therefore predispose to

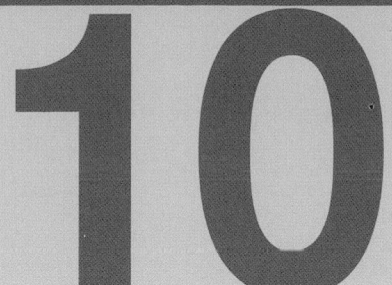

dental caries and obesity, respectively. They also have a low fibre content, and dietary fibre can help in the prevention of a number of diseases (see p. 188).

- ***Long-term under-nutrition is implicated in disease*** by some epidemiological studies; for example, low growth rates *in utero* are associated with high death rates from cardiovascular disease in adult life.

In the UK, dietary reference values for food, energy and nutrients are stated as ***reference nutrient intakes*** (RNIs), on the basis of data from the Food and Agriculture Organization (FAO-WHO), United Nations University (UNU) expert committee and elsewhere. The RNI is sufficient, or more than sufficient, to meet the nutritional needs of 97.5% of healthy people in a population. Most people's daily requirements are less than this, and so an ***estimated average requirement*** (EAR) is also given, which will certainly be adequate for most. A lower reference nutrient intake (LRNI), which fails to meet the requirements of 97.5% of the population, is also given. The RNI figures quoted in this chapter are for the age group 19–50 years. These represent values for healthy subjects and are not always appropriate for patients with disease.

WATER AND ELECTROLYTE BALANCE

Water and electrolyte balance is dealt with fully in Chapter 9. About 1 L of water is required in the daily diet to balance insensible losses but much more is usually drunk, the kidneys being able to excrete large quantities. The daily RNI for sodium is 70 mmol (1.6 g) but daily sodium intake varies in the range 90–440 mmol (2–10 g). These are needlessly high intakes of sodium, which are thought by some to play a role in causing hypertension (see p. 1046). The World Health Organization (WHO) also recommends at least 90 mmol (3.5 g) potassium, which would reduce blood pressure and cardiovascular risk of stroke and coronary artery disease.

DIETARY REQUIREMENTS

Energy

Food is necessary to provide the body with energy ***(Fig. 10.1)***. The SI unit of energy is the joule (J), and 1 kJ = 0.239 kcal. The conversion factor of 4.2 kJ, equivalent to 1.00 kcal, is used in clinical nutrition.

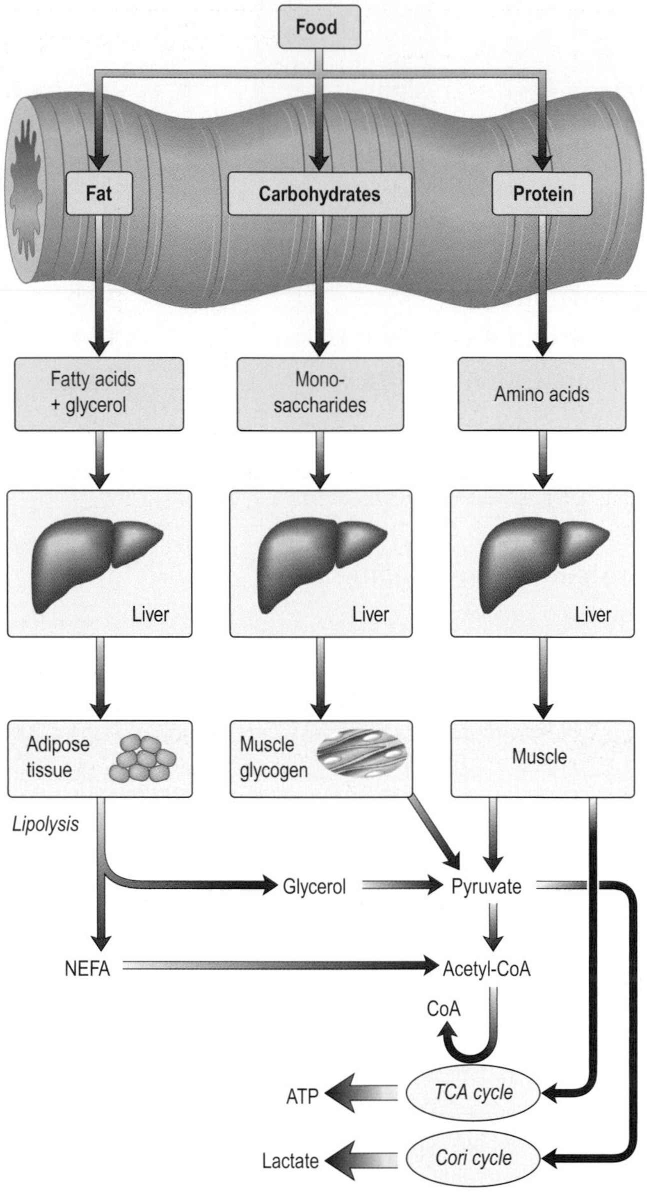

Figure 10.1 The production of energy from the main constituents of food. Alcohol produces up to 5% of total calories but the variation between individuals is wide. One mol of glucose produces 36 mol of adenosine triphosphate (ATP). CoA, coenzyme A; NEFA, non-esterified fatty acids; TCA, tricarboxylic acid.

Energy balance

Energy balance is the difference between energy intake and energy expenditure. Weight gain or loss is a simple but accurate way of indicating differences in energy balance.

Energy requirements

There are two approaches to assessing energy requirements for subjects who are weight-stable and close to energy balance:

- assessment of energy intake
- assessment of total energy expenditure.

Energy intake

Energy intake can be estimated from dietary surveys and, in the past, this has been used to decide daily energy requirements. However, measurement of energy expenditure gives a more accurate assessment of requirements.

Energy expenditure

Daily energy expenditure ***(Fig. 10.2)*** is the sum of:

- the basal metabolic rate (BMR)
- the thermic effect of food eaten
- occupational activities
- non-occupational activities.

Total energy expenditure can be measured using a double-labelled water technique. Water containing the stable isotopes ^{2}H and ^{18}O is given orally. As energy is expended, carbon dioxide and water are produced. The difference between the rates of loss of the two isotopes is used to calculate the carbon dioxide production,

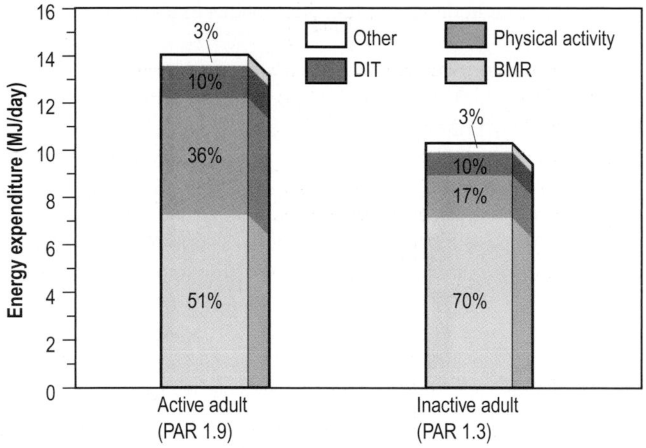

Figure 10.2 Daily energy expenditure in an active and a sedentary 70-kg adult. BMR, basal metabolic rate; DIT, dietary-induced thermogenesis; PAR, physical activity ratio.

Box 10.1 Equations for the prediction of basal metabolic rate (BMR) (in MJ/day)

Age range (years)	Equation for predicting BMR[a]	95% confidence limits
Men		
10–17	0.0740×(wt)+2.754	±0.88
18–29	0.0630×(wt)+2.896	±1.28
30–59	0.0480×(wt)+3.653	±1.40
60–74	0.0499×(wt)+2.930	N/A
75+	0.0350×(wt)+3.434	N/A
Women		
10–17	0.0560×(wt)+2.898	±0.94
18–29	0.0620×(wt)+2.036	±1.00
30–59	0.0340×(wt)+3.538	±0.94
60–74	0.0386×(wt)+2.875	N/A
75+	0.0410×(wt)+2.610	N/A

[a]Body weight (wt) in kg.
(Data from Department of Health, 1991.)

which is then used to calculate energy expenditure. This can be done on urine samples over a 2–3-week period with the subject ambulatory. The technique is accurate, but it is expensive and requires the availability of a mass spectrometer. An alternative tracer technique for measuring total energy expenditure is to estimate CO_2 production by isotopic dilution. A subcutaneous infusion of labelled bicarbonate is administered continuously by a minipump, and urine is collected to measure isotopic dilution by urea, which is formed from CO_2. Other methods for estimating energy expenditure, such as heart rate monitors or activity monitors, are also available but are less accurate.

Basal metabolic rate can be calculated by measuring oxygen consumption and CO_2 production, but it is more usually taken from standardized tables ***(Box 10.1)*** that only require knowledge of the subject's age, weight and sex.

Box 10.2 Physical activity ratio (PAR) for various activities (expressed as multiples of BMR)

Activity	PAR
Professional/housewife	1.7
Domestic helper/salesperson	2.7
Labourer	3.0
Reading/eating	1.2
Household/cooking	2.1
Gardening/golf	3.7
Jogging/swimming/football	6.9

The ***physical activity ratio*** (PAR) is expressed as multiples of the BMR for both occupational and non-occupational activities of varying intensities ***(Box 10.2)***.

Total daily energy expenditure

$$= \text{BMR} \times [\text{Time in bed} + (\text{Time at work} \times \text{PAR}) + (\text{Non-occupational time} \times \text{PAR})]$$

Thus, for example, to determine the daily energy expenditure of a 73-year-old, 50-kg female doctor, with a BMR of 4805 kJ/day, who spends one-third of a day sleeping, working and engaged in non-occupational activities, the latter at a PAR of 2.1, the following calculation ensues:

$$= (4805\ \text{kJ/day}) \times [0.3 \times 1.7) + (0.3 \times 2.10)] = 6919\ \text{kJ}\ (1655\ \text{kcal/day})$$

In the UK, the estimated 'average' daily energy requirement is:

- for a 55-year-old female – 8100 kJ (1940 kcal)
- for a 55-year-old male – 10 600 kJ (2550 kcal).

This is at present made up of about 50% carbohydrate, 35% fat, 15% protein±5% alcohol. In developing countries, however, carbohydrate may be >75% of the total energy input, and fat <15% of the total energy input.

Energy requirements increase during the growing period, with pregnancy and lactation, and sometimes following infection or trauma. In general, the increased BMR associated with inflammatory or traumatic conditions is counteracted or more than counteracted by a decrease in physical activity, so that total energy requirements are not increased.

In the basal state, energy demands for resting muscle are 20% of the total energy required, those for abdominal viscera 35–40%, those for brain 20% and those for heart 10%. There can be more than a 50-fold increase in muscle energy demands during exercise.

Energy stores

Although virtually all body fat and glycogen are available for oxidation, less than half the protein is available for oxidation. Figure 10.3 shows that fat accounts for the largest reserves of energy in both lean and obese subjects. The size of the stores determines survival during starvation.

Body weight

Body weight depends on energy balance. Intake depends not only on food availability but also on a number of complex interrelationships that include the stimulus of good food, the role of hunger, metabolic changes (e.g. hypoglycaemia), and the pleasure and habit of eating. Some people are able to keep their body weight

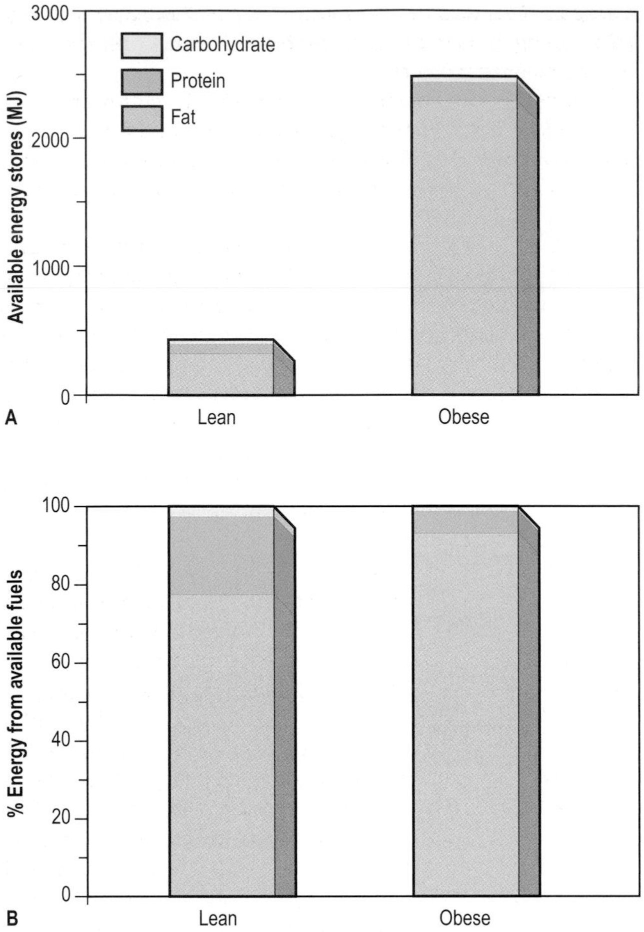

Figure 10.3 Available energy reserves from different fuels. Values are shown for a lean hypothetical 70-kg adult and an obese 140-kg adult. **A.** Expressed in MJ. **B.** Expressed as a percentage of the total.

constant within a few kilograms for many years, but most gradually increase their weight owing to a small but continuous increase of intake over expenditure. A gain or loss of energy of 25–29 MJ (6000–7000 kcal) would, respectively, increase or decrease body weight by approximately 1 kg.

Protein

In the UK, the adult daily RNI for protein is 0.75 g/kg, with protein representing at least 10% of the total energy intake. Most affluent people eat more than this, consuming 80–100 g of protein per day.

The total amount of nitrogen excreted in the urine represents the balance between protein breakdown and synthesis. In order to maintain nitrogen balance, at least 40–50 g of dietary protein are needed. The amount of protein oxidized can be calculated from the amount of nitrogen excreted in the urine over 24 hours using the following equation:

$$\text{Grams of protein required} = \text{Urinary nitrogen} \times 6.25$$

(most proteins contain about 16% of nitrogen)

In practice, urinary urea is more easily measured and forms 80–90% of the total urinary nitrogen (N). In healthy individuals, urinary nitrogen excretion reflects protein intake. However, excretion does not match intake in catabolic conditions (negative N balance), or during growth or repletion following an illness (positive N balance).

Protein contains many ***amino acids***:

- ***Indispensable (essential)***. There are nine amino acids that cannot be synthesized and must be provided in the diet: tryptophan, histidine, methionine, threonine, isoleucine, valine, phenylalanine, lysine and leucine.
- ***Dispensable (non-essential)***. These are amino acids that can be synthesized in the body (some may still be needed in the diet unless adequate amounts of their precursors are available).

Animal proteins (e.g. in milk, meat and eggs) contain a good balance of all the indispensable amino acids, but many proteins from vegetables are deficient in at least one indispensable amino acid. In developing countries, protein intake derives mainly from vegetable proteins. By combining foodstuffs with different low concentrations of indispensable amino acids (e.g. maize with legumes), protein intake can be adequate, provided enough vegetables are available.

Loss of protein from the body (negative N balance) occurs not only because of inadequate protein intake, but also because of inadequate energy intake. When there is loss of energy from the body, more protein is directed towards oxidative pathways and, eventually, gluconeogenesis for energy.

Role of amino acids

- ***Glutamine*** is quantitatively the most significant amino acid in the circulation and in inter-organ exchange.
- ***Alanine*** is released from muscle; it is deaminated and converted into pyruvic acid before entering the citric acid cycle.
- ***Homocysteine*** is a sulphur-containing amino acid that is derived from methionine in the diet. A raised plasma concentration is an independent risk factor for vascular disease.

Amino acids are utilized to synthesize products other than protein or urea. For example:

- ***Glycine*** is required for haem production.
- ***Tyrosine*** is required for melanin and thyroid hormones.
- ***Glutamine, aspartate and glycine*** are required for nucleic acid bases.
- ***Glutamate, cysteine and glycine*** are required for glutathione, which is part of the defence system against free radicals.

Fat

Dietary fat is chiefly in the form of triglycerides, which are esters of glycerol and free fatty acids. Fatty acids vary in chain length and in saturation ***(Box 10.3)***. The hydrogen molecules related to the double bonds can be in the *cis* or the *trans* position; most natural fatty acids in food are in the *cis* position ***(Box 10.4)***.

The ***essential fatty acids*** (EFAs) are linoleic and α-linolenic acid, both of which are precursors of prostaglandins. Eicosapentaenoic and docosahexaenoic acid are also necessary, but can be made to a limited extent in the tissues from linoleic and linolenic acid, and thus a dietary supply is not essential.

Synthesis of triglycerides, sterols and phospholipids is very efficient. Even with low-fat diets, subcutaneous fat stores can be normal.

Dietary fat provides 37 kJ (9 kcal) of energy per gram. A high-fat intake has been implicated in the causation of:

- cardiovascular disease
- cancer (e.g. breast, colon and prostate)

Box 10.3 The main fatty acids in foods

Fatty acid	No. of carbon atoms:no. of double bonds	Position of double bonds[a]
Saturated		
Lauric	C12:0	
Myristic	C14:0	
Palmitic	C16:0	
Stearic	C18:0	
Monounsaturated		
Oleic	C18:1	*n*-9
Elaidic	C18:1	*n*-9 *trans*
Polyunsaturated		
Linoleic	C18:2	*n*-6
α-Linolenic	C18:3	*n*-3
Arachidonic	C20:4	*n*-6
Eicosapentaenoic	C20:5	*n*-3
Docosahexaenoic	C22:6	*n*-3

[a]Positions of the double bonds (designated either *n* as here or ω) are shown counted from the methyl end of the molecule. All double bonds are in the *cis* position except that marked *trans*.

Box 10.4 Dietary sources of fatty acids

Type of acid	Sources
Saturated fatty acids	Mainly animal fat
***n*-6 fatty acids**	Vegetable oils and other plant foods
***n*-3 fatty acids**	Vegetable foods, rapeseed oil, fish oils
***trans* fatty acids**	Hydrogenated fat or oils, e.g. in margarine, cakes, biscuits

- obesity
- type 2 diabetes.

The data on causation are largely epidemiological and disputed by many. Nevertheless, it is often suggested that the consumption of saturated fatty acids should be reduced, accompanied by an increase in monounsaturated fatty acids, such as those in olive oil (the 'Mediterranean diet'), or polyunsaturated fatty acids. Any increase in polyunsaturated fats should not, however, exceed 10% of the total food energy, particularly as this requires a big dietary change.

Trans fats (partly hydrogenated fatty acids)

Increased consumption of hydrogenated vegetable and fish oils in margarines has led to increased *trans* fatty acid consumption. *Trans* fatty acids (also called *trans* fats) behave as if they were saturated fatty acids, increasing circulating low-density lipoprotein (LDL) and decreasing high-density lipoprotein (HDL) cholesterol concentrations, which, in turn, raise the risk of cardiovascular disease. In most countries, nutrition labels for all conventional foods and supplements must indicate the *trans* fatty acid content. The usage of *trans* fatty acids from partially hydrogenated oils has now been banned in many countries.

Polyunsaturated fatty acids

The ***n*-6 polyunsaturated fatty acids (PUFAs)** are components of membrane phospholipids, influencing membrane fluidity and ion transport. They also have antiarrhythmic, antithrombotic and anti-inflammatory properties, all of which are potentially helpful in preventing cardiovascular disease.

The ***n*-3 PUFAs** increase circulating HDL cholesterol and lower triglycerides, both of which might reduce cardiovascular risk. Some of the actions of *n*-3 PUFAs are mediated by a range of leukotrienes and eicosanoids, which differ in pattern and functions from those produced from *n*-6 PUFAs.

Epidemiological studies and clinical intervention studies suggest that *n*-3 PUFAs may have effects in the secondary prevention of cardiovascular disease and 'all-cause mortality' (e.g. a 20–30% reduction in mortality from cardiovascular disease, according to some studies). The benefits, which have been noted as early as 4 months after intervention, have been attributed largely to the antiarrhythmic effects of *n*-3 PUFAs, but some work suggests that *n*-3 PUFAs, administered as capsules, can be rapidly incorporated into atheromatous plaques, stabilizing them and preventing rupture. Whether these effects are due directly to *n*-3 PUFAs or other changes in the diet is still debated.

The ***GISSI Prevention Trial***, which followed over 11 000 patients for 3.5 years after a myocardial infarction, administered fish oils (eicosapentaenoic acid, EPA, and docosahexaenoic acid, DHA) in the form of capsules and demonstrated a striking benefit in reducing mortality. In contrast, a more recent study in patients with cardiovascular risk factors and no history of myocardial infarction found no effect of *n*-3 PUFAs on cardiovascular mortality and morbidity. The reasons for the discrepancy between these two studies are unclear, but the beneficial effect of *n*-3 PUFAs in those with a history of myocardial infarction may have been due to the antiarrhythmic effects of *n*-3 PUFAs, averting fatal ventricular arrhythmias. Another recent study in patients with glucose intolerance/diabetes and cardiovascular risk factors also did not find a beneficial effect of *n*-3 PUFAs on cardiovascular events.

Recommendations for fat intake

The British Nutrition Foundation and the American Heart Association presently recommend a two-fold increase of the current intake of total *n*-3 PUFAs (a several-fold increase in the intake of fish oils, and a 50% increase in the intake of α-linolenic acid). Implementing this recommendation will mean either a major change in the dietary habits of populations that eat little fish, or ingestion of capsules containing fish oils. Some government agencies have warned of the hazards of eating certain types of fish, which increase the risk of mercury poisoning and possibly other toxicities.

The current recommendations for fat intake for the UK are shown in ***Box 10.5***.

Cholesterol

Cholesterol is found in all animal products. Eggs are particularly rich in cholesterol, which is virtually absent from plants. The average daily intake in the UK is 300–500 mg. Cholesterol is also synthesized (see ***Fig. 14.4***), and only very high or low dietary intakes will significantly affect blood levels.

Essential fatty acid deficiency

Essential fatty acid deficiency may accompany PEM, but it has been clearly defined as a clinical entity only in patients on long-term parenteral nutrition given glucose, protein and no fat. Alopecia, thrombocytopenia, anaemia and dermatitis occur within weeks, with an increased ratio of triene (*n*-9) to tetraene (*n*-6) in plasma fatty acids.

Box 10.5 Recommended healthy dietary intake

Dietary component	Approximate amounts (% of total energy unless otherwise stated)	General hints
Total carbohydrate	55 (55–75)	Increase fruit, vegetables, beans, pasta, bread
Free sugar	10 (<10)*	Decrease sugary drinks
Protein	15 (10–15)	Decrease red meat (see 'Fat' below)
Total fat	30 (15–30)	Increase vegetable (including olive oil) and fish oil and decrease animal fat
Saturated fatty acids	10 (<10)	
Cis-monounsaturated fatty acids	20	Mainly oleic acid (*n*-6)
Cis-polyunsaturated fatty acids	6	Both *n*-6 and *n*-3 PUFAs
Approximate amounts		
Cholesterol	<300 (<300) mg/day	Decrease meat and eggs
Salt	<6 (<5) g/day	Decrease prepared meats and do not add extra salt to food
Total dietary fibre	30 (>25) g/day	Increase fruit, vegetables and wholegrain foods

Values in parentheses are goals for the intake of populations, as given by the World Health Organization (including populations who are already on low-fat diets). Some of the extreme ranges are not realistic short-term goals for developed countries, e.g. 75% of total energy from carbohydrate and 15% fat. When total energy intake is 2500 kcal (10 500 kJ) per day, 55% of intake comes from carbohydrate (344 g, i.e. 1376 kcal (5579 kJ)) and 30% from fat (83 g, i.e. 747 kcal (3137 kJ)). PUFAs, polyunsaturated fatty acids.
*Recent recommendations suggest <5% of total energy consumption.

Carbohydrate

Carbohydrates are readily available in the diet, providing 17 kJ (4 kcal) per gram of energy (15.7 kJ (3.75 kcal) per gram monosaccharide equivalent). Carbohydrate intake comprises:

- polysaccharide starch
- disaccharides (mainly sucrose)
- monosaccharides (glucose and fructose).

Carbohydrate is cheap, compared with other foodstuffs; a great deal is therefore eaten, usually more than required. WHO suggests that sugar intake should be <5% of a person's total energy consumption.

Dietary fibre

Dietary fibre, which is largely ***non-starch polysaccharide*** (NSP; entirely NSP according to some authorities), is often removed in the processing of food. This leaves highly refined carbohydrates, such as sucrose, which contribute to the development of dental caries and obesity. Lignin is included in dietary fibre in some classification systems but it is not a polysaccharide. It is only a minor component of the human diet.

The principal classes of NSP are:

- cellulose
- hemicelluloses
- pectins
- gums.

None of these is digested by gut enzymes. However, NSP is partly broken down in the gastrointestinal tract, mainly by colonic bacteria, producing gas and volatile fatty acids, e.g. butyrate.

All plant food, when unprocessed, contains NSP, so that all unprocessed food eaten will increase the NSP content of the diet. Bran, the fibre from wheat, provides an easy way of adding additional fibre to the diet; it increases faecal bulk and is helpful in the treatment of constipation.

The average daily intake of NSP in the diet is approximately 16 g. NSP deficiency is accepted as an entity by many authorities and it is suggested that the total NSP be increased to up to 30 g daily. This could be achieved by increased consumption of bread, potatoes, fruit and vegetables, with a reduction in sugar intake in order not to increase total calories. Each extra gram of fibre daily adds approximately 3–5 g to the daily stool weight. Pectins and gums have also been added to food to slow down monosaccharide absorption, and this is particularly useful in type 2 diabetes.

Eating a diet rich in plant foods (fruits, vegetables, cereals and whole grain – the main sources of dietary fibre) is broadly recommended for general health promotion, including protection against ischaemic heart disease, stroke and certain types of cancers. This has been attributed to a lipid-lowering effect and to the presence of protective substances, such as vitamin and non-vitamin antioxidants and other vitamins such as folic acid, which is linked to homocysteine metabolism, a risk factor for cardiovascular disease. Fermentation of fibre in the colon may protect against the development of colonic cancer. However, associated lifestyle factors, such as low physical activity, may also help explain some of those associations.

Health promotion

Many chronic diseases – particularly obesity, diabetes mellitus and cardiovascular disease – cause premature mortality and morbidity, and are potentially preventable by dietary change. This is a global problem; for example, obesity affects 1 in 9 adults in the world, and the body mass index (BMI) is now similar in high- and middle-income groups. Reduction in salt and fat intake, combined with exercise and stopping smoking, would have a major effect on the health of the population.

Box 10.5 suggests the composition of the 'ideal healthy diet'. The values given are based on the principle of:

- reducing total fat in the diet, particularly saturated fat
- increasing consumption of fish, which contains *n*-3 (or ω-3) PUFAs
- increasing intake of whole-grain cereals and green and orange vegetables and fruits, leading to an increase in fibre and antioxidants.

Reductions in dietary sodium and cholesterol have also been suggested. There would be no disadvantage in this, and most studies have suggested some benefit.

Fortification of foods

Fortification of foods with specific nutrients is common. In the UK, ***margarine*** and ***milk*** are fortified with vitamins A and D, ***flour*** with calcium, iron, thiamine and niacin, and ***breakfast cereals*** with several vitamins and iron. Not all substances used in fortification have nutritive value. For example, ***Olestra***, a polymer of sucrose and six or more triglycerides, has been used to combat obesity. It is not absorbed and is therefore used particularly in savoury snack foods (where it has FDA approval) as a 'fake fat'. Therefore, it results in a reduction in total calories. It has side-effects, such as loose stools and abdominal cramps, and its use is being carefully monitored.

Nutrient goals and dietary guidelines

The interests of the individual are often different from those associated with government policy. A distinction needs to be made between nutrient goals and dietary guidelines:

- ***Nutrient goals*** refer to the national intakes of nutrients that are considered appropriate for optimal health in the population.
- ***Dietary guidelines*** refer to the dietary methods used to achieve these goals.

Since dietary habits vary in different countries, dietary guidelines may also differ, even when the nutrient goals are the same. Nutrient goals are based on scientific information that links nutrient intake to disease. Although the information is incomplete, it includes evidence from a wide range of sources, including experimental animal studies, clinical studies, and both short-term and long-term epidemiological studies.

Further reading

Black RE, Victora CG, Walker SP et al. Maternal and child undernutrition and overweight in low-income and middle-income countries. *Lancet* 2013; 382:427–451.

Bosch J, Gerstein HC, Dagenais GR et al. n-3 fatty acids and cardiovascular outcomes in patients with dysglycemia. *N Engl J Med* 2012; 367:309–318.

Estruch R, Ros E, Salas-Salvado J et al. Primary prevention of cardiovascular disease with a Mediterranean diet. *N Engl J Med* 2013; 368:1279–1290.

Institute of Medicine. *Dietary Reference Intakes for Energy, Carbohydrate, Fiber, Fat, Fatty Acids, Protein, and Amino Acids*. Washington DC: National Academies Press; 2005.

Panel on Dietary Reference Values of the Committee on Medical Aspects of Food Policy. *Dietary Reference for Food Energy and Nutrients for the United Kingdom (Report 41DOH)*. London: HMSO; 1991.

Roncaglioni MC, Tombesi M, Avanzini F et al. n-3 fatty acids in patients with multiple cardiovascular risk factors. *N Engl J Med* 2013; 368:1800–1808.

Scientific Advisory Committee on Nutrition 2011. *Dietary Reference Values for Energy*. London: Stationery Office; 2012.

PROTEIN–ENERGY MALNUTRITION

Developed countries

Starvation uncomplicated by disease is relatively uncommon in developed countries, although some degree of under-nourishment is seen in very poor areas. Most nutritional problems occurring in the population at large are due to eating wrong combinations of foodstuffs, such as an excess of refined carbohydrate or a diet low in fresh vegetables. Under-nourishment associated with disease is common in hospitals and nursing homes, and ***Box 10.6*** gives a list of conditions in which malnutrition is often seen. Surgical complications, with sepsis, are a common cause. Many patients are admitted to hospital under-nourished, and a variety of chronic conditions predispose to this state ***(Box 10.7)***.

The majority of the weight loss, leading to malnutrition, is due to ***poor intake secondary to the anorexia associated with the underlying condition***. Disease may also contribute by causing malabsorption and increased catabolism, which is mediated by complex changes in cytokines, hormones, side-effects of drugs, and immobility. The elderly are particularly at risk of malnutrition because they often suffer from diseases and psychosocial problems, such as social isolation or bereavement ***(Box 10.7)***.

Pathophysiology of starvation

In the first 24 h following low dietary intake, the body relies for energy on the breakdown of hepatic glycogen to glucose

Box 10.6 Common conditions associated with protein–energy malnutrition

- Sepsis
- Trauma
- Surgery, particularly of the gastrointestinal tract with complications
- Gastrointestinal disease, particularly involving the small bowel
- Dementia
- Malignancy
- Any very ill patient
- Severe chronic inflammatory diseases
- Psychosocial: poverty, social isolation, anorexia nervosa, depression

Box 10.7 Nutritional consequences of disease and the underlying risk factors (physical/psychosocial problems)

Risk factors	Consequence
Underlying disease	
Almost any moderate/severe chronic disease Recovery from severe acute/subacute disease	Anorexia, increased requirements for some nutrients, and other effects indicated below (depending on condition)
Physical problems	
Muscle weakness (respiratory and peripheral muscles) and/or incoordination Severe arthritis in hands and arms	Problems with shopping, cooking and eating
Swallowing problem (neurological causes), painful or obstructive conditions of mouth and GIT*	Inadequate food intake, and/or risk of aspiration pneumonia
GIT symptoms (e.g. nausea, vomiting, diarrhoea, jaundice)	Food aversion, malabsorption (small bowel disease), anorexia
Sensory deficit (e.g. impaired sight, hearing and other deficits)	Difficulties in shopping, cooking and/or decreased intake of food
Psychosocial problems	
Loneliness, depression, bereavement, confusion, living alone, poverty, alcoholism, drug addiction	Self-neglect, inadequate intake of food or quality of food
Multiple drug use (polypharmacy)	Indication of severe disease or multiple physical and psychosocial problems; drugs may lead to confusion, sedation, depression and GIT side-effects (including malabsorption of nutrients)

*GIT, gastrointestinal tract.

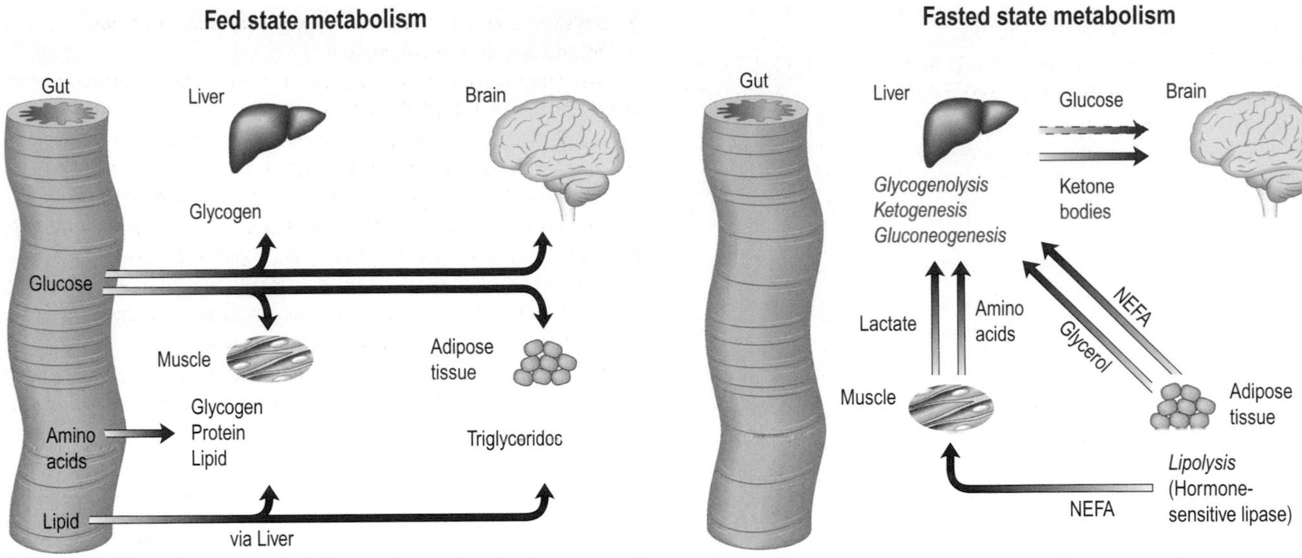

Figure 10.4 Metabolism in the fed and the fasted state. NEFA, non-esterified fatty acids.

(Fig. 10.4). Hepatic glycogen stores are small and therefore gluconeogenesis is soon necessary to maintain glucose levels. Gluconeogenesis takes place mainly from pyruvate, lactate, glycerol and amino acids, especially alanine and glutamine. The majority of protein breakdown takes place in muscle, with eventual loss of muscle bulk.

Lipolysis, the breakdown of the body's fat stores, also occurs. It is inhibited by insulin, but the level of this hormone falls off as starvation continues. The stored triglyceride is hydrolysed by lipase to glycerol, which is used for gluconeogenesis, and also to non-esterified fatty acids, which can be used directly as a fuel or oxidized in the liver to ketone bodies.

Adaptive processes take place as starvation continues, to prevent the body's available protein being completely utilized. There is a decrease in metabolic rate and total body energy expenditure. Central nervous metabolism changes from glucose as a substrate to ketone bodies. Gluconeogenesis in the liver decreases, as does protein breakdown in muscle, both of these processes being inhibited directly by ketone bodies. Most of the energy at this stage comes from adipose tissue, with some gluconeogenesis from amino acids, particularly from alanine in the liver and glutamine in the kidney.

The ***metabolic response to prolonged starvation*** differs between lean and obese individuals. One of the major differences concerns the proportion of energy derived from protein oxidation, which determines the proportion of weight loss from lean tissues. This proportion may be up to three times smaller in obese subjects than lean subjects. It can be regarded as an adaptation that depends on the composition of the initial reserves (see ***Fig. 10.3***). This means that deterioration in body function is more rapid in lean subjects, and survival time shorter in lean subjects (approximately 2 months) compared to the obese (in whom it can be at least several months).

Following trauma or shock, some of the adaptive changes do not take place. Glucocorticoids and cytokines (see below) stimulate the ubiquitin–proteasome pathway in muscle, which is responsible for accelerated proteolysis in muscle in many catabolic illnesses. In starvation, there is a decrease in BMR, while in inflammatory and traumatic disease, there is often an increase in BMR. These changes all result in continuing gluconeogenesis with massive muscle breakdown, and further reduction in survival time.

Regulation of metabolism

Tissue metabolism is regulated by multiple coordinated processes. Some are rapid, involving nerves, whilst others are slower, involving circulating substrates and hormones. Factors include:

- ***Circulating substrate concentrations***. The uptake and metabolism of ketone bodies, which serve as the major fuel for the brain during prolonged starvation, are primarily determined by the circulatory concentration, which can increase up to 5 mmol/L or more. The liver is responsible for the production of ketone bodies, which is, in turn, controlled by the availability of fatty acids derived from adipose tissue. Substrates may also compete with each other for metabolism; e.g. glucose competes with non-esterified fatty acids for uptake and metabolism in muscle and heart (the glucose–fatty acid cycle), and this is independent of hormones.
- ***Blood flow***. The delivery of substrates (and other signals) to tissues depends not only on their circulating concentration but also on the blood flow to tissues. In many tissues, there is coupling between metabolic activity and blood flow, with arterioles regulating blood flow to the tissue according to demand; e.g. blood flow to muscle increases during exercise.
- ***Signals***. Hormones and other signals, such as cytokines (see below), regulate intracellular metabolism.

Insulin/glucagon ratios in the fed and fasted state

In the fed state, insulin/glucagon ratios are high. Insulin promotes synthesis of glycogen, protein and fat, and inhibits lipolysis and gluconeogenesis.

In the fasted state, insulin/glucagon ratios are low. Glucagon acts mainly on the liver and has no action on muscle. It increases glycogenolysis and gluconeogenesis, as well as increasing ketone body production from fatty acids. It also stimulates lipolysis in adipose tissue. Catecholamines have a similar action to glucagon but also affect muscle metabolism. These agents both act via cyclic adenosine monophosphate (cAMP) to stimulate lipolysis, producing free fatty acids that can then act as a major source of energy.

Proportion of lean to fat tissue

During weight loss uncomplicated by disease, the proportion of lean to fat tissue loss (or proportion of energy derived from protein metabolism) is greater in lean than overweight/obese individuals.

During acute disease, loss of lean tissue, which is associated with protein oxidation, can be particularly rapid. Hormones such as corticosteroids, pro-inflammatory cytokines and insulin resistance are all involved.

Role of cytokines

The metabolic response to trauma, injury and inflammation depends on the balance between *pro*-inflammatory (e.g. tumour necrosis factor, TNF; interleukin-2, IL-2) and *anti*-inflammatory cytokines (e.g. IL-10), and the production of many of these cytokines is influenced by genetic polymorphisms. Since many chronic diseases, including atherosclerosis, have an inflammatory component, these changes have wide-reaching metabolic implications.

Cytokines such as IL-1, IL-6 and TNF play a significant role in regulating metabolism. In acute diseases, they contribute to the catabolic process, glycogenolysis, and acute phase protein synthesis. TNF, which inhibits lipoprotein lipase, is one of a number of 'cachexia factors' in patients with cancer.

It is unclear how these cytokines interact with central feeding pathways to cause anorexia. However, in animal models of both cancer and inflammatory bowel disease, many peripheral and central mediators of appetite are involved. For example, neuropeptide Y levels in the hypothalamus are often inappropriately low, so there is a reduced drive to feed.

Clinical features

Patients are sometimes seen with loss of weight or malnutrition (failure to thrive in children) as the primary symptom. Mostly, however, malnourishment is only seen as an accompaniment of some other disease process, such as malignancy. Severe malnutrition is seen mainly with advanced organic disease or after surgical procedures followed by complications. Three key features that help in the detection of chronic protein–energy malnutrition (PEM) in adults are listed in ***Box 10.8***.

Other factors that may suggest PEM include:

- history of decreased food intake/loss of appetite
- clothes becoming loose-fitting (weight loss) and a general appearance indicating obvious wasting
- physical and psychosocial disturbances likely to have contributed to the weight loss.

The factors listed in ***Box 10.8*** act as a link between detection and management (see also ***Fig. 10.5***, the Malnutrition Universal Screening Tool). If the underlying physical or psychosocial problems are not addressed adequately, treatment may not be successful.

PEM leads to a depression of the immunological defence mechanism, resulting in a decreased resistance to infection. It also detrimentally affects muscle strength and fatigue, reproductive function (e.g. in anorexia nervosa, which is common in adolescent girls; see pp. 927–928), wound healing and psychological function (depression, anxiety, hypochondriasis, loss of libido).

In children, growth failure is a key element in the diagnosis of PEM. WHO standards for optimal growth in children of 0–4 years

Box 10.8 Keys to detecting chronic protein–energy malnutrition (PEM) in developed countries

1. Body mass index (BMI)
- Probable chronic PEM: <18.5 kg/m²
- Possible chronic PEM: 18.5–20 kg/m²
- Little or no risk of chronic PEM: >20 kg/m²

In patients with oedema or dehydration the BMI may be somewhat misleading.

2. Weight loss in previous 3–6 months
- >10%: high risk of developing PEM
- 5–10%: possible risk of developing PEM
- <5%: low/no risk of developing PEM

3. Acute disease effect
- Diseases that have resulted or are likely to result in no dietary intake for >5 days (e.g. prolonged unconsciousness, persistent swallowing problems after a stroke, or prolonged ileus after abdominal surgery): high risk of malnutrition

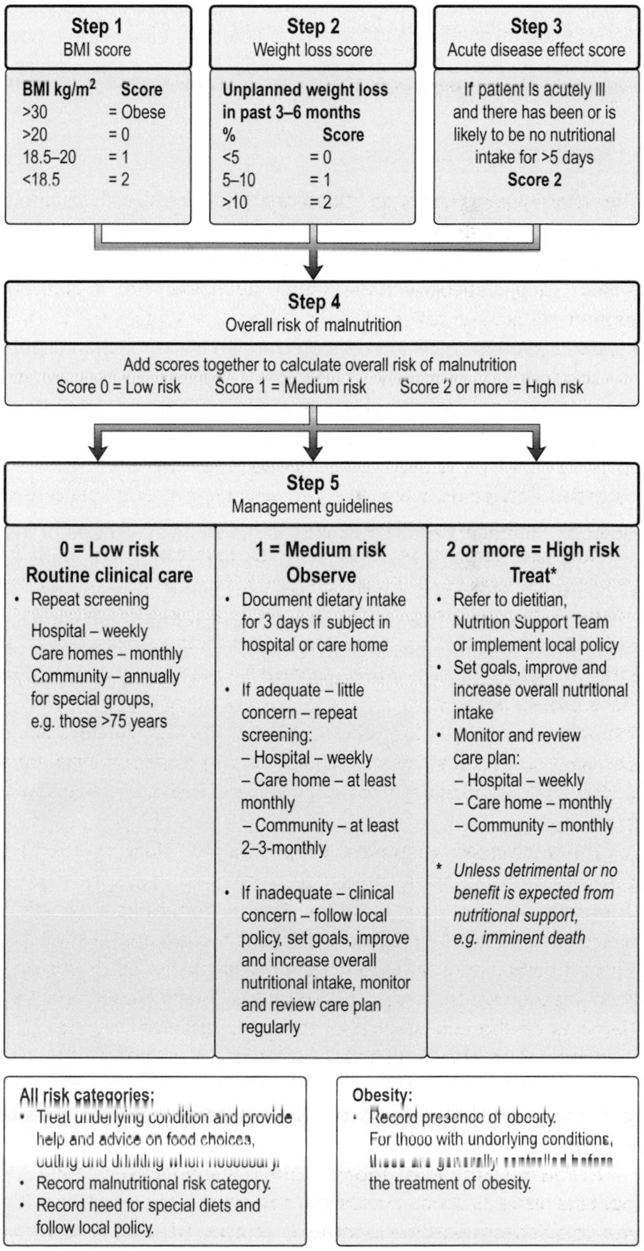

Figure 10.5 **Malnutrition Universal Screening Tool (MUST).** BMI, body mass index. *(With permission from the British Association for Parenteral and Enteral Nutrition (BAPEN), at:* http://www.bapen.org.uk.*)*

have been adopted by developing and developed countries. They aim to reflect optimal rather than prevailing growth in both developed and developing countries, since they involved a healthy pregnancy and children born to non-smoking, relatively affluent mothers who breast-fed their children exclusively or predominantly for the first 6 months of life. The general principles of management of severe PEM in children are similar in developed and developing countries but resources are required to manage the problems once they have been identified (see p. 194).

Management

When malnutrition is obvious and the underlying disease cannot be corrected at once, some form of nutritional support is necessary (see also pp. 212 and 214). Nutrition should be given enterally if the gastrointestinal tract is functioning adequately. This can be done most easily by encouraging the patient to eat more often and by giving a high-calorie supplement. If this is not possible, a liquefied diet may be given intragastrically via a fine-bore tube or by a percutaneous endoscopic gastrostomy (PEG). If both of these measures fail, parenteral nutrition is given.

Developing countries

The International Union of Nutritional Sciences, with support from the International Pediatric Association, launched a global Malnutrition Task Force in 2005 to ensure that an integrated system of prevention and treatment of malnutrition is actively supported.

In many areas of the world, people are on the verge of malnutrition due to extreme poverty. In addition, if events such as drought, war or changes in political climate occur, millions suffer from starvation.

Clinical features

Although the basic condition of PEM is the same in all parts of the world, whatever the cause, malnutrition resulting from long periods of near-total starvation produces unique clinical appearances in children that are virtually never seen in high-income countries. The term 'protein–energy malnutrition' covers the spectrum of clinical conditions seen in adults and children. Children under 5 years may present with the following:

- ***Kwashiorkor*** occurs typically in a young child displaced from breast-feeding by a new baby. It is often precipitated by infections such as measles, malaria and diarrhoeal illnesses. The child is apathetic and lethargic with severe anorexia. There is generalized oedema with skin pigmentation and thickening ***(Fig. 10.6B)***. The hair is dry and sparse, and may become reddish or yellow in colour. The abdomen is distended owing to hepatomegaly and/or ascites. The serum albumin is always low. The exact cause is unknown, but theories related to diet (low in protein and high in carbohydrate) and free radical damage in the presence of inadequate antioxidant defences have been proposed.
- ***Marasmus*** is the childhood form of starvation, which is associated with obvious wasting. The child looks emaciated, and there is obvious muscle wasting and loss of body fat. There is no oedema. The hair is thin and dry ***(Fig. 10.6A)***. The child is not so apathetic or anorexic as with kwashiorkor. Diarrhoea is frequently present and signs of infection must be looked for carefully.

The ***WHO classification of severe malnutrition (Box 10.9)*** makes no distinction between kwashiorkor and marasmus because

Box 10.9 Classification of childhood malnutrition

	Moderate malnutrition	Severe malnutrition[a]
Symmetrical oedema	No	Yes: oedematous malnutrition[b]
Weight-for-height SD score	–3 to –2 (70–79%)[c]	<–3 (<70%)[c] (severe wasting)[d]
Height-for-age SD score	–3 to –2 (85–89%)[c]	<–3 (<85%)[c] (severe stunting)

[a]The diagnoses are not mutually exclusive. [b]Older classifications use the terms kwashiorkor and marasmic kwashiorkor instead. [c]Percentage of the median National Centre for Health Statistics/WHO reference. [d]Called marasmus (without oedema) in the Wellcome classification and grade II in the Gomez classification.

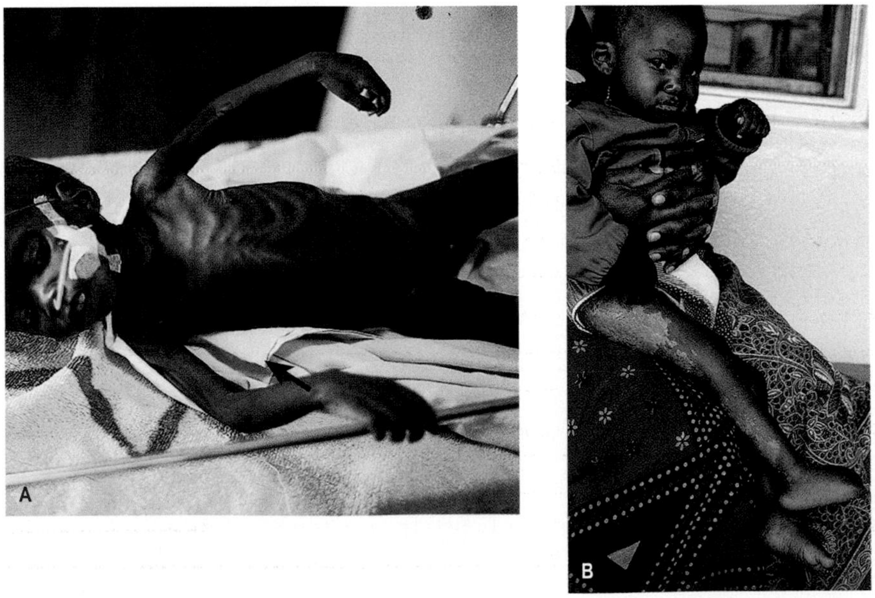

Figure 10.6 **Malnourished children. A.** Marasmus. **B.** Kwashiorkor. *(Courtesy of Dr Paul Kelly.)*

the approach to treatment is similar in both. The WHO classification of chronic under-nutrition in children is based on standard deviation (SD) scores. Thus, children with an SD score between –2 and –3 (between 3 and 2 SD scores below the median, corresponding to a value between 0.13 and 2.3 centiles) can be regarded as being at moderate risk of under-nutrition; below an SD score of –3, there is a risk of severe malnutrition. A low weight-for-height is a measure of thinness (wasting when pathological) and a low height-for-age is a measure of shortness (stunting when pathological). Those with oedema and clinical signs of severe malnutrition are classified as having oedematous malnutrition.

Starvation in adults may lead to extreme loss of weight, depending on the severity and duration. They may crave food, are apathetic, and complain of cold and weakness with a loss of subcutaneous fat and muscle wasting. The WHO classification is based on BMI, with a value <18.5 kg/m^2 indicating malnutrition (severe malnutrition if <16.0 kg/m^2).

Severely malnourished adults and children are very susceptible to respiratory and gastrointestinal infections, leading to an increased mortality in these groups.

Investigations

These are not always practicable in certain settings in the developing world.

- ***Blood tests*** may demonstrate the following results:
  - Anaemia due to folate, iron and copper deficiency is often present, but the haematocrit may be high owing to dehydration.
  - Eosinophilia suggests parasitic infestation.
  - Electrolyte disturbances are common.
  - Malarial parasites should be sought.
  - Human immunodeficiency (HIV) tests should be performed.
- ***Stools*** should be examined for parasitic infestations.
- ***Chest X-ray*** may reveal tuberculosis, which is common and easily missed if a chest X-ray is not performed.

Management

Management must involve the provision of protein and energy supplements and the control of infection. The approach to the treatment of children is described below. Adults do not usually suffer such severe malnutrition but the same general principles of treatment should be followed.

Resuscitation and stabilization

The severely ill child will require:

- correction of fluid and electrolyte abnormalities, avoiding intravenous therapy, if possible, because of the danger of fluid overload
- treatment of shock with oxygen
- treatment of hypoglycaemia (blood glucose <3 mmol/L), hypothermia (reduce heat loss, and provide additional heat if necessary) and infection (antibiotics) – these often co-exist.

The standard WHO ***oral hydration solution*** has a high sodium and low potassium content and is not suitable for severely malnourished children. Instead, the rehydration solution for malnutrition (ReSoMal) is recommended. It is commercially available but can also be produced by modification of the standard WHO oral hydration solution.

Infection is common ***(Box 10.10)***. Diarrhoea is often due to bacterial or protozoal overgrowth; metronidazole is very effective and is often given routinely. Parasites are also common and, as facilities for stool examination are usually not available, mebendazole 100 mg twice daily should be given for 3 days. In high-risk areas, antimalarial therapy is given. A recent study in Malawi suggests that the addition of antibiotics to therapeutic regimes for uncomplicated severe acute malnutrition in children less than 5 years of age is associated with a significant improvement in recovery and mortality.

Large doses of ***vitamin A*** are also given because deficiency of this vitamin is common. After the initial resuscitation, further stabilization over the next few days is undertaken, as indicated in ***Box 10.11***.

Box 10.10 Infections seen in PEM in developing countries

- Diarrhoea
  - Bacteria
  - Protozoa
  - Helminths
- Malaria
- Tuberculosis
- HIV infection
- Measles
- Respiratory infections

Box 10.11 Timeframe for the management of the child with severe malnutrition (10-step approach recommended by WHO)

Management	Stabilization		Rehabilitation	Follow-up
	Days 1–2	*Days 3–7*	*Weeks 2–6*	*Weeks 7–26*
1. Treat or prevent hypoglycaemia	→			
2. Treat or prevent hypothermia	→			
3. Treat or prevent dehydration	→			
4. Correct electrolyte imbalance	→	→	→	
5. Treat infection	→	→		
6. Correct micronutrient deficiencies	Without iron		With iron →	
7. Begin feeding	→	→		
8. Increase feeding to recover lost weight			→	→
9. Stimulate emotional and sensorial development	→	→	→	→
10. Prepare for discharge			→	

Re-feeding

This needs to be planned carefully. During the initial management of the acute situation, a balanced diet with sufficient protein and energy is given to maintain a steady state. Large increases in energy can lead to heart failure, circulatory collapse and death (***re-feeding syndrome***). Initial feeding involves the administration of feeds that are low in osmolarity and low in lactose. WHO recommendations are 100 kcal/kg per day; 1.0–1.5 g protein/kg per day; and 130 mL liquid/kg per day (100 mL/kg per day if the child has marked oedema). Attempts should be made to give the feeds slowly and frequently (e.g. 2-hourly during days 1–2; 3-hourly during days 3–5; and 4-hourly thereafter), although anorexia is often a problem and can be exacerbated by excessive feeding. If necessary, fluids and food should be given by nasogastric tube. The child is then gradually weaned to liquids and then solids by mouth. All severely malnourished children have vitamin and mineral deficiencies. Although anaemia is common, the WHO recommends giving iron only after the child develops a good appetite and starts gaining weight, because of concern about detrimental effects during the acute phase of illness (iron is a pro-oxidant). The child should be given daily micronutrient supplements for at least 2 weeks. These should include a multivitamin supplement with folic acid, zinc and copper.

Rehabilitation

Gradually, as the child improves, more energy can be given, and during rehabilitation, weight gain is achieved by providing extra energy and protein ('catch-up weight gain'). Children who have been severely ill need constant attention right through the convalescent period, as home conditions are often poor and feeds are refused. Sensory stimulation and emotional support are major components of management during both the stabilization and the rehabilitation phases. The treatment of underlying chronic infective conditions, such as HIV, malaria and tuberculosis, is also necessary.

Care setting

There are not enough hospitals or therapeutic feeding centres to cope with the malnutrition problem (even acute malnutrition problems); this emphasizes the need for outpatient and community-based programmes, although these require investment and time to build to full capacity. The programmes may involve the use of ready-to-use therapeutic foods, such as energy-dense pastes with minerals and vitamins, without the need to add water, which could potentially contaminate the food.

Prognosis

Children with extreme malnutrition have a mortality of over 50%. By careful management, this can be reduced significantly to less than 10%, depending on the availability of facilities and trained staff. Treatment of underlying disease is essential. Brain development takes place in the first years of life, a time when severe PEM is frequently seen. There is evidence that intellectual impairment and behavioural abnormalities occur in severely affected children. Physical growth is also impaired. Probably both of these effects can be alleviated if it is possible to maintain a high standard of living with a good diet and freedom from infection over a long period.

Prevention

Prevention of PEM depends not only on the availability of adequate nutrients but also on the education of both governments and individuals in the importance of good nutrition and immunization

Box 10.12 Prevention of protein–energy malnutrition–GOBIF (a WHO priority programme)

- Growth monitoring: the WHO has a simple growth chart that the mother keeps
- Oral rehydration, particularly for diarrhoea
- Breast-feeding supplemented by food after 6 months
- Immunization: against measles, tetanus, pertussis, diphtheria, polio and tuberculosis (see also ***Box 11.19***)
- Family planning

(Box 10.12). Short-term programmes are useful for acute shortages of food, but long-term programmes involving improved agriculture are equally necessary. Bad feeding practices and infections are more prevalent than actual shortage of food in many areas of the world. However, good surveillance is necessary to avoid periods of famine.

Food supplements (and additional vitamins) should be given to 'at-risk' groups by adding high-energy food (e.g. milk powder, meat concentrates) to the diet. Pregnancy and lactation are times of high energy requirement and supplements have been shown to be beneficial.

Further reading

Black RE, Victora CG, Walker SP et al. Maternal and child undernutrition and overweight in low-income and middle-income countries. *Lancet* 2013; 382:427–451.

Cawood AL, Elia M, Stratton RJ. Systematic review and meta-analysis of the effects of high protein oral nutritional supplements. *Ageing Res Rev* 2012; 11:278–296.

Collins PF, Elia M, Stratton RJ. Nutritional support and functional capacity in chronic obstructive pulmonary disease: a systematic review and meta-analysis. *Respirology* 2013; 18:616–629.

Elia M. Multidisciplinary input is essential in the care of malnourished people. *Guidelines in Practice* 2013; 16:42–50.

Trehan I, Goldbach HS, Lacey N et al. Antibiotics as part of the management of severe acute malnutrition. *N Engl J Med* 2013; 368:425–435.

World Health Organization. *Guideline: Updates on the Management of Severe Acute Malnutrition in Infants and Children*. WHO: Geneva; 2013.

Wright CM, Williams AF, Ellman D et al. Using the new UK-WHO growth charts. *BMJ* 2010; 340:647–650 (charts and supporting materials: http://www.growthcharts.rcpch.ac.uk).

VITAMINS

Deficiencies due to inadequate intake associated with PEM ***(Box 10.13)*** are commonly seen in the developing countries. This is not, however, invariable. For example, vitamin A deficiency is not seen in Jamaica, but is common in PEM in Hyderabad, India. In the West, deficiency of vitamins is less common but prominent in the specific groups shown in ***Box 10.14***. The widespread use of vitamins as 'tonics' is unnecessary and should be discouraged. Toxicity from excess fat-soluble vitamins is occasionally seen.

FAT-SOLUBLE VITAMINS

Vitamin A

Vitamin A (retinol) is part of the family of retinoids, which is present in food and the body as esters combined with long-chain fatty acids. The richest food source is liver, but it is also found in milk, butter, cheese, egg yolks and fish oils. Retinol or carotene is added to margarine in the UK and other countries.

Box 10.13 Fat-soluble and water-soluble vitamins: UK reference nutrient intake (RNI) and lower reference nutrient intake (LRNI) for men aged 19–50 years[a]

Vitamin	RNI/day (sufficient)	LRNI/day (insufficient)	Major clinical features of deficiency	Dietary sources
Fat-soluble				
A (retinol)	700 µg	300 µg	Xerophthalmia, night blindness, keratomalacia, follicular hyperkeratosis	Oily fish, liver, dairy products (provitamin A carotenoids – carrots, dark green, leafy vegetables, corn, tomatoes)
D (cholecalciferol)	No dietary intake required	10 µg (living indoors)	Rickets, osteomalacia	Oily fish, fortified breakfast cereals and margarine, eggs, milk
K	(1 µg/kg body weight; safe and adequate)[b]		Coagulation defects	Green, leafy vegetables, liver, cheese, certain fruits (kiwi fruit, rhubarb)
E (α-tocopherol)	(15 mg)[c]		Neurological disorders, e.g. ataxia	Plant oils (soya, palm oil), animal fats, nuts, seeds, vegetables, wheatgerm
Water-soluble				
B_1 (thiamine)	0.4 mg/1000 kcal[d]	0.23 mg/1000 kcal[d]	Beriberi, Wernicke–Korsakoff syndrome	Wide range of animal and vegetable products. Fortified cereals, flour and bread, unrefined cereals, grain, nuts, legumes, organ meats
B_2 (riboflavin)	1.3 mg	0.8 mg	Angular stomatitis	Dairy products (major source), cereals grains, meat, fish, broccoli, spinach
Niacin	6.6 mg/1000 kcal	4.4 mg/1000 kcal	Pellagra	Meat, cereals
B_6 (pyridoxine)	15 µg/g of dietary protein	11 µg/g of dietary protein	Polyneuropathy	Meat, cereals
B_{12} (cobalamin)	1.5 µg	1.0 µg	Megaloblastic anaemia, neurological disorders	Meat, fortified breakfast cereals, eggs
Folate	200 µg	100 µg	Megaloblastic anaemia	Widely distributed in animal (especially liver) and plant foods (e.g. vegetables)
C (ascorbic acid)	40 mg	10 mg	Scurvy	Fresh vegetables, citrus fruits, strawberries, spinach, tomatoes

[a]Values vary with age and sex. For women, values are generally the same or lower than for men, except during pregnancy and lactation, when they are generally higher than for men. [b]No RNI. [c]No official RNI in the UK because the amount varies, depending on the polyunsaturated fatty acid content of the diet; 15 mg is the value from the National Academy of Sciences, USA. [d]Thiamine requirements are related to energy metabolism.

Box 10.14 Some causes of vitamin deficiency in developed countries

Decreased intake
- Alcohol dependency: chiefly B vitamins (e.g. thiamine)
- Small bowel disease: chiefly folate, occasionally fat-soluble vitamins
- Vegans: vitamin D (if no exposure to sunlight), vitamin B_{12}
- Elderly with poor diet: chiefly vitamin D (if no exposure to sunlight), folate
- Anorexia from any cause: chiefly folate

Decreased absorption
- Ileal disease/resection: only vitamin B_{12}
- Liver and biliary tract disease: fat-soluble vitamins
- Intestinal bacterial overgrowth: vitamin B_{12}
- Oral antibiotics: vitamin K

Miscellaneous
- Long-term enteral or parenteral nutrition: usually vitamin supplements are given
- Renal disease: vitamin D
- Drug antagonists (e.g. methotrexate interfering with folate metabolism)

Beta-carotene is the main carotenoid found in green vegetables, carrots and other yellow and red fruits. Other carotenoids, lycopene and lutein, are probably of little quantitative importance as dietary precursors of vitamin A.

Beta-carotene is cleaved in the intestinal mucosa by carotene dioxygenase, yielding retinaldehyde, which can be reduced to retinol. Between a quarter and a third of dietary vitamin A in the UK is derived from retinoids. Nutritionally, 6 µg of β-carotene is equivalent to 1 µg of preformed retinol; vitamin A activity in the diet is given as retinol equivalents.

Function

Retinol is stored in the liver and is transported in plasma bound to an α-globulin, retinol-binding protein (RBP). Vitamin A has several metabolic roles:

- Retinaldehyde in its *cis* form is found in the opsin proteins in the rods (rhodopsin) and cones (iodopsin) of the retina (see p. 1324). Light causes retinaldehyde to change to its *trans* isomer, and this leads to changes in membrane potentials that are transmitted to the brain.
- Retinol and retinoic acid are involved in the control of cell proliferation and differentiation.
- Retinyl phosphate is a co-factor in the synthesis of most glycoproteins containing mannose.

Vitamin A deficiency

Worldwide, vitamin A deficiency and xerophthalmia (see below) are the major causes of blindness in young children, despite intensive preventative programmes.

Xerophthalmia has been classified by the WHO ***(Box 10.15)***. Impaired adaptation, followed by night blindness, is the first effect. There is dryness and thickening of the conjunctiva and the cornea

Box 10.15 Classification of xerophthalmia (X) by ocular signs

Ocular signs	Classification
Night blindness	XN
Conjunctival xerosis	XIA
Bitot's spot	X2
Corneal xerosis	X2
Corneal ulceration/keratomalacia < ⅓ corneal surface	X3A
Corneal ulceration/keratomalacia > ⅓ corneal surface	X3B
Corneal scar	XS
Xerophthalmic fundus	XF

(From WHO/UNICEF/IVACG 1988.)

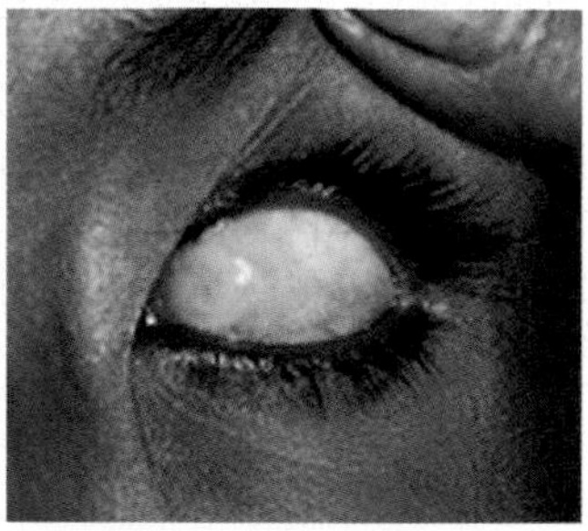

Figure 10.7 Vitamin A deficiency. Blindness due to vitamin A deficiency and corneal scarring. *(Courtesy of Ehrnstrom P. In: Bolognia J, Jorrizzo J, Rapini R (eds).* Dermatology, *2nd edn. St Louis: Mosby; 2008: Fig. 51.6.)*

(xerophthalmia occurs as a result of keratinization). Bitot's spots – white plaques of keratinized epithelial cells – are found on the conjunctiva of young children with vitamin A deficiency. These spots can, however, be seen without vitamin A deficiency, possibly caused by exposure. Corneal softening, ulceration and dissolution (keratomalacia) eventually occur, superimposed infection is a frequent accompaniment and both lead to blindness ***(Fig. 10.7)***. In PEM, retinol-binding protein is reduced, along with other proteins. This suggests vitamin A deficiency, although body stores are not necessarily reduced.

Vitamin A in malnourished children

Vitamin A supplementation (single oral dose of 60 mg retinol palmitate) appears to improve morbidity and mortality from measles. It has also been suggested that similar supplementation reduces morbidity and/or mortality from diarrhoeal diseases and respiratory infections, and improves growth. Despite low circulating concentrations of vitamin A in HIV-infected individuals, supplementation of HIV-infected pregnant women does not appear to reduce the risk of mother-to-child transmission of HIV.

Diagnosis

In parts of the world where deficiency is common, diagnosis is made on the basis of the clinical features, and deficiency should always be suspected if any degree of malnutrition is present. Blood levels of vitamin A will usually be low, but the best guide to diagnosis is a response to replacement therapy.

Management

Urgent treatment with retinol palmitate 30 mg orally should be given on two successive days. In the presence of vomiting and diarrhoea, 30 mg of vitamin A is given intramuscularly. Associated malnutrition must be treated, and superadded bacterial infection should be treated with antibiotics. Referral for specialist ophthalmic treatment is necessary in severe cases.

Prevention

Most Western diets contain enough dairy products and green vegetables, but vitamin A is added to foodstuffs (e.g. margarine) in some countries. Vitamin A is not destroyed by cooking.

In some developing countries, vitamin A supplements are given at the time a child attends for measles vaccination. Food fortification programmes are another approach. Education of the population is necessary and people should be encouraged to grow their own vegetables. In particular, pregnant women and children should be encouraged to eat green vegetables and yellow fruits.

Other effects of vitamin A

In a chronically malnourished population, maternal repletion with vitamin A before, during and after pregnancy may improve lung function in the offspring at 9–13 years. It may also reduce maternal mortality. Administration of vitamin A to young children at risk of deficiency reduces mortality, although to a lesser extent than previously thought. The effect of β-carotene in cardiovascular and other diseases is discussed below in the section entitled 'Dietary antioxidants' (see p. 201). Retinoic acid and some synthetic retinoids are used in dermatology (see ***Box 31.10***).

Possible adverse effects

- ***High intakes of vitamin A***. Chronic ingestion of retinol can cause liver and bone damage, hair loss, double vision, vomiting, headaches and other abnormalities. Single doses of 300 mg in adults or 100 mg in children can be harmful.
- ***Retinol is teratogenic***. The incidence of birth defects in infants is high with vitamin A intakes of >3 mg a day during pregnancy. In pregnancy, extra vitamin A or consumption of liver is not recommended in the UK. However, β-carotene is not toxic.

Vitamin D

Vitamin D is discussed in more detail in Chapter 19, where the most common manifestations of deficiency are discussed (rickets and osteomalacia). Vitamin D status is assessed by measurement of 25 hydroxyvitamin D in the serum. Vitamin D receptors are distributed widely in human tissues but their function in many non-musculoskeletal tissues still remains poorly understood. Vitamin D status has been linked to a wide range of diseases, including:

- cardiovascular disorders (ischaemic heart disease, heart failure, hypertension)
- respiratory disorders (chest infections)
- renal disorders (progression of renal disease)
- endocrine disorders (type 1 and type 2 diabetes)
- neuropsychiatric disorders (depression, cognitive deficits)
- cancer (e.g. prostate, breast, colon) and mortality from various causes.
- Multiple sclerosis (see p. 858)

It has therefore been suggested that vitamin D may have a role in global health, and not just the health of the musculoskeletal system. Studies of the relationship between vitamin D serum levels (25 hydroxyvitamin D) and the risk of the conditions listed above have led to different definitions of the optimal level of 25 hydroxyvitamin D for adequate status. This also implies that there are different requirements for vitamin D in different diseases. However, randomized controlled trials (RCTs) of vitamin D supplementation have not been as promising in averting some of these conditions as might have been anticipated from the observational relationships. Reduced circulating concentrations of vitamin D can result not only from lack of exposure to sunlight and a poor diet, but also from inflammation, smoking and obesity.

Vitamin K

Vitamin K is found as phylloquinone (vitamin K_1) in green, leafy vegetables, dairy products, rapeseed and soya bean oils. Intestinal bacteria can synthesize the other major form of vitamin K, menaquinone (vitamin K_2), in the terminal ileum and colon. Vitamin K is absorbed in a similar manner to other fat-soluble substances in the upper small gut. Some menaquinones must also be absorbed, as this is the major form found in the human liver.

Function

Vitamin K is a co-factor that is necessary for the production not only of blood clotting factors (II, VII, IX and X, and other proteins involved in coagulation; see p. 573), but also of proteins that are necessary for the formation of bone.

Vitamin K is a co-factor for the post-translational carboxylation of specific protein-bound glutamate residues in γ-carboxyglutamate (Gla). Gla residues bind calcium ions to phospholipid templates, and this action on factors II, VII, IX and X, and on proteins C and S, is required for coagulation to take place.

Bone osteoblasts contain three vitamin K-dependent proteins: osteocalcin, matrix Gla protein and protein S, which have a role in bone matrix formation. Osteocalcin contains three Gla residues, which bind tightly to the hydroxyapatite matrix, depending on the degree of carboxylation; this leads to bone mineralization. There is, however, no convincing evidence that vitamin K deficiency or antagonism affects bone other than rapidly growing bone.

Vitamin K deficiency

Vitamin K deficiency results in inadequate synthesis of clotting factors (see p. 573), which leads to an increase in the prothrombin time and haemorrhage. It has also been linked to bone health, but there is inadequate evidence to support the routine use of vitamin K to prevent osteoporosis and reduce fracture risk. Deficiency occurs in the newborn, in cholestatic jaundice, and with concomitant use of vitamin K antagonists.

The newborn

Deficiency occurs in the newborn owing to:

- poor placental transfer of vitamin K
- the fact that there is little vitamin K in breast milk
- the lack of hepatic stores of menaquinone (no intestinal bacteria in the neonate).

Deficiency leads to a haemorrhagic disease of the newborn, which can be prevented with prophylactic vitamin K. Vitamin K (phytomenadione 1 mg, i.m.) is given to all neonates after the risks have been discussed with parents and consent has been obtained.

Cholestatic jaundice

When bile flow into the intestine is interrupted, malabsorption of vitamin K occurs, as no bile salts are available to facilitate absorption and the prothrombin time increases. This can be corrected by giving 10 mg of phytomenadione intramuscularly. (Note that an increased prothrombin time caused by liver disease does not respond to vitamin K injection, there being no shortage of vitamin K – just poor liver function.) In patients with chronic cholestasis (e.g. primary biliary cholangitis), oral therapy with a water-soluble preparation, menadiol sodium phosphate 10 mg daily, is used.

Concomitant vitamin K antagonists

Oral anticoagulants, such as warfarin, antagonize vitamin K (see pp. 578–580). Antibacterial drugs also interfere with the bacterial synthesis of vitamin K.

Vitamin E

Vitamin E includes eight naturally occurring compounds that may be divided into tocopherols and tocotrienols. The most active compound and the most widely available in food is the natural isomer d-d-α-tocopherol (or RRR-α-tocopherol), which accounts for 90% of vitamin E in the human body. Vegetables and seed oils, including soya bean, saffron, sunflower, cereals and nuts, are the main sources. Animal products are poor sources of the vitamin. Vitamin E is absorbed with fat, transported in the blood largely in LDLs.

An individual's vitamin E requirement depends on the intake of polyunsaturated fatty acids (PUFAs). Since this varies widely, no daily requirement is given in the UK. The requirement stated in the USA is approximately 7–10 mg/day, but average diets contain much more than this. If PUFAs are taken in large amounts, more vitamin E is required.

Function

The biological activity of vitamin E results principally from its antioxidant properties. In biological membranes, it contributes to membrane stability. It protects cellular structures against damage from a number of highly reactive oxygen species, including hydrogen peroxide, superoxide and other oxygen radicals. Vitamin E may also affect cell proliferation and growth.

Vitamin E deficiency

The first deficiency to be demonstrated was a haemolytic anaemia described in premature infants. Infant formulations now contain vitamin E.

Deficiency is seen only in children with abetalipoproteinaemia (see p. 402) and in patients on long-term parenteral nutrition. The severe neurological deficit (gross ataxia) can be prevented with vitamin E injections.

Plasma or serum levels of α-tocopherol can be measured and should be corrected for the level of plasma lipids by expressing the value as milligrams per milligram of plasma lipid.

Epidemiological data and clinical trials

Animals fed an atherogenic diet supplemented with α-tocopherol develop far fewer new atheromatous lesions than those fed an atherogenic diet alone; there may be regression of existing lesions.

There is also evidence for vitamin E intake and blood α-tocopherol levels as an independent risk factor for the development of ischaemic heart disease in healthy, well-nourished individuals eating a Western diet. This has been shown in comparisons of different communities in the WHO 'MONICA' observational study.

Randomized trials involving vitamin E supplementation have produced conflicting results, possibly due to factors such as short duration of treatment, use of suboptimal doses or lack of concurrent administration of vitamin C. There are very few trials to assess the role of vitamin E in prevention of peripheral vascular disease and cancer.

WATER-SOLUBLE VITAMINS

Water-soluble vitamins are non-toxic and relatively cheap; they can therefore be given in large amounts if a deficiency is possible. The daily requirements for water-soluble vitamins are given in ***Box 10.13*** (on p. 195).

Thiamine (vitamin B_1)

Function

Thiamine diphosphate, often called thiamine pyrophosphate (TPP), is an essential co-factor, particularly in carbohydrate metabolism.

TPP is involved in the oxidative decarboxylation of acetyl coenzyme A (CoA) in mitochondria. In formation of acetyl CoA (from pyruvate) and in the Krebs cycle, TPP is the key enzyme for the decarboxylation of α-ketoglutarate to succinyl CoA. TPP is also the co-factor for transketolase, a key enzyme in the hexose monophosphate shunt.

Thiamine is found in many foodstuffs, including cereals, grains, beans and nuts, as well as pork and duck. It is often added to food (e.g. in cereals) in developed countries. The dietary requirement (see ***Box 10.13***) depends on energy intake, more being required if the diet is high in carbohydrates.

Following absorption, thiamine is found in all body tissues, the majority being in the liver. Body stores are small and signs of deficiency quickly develop with inadequate intake.

There is no evidence that a high oral intake is dangerous but ataxia has been reported after high parenteral therapy.

Thiamine deficiency

Thiamine deficiency is seen:

- As ***beriberi***, where the only staple food consumed is polished rice.
- In ***chronic alcohol-dependent patients*** who are consuming virtually no food at all.
- In ***starved patients*** (e.g. with carcinoma of the stomach), and in severe prolonged hyperemesis gravidarum, anorexia nervosa and prolonged total starvation in healthy subjects (e.g. fasts for political reasons). It can also occur in patients given parenteral nutrition with little or no thiamine, as large doses of glucose increase requirements for thiamine and can precipitate deficiency (e.g. during re-feeding).

Beriberi

This is now confined to the poorest areas of South-east Asia. It can be prevented by eating under-milled or parboiled rice, or by fortification of rice with thiamine. The prevention of beriberi needs a general increase in overall food consumption so that the staple diet is varied and includes legumes and pulses, which contain a large amount of thiamine. There are two main clinical types of beriberi, which, surprisingly, only rarely occur together.

- ***Dry beriberi*** usually presents insidiously with a symmetrical polyneuropathy. The initial symptoms are heaviness and stiffness of the legs, followed by weakness, numbness, and pins and needles. The ankle jerk reflexes are lost and eventually all the signs of polyneuropathy that may involve the trunk and arms are found (see p. 885). Cerebral involvement occurs, producing the picture of the Wernicke–Korsakoff syndrome (p. 885). In endemic areas, mild symptoms and signs may be present for years without unduly affecting the patient.
- ***Wet beriberi*** causes oedema. Initially, this is of the legs, but it can extend to involve the whole body, with ascites and pleural effusions. The peripheral oedema may mask the accompanying features of dry beriberi.

Thiamine deficiency impairs pyruvate dehydrogenase with accumulation of lactate and pyruvate, producing peripheral vasodilatation and eventually oedema. The heart muscle is also affected and heart failure occurs, causing a further increase in the oedema. Initially, there are warm extremities, a full, fast, bounding pulse and a raised venous pressure ('high-output state'), but eventually heart failure advances and a poor cardiac output ensues. The electrocardiogram may show conduction defects.

Infantile beriberi occurs, usually acutely, in breast-fed babies at approximately 3 months of age. The mothers show no signs of thiamine deficiency but presumably their body stores must be virtually nil. The infant becomes anorexic, develops oedema and has some degree of aphonia. Tachycardia and tachypnoea develop and, unless treatment is instituted, death occurs quickly.

Diagnosis

In endemic areas, the diagnosis of beriberi should always be suspected; if it is in doubt, treatment with thiamine should be instituted. A rapid disappearance of oedema after thiamine (50 mg i.m.) is diagnostic. Other causes of oedema must be considered (e.g. renal or liver disease), and the polyneuropathy is indistinguishable from that due to other causes. The diagnosis is confirmed by measurement of the circulating thiamine concentration or transketolase activity in red cells using fresh heparinized blood.

Management

Thiamine 50 mg i.m. is given for 3 days, followed by 50 mg of thiamine daily by mouth. The response in wet beriberi is seen in hours, providing a dramatic improvement, but in dry beriberi improvement is often slow to occur. In most cases, all the B vitamins are given because of multiple deficiency. Infantile beriberi is treated by giving thiamine to the mother, which is then passed on to the infant via the breast milk.

Thiamine deficiency in people with alcohol dependence or acute illness

In the developed world, alcohol-dependent people and those with severe acute illness receiving high-carbohydrate infusions without vitamins are the only major groups to suffer from thiamine deficiency. Rarely, they develop wet beriberi, which must be distinguished from alcoholic cardiomyopathy. More usually, however, thiamine deficiency presents with polyneuropathy or with the ***Wernicke–Korsakoff syndrome***.

This syndrome, which consists of dementia, ataxia, varying ophthalmoplegia and nystagmus (see p. 885), presents acutely and should be suspected in all heavy drinkers. If treated promptly it is reversible; if left, it becomes irreversible. It is a major cause of dementia in the USA.

Urgent treatment with thiamine 250 mg i.m. or i.v. infusion once daily is given for 3 days, often combined with other B-complex vitamins. Anaphylaxis can occur. Thiamine must always be given before any intravenous glucose infusion.

Riboflavin

Riboflavin is widely distributed throughout all plant and animal cells. Good sources are dairy products, offal and leafy vegetables. Riboflavin is not destroyed appreciably by cooking but is destroyed by sunlight. It is a flavo-protein that is a co-factor for many oxidative reactions in the cell.

There is no definite deficiency, although many communities have low dietary intakes. Studies in volunteers taking a low-riboflavin diet have produced:

- angular stomatitis or cheilosis (fissuring at the corners of the mouth)
- a red, inflamed tongue
- seborrhoeic dermatitis, particularly involving the face (around the nose) and the scrotum or vulva.

Conjunctivitis with vascularization of the cornea and opacity of the lens has also been described. It is probable, however, that many of the above features are due to multiple deficiencies rather than lack of riboflavin itself.

Riboflavin 5 mg daily can be tried for the above conditions, usually given as the vitamin B complex.

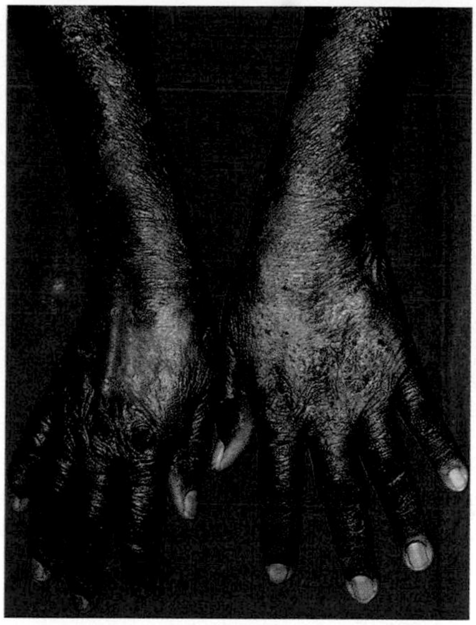

Figure 10.8 Pellagra. Hyperpigmentation with desquamation of the dorsal aspects of the hands and forearms. *(From Bolognia JL, Jorrizzo JL, Schaffer JV (eds).* Dermatology, *3rd edn. St Louis: Mosby; 2012, with permission.)*

Niacin

This is the generic name for the two chemical forms, nicotinic acid and nicotinamide, the latter being found in the two pyridine nucleotides, nicotinamide adenine dinucleotide (NAD) and nicotinamide adenine dinucleotide phosphate (NADP). Both act as hydrogen acceptors in many oxidative reactions, and in their reduced forms (NADH and NADPH) act as hydrogen donors in reductive reactions. Many oxidative steps in the production of energy require NAD and NADP.

Niacin is found in many foodstuffs, including plants, meat (particularly offal) and fish. Niacin is lost when bran is removed from cereals, but is added to processed cereals and white bread in many countries.

Niacin can be synthesized in humans from tryptophan, 60 mg of tryptophan being converted to 1 mg of niacin. The amount of niacin in food is given as the 'niacin equivalent', which is equal to the amount of niacin plus one-60th of the tryptophan content. Eggs and cheese contain tryptophan.

Kynureninase and kynurenine hydroxylase, key enzymes in the conversion of tryptophan to nicotinic acid, are both B_6 and riboflavin-dependent, and deficiency of these B vitamins can also produce pellagra.

Pellagra

This is rare but is found in people who eat virtually only maize: for example, in parts of Africa. Maize contains niacin in the form of niacytin, which is biologically unavailable and has a low content of tryptophan. In Central America, pellagra has always been rare because maize (for the cooking of tortillas) is soaked overnight in calcium hydroxide, which releases niacin. Many of the features of pellagra (*Fig. 10.8*) can be explained purely by niacin deficiency, but some are probably due to multiple deficiencies, including deficiencies of proteins and of other vitamins.

Clinical features

The classical features are dermatitis, diarrhoea and dementia. Although this is an easily remembered triad, not all features are always present and the mental changes are not a true dementia.

- ***Dermatitis***. In the areas of skin exposed to sunlight, there is redness initially, followed by cracks with occasional ulceration. Chronic thickening, dryness and pigmentation develop. The lesions are always symmetrical and often affect the dorsal surfaces of the hands. The perianal skin and vulva are frequently involved. Casal's necklace or collar is the term given to the skin lesion around the neck, which is confined to this area by the clothes worn.
- ***Diarrhoea***. This is often a feature but constipation is occasionally seen. Other gastrointestinal manifestations include a painful, red, raw tongue, glossitis and angular stomatitis. Recurring mouth infections occur.
- ***Dementia***. This occurs in chronic disease. In milder cases, there are symptoms of depression, apathy and sometimes thought disorders. Tremor and an encephalopathy frequently occur. Hallucinations and acute psychosis are also seen with more severe cases.

Pellagra may also occur in the following circumstances:

- *Isoniazid therapy.* This can lead to a deficiency of vitamin B_6, which is needed for the synthesis of nicotinamide from tryptophan. Vitamin B_6 is now given concomitantly with isoniazid.
- *Hartnup's disease*, a rare inborn error in which basic amino acids, including tryptophan, are not absorbed by the gut. There is also loss of this amino acid in the urine.
- *Generalized malabsorption* (rare).
- *Alcohol-dependent patients* who eat little.
- *Very-low-protein diets* given for renal disease or taken as a food fad.
- *Carcinoid syndrome and phaeochromocytomas*. In these disorders, tryptophan metabolism is diverted away from the formation of nicotinamide to form amines.

Diagnosis and management

In endemic areas, diagnosis and management are based on the clinical features, remembering that other vitamin deficiencies can produce similar changes (e.g. angular stomatitis). Nicotinamide (approximately 300 mg daily by mouth) is given, with a maintenance dose of 50 mg daily, and produces a dramatic improvement in the skin and diarrhoea. Mostly, however, vitamin B complex is given, as other deficiencies are often present.

An increase in the protein content of the diet, and treatment of malnutrition and other vitamin deficiencies, are essential.

Vitamin B_6

Vitamin B_6 exists as pyridoxine, pyridoxal and pyridoxamine, and is found widely in plant and animal foodstuffs. Pyridoxal phosphate is a co-factor in the metabolism of many amino acids. Dietary deficiency is extremely rare. Some drugs (e.g. isoniazid, hydralazine and penicillamine) interact with pyridoxal phosphate, producing B_6 deficiency. The polyneuropathy occurring after isoniazid usually responds to vitamin B_6.

Sideroblastic anaemia may respond to vitamin B_6 (see p. 526).

A polyneuropathy has occurred after high doses (>200 mg) given over many months. Vitamin B_6 is used for premenstrual tension; a daily dose of 10 mg should not be exceeded.

Biotin and pantothenic acid

Biotin is involved in a number of carboxylase reactions. It occurs in many foodstuffs and the dietary requirement is small. Deficiency is extremely rare and is confined to a few people who consume raw eggs, which contain an antagonist (avidin) to biotin. It has also been reported in patients receiving long-term parenteral nutrition without adequate amounts of biotin. It causes a dermatitis that responds to biotin replacements.

Pantothenic acid is widely distributed in all foods and deficiency in humans has not been described.

Vitamin C

Ascorbic acid is a powerful reducing agent that controls the redox potential within cells. It is involved in the hydroxylation of proline to hydroxyproline, which is necessary for the formation of collagen. The failure of this biochemical pathway in vitamin C deficiency accounts for virtually all of the clinical effects seen.

Humans, along with a few other animals (e.g. primates and the guinea-pig), are unusual in not being able to synthesize ascorbic acid from glucose.

Vitamin C is present in all fresh fruit and vegetables. Unfortunately, ascorbic acid is easily leached out of vegetables when they are placed in water and it is also oxidized to dehydro-ascorbic acid during cooking or exposure to copper or alkalis. Potatoes are a good source, as many people eat a lot of them, but vitamin C is lost during storage.

It has been suggested that ascorbic acid in high dosage (1–2 g daily) will prevent the common cold. While there is some scientific support for this, clinical trials have shown no significant effect. Vitamin C supplements have also been advocated to prevent atherosclerosis and cancer, but again a clear benefit has not been demonstrated.

Vitamin C deficiency is seen mainly in infants fed boiled milk and in the elderly and single people who do not eat vegetables. In the UK, it is also seen in Asians eating only rice and chapattis and also in food faddists.

Box 10.16 Clinical features of vitamin C deficiency (scurvy)

- Keratosis of hair follicles with 'corkscrew' hair
- Perifollicular haemorrhages
- Swollen, spongy gums with bleeding and superadded infection, loosening of teeth
- Spontaneous bruising
- Spontaneous haemorrhage
- Anaemia
- Failure of wound healing

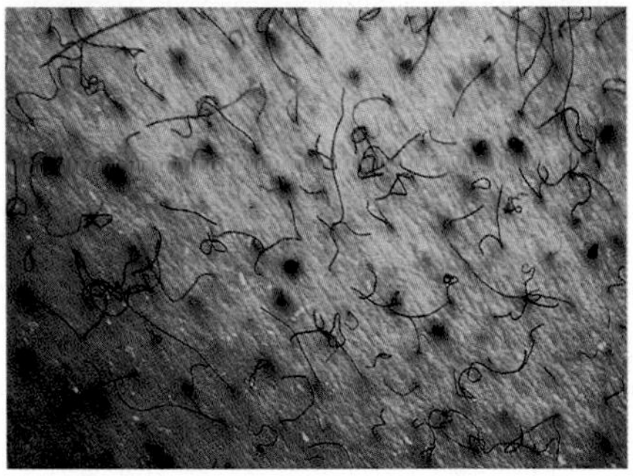

Figure 10.9 Scurvy. Corkscrew hairs and perifollicular haemorrhage on the lower extremity. *(From Bolognia JL, Jorrizzo JL, Schaffer JV (eds).* Dermatology, *3rd edn. St Louis: Mosby; 2012, with permission.)*

Scurvy

In adults, the early symptoms of vitamin C deficiency may be non-specific, with weakness and muscle pain. Other features are shown in ***Box 10.16***. Parafollicular haemorrhages and corkscrew hairs ***(Fig. 10.9)*** occur. In infantile scurvy, there is irritability, painful legs, anaemia and characteristic subperiosteal haemorrhages, particularly into the ends of long bones.

Diagnosis

The anaemia is usually hypochromic but, occasionally, a normochromic or megaloblastic anaemia is seen. The type of anaemia depends on whether iron deficiency (owing to decreased absorption or loss due to haemorrhage) or folate deficiency (folate being largely found in green vegetables) is present.

Plasma ascorbic acid is very low in obvious deficiency and a vitamin C level of <11 µmol/L (0.2 mg/100 mL) indicates vitamin C deficiency. The leucocyte-platelet layer (buffy coat) of centrifuged blood corresponds to vitamin C concentrations in other tissues. The normal level of leucocyte ascorbate is 1.1–2.8 pmol/10^6 cells.

Management

Initially, the patient is given 250 mg of ascorbic acid daily and encouraged to eat fresh fruit and vegetables. Subsequently, 40 mg daily will maintain a normal exchangeable body pool of about 900 mg (5.1 mmol).

Prevention

Orange juice should be given to bottle-fed infants. The intake of breast-fed infants depends on the mother's diet. In the elderly, eating adequate fruit and vegetables is the best way to avoid scurvy. Careful surveillance of the elderly, particularly those who live alone, is necessary. Ascorbic acid supplements should be necessary only occasionally.

Vitamin B_{12} and folate

These are dealt with on page 527 and daily requirements are shown in ***Box 10.13*** on p. 195.

Folate

In many developed countries, up to 15% of the population have a partial deficiency of 5,10-methylene tetrahydrofolate reductase, a key folate-metabolizing enzyme. This is due to a point mutation and is associated with an increase in neural tube defects and hyperhomocysteinaemia, which has been linked to cardiovascular disease. Autoantibodies against folate receptors have been found in serum from women who have had a pregnancy complicated by neural tube defects. However, the role of this in the pathogenesis is unclear.

In the USA and some other countries, enriched cereals are fortified with 1.4 mg/kg grain of folic acid to increase daily intake.

DIETARY ANTIOXIDANTS

Free radicals are generated during inflammatory processes, radiotherapy, smoking, and in the course of a wide range of diseases. They may cause uncontrolled damage of multiple cellular components, the most sensitive of which are unsaturated lipids, proteins and DNA, and they also disrupt the normal replication process. They have been implicated as a cause of a wide range of diseases, including malignant, acute inflammatory and traumatic diseases, cardiovascular disease, neurodegenerative conditions such as Alzheimer's disease, senile macular degeneration, and cataract. Defence against uncontrolled damage by free radicals is provided by antioxidant enzymes (e.g. catalase, superoxide dismutase) and antioxidants, which may be endogenous (e.g. glutathione) or exogenous (e.g. vitamins C and E, carotenoids). A possible causal link between lack of antioxidants and cardiovascular disease has emerged from epidemiological studies, although several RCTs have not confirmed this.

Epidemiology

Dietary intake

- A high intake of fruits and vegetables has been linked to a reduced risk of heart disease, cerebrovascular disease and total cardiovascular morbidity and mortality.
- A high intake of nuts (rich in vitamin E) and dietary components, such as red wine, onions and apples (rich in flavonoids), which are strong scavengers of free radicals, has also been linked to a reduced risk of cardiovascular disease.
- The seasonal variation in cardiovascular disease, which is higher in winter, has been related to a decreased intake of fresh fruit and vegetables at that time of year.
- The decline in cardiovascular disease in the USA since the 1950s has been associated with a simultaneous increase in the intake of fresh fruit and vegetables.

Status of antioxidant nutrients

The level of antioxidant nutrients in the circulation has been reported to be inversely related to cardiovascular morbidity and mortality, the extent of atherosclerosis as assessed by intra-arterial ultrasound, and clinical signs of ischaemic heart disease. The tissue content of lycopene, a marker of vegetable intake, has been reported to be low in patients with myocardial infarction.

Antioxidants, especially vitamin E, have been shown to prevent the initiation and progression of atherosclerotic disease in animals. They also reduce the oxidation of LDL in the arterial wall *in vitro*. Oxidation of LDL is an initial event in the atherosclerotic process (see pp. 992–993). However, these epidemiological studies show an association rather than a causal link, and RCTs comparing the antioxidant against a control group are necessary.

The results of ***RCTs*** (see also p. 26) have been formally evaluated through a series of systematic reviews and meta-analyses.

- For ***primary or secondary prevention*** of cardiovascular disease, intervention with β-carotene, α-tocopherol (vitamin E) and ascorbic acid (vitamin C) has demonstrated no significant benefit.
- Vitamin E or β-carotene given in, for example, stroke and fatal and non-fatal myocardial infarction has also not yielded benefits.
- There is a report of increased risk of intracerebral and subarachnoid haemorrhage in healthy individuals receiving carotene and α-tocopherol.
- A meta-analysis has shown a small but significant overall increased risk of cardiovascular death and all-cause mortality in individuals treated with β-carotene (compared to the control group).
- There is an increased risk of developing lung cancer when large doses of β-carotene are administered to subjects with a history of heavy smoking.
- Although administration of antioxidant nutrients has been proposed in a wide range of acute (e.g. critical illness, pancreatitis) and chronic diseases, the evidence base from RCTs is generally not strong.
- In some cases, improvement in indices of free radical damage has been demonstrated (e.g. in acute inflammatory conditions), but with little evidence of clinical benefit.

Epidemiological studies are also confounded by other associated variables, such as eating a low-fat diet or undertaking more exercise. The latter may be more valuable in the causal pathway than the intake of antioxidants. Diets rich in fresh fruit and vegetables also contain a range of antioxidants that were not tested in the clinical trials. Therefore, the results of large-scale RCTs using various combinations and doses of antioxidant nutrients are awaited. In the meantime, the policy of encouraging 'healthy' behaviour, which includes increased physical activity and a varied diet rich in fresh fruit and vegetables, and nuts, is still generally recommended both for the population as a whole and for those at risk of cardiovascular disease.

HOMOCYSTEINE, CARDIOVASCULAR DISEASE AND B VITAMINS

The circulating concentration of the amino acid homocysteine is an independent risk factor for cardiovascular disease. A high concentration is related to ischaemic heart disease, stroke, thrombosis, pulmonary embolism, coronary artery stenosis and heart failure. The strength of the association is similar to that in smoking or hyperlipidaemia.

Proposed mechanisms, based on experimental evidence, by which homocysteine detrimentally affects vascular function, include:

- the direct damaging effects of homocysteine on endothelial cells of blood vessels

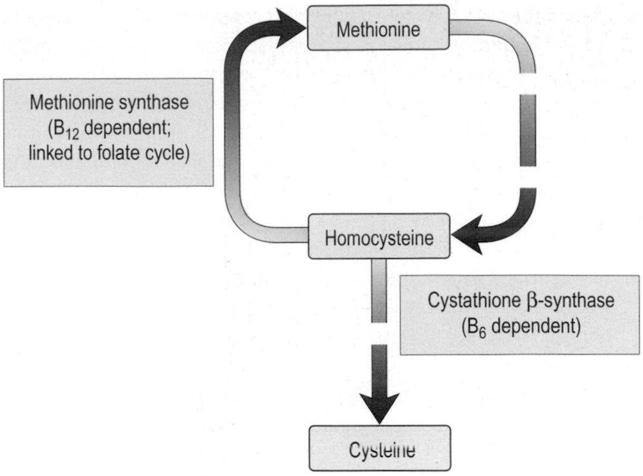

Figure 10.10 Homocysteine metabolism.

- an increase in blood vessel stiffness
- an increase in blood coagulation.

Homocysteine is not found in food, but results from metabolism within the body, which depends on folic acid, vitamin B_{12} and pyridoxine (vitamin B_6) ***(Fig. 10.10)***. Deficiency of one or more of these vitamins is common in the elderly, which would increase the concentration of homocysteine. If an elevated homocysteine concentration were causally linked to cardiovascular disease, then it should be possible to lower the risk by administering one or more of these vitamins to decrease the homocysteine concentration. However, several studies suggest that lowering homocysteine concentrations in this way does not reduce the risk of cardiovascular disease.

Further reading

Awasthi S, Peto R, Read S et al. Vitamin A supplementation every 6 months with retinol in 1 million pre-school children in north India: DEVTA, a cluster-randomised trial. *Lancet* 2013; 381:1469–1477.

Checkley W, West KP, Wise RA et al. Maternal vitamin supplementation and lung function in offspring. *N Engl J Med* 2010; 362:1784–1794.

Clarke R, Halsey J, Lewington S et al. Effects of lowering homocysteine levels with B vitamins on cardiovascular disease, cancer, and cause-specific mortality: meta-analysis of 8 randomized trials involving 37 485 individuals. *Arch Intern Med* 2010; 170:1622–1631.

Institute of Medicine. *Dietary Reference Intakes for Thiamin, Riboflavin, Niacin, Vitamin B6, Folate, Vitamin B12, Pantothenic Acid, Biotin, and Choline*. Washington DC: National Academies Press; 2000.

Marti-Carvajal AJ, Sola I, Lathyris D et al. Homocysteine-lowering interventions for preventing cardiovascular events. *Cochrane Database of Systematic Reviews (Online)* 2013; 1:CD006612.

Welsh P, Sattar N. Vitamin D and chronic disease prevention. *BMJ* 2014; 348:g228.

MINERALS

A number of minerals have been shown to be essential in animals, and an increasing number of deficiency syndromes are becoming recognized in humans. Long-term total parenteral nutrition allowed trace element deficiency to be studied in controlled conditions; now trace elements are always added to long-term parenteral nutrition regimens. It is highly probable that trace-element deficiency is also a frequent accompaniment of all PEM states, but this is difficult to study because of multiple deficiencies. Sodium, potassium, magnesium and chloride are discussed in Chapter 9. Reference nutrient intake (RNI) values are shown in ***Box 10.17***. However, in disease, the requirements of specific nutrients may increase (e.g. sodium potassium, magnesium and zinc in patients with persistent diarrhoea or other gastrointestinal fluid losses) or decrease (e.g. phosphate, potassium and sodium in chronic kidney disease).

Box 10.17 Daily reference nutrient intake (RNI) values for some elements

Element	Daily RNI	Dietary sources
Sodium	1.6 g (70 mmol)	Mostly in processed food (e.g. meat products, bread cereal) but contribution from added salt
Chloride	2.5 g (70 mmol)	As for sodium
Potassium	3.5 g (90 mmol)	Vegetables, fruit, juices, meat and milk
Calcium	700 mg (17.5 mmol)[a]	In many foodstuffs; two-thirds of intake comes from milk and milk products, and only 5% from vegetables[b]
Phosphate	550 mg (17.5 mmol)	All natural foods, e.g. milk, meat, bread, cereals
Magnesium	300 mg (12.3 mmol) for men 270 mg (10.9 mmol) for women	Milk, bread, cereal products, potatoes and other vegetables
Iron	160 μmol (8.7 mg) for men 260 μmol (14.8 mg) for women	Meat, bread, flour, cereal products, potatoes and vegetables
Copper	1.2 mg (19 μmol)	Shellfish, legumes, cereals and nuts
Zinc	9.5 mg (145 μmol) for men 7 mg (110 μmol) for women	Widely available in food
Iodine	140 μg (1.1 μmol)	Milk, meat and seafoods
Fluoride	None	Little fluoride in food except sea fish and tea (tea provides 70% of daily intake)
Selenium	75 μg (0.9 μmol) for men 60 μg (0.8 μmol) for women	Cereals, fish, meat, cheese, eggs, milk

[a]UK value; a substantially higher value is recommended in the USA. [b]In the UK, most flour is fortified.

Iron

Iron deficiency (see also pp. 524–526) is common worldwide, affecting both developing and developed countries. It is particularly prevalent in women of reproductive age. Dietary iron overload is seen in South African men who cook and brew in iron pots.

Copper

Copper deficiency

Menkes' kinky hair syndrome is a rare condition caused by malabsorption of copper. The Menkes' disease gene (*ATP7A*) encodes a copper-transporting ATPase and has a homology to the gene in Wilson's disease. Infants with this sex-linked recessive abnormality develop growth failure, mental retardation, bone lesions and brittle hair. Anaemia and neutropenia also occur. This condition, which serves as a model for copper deficiency, supports the idea that some of the clinical features seen in PEM are due to copper deficiency. Breast and cow's milk are low in copper, and supplementation is occasionally necessary when first treating PEM.

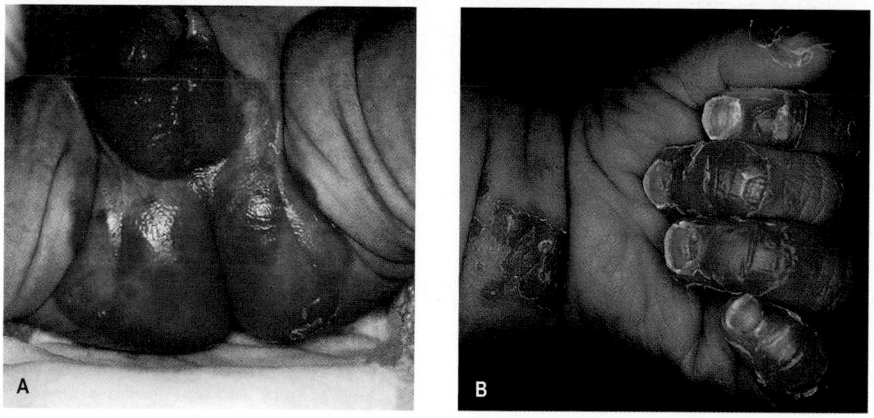

Figure 10.11 **Zinc deficiency (genetic). A.** Erythema and erosions. **B.** Crusting and desquamation. *(From Bolognia JL, Jorrizzo JL, Schaffer JV (eds).* Dermatology, *3rd edn. St Louis: Mosby; 2012, with permission.)*

Copper toxicity

This occurs in Wilson's disease; see page 479.

Zinc

Zinc is involved in many metabolic pathways, often acting as a coenzyme; it is essential for the synthesis of RNA and DNA. In young children in developing countries, death attributable to zinc deficiency is lower than previously thought. One study found significant improvements when extra zinc was provided with several other micronutrients.

Zinc deficiency

Acrodermatitis enteropathica is an inherited disorder caused by malabsorption of zinc. Infants develop growth retardation, severe diarrhoea, hair loss and a skin rash, which can occur anywhere on the body but is most often found around the mouth, genitalia and hands (a similar rash occurs in adults suffering from zinc deficiency due to other causes; see below). There are also associated *Candida* and bacterial infections ***(Fig. 10.11)***. This condition provides a model for zinc deficiency. Zinc supplementation results in a complete cure. Zinc deficiency probably also plays a role in PEM and in many diseases in children in the developing world. Zinc supplementation has been demonstrated as being of some benefit in, for example, the prevention of diarrhoeal diseases and acute respiratory infections; it also improves growth.

Levels of zinc have also been shown to be low in some patients with malabsorption or skin disease, and in patients with the acquired immunodeficiency syndrome (AIDS), but its exact role in these situations is disputed. Zinc has low toxicity, but high zinc levels from water stored in galvanized containers interfere with iron and copper absorption. Conversely, administration of copper or iron to treat deficiencies such as iron deficiency anaemia can precipitate zinc deficiency. Wound healing is impaired with moderate zinc deficiency and is improved by zinc supplements. Impaired taste and smell, hair loss and night blindness are also features of severe zinc deficiency.

Iodine

Iodine exists in foodstuffs as inorganic iodides, which are efficiently absorbed. Iodine is a constituent of the thyroid hormones (see pp. 1200–1201).

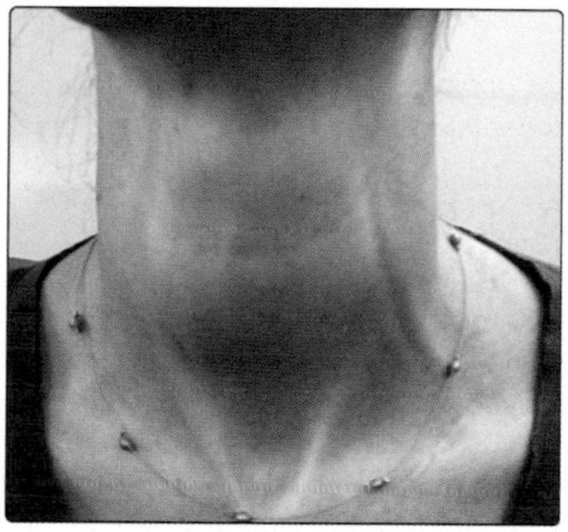

Figure 10.12 **Goitre due to iodine deficiency.** *(From Dhillon RS, East CA 2013 Ear, Nose and Throat and Head and Neck Surgery, 4th Edn, Elsevier, with permission.)*

Iodine deficiency

Many areas throughout the world lack iodine in the soil, and so iodine deficiency, which impairs brain development, is a WHO priority. Two billion people worldwide (one-third of whom are children) have insufficient iodine intake. Endemic goitre ***(Fig. 10.12)*** occurs in remote areas where the daily intake is below 70 μg, and in those parts 1–5% of babies are born with congenital hypothyroidism (with severe stunting, learning difficulty and a goitre). In these areas, iodized oil should be given intramuscularly to all reproductive women every 3–5 years. Salt iodization is now practised in many countries and is a simple, cost-effective way to prevent deficiency.

Fluoride

In areas where the level of fluoride in drinking water is less than 1 p.p.m. (0.7–1.2 mg/L), dental caries is relatively more prevalent. Fluoridation of the water provides 1–2 mg daily, resulting in a reduction of about 50% of tooth decay in children. There is little fluoride in food. Fluoride-containing toothpaste may add up to 2 mg/day.

Excessive fluoride intake in areas where the water fluoride level is above 3 mg/L can result in fluorosis, in which there is infiltration into the enamel of the teeth, producing pitting and discoloration.

Selenium

Clinical deficiency of selenium is rare, except in areas of China where Keshan disease, a selenium-responsive cardiomyopathy,

Box 10.18 Other trace elements

Element	Deficiency
Chromium	Glucose intolerance
Cobalt	Anaemia (vitamin B_{12})
Manganese	Skin rash, ?osteoporosis, ?mood
Molybdenum	?(case study involving parenteral nutrition)
Nickel	?Animals only

occurs. Selenium deficiency may also cause a myopathy. Interactions between selenium and viruses have also been implicated. Toxicity has been described with very high intakes.

Calcium

Calcium absorption (see also p. 708) from the gastrointestinal tract is vitamin D-dependent. Some 99% of body calcium is in the skeleton.

Increased calcium is required in pregnancy and lactation, when dietary intake must be increased. Calcium deficiency is usually due to vitamin D deficiency.

Phosphate

Phosphates (see also p. 171) are present in all natural foods, and dietary deficiency has not been described. Patients taking large amounts of aluminium hydroxide can, however, develop phosphate deficiency owing to binding in the gut lumen. It can also be seen in total parenteral nutrition. Symptoms include anorexia, weakness and osteoporosis.

Other trace elements

The possible significance of chromium, cobalt, manganese, molybdenum and nickel is shown in ***Box 10.18***.

Further reading

Bauer DC. Calcium supplements and fracture prevention. *N Engl J Med* 2013; 369:1537–1543.

Institute of Medicine. *Dietary Reference Intakes for Vitamin A, Vitamin K, Arsenic, Chromium, Copper, Iodine, Iron, Manganese, Molybdenum, Silicon, Vanadium, and Zinc*. Washington DC: Institute of Medicine; 2001.

Kotchen TA, Cowley AW, Jr, Frohlich ED. Salt in health and disease – a delicate balance. *N Engl J Med* 2013; 368:1229–1237.

Loscalzo J. Keshan disease, selenium deficiency, and selenoproteome. *N Engl J Med* 2014;370;18:1756–1760.

Pearce SHS, Cheetam TD. Diagnosis and management of vitamin D deficiency. *BMJ* 2010; 340:141–147.

Pitta AG, Chung M, Trikalinos T et al. Systematic review: vitamin D and cardiometabolic outcomes. *Ann Intern Med* 2010; 152:307–314.

Soofi S, Cousens S, Iqbal SP et al. Effect of provision of daily zinc and iron with several micronutrients on growth and morbidity among young children in Pakistan: a cluster-randomised trial. *Lancet* 2013; 382:29–40.

NUTRITION AND AGEING

Many animal studies have shown that life expectancy can be extended by restricting food intake. It is, however, not known whether the ageing process in humans can be altered by nutrition.

The ageing process

The process of ageing is not well understood. While wear and tear may play a role, it is an insufficient explanation for the causation of ageing. The 'programmed' theories depend on inbuilt biological clocks that regulate lifespan, and involve genes that are responsible for controlling signals that influence various body systems. The 'error' theories involve environmental stressors that induce damage (e.g. mitochondrial DNA damage or cross-linking).

The search for a single cause of ageing, such as a single gene defect, has been replaced by the view that ageing is a complex multifactorial process that involves an interaction between genetic, environmental and stochastic (random damage to essential molecules) causes. The following theories have been suggested.

Molecular theories

- ***Genetic regulation***. Ageing results, for example, from changes in expression of genes that regulate both development and ageing. An insulin-like signalling pathway has been linked to the lifespan of worms, flies and mice (activation of a transcription factor in response to reduced insulin-like signalling prolongs lifespan).
- ***Epigenetic regulation***. Epigenetic modification, including DNA methylation and histone modification, can help explain why individuals with similar genetic backgrounds can age very differently.
- ***Codon restriction***. Inadequate messenger RNA (mRNA) translation results from inadequate decoding of codons in mRNA.
- ***Error catastrophe***. Errors in gene expression give rise to abnormal proteins.
- ***Somatic mutation***. There is cumulative molecular damage mainly to genetic material.
- ***Dysdifferentiation***. Cumulative random molecular damage detrimentally affects gene expression.

Mutations in genes encoding lamin A are found in fibroblasts of elderly people and in progeria syndromes.

Cellular theories

- ***Cellular senescence–telomere***. An increase in senescent cells is caused by:
  - ***Loss of telomeres***, which is known to occur with ageing (with each cell division, a small amount of DNA is necessarily lost at each end of the chromosome). Activation of the telomerase enzyme regenerates telomeres, prevents senescence (replicative senescence) and immortalizes cell cultures. Cancer cells are known to activate telomerase. Accelerated telomerase shortening occurs in ***progerias***, such as ***Werner syndrome***. One study has also found that telomere length in leucocytes predicts coronary artery disease in middle-aged men at high risk, and these individuals might benefit from statin treatment.
  - ***Damage*** due to a variety of other factors, including DNA damage (stress-induced senescence).
- ***Free radical***. Production of free radicals takes place during oxidative metabolism, which damages fat, protein and DNA.
- ***Wear and tear***. There is cumulative damage from normal injury/stress, which is unable to repair itself.
- ***Apoptosis***. Programmed cell death (see p. 105) is caused by genetic events.

System theories

These theories involve loss in the function of neuroendocrine or immune systems with consequent age-related physiological changes and an increase in autoimmunity.

Whole-body metabolism and energy expenditure theory proposes that there is a fixed limit to the cumulative energy expenditure and metabolism during a lifetime; if this limit is reached quickly, the lifespan is short. Energy restriction in rodents reduces energy expenditure and prolongs lifespan, but there is a lack of studies in primates or humans.

Evolutionary theories

- ***Cumulative mutation***. Mutations that accumulate during a lifetime act in older age rather than during the active reproductive period (for which there is evolutionary selection), producing pathology and senescence. The theory was initially based on the observation that in Huntington's disease, which is due to a dominant lethal mutation that typically presents itself between 35 and 55 years, allows affected individuals to reproduce prior to their clinical diagnosis.
- ***Disposable soma***. The somatic body is maintained to ensure reproductive success, after which it is disposable. Factors that may enhance reproductive success may have detrimental effects on ageing; a possible example is androgen secretion, which may be beneficial to reproduction but potentially detrimental, with development of prostatic cancer and cardiovascular disease in later life.

Nutritional components of theories of ageing

Several of the theories described above have strong nutritional components. ***Disability and dependency*** in older humans are, at least partly, due to poor nutrition, and correction of deficiencies or nutrient imbalances can prevent the decline in function from falling below the disability threshold ***(Fig. 10.13)***. In this way, some loss of function may be prevented or reversed, especially if other measures – such as physical activity, which increases muscle mass and strength – are undertaken.

Early origins of health and disease in older adults

A low birth weight (and/or length) is associated with reduced height, as well as reduced mass and fat-free mass in adult life. These relationships are independent of genetic factors; the smaller of identical twins becomes a shorter and lighter adult.

Relationships have also been reported between growth of the fetus and a variety of diseases and risk factors for disease in adults and older people. These include cardiovascular disease (especially ischaemic heart disease), hypertension, diabetes, and even obesity and fat distribution. However, the strength of association for some of these conditions is weak. Animal studies involving dietary modifications (e.g. protein and zinc, even within the normal range) during pregnancy or in early postnatal life have clearly demonstrated effects, such as hypertension. The effects can not only persist through the lifetime of the offspring, but also be passed through to their offspring.

The extent to which these findings apply to humans is uncertain and the mechanisms are poorly understood. Since relationships have been reported between cardiovascular disease in old age and growth in the first few years of life, as well as starvation during puberty, it is likely that cumulative environmental stresses, including nutritional stress, from the time of implantation of the fertilized egg, to fetal and postnatal growth and development, and into adult life, summate to produce an overall disease risk (see ***Fig. 10.13***). Although high birth weight and length are associated with a reduced risk of cardiovascular disease in later life, they may also be associated with an increased risk of cancer.

Nutritional requirements in the elderly

These are qualitatively similar to the requirements of younger adults; the diet should contain approximately the same proportions of nutrients, and essential nutrients are still needed. However, the RNIs stated earlier (see ***Boxes 10.13*** and ***10.17***) are intended for healthy people without disease; specific requirements in disease, which is common in older people, are less well defined. Furthermore, the extent to which muscle loss is due to ageing, malnutrition and disease continues to be debated, as do the boundaries between sarcopenia, cachexia, malnutrition and frailty. ***Sarcopenia*** is defined as loss of skeletal muscle bulk, accompanied by decreased strength; unlike cachexia, it occurs without an underlying illness. Sarcopenia leads to disability with an increase in falls.

Maintenance of physical activity continues to be necessary for overall health, regardless of age. However, energy expenditure by the elderly is less, so they have a lower energy requirement. For people aged 60 and above, irrespective of age, the daily energy requirement has been set at approximately 1.5 × BMR. Because they have reduced fat-free mass – from an average of 60 kg to 50 kg in men, and from 40 kg to 35 kg in women – their BMR is reduced.

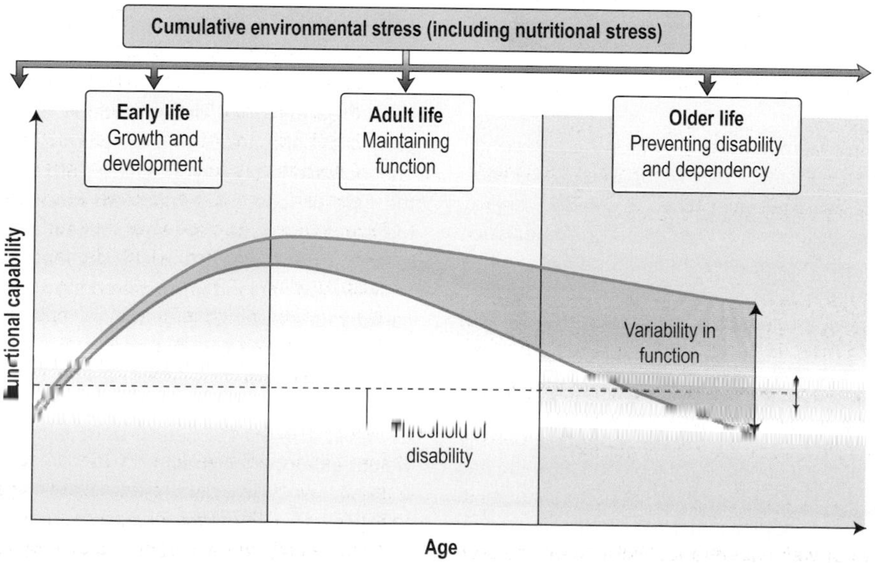

Figure 10.13 Nutrition and ageing. Nutrition is a contributory cause of the variability in function during the lifespan. Appropriate nutrition may improve function, or delay deterioration below the threshold of disability and dependence.

Nutritional deficits in the elderly are common and may be due to many factors, such as dental problems, lack of cooking skills (particularly in widowers), depression and lack of motivation. Significant malnourishment in developed countries is usually secondary to social problems or disease. In elderly people who are in institutions, multiple nutrient deficiencies are common. Vitamin D supplements (colecalciferol 20 μg (800 units) daily) may be required because of poor diet, and elderly people often do not go into the sunlight. Owing to the high prevalence of osteoporosis in elderly people, an increased daily calcium intake (1–1.5 g/day) is often recommended.

Further reading

Ali S, Garcia JM. Sarcopenia, cachexia and aging: diagnosis, mechanisms and therapeutic options – a mini-review. *Gerontology* 2014; 60:294–305.
Boyd-Kirkup JD, Green CD, Wu G et al. Epigenomics and the regulation of aging. *Epigenomics* 2013; 5:205–227.
Chatterji S, Byles J, Cutler D et al. Health, functioning, and disability in older adults – present status and future implications. *Lancet* 2015; 385:563–570.
Clegg A, Young J, Iliffe S et al. Frailty in elderly people. *Lancet* 2013; 381:752–762.
Cruz-Jentoft AJ, Landi F. Sarcopenia. *Clin Med* 2014; 14:183–186.
Mathers CD, Stevens GA, Boerma T et al. Causes of international increases in older age life expectancy. *Lancet* 2015: 385:540–548.
Prince MJ, Wu F, Guo Y et al. The burden of disease in older people and implications for health policy and practice. *Lancet* 2015; 385:549–562.
Xi H, Li C, Ren F et al. Telomere, aging and age-related diseases. *Aging Clin Exp Res* 2013; 25:139–146.

OBESITY

Obesity is almost invariable in developed countries and almost all people accumulate some fat as they get older. The WHO acknowledges that obesity (BMI >30 kg/m^2) is a worldwide problem that also affects many developing countries. Obesity implies an excess storage of fat and this can most easily be detected by looking at the undressed patient. Not all obese people eat more than the average person but all obviously eat more than they need.

The present obesity epidemic is mainly due to changes in lifestyle behaviour (although genetic factors may be involved in some individuals). There has been a trebling in the prevalence of obesity over the last three decades in the UK, as well as a vast increase in developing countries. The growing obesity problem in humans has affected children, adults and older people. Clinical and public health interventions require a multi-level approach: for example, by altering the cumulative environmental experience during the lifespan. Strategies to prevent and treat obesity in children can influence obesity in adults, and this in turn influences obesity in old age. Ultimately, all depend on changing energy balance through effects on food intake and/or energy expenditure.

Most patients suffer from simple obesity, but in certain conditions, obesity is an associated feature ***(Box 10.19)***. Even in the latter situation, the intake of calories must have exceeded energy expenditure over a prolonged period of time. Hormonal imbalance is often incriminated in women (e.g. after the menopause or when taking contraceptive pills), but most weight gain in such cases is usually small and due to water retention.

Pathophysiology

Genetic and environmental factors

These have always been difficult to separate in the study of obesity but there is little doubt that the recent obesity 'epidemic', which has developed over a few decades, is predominantly due to changes in lifestyle (various environmental factors) and unlikely to be caused by rapid changes in the gene pool over this period of time. This is consistent with the view that evolution during times of limited food resources has tended to defend more against under-nutrition than over-nutrition. However, observational studies in both monozygotic and dizygotic twins, reared together or apart, suggest that strong genetic influences account for the difference in BMI later in life, and that the influence of the childhood environment is weaker. These observations also showed that weight gain did not occur in all pairs of twins, suggesting that environmental factors operate.

Box 10.19 Conditions in which obesity is an associated feature

- Genetic syndromes associated with hypogonadism (e.g. Prader–Willi, Laurence–Moon–Biedl)
- Hypothyroidism
- Cushing syndrome
- Stein–Leventhal syndrome
- Drug-induced disorders (e.g. with corticosteroids)
- Hypothalamic damage (e.g. due to trauma, tumour)

A search for genetic factors led to the identification of a putative gene, first in the obese (*ob ob*) mouse and now in humans. The ***ob* gene** was shown to be expressed solely in both white and brown adipose tissue. The *ob* gene is found on chromosome 7 and produces a 16 kDa protein called **leptin**. In the *ob ob* mouse, a mutation in the *ob* gene leads to production of a non-functioning protein. Administration of normal leptin to these obese mice reduces food intake and corrects the obesity. A similar situation has been described in a very rare genetic condition that causes obesity in humans, in which leptin is not expressed.

In massively obese subjects, leptin mRNA in subcutaneous adipose tissue is 80% higher than in controls. Plasma levels of leptin are also very high, correlating with the BMI. Weight loss due to food restriction decreases plasma levels of leptin. However, in contrast to the *ob ob* mouse, the leptin structure is normal, and abnormalities in leptin are not the prime cause of human obesity.

Leptin secreted from fat cells was thought to act as a feedback mechanism between the adipose tissue and the brain, acting as a 'lipostat' (adipostat), and controlling fat stores by regulating hunger and satiety (see below). However, many other signals are involved and the human genome map has identified hundreds of genes that correlate with the presence of obesity. It is also interesting that obesity is largely restricted to humans and animals that are either domesticated or living in zoos.

Food intake

Many factors related to the home environment, such as finance and the availability of sweets and snacks, will affect food intake. Some individuals eat more during periods of heavy exercise or during pregnancy, and are unable to return to their former eating habits. The increase in obesity in social class 5 can usually be related to the type of food consumed (i.e. food containing sugar and fat). Measures to reduce the sugar content in popular foods and drinks are being introduced in various countries. Psychological factors and the way in which food is presented may override complex biochemical interactions.

It has been shown that obese patients eat more than they admit to eating, and over the years, a very small daily excess of intake over expenditure can lead to a large accumulation of fat. For example, a 44 kJ (10.5 kcal) daily excess would lead to a 10 kg weight gain over 20 years.

Control of appetite

Appetite is the desire to eat and this usually initiates food intake. Following a meal, satiation occurs. This depends on gastric and duodenal distension and the release of many substances peripherally and centrally.

Following a meal, cholecystokinin (CCK), bombesin, glucagon-like peptide 1 (GLP-1), enterostatin and somatostatin are released from the small intestine, and glucagon and insulin from the pancreas. All of these hormones have been implicated in the control of satiety. Centrally, the hypothalamus – particularly the lateral hypothalamic area and paraventricular and arcuate nuclei – plays a key role in integrating signals involved in appetite and body weight regulation *(Fig. 10.14)*.

Peripheral signals (1st order in *Fig. 10.14*)

- ***Peripheral appetite-suppressing signals***. ***Leptin*** and ***insulin*** act centrally to activate the ***appetite-suppressing pathway*** (while also inhibiting the appetite-stimulating pathway). Since these hormones circulate in proportion to adipose tissue mass, they can be regarded as long-term signals, although they probably also modulate short-term signals (insulin also responds acutely to meal ingestion). ***Peptide YY (PYY)*** is produced by the L cells of the large bowel and distal small bowel in proportion to the energy ingested. The release of this rapidly responsive (short-acting) signal begins shortly after food intake, suggesting that the initial response involves neural pathways, before ingested nutrients reach the site of PYY production. PYY is thought to reduce appetite, at least partly through inhibition of the ***appetite-stimulating pathway (NPY/AgRP-expressing neurones***). There are a large number of other peripheral appetite-suppressing signals, including GLP-1 and oxyntomodulin, which, like PYY, are produced by the gut in a nutrient-dependent manner.
- ***Peripheral appetite-stimulating signals***. Ghrelin is a 28-amino-acetylated peptide produced by the oxyntic cells of the fundus of the stomach. It is the first known gastrointestinal tract peptide that stimulates appetite by activating the central appetite-stimulating pathway. The circulatory concentration is high before a meal and is reduced rapidly by ingestion of a meal or glucose (compare PYY, which increases after a meal). It may also act as a long-term signal, as its circulating concentration in weight-stable individuals is inversely related to BMI over a wide range (compare insulin and leptin, which are positively related to BMI; see below). Ghrelin is also increased in several situations in which there is a negative energy balance, such as long-term exercise, very-low-calorie diets, anorexia nervosa, and both cancer and cardiac cachexia (an exception is vertical banded gastric bypass surgery, where its concentration is low rather than high). The peptide, obestatin, produced by the same gene that encodes ghrelin, counteracts the increase in food intake induced by ghrelin.

Central pathways (2nd order in *Fig. 10.14*)

There are two main pathways in the arcuate nucleus:

- The ***central appetite-stimulating (orexigenic) pathway*** in the ventromedial part of the arcuate nucleus, which expresses ***neuropeptide Y (NPY)*** and ***agouti pathway-related protein***

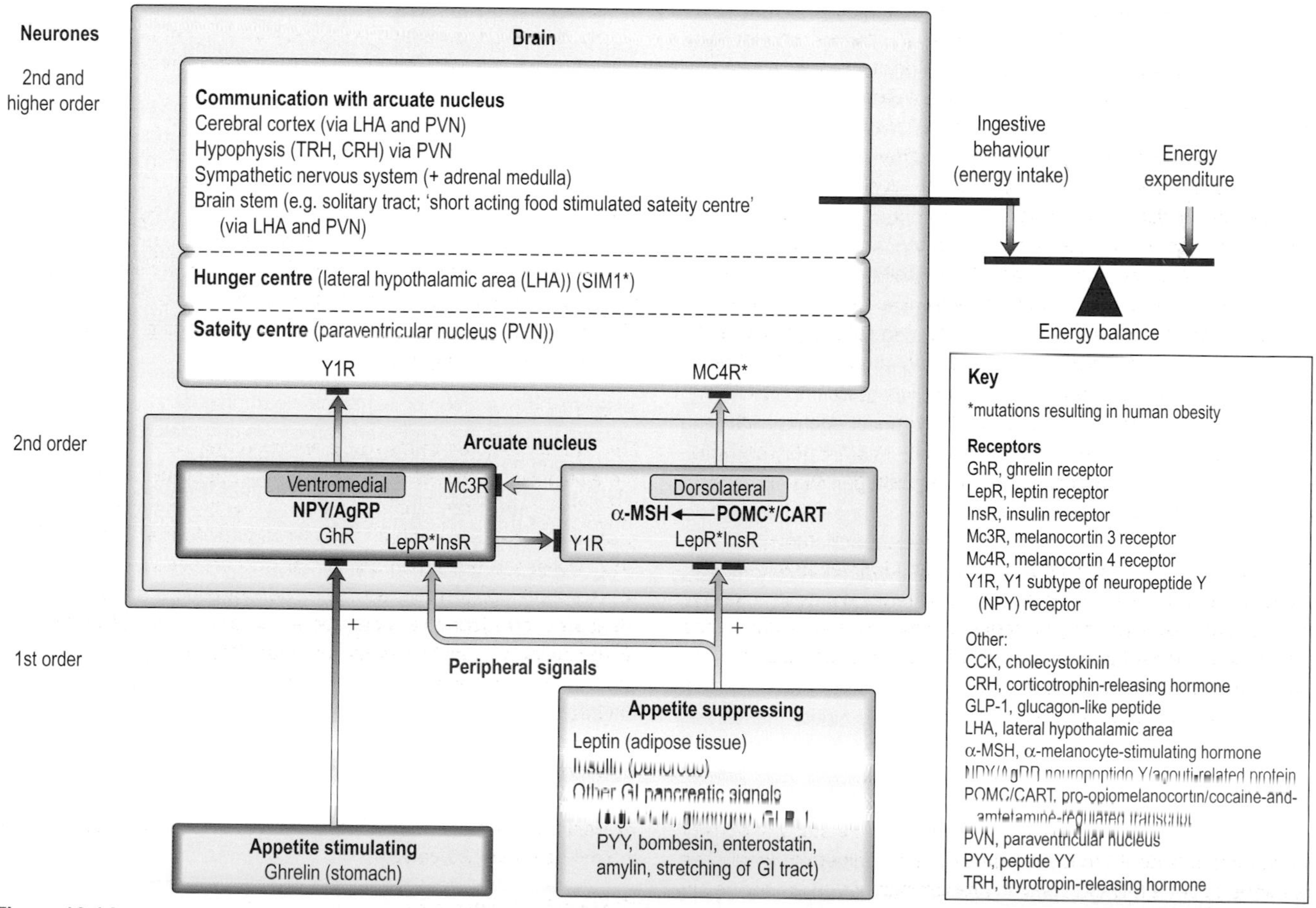

Figure 10.14 Peripheral signals and central pathways involved in the control of food intake. The stimulatory (orange) and suppressive (green) signals and pathways are shown. In the arcuate nucleus, POMC is converted to melanocortins, including α-MSH, through the action of prohormone convertase. The solid red areas represent receptors for a variety of signals (see list in the key).

(AgRP). Animal studies suggest that this pathway also decreases energy expenditure.

- The ***central appetite-suppressing pathway (anorexigenic pathway or leptin–melanocortin pathway)*** in the dorsolateral part of the arcuate nucleus, which expresses pro-opiomelanocortin/cocaine-and-amfetamine-regulated transcript (**POMC/CART**). In this pathway, α-melanocyte-stimulating hormone (α-MSH), formed by cleavage of POMC by prohormone convertase (PC1), exerts its appetite-suppressing effect via the melanocortin-4 receptors (Mc4R) in areas of the brain that regulate food intake and autonomic activity. Animal studies suggest that this pathway also increases energy expenditure.

These pathways interact with each other and feed into the lateral hypothalamus, which communicates with other parts of the brain, and influence the autonomic nervous system and ingestive behaviour.

These central pathways are in turn influenced by a variety of peripheral signals, which can also be classified as appetite-stimulating or appetite-suppressing.

Other factors

The single gene mutations affecting the appetite-suppressing pathway in humans, e.g. leptin, leptin receptor, *POMC*, *Mc4R*, *PC1* and *SIM1*, are rare and recessive, with the exception of *Mc4R*, which is common and dominant with incomplete penetrance. It appears that the ***Mc4R mutation*** accounts for 2–6% of human obesity. Affected individuals are obese without disturbances in pituitary function or resting energy expenditure, although children tend to be tall. However, these mutations are of little significance, as obesity is predominantly polygenic in origin (the human obesity gene map has already identified several hundreds of candidate genes).

The ***endocannabinoid system*** is also involved in both central and peripheral regulation of food intake and control of energy balance. There are two receptors: endocannabinoid (CB_1) in the brain and CB_2 in the periphery. CB_1 receptors are located in the cerebral cortex, cerebellum and hippocampus.

The control of appetite is extremely complex. To take just one signal, leptin, as an example, there can be leptin resistance, in which obese individuals have high circulating leptin but appetite is not reduced. In contrast, in acute starvation, leptin concentrations decrease to lower levels than could be expected from the prevailing adipose tissue mass. It is known that cytokines, such as TNF and IL-2, which are elevated in a wide range of inflammatory and traumatic conditions, also suppress appetite, although the exact pathways involved are not entirely clear. Finally, a range of transmitters in the central nervous system appear to affect appetite:

- appetite inhibitors: dopamine, serotonin, γ-aminobutyric acid
- appetite stimulators, e.g. opioids.

Energy expenditure

Basal metabolic rate

Basal metabolic rate (BMR) in obese subjects is higher than in lean subjects, which is not surprising since obesity is associated with an increase in lean body mass.

Physical activity

Obese patients tend to expend more energy during physical activity, as they have a larger mass to move. On the other hand, many obese patients decrease their amount of physical activity. The energy expended on walking at 3 miles/hour is only 15.5 kJ/min (3.7 kcal/min); therefore, a mild to moderate increase in physical activity plays only a small part in losing weight. Nevertheless, because increased body fat develops insidiously over many years, any change in energy balance is helpful.

Thermogenesis

About 10% of ingested energy is dissipated as heat and is unconnected with physical activity. This dietary-induced thermogenesis has been reported to be lower in obese and post-obese subjects than in lean subjects. This would tend to favour energy deposition in obesity and those predisposed to obesity. However, other reports have identified no difference in dietary-induced thermogenesis between lean and obese subjects.

When stimulated by cold or food, brown adipose tissue in animals dissipates the energy derived from ingested food into heat. This can be a major component of overall energy balance in small mammals but the effect is likely to be very small and of doubtful clinical significance in adult humans, even though brown adipose tissue is found in humans. The principal receptors mediating catecholamine-stimulated lipolysis in brown adipose tissue, and to a lesser extent at other sites, are the β_3-adrenergic receptors. Drugs with β_3-adrenergic activities have been developed but side-effects have limited their use.

Clinical features

Most patients recognize their own problems, although often they are unaware of the main foods that cause obesity. Many symptoms are related to psychological problems or social pressures, such as the woman who cannot find fashionable clothes to wear.

The degree of obesity can be assessed by comparing the patient with tables of ideal weight for height, calculating the BMI ***(Box 10.20)*** and measuring skinfold thickness. The latter should be measured over the middle of the triceps muscle; normal values are 20 mm in a man and 30 mm in a woman. A central distribution of body fat (a waist/hip circumference ratio of >1.0 in men and >0.9 in women) is associated with a higher risk of morbidity and mortality than a more peripheral distribution of body fat (waist/hip ratio <0.85 in men and <0.75 in women). This is because fat located centrally, especially inside the abdomen, is more sensitive to lipolytic stimuli, with the result that the abnormalities in circulating lipids are more severe.

Box 10.21 shows the conditions and complications that are associated with obesity. The relationship between cardiovascular disease (hypertension or ischaemic heart disease), hyperlipidaemia, smoking, physical exercise and obesity is complex. Difficulties arise in interpreting mortality figures because of the number of factors involved. Many studies do not differentiate between the types of physical exercise taken nor do they take into account the cuff-size

Box 10.20 BMI ranges used to classify degrees of overweight and associated risk of co-morbidities

WHO classification	BMI (kg/m^2)	Risk of co-morbidities
Overweight	25–30	Mildly increased
Obese	>30	
Class I	30–35	Moderate
Class II	35–40	Severe
Class III	>40	Very severe

BMI, body mass index; WHO, World Health Organization.

Box 10.21 Conditions and complications associated with obesity

- Psychological
- Osteoarthritis of knees and hips
- Varicose veins
- Hiatus hernia
- Gallstones
- Postoperative problems
- Back strain
- Accident proneness
- Obstructive sleep apnoea
- Hypertension
- Breathlessness
- Ischaemic heart disease
- Stroke
- Diabetes mellitus (type 2)
- Hyperlipidaemia
- Menstrual abnormalities
- Increased morbidity and mortality
- Increased cancer risk
- Heart failure
- Non-alcoholic fatty liver disease

Box 10.22 Potential benefits from loss of 10 kg in 100 kg patients with co-morbidities

Mortality
- 20–25% fall in total mortality
- 30–40% fall in diabetes-related deaths
- 40–50% fall in obesity-related cancer deaths

Blood pressure
- Fall of about 10 mmHg (systolic and diastolic)

Diabetes
- Reduction in risk of developing diabetes by >50%
- 30–50% fall in fasting blood glucose
- 15% fall in HbA_{1c}

Serum lipids
- 10% fall in total cholesterol
- 15% fall in LDL cholesterol
- 30% fall in triglycerides
- 8% increase in HDL cholesterol

HbA_{1c}, haemoglobin A_{1c}; HDL, high-density lipoprotein; LDL, low-density lipoprotein.

artefact in the measurement of blood pressure (an artefact will occur if a large cuff is not used in patients with a large arm). Nevertheless, obesity almost certainly plays a part in all of these diseases and should be treated. An exception is that stopping smoking, even if accompanied by weight gain, is more beneficial than any of the other factors. Physical fitness is also helpful, and there is some evidence to suggest that a fit obese person may have a similar cardiovascular risk to a leaner, unfit person, or even a lower risk.

Morbidity and mortality

Obese patients are at risk of early death, mainly from diabetes, coronary heart disease and cerebrovascular disease. The greater the obesity, the higher are the morbidity and mortality rates. For example, men who are 10% overweight have a 13% increased risk of death, while the increase in mortality for those 20% overweight is 25%. The rise is less in women, and in men over 65, obesity is not an independent risk factor. Weight reduction reduces this mortality and therefore should be strongly encouraged. The benefits are probably greater in more obese subjects ***(Box 10.22)***.

Metabolic syndrome

There are two classification systems, which are shown in ***Box 10.23***. The differences are as follows:

- A large waist is an absolute requirement for the International Diabetes Federation (IDF) but not for the Adult Treatment Panel 3 National Cholesterol Education Programme (ATP III NCEP).

Box 10.23 Classification systems for metabolic syndrome: NCEP ATP III and IDF

Risk factor	ATP III NCEP (any 3 of 5 features)	IDF (large waist + 2 features)
Waist circumference		
Men	>102 cm (40 in)	>94 cm (37 in)
Women	>88 cm (35 in)	>80 cm (35 in)
Triglycerides	>1.7 mmol/L (150 mg/dL)	≥1.7 mmol/L (150 mg/dL)
HDL cholesterol		
Men	<1.03 mmol/L (40 mg/dL)	<1.03 mmol/L (40 mg/dL)
Women	<1.29 mmol/L (50 mg/dL)	<1.29 mmol/L (50 mg/dL)
Blood pressure	>130/85 mmHg	>130/85 mmHg
Fasting glucose	≥6.1 mmol/L (110 mg/dL)	≥5.6 mmol/L (100 mg/dL)

ATP III, Adult Treatment Panel 3; HDL, high-density lipoprotein; IDF, International Diabetes Federation; NCEP, National Cholesterol Education Programme.

- The IDF criteria use lower cut-off values for waist circumference (close to values for people with a BMI of 25 kg/m^2) and lower fasting blood glucose concentrations.

This means that the prevalence of metabolic syndrome will be higher using the IDF criteria, and that the IDF criteria will identify at-risk patients at an earlier stage. This could lead to further investigations following on from the initial screening, and earlier institution of preventative as well as therapeutic measures.

Overweight/central obesity and insulin resistance, which causes glucose and lipid disturbances including non-alcoholic fatty liver disease, seem to form the basis of many features of the metabolic syndrome. Early treatment of obesity and the metabolic syndrome can prevent the development of clinical diabetes and its complications.

The metabolic syndrome is a combination of risk factors (***Box 10.23***). Its overall role in the prediction of the risk of cardiovascular disease has been questioned, as the sum of the combined risk factors involved in the syndrome does not offer more than the individual factors added together.

Management

Dietary control

This largely depends on a reduction in calorie intake. The most common diets allow a daily intake of approximately 4200 kJ (1000 kcal), although this may need to be nearer 6300 kJ (1500 kcal) for someone engaged in physical work. Very-low-calorie diets are also advocated by some, usually over shorter periods of time, but unless they are accompanied by changes in lifestyle, weight regain is likely. Patients must realize that prolonged dieting is necessary for large amounts of fat to be lost. Furthermore, a permanent change in eating habits is required to maintain the new low weight. It is relatively easy for most people to lose the first few kilograms but long term success in moderate obesity is poor (no more than 10%). Most obese people oscillate in weight, they often regain the lost weight but many manage to lose weight again. This 'cycling' in body weight may play a role in the development of coronary artery disease.

Many dietary regimens aim to produce a weight loss of approximately 1 kg/week. Weight loss will be greater initially owing

Box 10.24 Constituents of a diet for weight loss

- A total of 4200 kJ (1000 kcal) per day is allowed, made up of >50 g protein, approximately 100 g of carbohydrate and 40 g of fat
- Carbohydrate should be in the form of complex carbohydrates, such as vegetables and fruit, rather than simple sugars
- Alcohol should be discouraged (contains 29 kJ/g (7 kcal/g)); it can be substituted for other foods in the diet but it often reduces willpower
- With a varied diet, vitamin and mineral intake will be adequate and supplements are not necessary.

to accompanying protein and glycogen breakdown and consequent water loss. After 3–4 weeks, further weight loss may be very small because only adipose tissue is broken down and there is less accompanying water loss.

Patients must understand the principles of energy intake and expenditure, and the best results are obtained in educated, well-motivated patients. Constant supervision by healthcare professionals or close relatives, or through membership of a slimming club, helps to encourage compliance. It is essential to establish realistic aims. A 10% weight loss, which is regarded by some as a 'success' (see ***Box 10.22***), is a realistic initial aim.

An increase in exercise will increase energy expenditure and should be encouraged – provided there is no contraindication – since weight control is usually not achieved without exercise. The effects of exercise are complex and not entirely understood. However, exercise alone will usually produce little long-term benefit. On the other hand, there is evidence to suggest that, in combination with dietary therapy, it can prevent weight being regained. In addition, regular exercise (30 min daily) will improve general health.

The diet should contain adequate amounts of protein, vitamins and trace elements ***(Box 10.24)***.

A balanced diet, attractively presented, is of much greater value and is safer than any of the slimming regimens often advertised in magazines.

A wide range of diets are available, including low-fat or low-carbohydrate diets, and some suit certain individuals better than others. The following general statements can be made about them:

- All low-calorie diets produce loss of body weight and fat, irrespective of dietary composition. Short-term weight loss is faster on low-carbohydrate diets, as a result of greater loss of body water, which is regained after the end of dietary therapy.
- Very-low-fat diets are often low in vitamins E and B_{12}, and in zinc. Very-low-carbohydrate diets may be nutritionally inadequate and may lead to deficiencies.
- Low-fat diets decrease LDL triglycerides and increase HDL, whereas low-carbohydrate diets produce a greater decrease in HDL and triglyceride, with no change in LDL.
- There are some potential long-term concerns with low-carbohydrate diets (high in fat and protein), including increased risk of osteoporosis, renal stones and atheroma (due to high intake of saturated fat, high *trans* fat and cholesterol, and the lack of fruits, vegetables and whole grains), but long-term studies are lacking.
- Low-energy-density diets, often bulky and rich in fibre and complex carbohydrates, may be more satiating but they are often less palatable than high-energy-dense diets, which may affect long-term compliance.
- Liquids, such as soft drinks, appear to be less satiating than solid foods.
- A study has shown that Mediterranean and low-carbohydrate diets are as effective as a low-fat diet for weight loss.

Behavioural modification

The aim of behavioural modification is to encourage the patient to take personal responsibility for changing lifestyle, which will determine dietary habits and physical activity. Family therapy may also be useful, especially when it involves obese children, but can be time-consuming and expensive. Cognitive behavioural therapy is even more time-consuming and expensive.

Drug therapy

Drugs can be used in the short term (e.g. up to 3 months and then reviewed), as an adjunct to the dietary regimen, but they do not substitute for strict dieting. The pancreatic lipase inhibitor, orlistat, was the only licensed drug for obesity in the UK in 2015.

Centrally acting drugs are as follows:

- Drugs acting on both **serotoninergic and noradrenergic pathways**, e.g. sibutramine (now withdrawn in Europe due to side-effects). Other drugs are being evaluated.
- **Cannabinoid-1 receptor blockers**, e.g. rimonabant (now withdrawn due to depression/suicide risk), acting on the endocannabinoid system.
- **Drugs acting on the noradrenergic pathways**. These do suppress appetite but all have been withdrawn, at least in the UK, because of cardiovascular side-effects.

Peripherally acting drugs are as follows:

- ***Orlistat*** is an inhibitor of pancreatic and gastric lipases. It reduces dietary fat absorption and aids weight loss. Weight regain occurs after the drug is stopped. It has been used continuously in a large-scale trial for up to 2 years. Patients complain of diarrhoea during treatment and, to avoid this, take a low-fat diet, resulting in weight loss.
- ***GLP-1*** suppresses appetite; injections have been used to treat obesity (see ***Fig. 10.14***) and type 2 diabetes mellitus (see p. 1254).

A systematic review of long-term pharmacotherapy concluded that there was a paucity of long-term studies with anti-obesity agents, and that in weight loss trials of 1 year's duration, these agents appear to be only modestly effective in promoting weight loss (about 3 or 4 kg greater weight loss, respectively, than the control group). Other randomized trials show that a combination of lifestyle modification and pharmacotherapy produces greater weight loss than either treatment alone, but the withdrawal of several anti-obesity drugs suggests that a pharmacotherapeutic magic bullet to treat obesity without substantial short-term and long-term effects is not yet available; the search continues. Alternative forms of treatment should be considered (unless obesity and its risks are accepted as part of modern society).

Surgical management (bariatric surgery, metabolic surgery)

Surgery is now performed laparoscopically in patients with morbid obesity (BMI >40 kg/m^2), or in patients with a BMI >35 kg/m^2 and obesity-related complications, after conventional medical treatments have failed. It can be used as a first-line option for individuals with a BMI >50 kg/m^2. Fitness for surgery should be checked, especially in older people. Some centres may insert a balloon into the stomach to initiate weight loss prior to bariatric surgery for morbid obesity. A variety of gastrointestinal surgical procedures have been used, which fall into three main groups ***(Fig. 10.15)***:

- ***Restrictive procedures***, which restrict the ability to eat (e.g. adjustable gastric banding, vertical banded gastroplasty and sleeve gastroplasty).
- ***Malabsorptive procedures***, which reduce the ability to absorb nutrients (e.g. biliopancreatic diversion and Roux-en-Y gastric

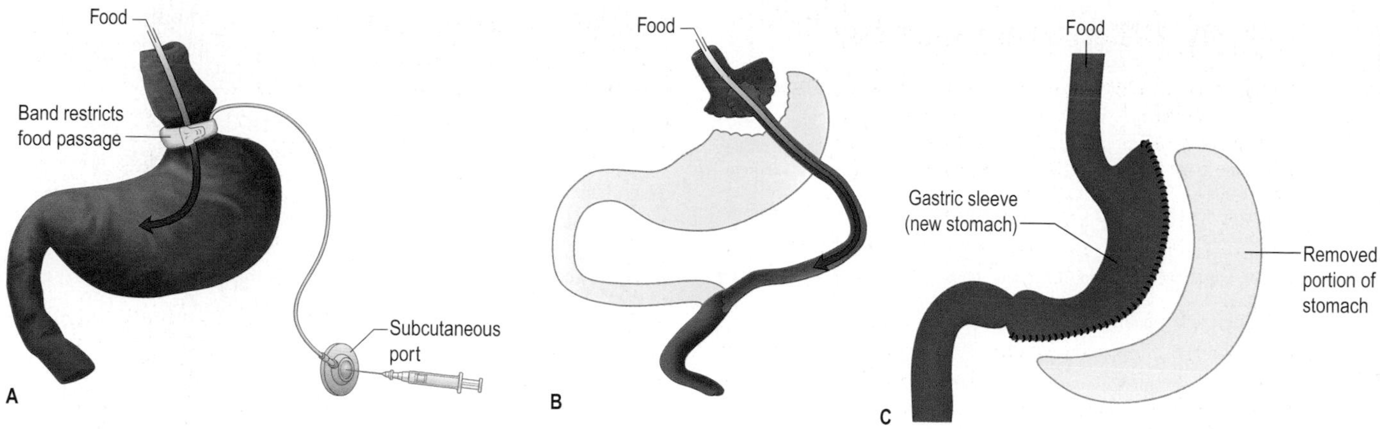

Figure 10.15 Examples of surgical procedures to treat morbid obesity. A. *Restrictive procedure*: gastric banding with a subcutaneous port attached to the anterior abdominal wall so that fluid can be injected into the adjustable band around the upper stomach. **B. *Restrictive plus malabsorptive procedure*:** Roux-en-Y gastric bypass, in which food bypasses through a small stomach pouch and bypasses the proximal small bowel. **C. *Gastric sleeve*.**

bypass). The malabsorptive procedures cause nutrient deficiencies, malnutrition and, in some cases, anastomotic leaks and the dumping syndrome (e.g. with the duodenal switch).

- ***Restrictive plus malabsorptive procedures*** (e.g. duodenal switch, Roux-en-Y gastric bypass, intragastric balloon.

The procedures all have advantages and disadvantages, and there is controversy about the procedure of choice for specific groups of patients. The restrictive procedures are more straightforward than the complex bypass procedures. The adjustable gastric banding procedure is attractive in concept, especially since it can be undertaken laparoscopically with a lower perioperative mortality (<0.3%) than the other procedures (approximately 1%); it can, however, be associated with erosion and slippage of the band, as well problems with the port, making repeat operations a frequent requirement (>10% of cases). The sleeve gastrectomy is associated with heartburn and greater risk of weight regain, but a biliary pancreatic diversion (duodenal switch) can be added at a later time.

There is a need to monitor nutrient status carefully with blood tests and to provide supplements of vitamins and minerals (including iron and calcium), as nutrient deficiencies are common. Weight loss following the combined restrictive and malabsorptive procedures tends to be greater than with either procedure alone.

A systematic analysis of several bariatric surgical procedures concluded that, in comparison to non-surgical treatments, they produced significantly more weight loss (23–37 kg), which was maintained up to 8 years and associated with improvement in quality of life and co-morbidities. There is now evidence showing that the risk of myocardial infarction, stroke, cardiovascular events and mortality is reduced by about half compared to non-surgical controls over a follow-up period of 2–15 years. Although fertility is improved after bariatric surgery, women are advised to delay pregnancy for a year or more after rapid and substantial weight loss, while the safety of pregnancy is being elucidated. A recent study has shown a reduction in risk of gestational diabetes and earlier than expected birth but the benefits and risks of bariatric surgery still need further study. The commissioning of specialist obesity services should be multidisciplinary and should not focus on the surgical treatment only.

Liposuction, the removal of large amounts of fat by suction (liposuction), does not deal with the underlying problem and weight regain frequently occurs. There appears to be no reduction in cardiovascular risk factors with the procedure.

Prevention

Preventing obesity must always be the goal because most obese people find it difficult to maintain any weight loss they have managed to achieve. All health professionals must be aware of the dangers of obesity and encourage children, and young as well as older adults, from gaining too much weight. A small gain each year over a long period produces an obese individual for whom treatment is difficult. Public health policies should consider the creation of public places to encourage physical activity and fitness, education about the benefits of losing weight or not gaining it, through healthy eating and physical activity, and changes in food composition (alternatives to high-fat, high-energy-dense foods and sugar reduction).

Since the present obesity epidemic has resulted from lifestyle changes, it is appropriate to promote lifestyle changes, not only as the first-line therapy for most overweight and obese individuals, but also in the prevention of overweight and obesity. Lifestyle modification would involve changes in the amount of time watching television and using computers, use of bicycle paths, dietary changes and educational activities for patients and public, parents and children. To prevent long-term weight gain after any of the therapies discussed above, each therapy should be part of a package that involves lifestyle modification.

Further reading

Caprio S. Calories from soft drinks – do they matter? *N Engl J Med* 2012; 367:1462–1463.

Casazza K, Pate R, Allison DB. Myths, presumptions, and facts about obesity. *N Engl J Med* 2013; 368:2236–2237.

Caughey AB. Bariatric surgery before pregnancy. *New Engl J Med* 2015: 372; 877–878.

Choban P, Dickerson R, Malone A et al. A.S.P.E.N. Clinical guidelines: nutrition support of hospitalized adult patients with obesity. *J Parenter Enteral Nutr* 2013; 37:714–744.

Dietz WH. Reversing the tide of obesity. *Lancet* 2011; 378:744 [illegible] plus series on obesity: 804–814; 815–825; 826–837; 838–847.

Eckel RH, Alberti KG, Grund SM. The metabolic syndrome. *Lancet* 2010; 375:181–183.

Grant P, Piya M, McGowan B et al. The bariatric physician. *Clin Med* 2014; 14:30–33.

Hawkes C, Smith TG, Jewell J et al. Smart food policies for obesity prevention. *Lancet* 2015; 385:2410–2421.

Huang TT-K, Cawley JH, Ashe M et al. Mobilisation of public support for policy actions to prevent obesity. *Lancet* 2015; 385:2422–2431.
Kwok CS, Pradhan A, Khan MA et al. Bariatric surgery and its impact on cardiovascular disease and mortality: a systematic review and meta-analysis. *Int J Cardiol* 2014; 173:20–28.
Lu Y, Hajifathalian K, Ezzati M et al. Metabolic mediators of the effects of body-mass index, overweight, and obesity on coronary heart disease and stroke: a pooled analysis of 97 prospective cohorts with 1.8 million participants. *Lancet* 2014; 383:970–983.
National Institute for Health and Care Excellence. *NICE Public Health Guideline 53: Managing Overweight and Obesity in Adults – Lifestyle Weight Management Services*. NICE 2014; http://www.nice.org.uk/guidance/ph53.
O'Rourke RW. Metabolic thrift and the genetic basis of human obesity. *Ann Surg* 2014; 259:642–648.
Ozanne SE. Epigenetic signatures of obesity. *New Engl J Med* 2015; 372:973–974.
Roberto CA, Swinburn B, Hawkes C et al. Patchy progress of obesity prevention: emerging examples, entrenched barriers, new thinking. *Lancet* 2015; 385:2400–2409.
Stein J, Stier C, Raab H et al. Review article: The nutritional and pharmacological consequences of obesity surgery. *Aliment Pharmacol Ther* 2014; 40:582–609.

NUTRITIONAL SUPPORT

Support in the hospital patient

Nutritional support is recognized as being necessary in many hospitalized patients. The pathophysiology and hallmarks of malnutrition have been described earlier (see pp. 189–191); here, the forms of nutritional support that are available are discussed, along with special nutritional requirements in some diseases.

Principles

Some form of nutritional supplementation is required in those patients who cannot eat, should not eat, will not eat or cannot eat enough. All patients should be screened for malnutrition on admission and the findings linked to a care plan, preferably under the supervision of a trained multidisciplinary team, including a registered dietician. Plans are discussed with patients and consent is taken for any invasive procedure (e.g. nasogastric tube, parenteral nutrition). If the patient is unable to give consent, the healthcare team should act in the patient's best interest, taking into account any previously expressed wishes of the patient and views of the family. It is usually necessary to provide nutritional support for:

- all severely malnourished patients on admission to hospital
- moderately malnourished patients who, because of their physical illness, are not expected to eat for more than 5 days
- normally nourished patients expected not to eat for more than 5 days or expected to eat less than half their intake for more than 8–10 days.

Enteral rather than parenteral nutrition should be used if the gastrointestinal tract is functioning normally.

In the ***re-feeding syndrome***, the shifts of water and electrolytes that occur during parenteral and enteral nutrition can be life-threatening. Carbohydrate intake stimulates insulin release, which leads to cellular uptake of phosphate, potassium and magnesium. *Complications* include hypophosphataemia, hypokalaemia, hypomagnesaemia and fluid overload because of sodium retention (decreased renal excretion of sodium and water). Biochemical abnormalities can result in cardiac arrhythmias and respiratory insufficiency, and are associated with a raised mortality. Any electrolyte deficiency should be replaced and monitored, and patients who have eaten little or nothing for more than 5 days should initially receive no more than 50% of their energy requirements (National Institute for Health and Care Excellence (NICE) guidelines). Patients at risk of the re-feeding syndrome should be given high potency vitamins daily for 10 days and oral or enteral thiamine 50 mg 4 times daily for 10 days, along with multivitamins.

Nutritional requirements for adults

The exact nutrient requirements in many disease states are not clearly defined and vary with the stage and severity of disease, as well as nutritional status. The optimal protein and energy intakes needed to produce the best clinical outcomes in acute critical illness continue to be debated. The following general guidance is provided for specific nutrients or groups of nutrients:

- ***Fluid***. Typical requirements are approximately 2–3 L/day (>60 years=30 mL/kg, 18–60 years=35 mL/kg). Requirements are increased in patients with large-output fistulae, nasogastric aspirates, diarrhoea and fever. Requirements are reduced in patients with oedema, hepatic failure, renal failure (oliguric and not dialysed) and brain oedema.
- ***Energy***. Typical requirements are approximately 7.5–10.0 MJ/day (1800–2400 kcal/day). Disease increases resting energy expenditure but decreases physical activity. Extra energy is given for repletion and reduced energy for obesity.
- ***Protein***. Typical requirements are 9–15 g N/day (56–94 g protein/day) or 0.15–0.25 g N/kg per day (0.94–1.56 g protein/kg per day). Extra protein may be needed in severely catabolic conditions, such as extensive burns, sepsis and major trauma.
- ***Major minerals***. Typical requirements for sodium and potassium are 60–100 mmol/day (1.0–1.5 mmol/kg). Requirements are increased in patients with gastrointestinal effluents. The excretion of these minerals in various effluents can provide an indication of the additional requirements (see ***Box 9.12***). Requirements may be low in patients with fluid overload (or those with hypernatraemia and hyperkalaemia). The requirements for calcium and magnesium are higher in enteral than in parenteral nutrition because only a proportion of these minerals is absorbed by the gut.
- ***Trace elements***. For trace elements such as iodine, fluoride and selenium, which are well absorbed, the requirements are similar in enteral and parenteral nutrition. For other trace elements, such as iron, zinc, manganese and chromium, the requirements in parenteral nutrition are substantially lower than in enteral nutrition ***(Fig. 10.16)***.
- ***Vitamins***. Many vitamins are given in greater quantities in patients receiving parenteral nutrition than in those receiving enteral nutrition ***(Fig. 10.17)***. This is because patients on parenteral nutrition may have increased requirements, partly because of severe disease, partly because they may already have depleted pools of vitamins, and partly because some vitamins degrade during storage. Vitamin K is usually absent from parenteral nutrition regimens and therefore it may need to be administered separately.

Enteral nutrition

In enteral nutrition, feeds can be given by various routes:

- By mouth (food can be supplemented with solid or liquid supplements with multiple benefits).
- By fine-bore nasogastric tube ***(Box 10.25)***.
- By percutaneous endoscopic gastrostomy (PEG). This is useful for patients who need enteral nutrition for a prolonged period (e.g. >30 days), such as those with swallowing problems following a head injury, or elderly people after a stroke.
  A catheter is placed percutaneously into the stomach under endoscopic control ***(Fig. 10.18)***.

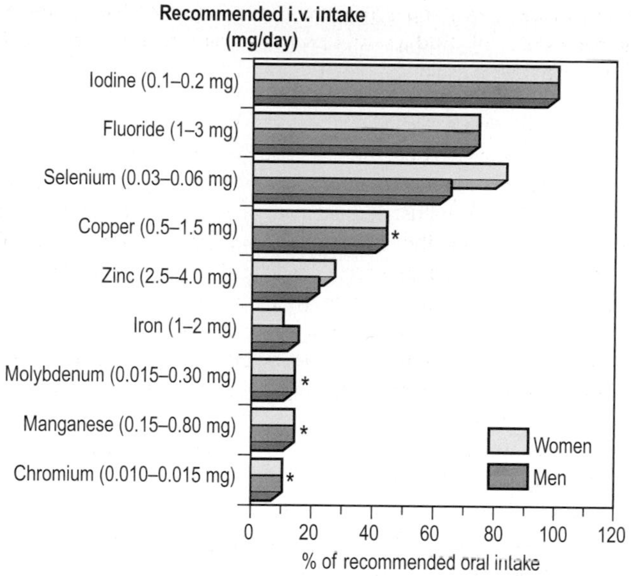

Figure 10.16 Trace elements. Recommended intravenous intake in absolute values and as a percentage of recommended oral intake. *Trace elements for which there is too little information to establish a recommended value for dietary oral intake; the midpoint of estimated safe and adequate oral intake is shown.

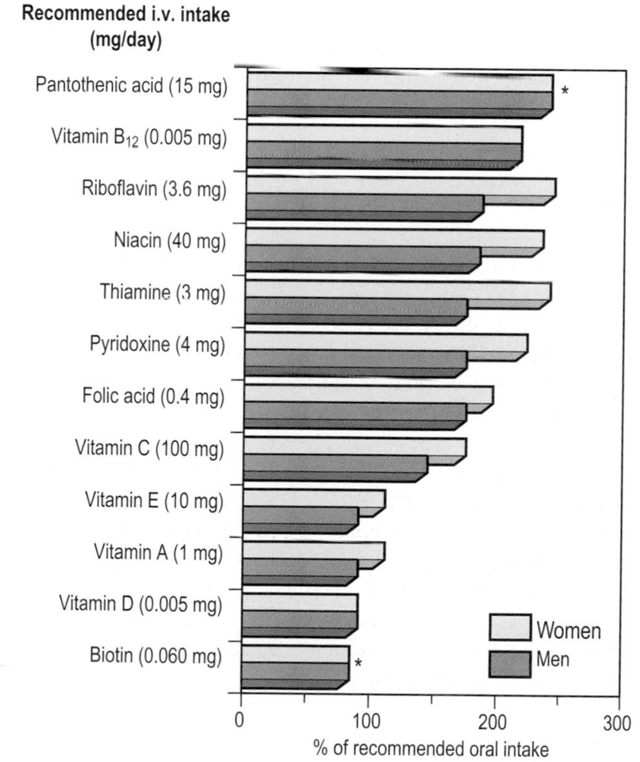

Figure 10.17 Vitamins. Recommended intravenous intake in absolute values and as a percentage of recommended oral intake. *Vitamins for which there is too little information to establish recommended dietary oral intake; the midpoint of estimated safe and adequate oral intake is shown.

Box 10.25 Enteral feeding via nasogastric tube

Explain the procedure to the patient and obtain consent.

Procedure
- Insert a fine-bore tube intranasally with a wire stylet.
- Confirm the position of the tube in the stomach by aspiration of gastric contents (check pH).
- Check by X-ray if aspiration is unsuccessful or pH <5.5 (pH <5 in some centres) is not definitive. Care should be taken in patients on strong acid suppressants such as proton pump inhibitors.

Problems
- No satisfactory way of keeping nasogastric tubes in place (up to 60% come out).

Main complications
- Regurgitation and aspiration into bronchus.
- Blockage of the nasogastric tube.
- Gastrointestinal side-effects, the most common being diarrhoea.
- Metabolic complications, including hyperglycaemia and hypokalaemia, as well as low levels of magnesium, calcium and phosphate.

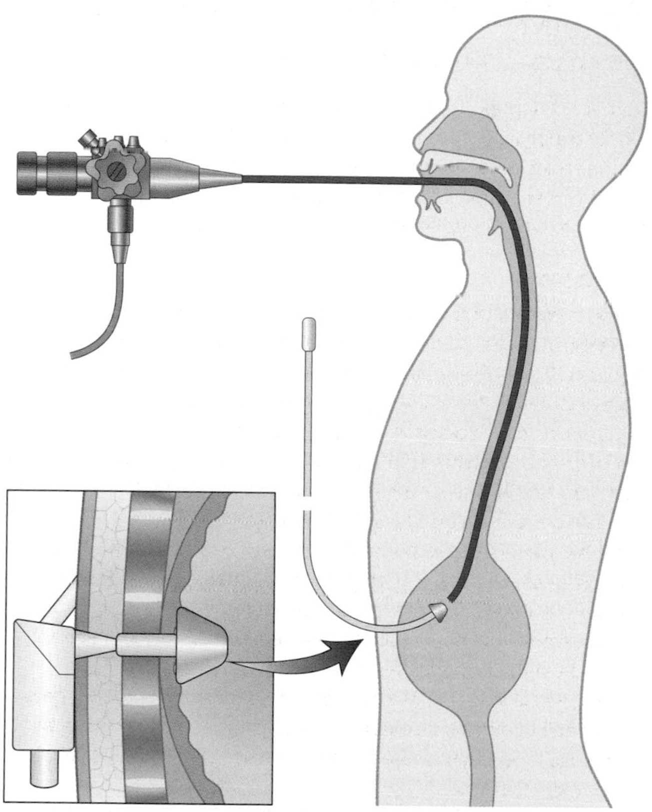

Figure 10.18 Percutaneous endoscopic gastrostomy (PEG).

- By needle catheter jejunostomy. In this technique, a fine catheter is inserted into the jejunum at laparotomy and brought out through the abdominal wall.

Diet formulation

A polymeric diet with whole protein and fat can be used (Box [illegible]) except in patients with severely impaired gastrointestinal function, who may require a pre-digested (i.e. semi-elemental/elemental) diet. In these patients, the nitrogen source is purified low-molecular-weight peptides or amino acid mixtures, the fat sometimes being given partly as medium-chain triglycerides (MCTs).

Box 10.26 Standard enteric diet, providing 8.4 MJ/day (=2000 kcal/day)

Energy
- Carbohydrate as glucose polymers (49–53% of total energy). Fat as triglycerides (30–35% of total energy)

Nitrogen
- Whole protein (10–14 g of nitrogen/day). Additional electrolytes, vitamins and trace elements

Features
- Ratio of energy to nitrogen kJ : g = 620 : 1 (kcal : g = 150 : 1). Osmolality = 285–300 mOsm/kg

Management of enteral nutrition

Daily amounts of fluid vary between 1.5 and 2.5 L, but small amounts are started in patients with suspected poor gastric emptying and severe malnutrition (to avoid the re-feeding syndrome).

Hypercatabolic patients require a high supply of nitrogen (0.25–0.35 g/kg daily) and often will not achieve positive nitrogen balance until the primary injury is resolved.

The success of enteral feeding depends on careful supervision of the patient, with monitoring of weight, biochemistry and diet charts.

Parenteral nutrition

This should only be used if the enteral route cannot be used. The need for major improvements in the practice of parenteral nutrition in UK hospitals has been emphasized by the National Confidential Enquiry into Patient Outcome and Death (NCEPOD). This included a requirement for improvements at every level: assessment, monitoring and follow-up, including appropriate care of lines to avoid catheter-related sepsis and documentation.

Peripheral parenteral nutrition

Specially formulated mixtures for peripheral use are available; these have a low osmolality (<800 mosmol/L) and contain lipid emulsions. Heparin and corticosteroids can be added to the infusion and local application of glyceryl trinitrate patches reduces the occurrence of thrombophlebitis and prolongs catheter life.

- A peripheral cannula can be inserted into a mid-arm vein (20 cm) and can be left for up to 5 days.
- A longer (60 cm), peripherally inserted central catheter (PICC) placed into an antecubital fossa vein has its distal end lying in a central vein; here, there is less risk of thrombophlebitis and hyperosmolar solutions can be given. With careful management, PICCs can be used for up to a month or so.

Peripheral parenteral nutrition is often preferred initially, allowing time to consider the necessity for insertion of a central venous catheter.

Parenteral nutrition via a central venous catheter

A silicone catheter is placed into a central vein, usually adopting an infraclavicular approach to the subclavian vein ***(Box 10.27)***. The skin-entry site should be dressed carefully and not disturbed unless there is a suggestion of catheter-related sepsis.

Complications of catheter placement include central vein thrombosis, pneumothorax and embolism, but one of the most common problems is catheter-related sepsis. Organisms, mainly staphylococci, enter along the side of the catheter, leading to septicaemia. Sepsis can be prevented by ensuring careful and sterile placement of the catheter, not removing the dressing over the catheter entry site, and not giving other substances (e.g. blood products, antibiotics) via the central vein catheter.

Box 10.27 Central catheter placement for parenteral nutrition

This should be performed only by experienced clinicians under aseptic conditions in an operating theatre.

Explain the procedure to the patient and obtain consent.

- Place the patient supine with 5° of head-down tilt to avoid air embolism.
- Infiltrate the skin below the midpoint of the right clavicle with 1–2% lidocaine and make a 1 cm skin incision.
- Insert a 20-gauge needle on a syringe beneath the clavicle and first rib, angling it towards the tip of a finger held in the suprasternal notch.
- When blood is aspirated freely, use the needle as a guide to insert the cannula through the skin incision and into the subclavian vein.
- Advance the catheter so that its tip lies in the distal part of the superior vena cava.
- Create a skin tunnel under local anaesthetic using an introducer inserted through a point about 10 cm below and medial to the incision and passed upwards to the incision.
- Pass the proximal end of the catheter (with hub removed) backwards through the introducer so that it emerges 10 cm below the clavicle; suture it to the chest wall.
- Now suture the original infraclavicular entry incision.

Sepsis should be suspected if the patient develops fever and leucocytosis. In two-thirds of cases, organisms can be grown from the catheter tip after removal. Treatment involves removal of the catheter and appropriate systemic antibiotics.

Nutrients

With parenteral nutrition, it is possible to provide sufficient nitrogen for protein synthesis and calories to meet energy requirements. Electrolytes, vitamins and trace elements are also necessary. All of these substances are infused simultaneously.

Nitrogen source

Most patients receive at least 11–15 g N/day, in the form of synthetic L-amino acids.

Energy source

Energy is supplied by glucose, with additional calories provided by a fat emulsion. Fat infusions give a greater number of calories in a smaller volume than can be provided by carbohydrate. Fat infusions are not hypertonic and they also prevent essential fatty acid deficiency, which has been reported in long-term parenteral nutritional regimens without fat emulsions. It causes a scaly skin, hair loss and a delay in healing.

Electrolytes, vitamins and trace elements

Initially, the electrolyte status should be monitored on a daily basis and electrolyte solutions given as appropriate. Fat- and water-soluble vitamins and minerals, including trace elements, should be given routinely (see ***Figs 10.16*** and ***10.17***).

Management of parenteral nutrition

Peripheral parenteral nutrition is administered via 3 L bags over 24 hours, the constituents being premixed under sterile conditions by the pharmacy. ***Box 10.28*** shows the composition that provides 9 g of nitrogen and 7206 kJ (1700 kcal) in 24 hours.

Box 10.28 Examples of parenteral nutrition regimens[a]

Peripheral

Nitrogen

- L-amino acids 9 g/L: 1 L

Energy

- Glucose 20%: 1 L
- Lipid 20%: 0.5 L
- + Trace elements, electrolytes, water-soluble and fat-soluble vitamins, heparin 1000 U/L and hydrocortisone 100 mg; insulin is added if required. Nitrogen 9 g, non-protein calories 7206 kJ (1700 kcal)

Central

Nitrogen

- L-amino acids 14 g/L: 1 L

Energy

- Glucose 50%: 0.5 L
- Glucose 20%: 0.5 L
- + Lipid 10% as either Intralipid or Lipofundin: 0.5 L; fractionated soya oil 100 g/L, soya oil 50 g, medium-chain triglycerides 50 g/L
- + Electrolytes, water-soluble and fat-soluble vitamins, trace elements; heparin and insulin may be added if required. Nitrogen 14 g, non-protein calories 9305 kJ (2250 kcal)

[a]All mixed in 3-L bags and infused over 24 h.

For a ***central venous parenteral nutrition regimen***, most hospitals now use premixed 3 L bags. A standard parenteral nutrition regimen that provides 14 g of nitrogen 9305 kJ (2250 kcal) over 24 hours is also given in ***Box 10.28***.

Monitoring includes:

- ***Blood tests***. Plasma electrolytes and glucose are checked daily (at least initially); full blood count, liver biochemistry and function, calcium and phosphate twice weekly; and magnesium, zinc and triglycerides weekly.
- ***Nutritional status***. Weight and skinfold thickness are monitored on a weekly basis if appropriate callipers are available. Daily weight changes reflect changes in fluid balance.
- ***Nitrogen balance assessment*** (see p. 186). This requires complete collections of urine.

Complications

- ***Mechanical***: insertional trauma and catheter-related (see above).
- ***Metabolic***: e.g. hyperglycaemia (insulin therapy is usually necessary), fluid and electrolyte disturbances, hypercalcaemia, nutrient deficiencies (if inadequately provided).
- ***Organ or tissue dysfunction***: e.g. abnormal liver dysfunction, respiratory distress and metabolic bone disease.
- ***Others***: e.g. rare allergic reactions to lipid, and psychological disturbances.

Support in the home patient

In both high- and low-income countries, there is considerably more undernutrition in the community than in hospital. However, the principles of care are very similar: detection of malnutrition and the underlying risk factors; treatment of underlying disease processes and disabilities; correction of specific nutrient deficiencies; and provision of appropriate nutritional support. This typically begins with dietary advice, and may involve the provision of 'meals on wheels' by social services. A systematic review of the use of nutritional supplements in the community came to the following conclusions:

- Supplements are generally of more value in ***patients with a BMI <20 kg/m² and children with growth failure*** (weight for height <85% of ideal) than in those with better anthropometric indices. They are likely to be of little or no value in patients with little weight loss and a BMI >20 kg/m². The supplemental energy intake in such subjects largely replaces oral food intake.
- Supplements may be of value in ***weight-losing patients*** (e.g. >10% weight loss compared to pre-illness) with a BMI >20 kg/m², and in ***children with deteriorating growth performance*** without chronic protein–energy under-nutrition.
- The functional benefits vary according to the patient group. In patients with ***chronic obstructive airways disease***, the observed functional benefits were increases in respiratory muscle strength, handgrip strength, and walking distance/duration of exercise. In the ***elderly***, the benefits were reduction in number of falls, or increase in activities of daily living, and reduction in pressure ulcer surface area. In patients with ***HIV/AIDS***, there were changes in immunological function and improved cognition. Patients with ***liver disease*** experienced a lower incidence of severe infections and had a lower frequency of hospitalization.
- ***Acceptability and compliance*** are likely to be better when a choice of supplements (of type, flavour, consistency) and the schedule are decided in conjunction with the patient and/or carer. Adjustments to these may be necessary when there is a change in patterns of daily activities, disease status, and 'taste fatigue' with prolonged use of the same supplement.
- Nutritional ***counselling and monitoring*** are recommended before and after the start of supplements (see below).

Some patients receive enteral tube feeding or parenteral nutrition at home. At any one point in time in developed countries, enteral tube feeding occurs more frequently at home than in hospital.

Home enteral nutrition

In adults, the most common reason for starting home tube feeding is for swallowing difficulties. This involves patients with neurological disorders, such as motor neurone disease, multiple sclerosis and Parkinson's disease, but the most common single diagnosis is cerebrovascular disease. Approximately 2% of patients who have had a stroke in the UK receive home enteral tube feeding (HETF). However, in a British Nutrition survey of patients with these disorders (apart from Parkinson's), only 15% in total were able to return to oral feeding after 1 year.

The swallowing capabilities of patients should be assessed regularly in order to avoid unnecessary tube feeding. The patients and/or carers should have adequate training, contacts with appropriate health professions, and a reliable delivery service for feeds and ancillary equipment. They should also be clear about how to manage simple problems associated with the feeding tube, which is usually a gastrostomy tube rather than a nasogastric tube.

Home parenteral nutrition

Home parenteral nutrition is practised much less frequently, and usually comes under the supervision of specialist centres. The potential value of intestinal transplantation in patients with long-term intestinal failure is still being assessed.

Further reading

Boateng AA, Sriram K, Meguid MM et al. Refeeding syndrome: treatment considerations based on collective analysis of literature case reports. *Nutrition* 2010; 26:156–167.
Casaer MP, Van den Berghe G. Nutrition in the acute phase of critical illness. *N Engl J Med* 2014; 370:2450–2451.
Elia M. Multidisciplinary input is essential in the care of malnourished people. *Guidelines in Practice* 2013; 16:42–50.
Elia M, Wheatley C. *Nutritional Care and the Patient Voice. Are We Being Listened To?* Redditch: BAPEN; 2014.
Malone A. Clinical guidelines from the American Society for Parenteral and Enteral Nutrition: best practice recommendations for patient care. *J Infus Nurs* 2014; 37:179–184.
Mirtallo JM. Consensus of parenteral nutrition safety issues and recommendations. *J Parenter Enteral Nutr* 2012; 36(2 Suppl):62S.
Russell CA, Elia M. *Nutrition Screening Surveys in Hospitals in England, 2007–2011: A Report Based on the Amalgamated Data from the Four Nutrition Screening Week Surveys Undertaken by BAPEN in 2007, 2008, 2010 and 2011.* BAPEN; 2014.

FOOD ALLERGY AND FOOD INTOLERANCE

Many people ascribe their various symptoms to food, and many such sufferers are seen and started on exclusion diets. The scientific evidence that food does harm is weak, in most instances, although adverse reactions to food certainly exist. These can be divided into those that involve immune mechanisms (***food allergy***) and those that do not (***food intolerance***).

Food allergy

Food allergy, which is estimated to affect up to 5–7% of young children and 1–2% of adults (with a rising prevalence), may be mediated by immunoglobulin E (IgE) or not mediated by IgE (T cell-mediated). The IgE-mediated reactions tend to occur early after a food challenge (within minutes to an hour). Adults tend to be allergic to fish, shellfish and peanuts, while children tend to be allergic to cow's milk, egg white, wheat and soy. Peanuts are very allergenic and peanut allergy persists throughout life. The following conditions can result from food allergy:

- ***Acute hypersensitivity***. An example is urticaria, vomiting or diarrhoea after eating nuts, strawberries or shellfish. These IgE-mediated reactions do not usually produce clinical problems, as the patients have already learned to avoid the suspected food. Inadvertent ingestion of the incriminating food can sometimes occur, leading to angioneurotic oedema (see pp. 1356–1357).
- ***Eczema and asthma***. These tend to affect young children; they are often due to egg and are IgE-mediated.
- ***Rhinitis and asthma***. These have been produced by foods such as milk and chocolate, mainly in atopic subjects.
- ***Chronic urticaria***. This has been treated successfully by an exclusion diet.
- ***Food-sensitive enteropathy***. This may manifest itself as coeliac disease (gluten (wheat) sensitive enteropathy) and cow's milk enteropathy (in infants); it is T cell-mediated.

Food intolerance

- ***Migraine***. This sometimes follows the intake of foods such as chocolate, cheese and alcohol, which are rich in certain amines, such as tyramine. Patients on monoamine oxidase inhibitors, which are involved in the metabolism of these amines, are particularly vulnerable.
- ***Irritable bowel syndrome***. In some patients, this seems to be related to ingestion of certain food items, such as wheat, but the mechanisms are not clearly defined.
- ***Chinese restaurant syndrome***. Monosodium glutamate, a flavour enhancer used in cooking Chinese food, may produce dizziness, faintness, nausea, sweating and chest pains.
- ***Lactose intolerance***. Patients develop abdominal bloating and diarrhoea following ingestion of lactose, which is present in milk (see p. 395). This is probably the most common form of food intolerance worldwide, and may be genetic in origin.
- ***Phenylketonuria***. This can also be classified as a form of food intolerance; it is due to lack of phenylalanine hydroxylase, which is necessary for the metabolism of phenylalanine present in dietary protein.

A number of other inborn errors of metabolism can also be regarded as forms of food intolerance.

Food intolerance may be caused by a constituent of food (e.g. the histamine in mackerel or canned food, or the tyramine in cheeses); by chemical mediators released by food (e.g. histamine may be released by tomatoes or strawberries); or by toxic chemicals found in food (e.g. the food additive tartrazine). Many other additives and compounds with certain E numbers have been implicated as causing reactions but the evidence is poor.

There is little or no evidence to suggest that diseases such as arthritis, behavioural and affective disorders, and Crohn's disease are due to ingestion of a particular food. Multiple vague symptoms, such as tiredness or malaise, are also not caused by food allergy. Most of the patients in this group are suffering from a psychiatric disorder (see pp. 901–902).

Management

- The history may help to delineate the causative agent, particularly when the effects are immediate.
- Skin-prick testing with allergen and measurement in the serum of antigen or antibodies have not correlated with symptoms and are usually misleading. Although widely advertised, 'fringe' techniques, such as hair analysis, are of no value.
- Diagnostic exclusion diets are sometimes used but are time-consuming. They can occasionally be of value in identifying a particular food that is causing problems.
- Dietary challenge consists of the food and the test being given sublingually or by inhalation in an attempt to reproduce the symptoms. Again, this may be helpful in a few cases.
- Most people who have acute reactions to food realize it and stop eating the food; they do not require medical attention. In the remainder of patients, a small minority seem to be helped by modifying their diet but there is no good scientific evidence to support these exclusion diets. A recent study showed that the introduction of peanuts decreased the frequency of peanut allergy in children at high risk of developing this allergy, and modulated immune responses to peanuts.
- Increasing evidence suggests that many children with milk and egg allergies are able to tolerate the food when heat-modified, and this may speed up resolution of the allergy.
- There is no good evidence to recommend that pregnant or breast-feeding women should change their diet to prevent allergies in infants at high risk or normal risk.

Further reading

de Silva D, Geromi M, Halken S et al. Primary prevention of food allergy in children and adults: systematic review. *Allergy* 2014; 69:581–589.

de Silva D, Geromi M, Panesar SS et al. Acute and long-term management of food allergy: systematic review. *Allergy* 2014; 69:159–167.

Gruchalla RS, Sampson HA. Preventing peanut allergy through early consumption. *New Engl J Med* 2015; 372:875–877.

Longo G, Berti I, Burks AW et al. IgE-mediated food allergy in children. *Lancet* 2013; 382:1656–1664.

Nwaru BI, Hickstein L, Panesar SS et al. The epidemiology of food allergy in Europe: a systematic review and meta-analysis. *Allergy* 2014; 69:62– 75.

Perry TT, Pesek RD. Clinical manifestations of food allergy. *Pediat Ann* 2013; 42:96– 101.

Sicherer SH, Sampson HA. Food allergy: epidemiology, pathogenesis, diagnosis, and treatment. *J Allergy Clin Immunol* 2014; 133:291–307; quiz 08.

Turner PJ, Boyle RJ. Food allergy in children: what is new? *Curr Opin Clin Nutr Metab Care* 2014; 17:285–293.

ALCOHOL

Although alcohol is not a nutrient, it is consumed in large quantities all over the world. In many countries, alcohol consumption is becoming a major medical and social problem (see pp. 920–922). It increases morbidity and mortality in a variety of ways, including effects on heart disease, stroke, cancers, liver and neurological/psychiatric problems, and is associated with nutritional deficiencies and abnormal metabolism of drugs.

Ethanol (ethyl alcohol) is oxidized, in the steps shown in ***Box 10.29***, to acetaldehyde. Acetaldehyde is then converted to acetate, 90% in the liver mitochondria. Acetate is released into the blood and oxidized by peripheral tissues to carbon dioxide and water.

Alcohol dehydrogenases are found in many tissues and it has been suggested that enzymes present in the gastric mucosa may contribute substantially to ethanol metabolism.

Ethanol itself produces 29.3 kJ/g (7 kcal/g), but many alcoholic drinks also contain sugar, which increases their calorific value. For example, 1 pint of beer provides about 1045 kJ (250 kcal), so heavy drinkers will be unable to lose weight if they continue to drink.

Effects of excess alcohol consumption

Excess consumption of alcohol leads to two major problems, both of which can be present in the same patient:

- alcohol dependence syndrome (see pp. 921–922)
- physical damage to various tissues.

Each unit of alcohol (defined as 10 mL (7.9 g) of pure ethanol) corresponds to about half a pint of normal beer, one single measure of spirit or half a glass of wine) ***(Fig. 10.19)***. An intake of less than 21 units per week in men and 14 units per week in women is generally considered to be safe, but recent UK guidelines suggest 14 units for women and men. All the long-term effects of excess alcohol consumption are due to excess ethanol, irrespective of the type of alcoholic beverage; that is, beer and spirits are no different in their long-term effects. Short-term effects, such as hangovers, depend on additional substances, particularly other alcohols such as isoamyl alcohol, which are known as congeners. Brandy and bourbon contain the highest percentage of congeners.

The amount of alcohol that produces damage varies and not everyone who drinks heavily will suffer physical damage. For example, only 20% of people who drink heavily develop cirrhosis of the liver. The effect of alcohol on different organs of the body is not the same; in some patients, the liver is affected; in others, the brain or muscle. The differences may be genetically determined.

Thiamin deficiency contributes to neurological (confusion, Wernicke–Korsakoff syndrome; see p. 885) and some of the non-neurological manifestations (cardiomyopathy). The susceptibility of different organs to damage is variable and the figures given in ***Box 10.30*** are provided only as a guide to sensible drinking. Heavy drinkers who persist for many years are at greater risk than heavy sporadic drinkers.

Box 10.29 The main pathways of ethanol oxidization

Alcohol dehydrogenase

$$\underset{\text{(ethanol)}}{CH_3CH_2OH} + NAD^+ \xrightarrow{ADH} \underset{\text{(acetaldehyde)}}{CH_3CHO} + NADH + H^+ \qquad [1]$$

Liver microsomal enzyme oxidizing system (MEOS)

- Includes the specific P450 enzyme, CYP2EI, which is induced by ethanol

$$CH_3CH_2OH + NADPH + H^+ + O_2 \xrightarrow{MEOS} CH_3CHO + NADP + 2H_2O \qquad [2]$$

Box 10.30 Guide to sensible alcohol drinking

Daily maximum

- 3 units for men; 2 units for women

To help achieve this

- Use a standard measure
- Do not drink during the daytime
- Have alcohol-free days each week

Remember

- Health can be damaged without being 'drunk'. Regular heavy intake is more harmful than occasional binges
- Do not drink to 'drown your sorrows'
- In the UK, the drink-before-driving limit of alcohol in the blood is 800 mg/L (80 mg%)
- 1 unit of alcohol is eliminated per hour; therefore spread drinking time
- Food decreases absorption and therefore results in a lower blood alcohol level
- 4–5 units are sufficient to put the blood alcohol level over the legal driving limit in a 70 kg man (less in a lighter person)

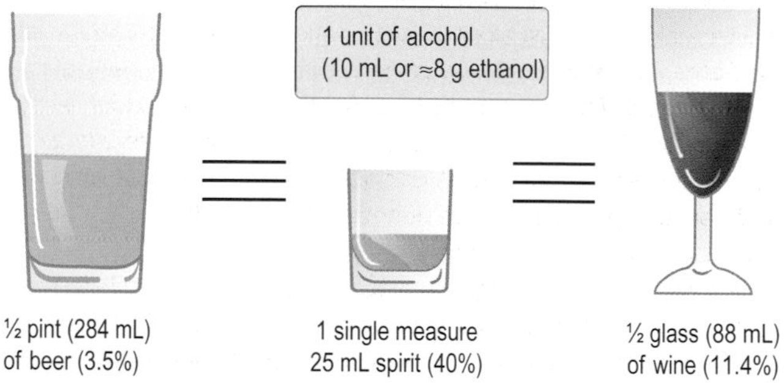

Figure 10.19 Measures containing 1 unit of alcohol. The percentage refers to the proportion of alcohol by volume (vol/vol). The alcohol content of beers, spirits and wines can vary substantially.

Liver disease

In general, the effects of a given intake of alcohol seem to be worse in women. The following figures are for men and should be reduced by about 30% for women:

- ***High risk***: 160 g ethanol per day (20 single drinks)
- ***Medium risk***: 80 g ethanol per day (10 single drinks)
- ***Little risk***: 40 g ethanol per day (5 single drinks).

Box 10.31 Physical effects of excess alcohol consumption

Central nervous system
- Epilepsy (see pp. 847–848)
- Wernicke–Korsakoff syndrome (see p. 885)
- Polyneuropathy (see p. 885)

Muscles
- Acute or chronic myopathy

Cardiovascular system
- Cardiomyopathy (see p. 1037)
- Beriberi heart disease (see p. 198)
- Cardiac arrhythmias
- Hypertension

Metabolism
- Hyperuricaemia (gout)
- Hyperlipidaemia
- Hypoglycaemia
- Obesity

Endocrine system
- Pseudo-Cushing syndrome

Respiratory system
- Chest infections

Gastrointestinal system
- Acute gastritis (including bleeding; see pp. 384–385)
- Carcinoma of the oesophagus or large bowel
- Pancreatic disease
- Liver disease (fatty liver, hepatitis, cirrhosis; see pp. 480–482)

Haemopoiesis
- Macrocytosis (due to direct toxic effect on bone marrow or folate deficiency)
- Thrombocytopenia
- Leucopenia

Bone
- Osteoporosis
- Osteomalacia

Alcohol consumption in pregnancy

Women are advised not to drink alcohol at all during pregnancy because consumption of even small amounts of alcohol can lead to 'small babies' and may also increase the risk of miscarriage. The fetal alcohol syndrome is characterized by mental retardation, dysmorphic features and growth impairment; it occurs in fetuses of alcohol-dependent women.

A summary of the physical effects of alcohol is given in ***Box 10.31***. Details of these diseases are discussed in the relevant chapters. The effects of alcohol withdrawal are discussed on page 922.

Specific public health and clinical guidance on prevention and management of alcohol-related disorders has been produced by NICE. The clinical guidelines specifically address alcohol withdrawal, Wernicke's encephalopathy, and both alcohol-related liver and pancreatic disease.

Further reading

Braglehole R, Bonita R. Alcohol and global health priority. *Lancet* 2009; 373:2173–2174.
National Institute for Health and Care Excellence. *NICE Clinical Guideline 115: Alcohol-use Disorders: Diagnosis, Assessment and Management of Harmful Drinking and Alcohol Dependence*. NICE 2011; http://www.nice.org.uk/guidance/cg115.
Stewart S, Swain S. Assessment and management of alcohol dependence and withdrawal in the acute hospital: concise guidance. *Clin Med* 2012; 12:266–271.

Bibliography

Elia M, Ljungqvist O, Stratton RJ et al. *Clinical Nutrition*, 2nd edn. Oxford: Wiley–Blackwell, 2013 (part of Nutrition Society textbook bundle; available at http://eu.wiley.com).

Significant websites

http://www.ajcn.org/ *American Journal of Clinical Nutrition*
http://www.ama-assn.org/ *American Medical Association; assessment and management of adult obesity*
http://www.fao.org/ *Food and Agriculture Organization; autonomous body within the United Nations aiming to improve health through nutrition and agricultural productivity, especially in rural populations*
http://www.foodstandards.gov.uk *UK information on food composition and dietary surveys*
http://www.ific.org/ *International Food Information Council; non-profit organization providing access to health and nutrition resources to improve communication of health and nutrition information to consumers*
http://www.nature.com/ejcn/ *European Journal of Clinical Nutrition*
http://www.nature.com/ijo *International Journal of Obesity*
https://www.nice.org.uk/search?q=obesity *NICE; various publications related to obesity*
https://www.nice.org.uk/search?q=alcohol *NICE; various publications related to prevention and treatment of alcohol-related problems*
http://jn.nutrition.org/ *Journal of Nutrition*
http://www.nutritioncare.org/ *Journal of Parenteral and Enteral Nutrition*
http://www.nutritionsociety.org/publications/ *British Journal of Nutrition*
http://www.nhlbi.nih.gov/health/educational/ *National Heart, Lung and Blood Institute: Aim for a Healthy Weight*
http://www.who.int/nut *WHO recommendations and intervention programmes for nutrient-related diseases*
http://www.who.int/nutgrowthdb/ *World Health Organization; provides information on worldwide nutritional issues, resources and research*

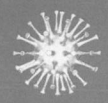

11 Infectious diseases and tropical medicine

Gavin Barlow, William L Irving, Peter J Moss

See your e-book for extra images, extra tables, MCQs and Special Topics from the International Advisory Board.

SITES OF INFECTION WITH COMMON ORGANISMS

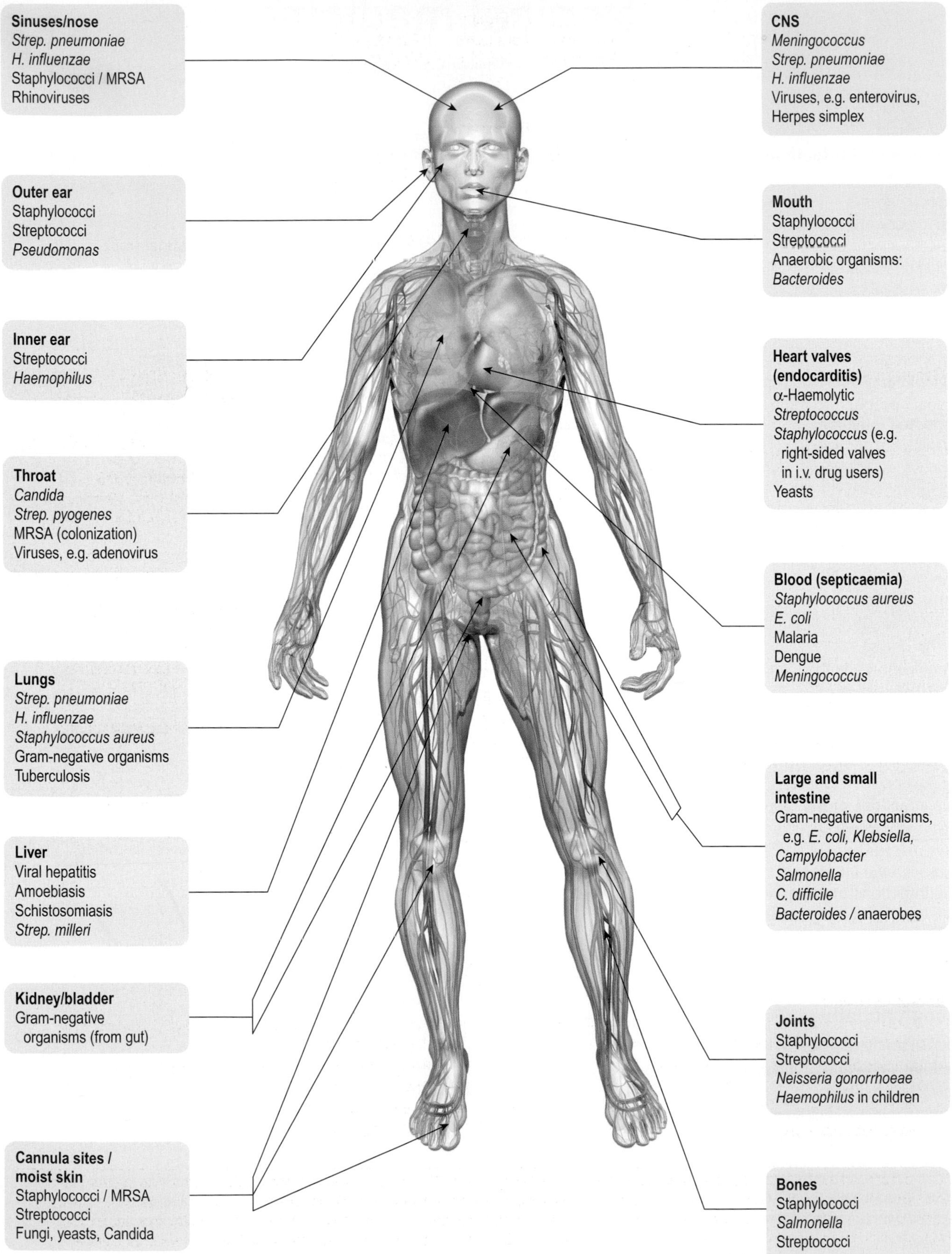
Sinuses/nose
Strep. pneumoniae
H. influenzae
Staphylococci / MRSA
Rhinoviruses
Outer ear
Staphylococci
Streptococci
Pseudomonas
Inner ear
Streptococci
Haemophilus
Throat
Candida
Strep. pyogenes
MRSA (colonization)
Viruses, e.g. adenovirus
Lungs
Strep. pneumoniae
H. influenzae
Staphylococcus aureus
Gram-negative organisms
Tuberculosis
Liver
Viral hepatitis
Amoebiasis
Schistosomiasis
Strep. milleri
Kidney/bladder
Gram-negative organisms (from gut)
Cannula sites / moist skin
Staphylococci / MRSA
Streptococci
Fungi, yeasts, Candida
CNS
Meningococcus
Strep. pneumoniae
H. influenzae
Viruses, e.g. enterovirus, Herpes simplex
Mouth
Staphylococci
Streptococci
Anaerobic organisms: *Bacteroides*
Heart valves (endocarditis)
α-Haemolytic *Streptococcus*
Staphylococcus (e.g. right-sided valves in i.v. drug users)
Yeasts
Blood (septicaemia)
Staphylococcus aureus
E. coli
Malaria
Dengue
Meningococcus
Large and small intestine
Gram-negative organisms, e.g. *E. coli, Klebsiella,*
Campylobacter
Salmonella
C. difficile
Bacteroides / anaerobes
Joints
Staphylococci
Streptococci
Neisseria gonorrhoeae
Haemophilus in children
Bones
Staphylococci
Salmonella
Streptococci

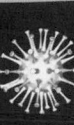

IN SUSPECTED INFECTION

History

Symptoms Travel (see p. 233, ***Box 11.11***)
Animal contact Occupation Sexual history
IV drugs use?

↓

Examination

Temperature Heart rate Respiration rate
Rash Blood pressure Confusion
A B C D E

↓

Patient suspected of sepsis

↓

Management (Sepsis Six)
(within first 60 min of admission)

1. High-flow O_2
2. Blood culture and source control
3. IV antibiotics
4. IV fluid resuscitation
5. Hb and serial lactates
6. Hourly urine output measurements

↓

Do quick SOFA (qSOFA)

- Respiratory rate ≥22/min
- Altered mentation ↓ (GCS)
- Systolic BP ≤100 mmHg

↓

If >2 refer to Outreach CCU

↓

Admit to CCU
Do SOFA (p. 1154)

↓

Sepsis

Give adequate fluid
if vasopressors required
to maintain MAP >65 mmHg
+
Serum lactate >2 mmol/L

↓

Redefine state

Septic shock

Infection
+
Hypovolaemia
+
SOFA >2

General Investigations

Bloods	FBC
	U+Es
	LFTs
	CRP/ESR
	Serum lactate
	Glucose
Urine	NAAT
	MSU
	Culture
Arterial blood gases	
Imaging	X-ray
	Ultrasound
	Echo
	CT/MRI
	PET
	Radionuclides
Bacteriological	Blood cultures × 3
	Culture of specific sites of infection
	PCR

Abnormalities in sepsis

FBC
- WBC >12,000 x 10^9/L or <4000 x 10^9/L
- Platelets < 100,000 x 10^9/L

UE ↑ creatinine >310 μmol/L
Acute oliguria (urine output <0.5 mL/kg/hr)

LFTs
- Hyperbilirubinaemia >70 mmol/L

Serum lactate >2 mmol/L

Blood gases
- Arterial hypoxaemia PaO_2/FiO_2 <30

Coagulation abnormalities

INR >1.5
or
PTT >60 secs

End-organ failure

- Systolic blood pressure (SBP) <90 mmHg or >40 mmHg fall from baseline or mean arterial pressure (MAP) <65 mmHg
- Bilateral pulmonary infiltrates with no new need for oxygen to maintain saturations >90% or with PaO_2/FiO_2 ratio <300 mmHg or 39.9 kPa
- Serum lactate >2.0 mmol/l
- Serum creatinine >176.8 μmol/L or urine output <0.5 mL/kg per hour for 2 successive hours
- INR >1.5 or an (activated) partial thromboplastin time (PTT) >60 sec
- Platelet count <100 × 10^9/L
- Bilirubin >34.2 μmol/L

CCU, critical care unit; CGS, glasgow coma scale; CRP, C-reactive protein; CT, computed tomography; ESR, erythrocyte sedimentation rate; FBC, full blood count; FiO_2, fraction of inspired oxygen; INR, International Normalized Ratio; LFTs, liver function tests; MAP, mean arterial pressure; MRI, magnetic resonance imaging; MSU, mid-stream specimen of urine; NAAT, nucleic acid amplification technique; PaO_2, arterial oxygen tension; PCR, polymerase chain reaction; PET, positron emission tomography; SOFA, sequential organ failure assessment; U+Es, urea and electrolytes.

(Modified from Singer M, Deutschman CS, Seymour CW, et al. The Third International Consensus Definitions for Sepsis and Septic Shock (Sepsis-3). *JAMA* 2016; 315(8):801–810.)

INFECTION AND INFECTIOUS DISEASE

INTRODUCTION

'Infection' is defined as the process of pathogenic organisms invading and multiplying in or on a host's tissues. The term should be reserved for situations in which this results in harm, rather than when an infectious agent simply colonizes the host without ill effect. The delicate balance between colonizing pathogenic and non-pathogenic organisms in health is increasingly being recognized in studies of the human microbiome. Infectious diseases remain one of the main causes of morbidity and mortality in humans, particularly in developing areas, where they are associated with poverty and overcrowding.

In the ***developed world***, increasing prosperity, hygiene, universal immunization and antibiotics have reduced the prevalence of infectious disease. Increasingly, however, antibiotic-resistant, and difficult-to-treat, strains of microorganisms are being isolated, and diseases such as human immunodeficiency virus (HIV) infection, variant Creutzfeldt–Jakob disease (vCJD), avian and pandemic H1N1 influenza, and Middle East respiratory syndrome (MERS) have emerged. There is increased global mobility, both enforced (as a result of war, civil unrest and natural disaster) and voluntary (for tourism and economic benefit). This has aided the spread of infectious disease and allowed previously localized pathogens, such as dengue, West Nile virus and chikungunya, to establish themselves across much wider territories. An increase in the movement of livestock and animals has enabled the spread of zoonotic diseases like monkeypox, while changes in farming and food-processing methods have contributed to an increase in the incidence of food- and water-borne diseases. Deteriorating social conditions in the inner city areas of our major conurbations have facilitated the resurgence of tuberculosis and other infections. Prisons and refugee camps, where large numbers of people are forced to live in close proximity, often in poor conditions, continue to provide a breeding ground for devastating epidemics of infectious disease. There are ongoing concerns about the deliberate release of infectious agents, such as smallpox or anthrax, by terrorist groups or national governments.

In the ***developing world***, successes such as the eradication of smallpox have been balanced or outweighed by the new plagues. Communicable, maternal, neonatal and nutritional conditions were responsible for 23% of deaths worldwide in 2012. Although, increasingly, the leading causes of deaths are non-communicable diseases, lower respiratory tract infections, HIV and diarrhoeal diseases still account for 11% of all deaths ***(Box 11.1)***. In low-income countries, these infections remain common causes of mortality, malaria and tuberculosis being the sixth and eighth most common causes of death, respectively. In 2012, 8.6 million people developed tuberculosis, 1.3 million died and there were 450 000 cases of multidrug-resistant tuberculosis; approximately 2.7 million people caught malaria with 627 000 deaths; and 42.1 million were treated for schistosomiasis. Some 240 million people are chronically infected with a hepatitis virus (either hepatitis B or C virus) and 35 million people are living with HIV or the acquired immunodeficiency syndrome (AIDS, or advanced HIV), with 2.1 million new HIV infections in 2013 (70% in sub-Saharan Africa). Infections are often multiple and there is synergy between different infections (e.g. tuberculosis and HIV) and other factors such as malnutrition. Many of the infectious diseases affecting developing countries are preventable or treatable, but continue to thrive owing to lack of money and political will. The surveillance of infectious diseases is generally poor in such countries, resulting in a slow response to emerging problems. It seems likely that the emergence of highly resistant Gram-negative pathogens will disproportionately affect the poor and vulnerable.

Box 11.1 Leading causes of mortality worldwide, 2012

Causes of death	Number/percentages of death	
	Millions (annual)	*%*
Ischaemic heart disease	7.4	13.2
Stroke	6.7	11.9
Chronic obstructive pulmonary disease	3.1	5.6
Lower respiratory infections	3.1	5.5
Trachea, bronchus, lung cancers	1.6	2.9
HIV/AIDS	1.5	2.8
Diarrhoeal diseases	1.5	2.7
Diabetes mellitus	1.5	2.7
Road injury	1.3	2.3
Hypertensive heart disease	1.1	2.0

(Data from World Health Organization, www.who.int.)

The World Health Organization (WHO) set eight Millennium Development Goals (MDGs; see p. 43), meant to be achieved by 2015; these included combating HIV/AIDS, malaria and other diseases. Subsequently, new HIV infections fell by 33% between 2001 and 2012, and approximately 10 million people in low- and middle-income countries are now receiving anti-retroviral therapy. Of the 97 countries with ongoing malaria transmission in 2013, 20 were classified as being in the pre-elimination or elimination phase. Whilst a lot has been achieved by public/private partnerships, such as the Global Fund, and other governmental, non-governmental and charitable funders, it is clear that there is still much to be done and it is likely that many countries will not achieve all of the goals.

The impact of global warming on the spread and incidence of infection remains uncertain. Both natural climatic events and the gradual global change in weather conditions can affect the spread and transmission of infectious diseases. Changes in temperature directly influence the behaviour of insect vectors, while changes in rainfall have an effect on water-borne disease. Climate change also triggers population movement and migration, indirectly affecting infection transmission.

Infectious agents

The causative agents of infectious diseases can be divided into four groups.

Prions are the most recently recognized and the simplest infectious agents, consisting of a single protein molecule. They contain no nucleic acid and therefore no genetic information; their ability to propagate within a host relies on inducing the conversion of endogenous prion protein PrP^{c} into an abnormal protease-resistant isoform referred to as PrP^{Sc} or PrP^{Res}.

Viruses contain both protein and nucleic acid, and so carry the genetic information for their own reproduction. However, they lack the apparatus to replicate autonomously, relying instead on 'hijacking' the cellular machinery of the host. They are small (usually less than 250 nanometres (nm) in diameter) and each virus possesses only one species of nucleic acid (either RNA or DNA).

Bacteria are usually, though not always, larger than viruses. Unlike the latter, they have both DNA and RNA, with the genome encoded by DNA. They are enclosed by a cell membrane, and even bacteria that have adopted an intracellular existence remain enclosed within their own cell wall. Bacteria are capable of fully autonomous reproduction and the majority are not dependent on host cells.

Eukaryotes are the most sophisticated infectious organisms, displaying sub-cellular compartmentalization. Different cellular functions are restricted to specific organelles: for example, photosynthesis takes place in the chloroplasts, DNA transcription in the nucleus and respiration in the mitochondria. Eukaryotic pathogens include unicellular protozoa, fungi (which can be unicellular or filamentous) and multicellular parasitic worms.

Other higher classes, notably the insects and the arachnids, also contain species that can parasitize humans and cause disease; these are discussed in more detail on page 316.

Host–organism interactions

Each of us is colonized by huge numbers of microorganisms (10^{14} bacteria, plus viruses, fungi, protozoa and worms), with which we coexist. The relationship with some of these organisms is symbiotic, in which both partners benefit, while other organisms are commensals, living on the host without causing harm. Infection and illness may be due to these normally harmless commensals and symbiotes evading the body's defences and penetrating into abnormal sites. Alternatively, disease may be caused by exposure to exogenous pathogenic organisms that are not part of our normal flora.

The symptoms and signs of infection are a result of the interaction between host and pathogen. In some cases, such as the early stages of influenza, symptoms are almost entirely due to killing of host cells by the invading organism. Usually, however, the harmful effects of infection are caused by a combination of direct microbial pathogenicity and the body's response to infection. In meningococcal septicaemia, for example, much of the tissue damage is caused by cytokines released in an attempt to fight the bacteria. The molecular mechanisms underlying host–pathogen interactions are discussed in more detail on pages 227–229.

Sources of infection

The endogenous skin and bowel commensals can cause disease in the host, either because they have been transferred to an inappropriate site (e.g. bowel coliforms causing urinary tract infection) or because host immunity has been attenuated (e.g. candidiasis in an immunocompromised host). Many infections are acquired from other people, who may be symptomatic themselves or be asymptomatic carriers. Some bacteria, like the meningococcus, are common transient commensals but cause invasive disease in a small minority of those colonized. Infection with other organisms, such as the hepatitis B virus, can be followed in some cases by an asymptomatic but potentially infectious carrier state.

Zoonoses are infections that can be transmitted from wild or domestic animals to humans. Infection can be acquired in a number of ways: direct contact with the animal, ingestion of meat or animal products, contact with animal urine or faeces, aerosol inhalation, via an arthropod vector or by inoculation of saliva in a bite wound. Many zoonoses can also be transmitted from person to person. Some zoonoses are listed in ***Box 11.2***.

Most microorganisms do not have a vertebrate or arthropod host but are free-living in the environment. The vast majority of these environmental organisms are non-pathogenic but a few can cause human disease ***(Box 11.3)***. Person-to-person transmission of these infections is rare. Some parasites may have a stage of their life cycle that is environmental (e.g. the free-living larval stage of *Strongyloides stercoralis* and the hookworms), even though the adult worm requires a vertebrate host. Other pathogens can survive for periods in water or soil and be transmitted from host to host via this route (see below); these should not be confused with true environmental organisms.

Routes of transmission

Endogenous infection

The body's own endogenous flora can cause infection if the organism gains access to a usually sterile site. This can happen by simple mechanical transfer, such as when colonic bacteria enter the female urinary tract. The non-specific host defences may be breached, for example, by cutting or scratching the skin and allowing surface commensals to gain access to deeper tissues; this is frequently the aetiology of cellulitis. There may be more serious defects in host immunity owing to disease or chemotherapy, allowing normally harmless skin and bowel flora to produce invasive disease.

Air-borne spread

Many respiratory tract pathogens are spread from person to person by aerosol or droplet transmission. Secretions containing the infectious agent are coughed, sneezed or breathed out and are then inhaled by a new victim. Some enteric viral infections may also be spread by aerosols of faeces or vomit. Environmental pathogens, such as *Legionella pneumophila*, and zoonoses, such as ornithosis, are also acquired by aerosol inhalation, while rabies virus may be inhaled in the dust from bat droppings.

Faeco-oral spread

Transmission of organisms by the faeco-oral route occur by direct transfer (usually in small children), by contamination of clothing or household items (usually in institutions or conditions of poor hygiene) or, most commonly, via contaminated food or water. Human and animal faecal pathogens get into the food supply at any stage. Raw sewage is used as fertilizer in many parts of the world, contaminating growing vegetables and fruit. Poor personal hygiene can result in contamination during production, packaging, preparation or serving of foodstuffs. In the Western world, the centralization of the food supply and increased processing of food have allowed the potential for relatively minor episodes of contamination to cause widely disseminated outbreaks of food-borne infection.

Water-borne faeco-oral spread is usually the result of inadequate access to clean water and safe sewage disposal, and is common throughout the developing world. Worldwide, 1.1 billion people have no access to clean water and 2.6 billion do not have basic sanitation.

Vector-borne disease

Many tropical infections, including malaria, are spread from person to person or from animal to person by an arthropod vector. Vector-borne diseases are also found in temperate climates but are relatively uncommon. In most cases, part of the parasite life cycle takes place within the body of the arthropod and each parasite species requires a specific vector. Simple mechanical transfer of infective

Box 11.2 Zoonotic infections

Disease	Pathogen	Animal reservoir	Mode of transmission
Prions			
vCJD	Prion protein	Cattle	Ingestion (CNS tissue)
Viruses			
Lassa fever	Arenavirus	Multimammate rats	Direct contact
Avian influenza	Influenza H5N1	Birds	Inhalation
Japanese encephalitis	Flavivirus	Pigs	Mosquito bite
Rabies	Rhabdovirus	Dogs and other mammals	Saliva, faeces (bats)
Yellow fever	Flavivirus	Primates	Mosquito bite
Monkeypox	Orthopox virus	Rodents, small mammals	Uncertain
SARS	Coronavirus	Unsure, most likely bats	Droplet
MERS	Coronavirus	Camels	Droplet
Bacteria			
Gastroenteritis	*Escherichia coli* *Salmonella enteritidis* and others *Campylobacter jejuni*	Cattle, chickens Chickens, cattle Various, e.g. chickens	Ingestion (contaminated food) Ingestion (meat, eggs) Ingestion (meat, milk, water)
Leptospirosis	*Leptospira interrogans*	Rodents	Ingestion (urine)
Brucellosis	*Brucella abortus* *Brucella melitensis*	Cattle Sheep, goats	Contact; ingestion of milk/cheese
Anthrax	*Bacillus anthracis*	Cattle, sheep	Contact; ingestion
Lyme disease	*Borrelia burgdorferi*	Deer	Tick bite
Cat-scratch disease	*Bartonella henselae*	Cats	Flea bite
Plague	*Yersinia pestis*	Rodents	Flea bite
Typhus	Various *Rickettsia* spp.	Various	Arthropod bite
Ornithosis (psittacosis)	*Chlamydia psittaci*	Psittacine and other birds	Aerosol
Others			
Toxoplasmosis	*Toxoplasma gondii*	Cats and other mammals	Ingestion (meat, faeces)
Hydatid disease	*Echinococcus granulosus*	Dogs	Ingestion (faeces)
Trichinosis	*Trichinella spiralis*	Pigs, bears	Ingestion (meat)
Toxocariasis	*Toxocara canis*	Dogs	Ingestion
Cutaneous larva migrans	*Ancylostoma caninum*	Dogs	Penetration of skin by larvae

CNS, central nervous system; MERS, Middle East respiratory syndrome; SARS, severe acute respiratory syndrome; vCJD, variant Creutzfeldt–Jakob disease.

organisms from one host to another can occur but is rare. Some vector-borne diseases are shown in ***Box 11.4***.

Direct person-to-person spread

Organisms can be passed on directly in a number of ways. Sexually transmitted infections are dealt with on pages 317–331. Skin infections such as ringworm, and ectoparasites such as scabies and head lice, can be spread by simple skin-to-skin contact. Other organisms are passed on by transmission from blood (or, occasionally, some other body fluid) to blood. Blood-to-blood transmission can occur during sexual contact; from mother to infant, either transplacentally or in the peripartum; between intravenous drug users sharing any part of their injecting equipment; when infected medical or other (e.g. tattoo needles) equipment is reused; if contaminated blood or blood products are transfused; or in any sporting or accidental contact when blood is spilled. Ingestion of infected breast milk is another route of person-to-person spread for some infections (e.g. HIV).

Indirect person-to-person spread

Many organisms can be spread from person to person indirectly by contamination of fomites (e.g. door handles), which are subsequently touched by another person. Common examples include respiratory viruses, such as influenza, and healthcare-associated pathogens, such as meticillin-resistant *Staphylococcus aureus* (MRSA) and the spores of *Clostridium difficile*. This is sometimes an overlooked route of transmission; minimization requires, for example, hand-washing immediately after sneezing or coughing and when moving from ward to ward in a hospital, and optimal cleaning regimens in institutions.

Direct inoculation

Infection can occur when pathogenic organisms breach the normal mechanical defences by direct inoculation. Some of the circumstances in which this can occur are covered under endogenous infection and blood-to-blood transmission above. Some environmental organisms may be inoculated by accident; this is a common mode of transmission of tetanus and certain fungal infections. Rabies virus may be inoculated by the bite of an infected animal.

Consumption of infected material

Although many food-related zoonotic infections are due to contamination of food with animal faeces (and are thus, strictly speaking, faeco-oral), several diseases are transmitted directly in animal products. These include some strains of *Salmonella* (eggs, chicken

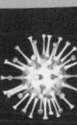

Box 11.3 Environmental organisms that can cause human infection

Organism	Disease (most common presentations)
Bacteria	
Burkholderia pseudomallei	Melioidosis
Burkholderia cepacia	Lung infection in cystic fibrosis
Pseudomonas spp.	Various
Legionella pneumophila	Legionnaires' disease (pneumonia)
Bacillus cereus	Gastroenteritis
Listeria monocytogenes	Various
Clostridium tetani	Tetanus
Clostridium perfringens	Gangrene, septicaemia
Mycobacteria other than tuberculosis (MOTT)	Pulmonary infections
Fungi	
Candida spp.	Local and disseminated infection
Cryptococcus neoformans	Meningitis, pulmonary infection
Histoplasma capsulatum	Pulmonary infection
Coccidioides immitis	Pulmonary infection
Mucor spp.	Mucormycosis (rhinocerebral, cutaneous)
Sporothrix schenckii	Lymphocutaneous sporotrichosis
Blastomyces dermatitidis	Pulmonary infections
Aspergillus fumigatus	Pulmonary infections

Box 11.4 Infections transmitted by arthropod vectors

Vector	Disease	Microorganism
Mosquito	Malaria	*Plasmodium* spp.
	Lymphatic filariasis	*Wuchereria bancrofti*, *Brugia malayi*
	Yellow fever	Flavivirus
	West Nile fever	Flavivirus
	Dengue	Flavivirus
	Zika	Flavivirus
Sandfly	Leishmaniasis	*Leishmania* spp.
	Bartonellosis	*Bartonella bacilliformis*
Blackfly	Onchocerciasis	*Onchocerca volvulus*
Tsetse fly	Sleeping sickness	*Trypanosoma brucei*
Flea	Plague	*Yersinia pestis*
	Endemic typhus	*Rickettsia typhi*
Reduviid bug	Chagas' disease	*Trypanosoma cruzi*
Louse	Epidemic typhus	*Rickettsia prowazekii*
	Louse-borne relapsing fever	*Borrelia recurrentis*
Hard tick	Lyme disease	*Borrelia burgdorferi*
	Typhus (spotted fever group)	*Rickettsia* spp.
	Babesiosis	*Babesia* spp.
	Tick-borne relapsing fever	*Borrelia duttonii*
	Tick-borne encephalitis	Flavivirus
	Congo–Crimean haemorrhagic fever	Nairovirus (Bunyavirus)

meat), brucellosis (unpasteurized milk), *E. coli*, and the prion diseases kuru and vCJD (neural tissue).

Prevention and control

Methods of preventing infection depend on the source and route of transmission.

- ***Infection control measures***. Poor infection control practice in hospitals and other healthcare environments can cause the transfer of infection from person to person. It is essential for all healthcare workers to wash or clean their hands before and after patient contact; whenever necessary, they should wear gloves, aprons and other protective equipment. This is particularly necessary when they are performing invasive procedures or manipulating indwelling devices. Care should also be taken with contact with a patient known to be colonized or infected with a resistant organism (e.g. carbapenemase-producing *Klebsiella pneumoniae*) or a communicable pathogen with high mortality (e.g. Ebola), or a patient who has diarrhoea (e.g. *Clostridium difficile* infection).
- ***Eradication of reservoir***. In a few diseases, for which humans are the only natural reservoir of infection, it may be possible to eliminate disease by an intensive programme of case-finding, ***treatment and immunization***. This has been achieved in the case of smallpox. If there is an animal or environmental reservoir, complete eradication is unlikely, but local control methods may decrease the risk of human infection (e.g. killing of rodents to control plague, leptospirosis and other diseases).
  - For ***arthropod–vector-borne infections***. It may be possible to destroy the vector species (which may be practical in certain circumstances) or to take measures to avoid being bitten (e.g. insect repellent sprays, impregnated bed nets).
  - For ***food-borne infections***. Improvements in food handling and preparation result in less contamination during processing, transport or preparation. Organisms intrinsically present in food can be killed by appropriate preparation and cooking. Improved surveillance and regulation of the food industry, as well as better health education for the public, are necessary.
  - For ***faeco-oral infections***. Improvements in water supply and sanitation (recognized in the Millennium Development Goals) could dramatically decrease the prevalence of faeco-oral infections.
  - For ***blood-borne infections***. Blood transfer may be prevented, e.g. in blood transfusions and contaminated medical equipment. Donated blood is routinely tested for infection in most developed countries.
  - For ***infections spread by air-borne and direct contact***. Some air-borne respiratory infections and some infections spread by direct contact can be controlled by isolating patients. This is often difficult, but isolation is useful in patients with severe immunodeficiency to protect them from infection.
- ***Immunization*** (see pp. 245–246).

Healthcare-associated infections

The burden of morbidity, mortality and cost attributed to healthcare-associated infection (HCAI) has been highlighted in many developed countries. Although data from low-income countries are lacking, the impact of HCAI is likely to be even greater. *Clostridium difficile*, *Staph. aureus* (especially MRSA), vancomycin-resistant enterococci and the increasingly difficult-to-treat, multiresistant, Gram-negative organisms are all strongly associated with healthcare contact and are a growing problem in hospitals worldwide. In 2011, the number of inpatients with an HCAI in acute hospitals in England decreased to 6.4%, compared to 8.2% in 2006, the most frequent infections affecting the respiratory tract, urinary tract and surgical sites. Over a similar period, there have also been notable declines in the incidences of, and mortality caused by, MRSA bloodstream and *C. difficile* infections. These have been due to higher standards of basic infection control, including rapid isolation of patients, hospital cleaning and universal MRSA screening (and decolonization therapy, if positive) on entry to acute hospitals and prior to surgery.

HCAI control measures

- The ***care bundle approach*** is used: a set (typically 3–5) of, ideally, highly evidence-based, simple actions that healthcare professionals should always take to minimize the risk of a negative outcome. As an example, see the *Matching Michigan* approach to reducing infections associated with central intravenous catheters ('Further reading').

Other infection control measures that health workers should focus on to reduce the risk of HCAI include:

- ***Hand hygiene***. Before and after all patient contacts, and after contact with body fluids, mucous membranes, non-intact skin or fomites in the patient's environment, soap and water (rather than an alcohol-based rub) should be used after visible contamination of hands and when patients are vomiting or have diarrhoea, even if gloves are used.
- ***Personal protective equipment***. Gloves should be worn for all invasive procedures, including venesection, and contact with sterile sites, mucous membranes, bodily fluids or non-intact skin. Disposable plastic aprons should be used when there is a risk of contamination of clothing or skin; if there is a risk of extensive contamination, surgical gowns should be worn.
- ***Aseptic technique***. This should be adopted for all invasive procedures, when using and manipulating invasive devices, and when in contact with all wounds.
- ***Urinary catheters***. Insert these only when it is essential to do so and remove them as soon as possible. Ensure that a clear care plan is in place for longer-term catheters.
- ***Vascular access devices***. Insert a vascular catheter only when there is a clear plan to use it; check the device daily and remove as soon as possible. Use 2% chlorhexidine gluconate in 70% isopropyl alcohol for skin decontamination prior to insertion and to clean the access port or hub prior to use. Ensure that a clear care plan is in place for medium- or long-term devices.

Classification of outbreaks

The type of outbreak has a bearing on the public health measures that need to be instituted for its control.

- ***Person-to-person*** is where infection is passed from one infected individual to another and outbreaks of infection are separated by the incubation period.
- ***Point source*** is where there is a single source of infection, e.g. food eaten at a social function. All those infected will develop symptoms at the same time, around the expected incubation period.
- ***Common source*** is where there is a single source of infection but infection is spread over a period of time, e.g. a symptomatic carrier of infection working with food preparation. Many people will be exposed over a long period of time.
- ***Epidemic*** is when there is an increased and unusually widespread infection in the community, causing waves of infection. Epidemics spread through communities and affect all people who have no active immunity to that infection.

Box 11.5 Notifiable diseases in England and Wales[a]

- Acute encephalitis
- Acute infectious hepatitis
- Acute meningitis
- Acute poliomyelitis
- Anthrax
- Botulism
- Brucellosis
- Cholera
- Diphtheria
- Ebola
- Enteric fever (typhoid and paratyphoid)
- Food poisoning
- Haemolytic uraemic syndrome (HUS)
- Infectious bloody diarrhoea
- Invasive group A streptococcus
- Legionnaires' disease
- Leprosy
- Malaria
- Measles
- Meningococcal septicaemia (without meningitis)
- MERS
- Mumps
- Plague
- Rabies
- Rubella
- Scarlet fever
- Severe acute respiratory syndrome (SARS)
- Smallpox
- Tetanus
- Tuberculosis
- Typhus
- Viral haemorrhagic fever
- Viral hepatitis
- Whooping cough
- Yellow fever
- Zika

[a]*Diseases are notifiable to Local Authority Proper Officers under the Health Protection (Notification) Regulations 2010. MERS, Middle East respiratory syndrome.*

- ***Pandemic*** is an epidemic, as defined above, occurring worldwide or over a very wide geographical area and crossing international boundaries, usually affecting a large number of people.

Some infectious diseases should be notified to the public health authorities, so that they are aware of cases and outbreaks and can respond accordingly. Diseases that are notifiable in England and Wales are listed in ***Box 11.5***.

Further reading

Farmer PE. Shattuck lecture. Chronic infectious disease and the future of health care delivery. *N Engl J Med* 2013; 369:2424–2436.
Fineberg HV, Hunter DJ. A global view of health – an unfolding series. *N Engl J Med* 2013; 368:78–79.
Fisman DN, Leung GM, Lipsitch M. Nuanced risk assessment for emerging infectious diseases. *Lancet* 2013; 383:189–190.
Hopkins DR. Global health: disease eradication. *N Engl J Med* 2013; 368:54–63.
Horton R, Das P. Indian health: the path from crisis to progress. *Lancet* 2011; 377:181–183.
Karesh WB, Dobson A, Lloyd-Smith JO et al. Ecology of zoonoses: natural and unnatural histories. *Lancet* 2012; 380:1936–1945.
Kilpatrick AM, Randolph SE. Drivers, dynamics, and control of emerging vector-borne zoonotic diseases. *Lancet* 2012; 380:1946–1955.
Loveday HP, Wilson JA, Pratta RJ et al. Epic3: national evidence-based guidelines for preventing healthcare-associated infections in NHS hospitals in England. *J Hosp Infect* 2014; 86S1:S1–S70.
Morse SS, Mazet JAK, Woolhouse M et al. Prediction and prevention of the next pandemic zoonosis. *Lancet* 2012; 380:1956–1965.
Murray CJ, Lopez AD. Measuring the global burden of disease. *N Engl J Med* 2013; 369:448–457.
[No authors listed]. The GAVI Alliance – successes and ongoing challenges. *Lancet* 2013; 382:1310.
Peleg AY, Hooper DC. Hospital-acquired infections due to Gram-negative bacteria. *N Engl J Med* 2010; 362:1804–1813.
Relman DA. Microbial genomics and infectious diseases. *N Engl J Med* 2011; 365:347–357.
Shurman EK. Global climate change and infectious disease. *N Engl J Med* 2010; 282:1061–1063.
Sultan F, Khan A. Infectious diseases in Pakistan: a clear and present danger. *Lancet* 2013; 381:2138–2139.
Infection parts 1, 2 and 3. *Medicine*, November and December 2013; 41:611–730 and January 2014; 42:1–64.
http://www.gov.uk/ *Public Health England.*
http://www.patientsafetyfirst.nhs.uk/ *Patient Safety First: Matching Michigan – Reducing CVC [central venous catheter] Bloodstream Infections.*
http://www.who.int/ *World Health Organization infectious diseases.*

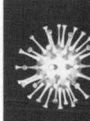

PRINCIPLES AND BASIC MECHANISMS

The majority of microorganisms cause no harm and some play a role in the normal functioning of the mouth, vagina and intestinal tract. However, many microorganisms have the potential to produce disease. This results from inoculation into damaged tissues, tissue invasion, a variety of virulence factors, or toxin production.

Specificity

Microorganisms are often highly specific with respect to the organ or tissue they infect (see p. 220). For example, a number of viruses are hepatotropic, such as those responsible for hepatitis A, B, C and E and for yellow fever. This predilection for specific sites in the body relates partly to the presence of appropriate receptors on different cell types and partly to the immediate environment in which the organism finds itself; for example, anaerobic organisms colonize the anaerobic colon, whereas aerobic organisms are generally found in the mouth, pharynx and proximal intestinal tract. Other organisms that show selectivity include:

- Streptococcus pneumoniae (respiratory tract)
- Escherichia coli (urinary and alimentary tract).

Even within a species of bacterium such as *E. coli*, there are clear differences between strains with regard to their ability to cause gastrointestinal disease (see p. 274), which, in turn, differ from uropathogenic *E. coli*, which are responsible for urinary tract infection.

Within an organ, a pathogen may show selectivity for a particular cell type. In the intestine, for example, rotavirus predominantly invades and destroys intestinal epithelial cells on the upper portion of the villus, whereas reovirus selectively enters the body through the specialized epithelial cells, known as M cells, which cover the Peyer's patches (see p. 393).

Pathogenesis

Figure 11.1 summarizes some of the steps that occur during the pathogenesis of infection. In addition, pathogens have developed a variety of mechanisms to evade host defences. For example, some pathogens produce toxins directed at phagocytes – *Staphylococcus aureus* (α-toxin), *Streptococcus pyogenes* (streptolysin) and *Clostridium perfringens* (α-toxin) – while others, such as *Salmonella* spp. and *Listeria monocytogenes*, can survive within macrophages. Several pathogens possess a capsule that protects against complement activation (e.g. *Strep. pneumoniae*). Antigenic variation is an additional mechanism for evading host defences that is recognized in viruses (antigenic shift and drift in influenza), bacteria (flagella of *Salmonella* and gonococcal pili) and protozoa (surface glycoprotein changes in *Trypanosoma*).

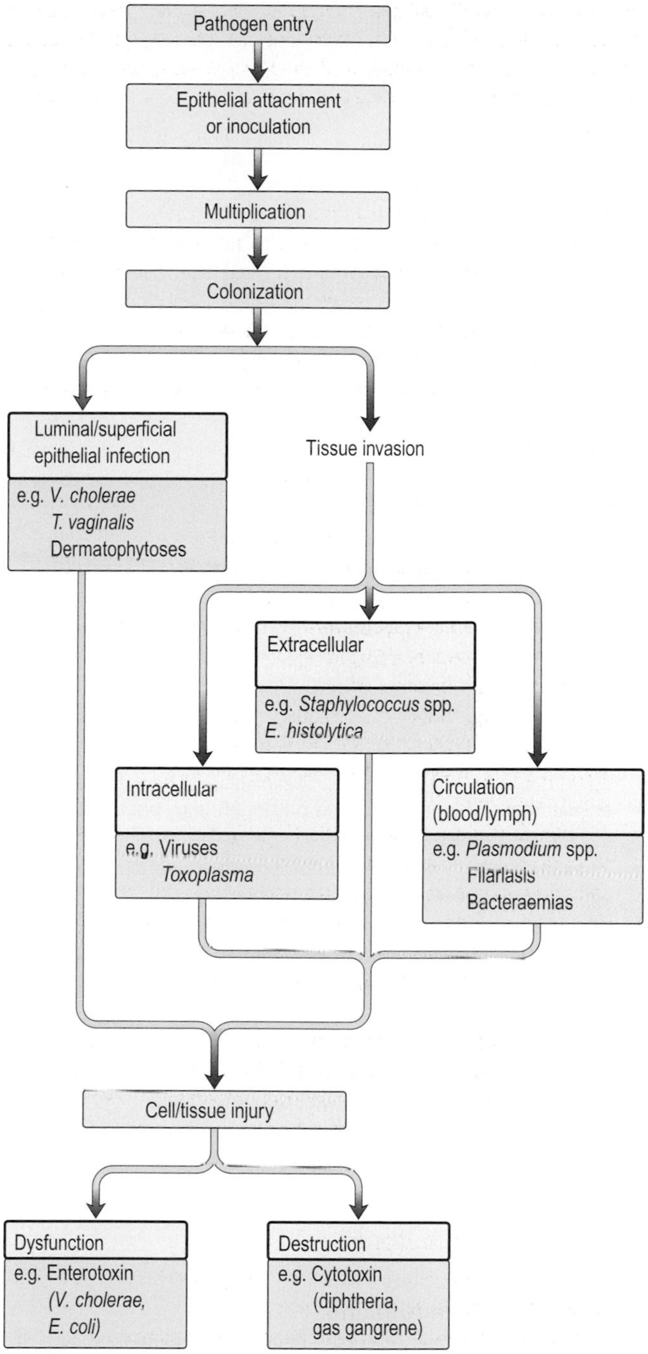

Figure 11.1 The pathogenesis of infection.

Epithelial attachment

Many bacteria attach to the epithelial substratum by specific organelles called pili (or fimbriae) that contain a surface lectin (or lectin) – a protein or glycoprotein that recognizes specific sugar residues on the host cell. This family of molecules is known as adhesins (see pp. 94–95). Following attachment, some bacteria, such as species of coagulase-negative staphylococci, produce an extracellular slime layer and recruit additional bacteria, which cluster together to form a biofilm. These biofilms can be difficult to eradicate and are a frequent cause of medical device-associated infections that affect prosthetic joints and heart valves, as well as indwelling catheters. Many viruses and protozoa (e.g. *Plasmodium* spp., *Entamoeba histolytica*) attach to specific epithelial target-cell receptors. Other parasites, such as hookworm, have specific attachment organs (buccal plates) that firmly grip the intestinal epithelium.

Colonization

Following epithelial attachment, pathogens may remain either on the surface epithelium or within the lumen of the organ they have colonized. Tissue invasion may follow.

Invasion may result in:

- an intracellular location for the pathogen (e.g. viruses, *Mycobacterium* spp., *Toxoplasma gondii*, *Plasmodium* spp.)

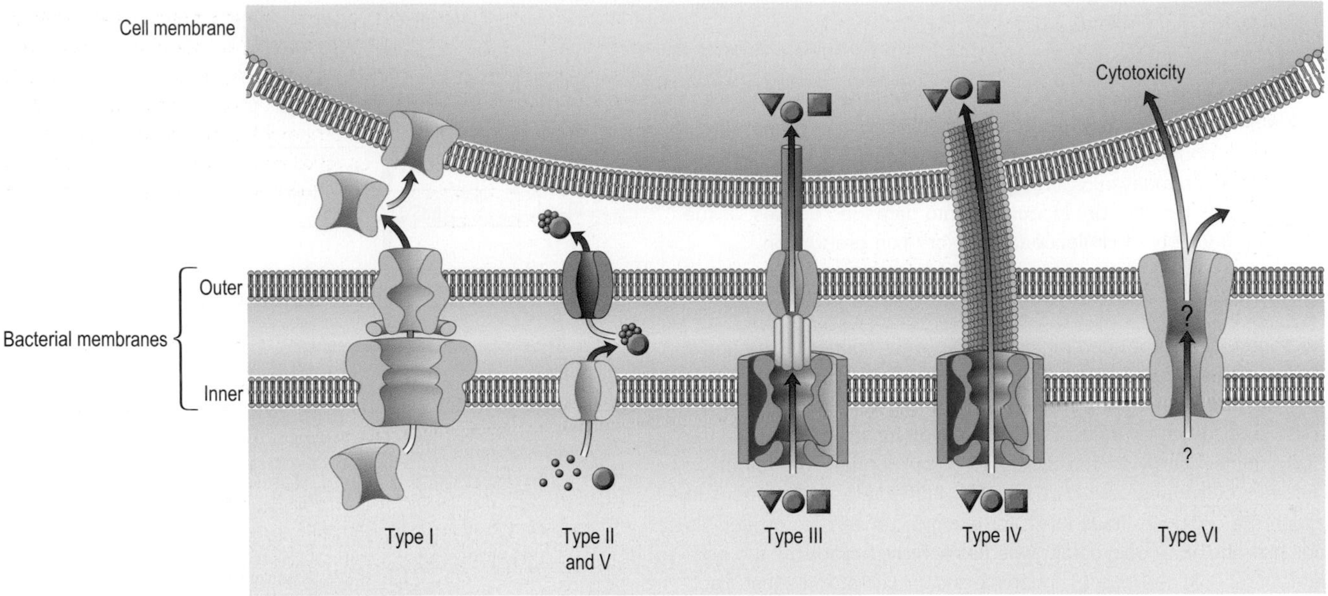

Figure 11.2 Protein secretion pathways for Gram-negative bacteria. These specialized pathways are necessary for virulence. *Types I and II* facilitate protein (toxin) secretion into the extracellular space (type I). Type II does this in two stages. *Types III and IV* pathways secrete toxins, as well as injecting toxins directly into the host cells via multiprotein complexes across the bacterial cell envelope and host-cell membrane. *Type V* is a minor variation of type II. The *type VI* pathway is unclear but is involved in cytotoxicity. *(Reproduced with permission from Yarh TL. A critical new pathway for toxin secretion?* New England Journal of Medicine *2006; 355:1171–1172. ©2006 Massachusetts Medical Society. All rights reserved.)*

- an extracellular location for the pathogen (e.g. pneumococci, *E. coli*, *Entamoeba histolytica*)
- invasion directly into the blood or lymph circulation (e.g. schistosome schistosomula and trypanosomes).

Once the pathogen is firmly established in its target tissue, a series of events follows that usually culminates in damage to the host.

Tissue dysfunction or damage

Microorganisms produce disease by a number of well-defined mechanisms, as described below.

Cell lysis

The presence of replicating viruses within a cell may interfere with host-cell metabolism, such that the cell dies – so-called cytolytic or cytocidal infection.

Exotoxins and endotoxins

- ***Exotoxins*** have many diverse activities, including inhibition of protein synthesis (diphtheria toxin), neurotoxicity (*Clostridium tetani* and *C. botulinum*) and enterotoxicity, which results in intestinal secretion of water and electrolytes (*E. coli*, *Vibrio cholerae*). Colonization and secretion in many classical diarrhoeal diseases are the result of virulence-associated genes that encode protein secretion systems ***(Fig. 11.2)***.
- ***Endotoxin*** is a lipopolysaccharide (LPS) in the cell wall of Gram-negative bacteria. It is responsible for many of the features of septic shock (see pp. 1154–1155), namely: hypotension, fever, intravascular coagulation and, at high doses, death. The effects of endotoxin are mediated predominantly by release of tumour necrosis factor.

The clinical expression of disease caused by ***Staphylococcus aureus*** varies according to site, invasion and toxin production and is summarized in ***Box 11.6***. Furthermore, host susceptibility to infection may be linked to genetic or acquired defects in host immunity that may complicate intercurrent infection, injury, ageing and metabolic disturbances ***(Box 11.7)***.

? Box 11.6 Clinical conditions produced by *Staphylococcus aureus*

Due to invasion

Skin
- Furuncles
- Cellulitis
- Impetigo
- Carbuncles

Lungs
- Pneumonia
- Lung abscesses

Heart
- Endocarditis
- Pericarditis

Central nervous system
- Meningitis
- Brain abscesses

Bones and joints
- Osteomyelitis, arthritis

Miscellaneous
- Parotitis
- Pyomyositis
- Septicaemia
- Enterocolitis

Due to toxin
- Staphylococcal food poisoning
- Scalded skin syndrome
- Bullous impetigo
- Staphylococcal scarlet fever
- Toxic shock syndrome

Host response to infection

Natural defences

The natural host defences to infection are those of an intact surface epithelium with local production of secretions, antimicrobial enzymes (e.g. lysozyme in the eye) and, in the stomach, gastric acidity. The latter is reduced by proton-pump inhibitors, increasing the risk of some gastroenteritic infections, including *C. difficile* infection. The mucociliary escalator of the large airways is unique to the lung but is destroyed by smoking.

Immunological defences

Antibody- and cell-mediated immune mechanisms play a vital role in combating infection. All organisms can initiate secondary

Box 11.7 Examples of host factors that increase susceptibility to staphylococcal infections[a]

Injury to skin or mucous membranes
- Abrasions
- Trauma (accidental or surgical)
- Burns
- Insect bites

Metabolic abnormalities
- Diabetes mellitus
- Uraemia

Foreign bodies[b]
- Intravenous and other indwelling catheters
- Cardiac and orthopaedic prostheses
- Tracheostomies

Abnormal leucocyte function
- Job syndrome
- Chédiak–Higashi syndrome
- Steroid therapy
- Drug-induced leucopenia

Postviral infections
- Influenza

Miscellaneous conditions
- Excess alcohol consumption
- Malnutrition
- Malignancies
- Old age
- Recent antibiotic therapy

[a]*Predominantly* Staphylococcus aureus. [b]*Often* Staph. epidermidis.

immunological mechanisms, such as complement activation, immune complex formation and antibody-mediated cytolysis of cells. The immunological response to infection is described on page 121.

Metabolic and immunological consequences

Fever

Body temperature is controlled by the thermoregulatory centre in the anterior hypothalamus in the floor of the third ventricle. Body temperature is maintained at 36.8°C in health, with a diurnal variation of ±0.5°C. Gram-negative bacteria contain LPS and peptidoglycan, which is also a component of Gram-positive bacterial cell walls. Toll-like receptors (TLRs; see p. 127) on monocytes and dendritic cells recognize these lipopolysaccharides and generate signals, leading to the formation of inflammatory cytokines, such as interleukin (IL)-1, IL-6, IL-12, tumour necrosis factor alpha (TNF-α) and many others. These cytokines act on the thermoregulatory centre by increasing prostaglandin (PGE_2) synthesis. The antipyretic effect of salicylates is brought about, at least in part, through their inhibitory effects on prostaglandin synthase.

Fever production has a positive effect on the course of infection. However, for every 1°C rise in temperature, there is a 13% increase in resting metabolic rate and oxygen consumption. Fever, therefore, leads to increased energy requirements at a time when anorexia leads to decreased food intake. The normal compensatory mechanisms in starvation (e.g. mobilization of fat stores) are inhibited in acute infections. This leads to an increase in skeletal muscle breakdown, releasing amino acids, which, via gluconeogenesis, are used to provide energy.

The inflammatory response

The inflammatory response is a fundamental biological response to a variety of stimuli, including microorganisms or their products, such as endotoxin, which acts on monocytes and macrophages. Non-phagocytic cells (lymphocytes, natural killer cells) are also involved. The release of cytokines, notably TNF-α, IL-1, IL-6 and interferon-γ, leads to the release of a cascade of other mediators involved in inflammation and tissue remodelling, such as interleukins, prostaglandins, leukotrienes and corticotropin.

The biological behaviour of the pathogen and the consequent host response are responsible for the clinical expression of disease that often allows clinical recognition. The incubation period following exposure can be helpful (e.g. 14–21 days for chickenpox). The site and distribution of a rash may be diagnostic (e.g. shingles), while symptoms of cough, sputum and pleuritic pain point to lobar pneumonia. Fever and meningismus characterize classical meningitis. Infection may remain localized or become disseminated and give rise to septic shock and disturbances of protein metabolism and acid–base balance.

Further reading

Eltzschig HK, Carmeliet P. Hypoxia and inflammation. *N Engl J Med* 2011; 364:656–665.

Fey PD, Olson ME. Current concepts in biofilm formation of Staphylococcus epidermidis. *Future Microbiol* 2010; 5:917–933.

Lemichez E, Lecuit M, Nassif X et al. Breaking the wall: targeting of the endothelium by pathogenic bacteria. *Nat Rev Microbiol* 2010; 8:93–104.

CLINICAL APPROACH TO THE PATIENT WITH A SUSPECTED INFECTION

Fever is often regarded as the cardinal feature of infection, but not all febrile illnesses are infections and not all infections present with a fever. Fever is usually intermittent, may not be present at the time of presentation and occurs less commonly in elderly patients. Infection can also present with hypothermia (temperature <36°C), which is a poor prognostic sign.

The three critical points in the assessment and management of a patient with infection or sepsis are:

- ***physiological assessment*** (severity of illness), which is predominantly based on systematic examination of key physiological markers at initial presentation
- ***diagnostic assessment***, which is predominantly based on history-taking, examination and review of those diagnostic tests available at presentation and subsequently performed (see below)
- ***management***, based on linkage of the above physiological and diagnostic assessments to key interventions; antibiotics and, when required, intravenous fluids, oxygen, infection source control (e.g. drainage of an abscess) and advanced physiological support.

A detailed history can be taken first in a physiologically stable patient but may need to be delayed until after a patient is stabilized in a case of sepsis.

Physiological assessment

Patients should initially be assessed according to the airway, breathing, circulation, disability and extremities (ABCDE) approach (see p. 1156). A succinct history can be taken as this is done. In particular, evidence suggesting sepsis or septic shock should be sought, according to the definitions:

Sepsis is defined as life-threatening organ dysfunction caused by dysregulated host response to infection.

Septic shock is defined as sepsis that has circulatory, cellular and metabolic abnormalities that are associated with a greater risk of mortality than sepsis alone.

Hypoperfusion is diagnosed if one or more of the following is present after the administration of at least 30 mL/kg body weight intravenous fluids *or* the patient has a serum lactate >4 mmol/L:

- systolic blood pressure of <90 mmHg
- mean arterial pressure (MAP) of <65 mmHg

- fall of >40 mmHg in the patient's usual systolic blood pressure that persists.

Diagnostic assessment

History-taking and examination should aim to identify the site(s) of infection and also the likely causative organism(s).

History

A detailed history is taken with specific questions about symptoms (see p. 221) and epidemiological risk factors for infection. The latter are based on sources of infection and routes of transmission (see p. 223).

- ***Symptoms***.
- ***Travel history***. Some diseases are more prevalent in certain geographical locations.
- ***Food and water history***. Include systemic, as well as gastroenteric, infections.
- ***Occupational history***. Healthcare workers may be exposed to certain infections by, for example, air-borne (e.g. chickenpox), person-to-person (e.g. MRSA) and needlestick injury (e.g. blood-borne viruses) routes of transmission.
- ***Animal contact***. Domestic, farm and wild animals can all be responsible.
- ***Sexual activity***. As well as the traditional sexually transmitted infections, HIV, hepatitis B and, occasionally, other blood-borne infections can be transmitted sexually. Some enteric infections are more common among men having sex with men.
- ***Intravenous drug use***. As well as blood-borne viruses, drug injectors are susceptible to a variety of bacterial and fungal infections due to inoculation. Other needle exposures, such as tattooing, body piercing and receipt of blood products (especially outside the UK), are also risk factors for blood-borne viruses.
- ***Leisure activities***. Certain pastimes may predispose to water-borne infections or zoonoses.
- ***Vaccination history***. Patients who have not received certain childhood (e.g. measles) or pre-travel (e.g. typhoid) vaccines are at higher risk if exposed.

Clinical examination

A thorough examination covering all systems is required. Skin rashes ***(Fig. 11.3)*** and lymphadenopathy are common features of infectious diseases and the ears, eyes, mouth and throat should also be inspected. Infections commonly associated with a rash are listed in ***Box 11.8***. Rectal, vaginal and penile examination is required in sexually transmitted infections. The fever pattern may occasionally be helpful: for example the tertian fever of falciparum malaria.

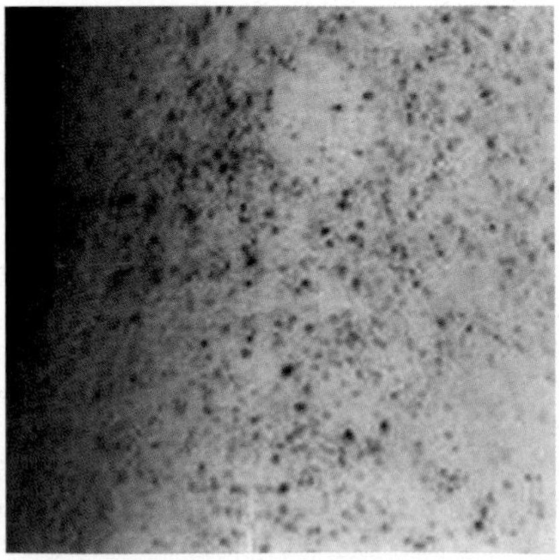

Figure 11.3 Skin rashes and lymphadenopathy are common non-specific features of infectious diseases.

Investigations

In some infections, such as chickenpox, the clinical presentation is so distinctive that no investigations are normally necessary to confirm the diagnosis. Many cases require further tests to determine the cause and site of the infection.

General investigations (to assess health and identify organ(s) involved)

These will vary depending on circumstances:

- ***Blood tests***. Routine blood count, erythrocyte sedimentation rate (ESR) (or plasma viscosity) and C-reactive protein (CRP), liver biochemistry and function, urea and electrolytes, and serum lactate. CRP is a non-specific marker of inflammation and is raised in many different infections; it is more useful in monitoring response to treatment than in making a diagnosis ***(Box 11.9)***. The exact role of procalcitonin in the diagnostic and prognostic assessment of bacterial infections is controversial; it may have a useful role in antibiotic stewardship (see pp. 234–235), particularly for respiratory tract infections and in the critical care environment, by detecting when it is safe to stop antibiotic therapy.
- ***Imaging***. X-ray, ultrasound, echocardiography, computed tomography (CT) and magnetic resonance imaging (MRI) are used to identify and localize infections. Positron emission tomography (PET) and single photon emission tomography (SPECT) have proved useful in localizing infection, especially when combined with CT scanning. However, the sensitivity and specificity of these tests in diagnosing infection have yet to be determined and their use remains limited. Biopsy or aspiration of tissue for microbiological examination is facilitated by ultrasound or CT guidance.

Box 11.8 Infections commonly associated with a rash

Macular/maculopapular
- Measles
- Rubella
- Enteroviruses
- Human herpesvirus 6
- Epstein–Barr virus
- Cytomegalovirus
- Human erythrovirus (parvovirus) B19
- Human immunodeficiency virus (HIV)
- Dengue
- Typhoid
- Secondary syphilis
- Rickettsial spotted fevers

Vesicular
- Chickenpox (varicella zoster virus)
- Shingles (varicella zoster virus)
- Herpes simplex virus
- Hand, foot and mouth disease (Coxsackie virus, enterovirus 71)
- Herpangina (Coxsackie virus)

Petechial/haemorrhagic
- Meningococcal septicaemia
- Any septicaemia with disseminated intravascular coagulation (DIC)
- Rickettsiae
- Viruses (see ***Box 11.33***)

Erythematous
- Scarlet fever
- Lyme disease (erythema chronicum migrans)
- Toxic shock syndrome
- Human erythrovirus (parvovirus) B19

Urticarial
- *Toxocara*
- *Strongyloides*
- *Schistosoma*
- Cutaneous larva migrans

Others
- Tick typhus (eschar)
- Primary syphilis (chancre)
- Anthrax (ulcerating papule)

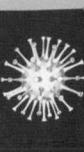

Box 11.9 General investigations for a patient with suspected infection

Investigation	Possible cause
Full blood count	
Neutrophilia	Bacterial infection
Neutropenia	Viral infection Brucellosis Typhoid Typhus Overwhelming sepsis
Lymphocytosis	Viral infection
Lymphopenia	HIV infection (not specific)
Atypical lymphocytes	Infectious mononucleosis
Eosinophilia	Invasive parasitic infection
Thrombocytopenia	Overwhelming sepsis Malaria
ESR or C-reactive protein	Elevated in many infections
Urea and electrolytes	Potentially deranged in severe illness from any cause
Procalcitonin	Elevated particularly in bacterial infection
Liver enzymes	
Minor elevation of transferases	Non-specific feature of many infections Mild viral hepatitis
High transferases, elevated bilirubin	Viral hepatitis (usually A, B or E)
Coagulation	May be deranged in hepatitis and in overwhelming infection of any type
Serum lactate	Used in the assessment of sepsis severity

- ***Radionuclide scanning*** after injection of indium- or technetium-labelled white cells (previously harvested from the patient) occasionally helps to localize infection. It is most effective when the peripheral white cell count is raised and is of particular value in localizing occult abscesses.

Microbiological investigations (to identify causative organism)

Diagnostic services range from simple microscopy to molecular probes. It is often helpful to discuss the clinical problem with a microbiologist to ensure that appropriate tests are performed and that specimens are collected and transported correctly.

Direct tests

Some microbiological tests rely on direct examination of a tissue specimen (e.g. blood, cerebrospinal fluid (CSF) or urine) for the presence of microorganisms: for example, microscopy and electron microscopy. Other direct tests identify specific microbial components, such as nucleic acids, cell wall molecules and other antigens. Specific genes from many pathogenic microorganisms have been cloned and sequenced.

Nucleic acid detection

Nucleic acid probes can be designed to detect these sequences, identifying pathogen-specific nucleic acid in body fluids or tissue. The use of nucleic acid amplification techniques (NAATs) such as the polymerase chain reaction (PCR) has increased the power of these tests to detect very small quantities of microbial material. Such techniques not only are exquisitely sensitive, but also may enable quantitation (e.g. viral load testing) and sub-speciation (e.g. at the genotype level). However, the ability to detect tiny amounts of nucleic acid in a sample means that there is a significant potential for false-positive results due to contamination. This is less likely when looking for viral nucleic acid and it is in the area of virology that NAAT tests are most widely used. Bacterial identification has been introduced to clinical practice with PCR tools for amplifying bacterial ribosome 16S subunits. This allows 'screening' of clinical samples for a wide range of organisms, but because of the risk of contamination results must be interpreted in the light of clinical findings.

Culture

Culture techniques can be applied to a wide variety of bacteria, fungi and viruses. However, some organisms are difficult to grow and may require special culture media and conditions. Viruses are particularly difficult (and in many cases impossible) to culture in the laboratory. Increasingly, traditional culture techniques are combined with subsequent molecular tests, such as Matrix-assisted laser desorption ionization time-of-flight (MALDTI-TOF) and PCR, to reduce the time to identification of pathogens, including, for example, whether a pathogen produces an extended-spectrum beta lactamase (ESBL) or carbapenemase (associated with multi-drug resistance in Gram-negative bacteria).

Specimens to be sent for microscopy and culture ***(Box 11.10)*** are as follows:

- ***Blood and urine*** should routinely be sent for bacterial culture if infection is suspected in hospitalized patients, regardless of whether fever is present at the time.
- ***CSF, sputum and biopsy*** specimens are sent if clinically indicated.
- ***Special culture techniques*** are required for fungi, mycobacteria and some other bacteria such as *Brucella* spp., and the laboratory must be informed.
- ***Faecal culture*** for viruses is not helpful in the investigation of gastroenteritis; the viruses responsible do not grow in routine tissue culture. Antigen or nucleic acid detection techniques (see below) are more appropriate, especially in the investigation of an outbreak of diarrhoea and vomiting (e.g. norovirus). Protozoa are a cause of diarrhoea in returning travellers, immunocompromised patients, toddlers and men having sex with men, farm workers and in any cases of prolonged unexplained diarrhoea. Detection of a specific clostridial toxin is a more reliable test for diarrhoea caused by *C. difficile* than culture of the organism itself. Routine stool culture is costly and is frequently unnecessary.

Immunodiagnostic tests

These can be divided into two types:

- tests that detect ***microbial components***, using a polyvalent antiserum or a monoclonal antibody
- tests that detect an ***antibody response*** to infection (serological tests).

These investigations are valuable in the identification of organisms that are difficult to culture, especially viruses and fungi, and can also be helpful when antibiotics have been administered before samples were obtained. Elevated antibody titres on a single occasion (especially of immunoglobulin (Ig) G) are rarely diagnostic and it may be difficult to distinguish between past and acute infection. Paired serological tests a few weeks apart, or specific assays for IgM antibodies (indicating an acute infection), are more helpful. Avidity testing may also enable distinction between recent infection (low-avidity antibodies) and historical infection (high-avidity antibodies). Numerous serological tests are available; they should only be used in light of the clinical picture.

Box 11.10 Specimens and indications for microscopy, culture and other microbiological tests

Specimen	Investigation	Indication
Blood	Giemsa stain for malaria Malaria antigen detection test	Any symptomatic traveller returning from a malarious area
	Stains for other parasites	Specific tropical infections
	Culture	All suspected bacterial infections
Urine	Microscopy and culture	All suspected bacterial infections
	TB culture	Suspected TB Unexplained leucocytes in urine
	NAAT	STIs
Faeces	Microscopy±iodine stain	Suspected protozoal diarrhoea
	Culture	All unexplained diarrhoea
	PCR/antigen detection (not usually necessary to do both)	Suspected viral diarrhoea in children
	Clostridium difficile toxin	Diarrhoea following hospital stay or antibiotic treatment
Throat swabs	Culture	Suspected bacterial tonsillitis and pharyngitis
	PCR	Viral meningitis
	PCR/antigen detection	Viral respiratory infections where urgent diagnosis is considered necessary
Sputum	Microscopy and culture	Unusual chest infections; pneumonia
	Auramine stain/TB culture (liquid culture; see p. 1110)	Suspected TB
	Other special stains/ cultures	Immunocompromised patients Suspected fungal infections
Cerebrospinal fluid	Microscopy and culture	Suspected meningitis
	Auramine stain/TB culture	Suspected TB, meningitis
	Other special stains/ cultures	Immunocompromised patients Suspected fungal infections
	PCR	Suspected encephalitis or viral or bacterial meningitis
Rash aspirate:		
Petechial	Microscopy and culture	Meningococcal disease
Vesicular	PCR/antigen detection/viral culture	Herpes simplex/zoster

NAAT, nuclear acid amplification test; PCR, polymerase chain reaction; STI, sexually transmitted infection; TB, tuberculosis.

Management of sepsis

Many infections, particularly those caused by viruses, are self-limiting and require no treatment. Patients who have sepsis, however, require immediate antibiotic and supportive therapies and commencement of investigations within 1 hour, as every hour delay increases the mortality by 8%.

Acute medical units (AMU) have a key role to play in early sepsis management. All patients must be assessed for sepsis and a clear clinical pathway defined. A qSOFA (see p. 1154) is a useful bedside assessment. This should include initiation of all investigations necessary to confirm or exclude organ dysfunction and include criteria for escalation/de-escalation of care.

The 'Sepsis Six' (or equivalent) can be used as a delivery method for early sepsis care (see algorithm on p. 221).

The '**Sepsis Six**' recommendations are:

- ***High-flow oxygen***. This is given via a facemask with a reservoir bag titrated to pulse oximetry readings or arterial blood gas results.
- ***Blood cultures*** (before antibiotic therapy; see above). ***Source control*** should be established as soon as possible (e.g. drainage of an abscess or removal of an infected intravenous access device).
- ***Intravenous antibiotics***. These should be given within 1 hour (see below)
- ***Intravenous fluid resuscitation***, e.g. 30 mL/kg of crystalloid (0.9% saline) for adult patients with evidence of end-organ dysfunction (see above). Septic shock is diagnosed if hypoperfusion persists after this fluid challenge.
- ***Haemoglobin and serial lactate measurement***. Transfuse blood when the haemoglobin concentration is <70 g/L, aiming for a target range of 70–90 g/L in adults; ***mortality*** correlates with serum lactate (<2 mmol/L = 15%; 2–4 mmol/L = 25%; >4 mmol/L = 38%).
- ***Hourly urine output measurement***. Aim for a urine output of >0.5 mL/kg per hour.

Patients initially managed on an acute medical unit (AMU) should achieve the following physiological goals by 6 h:

- MAP ≥65 mmHg
- urine output >0.5 mL/kg per hour
- other evidence of improving end-organ dysfunction (e.g. improved oxygen saturations, declining lactate).

Patients who fail to achieve these goals are referred to the ***critical care unit*** (see pp. 1156–1161) for advanced physiological support.

The choice of antibiotic should be governed by:

- the physiological assessment of the patient (see above)
- the likely cause of the infection (i.e. diagnostic assessment).

It is always preferable to have a definite microbial diagnosis before starting treatment, so that an antibiotic with the most appropriate site of action and narrowest spectrum of activity can be chosen. However, some patients are too unwell to wait for the results (which, in the case of culture, may take days). In diseases such as meningitis or severe sepsis, a delay in treatment may be fatal and broad-spectrum intravenous therapy must be started on an empirical basis. Ideally, appropriate samples for culture should be taken before the first dose of antibiotic, but therapy should not be delayed in potentially life-threatening infection to obtain, for example, a urine specimen. For patients who are physiologically stable, specific therapy is often deferred pending results.

Special circumstances

Returning travellers

A detailed travel itinerary, including any flight stopovers, should be taken from anyone who is unwell after arriving from another country. Previous travel should also be covered, as some infections may be chronic or recurrent. It is necessary to find out not just which countries were visited but also the type of environment; a stay in a remote jungle village carries different health risks from a holiday in an air-conditioned coastal holiday resort. Food and water consumption, bathing and swimming habits, animal and insect contact, and contact with human illness all need to be established. Enquiry should be made about sexual contacts, drug use and medical

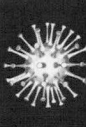

Box 11.11 Causes of febrile illness in travellers returning from the tropics and other countries

The World Health Organization advises that fever occurring in a traveller 1 week or more after entering a malaria risk area and up to 3 months after departure is a medical emergency

Developing countries
- Malaria
- Schistosomiasis
- Dengue
- Tick typhus
- Typhoid
- Tuberculosis
- Dysentery
- Hepatitis A
- Amoebiasis

Specific geographical areas (see text)
- Histoplasmosis
- Brucellosis

Worldwide
- Influenza
- Pneumonia
- Upper respiratory tract infection
- Urinary tract infection
- Traveller's diarrhoea
- Viral infection
- Systemic inflammatory response syndrome (SIRS)
- Ebola
- Middle Eastern respiratory syndrome (MERS)
- Zika

Box 11.12 Common causes of infection in immunocompromised patients

Deficiency	Causes	Organisms
Neutropenia	Chemotherapy Myeloablative therapy Immunosuppressant drugs	*Escherichia coli* *Klebsiella pneumoniae* *Staphylococcus aureus* *Staph. epidermidis* *Aspergillus* spp. *Candida* spp.
Cellular immune defects	HIV infection Lymphoma Myeloablative therapy Congenital syndromes	Respiratory syncytial virus Cytomegalovirus Epstein–Barr virus Herpes simplex and zoster *Salmonella* spp. *Mycobacterium* spp. (esp. *M. avium-intracellulare*) *Cryptococcus neoformans* *Candida* spp. *Cryptosporidium parvum* *Pneumocystis jiroveci* *Toxoplasma gondii*
Humoral immune deficiencies	Congenital syndromes Chronic lymphocytic leukaemia Corticosteroids	*Haemophilus influenzae* *Streptococcus pneumoniae* Enteroviruses
Terminal complement deficiencies (C5–C9)	Congenital syndromes	*Neisseria meningitidis* *N. gonorrhoeae*
Splenectomy	Surgery Trauma	*Strep. pneumoniae* *N. meningitidis* *H. influenzae* Malaria

treatment (especially parenteral). In some parts of the world, over 90% of professional sex workers are HIV-positive and hepatitis B and C are very common in parts of Africa and Asia. Special tests may be needed, depending on the epidemiological risks and clinical signs, and malaria films are mandatory in anyone who is unwell after being in a malarious area. Some of the more common causes of a febrile illness in returning travellers are listed in ***Box 11.11***.

Immunocompromised patients

Advances in medical treatment over the past three decades have led to a huge increase in the number of patients living with immunodeficiency states. Cancer chemotherapy, the use of immunosuppressive drugs and the worldwide AIDS epidemic have all contributed to this. The presentation may be very atypical in the immunocompromised patient with few, if any, localizing signs or symptoms. Infection can be due to organisms that are not usually pathogenic, including environmental bacteria and fungi. The normal physiological responses to infection (e.g. fever, neutrophilia) may be diminished or absent. The onset of symptoms may be sudden and the course of the illness fulminant. A high index of suspicion for infections in people who are known to be immunosuppressed is required. Common causes of infection in immunocompromised patients are shown in ***Box 11.12***. For neutropenic sepsis, see pages 604–605.

Injecting drug users

Parenteral drug use is associated with a variety of local and systemic infections. HIV, HBV and HCV infections can all be transmitted if injecting equipment is shared. Abscesses and soft tissue infections at the site of injection are common, especially in the groin, and may involve adjacent vascular and bony structures. Systemic infections are also common; they are most frequently caused by *Staph. aureus* and group A streptococci but a wide variety of other bacterial and fungal pathogens may be implicated.

Highly transmissible infections

Relatively few patients with infectious diseases present a serious risk to healthcare workers and other contacts. However, the appearance of diseases like the 'new' strains of influenza (such as H5N1 avian influenza and pandemic H1N1), the occasional importation of zoonoses like Lassa fever and Ebola (see p. 267), and concerns about the bioterrorist use of agents such as smallpox mean that there is still the potential for unexpected outbreaks of life-threatening disease. During the worldwide outbreak of severe acute respiratory syndrome (SARS) in 2003, scrupulous infection control procedures reduced the spread of infection. However, in the 'inter-epidemic' period, it is difficult to maintain the same level of alert. Healthcare workers should remain vigilant because the early symptoms of many of these diseases are non-specific. In Africa, many healthcare workers are developing multidrug-resistant tuberculosis from contact with HIV patients.

Pyrexia of unknown origin

History, clinical examination and simple investigation will reveal the cause of a fever in most patients. In a small number, however, no diagnosis is apparent, despite continuing symptoms. The term pyrexia (or fever) of unknown origin (PUO) is sometimes used to describe this problem. Various definitions have been suggested for PUO; a useful one is 'a fever persisting for >2 weeks, with no clear diagnosis despite intelligent and intensive investigation'. Patients who are known to have HIV or other immunosuppressive conditions are normally excluded from the definition of PUO, as the investigation and management of these patients are different.

Successful diagnosis of the cause of PUO depends on knowledge of the likely and possible aetiologies. These have been documented in a number of studies and are summarized in ***Box 11.13***.

A detailed history and examination is essential, taking into account the possible causes, and the examination should be repeated on a regular basis in case new signs appear. Investigative findings to date should be reviewed, obvious omissions amended

Box 11.13 Causes of pyrexia of unknown origin

Infection (20–40%)
- Pyogenic abscess
- Tuberculosis
- Infective endocarditis
- Toxoplasmosis
- Epstein–Barr virus infection
- Cytomegalovirus infection
- Primary HIV infection
- Brucellosis
- Lyme disease

Malignant disease (10–30%)
- Lymphoma
- Leukaemia
- Renal cell carcinoma
- Hepatocellular carcinoma

Vasculitides (15–20%)
- Adult Still's disease
- Systemic lupus erythematosus
- Granulomatosis with polyangiitis
- Giant cell arteritis
- Polymyalgia rheumatica

Miscellaneous (10–25%)
- Drug fevers
- Thyrotoxicosis
- Inflammatory bowel disease
- Sarcoidosis
- Granulomatous hepatitis
- Factitious fever
- Familial Mediterranean fever

Undiagnosed (5–25%)

and abnormalities followed up. Confirmation should be sought that the patient does have objective evidence of a raised temperature; this may require admission to hospital if the patient is not already under observation. Some people have an exaggerated circadian temperature variation (usually peaking in the evening), which is not pathological.

The range of tests available is discussed above. Obviously, investigation is guided by particular abnormalities on examination or initial test results, but in some cases 'blind' investigation is necessary. Some investigations, especially cultures, should be repeated regularly and serial monitoring of inflammatory markers such as CRP allows assessment of progress.

Ultrasound, echocardiography, CT, MRI, PET and labelled white-cell scanning can all help in establishing a diagnosis if used appropriately; the temptation to scan all patients with PUO from head to toe as a first measure should be avoided. Biopsy of the bone marrow (and, less frequently, liver) may be useful, even in the absence of obvious abnormalities, and temporal artery biopsy is helpful to confirm temporal arteritis in the elderly (see p. 701). Bronchoscopy can be used to obtain samples for microbiological and histological examination if sputum specimens are not adequate. Molecular and serological tests have greatly improved the diagnosis of infectious causes of PUO, but these tests should only be ordered and interpreted in the context of the clinical findings and epidemiology.

Management

Management of a patient with a persistent fever is aimed at the underlying cause; if possible, only symptomatic treatment should be given until a diagnosis is made. Blind antibiotic therapy may make diagnosis of an occult infection more difficult and empirical steroid therapy may mask an inflammatory response without treating the underlying cause. In a few patients, no cause of fever is found despite many months of investigation and follow-up. In most of these individuals, the symptoms do eventually settle spontaneously, and if no definite cause has been identified after 2 years, the long-term prognosis is good.

Further reading

Hrabák J, Chudácková E, Walková R. Matrix-assisted laser desorption ionization-time of flight (MALDI-TOF) mass spectrometry for detection of antibiotic resistance mechanisms: from research to routine diagnosis. *Clin Microbiol Rev* 2013; 26:103–114.

Ross AGP, Olds GR, Cripps AW et al. Enteropathogens and chronic illness in returning travelers. *N Engl J Med* 2013; 368:1817–1825.

http://www.labtestsonline.org.uk/ *Non-commercial advice on available laboratory tests.*

https://www.rcplondon.ac.uk/resources/ *UK Royal College of Physicians: 2014 Acute care toolkit 9: Sepsis.*

ANTIMICROBIAL CHEMOTHERAPY

Principles of use and antibiotic stewardship

Antibiotics have undoubtedly reduced the morbidity and mortality associated with life-threatening infections, major surgery and other interventions, such as chemotherapy for cancer. Unnecessary prescribing has resulted in patient harm and mortality through adverse effects such as *C. difficile* infection, as well as the ongoing evolution and spread of antibiotic-resistant pathogens. Antibiotic resistance is now a major worldwide problem and 'total resistance' has been described.

In particular, some Gram-negative bacteria, such as *E. coli* and *K. pneumoniae*, have developed an extended spectrum of antibiotic resistance, with some strains, such as those that produce New Delhi metallo-beta-lactamase-1 (NDM-1), now almost untreatable. In 2013, the Centers for Disease Control and Prevention estimated that there were over 2 million infections caused by resistant bacteria and fungi in the United States each year, with more than 23 000 deaths. In northern India, a recent study showed that 5% of clinical *E. coli* isolates from a tertiary hospital were NDM-1 producers. These bacteria typically infect vulnerable patient groups and retain sensitivity only to very few less familiar and infrequently used antibiotics, such as colistimethate (polymixin E) and tigecycline. These are now often used in combination when treating these infections, but have been associated with serious adverse effects or poorer patient outcomes; mortality associated with highly resistant infections is considerable.

Antibiotics increase the natural selection of resistant pathogens that are innately resistant. They also allow genetic mutations under an antibiotic resistance pressure and bacteria to acquire that code for resistance. They also facilitate person-to-person spread of resistant organisms by damaging the human microbiome that protects mucosal surfaces against colonization and subsequent infection. Good antibiotic stewardship, in the form of promotion of the appropriate use of antibiotics, the adoption of antibiotic guidelines, epidemiological surveillance of resistant pathogens and prescribing, and education and feedback to prescribers, has helped reduce resistance spread.

The core principle of antibiotic stewardship is that broad-spectrum antibiotics, which, in general, are more likely to cause *C. difficile* infection and contribute to resistance, should only be prescribed for life-, limb- or sight-threatening infections when the underlying microbial diagnosis is unclear. Neither should antibiotics be prescribed for self-limiting or viral infections.

In physiologically stable patients who are deemed to need an antibiotic or those with a clear microbiological diagnosis, the antibiotic with the narrowest spectrum that is effective should be chosen. Nevertheless, there were increases of 4% and 12% in antibiotic prescribing by general practitioners and hospitals, respectively, between 2010 and 2013.

The principles of the UK's *Start Smart and then Focus* antibiotic stewardship campaign are described below.

'Start smart'

- Do not start antibiotics in the absence of clinical evidence of bacterial infection.

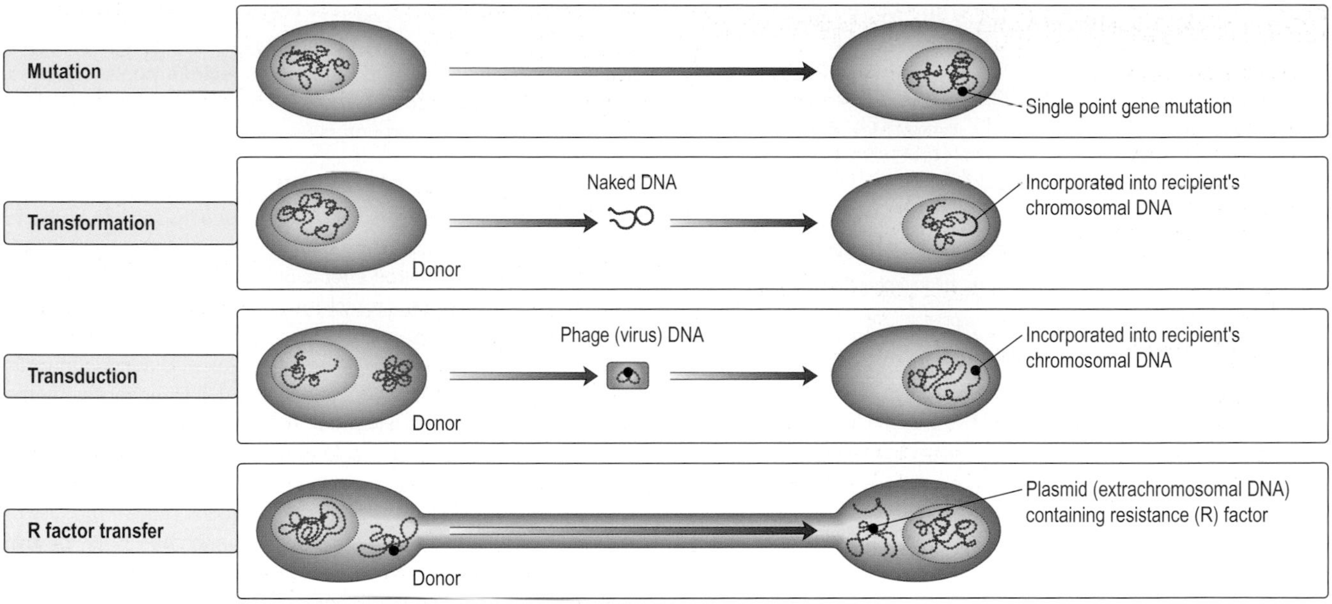

Figure 11.4 Some mechanisms for the development of resistance to antimicrobial drugs. These involve either a single point mutation or transfer of genetic material from another organism (transformation, transduction or R factor transfer).

- Take a thorough allergy history.
- Use local guidelines to initiate prompt and effective antibiotic treatment within 1 h of diagnosis (or as soon as possible) if there is evidence/suspicion of life-threatening bacterial infection.
- Document, on the drug chart and in the notes, the exact clinical indication, duration or review/stop date, route and dose.
- Obtain (appropriate) cultures first.
- Prescribe single-dose antibiotics for surgical prophylaxis within the 60 min *prior* to surgical incision or tourniquet inflation where antibiotics have been shown to be effective.

'Then focus'

- Review the clinical diagnosis and the continuing need for antibiotics by 48 h and make a clear plan of action – the 'Antimicrobial Prescribing Decision'.
- Remember that the five antimicrobial prescribing decision options are:
  - stop
  - switch from intravenous to oral antibiotics;
  - change to a more appropriate antibiotic
  - continue
  - give outpatient parenteral antibiotic therapy (OPAT).
- Document the clinical decisions described above in the notes and drug chart.

Mechanisms of action and resistance to antimicrobial agents

Antibiotics act at different sites of the bacterium, either inhibiting essential steps in metabolism or assembly, or destroying vital components such as the cell wall.

Resistance to an antibiotic can be the result of:

- impaired or altered permeability of the bacterial cell envelope, e.g. penicillins in Gram-negative bacteria
- active expulsion from the cell by membrane efflux systems
- alteration of the target site (e.g. single point mutations in *E. coli* or a penicillin-binding protein in *Strep. pneumoniae*, leading to acquired resistance; see below)
- over-production of the target site
- specific enzymes that inactivate the drug before or after cell entry (e.g. β-lactamases)
- development of a novel metabolic bypass pathway.

The development or acquisition of resistance to an antibiotic by bacteria involves either a mutation at a single point in a gene or transfer of genetic material from another organism ***(Fig. 11.4)***. Larger fragments of DNA may be introduced into a bacterium either by transfer of 'naked' DNA or via a bacteriophage (a virus) DNA vector. Both the former (transformation) and the latter (transduction) are dependent on integration of this new DNA into the recipient chromosomal DNA. This requires a high degree of homology between the donor and recipient chromosomal DNA.

Finally, antibiotic resistance can be transferred from one bacterium to another by conjugation, when extrachromosomal DNA (a plasmid) containing the resistance factor (R factor) is passed from one cell into another during direct contact. Transfer of such R factor plasmids can occur between unrelated bacterial strains and involve large amounts of DNA and often codes for multiple antibiotic resistance: for example, as for the fluoroquinolones.

Transformation is probably the least clinically relevant mechanism, whereas transduction and R factor transfer are usually responsible for the sudden emergence of multiple antibiotic resistances in a single bacterium. Increasing resistance to many antibiotics has developed ***(Box 11.14)***.

Empirical 'blind' therapy

Most antibiotic prescribing, especially in the community, is empirical. Even in hospital practice, microbiological documentation of the nature of an infection and the susceptibility of the pathogen is generally not available for a day or two. Initial choice of therapy relies on a clinical diagnosis and, in turn, a presumptive microbiological diagnosis. Such 'blind therapy' is directed at the most likely pathogen(s) responsible for a particular syndrome such as meningitis, urinary tract infection or pneumonia. Examples of 'blind therapy' for these three conditions are ceftriaxone, trimethoprim and amoxicillin (with or without a macrolide), respectively. Initial therapy in the severely ill patient is often broad-spectrum in order

Box 11.14 Examples of bacteria that have developed resistance to common antibiotics*

Pathogen	Previously sensitive to
Enterobacteriaceae (most common Gram-negative pathogens)	Amoxicillin, trimethoprim, ciprofloxacin, gentamicin, piperacillin/tazobactam, meropenem
Enterococcus **spp.**	Glycopeptides (GRE), vancomycin (VRE)
Helicobacter pylori	Metronidazole, clarithromycin
Haemophilus influenzae	Amoxicillin, chloramphenicol
Neisseria gonorrhoeae	Penicillin, ciprofloxacin, ceftriaxone
Pseudomonas aeruginosa	Ciprofloxacin, gentamicin, piperacillin/tazobactam, meropenem
Salmonella **spp.**	Amoxicillin, sulphonamides, ciprofloxacin
Shigella **spp.**	Amoxicillin, trimethoprim, tetracycline
Staphylococcus aureus	Penicillin, meticillin (MRSA), vancomycin (VRSA), ciprofloxacin, macrolides, tetracycline
Streptococcus pneumoniae	Penicillin, macrolides, cefotaxime
Streptococcus pyogenes	Macrolides, clindamycin, tetracycline
Vibrio cholerae	Fluoroquinolones, azithromycin

*For mycobacterial resistance, see pages 1111–1112.

to cover the range of possible pathogens but should be targeted once microbiological information becomes available. There is little firm evidence that bactericidal drugs (penicillins, cephalosporins, aminoglycosides) are more effective than bacteriostatic drugs (tetracyclines), but it is generally considered better to use the former in the treatment of bacterial endocarditis and in patients in whom host defence mechanisms are compromised, particularly in those with neutropenia. In patients with less severe infections, a narrower-spectrum agent can be used from the outset while awaiting culture results, as the potential consequences of initial inadequate coverage are less serious.

Combination therapy

Combinations of drugs are occasionally required for reasons other than providing broad-spectrum cover. Tuberculosis is initially treated with three or four agents to avoid the emergence of resistance. Synergistic inhibition is achieved by using penicillin and gentamicin in enterococcal endocarditis, or gentamicin and ceftazidime in life-threatening *Pseudomonas* infection. In general, combinations should be avoided because of the increased risk of adverse effects, including damage to the human microbiome, and drug interactions, but may need to be employed more in order to prevent or treat antibiotic-resistant infections.

Pharmacokinetic factors

To be successful, sufficient antibiotic must penetrate to the site of the infection. Knowledge of the standard pharmacokinetic considerations of absorption, distribution, metabolism and excretion for the various drugs is required. Difficult sites include the brain, eye and prostate, while loculated abscesses are inaccessible to most agents and therefore often require radiological or surgical drainage (i.e. source control).

Many mild to moderate infections can be treated effectively with oral antibiotics, provided that the patient is compliant. Parenteral administration is indicated in the severely ill patient to ensure rapid high and/or consistent blood and tissue concentrations of drug. Some antibiotics can only be administered parenterally, such as the aminoglycosides and extended-spectrum cephalosporins. Parenteral therapy is also required if the patient is unable to swallow or if gastrointestinal absorption is unreliable.

Dose and duration of therapy

These will vary according to the nature, severity and response to therapy. The need to clear the infection completely must be balanced against the undesired effects of prolonged antibiotic therapy (e.g. promotion of antimicrobial resistance, drug toxicity, superinfection with organisms such as *Candida* spp. or *C. difficile*, and cost). For many infections, 5–7 days of treatment is adequate, while for some (e.g. uncomplicated urinary tract infections and some forms of bacterial gastroenteritis) 1–3 days is enough. However, other infections require much longer: bacterial endocarditis normally needs 4–6 weeks, bone and prosthetic joint infections often need 6–12 weeks, and mycobacterial infections require months or even years of therapy. In a few conditions such as HIV or chronic hepatitis B infection, treatment is suppressive rather than curative, so lifelong antimicrobial treatment is needed. Even within a course of treatment, it may be possible to simplify or streamline therapy – for example, change from intravenous to oral, or from broad-spectrum to narrow-spectrum – as the patient improves.

Renal and hepatic insufficiency

Patients with renal impairment may require a reduction in dose or an increase in dosing interval in order to avoid the toxic accumulation of antibiotic. This applies to the β-lactams and especially the aminoglycosides and vancomycin. In those with hepatic insufficiency, dose reduction is often required for agents that rely on extensive hepatic metabolism for excretion. A full list of such drugs can be found in the national formularies (e.g. the *British National Formulary*, or BNF).

Therapeutic drug monitoring

To ensure therapeutic yet non-toxic drug concentrations, serum concentrations of drugs such as the aminoglycosides and vancomycin should be monitored, especially in those with impaired or changing renal function. Therapeutic drug monitoring of antibiotics not usually monitored, such as the β-lactams, may be necessary to optimize therapy in the fight against antibiotic resistance. Specific monitoring algorithms are available in national formularies but local guidelines should be followed when available.

Antibiotic chemoprophylaxis

The value of antibiotic chemoprophylaxis has been questioned, as there are relatively few controlled trials to prove efficacy (see pp. 1020–1021). The evidence for chemoprophylaxis against infective endocarditis is an example. National Institute for Health and Care Excellence (NICE) guidelines recognize that procedures can cause bacteraemia but without a significant risk of infective endocarditis. Even patients at 'high risk', such as those with previous infectious endocarditis, prosthetic heart valves and surgical shunts, do not always require prophylaxis ***(Box 11.15)***. However, there are a number of indications for which the prophylactic use of antibiotics is still advised. These include surgical procedures where the risk of infection is high (colon surgery) or the consequences of infection are serious (post-splenectomy sepsis). The choice of agent(s) is determined by the likely infectious risk and the established efficacy and safety of the regimen. Antibiotic prophylaxis for the vast majority of surgical or radiological procedures should not extend for more

Box 11.15 Antibiotic chemoprophylaxis

Clinical problem	Aim	Drug regimen[a]
General		
Splenectomy/ spleen malfunction	To prevent serious pneumococcal sepsis	Phenoxymethylpenicillin 500 mg 12-hourly
Rheumatic fever	To prevent recurrence and further cardiac damage	Phenoxymethylpenicillin 250 mg ×2 daily or sulfadiazine 1 g if allergic to penicillin
Meningitis:		
Due to meningococci	To prevent infection in close contacts	Adults: rifampicin 600 mg twice daily for 2 days (Children <1 year: 5 mg/kg; >1 year: 10 mg/kg) Alternative (single dose) ciprofloxacin 500 mg (p.o.) or ceftriaxone 250 mg (i.m.)
Due to *H. influenzae* type b	To reduce nasopharyngeal carriage and prevent infection in close contacts	Adults: rifampicin 600 mg daily for 4 days (Children: <3 months 10 mg/kg; >3 months 20 mg/kg)
Tuberculosis	To prevent infection in exposed (close contacts) tuberculin-negative individuals, infants of infected mothers, and immunosuppressed patients	Oral isoniazid 300 mg daily for 6 months (Children: 5–10 mg/kg daily)

Endocarditis[b]

Antibacterial prophylaxis and chlorhexidine mouthwash are *not* recommended for the prevention of endocarditis in patients undergoing dental procedures

Antibacterial prophylaxis is *not* recommended for the prevention of endocarditis in patients undergoing procedures of the:
- Upper and lower respiratory tract (including ear, nose and throat procedures and bronchoscopy)
- Genitourinary tract (including urological, gynaecological and obstetric procedures)
- Upper and lower gastrointestinal tract

Any infection in patients at risk of endocarditis should be investigated promptly and treated appropriately to reduce the risk of endocarditis

If patients at risk of endocarditis are undergoing a gastrointestinal or genitourinary tract procedure at a site where infection is suspected, they should receive appropriate antibacterial therapy that includes cover against organisms that cause endocarditis

Patients at risk of endocarditis should be:
- Advised to maintain good oral hygiene
- Told how to recognize signs of infective endocarditis and advised when to seek expert advice.

[a]Unless stated, doses are those recommended in adults. For surgical procedure, see individual procedures in text. [b]NICE guidelines for adults and children undergoing interventional procedures, March 2008.
(Adapted from Joint Formulary Committee. *British National Formulary*, 70th edn. London: BMJ Group and RPS Publishing; 2015.)

than 24 hours post procedure and, for most operations, a single dose at induction is all that is required.

Outpatient parenteral antibiotic therapy

Outpatient parenteral antibiotic therapy (OPAT) is an increasingly employed and safe approach to administering intravenous antibiotics, either in an outpatient clinic or at home, to clinically stable patients who require intravenous therapy. A wide range of acute and chronic infections can be managed in this way, including skin and soft tissue infections, bone/joint infections, pyelonephritis, endocarditis, organ and tissue abscesses, and multidrug-resistant tuberculosis. Usually, OPAT is either administered once daily by bolus or infusion (depending on the agent) using an antibiotic with a long half-life (e.g. teicoplanin, daptomycin, ertapenem), or given continuously by an elastomeric device (e.g. flucloxacillin, piperacillin/tazobactam), or is self-, carer- or nurse-administered at home. Careful patient selection and subsequent supervision and monitoring are mandatory.

Antibacterial drugs

β-Lactams (penicillins, cephalosporins, monobactams and carbapenems)

Penicillins

Structure. The β-lactams share a common ring structure (***Fig. 11.5***). Changes to the side-chain of benzylpenicillin (penicillin G) render the phenoxymethyl derivative (penicillin V) resistant to gastric acid and allow it to be orally absorbed. The presence of an amino group in the phenyl radical of benzylpenicillin increases its antimicrobial spectrum to include many Gram-negative and Gram-positive organisms. More extensive modification of the side-chain (e.g. as in flucloxacillin) renders the drug insensitive to bacterial penicillinase. This is useful in treating infections caused by penicillinase (β-lactamase)-producing staphylococci.

Mechanism of action. The β-lactams block bacterial cell-wall mucopeptide formation by binding to and inactivating specific penicillin-binding proteins (PBPs), which are peptidases involved in the final stages of cell-wall assembly and division. Meticillin-resistant *Staph. aureus* (MRSA; see p. 270) produces a low-affinity PBP that retains its peptidase activity, even in the presence of high concentrations of meticillin. Many bacteria are able to produce penicillinases and β-lactamases, which inactivate antibiotics of this class. The emergence of Gram-negative organisms producing extended-spectrum β-lactamases (ESBLs) and carbapenemases has rendered some bacteria potentially resistant to all β-lactam antibiotics and often to other classes of antibiotics as well.

Indications for use. Benzylpenicillin can only be given parenterally and is still the drug of choice for some serious infections. However, due to increasing antimicrobial resistance, it should not be used as monotherapy in serious infections without laboratory confirmation that the organism is penicillin-sensitive. Uses include serious streptococcal infections (including infective endocarditis), necrotizing fasciitis and gas gangrene (usually combined with other

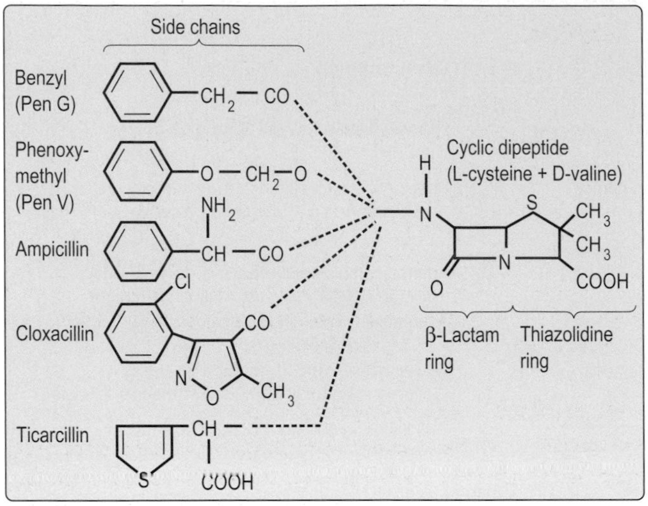

Figure 11.5 The structure of penicillins.

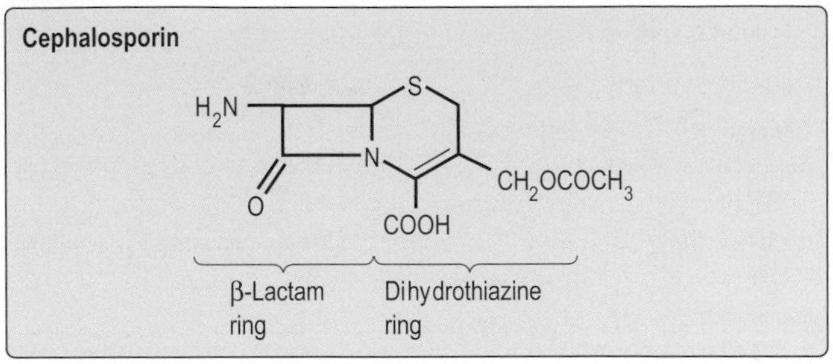

Figure 11.6 The structure of a cephalosporin.

antibiotics), actinomycosis, anthrax and spirochaetal infections (syphilis, yaws).

Phenoxymethylpenicillin (penicillin V) is an oral preparation that is used chiefly to treat streptococcal pharyngitis and as prophylaxis against rheumatic fever.

Flucloxacillin is used in infections caused by β-lactamase (penicillinase)-producing staphylococci and remains the drug of choice for serious infections caused by meticillin-sensitive *Staph. aureus* (MSSA).

Ampicillin is susceptible to β-lactamase but its antimicrobial activity includes streptococci, pneumococci and enterococci, as well as Gram-negative organisms such as *Salmonella* spp., *Shigella* spp., *E. coli*, *H. influenzae* and *Proteus* spp. Drug resistance has, however, eroded its efficacy against these Gram-negatives. It is widely used in the treatment of respiratory tract infections. Amoxicillin has similar activity to ampicillin but is better absorbed when given by mouth.

The extended-spectrum penicillin, ticarcillin, is active against *Pseudomonas* infections, as is the acylureidopenicillin piperacillin in combination with tazobactam.

Clavulanic acid is a powerful inhibitor of many bacterial β-lactamases and, when given in combination with an otherwise effective agent such as amoxicillin (co-amoxiclav) or ticarcillin, can broaden the spectrum of activity of the drug. Sulbactam acts similarly and is available combined with ampicillin, while tazobactam in combination with piperacillin is effective in appendicitis, peritonitis, pelvic inflammatory disease and complicated skin infections. The penicillin/β-lactamase inhibitor combinations are also active against β-lactamase-producing staphylococci.

Pivmecillinam is used for the treatment of urinary tract infection and has activity against Gram-negative bacteria, including ESBL-producing *E. coli*, *Klebsiella*, *Enterobacter* and *Salmonella*, but not against *Pseudomonas*.

Temocillin is active only against Gram-negative bacteria, including many ESBL producers; it appears to be relatively less likely to trigger *C. difficile* infection and is increasingly used because of resistance. It is not active against *Pseudomonas* or *Acinetobacter* spp.

Interactions. Penicillins inactivate aminoglycosides when mixed in the same solution.

Toxicity. Generally, the penicillins are safe. Hypersensitivity (skin rash (common), urticaria, anaphylaxis), encephalopathy and tubulointerstitial nephritis can occur. Ampicillin also produces a hypersensitivity rash in approximately 90% of patients with infectious mononucleosis (glandular fever) who receive this drug. Co-amoxiclav causes cholestatic jaundice six times more frequently than amoxicillin, as does flucloxacillin.

Cephalosporins

The cephalosporins ***(Fig. 11.6)*** have an advantage over the penicillins in that they are not inactivated by staphylococcal penicillinases (but are still inactive against meticillin-resistant staphylococci except the fifth-generation cephalosporins, ceftaroline and ceftobiprole) and have a broader range of activity that includes both Gram-negative and Gram-positive organisms, but excludes enterococci and anaerobic bacteria. Only certain cephalosporins (e.g. ceftazidime and cefpirome) are active against *Pseudomonas aeruginosa.*

Indications for use. These broad-spectrum antibiotics should be reserved for the treatment of specific serious infections, such as meningitis and meningococcal disease and acute epiglottitis. They may be used for severe sepsis secondary to a wide variety of other infections, but in the UK and many other countries they have largely been replaced by other agents because of their link with *C. difficile* infection.

Interactions. There are relatively few interactions.

Toxicity. The toxicity is similar to that of the penicillins but is less common. Some 10% of patients are allergic to both groups of drugs. The early cephalosporins caused proximal tubule damage, although the newer derivatives have fewer nephrotoxic effects. Second- and third-generation cephalosporins are strongly associated with *C. difficile* infection and alternative antibiotics should be used when possible.

Monobactams

Aztreonam is the only member of this class available. It is a synthetic β-lactam and, unlike the penicillins and cephalosporins, has no ring other than the β-lactam; hence its description as a monobactam.

It is not inactivated by most β-lactamases and is less likely to induce β-lactamase production.

Indications for use. Aztreonam's spectrum of activity is limited to aerobic Gram-negative bacilli. It is a useful alternative to aminoglycosides in combination therapy, largely for the treatment of intra-abdominal sepsis, has activity against many ESBL producers and is also used in Pseudomonas infection (including lung infection in cystic fibrosis).

Toxicity. This is as for the β-lactam antibiotics.

Carbapenems

The carbapenems are semisynthetic β-lactams and include imipenem, meropenem, doripenem and ertapenem. They currently have the broadest spectrum of the antibiotics, being active against

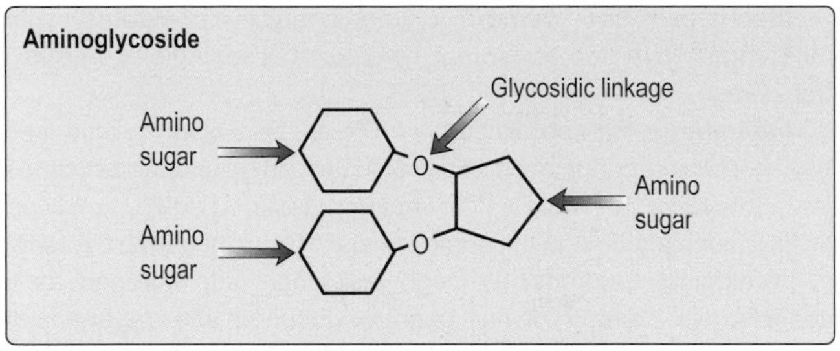

Figure 11.7 **The structure of an aminoglycoside.**

the majority of Gram-positive (but not MRSA) and Gram-negative, as well as anaerobic, bacterial pathogens. Ertapenem, unlike the others, is not active against *Pseudomonas* or *Acinetobacter* spp. They differ in their dosage and frequency of administration. Imipenem is partially inactivated in the kidney by enzymatic inactivation and is therefore administered in combination with cilastatin.

Indications for use. They are used for serious nosocomial infections when multidrug-resistant Gram-negative bacilli or mixed aerobe and anaerobe infections are suspected.

Toxicity. This is similar to that of β-lactam antibiotics. Nausea, vomiting and diarrhoea occur in less than 5% of cases. Imipenem may cause seizures and should not be used to treat meningitis; meropenem is safe for this indication.

Aminoglycosides

Structure. These antibiotics are polycationic compounds of amino sugars ***(Fig. 11.7)***.

Mechanism of action. Aminoglycosides interrupt bacterial protein synthesis by inhibiting ribosomal function (messenger and transfer RNA).

Indications for use. Streptomycin is bactericidal and is rarely used except for the treatment of tularaemia or plague. Neomycin is used only for the topical treatment of eye, ear and skin infections. Even though it is poorly absorbed, prolonged oral administration can produce ototoxicity.

Gentamicin and tobramycin are given parenterally. They are highly effective against many Gram-negative organisms, including *Pseudomonas* spp. They are synergistic at low doses with penicillins against *Enterococcus* spp. and viridans streptococci, and are therefore often used in endocarditis. Netilmicin and amikacin have a similar spectrum but are more resistant to the aminoglycoside-inactivating enzymes (phosphorylating, adenylating or acetylating) produced by some bacteria. Their use should be restricted to gentamicin-resistant organisms.

Interactions. Enhanced nephrotoxicity occurs with other nephrotoxic drugs, ototoxicity with some diuretics and neuromuscular blockade with curariform drugs.

Toxicity. This is dose-related. Aminoglycosides are nephrotoxic and ototoxic (vestibular and auditory), particularly in the elderly. The m.1555A>G mutation has been associated with gentamicin ototoxicity but appears to occur in less than 1% of the general population; rapid pre-treatment testing is not currently feasible. Therapeutic drug monitoring is necessary to ensure therapeutic and non-toxic drug concentrations. Once-daily dosing is used for most indications, with a serum drug level taken at 6–14 hours post dose, followed by application of an appropriate nomogram to determine the subsequent frequency of dosing (e.g. 24- or 48-hourly). When used for endocarditis, low doses are prescribed every 12 hours with different target pre- and post-dose level ranges than for once-daily dosing.

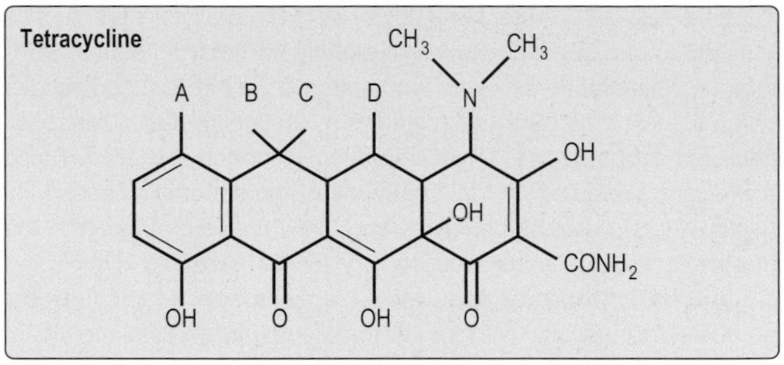

Figure 11.8 **The structure of a tetracycline.** Substitution of CH_3, OH or H at positions A–D produces variants of tetracycline.

Tetracyclines and glycylcyclines

Structure. These are bacteriostatic drugs possessing a four-ring hydronaphthacene nucleus ***(Fig. 11.8)***. Included among the tetracyclines are tetracycline, oxytetracycline, demeclocycline, lymecycline, doxycycline and minocycline. Tigecycline is an injectable glycylcycline, which is structurally related to the tetracyclines.

Mechanism of action. Tetracyclines inhibit bacterial protein synthesis by interrupting ribosomal function (transfer RNA).

Indications for use. Tetracyclines are active against Gram-positive and Gram-negative bacteria but their use for the latter is limited due to bacterial resistance. Tetracyclines are active against *V. cholerae, Rickettsia* spp., *Mycoplasma* spp., *Coxiella burnetii*, *Chlamydia* spp. and *Brucella* spp., and have good overall activity against community-acquired bacterial respiratory pathogens; they are low-risk for *C. difficile* infection and are therefore increasingly used for respiratory tract infections.

Tigecycline is active against many organisms resistant to tetracycline and other antibiotics. These include vancomycin-resistant enterococci, MRSA and Gram-negative bacilli, including *Acinetobacter* spp., but not *Pseudomonas* or *Proteus* spp.; tigecycline is increasingly used in combination with other antibiotics (e.g. colistimethate sodium) to treat infections due to highly resistant, carbapenemase-producing, Gram-negative bacteria. The licensed indications are complicated skin and soft tissue infections and intra-abdominal sepsis. However, a 2010 US Food and Drug Administration (FDA) alert raised concern about the efficacy of tigecycline in some serious infections (notably ventilator-associated pneumonia, VAP; see p. 1165) and it should be used only on expert advice.

Interactions. The efficacy of tetracyclines is reduced by antacids and oral iron-replacement therapy.

Toxicity. Tetracyclines are generally safe drugs, but they may enhance established or incipient renal failure, although doxycycline is safer than others in this group. They cause brown discoloration of growing teeth and thus these drugs are not given to children or pregnant women. Photosensitivity occurs in approximately 1 in 20 patients. Nausea and vomiting are the most frequent adverse effects of tigecycline.

Macrolides

Erythromycin and clarithromycin

Structure. Erythromycin and clarithromycin both consist of a lactone ring with two sugar side-chains, one of which is an aminosugar.

Mechanism of action. Macrolides inhibit protein synthesis by interrupting ribosomal function.

Indications for use. Erythromycin has a similar (but not identical) antibacterial spectrum to penicillin and may be useful in individuals with penicillin allergy, especially in the management of bacterial respiratory infections. It can be given orally or parenterally, but oral intake is associated with significant gastrointestinal side-effects, while the intravenous formulation is very irritant and causes phlebitis. For these reasons, clarithromycin (which has similar antimicrobial properties but fewer side-effects) is often preferred. These drugs are preferred in the treatment of pneumonias caused by *Legionella* spp. and *Mycoplasma* spp. They are also effective in the treatment of infections due to *Bordetella pertussis* (whooping cough), *Campylobacter* spp. and *Chlamydia* spp. Macrolides are otherwise not usually used for life-threatening or serious infections, such as endocarditis and meningitis.

Other macrolides

These include azithromycin and telithromycin. They have a broad spectrum of activity that includes selective Gram-negative organisms, mycobacteria and *Toxoplasma gondii*. Compared with erythromycin, they have superior pharmacokinetic properties with enhanced tissue and intracellular penetration and a longer half-life that allows once-daily dosage. Concern has been raised about the use of azithromycin in bloodstream infections (bacteraemia) because of low serum bioavailability. Azithromycin is also used for trachoma, cholera and for some sexually transmitted infections.

Interactions. Erythromycin and other macrolides interact with theophyllines, carbamazepine, digoxin and ciclosporin, occasionally necessitating dose adjustment of these agents.

Toxicity. Diarrhoea, vomiting and abdominal pain are the main side-effects of erythromycin (less with clarithromycin and azithromycin) as a consequence of the intestinal prokinetic properties of the macrolides. QT_c prolongation is a recognized cardiac effect of the macrolides and may lead to the potentially life-threatening syndrome of 'torsades de pointes' (see p. 975); concomitant use of other drugs that cause QT_c prolongation is avoided unless absolutely essential.

Fidaxomicin

Fidaxomicin is a macrocyclic antibacterial that is poorly absorbed from the intestine and is used for the treatment of *C. difficile* infection. It is thought to have a lower recurrence rate than vancomycin or metronidazole.

Chloramphenicol

Structure. Chloramphenicol is the only naturally occurring antibiotic containing nitrobenzene ***(Fig. 11.9)***. This structure probably accounts for its toxicity in humans and for its activity against bacteria.

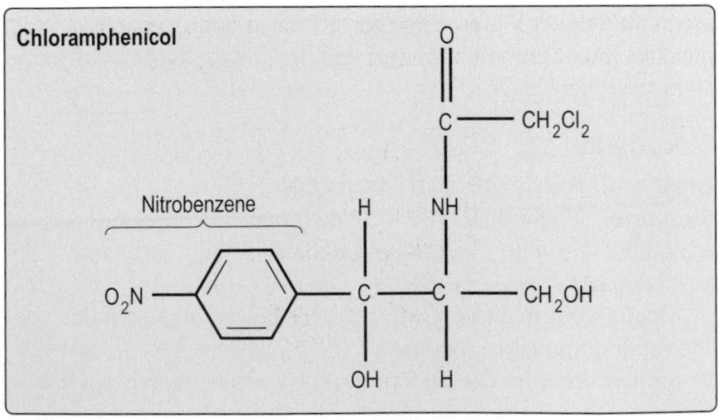

Figure 11.9 The structure of chloramphenicol.

Mechanism of action. Chloramphenicol competes with messenger RNA for ribosomal binding. It also inhibits peptidyl transferase.

Indications for use. Because of its adverse-effect profile (see below), chloramphenicol had been little used in developed countries for many years. It is increasingly being prescribed again, however, as it remains active against some resistant Gram-negative bacteria. In developing countries, although resistance has emerged as a considerable problem, it has been invaluable in the treatment of meningitis and severe infections caused by *Salmonella typhi* and *S. paratyphi* (enteric fevers), and is also active against *H. influenzae* (meningitis and acute epiglottitis) and *Yersinia pestis* (plague). It is used topically for the treatment of purulent conjunctivitis.

Interactions. Chloramphenicol enhances the activity of anticoagulants, phenytoin and some oral hypoglycaemic agents.

Toxicity. Severe irreversible bone marrow suppression is rare but nevertheless now restricts the usage of this drug where other options exist. Therapeutic drug monitoring, where available, is recommended: trough levels <15 mg/L, 2 h after administration 10–25 mg/L. Chloramphenicol should not be given to premature infants or neonates because of their inability to conjugate and excrete this drug; high blood levels lead to circulatory collapse and the often-fatal 'grey baby syndrome'.

Sodium fusidate

Structure. Sodium fusidate has a structure resembling that of bile salts.

Mechanism of action. It is a potent inhibitor of bacterial protein synthesis. Its entry into cells is facilitated by the detergent properties inherent in its structure.

Indications for use. Sodium fusidate is mainly used for penicillinase-producing *Staph. aureus* infections such as osteomyelitis (it is well concentrated in bone) or endocarditis, and for other staphylococcal infections accompanied by septicaemia. The drug is well absorbed orally but must be used in combination with another staphylococcal agent to prevent resistance emerging. Resistance may occur rapidly; sodium fusidate is available in topical preparations, but these should be avoided to limit the risk of resistance emerging.

Toxicity. Sodium fusidate commonly causes gastrointestinal adverse effects and may occasionally be hepatotoxic; however, it is generally a safe drug and can be given during pregnancy if necessary. Concomitant statin use is avoided.

Sulphonamides and trimethoprim

Structure. The sulphonamides are all derivatives of the prototype sulfanilamide. Trimethoprim is a 2,4-diaminopyrimidine.

Mechanism of action. Sulphonamides block thymidine and purine synthesis by inhibiting microbial folic acid synthesis. Trimethoprim prevents the reduction of dihydrofolate to tetrahydrofolate (see ***Fig. 16.12***).

Indications for use. Sulfamethoxazole is mainly used in combination with trimethoprim (as co-trimoxazole). Because of its adverse effect profile, use in developed countries was largely restricted to the treatment and prevention of *Pneumocystis jiroveci* infection and listeriosis, although it is increasingly being prescribed in hospitals again for other infections, such as acute exacerbations of chronic bronchitis and urinary tract infections, as it appears to be of relatively lower risk for triggering *C. difficile* infection and remains useful for some resistant Gram-negative infections. It may also be used for toxoplasmosis and nocardiosis. Trimethoprim alone is often used for urinary tract infections.

Resistance to sulphonamides is often plasmid-mediated and results from the production of sulphonamide-resistant dihydropteroate synthase from altered bacterial cell permeability to these agents.

Interactions. Sulphonamides potentiate oral anticoagulants and some hypoglycaemic agents.

Toxicity. The adverse effects of co-trimoxazole are most commonly due to the sulphonamide component. Sulphonamides cause a variety of skin eruptions, including toxic epidermal necrolysis, the Stevens–Johnson syndrome, thrombocytopenia, folate deficiency and megaloblastic anaemia with prolonged usage. They can provoke haemolysis in individuals with glucose-6-phosphate dehydrogenase deficiency and therefore should not be used in such people. Trimethoprim is similar in molecular structure to the potassium-sparing diuretic amiloride; monitoring of renal function is required when using trimethoprim or co-trimoxazole, particularly when the patient is prescribed other potassium-sparing drugs (e.g. angiotensin-converting enzyme (ACE) inhibitors) and during prolonged therapy to avoid hyperkalaemia.

Quinolones (ciprofloxacin, moxifloxacin, norfloxacin, ofloxacin, levofloxacin and gemifloxacin)

These are useful oral broad-spectrum antibiotics, related structurally to nalidixic acid. The latter achieves only low serum concentrations after oral administration and its use is limited to the urinary tract, where it is concentrated. Moxifloxacin, levofloxacin and gemifloxacin have greater activity against Gram-positive pathogens.

Mechanism of action. The quinolone group of bactericidal drugs inhibits bacterial DNA synthesis by inhibiting topoisomerase IV and DNA gyrase, the enzyme responsible for maintaining the superhelical twists in DNA.

Indications for use. The extended-spectrum quinolones such as ciprofloxacin have activity against Gram-negative bacteria, including some *Pseudomonas aeruginosa* and some Gram-positive bacteria (e.g. anthrax; see p. 287). They are useful in Gram-negative bloodstream infections, bone and joint infections, urinary and respiratory tract infections, meningococcal carriage, some sexually transmitted diseases such as gonorrhoea and non-specific urethritis due to *Chlamydia trachomatis*, and severe cases of travellers' diarrhoea (see pp. 277–279). The newer oral quinolones (e.g. moxifloxacin) provide an alternative to β-lactams in the treatment of community-acquired lower respiratory tract infections; cover against *Strep. pneumoniae*, *H. influenzae* and the atypical respiratory bacteria is provided. They are also being used for the treatment of tuberculosis (see pp. 1110–1113).

In many countries, a high proportion of *E. coli* and *Klebsiella* spp. are now resistant. Resistance is also a growing problem among *Salmonella*, *V. cholera*, *Strep. pneumoniae* and *Staph. aureus*; almost all healthcare-associated MRSA strains are resistant. Resistance also occurs in tuberculosis treatment (see pp. 1111–1112).

Interactions. Ciprofloxacin can induce toxic concentrations of theophylline.

Toxicity. Gastrointestinal disturbances, photosensitive rashes and occasional neurotoxicity can occur. Use should be avoided in pregnancy and, unless the benefit outweighs the risk, in childhood and patients taking corticosteroids. Tendon damage, including rupture, can occur within 48 hours of use and the drug should be stopped immediately; it should not be given in patients with tendonitis. MRSA and *C. difficile* infections in hospitals have been linked to high prescribing rates of quinolones and use is discouraged where an effective alternative is available. As with the macrolides, there is concern about QT_c prolongation; concomitant prescribing with other QT_c-prolonging drugs is avoided whenever possible.

Oxazolidinones

Structure. Linezolid was the first oxazolidinone antibacterial developed. Tedizolid has recently been approved for use in skin and skin structure infections.

Mechanism of action. Linezolid inhibits protein synthesis by binding to the bacterial 23S ribosomal RNA of the 59S subunit, thereby preventing the formation of a functional 70S complex essential to bacterial translation. Tedizolid has a similar mechanism of action.

Indications for use. Oxazolidinones are active against a variety of Gram-positive pathogens, including vancomycin-resistant *Enterococcus faecium* (although, unfortunately, resistant organisms have been reported), MRSA and penicillin-resistant *Strep. pneumoniae*. They are also active against group A and group B streptococci. Clinical experience with linezolid has demonstrated efficacy in a variety of hospitalized patients with severe to life-threatening infections, such as bacteraemia, hospital-acquired pneumonia, and skin and soft tissue and bone and joint infections. These drugs can be given both intravenously and by mouth, and are almost 100% bioavailable by the oral route in patients with normal gastrointestinal absorption.

Interactions. Oxazolidinones interact reversibly as non-selective inhibitors of monoamine oxidase and have the potential for interacting with serotoninergic and adrenergic agents.

Toxicity. Side-effects include gastrointestinal disturbances, headache, rash, hypertension, reversible but potentially severe cytopenias, and occasional reports of optic and peripheral neuropathy in patients receiving linezolid for longer than 28 days. Weekly monitoring of the full blood count for cytopenias, and for other serious adverse effects, is mandatory. Safety has not yet been shown in pregnancy but linezolid has been used successfully for serious infections in children.

Nitroimidazoles

Structure. These agents are active against anaerobic bacteria and some pathogenic protozoa. The most widely used drug is metronidazole ***(Fig. 11.10)***. Others include tinidazole and nimorazole.

Mechanism of action. After reduction of their 'nitro' group to a nitrosohydroxyl amino group by microbial enzymes, nitroimidazoles cause strand breaks in microbial DNA.

Indications for use. Metronidazole plays a major role in the treatment of anaerobic bacterial infections, particularly those due to *Bacteroides* spp. It is also used prophylactically in colonic surgery. It may be given orally, by suppository (well absorbed and cheap) or intravenously (more expensive). It is also the treatment of choice for mild *C. difficile* infection, amoebiasis, giardiasis and infection with *Trichomonas vaginalis*.

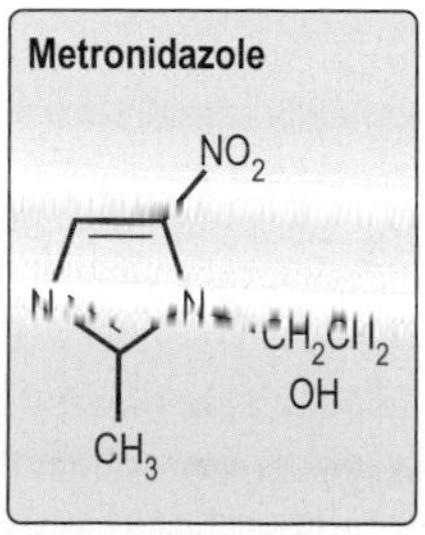

Figure 11.10 The structure of metronidazole, a nitroimidazole.

Interactions. Nitroimidazoles can produce a disulfiram-like reaction with ethanol and enhance the anticoagulant effect of warfarin; patients should be warned not to drink alcohol whilst taking them.

Toxicity. Nitroimidazoles are tumorigenic in animals and mutagenic for bacteria, although carcinogenicity has not been described in humans. They cause a metallic taste and polyneuropathy with prolonged use. High-dose regimens should be avoided in pregnancy and during breast-feeding, unless the benefit is deemed to outweigh the risk.

Glycopeptides

The glycopeptides are antibiotics active against Gram-positive bacteria and act by inhibiting cell wall synthesis.

Vancomycin

Vancomycin is given intravenously for MRSA and other multi-resistant, Gram-positive organisms. It is also used for treatment and prophylaxis against Gram-positive infections in penicillin-allergic patients. It is given in *Strep. pneumoniae* meningitis, in combination with other effective antibiotics, when disease is caused by penicillin-resistant strains. By mouth, it is not absorbed from the gastrointestinal tract and is the preferred therapy for moderate to severe *C. difficile* infection. Glycopeptide-resistant enterococci (GRE) and *Staphylococcus* spp. (see p. 270) are recognized but, in general, Gram-positive bacteria are more likely to become resistant to β-lactam antibiotics than glycopeptides.

Toxicity. Vancomycin can cause ototoxicity and nephrotoxicity, and thus pre-dose (trough) serum levels should be monitored regularly. Serum levels at 1 h post dose (peak) are also monitored to optimize drug efficacy (see p. 236). Care must be taken to avoid extravasation at the injection site, as this causes necrosis and thrombophlebitis. Too rapid infusion can produce symptomatic release of histamine (red man syndrome).

Teicoplanin

This glycopeptide antibiotic is less nephrotoxic than vancomycin. It has more favourable pharmacokinetic properties, allowing once-daily or thrice-weekly dosage. It is given intravenously and pre-dose (trough) serum levels are monitored to optimize efficacy.

Other antibiotics

Clindamycin. This is not widely used because of its strong association with *C. difficile* infection. It is active against Gram-positive cocci, including some penicillin-resistant staphylococci, and is a useful agent for severe streptococcal or staphylococcal cellulitis. It has the added effect of inhibiting staphylococcal toxic shock syndrome toxin 1 (TSST-1) and alpha toxin production and has a role in infections caused by *Staph. aureus* secreting Panton Valentine leucocidin (PVL). It is also active against anaerobes, especially *Bacteroides*. It is well concentrated in bone and used for osteomyelitis.

Mupirocin. Mupirocin prevents bacterial RNA and protein synthesis. It is only used topically, mainly for the nasal eradication of *Staph. aureus*, including MRSA, but can also be used for minor skin infections. Resistance can be a problem.

Streptogramins. A combination of quinupristin and dalfopristin is used for Gram-positive bacteria that have failed to respond to other antibacterials. It has found only limited use and is not available in the UK. Virginiamycin and pristinamycin are also available.

Daptomycin. This is a lipopeptide with a similar spectrum to vancomycin and is given by the intravenous route. It is used particularly for complicated skin and soft tissue infections, including those caused by MRSA, and is also a useful alternative agent for endocarditis, bone and joint infections, and Gram-positive bloodstream infections.

Fosfomycin is a relatively old antibiotic that has been used in some European countries for many years and is effective against many Gram-positive and Gram-negative bacteria, but has limited activity against *Pseudomonas* spp. It has a unique mechanism of action on the cell walls of bacteria, retains activity against many ESBL-producing organisms and is therefore the subject of renewed interest. It is increasingly used in the UK, particularly for resistant urinary tract infections, and is available in oral and intravenous formulations.

Colistimethate sodium (***polymixin E***). This is another old antibiotic that, until recently, was rarely used in clinical practice because of concerns about, usually reversible, neuro- and nephrotoxicity. The emergence of carbapenemase-producing Gram-negative bacteria, however, has resulted in increased use, often in combination with other antibiotics such as tigecycline and high doses of carbapenems. The mechanism of bacterial killing is thought to be due to disruption of the bacterial cell membrane following binding to the lipopolysaccharide component. It is active against most Gram-negative bacilli and is administered intravenously for serious infections. Plasmid-mediated resistance has recently been described.

Rifaximin. This is a rifamycin with poor gastrointestinal absorption. It is used in portosystemic encephalopathy (see p. 474) and to prevent traveller's diarrhoea; it may be of short-term benefit in irritable bowel syndrome.

Anti-tuberculosis drugs

These are described on pages 1110–1113. Rifampicin is also used in other infections apart from tuberculosis.

Antifungal drugs

See ***Box 11.16***.

Polyenes

Polyenes react with the sterols in fungal membranes, increasing permeability and thus damaging the organism. The most potent is amphotericin, which is used intravenously in severe systemic fungal infections. Nephrotoxicity is a major problem and dosage levels must take background renal function into account. Liposomal amphotericin is less toxic but very expensive. Nystatin is not absorbed through mucous membranes and is therefore useful for the treatment of oral and enteric candidiasis and for vaginal infection. It can only be given orally or as pessaries.

Box 11.16 Antifungal agents

Polyenes
- Amphotericin, nystatin

Echinocandins
- Caspofungin
- Anidulafungin
- Micafungin

Azoles
- Miconazole, ketoconazole, fluconazole, itraconazole, voriconazole, posaconazole, isavuconazole
- Topical clotrimazole, sulconazole, tolnaftate, econazole, tioconazole

Allylamines
- Terbinafine

Other antifungals
- Amorolfine (topical only)
- 5-Flucytosine
- Griseofulvin

Azoles

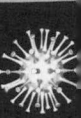

Imidazoles. Imidazoles, such as ketoconazole, miconazole and clotrimazole, are broad-spectrum antifungal drugs. They are predominantly fungistatic and act by inhibiting fungal sterol synthesis, resulting in damage to the cell wall. Ketoconazole is active orally but can produce liver damage. It is effective in candidiasis and deep mycoses, including histoplasmosis and blastomycosis, but not in aspergillosis and cryptococcosis.

Clotrimazole and miconazole are used topically for the treatment of ringworm and cutaneous and genital candidiasis. Econazole is used for the topical treatment of cutaneous and vaginal candidiasis and dermatophyte infections, while tioconazole is indicated for fungal nail infections.

Triazoles. These include fluconazole, voriconazole, posaconazole and itraconazole. Fluconazole is noted for its ability to enter CSF and is used for candidiasis and for the treatment of central nervous system (CNS) infection with *Cryptococcus neoformans*. Itraconazole fails to penetrate CSF. It is the agent of choice for non-life-threatening blastomycosis and histoplasmosis. It is also moderately effective in invasive aspergillosis. Toxicity is mild. Voriconazole has broad-spectrum activity that includes *Candida*, *Cryptococcus* and *Aspergillus* spp. and other filamentous fungi. It is available for oral and intravenous use. Adverse effects include rash, visual disturbance and abnormalities of liver enzymes. It is indicated for invasive aspergillosis and severe *Candida* infections unresponsive to amphotericin and fluconazole, respectively. Isavuconazole has recently been used for invasive mould disease.

Allylamines

Terbinafine has broad-spectrum antifungal and also anti inflammatory activity. It is well absorbed orally and accumulates in keratin. It is useful for the treatment of superficial mycoses, such as dermatophyte infections, onychomycosis and cutaneous candidiasis. A topical formulation is also available to treat fungal skin infections.

Echinocandins

These act by inhibiting the cell-wall polysaccharide, glucan. Caspofungin, which is administered intravenously, is active against *Candida* spp. and *Aspergillus* spp., and is indicated for invasive candidiasis and invasive aspergillosis unresponsive to other drugs. Other echinocandins include micafungin and anidulafungin, approved for the treatment of disseminated candidiasis. Severe hepatotoxicity has been reported with micafungin and liver biochemistry must be monitored.

Flucytosine

The fluorinated pyridine derivative, flucytosine, is used in combination with amphotericin B for cryptococcal meningitis. Side-effects are uncommon, although it may cause bone marrow suppression. It is active when given orally or parenterally.

Antiviral drugs

Drugs for HIV infection are discussed on pages 341–346, and the treatment of hepatitis C virus infections on pages 460–461.

Anti-herpesvirus drugs

Nucleoside analogues

Aciclovir. Aciclovir (***Fig. 11.11A***; also known as acycloguanosine) is an acyclic nucleoside analogue that acts as a chain terminator of herpesvirus DNA synthesis. This drug is converted to aciclovir monophosphate by a virus-encoded thymidine kinase produced by the alpha herpesviruses, herpes simplex types 1 and 2, and varicella zoster virus ***(Box 11.17)***. Conversion to the triphosphate is then achieved by cellular enzymes. Aciclovir triphosphate acts as a potent inhibitor of viral (but not cellular) DNA polymerase and also competes with deoxyguanine triphosphate for incorporation into the growing chains of herpesvirus DNA, thereby resulting in chain synthesis termination due to its acyclic structure. This highly

Box 11.17 Antiviral agents[a]

Virus	Structure/mode of action	Drug	Route of administration	Notes
Anti-herpesvirus	Nucleoside analogue	Aciclovir	Oral, i.v., topical	HSV, VZV
		Valaciclovir	Oral	HSV, VZV
		Famciclovir	Oral	HSV, VZV
		Ganciclovir	i.v.	CMV
		Valganciclovir	Oral	CMV
	Nucleotide analogue	Cidofovir	i.v.	CMV
		Brincidofovir	Oral	CMV
	Pyrophosphate analogue	Foscarnet	i.v.	CMV
	Helicase primase inhibitor	Pritelivir	Oral	HSV
	UL97 inhibitor	Maribavir		CMV
Anti-influenza	Neuraminidase inhibitor	Zanamivir	Inhaled	Influenza A, B
		Oseltamivir	Oral	Influenza A, B
Anti-hepatitis B virus	Nucleoside analogue	Lamivudine	Oral	Rapid resistance
		Telbivudine	Oral	Rapid resistance
		Entecavir	Oral	High barrier to resistance
	Nucleotide analogue	Adefovir	Oral	
		Tenofovir	Oral	High barrier to resistance
Other	Nucleoside analogue	Ribavirin	Oral, i.v.	Broad spectrum; RSV, HCV
	Interferons		i.m.	Pegylated

[a]For drugs used in HIV, see pp. 340–349; for drugs used in the treatment of hepatitis C virus infection, see pp. 460–461). CMV, cytomegalovirus; HCV, hepatitis C virus; HSV, herpes simplex virus; i.m., intramuscular; i.v., intravenous; RSV, respiratory syncytial virus; VZV, varicella zoster virus.

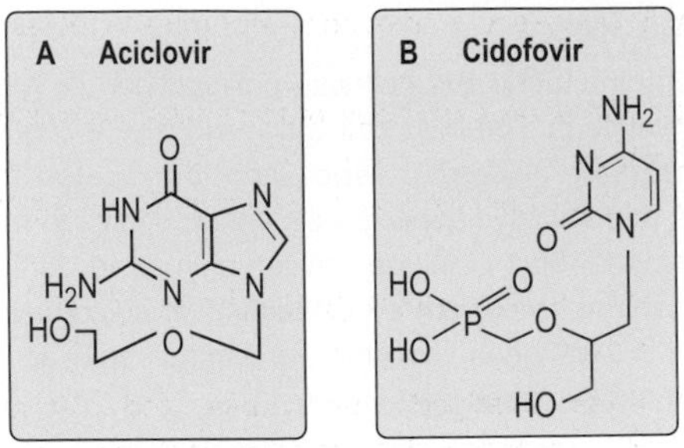

Figure 11.11 **The structure of antiviral drugs. A.** Aciclovir. **B.** Cidofovir.

specific mode of activity, targeted only to virus-infected cells, means that aciclovir has very low toxicity. Crystallization in the renal tubules is a well-recognized adverse effect, and patients should be well hydrated, particularly when high-dose intravenous therapy is being used. Intravenous, oral and topical preparations are available for the treatment of herpes simplex and varicella zoster virus infections. Treatment does not eliminate the virus so relapses do occur.

Valaciclovir. This is an oral pro-drug of aciclovir. Coupling of the amino acid valine to the acyclic side-chain of aciclovir allows better intestinal absorption. The valine is removed by enzymic action and aciclovir is released into the circulation. A similar pro-drug of a related nucleoside analogue (penciclovir) is the antiherpes drug, famciclovir. The mode of action and efficacy of famciclovir are similar to those of aciclovir.

Ganciclovir. This guanine analogue is structurally similar to aciclovir, with extension of the acyclic side-chain by a carboxymethyl group. It is active against herpes simplex viruses and varicella zoster virus by the same mechanism as aciclovir. In addition, phosphorylation by a protein kinase encoded by the *UL97* gene of cytomegalovirus renders it potently active against this virus. Thus, ganciclovir is currently the first-line treatment for cytomegalovirus disease. Intravenous and oral preparations are available, as is an oral pro-drug, valganciclovir. This is preferred for the initial treatment of CMV retinitis (see pp. 258–259). Unlike aciclovir, ganciclovir has a significant toxicity profile, including neutropenia, thrombocytopenia and, rarely, sterilization by inhibition of spermatogenesis. It is therefore reserved for the treatment or prevention of life- or sight-threatening cytomegalovirus infection in immunocompromised patients.

Nucleotide analogues

Cidofovir. This is a phosphonate derivative of an acyclic nucleoside that acts as a viral DNA polymerase inhibitor ***(Fig. 11.11B)***. It is administered intravenously for the treatment of severe cytomegalovirus infections in patients with advanced HIV infection for whom other drugs are inappropriate. It is given with probenecid and, as it is nephrotoxic, particular attention should be given to hydration and to monitoring of renal function.

Brincidofovir (also referred to as CMX001). This consists of cidofovir, which is bound to a lipid moiety, enabling an oral route of administration and avoiding renal toxicity. This drug shows great promise in clinical trials.

Pyrophosphate analogues

Foscarnet (sodium phosphonoformate). This is a simple pyrophosphate analogue that inhibits viral DNA polymerases. It is active against herpesviruses and its main roles are as a second-line treatment for severe cytomegalovirus disease and in the treatment of aciclovir-resistant herpes simplex infection. It is given intravenously and the potential for severe side-effects, particularly renal damage, limits its use.

Novel anti-herpesvirus agents

New drugs undergoing clinical trials include pritelivir, an inhibitor of the herpes simplex viral helicase-primase enzyme complex; maribavir, an inhibitor of the product of the *UL97* gene of cytomegalovirus, which plays a key role in allowing viral egress from an infected cell; and letermovir, an inhibitor of the cytomegalovirus terminase enzyme complex, which cuts the string of cytomegalovirus genomes synthesized in an infected cell into unit-length genomes for packaging in the capsid.

Anti-influenza drugs

Adamantanes

Amantadine. The use of amantadine and derivatives in the treatment and prophylaxis of influenza has largely been superseded by the neuraminidase inhibitors. Amantadine is active prophylactically and therapeutically against influenza A virus (it is inactive against influenza B virus). CNS side-effects, such as insomnia, dizziness and headache, may occur (amantadine is also used as a treatment for Parkinson's disease) and the drug is poorly tolerated, especially in the elderly.

Neuraminidase inhibitors

Zanamivir (administered by inhalation) and ***oseltamivir*** (an oral preparation). These drugs inhibit the action of the neuraminidase of influenza A and B. Both have been shown to be effective in reducing the duration of illness in influenza if given within the first 48 hours. Oseltamivir is also available for the prophylaxis of influenza among household contacts of an index case. Intravenous peramivir and zanamivir were both reported to be effective in treating patients during the 2010 influenza pandemic, but neither is currently licensed for routine use in this way.

Anti-hepatitis B drugs

A number of nucleoside and nucleotide analogues have been shown to inhibit the reverse transcriptase function of hepatitis B virus and thereby suppress viral replication (see p. 458). The first such agents, ***lamivudine*** and ***adefovir***, have largely been superseded by the more potent drugs ***entecavir*** and ***tenofovir***, both of which also have a considerably higher barrier to resistance.

Telbivudine and ***emtricitabine*** are also nucleoside analogue inhibitors of HBV DNA polymerase activity.

Other drugs

Ribavirin. This synthetic purine nucleoside derivative, which interferes with 5′-capping of messenger RNA, is active against several RNA and DNA viruses, at least *in vitro*. Its major use is in the treatment of chronic hepatitis C infection in combination with pegylated interferon-alfa (IFN-α), although it has no effect when given alone (see pp. 460–461). It is administered orally. Haemolytic anaemia is the most frequent adverse reaction. It is also administered by a small-particle aerosol generator (SPAG) to infants with acute respiratory syncytial virus (RSV) infection. Another indication is in the treatment of Lassa fever virus infection.

Palivizumab. This monoclonal antibody is specifically indicated to prevent seasonal RSV infection in infants at high risk of this infection. It is administered by intramuscular injection.

Interferons

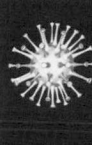

These are naturally occurring proteins with a multiplicity of actions, including antiviral, immunomodulatory and antiproliferative effects. Interferons are produced by virus-infected cells, macrophages and lymphocytes. They induce an antiviral state in uninfected cells, through activation of a complex set of biochemical pathways. They have been synthesized commercially, either by culture of lymphoblastoid cells or by recombinant DNA technology, and are licensed for therapeutic use.

The potency of INF-α has been enhanced by coupling the protein with polyethylene glycol. The resulting PEG interferon given once weekly has been shown to improve the response to, and reduce the side-effects from, treatment for hepatitis B and C (see pp. 457–458 and 460–461).

Further reading

Barr DA, Seaton RA. Outpatient parenteral antimicrobial therapy (OPAT) and the general physician. *Clin Med* 2013; 13:495–499.

Chandresekar P. Management of invasive fungal infections: a role for polyenes. *J Antimicrob Chemother* 2011; 66:457–465.

Chapman AL, Seaton RA, Cooper MA et al. Good practice recommendations for outpatient parenteral antimicrobial therapy (OPAT) in adults in the UK: a consensus statement. *J Antimicrob Chemother* 2012; 67:1053–1062.

Department of Health Advisory Committee on Antimicrobial Resistance and Healthcare Associated Infection (ARHAI). *Antimicrobial Stewardship: 'Start Smart – Then Focus' Guidance*. London: Department of Health; 2011.

Griffiths PD. A perspective on antiviral resistance. *J Clin Virol* 2009; 46:3–8.

Hand K. Antibiotic stewardship. *Clin Med* 2013; 13:499–503.

Llarrull LI, Testero SA, Fisher JF et al. The future of the β-lactams. *Curr Opin Microbiol* 2010; 13:551–557.

Masterton RG. Antibiotic de-escalation. *Crit Care Clin* 2011; 27:149–162.

Moellering RC Jr. NDM-1 – a cause for worldwide concern. *N Engl J Med* 2010; 363:2377–2379.

Rossi F, Diaz L, Wollam A et al. Brief report: transferable vancomycin resistance in a community-associated MRSA lineage. *N Engl J Med* 2014; 370:1524–1531.

Thornhill MH, Dayer MJ, Forde JM et al. Impact of the NICE guideline recommending cessation of antibiotic prophylaxis for prevention of infective endocarditis: before and after study. *BMJ* 2011; 342:d2392.

Yahav D, Farbman L, Leibovici L et al. Colistin: new lessons on an old antibiotic. *Clin Microbiol Infect* 2012; 18:18–29.

http://www.antibiotic-action.com/ *Antibiotic Action*.

http://www.bnf.org *British National Formulary (BNF)*.

http://www.bsac.org.uk/ *British Society for Antimicrobial Chemotherapy: NICHE campaign – your five moments of prescribing to prevent antibiotic resistance*.

http://www.cdc.gov/drugresistance/ *US Centers for Disease Control and Prevention: Antibiotic resistance threats in the United States in 2013*.

http://www.rcgp.org.uk/clinical-and-research/ *Royal College of General Practitioners: TARGET Antibiotics Toolkit*.

IMMUNIZATION AGAINST INFECTIOUS DISEASES

Although effective antimicrobial chemotherapy is available for many diseases, the ultimate aim of any infectious disease control programme is to prevent infection occurring. This is achieved either by:

- eliminating the source or mode of transmission of an infection (see p. 223), *or*
- reducing host susceptibility to environmental pathogens.

Immunization, immunoprophylaxis and immunotherapy

Immunization has changed the course and natural history of many infectious diseases. Passive immunization by administering preformed antibody, either in the form of immune serum or purified normal immunoglobulin, provides short-term immunity and has been effective in both the prevention (immunoprophylaxis) and treatment (immunotherapy) of a number of bacterial and viral diseases ***(Box 11.18)***. The active immunization schedule currently recommended is summarized in ***Box 11.19***. Long-lasting immunity is achieved only by active immunization with a live attenuated or an inactivated organism or a subunit thereof ***(Box 11.20)***. Active immunization may also be performed with microbial toxin (either native or modified): that is, a toxoid. Immunization should be kept up to date with booster doses throughout life. Travellers to developing countries, especially if visiting rural areas, should in addition enquire about further specific immunizations.

In 1974, the WHO introduced the Expanded Programme on Immunization (EPI). By 1994, more than 80% of the world's children had been immunized against tuberculosis, diphtheria, tetanus, pertussis, polio and measles. It is hoped that poliomyelitis will be eradicated worldwide in the near future, which will match the past success of global smallpox eradication. Introduction of conjugate vaccines against *Haemophilus influenzae* type b (Hib) and *Streptococcus pneumoniae* has proved highly effective in controlling invasive *H. influenzae* infection, notably meningitis, and reducing invasive pneumococcal disease ***(Fig. 11.12)***. A safe and immunogenic vaccine against *Neisseria meningitidis* serogroup B has recently been developed and included in childhood vaccination schedules in some countries. Childhood immunization (e.g. tetanus) should be maintained throughout adulthood; this is often overlooked by patients and healthcare professionals alike.

Protection for travellers to developing/tropical countries

There has been a huge increase in the number of people travelling to developing countries, mainly for recreation and leisure. The risk of infection depends on the area to be visited, the type of activity and the underlying health of the traveller. Advice should therefore always be based on an individual assessment.

Box 11.18 Examples of passive immunization available

Infection	Antibody	Indication	Efficacy
Bacterial			
Tetanus	Human tetanus immune globulin	Prevention and treatment	+
Diphtheria	Horse serum	Prevention and treatment	+
Botulism	Horse serum	Treatment	+
Viral			
Hepatitis A Measles	Human normal immune globulin	Prevention (rarely required since vaccine introduced)	+
Hepatitis B	Human hepatitis B immune globulin	Prevention	+
Varicella zoster	Human varicella zoster immune globulin	Prevention	+

Box 11.19 Recommended childhood immunization schedules

Time of immunization	Vaccine
UK[a]	
2 months old	Diphtheria, tetanus, pertussis, polio and Hib (DTaP/IPV/Hib) Pneumococcal conjugate (PCV) Rotavirus
3 months	Diphtheria, tetanus, pertussis, polio and Hib (DTaP/IPV/Hib) Meningococcal C conjugate (MenC), Meningococcal group B vaccine Rotavirus
4 months	Diphtheria, tetanus, pertussis, polio and Hib (DTaP/IPV/Hib) Pneumococcal conjugate (PCV)
12–13 months (i.e. within a month of first birthday)	Hib/MenC conjugate, Meningococcal group B vaccine (2 doses) Pneumococcal conjugate (PCV) Measles, mumps and rubella (MMR)
3 years and 4 months, or soon after	Diphtheria, tetanus, pertussis and polio (DTaP/IPV or dTaP/IPV) Measles, mumps and rubella (MMR)
2 years to <17 years annually	Influenza, by nasal spray (being phased in over several years)
Girls around 12–14 years	Human papillomavirus vaccine
Around 14 years old	Tetanus, diphtheria and polio (Td/IPV) Meningococcus group C conjugate
WHO for all children[b]	
As soon as possible after birth	BCG + HBV + (PV[c])
6 weeks	DPT + PV + HBV + Hib + PCV + Rotavirus
10 weeks	DPT + PV + HBV + (Hib[d]) + (PCV[d]) + Rotavirus
14 weeks	DPT + PV + Hib + PCV + (HBV[d]) + (Rotavirus[e])
9 or 12 months	Measles (second dose at 15–18 months in high-risk countries) + Rubella
As soon as possible after 9 years old	HPV (2 doses at least 6 months apart)

[a]Children at risk only. For more detailed advice about childhood immunization, see *The Green Book* (see 'Further reading' for details). [b]Model scheme for all children; additional vaccines are recommended in some locations: http://www.who.int/immunization/. [c]In high-risk countries. [d]Depending on schedule adopted. [e]Depending on formulation used. BCG, bacille Calmette–Guérin; DPT, adsorbed diphtheria, whole-cell pertussis, tetanus triple vaccine; HBV, hepatitis B vaccine; Hib, *Haemophilus influenzae* type b; HPV, human papillomavirus vaccine; PCV, pneumococcal conjugate vaccine; PV, polio vaccine. Mumps vaccine is also given in many developing countries.

Protection for travellers against infection can be divided into three categories:

- personal protection, e.g.:
  - insect repellents
  - impregnated bed netting
  - avoidance of animals
  - care with food and drink
  - condoms
- chemoprophylaxis, e.g. antimalarials
- immunization, e.g.:
  - yellow fever
  - hepatitis A and B
  - typhoid.

Box 11.20 Examples of active immunization available

Live attenuated vaccines
- Oral polio (Sabin) (not recommended, only used for outbreaks)
- MMR (measles, mumps, rubella)[a]
- Rotavirus
- Varicella zoster
- Yellow fever
- BCG
- Typhoid

Toxoids
- Diphtheria
- Tetanus

Recombinant vaccines
- Hepatitis B

Inactivated and/or conjugate vaccines
- Hepatitis A
- Pertussis
- Typhoid – whole cell and Vi antigen
- Polio (Salk) for routine use
- Influenza
- Human papillomavirus (HPV)
- Cholera (oral) – includes toxoid
- Meningococcus groups A, C W135 and Y
- Meningococcus groups B and C
- Rabies
- Anthrax
- Tick-borne encephalitis
- Japanese encephalitis
- Pneumococcal
- *Haemophilus influenzae* type b

[a]Individual vaccines for measles, mumps and rubella are not licensed in the UK. BCG, bacille Calmette–Guérin.

Because situations and risks can change rapidly, websites (which can be regularly updated) are often the best source of advice on travel health.

Further reading

Gossger N, Snape MD, Yu LM et al. Immunogenicity and tolerability of recombinant serogroup B meningococcal vaccine administered with or without routine infant vaccinations according to different immunization schedules: a randomized controlled trial. *JAMA* 2012; 307:573–582.

http://www.cdc.gov/travel *Centers for Disease Control (CDC) travel health site.*

http://www.gov.uk/government/collections/ *The Green Book – Immunisation Against Infectious Disease.*

http://www.gov.uk/government/publications/routine-childhood-immunisation-schedule *Public Health England: Routine Childhood Immunisations from Summer 2015.*

http://travelhealthpro.org.uk *National Travel Health Network and Centre.*

VIRAL INFECTIONS

Introduction

Viruses are much smaller than other infectious agents and contain either DNA or RNA – not both, as do bacteria and other microorganisms. Details of the structure, size and classification of human DNA and RNA viruses are shown in ***Boxes 11.21*** and ***11.22***, respectively. Since viruses are metabolically inert, they must live intracellularly, using the host cell for synthesis of viral proteins and nucleic acid. Viruses have a central nucleic acid core surrounded by a protein coat (capsid) that is antigenically unique for a particular virus. The capsid imparts a helical or icosahedral structure to the virus. Some viruses also possess an outer envelope consisting of lipid and protein.

Outcomes of virus infection of a cell

Replication of viruses within a cell may result in sufficient distortion of normal cell function so as to result in cell death – a ***cytocidal*** or ***cytolytic*** infection. However, acute cell death is not an inevitable consequence of virus infection of a cell. In a ***chronic***, or ***persistent***,

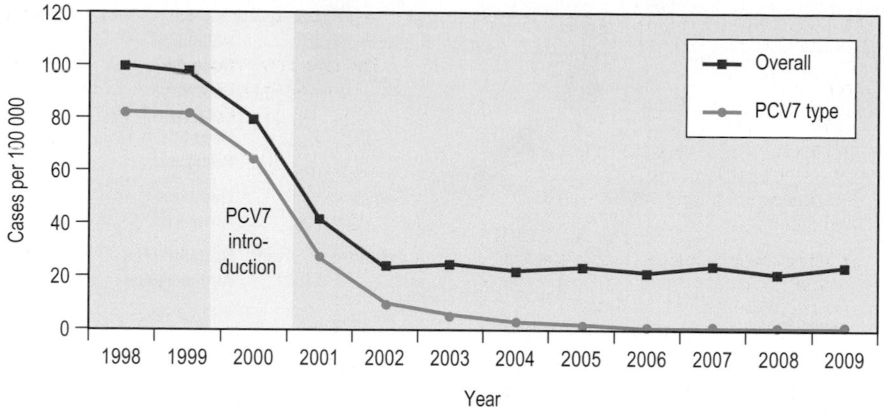

Figure 11.12 **Decline in invasive pneumococcal disease in young children following introduction of a pneumococcal conjugate vaccine (PCV) in the USA.** *(From the Centers for Disease Control and Prevention (*http://www.cdc.gov/pneumococcal/surveillance.html*), with permission.)*

Box 11.21 Human DNA viruses

Structure		Approximate size	Family	Viruses
Symmetry	*Envelope*			
Icosahedral	–	80nm	Adenovirus	**Adenoviruses** (>50 serotypes)
Icosahedral	+	100nm (160nm with envelope)	Herpesvirus	**Herpes simplex virus (HSV) types 1 and 2** **Varicella zoster virus** **Cytomegalovirus** **Epstein–Barr virus (EBV)** **Human herpesvirus type 6 (HHV-6)** **Human herpesvirus type 7 (HHV-7)** **Human herpesvirus type 8 (HHV-8)**
Icosahedral	+	42nm	Hepadnavirus	**Hepatitis B virus (HBV)**
Icosahedral	–	50nm	Papovavirus	**Human papillomaviruses** (>100 types)
Icosahedral	–	40–45nm	Polyomavirus	**Polyomaviruses JC and BK**
Icosahedral	–	23nm	Parvovirus	**Erythrovirus B19, bocavirus**
Complex	+	300nm×200nm	Poxvirus	**Variola virus** **Vaccinia virus** **Monkeypox** **Cowpox** **Orf** **Molluscum contagiosum**

infection, virus replication continues throughout the lifespan of the cell but does not interfere with the normal cellular processes necessary for cell survival. Hepatitis B and C viruses may interact with cells in this way. Some viruses, such as those of the herpesvirus family, are able to go ***latent*** within a cell; in such a state, the virus genome is present within the cell, but there is very little, if any, production of viral proteins and no production of mature virus particles. Finally, some viruses are able to ***transform*** cells, leading to uncontrolled cell division – for example, Epstein–Barr virus infection of B lymphocytes – resulting in the generation of an immortal lymphoblastoid cell line.

VIRUS INFECTIONS OF THE SKIN AND MUCOUS MEMBRANES

A number of different virus infections are associated with skin rashes (exanthems) or eruptions on the mucous membranes (enanthems) (see ***Box 11.8***). Rashes may be ***vesicular*** (i.e. consisting of fluid-filled vesicles) or ***maculopapular***.

Vesicular viral rashes

Herpes simplex virus infection

Members of the *Herpesviridae* family are causes of a wide range of human diseases ***(Box 11.23)***. The hallmark of all herpesvirus infections is the ability of the viruses to establish latent infections that then persist for the life of the individual.

Two types of herpes simplex virus (HSV; ***Fig. 11.13***) have been identified: HSV-1 is the major cause of herpetic stomatitis, herpes labialis ('cold sore'), keratoconjunctivitis and encephalitis, whereas HSV-2 causes genital herpes and may also be responsible for systemic infection in the immunocompromised host. These divisions are not rigid, however, for HSV-1 can give rise to genital herpes and HSV-2 can cause infections in the mouth. The site of latency for both HSV-1 and 2 is the nerve cell body.

HSV-1

The portal of entry of HSV-1 infection is usually via the mouth or, occasionally, the skin. The primary infection may go unnoticed, or may produce a severe inflammatory reaction with vesicle formation

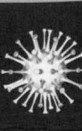

Box 11.22 Human RNA viruses

Structure		Approximate size	Family	Viruses
Symmetry	*Envelope*			
Icosahedral	–	30 nm	Picornavirus	**Poliovirus** **Coxsackievirus** **Echovirus** **Enterovirus 68–71** **Hepatitis A virus (HAV)** **Rhinovirus**
Icosahedral	–	80 nm	Reovirus	**Reovirus** **Rotavirus**
Icosahedral	+	50–80 nm	Togavirus	**Rubella virus** **Alphaviruses**
Icosahedral	+	50–80 nm	Flavivirus	**Yellow fever virus** **Dengue virus** **Zika virus** **Japanese encephalitis virus** **West Nile virus** **Hepatitis C virus (HCV)** **Tick-borne encephalitis virus**
Spherical	+	80–100 nm	Bunyavirus	**Congo–Crimean haemorrhagic fever** **Hantavirus** **Rift Valley fever virus**
Spherical	–	35–40 nm	Calicivirus	**Norovirus** **Sapovirus**
Spherical	–	28–30 nm	Astrovirus	**Astrovirus**
Spherical	–	30–34 nm	Hepevirus	**Hepatitis E virus (HEV)**
Helical	+	80–120 nm	Orthomyxovirus	**Influenza viruses A, B and C**
Helical	+	100–300 nm	Paramyxovirus	**Parainfluenza viruses 1–4** **Measles virus** **Mumps virus** **Respiratory syncytial virus (RSV)** **Human metapneumovirus** **Nipah virus** **Hendra virus**
Helical	+	80–220 nm	Coronavirus	**229E, OC43, NL63, HK1, SARS, MERS**
Helical	+	60–175 nm	Rhabdovirus	**Lyssavirus – rabies**
Helical	+	100 nm	Retrovirus	**Human immunodeficiency viruses (HIV-1 and 2)** **Human T-cell lymphotropic viruses (HTLV-1 and 2)**
Helical	+	100–300 nm	Arenavirus	**Lassa virus** **Lymphocytic choriomeningitis virus**
Pleomorphic	+	Filaments or circular forms; 100×130–2600 nm	Filovirus	**Marburg virus** **Ebola virus**

MERS, Middle East respiratory syndrome; SARS, severe acute respiratory syndrome.

Box 11.23 Major diseases caused by human herpesviruses

Sub-family	Virus	Children	Adults	Immunocompromised
α-Herpesvirus	Herpes simplex type 1	Stomatitis[a] Herpes simplex encephalitis	Cold sores Herpes simplex encephalitis Keratitis Erythema multiforme	Dissemination
	Herpes simplex type 2	Neonatal herpes[a]	Primary genital herpes[a] Recurrent genital herpes	Dissemination
	Varicella zoster virus	Chickenpox[a]	Shingles	Dissemination
β-Herpesvirus	Cytomegalovirus	Congenital[a]		Pneumonitis Retinitis Gastrointestinal
	Human herpesvirus type 6	Roseola infantum[a]		Pneumonitis
	Human herpesvirus type 7	Roseola infantum[a]		
γ-Herpesvirus	Epstein–Barr virus		Infectious mononucleosis[a] Burkitt's lymphoma Nasopharyngeal carcinoma	Lymphoma
	Human herpesvirus type 8		Kaposi's sarcoma	Kaposi's sarcoma

[a]Signifies primary infection.

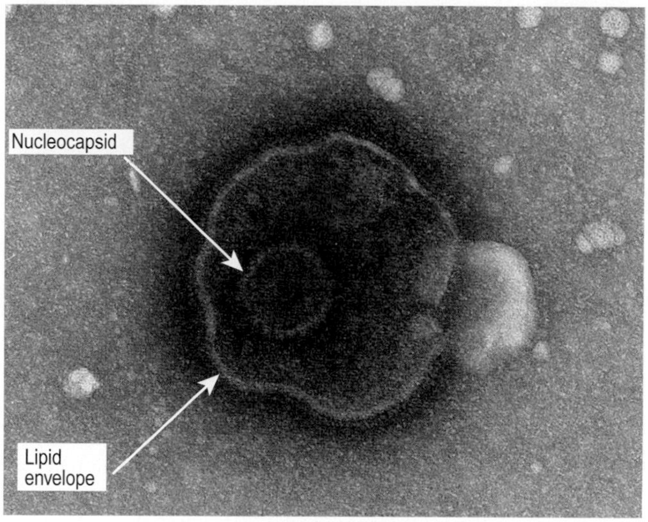

Figure 11.13 **Electron micrograph of herpes simplex virus.**

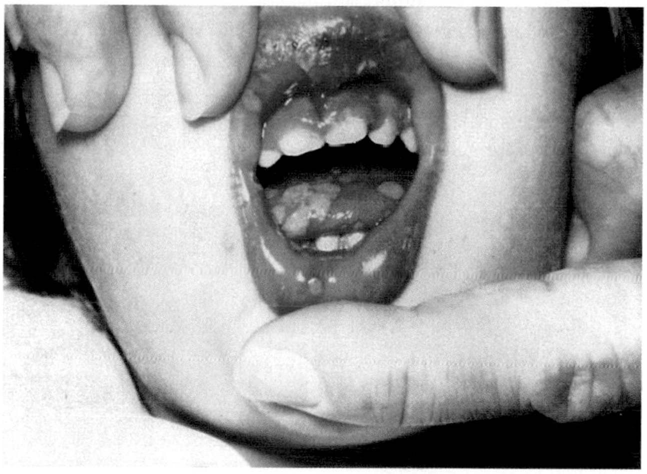

Figure 11.14 **Primary herpes simplex type 1 (gingivostomatitis).**

leading to painful ulcers (gingivostomatitis; ***Fig. 11.14***). Virus may be reactivated from the trigeminal ganglion by stress, trauma, febrile illnesses and ultraviolet radiation, producing the recurrent form of the disease known as herpes labialis ('cold sore'). Approximately 70% of the population is infected with HSV-1 and recurrent infections occur in one-third of individuals. Reactivation often produces localized paraesthesiae in the lip before the appearance of a cold sore.

Complications of HSV-1 infection include transfer to the eye (dendritic ulceration, keratitis), acute encephalitis (see p. 865), nail-bed infections (herpetic whitlow) and erythema multiforme (p. 1363).

HSV-2

The clinical features, diagnosis and management of genital herpes are described on pages 327–328. The virus remains latent in the sacral ganglia and, during recurrence, can produce a radiculomyelopathy, with pain in the groin, buttocks and upper thighs. Primary anorectal herpes infection is common in men having sex with men (see p. 327).

Neonates may develop primary HSV infection following vaginal delivery in the presence of active genital HSV infection in the mother, particularly if the maternal disease is a primary, rather than a recurrent, infection. The disease in the baby varies from localized skin lesions (about 10–15%) to widespread visceral disease most often affecting the lungs, liver and brain, with a poor prognosis. Caesarean section should therefore be performed if active genital HSV infection is present during labour.

Immunocompromised patients, such as those receiving intensive cancer chemotherapy or those with AIDS, may develop disseminated HSV infection involving many of the viscera. In severe cases, death may result from hepatitis and encephalitis. Eczema herpeticum is a serious complication in individuals with eczema, where the non-intact skin allows spread of lesions across large areas and bloodstream access, which may lead to herpetic involvement of internal organs.

Diagnosis and management

Confirmation of clinical diagnosis is most commonly obtained by detection of HSV DNA in vesicle fluid by PCR. Treatment of HSV-associated disease is with aciclovir and derivatives.

Varicella (chickenpox) and herpes zoster (shingles)

Infection with varicella zoster virus (VZV), another herpesvirus, produces two distinct diseases: varicella (chickenpox) and herpes zoster (shingles). The ***primary infection*** is chickenpox. It usually occurs in childhood, the virus entering through the mucosa of the upper respiratory tract. In some countries (e.g. the Indian subcontinent), a different epidemiological pattern exists, with most infections occurring in adulthood. Chickenpox rarely occurs twice in the same individual. Infectious virus is spread from the throat and from fresh skin lesions by air-borne transmission or direct contact. The period of infectivity in chickenpox extends from 2 days before the appearance of the rash until the skin lesions are all at the crusting stage. Following recovery from chickenpox, the virus remains latent in dorsal root and cranial nerve ganglia. ***Reactivation*** of infection then results in shingles.

Clinical features of chickenpox

Some 14–21 days after exposure to VZV, a brief prodromal illness of fever, headache and malaise heralds the eruption of chickenpox, characterized by the rapid progression of macules to papules to vesicles to pustules in a matter of hours ***(Fig. 11.15)***. In young children, the prodromal illness may be very mild or absent. The illness

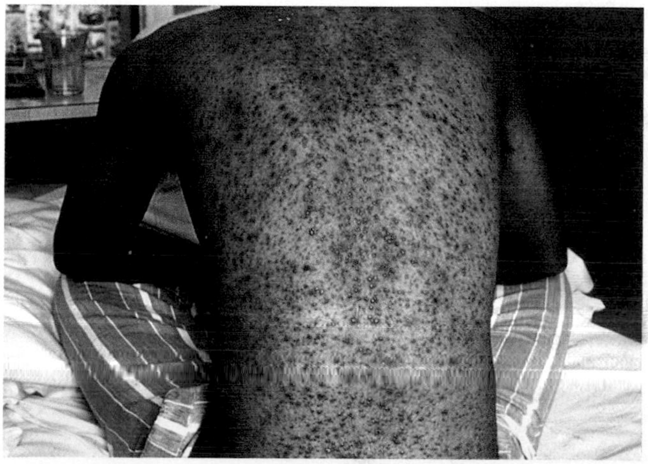

Figure 11.15 **Chickenpox in an adult.** Generalized varicella zoster virus (VZV) infection.

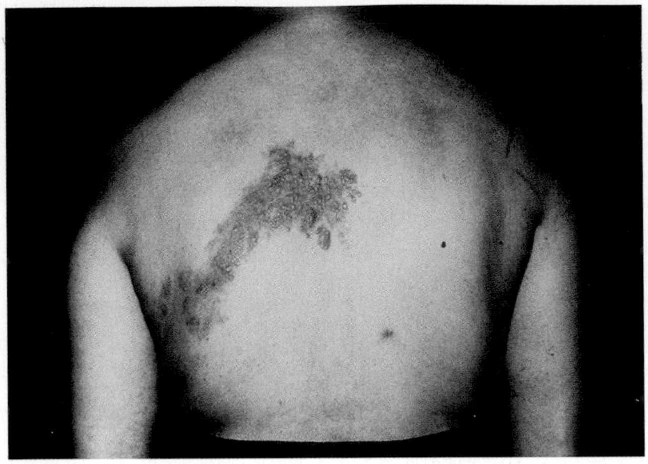

Figure 11.16 **Shingles.** Varicella zoster virus (VZV) affecting a dermatome. *(Reproduced with kind permission of the Imperial College School of Medicine.)*

tends to be more severe in older children and can be debilitating in adults. The lesions occur on the face, scalp, trunk and, to a lesser extent, on the extremities. It is characteristic to see skin lesions at all stages of development on the same area of skin. Fever subsides as soon as new lesions cease to appear. Eventually, the pustules crust and heal without scarring.

Complications of chickenpox include pneumonia, which generally begins 1–6 days after the skin eruption, and bacterial superinfection of skin lesions. Pneumonia is more common in adults than in children, and cigarette smokers are at particular risk. Pulmonary symptoms are usually more striking than the physical findings, although a chest X-ray usually shows diffuse changes throughout both lung fields. CNS involvement occurs in about 1 per 1000 cases and most commonly presents as an acute truncal cerebellar ataxia. The immunocompromised are susceptible to disseminated infection, with multiorgan involvement. Women in pregnancy are prone to severe chickenpox and, in addition, there is a risk of intrauterine infection with structural damage to the fetus (if maternal infection is within the first 20 weeks of pregnancy, the risk of varicella embryopathy is 1–2%).

Clinical features of shingles

Shingles (see p. 1344) arises from the reactivation of VZV latent within the dorsal root or cranial nerve ganglia. It may occur at any age but is most common in the elderly, producing skin lesions similar to those of chickenpox, although classically they are unilateral and restricted to a sensory nerve (i.e. dermatomal) distribution ***(Fig. 11.16)***. The onset of the rash of shingles is usually preceded by severe dermatomal pain, indicating the involvement of sensory nerves in its pathogenesis. Virus is disseminated from freshly formed vesicles and may cause chickenpox in susceptible contacts.

The most common complication of shingles is post-herpetic neuralgia (PHN; see p. 866).

Diagnosis

The diseases are usually recognized clinically but can be confirmed by detection of VZV DNA within vesicular fluid using PCR, electron microscopy, immunofluorescence or culture of vesicular fluid, and by serology.

Prevention and management

Chickenpox usually requires no treatment in healthy children and infection results in life-long immunity. Aciclovir and derivatives are, however, licensed for this indication in the USA, where the argument for treatment is that the sooner the child recovers, the sooner the carer can return to work. However, the disease may be fatal in the immunocompromised, who should therefore be offered protection, after exposure to the virus, with zoster-immune globulin (ZIG) and high-dose aciclovir at the first sign of development of the disease.

Anyone with chickenpox who is over the age of 16 years should be given antiviral therapy with aciclovir or a similar drug, if they present within 72 hours of onset. Prophylactic ZIG is recommended for susceptible pregnant women exposed to VZV and, if chickenpox develops, aciclovir treatment should be given. (N.B. Aciclovir has not been licensed for use in pregnant women.) If a woman has chickenpox at term, her baby should be protected by ZIG if delivery occurs within 7 days of the onset of the mother's rash. An effective live attenuated varicella vaccine is licensed as a routine vaccination of childhood in the USA; it is available on a named patient basis in the UK and also for susceptible healthcare workers.

Shingles involving motor nerves – for example, the VIIth cranial nerve, leading to facial palsy – is also treated with aciclovir (or derivatives thereof), as the duration of lesion formation and time to healing can be reduced by early treatment. Aciclovir, valaciclovir and famciclovir have all been shown to reduce the burden of PHN when treatment is given in the acute phase. Shingles involving the ophthalmic division of the trigeminal nerve has an associated 50% incidence of acute and chronic ophthalmic complications. Early treatment with aciclovir reduces this to 20% or less. As for chickenpox, all immunocompromised individuals should be given aciclovir at the onset of shingles, no matter how mild the attack appears when it first presents.

Vaccination of all adults over the age of 60 (USA) or 70 (UK), with a live vaccine at a dose higher than that used for chickenpox prophylaxis in childhood, reduces shingles-related morbidity and PHN, and is recommended.

Picornavirus infections

The picornaviruses (pico = small) are a large family of small RNA viruses, which includes the enteroviruses and rhinoviruses, and also hepatitis A virus (see p. 452). The term enterovirus refers to the enteric means of spread of these viruses: that is, via the faeco-oral route. The enteroviruses include poliovirus types 1–3, Coxsackie A and B viruses, echoviruses and enteroviruses (EV) 68–71. There are several newly described EVs yet to be officially classified.

Herpangina

This disease is mainly caused by Coxsackie A viruses and presents with a vesicular eruption on the fauces, palate and uvula. The lesions evolve into ulcers. The illness is usually associated with fever and headache but is short-lived, recovery occurring within a few days.

Hand, foot and mouth disease

This disease is mainly caused by Coxsackievirus A16 or A10. It is also the main feature of infection with EV71. Oral lesions are similar to those seen in herpangina but may be more extensive in the oropharynx. Vesicles and a maculopapular eruption also appear, typically on the palms of the hands and the soles of the feet, but also on other parts of the body. This infection commonly affects children. Recovery occurs within a week.

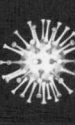

Poxvirus infections

Smallpox (variola)

This disease was eradicated in 1977 following an aggressive vaccination policy. Its possible use in bioterrorism has resulted in the re-introduction of smallpox vaccination in some countries (see p. 233).

Monkeypox

This is a rare zoonosis that occurs in small villages in tropical rainforests in several countries of West and Central Africa. Its clinical effects, including a generalized vesicular rash, are indistinguishable from those of smallpox, but person-to-person transmission is unusual. Most infections occur in children who have not been vaccinated against smallpox. Disease can be severe, with mortality rates of 10–15% in unvaccinated individuals. Serological surveys indicate that several species of squirrel are the likely animal reservoir. The virus was introduced into the USA in 2003 via West African small mammals illegally imported as pets. Widespread infection of prairie dogs resulted and there were 37 laboratory confirmed cases in humans.

Cowpox

Cowpox produces large vesicles that are classically found on the hands of individuals in contact with infected cows. The lesions are associated with regional lymphadenitis and fever. Cowpox virus has been found in a range of species, including domestic and wild cats, and the reservoir is thought to exist in a range of rodents.

Vaccinia virus

This is a laboratory virus and does not occur in nature in either humans or animals. Its origins are uncertain but it has been invaluable in its use as the vaccine to prevent smallpox.

Orf

This poxvirus causes contagious pustular dermatitis in sheep and hand lesions in humans (see p. 1345).

Molluscum contagiosum

This is discussed on pages 1344–1345.

Human papillomavirus infections

These cause warts (see p. 1344). They also cause cervical cancer (p. 265).

Maculopapular viral rashes

Measles (rubeola)

Measles virus is a paramyxovirus (see ***Box 11.22***). Measles is a highly communicable disease that occurs worldwide. With the introduction of aggressive immunization policies, the incidence of measles has fallen dramatically in the West but in 2012 there were 122 000 measles deaths globally, mostly in Africa and South-east Asia, with mortality being highest in children younger than 12 months of age. It is spread by droplet infection and the period of infectivity is from 4 days before until 2 days after the onset of the rash.

Clinical features

The incubation period is 8–14 days. Two distinct phases of the disease can be recognized.

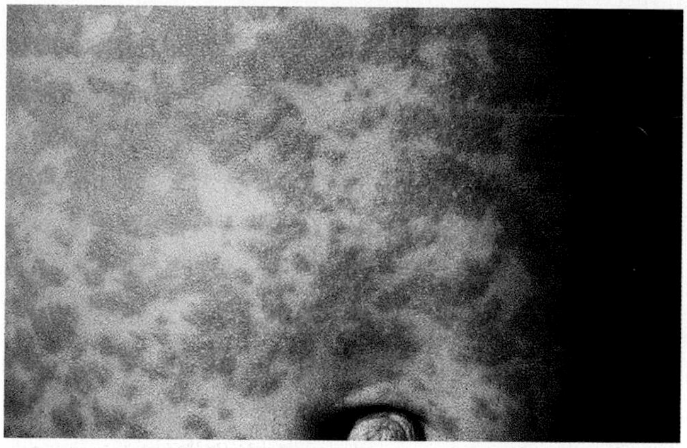

Figure 11.17 Measles. *(Courtesy of Dr MW McKendrick, Royal Hallamshire Hospital, Sheffield.)*

Typical measles

- ***Pre-eruptive and catarrhal stage***. This is the stage of viraemia and viral dissemination. Malaise, fever, rhinorrhoea, cough, conjunctival suffusion and the pathognomonic Koplik's spots are present during this stage. Koplik's spots are small, greyish, irregular lesions surrounded by an erythematous base and are found in greatest numbers on the buccal mucous membrane opposite the second molar tooth. They occur a day or two before the onset of the rash.
- ***Eruptive or exanthematous stage***. This is characterized by the presence of a maculopapular rash that initially occurs on the face, chiefly the forehead, and then spreads rapidly to involve the rest of the body ***(Fig. 11.17)***. At first, the rash is discrete but later it may become confluent and patchy, especially on the face and neck. It fades in about 1 week and leaves behind a brownish discoloration.

The most feared complication in an immunocompetent child is acute measles encephalitis, which has an incidence of 1/1000–1/5000 cases of measles. This is post-infectious – that is, virus is not present in the brain – and the encephalitis presumably arises through an aberrant cross-reaction of the host immune response to infection. Prognosis is poor, with a high mortality (30%), and severe residual damage in survivors.

Measles carries a high mortality in the malnourished and in those who have other diseases. Complications are common in such individuals and include bacterial pneumonia, bronchitis, otitis media and severe diarrhoea. Less commonly, myocarditis, hepatitis and encephalomyelitis occur. In those who are malnourished or those with defective cell-mediated immunity, the classical maculopapular rash may not develop and widespread desquamation may occur. The virus also causes the rare condition called subacute sclerosing panencephalitis, which may follow measles infection occurring early in life (<18 months of age). Persistence of the virus with reactivation before puberty results in accumulation of virus in the brain, progressive mental deterioration and a fatal outcome (see p. 867).

Maternal measles, unlike rubella, does not cause fetal abnormalities. It is, however, associated with spontaneous abortions and premature delivery.

Diagnosis and management

Most cases of measles are diagnosed clinically but detection of measles-specific IgM in blood or oral fluid, or genome or antigen detection from nasopharyngeal aspirates or throat swabs, should be used to confirm the diagnosis.

Management is supportive. Antibiotics are indicated only if secondary bacterial infection occurs.

Prevention

A previous attack of measles confers a high degree of immunity and second attacks are uncommon. Normal human immunoglobulin given within 5 days of exposure effectively aborts an attack of measles. It is indicated for previously unimmunized children below 3 years of age, during pregnancy and in those with debilitating disease.

Active immunization

Children in the UK are immunized with the combined mumps/measles/rubella (MMR) vaccine (see ***Box 11.19***). In developing countries, the first measles vaccination is given at 9 months. Measles vaccination resulted in a 78% drop in measles deaths between 2000 and 2012 worldwide.

Rubella

Rubella ('German measles') is caused by a spherical, enveloped RNA virus belonging to the rubivirus genus of the family Togaviridae, which is easily killed by heat and ultraviolet light. While the disease can occur sporadically, epidemics are not uncommon. It has a worldwide distribution. Spread of the virus is via droplets; maximum infectivity occurs before and during the time the rash is present.

Clinical features

The incubation period is 14–21 days, averaging 18 days. The clinical features are largely determined by age, symptoms being mild or absent in children under 5 years.

During the prodrome, the patient may develop malaise, fever, mild conjunctivitis and lymphadenopathy involving particularly the suboccipital, post-auricular and posterior cervical groups of lymph nodes. Small petechial lesions on the soft palate (Forchheimer spots) are suggestive but not diagnostic. Splenomegaly may be present.

The eruptive or exanthematous phase usually occurs within 7 days of the initial symptoms. The rash first appears on the forehead and then spreads to involve the trunk and limbs. It is pinkish red, macular and discrete, although some of these lesions may coalesce ***(Fig. 11.18)***. It usually fades by the second day and rarely persists beyond 3 days after its appearance.

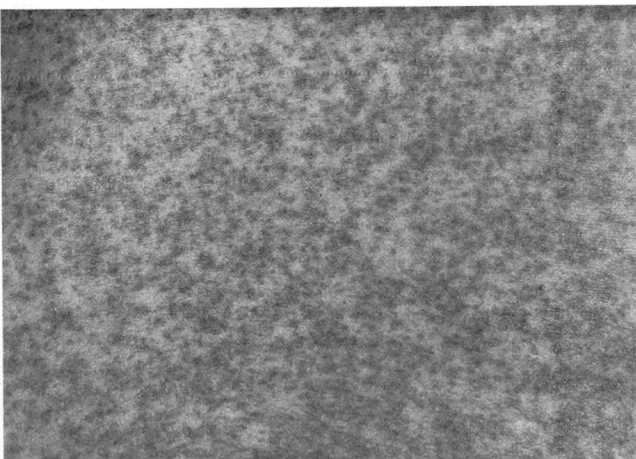

Figure 11.18 Rubella rash.

Complications

Complications are rare. They include superadded pulmonary bacterial infection, arthralgia (more common in females), haemorrhagic manifestations due to thrombocytopenia, and encephalitis. Maternal infection in pregnancy may result in the congenital rubella syndrome. Rubella affects the fetuses of up to 80% of all women who contract the infection during the first trimester of pregnancy. The incidence of congenital abnormalities diminishes in the second trimester and no ill-effects result from infection in the third trimester.

Congenital rubella syndrome is characterized by the presence of fetal cardiac malformations, especially patent ductus arteriosus and ventricular septal defect, eye lesions (especially cataracts), microcephaly, mental retardation and deafness. Hepatosplenomegaly, myocarditis, interstitial pneumonia and metaphyseal bone lesions also occur.

Diagnosis and management

Laboratory diagnosis is essential (especially in pregnancy) to distinguish the illness from other virus infections (e.g. erythrovirus B19, echovirus) and drug rashes. This is achieved by the detection of rubella-specific IgM by enzyme-linked immunosorbent assay (ELISA) in an acute serum sample, preferably confirmed by the demonstration of IgG seroconversion (or a rising titre of IgG) in a subsequent sample taken 14 days later. Viral genome can be detected in throat swabs (or oral fluid samples), urine and, in the case of intrauterine infection, the products of conception.

Management is supportive.

Prevention

Several live attenuated rubella vaccines have been used with great success in preventing this illness and these have been successfully combined with measles and mumps vaccines in the MMR vaccine. Use of the vaccine is contraindicated during pregnancy or if there is a likelihood of pregnancy within 3 months of immunization. Inadvertent use of the vaccine during pregnancy has not, however, revealed a risk of teratogenicity.

Erythrovirus infections

Human erythrovirus (also known as parvovirus) B19 causes erythema infectiosum (fifth disease), a common infection in schoolchildren. The rash is typically on the face (the '***slapped cheek***' appearance). The patient is well and the rash can recur over weeks or months. Asymptomatic infection occurs in 20% of children. Non-specific respiratory tract illness is another common manifestation of infection. In adults, the rash may be clinically indistinguishable from rubella. Moderately severe self-limiting polyarthropathy (see p. 691) is common if infection occurs in adulthood, especially in women (also true of rubella). The virus infects bone marrow cells, and aplastic crisis may occur in patients with chronic haemolysis (e.g. sickle cell disease). Chronic infection with anaemia occurs in immunocompromised subjects. Hydrops fetalis (3% risk) and spontaneous abortion (9% risk) may result from maternal infection in the first and second trimesters of pregnancy.

Diagnosis of acute infection is by detection of parvovirus-specific IgM and/or DNA.

Human herpesvirus types 6 and 7 infection

These human herpesvirus occur worldwide and exist as latent infections in over 85% of the adult population. They are spread by contact with oral secretion. Human herpesvirus type 6 (HHV-6) causes roseola infantum (exanthem subitum), which presents as a high fever followed by a generalized macular rash in infants. HHV-6 is a common cause of febrile convulsions, and aseptic meningitis or encephalitis occurs as a rare complication. Reactivation in the immunocompromised may lead to severe pneumonia.

The full spectrum of disease due to HHV-7 has not yet been fully characterized but, like HHV-6, it may cause roseola infantum in infants.

Management

Supportive management only is recommended for the common infantile disease. Ganciclovir can be used in the immunocompromised.

Further reading

Cohen JI. Herpes zoster. *New Engl J Med* 2013; 369:255–263.
Moss WJ, Griffin DE. Measles. *Lancet* 2012; 379:153–162.

VIRUS INFECTIONS OF THE RESPIRATORY TRACT

There are many viruses that can cause upper respiratory tract infection (URTI): for example, in the nose (rhinitis), throat (tonsillitis, pharyngitis), sinuses (sinusitis), ear (otitis media), eye (conjunctivitis) or larynx (laryngitis) ***(Box 11.24)***. Infections below the larynx are referred to as lower respiratory tract infections (LRTIs). URTIs are common but relatively trivial; LRTIs are less common but may result in hospitalization and even death.

Upper respiratory tract infections

The common cold – coryza, rhinitis

Rhinovirus infection is the most common cause of the common cold (see pp. 1075–1076). Peak incidence rates occur in the colder months, especially spring and autumn. There are multiple rhinovirus serotypes (>100), which explains why infection occurs throughout life and makes vaccine control impracticable. In contrast to enteroviruses, which replicate at 37°C, rhinoviruses grow best at 33°C (the temperature of the upper respiratory tract), which explains the localized disease characteristic of common colds.

Human coronaviruses were first isolated in the mid-1960s and the majority of isolates (related to the reference strains 229E and OC43) have been associated with common colds. In 2004 and 2005, two new coronavirus infections of humans were described: NL63 and HKU1. These are also associated with coryzal symptomatology. Coronaviruses have recently become of interest owing to the discovery of two new viruses causing life-threatening LRTI (see below).

Box 11.24 Virus infections of the respiratory tract

Virus	Disease
Upper respiratory tract infections	
Rhinoviruses (>100 serotypes)	Common cold, rhinitis
Parainfluenza viruses 1–4	Croup
Coronaviruses OC43, 229E	Common cold
Respiratory syncytial virus	Cough, sore throat
Human metapneumovirus	Cough, sore throat
Adenoviruses (>50 serotypes)	Pharyngitis, conjunctivitis Common cold (see pp. 1075–1076)
Enteroviruses (Coxsackie, echo)	Bronchiolitis in young babies
Lower respiratory tract infections	
Influenza A, B	Epidemics and pandemics of influenza
Respiratory syncytial virus	Bronchiolitis, pneumonia in young babies
Rarely	
Cytomegalovirus	Pneumonitis in immunocompromised
Varicella zoster virus	Pneumonia in adults with primary infection
Measles	Giant-cell pneumonia in immunocompromised
MERS-coronavirus	Pneumonia, geographically restricted

MERS, Middle East respiratory syndrome.

Parainfluenza

Parainfluenza is caused by the parainfluenza viruses types I–IV; these have a worldwide distribution and cause acute respiratory disease. Type IV appears to be less virulent than the other types and has been linked only to mild upper respiratory diseases in children and adults.

Parainfluenza is essentially a disease of children and presents with features similar to those of the common cold. When severe, a brassy cough with inspiratory stridor and features of laryngotracheitis (croup) are present. Fever usually lasts for 2–3 days and may be more prolonged if pneumonia develops. The development of croup is due to sub-mucosal oedema and consequent airway obstruction in the subglottic region. This may lead to cyanosis, subcostal and intercostal recession and progressive airway obstruction. Infection in the immunocompromised is usually prolonged and may be severe. Management is supportive with oxygen, humidification and sedation when required. The role of steroids and the antiviral agent ribavirin is controversial.

Adenovirus infection

Over 50 adenovirus serotypes have been identified as human pathogens, infecting a number of different cell types and therefore resulting in different clinical syndromes. Adenovirus infection commonly presents as an acute pharyngitis, and extension of infection to the larynx and trachea in infants may lead to croup. By school age, the majority of children show serological evidence of previous infection. Certain subtypes produce an acute conjunctivitis associated with pharyngitis. In adults, adenovirus causes acute follicular conjunctivitis and, rarely, pneumonia that is clinically similar to that produced by *Mycoplasma pneumoniae* (see p. 1104). Certain adenoviruses cause gastroenteritis (see pp. 273–279) without respiratory disease, and adenovirus infection may be responsible for acute mesenteric lymphadenitis in children and young adults. Mesenteric adenitis due to adenoviruses may lead to intussusception in infants. Infection in an immunocompromised host, such as a bone marrow transplant recipient, may result in multisystem failure and fatal disease.

Other viral causes of URTI

Human erythrovirus B19 infection may present as a URTI. Bocavirus is a recently identified erythrovirus, which accounts for around 1.5% of respiratory tract infections in young children. Coxsackie and echoviruses, which both belong to the enterovirus family, are occasionally found in respiratory tract secretions of young babies. WU and KI polyomaviruses have been recently identified. These may be associated with respiratory tract infections in young children.

Lower respiratory tract infections

Viral infections resulting in life-threatening LRTIs are influenza, respiratory syncytial virus and the Middle East respiratory syndrome coronavirus. However, other causes of viral pneumonia occasionally arise, and these are listed in ***Box 11.24***.

Influenza

Influenza viruses belong to the family orthomyxoviridae, having a segmented negative strand RNA genome. The influenza virus is a spherical or filamentous enveloped virus. Haemagglutinin (H), a surface glycoprotein, aids attachment of the virus to the surface of susceptible host cells at specific sialic acid receptor sites. Release of replicated viruses from the cell surface, effected by budding through the cell membrane, is facilitated by the action of the enzyme neuraminidase (N), which is also present on the viral envelope. Three types of influenza virus are recognized – A, B and C – distinguishable by the nature of their internal proteins. In addition, sixteen H subtypes (H1–H16) and nine N subtypes (N1–N9) have been identified for influenza A viruses but only H1, H2, H3, N1 and N2 have established stable lineages in the human population since 1918.

- ***Influenza A*** is generally responsible for pandemics and epidemics.
- ***Influenza B*** often causes smaller or localized and milder outbreaks, such as in camps or schools. There are no subtypes of influenza B.
- ***Influenza C*** rarely produces disease in humans.

Antigenic shift generates new influenza A subtypes, which emerge at irregular intervals and give rise to influenza pandemics. Possible mechanisms include:

- Genetic reassortment of the RNA of the virus (which is arranged in eight segments) with that of an avian influenza virus. This requires co-infection of a host with both human and avian viruses. The pig is one animal in which this may occur. Alternatively, humans may act as the mixing vessel.
- Trans-species transmission of an avian influenza virus to humans. Viruses transmitted in this way are usually not well adapted to growth in their new host but adaptation may occur as a result of spontaneous mutations, leading to the emergence of a pandemic strain.

Antigenic drift (minor changes in influenza A and B viruses) results from point mutations leading to amino acid changes in the two surface glycoproteins, haemagglutinin and neuraminidase, which induce humoral immunity. This enables the virus to evade previously induced immune responses and is the process whereby annual influenza epidemics arise.

Thus, changes due to antigenic shift or drift render the individual's immune response less able to combat the new variant.

The incidence of infection increases during the winter months. Spread is mainly by droplet infection but fomites and direct contact have also been implicated. Influenza pandemics of the 20th century are listed in ***Box 11.25***.

In 1997, avian influenza A/H5N1 viruses were first isolated from humans, raising the spectre of another pandemic. As of January 2014, over 650 sporadic human A/H5N1 infections have been reported from 15 countries, mostly in Asia (Indonesia, China and Vietnam) and almost always arising from direct contact with infected chickens, with a mortality of >50%. While this virus is highly pathogenic to humans, due to the induction of a cytokine storm within the lungs, it still has not evolved to replicate well in human cells and human-to-human spread is unusual. However, anxieties remain that either genetic re-assortment will occur in a human co-infected with human A/H1N1 or A/H3N2 viruses, or adaptive mutations will occur within infected human hosts, such that a truly pandemic strain will emerge.

In April 2009, a novel influenza A virus, now referred to as A(H1N1) pdm09, was identified in patients with severe respiratory illness in Mexico and North America. The virus quickly spread across the world, with the WHO declaring an official pandemic on 11 June 2009. The virus was the end-product of several re-assortments between pre-existing swine, avian and human virus lineages, with the swine H1 protein showing around 20% amino acid sequence divergence from previously circulating human seasonal H1N1 influenza viruses. Although unquestionably highly transmissible (with estimates of millions of infections worldwide within 1 year), this pandemic virus was (perhaps fortunately) not especially virulent. Most infections occurred in children; adults over 50 years of age had evidence of pre-existing protective immunity. A minority of infections resulted in serious disease, with an estimated 200 000 deaths worldwide. Risk factors for serious disease included pre-existing underlying medical conditions, age <5 years, obesity and pregnancy. The pandemic was declared officially over by the WHO in August 2010, the virus now behaving as a normal seasonal influenza virus, and replacing the previously circulating A H1N1 virus.

Novel influenza viruses may continue to infect humans sporadically, raising the possibility of a new pandemic. In 2013, over 100 cases of infection with an H7N9 virus were reported from China, a third of whom died. Most cases gave a history of exposure to live animals, including chickens.

Purified haemagglutinin and neuraminidase from recently circulating strains of influenza A and B viruses are incorporated in current vaccines.

The clinical features, diagnosis, treatment and prophylaxis of influenza are discussed on page 1078.

Box 11.25 Influenza pandemics of the 20th century

Year	Virus subtype	Comments
1918–19	H1N1	>40 million deaths
1957	H2N2	'Asian' influenza
1968	H3N2	
1976[a]	H1N1	'Russian' influenza
2009	H1N1pdm	Derived from swine influenza

[a]Not thought to be a natural occurrence.

Respiratory syncytial virus infection

Respiratory syncytial virus (RSV) is a paramyxovirus that causes many respiratory infections in epidemics each winter. It is a common cause of bronchiolitis in infants, complicated by pneumonia in approximately 10% of cases. The infection normally starts with upper respiratory symptoms. After an interval of 1–3 days, a cough and low-grade fever may develop. The onset of bronchiolitis is characterized by dyspnoea and hyperexpansion of the chest with subcostal and intercostal recession. The disease may be severe and potentially fatal in babies with underlying cardiac, respiratory (including prematurity) or immunodeficiency disease. The virus undergoes antigenic drift and, consequently, re-infection occurs throughout life. RSV is occasionally the cause of outbreaks of influenza-like illness or pneumonia in the elderly (in residential homes) and in the immunocompromised.

Transfer of infection between children in hospital (hospital-acquired infection) commonly occurs unless infected patients are isolated or cohorted. Meticulous attention to hand-washing and other infection control measures reduces the risk of transmission by staff members (see p. 224).

Diagnosis and management

Genome detection or immunofluorescence on nasopharyngeal aspirates, virus culture and serology are the usual ways of confirming the diagnosis.

Management is generally supportive, but aerosolized ribavirin can be given to severe cases, particularly those with underlying cardiac or respiratory disease.

Prevention

No vaccine is currently available for RSV but high-risk children (including those with bronchopulmonary dysplasia and congenital heart disease) can be protected against severe disease by monthly administration of either a hyperimmune globulin against RSV, or a humanized monoclonal antibody (palivizumab) during the winter months.

Metapneumovirus

Human metapneumovirus (hMPV) belongs to the same virus family as RSV, and causes approximately 10% of LRTIs in infants and young children. Infection is clinically indistinguishable from that caused by RSV.

Coronavirus infection – severe acute respiratory and Middle East respiratory syndromes

In November 2002, an apparently new LRTI occurred in China and spread rapidly in other parts of the Far East and across the world.

This disease, known as 'severe acute respiratory syndrome' (SARS), of which bronchopneumonia is a major feature, was caused by a previously unknown coronavirus (SARS-CoV). Similarity of this virus to coronaviruses isolated from civet cats, raccoons and ferret badgers indicates the likelihood that SARS is a zoonotic disease. Bats are the likely host species for this virus. The epidemic was finally brought under control in the summer of 2003, by which time there had been >8000 cases with approximately 800 deaths. Naturally acquired infection has not been reported since.

In 2012, a new coronavirus, Middle East respiratory syndrome coronavirus (MERS-CoV), was identified in a patient who died of acute respiratory failure in Saudi Arabia. There have been over 750 cases since, with a mortality of around 40%, almost all acquired in the Middle East, the most likely source being a virus from camels. Person-to-person spread has been described but has not been sufficient to cause large-scale outbreaks.

Further reading

Fineberg HV. Pandemic preparedness and response – lessons from the H1N1 influenza of 2009. *New Engl J Med* 2014; 370:1335–1342.

Hall CB. Respiratory syncytial virus in young children. *Lancet* 2010; 375:1500–1501.

Pebody R, Watson JM, Zambon M. Novel coronavirus: how much of a threat? *BMJ* 2013; 346:f1301.

Uyeki TM. Preventing and controlling influenza with available interventions. *New Engl J Med* 2014; 370:789–791.

SYSTEMIC VIRAL INFECTIONS

Dengue

This is the most common arthropod-borne viral infection in humans; over 100 million cases occur every year in the tropics, with over 10 000 deaths from dengue haemorrhagic fever ***(Fig. 11.19)***. Dengue is caused by a flavivirus. The disease is endemic in all tropical regions, including northern Australia, most South-east Asian countries, tropical Africa and the Middle East, and Caribbean countries. Cases of dengue are also imported into the continental USA and Europe (e.g. Italy) via tourists returning from endemic countries.

Four different antigenic varieties of dengue virus are recognized and all are transmitted by the daytime-biting *Aedes aegypti*, which breeds in standing water in refuse dumps in inner cities. *A. albopictus* is a less common transmitter. Humans are infective during the first 3 days of the illness (the viraemic stage; ***Fig. 11.20***). Mosquitoes become infective about 2 weeks after feeding on an infected individual and remain so for life. The disease is usually endemic. Heterotypic immunity between serotypes after the illness is partial and lasts only a few months, although homotype immunity is life-long.

Clinical features

The incubation period is 5–6 days following the mosquito bite. Asymptomatic or mild infections are common. Two clinical forms are recognized ***(Fig. 11.20)***.

Classic dengue fever

Classic dengue fever is characterized by the abrupt onset of fever, malaise, headache, facial flushing, retrobulbar pain that worsens on eye movements, conjunctival suffusion and severe backache, which is a prominent symptom. Lymphadenopathy, petechiae on the soft palate and transient, morbilliform skin rashes may also appear on the limbs with subsequent spread to involve the trunk. Desquamation occurs subsequently. Cough is uncommon. The fever subsides after 3–4 days, the temperature returns to normal for a couple of days and then the fever returns, together with the features already mentioned, but milder. This biphasic or 'saddleback' pattern is considered characteristic. Severe fatigue, a feeling of being unwell and depression are common for several weeks after the fever has subsided.

Dengue haemorrhagic fever

Dengue haemorrhagic fever (DHF) is a severe form of dengue fever and is believed to be the result of two or more sequential infections with different dengue serotypes. It is characterized by the capillary leak syndrome, thrombocytopenia, haemorrhage, hypotension and shock. It is characteristically a disease of children, occurring most commonly in South-east Asia. The disease has a mild start, often with symptoms of an URTI. This is then followed by the abrupt onset of shock and haemorrhage into the skin and ear, epistaxis, haematemesis and melaena, known as the ***dengue shock syndrome***. This has a mortality of up to 44%. Serum complement levels are depressed and there is laboratory evidence of disseminated intravascular coagulation (DIC; see pp. 573–574).

Diagnosis and management

- Isolation of dengue virus by tissue culture, or detection of viral RNA by PCR in sera obtained during the first few days of illness, is diagnostic.

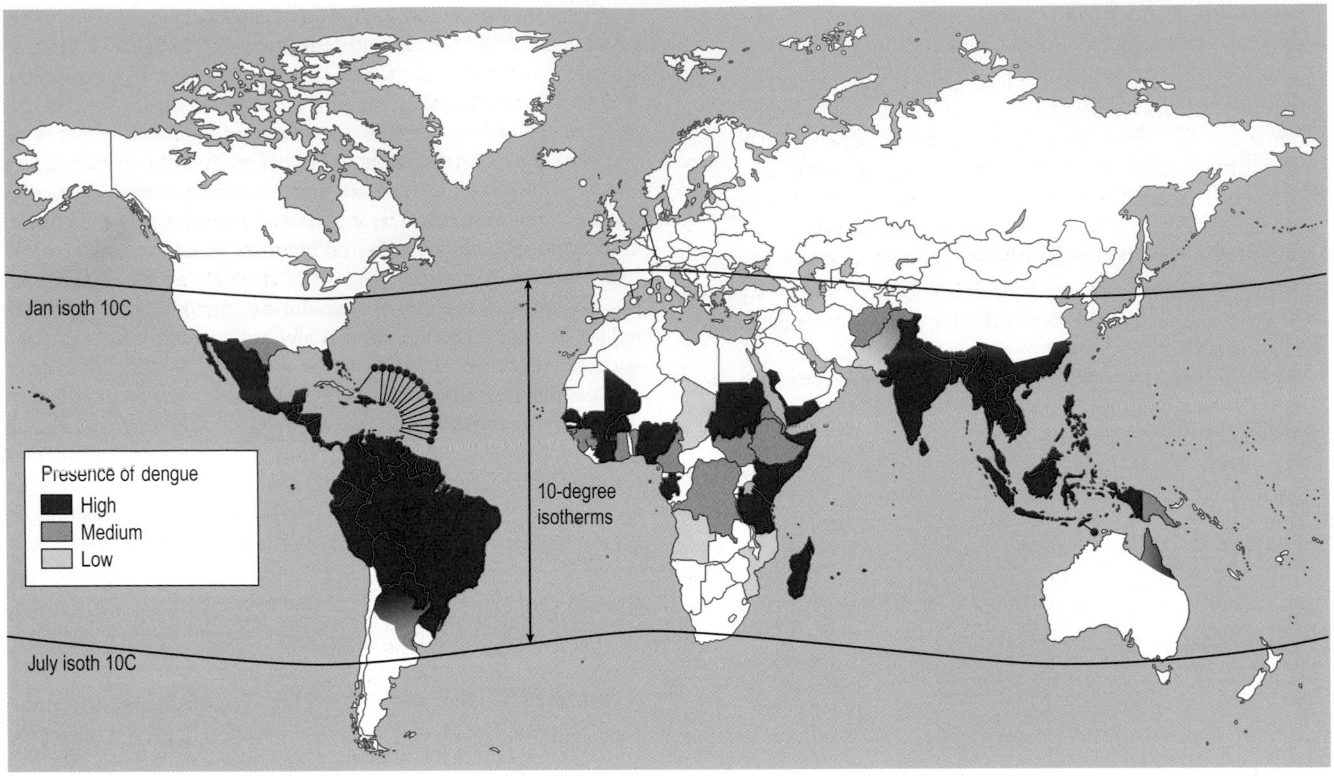

Figure 11.19 **Global dengue burden.**

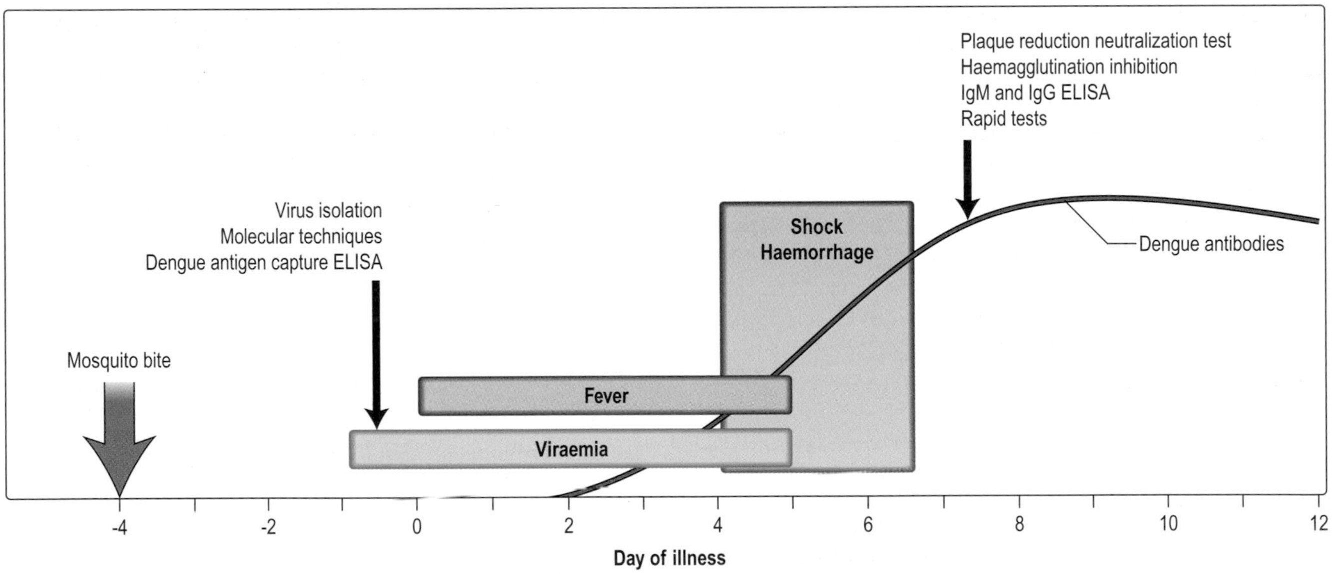

Figure 11.20 **Dengue infection – course and timing of diagnosis.** ELISA, enzyme-linked immunosorbent assay; Ig, immunoglobulin. *(From Halstead SB. Dengue.* Lancet *2007; 370:1644–1652, with permission.)*

- Detection of virus-specific IgM antibodies, or of rising IgG titres in sequential serum samples, haemagglutination inhibition, ELISA or complement-fixation assays confirm the diagnosis.
- Blood tests show leucopenia and thrombocytopenia.

Management is supportive with analgesics and adequate fluid replacement. Corticosteroids are of no benefit and convalescence can be slow. In DHF, blood transfusion may be necessary, as well as intensive care support.

Prevention

Travellers should be advised to sleep under impregnated nets but this is not very effective, as the mosquito bites in daytime. Topical insect repellents should be used. Adult mosquitoes should be destroyed by sprays and breeding sites, such as small pools of stagnant water, should be eradicated. There is no effective vaccine yet, although some are being trialled.

Zika virus infection

Zika virus, a flavivirus closely related to dengue viruses, has come to prominence in 2016 following an explosive pandemic throughout South and Central America, and the Caribbean. Like dengue, Zika is an arbovirus, transmitted to humans by Aedes mosquitoes. Illness, when it arises, is usually unremarkable, with fever, myalgia, eye pain, prostration and maculopapular rash, with spontaneous resolution. However, the epidemiological association of the emergence of Zika virus outbreaks with subsequent dramatic increases in the number of cases of microcephaly in infants (e.g. Brazil reported a 20-fold increase in incidence from 2014–2015) has led the WHO to declare Zika a public health emergency of international concern. The link between Zika infection in pregnancy and subsequent microcephaly is not yet proven beyond doubt, but the circumstantial evidence is suggestive, and there are recent reports of findings of Zika virus RNA in the brain tissue of an affected neonate. There are also data suggesting an increase in Guillain–Barré syndrome following Zika virus epidemics. Accurate diagnosis of infection is complicated by serological cross-reactivity with dengue viruses. Further research on the consequences of infection with Zika virus is urgently needed.

Chikungunya

Chikungunya virus is an alphavirus, a genus within the Togavirus family. Viruses spread by insects are collectively referred to as arthropod-borne viruses, or arboviruses (***Boxes 11.26*** and ***11.27***). There are eight alphaviruses that result in human disease. These are transmitted by mosquitoes, are globally distributed and tend to acquire their names from the location where they were first isolated (such as Ross River, Eastern, Venezuelan and Western equine encephalitis viruses) or from the local expression for a major symptom caused by the virus (such as chikungunya, meaning 'doubled up'). Infection is characterized by fever, headache, maculopapular skin rash, arthralgia, myalgia and sometimes encephalitis. After 1 year, at least 20% of patients still suffer recurrent joint pains. Mortality is around 0.1%, mostly in the elderly or very young.

Major epidemics of chikungunya, spread via *A. aegypti* or *A. albopictus*, have been reported in India, Sri Lanka and islands in the Indian Ocean (including Reunion, Mauritius and the Seychelles) in 2005 and 2006, with at least 1 million cases and several hundred deaths. The severity of these epidemics is possibly due to a viral strain with mutations resulting in a higher neurovirulence. Several European countries reported cases of chikungunya in returning travellers, including 133 cases in the UK in 2006. The virus may now populate the local *Aedes* mosquito via increased numbers of travellers, who may import virus into countries where it has not previously been described; for example, an outbreak in Italy in 2007 involved over 150 cases with one death, and two locally acquired confirmed cases were reported from the French mainland in 2010. In 2013, an outbreak in the Caribbean islands spread to contiguous Central and South American countries, and over 200 cases were reported in 2014 in the USA.

A chikungunya virus-like particle vaccine is in clinical trial.

Box 11.26 Arbovirus (arthropod-borne) infection

Defining features of arboviruses

- Arboviruses are zoonotic viruses, transmitted through the bites of insects, especially mosquitoes and ticks
- >385 viruses are classified as arboviruses
- Most are members of the Togavirus, Flavivirus and Bunyavirus families (see ***Box 11.27***)
- *Culex*, *Aedes* and *Anopheles* mosquitoes account for transmission of the majority of these viruses

Clinical features of arbovirus infection

- Most arbovirus diseases are generally mild; epidemics are frequent and when these occur, the mortality is high
- In general, the incubation period is short (<10 days). Common features include a biphasic illness, pyrexia, conjunctival suffusion, a rash, retro-orbital pain, myalgia and arthralgia. Lymphadenopathy is seen in dengue
- ***Haemorrhage*** (from increased vascular permeability, capillary fragility, consumptive coagulopathy) is a feature of some arbovirus infections (see ***Box 11.33***)
- ***Encephalitis*** resulting from cerebral invasion may be prominent in some arbovirus fevers.

Box 11.27 Some arboviruses

Family	Genus	Viruses	Transmission	Predominant clinical syndrome
Togaviridae	Alphaviruses	Eastern, Western, Venezuelan equine encephalitis viruses	All are mosquito-borne	E
		Chikungunya		F
		Ross River		F
Flaviviridae	Flaviviruses	St Louis encephalitis	Mosquito-borne	E
		Japanese encephalitis		E
		Murray valley encephalitis		E
		Yellow fever (see pp. 265–266)		Yellow fever
		Dengue (see pp. 255–256)		Dengue, H
		Zika virus		F
		West Nile		E
		Louping ill	Tick-borne	E
		Tick-borne encephalitis		E
		Kyasanur Forest		H
		Omsk haemorrhagic fever		H
Bunyaviridae	Orthobunyaviruses	La Crosse	Mosquito-borne	E
	Phleboviruses	Rift Valley fever	Mosquito-borne	F
	Nairoviruses	Congo–Crimean haemorrhagic fever	Tick-borne	H

E, encephalitis or aseptic meningitis; F, tropical fever, often with headache, myalgia, rash, arthralgia; H, haemorrhagic fever.

Infectious mononucleosis: Epstein–Barr virus infection

Globally, most individuals are infected with Epstein–Barr virus (EBV) at an early age (0–5 years), at which time clinical symptoms are unusual. Infection at an older age is associated with an acute febrile illness known as infectious mononucleosis (glandular fever), which occurs worldwide in adolescents and young adults. EBV is probably transmitted in saliva and by aerosol.

Clinical features

The predominant symptoms of infectious mononucleosis are fever, headache, malaise and sore throat. Palatal petechiae and a transient macular rash are common, the latter occurring in 90% of patients who have received ampicillin (inappropriately) for the sore throat. Cervical lymphadenopathy, particularly of the posterior cervical nodes, and splenomegaly are characteristic. Mild hepatitis is common, but other complications such as myocarditis, meningitis, encephalitis, cerebellar ataxia, mesenteric adenitis and splenic rupture are rare. Splenic rupture may occur in the first 3 weeks of illness and contact sport should be avoided during this period.

Although some young adults remain debilitated and depressed for some months after infection, the evidence for reactivation of latent virus in healthy individuals is controversial, although this is thought to occur in immunocompromised patients. The site of EBV latency is in resting memory B lymphocytes. Severe, often fatal, infectious mononucleosis may result from a rare X-linked lymphoproliferative syndrome affecting young boys. Those who survive have an increased risk of hypogammaglobulinaemia and/or lymphoma. EBV is the cause of oral hairy leucoplakia in AIDS patients and is intimately linked to the generation of a number of malignancies (see below). EBV is a cause of haemophagocytic lymphohistiocytosis (HLH), a rare condition presenting with fever, rash, jaundice, hepatosplenomegaly and enlarged lymph nodes. Blood tests show cytopenia and a high ferritin, and the bone marrow shows haemophagocytosis. HLH can be primary (inherited) or secondary (e.g. to EBV), and has a high mortality.

Diagnosis

EBV infection should be strongly suspected if atypical mononuclear cells (activated CD8-positive T lymphocytes) are found in the peripheral blood in large numbers. It can be confirmed during the second week of infection by a positive Paul–Bunnell reaction, which detects heterophile antibodies (IgM) that agglutinate sheep erythrocytes, in around 90% of cases. False-positives can occur in other conditions, such as viral hepatitis, Hodgkin's lymphoma and acute leukaemia. The Monospot test is a sensitive and easily performed screening test for heterophile antibodies. Specific EBV IgM antibodies indicate recent infection by the virus. Clinically similar illnesses are produced by cytomegalovirus, toxoplasmosis and acute HIV infection (the so-called seroconversion illness) but these can be distinguished serologically.

Management

The majority of cases require no specific treatment and recovery is rapid. Corticosteroid therapy is advised when there is neurological involvement (e.g. encephalitis, meningitis, Guillain–Barré syndrome), when there is marked thrombocytopenia or haemolysis, or when the tonsillar enlargement is so marked as to cause respiratory obstruction.

Cytomegalovirus infection

Clinically significant cytomegalovirus (CMV) infection arises particularly in two patient groups: fetuses who acquire the infection transplacentally and are born congenitally infected, and patients who are immunosuppressed, such as transplant recipients or people with HIV infection. As with all herpesviruses, the virus persists for life, usually as a latent infection but one that may become reactivated, especially in immunocompromised patients. Over 50% of the adult population has serological evidence of latent CMV infection.

Clinical features

In healthy children and adults, CMV infection is usually asymptomatic but may cause an illness similar to infectious mononucleosis, with fever, occasionally lymphocytosis with atypical lymphocytes, and hepatitis with or without jaundice. The Paul–Bunnell test for heterophile antibody is negative. Infection may be spread in saliva (accounting for extensive person-to-person spread in childcare units), sexual intercourse or blood transfusion, and transplacentally to the fetus. Disseminated fatal infection with widespread visceral involvement occurs in the immunocompromised (see p. 352) and may cause encephalitis, retinitis, pneumonitis and diffuse involvement of the gastrointestinal tract.

Intrauterine infection may arise from either primary or reactivated maternal infection. CMV is, by far, the most common congenital infection; in developed countries, such as the UK, 0.3–1% of all babies are born congenitally infected with CMV. Around 5–10% of such babies have severe disease evident at birth, with a poor prognosis. CNS involvement may cause microcephaly and motor disorders. Jaundice and hepatosplenomegaly are common and thrombocytopenia and haemolytic anaemia also occur. Periventricular calcification is seen on skull X-ray. A further 5–10% of infected babies are normal at birth but developmental abnormalities become apparent later: for example, sensorineural nerve deafness. The remaining 80–85% of infected babies are normal at birth and develop normally.

Diagnosis

Serological tests can identify latent (IgG) or primary (IgM) infection. However, most infections are now diagnosed by detection and quantification of CMV DNA or RNA using molecular amplification techniques, in blood or other body fluid samples. The virus can also be identified in tissues by the presence of characteristic intranuclear 'owl's eye' inclusions ***(Fig. 11.21)*** on histological staining and by direct immunofluorescence.

Management

In the immunocompetent, infection is usually self-limiting and no specific treatment is required. In the immunosuppressed, ganciclovir (5 mg/kg twice daily for 14–21 days) reduces retinitis and gastrointestinal damage, and can eliminate CMV from blood, urine and respiratory secretions. It is less effective against pneumonitis. In patients who are continually immunocompromised, maintenance therapy may be necessary. Drug resistance may arise during long-term therapy, such as in transplant recipients. Bone marrow toxicity is common. Valganciclovir, foscarnet and cidofovir are also available, and there are promising new drugs undergoing clinical trial including brincidofovir, maribavir and letermovir (see p. 244). Treatment of CMV in neonates is difficult, but therapy of infected babies with evident CNS involvement has been shown to improve

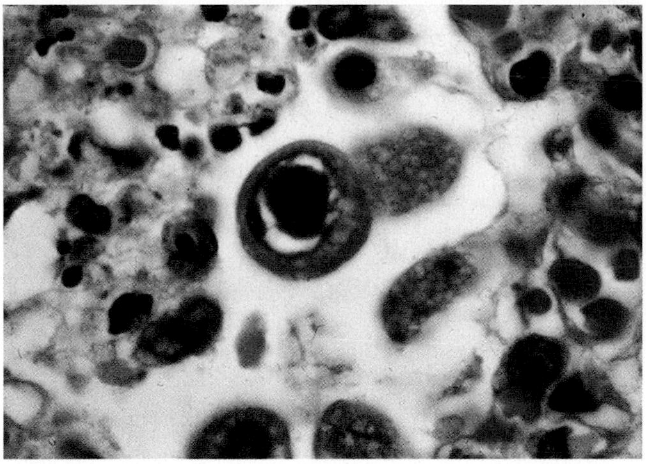

Figure 11.21 **Typical 'owl's eye' inclusion-bearing cell infected with cytomegalovirus.**

long-term hearing outcome, and 6 months of valganciclovir therapy is now recommended.

Mumps

Mumps is the result of infection with a paramyxovirus. It is spread by droplet infection, by direct contact or through fomites. Humans are the only known natural hosts. The peak period of infectivity is 2–3 days before the onset of the parotitis and for 3 days afterwards.

Clinical features

The incubation period averages 18 days. Although no age is exempt, it is primarily a disease of school-aged children and young adults; it is uncommon before the age of 2 years. The prodromal symptoms are non-specific and include fever, malaise, headache and anorexia. This is usually followed by severe pain over the parotid glands, with either unilateral or bilateral parotid swelling ***(Fig. 11.22)***. These enlarged glands obscure the angle of the mandible and may elevate the ear lobe, which does not occur in cervical lymph node enlargement. Trismus due to pain is common at this stage. Submandibular gland involvement occurs less frequently.

Complications

CNS involvement is the most common extrasalivary gland manifestation of mumps. Clinical meningitis occurs in 5% of all infected patients, and 30% of patients with CNS involvement have no evidence of parotid gland involvement.

Epididymo-orchitis develops in about one-third of patients who develop mumps after puberty. Bilateral testicular involvement results in sterility in only a small percentage of these patients. Pancreatitis, oophoritis, myocarditis, mastitis, hepatitis and polyarthritis may also occur.

Diagnosis and management

The diagnosis of mumps is on the basis of the clinical features. Viral RNA can be demonstrated by genome detection assays in saliva, throat swabs, urine and CSF. Serological demonstration of a mumps-specific IgM response in an acute blood or oral fluid sample is also diagnostic.

Treatment is supportive. Attention should be given to adequate nutrition and mouth care. Analgesics should be used to relieve pain.

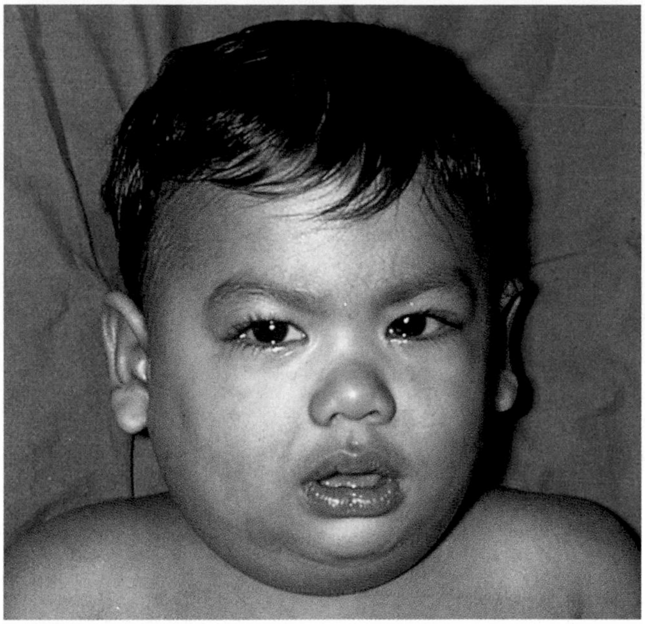

Figure 11.22 **Mumps: a child with a swollen face.** *(From Chaudhry B, Harvey DR.* Mosby's Color Atlas and Text of Paediatrics and Child Health. *Edinburgh: Mosby; 2001. ©Elsevier 2001.)*

Box 11.28 Human lymphotropic retroviruses

Sub-family	Virus	Disease
Lentivirus	HIV-1	AIDS
	HIV-2	AIDS
Oncovirus	HTLV-1	Adult T-cell leukaemia/lymphoma Tropical spastic paraparesis
	HTLV-2	Myelopathy

AIDS, acquired immunodeficiency syndrome; HIV, human immunodeficiency virus; HTLV, human T-cell lymphotropic virus.

Prevention

Children in the UK are immunized with the live attenuated MMR vaccine (see ***Box 11.19***) and the mumps vaccine is given in most developing countries. Vaccination is contraindicated in immunosuppressed individuals, during pregnancy, or in those with severe febrile illnesses.

HIV infections

The human immunodeficiency viruses (HIV) belong to the Retrovirus family ***(Box 11.28)***, and are characterized by their ability to replicate through a DNA intermediate using the enzyme reverse transcriptase.

HIV-1 and the related virus, HIV-2, are further classified as lentiviruses ('slow' viruses) because of their slowly progressive clinical effects.

HIV-1 and HIV-2 give rise to the acquired immunodeficiency syndrome (AIDS) and are discussed on page 333.

Human T cell lymphotropic virus type 1 (HTLV-1) causes adult T-cell leukaemia/lymphoma and tropical spastic paraparesis.

Myocarditis and skeletal muscle infection

Enterovirus infection is a cause of acute myocarditis and pericarditis, from which, in general, there is complete recovery. However, these viruses can also cause chronic congestive cardiomyopathy and, rarely, constrictive pericarditis. Skeletal muscle involvement, particularly of the intercostal muscles, is a feature of Bornholm disease, a febrile illness usually due to Coxsackievirus B. The pain may be of such an intensity as to mimic pleurisy or an acute abdomen. The infection affects both children and adults and may be complicated by meningitis or cardiac involvement. Myocarditis and pericarditis are also discussed on pages 1036-1037 and 1043.

Postviral/chronic fatigue syndrome

Many viral infections have been implicated aetiologically, including EBV, Coxsackie B viruses, echoviruses, CMV and hepatitis A virus. Non-viral causes, such as allergy to *Candida* spp., have also been proposed. Only a minority of patients have an identifiable precipitating infectious illness (see also p. 900).

Further reading

Fauci AS, Morens DM. Zika virus in the Americas – yet another Arbovirus threat. *New Engl J Med* 2016; 374:601–604.
Guzman MG, Harris E. Dengue. *Lancet* 2015; 385:453–465.
Hviid A, Rubin S, Muhlemann K. Mumps. *Lancet* 2008; 371:932–944.
Luzuriaga K, Sullivan JL. Infectious mononucleosis. *N Engl J Med* 2010; 362:1993–2000.
Massad E, Bezerra Coutinho FA. The cost of dengue control. *Lancet* 2011; 377:1630–1631.
Simmons CP, Farrar JJ, Chau NV et al. Current concepts: dengue. *New Engl J Med* 2012; 366:1423–1432.
Weaver SC, Lecuit M. Chikungunya virus and the global spread of a mosquito-borne disease. *N Engl J Med* 2015; 372:1231–1239.

VIRUS INFECTIONS OF THE NERVOUS SYSTEM

Poliovirus infection (poliomyelitis)

Poliomyelitis occurs when a susceptible individual is infected with poliovirus type 1, 2 or 3. These viruses have a propensity for the nervous system, especially the anterior horn cells of the spinal cord and cranial motor neurones. Spread is usually via the faeco-oral route, as the virus is excreted in the faeces.

Clinical features

The incubation period is 7–14 days. Although polio is essentially a disease of childhood, no age is exempt. The clinical manifestations vary considerably. The most common outcome (95% of individuals) is asymptomatic seroconversion.

- ***Abortive poliomyelitis*** occurs in approximately 4–5% of cases, characterized by the presence of fever, sore throat and myalgia. The illness is self-limiting and of short duration.
- ***Non-paralytic poliomyelitis*** (poliovirus meningitis) has features of abortive poliomyelitis, as well as signs of meningeal irritation, but recovery is complete.
- ***Paralytic poliomyelitis*** occurs in approximately 0.1% of infected children (1.3% of adults). Factors predisposing to the development of paralysis include male sex, exercise early in the illness, trauma, surgery or intramuscular injection, which localize the paralysis, and recent tonsillectomy (bulbar poliomyelitis).

The paralytic form of the disease follows about 4–5 days after an initial illness simulating abortive poliomyelitis. Meningeal irritation and muscle pain recur and are followed by the onset of asymmetric flaccid paralysis without sensory involvement.

Aspiration pneumonia, myocarditis, paralytic ileus and urinary calculi are late complications of poliomyelitis.

Diagnosis

The diagnosis is a clinical one. Distinction from Guillain–Barré syndrome is easily made by the absence of sensory involvement and the asymmetrical nature of the paralysis in poliomyelitis. Laboratory confirmation and distinction between the wild virus and vaccine strains is achieved by genome detection techniques, virus culture, neutralization and temperature marker tests.

Management

Management is supportive. Bed rest is essential during the early course of the illness. Respiratory support with intermittent positive-pressure respiration is required if the muscles of respiration are involved.

Prevention and control

In 1988, the World Health Assembly adopted the goal of eliminating poliomyelitis worldwide. Since then, the estimated 350 000 annual cases arising in 125 countries have been reduced by over 99%, with only Pakistan, Nigeria and Afghanistan never having terminated indigenous transmission. The eradication campaign has relied on improvements in sanitation, hygiene and the widespread use of polio vaccines. However, spread of infection via travel from endemic countries has led to the disease reappearing in a number of states, including China, Cameroon, Syria and Somalia, and in 2014, the WHO declared the spread of poliomyelitis to be a global public health emergency. The creation of a poliomyelitis-free world remains the goal, with a revised strategic plan to achieve this by 2018. Vaccination remains the bedrock of the campaign. New preparations of inactivated IM poliovirus vaccine (IPV) have greater potency than the original Salk IPV. The greater reliability of IPV in hot climates and the scientific and ethical problems of continuing to use oral polio vaccine (OPV) in countries free from poliomyelitis mean that IPV has replaced OPV in the routine immunization schedules in many countries.

Coxsackievirus, echovirus and other enterovirus infections

These viruses are also spread by the faeco-oral route. They each have a number of different types and are responsible for a broad spectrum of disease involving the skin and mucous membranes, muscles, nerves, heart ***(Box 11.29)*** and, rarely, other organs, such as the liver and pancreas. They are frequently associated with pyrexial illnesses and are the most common cause of aseptic meningitis.

Clinical features

- ***Neurological disease***. Other enteroviruses in addition to poliovirus can cause a broad range of neurological disease, including meningitis, encephalitis and a paralytic disease similar to poliomyelitis. EV71, more usually associated with hand, foot and mouth disease, has a particular predilection for neuroinvasion. Epidemics of EV71 are not infrequent; an estimated 6 million cases have occurred globally in the past 10 years, with over 2000 deaths from a variety of serious neuromotor syndromes. An inactivated EV71 vaccine has shown promising results in recent trials in China.
- ***Meningitis and encephalitis***. Many virus infections may result in either meningitis or an encephalitic illness ***(Box 11.30)***. The latter may arise by direct virus invasion of nervous tissue, or by induction of an aberrant cross-reactive immune response (post-infectious encephalitis). Encephalitis due to herpes simplex virus is described on page 865.

Box 11.29 Picornavirus infections (excluding poliovirus and rhinovirus)

Disease	Coxsackievirus		Echovirus	Enterovirus
	A (Types A1–A22, A24)	*B (Types B1–B6)*	*(Types 1–9, 11–17, 29–33)*	*(Types 68–71)*
Cutaneous and mucosal				
Herpangina	+++	+	+	
Hand, foot and mouth	+++	+	+	++
Erythematous rashes	+	+	+++	
Conjunctivitis	+			
Neurological				
Paralytic	+	±	+	
Meningitis	++	++	+++	+
Encephalitis	++	++	±	+
Cardiac				
Myocarditis and pericarditis	+	+++	+	
Muscular				
Myositis (Bornholm disease)	+	+++	+	

+++, often causes; ++, sometimes causes; +, rarely causes; ±, possibly causes.

Box 11.30 Viral causes of meningitis and encephalitis

Virus	Comments	Outcome
Meningitis		
Enteroviruses, esp. Coxsackie B and echoviruses		
Mumps virus		
Herpes simplex virus		
Encephalitis, direct invasion		
Herpes simplex viruses	Most common cause of sporadic encephalitis. Any age	High morbidity and mortality
Mumps virus	Spread from meninges resulting in meningoencephalitis	Most patients recover
Measles virus	Subacute sclerosing encephalitis	Rare, high mortality
Varicella zoster virus	May cause vasculitis	May arise with reactivation (shingles)
Cytomegalovirus	Only in immunocompromised	Poor prognosis
Enteroviruses	EV71; otherwise usually only in immunocompromised	
HIV	Dementia is main feature	
Japanese encephalitis virus	Flavivirus, mosquito-borne	
West Nile encephalitis virus	Flavivirus, mosquito-borne	Birds are primary host. Higher mortality in elderly
Tick-borne encephalitis viruses	Flaviviruses, tick-borne	
Lymphocytic choriomeningitis virus	Arenavirus	House mouse is primary host
Hendra, Nipah viruses	Paramyxoviruses	Zoonotic infections from horses, pigs
Rabies virus	Acquired from animal or bat bite	Almost always fatal
JC virus	Only in immunocompromised	Results in progressive multifocal leucoencephalopathy
Eastern, Venezuelan encephalitis viruses	Alphaviruses, mosquito-borne	Geographically restricted to the Americas
Encephalitis, post-infectious		
May arise from a number of different virus infections including measles (1 in 1000–5000 cases of measles), influenza, varicella zoster		

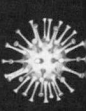

Japanese encephalitis

Japanese encephalitis is a mosquito-borne encephalitis caused by a flavivirus. It has been reported most frequently from the rice-growing countries of South-east Asia and the Far East. *Culex tritaeniorhynchus* is the usual vector and this feeds mainly on pigs, as well as birds such as herons and sparrows. Humans are accidental hosts.

The incubation period is 5–15 days. Most infections are asymptomatic. When disease arises, the onset is heralded by severe rigors. Fever, headache and malaise last 1–6 days. Weight loss is prominent. In the acute encephalitic stage, the fever is high (38–41°C), neck rigidity occurs and neurological signs, such as altered consciousness, hemiparesis and convulsions, develop. Mental deterioration occurs over a period of 3–4 days and culminates in coma. Mortality varies from 7% to 40% and is higher in children. Residual neurological defects, such as deafness, emotional lability and hemiparesis, occur in about 70% of patients who have had CNS involvement. Convalescence is prolonged. Antibody detection in serum and CSF by IgM capture ELISA is a useful rapid diagnostic test. Vaccines containing formalin-inactivated viruses derived from mouse brain are effective and available. Management is supportive.

West Nile encephalitis

In 1999, West Nile virus was first recognized in the Western hemisphere (New York, USA) having been previously reported in Africa, Asia and parts of Europe. By the end of 2009, the US outbreak had resulted in over 25 000 human cases and over 1100 deaths. The vast majority of infections are asymptomatic. In a minority of cases, infection presents as a febrile illness with a maculopapular rash, 1% resulting in severe encephalitis. Disease severity and mortality are age-related, being greatest in the elderly. The primary hosts of infection are birds. It is spread by mosquitoes and may also infect humans and horses. It can also be transmitted by blood transfusions, breast-feeding and organ donation from an infected individual. Diagnosis is by genome detection in appropriate samples, or specialized serology for the detection of IgM virus-specific antibodies.

Tick-borne encephalitis

This arises from infection with a flavivirus (actually a series of closely related viruses) transmitted by *Ixodes* spp. ticks. It occurs in an area extending from Western Europe to Japan. The tick is the main reservoir for the virus, which is transmitted when it feeds on mice and other rodents.

The disease starts 4–28 days after a bite from an infected tick and is biphasic in 80% of patients. Fever, malaise, headache and fatigue are followed, after a symptom-free period of about 7 days, by encephalitis. There may be associated limb paralysis, which is due to anterior horn cell involvement mainly of the cervical region. Cranial nerve involvement also occurs. Tick-borne encephalitis virus (TBEV) IgM and IgG antibodies are present and the virus can be detected in blood by reverse transcription polymerase chain reaction (RT-PCR). Overall mortality is about 1% (but can be considerably higher for certain strains); 30% have impairment in neurological function with persistent paralysis in 6%. A preventative vaccine is available.

Lymphocytic choriomeningitis

This infection is a zoonosis, the natural reservoir of lymphocytic choriomeningitis (LCM) virus (an arenavirus; see **Box 11.22**) being the house mouse. Infection is by inhalation from urine-contaminated rubbish and is characterized by:

- non-nervous-system illness, with fever, malaise, myalgia, headache, arthralgia and vomiting
- ***meningitis*** in addition to the above symptoms.

Occasionally, a more severe form occurs, with encephalitis leading to disturbance of consciousness.

This illness is generally self-limiting and requires no specific treatment.

Hendra and Nipah virus infection

Hendra virus and Nipah virus are zoonotic viruses that have caused disease in humans who have been in contact with infected animals (horses and pigs, respectively). The viruses are named after the locations where they were first isolated – Hendra in Australia and Nipah in Malaysia – and both are classified as paramyxoviruses. Hendra virus has caused severe respiratory distress in horses and humans, and Nipah virus caused a major outbreak of viral encephalitis (265 cases and 105 deaths) in Malaysia between September 1998 and April 1999. Management of these conditions is largely supportive, although there is some evidence that early treatment with ribavirin may reduce their severity.

Rabies

Rabies is a major problem in some countries, with an estimated 55 000 deaths per year worldwide. Established infection is almost invariably fatal; there are only a handful of recorded cases of survival from clinical rabies. It is caused by the rabies virus, a single-stranded RNA virus of the Lyssavirus genus. The virus is bullet-shaped and has spike-like structures arising from its surface containing glycoproteins that cause the host to produce neutralizing, haemagglutination-inhibiting antibodies. The virus has a marked affinity for nervous tissue and the salivary glands. It exists in two major epidemiological settings:

- ***Urban rabies*** is most frequently transmitted to humans through rabid dogs and, less frequently, cats.
- ***Sylvan (wild) rabies*** is maintained in the wild by a host of animal reservoirs such as foxes, skunks, jackals, mongooses and bats.

With the exception of Australia, New Zealand and the Antarctic, human rabies has been reported from all continents. Transmission is usually through the bite of an infected animal. However, the percentage of rabid bites leading to clinical disease ranges from 10% (on the legs) to 80% (on the head). Other forms of transmission, if they occur, are rare.

Virus replicates in the muscle cells near the entry wound. It penetrates the nerve endings and travels in the axoplasm to the spinal cord and brain. In the CNS, the virus again proliferates before spreading to the salivary glands, lungs, kidneys and other organs via the autonomic nerves.

Clinical features

The incubation period is variable, ranging from a few weeks to several years; on average, it is 1–3 months. In general, bites on the head, face and neck have a shorter incubation period than those elsewhere. In humans, two distinct clinical varieties of rabies are recognized:

- ***Furious rabies*** – the classic variety. The only characteristic feature in the prodromal period is the presence of pain and tingling at the site of the initial wound. Fever, malaise and headache are also present. About 10 days later, marked anxiety and agitation or depressive features develop. Hallucinations, bizarre behaviour and paralysis may also occur. Hyperexcitability, the hallmark of this form of rabies, is precipitated by auditory or visual stimuli. Hydrophobia (fear of water) is present in 50% of patients and is due to severe pharyngeal spasms on attempting to eat or drink. Aerophobia (fear of air) is considered pathognomonic of rabies. Examination reveals hyper-reflexia, spasticity and evidence of sympathetic overactivity indicated by pupillary dilatation and diaphoresis. The patient goes on to develop convulsions, respiratory paralysis and cardiac arrhythmias. Death usually occurs in 10–14 days.

- ***Dumb rabies*** – the paralytic variety. Dumb rabies, or paralytic rabies, presents with a symmetrical ascending paralysis resembling the Guillain–Barré syndrome. This variety of rabies commonly occurs after bites from rabid bats.

Diagnosis

The diagnosis of rabies is generally made clinically. Skin-punch biopsies are used to detect antigen with an immunofluorescent antibody test on frozen section. Viral RNA can be isolated using RT-PCR. Isolation of viruses from saliva or the presence of antibodies in blood or CSF may establish the diagnosis. The corneal smear test is not recommended, as it is unreliable. The classic Negri bodies are detected at postmortem in 90% of all patients with rabies; these are eosinophilic, cytoplasmic, ovoid bodies, 2–10 nm in diameter, seen in greatest numbers in the neurones of the hippocampus and the cerebellum. The diagnosis should be made pathologically on the biting animal using RT-PCR, immunofluorescence assay (IFA) or tissue culture of the brain.

Management

Once the CNS disease is established, therapy is symptomatic, as death is virtually inevitable. The patient should be nursed in a quiet, darkened room. Nutritional, respiratory and cardiovascular support may be necessary.

Drugs such as morphine, diazepam and chlorpromazine should be used liberally in patients who are excitable.

Prevention and control

Pre-exposure prophylaxis

This is given to individuals with a high risk of contracting rabies, such as laboratory workers, animal handlers and veterinarians. Three doses of human diploid (HDCV) or chick embryo cell vaccine, given by deep subcutaneous or intramuscular injection on days 0, 7 and 28, provide effective immunity. A reinforcing dose is given after 12 months and additional reinforcing doses are given every 3–5 years, depending on the risk of exposure. Vaccines of nervous tissue origin are still used in some parts of the world. These, however, are associated with significant side-effects and should not be used if HDCV is available.

Post-exposure prophylaxis

The wound should be cleaned carefully and thoroughly with soap and water, and left open. Human rabies immunoglobulin should be given immediately (20 IU/kg); half should be injected around the area of the wound and the other half should be given intramuscularly. Five 1.0-mL doses of HDCV should be given intramuscularly: the first dose is given on day 0 and is followed by injections on days 3, 7, 14 and 28. Reaction to the vaccine is uncommon.

Control

Domestic animals should be vaccinated if there is any risk of rabies in the country. In the UK, control has been by quarantine of imported animals for 6 months and no indigenous case of rabies has been reported for many years. The Pet Travel Scheme (PETS) enables certain pet animals to enter or re-enter Great Britain without quarantine if they come from qualifying countries via designated routes, are carried by authorized transport companies and meet the conditions of the scheme. Wild animals in 'at-risk' countries must be handled with great care.

Progressive multifocal leucoencephalopathy

JC virus, a polyomavirus, is the cause of progressive multifocal leucoencephalopathy (PML), which presents as dementia in the immunocompromised and is due to progressive cerebral destruction resulting from accumulation of the virus in brain tissue. The virus is acquired usually in childhood, and may reactivate if the host immune system becomes compromised in later life. Reactivation of JC virus and development of PML have recently been described in multiple sclerosis patients treated with the monoclonal antibody, natalizumab, directed against the cell adhesion molecule, $\alpha 4$ integrin.

Further reading

Lindquist L, Vapalahti O. Tick-borne encephalitis. *Lancet* 2008; 371:1861–1871.

Mundel T, Orenstein WA. No country is safe without global eradication of poliomyelitis. *New Engl J Med* 2013; 369:2045–2046.

Petersen LR, Fischer M. Unpredictable and difficult to control – the adolescence of West Nile virus. *New Engl J Med* 2012; 367:1281–1284.

VIRUS INFECTIONS OF THE GASTROINTESTINAL TRACT

Virus infections that commonly result in acute gastroenteritis (diarrhoea and vomiting) are listed in ***Box 11.31***.

Rotavirus infection

Rotaviruses are a major cause of infantile gastroenteritis worldwide. The virus (Latin *rota* = wheel) is so named because of its electron microscopic appearance with a characteristic circular outline and radiating spokes ***(Fig. 11.23)***. It belongs to the reovirus family, which have double-stranded RNA segmented genomes. More than

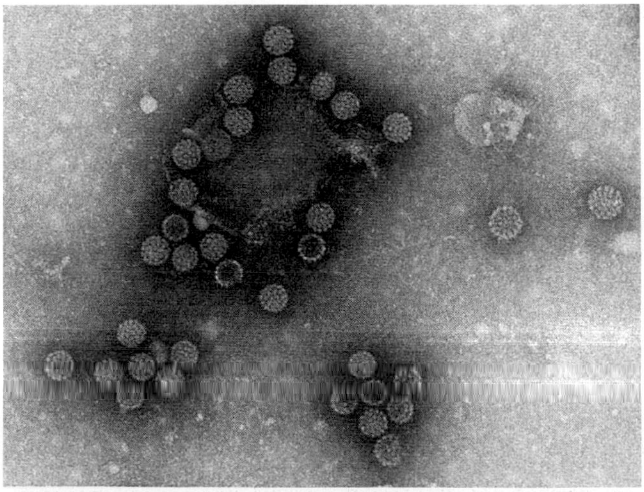

Figure 11.23 Electron micrograph of human rotavirus.

500 000 infected children under the age of 5 years are estimated to die annually in resource-deprived countries, compared with 75–150 in the USA. The prevalence is higher during the winter months in non-tropical areas. Asymptomatic infections are common and bottle-fed babies are more likely to be symptomatic than those that are breast-fed.

Adults may become infected with rotavirus but symptoms are usually mild or absent. The virus may, however, cause diarrhoea in immunosuppressed adults, or outbreaks in patients on care of the elderly wards.

Clinical features

The illness is characterized by vomiting, fever, diarrhoea and the metabolic consequences of water and electrolyte loss.

Diagnosis and differential diagnosis

The diagnosis can be established by PCR for genome detection, or ELISA for the detection of rotavirus antigen in faeces and by electron microscopy of faeces. Histology of the jejunal mucosa in children shows shortening of the villi, with crypt hyperplasia and mononuclear cell infiltration of the lamina propria.

Management and prevention

Management is directed at overcoming the effects of water and electrolyte imbalance with adequate oral rehydration therapy and, when indicated, intravenous fluids ***(Box 11.32)***. Antibiotics should not be prescribed. A controlled trial in Egypt in children with rotavirus diarrhoea demonstrated faster recovery (31 h versus 75 h) in those given nitazoxanide, a broad-spectrum anti-infective agent, for 3 days compared with placebo.

Box 11.31 Viruses associated with gastroenteritis

- Rotaviruses (groups A, B and C)
- Enteric adenoviruses (types 40 and 41)
- Caliciviruses (includes noroviruses and sapoviruses)
- Astroviruses

Rotavirus vaccines

Despite a major setback when the first licensed rotavirus vaccine was rapidly withdrawn from the market in 1999 following reports of increased rates of intussusception, two new vaccines have been developed and are now used in many countries. Both are live vaccines. One (Rotarix) contains an attenuated human strain, the relevant antigens being P[8] and G1; the other (Rotateq) is based on a bovine parent strain and comprises five single-gene reassortants, each containing a human-strain outer capsid gene encoding the most common human antigenic types (P[8] and G1–4). Routine rotavirus vaccination was introduced in the UK in 2012, following which the first full year's data demonstrated a 71% drop in laboratory-confirmed cases.

Calicivirus infection

The caliciviruses are an extensive virus family, named after the cup-shaped (Latin *calyx* = cup) indentations on their viral surface seen by electron microscopy. The family contains four genera, two of which, the noroviruses and sapoviruses, infect humans and cause gastroenteritis.

Norovirus is the major cause of acute non-bacterial gastroenteritis, causing outbreaks in nursing homes, hospitals, schools, leisure centres, restaurants and cruise ships. In countries that have adopted routine rotavirus vaccination of infants, norovirus has become the leading cause of clinically significant acute gastroenteritis in children. Transmission is mostly faeco-oral with outbreaks suggesting a common source, such as food and water, and fomites. Aerosol transmission also occurs and noroviruses can be detected in vomit. Illness is usually self-limiting (12–48 h) and mild, consisting of nausea, headache and abdominal cramps, followed by diarrhoea and vomiting, which may be the only feature (winter vomiting). Diagnosis is by demonstration of viral nucleic acid or antigen in diarrhoeal faeces. Treatment is with oral rehydration solutions. Prevention can be difficult but hand-washing and good hygienic food preparation are required.

Sapovirus causes gastroenteritis, mainly in children.

Further reading

Desselberger U, Gray J. Viral gastroenteritis. *Medicine* 2013; 41:700–703.
Iturriza-Gomara M, Cunliffe N. Welcoming rotavirus vaccine to the UK immunization schedule. *BMJ* 2013; 346:7.

Box 11.32 Oral rehydration solutions (ORS) and intravenous solutions used in moderate and severe diarrhoea

Solution	Salts (mmol/L)				Substance added (per L of water)	
	Na^+	K^+	Cl^-	Glucose	Substance	Quantity
Oral						
World Health Organization Hypo-osmolar formulation	75	20	65	75	NaCl Na citrate KCl Glucose	2.6 g 2.9 g 1.5 g 13.5 g
Cereal-based	85	–	80	–	Cooked rice Salt (NaCl)	80 g 5 g
Household	85	–	80	111	Glucose Salt (NaCl)	20 g 5 g
UK/Europe	35–60	20	37	90–200	Pre-prepared solutions	
Intravenous						
Ringer's lactate[a]	131	5	111	0	Pre-prepared	

[a]Contains Ca^{2+} 2 mmol and HCO_3^- (as lactate).

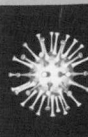

Parashar UD, Nelson EAS, Kang G. Diagnosis, management and prevention of rotavirus gastroenteritis in children. *BMJ* 2014; 348:29–34.

VIRAL HEPATITIS

A number of distinct virus infections may result in inflammation of the liver (hepatitis). The viruses belong to different virus families, are spread by different routes, and may have differing clinical consequences (see ***Box 14.5***). Viral hepatitis is discussed further on pages 452-461.

VIRUSES AND MALIGNANT DISEASE

Around 15–20% of all human malignant disease arises from infection. Recognition of the infectious cause of a particular cancer raises the possibility of developing an anti-cancer vaccine, as has now happened for both hepatitis B virus and human papillomavirus.

Hepatitis viruses and primary hepatocellular carcinoma

Globally, hepatocellular carcinoma is amongst the most common causes of death due to malignant disease. A high percentage arises in patients infected with either hepatitis B or C viruses. These are discussed in more detail on page 485.

Human papillomaviruses and cancer of the uterine cervix

Papillomaviruses tend to produce chronic infections (see also p. 318). Human papillomaviruses (HPVs), of which there are at least 100 types, are responsible for the common skin and genital warts, and certain types (mainly 16 and 18) are the cause of carcinoma of the cervix and some oral cancers (type 16). Vaccines against HPV types 16 and 18 are available. The current recommendations in many countries are for vaccination of all girls at age 9–14 years. It may also be sensible to vaccinate boys but this strategy is much less cost-effective. (For ***genital warts***, see p. 326.)

Epstein–Barr virus and malignant disease

EBV infection has been associated with a number of malignant diseases, including Burkitt's lymphoma, undifferentiated nasopharyngeal carcinoma, post-transplant lymphoma, the immunoblastic lymphoma of AIDS patients, some forms of Hodgkin's lymphoma and gastric cancer. Different levels of expression of EBV latency genes occur in these proliferative conditions caused by the virus, and various co-factors are also involved in their pathogenesis; for example, in Burkitt's lymphoma, the most common tumour of childhood in sub-Saharan Africa, epidemiological evidence points to an interplay between EBV infection and the presence of hyperendemic (i.e. present all year round) malaria.

Kaposi's sarcoma and human herpesvirus type 8

HHV-8 is strongly associated with the aetiology of all forms of Kaposi's sarcoma. Antibody prevalence is high in those with tumours but relatively low in the general population of most industrialized countries. High rates of infection (>50% population) have been described in Central and Southern Africa, and this matches the geographical distribution of classical Kaposi's sarcoma before the era of AIDS. HHV-8 is transmitted sexually and through exposure to blood from needle sharing. It is thought that salivary transmission may be the predominant route in Africa. HHV-8 RNA transcripts have been detected in Kaposi's sarcoma cells and in circulating mononuclear cells from patients with the tumour. This virus also has an aetiological role in two rare lymphoproliferative diseases: multicentric ***Castleman's disease*** (a disorder of the plasma cell type) and ***primary effusion lymphoma*** (body-cavity-based lymphoma), which is characterized by pleural, pericardial or peritoneal lymphomatous effusions in the absence of a solid tumour mass.

Other rare malignancies due to virus infection

HTLV-1, a lentivirus belonging to the same virus family as HIV, is the aetiological agent of adult T-cell leukaemia/lymphoma. Merkel cell polyomavirus has been identified in the malignant tissue of the rare Merkel cell carcinoma of the skin.

Further reading

Barton S, O'Mahony C. HPV vaccination – reaping the rewards of the appliance of science. *BMJ* 2013; 346:f2184.

VIRAL HAEMORRHAGIC FEVERS

These comprise infection with a range of different viruses ***(Box 11.33)***, which have in common the clinical feature of haemorrhagic manifestations.

Yellow fever

Yellow fever, caused by a flavivirus, is an illness of widely varying severity. It is confined to Africa (90% of cases) and South America between latitudes 15°N and 15°S. For poorly understood reasons, yellow fever has not been reported from Asia, despite the fact that climatic conditions are suitable and the vector, *Aedes aegypti*, is common. The infection is transmitted in the wild by *A. africanus* in Africa and the *Haemagogus* species in South and Central America. Extension of infection to humans (via the mosquito from monkeys) leads to the occurrence of 'jungle' yellow fever. *A. aegypti*, a domestic mosquito that lives in close relationship to humans, is responsible for human-to-human transmission in urban areas (urban yellow fever). Once infected, a mosquito remains so for life.

Clinical features

The incubation period is 3–6 days. Mild infection is indistinguishable from other viral fevers such as influenza or dengue.

Box 11.33 Viral infections associated with haemorrhagic manifestations[a]

Flavivirus
- Yellow fever (urban and sylvan)
- Dengue haemorrhagic fever
- Kyasanur Forest disease
- Omsk haemorrhagic fever

Bunyavirus
- Rift Valley fever
- Congo Crimean haemorrhagic fever
- Hantavirus infections

Arenavirus
- Argentinian haemorrhagic fever
- Bolivian haemorrhagic fever
- Lassa fever
- Epidemic haemorrhagic fever

Filovirus
- Marburg
- Ebola

[a]*Most of these are arboviruses. Some (e.g. Hantavirus, Lassa fever) have a rodent vector. The source and transmission route of filoviruses are not known.*

Three phases in the severe (classical) illness are recognized. Initially, the patient presents with a high fever of acute onset, usually 39–40°C, which then returns to normal in 4–5 days. During this time, headache is prominent. Retrobulbar pain, myalgia, arthralgia, a flushed face and suffused conjunctivae are common. Epigastric discomfort and vomiting are present when the illness is severe. Relative bradycardia (Faget's sign) is present from the second day of illness. The patient then makes an apparent recovery and feels well for several days. Following this 'phase of calm', the patient again develops increasing fever, deepening jaundice and hepatomegaly. Ecchymosis, bleeding from the gums, haematemesis and melaena may occur. Coma, which is usually a result of uraemia or haemorrhagic shock, occurs for a few hours preceding death. The mortality rate is up to 40% in severe cases. The pathology of the liver shows mid-zone necrosis and eosinophilic degeneration of hepatocytes (Councilman bodies; see pp. 451–452).

Diagnosis and management

The diagnosis is established by a history of travel and vaccination status and by isolation of the virus (when possible) from blood during the first 3 days of illness. Serodiagnosis is possible, but in endemic areas cross-reactivity with other flaviviruses is a problem.

Management is supportive. Bed rest (under mosquito nets), analgesics and maintenance of fluid and electrolyte balance are required.

Prevention and control

Yellow fever is an internationally notifiable disease. It is easily prevented by using the attenuated 17D chick embryo vaccine but concerns over safety have arisen because of infection with the 17D virus. Vaccination is not recommended for children under 9 months or immunosuppressed patients, unless there are compelling reasons. For the purposes of international certification, immunization is valid for 10 years, but protection lasts much longer than this and probably for life. The WHO Expanded Programme of Immunization includes yellow fever vaccination in endemic areas.

Congo–Crimean haemorrhagic fever

Congo–Crimean haemorrhagic fever (CCHF) virus belongs to the *Nairovirus* genus of the family Bunyaviridae. This family contains more than 200 viruses, grouped into a number of genera, most of which are arthropod-borne.

The disease CCHF is found mainly in Asia and Africa. The primary hosts are cattle and hares, and the vectors are the *Hyalomma* ticks. Following an incubation period of 3–6 days, there is an influenza-like illness with fever and haemorrhagic manifestations. The mortality is 10–50%.

Hantavirus infection

Hantaviruses belong to the Hantavirus genus of Bunyaviridae and are enzootic viruses of wild rodents, which are spread by aerosolized excreta and not by insect vectors. The most severe form of this infection is Korean haemorrhagic fever (also known as haemorrhagic fever with renal syndrome, HFRS). This condition has a mortality of 5–10% and is characterized by fever, shock and haemorrhage followed by an oliguric phase. Milder forms of the disease are associated with related viruses (e.g. Puumala virus) and may present as nephropathia epidemica, an acute fever with renal involvement, seen in Scandinavia and in other European countries in people who have been in contact with bank voles. In the USA, a hantavirus (transmitted by the deer mouse) termed Sin Nombre was identified as the cause of outbreaks of acute respiratory disease (hantavirus pulmonary syndrome, HPS) in adults. Other hantavirus types and rodent vector systems have been associated with this syndrome.

Diagnosis of hantavirus infection is made by an ELISA technique for specific antibodies.

Rift Valley fever

Rift Valley fever, caused by a virus from the Phlebovirus genus of the Bunyaviridae, is primarily an acute febrile illness of livestock: sheep, goats and camels. It is found in southern and eastern Africa. The vector in East Africa is *Culex pipiens* and in southern Africa, *Aedes caballus*, but disease can be transmitted by the bite of an infected animal. Following an incubation period of 3–6 days, the patient has an acute febrile illness that is difficult to distinguish clinically from other viral fevers. The temperature pattern is usually biphasic. The initial febrile illness lasts 2–4 days and is followed by a remission and a second febrile episode. Complications are indicative of severe infection and include retinopathy, meningoencephalitis, haemorrhagic manifestations and hepatic necrosis. Mortality approaches 50% in severe forms of the illness. Management is supportive. Animals can be vaccinated.

Lassa fever

Lassa fever virus belongs to the Arenavirus family. Arenaviruses are pleomorphic, round or oval viruses with diameters ranging from 50 to 300 nm. The virion surface has club-shaped projections and the virus itself contains a variable number of characteristic electron-dense granules that represent residual, non-functional host ribosomes. The illness called Lassa fever was first documented in the town of Lassa, Nigeria, in 1969 and is confined to sub-Saharan West Africa (Nigeria, Liberia and Sierra Leone). The multimammate rat, *Mastomys natalensis*, is known to be the reservoir. Humans are infected by ingesting foods contaminated by rat urine or saliva containing the virus. Person-to-person spread by body fluids also occurs. Only 10–30% of infections are symptomatic. Related arenaviruses are the causative agents of Argentinian and Bolivian haemorrhagic fevers.

Clinical features

The incubation period is 7–18 days. The disease is insidious in onset and is characterized by fever, myalgia, severe backache, malaise and headache. A transient maculopapular rash may be present. A sore throat, pharyngitis and lymphadenopathy occur in over 50% of patients. In severe cases, epistaxis and gastrointestinal bleeding may occur, hence the classification of Lassa fever as a viral haemorrhagic fever. The fever usually lasts 1–3 weeks, and recovery within 1 month of the onset of illness is usual. However, death occurs in 15–20% of hospitalized patients, usually from irreversible hypovolaemic shock.

Diagnosis

The diagnosis is established by serial serological tests (including the Lassa virus-specific IgM titre) or by genome detection by means of RT-PCR in throat swab, serum or urine.

Management

Management is supportive. In addition, clinical benefit and reduction in mortality can be achieved with ribavirin therapy, if given in the first week.

In non-endemic countries, strict isolation procedures should be used, the patient ideally being nursed in a flexible-film isolator. Specialized units for the management of Lassa fever and other haemorrhagic fevers have been established in the UK. As Lassa fever virus and other causes of haemorrhagic fever (Marburg/Ebola and Congo–Crimean haemorrhagic fever viruses; ***Box 11.33***) have been transmitted from patients to staff in healthcare situations, great care should be taken in handling specimens and clinical material from these patients.

Marburg virus disease and Ebola virus disease

These severe haemorrhagic, febrile illnesses are discussed together because their clinical manifestations are similar, and the causative negative-strand RNA viruses belong to the same virus family, the Filoviridae, so called because the viruses have a filamentous appearance on electron microscopy. The diseases are named after Marburg in Germany and the Ebola river region in the Sudan and Zaire, where these viruses first appeared. The natural reservoir for these viruses has not been identified and the precise mode of spread from one individual to another has not been elucidated. Five distinct species of Ebola virus have been identified, which vary in terms of case fatality rates: less than 40% for Bundibugyo, 50% for Sudan, and 70–90% for Zaire Ebola viruses. There has only been one (non-fatal) case of Tai Forest Ebola virus infection. Reston Ebola virus, the only Asian species, has not been associated with human mortality.

Epidemics have occurred periodically in recent years, mainly in sub-Saharan Africa. Ebola viruses are zoonotic pathogens, with fruit bats thought to be the natural host. The illness is characterized by the acute onset of severe headache, myalgia, vomiting and high fever, followed by prostration. On about the fifth day of illness, a non-pruritic maculopapular rash develops on the face and then spreads to the rest of the body. Diarrhoea is profuse and is associated with abdominal cramps and vomiting. Haematemesis, melaena or haemoptysis may occur between the seventh and sixteenth days. Hepatosplenomegaly and facial oedema are usually present. In Ebola virus disease, chest pain and a dry cough are prominent symptoms.

In August 2014, the WHO declared the ongoing outbreak of Zaire Ebola virus infection in West Africa a public health emergency of international concern, with an estimated several thousand deaths. Guinea, Sierra Leone and Liberia were the worst affected countries. Treatment is symptomatic, although a number of experimental therapies, mostly focused on monoclonal antibodies, are being tried. Experimental vaccines are also being developed. In the absence of effective therapy, accurate diagnosis and infection control precautions are the only intervention strategies. Lack of infrastructure to support rapid molecular diagnostic techniques, and to allow institution of the meticulous patient isolation necessary to interrupt human-to-human transmission of infection, has contributed to generating the largest outbreak yet recorded. Asymptomatic people may be infected but have a low viral count, making transmission unlikely.

Further reading

Drazen JM. Ebola in West Africa at one year – from ignorance to fear to roadblocks. *New Engl J Med* 2015; 372:563–564.
Frieden TR, Damjon I, Bell BP et al. Ebola 2014 – new challenges, new global response and responsibility. *New Engl J Med* 2014; 371:1177–1180.

TRANSMISSIBLE SPONGIFORM ENCEPHALOPATHIES (PRION DISEASES)

Transmissible spongiform encephalopathies (TSEs) are caused by the accumulation in the nervous system of a protein, termed a 'prion', which is an abnormal isoform (PrP^{Sc}) of a normal host protein (PrP^{c}).

Although familial forms of prion disease are known to exist, these conditions can be transmissible, particularly if brain tissue enters another host. There is no convincing evidence for the presence of nucleic acid in association with prions; thus these agents cannot be considered orthodox viruses and it is the abnormal prion protein itself that is infectious and can trigger a conversion of the normal protein into the atypical isoform. After infection, a long incubation period is followed by CNS degeneration associated with dementia or ataxia, which invariably leads to death. Histology of the brain reveals spongiform change with an accumulation of the abnormal prion protein in the form of amyloid plaques.

The human prion diseases are Creutzfeldt–Jakob disease, including the sporadic, familial, iatrogenic and variant forms of the disease, Gerstmann–Straussler–Scheinker syndrome, fatal familial insomnia and kuru.

- ***Creutzfeldt–Jakob disease*** (***CJD***). CJD usually occurs sporadically worldwide with an annual incidence of 1 per million of the population. Although, in most cases, the epidemiology remains obscure, iatrogenic transmission to others has occurred as a result of administration of human cadaveric growth hormone or gonadotrophin, from dura mater and corneal grafting and in neurosurgery from reuse of contaminated instruments and electrodes (iatrogenic CJD).
- ***Variant CJD*** (***vCJD***). In the UK, knowledge that large numbers of cattle with the prion disease, bovine spongiform encephalopathy (BSE), had gone into the human food chain, led to enhanced surveillance for emergence of the disease in humans. Based on transmission studies in mice and on glycosylation patterns of prion proteins, the evidence is convincing that this has occurred and, to date, there have been approximately 170 confirmed and suspected cases of vCJD (human BSE) in the UK and 40 in the rest of the world. In contrast to sporadic CJD, which presents with dementia at a mean age of onset of 60 years, vCJD presents with ataxia, dementia, myoclonus and chorea at a mean age of onset of 29 years. The epidemic curves of BSE and vCJD in the UK and Europe are shown in ***Figure 11.24***, with very few UK cases identified in the last 5 years.
- ***Gerstmann–Straussler–Scheinker syndrome*** and ***fatal familial insomnia***. These are rare prion diseases, usually occurring in families with a positive history. The pattern of inheritance is autosomal dominant with some degree of variable penetrance. The gene encoding PrP^{C} in these families often contains mutations.
- ***Kuru***. This disease was described and characterized in the Fore highlanders in north-east New Guinea. Transmission was associated with ritualistic cannibalism of deceased relatives. With the cessation of cannibalism by 1960, the disease has gradually diminished and recent cases had all been exposed to the agent before 1960.

The infectious agents of prion disease have remarkable characteristics. In the infected host there is no evidence of inflammatory,

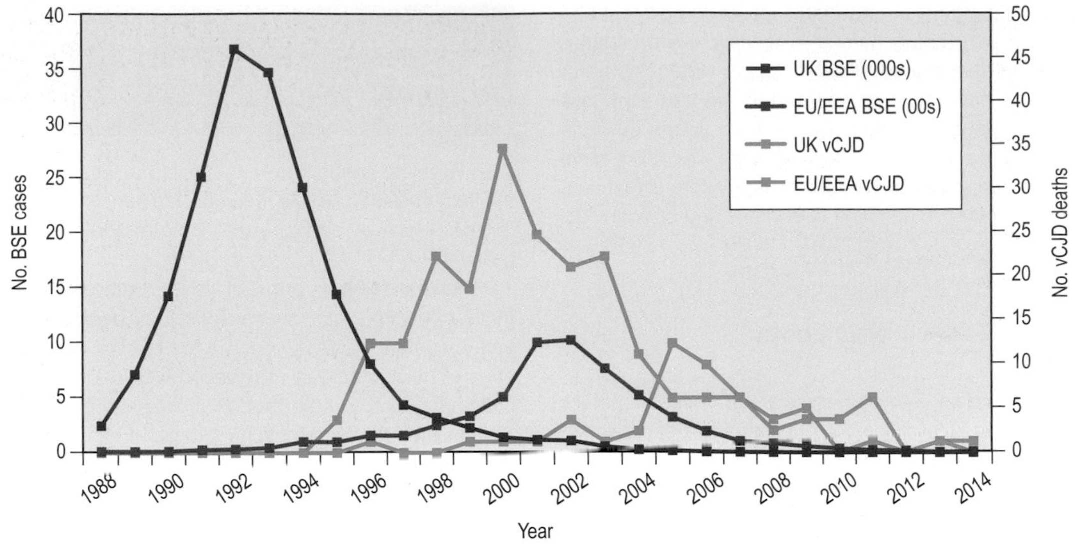

Figure 11.24 Creutzfeldt–Jakob disease. Number of reported cases of bovine spongiform encephalitis (BSE) and variant Creutzfeldt–Jakob disease (vCJD) in the European Union (EU)/European Economic Area (EEA) and the UK, 1988–2014. *(From the National CJD Research and Surveillance Unit (NCJDRSU), with permission; source data available courtesy of NCJDRSU, CJD International Surveillance Network and World Organisation for Animal Health.)*

cytokine or immune reactions. The agent is highly resistant to decontamination, and infectivity is not reliably destroyed by autoclaving or by treatment with formaldehyde and most other gas or liquid disinfectants. It is very resistant to γ-irradiation. Autoclaving at a high temperature (134–137°C for 18 min) is used for decontamination of instruments and hypochlorite (20 000 p.p.m. available chlorine) or 1 molar sodium hydroxide is used for liquid disinfection. Uncertainty about the reliability of any methods for safe decontamination of surgical instruments has necessitated the introduction of guidelines for patient management.

Further reading

Salmon R. How widespread is variant Creutzfeldt–Jakob disease? *BMJ* 2013; 347:f5994.

BACTERIAL INFECTIONS

Classification of bacteria

Bacteria are unicellular organisms (prokaryotes), of which only a small fraction are of medical relevance. They have traditionally been classified according to the Gram stain, which distinguishes Gram-positive from Gram-negative organisms. Using light microscopy, these can then largely be divided into cocci (spheres) and bacilli (rods). Some have a spiral appearance (spirochaetes) while others, such as *Clostridium* spp., may produce spores ***(Box 11.34)***.

- ***Gram-positive organisms***. The cell-wall arrangement of Gram-positive cocci contains a phospholipid bilayer surrounded by peptidoglycan made up of repeating units of *N*-acetylglucosamine and *N*-acetylmuramic acid.
- ***Gram-negative organisms***. Gram-negative bacilli possess a second outer lipid bilayer containing protein and lipopolysaccharide (endotoxin).

Genetic classification is redefining bacteria in terms of DNA sequence information and has led to the reclassification of several bacterial species.

Culturing bacteria

Bacteria can often be cultured in broth or on solid agar. Those growing in the absence of oxygen are strict anaerobes (e.g. *Bacteroides* spp.), while oxygen-dependent bacteria are known as aerobes (e.g. *Pseudomonas* spp.). Many pathogens can tolerate reduced concentrations of oxygen (e.g. *E. coli*). Some organisms are more demanding in their growth requirements and require special laboratory media (e.g. *Mycoplasma* spp. and *Mycobacterium* spp.); others require more prolonged incubation (e.g. *Brucella* spp.).

Diagnosis and management of bacterial infections

The history and examination usually localize the infection to a specific organ or body site. A systemic response may accompany such localized disease or, in the case of bloodstream infections, be the primary mode of presentation. The microbiological diagnosis is difficult to establish in most community-managed infections; even in hospital, where there is ready access to diagnostic laboratories, only a minority of infections are identified. In practice, most bacterial infections are initially diagnosed and managed empirically, with a precise microbiological diagnosis made later, if at all.

BACTERIAL INFECTIONS OF THE SKIN AND SOFT TISSUES

Superficial infections

Infections of the skin and the soft tissues beneath are common. These are usually bacterial or fungal (see pp. 1345–1347). Most skin and soft tissue infections are caused by the Gram-positive cocci *Staphylococcus aureus* and *Streptococcus pyogenes*, although many other species have been implicated ***(Box 11.35)***.

The classification of soft tissue infections is complex, because imprecise and overlapping terms are in use. (The commonly encountered infections are described in more detail on pp. 285–288.)

The majority of skin and superficial soft tissue infections are due to bacteria on the skin surface penetrating the dermis or the

Box 11.34 Classification of bacteria affecting humans

Bacteria	Cocci	Bacilli	Others
Aerobic			
Gram-positive	*Staphylococcus aureus* *Staph. epidermidis* *Streptococcus pneumoniae* *Strep. pyogenes* (group A) *Strep. agalactiae* (group B) Enterococci *Viridans* streptococci	*Listeria monocytogenes* *Corynebacterium diphtheriae* *Bacillus anthracis* *B. cereus*	
Gram-negative	*Neisseria gonorrhoeae* *N. meningitidis* *Moraxella catarrhalis* *Bordetella pertussis*	*Escherichia coli* *Klebsiella* spp. *Proteus* spp. *Haemophilus influenzae* *Legionella* spp. *Salmonella* spp. *Shigella* spp. *Campylobacter jejuni* *Helicobacter pylori* *Pseudomonas* spp. *Brucella* spp. *Acinetobacter* spp. *Burkholderia* spp. *Vibrio cholerae* *Yersinia pestis*	
Anaerobic			
Gram-positive	Peptococci Peptostreptococci	*Actinomyces* spp. *Clostridium perfringens* *C. difficile* *C. botulinum* *C. tetani*	
Gram-negative		*Bacteroides fragilis* group *Fusobacterium* spp.	
Spirochaetes			*Treponema pallidum* *Leptospira* spp. *Borrelia* spp.
Others			*Mycobacterium* spp. *Mycoplasma pneumoniae* *Ureaplasma* spp. *Chlamydia* spp.

subcutaneous tissues. Infection can take place via hair follicles, insect bites, cuts and abrasions or skin damaged by superficial fungal infection. Sometimes infection is introduced by an animal bite or a penetrating foreign body; in these cases, more unusual organisms may be found. A number of factors predispose to cellulitis and other soft tissue infections ***(Box 11.36)***.

Staphylococcus aureus infection

Staphylococci are part of the normal microflora of the human skin and nasopharynx; up to 25% of people are carriers of *Staph. aureus*, the species responsible for the majority of staphylococcal infections. Other species of staphylococci are only rarely pathogenic. Although soft tissue infections are the most common manifestation of *Staph. aureus* disease, numerous other sites can be affected (see ***Box 11.6***).

Box 11.35 Bacterial causes of superficial skin and soft tissue infection

Specific risk factors	Likely organisms
None	*Staphylococcus aureus* *Streptococcus pyogenes*
Diabetes, peripheral vascular disease	Group B streptococci
Animal bite	*Pasteurella multocida, Capnocytophaga canimorsus*
Fresh water exposure	*Aeromonas hydrophila*
Sea water exposure	*Vibrio vulnificans*
Lymphoedema, stasis dermatitis	Groups A, C and G streptococci
Hot tub exposure	*Pseudomonas aeruginosa*
Malignant otitis externa	*Pseudomonas aeruginosa*
Human bite	*Fusobacterium* spp.

Box 11.36 Predisposing factors for skin and soft tissue infection

- Diabetes mellitus
- Chronic lymphoedema
- Peripheral vascular disease
- Venous ulcers
- Steroid treatment
- Malnutrition
- Some immunodeficiency states (e.g. Job syndrome)
- Nasal carriage of *Staphylococcus aureus*

Invasive staphylococcal infection

Invasive staphylococcal infection is often associated with breaches in the skin: for example, due to injecting drug use, iatrogenic cannulation, surgery or trauma. In clinical situations, scrupulous attention to disinfection and hygiene when performing invasive procedures can minimize the risk of infection (see the Matching Michigan programme, 'Further reading'). Although *Staph. aureus* is the most common species of staphylococci implicated in catheter-related infections, other normally non-pathogenic species, such as *Staph. epidermidis* (which is often intrinsically resistant to flucloxacillin), may be found. Flucloxacillin remains the first-choice antibiotic in staphylococcal infection when the organism is known to be sensitive, but with the increasing prevalence of meticillin-resistant *Staph. aureus* (MRSA), other agents are often needed. Other options in uncomplicated cellulitis include clindamycin and clarithromycin, while, for more serious infections (or when MRSA is suspected), agents include glycopeptides, linezolid and daptomycin.

Staphylococcal virulence factors

Staph. aureus can produce a variety of toxins and virulence factors that affect the type and severity of infection. These include staphylococcal enterotoxin A, superantigenic staphylococcal exotoxins, toxic shock toxin 1 and Panton Valentine leucocidin (PVL). The last of these has been found mainly in community-associated strains of *Staph. aureus* (both MRSA and meticillin-sensitive MSSA), rather than in hospital-acquired or epidemic strains. Community-associated PVL-producing MRSA and MSSA are becoming an increasingly common cause of invasive soft tissue and lung infections in some countries (notably the USA), although it is unclear whether PVL itself is directly responsible for the increased virulence.

Meticillin-resistant *Staphylococcus aureus*

Staph. aureus is commonly resistant to penicillin, and isolated resistance to other β-lactam antibiotics, such as meticillin (now rarely used) and flucloxacillin, has been recognized since the development of the first semi-synthetic penicillins in the early 1960s. However, in the last 40 years, strains of meticillin-resistant *Staphylococcus aureus* (MRSA) with resistance to a much wider range of antibiotics have emerged. In some cases, only the glycopeptide antibiotics, vancomycin and teicoplanin, are effective (along with the new agents discussed below) and a few organisms have been isolated with decreased sensitivity even to these.

Vancomycin-insensitive *Staph. aureus* (VISA) develops because the organism produces a thick cell wall by changing the synthesis of cell-wall material. Vancomycin-resistant *Staph. aureus* (VRSA) acquires resistance by receiving the *van A* gene from vancomycin-resistant enterococci (see ***Fig. 11.4***).

Apart from the glycopeptides, such as vancomycin, four other ***classes of antibiotic*** are effective against β-lactam resistant Gram-positive bacteria, including MRSA: these are the oxazolidinones (e.g. linezolid), tigecycline, daptomycin, and the lesser used streptogramins (e.g. quinupristin with dalfopristin).

MRSA is usually found as a skin commensal, especially in hospitalized patients or nursing home residents. However, it can cause a variety of infections in soft tissues and elsewhere, and can lead to death. It is particularly associated with surgical wound infections. Eradication of the organism is difficult and people who are known to be colonized should be isolated from those at risk of significant infection. Topical decolonization is often used but is of limited efficacy. Hand-washing is more effective at controlling spread (see p. 224).

Although MRSA is generally regarded as a hospital-associated organism, it is commonly seen in people away from the hospital setting, both as a colonizer and as a cause of disease. Often the organisms are the typical 'hospital' strains of MRSA and have been acquired directly or indirectly from a healthcare setting (e.g. in workers in care homes). However, there is an increasing prevalence in some countries of true community-associated MRSA (CA-MRSA), with no discernible links to hospital or residential care. These CA-MRSA have different resistance profiles to typical hospital strains (often retaining sensitivity to tetracyclines, clindamycin and co-trimoxazole) and are more likely to produce PVL.

Detection

Culture takes 24 hours. A rapid (2-h) real-time PCR assay is also available.

Pasteurellosis

Pasteurella multocida is found in the oropharynx of up to 90% of cats and 70% of dogs. It can cause soft tissue infections following animal bites. Although the infection initially resembles other forms of cellulitis, there is a greater tendency to spread to deeper tissues, resulting in osteomyelitis, tenosynovitis or septic arthritis. The organism is sensitive to penicillin, but as infections following animal bites are often polymicrobial, co-amoxiclav is a better choice.

Cat-scratch disease

Cat-scratch disease is a zoonosis caused by *Bartonella henselae*. Asymptomatic bacteraemia is relatively common in domestic and, especially, feral cats, and human infection is probably due to direct inoculation from the claws or via cat flea bites. Regional lymphadenopathy appears 1–2 weeks after infection; the nodes become tender and may suppurate. Histology of the nodes shows granuloma formation and the illness may be mistaken for mycobacterial infection or lymphoma. There are usually few systemic symptoms in immunocompetent patients, although more severe disease may be seen in the immunocompromised. In these patients, tender cutaneous or subcutaneous nodules are seen (***bacillary angiomatosis***), which may ulcerate. The lymphadenopathy resolves spontaneously over weeks or months, although surgical drainage of very large suppurating nodes may be necessary. *B. henselae* is sensitive to azithromycin, doxycycline and ciprofloxacin, but drug selection and clinical benefit of treatment are variable according to the primary site of the infection.

Toxin-mediated skin disease

A number of skin conditions, although caused by bacteria, are mediated by exotoxins rather than direct local tissue damage.

Staphylococcal scalded skin syndrome

The scalded skin syndrome is caused by a toxin-secreting strain of *Staph. aureus*. It principally affects children under the age of 5. The toxin, exfoliatin, causes intra-epidermal cleavage at the level of the stratum corneum, leading to the formation of large, flaccid blisters that shear readily. It is a relatively benign condition and responds to treatment with flucloxacillin.

Toxic shock syndrome

Toxic shock syndrome (TSS) is usually due to toxin-secreting staphylococci but toxin-secreting streptococci have also been implicated. Although historically associated with vaginal colonization and tampon use in women, this is not always the case. The exotoxin (normally toxic shock syndrome toxin 1, TSST-1) causes cytokine release with abrupt onset of fever and shock, with a diffuse macular rash and desquamation of the palms and soles. Many patients are severely ill and mortality is about 5%. Management is mainly supportive, although the organism should be eradicated.

Scarlet fever

See pages 271–272.

Deep soft tissue infections

Infections of the deeper soft tissues are much less common than superficial infections and tend to be more serious. Usually, they are related to penetrating injuries (including injecting drug use) or to surgery, and the causative organisms relate to the nature of the wound.

Necrotizing fasciitis

Necrotizing fasciitis is a fulminant, rapidly spreading infection associated with widespread tissue destruction (through all tissue planes) and a high mortality. Historically, two forms are described. Type 1, caused by a mixture of aerobic and anaerobic bacteria, is usually seen following abdominal surgery or in diabetics. Type 2, caused by group A streptococci (GAS), arises spontaneously in previously healthy people. Other organisms are now also recognized as causing necrotizing fasciitis, most notably *Vibrio* species (*V. vulnificans*), associated with sea water in the tropics. All types are characterized by severe pain at the site of initial infection, rapidly followed by tissue necrosis. Infection tracks rapidly along the tissue

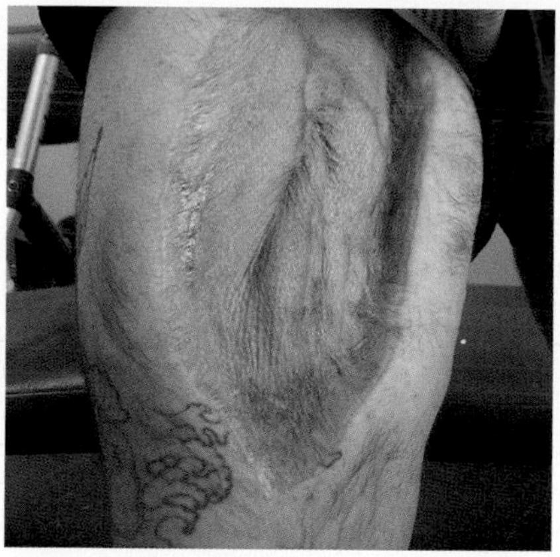

Figure 11.25 Necrotizing fasciitis with widespread tissue destruction (following treatment).

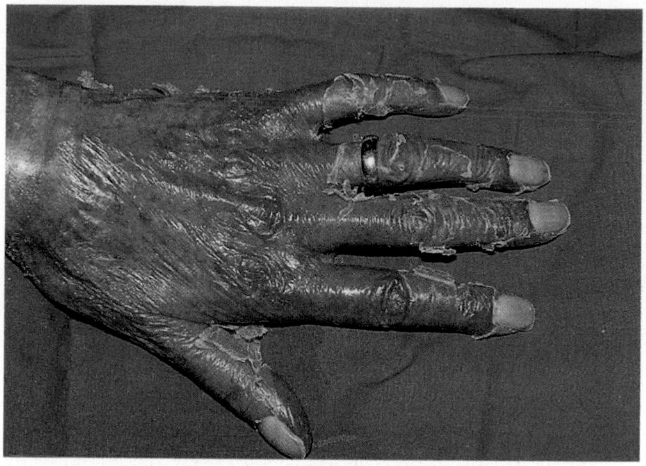

Figure 11.26 Scarlet fever rash, showing desquamation.

planes, causing spreading erythema, pain and sometimes crepitus. In patients with fever, toxicity and pain that is out of proportion to the skin findings, necrotizing fasciitis should be suspected and must be treated aggressively and promptly with antibiotics and urgent surgical exploration, with extensive debridement or amputation if necessary ***(Fig. 11.25)***. Laboratory investigations show a high CRP and a very raised white count (often $>25 \times 10^9$/L). Imaging with ultrasound/CT may be helpful but should not delay urgent surgical exploration. Multiorgan failure is common and mortality is high.

Confirmed GAS necrotizing fasciitis is treated with high doses of benzylpenicillin and clindamycin; mixed- or unknown-organism infection is treated with a broad-spectrum combination, which should include metronidazole.

Gas gangrene

Gas gangrene is caused by deep tissue infection with *Clostridium* spp., especially *C. perfringens*, and follows contaminated penetrating injuries. It is historically associated with battlefield wounds but is also seen in intravenous drug users and following abdominal surgery. The initial infection develops in an area of necrotic tissue caused by the original injury; toxins secreted by the bacteria kill surrounding tissue and enable the anaerobic organism to spread rapidly. Toxins are also responsible for the severe systemic features of gas gangrene. Treatment consists of urgent surgical removal of necrotic tissue and treatment with benzylpenicillin and clindamycin.

Further reading

Bion J, Richardson A, Hibbert P et al. 'Matching Michigan': a 2-year stepped interventional programme to minimise central venous catheter-blood stream infections in intensive care units in England. *BMJ Quality and Safety 2012* (open access online: bmjqs-2012-001325).

Gardete S, Tomasz A. Mechanisms of vancomycin resistance in *Staphylococcus aureus*. *J Clin Invest* 2014; 124:2836–2840.

Lowy FD. How Staphylococcus aureus adapts to its host. *N Engl J Med* 2011; 364:1987–1990.

Marimuthu K, Harbarth S. Screening for methicillin-resistant Staphylococcus aureus – all doors closed? *Curr Opin Infect Dis* 2014; 27:356–362.

Stevens DL, Bisno AL, Chambers HF et al. Practice guidelines for the diagnosis and management of skin and soft tissue infections: 2014 update by the Infectious Diseases Society of America. *Clin Infect Dis* 2014; 59:10–52.

BACTERIAL INFECTIONS OF THE RESPIRATORY TRACT

Infections of the respiratory tract are divided into those affecting the upper and respiratory tract and those affecting the lower respiratory tract, which are separated by the larynx. In health, the lower respiratory tract is normally sterile owing to a highly efficient defence system (see pp. 1064–1065). Infections of the upper respiratory tract are particularly common in childhood, when they are usually the result of virus infection. The paranasal sinuses and middle ear are contiguous structures and can be involved secondary to viral infections of the nasopharynx. The lower respiratory tract is frequently compromised by smoking, air pollution, aspiration of upper respiratory tract secretions and chronic lung disease, notably chronic obstructive pulmonary disease. Infections of the respiratory tract are defined clinically, sometimes radiologically (as in the case of pneumonia), and by appropriate microbiological sampling.

Upper respiratory tract infections

- The common cold (acute coryza) (viral; see pp. 1075–1076).
- Sinusitis (see p. 1319).
- Rhinitis (see pp. 1076–1077).
- Pharyngitis (see pp. 1077–1078).

Scarlet fever

Scarlet fever occurs when the infectious organism (usually a group A streptococcus but occasionally C and G) produces erythrogenic toxin in an individual who does not possess neutralizing antitoxin antibodies. Infections may be sporadic or epidemic, occurring in residential institutions such as schools, prisons and military establishments.

Clinical features

The onset of this relatively mild disease, which mainly affects children, is 2–4 days following a streptococcal infection (usually in the pharynx). Regional lymphadenopathy, fever, rigors, headache and vomiting are present. The rash, which blanches on pressure, usually appears on the second day of illness. It is generalized, but typically absent from the face, palms and soles. The rash usually lasts about 5 days and is followed by extensive desquamation of the skin ***(Fig. 11.26)***. The face is flushed, with characteristic circumoral pallor. Early in the disease, the tongue has a white coating, through which prominent bright red papillae can be seen ('strawberry tongue'). Later, the white coating disappears, leaving a raw-looking, bright red colour ('raspberry tongue'). The patient is infective for 10–21 days after the onset of the rash, unless treated with penicillin.

Scarlet fever may be complicated by peritonsillar or retropharyngeal abscesses and otitis media.

Diagnosis

The diagnosis is established by the typical clinical features and culture of a throat swab.

Management

Treatment of the underlying infection is with phenoxymethylpenicillin 500 mg 6-hourly for 10 days, or parenteral benzylpenicillin if necessary.

Diphtheria

Diphtheria (caused by *Corynebacterium diphtheriae*) occurs worldwide. Its incidence in the West has fallen dramatically following widespread active immunization, but has re-emerged in Eastern Europe. Transmission is mainly through air-borne droplet infection. *C. diphtheriae* is a Gram-positive bacillus; only strains that carry the *tox+* gene are capable of toxin production.

Clinical features

Diphtheria was formerly a disease of childhood but may affect adults in countries where childhood immunization has been interrupted or uptake is poor. The incubation period is 2–7 days. The manifestations are local (due to the membrane) or systemic (due to exotoxin). The presence of a membrane, however, is not essential to the diagnosis. The illness is insidious in onset but co-infection with other bacteria, such as *Strep. pyogenes*, occurs.

Nasal diphtheria is characterized by the presence of a unilateral, serosanguineous nasal discharge that crusts around the external nares.

Pharyngeal diphtheria is associated with the greatest toxicity and is characterized by marked tonsillar and pharyngeal inflammation and the presence of a membrane. The tough, greyish yellow membrane is formed by fibrin, bacteria, epithelial cells, mononuclear cells and polymorphs, and is firmly adherent to the underlying tissue. Regional lymphadenopathy, often tender, is prominent and produces the so-called 'bull-neck'.

Laryngeal diphtheria is usually a result of extension of the membrane from the pharynx. A husky voice, a brassy cough and, later, dyspnoea and cyanosis due to respiratory obstruction are common features.

Clinically evident myocarditis occurs, often weeks later, in patients with pharyngeal or laryngeal diphtheria. Acute circulatory failure due to myocarditis may occur in convalescent individuals around the tenth day of illness and is usually fatal. Neurological manifestations occur either early in the disease (palatal and pharyngeal wall paralysis) or several weeks after its onset (cranial nerve palsies, paraesthesiae, polyneuropathy or, rarely, encephalitis).

Cutaneous diphtheria is uncommon but seen in association with burns and in individuals with poor personal hygiene. Typically, the ulcer is punched-out with undermined edges and is covered with a greyish white to brownish adherent membrane. Constitutional symptoms are uncommon.

Diagnosis

This must be made on clinical grounds since therapy is usually urgent; the mortality rate is about 10%. It is confirmed by bacterial culture and toxin studies.

Management

Antitoxin therapy is the only specific treatment. It must be given promptly to prevent further fixation of toxin to tissue receptors, since fixed toxin is not neutralized by antitoxin. Depending on the severity, 20 000–100 000 units of horse-serum antitoxin should be administered intramuscularly, after an initial test dose to exclude any allergic reaction. Intravenous therapy may be required in a very severe case. There is a risk of acute anaphylaxis after antitoxin administration and of serum sickness 2–3 weeks later ***(Box 11.37)***. However, the risk of death outweighs the problems of anaphylaxis. Antibiotics should be administered concurrently to eliminate the organisms and thereby remove the source of toxin production. Benzylpenicillin 1.2 g four times daily is given for 1 week, or amoxicillin 500 mg three times daily.

The cardiac and neurological complications need intensive therapy. Recovery and rehabilitation can take many weeks.

Box 11.37 Antitoxin administration

- Many antitoxins are heterologous and therefore dangerous
- Hypersensitivity reactions are common

Prior to treatment

- Question the patient about:
  - allergic conditions (e.g. asthma, hay fever)
  - previous antitoxin administration
- Read the instructions on the antitoxin package carefully
- Always give a subcutaneous test dose
- Have adrenaline (epinephrine) available

Prevention

Patients with suspected diphtheria must be isolated, and the local public health authorities should be informed. Staff caring for the patient should have documented immunization status. All contacts of the patient should have throat swabs sent for culture; those with a positive result should be treated with penicillin or a macrolide, and be given active immunization or a booster dose of diphtheria toxoid. Diphtheria is prevented by active immunization in childhood (see p. 245). Booster doses should be given to those travelling to endemic areas if more than 10 years have elapsed following their primary course of immunization.

Pertussis (whooping cough)

Pertussis occurs worldwide. Humans are both the natural hosts and reservoirs of infection. The disease is caused by *Bordetella pertussis*, a Gram-negative coccobacillus. *B. parapertussis* and *B. bronchiseptica* produce milder infections. Pertussis is highly contagious and is spread by droplet infection. In its early stages, it is indistinguishable from other types of upper respiratory tract infection. Epidemic disease occurred in the UK when the safety of the whooping cough vaccine was questioned; currently, uptake exceeds 95% and the disease is uncommon.

Clinical features

The incubation period is 7–10 days. Whooping cough is mainly a disease of childhood, with 90% of cases occurring below 5 years of age. However, no age is exempt, as the antibody levels fall over the years, although in adults mild infection may not be recognised.

During the ***catarrhal stage***, the patient is highly infectious and cultures from respiratory secretions are positive in over 90% of patients. Malaise, anorexia, mucoid rhinorrhoea and conjunctivitis are present. The ***paroxysmal stage***, so called because of the characteristic paroxysms of coughing, begins about 1 week later. Paroxysms with the classic inspiratory whoop are seen only in younger individuals in whom the lumen of the respiratory tract is compromised by mucus secretion and mucosal oedema. These paroxysms usually terminate in vomiting. Conjunctival suffusion and petechiae, and ulceration of the frenulum of the tongue, are common. Lymphocytosis due to the elaboration of a lymphocyte-promoting factor by *B. pertussis* is characteristic. This stage lasts approximately 2 weeks and may be associated with several complications, including pneumonia, atelectasis, rectal prolapse and inguinal hernia. Cerebral anoxia may occur, especially in younger children, resulting in convulsions. Bronchiectasis is a rare sequel.

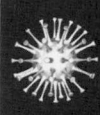

Diagnosis

The diagnosis is suggested clinically by the characteristic whoop and a history of contact with an infected individual. PCR tests are rapid and highly sensitive, but culture of a nasopharyngeal swab remains necessary for definitive diagnosis.

Management

If the disease is recognized in the catarrhal stage, macrolides will abort or decrease the severity of the infection (although resistance to these agents has been reported in the USA). Azithromycin for 5 days is frequently used. In the paroxysmal stage, antibiotics have little role to play in altering the course of the illness.

Prevention and control

Affected individuals should be isolated. Pertussis is an easily preventable disease and effective active immunization is available (see ***Box 11.19***). Convulsions and encephalopathy have been reported as rare complications of vaccination but they are probably less frequent than after whooping cough itself. Any exposed susceptible infant should receive prophylactic clarithromycin.

Acute epiglottitis

Acute epiglottitis (see p. 1078) has been virtually eliminated among children in those countries that have introduced *Haemophilus influenzae* vaccine, as in the UK. Occasionally, infections are seen in adults. The clinical features are described on page 1078.

Acute laryngotracheobronchitis (croup)

See page 1078.

Influenza

Influenza is a viral infection; see page 1078.

Lower respiratory tract infections

Pneumonia

For community-acquired pneumonia, see pages 1100–1104; hospital-acquired pneumonia, pages 1105-1106; and pneumonia in immunocompromised persons, page 1106.

Ornithosis (psittacosis)

Although originally thought to be limited to the psittacine birds (parrots, parakeets and macaws), it is known that the disease is widely spread among many species of birds, including pigeons, turkeys, ducks and chickens (hence the broader term 'ornithosis'). Human infection is related to exposure to infected birds and is therefore a true zoonosis. The causative organism, *Chlamydia psittaci*, is excreted in avian secretions; it can be isolated for prolonged periods from birds that have apparently recovered from infection. The organism gains entry to the human host by inhalation. (For clinical features and treatment, see p. 1105.)

Acinetobacter infection

This Gram-negative coccobacillus is becoming increasingly prominent in hospital-acquired infections, particularly as a cause of ventilator-associated pneumonia (see p. 1165) and vascular catheter infections. It is a cause of community-acquired infections in tropical countries and is associated with wars and natural disasters. The organism is resistant to many antibiotics, including carbapenems. Polymyxin and tigecycline are being used but resistance is still a problem.

Other respiratory infections

Chlamydophila pneumoniae causes a relatively mild pneumonia in young adults, clinically resembling infection caused by *Mycoplasma pneumoniae*. Diagnosis can be confirmed by specific IgM serology. Treatment is with clarithromycin 500 mg 12-hourly, tetracycline 500 mg every 6–8 h or a fluoroquinolone (see also p. 1103).

Other *Chlamydophila* infections include trachoma (see p. 288), lymphogranuloma venereum (p. 330) and other genital infections.

Legionnaires' disease is caused by *Legionella pneumophila* and other *Legionella* spp. It is described on page 1103.

Lung abscess is described on pages 1104–1105.

Tuberculosis is described on page 1106–1113.

Further reading

Barlow RS, Reynolds RE, Cieslak PR et al. Vaccinated children and adolescents with pertussis infections experience reduced illness severity and duration. *Clin Infect Dis* 2014; 58:1523–1529.

Kole A, Roy R, Kar S. Cardiac involvement in diphtheria. *Ann Trop Med Public Health* 2012; 5:302–306.

BACTERIAL INFECTIONS OF THE GASTROINTESTINAL TRACT

Gastroenteritis

The most common form of acute gastrointestinal infection is gastroenteritis, causing diarrhoea with or without vomiting. Children in the developing world can expect, on average, 3–6 bouts of severe diarrhoea every year. Although oral rehydration programmes have cut the death toll significantly, up to 2 million people die every year as a direct result of diarrhoeal disease. In the Western world, diarrhoea is both less common and less likely to cause death. However, it remains a major cause of morbidity, especially in the elderly. Other groups who are at increased risk of infectious diarrhoea include travellers to developing countries, men having sex with men, and infants in day-care facilities.

Aetiology

Viral gastroenteritis (see pp. 263–265) is a common cause of diarrhoea and vomiting in young children but is less commonly seen in adults, other than in the context of common source outbreaks (usually due to norovirus). It is a major cause of morbidity and mortality among infants in low-income countries. Protozoal and helminthic gut infections (see pp. 305–307) are rare in the West but relatively common in developing countries. However, the most common cause of significant adult gastroenteritis worldwide is bacterial infection.

Box 11.38 Pathogenic mechanisms of bacterial gastroenteritis

Pathogenesis	Mode of action	Clinical presentation	Examples
Mucosal adherence	Effacement of intestinal mucosa	Moderate watery diarrhoea	Enteropathogenic *E. coli* (EPEC) Enteroaggregative *E. coli* (EAggEC) *E. coli* O14:H4 Diffusely adhering *E. coli* (DAEC)
Mucosal invasion	Penetration and destruction of mucosa	Dysentery	*Shigella* spp. *Campylobacter* spp. Enteroinvasive *E. coli* (EIEC)
Toxin production			
Enterotoxin	Fluid secretion without mucosal damage	Profuse watery diarrhoea	*Vibrio cholerae* *Salmonella* spp. *Campylobacter* spp. Enterotoxigenic *E. coli* (ETEC) *Bacillus cereus* *Staphylococcus aureus* producing enterotoxin B *Clostridium perfringens* type A
Cytotoxin	Damage to mucosa	Dysentery	*Salmonella* spp. *Campylobacter* spp. Enterohaemorrhagic *E. coli* O157 (EHEC) *E. coli* O104:H4

Mechanisms

Bacteria can cause diarrhoea in three different ways ***(Box 11.38)***. Some species may employ more than one of these methods. In addition to these direct mechanisms, a proportion of people develop post-infectious irritable bowel syndrome, a functional bowel disorder triggered by infection but persisting after resolution of the inflammation (see p. 431).

Mucosal adherence

Most bacteria causing diarrhoea must first adhere to specific receptors on the gut mucosa. A number of different molecular adhesion mechanisms have been elaborated: for example, adhesions at the tip of the pili or fimbriae that protrude from the bacterial surface aid adhesion. For some pathogens, this is merely the prelude to invasion or toxin production but others, such as enteropathogenic *Escherichia coli* (EPEC), cause attachment–effacement mucosal lesions on electron microscopy and produce a secretory diarrhoea directly as a result of adherence. Enteroaggregative *E. coli* (EAggEC) adhere in an aggregative pattern, with the bacteria clumping on the cell surface, and its toxin causes persistent diarrhoea. Diffusely adhering *E. coli* (DAEC) adheres in a uniform manner and may also cause diarrhoea. Both are mainly seen in low-income countries with poor hygiene and inadequate clean water supply.

E. coli O104:H4, which was responsible for a huge outbreak of gastroenteritis in Germany in 2011, has two different diarrhoea-causing *E. coli* pathotypes: typical enteroaggregative *E. coli* and Shiga-toxin-producing *E. coli*.

Mucosal invasion

Invasive pathogens, such as *Shigella* spp., enteroinvasive *E. coli* (EIEC) and *Campylobacter* spp., penetrate into the intestinal mucosa. Initial entry into the mucosal cells is facilitated by the production of 'invasins', which disrupt the host-cell cytoskeleton. Subsequent destruction of the epithelial cells allows further bacterial entry, which also causes the typical symptoms of dysentery: low-volume bloody diarrhoea, with abdominal pain.

Box 11.39 Bacterial causes of watery diarrhoea and dysentery

Watery diarrhoea

- *Bacillus cereus* } plus profuse vomiting
- *Staphylococcus aureus* } plus profuse vomiting
- *Vibrio cholerae*
- Enterotoxigenic *Escherichia coli* (ETEC)
- Enteropathogenic *Escherichia coli* (EPEC)
- *Salmonella* spp.
- *Campylobacter jejuni*
- *Clostridium perfringens*
- *Clostridium difficile*

Dysentery

- *Shigella* spp.
- *Salmonella* spp.
- *Campylobacter* spp.
- Enteroinvasive *Escherichia coli* (EIEC)
- Enterohaemorrhagic *Escherichia coli* (EHEC)
- *Yersinia enterocolitica*
- *Vibrio parahaemolyticus*
- *Clostridium difficile*

Toxin production

Gastroenteritis can be caused by different types of bacterial toxins (see ***Fig. 11.2***):

- ***Enterotoxins***, produced by the bacteria adhering to the intestinal epithelium, induce excessive fluid secretion into the bowel lumen, leading to watery diarrhoea, without physically damaging the mucosa (e.g. cholera, enterotoxigenic *E. coli* (ETEC)). Some enterotoxins pre-formed in the food primarily cause vomiting (e.g. *Staph. aureus* and *Bacillus cereus*). A typical example of this is 'fried rice poisoning', in which *B. cereus* toxin is present in cooked rice left standing overnight at room temperature.
- ***Cytotoxins*** damage the intestinal mucosa and, in some cases, vascular endothelium as well (e.g. *E. coli* O157).

Clinical syndromes

Bacterial gastroenteritis can be divided on clinical grounds into two broad syndromes: ***watery diarrhoea*** (usually due to enterotoxins or adherence) and ***dysentery*** (usually due to mucosal invasion and damage) ***(Box 11.39)***. With some pathogens, such as *Campylobacter jejuni*, there may be overlap between the two syndromes.

Management

Bacterial gastroenteritis is usually self-limiting and does not require antibacterials unless the infection is severe or the patient is immunocompromised. Details are given on page 275.

Salmonella

Gastroenteritis can be caused by many of the numerous serotypes of *Salmonella* (all of which are members of a single species, *S. choleraesuis*), but the most commonly implicated are *S. enteritidis* and *S. typhimurium*. These organisms, which are found all over the world, are commensals in the bowels of livestock (especially poultry) and in the oviducts of chicken (where the eggs can become infected). They are usually transmitted to humans in contaminated foodstuffs and water.

Salmonellae can affect both the large and small bowel, and induce diarrhoea both by production of enterotoxins and by invasion. The typical symptoms commence abruptly 12–48 h after infection and consist of nausea, cramping abdominal pain, diarrhoea and, sometimes, fever. The diarrhoea can vary from profuse and watery to a bloody dysentery syndrome. Spontaneous resolution usually occurs in 3–6 days, although the organism may persist in the faeces for several weeks. Bacteraemia occurs in 1–4% of cases and is more common in the elderly and the immunosuppressed. Occasionally, bacteraemia is complicated by metastatic infection, especially of atheroma on vascular endothelium, with potentially devastating consequences. In healthy adults, *Salmonella* gastroenteritis is usually a relatively minor illness, but young children and the elderly are at risk of significant dehydration.

Specific diagnosis is made by culturing the organism from blood or faeces, but management is usually empirical and includes oral rehydration (see **Box 11.32**).

Campylobacter jejuni

C. jejuni is also a zoonotic infection, existing as a bowel commensal in many species of livestock, such as poultry and cattle. It is found worldwide and is a common cause of childhood gastroenteritis in developing countries. Adults in these countries may be tolerant of the organism, excreting it asymptomatically. In the West, it is a common cause of sporadic food-borne outbreaks of diarrhoea (with about 450 000 cases per year in the UK). The most common sources are undercooked meat (especially beefburgers and chicken) and contaminated milk products and water.

Like *Salmonella*, *Campylobacter* can affect the large and small bowel and can cause a wide variety of symptoms. The incubation period is usually 2–4 days, after which there is an abrupt onset of nausea, diarrhoea and severe abdominal cramps. The diarrhoea is usually profuse and watery, but an invasive haemorrhagic colitis is sometimes seen. Bacteraemia is very rare and infection is usually self-limiting in 3–5 days. Diagnosis is made from stool cultures. Quinolone resistance is now widespread (30% in the UK) and, if symptoms are severe, azithromycin 500 mg once daily is the drug of choice (**Box 11.40**).

Shigella

Shigellae are enteroinvasive bacteria, which cause classical bacillary dysentery. The principal species causing gastroenteritis are *S. dysenteriae*, *S. flexneri* and *S. sonnei*, which are found with varying prevalence in different parts of the world. All cause a similar syndrome, as a result of damage to the intestinal mucosa. Some strains of *S. dysenteriae* also secrete a cytotoxin affecting vascular endothelium. Although shigellae are found worldwide, transmission is strongly associated with poor hygiene. The organism is spread from person to person and only small numbers need to be ingested to cause illness (<200, compared with 10^4 for *Campylobacter* and $>10^5$ for *Salmonella*). Bacillary dysentery is far more prevalent in the developing world, where the main burden falls on children.

Symptoms start 24–48 h after ingestion and typically consist of frequent, small-volume stools containing blood and mucus. Dehydration is not as significant as in the secretory diarrhoeas, but systemic symptoms and intestinal complications are worse. The

Box 11.40 Antibiotics in adult acute bacterial gastroenteritis

Condition	Indications	Drug of choice	Other drugs	Benefits
Dysentery **Suspected or confirmed shigellosis**	Most patients	Ciprofloxacin 500 mg twice daily	Ampicillin 500 mg four times daily Azithromycin 500 mg once daily Co-trimoxazole 960 mg twice daily	Relieve symptoms Shorten illness Reduce mortality in children Decrease transmission
Cholera	All patients	Ciprofloxacin 500 mg twice daily	Tetracycline 250 mg four times daily Azithromycin 1 g single dose Doxycycline 300 mg single dose	Relieve symptoms Shorten illness Decrease transmission
Empirical therapy of watery diarrhoea[a]	Severe symptoms Prolonged illness Elderly patients Immunosuppressed	Ciprofloxacin 500 mg twice daily	Azithromycin 500 mg once daily Co-trimoxazole 960 mg twice daily	Relieve symptoms Shorten illness May decrease complications
Travellers' diarrhoea[a]	Rarely used	Ciprofloxacin 500 mg twice daily	Co-trimoxazole 960 mg twice daily	Relieve symptoms Shorten illness
Treatment of confirmed *Salmonella*[a]	Symptoms not improving (rarely needed)	Ciprofloxacin 500 mg twice daily	Azithromycin 500 mg once daily	May shorten illness
Treatment of confirmed *Campylobacter*[a]	Symptoms not improving (rarely needed)	Azithromycin 500 mg once daily	Co-trimoxazole 960 mg twice daily	May shorten illness
Clostridium difficile	Most cases (unless symptoms resolved)	Metronidazole 400 mg three times daily	Vancomycin 125–250 mg four times daily Fidaxomicin 200 mg twice daily	Relieve symptoms Shorten illness May reduce relapse rate

[a]Antibiotics are not needed for the majority of adult cases in developed countries.

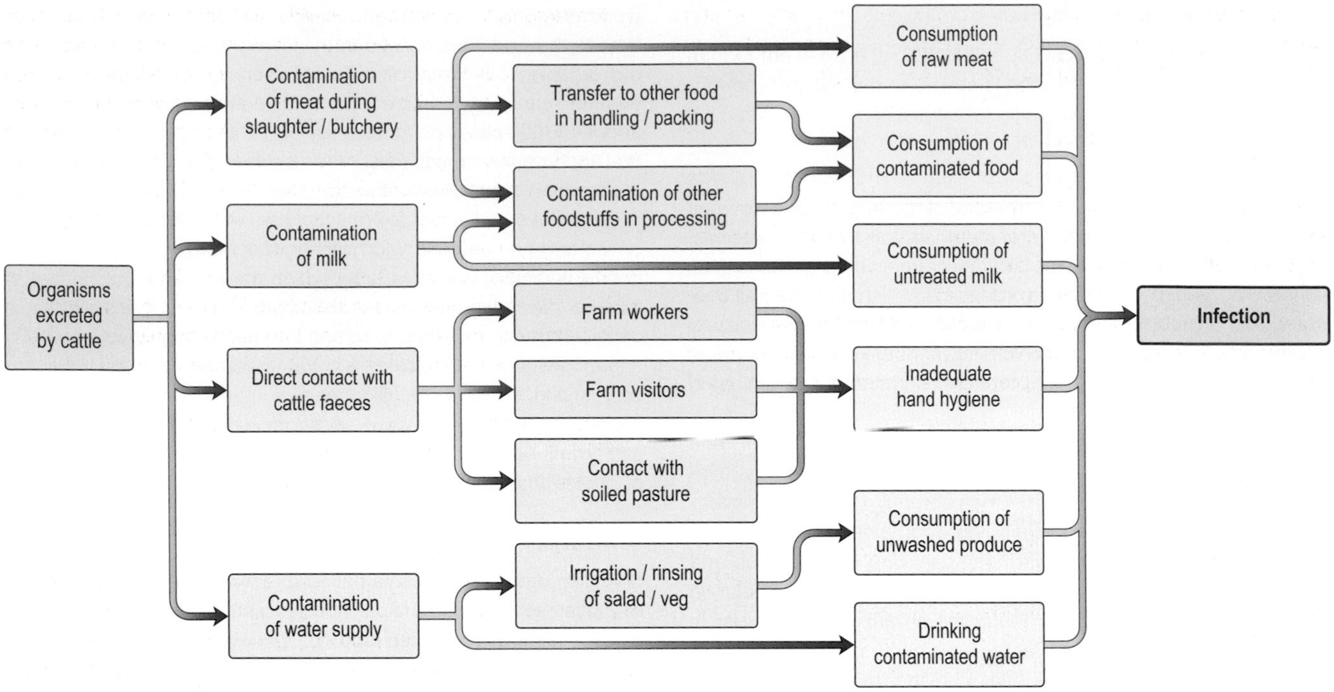

Figure 11.27 Routes of human infection with *E. coli* O157.

illness is usually self-limiting in 7–10 days, but in children in developing countries the mortality may be as high as 20%.

Antibiotic treatment decreases the severity and duration of diarrhoea, reduces mortality in children and possibly lowers the risk of further transmission. Resistance to antibiotics is widespread and, wherever possible, treatment should be based on known local sensitivity patterns. In some areas, amoxicillin or co-trimoxazole may still be effective but in many places ciprofloxacin is needed, although resistance to this agent is increasing.

Enteroinvasive *Escherichia coli*

Enteroinvasive *Escherichia coli* (EIEC) causes an illness indistinguishable from shigellosis. Definitive diagnosis is made by stool culture but most cases are probably treated empirically as shigellosis.

Enterohaemorrhagic *Escherichia coli*

Enterohaemorrhagic *Escherichia coli* (EHEC; usually serotype O157:H7 and also known as verotoxin-producing *E. coli*, or VTEC) is a well-recognized cause of gastroenteritis in humans. It is a zoonosis that is usually associated with cattle and there have been a number of major outbreaks (notably in Scotland and Japan) associated with contaminated food. A variety of modes of transmission have been reported and EHEC is a paradigm for all enteric livestock-associated zoonoses ***(Fig. 11.27)***. EHEC secretes a toxin (Shiga-like toxin 1), which affects vascular endothelial cells in the gut and in the kidney. After an incubation period of 12–48 h, it causes diarrhoea (frequently bloody), associated with abdominal pain and nausea. Some days after the onset of symptoms, the patient may develop thrombotic thrombocytopenic purpura (see pp. 570–571) or haemolytic uraemic syndrome (HUS; see pp. 749–750). This is more common in children and may lead to permanent renal damage or death. Non-O157 serotypes are of increasing concern.

Between May and June 2011, the largest ever recorded outbreak of Shiga toxin-producing *E. coli* (STEC) causing HUS was recorded in Germany. The outbreak was caused by the O104 serotype and over 2000 people were affected. High rates of HUS were observed in adults not in the typical 'at-risk' age range. The increased virulence of this strain is possibly due to it having two different pathotypes (see p. 274).

Treatment is mainly supportive; there is evidence that antibiotic therapy might precipitate HUS by causing increased toxin release, although this remains controversial.

Enterotoxigenic *Escherichia coli*

Enterotoxigenic *Escherichia coli* (ETEC) produce both heat-labile and heat-stable enterotoxins, which stimulate secretion of fluid into the intestinal lumen. The result is watery diarrhoea of varying intensity, which usually resolves within a few days. Transmission is normally from person to person via contaminated food and water. The organism is common in developing countries and is a major cause of travellers' diarrhoea (see below).

Vibrio

Cholera, due to *Vibrio cholerae*, is the prototypic pure enterotoxigenic diarrhoea; it is described on pages 288–289.

V. parahaemolyticus causes acute watery diarrhoea after raw fish or shellfish is eaten that has been kept for several hours without refrigeration. Explosive diarrhoea, abdominal cramps and vomiting occur, with a fever in 50%. It is self-limiting, lasting up to 10 days.

Yersiniosis

Yersinia enterocolitica infection is a zoonosis of a variety of domestic and wild mammals. Human disease can arise either via contaminated food products, such as pork, or from direct animal contact. *Y. enterocolitica* can cause a range of gastroenteric symptoms, including watery diarrhoea, dysentery and mesenteric adenitis. The illness is usually self-limiting but ciprofloxacin may shorten the duration. *Y. pseudotuberculosis* is a much less common human pathogen; it causes mesenteric adenitis and terminal ileitis.

Staphylococcus aureus

Some strains of *Staph. aureus* can produce a heat-stable toxin (enterotoxin B), which causes massive secretion of fluid into the intestinal lumen. It is a common cause of food-borne gastroenteritis in Europe and the USA, outbreaks usually occurring as a result of poor food hygiene. Because the toxin is pre-formed in the contaminated food, onset of symptoms is rapid, often within 2–4 hours of consumption. There is violent vomiting, followed within hours by profuse watery diarrhoea. Symptoms have usually subsided within 24 hours.

Bacillus cereus

B. cereus produces two toxins. The first one causes vomiting 2–4 hours after ingesting pre-formed heat stable exotoxins. The second causes watery diarrhoea up to 12 hours after uncooked food is ingested that contains spores or viable bacteria that multiply and produce a toxin within the bowel. The cause is germination of spores, often in semi-cooked rice stored in warm temperatures prior to ingestion. Rarely liver failure occurs (see p. 486).

Clostridial infections

Clostridium difficile

Clostridium difficile causes watery diarrhoea, colitis and pseudomembranous colitis. It is a Gram-positive, anaerobic, spore-forming bacillus and is found as part of the normal bowel flora in 3–5% of the population and even more commonly (up to 20%) in hospitalized people.

Pathogenesis. *C. difficile* produces two toxins: toxin A is an enterotoxin while toxin B is cytotoxic and causes bloody diarrhoea. It causes illness either in patients who have been given antibiotic therapy that has eliminated other bowel commensals, or in those who are debilitated for other reasons. Almost all antibiotics have been implicated but an increase in cases has been attributed in part to the overuse of quinolones (e.g. ciprofloxacin). Hospital-acquired infections remain common, partly due to increased spread from person to person and via fomites. Strains of *C. difficile* with greater capacity for toxin production have been reported (e.g. the ribotype NAP1/BI/027) in a number of hospital outbreaks with a high mortality.

Clinical features. *C. difficile*-associated diarrhoea (CDAD) can begin anything from 2 days to some months after taking antibiotics. Elderly hospitalized patients are most frequently affected. It is unclear why some carriers remain asymptomatic. Symptoms can range from mild diarrhoea to profuse, watery, haemorrhagic colitis, along with lower abdominal pain. The colonic mucosa is inflamed and ulcerated, and can be covered by an adherent membrane-like material (pseudomembranous colitis). The disease is usually more severe in the elderly and can cause intractable diarrhoea, leading to toxic megacolon and death. Markers of severity include:

- temperature >38.5°C
- white cell count >15 × 10^9
- serum creatinine >50% above baseline
- raised serum lactate
- severe abdominal pain.

Diagnosis. Diagnosis is made by detecting A or B toxins in the stools using ELISA or PCR for C. *difficile* nucleic acid.

Management. Treatment is with metronidazole 400 mg three times daily (mild or moderate disease) or oral vancomycin 125–500 mg four times daily (in more severe or relapsing cases). Fidaxomicin is also effective. Causative antibiotics should be discontinued if possible. In refractory or relapsing cases, instilling faeces from the bowel of a healthy donor (faecal transplant) can restore normal bowel flora and eradicate the *C. difficile* infection. This therapy may become the standard for *C. difficile* infections.

Prevention. Infection control relies on:

- Responsible use of antibiotics (see pp. 234–235).
- Hygiene, which should involve all health workers, as well as patients and relatives. Washing hands thoroughly using soap and water is essential, as alcohol disinfectants do not kill spores (see pp. 224–247).
- Hospital cleaning of surfaces should be performed regularly to try to reduce transmission from fomites.
- Isolation of patients with *C. difficile*.

Clostridium perfringens

C. perfringens infection is due to inadequately cooked food, usually meat or poultry allowed to cool for a long time, during which period the spores germinate. The ingested organism produces an enterotoxin that causes watery diarrhoea with severe abdominal pain, usually without vomiting.

Travellers' diarrhoea

Travellers' diarrhoea is defined as the passage of three or more unformed stools per day in a resident of an industrialized country travelling in a developing nation. Infection is usually food- or water-borne, and younger travellers are most often affected (probably reflecting behaviour patterns). Reported attack rates vary from country to country but approach 50% for a 2-week stay in many tropical countries. The disease is usually benign and self-limiting; treatment with quinolone antibiotics may hasten recovery but is not normally necessary. Prophylactic antibiotic therapy may also be effective for short stays but should not be used routinely. The common causative organisms are listed in **Box 11.41**.

Management of acute gastroenteritis *(Fig. 11.28)*

In children in low-income countries, untreated diarrhoea has a high mortality due to dehydration, often on a background of malnutrition and other chronic infection. Death and serious morbidity are less common in adults but still occur, particularly in developing countries and in the elderly.

The mainstay of treatment for all types of gastroenteritis is oral rehydration solutions (ORS) (see **Box 11.32**). The use and formulation

Box 11.41 Commonly identified causes of travellers' diarrhoea[a]

Organism	Frequency (varies from country to country)
Enterotoxigenic *Escherichia coli*	30–70%
Shigella spp.	0–15%
Salmonella spp.	0–10%
Campylobacter spp.	0–15%
Viral pathogens	0–10%
Giardia intestinalis	0–3%

[a]In most cases, no microbiological diagnosis is made.

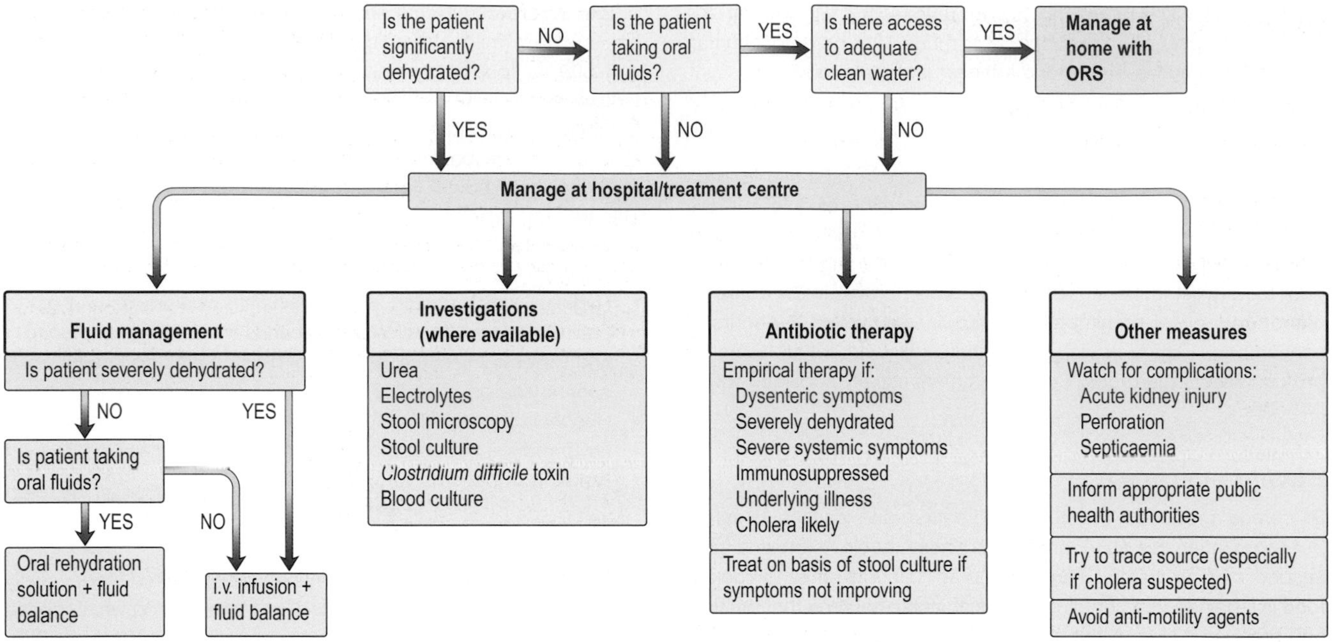

Figure 11.28 **Gastroenteritis: management plan.** ORS, oral rehydration solution.

Box 11.42 Bacterial causes of food poisoning

Organism	Source/vehicles	Incubation period	Symptoms	Diagnosis	Recovery
Staphylococcus aureus	Humans – contaminated food and water	2–4 h	Diarrhoea, vomiting and dehydration	Culture of organism in vomitus or remaining food	<24 h
***E. coli* (ETEC)**	Salads, water, ice	24 h	Watery diarrhoea	Stool culture	1–4 days
***E. coli* O157:H7**	Cattle – contaminated foodstuffs	12–48 h	Watery diarrhoea ± haemorrhagic colitis, HUS	Stool culture	10–12 days
Yersinia enterocolitica	Milk, pork	2–14 h	Abdominal pain, vomiting, diarrhoea	Stool culture	2–30 days
Bacillus cereus	Environment – rice, ice cream, chicken	1–6 h 6–14 h	Vomiting Diarrhoea	Culture of organism in faeces and food	Rapid
Clostridium perfringens	Environment – contaminated food	8–22 h	Watery diarrhoea and cramping pain	Culture of organism in faeces and food	2–3 days
Listeria monocytogenes	Environment – milk, raw vegetables, dairy products, unpasteurized cheese	Variable	Colic, diarrhoea and vomiting	Stool culture	Variable
Vibrio parahaemolyticus	Seafood	2–48 h	Diarrhoea, vomiting	Stool, food	2–10 days
Clostridium botulinum	Environment – bottled or canned food	18–24 h	Brief diarrhoea and paralysis due to neuromuscular blockade	Demonstration of toxin in food or faeces	10–14 days
***Salmonella* spp.**	Cattle and poultry – eggs, meat	12–48 h	Abrupt diarrhoea, fever and vomiting	Stool culture	Usually 3–6 days but may be up to 2 weeks
Campylobacter jejuni	Cattle and poultry – meat, milk	48–96 h	Diarrhoea ± blood, fever, malaise and abdominal pain	Stool culture	3–5 days
***Shigella* spp.**	Humans – contaminated food and water	24–48 h	Acute watery, bloody diarrhoea	Stool culture	7–10 days

ETEC, enterotoxigenic *Escherichia coli*; HUS, haemolytic uraemic syndrome.

Box 11.43 Organic toxins causing food poisoning[a]

Toxin	Source	Illness
Scombrotoxin	Tuna, mackerel	Histamine fish poisoning
Ciguatoxin	Barracuda, snapper	Ciguatera (diarrhoea and paraesthesia)
Dinoflagellate plankton toxin	Shellfish	Neurotoxic shellfish poisoning
Haemagglutinins	Inadequately prepared dried kidney beans	Diarrhoea and vomiting
Unknown	Buffalo fish	Haff disease (toxic rhabdomyolysis)
Phallotoxins, amatoxins	Mushrooms	Various

[a]See pages 81–83.

of ORS are discussed on pages 264 and 288–289. It is also important to remember that other diseases, notably urinary tract infections and chest infections in the elderly, and malaria at any age, can present with acute diarrhoea. Most cases of acute gastroenteritis (especially in developed countries) resolve within 10 days; if symptoms persist, other causes, such as colitis, are more likely.

Food poisoning

Food poisoning is a legally notifiable condition in England and Wales. There is some overlap between food poisoning (defined as 'any disease of an infective or toxic nature caused by or thought to be caused by the consumption of food and water') and gastroenteritis. However, not all cases of gastroenteritis are due to food poisoning, as the pathogens are not always food- or water-borne. Conversely, some types of food poisoning (e.g. botulism) do not primarily cause gastroenteritis. Common bacterial causes of food poisoning are listed in ***Box 11.42***. Food poisoning may also be caused by a number of non-infectious organic and inorganic toxins ***(Box 11.43)***. (Listeriosis is described on see pp. 283–284.)

The increase in reported food poisoning in developed countries is due, at least in part, to changes in the production and distribution of food. Livestock raised and slaughtered under modern intensive farming conditions is frequently contaminated with *Salmonella* or *Campylobacter*. However, the main problem is not at this stage. Only 0.02–0.1% of the eggs from a flock of chickens infected with *S. enteritidis* will be affected and then only at a level of less than 20 cells per egg – harmless to most healthy individuals. It is flaws in the processing, storage and distribution of food products that allow massive amplification of the infection, resulting in extensive contamination. The internationalization of the food supply encourages widespread and distant transmission of the resulting infections.

Enteric fever

See page 289.

Other gastrointestinal infections

Gastric infection with ***Helicobacter pylori*** is discussed on pages 378–381, ***Whipple's disease*** on page 400 and ***bacterial peritonitis*** on pages 434–435.

Further reading

Blaser MJ. Deconstructing a lethal foodborne epidemic. *N Engl J Med* 2011; 365:1835–1836.

Dallman TJ, Chattaway MJ, Cowley LA et al. An investigation of the diversity of strains of EAEC isolated from case of a large multi-pathogen foodborne outbreak in the UK. *PLoS One* 2014; 9:98–103.

Debast SB, Bauer MP, Kuiper EJ et al. ESCMID: Update of the treatment guidance document for Clostridium difficile infection. *Clin Microbiol Infect* 2014; 20:1–26.

Klontz ES, Das SK, Ahmed D et al. Long term comparison of antibiotic resistance in Vibro cholerae O1 and Shigella species between urban and rural Bangladesh. *Clin Infect Dis* 2014; 58:e133–136.

Leffler DA, Lamont JT. Clostridium difficile infection. *N Engl J Med* 2015; 372:1539-1548.

Smith KE, Wilker PR, Reiter PL et al. Antibiotic treatment of Escherichia coli O157 infection and the risk of hemolytic uremic syndrome. *Paediatr Infect Dis J* 2012; 31:37–41.

van Nood E, Vrieze A, Nieuwdorp M et al. Duodenal infusion of donor feces for recurrent *Clostridium difficile*. *N Engl J Med* 2013; 368:407–415.

Wagenaar JA, French NP, Havelaar AH. Preventing Campylobacter at the source: why is it so difficult? *Clin Infect Dis* 2013; 57:1600–1606.

BACTERIAL INFECTIONS OF THE CARDIOVASCULAR SYSTEM

Infective endocarditis is discussed on pages 1017–1021.

BACTERIAL INFECTIONS OF THE NERVOUS SYSTEM

The central and peripheral nervous systems can be affected by a variety of microorganisms, including bacteria, viruses (see p. 862) and protozoa (p. 267), which cause disease by direct invasion or via toxins. The nervous system is also vulnerable to prion disease (see pp. 267–268 and 434–435).

Bacterial meningitis

The most common bacterial disease affecting the CNS is acute meningitis (see pp. 862–865), which causes about 175 000 deaths per year, predominantly in the developing world. Epidemic meningitis due to *Neisseria meningitidis* (usually group A) is common in a broad belt across sub-Saharan Africa and is also seen in parts of Asia. In Europe and North America, bacterial meningitis is usually sporadic, with serogroup B predominating. A conjugate vaccine for serogroup C meningococcus has resulted in a fall in the number of cases of group C meningitis in those countries where it is now part of the childhood immunization schedule. Vaccines against group B meningococcus have been approved in many countries.

Streptococcus pneumoniae is the other major cause of meningitis throughout the world, while tuberculous meningitis (see pp. 864–865) is common in sub-Saharan Africa and parts of Asia.

Haemophilus influenzae type b (Hib) was once a common cause of meningitis in children, but since an effective vaccine has been available, serious *H. influenzae* infections have become rare in countries that have also instituted immunization programmes; however, invasive *H. influenzae* infection remains common in some parts of the world.

Other less common causes of meningitis in adults include group B streptococci, *Listeria monocytogenes* (see pp. 283–284), *Staph. aureus* and Gram-negative bacilli. These organisms are usually associated with an underlying illness or immunocompromising condition, or with a CSF leak.

Cerebral abscess

This is covered on page 867.

Toxin-mediated infections

Botulism

Clostridium botulinum is a common environmental organism that produces spores that can survive heating to 100°C. It causes illness by contaminating canned or bottled foodstuffs, in which the anaerobic organism can multiply and elaborate a neurotoxin. After ingestion, the toxin causes profound neuromuscular blockade, leading to autonomic and motor paralysis. The first symptoms, occurring 18–24 hours after ingestion, are nausea and diarrhoea. These are followed by cranial nerve palsies and then progressive symmetrical paralysis, leading to respiratory failure.

The diagnosis is usually clinical and is confirmed by detection of toxin in faeces or in the contaminated food. Management is mainly supportive, with mechanical ventilation if necessary. Antitoxin is available in some countries (including the UK); the risk of anaphylaxis is relatively high and antitoxin should only be used in severe cases. A subcutaneous test dose should be given before intravenous or intramuscular injection. Antibiotics have no proven role. The overall mortality from botulism is high, but patients who survive the acute paralysis can make a full recovery.

Botulism may also follow the contamination of wounds and injection of street heroin contaminated with *C. botulinum*; in infants, botulism may be related to bowel colonization by the organism.

Tetanus

Tetanus is also due to a toxin-secreting clostridium: *C. tetani*. The organism is found in soil, and illness usually results from a contaminated wound. The injury itself may be trivial and disregarded by the individual. Tetanus can also complicate injecting drug use. In developing countries, neonatal tetanus follows contamination of the umbilical stump, often after the area is dressed with dung. The overall incidence of tetanus across the world has fallen significantly in the past 20 years, due mainly to active immunization.

The organism is not invasive and clinical manifestations of the disease are due to the potent neurotoxin, tetanospasmin. Tetanospasmin acts on both the α and δ motor systems at synapses, resulting in disinhibition. It also produces neuromuscular blockade and skeletal muscle spasm, and acts on the sympathetic nervous system. The end result is marked flexor muscle spasm and autonomic dysfunction.

Clinical features

The incubation period varies from a few days to several weeks. The most common form of the disease is generalized tetanus. General malaise is rapidly followed by trismus (lockjaw) due to masseter muscle spasm. Spasm of the facial muscles produces the characteristic grinning expression known as risus sardonicus. If the disease is severe, painful reflex spasms develop, usually within 24–72 hours of the initial symptoms. The interval between the first symptom and the first spasm is referred to as the 'onset time'. The spasms may occur spontaneously but are easily precipitated by noise, handling of the patient, or light. Respiration may be impaired because of laryngeal spasm; oesophageal and urethral spasm lead to dysphagia and urinary retention, respectively, and there is arching of the neck and back muscles (opisthotonus). Autonomic dysfunction produces tachycardia, a labile blood pressure, sweating and cardiac arrhythmias. Patients with tetanus are mentally alert.

Death results from aspiration, hypoxia, respiratory failure, cardiac arrest or exhaustion. Mild cases with rigidity usually recover. Poor prognostic indicators include a short incubation period, short onset time and extremes of age.

Localized tetanus is a milder form of the disease. Pain and stiffness are confined to the site of the wound, with increased tone in the surrounding muscles. Recovery is usual.

Cephalic tetanus is uncommon but invariably fatal. It usually occurs when the portal of entry of *C. tetani* is the middle ear. Cranial nerve abnormalities, particularly of the VIIth nerve, are usual. Generalized tetanus may or may not develop.

Neonatal tetanus is characterized by failure to thrive, poor sucking, grimacing and irritability, followed by the rapid development of intense rigidity and spasms. Mortality approaches 100%. One aim of the WHO Expanded Programme on Immunization (EPI) is to eliminate this condition by immunizing all women of childbearing age, providing clean delivery facilities and strengthening surveillance in high-risk areas.

Diagnosis

Few diseases resemble tetanus in its fully developed form and the diagnosis is therefore usually clinical. Rarely, *C. tetani* is isolated from wounds. Phenothiazine overdosage, strychnine poisoning, meningitis and tetany can occasionally mimic tetanus.

Management

Suspected tetanus

Any wound must be cleaned and debrided to remove the source of toxin. Human tetanus immunoglobulin 250 units should be given, along with an intramuscular injection of tetanus toxoid. If the patient is already protected, a single booster dose of the toxoid is given; otherwise, the full three-dose course of adsorbed vaccine is given (see below).

Established tetanus

Management is supportive medical and nursing care. Improvement in this area has contributed, more than any other single measure, to the decrease in the mortality rate from 60% to nearer 20%. Patients are nursed in a quiet, isolated, well-ventilated, darkened room. Benzodiazepines are used to control spasms and sedate the patient; if the airway is compromised, intubation and mechanical ventilation may be necessary. Magnesium sulphate infusion may decrease the need for antispasmodics.

Antibiotics and antitoxin should be administered, even in the absence of an obvious wound. Intravenous metronidazole for 7–10 days is the drug of choice, although penicillin is also effective. Human tetanus immunoglobulin (HTIG) should be given as soon as possible, by either intravenous infusion or intramuscular injection to neutralize any circulating toxin. If HTIG is not available, human normal immunoglobulin (HNIG) can be used. If the patient recovers, active immunization should be instituted, as immunity following tetanus is incomplete.

Prevention

An effective, safe and relatively cheap vaccine means that tetanus is an eminently preventable disease. After initial active immunization, boosters are recommended at 10-year intervals for all adults. Infant immunization schedules in all countries include tetanus (see ***Box 11.19***). Protection by passive immunization with HTIG or HNIG is short-lived, lasting only about 2 weeks.

Further reading

Dimecheli V, Barale A, Rivetti A. Vaccines for women to prevent neonatal tetanus. *Cochrane Database Syst Rev (Online)* 2013; CD002959.

Rodrigo C, Fernando D, Rajapakse S. Pharmacological management of tetanus: an evidence-based review. *Crit Care* 2014; 18:217.

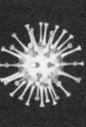

BACTERIAL BONE AND JOINT INFECTIONS

- Infective arthritis (see pp. 690–692)
- Osteomyelitis (see p. 718).

BACTERIAL INFECTIONS OF THE URINARY TRACT

- Complicated versus uncomplicated infections (see p. 764)
- Acute pyelonephritis (see p. 764)
- Reflux nephropathy (see pp. 764–765)
- Perinephric abscess (renal carbuncle; see p. 766)
- Bacterial prostatitis (see p. 766)
- Tuberculosis of the urinary tract (see pp. 766–767).

SYSTEMIC/MULTISYSTEM BACTERIAL INFECTIONS

Many infections are confined to a particular body organ or system, owing to the metabolic requirements of the organism, the route of infection or the response of host defences. Other infections can potentially affect several systems or the entire body. Under unusual circumstances, such as altered host immunity, infections that are normally circumscribed may become systemic. This section describes those infections that commonly cause multisystem disease in an immunocompetent host.

Bacteraemia and sepsis syndrome

(See also pp. 1150–1161.)

Bacteraemia, the transient presence of organisms in the blood, can occur in healthy people without causing symptoms. It can follow surgery, dental treatment and even tooth-brushing. Bacteraemia can also occur from the bowel or bladder, especially in the presence of local inflammation. Unless a site of metastatic infection is established (such as the heart valves), most organisms are rapidly cleared from the blood.

Sepsis is the term used to describe the signs and symptoms of a systemic inflammatory response syndrome (SIRS; see p. 221) to a localized primary site of infection. Viral, bacterial, fungal and parasitic disease can all trigger the sepsis syndrome.

SIRS is not unique to infection and may complicate a variety of events and conditions such as trauma, chronic inflammatory diseases and malignancy (e.g. lymphoma).

Severe sepsis and septic shock are described on pages 1154–1155.

Meningococcal sepsis

Neisseria meningitidis is found worldwide, in five major sero-groups. In sub-Saharan Africa and parts of Asia, where group A meningococcus is prevalent, it usually causes epidemic disease. Groups Y and W can also cause epidemic infection, while groups B and C (the predominant strains in Europe and North America) tend to be sporadic.

Humans are the only known reservoir for the organism, which is carried asymptomatically in the nasopharynx of 5–20% of the general population. Meningococcal disease occurs when the bacteria invade the nasal mucosa and enter the bloodstream; this only happens in a small percentage of those colonized. Invasion depends on both host and bacterial factors. It is more likely to take place soon after colonization has occurred and following viral upper respiratory infections.

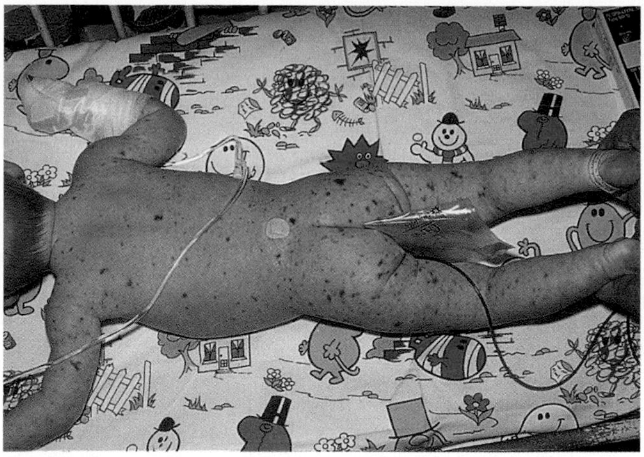

Figure 11.29 Meningococcal infection, showing a purpuric rash.

Clinical features

Invasive meningococcal infection may cause meningitis, the meningococcal sepsis syndrome or both. Meningitic disease (see p. 863) usually presents with the classical triad of headache, fever and neck stiffness. Vomiting, diminished consciousness and focal neurological signs occur, although some patients, especially in the early stages, only have mild symptoms. Meningococcal septicaemia causes the typical features of septic shock, such as fever, myalgia and hypotension (see pp. 1154–1155), and may be accompanied by a petechial or haemorrhagic rash ***(Fig. 11.29)***. In some cases, the patient can deteriorate rapidly, with shock, disseminated intravascular coagulation and multiorgan failure.

Diagnosis

The presence of meningitis and sepsis syndrome with a typical rash is strongly suggestive of meningococcal disease. Gram-negative diplococci may be seen on Gram stain of CSF or of aspirate from petechiae; meningococci can also be cultured from CSF or blood, or detected by PCR.

Management

N. meningitidis is sensitive to benzylpenicillin (in most cases), third-generation cephalosporins and chloramphenicol; cefotaxime or ceftriaxone is the recommended treatment in the UK (see ***Box 21.57***). Meningococcal sepsis should be managed in the same way as any other form of bacterial sepsis. The mortality from meningococcal sepsis in developed countries is currently approximately 10%, while that from meningococcal meningitis alone is less than 5% (see below). Mild neurological sequelae (especially vestibular nerve damage) are common but serious brain damage is relatively unusual.

The meningococcal C conjugate vaccine has contributed to an overall reduction of invasive meningococcal disease in the UK: 800 cases were reported in England and Wales in 2013, compared with 2784 in 1999 (when the group C meningococcal immunization programme began). Group B vaccines were licensed and approved for use in the UK in 2014, and from the start of 2016 are being introduced into the routine childhood/young adult immunization programme. A combined A/C/W135/Y vaccine is available for control of outbreaks caused by these strains and for travellers to endemic areas.

Close contacts of a case of meningococcal disease should be given prophylaxis with oral rifampicin or ciprofloxacin to eradicate the bacteria from the nasopharynx and reduce the risk of onward spread. In the case of group C disease, contacts should be offered immunization.

Rheumatic fever

Rheumatic fever is an inflammatory disease that occurs in children and young adults (the first attack usually takes place between 5 and 15 years of age) as a result of infection with group A streptococci (GAS). It affects the heart, skin, joints and CNS. It is relatively common in the Middle and Far East, Eastern Europe and South America, but is now rare in Western Europe and North America. This decline in the incidence of rheumatic fever in the developed world (from 10% of children in the 1920s to 0.01% today) parallels the reduction in all streptococcal infections and is largely due to improved hygiene and the use of antibiotics.

Pharyngeal infection with GAS is followed, in a small proportion of cases, by the clinical syndrome of rheumatic fever. This is thought to develop because of an autoimmune reaction triggered by molecular mimicry between the cell-wall M proteins of the infecting *Streptococcus pyogenes* and cardiac myosin and laminin. The condition is not due to direct infection of the heart or to the production of a toxin.

Clinical features

The disease presents suddenly, with fever, joint pains and malaise. Diagnosis relies on the presence of two or more major clinical manifestations, or one major manifestation plus two or more minor features, in addition to evidence of current or recent streptococcal infection. These are known as the modified Jones criteria ***(Box 11.44)***.

Carditis manifests as:

- new or changed heart murmurs
- development of cardiac enlargement or cardiac failure
- appearance of a pericardial effusion and electrocardiographic (ECG) changes of pericarditis, myocarditis, AV block or other cardiac arrhythmias.

Non-cardiac features include the following:

- Fever.
- The arthritis associated with rheumatic fever (see pp. 703–704) is classically a fleeting migratory polyarthritis affecting large joints such as the knees, elbows, ankles and wrists. Once the acute inflammation disappears, the rheumatic process leaves the joints normal
- Sydenham's chorea (or St Vitus' dance; see p. 856) is involvement of the CNS that develops late after a streptococcal infection. Sufferers are noticeably 'fidgety' and display spasmodic, unintentional, choreiform movements. Speech is often affected
- Skin manifestations include erythema marginatum, a transient pink rash with slightly raised edges, which occurs in 20% of cases. The erythematous areas found mostly on the trunk and limbs coalesce into crescentic ring-shaped patches. Subcutaneous nodules, which are painless, pea-sized, hard nodules beneath the skin, may also occur.

Box 11.44 Modified Jones criteria for the diagnosis of rheumatic fever

Evidence of antecedent streptococcal infection
- Positive throat culture for group A streptococcus
- Good clinical history (e.g. of scarlet fever)
- Elevated antistreptolysin O titre (or other serological assay for streptococci)

Major criteria
- Carditis
- Polyarthritis
- Chorea
- Erythema marginatum
- Subcutaneous nodules

Minor criteria
- Fever
- Arthralgia (unless arthritis counted as major criterion)
- Previous rheumatic fever
- Raised ESR/C-reactive protein
- Leucocytosis
- Prolonged PR interval on ECG (unless carditis counted as major criterion)

ESR, erythrocyte sedimentation rate.

Investigations

- ***Throat swabs*** for GAS.
- ***Antistreptolysin O titre*** and ***anti-DNAse B***.
- ***Cardiac investigations***, e.g. ECG, echocardiogram.

Management

Absolute bed rest is usually recommended, although the evidence for this dates from the pre-antibiotic era. It is probably reasonable to start mobilizing the patient when acute symptoms start to improve.

Residual streptococcal infections should be eradicated with oral phenoxymethylpenicillin 500 mg four times daily for 1 week. This therapy should be administered even if nasal or pharyngeal swabs do not culture the streptococci.

The arthritis of rheumatic fever usually responds to non-steroidal anti-inflammatory drugs (NSAIDs), although these have no impact on long-term cardiac sequelae. There is no good evidence that steroids are of benefit, although some experts give high-dose prednisolone if there is severe carditis. Recurrences are most common when persistent cardiac damage is present and are prevented by the continued administration of oral phenoxymethylpenicillin 250 mg twice daily or i.m. benzathine penicillin G 1.2 million units monthly until the age of 20 years or for 5 years after the latest attack (see p. 293). Erythromycin or clarithromycin is used if the patient is allergic to penicillin. Any streptococcal infection that does develop should be treated promptly.

Prognosis

More than 50% of those who suffer acute rheumatic fever with carditis will later (after 10–20 years) develop chronic rheumatic valvular disease, predominantly affecting the mitral and aortic valves.

Leptospirosis

Leptospirosis is a zoonosis caused by the spirochaete *Leptospira interrogans*. There are over 200 serotypes. The main types affecting humans are:

- *L. i. icterohaemorrhagiae* (normal host: rodents)
- *L. i. canicola* (dogs and pigs)
- *L. i. hardjo* (cattle)
- *L. i. pomona* (pigs and cattle).

Leptospires are excreted in the animal's urine and enter the host through a skin abrasion or through intact mucous membranes. Leptospirosis can also be caught by ingestion of contaminated water. The organism can survive for many days in warm fresh water and for up to 24 h in sea water.

In England and Wales, only about 50 cases of leptospirosis are reported every year (although many mild infections probably go undiagnosed) and it remains largely an occupational disease of farmers, vets and others who work with animals. In some parts of the world (e.g. Hawaii, where the annual incidence is high), it is associated with a variety of recreational activities that bring people into closer contact with rodents. Outbreaks of leptospirosis have also been associated with flooding.

Clinical features

In 1896, Weil described a severe illness consisting of jaundice, haemorrhage and renal impairment caused by *L. i. icterohaemorrhagiae*, but fortunately 90–95% of infections are subclinical or cause only a mild fever. The incubation period of leptospirosis is usually 7–14 days and the illness typically has two phases. A leptospiraemic phase, which lasts for up to a week, is followed after a couple of days' interval by an immunological phase. The first phase is characterized by severe headache, malaise, fever, anorexia and myalgia. Most patients have conjunctival suffusion. Hepatosplenomegaly, lymphadenopathy and various skin rashes are sometimes seen. The second phase is usually mild. Half of patients have meningism, about a third of whom have a CSF lymphocytosis. The majority of patients recover uneventfully at this stage.

In severe disease, there may not be a clear distinction between phases. Following the initial symptoms, patients progressively develop hepatic and kidney injury, haemolytic anaemia and circulatory collapse. Cardiac failure and pulmonary haemorrhage may also occur. Even with full supportive care, the mortality is around 10%, rising to 15–20% in the elderly.

Diagnosis

The diagnosis is usually a clinical one. Leptospires can be cultured from blood or CSF during the first week of illness, but culture requires special media and may take several weeks. Leptospiral DNA can be detected by PCR in the blood and urine. A minority of patients may also excrete the organism in their urine from the second week onwards. Confirmation is usually serological. Specific IgM antibodies start to appear from the end of the first week and the diagnosis is often made retrospectively with a microscopic agglutination test (MAT) showing a fourfold rise. There is typically a leucocytosis and, in severe infection, thrombocytopenia and an elevated creatine phosphokinase.

Management

Early antibiotic therapy may limit the progress of the disease; if antibiotics are used, they should be started as quickly as possible. The efficacy of antibiotics in mild disease is debated; if they are used, oral doxycycline is the best choice. Intravenous penicillin or ceftriaxone should be given in more severe cases. Intensive supportive care is needed for those patients who develop hepatorenal failure.

Brucellosis

Brucellosis (Malta fever, undulant fever) is a zoonosis and has a worldwide distribution, although it has been virtually eliminated from cattle in the UK, where there have been few infections – mainly imported – in recent years. The highest incidence is in the Mediterranean countries, the Middle East and the tropics; there are about 500 000 new cases diagnosed per year worldwide.

The organisms usually gain entry into the human body via the mouth; less frequently, they may enter via the respiratory tract, genital tract or abraded skin. The bacilli travel in the lymphatics and infect lymph nodes. This is followed by haematogenous spread with ultimate localization in the reticulo-endothelial system. Acquisition is usually by the ingestion of raw milk from infected cattle or goats, although occupational exposure is also common. Person-to-person transmission is rare.

Clinical features

The incubation period of acute brucellosis is 1–3 weeks. The onset is insidious, with malaise, headache, weakness, generalized myalgia and night sweats. The fever pattern is classically undulant, although continuous and intermittent patterns are also seen. Lymphadenopathy and hepatosplenomegaly are common; sacroiliitis, arthritis, osteomyelitis, epididymo-orchitis, meningoencephalitis and endocarditis have all been described.

Untreated brucellosis can give rise to chronic infection, lasting a year or more. This is characterized by easy fatigability, myalgia and occasional bouts of fever and depression. Splenomegaly is usually present. Occasionally, infection can lead to localized brucellosis, which may not be associated with systemic symptoms. Bones and joints, spleen, endocardium, lungs, urinary tract and nervous system may be involved.

Diagnosis

Blood (or bone marrow) cultures are positive during the acute phase of illness in 50% of patients (higher in *B. melitensis*), but prolonged culture is needed. In chronic disease, serological tests are of greater value. The *Brucella* agglutination test, which demonstrates a fourfold or greater rise in titre (>1 in 160) over a 4-week period, is highly suggestive of brucellosis. An elevated serum IgG level is evidence of current or recent infection; a negative test excludes chronic brucellosis. In localized brucellosis, antibody titres are low and the diagnosis is usually established by culturing the organisms from the involved site. Species-specific PCR tests are also available.

Management and prevention

Brucellosis should be treated with a combination of doxycycline, rifampicin and an aminoglycoside (usually gentamicin). Prevention and control involve careful attention to hygiene when handling infected animals, eradication of infection in animals through vaccination, and the pasteurization of milk. No vaccine is available for use in humans.

Listeriosis

Listeria monocytogenes is an environmental organism that is widely disseminated in soil and decayed matter. It affects both animals and humans; the most common route of human infection is in contaminated foodstuffs. The organism can grow at temperatures as low as 4°C and the most commonly implicated foods are unpasteurized soft cheeses, raw vegetables and chicken pâtés. Listeriosis is a rare but serious infection affecting mainly neonates, pregnant women, the elderly and the immunocompromised. *L. monocytogenes* has also been recognized as a cause of self-limiting, food-borne gastroenteritis in healthy adults, but the incidence of this is unknown.

In pregnant women, *Listeria* causes an influenza-like illness, but infection of the fetus can lead to septic abortion, premature labour and stillbirth. Early treatment of *Listeria* in pregnancy may prevent this but the overall fetal loss rate is about 50%. In the elderly and the immunocompromised, *Listeria* can cause meningoencephalitis. Bacteraemia and a variety of focal infections have also been described.

The diagnosis is established by culture of blood, CSF or other body fluids. The treatment of choice for adult listeriosis is ampicillin plus gentamicin. Co-trimoxazole is also effective but the organism is resistant to cephalosporins.

Q fever

Q fever is a zoonosis caused by *Coxiella burnetii*. Infection is widespread in domestic, farm and other animals, birds and arthropods; spread is mainly by ticks. Modes of transmission to humans are by dust, aerosol and unpasteurized milk from infected cows. The formation of spores means that *C. burnetii* can survive in extreme environmental conditions for long periods. The infective dose is very small, so that minimal animal contact is required. One reported outbreak occurred among inhabitants of a village through which infected sheep had passed. Infection in the UK is rare and is usually associated with farm and abattoir workers. A large outbreak in the Netherlands (with 4000 human cases) has been linked to intensive goat farming.

Clinical features

Symptoms begin insidiously 2–4 weeks after infection. Fever is accompanied by influenza-like symptoms with myalgia and headache. The acute illness usually resolves spontaneously but pneumonia or hepatitis may develop. Occasionally, infection can become chronic, with endocarditis, myocarditis, uveitis, osteomyelitis or other focal infections.

C. burnetii is an obligate intracellular organism and does not grow on standard culture media. Diagnosis is made serologically using an immunofluorescent assay. Antibody tests for two different bacterial antigens, caused by an antigenic shift, allow distinction between acute and chronic infection. A PCR assay is available but the sensitivity is low.

Management

Treatment with doxycycline or azithromycin shortens the duration of the acute illness, and there is emerging evidence that it may reduce the incidence of chronic sequelae. For chronic Q fever, including endocarditis, doxycycline is often combined with rifampicin or hydroxychloroquine. Even prolonged courses of treatment may not clear the infection. A vaccine is available for those at high risk.

Lyme disease

Lyme disease is caused by spirochaetes of the genus *Borrelia. B. burgdorferi* is the sole cause of Lyme disease in the USA. In Europe, *B. afzelii* and *B. garinii* are also implicated. Lyme disease is a zoonosis of deer and other wild mammals. It has increased in both incidence and detection; it is now known to be widespread in the USA, Europe, Russia and the Far East. About 800 autochthonous cases are seen in England and Wales each year. Infection is transmitted from animal to humans by ixodid ticks and is most likely to occur in rural wooded areas in spring and early summer ***(Fig. 11.30)***. Co-infection with other organisms, such as ehrlichiosis, occurs.

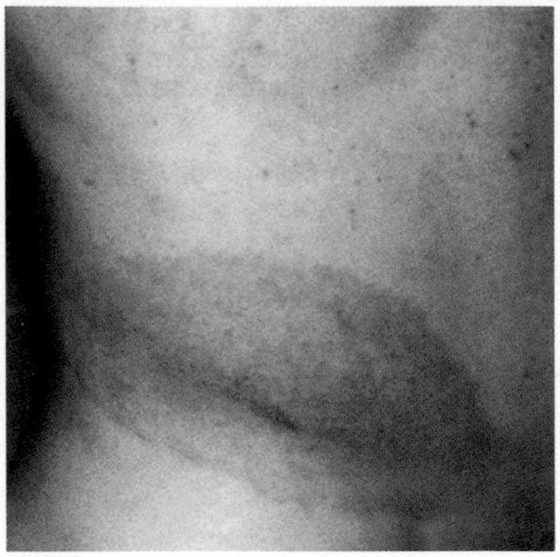

Figure 11.30 **The skin lesion, erythema migrans, at the site of a tick bite.**

Clinical features

There are three stages of Lyme infection:

- Early localized disease presents about a week after the tick bite with erythema migrans (a macular rash), lymphadenopathy, and associated fever and headache. Many people recover spontaneously at this stage.
- Early disseminated disease occurs days to weeks after the appearance of erythema migrans. Some patients may develop a more widespread rash, and after several weeks or months a small proportion of untreated cases may develop neurological complications such as meningitis, encephalitis, cranial or peripheral neuritis, or radiculopathies. Cardiac involvement is seen in the USA but is rare elsewhere. Myalgia and arthritis may also occur at this stage.
- Late Lyme disease, which is rare, can cause chronic arthritis, encephalomyelitis and other neurological disorders, and acrodermatitis chronica atrophicans. There is little evidence for persistent infection at this stage and extended antibiotic therapy is unjustified.

Diagnosis

The clinical features and epidemiological considerations are usually strongly suggestive. The diagnosis can be confirmed only rarely by isolation of the organisms from blood, skin lesions or CSF. IgM antibodies are detectable in the first month and IgG antibodies are invariably present late in the disease. Sensitive antibody detection tests are available but false-positive results occur and an initial positive test should always be followed by a confirmatory immunoblot assay. Even a genuine positive IgG result may be a marker of previous exposure rather than of ongoing infection.

Management

Amoxicillin or doxycycline given early in the course of the disease shortens the duration of the illness in approximately 50% of patients. Disseminated or late disease should be treated with 2–4 weeks of intravenous ceftriaxone. However, treatment is unsatisfactory and preventative measures are recommended. In tick-infested areas, repellents and protective clothing should be worn. Prompt removal of any tick is essential, as infection is unlikely to take place unless the tick has been attached for more than 48 hours. Ticks should be grasped with forceps near to the point of attachment to the skin and then withdrawn by gentle traction. Antibiotic prophylaxis following a tick bite is not usually justified, even in areas where Lyme disease is common. There is currently no effective vaccine.

Tularaemia

Tularaemia is due to infection caused by *Francisella tularensis*, a Gram-negative coccobacillus. It is primarily a zoonosis, acquired mainly from rodents. Infection can be transmitted by arthropod vectors or by the handling of infected animals, when the microorganisms enter through minor abrasions or mucous membranes. Occasionally, infection occurs from contaminated water or from uncooked meat. The disease is widely distributed in North America, Northern Europe and Asia, but the particularly virulent type A subspecies is only seen in the USA. It is relatively rare, occurring mainly in hunters, trappers and others in close contact with animals.

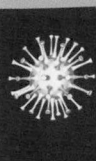

The incubation period of 2–7 days is followed by a generalized illness. The most common presentation is ulceroglandular tularaemia. A papule occurs at the site of inoculation. This ulcerates and is followed by tender, suppurative lymphadenopathy. Rarely, this can be followed by bacteraemia, leading to septicaemia, pneumonia or meningitis. These forms of the disease carry a high mortality if untreated.

Diagnosis is by a rising titre seen on a bacterial agglutination test, which is positive after 2 weeks. Routine cultures are often negative. PCR is now becoming the standard diagnostic test.

Tularaemia should be treated with streptomycin or gentamicin, although doxycycline is used in mild disease.

Further reading

Edouard S, Million M, Royer G et al. Reduction in incidence of Q fever endocarditis: 27 years of experience of a national reference center. *J Infection* 2014; 68:141–148.

Halperin SA, Bettinger JA, Greenwood B et al. The changing and dynamic epidemiology of meningococcal disease. *Vaccine* 2012; 30:73–77.

Kassegne K, Hu W, Ojcius DM et al. Identification of collagenase as a critical virulence factor for invasiveness and transmission of pathogenic Leptospira species. *J Infect Dis* 2014; 209:1105–1115.

Rubach MP, Halliday JEB, Cleaveland S et al. Brucellosis in low-income and middle-income countries. *Curr Opin Infect Dis* 2013; 26:404–412.

Shapiro ED. Lyme disease. *N Engl J Med* 2014; 370:1724–1731.

BACTERIAL INFECTIONS SEEN IN DEVELOPING AND TROPICAL COUNTRIES

Skin, soft tissue and eye disease

Leprosy

Leprosy is caused by the acid-fast bacillus *Mycobacterium leprae*. Unlike other mycobacteria, this does not grow in artificial media or even in tissue culture. Apart from the nine-banded armadillo, humans are the only natural host of *M. leprae*, although it can be grown in the footpads of mice.

The WHO campaign to control leprosy has been hugely successful, more than 14 million people having been cured of the disease. The number of people with active leprosy has fallen from 5.4 million in 1985 to about 190 000 at the end of 2013, largely as the result of supervised multidrug treatment regimens. The majority of the remaining cases are in India and Brazil and, despite the successes, many new infections are occurring in these countries. The WHO has announced a 'Final Push' strategy to attempt to eradicate the disease completely.

The precise mode of transmission of leprosy is still uncertain but it is likely that nasal secretions play a role. Infection is related to poverty and overcrowding. Once an individual has been infected, subsequent progression to clinical disease appears to be dependent on several factors. Males appear to be more susceptible than females and there is evidence from twin studies of a genetic susceptibility. The main factor, however, is the response of the host's cell-mediated immune system.

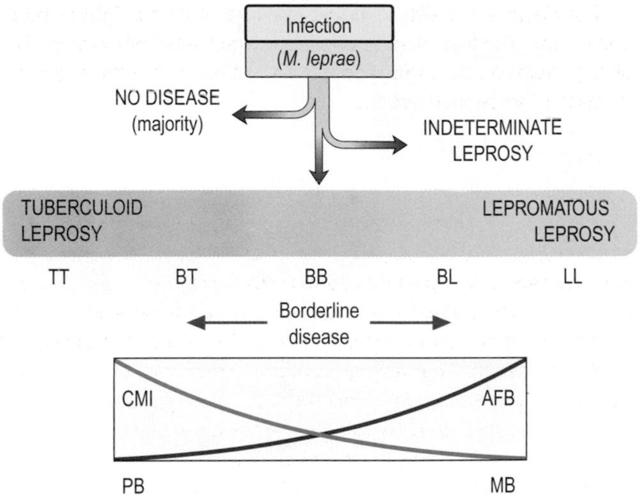

Figure 11.31 Clinical spectrum of leprosy with the combined Ridley–Jopling and WHO classification. AFB, acid-fast bacilli; BB, borderline; BL, borderline lepromatous; BT, borderline tuberculoid; CMI, cell-mediated immunity; LL, lepromatous leprosy; MB, multibacillary; PB, paucibacillary; TT, tuberculoid leprosy.

Two ***polar types*** of leprosy are recognized ***(Fig. 11.31)***:

- ***Tuberculoid leprosy***, a localized disease that occurs in individuals with a high degree of cell-mediated immunity (CMI). The T-cell response to the antigen releases interferon, which activates macrophages to destroy the bacilli (Th1 response) but with associated destruction of the tissue.
- ***Lepromatous leprosy***, a generalized disease that occurs in individuals with impaired CMI ***(Fig. 11.31)***. Here the tissue macrophages fail to be activated and the bacilli multiply intracellularly. Th2 cytokines are produced.

The WHO classification of leprosy depends on the number of skin lesions and the number of bacilli detected on the skin smears: ***paucibacillary leprosy*** has five or fewer skin lesions with no bacilli; ***multibacillary leprosy*** has six or more lesions that may have bacilli.

In practice, many patients will fall between these two extremes and some may move along the spectrum as the disease progresses or is treated.

Clinical features

The incubation period is typically from 2 to 6 years, although it may be as short as a few months or as long as 20 years. The onset of leprosy is generally insidious (although acute onset is known to occur). Patients may present with a transient rash, features of an acute febrile illness, evidence of nerve involvement, or with any combination of these.

The spectrum of disease can be divided into five clinical groups ***(Fig. 11.32)***.

Diagnosis

The diagnosis of leprosy is essentially clinical with:

- hypopigmented/reddish patches with loss of sensation
- thickening of peripheral nerves
- acid-fast bacilli (AFB) seen on skin slit smears/biopsy. Small slits are made in pinched skin and the fluid obtained is smeared on a slide and stained for AFB.

Patients should be examined for skin lesions in adequate natural light. Occasionally, nerve biopsies are helpful. Detection of *M.*

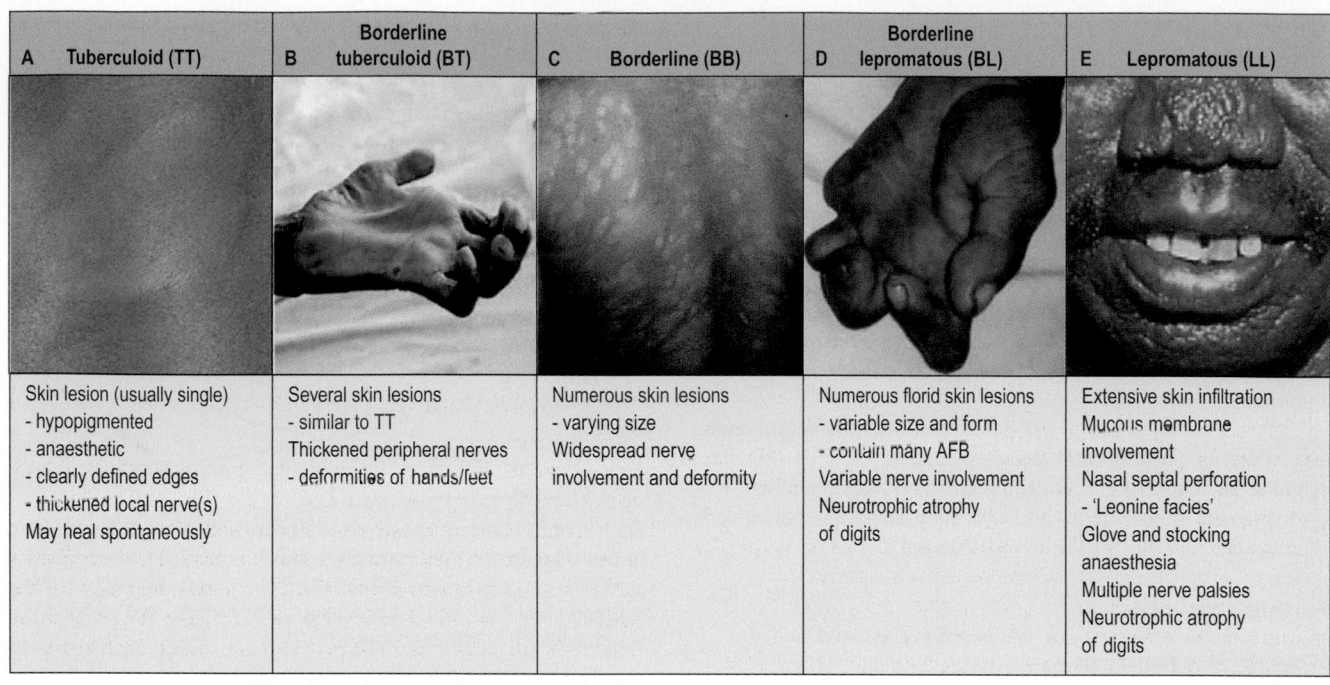

A Tuberculoid (TT)	B Borderline tuberculoid (BT)	C Borderline (BB)	D Borderline lepromatous (BL)	E Lepromatous (LL)
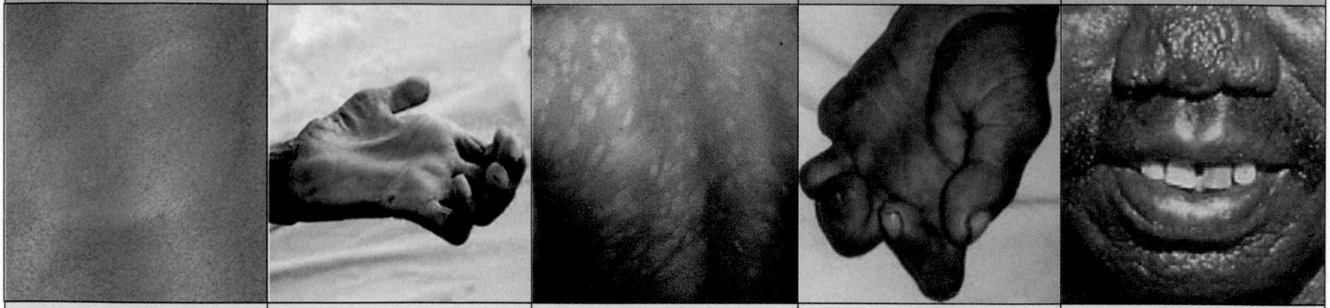				
Skin lesion (usually single) - hypopigmented - anaesthetic - clearly defined edges - thickened local nerve(s) May heal spontaneously	Several skin lesions - similar to TT Thickened peripheral nerves - deformities of hands/feet	Numerous skin lesions - varying size Widespread nerve involvement and deformity	Numerous florid skin lesions - variable size and form - contain many AFB Variable nerve involvement Neurotrophic atrophy of digits	Extensive skin infiltration Mucous membrane involvement Nasal septal perforation - 'Leonine facies' Glove and stocking anaesthesia Multiple nerve palsies Neurotrophic atrophy of digits

Figure 11.32 The spectrum of disease in leprosy. AFB, acid-fast bacilli. *(C, From Cohen J, Powderly JG.* Infectious Diseases, *3rd edn. London: Mosby; 2010, with permission. E, From Goering R et al.* Mims' Medical Microbiology, *5th edn. London: Mosby; 2013, courtesy of DA Lewis, with permission.)*

Box 11.45 Recommended treatment regimens for leprosy in adults (modified WHO guidelines)

Multibacillary leprosy (LL, BL, BB)
- Rifampicin 600 mg once monthly, supervised
- Clofazimine 300 mg once monthly, supervised
- Clofazimine 50 mg daily, self-administered
- Dapsone 100 mg daily, self-administered
- Treatment continued for 12 months

Paucibacillary leprosy (BT, TT)
- Rifampicin 600 mg once monthly, supervised
- Dapsone 100 mg daily, self-administered
- Treatment continued for 6 months

Single-lesion paucibacillary leprosy
- Rifampicin 600 mg
- Ofloxacin 400 mg
- Minocycline 100 mg

} (as a single dose)

BB, borderline; BL, borderline lepromatous; BT, borderline tuberculoid; LL, lepromatous; TT, tuberculoid.

Box 11.46 Lepra reactions following commencement of anti-mycobacterial treatment

Type 1
- Occurs in borderline disease
- Type IV hypersensitivity reaction
- Lasts for many months
- Upgrading (→TT) or downgrading (→BB)
- Abrupt onset of nerve palsies in upgrading
- Treatment:
  - Prednisolone

Type 2 (erythema nodosum leprosum)
- Occurs in lepromatous disease
- Type III (immune complex) hypersensitivity reaction
- Last days to weeks:
  - Fever
  - Arthralgia
  - Subcutaneous nodules
  - Iridocyclitis
- Rare since clofazimine included in treatment
- Treatment:[a]
  - Analgesia
  - Clofazimine (if not already started)
  - Prednisolone if eye involvement
  - Continuation of anti-mycobacterial treatment

[a]Thalidomide no longer has any role in the management of lepra reactions. BB, borderline; TT, tuberculoid.

leprae DNA is possible in all forms of leprosy using PCR and can be used to assess the efficacy of treatment.

Management

Multidrug therapy (MDT) is essential because of developing drug resistance (up to 40% of bacilli in some areas are resistant to dapsone). Much shorter courses of treatment are now being used; the current WHO recommended drug regimens for leprosy are shown in ***Box 11.45*** but longer therapy is required in severe cases. Follow-up, including skin smears, is obligatory. Immunological reactions ('lepra reactions') can occasionally occur after treatment is started, especially in borderline and lepromatous disease ***(Box 11.46)***.

Patient education is essential. Patients should be taught self-care of their anaesthetic hands and feet to prevent ulcers. If ulcers develop, no weight-bearing should be permitted. Cheap canvas shoes with cushioned insoles are protective.

Leprosy should be treated in specialist centres with adequate physiotherapy and occupational therapy support. Surgery and physiotherapy also play a role in the management of trophic ulcers and deformities of the hands, feet and face.

Prognosis in tuberculoid leprosy is good, even if untreated; lepromatous leprosy is progressive if untreated.

Prevention

The prevention and control of leprosy depend on rapid treatment of infected patients, particularly those with lepromatous and borderline lepromatous types, to decrease the bacterial reservoir.

Anthrax

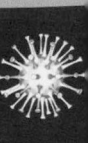

Anthrax is caused by *Bacillus anthracis*. The spores of these Gram-positive bacilli are extremely hardy and withstand extremes of temperature and humidity. The organism is capable of toxin production and this property correlates most closely with its virulence. The disease occurs worldwide but it is most common in Africa and Southern Asia. Transmission is through direct contact with an infected animal; infection is most frequently seen in farmers, butchers and dealers in wool and animal hides. Spores can also be ingested or inhaled. There have been cases in the USA due to the deliberate release of anthrax spores as a bioterrorist weapon (see p. 60).

Clinical features

The incubation period is 1–10 days.

- ***Cutaneous anthrax*** is the most common form. The small, erythematous, maculopapular lesion is initially painless. It may subsequently vesiculate and ulcerate, with formation of a central black eschar. The illness is self-limiting in the majority of patients but, occasionally, perivesicular oedema and regional lymphadenopathy may be marked and toxaemia can occur.
- ***Inhalational anthrax*** (wool-sorter's disease) follows inhalation of spores. A febrile illness is accompanied by a non-productive cough and retrosternal discomfort; pleural effusions are common. Untreated, the mortality is about 90%; in the bioterrorism cases in the USA, it was 45% despite treatment.
- ***Gastrointestinal anthrax*** is due to consumption of undercooked, contaminated meat. It presents as severe gastroenteritis; haematemesis and bloody diarrhoea can occur. Toxaemia, shock and death may follow.

Diagnosis

The diagnosis is established by demonstration of the organism in smears from cutaneous lesions or by culture of blood and other body fluids. Serological confirmation can be obtained using ELISAs that detect antibodies to both the organism and a toxin.

Management

Ciprofloxacin is considered the best treatment. In mild cutaneous infections, oral therapy for 2 weeks is adequate but therapy for 60 days was used in the recent outbreaks in the USA. In more severe infections, high doses of intravenous antibiotics are needed, along with appropriate supportive care. The monoclonal antibody, raxibacumab, has been shown in animal studies to improve survival in inhalational anthrax. Any suspected case should be reported to the relevant authority.

Control

Any infected animal that dies should be burned and the area in which it was housed disinfected. Where animal husbandry is poor, mass vaccination of animals may prevent widespread contamination but needs to be repeated annually. A human vaccine is available for those at high risk, and prophylactic ciprofloxacin is used following exposure. Some countries are establishing public health policies to deal with the deliberate release of anthrax spores.

Mycobacterial ulcer (buruli ulcer)

Buruli ulcer, caused by *Mycobacterium ulcerans*, is seen in humid rural areas of the tropics, especially in Africa. The mode of transmission is thought to be via infected water bugs living in pools and muddy fields. A small subcutaneous nodule at the site of infection gradually ulcerates, involving subcutaneous tissue, muscle and fascial planes. The ulcers are usually large with undermined edges and markedly necrotic bases due to mycolactone (a toxin produced by the mycobacterium). Smears taken from necrotic tissue generally reveal numerous acid-fast bacilli. The only effective treatment was wide surgical excision with skin grafts, but this is often unavailable in areas where the disease is prevalent. However, there is now good evidence that combination therapy with rifampicin plus one of streptomycin, clarithromycin or moxifloxacin given for 8 weeks, will heal ulcers in many cases.

Endemic treponematoses (bejel, yaws and pinta)

These diseases are found in various parts of the tropics and subtropics, mainly in impoverished rural areas.

They are easy to treat with antibiotics, and in the absence of an animal reservoir it may be possible to eradicate them completely (India declared itself free of yaws in 2006). Improvements in sanitation and an increase in living standards will speed this process, as organisms are transmitted by bodily contact, usually in children, the organism entering through damaged skin.

Clinical features

Yaws

Yaws (caused by *Treponema pertenue*) is the most widespread and common of the endemic treponemal diseases. It is transmitted by skin-to-skin contact, often in children. After an incubation period of weeks or months, a primary inflammatory reaction occurs at the inoculation site, from which organisms can be isolated. Dissemination of the organism leads to multiple papular lesions containing treponemes; these skin lesions usually involve the palms and soles. There may also be bone involvement, particularly affecting the long bones and those of the hand.

Approximately 10% of those infected go on to develop late yaws. Bony gummatous lesions may progress to cause gross destruction and disfigurement, particularly of the skull and facial bones, the interphalangeal joints and the long bones. Plantar hyperkeratosis is characteristic. As in syphilis, there may be a latent period between the early and late phases of the disease but visceral, neurological and cardiovascular problems do not occur.

Bejel (endemic syphilis)

Bejel is seen in Africa, the Middle East and Central Asia. The causative organism (*Treponema endemicum*) enters through abrasions in the skin directly or by mouth-to-mouth or skin-to-skin contact indirectly, often between children. Bejel differs from venereal syphilis in that the primary lesion is small and often in the mouth and not commonly seen. The late stages resemble syphilis but cardiological and neurological manifestations are rare.

Pinta

Pinta (caused by *Treponema carateum*) is restricted mainly to Central and South America. It is milder than the other treponematoses and is confined to the skin. The primary lesion is a pruritic red papule, usually on the hand or foot. It may become scaly but never ulcerates, and is generally associated with regional lymphadenopathy. In the later stages, similar lesions can continue to occur for up to 1 year, associated with generalized lymphadenopathy. Eventually, the lesions heal, leaving hyperpigmented or depigmented patches.

Diagnosis and management

In endemic areas, the diagnosis is usually clinical. The causative organism can be identified from the exudative lesions under dark-ground microscopy. Serological tests for syphilis are positive and do not differentiate between the conditions.

Single-dose oral azithromycin has now replaced intramuscular benzathine penicillin as the treatment of choice.

Mass treatment with azithromycin is part of the WHO strategy to eradicate yaws.

Trachoma

Trachoma, caused by the intracellular bacterium *Chlamydia trachomatis*, is the most common infectious cause of blindness in the world. It is estimated that there are 85 million active infections and 8 million people who have been blinded by trachoma. It is a disease of poverty, which is found mainly in the tropics and the Middle East; it is entirely preventable. Trachoma commonly occurs in children and is spread by direct transmission or by flies. Isolated infection is probably self-limiting and it is repeated infection that leads to chronic eye disease.

Clinical features

Infection is bilateral and begins in the conjunctiva, with marked follicular inflammation and subsequent scarring. Scarring of the upper eyelid causes entropion, leaving the cornea exposed to further damage with the eyelashes rubbing against it (trichiasis). The corneal scarring that eventually occurs leads to blindness.

Trachoma may also occur as an acute ophthalmic infection in the neonate.

Diagnosis and management

The diagnosis is generally made clinically.

Systemic therapy with a single dose of azithromycin 20 mg/kg is the treatment of choice, but reinfection is common and repeated treatments are often needed. In some endemic areas, routine mass drug administration is used in children. Once infection has been controlled, surgery may be required for eyelid reconstruction and for treatment of corneal opacities.

Prevention

Community health education, improvements in water supply and sanitation (pit latrines), and earlier case reporting could have a substantial impact on disease prevalence. This is reflected in the 'SAFE' approach to trachoma:

- surgery
- antibiotics
- facial cleanliness
- environmental improvement.

The WHO target is global eradication by 2020.

Further reading

Kummerfeldt CE. Raxibacumab: potential role in the treatment of inhalational anthrax. *Infect Drug Resist* 2014; 7:101–109.

West SK, Moncada J, Munoz B. Is there evidence for resistance of ocular Chlamydia trachomatis to azithromycin after mass treatment for trachoma control? *J Infect Dis* 2014; 210:65–71.

Gastrointestinal infections

Cholera

Cholera is caused by the curved, flagellated, Gram-negative bacillus, *Vibrio cholerae*. The organism is killed by temperatures of 100°C in a few seconds but can survive in ice for up to 6 weeks. One major pathogenic serogroup possesses a somatic antigen (O1) with two biotypes: classical and El Tor. The El Tor biotype replaced the classical biotype as the major cause of the seventh pandemic, which began in the 1960s and spread into South and Central America. Infection with the El Tor biotype is generally associated with milder symptoms but can still cause severe and life-threatening disease.

The fertile, humid Gangetic plains of West Bengal have traditionally been regarded as the home of cholera. However, a series of pandemics have spread the disease across the world, usually following trade routes. The seventh pandemic currently affects large areas of Asia and sub-Saharan Africa. A new serogroup (O139 Bengal) is responsible for many cases in Bangladesh, India and South-east Asia.

Transmission is by the faeco-oral route. Contaminated water plays a major role in the dissemination of cholera, although contaminated foodstuffs and contact carriers may contribute in epidemics. Achlorhydria or hypochlorhydria facilitates passage of the cholera bacilli into the small intestine. Here they proliferate, elaborating an exotoxin that produces massive secretion of isotonic fluid into the intestinal lumen (see p. 426). Cholera toxin also releases serotonin (5-hydroxytryptamine, 5-HT) from enterochromaffin cells in the gut, which activates a neural secretory reflex in the enteric nervous system. This may account for at least 50% of cholera toxin's secretory activity. *V. cholerae* also produces other toxins (zona occludens toxin (ZOT) and accessory cholera toxin (ACT)), which contribute to its pathogenic effect.

Clinical features

The incubation period varies from a few hours to 6 days. The majority of patients with cholera have a mild illness that cannot be distinguished clinically from diarrhoea due to other infective causes. In severe cases, there is abrupt onset of profuse painless diarrhoea, followed by vomiting. As the illness progresses, the typical 'rice water' stool, flecked with mucus, may be seen. There is massive fluid loss, and if this is not replaced, the features of hypovolaemic shock (cold clammy skin, tachycardia, hypotension and peripheral cyanosis) and dehydration (sunken eyes, hollow cheeks and a diminished urine output) appear. The patient, though apathetic, is usually lucid. Muscle cramps may be severe. Children may present with convulsions owing to hypoglycaemia.

With adequate treatment the prognosis is good, with a gradual return to normal clinical and biochemical parameters in 1–3 days.

Diagnosis

This is largely clinical. Examination of freshly passed stools may demonstrate rapidly motile organisms (although this is not diagnostic, as *Campylobacter jejuni* may give a similar appearance). A rapid dipstick test is also available. Stool and rectal swabs should be taken for culture to confirm the diagnosis and to establish antibiotic sensitivity. Cholera should always be reported to the appropriate public health authority.

Management

The mainstay of treatment is rehydration, and with appropriate and effective rehydration therapy, mortality has decreased to less than 1%. Oral rehydration is usually adequate, but intravenous therapy is sometimes required ***(Fig. 11.33)***.

Oral rehydration solutions (***ORS***) are based on the observation that glucose (and other carbohydrates) enhance sodium and water

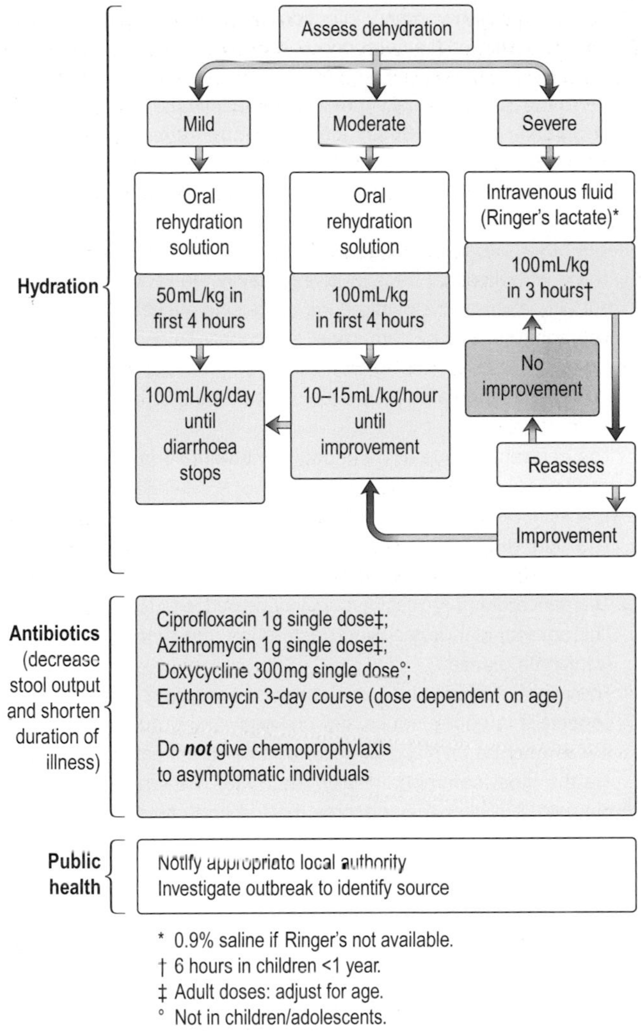

Figure 11.33 The management of cholera.

absorption in the small intestine, even in the presence of secretory loss due to toxins. Additions such as amylase-resistant starch to glucose-based ORS have been shown to increase the absorption of fluid. Cereal-based electrolyte solutions have been found to be as effective as sugar/salt ORS and actually reduce stool volume as well as rehydrating. The WHO recommends the use of reduced-osmolarity ORS for all types of diarrhoea, although concerns remain about the risk of hyponatraemia. Suitable solutions for rehydration are listed in ***Box 11.32***.

Immunization is now recommended by the WHO in potential or actual outbreak situations. Two killed oral vaccines are available. The best preventative measures, however, are good hygiene and improved sanitation.

Enteric fever

Over 17 million new cases of enteric fever occur annually worldwide, mainly in India and Africa, causing 600 000 deaths per year. Enteric fever is an acute systemic illness characterized by fever, headache and abdominal discomfort. ***Typhoid***, the typical form of enteric fever, is caused by *Salmonella typhi*. A similar but generally less severe illness known as ***paratyphoid*** is due to infection with *S. paratyphi* A, B or C. Humans are the only natural host for *S. typhi*, which is transmitted in contaminated food or water. The incubation period is 10–14 days.

Clinical features

After ingestion, the bacteria invade the small bowel wall via Peyer's patches, from where they spread to the regional lymph nodes and then to the blood. The onset of illness is insidious and non-specific, with intermittent fever, headache and abdominal pain. Physical findings in the early stages include abdominal tenderness, hepatosplenomegaly, lymphadenopathy and a scanty maculopapular rash ('rose spots'). Without treatment (and occasionally even after treatment), serious complications can arise, usually in the third week of illness. These include meningitis, lobar pneumonia, osteomyelitis, intestinal perforation and intestinal haemorrhage. The fourth week of the illness is characterized by gradual improvement but, in developing countries, up to 30% of those infected will die and 10% of untreated survivors will relapse. This compares with a mortality rate of 1–2% in the USA.

After clinical recovery, 5–10% of patients will continue to excrete *S. typhi* for several months: these are termed convalescent carriers. Between 1% and 4% will continue to carry the organism for more than a year: this is chronic carriage. The usual site of carriage is the gall bladder and chronic carriage is associated with the presence of gallstones. However, in parts of the Middle East and Africa where urinary schistosomiasis is prevalent, chronic carriage of *S. typhi* in the urinary bladder is also common.

Paratyphoid fever is associated with a milder and shorter illness, and complications are uncommon.

Diagnosis

The definitive diagnosis of enteric fever requires the culture of *S. typhi* or *S. paratyphi* from the patient. Blood culture is positive in most cases in the first 2 weeks. Culture of intestinal secretions, faeces and urine is also used, although care must be taken to distinguish acute infection from chronic carriage. Bone marrow culture is more sensitive than blood culture but is rarely required, except in patients who have already received antibiotics. Leucopenia is common but non-specific. Serological investigations, such as the Widal antigen test, are of little practical value, are easily misinterpreted and should not be used.

Management

Increasing antibiotic resistance is seen in isolates of *S. typhi*, especially in the Indian subcontinent. Chloramphenicol, co-trimoxazole and amoxicillin may all still be effective in some cases, but quinolones (e.g. ciprofloxacin 500 mg twice daily) are now the treatment of choice. Some resistance is starting to appear to ciprofloxacin; ideally, treatment should be based on known local resistance patterns. Azithromycin is the best choice in quinolone-resistant cases; ceftriaxone has also been shown to be effective. The patient's temperature may remain elevated for several days after antibiotics are started and this alone is not a sign of treatment failure. Prolonged antibiotic therapy may eliminate the carrier state, but in the presence of gall bladder disease it is rarely effective. Cholecystectomy is not usually justified on clinical or public health grounds.

Prevention

This is mainly through improved sanitation and clean water. Travellers should avoid drinking untreated water, taking ice in drinks and eating ice creams. Vaccination with either injectable inactivated or oral live attenuated vaccines gives partial protection.

Further reading

Harris JB, LaRocque RC, Qadri F. Cholera. *Lancet* 2012; 379:2466–2467.
Park SE, Marks F. A conjugate vaccine against typhoid fever. *Lancet Infect Dis* 2014; 14:90–91.
Pastor M, Pedraz JL, Esquisabel A. The state-of-the-art of approved and under-development cholera vaccines. *Vaccine* 2013; 31:4069–4078.

Systemic infections

Tuberculosis

Tuberculosis (TB) is caused by *Mycobacterium tuberculosis* and, occasionally, *M. bovis* or *M. africanum*. These are slow-growing bacteria and, unlike other mycobacteria, are facultative intracellular organisms. The prevalence of TB increases with poor social conditions, inadequate nutrition and overcrowding. In developing countries, it is most commonly acquired in childhood.

The impact of TB in the developing world has been magnified in the past 20 years by the emergence of the HIV pandemic (see pp. 331–334) ***(Fig. 11.34)***.

Widespread misuse of antibiotics, combined with the breakdown of healthcare systems in parts of Africa and Eastern Europe, has led to the emergence of drug-resistant TB. Multidrug-resistant tuberculosis (MDR-TB) is caused by bacteria that are resistant to both rifampicin and isoniazid, two drugs that form the mainstay of treatment. MDR-TB is now widespread in many parts of the world (see ***Fig. 24.37***), including Asia, Eastern Europe and Africa. Extensively drug-resistant tuberculosis (XDR-TB) is additionally resistant to quinolones and injectable second-line agents. MDR-TB and, especially, XDRTB are very difficult to treat and carry significant mortality, even with the best medical care (see pp. 1111–1112).

In most people, the initial primary TB is asymptomatic or causes only a mild illness. The focus of the disease heals.

Occasionally, the primary infection progresses locally to a more widespread lesion. Haematogenous spread at this stage may give rise to miliary TB.

TB in the adult is usually the result of reactivation of old disease (post-primary TB) but primary infection or, more rarely, reinfection also occurs.

Pulmonary TB is the most common form; this is described on page 1108, along with the chemotherapeutic regimens. TB also affects other parts of the body.

- The gastrointestinal tract, involving mainly the ileocaecal area but occasionally the peritoneum, producing ascites (see p. 436)
- The genitourinary system, most commonly involving the kidneys but also causing painless, craggy swellings in the epididymis and salpingitis, tubal abscesses and infertility in females.
- The central nervous system, causing tuberculous meningitis and tuberculomas (see p. 867).
- The skeletal system, causing septic arthritis and osteomyelitis.
- The skin, giving rise to lupus vulgaris.
- The eyes, where it can cause choroiditis or iridocyclitis.
- The pericardium, producing constrictive pericarditis (see p. 1043).
- The adrenal glands, causing destruction and producing Addison's disease.
- The lymph nodes, which is a common mode of presentation, especially in young adults and children. Any group of lymph nodes may be involved but hilar and paratracheal lymph nodes are the most common. Initially, the nodes are firm and discrete, but later they become matted and can suppurate with sinus formation. Scrofula is the term used to describe massive cervical lymph node enlargement with discharging sinuses. Mycobacterial lymph node disease may also be caused by non-tuberculous mycobacteria.

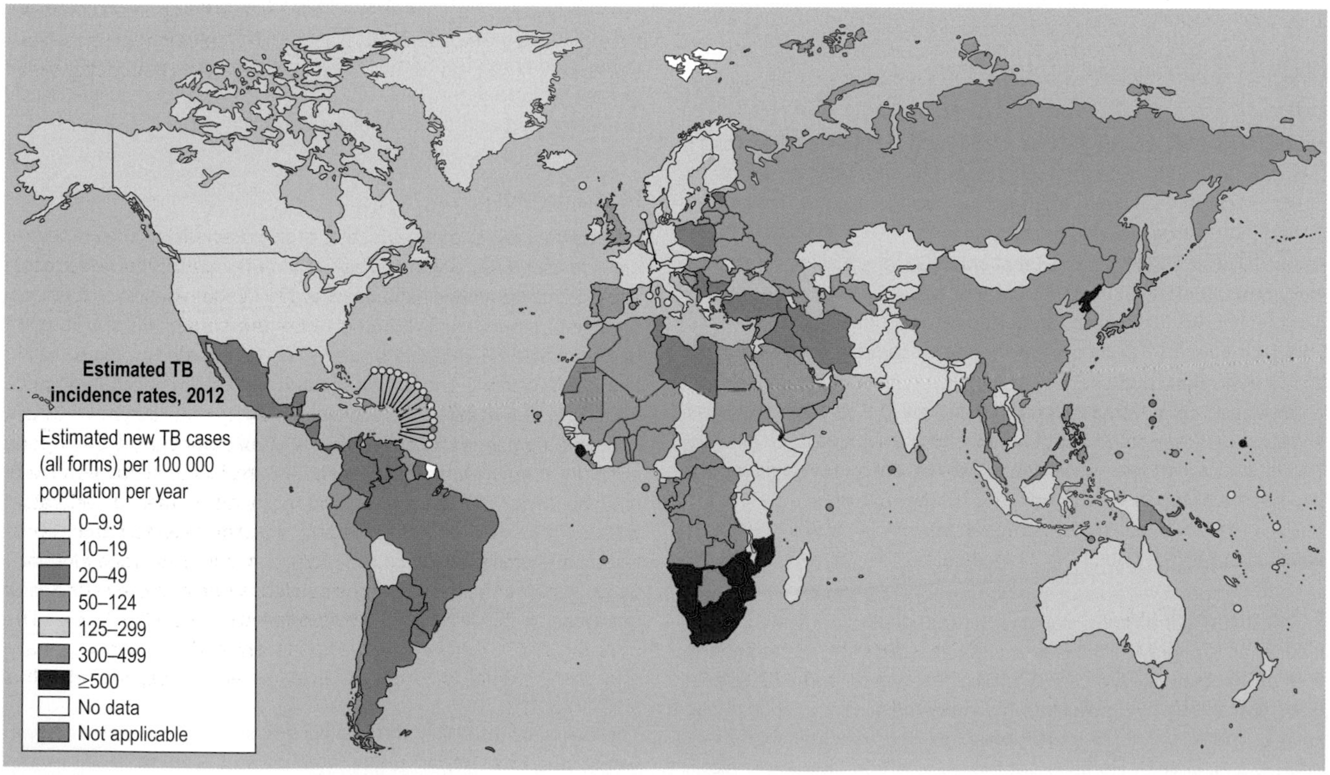

Figure 11.34 Tuberculosis: geographical distribution. *(From World Health Organization.* Global Tuberculosis Report, 2013. *Geneva: WHO; 2013, with permission.)*

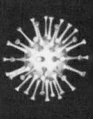

Box 11.47 Examples of non-tuberculous mycobacteria causing disease in humans

Clinical	Common cause	Rare cause
Chronic lung disease	*Mycobacterium avium-intracellulare* *M. kansasii*	*M. malmoense* *M. xenopi*
Local lymphadenitis	*M. avium-intracellulare* *M. scrofulaceum*	*M. malmoense* *M. fortuitum*
Skin and soft tissue infection		
Fish tank granuloma	*M. marinum*	
Abscesses, ulcers, sinuses	*M. fortuitum* *M. chelonae*	*M. haemophilum*
Bone and joint infection	*M. kansasii* *M. avium-intracellulare*	*M. scrofulaceum*
Disseminated infection (in HIV)	*M. avium-intracellulare*	

Non-tuberculous mycobacterial infections

The majority of mycobacterial species are environmental organisms and are rarely pathogenic. Some have been found to cause disease in humans, particularly in immunocompromised patients or those with pre-existing chronic lung disease ***(Box 11.47)***.

Plague

Plague is caused by *Yersinia pestis*, a Gram-negative bacillus. Sporadic cases of plague (as well as occasional epidemics) occur worldwide: about 2000 cases per year are reported to the WHO, with a 10% mortality. The majority of cases are in sub-Saharan Africa, although the disease is occasionally seen in developed countries in people undertaking outdoor pursuits. The main reservoirs are woodland rodents, which transmit infection to domestic rats (*Rattus rattus*). The usual vector is the rat flea, *Xenopsylla cheopis*. These fleas bite humans when there is a sudden decline in the rat population. Occasionally, spread of the organisms may be through infected faeces being rubbed into skin wounds, or through inhalation of droplets.

Clinical features

Four clinical forms are recognized: bubonic, pneumonic, septicaemic and cutaneous.

Bubonic plague

This is the most common form and occurs in about 90% of infected individuals. The incubation period is 2–7 days. The onset of illness is acute, with high fever, chills, headache, myalgia, nausea, vomiting and, when severe, prostration. This is rapidly followed by the development of lymphadenopathy (buboes), most commonly involving the inguinal region. Characteristically, these are matted and tender, and suppurate in 1–2 weeks.

Pneumonic plague

This is characterized by the abrupt onset of features of a fulminant pneumonia with bloody sputum, marked respiratory distress, cyanosis and death in almost all affected patients.

Septicaemic plague

This presents as an acute fulminant infection with evidence of shock and disseminated intravascular coagulation (DIC). If it is left untreated, death usually occurs in 2–5 days. Lymphadenopathy is unusual.

Cutaneous plague

This presents either as a pustule, eschar or papule, or as extensive purpura, which can become necrotic and gangrenous.

Diagnosis

This is based on clinical, epidemiological and laboratory findings. Microscopy (on blood or lymph node aspirate) or a rapid antigen detection test can provide a presumptive diagnosis in an appropriate clinical setting. Blood or lymph node culture, or paired serological tests, are required for confirmation. Rapid diagnosis can be made in 15 minutes using *Y. pestis* F1 antigen in serum or sputum.

Management

Treatment is urgent and should be instituted before the results of culture studies are available. The treatment of choice is gentamicin 1 mg/kg i.v. three times daily for 10 days. Oral doxycycline 500 mg four times daily and chloramphenicol are also effective.

Prevention

Prevention of plague is largely dependent on control of the flea population. Outhouses or huts should be sprayed with insecticides that are effective against the local flea. During epidemics, rodents should not be killed until the fleas are under control, as the fleas will leave dead rodents to bite humans. Tetracycline 500 mg four times daily for 7 days is an effective chemoprophylactic agent. Both killed and attenuated vaccines have been available for many years but have limited efficacy.

Relapsing fevers

These conditions are so named because, after apparent recovery from the initial infection, one or more recurrences may occur after a week or more without fever. They are caused by spirochaetes of the genus *Borrelia*.

Clinical features

Louse-borne relapsing fever

This condition (caused by *B. recurrentis*) is spread by body lice and only humans are affected. Classically, it is an epidemic disease of armies and refugees, although it is also endemic in the highlands of Ethiopia, Yemen and Bolivia. Lice are spread from person to person when humans live in close contact in impoverished conditions. Infected lice are crushed by scratching, allowing the spirochaete to penetrate through the skin. Symptoms begin 3–10 days after infection and consist of a high fever of abrupt onset with rigors, generalized myalgia and headache. A petechial or ecchymotic rash may be seen. The patient's general condition then deteriorates, with delirium, hepatosplenomegaly, jaundice, haemorrhagic problems and circulatory collapse. Although complete recovery may occur at this time, the majority experience one or more relapses of diminishing intensity over the weeks following the initial illness. The severity of the illness varies enormously and some cases have only mild symptoms. However, in some epidemics, mortality has exceeded 50%.

Tick-borne relapsing fever

This is caused by *B. duttoni* and other *Borrelia* species, spread by soft (argasid) ticks. Rodents are also infected and humans are incidental hosts, acquiring the spirochaete from the saliva of the infected tick. This disease is found mainly in countries where traditional mud huts are the form of shelter and is a common cause of febrile illness in parts of Africa. The illness is generally similar to the louse-borne disease, although neurological involvement is more common.

Diagnosis and management

Spirochaetes can be demonstrated microscopically in the blood during febrile episodes; organisms are more numerous in louse-borne relapsing fever. Treatment is usually with tetracycline or doxycycline. A severe Jarisch–Herxheimer reaction (see p. 329) occurs in many patients.

Prevention

Control of infection relies on elimination of the vector. Ticks live for years and remain infected, passing the infection to their progeny. These reservoirs of infection should be controlled by spraying houses with insecticides and by reducing the number of rodents. Post-exposure prophylaxis has been shown to be effective in areas where tick-borne disease is highly endemic. Patients infested with lice should be deloused by washing with a suitable insecticide. All clothes must be thoroughly disinfected.

Rickettsial diseases

Rickettsiae (and the closely related *Orientiae)* are small, intracellular bacteria that are spread to humans by arthropod vectors, including body lice, fleas, hard ticks and larval mites. Rickettsiae inhabit the alimentary tract of these arthropods and the disease is spread to the human host by inoculation of their faeces through broken human skin, generally produced by scratching ***(Fig. 11.35)***. Rickettsiae multiply intracellularly and can enter most mammalian cells, although the main lesion produced is a vasculitis caused by invasion of endothelial cells of small blood vessels ***(Fig. 11.36)***. Multisystem involvement is usual.

Typhus group

Typhus is the collective name given to a group of diseases caused by *Rickettsia* species. ***Box 11.48*** shows a list of rickettsial diseases; with the advent of molecular techniques, many new species of rickettsia causing human disease have been identified.

Clinical features

Typhus fever group

Epidemic typhus

The vector of epidemic typhus is the human body louse and, as with louse-borne relapsing fever, epidemics are associated with war and refugees. Outbreaks have occurred in Africa, Central and South America, and Asia.

The incubation period of 1–3 weeks is followed by an abrupt febrile illness associated with profound malaise and generalized myalgia. Headache is severe and there may be conjunctivitis with orbital pain. A measles-like eruption appears around the fifth day. At the end of the first week, signs of meningoencephalitis appear and CNS involvement may progress to coma. At the height of the illness, splenomegaly, pneumonia, myocarditis and gangrene at the peripheries may be evident. Oliguric acute kidney injury occurs in fulminating disease, which is usually fatal. Recovery begins in the third week but is generally slow. The disease may recur many years after the initial attack owing to rickettsiae that lie dormant in lymph nodes. The recrudescence is known as Brill–Zinsser disease. The factors that precipitate recurrence are not clearly defined, although other infections may play a role.

Box 11.48 Infections caused by rickettsiae

Disease	Organism	Reservoir	Vector
Typhus fever group			
Epidemic typhus	*Rickettsia prowazekii*	Human	Human body louse
Endemic (murine) typhus	*R. typhi*	Rodent	Rat flea
Scrub typhus	*Orientia tsutsugamushi*	Trombiculid mite	Trombiculid mite
Spotted fever group			
African tick typhus	*R. africae*	Various mammals	Hard tick
Mediterranean spotted fever	*R. conorii*	Rodent, dog	Hard tick
Rocky Mountain spotted fever	*R. rickettsii*	Rodent, dog	Hard tick
Rickettsial pox	*R. akari*	Rodent	Mite
Flea-borne spotted fever	*R. felis*	Various mammals	Flea

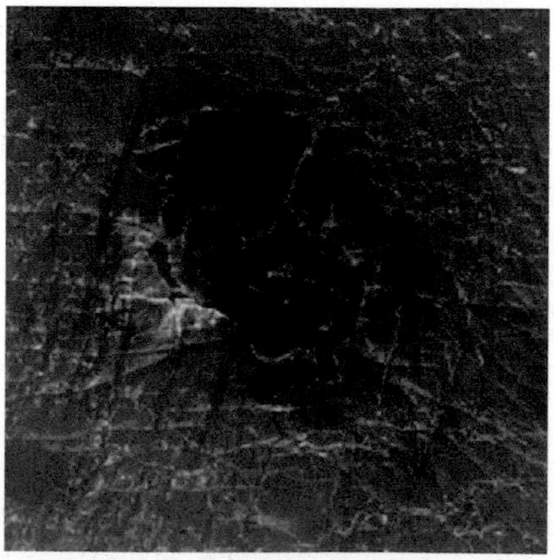

Figure 11.35 An eschar developing at the site of the bite in rickettsial disease.

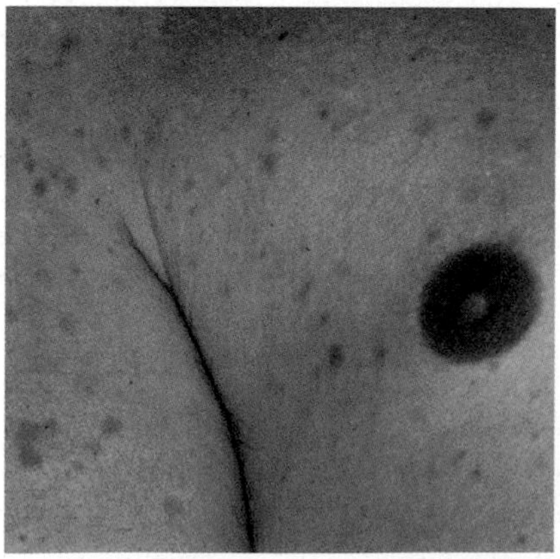

Figure 11.36 The petechial rash of rickettsial spotted fever.

Endemic (murine) typhus

This is an infection of rodents that is inadvertently spread to humans by rat fleas. The disease closely resembles epidemic typhus but is much milder and rarely fatal.

Scrub typhus

Found throughout Asia and the Western Pacific, this disease is spread by larval trombiculid mites (chiggers). An eschar (a black, crusted, necrotic papule) can often be found at the site of the bite. The clinical illness is very variable, ranging from a mild illness to fulminant and potentially fatal disease. The more severe cases resemble epidemic typhus. Unlike other types of typhus, the organism is passed on to subsequent generations of mites, which consequently act as both reservoir and vector.

Spotted fever group

A variety of *Rickettsia* species, collectively known as the spotted fever group rickettsiae, cause the illnesses known as spotted fevers. In most cases, the vector is a hard tick. Although the causative organism and the name of the illness vary from place to place, the clinical course is common to all.

The typical feature of the spotted fevers is a widespread petechial rash, although a variety of other types of skin lesion are seen especially in Rocky Mountain spotted fever. The form of African tick typhus caused by *R. africae* often presents without a rash.

After an incubation period of 4–10 days, an eschar may develop at the site of the bite in association with regional lymphadenopathy. There is abrupt onset of fever, myalgia and headache, accompanied by a maculopapular rash that may become petechial. Neurological, haematological and cardiovascular complications occur as in epidemic typhus, although these are uncommon.

Diagnosis

The diagnosis is generally made on the basis of the history and clinical course of the illness. It can be confirmed serologically or by PCR.

Management and prevention

Doxycycline or tetracycline given for 5–7 days is the treatment of choice. Ciprofloxacin is also effective. Doxycycline 200 mg weekly protects against scrub typhus; it is reserved for highly endemic areas. Rifampicin is also used when resistance to tetracycline is present. Seriously ill patients need intensive care. Control of typhus is achieved by eradication of the arthropod vectors. Lice and fleas can be eradicated from clothing by insecticides (0.5% malathion or DDT). Control of rodents is necessary in endemic typhus and some of the spotted fevers. Areas of vegetation infested with trombiculid mites can be cleared by chemical spraying from the air. Bites from ticks and mites should be avoided by wearing protective clothing on exposed areas of the body. The likelihood of infection from ticks is related to the duration of feeding; in high-risk areas, the body should be inspected twice a day, as the bites are painless, and any ticks should be removed (see p. 284).

Bartonellosis

Bartonella spp. are intracellular bacteria closely related to the rickettsiae. A number of human diseases can be caused by these organisms; as in rickettsial disease, infection is usually spread from animals via an arthropod vector ***(Box 11.49)***.

Box 11.49 Human infections caused by *Bartonella* spp. and *Ehrlichia* spp.

Disease	Organism	Reservoir	Vector
Bartonella			
Carrion's disease	*Bartonella bacilliformis*	Unknown	Sandfly
Cat-scratch disease	*B. henselae*	Cat	Cat flea
Bacillary angiomatosis	*B. henselae*	Cat	Cat flea
Trench fever	*B. quintana*	Human	Body louse
Ehrlichia			
Human monocytic ehrlichiosis (HME)	*Ehrlichia chaffeensis*	Deer	Hard tick
Human granulocytic ehrlichiosis (HGE)[a]	*Ehrlichia ewingii* *Anaplasma phagocytophilum*[b]	Small mammals and deer	Hard tick

[a]Also known as human granulocytic anaplasmosis. [b]Formerly known as *Ehrlichia phagocytophilia*.

Carrion's disease (*Bartonella bacilliformis*)

This disease is restricted mainly to the habitat of its main vector, the sandfly, in the river valleys of the Andes mountains at an altitude of 500–3000 m. Two clinical presentations are seen, which may occur alone or consecutively. ***Oroya fever*** is an acute febrile illness causing myalgia, arthralgia, severe headache and confusion, followed by a haemolytic anaemia. ***Verruga peruana*** consists of eruptions of reddish-purple haemangiomatous nodules, resembling bacillary angiomatosis. It may follow 4–6 weeks after Oroya fever or be the presenting feature of infection. Spontaneous resolution may occur over a period of months or years. Carrion's disease is frequently complicated by superinfection, especially with *Salmonella* spp.

The diagnosis is made by culturing bacilli from blood or peripheral lesions. Serological tests have been developed but are not widely available.

Treatment with chloramphenicol or tetracycline is very effective in acute disease, but less so in verruga peruana.

Cat-scratch disease and bacillary angiomatosis (*Bartonella henselae*)

These are described on page 270.

Trench fever

Trench fever is caused by *Bartonella quintana* and transmitted by human body lice. It is mainly seen in refugees and the homeless. It is characterized by cyclical fever (typically, every 5 days), chills and headaches, accompanied by myalgia and pretibial pain. The disease is usually self-limiting but it can be treated with erythromycin or doxycycline if symptoms are severe.

Ehrlichiosis

Ehrlichiosis and anaplasmosis are infections caused by tick-borne, rickettsia-like bacteria. At least three species have been implicated: *Ehrlichia chaffeensis*, which causes human monocytic ehrlichiosis (HME), and *E. ewingii* and *Anaplasma phagocytophilum* (formerly known as *E. phagocytophilum*), which cause human granulocytic ehrlichiosis (HGE, also known as human granulocytic anaplasmosis). All cause a rather non-specific febrile illness with fever, myalgia and headache. Treatment is with doxycycline. The vectors are hard ticks and the main reservoir hosts are deer. As with most tick-borne zoonoses, the avoidance of tick bites and the prompt removal of feeding ticks are the best forms of prevention.

Melioidosis

The term melioidosis refers to infections caused by the Gram-negative bacterium *Burkholderia pseudomallei*. This environmental organism, which is found in soil and surface water, is distributed widely in the tropics and subtropics. The majority of clinical cases of melioidosis occur in South-east Asia. Infection follows inhalation or direct inoculation. More than half of all patients with melioidosis have predisposing underlying disease; it is particularly common in diabetics.

B. pseudomallei causes a wide spectrum of disease and the majority of infections are probably subclinical. Illness may be acute or chronic, and localized or disseminated, but one form of the disease may progress to another and individual patients may be difficult to categorize. The most serious form is septicaemic melioidosis, which is often complicated by multiple metastatic abscesses; this is frequently fatal. Serological tests are available but definitive diagnosis depends on isolating the organism from blood or appropriate tissue. *B. pseudomallei* has extensive intrinsic antibiotic resistance. The most effective agent is ceftazidime, which is given intravenously for 2–4 weeks; this should be followed by several months of co-amoxiclav or co-trimoxazole to prevent relapses.

Actinomycosis

Actinomyces spp. are branching, Gram-positive higher bacteria, which are normal mouth and intestine commensals; they are particularly associated with poor mouth hygiene. *Actinomyces* have a worldwide distribution but are a rare cause of disease in the West.

Clinical features

- ***Cervicofacial actinomycosis***, the most common form, usually occurs following dental infection or extraction. It is often indolent and slowly progressive, is associated with little pain, and results in induration and localized swelling of the lower part of the mandible. Sinuses and tracts develop, with discharge of 'sulphur' granules.
- ***Thoracic actinomycosis*** follows inhalation of organisms, usually into a previously damaged lung. The clinical picture is not distinctive and is often mistaken for malignancy or tuberculosis. Symptoms such as fever, malaise, chest pain and haemoptysis are present. Empyema occurs in 25% of patients and local extension produces chest-wall sinuses with discharge of 'sulphur' granules.
- ***Abdominal actinomycosis*** most frequently affects the caecum. Characteristically, an indurated mass is felt in the right iliac fossa. Later, sinuses develop. The differential diagnosis includes malignancy, tuberculosis, Crohn's disease and amoeboma. The incidence of pelvic actinomycosis appears to be increasing with wider use of intrauterine contraceptive devices.

Occasionally, actinomycosis becomes disseminated to involve any site.

Diagnosis and management

Diagnosis is by microscopy and culture of the organism. Treatment often involves surgery, as well as antibiotics. Penicillin is the drug of choice. Intravenous penicillin 2.4 g 4-hourly is given for 4–6 weeks, followed by oral amoxicillin for at least 3–4 months after clinical resolution. Tetracyclines are also effective.

Nocardia infections

Nocardia spp. are Gram-positive branching bacteria, which are found in soil and decomposing organic matter. *N. asteroides* and, less often, *N. brasiliensis* are the main human pathogens.

Clinical features

Mycetoma is the most common illness. This is a result of local invasion by *Nocardia* spp. and presents as a painless swelling, usually on the sole of the foot (Madura foot). The swelling of the affected part of the body continues inexorably. Nodules gradually appear, which eventually rupture and discharge characteristic 'grains', which are colonies of organisms. Systemic symptoms and regional lymphadenopathy are rare. Sinuses may occur several years after the onset of the first symptom. A similar syndrome may be produced by other branching bacteria and also by species of eumycete fungi, such as *Madurella mycetomi* (see p. 297).

Pulmonary disease, which follows inhalation of the organism, presents with cough, fever and haemoptysis; it is usually seen in the immunocompromised. Pleural involvement and empyema occur. In severely immunosuppressed patients, initial pulmonary infection may be followed by disseminated disease.

Diagnosis and management

The diagnosis is often delayed, partly because of inadequate specimens and partly because *Nocardia* requires prolonged culture on standard media. Severe pulmonary or disseminated infection may require parenteral treatment. Co-trimoxazole, linezolid, ceftriaxone and amikacin have all been used successfully, but *in vitro* sensitivities are variable and there is no consensus on the best treatment.

Further reading

Bitam I, Dittmar K, Parola P et al. Fleas and flea-borne diseases. *Int J Infect Dis* 2010; 14:e667–e676.

Elbir H, Raoult D, Drancourt M. Relapsing fever borreliae in Africa. *Am J Trop Med Hyg* 2013; 89:288–192.

Oyston P, Williamson ED. Prophylaxis and therapy of plague. *Expert Rev Anti Infect Ther* 2013; 11:817–829.

Parola P, Paddock CD, Dance D. Treatment and prophylaxis of melioidosis. *Int J Antimicrob Agents* 2014; 43:310–318.

Simpson RS, Read RC. Nocardiosis and actinomycosis. *Medicine (UK)* 2014; 42:23–25.

Socolovschi C. Update on tick-borne rickettsioses around the world: a geographic approach. *Clin Microbiol Rev* 2013; 26:657–702.

FUNGAL INFECTIONS

Morphologically, fungi can be grouped into three major categories:

- yeasts and yeast-like fungi, which reproduce by budding
- moulds, which grow by branching and longitudinal extension of hyphae
- dimorphic fungi, which behave as yeasts in the host but as moulds *in vitro*.

Despite the fact that fungi are ubiquitous, systemic fungal infections are relatively rare (in contrast to superficial fungal infections of the skin, nails and orogenital mucosae; see pp. 1345–1347). Systemic mycoses are usually seen in immunocompromised patients and in critical care settings, and are becoming more prevalent as this population of patients increases.

Box 11.50 Common fungal infections

Systemic
- Histoplasmosis
- Cryptococcosis
- Coccidioidomycosis
- Blastomycosis
- Zygomycosis (mucormycosis)
- Candidiasis
- Aspergillosis
- *Pneumocystis jiroveci* (formerly *P. carinii*)

Subcutaneous
- Sporotrichosis
- Subcutaneous zygomycosis
- Chromoblastomycosis
- Mycetoma

Superficial
- Dermatophytosis
- Superficial candidiasis
- *Malassezia* infections

Fungal infections are transmitted by inhalation of spores, contact with the skin or direct inoculation. This last can occur through penetrating injuries, injecting drug use or iatrogenic procedures. Fungi may also produce allergic pulmonary disease. Some fungi, such as *Candida albicans*, are human commensals. Fungal infections are usually divided into systemic, subcutaneous or superficial ***(Box 11.50)***. However, these divisions can be misleading, as many fungi that cause superficial infection in the healthy host can cause invasive or disseminated infection in immunocompromised patients, while 'deep' subcutaneous infections can invade other organs to cause systemic disease (see 'Further reading').

SYSTEMIC FUNGAL INFECTIONS

Candidiasis

Candidiasis is the most common fungal infection in humans and is predominantly caused by *Candida albicans*, although other species of *Candida* are increasingly recognized. *Candida* are small asexual yeasts. They are found worldwide, and most species that are pathogenic to humans are normal oropharyngeal and gastrointestinal commensals.

Clinical features

Most human candidiasis is superficial. Vaginal and oral thrush are the most common forms; these are typically seen in the very young, the elderly, patients on antibiotic therapy and those who are immunosuppressed. Candidal oesophagitis presents with painful dysphagia. Cutaneous candidiasis typically occurs in intertriginous areas. It is also a cause of paronychia.

Invasive candidiasis is usually associated with intravascular devices (especially in intensive care units) and with profound immunosuppression. Dissemination can lead to meningitis, visceral and pulmonary abscesses, endophthalmitis and osteomyelitis.

Diagnosis and management

The fungi can be demonstrated in scrapings from infected lesions, tissue secretions or, in invasive disease, from blood cultures.

Treatment varies, depending on the site and severity of infection, and on the sensitivity of the organism. Superficial lesions may respond to topical nystatin or amphotericin B, although systemic agents may be needed for more extensive infection. For invasive infection, parenteral therapy with amphotericin B, fluconazole, voriconazole or echinocandins is necessary. Many non-*albicans* species are intrinsically resistant to many antifungals, and even *C. albicans* can develop extensive resistance (especially to azoles).

Histoplasmosis

Histoplasmosis is caused by *Histoplasma capsulatum* (see p. 348). Spores can survive in moist soil for several years, particularly when it is enriched by bird and bat droppings. Histoplasmosis occurs worldwide but is commonly seen only in Ohio and the Mississippi river valleys, where over 80% of the population have been subclinically exposed. Transmission is mainly by inhalation of the spores, particularly when clearing out attics, barns and bird roosts or exploring caves.

Clinical features

Primary pulmonary histoplasmosis is usually asymptomatic. Calcification in the lungs, spleen and liver occurs in patients from areas of high endemicity. When symptomatic, primary pulmonary histoplasmosis generally presents as a mild influenza-like illness, with fever, chills, myalgia and cough. The systemic symptoms are pronounced in severe disease.

Complications, such as atelectasis, secondary bacterial pneumonia, pleural effusions, erythema nodosum and erythema multiforme, also occur.

Chronic pulmonary histoplasmosis is clinically similar to pulmonary tuberculosis (see p. 1108). It is usually seen in American white males over the age of 50 years. Disseminated histoplasmosis resembles disseminated tuberculosis, with fever, lymphadenopathy, hepatosplenomegaly, weight loss, leucopenia and thrombocytopenia. Rarely, features of meningitis, hepatitis, hypoadrenalism, endocarditis and peritonitis may dominate the clinical picture.

Diagnosis

Definitive diagnosis is possible by culturing the fungi (e.g. from sputum) or by demonstrating them on histological sections. *H. capsulatum* glycoprotein can be detected in the urine and serum in those with acute pulmonary and disseminated infection. Antibodies usually develop within 3 weeks of the onset of illness and are best detected by complement fixation or immunodiffusion (sensitivity of 95% and 90%, respectively).

Management

Only symptomatic acute pulmonary histoplasmosis, chronic histoplasmosis and acute disseminated histoplasmosis require therapy. Itraconazole is effective in mild to moderate disease. Severe infection is treated with intravenous amphotericin B for 1–2 weeks, followed by itraconazole for a total of 12 weeks, or with voriconazole. Surgical excision of histoplasmomas (pulmonary granuloma due to *H. capsulatum*) or chronic cavitatory lung lesions and release of adhesions following mediastinitis are often required.

African histoplasmosis

This is caused by *Histoplasma duboisii*, the spores of which are larger than those of *H. capsulatum*. Skin lesions (e.g. abscesses, nodules, lymph node involvement and lytic bone lesions) are prominent. Pulmonary lesions do not occur. Treatment is similar to that for *H. capsulatum* infection.

Aspergillosis

Aspergillosis is caused by one of several species of dimorphic fungi of the genus *Aspergillus*. Of these, *A. fumigatus* is the most common, although *A. flavus* and *A. niger* are also recognized. These fungi are ubiquitous in the environment and are commonly found on decaying leaves and trees. Humans are infected by inhalation of the spores.

Disease manifestation depends on the dose of the spores inhaled, as well as the immune response of the host. Three major forms of the disease are recognized: bronchopulmonary allergic aspergillosis, aspergilloma and invasive aspergillosis (see p. 1123).

The diagnosis and treatment are described in more detail on pages 1122–1123.

Cryptococcosis

Cryptococcosis is caused by the yeast-like fungus *Cryptococcus neoformans*. It has a worldwide distribution and appears to be spread by birds, especially pigeons, in their droppings. The spores gain entry into the body through the respiratory tract, where they elicit a granulomatous reaction. Pulmonary symptoms are, however, uncommon; meningitis, which usually occurs in those with HIV infection or lymphoma, is the usual mode of presentation and often develops subacutely. Less commonly, lung cavitation, hilar lymphadenopathy, pleural effusions and, occasionally, pulmonary fibrosis occur. Skin and bone involvement is rare.

Diagnosis and management

Diagnosis is established by demonstrating the organisms in appropriately stained tissue sections. A positive latex cryptococcal agglutinin test performed on the CSF is diagnostic of cryptococcosis.

Liposomal amphotericin B alone or in combination with flucytosine for 2 weeks is followed by oral fluconazole 400 mg daily. Therapy should be continued for 8 weeks if meningitis is present. Fluconazole has greater CSF penetration and is used when toxicity is encountered with amphotericin B and flucytosine, and as maintenance therapy in immunocompromised patients, especially those with HIV infection (see pp. 349–350).

Coccidioidomycosis

Coccidioidomycosis is caused by the non-budding spherical form (spherule) of *Coccidioides immitis*. This is a soil saprophyte and is found in the southern USA, Central America and parts of South America. Humans are infected by inhalation of the thick-walled, barrel-shaped spores called arthrospores. Occasionally, epidemics of coccidioidomycosis have been documented following dust storms.

Clinical features

The majority of patients are asymptomatic and the infection is only detected by the conversion of a skin test using coccidioidin (extract from a culture of mycelial growth of *C. immitis*) from negative to positive. Acute pulmonary coccidioidomycosis presents, after an incubation period of about 10 days, with fever, malaise, cough and expectoration. Erythema nodosum, erythema multiforme, phlyctenular conjunctivitis and, less commonly, pleural effusions may occur. Complete recovery is usual.

Pulmonary cavitation with haemoptysis, pulmonary fibrosis, meningitis, lytic bone lesions, hepatosplenomegaly, skin ulcers and abscesses may occur in severe disease.

Diagnosis

The organism can be identified in respiratory secretions and can be cultured in specialist laboratories. Serological tests are also widely used for diagnosis. These include the highly specific latex agglutination and precipitin tests (IgM), which are positive within 2 weeks of infection and decline thereafter. Other tests include complement fixation, ELISA and radioimmunoassay.

A complement-fixation test (IgG) performed on the CSF is diagnostic of coccidioidomycosis meningitis; it becomes positive within 4–6 weeks and remains so for many years.

Management

Mild pulmonary infections are self-limiting and require no treatment, but progressive and disseminated disease requires urgent therapy. Ketoconazole, itraconazole or fluconazole for 6 months is the treatment of choice for primary pulmonary disease, with more prolonged courses for cavitating or fibronodular disease. Fluconazole in high dose (600–1000 mg daily) is given for meningitis. Itraconazole provides an alternative. Voriconazole and posaconazole are used for poor responders. Surgical excision of cavitatory pulmonary lesions or localized bone lesions may be necessary.

Blastomycosis

Blastomycosis is a systemic infection caused by the biphasic fungus *Blastomyces dermatitidis*. Although initially believed to be confined to certain parts of North America, it has been reported from South America, India and the Middle East.

Clinical features

Blastomycosis primarily involves the skin, where it presents as non-itchy papular lesions that later develop into ulcers with red verrucous margins. The ulcers are initially confined to the exposed parts of the body but later involve the unexposed parts as well. Atrophy and scarring may occur. Pulmonary involvement presents as a solitary lesion resembling a malignancy or gives rise to radiological features similar to the primary complex of tuberculosis. Systemic symptoms, such as fever, malaise, cough and weight loss, are usually present. Bone lesions are common and present as painful swellings.

Diagnosis and management

The diagnosis is confirmed by demonstrating the organism in histological sections or by culture, although results can be negative in 30–50% of cases. Enzyme immunoassay may be helpful, although there is some cross-reactivity of antibodies to *Blastomyces* with *Histoplasma*.

Itraconazole is preferred for treating mild to moderate disease in the immunocompetent for periods up to 6 months. Ketoconazole or fluconazole is also used. In severe or unresponsive disease and in the immunocompromised, amphotericin B is indicated.

Mucormycosis

The terminology of mucormycosis and zygomycosis is confusing. ***Invasive zygomycosis*** (also known as ***mucormycosis***) is rare and is caused by several fungi, including *Mucor* spp., *Rhizopus* spp. and *Absidia* spp. It usually occurs in immunocompromised or severely ill patients, and has a high mortality. The hallmark of the disease is vascular invasion with marked haemorrhagic necrosis.

Rhinocerebral mucormycosis is a specific, locally invasive form of the condition. Nasal stuffiness, facial pain and oedema, and necrotic, black nasal turbinates are characteristic. It is rare and is mainly seen in diabetics with ketoacidosis.

Other forms of invasive zygomycosis include pulmonary and disseminated infection (in immunosuppressed patients) and gastrointestinal infection (in malnutrition).

Subcutaneous zygomycosis is described below.

Management of locally invasive and systemic disease is with amphotericin B and surgical debridement, but even with the best care, mortality exceeds 50%.

Further reading

Arenas R, Moreno-Couteno G, Welsh O. Classification of subcutaneous and systemic mycoses. *Clin Dermatol* 2012; 30:369–371.

Gamaletsou MN, Walsh TJ, Zaoutis T. A prospective, cohort, multicentre study of candidaemia in hospitalized adult patients with haematological malignancies. *Clin Microbiol Infect* 2014; 20:O50–O57.

Kullberg BJ, Arendrup MC. Invasive Candidiasis. *N Engl J Med* 2015; 373:1445–1456.

SUBCUTANEOUS FUNGAL INFECTIONS

Sporotrichosis

Sporotrichosis is caused by the saprophytic fungus *Sporothrix schenckii*, which is found worldwide. Infection usually follows cutaneous inoculation, at the site of which a reddish, non-tender, maculopapular lesion develops; this is referred to as 'plaque sporotrichosis'. Pulmonary involvement and disseminated disease rarely occur.

Treatment with itraconazole 100–200 mg/day for 3–6 months is usually curative.

Subcutaneous zygomycosis

Subcutaneous zygomycosis can be seen as a form of mucormycosis in immunocompromised patients, as described above. However, the term is also used to describe a largely tropical condition caused by filamentous fungi of the *Basidiobolus* genus, and typically associated with inoculation injuries and trauma. The disease usually remains confined to the subcutaneous tissues and muscle fascia. It presents as a brawny, woody infiltration involving the limbs, neck and trunk. Amphotericin B is the drug of choice, usually in combination with surgical debridement. Even the cutaneous/subcutaneous form of the infection carries a significant mortality.

Chromoblastomycosis

Chromoblastomycosis (chromomycosis) is caused by fungi of various genera, including *Phialophora*, *Wangella* and *Fonsecaea*. These are found mainly in tropical and subtropical countries. Chromoblastomycosis presents initially as a small papule, usually at the site of a previous injury, which persists for several months before ulcerating. The lesion later becomes warty and encrusted, and gradually spreads. Satellite lesions may be present. Itching is frequent. The drug of choice is amphotericin B in combination with itraconazole or voriconazole. Cryosurgery is used to remove local lesions.

Mycetoma (Madura foot)

Mycetoma may be due to subcutaneous infection with fungi (*Eumycetes* spp.) or bacteria (see p. 294). It is largely confined to the tropics. Infection results in local swelling, which may discharge through sinuses. Bone involvement may follow.

Management consists of surgical debridement, combined with antimicrobials chosen according to the aetiological agent.

Pneumocystis jiroveci infection

Genetic analysis has shown *P. jiroveci* to be homologous with fungi. *Pneumocystis jiroveci* disease is almost invariably associated with immunodeficiency states, particularly AIDS, and is discussed on page 349.

Further reading

Queiroz-Telles F, Nucci M, Colombo AL et al. Mycoses of implantation in Latin America: an overview of epidemiology, clinical manifestations, diagnosis and treatment. *Med Mycol* 2011; 49:225–236.

SUPERFICIAL FUNGAL INFECTIONS

Dermatophytosis

Dermatophytoses are chronic fungal infections of keratinous structures, such as the skin, hair or nails. *Trichophyton* spp., *Microsporum* spp., *Epidermophyton* spp. and *Candida* spp. can also infect keratinous structures.

Malassezia infection

Malassezia spp. are found on the scalp and greasy skin, and are responsible for seborrhoeic dermatitis, pityriasis versicolor (hypo- or hyperpigmented rash on the trunk) and *Malassezia* folliculitis (itchy rash on the back).

Treatment is with topical antifungals, or oral ketoconazole if infection is refractory or more extensive.

PROTOZOAL INFECTIONS

Protozoa are unicellular eukaryotic organisms. They are more complex than bacteria and belong to the animal kingdom. Although many protozoa are free-living in the environment, some have become parasites of vertebrates, including humans, often developing complex life cycles involving more than one host species. In order to be transmitted to a new host, some protozoa transform into hardy cyst forms, which can survive harsh external conditions. Others are transmitted by an arthropod vector, in which a further replication cycle takes place before infection of a new vertebrate host.

BLOOD AND TISSUE PROTOZOA

Malaria

Human malaria is usually caused by one of four species of the genus *Plasmodium*: *P. falciparum*, *P. vivax*, *P. ovale* and *P. malariae*. Occasionally, other species of malaria usually found in primates (e.g. *P. knowlesi*) can affect humans. Malaria probably originated from animal malarias in Central Africa but was spread around the globe by human migration. Public health measures and changes in land use have eradicated malaria in most developed countries, although the potential for malaria transmission still exists in many areas. Some 220 million people were infected in 2010, with 650 000 deaths (mainly in African children). Over 25 000 infections per year occur in travellers from non-malarious countries.

Epidemiology

Malaria is transmitted by the bite of female anopheline mosquitoes. The parasite undergoes a temperature-dependent cycle of development in the gut of the insect and its geographical range therefore depends on the presence of the appropriate mosquito species and an adequate temperature. The disease occurs in endemic or epidemic form throughout the tropics and subtropics, except for some areas above 2000 m (*Fig. 11.37*).

In areas of so-called ***stable transmission*** (including much of sub-Saharan Africa), transmission occurs consistently year round. The bulk of mortality is seen in children, while those who survive to adulthood acquire significant immunity; low-grade parasitaemia is still present but causes few symptoms. ***Unstable transmission***

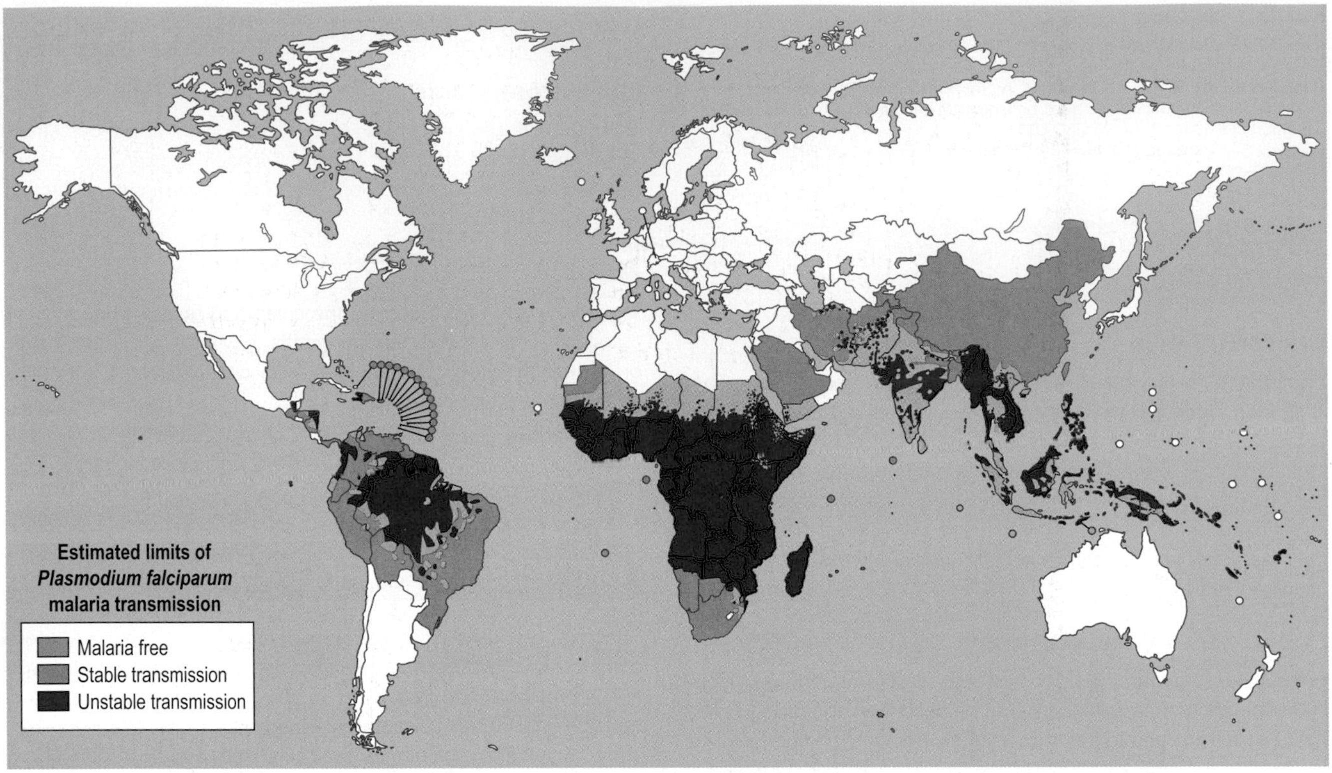

Figure 11.37 ***Plasmodium falciparum*** **malaria transmission: geographical distribution.** ***Grey areas*** are likely to be risk-free. This arises either because health surveillance reports 0 cases for 3 years, because low temperatures or high aridity are likely to preclude transmission, or because specific medical intelligence exists defining the area as risk-free. ***Pink areas*** are where local transmission cannot be ruled out but levels of risk are extremely low, with annual case incidence reported at less than 1 per 10 000. ***Red areas*** are at risk of stable malaria transmission. This is a very broad classification of risk, including any regions where the annual case incidence is likely to exceed 1 per 10 000. *(From Malaria Atlas Project, with permission; http://www.map.ox.ac.uk/browse-resources/transmission-limits/Pf_limits/world/.)*

occurs when there is erratic, seasonal or low-level transmission (e.g. in the Sahel belt, mosquitoes feed only in the rainy season). In these circumstances, little protective immunity develops and symptomatic malaria occurs at all ages. Changes in environmental or social conditions in such areas can lead to epidemics with substantial mortality in all age groups.

Malaria can also be transmitted in contaminated blood transfusions. It has occasionally been seen in injecting drug users sharing needles and in patients with a hospital-acquired infection related to contaminated equipment. Rare cases are acquired outside the tropics when mosquitoes are transported from endemic areas ('airport malaria'), or when the local mosquito population becomes infected by a returning traveller.

Parasitology

The female mosquito becomes infected after taking a blood meal containing gametocytes, the sexual form of the malarial parasite ***(Fig. 11.38)***. The developmental cycle in the mosquito usually takes 7–20 days (depending on temperature), culminating in the migration of infective sporozoites to the insect's salivary glands. The sporozoites are inoculated into a new human host and those not destroyed by the immune response are rapidly taken up by the liver. Here they multiply inside hepatocytes as merozoites: this is pre-erythrocytic (or hepatic) sporogeny. After a few days, the infected hepatocytes rupture, releasing merozoites into the blood, from where they are rapidly taken up by erythrocytes. In the case of *P. vivax* and *P. ovale*, a few parasites remain dormant in the liver as hypnozoites. These may reactivate at any time subsequently, causing relapsing infection.

Inside the red cells, the parasites again multiply, changing from merozoite, to trophozoite, to schizont and finally appearing as 8–24 new merozoites. The erythrocyte ruptures, releasing the merozoites to infect further cells. Each cycle of this process, which is called erythrocytic schizogony, takes about 48 hours in *P. falciparum*, *P. vivax* and *P. ovale* disease and about 72 hours in *P. malariae* disease. *P. vivax* and *P. ovale* mainly attack reticulocytes and young erythrocytes, while *P. malariae* tends to attack older cells; *P. falciparum* will parasitize any stage of erythrocyte.

A few merozoites develop not into trophozoites but into gametocytes. These are not released from the red cells until taken up by a feeding mosquito to complete the life cycle.

Pathogenesis

The pathology of malaria is related to anaemia, cytokine release and, in the case of *P. falciparum*, widespread organ damage due to impaired microcirculation. The anaemia seen in malaria is multifactorial ***(Box 11.51)***. In *P. falciparum* malaria, red cells containing schizonts adhere to the lining of capillaries in the brain, kidneys, gut, liver and other organs. As well as causing mechanical obstruction, these schizonts rupture, releasing toxins and stimulating further cytokine release.

After repeated infections, partial immunity develops, allowing the host to tolerate parasitaemia with minimal ill effects. This immunity is largely lost if there is no further infection for a couple of years.

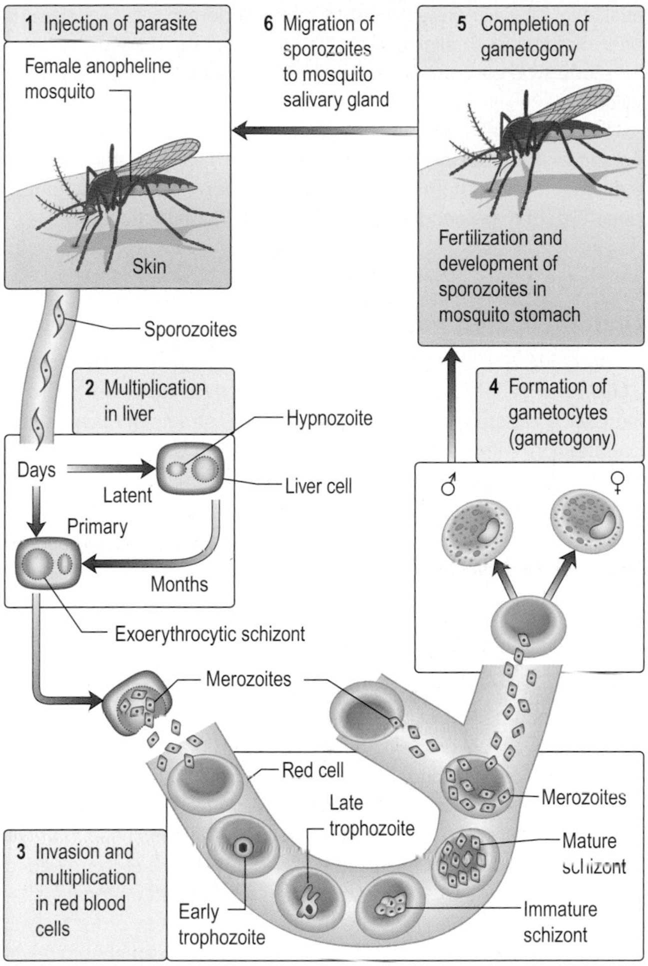

Figure 11.38 A schematic life cycle of *Plasmodium vivax*.

Box 11.51 Causes of anaemia in malaria infection

- Haemolysis of infected red cells
- Haemolysis of non-infected red cells (blackwater fever)
- Dyserythropoiesis
- Splenomegaly and sequestration
- Folate depletion

Certain genetic traits also confer some immunity to malaria. People who lack the Duffy antigen on the red cell membrane (a common finding in West Africa) are not susceptible to infection with *P. vivax*. Certain haemoglobinopathies (including sickle cell trait) also give some protection against the severe effects of malaria; this may account for the persistence of these otherwise harmful mutations in tropical countries. Iron deficiency may also have some protective effect. The spleen appears to play a role in controlling infection and splenectomized people are at risk of overwhelming malaria. Some individuals appear to have a genetic predisposition for developing cerebral malaria following infection with *P. falciparum*. Pregnant women are especially susceptible to severe disease.

Clinical features

Typical malaria is seen in non-immune individuals. This includes children in any area, adults in areas of unstable transmission, and any visitors from a non-malarious region.

The normal incubation period is 10–21 days but can be longer. The most common symptom is fever, although malaria may present initially with general malaise, headache, vomiting or diarrhoea. At first, the fever may be continual or erratic; the classical tertian or quartan fever appears only after some days. The temperature often reaches 41°C and is accompanied by rigors and drenching sweats.

P. *vivax* or *P. ovale* infection

The illness is usually relatively mild (although *P. vivax* can occasionally cause severe disease). Anaemia develops slowly and there may be tender hepatosplenomegaly. Spontaneous recovery usually occurs within 2–6 weeks but hypnozoites in the liver can cause relapses for many years after infection. Repeated infections often cause chronic ill health due to anaemia and hyper-reactive splenomegaly.

P. *malariae* infection

This also causes a relatively mild illness but tends to run a more chronic course. Parasitaemia may persist for years, with or without symptoms. In children, *P. malariae* infection is associated with glomerulonephritis and nephrotic syndrome.

P. *falciparum* infection

This causes, in many cases, a self-limiting illness similar to the other types of malaria, although the paroxysms of fever are usually less marked. However, it may also cause serious complications ***(Fig. 11.39)*** and the vast majority of malaria deaths are due to *P. falciparum*. Patients can deteriorate rapidly, and children in particular progress from reasonable health to coma and death within hours. A high parasitaemia (>1% of red cells infected) is an indicator of severe disease, although patients with apparently low parasite levels may also develop complications (peripheral parasite counts can be misleading, as many parasitized cells are sequestered in the microcirculation). ***Cerebral malaria*** is marked by diminished consciousness, confusion and convulsions, often progressing to coma and death. Untreated, it is universally fatal. ***Blackwater fever*** is due to widespread intravascular haemolysis, affecting both parasitized and unparasitized red cells, giving rise to dark urine.

Hyper-reactive malarial splenomegaly (tropical splenomegaly syndrome)

This is seen in older children and adults in areas where malaria is hyperendemic. It is associated with an exaggerated immune response to repeated malaria infections and is characterized by anaemia, massive splenomegaly and elevated IgM levels. Malaria parasites are scanty or absent. Tropical splenomegaly syndrome usually responds to prolonged treatment with prophylactic antimalarial drugs.

Diagnosis

Malaria should be in the differential diagnosis of anyone who presents with a febrile illness in, or having recently left, a malarious area. *Falciparum* malaria is unlikely to present more than 3 months after exposure, even if the patient has been taking prophylaxis, but *vivax* malaria may cause symptoms for the first time up to a year after leaving a malarious area.

Diagnosis is usually made by identifying parasites on a Giemsa-stained thick or thin blood film (thick films are more difficult to interpret and it may be difficult to speciate the parasite, but they have a higher yield). At least three films should be examined before malaria is declared unlikely. Rapid antigen detection tests are

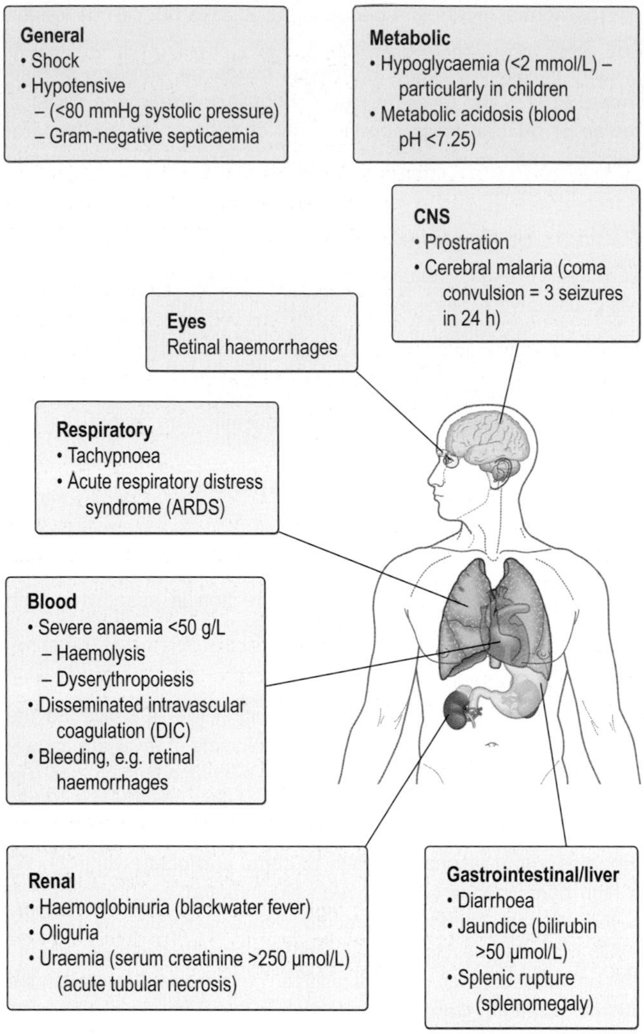

Figure 11.39 Features of severe *falciparum* malaria.

available for near-patient use. In many endemic areas, malaria is over-diagnosed on clinical grounds and a definite diagnosis should be made wherever possible. Serological tests are of no diagnostic value.

Parasitaemia is common in endemic areas and the presence of parasites does not necessarily mean that malaria is the cause of the patient's symptoms. Further investigation, including a lumbar puncture, may be needed to exclude bacterial infection.

Management

Uncomplicated malaria

Chloroquine is still widely used to treat non-*falciparum* malaria ***(Box 11.52)***, and in many areas it remains effective. However, there is increasing resistance to chloroquine in some strains of *P. vivax*, and co-infection with *P. falciparum* is common in some parts of the world. It is therefore sensible to use oral artemisinin combination therapy, where available, for all cases of malaria. Following successful treatment of *P. vivax* or *P. ovale* malaria, it is necessary to give a 2- to 3-week course of primaquine (0.25–0.5 mg daily) to eradicate the hepatic hypnozoites and prevent relapse. This drug can precipitate haemolysis in patients with glucose-6-phosphate dehydrogenase deficiency (see pp. 541–543).

The artemisinin-based drugs are the most effective treatment for both uncomplicated and severe infections with *P. falciparum*, in adults and in children. Artemisinin-based combination therapy (ACT) is the recommended oral treatment for uncomplicated *falciparum* malaria worldwide. These drugs are now quite widely available, partly through the efforts of the Global Fund (see 'Further reading'). Five different fixed-dose combinations are recommended by the WHO ***(Box 11.53)***; the choice should be based on local resistance to the 'partner' drug (see 'Further reading'). In order to limit the development of resistance, artemisinin derivatives should never be given as monotherapy; some resistance has already been reported in parts of South-east Asia, although, at present, this can usually be overcome by using longer courses of treatment. The WHO recommends that a single dose of primaquine should be given as a gametocide, to decrease transmission.

Box 11.52 Drug treatment of uncomplicated malaria

Parasite	Drugs	Regimen	Plus	Regimen
P. vivax *P. ovale* *P. malariae*	Chloroquine	600 mg[a] 300 mg[b] 6 h later 300 mg 24 h later 300 mg 24 h later	Primaquine	0.25–0.5 mg/kg/day for 2–3 weeks
	or (if known resistance to chloroquine, or dual infection with P. falciparum*)*			
	ACT (not artesunate + SP)	3 days	Primaquine	0.25–0.5 mg/kg/day for 2–3 weeks
P. falciparum (adults, endemic zone)	ACT	3 days	Primaquine	0.75 mg/kg single dose
	or (if not available)			
	Quinine + doxycycline	7 days	Primaquine	0.75 mg/kg single dose
P. falciparum (pregnant women)	First trimester: quinine + doxycycline[c] Second/third trimesters: ACT	7 days 3 days		
P. falciparum (infants)	ACT	3 days; appropriate dose for body weight	Primaquine	0.75 mg/kg single dose
P. falciparum (returning traveller)	Atovaquone-proguanil or quinine + doxycycline	7 days		

[a]10 mg/kg in children. [b]5 mg/kg in children. [c]Only use ACT if quinine not available. ACT, artemisinin-based combination therapy; SP, sulfadoxine–pyrimethamine.

Severe *falciparum* malaria

Severe malaria, indicated by the presence of any of the complications discussed above, or a parasite count >1% in a non-immune patient, is a medical emergency ***(Box 11.54)***. Anyone involved in managing patients with malaria should be familiar with the latest WHO guidelines.

- Intravenous artesunate is more effective than intravenous quinine and should be used where available. Absorption from intramuscular injection is less reliable than that from intravenous injection.
- Intensive care facilities may be needed, including mechanical ventilation and dialysis.
- Severe anaemia may require transfusion.
- Careful monitoring of fluid balance is essential; both pulmonary oedema and pre-renal failure are common.
- Hypoglycaemia can be induced both by the infection itself and by quinine treatment.
- Superadded bacterial infection is common.

Box 11.53 Suitable artemisinin combination therapies (ACT) for malaria

Drugs	Regimen
Fixed-dose combination tablets available	
Artemether–lumefantrine	4 tablets twice daily for 3 days[a]
Artesunate–amodiaquine	4 mg/kg per day artesunate for 3 days
Dihydroartemisinin–piperaquine	4 mg/kg per day dihydroartemisinin for 3 days
Available as fixed-dose, co-packaged, separate tablets	
Artesunate–mefloquine[b]	4 mg/kg per day artesunate for 3 days
Artesunate–sulfadoxine–pyrimethamine[c]	4 mg/kg per day artesunate for 3 days
Alternatives where no combination packages are available	
Artesunate + clindamycin	2 mg/kg per day + 10 mg/kg twice daily for 7 days
Artesunate + doxycycline	2 mg/kg per day + 3.5 mg/kg per day for 7 days

[a]Adult dose: reduce dose by body weight for children. [b]Combination tablet available soon. [c]Not suitable for *P. vivax* or mixed infections. Different fixed-dose combinations available.

Prevention and control

Malaria is a priority for the WHO, which announced its 'Roll Back Malaria campaign' in 1998. This has had considerable success, and global malaria-specific mortality decreased by 25% between 2000 and 2010. Some countries either have eradicated malaria or plan to do so soon, but for much of Africa the aim remains control rather than eradication. A three-part strategy is now widely endorsed and supported by governments and non-governmental organizations ***(Box 11.55)***.

As with many vector-borne diseases, control of malaria relies on a combination of case treatment, vector eradication and personal protection from vector bites, such as that provided by insecticide (permethrin)-treated nets. Mosquito eradication is usually achieved by a combination of insecticide use (e.g. house spraying with DDT) and manipulation of the habitat (e.g. marsh drainage). Alongside these elements, there has been renewed interest in chemoprevention, in which children in endemic areas are given monthly doses of antimalarials during the rainy season. This has been shown to reduce the incidence of malaria but may lead to an increased risk of drug resistance. Pregnant women, who are at greater risk of complications from malaria, may also be offered chemoprevention (although drug options are limited). Enormous effort (and resource) has been devoted to the search for a malaria vaccine. A new vaccine may soon be available, as it has shown benefit in a phase 3 study.

Non-immune travellers to malarious areas should take measures to avoid insect bites, such as using insect repellent (diethyltoluamide (DEET) 20–50% in lotions and sprays) and sleeping under mosquito nets. Antimalarial prophylaxis should also be taken in most cases, although this is never 100% effective ***(Box 11.56)***. The precise choice of prophylactic regimen depends both on the individual traveller and on the specific itinerary; further details can be found in national formularies or travel advice centres.

Box 11.55 Strategy for controlling malaria

1. Aggressive control in highly endemic countries, to reduce mortality and decrease transmission
2. Progressive eradication at the endemic margins, to shrink the 'malaria map'
3. Research into new vaccines, new drugs, new diagnostics and better ways of delivering malaria care

Box 11.54 Drug treatment of severe *falciparum* malaria in adults and children

Drug/route	Immediate dose	Subsequent doses
Severe malaria is an emergency: after rapid assessment and confirmation of diagnosis, if possible, treatment should be started with whatever parenteral treatment is available. The options, in order of preference, are:		
1. Intravenous artesunate	2.4 mg/kg	2.4 mg/kg at 12 and 24 h, then daily (up to 7 days)
2. Intravenous quinine	20 mg/kg[a]	10 mg/kg 8-hourly (up to 7 days)
3. Intramuscular artesunate	2.4 mg/kg	2.4 mg/kg at 12 and 24 h, then daily (up to 7 days)
4. Intramuscular artemether	3.2 mg/kg	1.6 mg/kg daily
5. Rectal artesunate	10 mg/kg	Transfer to centre where parenteral therapy available
Continue parenteral treatment for at least 24 h, regardless of improvement in condition. After this, if the patient is improving, switch to oral therapy to complete 7 days with:		
ACT *Or* Quinine + doxycycline	*Plus*	Primaquine 0.75 mg/kg single dose

[a]10 mg/kg if patient has already received oral quinine or mefloquine. ACT, artemisinin-based combination therapy.

Box 11.56 Malaria prophylaxis for adult travellers

Area visited	Prophylactic regimen	Alternative
No chloroquine resistance	Chloroquine 300 mg weekly	Proguanil 200 mg daily
Limited chloroquine resistance	Chloroquine 300 mg weekly *plus* Proguanil 200 mg daily	Doxycycline 100 mg daily *or* Malarone 1 tablet daily *or* Mefloquine 250 mg weekly
Significant chloroquine resistance	Mefloquine 250 mg weekly	Doxycycline 100 mg daily *or* Malarone 1 tablet daily

Trypanosomiasis

African trypanosomiasis (sleeping sickness)

Sleeping sickness is caused by trypanosomes transmitted to humans by the bite of the tsetse fly (genus *Glossina*). It is endemic in a belt across sub-Saharan Africa, extending to about 14°N and 20°S: this marks the natural range of the tsetse fly. Two subspecies of trypanosome cause human sleeping sickness: *Trypanosoma brucei gambiense* ('Gambian sleeping sickness') and *T. b. rhodesiense* ('Rhodesian sleeping sickness').

Epidemiology

Sleeping sickness due to T. b. gambiense is found in an area stretching from Uganda in Central Africa, west to Senegal and south as far as Angola. Humans are the major reservoir and infection is transmitted by riverine *Glossina* species (e.g. *G. palpalis*).

Sleeping sickness due to T. b. rhodesiense occurs in East and Central Africa from Ethiopia to Botswana. It is a zoonosis of both wild and domestic animals. In endemic situations, it is maintained in game animals and transmitted by savannah flies such as *G. morsitans*. Epidemics are usually related to cattle and the vectors are riverine flies.

Political upheavals during the 1990s disrupted established treatment and control programmes, resulting in major epidemics in Angola, the Democratic Republic of Congo (DRC) and Uganda. By 1997, as many as 500 000 people were affected by sleeping sickness. A concerted control programme has brought this number down to below 30 000, most of whom are in DRC and the Central African Republic.

Parasitology

Tsetse flies bite during the day and, unlike most arthropod vectors, both males and females take blood meals. An infected insect may deposit metacyclic trypomastigotes (the infective form of the parasite) into the subcutaneous tissue. These cause local inflammation ('trypanosomal chancre') and regional lymphadenopathy. Within 2–3 weeks, the organisms invade the bloodstream, subsequently spreading to all parts of the body, including the brain.

Clinical features

T. b. gambiense causes a chronic, slowly progressive illness. Episodes of fever and lymphadenopathy occur over months or years and hepatosplenomegaly may develop. Eventually, infection reaches the CNS, causing headache, behavioural changes, confusion and daytime somnolence. As the disease progresses, patients may develop tremors, ataxia, convulsions and hemiplegias; eventually, coma and death supervene. Histologically, there is a lymphocytic meningoencephalitis, with scattered trypanosomes visible in the brain substance.

T. b. rhodesiense sleeping sickness is a much more acute disease. Early systemic features may include myocarditis, hepatitis and serous effusions, and patients can die before the onset of CNS disease. If they survive, cerebral involvement occurs within weeks of infection and is rapidly progressive.

Box 11.57 Drugs used in the treatment of African trypanosomiasis

Disease stage	*Trypanosoma brucei gambiense*	*Trypanosoma brucei rhodesiense*
1	Pentamidine	Suramin[a]
2 (CNS)	Eflornithine + nifurtimox Eflornithine monotherapy (melarsoprol)	Melarsoprol

[a]Severe allergic reactions common: give test dose.

Diagnosis

Trypanosomes may be seen on Giemsa-stained smears of thick or thin blood films, or of lymph node aspirate. Blood films are usually positive in *T. b. rhodesiense* infection but may be negative in *T. b. gambiense* disease; concentration techniques may increase the yield. Serological tests are useful for screening for infection; the card agglutination test for trypanosomiasis (CATT) is a robust and easy-to-use field assay. Examination of CSF is essential in patients with evidence of trypanosomal infection. CNS involvement causes lymphocytosis and elevated protein in the CSF, and parasites may be seen in concentrated specimens.

Management

The treatment of sleeping sickness had remained largely unchanged for more than 40 years, but better drugs are now available for *T. b. gambiense* infection and further new agents are undergoing clinical trials. In both forms of disease, treatment is usually effective if given before the onset of CNS involvement ***(Box 11.57)***. A single dose of suramin should be given to patients with parasitaemia prior to lumbar puncture, to avoid inoculation into the CSF. The treatment of choice for second-stage (CNS) disease in *T. b. gambiense* is a combination of eflornithine and nifurtimox, a therapy introduced in 2009 and provided free of charge via the WHO. Melarsoprol remains the only treatment for CNS infection with *T. b. rhodesiense*. It is extremely toxic: 2–10% of patients develop an acute encephalopathy, with a 50–75% mortality; peripheral neuropathy and hepatorenal toxicity are also common. Between 3% and 6% of patients relapse following melarsoprol treatment.

Control

Control programmes coordinated by the WHO have been effective in many areas. As in many vector-borne diseases, prevention depends largely on elimination, control or avoidance of the vector.

South American trypanosomiasis (Chagas' disease)

Chagas' disease is widely distributed in rural areas of South and Central America, where up to 8 million people are infected. It is caused by *Trypanosoma cruzi*, which is transmitted to humans in the faeces of blood-sucking reduviid bugs (also called cone-nose or assassin bugs). Faeces infected with *T. cruzi* trypomastigotes are rubbed in through skin abrasions, mucosa or conjunctiva. The bugs, which live in mud or thatch buildings, feed on a variety of vertebrate hosts (e.g. rats, opossums) at night, defecating as they do so.

The parasites spread in the bloodstream before entering host cells and multiplying. Cell rupture releases them back into the circulation, where they can be taken up by a feeding bug. Further multiplication takes place in the insect gut, completing the trypanosome life cycle. Human infection can also occur via contaminated blood transfusion or, occasionally, by transplacental spread.

Clinical features

Acute infection

This usually occurs in children and often passes unnoticed. A firm, reddish papule is sometimes seen at the site of entry, associated with regional lymphadenopathy. In the case of conjunctival infection, there is swelling of the eyelid, which may close the eye (Romaña's sign). There may be fever, lymphadenopathy, hepatosplenomegaly and, rarely, meningoencephalitis. Acute Chagas' disease is occasionally fatal in infants but normally there is full recovery within a few weeks or months.

Chronic infection

Some 10–30% of people go on to develop ***chronic Chagas' disease*** after a latent period of many years. The pathogenesis is unclear: it is possibly due to an autoimmune response triggered by the initial infection, although some evidence has thrown doubt on this mechanism. The heart is commonly affected, with conduction abnormalities, arrhythmias, aneurysm formation and cardiac dilatation. Gastrointestinal involvement leads to progressive dilatation of parts of the gastrointestinal tract; this commonly results in mega-oesophagus (causing dysphagia and aspiration pneumonia) and megacolon (causing severe constipation).

Diagnosis

Trypanosomes may be seen on a stained blood film during the acute illness. PCR is also sensitive in diagnosis in the acute phase. In chronic disease, parasites may be detected by xenodiagnosis; infection-free reduviid bugs are allowed to feed on the patient and the insect gut subsequently examined for parasites. Serological tests can detect both acute and chronic Chagas' disease.

Management and control

Nifurtimox and benznidazole are the main drugs used in Chagas' disease. Both are highly effective in acute infection, with a cure rate of over 90%, but much less so in chronic disease. They are relatively toxic, with adverse reactions in up to 40% of patients, and new drugs are urgently needed. Antiarrhythmic drugs and pacemakers may be needed in cardiac disease and surgical treatment is sometimes required for gastrointestinal complications.

In the long term, prevention of Chagas' disease relies on improved housing and living conditions. Several coordinated multinational vector control programmes have been implemented, with some success in reducing transmission.

Leishmaniasis

This group of diseases is caused by protozoa of the genus *Leishmania*, which are transmitted by the bite of the female phlebotomine sandfly ***(Box 11.58)***. Leishmaniasis is seen in localized areas of Africa, Asia (particularly India and Bangladesh), Europe, the Middle East and South and Central America. Certain parasite species are specific to each geographical area. The clinical picture is dependent on the species of parasite and on the host's cell-mediated immune response. Asymptomatic infection, in which the parasite is suppressed or eradicated by a strong immune response, is common in endemic areas, as demonstrated by a high incidence of positive leishmanin skin tests. Symptomatic infection may be confined to the skin (sometimes with spread to the mucous membranes; ***Fig. 11.40***) or widely disseminated throughout the body (visceral leishmaniasis). Relapse of previously asymptomatic infection is seen in patients who become immunocompromised, especially those with HIV infection.

In some areas, leishmaniasis is primarily zoonotic, whereas in others humans are the main reservoir of infection. In the vertebrate host, the parasites are found as oval amastigotes (Leishman–Donovan bodies). These multiply inside the macrophages and cells of the reticuloendothelial system and are then released into the circulation as the cells rupture. Parasites are taken into the gut of a feeding sandfly (genus *Phlebotomus* in the Old World, genus

Box 11.58 *Leishmania* species causing visceral and cutaneous disease in humans

Disease type	Species complex	Species
Visceral leishmaniasis	*L. donovani*	*L. donovani* *L. infantum* *L. chagasi*
Cutaneous leishmaniasis	*L. tropica* *L. major* *L. aethiopica* *L. mexicana*	*L. tropica* *L. major* *L. aethiopica* *L. mexicana* *L. amazonensis* *L. garnhami* *L. pifanoi* *L. venezuelensis*
	L. braziliensis	*L. braziliensis* *L. guyanensis* *L. panamanensis* *L. peruviana*
Mucocutaneous leishmaniasis		*L. braziliensis*

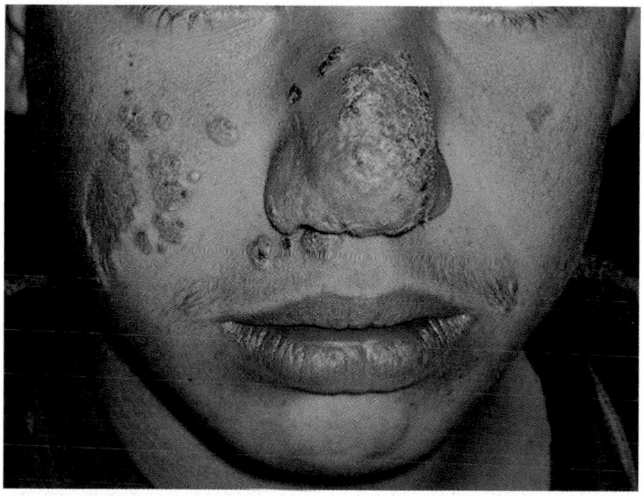

Figure 11.40 Hyperkeratotic nodular cutaneous leishmaniasis lesions and leishmaniasis recidivans (on right cheek) due to L. tropica. *(Source: Bailey MS, Lockwood DNJ. Cutaneous leishmaniasis. Clinics in Dermatology 2007; 25:203–211.)*

Lutzomyia in the New World), where they develop into the flagellate promastigote form. These migrate to the salivary glands of the insect, where they can be inoculated into a new host.

Visceral leishmaniasis

Clinical features

Visceral leishmaniasis (kala azar) is caused by *L. donovani*, *L. infantum* or *L. chagasi*, and is prevalent in localized areas of Asia, Africa, the Mediterranean littoral and South America. In parts of India, where humans are the main host, the disease occurs in epidemics. In most other areas, it is endemic, and it is mainly children and visitors to the area who are at risk. The main animal reservoirs in Europe and Asia are dogs and foxes, while in Africa it is carried by various rodents. About 300 000 people are currently infected, with more than 20 000 deaths per year.

The incubation period is usually 1–2 months but may be several years. The onset of symptoms is insidious and the patient may feel quite well, despite markedly abnormal physical findings. Fever is common and, although usually low-grade, may be high and intermittent. The liver and especially the spleen become enlarged; lymphadenopathy is common in African kala azar. The skin becomes rough and pigmented. If the disease is not treated, profound pancytopenia develops and the patient becomes wasted and immunosuppressed. Death usually occurs within a year and is normally due to bacterial infection or uncontrolled bleeding.

Diagnosis

Specific diagnosis is made by demonstrating the parasite in stained smears of aspirates of bone marrow, lymph node, spleen or liver. The organism can also be cultured from these specimens. Specific serological tests are positive in 95% of cases. Pancytopenia, hypoalbuminaemia and hypergammaglobulinaemia are common. The leishmanin skin test is negative, indicating a poor cell-mediated immune response.

Management

The most widely used drugs for visceral leishmaniasis remain the pentavalent antimony salts (e.g. sodium stibogluconate and meglumine antimoniate), despite toxicity and increasing resistance. Intravenous amphotericin B (preferably liposomal, which may be curative as a single-dose treatment) is effective but expensive; intramuscular paromomycin is cheaper and also has a good cure rate. The oral drug miltefosine has been shown in India to be highly effective, especially in combination with liposomal amphotericin; this and other combination therapies are being increasingly used to shorten treatment courses and limit resistance.

Successful treatment may be followed in a small proportion of patients by a skin eruption called ***post-kala azar dermal leishmaniasis*** (PKDL). It starts as a macular or maculopapular nodular rash, which spreads over the body. It is most often seen in Sudan and India, and is difficult to treat, although it may improve with miltefosine.

HIV co-infection

Visceral leishmaniasis is strongly associated with HIV-related immunosuppression, and the two infections may be passed on together through injecting drug use. In Southern Europe, antiretroviral therapy has largely controlled the problem, but increasing numbers of cases are being seen in Brazil and India (see p. 350).

Cutaneous leishmaniasis

Cutaneous leishmaniasis is caused by a number of geographically localized species, which may be zoonotic or anthroponotic. Following a sandfly bite, *Leishmania* amastigotes multiply in dermal macrophages. The local response depends on the species of *Leishmania*, the size of the inoculum and the host immune response. Single or multiple painless nodules occur on exposed areas 1 week to 3 months following the bite. These enlarge and ulcerate with a characteristic erythematous raised border. An overlying crust may develop. The lesions heal slowly over months or years, sometimes leaving a disfiguring scar.

L. major and *L. tropica* are found in Russia and Eastern Europe, the Middle East, Central Asia, the Mediterranean littoral and sub-Saharan Africa. The reservoir for *L. major* is desert rodents, while *L. tropica* has a mainly urban distribution with dogs and humans as reservoirs. *L. aethiopica* is found in the highlands of Ethiopia and Kenya, where the animal reservoir is the hyrax. The skin lesions usually heal spontaneously with scarring; this may take a year or more in the case of *L. tropica*. Leishmaniasis recidivans is a rare chronic relapsing form caused by *L. tropica*.

L. mexicana is found predominantly in Mexico, Guatemala, Brazil, Venezuela and Panama; infection usually runs a benign course with spontaneous healing within 6 months. *L. braziliensis* infections (which are seen throughout tropical South America) also usually heal spontaneously but may take longer.

L. mexicana amazonensis and *L. aethiopica* may occasionally cause diffuse cutaneous leishmaniasis. This is rare and is characterized by diffuse infiltration of the skin by Leishman–Donovan bodies. Visceral lesions are absent.

Diagnosis and management

The diagnosis can often be made clinically in a patient who has been in an endemic area. Giemsa stain on a split-skin smear will demonstrate *Leishmania* parasites in 80% of cases. Biopsy tissue from the edge of the lesion can be examined histologically and parasites identified by PCR; culture is less often successful. The leishmanin skin test is positive in over 90% of cases but does not distinguish between active and resolved infection. Serology is unhelpful.

Small lesions usually require no treatment. Large lesions or those in cosmetically sensitive sites can sometimes be treated locally by curettage, cryotherapy or topical antiparasitic agents. In other cases, systemic treatment (as for visceral leishmaniasis) is required.

Mucocutaneous leishmaniasis

Mucocutaneous leishmaniasis occurs in 3–10% of infections with *L. b. braziliensis* and is most common in Bolivia and Peru. The cutaneous sores are followed months or years later by indurated or ulcerating lesions affecting mucosa or cartilage, typically on the lips or nose ('espundia'). The condition can remain static, or there may be progression over months or years affecting the nasopharynx, uvula, palate and upper airways.

Diagnosis and management

Biopsies usually show only very scanty organisms, although parasites can be detected by PCR; serological tests are frequently positive.

Amphotericin B is the treatment of choice, if available, although systemic antimonial compounds are widely used; miltefosine may also be effective. Relapses are common following treatment.

Patients may die because of secondary bacterial infection or, occasionally, laryngeal obstruction.

Prevention

Prevention of leishmaniasis relies on control of vectors and/or reservoirs of infection. Insecticide spraying, control of host animals and treatment of infected humans may all be helpful. Personal protection against sandfly bites is also necessary, especially in travellers visiting endemic areas. Sandflies are poor fliers and sleeping off the ground helps prevent bites.

Other protozoal diseases of the blood and tissues

Toxoplasmosis

Toxoplasmosis is caused by the intracellular protozoan parasite *Toxoplasma gondii*. The sexual form of the parasite lives in the gut of the definitive host, the cat, where it produces oocysts. After a period of maturing in the environment, these oocysts become the source of infection for secondary hosts, which may ingest them. In the secondary hosts (which include humans, cattle, sheep, pigs, rodents and birds), there is disseminated infection. Following a successful immune response, the infection is controlled, but dormant parasites remain encysted in host tissue for many years. The life cycle is completed when carnivorous felines eat infected animal tissue. Humans are infected either from contaminated cat faeces, or by eating undercooked infected meat; transplacental infection may also occur.

Clinical features

Toxoplasmosis is common: seroprevalence in adults in the UK is about 25%, rising to 90% in some parts of Europe. Most infections are asymptomatic or trivial. Symptomatic patients usually present with lymphadenopathy, mainly in the head and neck. There may be fever, myalgia and general malaise; occasionally, there are more severe manifestations, including hepatitis, pneumonia, myocarditis and choroidoretinitis. Lymphadenopathy and fatigue can sometimes persist for months after the initial infection.

Congenital toxoplasmosis may also be asymptomatic but can produce serious disease. Clinical manifestations include microcephaly, hydrocephalus, encephalitis, convulsions and mental retardation. Choroidoretinitis is common; occasionally, this may be the only feature.

Immunocompromised patients, especially those with HIV infection, are at risk of serious infections with *T. gondii*. In acquired immunodeficiency states, this is usually due to reactivation of latent disease (see p. 350).

Diagnosis

Diagnosis is usually made serologically. IgG antibodies detectable by the Sabin–Feldman dye test remain positive for years; acute infection can be confirmed by demonstrating a rising titre of specific IgM.

Management

Acquired toxoplasmosis in an immunocompetent host rarely requires treatment. In those with severe disease (especially eye involvement), sulfadiazine 2–4 g daily and pyrimethamine 25 mg daily are given for 4 weeks, along with folinic acid. The management of pregnant women with toxoplasmosis aims to decrease the risk of fetal complications. However, there is little good evidence that giving spiramycin, either alone or in combination with sulfadiazine (which is the recommended treatment), has any significant effect on the frequency or severity of fetal damage. Infected infants should be treated from birth. The treatment of toxoplasmosis in HIV-positive patients is covered on page 350.

Babesiosis

Babesiosis is a tick-borne parasitic disease, diagnosed most commonly in North America and Europe. It is a zoonosis of rodents and cattle, and is occasionally transmitted to humans; infection is more common and more severe in those who are immunocompromised following splenectomy. The causative organisms are the *Plasmodium*-like *Babesia microti* (rodents) and *B. divergens* (cattle).

The incubation period averages 10 days. In patients with normal splenic function, the illness is usually mild. In splenectomized individuals, systemic symptoms are more pronounced and haemolysis is associated with haemoglobinuria, jaundice and acute kidney injury. Examination of a peripheral blood smear may reveal the characteristic *Plasmodium*-like organisms.

The standard treatment of severe babesiosis is a combination of quinine 650 mg and clindamycin 600 mg orally three times daily for 7 days. Atovaquone and azithromycin plus doxycycline are used for persistent or relapsing disease.

Further reading

Bern C. Antitrypanosomal therapy for chronic Chagas' disease. *N Engl J Med* 2011; 364:2527–2534.
Moorthy VS, Okwo-Bele JM. Final results from a pivotal phase 3 malaria vaccine trial. *Lancet* 2015; 386:5–7.
Noor AM, Kinyoki DK, Mundia CN et al. The changing risk of P. falciparum malaria infections in Africa 2000–2010. *Lancet* 2014; 383:1739–1747.
Phompradit P, Muhamad P, Wisedpanichkij R. Four years' monitoring of in vitro sensitivity and candidate molecular markers of resistance of Plasmodium falciparum to artesunate–mefloquine combination in the Thai–Myanmar border. *Malaria J* 2014; 13:article 23.
Simarro PP, Diarra A, Postigo JAR et al. The human African trypanosomiasis control and surveillance programme of the WHO 2000–2009: the way forward. *PLoS Negl Trop Dis* 2015; 9:e0003785.
Somé AF, Zongo I, Compaoré Y-D et al. Selection of drug resistance-mediating Plasmodium falciparum genetic polymorphisms by seasonal malaria chemoprevention in Burkina Faso. *Antimicrob Agents Chemother* 2014; 58:3660–3665.
Sudarshi D, Brown M. Human African trypanosomiasis in non-endemic countries. *Clin Med* 2015; 15:70–73.
Sundar S, Chakravarty J. Leishmaniasis: an update of current pharmacotherapy. *Expert Opin Pharmacother* 2013; 14:53–63.
Tarral A, Blesson S, Mordt OV et al. Determination of an optimal dosing regimen for fexinidazole, a novel oral drug for the treatment of human African trypanosomiasis: first-in-human studies. *Clin Pharmacokinet* 2014; 53:565–580.
Whie NJ, Pukrittayakamee S, Hien TT et al. Malaria. *Lancet* 2014; 383:723–735.
http://www.theglobalfund.org *The Global Fund.*
http://www.who.int/leishmaniasis/resources/en/ *WHO Technical Report 949 Control of the leishmaniases.*
http://www.who.int/malaria/publications/ *WHO guidelines for the treatment of malaria.*
http://www.who.int/mediacentre/en *Factsheets on many infections of the tropics and subtropics (including all the protozoal diseases).*
http://www.wwarn.org *Up-to-date information on resistance to all antimalarials.*

GASTROINTESTINAL PROTOZOA

The major gastrointestinal parasites of humans are shown in Box 11.59.

Amoebiasis

Amoebiasis is caused by *Entamoeba histolytica*. There are three morphologically identical species of amoeba, which can be distinguished by molecular techniques after culture of the trophozoite: *E.*

Box 11.59 Pathogenic human intestinal protozoa

Amoebae
- *Entamoeba histolytica*

Flagellates
- *Giardia intestinalis*

Ciliates
- *Balantidium coli*

Coccidia
- *Cryptosporidium parvum*
- *Isospora belli*
- *Sarcocystis* spp.
- *Cyclospora cayetanensis*

Microspora
- *Enterocytozoon bieneusi*
- *Encephalitozoon* spp.

histolytica, which is pathogenic; *E. dispar*, which is non-pathogenic; and *E. moshkovskii*, which is of uncertain significance. Amoebiasis occurs worldwide, although much higher incidence rates are found in the tropics and subtropics.

The organism exists both as a motile trophozoite and as a cyst that can survive outside the body. Cysts are transmitted by ingestion of contaminated food or water, or spread directly by person-to-person contact. Trophozoites emerge from the cysts in the small intestine and then pass on to the colon, where they multiply.

Clinical features

It is believed that many individuals can carry the pathogen without obvious evidence of clinical disease (asymptomatic cyst passers). However, this may be due, in some cases, to the misidentification of non-pathogenic *E. dispar* as *E. histolytica*, and it is not clear how often true *E. histolytica* infection is symptomless. In affected people, *E. histolytica* trophozoites invade the colonic epithelium, probably with the aid of their own cytotoxins and proteolytic enzymes. The parasites continue to multiply and, finally, frank ulceration of the mucosa occurs. If penetration continues, trophozoites may enter the portal vein, via which they reach the liver and cause intrahepatic abscesses. This invasive form of the disease is serious and may even be fatal.

The incubation period of intestinal amoebiasis is highly variable and may be as short as a few days or as long as several months. The usual course is chronic, with mild intermittent diarrhoea and abdominal discomfort. This may progress to bloody diarrhoea with mucus and is sometimes accompanied by systemic symptoms, such as headache, nausea and anorexia. Less commonly, infection may present as acute amoebic dysentery, resembling bacillary dysentery or acute ulcerative colitis.

Complications are unusual but include toxic dilatation of the colon, chronic infection with stricture formation, severe haemorrhage, amoeboma and amoebic liver abscess. Amoebic liver abscesses often develop in the absence of a recent episode of colitis. Tender hepatomegaly, a high swinging fever and profound malaise are characteristic, although early in the course of the disease both symptoms and signs may be minimal. The clinical features are described in more detail on page 484.

Diagnosis

Microscopic examination of fresh stool or colonic exudate obtained at sigmoidoscopy is the simplest way of diagnosing colonic amoebic infection. To confirm the diagnosis, motile trophozoites containing red blood cells must be identified; the presence of amoebic cysts alone does not imply disease. Sigmoidoscopy and barium enema examination may show colonic ulceration but are rarely diagnostic.

The amoebic fluorescent antibody test is positive in at least 90% of patients with liver abscess and in 60–70% with active colitis. Seropositivity is low in asymptomatic cyst passers.

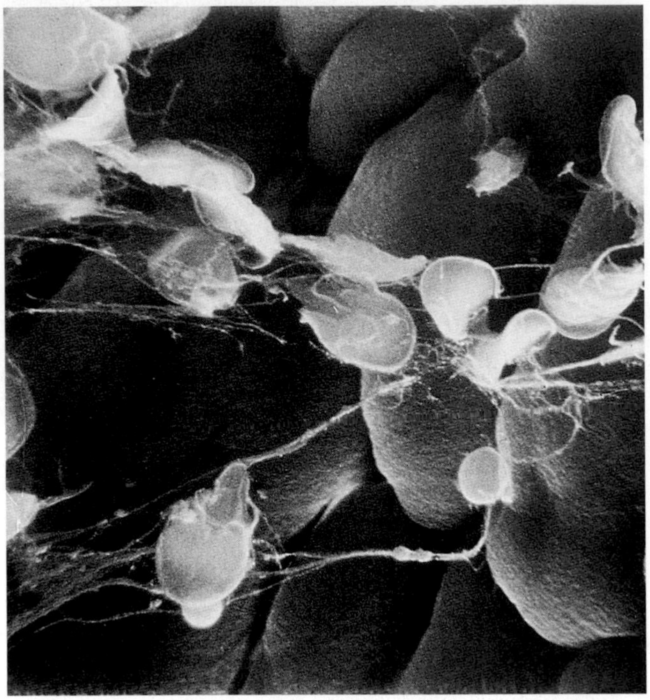

Figure 11.41 ***Giardia intestinalis*** **on small intestinal mucosa.** *(Courtesy of Dr A Phillips, Department of Electron Microscopy, Royal Free Hospital, London.)*

Management

Metronidazole 800mg three times daily for 5days is given in amoebic colitis; a lower dose (400mg three times daily for 5days) is usually adequate in liver abscess. Tinidazole is also effective. After treatment of the invasive disease, the bowel should be cleared of parasites with a luminal amoebicide such as diloxanide furoate.

Prevention

Amoebiasis is difficult to eradicate because of the substantial human reservoir of infection. The only progress will be through improved standards of hygiene, sanitation and better access to clean water. Cysts are destroyed by boiling but chlorine and iodine sterilizing tablets are not always effective.

Giardiasis

Giardia intestinalis is a flagellate ***(Fig. 11.41)*** that is found worldwide. It causes small intestinal disease, with diarrhoea and malabsorption. Prevalence is high in many developing countries and it is the most common parasitic infection in travellers returning to the UK. In certain parts of Europe and in some rural areas of North America, large water-borne epidemics have been reported. Person-to-person spread may occur in day nurseries and residential institutions. The organism exists as both a trophozoite and a cyst, the latter being the form in which it is transmitted.

The organism sometimes colonizes the small intestine and may remain there without causing detriment to the host. In other cases, severe malabsorption may occur, which is thought to be related to morphological damage to the small intestine. The changes in villous architecture are usually mild partial villous atrophy; subtotal villous atrophy is rare. The mechanism by which the parasite causes alteration in mucosal architecture and produces diarrhoea and intestinal malabsorption is unknown; there is evidence that the morphological damage is immune-mediated. Bacterial overgrowth has also been found in association with giardiasis and may contribute to fat malabsorption.

Clinical features

Many individuals excreting *Giardia* cysts have no symptoms. Others become ill within 1–3 weeks of ingesting cysts; symptoms include diarrhoea, often watery in the early stage of the illness, nausea, anorexia, and abdominal discomfort and bloating. In most people affected, these symptoms resolve after a few days, but in some they persist. Stools may then become paler, with the characteristic features of steatorrhoea. If the illness is prolonged, weight loss occurs and can be marked. Chronic giardiasis, frequently seen in developing countries, can result in growth retardation in children.

Diagnosis

Both cysts and trophozoites can be found in the stool, but negative stool examination does not exclude the diagnosis since the parasite may be excreted at irregular intervals. The parasite can also be seen in duodenal aspirates (obtained with either an endoscope or a luminal capsule) and in histological sections of jejunal mucosa.

Management

Metronidazole 2 g as a single dose on three successive days will cure the majority of infections, although sometimes a second or third course is necessary. Alternative drugs include tinidazole, mepacrine and albendazole. Preventative measures are similar to those outlined above for *E. histolytica*.

Cryptosporidiosis

This organism is found worldwide, cattle being the major natural reservoir. It has also been demonstrated in supplies of drinking water in the UK. The parasite is able to reproduce both sexually and asexually; it is transmitted by oocysts excreted in the faeces.

In healthy individuals, cryptosporidiosis is a self-limiting illness. Acute watery diarrhoea is associated with fever and general malaise lasting for 7–10 days. In immunocompromised patients, especially those with HIV, diarrhoea is severe and intractable (see p. 350).

Diagnosis is usually made by faecal microscopy, although the parasite can also be detected in intestinal biopsies. There is no reliable treatment but nitazoxanide may be of benefit.

Balantidiasis

Balantidium coli is the only ciliate that produces clinically significant infection in humans. It is found throughout the tropics, particularly in Central and South America, Iran, Papua New Guinea and the Philippines. It is usually carried by pigs, and infection is most common in those communities that live in close association with swine. Its life cycle is identical to that of *E. histolytica*. *B. coli* causes diarrhoea and sometimes a dysenteric illness with invasion of the distal ileal and colonic mucosa. Trophozoites rather than cysts are found in the stool. Treatment is with tetracycline or metronidazole.

Blastocystis hominis infection

B. hominis is a strictly anaerobic protozoan pathogen that inhabits the colon. The pathogenicity for humans remains controversial, despite many studies looking at response to chemotherapy.

Cyclospora cayetanensis infection

C. cayetanensis, a coccidian protozoal parasite, was originally recognized as a cause of diarrhoea in travellers to Nepal. It has been detected in stool specimens from immunocompetent and immunodeficient people worldwide. Infection is usually self-limiting but can be treated with co-trimoxazole.

Microsporidiosis

Protozoa of the phylum *Microsporea* can cause diarrhoea in patients with HIV/AIDS (see p. 350).

Further reading

Wright SG. Protozoan infections of the gastrointestinal tract. *Infect Dis Clin North Am* 2012; 26:323–339.

HELMINTHIC INFECTIONS

Worm infections are very common in developing countries, causing much disease in both humans and domestic animals. Worms are frequently imported into industrialized countries. The most common human helminth infections are listed in ***Box 11.60***. Three in particular – ascariasis, hookworm and trichuriasis – are included in a list of 13 'neglected tropical diseases', which the WHO has identified as causing major disability among the poorest people in the world.

Helminths are the largest internal human parasite. They reproduce sexually, generating millions of eggs or larvae. ***Nematodes***

Box 11.60 Helminths commonly infecting humans

	Helminth	Common name/ disease caused
Nematodes (roundworms)		
Tissue-dwelling worms	*Wuchereria bancrofti*	Filariasis
	Brugia malayi/timori	Filariasis
	Loa loa	Loiasis
	Onchocerca volvulus	River blindness
	Dracunculus medinensis	Dracunculiasis
	Mansonella perstans	Mansonellosis
Intestinal human nematodes	*Enterobius vermicularis*	Threadworm
	Ascaris lumbricoides	Roundworm
	Trichuris trichiura	Whipworm
	Necator americanus	Hookworm
	Ancylostoma duodenale	Hookworm
	Strongyloides stercoralis	Strongyloidosis
Zoonotic nematodes	*Toxocara canis*	Toxocariasis
	Trichinella spiralis	Trichinellosis
Trematodes (flukes)		
Blood flukes	*Schistosoma* spp.	Schistosomiasis
Lung flukes	*Paragonimus* spp.	Paragonimiasis
Intestinal/hepatic flukes	*Fasciolopsis buski*	
	Fasciola hepatica	
	Clonorchis sinensis	
	Opisthorchis felineus	
Cestodes (tapeworms)		
Intestinal adult worms	*Taenia saginata*	Beef tapeworm
	Taenia solium	Pork tapeworm
	Diphyllobothrium latum	Fish tapeworm
	Hymenolepis nana	Dwarf tapeworm
Larval tissue cysts	*Taenia solium*	Cysticercosis
	Echinococcus granulosus	Hydatid disease
	Echinococcus multilocularis	Hydatid disease
	Spirometra mansoni	Sparganosis

and ***trematodes*** have a mouth and intestinal tract, while ***cestodes*** absorb nutrients directly through the outer tegument. All worms are motile, although once the adults are established in their definitive site, they rarely migrate further. Adult helminths may be very long-lived: up to 30 years in the case of the schistosomes.

Many helminths have developed complex life cycles, involving more than one host. Both primary and intermediate hosts are often highly specific to a particular species of worm. In some cases of human infection, humans are the primary host, while in others, humans are a non-specific intermediary or are coincidentally infected. Multiple infections with different helminths are common in endemic areas. Mass treatment programmes, in which one or more anthelminthic drugs are given on a regular (usually annual) basis, are used to keep the total worm load down, and the WHO recommends treating all schoolchildren at regular intervals in areas where helminth infections are common ***(Box 11.61)***.

NEMATODES

Human infections can be divided into:

- ***Tissue-dwelling worms***, including the filarial worms and the Guinea worm *Dracunculus medinensis*.
- ***Human intestinal worms***, including the human hookworms, the common roundworm (*Ascaris lumbricoides*) and *Strongyloides stercoralis*, which are the most common helminthic parasites of humans. The adult worms live in the human gut and do not usually invade tissues, but many species have a complex life cycle involving a migratory larval stage.
- ***Zoonotic nematodes***, which accidentally infect humans and are not able to complete their normal life cycle. They often become 'trapped' in the tissues, causing a potentially severe local inflammatory response.

Box 11.61 Drugs used in mass treatment of helminth infections

Drug	Infection
Diethylcarbamazine (DEC)	Loiaisis Filariasis
Ivermectin	Loiaisis Filariasis Onchocerciasis Strongyloidiasis
Albendazole	Filariasis (with DEC) Intestinal helminths
Praziquantel	Schistosomiasis

Tissue-dwelling worms

Filariasis

Several nematodes belonging to the superfamily Filarioidea can infect humans. The adult worms are long and thread-like, ranging from 2 cm to 50 cm in length; females are generally much larger than males. Larval stages are inoculated into humans by various species of biting flies (each specific to a particular parasite). The adult worms that develop from these larvae mate, producing millions of offspring (microfilariae), which migrate in the blood or skin. These are ingested by feeding flies, in which the remainder of the life cycle takes place. Disease, which may be caused either by the adult worms or by microfilariae, is caused by the host immune response to the parasite and is characterized by massive eosinophilia. Adult worms are long-lived (10–15 years) and re-infection is common, so that disease tends to be chronic and progressive.

Lymphatic filariasis

Lymphatic filariasis, which may be caused by different species of filarial worm, has a scattered distribution in the tropics and subtropics ***(Box 11.62)***. More than 1 billion people in developing countries are at risk. *Wuchereria bancrofti* is transmitted to humans by a number of mosquito species, mainly *Culex fatigans*. Adult female worms (which are 5–10 cm long) live in the lymphatics, releasing large numbers of microfilariae into the blood. Generally, this occurs at night, coinciding with the nocturnal feeding pattern of *C. fatigans*. Non-periodic forms of *W. bancrofti*, transmitted by day-biting species of mosquito, are found in the South Pacific. *Brugia malayi* (and the closely related *B. timori*) is very similar to *W. bancrofti*, exhibiting the same nocturnal periodicity. The usual vectors are mosquitoes of the genus *Mansonia*, although other mosquitoes have been implicated.

Many filarial worms coexist with symbiotic *Wolbachia* bacteria, which are, in themselves, a cause of inflammation in the human host.

Clinical features

Following the bite of an infected mosquito, the larvae enter the lymphatics and are carried to regional lymph nodes. Here, they grow and mature for 6–18 months.

Box 11.62 Diseases caused by the filarial worms

Organism	Adult worm	Microfilariae	Major vector	Clinical signs	Distribution
Wuchereria bancrofti	Lymphatics	Blood	*Culex* spp.	Fever Lymphangitis Elephantiasis	Tropics
Brugia timori/malayi	Lymphatics	Blood	*Mansonia* spp.	Fever Lymphangitis Elephantiasis	East and South-east Asia, South India, Sri Lanka
Loa loa	Subcutaneous	Blood	*Chrysops* spp.	'Calabar' swellings Urticaria	West and Central Africa
Onchocerca	Subcutaneous	Skin, eye	*Simulium* spp.	Subcutaneous nodules Eye disease	Africa, South America
Mansonella perstans	Retroperitoneal	Blood	*Culicoides* spp.	Allergic eosinophilia	Sub-Saharan Africa, South America

Adult worms produce allergic lymphangitis. The clinical picture depends on the individual immune response, which in turn may depend on factors such as age at first exposure. In endemic areas, many people have asymptomatic infection. Sometimes, early infection is marked by bouts of fever accompanied by pain, tenderness and erythema along the course of affected lymphatics. Involvement of the spermatic cord and epididymis are common in Bancroftian filariasis. These acute attacks subside spontaneously in a few days but usually recur. Recurrent episodes cause intermittent lymphatic obstruction, which in time can become fibrotic and irreversible. Obstructed lymphatics may rupture, causing cellulitis and further fibrosis; there may also be chylous pleural effusions and ascites. Over time, there is progressive enlargement, coarsening and fissuring of the skin, leading to the classical appearances of elephantiasis. The limbs or scrotum may become hugely swollen. Eventually, the adult worms will die, but the lymphatic obstruction remains and tissue damage continues. Elephantiasis takes many years to develop and is only seen in association with recurrent infection in endemic areas.

Occasionally, the predominant features of filarial infection are pulmonary. Microfilariae become trapped in the pulmonary capillaries, generating an intense local allergic response. The resulting pneumonitis causes cough, fever, weight loss and shifting radiological changes, associated with a high peripheral eosinophil count. This is known as ***tropical pulmonary eosinophilia***.

Diagnosis

The clinical picture in established disease is usually diagnostic, although similar lymphatic damage may occasionally be caused by silicates absorbed through the feet from volcanic soil (podoconiosis). Parasitological diagnosis has traditionally relied on detecting microfilariae in blood films or skin snips, but rapid and sensitive near-patient antigen detection tests are now available.

Management

Diethylcarbamazine (DEC) kills both adult worms and microfilariae. Serious allergic responses may occur as the parasites are killed and particular care is needed when using DEC in areas endemic for loiasis. Mass treatment programmes using combinations of DEC, ivermectin and albendazole to target various helminthic infections are used in many parts of the world; the exact regimens depend on local situations. Over 500 million people have already received such treatment. There is currently much interest in using doxycycline to kill the symbiotic *Wolbachia* bacteria, without which the adult worm will eventually die. However, the best way of incorporating this into the overall management strategy remains unclear. Vector control with insecticide bed nets is helpful in certain areas.

Loiasis

Loiasis is found in the humid forests of West and Central Africa. The causative parasite, *Loa loa*, is a small (3–7 cm) filarial worm, which is found in the subcutaneous tissues. The microfilariae circulate in the blood during the day but cause no direct symptoms. The vectors are day-biting flies of the genus *Chrysops*.

Adult worms migrate around the body in subcutaneous tissue planes. Worms may be present for years, frequently without causing symptoms. From time to time, localized, tender, hot, soft tissue swellings occur due to hypersensitivity (Calabar swellings), often near to a joint. These are produced in response to the passage of a worm and usually subside over a few days or weeks. There may also be more generalized urticaria and pruritus. Occasionally, a worm may be seen crossing the eye under the conjunctiva; it may also enter retro-orbital tissue, causing severe pain. Short-term residents of endemic areas often have more severe manifestations of the disease.

Microfilariae may be seen on stained blood films, although these are often negative. Serological tests are relatively insensitive and cross-react with other microfilariae. There is usually massive eosinophilia. DEC may cause severe allergic reactions associated with parasite killing and is being replaced by newer agents. Ivermectin in single doses of 200–400 μg/kg is effective: it may occasionally cause severe reactions. Albendazole, which causes a more gradual reduction in microfilarial load, may be preferable in heavily infected patients. Mass treatment with either DEC or ivermectin can decrease the transmission of infection but the mainstay of prevention is vector avoidance and control.

Onchocerciasis

Onchocerciasis (river blindness) affects 37 million people worldwide, of whom 250 000 are blind and 500 000 visually impaired; most of these are in West and Central Africa, with small foci in the Yemen, and in Central and South America. It is the result of infection with *Onchocerca volvulus*. Infection is transmitted by day-biting flies of the genus *Simulium*.

Pathogenesis

Infection occurs when larvae are inoculated into humans by the bite of an infected fly. The worms mature in 2–4 months and can live for more than 15 years. Adult worms, which can reach lengths of 50 cm (although they are <0.5 mm in diameter), live in the subcutaneous tissues. They may form fibrotic nodules, especially over bony prominences and sites of trauma. Huge numbers of microfilariae are distributed in the skin and may invade the eyes. Live microfilariae cause relatively little harm, but dead parasites may cause severe allergic reactions, with hyaline necrosis and loss of tissue collagen and elastin. In the eye, a similar process causes conjunctivitis, sclerosing keratitis, uveitis and secondary glaucoma. Choroidoretinitis is also occasionally seen.

Clinical features

Symptoms usually start about a year after infection. Initially, there is generalized pruritus, with urticaria and fleeting oedema. Subcutaneous nodules (which can be detected by ultrasound) start to appear, and in dark-skinned individuals, there is hypo- and hyperpigmentation from excoriation and inflammatory changes. Over time, more chronic inflammatory changes appear, with roughened, inelastic skin. Superficial lymph nodes become enlarged and, in the groin, may hang down in loose folds of skin ('hanging groin'). Eye disease, which is associated with chronic heavy infection, usually first manifests as itching and conjunctival irritation. This gradually progresses to more extensive eye disease and eventually to blindness.

Diagnosis

In endemic areas, the diagnosis can often be made clinically, especially if supported by finding eosinophilia on a blood film. In order to identify parasites, skin snips taken from the iliac crest or shoulder are placed in saline under a cover slip. After 4 hours, microscopy will show microfilariae wriggling free on the slide. If this is negative, DEC can be applied topically under an occlusive dressing and will provoke an allergic rash in the majority of infected people (modified Mazzotti reaction); this should not be routinely performed, as it is unpleasant. Slit-lamp examination of the eyes may reveal the microfilariae. Rapid near-patient serological card tests are under evaluation.

Management and prevention

Ivermectin, in a single dose of 150 µg/kg, kills microfilariae and prevents their return for 6–12 months. There is little effect on adult worms, so annual (or more frequent) retreatment is needed. In patients co-infected with *Loa loa*, ivermectin may occasionally induce severe allergic reactions, including a toxic encephalopathy.

The WHO Onchocerciasis Control Programme (OCP), which started in 1974, had a considerable impact on onchocerciasis in West Africa. A combination of vector control measures and, more recently, mass treatment with ivermectin led to a decrease in both infection rates and progression to serious disease. The control programme has been handed over to local governments by the WHO, and local mass treatment programmes are still running in most endemic countries. Eradication may eventually be possible, as humans are the only host, but measures are required over a long period because of the longevity of the worm (10–15 years).

Mansonellosis

Mansonella perstans is a filarial worm transmitted by biting midges of the genus *Culicoides*. Small numbers of microfilariae are found in the blood, and although they do not cause serious disease, there may be minor allergic reactions and an eosinophilia.

Dracunculiasis

Infection with the Guinea worm, *Dracunculus medinensis*, occurs when water fleas (copepods) containing the parasite larvae are swallowed in contaminated drinking water. Ingested larvae mature and the female worm, which can reach over 1 metre in length, migrates through connective and subcutaneous tissue for 9–18 months before surfacing on the skin. The uterus of the worm ruptures, releasing larvae that are ingested by the small crustacean water fleas, and the cycle is completed.

The ***diagnosis*** is clinical. The traditional ***management***, extracting the worm over several days by winding it round a stick, is probably still the most effective. The worm should not be damaged. Antibiotics may be needed to control secondary infection.

Prevention and control of dracunculiasis has been one of the success stories in tropical medicine. Large-scale eradication programmes (involving removal of water fleas, and thus infective larvae, by chemical treatment or simple filtration) have been in place for several years. The number of reported cases has fallen from over 3 million in 1985 to just 148 in 2013. The disease is now confined to a handful of small areas of Africa, mainly in south Sudan. Humans are the only host of *D. medinensis* and it should therefore be possible to eradicate this parasite completely.

Human intestinal nematodes

Adult intestinal nematodes (also sometimes referred to as soil-transmitted helminths, or geohelminths) live in the human gut. There are two main types of life cycle, both usually including a soil-based stage. In some species, infection is spread by ingestion of eggs (which often require a period of maturation in the environment); in others, the eggs hatch in the soil and larvae penetrate directly through the skin of a new host. *Strongyloides* is unusual, in that it is the only nematode that is able to complete its life cycle in humans. Larvae may hatch before leaving the colon and so are able to re-infect the host by penetrating the intestinal wall and entering the venous system.

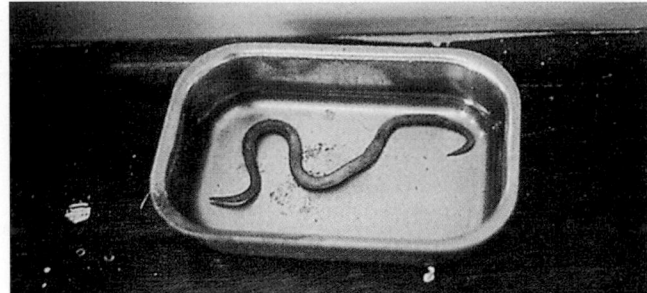

Figure 11.42 ***Ascaris lumbricoides*****.** The worm is approximately 20 cm long.

Ascariasis (roundworm infection)

Ascaris lumbricoides is a pale yellow worm, 20–35 cm in length ***(Fig. 11.42)***. It is found worldwide but is particularly common in poor rural communities, where there is heavy faecal contamination of the immediate environment. Larvae hatch and penetrate the duodenum, migrating through the tissues to the lungs before being expectorated and swallowed. The adult worms live in the small intestine. Ova are deposited in faeces and require a 2–4-month maturation in the soil before they are infective.

Infection is usually asymptomatic, although heavy infections are associated with nausea, vomiting, abdominal discomfort and anorexia. Worms can sometimes obstruct the small intestine, the most common site being the ileocaecal valve. They may also occasionally invade the appendix, causing acute appendicitis, or the bile duct, resulting in biliary obstruction and suppurative cholangitis. Larvae in the lung may produce pulmonary eosinophilia. Heavy infection in children, especially those who are already malnourished, may have significant effects on nutrition and development. Serious morbidity and mortality are rare in ascariasis, but the huge number of people infected means that, on a global basis, roundworm infection causes a significant burden of disease, especially in children.

Ascaris eggs can be identified in the stool and, occasionally, adult worms emerge from the mouth or the anus. They may also be seen on barium enema studies. Appropriate drug treatments are shown in ***Box 11.63***. Very rarely, surgical or endoscopic intervention may be required for intestinal or biliary obstruction.

Threadworm (*Enterobius vermicularis*)

E. vermicularis is a small (2–12 mm) worm, which is common throughout the world. Larval development takes place mainly in the small intestine and adult worms are normally found in the colon. The gravid female deposits eggs around the anus, causing intense itching, especially at night. Unlike those of *A. lumbricoides*, the eggs do not require a maturation period in soil, and infection is often directly transmitted from anus to mouth via the hands. Eggs may also be deposited on clothing and bed linen, and are subsequently either ingested or inhaled. Apart from discomfort and local excoriation, infection is usually harmless.

Ova can be collected either by using a moistened perianal swab, or by applying adhesive cellophane tape to the perianal skin. They can then be identified by microscopy.

The most commonly used drugs are mebendazole and piperazine ***(Box 11.63)***. However, isolated treatment of an affected person is often ineffective. Other family members (especially small children) may also need to be treated and the whole family should be given advice about personal hygiene. Two courses of treatment 2 weeks apart may break the cycle of autoinfection.

Box 11.63 Drugs used for treating human intestinal nematodes[a]

Drug	Dosage	*Ascaris*	Hookworm	*Enterobius*	*Trichuris*	*Strongyloides*
Piperazine	75 mg/kg	++	+	++	–	–
Pyrantel pamoate	10 mg/kg	++	+	++	–	–
Oxantel pamoate	10 mg/kg	++	+	n/a	++	–
Albendazole	400 mg[b]	++	++	++	+	+
Mebendazole	500 mg[c]	++	++	++	+	+
Tiabendazole	25 mg/kg[b]	n/a	n/a	n/a	n/a	++
Levamisole	2.5 mg/kg	++	+	n/a	n/a	–
Ivermectin	200 µg/kg[d]	n/a	n/a	n/a	n/a	++

++, highly effective; +, moderately effective; –, ineffective; n/a, drug not used for this indication/no data available. [a]Single dose unless otherwise stated. [b]Twice daily for 3 days in strongyloidiasis. [c]WHO recommended dose for developing countries; in the UK, commonly given as 100 mg single dose for threadworm or 100 mg twice daily for 3 days for whipworm. [d]Once daily for 2 days.

Whipworm (*Trichuris trichiura*)

Infections with whipworm are common worldwide, especially in poor communities with inadequate sanitation. Adult worms, which are 3–5 cm long, inhabit the terminal ileum and caecum, although in heavy infection they are found throughout the large bowel. The head of the worm is embedded in the intestinal mucosa. Ova are deposited in the faeces and require a maturation period of 3–4 weeks in the soil before becoming infective.

Infection is usually asymptomatic, but mucosal damage can occasionally be so severe that there is colonic ulceration, dysentery or rectal prolapse.

Diagnosis is made by finding ova on stool microscopy, or occasionally by seeing adult worms on sigmoidoscopy. Drug treatment is shown in ***Box 11.63***.

Hookworm

Hookworm infections, caused by the human hookworms *Ancylostoma duodenale* and *Necator americanus*, are found worldwide. They are relatively rare in developed countries but very common in areas with poor sanitation and hygiene; overall, about 25% of the world's population is affected. Hookworm infection is a major contributing factor to anaemia in the tropics. *A. duodenale* is found mainly in East Asia, North Africa and the Mediterranean, while *N. americanus* is the predominant species in South and Central America, South-east Asia and sub-Saharan Africa.

Adult worms (which are about 1 cm long) live in the duodenum and upper jejunum, where they are often found in large numbers. They attach firmly to the mucosa using the buccal plate, feeding on blood. Eggs passed in the faeces develop in warm, moist soil, producing infective filariform larvae. These penetrate directly through the skin of a new host and are carried in the bloodstream to the lungs. Having crossed into the alveoli, the parasites are expectorated and then swallowed, thus arriving at their definitive home.

Clinical features

Local irritation as the larvae penetrate the skin ('ground itch') may be followed by transient pulmonary signs and symptoms, often accompanied by eosinophilia. Light infections, especially in a well-nourished person, are often asymptomatic. Heavier worm loads may be associated with epigastric pain and nausea, resembling peptic ulcer disease. Chronic heavy infection, particularly on a background of malnourishment, may cause iron deficiency anaemia and hypoproteinaemia. Heavy infection in children is associated with delays in physical and mental development.

Diagnosis and management

The diagnosis is made by finding eggs on faecal microscopy. In infections heavy enough to cause anaemia, these will be present in large numbers. The aim of treatment in endemic areas is reduction of worm burden rather than complete eradication; albendazole given as a single dose is the best drug ***(Box 11.63)***. The WHO is promoting mass treatment programmes for schoolchildren in many parts of the world, together with treatment for schistosomiasis where appropriate.

Strongyloidiasis

Strongyloides stercoralis is a small (2 mm long) worm that lives in the small intestine. It is found in many parts of the tropics and subtropics, and is especially common in Asia. Eggs hatch in the bowel and larvae are found in the stool. Usually, these are non-infective rhabditiform larvae, which require a further period of maturation in the soil before they can infect a new host, but sometimes this maturation can occur in the large bowel. Infective filariform larvae can therefore penetrate directly through the perianal skin, re-infecting the host. In this way, autoinfection may continue for years or even decades. Some war veterans who were imprisoned in the Far East during the Second World War were found to have active strongyloidiasis over 50 years later. After skin penetration, the life cycle is similar to that of the hookworm, except that the adult worms may burrow into the intestinal mucosa, causing a local inflammatory response.

Clinical features

S. stercoralis, following skin penetration, causes a similar local dermatitis to hookworm. In autoinfection, this manifests as a migratory linear weal around the buttocks and lower abdomen (cutaneous larva currens). In heavy infections, damage to the small intestinal mucosa can cause malabsorption, diarrhoea and even perforation. There is usually a persistent eosinophilia.

In patients who are ***immunosuppressed*** (e.g. by corticosteroid therapy or intercurrent illness), filariform larvae may penetrate directly through the bowel wall in huge numbers, causing an overwhelming and usually fatal generalized infection (the strongyloidiasis hyperinfestation syndrome). This condition is often complicated by Gram-negative septicaemia due to bowel organisms.

Diagnosis and management

Motile larvae may be seen on stool microscopy, especially after a period of incubation. Serological tests are also useful. The best drug for treating strongyloidiasis is ivermectin (200 μg/kg daily for 2 days); albendazole (15 mg/kg 12-hourly for 3 days) is also effective. In hyperinfection, antibiotics against Gram-negative organisms should be given.

Zoonotic nematodes

A number of nematodes that are principally parasites of animals may also affect humans. The most common are described below.

Trichinosis

The normal hosts of *Trichinella spiralis*, the cause of trichinosis, include pigs, bears and warthogs. Humans are infected by eating undercooked meat from these animals. Ingested larvae mature in the small intestine, where adults release new larvae that penetrate the bowel wall and migrate through the tissues. Eventually, these larvae encyst in striated muscle.

Light infections are usually asymptomatic. Heavier loads of worms produce gastrointestinal symptoms as the adults establish themselves in the small intestine, followed by systemic symptoms as the larvae invade. The latter include fever, oedema and myalgia. Massive infection may occasionally be fatal but usually the symptoms subside once the larvae encyst.

The ***diagnosis*** can usually be made from the clinical picture, associated eosinophilia and serological tests. If necessary, it can be confirmed by muscle biopsy a few weeks after infection. Long-standing infection may be revealed by the presence of numerous calcified cysts on X-ray. Albendazole (20 mg/kg for 7 days), given early in the course of the illness, will kill the adult worms and decrease the load of larvae reaching the tissues. Analgesia and steroids may be needed for symptomatic relief.

Toxocariasis (visceral larva migrans)

Eggs of the dog roundworm, *Toxocara canis*, are occasionally ingested by humans, especially children. The eggs hatch and the larvae penetrate the small intestinal wall and enter the mesenteric circulation, but are then unable to complete their life cycle in a 'foreign' host. Many are held up in the capillaries of the liver, where they generate a granulomatous response, but some may migrate into other tissues, including lungs, striated muscle, heart, brain and eye. In most cases, infection is asymptomatic and the larvae die without causing serious problems. In heavy infections, there may be generalized symptoms (fever and urticaria) and eosinophilia, as well as focal signs related to the migration of the parasites. Pulmonary involvement may cause bronchospasm and chest X-ray changes. Ocular infection may produce a granulomatous swelling mimicking a retinoblastoma, while cardiac or neurological involvement is occasionally fatal. Rarely, larvae survive in the tissues for many years, causing symptoms long after infection.

Isolation of the larvae is difficult and the diagnosis is usually made serologically. Albendazole 400 mg daily (5–10 mg/kg in children) for a week is the most effective treatment.

Cutaneous larva migrans

Cutaneous larva migrans is caused by the larvae of the non-human hookworms, *Ancylostoma braziliense* and *A. caninum*. Like human hookworms, these hatch in warm, moist soil and then penetrate the skin. In humans, they are unable to complete a normal life cycle and instead migrate under the skin for days or weeks until they eventually die. The wandering of the larva is accompanied by a clearly defined, serpiginous, itchy rash, which progresses at the rate of about 1 cm per day. There are usually no systemic symptoms. The diagnosis is purely clinical. Single larvae may be treated with a 15% solution of topical tiabendazole; multiple lesions require systemic therapy with a single dose of albendazole 400 mg or ivermectin 150–200 μg/kg.

TREMATODES

Trematodes (flukes) are flat, leaf-shaped worms. They have complex life cycles, often involving fresh-water snails and intermediate mammalian hosts. Disease is caused by the inflammatory response to eggs or to the adult worms.

Water-borne flukes

Schistosomiasis

Schistosomiasis affects nearly 240 million people in the tropics and subtropics, mostly in sub-Saharan Africa. Chronic infection causes significant morbidity and, after malaria, it has the most socioeconomic impact of any parasitic disease. Schistosomiasis is largely a disease of the rural poor but has also been associated with major development projects, such as dams and irrigation schemes.

Parasitology and pathogenesis

There are three species of schistosome that commonly cause disease in humans: *Schistosoma mansoni*, *S. haematobium* and *S. japonicum*. *S. mekongi* and *S. intercalatum* also affect humans but have a very restricted distribution ***(Fig. 11.43)***. Eggs are passed in the urine or faeces of an infected person and hatch in fresh water to release the miracidia. These ciliated organisms penetrate the tissue of the intermediate host, a species of water snail specific to each species of schistosome. After multiplying in the snail, large numbers of fork-tailed cercariae are released back into the water, where they can survive for 2–3 days. During this time, the cercariae can penetrate the skin or mucous membranes of the definitive host, humans. Transforming into schistosomulae, they pass through the lungs before reaching the portal vein, where they mature into adult worms (the male is about 20 mm long and the female a little larger). Worms pair in the portal vein before migrating to their final destination: mesenteric veins in the case of *S. mansoni* and *S. japonicum*, and the vesicular plexus for *S. haematobium*. Here, they may remain for many years, producing vast numbers of eggs. The majority of these are released in urine or faeces, but a small number become embedded in the bladder or bowel wall and a few are carried in the circulation to the liver or other distant sites.

The pathology of schistosome infection varies with species and stage of infection. In the early stages, there may be local and systemic allergic reactions to the migrating parasites. As eggs start to be deposited, there may be a local inflammatory response in the bowel or bladder, while ectopic eggs may produce granulomatous lesions anywhere in the body. Chronic heavy infection, in which large numbers of eggs accumulate in the tissues, leads to fibrosis, calcification and, in some cases, dysplasia and malignant change. Morbidity and mortality are related to duration of infection and worm load, as well as to the species of parasite. Children in endemic

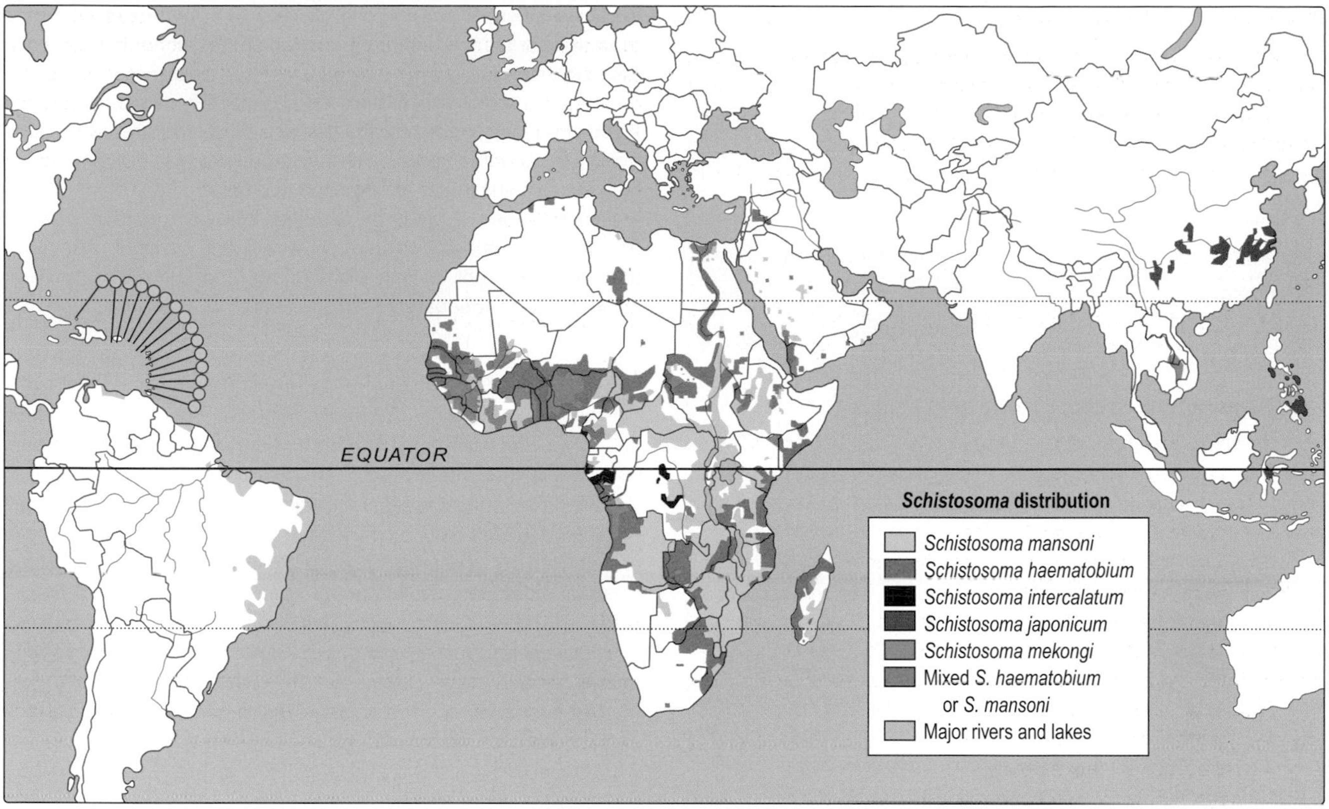

Figure 11.43 Schistosomiasis: geographical distribution. *(From Colley DG, Bustinduy AL, Secor WE, King CH. Human schistosomiasis. Lancet 2014; 383:2253–2264, with permission.)*

areas tend to have the heaviest worm load because of both increased exposure to infection and differences in the immune response between adults and children.

Clinical features

Cercarial penetration of the skin may cause local dermatitis ('swimmer's itch'). After a symptom-free period of 3–4 weeks, systemic allergic features may develop, including fever, rash, myalgia and pneumonitis (Katayama fever). These allergic phenomena are common in non-immune travellers but are rarely seen in local populations, who are usually exposed to infection from early childhood onwards. If infection is sufficiently heavy, symptoms from egg deposition may start to appear 2–3 months after infection.

S. *haematobium* infection (bilharzia)

The earliest symptom is usually painless terminal haematuria. As bladder inflammation progresses, there is increased urinary frequency and groin pain. Obstructive uropathy develops, leading to hydronephrosis, chronic kidney disease and recurrent urinary infection. There is a strong association between chronic urinary schistosomiasis and squamous cell bladder carcinoma. The genitalia may also be affected and ectopic eggs may cause pulmonary or neurological disease.

S. *mansoni*

This usually affects the large bowel. Early disease produces superficial mucosal changes, accompanied by blood-stained diarrhoea. Later, the mucosal damage becomes more marked, with the formation of rectal polyps, deeper ulceration and, eventually, fibrosis and stricture formation. Ectopic eggs are carried to the liver, where they cause an intense granulomatous response. Hepatitis is followed by progressive periportal fibrosis, leading to portal hypertension, oesophageal varices and splenomegaly (see p. 484). Hepatocellular function is usually well preserved.

S. *japonicum*

Unlike the other species, *S. japonicum* infects numerous other mammals apart from humans. It is similar to *S. mansoni* but infects both large and small bowel and produces a greater number of eggs. Disease therefore tends to be more severe and rapidly progressive. Hepatic involvement is more common and neurological involvement is seen in about 5% of cases.

Diagnosis

Schistosomiasis is suggested by relevant symptoms following fresh-water exposure in an endemic area. In the early allergic stages, the diagnosis can only be made clinically. When egg deposition has started, the characteristic eggs (with a terminal spine in the case of *S. haematobium* and a lateral spine in the other species) can be detected on microscopy. In *S. haematobium* infection, the best specimen for examination is a filtered midday urine sample. Parasites may also be found in semen and in rectal snip preparations. *S. mansoni* and *S. japonicum* eggs can usually be found in faeces or in a rectal snip. Serological tests are available and may be useful in the diagnosis of travellers returning from endemic areas, although the test may not become positive for 12 weeks after infection; a parasitological diagnosis should always be made, if possible. In chronic disease, X-rays, ultrasound examinations and

Box 11.64 Treatment of trematode infections

Parasite	Drug and dose
Schistosoma mansoni	Praziquantel 40 mg/kg single dose[a]
S. haematobium	Praziquantel 40 mg/kg single dose[a]
S. japonicum	Praziquantel 60 mg/kg single dose[a]
Paragonimus spp.	Praziquantel 25 mg/kg 8-hourly for 3 days
Clonorchis sinensis	Praziquantel 25 mg/kg 8-hourly for 1–3 days[c]
Opisthorchis spp.	Praziquantel 25 mg/kg 8-hourly for 1–3 days[c]
Fasciolopsis buski	Praziquantel 25 mg/kg 8-hourly for 1 day
Fasciola hepatica	Triclabendazole 10 mg/kg single dose[b]

[a]May be split to minimize nausea. [b]Repeated if necessary. [c]Depending on worm load.

endoscopy may show abnormalities of the bowel or urinary tract, although these are non-specific. Liver biopsy may show the characteristic periportal fibrosis.

Management

The aim of treatment in endemic areas is to decrease the worm load and therefore minimize the chronic effects of egg deposition. It may not always be possible (or even desirable) to eradicate adult worms completely and re-infection is common. However, a 90% reduction in egg output has been achieved in mass treatment programmes, and in light infections where there is no risk of re-exposure, the drugs are usually curative. The most widely used is praziquantel ***(Box 11.64)***, which is effective against all species of schistosome, well tolerated and reasonably cheap.

Prevention

Prevention of schistosomiasis is difficult and relies on a combination of approaches. Mass treatment of the population (especially children) will decrease the egg load in the community. Health education programmes, the provision of latrines and access to a safe water supply should decrease contact with infected water. Attempts to eradicate the snail host have generally been unsuccessful, although man-made bodies of water can often be made less 'snail-friendly'. Travellers should be advised to avoid potentially infected water.

Food-borne flukes

Many flukes infect humans via ingestion of an intermediate host, often fresh-water fish.

Paragonimiasis

Over 20 million people are infected with lung flukes of the genus *Paragonimus*. The adult worms (of which the major species is *P. westermani*) live in the lungs, producing eggs that are either expectorated, or swallowed and passed in the faeces. Miracidia emerging from the eggs penetrate the first intermediate host, a fresh-water snail. Larvae released from the snail seek out the second intermediate host, fresh-water crustacea, in which they encyst as metacercariae. Humans and other mammalian hosts become infected after consuming uncooked shellfish. Cercariae penetrate the small intestinal wall and migrate directly from the peritoneum to the lungs across the diaphragm. Having established themselves in the lung, the adult worms may survive for 20 years.

The common clinical features are fever, cough and mild haemoptysis. In heavy infections, the disease may progress, sometimes mimicking pneumonia or pulmonary tuberculosis. Ectopic worms may cause signs in the abdomen or the brain.

The diagnosis is made by detection of ova on sputum or stool microscopy. Radiological appearances are variable and non-specific. Treatment is with praziquantel and prevention involves avoidance of inadequately cooked shellfish.

Liver flukes

The human liver flukes, *Clonorchis sinensis*, *Opisthorchis felineus* and *O. viverrini*, are almost entirely confined to East and South-east Asia, where they infect more than 20 million people. Adults live in the bile ducts, releasing eggs into the faeces. The parasite requires two intermediate hosts, a fresh-water snail and a fish, and humans are infected by consumption of raw fish. The cycle is completed when excysted worms migrate from the small intestine into the bile ducts.

Infection is often asymptomatic but may be associated with cholangitis and biliary carcinoma. The diagnosis is made by identifying eggs on stool microscopy. Treatment is with praziquantel, and infection can be avoided by cooking fish adequately.

Other fluke infections

Humans can also be infected with a variety of animal flukes: notably, the liver fluke, *Fasciola hepatica*, and the intestinal fluke, *Fasciolopsis buski*. Both require a water snail as an intermediate host; cercariae encyst on aquatic vegetation and then are consumed by animals or humans. After ingestion, *F. hepatica* penetrates the intestinal wall before migrating to the liver: during this stage, it causes systemic allergic symptoms. After reaching the bile ducts, it causes similar problems to those caused by the other liver flukes. *F. buski* does not migrate after it excysts and causes mainly bowel symptoms.

Management of trematode infections

For treatment, see ***Box 11.64***.

CESTODES

Cestodes (tapeworms) are ribbon-shaped worms, which vary from a few millimetres to several metres in length. Adult worms live in the human intestine, where they attach to the epithelium using suckers on the anterior portion (scolex). From the scolex arises a series of progressively developing segments, called proglottids. The mature distal segments contain eggs, which either may be released directly into the faeces, or are carried out with an intact detached proglottid. The eggs are consumed by intermediate hosts, after which they hatch into larvae (oncospheres). These penetrate the intestinal wall of the host (pig or cattle) and encyst in the tissues. Humans ingest the cysts in undercooked meat and the cycle is completed when the parasites excyst in the stomach and develop into adult worms in the small intestine. Infections are usually solitary but several adult tapeworms may coexist. The exceptions to this life cycle are the dwarf tapeworm, *Hymenolepis nana*, which has no intermediate host and is transmitted from person to person by the faeco-oral route; and *Taenia solium*, which can cause either normal tapeworm infection (when humans are the definitive host) or cysticercosis (when humans are the intermediate host).

Taenia saginata

T. saginata, the beef tapeworm, may reach a length of several metres. It is found in all countries where under-cooked beef is eaten. The adult worm causes few, if any, symptoms. Infection is usually discovered when proglottids are found in faeces or on underclothing, often causing considerable anxiety. Ova may also be seen on stool microscopy. Infection can be cleared with a single dose of praziquantel (10 mg/kg). It can be prevented by careful meat inspection or by thorough cooking of beef.

Taenia solium and cysticercosis

T. solium, the pork tapeworm, is generally smaller than *T. saginata*, although it can still reach 6 metres in length. It is particularly common in South America, South Africa, China and parts of South-east Asia. As with *T. saginata*, infection is usually asymptomatic. The ova of the two species are identical but the proglottids can be distinguished on inspection.

Pork tapeworm infection is acquired by eating uncooked pork. ***Treatment*** is with praziquantel or niclosamide. Drug treatment should not be accompanied by a purgative, as was previously believed.

Cysticercosis occurs when humans become the intermediate host of the parasite, and is caused by cysts rather than the adult worm. It follows the ingestion of eggs from contaminated food and water. Faeco-oral autoinfection can occur but is rare. Patients with tapeworms do not usually develop cysticercosis and individuals with cysticercosis do not usually harbour tapeworms. Following the ingestion of eggs, the larvae are liberated, penetrate the intestinal wall, and are carried to various parts of the body where they develop into cysticerci. These are cysts, 0.5–1 cm in diameter, containing the scolex of a new adult worm. Common sites for cysticerci include subcutaneous tissue, skeletal muscle and brain.

Superficial cysts may be felt under the skin but usually cause no significant symptoms. Cysts in the brain can cause a variety of problems, including epilepsy, personality change, hydrocephalus and focal neurological signs (see pp. 866-867). These may only appear many years after infection.

Muscle cysts tend to calcify and are often visible on X-rays. Cutaneous cysts can be excised and examined. Brain cysts are less prone to calcification and are often seen only on CT or MRI scan. Serological tests may support the diagnosis.

Management of cysticercosis

Following years of controversy, recent studies do suggest that anthelminthic drugs are of benefit in most cases of neurocysticercosis, although the role of these drugs in other forms of cysticercosis remains unproven. Albendazole 15 mg/kg daily for 8–20 days is the drug of choice; the alternative is praziquantel 50 mg/kg daily (in divided doses) for 15 days.

Successful treatment is accompanied by increased local inflammation, and corticosteroids should be given during and after the course of anthelminthic. Prevention of cysticercosis depends mainly on good hygiene.

Cerebral cysticercosis

Anticonvulsants should be given for epilepsy, and surgery may be indicated if there is hydrocephalus (see pp. 870–871).

Diphyllobothrium latum

Infection with the fish tapeworm, *D. latum*, is common in Northern Europe and Japan, owing to the consumption of raw fish. The adult worm reaches a length of several metres but, like the other tapeworms, usually causes no symptoms. A megaloblastic anaemia (due to competitive utilization of vitamin B_{12} by the parasite) may occur. Diagnosis and treatment are the same as for *Taenia* species.

Hydatid disease

Hydatid disease occurs when humans become an intermediate host of the dog tapeworm, *Echinococcus granulosus*. The adult worm lives in the gut of domestic and wild canines and the larval stages are usually found in sheep, cattle and camels. Humans may become infected either from direct contact with dogs, or from food or water contaminated with dog faeces. After ingestion, the parasites excyst, penetrate the small intestine wall, and are carried to the liver and other organs in the bloodstream. A slow-growing, thick-walled cyst is formed, inside which further larval stages of the parasite develop. The life cycle cannot be completed unless the cyst is eaten by a dog. Hydatid disease is prevalent in areas where dogs are used in the control of livestock, especially sheep. It is common in Australia, Argentina, the Middle East and parts of East Africa.

Symptoms depend mainly on the site of the cyst. The liver is the most common organ affected (60%), followed by the lung (20%), kidneys (3%), brain (1%) and bone (1%). The symptoms are those of a slowly growing benign tumour. Pressure on the bile ducts may cause jaundice. Rupture into the abdominal cavity, pleural cavity or biliary tree may occur. In the latter situation, intermittent jaundice, abdominal pain and fever associated with eosinophilia result. A cyst rupturing into a bronchus may result in its expectoration and spontaneous cure, but if secondary infection supervenes, a chronic pulmonary abscess will form. Focal seizures can occur if cysts are present in the brain. Renal involvement produces lumbar pain and haematuria. Calcification of the cyst occurs in about 40% of cases.

A related parasite of foxes, *E. multilocularis*, causes a similar but more severe infection, alveolar hydatid disease. These cysts are invasive and metastases may occur.

The diagnosis and treatment of hydatid liver disease are described on page 484.

Further reading

Adegnika AA, Zinsou JF, Issifou S et al. Randomized, controlled, assessor-blind clinical trial to assess the efficacy of single- versus repeated-dose albendazole to treat Ascaris lumbricoides, Trichuris trichiura, and hookworm infection. *Antimicrob Agents Chemother* 2014; 58:2535–2540.

Anderson R, Hollingsworth TD, Truscott J et al. Optimisation of mass chemotherapy to control soil-transmitted helminth infection. *Lancet* 2012; 379:289–290.

Colley DG, Bustinduy AL, Secor WE et al. Human schistosomiasis. *Lancet* 2014; 383:2253–2264.

Lustigman S, Prichard RK, Gazzinelli A et al. A research agenda for helminth diseases of humans: the problem of helminthiasis. *PLoS Negl Trop Dis* 2012; 6:e1582.

Molyneux DH. Tropical lymphedemas – control and prevention. *N Engl J Med* 2012; 366:1169–1171.

Papier K, Williams GM, Luceres-Catubig R et al. Childhood nutrition and parasitic helminth infections. *Clin Infect Dis* 2014; 59:234–243.

Qian MB, Utzinger J, Keiser J, Zhou XN. Clonorchiasis. *Lancet* 2016; 387:800–810.

Zea-Vera A, Cordova EG, Rodriguez S et al. Parasite antigen in serum predicts the presence of viable brain parasites in patients with apparently calcified cysticercosis only. *Clin Infect Dis* 2013; 57:e154–e159.

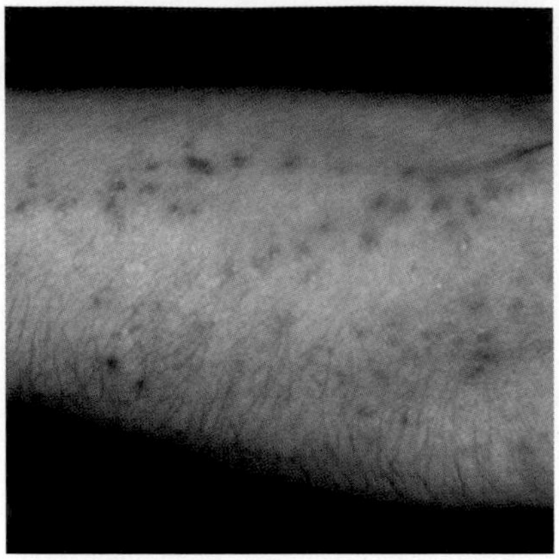

Figure 11.44 Papular urticaria due to bedbug bites.

http://www.plosntds.org *PLoS Neglected Tropical Diseases: the Anti-*Wolbachia *Consortium is coordinating research.*

ARTHROPOD ECTOPARASITES

Arthropods, which include the arachnid ticks and mites as well as insects, may be responsible for human disease in several ways.

Local hypersensitivity reactions

Local lesions may be caused by hypersensitivity to allergens in arthropod saliva. This common reaction, known as papular urticaria, is non-specific and is seen in the majority of people in response to the bite of a variety of blood-sucking arthropods, including mosquitoes, bugs, ticks, lice and mites ***(Fig. 11.44)***. Occasionally, tick bites may cause a more severe systemic allergic response, especially in previously sensitized individuals.

Most of these parasites alight on humans only to feed but some species of lice live in very close proximity to the skin: body lice in clothing, and head and pubic lice on human hairs (see p. 331).

Resident ectoparasite infections

Other ectoparasites are actually resident within the skin, causing more specific local lesions.

Scabies

See page 1347.

Jiggers

Jiggers is due to infection with the jigger flea, *Tunga penetrans*, and is common throughout South America and Africa. The pregnant female flea burrows into the sole of the foot, often between the toes. The egg sac grows to about 0.5 cm in size, before the eggs are discharged on to the ground. The main danger is bacterial infection or tetanus. The flea should be removed with a needle or scalpel and the area kept clean until it heals.

Myiasis

Myiasis is caused by invasion of human tissue by the larva of certain flies, principally the Tumbu fly, *Cordylobia anthropophaga* (found in sub-Saharan Africa), and the human botfly, *Dermatobia hominis* (Central and South America). The larvae, which hatch from eggs laid on laundry and linen, burrow into the skin to form boil-like lesions; a central breathing orifice may be visible. Again, the main risk is secondary infection. It is not always easy to extract the larva; covering it with petroleum jelly may bring it up in search of air.

Systemic envenoming

Many arthropods can cause local or systemic illness through envenoming: that is, injection of venom.

The main role of arthropods in causing human disease is as vectors of parasitic and viral infections. Some of these infections are shown in ***Box 11.4*** and discussed in detail elsewhere.

12 Sexually transmitted infections and human immunodeficiency virus

Janet D Wilson, Jane Anderson

See your e-book for key learning points, summaries, clinical tips, drug tips, extra tables, extra images, interactive Figures, MCQs and Special Topics from the International Advisory Board.

SEXUALLY TRANSMITTED INFECTIONS

Sexually transmitted infections (STIs) are among the most common causes of illness in the world and remain endemic in all societies. They have a profound impact on sexual and reproductive health, and rank among the top five disease categories for which adults seek healthcare worldwide.

The World Health Organization (WHO) estimated that in 2008 there were over 498 million new cases of the four major curable STIs in adults aged 15–49 throughout the world. These included 10.6 million cases of syphilis, 106.1 million of gonorrhoea, 105.7 million of chlamydia and 276.4 million of trichomoniasis. The estimates suggest that the vast majority of these infections were in low-income countries. The pattern of STIs is usually different in high-income countries: for example, in England in 2013, the most common STIs were chlamydia (208 755; 47%), genital warts (73 418; 17%), genital herpes (32 279; 7%) and gonorrhoea (29 291; 7%). The public health, social and economic consequences of STIs are extensive, both for acute infections and for their longer-term sequelae. The inflammation caused by one STI can increase the risk of acquisition of others, and most infections increase the acquisition and transmission of the human immunodeficiency virus (HIV).

The highest prevalence of STIs is in young people, men having sex with men (MSM) and bisexual men, and black and ethnic minority populations. STIs are associated with high-risk sexual behaviour, more frequent partner change and inconsistent use of condoms. Increased travel, both within and between countries, recreational drug use and alcohol are also implicated.

All STIs can be asymptomatic and multiple infections frequently coexist; hence many people without symptoms attend sexual health clinics to seek sexual health checks and advice.

CLINICAL APPROACH TO THE PATIENT WITH AN STI

Patients presenting with possible STIs are frequently anxious, embarrassed and concerned about confidentiality. Staff must be alert to these issues and respond sensitively. The clinical setting must ensure privacy and reinforce confidentiality.

History

The history of the presenting complaint usually focuses on genital symptoms, the most common being:

- urethral discharge in males ***(Box 12.1)***
- vaginal discharge ***(Box 12.2)***
- lower abdominal pain ***(Box 12.3)*** in females
- genital lumps ***(Box 12.4)***
- genital ulceration ***(Box 12.5)***
- genital itching ***(Box 12.6)***
- anal symptoms ***(Box 12.7)***

Details should be obtained of any associated pain, malodour, genital swelling and any abnormal bleeding. Systemic symptoms of fever, skin rash, joint pains and eye symptoms may also be present. Enquiries should be made as to any previous STIs, including dates and treatment received, HIV testing and results, and hepatitis B vaccination status if appropriate (see pp. 320–321).

Box 12.1 Causes of urethral discharge

- Urethritis in men usually presents with a urethral discharge and dysuria
- Usually divided into gonococcal (due to *N. gonorrhoeae*) or non-gonococcal urethritis (NGU)

Infective causes
- *Chlamydia trachomatis*[a]
- *Mycoplasma genitalium*[b]
- *Ureaplasma urealyticum*
- *Neisseria gonorrhoeae*
- *Trichomonas vaginalis* (TV)[c]
- Herpes simplex virus (HSV)[c]
- Urinary tract infection (UTI)[d]
- Adenoviruses (often associated with conjunctivitis)[c]

Non-infective causes
- Non-specific urethritis (where no cause can be identified)
- Physical or chemical trauma
- Urethral stricture

Questions that help discriminate between causes
- Colour of discharge
- Any dysuria, urinary frequency, nocturia or haematuria?
- Any testicular pain or swelling?
- Any other symptoms, e.g. genital sores or rash, sore eyes?

Investigations
- Microscopy of urethral discharge, nucleic acid amplification test (NAAT) and culture for *N. gonorrhoeae*, NAAT for *C. trachomatis*, serology for syphilis and HIV
- Tests for TV and HSV are not usually performed routinely
- There are no commercial tests available for *M. genitalium* and *U. urealyticum*
- A mid-stream specimen of urine (MSU) should be taken if symptoms are suggestive of UTI

[a]Most common cause of NGU. [b]Second most common cause of NGU. [c]Rarer causes of NGU. [d]Most frequent non-sexually transmitted cause of NGU.

Box 12.2 Causes of vaginal discharge

Infective causes
Vaginal infections
- Bacterial vaginosis (BV)[a]
- *Candida albicans*[a]
- *Trichomonas vaginalis* (TV)[b]

Cervical infections
- *Chlamydia trachomatis*
- *Neisseria gonorrhoeae*
- Herpes simplex virus

Non-infective causes
- Physiological discharge/cervical ectopy[c]
- Cervical polyps
- Neoplasms
- Retained products (e.g. of conception, tampons)
- Chemical irritation

Questions that help discriminate between causes
- Does the discharge have an offensive odour?
- Any vulval itching or soreness?
- Any other symptoms, e.g. dysuria, intermenstrual or postcoital bleeding, abdominal pain?

Investigations
- Microscopy of vaginal discharge for BV, candida and TV, culture for candida, nucleic acid amplification test (NAAT; if available) or culture for TV, NAAT for *N. gonorrhoeae* and *C. trachomatis*, serology for syphilis and HIV

[a]The most common causes of altered vaginal discharge but C. trachomatis *and* N. gonorrhoeae *infections must also be considered. [b]The most common cause worldwide but rarer in high-income countries. [c]Also a common cause (diagnosis usually made on the basis of exclusion of infective causes).*

Box 12.3 Causes of lower abdominal pain

Infective causes
- Pelvic inflammatory disease (PID)[a,b]
  - *Chlamydia trachomatis*[c]
  - *Neisseria gonorrhoeae*
  - *Mycoplasma genitalium*
  - Bacterial vaginosis (BV)
- Urinary tract infection (UTI)

Non-infective causes
- Ectopic pregnancy
- Acute appendicitis
- Endometriosis
- Irritable bowel syndrome
- Neoplasms
- Torsion or haemorrhage of ovarian cyst

Questions that help discriminate between causes
- Site, character and duration of pain?
- Any vaginal discharge, postcoital or intermenstrual bleeding, or deep dyspareunia?
- Date of last menstrual period (LMP) and contraception used? Is pregnancy possible?
- Any dysuria, urinary frequency, nocturia or haematuria?
- Any nausea, vomiting, diarrhoea or constipation?

Investigations
- Microscopy of vaginal discharge for BV and TV, nucleic acid amplification test (NAAT; if available) or culture for TV, NAAT and culture for *N. gonorrhoeae*, NAAT for *C. trachomatis*, serology for syphilis and HIV
- There are no commercial tests available for *M. genitalium*
- A pregnancy test should be performed, as ectopic pregnancy is a differential diagnosis
- A mid-stream specimen of urine (MSU) should be taken if symptoms are suggestive of UTI

[a]Most common in young (under 25 years) sexually active women. [b]Symptoms of abnormal vaginal discharge and/or abnormal bleeding are usually present with PID, and BV is also often present. [c]The most common cause of PID.

A full general medical history should be obtained, including a history of allergies and a drug history, particularly of any recent antibacterial or antiviral treatment. In women, a menstrual, obstetric and cervical cytology screening history should be obtained, as well as details of current contraception. Any past or current history of drug (including recreational use) and/or alcohol misuse should be explored.

A ***sexual history*** should be taken that includes:
- number and types of recent sexual contacts with dates
- gender of partners
- whether the partner is regular or casual; if regular, how long the couple has been having sex
- use of condoms
- any known symptoms or STI diagnosis in the partner
- sexual practices, e.g. insertive or receptive vaginal, insertive or receptive anal, insertive or receptive pharyngeal, and insertive or receptive oroanal sex
- number of partners over the past 3 months, particularly in people who frequently change partners
- number of sexual partners over the past 12 months, in those at higher risk of STIs, such as young people and men having sex with men (MSM)
- whether the patient has ever paid, or has been paid, for sex
- country of origin of any sexual partners, in view of the differences in prevalence of HIV, hepatitis B and C, certain

Box 12.4 Causes of genital lumps

Infective causes

- Human papillomavirus (HPV; anogenital warts)[a,b]
- Molluscum contagiosum
- *Sarcoptes scabiei* (scabies – excoriated lesions)[c]
- *Treponema pallidum*
  - Secondary condylomata lata[d]

Non-infective causes

- Normal anatomical variants (e.g. papillae, sebaceous glands and skin tags)
- Sebaceous cysts
- Neoplasms

Questions that help discriminate between causes

- Where are the lumps?
- Are they single or multiple?
- Are they itchy or painful?
- How long have they been present?
- Are there any lumps or rashes elsewhere on the skin?

Investigations

- Nucleic acid amplification test (NAAT) for *N. gonorrhoeae* and NAAT for *C. trachomatis*, serology for syphilis and HIV
- Diagnoses of anogenital warts and molluscum contagiosum are made on clinical appearances; HPV testing is not appropriate for diagnosing anogenital warts

[a]Most common infective causes, followed by molluscum contagiosum. [b]Lumps present on the mucous membranes are more likely to be anogenital warts, as molluscum contagiosum does not occur there. [c]Can present with excoriated papules on the genital area due to excessive scratching. [d]Moist papules present in secondary syphilis – rare but easily misdiagnosed as anogenital warts.

STIs such as chancroid and donovanosis, and the patterns of gonococcal antibiotic resistance worldwide.

An STI and HIV acquisition risk assessment should be routinely undertaken. Those identified as being at high risk of STIs (e.g. frequent partner change, unprotected sex, use of drugs and/or alcohol to a level that reduces safer sex) and those with ongoing higher risk of HIV (e.g. MSM, sexual partners from countries with high HIV prevalence) should be offered risk reduction advice based on motivational interview techniques and be made aware of the availability of post-exposure HIV prophylaxis following sexual exposure (PEPSE). See page 347 for more details.

Examination

The inguinal, genital and perianal areas should be examined using a good light source. The groins should be palpated for lymphadenopathy, and the pubic hair and skin examined for nits and lice and any skin rashes or lumps. The external genitalia and perianal area should be examined for signs of erythema, fissures, lumps, ulcers, pigmented or hypopigmented areas. A rectal examination/proctoscopy should be performed in patients with rectal symptoms, in those with perianal warts extending into the anal canal, and in men with prostatic symptoms.

In men, the skin of the penile shaft (retracting the prepuce if present) should be examined for rashes, lumps, or ulcers, and the urethral meatus should be inspected for erythema and discharge ***(Fig. 12.1)***. The scrotal contents should be palpated, noting any tenderness or lumps, as well as the consistency of the testes.

In women, the labia majora, labia minora, clitoris, urethra, introitus and perineum should be examined for rashes, lumps or ulcers. Any evidence of female genital mutilation (FGM) should be documented. A bivalve vaginal speculum should be inserted and the

Box 12.5 Causes of genital ulceration

Infective causes

- Herpes simplex virus (HSV) types 1 and 2[a]:
  - Primary
  - Recurrent
- *Treponema pallidum*[b]
  - Primary chancre
  - Secondary mucous patches
  - Tertiary gumma
- Herpes zoster[c]
- Lymphogranuloma venereum (LGV)[d]
- Chancroid[d]
- Donovanosis (granuloma inguinale)[d]

Non-infective causes

- Trauma
- Aphthous ulceration (e.g. as in Behçet syndrome)[e]
- Lichen sclerosus
- Erosive lichen planus
- Fixed drug eruptions
- Stevens–Johnson syndrome
- Crohn's disease
- Neoplasms

Questions that help distinguish between causes

- Are the ulcers painful?
- Are they single or multiple?
- How long have they been present?
- Is there any external dysuria?
- Are there any ulcers or rash elsewhere on the skin?
- Are there any systematic symptoms?

Investigations

- Ulcer swab for HSV polymerase chain reaction (PCR). Some laboratories also test these swabs for *T. pallidum* using PCR. Nucleic acid amplification test (NAAT) for *N. gonorrhoeae*, NAAT for *C. trachomatis*, serology for syphilis and HIV. Syphilis serology should be repeated after the 3-month window period if appropriate
- In men who have sex with men (MSM), consider an ulcer swab for *C. trachomatis* and NAAT with genotyping for LGV if positive

[a]Most common cause of multiple painful ulcers. [b]Syphilis ulcers are usually single and non-painful. [c]Much rarer than HSV and characterized by unilateral presentation. [d]LGV rare except in MSM; chancroid and donovanosis extremely rare. [e]Most common non-infective cause; usually, there is a history of similar lesions in the mouth.

Box 12.6 Causes of genital itching

Infective causes

- *Candida albicans*[a]
- *Trichomonas vaginalis* (TV)
- *Phthirus pubis* (pubic lice)[b]
- *Sarcoptes scabiei* (scabies)[c]

Non-infective causes[d]

- Irritant dermatitis
- Genital eczema
- Lichen sclerosus
- Lichen planus

Questions that help distinguish between causes

- Site and duration of itching?
- Any vaginal discharge, offensive odour or vulval swelling?
- Any itching or rash elsewhere on the skin, or any known skin problems?

Investigations

- Microscopy of vaginal discharge for candida and TV, culture for candida, nucleic acid amplification test (NAAT; if available) or culture for TV, NAAT for *N. gonorrhoeae* and *C. trachomatis*, serology for syphilis and HIV

[a]The most frequent symptom in females is vulval itching rather than vaginal discharge. [b]Relatively rare but easily visible in the hair area. [c]Can cause genital itching and may present with excoriated papules due to excessive scratching. [d]Genital dermatoses are common causes of genital itching and are frequently misdiagnosed as candida.

Box 12.7 Causes of rectal symptoms

- Symptoms of proctitis are rectal pain, mucopurulent anal discharge, rectal bleeding, constipation and tenesmus
- Proctoscopy may reveal mucosal erythema, oedema, contact bleeding and a mucopurulent discharge, with ulceration in severe cases

Infective causes

Rectal infections

- *Neisseria gonorrhoeae*[a]
- *Chlamydia trachomatis*[a]
- Lymphogranuloma venereum (LGV)[b]
- Herpes simplex virus (HSV)[c]
- *Treponema pallidum*[c]

Intestinal infections

- *Shigella* spp.[b]
- *Campylobacter* spp.
- *Entamoeba histolytica*
- *Salmonella* spp.
- *Escherichia coli*
- *Cryptosporidium* spp.

Non-infective causes

- Ulcerative colitis
- Crohn's disease
- Neoplasms

Questions that help distinguish between causes

- Any irritation or pain around the anus or in the rectum?
- Any discharge or bleeding from the anus?
- Any abdominal pain, diarrhoea or blood in the stool?
- Any feeling of incomplete bowel evacuation or constipation?
- Any systematic symptoms?

Investigations

- Microscopy of a rectal smear, rectal culture and nucleic acid amplification test (NAAT) for *N. gonorrhoeae*, NAAT for *C. trachomatis*, serology for syphilis and HIV. If positive for *C. trachomatis*, genotyping for LGV should be requested
- If there is severe proctitis, a swab for HSV and *T. pallidum* polymerase chain reaction (PCR) should be performed
- LGV should be considered in MSM with suspected inflammatory bowel disease, as the clinical presentation can be very similar
- Cultures for enteric pathogens should be performed if symptoms of enteritis are present

[a]*Most common causes of proctitis in women and MSM.* [b]*Outbreaks occurring in Europe in MSM.* [c]*Rarer causes than* N. gonorrhoeae *and* C. trachomatis*; mainly seen in MSM.*

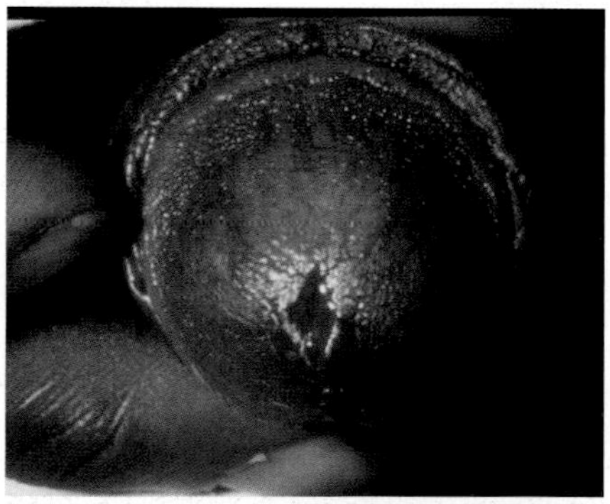

Figure 12.1 **Mucopurulent urethral discharge.**

vagina examined for erythema, discharge, lumps or ulcers. The cervix should be inspected and any ectopy noted, as well as any discharge ***(Fig. 12.2A)***, contact bleeding ***(Fig. 12.2B)***, ulceration or raised lesions. A bimanual pelvic examination should be performed in those complaining of abdominal pain to determine the size and any tenderness of the uterus, as well as any cervical motion or adnexal tenderness and the presence of any masses.

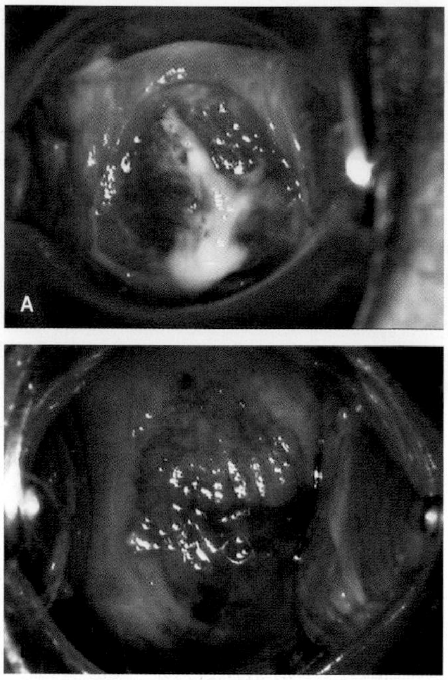

Figure 12.2 **Cervicitis.** A. Purulent discharge. B. Contact bleeding.

If systemic symptoms have been identified, a general examination should be performed with inspection of the skin, mouth, pharynx and lymph nodes. Signs of HIV infection are covered on p. 336.

Investigation of STIs

Although the history and examination will guide investigations, it should be remembered that multiple infections may coexist and may be asymptomatic. Tests for all STIs are indicated in any patient with a known STI or in those who have been in contact with an STI. The recommended tests for specific infections are indicated in the sections below.

Asymptomatic STI screening

The minimum investigations should include tests for chlamydia, gonorrhoea, syphilis and HIV. HIV antibody testing should be performed on an 'opt out' basis. If it is declined, the reasons why should be documented. Screening for hepatitis viruses should be performed in those at increased risk, as indicated below.

Screening for hepatitis A and vaccination. Test for antibodies to hepatitis A (with vaccination if negative) should be performed in injecting drug users, people with chronic hepatitis B or C, or HIV, and MSM in areas where an outbreak of hepatitis A has been reported.

Screening for hepatitis B and vaccination. The recommended screening test in those who have not been immunized is immunoglobulin G (IgG) anti-hepatitis B core (anti-HBc), which is a marker of past infection. If positive, hepatitis B surface antigen (HBsAg) testing should be performed, as this identifies currently infected individuals. Screening is recommended for the following: sexual partners of those who are HBsAg-positive, MSM and their sexual partners, people who have been sexually assaulted, sex workers, injecting drug users and their sexual partners, individuals or those with a sexual partner from countries with a high prevalence of hepatitis B (which are countries outside Western Europe, North America and Australasia), needle-stick recipients, people with chronic hepatitis C or HIV, and those born to a mother infected with hepatitis B. Patients who are negative and have ongoing increased risk should be offered vaccination.

Screening for hepatitis C (HCV). Screening for antibodies to hepatitis C is recommended in the sexual partners of HCV-positive people, injecting drug users, needle-stick recipients, people with chronic hepatitis B or HIV, and those born to a mother infected with HCV.

Investigations for symptomatic patients

The investigations will depend on the clinical presentation but should always include tests for chlamydia, gonorrhoea, syphilis and HIV. The recommended investigations for these presentations are shown in ***Boxes 12.1–12.7***.

Management, prevention and control

The treatment of specific conditions is covered in the appropriate sections. Most sexual health clinics give directly observed therapy where possible or dispense medication directly to the patient to improve adherence in order to prevent onward transmission.

Tracing the sexual partners of patients is crucial in controlling the spread of STIs. The aims are to identify and treat those with infections (particularly those with asymptomatic infections) in order to prevent the spread within the community. Also, appropriate antibiotic therapy is usually offered to recent sexual partners of those known to have an active infection (epidemiological treatment). Interviewing people about their sexual partners requires considerable tact and sensitivity, and specialist health advisers are available in sexual health clinics.

Many STI diagnoses are in young adults (16–24 years). Prevention starts with education and information. People begin sexual activity at ever-younger ages and education programmes need to include school pupils, as well as young adults. Education of health professionals is also crucial. Primary public health prevention aimed at informing groups at particular risk in order to modify sexual behaviour should be implemented at a national level. Secondary interventions include the prompt diagnosis and appropriate management of STIs in order to reduce complications and onward transmission. The National Chlamydia Screening Programme (NCSP) in England aims to provide earlier detection and treatment for chlamydia by providing easy access for under-25-year-olds to chlamydia testing in community settings.

Reducing the numbers of sexual partners, avoiding overlapping relationships, using condoms correctly and consistently, and avoiding sex if symptoms are present can reduce the risks of acquiring and transmitting an STI. For those who change their sexual partners frequently, regular check-ups (approximately 3-monthly) are advisable. Once people develop symptoms, they should be encouraged to seek medical advice as soon as possible to reduce complications and spread to others.

Further reading

British Association for Sexual Health and HIV (BASHH). *BASHH Clinical Effectiveness Guidelines*. BASHH; available online at http://www.bashh.org/.

Mercer CH, Tanton C, Prah P et al. Changes in sexual attitudes and lifestyles in Britain through the life course and over time: findings from the National Surveys of Sexual Attitudes and Lifestyles (Natsal). *Lancet* 2013; [illegible]

Sonnenberg P, Clifton S, Beddows S et al. Prevalence, risk factors, and uptake of interventions for sexually transmitted infections in Britain: findings from the National Surveys of Sexual Attitudes and Lifestyles (Natsal). *Lancet* 2013; 382:1795–1806.

Winter A, Ross J (eds). Sexually transmitted infections – Parts 1 and 2. *Medicine* 2014; 42:281–404.

World Health Organization. *Global Incidence and Prevalence of Selected Curable Sexually Transmitted Infections – 2008*. Geneva: WHO; 2012.

SPECIFIC INFECTIONS

HIV/AIDS

This is discussed on pages 331–355.

Hepatitis B

This is discussed on pages 454-457. Sexual contacts should be screened and immunized if they are not immune.

Chlamydia trachomatis

C. trachomatis (CT) is the most common STI in the UK; up to 10% of sexually active people below the age of 25 years are infected. It infects the urethra, endocervix, rectum, pharynx and conjunctiva, and is transmitted by direct inoculation of infected secretions from one mucous membrane to another. As up to 80% of women and 50% of men may be asymptomatic, it is frequently unrecognized and therefore untreated. Pelvic inflammatory disease, the main complication of CT, can result in tubal infertility, ectopic pregnancy and chronic pelvic pain, causing significant morbidity and cost to health services.

Clinical features

The exact incubation period is unclear but is thought to be between 7 and 21 days.

In men, it can cause an anterior urethritis with a mucoid or mucopurulent urethral discharge (which may be worse on waking, when there may be crusting at the meatus) and dysuria. The infection can ascend along the vas deferens, leading to epididymo-orchitis.

In women, the most common site of infection is the endocervix but the urethra can also be infected. Symptoms may include increased vaginal discharge, dysuria, postcoital or intermenstrual bleeding, and lower abdominal pain. Examination of the cervix may reveal mucopurulent cervicitis and/or contact bleeding. Ascending infection into the uterus and fallopian tubes causes endometritis and acute salpingitis (pelvic inflammatory disease). In pregnancy, CT is associated with preterm birth, postpartum infection, and neonatal mucopurulent conjunctivitis and pneumonia due to vertical transmission during vaginal delivery.

Rectal infection, through receptive anal sex, may be asymptomatic but can cause proctitis. Reactive arthritis (see p. 686) can occur with CT infection, particularly in human leucocyte antigen (HLA)-B27-positive individuals.

Diagnosis

Nucleic acid amplification tests (NAATs) are the diagnostic tests of choice for CT, as they have sensitivities of 90–99%. In men, first-voided urine (FVU) samples or urethral swabs, and in women vulvovaginal swabs (VVSs) or endocervical swabs, are taken. Self-taken VVSs are as sensitive at detecting CT as clinician-taken VVSs but FVU samples in women are less sensitive than VVSs and endocervical swabs. The advantages of male FVU samples and self-taken VVSs is that they are non-invasive (meaning they can be obtained by the patient without the need for an examination), so are ideal for asymptomatic chlamydia screening.

MSM who practise receptive anal sex and receptive oral sex should have rectal and pharyngeal swabs for CT NAAT performed.

Management

Macrolide or tetracycline antibiotics are most commonly used to treat CT. Azithromycin 1 g as a single dose or doxycycline 100 mg ×2 daily for 7 days is the recommended regimen for uncomplicated infection. Both of these drugs have similar efficacies of more than 95%. Azithromycin 1 g as a single dose is recommended in pregnant or lactating women by WHO, USA, UK and Australian guidelines but the manufacturers advise use only if adequate alternatives are not available. Tetracyclines are contraindicated in pregnancy. Longer courses of antibiotics are required for complicated infections (see pelvic inflammatory disease and epididymo-orchitis below). Epidemiological treatment pending test results is usually offered to those who have had recent sexual intercourse with someone who has confirmed CT infection, as the infection rate can be up to 50%. Abstinence from sex for at least 7 days, or until treatment is completed, should be advised. Sexual contacts must be traced, notified and treated, particularly as many infections are asymptomatic.

A follow-up interview (possibly by telephone) should be held in order to assess adherence to therapy and partner notification. A routine test of cure is not necessary after treatment with azithromycin or doxycycline, except in pregnant women or where symptoms persist or re-infection is suspected. NAATs may remain positive for some time after treatment, as they detect non-viable organisms, so a test of cure should be deferred until 6 weeks after the start of treatment.

Gonorrhoea

Neisseria gonorrhoeae is a Gram-negative intracellular diplococcus ***(Fig. 12.3)***, which infects the urethra, endocervix, rectum, pharynx and conjunctiva. It is transmitted by direct inoculation of infected secretions from one mucous membrane to another. Up to 50% of infected women and 10% of infected men are asymptomatic. Co-infection with CT is common, occurring in 20% of men and 40% of women with gonorrhoea (GC).

Clinical features

The incubation period is 2–14 days, with most symptoms in males occurring between 2 and 5 days.

In men, GC can cause anterior urethritis with mucopurulent or purulent urethral discharge and dysuria ***(Fig. 12.4)***. The discharge can be profuse, causing staining of underwear. Complications include ascending infection, leading to epididymo-orchitis and acute prostatitis.

In women, symptoms may include increased vaginal discharge, dysuria, postcoital or intermenstrual bleeding, and lower abdominal pain. Examination of the cervix may reveal mucopurulent or purulent cervicitis and/or contact bleeding. Complications include Bartholin's abscesses, and ascending infection into the uterus and fallopian tubes causes endometritis and acute salpingitis (pelvic inflammatory disease). In pregnancy, GC is associated with preterm birth, postpartum infection, and neonatal purulent conjunctivitis due to vertical transmission during vaginal delivery.

Rectal infection, through receptive anal sex, may be asymptomatic but can cause proctitis. GC septicaemia (disseminated gonococcal infection, DGI) is a rare complication presenting as fever, tenosynovitis, arthritis and characteristic erythematous skin lesions with necrotic centres.

Diagnosis

NAATs are the diagnostic test of choice for *N. gonorrhoeae*, as they have better sensitivity than culture. However, as *N. gonorrhoeae* antimicrobial resistance is increasing, culture on selective media should be performed prior to any treatment for GC being given. In men, FVU samples or urethral swabs, and in women VVSs or endocervical swabs, are the specimens of choice for GC NAATs. Self-taken VVSs are as sensitive at detecting GC as clinician-taken VVSs. FVU samples in women should not be used as they are less sensitive than VVSs and endocervical swabs. As male FVU samples and self-taken VVSs are non-invasive samples, they are ideal for asymptomatic screening. MSM who practise receptive anal sex and receptive oral sex should have rectal and pharyngeal swabs for GC NAATs performed. A urethral swab in men, an endocervical swab in women, and rectal and pharyngeal swabs in both are the specimens to use for culture.

Microscopy of Gram-stained urethral and endocervical secretions may demonstrate intracellular, Gram-negative diplococci, allowing rapid diagnosis. The sensitivity ranges from 90% in urethral specimens from symptomatic men to 50% in endocervical specimens. Microscopy should not be used for pharyngeal specimens. The sensitivity of blood and synovial fluid cultures is poor, so NAATs from the genital tract, rectum and pharynx remain the tests of choice for investigations of DGI.

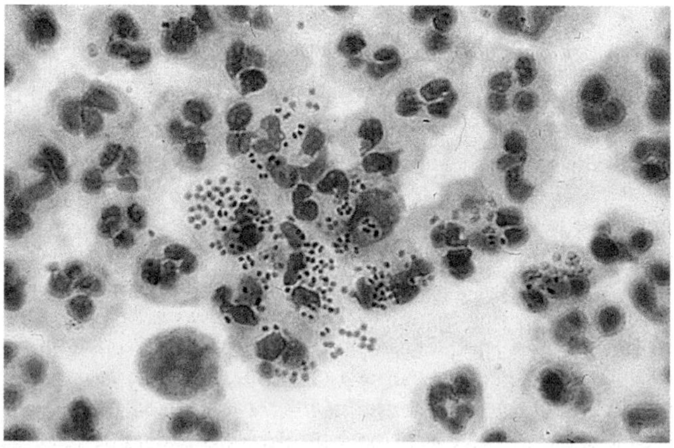

Figure 12.3 ***Neisseria gonorrhoeae.*** Gram-negative intracellular diplococci. *(Courtesy of Dr B. Goh.)*

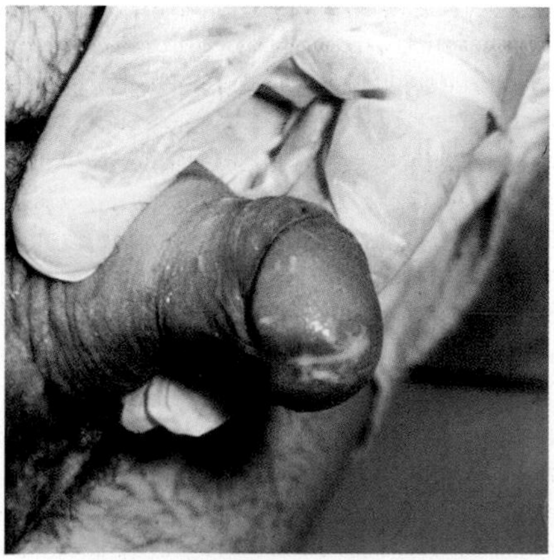

Figure 12.4 ***Neisseria gonorrhoeae.*** Mucopurulent urethral discharge.

Management

Treatment should be given to those who have positive microscopy, a positive NAAT or a positive culture for GC. Antibiotic-resistant strains of *N. gonorrhoeae* are increasing and dual antibiotic therapy should always be used in order to reduce development of further resistance. Single-dose ceftriaxone 500 mg i.m. with azithromycin 1 g is recommended in the UK. If there is a history of penicillin anaphylaxis or established cephalosporin allergy, spectinomycin 2 g i.m. with azithromycin 1 g should be used. Both of these regimens can be used in pregnancy. Epidemiological treatment pending test results is usually offered to those who have had recent sexual intercourse with someone with confirmed GC infection, as the infection rate is usually about 50%. Longer courses of antibiotics are required for complicated infections (see pelvic inflammatory disease and epididymo-orchitis below). Abstinence from sex for at least 7 days, or until treatment has been completed, should be advised. All sexual contacts should be notified, examined and treated.

A follow-up assessment and test of cure using GC NAAT should take place 14 days after treatment.

Non-gonococcal urethritis

Non-gonococcal urethritis (NGU) in men is usually characterized by a urethral discharge and dysuria. There are a number of causes, many of which are sexually transmitted; the most common of these is *C. trachomatis*, which is discussed above. Other causes are *Mycoplasma genitalium*, *Ureaplasma urealyticum*, *Trichomonas vaginalis* (TV), herpes simplex virus (HSV) 1 and 2, and adenoviruses, in that order of frequency. Studies investigating the aetiology of NGU have consistently identified no known cause in over 60% of cases. Non-sexually transmitted causes of NGU may be urinary tract infections (UTIs), foreign bodies and strictures.

Clinical features

The incubation period is usually 2–3 weeks. The main symptom is a mucoid or mucopurulent urethral discharge, which may be worse on waking, when there may be crusting at the meatus. Dysuria is common but not universal. Discomfort or itching within the urethra may be present.

Diagnosis

NAAT for *N. gonorrhoeae* and for *C. trachomatis* should be performed in all men with symptoms of urethritis on either an FVU sample or urethral swab. Microscopy of Gram-stained urethral secretion showing five or more polymorphonuclear leucocytes per high-power (×1000 oil-immersion lens) field is diagnostic. Men who are symptomatic but have no objective evidence of urethritis should be re-examined and tested after holding their urine overnight. Testing for TV and HSV is not routinely performed and there are no commercial tests available for *M. genitalium* and *U. urealyticum*. A mid-stream specimen of urine (MSU) should be taken if symptoms are suggestive of a UTI (urinary frequency, nocturia, urgency, haematuria).

Management

Therapy for NGU is with either doxycycline 100 mg ×2 daily for 7 days or azithromycin 1 g orally as a single dose. Abstinence from sex for at least 7 days should be advised. All sexual contacts should be notified, examined and treated. Follow-up is only indicated if CT is confirmed or if symptoms persist.

Recurrent/persistent NGU

This is defined as persistent or recurrent symptomatic urethritis occurring 30–90 days following treatment of acute NGU, and occurs in 10–20% of cases. The aetiology is probably multifactorial but *M. genitalium* and *T. vaginalis* are likely causes. It is necessary to ensure that there is still objective evidence of urethritis, that there was good adherence to NGU treatment with sexual abstinence, and that sexual partners were also treated. If there is no objective evidence of urethritis, patients should be reassured and further antibiotic therapy avoided. Subsequent treatment needs to cover *M. genitalium* and *T. vaginalis*. The recommended treatment is azithromycin 500 mg orally as a single dose, followed by 250 mg daily for 4 days with metronidazole 400 mg ×2 daily for 5 days.

Pelvic inflammatory disease

Pelvic inflammatory disease (PID) results when infections ascend from the cervix or vagina into the upper genital tract. It is most frequent in young (under 25 years) sexually active women. It includes endometritis, salpingitis, tubo-ovarian abscess and pelvic peritonitis. The main causes are *C. trachomatis* and *N. gonorrhoeae*, but these are identified in less than half of the cases of PID in the UK. *M. genitalium* has been associated with PID and anaerobes have also been implicated. Even in women with laparoscopically proven PID, often no bacterial cause is found. PID has serious long term sequelae due to tubal damage and pelvic adhesions, resulting in tubal infertility, increased risk of ectopic pregnancy and chronic pelvic pain. The risk of sequelae increases with more severe and multiple episodes of PID. Tubal infertility occurs in 10–12% of women after one episode of PID and increases to 50–60% after three or more episodes. The risk of ectopic pregnancy is increased 6–10-fold and abdominal or pelvic pain for longer than 6 months occurs in 18% of women.

Clinical features

The onset of symptoms often occurs in the first part of the menstrual cycle. Lower abdominal pain, usually bilateral, is the most common symptom, with increased vaginal discharge, irregular bleeding, deep dyspareunia and dysuria being present in some women. There may be a mucopurulent cervical discharge with contact bleeding. Lower abdominal tenderness and adnexal and cervical motion tenderness on bimanual examination are the most common signs.

Diagnosis

The diagnosis is usually made on the clinical findings of lower abdominal pain, with supportive symptoms of increased vaginal discharge and abnormal bleeding, and cervical motion and/or adnexal tenderness on bimanual examination. However, such a clinical diagnosis has a specificity of only 65–70%. The differential diagnosis includes ectopic pregnancy, acute appendicitis, endometriosis, UTI and irritable bowel disease.

Investigations should include microscopy of Gram-stained vaginal discharge for bacterial vaginosis (BV), NAAT and culture for *N. gonorrhoeae*, and NAAT for *C. trachomatis*. There are no commercial tests available for *M. genitalium*. A pregnancy test should be performed on all women suspected of having PID, as ectopic pregnancy is a differential diagnosis. An MSU should be taken if symptoms are suggestive of a UTI (urinary frequency, nocturia, urgency, haematuria).

Management

Early diagnosis and treatment reduce the risk of long-term sequelae, so empirical treatment should be started before microbiology results are known. A broad-spectrum antibiotic regimen is needed to cover the main bacterial causes. The recommended regimens are: single-dose ceftriaxone 500 mg i.m. with doxycycline 100 mg ×2 daily and metronidazole 400 mg ×2 daily for 14 days; or ofloxacin 400 mg ×2 daily and metronidazole 400 mg ×2 daily for 14 days. Abstinence from sex for at least 14 days should be advised. All sexual contacts should be notified, examined and treated.

Those with moderate or severe clinical findings should be reviewed within 2–3 days to ensure they are improving on treatment. Lack of response requires further investigation and possible admission for intravenous therapy and/or surgical intervention. All women should be seen after 2 weeks in order to assess symptom resolution, adherence to therapy and partner notification.

Epididymo-orchitis

Acute epididymo-orchitis is a clinical syndrome consisting of pain, swelling and inflammation of the epididymis that can extend into the testis. It is caused mainly by extension of infection from the urethra or the bladder. In men under 35 years, *C. trachomatis* and *N. gonorrhoeae* are the main causes, but in men over 35 years, it is more commonly a complication of a UTI. Mumps is another cause of epididymo-orchitis in non-immune men. The most common differential diagnosis is torsion of the spermatic cord, which is a urological emergency.

Clinical features

The typical presentation is subacute onset of unilateral scrotal pain and swelling. There may also be symptoms of a urethral discharge and dysuria but these are often absent. On examination, there is tenderness and usually palpable swelling of the epididymis. There may also be some tenderness and swelling of the testicle, with oedema and erythema of the overlying scrotal skin. A urethral discharge may be present.

Diagnosis

The diagnosis is usually made on the above clinical findings. The main differential diagnosis is testicular torsion.

Investigations include a NAAT and culture for *N. gonorrhoeae* and a NAAT for *C. trachomatis*. If microscopy of Gram-stained urethral secretions shows five or more polymorphonuclear leucocytes per high-power (×1000 oil-immersion lens) field, this indicates the diagnosis of NGU. If intracellular Gram-negative diplococci are present, this is suggestive of GC. An MSU should be taken if symptoms are suggestive of a UTI (urinary frequency, nocturia, urgency, haematuria) and in older men.

Management

As empirical treatment should be started before microbiology results are known, a broad-spectrum antibiotic regimen is needed to cover the main bacterial causes. In younger men, where an STI is the likely diagnosis, the recommended regimen is single-dose ceftriaxone 500 mg i.m. with doxycycline 100 mg ×2 daily for 14 days. Where a UTI is the more likely diagnosis, ofloxacin 200 mg ×2 daily for 14 days should be prescribed. Abstinence from sex for at least 14 days should be advised. All sexual contacts should be notified, examined and treated.

Patients should be reassessed after 3 days if there is no improvement in their symptoms, as such lack of response requires further investigations. All should be seen after 2 weeks in order to assess symptom resolution, adherence to therapy and partner notification.

Bacterial vaginosis

Bacterial vaginosis (BV) is the most frequent cause of vaginal discharge among women of childbearing age. A BV prevalence of 9% has been reported in women attending general practice for cervical cytology screening and in 15% of pregnant women in the UK. BV develops when the normal *Lactobacilli*-dominant vaginal flora are replaced by an overgrowth of other bacteria, including *Gardnerella vaginalis*, anaerobes, mycoplasmas and *Mobiluncus* spp. It is not regarded as a sexually transmitted disease. BV in pregnancy is associated with an increased risk of miscarriage and preterm birth. It also increases the risk of acquisition and transmission of HIV. Up to 50% of women with BV have no symptoms and, as it is not regarded as an STI, it is not necessary to look for or treat asymptomatic BV.

Clinical features

The symptoms are an increased vaginal discharge and offensive fishy odour. On examination, there is a creamy-white homogeneous discharge, which may be slightly frothy (due to the volatile amine production by the bacteria, and which is responsible for the characteristic odour) and adherent to the vaginal walls ***(Fig. 12.5)***. Visible inflammatory changes are not seen with BV, so there should be no vaginal inflammation.

Diagnosis

The most accurate method of diagnosis is microscopy of Gram-stained vaginal discharge, as the characteristic pattern of the BV bacteria is easily distinguished from the normal *Lactobacilli*-dominant vaginal flora. It is possible to diagnose BV just on clinical criteria but this is less specific. All three of the following should be present for the diagnosis to be made:

- characteristic creamy-white homogeneous vaginal discharge
- raised vaginal pH of >4.5 (measured using narrow-range pH paper)
- characteristic fishy odour, which can be released by mixing the vaginal discharge with 10% potassium hydroxide.

Management

The recommended treatment is oral metronidazole 400 mg ×2 daily for 5–7 days. A single dose of metronidazole 2 g can also be used

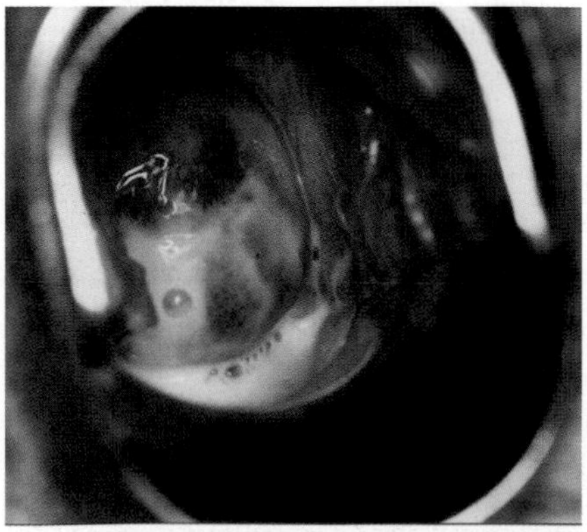

Figure 12.5 Bacterial vaginosis. Homogenous creamy-white vaginal discharge, which may be slightly frothy and adherent to the vaginal walls.

but this is slightly less effective. Alternative topical treatments are intravaginal metronidazole 0.75% gel for 5 nights, or intravaginal clindamycin 2% cream for 7 nights. High-dose metronidazole should be avoided in pregnancy but the 5–7-day oral course can be safely prescribed, as can either of the intravaginal regimens.

BV recurrences are frequent, with about 50% of women experiencing a recurrence within 12 months of completing metronidazole therapy. Simultaneous treatment of the male partner does not reduce the rate of recurrence, and treatment of male partners is not indicated.

Candidiasis

Candida is a ubiquitous organism and is not classified as an STI. Vulvovaginal *Candida* infection is extremely common; about 75% of women have at least one episode of symptomatic candidiasis in their lifetime. About 20% of asymptomatic women are colonized with *Candida*, and this figure rises to 30–40% in pregnancy and uncontrolled diabetes. Predisposing factors for symptomatic infection include pregnancy, diabetes, the use of broad-spectrum antibiotics and corticosteroids, and immunosuppression. *Candida albicans* causes 90% of vaginal yeast infections, with *Candida glabrata* and other *Candida* species causing the remainder. Male sexual partners of women with candidiasis can contract transient penile colonization (and may develop penile rashes) following sex due to direct inoculation from the vagina.

Clinical features

In women, the main symptom is vulval itching, which is present in nearly all symptomatic women. An increased thick, white vaginal discharge, vulval burning, external dysuria and superficial dyspareunia may also be present. On examination, vulval erythema, fissuring and oedema may be present. There may be the typical white, curdy, adherent plaques on the vaginal walls ***(Fig. 12.6)*** but the discharge may be minimal.

In men, there may be a transient penile irritation and rash immediately following sex, but some men experience more persistent balanoposthitis. On examination, there may be erythema of the foreskin and glans penis, or a spotty, red, itchy rash on the glans, with an accumulation of white discharge under the foreskin. In severe cases, there may be fissuring and phimosis of the foreskin.

Diagnosis

Microscopy of a Gram-stained vaginal smear, or a sub-preputial smear, identifies the fungal pseudohyphae and spores in 50% of cases of candidiasis. Culture of vaginal, or sub-preputial, swabs has almost 100% sensitivity. Diabetes should be excluded in men with severe balanoposthitis.

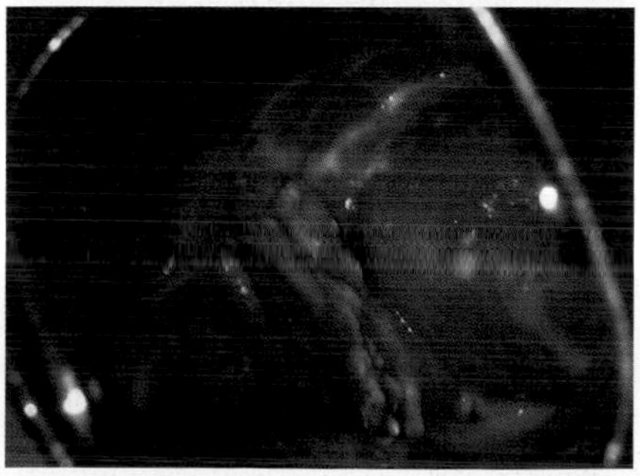

Figure 12.6 Candidiasis. Adherent plaques of discharge on the vaginal walls.

Management

There are a number of short-course oral and intravaginal antifungal agents available, all with efficacies of 80–85%. Recommended treatments are the oral triazole drugs, such as fluconazole 150 mg as a single dose or itraconazole 200 mg ×2 daily for 1 day, and intravaginal imidazole pessaries or creams such as clotrimazole pessary 500 mg as a single dose, miconazole vaginal ovule 1.2 g as a single dose or econazole pessary 150 mg nightly for 1–3 nights. These treatments can be supplemented with antifungal cream applied to the vulva. Males can be treated with either oral therapy or topical antifungal cream. Nystatin pessaries 200 000 units nightly for 14 nights are the treatment of choice for *C. glabrata* and other non-*albicans* yeasts. Intravaginal treatment is safe in pregnancy but oral therapies should not be used.

Recurrent candidiasis (four or more symptomatic episodes in 1 year) occurs in up to 5% of healthy women of reproductive age. It frequently requires weekly oral fluconazole 150 mg, or clotrimazole pessary 500 mg, for up to 6 months in order to prevent recurring symptoms. There is no evidence that treatment of male partners reduces recurrences in women, so male partners do not need treatment unless they also have symptoms.

Trichomoniasis

Trichomonas vaginalis (TV) is the most common STI worldwide but it is much rarer in Western Europe and Australasia. The organism is a flagellated protozoon that is sexually transmitted. In women, it infects the vagina and urethra; in men, it infects the urethra and sub-preputial sac. Nearly all infected men are asymptomatic, as are 10–50% of women. TV in pregnancy is associated with an increased risk of preterm birth and low birth weight, and it increases the risk of acquisition of HIV.

Clinical features

In women, the most common symptoms are an increased purulent vaginal discharge and malodour. There may also be vulval pruritus, external dysuria and dyspareunia. On examination, there may be vulval erythema and the vaginal mucosa is often inflamed. The discharge is yellow or grey and frothy, and can be profuse. The cervix may have multiple small haemorrhagic areas, which have given rise to the description 'strawberry cervix'.

In men, the majority have no symptoms, although they may complain of urethral discharge, irritation and dysuria.

Diagnosis

Phase-contrast microscopy of vaginal discharge identifies the motile protozoa in 50% of infected females. The sensitivity of microscopy of urethral discharge in males is much lower. Culture will detect 70–80% of infections but NAATs of vaginal swabs in women, and first-pass urine (FPU) or urethral swabs in males, will detect over 90%.

Management

The treatment of choice is metronidazole 2 g orally as a single dose or 400 mg ×2 daily for 7 days. Single dose treatment has the advantage of improved adherence. However, in women who are HIV-positive, the 7-day course of metronidazole has better efficacy than single-dose treatment. As TV infects areas beyond the vagina (e.g. the urethra), intravaginal metronidazole gel has poor cure rates and should not be used. High-dose metronidazole should be avoided in pregnancy but the 7-day oral course can be safely prescribed.

Abstinence from sex for at least 7 days should be advised. All sexual contacts should be notified, examined and treated. Tests of cure are only recommended if the patient remains symptomatic following treatment, or if symptoms recur.

Occasionally, TV can become resistant to metronidazole and other nitroimidazoles. This is usually relative rather than absolute and may be overcome by high-dose metronidazole or tinidazole therapy.

Human papillomavirus – anogenital warts

Anogenital warts are painless, benign, epithelial tumours and are a common STI. The causative agent is human papillomavirus (HPV) types 6 and 11. Genital HPV infection is acquired by direct skin-to-skin contact during sex with a person who has either clinical or subclinical infection. Subclinical infection is very common in young sexually active people, with rates of up to 20%. Anogenital warts are the 'tip of the iceberg', occurring in only about 1% of those with subclinical infection.

Warts due to HPV 6 and 11 do not undergo malignant transformation. The main oncogenic HPV types are 16 and 18. These lead to subclinical infection, not genital warts, and cause the majority of cases of cervical and other anogenital cancers (see p. 265). Neonates may acquire HPV from an infected birth canal, which may result either in anogenital warts or in laryngeal papillomatosis.

Clinical features

Anogenital warts have a long incubation period; the average is 3 months but it can extend to years. The warts first appear at sites of trauma during sex, so in males they tend to appear around the prepuce and glans; from there, they can spread to the urethra and down the penile shaft. In women, they usually start at the fourchette and then spread to the vulva and perineum ***(Fig. 12.7)***. Perianal lesions are common in both sexes but are more common in MSM. Warts on mucous membranes tend to be soft and non-keratinized, whereas those on the hair-bearing skin tend to be firm and keratinized.

Warts tend to increase in size and number during pregnancy or in immunosuppressed patients.

Diagnosis

The diagnosis is made on the clinical appearances. HPV testing is not appropriate for diagnosing anogenital warts. The main differential diagnoses are molluscum contagiosum and the condylomata lata of secondary syphilis. Atypical lesions should be biopsied, particularly in older patients, as pre-malignant and malignant lesions can look similar to warts. Investigations should include NAAT for *N. gonorrhoeae* and NAAT for *C. trachomatis*, serology for syphilis and HIV, as co-infection with other STIs is common.

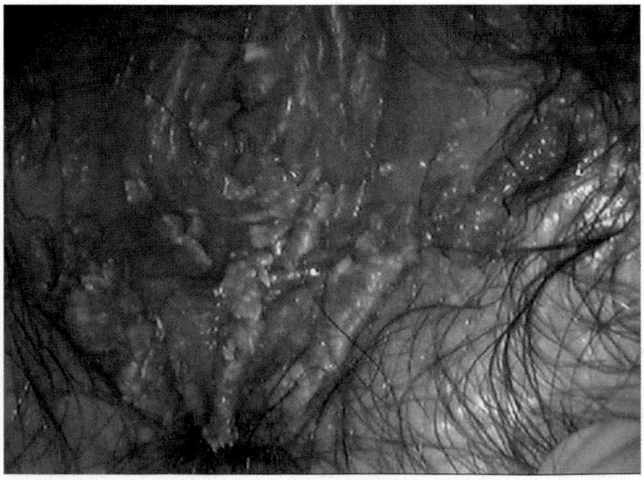

Figure 12.7 Genital warts on the fourchette and perineum.

Management

There are a number of treatments available for anogenital warts but all of them have significant failure and relapse rates. The choice of treatment depends on the number, type and distribution of lesions. Topical podophyllotoxin (0.5% solution or 0.15% cream used twice daily for 3 consecutive days per week) acts as a cytotoxic agent and is useful for non-keratinized warts; keratinized warts respond better to ablative therapy, such as cryotherapy or electrocautery. Imiquimod enhances the local immune response when applied to skin infected with HPV (5% cream used daily, three times a week) and is effective in both types of warts. Podophyllotoxin and imiquimod have the advantage of being self-applied home therapies.

Podophyllotoxin and imiquimod should not be used in pregnancy. Pregnant women, those co-infected with HIV and those with other causes of immunosuppression may have a poorer response to treatment.

The use of condoms should be advised in new relationships, as they protect against the transmission of HPV infection and genital warts. Current sexual partners may have undetected genital warts so may benefit from a sexual health assessment.

Follow-up is recommended in order to monitor the response to treatment and to assess the need for any change of therapy.

Prevention and vaccination

There are two very effective vaccines against HPV. One protects against HPV types 16 and 18 (the bivalent vaccine, which covers the most common high-risk types) and the other protects against types 6, 11, 16 and 18 (the quadrivalent vaccine, which covers the most common high-risk types and those that cause genital warts). They are given over 6 months in three divided doses and have excellent safety profiles, with almost 100% serological response that is maintained over a number of years. Vaccination is most beneficial in those who have not yet been exposed to HPV infection; hence most programmes target those aged 12–13 years.

The best evidence of the effect of HPV vaccination is from Australia, where there has been a school-based quadrivalent HPV vaccination programme in girls since 2007. The programme has recently been extended to include boys. There has been a rapid reduction of more than 90% in genital warts and a reduction of high-grade cervical lesions.

Molluscum contagiosum

Molluscum contagiosum (see pp. 1344–1345) is a large DNA virus. It causes small (typically 2–5 mm in diameter), benign, smooth papules with central umbilication. It is spread via direct skin-to-skin contact. When it is transmitted sexually, the lesions are usually multiple and present on the labia majora, penile shaft, pubic region, lower abdomen and upper inner thighs.

Diagnosis

The diagnosis is made on the characteristic clinical appearance. As it is a sexually acquired condition, investigations for other STIs should include NAAT for *N. gonorrhoeae* and NAAT for *C. trachomatis*, and serology for syphilis and HIV.

Management

Molluscum infection is often self-limiting, resolving naturally. Treatment options, if required, are cryotherapy, podophyllotoxin cream or imiquimod cream. The creams have the advantage of being self-applied home therapies. Podophyllotoxin and imiquimod should be avoided in pregnancy. Patients should be advised about the risks of autoinoculation of the virus and discouraged from shaving or waxing the pubic hair in order to prevent further spread. No routine follow-up or partner notification is required unless any other STIs are identified.

Herpes simplex

Genital herpes (also see pp. 247–249) is the most common cause of genital ulceration in all countries worldwide. The peak incidence for primary infection is in 16–24-year-olds. Women acquire the infection more frequently than men, probably because of the larger surface area of susceptible mucous membrane on the vulva. Transmission occurs from the mucous membrane of a person who is shedding herpes simplex virus (HSV), many of whom will be asymptomatic. Only about 20% of people with serological evidence of genital herpes give a clinical history of herpes, suggesting that many individuals have subclinical infection.

Genital herpes can be due to HSV type 1 or type 2. It is possible to be co-infected with both HSV-1 and HSV-2. HSV-1 infection may be spread from an infected genital tract or from orolabial lesions via orogenital sex. HSV-2 is almost always transmitted via genital-to-genital contact. In the UK, more than 50% of primary HSV is due to HSV-1.

During the primary infection, the virus ascends the peripheral sensory nerves supplying the area of inoculation and establishes latency in the dorsal root ganglia, thus allowing future reactivation and recurrences.

Clinical features

Initial episode is the first occurrence of either HSV-1 or HSV-2. This is sub-divided as below, depending on whether or not the person has had prior exposure to the other HSV type.

Primary genital infection is the first ever exposure to either HSV type 1 or 2. It typically presents with multiple painful, shallow ulcers ***(Fig. 12.8)***. There is usually tender inguinal lymphadenopathy and systemic symptoms of viraemia, including fever, myalgia and headache. In women, external dysuria and vulval pain are the main symptoms. Ulcers may be present on the cervix and can have the appearance of a malignancy. Rectal infection may lead to severe proctitis with pain and bleeding (this is mainly seen in MSM). The lesions start to heal over a period of 10–21 days, even without treatment. Neurological complications can include aseptic meningitis and autonomic neuropathy leading to urinary retention. However, primary infection can be asymptomatic.

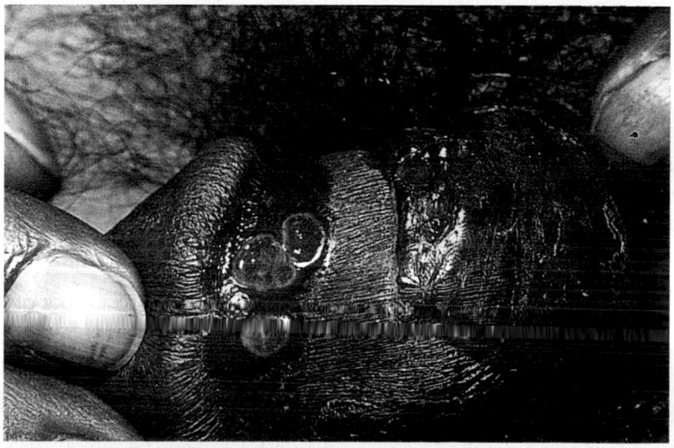

Figure 12.8 Herpes simplex rash on the penis. *(Courtesy of Dr B. Goh.)*

Non-primary genital infection occurs in people with previous HSV-1 or HSV-2 who then acquire the other type of genital HSV. There is some cross-protection from the prior HSV infection, resulting in a milder illness than in primary infection. Non-primary genital infections are more likely to be asymptomatic than primary infections.

Recurrent genital herpes is due to reactivation of previous HSV-1 or HSV-2 infection. HSV-2 recurs more frequently than HSV-1. The median recurrence rate in the subsequent year following a primary or non-primary infection is about one recurrence for HSV-1 and about four recurrences for HSV-2. The recurrences may be preceded by a prodrome of tingling, itching or pain in the area. On examination, there are usually a few ulcers confined to a small area and systemic symptoms are rare. Recurrences are not always noticed and asymptomatic, subclinical viral shedding can occur. However, all of these reactivated episodes are potentially infectious. Long-term studies show that symptomatic recurrences and subclinical viral shedding gradually decrease with time.

The clinical presentation of primary infection in immunosuppressed patients (including those with HIV and pregnant women) is usually more severe, with increased frequency of symptomatic and subclinical recurrences. Rarely, the infection can disseminate, causing a systemic life-threatening condition.

Genital herpes increases the acquisition and transmission of HIV and is an attributable risk in the spread of HIV. Many people with recurrent HSV develop psychological and psychosexual problems and fear rejection on disclosure of their infection to sexual partners.

Diagnosis

HSV DNA detection using polymerase chain reaction (PCR) on a swab taken from the ulcer is the diagnostic method of choice. This can distinguish between HSV-1 and HSV-2. Tests for other STIs should be performed, including NAAT for *N. gonorrhoeae* and NAAT for *C. trachomatis*, NAAT (if available) or culture for TV, and serology for syphilis and HIV.

Blood tests for HSV type-specific antibodies can be used to diagnose prior HSV-1 and HSV-2 infections when the clinical history is suggestive of genital herpes but confirmation by HSV DNA detection has not been possible. The presence of HSV-2 antibodies is indicative of genital herpes but the presence of HSV-1 antibodies cannot differentiate between genital and orolabial infections.

Management

Initial episode

Saltwater bathing or sitting in a warm bath is soothing and may allow women to pass urine more comfortably. Topical anaesthetic agents can also be used to ease micturition. Recommended antiviral therapies are aciclovir 400 mg ×3 daily, valaciclovir 500 mg ×2 daily or famciclovir 250 mg ×3 daily, all for 5 days. Aciclovir is the drug of choice in pregnancy and breast-feeding. If lesions are already healing, antiviral therapy will have little added effect. Secondary bacterial infection occasionally occurs and should be treated.

The natural history of HSV infection should be explained, including recurrences, subclinical viral shedding, and the potential for sexual transmission with both of these infections. Patients should be advised to avoid sex during the prodrome and recurrences. Subclinical viral shedding is most common during the first 12 months following initial HSV-2 infection and in those with frequent symptomatic recurrences. Condoms and suppressive treatment reduce the risk of transmission from subclinical viral shedding but neither completely prevents it. Consequently, disclosure should be advised in all relationships.

Recurrence

The appropriate management will depend on the number and severity of recurrences. As recurrences tend to be less severe and self-limiting, they can sometimes be managed with saltwater bathing and topical anaesthetic agents.

Episodic treatment

When recurrences are infrequent but severe, episodic antiviral therapy, started early by the patient, will reduce the duration and severity but will not reduce the number of recurrences. Recommended episodic regimens are aciclovir 400 mg ×3 daily, valaciclovir 500 mg ×2 daily, or famciclovir 250 mg ×3 daily, all for 5 days. Shorter-course therapies are also effective: aciclovir 800 mg ×3 daily for 2 days, famciclovir 1 g ×2 daily for 1 day or valaciclovir 500 mg ×2 daily for 3 days can be used.

Suppressive treatment

In those with six or more recurrences per year, long-term suppressive therapy is effective at stopping, or reducing, the recurrences. The decision whether to start suppressive treatment depends on the number of recurrences and the inconvenience of taking daily treatment. Recommended regimens are aciclovir 400 mg ×2 daily, valaciclovir 500 mg daily or famciclovir 250 mg ×2 daily for a maximum of 12 months. Therapy should then be discontinued in order to assess the frequency of recurrences. If they are still frequent, suppressive treatment can be restarted.

Frequent recurrences are associated with psychological and psychosexual morbidity; support and counselling are often needed.

HSV in pregnancy

The main risk of HSV in pregnancy is vertical transmission. Despite antiviral treatment, neonatal HSV has a high mortality rate and high morbidity in those who survive. The primary episode of genital HSV in late pregnancy poses the highest risk of transmission, and women within 6 weeks of the expected delivery date should be offered caesarean section. Women who present with an initial episode of HSV in the first or second trimester can be given suppressive aciclovir from 36 weeks' gestation. This reduces recurrences and subclinical viral shedding, and therefore the need for a caesarean section. The dose of suppressive treatment should be aciclovir 400 mg ×3 daily due to the altered pharmacokinetics of the drug in late pregnancy.

The risk of neonatal herpes with recurrent HSV is small, even if lesions are present at the time of delivery. The Royal College of Obstetricians and Gynaecologists in the UK suggests that caesarean section is not indicated in such women, but daily suppressive aciclovir from 36 weeks' gestation should be started.

Syphilis

Syphilis is a chronic systemic disease caused by *Treponema pallidum* (TP), a motile spirochaete. It is mainly transmitted by direct contact with an infectious lesion and enters the new host through breaches in squamous or columnar epithelium, usually during sex. Primary infection of non-genital sites may occur but is rare. It can also be transmitted by infected blood products or from mother to child during pregnancy. Hence syphilis is classified as acquired or congenital. ***Acquired syphilis*** is further subdivided into primary, secondary and early latent (all are also referred to as early or infectious syphilis, and indicate that infection has been acquired during the last 2 years), late latent (infection for more than 2 years) and tertiary syphilis (the most destructive stage, which includes cardiovascular and neurological syphilis and gummatous lesions of any organ). ***Congenital syphilis*** is also further subdivided into early (diagnosed within the first 2 years of life) and late (diagnosed over the age of 2).

The incidence varies significantly with geographic location. It is more common in low- and middle-income countries; in high-income countries, it is mainly confined to MSM. For instance, diagnoses of infectious syphilis in England between 2004 and 2013 increased by 36% in men with 74% of the infections being in MSM, whereas they decreased by 37% in women. However, syphilis still affects large numbers of pregnant women worldwide. It was estimated that, in 2008, 1.4 million pregnant women were infected worldwide, causing approximately 520 000 adverse pregnancy outcomes, including 215 000 stillbirths, 90 000 neonatal deaths, 65 000 preterm or low-birth-weight babies, and 150 000 babies with congenital infections. Antenatal screening for syphilis, followed by adequate treatment during pregnancy, can prevent many of these adverse outcomes.

Clinical features

Primary syphilis

Between 10 and 90 days (mean 21 days) after exposure, a papule develops at the site of inoculation. This ulcerates to become a painless, firm ulcer (chancre). There is usually also a painless regional lymphadenopathy. The primary lesion may go unnoticed, especially if it is on the cervix or within the rectum. Healing occurs spontaneously within 2–6 weeks.

Secondary syphilis

Between 6 and 10 weeks after the appearance of the primary lesion, constitutional symptoms with fever, sore throat, malaise and arthralgia may appear due to septicaemia. Hence, any organ may be affected and hepatitis, nephritis, arthritis and meningitis have all been described.

Common signs include:

- widespread skin rash (present in 75%), which can involve the whole body, including the palms and soles – typically, a non-itchy, maculopapular rash that may have a coppery colour ***(Fig. 12.9)***
- generalized lymphadenopathy (present in 50%)
- condylomata lata, which are moist, wart-like plaques found in the perianal area and other moist body sites
- mucosal lesions in the mouth and on the genitalia presenting as distinct mucous patches or becoming confluent to form 'snail-track ulcers'.

Without treatment, the symptoms and signs of secondary syphilis resolve but may recur, especially in the first year of infection.

Latent syphilis

Latent syphilis is diagnosed on the basis of reactive syphilis serology in someone who has no symptoms and has not been treated.

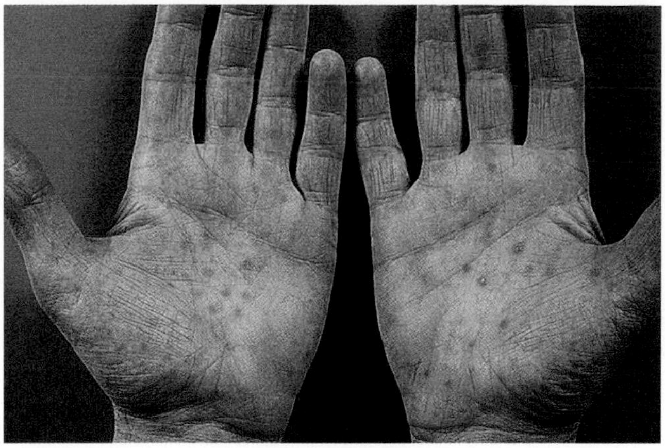

Figure 12.9 Rash of secondary syphilis on the palms. *(Courtesy of Dr B. Goh.)*

It is divided into early latent (defined as within 2 years of acquiring the infection, or within 1 year in USA) and late latent syphilis (present for 2 or more years), as sexual transmission can occur in early latency but not in late latent disease. Latent syphilis may persist for years or may even be life-long.

Tertiary syphilis

About one-third of people with untreated latent syphilis will develop tertiary syphilis within 2 to 30 or more years of contracting the infection. Gummatous syphilis (with inflammatory, granulomatous, destructive lesions) is the most benign and commonly involves the skin and bones, but lesions can occur in any organ. Cardiovascular syphilis causes aortitis, aortic regurgitation, aneurysm of the ascending aorta and stenosis of the coronary artery ostia. Neurosyphilis causes chronic meningovascular damage and endarteritis of the small vessels of the brain and spinal cord, presenting as 'general paralysis of the insane' and tabes dorsalis.

Syphilis in pregnancy and congenital syphilis

Syphilis can be transmitted transplacentally at any stage of pregnancy. The risk of transmission is dependent on the stage of maternal infection and can be up to 100% in early syphilis, and even up to 10% with late infection. The WHO estimates that untreated early syphilis in pregnancy results in rates of second-trimester miscarriage or stillbirth of 25%, preterm birth before 32 weeks' gestation of 13%, neonatal death of 11% and congenital syphilis amongst the infants born of 20%. Detection and treatment of syphilis early in pregnancy prevent congenital syphilis and neonatal death at term, and reduce adverse pregnancy outcomes.

Signs of early congenital syphilis occur in the neonatal period and include a rash, condylomata lata, mucous patches, nasal discharge, hepatosplenomegaly and periostitis. Late syphilis (occurring after 2 years of age) can present with neurological or gummatous lesions but also includes the 'stigmata of congenital syphilis', resulting from early damage to developing structures, particularly teeth and bones. These are Hutchinson's teeth, sabre tibia, bossing of the frontal and parietal bones, and saddle nose.

Diagnosis

T. pallidum cannot be cultured but it can be identified by darkground microscopy of secretions from a primary chancre or condylomata lata; however, sensitivity is dependent on highly skilled microscopists. Some laboratories are able to test swabs for TP using PCR but serological testing remains the main laboratory diagnosis.

Most laboratories use a treponemal enzyme immunoassay (EIA) to detect IgG and IgM as a screening test. If this is positive, a further treponemal test and a non-treponemal test are performed.

Treponemal tests

T. pallidum haemagglutination (TPHA) and *T. pallidum* particle agglutination (TPPA) assays are highly specific for treponemal disease but usually remain positive for life, even after treatment, so are unable to differentiate between prior treated infection and re-infection.

Non-treponemal tests

The Venereal Disease Research Laboratory (VDRL) and rapid plasma reagin (RPR) tests become positive within 3–4 weeks of the primary infection. They are quantifiable tests that can be used to monitor treatment response and evidence of re-infection. These tests are not specific to syphilis and false-positive results may occur in other conditions, particularly in other infections and autoimmune diseases.

Examination of the cerebrospinal fluid (CSF) for evidence of neurosyphilis is indicated in those patients with positive syphilis serology who demonstrate neurological signs and symptoms.

Management

Treponemocidal levels of an antibiotic are required for at least 7 days in early syphilis to cover the slow division time of the organism (30 h). In late syphilis, treponemes may divide even more slowly, so longer therapy is required. Ideally, a long-acting penicillin should be given intramuscularly.

Early syphilis (primary, secondary and early latent)

- Benzathine penicillin G 2.4 MU i.m. single dose.

  In penicillin allergy:
- Doxycycline 100 mg ×2 daily for 14 days.

The ***Jarisch–Herxheimer reaction*** is caused by release of inflammatory cytokines and occurs in 50% of patients with primary syphilis and up to 90% with secondary syphilis. It occurs about 8 hours after the injection and usually consists of mild fever, malaise and headache lasting several hours.

Late latent, cardiovascular and gummatous syphilis

- Benzathine penicillin G 2.4 MU i.m. three doses at weekly intervals.

  In penicillin allergy:
- Doxycycline 100 mg ×2 daily for 28 days.

Neurosyphilis

- Procaine penicillin 2.4 MU i.m. daily plus probenecid 500 mg orally ×4 daily for 14–17 days.

  In penicillin allergy:
- Doxycycline 200 mg ×2 daily for 28 days.

Pregnancy

- Penicillin can be safely used in pregnancy but doxycycline should not be used.

Syphilis and HIV

The diagnosis and management of syphilis in HIV-co-infected patients remains unaltered; however, if untreated, it may advance more rapidly than in HIV-negative patients and has a higher incidence of neurosyphilis.

Prognosis and follow-up

Those being treated for early syphilis should abstain from sex for at least 14 days and sexual contacts must be traced and investigated. There should be regular follow-up within the first year using repeat VDRL/RPR titres to establish the 'fourfold fall', which demonstrates adequately treated syphilis.

The prognosis of syphilis depends on the stage at which the infection is treated. Early syphilis has an excellent outlook, but once permanent damage has occurred in tertiary syphilis, the damage will not be reversed, although further progression will be halted.

Lymphogranuloma venereum

Lymphogranuloma venereum (LGV) is an STI caused by the invasive serovars, L1, L2 and L3, of *Chlamydia trachomatis*. It is endemic in several tropical areas, including southern Africa, India, South-east Asia and the Caribbean. It used to be rare in Western Europe but since 2003 it has become hyper-endemic among MSM, particularly those with HIV. It is frequently associated with other STIs and acute hepatitis C infection. The main presentation in MSM is with rectal symptoms. LGV should be considered in MSM with suspected inflammatory bowel disease, as the clinical presentation can be very similar and the histological findings of LGV proctitis are similar to other causes of granulomatous proctitis, such as Crohn's disease.

Clinical features

There are three clinical stages. The primary lesion may be transient and is frequently unnoticed. In the genital area, it takes the form of a painless papule or shallow ulcer appearing at the area of inoculation, 3–30 days after exposure. The main presentation in MSM is proctitis with symptoms of rectal pain, mucopurulent discharge, rectal bleeding, constipation and tenesmus. Some also report systemic symptoms, such as fever and malaise.

The secondary lesions are enlarged, tender regional lymph nodes. With genital LGV, they are usually unilateral and affect the inguinal and femoral nodes. When both are involved, the 'groove sign' develops due to the inguinal ligament separating the two enlarged lymph node systems. The nodes may become matted with bubo formation, which may rupture.

The tertiary stage is a chronic inflammatory response with tissue destruction. In the rectum, it can cause fistulae, strictures and granulomatous fibrosis, mimicking Crohn's disease. There may also be scarring of the genital area, and destruction of local lymph nodes can lead to genital lymphoedema.

Diagnosis

Genital LGV

A swab should be taken from the ulcer base for *C. trachomatis* NAAT. If this is positive for *C. trachomatis*, genotyping for LGV should be requested. Testing for the other causes of genital ulcers should be undertaken (see ***Box 12.5***) and should include an ulcer swab for HSV and TP PCR, and serology for syphilis, which should be repeated after the 3-month window period. A NAAT for *N. gonorrhoeae*, NAAT for *C. trachomatis* and serology for HIV should also be carried out.

Rectal LGV

A swab should be taken from the rectal mucosa for *C. trachomatis* NAAT. If this is positive for *C. trachomatis*, genotyping for LGV should be requested. Swabs should also be taken for *N. gonorrhoeae* NAAT, and HSV and TP PCR. Serology for syphilis and HIV should be performed, and serology for hepatitis C should be considered in view of the frequent co-infection of acute hepatitis C with LGV.

Management

First-choice treatment is doxycycline 100 mg ×2 daily for 21 days or erythromycin 500 mg ×4 daily for 21 days. Symptoms should start to resolve within 1–2 weeks of commencing therapy. Patients should be advised to abstain from sex until completion of treatment. Sexual contacts should be notified, examined, tested and treated. Follow-up should continue until all symptoms and signs have resolved, which is usually by 3–6 weeks.

Chancroid

Chancroid is caused by *Haemophilus ducreyi*. It used to be one of the most common causes of genital ulcers worldwide but its incidence has now decreased markedly. One of the drivers for its improved control and reduced incidence is its association with the acquisition of HIV infection. It is extremely rare in high-income countries.

Clinical features

Chancroid has a short incubation period of 4–7 days. A tender papule develops at the site of inoculation, which breaks into a painful, ragged-edged ulcer with a necrotic base that bleeds easily. The usual sites of infection are the prepuce and glans penis in men and the labia minora and fourchette in women. There is often painful inguinal lymphadenopathy, which can develop into large buboes that suppurate.

Diagnosis and management

Detection of *H. ducreyi* DNA using PCR is the most sensitive diagnostic test but there are no commercial assays available for this. A 'probable diagnosis' may be made if the patient presents the appropriate clinical picture, without evidence of syphilis or HSV.

Testing for the other causes of genital ulcers should be undertaken (see ***Box 12.5***) and should include an ulcer swab for HSV and TP PCR, an ulcer swab for *C. trachomatis* NAAT with genotyping for LGV if positive, and serology for syphilis, which should be repeated after the 3-month window period. A NAAT for *N. gonorrhoeae*, NAAT for *C. trachomatis* and serology for HIV should also be performed.

Single-dose regimens include azithromycin 1 g orally or ceftriaxone 250 mg i.m. Multiple-dose regimens are ciprofloxacin 500 mg ×2 daily for 3 days or erythromycin 500 mg ×4 daily for 7 days. Multiple-dose regimens should be used in HIV patients as treatment failures have been reported with single-dose therapy. Patients should be advised to abstain from sex for at least 7 days and be followed up at 3–7 days, when the ulcers should be healing. HIV-infected patients should be monitored closely, as healing may be slower. Sexual partners should be notified, examined and treated epidemiologically, as asymptomatic carriage has been reported.

Donovanosis

Donovanosis (also known as granuloma inguinale) is exceedingly rare and is confined to a few countries in South-east Asia, South America and the Caribbean. It is caused by *Klebsiella granulomatis*.

Clinical features

Nodules at the site of inoculation develop into friable, non-painful ulcers or hypertrophic lesions that increase in size. There is enlargement of the inguinal lymph nodes, which may ulcerate.

Diagnosis and management

The diagnosis is made on the presence of Donovan bodies in scrapings or biopsies of the lesions. Donovan bodies are the encapsulated intracellular Gram-negative rods of *Klebsiella granulomatis* that are visible within histiocytes in the tissue samples. They appear deep purple when stained with Giemsa, Wright's or Leishman stains. Screening for all other STIs should be undertaken.

Antibiotic treatment should be given for a minimum of 3 weeks and until the lesions have healed. Regimens include azithromycin 1 g weekly or 500 mg daily, or ciprofloxacin 750 mg ×2 daily. Patients should be advised to abstain from sex for at least 3 weeks and be followed up until the lesions have fully resolved. Sexual partners should be notified, examined and treated if necessary.

Pediculosis pubis

The pubic louse (*Phthirus pubis*) is able to attach tightly to the pubic and coarse body hair. It can also attach to eyelashes and eyebrows. It is host-specific and is transferred by close bodily contact. Although infestation may be asymptomatic, the most common complaint is of itch due to hypersensitivity to the louse bites.

Diagnosis and management

Lice may be seen on the pubic and body hairs. They resemble small scabs or freckles but can be seen moving. The eggs (nits) are laid at the hair base and are strongly adherent to the hairs. Screening for other STIs should include NAAT for *N. gonorrhoeae*, NAAT for *C. trachomatis* and serology for syphilis and HIV.

Treatment should be applied to all areas of the body, including facial hair if present. Malathion 0.5% should be left on for at least 2 hours, and permethrin 1% left on for 10 minutes. A second application is usually advised after 3–7 days. Permethrin is safe in pregnancy. Sexual partners should be examined and treated if infected.

Scabies

This is discussed on page 1347.

Further reading

Brunham RC, Gottlieb SL, Paavonen J. Pelvic inflammatory disease. *New Engl J Med* 2015; 372:2039–2208.

Chow EP, Read TR, Wigan R et al. Ongoing decline in genital warts among young heterosexuals 7 years after the Australian human papillomavirus (HPV) vaccination programme. *Sex Transm Infect* 2015; 91:214–219.

Garland SM. The Australian experience with the human papillomavirus vaccine. *Clin Ther* 2014; 36:17–23.

Hawkes SJ, Gomez GB, Broutet N. Early antenatal care: does it make a difference to outcomes of pregnancy associated with syphilis? *PLoS One* 2013; 8:e56713.

Hofstetter AM, Rosenthal SL, Stanberry LR. Current thinking on genital herpes. *Curr Opin Infect Dis* 2014; 27:75–83.

Ingles DJ, Pierce Campbell CM, Messina JA et al. Human papillomavirus virus (HPV) genotype- and age-specific analyses of external genital lesions among men in the HPV Infection in Men (HIM) study. *J Infect Dis* 2015; 211:1060–1067.

Kreimer AR, Pierce Campbell CM, Lin H-Y et al. Incidence and clearance of oral human papillomavirus infection in men: the HIM cohort study. *Lancet* 2013; 382:877.

Merin A, Pachankis JE. The psychological impact of genital herpes stigma. *J Health Psychol* 2011; 16:80–90.

Mitchell C, Prabhu M. Pelvic inflammatory disease: current concepts in pathogenesis, diagnosis and treatment. *Infect Dis Clin North Am* 2013; 27:793–809.

HUMAN IMMUNODEFICIENCY VIRUS AND ACQUIRED IMMUNODEFICIENCY SYNDROME

EPIDEMIOLOGY AND PATHOGENESIS

Epidemiology

Since the first description of AIDS in 1981 and the identification of the causative organism, HIV, in 1983, more than 78 million people are estimated to have been infected and 39 million people have died. At least 35 million people worldwide are living with HIV infection. Highly active anti-retroviral therapy (ART) has dramatically reduced mortality for those who are able to access care, transforming HIV from a universally fatal infection into a long-term manageable condition, with a consequent rise in global prevalence. Effective therapy since 2001 has also reduced infectiousness, and new infections globally have fallen by 38%, although there is considerable geographical diversity. Sub-Saharan Africa remains the most seriously affected, and in Eastern Europe and parts of central Asia, infection rates continue to rise. The human, societal and economic costs are huge. HIV is a major contributor to the global burden of disease, being the leading cause of disability-adjusted life-years for people aged 30–45 years. Demographics of the epidemic have varied greatly, influenced by social, behavioural, cultural and political factors. Current global estimates suggest that 38% of people living with HIV are on ART, but that, for each individual starting therapy, there are two new infections, highlighting the size of the problem and the global inequalities that exist in healthcare.

In the UK, falling death rates and sustained new infections mean that the total number of people living with HIV continues to rise. In 2013, 107 000 people were estimated to be living with HIV and 6000 were newly diagnosed. Individuals accessing care almost doubled in number from a decade earlier, and MSM and culturally diverse heterosexual populations from sub-Saharan Africa are the two largest groups of people living with HIV. Of those diagnosed with HIV in the UK, 30% are women. As mortality rates fall, the population living with HIV is becoming older, with 1 in 4 now aged 50 years and over.

Approximately one-quarter of those with HIV infection in the UK are undiagnosed and unaware of their infection, which contributes to late diagnosis, poorer clinical outcomes and onward transmission. Late diagnosis is now the most common cause of HIV-related morbidity and mortality in the UK. The proportion and number of people diagnosed late (with a CD4 count of <350 cells/mm^3 within 3 months of their diagnosis) declined from 57% in 2004 to 42% in 2013. Reducing late and undiagnosed HIV through wider testing, particularly in patients presenting with clinical conditions that are associated with HIV and those in areas with high seroprevalence, is critical to both the individual and public health ***(Box 12.8)***.

Routes of acquisition

Despite the fact that HIV can be isolated from a wide range of body fluids and tissues, the majority of infections are transmitted via semen, cervical secretions and blood. The most significant marker for transmission risk is the HIV viral load, which is highest in acute infection, and reduced by effective ART. HIV-associated stigma and discrimination, gender-based violence and, in some countries of the world, the legal position for those at especially high risk can all

Box 12.8 HIV testing: UK guidelines on where and who to test

Universal: clinical settings in which all patients should be offered HIV testing:
- Genitourinary medicine/sexual health clinics
- Antenatal services
- Termination of pregnancy services
- Drug dependency programmes
- Healthcare services for tuberculosis, hepatitis B, hepatitis C and lymphoma
- High-prevalence areas where diagnosed HIV infection is ≥2 per 1000 resident population
- People in prison

People in whom HIV testing is recommended
- All patients diagnosed with a sexually transmitted infection
- Sexual partners of men and women known to be HIV-positive
- Men who have disclosed sexual contact with other men
- Female sexual contacts of men who have sex with men
- People reporting a history of injecting drug use
- Men and women known to be from a country of high HIV prevalence (>1%)
- Men and women who report sexual contact abroad or in the UK with individuals from countries of high HIV prevalence
- Patients presenting for healthcare where HIV enters the differential diagnosis (see **_Box 12.9_**)

HIV-associated indicator conditions

Respiratory
- Tuberculosis, pneumocystis[a], bacterial pneumonia, aspergillosis

Neurology
- Cerebral toxoplasmosis[a], primary cerebral lymphoma[a], cryptococcal meningitis[a], progressive multifocal leucoencephalopathy[a], aseptic meningitis/encephalitis, cerebral abscess, space-occupying lesion of unknown cause, Guillain–Barré syndrome, transverse myelitis, peripheral neuropathy, dementia

Dermatology
- Kaposi's sarcoma[a], severe/recalcitrant seborrhoeic dermatitis, severe/recalcitrant psoriasis, multidermatomal/recurrent herpes zoster

Gastroenterology
- Persistent cryptosporidiosis[a], oral candidiasis, oral hairy leukoplakia, chronic diarrhoea of unknown cause, weight loss of unknown cause, *Salmonella*, *Shigella*, *Campylobacter*, hepatitis B infection, hepatitis C infection

Oncology
- Non-Hodgkin's lymphoma[a], anal cancer, anal intraepithelial dysplasia, lung cancer, seminoma, head and neck cancer, Hodgkin's lymphoma, Castleman's disease

Gynaecology
- Cervical cancer[a], vaginal intraepithelial neoplasia, cervical intraepithelial neoplasia, grade 2 or above

Haematology
- Any unexplained blood dyscrasia, including thrombocytopenia, neutropenia and lymphopenia

Ophthalmology
- Cytomegalovirus retinitis, infective retinal diseases including herpesviruses and toxoplasma, any unexplained retinopathy

ENT
- Lymphadenopathy of unknown cause, chronic parotitis, lymphoepithelial parotid cysts

Other
- Mononucleosis-like syndrome (primary HIV infection), pyrexia of unknown origin, any lymphadenopathy of unknown cause, any sexually transmitted infection

[a]*AIDS-defining condition.*

(From http://guidance.nice.org.uk/PH33 ; http://www.nice.org.uk/guidance/PH34; http://www.bhiva.org/HIVTesting2008.aspx.)

impede access to appropriate services and increase the risks of transmission and acquisition of HIV.

Sexual intercourse (vaginal and anal)

Globally, heterosexual intercourse accounts for the vast majority of infections, and coexistent STIs, especially those causing genital ulceration, enhance transmission. Passage of HIV appears to be more efficient from men to women, and to the receptive partner in anal intercourse, than vice versa. In the UK, sex between men accounts for over half of the new diagnoses reported, but there is a consistent rate of heterosexual transmission. In Central and sub-Saharan Africa, the epidemic has always been heterosexual and more than half of infected adults in these regions are women. South-east Asia and the Indian subcontinent are experiencing an explosive epidemic, driven by heterosexual intercourse and a high incidence of other STIs.

Mother-to-child transmission (transplacental, perinatal, breast-feeding)

Vertical transmission is the most common route of HIV infection in children. European studies suggest that, without intervention, 15% of babies born to HIV-positive mothers are likely to be infected, although rates of up to 40% have been reported from Africa and the USA. Increased vertical transmission is associated with advanced disease in the mother, maternal viral load, prolonged and premature rupture of membranes, and chorioamnionitis. Transmission can occur *in utero*, although the majority of infections take place perinatally. Breast-feeding has been shown to double the risk of vertical transmission. In the developed world, interventions to reduce vertical transmission, including screening for infection in pregnancy, the use of anti-retroviral agents (ARVs) and the avoidance of breast-feeding, have led to a dramatic fall in the numbers of infected children. In the UK, the risk of vertically transmitted infection is 1 : 1000. The lack of access to these interventions in resource-poor countries in which 90% of infections occur is a major global issue.

Contaminated blood, blood products and organ donations

Screening of blood and blood products was introduced in 1985 in Europe and North America. Prior to this, HIV infection was associated with the use of clotting factors (for haemophilia) and with blood transfusions. In some parts of the world where blood products may not be screened and in areas where the rate of new HIV infections is very high, transfusion-associated transmission continues to occur.

Contaminated needles (intravenous drug misuse, injections and needle-stick injuries)

The practice of sharing needles and syringes for intravenous drug use continues to be a major route of transmission of HIV in parts of South-east Asia, Latin America and Eastern Europe. In some areas, including the UK, successful education and needle exchange schemes have reduced the rate of transmission by this route. Iatrogenic transmission from needles and syringes used in developing countries is reported. Healthcare workers have a risk of approximately 0.3% following a single needle-stick injury with known HIV-positive blood.

There is no evidence that HIV is spread by social or household contact or by blood-sucking insects such as mosquitoes and bed bugs.

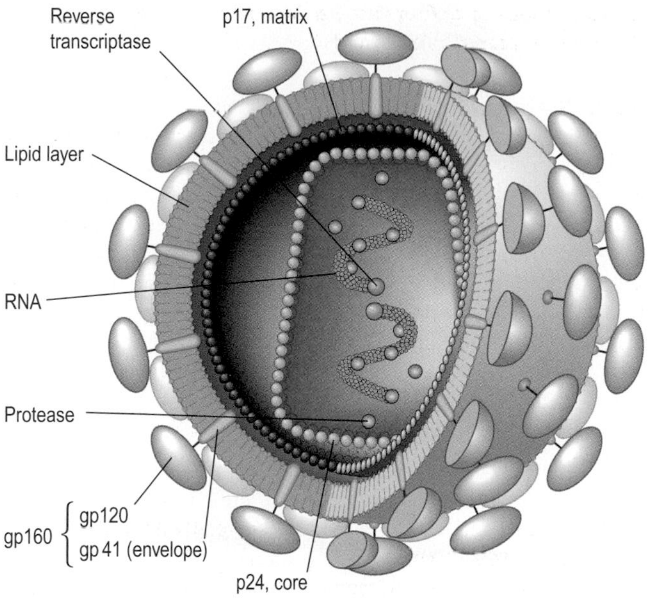

Figure 12.10 Structure of HIV. Two molecules of single-stranded RNA are shown within the nucleus. The reverse transcriptase polymerase converts viral RNA into DNA (a characteristic of retroviruses). The protease includes integrase (p32 and p10). The p24 (core protein) levels can be used to monitor HIV disease. p17 is the matrix protein; gp120 is the outer envelope glycoprotein, which binds to cell surface CD4 molecules; and gp41, a transmembrane protein, influences infectivity and cell fusion capacity.

Pathology

The virus

HIV belongs to the lentivirus group of the retrovirus family. There are two types, HIV-1 and HIV-2. HIV-1 is the most frequently occurring strain globally. HIV-2 is almost entirely confined to West Africa, although there is some spread to Europe, particularly France and Portugal. HIV-2 has only 40% structural homology with HIV-1 and, although it is associated with immunosuppression and AIDS, it appears to take a more indolent course than HIV-1. Many of the drugs that are used in HIV-1 are ineffective in HIV-2. The structure of HIV is shown in ***Figure 12.10***.

Retroviruses are characterized by possession of the enzyme reverse transcriptase, which allows viral RNA to be transcribed into DNA and thence incorporated into the host cell genome. Reverse transcription is an error-prone process with a significant rate of mis-incorporation of bases. This, combined with a high rate of viral turnover, leads to considerable genetic variation and a diversity of viral subtypes or clades. On the basis of DNA sequencing, HIV-1 is divided into four distinct strains, which represent four independent cross-species transfers: three (M, N and O) based on the chimpanzee-related strains of simian immunodeficiency virus (SIV) and one (P) that may represent chimpanzee to gorilla to human transmission.

- ***Group M (major) subtypes*** (98% of infections worldwide) exhibit a high degree of diversity, with subtypes (or clades), denoted A–K. There is a predominance of subtype B in Europe, North America and Australia, but areas of Central and sub-Saharan Africa have multiple M subtypes, clade C being the most common. Recombination of viral material generates an array of circulating recombinant forms (CRFs), which increase the genetic diversity and are becoming more common.
- ***Group N (new)*** is mostly confined to parts of west Central Africa (e.g. Gabon).
- ***Group O (outlier) subtypes*** are highly divergent from group M and are largely confined to small numbers centred on Cameroon.
- ***Group P***, related to gorilla strains of SIV, has been identified from a patient from Cameroon.

Pathogenesis

The interrelationship between HIV and the host immune system is the basis of the pathogenesis of HIV disease. At the time of initial exposure, the virus is transported by dendritic cells from mucosal surfaces to regional lymph nodes, where permanent infection is established, usually by one ‘founder virus’. The host cellular receptor that is recognized by HIV surface glycoprotein gp120 is the CD4 molecule, which defines the cell populations that are susceptible to infection ***(Fig. 12.11)***. The interaction between CD4 and HIV gp120 surface glycoprotein, together with host chemokine CCR5 or CXCR4 co-receptors, is responsible for HIV entry into cells. Although CCR5 CD4 memory T lymphocytes within all body systems are susceptible to infection and depletion, those found in the gastrointestinal tract are heavily infected early in the process. These lymphocytes become rapidly depleted, leading to compromised mucosal immune function, and thus allowing microbial lipopolysaccharides to enter the circulation. HIV infection that is independent of CD4 receptors can occur in astrocytes and renal epithelial cells, leading to end-organ damage.

Studies of viral turnover have demonstrated a virus half-life in the circulation of about 6 hours. To maintain observed levels of plasma viraemia, 10^8–10^9 virus particles need to be released and cleared daily. Virus production by infected cells lasts for about 2 days and is probably limited by the death of the cell, owing to direct HIV effects. This links HIV replication to the process of CD4 destruction and depletion. Progressive loss of activated CD4 T lymphocytes due to killing by CD8 cells is a key factor in the immunopathogenesis of HIV. Natural killer cells are involved in the host immune response, although escape mutations within the virus population compromise their antiviral effects. The production of neutralizing antibodies, which, in some people, can be against several viral subtypes, occurs at about 12 weeks after infection.

Resulting cell-mediated immunodeficiency leaves the host open to infections with intracellular pathogens, while coexisting antibody abnormalities predispose to infections with capsulated bacteria. HIV is associated with immune activation, a long-term inflammatory state, which is a key driver of disease progression. T-cell activation is observed from the earliest stages of infection, which, in turn, leads to an increase in the numbers of susceptible CD4-bearing target cells that can become infected and destroyed. This inflammatory state is associated with HIV itself, with co-pathogens such as cytomegalovirus, and with the translocation of microbial products, in particular lipopolysaccharides, from the gut into the systemic circulation following HIV destruction of normal mucosal immunity. Raised levels of inflammatory cytokines and coagulation system activation occur. These inflammatory responses may remain, despite effective ART, and play a role in HIV-associated end-organ damage, as well as raising the risks of myocardial infarction and some malignancies.

Further reading

Jones A, Cremin I, Abdullah F et al. Transformation of HIV from pandemic to low-endemic levels: a public health approach to combination prevention. *Lancet* 2014; 384:272–279.

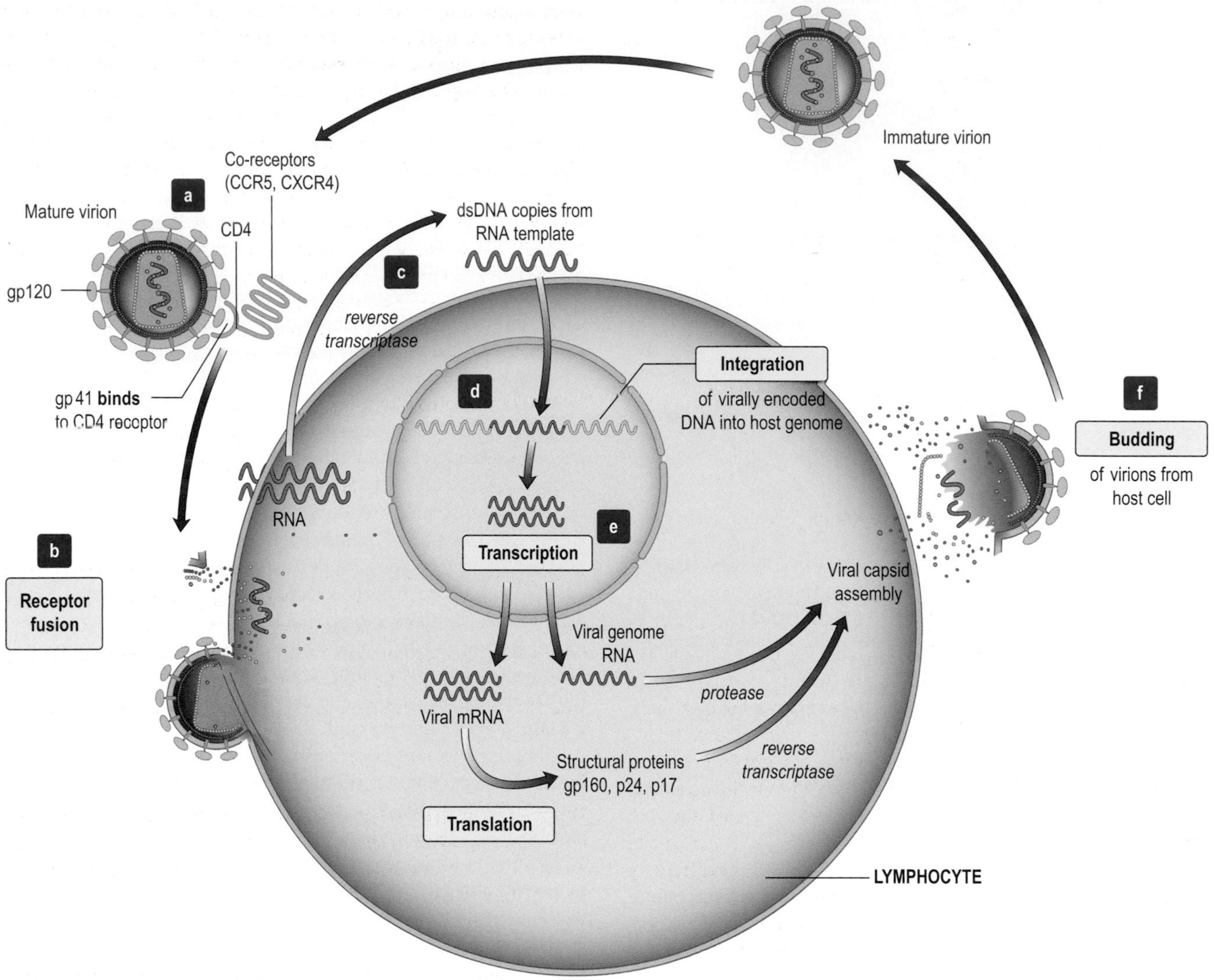

Figure 12.11 **HIV entry and replication in CD4 T lymphocytes.**
(a) ***Binding***: the virus binds to host CD4 receptor molecules via the envelope glycoprotein gp120 and co-receptors CCR5 and CXCR4.
(b) ***Fusion***: a subsequent conformational change results in fusion between gp41 and the cell membrane.
(c) ***Reverse transcription***: entry of the viral capsid is followed by uncoating of the RNA. DNA copies are made from both RNA templates. DNA polymerase from the host cell leads to the formation of double-stranded DNA (dsDNA).
(d) ***Integration***: in the nucleus, virally encoded DNA is inserted into the host genome.
(e) ***Transcription***: regulatory proteins control transcription (an RNA molecule is now synthesized from the DNA template).
(f) ***Budding***: the virus is re-assembled in the cytoplasm and budded out from the host cell.

National AIDS Trust. *HIV and Black African Communities in the UK*. London: National AIDS Trust; 2014.
Public Health England. *HIV in the United Kingdom: 2014 Report*. London: Public Health England; 2014.
Punyacharoensin N, Edmunds WJ, De Angelis D et al. Modelling the HIV epidemic among MSM in the United Kingdom: quantifying the contributions to HIV transmission to better inform prevention initiatives. *AIDS* 2015; 29:339–349.

CLINICAL APPROACH TO THE PATIENT WITH HIV

Diagnosis and natural history

HIV is now a manageable chronic condition with a life expectancy that can match that of the general population, in those who start effective ART early enough. Starting treatment when disease is more advanced compromises clinical outcomes. In 2013, 24% of those living with HIV in the UK were unaware of their infection; 42% of people newly diagnosed in the UK in 2013 were 'late presenters' – that is, they had a CD4 count below the threshold to start therapy (<350 cells/mm^3); and in 33%, the CD4 count was <200 cells/mm^3, putting them at high risk of HIV-associated pathology ***(Fig. 12.12)***. Increasing the uptake of HIV testing is a major public health objective. Guidelines on HIV testing from the British HIV Association (BHIVA) and the National Institute for Health and Care Excellence (NICE) include clinical settings in which HIV testing should be universally offered, together with a list of clinical situations and diagnoses (indicator conditions) that are highly predictive of HIV infection and in which HIV testing should be recommended ***(Box 12.8)***. Testing should be recommended for all new registrants in primary care and patients admitted to acute medical care in areas of the UK where HIV seroprevalence is >2/1000 population.

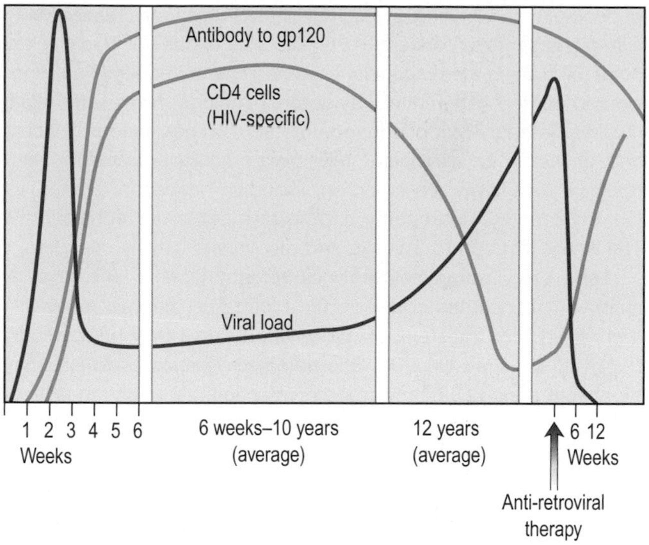

Figure 12.12 The immune response to HIV (seroconversion).

Discussion about HIV testing and the consent required is straightforward and within the competencies of a wide range of healthcare professionals. Sensitive and specific point-of-care HIV antibody tests using either blood or oral fluids can give results within minutes and have extended the possibilities for diagnosis. Home sampling approaches, with specimens sent to a central laboratory and results given over the telephone, have been shown to increase testing rates in some populations. Changes in legislation in the UK now allow for the sale of home testing kits for HIV, although 'kite-marked' kits are not yet available. It is crucial for all reactive point-of-care tests to be followed up with confirmatory serological assays and for appropriate arrangements to be made to ensure that patients receive their test results and those who are found to be HIV-positive have rapid routes into specialist care.

Investigation of HIV

HIV infection is diagnosed either by detection of virus-specific antibodies (anti-HIV) or by direct identification of viral material. The recommended UK first-line assay is one that tests for HIV antibody *and* p24 antigen simultaneously. These fourth-generation assays have the advantage of reducing the time between infection and an HIV-positive test result to 1 month, which is several weeks earlier than with sensitive third-generation (antibody-only detection) assays.

Detection of IgG antibody to envelope components

This is the most commonly used marker of infection. The routine tests used for screening are based on enzyme-linked immunosorbent assay (ELISA) techniques, which may be confirmed with Western blot assays. Up to 3 months (mean 6 weeks) may elapse from initial infection to antibody detection (serological latency, or window period). These antibodies to HIV have no protective function and persist for life. As with all IgG antibodies, anti-HIV will cross the placenta. All babies born to HIV-positive women will thus have the antibody at birth. In this situation, anti-HIV antibody is not a reliable marker of active infection, and in uninfected babies will be gradually lost over the first 18 months of life.

Simple and rapid HIV antibody assays are increasingly available, giving results within minutes. Assays that can utilize alternative body fluids to serum/plasma, such as oral fluid, whole blood and urine, are now available and home testing kits are being developed. These tests are extremely sensitive and may give false-positive results, making it necessary to perform a confirmatory test.

A serologic testing algorithm for recent HIV seroconversions (STARHS) can be used to identify recently acquired infection. A highly sensitive ELISA that is able to detect HIV antibodies 6–8 weeks after infection is used on blood in patients with a positive oral fluid test, in parallel with a less sensitive (detuned) test that identifies later HIV antibodies within 130 days. A positive result on the sensitive test and a negative 'detuned' test are indicative of recent infection, while positive results on both tests point to an infection that is more than 130 days old. The major application of this is in epidemiological surveillance and monitoring.

Detection of IgG antibody to p24 (anti-p24)

This can be detected from the earliest weeks of infection and through the asymptomatic phase. It is frequently lost as the disease progresses.

Genome detection assays

Nucleic acid-based assays that amplify and test for components of the HIV genome are available. These assays are used to aid the diagnosis of HIV in the babies of HIV-positive mothers or in situations where serological tests may be inadequate, such as in early infection when antibody may not be present, or in subtyping HIV variants for medico-legal reasons. (See the discussion of viral load monitoring on p. 339.)

Detection of viral p24 antigen (p24ag)

This is detectable shortly after infection but has usually disappeared by 8–10 weeks after exposure. It can be a useful marker in individuals who have been infected recently but have not had time to mount an antibody response.

Isolation of virus in culture

This is a specialized technique available in some laboratories as a diagnostic aid and a research tool.

Clinical features of untreated HIV

The spectrum of illnesses associated with HIV infection is broad and is the result of direct HIV effects, HIV-associated immune dysfunction, and the drugs used to treat the condition, as well as coexisting morbidity and co-infections. Since the introduction of effective therapy, the majority of people with HIV in resource-rich settings begin treatment whilst asymptomatic, before the onset of significant immunosuppression or progression to an AIDS-defining event.

Several classification systems exist, the most widely used being the 1993 Centers for Disease Control (CDC) classification ***(Box 12.9)***. This classification depends, to a large extent, on definitive diagnoses of infection, which makes it more difficult to apply in those areas of the world without sophisticated laboratory support.

As immunosuppression progresses, the patient is susceptible to an increasing range of opportunistic infections and tumours, certain of which meet the criteria for the diagnosis of AIDS ***(Box 12.10)***.

The definition of AIDS differs between the USA and Europe. The US definition includes individuals with CD4 counts of <200 cells/mm^3, in addition to the clinical classification based on the presence of specific indicator diagnoses shown in ***Box 12.9***. In Europe, the definition remains based on the diagnosis of specific clinical

Box 12.9 Summary of the Centers for Disease Control (CDC) classification of HIV infection

Absolute CD4 count (/mm³)	A	B	C
	Asymptomatic or persistent generalized lymphadenopathy or acute seroconversion illness	*HIV-related conditions,*[a] *not A or C*	*Clinical conditions listed in AIDS surveillance case definition (see Box 12.10)*
>500	A1	B1	C1
200–499	A2	B2	C2
<200	A3	B3	C3

[a]Examples of category B conditions include: bacillary angiomatosis, candidiasis (oropharyngeal), constitutional symptoms, oral hairy leukoplakia, herpes zoster involving more than one dermatome, idiopathic thrombocytopenic purpura, listeriosis, pelvic inflammatory disease, especially if complicated by tubo-ovarian abscess, peripheral neuropathy.

Box 12.10 AIDS-defining conditions

- Candidiasis of bronchi, trachea or lungs
- Candidiasis, oesophageal
- Cervical carcinoma, invasive
- Coccidioidomycosis, disseminated or extrapulmonary
- Cryptococcosis, extrapulmonary
- Cryptosporidiosis, chronic intestinal (1-month duration)
- Cytomegalovirus (CMV) disease (other than liver, spleen or nodes)
- CMV retinitis (with loss of vision)
- Encephalopathy, HIV-related
- Herpes simplex, chronic ulcers (1-month duration), or bronchitis, pneumonitis or oesophagitis
- Histoplasmosis, disseminated or extrapulmonary
- Isosporiasis, chronic intestinal (1-month duration)
- Kaposi's sarcoma
- Lymphoma, Burkitt's
- Lymphoma, immunoblastic (or equivalent term)
- Lymphoma (primary) of brain
- *Mycobacterium avium-intracellulare* complex or *M. kansasii*, disseminated or extrapulmonary
- *Mycobacterium tuberculosis*, any site
- *Mycobacterium*, other species or unidentified species, disseminated or extrapulmonary
- *Pneumocystis jiroveci* pneumonia
- Pneumonia, recurrent
- Progressive multifocal leucoencephalopathy
- *Salmonella* septicaemia, recurrent
- Toxoplasmosis of brain
- Wasting syndrome, due to HIV

conditions with no inclusion of CD4 lymphocyte counts. Where ART is available and started before the development of severe immunosuppression, progression to AIDS is now uncommon.

Incubation, seroconversion and primary illness

Primary HIV infection (PHI) refers to the first 6-month period following HIV acquisition. This is a period of uncontrolled viral replication resulting in high levels of HIV circulating in the plasma and genital tract, and consequently of high infectiousness. At a population level, PHI is increasingly recognized as a contributor to onward transmission. In the UK, up to 20% of all newly diagnosed individuals are recently infected. The 2–4 weeks immediately following infection may be silent, both clinically and serologically. In a number of people, a self-limiting acute viral illness, which may be confused with glandular fever, occurs 3–6 weeks after exposure. This is a key point for making the diagnosis; however, HIV is frequently not considered in the differential. Symptoms include fever, arthralgia, myalgia, lethargy, lymphadenopathy, sore throat, mucosal ulcers and, occasionally, a transient, faint pink, maculopapular rash. Neurological symptoms are common, including headache, photophobia, myelopathy, neuropathy and, in rare cases, encephalopathy. The illness lasts up to 3 weeks and recovery is usually complete.

Laboratory abnormalities include lymphopenia with atypical reactive lymphocytes noted on the blood film, thrombocytopenia and raised liver transferases. CD4 lymphocytes may be markedly depleted and the CD4:CD8 ratio reversed. Antibodies to HIV may be absent during this early stage of infection, although the level of circulating viral RNA is high and p24 core protein may be detectable. NAAT assays of HIV RNA may be diagnostic 7 days before a p24 antigen test and 12 days before a sensitive HIV antibody test. If PHI is suspected but standard diagnostic tests are negative, then repeat testing in 7 days and referral for expert advice is recommended.

Clinical latency

The rate of clinical progression of untreated HIV is variable. The majority of people with HIV infection are asymptomatic for a substantial but variable length of time. However, the virus continues to replicate and the person is infectious. Most people with HIV have a gradual decline in CD4 count over a period of approximately 10 years before progression to symptomatic disease or AIDS. Others progress much more rapidly, with continued high levels of viral RNA and a rapid decline in CD4 count over 2–5 years. Other long-term non-progressors may continue with a normal CD4 count over many years. Within this group, a small sub-population of elite controllers maintain a viral load <2000 copies/mL or even undetectable levels without therapy.

Older age is associated with more rapid progression. Gender and pregnancy *per se* do not appear to influence the rate of progression, although women may fare less well for a variety of reasons. A subgroup of patients with asymptomatic infection have ***persistent generalized lymphadenopathy*** (PGL), defined as lymphadenopathy (>1 cm) at two or more extra-inguinal sites for more than 3 months in the absence of causes other than HIV infection. The nodes are usually symmetrical, firm, mobile and non-tender. There may be associated splenomegaly. The architecture of the nodes shows hyperplasia of the follicles and proliferation of the capillary endothelium. Biopsy is rarely indicated. Similar disease progression has been noted in asymptomatic patients with or without PGL. Nodes may disappear with disease progression.

Symptomatic HIV infection

As HIV infection progresses, the viral load rises, the CD4 count falls and the patient develops an array of symptoms and signs. The clinical picture is the result of direct HIV effects and of the associated immunosuppression.

In an individual patient, the clinical consequences of HIV-related immune dysfunction will depend on at least three factors:

- ***The microbial exposure of the patient throughout life***. Many clinical episodes represent reactivation of previously acquired infection, which has been latent. Geographical factors determine the microbial repertoire of an individual patient. Those organisms requiring intact cell-mediated immunity for their control are most likely to cause clinical problems.

- ***The pathogenicity of organisms encountered***. High-grade pathogens, such as *Mycobacterium tuberculosis*, *Candida* and the herpesviruses, are clinically relevant, even when immunosuppression is mild, and will thus occur earlier in the course of the disease. Less virulent organisms occur at later stages of immunodeficiency.
- ***The degree of immunosuppression of the host***. When patients are severely immunocompromised (CD4 count <100 cells/mm^3), disseminated infections with organisms of very low virulence, such as *M. avium-intracellulare* (*MAI*) and *Cryptosporidium*, are able to establish themselves. These infections are very resistant to treatment, mainly because there is no functioning immune response to clear organisms. This hierarchy of infection allows for appropriate intervention with prophylactic drugs.

Box 12.11 Some mucocutaneous manifestations of HIV infection[a]

Skin
- Dry skin and scalp
- Onychomycosis
- Seborrhoeic dermatitis
- Tinea: cruris, pedis
- Pityriasis: versicolor, rosea
- Folliculitis
- Acne
- Molluscum contagiosum
- Warts
- Herpes zoster: multi-dermatomal disseminated
- Papular pruritic eruption
- Scabies
- Ichthyosis
- Kaposi's sarcoma

Mucous membranes
- Candidiasis: oral, vulvovaginal
- Oral hairy leukoplakia
- Aphthous ulcers
- Herpes simplex: genital, oral, labial
- Periodontal disease
- Warts: oral, genital

[a]*See also pages 1384–1385.*

End-organ effects of HIV

Neurological disease

Infection of the nervous tissue occurs at an early stage but clinical neurological involvement increases as HIV advances. This includes ***AIDS dementia complex*** (***ADC***), ***sensory polyneuropathy*** and ***aseptic meningitis*** (see p. 866). These conditions are much less common since the introduction of ART. The pathogenesis is thought to be due both to the release of neurotoxic products by HIV itself and to cytokine abnormalities secondary to immune dysregulation.

ADC has varying degrees of severity, ranging from mild memory impairment and poor concentration through to severe cognitive deficit, personality change and psychomotor slowing. Changes in affect are common and depressive or psychotic features may be present. The spinal cord may show vacuolar myelopathy histologically. In severe cases, computed tomography (CT) scanning of the brain shows atrophic change of varying degrees. Magnetic resonance imaging (MRI) changes consist of white matter lesions of increased density on T2-weighted sections. Electroencephalography (EEG) shows non-specific changes consistent with encephalopathy. The CSF is usually normal, although the protein concentration may be raised. Patients with mild neurological dysfunction may be unduly sensitive to the effects of other insults, such as fever, metabolic disturbance or psychotropic medication, any of which may lead to a marked deterioration in cognitive functioning.

Sensory polyneuropathy is seen in advanced HIV infection, mainly in the legs and feet, although hands may be affected. Severe forms cause intense pain, usually in the feet, which disrupts sleep, impairs mobility and generally reduces the quality of life.

Autonomic neuropathy may also occur with postural hypotension and diarrhoea. Autonomic nerve damage is found in the small bowel.

ARVs that penetrate the central nervous system (CNS) can lead to significant improvements in cognitive function in many patients with ADC. They may also have a neuroprotective role.

Eye disease

Eye pathology may occur in the later stages. The most serious condition is cytomegalovirus retinitis (see p. 258), which is sight-threatening. Retinal cotton wool spots due to HIV *per se* are rarely troublesome but they can be confused with cytomegalovirus retinitis. Anterior uveitis can present as acute red eye associated with rifabutin therapy for mycobacterial infections in HIV. Steroids used topically are usually effective but modification of the dose of rifabutin is required to prevent relapse. Pneumocystis, toxoplasmosis, syphilis and lymphoma can all affect the retina and the eye may be the site of first presentation.

Mucocutaneous manifestations

The skin is a common site for HIV-related pathology ***(Box 12.11)***, as the function of dendritic and Langerhans cells, both target cells for HIV, is disrupted. Delayed-type hypersensitivity, a good indicator of cell-mediated immunity, is frequently reduced or absent, even before clinical signs of immunosuppression appear. Pruritus is a common complaint at all stages of HIV. Generalized dry, itchy, flaky skin is typical and the hair may become thin and dry. An intensely pruritic papular eruption favouring the extremities may be found, particularly in patients from African backgrounds. Eosinophilic folliculitis presents with urticarial lesions, particularly on the face, arms and legs.

Drug reactions with cutaneous manifestations are frequent, rashes developing notably to sulphur-containing drugs, amongst others (see ***Fig. 31.52***). Recurrent aphthous ulceration, which is severe and slow to heal, may impair the patient's ability to eat. Biopsy may be indicated to exclude other causes of ulceration. Topical steroids are useful and resistant cases may respond to thalidomide. In addition to the above, the skin is a common site of opportunistic infections (see pp. 1384–1385).

Haematological complications

These are common in advanced HIV infection.

- ***Lymphopenia*** progresses as the CD4 count falls.
- ***Anaemia of chronic HIV infection*** is usually mild, normochromic and normocytic.
- ***Neutropenia*** is common and usually mild.
- ***Isolated thrombocytopenia*** may occur early in infection and be the only manifestation of HIV for some time. Platelet counts are often moderately reduced but can fall dramatically to 10–20 × 10^9/L, producing easy bleeding and bruising. Circulating antiplatelet antibodies lead to peripheral destruction. Megakaryocytes are increased in the bone marrow but their function is impaired. Effective ART usually produces a rise in platelet count. Thrombocytopenic patients undergoing dental, medical or surgical procedures may need therapy with human immunoglobulin, which gives a transient rise in platelet count, or with platelet transfusion. Steroids are best avoided.

- ***Pancytopenia*** occurs because of underlying opportunistic infection or malignancies, in particular *M. avium-intracellulare*, disseminated cytomegalovirus and lymphoma.
- ***Other complications*** involve myelotoxic drugs, which include zidovudine (megaloblastic anaemia, red cell aplasia, neutropenia), lamivudine (anaemia, neutropenia), ganciclovir (neutropenia), systemic chemotherapy (pancytopenia) and co-trimoxazole (agranulocytosis).

Gastrointestinal effects

Weight loss and diarrhoea are common in people with advanced untreated HIV infection (see ***Box 13.19***). Wasting is a common feature of advanced HIV infection, which, although originally attributed to direct HIV effects on metabolism, is usually a consequence of anorexia. There is a small increase in resting energy expenditure in all stages of HIV, but weight and lean body mass usually remain normal during periods of clinical latency when the patient is eating normally.

HIV enteropathy with varying degrees of villous atrophy has been described with chronic diarrhoea when no other pathogen has been found.

Hypochlorhydria is reported in patients with advanced HIV disease and may have consequences for drug absorption and bacterial overgrowth in the gut.

Rectal lymphoid tissue cells are the targets for HIV infection during penetrative anal sex and may be a reservoir for infection to spread through the body.

Renal complications

HIV-associated nephropathy (***HIVAN***; see p. 737), although rare, can cause significant renal impairment, particularly in more advanced disease. It is most frequently seen in black male patients and can be exacerbated by heroin use.

Nephrotic syndrome subsequent to focal glomerulosclerosis is the usual pathology, which may be a consequence of HIV cytopathic effects on renal tubular epithelium. The course is usually relentlessly progressive and dialysis may be required.

Many ***nephrotoxic drugs*** are used in the management of HIV-associated pathology, particularly foscarnet, amphotericin B, pentamidine and sulfadiazine. Tenofovir is associated with Fanconi syndrome (see p. 1286).

Respiratory complications

The upper airway and lungs serve as a physical barrier to air-borne pathogens and any damage will decrease the efficiency of protection, leading to an increase in upper and lower respiratory tract infections. The sinus mucosa may also function abnormally in HIV infection and is frequently the site of chronic inflammation. Response to antibacterial therapy and topical steroids is usual but some patients require surgical intervention. A similar process is seen in the middle ear, which can lead to chronic otitis media.

Lymphoid interstitial pneumonitis (***LIP***) is well described in paediatric HIV infection but is uncommon in adults. There is an infiltration of lymphocytes, plasma cells and lymphoblasts in alveolar tissue. Epstein–Barr virus may be present. The patient presents with dyspnoea and a dry cough, which may be confused with pneumocystis infection (see p. 349). Reticular nodular shadowing is seen on chest X-ray. Therapy with steroids may produce clinical and histological benefit in some patients.

Endocrine complications

Various endocrine abnormalities have been reported, including reduced levels of testosterone and abnormal adrenal function. The latter assumes clinical significance in advanced disease when intercurrent infection superimposed on borderline adrenal function precipitates clear adrenal insufficiency, requiring replacement doses of gluco- and mineralocorticoid. Cytomegalovirus is also implicated in adrenal-deficient states.

Cardiac complications

Cardiovascular pathology is increasingly recognized as a cause of morbidity in people with HIV. Although lipid dysregulation has been associated with ARV medication, the observation has been made that high-density lipoprotein (HDL) levels are lower in those with untreated HIV infection than in HIV-negative controls. In a large international study (SMART), ischaemic heart disease was more common in those who took intermittent ARV therapy than in those who maintained viral suppression. Cardiomyopathy, although rare, is associated with HIV and may lead to congestive cardiac failure. Lymphocytic and necrotic myocarditis has been described. Ventricular biopsy should be performed to ensure that other treatable causes of myocarditis are excluded.

Conditions associated with HIV immunodeficiency

Immunodeficiency (see pp. 138–142) allows the development of opportunistic infections (***Box 12.12*** and see also ***Box 12.21***). These are diseases caused by organisms that are not usually considered pathogenic, unusual presentations of known pathogens, and the occurrence of tumours that may have an oncogenic viral aetiology. Susceptibility increases as the patient becomes more immunosuppressed. CD4 T-lymphocyte numbers are used as markers to predict the risk of infection. Patients with CD4 counts of >200 cells/mm^3 are at low risk for the majority of AIDS-defining opportunistic infections. A hierarchy of thresholds for specific infectious risks can be constructed. Mechanisms include defective T-cell function against protozoa, fungi and viruses, impaired macrophage function against intracellular bacteria such as *Mycobacteria* and *Salmonella*, and defective B-cell immunity against capsulated bacteria such as *Streptococcus pneumoniae* and *Haemophilus*. Many of the

Box 12.12 Major HIV-associated pathogens

Protozoa
- *Toxoplasma gondii*
- *Cryptosporidium parvum*
- *Microsporidia* spp.
- *Leishmania donovani*
- *Isospora belli*

Viruses
- *Cytomegalovirus*
- *Herpes simplex*
- *Varicella zoster*
- *Human papillomavirus*
- *JC polyomavirus*

Fungi and yeasts
- *Pneumocystis jiroveci*
- *Cryptococcus neoformans*
- *Candida* spp.
- Dermatophytes (*Trichophyton*)
- *Aspergillus fumigatus*
- *Histoplasma capsulatum*
- *Coccidioides immitis*

Bacteria
- *Salmonella* spp.
- *Mycobacterium tuberculosis*
- *M. avium-intracellulare*
- *Streptococcus pneumoniae*
- *Staphylococcus aureus*
- *Haemophilus influenzae*
- *Moraxella catarrhalis*
- *Rhodococcus equii*
- *Bartonella quintana*
- *Nocardia*

organisms causing clinical disease are ubiquitous in the environment or are already carried by the patient.

Diagnosis in an immunosuppressed patient may be complicated by a lack of typical signs, as the inflammatory response is impaired. Examples are lack of neck stiffness in cryptococcal meningitis or minimal clinical findings in early *Pneumocystis jiroveci* pneumonia. Multiple pathogens may coexist. Indirect serological tests are frequently unreliable. Specimens should be obtained from the appropriate site for examination and culture in order to make a diagnosis.

Assessment and monitoring of HIV-positive patients

Initial assessment

People are newly diagnosed with HIV in an increasingly wide range of settings and need to be transferred appropriately into effective care. All those with a new diagnosis of HIV should be reviewed by an HIV clinician within 2 weeks of diagnosis, or earlier if the patient is symptomatic or has other acute needs. A full medical history, physical examination and laboratory evaluation should be undertaken in all newly diagnosed patients to determine the stage of infection and the presence of co-morbidities and co-infections, and to assess overall physical, mental and sexual health. The initial assessment should also include details of the patient's socioeconomic situation, relationships, family and social support networks, and substance misuse, together with contact tracing and partner notification. Specialist advice should be sought if there are children who require testing. Baseline investigations will depend on the clinical setting, but those appropriate for an asymptomatic person in the UK are shown in ***Box 12.13***.

Box 12.13 Baseline assessment investigations for a newly diagnosed asymptomatic patient with HIV infection

History of all other coexisting conditions, including sexual, psychiatric and reproductive health
- Full drug history, including recreational substances
- Vaccination history
- Social circumstances to include relationships, disclosure, support

Haematology
- Full blood count, differential count and film

Biochemistry
- Serum, liver and renal function, including estimated glomerular filtration rate (eGFR)
- Fasting serum lipid profile, total cholesterol, high-density lipoprotein (HDL) cholesterol
- Fasting blood glucose
- Serum bone profile, including 25-OH-vitamin D
- Urinalysis
- Dipstick for blood, protein and glucose
- Urine protein:creatinine ratio

Immunology
- Lymphocyte subsets (repeat to confirm baseline within 1–3 months)
- HLA-B*5701 status

Virology
- HIV antibody (confirmatory)
- HIV viral load
- HIV genotype and subtype determination
- Hepatitis A IgG
- Hepatitis B surface antigen and full profile
- Hepatitis C antibody (followed by hepatitis C RNA testing if antibody-positive, and confirmation of antibody-positive status if RNA negative)

Microbiology
- Toxoplasmosis serology
- Syphilis serology
- Tuberculosis status
- Screen for other sexually transmitted infections

Other
- Cervical cytology
- Chest X-ray if indicated
- 10-year cardiovascular risk assessment
- Fracture risk assessment
- Body mass index (BMI)

Monitoring

Patients are regularly monitored, depending on infection and treatment stage.

For people who are not yet on therapy, monitoring should take place 2–4 times per year, with longer intervals for those with higher CD4 counts, to assess progression of the infection and the need for treatment. Decisions about appropriate intervention can be made.

For people starting therapy and those on established effective therapy, monitoring is described in on page 344.

Immunological monitoring

CD4 lymphocytes. The absolute CD4 count and its percentage of total lymphocytes fall as HIV progresses. These figures bear a relationship to the risk of occurrence of HIV-related pathology, and patients with counts <200 cells/mm^3 are at greatest risk. Rapidly falling CD4 counts and those at or below 350 are an indication for immediate initiation of ART. Factors other than HIV (e.g. smoking, exercise, intercurrent infections and diurnal variation) also affect CD4 numbers. CD4 counts are performed at approximately 4–6-monthly intervals unless values are approaching critical levels for intervention, in which case they are performed more frequently.

Virological monitoring

Viral load (***HIV RNA***). HIV replicates at a high rate throughout the course of infection, many billions of new virus particles being produced daily. The rate of viral clearance is relatively constant in any individual and thus the level of viraemia is a reflection of the rate of virus replication. This has both prognostic and therapeutic value.

The commonly used term 'viral load' encompasses viraemia and HIV RNA levels. Three ***HIV RNA assays for viral load*** are in current use:

- branched-chain DNA (bDNA)
- reverse transcription polymerase chain reaction (RT-PCR)
- nucleic acid sequence-based amplification (NASBA).

Results are given in copies of viral RNA/mL of plasma, or converted to a logarithmic scale, and there is good correlation between tests. The most sensitive test is able to detect as few as 20 copies of viral RNA/mL. Transient increases in viral load are seen following immunizations (e.g. for influenza and *Pneumococcus*) or during episodes of acute intercurrent infection (e.g. tuberculosis), and viral load measurements should not be carried out within a month of these events.

By about 6 months after seroconversion to HIV, the viral set-point for an individual is established and there is a correlation between HIV RNA levels and long-term prognosis, independent of the CD4 count. Those patients with a viral load consistently >100 000 copies/mL have a 10 times higher risk of progression to AIDS over the ensuing 5 years than those consistently <10 000 copies/mL.

HIV RNA is the standard marker of treatment efficacy (see below). Both duration and magnitude of virus suppression are pointers to clinical outcome. The aim of therapy is to secure long-term virological suppression, and a rising viral load in a patient whose adherence is assured indicates drug failure.

Baseline measurements are followed by repeat estimations at intervals of 4–6 months, ideally in conjunction with CD4 counts, to allow both pieces of evidence to be used together in decision-making. Following initiation of ART or changes in therapy, a reduction in viral load should be seen by 4 weeks, reaching a maximum at 10–12 weeks, when repeat viral load testing should be carried out (see ***Fig. 12.12***).

Genotype determination

Clear genotype variations exist within HIV; not only are there variations between viral subtypes but also well-identified point mutations are associated with resistance to ARVs. New infections with drug-resistant variants of HIV may be seen. Viral genotype analysis is recommended for all newly diagnosed patients with HIV. The most appropriate sample is the one closest to the time of diagnosis and the results are used to guide the selection of ART agents.

Further reading

Asboe D, Aitken C, Boffito M et al. British HIV Association guidelines for the routine investigation and monitoring of adult HIV-1-infected individuals 2011. *HIV Med* 2012; 13:1–44.

Deeks SG, Lewin SR, Havlir DV. The end of AIDS: HIV infection as a chronic disease. *Lancet* 2013; 382:1525–1533.

May MT, Gompels M, Delpech V et al. Impact on life expectancy of HIV-1 positive individuals of CD4+ cell count and viral load response to antiretroviral therapy: UK cohort study. *AIDS* 2014; 28:1193–1202.

Box 12.14 An approach to sick HIV-positive patients

Potential problems

- Adverse drug reactions
- Drug–drug interactions
- Presentation or complications of malignancy
- Immune reconstitution phenomenon
- Infection in an immunocompromised host
- Acute opportunistic infections
- Organic or functional brain disorders
- Non-HIV-related pathology

Full medical history

- Anti-retroviral drugs, recreational drugs, prophylaxis, travel, previous HIV-related pathology, potential source of infectious agents (food hygiene, pets, contacts with acute infections, contact with tuberculosis, sexually transmitted infections)
- Secure confidentiality; ask the patient who is aware of the HIV diagnosis

Full physical examination

- Signs of adverse drug reactions, e.g. skin rashes, oral ulceration
- Signs of disseminated sepsis
- Clinical evidence of immunosuppression, e.g. oral candida, oral hairy leukoplakia
- Focal neurological signs and/or meningism
- Evidence of altered mental state – organic or functional
- Examine:
  - Genitalia, e.g. herpes simplex, syphilis, gonorrhoea
  - Fundi, e.g. cytomegalovirus retinitis
  - Mouth
- Lymphadenopathy

Immediate investigations[a]

- Full blood count and differential count
- Liver and renal function tests
- Plasma glucose
- Blood gases, including acid–base balance
- Blood cultures, including specimens for mycobacterial culture
- Microscopy and culture of available/appropriate specimens: stool, sputum, urine, cerebrospinal fluid
- Malaria screen in recent travellers from malaria areas
- Serological tests for cryptococcal antigen, toxoplasmosis; save serum for viral studies
- Chest X-ray
- CT/MRI scan of brain if there are focal neurological signs and *always* before lumbar puncture

[a]*Lymphocyte subsets and HIV viral load assays may yield misleading results during intercurrent illness.*

MANAGEMENT OF HIV-POSITIVE PATIENTS

Effective ART has transformed the clinical outcomes for people with HIV, extending life expectancy towards that of the general population, bringing down morbidity and cutting infectiousness to people who are HIV-negative. Current management strategies aim to maximize wellbeing with long-term, effective suppressive therapy within a chronic condition model, beginning before the patient is symptomatic ***(Box 12.14)***. The treatment of opportunistic conditions in immunosuppressed patients is most commonly seen either in situations where ART is not available or in previously undiagnosed patients presenting with advanced infection. With access and adherence to potent, tolerable ARVs within a managed clinical setting, life expectancy for people with HIV can approach that of the general population. Nevertheless, there is still no cure for HIV and patients live with a chronic, potentially infectious and unpredictable condition. Limitations on ART efficacy include the inability of existing drugs to clear HIV from certain intracellular pools, the occurrence of drug side-effects, adherence requirements, complex drug–drug interactions and the emergence of resistant viral strains. Even with complete viral suppression, ART does not fully restore health, and treated infection is associated with a variety of non-AIDS complications, including cardiovascular disease and some cancers.

The ***aims of management*** in HIV infection are to:

- maintain physical and mental health
- improve the quality of life
- increase survival rates
- restore and improve immune function
- avoid onward transmission of the virus
- provide appropriate clinical care as needed.

This requires long-term, maximal suppression of HIV activity using ARV medication and management adopting a multidisciplinary team approach. Regular assessment is needed to obtain details of intercurrent medical problems, medications, vaccinations, any recreational drug use, sexual history, reproductive decision-making, cervical cytology, and social situation to include support networks, employment, benefits and accommodation. Depression and anxiety are common among people living with HIV and can have a deleterious impact on adherence to medication regimens, making it important for mood and cognitive function to be routinely and regularly assessed. Psychological support may be needed, not only for the patient but also for family, friends and carers. Regular reviews of sexual and reproductive health, together with advice on reducing the risk of HIV transmission, must be provided and future

Box 12.15 Anti-retroviral drugs (ARVs) commonly used in clinical practice

Drug class	Drugs	Comments
Nucleoside and nucleotide reverse transcriptase inhibitors (NRTIs)	Tenofovir, abacavir, zidovudine[a], stavudine[a], lamivudine, emtricitabine	Tenofovir associated with renal dysfunction Abacavir associated with hypersensitivity reactions in at-risk individuals (HLA-B*5701) Zidovudine and stavudine (both now rarely used in the UK) are associated with fat redistribution (lipoatrophy) Abacavir plus lamivudine should only be used when baseline VL is <100 000 copies/mL The combination of tenofovir plus emtricitabine is a preferred first-line regimen in most regions
Non-nucleoside reverse transcriptase inhibitors (NNRTIs)	Efavirenz, nevirapine[a], etravirine, rilpivirine	Efavirenz can cause central nervous system toxicity (usually time-limited) Nevirapine can cause severe hepatotoxicity in patients with higher CD4 cell counts (>250 cells/mm^3 for women and >400 cells/mm^3 for men) Rilpivirine should only be used when baseline VL is <100 000 copies/mL Etravine is given twice daily and has generally been used as a second-line regimen
Integrase inhibitors or integrase strand transfer inhibitors (INSTIs)	Raltegravir, dolutegravir, elvitegravir	Integrase inhibitors are generally well tolerated and have fewer adverse effects than other ARV classes Raltegravir is taken twice daily Elvitegravir requires boosting by cobicistat
Protease inhibitors	Fosamprenavir, atazanavir, darunavir, lopinavir, saquinavir (ritonavir)	Most protease inhibitors are extensively metabolized by the cytochrome P450 3A system; ritonavir is generally given at low doses (100–200 mg per day) to inhibit P450 and boost the co-administered protease inhibitors Most protease inhibitors are associated with hyperlipidaemia and other metabolic abnormalities such as insulin resistance Long-term protease inhibitor exposure has been associated with increased risk of cardiovascular disease
CCR5 inhibitors	Maraviroc	Maraviroc is only active in patients who do not have virions that use CXCR4 for cell entry. A specialized assay is therefore needed to screen for co-receptor tropism. By contrast with other ARVs, maraviroc binds to a host rather than a viral target
Fusion inhibitors	Enfuvirtide	Enfuvirtide must be given subcutaneously twice daily and is very expensive; generally used only in patients who have no other therapeutic options

[a]Some drugs, such as zidovudine, stavudine and nevirapine, are generally used in resource-limited regions because of cost considerations. These are not recommended as preferred agents in resource-rich regions in view of their potential toxic effects. VL, viral load.
(Modified from: Volberding PA, Deeks SG. Antiretroviral therapy and management of HIV infection. *Lancet* 2010; 376(9734):49–62.)

sexual practices discussed. Information is required to allow people to make informed choices about childbearing. The implications for sexual partners and existing family members should be considered and diagnostic testing offered as necessary. Regular monitoring of weight, body mass index, blood pressure and cardiovascular risk is required. Dietary assessment and advice should be freely accessible. General health promotion advice on smoking, alcohol, diet, drug misuse and exercise should be given, particularly in light of the cardiovascular, metabolic and hepatotoxicity risks associated with HIV and its treatment.

Anti-retroviral drugs

The treatment of HIV using anti-retroviral therapy (ART; ***Box 12.15***) continues to evolve and improve. Increased potency, reduced toxicity, greater convenience of formulation, and availability of compounds with different mechanisms of action, coupled with an improved understanding of drug resistance, have combined to improve HIV clinical and virological outcomes consistently. An increase in the numbers of compounds, and the array of drug–drug interactions, for example, combine to make HIV treatment complex, and better clinical outcomes have been linked closely to physician expertise and the numbers of patients under direct care. With several of the older compounds now available as generics, some drug costs are likely to fall, and commissioners are increasingly focusing on the cost-effectiveness of the newer agents to justify their use. Regularly updated treatment guidelines are produced in the UK by the British HIV Association and in the USA by the Department of Health and Human Services. The most up-to-date versions can be found on their websites (see 'Further reading') and the current version must be used.

The key practical principles of prescribing ARVs are given in ***Box 12.16***.

Reverse transcriptase inhibitors

Nucleoside/nucleotide analogues

Nucleoside reverse transcriptase inhibitors (NRTIs) inhibit the synthesis of DNA by reverse transcription and also act as DNA chain terminators. NRTIs need to be phosphorylated intracellularly for activity to occur. These were the first group of agents to be used against HIV. Usually, two drugs of this class are combined to provide the 'backbone' of an ART regimen. Several fixed-dose NRTI combinations are available, which helps reduce the pill burden. NRTIs have been associated with mitochondrial toxicity (see p. 346), a consequence of their effect on the human mitochondrial DNA polymerase. Lactic acidosis is a recognized complication of the older members this group of drugs. Nucleotide analogues (nucleotide reverse transcriptase inhibitors, NtRTIs) have a similar mechanism of action but require only two intracellular phosphorylation steps for activity (as opposed to the three steps for nucleoside analogues).

Box 12.16 Prescribing anti-retroviral drugs (ARVs): practice points

Characteristics of ARVs	Practice points
Adherence for the long term is key to success	Make treatment decisions in partnership with the patient. Check for any factors that may compromise accurate adherence Ensure that the proposed drug regimen fits with lifestyles Clarify that the patient is fully conversant with the requirements and understands the reasons for strict adherence Check access to appropriate storage conditions for some agents
Should not be stopped suddenly	Make sure that mechanisms are in place to ensure adequate drug supplies, e.g. regular clinic appointments, repeat prescriptions, home delivery of medications Beware unexpected time away from home, e.g. holidays, intercurrent hospital admissions, immigration detention, police detention If there is an urgent medical indication to stop, obtain advice from specialist physician or pharmacist
Can be compromised by the introduction of other medications, including other ARVs and vice versa	Take care with DDA therapies in hepatitis C (expert advice required) Be careful with enzyme inducers, e.g. rifampicin, rifabutin, warfarin, nevirapine, which will reduce the effective levels of some ARVs Remember that methadone levels may be reduced by efavirenz Note that some ARVs block the metabolism of other agents, which may reach toxic levels, e.g. steroids, statins Always check potential interactions before adding new agents; see www.hiv-druginteractions.org Remember that therapeutic drug monitoring is necessary
Can interact adversely with some herbal, complementary and recreational agents	Note that herbal remedies that induce cytochrome P450, e.g. St John's wort and Chinese herbal remedies, will reduce levels of some ARVs Check potential interactions before adding new agents; see www.hiv-druginteractions.org Remember that therapeutic drug monitoring is necessary
May produce additive toxicities when given with other medications	For example, note that corticosteroid (inhaled and systemic) levels may be elevated, statins, hepatotoxicity with anti-tuberculosis medication, myelosuppression with chemotherapy or high-dose co-trimoxazole
Are associated with a range of adverse drug reactions, which may be confused with other pathology	For example, note that rash, fever, nausea, diarrhoea may all be caused by intercurrent pathology and/or ARVs
May exacerbate co-morbidities	Remember immune reconstitution inflammatory syndrome (IRIS). Examples include hepatic dysfunction due to hepatitis B and C, cardiovascular risk, osteoporosis

Non-nucleoside analogues

Non-nucleoside reverse transcriptase inhibitors (NNRTIs) interfere with reverse transcriptase by direct binding to the enzyme. They are generally small molecules that are widely disseminated throughout the body and have a long half-life. NNRTIs affect cytochrome P450. They are ineffective against HIV-2. The level of cross-resistance across the class is very high. All have been associated with rashes and elevation of liver enzymes. Second-generation NNRTIs, such as etravirine and rilpivirine, which have fewer adverse effects, have some activity against viruses resistant to other compounds of the NNRTI class.

Protease inhibitors

Protease inhibitors (PIs) act competitively on the HIV aspartyl protease enzyme, which is involved in the production of functional viral proteins and enzymes. As a consequence, viral maturation is impaired and immature dysfunctional viral particles are produced. Most of the PIs are active at very low concentrations and *in vitro* are found to have synergy with reverse transcriptase inhibitors. However, there are differences in toxicity, pharmacokinetics, resistance patterns and also cost, which influence prescribing. Cross-resistance can occur across the PI group. There appears to be no activity against human aspartyl proteases (e.g. renin), although there are clinically significant interactions with the cytochrome P450 system. This is used to therapeutic advantage, 'boosting' blood levels of PI by blocking drug breakdown with small doses of ritonavir or cobicistat. PIs have been linked with abnormalities of fat metabolism and control of blood sugar, and some have been linked with deterioration in clotting function in people with haemophilia. In general, PIs have a higher genetic barrier to resistance than other drug classes, and newer PIs such as darunavir have activity against viruses resistant to the older drugs in the class.

Integrase inhibitors

These drugs act as a selective inhibitor of HIV integrase, which blocks viral replication by preventing insertion of HIV DNA into the human DNA genome. Three compounds are in clinical use and are effective in treatment of both drug-experienced and drug-naive patients, with tolerability and safety profiles that are superior to those of NNRTIs and PIs. For these reasons, dolutegravir, a second-generation integrase inhibitor, has been shown to be superior to both efavirenz and darunavir, and also has a high genetic barrier to resistance.

Co-receptor blockers

Maraviroc is a chemokine receptor antagonist that blocks the cellular CCR5 receptor entry by CCR5 tropic strains of HIV. These strains are found in earlier HIV infection and, with time adaptations (against which maraviroc is ineffective), allow the CXCR4 receptor to become the more dominant form. The drug is metabolized by cytochrome P450 (3A), giving the potential for drug–drug interactions. Tropism assays to establish that the patient is carrying a CCR5 tropic virus are required before treatment is used.

Fusion inhibitors

Enfuvitide is the only licensed compound in this class of agents. It is an injectable peptide derived from HIV gp41 that inhibits gp41-mediated fusion of HIV with the target cell. It is synergistic with NRTIs and PIs. Although resistance to enfuvitide has been described, there is no evidence of cross-resistance with other drug

Box 12.17 When to start anti-retroviral therapy (ART)

Primary HIV infection

- *Treatment* is recommended if any one of the following criteria is met:
  - There is neurological involvement
  - The CD4 count is <350 cells/mm^3
  - Any AIDS-defining illness is present (see ***Box 12.10***)

Established HIV infection

- *CD4 <250 cells/mm^3*
  - Treat
- *CD4 251–350 cells/mm^3*
  - Treat as soon as patient is ready
- *CD4 >350 cells/mm^3*
  - Consider enrolment into a 'when to start' trial
- *Treatment to prevent onward transmission*
  - The evidence that treatment with ART lowers the risk of transmission should be discussed with all patients, and an assessment of the current risk of transmission to others made at the time of this discussion. If, following discussion, a patient with a CD4 cell count >350 cells/mm^3 wishes to start ART to reduce the risk of transmission to partners, ART should be initiated
- *AIDS diagnosis/CDC stage C*
  - Treat (except for tuberculosis when CD4 is >350 cells/mm^3)

CDC, Centers for Disease Control.

(Modified from Williams I, Churchill D, Anderson J et al. British HIV Association guidelines for the treatment of HIV-1-positive adults with antiretroviral therapy 2012. Updated November 2013. HIV Medicine *2014; 15(Suppl. 1):1–85. http://www.bhiva.org/documents/Guidelines/Treatment/2012/hiv1029_2.pdf.)*

Box 12.18 Initial ART regimens: choice of initial therapy and preferred regimens[a]

Therapy-naive patients should start with a regimen that contains two nucleoside reverse transcriptase inhibitors and a third agent, either a ritonavir-boosted protease inhibitor, a non-nucleoside reverse transcriptase inhibitor or an integrase inhibitor

Preferred	Alternative
Nucleoside reverse transcriptase inhibitor	
Emtricitabine[b]	Abacavir[c,d,e]
Tenofovir[b]	Lamivudine[c]
Third agent	
Atazanavir/ritonavir	Fosamprenavir/ritonavir
Darunavir/ritonavir	Lopinavir/ritonavir
Efavirenz	Nevirapine[f]
Elvitegravir/cobicistat	Rilpiverine[e]
Raltegravir	

[a]Drugs listed in alphabetical order. [b]Co-formulated as Truvada. [c]Co-formulated as Kivexa. [d]Abacavir is contraindicated if patient is HLA-B*5701-positive. [e]Use recommended only if baseline viral load is <100 000 copies/mL. [f]Nevirapine is contraindicated if baseline CD4 is >250 cells/mm^3 in women or >400 cells/mm^3 in men.

(Modified from Williams I, Churchill D, Anderson J et al. British HIV Association guidelines for the treatment of HIV-1-positive adults with antiretroviral therapy 2012. Updated November 2013. *HIV Medicine* 2014; 15(Suppl. 1):1–85. http://www.bhiva.org/documents/Guidelines/Treatment/2012/hiv1029_2.pdf.)

classes. Because it has an extracellular mode of action there are few drug–drug interactions. Side-effects relate to the subcutaneous route of administration in the form of injection site reactions.

Starting therapy

Although the benefits of ART in HIV infection are indisputable, treatment regimens require a long-term commitment to high levels of adherence. Risks of therapy include short- and longer-term side-effects, drug–drug interactions and the potential for development of resistant viral strains, although, with newer agents and improved formulations, the difficulties associated with treatment have diminished. The full involvement of patients in therapeutic decision-making is essential for success. Various national guidelines and treatment frameworks exist (e.g. guidelines from BHIVA, guidelines from the US Department of Health and Human Services (DHHS), recommendations from the International Antiviral Society (IAS)). Laboratory marker data, including viral load, genotype and CD4 counts, together with individual circumstances, underpin therapeutic decision-making. The current UK recommendations are shown in ***Box 12.17***. In situations where therapy is recommended but the patient elects not to start, then more intensive clinical and laboratory monitoring is advisable.

Questions still remain about the best time to start therapy. Unequivocal clinical benefit has been demonstrated with the use of ARVs in advanced HIV disease. In all patients with symptomatic HIV disease, HIV-related co-morbidity, AIDS or a CD4 count that is consistently <200 cells/mm^3, treatment should be initiated as soon as possible. In such situations, there is a significant risk of serious HIV-associated morbidity and mortality, and the longer-term prognosis for patients initiating therapy <200 cells/mm^3 is not as good as for those who start at higher counts.

In asymptomatic patients, the absolute CD4 count is the key investigation used to guide treatment decisions. The UK recommendation is that therapy should be started at or around a CD4 count of 350 cells/mm^3. Treatment should not be delayed if the CD4 count is close to this threshold.

Debate persists around starting therapy at higher CD4 counts. The risk of disease progression for individuals with a count >350 cells/mm^3 is low and has to be balanced against ARV therapy toxicity and the development of resistance. However, there is growing appreciation of the long-term inflammatory effects of HIV that predispose to non-AIDS illnesses, which, together with the reduction in infectiousness for those on effective therapy, is shifting opinion towards starting sooner. Earlier intervention at higher CD4 counts may be considered in those with a higher risk of disease progression: for example, with high viral loads (>60 000 copies/mL) or rapidly falling CD4 count (losing more than 80 cells/year). Co-infection with hepatitis B and C virus may be an indication for earlier intervention (see p. 351). Patients with primary HIV infection and neurological involvement, an AIDS-defining illness or a CD4 count <350 cells/mm^3 should start therapy, which should be continued indefinitely. Special situations (seroconversion, pregnancy, post-exposure prophylaxis) in which ARV agents may be used are described on pages 346–347.

The evidence that treatment reduces infectiousness should be discussed with all patients with HIV; those who wish to start treatment to reduce the risk of transmission to others should do so, irrespective of CD4 count.

Choice of drugs

The drug regimen used for starting therapy must be individualized to suit each patient's needs. As differences in drug efficacy become less marked, tailoring treatment to the patient's needs and lifestyle is key to success. Treatment is initiated with three drugs: two NRTIs in combination, with a third agent – either an NNRTI, a boosted PI or an integrase inhibitor (***Boxes 12.15*** and ***12.18***). The development of fixed-dose co-formulations reduces pill burden, increases convenience and facilitates adherence.

Nucleoside reverse transcriptase inhibitor

The choice of two NRTIs to form the backbone of therapy is influenced by efficacy, toxicity and ease of administration. The availability of once-daily, one-tablet, fixed-dose combinations, Truvada (tenofovir/emtricitabine) and Kivexa (abacavir/lamivudine), has led to the prescription of one of these as the two-NRTI backbone for the majority of patients who are naive to medication. Kivexa should be used only in those who are HLA-B*5701-negative. Data comparing Truvada and Kivexa in naive patients have demonstrated the non-inferiority of Kivexa at viral levels <100 000 copies/mL. In patients with high viral levels, Kivexa should be reserved for use when Truvada is contraindicated.

Non-nucleoside reverse transcriptase inhibitor

The decision about whether to use an NNRTI, a boosted PI or an integrase inhibitor will depend on the particular circumstances of each patient. In the UK, however, an NNRTI-based regimen is still the most commonly prescribed for patients starting treatment.

Efavirenz is the recommended option in the UK, having demonstrated good durability over time, and potency at low CD4 counts and in high viral loads. It is associated with CNS side-effects, such as dysphoria and insomnia. Rilpivirine has fewer side-effects and is better tolerated than efavirenz, but is less effective when the viral load is >100 000 copies/mL, making it an alternative rather than a preferred first-line drug. Single-tablet, fixed-dose preparation of efavirenz co-formulated with Truvada (Atripla) and rilpivirine with Truvada (Eviplera) allows for a 'one pill once a day' regimen.

Nevirapine is of equivalent potency to efavirenz but has a higher incidence of hepatotoxicity and rash. Toxicity is greater in women and in those with higher CD4 counts. It is contraindicated in women with CD4 counts >250 cells/mm^3 and in men with counts >400 cells/mm^3. It can be a useful alternative to efavirenz if CNS side-effects are troublesome, and in women with lower CD4 counts who wish to conceive.

Etravirine is a second-generation NNRTI with some activity against drug-resistant strains, and is useful in the treatment of experienced patients.

Protease inhibitors

This class of drugs has demonstrated excellent efficacy in clinical practice. PIs are usually combined with a low dose of ritonavir (a 'boosting' PI), which provides a pharmacokinetic advantage by blocking cytochrome P450 metabolism. If this approach is used, the half-life of the active drug is increased, allowing greater drug exposure, fewer pills, enhanced potency and a minimized risk of resistance. The disadvantages include a greater pill burden and increased risk of greater lipid abnormalities, particularly raised fasting triglycerides. Cobicistat, a novel cytochrome P450 inhibitor with no intrinsic anti-HIV activity, is an alternative.

Atazanavir, darunavir and lopinavir, boosted with ritonavir, are most commonly used as first-line therapy. All three can cause gastrointestinal disturbance and lipid abnormalities. Atazanavir increases unconjugated bilirubin levels and may produce icterus. All have interactions with cytochrome P450.

Integrase inhibitors

The potency of this class of drug, coupled with the relatively favourable side-effect profile in comparison to efavirenz and fewer drug interactions in comparison to PIs, makes it an increasingly popular third agent.

Raltegravir, the first licensed compound in this drug class, has high anti-HIV activity for both treatment-naive and treatment-experienced patients, with a favourable side-effect profile and few drug interactions. The genetic barrier for resistance is relatively low, twice daily dosing is required and there are no single-tablet co-formulations available.

Elvitegravir is metabolized via the cytochrome P450 pathway, requiring co-administration of a cytochrome-P450 blocker to secure adequate plasma concentrations, thus increasing the drug–drug interaction potential. Single-tablet co-formulations exist with tenofovir, emtricitabine and cobicistat (Stribild). Dolutegravir, a second-generation integrase inhibitor with a good side-effect profile, has a higher genetic barrier to resistance than raltegravir and can be dosed once daily. A fixed-dose tablet of dolutegravir co-formulated with abacavir and lamivudine has recently been approved.

Box 12.19 Monitoring patients on ART

Clinical history
- Assessment of adherence to medication
- Evidence of ART toxicity
- Documentation of any new clinical conditions occurring since last assessment
- Drug history, including all co-medications (prescribed, recreational, over-the-counter, complementary and herbal)

Physical examination
- Blood pressure
- Weight
- HIV viral load
- Lymphocyte subsets
- Full blood count
- Urinalysis if tenofovir is being used
- Liver and renal function
- Fasting lipid profile
- Fasting blood glucose

Additional investigations (depending on the clinical picture)
- HIV genotype if there is evidence of virological failure
- Therapeutic drug level monitoring

Monitoring therapy

Success rates for initial therapy using modern ARVs, as judged by virological response, are very high. By 4 weeks of therapy, the viral load should have dropped by at least 1 log10 copies/mL and by 12–24 weeks should be below 50 copies/mL. A suboptimal response at either time point demands a full assessment and possible change in therapy. Once stable on therapy, the viral load should be routinely measured every 3–6 months. CD4 count should be repeated at 1 and 3 months after starting ART and then every 3–4 months. Once the viral load is <50 copies/mL and the CD4 count has been <350 cells/mm^3 for at least 12 months, monitoring frequency may fall to 6-monthly or even longer ***(Box 12.19)***. Impaired immunological recovery is associated with treatment initiation in advanced infection (a low CD4 count and late presentation) and with older age.

Regular clinical assessment should include review of adherence to, and tolerability of, the regimen, weight, blood pressure and urinalysis. Patients should be monitored for drug toxicity, including full blood count, liver and renal function, and fasting lipids and glucose levels.

Drug resistance

Resistance to ARVs ***(Box 12.20)*** results from mutations in the protease reverse transcriptase and integrase genes of the virus. HIV has a rapid turnover, with 10^8 replications occurring per day. The error rate is high, resulting in genetic diversity within the population of virus in an individual, which will include drug-resistant mutants. When drugs only partially inhibit virus replication, there will be a selection pressure for the emergence of drug-resistant strains. The rate at which resistance develops depends on the frequency of

Box 12.20 Mechanisms and implications of HIV drug resistance

1. HIV replicates rapidly and inaccurately. Replication in the presence of anti-retroviral (ARV) drugs leads to a selection pressure for those mutations that can survive, i.e. selects for drug resistance
2. Specific point mutations in the viral reverse transcriptase, protease and integrase genes correlate with reduced drug sensitivity and can be identified by genotyping the virus
3. Inadequate ARV drug levels both fail to suppress viral replication/viral load and precipitate drug resistance
4. Inadequate drug levels can result from poor adherence, altered gastrointestinal tract absorption, increased drug breakdown and drug–drug interactions
5. Some ARVs, especially NNRTIs and integrase inhibitors, have a low genetic barrier, i.e. a small number of mutations that occur rapidly can quickly result in high levels of resistance
6. Stopping drugs with a long half-life can leave a sub-therapeutic drug tail for long enough for resistant strains to develop
7. In patients on stable ARV therapy, the introduction of new drugs that have an impact on cytochrome P450 pathways can lead to dangerous alterations in ARV drug levels
8. Therapeutic drug monitoring (TDM) may be a useful investigation for some drugs in some circumstances
9. Without drug selection pressure, wild-type virus reasserts itself; resistant variants no longer make up the major circulating viral strains and may not be found on investigation. This means that genotyping should, if possible, be carried out on specimens obtained whilst the patient is on therapy
10. Resistant variants survive and are archived. They reappear if the drug selection pressure is re-introduced. This means that all previous genotypes need to be considered when assessing virological failure and planning new therapy

pre-existing variants and the number of mutations required. Resistance to most NRTIs and PIs occurs with an accumulation of mutations, whilst a single-point mutation will confer high-level resistance to NNRTIs. There is evidence for the transmission of HIV strains that are resistant to all or some classes of drugs. Studies of primary HIV infection have shown prevalence rates of between 2% and 20%. Prevalence of primary mutations associated with drug resistance in chronically infected patients not on treatment ranges from 3% to 10% in various studies.

HIV anti-retroviral drug resistance testing has become routine clinical management in patients at diagnosis/before starting therapy and for whom therapy is failing. The tests are based on PCR amplification of virus and give an indirect measure of drug susceptibility in the predominant variants. Such assays are limited by both the starting concentration of virus and their ability to detect minority strains.

For results to be useful in situations where therapy is failing, samples must be analysed when the patient is on therapy, as once the selection pressure of therapy is withdrawn, wild-type virus becomes the predominant strain and resistance mutations present earlier may no longer be detectable.

Databases containing nearly all published HIV (amongst others) and protease sequences and associated resistance patterns are maintained in real time by Stanford University (see 'Further reading').

Phenotypic assays provide a more direct measure of susceptibility but the complexity of the assays limits availability.

Drug interactions

Drug therapy in HIV is complex and the potential for clinically relevant drug interactions is substantial. Both PIs and NNRTIs are able to inhibit and induce cytochrome P450 variably, influencing both their own metabolic rates and those of other drugs. Both inducers and inhibitors of cytochrome P450 are sometimes prescribed simultaneously. Induction of metabolism may result in sub-therapeutic ARV levels with the risk of treatment failure and development of viral resistance, whilst inhibition can raise drug levels to toxic values and precipitate adverse reactions.

Conventional (e.g. rifamycins) and complementary therapies (e.g. St John's wort) affect cytochrome P450 activity and may precipitate substantial drug interactions. Therapeutic drug monitoring (TDM), indicating peak and trough plasma levels, may be useful in certain settings.

Potential interactions can be checked using the online tool maintained by Liverpool University (see 'Further reading').

Adherence

Patients' beliefs about their personal need for medicines and their concerns about treatment affect how and whether they take them. Adherence to treatment is pivotal to success. Levels of adherence below 95% have been associated with poor virological and immunological responses, although some of the newer ARVs are more forgiving. Poor absorption and low bioavailability mean that, for some compounds, trough levels are barely adequate to suppress viral replication, and missing even a single dose will result in plasma drug levels falling dangerously low. Patchy adherence facilitates the emergence of drug-resistant variants, which, in time, will lead to virological treatment failure.

Factors implicated in poor adherence may be associated with the medication, with the patient or with the provider. The former include side-effects linked with medications, the degree of complexity and pill burden, and inconvenience of the regimen. Patient factors include the level of motivation and commitment to the therapy, psychological wellbeing, the level of available family and social support, and health beliefs. Supporting adherence is a key part of clinical care and specific guidelines are available (BHIVA 2004). Education of patients about their condition and treatment is a fundamental requirement for good adherence, as is education of clinicians in adherence support techniques. The acceptability and tolerability of the regimen, together with an assessment of adherence, should be documented at each visit. Provision of acute and ongoing multidisciplinary support for adherence within clinical settings should be universal. Medication-alert devices may be useful for some patients.

Treatment failure

Failure of ART – that is, persistent viral replication causing immunological deterioration and eventual clinical evidence of disease progression – is caused by a variety of factors, such as poor adherence, limited drug potency, and food or other medication that may compromise drug absorption. There may be drug interactions or limited penetration of drug into sanctuary sites such as the CNS, permitting viral replication. Side-effects and other patient-related elements contribute to poor adherence.

Changing therapy

A rise in viral load, a falling CD4 count or new clinical events that imply progression of HIV disease are all reasons to review therapy. Reasons for treatment failure include the emergence of resistant viral strains, poor patient adherence and intolerance/adverse drug reactions. Virological failure – that is, two consecutive viral loads of >400 copies/mL in a previously fully suppressed patient – requires investigation. Viral genotyping should be used to help select future therapy, choosing at least two new agents to which the virus is fully sensitive. If a new suitable treatment option is available, it should be started as soon as possible.

Treatment failure in highly treatment-experienced patients poses considerable challenges but new classes of ARVs, with activity against drug-resistant strains of HIV, make long-term virological suppression a realistic objective, even in heavily pre-treated patients. However, in some situations, it may be better to hold back a new drug and await development of another new agent to give the maximum chance of success.

If the patient has a viral load below the limit of detection and a change needs to be made because of intolerance of a particular drug, then a switch should be made to another sensitive drug within the same class. Simplification of complex regimens may be considered if adherence is problematic.

Stopping therapy

ARVs may have to be stopped in, for example, cumulative toxicity, or when there are potential drug interactions with medications needed to deal with another more pressing problem. If adherence is poor, stopping completely may be preferable to continuing with inadequate dosing, in order to reduce the development of viral resistance. Poor quality of life and the view of the patient should be discussed.

The NRTIs efavirenz and nevirapine have long half-lives and, depending on the other components of the regimen, may need be stopped *before* the other drugs in the mixture to reduce the risk of drug resistance. If this is not possible, a boosted PI may be used, either as a substitute for the NNRTI or as monotherapy, for several weeks to cover the period of sub-therapeutic levels.

Complications of anti-retroviral therapy

Side-effects are a common problem in ART (see ***Box 12.15***). Some are acute and associated with initiation of medication, whilst others emerge after longer-term exposure to drugs.

Allergic reactions

Allergic reactions occur with greater frequency in HIV infection and have been documented with all the ARVs. Abacavir is associated with a potentially fatal hypersensitivity reaction, strongly associated with the presence of HLA-B*5701, usually within the first 6 weeks of treatment. There may be a discrete rash and often a fever, coupled with general malaise and gastrointestinal and respiratory symptoms. The diagnosis is clinical and symptoms resolve when abacavir is withdrawn. Re-challenge with abacavir can be fatal and is contraindicated. In the UK, routine screening for the HLA-B*5701 allele has reduced the incidence of abacavir hypersensitivity. Allergies to NNRTIs (often in the second or third week of treatment) usually present with a widespread maculopapular pruritic rash, often with a fever and disordered liver biochemical tests. Reactions can resolve, even with continuing therapy, but drugs should be stopped immediately in any patient with mucous membrane involvement or severe hepatic dysfunction.

Lipodystrophy and metabolic syndrome

A syndrome of lipodystrophy occurs in patients with HIV on ART, comprising characteristic morphological changes and metabolic abnormalities. The main characteristics include a loss of subcutaneous fat in the arms, legs and face (lipoatrophy), deposition of visceral, breast and local fat, raised total cholesterol, HDL cholesterol and triglycerides, and insulin resistance with hyperglycaemia. The syndrome is potentially associated with increased cardiovascular morbidity. The highest incidence occurs in those taking combinations of NRTIs and PIs. The older drugs, stavudine and zidovudine, are associated with the lipoatrophy component of the process. Dietary advice and increase in exercise may improve some of the metabolic problems and help body shape. Statins and fibrates are recommended to reduce circulating lipids. Simvastatin is contraindicated, as it has high levels of drug interactions with PIs.

Mitochondrial toxicity and lactic acidosis

Mitochondrial toxicity, mostly involving the older drugs, stavudine and didanosine, in the nucleoside analogue class, leads to raised lactate and lactic acidosis, which has, in some cases, been fatal. NRTIs inhibit gamma-DNA polymerase and other enzymes that are necessary for normal mitochondrial function. Symptoms are often vague and insidious, and include anorexia, nausea, abdominal pain and general malaise. Venous lactate is raised and the anion gap is typically widened. This is a serious condition, requiring immediate cessation of ART and provision of appropriate supportive measures until normal biochemistry is restored. All patients should be alerted to the possible symptoms and encouraged to attend hospital promptly.

Bone metabolism

A variety of bone disorders have been reported in HIV: in particular, osteopenia, osteoporosis and avascular necrosis. The prevalence of these conditions has varied widely in different studies. ARVs, particularly PIs, have been implicated in the aetiology, although untreated HIV is believed to have a direct impact on bone metabolism.

IRIS

Paradoxical inflammatory reactions (immune reconstitution inflammatory syndrome, IRIS) may occur on initiating ART. This occurs usually in people who have been profoundly immunosuppressed and begin therapy. As their immune system recovers, they are able to mount an inflammatory response to a range of pathogens, which can include exacerbation of symptoms with new or worsening clinical signs. Examples include unusual mass lesions or lymphadenopathy associated with mycobacteria, including deteriorating radiological appearances associated with tuberculosis infection. Inflammatory retinal lesions in association with cytomegalovirus, deterioration in liver function in chronic hepatitis B carriers, and vigorous vesicular eruptions with herpes zoster have also been described. To avoid this situation, certain pathogens, in particular *Mycobacterium tuberculosis* and *Cryptococcus*, should be treated for several weeks to reduce the microbiological burden before ARVs are initiated.

Specific therapeutic situations

Acute seroconversion

ART in patients presenting with an acute seroconversion illness is controversial. This stage of disease may represent a unique opportunity for therapy, as there is less viral diversity and the host immune capacity is still intact. There is evidence to show that the viral load can be reduced substantially by aggressive therapy at this stage, although it rises when treatment is withdrawn. The longer-term clinical sequelae of treatment at this stage remain uncertain. People with severe symptoms during primary HIV infection may gain a clinical improvement on ARVs. If treatment is contemplated in this situation, then it should be assumed that it will be continued for the long term.

Pregnancy

In the UK, the mother-to-child HIV transmission rate is 1% for all women diagnosed prior to delivery and 0.1% for women on ART with a viral load of <50 copies/mL. Management of HIV-positive pregnant women requires close collaboration between obstetric, medical and paediatric teams. The management aim is to deliver a healthy, uninfected baby to a healthy mother without prejudicing the future treatment options of the mother. Although considerations of pregnancy must be factored into clinical decision-making, pregnancy *per se* should not be a contraindication to providing optimum HIV-related care for the woman. HIV-positive women are advised against breast-feeding, which doubles the risk of vertical transmission. Delivery by caesarean section reduced the risk of vertical transmission in the pre-highly active anti-retroviral therapy (HAART) era, but if the woman is on effective ART and the labour is uncomplicated, vaginal delivery carries no additional risk. Women conceiving on an effective ART regimen should continue on their medication. For women naive to therapy who require treatment of their own HIV, whether pregnant or not, triple therapy is the regimen of choice. Risk of vertical transmission increases with viral load. Although the fetus will be exposed to more drugs, the chances of reducing the viral load, and hence preventing infection, are greatest with a potent triple therapy regimen in the mother. In this situation, ***treatment*** should start as soon as possible and continue during delivery. The baby should receive zidovudine for 4 weeks postpartum and the mother should remain on ARVs with appropriate monitoring and support.

Women who do not need treatment for themselves should be prescribed a short course of ART, initiated at the beginning of the second trimester if the baseline viral load is >30 000 HIV RNA copies/mL. Consideration should be given to starting earlier if the viral load is >100 000 HIV RNA copies/mL.

Post-exposure prophylaxis

The time taken for HIV infection to become established after exposure offers an opportunity for prevention. Animal models provide support for the use of triple ARVs for post-exposure prophylaxis (PEP) but there are no prospective trials to inform the best approach and each situation should be evaluated on a case-by-case basis to estimate the potential risk of infection and potential treatment benefit.

Healthcare workers may be treated following occupational exposure to HIV, as may those exposed sexually. The risk of acquisition of HIV following exposure is dependent on the risk that the source is HIV-positive (if this is unknown in a sexual exposure) and the risk of transmission of the particular exposure. PEP may be useful up to 72 hours after possible exposure. In the UK, the standard regimen is Truvada plus raltegravir, although this may be varied depending on what is known about the source. When the source patient is known to have an undetectable HIV viral load (<200 copies HIV RNA/mL), PEP is not recommended.

Treatment is given for 4 weeks and the recipient should be monitored for toxicity. The at-risk patient should be tested for established HIV infection before PEP is dispensed. Rapid point-of-care tests are particularly useful in this setting. PEP following sexual exposure should not be seen as a substitute for other methods of prevention. Pre-exposure prophylaxis is discussed on page 355.

Towards cure

Current therapy, although effective, is life-long, expensive and complex. There is increasing interest in the possibilities of a cure for HIV: either a 'functional' cure, which would mean long-term control of the virus without the use of drugs, or a 'sterilizing' cure, which would require all HIV-containing cells to be eliminated. Several reports of successful interventions exist. These include a patient with HIV infection who underwent bone marrow transplantation for acute myeloid leukaemia (the 'Berlin Patient'), interventions very early in the course of the infection, which may allow immune function to be preserved. Ways are being explored in which latently infected T cells could be purged. The possibilities are being studied of making cells resistant to new HIV infection, using gene manipulation to alter the CCR5 receptor that mediates viral entry into the cell. Despite some early encouraging results, it is clear that there is still a very long way to go and that, at least for the moment, there is no realistic alternative to life-long ART.

Opportunistic infections in the ART era

Although effective ART has resulted in a remarkable decline in opportunistic infections in patients with HIV, not all those at risk may be either on or adhering to effective treatment. In 2009, 19% of those newly diagnosed with HIV in the UK had a CD4 count of <200 cells/mm^3 at presentation, and over 25% of those living with HIV remain undiagnosed, making late presentation and opportunistic infections more likely. In parallel, the types of infection seen in the context of HIV have altered, with fewer episodes of the 'classic' opportunistic infections, such as *Pneumocystis* pneumonia and cytomegalovirus, but an increase in community-acquired infections such as *Strep. pneumoniae* and *Haemophilus influenzae* ***(Box 12.21)***.

Immune reconstitution with ART may produce unusual responses to opportunistic pathogens and confuse the clinical picture. Thus, prevention and treatment of opportunistic infections remains an integral part of the management of HIV infection.

Prevention of opportunistic infection in patients with HIV

Avoidance of infection

Exposure to certain organisms can be avoided in those known to be HIV-positive and immunosuppressed. Attention to food hygiene will reduce exposure to *Salmonella*, toxoplasmosis and *Cryptosporidium*, and protected sexual intercourse will reduce exposure to herpes simplex virus (HSV), hepatitis B and C viruses, and papillomaviruses. Cytomegalovirus-negative patients should be given cytomegalovirus-negative blood products. Travel-related infection can be minimized with appropriate advice.

Immunization strategies

Guidance on the appropriate use of vaccines in HIV ***(Box 12.22)*** is available from BHIVA (see 'Further reading'). Immunization may not be as effective in HIV-positive individuals.

Hepatitis A and B vaccines should be given to those without natural immunity who are at risk, particularly if there is coexisting liver pathology, such as hepatitis C.

Chemoprophylaxis

In the absence of a normal immune response, many opportunistic infections are hard to eradicate using antimicrobials and the recurrence rate is high. Primary and secondary chemoprophylaxis has reduced the incidence of many opportunistic infections. Advantages must be balanced against the potential for toxicity, drug interactions and cost, with each medication added to what are often complex drug regimens.

Box 12.21 Some causes of opportunistic pneumonia in immunocompromised patients[a]

Pathogen	Affected patient population	Clinical and radiographic features
Pneumocystis jiroveci	Impaired cell-mediated immunity: HIV infection with CD4 <200 cells/mm^3, long-term corticosteroid use, immunosuppressant drugs	*Pneumocystis* pneumonia Perihilar ground-glass shadowing, cysts
Non-tuberculous mycobacterial species	Impaired cell-mediated immunity: HIV infection CD4 usually <200 cells/mm^3 Structural lung disease: bronchiectasis, cystic fibrosis, severe COPD	Varied clinical presentation (see p. 1113): Non-specific fevers, cough, malaise Lymphadenopathy or hepatosplenomegaly CT findings: nodules, cavitation, thickened airways, 'tree-in-bud' small airways
***Nocardia* spp.**	Impaired cell-mediated immunity: HIV infection CD4 usually <150 cells/mm^3, chronic corticosteroid use, post-solid-organ transplantation, post-stem-cell transplantation Structural lung disease: bronchiectasis, cystic fibrosis, severe COPD	Acute, subacute or chronic pneumonia Multiple radiographic presentations including lobar infiltrates, abscesses, cavities, pleural effusion, pulmonary nodules
***Aspergillus* spp.** ***Zygomycetes* spp.** ***Penicillium* spp.**	Prolonged neutropenia: post-chemotherapy for haematological malignancy, post-stem-cell transplant (myeloablative transplants are at particular risk) Impaired cell-mediated immunity: graft-versus-host disease, immunosuppressant therapy Chronic granulomatous disease	Invasive fungal pneumonia characterized by cough ± haemoptysis, pleuritic pain and fevers CT findings are any of: cavitating consolidation, 'tree-in-bud', nodules with ground-glass halo and, in later stages, air-crescent sign (caused by lung necrosis)
***Cryptococcus* spp.**	Impaired cell-mediated immunity: HIV infection CD4 usually <200 cells/mm^3, chronic corticosteroid use, post-solid-organ transplantation, post-stem-cell transplantation	Non-specific respiratory symptoms of fever, cough, breathlessness Usually associated with neurological involvement but isolated pulmonary disease does occur Progresses to disseminated disease in immunocompromised patients CT findings are any of: cavities, nodules, infiltrates
Histoplasma capsulatum	Impaired cell-mediated immunity: HIV infection CD4 usually <50 cells/mm^3	Fever, fatigue, weight loss Cough and dyspnoea are the most common respiratory symptoms Chest X-ray can be normal in disseminated disease CT findings: diffuse reticular/reticulonodular infiltrates, miliary infiltrates, occasionally mediastinal lymphadenopathy
Coccidioides ***Paracoccidioides*** ***Blastomyces***	Impaired cell-mediated immunity: HIV infection CD4 usually <50 cells/mm^3	Often presents as disseminated disease (chest X-ray often normal) Focal or diffuse pneumonia CT findings: diffuse reticulonodular infiltrates, consolidation, nodules (multiple or single), cavities, mediastinal lymphadenopathy
Cytomegalovirus (uncommon – usually presents with retinitis or colitis)	Impaired cell-mediated immunity: HIV infection CD4 usually <50 cells/mm^3, post-transplantation on immunosuppressant therapy	Cough, dyspnoea and fever CT findings: reticular or ground-glass opacities, alveolar infiltrates, nodules/nodular opacities, pleural effusions
Respiratory syncytial virus, human metapneumovirus, influenza, parainfluenza	Impaired cell-mediated immunity: HIV infection CD4 usually <200 cells/mm^3, chronic corticosteroid use, post-solid-organ transplantation, post-stem-cell transplantation	Cough, dyspnoea and fever CT findings: ground-glass opacification, air-space shadowing, 'tree-in-bud', airway dilatation and wall thickening
Toxoplasma gondii	Impaired cell-mediated immunity: HIV infection CD4 usually <100 cells/mm^3	Isolated pulmonary or disseminated disease Dry cough, fever, dyspnoea CT findings: appearance similar to those of *Pneumocystis jiroveci* or fungal pneumonia; pleural effusion

[a]See ***Box 24.33***. COPD, chronic obstructive pulmonary disease; CT, computed tomography.

- Primary prophylaxis is effective in reducing the risk of *Pneumocystis jiroveci*, toxoplasmosis and *Mycobacterium avium-intracellulare*.
- Primary prophylaxis is ***not*** normally recommended against cytomegalovirus, herpesviruses or fungi.

With the introduction of ART and immune reconstitution, ongoing chemoprophylaxis can be discontinued in those patients with CD4 counts that remain consistently >200 cells/mm^3. In areas where effective ART may not be available, long-term secondary prophylaxis still has a role. Other less severe but recurrent infections may also warrant prophylaxis (e.g. herpes simplex, candidiasis).

Further reading

Ananworanich J, Fauci AS. HIV cure research: a formidable challenge. *J Virus Erad* 2015; 1:1–3.

British HIV Association. *British HIV Association Standards of Care for People Living with HIV 2013*. London: BHIVA; 2012.

British HIV Association. *British HIV Association Guidelines for the Management of HIV Infection in Pregnant Women 2012*. London: BHIVA; 2012.

Deeks SG, Hunt PW. Antiretroviral therapy: stubborn limitations persist. *Lancet* 2014; 384:214–216.

Box 12.22 Use of vaccines in HIV-infected adults

Vaccines for use in all HIV-infected adults (all inactivated)

- Anthrax
- Cholera – WC/rBS
- *Haemophilus influenzae* b (Hib)
- Hepatitis A
- Hepatitis B
- Influenza – parenteral
- Japanese encephalitis
- Meningococcus – MenC
- Meningococcus – ACWY
- Pneumococcus – PPV23
- Poliomyelitis – parenteral (IPV)
- Rabies
- Tetanus–diphtheria (Td)
- Tick-borne encephalitis
- Typhoid – ViCPS

Vaccines contraindicated in all HIV-infected adults

- Cholera – CVD103-HgR (live)
- Influenza – intranasal (live)
- Poliomyelitis – oral (OPV) (live)
- Smallpox (vaccinia) (live)
- Tuberculosis (BCG) (live)
- Typhoid – Ty21a (live)

Vaccines for use only in asymptomatic HIV-infected adults with a current CD4 count >200 cells/mm^3

- Measles, mumps, rubella (MMR)
- Varicella
- Yellow fever

(Based on BHIVA Guidelines 2006: www.bhiva.org.)

Fidler S, Anderson J, Azad Y et al. Position statement on the use of antiretroviral therapy to reduce HIV transmission, January 2013: the British HIV Association (BHIVA) and the Expert Advisory Group on AIDS (EAGA). *HIV Med* 2013; 14:259–262.

Geretti AM, Tsakiroglou M. HIV: new drugs, new guidelines. *Curr Opin Inf Dis* 2014; 27:545–553.

Lewin SR, Deeks SG, Barré-Sinoussi F. Towards a cure for HIV – are we making progress? *Lancet* 2014; 384:209–211.

Passaes CP, Sáez-Cirión A. HIV cure research: advances and prospects. *Virology* 2014; 454–455:340–352.

Sabin CA, Schwenk A, Johnson MA et al. Late diagnosis in the HAART era: proposed common definitions and associations with mortality. *AIDS* 2010; 24:723–727.

Williams I, Churchill D, Anderson J et al. British HIV Association guidelines for the treatment of HIV-1-positive adults with antiretroviral therapy 2012 (Updated November 2013). *HIV Med* 2014; 15(S1):1–6.

Young B, Zuniga JM, Montaner J et al. Controlling the HIV epidemic with antiretrovirals: moving from consensus to implementation. *Clin Infect Dis* 2014; 59(Suppl 1):S1–S2.

http://hivdb.stanford.edu *Stanford University HIV drug resistance database.*

http://www.aidsinfo.nih.gov/guidelines *US Department of Health and Human Services guidelines on the use of ARVs in HIV-1-infected adults and adolescents.*

http://www.apregistry.com *Details of adverse effects associated with ARVs in pregnancy; maintained by the Antiretroviral Pregnancy Registry, which holds prospective international data and is regularly updated.*

http://www.gov.uk/ *Guidance on HIV post-exposure prophylaxis.*

http://www.hiv-druginteractions.org *Potential HIV drug interactions can be checked using the online tool maintained by Liverpool University.*

SPECIFIC CONDITIONS ASSOCIATED WITH HIV INFECTION

Fungal infections

Pneumocystis jiroveci infection

Pneumocystis jiroveci most commonly causes pneumonia (PCP; see p. 1106) but can cause disseminated infection. It is not usually seen until patients are severely immunocompromised with a CD4 count <200 cells/mm^3. The introduction of effective ART and primary prophylaxis in patients with CD4 counts of <200 cells/mm^3 has significantly reduced the incidence in the UK. The organism damages alveolar epithelium, which impedes gas exchange and reduces lung compliance.

The onset is often insidious over a period of weeks, with a prolonged period of increasing shortness of breath (usually on exertion), non-productive cough, fever and malaise. ***Clinical features*** on examination include tachypnoea, tachycardia, cyanosis and signs of hypoxia. Fine crackles are heard on auscultation, although in mild cases there may be no auscultatory abnormality. In early infection, the chest X-ray is normal but the typical appearances are of bilateral perihilar interstitial infiltrates, which can progress to confluent alveolar shadows throughout the lungs. High-resolution CT scans of the chest demonstrate a characteristic ground-glass appearance, even when there is little to see on the chest X-ray. The patient is usually hypoxic and desaturates on exercise. Definitive diagnosis rests on demonstrating the organisms in the lungs via bronchoalveolar lavage or by PCR amplification of the fungal DNA from a peripheral blood sample. As the organism cannot be cultured *in vitro*, it must be directly observed either with silver staining or with immunofluorescent techniques.

Treatment should be instituted as early as possible. First-line therapy is with intravenous co-trimoxazole (120 mg/kg daily in divided doses) for 21 days. Up to 40% of patients receiving this regimen will develop some adverse drug reaction, including a typical allergic rash. If the patient is sensitive to co-trimoxazole, intravenous pentamidine (4 mg/kg per day) or dapsone and trimethoprim is given for the same duration. Atovaquone or a combination of clindamycin and primaquine is also used. In severe cases (P_aO_2 <9.5 kPa), systemic corticosteroids reduce mortality and should be added. Continuous positive airways pressure (CPAP) or mechanical ventilation (see pp. 1165–1166) is required if the patient remains severely hypoxic or becomes too tired. Pneumothorax may complicate the clinical course in an already severely hypoxic patient. If not already on ART, this should be initiated early in the course of infection.

Secondary prophylaxis is required in patients whose CD4 count remains <200 cells/mm^3, to prevent relapse, the usual regimen being co-trimoxazole 960 mg three times a week. Patients sensitive to sulphonamide are given dapsone, pyrimethamine or nebulized pentamidine. The last protects only the lungs and does not penetrate the upper lobes particularly efficiently; hence, if relapses occur on this regimen, they may be either atypical or extrapulmonary.

Cryptococcosis

The most common presentation of cryptococcal infection (see p. 296) in the context of HIV is meningitis, although pulmonary and disseminated infections can also occur. The organism, *C. neoformans*, is widely distributed, often in bird droppings, and is usually acquired by inhalation. The onset may be insidious with non-specific fever, nausea and headache. As the infection progresses, the conscious level is impaired and changes in affect may be noted. Fits or focal neurological presentations are uncommon. Neck stiffness and photophobia may be absent, as these signs depend on the inflammatory response of the host, which, in this setting, is abnormal.

Diagnosis is made on examination of the CSF (perform a CT scan before lumbar puncture to eliminate space-occupying pathology). Indian ink staining shows the organisms directly and CSF cryptococcal antigen is positive at variable titre. It is unusual for the cryptococcal antigen to become negative after treatment, although the levels should fall substantially. Cryptococci can also be cultured from CSF and/or blood.

Factors associated with a poor prognosis include a high organism count in the CSF, a low white cell count in the CSF, and an impaired consciousness level at presentation.

Initial ***treatment*** is usually with intravenous liposomal amphotericin B (4.0 mg/kg per day) with or without flucytosine as induction, although intravenous fluconazole (400 mg daily) is useful if renal function is impaired or if amphotericin side-effects are troublesome.

Patients diagnosed with cryptococcal disease should receive ART, starting at approximately 2 weeks after commencement of cryptococcal treatment, to minimize the risk of IRIS.

Candidiasis

Mucosal infection, particularly oral, with *Candida* (see p. 295) is common in immunosuppressed HIV-positive patients. *C. albicans* is the usual organism, although *C. krusei* and *C. glabrata* occur. Pseudomembranous candidiasis, consisting of creamy plaques in the mouth and pharynx, is easily recognized but erythematous *Candida* appears as reddened areas on the hard palate or as atypical areas on the tongue. Angular cheilitis can occur in association with either form. Vulvovaginal *Candida* may be difficult to treat.

Oesophageal *Candida* infection produces odynophagia (see p. 366). Fluconazole or itraconazole is the agent of choice for ***treatment***. Disseminated *Candida* is uncommon in the context of HIV infection, but if present, fluconazole is the preferred drug; amphotericin, voriconazole or caspofungin is also used. *C. krusei* may colonize patients who have been treated with fluconazole, as it is fluconazole-resistant. Amphotericin is useful in the treatment of this infection, and an attempt to type *Candida* from clinically azole-resistant patients should be made. The most successful strategy for managing HIV-positive patients with candidiasis is effective ART.

Aspergillosis

Infection with *Aspergillus fumigatus* (see pp. 295–296) is rare in HIV, unless there are coexisting factors, such as lung pathology, neutropenia, transplantation or glucocorticoid use. Spores are airborne and ubiquitous. Following inhalation, lung infection proceeds to haematogenous spread to other organs. Sinus infection occurs.

Voriconazole is the preferred ***treatment***, with liposomal amphotericin B (3 mg/kg i.v. daily) as an alternative. Caspofungin is also effective.

Histoplasmosis, blastomycosis, coccidioidomycosis and *Penicillium marneffei* infection

These fungal infections are geographically restricted but should be considered in HIV-positive patients who have travelled to areas of high risk. The most common manifestation is with pneumonia, which may be confused with *Pneumocystis jiroveci* in its presentation (see above), although systemic infection is reported, particularly with *Penicillium*, which can also produce papular skin lesions. ***Treatment*** is with amphotericin B.

Protozoal infections

Toxoplasmosis

Toxoplasma gondii (see p. 305) most commonly causes encephalitis and cerebral abscess in the context of HIV, usually as a result of reactivation of previously acquired infection. The incidence depends on the rate of seropositivity to toxoplasmosis in the particular population. High antibody levels are found in France (90% of the adult population). About 25% of the adult UK population is seropositive to *Toxoplasma*.

Clinical features include a focal neurological lesion and convulsions, fever, headache and possible confusion. Examination reveals focal neurological signs in more than 50% of cases. Eye involvement with chorioretinitis may also be present. In most, but not all, cases of *Toxoplasma*, serology is positive. Typically, contrast-enhanced CT scan of the brain shows multiple ring-enhancing lesions. A single lesion on CT may be found to be one of several on MRI. A solitary lesion on MRI, however, makes a diagnosis of toxoplasmosis unlikely.

Diagnosis is by characteristic radiological findings on CT and MRI. Single photon emission computed tomography (SPECT) may also be helpful differentiating toxoplasmosis from primary CNS lymphoma. In most cases, an empirical trial of anti-toxoplasmosis therapy is instituted; if this leads to radiological improvement within 3 weeks, this is considered diagnostic. The differential diagnosis includes cerebral lymphoma, tuberculoma or focal cryptococcal infection.

Treatment is with pyrimethamine for at least 6 weeks (loading dose 200 mg, then 50 mg daily), combined with sulfadiazine and folinic acid. Clindamycin and pyrimethamine may be used in patients allergic to sulphonamide.

ART should be initiated as soon as the patient is clinically stable, approximately 2 weeks after acute treatment has begun to minimize the risk of IRIS.

Cryptosporidiosis

Cryptosporidium parvum (see p. 307) can cause a self-limiting acute diarrhoea in an immunocompetent individual. In HIV infection, it can cause severe and progressive watery diarrhea, which may be associated with anorexia, abdominal pain, and nausea and vomiting. In the era of ART, the infection is rare. Cysts attach to the epithelium of the small bowel wall, causing secretion of fluid into the gut lumen and failure of fluid absorption. It is also associated with sclerosing cholangitis (see pp. 476–477). The cysts are seen on stool specimen microscopy using Kinyoun acid-fast stain and are readily identified in small bowel biopsy specimens. ART is associated with complete resolution of infection following restoration of immune function; otherwise, ***treatment*** is largely supportive. Nitazoxanide may have some effect.

Microsporidiosis

Enterocytozoon bieneusi and *Septata intestinalis* are causes of diarrhoea. Spores can be detected in stools using a trichrome or fluorescent stain that attaches to the chitin of the spore surface. ART and immune restoration constitute the ***treatment*** of choice and can have a dramatic effect.

Leishmaniasis

Leishmaniasis (see pp. 303–305) occurs in immunosuppressed HIV-positive individuals who have been in endemic areas, which include South America, tropical Africa and much of the Mediterranean. Symptoms are frequently non-specific, with fever, malaise, diarrhoea and weight loss. Splenomegaly, anaemia and thrombocytopenia are significant findings. Amastigotes may be seen on bone marrow biopsy or from splenic aspirates. Serological tests exist for *Leishmania* but they are not reliable in this setting.

Treatment is with liposomal amphotericin, the drug of choice, and ART once the patient is stable. Relapse is common without ART, in which case long-term secondary prophylaxis may be given.

Viral infections

Hepatitis B and C virus co-infection with HIV

Because of the comparable routes of transmission of hepatitis viruses (see pp. 454–455 and 459) and HIV, co-infection is common, particularly in MSM, drug users and those infected by blood products. A higher prevalence of hepatitis viruses is found in those with HIV infection than in the general population. Globally, estimates suggest that 5–15% of people with HIV have chronic hepatitis B virus (HBV) infection and about one-third have hepatitis C virus (HCV) infection. In the UK, 6.9% of adults with HIV are also estimated to be HBsAg-positive. A global epidemic of acute hepatitis C has been observed over the past decade amongst HIV-positive MSM.

As treatment advances have improved HIV prognosis, hepatitis virus co-infection has become an increasingly significant cause of morbidity and mortality, making the management of HIV and hepatitis co-infection a necessary aspect of clinical care.

All those with newly diagnosed HIV should be screened for hepatitis A, B and C; for those without evidence of immunity, hepatitis A and B vaccines should be provided.

Patients with HIV and hepatitis co-infection are more likely to have rapid liver disease progression than people with mono-infection. In all patients with chronic HCV/HIV and HBV/HIV infections, liver disease should be staged (see p. 452) For those who are likely to have cirrhosis, appropriate monitoring for complications of portal hypertension and HCV screening should be performed. Patients with HIV and liver disease should be jointly managed by clinicians from HIV and hepatitis backgrounds. For people with end-stage liver disease, care should be based in specialist centres, ideally with link to a transplant unit.

In co-infected patients, the hepatotoxicity associated with certain ARVs may be potentiated. Advice on alcohol use and safer sexual practices should be given to all co-infected patients.

Hepatitis B infection

Hepatitis B infection (see pp. 454–457) does not appear to influence the natural history of HIV or responses to anti-HIV treatment; however, in HIV co-infected patients, there is a significantly reduced rate of hepatitis B e antigen (HBeAg) clearance, the HBV viral load is higher, and the risk of developing chronic infection is increased. In those with resolved or controlled hepatitis B infection, disease may reactivate. Liver disease occurs most commonly in those with high HBV DNA levels indicative of continuing replication. In HBV infection, detection and quantification of HBV DNA act as a marker of viral activity and are predictive of response to treatment. Baseline HBV resistance testing may guide interventions in those previously exposed to antiviral drugs.

Decisions about whether HBV and/or HIV require ***treatment*** must be based on assessment of both viruses. All treatments for HBV that include agents with concomitant anti-HIV activity, including tenofovir and emtricitabine, must be used within an effective anti-HIV regimen. UK guidelines recommend that ART inclusive of anti-HBV-active agents should be initiated in all co-infected patients with a CD4 count of <500 cells/mm^3, or with evidence of fibrotic liver damage or with active HDV replication. Patients with a CD4 of ≥500 cells/mm^3, an HBV DNA of <2000 IU/mL, and minimal or no evidence of fibrosis can be given the option to commence treatment or to be monitored not less than 6-monthly with HBV DNA and measurement of alanine aminotransferase (ALT), and at least yearly for evidence of fibrosis. Initiation of ART may result in a flare of HBV resulting from the improved immune function. If ART is not indicated for HIV and the CD4 count is ≥500 cells/mm^3, the approach to HBV treatment may include the use of HBV-exclusive agents pegylated interferon and adefovir to avoid inducement of HIV resistance.

Hepatitis C infection

Hepatitis C is associated with more rapid progression of HIV infection and the CD4 responses to ART in co-infected patients may be blunted. Hepatitis C progression is both more likely and more rapid in the presence of HIV infection, and the hepatitis C viral load tends to be elevated. The drug-related hepatotoxicity may be worse in those with HCV co-infection. Assessment of co-infected patients requires full clinical and laboratory evaluation and staging of both infections. For HCV, both viral load and genotype will influence therapeutic decision-making.

Treatment is a rapidly changing and complex field with increasing availability of direct-acting antivirals (DAAs) for the treatment of hepatitis C.

All HIV/HCV co-infected patients should be given the option to commence ART. For those with CD4 cell counts of <500 cells/mL, irrespective of whether HCV treatment is planned or not, ART should be initiated. If HCV therapy is planned, then for those with CD4 cell counts between 350 and 500 cells/mL, ART should be started first. Patients with a CD4 cell count of >500 cells/mL, including those who defer hepatitis C therapy, should be given the option to commence ART. If they opt to defer, they should be monitored closely for HIV or hepatitis C disease progression, including at least an annual assessment of liver fibrosis.

All patients with HCV/HIV infection should be assessed for suitability for treatment of hepatitis C. The drug options for HCV in individuals with co-infection are similar to the choices for those infected with HCV alone (see pp. 460–461), depending on the stage of disease, HCV genotype and co-administered ART. The introduction of DAAs for HCV has changed the treatment landscape. The latest HCV agents (see pp. 460–461) are given for 12 weeks with response rates of more than 90%.

When DAAs are chosen, some restriction on first-line ARV choice exists due to drug–drug interactions. The ritonavir-boosted AbbVie regimen may interact with commonly used HIV medications and there are reports of an interaction between tenofovir and sofosbuvir. Careful selection of the most effective combination of antivirals is required and expert opinion should be sought. Online information resources (see 'Further reading') provide data on possible interactions.

All those with HIV/HCV co-infection who defer treatment should undergo hepatic elastography (see p. 446) or an alternative non-invasive form of monitoring at least annually.

Acute hepatitis C has increased in people with HIV, particularly MSM, and recognized epidemics have been reported in a number of countries, including the UK. UK guidelines recommend that patients without a decrease of 2log10 in HCV RNA at week 4 post diagnosis of acute infection, or with a positive HCV RNA at week 12 post diagnosis of acute infection, be offered therapy for 24 weeks with pegylated interferon and ribavirin. Immune responses to HCV do not protect against re-infection, and high rates have been reported following both therapeutic and spontaneous clearance. Patients who initially clear HCV but have evidence of re-emergent virus should be assessed for relapse or re-infection; relapse is treated as for chronic HCV and re-infection is managed as for acute hepatitis C. The benefits and cost-effectiveness of the new all-oral HCV regimens in patients with acute hepatitis C have not yet been assessed but the drugs are likely to be effective, although very costly.

Cytomegalovirus infection

Cytomegalovirus (CMV; see pp. 258–259) has been the cause of considerable morbidity in HIV-positive individuals, especially in the later stages of disease when the CD4 count is consistently <100 cells/mm^3. The availability of ART has dramatically altered the epidemiology, as a majority of patients start ARVs before they are at risk for CMV disease. The major problems encountered are retinitis, colitis, oesophageal ulceration, encephalitis and pneumonitis. CMV infection is associated with an arteritis, which may be the major pathogenic mechanism. CMV also causes polyradiculopathy and adrenalitis.

CMV retinitis

This occurs once the CD4 count is <50 cells/mm^3. Although usually unilateral to begin with, the infection may progress to involve both eyes. Presenting features depend on the area of retina involved (loss of vision being most common with macular involvement) and include floaters, loss of visual acuity, field loss and scotomata, orbital pain and headache.

Examination of the fundus ***(Fig. 12.13)*** reveals haemorrhages and exudates, which follow the vasculature of the retina (so-called 'pizza pie' appearances). The features are highly characteristic and the diagnosis is made clinically. Retinal detachment and papillitis may occasionally occur. If untreated, retinitis spreads within the eye, destroying the retina within its path. Routine fundoscopy should be carried out on all HIV-positive patients to look for evidence of early infection. Any patient with symptoms of visual disturbance should have a thorough examination with pupils dilated; if no evident pathology is seen, a specialist ophthalmological opinion should be sought.

Treatment for CMV should be started as soon as possible, with either oral valganciclovir (900 mg twice daily), i.v. ganciclovir (5 mg/kg twice daily), or foscarnet (90 mg/kg twice daily) given intravenously for at least 3 weeks or until retinitis is quiescent. If immunosuppression is not reversed, reactivation is common, leading to blindness. The major side-effect of ganciclovir is myelosuppression, and foscarnet is nephrotoxic. Maintenance therapy may be required until ART is instituted and has improved immune competence. Valganciclovir, an oral prodrug of ganciclovir, has some long-term benefit when used as maintenance therapy, but a lower efficacy than intravenous ganciclovir. Ganciclovir can be given directly into the vitreous cavity but regular injections are required. A sustained-release implant of ganciclovir can be surgically inserted into the affected eye. Cidofovir is available for use when the above drugs are contraindicated. It has renal toxicity.

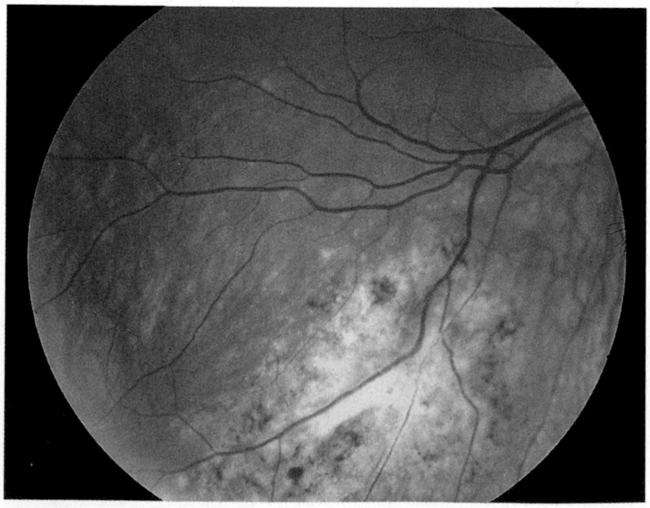

Figure 12.13 Untreated cytomegalovirus retinitis.

CMV gastrointestinal conditions

CMV colitis usually presents with abdominal pain, often generalized or in the left iliac fossa, diarrhoea that may be bloody, generalized abdominal tenderness and a low-grade fever. Dilated large bowel may be seen on abdominal X-ray. Sigmoidoscopy shows a friable or ulcerated mucosa; histology shows the characteristic 'owl's eye' cytoplasmic inclusion bodies (see ***Fig. 11.21***).

Treatment is with i.v. ganciclovir (5 mg/kg twice daily) for 14–28 days; when stable, optimization of ART improves symptoms and the histological changes are reversed. Restoration of immune competence with ART removes the need for maintenance therapy.

Other sites along the gastrointestinal tract are also prone to CMV infection: for example, ulceration of the oesophagus, usually in the lower third, causes odynophagia. CMV can also cause hepatitis.

CMV neurological conditions

CMV encephalopathy has clinical similarities to that caused by HIV itself, although it tends to be more aggressive in its course. ***CMV polyradiculopathy*** can affect the lumbosacral roots, leading to muscle weakness and sphincter disturbance. The CSF has an increase in white cells, which, surprisingly, are almost all neutrophils. Although progression may be arrested by anti-CMV medication, functional recovery may not occur. Diagnosis may be based on MRI and CSF PCR. ***Treatment*** is with ganciclovir. ART should be started after anti-CMV treatment.

Herpesvirus infection

Herpes simplex primary infection (see pp. 247–249) occurs with greater frequency and severity, presenting in an ulcerative rather than vesicle form in profoundly immunosuppressed individuals. Genital, oral and occasionally disseminated infection is seen. Viral shedding may be prolonged in comparison with immunocompetent patients.

Varicella zoster virus infection

Varicella zoster can occur at any stage of HIV but tends to be more aggressive and longer-lasting in the more immunosuppressed patient. Multidermatomal zoster may occur.

Treatment with aciclovir is usually effective. Frequent recurrences need suppressive therapy. Aciclovir-resistant strains (usually due to thymidine kinase-deficient mutants) in HIV-positive patients have become more common. Such strains may respond to foscarnet.

Herpesvirus 8 (***HHV-8***) is the causative agent of Kaposi's sarcoma (see p. 265).

Epstein–Barr virus infection

Patients with HIV have been shown to have high levels of Epstein–Barr virus (EBV) colonization (see p. 258). There are increased EBV titres in oropharyngeal secretions and high levels of EBV-infected B cells. The normal T-cell response to EBV is depressed in HIV. EBV is strongly associated with primary cerebral lymphoma and non-Hodgkin's lymphoma (see below). Oral hairy leukoplakia caused by EBV is a sign of immunosuppression first noted in HIV but now also recognized in other conditions. It appears intermittently on the lateral borders of the tongue or the buccal mucosa as

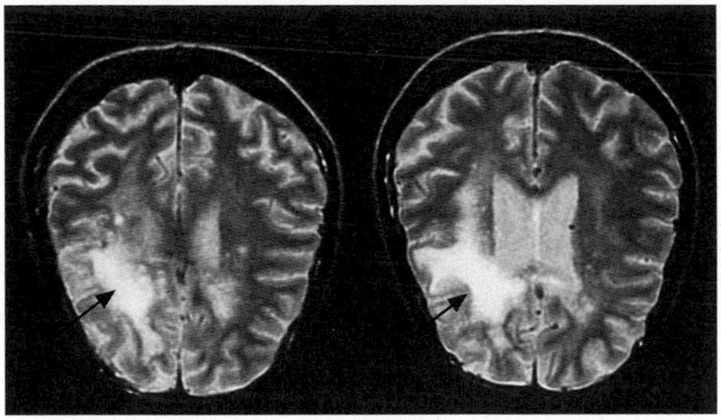

Figure 12.14 **MRI scans showing progressive multifocal leucoencephalopathy.**

a pale, ridged lesion. Although it is usually asymptomatic, patients may find it unsightly and occasionally painful. The virus can be identified histologically and on electron microscopy. There is a variable response to ***treatment*** with aciclovir.

Human papillomavirus infection

Human papillomavirus (HPV; see p. 326) produces genital, plantar and occasionally oral warts, which may be slow to respond to therapy and recur repeatedly. HPV is associated with the more rapid development of cervical and anal intraepithelial neoplasia, which in time may progress to squamous cell carcinoma of the cervix or rectum in HIV-positive individuals. HPV vaccination is now available (see p. 326).

Polyomavirus infection

JC virus, a member of the papovavirus family, which infects oligodendrocytes, causes progressive multifocal leucoencephalopathy (PML; see p. 263). This leads to demyelination, particularly within the white matter of the brain. The features are of progressive neurological and/or intellectual impairment, often including hemiparesis or aphasia. The course is usually inexorably progressive but a stuttering course may be seen. Radiologically, the lesions are usually multiple and confined to the white matter. They do not enhance with contrast and do not produce a mass effect. MRI ***(Fig. 12.14)*** is more sensitive than CT and reveals enhanced signal on T2-weighted images of the lesions. MRI appearances and JC virus detection by PCR in a CSF sample are usually sufficient for diagnosis and avoid the need for a tissue diagnosis requiring brain biopsy. There is no specific ***treatment***. Effective ART is the only intervention that has been shown to deliver both clinical and radiological remission.

Bacterial infections

Bacterial infection in HIV is common. Cell-mediated immune responses normally control infection against intracellular bacteria, e.g. mycobacteria. The abnormalities of B-cell function associated with HIV lead to infections with encapsulated bacteria, as reduced production of IgG2 cannot protect against the polysaccharide coat of such organisms. These functional abnormalities may be present well before there is a significant decline in CD4 numbers and so bacterial sepsis may be seen at early stages of HIV infection. *Streptococcus pneumoniae*, *Haemophilus influenzae* and *Moraxella catarrhalis* infections are examples. Bacterial infection is often disseminated and, although usually amenable to standard antibiotic therapy, may reoccur. Long-term prophylaxis is required if recurrent infection is frequent.

Mycobacterium tuberculosis infection

Many parts of the world, such as Africa, that have a high prevalence of tuberculosis (TB; see p. 290) also have high rates of HIV infection, both of which are increasing. The respiratory transmission of TB means both HIV-positive and HIV-negative people are being infected. TB can cause disease when there is only minimal immunosuppression and thus often appears early in the course of HIV infection. HIV-related TB frequently represents reactivation of latent TB, but there is also clear evidence of newly acquired infection and hospital-acquired spread in HIV-positive populations.

The pattern of disease differs with immunosuppression:

- Patients with relatively well-preserved CD4 counts have a clinical picture similar to that seen in HIV-negative patients with pulmonary infection.
- In more advanced HIV disease, atypical pulmonary presentations occur without cavitation and prominent hilar lymphadenopathy, or extrapulmonary TB affecting lymph nodes, bone marrow or liver. Bacteraemia may be present.

Diagnosis depends on demonstrating the organisms in appropriate tissue specimens. The response to tuberculin testing is blunted in HIV-positive individuals and is unreliable. Sputum microscopy may be negative, even in pulmonary infection, and culture techniques are the best diagnostic tool.

M. tuberculosis infection usually responds well to standard ***treatment*** regimens, although the duration of therapy may be extended, especially in extrapulmonary infection. Multidrug resistant and extensive drug-resistant TB (see p. 290) is becoming a problem, particularly in the USA, where it is developing into a health danger. Cases from HIV units in the UK have been reported. Compliance with anti-tuberculous therapy needs to be emphasized. Treatment of TB (see below) is not curative and long-term isoniazid prophylaxis may be given. In patients from TB-endemic areas, primary prophylaxis may prevent the emergence of infection.

Drug–drug interactions between anti-retroviral and anti-tuberculous medications are complex and are a consequence of enzyme induction or inhibition. Rifampicin is a potent inducer of cytochrome P450, which is also the route for metabolism of HIV PIs. Using both drugs together results in a reduction in circulating PI with reduced efficacy and increased potential for drug resistance. Some PIs themselves block cytochrome P450, which leads to potentially toxic levels of rifampicin and problems such as uveitis and hepatotoxicity. The NNRTI class also interacts variably with rifamycins, requiring dose alterations. Additionally, there are overlapping toxicities between ART regimens and anti-tuberculous drugs, in particular hepatotoxicity, peripheral neuropathy and gastrointestinal side-effects. Rifabutin has a weaker effect on cytochrome P450 and may be substituted for rifampicin. Dose adjustments must be made for drugs used in this situation to take account of these interactions.

Paradoxical inflammatory reactions (IRIS), which can include exacerbation of symptoms, new or worsening clinical signs, and deteriorating radiological appearances, have been associated with the improvement of immune function seen in HIV-positive patients starting ART in the face of *M. tuberculosis* infection. They are most commonly seen in the first few weeks after initiation of ART in patients recovering from TB and can last several weeks or months. The syndrome does not reflect inadequate TB therapy and is not confined to any particular combination of ARVs. It is vital to exclude new pathology in this situation. However, delaying ART increases the risks of further opportunistic events. Allowing at least 2 weeks of anti-tuberculous therapy before commencing ART allows some reduction in the burden of mycobacteria. If the CD4 count is <100 cells/mm^3, then ARVs should be started at about 2 weeks of anti-tuberculous medication. If the CD4 count is >200 cells/mm^3, then initiation of ART may be delayed for at least 6 weeks after the start of anti-tuberculous therapy.

Mycobacterium avium-intracellulare infection

Atypical mycobacteria, particularly *M. avium-intracellulare* (MAI), generally appear only in the very late stages of HIV infection when patients are profoundly immunosuppressed. MAI is a saprophytic organism of low pathogenicity that is ubiquitous in soil and water. Entry may be via the gastrointestinal tract or lungs with dissemination via infected macrophages.

The major ***clinical features*** are fevers, malaise, weight loss, anorexia and sweats. Dissemination to the bone marrow causes anaemia. Gastrointestinal symptoms may be prominent with diarrhoea and malabsorption. At this stage of disease, patients frequently have other concurrent infections, so differentiating MAI is difficult on clinical grounds. Direct examination and culture of blood, lymph node, bone marrow or liver give the diagnosis most reliably.

MAI is typically resistant to standard anti-tuberculous ***treatments***, although ethambutol may be useful. Drugs such as rifabutin in combination with clarithromycin or azithromycin reduce the burden of organisms and, in some, ameliorate symptoms. A common combination is ethambutol, rifabutin and clarithromycin. Addition of amikacin to a drug regimen may produce a good symptomatic response. Primary prophylaxis with rifabutin or azithromycin may delay the appearance of MAI, but no corresponding increase in survival has been shown.

Infections due to other organisms

Influenza virus A (IVA) is no more frequent in HIV-positive people, but has been associated with an increased severity and complication rate in those with HIV, in particular when CD4 counts are low. Oseltamivir oral 75 mg twice daily for 5 days should be used as treatment. People with HIV should be vaccinated annually against IVA. Prophylaxis with oseltamivir is used in unvaccinated individuals with a CD4 count <200 cells/mm^3.

Salmonellae (non-typhoidal; see p. 275) are much less frequent pathogens in HIV infection if effective ART is being used. Salmonellae are able to survive within macrophages, this being a major factor in their pathogenicity. Organisms are usually acquired orally and frequently result in disseminated infection. Gastrointestinal disturbance may be disproportionate to the degree of dissemination, and once the pathogen is in the bloodstream, any organ may be infected. *Salmonella* osteomyelitis and cystitis have been reported. Diagnosis is from blood and stool cultures. Despite increasing reports of resistance, a majority of isolates are sensitive to oral ciprofloxacin 500 mg twice daily for 5 days. Education on food hygiene should be provided.

Skin conditions, such as folliculitis, abscesses and cellulitis, are common and are usually caused by *Staph. aureus.* Periodontal disease, which may be necrotizing, causes pain and damage to the gums. It is more common in smokers but no specific causative agent has been identified. Therapy is with local debridement and systemic antibiotics.

Strongyloides (see pp. 311–312), a nematode found in tropical areas, may produce a hyper-infection syndrome in HIV-positive patients. Larvae are produced, which invade through the bowel wall and migrate to the lung and occasionally to the brain. Albendazole or ivermectin may be used to control infection. Gram-negative septicaemia can develop (see p. 311).

Scabies (see p. 1347) may be much more severe in HIV infection. It may be widely disseminated over the body and appear as atypical, crusted papular lesions known as 'Norwegian scabies', from which mites are readily demonstrated. Superadded staphylococcal infection may occur. Treatment with conventional agents, such as lindane, may fail and ivermectin has been used to good effect in some patients.

Neoplasms

HIV infection is associated with an increased risk of cancer, the most tightly linked being Kaposi's sarcoma, non-Hodgkin's lymphoma and cervical cancer, which are AIDS-defining. Other cancers that have an association with infectious agents, such as liver and anal cancer and Hodgkin's lymphoma, although not AIDS-defining, are significantly more common in HIV-positive patients. Patterns are changing and there has been a marked reduction in AIDS-defining malignancy in association with effective ART. The increased longevity for people with HIV increases the risks for development of cancers that are associated with older age. Some data suggest that ART may provide some prevention benefits for non-AIDS-defining malignancies.

Kaposi's sarcoma

Kaposi's sarcoma (KS; see pp. 1374–1375) in association with HIV (epidemic KS) behaves more aggressively than that associated with HIV-negative populations (endemic KS). The incidence has fallen significantly since the introduction of ART. Human herpesvirus 8 (HHV-8) is involved in the pathogenesis. KS skin lesions are characteristically pigmented and well circumscribed, occurring in multiple sites. KS is a multicentric tumour consisting of spindle cells and vascular endothelial cells, which together form slit-like spaces in which red blood cells become trapped. This process is responsible for the characteristic purple hue of the tumour. In addition to the skin lesions, KS affects lymphatics and lymph nodes, the lung and gastrointestinal tract, giving rise to a wide range of symptoms and signs. Most patients with visceral involvement also have skin or mucous membrane lesions. Visceral KS carries a worse prognosis than disease confined to the skin. KS is seen around the eye ***(Fig. 12.15)***, particularly in the conjunctivae, which can lead to periorbital oedema.

ART leads to regression of lesions. Local radiotherapy gives good results in skin lesions and is helpful in lymph node disease. In aggressive disease, systemic chemotherapy is indicated.

Lymphoma

A significant proportion of patients with HIV develop lymphoma, mostly of the non-Hodgkin's, large B-cell type. These are frequently extranodal, often affecting the brain, lung and gastrointestinal tract. Many of these tumours are strongly associated with Epstein–Barr virus, with evidence of expression of latent gene nuclear antigens such as EBNA 1–6, some of which are involved in the immortalization of B cells and drive a neoplastic pathway.

HIV-associated lymphomas are frequently very aggressive. Patients often present with systemic 'B' syndromes and progress rapidly, despite chemotherapy. Primary cerebral lymphoma is variably responsive to radiotherapy but overall carries a poor prognosis. Lymphomas occurring early in the course of HIV infection tend to

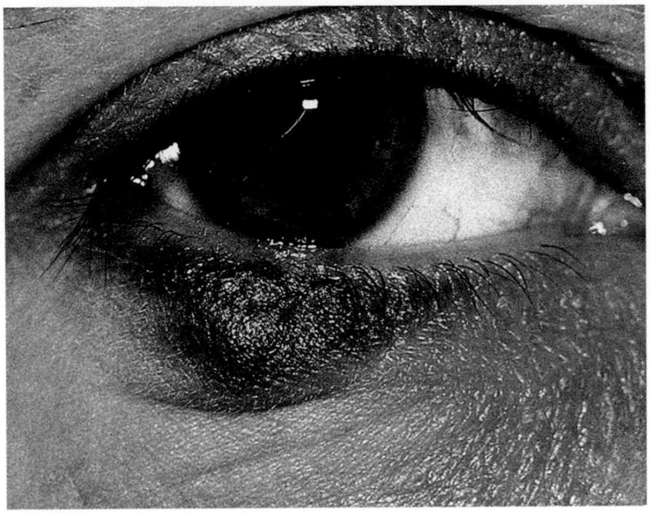

Figure 12.15 Kaposi's sarcoma of the eyelid.

respond better to therapy and carry a better prognosis, occasionally going into complete remission.

Cervical carcinoma

Women with HIV are at increased risk of cervical cancer caused by oncogenic subtypes of human papillomavirus. Annual cervical cytology is indicated to monitor for pre-malignant changes.

Further reading

Bichoupan K, Dieterich D, Martel-Laferrière V. HIV-hepatitis C virus co-infection in the era of direct-acting antivirals. *Curr HIV/AIDS Rep* 2014; 11:241–249.
Boulware DR, Meya DB, Muzoora C et al. Timing of antiretroviral therapy after diagnosis of cryptococcal meningitis. *New Engl J Med* 2014; 370:2487–2498.
Bradshaw D, Matthews G, Danta M. Sexually transmitted hepatitis C infection: the new epidemic in MSM? *Curr Opin Infect Dis* 2013; 26:66–72.
Joshi D, O'Grady J, Dieterich D et al. Increasing burden of liver disease in patients with HIV infection. *Lancet* 2011; 377:1198–1209.
Lacombe K, Bottero J, Lemoine M et al. HIV/hepatitis B virus co-infection: current challenges and new strategies. *J Antimicrob Chemother* 2010; 65:10–17.
Munteanu DI, Rockstroh JK. New agents for the treatment of hepatitis C in patients co-infected with HIV. *Therapeut Adv Infect Dis* 2013; 1:71–80.
Nelson M, Dockrell D, Edwards S. British HIV Association and British Infection Association guidelines for the treatment of opportunistic infection in HIV-seropositive individuals 2011. *HIV Med* 2011; 12(S2):1–5.
Rockstroh JK, Bhagani S. Managing HIV/hepatitis C co-infection in the era of direct acting antivirals. *BMC Med* 2013; 11:234.
Wilkins E, Nelson M, Agarwal K et al. British HIV Association guidelines for the management of hepatitis viruses in adults infected with HIV 2013. *HIV Med* 2013; 14(S4):1–71.
http://www.euro.who.int/ *Guidelines on the management of hepatitis C and HIV co-infection.*
http://www.hep-druginteractions.org *Potential hepatitis drug interactions can be checked using the online tool maintained by Liverpool University.*

PREVENTION AND CONTROL OF HIV INFECTION

HIV is a completely preventable infection, yet rates of new HIV infection continue and prevention measures remain fundamental to the control of the epidemic. Combinations of behavioural, biomedical and structural approaches with interventions appropriate for the particular population at risk are required. Models of the epidemic in the UK suggest that a majority of new infections are transmitted from people who are unaware of their HIV status. Reducing the high rates of undiagnosed infection through scaling-up of testing and treatment is therefore central to an effective prevention response. For those at high risk of acquisition, there needs to be an additional emphasis on the need for repeat testing, as those with early infection and a high viral load are particularly infectious. Vaccine development has been hampered by the genetic variability of the virus and the complex immune response that is required from the host, with disappointing results from trials of candidate agents.

Consistent condom use and education for behaviour change have been key strategies. Provision of clean injecting equipment has been successful in those countries where it has been implemented.

Medically performed circumcision has been shown in African studies of HIV-negative heterosexual men to reduce the female-to-male transmission of HIV by at least 50%. A more modest reduction in HIV incidence in HIV-negative women following circumcision of HIV-positive male partners has been demonstrated but only at 2 years after the procedure.

The role of ART in the prevention of infection has grown enormously in the past few years. Initiation of ART by people with HIV substantially reduces onward transmission. A 96% reduction in risk of HIV transmission from HIV-positive people to their HIV-uninfected heterosexual sexual partners has been demonstrated. Vertical transmission can be reduced to negligible levels by the use of effective ART in pregnant women.

Post-exposure prophylaxis (PEP) following sexual or occupational exposure can reduce the risk of infection if implemented promptly. The use of ARVs by people who are HIV-negative prior to potential exposure (pre-exposure prophylaxis, PrEP), to prevent acquisition of infection, has been shown to be successful in a number of clinical trial settings in MSM, although the results from similar studies amongst heterosexual women have been less successful. Daily Truvada (see p. 344) demonstrated an 86% decrease in the risk of HIV infection amongst MSM in the UK PROUD study, and a similar rate of protection when taken intermittently in the French IPERGAY trial. On the basis of these results, work is required that will allow the scaling-up of access to PrEP in the UK.

Partner notification schemes are helpful but are sensitive and controversial. Availability and accessibility of confidential HIV testing provide an opportunity for individual health education and risk reduction to be discussed.

Understanding and changing behaviour is crucial but notoriously difficult, especially in areas that carry as many taboos as sex, HIV and AIDS. Stigma, poverty, punitive legislation, social unrest and war all contribute to the spread of HIV. Political will, not always readily available, is required if progress in these areas is to be seen.

Further reading

Mayer KH. Antiretroviral chemoprophylaxis: new successes and questions. *Lancet* 2015; 385:2236–2237.
McCormack SM, Gafos M, Desai M et al. Biomedical prevention: state of the science. *Clin Infect Dis* 2014; 59(Suppl 1):S41–46.
http://www.BHIVA.org.uk *British HIV Association guidance on the appropriate use of vaccines in HIV.*

Bibliography

Aral S, Fenton KA, Lipshutz JA. *The New Public Health and STD/HIV Prevention: Personal, Public and Health Systems Approaches.* New York: Springer; 2013.
Ferreira A, Young T, Mathews C et al. *Strategies for Partner Notification for Sexually Transmitted Infections, Including HIV (Cochrane Review).* Chichester: Cochrane Library; 2013; Issue 10.
Fowler N. *AIDS. Don't Die of Prejudice.* London: Bite Back; 2014.
Maartens G, Celum C, Lewin SR. HIV infection: epidemiology, pathogenesis, treatment, and prevention. *Lancet* 2014; 384:258–271.
Smith CJ, Ryom L, Weber R et al. Trends in underlying causes of death in people with HIV from 1999 to 2011 (D:A:D): a multicohort collaboration. *Lancet* 2014; 384:241–248.
World Health Organization. *Consolidated Guidelines on HIV Prevention, Diagnosis, Treatment and Care for Key Populations.* Geneva: WHO; 2014.

13 Gastrointestinal disease

James Lindsay, Louise Langmead, Sean L Preston

See your e-book for key learning points, clinical tips, drug tips, extra tables, extra images, videos, learning challenges, MCQs and Special Topics from the International Advisory Board.

INTRODUCTION

The gastrointestinal tract has many functions, such as digestion, absorption and excretion, as well as the synthesis of hormones, growth factors and cytokines. In addition, a complex enteric nervous system controls its function and communicates with the central and peripheral nervous systems. Finally, as the gastrointestinal tract contains the largest source of foreign antigens, it has very well-developed arms of both the innate and the acquired immune systems. The intestinal microbiota exerts a range of beneficial functions aiding nutrition, absorption and the development of a mature immune system. Disruption of the composition and diversity of the microbiota is associated with the development of gastrointestinal and systemic disease.

In ***developed countries***, gastrointestinal symptoms are a common reason for attendance at primary care clinics and at hospital outpatient departments. Approximately 75% of these consultations are for non-organic symptoms. The clinician's main task is therefore to recognize when organic disease must be sought or excluded, remembering that 20% of all cancers occur in the gastrointestinal tract ***(Fig. 13.1)***. In ***developing countries***, malnutrition and poor hygiene make infection a more probable diagnosis. The clinician needs to recognize and treat these infections promptly and also help with prevention.

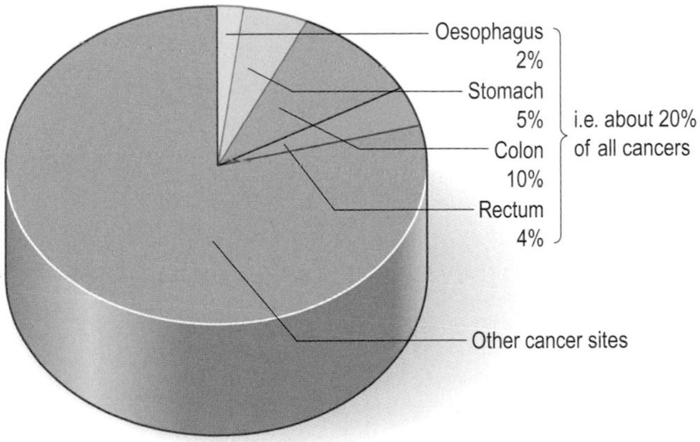

Figure 13.1 Relative contribution of gastrointestinal sites to all cancers.

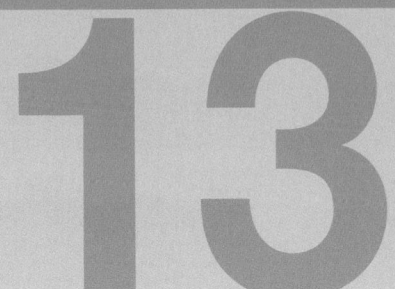

GASTROINTESTINAL DISEASE

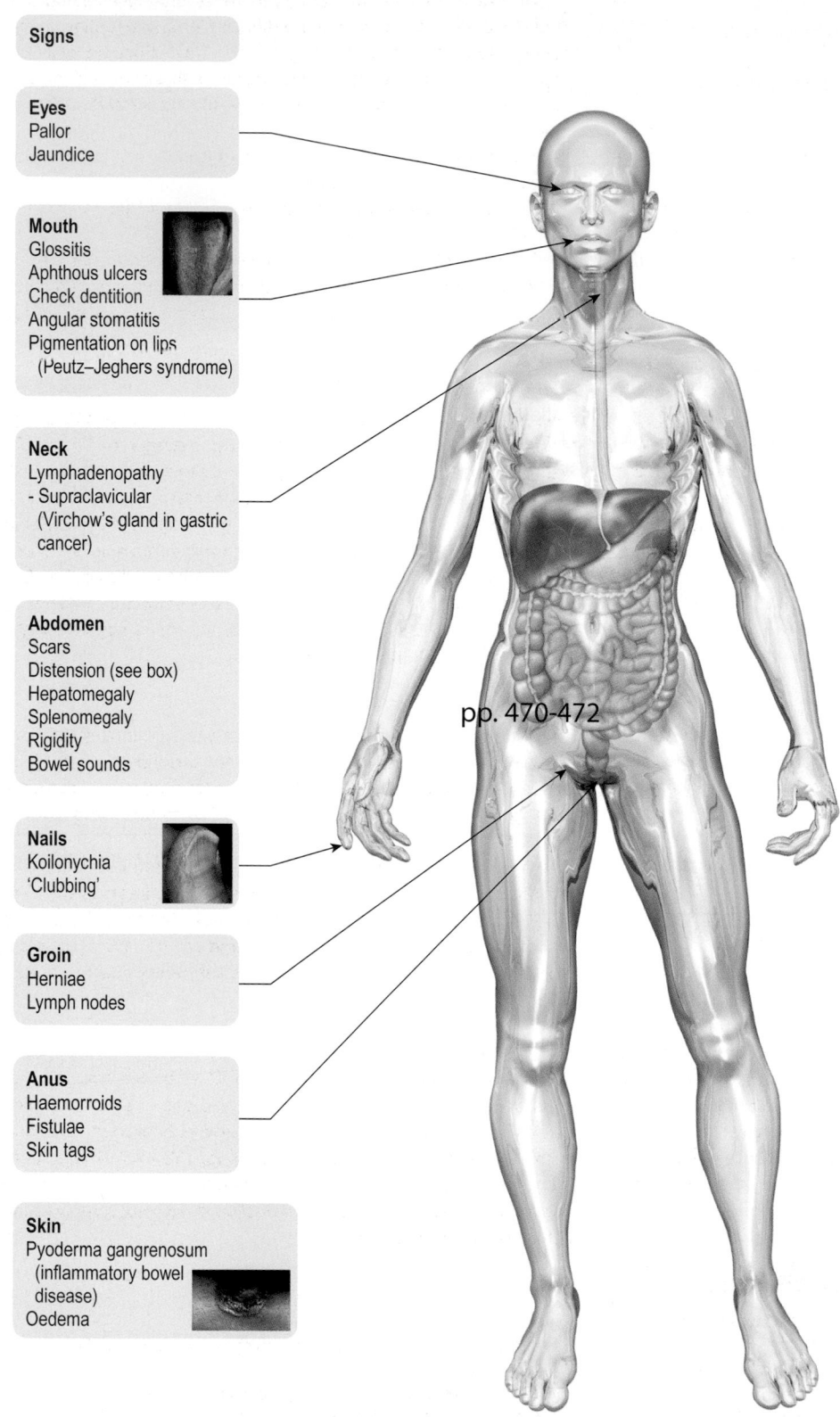

Signs

Eyes
Pallor
Jaundice

Mouth

Glossitis
Aphthous ulcers
Check dentition
Angular stomatitis
Pigmentation on lips
(Peutz–Jeghers syndrome)

Neck
Lymphadenopathy
- Supraclavicular
  (Virchow's gland in gastric cancer)

Abdomen
Scars
Distension (see box)
Hepatomegaly
Splenomegaly
Rigidity
Bowel sounds

Nails

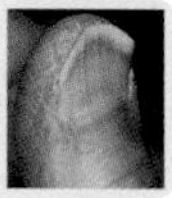

Koilonychia
'Clubbing'

Groin
Herniae
Lymph nodes

Anus
Haemorroids
Fistulae
Skin tags

Skin
Pyoderma gangrenosum
(inflammatory bowel disease)
Oedema

General
Colour
In pain?
Temperature
Dehydrated
Weight loss?

Symptoms
Nausea
Vomiting
- Haematemesis
- Peptic ulcer
- Oesophageal
  - Mallory–Weiss
  - Varices (pp. 470–472)
Dysphagia
- Odynophagia
Abdominal
- Distension (see box)
- Tenderness
- Rigidity
- Bowel Sounds
Oedema

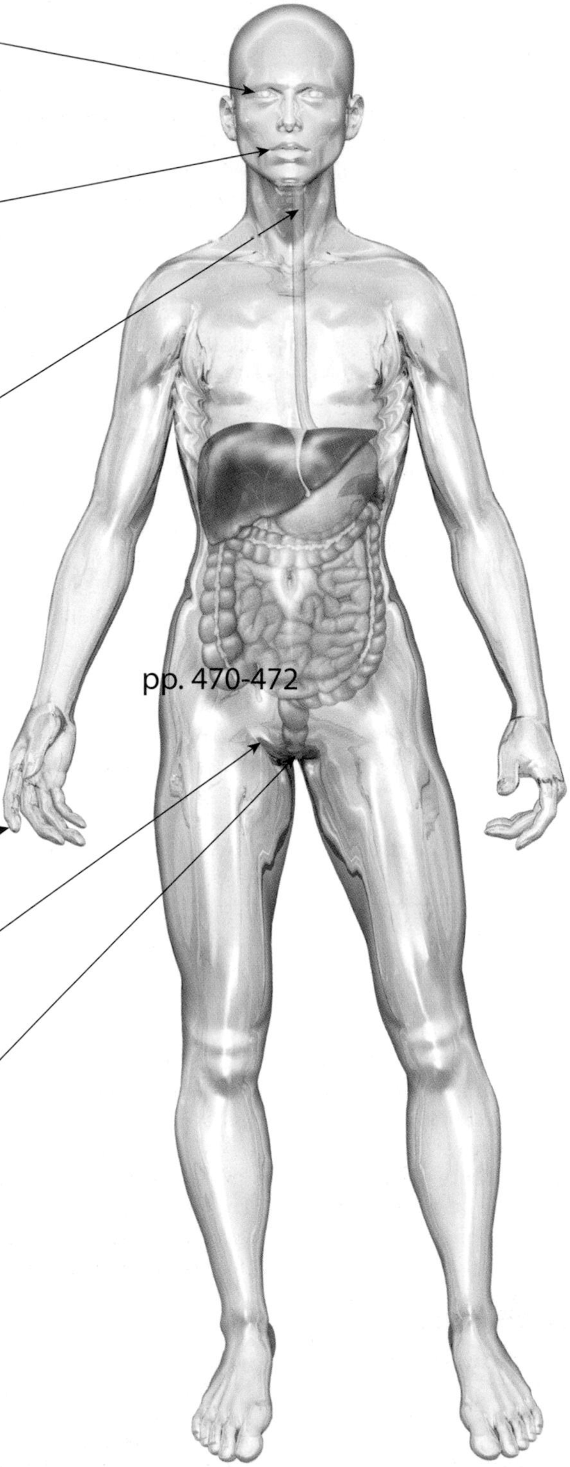

CLINICAL APPROACH TO THE PATIENT WITH GASTROINTESTINAL DISEASE

Clinical features of gastrointestinal disease

Stomatitis and halitosis

Stomatitis is inflammation in the mouth from any cause. Angular stomatitis is inflammation of the corners of the mouth.

Halitosis (bad breath) is a common symptom and is due to poor oral hygiene, anxiety (often when halitosis is more apparent to the patient than real) or rarer causes, such as oesophageal stricture and pulmonary sepsis.

Dyspepsia and indigestion

'Indigestion' is common: 80% of the population will suffer from this symptom at some time. Dyspepsia is an inexact term used to describe a number of upper abdominal symptoms such as heartburn, acidity, pain or discomfort, nausea, wind, fullness or belching. Patients who use the term 'indigestion' may also be describing lower gastrointestinal symptoms such as constipation or the presence of undigested vegetable material in the stool, so obtaining a precise history is necessary.

Features of dyspepsia that are suggestive of serious diseases such as cancer are known as ***'alarm' symptoms***. They include:

- dysphagia
- weight loss
- vomiting
- anorexia
- haematemesis or melaena.

Patients aged ≥55 years who demonstrate these features have a higher possibility of significant gastrointestinal pathology and should be investigated on an urgent basis.

Dysphagia and odynophagia

These symptoms are described on pages 365–366.

Vomiting

Many gastrointestinal (and non-gastrointestinal) conditions are associated with vomiting ***(Box 13.1)***.

Vomiting is regulated by a complex reflex involving central neural control centres, located in the lateral reticular formation of the medulla, which are stimulated by the chemoreceptor trigger zones (CTZs) in the floor of the fourth ventricle, and also by vagal afferents from the gut. The central zones are directly stimulated by toxins, drugs, motion sickness and metabolic disturbances. Raised intracranial pressure has a direct effect on the vomiting centre, leading to vomiting. Luminal toxins, inflammation and mechanical obstruction are local gastrointestinal causes of vomiting.

Nausea is a feeling of wanting to vomit, often associated with autonomic effects, including salivation, pallor and sweating. It frequently precedes actual vomiting. Retching is a strong, involuntary, unproductive effort to vomit, associated with abdominal muscle contraction but without expulsion of gastric contents through the mouth.

Faeculent vomiting suggests low intestinal obstruction or the presence of a gastrocolic fistula.

Haematemesis is vomiting of fresh or altered blood ('coffee-grounds') (see pp. 384–387).

Early morning nausea and vomiting are seen in pregnancy, alcohol dependence and some metabolic disorders (e.g. uraemia).

Persistent nausea alone is often stress-related and is not due to gastrointestinal disease.

Flatulence

This term describes excessive wind. It is used to indicate belching, abdominal distension, gurgling and the passage of flatus per rectum. Swallowing air (aerophagia) is described on page 430. Some of the swallowed air passes into the intestine, where most of it is absorbed, but some remains to be passed rectally. Colonic bacterial breakdown of non-absorbed carbohydrate also produces gas. Rectal flatus thus consists of nitrogen, carbon dioxide, hydrogen and methane. It is normal to pass rectal flatus up to 20 times/day. Causes of increased gas production and intake include a high-fibre diet and carbonated drinks.

Diarrhoea and constipation

These are common complaints and in the community are not usually due to serious disease. They are described in detail on pages 425–428 and 415–417, respectively. Some general rules concerning the aetiology and investigation of diarrhoea are shown in ***Box 13.2***.

Patients often consider themselves constipated if their bowels are not open on most days, though normal stool frequency is very variable, from 3 times daily to 3 times a week. The difficult passage of hard stool is also regarded as constipation, irrespective of stool frequency. Constipation with hard stools is rarely due to organic colonic disease.

Abdominal pain

Organic abdominal pain is stimulated mainly by the stretching of smooth muscle or organ capsules. Severe acute abdominal pain can be caused by a large number of gastrointestinal conditions, and normally presents as an emergency (see pp. 432–435). An apparent 'acute abdomen' can occasionally be due to referred pain from the chest, as in pneumonia, or to metabolic causes, such as diabetic ketoacidosis or porphyria.

Box 13.1 Causes of vomiting: some examples

- Any gastrointestinal disease
- Infections:
  - Viral (influenza, norovirus)
  - Bacterial (pertussis, urinary infection)
- Central nervous system disease:
  - Raised intracranial pressure
  - Vestibular disturbance, e.g. motion sickness
  - Migraine
- Metabolic:
  - Uraemia
  - Hypercalcaemia

Box 13.2 Simple rules in diarrhoea

- A single episode of diarrhoea is commonly due to dietary indiscretion or anxiety.
- Large-volume, watery stools always have an organic cause.
- Bloody diarrhoea implies colonic and/or rectal disease.
- Acute diarrhoea lasting 2–3 days is most often due to an infective cause.
- Inflammatory bowel disease should be considered for severe or prolonged symptoms.
- Stool cultures should be taken to exclude an infective cause.

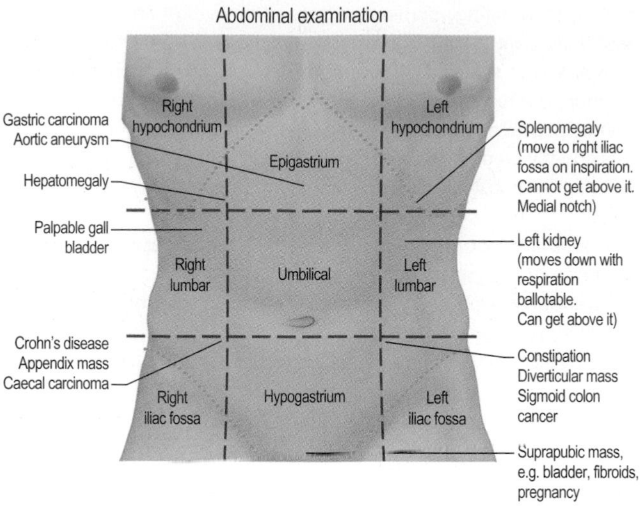

Figure 13.2 The abdominal quadrants.

Check:

- site *(Fig. 13.2)*, intensity, character, duration and frequency of the pain
- aggravating and relieving factors
- associated symptoms, including non-gastrointestinal symptoms.

Upper abdominal pain

Epigastric pain is very common and is often related to food intake. Although functional dyspepsia is the most common diagnosis, the symptoms of peptic ulcer disease can be identical. ***Heartburn*** (a burning pain behind the sternum) is a common symptom of gastro-oesophageal reflux.

Right hypochondrial pain may originate from the gall bladder or biliary tract. Biliary pain can also be epigastric. ***Biliary pain*** is typically intermittent and severe, lasts a few hours and remits spontaneously, to recur weeks or months later. Hepatic congestion (e.g. in hepatitis or cardiac failure) and sometimes peptic ulcer disease can present with pain in the right hypochondrium. Chronic, persistent or constant pain in the right (or left) hypochondrium in a well-looking patient is a frequent functional symptom; this chronic pain is not due to gall bladder disease (see pp. 491–492).

Lower abdominal pain

Pain in the left iliac fossa may be colonic in origin (e.g. acute diverticulitis) but chronic pain is most commonly associated with functional bowel disorders.

Lower abdominal pain in women occurs in a number of gynaecological disorders and the differentiation from gastrointestinal disease may be difficult.

Pain in the right iliac fossa may be due to acute appendicitis or ileocaecal disease, but may also commonly be functional.

Proctalgia fugax is a severe pain deep in the rectum that comes on suddenly but lasts only for a short time. It is not due to organic disease.

Abdominal wall pain

Persistent abdominal pain with localized tenderness, which is not relieved by tensing the abdominal muscles, is probably from the abdominal wall itself. Causes are thought to include nerve entrapment, external hernias, and entrapment of internal viscera (commonly omentum) within traumatic or surgical alterations of abdominal wall musculature.

Anorexia and weight loss

Anorexia describes reduced appetite. It is common in systemic disease and may be seen in psychiatric disorders. Anorexia often accompanies cancer but is usually a late symptom and not of diagnostic help. Weight loss is almost always due to reduced food intake and is a frequent accompaniment of gastrointestinal diseases. Weight loss in malabsorption disorders is primarily due to anorexia. Weight loss with a normal or increased dietary intake only occurs with hyperthyroidism and other catabolic states. Weight loss should always be assessed objectively, as patients' impressions are unreliable.

Examination of the gastrointestinal system

Examination of the abdomen

Inspection

Look for abdominal distension. Common causes ('the five Fs') are: flatus, fat, fetus, fluid and faeces. Intermittent distension is most commonly a feature of functional bowel disorders.

Palpation

Feel for palpable masses or abdominal tenderness. All abdominal quadrants should be palpated in turn, followed by deeper palpations; remember to watch the patient's face for signs of pain or discomfort. Evaluate any palpable mass and note its size, shape and consistency and whether it moves with respiration, to decide which organ is involved. Some abdominal organs may be just palpable normally, usually in thin people *(Fig. 13.3)*. Riedel's lobe is an anatomical variant consisting of a palpable enlargement of the lateral portion of the right lobe of the liver. The hernial orifices should be examined if intestinal obstruction is suspected.

Percussion

Abdominal percussion detects the areas of dullness caused by the liver and spleen, those due to ascites or those over masses. It can also detect a full bladder. ***Ascites*** is a term for excess fluid in the peritoneal cavity. It is detected clinically by central abdominal resonance caused by gas within small bowel loops, with dullness in the flanks that shifts when the patient lies on their side. This 'shifting dullness' is a reliable physical sign, if 1–2 L of fluid are present.

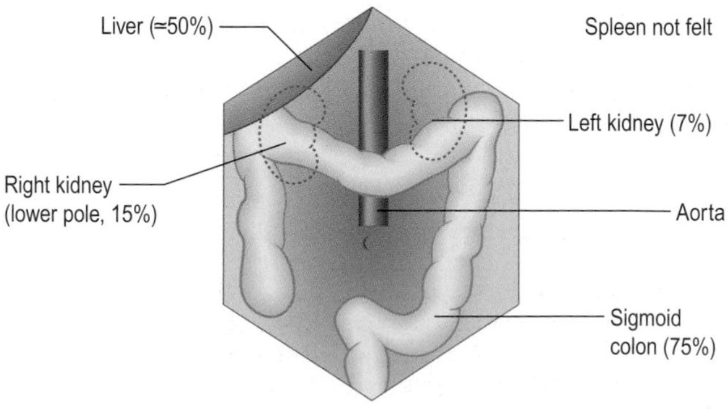

Figure 13.3 The organs that are sometimes palpable in thin subjects.

Auscultation

Auscultation is not of great value in abdominal disease, except for evaluation of bowel sounds in the acute abdomen (see p. 433). Abdominal bruits are often present in normal subjects and are rarely clinically significant.

A succussion splash suggests gastric outlet obstruction if the patient has not drunk for 2–3 hours. The splash of fluid in the stomach can be heard with a stethoscope laid on the abdomen when the patient is moved.

Examination of the rectum and sigmoid colon

A digital examination of the rectum should be performed in all patients with a change in bowel habit or rectal bleeding, and prior to endoscopic examination of the rectum.

- ***Proctoscopy (Box 13.3)*** is performed in all patients with a history of bright red rectal bleeding to look for anorectal pathology such as haemorrhoids; a rigid sigmoidoscope is too narrow and long to enable adequate examination of the anal canal.
- ***Sigmoidoscopy***, either flexible or rigid, is part of the routine hospital examination in cases of diarrhoea and in patients with lower abdominal symptoms such as a change in bowel habit or rectal bleeding. ***Rigid sigmoidoscopy*** can visualize the distal 20–25 cm of large bowel, whereas ***flexible sigmoidoscopy*** (*FS*) can reach up to the splenic flexure (60 cm), and is typically performed in the endoscopy unit after evacuation of the distal colon using an enema or suppository. Rigid sigmoidoscopy is more mobile and is easily performed on the ward or in the outpatient department. Most rectal bleeding is due to benign anorectal disease (haemorrhoids or fissure *in ano*) and an otherwise normal FS can be reassuring and avoids over-investigation. Up to 60% of colonic neoplasms occur within the range of FS and FS is therefore used as screening test for colorectal cancer in asymptomatic average-risk individuals.

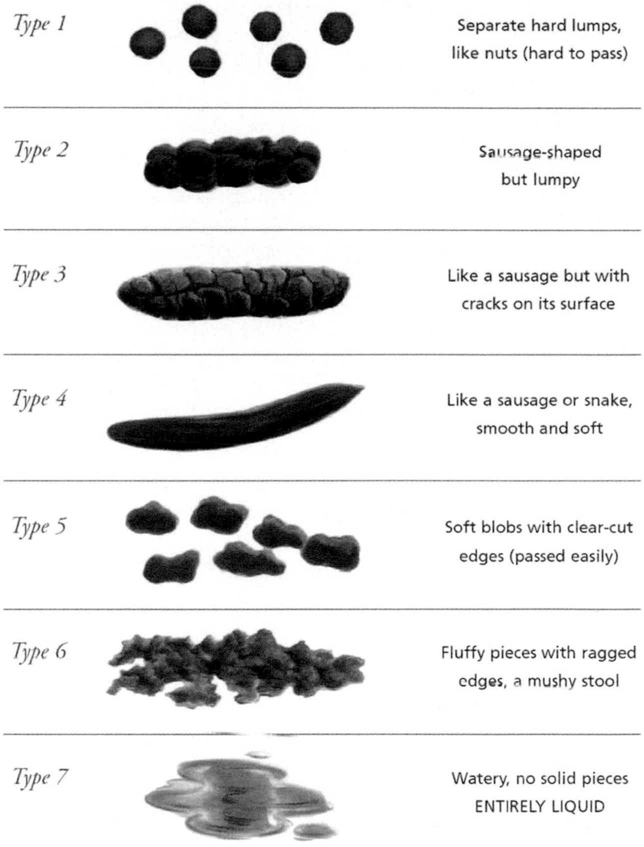

Type 1
Separate hard lumps, like nuts (hard to pass)
Type 2
Sausage-shaped but lumpy
Type 3
Like a sausage but with cracks on its surface
Type 4
Like a sausage or snake, smooth and soft
Type 5
Soft blobs with clear-cut edges (passed easily)
Type 6
Fluffy pieces with ragged edges, a mushy stool
Type 7
Watery, no solid pieces ENTIRELY LIQUID

Figure 13.4 The Bristol Stool Chart. *(Reproduced by kind permission of Dr K W Heaton, Reader in Medicine at the University of Bristol. © 2000 Norgine Pharmaceuticals Ltd.)*

Stool examination

It is useful to confirm a patient's account (e.g. passing of blood or steatorrhoea). The shape and size may be helpful (e.g. 'rabbit dropping' or ribbon-like stools in irritable bowel syndrome). Stool charts for recording consistency and frequency of defecation are useful in inpatients to follow the progress of diarrhoea, particularly in the management of severe colitis. The Bristol Stool Chart is commonly used in the UK ***(Fig. 13.4)***.

Investigation of gastrointestinal disease

Routine haematology and biochemistry, followed by endoscopy and radiology, are the principal investigations. The investigation of small bowel disease is discussed in more detail on pages 394–395. Manometry is mainly used in oesophageal disease (see p. 366) and anorectal disorders (see pp. 419–420).

Box 13.3 Proctoscopy

- The proctoscope is passed into the anus and the obturator is removed.
- The patient strains down as the proctoscope is removed.
- Haemorrhoids are seen as purplish veins in the left lateral, right posterior or right anterior position.
- Fissures may also be seen, but pain often prevents the procedure from being performed.

Endoscopy

Video endoscopes relay colour images to a high-definition television monitor. The tip of the endoscope can be angulated in all directions, and channels in the instrument are used for air insufflation, water injection, suction, and the passage of accessories such as biopsy forceps or brushes for obtaining tissue, snares for polypectomy and needles for injection therapies. Permanent photographic or video records of the procedure are obtained.

- ***Oesophagogastroduodenoscopy*** (***OGD***, 'gastroscopy') is the investigation of choice for upper gastrointestinal disorders with the possibility of therapy and mucosal biopsy. Findings include reflux oesophagitis, gastritis, ulcers and cancer. Therapeutic OGD is used to treat upper gastrointestinal haemorrhage and both benign and malignant obstruction. The mortality for diagnostic endoscopy is 0.001% with significant complications in 1 : 10 000, usually when performed as an emergency (e.g. gastrointestinal haemorrhage).
- ***Colonoscopy*** allows good visualization of the whole colon and terminal ileum. Biopsies can be obtained and polyps removed. Benign strictures can be dilated and malignant strictures stented. The success rate for reaching the caecum should be at least 90% after training. Cancer, polyps and diverticular disease are the most common significant findings. Perforation occurs in 1 : 1000 examinations but this is higher (up to 2%) after polypectomy and endoscopic mucosal resection ***(Box 13.4)***.

Box 13.4 Gastroscopy and colonoscopy

- Explain the procedure to the patient, including benefits and risks.
- Discuss the need for sedation.
- Obtain written informed consent.

Gastroscopy

- The patient should be fasted for at least 4 h.
- Give oxygen and monitor oxygen saturation with an oximeter.
- Give lidocaine throat spray or sedation (midazolam ± opiate if required).
- Pass the gastroscope to the duodenum under direct vision.
- Examine during insertion and withdrawal.
- Gastroscopy takes 5–15 min, depending on the indication and findings.
- Withhold fluid and food until local anaesthetic/sedation wears off.
- Complications are rare but beware of over-sedation, perforation and aspiration.
- The patient must be accompanied home if sedation has been given.

Colonoscopy

- Stop oral iron a week before the procedure.
- Restrict the diet to low-residue foods for 48 h; clear fluids only for 24 h.
- Use a local bowel-cleansing regime, usually starting 24 h beforehand (e.g. two sachets of sodium picosulfate with magnesium citrate and 2–4 bisacodyl tablets, or macrogols 2–4 L, or local alternative; more if constipated).
- Give oxygen and monitor O_2 levels.
- Give sedation (midazolam ± opiate) if required by the patient.
- Pass the colonoscope to the caecum or ileum under direct vision.
- Examine in detail during withdrawal.
- Colonoscopy takes 15–30 min, depending on the colon anatomy, indication and findings.
- Withhold fluid and food until sedation wears off.
- Observe the patient for at least an hour after sedation has been given.
- Complications are rare but beware of over-sedation, perforation and aspiration.
- The patient must be accompanied home if sedation has been given.

For patients on antiplatelet therapy and anticoagulants (including antithrombotic agents), see Veitch AM, Vanbiervliet G, Gershlick AH et al. Endoscopy in patients on antiplatelet or anticoagulant therapy including direct oral anticoagulants. British Society of Gastroenterology (BSG) and European Society of Gastrointestinal Endoscopy (ESGE) guidelines. Gut *2016; 65:374–389.*

- ***Endoscopic retrograde cannulation of biliary and pancreatic duct (ERCP)*** combines endoscopy and fluoroscopy to visualize the pancreaticobiliary tree. It is not used diagnostically but is employed for interventions such as gall stone extraction and stenting of benign and malignant strictures in the common bile duct. Complications include perforation, pancreatitis and sepsis.
- ***Endoscopic ultrasound*** (***EUS***) is performed with a gastroscope incorporating an ultrasound probe at the tip. It is used diagnostically for lesions in the oesophageal or gastric wall, including the detailed TNM staging (see pp. 375–376) of oesophageal/gastric cancer, and for the detection and biopsy of pancreatic tumours and cysts.
- ***Endoanal and endorectal ultrasonography*** are performed to define the anatomy of the anal sphincters (see p. 418), to detect perianal disease and to stage superficial rectal tumours.
- ***Balloon enteroscopy***, either double- or single-balloon, can examine the small bowel from the duodenum to the ileum, adopting both cranial and caudal approaches, and using specialized enteroscopes in expert centres.
- ***Capsule endoscopy*** is used for the evaluation of obscure gastrointestinal bleeding (after negative gastroscopy and colonoscopy) and for the detection of small bowel tumours and occult inflammatory bowel disease. It should be avoided if strictures are suspected.

Imaging

Full clinical information must be provided before the examination, and ideally, the images obtained should be reviewed with the radiologist to aid interpretation. The optimal technique to be used will depend on local expertise.

Plain X-rays

Plain X-rays of the chest and abdomen are chiefly used in the investigation of an acute abdomen. Interpretation depends on analysis of gas shadows inside and outside the bowel. Plain films are particularly useful where obstruction or perforation is suspected, to exclude toxic megacolon in colitis, and to assess faecal loading in constipation. Calcification may be seen with gall-bladder stones and in chronic pancreatitis, though computed tomography is more sensitive for both.

Ultrasound

Ultrasonography involves no radiation and is the first-line investigation for abdominal distension: for example, in ascites, a mass or suspected inflammatory conditions. It can show dilated, fluid-filled loops of bowel in obstruction, and thickening of the bowel wall. It can be used to guide biopsies or percutaneous drainage. In an acute abdomen, ultrasound can diagnose cholecystitis, appendicitis, enlarged mesenteric glands and other inflammatory conditions.

Computed tomography

Computed tomography (CT) involves a significant dose of radiation (approximately 10 millisieverts). Modern multislice fast scanners and techniques, involving intraluminal and intravenous contrast, enhance diagnostic capability. Intraluminal contrast may be positive (Gastrografin or Omnipaque) or negative (usually water). The bowel wall and mesentery are well seen after intravenous contrast, especially with negative intraluminal contrast. Clinically unsuspected diseases of other abdominal organs are quite often also revealed ***(Fig. 13.5A)***.

CT is widely used as a first-line investigation for the acute abdomen. It is sensitive for small volumes of gas from a perforated viscus, as well as leakage of contrast from the gut lumen.

Inflammatory conditions, such as abscesses, appendicitis, diverticulitis, Crohn's disease and its complications, are well demonstrated. In high-grade bowel obstruction, CT is usually diagnostic of both the presence and the cause of the obstruction.

CT is widely used in cancer staging and as guidance for biopsy of tumour or lymph nodes.

CT pneumocolon/CT colonography (virtual colonoscopy) after CO_2 insufflation into a previously cleansed colon provides an alternative to colonoscopy for diagnosis of colonic mass lesions ***(Fig. 13.5B)***. It is being evaluated as a screening test for colon pathology with sensitivities of over 90% for >10 mm polyps.

Unprepared CT is a good test for colon cancer in the frail (often elderly) patient who would have problems with bowel preparation.

Magnetic resonance imaging

Magnetic resonance imaging (MRI) uses no radiation and is particularly useful in the evaluation of rectal cancers and of abscesses and fistulae in the perianal region. It is also useful in small bowel disease (MR enteroclysis) and in hepatobiliary and pancreatic disease.

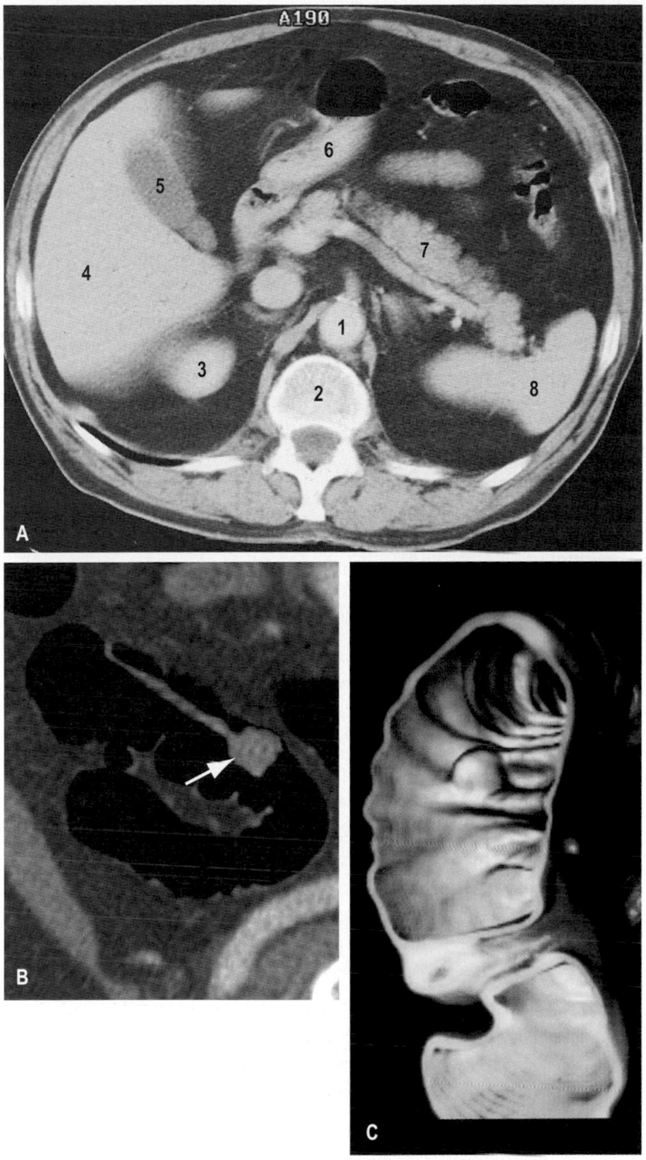

Figure 13.5 Computed tomography in gastrointestinal disease.
A. CT scan of the normal abdomen at the level of T12. (1) Aorta; (2) spine; (3) top of right kidney; (4) liver; (5) gall bladder; (6) stomach (containing air); (7) pancreas; (8) spleen.
B. CT cross-sectional (two-dimensional) image of a colonic polyp on a long stalk. The colon has been emptied as for visual colonoscopy. The pedunculated polyp and its stalk show enhancement after intravenous contrast.
C. Three-dimensional reconstruction of part of the colon (false colour) generated by a computer program from multiple axial CT images. A sessile polypoid lesion is shown. *(B and C: Courtesy of Dr Paul Jenkins.)*

Positron emission tomography

Positron emission tomography (PET) relies on detection of the metabolism of fluorodeoxyglucose. It is used for staging oesophageal, gastric and colorectal cancer and in detecting metastatic and recurrent disease. PET/CT adds additional anatomical information.

Contrast studies

- ***Barium swallow*** examines the oesophagus and proximal stomach. Its main use is for investigating dysphagia.
- ***Double-contrast barium meal*** examines the oesophagus, stomach and duodenum. Barium is given to produce mucosal coating, and effervescent granules producing carbon dioxide in the stomach create a double contrast between gas and barium. This test has high accuracy for the detection of significant pathology, such as ulcers and cancer, but requires good technique. Gastroscopy is a more sensitive test and enables biopsy of suspicious areas.
- ***Small bowel meal or follow-through*** specifically examines the small bowel. Ingested barium passes through the small bowel into the right colon. The fold pattern and calibre of the small bowel are assessed. Specific views of the terminal ileum can be obtained and are used to identify early changes in patients with suspected Crohn's disease. MRI is being used more frequently, as it does not involve radiation.
- ***Absorbable water-soluble*** (***Gastrografin or Omnipaque***) ***contrast agents*** should be used in preference to barium when perforation is suspected anywhere in the gut.

Radioisotopes

Radionuclides are used to a varying degree, depending on availability and expertise. Some of the more common indications and techniques are as follows:

- Detection of the urease activity of ***Helicobacter pylori*** – ^{13}C urea breath test (see p. 379).
- Measurement of the ***rate of gastric emptying*** – sequential gamma camera scans after oral [^{99m}Tc]technetium-sulphur colloid or indium-labelled diethylene triamine penta-acetic acid (^{111}In-DTPA).
- Demonstration of a ***Meckel's diverticulum*** – gamma camera scan after intravenous [^{99m}Tc]pertechnetate, which has affinity for gastric mucosa.
- Assessment of the extent of ***inflammation*** and presence of inflammatory collections in inflammatory bowel disease – gamma camera scan after intravenous injection of white cells labelled with ^{99m}Tc-hexamethylpropyleneamine oxime (HMPAO).
- Evaluation of ***neuroendocrine tumours*** and their metastases – gamma camera scan after intravenous radiolabelled octreotide or meta-iodobenzylguanidine (MIBG).
- Assessment of ***obscure gastrointestinal bleeding*** – gamma camera abdominal scan after intravenous injection of red cells labelled with ^{99m}Tc (only useful if the bleeding is >2 mL/min).
- Measurement of ***albumin loss*** in the stools (in ***protein-losing enteropathy***) – following albumin labelled *in vivo* with intravenous $^{51}CrCl_3$. This test has largely been replaced by the measurement of the intestinal clearance of ***α_1-antitrypsin***.
- Assessment of ***bile salt malabsorption*** (in patients with unexplained diarrhoea) – gamma camera scan to measure both isotope retention and faecal loss of orally administered ^{75}Selenium-homocholic acid taurine (SeHCAT) (see p. 427).
- Detection of ***bacterial overgrowth*** in the small bowel – measurement of $^{14}CO_2$ in breath following oral ^{14}C glycocholic acid.

THE MOUTH

The oral cavity extends from the lips to the pharynx and contains the tongue, teeth and gums. Its primary functions are mastication, swallowing and speech. Problems in the mouth are extremely common and, although they may be trivial, they can produce severe symptoms. Poor dental hygiene is often a factor.

Box 13.5 Causes of mouth ulcers

- Idiopathic aphthous ulceration (most common)
- Gastrointestinal disease:
  - Inflammatory bowel disease
  - Coeliac disease
- Infection:
  - Viral – herpes simplex virus (HSV), human immunodeficiency virus (HIV), Coxsackie
  - Fungal – candidiasis
  - Bacterial – syphilis, tuberculosis
- Systemic disease:
  - Reactive arthritis (see p. 686)
  - Behçet syndrome
  - Systemic lupus erythematosus
- Trauma:
  - e.g. Dentures
- Neoplasia:
  - e.g. Squamous cell carcinoma
- Drugs:
  - In erythema multiforme major, toxic epidermal necrolysis
  - Chemotherapy, antimalarials
- Skin disease:
  - Pemphigoid
  - Pemphigus
  - Lichen planus

Recurrent aphthous ulceration

Idiopathic aphthous ulceration is common and affects up to 25% of the population. Recurrent painful round or ovoid mouth ulcers are seen with inflammatory halos. They are more common in females and non-smokers, usually appear first in childhood, and tend to reduce in number and frequency before the age of 40. Other family members may be affected. There is no sign of systemic disease.

- ***Minor aphthous ulcers*** are the most common; they are <10 mm diameter, have a grey/white centre with a thin erythematous halo, and heal within 14 days without scarring. They rarely affect the dorsum of the tongue or hard palate.
- ***Major aphthous ulcers*** (>10 mm diameter) often persist for weeks or months and heal with scarring.

The cause is not known. Deficiencies of iron, folic acid or vitamin B_{12} (with or without gastrointestinal disorders) are sometimes found but are not causally linked. Secondary causes, such as Crohn's disease, should be excluded ***(Box 13.5)***.

There are no specific effective therapies. Sufferers should avoid oral trauma, and acidic foods or drinks that cause pain. Topical (1% triamcinolone) or systemic corticosteroids may lessen the duration and severity of the attacks. Chlorhexidine gluconate or tetracycline mouthwash, dapsone, colchicine, thalidomide and azathioprine have all been used with variable effect.

Neoplasia (squamous cell carcinoma)

Malignant tumours of the mouth account for 1% of all malignant tumours in the UK. The majority develop on the floor of the mouth or lateral borders of the tongue. Early lesions may be painless, but advanced tumours are easily recognizable as hard, indurated ulcers with raised and rolled edges. Aetiological agents include tobacco, heavy alcohol consumption and the areca nut. Human papillomavirus 16 causes some oral cancers. Pre-malignant lesions include leucoplakia (single adherent white patch), lichen planus, submucous fibrosis and erythroplakia (a red patch).

Management

Treatment is by surgical excision, which may require extensive neck dissection to remove involved lymph nodes and/or radiotherapy. Ablative treatment with photodynamic therapy is being pioneered for early lesions.

Pigmented neoplastic lesions

These include melanotic naevi on the hard palate and buccal mucosa. These are rarer in the mouth than on the skin. Malignant melanomas are rare, but more common in males, and occur mainly on the upper jaw. The 5-year survival is only 5%.

Non-neoplastic lesions

Oral white patches

Transient white patches either are due to *Candida* infection or are very occasionally found in systemic lupus erythematosus. Local causes include mechanical, irritative or chemical trauma from drugs (e.g. ill-fitting dentures or aspirin). Oral candidiasis in adults is seen following therapy with broad-spectrum antibiotics or inhaled steroids, and in people with diabetes, patients who are seriously ill or those who are immunocompromised.

Persistent white patches can be due to ***leucoplakia***, which is associated with alcohol and (particularly) smoking; it is premalignant. A biopsy should always be taken; histology shows alteration in the keratinization and dysplasia of the epithelium. Treatment is unsatisfactory. Isotretinoin possibly reduces disease progression. ***Oral lichen planus*** presents as white striae, which can rarely extend into the oesophagus.

Oral pigmented lesions

Racial pigmentation is scattered and symmetrically distributed. Amalgam tattoo is the most common form of localized oral pigmentation and consists of blue–black macules involving the gingivae; it results from dental amalgam sequestering into the tissues. Diseases causing pigmentation include Peutz–Jeghers syndrome and Addison's disease. Heavy metals (e.g. lead, bismuth and mercury) and drugs (e.g. phenothiazines and antimalarials) all cause pigmentation of the gums.

The tongue

The tongue may be affected by inflammatory or malignant processes, with similar lesions to those described above.

Glossitis

Glossitis is a red, smooth, sore tongue associated with vitamin B_{12}, folate, iron, riboflavin and nicotinic acid deficiency. It is also seen in infections due to *Candida*.

Black hairy tongue

A black hairy tongue is due to a proliferation of chromogenic microorganisms causing brown staining of elongated filiform papillae. The causes are unknown, but heavy smoking and the use of antiseptic mouthwashes have been implicated.

Geographic tongue

A geographic tongue is an idiopathic condition occurring in 1–2% of the population and may be familial. There are erythematous areas surrounded by well-defined, slightly raised irregular margins. The lesions are usually painless and the patient should be reassured.

The gums

The gums (gingivae) are the mucous membranes covering the alveolar processes of the mandible and the maxilla. Diseases of the gum are shown in ***Box 13.6***.

Box 13.6 Gum diseases

	Cause	Management
Chronic gingivitis	Bacterial plaque	Plaque removal
Acute (necrotizing) ulcerative gingivitis (Vincent's angina)	Spirochaete and fusiform bacteria (poor hygiene and smoking)	Oral metronidazole 200 mg 3 times daily for 3 days Chlorhexidine mouthwash
Desquamative gingivitis (smooth red atrophic gingivae)	Lichen planus or mucous membrane pemphigoid	Confirmation with biopsy
Gingival swelling	Inflammation (e.g. pregnancy, scurvy) infiltrations (leukaemia) or fibrous hyperplasia (e.g. drug-induced – phenytoin, ciclosporin, nifedipine)	

Box 13.7 Diseases of the salivary glands

- Dry mouth (xerostomia):
  - Sjögren syndrome
  - Drugs (e.g. antimuscarinic, anti-parkinsonian, lithium, tricyclics, monoamine oxidase inhibitors (MAOIs))
  - Radiotherapy
  - Psychogenic
  - Dehydration
- Acute sialadenitis:
  - Viral (e.g. mumps)
  - Bacterial (e.g. *Staphylococcus, Streptococcus*)
- Salivary duct obstruction:
  - Calculus
- Sarcoidosis (see pp. 1118–1120)
- Neoplasms (3% of all tumours worldwide):
  - Pleomorphic adenoma (15% become malignant and can cause VII lower motor neurone signs)

The teeth

Dental caries occur as a result of bacterial damage to tooth structures leading to tooth decay and 'cavities'. The main cause in humans is *Streptococcus mutans*, which is cariogenic only in the presence of dietary sugar. Dental caries can progress to pulpitis and pulp necrosis, and spreading infection can cause dentoalveolar abscesses. If there is soft tissue swelling, antibiotics (e.g. amoxicillin or metronidazole) should be prescribed prior to dental intervention.

Erosion of the teeth can result from exposure to acid (e.g. in bulimia nervosa) or, very occasionally, from severe gastro-oesophageal reflux disease.

Oral manifestations of human immunodeficiency virus infection

Patients infected with human immunodeficiency virus (HIV) often have characteristic oral lesions. Lesions strongly associated with HIV infection include candidiasis (with erythema and/or white exudates), erythematous candidiasis, oral hairy leucoplakia, Kaposi's sarcoma, non-Hodgkin's lymphoma, necrotizing ulcerative gingivitis and necrotizing ulcerative periodontitis; these are described elsewhere.

All oral lesions are much less common since the introduction of anti-retroviral therapy (ART; see pp. 341–346).

THE SALIVARY GLANDS

Diseases of the salivary glands are shown in ***Box 13.7***.

THE PHARYNX AND OESOPHAGUS

Anatomy and physiology

The ***pharynx*** consists of the nasal, oral and laryngeal sections. The latter is the part of the throat that connects to the oesophagus.

The ***oesophagus*** is a muscular tube approximately 20 cm long that connects the pharynx to the stomach just below the diaphragm. Its only function is to transport food from the mouth to the stomach. In the upper portion of the oesophagus, both the outer longitudinal layer and inner circular muscle layers are striated. In the lower two-thirds of the oesophagus, including the thoracic and abdominal parts containing the lower oesophageal sphincter, both layers are composed of smooth muscle.

The oesophagus is lined by stratified squamous epithelium, which extends distally to the squamocolumnar junction where the oesophagus joins the stomach, recognized endoscopically by a zigzag ('Z') line, just above the most proximal gastric folds.

The oesophagus is separated from the pharynx by the ***upper oesophageal sphincter*** (UOS), which is normally closed due to tonic activity of the nerves supplying the oricopharyngeus. The ***lower oesophageal sphincter*** (LOS) consists of a 2–4 cm zone in the distal end of the oesophagus that has a high resting tone and, assisted by the diaphragmatic sphincter, is largely responsible for the prevention of gastric reflux.

Swallowing

During swallowing, the bolus of food is voluntarily moved from the mouth to the pharynx. This process is mediated by a complex reflex involving a swallowing centre in the dorsal motor nucleus of the vagus in the brainstem. Once activated, the swallowing centre neurones send pre-programmed discharges of inhibition followed by excitation to the motor nuclei of the cranial nerves. This results in initial relaxation, followed by distally progressive activation of neurones to the oesophageal smooth muscle and LOS. Pharyngeal and oesophageal peristalsis mediated by this swallowing reflex causes ***primary peristalsis***. ***Secondary peristalsis*** arises as a result of stimulation by a food bolus in the lumen, mediated by a local intra-oesophageal reflex. ***Tertiary contractions*** indicate pathological non-propulsive contractions resulting from aberrant activation of local reflexes within the myenteric plexus.

The smooth muscle of the thoracic oesophagus and LOS is supplied by vagal autonomic motor nerves consisting of extrinsic preganglionic fibres and intramural postganglionic neurones in the myenteric plexus ***(Fig. 13.6)***. There are parallel excitatory and inhibitory pathways.

Clinical features of oesophageal disorders

Symptoms

Major oesophageal symptoms are:

- ***Dysphagia***. Difficulty in swallowing is defined as a sensation of obstruction during the passage of liquid or solid through the pharynx or oesophagus: that is, within 15 s of food leaving the

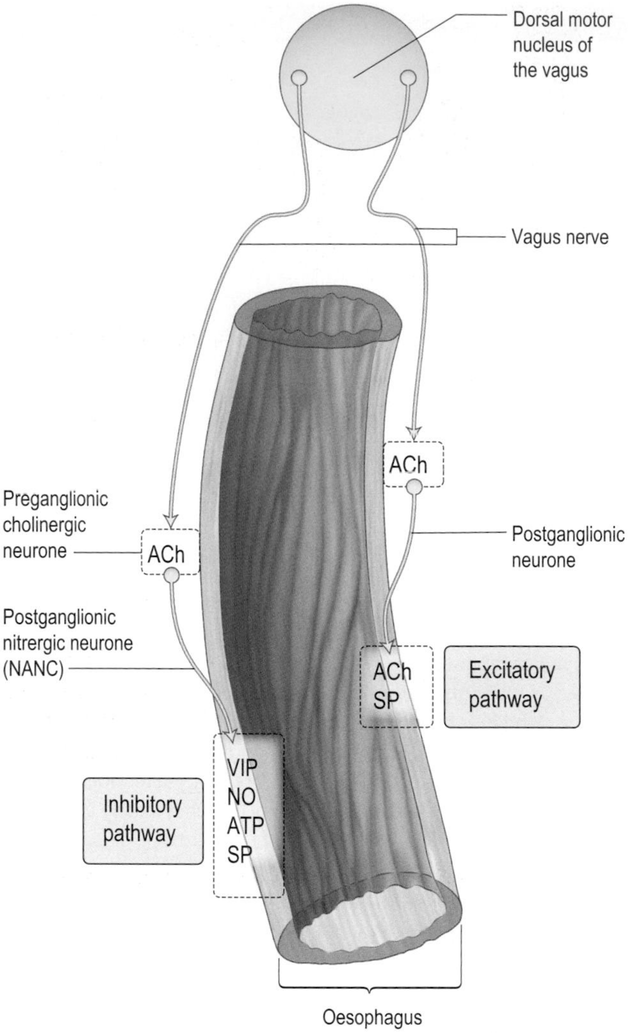

Figure 13.6 Innervation of the oesophagus. The excitatory pathway consists of vagal preganglionic neurones releasing acetylcholine (ACh), connecting to postganglionic neurones that release ACh and substance P (SP). The inhibitory pathway consists of vagal preganglionic neurones releasing ACh, connecting to postganglionic neurones that release nitric oxide (NO), vasoactive intestinal peptide (VIP), adenosine triphosphate (ATP) and SP.

mouth. The characteristics of the progression of dysphagia to solids can be helpful. For example, intermittent slow progression with a history of heartburn suggests a benign peptic stricture; relentless progression over a few weeks suggests a malignant stricture. The slow onset of dysphagia for solids and liquids at the same time suggests a motility disorder, such as achalasia (see pp. 371–372). The causes are shown in ***Box 13.8***.
- ***Odynophagia***. This term describes pain during the act of swallowing and is suggestive of oesophagitis. Causes include reflux, infection, chemical oesophagitis due to drugs such as bisphosphonates or slow-release potassium, or oesophageal stenosis.
- ***Substernal discomfort/heartburn***. This is a common symptom of reflux of gastric contents into the oesophagus. It is usually a retrosternal burning pain that can spread to the neck, across the chest; when severe, it can be difficult to distinguish from the pain of ischaemic heart disease. It is often worst lying down at night, when gravity promotes reflux, or on bending or stooping.
- ***Regurgitation***. This is the effortless reflux of oesophageal contents into the mouth and pharynx. Uncommon in normal subjects, it occurs frequently in patients with gastro-oesophageal reflux disease or organic stenosis.

? Box 13.8 Causes of dysphagia

Disease of mouth and tongue
- e.g. Candidiasis

Neuromuscular disorders
- Pharyngeal disorders
- Bulbar palsy (e.g. motor neurone disease, stroke)
- Myasthenia gravis

Oesophageal motility disorders
- Achalasia
- Scleroderma
- Diffuse oesophageal spasm
- Presbyoesophagus
- Diabetes mellitus
- Chagas' disease

Extrinsic pressure
- Mediastinal glands
- Goitre
- Enlarged left atrium

Intrinsic lesion
- Foreign body
- Stricture:
  - Benign – peptic, corrosive
  - Malignant – carcinoma
- Lower oesophageal ring
- Oesophageal web
- Pharyngeal pouch

Signs

The main sign of oesophageal disease is weight loss due to reduced food intake. Cervical lymphadenopathy with cancer is uncommon. Very rarely, a pharyngeal pouch may be seen to swell the neck during drinking.

Investigation of oesophageal disorders

- ***Barium swallow and meal***. A radiological contrast study of the oesophagus can give both anatomical and functional information, but on the whole has been superseded by gastroscopy as the initial investigation of choice.
- ***Gastroscopy***. This is the usual first-line investigation for suspected oesophageal disorders.
- ***Manometry (Fig. 13.7)***. This is performed by passing a catheter through the nose into the oesophagus and measuring the pressures generated within the oesophagus. It is used to assess oesophageal motor activity and measure pressures within the sphincters. It is not a primary investigation and should be performed only when the diagnosis has not been achieved by history, radiological imaging or endoscopy. It is the gold standard investigation for motility disorders of the oesophagus such as achalasia. Recordings are usually made over a short time period or, much more rarely, for up to 72 h. High-resolution manometry has superseded conventional manometry and the greater concentration of pressure sensors enables the identification of a wider range of abnormalities of oesophageal function with a greater diagnostic accuracy.
- ***Ambulatory pH monitoring***. A pH-sensitive probe is positioned in the lower oesophagus and is used to identify acid reflux episodes (pH <4). Catheter and implantable sensors are available, with devices in place for 24 h, up to 96 h; both are insensitive to alkali. Although only 5–10% of recorded acid reflux episodes are perceived by the patient, pH is a valuable means of correlating episodes of acid reflux with patient's symptoms.

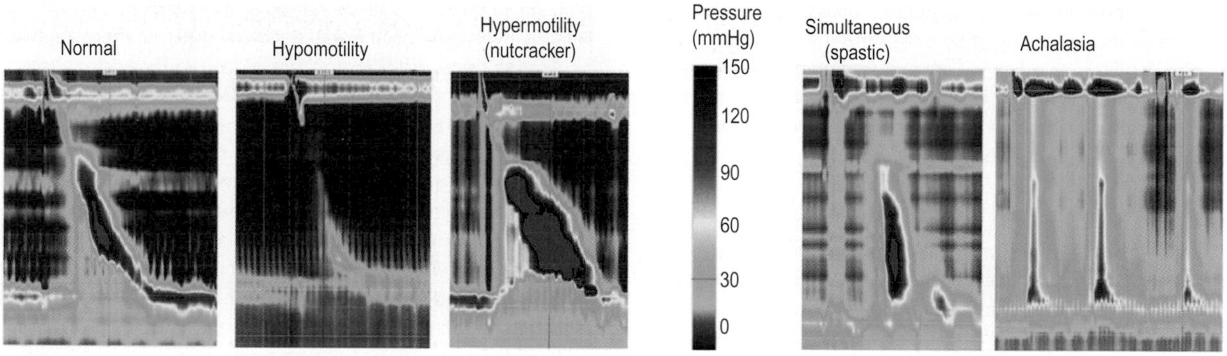

Figure 13.7 High-resolution manometry of the oesophagus. Results are shown in the normal subject and in patients with hypomotility, hypermotility, simultaneous (spastic) contractions and achalasia. Changes in colour reflect changes in pressure.

- ***Impedance***. A catheter is used to measure the resistance to flow of 'alternating current' in the contents of the oesophagus. Combined with measurement of pH, it allows assessment of acid, weakly acid, alkaline and gaseous reflux, which is helpful in understanding the symptoms that are produced by a non-acid reflux, particularly in those patients who continue to have symptoms while on proton pump inhibition. Treatment is, however, difficult in these conditions and usually involves either alginates or pro-motility agents, or a combination of the two.

Gastro-oesophageal reflux disease (GORD)

Pathophysiology

The reflux of gastric acid, pepsin, bile and duodenal contents back into the oesophagus can be influenced by many factors that overcome the innate defence mechanisms, primarily the lower oesophageal sphincter. Between swallows, the muscles of the oesophagus are relaxed, except for those of the two sphincters. The LOS in the distal oesophagus remains closed because of the unique property of the muscle, and relaxes when swallowing is initiated (see p. 365). ***Transient lower (o)esophageal sphincter relaxations*** (TLESRs) are part of normal physiology, but occur more frequently in patients with gastro-oesophageal reflux disease (GORD), allowing gastric acid to flow back into the oesophagus ***(Fig. 13.8)***. Increased abdominal pressure (pregnancy) and low LOS pressure also predispose to GORD.

Other anti-reflux mechanisms involve the intra-abdominal segment of the oesophagus, which acts as a flap valve. In addition, the mucosal rosette, formed by folds of the gastric mucosa, and the crural diaphragm at the LOS, which contracts and acts like a pinchcock, prevent acid reflux. A hiatus hernia can impair this mechanism ***(Box 13.9)***. Normally, the oesophagus is also 'cleared' rapidly of refluxate by secondary peristalsis, gravity and salivary bicarbonate.

The clinical features of reflux occur when the anti-reflux mechanisms fail, allowing acidic gastric contents to make prolonged contact with the lower oesophageal mucosa. The sphincter relaxes transiently, independently of a swallow, after meals, and this is the cause of almost all reflux in normals and about two-thirds of GORD patients.

The role of the ***acid pocket*** in GORD has gained more credence in the last 5 years. Food and fluid generally increase the gastric pH, but the acid pocket is an area of unbuffered gastric acid that accumulates postprandially in the proximal stomach. It serves as a reservoir for acid reflux, particularly in individuals with a hiatus hernia where the distal oesophagus is supradiaphragmatic, especially on lying flat. This can be specifically targeted with an antacid–alginate combination.

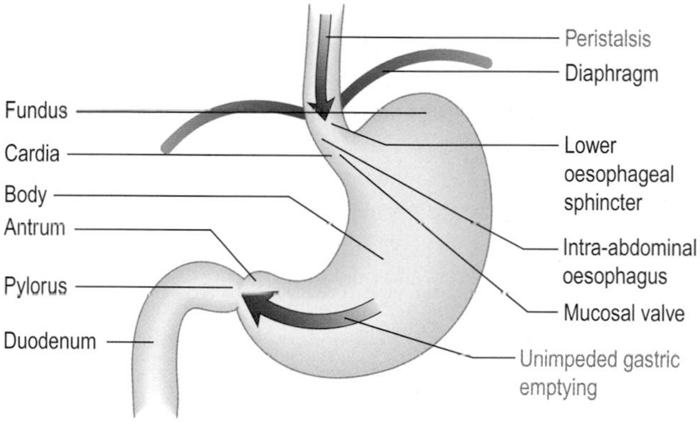

Figure 13.8 The main anti-reflux mechanisms. These are shown on the right.

Box 13.9 Hiatus hernia

Sliding hiatus hernia

The oesophageal–gastric junction and part of the stomach 'slide' through the hiatus so that it lies above the diaphragm.

- Present in 30% of people over 50 years
- Produces no symptoms – any symptoms are due to reflux

Rolling or para-oesophageal hernia

Part of the fundus of the stomach prolapses through the hiatus alongside the oesophagus.

- The lower oesophageal sphincter remains below the diaphragm and remains competent
- Occasionally, severe pain occurs due to volvulus or strangulation

Oesophageal mucosal defence mechanisms

- ***Surface***. Mucus and the unstirred water layer trap bicarbonate. This mechanism is a weak buffering mechanism compared to that in the stomach and duodenum.
- ***Epithelium***. The apical cell membranes and the junctional complexes between cells act to limit diffusion of H^+ into the cells. In oesophagitis, the junctional complexes are damaged, leading to increased H^+ diffusion and cellular damage.
- ***Postepithelium***. Bicarbonate normally buffers acid in the cells and intracellular spaces. Hydrogen ions impair the growth and replication of damaged cells.

- ***Sensory mechanisms***. Acid stimulates primary sensory neurones in the oesophagus by activating the vanilloid receptor-1 (VR1). This can initiate inflammation and release of pro-inflammatory substances from the tissue and produce pain. Pain can also be due to contraction of longitudinal oesophageal muscle.

Clinical features

Heartburn is the major feature. The burning chest pain is aggravated by bending, stooping and lying down, which promote acid exposure, and may be relieved by oral antacids and alginates. The patient typically complains of pain on drinking hot liquids or alcohol.

Factors associated with GORD are shown in ***Box 13.10***.

The correlation between heartburn and oesophagitis is poor. Some patients have mild oesophagitis but severe heartburn, while others have severe oesophagitis in the absence of symptoms, and can present with haematemesis or iron deficiency anaemia from chronic blood loss. Psychosocial factors are often determinants of symptom severity, with heartburn increased during times of stress.

Differentiation of cardiac and oesophageal pain can be difficult; 20% of cases seen in emergency departments have GORD ***(Box 13.11)***. A trial of antacid therapy is often useful, resolving reflux-induced pain, before progressing to 24-hour pH studies only if symptoms persist.

Regurgitation of food and acid into the mouth occurs, particularly on bending or lying flat. Aspiration pneumonia is unusual without an accompanying obstruction, but cough and asthma can occur and respond slowly (1–4 months) to a proton pump inhibitor (PPI).

Laryngopharyngeal reflux disease (LPRD) is the transport of gastric contents into the larynx and pharynx, usually, although not exclusively, in the context of GORD. Heartburn may be one of the associated symptoms but cough, hoarse voice, postnasal drip and asthma are more frequently seen, but are not common.

Diagnosis and investigations

The ***clinical*** diagnosis can usually be made without investigation. Unless there are alarm signs, especially dysphagia (see p. 365–366), patients under the age of 45 years can safely be treated initially without investigations. If investigation is required, there are two aims:

- ***Assess oesophagitis and hiatal hernia by endoscopy***. If there is oesophagitis ***(Fig. 13.9)*** or Barrett's oesophagus (see pp. 370–371), reflux is confirmed.
- ***Document reflux by intraluminal monitoring (Fig. 13.10)***. Twenty-four-hour intraluminal pH monitoring or impedance combined with manometry is helpful if there is no response to PPIs and should always be performed to confirm reflux before surgery. A DeMeester score is calculated, each reflux episode being defined as an oesophageal pH of <4; a score of >14.72 indicates reflux. There should also be a good correlation between reflux (pH <4.0) and symptoms. It is also helpful to

Box 13.10 Factors associated with gastro-oesophageal reflux

- Pregnancy or obesity
- Fat, chocolate, coffee or alcohol ingestion
- Large meals
- Cigarette smoking
- Drugs – antimuscarinic, calcium-channel blockers, nitrates
- Systemic sclerosis
- Treatment for achalasia
- Hiatus hernia

Box 13.11 Classic features of the pain of gastro-oesophageal reflux and cardiac ischaemia

Reflux pain: burning, worse on bending, stooping or lying down

- Seldom radiates to the arms
- Worse with hot drinks or alcohol
- Relieved by antacids

Cardiac ischaemic pain

- Gripping or crushing
- Radiates to neck or left arm
- Worse with exercise
- Accompanied by dyspnoea

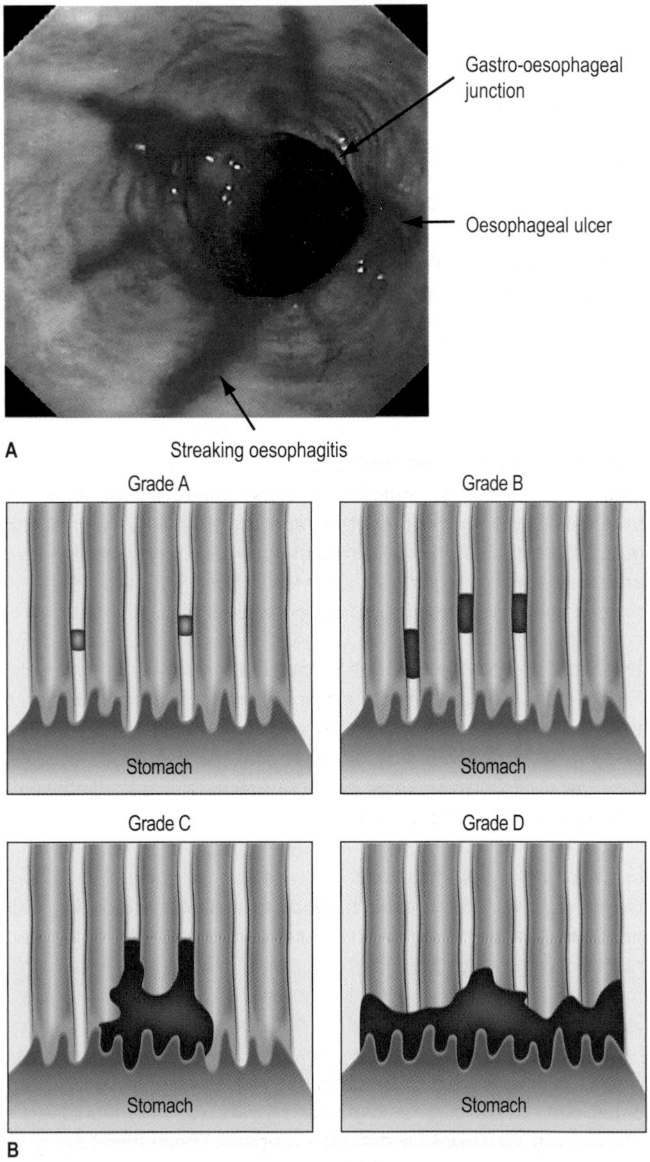

Figure 13.9 Oesophagitis. A. Oesophagitis seen on endoscopy. **B.** Los Angeles classification of oesophagitis. *Grade A*=mucosal breaks confined to the mucosal folds, each no longer than 5 mm. *Grade B*=at least one mucosal break longer than 5 mm confined to the mucosal fold but not continuous between two folds. *Grade C*=mucosal breaks that are continuous between the tops of mucosal folds but not circumferential. *Grade D*=extensive mucosal breaks engaging at least 75% of the oesophageal circumference.

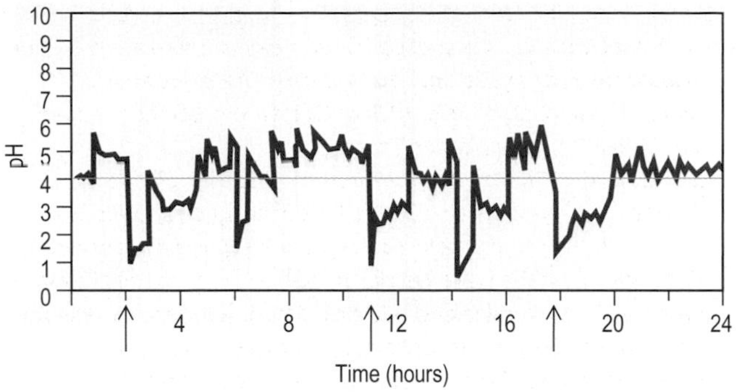

Figure 13.10 Twenty-four-hour intraluminal pH monitoring. Five reflux episodes (pH <4) occurred but only three produced symptoms (arrowed).

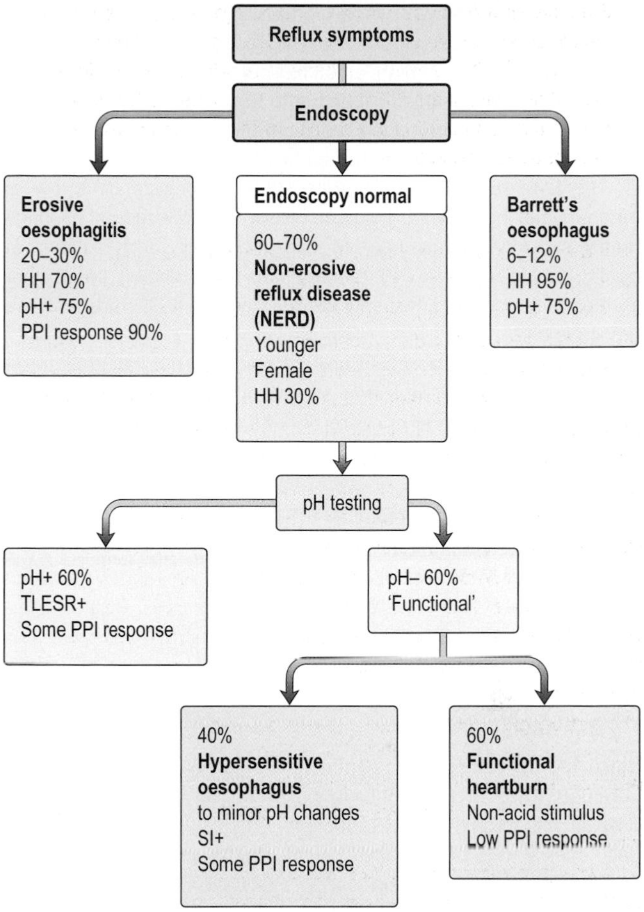

Figure 13.11 Outcome of patients with reflux symptoms. HH, hiatus hernia; pH+, meets standard criteria for excessive acid reflux on intraluminal testing; pH–, does not meet standard criteria for excessive acid reflux; PPI, proton pump inhibitor SI+, symptom index; TLESR, transient lower (o)esophageal sphincter relaxation.

assess oesophageal dysmotility as a potential cause of the symptoms, leading to impaired oesophageal clearance.

Management

Approximately half of patients with reflux symptoms in primary care can be treated successfully with simple antacids, loss of weight and raising the head of the bed at night. Precipitating factors should be avoided, with dietary measures, reduction in alcohol and caffeine consumption, and cessation of smoking. These measures are simple to say but difficult to carry out, though they are useful in mild disease in compliant patients.

Drugs

Alginate-containing antacids

Alginate-containing antacids (10 mL three times daily) are the most frequently used 'over-the-counter' agents for GORD. They form a gel or 'foam raft' with gastric contents to reduce reflux. Magnesium-containing antacids tend to cause diarrhoea while aluminium-containing compounds may cause constipation.

Dopamine antagonist prokinetic agents

The dopamine antagonist prokinetic agents metoclopramide and domperidone are occasionally helpful, as they enhance peristalsis and speed gastric emptying, but there are few data to substantiate this. The role of domperidone has been limited still further following reports of serious cardiac side-effects.

H_2-receptor antagonists

H_2-receptor antagonists (e.g. cimetidine, ranitidine, famotidine and nizatidine) are frequently used for acid suppression if antacids fail, as they can easily be obtained.

Proton pump inhibitors

Proton pump inhibitors (PPIs; omeprazole, rabeprazole, lansoprazole, pantoprazole, esomeprazole) inhibit gastric hydrogen/potassium-adenosine triphosphatase. PPIs reduce gastric acid secretion by up to 90% and are the drugs of choice for all but mild cases. Most patients with GORD will respond well, with approximately 60% symptom-free after 4 weeks of a once-daily PPI. Patients with severe symptoms may need twice-daily PPIs and prolonged treatment, often for years. Once oesophageal sensitivity has normalized, a lower dose, e.g. omeprazole 10 mg, may be sufficient for maintenance. Long-term PPI prescription is not uncommon, and although some recent data have suggested side-effects such as osteoporosis, and an increase in gastrointestinal infections such as *Clostridium difficile*, these are uncommon and tend to occur in at-risk patients.

Patients who do not respond to a PPI and have continuing symptoms with a normal endoscopy are described as having ***non-erosive reflux disease (NERD) (Fig. 13.11)***. These patients are usually female and often the symptoms are functional, although a small group have a 'hypersensitive' oesophagus, giving discomfort with only slight changes in pH. Isomers of some of the original PPIs (e.g. dexlansoprazole) have the benefit of more effective gastric acid inhibition over a longer time period, as their metabolism of the active metabolite is slower.

Endoluminal gastroplication

In this endoscopic procedure, multiple plications or pleats are made below the gastro-oesophageal junction. Randomized controlled trials have shown benefit with reduction in heartburn, acid reflux episodes and PPI usage, but not sustained improvements in the oesophageal pH measurements.

Surgery

Surgery should never be performed for a hiatus hernia alone. The best predictors of a good surgical result are typical reflux symptoms with documented acid reflux, which correlates with symptoms and response to a PPI. With such highly selected cases in experienced hands, the laparoscopic Nissen fundoplication has a satisfaction rate of over 90% at 5 years, and available 10-year data show satisfaction rates remain high at 88%. Current surgical techniques return the oesophagogastric junction to the abdominal cavity, mobilize the gastric fundus, close the diaphragmatic crura snugly and involve a short, tension-free fundoplication.

The ***Linx reflux management system*** consists of a row of magnets that increase LOS closure pressure, allowing food passage during swallowing; it is inserted laparoscopically. Improvement in quality of life with no PPI therapy has been shown but further studies are necessary. Patients cannot have an MRI study with the device *in situ*.

Indications for operation are not clear-cut but include intolerance to medication, the desire for freedom from medication, the expense of therapy and concern about long-term side-effects.

The most common cause of mechanical fundoplication failure is recurrent hiatus hernia.

Patients with oesophageal dysmotility unrelated to acid reflux, those with no response to PPIs and those with underlying functional bowel disease should rarely have surgery.

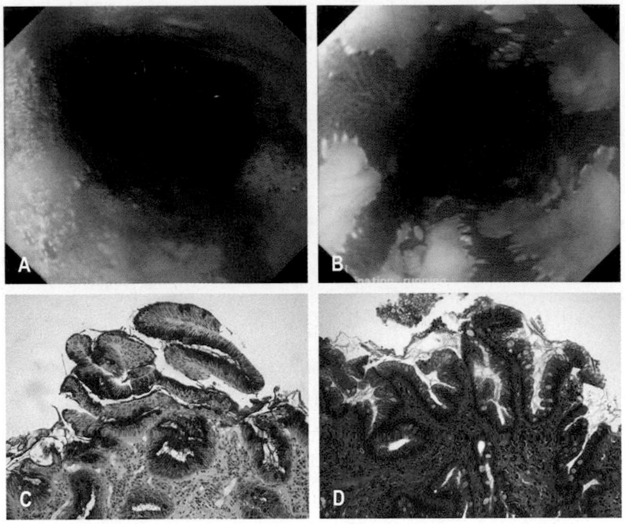

Figure 13.12 Barrett's oesophagus. A. Endoscopic picture of Barrett's oesophagus. **B.** Endoscopic narrow band imaging of Barrett's mucosa. **C.** Alcian blue staining of Barrett's mucosa highlighting the blue-staining goblet cells. **D.** Haematoxylin and eosin staining of Barrett's columnar mucosa.

Complications of gastro-oesophageal reflux disease

Peptic stricture

Since the advent of PPIs, peptic strictures have become far less common. They usually occur in patients over the age of 60 and present with intermittent dysphagia for solids, which worsens gradually over a long period. Mild cases may respond to PPIs alone. More severe cases need endoscopic dilatation and long-term PPI therapy. Surgery is required if medical treatment fails.

Barrett's oesophagus

Barrett's oesophagus ***(Fig. 13.12)*** is a condition in which part of the normal oesophageal squamous epithelium is replaced by metaplastic columnar mucosa to form a segment of 'columnar-lined oesophagus' (CLO). It is a complication of GORD and there is almost always a hiatus hernia present.

Diagnosis and classification

The diagnosis is made if endoscopy shows proximal displacement of the squamocolumnar mucosal junction and biopsy demonstrates columnar lining above the proximal gastric folds (>1 cm); intestinal metaplasia is no longer a requirement of the British Society of Gastroenterology definition but is central to the American College of Gastroenterology guidelines. Barrett's oesophagus may be seen as a continual circumferential sheet, as finger-like projections extending upwards from the squamocolumnar junction or as islands of columnar mucosa interspersed with areas of squamous mucosa. The Prague classification ***(Fig. 13.13)*** is used for recording the endoscopic distribution, stating both the length of circumferential CLO (C measurement) and the maximum length (M measurement), the distance from the top of the gastric folds to the most proximal tongue of the columnar mucosa.

Central obesity increases the risk of Barrett's by 4.3 times. Long-segment (>3 cm) and short-segment (<3 cm) Barrett's is found, respectively, in 5% and 15% of patients undergoing endoscopy for reflux symptoms. Barrett's is also often found incidentally in endoscoped patients without reflux symptoms. It is most common in middle-aged obese men. The major concern is that approximately 0.12–0.5% of Barrett's patients develop oesophageal adenocarcinoma per year, the majority, probably, through a gradual transformation from intestinal metaplasia to low-grade then high-grade dysplasia, before invasive adenocarcinoma. Barrett's increases the chance of developing oesophageal adenocarcinoma 30- to 50-fold in early studies but recent studies have shown the risk to be much lower and closer to a 1% lifetime risk in the typical patient.

Because of the poor correlation between Barrett's oesophagus and symptoms, screening is not recommended; however, in the absence of high-quality trial evidence, endoscopic surveillance is recommended by some. This involves inspection of the oesophageal mucosa with a high-definition gastroscope, and the taking of targeted biopsies of any focally abnormal tissue in addition to random biopsies from all four quadrants (every 1–2 cm) of the CLO. The interval between endoscopies is determined by the length of the CLO and the degree of cellular disturbance within it. High-grade dysplasia (HGD) is usually associated with endoscopically visible nodules or ulceration, optimally visualized with a high-definition endoscope. Chromo-endoscopy (the topical application of stains or pigments via the endoscope), narrow band and autofluorescence imaging may aid the diagnosis of dysplasia and carcinoma. Endoscopic technology has improved the detection of pre-malignant lesions, enabling their removal by either endoscopic mucosal resection (EMR) or endoscopic submucosal dissection, therefore preventing surgical oesophagectomy.

If ***low-grade dysplasia*** is found on endoscopic surveillance, a repeat endoscopy with quadrantic biopsies every 1 cm is usually performed within 6 months, while on high-dose proton pump inhibition. Long-term surveillance and more aggressive endoscopic treatment of this group are the subjects of ongoing research.

If ***high-grade dysplasia*** is found, it is usually in the context of an endoscopically visible lesion, which, if nodular, is removed by endoscopic mucosal resection for more accurate histological staging. If high-grade dysplasia is detected in the absence of any endoscopically visible lesion, high-dose proton pump inhibition is started and repeat biopsies taken within 3 months. Endoscopic ultrasound is frequently used to stage this patient group more

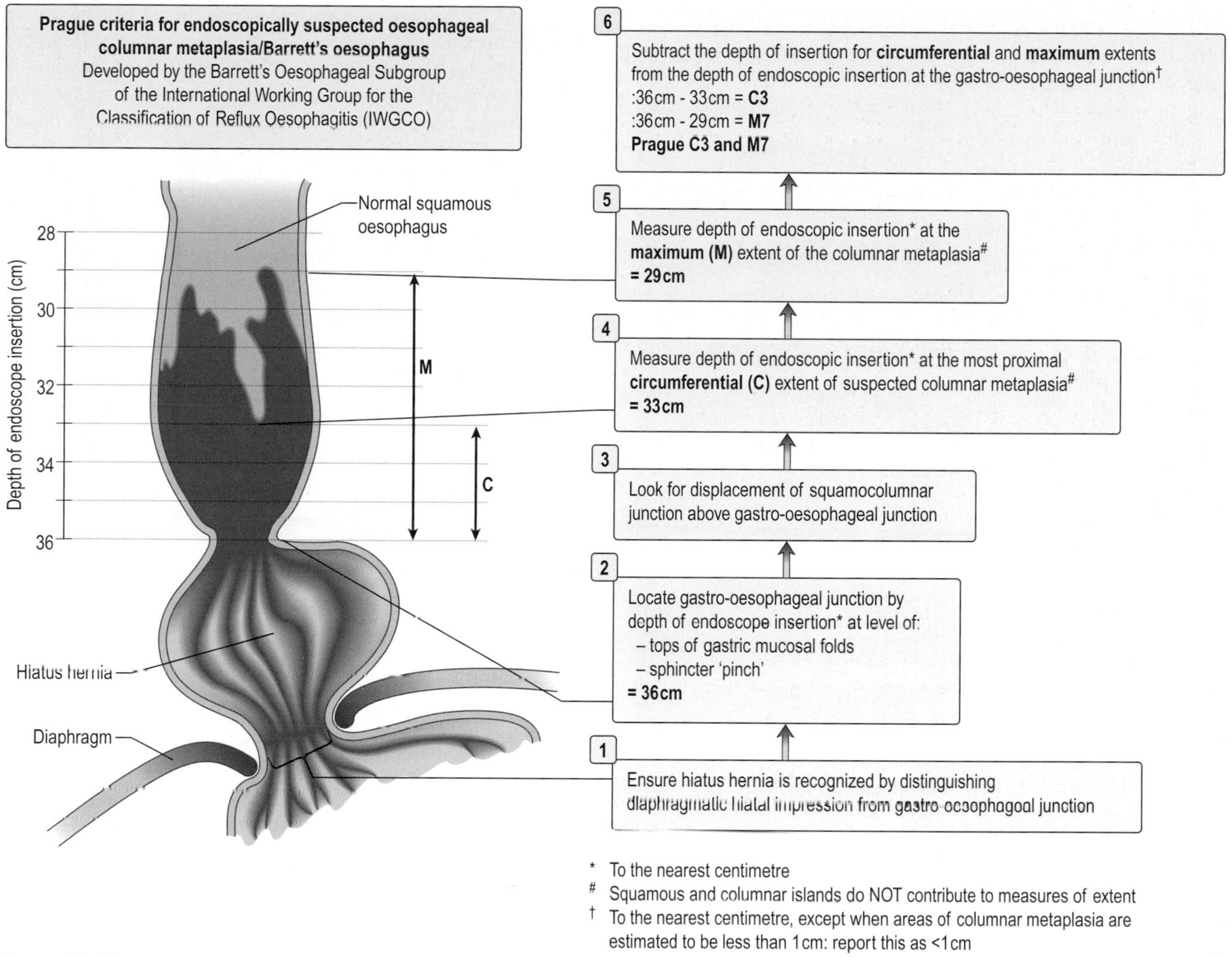

Figure 13.13 The Prague criteria for endoscopically suspected oesophageal columnar metaplasia/Barrett's oesophagus.

accurately, in order to exclude cancer and associated significant lymphadenopathy.

Radiofrequency ablation (RFA) has superseded photodynamic therapy as the technique of choice for endoscopic treatment of dysplasia within Barrett's segments following removal of any nodular lesions, returning the oesophagus to squamous lining. The benefit of RFA in low-grade dysplasia is currently under evaluation.

Motility disorders

Achalasia

Achalasia is characterized by oesophageal aperistalsis and impaired relaxation of the lower oesophageal sphincter. The lower oesophageal pressure is elevated in more than half of patients.

Clinical features

The incidence of achalasia is 1:100 000 and is equal in males and females. It occurs at all ages but is rare in childhood. Patients usually have a long history of intermittent dysphagia, characteristically for both liquids and solids from the onset. Regurgitation of food from the dilated oesophagus occurs, particularly at night, and aspiration pneumonia is a complication. Spontaneous chest pain occurs and is said to be due to oesophageal 'spasm'; it may be misdiagnosed as cardiac pain. Dysphagia may be mild and accepted by the patient as normal; weight loss is usually minimal.

Pathogenesis

The aetiology of achalasia is unknown, with autoimmune, neurodegenerative and viral aetiologies all being postulated. A similar clinical picture is seen in chronic Chagas' disease (American trypanosomiasis; see pp. 302–303), where there is damage to the neural plexus of the gut.

Histopathology shows inflammation of the myenteric plexus of the oesophagus with reduction of ganglion cell numbers. Cholinergic innervation appears to be preserved. Reduction in nitric oxide synthase-containing neurones has been shown by immunohistochemical staining. Pharmacological studies in patients with achalasia support the selective loss of ***inhibitory***, nitrergic neurones.

Differential diagnosis

The differential diagnosis of achalasia worldwide includes genetic syndromes, infectious diseases, neoplasms and chronic inflammatory conditions.

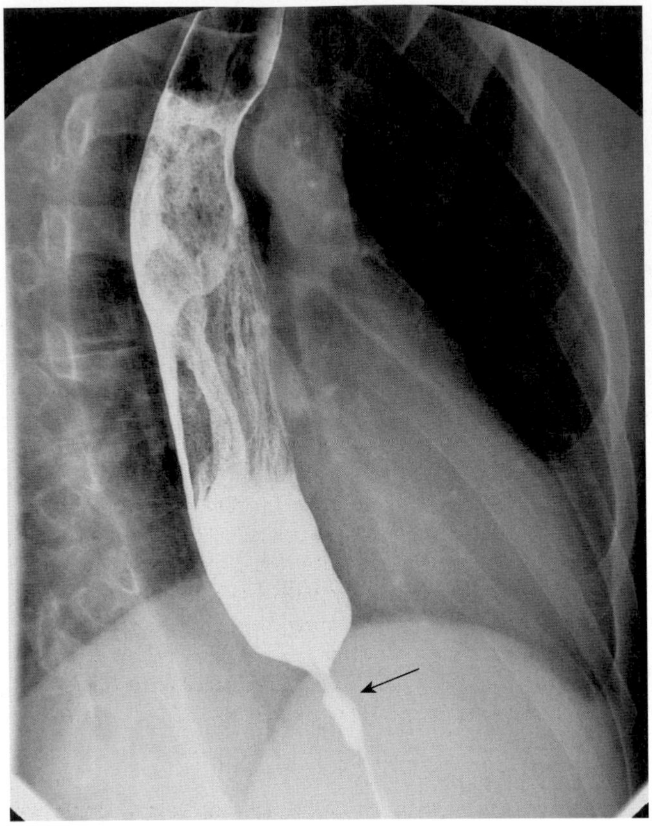

Figure 13.14 Barium swallow showing achalasia. There is an atonic body of the oesophagus and a narrowed distal end (arrowed). Note the food residue in the dilated oesophagus.

Investigations

- ***Chest X-ray*** shows a dilated oesophagus, sometimes with a fluid level seen behind the heart. The fundal gas shadow is absent.
- ***Barium swallow*** shows lack of peristalsis and often synchronous contractions in the body of the oesophagus, sometimes with dilatation. The lower end shows a 'bird's beak' due to failure of the sphincter to relax ***(Fig. 13.14)***.
- ***Oesophagoscopy*** is performed to exclude a carcinoma at the lower end of the oesophagus, as this can produce a similar X-ray appearance. When there is marked dilatation, a 24-h liquid-only diet and a washout, prior to endoscopy, are useful to remove food debris. In true achalasia, the endoscope passes through the LOS with little resistance.
- ***CT scan*** excludes distal oesophageal cancer.
- ***Manometry*** shows aperistalsis of the oesophagus and failure of relaxation of the LOS (see ***Fig. 13.7***).

Management

All current forms of treatment for achalasia are ***palliative***. Drug therapy rarely produces satisfactory or durable relief; nifedipine (20 mg sublingually), nitrates or sildenafil can be tried initially.

Endoscopic and surgical therapies are equally effective. Endoscopic dilatation of the LOS, using a pneumatic balloon under X-ray control, weakens the sphincter and is initially successful in 80% of cases. About 50% of patients require a second or third dilatation in the first 5 years. There is a low but significant risk of perforation. Intrasphincteric injection of botulinum toxin A produces satisfactory initial results but the effects wear off within months. Further injections can be given. It is safer and simpler than dilatation, so may be valuable in patients at risk of death if a perforation occurs. Neither pneumatic dilatation nor botulinum toxin works as well in younger patients.

Surgical division of the LOS, Heller's operation, usually performed laparoscopically, is the surgical treatment of choice. Per oral endoscopic myotomy (POEM) is a novel technique, which is a division of the LOS using a gastroscope. The early results show great promise.

Reflux oesophagitis complicates all procedures and aperistalsis of the oesophagus remains.

Complications

There is a slight increase in the incidence of squamous carcinoma of the oesophagus in both treated and untreated cases (7% after 25 years).

Systemic sclerosis

The oesophagus is involved in almost all patients with this disease. Diminished peristalsis and oesophageal clearance, detected manometrically (see ***Fig. 13.7***) or by barium swallow, is due to replacement of the smooth muscle by fibrous tissue. LOS pressure is decreased, allowing reflux with consequent mucosal damage. Strictures may develop. Initially, there are no symptoms, but dysphagia and heartburn occur as the oesophagus becomes more severely involved. Similar motility abnormalities may be found in other autoimmune rheumatic disorders, particularly if Raynaud's phenomenon is present. Treatment is as for reflux disease (see pp. 369–370) and benign stricture.

Diffuse oesophageal spasm

This is a severe form of oesophageal dysmotility that can sometimes produce retrosternal chest pain and dysphagia. It can accompany GORD. Swallowing is accompanied by bizarre and marked contractions of the oesophagus without normal peristalsis (see ***Fig. 13.7***). On barium swallow, the appearance may be that of a 'corkscrew' oesophagus. However, asymptomatic oesophageal 'dysmotility' is not infrequent, particularly in patients over the age of 60 years.

A variant of diffuse oesophageal spasm is the 'nutcracker' oesophagus, which is characterized by very high-amplitude peristalsis (pressures >200 mmHg) within the oesophagus. Chest pain is more common than dysphagia.

Management

True oesophageal spasm producing severe symptoms is uncommon and treatment is often difficult. PPIs may be successful if reflux is a factor. Antispasmodics, nitrates, calcium-channel blockers and γ-aminobutyric acid (GABA) receptor agonists (e.g. baclofen) are used. Occasionally, balloon dilatation or even longitudinal oesophageal myotomy is necessary.

Miscellaneous motility disorders

Abnormalities of motility that occasionally produce dysphagia are found in the elderly, and in diabetes mellitus, myotonic dystrophy, oculopharyngeal muscular dystrophy and myasthenia gravis, as well as neurological disorders involving the brainstem.

Other oesophageal disorders

Oesophageal diverticulum

Diverticula occur:

- immediately ***above*** the upper oesophageal sphincter (pharyngeal pouch – Zenker's diverticulum; see p. 1322).
- near the ***middle*** of the oesophagus (traction diverticulum due to inflammation, or associated with diffuse oesophageal spasm or mediastinal fibrosis)
- just above the ***lower*** oesophageal sphincter (epiphrenic diverticulum – associated with achalasia).

Usually detected incidentally on a barium swallow performed for other reasons, these are often asymptomatic. Dysphagia and regurgitation can occur with a pharyngeal pouch, becoming more problematic as the diverticula increase in size (see p. 1322). These can be treated surgically and endoscopically.

Rings and webs

An oesophageal web is a thin, membranous tissue flap covered with squamous epithelium. Most acquired webs are located anteriorly in the postcricoid region of the cervical oesophagus and are well seen on barium swallow. They may produce dysphagia. In the ***Plummer–Vinson syndrome*** (or ***Paterson–Brown–Kelly syndrome***), a web is associated with chronic iron deficiency anaemia, glossitis and angular stomatitis. This rare syndrome affects mainly women and its aetiology is not understood. The web may be difficult to see at endoscopy and is often ruptured unintentionally by the passage of the endoscope. Dilatation of the web is rarely necessary. Iron is given for the iron deficiency.

Lower oesophageal rings

Lower oesophageal rings are of two types:

1. ***Mucosal (Schatzki's ring, also called B ring)*** is located at the squamocolumnar mucosal junction and is common ***(Fig. 13.15)***. It is associated with a characteristic history of intermittent bolus obstruction.
2. ***Muscular (A ring)*** is located proximal to the mucosal ring and is uncommon. It is covered by squamous epithelium and may cause dysphagia.

Management for these rings is usually with reassurance and dietary advice, but dilatation is occasionally necessary. After a single dilatation, 68% of patients with Schatzki's rings are symptom-free at 1 year and 35% remain symptom-free after 2 years, but only 11% are symptom-free at 3 years. Many also respond to oral PPI, either alone or with dilatation.

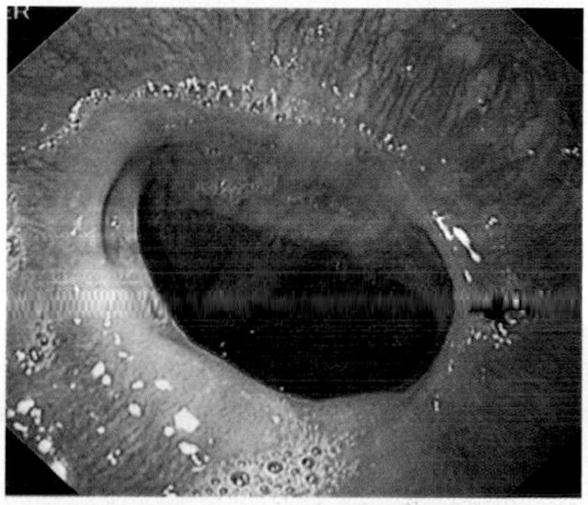

Figure 13.15 Schatzki's ring. Endoscopic view.

Benign oesophageal stricture

Peptic stricture ***(Fig. 13.16)*** secondary to reflux is the most common cause of benign strictures (for treatment, see p. 370). They also occur after the ingestion of corrosives, radiotherapy, sclerotherapy of varices and prolonged nasogastric intubation. Dysphagia is usually treated by endoscopic dilatation. Surgery is sometimes required.

Oesophageal infections

Infection is a cause of painful swallowing and is seen particularly in immunosuppressed (e.g. on chemotherapy) and debilitated patients, and in those with acquired immunodeficiency syndrome (AIDS). Infection can occur with:

- *Candida*
- herpes simplex
- cytomegalovirus
- *Mycobacterium tuberculosis*.

It is occasionally difficult to distinguish between these disorders on oesophagoscopy, as only widespread ulceration is seen. In candidiasis, the characteristic white plaques are frequently found; oral candidiasis is not always present. The diagnosis of *Candida* infection can be confirmed by examining a direct smear taken at endoscopy, but often infections are mixed and cultures and biopsies must be performed. Tuberculosis causes deep ulceration with associated mediastinal lymphadenopathy.

Management

Most patients on large doses of immunosuppressive agents are treated prophylactically for candidiasis with nystatin, fluconazole or amphotericin. Antifungal or antiviral treatment is prescribed appropriately for other infections.

Mallory–Weiss syndrome

This is described on page 387.

Eosinophilic oesophagitis

Eosinophils can be seen in the oesophageal mucosa (which is usually devoid of eosinophils microscopically) due to a variety of causes, such as eosinophilic (or allergic) oesophagitis and GORD.

Eosinophilic oesophagitis ***(Fig. 13.17)*** is increasingly recognized but its pathogenesis is unknown. There may be a personal or family history of allergic disorders, such as food allergy, eczema or asthma.

Patients present with a long history of dysphagia, food impaction, 'heartburn' and oesophageal pain caused by the

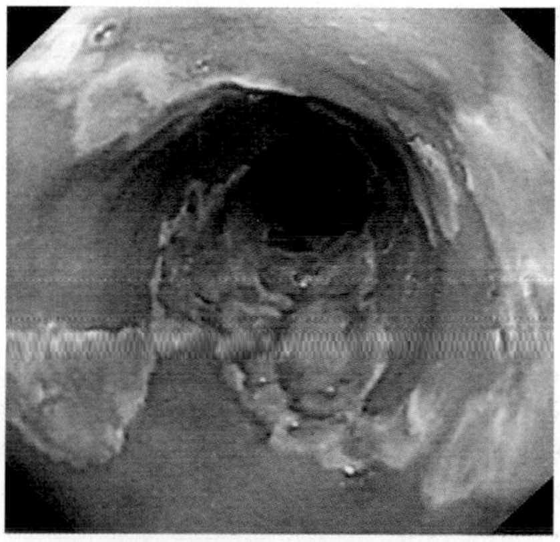

Figure 13.16 Benign oesophageal reflux stricture. Endoscopic view.

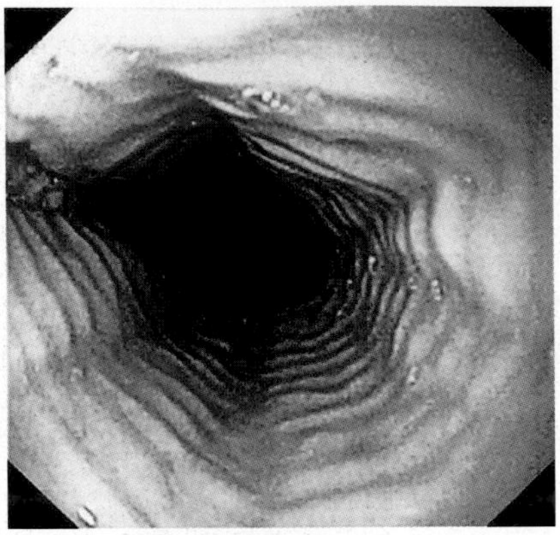

Figure 13.17 Eosinophilic oesophagitis.

eosinophil-induced oesophageal inflammation. Usually, the patient is male and white, and has an average age at diagnosis of 35, but eosinophilic oesophagitis is becoming more common in children.

Typical endoscopic abnormalities include mucosal furrowing, loss of vascular pattern due to a thickened mucosa, plaques of eosinophilic surface exudate and prominent circular folds, but the oesophagus may appear macroscopically normal. Reflux oesophagitis and Schatzki's rings may coexist. Endoscopic forceps biopsies should be taken throughout the oesophagus for histology and eosinophil numbers calculated.

The eosinophilic infiltration of the oesophagus due to ***reflux disease*** tends to have a different microscopic appearance and fewer eosinophils.

Management

First-line treatment is with topical steroids, such as swallowing fluticasone spray or budesonide syrup. If this is not effective, systemic steroids or empirical elimination diets may also be used (dietary treatment is more beneficial in children). A cohort of patients respond to PPIs in the absence of GORD. Dilatation is sometimes necessary, with a risk of perforation of 2%.

Oesophageal perforation

Oesophageal perforation most commonly occurs at the time of endoscopic dilatation and, rarely, following insertion of a nasogastric tube, gastroscope or transoesophageal echoprobe. Patients with malignant, corrosive or post-radiotherapy strictures are more likely to perforate than those with a benign peptic stricture.

Management

This normally involves placement of an expanding covered oesophageal stent (see p. 376), which usually seals the hole. A water-soluble contrast X-ray is performed after 2–3 days to check the perforation has sealed.

Oesophageal rupture

'Spontaneous' oesophageal rupture occurs with violent vomiting (Boerhaave syndrome), producing severe chest pain and collapse in typical cases. Diagnosis can be difficult because classic symptoms are absent in about one-third of cases, and delays in presentation for medical care are common. Rupture may follow alcohol ingestion. A chest X-ray shows a hydropneumothorax. The diagnosis is made with a water-soluble contrast swallow or on CT. The mortality rate is approximately 35%, making it the most lethal perforation of the gastrointestinal tract. The best outcomes are associated with early diagnosis and definitive surgical management within 12 hours of rupture. If intervention is delayed longer than 24 hours, the mortality rate (even after surgery) rises to above 50%, and to nearly 90% after 48 hours.

Box 13.12 Risk factors for cancer of the oesophagus

Squamous cell carcinoma
- Tobacco smoking
- High alcohol intake
- Plummer–Vinson syndrome
- Achalasia
- Corrosive strictures
- Coeliac disease
- Breast cancer treated with radiotherapy
- Tylosis[a]

Adenocarcinoma
- Longstanding heartburn
- Barrett's oesophagus
- Tobacco smoking
- Obesity
- Breast cancer treated with radiotherapy
- Older age

[a] *Tylosis is a rare autosomal dominant condition with hyperkeratosis of the palms and soles.*

Oesophageal tumours

Cancer of the oesophagus

This is the sixth most common cancer worldwide. Squamous cancers occurring in the middle third account for 40% of tumours, and for 15% in the upper third. Adenocarcinomas occur in the lower third of the oesophagus and at the cardia, and represent approximately 45% of tumours. Primary small cell cancer of the oesophagus is extremely rare.

Epidemiology and aetiology

Squamous cell carcinoma

The geographic variation in incidence is greater than for any other carcinoma – often in regions very close to one another. Squamous cell carcinoma (SCC) is common in Ethiopia, China, South and East Africa, and the Caspian regions of Iran. By contrast, North, Central and West Africa have low rates.

In the UK, the incidence is 5–10 per 100 000 and SCC represents 2.2% of all malignant disease. The incidence is decreasing, in contrast to that of adenocarcinoma. SCC of the oesophagus is more common in men (2 : 1). Risk factors are shown in ***Box 13.12***.

High levels of alcohol consumption increase the risk of squamous cell cancer of the oesophagus, while tobacco use is associated with an increased incidence of both squamous cell and adenocarcinomas of the oesophagus. Smoking, obesity and low fruit and vegetable consumption are implicated in approximately 9 in 10 squamous cell cancers of the oesophagus.

Diets rich in fibre, carotenoids, folate, vitamin C and non-starchy vegetables probably decrease the risk of oesophageal cancer, whereas diets high in saturated fat, cholesterol and refined cereals have been associated with an increased risk. Red and processed meat intake has been associated with an increased risk of both oesophageal SCC and adenocarcinoma. Conversely, fish and white meat consumption have been inversely associated with risk of oesophageal SCC in case–control studies from Italy, Switzerland and Uruguay.

Adenocarcinoma

These tumours primarily arise in columnar-lined epithelium in the lower oesophagus (see Barrett's oesophagus, pp. 370–371). The

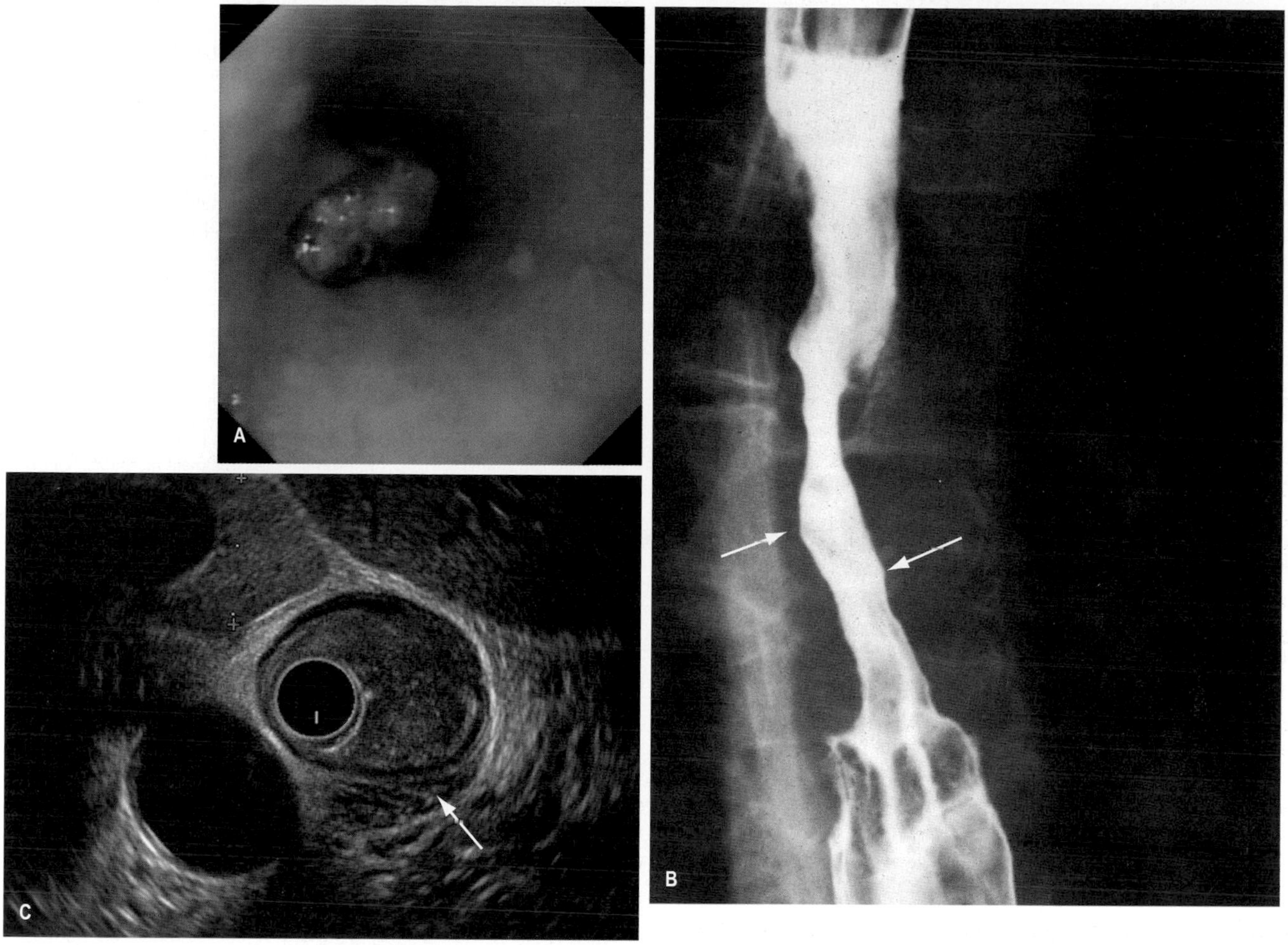

Figure 13.18 Carcinoma of the oesophagus. A. Endoscopic image. **B.** Barium swallow, showing an irregular narrowed area (arrowed) at the lower end of the oesophagus. **C.** Endoscopic ultrasound. The central concentric circles are the probe. The arrow points to a break in the muscle layer and the soft tissue mass of the carcinoma.

incidence of this tumour is increasing in western industrialized countries). It currently accounts for more than 70% of all new oesophageal cancer diagnoses. Extension of an adenocarcinoma of the gastric cardia into the oesophagus can present with the same symptoms. Previous reflux symptoms increase the risk up to eight-fold and the risk is proportional to their severity.

Clinical features

Carcinoma of the oesophagus occurs mainly in those aged 60–70 years. Dysphagia is progressive and unrelenting. Initially, there is difficulty in swallowing solids but, typically, dysphagia for liquids follows within weeks. Impaction of food causes pain but more persistent pain implies infiltration of adjacent structures.

The lesion may be ulcerative, proliferative or scirrhous, extending variably around the wall of the oesophagus to produce a stricture. Direct invasion of the surrounding structures and metastases to lymph nodes are more common than disseminated metastases. Weight loss, due to the dysphagia as well as to anorexia, is frequent. Oesophageal obstruction eventually causes difficulty in swallowing saliva, coughing and aspiration into the lungs.

Weight loss, anorexia and lymphadenopathy are the most common physical signs.

Investigations

Diagnosis

- ***Endoscopy*** provides histological proof of the carcinoma ***(Fig. 13.18A)***.
- ***Barium swallow*** can be useful where the differential diagnosis of dysphagia includes a motility disorder such as achalasia ***(Fig. 13.18B)***.

Staging

The TNM staging system is used (see p. 383); it is similar to the one used for gastric cancer. Tumour invasion of the wall of the oesophagus (T), presence of tumour in lymph nodes (N) and metastases (M) are combined into stage categories. Tumours arising in the cervical, thoracic or abdominal oesophagus, including those that arise from within 5 cm from the gastro-oesophageal junction, share the same TNM staging criteria, but recent reclassification has differentiated between ***squamous*** and ***adenocarcinoma*** cancers.

- ***CT scan*** of the thorax and upper abdomen shows the volume of the tumour, local invasion, peritumoral and coeliac lymph node involvement, and metastases in the lung and elsewhere.

- ***MRI*** is equivalent to CT in local staging but not as good for pulmonary metastases.
- ***Endoscopic ultrasound*** has an accuracy rate of nearly 90% for assessing depth of tumour and infiltration, and of 80% for staging lymph node involvement. It is useful if CT has not already demonstrated that a cancer is too advanced for surgery. A fine-needle aspiration (FNA) of lymph nodes improves staging accuracy. Accurate T staging is necessary, as cancers confined to the superficial mucosa can be removed endoscopically ***(Fig. 13.18C)***.
- ***Laparoscopy*** is useful if the tumour is at the cardia, to look for peritoneal and node metastases.
- ***PET*** after fluorodeoxyglucose is used principally to confirm distant metastases suspected on CT.

Management

Although oesophageal SCC and adenocarcinoma are undoubtedly two different disease processes with independent tumour biology, the majority of trial data do not discriminate between the two. The influence of histology on treatment is therefore unclear and varies around the globe.

Treatment is dependent on the age and performance status of the patient and the stage of the disease, with approximately 40% of all patients still alive 1 year after diagnosis. Five-year survival with stage 1 disease is 80% (T_1/T_2, N_0, M_0), stage 2 is 30%, stage 3 is 18% and stage 4 is 4%. Some 70% of patients present with stage 3 or greater disease, so that overall survival is 40% at 1 year and around 15% at 5 years. Management should be undertaken by multidisciplinary teams, including gastroenterologists, upper gastrointestinal surgeons, oncologists, palliative care physicians and dieticians.

- ***Surgery*** provides the best chance of a cure but should only be used when imaging (see above) has shown that the tumour has not infiltrated outside the oesophageal wall. Less than 40% of patients will have potentially resectable disease at the time of presentation. Patients must be evaluated preoperatively, particularly with regard to performance status (see p. 383), and surgery should be undertaken in designated units. Poor outcome data from surgery alone have challenged its role as monotherapy and it is more often used in conjunction with neo-adjuvant (preoperative) and adjuvant (postoperative) treatment. The role of surgery in early oesophageal SCC is less clear. As mentioned previously, endoscopic mucosal resection may be appropriate for early mucosal disease.
- ***Preoperative ('neo-adjuvant') chemoradiation therapy*** may benefit patients with stage 2b and 3 disease. Prolongation of survival has been shown in some studies. In the USA, neo-adjuvant chemoradiotherapy is preferred to the neo-adjuvant chemotherapy that is typically used in the UK.
- ***Palliative therapy*** is often the only realistic possibility. Dilatation is only of short-term benefit and the perforation risk is higher than for benign strictures. Combination of endoscopic dilatation with laser or brachytherapy (see p. 603) prolongs luminal patency and gives as good, if not better, functional results than stenting. Insertion of an expanding metal stent allows liquids and soft foods to be eaten.
- ***Chemoradiation alone*** is sometimes given but evidence of benefit is poor, except in early-stage SCC.
- ***Nutritional support***, as well as support for the patient and their family, is vital in this distressing condition.

Other oesophageal tumours

Most other tumours are rare. ***Gastrointestinal stromal tumours*** (see p. 384) and ***leiomyomas*** (both submucosal tumours) are found usually by chance; 10% cause dysphagia or bleeding. Surgical removal is performed for symptomatic lesions or those over 3 cm, which are more likely to harbour malignancy. Small, benign tumours are relatively common and often do not require treatment.

Kaposi's sarcoma is found in the oesophagus as well as the mouth (see p. 354) and hypopharynx in patients with AIDS.

Further reading

Boeckxstaens GE, Annese V, des Varannes SB et al., for the European Achalasia Trial Investigators. Pneumatic dilation versus laparoscopic Heller's myotomy for idiopathic achalasia. *N Engl J Med* 2011; 364:1807–1816.
Furuta GT, Katzka DA. Eosinophilic esophagitis. *N Engl J Med* 2015; 373:1640–1648.
Galmiche J-P, Hatlebakk J, Attwood S et al., for the LOTUS Trial Collaborators. Laparoscopic antireflux surgery vs esomeprazole treatment for chronic GERD: the LOTUS Randomized Clinical Trial. *JAMA* 2011; 305:1969–1977.
Hvid-Jensen F, Pedersen L, Drewes AM et al. Incidence of adenocarcinoma among patients with Barrett's esophagus. *N Engl J Med* 2011; 365:1375–1383.
Kahrilas PJ, McColl K, Fox M et al. The acid pocket: a target for treatment in reflux disease? *Am J Gastroenterol* 2013; 108:1058–1064.
Kandulski A, Malfertheiner P. GERD in 2010: diagnosis, novel mechanisms of disease and promising agents. *Nat Rev Gastroenterol Hepatol* 2011; 8:73–74.
Okines A, Sharma B, Cunningham D. Perioperative management of esophageal cancer. *Nat Rev Clin Oncol* 2010; 7:231–238.
Richter JE, Boeckxstaens GE. Management of achalasia: surgery or pneumatic dilation. *Gut* 2011; 60:869–876.
Rustgi AK, El-Serag HB. Esophageal carcinoma. *N Engl J Med* 2014: 371:2499–2509.
Sharma P. Barrett's esophagus. *N Engl J Med* 2009; 361:2548–2556.
http://www.cancerresearchuk.org *Cancer Research UK.*

THE STOMACH AND DUODENUM

Anatomy

The stomach occupies a small area immediately distal to the oesophagus (the cardia), the upper region (the fundus, under the left diaphragm), the mid-region or body and the antrum, which extends to the pylorus (see ***Fig. 13.8***). It serves as a reservoir where food can be retained and broken up before being actively expelled into the proximal small intestine.

The smooth muscle of the wall of the stomach has three layers: outer longitudinal, inner circular and innermost oblique layers. There are two sphincters: the gastro-oesophageal sphincter and the pyloric sphincter. The latter is largely made up of a thickening of the circular muscle layer and controls the exit of gastric contents into the duodenum.

The duodenum has outer longitudinal and inner smooth muscle layers. It is C-shaped and the pancreas sits in the concavity. It terminates at the duodenojejunal flexure, where it joins the jejunum.

- The ***mucosal lining*** of the stomach can stretch in size with feeding. The greater curvature of the undistended stomach has thick folds or rugae. The mucosa of the upper two-thirds of the stomach contains ***parietal cells***, which secrete hydrochloric acid, and ***chief cells***, which secrete pepsinogen (which initiates proteolysis). There is often a colour change at the junction between the body and the antrum of the stomach, which can be seen macroscopically and confirmed by measuring surface pH.
- The ***antral mucosa*** secretes bicarbonate and contains mucus-secreting cells and ***G cells***, which secrete gastrin, stimulating acid production. There are two major forms of gastrin, G17 and G34, depending on the number of amino-acid residues. G17 is the major form found in the antrum.

Somatostatin, a suppressant of acid secretion, is also produced by specialized antral cells (***D cells***).

- ***Mucus-secreting cells*** are present throughout the stomach and secrete mucus and bicarbonate. The mucus is made of glycoproteins called mucins.
- The ***'mucosal barrier'***, made up of the plasma membranes of mucosal cells and the mucus layer, protects the gastric epithelium from damage by acid and, for example, alcohol, aspirin, non-steroidal anti-inflammatory drugs (NSAIDs) and bile salts. Prostaglandins stimulate secretion of mucus, and their synthesis is inhibited by aspirin and NSAIDs, which inhibit cyclo-oxygenase (see ***Fig. 24.30***).
- The ***duodenal mucosa*** has villi like the rest of the small bowel, and also contains Brunner's glands, which secrete alkaline mucus. This, along with the pancreatic and biliary secretions, helps to neutralize the acid secretion from the stomach when it reaches the duodenum.

Physiology

Acid secretion is central to the functionality of the stomach; factors controlling acid secretion are shown in ***Figure 13.19***. Acid is not essential for digestion but does prevent some food-borne infections. It is under neural and hormonal control, and both stimulate acid secretion through the direct action of histamine on the parietal cell. Acetylcholine and gastrin also release histamine via the enterochromaffin cells. Somatostatin inhibits both histamine and gastrin release, and therefore acid secretion.

Other major gastric functions are:

- reservoir for food
- emulsification of fat and mixing of gastric contents
- secretion of intrinsic factor
- absorption (of only minimal importance).

Gastric emptying depends on many factors. There are osmoreceptors in the duodenal mucosa, which control gastric emptying by local reflexes and the release of gut hormones. In particular, intraduodenal fat delays gastric emptying by negative feedback through duodenal receptors.

Gastritis and gastropathy

'***Gastritis***' indicates inflammation associated with mucosal injury (although the term is often used loosely by endoscopists to describe 'redness'), and '***gastropathy***' indicates epithelial cell damage and regeneration without inflammation.

Gastritis

Several classifications of gastritis (e.g. Sydney classification) have been proposed but are controversial due to lack of correlation between endoscopic and histological findings. *H. pylori* infection is the most common cause of gastritis, with autoimmune gastritis being seen in 5% of cases; the remaining causes include viruses (e.g. cytomegalovirus and herpes simplex), duodenogastric reflux and specific causes, e.g. Crohn's, more common in children than adults. Chronic inflammation, particularly if induced by *H. pylori*, can lead to gastric intestinal metaplasia, a precursor to gastric cancer. The role of surveillance in these patients is unclear.

Autoimmune gastritis

This affects the fundus and body of the stomach (pangastritis), leading to atrophic gastritis and loss of parietal cells, with achlorhydria and intrinsic factor deficiency causing the clinical syndrome

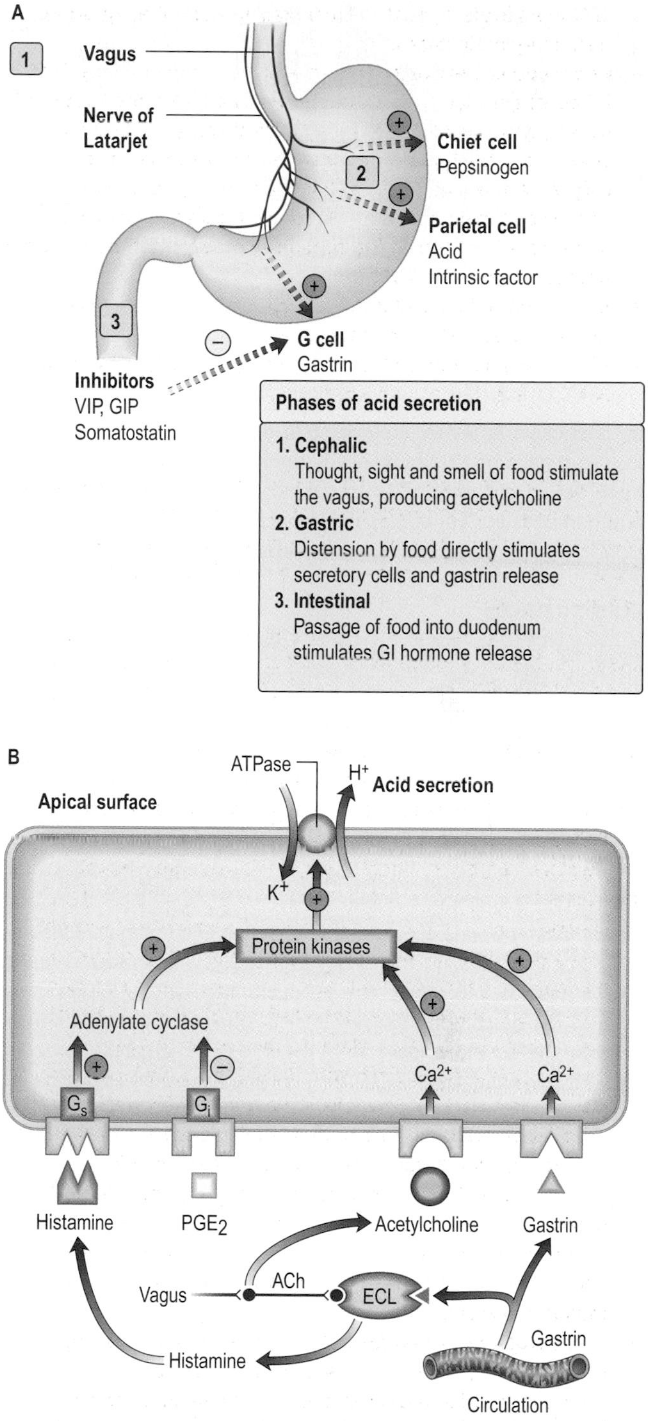

Figure 13.19 Pathophysiology of acid secretion. A. Control of acid secretion. **B.** Mechanisms involved in acid secretion. Histamine stimulates the G_s protein via the H_2 receptors and acts via cyclic adenosine monophosphate (cAMP). Prostaglandin E_2 (PGE_2) activates the G_i protein and *inhibits* acid secretion. Acetylcholine (ACh) acts via the vagus M_3 receptors. ACh also acts via the enterochromaffin cell (ECL). Gastrin acts via the cholecystokinin B (CCKBB)–gastrin receptor, increasing the intracellular free calcium, and also via the ECL cell, stimulating histamine. Gs and Gi, stimulating and inhibiting G-proteins; GIP, gastric inhibitory polypeptide; VIP, vasoactive intestinal polypeptide.

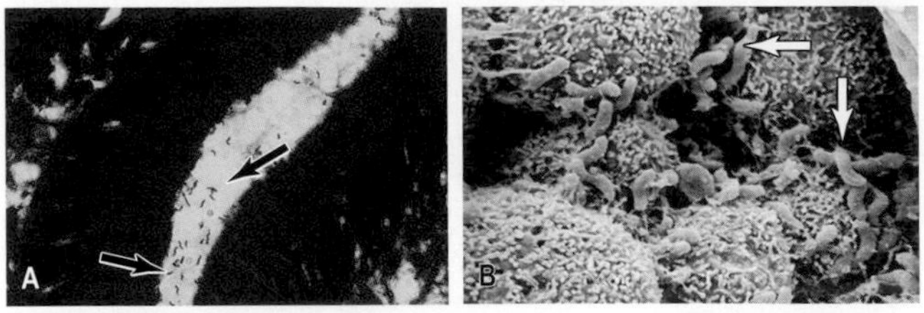

Figure 13.20 ***Helicobacter pylori*. A.** Organisms (arrowed) are shown on the gastric mucosa (cresyl fast violet (modified Giemsa) stain). **B.** Scanning electron microscopy, showing the spiral-shaped bacterium (arrowed). *(**A,** Courtesy of Dr Alan Phillips, Department of Paediatric Gastroenterology, Royal Free Hospital.)*

of 'pernicious anaemia' (see pp. 528–529). Metaplasia, usually of the intestinal type, is almost always in the context of atrophic gastritis. Serum autoantibodies to gastric parietal cells are common and non-specific; antibodies to intrinsic factor are rarer and more significant (see p. 528).

Gastropathy

Gastropathy is usually caused by irritants (drugs, NSAIDs and alcohol), bile reflux and chronic congestion. Acute erosive/haemorrhagic gastropathy can also be seen after severe stress (stress ulcers); secondary to burns (Curling ulcers), trauma, shock or renal failure; and in portal hypertension (called portal gastropathy). The underlying mechanism for these ulcers is unknown but may be related to an alteration in mucosal blood flow.

Helicobacter pylori infection

Helicobacter pylori is a slow-growing, spiral, Gram-negative, flagellate, urease-producing bacterium ***(Fig. 13.20)***, which plays a major role in gastritis and peptic ulcer disease. It colonizes the mucous layer in the gastric antrum, but is also found in the duodenum in areas of gastric metaplasia. *H. pylori* is found in greatest numbers under the mucous layer in gastric pits, where it adheres specifically to gastric epithelial cells. It is protected from gastric acid by the juxtamucosal mucous layer which traps bicarbonate secreted by antral cells, and ammonia produced by bacterial urease.

Epidemiology

The prevalence of *H. pylori* is high in developing countries (80–90% of the population) and much lower (20–50%) in developed countries. Infection rates are highest in lower-income groups. Infection is usually acquired in childhood; although the exact route is uncertain, it may be faecal–oral or oral–oral. The incidence increases with age, probably due to acquisition in childhood when hygiene was poorer (cohort effect) rather than infection in adult life, which is most likely far less than 1% per year in developed countries.

Pathogenesis

The pathogenetic mechanisms are not fully understood, with the majority of the colonized population remaining asymptomatic throughout their life. *H. pylori* is highly adapted to the stomach environment, exclusively colonizing gastric epithelium and inhabiting the mucous layer, or just beneath. It adheres by a number of adhesion molecules including BabA, which binds to the Lewis antigen expressed on the surface of gastric mucosal cells and causes gastritis in all infected subjects. Damage to the gastric epithelial cell is caused by the release of enzymes and the induction of apoptosis through binding to class II major histocompatibility complex (MHC) molecules. The production of urease enables the conversion of urea to ammonium and chloride, which are directly cytotoxic. Ulcers are most common when the infecting strain expresses *CagA* (cytotoxic-associated protein) and *VacA* (vacuolating toxin) genes secondary to a more pronounced inflammatory and immune response. Expression of *CagA* and *VacA* is associated with greater induction of interleukin 8 (IL-8), a potent mediator of gastric inflammation. Genetic variations in the host are also thought to be involved; for example, polymorphisms leading to increased levels of IL-1β are associated with atrophic gastritis and cancer.

Results of *H. pylori* infection

- Inflammation (antral gastritis and gastric intestinal metaplasia).
- Peptic ulcers (duodenal and gastric).
- Gastric cancer (see pp. 381–382).

Antral gastritis

Antral gastritis is the usual effect of *H. pylori* infection. It is normally asymptomatic, although patients without ulcers do sometimes experience relief of dyspeptic symptoms after *Helicobacter* eradication. Chronic antral gastritis causes hypergastrinaemia due to gastrin release from antral G cells. The subsequent increase in acid output is usually asymptomatic but can lead to duodenal ulceration.

Duodenal ulcer

The prevalence of *H. pylori* infection in patients with duodenal ulcers (DUs; see ***Fig. 13.22A***) is falling and in the developed world is now between 50% and 75%, whereas duodenal ulceration was once rare in the absence of *H. pylori* infection. This has been attributed to a decrease in prevalence of the bacterium and an increase in NSAID use. Eradication of the infection improves ulcer healing and decreases the incidence of recurrence.

The precise mechanism of duodenal ulceration is unclear, as only 15% of patients infected with *H. pylori* (50–60% of the adult population worldwide) develop duodenal ulcers. Factors that have been implicated include increased gastrin secretion, smoking, bacterial virulence and genetic susceptibility.

Gastric ulcer

Gastric ulcers (GUs; see ***Fig. 13.22B***) are associated with a gastritis affecting the body as well as the antrum of the stomach (pangastritis), causing parietal cell loss and reduced acid production. The ulcers are thought to occur because of a reduction of gastric mucosal resistance due to cytokine production caused by the infection, or perhaps because of alterations in gastric mucus.

Peptic ulcer disease

A ***peptic ulcer*** consists of a break in the superficial epithelial cells penetrating down to the muscularis mucosa of either the stomach or the duodenum; there is a fibrous base and an increase in inflammatory cells. ***Erosions***, by contrast, are superficial breaks in the mucosa alone. DUs are most commonly found in the duodenal cap; the surrounding mucosa appears inflamed, haemorrhagic or friable (duodenitis). GUs are most commonly seen on the lesser curve near the incisura, but can be found in any part of the stomach.

Epidemiology of peptic ulcer disease

DUs affect approximately 10% of the adult population and are 2–3 times more common than GUs.

Ulcer rates are declining rapidly for younger men and increasing for older individuals, particularly women. Both DUs and GUs are common in the elderly. There is considerable geographical variation, with peptic ulcer disease being more prevalent in developing countries related to the high *H. pylori* infection. In the developed world, the percentage of NSAID-induced peptic ulcers is increasing as the prevalence of *H. pylori* declines.

Clinical features of peptic ulcer disease

The characteristic feature of peptic ulcer is recurrent, burning epigastric pain. It has been shown that if a patient points with a single finger to the epigastrium as the site of the pain, this is strongly suggestive of peptic ulcer disease. The relationship of the pain to food is variable and, on the whole, not helpful in diagnosis. The pain of a DU classically occurs at night (as well as during the day) and is worse when the patient is hungry, but this is not reliable. The pain of both GUs and DUs may be relieved by antacids.

Nausea may accompany the pain; vomiting is infrequent but can relieve the pain. Anorexia and weight loss may occur, particularly with GUs. Persistent and severe pain suggests complications, such as penetration into other organs. Back pain suggests a penetrating posterior ulcer. Severe ulceration can occasionally be symptomless, as many who present with acute ulcer bleeding or perforation have no preceding ulcer symptoms.

Untreated, the symptoms of a DU relapse and remit spontaneously. The natural history is for the disease to remit over many years due to the onset of atrophic gastritis and a decrease in acid secretion.

Epigastric tenderness is common in both ulcer and non-ulcer dyspepsia.

Diagnosis of *Helicobacter pylori* infection

Diagnosis of *H. pylori* is necessary if the clinician plans to treat a positive result. This is usually in the context of active peptic ulcer disease, previous peptic ulcer disease or mucosa-associated lymphoid tissue (MALT) lymphoma, or to 'test and treat' patients with dyspepsia under the age of 55 with no alarm symptoms (i.e. weight loss, anaemia, dysphagia, vomiting or family history of gastrointestinal cancer). ***Examination*** is usually unhelpful.

Non-invasive methods

- ***Serological tests*** detect immunoglobulin G (IgG) antibodies and are reasonably sensitive (90%) and specific (83%). They have been used in diagnosis and in epidemiological studies. IgG titres may take up to 1 year to fall by 50% after eradication therapy and therefore are not useful for confirming eradication or the presence of a current infection. Antibodies can also be found in the saliva but tests are not as sensitive or specific as serology.
- ***^{13}C-Urea breath test (Fig. 13.21)*** is a quick and reliable test for *H. pylori* and can be used as a screening test. The measurement of $^{13}CO_2$ in the breath after ingestion of ^{13}C-urea requires a mass spectrometer. The test is sensitive ([illegible]) and specific ([illegible]), but the sensitivity can be improved by ensuring the patient has not taken antibiotics in the 4 weeks before the test and PPIs in the previous 2 weeks.
- ***Stool antigen test*** is beginning to supersede breath testing as the method used to determine *H. pylori* status. A specific immunoassay, using monoclonal antibodies for the qualitative detection of *H. pylori* antigen, is now widely available. The overall sensitivity is 97.6% and specificity is 96%. The test is useful in the diagnosis of *H. pylori* infection and for monitoring efficacy of eradication therapy. Patients should be off PPIs for 2 weeks but can continue with H_2-blockers. Newer stool antigen tests are being developed that can be performed in the clinic setting, although at present the sensitivity and specificity are not as good as for those performed in the laboratory.

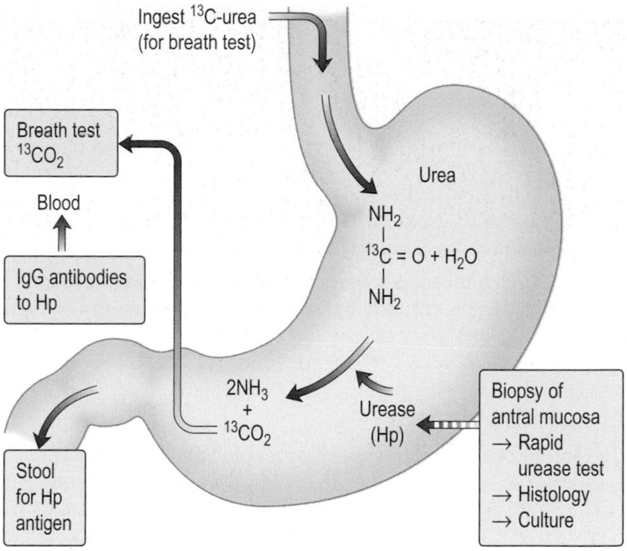

Figure 13.21 Metabolism of urea by *Helicobacter pylori* (Hp). The different tests available for the detection of *H. pylori* are shown.

Invasive methods (endoscopy)

- ***Biopsy urease test***. Gastric biopsies, usually antral unless additional material is needed to exclude proximal migration, are added to a substrate containing urea and phenol red. If *H. pylori* is present, the urease enzyme that the bacteria produce splits the urea to release ammonia, which raises the pH of the solution and causes a rapid colour change (yellow to red). This enables patients' *H. pylori* status to be determined before they leave the endoscopy suite. The test may be falsely negative if patients are taking PPIs or antibiotics at the time.
- ***Histology***. *H. pylori* can be detected histologically on routine (Giemsa) stained sections of gastric mucosa obtained at endoscopy. The sensitivity is reduced if a patient is on PPIs, but less so than with the urease test. Sensitivity can be improved with immunohistochemical staining using an anti-*H. pylori* antibody.
- ***Culture***. Biopsies obtained can be cultured on a special medium, and *in vitro* sensitivities to antibiotics can be tested. This technique is typically used for patients with refractory *H. pylori* infection to identify the appropriate antibiotic regimen; routine culture is rare.

Investigation of suspected peptic ulcer disease

- ***Patients under 55 years of age***, with typical symptoms of peptic ulcer disease who test positive for *H. pylori*, can start eradication therapy without further investigation.
- ***Older patients*** require endoscopic diagnosis ***(Fig. 13.22)*** and exclusion of cancer. All gastric ulcers must be biopsied to exclude an underlying malignancy and should be followed up endoscopically until healing has taken place.
- ***All patients with 'alarm symptoms'*** should undergo endoscopy.

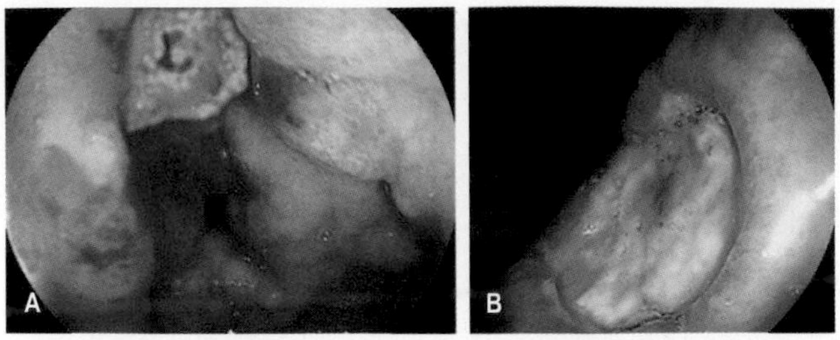

Figure 13.22 **Endoscopic views in *Helicobacter pylori* infection.** **A.** Duodenal ulcer with inflamed duodenal folds. **B.** Benign gastric ulcer.

Management

Eradication therapy

Current recommendations are that all patients with duodenal and gastric ulcers should have *H. pylori* eradication therapy if the bacteria are present. Many patients have incidental *H. pylori* infection with no GU or DU. On balance, whether all such patients should have eradication therapy is controversial (see 'Functional dyspepsia', pp. 429–430).

The increase in the prevalence of GORD and adenocarcinoma of the lower oesophagus in the last few years is currently unexplained, but has been postulated to be linked to eradication of *H. pylori*; this seems unlikely but is not disproven.

Depending on local antibacterial resistance patterns, standard eradication therapies in the developed world are successful in approximately 90% of patients. Re-infection is very uncommon (1%) in developed countries. In developing countries, re-infection is more common, compliance with treatment may be poor and metronidazole resistance is high (>50%, as it is frequently used for parasitic infections), so failure of eradication is common.

There are many regimens for eradication, but all must take into account that:

- Good compliance is essential.
- There is a high incidence of resistance to metronidazole and clarithromycin, particularly in some populations. Clarithromycin resistance has doubled in Europe in the last decade.
- Oral metronidazole has frequent side-effects.
- Bismuth chelate is unpleasant to take, even as tablets.

Metronidazole, clarithromycin, amoxicillin, tetracycline and bismuth are the most widely used agents. Resistance to amoxicillin (1–2%) and tetracycline (<1%) is low, except in countries where they are available without prescription, where resistance may exceed 50%. Quinolones (such as ciprofloxacin), furazolidone and rifabutin are also used when standard regimens have failed ('rescue therapy'). None of these drugs is effective alone; eradication regimens therefore usually comprise two antibiotics, given with powerful acid suppression in the form of a PPI. Bismuth-containing quadruple therapy is advocated as first-line treatment because of increasing clarithromycin resistance; the standard clarithromycin-based triple therapy has been replaced as the treatment of choice in areas where resistance is high.

Example regimens

- Omeprazole 20 mg+clarithromycin 500 mg and amoxicillin 1 g – all twice daily
- Omeprazole 20 mg+metronidazole 400 mg and clarithromycin 500 mg – all twice daily.

These should be given for 7 or 14 days. Two-week treatments increase the eradication rates but increased side-effects may reduce compliance.

In ***eradication failures*** and in areas of clarithromycin resistance, bismuth chelate (120 mg 4 times daily), metronidazole (400 mg 3 times daily), tetracycline (500 mg 4 times daily) and a PPI (20–40 mg twice daily) for 14 days is used. Sequential courses of therapy are also used in such cases (5 days of PPI and amoxicillin, followed by a 5-day period of PPI with clarithromycin and tinidazole). With the increase in clarithromycin resistance, many are using this quadruple therapy for initial treatment.

Prolonged therapy with a PPI after a course of PPI-based 7-day triple therapy is not necessary for ulcer healing in most *H. pylori*-infected patients. The effectiveness of treatment for uncomplicated duodenal ulcer should be assessed symptomatically. If symptoms persist, breath or stool testing should be performed to check eradication (off PPI therapy).

Patients with a risk of bleeding or those with complications, such as haemorrhage or perforation, should always have a ^{13}C-urea breath test or stool test for *H. pylori* 6 weeks after the end of treatment to be sure that eradication has been successful. Long-term PPIs may be necessary if a rebleed would be likely to be fatal.

General measures

Stopping smoking should be strongly encouraged, as smoking slows mucosal healing.

Patients with gastric ulcers should be routinely re-endoscoped at 6 weeks to confirm mucosal healing and exclude an underlying gastric cancer. Repeat biopsies may be necessary.

Complications of peptic ulcer disease

Haemorrhage

See page 386.

Perforation

The frequency of perforation (see also pp. 432–435) of peptic ulceration is decreasing, partly because of medical therapy. DUs perforate more commonly than GUs, usually into the peritoneal cavity; perforation into the lesser sac also occurs. Detailed management of perforation is described on pages 432-435. Laparoscopic surgery is usually performed to close the perforation and drain the abdomen. Conservative management using nasogastric suction, intravenous fluids and antibiotics is occasionally used in elderly and very sick patients.

Gastric outlet obstruction

The obstruction may be pre-pyloric, pyloric or duodenal. The obstruction occurs either because there is an active ulcer with surrounding oedema or because the healing of an ulcer has been followed by scarring. However, obstruction due to peptic ulcer disease and gastric malignancy are now uncommon; Crohn's disease or external compression from a pancreatic carcinoma is a more common cause. Adult hypertrophic pyloric stenosis is a very rare cause.

After gastric outlet obstruction, the stomach becomes full of gastric juice and ingested fluid and food, giving rise to the main symptom of vomiting, usually without pain, as the characteristic ulcer pain has abated owing to healing.

Vomiting is infrequent, projectile and large in volume; the vomitus contains particles of previous meals. On examination of the abdomen, there may be a succussion splash. The diagnosis is made by endoscopy but can be suspected from the nature of the vomiting; by contrast, psychogenic vomiting is frequent, small-volume and usually noisy.

Severe or persistent vomiting causes loss of acid from the stomach and a hypokalaemic metabolic alkalosis (see pp. 180–181). Vomiting will often settle with intravenous fluid and electrolyte replacement, gastric drainage via a nasogastric tube, and potent acid suppression therapy. Endoscopic dilatation of the pyloric region is useful, as is luminal stenting, and overall, 70% of patients can be managed without surgery.

Surgical treatment and its long-term consequences

Once the mainstay of treatment, surgery is now used in peptic ulcer disease only for complications including:

- recurrent uncontrolled haemorrhage
- perforation, which is oversewn.

No other procedure, such as gastrectomy or vagotomy, is required.

In the past, two types of operation were performed: a partial gastrectomy or a vagotomy. In the latter, either a truncal vagotomy with a pyloroplasty or gastro-jejunostomy was performed, or highly selective vagotomy or proximal gastric vagotomy, which did not require a bypass procedure.

Long-term complications of surgery, which are still seen occasionally, include:

- ***Recurrent ulcer***. If this occurs, check for *H. pylori*; rule out Zollinger–Ellison syndrome (see p. 512). Malignancy needs to be excluded in all cases.
- ***Dumping***. This term describes a number of upper abdominal symptoms (e.g. nausea and distension associated with sweating, faintness and palpitations) that occur in patients following gastrectomy or gastroenterostomy. It is due to 'dumping' of food into the jejunum, causing rapid fluid shifts from plasma to dilute the high osmotic load with reduction of blood volume. The symptoms are usually mild and patients adapt to them. It is rare for it to be a long-term problem, and if so, the symptoms usually have a functional element. Hypoglycaemia can also occur.
- ***Diarrhoea***. This was chiefly seen after vagotomy. Recurrent severe episodes occurred in about 1% of patients. Antidiarrhoeals are the usual treatment.
- ***Nutritional complications***. In the long term, almost any gastric surgery, but particularly gastrectomy, may be followed by:
  - iron deficiency, due to poor absorption
  - folate deficiency, usually due to poor intake
  - vitamin B_{12} deficiency, due to intrinsic factor deficiency
  - weight loss, usually due to reduced intake.

Other *H. pylori*-associated diseases

- ***Gastric adenocarcinoma***. The incidence of distal (but not proximal) gastric cancer parallels that of *H. pylori* infection in countries with a high incidence of gastric cancer. Serological studies show that people infected with *H. pylori* have a higher incidence of distal gastric carcinoma (see p. 382).
- ***Gastric B cell lymphoma***. Over 70% of patients with gastric B cell lymphomas (MALT) have *H. pylori*. *H. pylori* gastritis has been shown to contain the clonal B cell that eventually gives rise to the MALT lymphoma (see pp. 384 and 382).

NSAIDs, *Helicobacter* and ulcers

Aspirin and other NSAIDs deplete mucosal prostaglandins by inhibiting the cyclo-oxygenase (COX) pathway, which leads to mucosal damage. Cyclo-oxygenase occurs in two main forms: COX-1, the constitutive enzyme; and COX-2, inducible by cytokine stimulation in areas of inflammation. COX-2-specific inhibitors have less effect on the COX-1 enzyme in the gastric mucosa; they still produce gastric mucosal damage but less than with other conventional NSAIDs. Their use is limited by concern regarding cardiovascular side-effects.

Some 50% of patients taking regular NSAIDs will develop gastric mucosal damage and approximately 30% will have ulcers on endoscopy. Only a small proportion of patients have symptoms (about 5%) and only 1–2% have a major problem: that is, gastrointestinal bleed or perforation. Because of the large number of patients on NSAIDs, including low-dose aspirin for vascular prophylaxis, this is a significant problem, particularly in the elderly.

H. pylori and NSAIDs are independent and synergistic risk factors for the development of ulcers. In a meta-analysis, the odds ratio (OR) for the incidence of peptic ulcer was 61.1 in patients infected with *H. pylori* and also taking NSAIDs, compared with uninfected controls not taking NSAIDs.

Management

- Stop the ingestion of NSAIDs.
- Give a PPI.
- Start *H. pylori* eradication therapy if the patient is *H. pylori*-positive.

In many people with severe arthritis, stopping NSAIDs may not be possible. Therefore use:

- ***An NSAID*** with low GI side-effects at the lowest dose possible (see pp. 665–666). If there is no cardiovascular risk, a COX-2 NSAID can be used (see p. 666).
- ***Prophylactic cytoprotective therapy***, e.g. PPI or misoprostol (a synthetic analogue of prostaglandin E_1 800 μg/day) for all high-risk patients, i.e. over 65 years, those with a peptic ulcer history, particularly with complications, and those on corticosteroid or anticoagulant therapy. PPIs reduce the risk of endoscopic duodenal and gastric ulcers and are better tolerated than misoprostol, which causes diarrhoea.

Gastric tumours

Adenocarcinoma

Gastric cancer is currently the fourth most common cancer found worldwide and the second leading cause of cancer-related mortality. The incidence increases with age (peak incidence 50–70 years), and it is rare under the age of 30 years. The highest incidence of the disease is found in Eastern Asia, Eastern Europe and South America. The incidence in men is twice that in women and varies throughout the world, being high in Japan (M: 53/100 000, F: 21.3/100 000) and Chile, and relatively low in the USA (M: 7/100 000, F: 2.9/100 000). In the UK, carcinoma of the stomach (see ***Fig. 13.1***) is the eighth most common cancer (M: 16/100 000, F 9/100 000). The overall worldwide incidence of gastric carcinoma is falling, even in Japan, probably due to reductions in the incidence of *Helicobacter* and, before this, improvements in food storage. However, the incidence of proximal gastric cancers is increasing in the West and they have very similar demographic and pathological features to Barrett's-associated oesophageal adenocarcinoma.

Epidemiology and pathogenesis

- ***H. pylori infection*** and distal gastric cancer are strongly linked. *H. pylori* is recognized by the International Agency for Research in Cancer (IARC) as a group 1 (definite) gastric

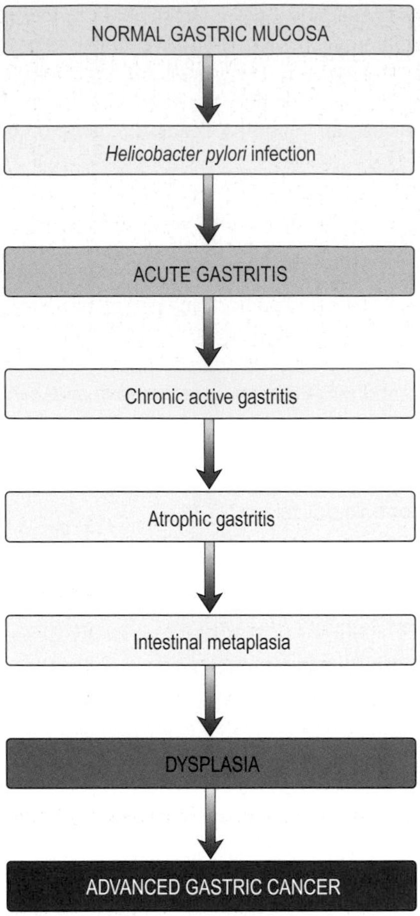

Figure 13.23 **Flow diagram showing the development of gastric cancer associated with *H. pylori* infection.**

carcinogen. *H. pylori* infection causes chronic gastritis, which eventually leads to atrophic gastritis and pre-malignant intestinal metaplasia ***(Fig. 13.23)***. Much of the earlier epidemiological data (i.e. the increase of cancer in lower socioeconomic groups) can be explained by the intrafamilial spread of *H. pylori*. Epstein–Barr virus is detected in 2–16% of gastric cancers worldwide, but its role in aetiology is not well understood.

- ***Dietary factors*** may also be involved (as both initiators and promoters) and have separate roles in carcinogenesis. Diets high in salt probably increase the risk. Dietary nitrates can be converted into nitrosamines by bacteria at neutral pH; nitrosamines are known to be carcinogenic in animals but the evidence in human carcinogenesis is limited. Nitrosamines are also present in the stomach of patients with achlorhydria, who have an increased cancer risk.
- ***Tobacco smoking*** is associated with an increased incidence of stomach cancer.
- ***Genetic abnormality*** is also a factor. The most common abnormality is a loss of heterozygosity (LOH) of tumour suppressor genes such as *p53* (in 50% of cancers, as well as in pre-cancerous states) and the gene encoding adenomatous polyposis coli (*APC*) (in over one-third of gastric cancers). These abnormalities are similar to those found in colorectal cancers. Some rare families with diffuse gastric cancer have been shown to have mutations in the E-cadherin gene (*CDH-1*). There is a higher incidence of gastric cancer in blood group A patients.
- ***First-degree relatives*** of patients with gastric cancer have 2–3-fold increased relative risk of developing the disease, but this may be environmental rather than inherited.
- ***Pernicious anaemia*** carries a small increased risk of gastric carcinoma due to the accompanying atrophic gastritis.
- ***Partial gastrectomy*** (postoperative stomach) carries an increased risk of gastric cancer, whether performed for a GU or DU; this is probably due to untreated *H. pylori* infection.

Screening

Earlier diagnosis has been advocated in an attempt to improve the poor prognosis of gastric cancer. (Screening is discussed on pp. 591–592.) Although the incidence of gastric cancer is falling in Japan, where aggressive screening by barium studies is followed by endoscopy if there is doubt, there is no evidence that screening has had an effect on overall mortality. Similarly, early investigation of dyspepsia has had little effect on mortality, possibly because of the relatively low prevalence of cancer.

Early gastric cancer

Early gastric cancer is defined as a carcinoma that is confined to the mucosa or submucosa, regardless of the presence of lymph node metastases. It is associated with 5-year survival rates of approximately 90%, but many of these patients would have survived 5 years without treatment. In Japan, mass screening with mobile units has increased the proportion of early gastric cancers (EGC) diagnosed. In a large series of patients from the UK with gastric cancer, only 0.7% were identified as having EGC. They are usually detected by chance, as although EGC exists in Western populations, endoscopists do not readily recognize it at present.

Pathology

There are two major types of gastric cancer:

- ***Intestinal*** (***type 1***) with well-formed glandular structures (differentiated). The tumours are polypoid or ulcerating lesions with heaped-up, rolled edges. Intestinal metaplasia is seen in the surrounding mucosa, often with *H. pylori*. This type is more likely to involve the distal stomach and occur in patients with atrophic gastritis. It has a strong environmental association.
- ***Diffuse*** (***type 2***) with poorly cohesive cells (undifferentiated) that tend to infiltrate the gastric wall. It may involve any part of the stomach, especially the cardia, and has a worse prognosis than the intestinal type. Loss of expression of the cell adhesion molecule E-cadherin is the key event in the carcinogenesis of diffuse gastric cancers. Unlike type 1 gastric cancers, type 2 cancers have similar frequencies in all geographic areas and occur in a younger population.

Some 50% of gastric cancers in Western countries occur in the proximal stomach.

Clinical features

Symptoms

Around 50% of patients with EGC discovered at screening have no symptoms. Most patients with carcinoma of the stomach have advanced disease at the time of presentation. The most common symptom of advanced disease is epigastric pain, indistinguishable from the pain of peptic ulcer disease; it may be relieved by food and antacids. The pain can vary in intensity but may be constant and

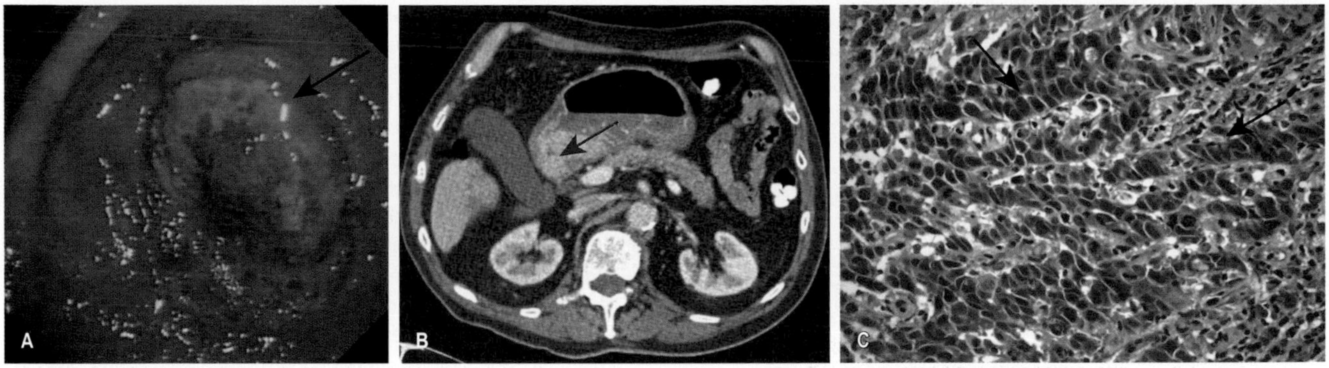

Figure 13.24 **Carcinoma of the stomach. A.** Endoscopic picture showing a large, irregular ulcer with rolled edges (arrowed). **B.** Axial CT scan (ulcer arrowed). **C.** Histopathology showing an adenocarcinoma (arrowed).

severe, and there may also be nausea, anorexia and weight loss. Vomiting is frequent and can be severe if the tumour encroaches on the pylorus. Dysphagia can occur with tumours involving the fundus. Gross haematemesis is unusual but anaemia from occult blood loss is frequent. No pattern of symptoms is suggestive of EGC.

Widely spreading submucosal gastric cancer causes diffuse thickening and rigidity of the stomach wall and is called 'linitis plastica'.

Patients can present at a late stage with malignant ascites or jaundice due to liver involvement. Metastases also occur in bone, brain and lung, producing appropriate symptoms.

Signs

Weight loss is often the dominant feature. Nearly 50% of patients have a palpable epigastric mass with abdominal tenderness. A palpable lymph node is sometimes found in the supraclavicular fossa (Virchow's node, usually on the left side), and metastases are present in up to one-third of patients at presentation. This cancer is the most frequently associated with dermatomyositis (see p. 698) and acanthosis nigricans.

Diagnosis

- ***Gastroscopy (Fig. 13.24)*** allows biopsies to be taken for histological assessment. Positive biopsies can be obtained in almost all cases of obvious carcinoma, but a negative biopsy does not necessarily rule out the diagnosis. For this reason, 8–10 biopsies should be taken from suspicious lesions. Diffuse type gastric cancer infiltrates the submucosa and muscularis propria and can be undetected on endoscopy; multiple deep biopsies help.

Staging

- ***CT scan of the chest and abdomen*** with a gastric water load can demonstrate gastric wall thickening, lymphadenopathy and lung and liver secondaries, but has limited ability to determine the depth of local tumour invasion.
- ***Endoscopic ultrasound*** is useful for local staging to demonstrate the depth of penetration of the cancer through the gastric wall and extension into local lymph nodes. It complements CT and ultrasound but is most relevant to confirm that a cancer is confined to the superficial mucosa, before endoscopic resection.
- ***Laparoscopy*** is useful in patients being considered for surgery to exclude serosal disease.

Box 13.13 Gastric cancer – staging and 5-year survival rates

Stage	TNM[a] stage	5-year survival (%)
1	T1N0M0, T1N1M0 or T2N0M0	88
2	T1N2M0, T2N1M0 or T3N0M0	65
3a	T2N2M0, T3N1M0 or T4N0M0	35
3b	T3N2M0	35
4	T4N1–3M0, TxN3M0 or TxNxM1[b]	5

[a]T, tumour; N, nodes; M, metastases. [b]Tx indicates any T stage; Nx, any N stage.

- ***PET and CT/PET*** can be helpful in further delineation of the cancer.

The TNM classification is used. The tumour grade (T) indicates depth of tumour invasion, N denotes the presence or absence of lymph nodes, and M indicates presence or absence of metastases. TNM classification is then combined into stage categories 0–4. At presentation, two-thirds of patients are at stage 3 or 4: that is, advanced disease ***(Box 13.13)***. The histological grade of the tumour also determines survival.

Management

As with all cancers, treatment is discussed with a multidisciplinary team. Early non-ulcerated mucosal lesions can be removed endoscopically by either endoscopic mucosal resection or endoscopic submucosal dissection.

Surgery remains the most effective form of treatment if the patient is an operative candidate. Careful selection has reduced the numbers undergoing surgery and has improved the overall surgical 5-year survival rates to around 30%. Five-year survival rates in 'curative' operations are as high as 50%. Surgery, combined chemoradiotherapy and treatment of advanced disease are described on pages 635–636. The multinational MAGIC trial demonstrated the benefits of perioperative chemotherapy with epirubicin, cisplatin and infusional 5-fluorouracil (ECF) (see p. 636), where 5-year survival in operable gastric and lower oesophageal adenocarcinomas increased from 23% to 36%. An alternative regimen is oral epirubicin, oxaliplatin and capecitabine. Despite the improved results, the overall survival rate for a patient with gastric carcinoma has not dramatically improved, with a maximum 5-year survival rate of 10% overall. Palliative care, with relief of pain and counselling, is usually required.

Gastrointestinal stromal tumours (GIST)

Gastrointestinal stromal tumours (GISTs) are a subset of gastrointestinal mesenchymal tumours of varying differentiation. They are usually asymptomatic and found by chance but occasionally they can ulcerate and bleed. There are 200–900 new cases each year in the UK. GISTs mostly affect people between 55 and 65 years of age.

These tumours were previously classified as gastrointestinal leiomyomas, leiomyosarcomas, leiomyoblastomas or schwannomas. Truly benign leiomyomas do occur, mainly in the oesophagus, but GISTs are now recognized as a distinct group of mesenchymal tumours and comprise about 80% of gastrointestinal mesenchymal tumours. They are of stromal origin and are thought to share a common ancestry with the interstitial cells of Cajal. They have varying differentiation, with mutations occurring in the cellular proto-oncogene *KIT* (which leads to activation and cell-surface expression of the tyrosine kinase KIT (CD 117)) in 80%, and also in platelet-derived growth factor receptor-α (PDGFRA) in up to 10% of patients.

Management

Treatment is surgical as far as possible. These tumours generally grow slowly but may be malignant. Imatinib, a tyrosine kinase inhibitor (see pp. 601–602), is chosen for unresectable or metastatic disease, and is now used as adjunctive therapy after surgical removal of the primary in the absence of metastatic disease. Some patients are resistant to this; sunitinib can be used as an alternative agent over a short time period.

Primary gastric lymphoma

Mucosa-associated lymphatic tissue (MALT) lymphomas are indolent B-cell marginal zone lymphomas that primarily involve sites other than lymph nodes (gastrointestinal tract, thyroid, breast or skin). They constitute about 10% of all types of non-Hodgkin's lymphoma (NHL).

Aetiology

About 90% of cases are due to *H. pylori* infection. Chromosome abnormalities t(1;14)(p22; q32) and t(11;18)(q21; q21) have also been noted in this form of NHL.

Clinical features

Most patients are diagnosed in their 60s with stage I or stage II disease outside the lymph nodes. Patients have stomach pain, ulcers or other localized symptoms, but rarely have systemic complaints such as fatigue or fever.

Management

Eradication of *H. pylori* infection may resolve cases of local gastric involvement. After standard eradication regimens, 50% of patients show resolution at 3 months. Other patients may resolve after 12–18 months of observation. Stage III or IV disease is treated with surgery or chemotherapy with or without radiation. The prognosis is good, with an estimated 90% 5-year survival.

Gastric polyps

Gastric polyps are found in about 1% of endoscopies, usually by chance. They rarely produce symptoms, but larger lesions can result in anaemia or haematemesis.

Endoscopic biopsy is the usual approach to diagnosis and treatment is possible polypectomy based on histological finding. Occasional large or multiple polyps may require surgery.

- ***Hyperplastic polyps*** are by far the most common type. Most are <2 cm. The polyps are rarely pre-malignant, but may be accompanied by pre-malignant atrophic gastritis.
- ***Adenomatous polyps*** are usually solitary lesions in the antrum. Approximately 3% progress to gastric cancer, especially if >2 cm in diameter, but they are not a common cause of gastric cancer (compare this with colorectal cancer).
- ***Cystic gland polyps*** contain microcysts that are lined by fundic-type parietal and chief cells. They are located in the fundus and body of the stomach. They are found in otherwise normal subjects, but are especially common in familial polyposis syndromes and patients on PPIs. Their malignant potential is negligible, although low-grade dysplasia is seen in the absence of familial adenomatous polyposis coli (FAP), and high-grade dysplasia exclusively in its presence.
- ***Inflammatory fibroid polyps*** are benign spindle cell tumours infiltrated by eosinophils. Excision of these polyps is indicated because of their propensity to enlarge and cause obstruction.

Further reading

Downs-Kelly E, Rubin BP. Gastrointestinal stromal tumors: molecular mechanisms and targeted therapies. *Pathol Res Int* 2011; 708596.

Gisbert JP, Calvet X, O'Connor JP et al. The sequential therapy regimen for *Helicobacter pylori* eradication. *Expert Opin Pharmacother* 2010; 11:905–918.

Malfertheiner P, Bazzoli F, Delchier JC et al. *Helicobacter pylori* eradication with a capsule containing bismuth subcitrate potassium, metronidazole, and tetracycline given with omeprazole versus clarithromycin-based triple therapy: a randomised, open-label, non-inferiority, phase 3 trial. *Lancet* 2011; 377:905–913.

McColl KE. *Helicobacter pylori* infection. *N Engl J Med* 2010; 362:1597–1604.

Rostom A. *Prevention of NSAID Induced Gastrointestinal Ulcers* (Cochrane Reviews Abstract). Chichester: Cochrane Library; 2007.

ACUTE AND CHRONIC GASTROINTESTINAL BLEEDING

This section should be read in conjunction with the descriptions of the specific conditions mentioned.

Acute upper gastrointestinal bleeding

The cardinal features are haematemesis (the vomiting of blood) and melaena (the passage of black tarry stools, the black colour being due to blood altered by passage through the gut). Melaena can occur with bleeding from any lesion proximal to the right colon. Rarely, melaena can also result from bleeding from the right colon.

Following a bleed from the upper gastrointestinal tract, unaltered blood can appear *per rectum*, but the bleeding must be massive and is almost always accompanied by shock. The passage of dark blood and clots without shock is always due to lower gastrointestinal bleeding.

Aetiology

Peptic ulceration is the most common cause of serious and life-threatening gastrointestinal bleeding ***(Fig. 13.25)***. The relative incidence of causes depends on the patient population; overall, incidence has fallen. In the developing world, haemorrhagic viral infections (see ***Box 11.33***) can cause significant gastrointestinal bleeding.

Drugs

Aspirin (even 75 mg/day) and other NSAIDs can produce ulcers and erosions. These agents are also responsible for gastrointestinal haemorrhage from both duodenal and gastric ulcers, particularly in the elderly. They are available over the counter in the UK and patients may not be aware that they are taking aspirin or an NSAID.

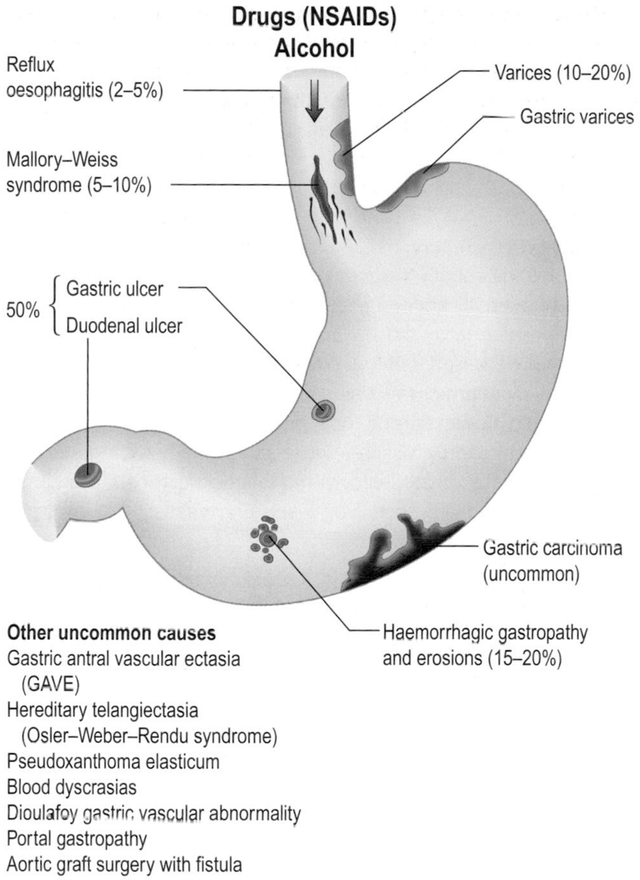

Figure 13.25 Causes of upper gastrointestinal haemorrhage. The approximate frequency is also given. NSAID, non-steroidal anti-inflammatory drug.

Corticosteroids in the usual therapeutic doses have no influence on gastrointestinal haemorrhage. Anticoagulants and antiplatelet agents do not cause acute gastrointestinal haemorrhage *per se*, but bleeding from any cause is greater if the patient is anticoagulated.

Clinical approach to the patient

All cases with a recent (i.e. within 48 hours) significant gastrointestinal bleed should be seen in hospital. In many, no immediate treatment is required, as there has been only a small amount of blood loss. Approximately 85% of patients stop bleeding spontaneously within 48 hours.

Scoring systems have been developed to assess the risk of rebleeding or death.

Boxes 13.14 and ***13.15*** show the Rockall score, which is based on clinical and endoscopy findings. The Blatchford score uses the level of plasma urea, haemoglobin and clinical markers, but not endoscopic findings, to determine the need for intervention such as blood transfusion or endoscopy in gastrointestinal bleeding.

The following factors affect the risk of rebleeding and death:

- age
- evidence of co-morbidity, e.g. cardiac failure, ischaemic heart disease, chronic kidney disease and malignant disease
- presence of the classical clinical features of shock (pallor, cold peripheries, tachycardia and low blood pressure)
- endoscopic diagnosis, e.g. Mallory–Weiss tear, peptic ulceration, gastric antral vascular ectasia (GAVE; ***Fig. 13.26***)
- endoscopic stigmata of recent bleeding, e.g. adherent blood clot, spurting vessel
- clinical signs of chronic liver disease.

Bleeding associated with liver disease is often severe and recurrent if it is from varices. Liver failure can develop.

Box 13.14 Rockall risk assessment score in non-variceal upper gastrointestinal haemorrhage

Variable	Score			
	0	*1*	*2*	*3*
Age (years)	<60	60–79	>79	–
Circulation	BP >100 mmHg Pulse <100 b.p.m.	BP >100 mmHg Pulse >100 b.p.m.	BP <100 mmHg Pulse >100 b.p.m.	–
Co-morbidity	None	–	Cardiac disease, any other major co-morbidity	Chronic kidney disease, liver failure, disseminated malignancy
Endoscopic diagnosis	Mallory–Weiss tear, no lesion	All other diagnoses	Malignancy of the upper gastrointestinal tract	–
Major SRH	None, or dark spots	–	Blood in the upper gastrointestinal tract, adherent clot or spurting vessel	–

BP, blood pressure (systolic); SRH, stigmata of recent haemorrhage.

Box 13.15 Rockall scores post-endoscopy

Risk score	Predicted mortality (%)	
	Rebleed	*No rebleed*
0	5	0
1	3	0
2	5	0
3	11	3
4	14	5
5	24	11
6	33	17
7	44	27
8+	42	41

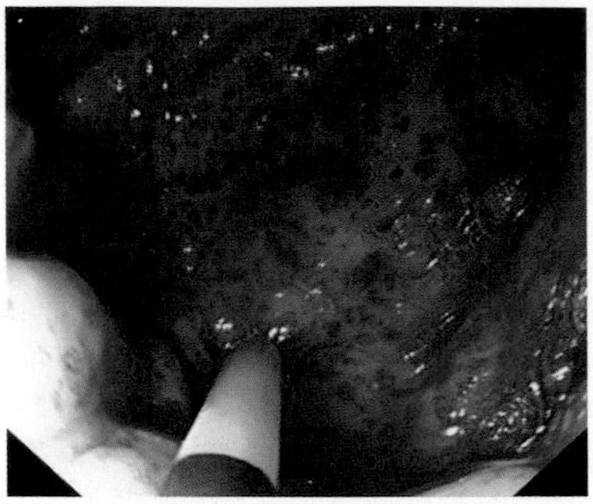

Figure 13.26 **Endoscopic view of gastric antral vascular ectasia (GAVE).** An argon plasma coagulation catheter is shown at 6 o'clock.

Box 13.16 Management of acute gastrointestinal bleeding

- Take history and perform examination. Note co-morbidity
- Monitor pulse and BP half-hourly
- Take blood for haemoglobin, urea, electrolytes, liver biochemistry, coagulation screen, group and crossmatching (2 units initially)
- Establish intravenous access – two large-bore i.v. cannulae
- Give blood transfusion/colloid if necessary. Indications for blood transfusion are:
  - a. Shock (pallor, cold nose, systolic BP below 100 mmHg, pulse >100 b.p.m.)
  - b. Haemoglobin <100 g/L in patients with recent or active bleeding
- Give oxygen therapy
- Perform urgent endoscopy in shocked patients/liver disease
- Continue to monitor pulse and BP
- Re-endoscope for continued bleeding/hypovolaemia
- Arrange surgery if bleeding persists

Management

Immediate management

This is shown in ***Box 13.16***. In addition, stop NSAIDs, aspirin, clopidogrel and warfarin if patients are taking them. Stopping antiplatelets can be dangerous and may produce thrombosis; discuss this urgently with a cardiologist.

Many hospitals have multidisciplinary specialist teams with agreed protocols and the latter should be followed. Patients should be managed in high-dependency beds. Oxygen should be given and the patient should be kept nil by mouth until an endoscopy has been performed.

Patients with large bleeds and clinical signs of shock require urgent resuscitation. Details of the management of shock are given in ***Figure 25.24***.

Blood volume

The major principle is to restore the blood volume rapidly to normal via one or more large-bore intravenous cannulae; plasma expanders or 0.9% saline are given until the blood becomes available (see pp. 1157–1158). Transfusion of red cell concentrates is used with a proposed transfusion threshold of 70 g/L. This has yet to be universally adopted.

Transfusion must be monitored to avoid overload leading to heart failure, particularly in the elderly. The pulse rate and venous pressure are guides to adequacy of transfusion. A central venous pressure line is inserted for patients with organ failure who require blood transfusion, and in those most at risk of developing heart failure.

Haemoglobin levels are generally a poor indicator of the need to transfuse because anaemia does not develop immediately as haemodilution has not taken place. In most patients, the bleeding stops, albeit temporarily, so that further assessment can be made.

Endoscopy

Endoscopy will usually diagnose, stratify risk, and enable therapy to be performed if needed. Endoscopy should be carried out as soon as possible after the patient has been resuscitated. Patients with Rockall scores of 0 or 1 pre-endoscopy may be candidates for immediate discharge (see below) and outpatient endoscopy the following day, depending on local policy.

Endoscopy can detect the cause of the haemorrhage in 80% or more of cases. In patients with a peptic ulcer, if the stigmata of a recent bleed are seen (i.e. a spurting vessel, active oozing, fresh or organized blood clot or black spots), the patient is more likely to rebleed. Calculation of the post-endoscopy Rockall score (see ***Box 13.15***) gives an indication of the risk of rebleeding and death.

At first endoscopy:

- Varices should be treated, usually with banding.
- Stenting is also used for bleeding varices but is not yet widely available (see p. 471). It is an alternative to a Sengstaken tube.
- Bleeding ulcers and those with stigmata of recent bleeding should be treated using two or three haemostatic methods: injection with adrenaline (epinephrine) and thermal coagulation (with heater probe, bipolar probe, or laser or argon plasma coagulation) or endoscopic clipping; dual and triple therapy is more effective than monotherapy in reducing rebleeding. Haemostatic powders have recently been developed that can be sprayed through a catheter during gastroscopy. These are useful in the more difficult bleeds, such as cancer-related bleeding and challenging ulcers.
- Antral biopsies should be taken to look for *H. pylori*. A positive biopsy urease test is valid but a negative test is not reliable. If the urease test is negative, gastric histology should always be performed.

Drug therapy

After diagnosis at endoscopy, an intravenous PPI (e.g. omeprazole 80 mg followed by infusion 8 mg/h for 72 h) should be given to all patients with actively bleeding ulcers or ulcers with a visible vessel, as it reduces rebleeding rates and the need for surgery.

Uncontrolled or repeat bleeding

Endoscopy should be repeated to assess the bleeding site and to treat, if possible. Embolization by an interventional radiologist may be necessary if the bleeding persists. If this is not available locally or is unsuccessful, surgery is used to control the haemorrhage primarily.

Discharge policy

The patient's age, diagnosis on endoscopy, co-morbidity, the presence or absence of shock and the availability of support in the community should be taken into consideration. In general, all patients who are haemodynamically stable and have no stigmata of recent haemorrhage on endoscopy (Rockall score pre-endoscopy 0, post-endoscopy <1) can be discharged from hospital within

24 hours. All shocked patients and patients with co-morbidity need longer inpatient observation.

Specific conditions

Oesophageal varices

These are discussed on page 471.

Mallory–Weiss tear

This is a linear mucosal tear occurring at the oesophagogastric junction and produced by a sudden increase in intra-abdominal pressure. It often follows a bout of coughing or retching, and is classically seen after alcoholic 'dry heaves'. There may, however, be no antecedent history of retching. Most bleeds are minor and discharge is usual within 24 hours. The haemorrhage may be large but most patients stop spontaneously. Early endoscopy confirms diagnosis and allows therapy such as clipping if necessary. Surgery with oversewing of the tear is rarely needed.

Chronic peptic ulcer

Eradication of *H. pylori* is started as soon as possible (see p. 380). A PPI is continued for 4 weeks to ensure ulcer healing. Eradication of *H. pylori* should always be checked in a patient who has bled, and long-term acid suppression is given if *H. pylori* eradication cannot be achieved. If bleeding is not controlled, the patient should either undergo angiography and embolization or be referred directly for surgery.

Gastric carcinoma

Most of these patients do not have large bleeds but surgery is occasionally necessary for uncontrolled or repeat bleeding. Usually, surgery can be delayed until the patient has been fully evaluated (see p. 383). Oozing from gastric cancer is very difficult to control endoscopically. Radiotherapy can occasionally be successful but its effects are not immediate.

Bleeding after percutaneous coronary intervention

In the era of ever more aggressive percutaneous coronary intervention (PCI), the list of antithrombotic medication grows longer: glycoprotein IIb/IIIa inhibitors, unfractionated heparin, low-molecular-weight heparin, fondaparinux and platelet inhibitors (e.g. clopidogrel, prasugrel and ticagrelor). Taken in addition to the oral anticoagulants that this group of patients are often taking, these give rise to a gastrointestinal bleeding rate of approximately 2% of patients undergoing PCI (who are on antiplatelet therapy, e.g. clopidogrel), and there is a high mortality of 5–10%. It has become increasingly evident in this patient group that gastroscopy should be performed on an urgent basis and not deferred for days or weeks. A bolus of intravenous PPI is administered, followed by an infusion; platelet infusion is given to counter the effect of clopidogrel. Management is difficult, as cessation of antiplatelet therapy has a high risk of acute stent thrombosis and also an associated high mortality. Using a risk assessment score (e.g. Blatchford), a reasonable approach is to stop all antiplatelet therapy in high-risk patients but continue it in low-risk ones. Co-prescribed proton pump inhibition does not decrease the antiplatelet effect of clopidogrel, as was first thought. These patients should be under the combined care of a cardiologist and a gastroenterologist.

Prognosis

The mortality from gastrointestinal haemorrhage has not changed from 5–12% over the years, despite many changes in management, mainly because of a demographic shift to more elderly patients with co-morbidity. The lowest mortality rates are achieved in dedicated medical/surgical gastrointestinal units.

Acute lower gastrointestinal bleeding

Massive bleeding from the lower gastrointestinal tract is rare and is usually due to diverticular disease or ischaemic colitis. Common causes of small bleeds are haemorrhoids and anal fissures. The causes of lower gastrointestinal bleeding are shown in ***Figure 13.27***.

Management

Most acute lower gastrointestinal bleeds start and stop spontaneously. The few patients who continue bleeding and are haemodynamically unstable need resuscitation using the same principles as for upper gastrointestinal bleeding (see p. 386). Surgery is rarely required.

A diagnosis is made using the history and examination, including rectal examination and the following investigations as appropriate:

- ***Proctoscopy*** (e.g. anorectal disease, particularly haemorrhoids)
- ***Flexible sigmoidoscopy or colonoscopy*** (e.g. inflammatory bowel disease, cancer, ischaemic colitis, diverticular disease, angiodysplasia)
- ***Video capsule endoscopy (Fig. 13.28)***
- ***Angiography*** to seek vascular abnormality (e.g. angiodysplasia). The yield of angiography is low, so it is a test of last resort.

Isolated episodes of rectal bleeding in the young (<45 years) usually only require rectal examination and flexible sigmoidoscopy because the probability of a significant proximal lesion is very low, unless there is a strong family history of colorectal cancer at a young age. Individual lesions are treated as appropriate.

Chronic gastrointestinal bleeding

Patients with chronic bleeding usually present with iron deficiency anaemia (see pp. 524–526).

Chronic blood loss producing iron deficiency anaemia in all men, and all women after the menopause, is always due to bleeding from the gastrointestinal tract. The primary concern is to exclude cancer,

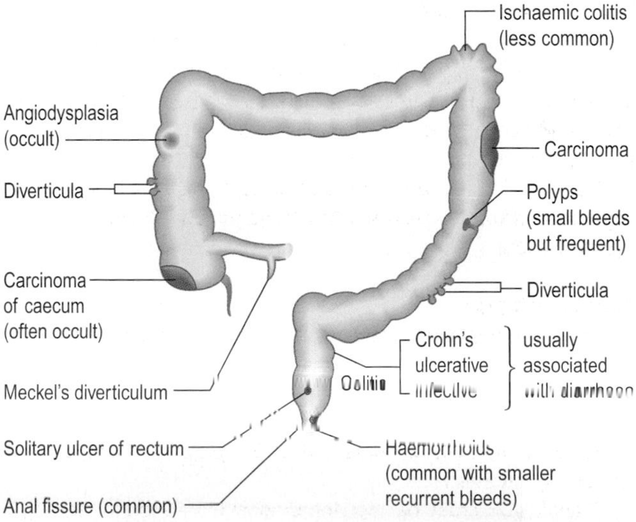

Figure 13.27 Causes of lower gastrointestinal bleeding. The sites shown are illustrative – many of the lesions can be seen in other parts of the colon.

particularly of the stomach or right colon, and coeliac disease. Occult stool tests are unhelpful.

Diagnosis

Chronic blood loss can occur with any lesion of the gastrointestinal tract that produces acute bleeding (see ***Figs 13.25*** and ***13.27***). However, oesophageal varices usually bleed overtly and rarely present as chronic blood loss. Although uncommon in developed countries, hookworm is the most common worldwide cause of chronic gastrointestinal blood loss.

History and examination may indicate the most likely site of the bleeding, but if no clue is available, it is usual to investigate both the upper and lower gastrointestinal tract endoscopically at the same session ('top and tail'), especially in males and postmenopausal females:

- ***Upper gastrointestinal endoscopy*** is usually performed first. Duodenal biopsies should always be taken to diagnose coeliac disease, even if coeliac serology has been performed.
- ***Colonoscopy*** follows and any lesion should be biopsied or removed, though it is unsafe to assume that colonic polyps are the cause of chronic blood loss.
- ***Unprepared CT*** scanning is a reasonable test to look for colon cancer in frail patients.
- ***CT colonography*** can be used as an alternative to colonoscopy.

If gastroscopy, colonoscopy and duodenal biopsy have not revealed the cause, investigation of the small bowel is necessary. ***Capsule endoscopy*** is the diagnostic investigation of choice but currently has no therapeutic ability. Positive diagnostic yield varies from 60% to 85%, depending on series. Bleeding lesions can be identified and later treated with balloon-assisted enteroscopy.

Occasionally, intravenous technetium-labelled colloid may be used to demonstrate a potential bleeding site in a Meckel's diverticulum.

Management

The cause of the bleeding should be dealt with, if found. Oral iron is given to treat anaemia (see pp. 525–526), although intravenous infusions are occasionally required. Some patients will require maintenance with regular transfusion as a last resort.

Further reading

Banerjee S, Cash BD, Dominitz JA et al. and the ASGE Standards of Practice Committee. The role of endoscopy in the management of patients with peptic ulcer disease. *Gastrointest Endosc* 2010; 71:663–668.

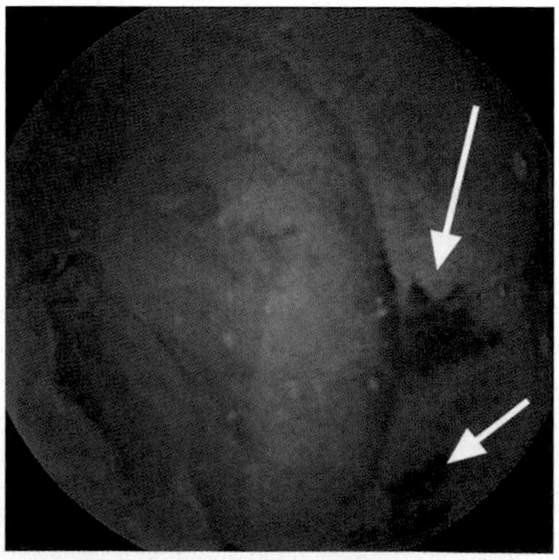

Fig. 13.28 Angiodysplastic lesions (arrows) seen on video capsule endoscopy.

Blatchford O, Murray WR, Blatchford M. A risk score to predict need for treatment for upper-gastrointestinal haemorrhage. *Lancet* 2000; 356:1318–1321.
Herbert FC, Carson JL. Transfusion threshold of 7 g per deciliter – the new normal. *N Engl J Med* 2014; 371:1459–1461.
[No authors listed]. Managing acute upper gastrointestinal bleeding. *Lancet* 2011; 377:1048.
Sidhu R, Sanders DS, Morris AJ et al. Guidelines on small bowel enteroscopy and capsule endoscopy in adults. *Gut* 2008; 57:125–136.
http://www.rcplondon.ac.uk/resources/upper-gastrointestinal-bleeding-toolkit *British Society of Gastroenterology toolkit for managing upper GI bleeding.*

THE SMALL INTESTINE

Anatomy

The small intestine extends from the duodenum to the ileocaecal valve. It is 3–6 m in length, and 300 m^2 in surface area. The upper 40% is the duodenum and jejunum; the remainder is the ileum. Its surface area is enormously increased by circumferential mucosal folds that bear multiple finger-like projections called villi. On the villi, the surface area is further increased by microvilli on the luminal side of the epithelial cells (enterocytes) ***(Fig. 13.29)***.

Each villus consists of a core containing blood vessels, lacteals (lymphatics) and cells (e.g. plasma cells and lymphocytes). The lamina propria contains plasma cells, lymphocytes, macrophages, eosinophils and mast cells. The crypts of Lieberkühn are the spaces between the bases of the villi.

Enterocytes are formed at the bottom of the crypts and migrate toward the tops of the villi, where they are shed. This process takes 3–4 days. On its luminal side, the enterocyte is covered by microvilli and a gelatinous layer called the glycocalyx. Scattered between the epithelial cells are mucin-secreting goblet cells and occasional intraepithelial lymphocytes and Paneth cells. Most of the blood supply to the small intestine is via branches of the superior

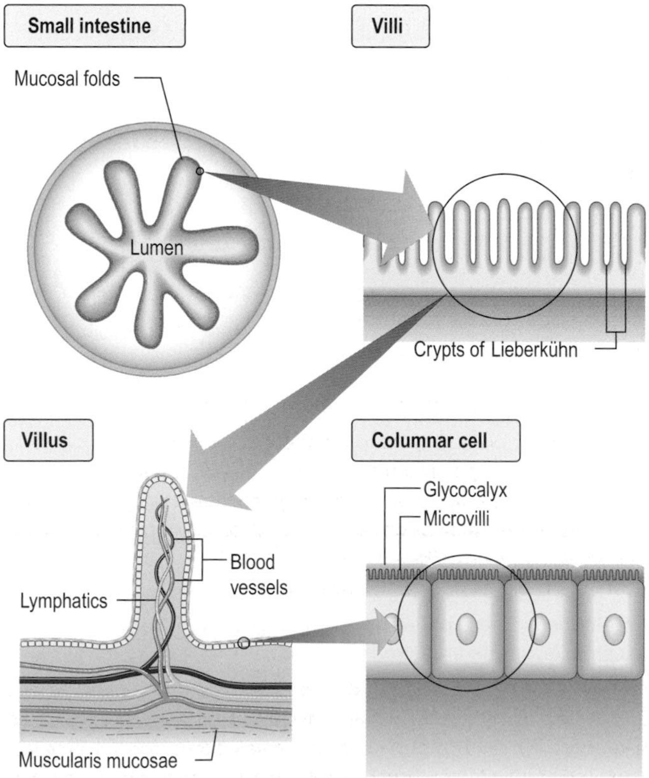

Figure 13.29 Structure of the small intestine.

mesenteric artery. The terminal branches are end arteries; there are no local anastomotic connections.

Enteric nervous system

The enteric nervous system (ENS) controls the functioning of the small bowel; it is an independent system that coordinates absorption, secretion, blood flow and motility. It is estimated to contain 10^8 neurones (as many as the spinal cord), organized in two major ganglionated plexuses: the *myenteric plexus* between the muscular layers of the intestinal wall, and the *submucosal plexuses* associated with the mucosa. The ENS communicates with the central nervous system (CNS) via autonomic afferent and efferent pathways but can operate autonomously.

Coordination of small intestinal function involves a complex and only partly understood interplay between many neuroactive mediators and their receptors, ion channels, gastrointestinal hormones, nitric oxide and other transmitters. Acetylcholine, adrenaline (epinephrine), adenosine triphosphate (ATP), vasoactive intestinal peptide (VIP), and other hormones and opioids have been shown to have actions in the small bowel but the exact role of each is not yet clear.

Gut motility

The contractile patterns of the small intestinal muscular layers are primarily determined by the ENS. The CNS and gut hormones also have a modulatory role in motility. The interstitial cells of Cajal, which lie within the smooth muscle, appear to govern rhythmic contractions.

During fasting, a distally migrating sequence of motor events, termed the migrating motor complex (MMC), occurs in a cyclical fashion. The MMC consists of:

- a period of motor quiescence (*phase I*)
- a period of irregular contractile activity (*phase II*)
- a short (5–10-min) burst of regular phasic contractions (*phase III*).

Each MMC cycle lasts for approximately 90 minutes. In the duodenum, phase III is associated with increased gastric, pancreatic and biliary secretions. The role of the MMC is unclear, but the strong phase III contractions propel secretions, residual food and desquamated cells towards the colon. It is named the 'intestinal housekeeper'.

After a meal, the MMC pattern is disrupted and replaced by irregular contractions. This seemingly chaotic pattern lasts typically for 2–5 hours after feeding, depending on the size and nutrient content of the meal. The irregular contractions of the fed pattern have a mixing function, moving intraluminal contents to and fro and aiding the digestive process.

Neuroendocrine peptide production

The hormone-producing cells of the gut are scattered diffusely throughout its length and also occur in the pancreas.

Gut hormones play a part in the regulation and integration of the functions of the small bowel and other metabolic activities, including appetite. Their actions are complex and interactive, both with each other and with the ENS ***(Box 13.17)***.

Physiology

In the small bowel, digestion and absorption of nutrients and ions takes place, as does the regulation of fluid absorption and secretion. The epithelial cells of the small bowel form a physical barrier that is selectively permeable to ions, small molecules and macromolecules. Digestive enzymes, such as proteases and disaccharidases, are produced by intestinal cells and expressed on the surface of microvilli; others, such as lipases produced by the pancreas, are associated with the glycocalyx. Some nutrients are absorbed most actively in specific parts of the small intestine: iron and folate in the duodenum and jejunum, and vitamin B_{12} and bile salts in the terminal ileum, where they have specific receptors.

General principles of absorption

Simple diffusion

This process is non-specific, requires no carrier molecule or energy, and takes place if there is a concentration gradient from the intestinal lumen (high concentration) to the bloodstream (low concentration). Vitamin B_{12} can be absorbed from the jejunum by this means.

Facilitated diffusion

Absorption takes place down a concentration gradient but a membrane carrier protein is involved, conferring specificity on the process. Fructose transport is an example.

Active transport

Absorption occurs via a specific carrier protein, powered by cellular energy, allowing a substance to be transported against a concentration gradient. Many carrier proteins are powered by ion gradients across the enterocyte wall. For example, glucose crosses the enterocyte microvillous membrane from the lumen into the cell against a concentration gradient by using a ***co-transporter*** carrier molecule. This is the sodium/glucose co-transporter, SGLT1 ***(Fig. 13.30)***.

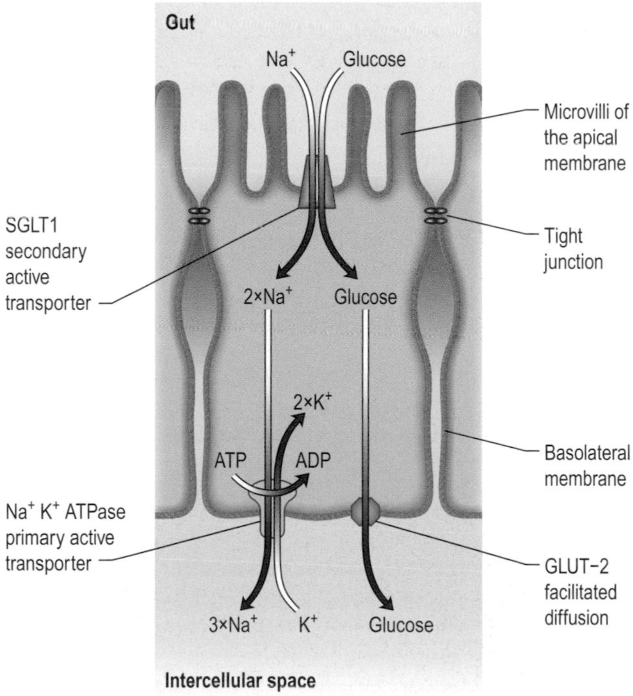

Figure 13.30 Transcellular uptake of glucose across the intestinal epithelia. Glucose is co-transported across the apical membrane with sodium ions by the sodium-dependent glucose transporter (SGLT). This is secondary active transport, as the sodium is travelling down its electrochemical gradient. The sodium gradient is maintained by the primary active transport of sodium across the basolateral membrane by the Na^+/K^+ ATPase (thus intracellular Na^+ is kept low). Transcellular transport of glucose is achieved by facilitated diffusion across the basolateral membrane as glucose is moved down its concentration gradient by GLUT-2.

Box 13.17 Gut regulatory peptides

Peptide	Localization	Main actions
Gastrin/cholecystokinin family		
Cholecystokinin (CCK): multiple forms from CCK8 (8 amino acids) to CCK83; 8, 33 and 58 are predominant. Terminal 5 amino acids same as gastrin	Duodenum and jejunum (I cells) Enteric nerves CNS	Causes gall bladder contraction and sphincter of Oddi relaxation. Trophic effects on duodenum and pancreas. Pancreatic secretion (minor role). Role in satiety – acting on CNS
Gastrin	G cells in gastric antrum and duodenum	Stimulates acid secretion. Trophic to mucosa
Secretin-glucagon family		
Secretin	Duodenum and jejunum (S cells)	Stimulates pancreatic bicarbonate secretion
Glucagon	Alpha cells of pancreas	Opposes insulin in blood glucose control
Vasoactive intestinal polypeptide (VIP)	Enteric nerves	Intestinal secretion of water and electrolytes. Neurotransmitter. Splanchnic vasodilatation, stimulates insulin release
Glucose-dependent insulinotropic peptide (GIP)	Duodenum (K cells) Gastric antrum Ileum	Release by intraduodenal glucose causes greater insulin release by islets than i.v. glucose (incretin effect)
Glucagon-like peptide-1 (GLP-1)	Ileum and colon (L cells)	Incretin. Stimulates insulin synthesis. Trophic to islet cells. Inhibits glucagon secretion and gastric emptying Stimulates growth of enterocytes
Glicentin	L cells, A cells	Stimulates insulin secretion and gut growth, inhibits gastric secretion
Growth hormone-releasing factor (GHRF)	Small intestine	Unclear
Pancreatic polypeptide family		
Pancreatic polypeptide (PP)	Pancreas (PP cells)	Inhibits pancreatic and biliary secretion
Peptide YY (PYY)	Ileum and colon (L cells)	Inhibits pancreatic exocrine secretion. Slows gastric and small bowel transit ('ileal brake'). Reduces food intake and appetite
Neuropeptide Y (NPY)	Enteric nerves	Stimulates feeding. Regulates intestinal blood flow
Other		
Motilin	Whole gut	Increases gastric emptying and small bowel contraction
Ghrelin	Stomach	Stimulates appetite, increases gastric emptying
Obestatin	Stomach and small intestine	Opposes ghrelin
Oxyntomodulin	Colon	Inhibits appetite
Gastrin releasing-polypeptide (bombesin)	Whole gut and pancreas	Stimulates pancreatic exocrine secretion and gastric acid secretion
Somatostatin	Stomach and pancreas (D cells) Small and large intestine	Inhibits secretion and action of most hormones
Substance P	Enteric nerves	Enhances gastric acid secretion, smooth muscle contraction
Neurotensin	Ileum	Affects gut motility. Increases jejunal and ileal fluid secretion
Insulin	Pancreatic β cells	Increases glucose utilization
Chromogranins	Neuroendocrine cells	Precursor for other regulatory peptides that inhibit neuroendocrine secretion

The process is powered by the energy derived from the flow of Na^+ ions from a high concentration outside the cell to a low concentration inside. The sodium gradient across the cell wall is maintained by a separate ATP-consuming Na^+/K^+ exchanger in the basolateral membrane. Glucose leaves the cell on the serosal side by facilitated diffusion via a sodium-independent carrier (GLUT-2) in the basolateral membrane.

Another active transport mechanism operates for Na^+ absorption in the ileum using an Na^+/H^+ ***exchange*** mechanism, powered by the outwardly directed gradient of H^+ across the cell membrane.

Absorption of nutrients in the small intestine

Carbohydrate

Dietary carbohydrate consists mainly of starch, with some sucrose and a small amount of lactose. Starch is a polysaccharide made up of numerous glucose units. In order to have a nutrient value, starch must be digested into smaller oligo-, di- and finally monosaccharides, which may then be absorbed. Polysaccharide hydrolysis begins in the mouth and is catalysed by salivary amylase, though the majority takes place under the action of pancreatic amylase in the upper intestine. The breakdown products of starch digestion are maltose and maltotriose, together with sucrose and lactose. These are further hydrolysed on the microvillous membrane by specific oligo- and disaccharidases to form glucose, galactose and fructose. These monosaccharides are then able to be transported across the enterocytes into the blood (see ***Fig. 13.30***).

Protein

Dietary protein is digested by pancreatic proteolytic enzymes to amino acids and peptides prior to absorption. These enzymes are

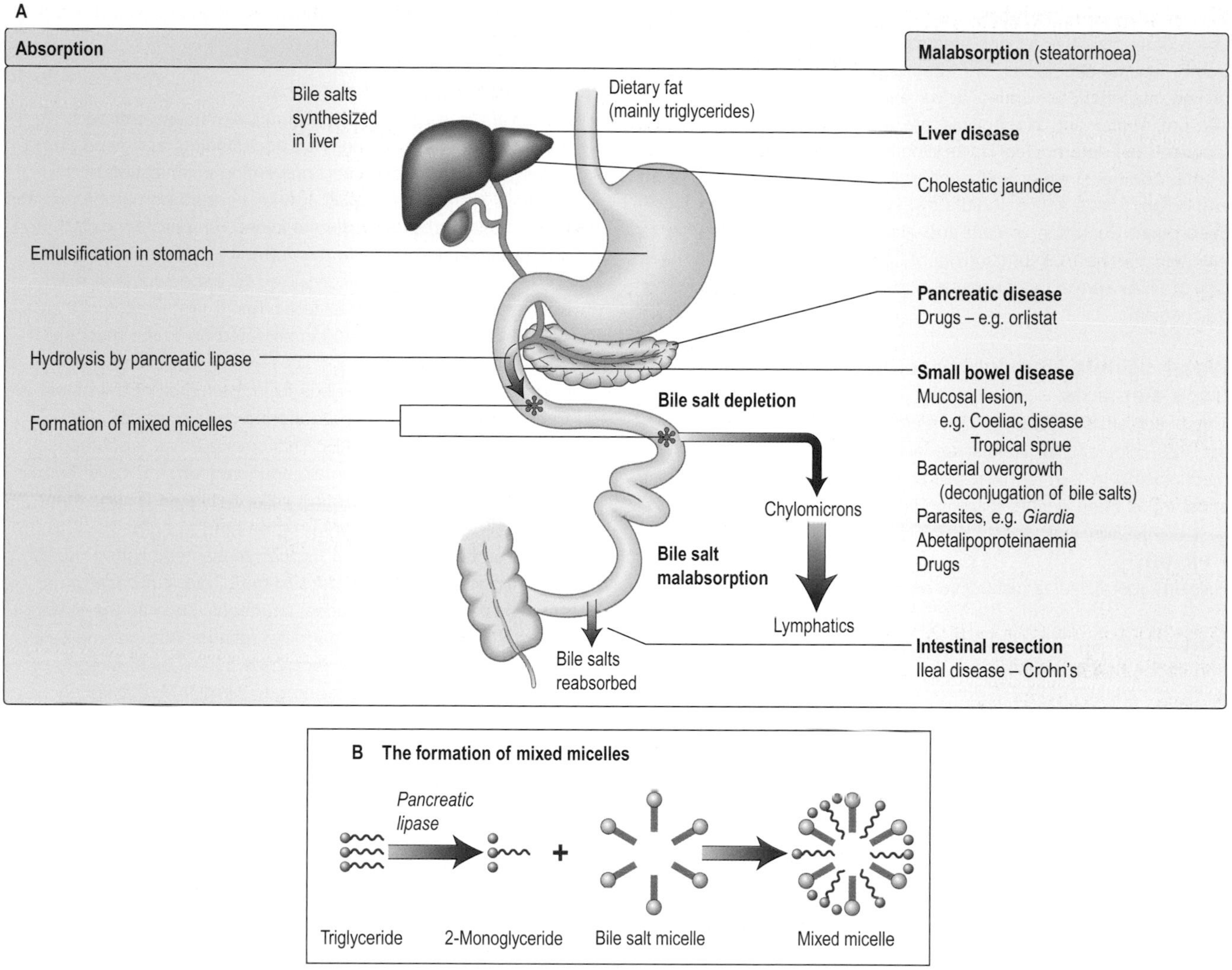

Figure 13.31 **Fat absorption in the small intestine. A.** The pathophysiology of fat absorption. **B.** The formation of mixed micelles.

secreted by the pancreas as pro-enzymes and transformed to active forms in the lumen. Protein in the duodenal lumen stimulates the enzymatic conversion of trypsinogen to trypsin, and this, in turn, activates the other pro-enzymes, chymotrypsin and elastase.

These enzymes break down protein into oligopeptides. Some di- and tripeptides are absorbed intact by carrier-mediated processes, while the remainder are broken down into free amino acids by peptidases on the microvillous membranes of the enterocytes, prior to absorption into the cell by a variety of amino acid and peptide carrier systems.

Fat

Dietary fat consists mainly of triglycerides with some cholesterol and fat-soluble vitamins. Fat is emulsified by mechanical action in the stomach. Bile containing the amphipathic detergents, bile acids and phospholipids enters the duodenum following gall bladder contraction. These substances act to solubilize fat and promote hydrolysis of triglycerides in the duodenum by pancreatic lipase to yield fatty acids and monoglycerides. Bile acids, phospholipids and the products of fat digestion cluster together with their hydrophilic ends on the outside to form aggregations called mixed micelles. Trapped in the centre of the micelles are the hydrophobic monoglycerides, fatty acids and cholesterol. At the cell membrane, the lipid contents of the micelles are absorbed, while the bile salts remain in the lumen. Inside the cell, the monoglycerides and fatty acids are re-esterified to triglycerides. The triglycerides and other fat-soluble molecules (e.g. cholesterol, phospholipids) are then incorporated into chylomicrons to be transported into the lymph.

Any unabsorbed lipids that reach the ileum delay gastric emptying via peptide YY, which is secreted by the ileum (called the **'ileal brake'**). This delay allows more time for absorption of lipids in the small intestine.

Medium-chain triglycerides (MCTs, fatty acids of chain length 6–12) are transported via the portal vein with a small amount of long-chain fatty acid. Patients with pancreatic exocrine or bile salt insufficiency can therefore supplement their fat absorption with MCTs.

Bile salts are not absorbed in the jejunum, so the intraluminal concentration in the upper gut is high. They pass down the intestine to be absorbed in the terminal ileum and are transported back to the liver. This enterohepatic circulation prevents excess loss of bile salts (see p. 443).

The pathophysiology of fat absorption is shown in ***Figure 13.31***. Interference with absorption can occur at all stages, as indicated, giving rise to steatorrhoea (>17 mmol or 6 g of faecal fat per day).

Water and electrolytes

Large amounts of water and electrolytes, partly dietary but mainly from intestinal secretions, are absorbed, coupled with absorption of monosaccharides, amino acids and bicarbonate in the upper jejunum. Water and electrolytes are also absorbed paracellularly (between the enterocytes) down electrochemical and osmotic gradients. Additional water and electrolytes are absorbed in the ileum and colon, where active sodium transport is not coupled to solute absorption. Secretion of fluid and electrolytes occurs together to maintain the normal functioning of the gut. Secretory diarrhoea (see p. 426) can occur because of defects in intestinal secretory mechanisms.

Water-soluble vitamins, essential metals and trace elements

These are all absorbed in the small intestine. Vitamin B_{12} (see pp. 529–530) and bile salts are absorbed by specific transport mechanisms in the terminal ileum; malabsorption of both these substances often occurs following ileal resection.

Calcium

Calcium absorption is discussed on page 708.

Iron

Iron absorption is discussed on pages 523–524.

Response of the small bowel to antigens and pathogens

The small bowel has a number of mechanisms to prevent colonization and invasion by pathogens while simultaneously preventing inappropriate responses to foreign antigens or the indigenous bacterial population. At the same time, commensal bacteria maintain the integrity of the small bowel and play a major role in host physiology.

Mechanisms

Physical defence

- The mucus layer.
- Continuous shedding of surface epithelial cells.
- The physical movement of the luminal contents.
- Colonization resistance – the ability of the indigenous microbiota to outcompete pathogens for a survival niche in the gut.

Innate chemical defence

- ***Enzymes*** such as lysozyme and phospholipase A_2, secreted by Paneth cells at the base of the crypts, help ensure an infection-free environment in the gut, even in the presence of commensal bacteria.
- ***Antimicrobial peptides*** are secreted from enterocytes and Paneth cells in response to pathogenic bacteria. These include ***defensins***, which are 15–20 amino-acid peptides with potent activity against a broad range of pathogens, including Gram-positive and Gram-negative bacteria, fungi and viruses.
- ***Trefoil peptides*** are a family of small proteins secreted by goblet cells. They consist of a three-loop structure with intra-chain disulphide bonds, which makes the molecules highly resistant to digestion. Their actions include stabilization of mucus, promotion of cell migration to injured areas, and promotion of repair. Three trefoil factors (TFFs) are found in humans (TFF1, TFF2 and TFF3), all of which have been implicated in the response to gastrointestinal injury in experimental models. Their molecular mode of action is not yet known.

Innate immunological defence

- ***Humoral defence***. IgA is the principal mucosal antibody. It mediates mucosal immunity by agglutinating and neutralizing pathogens in the lumen and preventing colonization of the epithelial surface ***(Fig. 13.32)***. IgA is secreted from immunocytes in the lamina propria as dimers joined by a protein called the 'joining chain' (J-chain); in this form, it is known as polymeric IgA (pIgA). This pIgA is internalized by endocytosis at the basolateral membrane of enterocytes. It crosses the cell as a complex of pIgA/pIgAR and is secreted on to the mucosal surface.
- ***B-cell sensitization***. Antigens from the lumen of the bowel are transported by M cells and dendritic cells in the follicle-associated epithelium (FAE). This covers Peyer's patches in the 'dome' region that contain abundant virgin B cells, helper T cells and antigen-presenting cells. Activated B cells then produce IgA locally and are programmed to home back to the lamina propria. They travel through mesenteric lymph nodes and then via the thoracic duct to the blood and back to the small bowel and other mucosal surfaces (such as the airways), where they undergo terminal differentiation into plasma cells. Homing back to the gut is facilitated by the $\alpha4\beta7$-integrin on gut-derived lymphocytes binding to MAdCAM-1, uniquely expressed on blood vessels in the gut.
- ***Cellular defence***. T lymphocytes also provide host defence and initiate, activate and regulate adaptive immune responses. ***Intestinal T lymphocytes*** occur principally in three major compartments:
  - *Organized gut-associated lymphoid tissue (GALT)*, such as Peyer's patches, where mucosal T cell responses are generated, and after which cells leave the organized lymphoid tissue and home back to the mucosa.
  - *The lamina propria*, containing mostly CD4 cells.
  - The *surface epithelium*, where these lymphocytes are known as intraepithelial lymphocytes (IELs) and are mostly CD8 cells. T cells are sensitized to antigen in the Peyer's patch lymphoid tissue in a similar fashion to B cells, and pass through mesenteric lymph nodes into the thoracic duct and into the circulation, homing back to the small bowel to end up in the lamina propria or the epithelium. It is probable that IELs are cytotoxic cells, capable of killing virally or bacterially infected epithelial cells. CD4 cells in the lamina propria of healthy individuals are highly activated cells, probably protecting against low-grade infections, since loss of these cells, as in HIV infection, leads to colonization of the gut by protozoa such as cryptosporidia.

Commensal bacteria

The relationship between the hundred thousand billion microbes in the human gut and the host are only beginning to be appreciated. New molecular sequencing techniques have allowed the identification and classification of the gut microbiota. The use of metabonomics has aided the assessment of its functional output. There is increasing evidence that a reduction in the diversity of the gut microbiota is associated with a range of conditions, including inflammatory bowel disease and metabolic syndrome. Germ-free mice have essentially no mucosal immune system, showing that the abundant and activated immune system seen in healthy

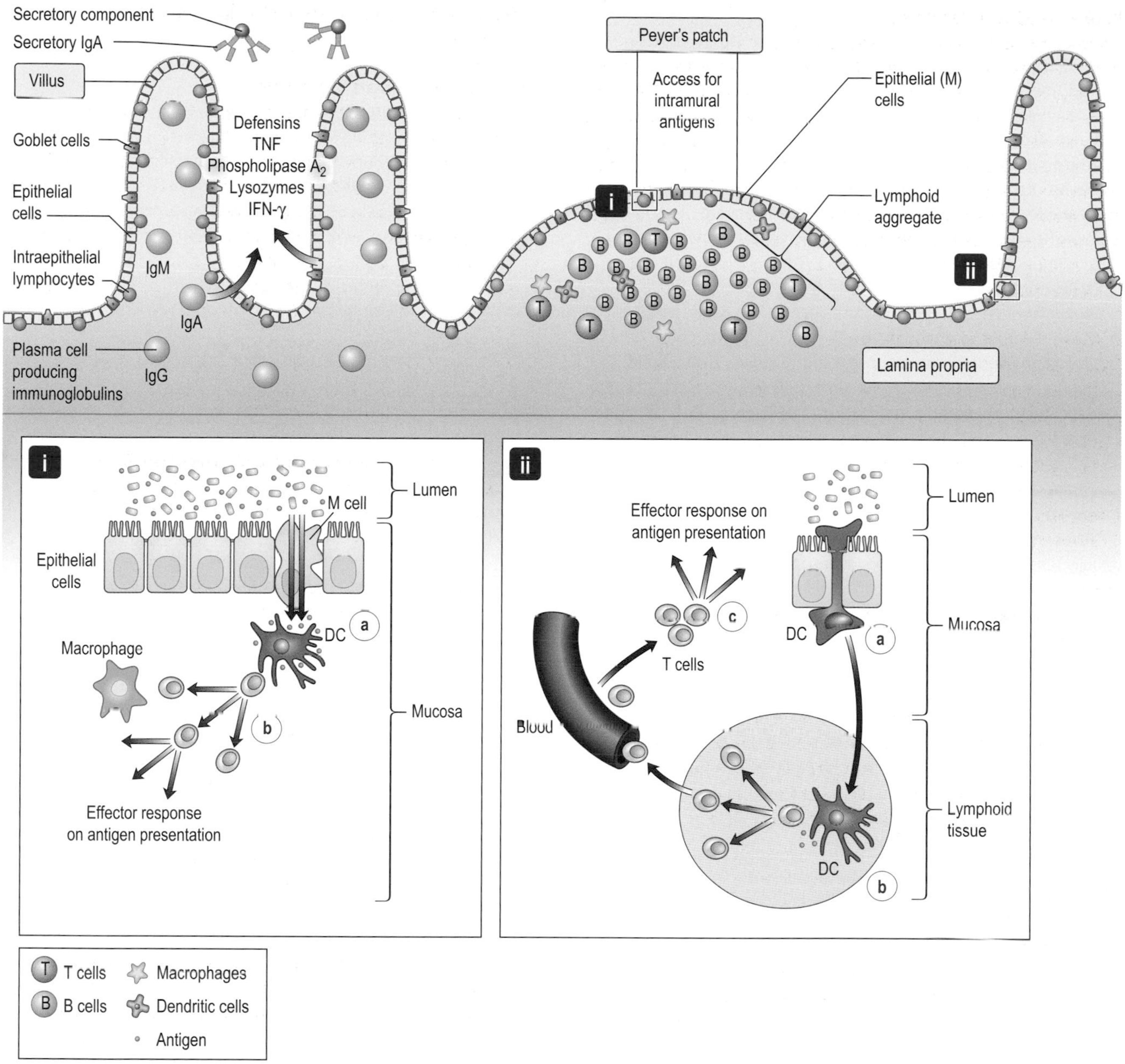

Figure 13.32 Small intestinal mucosa with a Peyer's patch, showing the gut-associated lymphoid tissue (GALT).
Inset i: **(a)** Specialized 'M' cells within a lymphoid follicle pass antigen to underlying antigen-presenting cells (APCs), such as dendritic cells (DCs). **(b)** DCs present antigen to T cells, resulting in activation and effector responses.
Inset ii: **(a)** DCs pass dendrites through epithelial tight junctions to sample luminal antigen. **(b)** DCs traffic to the mesenteric lymph node and present antigen to naive T cells, which differentiate into effector or regulatory subtypes and are imprinted with a gut homing integrin. **(c)** On subsequent antigen presentation, activated T cells home to lamina propria and exert a regulatory or inflammatory effect, depending on their phenotype. IFN-γ, interferon-gamma; Ig, immunoglobulin; TNF, tumour necrosis factor.

individuals is driven by the flora, without adverse effects. Bacteria also release chemical signals, such as lipopolysaccharide (LPS) and lipoteichoic acid, which are recognized by Toll-like receptors (TLRs) (see p. 127) present on a variety of intestinal cells, priming repair processes and enhancing the ability of the epithelium to respond to injury.

Oral tolerance

The immune system must guard against pathogens and toxins while avoiding an excessive response to the multiplicity of food antigens and commensal bacteria. The mechanisms by which tolerance occurs are undoubtedly multiple, including maintenance of barrier function to prevent excess antigen uptake, active inhibition via regulatory T cells, and dendritic cells that promote tolerogenic rather than immunogenic T-cell responses. All of these are likely to play a role in diseases such as coeliac disease, caused by an excessive T-cell response to gluten, or Crohn's disease, where tolerance to the indigenous bacterial population is defective.

Clinical features of small bowel disease

Regardless of the cause, the common presenting features of small bowel disease are listed below. However, 10–20% of patients will have no diarrhoea or any other gastrointestinal symptoms.

- ***Diarrhoea*** is common and may be watery.
- ***Steatorrhoea*** occurs when the stool fat is >17 mmol/day (or 6 g/day). The stools are pale, bulky and offensive, and float (because of their increased air content), leaving a fatty film on the water in the pan and proving difficult to flush away.
- ***Abdominal pain*** and discomfort. Abdominal distension can cause discomfort and flatulence. The pain has no specific character or periodicity and is not usually severe.
- ***Weight loss*** is largely due to the anorexia that invariably accompanies small bowel disease. The calorie deficit due to malabsorption is small relative to the reduction in intake.
- ***Nutritional deficiencies*** of iron, vitamin B_{12}, folate or all of these, leading to anaemia, are the only common deficiencies. Occasionally, malabsorption of other vitamins or minerals occurs, causing bruising (vitamin K deficiency), tetany (calcium deficiency), osteomalacia (vitamin D deficiency), or stomatitis, sore tongue and aphthous ulceration (multiple vitamin deficiencies). Oedema due to hypoproteinaemia is due to low intake and intestinal loss of albumin (protein-losing enteropathy).

Physical signs are few and non-specific. If present, they are usually associated with anaemia and the nutritional deficiencies described above.

Abdominal examination is often normal, but sometimes distension or, rarely, hepatomegaly or an abdominal mass is found. Visible peristalsis and high-pitched bowel sounds can indicate chronic subacute obstruction of the small intestine: for example, that due to stricturing Crohn's disease. Gross weight loss, oedema and muscle wasting are seen only in severe cases. A neuropathy, not always due to B_{12} deficiency, can be present.

Investigation of small bowel disease

The emphasis in the investigation of malabsorption ***(Fig. 13.33)*** is on the structural features of the underlying disorder, rather than on the documentation of malabsorption itself.

Blood tests

- ***Full blood count (FBC) and film***. Anaemia can be microcytic, macrocytic or normocytic, and the blood film may be dimorphic. Other abnormal cells (e.g. Howell–Jolly bodies, p. 553) may be seen in splenic atrophy associated with coeliac disease.
  - *Serum ferritin and iron saturation* should be measured to differentiate iron deficiency from anaemia of chronic disorder (see p. 525). Remember that ferritin is an acute phase protein and is therefore difficult to interpret in the context of an inflammatory response for any reason.
  - *Serum B_{12} and serum and red cell folate* should be measured. Red cell folate is a good indicator of the presence of small bowel disease. It is frequently low in both coeliac disease and Crohn's disease, which are the two most common causes of small bowel disease in developed countries.
- ***Inflammatory markers***. The erythrocyte sedimentation rate (ESR) and C-reactive protein (CRP) should be assessed.
- ***Serum calcium*** and alkaline phosphatase. Low serum calcium and raised alkaline phosphatase may indicate the presence of osteomalacia due to vitamin D deficiency.
- ***Liver biochemistry*** and serum albumin. Prothrombin time is also measured.

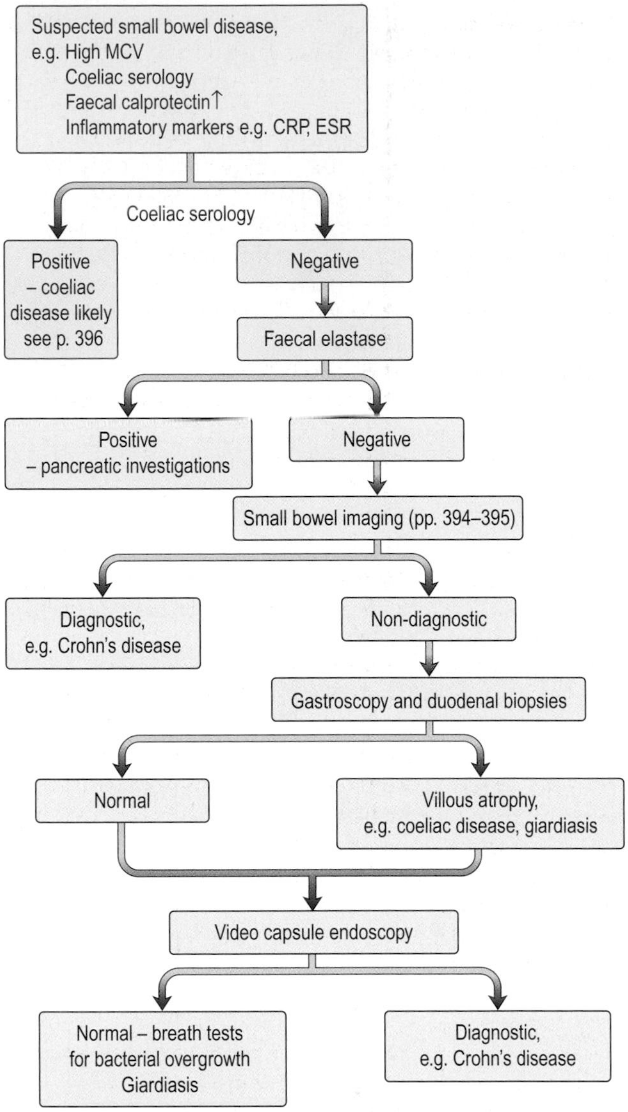

Figure 13.33 Flow diagram for the investigation of patients with suspected small bowel disease. BaFT, barium follow-through; CRP, C-reaction protein; ESR, erythrocyte sedimentation rate; MCV, mean cell volume; MRI, magnetic resonance imaging.

- ***Immunological tests***. Measurement of serum antibodies to endomysium and tissue transglutaminase is useful for the diagnosis of coeliac disease. These should always be accompanied by an assessment of total immunoglobulin levels.
- ***Human leukocyte antigen (HLA) testing***. This is useful in coeliac disease, particularly if doubt exists about the diagnosis.

Investigation of small bowel anatomy

- ***MRI enteroclysis***. This is cross-sectional imaging that does not involve radiation. It uses oral loading with water or a hypertonic solution to distend the small bowel lumen.
- ***Small bowel barium follow-through*** (see p. 363). This detects gross anatomical defects such as diverticula, strictures and Crohn's disease. Dilatation of the bowel and a changed fold pattern may suggest malabsorption but these are non-specific findings. Gross dilatation is seen in myopathic pseudo-obstruction. This is less used because of radiation.

- ***Small bowel biopsy***. This is used to assess the microanatomy of the small bowel mucosa. Biopsies are usually obtained via an endoscope passed into the duodenum and should be well orientated for correct evaluation. The histological appearances are described in the sections on individual diseases. A smear of the jejunal juice or a mucosal impression should also be made when *Giardia intestinalis* infection is suspected.
- ***Ultrasound***. This is a useful preliminary investigation, which can show thickened small bowel or distended loops.
- ***CT scanning***. CT is used to look for small bowel wall thickening, diverticula, and extraintestinal features such as abscesses (e.g. in Crohn's disease).
- ***Video capsule enteroscopy***. This technique is being widely used to visualize the small bowel lumen and mucosa directly along its entire length. It is particularly useful in the diagnosis of occult gastrointestinal bleeding.

Tests of absorption

These are required only in *complicated* cases:

- ***Fat malabsorption***. The confirmation of the presence of steatorrhoea is only occasionally necessary. Three-day faecal fat analysis, triglyceride breath tests and serum β carotene are now rarely performed. In rare cases when it is essential to confirm steatorrhoea, Sudan III staining of a faecal sample can be used.
- ***Lactose tolerance test***. Testing is of little use in adults because lactose intolerance is rarely a clinical problem; patients who are upset by milk usually avoid it. (Note: 500 mL of milk contain 20 g of lactose). Formal testing involves giving an oral dose of 50 g of lactose and serial measurement of blood glucose over 2 h. There is a high incidence of lactase deficiency in many parts of the world (e.g. the Mediterranean countries and parts of Africa and Asia).

Other tests

- ***Hydrogen breath test***. This is frequently used as a screening test to measure transit time and to detect small bowel bacterial overgrowth. Bacteria are present in the oral cavity so the mouth should be rinsed out with an antiseptic mouthwash beforehand. The appearance of a breath hydrogen peak after ***oral glucose*** is used to estimate mouth-to-caecum transit time. An earlier rise in the breath hydrogen after glucose indicates bacterial breakdown in the small intestine. This test is simple to perform and does not involve radioisotopes. However, interpretation is often difficult and sensitivity and specificity are low.
- ***Tests for pancreatic insufficiency***. These are used in the differential diagnosis of steatorrhoea. Human pancreatic elastase 1 (E1) remains undegraded during intestinal transit so its concentration in faeces reflects exocrine pancreatic function. The ***faecal elastase*** test quantifies E1 in stool, allowing the diagnosis or exclusion of severe pancreatic exocrine insufficiency (see p. 500).
- ***Other blood tests***. ***Serum immunoglobulins*** are measured to exclude immune deficiencies: in particular, IgA deficiency, which may lead to false-negative coeliac antibody tests. ***Gut peptides*** (e.g. VIP) are measured in high-volume secretory diarrhoea, and ***chromogranins*** A and B are raised in endocrine tumours.
- ***Tests for protein-losing enteropathy (PLE)*** (see p. 363). These tests are rarely required unless a low serum albumin is a major clinical feature.
- ***Measurement of α_1-antitrypsin clearance***. This is used to confirm protein-losing enteropathy (see p. 363). It does not require an isotope. Alpha$_1$-antitrypsin is a large molecule (>50 000 daltons), which is resistant to proteolysis. Simultaneous measurements of serum and stool concentration (24-h collection) are made.
- ***Bile salt loss***. This can be demonstrated by giving oral ***SeHCAT*** (a synthetic taurine conjugate) and measuring the retention of the bile acid by whole-body counting at 7 days.
- ***Stool tests***. ***Faecal calprotectin*** is 93% sensitive and 96% specific for inflammatory bowel disease in adults. Faecal lactoferrin is also an inflammatory marker.

Malabsorption

In many small bowel diseases, malabsorption of specific substances occurs, but these deficiencies do not usually dominate the clinical picture. An example is Crohn's disease, in which malabsorption of vitamin B_{12} can be demonstrated, but this is not usually the major problem; diarrhoea and general ill-health are the major features.

The major disorders of the small intestine that cause malabsorption are shown in ***Box 13.18***.

Coeliac disease (gluten-sensitive enteropathy)

Coeliac disease is a condition in which there is inflammation of the mucosa of the upper small bowel that improves when gluten is withdrawn from the diet and relapses when gluten is reintroduced. Up to 1% of many populations are affected, though most have clinically silent disease.

Aetiology

Gluten is the entire protein content of the cereals wheat, barley and rye. Prolamins (gliadin from wheat, hordeins from barley, secalins from rye) are damaging factors. These proteins are resistant to digestion by pepsin and chymotrypsin because of their high glutamine and proline content and remain in the intestinal lumen, triggering immune responses.

Immunology

Gliadin peptides pass through the epithelium (para- and/or intracellularly) and are deaminated by tissue transglutaminase, which increases their immunogenicity. Gliadin peptides then bind to antigen-presenting cells, which interact with CD4$^+$ T cells in the lamina propria via HLA class II molecules DQ2 or DQ8. These T cells produce pro-inflammatory cytokines, particularly interferon-γ. CD4$^+$ T cells also interact with B cells to produce endomysial and tissue transglutaminase antibodies. Gliadin peptides also cause release of IL-15 from enterocytes, activating intraepithelial lymphocytes with a natural killer cell marker. This inflammatory cascade releases metalloproteinases and other mediators, which contribute to the villous atrophy and crypt hyperplasia that are typical of the disease.

? Box 13.18 Disorders of the small intestine causing malabsorption

- Coeliac disease
- Dermatitis herpetiformis
- Tropical sprue
- Bacterial overgrowth
- Intestinal resection
- Whipple's disease
- Radiation enteropathy
- Parasite infestation (e.g. *Giardia intestinalis*)

The mucosa of the proximal small bowel is predominantly affected, the mucosal damage decreasing in severity towards the ileum as gluten is digested into smaller 'non-toxic' fragments.

Genetic factors

There is an increased incidence of coeliac disease within families but the exact mode of inheritance is unknown; 10–15% of first-degree relatives will have the condition, although it may be asymptomatic. The concordance rate in identical twins is about 70%.

HLA-DQ2 (DQAI*0501, DQBI*0201) and HLA-DQ8 (DQAI*0301, DQBI*0302) are associated with coeliac disease. Over 90% of patients will have HLA-DQ2, compared with 20–30% of the general population. Studies in twins and siblings indicate that HLA genes are responsible for <50% of the genetic cause of the disease. Many unaffected people also carry these genes, so other factors must also be involved. Non-HLA genes may also contribute to coeliac disease: for example, chromosome regions 19p13.1, 11q, 5q31–33 and 6q21–22. The *CD28/CTLA4/ILO5* gene cluster has also shown linkage with coeliac disease.

Environmental factors

Breast-feeding and the age of introduction of gluten into the diet are significant. Rotavirus infection in infancy also increases the risk; adenovirus-12, which has sequence homology with α-gliadin, was suspected as a causative agent but this is now thought to be unlikely.

Clinical features

Coeliac disease can present at any age. In infancy, it sometimes appears after weaning on to gluten-containing foods. The peak period for diagnosis in adults is in the fifth decade, with a female preponderance. Many patients are asymptomatic (silent) and come to attention because of routine blood tests: for example, a raised MCV, or iron deficiency in pregnancy. The symptoms are very variable and often non-specific; they include tiredness and malaise, often associated with anaemia.

Gastrointestinal symptoms may be absent or mild. Coeliac disease should be tested for in all patients with symptoms suggestive of irritable bowel syndrome. Diarrhoea or steatorrhoea, abdominal pain and weight loss suggest more severe disease. Mouth ulcers and angular stomatitis are frequent and can be intermittent. Infertility and neuropsychiatric symptoms of anxiety and depression occur.

Rare complications include tetany, osteomalacia or gross malnutrition with peripheral oedema. Neurological symptoms, such as paraesthesia, ataxia (due to cerebellar calcification), muscle weakness or a polyneuropathy occur; the prognosis for these symptoms is variable. There is an increased incidence of atopy and autoimmune disease, including thyroid disease, type 1 diabetes and Sjögren syndrome. Other associated diseases include inflammatory bowel disease, primary biliary cholangitis, chronic liver disease, interstitial lung disease and epilepsy. IgA deficiency is more common than in the general population. Long-term problems include osteoporosis, which occurs even in patients on long-term gluten-free diets.

Physical signs are usually few and non-specific, and are related to anaemia and malnutrition.

Diagnosis

Small bowel biopsy is still considered to be the 'gold standard' for positive diagnosis and is therefore desirable in all but the most clear-cut cases, because treatment involves a life-long diet that is both expensive and socially limiting. However, with the increasing accuracy of serological tests, it is no longer necessary to take duodenal biopsies for suspected coeliac disease in patients without antibodies. For example, in patients undergoing endoscopy for iron deficiency anaemia with negative coeliac serology, the pretest value of small bowel histology is <0.03%.

If biopsies are to be taken, 4–6 forceps biopsies should be taken from the second part of the duodenum and the bulb because the disease is sometimes patchy and it can be difficult to orientate endoscopic biopsies for histological section. Endoscopic signs, including absence of mucosal folds, mosaic pattern of the surface and scalloping of mucosal folds, are often present; however, their absence is not conclusive because they are markers of relatively severe disease.

Histology

Histological changes ***(Fig. 13.34)*** are of variable severity and, though characteristic, are not specific. Villous atrophy can be caused by other conditions, but coeliac disease is the most common cause of subtotal villous atrophy.

Histological examination shows crypt hyperplasia with chronic inflammatory cells in the lamina propria, and villous atrophy. The enterocytes become cuboidal with an increase in the number of intraepithelial lymphocytes. In the lamina propria, there is an increase in lymphocytes and plasma cells. The most severe histological change involving mucosal atrophy and hypoplasia is seen in patients who do not respond to a gluten-free diet.

In mild cases, the villous architecture is almost normal but there are increased numbers of intraepithelial lymphocytes.

Serology

Indications for testing include persistent diarrhoea, folate or iron deficiency, unexplained abnormal liver biochemistry, a family history of coeliac disease and associated autoimmune disease.

The most sensitive tests are for endomysial (EMA) and tissue transglutaminase (tTG) antibodies (95% sensitivity). Titres of either of these correlate with the severity of mucosal damage and so they can be used for dietary monitoring. Standard tests use IgA class antibodies. Selective IgA deficiency occurs in 2.5% of coeliac disease patients but only 0.25% of normals. In a few cases, this may render these tests falsely negative. In situations in which CD is strongly suspected in a patient negative for EMA antibodies, IgA levels should be measured; if low, IgG-based tests should then be used (e.g. deaminated gliadin peptide (DGP) antibody).

HLA typing

HLA-DQ2 is present in 90–95% of coeliac disease patients and HLA-DQ8 in about 8% – most of the rest. The *absence* of both alleles has a high negative predictive value for coeliac disease. HLA typing can be useful for risk assessment: for example, in patients already on a gluten-free diet, in whom serology would be negative.

Other investigations

- ***Haematology***. Mild or moderate anaemia is present in 50% of cases. Folate deficiency is common, often causing macrocytosis. Vitamin B_{12} deficiency is rare. Iron deficiency, due to malabsorption of iron and increased loss of desquamated cells, is common. A blood film may therefore show microcytes and macrocytes (i.e. a dimorphic picture), as well as hypersegmented polymorphonuclear

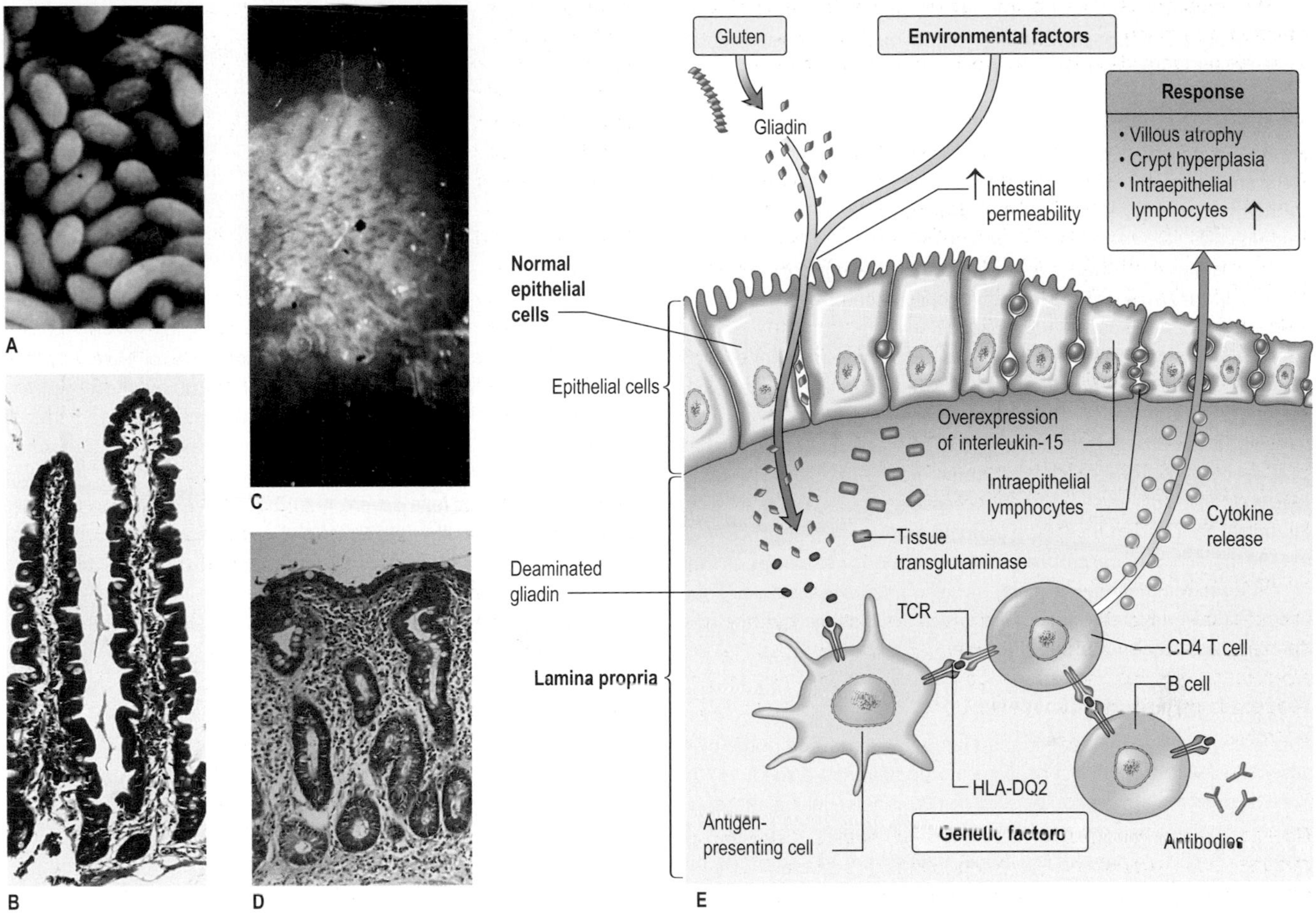

Figure 13.34 **Small bowel mucosal appearances – macroscopic and microscopic. A.** Normal mucosa under the dissecting microscope (DM). **B.** Normal mucosal histology. **C.** Coeliac disease – flattened mucosa. **D.** Coeliac disease – showing subtotal villous atrophy. **E.** Immune and genetic mechanisms in coeliac disease. TCR, T cell receptor. *(After Green PH, Cellier C. Coeliac disease.* New England Journal of Medicine *2007; 357:1731–1743.)*

leucocytes and Howell–Jolly bodies (see p. 553) due to splenic atrophy.

- ***Biochemistry***. *In severe cases*, biochemical evidence of osteomalacia may be seen (low calcium and high phosphate) and there is hypoalbuminaemia.
- ***Imaging***. A small bowel barium follow-through or MRI enteroclysis may show dilatation of the small bowel with slow transit. Folds become thicker, and in severe disease, total effacement is seen. Imaging is mainly used when a complication, such as lymphoma, is suspected.
- ***Bone densitometry***. Dual energy X-ray absorptiometry (DXA) should be performed on all patients because of the risk of osteoporosis.
- ***Capsule endoscopy*** (see p. 362). This is used to look for gut abnormalities when a complication is suspected.

Management

Replacement minerals and vitamins, such as iron, folic acid, calcium and vitamin D, may be needed initially to replace body stores.

Management is with a gluten-free diet for life. Dietary elimination of wheat, barley and rye usually produces a clinical improvement within days or weeks. Morphological improvement often takes months, especially in adults. Oats are tolerated by most coeliacs but must not be contaminated with flour during their production. Meat, dairy products, fruits and vegetables are naturally gluten-free and are all safe.

Gluten-free products can be expensive, unless subsidized by national health services. Patient support organizations, such as the Coeliac Society (UK), are valuable as information sources and for advice about diet, recipes and gluten-free processed foods. Despite advice, many patients do not keep to a strict diet but maintain good health. The long-term effects of this low gluten intake are uncertain but osteoporosis can occur, even in treated cases.

The usual cause of ***failure to respond*** to the diet is poor compliance. Dietary adherence can be monitored by serial tests for EMA and tTG. If clinical progress is suboptimal, then a repeat intestinal biopsy should be taken. If the diagnosis is equivocal on the diagnostic mucosal biopsy, or if the patient has already started on a gluten-free diet, then a gluten challenge, i.e. re-introduction of oral gluten, with evidence of jejunal morphological change, can confirm the diagnosis.

Patients should have ***pneumococcal vaccinations*** (because of splenic atrophy) once every 5 years (see p. 553).

Complications

A few patients do not improve on a strict diet and are said to have ***non-responsive coeliac disease***. Many of these patients are still ingesting gluten. A few of the others may have concomitant problems, such as microscopic colitis, inflammatory bowel disease, small bowel bacterial overgrowth or lactase deficiency.

A very small percentage will have the rare complication of ***refractory coeliac disease*** (RCD). In type 1 RCD, the lymphocytes are normal and the T-cell receptors are polyclonal, whilst in type 2, there are abnormal clonal lymphocytes with loss of CD8 and CD3 surface markers. The 5-year survival rates are 93% and 40–60%, respectively.

Very rarely, enteropathy-associated ***T-cell lymphoma (EATCL)*** (8–20% 5-year survival) or ulcerative jejunitis can occur as part of a spectrum of neoplastic T-cell disorders.

Small bowel adenocarcinoma is also increased in coeliac disease. ***Ulcerative jejunitis*** presents with fever, abdominal pain, perforation and bleeding.

Diagnosis of these conditions is with MRI or barium studies, but laparoscopy with full-thickness small bowel biopsies is often required. Steroids and immunosuppressive agents, such as azathioprine, are used in ulcerative jejunitis.

The incidence of ***carcinoma of the oesophagus***, as well as that of extragastrointestinal cancers, is also increased. Malignancy seems to be unrelated to the duration of the disease but the incidence is reduced by a gluten-free diet.

Dermatitis herpetiformis

This is an uncommon, blistering, subepidermal eruption of the skin associated with a gluten-sensitive enteropathy (see also p. 1370). Rarely, gross malabsorption occurs, but usually the jejunal morphological abnormalities are not as severe as in coeliac disease. The inheritance and immunological abnormalities are the same as for coeliac disease. The skin condition responds to dapsone but a gluten-free diet improves both the enteropathy and the skin lesion, and is recommended for long-term benefit.

Non-coeliac gluten intolerance

There is a recognized group of patients who are sensitive to dietary wheat and gluten-containing foods but do not have coeliac disease, in so far as their coeliac serology is negative and duodenal biopsies are normal. These patients have a range of symptoms, including diarrhoea, bloating and abdominal pain, which improve on avoidance of gluten. The mechanism is not yet clear.

Tropical sprue

This condition presents with chronic diarrhoea and malabsorption, and occurs in residents of or visitors to tropical areas where the disease is endemic: most of Asia, some Caribbean islands, Puerto Rico and parts of South America. Epidemics occur, lasting up to 2 years; in some areas, repeated epidemics are seen at varying intervals of up to 10 years.

The term tropical sprue is reserved for severe malabsorption (of two or more substances) accompanied by diarrhoea and malnutrition. A mild degree of malabsorption, sometimes following an enteric infection, is quite common in the tropics; it is usually asymptomatic and is sometimes called tropical malabsorption.

Aetiology

The aetiology is unknown but is likely to be infective because the disease occurs in epidemics and patients improve on antibiotics. A number of agents have been suggested but none has been unequivocally shown to be responsible. Different agents could be involved in different parts of the world.

Clinical features

These vary in intensity and consist of diarrhoea, anorexia, abdominal distension and weight loss. The onset is sometimes acute and occurs either a few days or many years after being in the tropics. Epidemics can break out in villages, affecting thousands of people at the same time. The onset can also be insidious, with chronic diarrhoea and evidence of nutritional deficiency. The clinical features of tropical sprue vary in different parts of the world, particularly as different criteria are used for diagnosis.

Diagnosis

Acute infective causes of diarrhoea must be excluded (see ***Box 13.23***), particularly *Giardia*, which can produce a syndrome very similar to tropical sprue. Malabsorption should be demonstrated, particularly of fat and vitamin B_{12}. The jejunal mucosa is abnormal, showing some villous atrophy (partial villous atrophy). In most cases, the lesion is less severe than that found in coeliac disease, although it affects the whole of the small bowel. Mild mucosal changes can be seen in asymptomatic individuals in the tropics.

Management

Many patients improve when they leave the sprue area and take folic acid (5 mg daily). Most patients also require an antibiotic to ensure a complete recovery (usually tetracycline 1 g daily for up to 6 months).

Severely ill patients require resuscitation with fluids and electrolytes for dehydration, and nutritional deficiencies should be corrected. Vitamin B_{12} (1000 μg) is also given to all acute cases.

Prognosis

The prognosis is excellent. Mortality is usually associated with water and electrolyte depletion, particularly in epidemics.

Bacterial overgrowth

The gut contains many resident bacteria in the terminal ileum and colon. Anaerobic bacteria, e.g. *Bacteroides*, bifidobacteria, are 100–1000 times more abundant than aerobic bacterial (facultative anaerobes), such as *Escherichia, Enterobacter* and *Enterococcus*. This gut microflora has major functions, including metabolic ones, such as fermentation of non-digestible dietary residues into short-chain fatty acids as an energy source in the colon.

The microflora that influences epithelial cell proliferation is involved in the development and maintenance of the immune system and protects the gut mucosa from colonization by pathogenic bacteria. Bacteria also initiate vitamin K production.

The upper part of the small intestine is almost sterile, containing only a few organisms derived from the mouth. Gastric acid kills some ingested organisms and intestinal motility keeps bacterial counts in the jejunum low. The normal terminal ileum contains faecal-type organisms, mainly *Escherichia coli* and anaerobes, and the colon has abundant bacteria.

Bacterial overgrowth is normally found in association with a structural abnormality of the small intestine, such as a stricture or diverticulum, although it can occur occasionally in the elderly without such an abnormality. *E. coli* and/or *Bacteroides*, both in concentrations of greater than 10^6/mL, are found as part of a mixed flora. These bacteria are capable of deconjugating and dehydroxylating bile salts, so that unconjugated and dehydroxylated bile salts can be detected in small bowel aspirates.

Clinical features

The clinical features of overgrowth are chiefly diarrhoea and steatorrhoea. There may also be symptoms caused by the underlying small bowel pathology. Steatorrhoea (see p. 394) occurs because of conjugated bile salt deficiency. Some bacteria can metabolize vitamin B_{12} and interfere with its binding to intrinsic factor, leading to mild B_{12} deficiency (see p. 528); it is rarely severe enough to produce a neurological deficit. Some bacteria produce folic acid, giving a high serum folate. Bacterial overgrowth has only minimal effects on the absorption of other substances. Confirmation of bacterial overgrowth is with the hydrogen breath test (see p. 395).

Management

If possible, the underlying lesion should be corrected (e.g. a stricture should be resected). Where this is not possible, rotating courses of antibiotics are necessary, such as metronidazole, a tetracycline or ciprofloxacin. The response to antibiotics is unpredictable.

Small intestinal resection

Small intestinal resection is usually well tolerated, but massive resection leaving less than 1 m of small bowel in continuity is followed by the short bowel syndrome. The effects of resection depend on the amount and location of the resection and the presence or absence of the colon. Resection of the jejunum is better tolerated than ileal resection, where there is less adaptation, probably due to low levels of glucagon-like peptide 2 (GLP-2), which is a specific growth hormone for the enterocyte. Patients with an anatomically short small bowel after surgical resection should have close follow-up to ensure they do not become depleted of electrolytes or develop malnutrition. Management will depend on investigations, but might include the use of loperamide and codeine to reduce small intestinal transit time, high-dose PPI therapy to reduce gastric secretion, oral rehydration solution and, where necessary, parenteral electrolyte and calorie replacement.

Ileal resection

The ileum is the site of specific mechanisms for the absorption of bile salts and vitamin B_{12}. Relatively small resections lead to malabsorption of these substances. Loss of the ileal brake (see p. 391) leads to diarrhoea. Removal of the ileocaecal valve increases the incidence of diarrhoea ***(Fig. 13.35)***.

The following occur after ileal resection:

- ***Bile-salt-induced diarrhoea***. Bile salts and fatty acids enter the colon and cause malabsorption of water and electrolytes (see pp. 426–427).
- ***Steatorrhoea and gallstone formation***. Increased bile salt synthesis can compensate for loss of approximately one-third of the bile salts in the faeces. Greater loss than this results in decreased micelle formation and steatorrhoea, and lithogenic bile and gallstone formation.
- ***Oxaluria and oxalate stones***. Bile salts in the colon cause increased oxalate absorption with oxaluria, leading to urinary stone formation.
- ***B_{12} deficiency***. Low serum B_{12}, macrocytosis and other effects of B_{12} deficiency are seen.

Investigations

These include imaging of the small bowel (see pp. 362–363), measurement of B_{12}, and a bile salt retention (SeHCAT) test (p. 395). A hydrogen breath test may show rapid transit (p. 395). Many patients require B_{12} replacement and some need a low-fat diet if there is steatorrhoea. Diarrhoea is often improved by colestyramine, which binds bile salts and reduces the level of diarrhoeogenic bile salts in the colon.

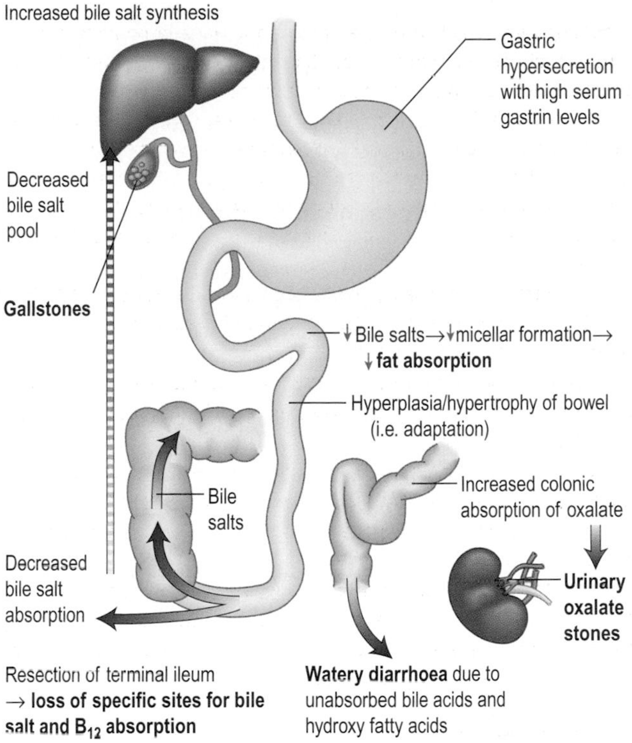

Figure 13.35 The effects of resecting the distal small bowel.

Jejunal resection

The ileum can compensate for loss of jejunal absorptive function. Jejunal resection may lead to gastric hypersecretion with high gastrin levels; the exact mechanism is unclear. Structural and functional intestinal adaptation takes place over the course of a year, with an increase in the absorption per unit length of bowel in both jejunum and ileum.

Massive intestinal resection (short bowel syndrome)

Intestinal failure results from obstruction, dysmotility, surgical resection, congenital defect, or disease-associated loss of absorption. It is characterized by the inability to maintain protein-energy, fluid, electrolyte or micronutrient balance. This most often occurs following resection for Crohn's disease, mesenteric vessel occlusion (see p. 402), radiation enteritis (see below) or trauma. There are two common situations.

Shortened small intestine ending at a terminal small bowel stoma

The major problem is sodium and fluid depletion; the majority of patients with ≤100 cm of jejunum remaining will require parenteral supplements of fluid and electrolytes, often with nutrients. Sodium losses can be minimized by increasing salt intake, restricting hypotonic fluids between meals, and administering oral glucose–electrolyte mixture with a sodium concentration of 90 mmol/L. Jejunal transit time can be increased and stomal effluent loss reduced by treatment with the somatostatin analogue octreotide, often used in combination with a PPI, loperamide and codeine phosphate. There is no benefit from a low-fat diet, but fat assimilation can be increased on treatment with colestyramine and synthetic bile acids.

Teduglutide, as GLP-2 analogue, reduces stomal output and the number of days of parenteral nutrition. More studies are needed.

Shortened small intestine in continuity with colon

Because of the absorptive capacity of the colon for fluid and electrolytes, only a small proportion of these patients require parenteral supplementation. Unabsorbed fat results in impairment of colonic fluid and electrolyte absorption, and so patients should be on a low-fat diet. A high carbohydrate intake is advised, as unabsorbed carbohydrate is metabolized anaerobically to short-chain fatty acids (SCFAs), which are absorbed; they also stimulate fluid and electrolyte absorption in the colon and act as an energy source (1.6 kcal/g). Patients are often treated with colestyramine to reduce diarrhoea and colonic oxalate absorption.

Whipple's disease

Whipple's disease is a rare infectious bacterial disease caused by *Tropheryma whipplei*. Some 87% of patients are males, and are usually white and middle-aged. Whipple's presents with arthritis and arthralgia, progressing over years to weight loss and diarrhoea with abdominal pain, and systemic symptoms of fever and weight loss. Peripheral lymphadenopathy and involvement of the heart, lung, joints and brain occur, simulating many neurological conditions.

Blood tests show features of chronic inflammation and malabsorption. Endoscopy typically shows pale, shaggy duodenal mucosa with eroded, red, friable patches.

Diagnosis

Diagnosis is made by small bowel biopsy. Periodic acid–Schiff (PAS)-positive macrophages are present but are non-specific. On electron microscopy, the characteristic trilaminar cell wall of *T. whipplei* can be seen within macrophages. *T. whipplei* antibodies can be identified by immunohistochemistry. A confirmatory polymerase chain reaction (PCR)-based assay is available.

Management

Treatment is with antibiotics that cross the blood–brain barrier, such as 160 mg trimethoprim and 800 mg sulfamethoxazole (co-trimoxazole) daily for 1 year. This is preceded by a 2-week course of streptomycin and penicillin or ceftriaxone. Treatment periods of less than 1 year are associated with relapse in about 40%.

Radiation enteritis

Radiation of >40 Gy will damage the intestine. The chronic effects of radiation are muscle fibre atrophy, ulcerative changes due to ischaemia, and obstruction due to radiation-induced fibrotic strictures.

Pelvic irradiation is frequently used for gynaecological and urinary tract malignancies, and so the ileum and rectum are the areas most often involved.

At the time of the irradiation, there may be nausea, vomiting, diarrhoea and abdominal pain, usually improving within 6 weeks of completion of therapy.

Chronic radiation enteritis is diagnosed if symptoms persist for ≥3 months. The prevalence is >15% of patients receiving radiotherapy that includes the abdomen. Abdominal pain due to obstruction is the main symptom. Malabsorption can be due to bacterial overgrowth in dilated segments and mucosal damage. Many patients suffer from increased bowel frequency. ***Management*** is symptomatic, although often unsuccessful in chronic radiation enteritis. Surgery should be avoided if possible, being reserved for obstruction or perforation.

Acute radiation damage to the rectum produces a ***radiation proctitis*** with diarrhoea and tenesmus, with or without blood. Local steroids sometimes help initially. When the acute phase heals, mucosal telangiectases form and may cause persistent bleeding. If there is resistant anaemia, these can be treated with argon plasma coagulation or, under a light anaesthetic, by packing the rectum with a formalin-soaked swab for 2 minutes, both of which destroy the telangiectases.

Parasite infestation

- ***Giardia intestinalis*** (see pp. 306–307) not only produces diarrhoea but also can produce malabsorption with steatorrhoea. Minor changes are seen in the jejunal mucosa and the organism can be found in the jejunal fluid or mucosa.
- ***Cryptosporidiosis*** (see p. 307) can also produce malabsorption.
- ***HIV infection*** causes patients to be particularly prone to parasitic infestation (Box 13.19).

Other causes of malabsorption

- ***Drugs that bind bile salts*** (e.g. colestyramine) and some antibiotics (e.g. neomycin) produce steatorrhoea.

Box 13.19 Gastrointestinal problems in patients with AIDS

Symptoms	Causes
Mouth/oesophagus	
Dysphagia	Herpes simplex virus (HSV)
Retrosternal discomfort	Cytomegalovirus (CMV)
Oral ulceration	Candidiasis
Small bowel/colon	
Chronic diarrhoea Steatorrhoea Weight loss	Parasites: *Entamoeba histolytica* *Giardia intestinalis* *Cryptosporidium* *Blastocystis hominis* *Isospora belli* *Microsporidia* *Cyclospora cayetanensis* Viruses: Cytomegalovirus, herpes simplex virus, adenovirus Bacteria: *Salmonella* *Campylobacter* *Shigella* *Mycobacterium avium-intracellulare* Non-infective enteropathy – cause unknown
Rectum/colon	
Bloody diarrhoea	Bacterial infection (e.g. *Shigella*)
Any site	
Weight loss Diarrhoea	Neoplasia: Kaposi's sarcoma Lymphoma Squamous carcinoma Infection – disseminated, e.g. *Mycobacterium avium-intracellulare* Anti-retroviral therapy (ART)

- ***Orlistat*** (see p. 210) is used in obesity to reduce fat absorption by inhibiting gastric and pancreatic lipase, so causing diarrhoea and steatorrhoea. A low-fat diet is also necessary, which leads to weight loss.
- ***Thyrotoxicosis*** causes diarrhoea, rarely with steatorrhoea, owing to increased gastric emptying and increased motility.
- ***Zollinger–Ellison syndrome*** is described on page 512.
- ***Intestinal lymphangiectasia*** produces diarrhoea and, rarely, steatorrhoea (see p. 402).
- ***Lymphoma*** that has infiltrated the small bowel mucosa causes malabsorption.
- ***Diabetes mellitus*** (see p. 1271) causes diarrhoea, malabsorption and steatorrhoea, sometimes due to bacterial overgrowth from autonomic neuropathy that leads to small bowel stasis.
- ***Hypogammaglobulinaemia***, which is seen in a number of conditions including lymphoid nodular hyperplasia, causes steatorrhoea due either to an abnormal jejunal mucosa or to secondary infestation with *Giardia intestinalis*.

Miscellaneous intestinal diseases

Protein-losing enteropathy

Protein-losing enteropathy refers to intestinal conditions that lead to protein loss, and usually manifest with hypoalbuminaemia. The causes include Crohn's disease, tumours, Ménétrier's disease, a condition with giant rugal folds ***(Fig. 13.36)***, coeliac disease and lymphatic disorders (e.g. lymphangiectasia).

Usually, protein-losing enteropathy forms a minor part of the generalized disorder but, occasionally, hepatic synthesis of albumin cannot compensate for the protein loss, and peripheral oedema dominates the clinical picture. The investigations are described on page 395 and treatment is that of the underlying disorder.

Meckel's diverticulum

This is the most common congenital abnormality of the gastrointestinal tract, affecting 2–3% of the population. The diverticulum projects from the wall of the ileum approximately 60 cm from the ileocaecal valve. It is usually symptomless. However, 50% contain gastric mucosa that secretes hydrochloric acid, and peptic ulcers can occur and may bleed (see p. 384) or perforate.

Acute inflammation of the diverticulum also occurs and is indistinguishable clinically from acute appendicitis. Rarely, there is obstruction from an associated band.

Management is surgical removal, often laparoscopically.

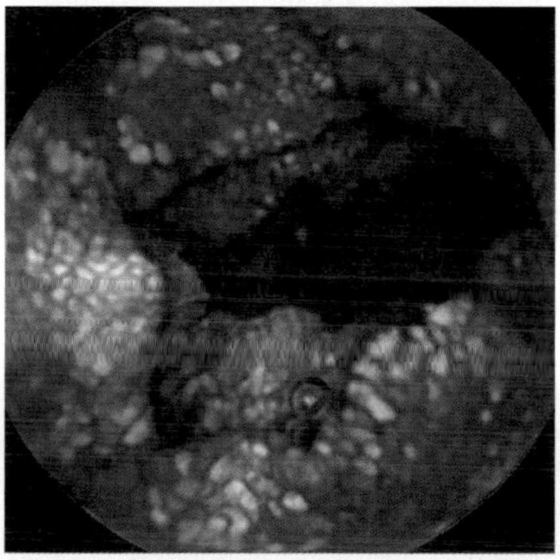

Figure 13.36 Protein-losing enteropathy showing giant rugal folds.

Tuberculosis

Tuberculosis (TB; see also pp. 1106–1113) can affect the intestine, as well as the peritoneum (see p. 436). In developed countries, most patients are from ethnic minority groups, or are immunocompromised because of HIV or drugs. Intestinal TB is due to reactivation of primary disease caused by *Mycobacterium tuberculosis*. Bovine TB occurs in areas where milk is unpasteurized and is rare in Western countries.

Clinical features

These are abdominal pain, weight loss, anaemia, fever with night sweats, obstruction, right iliac fossa pain or a palpable mass. The ileocaecal area is most commonly affected, but the colon – and, rarely, other parts of the gastrointestinal tract – can be involved. One-third of patients present acutely with intestinal obstruction or generalized peritonitis; 50% have X-ray evidence of pulmonary TB.

Diagnosis

Differential diagnosis includes Crohn's disease and caecal carcinoma.

- ***Small bowel follow-through*** may show transverse ulceration, and diffuse narrowing of the bowel with shortening of the caecal pole.
- ***Ultrasound, MRI or CT*** shows additional mesenteric thickening and lymph node enlargement.
- ***Histology and culture of tissue*** is desirable but not always possible. Specimens can be obtained by colonoscopy or laparoscopy but laparotomy is required in some cases. The histological findings include chronic inflammation with caseating granuloma. Acid-fast bacilli may be seen on dedicated stains. However, the histology is not always distinguishable from that of Crohn's disease.

Management

Drug treatment is similar to that for pulmonary TB (see pp. 1110–1113). Treatment should be started if there is a high degree of suspicion.

Amyloidosis

Systemic amyloidosis may affect any part of the gastrointestinal tract (see also pp. 1288–1289). Rectal biopsy may be diagnostic. Occasionally, amyloid deposits occur as polypoid lesions. The symptoms depend on the site of involvement; amyloidosis in the small intestine gives rise to diarrhoea.

Autoimmune rheumatic diseases

Systemic sclerosis (see pp. 695–697) most commonly affects the oesophagus (see p. 372), although the small bowel and colon are often found to be involved if investigated. There may be no symptoms of this involvement, but diarrhoea and steatorrhoea can occur due to bacterial overgrowth caused by reduced motility, dilatation and the presence of diverticula.

Intestinal ischaemia

Intestinal ischaemia results from occlusion of arterial inflow, occlusion of venous outflow or failure of perfusion; these factors may act alone or in combination and usually occur in the elderly.

- ***Arterial inflow occlusion*** can be caused by atheroma, thrombosis and embolism (cardiac arrhythmia), including cholesterol emboli (see pp. 753–754), aortic disease (occluding

ostia of mesenteric vessels) or vasculitis (see pp. 699–702), thromboangiitis and Takayasu syndrome (see pp. 1054–1055).
- ***Venous outflow occlusion*** occurs in 5–15% of cases, usually in sick patients with circulatory failure.
- ***Infarction without occlusion*** can occur due to reduced cardiac output, hypotension and shock, causing reduced intestinal blood flow.

Acute small intestinal ischaemia

An embolus from the heart in a patient with atrial fibrillation is the most common cause and usually occludes the superior mesenteric artery. Patients present with sudden abdominal pain and vomiting, with a distended and tender abdomen and absent bowel sounds. The patient is hypotensive and ill. Surgery is necessary to resect the gangrenous bowel. Mortality is high (up to 90%) and is related to coexisting disease, the development of multiorgan failure (MOF; see p. 1155) and massive fluid and electrolyte losses in the postoperative period. Survivors may go on to develop nutritionally inadequate short bowel syndrome (see pp. 399–400).

Ischaemic colitis

See page 418.

Chronic small intestinal ischaemia

This is due to atheromatous occlusion or cholesterol emboli of the mesenteric vessels, and is found particularly in the elderly. Good collateral circulation can minimize clinical effects. The characteristic symptom is postprandial abdominal pain and weight loss. Loud bruits may be heard but, as these are heard in normal subjects, they are of doubtful significance. The diagnosis is made using angiography.

Eosinophilic gastroenteritis

In this condition of unknown aetiology there is eosinophilic infiltration and oedema of any part of the gastrointestinal mucosa. The gastric antrum and proximal small intestine are usually involved, hosting either a localized lesion (eosinophilic granuloma) or diffuse sheets of eosinophils in the serosal and submucosal layers. There is an association with asthma, eczema and urticaria.

The condition occurs mainly in the third decade. The clinical presentation depends on the site of gut involvement. Abdominal pain, nausea and vomiting, and upper gastrointestinal bleeding occur. Peripheral eosinophilia is present in only 20% of patients. Endoscopic biopsy is useful for making the diagnosis histologically. Radiology may demonstrate mass lesions.

Treatment is with corticosteroids for the widespread infiltration, particularly if peripheral eosinophilia is present.

In some adults, the condition appears to be allergic (allergic gastroenteritis) and is associated with peripheral eosinophilia and high levels of plasma and tissue IgE. The relationship of eosinophilic oesophagitis (see pp. 373–374) to eosinophilic gastroenteritis is unclear.

Intestinal lymphangiectasia

Dilatation of the lymphatics may be primary or secondary to lymphatic obstruction, such as occurs in malignancy or constrictive pericarditis. Hypoproteinaemia with ankle oedema is the main feature. The rare primary form may be detected incidentally as dilated lacteals on a jejunal biopsy or it can produce steatorrhoea of varying degrees. White-tipped villi are seen on capsule endoscopy. Serum immunoglobulin levels are reduced, with low circulating lymphocytes. Management is with a low-fat diet, mid-chain triglycerides and fat-soluble vitamin supplements as required. Octreotide has a dramatic effect in a few primary cases, although the mechanism of action is unknown.

Abetalipoproteinaemia

This rare congenital disorder is due to a failure of apo B-100 synthesis in the liver and apo B-48 in the intestinal cell, so that chylomicrons are not formed. This leads to fat accumulation in the intestinal cells, lending a characteristic histological appearance to the jejunal mucosa. Clinical features include acanthocytosis (spiky red cells owing to membrane abnormalities), a form of retinitis pigmentosa, and mental and neurological abnormalities. The latter can be prevented by vitamin E injections.

Tumours of the small intestine

The small intestine is relatively resistant to the development of neoplasia and only 3–6% of all gastrointestinal tumours and less than 1% of all malignant lesions occur here. The reason for the rarity of tumours is unknown. Explanations include the fluidity and relative sterility of small bowel contents and the rapid transit time, reducing the time of exposure to potential carcinogens. It is also possible that the high population of lymphoid tissue and secretion of IgA in the small intestine protect against malignancy.

Adenocarcinoma and lymphoma

Adenocarcinoma of the small intestine is rare and found most frequently in the duodenum (in the periampullary region) and in the jejunum. It is the most common tumour of the small intestine, accounting for up to 50% of primary tumours.

Lymphomas are most frequently found in the ileum. These are of the non-Hodgkin's type and must be distinguished from peripheral or nodal lymphomas involving the gut secondarily.

In developed countries, the most common type of lymphoma is the B cell type arising from MALT (see pp. 395–396). These lymphomas tend to be annular or polypoid masses in the distal or terminal ileum, whereas most T cell lymphomas are ulcerated plaques or strictures in the proximal small bowel.

A tumour similar to Burkitt's lymphoma also occurs and commonly affects the terminal ileum of children in North Africa and the Middle East.

Predisposing factors for adenocarcinoma and lymphoma

Coeliac disease

There is an increased incidence of lymphoma of the T cell type and adenocarcinoma of the small bowel, as well as an unexplained increase in all malignancies, both in the gastrointestinal tract and elsewhere. The reason for the local development of malignancy is unknown. It is now accepted that coeliac disease is a pre-malignant condition but there is no association with the length of the symptoms. Management with a gluten-free diet can reduce the risk of both lymphoma and carcinoma.

Crohn's disease

There is a small increase in the incidence of adenocarcinoma of the small bowel in Crohn's disease.

Immunoproliferative small intestinal disease

Immunoproliferative small intestinal disease (IPSID) is a rare B cell disorder in which there is proliferation of plasma cells in the lamina propria of the upper small bowel, producing truncated monoclonal heavy chains, without associated light chains. The α heavy chains are found in the gut mucosa on immunofluorescence and can also be detected in the serum. IPSID usually occurs in countries surrounding the Mediterranean, but it has also been found in developing countries in South America and the Far East. It predominantly affects people in lower socioeconomic groups in areas with poor hygiene and a high incidence of bacterial and parasitic infection of the gut. IPSID presents as a malabsorptive syndrome associated with diffuse lymphoid infiltration of the small bowel and neighbouring lymph nodes, progressing in some cases to a lymphoma. The condition has also been documented in the developed world.

Clinically, patients present with abdominal pain, diarrhoea, anorexia, weight loss and symptoms of anaemia. There may be a palpable mass, and an ultrasound followed by an MRI scan may detect a mass lesion. Endoscopic biopsy is useful where lesions are within reach. Ultrasound and CT may show bowel wall thickening and the involvement of lymph nodes, which is common with lymphoma. Wireless capsule endoscopy can be used where obstruction by the capsule is not likely, but cannot deliver histology.

Management of small intestinal tumours

Adenocarcinoma

Most patients are treated surgically with a segmental resection. The overall 5-year survival rate is 20–35%; this varies with the histological grade and the presence or absence of lymph node involvement. Radiotherapy and chemotherapy are used in addition.

IPSID

If there is no evidence of lymphoma, antibiotics, such as tetracycline, should be tried initially. In the presence of lymphoma, combination chemotherapy is used; in one series, the 3–5-year survival rate was 58%.

Lymphoma

Most patients require surgery and radiotherapy with chemotherapy for more extensive disease. The prognosis varies with the type. The 5-year survival rate for T cell lymphomas is 25% but is better for B cell lymphomas, varying from 50% to 75%, depending on the grade of lymphoma.

Carcinoid tumours

These originate from the enterochromaffin cells (APUD cells) of the intestine. They make up 10% of all small bowel neoplasms, the most common sites being the appendix and terminal ileum. It is often difficult to be certain histologically whether a particular tumour is benign or malignant. A total of 10% of carcinoid tumours in the appendix present as acute appendicitis, secondary to obstruction. Surgical resection of the tumour is usually performed.

Most carcinoids do not secrete hormones or vasoactive compounds, and may present with liver enlargement due to metastases.

Carcinoid syndrome occurs in only 5% of patients with carcinoid tumours and only when there are liver metastases. Patients complain of spontaneous or induced bluish-red flushing, predominantly on the face and neck, sometimes leading to permanent changes with telangiectases.

Gastrointestinal symptoms consist of abdominal pain and recurrent watery diarrhoea. Cardiac abnormalities are found in 50% of patients and take the form of pulmonary stenosis or tricuspid incompetence. Examination of the abdomen reveals hepatomegaly. The tumours secrete a variety of biologically active amines and peptides, including serotonin (5-hydroxytryptamine, 5-HT), bradykinin, histamine, tachykinins and prostaglandins. The diarrhoea and cardiac complications are probably caused by 5-HT itself, but the cutaneous flushing is thought to be produced by one of the kinins, such as bradykinin. This is known to cause vasodilatation, bronchospasm and increased intestinal motility.

Diagnosis of carcinoid syndrome

- ***Ultrasound examination*** confirms the presence of liver secondary deposits.
- ***Urine*** shows a high concentration of 5-hydroxyindoleacetic acid (5-HIAA), which is the major metabolite of 5-HT.
- ***Serum chromogranin A*** is raised in nearly all hindgut tumours and 80–90% of symptomatic foregut and midgut tumours.

Management of carcinoid syndrome

Treatment is with octreotide and lanreotide; both are octapeptide somatostatin analogues that inhibit the release of many gut hormones. They alleviate flushing and diarrhoea, and can control a carcinoid crisis. Interferon and other chemotherapeutic regimens also occasionally reduce tumour growth, but have not been shown to increase survival.

Most patients survive for 5–10 years after diagnosis.

Peutz–Jeghers syndrome

This consists of mucocutaneous pigmentation (circumoral in 95% of patients, and on the hands in 70% and feet in 60%) and gastrointestinal polyps. It has an autosomal dominant inheritance. The gene *STK11* (also known as *LKB1*) that is responsible for Peutz–Jeghers codes for a serine protein kinase and can be used for genetic analysis. The brown buccal pigment is characteristic of the condition. The polyps, which are hamartomas, can occur anywhere in the gastrointestinal tract but are most frequent in the small bowel. They may bleed or cause small bowel obstruction or intussusception (50% of patients).

Management

Management is by endoscopic polypectomy. Balloon enteroscopy may be necessary to reach all the small bowel polyps. Bowel resection should be avoided if possible, but may be necessary in patients presenting with gangrenous bowel due to intussusception. Follow-up is with yearly pan-endoscopy. There is an increased incidence of gastrointestinal cancers. Non-gastrointestinal cancers also occur with increased frequency, so yearly screening for uterine, ovarian and cervical cancer should start in the teens, and breast and testicular screening by the age of 20.

Other tumours

Adenomas, lipomas and stromal tumours (see p. 384) are rarely found and are usually asymptomatic and picked up incidentally. They occasionally present with iron deficiency anaemia. In familial adenomatous polyposis (FAP), duodenal adenomas form in one-third of patients and may progress to adenocarcinoma. This is the most common cause of death in FAP patients who have been treated by prophylactic colectomy.

Further reading

Abrahams C, Medzhitov R. Interactions between the host innate immune system and microbes in inflammatory bowel disease. *Gastroenterology* 2011; 140:1720–1728.

Aikou S, Ohmoto Y, Gunji T. Tests for serum levels of trefoil factor family proteins can improve gastric cancer screening. *Gastroenterology* 2011; 141:837–845.
Fenollar F, Puéchal X, Raoult D. Whipple's disease (review). *N Engl J Med* 2007; 356:55–66.
Lundin KE, Sollid LM. Advances in coeliac disease. *Curr Opin Gastroenterol* 2014; 30:154–162.
Malamut G, Cellier C. Refractory celiac disease. *Expert Rev Gastroenterol Hepatol* 2014; 8:323–328.
Mooney PD, Hadjivassiliou M, Sanders DS. Coeliac disease. *BMJ* 2014; 348:g1561.

INFLAMMATORY BOWEL DISEASE

Two major forms of inflammatory bowel disease (IBD) are recognized:

- Crohn's disease (CD), which can affect any part of the gastrointestinal tract
- Ulcerative colitis (UC), which affects only the colon.

There is a degree of overlap between these two conditions in their aetiopathogenesis, clinical features, histological and radiological abnormalities; in 10% of cases of IBD causing colitis, a definitive diagnosis of either UC or CD is not possible and the diagnosis is termed colitis of undetermined type and (a)etiology (CUTE). It is clinically useful to distinguish between UC and CD because of differences in their management, although, in reality, they may represent two aspects of the same disease.

Another form of colitis related to microscopic inflammation is termed microscopic colitis; this is subdivided into lymphocytic and collagenous types (see pp. 414–415). The distinction between this and IBD is the absence of macroscopic evidence of inflammation.

Epidemiology

- The incidence of CD varies from country to country but is approximately 4–10 per 100 000 annually, with a prevalence of 25–100/100 000.
- The incidence of UC is stable at 6–15/100 000 annually, with a prevalence of 80–150/100 000.

Although both conditions have a worldwide distribution, the highest incidence rates and prevalence have been reported from Northern Europe, the UK and North America. Both race and ethnic origin affect the incidence and prevalence of CD and UC. Thus, in North America, prevalence rates of CD are lower in Hispanic and Asian people (4.1/100 000 and 5.6/100 000, respectively) compared with white individuals (43.6/100 000). Jewish people are more prone to IBD than any other ethnic group. Prevalence rates also change after migration; thus there is an increasing incidence of CD in the UK-born children of migrants from South-east Asia. Recent studies suggest that the incidence of both CD and UC is increasing in traditional low-prevalence areas such as South-east Asia.

Approximately 25% of patients are diagnosed before their 18th birthday and there is evidence that disease commencing in youth is more extensive and more aggressive than that occurring in older patients.

Aetiology and pathogenesis

Although the aetiology of IBD is unknown, it is increasingly clear that IBD represents the interaction between several co-factors: genetic susceptibility, the environment, the intestinal microbiota and host immune response ***(Fig. 13.37)***.

Genetic factors

CD and UC are complex polygenic diseases and having a positive family history is the largest independent risk factor for development of IBD. Up to 1 in 5 patients with CD and 1 in 6 patients with UC will have a first-degree relative with the disease. The monozygotic and dizygotic twin concordance rates for CD are 20–50% and 10%, respectively.

Genome-wide association studies have identified multiple susceptibility loci, and many of the underlying risk variants have been identified. The major genetic factors for CD include the *NOD2* (*CARD 15*) gene (nucleotide oligomerization domain 2), the autophagy genes and the Th17 pathway (IL-23-type 17 helper T cells). The NOD2 protein on chromosome 16 is an intracellular

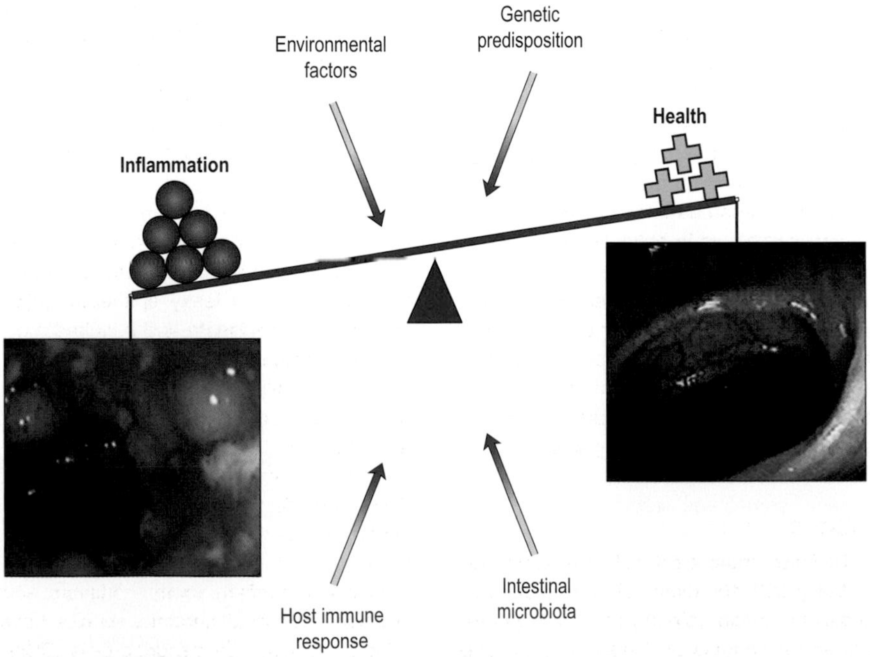

Figure 13.37 The aetiopathogenesis of inflammatory bowel disease.

sensor of bacterial peptidoglycan, present in bacterial cell walls (see below). NOD2 is expressed in epithelial cells, macrophages and endothelial cells. Individuals who are homozygote or compound heterozygote for one of several mutations in the *NOD2* gene have a significantly increased risk of developing ileal CD. Likewise, mutations in the autophagy genes *ATG16L1* and *IRGM* (immunity-related GTP-ase M-protein) and IL-23 receptor gene increase CD risk, and mutations in genes associated with the mucosal barrier increase UC risk. However, the presence of IBD-associated genes in many unaffected individuals and the failure of the approximately 71 genetic susceptibility loci identified thus far to explain more than around one-fifth of the genetic risk of CD highlight the complexity of the genetic basis of IBD. Specific genetic defects in the IL-10 receptor pathway are associated with a severe form of extremely early-onset colitis and perianal disease in children.

Apart from susceptibility, HLA genes on chromosome 6 also appear to have a role in modifying the disease. The *DRB*0103* allele is linked to a particularly aggressive course of UC and the need for surgery, as well as with colonic CD. *DRB*0103* and *MICA*010* are associated with perianal disease, and *DRB*0701* with ileal CD. For the extraintestinal disease complications and HLA links, see page 407.

Environmental and other factors

- ***Smoking***. Patients with CD are more likely to be smokers, and smoking has been shown to exacerbate CD and increase the risk of disease recurrence after surgery. By contrast, there is an increased risk of UC in non- or ex-smokers and nicotine has been shown to be an effective treatment in one small clinical trial.
- ***NSAIDs***. NSAID ingestion is associated with both the onset of IBD and flares of disease in patients with an established diagnosis.
- ***Hygiene***. Poor and large families living in crowded conditions have a lower risk of developing CD. A 'clean' environment may not expose the intestinal immune system to pathogenic or non-pathogenic microorganisms such as helminths, which seems to alter the balance between effector and regulatory immune responses.
- ***Nutritional factors***. Many foods and food components have been suggested as playing a role in the aetiopathogenesis of IBD (e.g. high sugar and fat intake) but, unfortunately, the results of numerous studies designed to define risk have been equivocal. However, breast-feeding may provide protection against the development of IBD in offspring.
- ***Psychological factors***. Factors such as chronic stress and depression seem to increase relapses in patients with quiescent disease.
- ***Appendicectomy***. This appears to be 'protective' against the development of UC, particularly if performed for appendicitis or for mesenteric lymphadenitis before the age of 20. It also influences the clinical course of UC, with a lower incidence of colectomy and reduced need for immunosuppressive therapy. By contrast, appendicectomy may increase the risk of development of CD.

The intestinal microbiota

The gut is colonized by 10 times more bacterial organisms than there are host cells, there being 300–400 distinct bacterial species. The intestinal microbiota plays a crucial role in perpetuating intestinal inflammation, in both animal models of disease and patients with IBD. The number of mucosal adherent bacteria is increased in patients with CD compared to healthy subjects, and diversion of the bacterial component of the faecal stream induces clinical remission. However, there is also evidence of an immunoregulatory role for the commensal microbiota, which protects against intestinal inflammation and upregulates epithelial defence mechanisms in animal models of colitis.

Mechanisms by which the intestinal microbiota may relate to the aetiology of IBD include:

- ***Intestinal dysbiosis***. There is an alteration in the bacterial flora in patients with CD. Although results vary due to differences in both the patient groups studied and the microbiological method utilized, the most consistent finding in patients with IBD is a reduced diversity of microbial species. In addition, higher concentrations of *Bacteroides* and *E. coli*, and lower concentrations of bifidobacteria and *Faecalibacterium prausnitzii* have been reported in faecal and mucosal samples from patients with CD compared to healthy controls. Lower concentrations of *F. prausnitzii* have been found in patients with active compared with quiescent disease, and low levels of this organism in CD resection specimens predict subsequent endoscopic disease recurrence.
- ***Specific pathogenic organisms***. It has been shown that there is increased *E. coli* adherence to the ileal epithelial cells in CD, with evidence of invasion into the mucosa. *E. coli*'s type 1 pili adhere to a protein called carcinoembryonic antigen-related cell adhesion molecule 6 (CEACAM6). Many authors have also suggested a link between CD and *Mycobacterium paratuberculosis* (MAP), although recent PCR-based studies have failed to confirm this and therapeutic trials of anti-*Mycobacterium tuberculosis* (MTB) therapy were not effective.
- ***Bacterial antigens***. Bacteria exert their influence by the interaction of ligands such as peptidoglycan-polysaccharides (PG-PS) and lipopolysaccharides (LPS) with host pattern recognition receptors such as the Toll-like receptor family (cell surface) and the NOD family (intracellular).
- ***Defective chemical barrier or intestinal defensins*** (see p. 392). Evidence suggests a decrease in human α defensin-1 (HD-1) in the mucosa of both CD and UC, and a lack of induction of HD-2, HD-3 and HD-5 in CD.
- ***Impaired mucosal barrier function***. This may explain the presence of unusual and potentially pathogenic bacteria, such as MAP, *Listeria* and mucosal adherent *E. coli*. However, their presence does not necessarily imply causation of the disease, and they may reflect previous disease activity.

The intestinal immune system

IBD occurs when the mucosal immune system exerts an inappropriate response to luminal antigens, such as bacteria, which may enter the mucosa via a leaky epithelium ***(Fig. 13.38)***. Bacterial ligands interact with the innate and acquired mucosal immune system via Toll-like receptors expressed on both epithelial and antigen-presenting cells. Deficiencies occur in the clearance of invading bacteria by aspects of the innate immune system, such as neutrophils, which may allow inappropriate activation of the acquired immune system. In keeping with the genetic susceptibility loci identified, these findings highlight a deficiency in patients with IBD in a component of the inflammasome (an intracellular danger sensor of the innate immune system that can trigger caspase-1-dependent processing of inflammatory mediators, such as IL-1β and IL-18). In addition, individual bacterial species have distinct immunological effects mediated by dendritic cells (DCs), which sample bacteria from the intestinal lumen and direct the subsequent functional

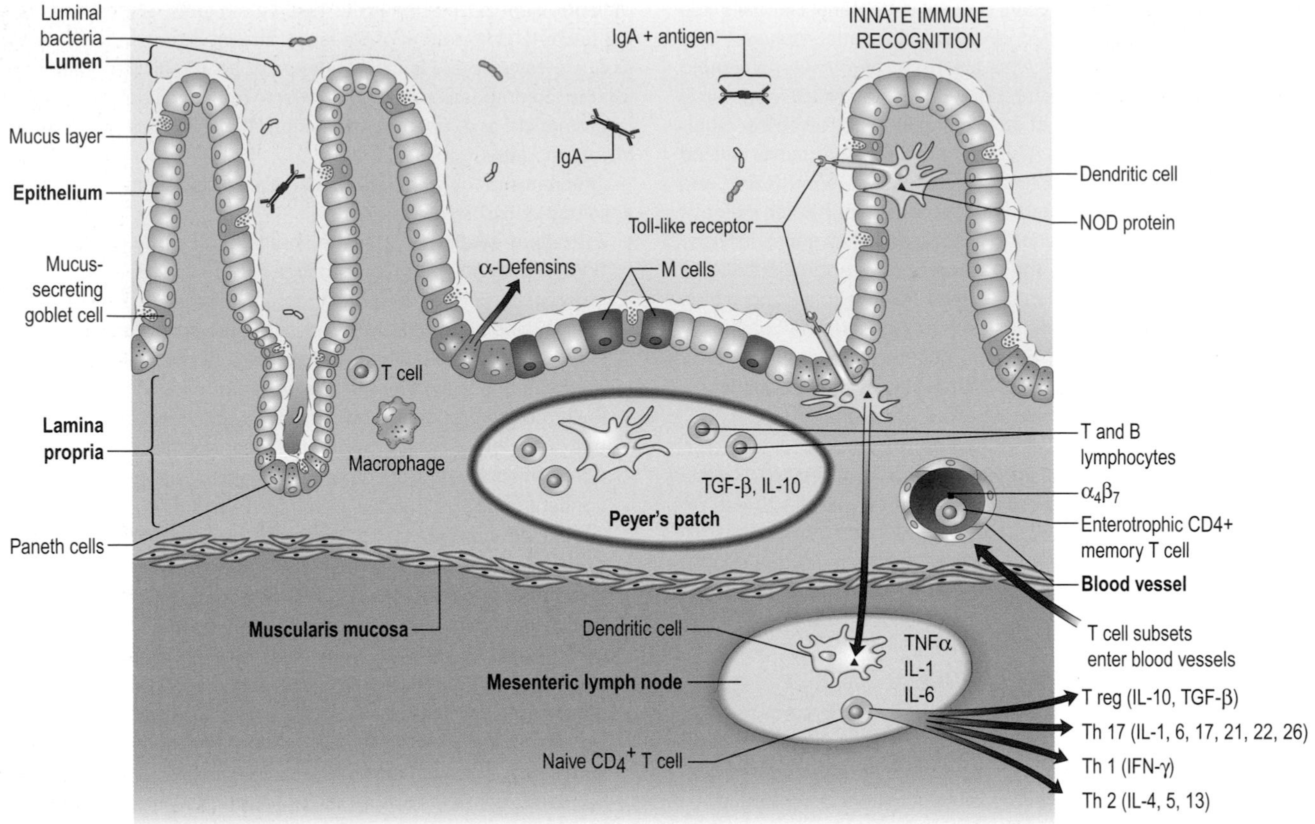

Figure 13.38 Cellular intestinal processes involved in inflammatory bowel disease. Bacterial ligands attach to the epithelium and antigen-presenting cells (e.g. dendritic cells and macrophages) via Toll-like receptors and the NOD protein. The dendritic cells migrate to the Peyer's patches and mesenteric lymph nodes. They present antigens to naive T cells, releasing a number of cytokines that cause damage. The T-cell subsets enter the blood vessels, where the enterotropic molecules α4-β7 are induced and allow homing back to the gut, causing further damage. IFN-γ, interferon-gamma; IL, interleukin; TGF-β, transforming growth factor-beta; TNF-α, tumour necrosis factor-alpha. *(Modified from Abraham C, Cho JH. Inflammatory bowel disease.* N Engl J Med *2009; 361:2066–2078.)*

differentiation of naive T cells into effector or regulatory populations. IBD is associated with an imbalance in the relative numbers of intestinal homing effector (Th1 and Th17) and regulatory T cell populations, which disturbs the normal tolerance to the luminal antigenic load.

The pro-inflammatory cytokines released by these activated effector T cells stimulate macrophages to secrete pro-inflammatory cytokines, such as tumour necrosis factor-alpha (TNF-α), IL-1 and IL-6 in large quantities. These mechanisms result in increased adhesion molecule expression on the intestinal vascular endothelium, which facilitates the recruitment of leucocytes from the circulation and the release of chemokines, all of which lead to tissue damage and also attract more inflammatory cells in a vicious circle.

Pathology

CD is a chronic inflammatory condition that may affect any part of the gastrointestinal tract from the mouth to the anus but has a particular tendency to affect the terminal ileum and ascending colon (ileocolonic disease) ***(Fig. 13.39)***. The disease can involve one small area of the gut, such as the terminal ileum, or multiple areas with relatively normal bowel in between (skip lesions). It may also involve the whole of the colon (total colitis), sometimes without macroscopic small bowel involvement. It is also associated with the development of perianal fistulae and fissures ***(Box 13.20)***.

UC can affect the rectum alone (proctitis), can extend proximally to involve the sigmoid and descending colon (left-sided colitis), or

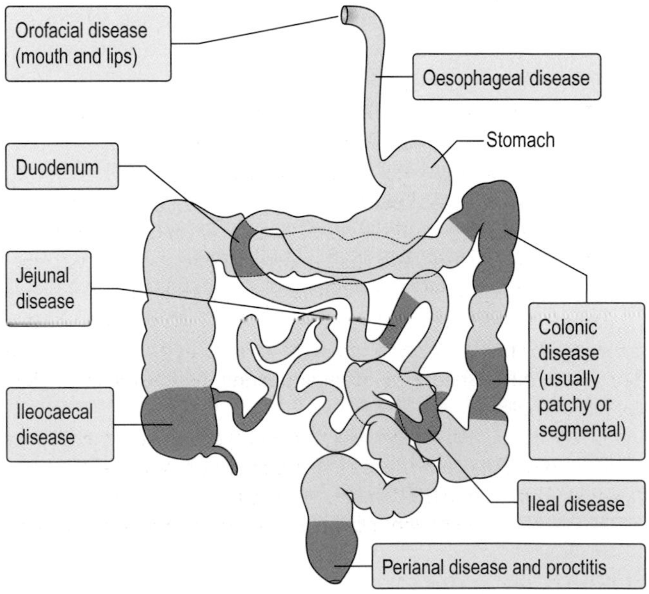

Figure 13.39 Sites of Crohn's disease.

Box 13.20 Anal and perianal complications of Crohn's disease

- Fissure *in ano* (multiple and indolent)
- Haemorrhoids
- Skin tags
- Perianal abscess
- Ischiorectal abscess
- Fistula *in ano* (may be multiple)
- Anorectal fistulae

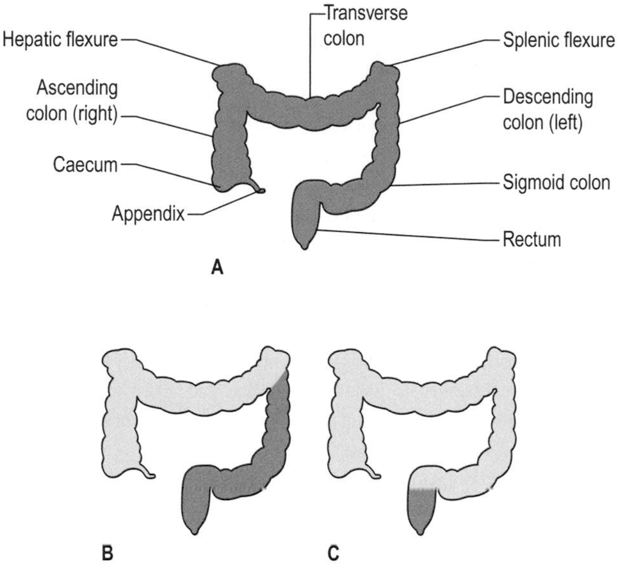

Figure 13.40 Sites of ulcerative colitis (Montreal classification). **A.** *Extensive colitis (E3)*: pancolitis, total colitis: entire colon and rectum inflamed. **B.** *Distal colitis (E2)*: left-sided colitis: rectum, sigmoid and descending colon inflamed. **C.** *Proctitis (E1)*: rectum only inflamed.

may involve the whole colon (extensive colitis) ***(Fig. 13.40)***. In a few of these patients, there is also inflammation of the distal terminal ileum (backwash ileitis).

Macroscopic changes

In ***CD***, the involved bowel is usually thickened and is often narrowed. Deep ulcers and fissures in the mucosa produce a cobblestone appearance. Intra-abdominal fistulae and abscesses may be seen, which reflect penetrating disease. An early feature is aphthoid ulceration in the colon, usually seen at colonoscopy ***(Fig. 13.41)***; later, larger and deeper ulcers appear in a patchy distribution, again producing a cobblestone appearance.

In ***UC***, the mucosa looks reddened and inflamed, and bleeds easily (friability). In severe disease, there may be extensive ulceration, with the adjacent mucosa appearing as post-inflammatory (pseudo-) polyps.

In ***fulminant colonic disease*** of either type, most of the mucosa is lost, leaving a few islands of oedematous mucosa (mucosal islands), and toxic dilatation occurs. On healing, the mucosa can return to normal, although there is usually some residual scarring.

Microscopic changes

In ***CD***, the inflammation extends through all layers (transmural) of the bowel, whereas in UC superficial inflammation limited to the mucosa is seen. In CD, there is an increase in chronic inflammatory cells and lymphoid hyperplasia, and in 50–60% of patients granulomas are present. These granulomas are non-caseating epithelioid cell aggregates with Langhans' giant cells.

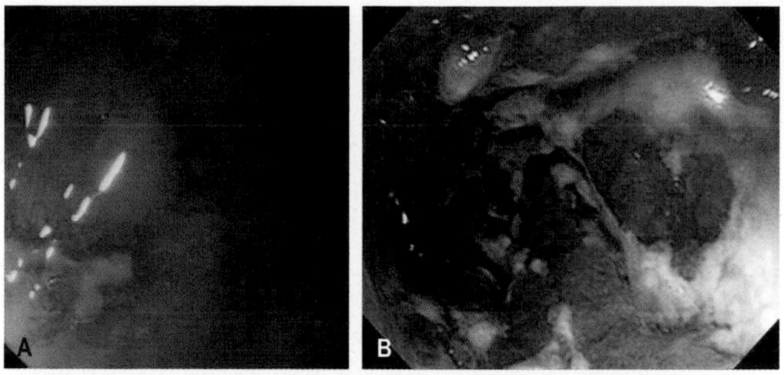

Figure 13.41 Crohn's disease: colonoscopic appearances. **A.** Aphthoid ulcers typical of Crohn's disease. **B.** Deep, serpiginous ulceration in colonic Crohn's disease.

Box 13.21 Histological differences between Crohn's disease and ulcerative colitis

Histological feature	Crohn's disease	Ulcerative colitis
Inflammation	Deep (transmural) patchy	Mucosal continuous
Granulomas	++	Rare
Goblet cells	Present	Depleted
Crypt abscesses	+	++

In ***UC***, the mucosa shows a chronic inflammatory cell infiltrate in the lamina propria. Crypt abscesses and goblet cell depletion are also seen.

These two diseases can usually be differentiated not only on the basis of clinical and radiological data but also on the histological differences seen in the rectal and colonic mucosa obtained by biopsy ***(Box 13.21)***.

It is occasionally not possible to distinguish between the two disorders, particularly if biopsies are obtained in the acute phase, and such patients are considered to have CUTE. Serological testing for anti-neutrophil cytoplasmic antibodies (ANCA) in UC and anti-*Saccharomyces cerevisiae* antibodies (ASCA) in CD may be of value in differentiating the two conditions (see pp. 408–409), although an exact diagnosis can sometimes be made only after examining a surgical colectomy specimen. Occasionally, examination of the colectomy specimen still does not lead to a diagnosis of CD or UC and the patient is labelled as having indeterminate colitis.

Extraintestinal manifestations

These occur with both diseases ***(Box 13.22)***. Joint complications are most common; the peripheral arthropathies are classified as:

- ***Type 1 (pauciarticular)*** attacks are acute and self-limiting (<10 weeks), and occur with IBD relapses; they are associated with other extraintestinal manifestations of IBD activity.
- ***Type 2 (polyarticular)*** arthropathy lasts longer (months to years), is independent of IBD activity and usually associated with uveitis.

Joint and other extragastrointestinal manifestations of IBD are shown in ***Box 13.22***. There is an association of HLA *DRB1*0103* with pauciarticular large-joint arthritis in UC and CD, and HLA-B44 with small-joint symmetrical arthritis. HLA-B27 is associated with sacroiliitis.

Differential diagnosis

Alternative causes of diarrhoea should be excluded ***(Box 13.23)*** and stool cultures (including *Clostridium difficile* toxin assay) must

Box 13.22 Extragastrointestinal manifestations of inflammatory bowel disease

- **Eyes:**
  - Uveitis
  - Episcleritis, conjunctivitis
- **Joints:**
  - Type I (pauciarticular) arthropathy
  - Type II (polyarticular) arthropathy
  - Arthralgia
  - Ankylosing spondylitis
  - Inflammatory back pain
- **Skin:**
  - Erythema nodosum
  - Pyoderma gangrenosum
- **Liver and biliary tree:**
  - Sclerosing cholangitis
  - Fatty liver
  - Chronic hepatitis
  - Cirrhosis
  - Gallstones
- **Nephrolithiasis**
- **Venous thrombosis**

Box 13.23 Causes of diarrhoea

Non-infective causes

- Inflammatory bowel disease
- Radiation proctitis or colitis
- Behçet's disease
- Diverticular disease
- Ischaemic colitis
- Gastrointestinal lymphoma
- Carcinoma of the colon (change in bowel habit)
- Malabsorption
- Gut resection
- Bile acid malabsorption
- Drugs – many, including
  - Laxatives
  - Metformin
  - Anti-cancer drugs
  - Statins
  - Proton pump inhibitors
- Faecal impaction with overflow
- Irritable bowel syndrome and functional diarrhoea
- Endocrine causes:
  - Zollinger–Ellison syndrome
  - VIPoma
  - Somatostatinoma
  - Glucagonoma
  - Carcinoid syndrome
  - Thyrotoxicosis
  - Medullary carcinoma of thyroid
  - Diabetic autonomic neuropathy
- Factitious diarrhoea:
  - Purgative abuse
  - Dilutional diarrhoea

Infective causes

- Bacterial, e.g.
  - *Campylobacter jejuni*
  - *Salmonella* spp.
  - *Shigella*
  - *Escherichia coli* (see p. 276)
  - Staphylococcal enterocolitis
  - *Bacillus cereus*
  - *Clostridium perfringens, C. botulinum, C. difficile*
  - Gastrointestinal tuberculosis
- Viral, e.g.
  - Rotavirus
- Fungal, e.g.
  - Histoplasmosis
- Parasitic, e.g.
  - Amoebic dysentery (*Entamoeba histolytica*)
  - Schistosomiasis
  - *Giardia intestinalis*

always be performed. However, symptoms persisting beyond 5 days are unlikely to be caused by infective gastroenteritis. Stool microscopy for parasitic diseases such as amoebiasis should be carried out in patients with a relevant travel history. CD should be considered in all individuals with evidence of vitamin malabsorption (e.g. megaloblastic anaemia) or malnourishment, as well as in children with reduced growth velocity. Ileocolonic tuberculosis (see p. 401) is common in developing countries, such as India, which makes a diagnosis of CD difficult. Microscopy and culture for TB of any available tissue is essential in these countries. A therapeutic trial of anti-TB therapy may be required. Lymphomas can occasionally involve the ileum and caecum, although they are rare in the patient population at risk from IBD.

Crohn's disease

Clinical features

The major symptoms are diarrhoea, abdominal pain and weight loss. Constitutional symptoms of malaise, lethargy, anorexia, nausea, vomiting and low-grade fever may be present and in 15% of these patients there are no gastrointestinal symptoms. Reduced growth velocity and delayed puberty may be the main presenting features in children. Despite the recurrent nature of this condition, some patients have an almost normal lifestyle. However, patients with extensive disease have frequent recurrences and progress from inflammatory to stricturing and penetrating disease. Approximately 50% of patients will require an intestinal resection within 5 years of diagnosis.

Clinical features are very variable and depend partly on the region of the bowel that is affected. The disease may present insidiously or acutely. Abdominal pain can be colicky, suggesting obstruction, but it usually has no special characteristics and sometimes in colonic disease only minimal discomfort is present. Diarrhoea occurs in 80% of all cases and in colonic disease it usually contains blood, making it difficult to differentiate from UC. Steatorrhoea can be present in small bowel disease. Diarrhoea can also be due to bile acid malabsorption, occurring as a consequence of ileal resection or ileal disease.

CD can also present as an emergency with acute right iliac fossa pain mimicking appendicitis. If laparotomy is undertaken, an oedematous, reddened terminal ileum is found. Other causes of an acute ileitis include infections such as *Yersinia* and TB.

CD is complicated by anal and perianal disease, and this is the presenting feature in 25% of cases, often preceding colonic and small intestinal symptoms (see ***Box 13.20***). Enteric fistulae – for example, to bladder, vagina or abdominal wall – occur in 20–40% of cases.

Examination

Physical signs are few, apart from loss of weight and signs of malnutrition. Aphthous ulceration of the mouth is often seen. Abdominal examination may be normal, although tenderness and/or a right iliac fossa mass are occasionally found. The mass is due either to inflamed loops of bowel that are matted together or to an abscess, which may also cause psoas muscle irritation. The anus should always be examined to look for oedematous anal tags, fissures or perianal abscesses.

The presence of extraintestinal features of IBD should be assessed (see ***Box 13.22***).

Investigations

Blood tests

- ***Anaemia*** is common and may be the normocytic, normochromic anaemia of chronic disease. However, deficiency of iron and/or folate also occurs. Despite terminal ileal involvement in CD, megaloblastic anaemia due to vitamin B_{12} deficiency is unusual, although serum B_{12} levels can be below the normal range.
- ***Raised ESR and CRP*** are found, as are raised white cell and platelet counts.
- ***Hypoalbuminaemia*** is present in severe disease as part of an acute phase response to inflammation associated with a raised CRP.

- ***Liver biochemistry*** may be abnormal.
- ***Blood cultures*** are required if septicaemia is suspected.
- ***Serological tests*** may reveal negative perinuclear ANCA (pANCA) and positive ASCA (see p. 407).

Stool tests

Stool cultures, including *C. difficile* toxin assay, should always be performed if diarrhoea is present. Microscopy for parasites is essential in patients with a relevant travel history. Faecal calprotectin and lactoferrin are raised in active intestinal disease.

Endoscopy and radiological imaging

- ***Colonoscopy*** is performed if colonic involvement is suspected, except in patients presenting with severe disease (in whom a limited unprepared sigmoidoscopy should be carried out). The findings vary from mild, patchy, superficial (aphthoid) ulceration to more widespread, larger and deeper ulcers that produce a cobblestone appearance (see ***Fig 13.41***). Endoscopic assessment of the terminal ileum is essential in all patients with suspected CD. Two biopsies should be performed in five areas, including the rectum and terminal ileum.
- ***Upper gastrointestinal endoscopy*** is required to exclude oesophageal and gastroduodenal disease in patients with relevant symptoms and is increasingly being performed in all patients at diagnosis to define the extent of disease accurately as a guide to prognosis.
- ***Small bowel imaging*** is mandatory in patients with suspected CD. The technique used will depend on availability and local expertise. Techniques include barium follow-through, CT scan with oral contrast, small bowel ultrasound or MRI enteroclysis. An asymmetrical alteration in the mucosal pattern with deep ulceration, and areas of narrowing or structuring may be found. Although disease is commonly confined to the terminal ileum ***(Fig. 13.42)***, other areas of the small bowel can be involved, and skip lesions with normal bowel are seen between affected sites. Axial imaging allows the diagnosis of extraintestinal sepsis in patients presenting acutely and is therefore preferred in this situation.
- ***Ultrasound scanning*** provides a convenient radiation-free method for assessing disease activity in the ileum and colon and can be performed by appropriately trained gastroenterologists at the bedside.
- ***Perianal MRI or endoanal ultrasound*** is used to evaluate perianal disease.
- ***Capsule endoscopy*** is used in CD patients when radiological examination is normal. A patency capsule assessment is often performed first to exclude strictures of the small bowel that would constitute a contraindication to subsequent capsule endoscopy.
- ***Radionuclide scans*** with indium- or technetium-labelled leucocytes are used in some centres to identify small intestinal and colonic disease inflammation and to localize extraintestinal abscesses.

Disease activity

This can be assessed using simple parameters such as haemoglobin, white cell count, inflammatory markers (raised ESR, CRP and platelet count) and serum albumin. Formal clinical activity indices (e.g. CD Activity Index or Harvey Bradshaw Index) are used in research studies. Faecal calprotectin or lactoferrin has the potential to be a simple, cheap, non-invasive marker of disease activity in IBD and these tests are of value in predicting response to and failure of treatment.

Box 13.24 Options for the medical treatment of Crohn's disease

Induction of remission
- Oral or i.v. glucocorticosteroids
- Enteral nutrition
- Anti-tumour necrosis factor (TNF) antibodies

Maintenance of remission
- Azathioprine, mercaptopurine, methotrexate
- Anti-TNF antibodies

Perianal disease
- Surgical drainage of sepsis
- Ciprofloxacin and metronidazole
- Azathioprine
- Anti-TNF antibodies

Medical management of Crohn's disease

See ***Box 13.24***.

General considerations

The aims of management are to induce and then maintain clinical remission and to achieve mucosal healing in order to prevent disease progression and complications. Alternative causes for symptoms, such as gastroenteritis, extraintestinal sepsis, stricture formation, functional gastrointestinal disease or bile salt malabsorption, must be excluded before commencing immunosuppressive therapy. Patients with mild symptoms and no evidence of extensive disease may require symptomatic treatment only. Cigarette smoking should be stopped. Anaemia, if due to vitamin B_{12}, folic acid or iron deficiency, should be treated with the appropriate replacement. Patients who are intolerant of oral iron should receive an intravenous iron infusion. Most patients can be treated as outpatients, although severe attacks may require admission, and prophylaxis for thromboembolism (see p. 1056) should be given to all inpatients.

Induction of remission

Glucocorticosteroids

These are commonly used to induce remission in moderate and severe attacks of CD (oral prednisolone 30–60 mg/day). Mild to moderate ileocaecal disease should be treated with controlled-release corticosteroids, such as budesonide, which has reduced systemic availability and is associated with a lower frequency and intensity of steroidal side-effects.

Overall remission/response rates vary from 60% to 90%, depending on type, site and extent of disease. Steroids should be avoided in patients with penetrating intestinal disease or perianal sepsis.

Aminosalicylates

These have been used but there is little evidence to support their efficacy in CD.

Antibiotics

Antibiotics (ciprofloxacin and metronidazole) are used for treating secondary complications of CD (e.g. abscess and perianal disease).

Exclusive enteral nutrition

This is the traditional treatment for moderate to severe attacks of CD in paediatric practice, but is under-utilized in adults due to

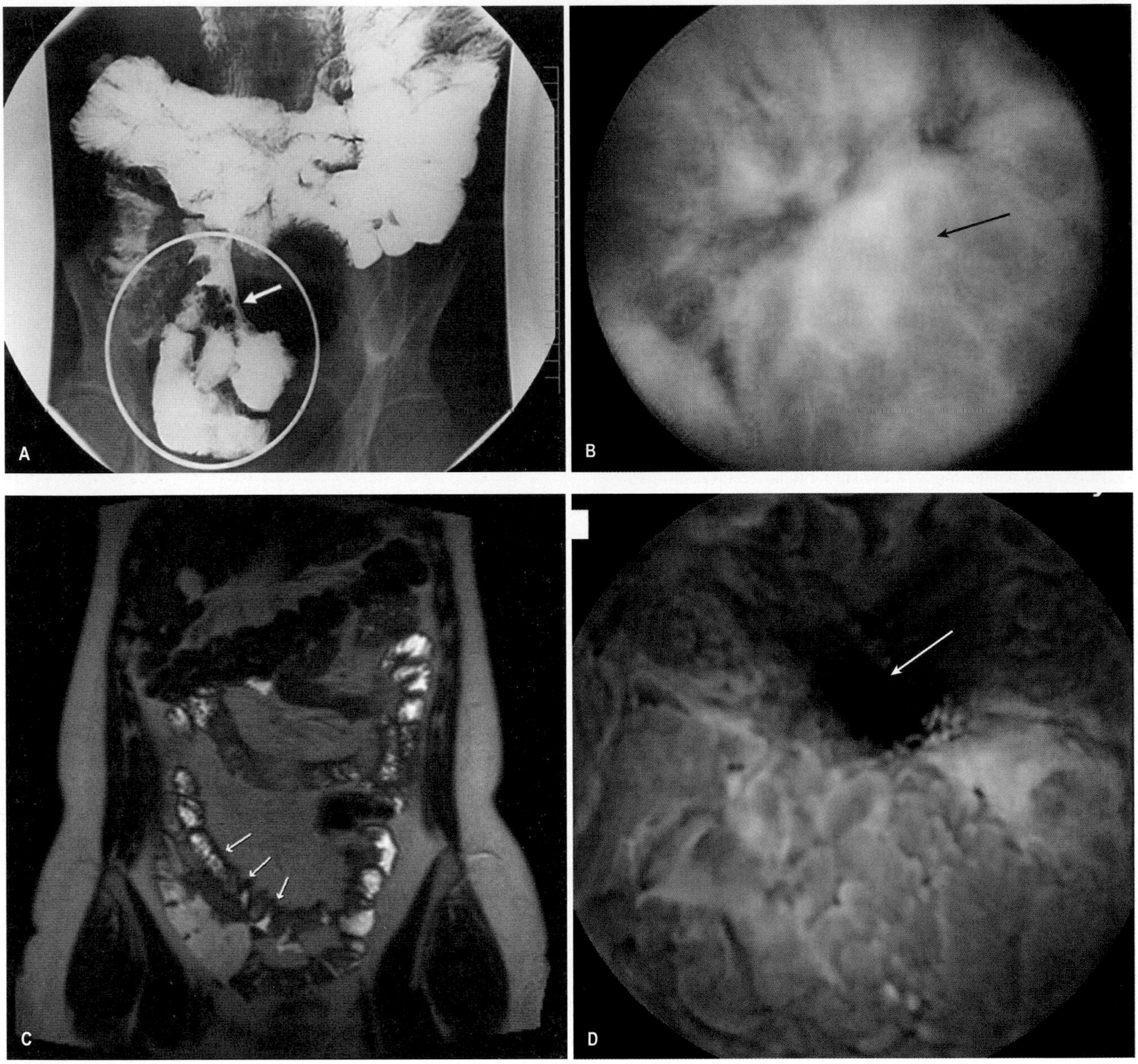

Figure 13.42 Imaging of the small bowel in Crohn's disease. A. Barium follow-through showing an ulcerated stricture (arrowed), pre-stenotic dilatation and separation of the small bowel loops due to fibro-fatty proliferation. **B.** Capsule endoscopy picture of an ileal ulcer in a patient with Crohn's disease (arrowed). **C.** MRI showing a thick-walled segment of ileal inflammation (arrowed). **D.** Capsule endoscopy showing an ileal Crohn's disease stricture (arrowed).

issues with compliance to the diet. If administered as the sole source of nutrition for 28 days, rates of induction of remission are similar to those obtained with steroids. Relapse rates are high, however, particularly in those with colonic involvement.

Refractory or fulminant disease

Patients with symptoms that do not respond to conventional therapy should be re-assessed to exclude an alternative diagnosis such as a stricture or penetrating abscess. In patients with disease limited to the terminal ileum, surgical resection may be appropriate. In those with more extensive disease, remission should be induced with an anti-TNF agent, either as monotherapy or preferably in combination with an immunosuppressant such as azathioprine (see below).

Maintenance of remission

All patients require regular monitoring to exclude persistent intestinal inflammation. Patients with disease that has a good prognosis (older age at diagnosis, no perianal disease, limited ulceration at index investigations, non-smoker) may not require maintenance therapy. Patients with disease that has a poor prognosis (young age at diagnosis, extensive small bowel disease, deep colonic ulceration, perianal/rectal disease, smoker) or that flares up after induction therapy is withdrawn require long-term maintenance immunosuppression. The goal of maintenance therapy is to prevent disease progression, as well as to reduce the need for corticosteroids, which are associated with a high burden of side-effects. Therapies that induce mucosal healing result in better outcomes. All maintenance therapies require careful monitoring to ensure optimal disease control and prevent side-effects. If there is ongoing evidence of disease activity, adherence should be confirmed and dose optimization or therapy escalation undertaken.

Conventional maintenance therapies

These include ***azathioprine*** (AZA, 2.5 mg/kg per day), ***mercaptopurine*** (MP, 1.5 mg/kg per day) and ***methotrexate*** (25 mg **once a week** until remission, then reduced to 15 mg per week) ***(Box 13.24)***. Long-term treatment with these drugs is necessary, as the rate of relapse on discontinuation is high. Patient education regarding side-effects and appropriate monitoring for complications is essential and may increase adherence. The key enzyme involved in AZA and MP metabolism is thiopurine methyl transferase (TPMT). This enzyme has a significant genetic variation and deficiencies can result in high circulating levels of thioguanine nucleotides with an increased risk of bone marrow depression. Assays of TPMT activity are available and should be performed before treatment. TPMT deficiency is not the only cause of bone marrow depression so 3-monthly blood counts should be performed on all patients. Metabolite measurement can be undertaken to assess adherence and ensure optimal dosing.

Anti-TNF agents

These have clear evidence of benefit in the induction and maintenance of remission in patients with CD. They are indicated in patients with disease refractory to conventional immunosuppressive therapy. Early use of anti-TNF therapy is indicated in selected patients with disease that has a poor prognosis (see above). They are also used to treat complex perianal/rectal disease once sepsis has been drained. Available anti-TNF agents include ***infliximab*** (a chimeric anti-TNF-α IgG1 monoclonal antibody), ***adalimumab*** (a fully humanized anti-TNF IgG1 monoclonal antibody) and ***certolizumab pegol*** (a PEGylated Fab′ fragment of a humanized anti-TNF antibody). They neutralize soluble TNF-α, bind to membrane bound TNF-α and induce immune cell apoptosis, although the exact mechanism of action is not defined. In clinical trials, they have been shown to exert a steroid-sparing effect and bring about complete mucosal healing in up to one-third of patients in the long term. This results in a reduced need for hospital admission and surgery. These agents should always be used on a regular basis as maintenance therapy, as they are less effective and induce anti-drug antibodies if used episodically. In patients who are naive to azathioprine, combination therapy increases efficacy and reduces immunogenicity. Their use should be limited to clinicians experienced in the management of CD, as they are associated with significant complications, including opportunistic infections (such as TB), demyelination and malignancy.

Novel biological therapies

Novel therapies for the treatment of CD include the anti-α4β7 integrin therapy, vedolizumab, which acts to reduce leucocyte recruitment to the inflamed intestine. Therapies that target the IL-12/IL-23 pathway, such as ustekinumab, are currently in phase III trials. Recent preliminary studies using the oral anti-sense oligonucleotide, Mongersen, have shown promise. This agent binds to, and causes degradation of, *SMAD7* messenger RNA, thereby [illegible] inflammatory markers.

Surgical management of Crohn's disease

Studies prior to the introduction of biological agents suggest that up to 80% of patients will require an operation at some time during the course of their disease. Nevertheless, surgery should be avoided if possible and only minimal resections undertaken, as recurrence (15% per year) is almost inevitable without prophylactic maintenance therapy. The *indications for surgery* are:

- failure of medical therapy, with acute or chronic symptoms producing ill-health
- complications (e.g. toxic dilatation, obstruction, perforation, abscesses, enterocutaneous fistula)
- failure to grow in children despite medical treatment
- presence of perianal sepsis: an examination is performed under anaesthetic, the sepsis is drained, and a seton is inserted to ensure ongoing drainage.

In patients with small bowel disease, some strictures can be widened (stricturoplasty), whereas others require resection and anastomosis. It is essential to consider postoperative maintenance therapy in patients undergoing ileocolonic resection and anastamosis. All patients should refrain from smoking. There is some evidence that a 3-month course of metronidazole reduces relapse rates. Patients with a high risk of relapse (previous surgery, smoker, penetrating disease at the time of index surgery) should be evaluated for maintenance immunosuppressive therapy. Patients should undergo an ileocolonoscopy to assess the anastamosis for disease recurrence 6 months after surgery, when further therapy can be agreed with the patient.

When colonic CD involves the entire colon and the rectum is spared or minimally involved, a subtotal colectomy and ileorectal anastomosis may be performed. An eventual recurrence rate of 60–70% in the ileum, rectum or both is to be expected; however, two-thirds of these patients retain a functional rectum for 10 years. If the whole colon and rectum are involved, a panproctocolectomy with an end ileostomy is the standard operation. CD patients are not suitable for a pouch operation (see p. 413), as recurrence in the pouch is high.

Problems associated with ileostomies include:

- mechanical problems
- dehydration, particularly if there is a short length of small bowel remaining
- psychosexual problems
- erectile dysfunction in men and reduced fecundity in women (due to prior pelvic surgery)
- recurrence of CD.

Prognosis

The majority of patients have inflammatory disease at diagnosis, although up to 20% will present with complicated disease, including strictures and penetrating disease. If disease is left untreated, its natural history is progression from inflammatory to stricturing and penetrating disease that may require surgery. Up to 50% of patients will require a surgical resection within the first 5 years of disease. The goal of therapy is to target early aggressive therapy at those patients with a poor prognosis. However, predicting disease prognosis at diagnosis is not easy. Features that imply a poor prognosis include young age at diagnosis (<20 years of age), extensive small bowel disease, complex perianal disease and deep ulceration at index colonoscopy.

Ulcerative colitis

Clinical features

The major symptom in UC is diarrhoea with blood and mucus, sometimes accompanied by lower abdominal discomfort. General

Box 13.25 Definition and management of a severe attack of ulcerative colitis

Definition

- Stool frequency: >6 stools/day with blood +++
- Fever: >37.5°C
- Tachycardia: >90 b.p.m.
- Erythrocyte sedimentation rate: >30 mm/h
- Anaemia: <100 g/L haemoglobin
- Albumin: <30 g/L

Management

- Admit to hospital
- Exclude enteric infection
- Confirm diagnosis with unprepared limited flexible sigmoidoscopy
- Assess fluid status
- Give prophylactic anticoagulation
- I.v. hydrocortisone 100 mg qds
- Monitor daily:
  - Stool frequency
  - Abdominal X-ray
  - Bloods (FBC/CRP/albumin)

features include malaise, lethargy and anorexia with weight loss, although these features are not as severe as with CD. Aphthous ulceration in the mouth may be seen. The disease can be mild, moderate or severe ***(Box 13.25)***, and in most patients runs a course of remissions and exacerbations. Disease extent is defined as limited to the rectum (proctitis), left-sided or extensive (see ***Fig. 13.40***).

Proctitis is characterized by the frequent passage of blood and mucus, urgency and tenesmus. There are normally few constitutional symptoms and the stool, when passed, may be solid. Patients are nevertheless greatly inconvenienced by the frequency of defecation.

In an acute attack of left-sided or extensive UC, patients have bloody diarrhoea, passing up to 10–20 liquid stools per day. Diarrhoea also occurs at night, with urgency and incontinence that is severely disabling for the patient. Patients with an acute severe flare of colitis ***(Box 13.25)*** require urgent admission for intensive therapy.

Toxic megacolon is a serious complication associated with acute severe colitis. The plain abdominal X-ray shows a dilated, thin-walled colon with a diameter of >6 cm; it is gas-filled and contains mucosal islands ***(Fig. 13.43)***. It is a particularly dangerous stage of advanced disease, with impending perforation and a high mortality (15–25%). Urgent surgery is required in all patients in whom toxic dilatation has not resolved within 48 hours, with intensive therapy as above. The differential diagnosis includes an infectious colitis, e.g. with *C. difficile* and cytomegalovirus.

Examination

In general, there are no specific signs in UC. The abdomen may be slightly distended or tender to palpation. Tachycardia and pyrexia are signs of severe colitis and mandate admission. The anus is usually normal. Rectal examination will reveal the presence of blood. Sigmoidoscopy is usually abnormal, showing an inflamed, bleeding, friable mucosa. Very occasionally, rectal sparing occurs, with normal proctoscopy.

Investigations

Blood tests

- ***White cell and platelet counts*** are commonly raised in moderate to severe attacks, and iron deficiency anaemia is present.

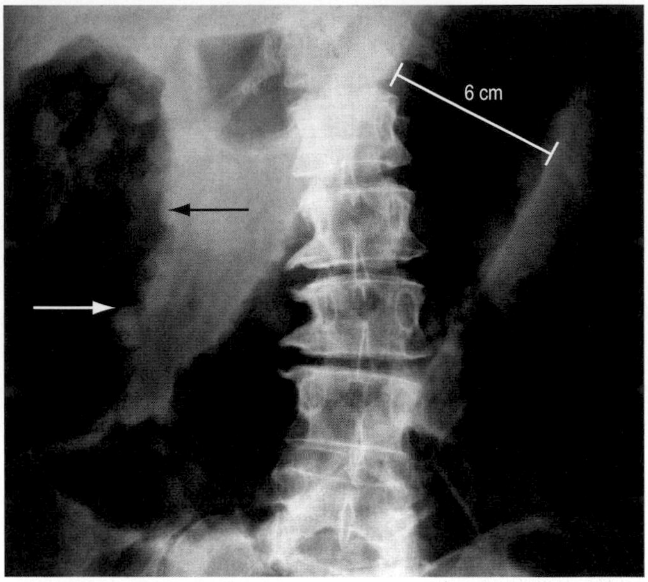

Figure 13.43 **Plain abdominal X-ray showing toxic dilatation.** The arrows indicate mucosal islands.

- ***ESR and CRP*** are often raised; liver biochemistry may be abnormal, with hypoalbuminaemia occurring in severe disease.
- ***pANCA*** may be positive. This is contrary to CD, where pANCA is usually negative (see p. 409).

Stool tests and *C. difficile* toxin

These should always be performed to exclude infective causes of colitis. Stool microscopy to exclude amoebiasis is mandated in patients with a relevant travel history. Faecal calprotectin/lactoferrin will be elevated.

Colonoscopy

Endoscopy with mucosal biopsy is the 'gold standard' investigation for the diagnosis of UC. Colonoscopy also allows assessment of disease activity and extent. In patients with long-term colitis, chromoendoscopy is used to diagnose dysplasia. Full colonoscopy should not be performed in severe attacks of disease for fear of perforation; instead, a limited unprepared flexible sigmoidoscopy should be used to confirm diagnosis.

Imaging

A plain abdominal X-ray is essential in patients suffering acute severe attacks to exclude colonic dilatation. However, the extent of disease is not reliably assessed using this investigation. Other imaging modalities are rarely used in the assessment of patients with UC, as endoscopy is preferred. However, inflammation of the colonic wall is detected on ultrasound, as is the presence of free fluid within the abdominal cavity.

Medical management of ulcerative colitis

Wherever possible, patients with IBD should be managed in patient-focused IBD clinics with access to a full multidisciplinary team. The mainstay of treatment for mild and moderate disease of any extent is an aminosalicylate, which acts topically in the colonic lumen. The active moiety of these drugs is 5-aminosalicylic acid (5-ASA), which is absorbed in the small intestine. Therefore, the various aminosalicylate preparations are designed to deliver the active 5-ASA to the colon. This is achieved by binding of 5-ASA with an azo bond to sulfapyridine (sulfasalazine), 4-aminobenzoyl-β-alanine (balsalazide) or to 5-ASA itself (olsalazine), coating with a pH-sensitive polymer, packaging of 5-ASA in microspheres, or a combination of these. The azo bonds are broken down by colonic bacteria to release 5-ASA within the colon.

The mode of action of 5-ASA in IBD is unknown, although it may involve the intracellular peroxisome proliferator-activated receptor (PPAR)-γ signalling pathway. The aminosalicylates have been shown to be effective in inducing remission in mild to moderately active disease, and maintaining remission in all forms of disease. There is also evidence that they are chemopreventive for UC-associated colorectal cancer. 5-ASA can rarely cause renal disease.

Proctitis

Rectal 5-ASA suppositories are the first-line treatment. Topical steroids are less effective than 5-ASA preparations. Oral 5-ASA can be added to increase remission rates. Some cases of proctitis do not respond to 5-ASA treatment and require oral prednisolone.

Left-sided colitis

Topical 5-ASA enemas are the first-line treatment. The addition of an oral 5-ASA will increase remission rates. Patients who do not respond to this or have worsening symptoms require oral prednisolone.

Extensive colitis

Patients with mild to moderate symptoms can be treated with an oral 5-ASA at an adequate dose. The additional of a 5-ASA enema increases remission rates. Patients who do not respond to this or have worsening symptoms require oral prednisolone.

Refractory/severe colitis of any extent

Patients with colitis that is refractory to standard conventional therapies should be investigated to ensure adherence to therapy, confirm active colitis and exclude infection, including biopsies to exclude reactivation of CMV colitis. They should then receive biological therapy with either an anti-TNF agent (infliximab, adalimumab or golimumab) or an anti-integrin therapy (vedolizumab).

Patients with severe colitis (Box 13.25) and those who do not respond to oral prednisolone should be admitted to hospital and treated initially with hydrocortisone 100 mg i.v. 6-hourly, with s.c. low-molecular-weight heparin to prevent thromboembolism. Investigations to confirm the diagnosis and exclude enteric infection (see above) should be performed and full supportive therapy administered (intravenous fluids, and nutritional support via the enteral route if required). The incidence of concomitant *C. difficile* infection in patients admitted for severe colitis is increasing. This is associated with a significant increase in morbidity and must be excluded. The clinical status of patients should be monitored daily (fever, tachycardia, stool frequency), and daily FBC, CRP, and urea and electrolytes should be performed. Repeat abdominal X-rays are required if patients are not improving. Success or failure of medical treatment of a severe attack of UC must be judged by an experienced gastroenterologist and colorectal surgeon. If patients have not responded to intravenous steroids within 3 days, either salvage [illegible] venous steroids, they should be switched to oral prednisolone after approximately 5 days, which they can be weaned off over 8–10 weeks. All patients who have been admitted for severe colitis should commence long-term maintenance therapy with a thiopurine (azathioprine/mercaptopurine).

Salvage therapy

Salvage therapy to avoid colectomy is required for patients with a CRP >45 mg/L or more than eight bowel motions after 3 days of intravenous hydrocortisone. Continuing steroid therapy alone in this situation will delay the inevitable colectomy and increase mortality. Salvage medical therapies with clear evidence of benefit in controlled clinical trials are intravenous ciclosporin 2 mg/kg per day as a continuous infusion or infliximab induction and maintenance therapy. Patients with extensive ulceration may require higher doses of induction infliximab. Patients with a low albumin level have been shown to have a lower response rate to salvage therapy. These agents should only be used by experienced gastroenterologists who are part of a multidisciplinary team with colorectal surgeons. Patients should be weaned off steroids rapidly, once salvage therapy has commenced, to reduce morbidity. Those who respond should be treated with oral ciclosporin or further infliximab infusions, as appropriate, while maintenance thiopurine therapy is commenced.

Surgical management of ulcerative colitis

While the treatment of UC remains primarily medical, surgery continues to have a central role because it may be life-saving, is curative and eliminates the long-term risk of cancer. The main indications for surgery are severe colitis that fails to respond to medical therapy, and chronic active therapy-refractory disease. Other indications are listed in **Box 13.26**. In expert centres, laparoscopic surgery is often used to improve postoperative pain, recovery time and cosmesis.

In acute disease, subtotal colectomy with end ileostomy and preservation of the rectum is the operation of choice. At a later date, a number of surgical options are available and are best carried out in a specialist colorectal centre. These include proctectomy with a permanent ileostomy; to avoid a permanent ileostomy, an ileo-anal pouch procedure can be performed ***(Fig. 13.44)***. The ileo-anal pouch is anastomosed to the anus at the dentate line following excision of the remaining rectum. One-third of patients, however, will experience '***pouchitis***', inflammation of the pouch mucosa with clinical symptoms of diarrhoea, bleeding, fever and, at times, exacerbation of extracolonic manifestations ***(Fig. 13.45)***. The incidence of pouchitis is twice as high in patients with primary sclerosing cholangitis and is also raised in patients with a positive ANCA and backwash ileitis prior to colectomy. Two-thirds of pouchitis cases will recur as either acute relapsing or chronic unremitting forms. The mainstay of treatment is antibiotics (metronidazole with or without ciprofloxacin). Treatment is not always satisfactory and steroids may be required. The probiotic VSL#3 has been shown to be effective in preventing the onset of pouchitis and in maintaining remission in patients with antibiotic-treated pouchitis to induce mucosal healing.

Course and prognosis

One-third of patients with distal inflammatory proctitis due to UC will develop more proximal disease, with 5–10% developing total

Box 13.26 Indications for surgery in ulcerative colitis

[illegible]
- Failure of medical treatment
- Toxic dilatation
- Haemorrhage
- Imminent perforation

[illegible]
- Incomplete response to medical treatment/ steroid-dependent
- Dysplasia on surveillance colonoscopy

colitis. One-third of patients with UC will have a single attack and the others will follow a relapsing course. One-third of patients with UC will undergo colectomy within 20 years of diagnosis.

Cancer in inflammatory bowel disease

Patients with UC and extensive Crohn's colitis have an increased incidence of developing dysplasia and subsequent colon cancer. The risk of dysplasia is related to the extent and duration of disease, as well as the presence of untreated mucosal inflammation. A family history of colorectal cancer and the presence of primary sclerosing cholangitis also increase the risk. Appropriate colonoscopic screening strategies according to guidelines are used by many, although evidence for overall benefit is still uncertain. A 40-year analysis of colonoscopy surveillance for neoplasia in UC, conducted at St Mark's Hospital in the UK, suggested that surveillance may have a significant role in reducing the risk of advanced and interval colorectal cancer.

Mortality in inflammatory bowel disease

Population-based studies demonstrate that mortality in UC is similar to that in the general population. The two exceptions are patients with severe colitis, who have a slightly higher mortality in the first year after diagnosis, and patients aged over 60 at the time of diagnosis. Although it is currently unclear whether there is a slightly higher overall mortality in patients with CD, those with extensive jejunal and ileal disease and those with gastric and duodenal disease have been shown to have a relatively higher mortality.

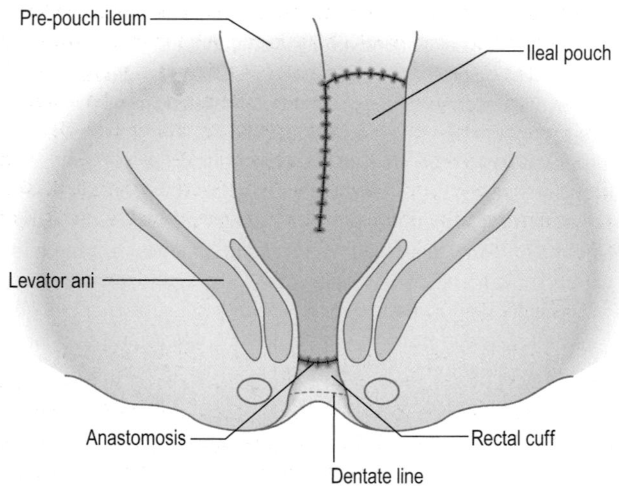

Figure 13.44 **An ileo-anal pouch for ulcerative colitis.**

Microscopic colitis

Patients with this group of disorders present with chronic or fluctuating watery diarrhoea. Although the macroscopic features on colonoscopy are normal, the histopathological findings on biopsy are abnormal. There are three distinct forms of microscopic inflammatory colitis:

- ***Microscopic UC***. There is a chronic inflammatory cell infiltrate in the lamina propria, with deformed crypt architecture and goblet cell depletion, with or without crypt abscesses. Treatment is as for UC; many patients respond to treatment with aminosalicylates alone.
- ***Microscopic lymphocytic colitis***. There is surface epithelial injury, prominent lymphocytic infiltration in the surface epithelium and increased lamina propria mononuclear cells.
- ***Microscopic collagenous colitis***. There is a thickened subepithelial collagen layer (>10 μm) adjacent to the basal membrane, and increased infiltration of the lamina propria with lymphocytes and plasma cells, and surface epithelial cell damage. It is predominantly a disorder of middle-aged or elderly females, and is associated with a variety of autoimmune disorders (arthritis, thyroid disease, limited cutaneous scleroderma and primary biliary cirrhosis).

The incidence of both microscopic lymphocytic and collagenous colitis is increased in patients with coeliac disease and this must be excluded. Treatment of microscopic and collagenous colitis is usually with budesonide. There is also evidence of benefit for aminosalicylates, bismuth-containing preparations and, if refractory, prednisolone and azathioprine. A small number of patients with microscopic lymphocytic and collagenous colitis have coexisting bile acid malabsorption and can thus respond to colestyramine. Prognosis is good.

Further reading

Ananthakrishnan AN. Epidemiology and risk factors for IBD. *Nat Rev Gastroenterol Hepatol* 2015; 12:205–217.
Cho JH, Gregersen PK. Genomics and the multifactorial nature of human autoimmune disease. *N Engl J Med* 2011; 365:1612–1623.
Choi CH, Rutter MD, Askara A et al. Forty-year analysis of colonoscopic surveillence programme for neoplasia in ulcerative colitis: an updated overview. *Am J Gastroenterol* 2015; 110:1022–1034.
Danese S, Fiocchi C. Ulcerative colitis. *N Engl J Med* 2011; 365:1713–1725.
Dignass A, Lindsay JO, Sturm A et al. Second European evidence-based consensus on the diagnosis and management of ulcerative colitis: current management. *J Crohns Colitis* 2012; 6:991–1030.
Ek WE, D'Amato M, Halfvarson J. The history of genetics in inflammatory bowel disease. *Ann Gastroenterol* 2014; 27:294–303.
Kalla R, Ventham NT, Satsangi J et al. Crohn's disease. *BMJ* 2014; 349:g6670.

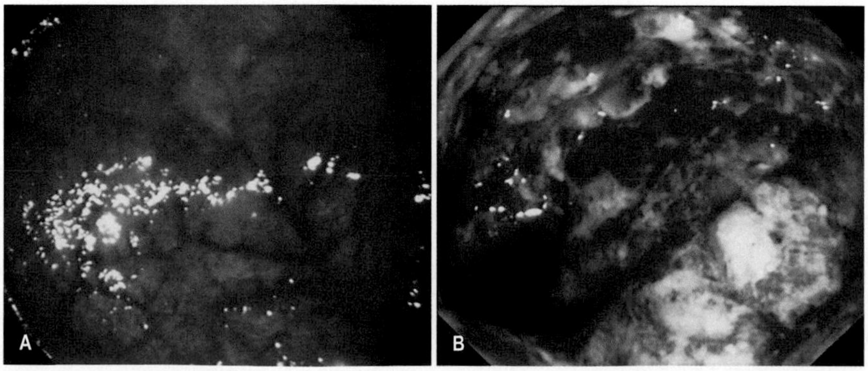

Figure 13.45 **Pouchitis: fibreoptic sigmoidoscopic appearances. A.** Mild changes. **B.** Severe haemorrhagic ulceration.

Kaser A, Zeissig S, Blumberg RS. Inflammatory bowel disease. *Annu Rev Immunol* 2010; 28:573–621.
Leiman DA, Lichtenstein GR. Therapy of inflammatory bowel disease: what to expect in the next decade. *Curr Opin Gastroenterol* 2014; 30:385–390.
Monteleone G, Neurath MF, Ardizzone S. Mongersen, an oral *SMAD7* antisense oligonucleotide, and Crohn's disease. *N Engl J Med* 2015; 372:1104–1113.
Mowat C, Cole A, Windsor A et al and IBD Section of the British Society of Gastroenterology. Guidelines for the management of inflammatory bowel disease in adults. *Gut* 2011; 60:571.
Nandivada P, Poylin V, Nagle D. Advances in the surgical management of inflammatory bowel disease. *Curr Opin Gastroenterol* 2012; 28:47–51.
Satangi J, Silverberg MS, Vermeire S et al. The Montreal classification of inflammatory bowel disease: controversies, consensus, and implications. *Gut* 2006; 55:749–753.
Strober W, Fuss IJ. Proinflammatory cytokines in the pathogenesis of inflammatory bowel disease. *Gastroenterology* 2011; 140:1756–1767.
Tilg H. Diet and intestinal immunity. *N Engl J Med* 2012; 366:181–183.
Van Assche G, Dignass A, Reinisch W et al and European Crohn's and Colitis Organisation (ECCO). The second European evidence-based Consensus on the diagnosis and management of Crohn's disease: special situations. *J Crohns Colitis* 2010; 4:63–101.
Van Assche G, Vermeire S, Rutgeerts P. Management of acute severe ulcerative colitis. *Gut* 2011; 60:130–133.
Van Assche G, Vermeire S, Rutgeerts P. The potential for disease modification in Crohn's disease. *Nat Rev Gastroenterol Hepatol* 2010; 7:79–85.

THE COLON AND RECTUM

Anatomy

The large intestine starts at the caecum, on the posterior medial wall of which is the appendix.

The ***colon*** is made up of ascending, transverse, descending and sigmoid parts, which join the rectum at the rectosigmoid junction ***(Fig. 13.46)***.

The muscle wall consists of an inner circular layer and an outer longitudinal layer. The outer layer is incomplete, coming together to form the taeniae coli, which produce the haustral pattern seen in the normal colon.

The mucosa of the colon is lined with epithelial cells and goblet cells. There are crypts but no villi, so that the surface is flat. A variety of cells, mainly lymphocytes and macrophages, are found in the lamina propria.

The blood supply to the colon is from the superior and inferior mesenteric vessels. The colon is innervated mainly by the enteric nervous system with input from the parasympathetic and sympathetic pathways. Spinal afferent neurones from the dorsal root ganglia innervate the entire colon.

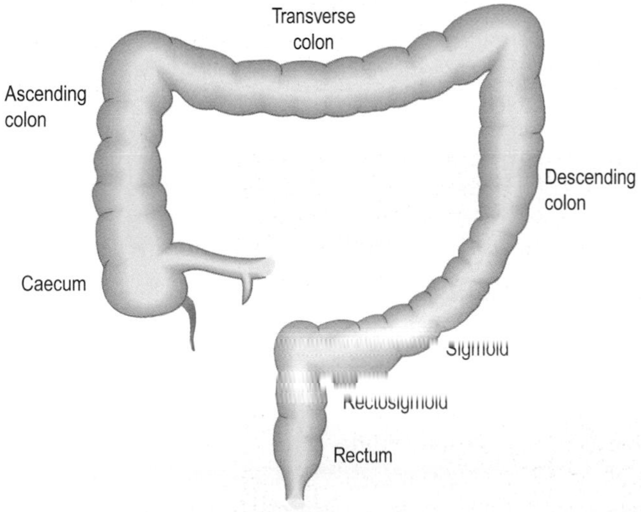

Figure 13.46 Structure of the large intestine.

The ***rectum*** is about 12 cm long. Its interior is divided by three crescentic circular muscles that produce shelf-like folds. These are the rectal valves, which can be seen at sigmoidoscopy. The anal canal has an internal and an external sphincter.

Physiology of the colon

The main roles of the colon are the absorption of water and electrolytes ***(Box 13.27)*** and the propulsion of contents from the caecum to the anorectal region. Approximately 1.5–2 L of fluid pass the ileocaecal valve each day. Absorption is stimulated by short-chain fatty acids, which are produced predominantly in the right colon by the anaerobic metabolism of dietary fibre by bacterial polysaccharidase enzyme systems. Colonic contents are mixed, aiding absorption by non-propagative segmenting muscular contractions. High-amplitude propagative colonic contractions cause propulsion. Peristalsis is induced by the release of serotonin (5-HT) from neuroendocrine cells in response to luminal distension. Serotonin activates the HT_4 receptors, which, in turn, results in the activation of sensory (calcitonin gene-related peptide, CGRP) neurones. Normal colonic transit time is 24–48 hours with normal stool weights of up to 250 g/day.

Physiology of defecation

The role of the rectum and anus in defecation is complex. The rectum is normally empty. Stool is propelled into the rectum by propagated colonic contractions. A sensation of fullness, a desire to defecate and urgency to defecate are experienced with increasing volumes of rectal content (threshold 100 mL). The sensations are associated with rectal contraction and a relaxation of the internal anal sphincter, both of which serve to push the stool down into the proximal anal canal. This increases the defecatory urge, which can only be suppressed by vigorous contraction of the external sphincter and puborectalis. If conditions are appropriate for defecation, the subject sits or squats, contracts the diaphragm and abdominal muscles, and relaxes the pelvic floor muscles, including puborectalis, and the anal sphincter muscles, with the result that stool is expelled.

Constipation

'Constipation' is a very common symptom, particularly in women and the elderly. A consensus definition used in research (the Rome III criteria) defines constipation as having two or more of the following for at least 12 weeks: infrequent passage of stools (<3/week), straining >25% of time, passage of hard stools, incomplete evacu-

Box 13.27 Input and output of water and electrolytes in the gastrointestinal tract over 24 hours

	Water (mL)	Sodium (mmol)	Potassium (mmol)
Input			
Diet	1500	150	80
Gastrointestinal secretions	7500	1000	40
[illegible]	[illegible]	[illegible]	[illegible]
Output			
Faeces	150	5	12
Ileostomy (adapted)	500–1000	60–120	4

Box 13.28 Causes of constipation

General
- Inadequate fibre intake
- Immobility

Metabolic/endocrine
- Diabetes mellitus
- Hypercalcaemia
- Hypothyroidism
- Porphyria

Functional
- Irritable bowel syndrome
- Idiopathic slow transit

Drugs
- Opiates
- Antimuscarinics
- Calcium-channel blockers, e.g. verapamil
- Antidepressants, e.g. tricyclics
- Iron

Neurological
- Spinal cord lesions
- Parkinson's disease

Psychological
- Depression
- Anorexia nervosa
- Repressed urge to defecate

Gastrointestinal disease
- Intestinal obstruction and pseudo-obstruction
- Colonic disease, e.g. carcinoma, diverticular disease
- Aganglionosis, e.g. Hirschsprung's disease, Chagas' disease
- Painful anal conditions, e.g. anal fissure

Defecatory disorders
- Rectal prolapse, mucosal prolapse intussusception and solitary rectal ulcer syndrome
- Large rectocele
- Pelvic floor dyssynergia/anismus
- Megarectum

ation and sensation of anorectal blockage. According to these definitions, 'constipation' affects more than 1 in 5 of the population.

Other symptoms include abdominal bloating and/or discomfort (undistinguishable from the irritable bowel syndrome), as well as local and perianal pain. The causes of constipation are shown in ***Box 13.28***.

Diagnosis

This relies on the history. When there has been a recent change in bowel habit in association with other significant symptoms (e.g. rectal bleeding), a colonoscopy or CT of the pneumocolon is indicated. By these means, gastrointestinal causes, such as colorectal cancer and narrowed segments due to diverticular disease, can be excluded.

Constipation can be classified into three broad categories but there is much overlap:

- normal transit through the colon (59%)
- defecatory disorders (25%)
- slow transit (13%).

Defecatory disorders with slow transit can occur together (3%).

Normal-transit constipation

In normal-transit constipation, stool traverses the colon at a normal rate, the stool frequency is normal and yet patients believe they are constipated. This is likely to be due to perceived difficulties of evacuation or the passage of hard stools. Patients may complain of abdominal pain or bloating. Normal-transit constipation can be distinguished from slow-transit constipation by undertaking marker studies of colonic transit. Capsules containing 20 radio-opaque shapes are swallowed on days 1, 2 and 3 and an abdominal X-ray obtained 120 hours after ingestion of the first capsule. Each capsule contains shapes of different configuration and the presence of more than 4 shapes from the first capsule, 6 from the second and 12 from the third denotes moderate to severe slow transit ***(Fig. 13.47)***.

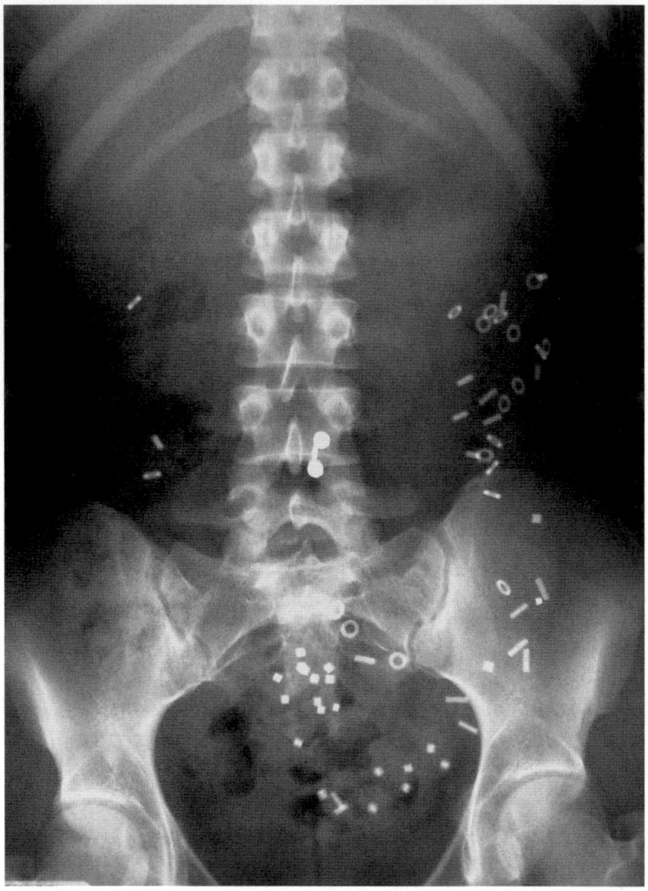

Figure 13.47 Slow-transit constipation. Straight abdominal X-ray taken on day 6 after ingestion of capsules, each containing 20 radio-opaque shapes, which were administered daily on days 1, 2 and 3. All the markers are retained, confirming the diagnosis of severe slow-transit constipation.

Defecatory disorders

A 'paradoxical' contraction, rather than the normal relaxation of puborectalis and the external anal sphincter and associated muscles during straining, may prevent evacuation (pelvic floor dyssynergia, anismus). These are mainly due to dysfunction of the anal sphincter and pelvic floor. An anterior rectocele is a common problem where there is a weakness of the rectovaginal septum, resulting in protuberance of the anterior wall of the rectum with trapping of stool if the diameter is >3 cm. In some patients, the mucosa of the anterior rectal wall prolapses downwards during straining (see p. 420), impeding the passage of stool, while in others there may be a higher mucosal intussusception.

In some patients, the rectum can become unduly sensitive to the presence of small volumes of stool, resulting in the urge to pass frequent amounts of small-volume stool and the sensation of incomplete evacuation.

The defecatory disorders can often be characterized by performing evacuation proctography and tests of anorectal physiology.

Slow-transit constipation

Slow-transit constipation occurs predominantly in young women who have infrequent bowel movements (usually less than once a week). The condition often starts at puberty and the symptoms

Box 13.29 Laxatives and enemas

Bulk-forming laxatives
- Dietary fibre
- Wheat bran
- Methylcellulose
- Mucilaginous gums – sterculia
- Mucilaginous seeds and seed coats, e.g. ispaghula husk

Stimulant laxatives
(Stimulate motility and intestinal secretion)
- Phenolphthalein
- Bisacodyl
- Anthraquinones – senna and dantron (only for the terminally ill)
- Docusate sodium
- Methylnaltrexone (for opioid-induced constipation)
- Lubiprostone
- Prucalopride
- Linaclotide
- Sodium picosulfate

Osmotic laxatives
- Magnesium sulphate
- Lactulose
- Macrogols

Suppositories
- Bisacodyl
- Glycerol

Enemas
- Arachis oil
- Docusate sodium
- Hypertonic phosphate
- Sodium citrate

include an infrequent urge to defecate, bloating, abdominal pain and discomfort. Some patients with severe slow-transit constipation have delayed emptying of the proximal colon and others a failure of 'meal-stimulated' colonic motility. Histopathological abnormalities have been demonstrated in the colons of some patients with severe slow-transit constipation, and some patients have coexisting disorders of small intestinal motility, consistent with a diagnosis of chronic idiopathic intestinal pseudo-obstruction (see p. 435).

Management

Any underlying cause should be treated. In patients with normal and slow-transit constipation, the main focus should be directed towards increasing the fibre content of the diet in conjunction with increasing fluid intake.

The use of laxatives should be restricted to cases where symptoms impact on the patient's quality of life. The types of laxatives available are listed in ***Box 13.29***. *Osmotic laxatives* act by increasing the colonic inflow of fluid and electrolytes; this acts not only to soften the stool but also to stimulate colonic contractility. The *polyethylene glycols (macrogols)* have the advantage over the synthetic disaccharide lactulose in that they are not fermented anaerobically in the colon to gas that can distend the colon and cause pain. The osmotic laxatives are preferred to the stimulatory laxatives, which act by stimulating colonic contractility and by causing intestinal secretion. *Prucalopride* is a high-affinity 5-HT_4 agonist that increases colonic transit and is an effective therapy for refractory constipation.

Linaclotide, a minimally absorbed peptide agonist of guanylate cyclase-C receptor, works by activating the cystic fibrosis transmembrane conductance regulator to stimulate chloride secretion and increase gastrointestinal fluid secretion. Significant benefit over placebo has been shown in clinical trials. *Lubiprostone* is an orally active agonist for type 2 chloride channels and therefore also increases gastrointestinal fluid secretion.

Patients with defecatory disorders should be referred to a specialist centre, as surgery may be indicated: for example, for anterior rectocele or internal anal mucosal intussusception. Anterior mucosal prolapse can be treated by injection, and those with pelvic floor dyssynergia (anismus) can benefit from biofeedback therapy.

Box 13.30 Aetiology of faecal incontinence

- **Congenital:**
  - e.g. surgery for imperforate anus
- **Anal sphincter dysfunction:**
  - Structural damage: surgery – anorectal, vaginal hysterectomy; obstetric injury during childbirth; trauma; radiation; perianal Crohn's disease
  - Pudendal nerve damage: childbirth
  - Perineal descent: prolonged straining at stool
- **Rectal prolapse**
- **Faecal impaction** with overflow diarrhoea
- **Severe diarrhoea:**
  - e.g. ulcerative colitis, functional diarrhoea, irritable bowel syndrome
- **Neurological and psychological disorders:**
  - Spinal trauma (S2–S4)
  - Spina bifida
  - Stroke
  - Multiple sclerosis
  - Diabetes mellitus (with autonomic involvement)
  - Dementia
  - Psychological illness

Miscellaneous colonic conditions

Megacolon

The term 'megacolon' is used to describe a number of congenital and acquired conditions in which the colon is dilated. In many instances, it is secondary to chronic constipation; in some parts of the world, Chagas' disease is a common cause.

In all young patients with megacolon, Hirschsprung's disease should be excluded. In this condition, which presents in the first years of life, an aganglionic segment of the rectum (megarectum) gives rise to constipation and subacute obstruction. Occasionally, Hirschsprung's disease affecting only a short segment of the rectum can be missed in childhood. A preliminary rectal biopsy is performed and stained for ganglion cells in the submucosal plexus. In doubtful cases, a full-thickness biopsy should be obtained. A frozen section is stained for acetylcholinesterase, which is elevated in Hirschsprung's disease. Manometric studies show failure of relaxation of the internal sphincter, which is diagnostic of Hirschsprung's disease. This condition can be successfully treated surgically.

Treatment of other causes of a megacolon is similar to that of slow-transit constipation, but saline washouts and manual removal of faeces are sometimes required.

Faecal incontinence

Of the healthy population over the age of 65, 7% experience a degree of incontinence. Incontinence is classified as minor (inability to control flatus or liquid stool, causing soiling) or major (frequent and inadvertent evacuation of stool of normal consistency). The common causes of incontinence are shown in ***Box 13.30***. Obstetric injury is a common cause and sphincter defects have been found in up to 30% of primiparous women. Endoanal ultrasonography or pelvic MRI is the investigation of choice in the assessment of anal sphincter damage ***(Fig. 13.48)***. Neurophysiological investigation of pudendal nerve function, anal sensation and anal sphincter function may be required to elicit the cause of the problem.

Initial ***management*** of minor incontinence is bowel habit regulation. Loperamide is the most potent antidiarrhoeal agent, which also increases internal sphincter tone.

Biofeedback is effective in some people with faecal incontinence associated with impaired function of the puborectalis muscle and the external anal sphincter. Sacral spinal nerve stimulation has been shown to be effective in the treatment of patients with a functionally

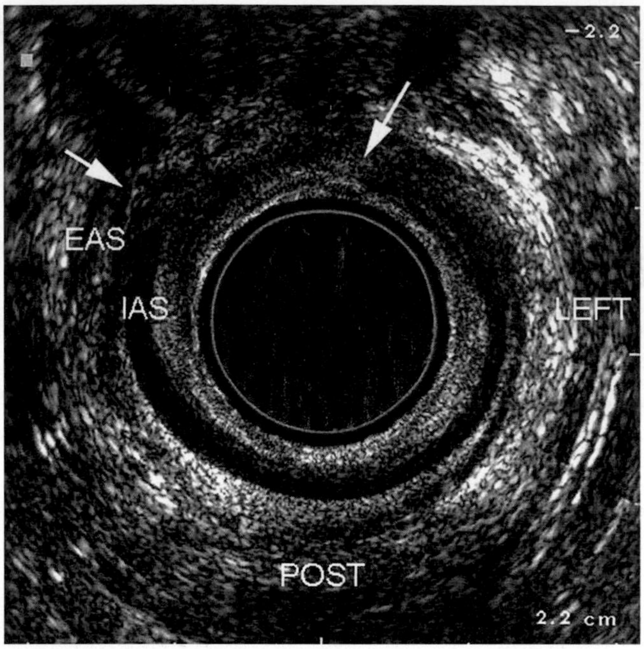

Figure 13.48 Endoanal ultrasound scan. Axial mid-canal image, showing a large tear between 10 and 1 o'clock (arrowed) following vaginal delivery, involving the external anal sphincter (EAS) and internal anal sphincter (IAS), and resulting in faecal incontinence. *(Courtesy of Professor Clive Bartram, Princess Grace Hospital, London.)*

deficient but morphologically intact external anal sphincter. Surgery may be required for anal sphincter trauma and should only be carried out in specialist centres.

Ischaemic disease of the colon (ischaemic colitis)

Occlusion of branches of the superior mesenteric artery (SMA) or inferior mesenteric artery (IMA), often in the older age group, commonly presents with sudden onset of abdominal pain and the passage of bright red blood *per rectum*, with or without diarrhoea. There may be signs of shock and evidence of underlying cardiovascular disease. The anatomy of the vascular supply to the colon results in a watershed area at the splenic flexure, which is therefore the most common site affected. This condition has also been described in women taking the contraceptive pill, patients on nicorandil, and those with thrombophilia and small- or medium-vessel vasculitis.

Examination

On examination, the abdomen may be distended and tender. A straight abdominal X-ray often shows thumb-printing (a characteristic sign of ischaemic disease) at the splenic flexure. Patients are likely to display signs of cardiovascular shock and may have a lactic acidosis.

Differential diagnosis and investigations

The differential diagnosis includes other causes of acute colitis. Patients often require an urgent CT scan to exclude perforation. An unprepared flexible sigmoidoscopy is the diagnostic investigation of choice; biopsies showing epithelial cell apoptosis and lamina propria fibrosis are characteristic. A colonoscopy should be performed when the patient has fully recovered to exclude the formation of a stricture at the site of disease and confirm mucosal healing. Patients without evidence of underlying cardiovascular disease should be screened for thrombophilia and vasculitis.

Management

Most patients settle on symptomatic treatment. A few patients show progressive signs of peritonism and imminent perforation, and require urgent surgery.

Diverticular disease

Diverticula are frequently found in the colon and occur in 50% of patients over the age of 50 years. They are most frequent in the sigmoid, but can be present throughout the whole colon.

The term ***diverticulosis*** indicates the presence of diverticula; ***diverticulitis*** implies that these diverticula are inflamed; ***diverticular colitis*** refers to crescentic inflammation on the folds in areas of diverticulosis. It is perhaps better to use the more general term diverticular disease, as it is often difficult to be sure whether the diverticula are inflamed. The precise mechanism of diverticula formation is not known. There is thickening of the muscle layer and, because of high intraluminal pressures, pouches of mucosa extrude through the muscular wall through weakened areas near blood vessels to form diverticula. An alternative explanation is cholinergic denervation with increasing age, which leads to hypersensitivity and increased uncoordinated muscular contraction. Diverticular disease seems to be related to the low-fibre diet eaten in developed countries and is rare in rural Africa.

Diverticulitis occurs when faeces obstruct the neck of the diverticulum, causing stagnation and allowing bacteria to multiply and produce inflammation. This can then lead to bowel perforation (peridiverticulitis), abscess formation, fistulae into adjacent organs, haemorrhage and even generalized peritonitis.

Clinical features and investigations

Diverticular disease is asymptomatic in 95% of cases and is usually discovered incidentally on colonoscopy or barium enema examination. No treatment other than advice to increase dietary fibre is required in those patients. In symptomatic patients, intermittent left iliac fossa pain or discomfort and an erratic bowel habit commonly occur, which are difficult to differentiate from the irritable bowel syndrome. In severe disease, luminal narrowing results in severe pain and constipation. In the absence of clinical signs of acute diverticulitis, a colonoscopy or 'virtual colonoscopy' (see p. 362) is the investigation of choice. Barium enema ***(Fig. 13.49)*** combined with flexible sigmoidoscopy is also used.

Management

Management of uncomplicated symptomatic disease is with a well-balanced (soluble and insoluble) fibre diet (20 g/day), with smooth muscle relaxants if required. Antibiotics and admission to hospital are not required for uncomplicated disease.

Acute diverticulitis

The pathophysiology of diverticulitis is associated with altered gut motility, increased luminal pressure and a disordered colonic micro-environment. Acute diverticulitis most commonly affects diverticula in the sigmoid colon. It presents with severe pain in the left iliac fossa, often accompanied by fever and constipation. These symptoms and signs are similar to those of appendicitis but are located on the left side. On examination, the patient is often febrile with a tachycardia. ***Abdominal examination*** shows tenderness, guarding

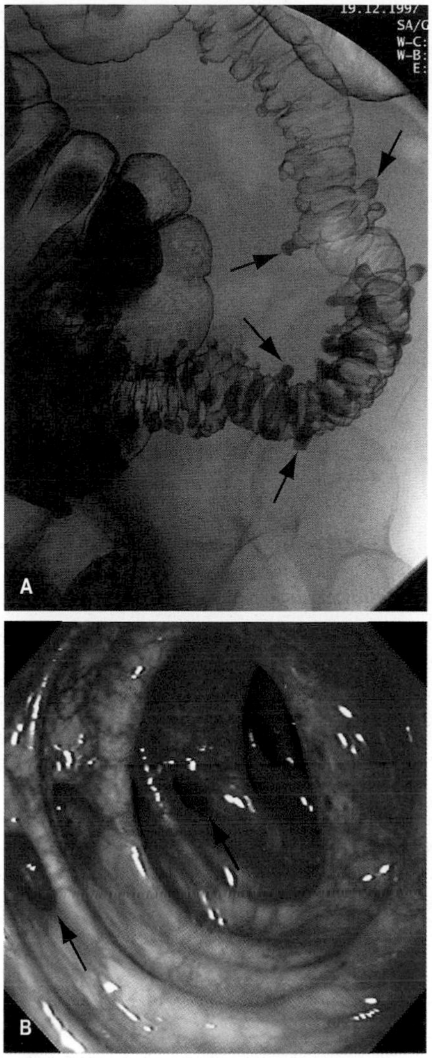

Figure 13.49 Diverticular disease. A. Double-contrast enema showing diverticula (arrowed). The barium is black on these films. **B.** Diverticula (arrowed) seen on colonoscopy.

and rigidity on the left side of the abdomen. A palpable tender mass is sometimes felt in the left iliac fossa.

Investigations

- ***Blood tests*** often reveal a polymorphonuclear leucocytosis. The ESR and CRP are raised.
- ***CT colonography (Fig. 13.50)*** will show colonic wall thickening, diverticula and often pericolic collections and abscesses. There is usually a streaky increased density extending into the immediate pericolic fat with thickening of the pelvic fascial planes. These findings are diagnostic of acute diverticulitis (95% sensitivity and specificity) and differ from those of malignant disease. Sigmoidoscopy and colonoscopy are not performed during an acute attack.
- ***Ultrasound examination*** is often more readily available and is cheaper. It can demonstrate thickened bowel and large pericolic collections, but is less sensitive than CT.

Management

Mild attacks can be treated on an outpatient basis using oral antibiotics such as ciprofloxacin and metronidazole. Patients with signs

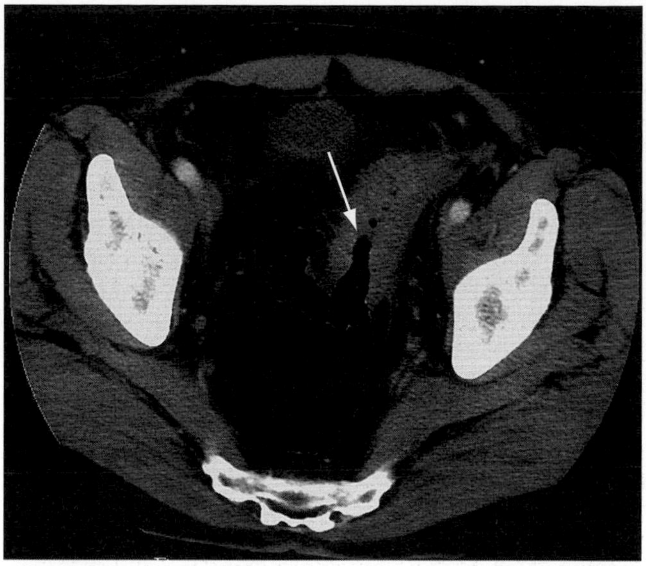

Figure 13.50 CT of lower abdomen, showing acute diverticulitis (arrowed). The bowel wall is thickened and there is loss of clarity of the pericolic fat. A narrow segment of bowel is seen to the left of the diseased segment.

of systemic upset (fevers, tachycardia), significant abdominal pain or co-morbidity require bowel rest, intravenous fluids and intravenous antibiotic therapy. Recent large trials of 5-ASA therapy have shown minor benefit in preventing recurrent diverticulitis. Repeat attacks often require surgery.

Complications of diverticular disease

- ***Perforation*** usually occurs in association with acute diverticulitis, and can lead to formation of a paracolic or pelvic abscess or generalized peritonitis. Surgery may be required.
- ***Fistula formation*** into the bladder, causing dysuria or pneumaturia, or into the vagina, causing discharge.
- ***Intestinal obstruction*** (see p. 435), usually after repeated episodes of acute diverticulitis.
- ***Bleeding*** is sometimes massive. In most cases, the bleeding stops and the cause of the bleeding can be established by colonoscopy and sometimes angiography. In rare cases, emergency segmental colectomy is required.
- ***Mucosal inflammation*** occurs in areas of diverticula, giving the appearance of a segmental colitis at endoscopy that may resemble Crohn's disease.

Anorectal disorders

Pruritus ani

Pruritus ani, or an itchy bottom, is common. Perianal excoriation results from scratching. Usually, the condition results from haemorrhoids or overactivity of sweat glands. ***Management*** consists of enhancing toilet hygiene, keeping the area dry and avoiding the use of perfumed moisturizing creams. Secondary causes include threadworm (*Enterobius vermicularis*) infestation, fungal infections (e.g. candidiasis) and perianal eczema, which should be treated appropriately.

Haemorrhoids

Haemorrhoids (primary – internal; second degree – prolapsing; third degree – prolapsed) usually cause rectal bleeding, discomfort and pruritus ani. Patients may notice red blood on their toilet paper and blood on the outside of their stools. They are the most common cause of rectal bleeding (see ***Fig. 13.27***).

Diagnosis is made by inspection, rectal examination and proctoscopy.

Management

If symptoms are minor, no treatment is required apart from advice about avoiding constipation. Suppositories containing a local anaesthetic and corticosteroids are helpful. If symptoms are more severe, rubber band ligation or injection of a sclerosant can be used. Haemorrhoidal artery ligation operation (HALO) uses Doppler ultrasound to identify and ligate feeding arteries to the haemorrhoids. This technique may replace surgery.

Anal fissures

An anal fissure is a tear in the sensitive skin-lined lower anal canal distal to the dentate line, which produces pain on defecation. It can be an isolated primary problem in young to middle-aged adults or may occur in association with Crohn's disease or ulcerative colitis, in which case perianal abscesses and anal fistulae can complicate the fissure.

Diagnosis can usually be made on the history alone and confirmed on perianal inspection. Rectal examination is often not possible because of pain and sphincter spasm. The spasm not only causes pain but also impairs wound healing. In severe cases, proctoscopy and sigmoidoscopy should be performed under anaesthesia to exclude other anorectal disease. Initial treatment is with local anaesthetic gel and stool softeners. Use of 0.4% glyceryl trinitrate and 2% diltiazem ointments is of benefit. Botulinum toxin is used in chronic fissures but lateral subcutaneous internal sphincterotomy is also employed for severe cases.

Fistula *in ano* and anorectal abscesses

The anatomy of perianal fistulae may be simple or complex ***(Fig. 13.51)***. The fistulae usually present as abscesses and heal after the abscess is incised. In other cases, a small, discharging pilonidal sinus may be noted by the patient.

Endoanal ultrasonography, MRI and/or examination under anaesthetic are usually required to define the primary and any secondary tracks, exclude sepsis and detect any associated disease, such as Crohn's disease and tuberculosis. Management is with surgical incision and drainage with antibiotics.

Rectal prolapse, intussusception and solitary rectal ulcer syndrome

All these conditions are thought to be related, rectal prolapse being the unifying pathology. Some patients with solitary rectal ulcer syndrome (SRUS) do not have prolapse but strain excessively and ulcerate the anterior rectal wall, which is forced into the anus during attempts at defecation. Constipation and chronic straining may be precipitating causes. Patients commonly present with slight bleeding and mucus on defecation, tenesmus and a sensation of anal obstruction.

SRUS is commonly located on the anterior wall of the rectum within 13 cm of the anal verge, and is sometimes difficult to distinguish from cancer and Crohn's disease during endoscopic examination. SRUS has typical histological features of non-specific inflammatory changes with bands of smooth muscle extending into the lamina propria.

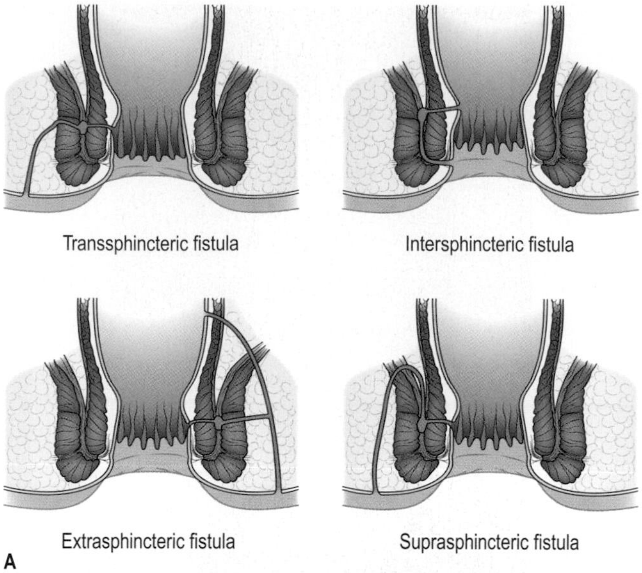

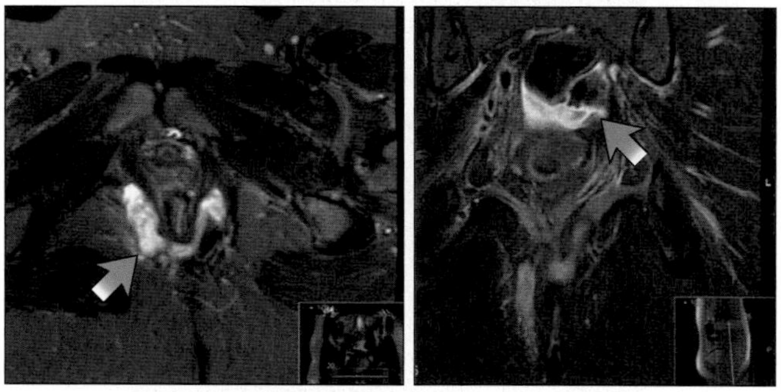

Figure 13.51 Perianal fistulae. A. Common sites. **B.** Fistulae and sepsis in Crohn's disease (arrowed). An MRI of the pelvis showing a complex extrasphincteric horseshoe tract with extension to the ischio-anal fossae (right; arrowed).

Asymptomatic SRUS should not be treated. Symptomatic patients should be advised to stop straining and measures should be taken to soften the stool. If rectal prolapse can be demonstrated during defecation, this should be repaired; in severe cases, surgical treatment by rectopexy may be indicated. Surgical treatment for complete rectal prolapse is also required.

Colonic tumours

Colon polyps and polyposis syndromes

A colonic polyp is an abnormal growth of tissue projecting from the colonic mucosa. Polyps range from a few millimetres to several centimetres in diameter and are single or multiple, pedunculated, sessile or 'flat' ***(Fig. 13.52)***.

Many histological types of polyp are found in the colon ***(Box 13.31)***. However, adenomas are the precursor lesions in most cases of colon cancer.

Classification of colorectal polyps

Classification is summarized in ***Box 13.31***.

Sporadic adenomas

An adenoma is a benign, dysplastic tumour of columnar cells or glandular tissue. Adenomas have tubular, tubulovillous or villous

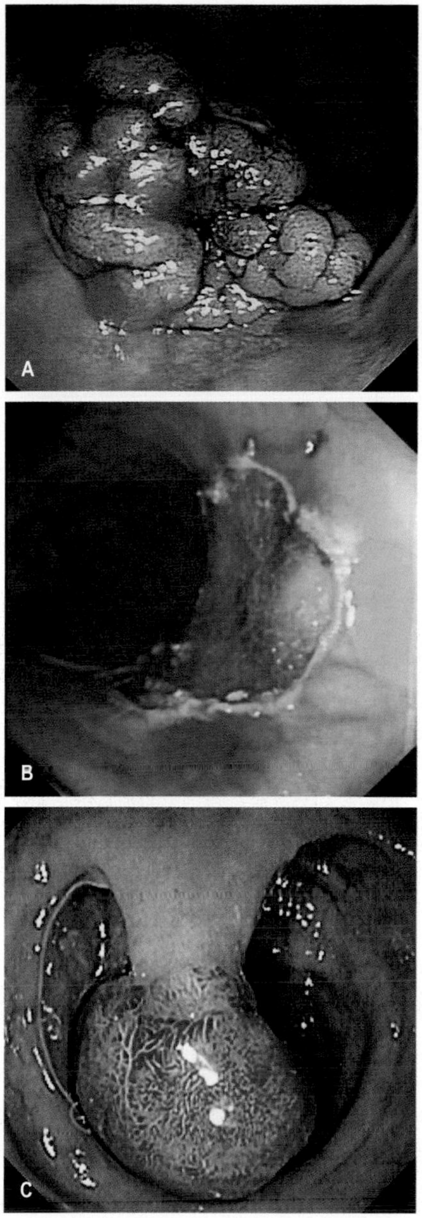

Figure 13.52 Colonoscopic appearance of sessile and pedunculated polyps. A. A sessile flat polyp with Indigo carmine. **B.** Colon after resection of a sessile polyp. **C.** A large pedunculated polyp.

morphology. The vast majority of adenomas are not inherited and are termed 'sporadic'. Although many sporadic adenomas do not become malignant in the patient's lifetime, they have a tendency to progress to cancer via increasing grades of dysplasia due to progressive accumulation of genetic changes (adenoma–carcinoma sequence). Factors favouring malignant transformation in colorectal polyps, and the relation between adenoma size and likelihood of cancer, are shown in ***Box 13.32***.

The progression from benign polyp to cancer is shown in Figure [illegible]

The likelihood of an adenoma being present increases with age; it is rare before the age of 30 years. By the age of 60–70, 5% of asymptomatic subjects will have a polyp of ≥1 cm, or cancer with no symptoms, and up to 50% will have at least one small <1 cm adenoma. Removal of polyps at colonoscopy and subsequent surveillance reduce the risk of development of colon cancer by approximately 80%. Techniques such as chromoscopy, using dye spray or narrow band imaging, are being used to assist in their detection (flat adenomas account for approximately 12% of all adenomas).

Polyps in the rectum and sigmoid often present with rectal bleeding. More proximal lesions rarely produce symptoms and most are diagnosed on barium enema, CT colonography or on colonoscopy performed for screening or for other reasons. Large villous adenomas can present with profuse diarrhoea with mucus and hypokalaemia.

Once a polyp has been found, it is almost always possible to remove it endoscopically. Surveillance guidelines dictate the frequency of repeat investigations:

- at 5 years, if 1 or 2 adenomas <1 cm are found
- at 3 years, if there are 3–4 small adenomas or at least 1 that is >1 cm
- at 1 year, if there are ≥5 small adenomas or there are ≥3, at least 1 of which is >1 cm.

If any doubt exists about the completeness of excision of any polyp, then an earlier repeat examination is suggested.

Sessile serrated adenomas

Serrated polyps form a heterogeneous group of colorectal lesions that includes the benign hyperplastic polyps (HPs), and the premalignant sessile serrated adenoma (SSA) and traditional serrated adenoma (TSA). They are characterized by the saw-tooth appearance of the crypt epithelium. It is now recognized that approximately 30% of colorectal cancers (particularly those in the right colon) originate from these lesions. Progression of serrated polyps is thought to occur via a distinct pathway from the adenoma–carcinoma sequence, with involvement of *BRAF* gene mutations and gene promoter hypermethylation (CpG island methylator phenotype, or CIMP; see p. 423). Microsatellite instability can be detected in both the adenoma–carcinoma and the serrated pathways. Endoscopic resection of SSAs and TSAs with appropriate surveillance is recommended.

Inherited polyposis syndromes

About 5% of colorectal cancers have a well-defined single-gene basis.

Familial adenomatous polyposis

Familial adenomatous polyposis (FAP) is an autosomal dominant condition arising from germline mutations of the *APC* gene, located on chromosome 5q21–q22. More than 825 different mutations have been identified. Penetrance is virtually 100%. It is characterized by the presence of hundreds to thousands of colorectal and duodenal adenomas. The mean age of adenoma development is 16 years; the average age at which colorectal cancer develops is 39 years. Tracing and screening of relatives are essential, and affected individuals should be offered a prophylactic colectomy. Surgical options include colectomy and ileorectal anastomosis, which requires lifelong surveillance of the rectal stump, or a restorative proctocolectomy or pouch procedure with complete removal of rectal mucosa.

Cystic gland polyps, predominantly in the proximal stomach, and duodenal adenomas are frequently found in FAP, as well as other extraintestinal lesions such as osteomas, epidermoid cysts and desmoid tumours. The duodenal adenomas may progress to cancer and are the most common cause of death in colectomized patients with FAP. Congenital hypertrophy of the retinal pigment

Box 13.31 Classification of colorectal polyps and polyposis syndromes

Histology	Polyposis syndrome	Defective gene	Inheritance	CRC risk
Hyperplastic	Hyperplastic polyposis	*BRAF*		Yes
Hamartoma	Juvenile polyposis	*MADH4* or *BMPR1A*	AD	10–70%
	Peutz–Jeghers syndrome	*STK11*	AD	Yes
	Cowden syndrome	*PTEN*	AD	10%?
	Lhermitte–Duclos disorder	*PTEN*	AD	
	Bannayan–Riley–Ruvalcaba syndrome	*PTEN*	AD	
Inflammatory	None	None		No
Lymphoid	Benign lymphoid polyposis	Unknown		No
Adenoma	FAP	*APC*	AD	100%
	AFAP			Yes
	Gardner syndrome			Yes
	Turcot syndrome			Yes
	MYH-AP	*MYH-AP*	AR	
Adenoma	Lynch syndrome (HNPCC)	Mismatch repair genes (*MSH-2, MLH-1*)	AD	70–80%

AD, autosomal dominant; AFAP, attenuated FAP; APC, adenomatous polyposis coli; AR, autosomal recessive; CRC, colorectal cancer; FAP, familial adenomatous polyposis; HNPCC, hereditary non-polyposis colorectal cancer; MLH-1, MutL homologue 1; MSH-2, MutS homologue 2; MYH-AP, MUT Y homologue-associated polyposis; PTEN, phosphatase and tensin homologue.

Box 13.32 Factors affecting risk of malignant change in an adenoma

Factor	Higher risk	Lower risk
Size	>1.5 cm	<1 cm
Type	Sessile or flat	Pedunculated
Histology	Severe dysplasia Villous architecture Squamous metaplasia	Mild dysplasia Tubular architecture
Number	Multiple polyps	Single polyp

epithelium (CHRPE) occurs in many families with FAP. Other cancers in FAP include thyroid, pancreatic and hepatoblastomas.

APC gene mutations can be found in about 80% of families with FAP. Once the mutation has been identified in an index case, other family members can be tested for the mutation, and screening can then be directed at mutation carriers. If a mutation cannot be found in a known FAP case, all family members should undergo clinical screening with regular colonoscopy.

Attenuated FAP may be missed as it presents later (average age 44 years) and has fewer polyps (<100), which tend to occur on the right side of the colon rather than on the left. It may be indistinguishable from sporadic cases but the gene mutation is in the *APC* germline.

MYH-associated polyposis

MUT Y homologue-associated polyposis (MYH-AP) is an autosomal recessive inherited syndrome of multiple colorectal adenomas and cancer. *MYH* is a base-excision-repair gene that corrects oxidative DNA damage. MYH-AP may account for 7–8% of families with the FAP phenotype in whom *APC* mutations cannot be found. Subjects with multiple adenomas or an FAP phenotype without *APC* mutations and with a family history compatible with a recessive pattern of inheritance should be tested for MYH-AP.

Lynch syndrome

In Lynch syndrome (previously called hereditary non-polyposis colon cancer, HNPCC), polyps are formed in the colon and may progress rapidly to colon cancer. It affects 1 : 5000 people, causing 3–10% of colorectal cancer cases.

The disease is caused by a mutation in one of the DNA mismatch repair genes, usually *hMSH2* or *hMLH1*, although others (*hMSH6, PMS1* and *PMS*) have been reported. Mismatch repair genes are responsible for maintaining the stability of DNA during replication. Inheritance is autosomal dominant. The defect in function of the mismatch repair mechanism causes naturally occurring, highly repeated, short DNA sequences known as microsatellites to be shorter or longer than normal, a phenomenon called microsatellite instability (MSI).

Onset of cancer is earlier than in sporadic cases, at age 40–50 or younger. Tumours have a predilection for the right colon, in contrast to sporadic cases. In contrast to FAP, the lifetime risk of colon cancer (penetrance of the gene) in mutation carriers is 70–80%. Other cancers are also more common in Lynch syndrome: stomach, small intestine, bladder, skin, brain and hepatobiliary system. Female patients are at risk for endometrial and ovarian cancer.

The diagnosis is made from the family history of colon cancer at a young age and the presence of associated cancers in the family. These are formalized in the various editions of the Amsterdam and the Bethesda criteria ***(Box 13.33)***.

Turcot syndrome

This consists of FAP or Lynch syndrome (HNPCC) with brain tumours.

Gardner syndrome

This involves, in addition to FAP, desmoid tumours, osteomas of the skull and other lesions.

Hamartomatous polyps

These are commonly large and stalked. The inherited syndromes show autosomal dominant inheritance and include:

- ***Juvenile polyps***, which occur mainly in children and teenagers, and are found mainly in the colon; histologically, they show mucus retention cysts. Most are sporadic, but a syndrome of juvenile polyposis is defined as: >3–5 juvenile colonic polyps, juvenile polyps throughout the gastrointestinal

Box 13.33 Diagnostic criteria for Lynch syndrome

Modified Amsterdam criteria
- One individual diagnosed with CRC (or extracolonic Lynch tumours) before age 50 years
- Two affected generations
- Three affected relatives, one a first-degree relative of the other two
- FAP excluded
- Tumours verified by pathological examination

Bethesda guidelines
- CRC diagnosed in patient who is younger than 50 years
- Presence of synchronous, metachronous CRC, or other Lynch tumours, irrespective of age
- CRC with the MSI-H histology diagnosed in a patient who is younger than 60 years
- CRC diagnosed in one or more first-degree relative with a Lynch-related tumour, with one of the cancers being diagnosed under the age 50 years
- CRC diagnosed in two or more first- or second-degree relatives with Lynch-related tumours, irrespective of age

CRC, colorectal cancer; MSI-H, microsatellite instability – high.

Box 13.34 Risk factors in colorectal cancer

Increased risk
- Increasing age
- Animal fat (saturated) and red meat consumption
- Sugar consumption
- Colorectal polyps
- Family history of colon cancer or colonic polyps
- Chronic inflammatory bowel disease
- Obesity (body and abdominal)
- Smoking
- Acromegaly
- Abdominal radiotherapy
- Ureterosigmoidostomy

Decreased risk
- Vegetable, garlic, milk, calcium consumption
- Exercise (colon only)
- Aspirin (including low-dose) and other NSAIDs

NSAIDs, non-steroidal anti-inflammatory drugs.

tract, or any number of polyps with a family history. This is an autosomal dominant condition and the relevant gene has been identified (see ***Box 13.31***). The polyps are a cause of bleeding and intussusception in the first decade of life. There is also an increased risk of colonic cancer (relative risk (RR) of 34), and surveillance and removal of polyps must be undertaken.

- ***Peutz–Jeghers syndrome*** (see p. 403).
- ***PTEN hamartoma–tumour syndrome*** (PHTS), which includes Cowden syndrome, Bannayan–Riley–Ruvalcaba syndrome and all syndromes caused by germline phosphatase and tensin homologue (*PTEN*) mutations. Cowden (multiple hamartoma) syndrome is associated with characteristic skin stigmata, and by intestinal polyps regarded as hamartomas but with a mixture of cell types. These patients have an increased risk of various extraintestinal malignancies (thyroid, breast, uterine and ovarian). These syndromes are uncommon and together account for <1% of colon cancer cases.

Colorectal carcinoma

Colorectal cancer (CRC) is the third most common cancer worldwide and the second most common cause of cancer death in the UK.

Each year approximately, 40 000 new cases are diagnosed in England and Wales (68% colon, 32% rectal cancer), and CRC is registered as the cause of death in about half this number. The prevalence rate per 100 000 (at all ages) is 53.5 for men and 36.7 for women. The incidence increases with age; the average age at diagnosis is 60–65 years. Approximately 20% of patients in the UK have distant metastases at diagnosis. The disease is much more common in westernized countries than in Asia or Africa.

Factors related to risk of colorectal cancer are shown in ***Box 13.34***.

Genetics

Most colorectal cancers develop as a result of progression from normal mucosa to adenoma to invasive cancer. This progression is controlled by the accumulation of abnormalities in a number of critical growth-regulating genes and can be divided into three main pathways:

- ***Chromosomal instability (CIN)***. CIN is the most common cause of conventional adenomas throughout the colon. This pathway involves the sequential accumulation of genetic mutations in tumour suppressor genes, usually initiated by a mutation in the gene encoding adenomatous polyposis coli (*APC*).
- ***CpG island methylator phenotype***. CpG island methylator phenotype (CIMP) tumours arise via the serrated neoplasia pathway and have a marked predilection for the proximal colon. Following an initiating genetic mutation in the genes encoding *BRAF* or *KRAS*, these lesions progress via *epigenetic* silencing of tumour suppressor and mismatch repair (MMR) genes by promoter methylation (p. 421). This pathway is epitomized by the serrated polyposis syndrome.
- ***Microsatellite instability***. Microsatellite instability (MSI) tumours are also more commonly located in the proximal colon. They arise from defective DNA repair through inactivation of mismatch repair genes, epitomised by the germline mutation of MMR genes seen in Lynch syndrome (HNPCC).

This molecular classification can help to distinguish clinical characteristics, such as patient demographics, tumour distribution, response to therapy and prognosis.

Cancer families

A family history of CRC confers an increased risk to relatives. Family history is, next to age, the most common risk factor for CRC. FAP ***(Fig. 13.53)*** is the best-recognized syndrome predisposing to CRC but represents less than 1% of all colorectal cancers. Lynch syndrome (HNPCC) accounts for 3–10% of familial cancer (see p. 422).

Additionally, some colon cancers arise, at least in part, from an inherited predisposition, so-called familial risk ***(Box 13.35)***. Estimates of their frequency range from 10% to 30% of all CRC but the genes involved have yet to be identified. The risk of CRC can be estimated from a family history matched with empirical risk tables, so that appropriate advice regarding screening can be offered.

Most CRCs are, however, sporadic and occur in individuals without a strong family history. Their distribution is shown in ***Figure 13.54***.

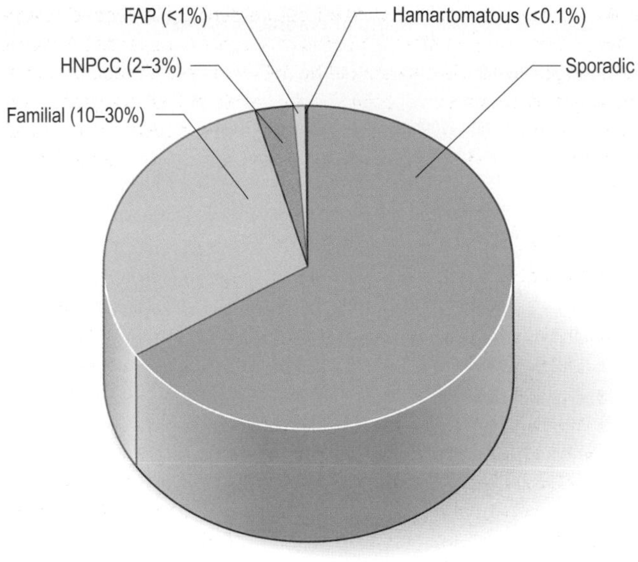

Figure 13.53 Percentages of colon cancer according to family risk. FAP, familial adenomatous polyposis; HNPCC, hereditary non-polyposis colorectal cancer (Lynch syndrome).

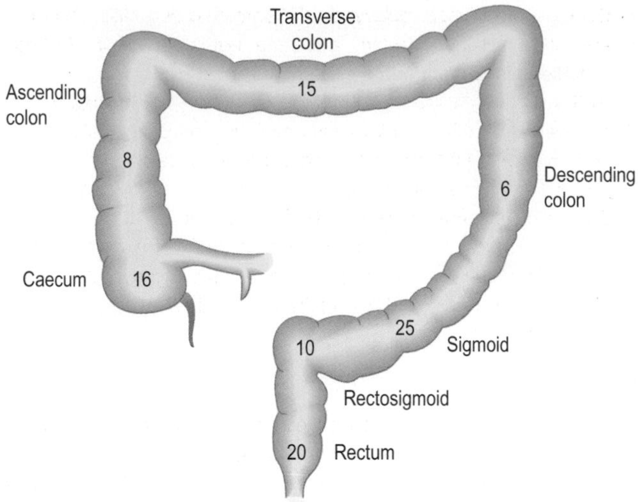

Figure 13.54 Distribution of sporadic colorectal cancer. Only 60% are in the range of flexible sigmoidoscopy.

Box 13.35 Lifetime risk of colorectal cancer (CRC) in first-degree relatives of a CRC patient

Individuals affected	Risk
Population risk	1 in 50
One first-degree relative affected (any age)	1 in 17
One first-degree and one second-degree relative affected	1 in 12
One first-degree relative affected (age <45)	1 in 10
Two first-degree relatives affected	1 in 6
Autosomal dominant pedigree	1 in 2

(From: Houlston RS, Murday V, Harocopos C et al. Screening and genetic counselling for relatives of patients with colorectal cancer in a family cancer clinic. *British Medical Journal* 1990; 301:366–368.)

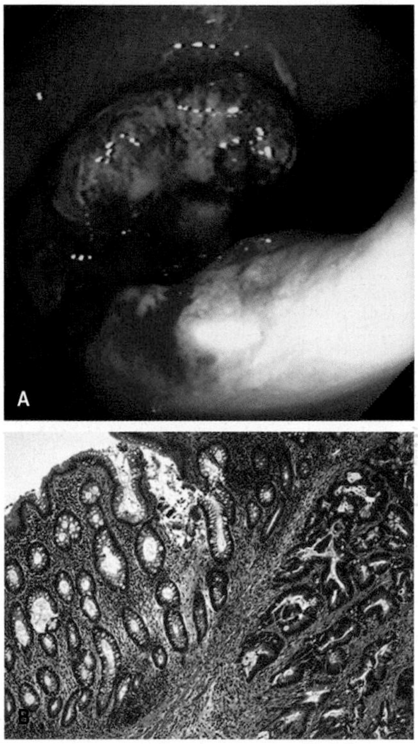

Figure 13.55 Carcinoma in the ascending colon. A. Colonoscopic appearance of a large irregular ulcer. **B.** Histopathology showing an adenocarcinoma.

Pathology

CRC, which usually takes the form of a polypoid mass with ulceration, spreads by direct infiltration through the bowel wall. It involves lymphatics and blood vessels with subsequent spread, most commonly to the liver and lung. Synchronous cancers are present in 2% of cases. Histology is adenocarcinoma with variably differentiated glandular epithelium and mucin production. 'Signet ring' cells, in which mucin displaces the nucleus to the side of the cell, are relatively uncommon and generally have a poor prognosis.

Clinical features

Symptoms suggestive of colorectal cancer include change in bowel habit with looser and more frequent stools, rectal bleeding, tenesmus and symptoms of anaemia. A rectal or abdominal mass may be palpable. Cancers arising in the caecum and right colon are often asymptomatic until they present as an iron deficiency anaemia. Cancer may present with intestinal obstruction.

Patients aged over 35–40 years presenting with new large bowel symptoms should be investigated. Digital examination of the rectum is essential and examination of the colon should be performed in all cases.

Investigations

- ***Colonoscopy*** is the 'gold standard' for investigation and allows biopsy for histology. Biopsy of the tumour is mandatory, usually at endoscopy ***(Fig. 13.55)***.
- ***Double-contrast barium enema*** can visualize the large bowel but has now been superseded by CT colonography.
- ***Endoanal ultrasound and pelvic MRI*** are used for staging rectal cancer.

- ***Chest, abdominal and pelvic CT*** scanning evaluate tumour size, local spread, and liver and lung metastases, contributing to tumour staging.
- ***PET scanning*** is useful for detecting occult metastases and for evaluation of suspicious lesions found on CT or MRI.
- ***MRI*** is also useful for evaluating suspicious lesions found on CT or ultrasound, especially in the liver.
- ***Serum carcinoembryonic antigen*** (***CEA***) is of little use for primary diagnosis and should not be performed as a screening test. It is useful for follow-up; rising levels suggest recurrence.
- ***Faecal occult blood (FOB) tests*** are used for mass population screening.

Management

Management should be undertaken by multidisciplinary teams working in specialist units. About 80% of patients with CRC undergo surgery (often laparoscopically). The operative procedure depends on the cancer site. Long-term survival relates to the stage of the primary tumour and the presence of metastatic disease. There has been a gradual move from using Dukes' classification to the TNM classification system (see ***Box 24.58***). Long-term survival is only likely when the cancer is completely removed by surgery with adequate clearance margins and regional lymph node clearance.

- ***Total mesorectal excision*** (***TME***) is required for rectal cancers and removes the entire package of mesorectal tissue surrounding the cancer. A low rectal anastomosis is then performed. Abdomino-perineal excision, which requires a permanent colostomy, is reserved for very low tumours within 5 cm of the anal margin. TME combined with preoperative radiotherapy reduces local recurrence rates in rectal cancer to around 8% and improves survival. Pre- or postoperative chemotherapy reduces local recurrence rates but had no effect on survival in a recent study.
- ***Segmental resection*** and restorative anastomosis, with removal of the draining lymph nodes as far as the root of the mesentery, is used for cancer elsewhere in the colon. Surgery in patients with obstruction carries greater morbidity and mortality. Where technically possible, preoperative decompression by endoscopic stenting with a mesh-metal stent relieves obstruction, so surgery can be elective rather than emergency, and is probably associated with a decrease in morbidity and mortality.
- ***Local transanal surgery*** is very occasionally used for early superficial rectal cancers.
- ***Surgical or ablative treatment of liver and lung metastases*** prolongs life where treatment is technically feasible and the patient is fit enough to undergo the treatment.
- ***Radiotherapy is not helpful*** for colonic cancers proximal to the rectum because of difficulties in delivering a sufficient dose to the tumour without excess toxicity to adjacent structures, particularly the small bowel.
- ***Adjuvant postoperative chemotherapy*** improves disease-free survival and overall survival in stage III colon cancer (see pp. 636–637). Those with stage II tumours and advanced features such as vascular invasion may also benefit.

Management of ***advanced colorectal cancer*** is discussed on pages 636–637.

Follow-up

All patients who have surgery should have a total colonoscopy performed before surgery to look for additional lesions. If total colonoscopy cannot be achieved before surgery, a second 'clearance' colonoscopy within 6 months of surgery is essential. Patients with stage II or III disease should be followed up with regular colonoscopy and CEA measurements; rising levels of CEA suggest recurrence. Annual CT scanning of the chest and abdomen to detect operable liver metastases should be performed for up to 3 years post surgery.

Screening for CRC

- ***FOB tests*** have been studied as a screening test for colorectal cancer. Several large randomized studies have demonstrated a reduction in cancer-related mortality of 15–33%. Immunologically based FOB tests are superior to the conventional guaiac-based systems. The disadvantage of screening with FOB is its relatively low sensitivity, which means many negative colonoscopies. In FOB test screen-positive patients in the UK National Bowel Cancer Screening Programme (NHS BCSP), about 10% have cancer, 40% have adenomas and the colon is normal in 50%.
- ***Flexible sigmoidoscopy*** screening has been shown to reduce the mortality from CRC, but not overall mortality.
- ***Colonoscopy*** is the 'gold standard' technique for examination of the colon and rectum and is the investigation of choice for high-risk patients. Universal screening strategies have been implemented in the UK for subjects between 60 and 69 who have a positive FOB. Cancer has been detected in 8–12% of patients, 75% of which was located in the left colon; 72% of detected cancers are at an 'early' stage (10% polyp cancer, 32% stage I and 30% stage II).
- ***CT colonography*** ('virtual colonoscopy'; see ***Fig. 13.5***) is increasingly being used.

Further reading

Atkin WS, Edwards R, Kralj-Hans I et al and UK Flexible Sigmoidoscopy Trial Investigators. Once-only flexible sigmoidoscopy screening in prevention of colorectal cancer: a multicentre randomised controlled trial. *Lancet* 2010; 375:1624–1633.

Camilleri M, Bharucha AE. Behavioural and new pharmacological treatments for constipation: getting the balance right. *Gut* 2010; 59:1288–1296.

Cunningham D, Atkin W, Lenz HJ et al. Colorectal cancer. *Lancet* 2010; 375:1030.

Markowitz SD, Bertagnolli MM. Molecular origins of cancer: molecular basis of colorectal cancer. *N Engl J Med* 2009; 361:2449–2460.

Morris AM, Regenbogen SE, Hardiman KM et al. Sigmoid diverticulitis: a systematic review. *JAMA* 2014; 311:287–297.

National Institute for Health and Care Excellence. *NICE Clinical Guideline 49: Faecal Incontinence: The Management of Faecal Incontinence*. NICE 2007; http://www.nice.org.uk/guidance/CG49.

Norton C. Treating faecal incontinence with bulking-agent injections. *Lancet* 2011; 377:971–972.

Tursi A. Diverticular disease: what is the best long-term treatment? Nature Reviews. *Gastroenterol Hepatol* 2010; 7:77–78.

http://www.bsg.org.uk *British Society of Gastroenterology*.

DIARRHOEA

Diarrhoea is a common clinical problem and yet there is no uniformly accepted definition. Organic causes (stool weights >250 g/day) have to be distinguished from functional causes such as irritable bowel syndrome. Sudden onset of bowel frequency associated with crampy abdominal pains, and a fever, will point to an *infective cause*; bowel frequency with loose, blood-stained stools to an *inflammatory basis*; and the passage of pale, offensive stools that float, often accompanied by loss of appetite and weight loss, to *steatorrhoea*. Nocturnal bowel frequency and urgency usually point to an *organic* cause. Passage of frequent, small-volume stools (often formed) points to a *functional* cause (see pp. 428–432).

Pathophysiology

Osmotic diarrhoea

The gut mucosa acts as a semipermeable membrane and fluid enters the bowel if there are large quantities of non-absorbed hypertonic substances in the lumen. This occurs because the patient:

- has ingested a non-absorbable substance (e.g. a purgative, such as magnesium sulphate or magnesium-containing antacid)
- has generalized malabsorption, so that high concentrations of solute (e.g. glucose) remain in the lumen
- has a specific absorptive defect (e.g. disaccharidase deficiency or glucose-galactose malabsorption).

The volume of diarrhoea produced by these mechanisms is reduced by the absorption of fluid by the ileum and colon. The diarrhoea stops when the patient stops eating or the malabsorptive substance is discontinued.

Secretory diarrhoea

In this disorder, there is both active intestinal secretion of fluid and electrolytes, and decreased absorption. The mechanism of intestinal secretion is shown in ***Figure 13.56A***.

Common causes of secretory diarrhoea are:

- enterotoxins (e.g. cholera, *E. coli* thermolabile or thermostable toxin, *C. difficile* toxin)
- hormones (e.g. vasoactive intestinal peptide in Verner–Morrison syndrome; see p. 512)
- bile salts (in the colon) following ileal resection
- fatty acids (in the colon) following ileal resection
- some laxatives (e.g. docusate sodium).

Inflammatory diarrhoea (mucosal destruction)

Diarrhoea occurs because of damage to the intestinal mucosal cell so that there is a loss of fluid and blood ***(Fig. 13.56B)***. In addition, there is defective absorption of fluid and electrolytes. Common causes are infective conditions (e.g. dysentery due to *Shigella*) and inflammatory conditions (e.g. ulcerative colitis and Crohn's disease).

Abnormal motility

Diabetic, post-vagotomy and hyperthyroid diarrhoea are all due to abnormal motility of the upper gut. Symptoms may be exacerbated by small bowel bacterial overgrowth.

Causes of diarrhoea are shown in ***Box 13.23***. It should be noted that the irritable bowel syndrome, colorectal cancer, diverticular disease and faecal impaction with overflow in the elderly do not cause 'true' organic diarrhoea (i.e. >250 g/day), even though patients may complain of diarrhoea. Worldwide, infection and infestation are major problems and these are discussed under the causative organisms in Chapter 11.

Acute diarrhoea

Diarrhoea of sudden onset is very common, is often short-lived and requires no investigation or treatment. Although dietary causes should be considered, diarrhoea due to viral agents may also last 24–48 hours (see pp. 263–265). The causes of other infective diarrhoeas are shown on pages 273–279. Travellers' diarrhoea, which affects people travelling outside their own countries, particularly to developing countries, usually lasts 2–5 days; it is discussed on pages 277–279. Cholera is described on pages 288–289.

Clinical features

Clinical features associated with the acute diarrhoeas include fever, abdominal pain and vomiting. If the diarrhoea is particularly severe, dehydration can be a problem; the very young and very old are at special risk from this.

Investigations

Investigations are necessary if the diarrhoea has lasted more than 5–7 days. Stools (up to three) should be sent immediately to the laboratory for culture and examination for ova, cysts and parasites and for *C. difficile* toxin assay. If the diagnosis has still not been made, a sigmoidoscopy and rectal biopsy should be performed, with colonoscopy if necessary. Viral and bacterial infective diarrhoeas do not last more than 7–10 days; in this case, inflammatory bowel disease as a cause of the diarrhoea is a more likely diagnosis.

Management

Oral fluid and electrolyte replacement is often necessary. Special oral rehydration solutions (e.g. sodium chloride and glucose powder) are available for use in severe episodes of diarrhoea, particularly in infants. Antidiarrhoeal drugs are thought to impair the clearance of any pathogen from the bowel but may be necessary for short-term relief (e.g. codeine phosphate 30 mg four times daily or loperamide 2 mg three times daily). Antibiotics are occasionally necessary for infective gastroenteritis, depending on the organism.

Chronic diarrhoea

This always needs investigation. The flow diagram in ***Figure 13.57*** is illustrative; whether the large or the small bowel is investigated first will depend on the clinical story of, for example, bloody diarrhoea or steatorrhoea. The investigations and treatment are described in detail under the individual diseases. Colonoscopy with ileoscopy is usually the first investigation if stool cultures are negative and small bowel disease is not suspected.

Clostridium difficile-associated diarrhoea (pseudomembranous colitis)

Pseudomembranous colitis (see p. 277) may develop following the use of any antibiotic. Diarrhoea occurs in the first few days after taking the antibiotic or even up to 6 weeks after stopping the drug. The causative agent is *C. difficile* (see p. 277).

Bile acid malabsorption

Bile acid malabsorption is an under-diagnosed cause of chronic diarrhoea and many patients with this disorder are assumed to have the irritable bowel syndrome. Bile acid diarrhoea occurs when the terminal ileum fails to reabsorb bile acids. When present in increased concentrations in the colon, bile acids (particularly the dihydroxy bile acids: deoxycholate and chenodeoxycholate) lead to diarrhoea by reducing absorption of water and electrolytes and, at higher concentrations, inducing secretion as well as increasing colonic motility. A variety of causes of bile acid malabsorption are recognized ***(Box 13.36)***.

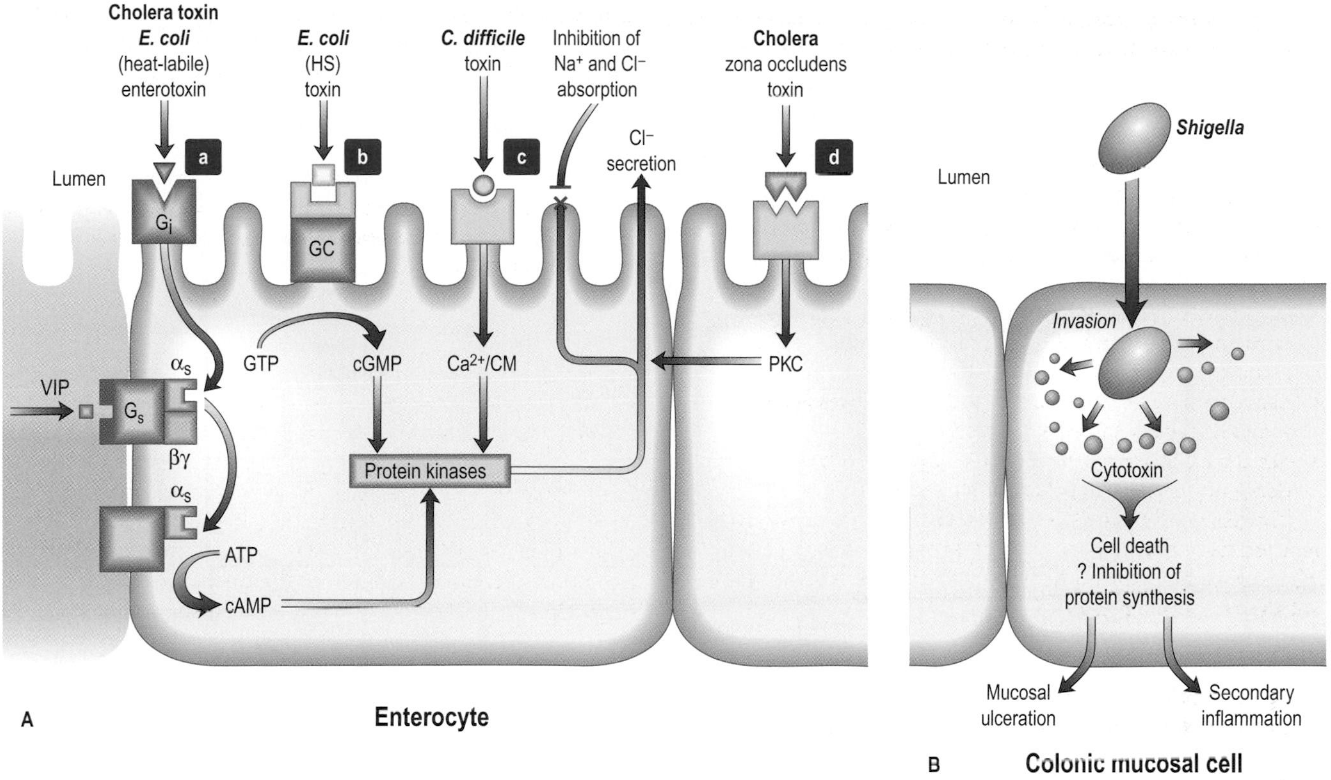

Figure 13.56 Mechanisms of diarrhoea.
A. ***Small intestinal secretion of water and electrolytes***. **(a)** *Cholera toxin* binds to its receptor (monosialoganglioside G_i) via fimbria (toxin co-regulated pili) on its β-subunit. This activates the α_s subunit (of the G_s protein), which in turn dissociates and activates cyclic AMP (cAMP). The increase in cAMP activates intermediates (e.g. protein kinase and Ca^{2+}), which then act on the apical membrane, causing Cl^- secretion (with water) and inhibition of Na^+ and Cl^- absorption. *Heat-labile E. coli enterotoxin* shares a receptor with cholera toxin. **(b)** *Heat-stable (HS) E. coli toxin* binds to its own receptor and activates guanylate cyclase (cGMP), producing the same effect on secretion.
(c) *Clostridium difficile* activates the protein kinases via Ca^{2+}/calmodulin (Ca^{2+}/CM). **(d)** *Zona occludens toxin* is the product of the *ZOT* gene, which loosens tight junctions and is required for function of the cholera toxin. It has enterotoxic activity, producing secretion. Cholera and *E. coli* cause these effects without invasion of the cell.
B. ***Colonic mucosal cell***. This demonstrates one of the mechanisms by which an invasive pathogen (e.g. *Shigella*) acts. Following penetration, the pathogens generate cytotoxins, which leads to mucosal ulceration and cell death. ATP, adenosine triphosphate; G, G protein consisting of subunits α, β, γ; GC, guanyl cyclase; GMP, guanosine monophosphate; GTP, guanosine triphosphate;
i, inhibitory; PKC, protein kinase C; s, stimulatory; VIP, vasoactive intestinal polypeptide.

? Box 13.36 Causes of bile acid diarrhoea

- Ileal resection
- Ileal disease, e.g. active or inactive Crohn's disease
- Primary bile acid diarrhoea
- Post-infective gastroenteritis
- Rapid small bowel transit
- Post-cholecystectomy

Bile acid malabsorption should be considered not only in patients with chronic diarrhoea of unknown cause, but also in those with diarrhoea and associated disease who are not responding to standard therapy (e.g. patients with terminal ileal Crohn's disease or microscopic inflammatory colitis).

Diagnosis is made using the SeHCAT test, in which a radiolabelled bile acid analogue is administered and percentage retention at 7 days calculated (<19% retention abnormal). Treatment is with bile salt sequestrants such as colestyramine, a resin that binds and inactivates the action of bile acids in the colon. The best treatment results are obtained in patients with a SeHCAT retention of <5%.

Factitious diarrhoea

Factitious diarrhoea accounts for up to 4% of new patients with diarrhoea attending gastroenterology clinics.

Purgative abuse

This is most commonly seen in females who surreptitiously take high-dose purgatives and are often extensively investigated for chronic diarrhoea. The diarrhoea is usually of high volume (>1 L daily) and patients may have a low serum potassium. Biochemical analysis of the stool may help diagnose laxative abuse. Management is difficult, as most patients deny purgative ingestion. Purgative abuse often occurs in association with eating disorders and patients may need psychiatric help.

Dilutional diarrhoea

In this condition, raised stool weights occur as a consequence of patients deliberately diluting their stool with urine or tap water. The diagnosis is made by measuring stool osmolality and electrolyte concentrations in order to calculate the faecal osmolar gap.

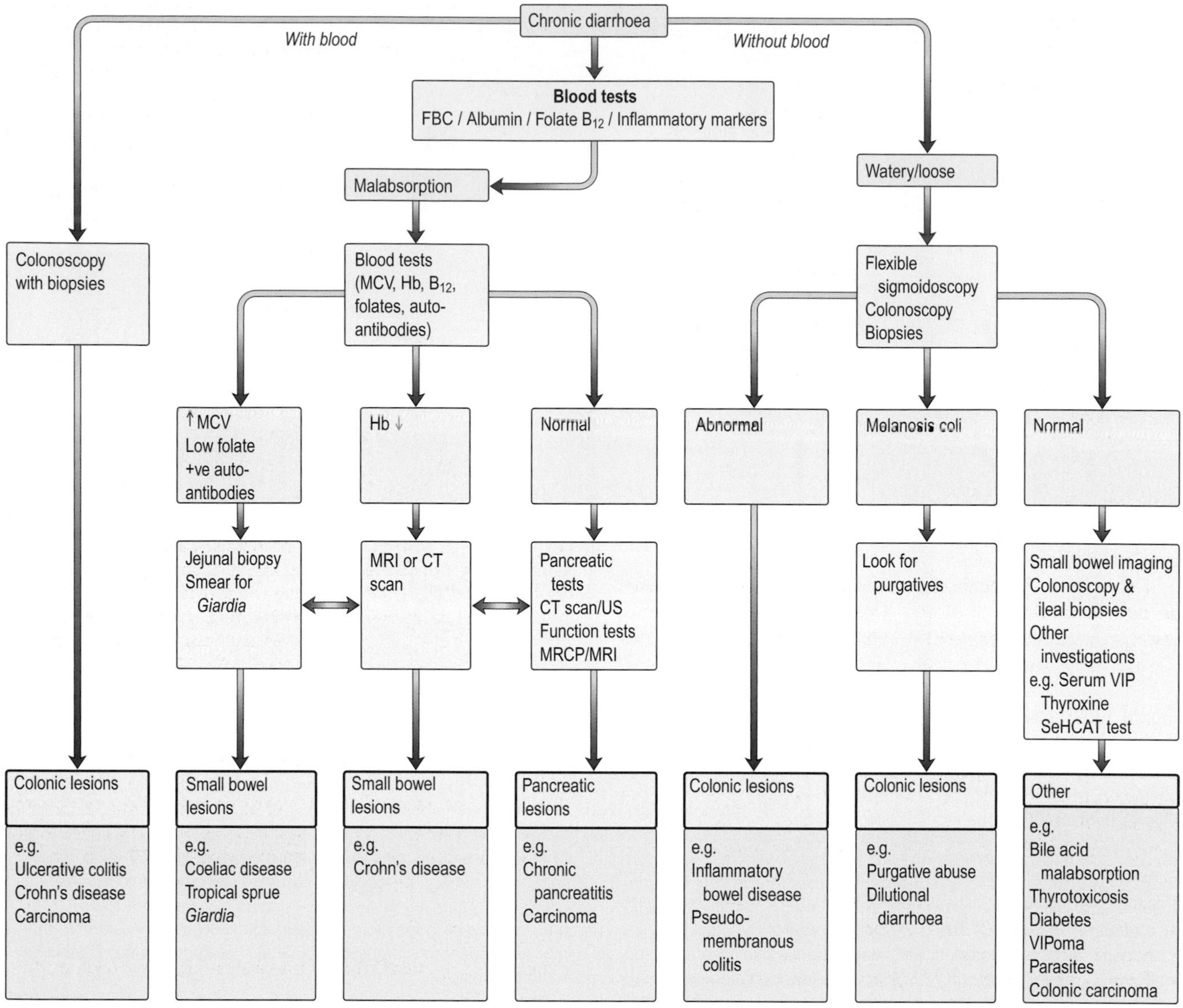

Figure 13.57 Flow diagram for the investigation of chronic diarrhoea. Note: **All patients should have had stool cultures with toxin testing for *Clostridium difficile*.** CT, computed tomography; FBC, full blood count; Hb, haemoglobin; MCV, mean cell volume; MRCP, magnetic resonance cholangiopancreatography; MRI, magnetic resonance imaging; SeHCAT, ^{75}Selenium-homocholic acid taurine; US, ultrasound; VIP, vasoactive intestinal polypeptide.

Diarrhoea in patients with HIV infection

Chronic diarrhoea is a common symptom in HIV infection, but HIV's role in the pathogenesis of diarrhoea is unclear. *Cryptosporidium* (see p. 350) is the pathogen most commonly isolated. *Isospora belli* and microsporidia have also been found.

The cause of the diarrhoea is often not found and treatment is symptomatic. ***Box 13.19*** shows the conditions affecting the gastrointestinal tract in patients with AIDS.

Box 13.37 Chronic gastrointestinal symptoms suggestive of a functional gastrointestinal disorder

- Nausea alone
- Vomiting alone
- Belching
- Chest pain unrelated to exercise
- Postprandial fullness
- Abdominal bloating
- Abdominal discomfort/pain (right or left iliac fossa)
- Passage of mucus *per rectum*
- Frequent bowel actions with urgency first thing in morning

FUNCTIONAL GASTROINTESTINAL DISORDERS

There is a large group of gastrointestinal disorders that are termed 'functional' because symptoms occur in the absence of any demonstrable abnormalities in the digestion and absorption of nutrients, fluid and electrolytes, and no structural abnormality can be identified in the gastrointestinal tract, although there may be discernible abnormalities in neuromuscular function, such as dysmotility and visceral hypersensitivity, which are not routinely investigated.

Box 13.37 lists some of the symptoms that are suggestive of a functional gastrointestinal disorder. Modern classification systems are based on the premise that, for each disorder, there is a symptom

Box 13.38 Modified Rome III functional gastrointestinal disorders

A. **Functional oesophageal disorders:**
- Heartburn
- Chest pain of presumed oesophageal origin
- Dysphagia
- Globus

B. **Functional gastroduodenal disorders:**
- Non-ulcer dyspepsia
- Belching disorders
- Nausea and vomiting disorders
- Rumination syndrome in adults

C. **Functional bowel disorders:**
- Irritable bowel syndrome
- Functional bloating
- Functional constipation
- Functional diarrhoea
- Unspecified functional bowel disorder

D. **Functional abdominal pain syndrome**

E. **Functional gall bladder and sphincter of Oddi disorders**

cluster that 'breeds true' across clinical and population groups. There is inevitably overlap, some symptoms being common to more than one disorder.

Box 13.38 lists the common functional gastrointestinal disorders, as defined by Rome III criteria. These conditions are extremely common worldwide, comprising 80% of patients seen in the gastroenterology clinic.

Pathophysiology and brain–gut interactions

People with functional gastrointestinal disorders (FGIDs) are characterized by having a greater gastrointestinal motility response to life events than normal subjects. There is, however, a poor association between measured gastrointestinal motility changes and symptoms in many of the FGIDs. Patients with FGID have been shown to have abnormalities in visceral sensation and to have a lower pain threshold when tested with balloon distension (visceral hyperalgesia). Visceral hypersensitivity possibly relates to:

- altered receptor sensitivity at the viscus itself
- increased excitability of the spinal cord dorsal horn neurones
- altered central modulation of sensations.

A systematic review of published studies suggests that 10% of patients who experience an acute infective gastroenteritis develop a degree of FGID. It is not clear whether this is caused by post-infectious bile salt malabsorption, alterations in the mucosal immune system or the use of antibiotics to treat the index infection

The brain–gut axis describes a combination of intestinal motor, sensory and activities ***(Fig. 13.58)***. Thus, extrinsic (e.g. vision, smell) and intrinsic (e.g. emotion, thought) information can affect gastrointestinal sensation because of the neural connections from higher centres. Conversely, viscerotropic events can affect central pain perception, mood and behaviour.

Psychological stress can exacerbate gastrointestinal symptoms, and psychological disturbances are more common in patients with FGIDs. These disturbances alter attitude to illness, promote health-care seeking, and often lead to a poor clinical outcome. They have psychosocial consequences with poor quality of life at home and work. Early in life, genetic and environmental influences (e.g. family attitudes towards bowel training, verbal or sexual abuse, exposure to an infection) may affect psychosocial development (susceptibility to life stress, psychological state, coping skills, development of social support) or the development of gut dysfunction (abnormal motility or visceral hypersensitivity). Therefore, FGID should be regarded as a dysregulation of brain–gut function.

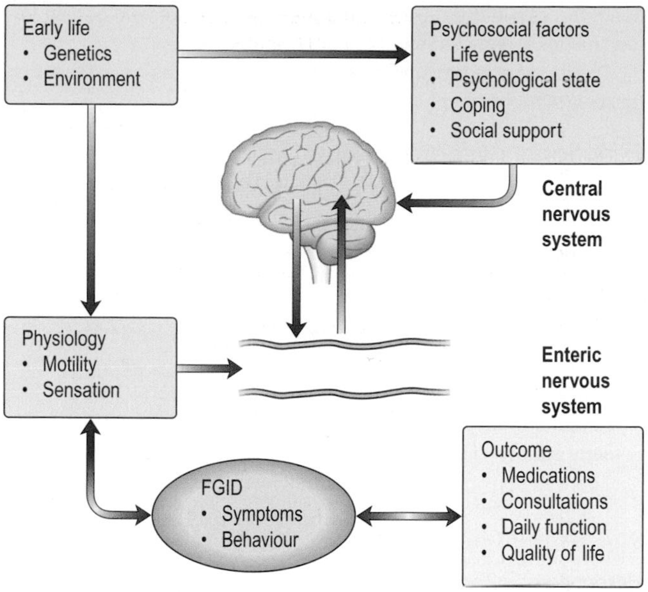

Figure 13.58 A biopsychosocial conceptualization of the pathogenesis and clinical expression of functional gastrointestinal disorders (FGIDs). Genetic, environmental and psychological factors may interact to cause dysregulation of brain–gut function. *(Modified from Drossman DA. The functional gastrointestinal disorders and the Rome III process. Gastroenterology 2006; 130:1377–1390, with permission from Elsevier.)*

Functional oesophageal disorders

The criteria for diagnosis rest mainly on compatible symptoms. However, pathological gastro-oesophageal reflux and eosinophilic oesophagitis may need to be excluded (see pp. 373–374).

Globus

This presents as:

- persistent or intermittent sensation of a lump or foreign body in the throat
- occurrence of the sensation between meals
- absence of dysphagia and pain on swallowing (odynophagia).

Management is with explanation and reassurance, and a trial of anti-reflux therapy. Antidepressants may be tried.

Functional chest pain of presumed oesophageal origin

This is characterized by episodes of mainly midline chest pain, not burning in nature, that are potentially of oesophageal origin and occur in the absence of a cardiological cause, gastro-oesophageal reflux and achalasia.

More than half of patients will respond to high-dose acid-suppression therapy in the first week; some will respond to nitrates and calcium-channel blockers.

Antidepressant therapy, e.g. amitriptyline or the selective serotonin reuptake inhibitor (SSRI) citalopram, have been shown to be effective.

Functional gastroduodenal disorders

Functional dyspepsia

This is the second most common functional gastrointestinal disorder (after irritable bowel syndrome). Patients can present with a spectrum of symptoms, including upper abdominal pain or discomfort, fullness, early satiety, bloating and nausea.

These patients have no structural abnormality as an explanation for their symptoms.

Functional dyspepsia subgroups

Two subgroups, based on the predominant (or most bothersome) single symptom, are suggested:

- ***Epigastric pain syndrome***, with pain centred in the upper abdomen as the predominant (most bothersome) symptom.
- ***Postprandial distress syndrome***, with an unpleasant or troublesome, non-painful sensation (discomfort) centred in the upper abdomen being the predominant symptom. This sensation may be associated with upper abdominal fullness, early satiety, bloating and nausea.

There is considerable overlap between these two groups.

Investigations

Helicobacter pylori infection should be excluded using a stool antigen test, but many young patients (<50 years) require no further investigation. Older patients or those with alarm symptoms require endoscopy. Gastroscopy often shows gastritis but it is doubtful whether this is the cause of the symptoms.

Management

The range of therapies prescribed for functional dyspepsia reflects the uncertain pathogenesis and the lack of satisfactory treatment options. Management is further confounded by high placebo response rates (20–60%). A proportion of patients will respond satisfactorily to reassurance, explanations and lifestyle changes. Proton pump inhibitors and prokinetic agents are used for patients with epigastric pain syndrome and postprandial distress syndrome, respectively. Reducing intake of fat, coffee and alcohol and stopping cigarette smoking help. SSRI medication is tried in refractory cases.

H. pylori eradication therapy has been shown to be effective in some patients with functional dyspepsia.

Aerophagia

Aerophagia refers to a repetitive pattern of swallowing or ingesting air and belching. It is usually an unconscious act unrelated to meals. Usually, no investigation is required. Explanation that the symptoms are due to swallowed air, and reassurance are necessary, as is treatment of associated psychiatric disease.

Functional vomiting

Functional vomiting is a rare condition in clinical practice, although chronic nausea is a frequent accompaniment in all functional gastrointestinal disorders. CNS pathology and migrainous syndromes (cyclical vomiting syndrome) should be considered and treated.

Clinical features

Clinically, functional vomiting is characterized by:

- frequent episodes of vomiting, occurring on at least 1 day a week
- absence of criteria for an eating disorder, rumination or major psychiatric disease
- absence of self-induced and medication-induced vomiting
- absence of abnormalities in the gut or CNS and of metabolic disease to explain the recurrent vomiting.

Investigations

Investigation is often not required but non-gastrointestinal disorders should always be excluded (see ***Box 13.1***).

Management

Treatment is with anti-nausea drugs and antidepressants; behavioural therapy and psychotherapy are helpful. Dietary changes occasionally help.

Cyclical vomiting syndrome

This syndrome is characterized by typical bouts of intense vomiting lasting for hours to days, separated by periods with no symptoms. It can occur in children or adults. There is a link to migraine headaches but the cause is not known. In some cases, provocative triggers can be identified; for example, there is a specific syndrome associated with frequent cannabis use – cannabinoid hyperemesis syndrome.

Diagnosis of cyclical vomiting syndrome is by recognition of the pattern of symptoms and ruling out of other causes.

Management

Treatment is with antiemetics and intravenous rehydration and electrolyte replacement during bouts, with avoidance of triggers where these are known. Prophylactic treatment of migraine, when it coexists, may help.

Gastroparesis

Gastroparesis results when there is delayed gastric emptying. There are a number of known associations, such as diabetes, but many cases are primary. Symptoms include nausea, vomiting, early satiety, fullness, bloating and upper abdominal pain.

Management is directed at relief of symptoms and correction of nutritional deficiencies. Improvement of gastric emptying can sometimes be achieved by medical or surgical treatments, such as pro-motility agents or gastric pacemaker insertion. In diabetics, glycaemic control is helpful.

Functional bowel disorders

Irritable bowel syndrome

Irritable bowel syndrome (IBS) is the most common FGID. In Western populations, up to 1 in 5 people report symptoms consistent with IBS. Approximately 50% will consult their doctors and, of these, up to 30% will be referred by their doctor to a hospital specialist. Up to 40% of all patients seen in specialist gastroenterology clinics will have IBS. Estimates in the UK put the annual cost of IBS to healthcare resources as £45.6 million; in the USA, the cost is higher at $8 billion. In the UK, approximately one-quarter of IBS patients take time off work for periods ranging from 7 to 13 days each year.

The factors that determine whether an IBS sufferer in the community seeks medical advice include higher illness attitude scores and higher anxiety and depression scores than non-consulters. Consulters perceive that their symptoms are more severe than those of non-consulters, and consulting behaviour may be determined by the number of presenting symptoms. Female consulters outnumber male consulters by a factor of 2–3 to 1.

Box 13.39 Non-gastrointestinal features of irritable bowel syndrome

Gynaecological symptoms
- Painful periods (dysmenorrhoea)
- Pain following sexual intercourse (dyspareunia)

Urinary symptoms
- Frequency
- Urgency
- Passing urine at night (nocturia)
- Incomplete emptying of bladder

Other symptoms
- Joint hypermobility
- Back pain
- Headaches
- Bad breath, unpleasant taste in the mouth
- Poor sleeping
- Fatigue

Box 13.40 Some factors that can trigger onset of irritable bowel symptoms

- Affective disorders, e.g. depression, anxiety
- Psychological stress and trauma
- Gastrointestinal infection
- Antibiotic therapy
- Sexual, physical or verbal abuse
- Pelvic surgery
- Eating disorders

IBS – a multisystem disorder

IBS patients suffer from a number of non-intestinal symptoms ***(Box 13.39)***, which may be more intrusive than the classical features. IBS coexists with chronic fatigue syndrome (see pp. 899–900), fibromyalgia (see pp. 664–665) and temporomandibular joint dysfunction.

The biopsychosocial conceptualization of the pathogenesis and clinical expression of FGIDs ***(Fig. 13.58)*** is particularly relevant to IBS, and ***Box 13.40*** lists some common factors that have been shown to trigger IBS symptoms. Infectious diarrhoea precedes the onset of IBS symptoms in 7–30% of patients. Whether this is a factor for all patients or just a small subgroup remains controversial. Risk factors in these patients have been shown to include female gender, severity and duration of diarrhoea, pre-existing adverse life events and high hypochondriacal anxiety and neurotic scores at the time of the initial illness. Symptoms of anxiety and depression are more common in IBS patients, and stress or adverse life events often precede the onset of chronic bowel symptoms.

Diagnosis

Diagnostic criteria (Rome III 2006) state that, in the preceding 3 months, there should be at least 3 days/month of recurrent abdominal pain or discomfort associated with two or more of the following for at least 25% of the time:

1. improvement with defecation
2. onset associated with a change in frequency of stool
3. onset associated with a change in form (appearance) of stool.

These are useful for comparative studies.

Subgroups of IBS patients can be identified according to the criteria listed in ***Box 13.41***.

The decision as to whether to investigate and the choice of investigations should be based on clinical judgement. Pointers to the need for thorough investigation are the presence of the above symptoms in association with rectal bleeding, nocturnal pain, fever and weight loss, and a clinical suspicion of organic diarrhoea. A raised stool calprotectin or lactoferrin would suggest inflammation needing further investigation.

Box 13.41 Subtyping irritable bowel syndrome by predominant stool pattern

Type	Description
IBS with constipation (IBS-C)	Hard lumpy stools >25% and loose (mushy) or watery stools <25% of bowel movements
IBS with diarrhoea (IBS-D)	Loose (mushy) or watery stools >25% and hard or lumpy stools <25% of bowel movements
Mixed IBS (IBS-M)	Hard or lumpy stools >25% and loose (mushy) or watery stools >25% of bowel movements
Unsubtyped IBS	Insufficient abnormality of stool consistency to meet criteria for IBS-C, D or M

Management

Current strategies for the treatment of IBS include therapies that target central and end-organ pathways ***(Box 13.42)***; these are not mutually exclusive.

Patients with IBS are often worried that their symptoms are due to a serious disease such as cancer. A positive diagnosis of IBS with an explanation of the symptoms and reassurance is often helpful and may require no further treatment. ***Box 13.42*** shows the overall management strategies used in IBS for those with severe and longstanding problems. Patients should be treated sympathetically and some may require psychiatric support.

Pain/gas/bloat syndrome/midgut dysmotility

Disordered motility and visceral sensation that predominantly affects the small intestine or midgut result in symptoms of pain and bloating without altered defecation. Other symptoms include postprandial fullness, nausea and, on occasions, anorexia and weight loss.

Management of patients with pain/gas/bloat syndrome is not easy, and in some, pain can be chronic and severe. Narcotics should always be avoided. Central and end-organ-targeted treatment approaches should be combined: for example, the SSRI paroxetine combined with a prokinetic agent, such as domperidone, or a smooth muscle relaxant, such as mebeverine. Small bowel bacterial overgrowth can be a contributory feature that can be treated with non-absorbed antibiotics such as rifaximin. Recent research has highlighted the benefit of altering the fermentable components of the diet. A diet with reduced fermentable oligo-, di- and monosaccharides and polyols (**FODMAP**) will exclude a range of food types, including garlic, onions, specific beans, fructose-containing fruit, wheat-containing products, and certain natural and synthetic sweeteners. Small sham-diet-controlled clinical trials have shown significant benefit in patients with functional symptoms but long-term randomized controlled studies are necessary.

Some patients with pain/gas/bloat syndrome have particularly severe and chronic symptoms, which may be nocturnal. A small subgroup of these has been shown to have manometric features consistent with a diagnosis of *chronic idiopathic intestinal pseudo-obstruction (CIIP)*, and specifically of an enteric neuropathy. Full-thickness small intestinal biopsies confirm this diagnosis by showing a deficiency of α actin staining in the inner circular layer of smooth muscle. More appropriately, these patients should be considered as having a gastrointestinal neuromuscular disorder of the gut. About 10% of these individuals are subsequently found to have an underlying autoimmune overlap disorder (see p. 699).

Management of patients with neuromuscular disorders of the gut requires a multidisciplinary approach, with an emphasis on

Box 13.42 Approaches to the management of the irritable bowel syndrome

Treatment modality	Action
End-organ treatment	
Exploration of dietary triggers	Refer to dietitian
High-fibre diet ± fibre supplements for constipation, low FODMAP diet for bloating	Refer to dietitian
Alteration of microbiota	Rifaximin has shown short-term benefit in IBS patients without constipation (target I and II trials) Pro- and prebiotics
Anti-diarrhoeal drugs for bowel frequency	Loperamide Codeine phosphate Co-phenotrope Eluxadoline[a]
Constipation	5-HT_4 receptor agonist, e.g. prucalopride
Smooth muscle relaxants for pain	Mebeverine hydrochloride Dicycloverine hydrochloride Peppermint oil
Central treatment	
Explanation of physiology and symptoms	At consultation (leaflets with diagrams help)
Psychotherapy	Refer to clinical psychologist (see p. 900)
Hypnotherapy	
Cognitive behavioural therapy	Refer to psychiatrist
Antidepressants	Functional diarrhoea – clomipramine Diarrhoea-predominant IBS – tricyclic group, e.g. amitriptyline Constipation-predominant IBS – SSRI, e.g. paroxetine

[a]Eluxadoline – a μ- and κ-opioid receptor agonist and δ-opioid receptor antagonist.
FODMAP, fermentable oligo-, di- and monosaccharides and polyols; SSRI, selective serotonin reuptake inhibitor.

the management of pain, psychological state and nutrition. Patients with underlying autoimmune inflammatory mixed connective tissue disorders may benefit from primary treatment of these. Patients with intestinal failure as a result of CIIP need long-term parenteral nutrition.

Functional diarrhoea

In this form of functional bowel disease, symptoms occur in the absence of abdominal pain. They commonly include:

- the passage of several stools in rapid succession, usually first thing in the morning; no further bowel action may occur that day, or defecation takes place only after meals
- a first stool of the day that is usually formed, the later ones being mushy, looser or watery
- urgency of defecation
- anxiety, and uncertainty about bowel function with restriction of movement (e.g. travelling)
- exhaustion after defecation.

Chronic diarrhoea without pain is caused by many diseases that are indistinguishable by history from functional diarrhoea. Features that are atypical of a functional disorder (e.g. large-volume stools, rectal bleeding, nutritional deficiency and weight loss) call for more extensive investigations.

Treatment of functional diarrhoea is with loperamide, often combined with a tricyclic antidepressant prescribed at night (e.g. clomipramine 10–30 mg).

Further reading

Chang L. The role of stress on physiologic responses and clinical symptoms in irritable bowel syndrome. *Gastroenterology* 2011; 140:761–765.
Drossman DA. The functional gastrointestinal disorders and the Rome III process. *Gastroenterology* 2006; 130:1377–1390.
Ford AC, Talley NJ. IBS in 2010: advances in pathophysiology, diagnosis and treatment. *Nat Rev Gastroenterol Hepatol* 2011; 8:76–78.
Manabe N, Rao AS, Wong BS et al. Emerging pharmacologic therapies for irritable bowel syndrome. *Curr Gastroenterol Rep* 2010; 12:8–16.
Moayyedi P, Ford AC, Talley NJ et al. The efficacy of probiotics in the treatment of irritable bowel syndrome: a systematic review. *Gut* 2010; 59:325–332.
National Institute for Health and Care Excellence. *NICE Clinical Guideline 61: Irritable Bowel Syndrome in Adults: Diagnosis and Management of Irritable Bowel Syndrome in Primary Care.* NICE 2008; http://www.nice.org.uk/guidance/cg61.

THE ACUTE ABDOMEN

This section deals with the acute abdominal conditions that cause the patient to be hospitalized within a few hours of the onset of pain ***(Box 13.43)***. If they are recognized quickly as an emergency, a reduction in morbidity and mortality can be achieved. Although a specific diagnosis should be attempted, the immediate problem in management is to decide whether an 'acute abdomen' exists and whether surgery is required.

Diagnosis

History

This should include previous operations, any gynaecological problems and presence of any concurrent medical condition.

Pain

The onset, site, type and subsequent course of the pain should be determined as accurately as possible. In general, the pain of an acute abdomen can be either constant (usually owing to inflammation) or colicky (because of a blocked 'tube'). The inflammatory nature of a constant pain will be supported by a raised temperature, tachycardia and/or a raised white cell count. If these are normal, then other causes (e.g. musculoskeletal, aortic aneurysm), even rare ones (e.g. porphyria), should be considered. Colicky pain can be due to an obstruction of the gut, biliary system, urogenital system or uterus. These cases will probably require conservative management initially,

Box 13.43 Common causes of acute abdominal pain

Diagnosis	%[a]
Non-specific abdominal pain	35
Acute appendicitis	30
Gall bladder disease	10
Gynaecological disorders	5
Intestinal obstruction	5
Perforated ulcer/dyspepsia	5
Renal colic	2
Urinary tract infection	2
Diverticular disease	2
Other diagnoses	4

[a]Percentages are approximate and vary in different communities.

along with analgesics. If a colicky pain becomes a constant pain, then inflammation of the organ may have supervened (e.g. strangulated hernia, ascending cholangitis or salpingitis).

A ***sudden onset*** of pain suggests:

- perforation (e.g. of a duodenal ulcer)
- rupture (e.g. of an ectopic pregnancy)
- torsion (e.g. of an ovarian cyst)
- acute pancreatitis
- infarction (e.g. mesenteric).

Back pain suggests:

- pancreatitis
- rupture of an aortic aneurysm
- renal tract disease.

Inflammatory conditions (e.g. appendicitis) produce a more gradual onset of pain. With peritonitis, the pain is continuous and may be made worse by movement. Many inflammatory conditions can progress to those listed as having a sudden onset due to complications.

Vomiting

Vomiting may accompany any acute abdominal pain but, if persistent, suggests an obstructive lesion of the gut. The character of the vomit should be asked about. Does it contain blood, bile or small bowel contents?

Other symptoms

Any change in bowel habit or of urinary frequency should be documented and, in females, a gynaecological history, including last menstrual period, should be taken.

Physical examination

The general condition of the person should be noted. Does he or she look ill or shocked? Large volumes of fluid may be lost from the vascular compartment into the peritoneal cavity or into the lumen of the bowel, giving rise to hypovolaemia: that is, a pale, cold skin, a weak, rapid pulse and hypotension.

The abdomen

- ***Inspection***. Look for the presence of scars, distension or masses.
- ***Palpation***. The abdomen should be examined gently for sites of tenderness and the presence or absence of guarding. Guarding is involuntary spasm of the abdominal wall and indicates peritonitis. This can be localized to one area or may be generalized, involving the whole abdomen.
- ***Bowel sounds***. Increased high-pitched, tinkling bowel sounds indicate fluid obstruction; this occurs because of fluid movement within the dilated bowel lumen. Absent bowel sounds suggest peritonitis. In an obstructed patient, absent bowel sounds may be due to strangulation, ischaemia or ileus. It is essential for the hernial orifices to be examined if intestinal obstruction is suspected.

Vaginal and rectal examination

Vaginal examination can be very helpful, particularly in diagnosing gynaecological causes of an acute abdomen (e.g. a ruptured ectopic pregnancy). Rectal examination is less helpful, as localized tenderness may be due to any cause; it may show blood on the glove.

Other observations

- ***Temperature***. Fever is more common in acute inflammatory processes.

Box 13.44 Medical causes of acute abdomen

- **Referred pain:**
  - Pneumonia
  - Myocardial infarction
- **Functional gastrointestinal disorders**
- **Renal causes:**
  - Pelviureteric colic
  - Acute pyelonephritis
- **Metabolic causes:**
  - Diabetes mellitus
  - Acute intermittent porphyria
  - Lead poisoning
  - Familial Mediterranean fever
- **Haematological causes:**
  - Haemophilia and other bleeding disorders
  - Henoch–Schönlein purpura
  - Sickle cell crisis
  - Polycythaemia vera
  - Paroxysmal nocturnal haemoglobinaemia
- **Vasculitis**

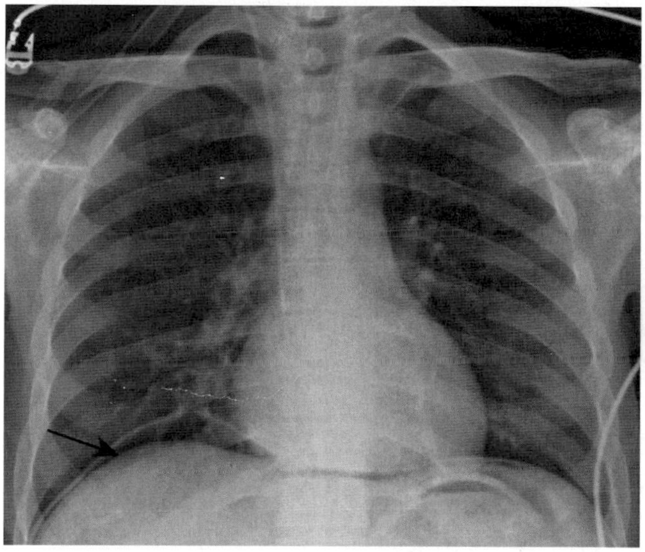

Figure 13.59 X-ray showing air under the diaphragm (arrowed).

- ***Urine***. Examine for:
  - blood – suggests urinary tract infection or renal colic
  - glucose and ketones – ketoacidosis can present with acute pain
  - protein and white cells – to exclude acute pyelonephritis.
- ***Medical causes***. These should be borne in mind ***(Box 13.44)***.

Investigations

- ***Blood count***. A raised white cell count occurs in inflammatory conditions.
- ***Serum amylase***. High levels (more than five times normal) indicate acute pancreatitis. Raised levels below this can occur in any acute abdomen and should not be considered diagnostic of pancreatitis.
- ***Serum electrolytes***. These are not particularly helpful for diagnosis but are useful for general evaluation of the patient.
- ***Pregnancy test***. A urine dipstick is used for women of childbearing age.
- ***X-rays***. An erect chest X-ray is useful to detect air under the diaphragm caused by a perforation ***(Fig. 13.59)***. Dilated loops of bowel or fluid levels are suggestive of obstruction on abdominal X-ray ***(Fig. 13.60)***.

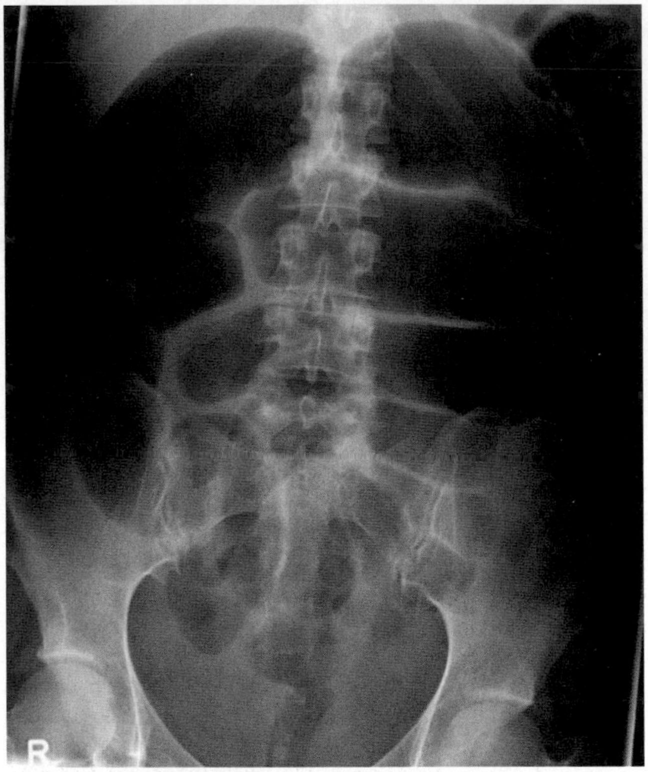

Figure 13.60 X-ray showing small bowel obstruction.

- ***Ultrasound***. This is useful in the diagnosis of acute cholangitis, cholecystitis and aortic aneurysm, and in expert hands is reliable in the diagnosis of acute appendicitis. Gynaecological and other pelvic causes of pain can be detected.
- ***CT scan***. Spiral CT of the abdomen and pelvis is the most accurate investigation in most acute emergencies. It should be used more often to avoid unnecessary laparotomies.
- ***Laparoscopy***. This is used increasingly as a diagnostic tool prior to proceeding with surgery, particularly in men and women over the age of 50 years. In addition, therapeutic manœuvres, such as appendicectomy, can be performed.

Acute appendicitis

This is a common surgical emergency and affects all age groups. Appendicitis should always be considered in the differential diagnosis if the appendix has not been removed.

Acute appendicitis mostly occurs when the lumen of the appendix becomes obstructed with a faecolith; however, in some cases, there is only generalized acute inflammation. If the appendix is not removed at this stage, gangrene occurs with perforation, leading to a localized abscess or to generalized peritonitis.

Clinical features

Most patients present with abdominal pain; in many, it starts vaguely in the centre of the abdomen, becoming localized to the right iliac fossa in the first few hours. Nausea, vomiting, anorexia and occasional diarrhoea can occur.

Examination of the abdomen usually reveals tenderness in the right iliac fossa, with guarding due to the localized peritonitis. There may be a tender mass in the right iliac fossa. Although raised white cell counts, ESR and CRP are helpful, other laboratory tests can be less valuable. An ultrasound scan can detect an inflamed appendix and can also indicate an appendix mass or other localized lesion. CT is highly sensitive (98.5%) and specific (98% negative predictive value; 99.5% positive predictive value), and reduces the incidence of removal of a 'normal' appendix. With the use of these investigations, the incidence of 'normal' appendix histology has fallen to 15–20%.

Differential diagnosis

- Non-specific mesenteric lymphadenitis – may mimic appendicitis.
- Acute terminal ileitis due to Crohn's disease or *Yersinia* infection.
- Gynaecological causes:
  - Inflamed Meckel's diverticulum
  - Functional bowel disease.

Management

The appendix is removed by laparoscopic surgery. If an appendix mass is present, the patient is usually treated conservatively with intravenous fluids and antibiotics. The pain subsides over a few days and the mass usually disappears over a few weeks. Interval appendicectomy is recommended at a later date to prevent further acute episodes.

Gynaecological causes of an acute abdomen

Ruptured ectopic pregnancy

The fallopian tube is the most common extrauterine site of implantation. Delayed diagnosis is the major cause of morbidity. Most patients will present with recurrent low abdominal pain associated with vaginal bleeding. Diagnosis is usually made with abdominal and transvaginal ultrasound. Most patients can be managed by laparoscopic salpingostomy or salpingectomy.

Ovarian causes

- Rupture of 'functional' ovarian cysts in the middle of the cycle (Mittelschmerz).
- Torsion or rupture of ovarian cysts.

Acute salpingitis

Most cases are associated with sexually transmitted infection. Patients commonly present with bilateral low abdominal pain, a fever and vaginal discharge. In the ***Fitz-Hugh–Curtis syndrome***, *Chlamydia* infection tracks up the right paracolic gutter to cause a perihepatitis. Patients can present with acute right hypochondrial pain, fever and mildly abnormal liver biochemistry.

Acute peritonitis

Localized peritonitis

There is virtually always some degree of localized peritonitis with all acute inflammatory conditions of the gastrointestinal tract (e.g. acute appendicitis, acute cholecystitis). Pain and tenderness are largely features of this localized peritonitis. The treatment is for the underlying disease.

Generalized peritonitis

This is a serious condition, resulting from irritation of the peritoneum owing to infection (e.g. perforated appendix) or from chemical irritation due to leakage of intestinal contents (e.g. perforated ulcer). In the latter case, superadded infection gradually occurs; *E. coli* and *Bacteroides* are the most common organisms.

The peritoneal cavity becomes acutely inflamed, with production of an inflammatory exudate that spreads throughout the peritoneum, leading to intestinal dilatation and paralytic ileus.

Clinical features

In perforation, the onset is sudden with acute, severe abdominal pain, followed by general collapse and shock. The patient may improve temporarily, only to become worse later as generalized toxaemia occurs.

When peritonitis is secondary to inflammatory disease, the onset is less rapid, the initial features being those of the underlying disease.

Investigations

Investigations should always include an erect chest X-ray. X-ray is used to detect free air under the diaphragm, and serum amylase is measured to diagnose acute pancreatitis, which is treated conservatively. Imaging with ultrasound and/or CT should always be performed for diagnosis.

Management

Peritonitis is treated surgically after adequate resuscitation and the re-establishment of a good urinary output. This includes insertion of a nasogastric tube, intravenous fluids and antibiotics. Surgery has a two-fold objective:

- peritoneal lavage of the abdominal cavity
- specific treatment of the underlying condition.

Complications

Any delay in the treatment of peritonitis produces more profound toxaemia and septicaemia, which may lead to development of multiorgan failure (see p. 1155). Local abscess formation can occur and should be suspected if a patient continues to remain unwell postoperatively, with a swinging fever, high white cell count and continuing pain. Abscesses are commonly pelvic or subphrenic, and can be localized and drained using ultrasound and CT scanning techniques.

Intestinal obstruction

Most intestinal obstruction is due to a mechanical block. Sometimes, the bowel does not function, leading to a paralytic ileus. This occurs temporarily after most abdominal operations and with peritonitis. Some causes of intestinal obstruction are shown in ***Box 13.45***. The most common cause in adults is adhesions.

Obstruction of the bowel leads to bowel distension above the block, with increased secretion of fluid into the distended bowel. Bacterial contamination takes place in the distended stagnant bowel. In strangulation, the blood supply is impeded, leading to gangrene, perforation and peritonitis unless urgent treatment of the condition is undertaken.

? Box 13.45 Causes of intestinal obstruction

Small intestinal obstruction

- Adhesions (80% in adults)
- Hernias
- Crohn's disease
- Intussusception
- Obstruction due to extrinsic involvement by cancer

Colonic obstruction

- Carcinoma of the colon
- Sigmoid volvulus
- Diverticular disease

Clinical features

The patient complains of abdominal colic, vomiting and constipation without passage of wind. In upper gut obstruction the vomiting is profuse, but in lower gut obstruction it may be absent.

Examination of the abdomen reveals distension with increased bowel sounds. Marked tenderness suggests strangulation, and urgent surgery is necessary. Examination of the hernial orifices and rectum must be performed. X-ray of the abdomen reveals distended loops of bowel proximal to the obstruction. Fluid levels are seen in small bowel obstruction on an erect film. In large bowel obstruction, the caecum and ascending colon are distended. An instant, water-soluble Gastrografin enema without air insufflation may help to demonstrate the site of the obstruction. CT can localize the lesion accurately and is the investigation of choice.

Management

Initial management is by resuscitation with intravenous fluids (mainly 0.9% saline with potassium) and decompression. Many cases will settle on conservative management, but an increasing temperature, raised pulse rate, increasing pain and a rising white cell count require urgent scanning and possible exploratory laparotomy.

Laparotomy with removal of the obstruction will be necessary in some cases of small bowel obstruction. If the bowel is gangrenous owing to strangulation, gut resection will be required. A few patients (e.g. those with Crohn's disease) may have recurrent episodes of incomplete intestinal obstruction that can be managed conservatively. In large bowel obstruction due to malignancy, a self-expanding metal stent can be used, followed by elective surgery. In critically ill patients, a defunctioning colostomy may be needed. Volvulus of the sigmoid colon can be managed by the passage of a flexible sigmoidoscope or a rectal tube to un-kink and deflate the bowel, but recurrent volvulus may require sigmoid resection.

Acute colonic pseudo-obstruction

A clinical picture mimicking mechanical obstruction may develop in patients who do not have a mechanical cause. In more than 80% of cases, it complicates other clinical conditions, such as:

- intra-abdominal trauma, pelvic, spinal and femoral fractures
- postoperative states (abdominal, pelvic, cardiothoracic, orthopaedic, neurosurgical)
- intra-abdominal sepsis
- pneumonia
- metabolic disorders (e.g. electrolyte disturbances, malnutrition, diabetes mellitus, Parkinson's disease)
- drugs – opiates (particularly after orthopaedic surgery), antidepressants, antiparkinsonian drugs.

Patients present with rapid and progressive abdominal distension and pain. X-ray shows a gas-filled large bowel. Management is of the underlying problem (e.g. withdrawal of opiate analgesia), together with a trial of intravenous neostigmine therapy. Patients should be monitored and consideration should be given to surgery if the diameter of the caecum exceeds 14 cm.

THE PERITONEUM

Anatomy and physiology

The peritoneal cavity is a closed sac lined by mesothelial cells; these produce surfactant, which acts as a lubricant within the peri-

Box 13.46 Diseases of the peritoneum

Infective (bacterial) peritonitis
- Secondary to gut disease, e.g. appendicitis
- Perforation of any organ
- Chronic peritoneal dialysis
- Spontaneous, usually in ascites with liver disease
- Tuberculosis

Neoplasia
- Secondary deposits (e.g. from ovary, stomach)
- Primary mesothelioma

Vasculitis
- Rheumatic autoimmune disease
- Polyserositis (e.g. familial Mediterranean fever)

toneal cavity. The cavity contains <100 mL of serous fluid containing <30 g/L of protein.

The mesothelial cells lining the diaphragm have gaps that allow communication between the peritoneum and the diaphragmatic lymphatics. Approximately one-third of fluid drains through these lymphatics, the remainder through the parietal peritoneum. These mechanisms allow particulate matter to be removed rapidly from the peritoneal cavity.

Complement activation is an early defence mechanism and is followed rapidly by upregulation of the peritoneal mesothelial cells and migration of polymorphonuclear neutrophils and macrophages into the peritoneum.

Mast cells release potent mediators of inflammation, including histamine and eicosanoids, and interact with T cells to generate an immune response.

The peritoneum-associated lymphoid tissue includes the omental milky spots, the lymphocytes within the peritoneal cavity and the draining lymph nodes. B cells with a unique $CD5^+$ are common. This defence system plays a major role in localizing peritoneal infection.

Disorders affecting the peritoneum

Conditions that can affect the peritoneum are shown in ***Box 13.46***.

Peritonitis can be acute or chronic, as seen in TB. Most cases of infective peritonitis are secondary to gastrointestinal disease, but it occurs occasionally without intra-abdominal sepsis in ascites due to liver disease. Very rarely, fungal and parasitic infections (e.g. amoebiasis, candidiasis) can also cause primary peritonitis. Peritonitis is discussed further on pages 434-435.

The peritoneum can be involved by secondary malignant deposits, and the most common cause of ascites in a young to middle-aged woman is an ovarian carcinoma.

A ***subphrenic abscess*** is usually secondary to infection in the abdomen and is characterized by fever, malaise, pain in the right or left hypochondrium and shoulder-tip pain. An erect chest X-ray may show gas under the diaphragm, impaired movement of the diaphragm on screening and/or a pleural effusion. Ultrasound is usually diagnostic. Percutaneous catheter drainage inserted under CT or ultrasound guidance and antibiotics constitute highly successful therapy.

Ascites is associated with all diseases of the peritoneum. The fluid that collects is an exudate with a high protein content. It is also seen in liver disease. The mechanism, causes and investigation of ascites are discussed on pages 472–474.

Peritoneal adhesions

Adhesions form as a result of abdominal or pelvic surgery, or inflammation in the abdominoperitoneal cavity. They cause a variety of conditions, including adhesive small bowel obstruction (ASBO), chronic abdominal pain, complications during future surgery, and female infertility when they involve the fallopian tubes or ovaries. There is no satisfactory medical or surgical treatment and so surgical techniques have been developed to minimize peritoneal injury,

Retroperitoneal fibrosis (peri-aortitis)

This is a rare condition, in which there is a marked fibrosis over the posterior abdominal wall and retroperitoneum. It is associated with raised serum IgG4 levels (see p. 145) and is described on pages 760–761.

Tuberculous peritonitis

This is the second most common form of abdominal TB. Three subgroups can be identified: wet, dry and fibrous.

- In patients with the ***wet*** type, ascitic fluid should be examined for protein concentration (>20 g/L) and tubercle bacilli (rarely found).
- In the ***dry*** form, patients present with subacute intestinal obstruction, which is due to tuberculous small bowel adhesions.
- In the ***fibrous*** form, patients present with abdominal pain, distension and ill-defined, irregular, tender abdominal masses.

The diagnosis of peritoneal TB can be supported by findings on ultrasound or CT screening (mesenteric thickening and lymph node enlargement). A histological diagnosis is not always required before instituting treatment. In some patients, careful laparoscopy (to avoid perforation) may have to be performed, and rarely laparotomy.

Management

Drug treatment is similar to that for pulmonary TB (see pp. 1110–1113) and should be supervised by chest physicians who have experience in dealing with contacts.

Bibliography

Feldman M, Friedman LS, Brandt LL. *Sleisenger and Fordtran's Gastrointestinal and Liver Disease*, 10th edn. Philadelphia: WB Saunders; 2015.

Significant websites

http://www.bsg.org.uk *British Society of Gastroenterology.*
http://www.coeliac.co.uk *Coeliac UK.*
http://www.corecharity.org.uk/Information.html *Gastric ulcer and GORD.*
http://www.nacc.org.uk UK *Crohn's and Colitis UK.*

14 Liver disease

Graham Foster, Alastair O'Brien

See your e-book for key learning points, clinical tips, drug tips, extra tables, extra images, interactive Figures, MCQs and Special Topics from the International Advisory Board.

INTRODUCTION

The aetiology of liver disease differs from region to region. In the developed world, liver inflammation is most often due to obesity, the metabolic syndrome (non-alcoholic fatty liver disease, NAFLD), non-alcoholic steatohepatitis (NASH) and alcohol excess. In the developing world, chronic viral infection with either hepatitis B or hepatitis C is the leading cause of liver mortality. In England, liver disease is the fifth most common cause of premature mortality. Globally, about half a billion people suffer from chronic viral hepatitis. Health education and the improvement in public health, along with vaccination programmes, should help to stop the spread of viral infections and reduce risk factors for the metabolic syndrome.

Cirrhosis represents the final common pathway for liver diseases and is characterized by progressive fibrosis of the liver parenchyma, which leads to portal hypertension and deterioration of liver function. In decompensated cirrhosis, the median overall survival is 2 years, which is a far worse prognosis than for many cancers.

Imaging techniques enable the liver, biliary tree and pancreas to be visualized with precision, resulting in earlier diagnosis. Liver transplantation is an established therapy for both acute and chronic liver disease.

LIVER

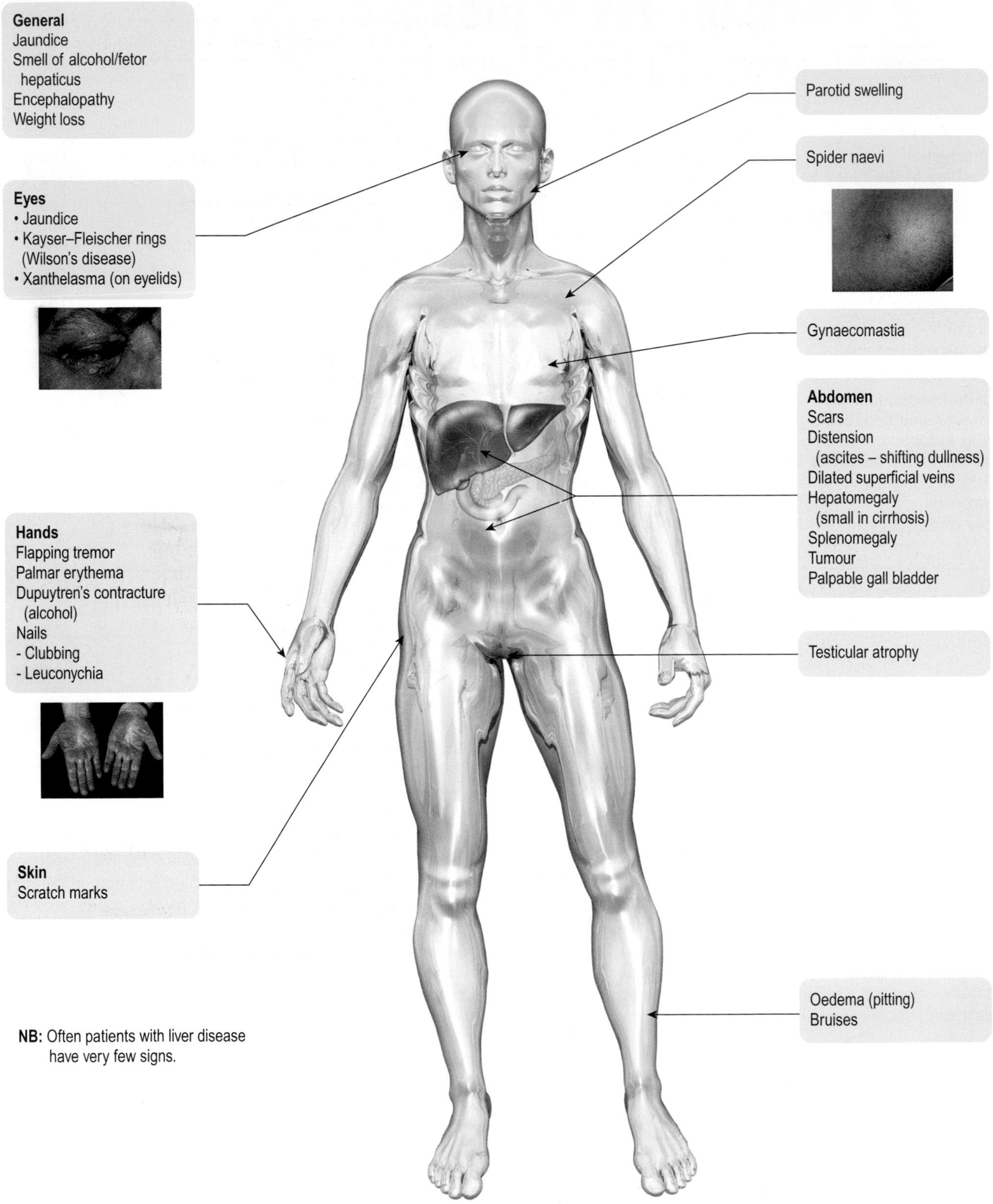

NB: Often patients with liver disease have very few signs.

LIVER

Functions

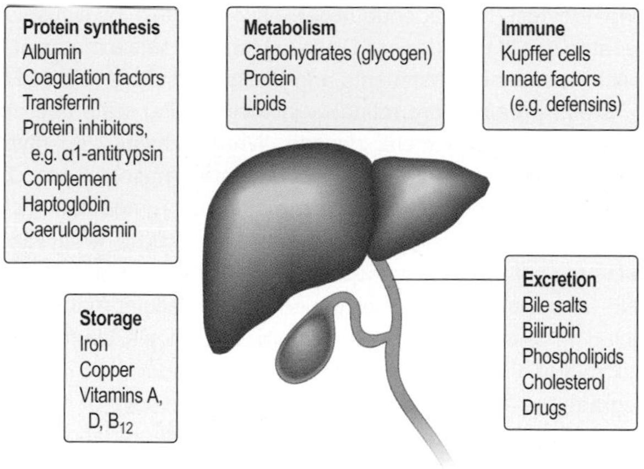

Palpation of liver and spleen

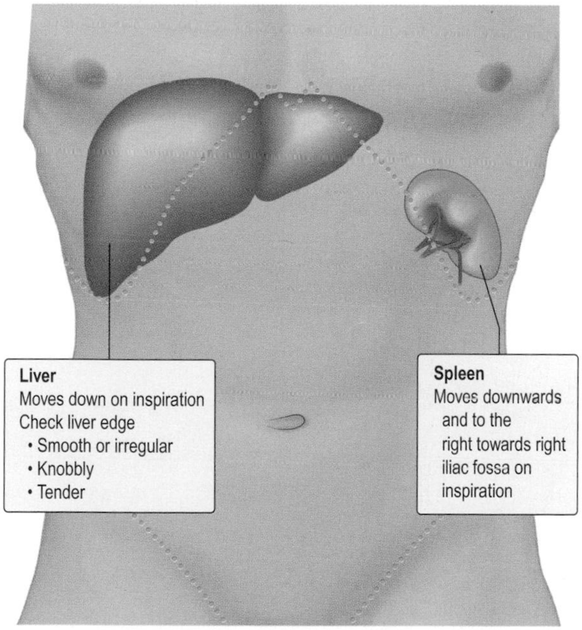

Liver biochemistry and function tests: serum levels

Biochemistry
- ***From hepatocytes***
  - ALT (alanine transferase)
  - AST (aspartate transferase)
  - γGT (gamma glutamyl transpeptidase)
- ***From bile canalicular membranes***
  - ALK (alkaline phosphate)

Function
- Albumin
- Prothrombin time

ADDITIONAL TESTS

Acute liver disease – blood tests and imaging

- **Viral**
  - HBsAg, IgM anti-HBc
  - IgM HAV
  - Anti-HEV
  - Anti-HCV
  - Cytomegalovirus
  - Epstein–Barr
  - Herpes simplex
- **Autoantibodies**
  - Anti-nuclear antibody (ANA)
  - Anti-smooth muscle antibody (ASMA)
  - Liver, kidney, muscle (LKM)
- **Immunoglobulins**
- **Ultrasound of liver**

Chronic liver disease – screening tests

- **Viral**
  - Hepatitis B surface antigen (HBsAg)
  - Hepatitis C antibody
- **Autoantibodies**
  - Anti-nuclear antibody
  - Smooth muscle antibody
  - Anti-mitochondrial antibody (primary biliary cholangitis)
- **Immunoglobulins**
- **Ferritin** - ↑↑ in haemochromatosis
- **Caeruloplasmin ↓, serum copper ↓, urine copper ↑**
  - Wilson's disease
  - α-fetoprotein for hepatocellular carcinoma
- **Ultrasound**

ANATOMY OF THE LIVER AND BILIARY SYSTEM

The liver

The liver is the body's largest internal organ (1.2–1.5 kg) and is situated in the right hypochondrium. A functional division into the larger right lobe (containing caudate and quadrate lobes) and the left lobe is made by the middle hepatic vein. The liver is further subdivided into eight segments ***(Fig. 14.1)*** by divisions of the right, middle and left hepatic veins. Each segment has its own portal pedicle, permitting individual segment resection at surgery.

The hepatic blood supply constitutes 25% of the resting cardiac output and is delivered via two main vessels, entering via the liver hilum (porta hepatis):

- ***The hepatic artery***, a branch of the coeliac axis, supplies 25% of the hepatic blood flow. The hepatic artery autoregulates flow, ensuring a constant total blood flow.
- ***The portal vein*** drains most of the gastrointestinal tract and the spleen. It supplies 75% of hepatic blood flow. The normal portal pressure is 5–8 mmHg; flow increases after meals.

The blood from these vessels is distributed to the segments and flows into the sinusoids via the portal tracts.

Blood leaves the sinusoids, entering branches of the hepatic vein, which join into three main branches before entering the inferior vena cava.

The ***caudate lobe*** is an autonomous segment, as it receives an independent blood supply from the portal vein and hepatic artery, and its hepatic vein drains directly into the inferior vena cava.

Lymph, formed mainly in the perisinusoidal space, is collected in lymphatics that are present in the portal tracts. These small lymphatics enter larger vessels, which eventually drain into the portal system.

The ***acinus*** is the functional hepatic unit. This consists of parenchyma supplied by the smallest portal tracts containing portal vein radicles, hepatic arterioles and bile ductules ***(Fig. 14.2)***. The hepatocytes near this triad (zone 1) are well supplied with oxygenated blood and are more resistant to damage than the cells nearer the terminal hepatic (central) veins (zone 3).

The ***sinusoids*** lack a basement membrane and are loosely surrounded by specialist fenestrated endothelial cells and Kupffer cells (phagocytic cells). Sinusoids are separated by plates of liver cells (hepatocytes). The subendothelial space between the sinusoids and hepatocytes is the space of Disse, which contains a matrix of basement membrane constituents and stellate cells (see ***Fig. 14.21***).

Stellate cells store retinoids in their resting state and contain the intermediate filament, desmin. When activated (to myofibroblasts), they are contractile and regulate sinusoidal blood flow. Endothelin and nitric oxide play a major role in modulating stellate cell contractility. Stellate cells are activated by a wide variety of inflammatory cytokines (such as tumour necrosis factor-alpha, TNF-α); once activated, they generate extracellular matrix proteins, including collagen, leading, eventually, to cirrhosis. Under appropriate conditions, stellate cells can also produce proteases that degrade the extracellular matrix, leading to reversal of fibrosis. The balance between collagen production and degradation is critical to the progression of liver scarring and cirrhosis development/resolution (see p. 466).

The biliary system

Bile canaliculi form a network between the hepatocytes. These join to form thin bile ductules near the portal tract, which, in turn, enter the bile ducts in the portal tracts. These then combine to form the right and left hepatic ducts, which leave each liver lobe. The hepatic ducts join at the porta hepatis to form the common hepatic duct. The cystic duct connects the gall bladder to the lower end of the

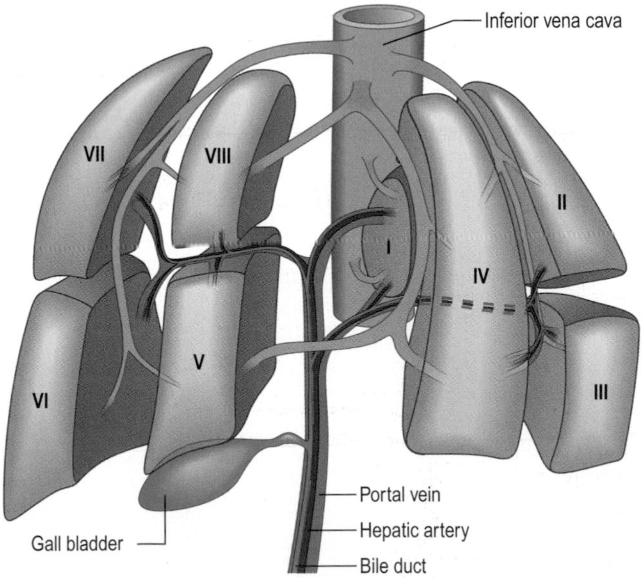

Figure 14.1 Segmental anatomy of the liver. The eight hepatic segments are shown: I, caudate lobe; II–IV, left hemiliver; V–VIII, right hemiliver.

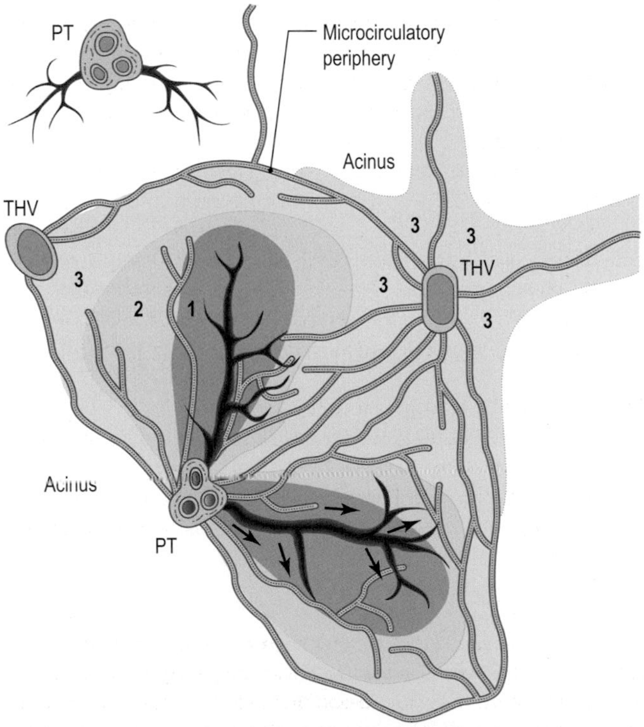

Figure 14.2 The acinus. *Zones 1, 2 and 3* represent areas supplied by blood, with zone 1 being best oxygenated. *Zone 3* is supplied by blood remote from afferent vessels and is in the microcirculatory periphery of the acinus. The perivascular area (the star-shaped green area around the terminal hepatic venule (THV)) is formed by the most peripheral parts of zone 3 and is made up of several adjacent acini; it is the least well oxygenated area. PT, portal triad.

common hepatic duct. The gall bladder lies under the right lobe of the liver and stores and concentrates hepatic bile; its capacity is approximately 50 mL. The common bile duct is formed at the junction of the cystic and common hepatic ducts and is 8 mm in diameter or less, passing through the head of the pancreas, and narrowing at its lower end to pass into the duodenum. The common bile duct and pancreatic duct open into the second part of the duodenum, most often through a common channel at the ampulla of Vater, which contains the muscular sphincter of Oddi. This contracts rhythmically and prevents all of the bile from entering the duodenum, by maintaining a higher pressure than the gall bladder in the fasting state.

FUNCTIONS OF THE LIVER

Protein metabolism (see also page 186)

Synthesis and storage

The liver is the principal site of synthesis of all circulating proteins, apart from γ-globulins (produced in the reticuloendothelial system). The liver receives amino acids from the intestine and muscles and, by controlling the rate of gluconeogenesis and transamination, regulates plasma levels. Plasma contains 60–80 g/L of protein, mainly albumin, globulin and fibrinogen.

Albumin has a half-life of 16–24 days, and 10–12 g is synthesized daily. Its main functions are to maintain intravascular oncotic (colloid osmotic) pressure, and to transport water-insoluble substances such as bilirubin, hormones, fatty acids and drugs. Reduced synthesis of albumin over prolonged periods produces hypoalbuminaemia and is seen in chronic liver disease and malnutrition. Hypoalbuminaemia is also found in hypercatabolic states (e.g. trauma, burns and sepsis) and in diseases associated with an excessive loss (e.g. nephrotic syndrome or protein-losing enteropathy).

Transport or carrier proteins, such as transferrin and caeruloplasmin, acute phase and other proteins (e.g. α_1-antitrypsin and α-fetoprotein) are also produced in the liver.

The liver also synthesizes all coagulation factors (except for one-third of factor VIII) – that is, fibrinogen, prothrombin, factors V, VII, IX, X and XIII, proteins C and S, and antithrombin (see pp. 565–567), as well as components of the complement system. The liver stores large amounts of certain vitamins, particularly A, D and B_{12}, lesser amounts of others (vitamin K and folate), and minerals – iron in ferritin and haemosiderin, and copper.

Degradation (nitrogen excretion)

Amino acids are degraded by transamination and oxidative deamination to produce ammonia, which is then converted to urea and excreted by the kidneys. This is the major pathway for the elimination of nitrogenous waste. Failure of this process occurs in severe liver disease.

Carbohydrate metabolism

Glucose homeostasis and maintenance of blood sugar are major functions of the liver. It stores approximately 80 g of glycogen. In the immediate fasting state, blood glucose is maintained either by glucose release from glycogen breakdown (glycogenolysis) or by synthesis of new glucose (gluconeogenesis). Sources for gluconeogenesis are lactate, pyruvate, amino acids from muscles (mainly alanine and glutamine), and glycerol from lipolysis of fat stores. In prolonged starvation, ketone bodies and fatty acids are used as alternative sources of fuel as body tissues adapt to a lower glucose requirement (see p. 190).

Lipid metabolism

Fats are insoluble in water and are transported in plasma as protein–lipid complexes (lipoproteins). These are discussed in detail on pages 1277–1279.

The liver has a major role in the metabolism of lipoproteins. It synthesizes very-low-density lipoproteins (VLDLs) and high-density lipoproteins (HDLs). HDLs are the substrate for lecithin-cholesterol acyltransferase (LCAT), which catalyses the conversion of free cholesterol to cholesterol ester (see below). Hepatic lipase removes triglyceride from intermediate-density lipoproteins (IDLs) to produce low-density lipoproteins (LDLs) which are degraded by the liver after uptake by specific cell-surface receptors (see ***Fig. 28.3***).

Triglycerides are mainly of dietary origin but are also formed in the liver from circulating free fatty acids (FFAs) and glycerol, and incorporated into VLDLs. Oxidation or *de novo* synthesis of FFAs occurs in the liver, depending on availability of dietary fat.

Cholesterol may be of dietary origin but most is synthesized from acetyl-coenzyme A (acetyl-CoA) in the liver, intestine, adrenal cortex and skin. It either occurs as free cholesterol or is esterified with fatty acids; this reaction is catalysed by LCAT. This enzyme is reduced in severe liver disease, increasing the ratio of free cholesterol to ester, which alters membrane structures. One result of this is the red cell abnormalities (e.g. target cells) seen in chronic liver disease. Phospholipids (e.g. lecithin) are synthesized in the liver. The complex interrelationships between protein, carbohydrate and fat metabolism are shown in ***Figure 14.3***.

Formation of bile

Bile secretion and bile acid metabolism

Bile consists of water, electrolytes, bile acids, cholesterol, phospholipids and conjugated bilirubin. Two processes are involved in bile secretion across the canalicular membrane of the hepatocyte – ***bile salt-dependent*** and ***bile salt-independent*** processes – each

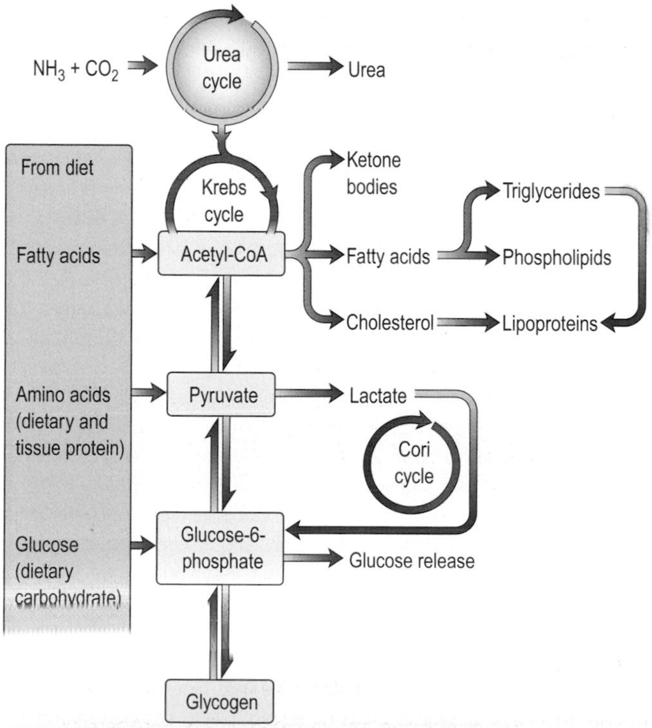

Figure 14.3 Interrelationships of protein, carbohydrate and lipid metabolism in the liver.

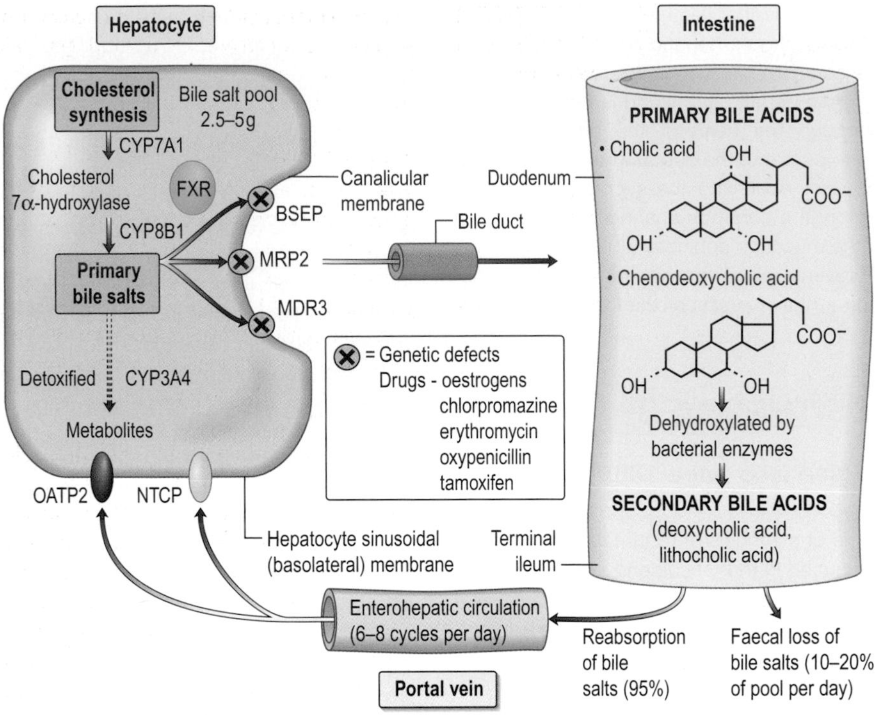

Figure 14.4 Cholesterol synthesis and its conversion to primary and secondary bile acids. All bile acids are normally conjugated with glycine or taurine. BSEP, bile salt export pump; FXR, nuclear farnesoid X receptor; MDR3, multidrug-resistant protein 3; MRP2, multidrug-resistant protein 2; NTCP, sodium taurocholate co-transporting polypeptide; OATP2, sodium-independent organic anion-transporting polypeptide 2.

contributing about 230 mL/day. Another 150 mL/day is produced by bile ductule epithelial cells.

Bile formation requires uptake of bile acids and other organic and inorganic ions across the basolateral (sinusoidal) membranes by multiple transport proteins (sodium taurocholate co-transporting polypeptide (NTCP) and sodium-independent organic anion-transporting polypeptide 2 (OATP2); ***Fig. 14.4***). This process is driven by sodium/potassium adenosine triphosphatase (Na^+/K^+-ATPase) in the basolateral membranes. Intracellular transport across hepatocytes is partly through microtubules and partly by cytosol transport proteins.

Bile acids are also synthesized in hepatocytes from cholesterol, the rate-limiting step being those catalysed mainly by cholesterol-7α-hydroxylase and the P450 enzymes (CYP7A1 and CYP8B1).

The bile acid receptor, farnesoid X, blocks bile acid formation from cholesterol and also regulates the transport proteins (NTCP, OATP2) that increase bile acid uptake by the liver. It is a target for a new class of therapeutic drugs, farnesoid X receptor (FXR) agonists (see pp. 442–443).

The canalicular membrane contains multispecific organic anion transporters, mainly ATPase-dependent (ATP binding cassette), the multidrug-resistant protein 2 (MRP2), multidrug-resistant protein 3 (MDR3) and the bile salt excretory pump (BSEP), which carry a broad range of compounds including bilirubin diglucuronide, glucuronidated and sulphated bile acids, and other organic anions against a concentration gradient into the biliary canaliculus. Na^+ and water follow the passage of bile salts by diffusion across the tight junction between hepatocytes (a bile salt-dependent process). In the bile salt-independent process, water flow is due to other osmotically active solutes such as glutathione and bicarbonate.

Secretion of a bicarbonate-rich solution is stimulated mainly by secretin and inhibited by somatostatin. This involves several membrane proteins, including the Cl^-/HCO_3^- exchanger and the cystic fibrosis transmembrane conductance regulator that controls Cl^- secretion, and water channels (aquaporins) in cholangiocyte membranes.

The bile acids are excreted into bile and pass via the common bile duct into the duodenum. The two primary bile acids – cholic acid and chenodeoxycholic acid ***(Fig. 14.4)*** – are conjugated with glycine or taurine, which increases their solubility. Intestinal bacteria convert these acids into secondary bile acids, deoxycholic and lithocholic acid. ***Figure 14.5*** shows the enterohepatic circulation of bile acids.

The average total bile flow is 600 mL/day. When fasting, half flows into the duodenum and half is diverted into the gall bladder. The gall bladder mucosa absorbs 80–90% of the water and electrolytes, but is impermeable to bile acids and cholesterol. Following a meal, the I cells of the duodenal mucosa secrete cholecystokinin, which stimulates contraction of the gall bladder and relaxation of the sphincter of Oddi, allowing bile to enter the duodenum. An adequate bile flow is dependent on bile salts being returned to the liver by the enterohepatic circulation.

Bile acids act as detergents; their main function is lipid solubilization. Bile acid molecules have both a hydrophilic and a hydrophobic end. In aqueous solutions they form micelles, with their hydrophobic (lipid-soluble) ends in the centre. Micelles are expanded by cholesterol and phospholipids (mainly lecithin), forming mixed micelles.

Bile acid receptors in liver disease

Bile acids have been identified as crucial cell signalling molecules that regulate multiple biological processes. Bile acids are endogenous ligands for FXR and TGR5, a G-protein coupled receptor. Gain- and loss-of-function studies have demonstrated that both are involved in the regulation of lipid and carbohydrate metabolism and inflammatory responses. These receptors may therefore be potential targets for treatment of non-alcoholic fatty liver disease (NAFLD). Furthermore,

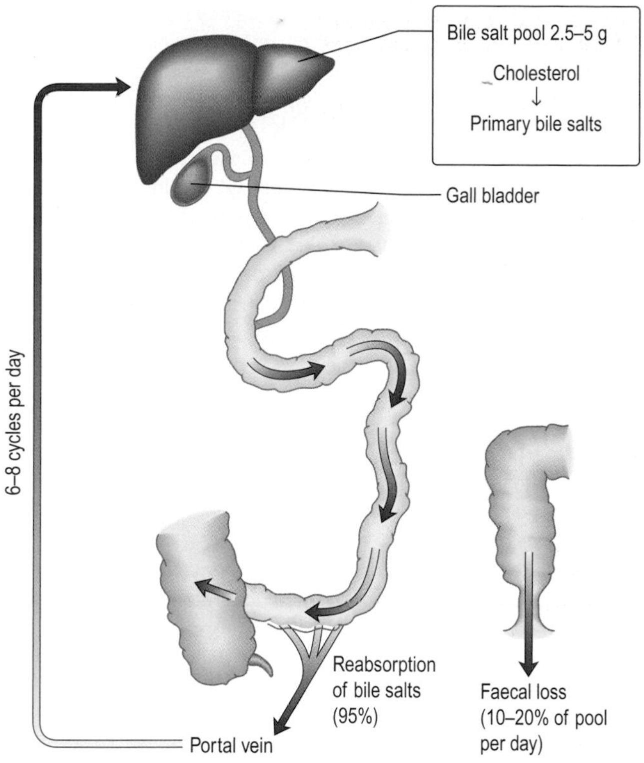

Figure 14.5 Recirculation of bile acids. The bile salt pool is relatively small and the entire pool recycles 6–8 times via the enterohepatic circulation. Synthesis of new bile acids compensates for faecal loss.

recent experimental and phase II studies have shown that the FXR agonist, obeticholic acid, may be beneficial in primary biliary cholangitis (PBC). Obeticholic acid also improves portal hypertension in rodents. It is hoped that these experimental and early-phase findings will translate into new treatments.

Bilirubin metabolism

Bilirubin is produced mainly from the breakdown of mature red cells by Kupffer cells in the liver and reticuloendothelial system; 15% of bilirubin is formed from catabolism of other haem-containing proteins, such as myoglobin, cytochromes and catalases.

Normally, 250–300 mg (425–510 mmol) of bilirubin are produced daily. The iron and globin are removed from haem and reused. Biliverdin is formed from haem and reduced to form bilirubin (see p. 521). The bilirubin produced is unconjugated and water-insoluble, due to internal hydrogen bonding, and is transported to the liver attached to albumin. Bilirubin dissociates from albumin and is taken up by hepatic cell membranes and transported to the endoplasmic reticulum by cytoplasmic proteins, where it is conjugated with glucuronic acid and excreted into bile. The microsomal enzyme, uridine diphosphoglucuronosyl transferase, catalyses the formation of bilirubin monoglucuronide and then diglucuronide. This conjugated bilirubin is water-soluble; it is actively secreted into biliary canaliculi and excreted into the intestine within bile (see ***Fig. 16.5***). It is not absorbed from the small intestine because of its large molecular size. In the terminal ileum, bacterial enzymes hydrolyse the molecule, releasing free bilirubin, which is then reduced to urobilinogen; some of this is excreted in the stools as stercobilinogen. The remainder is absorbed by the terminal ileum, passes to the liver via the enterohepatic circulation, and is re-excreted into bile. Urobilinogen bound to albumin enters the circulation and is excreted in urine via the kidneys. When hepatic excretion of conjugated bilirubin is impaired, a small amount is strongly bound to serum albumin and is not excreted by the kidneys; it accounts for persisting hyperbilirubinaemia after cholestasis has resolved.

Hormone and drug inactivation

The liver catabolizes hormones such as insulin, glucagon, oestrogens, growth hormone, glucocorticoids and parathyroid hormone. It is also the prime target organ for many hormones (e.g. insulin). It is the major site for the metabolism of drugs (see p. 487) and alcohol (see pp. 217–218). Fat-soluble drugs are converted to water-soluble substances that facilitate their excretion in the bile or urine. Cholecalciferol is converted to 25-hydroxycholecalciferol.

Immunological function

The liver plays a key role in the innate immune response and acts as a 'sieve' for bacterial and other antigens carried to it by the portal vein from the gastrointestinal tract (see p. 468).

Hepatocytes are responsible for biosynthesis of 80–90% of innate immune proteins, including complement components and many secreted pattern-recognition receptors (PRRs) expressed by host cells. Kupffer cells (KCs), which account for 80–90% of the total population of fixed tissue macrophages, are a critical component of the mononuclear phagocytic system and are central to both the hepatic and the systemic responses to pathogens. Following stimulation by endotoxin, the Kupffer cells release interleukin (IL)-6, IL-8 and TNF-α, and, in combination with liver sinusoidal cells, are responsible for the elimination of molecular wastes from the body.

In addition, liver lymphocytes are rich in innate immune cells, including natural killer and T cell receptor γδ T cells. Finally, nonparenchymal liver cells express high levels of membrane-bound PRRs, such as Toll-like receptor cells (TLRs). Not only does innate immunity in the liver play a key role in host defence against microbial infection and tumour formation, but it also contributes to the pathogenesis of acute and chronic liver diseases, including alcoholic liver disease (see pp. 480–482).

Further reading

Dooley J, Lok A, Burroughs AK et al. Anatomy and function. In: *Sherlock's Diseases of the Liver and Biliary System*, 12th edn. London: Wiley–Blackwell; 2011.

Li Y, Jadhav K, Zhang Y. Bile acid receptors in non-alcoholic fatty liver disease. *Biochem Pharmacol* 2013; 86:1517–1524.

CLINICAL APPROACH TO THE PATIENT WITH LIVER DISEASE

Investigations

Investigative tests can be divided into:

- ***Blood tests***:
  - Liver 'function' tests: serum albumin and bilirubin; prothrombin time (PT)
  - Liver biochemistry: serum aspartate (AST) and alanine aminotransferases (ALT) – an increase reflects hepatocellular damage; serum alkaline phosphatase (ALP) and gamma-glutamyl transpeptidase (γ-GT) – an increase reflects cholestasis; total protein.
  - Viral markers.
  - Additional blood investigations; haematological, biochemical, immunological, markers of liver fibrosis and genetic analysis.

Box 14.1 Useful blood and urine tests for certain liver diseases

Test	Disease
Anti-mitochondrial antibody	Primary biliary cholangitis
Anti-nuclear, smooth muscle (actin), liver/kidney microsomal antibody	Autoimmune hepatitis
Raised serum immunoglobulins:	
IgG	Autoimmune hepatitis
IgG4	Autoimmune hepatitis/ cholangiopathy and pancreatitis
IgM	Primary biliary cholangitis
Viral markers	Hepatitis A, B, C, D, E and others
α-Fetoprotein	Hepatocellular carcinoma
Serum iron, transferrin saturation, serum ferritin	Hereditary haemochromatosis
Serum and urinary copper, serum caeruloplasmin	Wilson's disease
α_1-Antitrypsin	α_1-Antitrypsin deficiency (cirrhosis (± emphysema))
Anti-nuclear cytoplasmic antibodies (ANCA)	Primary sclerosing cholangitis
Markers of liver fibrosis (p. 445)	Non-alcoholic fatty liver disease
	Hepatitis C
Genetic analyses	e.g. *HFE* gene (hereditary haemochromatosis), α_1-antitrypsin

- ***Urine tests*** – for bilirubin and urobilinogen.
- ***Imaging techniques*** – to define gross anatomy.
- ***Liver biopsy*** – for histology.

Blood tests ordered for 'liver function' are usually processed by an automated multichannel analyser to produce serum levels of bilirubin, aminotransferases, alkaline phosphatase, γ-GT and total proteins. These routine tests are markers of liver damage but not actual tests of 'function' *per se*. Subsequent investigations are often based on these tests.

Blood tests

Useful blood tests for certain liver diseases are shown in ***Box 14.1***.

Liver function tests

Serum albumin

This is a marker of synthetic function and is useful for gauging the severity of chronic liver disease: a falling serum albumin is a bad prognostic sign. In acute liver disease, initial albumin levels may be normal. Interpretation of a low albumin can be difficult when other causes of hypoalbuminaemia (e.g. malnutrition, urinary protein loss or sepsis) are present.

Bilirubin

Serum bilirubin is normally almost all unconjugated. In liver disease, increased serum bilirubin is usually accompanied by other abnormalities in liver biochemistry. Differentiation between conjugated or unconjugated bilirubin is only necessary in congenital disorders of bilirubin metabolism (see below) or to exclude haemolysis.

Prothrombin time

Prothrombin time (PT) is also a marker of synthetic function. Because of its short half-life, it is a sensitive indicator of both acute and chronic liver disease. Vitamin K deficiency should be excluded as the cause of a prolonged PT by giving an intravenous bolus (10 mg) of vitamin K. Vitamin K deficiency commonly occurs in biliary obstruction, as the low intestinal concentration of bile salts results in poor absorption of vitamin K.

Prothrombin times vary in different laboratories, depending upon the thromboplastin used in the assay. The International Normalized Ratio (INR) was developed to standardize anticoagulation with coumarin derivatives but is very variable in liver disease, and causes large differences when included in prognostic scores for cirrhosis across different centres. A rising INR in patients with liver disease that is not corrected by vitamin K is a poor prognostic sign.

Liver biochemistry

Aminotransferases

These enzymes (often referred to as transaminases) are contained in hepatocytes and leak into the blood with liver cell damage. Two enzymes are measured:

- ***Aspartate aminotransferase*** (AST) is primarily a mitochondrial enzyme (80%; 20% in cytoplasm) and is also present in heart, muscle, kidney and brain. High levels are seen in hepatic necrosis, myocardial infarction, muscle injury and congestive cardiac failure.
- ***Alanine aminotransferase*** (ALT) is a cytosol enzyme, more specific to the liver, so that a rise only occurs with liver disease.

  The ALT : AST ratio is a useful clinical indicator.
  - In viral hepatitis, ALT is greater than AST unless cirrhosis is present, in which case AST is greater than ALT.
  - In alcoholic liver disease and steatohepatitis, the AST is often greater than the ALT.
  - In patients with viral hepatitis, an AST : ALT ratio of more than 1 indicates cirrhosis.
  - In patients with liver disease without cirrhosis, in whom AST is greater than ALT, alcohol or obesity is the most likely aetiological agent.

Alkaline phosphatase

Alkaline phosphatase (ALP) is present in hepatic canalicular and sinusoidal membranes, and also in bone, intestine and placenta. If necessary, its origin can be determined by electrophoretic separation of isoenzymes or bone-specific monoclonal antibodies. In clinical practice, if the γ-GT is also abnormal, the ALP is presumed to come from the liver.

Serum ALP is raised in both intrahepatic and extrahepatic cholestatic disease of any cause, due to increased synthesis. In cholestatic jaundice, levels may be 4–6 times the normal limit. Raised levels also occur with hepatic infiltrations (e.g. metastases) and in cirrhosis, frequently in the absence of jaundice. The highest serum levels due to liver disease (>1000 IU/L) are seen with hepatic metastases and PBC.

γ-Glutamyl transpeptidase

This is a microsomal enzyme present in liver, and also in many tissues. Its activity can be induced by many drugs such as phenytoin, warfarin and rifampicin, and by alcohol. If the ALP is normal, a raised serum γ-GT can be a useful guide to alcohol intake (see p. 921). However, mild elevations of γ-GT are common, even with minimal alcohol consumption, and it is also raised in fatty liver disease. In the absence of other liver function test abnormalities, a slightly raised γ-GT can safely be ignored. In cholestasis, the γ-GT rises in parallel with the ALP, as it has a similar pathway of excretion. This is also true of 5-nucleotidase, another microsomal enzyme that can be measured in blood.

Total proteins and globulin fraction

The globulin fraction is often raised in autoimmune hepatitis; if it falls, it indicates successful therapy.

Viral markers

Viruses are a major cause of liver disease. Virological studies have a key role in diagnosis; markers are available for most common viruses that cause hepatitis.

Additional blood investigations

Haematological tests

A full blood count may show thrombocytopenia. Thrombocytopenia is a common finding in cirrhosis and is often aggravated by alcohol-induced bone marrow suppression. A low platelet count (below the lower limit of normal – 150×10^9/L) should be regarded as indicative of cirrhosis, unless another cause can be found. In alcohol excess, red blood cells are often macrocytic.

Biochemical tests

- ***α_1-Antitrypsin*** enzyme deficiency can produce cirrhosis.
- ***α-Fetoprotein*** is normally produced by the fetal liver. Its reappearance in increasing and high concentrations in adults indicates hepatocellular carcinoma. Increased concentrations in pregnancy in blood and amniotic fluid suggest fetal neural tube defects. Blood levels are also slightly raised with regenerative liver tissue in patients with hepatitis, chronic liver disease and also teratomas.
- ***Urinary copper*** is raised, and serum copper and caeruloplasmin are low in Wilson's disease (see p. 479).

Immunological tests

Serum immunoglobulins Increased γ-globulins are thought to result from reduced phagocytosis by sinusoidal and Kupffer cells of the gut-absorbed antigens. These antigens then stimulate antibody production in the spleen, lymph nodes and portal tract lymphoid and plasma cell infiltrates. In PBC, the predominant raised serum immunoglobulin is IgM, while in autoimmune hepatitis it is IgG. IgG4 is raised in autoimmune pancreatitis/cholangitis (see p. 506 and ***Box 8.12***).

Serum autoantibodies

- ***Anti-mitochondrial antibody (AMA)*** in serum is found in over 95% of patients with PBC (see p. 475). Several different AMA subtypes are described, depending on their antigen specificity, and are also found in autoimmune hepatitis and other autoimmune diseases. AMA is demonstrated by an immunofluorescent technique and is neither organ- nor species-specific. The M2 subtype is specific for PBC.
- ***Nucleic, smooth muscle (actin), liver/kidney microsomal antibodies*** can be found in serum, often in high titre, in patients with autoimmune hepatitis. These serum antibodies are also present in other autoimmune conditions and other liver diseases.
- ***Anti-nuclear cytoplasmic antibodies (ANCA)*** can be found in the serum of patients with primary sclerosing cholangitis (see pp. 476–477).

Markers of liver fibrosis

Fibrosis plays a key role in the outcome of many chronic liver diseases, and accurate assessment of fibrosis is critical for the appropriate management of many liver disorders. A variety of different systems have been developed to assess the extent of liver fibrosis and these range from algorithms of varying degrees of complexity that use standard haematological and biochemical tests, to novel biomarkers. Simple algorithms include the **APRI** (***a***spartate aminotransferase to ***p***latelet ***r***atio ***i***ndex) score, while more complex commercial tests include the **fibrotest algorithm**. Novel biomarker-based algorithms include those based on measurements of hyaluronic acid, procollagen III amino terminal peptide and tissue inhibitor of metalloproteinase I (TIMP-1), all combined in the **enhanced liver fibrosis (ELF) test**. In general, these markers have been developed for chronic hepatitis C but they are often successfully applied to other liver disorders. The current assays have a high sensitivity/specificity for the detection or absence of cirrhosis but are less effective at detecting intermediate levels of fibrosis. Combining mechanical non-invasive fibrosis tests, such as transient elastography (see p. 446), with fibrosis markers allows many patients to avoid a liver biopsy to assess fibrosis.

Genetic analysis

These tests are performed routinely for haemochromatosis (*HFE* gene) and for α_1-antitrypsin deficiency. Markers are also available for the most frequent abnormal genes in Wilson's disease (see p. 479).

Urine tests

Dipstick tests are available for ***bilirubin*** and ***urobilinogen***. Bilirubinuria is due to the presence of conjugated (soluble) bilirubin; it is found in patients with jaundice due to hepatobiliary disease, but is absent if unconjugated bilirubin is the major cause of jaundice. The presence of urobilinogen in urine is of little value in practice but suggests haemolysis or hepatic dysfunction.

Imaging techniques

Ultrasound examination

This is a non-invasive, safe and relatively cheap technique. It involves the analysis of the reflected ultrasound beam detected by a probe moved across the abdomen. The normal liver appears as a relatively homogeneous structure. The gall bladder, common bile duct, pancreas, portal vein and other structures in the abdomen can be visualized. **Abdominal ultrasound is useful in**:

- Detection of extrahepatic obstruction (the bile duct is usually dilated, particularly in advanced disease). Note that opiates may cause biliary dilatation without obstruction, and so scans in injecting drug users often show extrahepatic biliary dilatation.
- Assessment of a jaundiced patient (to exclude obstruction) (see p. 450).
- Assessment of hepatomegaly/splenomegaly.
- Detection of gallstones (see ***Fig. 15.2***).
- Assessment of focal liver disease – lesions >1 cm.
- Assessment of portal and hepatic vein patency.
- Assessment of the hepatic parenchyma – diffuse fatty infiltration often leads to a 'bright' appearance on ultrasound but experience is required to distinguish this from normal variation.
- Identification of cirrhosis – in advanced cirrhosis, the liver edge is irregular and the spleen is often enlarged. Note that a normal ultrasound does not exclude cirrhosis.
- Assessment of lymph node enlargement.

Other abdominal masses can be delineated and biopsies obtained under ultrasonic guidance.

Colour Doppler ultrasound

This will demonstrate vascularity within a lesion, and the direction of portal and hepatic vein blood flow.

Ultrasound contrast agents

These are mostly based on the production of microbubbles within flowing blood. They enhance the detection of vascularity, allowing the detection of abnormal circulation within liver nodules, and giving a more specific diagnosis of hepatocellular carcinoma.

Hepatic stiffness (transient elastography)

Using an ultrasound transducer, a vibration of low frequency and amplitude is passed through the liver, the velocity of which correlates with hepatic stiffness. Stiffness (measured in kPa) increases with worsening liver fibrosis (sensitivity and specificity 80–95%, compared to liver biopsy). Elastography can reliably exclude cirrhosis and there is some evidence to show that, in cirrhosis, increasing liver stiffness is associated with a higher risk of complications. Elastography is less effective for determining lesser degrees of fibrosis but, particularly when combined with non-invasive fibrosis tests (see above), it can be used to exclude cirrhosis reliably. It cannot be employed in the presence of ascites and morbid obesity, and is affected by inflammatory tissue and congestion.

Acoustic radiation force impulse is incorporated into standard B mode ultrasonography and has similar physical principles to transient elastography.

Computed tomography examination

Computed tomography (CT), during or immediately after intravenous contrast, shows both arterial and portal venous phases of enhancement, enabling more precise characterization of a lesion and its vascular supply ***(Fig. 14.6)***. Retrospective analysis of data allows multiple overlapping slices to be obtained with no increase in the radiation dose, providing excellent visualization of the size, shape and density of the liver, pancreas, spleen, lymph nodes and lesions in the porta hepatis. Multiplanar and three-dimensional reconstruction in the arterial phase can create a CT angiogram, often making formal invasive angiography unnecessary. CT also provides guidance for biopsy. It has advantages over ultrasound in detecting calcification and is useful in obese subjects, although ultrasound is usually the imaging modality used first to investigate liver disease.

Magnetic resonance imaging

Magnetic resonance imaging (MRI) produces cross-sectional images in any plane within the body and does not involve radiation. It is the most sensitive investigation for focal liver disease but can also assess fibrosis. Diffuse liver disease alters the T1 and T2 characteristics. Other fat-suppression modes, such as ***short T1 inversion recovery (STIR)***, allow good differentiation between haemangiomas and other lesions. Contrast agents such as intravenous gadolinium, which allow further characterization of lesions, are suitable for those with iodine allergy, and provide angiography and venography of the splanchnic circulation. Use of these agents has superseded direct arteriography.

Magnetic resonance cholangiopancreatography

Magnetic resonance cholangiopancreatography (MRCP) involves the manipulation of data acquired by MRI. A heavily T2-weighted sequence enhances visualization of the 'water-filled' bile ducts and pancreatic ducts to produce high-quality images of ductal anatomy. This non-invasive technique is replacing diagnostic (but not therapeutic) endoscopic retrograde cholangiopancreatography

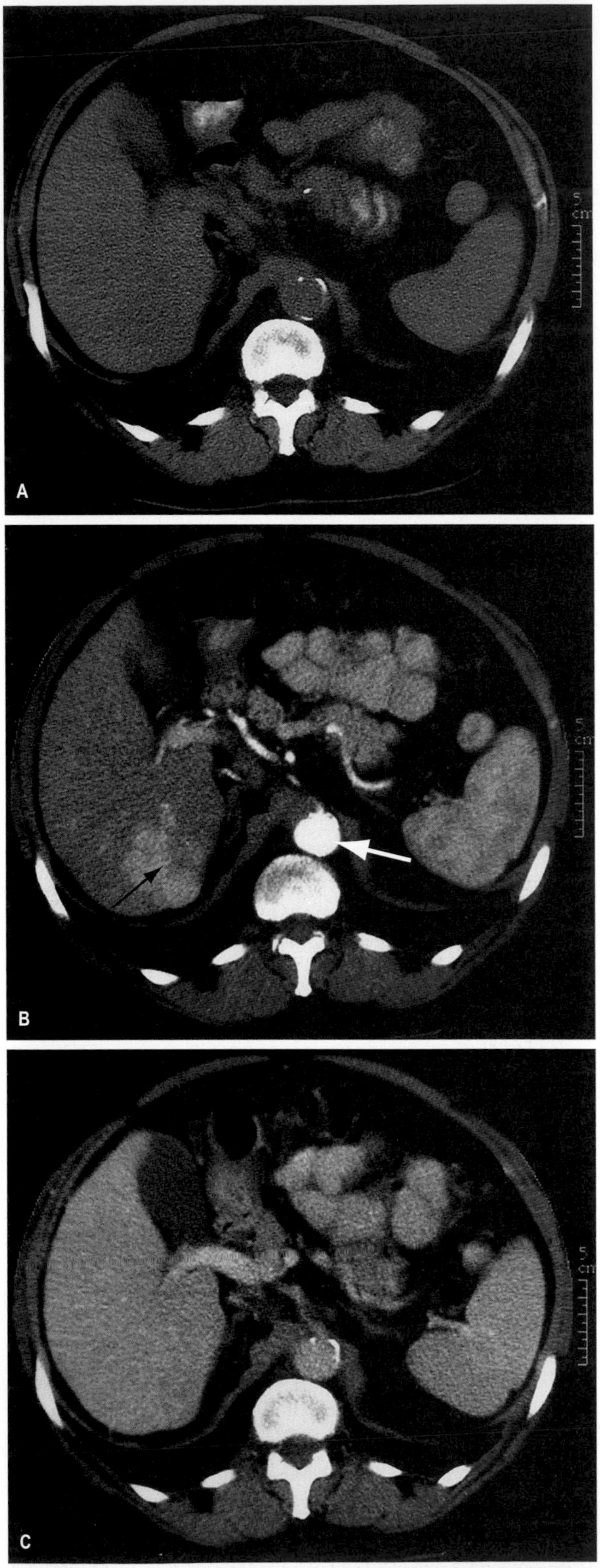

Figure 14.6 Use of contrast-enhanced spiral CT. A. Unenhanced. B. Arterial phase (note high-density contrast in the aorta (thick arrow)). There is an irregular mass (thin arrow) in the posterior aspect of the right lobe of the liver, which is only well seen on this early arterial phase enhanced scan. **C. Portal venous phase** scan through the right lobe of the liver.

(see p. 501), and is usually the next test to be applied if a biliary abnormality is present on ultrasound examination.

Plain X-rays of the abdomen

These are rarely requested but may show:

- gallstones – 10% contain enough calcium to be seen
- air in the biliary tree owing to its recent instrumentation, surgery, or a fistula between the intestine and the gall bladder
- pancreatic calcification
- rarely, calcification of the gall bladder (porcelain gall bladder).

Radionuclide imaging – scintiscanning

In a ^{99m}Tc-IODIDA scan, technetium-labelled iododiethyl IDA is taken up by the hepatocytes and excreted rapidly into the biliary system. Its main uses are in the diagnosis of:

- acute cholecystitis
- jaundice due to either biliary atresia or hepatitis in the neonatal period.

Endoscopy

Upper gastrointestinal endoscopy is used for diagnosis and treatment of varices, detection of portal hypertensive gastropathy, and for detection of associated lesions such as peptic ulcers. Colonoscopy may show portal hypertensive colopathy. Capsule endoscopy can identify small intestinal varices.

Endoscopic retrograde cholangiopancreatography

Endoscopic retrograde cholangiopancreatography (ERCP) outlines the biliary and pancreatic ducts (see p. 501).

Angiography

This is performed by selective catheterization of the coeliac axis and hepatic artery. It outlines the hepatic vasculature and the abnormal vasculature of hepatic tumours, but spiral CT and MRI have replaced diagnostic angiography. The portal vein can be demonstrated with increased definition using subtraction techniques that have replaced splenoportography (by direct splenic puncture).

In ***digital vascular imaging*** (DVI), contrast given intravenously or intra-arterially can be detected in the portal system using computerized subtraction analysis.

Hepatic venous cannulation allows abnormal hepatic veins to be diagnosed in patients with Budd–Chiari syndrome and is also used to measure portal pressure indirectly. There is a 1 : 1 relationship of occluded (by balloon) hepatic venous pressure with portal pressure in patients with alcoholic or viral-related cirrhosis. The height of portal pressure has prognostic value for survival in cirrhosis: a difference of the occluded minus the free hepatic venous pressure (hepatic venous pressure gradient, HVPG) of 20% or more from baseline values, or <12 mmHg, has been associated with protection from rebleeding, and prevention of other complications of cirrhosis.

Liver biopsy

Histological examination of the liver is valuable in the differential diagnosis of diffuse or localized parenchymal disease and its severity. Liver biopsy can be performed on a day-case basis. The indications and contraindications are shown in ***Box 14.2***. The mortality rate is less than 0.02% when the technique is performed by experienced operators.

Liver biopsy guided by ultrasound or CT is performed under a local anaesthetic via a percutaneous approach in the right intercostal space. A transjugular approach is used when liver histology is essential for management but coagulation abnormalities or ascites prevent the percutaneous approach.

Most ***complications*** of liver biopsy occur within 24 hours (usually in the first 2 hours). They are often minor, and include abdominal or shoulder pain that settles with analgesics. Minor intraperitoneal bleeding can occur but this settles spontaneously. Rare complications include major intraperitoneal bleeding, haemothorax and pleurisy, biliary peritonitis, haemobilia and transient septicaemia. Haemobilia produces biliary colic, jaundice and melaena within 3 days of the biopsy.

Box 14.2 Indications for and contraindications to liver biopsy

Diagnosis
- Multiple parenchymal liver diseases
- Abnormal liver tests of unknown aetiology
- Fever of unknown origin
- Focal or diffuse abnormalities on imaging studies (rarely for HCC)
- Unexplained hepatomegaly
- Drug-related liver disease
- Post liver transplant

Prognosis
- Staging of known parenchymal liver disease, e.g. hepatitis B/C, NAFLD, PBC, AIH, PSC
- Haemochromatosis and alcohol-induced liver disease

Management
- Development of treatment plans based on histological analysis

Usual contraindications to percutaneous needle biopsy
- Uncooperative patient
- Prolonged INR (>1.5)*
- Platelets $<60 \times 10^9$/L*
- Ascites
- Extrahepatic cholestasis

AIH, autoimmune hepatitis; HCC, hepatocellular carcinoma; INR, International Normalized Ratio; NAFLD, non-alcoholic fatty liver disease; PBC, primary biliary cholangitis; PSC, primary sclerosing cholangitis.

Further reading

Tripodi A, Mannucci PM. The coagulopathy of chronic liver disease. *N Engl J Med* 2011; 365:147–156.

Clinical features of liver disease

Symptoms

Acute liver disease

This may be asymptomatic and anicteric. Symptomatic disease, often viral, produces malaise, anorexia and fever. Jaundice (see below) may appear as the illness progresses.

Chronic liver disease

Patients may be asymptomatic or experience non-specific symptoms, particularly weakness, anorexia and fatigue. Specific symptoms include:

- right hypochondrial pain due to liver distension
- abdominal distension due to ascites
- ankle swelling due to fluid retention
- haematemesis and melaena from gastrointestinal haemorrhage
- pruritus due to cholestasis – often an early symptom of PBC
- gynaecomastia, loss of libido and amenorrhoea due to endocrine dysfunction

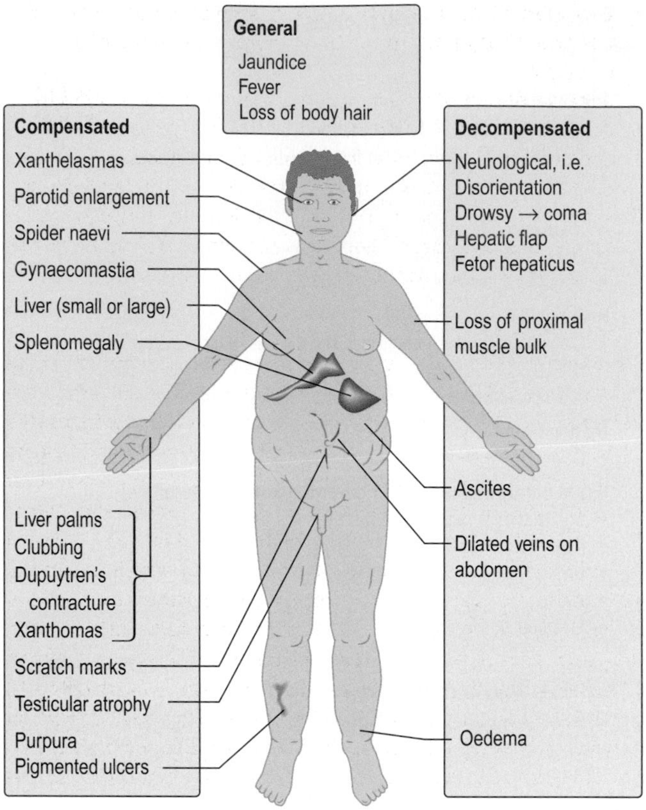

Figure 14.7 Physical signs in chronic liver disease.

- confusion and drowsiness due to neuropsychiatric complications (portosystemic encephalopathy).

Signs

Acute liver disease

There may be few signs, apart from jaundice and an enlarged liver. Jaundice is a yellow discoloration of the skin and mucous membranes, and is best seen in the conjunctivae and sclerae. In the cholestatic phase of the illness, pale stools and dark urine are present. Spider naevi and palmar erythema usually indicate chronic disease but can occur in severe acute disease.

Chronic liver disease

The physical signs are shown in ***Figure 14.7***. However, physical examination is occasionally normal in patients with advanced chronic liver disease.

The skin

The chest and upper body may show ***spider naevi***. These are telangiectases that consist of a central arteriole with radiating small vessels (resembling a spider's legs). They are found in the distribution of the superior vena cava and more than five are diagnostic. They may also occur in pregnancy.

In haemochromatosis, the skin may have a slate-grey appearance.

The hands may show ***palmar erythema***, indicative of a hyperdynamic circulation; it is also seen in pregnancy, thyrotoxicosis or rheumatoid arthritis. Clubbing occasionally occurs, and a Dupuytren's contracture is often seen in alcoholic cirrhosis, though the association is with alcohol consumption rather than liver disease itself.

Xanthomas (cholesterol deposits) are seen in the palmar creases or above the eyes in PBC.

The abdomen

Initial hepatomegaly will be followed by a small liver in well-established cirrhosis. Splenomegaly occurs with portal hypertension.

The endocrine system

Gynaecomastia (occasionally unilateral) and testicular atrophy may be found in males. Gynaecomastia is probably related to altered oestrogen metabolism, often combined with spironolactone treatment.

Additional physical signs in decompensated cirrhosis are shown in ***Figure 14.7***.

JAUNDICE

Jaundice (icterus) is detectable clinically when the serum bilirubin is >50 µmol/L (3 mg/dL). It may be divided into:

- ***haemolytic jaundice*** – increased bilirubin load for the liver cells
- ***congenital hyperbilirubinaemias*** – defects in conjugation
- ***cholestatic jaundice*** – including hepatocellular (parenchymal) liver disease and large duct obstruction.

Haemolytic jaundice

The increased breakdown of red cells (see p. 521) leads to an increase in production of bilirubin. The resulting jaundice is usually mild (serum bilirubin of 68–102 µmol/L, or 4–6 mg/dL), as normal liver function can easily manage the increased bilirubin. Unconjugated bilirubin is not water-soluble and therefore does not pass into urine: hence 'acholuric jaundice'. Urinary urobilinogen is increased.

The causes are those of haemolytic anaemia (pp. 531–533), and clinical features of anaemia, jaundice, splenomegaly, gallstones and leg ulcers may be seen.

Investigations show haemolysis (p. 532) and elevated unconjugated bilirubin, but normal serum ALP, transferases and albumin. Serum haptoglobulins are low.

Congenital hyperbilirubinaemias (non-haemolytic)

Unconjugated types

Gilbert syndrome

This is the most common familial conjugated hyperbilirubinaemia and affects 2–7% of the population. It is asymptomatic and usually detected incidentally with a raised bilirubin (17–102 µmol/L, or 1–6 mg/dL). All other liver biochemistry is normal and there are no signs of liver disease. There is a family history of jaundice in 5–15% of patients. Most patients have reduced levels of UDP-glucuronosyl transferase (UGT-1) activity, the enzyme that conjugates bilirubin with glucuronic acid.

Mutations occur in the gene (UGT1A1 promoter region) encoding this enzyme, with an expanded nucleotide repeat consisting of two extra bases in the upstream 5′ promoter element. This abnormality appears to be necessary for the syndrome, but is not in itself sufficient for clinical manifestation (phenotypic expression).

Establishing the diagnosis is necessary to provide reassurance and prevent unnecessary investigations. The raised unconjugated bilirubin is diagnostic and rises on fasting and during mild illness. The reticulocyte count is normal, excluding haemolysis, and no treatment is necessary.

Crigler–Najjar syndrome

This is very rare. Only patients with type II (autosomal dominant) disease, with a decrease in rather than absence (type I – autosomal recessive) of UGT survive into adult life. Liver histology is normal. Transplantation is the only effective treatment.

Conjugated types

Dubin–Johnson and Rotor syndromes

Dubin–Johnson and Rotor syndromes (autosomal recessive) are due to defects in hepatic bilirubin handling. The prognosis is good in both. In the Dubin–Johnson syndrome, the liver is black owing to melanin deposition.

Benign recurrent intrahepatic cholestasis

This is rare and presents in early adulthood. Recurrent attacks of acute cholestasis occur without progression to chronic liver disease. Jaundice, severe pruritus, steatorrhoea and weight loss develop. Serum γ-GT is normal. Benign recurrent intrahepatic cholestasis may be associated with intrahepatic cholestasis of pregnancy (see p. 1304).

Progressive familial intrahepatic cholestasis syndromes

Progressive familial intrahepatic cholestasis (PFIC) syndromes are a heterogeneous group of autosomal recessive conditions defined by defective secretion of bile acids (see ***Figs 14.4*** and ***15.1***).

- In ***type 1*** (PFIC1), with cholestasis in the first weeks of life, the γ-GT is normal.
- In ***type 2*** (PFIC2), there is frequently a non-specific giant cell hepatitis that progresses to cholestasis; again, γ-GT is normal.
- In ***type 3*** (PFIC3), deficient canalicular phosphatidylcholine transport and accumulation of toxic bile acids cause liver damage, which can lead to cirrhosis.

Liver transplantation is the only cure for these syndromes.

Cholestatic jaundice (acquired)

This condition can be divided into extrahepatic and intrahepatic cholestasis. The causes are shown in ***Figure 14.8***.

- ***Extrahepatic cholestasis*** is due to large duct obstruction of bile flow at any point in the biliary tract distal to the bile canaliculi.
- ***Intrahepatic cholestasis*** occurs because of failure of bile secretion, which may be caused by intrinsic defects in bile secretion or inflammation in the intrahepatic ducts.

Clinically, in both types, there is jaundice with pale stools and dark urine, and the serum bilirubin is conjugated. However, intrahepatic and extrahepatic cholestatic jaundice must be differentiated, as their clinical management is entirely different.

Differential diagnosis of jaundice

Jaundice may occur in previously healthy people who have an acute hepatic illness or may develop in patients with cirrhosis who have 'decompensated' (see p. 448). The management of decompensated cirrhosis is described on page 467 but all patients with jaundice should be questioned closely about risk factors for chronic liver disease to determine whether this is a true acute presentation rather than an 'acute on chronic' illness. The history often gives a clue to the diagnosis. Certain causes of jaundice are more likely in particular categories of people. For example, a young person is more likely to have infectious hepatitis, so questions should be asked about drug and alcohol misuse, and sexual behaviour. An elderly person with gross weight loss is more likely to have a carcinoma. All patients may complain of malaise. Abdominal pain occurs in patients with biliary obstruction by gallstones, and sometimes with an enlarged liver there is pain resulting from distension of the capsule.

Questions should be appropriate to the particular situation, and the following aspects of the history should be covered:

- ***Country of origin***. The incidence of hepatitis B virus (HBV) and hepatitis C virus (HCV) infection is increased in many parts of the world (see pp. 454–455).
- ***Duration of illness***. A history of jaundice with prolonged weight loss in an older patient suggests malignancy. A short history, particularly with a prodromal illness of malaise, suggests an infectious hepatitis.
- ***Recent outbreak of jaundice***. An outbreak in the community suggests hepatitis A virus (HAV).

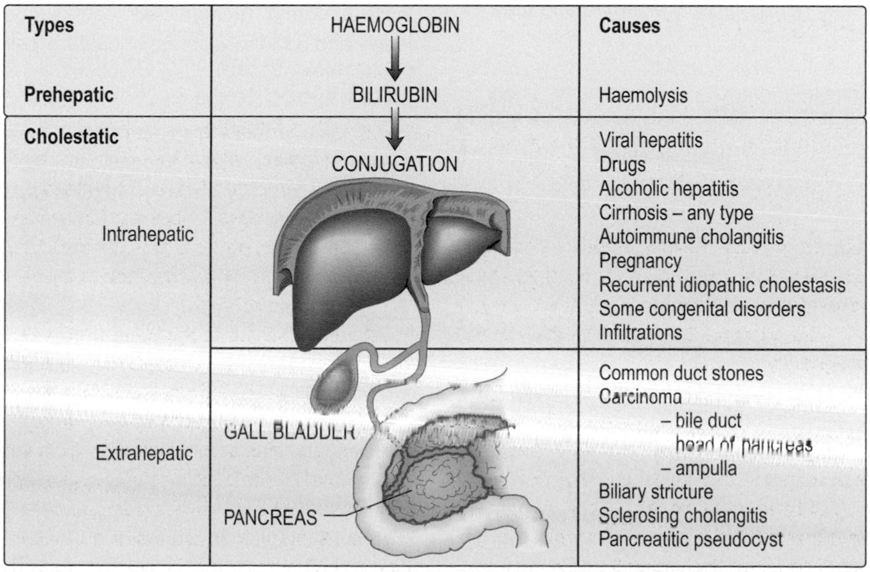
Types
HAEMOGLOBIN
Causes
Prehepatic
BILIRUBIN
Haemolysis
Cholestatic
CONJUGATION
Intrahepatic
Viral hepatitis
Drugs
Alcoholic hepatitis
Cirrhosis – any type
Autoimmune cholangitis
Pregnancy
Recurrent idiopathic cholestasis
Some congenital disorders
Infiltrations
Extrahepatic
GALL BLADDER
PANCREAS
Common duct stones
Carcinoma
– bile duct
head of pancreas
– ampulla
Biliary stricture
Sclerosing cholangitis
Pancreatitic pseudocyst

Figure 14.8 Causes of jaundice.

- ***Intravenous drug use, or recent injections or tattoos***. These all increase the chance of HBV and HCV infection.
- ***Men having sex with men***. This increases the chance of HBV and HCV infection.
- ***Female sex workers***. This increases the chance of HBV infection.
- ***Medical treatment in the developing world***. There is an increased risk of HBV and HCV due to poorly sterilized equipment or administration of unscreened blood or blood products.
- ***Alcohol consumption.*** A history of drinking habits should be taken, although many patients often understate their consumption.
- ***Drugs (particularly those taken in the previous 2–3 months)***. Many drugs, including over-the-counter and herbal preparations, cause jaundice (see pp. 487–488).
- ***Travel***. Certain areas have a high risk of hepatitis A virus (HAV) infection, as well as hepatitis E virus (HEV), but HAV is common in the UK and HEV is common in travellers to the Indian subcontinent.
- ***Family history***. Patients with, for example, Gilbert's disease may have family members who experience recurrent jaundice.
- ***Recent surgery***. Surgery on the biliary tract or for carcinoma is relevant.
- ***Environment***. People engaged in recreational activities in rural areas, as well as farm and sewage workers, are at risk for leptospirosis, hepatitis E and exposure to chemicals.
- ***Fevers or rigors***. These are suggestive of cholangitis or possibly a liver abscess.

Clinical features

The signs of acute and chronic liver disease should be looked for (see pp. 447–448). Certain additional signs may be helpful:

- ***Hepatomegaly***. A smooth, tender liver is seen in hepatitis and in extrahepatic obstruction, but a knobbly, irregular liver suggests metastases or cirrhosis. Causes of hepatomegaly are shown in **Box 14.3**.
- ***Splenomegaly***. This indicates portal hypertension when signs of chronic liver disease are present. The spleen can also be 'tipped' occasionally in viral hepatitis. In alcoholic cirrhosis, in particular, the spleen may not be grossly enlarged and may not be palpable

Box 14.3 Causes of hepatomegaly

Apparent
- Low-lying diaphragm
- Riedel's lobe
- Cirrhosis (early)

Inflammation
- Hepatitis
- Schistosomiasis
- Abscesses (pyogenic or amoebic)

Cysts
- Hydatid
- Polycystic

Metabolic
- Fatty liver
- Amyloid deposition
- Glycogen storage disease

Haematological
- Leukaemias
- Lymphoma
- Myeloproliferative disorders
- Thalassaemia

Tumours
- Primary and secondary carcinoma

Venous congestion
- Heart failure
- Constrictive pericarditis
- Hepatic vein occlusion

Biliary obstruction
- (Particularly extrahepatic)

- ***Ascites***. This is found in cirrhosis but can also be due to other causes (see **Box 14.19**).

A palpable gall bladder occurs with a carcinoma of the pancreas obstructing the bile duct. Generalized lymphadenopathy suggests a lymphoma.

Cold sores are often seen with a herpes simplex virus hepatitis.

Investigations

Jaundice is not itself a diagnosis and the cause should always be sought. The two most useful tests are the ***viral markers*** for HAV, HBV and HCV, with an ultrasound examination. Liver biochemistry confirms the jaundice and may help in the diagnosis.

An ***ultrasound examination*** should always be performed to exclude an extrahepatic obstruction, and to diagnose any features compatible with chronic liver disease. Ultrasound will demonstrate:

- the size of the bile ducts, which are dilated in extrahepatic obstruction **(Fig. 14.9)**
- the level of the obstruction
- the cause of the obstruction in virtually all patients with tumours and in 75% of patients with gallstones.

The pathological diagnosis of any mass lesion can be made by fine-needle aspiration cytology (sensitivity approximately 60%) or by needle biopsy (sensitivity approximately 90%).

A flow diagram for the general investigation of the jaundiced patient is shown in **Figure 14.10**.

Liver biochemistry

In hepatitis, serum AST and ALT tend to be high early in the disease, with only a small rise in serum ALP. Conversely, in extrahepatic obstruction, the ALP is high, with a smaller rise in aminotransferases. However, these findings alone cannot be relied upon to make a diagnosis in an individual case. The prothrombin time is often prolonged in longstanding liver disease, and the serum albumin is also low.

Haematological tests

In haemolytic jaundice, the bilirubin is raised and the other liver biochemistry is normal. A raised white cell count may indicate infection (e.g. cholangitis). A leucopenia often occurs in viral hepatitis, while abnormal mononuclear cells suggest infectious mononucleosis and a Monospot test should be performed.

Other blood tests

These include tests to confirm the presence of specific causes of acute or chronic liver disease, e.g. anti-mitochondrial antibody (AMA) for PBC. HIV status should be established.

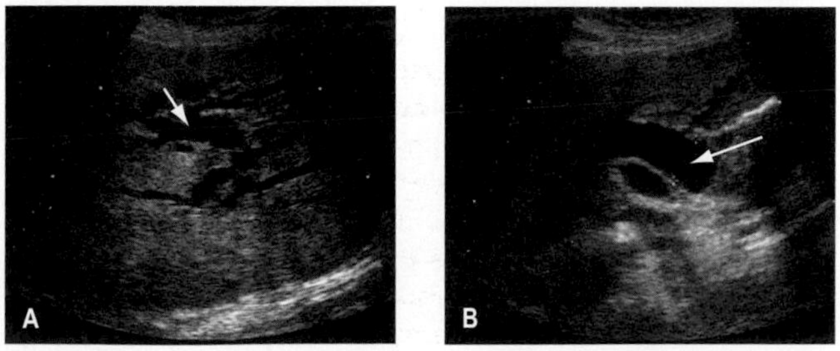

Figure 14.9 **Liver ultrasound. A.** Dilated intrahepatic bile ducts (arrowed). **B.** Common bile duct (arrowed). The normal bile duct measures 6 mm at the porta hepatis.

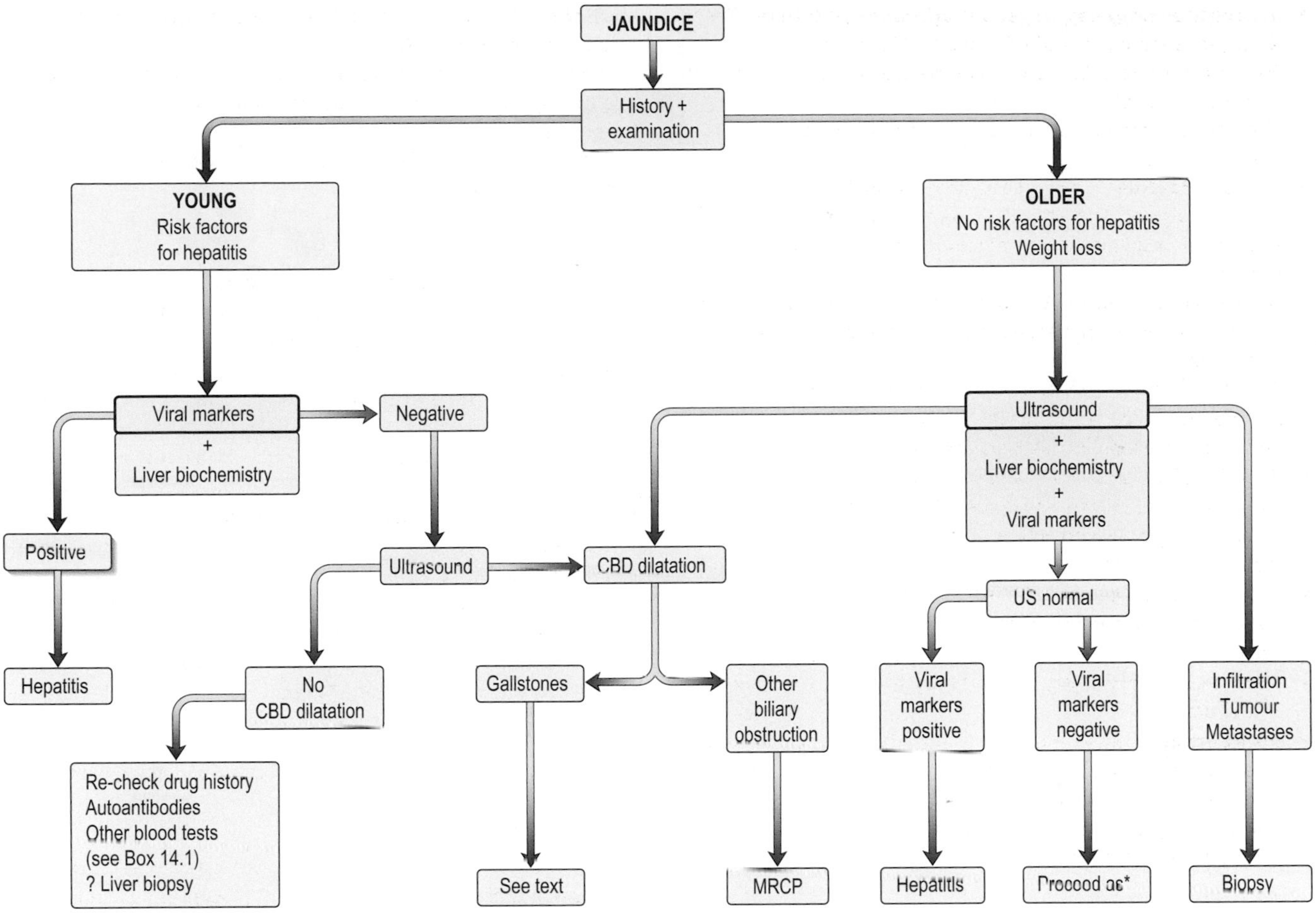

Figure 14.10 **Approach to the patient with jaundice.** CBD, common bile duct; MRCP, magnetic resonance cholangiopancreatography; US, ultrasound. *Proceed as in bottom left box (Re-check drug history ...).

HEPATITIS

- ***Acute parenchymal liver damage*** can be caused by many agents ***(Fig. 14.11)***.
- ***Chronic hepatitis*** is defined as any hepatitis lasting for 6 months or longer and is classified according to the aetiology ***(Box 14.4)***. Chronic viral hepatitis is the principal cause of chronic liver disease, cirrhosis and hepatocellular carcinoma worldwide.

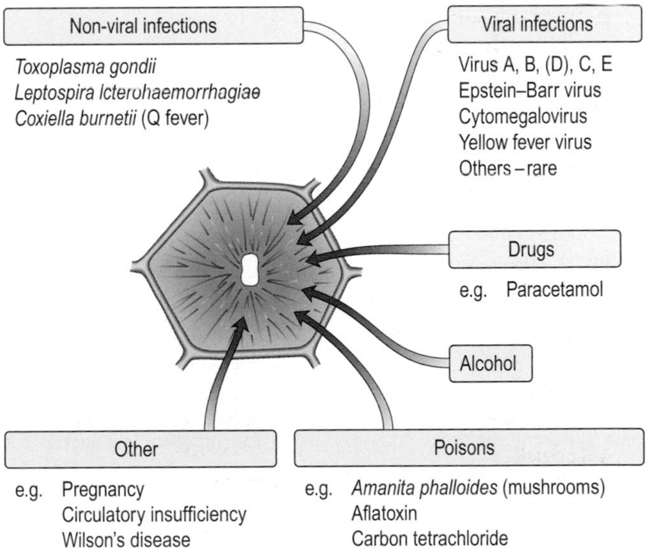

Figure 14.11 Some causes of acute parenchymal damage.

Acute hepatitis

Pathology

Although some histological features are suggestive of the aetiological factor, most changes are non-specific. Hepatocytes show degenerative changes (swelling, cytoplasmic granularity, vacuolation) and undergo necrosis (becoming shrunken, containing eosinophilic Councilman bodies). The distribution of these changes may vary with aetiology, but necrosis is usually maximal in zone 3. The extent of the damage is very variable between individuals, even when they are affected by the same agent; at one end of the spectrum, single and small groups of hepatocytes die (spotty or focal necrosis), while at the other end, there is multiacinar necrosis involving a substantial part of the liver (massive hepatic necrosis), resulting in acute hepatic failure. Between these extremes, there is limited confluent necrosis with collapse of the reticulin framework, leading to linking (bridging) between the central veins, between the central veins and portal tracts, and between the portal tracts. The extent of the inflammatory infiltrate is also variable, but portal tracts

Box 14.4 Causes of chronic hepatitis

- Metabolic:
  - Non-alcoholic fatty liver disease
- Alcohol-induced
- Viral:
  - Hepatitis B ± hepatitis D
  - Hepatitis C
  - Hepatitis E (immunosuppressed)
- Drugs:
  - (e.g. Methyldopa, isoniazid, ketoconazole, nitrofurantoin)
- Autoimmune
- Hereditary:
  - Wilson's disease, haemochromatosis.

Unusual causes include infections (syphilis, tuberculosis, various tropical infections), infiltrative diseases, including amyloidosis and lymphoma, and ingestion of toxins.

and lobules are infiltrated mainly by lymphocytes. Other variable features include cholestasis in zone 3 and fatty change, the latter being prominent in hepatitis that is due to alcohol or certain drugs.

Chronic hepatitis

Pathology

The pathological features are often diagnostic. Chronic inflammatory cell infiltrates, comprising lymphocytes, plasma cells and sometimes lymphoid follicles, are usually present in the portal tracts. The amount of inflammation varies from mild to severe. In addition, there may be:

- loss of definition of the portal/periportal limiting plate – interface hepatitis (damage is due to apoptosis rather than necrosis)
- lobular change, focal lytic necrosis, apoptosis and focal inflammation
- confluent necrosis
- fibrosis, which may be mild, bridging (across portal tracts) or severe cirrhosis.

The overall severity of the hepatitis is judged by the degree of hepatitis and inflammation (grading), and the severity of fibrosis or cirrhosis (staging). In chronic viral hepatitis, there are various scoring systems. For example, the ***Knodell Scoring System*** (histological activity index) uses the sum of four factors (periportal or bridging necrosis, intralobular degeneration and focal necrosis, portal inflammation and fibrosis). The ***Ishak score*** stages fibrosis from 0 (none) to 6 (cirrhosis). The ***METAVIR system*** has four stages. Scoring systems are used for drug trials and for assessing progression of disease, but are not quantitative measures of fibrosis and different systems may be used for different diseases (for example, the ***Brunt scoring system*** is usually applied to NAFLD, and the METAVIR system is reserved for hepatitis C).

Viral hepatitis

The differing features of the common forms of viral hepatitis are summarized in ***Box 14.5***. Two different patterns are recognized: acute hepatitis with rapid onset of infection and, usually, rapid resolution; and chronic viral hepatitis, which is asymptomatic and often detected on routine blood tests or during screening for infection. Hepatitis A always and E usually cause acute infections whilst hepatitis B, C and D may cause acute or chronic disease.

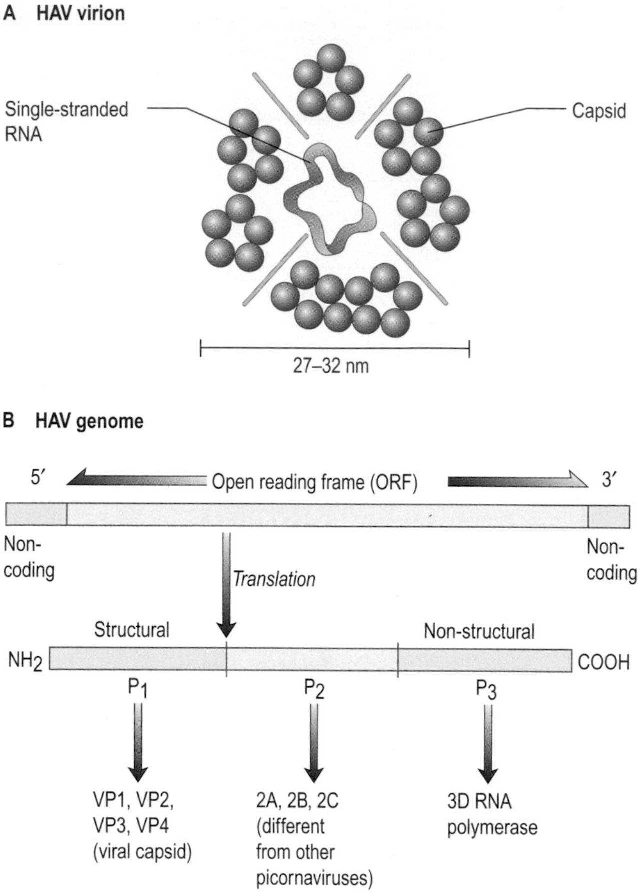

Figure 14.12 Hepatitis A. A. The hepatitis A (HAV) virion consists of four polypeptides (VP1–VP4), which form a tight protein shell, or capsid, containing the RNA. The major antigenic component is associated with VP1. **B.** Arrangement of the HAV genome.

Hepatitis A

Epidemiology

Hepatitis A is the most common acute viral hepatitis occurring worldwide, often in epidemics. The disease is commonly seen in the autumn and affects children and young adults. Spread of infection is mainly by the faeco-oral route and arises from the ingestion of contaminated food or water (e.g. shellfish). Overcrowding and poor sanitation facilitate spread. There is no carrier state. In the UK, it is a notifiable disease.

Hepatitis A virus (HAV)

Hepatitis A virus (HAV) is a picornavirus, having the structure shown in ***Figure 14.12***. It has a single serotype, as only one epitope is immunodominant. It replicates in the liver, is excreted in bile, and then excreted in the faeces for about 2 weeks before the onset of clinical illness and for up to 7 days after. The disease is maximally infectious just before the onset of jaundice. HAV particles can be demonstrated in the faeces by electron microscopy.

Clinical features

The viraemia causes the patient to feel unwell, with non-specific symptoms that include nausea and anorexia. Many recover at this stage and remain anicteric. An anicteric infection is common in

Box 14.5 Some features of viral hepatitis

	A	B	C	D	E
Virus	RNA	DNA	RNA	RNA	RNA
	27 nm	42 nm	Approx. 50 nm	36 nm (with HBsAg coat)	27–35 nm
	Picorna	Hepadna	Flaviviridae	Deltaviridae	Hepeviridae virus
Spread					
Faeco-oral	Yes	No	No	No	Yes
Blood/blood products	Rare	Yes	Yes	Yes	No
Vertical	No	Yes	Rare	Occasional	No
Saliva	Yes	Yes	Yes	? No	?
Sexual	Rare	Yes	Yes (rare)	Rare	No
Incubation	Short (2–3 weeks)	Long (1–5 months)	Long	Intermediate	Short
Age	Young	Any	Any	Any	Any
Carrier state	No	Yes	Yes	?	No[a]
Chronic liver disease	No	Yes	Yes	Yes	No[a]
Liver cancer	No	Yes	Yes	Yes	No
Mortality (acute)	<0.5%	<1%	<1%	<1%	1–2% (pregnant women 10–20%)
Immunization					
Passive	Normal immunoglobulin serum i.m. (0.04–0.06 mL/kg)	Hepatitis B immunoglobulin (HBIg)	No	No	No
Active	Vaccine	Vaccine	HBV vaccine to prevent co-infection	No	Vaccine

[a]Chronic hepatitis in immunosuppressed patients.
HBsAg, hepatitis B surface antigen.

children and leads to lifetime immunity. In the developing world, improvements in hygiene have reduced early infection and, paradoxically, led to an increase in symptomatic infection in exposed adults.

After 1 or 2 weeks, some patients become jaundiced and symptoms often improve. Persistence of nausea, vomiting or any mental confusion warrants assessment in hospital. As the jaundice deepens, the urine becomes dark and the stools pale, owing to intrahepatic cholestasis. The liver is moderately enlarged and the spleen is palpable in about 10% of patients. Occasionally, tender lymphadenopathy is seen, with a transient rash in some cases. Thereafter, the jaundice lessens and, in the majority of cases, the illness is over within 3–6 weeks. Extrahepatic complications are rare but include arthritis, vasculitis, myocarditis and acute kidney injury. A biphasic illness occasionally occurs, with the return of jaundice and, classically, a more severe 'second phase', which is cholestatic (cholestatic viral hepatitis) with an increase in the alkaline phosphatase rather than the aminotransferases; thus, it runs a prolonged course of 7–20 weeks. Rarely, the disease may be very severe with acute hepatitis, liver coma and death; this is more common in the elderly. The typical sequence of events after HAV exposure is shown in ***Figure 14.13***.

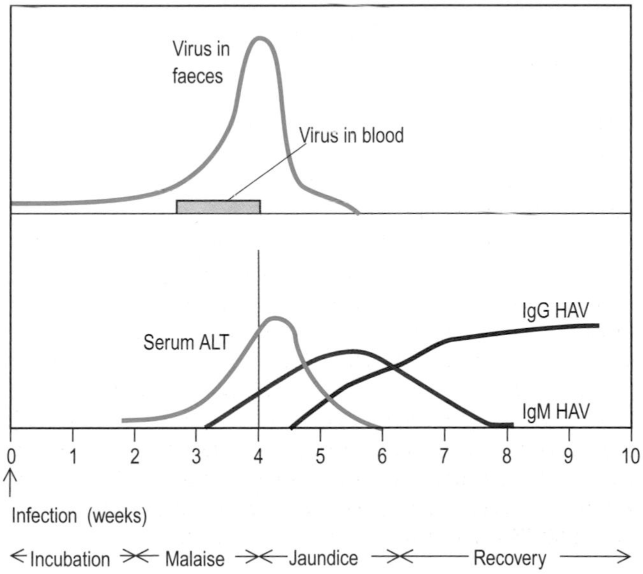

Figure 14.13 Hepatitis A virus (HAV): sequence of events after exposure. ALT, alanine aminotransferase; Ig, immunoglobulin.

Investigations

Liver biochemistry

- ***Prodromal stage***: The serum bilirubin is usually normal. However, there is bilirubinuria and increased urinary urobilinogen. A raised serum AST or ALT, which can sometimes be very high, precedes the jaundice.
- ***Icteric stage***: The serum bilirubin reflects the level of jaundice. Serum AST reaches a maximum 1–2 days after the appearance of jaundice, and may rise above 500 IU/L. Serum ALP is usually less than 300 IU/L.

After the jaundice has subsided, the aminotransferases may remain elevated for some weeks and occasionally for up to 6 months.

Haematological tests

There is leucopenia with a relative lymphocytosis. Very rarely, there is a Coombs'-positive haemolytic anaemia or an associated aplastic anaemia. The prothrombin time is prolonged in severe cases. The erythrocyte sedimentation rate (ESR) is raised.

Viral markers: antibodies to HAV

IgG antibodies are common in the general population over the age of 50 years, but an anti-HAV IgM means an acute infection. In areas of high prevalence, most children have antibodies by the age of 3 years following asymptomatic infection.

Other tests

Further tests are not necessary in the presence of an IgM antibody, but liver biochemistry must be followed to establish a return to normal levels.

Differential diagnosis

Differentiation must be made from all other causes of jaundice, but in particular from other types of viral and drug-induced hepatitis.

Prognosis

The prognosis is excellent, with most patients making a complete recovery. The mortality in young adults is 0.1% but increases with age. Death is due to acute hepatic necrosis. During convalescence, 5–15% of patients may suffer a relapse of the hepatitis but this settles spontaneously.

There is no reason to stop alcohol consumption, other than for the few weeks when the patient is ill. Patients may complain of debility for several months following resolution of the symptoms and biochemical parameters. This is known as the post-hepatitis syndrome and treatment is by reassurance. HAV hepatitis never progresses to chronic liver disease.

Management

There is no specific treatment, and rest and dietary measures are unhelpful. Corticosteroids have no benefit. Admission to hospital is not usually necessary.

Prevention

Control of hepatitis depends on good hygiene. The virus is resistant to chlorination but is killed by boiling water for 10 minutes.

Active immunization

A formaldehyde-inactivated HAV vaccine is given to people travelling frequently to endemic areas, patients with chronic liver disease, those with haemophilia, and workers in frequent contact with hepatitis cases (e.g. in residential institutions for patients with learning difficulties). Community outbreaks can be interrupted by vaccination. A single dose produces antibodies that persist for at least 1 year, with immunity lasting beyond 10 years. This obviates the need for a booster injection in healthy individuals.

Passive immunization

Normal human immunoglobulin (0.02 mL/kg i.m.) is used if exposure to HAV is <2 weeks. HAV vaccine should also be given.

Hepatitis B

Epidemiology

The hepatitis B virus (HBV) is present worldwide and there an estimated 220 million carriers. The UK and the USA have a low carrier rate (0.5–2%), but this rises to 10–20% in parts of Africa and the Middle and Far East.

Vertical transmission from mother to child, *in utero*, during parturition or soon after birth, is the usual means of transmission worldwide, although in Africa transmission from other infected children is very common during the early childhood years. HBV is not transmitted by breast-feeding.

Horizontal transmission occurs, particularly in children, through minor abrasions or close contact with other children, and HBV can survive on household articles, such as toys or toothbrushes, for prolonged periods. Childhood chronic HBV is associated with very high levels of viral replication (up to 10^{10} IU/mL), ensuring that high levels of virus are present in minute amounts of blood and thus facilitating viral spread.

HBV spread also occurs by the intravenous route (e.g. by transfusion of infected blood or blood products, or by contaminated needles used by drug users, tattooists or acupuncturists) or by close personal contact, such as during sexual intercourse, particularly in men who have sex with men. The virus can be found in semen and saliva.

Hepatitis B virus

The complete infective virion or Dane particle is a 42 nm particle comprising an inner core or nucleocapsid (27 nm), surrounded by an outer envelope of surface protein (hepatitis B surface antigen, HBsAg). This surface coat is produced in excess by the infected hepatocytes and can exist separately from the whole virion in serum and body fluid as 22 nm particles or tubules.

The hepatitis B virus (HBV) genome is variable, and genetic sequencing can be used to define the different HBV genotypes, A to H. There is a strong correlation between genotypes and geographical areas. **Genotype A** is found in north-west Europe, North America and Central Africa; **B** in South-east Asia (including China, Taiwan and Japan); genotype **C** in South-east Asia; **D** in southern Europe, India and the Middle East; **E** in West Africa; **F** in South and Central America, in American Indians and in Polynesia; **G** in France and the USA; and **H** in Central and South America. These genotypes may influence the chance of responding to interferon treatment (A more than B; C more than D) but all genotypes respond equally well to nucleoside analogues.

The core or nucleocapsid is formed of core protein (HBcAg), containing incompletely double-stranded circular DNA and DNA polymerase/reverse transcriptase. One strand is almost a complete circle and contains overlapping genes that encode both structural proteins (pre-S, surface (S), core (C)) and replicative proteins (polymerase and X). The other strand is variable in length. DR1 and DR2 are direct repeats necessary for HBV synthesis during viral replication ***(Fig. 14.14)***.

HBeAg is a protein formed via specific self-cleavage of the precore/core gene product, which is secreted separately by the cell.

Hepatitis B mutants

Mutations occur in the various reading frames of the HBV genome ***(Fig. 14.14)***. These mutants can emerge in patients with chronic HBV infection (escape mutants) or can be acquired by infection.

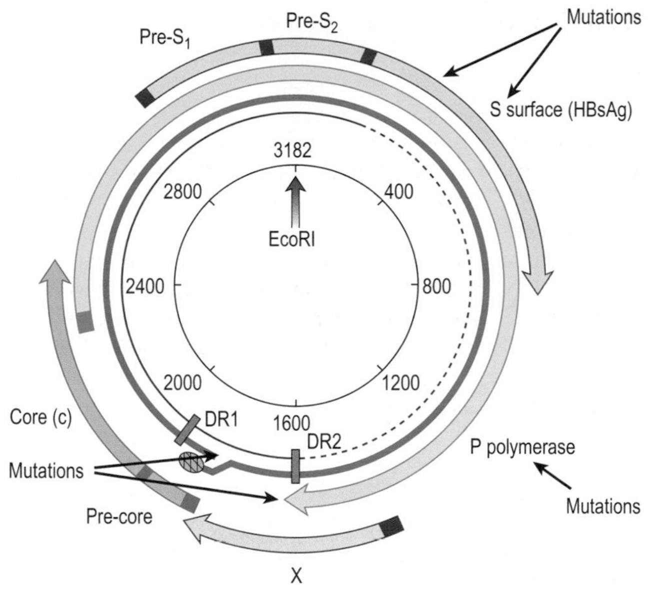

Figure 14.14 Hepatitis B virus (HBV) genome. The viral DNA is partially double-stranded (red incomplete circle and blue circle). The long strand (blue) encodes seven proteins from four overlapping reading frames (**S**, surface (**Pre-S_1**, **Pre-S_2**, S); **c**, core (Pre-C, C); **P**, polymerase (P); and X gene (**X**)). **EcoRI** restriction-enzyme-binding site is included as a reference point. **DR**, direct repeat; **HBsAg**, hepatitis B surface antigen.

HBsAg mutants are produced by alterations in the 'a' antigenic determinants of the HbsAg proteins, usually with a substitution of glycine for arginine at position 145. This results in changes in the antibody-binding domain and may confer resistance to the vaccine.

In patients with some HBV genotypes (particularly genotype D), a mutation in the ***pre-core region***, when a guanosine (G) to adenosine (A) change creates a stop codon (TAG), prevents the production of HBeAg (the secreted form of HBcAG), but the synthesis of HBcAg is unaffected. This mutation may be associated with HBeAg-negative disease but other mutations in the core promoter region of the virus also give rise to HBeAg-negative disease. To detect infectivity in HBeAg-negative disease, HBV DNA must always be measured, as no eAg will be present.

DNA polymerase mutants occur, particularly following treatment with the first generation of directly acting antiviral drugs, such as lamivudine.

Pathogenesis

Pre-S_1 and pre-S_2 regions are involved in attachment to the hepatocyte receptor, recently identified as the sodium taurocholate co-transporting polypeptide (NTCP). After penetration into the cell, the virus loses its coat and the virus core is transported to the nucleus without processing. The transcription of HBV into messenger RNA takes place when the HBV DNA is converted into a closed circular form (cccDNA), which acts as a template for RNA transcription.

Translation into HBV proteins (Box 14.6), as well as replication of the genome, takes place in the endoplasmic reticulum; the proteins are then packaged together and exported from the cell. There is an excess production of non-infective HBsAg particles, which are extruded into the circulation.

Box 14.6 Hepatitis B virus (HBV) proteins

HBV protein	Significance
Core	Protein of core particle; forms nucleocapsids
Pre-core (HBeAg)	Pre-core/core cleaves to HBeAg; good marker of active replication and role in inducing immunotolerance
Surface (HBsAg)	Envelope protein of HBV; basis of current vaccine
Pre-S_2 / Pre-S_1	HBV binding and entry into hepatocytes
Polymerase	Viral replication
X protein	Transcriptional and transactivator activity

The HBV is not usually directly cytopathic (although high replication levels in immunosuppressed individuals can lead to direct toxicity) and liver damage is produced by the host immune response.

HBV-specific cytotoxic CD8 T cells recognize the viral antigen via human leucocyte antigen (HLA) class I molecules on the infected hepatocytes. However, suppressor or regulatory T cells inhibit these cytotoxic cells, leading to viral persistence and chronic HBV infection. Th1 responses (IL-2, γ-interferon) are thought to be associated with viral clearance, and Th2 (IL-4, 5, 6, 10, 13) responses with the development of chronic infection and disease severity. Viral persistence in patients with a very poor cell-mediated response leads to an asymptomatic, inactive, chronic HBV infective state. However, a better response results in continuing hepatocellular damage, with the development of chronic hepatitis.

Chronic HBV infection progresses through a series of four distinct phases ***(Fig. 14.15)***.

- ***Immunotolerant phase***. The natural history of childhood-acquired HBV is shown in the figure. In this first early phase, high-level viral replication, with HBeAg, is not associated with an immune response and hence there is no damage to hepatocytes. Management is not indicated but close follow-up is required. This phase matures into the next adolescent phase.
- ***Immunoactive phase***. During adolescence, an immune response develops, leading to liver damage with fluctuating raised transferases (ALT) in the presence of high levels of HBeAg-positive infection. In some patients, this disease phase will progress to cirrhosis and therapy is therefore indicated to reduce the development of fibrosis. Management in this phase may lead to seroconversion from HBeAg-positive to HBeAg-negative.
- ***Immunosurveillance phase***. In many, the immunoactive phase is followed by a period of immune control (the 'inactive carrier' phase), when host immune responses suppress viral replication, leading to low-level HBV DNA (<2000 IU/mL), absence of HBeAg and normal ALTs.
  In some patients, the virus is eventually cleared with the loss of HBsAg.
- ***Immunoescape phase***. A proportion of patients with inactive HBV will reactivate their disease as they age, and this final phase of disease is characterized by high-level viral replication (HBV DNA $10^5/10^6$) but negative HBeAg and raised ALT. Note that, in this phase, fluctuating ALT levels may lead to a misdiagnosis and so the liver function tests and HBV DNA

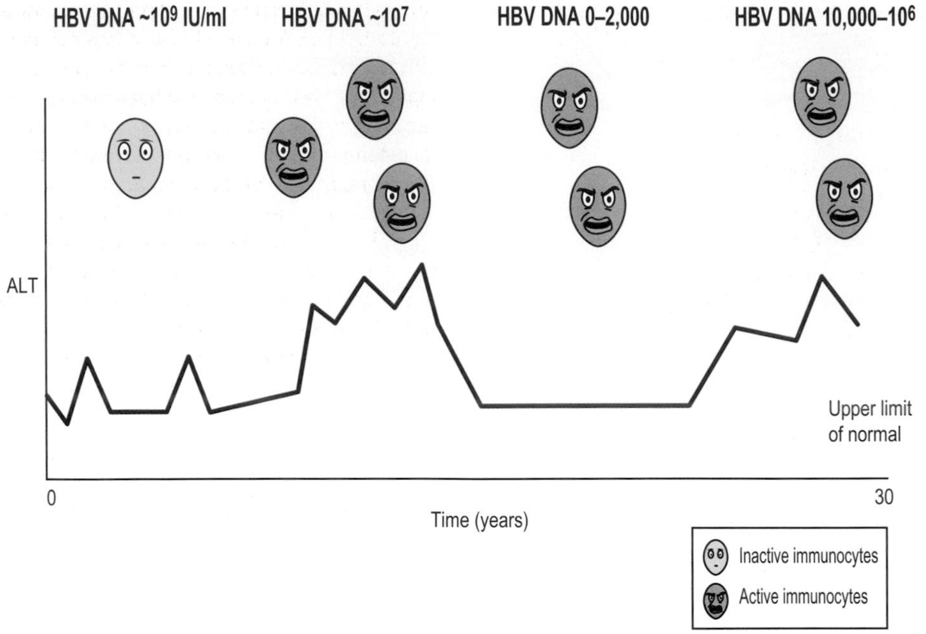

Figure 14.15 Natural history of childhood-acquired hepatitis B virus (HBV). Immunotolerant phase: Early disease is characterized by high-level viraemia with HBeAg (the secreted form of HBcAg) and a minimal immune response, leading to no significant liver damage. **Immunoactive phase:** Fluctuating liver function tests (ALTs) and ongoing liver damage that may lead to cirrhosis. Treatment in this phase may lead to seroconversion. In many, the immunoactive phase is followed by a period of immune control (the 'inactive carrier' phase), when host immune responses suppress viral replication, leading to low-level HBV DNA (<2000 IU/mL), absence of HBeAg and normal ALTs. In some patients, the virus is eventually cleared, with the loss of HBsAg; in many, however, viral reactivation occurs with viral mutations, leading to HBeAg-negative disease with high levels of viral replication (HBV DNA $10^5/10^6$) and alanine aminotransferase (ALT) in the absence of HBeAg. Note that, in this phase, fluctuating ALTs may lead to misdiagnosis, and so the ALTs and HBV DNA should be tested four times a year to establish the diagnosis in patients who are HBeAg-negative.

should be tested four times a year to establish the diagnosis in patients who are HBeAg-negative.

This disease phase is often associated with viral mutations (see above). Therapy for HBeAg-negative disease is indicated to prevent disease progression

Hepatocellular carcinoma (HCC) can develop in patients at all stages of disease but is more common in those with high levels of HBV DNA.

Immunosuppression, such as occurs during chemotherapy, aggravates all phases of HBV and a particular problem is seen in patients with HBeAg-negative, inactive disease, where the presence of normal liver biochemistry provides a false sense of security. HBV reactivation is common in such patients and has a high mortality. It is essential that all patients who are due to receive chemotherapy are screened for HBsAg, and those who have chronic HBV should receive prophylactic antiviral therapy, such as tenofovir or entecavir.

Clinical features of acute hepatitis B infection

The sequence of events following acute HBV infection is shown in ***Figure 14.16***. However, in many, the infection is subclinical. When HBV infection is acquired perinatally, an acute hepatitis does not usually occur and chronic infection develops. In adults, an acute infection is common and the virus is cleared in approximately 99% of patients. The clinical picture is the same as that found in HAV infection, although the illness may be more severe. In addition, a serum sickness-like immunological syndrome may be seen. This consists of rashes (e.g. urticaria or a maculopapular rash) and polyarthritis affecting small joints occurring in up to 25% of cases in the prodromal period. Fever is usual. Extrahepatic immune

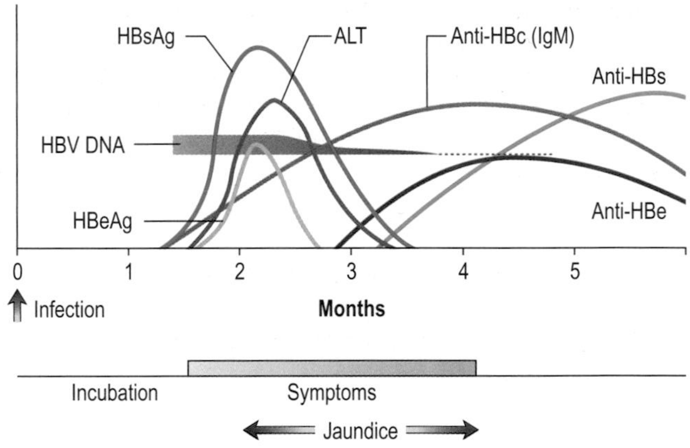

Figure 14.16 Time course of the events and serological changes seen following acute infection with hepatitis B virus (HBV). ***Antigens***: *HBsAg* appears in the blood from about 6 weeks to 3 months after an acute infection and then disappears. *HBeAg* rises early and usually declines rapidly. ***Antibodies***: *Anti-HBs* appears late and indicates immunity. *Anti-HBc* is the first antibody to appear and high titres of IgM anti-HBc suggest an acute and continuing viral replication. It persists for many months. *IgM anti-HBc* may be the only serological indicator of recent HBV infection in a period when HBsAg has disappeared and anti-HBs is not detectable in the serum. *Anti-HBe* appears after the anti-HBc and its appearance relates to a decreased infectivity: that is, a low risk. ALT, alanine aminotransferase.

Box 14.7 Significance of viral markers in hepatitis B

Marker	Significance
Antigens	
HBsAg	Acute or chronic infection
HBeAg	Acute hepatitis B Persistence implies: Continued infectious state Development of chronicity
HBV DNA	Implies viral replication Found in serum and liver Levels indicate response to antiviral treatment
Antibodies	
Anti-HBs	Immunity to HBV; previous exposure; vaccination
Anti-HBe	Seroconversion
Anti-HBc	
IgM	Acute hepatitis B (high titre) Chronic hepatitis B (low titre)
IgG	Past exposure to hepatitis B (HBsAg-negative)

complex-mediated conditions, such as an arteritis or glomerulonephritis, are occasionally seen.

Investigations

These are generally the same as for hepatitis A.

Specific tests

The markers for HBV are shown in ***Box 14.7***. HBsAg is looked for initially; if it is found, a full viral profile is then performed. In acute infection, as HBsAg may be cleared rapidly and anti-HBc IgM is diagnostic, patients must be tested for both HBsAg and anti-core antibodies if HBV is suspected. HBV DNA is the most sensitive index of viral replication.

Prognosis

The majority of patients recover completely, acute hepatic failure occurring in up to 1%. Some patients go on to develop chronic hepatitis and the outcome depends upon several factors, chiefly the age of the patient.

Management of acute hepatitis

This is mainly symptomatic. However, patients should have their HBV markers monitored. Several experts suggest that entecavir or tenofovir should be given for the persistent presence of HbeAg beyond 12 weeks, and in some patients who are very ill.

Prevention

Prevention depends on vaccination. In countries that do not vaccinate all citizens, prevention depends upon avoiding risk factors (see above). These include not sharing needles and having safe sex. Vertical transmission is discussed below. Infectivity is highest in those with the e antigen and/or HBV DNA in their blood.

Immunization

Vaccination is obligatory in most developed countries (but not the UK), as well as countries with high endemicity. Vaccination has been shown to reduce mortality and morbidity. In countries that do not have a universal vaccination policy, groups at high risk are vaccinated. These include all healthcare personnel; members of emergency and rescue teams; morticians and embalmers; children in high-risk areas; people with haemophilia; patients in some psychiatric units; patients with chronic kidney disease/on dialysis units; long-term travellers; men who have sex with men, bisexual men and sex workers; and intravenous drug users.

Active and passive (combined) prophylaxis with vaccination and immunoglobulin should be given to: healthcare staff with accidental needlestick injury; all newborn babies of HBsAg-positive mothers; and regular sexual partners of HBsAg-positive patients who have been found to be HBV-negative.

For adults, a dose of 500 IU of specific hepatitis B immunoglobulin (HBIG) (200 IU to newborns) is given; the vaccine (i.m.) is given at another site.

Active immunization

This is with a recombinant yeast vaccine, produced by insertion of a plasmid containing the gene of HBsAg into a yeast.

Dosage regimen

Three injections (at 0, 1 and 6 months) are given into the deltoid muscle; this gives short-term protection in over 90% of patients. People who are over 50 years of age or clinically ill and/or immunocompromised (including those with human immunodeficiency virus (HIV) infection or acquired immunodeficiency syndrome (AIDS)), have a poor antibody response; more frequent and larger doses are required. Antibody levels should be measured at 7–9 months after the initial dose in all at-risk groups. Antibody levels fall steadily after vaccination, and booster doses may be required after approximately 3–5 years. It is not cost-effective to check antibody levels prior to active immunization. There are few side-effects from the vaccine.

Chronic hepatitis B virus infection

Following an acute HBV infection, which may be subclinical, approximately 1–10% of patients will not clear the virus and will develop a chronic HBV infection. The features are described on pages 455–456.

Investigations

These may show a moderate rise in aminotransferases but infection with normal aminotransferases is common. The serum bilirubin is often normal. HBsAg and HBV DNA are found in the serum, sometimes with HBeAg.

Histologically, there is a full spectrum of changes, from near-normal with only a few lymphocytes and interface hepatitis to a full-blown cirrhosis. HBsAg may lend a 'ground-glass' appearance to the cytoplasm on haematoxylin and eosin staining, and this can be confirmed on orcein staining or, more specifically, with immunohistochemical staining. HBcAg can also be demonstrated in hepatocytes by appropriate immunohistochemical staining.

Management of chronic hepatitis B

Indications for therapy are similar for HBeAg-positive and negative patients with chronic hepatitis. **Three criteria** are used: serum HBV DNA levels, serum ALT levels and histological grade and stage:

- ***Patients with moderate to severe active necroinflammation*** and/or fibrosis in the liver biopsy, with HBV DNA above

2000 IU/mL (approximately 10 000 copies/mL) and/or ALT above the upper limit of normal are usually offered therapy. Age and co-morbidities also affect the decision to treat and the choice of agents.

- ***If cirrhosis is present***, treatment should be given, independent of ALT or HBV DNA levels. Patients with decompensated cirrhosis can also be treated with oral antiviral agents, but liver transplantation may be required.

All patients, regardless of disease phase, need long-term follow-up, as transition to an active phase is common; the lifetime risk of malignancy is increased in all patients who are HBsAg-positive.

Aim of therapy

This is to prevent disease progression and, ideally, to eliminate HBsAg.

- ***Interferon*** is an *immunostimulator* that induces an immune response, leading to prolonged remission after discontinuation of therapy.
- ***Oral nucleotides*** *suppress* viral replication and are used for prolonged periods of time.

In patients receiving long-term oral antiviral agents, liver fibrosis regresses. Even those patients with cirrhosis may recover, and the liver may remodel and lose all traces of fibrosis.

Antiviral agents

Interferon, *entecavir* and *tenofovir* are the most commonly used drugs.

Pegylated interferon-alfa-2a (180 μg once a week s.c.) is most often used in patients who are HBeAg-positive with active disease. Some patients (25–45%, depending on genotype – A and B respond best) lose HBeAg and move to the 'inactive' HBeAg-negative phase of disease. A proportion then goes on to lose HBsAg some years after treatment discontinuation. Patients with higher serum aminotransferase values (three times the upper limit of normal), who are younger, with viral loads <10^7 IU/mL, respond best to treatment. Patients with concomitant HIV respond poorly and those with cirrhosis should not receive interferon. Response can be assessed during therapy by measuring the serum levels of HBsAg: if these fall after 3 months, then a favourable outcome is likely, and most doctors stop therapy after 3 months if the HBsAg level remains unchanged. In patients with HBeAg-negative HBV, pegylated interferon-alfa-2a is increasingly used, as it offers a finite duration of therapy. A proportion of patients with active disease (high ALT, increased HBV DNA) convert to inactive disease, and response can be assessed by an early decline in HBsAg.

Side-effects of treatment include an acute influenza-like illness occurring 6–8 hours after the first injection. This usually disappears after subsequent injections but malaise, headaches and myalgia are common; depression, reversible hair loss and bone marrow depression and infection may also occur.

Oral antiviral therapy for HBV (entecavir, tenofovir and lamivudine) is very effective and almost all compliant patients respond with a decrease in HBV DNA to undetectable levels and a reduction in liver inflammation ***(Box 14.8)***. Both HBeAg-positive and HBeAg-negative patients respond equally well. Long-term viral suppression has been shown to reverse fibrosis, and even patients with cirrhosis respond with reversion of fibrosis. Resistance is rarely seen with third-generation drugs, and older, more resistance-prone drugs, like ***lamivudine***, are no longer recommended. A small proportion of patients develop an immune response leading to loss of HBeAg and, very rarely, loss of HBsAg. However, the majority of patients who commence oral antiviral agents will require very prolonged treatment, perhaps life-long. Studies to determine whether antiviral therapy can ever be safely discontinued are in progress. ***Entecavir*** and ***tenofovir*** are the drugs of choice for HBV, and both agents are associated with very few side-effects and an excellent response. Combination therapy has little benefit and a single drug should be used.

Box 14.8 Factors predictive of a sustained response to treatment in chronic hepatitis B

Duration of disease
- Short

Liver biochemistry
- High serum aminotransferases

Histology
- Active liver disease (mild to moderate)

Viral levels
- Low HBV DNA levels

Other
- Absence of immunosuppression
- Female gender
- Adult-acquired
- Delta virus negative
- Rapidity of response to oral therapy

Prognosis

The clinical course of hepatitis B is very variable; treatments have improved survival, stopped progression of fibrosis and enabled regression of fibrosis to occur. Established cirrhosis is associated with a poor prognosis. *Hepatocellular carcinoma (HCC)* is a frequent association and is one of the most common carcinomas in HBV-endemic areas such as the Far East. Surveillance for HCC must continue, even when HBV DNA is negative in patients who have HBsAg and are not treated, and also in these rendered negative by therapy. The incidence of HCC is being reduced by routine HBV vaccination of all children.

Hepatitis D

This is caused by the hepatitis D virus (HDV or delta virus), which is an incomplete RNA particle enclosed in a shell of HBsAg; it belongs to the Deltaviridae family. The virus is unable to replicate on its own but is activated by the presence of HBV. It is common in some parts of the world, including Eastern Europe (Romania, Bulgaria), North Africa and the Brazilian rainforest. Hepatitis D viral infection can occur either as a co-infection or as a superinfection.

- ***Co-infection*** of HDV and HBV is clinically indistinguishable from an acute icteric HBV infection, but a biphasic rise of serum aminotransferases may be seen. ***Diagnosis*** is confirmed by finding serum IgM anti-HDV in the presence of IgM anti-HBc. IgM anti-delta appears at 1 week and disappears by 5–6 weeks (occasionally 12 weeks), when serum IgG anti-delta is seen. The HDV RNA is an early marker of infection. The infection may be transient but the clinical course is variable.
- ***Superinfection*** results in an acute flare-up of previously quiescent chronic HBV infection. A rise in serum AST or ALT may be the only indication of infection. ***Diagnosis*** is made by finding HDV RNA or serum IgM anti-HDV at the same time as IgG anti-HBc. Active HBV DNA synthesis is reduced by delta superinfection and patients are usually negative for HBeAg with low HBV DNA.

Acute hepatic failure can follow both types of infection but is more common after co-infection. HDV RNA in the serum and liver can be measured and is found in acute and chronic HDV infection.

Chronic hepatitis D

This is a relatively infrequent chronic hepatitis, but spontaneous resolution is rare. Between 60% and 70% of patients will develop cirrhosis, and more rapidly than with HBV infection alone. In 15%, the disease is rapidly progressive, with development of cirrhosis in only a few years. The diagnosis is made by finding anti-delta antibody in a patient with chronic liver disease who is HBsAg-positive. It can be confirmed by finding HDV in the liver or HDV RNA in the serum by reverse transcription polymerase chain reaction (PCR).

Management

Treatment of patients with active liver disease (raised ALT levels and/or inflammation on biopsy) is with pegylated interferon-alfa-2a for 12 months, although response rates are very low.

Hepatitis C

Epidemiology

An estimated 240 million people are infected with this virus worldwide. The prevalence rate of infection ranges from 0.4% in Europe, 1–3% in Southern Europe (possibly linked to intramuscular injections of vaccines or other medicines) and 6% in Africa; in Egypt, the rates are as high as 19% owing to parenteral antimony treatment for schistosomiasis. The virus is transmitted by blood and blood products, and was common in people with haemophilia treated before screening of blood products was introduced. The incidence in intravenous drug users is high (50–60%). The low rate of hepatitis C virus infection in high-risk groups – such as men who have sex with men, sex workers and attendees at sexually transmitted infection clinics – suggests a limited role for sexual transmission. Vertical transmission from a healthy mother to child can occur but is rare (approximately 5%). Other routes of community-acquired infection (e.g. close contact) are extremely rare. In 20% of cases, the exact mode of transmission is unknown.

Hepatitis C virus (HCV)

Hepatitis C virus (HCV) is a single-stranded RNA virus of the Flaviviridae family. The RNA genome is approximately 10 kb in length, encoding a polyprotein product consisting of structural (capsid and envelope) and non-structural viral proteins ***(Fig. 14.17)***. Comparisons of subgenomic regions, such as E1, NS4 or NS5, have allowed variants to be classified into six genotypes, which have differing geographical distributions. Variability is distributed throughout the genome, with the non-structural gene of different genotypes showing 30–50% nucleotide sequence disparity. Genotypes 1a and 1b account for 70% of cases in the USA and 50% in Europe. There is a rapid change in envelope proteins, making it difficult to develop a vaccine. Antigens from the nucleocapsid regions have been used to develop enzyme-linked immunosorbent assays (ELISAs). The current assay, ELISA-3, incorporates antigens NS3, NS4 and NS5 regions.

Clinical features

Most acute infections are asymptomatic, about 10% of patients having a mild influenza-like illness with jaundice and a rise in serum aminotransferases. Most patients will not be diagnosed until they present, years later, with evidence of abnormal transferase values at health checks or with chronic liver disease.

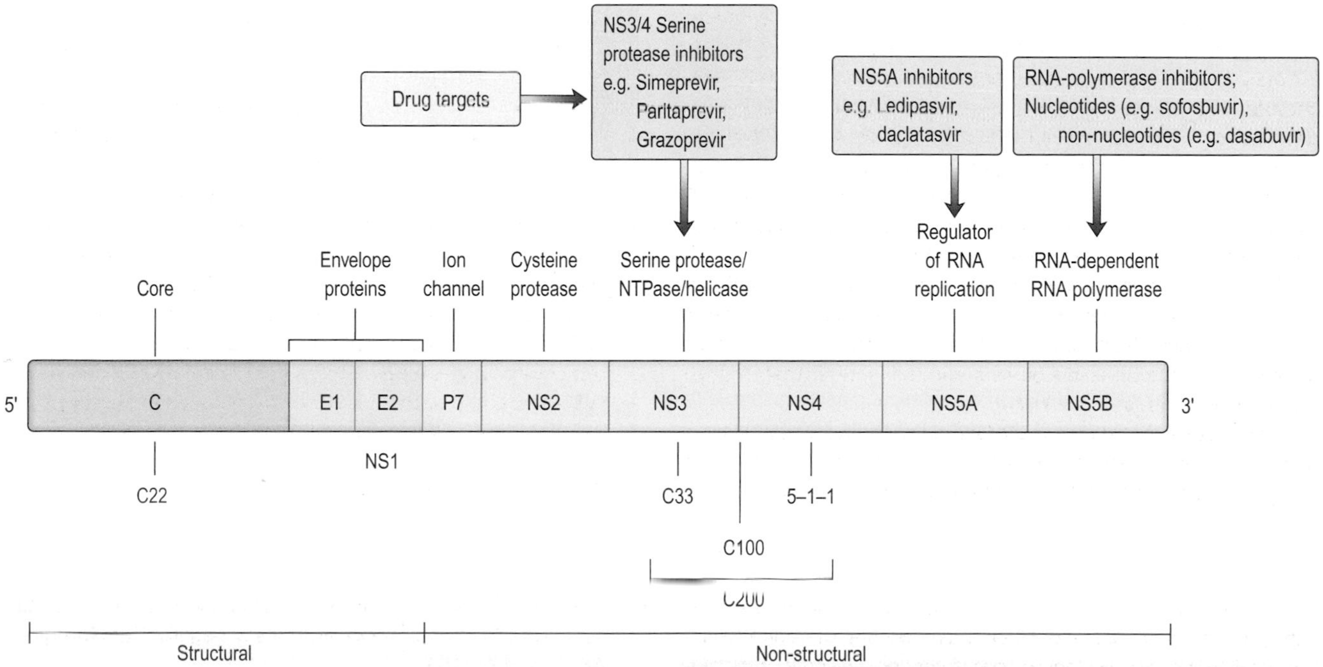

Figure 14.17 Hepatitis C virus. A single-stranded RNA virus with viral proteins. Targets for recent drugs are shown. C, core; E, envelope; NS, non-structural.

Investigations

This is by evaluation of HCV, RNA and HCV antibodies; HCV RNA can be detected from 1 to 8 weeks after infection. Anti-HCV tests are usually positive 8 weeks from infection. Patients with acute HCV infection should be tested on several occasions, as many have fluctuating viraemia during the first few months of infection, with periods of undetectable HCV RNA followed by virological relapse. Viral clearance is confirmed by multiple tests for HCV RNA over a period of many months.

Management

In acute infection, most experts recommend a period of monitoring for a few weeks with serial assessments of HCV RNA. If the viral load is falling, treatment may not be required, but the patient should be observed for several months to confirm true viral clearance. If the HCV RNA level does not decline, then therapy with interferon (with or without ribavirin) is indicated. Needle-stick injuries must be followed and treated early, although the vast majority (>97%) do not go on to develop viraemia. For treatment of patients with co-infection with HIV, see p. 351.

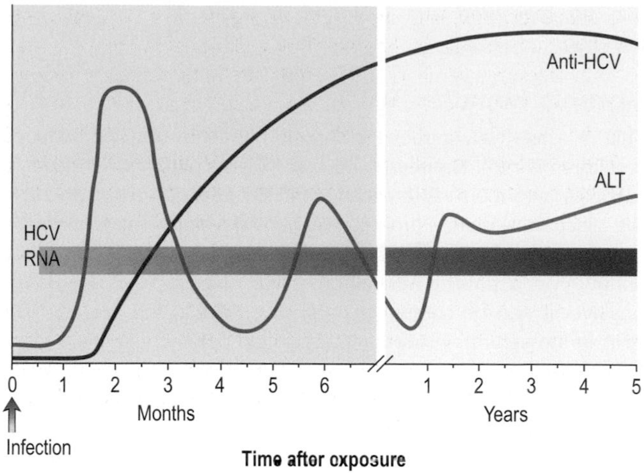

Figure 14.18 Time course of the events and serological changes seen following infection with hepatitis C virus. ALT, alanine aminotransferase.

Prognosis

Some 85–90% of asymptomatic patients develop chronic liver disease. A higher percentage of symptomatic patients 'clear' the virus, with only 48–75% going on to chronic liver disease (see pp. 447–448).

Chronic hepatitis C infection

Pathogenesis

As with hepatitis B infection, cytokines in the Th2 phenotypes are profibrotic and cause the development of chronic infection. A dominant CD4 Th2 response, with a weak CD8 interferon-gamma response, may lead to rapid fibrosis. Th1 cytokines are antifibrotic and thus a dominant CD4 Th1 and CD8 cytolytic response may cause less fibrosis.

Clinical features

Patients with chronic HCV infection are usually asymptomatic, the disease only being discovered following a routine biochemical test when mild elevations in the aminotransferases (usually ALT) are noticed (50%). The elevation in ALT may be minimal and fluctuating ***(Fig. 14.18)***, and some patients have a persistently normal ALT (25%), the disease being detected by checking HCV antibodies (e.g. in blood donors). Non-specific malaise and fatigue are common in chronic infection and often reverse following viral clearance. Extrahepatic manifestations are seen, including arthritis, cryoglobulinaemia with or without glomerulonephritis, and porphyria cutanea tarda. There is a higher incidence of diabetes, and associations with lichen planus, sicca syndrome and non-Hodgkin's lymphoma.

Chronic HCV infection causes slowly progressive fibrosis that leads, over decades, to cirrhosis. After 20 years of infection, 16% of patients have developed cirrhosis; the proportion that will ultimately develop cirrhosis after a lifetime of infection remains unknown but is likely to be higher than the proportions reported after short-term follow-up. Factors associated with rapid progression of HCV fibrosis include excess alcohol consumption, co-infection with HIV, obesity, diabetes and infection with genotype 3. Once cirrhosis has developed, some 3–4% per year will develop decompensated cirrhosis and approximately 1% will develop liver cancer. Unlike HBV infection, HCV does not cause liver cancer in the absence of cirrhosis. In most parts of the world, HCV was spread (either by injection drug use, or by poorly sterilized medical devices) in the 1970s. Given the slow development of cirrhosis, current mathematical models of disease burden predict a massive increase in HCV-related end-stage liver disease over the next decade.

Investigations

Diagnosis is made by finding HCV antibody in the serum using third-generation ELISA-3 tests. A small proportion of patients with spontaneous clearance will have undetectable HCV RNA in the serum (measured by PCR) but most individuals who are antibody-positive will be viraemic. The level of viraemia varies from a few thousand to many millions of viral copies per millilitre, although current practice is to present viral load measurements in international units (IU). Disease progression is not influenced by the viral load, but treatment outcome is modified in those with high levels of viraemia.

The HCV genotype should be characterized in patients who are to be given treatment (see below), and assessment of fibrosis (by either liver biopsy or non-invasive methods) is required in patients who would prefer to defer therapy. Cirrhosis should be excluded in all patients who have been infected for more than 20 years and a liver biopsy or non-invasive marker should be used.

Management

The aim of treatment is to eliminate the HCV RNA from the serum in order to:

- stop the progression of active liver disease
- prevent the development of HCC.

A clinical cure is determined by a sustained virological response (SVR), defined by a negative HCV RNA by PCR, 6 months after the end of therapy.

Antiviral agents

Treatment for HCV infection is undergoing a revolution, with treatments changing from interferon-based regimes to all-oral combination regimes using directly acting antiviral agents. The latter are expensive and currently are available and funded in a few countries only. However, new, less costly, all-oral regimes are expected and it is to be hoped that, in the near future, all patients can be cured without interferon, which is associated with numerous side-effects. Therapy for HCV is critically dependent upon the genotype of the infecting virus; current treatment algorithms are outlined below.

The direct-acting antiviral regimes for HCV target different viral replication enzymes, and inhibitors of the NS3 protease enzyme, the NS5A replication complex initiator and the NS5B polymerase are now available. NS5B polymerase can be inhibited by both nucleotide and non-nucleotidic inhibitors.

The optimal therapy for patients with ***genotype 1 infection*** is with a combination of direct-acting antiviral agents. Two regimes are available: one involves the nucleotide sofosbuvir, which, when combined with either a protease inhibitor (simeprevir) or an NS5A inhibitor (daclatasvir or ledipasvir), cures over 90% of patients. The preferred combination is likely to be an 8-week regime involving a combined tablet containing sofosbuvir plus ledipasvir, which showed SVR rates of 95% in clinical trials. Alternative regimes that do not involve a nucleotide usually require three agents; regimes involving a protease inhibitor, an NS5A inhibitor and a non-nucleotidic NS5B inhibitor have been shown to cure over 95% of patients following 12 weeks of treatment. Both regimes are effective in patients with cirrhosis and there is an on-going debate as to whether or not patients with cirrhosis should receive slightly longer durations of therapy.

Alternative interferon-based regimes for patients with genotype 1 HCV involve at least 24 weeks of a long-acting pegylated interferon (given by weekly injections), combined with the oral agent ribavirin and a protease inhibitor. Older protease inhibitors (telaprevir and boceprevir) are associated with high levels of anaemia but the newer protease inhibitors (such as simeprevir) are better tolerated.

For patients with ***genotype 2*** HCV, 12 weeks' therapy with sofosbuvir plus ribavirin cures over 90% and compares favourably to 24 weeks' therapy with pegylated interferon and ribavirin, which leads to an SVR in no more than 80% of individuals.

For ***genotype 3-infected patients***, 24 weeks of sofosbuvir plus ribavirin are required to achieve SVR rates of more than 80%; the cost of this regime has led many to suggest that interferon and ribavirin for 24 weeks should be used, as the response rate, approaching 70–80%, is not too dissimilar. Combining sofosbuvir with an NS5A inhibitor (such as ledipasvir or daclatasvir) allows the duration of therapy to be shortened to 12 weeks, and response rates approaching 90% are to be expected in patients without cirrhosis.

Patients with ***genotype 3 HCV and cirrhosis*** respond less well to current therapies; pegylated interferon combined with ribavirin and sofosbuvir for 12 weeks may be preferred, as response rates approaching 90% have been reported in large-scale clinical trials. Interferon-free regimes – sofosbuvir plus daclatasvir or ledipasvir – are effective alternatives, but ribavirin should be included in the regimen and therapy may need to be extended to 24 weeks. In the future, new drugs that are active against genotype 3 HCV may change this approach and allow effective, all-oral combination therapy for patients with cirrhosis. Novel NS5A inhibitors (5816) and protease inhibitors (grazoprevir) are expected in the near future and results of phase III trials are awaited with interest.

Side-effects of interferon are described on page 458. Ribavirin is usually well tolerated but side-effects include a dose-related haemolysis, pruritus and nasal congestion. Telaprevir causes a rash and anaemia, and boceprevir causes dysgeusia and anaemia. Pregnancy must be avoided with antiviral therapy. The new all-oral regimes are almost free of side-effects; they have not yet been widely used, however, so their full side-effect profile has not been clearly defined.

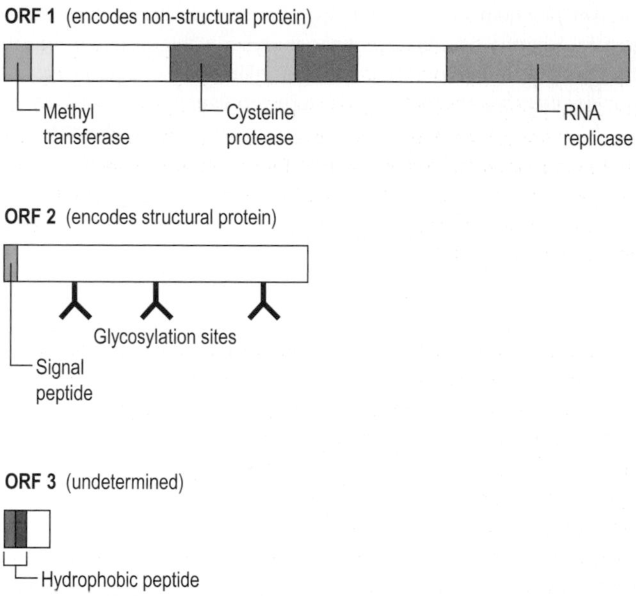

Figure 14.19 Hepatitis E genome. A single-stranded RNA genome is shown with three open reading frames (ORFs).

Hepatitis E

Hepatitis E virus (HEV) is an RNA virus (Hepeviridae virus; ***Fig. 14.19***); it causes a hepatitis that is clinically very similar to hepatitis A. It is enterally transmitted, usually by contaminated water, with 30% of dogs, pigs and rodents carrying the virus. Epidemics have been seen in many developing countries and sporadically in developed countries, in patients who have had contact with farm animals or have travelled abroad. In some developing countries, zoonotic infection from contaminated pork has led to acute HEV infection becoming relatively common. It has a mortality from fulminant hepatic failure of 1–2%, which rises to 20% in pregnant women. There is no carrier state and infection does not progress to chronic liver disease, except in some immunosuppressed patients. An ELISA for IgG and IgM anti-HEV is available for diagnosis. HEV RNA can be detected in the serum or stools by PCR. Prevention and control depend on good sanitation and hygiene; a vaccine has been developed and used successfully in China.

Hepatitis non-A–E

Approximately 10–15% of acute viral hepatitides cannot be typed and are described as hepatitis non-A–E. GB agent (hepatitis G virus, HGV) and transfusion-transmitted virus (TTV) agents have not been documented as causing disease in humans.

Acute hepatitis due to other infectious agents

Abnormal liver biochemistry is frequently found in a number of acute infections. The abnormalities are usually mild and have no clinical significance.

Infectious mononucleosis

Infectious mononucleosis (see also p. 258) is due to the Epstein–Barr (EB) virus. Mild jaundice, associated with minor abnormalities of liver biochemistry, is extremely common but 'clinical' hepatitis is rare. Hepatic histological changes occur within 5 days of onset; the sinusoids and portal tracts are infiltrated with large mononuclear cells but the liver architecture is preserved. A Paul–Bunnell or Monospot test is usually positive, and atypical lymphocytes are present in the peripheral blood. Treatment is symptomatic.

Cytomegalovirus

Cytomegalovirus (CMV; see also pp. 258–259) can cause acute hepatitis, usually a 'glandular fever-type syndrome', in healthy individuals, but is more severe in those with an impaired immune response. Only the latter need treatment with valganciclovir or ganciclovir (see pp. 258–259).

CMV DNA is positive in blood; CMV IgM is also positive, but there are false-positive reactions. Liver biopsy shows intranuclear inclusions and giant cells.

Herpes simplex

Very occasionally, the herpes simplex virus (see also pp. 247–249) causes a generalized acute infection, particularly in the immunosuppressed patient, and occasionally in pregnancy. Aminotransferases are usually massively elevated. Liver biopsy shows extensive necrosis. Aciclovir is used for treatment.

Toxoplasmosis

The clinical picture in toxoplasmosis (see also p. 305) is similar to that of infectious mononucleosis, with abnormal liver biochemistry, but the Paul–Bunnell test is negative.

Yellow fever

Yellow fever (see also pp. 265–266) is a viral infection carried by the mosquito *Aedes aegypti*; it can cause acute hepatic necrosis. There is no specific treatment.

Further reading

Amon JJ. Hepatitis in drug users: time for attention, time for action. *Lancet* 2011; 378:543–544.

European Association for the Study of the Liver. EASL Clinical Practice Guidelines: Management of chronic hepatitis B infection. *J Hepatol* 2012; 57:167–185.

European Association for the Study of the Liver. EASL Clinical Practice Guidelines: Management of hepatitis C virus infection. *J Hepatol* 2014; 60:392–420.

Hughes SA, Wedemeyer H, Harrison PM. Hepatitis delta virus. *Lancet* 2011; 378:73–85.

National Institute for Health and Care Excellence. *NICE Clinical Guideline 165: Hepatitis B (Chronic): Diagnosis and Management of Chronic Hepatitis B in Children, Young People and Adults*. NICE 2013; https://www.nice.org.uk/guidance/cg165.

Nelson PK, Mathers BM, Cowie B et al. Global epidemiology of hepatitis B and hepatitis C in people who inject drugs: results of systematic reviews. *Lancet* 2011; 378:578–583.

Razavi H, Waked I, Sarrazin C et al. The present and future disease burden of hepatitis C virus (HCV) infection with today's treatment paradigm. *J Viral Hepatitis* 2014; 21(Supplement S1):34–59.

Visvanathan K, Dusheiko G, Giles M et al. Managing HBV in pregnancy. *Gut* 2016; 65:340–350.

Wedemeyer H, Yurdaydìn C, Dalekos GN et al, for the HIDIT Study Group. Peginterferon plus adefovir versus either drug alone for hepatitis delta. *N Engl J Med* 2011; 364:322–331.

Zeuzem S. Decade in review – HCV: hepatitis C therapy – a fast and competitive race. *Nat Rev Gastroenterol Hepatol* 2014; 11:644–645.

Zhu FC, Zhang J, Zhang XF et al. Efficacy and safety of a recombinant hepatitis E vaccine in healthy adults: a large scale, randomized double blind placebo controlled phase 3 trial. *Lancet* 2010; 376:895–902.

http://www.easl.eu/_clinical-practice-guideline *European Association for the Study of the Liver: Clinical Practice Guidelines on viral hepatitis.*

ACUTE HEPATIC FAILURE

Acute liver failure is defined as acute liver injury with encephalopathy and dearranged coagulation (INR > 1.5) in a patient with a previously normal liver. The time intervals are variable. The development of jaundice to encephalopathy varies from 7 days (hyper-acute), 8–28 days (acute), and sub-acute (>21 and <26 weeks). Occasionally, patients may have previous liver damage: for example, D virus superinfection in a previous carrier of HBsAg, Budd–Chiari syndrome or Wilson's disease).

AHF is a rare but often life-threatening syndrome that is due to acute hepatitis from many causes ***(Box 14.9)***. These causes vary throughout the world; most cases are due to viral hepatitis, but paracetamol overdose is common in the UK (50% of cases). HCV does not usually cause acute hepatic failure, although exceptional cases have been reported from Japan and India.

Box 14.9 Causes of acute hepatic failure

Viruses
- HAV, HBV, (HDV), HEV; rarely, HCV
- Cytomegalovirus
- Haemorrhagic fever viruses
- Herpes simplex virus
- Paramyxovirus
- Epstein–Barr virus

Drugs (examples)
- Paracetamol (acetaminophen)
- Antibiotics (ampicillin-clavulanate, ciprofloxacin, doxycycline, erythromycin, isoniazid, nitrofurantoin, tetracycline)
- Antidepressants (amitriptyline, nortriptyline)
- Antiepileptics (phenytoin, valproate)
- Anaesthetic agents (halothane)
- Lipid-lowering medications (atorvastatin, lovastatin, simvastatin)
- Immunosuppressive agents (cyclophosphamide, methotrexate)
- NSAIDs
- Salicylates (as a result of Reye syndrome, p. 483)
- Disulfiram, flutamide, gold, propylthiouracil
- Illicit drugs (e.g. 'ecstasy' or cocaine)
- Herbal/alternative medicines (ginseng, pennyroyal oil, *Teucrium polium* chaparral or germander tea, kawa kawa)

Toxins
- *Amanita phalloides* mushroom toxin
- *Bacillus cereus* toxin
- Cyanobacteria toxin
- Organic solvents (e.g. carbon tetrachloride)
- Yellow phosphorus

Hepatic failure in pregnancy
- Acute fatty liver of pregnancy (AFLP)
- HELLP (*h*aemolysis, *e*levated *l*iver enzymes, *l*ow *p*latelets)

Vascular causes
- Ischaemic hepatitis
- Budd–Chiari syndrome
- Hepatic sinusoidal obstruction syndrome
- Portal vein thrombosis
- Hepatic arterial thrombosis (consider post transplant)

Metabolic causes
- α_1-antitrypsin deficiency
- Fructose intolerance
- Galactosaemia
- Lecithin–cholesterol acyltransferase deficiency
- Reye syndrome
- Tyrosinaemia
- Wilson's disease

Malignancies
- Primary (usually HCC, rarely cholangiocarcinoma)
- Secondary (extensive hepatic metastases or infiltration)

Miscellaneous
- Adult-onset Still's disease
- Heatstroke
- Primary graft non-function in liver transplant

HAV/HBV/HCV/HDV/HEV, hepatitis A/B/C/D/E virus; HCC, hepatocellular carcinoma; NSAIDs, non-steroidal anti-inflammatory drugs.

Box 14.10 Transfer criteria to specialized units for patients with acute liver injury

- INR >3.0
- Presence of hepatic encephalopathy
- Hypotension after resuscitation with fluid
- Metabolic acidosis
- Prothrombin time (seconds) > interval (hours) from overdose (paracetamol cases)

INR, International Normalized Ratio.

Histologically, there is multiacinar necrosis involving a substantial part of the liver. Severe fatty change is seen in pregnancy (see p. 1304) and Reye's syndrome (p. 486), or following intravenous tetracycline administration.

Clinical features

Examination shows a jaundiced patient with a small liver and signs of hepatic encephalopathy. The mental state varies from slight drowsiness, confusion and disorientation (grades I and II) to unresponsive coma (grade IV) with convulsions. Fetor hepaticus is common, but ascites and splenomegaly are rare. Fever, vomiting, hypotension and hypoglycaemia occur. Neurological examination shows spasticity and hyper-reflexia; plantar responses remain flexor until late. Cerebral oedema develops in 80% of patients with AHF but is far less common with subacute failure and its consequences of intracranial hypertension and brain herniation account for about 25% of the causes of death. Other complications include bacterial and fungal infections, gastrointestinal bleeding, respiratory arrest, kidney injury (hepatorenal syndrome and acute tubular necrosis) and pancreatitis.

Investigations

- Routine tests (see pp. 443–447)
- There is hyperbilirubinaemia, high serum aminotransferases and low levels of coagulation factors, including prothrombin and factor V. Aminotransferases are not useful indicators of the course of the disease, as they tend to fall along with the albumin with progressive liver damage.
- An electroencephalogram (EEG) is sometimes helpful in grading the encephalopathy.
- Ultrasound will define liver size and may indicate underlying liver pathology.

Management

There is no specific treatment but patients should be managed in a specialized unit. Transfer criteria to such units are shown in ***Box 14.10***. Supportive therapy as for hepatic encephalopathy is necessary (see p. 474). When signs of raised intracranial pressure (which is sometimes measured directly) are present, 20% mannitol (1 g/kg body weight) should be infused intravenously; this dose may need to be repeated. Dexamethasone is of no value. Hypoglycaemia, hypokalaemia, hypomagnesaemia, hypophosphataemia and hypocalcaemia should be anticipated and corrected with a 10% glucose infusion (checked by 2-hourly dipstick testing) and with potassium, calcium, phosphate and magnesium supplements. Hyponatraemia should be corrected with hypertonic saline (see p. 161). Coagulopathy is managed with intravenous vitamin K, platelets, blood or fresh frozen plasma. Haemorrhage may be a problem and patients are given a proton pump inhibitor (PPI) to prevent gastrointestinal bleeding. Prophylaxis against bacterial and fungal infection is routine, as infection is a frequent cause of death and may preclude liver transplantation. Suspected infection should be treated immediately with suitable antibiotics. Renal and respiratory failure should be treated as necessary. Liver transplantation has been a major advance for patients with AHF. It is difficult to judge the timing or the necessity for transplantation, but there are guidelines based on validated prognostic indices of survival (see below).

Box 14.11 Poor prognostic variables in acute hepatic failure indicating liver transplantation

Non-paracetamol (acetaminophen) causes

Three of following five:

- Drug or non-A, non-B hepatitis
- Age <10 and >40 years
- Interval from onset of jaundice to encephalopathy >7 days
- Serum bilirubin >300 μmol/L
- Prothrombin time >50 s (or >100 s in isolation)

Paracetamol overdose

- Arterial pH <7.3 (after resuscitation, 7.25 on acetylcysteine)

or

- Serum creatinine >300 μmol/L ***and***
- Prothrombin time >100 s ***and***
- Grade III–IV encephalopathy

Prognosis

In mild cases (grades I and II encephalopathy with drowsiness and confusion), two-thirds of the patients will survive. The outcome of severe cases (grades III and IV encephalopathy with stupor or deep coma) is related to the aetiology. In special units, 70% of patients with paracetamol overdosage and grade IV coma survive, as do 30–40% patients with HAV or HBV hepatitis. Poor prognostic variables indicating a need to transplant the liver are shown in ***Box 14.11***.

Further reading

Bernal W, Wendon J. Acute liver failure. *N Engl J Med* 2013; 369:2525–2534.

AUTOIMMUNE HEPATITIS

Autoimmune hepatitis (AIH) is a progressive inflammatory liver condition with a 75% female preponderance. Approximately 40% of AIH patients have a family history of autoimmune disease (e.g. pernicious anaemia, thyroiditis or coeliac disease), and at least 20% have concomitant autoimmune diseases or develop them during follow-up.

Pathogenesis

The pathogenesis of AIH is incompletely understood, although increasingly evidence demonstrates that genetic susceptibility, molecular mimicry and impaired immunoregulatory networks contribute to the initiation and perpetuation of the autoimmune attack. Liver damage is thought to be mediated primarily by T cell-mediated events (CD4+ T cells) against liver antigens, producing a progressive necroinflammatory process that leads to fibrosis and cirrhosis. However, no clear trigger mechanism has been found.

Clinical features

There are two peaks in presentation. In the peri- and postmenopausal group, patients may be asymptomatic, or present with fatigue and abnormalities in liver biochemistry or the presence of chronic liver disease on examination. In the teens and early twenties, the disease (often type II) presents as an acute hepatitis with jaundice and very high aminotransferases, which do not improve with time. This age group often has clinical features of cirrhosis and patients who are ill may also have features of an autoimmune disease, such as fever, migratory polyarthritis, glomerulonephritis, pleurisy, pulmonary infiltration or lung fibrosis.

There are rare overlap syndromes with primary biliary cholangitis and primary sclerosing cholangitis, existing concomitantly or developing consecutively.

Investigations

Liver biochemistry

The serum aminotransferases are high, with lesser elevations in the ALP and bilirubin. The serum γ-globulins are high: frequently twice normal, particularly the IgG. The biochemical pattern is similar in both types.

Haematology

A mild normochromic normocytic anaemia with thrombocytopenia and leucopenia is present, even before portal hypertension and splenomegaly. The prothrombin time is often high.

Autoantibodies

Two types of autoimmune hepatitis have been recognized:

- ***Type I with antibodies*** (titres >1 : 80):
  - anti-nuclear (ANA)
  - anti-smooth muscle (anti-actin).
- ***Type II with antibodies***: anti-liver/kidney microsomal (anti-LKM1). The main target is cytochrome P4502D6 (CYP2D6) on liver cell plasma membranes.
- A third type of AIH (AIH-3) was proposed, positive for anti-soluble liver antigen (SLA) and negative for conventional autoantibodies. However, subsequent studies showed that anti-SLA is also present in typical cases of AIH-1 and AIH-2. Patients positive for anti-SLA only, and therefore having *bona fide* AIH-3, are rare.

Approximately 13% of patients lack the autoantibodies listed above.

Liver biopsy

Since transferases and IgG levels do not reflect disease activity, liver biopsy is mandatory to confirm the diagnosis and evaluate disease severity. The biopsy ***(Fig. 14.20)*** commonly shows chronic active hepatitis with inflammation and interface hepatitis. This reflects the changes of chronic hepatitis described on page 452. The amount of interface hepatitis is variable, but tends to be high in untreated patients. Lymphoid follicles are less often seen than in hepatitis C, and plasma cell infiltration is frequent. Fibrosis is present in all but the mildest forms of the disease and approximately one-third of patients have cirrhosis at presentation.

Management

Prednisolone 30 mg is given daily for at least 2 weeks, followed by slow reduction to a maintenance dose of 5–15 mg daily. Azathioprine should be added, 1–2 mg/kg daily, as a steroid-sparing agent and, in some, as sole long-term maintenance therapy. Levels of thiopurine methyltransferase (TPMT) should be obtained before treatment is started (see p. 411). Other agents that have been used in resistant cases include budesonide (in non-cirrhotic patients), mycophenolate, ciclosporin and tacrolimus.

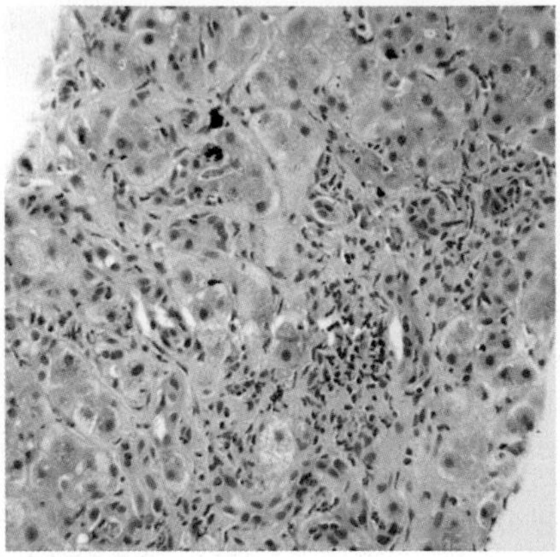

Figure 14.20 Chronic active hepatitis. Note the inflammation with interface hepatitis (×10).

Prognosis

Steroid and azathioprine therapy induce remission in over 80%; indeed, this response forms part of the diagnostic criteria. Treatment is life-long in most, although withdrawal may be considered after 2–3 years of biochemical remission. Those with initial cirrhosis are more likely to relapse following withdrawal and require indefinite therapy. Liver transplantation is performed if treatment fails, although the disease may recur. HCC occurs less frequently than with viral-induced cirrhosis. The risk of malignancy associated with chronic low-dose azathioprine therapy has been reported to be 1.4 times normal.

Further reading

Liberal R, Grant CR, Longhi MS et al. Diagnostic criteria of autoimmune hepatitis. *Autoimmun Rev* 2014; 13:435–440.

Liberal R, Grant CR, Mieli-Vergani G et al. Autoimmune hepatitis: a comprehensive review. *J Autoimmun* 2013; 41:126–139.

DRUG-INDUCED CHRONIC HEPATITIS

Several drugs can cause a chronic hepatitis similar to autoimmune hepatitis (see ***Box 14.23***). Patients are often female, present with jaundice and hepatomegaly, and have raised serum aminotransferases and globulin levels. Improvement follows drug withdrawal but exacerbations can occur with re-introduction. Isoniazid, amiodarone and methotrexate can cause chronic histological changes. With rare exceptions, patients with pre-existing chronic liver disease are not more susceptible to drug injury.

CHRONIC HEPATITIS OF UNKNOWN CAUSE

As increasing numbers undergo routine blood tests, mild elevations in serum aminotransferases and γ-GT are commonly found. Many will have no symptoms or signs of liver disease. All known aetiological agents should be excluded, risk factors for NAFLD evaluated, and tests carried out to exclude liver diseases. Liver biopsy should be performed if the elevation in aminotransferases (>100 IU/L) persists for over a year, but often only non-specific changes are found.

NON-ALCOHOLIC FATTY LIVER DISEASE

Non-alcoholic fatty liver disease (NAFLD) is now the most common cause of chronic liver disease in many developed countries. It is often detected on routine abdominal ultrasound examination, and steatosis is found in up to one-third of these patients. Traditionally, it was considered that the 10–30% of patients with non-alcoholic steatohepatitis (NASH) were considerably more likely than those with simple steatosis to develop cirrhosis, but a recent large study demonstrated no difference in liver-related adverse events between definite NASH and severe steatosis. However, patients with advanced fibrosis at presentation were much more likely to progress than those without. In this cohort, complications of cirrhosis were the third most common cause of death, following cardiovascular events and non-hepatic malignancies.

Risk factors for NAFLD are obesity, hypertension, type 2 diabetes and hyperlipidaemia, such that NAFLD is considered to be the liver component of the metabolic syndrome (see p. 209). Most patients are asymptomatic; hepatomegaly may be present. Mild increases in serum aminotransferases and/or γ-GT (with ALT greater than AST) are frequently the sole liver biochemical abnormality.

Pathogenesis

Histological changes follow a spectrum similar to those of alcohol-induced hepatic injury, and range from simple fatty change to fat and inflammation (NASH), fibrosis and cirrhosis.

Oxidative stress injury and other factors lead to lipid peroxidation in the presence of fatty infiltration and inflammation. Fibrosis may then occur, enhanced by insulin resistance, which induces connective tissue growth factor.

Investigations

- Diagnosis is usually by ***ultrasound*** demonstration of steatosis in the absence of other injurious causes, such as alcohol.
- ***Liver biopsy*** allows staging of the disease. Although no definitive guidelines exist, many clinicians perform a biopsy if a diagnosis of NASH or advanced fibrosis is considered likely.
- ***Elastography*** (see p. 446) is used to evaluate the degree of fibrosis but may not be technically possible in the morbidly obese.

Management

- All NAFLD patients require ***lifestyle advice*** aimed at weight loss, increased physical activity, and attention to cardiovascular risk factors. Calorie restriction is recommended, aimed at losing 0.5–1 kg per week until target weight is achieved. A reduction of more than 7–9% in body weight has been associated with reduced steatosis, hepatocellular injury and hepatic inflammation.
- ***Orlistat***, an enteric lipase inhibitor causing malabsorption of dietary fat, is used with a low-fat diet as an adjunct in subjects with a body mass index (BMI) of more than 30 kg/m^2. Only those achieving a loss of body weight of more than 5% in 3 months should continue orlistat, and then for only 1 year, as fat-soluble vitamin deficiency may occur.
- ***Pioglitazone*** or vitamin E may be used for those with biopsy-proven NASH, in whom lifestyle intervention has failed. Meta-analysis data demonstrated that pioglitazone significantly improved liver steatosis, inflammation and, to a lesser degree, fibrosis. However, it is associated with weight gain and reports of congestive cardiac failure, bladder cancer and reduced bone density. Conversely, pioglitazone reduces death, myocardial infarction and stroke in diabetes patients. The risks and benefits to each patient should be evaluated accordingly.
- ***Vitamin E*** (800 IU/day) is an antioxidant that improves steatohepatitis. However, a meta-analysis showed an increase in all-cause mortality at doses over 400 IU/day, and an increased risk of haemorrhagic stroke and prostate cancer has also been reported.
- Weight loss following ***bariatric surgery*** leads to reduced steatosis, steatohepatitis and fibrosis. The optimum technique is unknown and long-term data are lacking, although initial concerns about worsening fibrosis do not appear to have been borne out. Bariatric surgery should be avoided in those with advanced cirrhosis and portal hypertension, but gastric bypass and sleeve gastrectomy (pp. 210–211) have been shown to achieve weight loss and improve obesity-related co-morbidities in Child–Pugh A cirrhotic patients.

Hepatocellular carcinoma

The yearly cumulative incidence of HCC is 2.6% in patients with NASH cirrhosis, and ultrasound surveillance should therefore be performed 6-monthly. Hyperinsulinaemia and obesity are risk factors for many malignancies. Metformin and statin treatment may reduce the risk of HCC in patients with type 2 diabetes.

Liver transplantation

NASH cirrhosis is now the third most common indication for liver transplantation in the USA. Survival is comparable to that in other indications, and although recurrence occurs post transplant (4–25%), it does not appear to have an impact on graft survival. Patients frequently have multiple cardiovascular risk factors that should be managed aggressively. UK guidelines suggest that bariatric surgery could be considered at transplantation for the morbidly obese.

Further reading

Dyson JK, Anstee QM, McPherson S. Non-alcoholic fatty liver disease: a practical approach to treatment. *Frontline Gastroenterol* 2014; 5:277–286.
Gawrieh S, Chalasani N. NAFLD fibrosis score: is it ready for wider use in clinical practice and for clinical trials? *Gastroenterology* 2013; 145:717–719.
Newsome PN, Allison ME, Andrews PA et al. Guidelines for liver transplantation for patients with non-alcoholic steatohepatitis. *Gut* 2012; 61:484–500.

CIRRHOSIS

In cirrhosis, the liver architecture is diffusely abnormal and interferes with liver blood flow and function; this leads to the clinical manifestations of portal hypertension and liver failure.

Aetiology

Causes of cirrhosis are shown in ***Box 14.12***. Alcohol is currently the most common cause in the West, but likely to be superseded by NAFLD; viral infection the most common worldwide. Young patients with cirrhosis must be investigated to exclude treatable causes (e.g. Wilson's disease).

Box 14.12 Causes of cirrhosis

Common
- Alcohol
- Hepatitis B±D
- Hepatitis C
- Non-alcoholic fatty liver disease (NAFLD)

Others
- Primary biliary cholangitis
- Secondary biliary cirrhosis
- Autoimmune hepatitis
- Hereditary haemochromatosis
- Hepatic venous congestion
- Budd–Chiari syndrome
- Wilson's disease
- Drugs (e.g. methotrexate)
- α_1-Antitrypsin deficiency
- Cystic fibrosis
- Galactosaemia
- Glycogen storage disease
- Veno-occlusive disease
- Idiopathic (cryptogenic)
- ? Other viruses

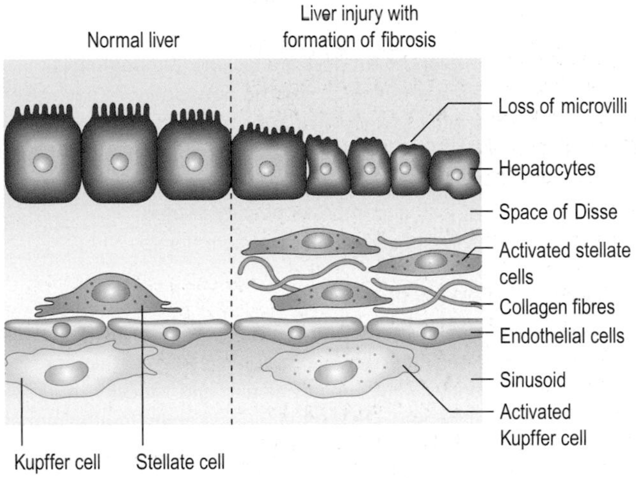

Figure 14.21 Pathogenesis of fibrosis. The normal liver is shown on the left. Activation of the stellate cell is followed by proliferation of fibroblasts and the deposition of collagen.

Pathogenesis

Although the liver has a remarkable capacity to adapt to injury through tissue repair, chronic injury results in inflammation, matrix deposition, necrosis and angiogenesis, all of which lead to fibrosis ***(Fig. 14.21)***. Liver injury causes necrosis and apoptosis, releasing cell contents and reactive oxygen species (ROS). This activates hepatic stellate cells and tissue macrophages through the CC-chemokine ligand 2–CC-chemokine receptor 2 (CCL2–CCR2) axis (see p. 440). These cells phagocytose necrotic and apoptotic cells and secrete pro-inflammatory mediators, including transforming growth factor-beta (TGF-β); this leads to transdifferentiation of stellate cells to myofibroblasts and platelet-derived growth factor (PDGF), which stimulates myofibroblast proliferation. Macrophages degrade scar matrix by secretion of matrix metalloproteinases (MMPs), but this is inhibited by concurrent myofibroblast and macrophage production of tissue inhibitors of metalloproteinases (TIMPs). This results in progressive matrix deposition and scar accumulation. Increased gut permeability and hepatic lipopolysaccharide–Toll-like receptor 4 (LPS–TLR4) signalling also promotes fibrogenesis. Repetitive or chronic injury and inflammation perpetuate this process.

If the cause of fibrosis is eliminated (e.g. treatment of viral hepatitis), resolution (complete reversal to near-normal liver architecture) of early fibrosis can occur. In cirrhosis, regression (improvement, not reversal) occurs, which improves clinical outcomes. Antifibrotic therapies are emerging (including stem cell transplant strategies) but currently liver transplantation is the only available treatment for liver failure.

Pathology

The characteristic features of cirrhosis are regenerating nodules separated by fibrous septa, and loss of lobular architecture within the nodules ***(Fig. 14.22A–C)***. Two types are described:

- ***Micronodular cirrhosis***. Regenerating nodules are usually <3 mm in size with uniform involvement of the liver; often caused by alcohol or biliary tract disease.
- ***Macronodular cirrhosis***. The nodules are of variable size and normal acini may be seen within larger nodules; often caused by chronic viral hepatitis.

A mixed picture with small and large nodules occurs occasionally.

Symptoms and signs are described on pages 447–448.

Investigations

Investigations aim to assess the severity and type of liver disease.

Severity

- ***Liver function***. Serum albumin and prothrombin time are the best indicators of liver function; the outlook is poor if the albumin level is <28 g/L. The degree to which the prothrombin time is prolonged is commensurate with disease severity.
- ***Liver biochemistry***. This may be normal, depending on the severity of disease. In most cases, there is a slight elevation in the serum ALP and serum aminotransferases. In decompensated cirrhosis, all biochemistry is deranged.
- ***Serum electrolytes***. A low sodium indicates severe liver disease due to a defect in free water clearance or excess diuretic therapy.
- ***Serum creatinine***. An elevated concentration >130 µmol/L is a marker of poor prognosis.
- ***Biomarkers***. In the Enhanced Liver Fibrosis (ELF™) test, which assesses fibrosis, a value of <7.7 indicates none to mild, 7.7–9.8 moderate, and ≥9.8 severe.

In addition, a serum α-fetoprotein of >200 ng/mL is strongly suggestive of HCC.

Type

This can be determined by:

- viral markers
- serum autoantibodies
- serum immunoglobulins
- iron indices and ferritin
- copper and caeruloplasmin (see p. 479)
- α_1-antitrypsin (see pp. 479–480).
- genetic markers.

Serum copper and serum α_1-antitrypsin should always be measured in young cirrhotics. Total iron-binding capacity (TIBC) and ferritin should be measured to exclude hereditary haemochromatosis; genetic markers are also available (see pp. 477–479).

Imaging

- ***Ultrasound examination*** can demonstrate changes in the size and shape of the liver. Fatty change and fibrosis produce a diffusely increased echogenicity. In established cirrhosis, there may be marginal nodularity of the liver surface and distortion of the arterial vascular architecture. The patency of the portal and hepatic veins can be evaluated. Ultrasound is useful for detecting HCC.
- ***Transient elastography*** is increasingly used to avoid liver biopsy (see p. 446). Technical limitations preclude its use in patients with ascites or morbid obesity, but it is suitable for most.

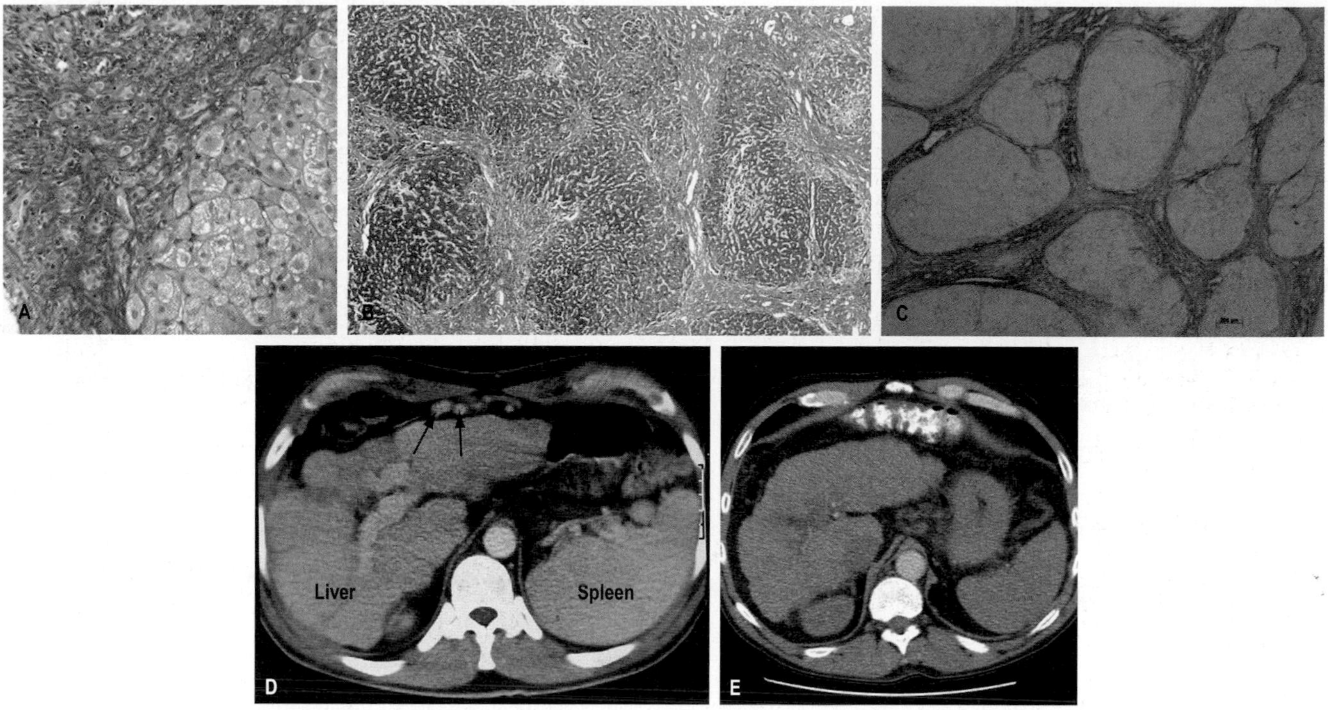

Figure 14.22 Pathology of cirrhosis. A. Haematoxylin and eosin histological view (×10). **B.** Histological appearance **(Giemsa stain)**, showing nodules of liver tissue of varying size, surrounded by fibrosis. **C. Picrosirius red stain of collagen** used for morphometric evaluation of fibrosis. **D. CT scan** showing an irregular lobulated liver. There is splenomegaly and enlargement of collateral vessels beneath the anterior abdominal wall (arrowed), caused by portal hypertension. **E. CT image showing cirrhosis**, with a patent portal vein and no space-occupying lesion.

- ***CT scanning*** (see p. 446) is also helpful. Figure 14.22D–E show hepatosplenomegaly and the dilated collaterals seen in chronic liver disease. Arterial phase-contrast-enhanced scans are useful for detecting of HCC.
- ***Endoscopy*** is performed for the detection and treatment of varices and portal hypertensive gastropathy. Colonoscopy is occasionally carried out for colopathy.
- ***MRI scanning*** is useful in the diagnosis of both malignant and benign tumours such as haemangiomas. MR angiography can demonstrate the vascular anatomy, and MR cholangiography the biliary tree.

Liver biopsy

This remains the 'gold standard' for confirming the type and severity of liver disease. Adequate samples, in terms of length and number of complete portal tracts, are necessary for diagnosis and staging/grading of chronic viral hepatitis; in macronodular cirrhosis, the core of liver may fragment, causing sampling errors. Immunocytochemical stains can identify viruses, bile ducts, angiogenic structures and oncogenic markers. Chemical measurement of iron and copper is necessary to confirm a diagnosis of iron overload or Wilson's disease. Digital image analysis of Picrosirius red staining can be used to quantitate collagen in biopsy specimens ***(Fig. 14.22C)***.

Management

Management is that of the complications of decompensated cirrhosis. Patients should undergo 6-monthly ultrasound to screen for the early development of HCC (see p. 485), as all therapeutic strategies work best with small, single tumours.

Treatment of the underlying cause may arrest or reverse cirrhosis. Patients with compensated cirrhosis should lead a normal life. Those at risk should receive hepatitis A and B vaccination. The only dietary restriction is to reduce salt intake (≤2 g sodium per day). Alcohol should be avoided, as should aspirin and non-steroidal anti-inflammatory drugs (NSAIDs), which may precipitate gastrointestinal bleeding or renal impairment.

Box 14.13 Poor prognostic indicators in cirrhosis

Blood tests

- Low albumin (<28 g/L)
- Low serum sodium (<125 mmol/L)
- Prolonged prothrombin time >6 s above normal value
- Raised creatinine >130 μmol/L

Clinical

- Persistent jaundice
- Failure of response to therapy
- Ascites
- Haemorrhage from varices, particularly with poor liver function
- Neuropsychiatric complications developing with progressive liver failure
- Small liver
- Persistent hypotension
- Aetiology (e.g. alcoholic cirrhosis, if the patient continues drinking)

Prognosis

Prognosis is extremely variable. In general, the 5-year survival rate is approximately 50%, depending on the stage at which diagnosis is made. Poor prognostic indicators are shown in ***Box 14.13***. Development of any complication usually worsens the prognosis.

There are a number of prognostic classifications based on modifications of Child's grading (A, B and C; ***Box 14.14***) and the Model for End-stage Liver Disease (MELD; ***Box 14.15***), based on serum bilirubin, creatinine and INR, which is widely used as a predictor of mortality in patients awaiting liver transplantation. Modifications of the MELD score (e.g. UKELD) are used in some countries.

Box 14.14 Scoring systems in cirrhosis: modified Child–Pugh classification

Score	1	2	3
Ascites	None	Mild	Moderate/severe
Encephalopathy	None	Mild	Marked
Bilirubin (μmol/L)	<34	34–50	>50
Albumin (g/L)	>35	28–35	<28
Prothrombin time (seconds over normal)	<4	4–6	>6

Add above scores for your patient for survival figures below:
Child's A (<7): 82% survival at 1 year, 45% at 5 years, 25% at 10 years
Child's B (7–9): 62% survival at 1 year, 20% at 5 years, 7% at 10 years
Child's C (10+): 42% survival at 1 year, 20% at 5 years, 0% at 10 years

Box 14.15 Scoring systems in cirrhosis: Model of End-stage Liver Disease (MELD)

3.8×LN (bilirubin in mg/dL)+9.6×LN (creatinine in mg/dL)+11.2×LN (INR)+6.4*
To convert:
- bilirubin from μmol/L to mg/dL, divide by 17
- creatinine from μmol/L to mg/dL, divide by 88.4

MELD scores (with no complications):
- Score <10: 97% survival at 1 year
- Score 30–40: 70% at 1 year

INR, International Normalized Ratio; LN, natural logarithm.
**Check online*

Acute-on-chronic liver failure

Acute-on-chronic liver failure (ACLF) refers to the condition of patients hospitalized for an acute complication of cirrhosis accompanied by organ failure(s); it has a high short-term mortality. ACLF is believed to be distinct from traditional decompensated cirrhosis, based not only on the presence of organ failure(s) and high mortality rate, but also on younger age, alcohol aetiology, higher prevalence of certain precipitating events (e.g. bacterial infections or active alcohol excess), and a higher level of systemic inflammation. It is estimated to occur in 31% of patients hospitalized with an acute complication of cirrhosis.

Liver assist devices

As the liver has great potential to regenerate, extracorporeal liver support devices may allow patients with liver failure to be bridged to recovery or even liver transplantation. Current approaches include the use of biological devices that contain hepatocytes and those that function as detoxification devices, and artificial liver support systems. However, no device is currently available routinely.

Gut–liver axis

The liver is exposed to gut-derived bacterial components that have little consequence in health, as an effective gut barrier limits the amount of bacterial components transported to the liver. In advanced liver disease, the intestinal barrier function is compromised due to changes in gut motility, an increase in intestinal permeability, and suppression of gut immunological functions. This leads to bacteria and components entering the portal circulation and being transported to the liver, activating Toll-like receptors and producing an inflammatory response. This cross-talk between the intestinal microbiota and the liver is referred to as the gut–liver axis; it is seen as a key pathophysiological mechanism in the progression of liver disease and development of the complications of cirrhosis. Antibiotics and non-selective β-blockers intercept the gut–liver axis by ***blocking bacterial translocation***, which is likely to account for their beneficial effects in reducing portal pressure, variceal haemorrhage and spontaneous bacterial peritonitis. However, absorbable antibiotics will lead to the selection of resistant bacteria. Rifaximin, a poorly absorbed antibiotic used for encephalopathy, specifically affects the gut flora and has a low risk for inducing resistance; it may therefore have a role in this indication.

Further reading

Leckie P, Davenport A, Jalan R. Extracorporeal liver support. *Blood Purif* 2012; 34:158–163.
Madsen BS, Havelund T, Krag A. Targeting the gut–liver axis in cirrhosis: antibiotics and non-selective β blockers. *Adv Ther* 2013; 30:659–670.
Moreau R, Jalan R, Gines P et al and the CANONIC Study Investigators of the EASL–CLIF Consortium. Acute-on-chronic liver failure is a distinct syndrome that develops in patients with acute decompensation of cirrhosis. *Gastroenterology* 2013; 144:1426–1437.
Pellicoro A, Ramachandran P, Iredale JP et al. Liver fibrosis and repair: immune regulation of wound healing in a solid organ. *Nat Rev Immunol* 2014; 14:181–194.

Liver transplantation

This is the only established treatment for advanced liver disease. Shortage of donors is a major problem in all developed countries and in some, such as Japan or South Korea, living related donors form the majority.

Indications

These include:
- ***Acute liver disease***: acute hepatic failure of any cause (see p. 463).
- ***Chronic liver disease***: usually for complications of cirrhosis that are no longer responsive to therapy.

The timing of transplantation depends on donor availability. All patients with end-stage cirrhosis (Child's grade C; MELD score ≥20; UKELD score ≥49) and those with debilitating symptoms should be referred to a transplant centre. In addition, specific extrahepatic complications of cirrhosis, even with preserved liver function, such as hepatopulmonary syndrome and porto-pulmonary hypertension, can be reversed by transplantation.

- ***Primary biliary cholangitis***. Patients should be transplanted when their serum bilirubin is persistently >100 μmol/L or when they have symptoms such as intractable pruritus.
- ***Chronic hepatitis B if HBV DNA-negative*** or levels are falling with therapy. Following transplantation, recurrence of hepatitis is prevented by hepatitis B immunoglobulin and nucleoside analogues in combination (see pp. 243–244).
- ***Chronic hepatitis C***. This is the most common indication. Universal HCV re-infection occurs with varying severity and cirrhosis occurs in 10–20% at 5 years. The new antiviral drugs are highly likely to improve these figures greatly.
- ***Autoimmune hepatitis***. In patients who have failed to respond to medical treatment, the disease can recur.
- ***Alcoholic liver disease***. Well-motivated patients who have stopped drinking without improvement of liver disease are offered a transplant, with frequent counselling. It has been shown that transplantation may represent life-saving treatment in patients with severe alcoholic hepatitis who are not responding to medical therapy. However, further studies are awaited.

- ***Primary metabolic disorders***. Examples are Wilson's disease, hereditary haemochromatosis and α_1-antitrypsin deficiency.
- ***NASH cirrhosis***. Now one of the most common causes of chronic liver disease in developed countries, this is likely to become the most frequent indication for transplantation.
- ***Other conditions***, such as primary sclerosing cholangitis (PSC), polycystic liver disease, and metabolic diseases such as primary oxaluria.

Contraindications

Absolute contraindications include active sepsis outside the hepatobiliary tree, malignancy outside the liver, liver metastases (except neuroendocrine), and a lack of psychological commitment on the part of the patient.

Relative contraindications are mainly anatomical considerations that make surgery more difficult, such as extensive splanchnic venous thrombosis. With exceptions, patients aged 70 years or over are not usually given a transplant. In HCC, the recurrence rate is high, unless there are fewer than three small (<3 cm) lesions or a solitary nodule of <5 cm (Milan criteria).

Preparation for surgery

Pre-transplant work-up includes confirmation of the diagnosis, ultrasound and cross-sectional imaging, and radiological demonstration of the hepatic arterial and biliary trees, as well as assessment of cardiorespiratory and renal status. In view of the ethical and financial implications of transplantation, regular psychosocial, and possibly psychiatric, support is vital.

The donor should be ABO-compatible (HLA matching is not necessary) and have no evidence of active sepsis, malignancy, or HIV, HBV or HCV infection. Younger donors (<50 years) experience better graft function. The donor liver is cooled and stored on ice; its preservation time may be up to 20 hours. The recipient operation takes approximately 8 hours and rarely requires a large blood transfusion. Cadaveric donor livers (from heart-beating or non-heart-beating donors) may consist of whole graft, split grafts (for two recipients) or reduced grafts. Live donors may be healthy individuals or patients with, for example, familial amyloid polyneuropathy, whose livers can be transplanted into others (domino transplant). The mortality of right lobe donors is between 1 in 200 and 1 in 400.

The operative mortality is low and most postoperative deaths occur in the first 3 months. Sepsis and haemorrhage can be serious complications. Opportunistic infections occur owing to immunosuppression. Various immunosuppressive agents have been used, but tacrolimus – alone or in combination with azathioprine or mycophenolate mofetil, steroids, sirolimus and microemulsified ciclosporin are the most common.

Rejection

- ***Acute or cellular rejection*** usually occurs 5–10 days post transplant; it can be asymptomatic or there may be a fever. On biopsy, a pleomorphic portal infiltrate is seen with prominent eosinophils, bile duct damage and endothelialitis of the blood vessels. This responds well to immunosuppressive therapy.
- ***Chronic ductopenic rejection*** is seen between 6 weeks and 9 months post transplant, with disappearing bile ducts (vanishing bile duct syndrome, VBDS), and an arteriopathy with narrowing and occlusion of the arteries. Early ductopenic rejection is rarely reversed by immunosuppression and often requires retransplantation.
- ***Graft-versus-host disease*** is extremely rare.

Prognosis

Elective liver transplantation in low-risk patients has a 90% 1-year survival and a 70–85% 5-year survival. Patients require life-long immunosuppression, although doses can be reduced over time without significant problems. Future strategies to reduce immunosuppression requirements after transplant may include infusion of autologous regulatory T cells. HCV cirrhosis, PSC and HCC are conditions in which long-term survival after transplantation is compromised by disease recurrence.

Further reading

Lucey MR. Liver transplantation for alcoholic liver diseases. *Nat Rev Gastroenterol Hepatol* 2014; 11:300–307.

Complications and effects of cirrhosis

These are shown in ***Box 14.16***.

Portal hypertension

The portal vein is formed by the union of the superior mesenteric and splenic veins. Normal pressure is 5–8 mmHg with only a small gradient across the liver to the hepatic vein, in which blood is returned to the heart via the inferior vena cava. Portal hypertension is classified according to the site of obstruction:

- ***Prehepatic*** – blockage of the portal vein before the liver
- ***Intrahepatic*** – distortion of the liver architecture, either pre-sinusoidal (e.g. schistosomiasis) or post-sinusoidal (e.g. cirrhosis)
- ***Post-hepatic*** – venous blockage outside the liver (rare).

As portal pressure rises above 10–12 mmHg, the compliant venous system dilates and collaterals form within the systemic venous system. The main sites of collaterals are the gastro-oesophageal junction, rectum, left renal vein, diaphragm, retroperitoneum and the anterior abdominal wall via the umbilical vein.

The collaterals at the gastro-oesophageal junction (varices) are superficial and tend to rupture. Portosystemic anastomoses at other sites rarely cause symptoms. Rectal varices are found frequently (30%) if looked for and can be differentiated from haemorrhoids, which are lower in the anal canal. The microvasculature of the gut becomes congested, giving rise to portal hypertensive gastropathy and colopathy, in which there is punctate erythema and erosions, which can bleed.

Pathophysiology

Following liver injury and fibrogenesis, the contraction of activated myofibroblasts (mediated by endothelin, nitric oxide and prostaglandins) contributes to increased resistance to blood flow. This increased resistance leads to portal hypertension and opening of portosystemic anastomoses in both pre-cirrhotic and cirrhotic livers. Neoangiogenesis also occurs. The hyperdynamic circulation of cirrhosis (caused by nitric oxide, cannabinoids and glucagon) leads to peripheral and splanchnic vasodilatation. This, combined with plasma volume expansion due to sodium retention (see

Box 14.16 Complications and effects of cirrhosis

- Portal hypertension and gastrointestinal haemorrhage
- Ascites
- Portosystemic encephalopathy
- Hepatocellular carcinoma
- Bacteraemias, infections
- Renal failure
- Hepatopulmonary syndrome

Box 14.17 Causes of portal hypertension

Prehepatic
- Portal vein thrombosis

Intrahepatic
- *Pre-sinusoidal*
  - Schistosomiasis; sarcoidosis
  - Primary biliary cholangitis
- *Sinusoidal*
  - Cirrhosis (e.g. alcoholic)
  - Partial nodular transformation
  - Congenital hepatic fibrosis
- *Post-sinusoidal*
  - Veno-occlusive disease
  - Budd–Chiari syndrome

Post-hepatic
- Right heart failure (rare)
- Constrictive pericarditis
- Inferior vena cava obstruction

'Ascites', pp. 472–473), has a significant effect in maintaining portal hypertension.

Aetiology

The most common cause is cirrhosis ***(Box 14.17)***. Others are described below.

Prehepatic causes

Extrahepatic blockage due to portal vein thrombosis can be caused by congenital portal venous abnormalities, neonatal sepsis of the umbilical vein, or inherited prothrombotic conditions, such as factor V Leiden or primary myeloproliferative disorders with or without *JAK2* mutations (see p. 97).

Patients present with gastrointestinal bleeding, often at a young age. They have normal liver function, and prognosis following bleeding is therefore excellent.

The portal vein blockage can be identified by ultrasound with Doppler imaging; CT and MR angiography are also used.

Treatment for variceal bleeding is usually repeated endoscopic therapy or non-selective beta-blockade. Splenectomy is only performed if there is isolated splenic vein thrombosis. Anticoagulation prevents further thrombosis and intestinal infarction, and does not increase the risk of bleeding.

Intrahepatic causes

Cirrhosis is by far the most common cause but others include:

- ***Non-cirrhotic portal hypertension*** is characterized by mild portal tract fibrosis on liver histology. The aetiology is unknown, but arsenic, vinyl chloride, antiretroviral therapy and other toxins have been implicated. A similar disease is frequently found in India. The liver lesion does not progress and prognosis is good.
- ***Schistosomiasis*** with extensive pipe-stem fibrosis in endemic areas such as Egypt and Brazil. Often, there is concomitant liver disease, such as HCV infection, which was transmitted by non-sterile equipment.
- ***Other causes*** include congenital hepatic fibrosis, and nodular regenerative hyperplasia and partial nodular transformation.

Post-hepatic causes

Prolonged severe heart failure with tricuspid incompetence or constrictive pericarditis can cause portal hypertension. The Budd–Chiari syndrome is described on page 482.

Clinical features

Patients are often asymptomatic, the only clinical evidence being splenomegaly, although features of chronic liver disease may exist (see pp. 447–448).

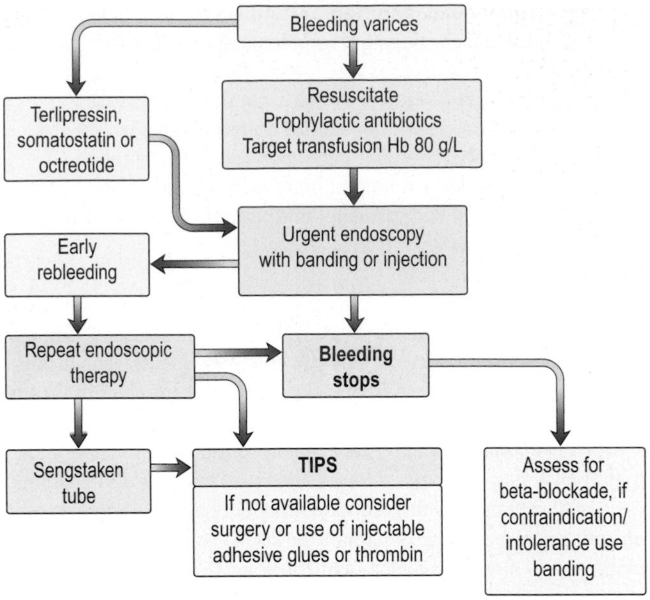

Figure 14.23 Management of gastrointestinal haemorrhage due to oesophageal varices. TIPS, transjugular intrahepatic portosystemic shunt.

Variceal haemorrhage

Approximately 90% of patients with cirrhosis will develop gastro-oesophageal varices over 10 years, but only one-third of these will bleed. Bleeding is likely to occur with large varices, or those with red signs at endoscopy, and in severe liver disease.

Management

Management can be divided into:

- the active bleeding episode
- prevention of rebleeding
- prophylactic measures to prevent the first haemorrhage.

Despite the therapeutic techniques available, prognosis ultimately depends on the severity of the underlying liver disease; overall 6-week mortality from variceal haemorrhage is 15–25%, reaching 50% in Child's grade C.

Initial management of acute variceal bleeding

See ***Figure 14.23***, and also the general management of gastrointestinal haemorrhage on page 385.

Resuscitation

- ***Assess*** the patient: pulse, blood pressure and conscious state.
- Insert a ***large-bore intravenous line*** and obtain ***blood*** for group and crossmatching, haemoglobin, prothrombin time/INR, urea, electrolytes, creatinine, liver biochemistry and blood cultures.
- ***Restore blood volume*** with plasma expanders or, if possible, blood transfusion. See the treatment of shock for more detail (pp. 1156–1161). Prompt correction, but not over-correction, of hypovolaemia is necessary in cirrhosis patients, as their baroreceptor reflexes are diminished. A target haemoglobin of 80 g/L is sufficient and this lessens the likelihood of early rebleeding.
- Carry out an ***ascitic tap***.
- ***Monitor for alcohol withdrawal***. Give intravenous thiamine.

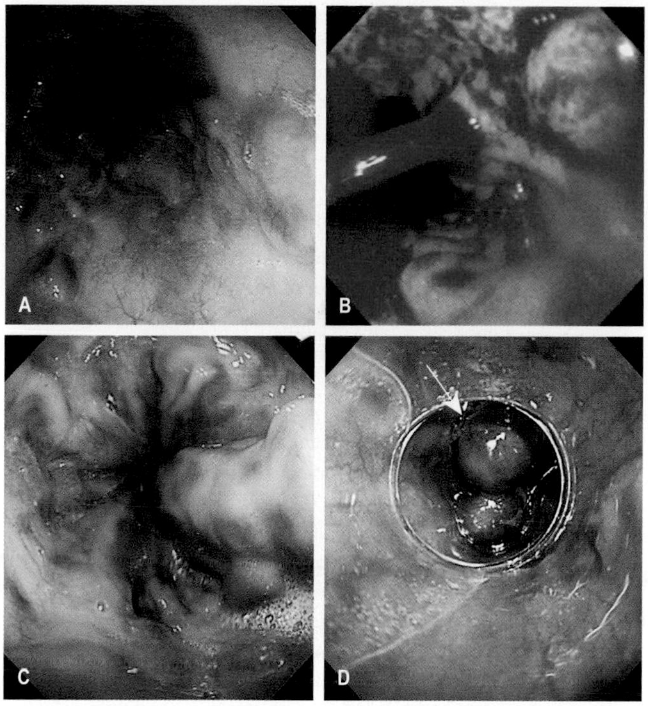

Figure 14.24 **Endoscopic views of oesophageal varices. A.** Gross varices. **B.** Blood spurting from a varix. **C.** Following a recent bleed. **D.** Varices with a band in place (arrowed). *(A, C and D Courtesy of Dr Peter Fairclough.)*

- Start ***prophylactic antibiotics***. These treat and prevent infection, and reduce early rebleeding and mortality.

Urgent endoscopy

Endoscopy ***(Fig. 14.24)*** should be performed to confirm the diagnosis and to exclude bleeding from other sites (e.g. gastric ulceration) and portal hypertensive gastropathy/**g**astric **a**ntral **v**ascular **e**ctasia (GAVE). The latter describes chronic gastric congestion, punctate erythema and gastric erosions, which may contribute to chronic anaemia. Portal hypertensive gastropathy and GAVE are distinct entities; management of portal hypertensive gastropathy is centred on reduction in portal pressures with β-blockers, whereas treatment of GAVE is endoscopic and uses various ablative techniques.

Variceal banding or injection sclerotherapy

Banding of oesophageal varices is performed by mounting a band on the tip of the endoscope, sucking the varix into the end of the scope, and dislodging the band over the varix using a trip-wire mechanism.

Between 15% and 20% of bleeding comes from gastric varices, which are associated with a greater mortality (up to 40%); endoscopic injection of cyanoacrylate is the best treatment.

Overall, haemostasis is achieved in 80–90% of patients. Best practice is to perform the endoscopy with the patient under general anaesthetic and to provide appropriate airway support.

Injection sclerotherapy is now rarely performed for oesophageal varices.

Other measures

Vasoconstrictor therapy

This is used to restrict portal inflow by splanchnic arterial constriction and has shown benefit when used in combination with endoscopic techniques.

- ***Terlipressin***. This is the only vasoconstrictor proven to reduce mortality. The dose is 2 mg 6-hourly, reducing to 1 mg 4-hourly after 48 h if a prolonged regimen is required (up to 5 days). Terlipressin should not be given to patients with ischaemic heart disease. The patient may complain of abdominal colic, and may defecate and have facial pallor owing to generalized vasoconstriction. If haemostasis has been achieved at endoscopy, there is probably little added benefit with this therapy and treatment should be tapered accordingly.
- ***Somatostatin***. This has few side-effects. An infusion of 250–500 μg/h reduces bleeding and is reserved for patients with contraindications to terlipressin. A recent prospective, multicentre study showed that haemostatic effects and safety at day 5 of treatment did not differ significantly between terlipressin, somatostatin and octreotide when utilized as adjuvants to endoscopic treatment.

Balloon tamponade

Balloon tamponade is used if endoscopic therapy has failed or if there is exsanguinating haemorrhage. The usual balloon tube is a four-lumen Sengstaken–Blakemore, which should be left in place for no more than 12 hours and removed in the endoscopy room prior to endoscopy. The tube is passed into the stomach and the gastric balloon inflated with air and pulled back. It should be positioned in close apposition to the gastro-oesophageal junction to prevent the cephalad variceal blood flow to the bleeding point. The oesophageal balloon should only be inflated if bleeding is not controlled by the gastric balloon alone.

Haemostasis is achieved in up to 90%. However, the balloon may cause serious complications, such as aspiration pneumonia, oesophageal rupture and mucosal ulceration. The procedure is also very unpleasant for the patient.

A self-expanding covered metal stent (Danis), which has a wire loop to enable removal, and is introduced orally or endoscopically, can be placed over the varices. This is effective and has the advantages that it does not impair swallowing, cannot be removed by uncooperative patients, and allows post-endoscopic investigation. The stent is removed 7 days after insertion. It is currently only used in specialist centres but early results are encouraging.

Additional management of the acute episode

- ***Measures to prevent encephalopathy***. Portosystemic encephalopathy (PSE) can be precipitated by a large bleed (blood contains protein). Management is as outlined on page 474.
- ***Nursing***. Patients require high-dependency/intensive care nursing. They should remain nil by mouth until bleeding has stopped.
- ***Reduction in acid secretion***. Ranitidine may be preferable to PPIs, as it lessens the risk of *Clostridium difficile* infection; PPIs are widely used, however. Sucralfate 1 g four times daily can reduce oesophageal ulceration following endoscopic therapy.

Management of an acute rebleed

Rebleeding occurs in about 15–20% within 5 days. The source should be established by endoscopy and is sometimes due to ulceration or slippage of a ligation band. Endoscopy should be performed once only to control *re*bleeding. If haemostasis cannot be achieved, then transjugular intrahepatic portocaval shunting will be necessary.

Transjugular intrahepatic portocaval shunt

Transjugular intrahepatic portocaval shunt (TIPS) is used when bleeding cannot be controlled either acutely or following a rebleed. Under X-ray guidance, a guidewire is passed from the jugular vein into the liver and the portal vein. After balloon expansion of the tract between the hepatic and portal veins, an expandable, covered metal shunt is placed over the wire to form a channel between the systemic and portal venous systems. It reduces the hepatic sinusoidal and portal vein pressure by creating a total shunt. There is an increased risk of portal systemic encephalopathy. Stent stenosis or thrombosis is far less frequent with 'covered', compared to 'bare', stents. Collaterals arising from the splenic or portal veins can be selectively embolized. These reduce rebleeding rates compared to endoscopic techniques, but do not improve survival and increase encephalopathy.

Emergency surgery

This is performed rarely when other measures fail or if TIPS is not available. Oesophageal transection and ligation of the feeding vessels to the bleeding varices is most commonly performed; an alternative is acute portosystemic shunt surgery.

Prevention of recurrent variceal bleeding (secondary prophylaxis)

The risk of bleeding recurring without prophylaxis is 60–80% over a 2-year period, with an approximate mortality of 20% per episode.

Prophylactic long-term measures

Non-selective beta-blockade

Oral propranolol or carvedilol to reduce the resting pulse rate by 25% decreases portal pressure. Portal inflow is reduced by a decrease in cardiac output (β_1) and by blockade of β_2 vasodilator receptors on the splanchnic arteries, leaving an unopposed vasoconstrictor effect. Significant reduction of hepatic venous pressure gradient (HVPG; measured by hepatic vein catheterization) is associated with very low rates of rebleeding, particularly if <12 mmHg. Data have emerged demonstrating that additional α_1-adrenergic blockade, causing vasodilatation with carvedilol, may increase the number of patients with a reduction in hepatic venous pressure gradient compared to propranolol.

Endoscopic treatment

Repeated courses of banding at 2-weekly intervals lead to obliteration of varices. This markedly reduces rebleeding, most instances occurring before the varices have been fully obliterated. Between 30% and 40% of varices return per year, so follow-up endoscopy should be performed at 1–3 months after obliteration and then every 6–12 months. Complications of banding include oesophageal ulceration, mediastinitis and, rarely, strictures.

Combination therapy reduces overall bleeding compared to endoscopic therapy alone but with no overall improvement in mortality. A pragmatic approach is therefore to give combination therapy to those who can tolerate beta-blockade, and band ligation alone to those who cannot.

Surgery

- ***Surgical portosystemic shunting*** is associated with an extremely low risk of rebleeding and is used if TIPS is not available. Hepatic encephalopathy is a significant complication. The 'shunts' are usually an end-to-side portocaval anastomosis or a selective distal splenorenal shunt (Warren shunt).
- ***Devascularization procedures***, including oesophageal transection, do not produce encephalopathy, and can be used when there is splanchnic venous thrombosis.
- ***Liver transplantation*** (see pp. 468–469) is the best option when there is poor liver function.

Prophylactic measures (primary prophylaxis)

Patients with cirrhosis and significant varices that have not bled should be prescribed non-selective β-blockers. This reduces the chances of upper gastrointestinal bleeding by approximately 50%, may increase survival, and is cost-effective. If there are contraindications, variceal banding is an option.

Ascites

Ascites, fluid within the peritoneal cavity, is a common complication of cirrhosis. Several factors underlie its pathogenesis:

- ***Sodium and water retention*** results from peripheral arterial vasodilatation (secondary to nitric oxide, atrial natriuretic peptide and prostaglandins), which causes a reduction in the effective blood volume. This reduction activates the sympathetic nervous system and the renin–angiotensin system, promoting salt and water retention (see ***Fig. 9.3***).
- ***Portal hypertension*** exerts a local hydrostatic pressure, leading to increased hepatic and splanchnic production of lymph, and transudation of fluid into the peritoneal cavity.
- ***Low serum albumin*** (due to poor liver function) may further contribute by reducing plasma oncotic pressure.

In patients with ascites, urine sodium excretion rarely exceeds 5 mmol in 24 hours. Loss of sodium from extrarenal sites accounts for approximately 30 mmol in 24 hours. Under these circumstances, a normal daily sodium intake of 120–200 mmol results in a positive sodium balance of approximately 90–170 mmol in 24 hours (equivalent to 600–1300 mL of fluid retained).

Clinical features

Abdominal swelling may develop over days or several weeks. Precipitating factors include a high-sodium diet or development of an HCC or splanchnic vein thrombosis. Mild abdominal pain and discomfort are common but, if more severe, should raise the suspicion of spontaneous bacterial peritonitis (see below). Respiratory distress and difficulty eating accompany tense ascites.

The presence of fluid is confirmed clinically by demonstrating shifting dullness. Many patients also have peripheral oedema. A pleural effusion (usually right-sided) may infrequently be found and arises from the passage of ascites through congenital diaphragmatic defects.

Investigations

A diagnostic aspiration of 10–20 mL of fluid should be obtained for:

- ***Cell count***. A neutrophil count >250 cells/mm^3 is indicative of an underlying (usually spontaneous) bacterial peritonitis.
- ***Gram stain and culture***.
- ***Protein measurement***. A high serum–ascites albumin gradient of >11 g/L suggests portal hypertension, and a low gradient <11 g/L is associated with non-liver disease-related abnormalities of the peritoneum, such as neoplasia ***(Box 14.18)***.
- ***Cytology***. A search should be made for malignant cells.
- ***Amylase*** Pancreatic ascites should be excluded.

The differential diagnosis of ascites is listed in ***Box 14.19***.

Box 14.18 The serum–ascites albumin gradient

High serum–ascites albumin gradient (>11 g/L)
- Portal hypertension, e.g. hepatic cirrhosis
- Hepatic outflow obstruction
- Budd–Chiari syndrome
- Hepatic veno-occlusive disease
- Tricuspid regurgitation
- Constrictive pericarditis
- Right-sided heart failure

Low serum–ascites albumin gradient (<11 g/L)
- Peritoneal carcinomatosis
- Peritoneal tuberculosis
- Pancreatitis
- Nephrotic syndrome

(Modified from Chung RT, Iafrate AJ, Amrein PC et al. Case records of the Massachusetts General Hospital. New England Journal of Medicine *2006; 354:2166–2175.)*

Box 14.19 Causes of ascites according to type of ascitic fluid

Straw-coloured
- Malignancy (most common cause)
- Cirrhosis
- Infective:
  - Tuberculosis
  - Following intra-abdominal perforation – any bacterium may be found (e.g. *Escherichia coli*)
  - Spontaneous in cirrhosis
- Hepatic vein obstruction (Budd–Chiari syndrome) – protein level high in fluid
- Chronic pancreatitis
- Congestive cardiac failure
- Constrictive pericarditis
- Meigs syndrome (ovarian tumour)
- Hypoproteinaemia (e.g. nephrotic syndrome)

Chylous
- Obstruction of main lymphatic duct (e.g. by carcinoma) – chylomicrons are present
- Cirrhosis

Haemorrhagic
- Malignancy
- Ruptured ectopic pregnancy
- Abdominal trauma
- Acute pancreatitis

Management

The aim is both to reduce sodium intake and to increase renal sodium excretion, producing a net reabsorption of fluid from the ascites into the circulating volume. The maximum rate at which ascites can be mobilized is 500–700 mL in 24 hours (see below).

- ***Serum electrolytes, creatinine and estimated glomerular filtration rate (eGFR)***. Check on alternate days; weigh the patient and measure urinary output daily.
- ***Bed rest***. This will cause a diuresis by improving renal perfusion, but is rarely helpful.
- ***Dietary sodium restriction***. It is possible to reduce sodium intake to 40 mmol in 24 h and still maintain an adequate protein and calorie intake with a palatable diet.
- ***Drugs***. Many contain significant amounts of sodium (up to 50 mmol daily). Examples include antacids and antibiotics (particularly penicillins and cephalosporins). Sodium-retaining drugs (NSAIDs, corticosteroids) should be avoided.
- ***Fluid restriction***. This is unnecessary unless the serum sodium is <128 mmol/L (see below).
- ***Diuretics***. The diuretic of choice is the aldosterone antagonist, spironolactone, starting at 100 mg daily. Chronic administration produces gynaecomastia. Eplerenone 25 mg once daily does not cause gynaecomastia.

The aim of diuretic therapy should be to produce a net loss of fluid approaching 700 mL in 24 hours (0.7 kg weight loss, or 1.0 kg if peripheral oedema is present). Although 60% of patients respond on this regimen, the spironolactone can be increased gradually to 400 mg daily if necessary, providing there is no hyperkalaemia. A loop diuretic, such as furosemide 20–40 mg or bumetanide 0.5 mg or 1 mg daily, is added if response is poor. These loop diuretics have several potential disadvantages, including hyponatraemia, hypokalaemia and volume depletion.

Diuretics should be temporarily discontinued if a rise in serum creatinine occurs, representing over-diuresis and hypovolaemia, or if there is hyperkalaemia or worsening encephalopathy. Hyponatraemia almost always represents haemodilution secondary to a failure to clear free water (usually a marker of reduced renal perfusion), and diuretics should be stopped if the sodium falls below 128 mmol/L. Vaptans (see p. 164), vasopressin V_2-receptor antagonists that increase free water clearance, have a small beneficial effect on hyponatraemia and ascites but do not affect mortality, complications of cirrhosis or renal failure; routine use in cirrhosis cannot be recommended.

Paracentesis

This is used to relieve symptomatic tense ascites or when diuretic therapy is insufficient to control accumulation of fluid. The main complications are hypovolaemia and renal dysfunction (post-paracentesis circulatory dysfunction), predominantly due to an accentuation of the arteriolar vasodilatation already present in these patients; this is more likely with >5 L removal and worse liver function. In patients with normal renal function and without hyponatraemia, this is overcome by infusing albumin (8 g/L of ascitic fluid removed). In practice, up to 20 L can be removed over 4–6 hours, with albumin infusion.

Shunts

A TIPS may be inserted to treat resistant ascites, providing there is no spontaneous portosystemic encephalopathy and there is minimal disturbance of renal function. Frequency of paracentesis and diuretic use is reduced and nutrition is enhanced. Survival may also improve.

A peritoneo-bladder conduit, by means of an implantable, rechargeable, battery-powered pump, has been developed for use in patients with advanced cirrhosis and resistant ascites (alfapump®). This removes ascites from the peritoneal cavity into the urinary bladder, to be eliminated through urination. Early studies have shown a reduction in the need for large-volume paracentesis but several complications, including pain and infection, occur.

Spontaneous bacterial peritonitis

Spontaneous bacterial peritonitis (SBP) represents a serious complication that is an indication for referral for transplant assessment; it occurs in up to 18% of patients with ascites who have undergone a decompensation. The infecting organisms gain access to the peritoneum by haematogenous spread; most are *Escherichia coli*, *Klebsiella* or enterococci. The condition should be suspected in any patient with ascites who deteriorates, as pain and pyrexia are frequently absent. Diagnostic aspiration should always be performed. A raised neutrophil count in ascites is sufficient evidence alone to start immediate treatment. A broad-spectrum antibiotic is used, with subsequent alteration according to culture results *in combination with infusions of human albumin solution*. Evidence has emerged that non-selective β-blockers should be stopped following diagnosis of SBP, as prescription increases the risk of renal impairment. Mortality is 10–15%. Recurrence is common (70% within a year) and secondary prevention – for example, with norfloxacin 400 mg daily – prolongs survival. Primary prophylaxis of SBP in patients with ascites protein <10 g/L or severe liver disease may prevent hepatorenal syndrome and improve survival.

Portosystemic encephalopathy

Portosystemic encephalopathy (PSE) is a chronic neuropsychiatric syndrome that is secondary to cirrhosis. Acute encephalopathy can occur in acute hepatic failure (see p. 462). PSE can arise in portal hypertensive patients due to spontaneous 'shunting', or in those with surgical or TIPS shunts.

Pathogenesis

In cirrhosis, the portal blood bypasses the liver via collaterals, and 'toxic' metabolites pass directly to the brain to produce encephalopathy. Ammonia-induced alteration of brain neurotransmitter balance, especially at the astrocyte–neurone interface, is considered to be the leading pathophysiological mechanism. Ammonia is produced by the breakdown of protein by intestinal bacteria. Other implicated substances are free fatty acids and mercaptans; accumulation of false neurotransmitters (octopamine) or activation of the γ-aminobutyric acid (GABA) inhibitory neurotransmitter system may also be responsible. Increased blood levels of aromatic amino acids (tyrosine and phenylalanine) and reduced branched-chain amino acids (valine, leucine and isoleucine) also occur. The factors precipitating PSE are shown in ***Box 14.20***.

Clinical features

An acute onset often has a precipitating factor ***(Box 14.20)***. The patient becomes increasingly drowsy and comatose.

Chronically, there is a disorder of personality, mood and intellect, with a reversal of normal sleep rhythm. These changes may fluctuate and a collateral history should be obtained. The patient is irritable, confused and disorientated, and has slow, slurred speech. General features include nausea, vomiting and weakness. There is hyper-reflexia and increased tone. Coma occurs as the encephalopathy becomes more marked. Convulsions are very rare, but if they do occur, other causes must be considered.

Signs include:

- fetor hepaticus (a sweet smell to the breath)
- a coarse flapping tremor seen when the hands are outstretched and wrists hyperextended (asterixis)
- constructional apraxia, with the patient being unable to write or draw a five-pointed star, for example
- decreased mental function, which can be assessed by using the serial sevens test or a trail-making (or connection) test.

Box 14.20 Factors precipitating portosystemic encephalopathy

- High dietary protein
- Gastrointestinal haemorrhage
- Constipation
- Infection, including spontaneous bacterial peritonitis
- Fluid and electrolyte disturbance due to diuretic therapy or paracentesis
- Drugs (e.g. any central nervous system depressant)
- Portosystemic shunt operations, TIPS
- Any surgical procedure
- Progressive liver damage
- Development of hepatocellular carcinoma

TIPS, transjugular intrahepatic portocaval shunt.

Investigations

Diagnosis is clinical.

Additional investigations

- ***EEG*** shows a decrease in the frequency of the normal α-waves (8–13 Hz) to 1.5–3 Hz. These changes occur before coma supervenes.
- ***Visual evoked responses*** (see p. 823) also detect subclinical encephalopathy.
- ***Arterial blood ammonia*** can be useful for the differential diagnosis of coma and for following a patient with PSE, but is not always available.

Management

- ***Identify and remove the possible precipitating cause***, such as cerebral depressant drugs, constipation or electrolyte imbalance due to over-diuresis.
- ***Give purgation and enemas*** to empty the bowels of nitrogenous substances. Lactulose (10–30 mL three times daily) is an osmotic purgative that reduces the colonic pH and limits ammonia absorption. Lactilol (β-galactoside sorbitol 30 g daily) is metabolized by colonic bacteria and is comparable in efficacy.
- ***Maintain nutrition***, if necessary via a fine-bore nasogastric tube, and do not restrict protein for more than 48 h.
- ***Give antibiotics***. Rifaximin is a poorly absorbed semisynthetic antibiotic based on rifamycin that has a beneficial effect on secondary prevention of PSE. Metronidazole (200 mg four times daily) may be effective acutely. Neomycin should be avoided.
- ***Stop or reduce diuretic therapy***.
- ***Give intravenous fluids*** as necessary (beware too much sodium).
- ***Treat infection***.
- ***Increase protein*** in the diet to the limit of tolerance as encephalopathy improves.

Prognosis

Acute encephalopathy in acute hepatic failure has a very poor prognosis associated with that of the disease itself. In cirrhosis, chronic PSE adversely affects prognosis but the course is very variable. Very rarely with chronic portosystemic shunting, an organic syndrome with cerebellar signs or choreoathetosis develops, as well as myelopathy leading to a spastic paraparesis due to demyelination. These patients require referral to a liver transplant centre.

Renal failure (hepatorenal syndrome)

The hepatorenal syndrome typically occurs in patients with advanced cirrhosis, portal hypertension, jaundice and ascites. The urine output is low with a low urinary sodium concentration, a maintained capacity to concentrate urine (i.e. intact tubular function) and almost normal renal histology. The renal failure is therefore described as 'functional'. It is often precipitated by over-vigorous diuretic therapy, NSAIDs, diarrhoea, paracentesis and infection, particularly spontaneous bacterial peritonitis.

The mechanism is similar to that of ascites, with extreme peripheral vasodilatation leading to decreased effective blood volume and consequent hypotension (see pp. 472–473). This causes increased plasma renin, aldosterone, noradrenaline (norepinephrine) and vasopressin, leading to renal vasoconstriction. There is an increased pre-glomerular vascular resistance that causes blood to be directed away from the renal cortex. This leads to a reduced glomerular filtration rate and plasma renin remains high. Salt and water retention occurs, with reabsorption of sodium from the renal tubules.

Eicosanoids have been incriminated in the pathogenesis, supported by precipitation of the syndrome by inhibitors of prostaglandin synthase, such as NSAIDs.

Diuretic therapy should be stopped and intravascular hypovolaemia corrected, preferably with albumin. Terlipressin or noradrenaline with intravenous albumin improves renal function in approximately 50%. Liver transplantation is the best option. In patients who are candidates for transplantation, haemodialysis can be used as a bridging option but is frequently difficult to perform, and survival is generally limited by the severity of the hepatic failure.

Hepatopulmonary syndrome

This is hypoxaemia in patients with advanced liver disease due to intrapulmonary vascular dilatation with no evidence of primary pulmonary disease. The patients have features of cirrhosis with spider naevi and clubbing, as well as cyanosis. Most are asymptomatic, but with more severe disease, patients are breathless on standing. Transthoracic echocardiography shows intrapulmonary shunting, and arterial blood gases confirm hypoxaemia. These changes are improved with liver transplantation.

Porto-pulmonary hypertension

This occurs in 1–2% of patients with cirrhosis and portal hypertension. It may respond to medical therapy (e.g. intravenous epoprostenol, or oral bosentan and sildenafil). Severe pulmonary hypertension is a contraindication to liver transplantation.

Primary hepatocellular carcinoma

This is discussed on page 485.

Further reading

Hadjihambi A, Khetan V, Jalan R. Pharmacotherapy for hyperammonemia. *Expert Opin Pharmacother* 2014; 15:1685–1695.

Kimer N, Krag A, Møller S et al. Systematic review with meta-analysis: the effects of rifaximin in hepatic encephalopathy. *Aliment Pharmacol Ther* 2014; 40:123–132.

Rodriguez-Roisin R, Krowka MJ. Hepatopulmonary syndrome. *N Engl J Med* 2008; 358:2378–2387.

Turon F, Casu S, Hernández-Gea V et al. Variceal and other portal hypertension related bleeding. *Best Pract Res Clin Gastroenterol* 2013; 27: 649–664.

Wong F, Nadim MK, Kellum JA et al. Working party proposal for a revised classification system of renal dysfunction in patients with cirrhosis. *Gut* 2011; 60:702–709.

Types of cirrhosis

Alcoholic cirrhosis

This is discussed in the section on alcoholic liver disease (see pp. 480–482).

Primary biliary cholangitis

Primary biliary cholangitis (PBC; ***Fig. 14.25***) is a chronic disorder with progressive destruction of small bile ducts, leading to cirrhosis. Women aged 40–50 years constitute 90% of patients. PBC is diagnosed increasingly frequently in its milder forms. The prevalence is approximately 7.5 per 100 000, with a 1–6% increase in first-degree relatives. PBC has been called 'chronic non-suppurative destructive cholangitis', a term more descriptive of the early lesion, which emphasizes the fact that true cirrhosis occurs only in the later stages.

Aetiology

The aetiology is unknown but an immunological basis is well described. Serum anti-mitochondrial antibodies (AMA) are found in almost all patients. The mitochondrial antigen M2 is specific to PBC and five M2-specific antigens have been identified. The presence of AMA in high titre is unrelated to the clinical or histological picture and its role in pathogenesis is unclear. Antibodies against nuclear antigens, e.g. anti-gp210, are present in 50% of patients and correlate with progression towards liver failure.

It seems likely that an environmental factor acts on a genetically predisposed host via molecular mimicry, initiating autoimmunity. *E. coli* and *Novosphingobium aromaticivorans* antibodies are present in high titre.

Synthesis of IgM is increased, thought to be due to failure of the switch from IgM to IgG antibody synthesis. No specific associated class II major histocompatibility complex (MHC) loci have been found.

Clinical features

Asymptomatic patients are discovered on routine examination or screening and may have hepatomegaly, a raised serum alkaline phosphatase or autoantibodies.

Pruritus is often the earliest symptom. Fatigue, which is frequently disabling, may accompany the pruritus, particularly in progressive cases. When jaundice appears, hepatomegaly is usually

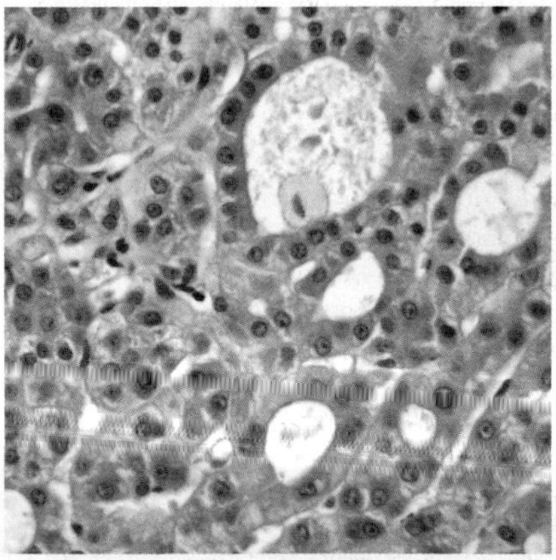

Figure 14.25 Primary biliary cholangitis. Portal tract inflammation with lymphocytes and plasma cells (×10).

present. Pigmented xanthelasma on eyelids or deposits of cholesterol in the creases of the hands may be seen.

Associated disorders

Autoimmune disorders (e.g. Sjögren syndrome, scleroderma, thyroid disease) occur with increased frequency. Keratoconjunctivitis sicca (dry eyes and mouth) is seen in 70% of cases. Renal tubular acidosis, membranous glomerulonephritis, coeliac disease and interstitial pneumonitis are also associations.

Investigations

- ***Mitochondrial antibodies*** – measured routinely by ELISA (in titres >1 : 160) – are present in over 95% of patients; M2 antibody is 98% specific. Other non-specific antibodies (e.g. anti-nuclear factor and smooth muscle) may also be present.
- ***High serum alkaline phosphatase*** is often the only liver biochemistry abnormality.
- ***Serum cholesterol*** is raised.
- ***Serum IgM*** may be very high.
- ***Ultrasound*** can show a diffuse alteration in liver architecture.
- ***Liver biopsy*** shows characteristic histological features of a portal tract infiltrate, mainly of lymphocytes and plasma cells; approximately 40% have granulomas. Most of the early changes are in zone 1. Later, there is damage to and loss of small bile ducts with ductular proliferation. Portal tract fibrosis and, eventually, cirrhosis are seen.

Hepatic granulomas are also seen in sarcoidosis, tuberculosis, schistosomiasis, drug reactions, brucellosis and parasitic infestation (e.g. strongyloidiasis).

Differential diagnosis

The classical picture presents little difficulty with diagnosis (and can be confirmed by biopsy, although this is only necessary in doubtful cases). A group of patients with the histological changes of PBC but the serology of autoimmune hepatitis are termed as having autoimmune cholangitis and respond to steroids and azathioprine.

In the jaundiced patient, extrahepatic biliary obstruction should be excluded by ultrasound or MRCP.

Management

- ***Ursodeoxycholic acid*** (10–15 mg/kg) improves bilirubin and aminotransferase levels. It should be given early in the asymptomatic phase, as these patients benefit, whereas no benefit is achieved in advanced disease.
- ***Steroids*** improve biochemical and histological disease but cause osteoporosis and other side-effects, and so should not be used.
- *Malabsorption* of ***fat-soluble vitamins (A, D and K)*** occurs and supplementation is required.
- ***Bisphosphonates*** are required for osteoporosis. Despite raised serum lipid concentrations, PBC is not associated with an increased cardiovascular disease risk and strategies for prevention of vascular events should be tailored to the individual.
- *Pruritus* is difficult to control; ***colestyramine*** is helpful, although unpalatable. ***Rifampicin***, and ***naloxone*** and ***naltrexone*** (opioid antagonists) have been shown to be of benefit. Intractable pruritus can be relieved by plasmapheresis or a molecular absorbent recirculating system (MARS).
- The lack of effective medical therapy has made PBC a major indication for ***liver transplantation*** (see p. 468).
- *Fatigue* is common and can be severely debilitating; there is no proven therapy and transplantation does not improve symptoms. Modafinil, used for narcolepsy, has shown promise but has yet to be evaluated in randomized studies; it may cause significant side-effects and has addictive potential.

Complications

The complications are those of cirrhosis. In addition, osteoporosis and, rarely, osteomalacia and a polyneuropathy occur.

Prognosis

Prognosis is very variable. Asymptomatic patients and those presenting with pruritus only will survive for more than 20 years. Symptomatic patients with jaundice have a more rapidly progressive course and may die of liver failure or bleeding varices within 5 years. Liver transplantation should therefore be offered when the serum bilirubin is persistently above 100 μmol/L.

Primary sclerosing cholangitis

Primary sclerosing cholangitis (PSC) is a chronic cholestatic liver disease characterized by fibrosing inflammatory destruction of both the intra- and extrahepatic bile ducts. In 75% of patients, PSC is associated with inflammatory bowel disease (usually ulcerative colitis); it is not unusual for PSC to predate the onset of inflammatory bowel disease. The causes are unknown but genetic susceptibility to PSC is associated with the HLA-A1-B8-DR3 haplotype. The autoantibody pANCA (anti-neutrophil cytoplasmic antibody) is found in the serum of 60% of cases. Seventy per cent of patients are men and the average age of onset is approximately 40 years. Secondary PSC is seen in patients with HIV and cryptosporidium (see p. 350) and may follow ketamine misuse.

Clinical features

With increasing screening of patients with inflammatory bowel disease, PSC is detected at an asymptomatic phase with abnormal liver biochemistry, usually a raised serum alkaline phosphatase. Symptomatic presentation is usually with fluctuating pruritus, jaundice and cholangitis.

Diagnosis

The typical biliary changes associated with PSC may be identified by MRCP. The cholangiogram characteristically shows irregularity of calibre of both intra- and extrahepatic ducts, although either may be involved alone ***(Fig. 14.26)***.

Pathology

Histology can be contributory; it shows inflammation of the intrahepatic biliary radicles with associated scar tissue, classically described as have the appearance of 'onion skin'. These changes range from minor inflammatory infiltrates to the level of established cirrhosis.

Management

PSC is a slowly progressive lesion (symptoms and biochemical tests may fluctuate), which ultimately leads to liver cirrhosis and associated decompensation. Recurrent cholangitis may be a feature before the onset of cirrhosis. Cholangiocarcinoma occurs in up to 15% of patients (see pp. 485–486 and 498).

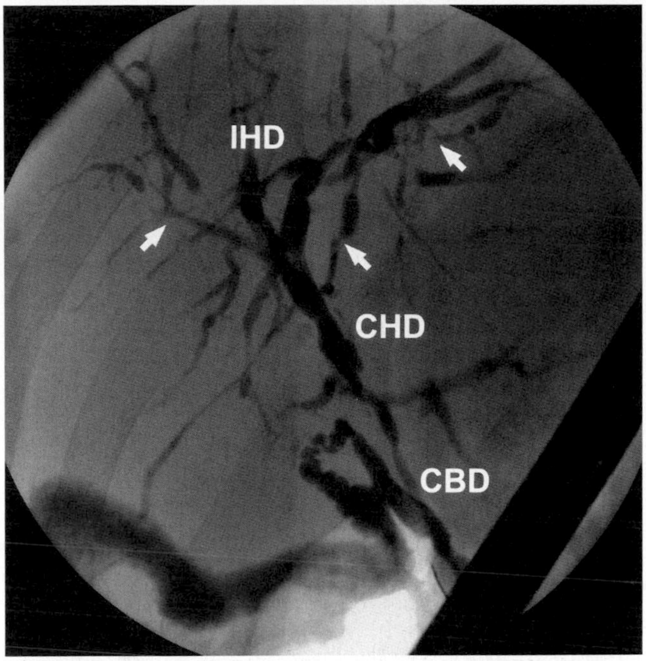

Figure 14.26 Primary sclerosing cholangitis. An endoscopic cholangiogram showing the typical features of primary sclerosing cholangitis. There are calibre irregularities of the intrahepatic ducts (**IHD**). There is also minor stricturing of the extrahepatic ducts at the confluence between the common bile duct (**CBD**) and the common hepatic duct (**CHD**).

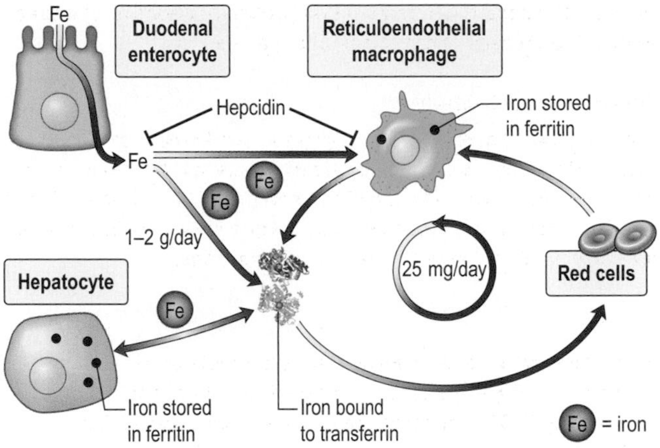

Figure 14.27 The circulation of iron from the duodenal enterocyte to and from the liver, red cells and reticuloendothelial macrophages. Some 1–2 g of iron is absorbed from the intestine (see ***Fig. 16.8***) and circulates bound to transferrin. The reticuloendothelial cells clear old erythrocytes and release iron to circulate and be stored as ferritin in the liver. The liver is the major site of production of the peptide hormone, hepcidin. **Hepcidin** blocks release of iron from the erythrocytes and macrophages by degrading the iron exporter transferrin. Fe, iron. *(Modified from Fleming RE, Ponka P. Iron overload in human disease.* N Engl J Med *2012; 366:348–359, with permission.)*

The only proven treatment is liver transplantation. The bile acid, ursodeoxycholic acid, has been evaluated extensively but there is no evidence of benefit. High-dose therapy (30 mg/kg) may be deleterious. In a small minority, the dominant lesion is sited in the extrahepatic ducts ***(Fig. 14.26)***. Such lesions may be amenable to endoscopic biliary intervention with balloon dilatation and temporary stent placement (see p. 497).

Secondary biliary cirrhosis

Cirrhosis can result from prolonged (for months) large duct biliary obstruction. Causes include bile duct strictures, gallstones and sclerosing cholangitis. An ultrasound examination and MRCP, sometimes followed by ERCP or percutaneous transhepatic cholangiography (where the ducts are cannulated under ultrasound guidance through the skin) if cannulation is difficult, is performed to outline the ducts, and any remedial cause is treated.

Hereditary haemochromatosis

Hereditary haemochromatosis (HH; see also p. 445) is an inherited disease characterized by excess iron deposition in various organs, leading to eventual fibrosis and functional organ failure. There are four main types of inherited disorders:

- ***type 1*** HFE: the ***HFE*** gene (mutation C282Y) is the most common and is on chromosome 6
- ***type 2A***: juvenile ***HJV*** gene (mutation G320V)
  type 2B: juvenile ***HAMP*** gene (mutation 93delG)
- ***type 3*** TfR2: the ***TfR2*** gene (mutation Y250X)
- ***type 4*** ferroportin: the ***SLC40A1*** gene (mutation V162del).

All are transmitted by an autosomal recessive gene, apart from the ferroportin iron overload, which is dominantly transmitted.

HH has a prevalence in Caucasians (homozygotes) of 1 in 400, but very variable phenotypic expression and a heterozygote (carrier) frequency of 1 in 10. It is the most common single-gene disorder in Caucasians.

Aetiology

Between 85% and 90% of patients with overt HH are homozygous for the Cys 282 Tyr (C282Y mutation): that is, type 1 *HFE*. A second mutation (His 63 Asp, H63D) occurs in about 25% of the population and is in complete linkage disequilibrium with Cys 282 Tyr.

Another form of haemochromatosis (type 3) occurs in southern Europe and is associated with TfR2, a transferrin receptor isoform. The other types, ferroportin-related (type 4) and juvenile forms (types 2A and 2B), are much rarer.

Dietary intakes of iron and chelating agents (ascorbic acid) may be relevant. Iron overload may be present in alcoholics; alcohol excess *per se* does not cause HH, although there is a history of excess alcohol intake in 25% of patients.

Mechanism of damage

The *HFE* gene protein interacts with the transferrin receptor 1, which is a mediator in intestinal iron absorption (see ***Fig. 16.8***). Iron is taken up by the mucosal cells inappropriately, exceeding the binding capacity of transferrin.

Hepcidin, a protein synthesized in the liver ***(Fig. 14.27)***, is central to the control of iron absorption; it is increased in iron deficiency states and decreased with iron overload. The mutations described above disrupt hepcidin expression, thereby internalizing ferroportin and leading to uninhibited iron overload.

Hepatic expression of the hepcidin gene is decreased in HFE haemochromatosis, facilitating liver iron overload. Excess iron is then gradually taken up by the liver and other tissues over a long period. It seems likely that it is the iron itself that precipitates fibrosis.

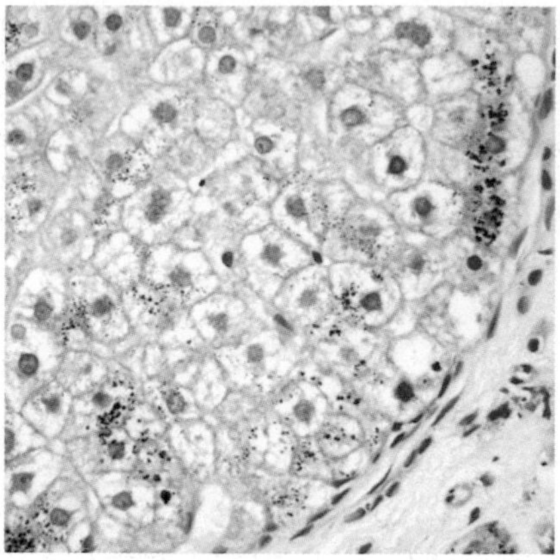

Figure 14.28 Cirrhotic nodule in haemochromatosis. Note the iron overload (blue) (Perls, ×25).

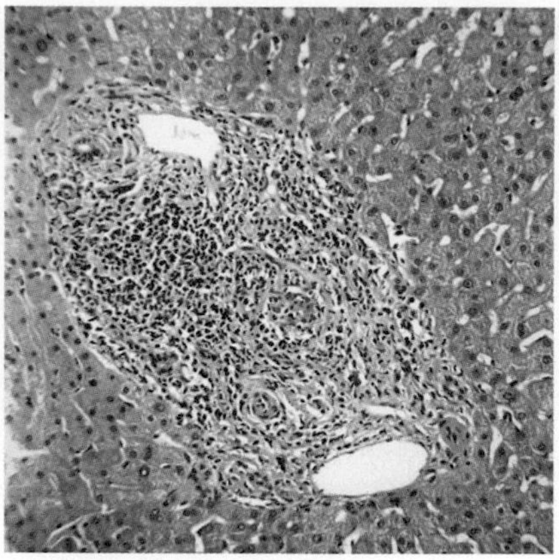

Figure 14.29 Hepatocellular carcinoma. (Haematoxylin and eosin, ×25.)

Pathology

In symptomatic patients, the total body iron content is 20–40g, compared with 3–4g in a normal person. The iron content is particularly increased in the liver ***(Fig. 14.28)*** and pancreas (50–100 times normal) but is also increased in other organs (e.g. the endocrine glands, heart and skin).

In established cases, the liver shows extensive iron deposition and fibrosis. Early in the disease, iron is deposited in the periportal hepatocytes (in pericanalicular lysosomes). Later, it is distributed widely throughout all acinar zones, biliary duct epithelium, Kupffer cells and connective tissue. Cirrhosis is a late feature.

Clinical features

The course of the disease depends on a number of factors, including gender, dietary iron intake, presence of associated hepatotoxins (especially alcohol) and genotypes. Overt clinical manifestations occur more frequently in men; the reduced incidence in women is probably explained by physiological blood loss and a smaller dietary intake of iron. Most affected individuals present in the fifth decade. The classic triad of bronze skin pigmentation (due to melanin deposition), hepatomegaly and diabetes mellitus is present only in cases of gross iron overload.

Hypogonadism secondary to pituitary dysfunction is the most common endocrine feature. Deficiency of other pituitary hormones is also found, but symptomatic endocrine deficiencies, such as loss of libido, are very rare. Cardiac manifestations, particularly heart failure and arrhythmias, are common, especially in younger patients. Calcium pyrophosphate is deposited asymmetrically in both large and small joints (chondrocalcinosis), leading to an arthropathy. The exact relationship of chondrocalcinosis to iron deposition is uncertain.

Complications

Some 30% of people with cirrhosis will develop primary hepatocellular carcinoma (HCC; ***Fig. 14.29***). HCC has been described only very rarely in non-cirrhotic patients in whom the excess iron stores have been removed. Early diagnosis is vital.

Investigations

Homozygotes

- ***Serum iron*** is elevated (>30 µmol/L) in 90% with a reduction in the TIBC and a transferrin saturation of >45%.
- ***Serum ferritin*** is elevated (usually >500 µg/L or 240 nmol/L).
- ***Liver biochemistry*** is often normal, even with established cirrhosis.

Heterozygotes

Heterozygotes may have normal biochemical tests or modest increases in serum iron transferrin saturation (>45%) or serum ferritin (usually >400 µg/L).

Genetic testing

If iron studies are abnormal, genetic testing is performed.

Liver biopsy

This is not required for diagnosis, but is useful to establish the extent of tissue damage, assess tissue iron, and measure the hepatic iron concentration (>180 µmol/g dry weight of liver indicates haemochromatosis).

Mild degrees of parenchymal iron deposition in patients with other forms of cirrhosis, particularly if due to alcohol, can often cause confusion with true homozygous HH.

Magnetic resonance imaging

MRI shows a dramatic reduction in the signal intensity of the liver and pancreas owing to the paramagnetic effect of ferritin and haemosiderin. A highly T2-weighted, gradient recalled echo (GRE) technique detects all clinically relevant liver iron overload (>60 µmol/g of liver). In secondary iron overload (haemosiderosis), which involves the reticuloendothelial cells, the pancreas is spared, enabling distinction between these two conditions.

Management

Venesection

This prolongs life and may reverse tissue damage; the risk of malignancy still remains if cirrhosis is present. All patients should have excess iron removed as rapidly as possible. This is achieved using venesection of 500 mL performed twice weekly for up to 2 years, i.e. 160 units with 250 mg of iron per unit, which equals 40 g removed. During venesection, serum iron and ferritin and the mean corpuscular volume (MCV) should be monitored. These fall only when available iron is depleted. Three or four venesections per year are required to prevent re-accumulation of iron. Serum ferritin should remain within the normal range.

Manifestations of the disease usually improve or disappear, except for diabetes, testicular atrophy and chondrocalcinosis. The requirements for insulin often diminish in diabetic patients. Testosterone replacement is often helpful.

In the rare patient who cannot tolerate venesection (because of severe cardiac disease or anaemia), chelation therapy with desferrioxamine, either intermittently or continuously by infusion, has been successful in removing iron.

Screening

In all cases of HH, all first-degree family members must be screened to detect early and asymptomatic disease. *HFE* mutation analysis is performed with measurement of transferrin saturation and serum ferritin.

In the general population, serum iron and transferrin saturation are the best and cheapest tests available.

Wilson's disease (progressive hepatolenticular degeneration)

Dietary copper is normally absorbed from the stomach and upper small intestine. Copper is transported to the liver loosely bound to albumin; in the liver, it is incorporated into apocaeruloplasmin, forming caeruloplasmin, a glycoprotein synthesized in the liver, and secreted into the blood. The remaining copper is normally excreted in the bile and excreted in faeces.

Wilson's disease is a very rare inborn error of copper metabolism that results in copper deposition in various organs, including the liver, the basal ganglia of the brain and the cornea. It is potentially treatable and all young patients with liver disease must be screened for this condition.

Aetiology

Wilson's disease is an autosomal recessive disorder with a molecular defect within a copper-transporting ATPase encoded by a gene (designated *ATP7B*) located on chromosome 13. It affects between 1 in 30 000 and 1 in 100 000 individuals. Over 300 mutations have been identified, the most frequent being His 1069 Gly (H1069Q), found in approximately 50% of Caucasian patients; compound heterozygotes are common. This mutation is rare in India and Asia. Wilson's disease occurs worldwide, particularly in countries where consanguinity is common. There is a failure of both incorporation of copper into procaeruloplasmin, which leads to low serum caeruloplasmin, and biliary excretion of copper. There is a low serum caeruloplasmin in over 80% of patients but this is not the cause of the copper deposition. The precise mechanism for the failure of copper excretion is not known.

Pathology

The liver histology is not diagnostic and varies from that of chronic hepatitis to macronodular cirrhosis. Stains for copper show a periportal distribution but this can be unreliable (see below). The basal ganglia are damaged and show cavitation, the kidneys show tubular degeneration, and erosions are seen in bones.

Clinical features

Children usually present with hepatic problems, whereas young adults have more neurological problems, such as tremor, dysarthria, involuntary movements and eventually dementia. The liver disease varies from episodes of acute hepatitis, especially in children (which can go on to acute hepatic failure), to chronic hepatitis or cirrhosis.

Typical signs are those of chronic liver disease with neurological signs of basal ganglia involvement (see p. 855). A specific sign is the Kayser–Fleischer ring, caused by copper deposition in Descemet's membrane in the cornea. It appears as a greenish-brown pigment at the corneoscleral junction and frequently requires slit-lamp examination for identification. It may be absent in young children.

Investigations

- ***Serum copper and caeruloplasmin*** are usually reduced but can be normal.
- ***Urinary copper*** is usually increased to 100–1000 μg in 24 h (1.6–16 μmol); normal levels <40 μg (0.6 μmol).
- ***Liver biopsy*** aids diagnosis, which depends on measurement of the amount of copper in the liver (>250 μg/g dry weight), although high levels of copper are also found in the liver in chronic cholestasis.
- ***Haemolysis and anaemia*** may be present.
- ***Genetic analysis*** is limited but selected exons are screened according to population groups.

Management

- Lifetime treatment with ***penicillamine***, 1–1.5 g daily, is effective in chelating copper. If treatment is started early, clinical and biochemical improvement can occur. Urinary copper levels should be monitored and the drug dose adjusted downwards after 2–3 years. Serious side-effects of the drug occur in 10% and include skin rashes, leucopenia, skin changes and renal damage.
- ***Trientine*** (1.2–1.8 g/day) and ***zinc acetate*** (150 mg/day) are used as maintenance therapy and for asymptomatic cases. All siblings and children of patients should be screened (*ATP7B* mutation analysis is useful) and treatment with zinc is given, even in the asymptomatic if there is evidence of copper accumulation. A diet low in copper (i.e. excluding chocolate and peanuts) is advised.

Prognosis

Early diagnosis and effective treatment have improved the outlook. Neurological damage is, however, permanent. Acute hepatic failure or decompensated cirrhosis should be treated by liver transplantation.

Alpha$_1$-antitrypsin deficiency

A deficiency of alpha$_1$-antitrypsin (α_1-AT; see also p. 1081) is sometimes associated with liver disease and pulmonary emphysema (particularly in smokers). Part of a family of serine protease inhibitors, or serpin superfamily, α_1-AT is a glycoprotein. Deficiency of α_1-AT is a genetic disorder and 1 in 10 northern Europeans carries an abnormal gene.

The protein is a 394-amino acid 52 kDa acute phase protein that is synthesized in the liver and constitutes 90% of the serum α_1-globulin seen on electrophoresis. Its main role is to inhibit the proteolytic enzyme, neutrophil elastase.

The gene is located on chromosome 14. The genetic variants of α_1-AT are characterized by their electrophoretic mobilities as medium (M), slow (S) or very slow (Z). The normal genotype is protease inhibitor MM (PiMM), the homozygote for Z is PiZZ, and the heterozygotes are PiMZ and PiSZ. S and Z variants are due to a single amino acid replacement of glutamic acid at positions 264 and 342 of the polypeptide, respectively. This results in decreased synthesis and secretion of the protein by the liver as protein–protein interactions occur between the reactive centre loop of one molecule and the β-pleated sheet of a second (loop sheet polymerization).

How this causes liver disease is uncertain. It is postulated that failure of secretion of the abnormal protein leads to an accumulation in the liver, causing liver damage.

Clinical features

The majority of patients with clinical disease are homozygotes with a PiZZ phenotype. Some may present in childhood and a few require transplantation. Approximately 10–15% of adult patients will develop cirrhosis, usually over the age of 50 years, and 75% will have respiratory problems. Approximately 5% of patients die of their liver disease. Heterozygotes (e.g. PiSZ or PiMZ) may develop liver disease but the risk is small.

Investigations

- ***Serum α_1-antitrypsin*** is low, at 10% of the normal level in the PiZZ phenotypes, and 60% of normal in the S variant.

Histologically, periodic acid–Schiff (PAS)-positive, diastase-resistant globules that contain α_1-AT are seen in periportal hepatocytes. Fibrosis and cirrhosis can be present.

Management

There is no treatment, apart from dealing with the complications of liver disease. Patients with hepatic decompensation should be assessed for liver transplantation, and should stop smoking (see p. 1081).

Further reading

Andrews NC. Closing the iron gate. *N Engl J Med* 2012; 366:376–370.
Bacon BR, Adams PC, Kowdley KV et al. Diagnosis and management of hemochromatosis: 2011 practice guideline by the American Association for the Study of Liver Diseases. *Hepatology* 2011; 54:328–343.
European Association for the Study of the Liver. EASL Clinical Practice Guidelines: Wilson disease. *J Hepatol* 2012; 56:671–685.
Gideon M et al. Primary sclerosing cholangitis. *Lancet* 2013; 382:1587–1599.
Pietrangelo A. Hereditary haemochromatosis: pathogenesis, diagnosis, and treatment. *Gastroenterology* 2010; 139:393–408.
Selmi C, Bowlus CL, Gershwin ME et al. Primary biliary cirrhosis. *Lancet* 2011; 377:1600–1609.

ALCOHOLIC LIVER DISEASE

This section describes the pathology and clinical features of alcoholic liver disease. The amounts needed to produce liver damage, alcohol metabolism, and other clinical effects of alcohol are described on pages 217–218.

Ethanol is metabolized in the liver by two pathways, resulting in an increase in the NADH/NAD ratio. The altered redox potential causes increased hepatic fatty acid synthesis with decreased fatty acid oxidation; both events lead to hepatic accumulation of fatty acid, which is then esterified to glycerides.

The changes in oxidation–reduction also impair carbohydrate and protein metabolism and are the cause of the centrilobular necrosis of the hepatic acinus that is typical of alcohol damage. TNF-α release from Kupffer cells causes the release of reactive oxygen species, leading, in turn, to tissue injury and fibrosis.

Acetaldehyde is formed by the oxidation of ethanol, and its effect on hepatic proteins may well be a factor in producing liver cell damage. The exact mechanism of alcoholic hepatitis and cirrhosis is unknown, but since only 10–20% of people who drink heavily will develop cirrhosis, a genetic predisposition is recognized. Immunological mechanisms have also been proposed, with the release of cytokines, particularly IL-8, which is a neutrophil chemoattractant; infiltration with neutrophils is a feature of alcoholic hepatitis.

Alcohol can enhance the effects of the toxic metabolites of drugs (e.g. paracetamol) on the liver, as it induces microsomal metabolism via the microsomal ethanol oxidizing system (MEOS; see p. 217).

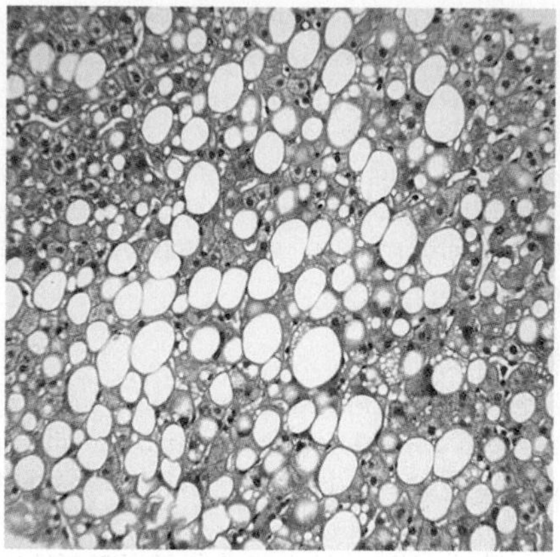

Figure 14.30 Liver steatosis (×10).

Pathology

Alcohol can produce a wide spectrum of liver disease from fatty change to hepatitis and cirrhosis.

Fatty liver

The metabolism of alcohol invariably produces fat in the liver ***(Fig. 14.30)***, mainly in zone 3. This is minimal with small amounts of alcohol, but with larger amounts the cells become swollen with fat (steatosis). There is no liver cell damage. The fat disappears on stopping alcohol. Steatosis is also seen in non-alcoholic fatty liver disease (NAFLD) (see p. 465).

In some cases, collagen is laid down around the central hepatic veins (perivenular fibrosis) and this can sometimes progress to cirrhosis without a preceding hepatitis. Alcohol directly affects stellate cells, transforming them into collagen-producing myofibroblast cells (see p. 440).

Alcoholic hepatitis

In addition to fatty change, there is infiltration by polymorphonuclear leucocytes and hepatocyte necrosis, mainly in zone 3. Dense cytoplasmic inclusions called Mallory bodies are sometimes seen in hepatocytes and giant mitochondria are also a feature. Mallory bodies are suggestive of, but not specific for, alcoholic damage, as they can be found in other liver disease, such as Wilson's disease and primary biliary cholangitis. If alcohol consumption continues, alcoholic hepatitis may progress to cirrhosis.

Alcoholic cirrhosis

This is classically of the micronodular type but a mixed pattern is also seen accompanying fatty change, and evidence of pre-existing alcoholic hepatitis may be present.

Clinical features

Fatty liver

There are often no symptoms or signs. Vague abdominal symptoms of nausea, vomiting and diarrhoea are due to the more general effects of alcohol on the gastrointestinal tract. Hepatomegaly, sometimes huge, can occur, together with other features of chronic liver disease.

Alcoholic hepatitis

The clinical features vary in degree:

- The patient may be well, with few symptoms, the hepatitis only being apparent on the liver biopsy in addition to fatty change.
- Mild to moderate symptoms of ill-health, occasionally with mild jaundice, may occur. Signs include all the features of chronic liver disease. Liver biochemistry is deranged and the diagnosis is made on liver histology.
- In the severe case, often superimposed on alcoholic cirrhosis, the patient is ill, with jaundice and ascites. Abdominal pain is frequently present, and a high fever is associated with the liver necrosis. On examination, there is deep jaundice, hepatomegaly, sometimes splenomegaly, and ascites with ankle oedema. The signs of chronic liver disease are also present.

Alcoholic cirrhosis

This represents the final stage of liver disease from alcohol use. Nevertheless, patients can be very well with few symptoms. On examination, there are usually signs of chronic liver disease (p. 448). The diagnosis is confirmed by liver biopsy.

The patient usually presents with one of the complications of cirrhosis. In many cases, there are features of alcohol dependency (see pp. 921–922), as well as evidence of involvement of other systems, such as polyneuropathy.

Investigations

Fatty liver

An elevated MCV often indicates heavy drinking. Liver biochemistry shows mild abnormalities with elevation of both serum aminotransferase enzymes. The γ-GT level is a useful test for determining whether the patient is taking alcohol. With severe fatty infiltration, marked changes in all liver biochemical parameters can occur. Ultrasound or CT will demonstrate fatty infiltration, as will liver histology. Elastography (p. 446) can be used to estimate the degree of fibrosis.

Alcoholic hepatitis

Investigations show a leucocytosis with markedly deranged liver biochemistry and elevated:

- serum bilirubin
- serum AST and ALT
- serum alkaline phosphatase
- prothrombin time.

A ***low serum albumin*** may also be found. Rarely, hyperlipidaemia with haemolysis (*Zieve syndrome*) may occur.

Liver biopsy, if required, is performed by the transjugular route because of the prolonged prothrombin time.

Alcoholic cirrhosis

Investigations are as for cirrhosis in general.

Management and prognosis

General management

All patients should stop drinking alcohol. Delirium tremens (a withdrawal symptom) is treated with diazepam. Intravenous thiamine should be given empirically to prevent Wernicke–Korsakoff encephalopathy. Bed rest is necessary, along with a diet high in protein and vitamin supplements. Dietary protein sometimes needs to be limited because of encephalopathy. Patients must be advised to participate in alcohol cessation programmes. The likelihood of abstention is dependent on many factors, particularly social and family ones.

Fatty liver

The patient is advised to stop drinking alcohol; the fat will disappear and the liver biochemistry usually returns to normal. Small amounts of alcohol can be drunk subsequently, as long as patients are aware of the problems and can control their consumption.

Alcoholic hepatitis

In severe cases, the patient requires admission to hospital. Nutrition must be maintained with enteral feeding, if necessary, and vitamin supplementation given. Steroid therapy has been widely used in patients with a discriminant function score of >32 but a recent multicentre UK study, which included over 1000 patients, suggested that there was no survival benefit.

Discriminant function (DF)

$$\text{DF} = [4.6 \times \text{prothrombin time above control in seconds}] + \text{bilirubin (mg/dL)}$$

Bilirubin mmol/L ÷ 17 to convert to mg/dL.
Severe = >32.

The response to steroid therapy can also be evaluated by the Lille score (>0.45 indicates poor response to steroids, which can therefore be stopped) and the Glasgow score (***Boxes 14.21*** and ***14.22***). A Glasgow score of >9 indicates that steroids are necessary because at >9 the 28-day mortality is 75%, while at <9 it is 50%. The MELD score (see p. 467) is also used but does not indicate which patients need steroid therapy.

Infection must be excluded or concomitantly treated. Treatment for encephalopathy and ascites is commenced. Antifungal prophylaxis should also be used.

Patients are advised to stop drinking for life, as this is undoubtedly a pre-cirrhotic condition. The prognosis is variable and, despite abstinence, the liver disease is progressive in many patients. Granulocyte-colony stimulating factor (G-CSF) for 5 days improves 90-day survival in preliminary studies.

Box 14.21 Lille score for alcoholic hepatitis

(*Calculator at http://www.lillemodel.com*)
R = 3.19 – (0.101 × age in years) + (0.147 × albumin on admission in g/L) + (0.0165 × change in bilirubin level from day 0 to day 7 in µmol/L) – (0.206 × renal insufficiency [0 if absent, 1 if present][a]) (0.0065 × bilirubin day 0 in µmol/L) – (0.0096 × INR)
A score of <0.16 indicates a 96% chance of survival at 28 days; ≥0.56 indicates a 55% chance of survival at 28 days.
Score = EXP(–R)/[1+EXP(–R)]

[a] *Creatinine >115 µmol/L.*

Box 14.22 Glasgow alcoholic hepatitis score

Score	1	2	3
Age	<50	>50	
White cell count ($\times 10^9$/L)	<15	>15	
Urea (nmol/L)	<5	>5	
Bilirubin (μmol/L)	<125	125–250	>250
INR	<1.5	1.5–2.0	>2.0

Poor prognosis = total score >9.

INR, International Normalized Ratio.

In severe cases, the mortality is at least 50%; with a prothrombin time twice normal, progressive encephalopathy and acute kidney injury, the mortality approaches 90%. Early transplantation for patients with severe alcoholic hepatitis has a survival rate of 78%, compared with 32% of those not transplanted. Unfortunately, many return to drinking.

Alcoholic cirrhosis

The management of cirrhosis is described on page 467. Again, all patients are advised to stop drinking for life. Abstinence from alcohol results in an improvement in prognosis, with a 5-year survival of 90%, but with continued drinking this falls to 60%. In advanced disease (i.e. jaundice, ascites and haematemesis) the 5-year survival rate falls to 35%, most of the deaths occurring in the first year. Liver transplantation results in good survival; recurrence of cirrhosis due to recidivism is rare. Patients often sign a contract with their clinicians regarding their abstinence, both before and after transplantation.

A trial of abstention to establish whether liver disease can improve is mandatory, but transplantation should not be denied if the patient continues to deteriorate. Specific follow-up regarding alcohol use is recommended.

HCC is a complication, particularly in men.

Further reading

Thursz MR, Richardson P, Allison M et al. Prednisolone or pentoxifylline for alcoholic hepatitis. *N Engl J Med* 2015; 372:1619–1628.

BUDD–CHIARI SYNDROME

In this condition, there is obstruction to the venous outflow of the liver owing to occlusion of the hepatic vein. In one-third of patients the cause is unknown, but specific causes include hypercoagulability states (e.g. paroxysmal nocturnal haemoglobinuria, polycythaemia vera) or thrombophilia (see p. 575), taking the contraceptive pill, or leukaemia. Other causes include occlusion of the hepatic vein owing to posterior abdominal wall sarcomas, renal or adrenal tumours, hepatocellular carcinoma, hepatic infections (e.g. hydatid cyst), congenital venous webs, radiotherapy or trauma to the liver.

Clinical features

The acute form presents with abdominal pain, nausea, vomiting, tender hepatomegaly and ascites (a fulminant form occurs particularly in pregnant women). In the chronic form, there is enlargement of the liver (particularly the caudate lobe), mild jaundice, ascites, a negative hepatojugular reflux, and splenomegaly with portal hypertension.

Investigations

Investigations show a high protein content in the ascitic fluid and characteristic liver histology with centrizonal congestion, haemorrhage, fibrosis and cirrhosis. Ultrasound, CT or MRI will demonstrate hepatic vein occlusion with diffuse abnormal parenchyma on contrast enhancement. The caudate lobe is spared because of its independent blood supply and venous drainage. There may be compression of the inferior vena cava. Pulsed Doppler sonography or colour Doppler is useful, as it shows abnormalities of flow in the hepatic vein. Thrombophilia screening is mandatory. Multiple defects of coagulation occur. Thrombosis of the portal vein is present in 2% of patients.

Differential diagnosis

A similar clinical picture can be produced by inferior vena caval obstruction, right-sided cardiac failure or constrictive pericarditis, and appropriate investigations should be performed.

Management

In the ***acute situation***, thrombolytic therapy can be given. Ascites should be treated, as should any underlying cause (e.g. polycythaemia). Congenital webs should be treated radiologically or resected surgically. A TIPS is the treatment of choice, as caval compression does not prejudice the efficacy of TIPS. Surgical portocaval shunts are reserved for those who fail this treatment, providing there is no caval obstruction or severe caval compression when a caval stent can be inserted. Liver transplantation is the first-choice treatment for ***chronic*** Budd–Chiari syndrome and for the fulminant form. Life-long anticoagulation is mandatory following TIPS and transplantation.

Prognosis

The prognosis depends on the aetiology but some patients can survive for several years.

Further reading

Mancuso A. An update on management of Budd–Chiari syndrome. *Ann Hepatol* 2014; 13:323–326.

HEPATIC SINUSOIDAL OBSTRUCTION SYNDROME

Hepatic sinusoidal obstruction syndrome (SOS; previously known as veno-occlusive disease) is due to injury of the hepatic veins and presents clinically like the Budd–Chiari syndrome. It was originally described in Jamaica, where the ingestion of toxic pyrrolizidine alkaloids in bush tea (made from plants of the genera *Senecio, Heliotropium* and *Crotalaria*) caused damage to the hepatic veins. It can be seen in other parts of the world. It also occurs as a complication of chemotherapy and total body irradiation, used before allogeneic bone marrow transplantation. The development of SOS after bone marrow transplantation carries a high mortality. Treatment is supportive, with control of ascites and hepatocellular failure. TIPS has been used in a few cases. Defibrotide is recommended for prophylactic use before bone marrow transplantation in children and adults with a high risk of SOS (e.g. pre-existing hepatic disease or prior treatment with gemtuzumab ozogamicin).

FIBROPOLYCYSTIC DISEASES

These diseases are usually inherited and lead to the presence of cysts or fibrosis in the liver, kidney and occasionally the pancreas, and other organs.

Polycystic disease of the liver

Multiple cysts can occur in the liver as part of autosomal dominant polycystic disease of the kidney (see pp. 789–790). These cysts are usually asymptomatic but occasionally cause abdominal pain and distension. Liver function is normal and complications such as oesophageal varices are very rare. The prognosis is excellent and depends on the kidney disease.

Solitary cysts

These are usually found by chance during imaging and are mainly asymptomatic.

Congenital hepatic fibrosis

In this rare condition, the liver architecture is normal but there are broad collagenous fibrous bands extending from the portal tracts. Congenital hepatic fibrosis is often inherited as an autosomal recessive condition but can also occur sporadically. It usually presents in childhood with hepatosplenomegaly, and portal hypertension is common. It may present later in life and can be misdiagnosed as cirrhosis.

A wedge biopsy of the liver may be required to confirm the diagnosis. The outlook is good and the condition should be distinguished from cirrhosis. Patients who bleed do well after endoscopic therapy of varices (or a portocaval anastomosis) because of their good liver function.

Congenital intrahepatic biliary dilatation (Caroli's disease)

In this rare, non-familial disease there are saccular dilatations of the intrahepatic or extrahepatic ducts. It can present at any age (although it usually does so in childhood) with fever, abdominal pain and recurrent attacks of cholangitis with Gram-negative septicaemia. Jaundice and portal hypertension are absent. Diagnosis is by ultrasound, percutaneous transhepatic cholangiography and MRCP. There is an increased risk of biliary malignancy.

LIVER ABSCESS

Pyogenic abscess

Pyogenic abscesses are uncommon; they may be single or multiple. The most common used to be a portal pyaemia from intra-abdominal sepsis (e.g. appendicitis or perforations), but now the aetiology is not known in many cases. In the elderly, biliary sepsis is a common cause. Other causes include trauma, bacteraemia and direct extension from, for example, a perinephric abscess.

The organism found most commonly is *E. coli*. *Streptococcus milleri* and anaerobic organisms such as *Bacteroides* are often seen. Other organisms include *Enterococcus faecalis*, *Proteus vulgaris* and *Staphylococcus aureus*. Often the infection is mixed.

Clinical features

Some patients are not acutely ill and present with malaise lasting several days or even months. Others can present with fever, rigors, anorexia, vomiting, weight loss and abdominal pain. In these patients, a Gram-negative septicaemia with shock can occur. On examination, there may be little to find. Alternatively, the patient may be toxic, febrile and jaundiced. In such patients, the liver is tender and enlarged, and there may be signs of a pleural effusion or a pleural rub in the right lower chest.

Investigations

Patients who are not acutely ill are often investigated as a case of 'pyrexia of unknown origin' (PUO) and most investigations will be normal. Often, the only clue to the diagnosis is a raised serum alkaline phosphatase.

- ***Serum bilirubin*** is raised in 25% of cases.
- ***Normochromic normocytic anaemia*** may occur, usually accompanied by a polymorphonuclear leucocytosis.
- ***Serum alkaline phosphatase, ESR and CRP*** are often raised.
- ***Serum vitamin B_{12}*** is very high, as it is stored in and subsequently released from the liver.
- ***Blood cultures*** are positive in only 30% of cases.

Imaging

Ultrasound is useful for detecting abscesses. A CT scan may be of value in complex and multiple lesions ***(Fig. 14.31)***. A chest X-ray will show elevation of the right hemidiaphragm with a pleural effusion in the severe case. Depending on age, imaging of the colon may be necessary to find the source of the infection.

Management

Aspiration of the abscess should be attempted under ultrasound control. Antibiotics should initially cover Gram-positive, Gram-negative and anaerobic organisms until the causative organism is identified.

Further drainage via a large-bore needle under ultrasound control or surgically may be necessary if resolution is difficult or slow. Any underlying cause must also be treated.

Prognosis

The overall mortality depends on the nature of the underlying pathology but has been reduced to approximately 16% with needle aspiration and antibiotics. A unilocular abscess in the right lobe has the best prognosis. Scattered multiple abscesses have a very high mortality, with only 1 in 5 patients surviving.

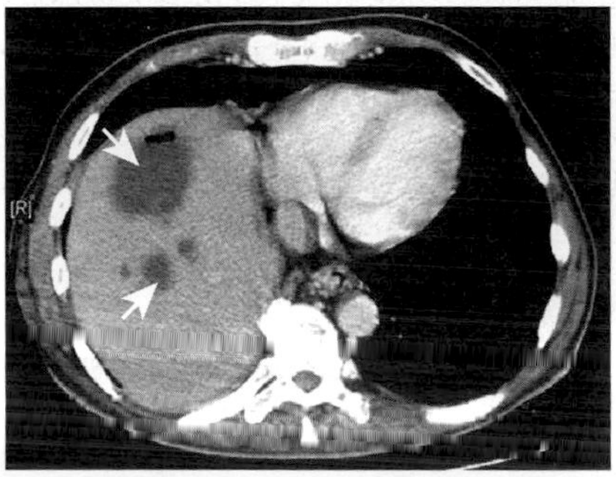

Figure 14.31 CT scan showing liver abscesses. Abscesses are shown in the right lobe of the liver (arrowed), secondary to partial biliary obstruction.

Amoebic abscess

This condition occurs worldwide and must be considered in patients travelling from endemic areas. *Entamoeba histolytica* (see pp. 305–306) can be carried from the bowel to the liver in the portal venous system, leading to portal inflammation, with the development of multiple microabscesses and, eventually, single or multiple large abscesses.

Clinically, the onset is usually gradual but may be sudden. There is fever, anorexia, weight loss and malaise. There is often no history of dysentery. On examination, the patient looks ill and has tender hepatomegaly and signs of an effusion or consolidation in the base of the right side of the chest. Jaundice is unusual.

Investigations

These are as for pyogenic abscess, plus:

- ***Serological tests for amoeba*** (e.g. haemagglutination, amoebic complement fixation test, ELISA). These are always positive, particularly if there are bowel symptoms; they remain positive after a clinical cure and therefore do not indicate current disease. A repeat negative test, however, is good evidence against an amoebic abscess.
- ***Diagnostic aspiration of fluid*** looking like anchovy sauce.

Management

Metronidazole 800 mg three times daily is given for 10 days. Aspiration is used in patients failing to respond, in those with multiple and sometimes large abscesses, and in those with abscesses in the left lobe of the liver or impending rupture.

Complications

Complications include rupture, secondary infection and septicaemia.

OTHER INFECTIONS OF THE LIVER

Schistosomiasis

Schistosoma mansoni and *S. japonicum* affect the liver, but *S. haematobium* rarely does so (see also pp. 312–314). During their life cycle, the ova reach the liver via the venous system and obstruct the portal branches, producing granulomas, fibrosis and inflammation, but not cirrhosis.

Clinical features and investigations

Clinically, there is hepatosplenomegaly and portal hypertension, which is particularly severe with *S. mansoni*. In Egypt, there is frequently concomitant chronic hepatitis C infection.

Investigations show a raised serum alkaline phosphatase, and ova can be found in the stools (centrifuged deposits) and in rectal and liver biopsies. Skin tests and other immunological tests often give false results and may also be positive because of past infection.

Management

Treatment is with praziquantel, but fibrosis still remains with a potential risk of portal hypertension, characteristically pre-sinusoidal due to intense portal fibrosis.

Hydatid disease

Cysts caused by *Echinococcus granulosus* are single or multiple. They usually occur in the lower part of the right lobe. The cyst has three layers: an outside layer derived from the host, an intermediate laminated layer, and an inner germinal layer that buds off brood capsules to form daughter cysts (see also pp. 315–316).

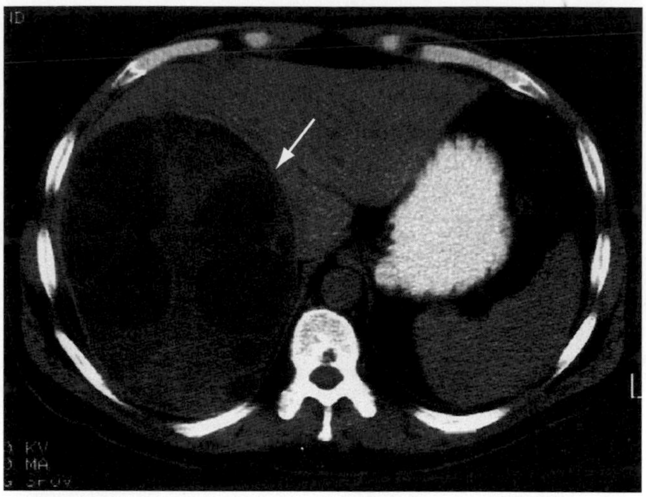

Figure 14.32 CT scan of liver showing a large hydatid cyst (arrowed). 'Daughter' cysts are also shown lying within it.

Clinical features and investigations

Clinically, there may be no symptoms or there may be a dull ache and swelling in the right hypochondrium.

Investigations show a peripheral eosinophilia in 30% of cases and usually a positive hydatid complement fixation test or haemagglutination (85%). Plain abdominal X-ray may show calcification of the outer coat of the cyst. Ultrasound and CT scan demonstrate cysts and may show diagnostic daughter cysts within the parent cyst ***(Fig. 14.32)***.

Management

Medical treatment (e.g. with albendazole 10 mg/kg, which penetrates into large cysts) results in cysts becoming smaller. Puncture, aspiration, injection, re-aspiration (PAIR) has been used since the 1980s. Fine-needle aspiration is undertaken under ultrasound control with chemotherapeutic cover. Surgery can be performed with removal of the cyst intact, if possible, after first sterilizing the cyst with alcohol, saline or cetrimide. Chronic calcified cysts can be left; there have been no well-designed clinical trials for any therapy.

Complications and prognosis

These include rupture into the biliary tree or other organs, or intraperitoneally, with spread of infection. The prognosis without any complications is good, although there is always a risk of rupture. ***Preventative measures*** include deworming of pet dogs and preventing pets from eating infected carcasses, as well as veterinary control programmes.

Echinococcus multilocularis causes alveolar echinococcosis and is almost exclusively a hepatic disease, with a high mortality if not treated. Early diagnosis enables radical surgery and then continued chemosuppression.

Acquired immunodeficiency syndrome

The liver is often involved in AIDS and is a significant cause of morbidity or mortality. HIV (see also pp. 331–355) itself is not the cause of the liver abnormalities. Clinical hepatomegaly is common (60% of patients). The following are seen, although less frequently in areas where anti-retroviral therapy (ART) is available:

- ***Pre-existing/coincidental viral hepatitis***. The hepatitis (HBV, HCV, HDV) progresses more rapidly and is a leading cause of death.
- ***Neoplasia***. Kaposi's sarcoma and non-Hodgkin's lymphoma may be seen, and there is an increased risk of HCC.
- ***Opportunistic infection*** (e.g. *Mycobacterium tuberculosis*, *M. avium-intracellulare*, *Cryptococcus*, *Candida albicans*, toxoplasmosis).
- ***Drug hepatotoxicity***.
- ***Secondary sclerosing cholangitis*** (see p. 350).
- ***Non-cirrhotic portal hypertension*** associated with anti-retroviral therapy.

Further reading

Joshi D, O'Grady J, Dieterich D et al. Increasing burden of liver disease in patients with HIV infection. *Lancet* 2011; 377:1198–1209.

LIVER DISEASE IN PREGNANCY

See pages 1303–1304.

LIVER TUMOURS

Secondary liver tumours

The most common liver tumour is a secondary (metastatic) tumour, particularly from the gastrointestinal tract (from the distribution of the portal blood supply), breast or bronchus. Secondary liver tumours are usually multiple.

Clinical features

These are variable but usually include weight loss, malaise, upper abdominal pain and hepatomegaly, with or without jaundice.

Diagnosis

Ultrasound is the primary investigation, with CT or MRI to define metastases and look for a primary. The serum alkaline phosphatase is almost invariably raised.

Management

This will depend on the site of the primary and the burden of liver metastases. The best results are obtained in colorectal cancer in patients with few hepatic metastases. If the primary tumour is removed and hepatic resection is performed, reasonable survival rates are possible. Chemotherapy is used, particularly with breast cancer (see p. 634). Radiofrequency ablation of the metastases is an alternative to surgery. Thermal therapy and cryotherapy are also used.

Primary malignant tumours

Primary liver tumours may be benign or malignant, but the most common are malignant.

Hepatocellular carcinoma

Hepatocellular carcinoma (HCC) is the fifth most common cancer worldwide.

Aetiology

Carriers of HBV and HCV have an extremely high risk of developing HCC. In areas where HBV is prevalent, 90% of patients with this cancer are positive for HBV. Cirrhosis is present in approximately 80% of these patients. The development of HCC is related to the integration of viral HBV DNA into the genome of the host hepatocyte (see p. 456), and to the degree of viral replication (>10 000 copies/mL). The risk of HCC in HCV is higher than in HBV (even higher with both HBV and HCV), despite no viral integration. Unlike HBV infection, cirrhosis is always present in HIV. Primary liver cancer is also associated with other forms of cirrhosis, such as alcoholic cirrhosis, non-alcoholic fatty liver disease (NAFLD)-associated cirrhosis, and haemochromatosis. Males are affected more than females. Other aetiological factors are aflatoxin (a metabolite of a fungus found in groundnuts) and androgenic steroids, and there is a weak association with the contraceptive pill.

Pathology

The tumour either is single or occurs as multiple nodules throughout the liver. Histologically, it consists of cells resembling hepatocytes. It can metastasize via the hepatic or portal veins to the lymph nodes, bones and lungs.

Clinical features

The clinical features include weight loss, anorexia, fever, an ache in the right hypochondrium and ascites. The rapid development of these features in a cirrhotic patient is suggestive of HCC. On examination, an enlarged, irregular, tender liver may be felt. Increasingly, due to surveillance, HCC is found without symptoms in patients with cirrhosis.

Investigations

- Routine liver biochemistry, full blood count, urea and electrolytes.
- ***Serum α-fetoprotein*** may be raised, but is normal in at least a third of patients.
- ***Ultrasound*** scans show filling defects in 90% of cases.
- ***Enhanced CT scans (Fig. 14.33)*** identify HCC but it is difficult to confirm the diagnosis in lesions smaller than 1 cm. An *MRI* can help to delineate lesions further.
- ***Tumour biopsy*** (see ***Fig. 14.29***), particularly under ultrasonic guidance, is now used less frequently for diagnosis as imaging techniques show characteristic appearances (hypervascularity of the nodule and lack of portal vein washout) and because seeding along the biopsy tract can occur.

Management and prognosis

See page 638.

Prevention

Persistent HBV infection, usually acquired after perinatal infection, is a high risk factor for HCC in many parts of the world, such as South-east Asia. Widespread vaccination against HBV is being used and this has reduced the annual incidence of HCC in Taiwan.

Cholangiocarcinoma

Cholangiocarcinomas are increasing in incidence and can be extrahepatic (see p. 498) or intrahepatic (see p. 638). Intrahepatic adenocarcinomas arising from the bile ducts account for approximately

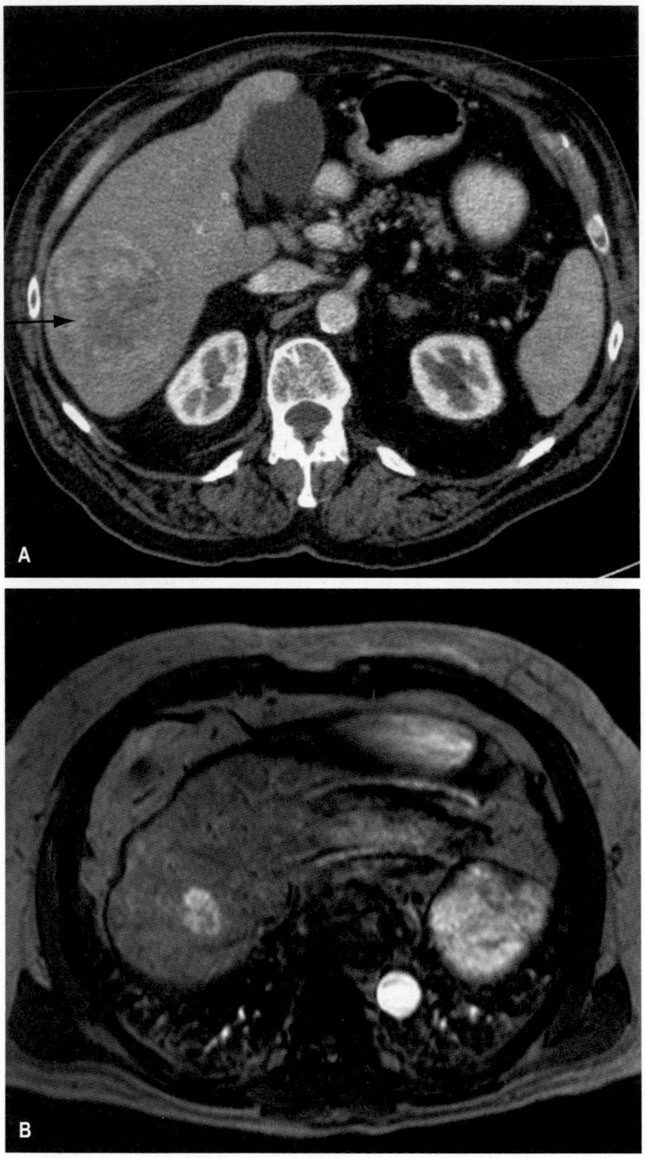

Figure 14.33 Hepatocellular carcinoma. A. CT showing cirrhosis with a hepatocellular carcinoma (arrowed). **B.** T2-weighted MRI of the liver following gadolinium contrast showing a hepatocellular carcinoma.

10% of primary tumours of the liver and biliary tract. They are not associated with cirrhosis or hepatitis B. In the Far East, they may be associated with infestation with *Clonorchis sinensis* or *Opisthorchis viverrini*. The clinical features are similar to those of primary HCC, except that jaundice is frequent with hilar tumours, and cholangitis is more common. There is an increased association with inflammatory bowel disease and primary sclerosing cholangitis (see pp. 476–477).

Surgical resection is rarely possible and patients usually die within 6 months. Transplantation is contraindicated, outside of specialized protocols.

Benign tumours

The most common benign tumour is a ***haemangioma***. It is usually small and single but can be multiple and large. Haemangiomas are usually found incidentally on ultrasound, CT or MRI, and have characteristic appearances. They require no treatment.

Hepatic adenomas are associated with oral contraceptives. They can present with abdominal pain or intraperitoneal bleeding. Resection is required only for symptomatic patients, those with tumours >5 cm in diameter, and in those in whom discontinuation of oral contraception does not result in shrinkage of the tumour. Immunohistochemical characteristics are helpful in indicating malignant potential, which is far more common in men.

Further reading

El-Serag HB. Hepatocellular carcinoma. *N Engl J Med* 2011; 365:1118–1127.
Forner A, Llovet JM, Bruix J et al. Hepatocellular carcinoma. *Lancet* 2012; 379:1245–1255.

MISCELLANEOUS CONDITIONS OF THE LIVER

Hepatic mitochondrial injury syndromes

These syndromes – in which there is mitochondrial damage with inhibition of β-oxidation of fatty acids – can be categorized as having the following causes:

- ***Genetic***, with abnormalities that include medium-chain acyl-coenzyme A dehydrogenase deficiency, leading to microsteatosis.
- ***Toxins*** leading to liver failure, which include aflatoxin and cerulide (produced by *Bacillus cereus*); the latter causes food poisoning (see p. 277).
- ***Drugs*** (e.g. i.v. tetracycline, valproic acid and nucleoside reverse-transcriptase inhibitors), which can produce a fatal microsteatosis.
- ***Idiopathic***, the best known being fatty liver of pregnancy (see p. 1304) and Reye syndrome. The latter, caused by inhibition of β-oxidation and uncoupling of oxidative phosphorylation in mitochondria, leads in children to an acute encephalopathy and diffuse microvesicular fatty infiltration of the liver. Aspirin ingestion and viral infections have been implicated as precipitating agents. Mortality is about 50%, usually due to cerebral oedema.

Idiopathic adult ductopenia

This unexplained condition is characterized by pruritus and cholestatic jaundice. Histology of the liver shows a decrease in intrahepatic bile ducts in at least 50% of the portal tracts, together with the features of cholestasis and marked fibrosis or cirrhosis. In most, the disease is progressive and the only treatment is liver transplantation.

Indian childhood cirrhosis

This condition of children is seen in the Indian subcontinent. The cause is unknown. Eventually, there is development of a micronodular cirrhosis with excess copper in the liver.

Hepatic porphyrias

These are dealt with on page 1290.

Cystic fibrosis

Cystic fibrosis (see also pp. 1088–1089) mainly affects the lung and pancreas, but patients can develop fatty liver, cholestasis and cirrhosis. The aetiology of the liver involvement is unclear.

Coeliac disease

Abnormal liver biochemical tests are common in coeliac disease (see also p. 396) and return to normal with a gluten-free diet. A tissue transglutaminase test should be performed if hepatic causes are not found when investigating abnormal liver biochemistry.

DRUGS AND THE LIVER

Drug metabolism

The liver is the major site of drug metabolism. Drugs are converted from fat-soluble to water-soluble substances that can be excreted in the urine or bile. This metabolism of drugs is mediated by a group of mixed-function enzymes (see p. 19).

Drug hepatotoxicity

Many drugs impair liver function. When abnormal liver biochemical tests are found, drugs should always be considered as a cause, particularly when other causes have been excluded. Damage to the liver by drugs is usually classified as being either predictable (or dose-related) or non-predictable (not dose-related) (see p. 22). However, there is considerable overlap and at least ***six mechanisms may be involved in the production of damage***:

1. disruption of intracellular calcium homeostasis
2. disruption of bile canalicular transport mechanisms
3. formation of non-functioning adducts (enzyme–drug), which may then lead to
4. presentation on the surface of the hepatocyte as new immunogens (attacked by T cells)
5. induction of apoptosis
6. inhibition of mitochondrial function, which prevents fatty acid metabolism and accumulation of both lactate and reactive oxygen species.

The predominant mechanism or combination of mechanisms determines the type of liver injury: that is, hepatitic, cholestatic or immunological (skin rashes, fever and arthralgia, i.e. serum-sickness syndrome). Eosinophilia and circulating immune complexes and antibodies are occasionally detected.

When a small amount of hepatotoxic drug whose effect is dose-dependent (e.g. paracetamol) is ingested, a large proportion of it undergoes conjugation with glucuronide and sulphate, while the remainder is metabolized by microsomal enzymes to produce toxic derivatives that are immediately detoxified by conjugation with glutathione. If larger doses are ingested, the former pathway becomes saturated and the toxic derivative is produced at a faster rate. Once the hepatic glutathione is depleted, large amounts of the toxic metabolite accumulate and produce damage (see p. 79).

The 'predictability' of drugs to produce damage can, however, be affected by metabolic events preceding their ingestion. For example, chronic alcohol users may become more susceptible to liver damage because of the enzyme-inducing effects of alcohol, or ill or starving patients may become susceptible because of the depletion of hepatic glutathione produced by starvation. Many other factors, such as environmental or genetic effects, may be involved in determining the 'susceptibility' of certain patients to certain drugs.

The incidence of drug hepatotoxicity is 14 per 100 000 population with a 6% mortality. It is the most common cause of acute liver failure in the USA. Liver transplantation is used.

Box 14.23 Liver damage produced by some drugs

Types of liver damage	Drugs	
Zone 3 necrosis	Carbon tetrachloride *Amanita* mushrooms Paracetamol	Salicylates Piroxicam Cocaine
Zone 1 necrosis	Ferrous sulphate	
Microvesicular fat	Sodium valproate	Tetracyclines
Steatohepatitis	Amiodarone Synthetic oestrogens	Nifedipine
Fibrosis	Methotrexate Other cytotoxic agents Arsenic	Vitamin A Retinoids
Vascular		
Sinusoidal dilatation	Contraceptive drugs	Anabolic steroids
Peliosis hepatis	Azathioprine Oral contraceptives Azathioprine	Anabolic steroids, e.g. Danazol
Veno-occlusive	Pyrrolizidine alkaloids (*Senecio* in bush tea)	Cytotoxics – cyclophosphamide
Acute hepatitis	Isoniazid Rifampicin Methyldopa Atenolol Enalapril Verapamil Ketoconazole	Cytotoxic drugs Clonazepam Disulfiram Niacin Volatile liquid anaesthetics, e.g. Halothane Infliximab
Chronic hepatitis	Methyldopa Nitrofurantoin	Fenofibrate Isoniazid
General hypersensitivity	Sulphonamides, e.g. Sulfasalazine Co-trimoxazole Fansidar Penicillins, e.g. Flucloxacillin Ampicillin Amoxicillin Co-amoxiclav NSAIDs, e.g. Salicylates Diclofenac	Allopurinol Anti-thyroid. e.g. Propylthiouracil Carbimazole Quinine, e.g. Quinidine Diltiazem Anticonvulsants, e.g. Phenytoin
Canalicular cholestasis	Sex hormones Ciclosporin Chlorpromazine Haloperidol Erythromycin Flucloxacillin	Fucidin Cimetidine/ranitidine Nitrofurantoin Imipramine Azathioprine Oral hypoglycaemics
Biliary sludge	Ceftriaxone	
Sclerosing cholangitis	Hepatic arterial infusion of 5-fluorouracil	
Hepatic tumours	Pills with high hormone content (adenomas)	
Hepatocellular carcinoma	Contraceptive pill	Danazol
Nodular regenerative hyperplasia	Azathioprine	Some anti-retroviral therapies

NSAID, non-steroidal anti-inflammatory drug. *Note*: Anti-HIV drugs, e.g. maraviroc, cause hepatic dysfunction.

Hepatitic damage

The type of damage produced by various drugs is shown in ***Box 14.23***. Most reactions occur within 3 months of starting the drug. Monitoring liver biochemistry in patients on long-term treatment, such as anti-tuberculosis therapy, is *mandatory*. If a drug is suspected of causing hepatic damage, it should be stopped immediately. Liver biopsy is of limited help in confirming the diagnosis, but occasionally, hepatic eosinophilia or granulomas may be seen. Diagnostic challenge with subtherapeutic doses of the drug is sometimes required after the liver biochemistry has returned to normal, to confirm the diagnosis.

Individual drugs

Paracetamol

In high doses, paracetamol produces liver cell necrosis (see above). The toxic metabolite binds irreversibly to liver cell membranes. Overdosage is discussed on pages 79–80.

Volatile liquid anaesthetics

Halothane, which was the first available drug in this class, is now not used in the UK because it produced hepatitis in patients with repeated exposures. Both sevoflurane and isoflurane also cause hepatotoxicity in those patients sensitized to halogenated anaesthetics; however, the risk is smaller than with halothane and remote with desflurane.

Steroid compounds

Cholestasis is caused by natural and synthetic oestrogens, as well as methyltestosterone. These agents interfere with canalicular biliary flow by blocking MRP2 and MDR3 (see ***Fig. 14.4***) and cause a pure cholestasis.

Cholestasis is rare with the contraceptive pill because of the low dosage used. However, the contraceptive pill is associated with an increased incidence of gallstones, hepatic adenomas (rarely, HCCs), the Budd–Chiari syndrome and peliosis hepatis. The latter condition, which also occurs with anabolic steroids, consists of dilatation of the hepatic sinusoids to form blood-filled lakes.

Phenothiazines

Phenothiazines (e.g. chlorpromazine) can produce a cholestatic picture owing to a hypersensitivity reaction. This occurs in 1% of patients, usually within 4 weeks of starting the drug. Typically, it is associated with a fever and eosinophilia. Recovery occurs on stopping the drug.

Anti-tuberculous chemotherapy

Isoniazid produces elevated aminotransferases in 10–20% of patients. Hepatic necrosis with jaundice occurs in a smaller percentage. The hepatotoxicity of isoniazid is related to its metabolites and is dependent on acetylator status. Rifampicin produces hepatitis, usually within 3 weeks of starting the drug, particularly in patients on high doses. Pyrazinamide produces abnormal liver biochemical tests and, rarely, liver cell necrosis.

Amiodarone

This leads to a steatohepatitis histologically, and liver failure if the drug is not stopped in time.

Sodium valproate

This causes mitochondrial injury with microvesicular steatosis. Intravenous carnitine should be used as an antidote.

Drug prescribing for patients with liver disease

The metabolism of drugs is impaired in severe liver disease (with jaundice and ascites), as the removal of many drugs depends on liver blood flow and the integrity of the hepatocyte. In general, therefore, the effect of drugs is prolonged by liver disease and also by cholestasis. This is further accentuated by portosystemic shunting, which diminishes the first-pass extraction of drugs. With hypoproteinaemia, there is decreased protein binding of some drugs, and bilirubin competes with many drugs for the binding sites on serum albumin. In patients with portosystemic encephalopathy, care must be taken in prescribing drugs with a central depressant action, such as narcotics, including codeine and anxiolytics. Other common drugs to be avoided in cirrhosis include angiotensin-converting enzyme (ACE) inhibitors (which cause hepatorenal failure) and NSAIDs (which cause bleeding).

Further reading

Björnsson E. Review article: drug-induced liver injury in clinical practice. *Aliment Pharmacol Ther* 2010; 32:3–13.

Bibliography

Ryder SD, Chapman RW (eds). Liver disorders: Parts 1 and 2. *Medicine* 2011; 39:507–634.

Williams R, Aspinall R, Bellis M et al. Addressing liver disease in the UK. *Lancet* 2014; 384:1953–1997.

15 Biliary tract and pancreatic disease

David Westaby, Christopher Wadsworth

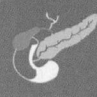

See your e-book for clinical tips, extra tables, learning challenges and MCQs.

INTRODUCTION

Biliary and pancreatic disease are a major burden on healthcare systems worldwide. In the West, acute pancreatitis and gallstone disease are the two most common gastrointestinal causes of urgent hospital admission. Pancreatic and biliary tree neoplasms carry a poor prognosis, pose significant diagnostic challenges and are increasing in incidence.

Current ultrasound, computed tomography (CT) and magnetic resonance imaging (MRI) technology enable the biliary tree and pancreas to be visualized with increasing resolution. Widespread use of such improved imaging has led to improved diagnosis but also to a burgeoning need to characterize and manage incidental, small, often asymptomatic lesions, particularly in the pancreas.

Endoscopic diagnosis of pancreatobiliary disease has been enhanced by improvements in endoscopic ultrasound technology, and the re-emergence of direct cholangioscopy for visualization of the bile duct. Therapeutic endoscopy and laparoscopic surgery are now widely available and permit a minimally invasive approach to the management of almost all gallstone disease, and to the resection or palliation of pancreatobiliary cancer.

THE GALL BLADDER AND BILIARY SYSTEM

The structure and function of the biliary system and the formation of bile are discussed on pages 441–443.

GALLSTONES

Gallstone disease represents a major cause of patient morbidity, particularly in the Western world, and has a major impact on health care economics. Gallstones may be present at any age but are unusual before the third decade. The prevalence of gallstones is strongly influenced by both age and gender. There is a progressive increase in the presence of gallstones with age but the prevalence is 2–3 times higher in women than in men, although this difference is less marked in the sixth and seventh decades. At this age, the prevalence ranges between 20% and 30%. The increase in life expectancy is reflected in an increased burden of symptomatic gallstone disease. There are considerable racial differences, gallstones being more common in Scandinavians, South Americans and Native North Americans but less common in Asian and African groups. These racial differences may reflect both genetic and dietary factors. Some of these differences are being eroded by the adoption of Western diets containing high cholesterol in countries with emerging economics.

Pathogenesis

Types of gallstones

The large majority of gallstones are of two types: cholesterol stones (containing >50% of the sterol) and, less frequently, 'pigment stones', predominantly composed of calcium bilirubinate or polymer-like complexes with calcium, copper and some cholesterol.

Cholesterol gallstones

This type of stone accounts for 85% of gallstones in the Western world. The formation of cholesterol stones is the consequence of cholesterol crystallization from gall bladder bile. This is dependent on three factors:

- cholesterol supersaturation of bile
- crystallization-promoting factors within bile
- motility of the gall bladder.

The majority of cholesterol is derived from hepatic uptake from dietary sources. However, hepatic biosynthesis may account for up to 20%. The rate-limiting step in cholesterol synthesis is β-hydroxy-β methyl glutaryl CoA (HMG-CoA) reductase, which catalyses the first step: that is, the conversion of acetate to mevalonate.

- The cholesterol formed is co-secreted with phospholipids into the biliary canaliculus as unilamellar vesicles.
- Cholesterol will only crystallize into stones when the bile is supersaturated with cholesterol relative to the bile salt and phospholipid content. This can occur as a consequence of excess cholesterol secretion into bile, which, in some instances, has been shown to be due to an increase in HMG-CoA reductase activity.

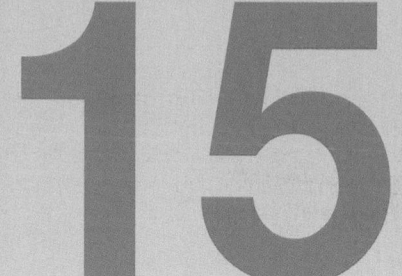

- Increased secretion of cholesterol into bile has also been associated with the insulin resistance associated with the metabolic syndrome.
- A high-cholesterol diet increases biliary cholesterol secretion and decreases bile salt synthesis and the bile salt pool in cholesterol gallstone subjects but not in controls.

These findings suggest that increased intestinal uptake of the sterol could play a role in gallstone pathogenesis. In support of this observation, pharmacological inhibition of cholesterol absorption prevents gallstone formation in a mouse model. Ezetimibe is a highly selective intestinal cholesterol absorption inhibitor, suppressing the uptake of dietary and biliary cholesterol across the brush border membrane of the enterocyte. This may offer a potential therapy for the management/prevention of gallstone formation in patients.

While cholesterol supersaturation of bile is essential for cholesterol stone formation, many individuals in whom such supersaturation occurs will never develop stones. It is the balance between cholesterol crystallizing and solubilizing factors that determines whether cholesterol will crystallize out of solution. A number of lipoproteins have been reported as putative crystallizing factors.

Statins are effective in the treatment of hypercholesterolaemia by competitively inhibiting HMG-CoA reductase. There is emerging evidence that statins reduce cholesterol secretion into bile and, by doing so, promote gallstone dissolution. The prevalence of gallstone disease in patient groups taking statins for the management of hypercholesterolaemia appears to be reduced.

Leptin (see p. 206) has been shown to increase cholesterol secretion into bile. Elevated levels of leptin during rapid weight loss may account for the increased incidence of cholesterol gallstones.

An alternative mechanism of supersaturation is a decreased bile salt content, which may occur as a consequence of bile salt loss (e.g. terminal ileal resection or ileal involvement with Crohn's disease).

The ***composition of the bile salt pool*** may also influence the ability to maintain cholesterol in solution. There is evidence that an increased proportion of the secondary hydrophobic bile acid (deoxycholic acid) in the bile acid pool may predispose to cholesterol stone formation. This has been linked with slow colonic transit, during which the primary bile acid, cholic acid, may undergo microbial enzyme metabolism, yielding deoxycholic acid, which is then absorbed back into the bile salt pool (see ***Fig. 14.4***).

Evidence from ***epidemiological***, family and twin studies points to the role of genetic factors in gallstone formation. A number of lithogenic genes have been identified, which may interact with environmental factors. The process of bile formation is maintained by a network of adenosine triphosphate-binding cassette (ABC) transporters in the hepatocyte canalicular membrane, which enables biliary secretion of cholesterol, bile salts and phospholipids. This process is regulated by the nuclear receptors farnesoid x receptor (*FXR*) and liver x receptor (*LXR*). Loss-of-function mutations in specific ABC transporter genes have been associated with cholesterol gallstones secondary to bile salt and phospholipid deficiencies within the nascent bile ***(Fig. 15.1)***. However, monogenic susceptibility appears uncommon. There are rare cases in which a single missense mutation of the multidrug-resistant (*MDR3*) gene has been associated with extensive intra- and extrahepatic cholelithiasis at an early age (<40 years).

Gall bladder motility represents a further factor that may influence the cholesterol crystallization from supersaturated bile. There is evidence from animal models that gall bladder stasis leads to cholesterol crystallization mediated by hypersecretion of mucin.

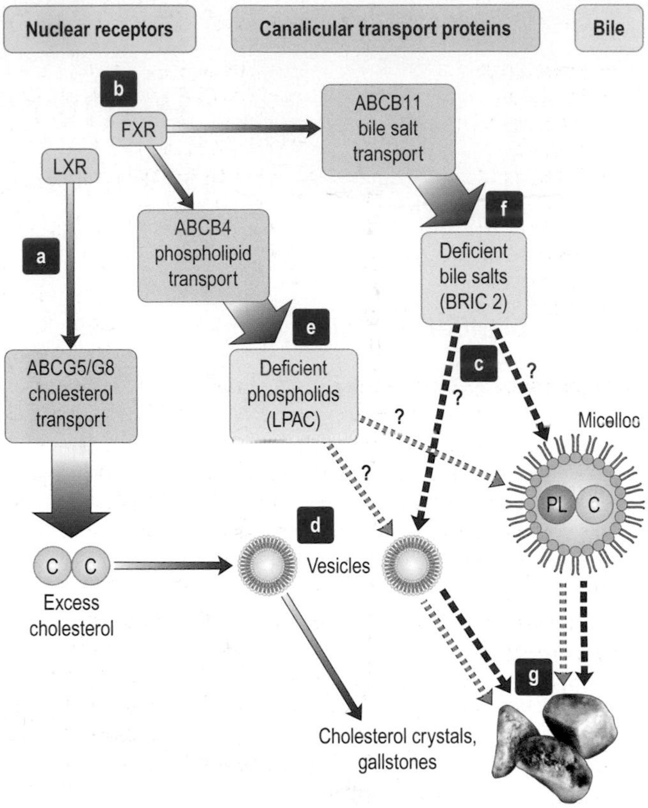

Figure 15.1 Nascent bile formation at the hepatocytic canalicular membrane, biliary cholesterol solubilization and gallstone formation.
(a) ABCG5/G8 transports cholesterol into bile (regulated by nuclear receptor *LXR*).
(b) ABCB11 and ABCB4 transport bile salts and phosphatidylcholine into bile (regulated by nuclear receptor *FXR*).
(c) Bile cholesterol is solubilized in mixed micelles or contained in cholesterol–phospholipid vesicles.
(d) Most gallstones are caused by excess biliary cholesterol secretion and subsequent crystallization from supersaturated vesicles (continuous lines).
(e) Low phospholipid-associated cholelithiasis (LPAC) occurs if there is deficient phospholipid in bile due to function mutations in gene *ABCB4*.
(f) Benign recurrent intrahepatic cholestasis (BRIC) type 2 is characterized by deficient bile salts in bile due to function mutations in gene *ABCB11*.
(g) In both LPAC and BRIC type 2, there is an increased risk of gallstone formation.

Abnormalities of gall bladder motility have been suggested as factors in such circumstances as pregnancy, multiparity and diabetes, as well as octreotide-related gall bladder stones (see p. 1194). Recognized risk factors for cholesterol gallstones are shown in ***Box 15.1***.

Bile pigment stones

The pathogenesis of pigment stones is entirely independent of cholesterol gallstones. There are two main types of pigment gallstones: black and brown.

Black pigment gallstones are composed of calcium bilirubinate and a network of mucin glycoproteins that interlace with salts, such as calcium carbonate and/or calcium phosphate. These stones range in colour from deep black to very dark brown and have a glass-like cross-sectional surface on fracturing. Because hyperbilirubinbilia is the critical risk factor, black stones are associated with

Box 15.1 Risk factors for cholesterol gallstones

- Increasing age
- Sex (F>M)
- Family history and genetics
- Multiparity
- Obesity ± metabolic syndrome
- Rapid weight loss
- Diet (e.g. high in animal fat/low in fibre)
- Drugs (e.g. contraceptive pill)
- Ileal disease or resection
- Cirrhosis
- Spinal cord injury
- Diabetes mellitus
- Acromegaly treated with octreotide
- Liver cirrhosis
- Total parental nutrition

all major ***haemolytic anaemias***, such as spherocytosis, sickle cell disease and thalassaemia, and also with subclinical haemolysis from prosthetic valve replacements, malaria, hypersplenism from hepatic cirrhosis, and foot trauma in long-distance runners. An increased prevalence of black pigment gallstones is also seen in Gilbert syndrome (see p. 448), which is associated with enhanced biliary secretion of monoglucuronosyl bilirubin.

There is evidence that bile salt loss into the colon (consequent on ileal resection or ileal disease) promotes solubilization and colonic reabsorption of bilirubin. This enhances the enterohepatic circulation and biliary secretion of bilirubin with the formation of gallstones. Pigment stones have also been linked with bacterial colonization of the biliary tree. Some pigment stones have been shown to contain bacteria, many of which produce glucuronidase and phospholipase, factors that are known to facilitate stone formation. It is speculated that this subclinical bacterial colonization of the bile duct is responsible for pigment stone formation.

Brown pigment stones are usually of a muddy hue and, on cross-section, seem to have alternating brown and tan layers. These stones are composed of calcium salts of fatty acids, as well as calcium bilirubinate. They are almost always found in the presence of bile stasis and/or biliary infection. Brown stones can form in any part of the biliary tree secondary to chronic stasis and the presence of anaerobic bacterial infection.

The ***Oriental hepatolithiasis syndrome (recurrent pyogenic cholangitis)*** is the most serious manifestation of pigment stone disease. Biliary strictures are formed, possibly due to nematode or fluke infestation within the extrahepatic and intrahepatic bile ducts. *Ascaris lumbricoides*, *Clonorchis sinensis* and *Opisthorchis viverrini* are the parasites most commonly recognized with this condition. The evidence for causation is unclear, as is the role of bacterial infection. Brown stones may also be the cause of recurrent bile duct stones following cholecystectomy, and are also found in the intrahepatic bile ducts in stenosing biliary disease such as Caroli syndrome and primary sclerosing cholangitis.

Clinical features

The majority of gallstones are asymptomatic and remain so during a person's lifetime. Gallstones are increasingly detected as an incidental finding at the time of either abdominal radiography or ultrasound scanning ***(Fig. 15.2)***. Over a 10–15-year period, approximately 20% of these stones will be the cause of symptoms and 10% will involve severe complications. Once gallstones have become symptomatic, there is a strong trend towards recurrent complications, often of increasing severity. Gallstones do not cause dyspepsia, fat intolerance, flatulence or other vague upper abdominal symptoms.

The clinical syndromes associated with gallstones are shown in ***Figure 15.3***.

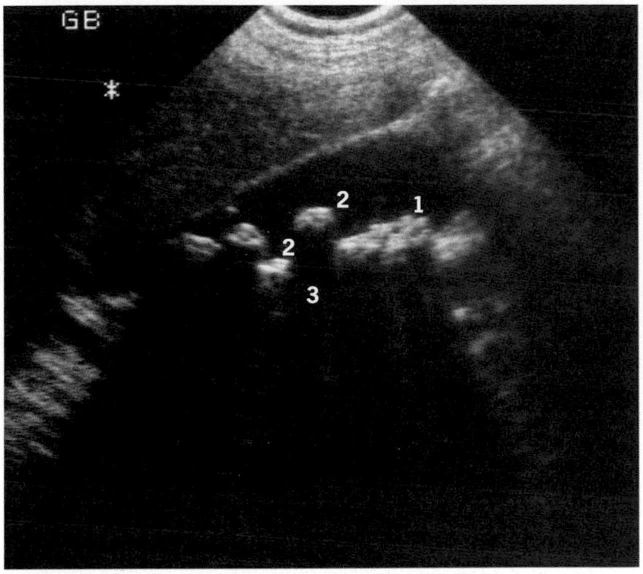

Figure 15.2 Gall bladder ultrasound with multiple echogenic gallstones causing well-defined acoustic shadowing. (1) Gall bladder. **(2)** Echogenic gallstones. **(3)** Acoustic shadow.

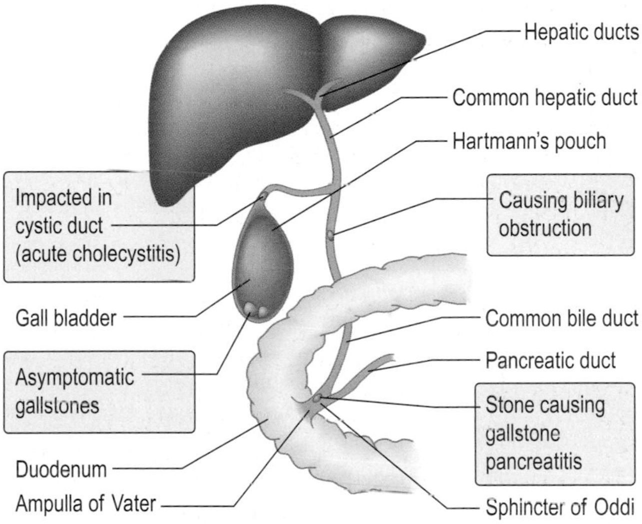

Figure 15.3 Clinical presentation of gallstones.

Biliary or gallstone colic

Biliary colic is the term used for the pain associated with the temporary obstruction of the cystic or common bile duct by a stone usually migrating from the gall bladder. Despite the term 'colic', the pain of stone-induced ductular obstruction is of sudden onset, severe but constant (not like a 'colic'), and has a crescendo characteristic. Some patients relate the symptoms to over-indulgence with food, particularly when this has a high fat content. The most common time of day for such an episode is in the mid-evening, lasting until the early hours of the morning.

The initial site of pain is usually in the epigastrium but there may be a right upper quadrant component. Radiation may occur over the right shoulder and right subscapular region.

Nausea and vomiting frequently accompany the more severe attacks. The attack may be terminated spontaneously after a number of hours or by the administration of opiate analgesia. More protracted pain, particularly when associated with fevers and rigors,

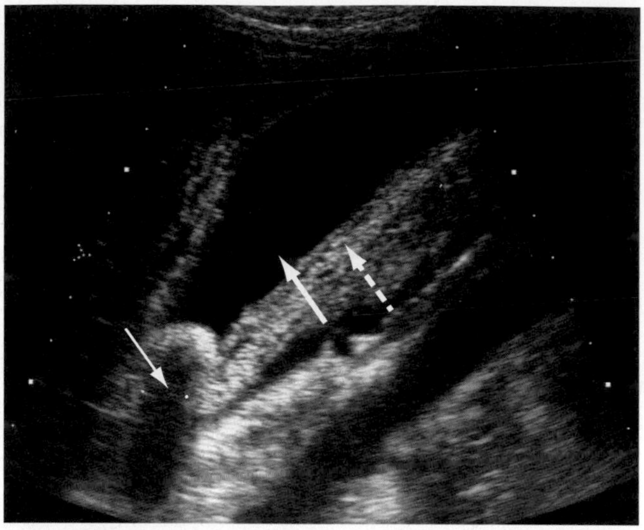

Figure 15.4 Ultrasound scan in a patient with acute cholecystitis. There is a ***stone*** (casting an acoustic shadow; ***thin arrow***) impacted in the gall bladder neck, with a ***distended gall bladder (thick arrow)*** and thickening and oedema of the gall bladder wall (dashed arrow).

suggests secondary complications such as cholecystitis, cholangitis or gallstone-related pancreatitis (see below).

Acute cholecystitis

The initial event in acute cholecystitis is the obstruction of gall bladder emptying. In 95% of cases, a gall bladder stone can be identified as the cause ***(Fig. 15.4)***. Such obstruction results in an increase of gall bladder glandular secretion, leading to progressive distension that, in turn, may compromise the vascular supply to the gall bladder.

There is also an inflammatory response secondary to retained bile within the gall bladder. Infection is a secondary phenomenon following the above vascular and inflammatory events.

The initial clinical features of an episode of cholecystitis are similar to those of biliary colic described above. However, over a number of hours, there is progression with severe localized right upper quadrant abdominal pain corresponding to parietal peritoneal involvement in the inflammatory process. The pain is associated with tenderness and muscle guarding or rigidity. This is frequently manifest by Murphy's sign, consisting of pain on taking a deep breath when the examiner's fingers are on the approximate location of the gall bladder. Occasionally, the gall bladder can become distended by pus (an empyema) and, rarely, an acute gangrenous cholecystitis develops, which can perforate, with generalized peritonitis.

Investigations

Biliary colic as a consequence of a stone in the neck of the gall bladder or cystic duct is unlikely to be associated with significant abnormality of laboratory tests. ***Abdominal ultrasound scan*** is the single most useful investigation for the diagnosis of gallstone-related disease (see ***Fig. 15.2***).

Acute cholecystitis is usually associated with:

- a moderate leucocytosis
- raised inflammatory markers (e.g. C-reactive protein, CRP).
- ***Serum bilirubin, alkaline phosphatase and aminotransferase levels*** may be marginally elevated in the presence of cholecystitis alone, even in the absence of bile duct obstruction. More significant elevation of the bilirubin and alkaline phosphatase is in keeping with bile duct obstruction.
- ***Abdominal ultrasound*** has a positive predictive value of 92% and a negative predictive value of 95% in patients with a clinical history of acute cholecystitis and Murphy's sign. Look for:
  - ***Gallstones*** within the gall bladder, particularly when these are obstructing the gall bladder neck or cystic duct.
  - ***Focal tenderness*** over the underlying gall bladder.
  - ***Thickening of the gall bladder wall***. This may also be seen with hypoalbuminaemia, portal hypertension and acute viral hepatitis.

Gallstones are a common finding in an ageing population, and in the absence of specific symptoms, great care should be taken when determining whether the gallstones are responsible for the symptoms.

Differential diagnosis

Typical cases of biliary colic are usually suspected on the clinical history. The differential diagnosis includes the irritable bowel syndrome (spasm of the hepatic flexure), carcinoma of the right side of the colon, atypical peptic ulcer disease, renal colic and pancreatitis.

The differential diagnosis of acute cholecystitis includes a number of other conditions marked by severe right upper quadrant pain and fever: for example, acute episodes of pancreatitis, perforated peptic ulceration or an intrahepatic abscess. Conditions above the right diaphragm, such as basal pneumonia, as well as myocardial infarction, may mimic the clinical picture on occasion.

Management

Cholecystectomy

Cholecystectomy is the treatment of choice for virtually all patients with symptomatic gall bladder stones. In patients admitted with specific gallstone-related complications (see below), cholecystectomy should be carried out during the period of that admission to prevent the risk of recurrence. For those presenting with pain alone, an elective procedure can be planned but the waiting time should be minimized to avoid the high risk of recurrent symptoms (approximately 30% over 4 months) and the need for another hospital admission.

Cholecystectomy should not be performed in the absence of typical symptoms just because stones are found on investigation. There is an ongoing debate as to whether prophylactic cholecystectomy is justified in young patients found to have small stones. Such patients have a long period over which they may develop symptomatic disease and small stones are an independent risk factor for the potentially serious complication of gallstone pancreatitis. The most recent guidance available does not recommend prophylactic surgery.

The laparotomy approach to cholecystectomy has now been replaced by the laparoscopic technique. Postoperative pain is minimized with only a short period of ileus and the early ability to mobilize the patient. Laparoscopic cholecystectomy can be safely carried out on a day-care basis in an elective setting in otherwise fit patients. This has considerable cost benefits over open cholecystectomy, which is now reserved for a small proportion of patients with contraindications, such as extensive previous upper abdominal surgery, ongoing bile duct obstruction or portal hypertension.

In approximately 5% of cases, a laparoscopic cholecystectomy is converted to an open operation because of technical difficulties: in particular, adhesions in the right upper quadrant or difficulty in identifying the biliary anatomy.

Acute cholecystitis

The initial management is conservative, consisting of nil by mouth, intravenous fluids, opiate analgesia and intravenous antibiotics. Bacteria that are commonly associated with cholecystitis include *Escherichia coli*, *Bacteroides fragilis*, *Klebsiella*, *Enterococcus* and *Pseudomonas* species. Antibiotic selection is dictated by local policy and is guided by the severity of any associated sepsis. Options include extended-spectrum cephalosporins (e.g. ceftriaxone) in combination with metronidazole, piperacillin/tazobactam or imipenem/meropenem.

Cholecystectomy is usually delayed for a few days to allow the symptoms to settle but can then be carried out quite safely in the majority of cases.

When the clinical situation fails to respond to this conservative management, particularly if there is increasing pain and fever, an empyema or gangrene of the gall bladder may have occurred. In this circumstance, urgent imaging (transabdominal ultrasound or CT scan) is required to define the pathology. Surgical intervention is usually required, although a radiologically placed gall bladder drain can be used as a temporizing measure for the management of an empyema. The placement of a drain is the best option in patients who are considered unfit for early surgery (because of ongoing sepsis or significant co-morbidity).

Specific complications of cholecystectomy

These include a biliary leak, either from the cystic duct or from the gall bladder bed. Injury to the bile duct itself occurs in up to 0.5% of laparoscopic operations and may have serious long-term sequelae in the form of a bile duct stricture and secondary biliary liver injury. Injuries to the extrahepatic biliary tree are more likely with variant duct anatomy, such as a low cystic duct insertion or draining of the cystic duct into the right posterior ducts rather than the common bile duct. There is an overall mortality of 0.2% associated with cholecystectomy.

Stone dissolution and shock wave lithotripsy

These non-surgical techniques for the management of gall bladder stones are used infrequently but still have a role in a few highly selected patients who may not be fit for cholecystectomy or have declined the surgical option.

Stone dissolution

Pure or near-pure cholesterol stones can be solubilized by increasing the bile salt content of bile. Most experience is with oral ursodeoxycholic acid. The approach requires long-term therapy and the recurrence rate of gallstones is high when therapy is stopped. Additional pharmacological tools for treating cholesterol gallstones include cholesterol-lowering agents that inhibit hepatic cholesterol synthesis (statins) or intestinal cholesterol absorption (ezetimibe), or drugs acting on specific nuclear receptors involved in cholesterol and bile acid homeostasis (see p. 442).

Extracorporeal shock wave lithotripsy

A shock wave can be directed either radiologically or by ultrasound on to gall bladder stones. This technique was highly successful but only in a restricted patient population. The cystic duct requires patency for stone fragments to pass. Recurrence rates are high but may be reduced by the pharmacological approaches discussed above.

The post-cholecystectomy syndrome

This refers to right upper quadrant pain, often biliary in type, which occurs a few months after the cholecystectomy but may be delayed for a number of years. The patients often comment that the pain is identical to that for which the original operation was carried out. In many cases, this syndrome is related to a functional large bowel disorder with colonic spasm at the hepatic flexure (hepatic flexure syndrome). It may be speculated that a functional gut disorder may have been responsible for the original pain that led to the cholecystectomy. In a small proportion of patients, the pain is the result of a retained common bile duct stone; in a further subsection of patients, sphincter of Oddi dysfunction is a potential cause.

Sphincter of Oddi dysfunction (SOD)

This is a clinical syndrome of biliary or pancreatic pain and is caused by either:

- sphincter of Oddi stenosis, e.g. following prior instrumentation or passage of stones
- sphincter of Oddi hypertension.

A full history of the type of pain, as well as an assessment of serum liver biochemistry and amylase during, and between, episodes of pain is performed.

Biliary SOD

In ***type I*** disease, patients have biliary-type pain with *both* raised serum bilirubin, alkaline phosphatase or aminotransferases during episodes *and* a distended common bile duct on imaging.

In ***type II*** disease, patients have biliary-type pain and *either* abnormal liver biochemistry during episodes *or* a distended common bile duct. In those with suspected type II SOD, sphincter of Oddi manometric studies can confirm the diagnosis and inform the decision as to whether to perform endoscopic sphincterotomy.

In ***type III*** disease, there is recurrent biliary-type pain but no abnormality in the liver biochemistry and a normal-calibre common bile duct.

Management is as follows:

- Type I SOD usually responds to endoscopic sphincterotomy.
- Type II SOD with demonstrable sphincter hypertension usually responds to endoscopic sphincterotomy.
- Type III SOD does not respond to endoscopic sphincterotomy and therefore this should not be performed.

Pancreatic SOD

In ***type I*** disease, patients have recurrent pancreatic pain, a raised serum amylase and a dilated pancreatic duct.

In ***type II*** disease, patients have recurrent pancreatic pain with *either* transient hyperamylasaemia *or* a dilated pancreatic duct.

In ***type III*** disease, patients have pain but neither an elevated amylase nor a dilated pancreatic duct.

Management is as follows:

- Types I and II SOD may respond to endoscopic sphincterotomy.
- Type III SOD with pain only does not respond to endoscopic sphincterotomy.

Common bile duct stones

The classical features of common bile duct (CBD) stones are biliary colic, fever and jaundice (acute cholangitis). This triad is present only in a minority of patients. Abdominal pain is the most common symptom and has the typical features of biliary colic (see above). Jaundice is a variable accompaniment and is almost always preceded by abdominal pain. A patient with bile duct stones may experience sequential episodes of pain, only some of which are accompanied by jaundice. In contrast to malignant bile duct obstruction, the level of jaundice associated with CBD stones characteristically tends to fluctuate. In the elderly or immunocompromised patient, cholangitis may present with very non-specific symptoms, and only associated abnormal liver biochemistry may point to the diagnosis.

Fever is present only in a minority of cases but indicates biliary sepsis and sometimes associated septicaemia. The presence of such biliary sepsis is a significant adverse prognostic factor.

A minority of patients with bile duct stones are discovered incidentally during imaging for gall bladder disease or other intra-abdominal pathology. Some 15% of patients undergoing cholecystectomy will have stones within the bile duct that are detected only at the time of operative cholangiography. The frequency of asymptomatic bile duct stones resulting in complications is not well documented. It is likely that many such stones will pass into the duodenum without causing symptoms. However, the potential for serious complication is well recognized; in most circumstances, incidentally identified bile duct stones are removed (see below).

Examination

If the patient is examined between episodes, there may be no abnormal physical finding. During a symptomatic episode, the patient may be jaundiced with a fever and associated tachycardia. There is tenderness in the right upper quadrant, varying from mild to extremely severe.

More widespread abdominal tenderness extending from the epigastrium to the left upper quadrant, associated with distension, may indicate associated stone-related pancreatitis (see below).

Investigations

Laboratory tests

- ***Full blood count*** is usually normal in the presence of uncomplicated bile duct stones.
- ***An elevated neutrophil count*** and raised inflammatory markers (erythrocyte sedimentation rate (ESR) and CRP) are frequent accompaniments of cholangitis.
- ***The raised serum bilirubin*** tends to be mild and often transient. Very high concentrations of bilirubin (>200 μmol/L) almost always reflect complete bile duct obstruction.
- ***Serum alkaline phosphatase and γ-glutamyl transpeptidase*** are similarly elevated in proportion to the degree of hyperbilirubinaemia.
- ***Aminotransferase levels*** are usually mildly elevated, but with complete bile duct obstruction there may be very marked rises to 10–15 times the normal value. The alanine aminotransferase is characteristically higher than the aspartate aminotransferase. These high levels may lead to an initial misdiagnosis of a hepatitic process.
- ***Serum amylase levels*** are often mildly elevated in the presence of bile duct obstruction but are markedly so if stone-related pancreatitis has occurred.
- ***Prothrombin time*** may be prolonged if bile duct obstruction has occurred and is sustained over several days; this reflects decreased absorption of vitamin K.

Imaging

- ***Transabdominal ultrasound*** is the initial imaging technique of choice. ***Bile duct obstruction*** is characterized by dilatation of intrahepatic biliary radicles, which are usually readily detected by the ultrasound scan. It may, however, not be possible to identify the cause of obstruction. Stones situated in the distal CBD are poorly visualized by transabdominal ultrasound and up to 50% are missed. The detection of stones within the gall bladder is poorly predictive of the cause of bile duct obstruction. Asymptomatic gallstones are common (up to 15%) in patients who are 65 years and older. Conversely, in 5–10% of patients with bile duct stones, no calculi can be seen within the gall bladder.
- ***Magnetic resonance cholangiography*** (***MRC***) delineates the fluid column within the biliary tree and is a sensitive technique for the detection of CBD stones in the presence of a dilated duct. The technique may be less accurate in the absence of duct dilatation (see the role of endoscopic ultrasound, below) ***(Fig. 15.5)***.
- ***CT scanning*** is an alternative way to detect bile duct dilatation. Opaque stones are more readily identifiable within the bile duct than radiolucent cholesterol stones. CT scanning also provides a means of excluding other causes of bile duct obstruction, such as carcinoma of the head of the pancreas.
- ***Endoscopic ultrasound scanning (Fig. 15.6)*** has enabled high-resolution imaging of the CBD, gall bladder and pancreas, although, unlike the preceding imaging techniques, it is an invasive procedure. The endoscopic ultrasound probe in the duodenum is in close proximity to the distal CBD and hence can identify the majority of stones at this level. This technique is particularly useful for identifying small calculi (microcalculi) in a non-dilated common bile duct.
- ***Endoscopic retrograde cholangiography***. In experienced hands, visualization of the CBD will be successful in 98% of cases, providing good documentation of bile duct stones ***(Figs 15.5*** and ***15.7***). However, small stones can still be missed. Endoscopic retrograde cholangiography (ERC) is an invasive procedure with recognized risks. In almost all circumstances, this is a therapeutic tool used to remove the stones that have been identified by the less invasive investigations described above.

Differential diagnosis

Cholangitis may occur independently of gallstones in any condition associated with impaired biliary drainage. It is commonly linked with primary abnormalities of the biliary tree, such as sclerosing cholangitis and Caroli syndrome (a congenital disorder leading to ectasia/dilatation of the intrahepatic bile ducts). Cholangitis may also complicate post-traumatic or surgery-associated bile duct strictures. It is unusual in malignant bile duct obstruction unless there has been prior endoscopic or surgical intervention. Jaundice may also be a feature of acute cholecystitis in the absence of bile duct stones. A stone impacted in the neck of the gall bladder (Hartmann's pouch) or the cystic duct itself may compress and obstruct the bile duct (Mirizzi syndrome). CBD stones may produce pain, but in the absence of jaundice, the differential diagnosis is that of biliary colic (see above).

Management

Acute cholangitis has a high morbidity and mortality, particularly in the elderly or those with serious co-morbidity. Successful management depends on intravenous antibiotics (as for acute cholecystitis) and urgent bile duct drainage. In most circumstances, the latter is achieved by the endoscopic retrograde approach (ERC, see above). Access to the bile duct is achieved by sphincterotomy, and

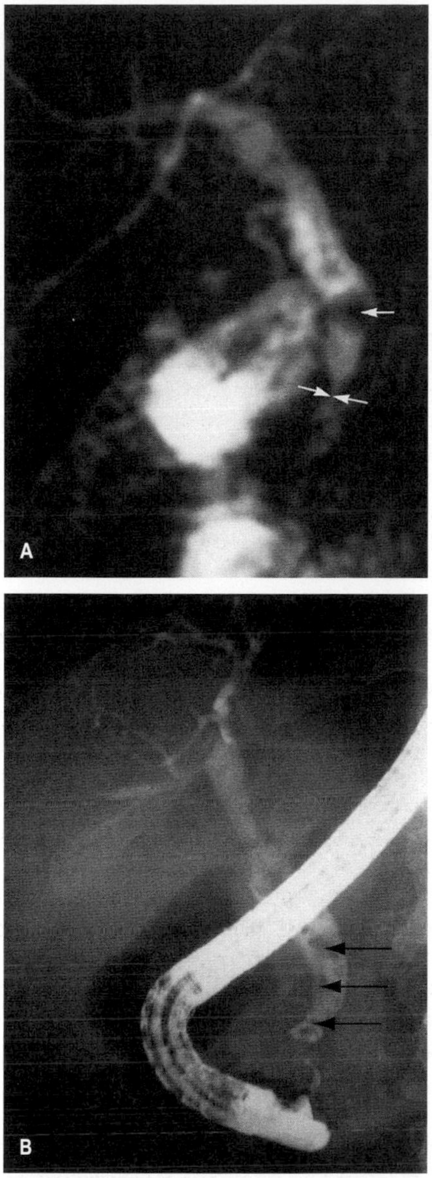

Figure 15.5 **A patient presenting with abdominal pain and jaundice. A. Magnetic resonance cholangiogram (MRC)** shows evidence of a distal common bile duct stricture (bottom arrows) with a stone in the bile duct proximal to this (top arrow). **B. An endoscopic retrograde cholangiopancreatogram (ERCP)** in the same patient confirms the details identified in the MRC scan. The stones (arrowed) were removed at the time of the ERCP after initial dilatation of the stricture.

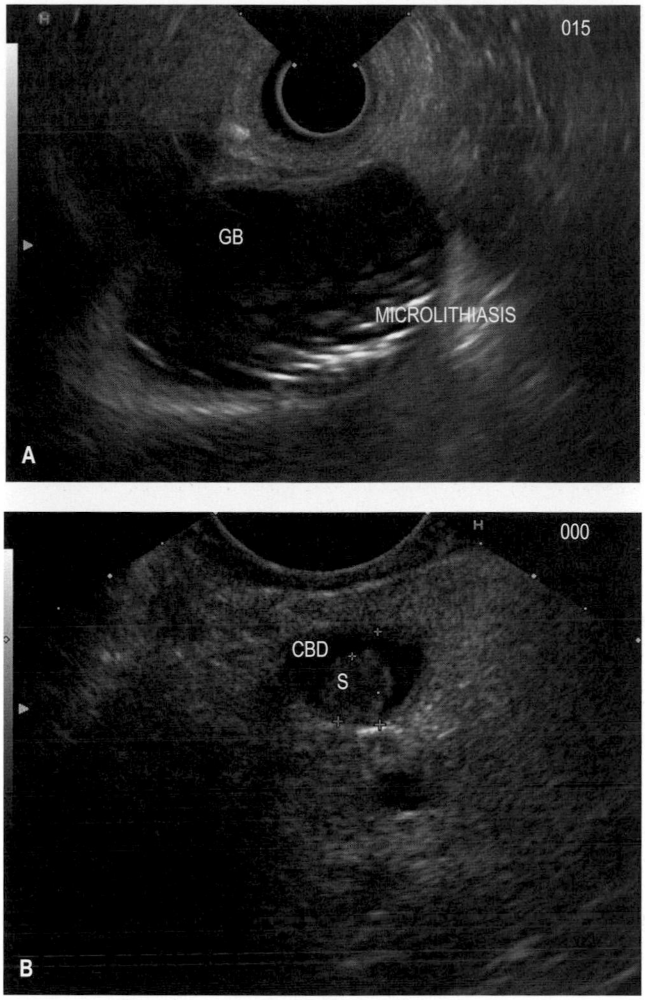

Figure 15.6 **An endoscopic ultrasound scan with the probe in the first part of the duodenum. A.** The gall bladder (GB) and multiple small, echo-poor stones within (microlithiasis). The patient had presented with recurrent episodes of unexplained abdominal pain. **B.** The common bile duct (CBD) and a stone (S) clearly identified within the lumen.

thereafter the stones can be removed by either balloon or basket catheters. In the severely ill patient, a piece of plastic tubing (termed a stent) can be inserted into the bile duct to maintain bile drainage without the need to remove the stones, hence minimizing the time required to complete the procedure. The residual stones can then be cleared and the stent removed endoscopically when the patient has recovered from the acute episode. If endoscopic drainage is not available or is prevented by an inability to access the second part of the duodenum, then a radiologically placed percutaneous biliary drain represents an alternative management option. Surgical drainage during an acute cholangitic episode has been associated with a high mortality and has been replaced by the endoscopic or percutaneous approach.

Urgent endoscopic bile duct clearance is also indicated in some patients with acute gallstone pancreatitis but only when this coexists with persisting bile duct obstruction (see below). Patients who have retained CBD stones after a previous cholecystectomy are also optimally managed by endoscopic clearance.

Patients shown to have CBD stones as well as gall bladder stones may be treated using different approaches:

- ***At the time of laparoscopic cholecystectomy***, which can also include exploration of the CBD via the cystic duct or via direct choledochotomy. By using these techniques, the surgeon can extract stones from the CBD. The skills and time required for bile duct exploration are considerably greater than those for laparoscopic cholecystectomy alone. This single-procedure approach minimizes the length of hospital admission. Concerns around an increased risk of bile duct injury with bile duct exploration have not been confirmed in controlled studies.

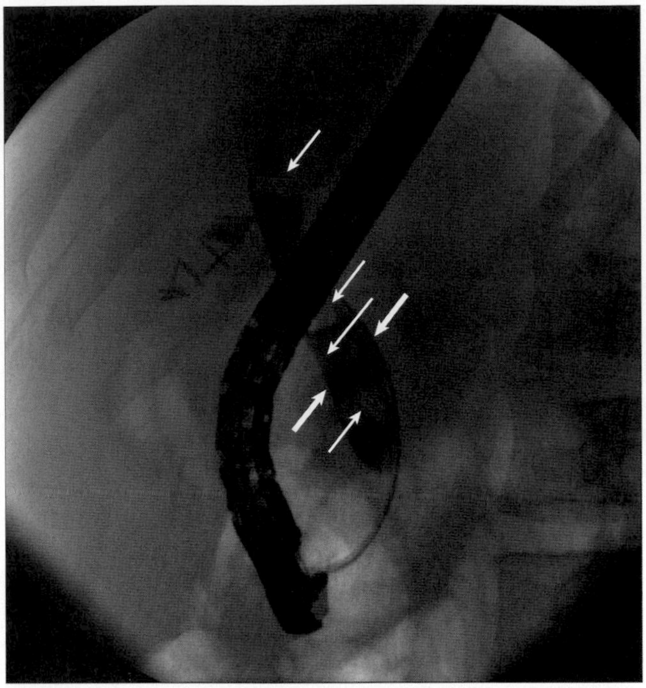

Figure 15.7 An endoscopic retrograde cholangiopancreatogram (ERCP) carried out in a patient with abdominal pain, fluctuating jaundice and fever. The cholangiogram shows a dilated common bile duct (between thick arrows) and multiple stones within (arrows). These stones were removed at the time of ERCP by means of balloon and basket retrieval. Note the multiple clips to the left of the upper bile duct, that were placed at a prior laparoscopic cholecystectomy.

- ***Independently timed endoscopic approach***, either immediately before or after the cholecystectomy. Removal of CBD stones by this method is preferred in the UK. Large bile duct stones (>10 mm) may present a significant challenge to endoscopic removal. Mechanical lithotripsy facilitates stone fragmentation and removal into the duodenum. Extracorporeal shock wave stone fragmentation has been used but is not widely available. The recent increased availability of endoscopic cholangioscopy (direct visualization of the bile duct) has facilitated intraductal shock wave lithotripsy, utilizing electrohydraulic or laser probes.
- ***A combined laparoscopic and endoscopic approach***, in which an ERC and duct clearance are carried out under the same anaesthetic used for the laparoscopic cholecystectomy. This approach is currently receiving support, based on a shortened hospital stay and the use of only one anaesthetic.

Complications of gallstones

- Acute cholecystitis and acute cholangitis have been discussed (see p. 492).
- Gallstone-related pancreatitis is discussed on pages 504–505.
- Gallstones can occasionally erode through the wall of the gall bladder into the intestine, giving rise to a biliary enteric fistula. Passage of a gallstone through to the small bowel can give rise to an ileus or true obstruction.
- There is little evidence that gallstones are associated with an increased risk of adenocarcinoma of the gall bladder (see pp. 497–498).

MISCELLANEOUS CONDITIONS OF THE BILIARY TRACT

Gall bladder

There are a number of non-calculous conditions of the gall bladder, some of which have been associated with symptoms.

Acalculous cholecystitis

Almost 10% of gall bladders removed for biliary symptoms are shown to have chronic inflammation within the wall but an absence of gallstones. Such cases are described as acalculous cholecystitis. In many instances, the gall bladder inflammation is minor and of doubtful significance. In some cases, chemical inflammation of the gall bladder may occur from reflux of pancreatic enzymes back into the biliary tree, usually through the common channel at the ampulla of Vater. Bacterial and viral infections of the gall bladder have been recognized as a cause of acalculous cholecystitis. The decision to carry out cholecystectomy in the absence of defined gall bladder stones should be guided by the specific features of the history and by evidence of a diseased gall bladder wall on ultrasound scanning.

A distinct subtype of acalculous cholecystitis is characterized by severe necroinflammation of the gall bladder and generally occurs in an elderly and already critically ill group of patients, usually after major trauma or surgery. Around 20% of these patients develop inflammatory masses with subsequent cholestasis and jaundice; gall bladder perforation is a frequent complication. Morbidity and mortality are very high, and aggressive management of sepsis with antibiotics and cholecystostomy (percutaneous gall bladder drainage) or urgent cholecystectomy is required.

Cholesterolosis of the gall bladder

In cholesterolosis, cholesterol and other lipids are deposited in macrophages within the lamina propria of the gall bladder wall. These may be diffusely situated, giving a granular appearance to the gall bladder wall, or on occasion may be more discrete, giving a polypoid appearance (see below). Cholesterolosis of the gall bladder may coexist with gallstones but also occurs independently. Some degree of gall bladder cholesterolosis is found in up to 26% of laparoscopic cholecystectomy specimens, and as an incidental finding in up to 12% of autopsies in an elderly population. Interestingly, in contrast to cholelithiasis, rates are equal in men and women. It is doubtful whether isolated gall bladder cholesterolosis is a cause of symptoms.

Adenomyomatosis of the gall bladder

Adenomyomatosis is a gall bladder abnormality characterized by hyperplasia of the mucosa, thickening of the muscle wall and multiple intramural diverticula (the so-called 'Rokitansky–Aschoff sinuses').

The condition is usually detected as an incidental finding during investigation for possible gall bladder disease. It has been suggested that this condition is secondary to increased intraluminal gall bladder pressure but this is not proven. Gallstones frequently coexist, particularly when the adenomyomatosis is in a segmental distribution, but there is no evidence to support a direct relationship. It is unlikely that adenomyomatosis alone is a cause of biliary symptoms and it is not considered a pre-malignant state.

Chronic cholecystitis

There are no symptoms or signs that can conclusively be shown to be due to chronic cholecystitis. Symptoms attributed to this condition are vague, such as indigestion, upper abdominal discomfort or distension. There is no doubt that gall bladders studied histologically can show signs of chronic inflammation and, occasionally, a small, shrunken gall bladder is found either radiologically or on ultrasound examination. However, these findings can be seen in asymptomatic people and therefore this clinical diagnosis should not be made. Most patients with chronic right hypochondrial pain suffer from functional bowel disease (see p. 360).

Extrahepatic biliary tract

Primary sclerosing cholangitis

In up to 40% of patients with primary sclerosing cholangitis (PSC; see also pp. 476–477), the clinical course is influenced by a dominant hilar or distal biliary stricture. This is relevant in those patients who do not have established advanced liver involvement, in whom maintaining bile flow may protect the liver from secondary biliary injury. Drainage with a surgical hepaticojejunostomy has been beneficial in some cases, but outcomes of such restricted surgery in PSC are generally inferior to orthotopic liver transplantation. Repeated endoscopic balloon dilatation of the dominant stricture, with or without temporary short-term stenting, has been associated with sustained improvement in jaundice, and even prolonged transplant-free survival. A significant minority of dominant strictures in PSC, particularly those at the hilum, represent development of an associated cholangiocarcinoma (see below). Development of cholangiocarcinoma in this context carries a very poor prognosis and surgical resection is rarely feasible. A benign dominant stricture in a non-cirrhotic patient, with recurrent cholangitis, refractory jaundice and pruritus, may be an indication for orthotopic liver transplantation. Conversely, superadded cholangiocarcinoma is currently an absolute contraindication to liver transplantation in most healthcare systems.

Autoimmune cholangitis

Immunoglobulin (Ig) G4-associated cholangitis is the biliary manifestation of a multisystem fibroinflammatory disorder in which affected organs have a characteristic lymphoplasmacytic infiltrate rich in IgG4-positive cells (see p. 145). The original description of this condition was in the context of autoimmune pancreatitis, and around 70% of these patients have evidence of IgG4 cholangiopathy (see p. 506). However, IgG4 cholangiopathy can exist in the absence of pancreatic involvement.

The large majority of cases are recognized in middle-aged or elderly men. Presentation is varied, depending on the systems involved, but may include abdominal pain and jaundice. Both intra- and extrahepatic biliary strictures may be seen and the findings may be misinterpreted as representing cholangiocarcinoma or PSC. The diagnosis relies on clinical suspicion, confirmation of an elevated serum IgG4 level, a typical lymphocytoplasmic infiltrate on histological examination of involved tissue, and clinical response to glucocorticosteroid treatment. The condition is almost always responsive to steroids but can lead to hepatic failure.

Biliary cysts (choledochal malformation)

Cystic malformations may occur anywhere in the biliary tree, although they are most commonly extrahepatic. The resulting dilatation of the bile duct may be of saccular, diverticular or fusiform configuration. In many cases, there is an associated abnormal pancreatobiliary junction – a congenital malunion where the pancreatic duct drains directly into the common bile duct. The majority of symptomatic cases present in childhood with features of cholangitis, jaundice or a palpable mass. The formation of stones and sludge within the cystic segment may predispose to acute relapsing pancreatitis. In adult life, choledochal cysts may be a differential diagnosis in patients presenting with symptoms suggestive of bile duct stones. Extrahepatic bile duct cysts must be fully resected to avoid recurrent biliary sepsis, as well as reducing the risk (approximately 15%) of subsequent cholangiocarcinoma.

Benign bile duct strictures

Benign strictures are a recognized complication of biliary surgery. They may result from inadvertent direct stapling of the duct, or may be a secondary consequence of ischaemic injury (often in association with a bile duct leak). Strictures may also occur at the level of any bile duct anastomosis, either enteric or duct-to-duct. Biliary stricturing is also a rare complication of major trauma to the right upper quadrant. The inflammation and fibrosis of chronic pancreatitis commonly impinges on the intrapancreatic common bile duct (see below). This can result in cholestasis, jaundice and cholangitis.

In most cases, initial therapy includes endoscopic balloon dilatation of the stricture and temporary bile duct stenting (see below). This may provide definitive management, but in some cases, surgical intervention with hepaticojejunostomy is required.

Haemobilia

Haemobilia describes blood in the biliary tree. This may be a consequence of liver trauma or a complication of liver surgery. Biopsy of the liver and erosion of a gallstone or hepatobiliary tumour into adjacent structures are also well-recognized causes. The end result is a fistula between a hepatic blood vessel and a bile duct.

Haemobilia may be a cause of significant gastrointestinal blood loss and should be suspected when melaena is accompanied by right-sided upper abdominal pain and jaundice, particularly in the context of recent hepatobiliary intervention. However, the bleeding may occur without any overt biliary symptoms. If the diagnosis is suspected, bleeding may be managed by occlusion of the feeding blood vessel by radiological embolization. Some patients will require surgery to control the bleeding point.

TUMOURS OF THE BILIARY TRACT

Gall bladder polyps

Polyps of the gall bladder are a common finding, being seen in approximately 4% of all patients referred for hepatobiliary ultrasonography. The vast majority of these are small (<5 mm) and non-neoplastic; they are inflammatory in origin or composed of cholesterol deposits (see above). Adenomas are the most common benign neoplasm of the gall bladder. Only a proportion of these have a cancerous potential. The only reliable predictor of malignant risk is polyp size (>10 mm). Cholecystectomy is recommended for any polyp of 10 mm in diameter or larger.

Carcinoma of the gall bladder

Adenocarcinoma of the gall bladder represents 1% of all cancers. The mean age of occurrence is the early sixties, with a female-to-male ratio of 3 : 1. Gall bladder stones are often found in association with gall bladder cancer; gallstones have been suggested as an aetiological factor but this relationship remains unproven. Diffuse calcification of the gall bladder (porcelain gall bladder), considered to be the end-stage of chronic cholecystitis, has also been associated with cancer of the gall bladder and is an indication for early cholecystectomy. Adenomatous polyps of the gall bladder in excess of 10 mm in diameter are also recognized as pre-malignant lesions (see above).

Carcinoma of the gall bladder may be detected incidentally at the time of planned cholecystectomy for gallstones; in such circumstances, resection of an early lesion may be curative. Radical surgery with negative resection margins offers the only potential cure. However, early lymphatic spread to the liver and adjacent biliary tract precludes curative resection in more advanced lesions. Palliative chemotherapy treatment may be given, usually with either 5-fluorouracil (5-FU)-based regimes, or gemcitabine (a nucleoside analogue) and cisplatin (a platinum-containing anticancer drug), with some evidence of a modest improvement in survival. A small proportion of cases are sensitive to radiotherapy. However, the generally advanced stage of disease at presentation means that the overall 5-year survival is less than 5%.

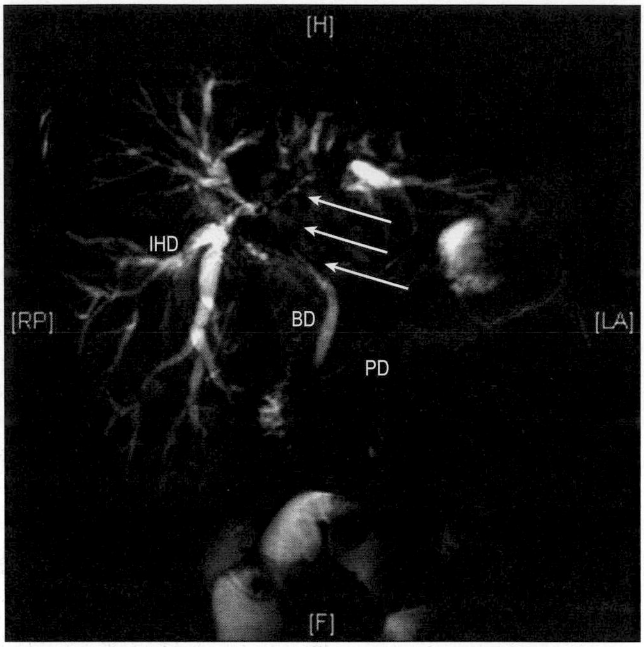

Figure 15.8 Magnetic resonance cholangiopancreatography (MRCP) image of hilar cholangiocarcinoma extending into left main duct. There is a normal-calibre distal bile duct (BD) and pancreatic duct (PD). The common hepatic duct and left main duct are strictured (arrowed). There is marked intrahepatic duct (IHD) dilatation.

Cholangiocarcinoma (see also pp. 485–486)

Cancers of the biliary tree are classified as intrahepatic (above the hilum of the liver) or extrahepatic (involving the hilum or bile duct distal to the hilum). The latter are classified either on the TMN classification or on the site of the lesion (Bismuth Corlette classification of biliary strictures). These malignancies represent approximately 1% of all cancers. A number of associations have been identified, such as that with choledochal malformation (see above) and with primary sclerosing cholangitis (see pp. 476–477). Chronic infection of the biliary tree with parasitic liver flukes, particularly *Opisthorchis viverrini* or *Clonorchis sinensis*, has also been strongly implicated in areas where they are endemic. Extrahepatic bile duct malignancy usually presents with jaundice and may be confirmed on imaging tests, initially ultrasound and thereafter CT and, in particular, magnetic resonance cholangiopancreatography (MRCP; ***Fig. 15.8***). Typical findings are of a bile duct stricture with proximal biliary dilatation, with or without a visible mass. Histopathological diagnosis often proves difficult because the malignant cells are few in number and contained within a dense stroma. Endoscopically obtained cytology specimens have only 30% sensitivity. This yield can be enhanced by using additional endoscopic sampling techniques, such as transpapillary biopsy, and analytical enhancements, such as fluorescent *in situ* hybridization and digital image analysis. The recent application of direct endoscopic cholangioscopy has enabled direct visualization of biliary lesions and targeted biopsy.

Cholangiocarcinoma is often detected at a late stage and is characterized by early perineural, vascular and lymphatic spread. In a minority of cases, complete surgical resection is feasible, offering the only chance of cure. Cholangiocarcinoma of the common bile duct may be amenable to a limited bile duct resection. Very distal lesions require a pancreatoduodenectomy (Whipple procedure), and perihilar lesions frequently require partial hepatic resection in addition to biliary resection. In some international centres, extensive neoadjuvant chemoradiation therapy, followed by liver transplantation, has been used to cure localized hilar cholangiocarcinoma. Results from this emerging technique show promise, but cholangiocarcinoma remains an absolute contraindication to liver transplantation in most healthcare systems worldwide due to early disease recurrence.

The majority of patients with cholangiocarcinoma are treated palliatively with biliary decompression (see below) and gemcitabine- and cisplatin-based chemotherapy regimes.

Secondary malignant involvement of the biliary tree

Carcinoma of the head of the pancreas frequently presents with common bile duct obstruction and jaundice. Metastases to the bile duct from distant cancers are uncommon. Melanoma is the most frequent neoplasm to do so. Infiltration of the bile duct is not uncommon in disseminated lymphoma. Other carcinomas that may give rise to bile duct metastases, in order of frequency, are those arising in the lung, breast and colon, as well as those from the pancreas (metastatic as compared to direct infiltration).

Management

Palliation of malignant bile duct obstruction

All patients must be fully staged for operability using the imaging techniques described above. However, in the greater proportion of patients, the treatment is palliative. Relief of bile duct obstruction has been shown to improve quality of life considerably and, with pain control, is the mainstay of effective palliation. Effective biliary decompression is also critical in jaundiced patients who wish to proceed with palliative chemotherapy. In recent years, endoscopic techniques have allowed the insertion of stents into the biliary tree to re-establish bile flow. The initial use of plastic stents has largely been replaced by self-expanding metal stents that have considerably longer periods of patency ***(Fig. 15.9)***. In the small proportion of patients in whom bile duct drainage is not possible endoscopically, the percutaneous route offers an alternative method of stent placement under radiological control.

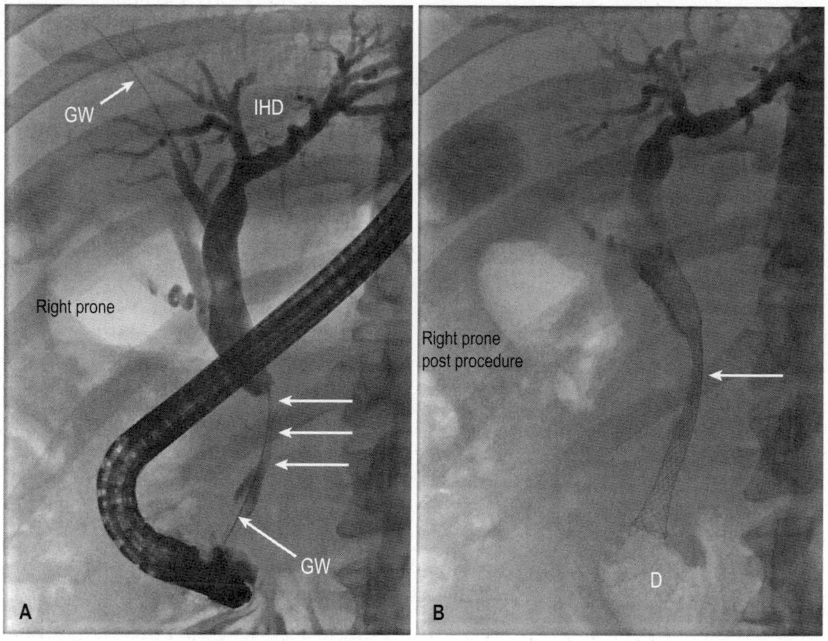

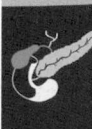

Figure 15.9 An ERCP in a patient presenting with painless jaundice. A. There is a ***tight stricture in the mid-common bile duct*** extending proximally over 4 cm (extent defined by arrows). The intrahepatic ducts (IHD) proximally are dilated. A guidewire (GW) has been place endoscopically across the stricture. **B.** A ***self-expanding metal stent*** has been placed across the stricture and released. The stent is compressed at the level of the stricture (arrow) but will open fully over 24 h. The contrast in the intrahepatic ducts has largely drained through the stent. The distal margin of the stent is in the duodenum (D).

Further reading

Khan SA, Davidson BR, Goldin RD et al. Guidelines for the diagnosis and treatment of cholangiocarcinoma: an update. *Gut* 2012; 61:1657–1669.
Razumilava N, Gores GJ. Cholangiocarcinoma. *Lancet* 2014; 383:2168–2179.

THE PANCREAS

Anatomy and function

Structure

The pancreas extends retroperitoneally across the posterior abdominal wall from the second part of the duodenum to the spleen. Anatomically, the pancreas is divided into a head, which rests within the concavity of the duodenum; a body, lying behind the base of the stomach; and a tail, which ends abutting the spleen. The neck of the pancreas lies between the body and head, and is in front of the superior mesenteric artery and vein. The head of the pancreas surrounds these two vessels. An uncinate process emerges from the lower part of the head, lying behind the superior mesenteric artery. The pancreas consists of exocrine and endocrine cells. The exocrine pancreas comprises 98% of the parenchyma.

The functional unit of the exocrine pancreas is composed of an acinus and its draining ductule. A ductule from the acinus drains into interlobular (intercalated) ducts, which, in turn, drain into the main pancreatic ductal system. The main pancreatic duct itself joins the common bile duct to enter the duodenum as a short single duct at the ampulla of Vater.

The endocrine component is scattered throughout the gland in the form of pancreatic islets (of Langerhans).

Exocrine function

The pancreatic acinar cells are responsible for the production of digestive enzymes. These include amylase, lipase, colipase, phospholipase and the proteases (trypsinogen and chymotrypsinogen). These enzymes are stored within the acinar cells in secretory granules and are released by exocytosis **(Fig. 15.10)**. The enzymes released by the acinar cells are transported into the duodenum by a high-volume pancreatic secretion, the majority of which is produced by the ductal cells. This fluid has a high concentration of bicarbonate, which neutralizes the gastric acid that has emptied into the duodenum. The neutralization of gastric acid is essential to facilitate pancreatic enzyme activity, which is pH-dependent (requiring a neutral pH).

After ingestion of a meal, pancreatic exocrine secretion is regulated by cephalic, gastric and intestinal stimuli. The cephalic phase is stimulated by behavioural cues related to the sight, smell and taste of food. The input from these sensory stimuli is integrated in the central nervous system at the dorsal vagal complex, and the output is transmitted to the exocrine pancreas via the vagus nerve. The gastric phase of pancreatic secretion results from the effects of the meal in the stomach. The major stimulus of pancreatic secretion in the gastric phase is gastric distension, which causes secretion of an enzyme-rich fluid with little secretion of water and bicarbonate. This phase is also under vagal control. The intestinal phase of pancreatic secretion starts when protein, fat and gastric acid from the stomach enters the duodenum and continues for the duration of the digestive period. It is mediated by both hormones and enteropancreatic vagovagal reflexes. Feedback regulatory events eventually terminate pancreatic secretion.

- ***Cholecystokinin*** (***CCK***) plays a major role in meal-stimulated digestive enzyme secretion during the intestinal phase of pancreatic secretion. The hormone is produced in *specialized gut endocrine cells (I cells)* of the mucosa of the small intestine and is secreted in response to intraluminal food. There are no CCK receptors in pancreatic cells of humans, and CCK acts via receptors on vagal afferent fibres to stimulate pancreatic secretion.

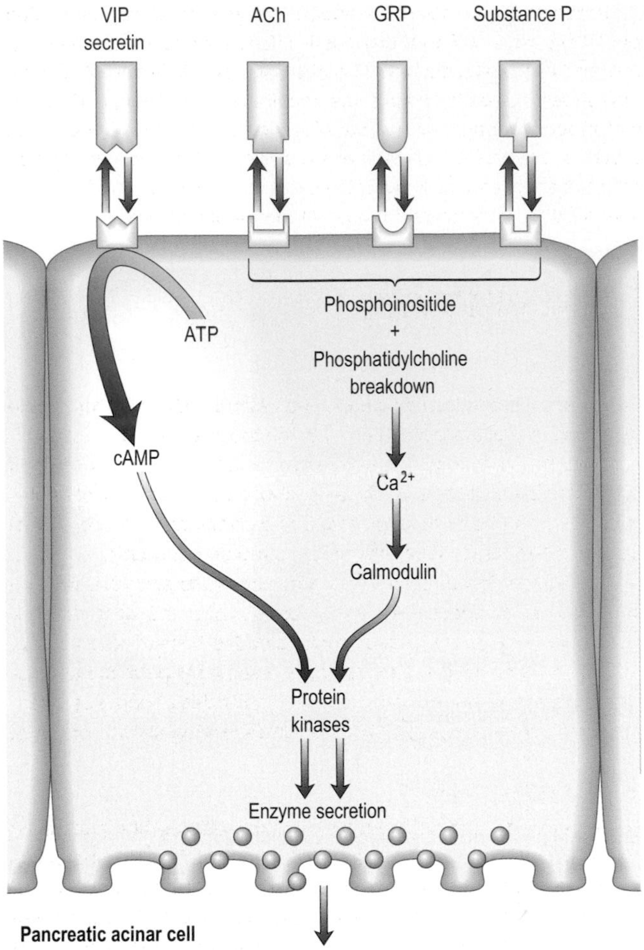

Figure 15.10 Stimulation of digestive enzyme secretion from the acinar cell. G-protein-coupled receptors have been identified for vasoactive intestinal peptide (VIP), secretin, acetylcholine (ACh), gastrin-releasing polypeptide (GRP) and substance P. There are no cholecystokinin (CCK) receptors in humans. ATP, adenosine triphosphate; cAMP, cyclic adenosine monophosphate.

- ***Secretin*** is also released from *specialized enteroendocrine cells* of the small intestine during a meal and, in particular, during duodenal acidification. Secretin has a direct effect on the pancreatic acinar cells, as well as the ductal cells. There is also a vagal-mediated secretory response. Secretin action is mediated via G-coupled receptors and calcium-mediated enzyme release. Secretin results in a bicarbonate-rich pancreatic secretion.

The efficiency of the digestive phase of pancreatic secretion requires a negative feedback mechanism to bring the process to a close. Completion of the postprandial secretory phase involves both neural and hormonal control.

- ***Pancreatic polypeptide*** is released from the *islet cells of the pancreas* in response to a meal and has an inhibitory effect on acinar enzyme secretion, via both a local effect and central receptors.
- ***Somatostatin***, present within the pancreas, stomach and central nervous system, also has an inhibitory effect. It is released in response to food and its effect is mediated by both direct pancreatic acinar inhibition and a central nervous system inhibitory component.
- ***Peptide YY*** (***PYY***), contained in *endocrine cells of the distal small intestine* is released by nutrients within the ileum and inhibits pancreatic secretion by acting on the acinar cells themselves, as well as centrally via the inhibitory regulation of vagal nerve.

There is also evidence that proteases within the duodenal lumen also have a negative feedback on acinar secretion. The gut-related peptides, leptin and ghrelin, as well as influencing appetite behaviour, are also regulatory factors in the exocrine function of the pancreas. This effect is believed to occur via hypothalamic centres.

The endocrine pancreas

This consists of hormone-producing cells arranged in nests or islets (islets of Langerhans). The hormones produced are secreted directly into the circulation and there is no access to the pancreatic ductular system. There are ***five main types of islet cell*** corresponding to different secretory components:

- The beta cells are the most common and are responsible for insulin production.
- The alpha cells produce glucagon.
- The D cells produce somatostatin.
- PP cells produce pancreatic polypeptide.
- Enterochromaffin cells produce serotonin.

A number of other hormones have been identified within the endocrine pancreas, including gastrin-releasing peptide, neuropeptide Y and galanin. These are believed to be neurotransmitters active in the neuro-gastrointestinal axis.

Investigations

Assessment of exocrine function

The assessment of pancreatic exocrine function is used in the investigation of patients with possible chronic pancreatic disease. Clinically evident fat malabsorption does not occur until there has been an 85–90% reduction in pancreatic lipase and is therefore a very late manifestation of pancreatic disease.

Direct tests of pancreatic function

These tests rely on the analysis of a duodenal aspirate following pancreatic stimulation.

The original test involved the oral administration of a specified meal (Lundh meal). Pancreatic stimulation is now achieved by intravenous secretin and cholecystokinin.

The aspirate is assessed for pancreatic enzymes and bicarbonate production. The procedure is time-consuming and requires a meticulous technique. There is good correlation with moderate to severe pancreatic function loss, but not with mild damage. These tests are not widely available.

The measurement of peak bicarbonate secretion following secretin stimulation is also performed using an endoscopic technique for aspirate collection. This method offers similar levels of predictive accuracy as seen with the secretin–cholecystokinin stimulation test but does require a 30-min endoscopic intubation.

Non-invasive indirect tests of pancreatic function

Faecal tests

- ***Faecal elastase*** is an enzyme produced in the pancreas; as it is not degraded in the intestine, it has high concentrations within the faeces. Diminished levels are seen in moderate and severe pancreatic insufficiency. This has replaced the faecal chymotrypsin test.
- ***Faecal fat estimation*** (rarely performed).

Oral pancreatic function tests

- ***N-benzoyl-L-tyrosyl-p-aminobenzoic acid*** (basis of the PABA test) and ***fluorescein dilaurate*** are oral compounds utilized in pancreatic function tests. Both are digested by pancreatic enzymes, releasing substrates that are excreted and measured in the urine. Both tests are commercially available and have good sensitivity in moderate to severe pancreatic exocrine failure.

Clinical application of pancreatic function tests

While the invasive duodenal aspiration tests represent the most sensitive and specific means of assessing pancreatic function, these are very rarely used outside specialized centres. The non-invasive tests are widely available but are only highly sensitive in the detection of severe pancreatic insufficiency. The faecal elastase test (in a commercially available form) provides similar sensitivity and specificity, and is the test of choice as a screening tool for pancreatic insufficiency.

Pancreatic imaging

Imaging (see pp. 445–447) has a pivotal role in the investigation and management of pancreatic disease, which covers the spectrum of acute, chronic and malignant conditions.

- ***A plain abdominal radiograph*** may show the calcification associated with chronic pancreatitis, particularly when alcohol is the aetiology.
- ***Transabdominal ultrasound*** of the pancreas usually offers reasonable views of the pancreas; it is a useful screening investigation for inflammation or neoplasia, and is reasonably sensitive for detection of gallstone disease in a patient with pancreatitis. Views may be limited by overlying bowel gas, and ultrasound should not be relied on in the exclusion of pancreatic neoplasia, if clinical suspicion exists.
- ***CT scan*** with contrast enhancement and following a specific pancreatic protocol remains the 'gold standard' imaging technique for the investigation of pancreatic disease.
- ***MRI scanning*** represents an alternative to CT. MRCP gives clear definition of the pancreatic duct, as well as the biliary tree. Gallstones (including microcalculi) may also be identified in the biliary tree using MRI/MRCP.
- ***Endoscopic ultrasound*** is very useful for identifying distal common bile duct stones, which may be the aetiology of an episode of acute pancreatitis. Endoscopic ultrasound can identify the early changes of chronic pancreatitis before these are evident with other imaging methods. There is also an increasing role for this technique to stage the operability of pancreatic adenocarcinoma, particularly with respect to vascular invasion. Endoscopic ultrasound is now considered the imaging technique of choice for investigating cystic lesions of the pancreas (see below). The technique allows fine-needle aspiration and histological sampling, as well as the therapeutic option of cyst drainage. Endoscopic ultrasound is a sensitive means of detecting small pancreatic tumours, particularly those of neuroendocrine origin.
- ***Endoscopic retrograde cholangiopancreatography*** (***ERCP***) is an invasive procedure and whilst having a good safety profile, is associated with a small risk of serious adverse events: in particular, the precipitation of acute pancreatitis. The availability of MRCP and endoscopic ultrasound has provided alternative means of defining pancreatic pathology. ERCP has an increasing therapeutic role in pancreatic disease (see below).

In summary, an initial transabdominal ultrasound, supplemented by CT, provides sufficient diagnostic information for most inflammatory and neoplastic conditions of the pancreas. MRI and MRCP are now widely available and provide additional information, particularly with respect to pancreatic ductular and biliary anatomy. Endoscopic ultrasound is a useful, albeit more invasive, tool for the investigation of both benign and malignant disease of the pancreas, and facilitates fine-needle aspiration and biopsy of targetable lesions.

PANCREATITIS

Classification

Pancreatitis is divided into ***acute*** and ***chronic***. By definition, acute pancreatitis is a process that occurs on the background of a previously normal pancreas and can return to normal after resolution of the episode. Nevertheless, acute alcoholic pancreatitis occurs only in chronic misuse of alcohol. In chronic pancreatitis, there is continuing inflammation with irreversible structural changes.

In practice, the differentiation between acute and chronic pancreatitis may be difficult. Any of the causes of acute pancreatitis, if untreated, may result in recurrent episodes, classified as ***acute relapsing pancreatitis*** and eventually resulting in permanent structural changes. In other cases, recurrent episodes of acute pancreatitis may represent exacerbations of an underlying chronic process.

Acute pancreatitis

Acute pancreatitis is a syndrome of inflammation of the pancreatic gland initiated by any acute injury. The causes of acute pancreatitis are listed in ***Box 15.2***. In the Western world, gallstones and alcohol account for the vast majority of episodes. Alcohol also causes chronic pancreatitis (see below). The severity of the pancreatitis may range from mild and self-limiting to extremely severe, with extensive pancreatic and peripancreatic necrosis, as well as haemorrhage. In the most severe form (approximately 10% of cases), the mortality is between 40% and 80%.

Box 15.2 Causes of acute pancreatitis

Common	Less common
Gallstones Alcohol Iatrogenic (post-ERCP, surgery) Idiopathic (<10%)	Trauma Infections, e.g. mumps, coxsackie B, HIV, adenovirus Pancreatic tumours Hereditary Congenital pancreatic abnormalities, e.g. pancreas divisum Metabolic, e.g. hypercalcaemia, hypertriglyceridaemia Venom, e.g. scorpion stings, spider Sphincter of Oddi dysfunction (see p. 493) Miscellaneous Drugs (see below)
Drugs	
Azathioprine/mercaptopurine	Aminosalicylates
Didanosine	Corticosteroids
Oestrogens	Metronidazole
Antibiotics, e.g. tetracycline	ACE inhibitors
Valproic acid	
Furosemide	
Sulphonamides	

ACE, angiotensin-converting enzyme; ERCP, endoscopic retrograde cholangiopancreatography.

Pathogenesis

This is still not completely understood. A precipitating event, such as gallstones or alcohol, is thought to induce the acute episode.

Gallstone pancreatitis

The inducing effect is obstruction to pancreatic drainage at the ampulla by a stone or associated oedema. In this pathological situation, trypsinogen is cleaved (by cathepsin B) to trypsin, and trypsin degradation by chymotrypsin C is impaired and quickly overwhelmed. Intracellular calcium also increases and may also cause early activation of trypsinogen with upregulation of nuclear factor kappa B, leading to extensive acinar cell damage.

Alcohol-induced pancreatitis

There is also evidence that alcohol interferes with calcium homeostasis in pancreatic acinar cells. In addition, activation of pancreatic stellate cells by acetaldehyde occurs, with production of collagen and then matrix proteins.

Whatever the nature of the initiating insult, the pancreatic inflammatory response is secondary to the premature and exaggerated activation of digestive enzymes, principally trypsin, within the pancreas itself. In severe cases, the subsequent cascade of autodigestion, microvascular injury, systemic inflammatory response and bacterial translocation can result in a devastating outcome.

Clinical features

Acute pancreatitis is a differential diagnosis in any patient with upper abdominal pain. The pain usually begins in the epigastrium, accompanied by nausea and vomiting. As inflammation spreads throughout the peritoneal cavity, the pain becomes more intense. Involvement of the retroperitoneum frequently leads to back pain.

The patient may give a history of previous similar episodes or be known to have gallstones. An attack may follow an alcoholic binge. However, in many cases, there are no obvious aetiological factors.

Physical examination at the time of presentation may show little more than a patient in pain with some upper abdominal tenderness but no systemic abnormalities. In severe disease, the patient has a tachycardia and hypotension, and is oliguric. Abdominal examination may show widespread tenderness with guarding, as well as reduced or absent bowel sounds. Specific clinical signs that support a diagnosis of severe necrotizing pancreatitis include periumbilical (*Cullen's sign*) and flank bruising (*Grey Turner's sign*). In patients with gallstone aetiology, the clinical picture may also include the features of jaundice or cholangitis.

Diagnosis

Blood tests

- ***Serum amylase*** is an extremely sensitive test if it is three times the upper limit of normal when measured within 24h of the onset of pain. A number of other conditions may occasionally cause a very elevated amylase ***(Box 15.3)***. Amylase levels gradually fall back towards normal over the next 3–5 days. With a late presentation, the serum amylase level may give a false-negative result.
- ***Urinary amylase*** levels may be diagnostic, as these remain elevated over a longer period of time.
- ***Serum lipase*** levels are also raised in acute pancreatitis and these remain elevated for a longer period of time than amylase levels. However, overall, the accuracy of serum lipase is not significantly greater than that of amylase and it is technically more difficult to measure.
- ***CRP level*** is useful in assessing disease severity and prognosis.
- ***Other baseline investigations*** include a full blood count, urea and electrolytes, blood glucose, liver biochemistry, plasma calcium and arterial blood gases. These are documented at presentation and then repeated at 24 and 48h, providing a basis for assessing the severity of an attack (see below).

> **Box 15.3 Elevation of serum amylase unrelated to pancreatitis**
>
> **Leakage of upper gastrointestinal contents into the peritoneum**
> - Upper gastrointestinal perforation
> - Biliary peritonitis
> - Intestinal infarction
>
> **Inherited abnormalities of amylase**
> - Macroamylasaemia

Radiology

- An erect ***chest X-ray*** is mandatory to exclude gastroduodenal perforation, which also raises the serum amylase ***(Box 15.3)***. A supine abdominal film may show gallstones or pancreatic calcification.
- An ***abdominal ultrasound scan*** is used as a screening test to identify a possible biliary (gallstone) cause of pancreatitis. Gallstones are difficult to detect in the distal common bile duct but dilated intrahepatic ducts may be present in the presence of bile duct obstruction. Stones within the gall bladder are not sufficient to justify a diagnosis of gallstone-related pancreatitis. The ultrasound may also demonstrate pancreatic swelling and necrosis, as well as peripancreatic fluid collections if present. In severe pancreatitis, the pancreas may be difficult to visualize because of gas-filled loops of bowel.
- ***Contrast-enhanced CT scanning*** is essential in all but the mildest attacks of pancreatitis. It should be performed after 72h to assess the extent of pancreatic necrosis. CT provides very valuable prognostic information. Later, repeated CT scans can detect other complications, including fluid collections, abscess formation and pseudocyst development ***(Fig. 15.11)***.
- ***MRI (MRCP***) assesses the degree of pancreatic damage and identifies gallstones within the biliary tree. MRI is particularly useful to differentiate between fluid and solid inflammatory masses.
- ***ERCP*** is used as a treatment measure to remove bile duct stones in selected cases of gallstone-related pancreatitis (see below).

Assessment of disease severity

The majority of cases of acute pancreatitis are mild and run a short, self-limiting course. However, approximately 25% run a more complicated course and in 10% this is life-threatening. The revised Atlanta criteria define mild, moderately severe or severe pancreatitis and are summarized in ***Box 15.4***; they require assessment of organ failure using the Modified Marshall scoring system ***(Box 15.5)***. In practice, patients with moderately severe acute pancreatitis should be managed as having severe disease until sustained improvement is seen.

In severe cases, mortality may be as high as 80%. The initial clinical course is marked by a systemic inflammatory response

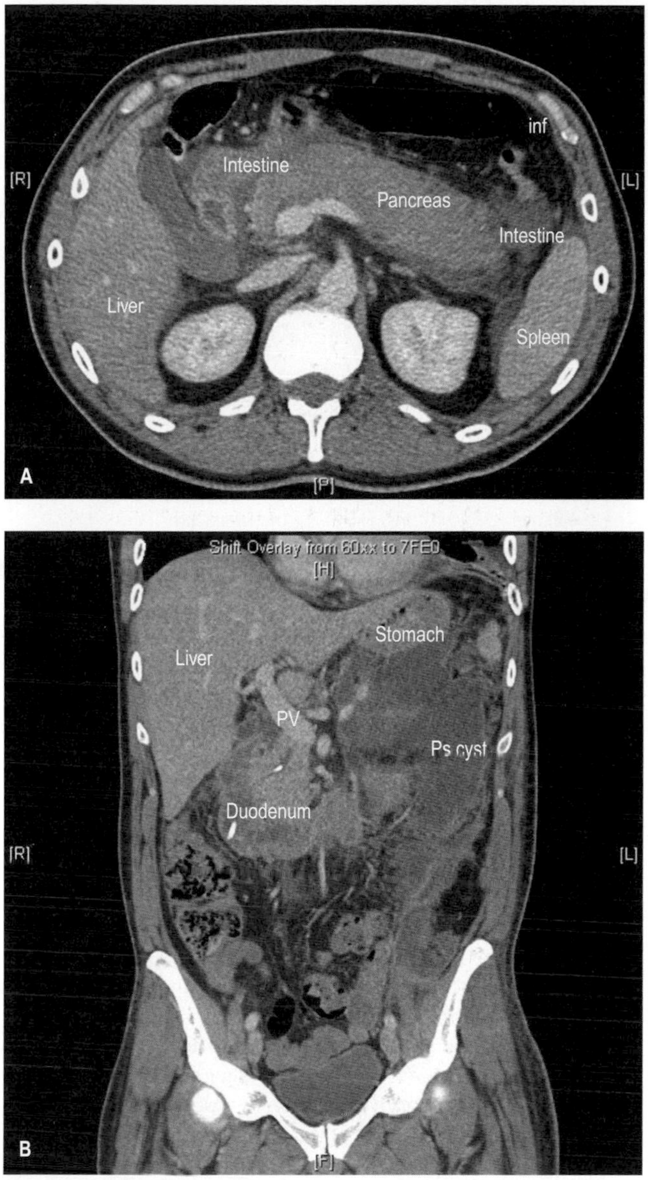

Figure 15.11 **Acute pancreatitis. A.** An ***abdominal CT scan*** with arterial phase contrast in a patient presenting with acute pancreatitis 48 h previously. The pancreas is swollen with very little uptake of contrast, suggesting a severe necrotizing process. There are peripancreatic inflammatory changes (inf). The liver and spleen are identified for reference. **B.** A ***coronal CT view*** in the same patient, carried out in second week after presentation. There is now a large fluid collection and debris within it. This is a precursor of a large pseudocyst (Ps), which extends down the left paracolic gutter into the pelvis. This has occurred as a consequence of a pancreatitis-induced ductal leak. The liver, stomach and duodenum are defined for reference. PV, portal vein.

syndrome (SIRS), haemodynamic instability and multiple organ failure. The consequences of SIRS, including respiratory and acute kidney injury, account for most of mortality within the first 7 days of an episode of severe acute pancreatitis. After 7 days, the majority of deaths are linked to delayed complications, such as sepsis due to infected collections or haemorrhage due to inflammatory erosion into major vessels.

Accurate identification of patients likely to progress to severe pancreatitis permits appropriate monitoring and intensive care to

Box 15.4 Severity of acute pancreatitis: revised Atlanta criteria 2013

Mild
- Absence of organ failure
- Absence of local complication

Moderate/severe
- Local complication and/or transient organ failure (<48 h)

Severe
- Persistent organ failure (>48 h), defined by the modified Marshall Score for the evolution of organ failure (see ***Box 15.5***)

be put in place. Early clinical assessment has been shown to have poor sensitivity for predicting a severe attack. Similarly, individual laboratory tests have very limited value. Therefore, multiple factors have been used to develop clinical scoring systems. The ***Glasgow and Ranson scoring systems*** (***Boxes 15.6*** and ***15.7***) are based on such parameters and have been shown to have 80% sensitivity for predicting a severe attack, although only after 48 hours from presentation. The ***Acute Physiology and Chronic Health Evaluation (APACHE II) score*** has been extensively adopted as a means of assessing the severity of a wide spectrum of illness. The APACHE scoring system is based on common physiological and laboratory values, patient age, and the presence or absence of a number of other chronic health problems, including obesity ***(Box 15.8)***. This scoring system appears to have a high sensitivity and can be applied as early as 24 hours after onset of symptoms. There is evidence that obesity affects the outcome of an episode of pancreatitis, perhaps because adipose tissue is a substrate for activated enzyme activity, worsening the inflammatory reaction. All scoring systems for predicting the severity of acute pancreatitis have their weaknesses and have proven to have modest utility in clinical practice. However, systematic classification tools can guide consistent clinical assessment, and are certainly necessary in clinical studies and audit of outcomes.

Management

The initial management of acute pancreatitis is similar for all causes. A multiple factor scoring system (ideally, APACHE II with a modification for obesity) should be used at the end of the first 24 hours after presentation to allow identification of patients with a predicted severe attack. This should be repeated at 48 hours to identify a further subgroup who appear to be moving into the severe category. These patients should be managed on a high-dependency or intensive care unit and the case should be discussed with a specialist pancreatic unit at an early stage. Even patients outside the severe category may require considerable supportive care.

Early fluid losses in acute pancreatitis may be large, requiring well-maintained intravenous access and a urinary catheter to monitor circulating volume and renal function. Arterial and central venous catheterization may be necessary to facilitate close monitoring of hemodynamic status and permit repeat sampling of arterial blood gases.

- ***Nasogastric suction***. This prevents abdominal distension and vomitus, and hence the risk of aspiration pneumonia.
- ***Baseline arterial blood gases***. These are a key predictive factor for severity of an episode and determine the need for continuous oxygen administration.
- ***Prophylactic antibiotics***. Controlled data for the use of antibiotics are available but the results are not uniform in showing benefit, particularly in demonstrating improved

Box 15.5 Modified Marshall scoring system[a]

Score system	0	1	2	3	4
Respiratory PO_2/FiO_2	>400	301–400	201–300	101–200	≤101
Renal Serum creatinine (μmol/L)	134	134–169	170–310	311–439	>439
Cardiovascular Systolic blood pressure (mmHg)	>90	<90 Fluid-responsive	<90 Not fluid-responsive	<90 pH <7.3	<90 pH <7.2

[a]A score of ≥2 in any system defines the presence of organ failure.

Box 15.6 Glasgow prognostic criteria in acute pancreatitis[a]

Criteria	Measurement
Age	>55 years
WBC	$>15\times10^9$/L
Blood glucose	>10 mmol/L
Serum urea	>16 mmol/L
Serum albumin	<30 g/L
Serum aminotransferase	>200 U/L
Serum calcium	<2 mmol/L
Serum LDH	>600 U/L
P_aO_2	<8.0 kPa (60 mmHg)

[a]More than 3 positive factors during the first 48 h suggests severe pancreatitis and a poorer prognosis. LDH, lactate dehydrogenase; WBC, white blood cell count.

Box 15.7 Ranson criteria in pancreatitis

Criteria	Measurement
At admission	
Age	>55 years
WBC	$>16\times10^9$/L
Blood glucose	>11 mmol/L
Serum LDH	>600 U/L
Serum aminotransferase	>250 U/L
Within 48 h	
Haematocrit fall	>10%
Serum aminotransferase	>200 U/L
Serum calcium	<2 mmol/L
Serum urea increase	>1.8 mmol/l
Base deficit	>4 Meq/L
P_aO_2	<8.0 kPa (60 mmHg)

LDH, lactate dehydrogenase; WBC, white blood cell count.

Box 15.8 The Acute Physiology and Chronic Health Evaluation (APACHE) II scoring system[a]

Physiological
- Temperature
- Heart rate
- Respiratory rate
- Mean arterial pressure
- Glasgow Coma Scale score
- Presence of acute kidney injury
- Age
- Organ insufficiency
- Immunocompromise

Laboratory
- Oxygenation (P_aO_2)
- Arterial pH
- Serum:
  - Sodium
  - Potassium
  - Creatinine
  - Haematocrit
  - White blood cell count

[a]APACHE is applied within 24 h of admission. Score can range from 0–71 (normal to abnormal). Higher scores correspond to more severe disease and a higher risk of death. Body mass index (BMI) is an additional parameter that can be added specifically in assessing severity of acute pancreatitis.

mortality. There is some evidence that the β-lactam imipenem reduces the incidence of infected pancreatic necrosis. Antibiotics should usually be reserved for cases where cholangitis or infected necrotic tissue is strongly suspected and, if possible, choice should be guided by blood culture results.

- ***Analgesia requirements***. Tramadol or other opiates are the drugs of choice for immediate post-presentation pain control. Unless there is prompt resolution of pain, a patient-controlled system of administration is indicated to provide continuous and adequate pain relief. Fentanyl has been used widely for this application. There is a theoretical risk that morphine and diamorphine might exacerbate pancreatic ductular hypertension by causing sphincter of Oddi contraction. Although there are no clinical data to support this risk, some clinicians therefore avoid these drugs in acute pancreatitis.
- ***Feeding***. In a severe episode, there is little likelihood of oral nutrition for a number of weeks. Total parenteral nutrition has been associated with a high risk of infection and has been replaced by enteral nutrition. In the absence of gastroparesis, most patients will tolerate nasogastric administration of feed without exacerbation of pain. In those with gastroparesis or poorly tolerated nasogastric feeding (exacerbation of pain or precipitation of nausea and vomitus), post-pyloric feeding should be instituted by the endoscopic placement of a nasojejunal tube.
- ***Anticoagulation***. Low-molecular-weight heparin should be given for prophylaxis of deep vein thrombosis.

In a small proportion of patients, multiorgan failure will develop in the first few days after presentation, reflecting the extent of SIRS. Such patients may require positive-pressure ventilation and renal support (see p. 1156).

Gallstone-related pancreatitis

In patients with gallstone-related pancreatitis and associated bile duct obstruction (particularly when complicated by cholangitis), endoscopic intervention with sphincterotomy and stone extraction

Box 15.9 Complications of acute pancreatitis

Systemic
- Systemic inflammatory response syndrome (SIRS)
- Multiorgan dysfunction

Pancreas
- Pancreatic fluid collections
- Necrosis ± infection
- Pancreatic abscess
- Pancreatic pseudocyst (after 4–6 weeks)

Lungs
- Pleural effusion
- Acute respiratory distress syndrome (ARDS)
  – hypoxia
- Pneumonia

Kidney
- Acute kidney injury

Gastrointestinal tract
- Gastrointestinal bleeding from gastric or duodenal erosions
- Paralytic ileus

Hepatobiliary
- Jaundice
- Common bile duct obstruction
- Portal vein thrombosis

Metabolic
- Hypoglycaemia
- Hyperglycaemia
- Hypocalcaemia

Haematological
- Disseminated intravascular coagulation (DIC)

is the treatment of choice. In the absence of bile duct obstruction, sphincterotomy and stone extraction are only of proven benefit when the episode of pancreatitis is predicted to be severe. In less severe cases of gallstone-related pancreatitis, the presence of residual bile duct stones can be assessed electively by MRCP or endoscopic ultrasound in the recovery phase of the acute episode; if stones are present, they can be removed at the time of ERCP. To prevent a recurrent episode of gallstone pancreatitis, cholecystectomy should be carried out as soon as feasible after the acute episode has resolved.

Complications

(See ***Box 15.9***.) After the first 7 days, the prognosis of acute pancreatitis is most closely related to the extent of pancreatic necrosis. This can be most accurately assessed by contrast-enhanced CT, which should be carried out in all patients with severe disease after the first week. Extensive necrosis (>50% of the pancreas) is associated with a high risk of further complicated disease, frequently requiring surgical intervention.

In this minority of patients with extensive necrosis of the pancreatic and peripancreatic tissues, superimposed infection is associated with a greatly increased risk of mortality. A 'step-up', minimally invasive approach is now preferred, with open surgical debridement avoided if at all possible. Long courses of antibiotics are given, and percutaneous drainage and endoscopic ultrasound-guided endoscopic necrosectomy are used to clear infected collections. The aims of such interventions are to control infection, evacuate devitalized tissues (the culture medium for invasive infection) and promote conditions for healing.

The best outcomes from intervention are achieved when debridement is delayed until at least 4 weeks after the onset of pancreatitis. When the damaged area has been walled off and liquefaction has begun, a pseudocyst develops. If necessary, acute sepsis may be controlled by percutaneous drainage of collections in the first instance.

Prognosis

The vast majority of patients with a mild to moderate episode of acute pancreatitis will make a full recovery with no long-term sequelae. Recurrent episodes of pancreatitis may occur, particularly if there has been any long-term pancreatic ductular damage. Patients with more severe acute pancreatitis may develop pancreatic insufficiency with respect to both exocrine (malabsorption) and endocrine function (diabetes); both of these carry their own significant, life-long morbidity.

Box 15.10 Causes of chronic pancreatitis

- Alcohol
- Chronic kidney disease
- Hereditary:
  – Cystic fibrosis
  – Trypsinogen and inhibitory protein defects
- Tropical
- Obstructive
- Trauma
- Idiopathic
- Hypercalcaemia
- Recurrent acute pancreatitis
- Autoimmune (IgG4)

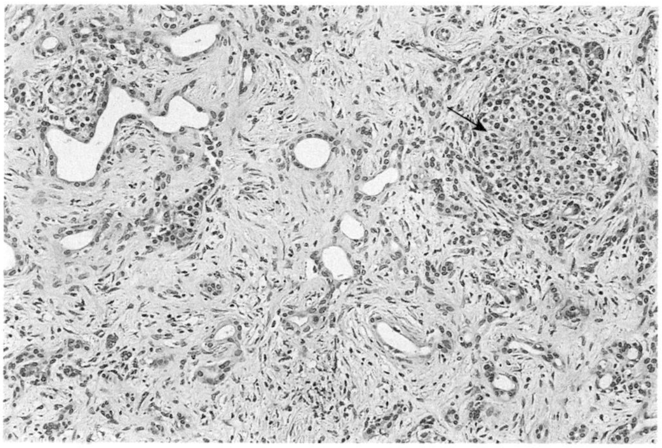

Figure 15.12 **Histology of chronic pancreatitis.** There is considerable loss of acini and replacement by fibrosis. Inflammatory cells are relatively inconspicuous at this late stage. Islets of Langerhans (one is arrowed) sometimes escape destruction but their loss can result in diabetes mellitus. *(From Underwood JC (ed.).* General and Systematic Pathology, *4th edn. Edinburgh: Churchill Livingstone; 2004, with permission.)*

Chronic pancreatitis

Aetiology

In developed countries, alcohol is reported to be the only aetiological factor in 60–80% of cases. There is a sizeable list of other reported aetiological factors, which can be categorized into toxic–metabolic, genetic, autoimmune, recurrent acute or severe acute pancreatitis, obstruction and idiopathic causes ***(Box 15.10)***.

Pathogenesis

There is increasing evidence that an increase in activated trypsin within the pancreas is a common pathway for the development of chronic pancreatitis. This may occur as a result of increased/premature activation of trypsinogen to trypsin, or of impaired inactivation/clearance of the activated enzyme from the pancreas. It is believed that the increased or prolonged intrapancreatic enzyme activity leads to the precipitation of proteins within the duct lumen in the form of plugs. These then form a nidus for calcification but are also the cause of ductal obstruction, leading to ductal hypertension and further pancreatic damage ***(Fig. 15.12)***.

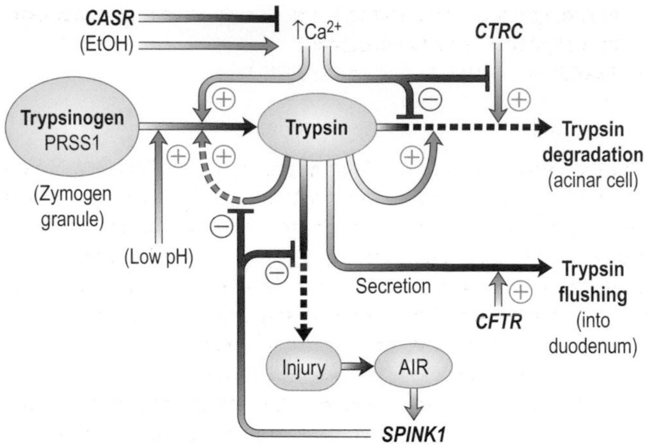

Figure 15.13 Genetic factors in trypsinogen activation and trypsin inactivation. Early activation of ***trypsinogen to trypsin*** within the pancreas is crucial in the development of pancreatitis. Trypsinogen activation is promoted by cationic trypsinogen mutations ***(PRSS1+)***, active trypsin, high calcium (Ca^{2+}) and low pH. Calcium levels are regulated in part by calcium-sensing receptor ***(CASR)*** and dysregulated by ethanol (EtOH). ***Active trypsin degradation*** is facilitated by ***CTRC*** and by other active trypsin molecules, but blocked by high calcium. Active trypsin within the pancreas leads to pancreatic injury, which causes an acute inflammatory response ***(AIR)***. AIR upregulates expression of serine protease inhibitor Kazal 1 ***(SPINK1)***, which blocks active trypsin and therefore prevents further activation of trypsinogens and limits further tissue injury. Cystic fibrosis transmembrane conductance regulator ***(CFTR)*** represents an extra-acinar cell mechanism to eliminate trypsin by flushing it out of the pancreatic duct and into the duodenum. *(Adapted from Whitcomb DC. Genetic aspects of pancreatitis. Annual Reviews of Medicine 2010; 61:413–424.)*

In the case of alcohol-related chronic pancreatitis, there is evidence that ethanol increases pro-enzyme activation, promoting trypsinogen activation, as well as diminishing the inactivation pathway. The observation that the vast majority of people drinking excess alcohol do not develop pancreatitis suggests that the disease process is a complex interaction of different mechanisms. It is proposed that the alcohol is only one factor that interacts with other environmental and/or genetic influences (see below).

Genetic aspects of chronic pancreatitis

A number of genetic factors have been identified that influence the process of trypsin activation and inactivation. Cationic trypsinogen is the major form of trypsinogen produced in the pancreas and encoded by the *PRSS1* gene ***(Fig. 15.13)***. Gain-of-function mutations of this gene are recognized as the major factor in hereditary pancreatitis, an autosomal dominant condition with variable penetrance.

Calcium levels within the pancreas have a role in the process of activation and inactivation of trypsinogen/trypsin and are, in part, modulated by the calcium-sensing receptor. Mutations coding for this receptor have been associated with pancreatitis and are believed to facilitate the damaging effects of alcohol on the pancreas.

The serine protease inhibitor Kazal type 1 (*SPINK-1*) is a specific trypsin inhibitor and is co-secreted with trypsinogen by the acinar cells. Loss-of-function mutations of the *SPINK-1* gene have been associated with the development of chronic pancreatitis and identified, in particular, as a factor in the development of tropical pancreatitis (almost certainly interacting with environmental triggers).

Chymotrypsin C is produced in trace amounts by the acinar cells and has also been shown to have a role in trypsin inactivation. Loss-of-function mutations of the encoding gene have been identified in patients with chronic pancreatitis.

The cystic fibrosis transmembrane conductance regulator (*CFTR*) is expressed on the apical surface of the acinar cells and is responsible for maintaining a high-volume, bicarbonate-rich pancreatic secretion. This high-volume secretion is responsible for flushing the activated trypsin into the duodenum. The homozygote or complex heterozygote *CFTR* mutations associated with the cystic fibrosis disease state are almost always manifest by perinatal/early pancreatic exocrine failure (see p. 508). An increased frequency of a single *CFTR* mutation in patients with idiopathic chronic pancreatitis has been identified.

The identification of a genetic component to the development of chronic pancreatitis has led to speculation that, in many cases, the evolution of the disease is dependent on the complex interaction of gene–gene and gene–environmental factors.

Autoimmune chronic pancreatitis

Two types of autoimmune chronic pancreatitis (ACP) have been identified. The **most common variant (type 1)** is seen predominantly in middle-aged men and is associated with raised serum and tissue levels of IgG4. Other autoantibodies, including those directed towards nuclear and smooth muscle antigens, are also observed. Extrapancreatic tissue involvement is common, including the biliary tree (autoimmune cholangitis; see above), as well as thyroid, salivary gland and renal tissue (see p. 760). In all these disorders, there is a raised serum IgG4 level and, pathologically, there is a dense lymphoplasmacytic infiltrate with many IgG4-positive plasma cells, a mild to moderate eosinophil infiltrate and an obliterative phlebitis in some organs. ACP is one of the few settings in which the pathogenesis of the disease may be independent of the activated trypsin pathways.

The **second variant (type 2)** tends to occur in early midlife with an equal sex distribution and does not have the autoimmune markers or IgG4-positive cells. Some 30% of cases are associated with inflammatory bowel disease. The disease is much more likely to be restricted to the pancreas and lacks the associations with other organ/tissue involvement seen with the type 1 variant. The hallmark of both types of autoimmune pancreatitis is evidence of responsiveness to steroids (see 'Management' below).

The presentation of autoimmune pancreatitis is varied, particularly in type 1, in which extrapancreatic disease may predominate. Abdominal pain and weight loss are common features; jaundice may be an early symptom, both secondary to bile duct obstruction by the inflamed head of pancreas, and a manifestation of the cholangitis seen in type 1 cases.

Clinical features

Pain is the most common presentation of chronic pancreatitis. It is usually epigastric and often radiates through into the back. The pattern of pain may be episodic, with short periods of severe pain, or is chronic and unremitting. For those with an alcohol-related aetiology, exacerbations of the pain may follow further alcohol excess, although this is not a uniform relationship. Alcohol excess or meals with a high fat content may also lead to exacerbations of pain, independent of the aetiology.

During periods of abdominal pain, anorexia is common and weight loss may be severe. This is particularly so in those patients with chronic, unremitting symptoms. Exocrine insufficiency may develop at any time and occasionally malabsorption is the presenting feature in the absence of abdominal pain. Diabetes occurs in approximately 30% of cases and is usually a late event in the disease process, almost always following the development of exocrine insufficiency. Jaundice secondary to obstruction of the common bile duct during its course through the fibrosed head of the pancreas may also occur and may be a presenting feature in a small proportion of patients.

Investigations

The extent to which investigations are required is dependent on the clinical setting.

- ***Serum amylase and lipase*** levels may be elevated, but in advanced disease there may not be sufficient residual acinar tissue to produce this elevation.
- ***Serum IgG4 levels*** should be measured in those cases with suspected autoimmune pancreatitis.
- ***Faecal elastase*** level will be abnormal in the majority of patients with moderate to severe pancreatic disease.
- ***Gene mutation analysis*** should be carried out in selected cases in whom the aetiology is uncertain. This is most relevant in patients presenting below the age of 40. Common mutations of the *PRSS1*, *SPINK-1* and *CFTR* encoding genes are available via reference centres.
- ***Transabdominal ultrasound scan*** is used for initial assessment.
- ***Contrast-enhanced CT scanning*** provides a more detailed assessment. In the presence of pancreatic calcification and a dilated pancreatic duct, the diagnosis of chronic pancreatitis can be readily established ***(Fig. 15.14)***. This may be much more difficult when these features are not present, and in particular with an atypical presentation such as steatorrhoea.
- ***MRI with MRCP*** is utilized to define more subtle abnormalities of the pancreatic duct, which may be seen in non-dilated chronic pancreatitis.
- ***Endoscopic ultrasound*** is used increasingly when doubt about the diagnosis remains after the above imaging, or specifically when complications of chronic pancreatitis, including pseudocyst formation and the possible development of malignancy, need assessment.
- ***MRCP*** has replaced diagnostic ERCP.

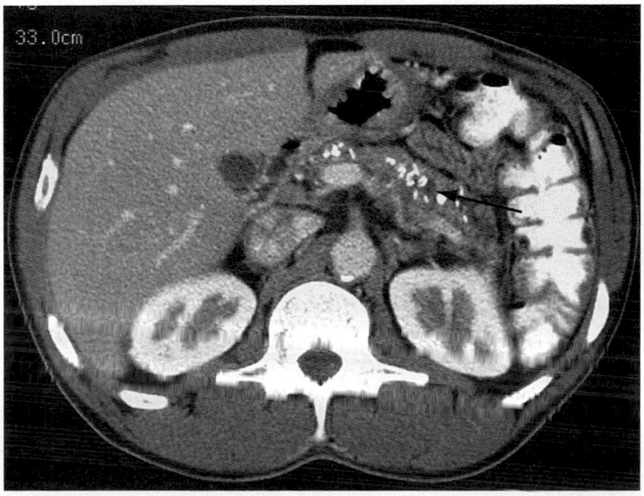

Figure 15.14 Contrast-enhanced CT scan in a patient with chronic pancreatitis. Multiple calcific densities (arrowed) are demonstrated along the line of the main pancreatic duct.

Differential diagnosis

The differential diagnosis is that of pancreatic malignancy. Carcinoma of the pancreas can reproduce many of the symptoms and imaging abnormalities that are commonly seen with chronic pancreatitis. The diagnosis of malignancy should be considered in patients with a short history in whom there is a localized pancreatic mass. Considerable difficulties may arise when a malignancy develops on the background of established chronic pancreatitis (the latter being a recognized pre-malignant lesion).

High-quality imaging is able to define malignant features with a localized mass lesion, local invasion and lymph node enlargement. Endoscopic ultrasound provides the most accurate assessment of a potential mass lesion.

Management

In patients with alcohol-related chronic pancreatitis, long-term abstinence is likely to be of benefit, although this has been difficult to prove. Autoimmune pancreatitis is steroid-responsive and failure to respond would put the diagnosis in question. Relapse is common when the steroids are withdrawn, and long-term immunomodulators (e.g. azathioprine) may be required.

Abdominal pain

For short-term flare-ups of pain, a combination of a non-steroidal anti-inflammatory drug (NSAID) and an opiate (tramadol) is usually sufficient for symptomatic relief. In patients with chronic unremitting pain, this may be inadequate and also risks opiate dependence.

Tricyclic antidepressants (e.g. amitriptyline) and membrane-stabilizing agents (e.g. pregabalin) are used for chronic pain and reduce the need for opiates. Coeliac axis nerve block may produce good pain relief but is unreliable in its extent and duration of action. In the majority of patients, some spontaneous improvement in pain control occurs with time. After a 6–10-year period, some 60% of patients will become pain-free. For patients with recurrent severe or debilitating chronic pain, both endoscopic and surgical intervention has been used. This is particularly the case in patients with chronic calcific disease with a dilated pancreatic duct upstream of a ductular stricture and/or stone. The endoscopic approach has centred on improving duct drainage by removing intraductal stones and duct stenting to maintain patency. Extracorporeal shock wave lithotripsy has been used to fragment stones within the head of the pancreas.

Surgical intervention usually involves a duct drainage procedure, which can be combined with partial resection of the diseased head of pancreas. Trials have reported improved pain control following surgical intervention, as compared with the endoscopic approach. However, many patients have a high level of debility (and often continued alcohol excess) and are unsuitable for major surgery. In such circumstances, endoscopic therapy is justified as a first measure and there is no evidence that this adversely influences subsequent surgery.

Malabsorption

The steatorrhoea associated with pancreatic insufficiency may be high, with up to 30 mmol of fat lost per 24 h. This will usually improve with pancreatic enzyme supplements. Current preparations are presented in the form of microspheres, which reduce the problems of acid degradation in the stomach. An acid suppressor (H_2-receptor antagonist or proton-pump inhibitor) is also given. Despite this, a proportion of patients continue to malabsorb, usually reflecting the inadequate mixing of the pancreatic supplements with the food, as well as the low pH in the duodenum secondary to inadequate pancreatic bicarbonate production. There is no justification to reduce fat intake below the recommended levels of a normal diet, as this will contribute to the malnutrition seen in patients with chronic pancreatitis. Dietetic input is valuable for the management of malabsorption and also for monitoring and alleviating the malnutrition that is often seen secondary to abdominal pain and food aversion.

Diabetes

Diabetes associated with pancreatic endocrine failure may be difficult to control, with a rapid progression from oral hypoglycaemic agents to an insulin requirement. Brittle control is a common problem secondary to inadequate glucagon production by the damaged pancreas.

Autoimmune pancreatitis

Most patients respond to glucocorticoid therapy, e.g. prednisolone 40 mg daily for 4–6 weeks. Relapses are treated with azathioprine.

Specific complications

The most common structural complication of chronic pancreatitis is a ***pancreatic pseudocyst***, a fluid collection surrounded by granulation tissue (see p. 505). These usually occur in relationship to a period of enhanced inflammatory activity within the pancreas giving abdominal pain but may develop silently during what would appear to be a stable phase. Intra- or retroperitoneal rupture, bleeding or cyst infection may occur. The larger cysts may occlude nearby structures, including the duodenum and the bile duct. In pseudocysts less than 6 cm in diameter, spontaneous resolution can be anticipated. In larger cysts that have been present for a period in excess of 6 weeks, resolution is less common and a long-term complication rate of approximately 30% can be anticipated. Many pseudocysts are closely opposed to the posterior wall of the stomach or duodenum, and can be successfully drained endoscopically using endoscopic ultrasound to identify the optimum drainage site. A direct fistula is created between the pseudocyst lumen and the gastric or duodenal lumen, which is then kept patent by the insertion of plastic stents. This approach will be successful in approximately 75% of cases. Surgical drainage is required for failures of endoscopic therapy or in circumstances where the pseudocyst anatomy does not allow endoscopic access.

Ascites and, occasionally, ***pleural effusions*** can be a direct consequence of chronic pancreatitis when there has been disruption of the main pancreatic duct. A high ascites or pleural fluid amylase will confirm the aetiology. Such disruptions of the main pancreatic duct require surgical intervention.

There is an increased risk of ***pancreatic cancer*** in patients with chronic pancreatitis. The risk of malignancy is closely related to the duration of the inflammatory process. The highest incidence has been reported in hereditary pancreatitis, with a 50-fold increase and a lifetime risk as high as 40%. This reflects the early onset (in childhood) of the disease. Increases of 20–30-fold have been described in patients carrying other gene mutations and early onset of disease. The lifetime risk of malignancy in other causes of chronic pancreatitis, such as alcohol, which develop much later is 10–15%. Cancer surveillance programmes have been proposed for the very high-risk groups (hereditary pancreatitis and other causes of early-onset disease), usually starting around the age of 40 years and relying on yearly imaging and tumour marker measurement.

Cystic fibrosis

Some 85% of people with cystic fibrosis (see pp. 1088–1089) will have pancreatic exocrine failure, and in the majority of these, this will develop *in utero* or the perinatal period. Malabsorption and failure to thrive are common presentations in the perinatal period and first year of life, and diabetes will develop subsequently in 30% of these cases during their lifetime.

In the remaining 15% of cases, there is an insufficiency of pancreatic exocrine secretion, which may persist throughout the patient's lifetime. This reflects residual *CFTR* function and is associated with class IV and V mutations. The patients tend to present later in life and have less severe pulmonary involvement, although this is not uniform. Some of these cases will progress to pancreatic exocrine insufficiency at variable times in the course of their disease. A small proportion develop symptomatic pancreatitis as part of this process.

The **management** of pancreatic exocrine insufficiency in cystic fibrosis is necessary to optimize growth and overall nutrition. ***Pancreatic enzyme supplements*** are closely titrated against the level of steatorrhoea. ***Fat intake*** should be maintained to avoid nutritional deficit. A daily ***lipase intake*** of up to 10 000 units/kg body weight is required. The efficacy of the supplements may be improved by the use of a ***proton-pump inhibitor***. These drugs reduce the risk of acid denaturation of the enzymes and also prevent acidification of the duodenum, which also impairs the enzymes' activity. Despite optimizing the use of enzyme supplements, a degree of fat malabsorption may persist. This reflects other luminal abnormalities of fat absorption in cystic fibrosis that are related to viscous mucus, small bowel bacterial colonization, and poor mixing of the food bolus with bile.

Further reading

Braganza JM, Lee SH, McCloy RF et al. Chronic pancreatitis. *Lancet* 2011; 377:1184–1197.

Johnson CD, Besselink MG, Carter R. Acute pancreatitis. *BMJ* 2014; 349:g4859.

Kamisawa T, Zen Y, Pillai J et al. IgG4-related disease. *Lancet* 2015; 385:1460–1471.

Lankisch PG, Apte M, Banks PA. Acute pancreatitis. *Lancet* 2015; 386:85–96.

PANCREATIC CANCER

The many types of pancreatic cancer can be divided into two main groupings. The vast majority of cases (about 99%) occur in the exocrine component of the pancreas. There are several subtypes of exocrine pancreatic cancer, but their diagnosis and treatment have much in common. A small minority of pancreatic cancers arise in the endocrine or hormone-producing tissue of the pancreas and have different clinical characteristics.

Pancreatic adenocarcinoma

The incidence of pancreatic cancer in the West has been estimated at approximately 10 cases per 100 000, with no increase over the last 20 years. The diagnosis is rarely made in persons younger than 40 years of age, and the median age at diagnosis is 71 years. Approximately 60% of patients with this condition are male. It is the eighth leading cause of death from cancer in men and the ninth leading cause of death from cancer in women throughout the world.

Some 96% of pancreatic cancers are adenocarcinoma in type and the large majority are of ductal origin.

Aetiology

Smoking is associated with a twofold increase. Excessive intake of alcohol or coffee and excessive use of aspirin have also been implicated. There is an increased incidence of pancreatic cancer among patients with a history of diabetes and chronic pancreatitis. The risk of developing pancreatic cancer is most marked in those patients with a genetic mutation predisposing to chronic pancreatitis (there is a 50 times increased risk in the presence of a *PRSS-1* mutation; see ***Fig. 15.13***). Although it is estimated that 5–10% of pancreatic cancers have an inherited component, the genetic basis for familial aggregation has not been identified in most cases. A subgroup of such high-risk kindreds carry germline mutations of DNA repair genes, such as *BRCA2* and the partner and localizer of *BRCA2*. Among people with a known family history of pancreatic cancer in a first-degree relative, the relative risk of the development of pancreatic cancer is increased by a factor of 2, 6 and 30 in people with one, two and three affected family members, respectively ***(Box 15.11)***.

Pathogenesis

Data suggest that pancreatic cancer results from the successive accumulation of gene mutations ***(Fig. 15.15)***. The cancer originates in the ductal epithelium and evolves from pre-malignant lesions to fully invasive cancer. The lesion called ***pancreatic intraepithelial neoplasia (PanIN)*** is the best-characterized histological precursor of pancreatic cancer. The progression from minimally dysplastic epithelium (PanIN grades 1A and 1B) to more severe dysplasia (grades 2 and 3) and finally to invasive carcinoma is paralleled by the successive accumulation of mutations. More than 90% of cases of pancreatic intraepithelial neoplasia of all grades have *KRAS* mutations. The mutational inactivation of the *CDKN2A*, *p53* and *SMAD* family member (*SMAD4*) tumour suppressors is detected with increasing frequency in type 2 and type 3 lesions of pancreatic intraepithelial neoplasia, suggesting that they are rate-limiting events for tumour progression. Exome-sequencing studies have identified additional loss-of-function mutations encoding components of the SWI/SNF nucleosome remodelling complex, which are cumulatively detected in approximately 10–15% of pancreatic adenocarcinomas, as well as other, less frequent, alterations.

A small percentage of pancreatic adenocarcinomas arise from cystic lesions, including ***intraductal papillary mucinous neoplasms (IPMN)*** and ***mucinous cystic neoplasia*** (see below). There is evidence that these cystic neoplasms demonstrate a similar multistep genetic and histological progression to invasive adenocarcinoma, although there are recognized differences in the mutational events that occur.

Box 15.11 Relative risks of pancreatic cancer in patients with a family history or associated gene mutations

Risk factor	Relative risk
Familial pancreatic cancer	
Two first-degree relatives affected	18
Three first-degree relatives affected	57
Hereditary pancreatic cancer syndromes	
BRCA2 mutation	5.9
Familial atypical multiple mole melanoma (FAMMM)	16
Peutz–Jeghers syndrome	36
Hereditary pancreatitis	50

Clinical features

Approximately two-thirds of pancreatic cancers are located in the head of the pancreas, and the remainder in the body and tail ***(Fig. 15.16)***. Patients with pancreatic cancer most commonly present with abdominal pain, anorexia and weight loss. Many patients have experienced low-grade symptoms for a number of months before they present for investigation. New onset of depressive symptoms has also been identified as an early manifestation. In many cases, the onset of these non-diagnostic symptoms is at a stage when there is already advanced local or metastatic disease. The pain associated with pancreatic cancer frequently radiates through into the back and, in some cases, is partially relieved by leaning forwards. Jaundice is a common, and maybe an early, manifestation of tumours of the ampulla and pancreatic head. This reflects the occlusion or compression of the distal common bile duct as it traverses the head of pancreas before entering the duodenum at the level of the ampulla. The patient may have noticed pale stools, dark urine and itching associated with bile duct obstruction in the absence (or prior to the onset) of detectable jaundice. Diabetes is

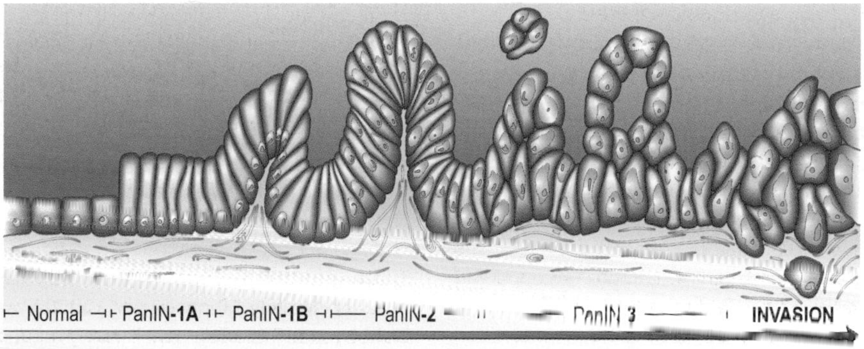

Figure 15.15 Genetic model for the development of pancreatic ductal adenocarcinoma. The stages indicate histological progression with specific gene alterations. ***PanIN,*** pancreatic intraepithelial neoplasia. *(Modified from Maitra A, Adsay NV, Argani P et al. Multicomponent analysis of the pancreatic adenocarcinoma progression model using a pancreatic intraepithelial neoplasia tissue microarray.* Modern Pathology *2003; 16:902–912, with permission from the Nature Publishing Group.)*

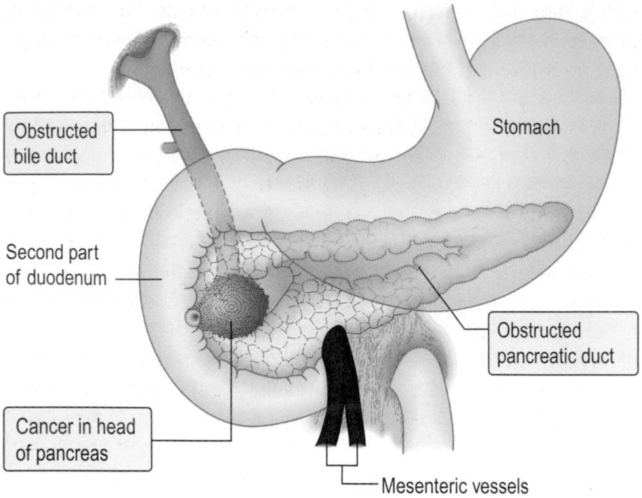

Figure 15.16 Carcinoma of the head of the pancreas. The close relationship of a carcinoma of the head of pancreas to the surrounding structures.

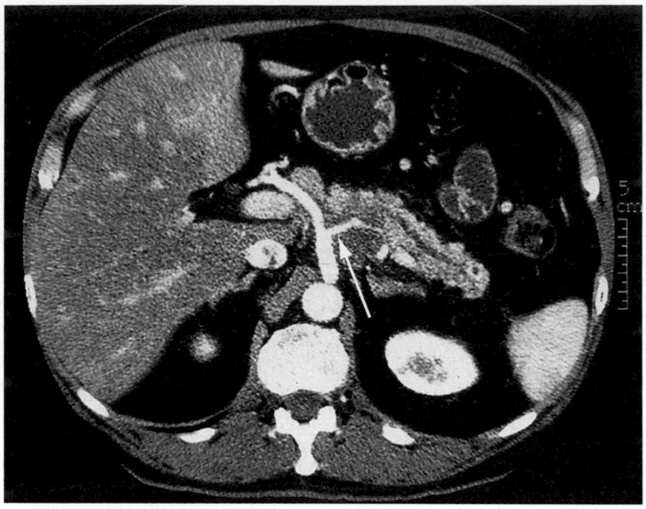

Figure 15.17 A contrast-enhanced CT scan showing a cancer of the body of the pancreas. There is retroperitoneal tumour extension enclosing the branches of the coeliac axis (arrowed).

present in at least 50% of patients with pancreatic cancer and may predate any other manifestation of disease. The obstruction of the pancreatic duct by the cancer may also lead to symptoms of malabsorption and overt steatorrhoea. An episode of symptomatic pancreatitis may, on occasion, be the presenting clinical picture. Other unusual presenting features can include thromboembolic phenomena, polyarthritis and skin nodules. These manifestations, distant to the tumour itself, have not been fully explained but may precede the development of a detectable pancreatic mass lesion by many months.

Signs

At the time of first presentation, there may be an absence of physical signs. Evidence of weight loss is common. Jaundice may be present with associated scratch marks prompted by pruritus. In a proportion of cases, the gall bladder will be palpable (***Courvoisier's sign***) secondary to an obstructed bile duct (or cystic duct). A palpable epigastric or central abdominal mass may be present as a reflection of advanced local disease. Liver metastases may be reflected in hepatomegaly.

Diagnosis and investigations

Patients with pancreatic adenocarcinoma frequently present for investigation at a stage in tumour development that precludes treatment of a curative nature. In many cases, symptoms have been present for a number of months but have not led to investigation that is specifically aimed at confirming/excluding a pancreatic cancer. To improve outcome from this cancer, there is increasing emphasis on earlier diagnosis. This is focused on targeted investigation for patients recognized as high-risk (see above). More emphasis is also placed on earlier referral for investigation in patients over the age of 40 who have low-grade symptoms that persist after initial assessment and empirical therapy. The upper gut symptoms frequently prompt referral for an upper gastrointestinal endoscopy. In most cases, this will not add diagnostic information and it is essential that a negative endoscopy does not delay further investigation – in particular, imaging.

- ***Transabdominal ultrasound*** is the initial imaging investigation in the majority of patients. In the presence of bile duct obstruction, this will confirm dilated intrahepatic bile ducts, as well as a mass in the head of the pancreas. Ultrasound is less reliable when the cancer is found in the body and tail of the pancreas because of overlying bowel gas, and has a sensitivity of detection of 60%. A negative transabdominal ultrasound scan should not be considered as excluding the diagnosis.
- ***Contrast-enhanced CT scan*** should confirm the presence of a mass lesion in most cases of pancreatic adenocarcinoma ***(Fig. 15.17)***. Lymph node involvement and metastatic disease will also be identified. If there is a high index of suspicion, a dual-phase pancreatic protocol CT scan should be requested from the outset. A high-quality pancreatic protocol CT is required as a staging procedure prior to planned curative surgery. Extending the CT to the chest will exclude pulmonary metastases.
- ***Endoscopic ultrasound*** is the most sensitive (>85%) non-surgical procedure for the detection of pancreatic cancer ***(Fig. 15.18)***. In most cases, it does not add to the diagnostic and staging information provided by the CT scan. However, the procedure is valuable for the definition of small (<2 cm) lesions of the pancreas, which may be missed on CT. Endoscopic ultrasound is now the approach of choice for obtaining cytological confirmation of the underlying malignancy. A histological/cytological diagnosis is essential prior to planned chemotherapy. There are concerns that needle sampling of the tumour prior to a planned curative resection might lead to cancer cell seeding. This has been reported as a rare event (1–2%).
- ***MRI and positron emission tomography (PET) scanning*** are techniques that are useful in a small proportion of patients when the local tumour or possibility of metastases has not been adequately defined.
- ***Several tumour markers*** have been evaluated for the diagnosis and monitoring of pancreatic cancer. The CA19–9 has reasonable sensitivity (80%) but a high false-positive rate. In individual patients, single values of these tumour markers may be of little help but a progressive elevation over time is often diagnostic; in such circumstances, tumour marker levels can be used to monitor response to treatment.

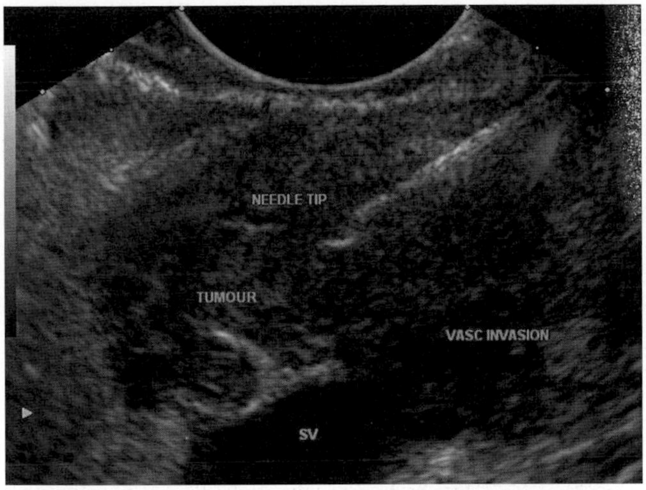

Figure 15.18 An endoscopic ultrasound scan with the probe in the distal stomach in a patient with pancreatic cancer. The patient presented with intractable periumbilical pain. A mass lesion of the pancreatic body is defined (***tumour***). There is invasion by the lesion into the splenic vein (***SV, vasc invasion***). The line of a transendoscopic needle is seen (***needle tip***), which has been placed under the guidance of the ultrasound probe to obtain a needle aspirate for cytological diagnosis.

Differential diagnosis

The diagnosis should not be difficult in the presence of painless jaundice or epigastric pain radiating into the back with progressive weight loss. Unfortunately, many patients present with very minor symptoms, including pain, change in bowel habit and weight loss. Imaging, particularly abdominal CT, should be performed if pancreatic cancer is suspected. IgG4-related autoimmune pancreatitis is now recognized as a differential diagnosis in patients presenting with abdominal pain, jaundice and an abnormal pancreas on imaging (localized or diffuse enlargement; see above). Pancreatic cancer may rarely present with recurrent episodes of typical acute pancreatitis.

Management

The 5-year survival rate for carcinoma of the pancreas is approximately 3%. Some 90% of patients with a diagnosis of pancreatic adenocarcinoma will have a cause of death directly related to the disease. Surgical intervention represents the only chance of long-term survival. Approximately 20% of all cases have a localized tumour suitable for resection, but in an elderly population, many of these have co-morbid factors that preclude such major surgery. Assessment of the primary tumour and involvement of local vessels, including the coeliac artery, superior mesenteric artery and vein, portal vein and hepatic artery, is critical in determining resectability. Strategies for management are optimally defined as part of a multidisciplinary team approach.

When treatment is considered of curative intent, a pancreatoduodenectomy (***Whipple procedure***) is required to remove tumours of the head and neck of the pancreas. Tumours of the body and tail are resected as part of a distal pancreatectomy, which is increasingly carried out by the laparoscopic approach. Adjuvant and neo-adjuvant chemotherapy (fluorouracil or gemcitabine) have been used in those undergoing attempted curative resection, with some evidence of improved survival. There is early evidence that more intensive multidrug regimes (the addition of irinotecan and oxaliplatin) may further improve outcome but at the expense of increased drug toxicity. Radiotherapy has been evaluated as adjuvant treatment but does not have an established role.

In the large majority of cases, therapy is considered non-curative. Chemotherapy (see above) is widely used in this setting, with increasing emphasis on multidrug regimens (see p. 638). The mainstay of palliative therapy is the attention to detail in managing the generalized and specific complications of pancreatic cancer.

- ***Pain*** is a debilitating feature in many cases. Management is best directed by dedicated pain teams. Opiates are a mainstay. There is some evidence that early intervention with coeliac axis block may have benefits.
- ***Nutritional deficit*** is a frequent feature at presentation and may be exacerbated by chemotherapy. Early dietetic support may alleviate this. Malabsorption is common with pancreatic cancer and can be managed by the introduction of pancreatic enzyme supplementation. The adverse metabolic effects of diabetes can be avoided by early detection and management.
- ***Obstructive jaundice*** will occur at some stage in 70% of cases and is frequently associated with anorexia and nausea, as well as pruritus. Endoscopic placement of endoprostheses (stents) offers excellent palliation (see pp. 498–499).
- ***Duodenal obstruction*** is seen in up to 20% of cases, particularly when the tumour is situated in the head or uncinate process of the pancreas. Endoscopic stenting is the treatment of choice with excellent palliation. Surgical bypass is an option in selected cases.

Pancreatic cystic neoplasms

Cystic lesions of the pancreas are common. Around 75% of these lesions will be pseudocysts (see p. 508) but, of the remainder, the majority are true cystic neoplasms. Careful characterization of lesions with CT and MRI, and discussion in a specialist pancreatic multidisciplinary team, are crucial. There is a high potential for the development of malignancy in true cystic neoplasms and therefore resection is generally recommended. The decision to operate may be difficult in patients with small (<3 cm) lesions of the head of the pancreas (in the absence of confirmed malignancy at presentation) and in those with significant co-morbidity. An initially conservative approach with follow-up imaging may be justified. Differentiation between pseudocysts and true cystic neoplasms may be difficult, even with multiple imaging techniques. Endoscopic ultrasound scanning and fine-needle aspiration are frequently helpful in characterizing cystic lesions of the pancreas. Endoscopic ultrasound appearance ***(Fig. 15.19)***, cytology, and the measurement of cyst fluid carcinoembryonic antigen and amylase may help to categorize cystic lesions and identify malignant change.

Serous cystadenomas are composed of multiple small, cystic cavities lined by cuboidal, glycogen-rich, mucin-poor cells. These lesions tend to occur in an elderly age group and are often an asymptomatic finding. Malignant transformation in a serous cystadenoma is extremely rare and so surgical resection is rarely required. Larger serous cystadenomas may cause local compressive complications, including pain, which may warrant surgical resection.

Solid pseudopapillary neoplasms are rare lesions, usually found in women in their fourth decade; they may occur anywhere in the pancreas. Resection is required, as around 20% show malignant features on histological examination.

Mucinous cystadenomas are almost exclusively found in women, usually in the fifth or sixth decade, and are sited in the

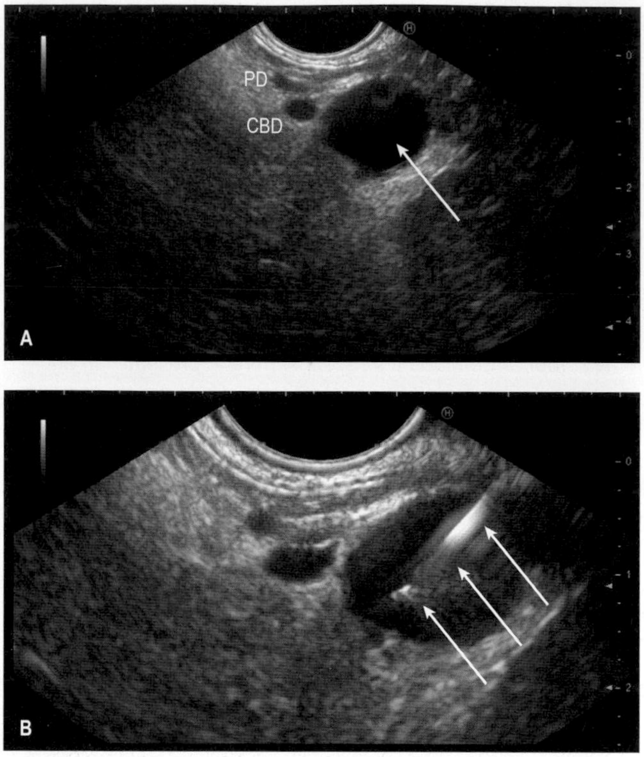

Figure 15.19 Linear endoscopic ultrasound images. A. A cystic lesion (arrowed) in the head of the pancreas; the common bile duct (CBD) and pancreatic duct (PD) are also visible. The lesion is an intraductal papillary mucinous neoplasm. **B.** The same lesion being sampled by fine needle aspiration for cytology, fluid amylase and fluid carcinoembryonic antigen estimation. The needle is arrowed.

pancreatic body and tail. Multilocular cysts are lined by tall, mucin-synthesizing cells. Around 20% of these lesions are malignant at the time of presentation and the majority appear to have malignant potential. Surgical resection is generally mandated.

Intraductal papillary mucinous neoplasm (IPMN) is a pancreatic cystic neoplasm that can arise in either the main pancreatic duct (main duct IPMN) or its side branches (branch duct IPMN). The majority are found in men between the ages of 60 and 70. Presentation is usually with pancreatic pain but branch duct IPMN is often an incidental finding. IPMNs are slowly progressive but carry a significant malignant potential. Generally, all main duct IPMNs and large branch duct IPMNs should be resected. Small branch duct IPMNs have a much lower malignant potential and are generally kept under radiological surveillance.

Cystic degeneration of a pancreatic adenocarcinoma or pancreatic neuroendocrine tumour can occur.

Pancreatic neuroendocrine tumour

Pancreatic neuroendocrine tumours (NETs) are thought to arise from the cells of the islets of Langerhans and can secrete a variety of active hormones, most frequently insulin. Pancreatic NETs have increased in incidence over the last two decades, reaching an incidence of 4–5/1 000 000 population. They represent a heterogeneous group of tumours with varying symptomology, tumour biology and prognosis. Between 25% and 50% of the patients present with symptoms related to hormones released from the tumour. The remainder have 'non-functioning' tumours that may be an incidental finding or present with symptoms related to tumour bulk, such as obstruction, jaundice, bleeding or abdominal mass. The increasing incidence of pancreatic NETs has been attributed to the widespread use of high-resolution cross-sectional imaging, leading to incidental detection of asymptomatic lesions.

In addition to insulin and glucagon, pancreatic NETs may synthesize ectopic hormones that are not usually found in the pancreas, such as gastrin, adrenocorticotrophin, vasoactive intestinal peptide and growth hormone. While many pancreatic endocrine tumours are multihormonal, one peptide tends to predominate and is responsible for any clinical syndrome (see below). Non-functioning pancreatic NETs often contain peptide hormone on immunostaining, but this remains functionally inactive. The majority of endocrine neoplasia pancreatic tumours are malignant in their behaviour. Between 10% and 15% of pancreatic NETs are linked to an inherited syndrome, such as the multiple endocrine neoplasia type 1 (MEN-1) or von Hippel–Lindau (VHL) syndrome (see p. 701).

Clinical syndromes

Insulinoma is described on pages 1275–1276.

A ***gastrinoma*** accounts for approximately 1 in 1000 cases of duodenal ulcer disease. This results from hypersecretion of gastric acid secondary to ectopic gastrin secretion within the endocrine pancreas (Zollinger–Ellison syndrome). Recurrent severe duodenal ulceration occurs, with only a partial response to acid suppression. The diagnosis is confirmed by an elevated gastrin level. High-dose proton-pump inhibitors are used to suppress symptoms.

A ***VIPoma*** is an endocrine pancreatic tumour producing vasoactive intestinal polypeptide (VIP). This causes secretory diarrhoea secondary to the stimulation of adenyl cyclase within the enterocyte (*Verner–Morrison or watery diarrhoea syndrome*). The clinical syndrome is one of profuse watery diarrhoea, hypokalaemia and a metabolic acidosis. To produce the syndrome, the tumours are usually in excess of 3 cm in diameter.

Glucagonomas are rare α-cell tumours that are responsible for a syndrome of migratory necrolytic dermatitis, weight loss, diabetes mellitus, deep vein thrombosis, anaemia and hypoalbuminaemia. The diagnosis is made by measuring pancreatic glucagon in the serum.

Somatostatinomas are rare malignant D-cell tumours of the pancreas. These tumours cause diabetes mellitus, gallstones and diarrhoea/steatorrhoea. They can be diagnosed by high serum somatostatin levels.

Investigations

Diagnosis is based on a combination of biochemical and histopathological markers. The biochemical diagnosis includes measurement of circulatory chromogranin A or specific hormones such as gastrin, insulin, glucagon and VIP. The histopathology includes features such as positive staining for chromogranin A and specific hormones such as gastrin, pro-insulin and glucagon.

Tumour localization depends on cross-sectional imaging, including CT and MRI scanning. The majority of NETs express somatostatin receptors, and a radiolabelled somatostatin analogue (such as octreotide) provides a means of tumour localization using scintigraphy. PET scanning with specific isotopes such as ^{11}C-5-hydroxytryptamine (^{11}C-5-HTP), fluorodopa and ^{68}Ga (DOTA)-octreotate has shown promise in the localization of disease.

Identification of the primary and possibly metastatic lesions may be difficult despite multiple imaging techniques. Endoscopic ultrasound is the most sensitive means of detecting small primary NETs in the pancreas. It also offers the opportunity to undertake fine

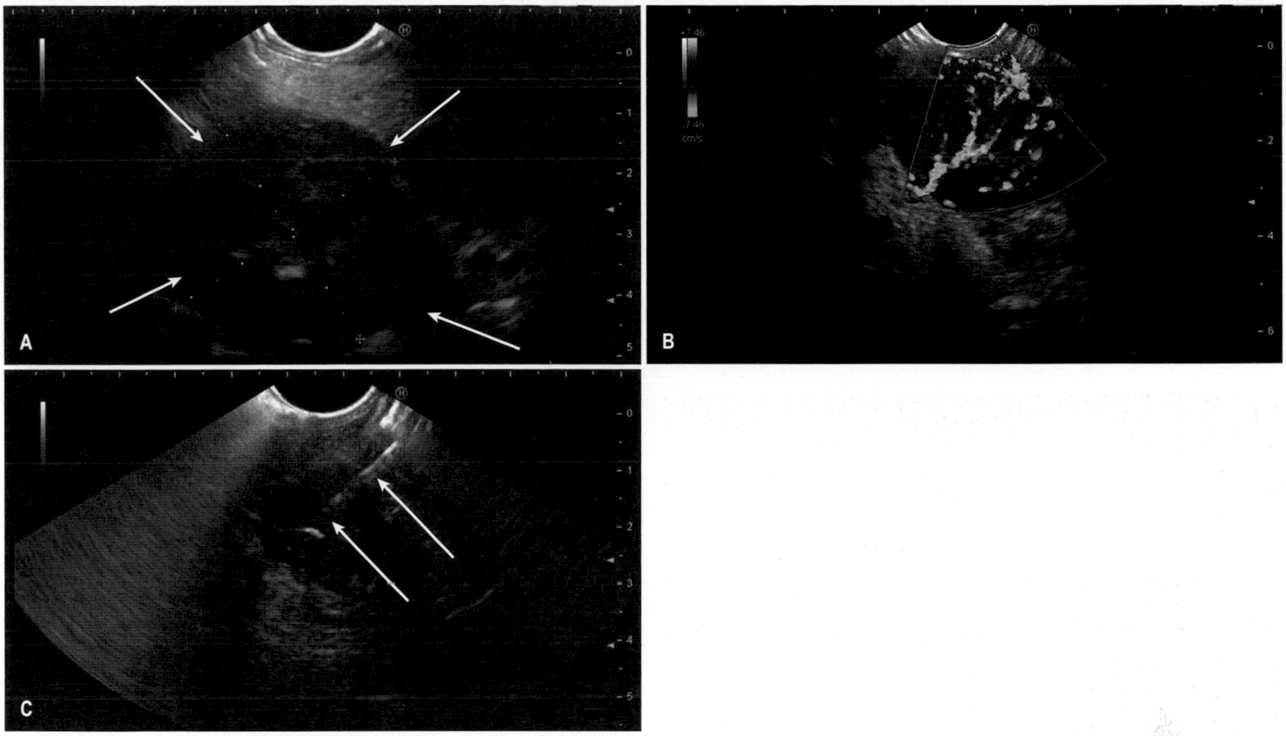

Figure 15.20 **Linear endoscopic ultrasound images. A.** A heterogeneous solid mass (arrowed) in the head of the pancreas with some central calcification. **B.** Doppler study demonstrating the vascularity of the lesion. **C.** Endoscopic ultrasound-guided fine needle aspiration (arrowed) of the same lesion, which confirmed the presence of a neuroendocrine tumour.

needle aspiration sampling of lesions, affording a cytopathological diagnosis ***(Fig. 15.20)***.

Management (see also pp. 638–639)

Treatment of pancreatic NETs requires a multidisciplinary approach and depends on the presence or absence of metastatic (usually hepatic) disease. Where possible, surgical resection of the primary lesion is the optimal management of pancreatic endocrine tumours, as it offers the only possible cure. The propensity of many endocrine tumours to metastasize early precludes cure in many cases. Debulking of the tumour, including liver metastases, is frequently carried out to facilitate systemic treatment.

Somatostatin analogues, such as octreotide and lanreotide, are used to control hormonal-related symptoms and also have a tumour-modulating effect. There is some evidence that somatostatin analogues combined with interferon-alfa also control tumour proliferation. Radionuclide therapy using somatostatin analogues has proven benefit in patients with tumours that express a high content of somatostatin receptors.

The ***chemotherapeutic agents***, streptozotocin, 5-fluorouracil and doxorubicin, produce partial remission in approximately 40% of cases. Recent advances include the introduction of tyrosine kinase and the mammalian target of rapamycin (mTOR) inhibitors. Pancreatic NETs show a very high degree of vascularization, as well as abundant production and secretion of growth factors. There is preliminary evidence of benefit from anti-angiogenesis therapy utilizing vascular endothelial growth factor (VEGF) antagonists.

In patients with extensive liver metastasis, occlusion of the arterial blood flow by hepatic arterial embolization may control hormone-related symptoms. In most cases, the tumours are slowly progressive and may allow a reasonable quality of life for many years.

Further reading

Ryan DP, Hong TS, Bardeesy N. Pancreatic adenocarcinoma. *N Engl J Med* 2014; 371:1039–1049.

Significant websites

http://www.bsg.org.uk *British Society of Gastroenterology guidelines.*
http://www.emedicine.medscape.com *Cholecystitis and cholelithiasis.*
http://www.gastrohep.com *Resources for gastroenterology, hepatology and endoscopy.*
http://www.gi.org *American College of Gastroenterology guidelines.*
http://www.nice.org.uk *Guidelines and service standards.*
http://www.ueg.eu/education *Online learning in gastroenterology.*

16 Haematological disease

Michael F Murphy, K John Pasi, Adam Mead

See your e-book for key learning points, clinical tips, drug tips, extra tables, interactive Figures, learning challenges and MCQs.

HAEMATOLOGY

General
Colour - Pale (e.g. anaemia)
- Plethoric (e.g. polycythaemia)
- Jaundice
Short of breath

Fundoscopy
Haemorrhage
(e.g. in thrombocytopenia)
Papilloedema
Enlarged veins

Purpura

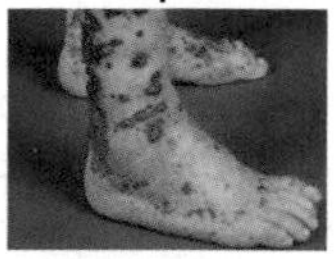

Petechiae

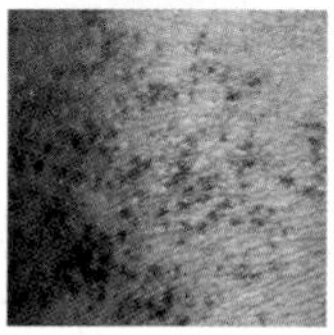

Skin
Purpura
Bruises
Petechiae
(thrombocytopenia)

Oedema

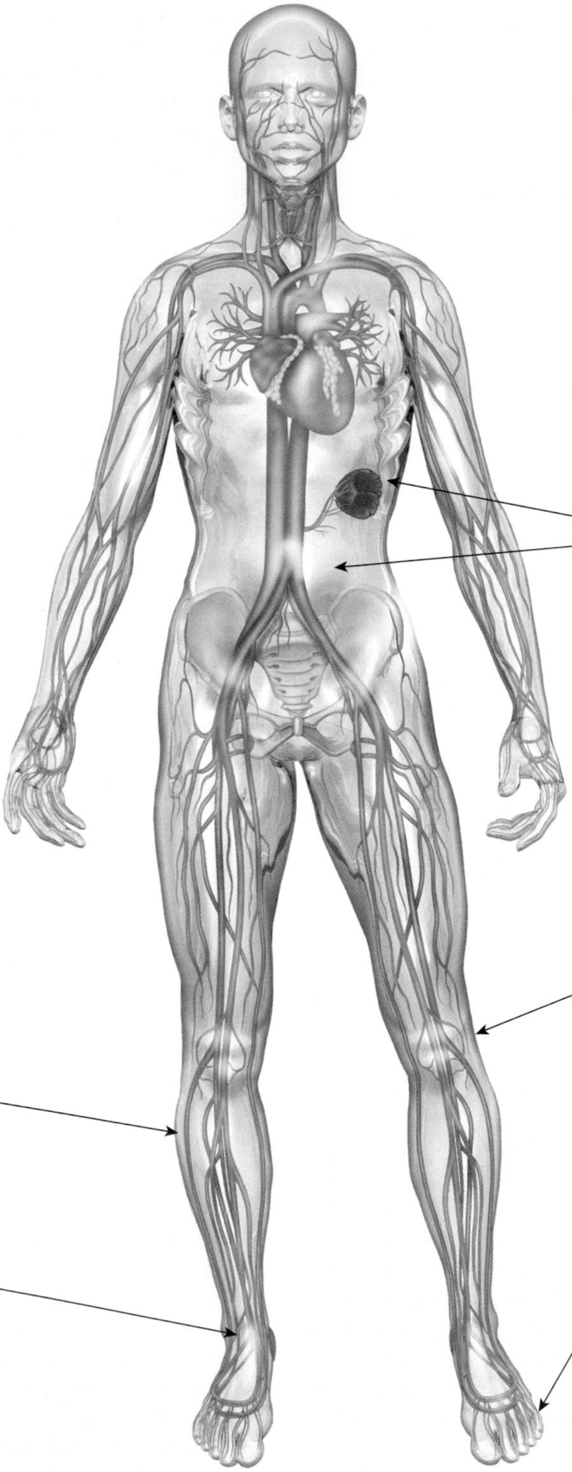

Angular stomatitis

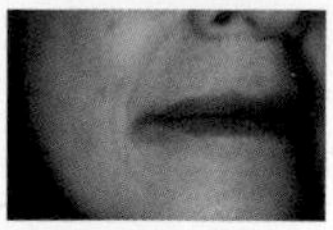

(From Epstein O 2008 Clinical Examination, 4th edn, with permission)

Mouth
Angular stomatitis
(iron deficiency)
Lips - telangiectasia
(hereditary haemorrhagic telangiectasia)
Tongue - Smooth/glossitis
Gum hypertrophy
(acute myeloid leukaemia)
Tonsils - enlarged

Abdomen
Hepatomegaly
Splenomegaly
Ascites
Masses
Inguinal lymph nodes

Hands
Koilonychia (iron deficiency)
Perfusion/circulation
Telangiectasia

Joints
Swelling
Deformity
Movements restricted

Check peripheral circulation
Toes - gangrene
(e.g. thrombocytosis)

Gangrene

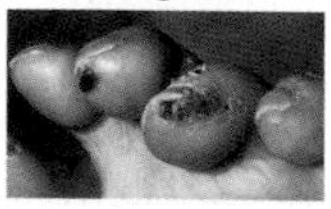

(From Epstein O 2008Clinical Examination, 4th Edn, Elsevier, with permission)

INTRODUCTION

Blood consists of:

- red cells
- white cells
- platelets
- plasma, in which the above elements are suspended.

Plasma is the liquid component of unclotted blood, which contains soluble fibrinogen. Serum is what remains after the formation of the fibrin clot.

The formation of blood cells (haemopoiesis)

The haemopoietic system includes the bone marrow, liver, spleen, lymph nodes and thymus. There is huge turnover of cells with the red cells surviving 120 days, platelets around 7 days but granulocytes only 7 hours. The production of as many as 10^{13} new myeloid cells (all blood cells except for lymphocytes) per day in the normal healthy state requires tight regulation according to the needs of the body.

Blood islands are formed in the yolk sac in the third week of gestation and produce primitive blood cells, which migrate to the liver and spleen. These organs are the chief sites of haemopoiesis from 6 weeks' to 7 months' gestation, when the bone marrow becomes the main source of blood cells. In childhood and adult life, the bone marrow is the only source of blood cells in a normal person.

At birth, haemopoiesis is present in the marrow of nearly every bone. As the child grows, the active red marrow is gradually replaced by fat (yellow marrow) so that haemopoiesis in the adult becomes confined to the central skeleton and the proximal ends of the long bones. Only if the demand for blood cells increases and persists do the areas of red marrow extend. Pathological processes interfering with normal haemopoiesis may result in resumption of haemopoietic activity in the liver and spleen, which is referred to as ***extramedullary haemopoiesis***.

All blood cells are derived from pluripotent stem cells. These stem cells have two key properties – the first is ***self-renewal***, i.e. the production of more stem cells, and the second is its ***proliferation and differentiation*** into progenitor cells, committed to one specific cell line. Pluripotential stem cells differentiate into mature blood cells through intermediate progenitor cells, which have lost the ability to self-renew but have high proliferative capacity. These progenitor cells can be broadly classified according to the blood cells that they are programmed to make ***(Fig. 16.1)***. For example, the common lymphoid progenitor (CLP) gives rise to T and B lymphoid cells; the former occurs in the thymus whereas B cell production primarily occurs in the bone marrow. The common myeloid progenitor gives rise to all non-lymphoid cells in the bone marrow via a series of intermediate progenitor cells. These cells cannot be recognized in bone marrow biopsies but are recognized by their ability to form colonies (reflecting their high proliferative capacity) when haemopoietic cells are immobilized in a soft gel matrix, the so-called colony-forming unit (CFU), which are named according to the type of cell they produce.

These haemopoietic stem and progenitor cells interact closely with a number of components contained within the specialized microenvironment of the bone marrow. This includes non-haemopoietic stromal cells, blood vessels and extracellular matrix, together creating a nurturing microenvironment for blood cell development. Central to this microenvironment are haemopoietic growth factors produced by stromal cells in the bone marrow and elsewhere, which are key regulators of blood cell production.

Haemopoietic growth factors

Haemopoietic growth factors are glycoproteins, which regulate the differentiation and proliferation of haemopoietic progenitor cells and the function of mature blood cells. Some growth factors are present in the circulation whereas other growth factors are produced within the bone marrow microenvironment by stromal cells such as fibroblasts, osteoblasts or endothelial cells or at sites of inflammation by activated T cells, monocytes and macrophages. Growth factors act on their respective cell surface receptors, expressed on haemopoietic cells at various stages of development, to maintain the haemopoietic progenitor cells and to stimulate increased production of one or more cell types in response to stresses such as blood loss and infection ***(Fig. 16.1)***.

These haemopoietic growth factors, including erythropoietin (EPO), interleukin (IL) 3, IL-6, IL-7, IL-11, IL-12, β-catenin, stem cell factor (SCF, Steel factor or C-kit ligand) and Fms-like tyrosine kinase 3 (Flt3), act via their specific receptor on cell surfaces to stimulate downstream signalling within the cell, such as the cytoplasmic Janus kinase (JAK) pathway (see pp. 96–97). This, in turn, activates signalling cascades within the cell, ultimately altering gene expression in the cell nucleus, and thus influencing behaviour of the cell: for example, to promote proliferation. Colony-stimulating factors (CSFs; the prefix indicates the cell type – see ***Fig. 16.1***), as well as interleukins and EPO, regulate the lineage-committed progenitor cells.

Thrombopoietin (TPO) is produced in the kidneys, liver and certain bone marrow stromal cells, and acts to control platelet production, along with IL-6 and IL-11. In addition to these factors, which stimulate haemopoiesis, there are other factors that inhibit the process; these include tumour necrosis factor (TNF) and transforming growth factor beta (TGF-β).

Uses in treatment

Many growth factors have been produced by recombinant DNA techniques and are being used clinically. Examples include granulocyte-colony-stimulating factor (G-CSF), which is used to accelerate haemopoietic recovery after chemotherapy and haemopoietic cell transplantation, and erythropoietin, which is used to treat anaemia in patients with chronic kidney disease and in patients with certain blood cancers. Thrombopoietin receptor agonists are being used to treat patients with immune thrombocytopenic purpura.

Peripheral blood

Automated cell counters are used to measure the haemoglobin (Hb) concentration and the number and size of red cells, white cells and platelets ***(Box 16.1)***. Other indices can be derived from these values. A blood film is still an essential adjunct to the above, as definitive abnormalities of cells can be seen.

- ***The mean corpuscular volume (MCV)*** of red cells is a useful index and is used to classify anaemia (see p. 522).
- ***The red cell distribution width (RDW)*** is calculated by dividing the *standard deviation* of the red cell width by the *mean cell width* × 100. An elevated RDW suggests variation in red cell size, i.e. anisocytosis, and this is seen in iron deficiency. In β-thalassaemia trait, the RDW is usually normal.
- ***The white cell count (WCC)*** (or white blood count, WBC) gives the total number of circulating leucocytes, and many

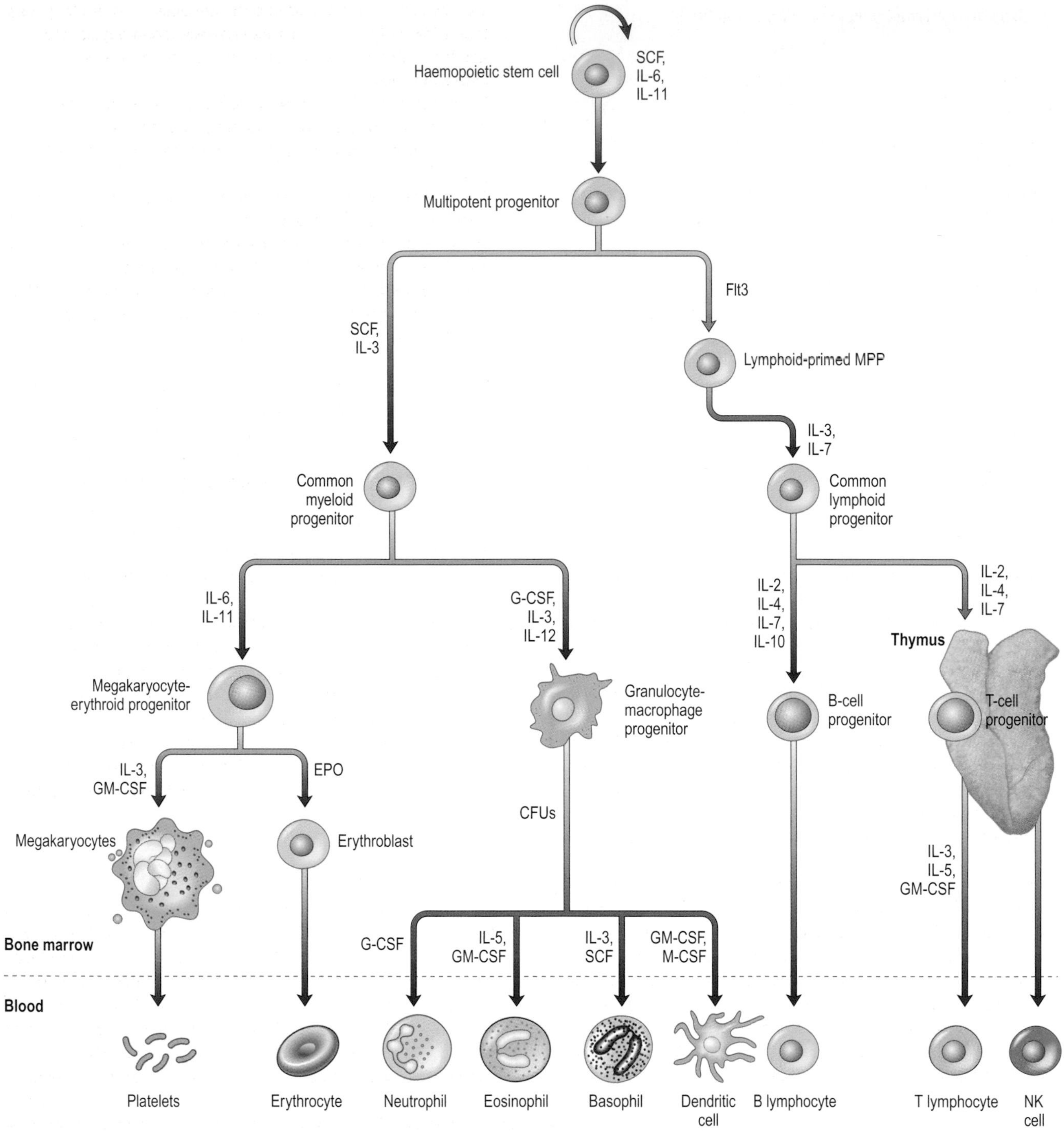

Figure 16.1 Roadmap of normal blood cell development. The process by which a haemopoietic stem cell develops into mature blood cells through a series of progenitor cell intermediates. The mature blood cells are platelets (P), erythrocytes (E), neutrophils (N), eosinophils (Eo), basophils (B), monocytes (**M**), B lymphocytes (**BL**) and T lymphocytes (**TL**). Some growth factors, which promote certain stages of blood cell development, are: **SCF** (stem cell factor), **TPO** (thrombopoietin), **G-CSF** (granulocyte-colony-stimulating factor), **EPO** (erythropoietin), **IL-7** (interleukin 7) and **Flt3** (Fms-like tyrosine kinase 3).

automated cell counters produce differential counts as well, specifically enumerating numbers of neutrophils, monocytes and lymphocytes.

- ***Reticulocytes*** are young red cells and usually comprise <2% of the red cells. The reticulocyte count gives a guide to the erythroid activity in the bone marrow. An increased count is seen with increased marrow maturity: for example, following haemorrhage or haemolysis, and during the response to treatment with a specific haematinic. A low count in the presence of anaemia indicates an inappropriate response by the bone marrow and may be seen in bone marrow failure (from whatever cause) or where there is a deficiency of a haematinic.
- ***Erythrocyte sedimentation rate*** **(*ESR*)** is the rate of fall of red cells in a column of blood and is a measure of the

Box 16.1 Normal values for peripheral blood

	Male	Female
Hb (g/L)	135–175	115–160
PCV (haematocrit; L/L)	0.4–0.54	0.37–0.47
RCC (10^{12}/L)	4.5–6.0	3.9–5.0
MCV (fL)	80–96	
MCH (pg)	27–32	
MCHC (g/L)	320–360	
RDW (%)	11–15	
WCC (10^9/L)	4.0–11.0	
Platelets (10^9/L)	150–400	
ESR (mm/h)	<20	
Reticulocytes	0.5–2.5% (50–100×10^9/L)	

ESR, erythrocyte sedimentation rate; Hb, haemoglobin; MCH, mean corpuscular haemoglobin; MCHC, mean corpuscular haemoglobin concentration; MCV, mean corpuscular volume of red cells; PCV, packed cell volume; RCC, red cell count; RDW, red blood cell distribution width; WCC, white cell count.

acute-phase response. The pathological process may be immunological, infective, ischaemic, malignant or traumatic. A raised ESR reflects an increase in the plasma concentration of large proteins, such as fibrinogen and immunoglobulins. These proteins cause rouleaux formation, with red cells clumping together and therefore falling more rapidly. The ESR increases with age, and is higher in females than in males.

- ***Plasma viscosity*** is a measurement used instead of the ESR in some laboratories. It is also dependent on the concentration of large molecules such as fibrinogen and immunoglobulins. It is not affected by the level of Hb.
- ***C-reactive protein* (*CRP*)** is a pentraxin, one of the proteins produced in the acute-phase response. It is synthesized exclusively in the liver and rises within 6 hours of an acute event. The CRP level rises with fever (possibly triggered by IL-1, IL-6, TNF-α and other cytokines), in inflammatory conditions and after trauma. It follows the clinical state of the patient much more rapidly than the ESR and is unaffected by the level of Hb, but it is less helpful than the ESR or plasma viscosity in monitoring chronic inflammatory diseases. The measurement of CRP is easy and quick to perform using an immunoassay that can be automated.

THE RED CELL

Erythropoiesis

Red cell precursors pass through several stages in the bone marrow. The earliest morphologically recognizable cells are pro-erythroblasts. Smaller erythroblasts result from cell divisions, and precursors at each stage progressively contain less RNA and more Hb in the cytoplasm. The nucleus becomes more condensed and is eventually lost from the late normoblast in the bone marrow when the cell becomes a reticulocyte.

- ***Reticulocytes*** contain residual ribosomal RNA and are still able to synthesize Hb. They remain in the marrow for about 1–2 days and are released into the circulation, where they lose their RNA and become mature red cells (erythrocytes) after another 1–2 days. Mature red cells are non-nucleated biconcave discs.
- Nucleated red cells (***late erythroblasts***) are not normally present in peripheral blood, but are present if there is extramedullary haemopoiesis and in some marrow disorders (see p. 563).
- About 10% of ***erythroblasts*** die in the bone marrow, even during normal erythropoiesis. Such ineffective erythropoiesis is substantially increased in some anaemias, such as thalassaemia major and megaloblastic anaemia.
- ***Erythropoietin*** is a hormone that controls erythropoiesis. The gene for erythropoietin is on chromosome 7 and codes for a heavily glycosylated polypeptide of 165 amino acids. Erythropoietin has a molecular weight of 30 400 and is produced in the peritubular cells in the kidneys (90%) and in the liver (10%). Its production is regulated mainly by tissue oxygen tension. Production is increased if there is hypoxia from whatever cause: for example, anaemia or cardiac or pulmonary disease. The erythropoietin gene is one of a number of genes that is regulated by the hypoxic sensor pathway. The 3′-flanking region of the erythropoietin gene has a hypoxic response element, which is necessary for the induction of transcription of the gene in hypoxic cells. Hypoxia-inducible factor 1 (HIF-1) is a transcription factor, which binds to the hypoxia response element and acts as a master regulator of several genes that are responsive to hypoxia. Erythropoietin stimulates an increase in the proportion of bone marrow precursor cells committed to erythropoiesis, and CFU-E are stimulated to proliferate and differentiate. Increased 'inappropriate' production of erythropoietin occurs in certain tumours such as renal cell carcinoma and from other causes (see ***Box 16.17***).

Haemoglobin synthesis

Haemoglobin performs the main functions of red cells, carrying O_2 to the tissues and returning CO_2 from the tissues to the lungs. Each normal adult Hb molecule (HbA) has a molecular weight of 68 000 and consists of two α and two β globin polypeptide chains ($\alpha_2\beta_2$). HbA comprises about 97% of the Hb in adults. Two other haemoglobin types, HbA_2 ($\alpha_2\delta_2$) and HbF ($\alpha_2\gamma_2$), are found in adults in small amounts (1.5–3.2% and <1%, respectively) (see pp. 534–535).

Haem synthesis occurs in the mitochondria of the developing red cell ***(Fig. 16.2)***. The major rate-limiting step is the conversion of glycine and succinic acid to δ-aminolaevulinic acid (ALA) by ALA synthase. Vitamin B_6 is a coenzyme for this reaction, which is inhibited by haem and stimulated by erythropoietin. Two molecules of δ-ALA condense to form a pyrrole ring (porphobilinogen). These rings are then grouped in fours to produce protoporphyrins and, with the addition of iron, haem is formed. Haem is then inserted into the globin chains to form a haemoglobin molecule. The structure of Hb is shown in ***Figure 16.3***.

Haemoglobin function

The biconcave shape of red cells provides a large surface area for the uptake and release of oxygen and carbon dioxide. Haemoglobin becomes saturated with oxygen in the pulmonary capillaries, where the partial pressure of oxygen is high and Hb has a high affinity for

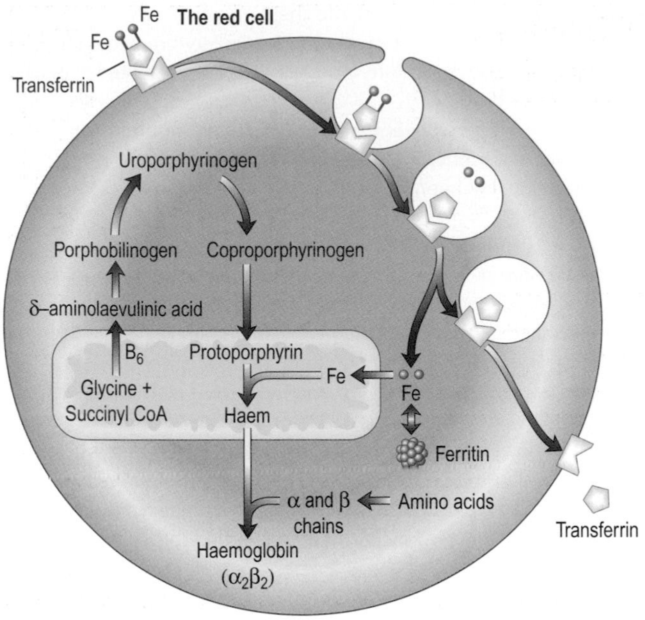

Figure 16.2 Haemoglobin synthesis. Transferrin attaches to a surface receptor on developing red cells. Iron is released and transported to the mitochondria, where it combines with protoporphyrin to form haem. Protoporphyrin itself is manufactured from glycine and succinyl CoA. Haem combines with α and β chains (formed on ribosomes) to make haemoglobin.

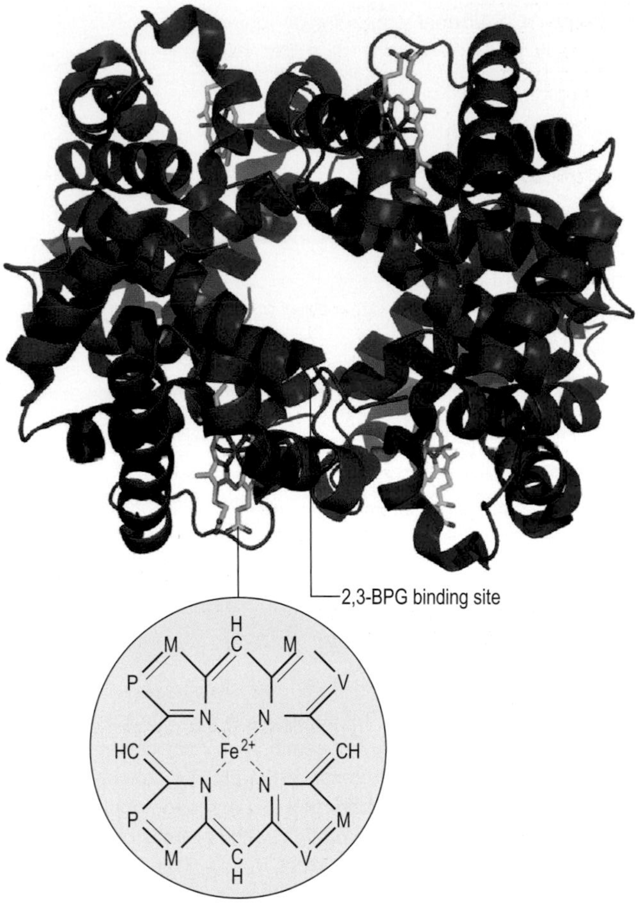

Figure 16.3 Model of the haemoglobin molecule showing α (red) and β (blue) chains. Bisphosphoglycerate (2,3-BPG) binds in the centre of the molecule and stabilizes the deoxygenated form by cross-linking the β chains (also see ***Fig. 16.4***). M, methyl; P, propionic acid; V, vinyl.

oxygen. Oxygen is released in the tissues, where the partial pressure of oxygen is low and Hb has a low affinity for oxygen.

In adult haemoglobin (Hb), a haem group is bound to each of the four globin chains; the haem group has a porphyrin ring with a ferrous atom, which can reversibly bind one oxygen molecule. The haemoglobin molecule exists in two conformations, Relaxed (R) and Taut (T), corresponding to oxyhaemoglobin and deoxyhaemoglobin, respectively ***(Fig. 16.4)***. The binding of one oxygen molecule to deoxyhaemoglobin increases the oxygen affinity of the remaining binding sites; this property is known as 'cooperativity' and is the reason for the sigmoid shape of the oxygen dissociation curve (see ***Figure 25.2***). The binding of oxygen can also be influenced by secondary effectors such as hydrogen ions, carbon dioxide and red cell 2,3-bisphosphoglycerate (2,3-BPG). Red cell metabolism produces 2,3-BPG from glycolysis, and the binding of 2,3-BPG stabilizes the T conformation, thus reducing its affinity for oxygen and increasing release of oxygen in the tissues. The P_{50} is the partial pressure of oxygen at which the haemoglobin is 50% saturated with oxygen. When the primary limitation to oxygen transport is in the periphery – for example, during heavy exercise or in anaemia – the P_{50} is increased to enhance oxygen unloading. Furthermore, hydrogen ions and carbon dioxide added to blood cause a reduction in the oxygen-binding affinity of haemoglobin (the Bohr effect), also helping the exchange of carbon dioxide and oxygen in the tissues. When the primary limitation is in the lungs – for example, in lung disease or high-altitude exposure – the P_{50} is reduced to enhance oxygen loading. A summary of normal red cell production and destruction is given in ***Figure 16.5***.

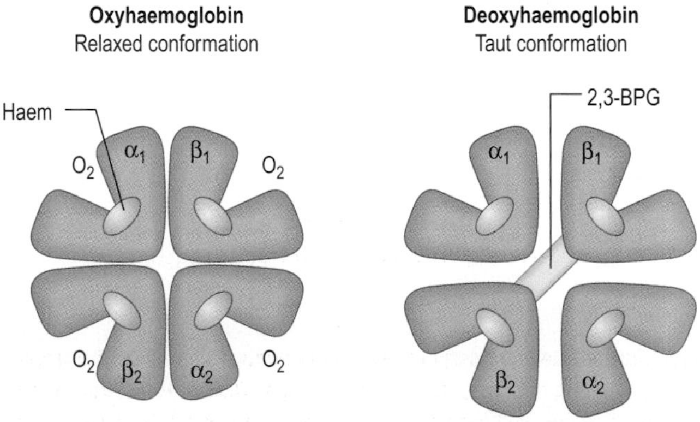

Figure 16.4 Oxygenated and deoxygenated haemoglobin molecule. The haemoglobin molecule is predominantly stabilized by α–β chain bonds rather than α–α and β–β chain bonds. The structure of the molecule changes during O_2 uptake and release. When O_2 is released, the β chains rotate on the $\alpha_1\beta_2$ and $\alpha_2\beta_1$ contacts, allowing the entry of 2,3-BPG, which causes a lower affinity of haemoglobin for O_2 and improved delivery of O_2 to the tissues.

ANAEMIA: AN INTRODUCTION

Anaemia is present when there is a decrease in Hb in the blood below the reference level for the age and sex of the individual

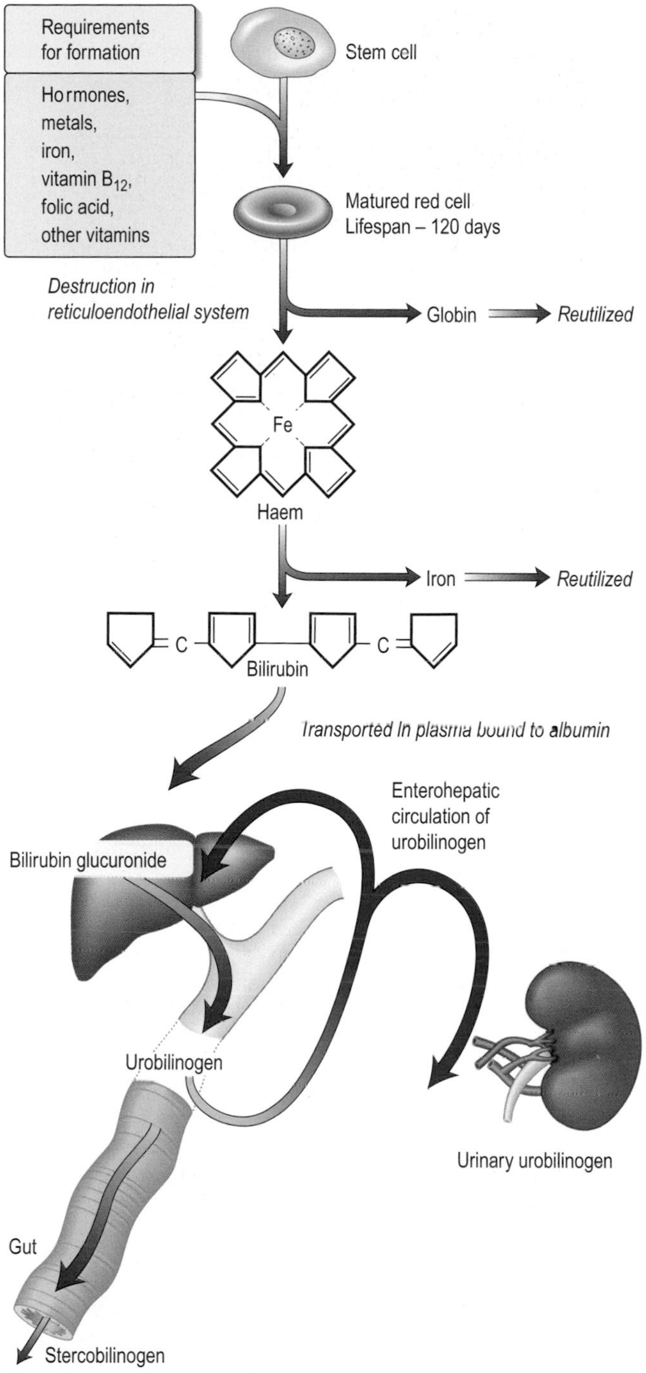

Figure 16.5 **Red cell production and breakdown.** (See p. 443.)

(see ***Box 16.1***). Alterations in the Hb may occur as a result of changes in the plasma volume, as shown in ***Figure 16.6***. A reduction in the plasma volume will lead to a spuriously high Hb; this is seen with dehydration and in the clinical condition of apparent polycythaemia (see p. 550). A raised plasma volume produces a spurious anaemia, even when combined with a small increase in red cell volume, as occurs in pregnancy.

The various types of anaemia, classified by MCV, are shown in ***Figure 16.7***. There are three major types:

- hypochromic microcytic with a low MCV
- normochromic normocytic with a normal MCV
- macrocytic with a high MCV.

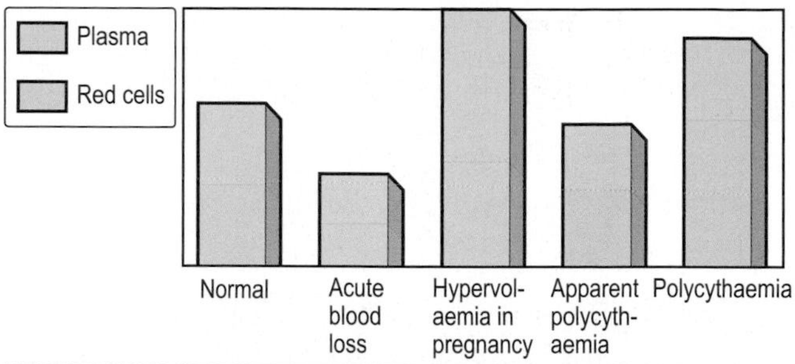

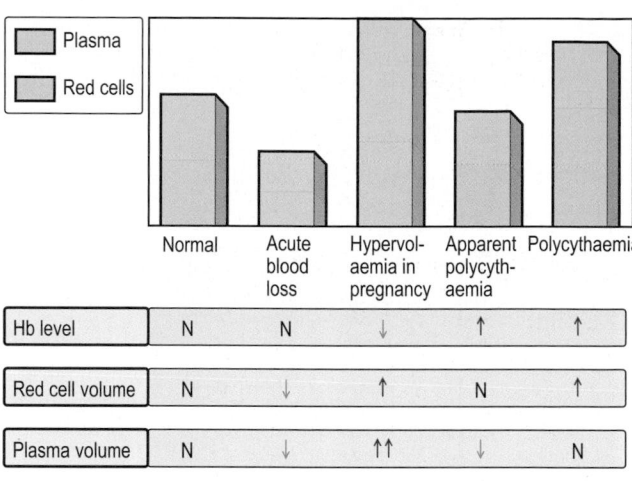

	Normal	Acute blood loss	Hypervolaemia in pregnancy	Apparent polycythaemia	Polycythaemia
Hb level	N	N	↓	↑	↑
Red cell volume	N	↓	↑	N	↑
Plasma volume	N	↓	↑↑	↓	N

Figure 16.6 **Alterations of haemoglobin in relation to plasma.**

Clinical features

Patients with anaemia may be asymptomatic. A slowly falling level of Hb allows for haemodynamic compensation and enhancement of the oxygen-carrying capacity of the blood. A rise in 2,3-BPG causes a shift of the oxygen dissociation curve to the right, so that oxygen is more readily given up to the tissues. Where blood loss is rapid, more severe symptoms will occur, particularly in elderly people.

Symptoms

These are all non-specific:

- fatigue, headaches and faintness
- breathlessness
- angina
- intermittent claudication
- palpitations.

Anaemia exacerbates cardiorespiratory problems especially in the elderly. For example, angina or intermittent claudication may be precipitated by anaemia. A good way to assess the effects of anaemia is to ask about breathlessness in relation to different levels of exercise (e.g. walking on the flat or climbing one flight of stairs).

Signs

- Pallor.
- Tachycardia.
- Systolic flow murmur.
- Cardiac failure.

Specific signs seen in the different types of anaemia will be discussed in the appropriate sections. Examples include:

- koilonychia – spoon-shaped nails seen in longstanding iron deficiency anaemia
- jaundice – found in haemolytic anaemia
- bone deformities – found in thalassaemia major
- leg ulcers – occur in association with sickle cell disease.

Anaemia is not a final diagnosis, and a cause should always be sought.

Investigations

Peripheral blood

A low Hb should always be evaluated with:

- The red cell indices.
- The WCC.

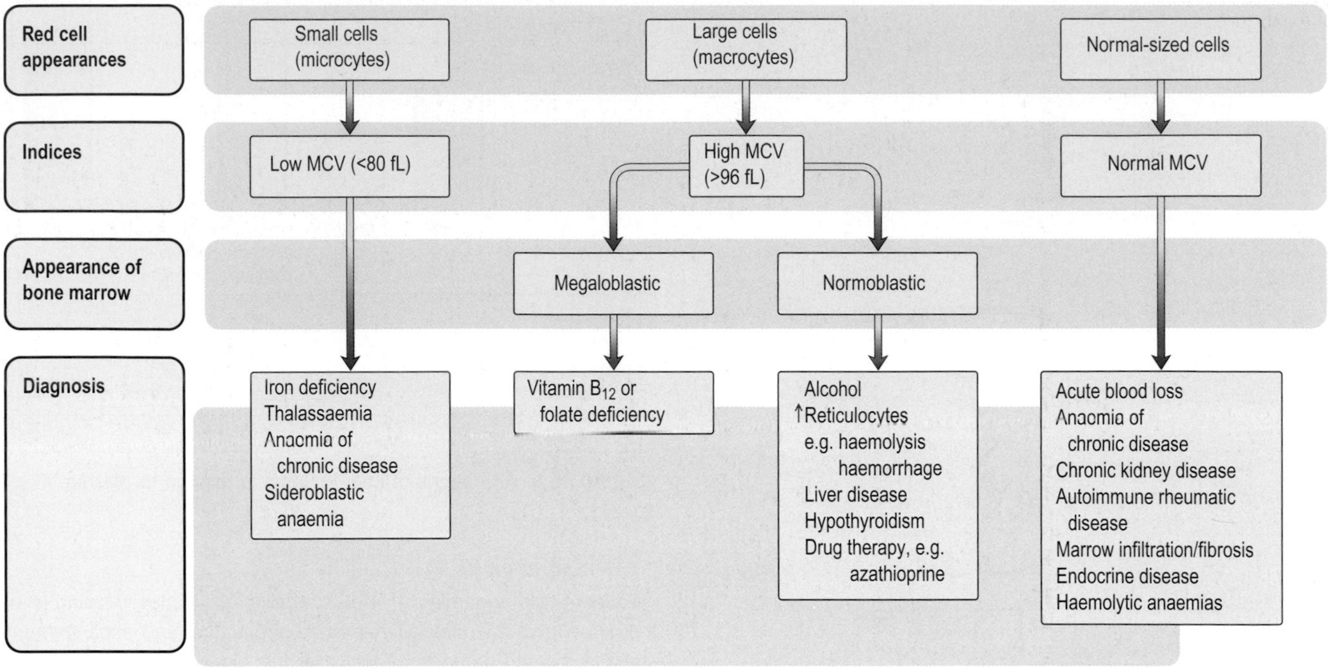

Figure 16.7 **Classification of anaemia.** MCV, mean corpuscular volume.

- The platelet count.
- The reticulocyte count (as this indicates marrow activity).
- The blood film, as abnormal red cell morphology (see ***Fig. 16.9***) may indicate the diagnosis. Where two populations of red cells are seen, the blood film is said to be dimorphic. This may, for example, be seen in patients with 'double deficiencies' (e.g. combined iron and folate deficiency in coeliac disease, or following treatment of anaemic patients with the appropriate haematinic).

Bone marrow

Techniques for obtaining bone marrow are shown in ***Box 16.2***.

Examination of the bone marrow is performed to investigate abnormalities found in the peripheral blood further ***(Box 16.2)***. Aspiration provides a film that can be examined by microscopy for the morphology of the developing haemopoietic cells. The trephine provides a core of bone that is processed as a histological specimen and allows an overall view of the bone marrow architecture, cellularity and presence/absence of abnormal infiltrates.

The following are assessed:

- cellularity of the marrow
- type of erythropoiesis (e.g. normoblastic or megaloblastic)
- cellularity of the various cell lines
- infiltration of the marrow, i.e. presence of non-haemopoietic cells such as cancer cells
- iron stores.

Special tests may be performed for further diagnosis: cytogenetic investigations, immunological investigations, cytochemical markers, biochemical analyses and microbiological culture.

Box 16.2 Techniques for obtaining bone marrow

The technique should be explained to the patient and consent obtained.

Aspiration

- Site – usually iliac crest
- Give local anaesthetic injection
- Use special bone marrow needle (e.g. Salah)
- Aspirate marrow
- Make smear with glass slide
- Stain with:
  - Romanowsky technique
  - Perls' reaction (acid ferrocyanide) for iron

Trephine

Indications include:

- 'Dry tap' obtained with aspiration
- Better assessment of cellularity, e.g. aplastic anaemia
- Better assessment of presence of infiltration or fibrosis

Technique

- Site – usually posterior iliac crest
- Give local anaesthetic injection
- Use special needle (e.g. Jamshidi – longer and wider than for aspiration)
- Obtain core of bone
- Fix in formalin; decalcify – this takes a few days
- Stain with:
  - Haematoxylin and eosin
  - Reticulin stain

MICROCYTIC ANAEMIA

Iron deficiency is the most common cause of anaemia in the world, affecting 30% of the world's population. This is because of the body's limited ability to absorb iron and the frequent loss of iron owing to haemorrhage. Although iron is abundant, most is in the insoluble ferric (Fe^{3+}) form, which has poor bioavailability. Ferrous (Fe^{2+}) iron is more readily absorbed.

The other causes of a microcytic hypochromic anaemia are anaemia of chronic disease, sideroblastic anaemia and thalassaemia. In thalassaemia (see pp. 535–538), there is a defect in globin synthesis, in contrast to the other three causes of microcytic anaemia, where the defect is in the synthesis of haem.

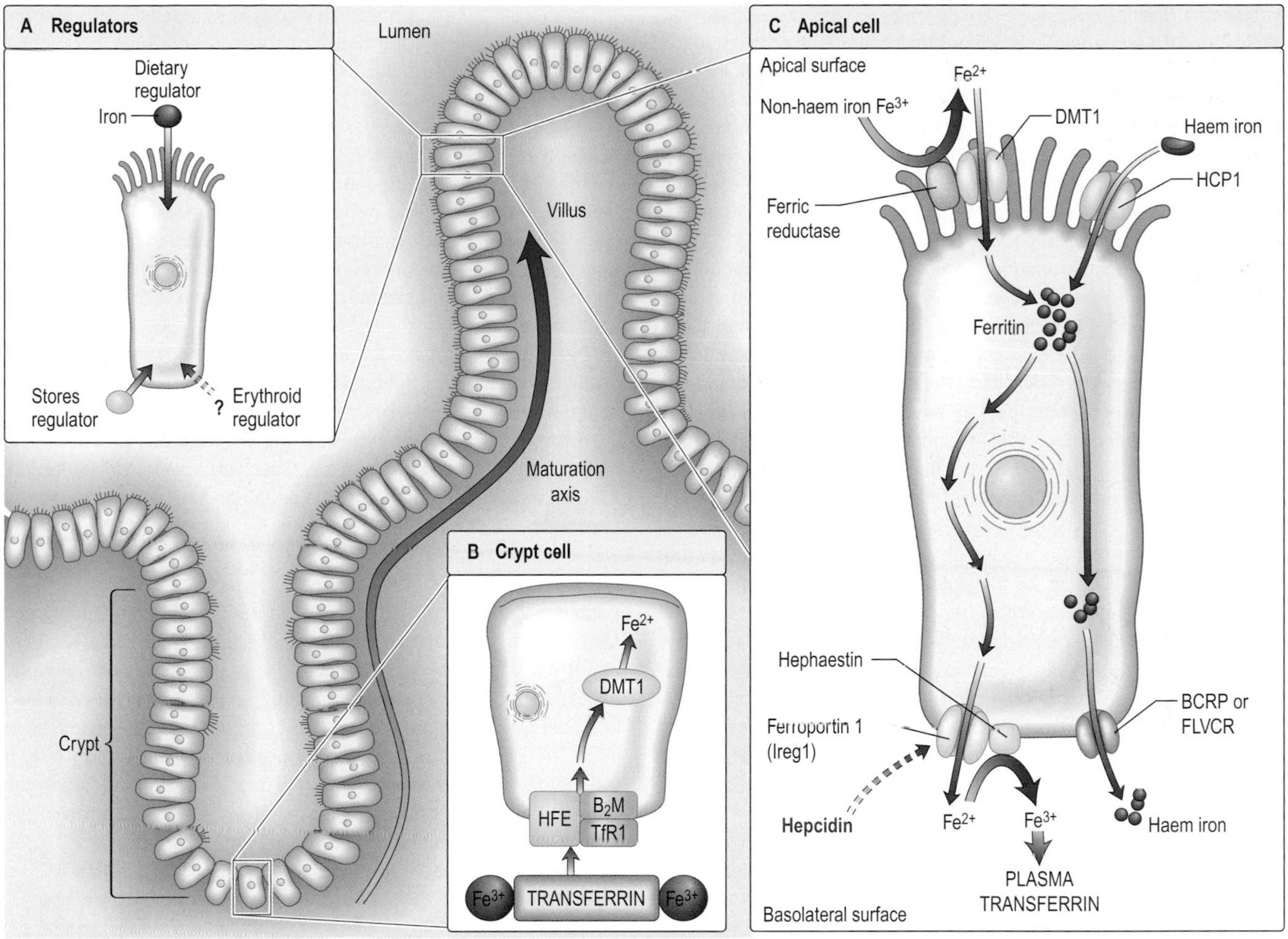

Figure 16.8 **Iron absorption.**
A. ***Regulation of the absorption of intestinal iron.*** The iron-absorbing cells of the duodenal epithelium originate in the intestinal crypts and migrate towards the tip of the villus as they differentiate (maturation axis). Absorption of intestinal iron is regulated by at least three independent mechanisms, although the **protein hepcidin is key.** First, iron absorption is influenced by recent dietary iron intake (*dietary regulator*). After a large dietary bolus, absorptive cells are resistant to iron uptake for several days. Second, iron absorption can be modulated considerably in response to body iron stores (*stores regulator*). Third, a signal communicates the state of bone marrow erythropoiesis to the intestine (*erythroid regulator*).
B. ***Duodenal crypt cells*** *sense body iron status through the binding of transferrin to the HFE/B_2M/TfR1 gene complex.* Cytosolic enzymes change the oxidative state of iron from ferric (Fe^{3+}) to ferrous (Fe^{2}+). A decrease in crypt cell iron concentration upregulates the divalent metal transporter (DMT1). This increases as crypt cells migrate up the villus and become mature absorptive cells.
C. ***Apical cell.*** Dietary iron is reduced from the ferric to the ferrous state by the brush border ferrireductase. ***DMT1*** facilitates iron absorption from the intestinal lumen. The export proteins, e.g. ferroportin 1 and hephaestin, transfer iron from the enterocyte into the circulation, depending on the *hepcidin* level. A second pathway absorbs intact haem iron into the circulation via BRCP and FLVCR.
BCRP, breast cancer resistant protein; B_2M, β_2-microglobulin; FLVCR, feline leukaemia virus subgroup C; HCP1, haem carrier protein-1; HFE, hereditary haemochromatosis gene; TfR1, transferrin receptor.

Iron

Dietary intake

The average daily diet in the UK contains 15–20 mg of iron, although normally only 10% of this is absorbed. Absorption may be increased to 20–30% in iron deficiency and pregnancy.

Non haem iron is mainly derived from cereals, which are commonly fortified with iron; it forms the main part of dietary iron. Haem iron is derived from haemoglobin and myoglobin in red or organ meats. Haem iron is better absorbed than non-haem iron, whose availability is more affected by other dietary constituents.

Absorption

Factors influencing iron and haem iron absorption ***(Fig. 16.8)*** are shown in ***Box 16.3***.

Box 16.3 Factors influencing iron absorption

- Haem iron is absorbed better than non-haem iron
- Ferrous iron is absorbed better than ferric iron
- Gastric acidity helps to keep iron in the ferrous state and soluble in the upper gut
- Formation of insoluble complexes with phytate or phosphate decreases iron absorption
- Iron absorption is increased with low iron stores and increased erythropoietic activity, e.g. bleeding, haemolysis, high altitude
- Absorption is decreased in iron overload, except in hereditary haemochromatosis, where it is increased

Dietary haem iron is more rapidly absorbed than non-haem iron derived from vegetables and grain. Most haem is absorbed in the proximal intestine, with absorptive capacity decreasing distally. The intestinal haem transporter HCP1 (haem carrier protein 1) has been identified and found to be highly expressed in the duodenum. It is upregulated by hypoxia and iron deficiency. Some haem iron may be reabsorbed intact into the circulation via the cell by two exporter proteins: BCRP (breast cancer resistant protein) and FLVCR (feline leukaemia virus subgroup C) ***(Fig. 16.8)***.

Non-haem iron absorption occurs primarily in the duodenum. Non-haem iron is dissolved in the low pH of the stomach and reduced from the ferric to the ferrous form by a brush border ferri-reductase. Cells in duodenal crypts are able to sense the body's iron requirements and retain this information as they mature into cells capable of absorbing iron at the tips of the villi. A protein, divalent metal transporter 1 (DMT1) or natural resistance-associated macrophage protein (NRAMP2), transports iron (and other metals) across the apical (luminal) surface of the mucosal cells in the small intestine.

Once inside the mucosal cell, iron may be transferred across the cell to reach the plasma, or be stored as ferritin; the body's iron status at the time the absorptive cell developed from the crypt cell is probably the crucial deciding factor. Iron stored as ferritin will be lost into the gut lumen when the mucosal cells are shed; this regulates iron balance. The mechanism of transport of iron across the basolateral surface of mucosal cells involves a transporter protein, ferroportin 1 (FPN 1) through its iron-responsive element (IRE). This transporter protein requires an accessory, multicopper protein, hephaestin ***(Fig. 16.8)***.

The body iron content is closely regulated by the control of iron absorption but there is no physiological mechanism for eliminating excess iron from the body. The key molecule regulating iron absorption is ***hepcidin***, a 25-amino acid peptide synthesized in the liver. Hepcidin acts by regulating the activity of the iron-exporting protein ferroportin by binding to ferroportin, causing its internalization and degradation, and thereby decreasing iron efflux from iron-exporting tissues into plasma. Therefore, high levels of hepcidin (occurring in inflammation states) via inflammatory cytokines, e.g. IL-6, will destroy ferroportin and limit iron absorption, and low levels of hepcidin (e.g. in anaemia, low iron stores, hypoxia) will encourage iron absorption. For example, in patients with haemochromatosis (see ***Fig. 14.27***), mutations in the genes *HFE*, *HJV* and *TfR2* will interrupt hepcidin synthesis. Therefore, in the intestinal cells, a deficiency of hepcidin would lead to less ferroportin being bound and thus more iron will be released into the plasma.

A longstanding mystery is why anaemias characterized by ineffective erythropoiesis, such as thalassaemia, are associated with excessive and inappropriate iron absorption. Preliminary evidence again suggests that the increased iron absorption in β-thalassaemia is mediated by downregulation of hepcidin and upregulation of ferroportin.

Transport in the blood

The normal serum iron level is about 13–32 μmol/L; there is a diurnal rhythm with higher levels in the morning. Iron is transported in the plasma bound to transferrin, a β-globulin that is synthesized in the liver. Each transferrin molecule binds two atoms of ferric iron and is normally one-third saturated. Most of the iron bound to transferrin comes from macrophages in the reticuloendothelial system and not from iron absorbed by the intestine. Transferrin-bound iron becomes attached by specific receptors to erythroblasts and reticulocytes in the marrow and the iron is removed (see ***Fig. 16.2***).

In an average adult male, 20 mg of iron, chiefly obtained from red cell breakdown in the macrophages of the reticuloendothelial system, is incorporated into Hb every day.

Iron stores

About two-thirds of the total body iron is in the circulation as haemoglobin (2.5–3 g in a normal adult man). Iron is stored in reticuloendothelial cells, hepatocytes and skeletal muscle cells (500–1500 mg). About two-thirds of this is stored as ferritin and one-third as haemosiderin in normal individuals. Small amounts of iron are also found in plasma (about 4 mg bound to transferrin), with some in myoglobin and enzymes.

Ferritin is a water-soluble complex of iron and protein. It is more easily mobilized than haemosiderin for Hb formation. It is present in small amounts in plasma.

Haemosiderin is an insoluble iron–protein complex found in macrophages in the bone marrow, liver and spleen. Unlike ferritin, it is visible by light microscopy in tissue sections and bone marrow films after staining by Perls' reaction.

Requirements

Each day, 0.5–1.0 mg of iron is lost in the faeces, urine and sweat. Menstruating women lose 30–40 mL of blood/month, an average of about 0.5–0.7 mg of iron/day. Blood loss through menstruation in excess of 100 mL will usually result in iron deficiency, as increased iron absorption from the gut cannot compensate for such losses of iron. The demand for iron also increases during growth (about 0.6 mg/day) and pregnancy (1–2 mg/day). In the normal adult, the iron content of the body remains relatively fixed. Increases in the body iron content (haemochromatosis) are classified into:

- hereditary haemochromatosis (see pp. 477–479), where a mutation in the *HFE* gene causes increased iron absorption
- secondary haemochromatosis (transfusion siderosis; see p. 537), due to iron overload in conditions treated by regular blood transfusion.

Iron deficiency

Iron deficiency anaemia develops when there is inadequate iron for haemoglobin synthesis. The causes are:

- blood loss
- increased demands such as growth and pregnancy
- decreased absorption (e.g. post-gastrectomy)
- poor intake.

Most iron deficiency is due to blood loss, usually from the uterus or gastrointestinal tract. Premenopausal women are in a state of precarious iron balance owing to menstruation. A common cause of iron deficiency worldwide is blood loss from the gastrointestinal tract resulting from parasites such as hookworm infestation. The poor quality of the diet, predominantly containing vegetables, also contributes to the high prevalence of iron deficiency in developing countries. Even in developed countries, iron deficiency is not uncommon in infancy, when iron intake is insufficient for the demands of growth. It is more prevalent in infants born prematurely or where the introduction of mixed feeding is delayed.

Clinical features

The symptoms of anaemia are described on page 521. The well-known clinical features of iron deficiency listed below are generally only seen in cases of very longstanding iron deficiency:

- brittle nails
- spoon-shaped nails (koilonychia)

- atrophy of the papillae of the tongue
- angular stomatitis
- brittle hair
- a syndrome of dysphagia and glossitis (Plummer–Vinson or Paterson–Brown–Kelly syndrome; see p. 373).

The diagnosis of iron deficiency anaemia relies on a clinical history, which should include questions about dietary intake, self-medication with non-steroidal anti-inflammatory drugs (NSAIDs; may give rise to gastrointestinal bleeding), and the presence of blood in the faeces (which may be a sign of haemorrhoids or carcinoma of the lower bowel). In women, a careful enquiry should be made about the duration of periods, the occurrence of clots and the number of sanitary towels or tampons used (normal 3–5 per day).

Investigations

- ***Blood count and film***. A characteristic blood film is shown in ***Figure 16.9***. The red cells are microcytic (MCV <80 fL) and hypochromic (mean corpuscular haemoglobin (MCH) <27 pg). There is poikilocytosis (variation in shape) and anisocytosis (variation in size).
- ***Serum iron and iron-binding capacity***. The serum iron falls and the total iron-binding capacity (TIBC) rises in iron deficiency compared with normal. Iron deficiency is regularly present when the transferrin saturation (i.e. serum iron divided by TIBC) falls below 19% ***(Box 16.4)***.

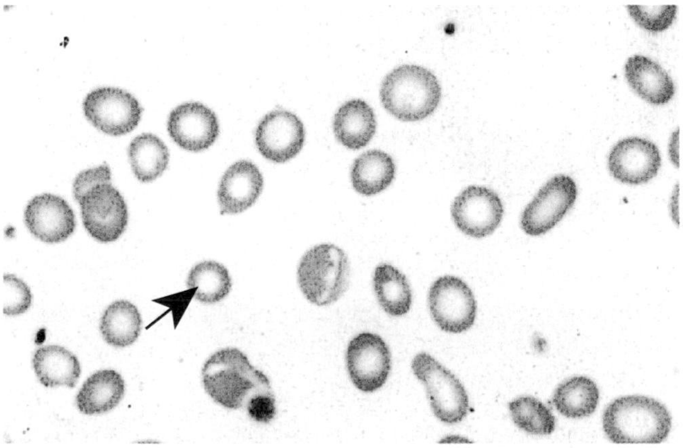

Figure 16.9 Hypochromic microcytic cells (arrow) on a blood film. Poikilocytosis (variation in shape) and anisocytosis (variation in size) are seen.

- ***Serum ferritin***. The level of serum ferritin reflects the amount of stored iron. The normal values for serum ferritin are 30–300 μg/L (11.6–144 nmol/L) in males and 15–200 μg/L (5.8–96 nmol/L) in females. In simple iron deficiency, a low serum ferritin confirms the diagnosis. However, ferritin is an acute-phase reactant, and levels increase in the presence of inflammatory or malignant diseases and also in the presence of liver damage. This can result in a normal ferritin level, even in the presence of iron deficiency. Very high levels of ferritin may be observed in hepatitis and in a rare disease, haemophagocytic lymphohistiocytosis (see p. 258).
- ***Serum soluble transferrin receptors***. The number of transferrin receptors increases in iron deficiency. The results of this immunoassay compare well with results from bone marrow aspiration at estimating iron stores. This assay can help to distinguish between iron deficiency and anaemia of chronic disease ***(Box 16.4)***, and may avoid the need for bone marrow examination, even in complex cases. It may sometimes be helpful in the investigation of complicated causes of anaemia.
- ***Other investigations***. These will be indicated by the clinical history and examination. Investigations of the gastrointestinal tract are often required to determine the cause of the iron deficiency (see p. 387).

Differential diagnosis

The presence of anaemia with microcytosis and hypochromia does not necessarily indicate iron deficiency. The most common of the other causes are thalassaemia, sideroblastic anaemia and anaemia of chronic disease, and in these disorders the iron stores are normal or increased. The differential diagnosis of microcytic anaemia is shown in ***Box 16.4***.

Management

The correct management of iron deficiency is to find and treat the underlying cause, and to give iron to correct the anaemia and replace iron stores. Patients with iron deficiency who are taking iron will increase their Hb level by approximately 10 g/L/week, unless of course other factors, such as bleeding, are present.

Oral iron is all that is required in most cases. The best preparation is ferrous sulphate (200 mg three times daily, a total of 180 mg ferrous iron), which is absorbed best when the patient is fasting. If the patient has side-effects such as nausea, diarrhoea or constipation, taking the tablets with food or reducing the dose using a preparation with less iron, such as ferrous gluconate (300 mg twice

Box 16.4 Microcytic anaemia: differential diagnosis

	Iron deficiency	Anaemia of chronic disease	Thalassaemia trait (α or β)	Sideroblastic anaemia
MCV	Reduced	Low normal or normal	Very low for degree of anaemia	Low in inherited type but often raised in acquired type
Serum iron	Reduced	Reduced	Normal	Raised
Serum TIBC	Raised	Reduced	Normal	Normal
Serum ferritin	Reduced	Normal or raised	Normal	Raised
Serum soluble transfer receptors	Increased	Normal	Normal or raised	Normal or raised
Iron in marrow	Absent	Present	Present	Present
Iron in erythroblasts	Absent	Absent or reduced	Present	Ring forms

MCV, mean corpuscular volume of red cells; TIBC, total iron binding capacity.

daily, only 70 mg ferrous iron), is all that is usually required to reduce the symptoms.

In developing countries, distribution of iron tablets and fortification of food are the main approaches for the alleviation of iron deficiency. However, iron supplementation programmes have been ineffective, probably mainly because of poor compliance.

Oral iron should be given for long enough to correct the Hb level and to replenish the iron stores; this can take 6 months. The most common causes of failure to respond to oral iron are:

- lack of compliance
- continuing haemorrhage
- incorrect diagnosis, e.g. thalassaemia trait.

These possibilities should be considered before parenteral (injected) iron is used. However, parenteral iron is required by occasional patients: for example, those who are intolerant to oral preparations, those with severe malabsorption and those with chronic disease (e.g. inflammatory bowel disease). Iron stores are replaced much faster with parenteral iron than with oral iron but the haematological response is no quicker. Parenteral iron can be given by slow intravenous infusion of low-molecular-weight iron dextran (test dose required), iron sucrose, ferric carboxymaltose or iron isomaltoside 1000; oral iron should be discontinued.

Anaemia of chronic disease

One of the most common types of anaemia, particularly in hospital patients, is the anaemia of chronic disease, occurring in individuals with chronic infections such as tuberculosis or chronic inflammatory disease such as Crohn's disease, rheumatoid arthritis, systemic lupus erythematosus (SLE), polymyalgia rheumatica and malignant disease. There is decreased release of iron from the bone marrow to developing erythroblasts, an inadequate erythropoietin response to the anaemia, and decreased red cell survival.

The exact mechanisms responsible for these effects are not clear but it seems likely that high levels of hepcidin expression play a key role (see above). Measurement of hepcidin levels is emerging as a useful test to help distinguish anaemia of chronic disease from iron deficiency anaemia.

The serum iron and the TIBC are low, and the serum ferritin is normal or raised because of the inflammatory process. The serum soluble transferrin receptor level is normal ***(Box 16.4)***. Stainable iron is present in the bone marrow but iron is not seen in the developing erythroblasts. Patients do not respond to iron therapy, and treatment is, in general, that of the underlying disorder. Recombinant erythropoietin therapy is used in the anaemia of renal disease (see p. 778), and occasionally in inflammatory disease (rheumatoid arthritis, inflammatory bowel disease).

Sideroblastic anaemia

Sideroblastic anaemias are inherited or acquired disorders characterized by a refractory anaemia, a variable number of hypochromic cells in the peripheral blood, and excess iron and ring sideroblasts in the bone marrow. The presence of ring sideroblasts is the diagnostic feature of sideroblastic anaemia. There is accumulation of iron in the mitochondria of erythroblasts owing to disordered haem synthesis, forming a ring of iron granules around the nucleus that can be seen with Perls' reaction. The blood film is often dimorphic; ineffective haem synthesis is responsible for the microcytic hypochromic cells. Sideroblastic anaemias can be inherited as an X-linked disease transmitted by females. Acquired causes include myelodysplasia, myeloproliferative disorders, myeloid leukaemia, drugs (e.g. isoniazid), alcohol misuse and lead toxicity. It can also occur in other disorders such as rheumatoid arthritis, carcinomas, and megaloblastic and haemolytic anaemias. A structural defect in δ-aminolaevulinic acid (ALA) synthase, the pyridoxine-dependent enzyme responsible for the first step in haem synthesis (see ***Fig. 16.2***), has been identified in one form of inherited sideroblastic anaemia. Primary acquired sideroblastic anaemia is one of the myelodysplastic syndromes (see pp. 551–552) and this is the cause of the vast majority of cases of sideroblastic anaemia in adults. Lead toxicity is described on page 77.

Management

Some patients respond when drugs or alcohol are withdrawn, if these are the causative agents. In occasional cases, there is a response to pyridoxine. Treatment with folic acid may be required to treat accompanying folate deficiency.

Further reading

Camaschella C. Iron-deficiency anemia. *N Engl J Med* 2015; 372:1832–1843.
Cullis JO. Diagnosis and management of anaemia of chronic disease. *Br J Haematol* 2011; 154:289–300.
DeLoughery TG. Microcytic anaemia. *N Engl J Med* 2014; 371:1324–1331.
Fleming RE, Ponka P. Iron overload in human disease. *N Engl J Med* 2012; 366:1548–1550.
Hentze MW, Muckenthaler MU, Galy B et al. Two to tango: regulation of mammalian iron absorption. *Cell* 2010; 142:24–38.

NORMOCYTIC ANAEMIA

Normocytic, normochromic anaemia is seen in anaemia of chronic disease, in some endocrine disorders (e.g. hypopituitarism, hypothyroidism and hypoadrenalism) and in some haematological disorders (e.g. aplastic anaemia and some haemolytic anaemias) (see ***Fig. 16.7***). In addition, this type of anaemia is seen acutely following blood loss.

MACROCYTIC ANAEMIAS

These can be divided into megaloblastic and non-megaloblastic types, depending on bone marrow findings.

Megaloblastic anaemia

Megaloblastic anaemia is characterized by the presence in the bone marrow of erythroblasts with delayed nuclear maturation because of defective DNA synthesis (megaloblasts). Megaloblasts are large and have large immature nuclei. The nuclear chromatin is more finely dispersed than normal and has an open, stippled appearance ***(Fig. 16.10)***. In addition, giant metamyelocytes are frequently seen in megaloblastic anaemia. These cells are about twice the size of normal cells and often have twisted nuclei. Megaloblastic changes occur in:

- vitamin B_{12} deficiency or abnormal vitamin B_{12} metabolism
- folic acid deficiency or abnormal folate metabolism
- other defects of DNA synthesis, such as congenital enzyme deficiencies in DNA synthesis (e.g. orotic aciduria), or those resulting from therapy with drugs interfering with DNA synthesis (e.g. hydroxycarbamide (hydroxyurea), azathioprine)
- myelodysplasia due to dyserythropoiesis.

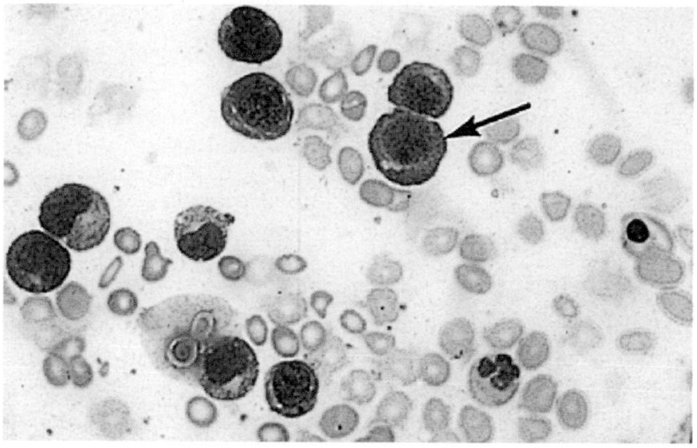

Figure 16.10 Megaloblasts (arrowed) in the bone marrow.

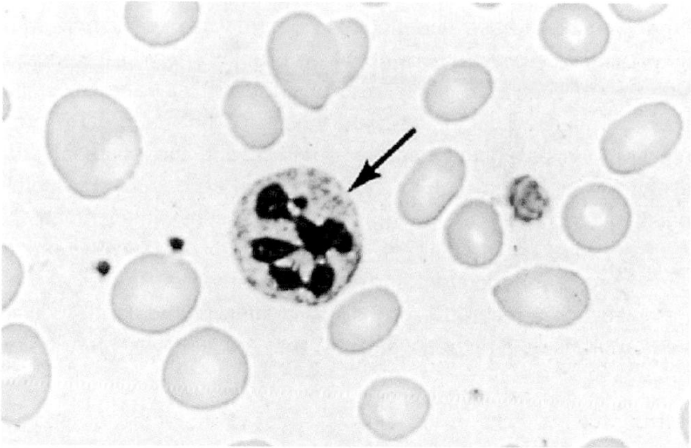

Figure 16.11 Macrocytes and a hypersegmented neutrophil (arrowed) on a peripheral blood film.

Haematological findings

- Anaemia may be present. The MCV is characteristically >96 fL unless there is a coexisting cause of microcytosis, in which case there may be a dimorphic picture with a normal/low average MCV.
- The peripheral blood film shows oval macrocytes with hypersegmented polymorphs with six or more lobes in the nucleus ***(Fig. 16.11)***.
- If severe, there may be leucopenia and thrombocytopenia.

Biochemical basis of megaloblastic anaemia

The key biochemical problem common to both vitamin B_{12} and folate deficiency is a block in DNA synthesis owing to an inability to methylate deoxyuridine monophosphate to deoxythymidine monophosphate, which is then used to build DNA ***(Fig. 16.12)***. The methyl group is supplied by the folate coenzyme, methylene tetrahydrofolate.

Deficiency of folate reduces the supply of this coenzyme; deficiency of vitamin B_{12} also reduces its supply by slowing the demethylation of methyltetrahydrofolate (methyl THF) and preventing cells receiving tetrahydrofolate for synthesis of methylene tetrahydrofolate polyglutamate.

Other congenital and acquired forms of megaloblastic anaemia are due to interference with purine or pyrimidine synthesis, causing an inhibition in DNA synthesis.

Vitamin B_{12} (cobalamin)

Vitamin B_{12} is synthesized by certain microorganisms, and humans are ultimately dependent on animal sources. It is found in meat,

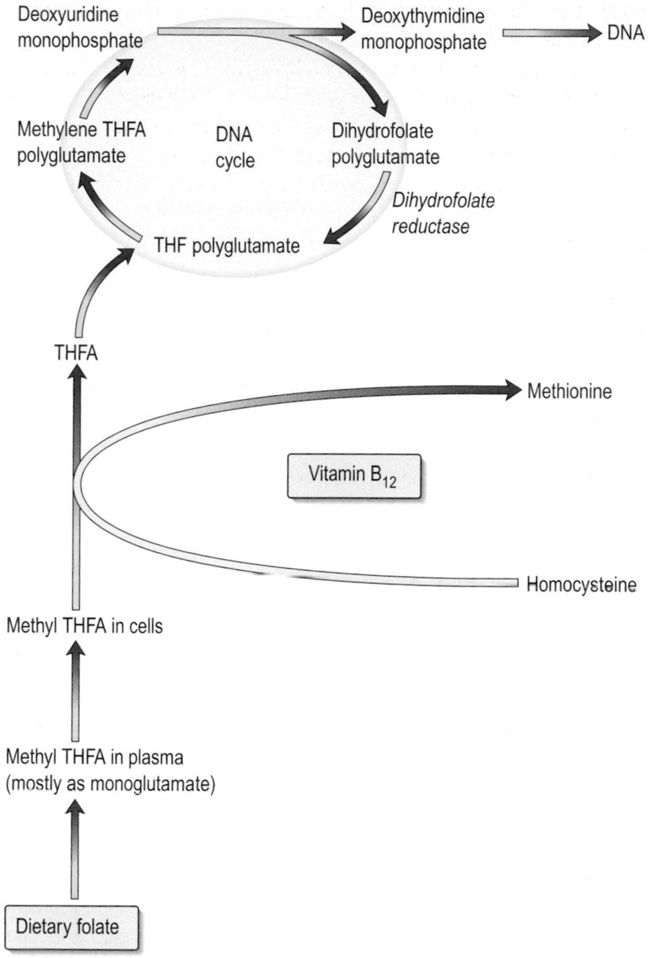

Figure 16.12 **Biochemical basis of megaloblastic anaemia.** The metabolic relationship between vitamin B_{12} and folate, and their role in DNA synthesis. THFA, tetrahydrofolate.

fish, eggs and milk, but not in plants. Vitamin B_{12} is not usually destroyed by cooking. The average daily diet contains 5–30 μg of vitamin B_{12}, of which 2–3 μg is absorbed. The average adult stores some 2–3 mg, mainly in the liver, and it may take 2 years or more after absorptive failure before vitamin B_{12} deficiency develops, as the daily losses are small (1–2 μg).

Vitamin B_{12} consists of a small group of compounds, the cobalamins, which are composed of a planar group with a central cobalt atom (corrin ring) and a nucleotide set at right angles. Vitamin B_{12} was first crystallized as cyanocobalamin, but the main natural cobalamins have deoxyadenosyl-, methyl- and hydroxocobalamin groups attached to the cobalt atom. Deoxyadenosylcobalamin is a coenzyme for the conversion of methylmalonyl CoA to succinyl CoA. Measurement of methylmalonic acid was used as a test for vitamin B_{12} deficiency but it is no longer carried out routinely.

Absorption and transport

Vitamin B_{12} is liberated from protein complexes in food by gastric enzymes and then binds to a vitamin B_{12}-binding protein ('R' binder), which is related to plasma transcobalamin I (TCI) and is derived from saliva. Vitamin B_{12} is released from the 'R' binder by pancreatic enzymes and then becomes bound to intrinsic factor.

Box 16.5 Vitamin B_{12} deficiency and abnormal B_{12} utilization: further causes[a]

Low dietary intake
- Veganism

Impaired absorption
Stomach
- Pernicious anaemia
- Gastrectomy
- Congenital deficiency of intrinsic factor

Small bowel
- Ileal disease or resection
- Bacterial overgrowth
- Tropical sprue
- Fish tapeworm (*Diphyllobothrium latum*)

Abnormal utilization
- Congenital transcobalamin II deficiency
- Nitrous oxide (inactivates B_{12})

[a]*See text.*

Intrinsic factor is a glycoprotein with a molecular weight of 45 000. It is secreted by gastric parietal cells along with H^+ ions. It combines with vitamin B_{12} and carries it to a specific receptor on the surface of the mucosa of the ileum, cubilin. Vitamin B_{12} enters the ileal cells and intrinsic factor remains in the lumen and is excreted. Vitamin B_{12} is transported from the enterocytes to the bone marrow and other tissues by the glycoprotein transcobalamin II (TCII). Vitamin B_{12} bound to TCII is known as holotranscobalamin or 'active B_{12}', as this is the form of vitamin B_{12} that is taken up by cells. Although TCII is the essential carrier protein for vitamin B_{12}, the amount of B_{12} on TCII is low. Vitamin B_{12} in plasma is mainly bound to TCI (70–90%). About 1% of an oral dose of B_{12} is absorbed 'passively' without the need for intrinsic factor.

Vitamin B_{12} deficiency

There are a number of causes of B_{12} deficiency and abnormal B_{12} metabolism ***(Box 16.5)***. The most common cause of vitamin B_{12} deficiency in adults is pernicious anaemia. Malabsorption of vitamin B_{12} because of pancreatitis, coeliac disease or treatment with metformin is mild and does not usually result in significant vitamin B_{12} deficiency.

Pernicious anaemia

Pernicious anaemia (PA) is an autoimmune disorder in which there is atrophic gastritis with loss of parietal cells in the gastric mucosa and consequent failure of intrinsic factor production and vitamin B_{12} malabsorption.

Pathogenesis

This disease is common in the elderly, about 1 in 8000 of the population aged over 60 years being affected in the UK. It can be seen in all races and is more common in females than males.

There is an association with other autoimmune diseases, particularly thyroid disease, Addison's disease and vitiligo. Approximately 50% of all patients with PA have thyroid antibodies. There is a higher incidence of gastric carcinoma with PA (1–3%) than in the general population.

Parietal cell antibodies are present in the serum in 90% of patients with PA – and also in 10% of normal individuals. Conversely, intrinsic factor antibodies, although found in only 50% of patients with PA, are specific for this diagnosis.

Pathology

Autoimmune gastritis (see pp. 377–378) affecting the fundus is present, with plasma cell and lymphoid infiltration. The parietal and chief cells are replaced by mucin-secreting cells. There is achlorhydria and absent secretion of intrinsic factor. The histological abnormality can be improved by corticosteroid therapy, which supports an autoimmune basis for the disease.

Clinical features

The onset of PA is insidious, with progressively increasing symptoms of anaemia. Patients are sometimes said to have a lemon-yellow colour owing to a combination of pallor and mild jaundice, caused by excess breakdown of haemoglobin. A red, sore tongue (glossitis) and angular stomatitis are sometimes present.

The neurological changes, if left untreated for a long time, can be irreversible. These neurological abnormalities occur only with very low levels of serum B_{12} (<60 ng/L or 50 pmol/L) and occasionally are seen in patients who are not clinically anaemic. The classical neurological features are those of a polyneuropathy progressively involving the peripheral nerves and the posterior and eventually the lateral columns of the spinal cord (subacute combined degeneration; see p. 886). Patients present with symmetrical paraesthesiae in the fingers and toes, early loss of vibration sense and proprioception, and progressive weakness and ataxia. Paraplegia may result. Dementia, psychiatric problems, hallucinations, delusions and optic atrophy may occur from vitamin B_{12} deficiency.

Investigations

- ***Haematological findings*** show the features of a megaloblastic anaemia, as described on page 527.
- ***Bone marrow*** shows the typical features of megaloblastic erythropoiesis (see ***Fig. 16.10***), although it is frequently not sampled in cases of straightforward macrocytic anaemia and a low serum vitamin B_{12}.
- ***Serum bilirubin*** and lactate dehydrogenase (LDH) may be raised as a result of ineffective erythropoiesis. Normally, a minor fraction of serum bilirubin results from premature breakdown of newly formed red cells in the bone marrow. In many megaloblastic anaemias, where the destruction of developing red cells is much increased, the serum bilirubin can be increased.
- ***Serum vitamin B_{12}*** is usually well below 160 ng/L, which is the lower end of the normal range. Serum vitamin B_{12} can be assayed using radioisotope dilution or immunological assays.
- ***Holotranscobalamin*** is the 'active' fraction of cobalamin, and its measurement may be a better marker for vitamin B_{12} deficiency than serum vitamin B_{12}.
- ***Serum methylmalonic acid (MMA) and homocysteine (HC)*** are raised in B_{12} deficiency but testing is only recommended in complex cases, such as those where there is a strong suspicion of vitamin B_{12} deficiency but where the vitamin B_{12} level is normal.

Absorption tests

Vitamin B_{12} absorption tests are no longer performed in the UK, as radioactive B_{12} is not available.

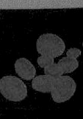

Gastrointestinal investigations

In PA, there is achlorhydria. Intubation studies can be performed to confirm this but are rarely carried out in routine practice. Endoscopy or barium meal examination of the stomach is performed only if gastric symptoms are present.

Differential diagnosis

Vitamin B_{12} deficiency must be differentiated from other causes of megaloblastic anaemia, principally folate deficiency, but usually this is quite clear from the blood levels of these two vitamins.

PA should be distinguished from other causes of vitamin B_{12} deficiency by testing for intrinsic factor antibodies ***(Box 16.5)***. Patients negative for intrinsic factor antibodies with no other cause of vitamin B_{12} deficiency may still have PA.

Management

See below.

Folic acid

Folic acid monoglutamate is not itself present in nature but occurs as polyglutamates. Folates are present in food as polyglutamates in the reduced dihydrofolate or tetrahydrofolate (THF) forms. Polyglutamates are broken down to monoglutamates in the upper gastrointestinal tract, and during the absorptive process these are converted to methyl THF monoglutamate, which is the main form in the serum. The methylation of homocysteine to methionine requires both methylcobalamin and methyl THF as coenzymes. This reaction is the first step in which methyl THF entering cells from the plasma is converted into folate polyglutamates. Intracellular polyglutamates are the active forms of folate and act as coenzymes in the transfer of single carbon units in amino acid metabolism and DNA synthesis ***(Fig. 16.12)***.

Dietary intake

Folate is found in green vegetables, such as spinach and broccoli, and offal, such as liver and kidney. Cooking causes a loss of 60–90% of the folate. The minimal daily requirement is about 100 µg.

Folate deficiency

The causes of folate deficiency are shown in ***Box 16.6***. The main cause is poor intake, which may occur alone or in combination with excessive utilization or malabsorption. The body's reserves of folate are about 10 mg. On a deficient diet, folate deficiency develops over the course of about 4 months, but folate deficiency may develop rapidly in patients who have both a poor intake and excess utilization of folate (e.g. patients in intensive care units).

Folic acid supplements at the time of conception and in the first 12 weeks of pregnancy reduce the incidence of neural tube defects. In the USA and Canada, mandatory fortification of grain products, such as bread, flour and rice, has substantially improved folate status and has been associated with a significant fall in neural tube defects. There is controversy about the role of folate supplementation in the reduction of cardiovascular and cerebrovascular disease by lowering homocysteine levels.

Clinical features

Patients with folate deficiency may be asymptomatic or may present with symptoms of anaemia or of the underlying cause. Glossitis can occur. Unlike with B_{12} deficiency, neuropathy does not occur.

? Box 16.6 Causes of folate deficiency

Nutritional (major cause)

Poor intake

- Old age
- Poor social conditions
- Starvation
- Alcohol excess (also causes impaired utilization)

Poor intake due to anorexia

- Gastrointestinal disease, e.g. partial gastrectomy, coeliac disease, Crohn's disease
- Cancer

Antifolate drugs

- Anticonvulsants:
  - Phenytoin
  - Primidone
- Methotrexate
- Pyrimethamine
- Trimethoprim

Excess utilization

Physiological

- Pregnancy
- Lactation
- Prematurity

Pathological

- Haematological disease with excess red cell production, e.g. haemolysis
- Malignant disease with increased cell turnover
- Inflammatory disease
- Metabolic disease, e.g. homocystinuria
- Haemodialysis or peritoneal dialysis

Malabsorption

- Occurs in small bowel disease, but the effect is minor compared with that of anorexia

Investigations

The haematological findings are those of a megaloblastic anaemia, as discussed on page 527.

Blood measurements

Serum folate reflects recent folate status and intake. It is usually measured using immunological methods; a level below 3 µg/L (7 nmol/L) is indicative of folate deficiency. The amount of folate in the red cells is a measure of tissue folate over the lifetime of red cells; a level below 150 µg/L (340 nmol/L) is consistent with folate deficiency, but measurement of the serum folate is usually sufficient to diagnose folate deficiency.

Further investigations

In many cases of folate deficiency, the cause is not obvious from the clinical picture or dietary history. Occult gastrointestinal disease should then be suspected and appropriate investigations, such as small bowel biopsy, should be performed.

Management and prevention of megaloblastic anaemia

Treatment depends on the type of deficiency. Blood transfusion is not usually indicated in chronic anaemia; indeed, it can be dangerous to transfuse elderly patients, as heart failure may be precipitated. Folic acid may produce a haematological response in vitamin B_{12} deficiency but may aggravate the neuropathy. Large doses of folic acid alone should not be used to treat megaloblastic anaemia unless the serum vitamin B_{12} level is known to be normal. In severely ill patients, it may be necessary to treat with both folic acid and vitamin B_{12} while awaiting serum levels.

Management of vitamin B_{12} deficiency

Hydroxocobalamin 1000 µg can be given intramuscularly to a total of 5–6 mg over the course of 2 weeks; 1000 µg is then necessary every 3 months for the rest of the patient's life.

Clinical improvement may occur within 48 hours and a reticulocytosis can be seen some 2–3 days after starting therapy, peaking at 5–7 days. Improvement of the polyneuropathy may occur over 6–12 months but longstanding spinal cord damage is irreversible. Hypokalaemia can occur and, if severe, supplements should be given. Iron deficiency often develops in the first few weeks of therapy. Hyperuricaemia also occurs but clinical gout is uncommon. In patients who have had a total gastrectomy or an ileal resection, vitamin B_{12} should be monitored; if levels are low, prophylactic vitamin B_{12} should be given. Vegans may require oral B_{12} supplements.

Oral treatment with vitamin B_{12} can also be used in patients but good compliance with treatment is required.

Management of folate deficiency

Folate deficiency can be corrected by giving 5 mg of folic acid daily; the same haematological response occurs as is seen after treatment of vitamin B_{12} deficiency. Treatment should be given for about 4 months to replace body stores. Any underlying cause, such as coeliac disease, should be treated.

Prophylactic folic acid (400 µg daily) is recommended for all women planning a pregnancy and in early pregnancy to reduce neural tube defects.

Women who have had a child with a neural tube defect should take 5 mg folic acid daily before and during a subsequent pregnancy.

Prophylactic folic acid, in a dose of 5 mg daily or weekly, is also given in chronic haematological disorders where there is rapid cell turnover and to patients undergoing renal dialysis.

Macrocytosis without megaloblastic changes

A raised MCV with macrocytosis on the peripheral blood film can occur with a normoblastic rather than a megaloblastic bone marrow.

A common ***physiological*** cause of macrocytosis is pregnancy. Macrocytosis may also occur in the newborn. Common ***pathological*** causes are:

- alcohol excess
- liver disease
- reticulocytosis (e.g. due to haemolysis)
- hypothyroidism
- some haematological disorders (e.g. aplastic anaemia, myelodysplasia, pure red cell aplasia, multiple myeloma)
- drugs (e.g. hydroxycarbamide, azathioprine)
- cold agglutinins due to autoagglutination of red cells (see p. 544) (the MCV decreases to normal with warming of the sample to 37°C).

In all these conditions, normal levels of vitamin B_{12} and folate will be found. The exact mechanisms in each case are uncertain, but in some there is increased lipid deposition in the red cell membrane.

An increased number of reticulocytes also leads to a raised MCV because they are large cells.

High alcohol consumption is a frequent cause of a raised MCV, and in such patients the MCV can be used as a surrogate marker for monitoring excessive alcohol consumption. A full-blown megaloblastic anaemia can also occur in people who use alcohol to excess; this is due to a toxic effect of alcohol on erythropoiesis and/or to dietary folate deficiency.

Further reading

British Committee for Standards in Haematology. Guidelines for the diagnosis and treatment of cobalamin and folate disorders. *Br J Haematol* 2014; 166:496–513.

ANAEMIA DUE TO MARROW FAILURE (APLASTIC ANAEMIA)

Aplastic anaemia is defined as pancytopenia with hypocellularity (aplasia) of the bone marrow; there are no leukaemic, cancerous or other abnormal cells in the peripheral blood or bone marrow. It is usually an acquired condition but may rarely be inherited.

Aplastic anaemia is due to a reduction in the number of pluripotential stem cells (see ***Fig. 16.1***), together with a fault in those remaining or an immune reaction against them so that they are unable to repopulate the bone marrow. Failure of only one cell line may also occur, resulting in isolated deficiencies such as the absence of red cell precursors in pure red cell aplasia. Evolution to myelodysplasia, paroxysmal nocturnal haemoglobinuria (PNH) or acute myeloid leukaemia occurs in some cases, probably owing to the emergence of an abnormal clone of haemopoietic cells.

Aetiology

A list of causes of aplasia is given in ***Box 16.7***. Immune mechanisms are probably responsible for most cases of idiopathic acquired aplastic anaemia and play a part in at least the persistence of many secondary cases. Activated cytotoxic T cells in blood and bone marrow are responsible for the bone marrow failure.

Many drugs may cause marrow aplasia, including cytotoxic drugs such as busulfan and doxorubicin, which are expected to cause transient aplasia as a consequence of their therapeutic use. However, some individuals develop aplasia due to sensitivity to non-cytotoxic drugs such as chloramphenicol, gold, carbimazole, chlorpromazine, phenytoin, ribavirin, tolbutamide, NSAIDs, and many others that have been reported to cause occasional cases of aplasia.

Inherited aplastic anaemias are rare. Multiple gene mutations have been identified. Several are tumour suppressor genes and have been seen in one-third of aplastic anaemias. Fanconi's anaemia is inherited as an autosomal recessive condition and is associated with skeletal, skin, eye, renal and central nervous system abnormalities. It usually presents between the ages of 5 and 10 years.

Clinical features

The clinical manifestations of marrow failure from any cause are anaemia, bleeding and infection. Bleeding is often the predominant

Box 16.7 Causes of aplastic anaemia

Primary
- Inherited, e.g. Fanconi's anaemia
- Idiopathic acquired (67% of cases)

Secondary
- Chemicals, e.g. benzene, toluene, glue sniffing
- Drugs:
  - e.g. Chemotherapeutic
  - Antibiotics, e.g. chloramphenicol, gold, penicillamine, phenytoin, carbamazepine, carbimazole, azathioprine
- Insecticides
- Ionizing radiation
- Infections:
  - Viral, e.g. hepatitis, Epstein–Barr virus, human immunodeficiency virus (HIV), erythrovirus
  - Other, e.g. tuberculosis
- Paroxysmal nocturnal haemoglobinuria
- Miscellaneous, e.g. pregnancy

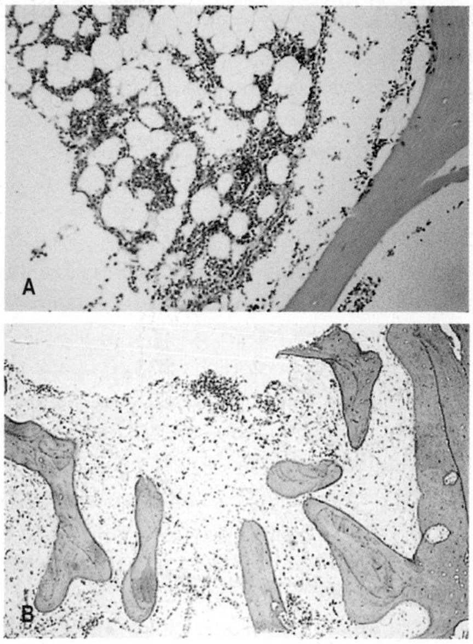

Figure 16.13 Bone marrow trephine biopsies in low-power view. **A.** Normal cellularity. **B.** Hypocellularity in aplastic anaemia.

Box 16.8 Causes of pancytopenia

- Aplastic anaemia (see *Box 16.7*)
- Drugs
- Megaloblastic anaemia
- Bone marrow infiltration or replacement:
  - Hodgkin's and non-Hodgkin's lymphoma
  - Acute leukaemia
  - Myeloma
  - Secondary carcinoma: myelofibrosis
- Hypersplenism
- Systemic lupus erythematosus
- Disseminated tuberculosis
- Paroxysmal nocturnal haemoglobinuria
- Overwhelming sepsis

initial presentation of aplastic anaemia with bruising and minimal trauma or blood blisters in the mouth. Physical findings include ecchymoses, bleeding gums and epistaxis. Mouth infections are common. Lymphadenopathy and hepatosplenomegaly are rare in aplastic anaemia.

Investigations

- Pancytopenia.
- The virtual absence of reticulocytes.
- A hypocellular or aplastic bone marrow with increased fat spaces *(Fig. 16.13)*.

Differential diagnosis

Aplastic anaemia must be differentiated from other causes of pancytopenia *(Box 16.8)*. A bone marrow trephine is essential for assessment of the bone marrow cellularity.

Management and prognosis

The treatment of aplastic anaemia depends on the underlying cause and the likelihood of spontaneous recovery of blood counts. Careful attention to supportive care is essential while awaiting bone marrow recovery and, in some cases, specific treatment can be used to accelerate marrow recovery.

The main danger is infection and stringent measures should be undertaken to avoid this (see also pp. 604–605). Any suspicion of infection in a severely neutropenic patient (neutrophil count of $<0.5\times10^9$/L) should lead to the immediate institution of broad-spectrum parenteral antibiotics. Supportive care, including transfusions of red cells and platelets, should be given as necessary. The cause of the aplastic anaemia must be eliminated if possible.

The course of aplastic anaemia can be variable, ranging from a rapid spontaneous remission to a persistent, increasingly severe pancytopenia, which may lead to death through haemorrhage or infection. The most reliable determinants for the prognosis are the number of neutrophils, reticulocytes and platelets, and the cellularity of the bone marrow.

A bad prognosis (i.e. severe aplastic anaemia) is associated with the presence of two of the following three features:

- neutrophil count of $<0.5\times10^9$/L
- platelet count of $<20\times10^9$/L
- reticulocyte count of $<40\times10^9$/L.

Haemopoietic stem cells are the treatment of choice for patients with severe aplastic anaemia under the age of 40 who have a human leucocyte antigen (HLA)-identical sibling donor, where it gives a 75–90% chance of long-term survival.

Immunosuppressive therapy is recommended for:

- patients with severe disease over the age of 40
- younger patients with severe disease who do not have an HLA-identical sibling donor
- patients who do not have severe disease but who are transfusion-dependent.

The standard immunosuppressive treatment is antithymocyte globulin (ATG) and ciclosporin, which results in response rates of 60–80% and 5-year survival rates of 75–85%.

Stem cell transplantation using matched unrelated donors is an option for patients under the age of 50 who have no matched sibling donor, and who have failed to respond to immunosuppression with ATG and ciclosporin; the results are improving (5-year survival of 65–73%). The main problems are graft rejection, graft-versus-host disease and viral infections.

Levels of haemopoietic growth factors (see *Fig. 16.1*) are normal or increased in most patients with aplastic anaemia, and are ineffective as primary treatment.

Steroids should not be used to treat severe aplastic anaemia except for serum sickness due to ATG. They are also used to treat children with congenital pure red cell aplasia (Diamond–Blackfan syndrome).

Adult pure red cell aplasia is associated with a thymoma in 5–15% of cases and thymectomy occasionally induces a remission. It may also be associated with autoimmune disease or be idiopathic. Steroids, cyclophosphamide, azathioprine and ciclosporin are effective treatments in some cases.

Further reading

British Committee for Standards in Haematology. Guidelines for the diagnosis and management of acquired aplastic anaemia. *Br J Haematol* 2009; 147:43–70.

HAEMOLYTIC ANAEMIAS: AN INTRODUCTION

Haemolytic anaemias are caused by increased destruction of red cells. The red cell normally survives about 120 days, but in haemolytic anaemias the red cell survival times are considerably shortened.

Breakdown of normal red cells occurs in the macrophages of the bone marrow, liver and spleen (see ***Fig. 16.5***).

Consequences of haemolysis (Fig. 16.14)

Shortening of red cell survival does not always cause anaemia, as there is a compensatory increase in red cell production by the bone marrow. If the red cell loss can be contained within the marrow's capacity for increased output, then a haemolytic state can exist without anaemia (***compensated haemolytic disease***). The bone marrow can increase its output by 6–8 times by increasing the proportion of cells committed to erythropoiesis (***erythroid hyperplasia***) and by expanding the volume of active marrow. In addition, immature red cells (***reticulocytes***) are released prematurely. These cells are larger than mature cells and stain with a light blue tinge on a peripheral blood film (the description of this appearance on the blood film is ***polychromasia***) due to the presence of residual ribosomal RNA. Reticulocytes may be counted accurately as a percentage of all red cells on a blood film using a supravital stain for residual RNA (e.g. new methylene blue).

Sites of haemolysis

Extravascular haemolysis

In most haemolytic conditions, red cell destruction is extravascular. The red cells are removed from the circulation by macrophages in the reticuloendothelial system, particularly the spleen.

Intravascular haemolysis

When red cells are rapidly destroyed within the circulation, haemoglobin is liberated. This is initially bound to plasma haptoglobins but these soon become saturated.

Excess free plasma haemoglobin is filtered by the renal glomerulus and enters the urine, although small amounts are reabsorbed by the renal tubules. In the renal tubular cell, haemoglobin is broken down and becomes deposited in the cells as ***haemosiderin***. This can be detected in the spun sediment of urine using Perls' reaction. Some of the free plasma haemoglobin is oxidized to ***methaemoglobin***, which dissociates into ***ferrihaem*** and globin. ***Plasma haemopexin*** binds ferrihaem, but if its binding capacity is exceeded, ferrihaem becomes attached to albumin, forming ***methaemalbumin***. On spectrophotometry of the plasma, methaemalbumin forms a characteristic band; this is the basis of ***Schumm's test***.

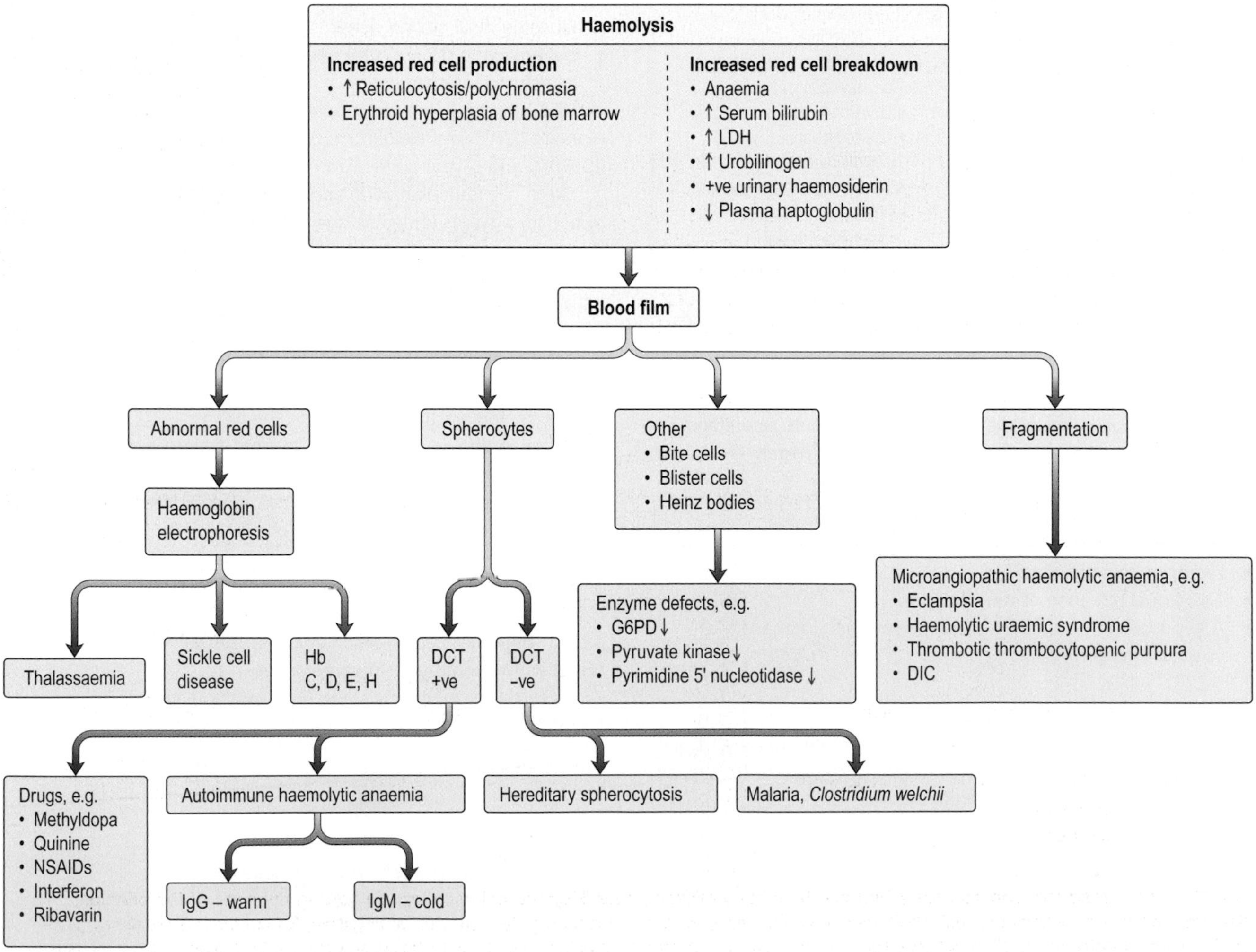

Figure 16.14 Haemolysis: diagnostic and haematological features. DCT, direct Coombs' test; DIC, disseminated intravascular coagulation; G6PD, glucose-6-phosphate dehydrogenase; LDH, lactate dehydrogenase; NSAIDs, non-steroidal anti-inflammatory drugs.

The **liver** plays a major role in removing haemoglobin bound to haptoglobin and haemopexin, and any remaining free haemoglobin.

Evidence for haemolysis

Increased red cell breakdown is accompanied by increased red cell production. This is shown in ***Figure 16.14***.

Demonstration of shortened red cell lifespan

Red cell survival can be estimated from ^{51}Cr-labelled red cells given intravenously but this is rarely performed.

Intravascular haemolysis

This is suggested by raised levels of plasma haemoglobin, haemosiderinuria, very low or absent haptoglobins, and the presence of methaemalbumin (positive Schumm's test).

Various laboratory studies will be necessary to determine the exact type of haemolytic anaemia present. The causes of haemolytic anaemias are shown in ***Box 16.9***.

INHERITED HAEMOLYTIC ANAEMIA

Red cell membrane defects

The normal red cell membrane consists of a lipid bilayer crossed by integral proteins with an underlying lattice of proteins (or cytoskeleton), including spectrin, actin, ankyrin and protein 4.1, attached to the integral proteins ***(Fig. 16.15)***.

Hereditary spherocytosis

Hereditary spherocytosis (HS) is the most common inherited haemolytic anaemia in Northern Europeans, affecting 1 in 5000. It is inherited in an autosomal dominant manner, but in 25% of patients neither parent is affected and it is presumed that HS has occurred by spontaneous mutation or is truly recessive. In the absence of a family history, the most important differential diagnosis is that of autoimmune haemolytic anaemia, which can usually be excluded by a negative direct antiglobulin test. HS is caused by defects in the red cell membrane, resulting in the cells losing part of the cell membrane as they pass through the spleen, possibly because the lipid bilayer is inadequately supported by the membrane skeleton. The best-characterized defect is a deficiency in the structural protein spectrin, but quantitative defects in other membrane proteins have been identified ***(Fig. 16.15)***, with ankyrin defects being the most common. The abnormal red cell membrane in HS is associated functionally with an increased permeability to sodium,

Box 16.9 Causes of haemolytic anaemia

Inherited

Red cell membrane defect
- Hereditary spherocytosis
- Hereditary elliptocytosis

Haemoglobin abnormalities
- Thalassaemia
- Sickle cell disease

Metabolic defects
- Glucose-6-phosphate dehydrogenase deficiency
- Pyruvate kinase deficiency
- Pyrimidine kinase deficiency

Acquired

Immune
- Autoimmune (see ***Box 16.16***)
  - Warm
  - Cold
- Alloimmune
  - Haemolytic transfusion reactions
  - Haemolytic disease of the newborn
  - After allogeneic bone marrow or organ transplantation
- Drug-induced

Non-immune
- Acquired membrane defects
  - Paroxysmal nocturnal haemoglobinuria
- Mechanical
  - Microangiopathic haemolytic anaemia
  - Valve prosthesis
  - March haemoglobinuria
- Secondary to systemic disease
  - Renal and liver failure
  - Miscellaneous section

Miscellaneous
- Infections, e.g. malaria, mycoplasma
- *Clostridium perfringens* (*welchii*), generalized sepsis
- Drugs and chemicals causing damage to the red cell membrane or oxidative haemolysis
- Hypersplenism
- Burns

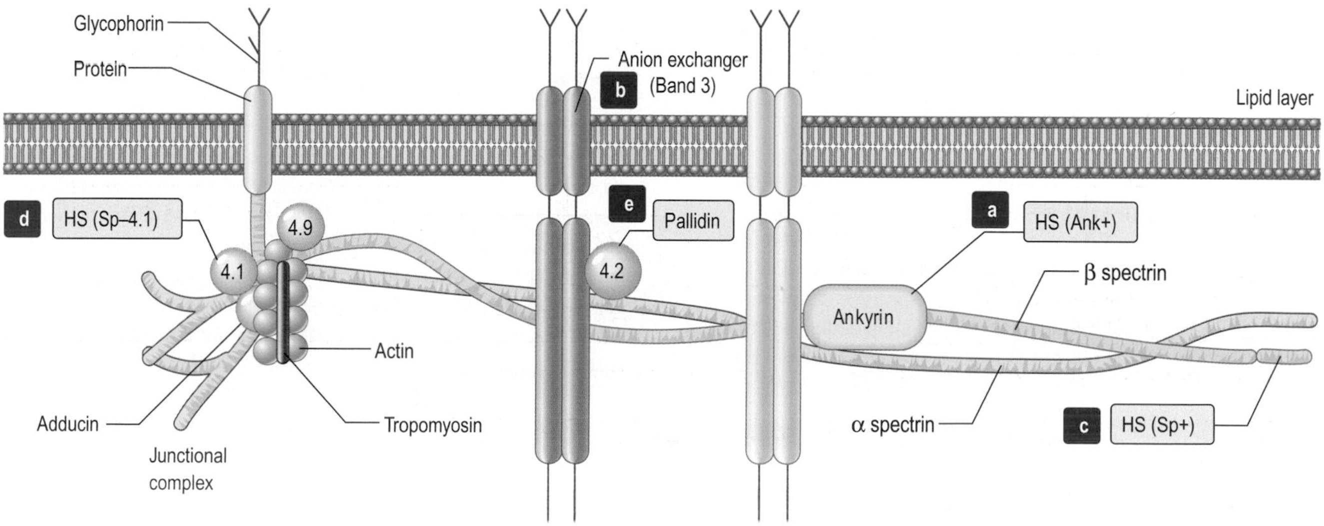

Figure 16.15 Hereditary spherocytosis (HS) and hereditary elliptocytosis (HE): red cell membrane showing the sites of the principal defects. Vertical interactions producing HS: **(a)** *ankyrin mutation*, HS (Ank+) producing deficiency (45% of cases); **(b)** HS *band 3 deficiency* (20%); **(c)** *β spectrin deficiency*, HS (Sp+) (<20%); **(d)** *abnormal spectrin/protein 4.1 binding*, HS (Sp–4.1); **(e)** *protein 4.2 (pallidin) deficiency* (Japanese). These produce various autosomal dominant and recessive forms of the disease. Horizontal interactions producing HE: α spectrin (80%), protein 4.1 (15%), β spectrin (5%).

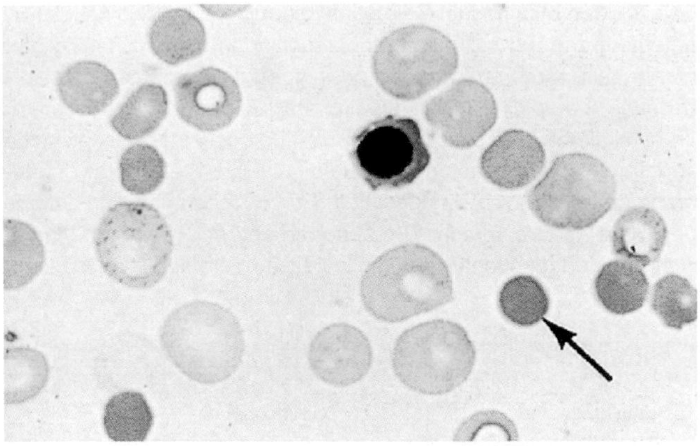

Figure 16.16 Spherocytes (arrowed). This blood film also shows reticulocytes, polychromasia and a nucleated erythroblast.

and this requires an increased rate of active transport of sodium out of the cells, which is dependent on adenosine triphosphate (ATP) produced by glycolysis. The surface-to-volume ratio decreases and the cells become spherocytic. Spherocytes are more rigid and less deformable than normal red cells. They are unable to pass through the splenic microcirculation so they have a shortened lifespan.

Clinical features

The condition may present with jaundice at birth. However, the onset of jaundice can be delayed for many years; some patients may go through life with no symptoms and are detected only during family studies. The patient may eventually develop anaemia, splenomegaly and ulcers on the leg. As in many haemolytic anaemias, the course of the disease may be interrupted by aplastic, haemolytic and megaloblastic crises. Aplastic anaemia usually occurs after infections, particularly with erythrovirus (parvovirus), whereas megaloblastic anaemia is the result of folate depletion caused by hyperactivity of the bone marrow. Chronic haemolysis leads to the formation of pigment gallstones (see pp. 490–491).

Investigations

- ***Anaemia***. This is usually mild but occasionally can be severe.
- ***Blood film***. This shows spherocytes ***(Fig. 16.16)*** and reticulocytes.
- ***Haemolysis***. This is evident (e.g. the serum bilirubin and urinary urobilinogen will be raised).
- ***Osmotic fragility***. When red cells are placed in solutions of increasing hypotonicity, they take in water, swell and eventually lyse. Spherocytes tolerate hypotonic solutions less well than do normal biconcave red cells. Osmotic fragility tests are infrequently carried out in routine practice but may be useful to confirm a suspicion of spherocytosis on a blood film.
- ***Direct antiglobulin (Coombs') test***. This is negative in hereditary spherocytosis, virtually ruling out autoimmune haemolytic anaemia, in which spherocytes are also commonly present.

Management

Splenectomy is indicated in hereditary spherocytosis to relieve symptoms due to anaemia or splenomegaly, reverse growth failure and prevent recurrent gallstones. It is best to postpone splenectomy until after childhood, as sudden overwhelming fatal infections, usually due to encapsulated organisms such as pneumococci, may occur (see p. 553). Splenectomy should be preceded by appropriate immunization and followed by life-long penicillin prophylaxis (see ***Box 16.20***). In addition to the well-known risk of bacterial infection, there is also a significant risk of adverse arterial and venous thromboembolic events after splenectomy and this needs to be taken into account when deciding whether to proceed to splenectomy.

Following splenectomy, the spherocytes persist but the Hb usually returns to normal, as the red cells are no longer destroyed.

Hereditary elliptocytosis

This disorder of the red cell membrane is inherited in an autosomal dominant manner and has a prevalence of 1 in 2500 in Caucasians. The red cells are elliptical due to deficiencies of protein 4.1 or the spectrin/actin/4.1 complex, which leads to weakness of the horizontal protein interaction and to the membrane defect (see ***Fig. 16.15***). *Clinically*, it is a similar condition to HS but milder. Only a minority of patients have anaemia and only occasional patients require splenectomy.

Rarely, hereditary spherocytosis or elliptocytosis may be inherited in a homozygous fashion, giving rise to a severe haemolytic anaemia sometimes necessitating splenectomy in early childhood.

Hereditary stomatocytosis

Stomatocytes are red cells in which the pale central area appears slit-like. Their presence in large numbers may occur in a hereditary haemolytic anaemia associated with a membrane defect, but excess alcohol intake is also a common cause. Although these hereditary conditions are very rare, a correct diagnosis is required – splenectomy is contraindicated, as it may result in fatal thromboembolic events.

Further reading

Bolton-Maggs PHB, Langer JC, Iolascon A et al. *Guidelines for the Diagnosis and Management of Hereditary Spherocytosis*. London: British Committee for Standards in Haematology; 2011; http://www.bcshguidelines.com.

Haemoglobin abnormalities

In early embryonic life, haemoglobins Gower 1, Gower 2 and Portland predominate. Later, fetal haemoglobin (HbF), which has two α and two γ chains, is produced ***(Fig. 16.17)***. There is increasing synthesis of β chains from 13 weeks' gestation and at term there is 80% HbF and 20% HbA. The haemoglobin switch from HbF to HbA occurs after birth, when the genes for γ chain production are further suppressed and there is rapid increase in the synthesis of β chains. BCL IIA, a zinc finger protein, is one of a number of proteins that suppress γ gene expression. There is little HbF produced (normally <1%) from 6 months after birth. The δ chain is synthesized just before birth and HbA_2 ($\alpha_2\delta_2$) remains at a level of about 2% throughout adult life ***(Box 16.10)***.

Globin chains are synthesized in the same way as any protein. A normal individual has four α-globin chain genes ***(Fig. 16.17)***, with two α-globin genes on each haploid genome (genes derived from one parent). These are situated close together on chromosome 16. The genes controlling the production of ε, γ, δ and β chains are close together on chromosome 11. The globin genes are arranged on chromosomes 16 and 11 in the order in which they are expressed

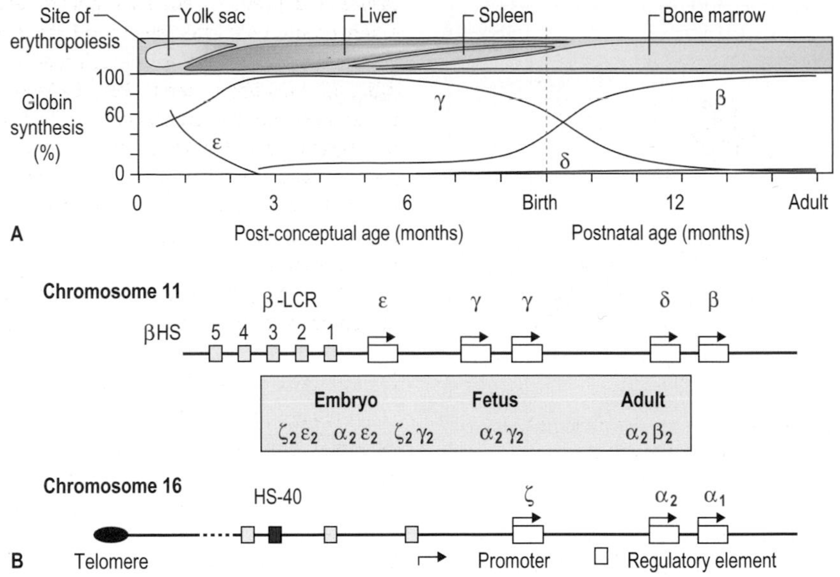

Figure 16.17 Normal development switches in globin expression. A. Sites of haemopoiesis and globin changes at various gestational ages. **B.** Structure of α-like and β-like globin gene clusters. HS, major upstream regulatory element; LCR, locus control region. *(From Higgs DR, Engel JD, Stamatoyannopoulos G. Thalassaemia.* Lancet *2012; 379:373–383, with permission.)*

Box 16.10 Some types of haemoglobin

	Haemoglobin	Structure	Comment
Normal	A	$\alpha_2\beta_2$	Comprises 97% of adult haemoglobin
	A_2	$\alpha_2\delta_2$	Comprises 2% of adult haemoglobin Elevated in β-thalassaemia
	F	$\alpha_2\gamma_2$	Normal haemoglobin in fetus from third to ninth month Increased in β-thalassaemia Comprises <1% of haemoglobin in adult
Abnormal chain production	H	β_4	Found in α-thalassaemia Biologically useless
	Barts	γ_4	Comprises 100% of haemoglobin in homozygous α-thalassaemia Biologically useless
Abnormal chain structure	SC	$\alpha_2\beta_2{}^S\alpha_2\beta_2{}^C$	Substitution of valine for glutamine acid in position 6 of β chain Substitution of lysine for glutamic acid in position 6 of β chain

and combine to give different haemoglobins. Normal haemoglobin synthesis is discussed on page 519.

Further reading

Forget BG. Progress in understanding the hemoglobin switch. *New Engl J Med* 2011; 365:852–854.

Haemoglobinopathies

Abnormalities occur in:

- globin chain production (e.g. thalassaemia)
- structure of the globin chain (e.g. sickle cell disease)
- combined defects of globin chain production and structure, e.g. sickle cell β-thalassaemia.

The thalassaemias

The thalassaemias affect people throughout the world ***(Fig. 16.18)*** and at least 60 000 severely affected individuals are born every year. Normally, there is balanced (1:1) production of α and β chains. The defective synthesis of globin chains in thalassaemia leads to 'imbalanced' globin chain production, causing precipitation of globin chains within the red cell precursors and resulting in ineffective erythropoiesis. Precipitation of globin chains in mature red cells leads to haemolysis.

Beta-thalassaemia

In ***homozygous*** β-thalassaemia, either no normal β chains are produced (β^0) or β-chain production is very reduced (β^+). There is an excess of α chains, which precipitate in erythroblasts and red cells, causing ineffective erythropoiesis and haemolysis. The excess α chains combine with whatever β, δ and γ chains are produced, resulting in increased quantities of HbA_2 and HbF and, at best, small amounts of HbA. In heterozygous β-thalassaemia, there is usually asymptomatic microcytosis with or without mild anaemia. ***Box 16.11*** shows the findings in the homozygote and heterozygote for the common types of β-thalassaemia.

Genetics

The molecular errors accounting for over 200 genetic defects leading to β-thalassaemia have been characterized. Unlike in

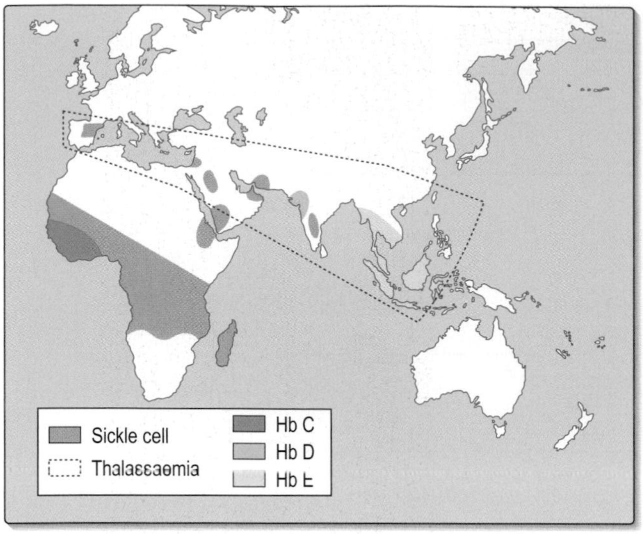

Figure 16.18 Major haemoglobin abnormalities: geographical distribution.

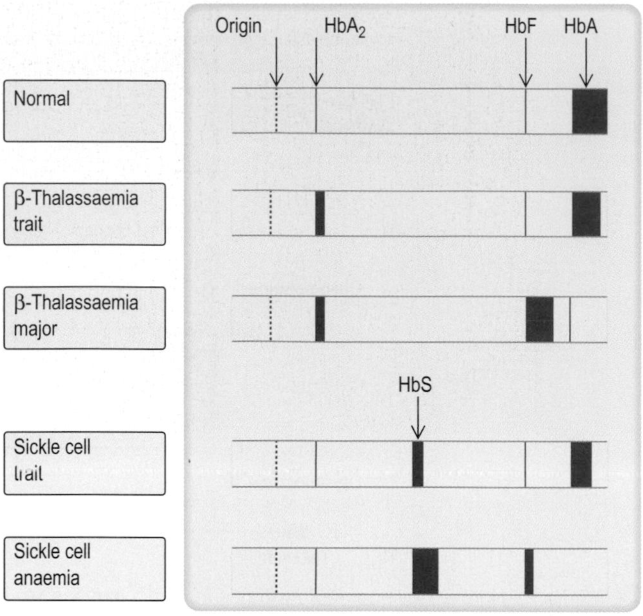

Figure 16.19 Patterns of haemoglobin electrophoresis.

Box 16.11 Beta-thalassaemia: common findings

Type of thalassaemia	Findings in homozygote	Findings in heterozygote
β^+	Thalassaemia major HbA+F+A_2	Thalassaemia minor HbA_2 raised
β^0	Thalassaemia major HbF+A_2	Thalassaemia minor HbA_2 raised
δβ	Thalassaemia intermedia	Thalassaemia minor HbF 5–15%
	HbF only	HbA_2 normal
$\delta\beta^+$ (Lepore)[a]	Thalassaemia major or intermedia	Thalassaemia minor
	HbF and Lepore	Hb Lepore 5–15% HbA_2 normal

[a]Hb Lepore is a cross-fusion product of δ and β globin genes.
(Adapted from Weatherall DJ. Disorders of the synthesis of function of haemoglobin. In: Weatherall DJ, Warrell DA, Cox TM, Firth JD (eds) *Oxford Textbook of Medicine*, 5th edn. Oxford: Oxford University Press; 2010.)

α-thalassaemia, the defects are mainly point mutations rather than gene deletions. The mutations result in defects in transcription, RNA splicing and modification, translation via frame shifts and nonsense codons producing highly unstable β-globin, which cannot be utilized.

Clinical syndromes

Clinically, β-thalassaemia can be divided into the following:

- thalassaemia minor (or trait), the symptomless heterozygous carrier state
- thalassaemia intermedia, a moderate anaemia not requiring regular transfusions (with a number of different genotypes)
- thalassaemia major (generally homozygous β-thalassaemia), a severe anaemia requiring regular transfusions.

Thalassaemia minor (trait)

This common carrier state (heterozygous β-thalassaemia) is asymptomatic. Anaemia is mild or absent. The red cells are hypochromic and microcytic with a low MCV and MCH, and the condition may be confused with iron deficiency. However, the two are easily distinguished, as in thalassaemia trait the serum ferritin and the iron stores are normal (see ***Box 16.4***). The RDW is usually normal (see p. 517). Hb electrophoresis usually shows a raised HbA_2 and often a raised HbF ***(Fig. 16.19)***. Iron should not be given to these patients unless they also have proven coincidental iron deficiency.

Thalassaemia intermedia

Thalassaemia intermedia patients include those who are symptomatic with moderate anaemia (Hb 70–100 g/L) and do not require regular transfusions.

Thalassaemia intermedia may be due to a combination of homozygous mild β+- and α-thalassaemia, where there is reduced α-chain precipitation, thus helping to reduce the degree of globin imbalance and having a consequent reduction in ineffective erythropoiesis and haemolysis. The inheritance of hereditary persistence of HbF with homozygous β-thalassaemia also results in a milder clinical picture than unmodified β-thalassaemia major because the excess α chains are partially removed by the increased production of γ chains.

Patients may have splenomegaly and bone deformities. Recurrent leg ulcers, gallstones and infections are also seen. It should be noted that these patients may be iron-overloaded despite a lack of regular blood transfusions. This is caused by excessive iron absorption, which results from the underlying dyserythropoiesis (see description of iron absorption, pp. 523–524).

Thalassaemia major

Most children affected by homozygous β-thalassaemia present during the first year of life with:

- failure to thrive and recurrent bacterial infections
- severe anaemia from 3 to 6 months, when the switch from γ- to β-chain production should normally occur
- extramedullary haemopoiesis that soon leads to hepatosplenomegaly and bone expansion, giving rise to the classical thalassaemic facies ***(Fig. 16.20A)***.

Skull X-rays in these children show the characteristic 'hair-on-end' appearance of bony trabeculation as a result of expansion

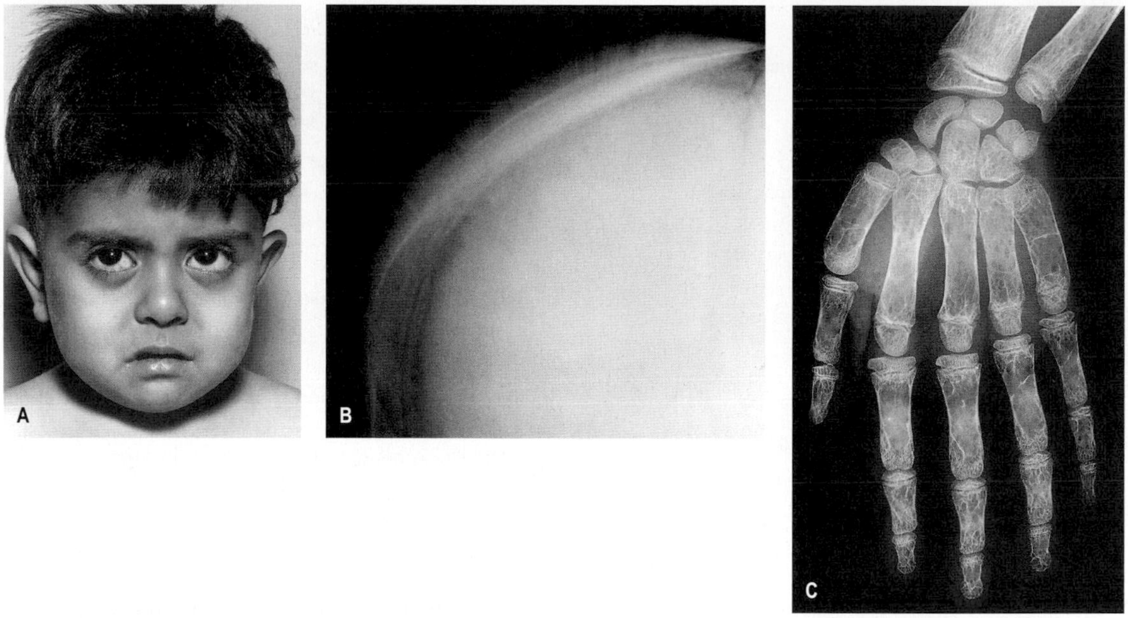

Figure 16.20 Thalassaemia. A. *Child with thalassaemia*, showing the typical facial features. B. *Skull X-ray* of a child with β-thalassaemia, showing the 'hair-on-end' appearance. C. X-*ray of a hand*, showing expansion of the marrow and a thinned cortex.

of the bone marrow into cortical bone ***(Fig. 16.20B)***. The expansion of the bone marrow is also shown in an X-ray of the hand ***(Fig. 16.20C)***.

The classic features of untreated thalassaemia major are generally only observed in patients from countries without good blood transfusion support.

Management

The aims of treatment are to suppress ineffective erythropoiesis, prevent bony deformities and allow normal activity and development.

- ***Long-term folic acid*** supplements are required.
- ***Regular transfusions*** should be given to keep the Hb above 100 g/L. Blood transfusions may be required every 4–6 weeks.
- If transfusion requirements increase, ***splenectomy*** may help, although this is usually delayed until after the age of 6 years because of the risk of infection. Prophylaxis against infection is required for patients undergoing splenectomy (see p. 553).
- ***Iron overload***, caused by repeated transfusions (transfusion haemosiderosis), may lead to damage to the endocrine glands, liver, pancreas and myocardium by the time patients reach adolescence. Among these complications of iron overload, cardiomyopathy and associated cardiac tachyarrhythmias are the leading causes of morbidity and mortality. Magnetic resonance imaging (MRI; myocardial T_2-relaxation time) is useful for monitoring iron overload in thalassaemia; both the heart and the liver can be monitored. The standard iron-chelating agent remains desferrioxamine, although it has to be administered parenterally. Desferrioxamine is given as an overnight subcutaneous infusion on 5–7 nights each week. Ascorbic acid 200 mg daily is given, as it increases the urinary excretion of iron in response to desferrioxamine. Often, young children have a very high standard of chelation, as it is organized by their parents. However, when the children become adults and take on this role themselves, they often rebel and chelation with desferrioxamine may become problematic. Deferiprone, an oral iron chelator, has been available for some years; results on a once-daily oral iron chelator, deferasirox, indicate that it is safe, similar in effectiveness to desferrioxamine and is being increasingly used.
- ***Intensive treatment with desferrioxamine*** has been reported to reverse damage to the heart in patients with severe iron overload, but excessive doses of desferrioxamine may cause cataracts, retinal damage and nerve deafness. Infection with *Yersinia enterocolitica* occurs in iron-loaded patients treated with desferrioxamine. Iron overload should be periodically assessed by measuring the serum ferritin and by assessing hepatic iron stores by MRI.
- ***Bone marrow transplantation*** has been used in young patients with HLA-matched siblings. It has been successful in patients in good clinical condition with a 3-year mortality of <5%, but there is a high mortality (>50%) in patients in poor condition with iron overload and liver dysfunction.
- ***Prenatal diagnosis and gene therapy*** are discussed on pages 116–117.
- ***Testing of patients' partners*** should be carried out. If both partners have β-thalassaemia trait, there is a 1 in 4 chance of such pregnancy resulting in a child having β-thalassaemia major. Therefore, couples in this situation must be offered prenatal diagnosis and counselling (see pp. 116–117).

Alpha-thalassaemia

Genetics

In contrast to β-thalassaemia, α-thalassaemia is often caused by gene deletions, although mutations of the α-globin genes may also occur. The gene for α-globin chains is duplicated on both chromosomes 16, that is, a normal person has a total of four α-globin genes. Deletion of one α-chain gene (α+) or both α-chain genes (α^0) on each chromosome 16 may occur ***(Box 16.12)***. The former is the most common of these abnormalities.

- ***Four-gene deletion*** (deletion of both genes on both chromosomes). There is no α-chain synthesis and only Hb

Box 16.12 The α-thalassaemias

Number of α-globin genes deleted	Genotype[a]	Haemoglobin type	Clinical picture
4	—/—	Hb Barts (γ4)	Hydrops fetalis
3	—/–α	HbH (α4)	Moderately severe anaemia Splenomegaly
2	–α/–α or —/αα	HbA Some HbH bodies	Mild anaemia
1	αα/–α	HbA	Very mild anaemia or no anaemia

[a]The normal α-globin genotype is αα/αα (i.e. four α-globin genes present).

Barts (γ4) is present. Hb Barts cannot carry oxygen and is incompatible with life (see ***Boxes 16.10*** and ***16.12***). Infants are either stillborn at 28–40 weeks or die very shortly after birth. They are pale and oedematous, and have enormous livers and spleens – a condition called hydrops fetalis.

- ***Three-gene deletion***. The severe reduction in α-chain synthesis results in HbH disease, which is common in parts of Asia. HbH has four β chains, although patients with HbH disease also have low levels of HbA and Hb Barts. HbA_2 is normal or reduced. HbH does not transport oxygen and precipitates in erythroblasts and erythrocytes. There is moderate anaemia (Hb 70–100 g/L) and splenomegaly (thalassaemia intermedia). The patients are not usually transfusion-dependent.
- ***Two-gene deletion*** (α-thalassaemia trait). There is microcytosis with or without mild anaemia. HbH bodies may be seen on staining a blood film with brilliant cresyl blue.
- ***One-gene deletion***. The blood picture is usually normal.

Globin chain synthesis studies for the detection of a reduced ratio of α to β chains may be necessary for the definitive diagnosis of α-thalassaemia trait.

Less commonly, α-thalassaemia may result from genetic defects other than deletions: for example, mutations in the stop codon producing an α chain with many extra amino acids (Hb Constant Spring). It has a more severe clinical course than HbH, with severe anaemia often precipitated by infection.

Further reading

Benz EJ, Jr. Newborn screening for α-thalassemia – keeping up with globalization. *N Engl J Med* 2011; 364:770–771.
Brittenham GM. Iron-chelating therapy for transfusional iron overload. *N Engl J Med* 2011; 364:146–156.
Higgs DR, Engel JD, Stamatoyannopoulos G. Thalassaemia. *Lancet* 2012; 379:373–383.
Piel FB, W eatherall DJ. The α thalassaemias. *New Engl J Med* 2014; 371:1908, 1916.
Taher AT, Musallam KM, Cappellini MD et al. Optimal management of β thalassaemia intermedia. *Br J Haematol* 2011; 152:512–523.

Sickle syndromes

Sickle cell haemoglobin (HbS) results from a single-base mutation of adenine to thymine, which produces a substitution of valine for glutamic acid at the sixth codon of the β-globin chain ($\alpha_2\beta_2{}^{6glu\rightarrow val}$). In the homozygous state (***sickle cell anaemia***), both genes are abnormal (HbSS), whereas in the heterozygous state (***sickle cell trait***, HbAS), only one chromosome carries the gene. As the synthesis of HbF is normal, the disease usually does not manifest itself until the HbF decreases to adult levels at about 6 months of age.

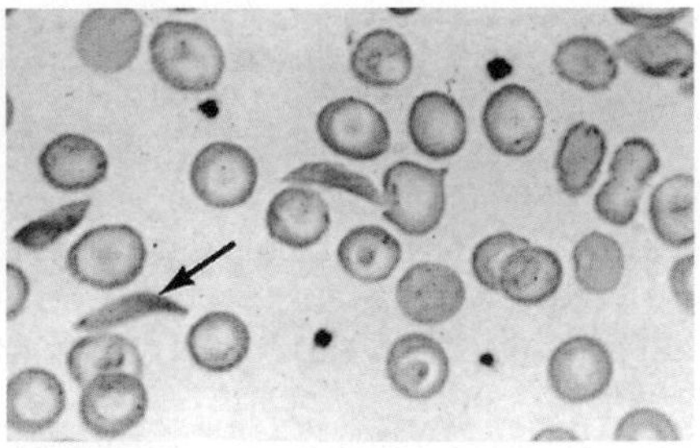

Figure 16.21 Sickle cells (arrowed) and target cells.

The sickle gene is most common in Africans (up to 25% gene frequency in some populations) but is also found in India, the Middle East and Southern Europe.

Pathogenesis

Deoxygenated HbS molecules are insoluble and polymerize. The flexibility of the cells is decreased and they become rigid and take up their characteristic sickle appearance ***(Fig. 16.21)***. This process is initially reversible but, with repeated sickling, the cells eventually lose their membrane flexibility and become irreversibly sickled. This is due to dehydration, partly caused by potassium leaving the red cells via a calcium-activated potassium channel called the Gardos channel. These irreversibly sickled cells are dehydrated and dense, and will not return to normal when oxygenated. Sickling can produce:

- a shortened red cell survival
- impaired passage of cells through the microcirculation, leading to obstruction of small vessels and tissue infarction.

Sickling is precipitated by infection, dehydration, cold, acidosis or hypoxia. In many cases, the cause is unknown, but adhesion proteins on activated endothelial cells (vascular cell adhesion molecule 1, or VCAM-1) may play a causal role, particularly in vaso-occlusion when rigid cells are trapped, facilitating polymerization. HbS releases its oxygen to the tissues more easily than does normal Hb, and patients therefore feel well despite being anaemic (except, of course, during crises or complications).

Depending on the type of haemoglobin chain combinations, three clinical syndromes occur:

- Homozygous HbSS patients have the most severe disease.
- Combined heterozygosity (HbSC) for HbS and C (see below) patients suffer intermediate symptoms.
- Heterozygous HbAS (sickle cell trait) patients have no symptoms (see pp. 540–541).

Sickle cell anaemia

Clinical features

Vaso-occlusive crises

An early presentation may be acute pain in the hands and feet (dactylitis) owing to vaso-occlusion of the small vessels. Severe pain in other bones, such as the femur, humerus, vertebrae, ribs and pelvis, occurs in older children and adults. These attacks vary greatly in frequency from patient to patient, and sometimes in the same patient from year to year; however, as a generalization, a patient with moderately severe sickle cell anaemia may have around three hospital admissions a year from painful vaso-occlusive crises. Fever often accompanies the pain.

Acute chest syndrome

This occurs in up to 30%, and pulmonary hypertension and chronic lung disease are the most common causes of death in adults with sickle cell disease. The acute chest syndrome is caused by infection, fat embolism from necrotic bone marrow or pulmonary infarction due to sequestration of sickle cells. It comprises shortness of breath, chest pain, hypoxia and new chest X-ray changes due to consolidation. The presentation may be gradual or very rapid, the latter leading to death in a few hours. Management is with pain relief, high-flow supplemental oxygen and antibiotics (cefotaxime and clarithromycin), which should be started immediately. Exchange transfusion will reduce the amount of HbS to <20% if there is no improvement. Ventilation (continuous positive airways pressure, or CPAP) may be necessary. Infections can be due to *Chlamydia* and mycoplasma, as well as *Streptococcus pneumoniae.*

Pulmonary hypertension

Pulmonary hypertension (defined as a mean pulmonary artery pressure >25 mmHg by right heart catheterization) is a known consequence of sickle cell anaemia, occurring in approximately 10% of patients. Its mechanism is not understood but contributory factors probably include sickle cell vasculopathy, damage from repeated chest crises, and repeated thromboembolism and intravascular haemolysis with consequent effects on reactive oxygen species and levels of scavenging nitric oxide. Development of pulmonary hypertension raises the risk of hypoxaemia and worsening sickle cell crises, and is an independent risk factor for mortality in patients with sickle cell anaemia. Diagnosis of pulmonary hypertension in patients with sickle cell anaemia should prompt consideration of therapies to reduce levels of HbS (see below) and also referral to a pulmonary hypertension specialist.

Anaemia

Chronic haemolysis produces a stable haemoglobin level, usually in the 60–80 g/L range, but an acute fall in the haemoglobin level can occur owing to:

- splenic sequestration
- bone marrow aplasia
- further haemolysis due to drugs, acute infection or associated glucose-6-phosphate dehydrogenase (G6PD) deficiency.

Splenic sequestration

Vaso-occlusion produces an acute painful enlargement of the spleen. There is splenic pooling of red cells and hypovolaemia, leading in some to circulatory collapse and death. The condition supervenes in childhood before multiple infarctions have occurred. The latter eventually lead to a fibrotic, non-functioning spleen. Liver sequestration can also occur.

Bone marrow aplasia

This most commonly follows infection with erythrovirus B19, which invades proliferating erythroid progenitors. There is a rapid fall in haemoglobin with no reticulocytes in the peripheral blood because of the failure of erythropoiesis in the marrow.

Long-term problems

- ***Growth and development***. Young children are short but regain their height by adulthood. However, they remain below the normal weight. Sexual maturation is often delayed and may require hormone therapy.
- ***Bones***. Bones are a common site for vaso-occlusive episodes, leading to chronic infarcts. Avascular necrosis of hips and shoulders, compression of vertebrae, and shortening of bones in the hands and feet occur. These episodes are the common cause for the painful crisis. Osteomyelitis is more frequent in sickle cell disease and is caused by *Staphylococcus aureus*, *Staph. pneumoniae* and salmonella (see p. 718). Occasionally, hip joint replacement may be required.
- ***Infections***. Infections are common in tissues susceptible to vaso-occlusion, such as bones, lungs and kidneys.
- ***Leg ulcers***. These occur spontaneously (vaso-occlusive episodes) or following trauma, and are usually found over the medial or lateral malleoli. They often become infected and are quite resistant to treatment; sometimes blood transfusion may facilitate ulcer healing.
- ***Cardiac problems***. Cardiac problems occur, with cardiomegaly, arrhythmias and iron overload cardiomyopathy. Myocardial infarctions are caused by thrombotic episodes, which are not secondary to atheroma.
- ***Neurological complications***. These occur in 25% of patients and include transient ischaemic attacks, fits, cerebral infarction, cerebral haemorrhage and coma. About 11% of patients under 20 years of age suffer strokes. The most common finding is obstruction of a distal intracranial internal carotid artery or a proximal middle cerebral artery. About 10% of children without neurological signs or symptoms have abnormal blood-flow velocity indicative of clinically significant arterial stenosis; such patients have a very high risk of stroke. It has been demonstrated that if children with stenotic cranial artery lesions, as demonstrated on transcranial Doppler ultrasonography, are maintained on a regular programme of transfusion that is designed to suppress erythropoiesis, so that no more than 30% of the circulating red cells are their own, about 90% of strokes in such children could be prevented.
- ***Cholelithiasis***. Pigment stones occur as a result of chronic haemolysis.
- ***Liver***. Chronic hepatomegaly and liver dysfunction are caused by trapping of sickle cells.
- ***Renal***. Chronic tubulointerstitial nephritis occurs (see pp. 768–769).
- ***Priapism***. An unwanted painful erection occurs from vaso-occlusion and can be recurrent. This requires urgent treatment, as it may result in impotence. Treatment is with an α-adrenergic blocking drug, analgesia and hydration.
- ***Eye***. Background retinopathy, proliferative retinopathy, vitreous haemorrhages and retinal detachments all occur. Regular yearly eye checks are required.
- ***Pregnancy***. Impaired placental blood flow causes spontaneous abortion, intrauterine growth retardation, pre-eclampsia and fetal death. Painful episodes, infections and severe anaemia occur in the mother.

Investigations

- ***Blood count***. The level of Hb is in the range 60–80 g/L with a high reticulocyte count (10–20%).
- ***Blood films***. These can show features of hyposplenism (see ***Fig. 16.26***) and sickling ***(Fig. 16.21)***.
- ***Sickle solubility test***. A mixture of HbS in a reducing solution such as sodium dithionite gives a turbid appearance because

Box 16.13 Complications of sickle cell disease requiring inpatient management

- Pain – uncontrolled by non-opiate analgesia
- Swollen, painful joints
- Acute sickle chest syndrome or pneumonia
- Mesenteric sickling and bowel ischaemia
- Splenic or hepatic sequestration
- Central nervous system deficit
- Cholecystitis (pigment stones)
- Cardiac arrhythmias
- Renal papillary necrosis resulting in colic or severe haematuria
- Hyphaema and retinal detachment
- Priapism

Box 16.14 Management of acute painful crisis in opioid-naive adults with sickle cell disease

Morphine/diamorphine
- 0.1 mg/kg i.v./s.c. every 20 min until pain controlled
- *Then* 0.05–0.1 mg/kg i.v./s.c. (or oral morphine) every 2–4 h

Patient-controlled analgesia (PCA)
(Example for adults >50 kg)

Diamorphine/morphine
- Continuous infusion: 0–10 mg/h
- PCA bolus dose: 2–10 mg
- Dose duration: 1 min
- Lockout time: 20–30 min

Adjuvant oral analgesia
- Paracetamol 1 g 6-hourly
- ± Ibuprofen[a] 400 mg 8-hourly
- *Or* diclofenac[a] 50 mg 8-hourly

Laxatives (all patients)
For example:
- Lactulose 10 mL × 2 daily
- Senna 2–4 tablets daily
- Sodium docusate 100 mg × 2 daily
- Macrogol 1 sachet daily
- Lubiprostone

Other adjuvants

Antipruritics
- Hydroxyzine 25 mg × 2 as required

Antiemetics
- Prochlorperazine 5–10 mg × 3 as required
- Cyclizine 50 mg × 3 as required

Anxiolytic
- Haloperidol 1–3 mg oral/i.m. × 2 as required

[a]*Caution advised with NSAIDs in renal impairment.*
(Adapted from Rees DC, Olujohungbe AD, Parker NE et al. Guidelines for the management of the acute painful crisis in sickle cell disease. British Journal of Haematology *2003; 120(5):744–752.)*

of precipitation of HbS, whereas normal Hb gives a clear solution. A number of commercial kits, such as Sickledex, are available for rapid screening for the presence of HbS: for example, before surgery in appropriate ethnic groups and in the Accident and Emergency department.

- ***Hb electrophoresis*** (see ***Fig. 16.19***). This is always needed to confirm the diagnosis. There is no HbA, 80–95% HbSS and 2–20% HbF.
- ***Patents.*** The parents of the affected child will show features of sickle cell trait.

Management

Precipitating factors (see above) should be avoided or treated quickly. The complications that require inpatient management are shown in ***Box 16.13***.

Acute painful attacks require supportive therapy with intravenous fluids, and adequate analgesia. Oxygen and antibiotics are only given if specifically indicated. Crises can be extremely painful and require strong, usually narcotic, analgesia. Morphine is the drug of choice. Milder pain can sometimes be relieved by codeine, paracetamol and NSAIDs ***(Box 16.14)***. Use of incentive spirometry is recommended for patients hospitalized for a vaso-occlusive crisis.

Infection prophylaxis is with penicillin 500 mg daily and vaccination with polyvalent pneumococcal and *Haemophilus influenzae* type b vaccine (see p. 553). Folic acid is given to all patients with haemolysis.

Anaemia

Blood transfusions should only be given when there are clear indications. Patients with steady state anaemia, those having minor surgery or those having painful episodes without complications should not be transfused. Transfusions should be given for acute chest syndrome and acute anaemia due to acute splenic sequestration or an aplastic crisis, aiming for an Hb of 100 g/L and HbS <30%. Before elective operations, transfusions given to increase the Hb to 100 g/L reduce the risk of perioperative complications. During pregnancy, repeated transfusions may be used to reduce the proportion of circulating HbS to <30% to prevent sickling. Following a stroke, there is a 90% chance of further episodes, which can be reduced by regular transfusion to keep HbS below 30%. Children with narrow intracerebral blood vessels detected by transcranial Doppler scans are at high risk of stroke, which has been shown to be reduced by 90% with regular transfusions to keep the HbS below 30%. Exchange transfusions may be necessary in patients with severe or recurrent crises, or before emergency surgery. Red cells for transfusion should be matched for Rhesus (Rh) and Kell blood groups to minimize the risk of alloimmunization. Ideally, patients requiring long-term transfusion, such as those with sickle cell anaemia and thalassaemia, should undergo molecular blood group typing before their first transfusion.

Hydroxycarbamide (hydroxyurea) has been widely used as therapy for sickle cell anaemia. It acts, at least in part, by increasing HbF concentrations. Hydroxycarbamide has been shown in trials to reduce the episodes of pain, the acute chest syndrome and the need for blood transfusions. Thus selected patients – for example, those who have three or more sickle cell-associated, moderate to severe vaso-occlusive crises in a 12-month period – should be offered hydroxycarbamide treatment.

Stem cell transplantation has been used to treat sickle cell anaemia, although in fewer numbers than for thalassaemia. Children and adolescents younger than 16 years of age who have severe complications (strokes, recurrent chest syndrome or refractory pain) and have an HLA-matched donor are the best candidates for transplantation.

Counselling

A multidisciplinary team should be involved, with regular clinic appointments to build up relationships. Adolescents require careful counselling over psychosocial issues and drug and birth control.

Prognosis

Some patients with HbSS die in the first few years of life from either infection or episodes of sequestration. However, there is marked individual variation in the severity of the disease and some patients have a relatively normal lifespan with few complications.

Sickle cell trait

These individuals have no symptoms unless extreme circumstances cause anoxia, such as flying in non-pressurized aircraft. Sickle cell trait gives some protection against *Plasmodium falciparum* malaria (see pp. 298–299), and consequently the sickle gene has been seen as an example of a balanced polymorphism (where the advantage of the malaria protection in the heterozygote is balanced by the mortality of the homozygous condition). Typically, there is 60% HbA and 40% HbS. It should be emphasized that, unlike with thalassaemia trait, the blood count and film of a person with sickle cell trait are normal. The diagnosis is made by a positive sickle test or by Hb electrophoresis (see ***Fig. 16.19***).

Other structural globin chain defects

There are very many Hb variants and most are not associated with any clinical manifestations. However, some Hb variants may interact with HbS; for example, compound heterozygosity for HbC and HbS gives rise to HbSC disease. The clinical course of HbSC disease is generally somewhat milder than that of HbSS disease, but there is an increased likelihood of thrombosis, which may lead to thrombosis in pregnancy and to retinopathy.

Combined defects of globin chain production and structure

Abnormalities of Hb structure (e.g. HbS, C) can occur in combination with thalassaemia. The combination of β-thalassaemia trait and sickle cell trait (sickle cell β-thalassaemia) resembles sickle cell anaemia (HbSS) clinically.

HbE ($\alpha_2\beta_2^{26glu \rightarrow lys}$) is the most common Hb variant in South-east Asia, and the second most prevalent haemoglobin variant worldwide. HbE heterozygotes are asymptomatic; the haemoglobin level is normal but red cells are microcytic. Homozygous HbE causes a mild microcytic anaemia, but the combination of heterozygosity for HbE and β-thalassaemia produces a variable anaemia, which can be as severe as β-thalassaemia major.

Prenatal screening and diagnosis of severe haemoglobin abnormalities

Of the offspring of parents who both have either β-thalassaemia or sickle cell trait, 25% will have β-thalassaemia major or sickle cell anaemia, respectively. Recognition of these heterozygous states in parent and family counselling provides a basis for antenatal screening and diagnosis (see pp. 116–117).

Pregnant women with either sickle cell trait or thalassaemia trait must be identified at antenatal booking either by selective screening of high-risk groups on the basis of ethnic origin or by universal screening of all pregnant women. Beta-thalassaemia trait can always be detected by a low MCV and MCH, and confirmed by haemoglobin electrophoresis. However, sickle cell trait is undetectable from a blood count and the laboratory needs a specific request to screen for sickle cell trait. Clearly, universal antenatal screening, as practised in the UK, avoids such problems.

If a pregnant woman is found to have a haemoglobin defect, her partner should be tested. Antenatal diagnosis is offered if both are affected, as there is a risk of a severe fetal Hb defect, particularly β-thalassaemia major. Fetal DNA analysis can be carried out using amniotic fluid, chorionic villus or fetal blood samples. Abortion is offered if the fetus is found to be severely affected. Chorionic villus biopsy has the advantage that it can be carried out in the first trimester, thus avoiding the need for second-trimester abortions.

Further reading

Howard J, Malfoy M, Llewelyn C et al. The transfusion alternatives preoperatively in sickle cell disease (TAPS) study: a randomised, controlled, multicentre clinical trial. *Lancet* 2013; 381:930–938.

Rees DC, Williams TN, Gladwin MT. Sickle-cell disease. *Lancet* 2010; 376:2018–2031.

Yawn BP, Buchanan GR, Afenyl-Annan AN et al. Management of sickle cell disease. *JAMA* 2014; 312:1033–1048.

Metabolic disorders of the red cell

Red cell metabolism

The mature red cell has no nucleus, mitochondria or ribosomes and is therefore unable to synthesize proteins. Red cells have only limited enzyme systems but they maintain the viability and function of the cells. In particular, energy is required in the form of ATP for maintenance of the flexibility of the membrane and the biconcave shape of the cells to allow passage through small vessels, and for regulation of the sodium and potassium pumps to ensure osmotic equilibrium. In addition, it is essential for Hb to be maintained in the reduced state.

The enzyme systems responsible for producing energy and reducing power ***(Fig. 16.22)*** are:

- the glycolytic (Embden–Meyerhof) pathway, in which glucose is metabolized to pyruvate and lactic acid with production of ATP
- the hexose monophosphate (pentose phosphate) pathway, which provides reducing power for the red cell in the form of NADPH (the reduced form of nicotinamide adenine dinucleotide phosphate).

About 90% of glucose is metabolized by the former and 10% by the latter. The hexose monophosphate shunt maintains glutathione (GSH) in a reduced state. Glutathione is necessary to combat oxidative stress to the red cell, and failure of this mechanism may result in:

- rigidity due to cross-linking of spectrin, which decreases membrane flexibility (see ***Fig. 16.15***) and causes 'leakiness' of the red cell membrane
- oxidation of the Hb molecule, producing methaemoglobin and precipitation of globin chains as Heinz bodies localized on the inside of the membrane; these bodies are removed from circulating red cells by the spleen.

2,3-BPG is formed from a side-arm of the glycolytic pathway ***(Fig. 16.22)***. It binds to the central part of the Hb tetramer, fixing it in the low-affinity state (see ***Fig. 16.4***). A decreased affinity with a shift in the oxygen dissociation curve to the right enables more oxygen to be delivered to the tissues.

In addition to the G6PD, pyruvate kinase and pyrimidine 5′ nucleotidase deficiencies described below, there are a number of rare enzyme deficiencies that need specialist investigation.

Glucose-6-phosphate dehydrogenase deficiency

The enzyme glucose-6-phosphate dehydrogenase (G6PD) holds a vital position in the hexose monophosphate shunt ***(Fig. 16.22)***, oxidizing glucose-6-phosphate to 6-phosphoglycerate with the reduction of NADP to NADPH. The reaction is necessary in red cells where it is the only source of NADPH, which is used via glutathione to protect the red cell from oxidative damage. G6PD deficiency is a common condition that presents with a haemolytic anaemia and affects millions of people throughout the world, particularly in Africa, around the Mediterranean, and in the Middle East (around 20%) and South-east Asia (up to 40% in some regions).

The gene for G6PD is localized to chromosome Xq28 near the factor VIII gene. The deficiency is therefore more common in males than in females. However, female heterozygotes can also have clinical problems due to Lyonization (see p. 109), whereby, because

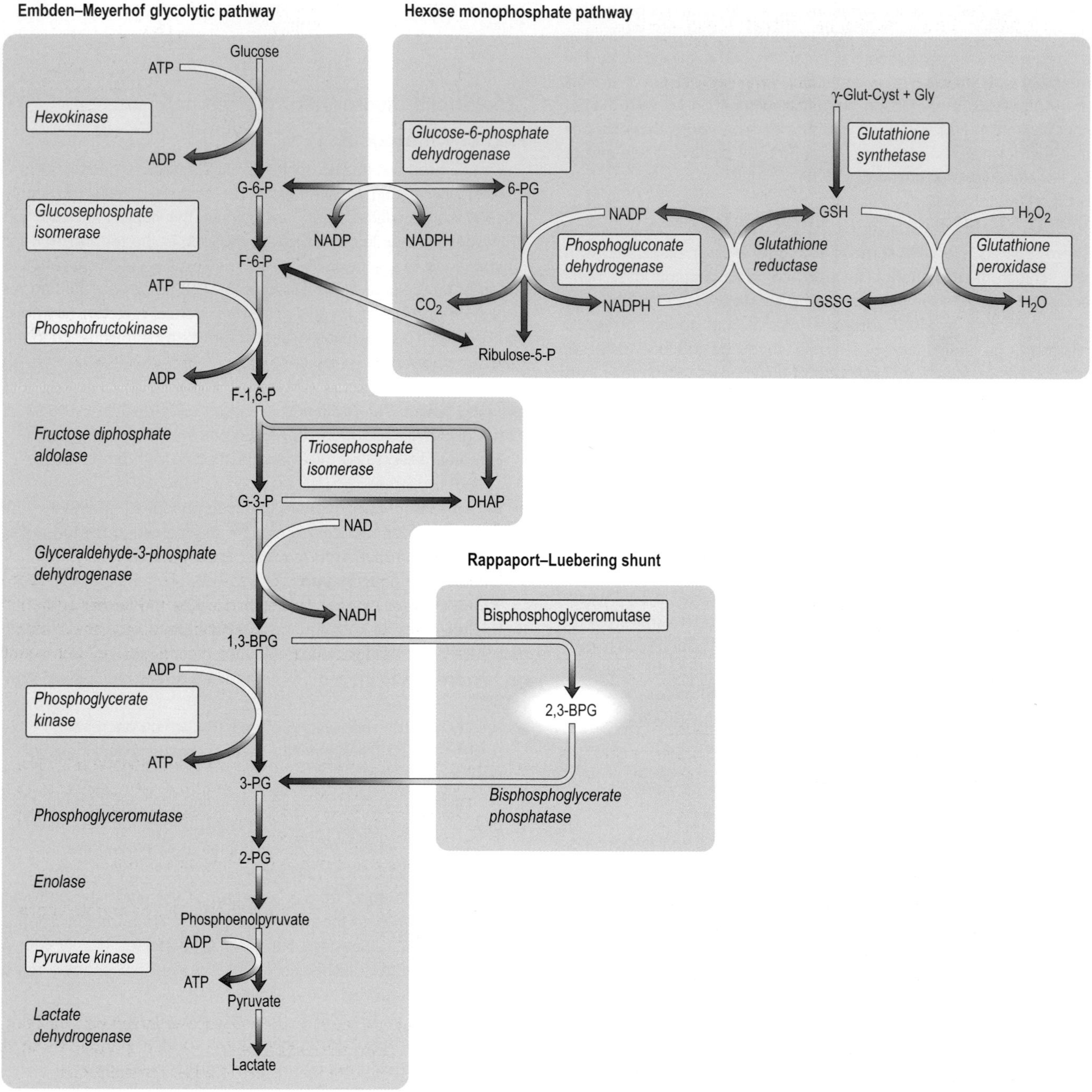

Figure 16.22 Glucose metabolism pathways. The enzymes in green boxes indicate documented hereditary deficiency diseases. ADP, adenosine diphosphate; ATP, adenosine triphosphate; BPG, bisphosphoglycerate; DHAP, dihydroxyacetone phosphate; F, fructose; G, glucose; GSH, reduced glutathione; GSSG, oxidized glutathione; NADH, reduced nicotinamide adenine dinucleotide; NADP, nicotinamide adenine dinucleotide phosphate; NADPH, reduced NADP; P, phosphate; PG, phosphoglycerate.

of random X-chromosome inactivation, female heterozygotes have two populations of red cells: a normal one and a G6PD-deficient one.

There are over 400 structural types of G6PD, and mutations are mostly single amino acid substitutions (missense point mutations). The World Health Organization (WHO) has classified variants by the degree of enzyme deficiency and severity of haemolysis. The most common types with normal activity are called type B^+, which is present in almost all Caucasians and about 70% of black Africans, and type A^+, which is present in about 20% of black Africans. There are many variants with reduced activity but only two are common. In the African or A^- type, the degree of deficiency is mild and more marked in older cells. Haemolysis is self-limiting, as the young red cells newly produced by the bone marrow have nearly normal enzyme activity. However, in the Mediterranean type, both young and old red cells have very low enzyme activity. After an oxidant shock, the Hb level may fall precipitously; death may follow unless the condition is recognized and the patient is transfused urgently.

Box 16.15 Drugs causing haemolysis in glucose-6-phosphate dehydrogenase deficiency

Analgesics, such as:
- Aspirin
- Phenacetin (withdrawn in the UK)

Antimalarials, such as:
- Primaquine
- Pyrimethamine
- Quinine
- Chloroquine
- Pamaquin

Antibacterials, such as:
- Most sulfonamides
- Nitrofurantoin
- Chloramphenicol
- Quinolones

Miscellaneous drugs, such as:
- Dapsone
- Vitamin K
- Probenecid
- Quinidine
- Dimercaprol
- Phenylhydrazine
- Methylene blue

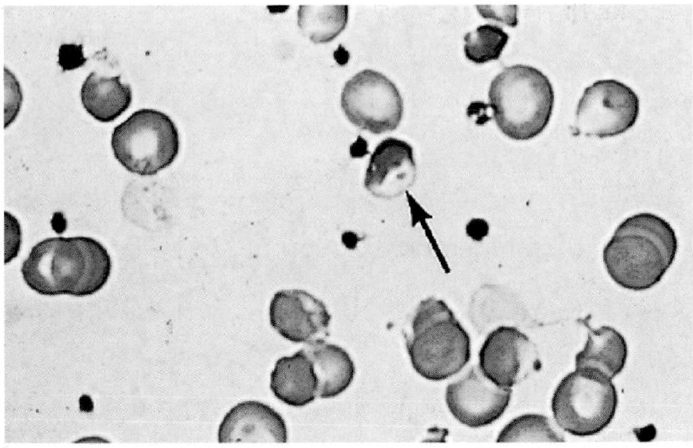

Figure 16.23 'Blister' cells (arrowed) in G6PD deficiency.

Clinical syndromes

- Acute drug-induced haemolysis ***(Box 16.15)*** – usually dose-related.
- Favism (ingestion of fava beans).
- Chronic haemolytic anaemia.
- Neonatal jaundice.
- Infections and acute illnesses – also precipitate haemolysis in patients with G6PD deficiency.

Mothballs containing naphthalene can also cause haemolysis.

The clinical features are due to rapid intravascular haemolysis with symptoms of anaemia, jaundice and haemoglobinuria.

Investigations

- ***Blood count*** is normal between attacks.
- ***During an attack***, the blood film may show irregularly contracted cells, bite cells (cells with an indentation in the membrane), blister cells (cells in which the Hb appears to have become partially detached from the cell membrane; ***Fig. 16.23***), Heinz bodies (red cell inclusions composed of denatured haemoglobin, best seen on films stained with methyl violet) and reticulocytosis.
- ***Haemolysis*** is evident (see p. 532).
- ***Several screening tests***, such as demonstration of the decreased ability of G6PD-deficient cells to reduce dyes, can be used to detect G6PD deficiency. The level of the enzyme may also be directly assayed. There are two diagnostic problems. Immediately after an attack, the screening tests may be normal (because the oldest red cells with least 6GPD activity are destroyed selectively). The diagnosis of heterozygous females may be difficult because the enzyme level may range from very low to normal, depending on Lyonization. However, the risk of clinically significant haemolysis is minimal in patients with borderline G6PD activity.

Management

- Any offending drugs should be stopped.
- Underlying infection should be treated.
- Blood transfusion may be life-saving.
- Splenectomy is not usually helpful.

Pyruvate kinase deficiency

This is the most common defect of red cell metabolism after G6PD deficiency; it affects thousands rather than millions of people worldwide. The site of the defect is shown in ***Figure 16.22***. Production of ATP is reduced, causing rigid red cells. Homozygotes have haemolytic anaemia and splenomegaly. It is inherited as an autosomal recessive condition.

Investigations

- ***Anaemia*** of variable severity is present (Hb 50–100 g/L). The oxygen dissociation curve is shifted to the right as a result of the rise in intracellular 2,3-BPG, and this reduces the severity of symptoms due to anaemia.
- ***Blood films*** show distorted ('prickle') cells and a reticulocytosis.
- ***Pyruvate kinase activity*** is low (affected homozygotes have levels of 5–20%).

Management

Blood transfusions may be necessary during infections and pregnancy. Splenectomy may improve the clinical condition and is usually advised for patients requiring frequent transfusions.

Pyrimidine 5′ nucleotidase deficiency

This autosomal recessive disorder produces a haemolytic anaemia with basophilic stippling of the red cells. The enzyme degrades pyrimidine nucleotides to cytidine and uridine (pentose phosphate shunt), which in turn leads to the degradation of RNA in the reticulocytes. Lack of the enzyme results in accumulation of partially degraded RNA, which shows as basophilic stippling in mature red cells. The enzyme is also inhibited by lead (see p. 77), and thus basophilic stippling is seen in lead poisoning. The hereditary form can be diagnosed by measuring the enzyme in erythrocytes. A screening test using the ultraviolet absorption spectrum of red cells is available.

Further reading

Cappellini MD, Fiorelli G. Glucose-6-phosphate dehydrogenase deficiency. *Lancet* 2008; 371:64–72.

ACQUIRED HAEMOLYTIC ANAEMIA

These anaemias may be divided into those due to immune, non-immune or other causes (see ***Box 16.9***).

Aetiology

Causes of immune destruction of red cells

- Autoantibodies.
- Drug-induced antibodies.
- Alloantibodies.

Causes of non-immune destruction of red cells

- Acquired membrane defects (e.g. paroxysmal nocturnal haemoglobinuria; see p. 548).
- Mechanical factors (e.g. prosthetic heart valves or microangiopathic haemolytic anaemia; see p. 548).
- Secondary to systemic disease (e.g. renal and liver disease).

Miscellaneous causes

- Various toxic substances can disrupt the red cell membrane and cause haemolysis (e.g. arsenic, and toxins produced by *Clostridium perfringens* (*welchii*)).
- Malaria frequently causes anaemia owing to the combination of a reduction in red cell survival and reduced production of red cells.
- Hypersplenism (see p. 553) results in a reduced red cell survival, which may also contribute to the anaemia seen in malaria.
- Extensive burns result in denaturation of red cell membrane proteins and reduced red cell survival.
- Some drugs (e.g. dapsone, sulfasalazine) cause oxidative haemolysis with Heinz bodies.
- Some ingested chemicals (e.g. weedkillers such as sodium chlorate) can cause severe oxidative haemolysis leading to acute kidney injury.

Autoimmune haemolytic anaemias

Autoimmune haemolytic anaemias (AIHAs) are acquired disorders resulting from increased red cell destruction due to red cell autoantibodies. These anaemias are characterized by the presence of a positive direct antiglobulin (Coombs') test, which detects the autoantibody on the surface of the patient's red cells ***(Fig. 16.24)***.

AIHA is divided into 'warm' and 'cold' types, depending on whether the antibody attaches better to the red cells at body temperature (37°C) or at lower temperatures. The major features and the causes of these two forms of AIHA are shown in ***Box 16.16***. In warm AIHA, IgG antibodies predominate and the direct antiglobulin test is positive with IgG alone, IgG and complement, or complement only. In cold AIHA, the antibodies are usually IgM. They easily elute off red cells, leaving complement, which is detected as C3d.

Immune destruction of red cells

IgM or IgG red cell antibodies, which fully activate the complement cascade, cause lysis of red cells in the circulation (intravascular haemolysis).

IgG antibodies frequently do not activate complement and the coated red cells undergo extravascular haemolysis ***(Fig. 16.25)***. They either are completely phagocytosed in the spleen through an interaction with Fc receptors on macrophages, or they lose part of the cell membrane through partial phagocytosis and circulate as

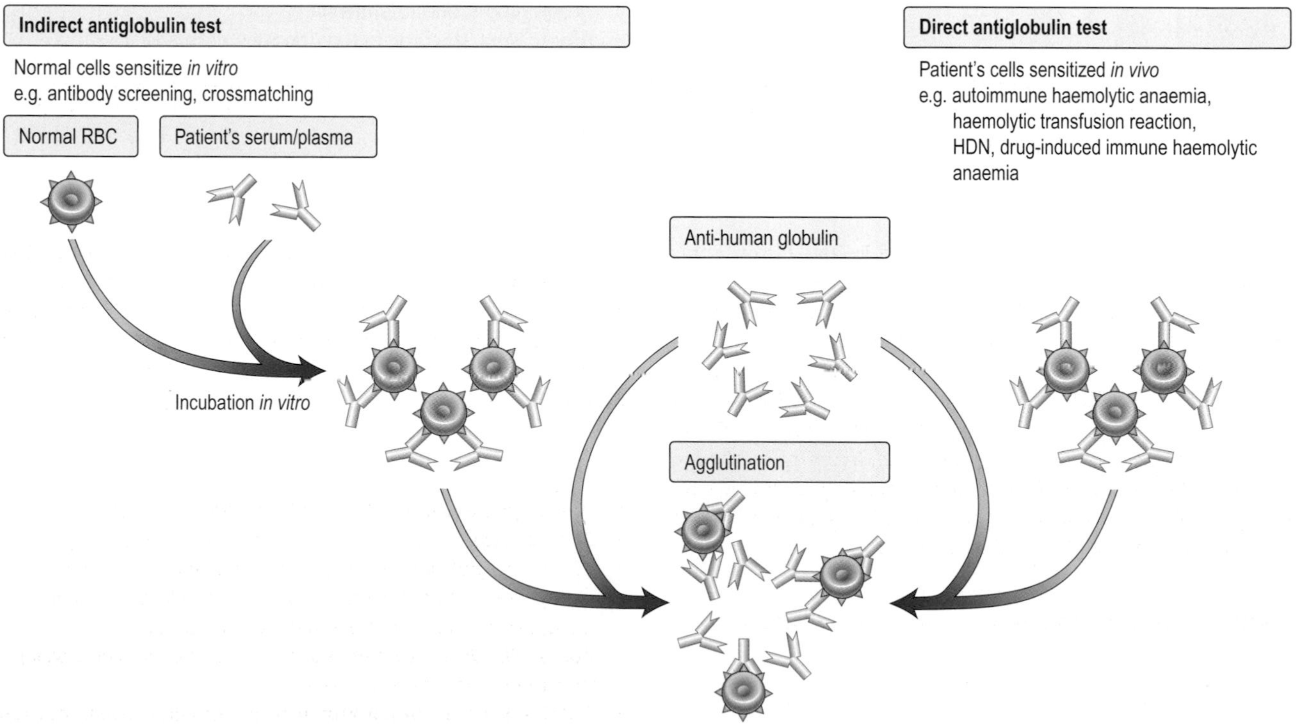

Figure 16.24 Antiglobulin (Coombs') tests. The anti-human globulin forms bridges between the sensitized cells, causing visible agglutination. The direct test detects patients' cells sensitized *in vivo*. The indirect test detects normal cells sensitized *in vitro*. HDN, haemolytic disease of newborn; RBC, red blood cell.

Box 16.16 Causes and major features of autoimmune haemolytic anaemias

	Warm	Cold
Temperature at which antibody attaches best to red cells	37°C	Lower than 37°C
Type of antibody	IgG	IgM
Direct Coombs' test	Strongly positive	Positive
Causes of primary conditions	Idiopathic	Idiopathic
Causes of secondary condition	Autoimmune rheumatic disorders, e.g. systemic lupus erythematosus Chronic lymphocytic leukaemia Lymphomas Hodgkin's lymphoma Carcinomas Drugs, many including methyldopa, penicillins, cephalosporins, NSAIDs, quinine, interferon	Infections, e.g. infectious mononucleosis, *Mycoplasma pneumoniae*, other viral infections (rare) Lymphomas Paroxysmal cold haemoglobinuria (IgG)

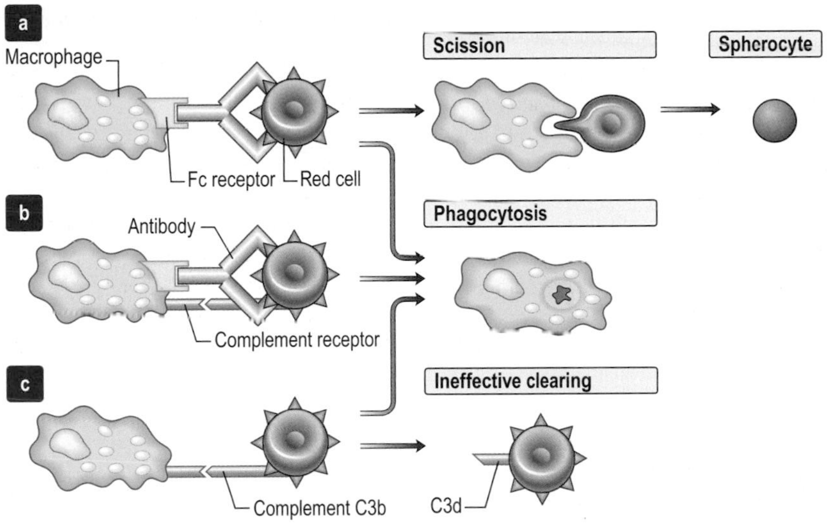

Figure 16.25 Extravascular haemolysis. This is due to interaction of antibody-coated cells with cells in the reticuloendothelial system, predominantly in the spleen. **(a)** Spherocytosis results from partial phagocytosis. **(b)** Complete phagocytosis may occur and this is enhanced if there is complement as well as antibody on the cell surface. **(c)** Cells coated with complement only are ineffectively removed and circulate with C3d or C3b on their surface.

spherocytes until they become sequestered in the spleen. Some IgG antibodies partially activate complement, leading to deposition of C3b on the red cell surface, and this may enhance phagocytosis, as macrophages also have receptors for C3b.

Non-complement-binding IgM antibodies are rare and have little or no effect on red cell survival. IgM antibodies, which partially rather than fully activate complement, cause adherence of red cells to C3b receptors on macrophages, particularly in the liver, although this is an ineffective mechanism of haemolysis. Most of the red cells are released from the macrophages when C3b is cleaved to C3d and then circulate with C3d on their surface.

'Warm' autoimmune haemolytic anaemias

Clinical features

These anaemias may occur at all ages and in both sexes, although they are most frequent in middle-aged females. They can present as a short episode of anaemia and jaundice but they often remit and relapse, and may progress to an intermittent chronic pattern. The spleen may be palpable. Infections or folate deficiency may provoke a profound fall in the haemoglobin level. Autoimmune haemolytic anaemias are primary or secondary. The most common underlying cause is a lymphoproliferative disorder ***(Box 16.16)***.

Investigations

- ***Haemolytic anaemia*** is evident (see pp. 533–543).
- ***Spherocytosis*** is present as a result of red cell damage.
- ***Direct antiglobulin test*** is positive, with either IgG alone (67%), IgG and complement (20%) or complement alone (13%) being found on the surface of the red cells.
- ***Autoantibodies*** may have specificity for the Rh blood group system (e.g. for the e antigen).
- ***Autoimmune thrombocytopenia*** and/or neutropenia may also be present (***Evans syndrome***; see p. 569).
- ***Abdominal CT scan*** should be carried out to detect abdominal lymphoma.

Management and prognosis

Corticosteroids (e.g. prednisolone in doses of 1 mg/kg daily) are effective in inducing a remission in about 80% of patients. Steroids reduce both production of the red cell autoantibodies and destruction of antibody-coated cells. Splenectomy is the most effective second-line therapy, but many patients prefer to avoid splenectomy because of the lack of a guarantee of a successful outcome, its potential complications and the need to take antibiotic prophylaxis (see p. 553). Other immunosuppressive drugs, such as azathioprine and rituximab, may be effective in patients who fail to respond to steroids and splenectomy. Blood transfusion may be necessary if there is severe anaemia, although compatibility testing is complicated by the presence of red cell autoantibodies.

'Cold' autoimmune haemolytic anaemias

Low titres of IgM cold agglutinins reacting at 4°C are normally present in plasma and are harmless. At low temperatures, these antibodies can attach to red cells and cause their agglutination in the cold peripheries of the body. In addition, activation of complement may cause intravascular haemolysis when the cells return to the higher temperatures in the core of the body.

After certain infections (such as those caused by *Mycoplasma*, cytomegalovirus or Epstein–Barr virus (EBV)), increased production of polyclonal cold agglutinins may occur, producing a mild to moderate transient haemolysis.

Chronic cold haemagglutinin disease

Chronic cold haemagglutinin disease (CHAD) usually occurs in the elderly with a gradual onset of haemolytic anaemia owing to the production of monoclonal IgM cold agglutinins. After exposure to cold, the patient develops an acrocyanosis similar to Raynaud's as a result of red cell autoagglutination.

Investigations

- ***Red cells*** agglutinate in the cold or at room temperature. Agglutination is sometimes seen in the sample tube after cooling but is more easily observed on the peripheral blood film made at room temperature. The agglutination is reversible after warming the sample. The agglutination may cause a spurious increase in the MCV (see p. 517).
- ***Cold agglutinin test*** demonstrates a markedly elevated titre in CHAD to >1:512.
- ***Direct antiglobulin test*** is positive with complement (C3d) alone.
- ***Monoclonal IgM antibodies*** have specificity for the Ii blood group system, usually for the I antigen but occasionally for the i antigen.

Management

Any underlying cause should be treated, if possible. Patients should avoid exposure to cold. Steroids, alkylating agents (chemotherapy) and splenectomy are usually ineffective. Treatment with anti-CD20 (rituximab) has been successful in some cases. Blood transfusion may be necessary, and if so, the patient should be in a warm environment; compatibility testing may be difficult due to the cold agglutinin.

Paroxysmal cold haemoglobinuria

Paroxysmal cold haemoglobinuria (PCH) is a rare condition associated with common childhood infections, such as measles, mumps and chickenpox. Intravascular haemolysis is associated with polyclonal IgG complement-fixing antibodies. These antibodies are biphasic, reacting with red cells in the cold in the peripheral circulation, with lysis occurring due to complement activation when the cells return to the central circulation. The antibodies have specificity for the P red cell antigen. The lytic reaction is demonstrated *in vitro* by incubating the patient's red cells and serum at 4°C and then warming the mixture to 37°C (Donath–Landsteiner test). Haemolysis is self-limiting but red cell transfusions may be necessary.

Drug-induced immune haemolytic anaemia

Drug-induced haemolytic anaemias are rare, although over 100 drugs have been reported to cause immune haemolytic anaemia. The interaction between a drug and red cell membrane may produce three types of antibodies:

- ***Antibodies to the drug*** only, e.g. quinidine, rifampicin. Immune complexes attach to red cells and may cause acute and severe intravascular haemolysis, sometimes associated with kidney injury. The haemolysis usually resolves quickly once the drug is withdrawn.
- ***Antibodies to the cell membrane*** only, e.g. methyldopa, fludarabine. There is extravascular haemolysis and the clinical course tends to be more protracted.
- ***Antibodies to part-drug, part-cell membrane***, e.g. penicillin. This develops only in patients receiving large doses of penicillin. The haemolysis typically develops over 7–10 days, and recovery is gradual after drug withdrawal.

Confirmation of the diagnosis of drug-induced immune haemolytic anaemia requires:

- A temporal association between administration of a drug and haemolytic anaemia.
- Recovery after withdrawal of the drug.
- A positive direct antiglobulin test.
- Drug-dependent red cell antibodies. These are detectable in the first and third mechanisms described above. In the second, the antibodies are not drug-dependent and are indistinguishable from autoantibodies.

Alloimmune haemolytic anaemia

Antibodies produced in one individual react with the red cells of another. This situation occurs in haemolytic disease of the newborn, in haemolytic transfusion reactions (see p. 557), and after allogeneic bone marrow, renal, liver, cardiac or intestinal transplantation when donor lymphocytes transferred in the allograft ('passenger lymphocytes') may produce red cell antibodies against the recipient and cause haemolytic anaemia.

Haemolytic disease of the newborn

Haemolytic disease of the newborn (HDN) is caused by fetomaternal incompatibility for red cell antigens. Maternal alloantibodies against fetal red cell antigens pass from the maternal circulation via the placenta into the fetus, where they destroy the fetal red cells. Only IgG antibodies are capable of transplacental passage from mother to fetus.

The most common type of HDN is that due to ABO incompatibility, where the mother is usually group O and the fetus group A.

HDN due to ABO incompatibility is usually mild and exchange transfusion is rarely needed. HDN due to RhD incompatibility has become much less common in developed countries following the introduction of anti-D prophylaxis (see below). HDN may be caused by antibodies against antigens in many blood group systems (e.g. other Rh antigens such as c and E, and Kell, Duffy and Kidd; see p. 554).

Sensitization occurs as a result of passage of fetal red cells into the maternal circulation (which most readily occurs at the time of delivery), so that first pregnancies are rarely affected. However, sensitization may occur at other times – for example, after a miscarriage, ectopic pregnancy or blood transfusion – or be due to episodes during pregnancy that cause transplacental bleeding, such as amniocentesis, chorionic villus sampling and threatened miscarriage.

Clinical features

These vary from a mild haemolytic anaemia of the newborn to intrauterine death from 18 weeks' gestation with the characteristic appearance of hydrops fetalis (hepatosplenomegaly, oedema and cardiac failure).

Kernicterus occurs owing to severe jaundice in the neonatal period, when the unconjugated (lipid-soluble) bilirubin exceeds 250 μmol/L and bile pigment deposition occurs in the basal ganglia. This can result in permanent brain damage, choreoathetosis and spasticity. In mild cases, it may present as deafness.

Investigations

Routine antenatal serology

All mothers should have their ABO and RhD groups determined and tested for atypical antibodies after attending the antenatal booking clinic. These tests should be repeated at 28 weeks' gestation.

If an antibody is detected, its blood group specificity should be determined and the mother should be retested at least monthly. A rising antibody titre of IgG antibodies or a history of HDN in a previous pregnancy is an indication for referral to a fetal medicine unit.

Antenatal assessment and treatment

If a clinically significant antibody capable of causing HDN, such as anti-D, anti-c or anti-K, is detected, the father's phenotype provides useful information for predicting the likelihood of the fetus carrying the relevant red cell antigen. If the father is heterozygous, the genotype of the fetus can be determined from fetal DNA obtained by amniocentesis, chorionic villus sampling or fetal blood sampling. Soluble fetal DNA in maternal plasma can also be used for RhD typing, avoiding an invasive procedure.

The severity of anaemia is assessed by Doppler flow velocity of the fetal middle cerebral artery; measurement of bile pigments in the amniotic fluid is no longer routinely used. If the infant appears to have severe anaemia on non-invasive monitoring, ultrasound-guided fetal blood sampling is used to confirm this directly; if necessary, an intravascular fetal transfusion of red cells is given.

Birth of an affected infant

A sample of cord blood is obtained at birth. This shows:

- anaemia with a high reticulocyte count
- a positive direct antiglobulin test
- a raised serum bilirubin.

Postnatal management

In mild cases, phototherapy may be used to convert bilirubin to water-soluble biliverdin. Biliverdin can be excreted by the kidneys and this therefore reduces the chance of kernicterus. In more severely affected cases, exchange transfusion may be necessary to replace the infant's red cells and to remove bilirubin. Indications for exchange transfusion include:

- a cord Hb of <120 g/L (normal cord Hb is 136–196 g/L)
- a cord bilirubin of >60 μmol/L
- a later serum bilirubin of >300 μmol/L
- a rapidly rising serum bilirubin level.

Further exchange transfusions may be necessary to remove the unconjugated bilirubin.

The blood used for exchange transfusions should be ABO-compatible with the mother and infant, lack the antigen against which the maternal antibody is directed, be fresh (no more than 5 days from the day of collection) and be cytomegalovirus (CMV)-seronegative to prevent transmission of CMV.

Prevention of RhD immunization in the mother

Anti-D should be given after delivery when all of the following conditions are fulfilled:

- The mother is RhD-negative.
- The fetus is RhD-positive.
- There is no maternal anti-D detectable in the mother's serum; that is, the mother is not already immunized.

The dose is 500 IU of IgG anti-D intramuscularly within 72 hours of delivery. The Kleihauer test is used to assess the number of fetal cells in the maternal circulation. A blood film prepared from maternal blood is treated with acid, which elutes HbA. HbF is resistant to this treatment and can be seen when the film is stained with eosin. If large numbers of fetal red cells are present in the maternal circulation, a higher or additional dose of anti-D will be necessary.

It may be necessary to give prophylaxis to RhD-negative women at other times when sensitization may occur, such as after an ectopic pregnancy, threatened miscarriage or termination of pregnancy. The dose of anti-D is 250 IU before 20 weeks' gestation and 500 IU after 20 weeks. A ***Kleihauer test*** should be carried out after 20 weeks to determine whether more anti-D is required.

Of previously non-immunized RhD-negative women carrying RhD-positive fetuses, 1–2% became immunized by the time of delivery. Antenatal prophylaxis with anti-D has been shown to reduce the incidence of immunization during pregnancy, and its routine use has been implemented in the UK. It can be given as two doses of anti-D immunoglobulin of either 500 IU or 1500 IU (one at 28 weeks' gestation and one at 34 weeks) or as a single dose of 1500 IU either at 28 weeks' gestation or between 28 and 30 weeks. Monoclonal anti-D could, in principle, replace polyclonal anti-D, which is collected from RhD-negative women immunized in pregnancy and deliberately immunized RhD-negative males, but it is likely to be some years before trials have been completed to confirm its safety and effectiveness.

Further reading

British Committee for Standards in Haematology (BCSH). Guideline for the use of anti-D immunoglobulin for the prevention of haemolytic disease of the fetus and newborn. *Transfus Med* 2014; 24:8–20.

Non-immune haemolytic anaemia

Paroxysmal nocturnal haemoglobinuria

Paroxysmal nocturnal haemoglobinuria (PNH) is a rare form of haemolytic anaemia that results from the clonal expression of haemopoietic stems cells that have mutations in the X-linked gene *PIG-A*. These mutations cause impaired synthesis of glycosylphosphatidylinositol (GPI), which anchors many proteins, such as decay accelerating factor (DAF; CD55), to the cell surface, and membrane inhibitor of reactive lysis (MIRL; CD59) to cell membranes. CD55, CD59 and other proteins are involved in complement degradation (at the C3 and C5 levels), and in their absence, the haemolytic action of complement continues.

Clinical features

The major clinical signs are intravascular haemolysis, venous thrombosis and haemoglobinuria. Haemolysis may be precipitated by infection, iron therapy or surgery. Characteristically, only the urine voided at night and in the morning on waking is dark in colour, although the reason for this phenomenon is not clear. In severe cases, all urine samples are dark. Urinary iron loss may be sufficient to cause iron deficiency. Some patients present insidiously with signs of anaemia and recurrent abdominal pains.

Venous thrombotic episodes may occur at atypical sites and severe thromboses may be a feature: for example, in hepatic (Budd–Chiari syndrome), mesenteric or cerebral veins. The cause of the increased predisposition to thrombosis is not known, but may be due to complement-mediated activation of platelets deficient in CD55 and CD59. Another suggestion is that intravascular haemolysis, which releases haemoglobin in the plasma, lowers plasma nitric oxide, causing the symptoms and venous thrombosis.

Investigations

- ***Intravascular haemolysis*** is evident (see p. 533).
- ***Flow cytometric analysis*** of red cells with anti-CD55 and anti-CD59 is undertaken.
- ***Bone marrow*** is sometimes hypoplastic (or even aplastic) despite haemolysis.

Management and prognosis

PNH is a chronic disorder requiring supportive measures such as blood transfusions, which are necessary for patients with severe anaemia. However, treatment with ***eculizumab*** has revolutionized therapy. The drug is administered intravenously every 7 days for the first 5 weeks and then every 2 weeks thereafter. It is a recombinant humanized monoclonal antibody that prevents the cleavage of C5 (and therefore formation of the membrane attack complex). It reduces intravascular haemolysis, haemoglobinuria and the need for transfusion, and gives an improved quality of life. Eculizumab also reduces the risk of thrombosis, the leading cause of mortality in PNH. It is now also being used in pregnancy. The most serious risk of terminal complement blockade is infection with *Neisseria meningitidis*; thus vaccination against *N. meningitidis* is recommended 2 weeks before commencing treatment.

Long-term anticoagulation may be necessary acutely for patients with recurrent thrombotic episodes. Its long-term value is unclear with the use of eculizumab. In patients with bone marrow failure, treatment options include immunosuppression with antilymphocyte globulin, ciclosporin or bone marrow transplantation. Eculizumab does not alleviate bone marrow failure. Bone marrow transplantation has been successfully carried out using either HLA-matched sibling donors in patients under the age of 50 or matched unrelated donors in patients under the age of 25.

The course of PNH is variable. PNH may transform into aplastic anaemia or acute leukaemia, but it may remain stable for many years and the PNH clone may even disappear, which must be taken into account if considering potentially dangerous treatments such as bone marrow transplantation. The median survival is 10–15 years.

Further reading

Brodsky RA. Paroxysmal nocturnal haemoglobinuria. *Blood* 2014; 124:2804–2811.

Mechanical haemolytic anaemia

Red cells may be injured by physical trauma in the circulation. Direct injury may cause immediate cell lysis or be followed by resealing of the cell membrane with the formation of distorted red cells or 'fragments'. These cells may circulate for a short period before being destroyed prematurely in the reticuloendothelial system.

The causes of mechanical haemolytic anaemia include:

- damaged artificial heart valves
- march haemoglobinuria, where there is damage to red cells in the feet associated with prolonged marching or running
- microangiopathic haemolytic anaemia (MAHA), where fragmentation of red cells occurs in an abnormal microcirculation because of malignant hypertension, eclampsia, haemolytic uraemic syndrome, thrombotic thrombocytopenic purpura, vasculitis or disseminated intravascular coagulation.

MYELOPROLIFERATIVE NEOPLASMS

Myeloproliferative neoplasms are clonal stem cell disorders characterized by uncontrolled proliferation of one or more of the cell lines in the bone marrow, usually erythroid, myeloid and/or megakaryocyte lines. Myeloproliferative disorders include:

- polycythaemia vera (PV)
- essential thrombocythaemia (ET)
- myelofibrosis – all of these three have a *JAK-2* molecular lesion
- chronic myeloid leukaemia (CML), a genetic *BCR-ABL* lesion.

These disorders are grouped together, as there can be transition from one disease to another; for example, PV can lead to myelofibrosis. They may also transform to acute myeloid leukaemia. The non-leukaemic myeloproliferative neoplasms (PV, ET and myelofibrosis) will be discussed in this section. CML is described on pages 612–613.

Polycythaemia

Polycythaemia (or erythrocytosis) is defined as an increase in haemoglobin, packed cell volume (PCV) and red cell count. PCV is a more reliable indicator of polycythaemia than is Hb, which may be disproportionately low in iron deficiency. Relative erythrocytosis is where the red cell volume is normal but there is a decrease in the plasma volume (see ***Fig. 16.6***).

Polycythaemia can be classified as primary polycythaemia (PV) or secondary polycythaemia. Secondary polycythaemia can be congenital or acquired. The latter is due to either an appropriate increase in erythropoietin in response to hypoxia, or an inappropriate increase in erythropoietin associated with ectopic production by tumours, such as a renal carcinoma. The causes of polycythaemia are given in ***Box 16.17***.

Primary polycythaemia: polycythaemia vera

Polycythaemia vera (PV) is a clonal stem cell disorder in which there is an excessive proliferation of erythroid, myeloid and/or megakaryocytic progenitor cells. Over 95% of patients with PV have acquired mutations of the gene Janus kinase 2 (*JAK2*), in the vast majority of cases a point mutation that causes the substitution of phenylalanine for valine at position 617 (JAK2V617F). JAK2 is a cytoplasmic tyrosine kinase that transduces signals, especially those triggered by haemopoietic growth factors such as erythropoietin, in normal and neoplastic cells. The significance of the discovery of the *JAK2* mutation in myeloproliferative neoplasms is two-fold: first, and of immediate significance, is the clinical utility of the detection of *JAK2* mutations for the diagnosis of PV, and second is the prospect of the development of new treatments for the myeloproliferative disorders based on targeting JAK2 activity.

Clinical features

The onset is insidious. PV usually presents in patients aged over 60 years with tiredness, itching, vertigo, headache and visual disturbance. It should be noted that these symptoms are also common in the normal population over the age of 60 and, consequently, PV is easily missed. Patients may also present with complications of the disease relating to thrombosis or haemorrhage. Increasingly, PV is detected on routine blood tests conducted for other reasons.

Severe itching is common after a hot bath or when the patient is warm. Gout due to increased cell turnover may be a feature, and peptic ulceration occurs in a minority of patients. Thrombosis and haemorrhage are the major complications of PV.

The patient is usually plethoric and has a deep dusky cyanosis. Injection of the conjunctivae is commonly seen. The spleen is palpable in 70% and is useful in distinguishing PV from secondary polycythaemia. The liver is enlarged in 50% of patients.

Diagnosis

JAK2 mutation screening is routine in the investigation of polycythaemia and is fully incorporated into diagnostic criteria. ***Box 16.18*** shows the revised WHO criteria for diagnosis in adults. The measurement of red cell and plasma volume is not routinely required. Measurement of serum ferritin can be useful to detect cases of iron-deficient PV. There may be a raised serum uric acid, leucocyte alkaline phosphatase and raised serum vitamin B_{12} and vitamin B_{12} binding protein (transcobalamin 1).

Management

Course and management

Treatment is designed to maintain a normal blood count and to prevent the complications of the disease, particularly thromboses and haemorrhage. Treatment is aimed at keeping the PCV below 0.45 L/L and the platelet count below 400×10^9/L.

There are three types of specific treatment:

- ***Venesection***. During initial phases of treatment, the removal of 400–500 mL of blood weekly will successfully relieve many of the symptoms of PV. Iron deficiency eventually limits erythropoiesis and only infrequent venesection is required. Venesection is often used as the sole treatment with the aim of maintaining a PCV of <0.45 L/L.

Box 16.17 Causes of polycythaemia

Primary
- Polycythaemia vera

Congenital
- Mutations in erythropoietin receptor
- High-oxygen-affinity haemoglobins
- Mutations in hypoxia-sensing pathways, e.g. Chuvash polycythaemia mutation in von Hippel–Lindau gene

Secondary

Due to an appropriate (hypoxic) increase in erythropoietin
- High altitude
- Chronic lung disease
- Cardiovascular disease (right-to-left shunt)
- Sleep apnoea
- Morbid obesity
- Heavy smoking

Due to an inappropriate increase in erythropoietin
- Renal disease: renal cell carcinoma, Wilms' tumour
- Hepatocellular carcinoma
- Adrenal tumours
- Cerebellar haemangioblastoma
- Massive uterine leiomyoma
- Over-administration of erythropoietin
- Treatment with androgen preparations

Relative
- Stress or spurious polycythaemia
- Dehydration
- Burns

Box 16.18 Polycythaemia vera: modified from revised WHO criteria

Major criteria
- Haemoglobin >185 g/L in men, >165 g/L in women or other evidence of increased red cell volume
- Presence of *JAK2* tyrosine kinase V617F or other functionally similar mutation such as *JAK2* exon 12 mutation

Minor criteria
- Bone marrow biopsy, showing hypercellularity for age with trilineage growth (panmyelosis) with prominent erythroid, granulocytic and megakaryocytic proliferation
- Serum erythropoietin level below the reference range for normal
- Endogenous erythroid colony (EEC) formation *in vitro*[a]

Diagnosis requires the presence of both major criteria and one minor criterion, or the presence of the first major criterion together with two minor criteria.

[a]*EEC testing is not routinely available but colony formation in the absence of exogenous erythropoietin in vitro is highly specific and sensitive in patients without previous treatment.*

(Research originally published in Tefferi A, Thiele J, Orazi A et al. Proposals and rationale for revision of the World Health Organization diagnostic criteria for polycythemia vera, essential thrombocythemia, and primary myelofibrosis: recommendations from an ad hoc international expert panel. Blood *2007; 110:1092–1097, ©American Society of Hematology.)*

- ***Chemotherapy***. Continuous or intermittent treatment with hydroxycarbamide (hydroxyurea) is used in patients who do not tolerate venesection or have other poorly controlled features of the disease, such as thrombocytosis, symptomatic splenomegaly or thrombosis. Interferon-alpha is also effective; it is administered by subcutaneous injection. Low-dose intermittent busulfan may be more convenient for elderly people but use must be weighed against the potential risk of long-term complications, such as the increased risk of leukaemia development with busulfan and related treatments.
- ***Low-dose aspirin***. Aspirin 75 mg daily with the above treatments is routinely used for patients with PV in the absence of contraindications
- ***Anagrelide***. This inhibits megakaryocyte differentiation and is useful for thrombocytosis.

Iron replacement should be avoided in patients with iron-deficient PV, as this can result in a dangerous rebound polycythaemia.

General measures

- ***Radioactive ^{32}P***. This is only given to patients over 70 years because of the increased risk of transformation to acute leukaemia.
- ***Allopurinol***. This can be given to block uric acid production. The pruritus is lessened by avoiding very hot baths.
- ***H1-receptor antagonists***. These have largely proved unsuccessful in relieving distressing pruritus but ***H2-receptor antagonists***, such as cimetidine, are occasionally effective.
- ***Surgery***. Polycythaemia should be controlled before surgery. Patients with uncontrolled PV have a high operative risk. In an emergency, reduction of the haematocrit by venesection and appropriate fluid replacement must be carried out.

Prognosis

PV develops into myelofibrosis in 30% of cases and into acute myeloblastic leukaemia in 5% as part of the natural history of the disease.

Secondary polycythaemias

Many high-oxygen affinity haemoglobin mutants (HOAHMs) have been described that lead to increased oxygen affinity but decreased oxygen delivery to the tissues, resulting in compensatory polycythaemia. A congenital autosomal recessive disorder (Chuvash polycythaemia) is due to a defect in the oxygen-sensing erythropoietin production pathway caused by a mutation of the von Hippel–Lindau (*VHL*) gene, resulting in an increased production of erythropoietin.

The causes of secondary polycythaemias are shown in ***Box 16.17***.

Serum erythropoietin (EPO) levels are normal or raised in secondary polycythaemia. Rarely, the discovery of a high EPO level may be the clue to the presence of an EPO-secreting tumour.

Management

The treatment is that of the precipitating factor; for example, renal or posterior fossa tumours need to be resected if possible. The most common cause is heavy smoking, which can produce as much as 10% carboxyhaemoglobin, and this can produce polycythaemia because of a reduction in the oxygen-carrying capacity of the blood. Heavy smokers also often have respiratory disease.

Complications of secondary polycythaemia are distinct to those seen in PV, and although hyperviscosity symptoms and thromboembolic episodes can occur, management depends on the underlying cause. Complications due to myeloproliferative disease, such as progression to myelofibrosis or acute leukaemia, do not develop. Venesection may be symptomatically helpful in the certain patients with secondary polycythaemia, particularly if the PCV is above 0.54 L/L.

'Relative' or 'apparent' polycythaemia (Gaisböck syndrome)

This condition was originally thought to be stress-induced. The red cell volume is normal, but as the result of a decreased plasma volume, there is a relative polycythaemia. 'Relative' polycythaemia is more common than PV and occurs in middle-aged men, particularly in association with smoking, high alcohol intake, obesity and high blood pressure. The condition may present with cardiovascular problems, such as myocardial or cerebral ischaemia. For this reason, it may be justifiable to venesect selected patients; management also requires modification of lifestyle factors, such as smoking and alcohol.

Essential thrombocythaemia

Essential thrombocythaemia (ET) is a myeloproliferative disorder, closely related to PV, which is characterized by a persistently raised platelet count. Patients usually have normal Hb levels, although mild anaemia may occur. The WCC is elevated in some patients. At diagnosis, the platelet count will usually be $>600\times10^9$/L, and may be as high as 2000×10^9/L, or rarely even higher. ET presents either symptomatically with thromboembolic or, less commonly, bleeding problems, or incidentally (e.g. at a routine medical check). Erythromelalgia, severe burning pain, erythema, and warmth of the extremities – primarily the feet and, to a lesser extent, the hands – may occur in some patients.

The diagnosis of ET is based on a sustained platelet count $\geq450\times10^9$/L in the absence of a possible reactive cause for thrombocytosis (see below), and absence of other haematological malignancy associated with thrombocytosis (e.g. PV, myelofibrosis). In selected cases, a bone marrow biopsy is required; however, the requirement for this has been largely replaced by molecular tests. The *JAK2* mutation test (see PV) is useful in that the gene is mutated in about half of all cases of ET, confirming a myeloproliferative neoplasm. For the remaining 50% of patients with a normal *JAK2* gene, testing for mutations in calreticulin (*CALR*) or the thrombopoietin receptor (*MPL*) will be informative in most cases, abrogating the need for a bone marrow biopsy. As a generalization, a person with a very high platelet count ($>1000\times10^9$/L), who is clinically normal with good health, will most likely prove to have ET. In a patient who has a lower platelet count (e.g. 600×10^9/L) and is in poor health, the diagnosis can be more difficult. Other disorders that may give rise to reactive high platelet counts include autoimmune rheumatic disorders and malignancy. Individuals who have been splenectomized (for any reason, including trauma) sometimes have high platelet counts.

Treatment

Treatment is with hydroxycarbamide (hydroxyurea), anagrelide or busulfan to control the platelet count to $<400\times10^9$/L.

Interferon-alpha is also effective; it is administered by subcutaneous injection. ET may eventually transform into PV, myelofibrosis or acute leukaemia, but the disease may not progress for many years. Aspirin is routinely used in patients with ET.

Myelofibrosis

Myelofibrosis is a very debilitating chronic myeloproliferative neoplasm. It may be primary or develop late in the course of essential thrombocythaemia or polycythaemia vera. There is clonal proliferation of stem cells and abnormal myeloid cells in the bone marrow, liver, spleen and other organs. Increased fibrosis in the bone marrow is caused by hyperplasia of abnormal megakaryocytes, which release fibroblast-stimulating factors such as platelet-derived growth factor.

Clinical features

The disease presents insidiously with lethargy, weakness and weight loss. Patients often complain of a 'fullness' in the upper abdomen due to splenomegaly, which is often massive. Severe pain related to respiration may indicate perisplenitis secondary to splenic infarction, and bone pain and attacks of gout can complicate the illness. Extramedullary haemopoiesis can develop, typically in the spleen but also affecting other organs. Bruising and bleeding occur because of thrombocytopenia or abnormal platelet function. Other physical signs include anaemia, fever and massive splenomegaly (for other causes, see p. 553).

Investigations

- ***Anaemia*** with leucoerythroblastic features is present (see p. 563). Poikilocytes and red cells with characteristic teardrop forms are seen. The WCC may be $>100\times10^9$/L, and the differential WCC may be very similar to that seen in chronic myeloid leukaemia; later, leucopenia may also develop.
- ***The platelet count*** may be very high but, in later stages, thrombocytopenia occurs.
- ***Bone marrow aspiration*** is often unsuccessful and this gives a clue to the presence of the condition. A bone marrow trephine is necessary to show the markedly increased fibrosis. Increased numbers of megakaryocytes may be seen.
- ***The Philadelphia chromosome*** is absent; this helps to distinguish myelofibrosis from most cases of chronic myeloid leukaemia.
- ***The JAK2 mutation*** is present in approximately half of the cases, and the *CALR* mutation in many of the cases without *JAK2* mutation.

Management

This consists of general supportive measures, such as blood transfusion, analgesics and allopurinol. Treatment for myelofibrosis is often difficult but an estimation of prognosis from a prognostic scoring system is a good basis on which to start planning a treatment strategy for the individual patient. This may range from observation alone in those with the best prognosis to drug treatment or allogeneic stem cell transplantation, offering a hope of cure for younger patients. Historically, symptomatic splenomegaly was managed using hydroxycarbamide, radiotherapy and, in some cases, splenectomy. However, the latter is associated with very significant morbidity and mortality in patients with myelofibrosis and the two former are largely ineffective. A new and very promising development in the treatment of myelofibrosis is targeted therapy with JAK inhibitors. Ruxolitinib is the first such JAK inhibitor treatment in routine clinical use. Ruxolitinib results in substantial spleen reduction and improvement in symptoms in many patients with higher-risk myelofibrosis. Although ruxolitinib may improve life expectancy in patients with myelofibrosis, it does not, however, eradicate the disease and underlying fibrosis remains in the vast majority of patients.

Prognosis

Patients may survive for ≥10 years; median survival is 4–5 years. Death may occur in 10–20% of cases from transformation to acute myeloid leukaemia. The other most common causes of death are progression of myelofibrosis, cardiovascular disease and infection.

Myelodysplasia

Myelodysplasia (MDS) describes a group of acquired bone marrow disorders that are due to a defect in stem cells. They are characterized by increasing bone marrow failure with quantitative and qualitative abnormalities in at least one of the three myeloid cell lines (red cells, granulocyte/monocytes and platelets). The natural history of MDS is variable, but there is a high morbidity and mortality owing to bone marrow failure, and transformation into acute myeloblastic leukaemia occurs in about 30% of cases. WHO classification of the myelodysplastic syndrome is shown in ***Box 16.19***.

Box 16.19 World Health Organization classification of myelodysplasia (MDS)

Disease	Marrow blasts (%)	Clinical presentation	Cytogenetic abnormalities (%)
Refractory anaemia (RA)	<5	Anaemia	25
RA with ring sideroblasts (RARS)	<5	Anaemia, ≥15% ringed sideroblasts in erythroid precursors	5–20
MDS with isolated del(5q) (5q– syndrome)	<5	Anaemia, normal platelets	100
Refractory cytopenia with multilineage dysplasia (RCMD)	<5	Bicytopenia or pancytopenia	50
Refractory anaemia with excess blasts-1 (RAEB-1)	5–9	Cytopenias + peripheral blood blasts (<5%)	30–50
Refractory anaemia with excess blasts-2 (RAEB-2)	10–19	Cytopenias, peripheral blood blasts present	50–70
Myelodysplastic syndrome, unclassified (MDS-U)	<5	Neutropenia or thrombocytopenia	50

(From: Vardiman JW, Brunning RD, Arber DA et al. Introduction and overview of the classification of myeloid neoplasms. In: Swerdlow SH, Campo E, Harris NL et al. (eds). *WHO Classification of Tumors of Haemopoietic and Lymphoid Tissues*. Geneva: WHO; 2008.)

Clinical features and investigations

MDS occurs mainly in the elderly, and presents with symptoms of anaemia, infection or bleeding due to pancytopenia. MDS should be suspected in patients with otherwise unexplained cytopenias or macrocytosis. Serial blood counts show evidence of increasing bone marrow failure with anaemia, neutropenia, monocytosis and thrombocytopenia, either alone or in combination. By contrast, in chronic myelomonocytic leukaemias, monocytes are $>1\times10^9$/L and the WCC is raised, in some cases markedly so ($>100\times10^9$/L).

The bone marrow cellularity can be increased, normal or reduced, irrespective of the pancytopenia. Dyserythropoiesis is usually present, and granulocyte precursors and megakaryocytes may also have abnormal morphology. The percentage of bone marrow blast cells is important for classification and prognostic risk stratification in MDS. Ring sideroblasts are present in some types. Cytogenetic abnormalities are common and are important for prognostic stratification. **Box 16.19** shows the classification and the clinical presentation.

Somatic point mutations are commonly seen. A poor survival rate is seen in those carrying mutations in *TP53*, *E2H2*, *ETV6*, *RUNX1* and *ASXL1*.

Management

MDS is a heterogeneous disease and management is dependent on clinical features and predicted prognosis; the latter can be estimated using international prognostic scoring systems that incorporate blood counts, bone marrow blast percentage and cytogenetics. Patients with lower-risk disease are usually managed conservatively with supportive care.

Patients with higher-risk disease should be considered for allogeneic transplantation, if eligible. Treatment options include the following:

- ***Supportive care*** is the mainstay for all patients with MDS and symptomatic low blood counts. Supportive care includes blood transfusion, and the prevention and treatment of MDS-associated bleeding and infection.
- ***Iron chelation*** should be considered for patients with good prognostic MDS who develop secondary iron overload (transfused with more than 20 units of red cells or serum ferritin >1000 μg/L).
- ***Erythropoietin*** can be used in selected patients with low-risk MDS, symptomatic anaemia and inappropriately low endogenous erythropoietin levels.
- ***Hypomethylating agents*** (e.g. azacitidine) is useful in selected patients.
- ***Immunosuppressive agents***, such as ciclosporin and antithymocyte globulin, can be used in selected patients, including patients with a hypocellular bone marrow. ***Intensive chemotherapy*** schedules used for acute myeloblastic leukaemia (see pp. 610–611) may be tried in selected patients with high-risk MDS and higher numbers of bone marrow blasts, but the remission rate is less than for acute myeloblastic leukaemia, and prolonged pancytopenia may occur owing to poor haemopoietic regeneration caused by the defect in stem cells.
- ***Lenalidomide*** (a thalidomide analogue) has been proven to be remarkably successful in the treatment of early-stage MDS with a chromosome 5q deletion (the 5q− syndrome). Avoid use in women of child-bearing age.
- ***Allogeneic stem cell transplantation*** offers the hope of cure for carefully selected MDS patients who have an HLA-identical sibling or an unrelated HLA-matched donor. Due to the potential morbidity and mortality associated with allogeneic stem cell transplantation, this procedure is usually restricted to patients without major co-morbidities who have higher-risk MDS and in whom the risk–benefit balance is clear.

Further reading

Adès L, Itzykson R, Fenaux P. Myelodysplastic syndromes. *Lancet* 2014; 383:2239–2252.
Bejar R, Stevenson K, Abdel-Wahab O et al. Clinical effect of point mutations in myelodysplastic syndromes. *N Engl J Med* 2011; 364:2496–2506.
British Committee for Standards in Haematology (BCSH). Guidelines for the diagnosis and management of adult myelodysplastic syndromes. *Br J Haematol* 2014; 164:503–525.
Geyer HL, Mesa RA. Therapy for myeloproliferative neoplasms: when, which agent and how? *Blood* 2014; 124:3529–3537.
Harrison CN, Bareford D, Butt N et al. Guideline for investigation and management of adults and children presenting with a thrombocytosis. *Br J Haematol* 2010; 149:352–375.
Reilly JT, McCullin MF, Beer PA et al. Guideline for the diagnosis and management of myelofibrosis. *Br J Haematol* 2012; 158:453–471.
Vannucchi AM. From palliation to targeted therapy in myelofibrosis. *New Engl J Med* 2010; 363:1180–1182.

THE SPLEEN

The spleen is the largest lymphoid organ in the body and is situated in the left hypochondrium. There are two anatomical components:

- the red pulp, consisting of sinuses lined by endothelial macrophages and cords (spaces)
- the white pulp, which has a structure similar to that of lymphoid follicles.

Blood enters via the splenic artery and is delivered to the red and white pulp. During the flow, the blood is 'skimmed', with leucocytes and plasma preferentially passing to white pulp. Some red cells pass rapidly through into the venous system while others are held up in the red pulp.

Function

Sequestration and phagocytosis

Normal red cells, which are flexible, pass through the red pulp into the venous system without difficulty. Old or abnormal cells are damaged by the hypoxia, low glucose and low pH found in the sinuses of the red pulp and are therefore removed by phagocytosis along with other circulating foreign matter. Howell–Jolly and Heinz bodies and sideroblastic granules have their particles removed by 'pitting' and are then returned to the circulation. IgG-coated red cells are removed through their Fc receptors by macrophages.

Extramedullary haemopoiesis

Pluripotential stem cells are present in the spleen and proliferate during severe haematological stress, such as in haemolytic anaemia, thalassaemia major and myelofibrosis.

Immunological function

About 25% of the body's T lymphocytes and 15% of B lymphocytes are present in the spleen. The spleen shares the function of production of antibodies with other lymphoid tissues.

Blood pooling

Up to one-third of the platelets are sequestrated in the spleen and can be rapidly mobilized. Enlarged spleens pool a significant percentage (up to 40%) of the red cell mass.

Splenomegaly

The spleen enlarges from under the left costal margin inferiorly and medially. It is dull to percussion and it may be possible to palpate a notch along its leading edge, which further differentiates the mass from an enlarged left kidney. The spleen typically measures 11 cm in its longest dimension. An enlarged spleen is only palpable if it is 1.5–2 times the size of a normal spleen. Ultrasound or CT scanning may be used to confirm splenomegaly and may also provide other useful information, such as the presence of abdominal lymphadenopathy.

Aetiology

A clinically palpable spleen can have many causes:

- ***Infection***:
  - acute, e.g. septic shock, infective endocarditis, typhoid, infectious mononucleosis
  - chronic, e.g. tuberculosis, brucellosis
  - parasitic, e.g. malaria, kala-azar and schistosomiasis.
- ***Inflammation***: rheumatoid arthritis, sarcoidosis, SLE.
- ***Haematological factors***: haemolytic anaemia, haemoglobinopathies and the leukaemias, lymphomas and myeloproliferative disorders.
- ***Portal hypertension***: liver disease.
- ***Miscellaneous***: storage diseases (e.g. Gaucher's disease), amyloidosis, primary and secondary neoplasias, tropical splenomegaly.

Massive splenomegaly is seen in myelofibrosis, chronic myeloid leukaemia, chronic malaria, kala-azar or, rarely, Gaucher's disease.

Hypersplenism

This can result from splenomegaly due to any cause. It is commonly seen with splenomegaly due to haematological disorders, portal hypertension, rheumatoid arthritis (Felty syndrome) and lymphoma. Hypersplenism produces:

- pancytopenia
- haemolysis due to sequestration and destruction of red cells in the spleen
- increased plasma volume.

Management

This is often dependent on the underlying cause, but splenectomy is sometimes required for severe anaemia or thrombocytopenia.

Problems after splenectomy

Splenectomy is performed mainly for:

- trauma
- immune thrombocytopenic purpura (see pp. 569–570)
- haemolytic anaemias (see p. 534)
- hypersplenism.

An immediate problem is an increased platelet count (usually 600–1000 × 10^9/L) for 2–3 weeks. Thromboembolic phenomena may occur. In the longer term, there is an increased risk of overwhelming infections, particularly pneumococcal infections.

Prophylaxis against infection after splenectomy or splenic dysfunction

See ***Box 16.20*** for prophylactic measures. All patients should be educated about the risk of infection and the importance of its early recognition and treatment. They should be given an information leaflet and should carry a card or bracelet to alert health professionals to their risk of overwhelming infection.

Box 16.20 Prophylaxis against infection after splenectomy or splenic dysfunction

Vaccinate 2–3 weeks before elective splenectomy

- A 23-valent unconjugated pneumococcal polysaccharide vaccine repeated every 5 years
- Meningococcal group C conjugate vaccine*
- Annual influenza vaccine
- *Haemophilus influenzae* type b (Hib) vaccine
- Long-term penicillin V 500 mg 12-hourly (if sensitive, use erythromycin)
- Meningococcal polysaccharide vaccine (ACWY) for travellers to Africa/Saudi Arabia, e.g. during Hajj and Umrah pilgrimages

**Men B vaccination is now available.*

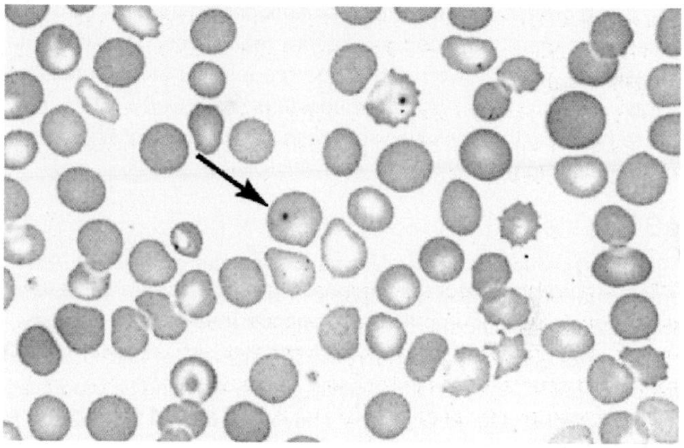

Figure 16.26 Post-splenectomy film with Howell–Jolly bodies (arrowed). Target cells and irregularly contracted cells are also shown.

Post-splenectomy haematological features

- ***Thrombocytosis*** persists in about 30% of cases.
- ***The WCC*** is usually normal but there may be a mild lymphocytosis and monocytosis.
- ***Abnormalities in red cell morphology*** are the most prominent changes and include Howell–Jolly bodies (contain basophilic nuclear remnants), Pappenheimer bodies (contain sideroblastic granules), target cells and irregular contracted red cells ***(Fig. 16.26)***. Pitted red cells can be counted.

Splenic atrophy

This is seen in sickle cell disease due to infarction. Hyposplenism is also seen in a wide range of non-haematological diseases, including coeliac disease, dermatitis herpetiformis and, occasionally, ulcerative colitis. Post-splenectomy haematological features are seen.

Further reading

Di Sabatino A, Carsetti R, Corazza GR. Post-splenectomy and hyposlenic states. *Lancet* 2011; 378:86–97.

BLOOD TRANSFUSION

The cells and proteins in the blood express antigens that are controlled by polymorphic genes; that is, a specific antigen may be present in some individuals but not in others. A blood transfusion may immunize the recipient against donor antigens that the recipient lacks (alloimmunization), and repeated transfusions increase the risk. Similarly, the transplacental passage of fetal blood cells during pregnancy may alloimmunize the mother against fetal antigens inherited from the father. Antibodies stimulated by blood transfusion or pregnancy, such as Rh antibodies, are termed ***immune antibodies*** and are usually IgG, in contrast to ***naturally occurring antibodies***, such as ABO antibodies, which are made in response to environmental antigens present in food and bacteria, and which are usually IgM.

BLOOD GROUPS

The blood groups are determined by antigens on the surface of red cells; more than 300 blood groups are recognized. The ABO and Rh systems are the two major blood groups, but incompatibilities involving many other blood groups (e.g. Kell, Duffy, Kidd) may cause haemolytic transfusion reactions and/or haemolytic disease of the newborn (HDN).

ABO system

This blood group system involves naturally occurring IgM anti-A and anti-B antibodies, which are capable of producing rapid and severe intravascular haemolysis of incompatible red cells.

The ABO system is under the control of a pair of allelic genes, *H* and *h*, and also three allelic genes, *A*, *B* and *O*, producing the genotypes and phenotypes shown in ***Box 16.21***. The A, B and H antigens are very similar in structure; differences in the terminal sugars determine their specificity. The *H* gene codes for enzyme H, which attaches fucose to the basic glycoprotein backbone to form H substance; this is the precursor for A and B antigens ***(Fig. 16.27)***.

The *A* and *B* genes control specific enzymes responsible for the addition to H substance of *N*-acetylgalactosamine for group A and d-galactose for group B. The *O* gene is amorphic and does not transform H substance; therefore O is not antigenic. The A, B and H antigens are present on most body cells. These antigens are also found in soluble form in tissue fluids, such as saliva and gastric juice, in the 80% of the population who possess secretor genes.

Box 16.21 The ABO system: antigens and antibodies

Phenotype	Genotype	Antigens	Antibodies	Frequency UK (%)
O	OO	None	Anti-A and anti-B	43
A	AA or AO	A	Anti-B	45
B	BB or BO	B	Anti-A	9
AB	AB	A and B	None	3

Rh system

There is a high frequency of development of IgG RhD antibodies in RhD negative individuals after exposure to RhD-positive red cells. The antibodies formed cause HDN and haemolytic transfusion reactions.

This system is coded by allelic genes: *C* and *c*, *E* and *e*, and *D* and no *D*, which is signified as *d*. They are inherited as triplets on each chromosome 1, one from each pair of genes (i.e. *CDE/cde*). RhD-negative individuals have no D protein in the red cell membrane, which explains why it is so immunogenic when RhD-negative individuals are exposed to RhD antigen through transfusion or pregnancy. In Caucasians, the RhD-negative phenotype almost always results from a complete deletion of the RhD gene; in black Africans, it can also result from an inactive gene containing stop codons in the reading frame.

PROCEDURE FOR BLOOD TRANSFUSION

The safety of blood transfusion depends on meticulous attention to detail at each stage leading to and during the transfusion. Avoidance of simple errors involving patient and blood sample identification at the time of collection of the sample for compatibility testing and at the time of transfusion would avoid most serious haemolytic transfusion reactions, almost all of which involve the ABO system.

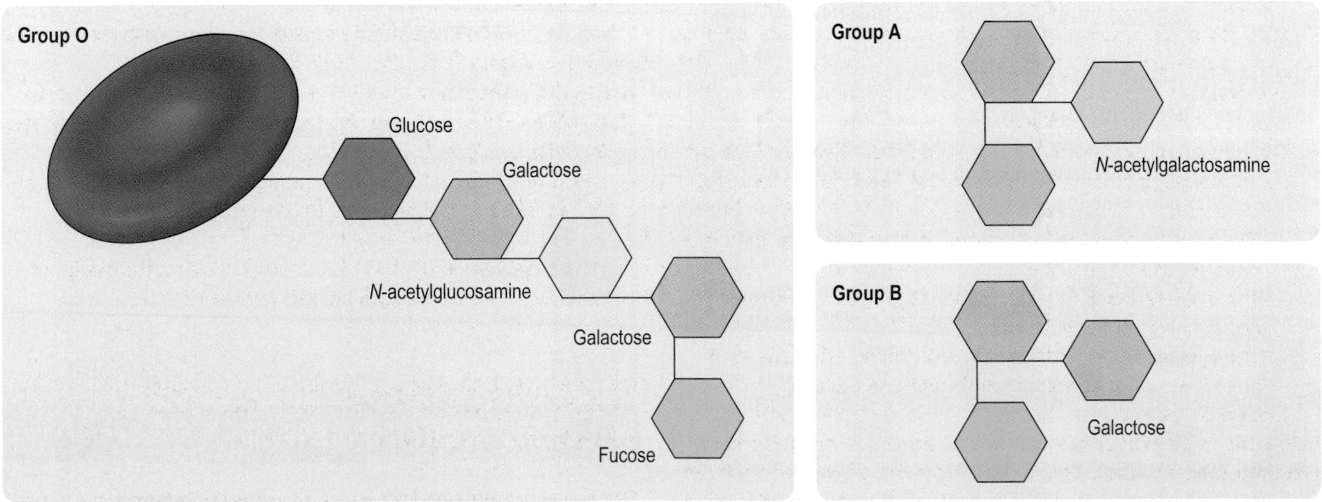

Figure 16.27 Sugar chains in the ABO blood group system.

Pre-transfusion compatibility testing

Blood grouping

The ABO and RhD groups of the patient are determined.

Antibody screening

The patient's serum or plasma is screened for atypical antibodies that may cause a significant reduction in the survival of the transfused red cells. The patient's serum or plasma is tested against red cells from at least two group O donors, expressing a wide range of red cell antigens, for detection of IgM red cell alloantibodies (using a direct agglutination test of cells suspended in saline) and IgG antibodies (using an indirect antiglobulin test, see p. 544). About 10% of patients have a positive antibody screening result; in this case, further testing is carried out using a comprehensive panel of typed red cells to determine the blood group specificity of the antibody (clinically significant red cell antibodies are detected in about 20% of patients with positive antibody screens).

Selection of donor blood and crossmatching

Selection procedures

Donor blood of the same ABO and RhD group as the patient is selected. Matching for additional blood groups is carried out for patients with clinically significant red cell antibodies (see below), and for patients who are likely to be multitransfused and are at high risk of developing antibodies, e.g. sickle cell disease; many hospitals routinely provide Kell-negative blood for women of child-bearing age to minimize the risk of alloimmunization and subsequent HDN.

Crossmatching procedures

Patients without atypical red cell antibodies

The full crossmatch involves testing the patient's serum or plasma against the donor red cells suspended in saline in a direct agglutination test, and also using an indirect antiglobulin test. In many hospitals, this serological crossmatch has been omitted, as a negative antibody screen makes it highly unlikely that there will be any incompatibility with the donor units. A greater risk is that of a transfusion error involving the collection of the patient sample or a mix-up of samples in the laboratory. Laboratories can use their information system to check the records of the patient and authorize the release of the donor units if a number of criteria are met (***computer or electronic crossmatching***), including the following:

- The system is automated for ABO and RhD grouping and antibody screening, including positive sample identification and electronic transfer of results.
- The patient's serum or plasma does not contain clinically significant red cell antibodies.
- The release of ABO-incompatible blood must be prevented by conformation of laboratory computer software to the following requirements:
  - The issue of blood is not allowed if the patient has only been grouped once.
  - The issue of blood is not allowed if the current group does not match the historical record.
  - The system must not allow the reservation and release of units that are ABO-incompatible with the patient.

Electronic issue can be extended to issue of previously unallocated blood at blood fridges remote from the main laboratory ('***remote blood issue***'). This is only possible using blood fridges that are electronically linked to the blood transfusion laboratory information system. The printing of compatibility labels for the blood and its collection are under electronic control, applying the same rules as electronic issue from the main laboratory. Issue of blood using this process reduces the time it takes to provide blood for patients needing it urgently, particularly at hospitals without a blood transfusion laboratory, because transport of blood from the central laboratory is not required. There are good examples of centralized transfusion services in cities such as Pittsburgh and Seattle in the USA, and this model is likely to be increasingly employed in other developed countries, including the UK.

Patients with atypical red cell antibodies

Donor blood should be selected that lacks the relevant red cell antigen(s), as well as being of the same ABO and RhD group as the patient. A full crossmatch should always be carried out.

Several other systems for blood grouping, antibody screening and crossmatching are available to hospital transfusion laboratories. They do not depend on agglutination of red cells in suspension, but rather on the differential passage of agglutinated and unagglutinated red cells through a column of dextran gel matrix (e.g. DiaMed and Ortho Biovue systems), or on the capture of antibodies by red cells immobilized on the surface of a microplate well (e.g. Capture-R solid phase system).

Blood ordering

Increasingly, hospitals are using electronic systems for blood ordering; some include algorithms for the appropriate use of blood, and 'alerts' if there is non-compliance with agreed blood count triggers for transfusion.

Elective surgery

Many hospitals have guidelines for the ordering of blood for elective surgery (maximum surgical blood ordering schedules). These are aimed at reducing unnecessary crossmatching and the amount of blood that eventually becomes outdated. Many operations in which blood is required only occasionally for unexpectedly high blood loss can be classified as '***group and save***'; this means that, where the antibody screen is negative, blood is not reserved in advance but can be made available quickly if necessary – that is, in a few minutes – using the electronic crossmatch procedure. If a patient has atypical antibodies, compatible blood should always be reserved in advance; this may take several days if the patient has multiple or unusual antibodies.

Emergencies

There may be insufficient time for full pre-transfusion testing. The options include:

- Blood required immediately – 2 units of O RhD-negative blood ('***emergency stock***') are used, to allow additional time for the laboratory to group the patient.
- Blood required in 10–15 min – blood of the same ABO and RhD groups as the patient is used ('***group compatible blood***').
- Blood required in 45 min – most laboratories will be able to provide fully crossmatched blood within this time.

COMPLICATIONS OF BLOOD TRANSFUSION

Reporting schemes under the term '***haemovigilance***' have been established in many countries, including the Serious Hazards of

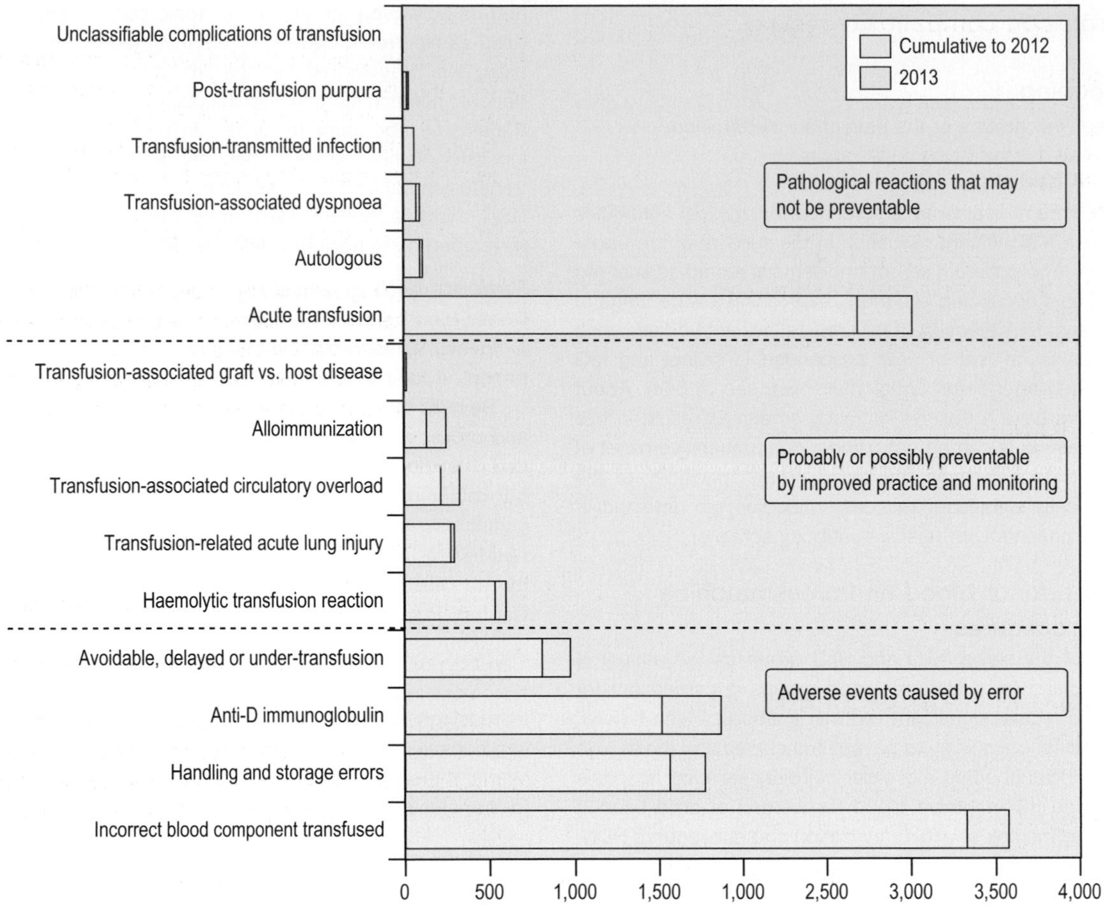

Figure 16.28 Overview of 13141 cases reported to the Serious Hazards of Transfusion (SHOT) scheme between 1996 and 2013. The adverse events are divided into pathological reactions that may not be preventable, those that are probably or possibly preventable, and those caused by error. Those reported in 2013 are indicated in pink at the right-hand side of each bar. *(From: PHB Bolton-Maggs (ed), D Poles, A Watt and D Thomas on behalf of the Serious Hazards of Transfusion Steering Group.* The 2013 SHOT Annual Report (2014)*, with permission.)*

Transfusion (SHOT) scheme in the UK, which produced its first report in the UK in 1997. ***Figure 16.28*** shows the reports to SHOT up to 2013, which indicate that '***incorrect blood component transfused***' is the most frequent type of serious incident, and is the second most frequent cause of mortality and serious morbidity after transfusion-related acute lung injury (TRALI). Errors in clinical areas, either in the collection of the blood sample for compatibility testing, the collection of blood from the fridge and/or the administration of blood (59%), were the most common source of error in 2012, and laboratory errors accounted for the remainder (41%). Death or serious morbidity can also be attributed to other complications of blood transfusion ***(Box 16.22)***, including transfusion-associated circulatory overload (TACO), transfusion-associated graft-versus-host disease (TA-GvHD) and bacterial infection of blood components.

Prevention of wrong blood transfusions

The serious consequences of such failures emphasize the need for meticulous checks at all stages in the procedure of blood transfusion. Written procedures and good training of staff are essential, and regular audit to ensure compliance is also required. New approaches are being used, including the use of barcode patient identification and new technology at the bedside. Handheld devices can be used to prompt staff through the key steps and check that the barcode on the patient's wristband matches the barcode on the unit of blood ***(Box 16.23)***.

Immunological complications

Alloimmunization

Blood transfusion carries a risk of alloimmunization to the many 'foreign' antigens present on red cells, leucocytes, platelets and plasma proteins. Alloimmunization also occurs during pregnancy – to fetal antigens inherited from the father and not shared by the mother (see pp. 546–547).

Alloimmunization does not usually cause clinical problems with the first transfusion but these may occur with subsequent transfusions. There may also be delayed consequences of alloimmunization, such as HDN and rejection of tissue or organ transplants.

Incompatibility

This may result in poor survival of transfused cells, such as red cells and platelets, and also in harmful effects of the antigen–antibody reaction.

Box 16.22 Complications of blood transfusion

Immunological

Alloimmunization and incompatibility

- Red cells:
  - Immediate haemolytic transfusion reactions
  - Delayed haemolytic transfusion reactions
- Leucocytes and platelets:
  - Non-haemolytic (febrile) transfusion reactions
  - Transfusion-related acute lung injury (TRALI)
  - Poor survival of transfused platelets and granulocytes
  - Post-transfusion purpura
  - Transfusion-associated graft-versus-host disease (TA-GvHD)
- Plasma proteins:
  - Urticarial and anaphylactic reactions

Non-immunological

Transmission of infection

- Viruses:
  - HAV, HBV, HCV, HEV
  - HIV
  - CMV, HTLV-1, WNV
- Parasites:
  - Malaria, trypanosomiasis, toxoplasmosis
- Bacteria
- Prions

Transfusion-associated circulatory overload (TACO)

Iron overload

- Due to multiple transfusions, see p. 537

Bleeding and electrolyte changes

- May be caused by massive transfusion of stored blood

CMV, cytomegalovirus; HAV/HBV/HCV/HEV, hepatitis A/B/C/E virus; HIV, human immunodeficiency virus; HTLV-1, human T cell leukaemia virus 1; WNV, West Nile virus.

Box 16.23 Bedside checks for blood unit compatibility

- The traditional pre-transfusion bedside checking required two nurses and checks of multiple items of written documentation.
- With barcode technology, a handheld computer scans a barcode on the patient wristband, corresponding to full patient details.
- The computer checks that the patient details match those on the unit's compatibility label barcode after pre-transfusion testing.
- This label also contains the unique number of the unit, and is matched with the number of the unit at the top left of the bag, to ensure that the blood bank has attached the right compatibility label.

Red cell complications: haemolytic transfusion reaction (immediate)

This is the most serious and life-threatening complication of blood transfusion and is usually due to ABO incompatibility. There is complement activation by the antigen–antibody reaction, usually caused by IgM antibodies and leading to rigors, lumbar pain, dyspnoea, hypotension, haemoglobinuria and renal failure. The initial symptoms may occur a few minutes after starting the transfusion. Activation of coagulation also occurs and bleeding due to disseminated intravascular coagulation (DIC) is a bad prognostic sign. Emergency treatment for shock (see pp. 1156–1161) is needed to maintain the blood pressure and renal function.

Diagnosis

This is confirmed by finding evidence of haemolysis (e.g. haemoglobinuria), and incompatibility between donor and recipient. All documentation should be checked to detect errors such as:

- failure to check the identity of the patient when taking the sample for compatibility testing (i.e. sample from the wrong patient)
- mislabelling of the blood sample with the wrong patient's name
- simple labelling or handling errors in the laboratory
- errors in the collection of blood, leading to delivery of the wrong blood to the ward/theatre
- failure to perform proper identity checks before the blood is transfused (i.e. blood transfused to the wrong patient).

Investigations

To confirm where the error occurred, blood grouping should be carried out on:

- the patient's original sample (used for the compatibility testing)
- a new sample taken from the patient after the reaction
- the donor units.

At the first suspicion of any serious transfusion reaction, the transfusion should always be stopped and the donor units returned to the blood transfusion laboratory with a new blood sample from the patient to exclude a haemolytic transfusion reaction.

Red cell complications: haemolytic transfusion reaction (delayed)

This occurs in patients alloimmunized by previous transfusions or pregnancies. The antibody level is too low to be detected by pre-transfusion compatibility testing but a secondary immune response occurs after transfusion, resulting in destruction of the transfused cells, usually by IgG antibodies.

Haemolysis is usually extravascular, as the antibodies are IgG, and the patient may develop anaemia and jaundice about a week after the transfusion, although most of these episodes are clinically silent. The blood film shows spherocytosis and reticulocytosis. The direct antiglobulin test is positive and detection of the antibody is usually straightforward.

Leucocyte complications: non-haemolytic (febrile) transfusion reactions

Febrile reactions are a common complication of blood transfusion in patients who have previously been transfused or pregnant. The usual causes are the presence of leucocyte antibodies in an alloimmunized recipient, which act against donor leucocytes in red cell concentrates, leading to release of pyrogens, or the release of cytokines from donor leucocytes in platelet concentrates. Typical signs are flushing and tachycardia, fever (>38°C), chills and rigors. Aspirin may be used to reduce the fever, although it should not be given to patients with thrombocytopenia. The routine introduction of leucocyte-depleted blood in the UK, to minimize the risk of transmission of variant Creutzfeldt–Jakob disease (vCJD) by blood transfusion (see below), has reduced the incidence of febrile reactions. Universal leucocyte depletion of all blood components is common in European countries, but the proportion of blood components that are leucocyte-depleted is variable across the USA.

Transfusion-related acute lung injury (TRALI)

Potent leucocyte antibodies in the plasma of donors, who are usually multiparous women, may cause TRALI, characterized by dyspnoea, fever, cough, and shadowing in the perihilar and lower lung fields on the chest X-ray. Prompt respiratory support is essential and mechanical ventilation is frequently necessary. TRALI usually resolves within 48–96 hours but the mortality was 13% in the 305 cases of TRALI reported to SHOT up to 2013. The avoidance of female plasma in the preparation of fresh frozen plasma (FFP) and pooled platelets and the testing of female plateletpheresis donors for leucocyte antibodies have been implemented in many developed countries to reduce the risk of TRALI and are lowering the number of reported cases.

Transfusion-associated graft-versus-host disease

Transfused donor lymphocytes that share an HLA haplotype with the patient are able to circulate, as they are not rejected; they may recognize the patient as 'foreign' and cause an acute GvHD reaction, including pancytopenia. It is usually fatal but no cases have occurred in the UK for many years, probably because of routine leucocyte depletion of blood components. However, certain groups of immunosuppressed patients at particular risk of TA-GvHD should receive irradiated blood to minimize the risk. Such patients include those with congenital or acquired immunodeficiencies: for example, individuals who have had treatment with purine analogue drugs, those who have undergone haemopoietic stem cell transplant, fetuses, and neonates who have received an intrauterine transfusion.

Platelet complications: post-transfusion purpura

See page 570.

Plasma protein complications: urticaria and anaphylaxis

Urticarial reactions are often attributed to plasma protein incompatibility but, in most cases, they are unexplained. They are common but rarely severe; stopping or slowing the transfusion and administering chlorphenamine 10 mg i.v. are usually sufficient treatment.

Anaphylactic reactions (see pp. 143–144) occasionally occur; severe reactions are seen in patients lacking IgA, who produce anti-IgA that reacts with IgA in the transfused blood. The transfusion should be stopped, and ***adrenaline*** (***epinephrine***) 0.5 mg i.m. and ***chlorphenamine*** 10 mg i.v. should be given immediately; endotracheal intubation may be required. Patients who have had severe urticarial or anaphylactic reactions should receive washed red cells, autologous blood or blood from IgA-deficient donors for patients with IgA deficiency.

Immunosuppression

Transfusions are known to have a favourable effect on the survival of subsequent renal allografts, due to transfusion-induced immunomodulation. The precise mechanism is unclear but may be associated with the transfusion of allogeneic leucocytes. Other possible clinical effects caused by transfusion-induced immunosuppression, such as an increase in postoperative infection and tumour recurrence, have been proposed but remain unproven.

Non-immunological complications

Transmission of infection

Viral transmission

Donor blood in the UK is currently tested for hepatitis B virus (HBV), hepatitis C virus (HCV), human immunodeficiency virus (HIV)-1 and human T-cell leukaemia virus 1 (HTLV-1). Cytomegalovirus (CMV)-seronegative tested blood is given to immunosuppressed patients who are susceptible to acquiring CMV. Blood services continue a vigilant search for new infectious agents ('emerging' infections) that may be transmitted by blood transfusion, and for methods to prevent their transmission, including donor screening, testing and pathogen inactivation. Donor questionnaires record recent travel to exclude possible risks of West Nile virus (WNV), the causal agent of meningoencephalitis, which has been transmitted by transfusion and transplantation in the USA.

The risk of transmission of viral infections by blood transfusion varies from country to country, depending on factors such as the underlying prevalence of transfusion-transmitted infections in the population and the measures taken to minimize the risk of transmission. Viral transmission via blood transfusion is still a major issue in the developing world. In the UK, the risk of transmission of HIV by blood transfusion is extremely low – <1 in 7 million units transfused. Prevention is based on self-exclusion of donors in 'high-risk' groups and testing of each donation for anti-HIV. The risk of transmission of HBV is <1 in 1.2 million units transfused. The incidence of HCV is <1 in 28 million units transfused since the introduction of testing of donor plasma for viral nucleic acid. A recent study found a high prevalence of HEV in the English population and in blood donors, but at present blood donations are not screened. Measures for inactivating viruses in plasma, such as coagulation factor concentrates or intravenous immunoglobulin, include treatment with solvents and detergents.

Bacterial transmission

Bacterial contamination of blood components is rare but it is one of the most frequent causes of death associated with transfusion. Some organisms, such as *Yersinia enterocolitica*, can proliferate in red cell concentrates stored at 4°C, but platelet concentrates stored at 22°C are a more frequent cause of this problem. Measures to avoid bacterial contamination include strict donor arm cleansing, diversion of the initial blood collection to samples for testing rather than into the collection bag, and bacterial detection systems for platelet concentrates, which have been implemented in most developed countries, including the USA. They were implemented in England in 2011.

Transfusion-transmitted syphilis is very rare. Spirochaetes do not survive for more than 72 hours in blood stored at 4°C, and each donation is tested using the ***Treponema pallidum haemagglutination assay*** (TPHA).

Variant Creutzfeldt–Jakob disease

In the UK, there continues to be concern about the risk of transmitting the prion protein that causes vCJD (see p. 267) by transfusion; four transmissions of vCJD have occurred following a blood transfusion in the UK. A number of measures have been taken in the UK, including universal leucocyte depletion of blood components in 1999, because the prion protein was thought to be primarily associated with lymphocytes. Blood donors are excluded if they have had a blood transfusion since 1980. UK donor plasma is not used for the manufacture of blood products; imported plasma from the USA is used instead. For children under the age of 16 years, FFP is sourced from plasma (from unremunerated donors) imported from the USA, on the basis that exposure to bovine spongiform encephalitis (BSE) from food was eliminated by 1 January 1996. FFP for this group is treated with methylthioninium chloride (methylene blue) to inactivate viruses.

While stringent measures are being taken to minimize the risk of transfusion-transmitted infection, it may never be possible to guarantee that donor blood is absolutely 'safe'. The current approach to the safety of blood components and plasma in the UK and other developed countries is cautious but it is not an absolute guarantee of safety. Clinicians should always consider the patient's requirement for transfusion carefully, and only transfuse if clinically appropriate (see below).

Transfusion-associated circulatory overload

See management of acute heart failure (pages 984–988).

Iron overload

See page 537.

Strategies for the avoidance of unnecessary transfusion

These include:

- Strict criteria for the use of blood components and blood products
- Stopping drug therapy (anticoagulants and antiplatelet drugs) that may potentiate bleeding in surgical patients
- The identification and treatment of anaemia prior to surgery and in pregnancy
- The use of antifibrinolytic drugs, e.g. tranexamic acid in major surgery
- The use of ***recombinant factor VIIa***, which is licensed to treat patients with haemophilia with inhibitors, and is being given 'off-licence' to treat patients with severe bleeding, such as after surgery, trauma or intracerebral haemorrhage. However, there is little evidence of its effectiveness for this latter indication and concerns about its safety remain.

Artificial haemoglobin solutions and other blood substitutes suitable for clinical use have not yet been developed. They generally have a short intravascular half-life, and a recent meta-analysis found a significant risk of mortality and myocardial infarction.

Autologous transfusion

An alternative to using blood from volunteer donors is to use the patient's own blood. There are three types of autologous transfusion:

- ***Predeposit***. The patient donates 2–5 units of blood at approximately weekly intervals before elective surgery.
- ***Preoperative haemodilution***. Immediately before surgery, 1 or 2 units of blood are removed from the patient and then retransfused to replace operative losses.
- ***Blood salvage***. Blood lost during or after surgery may be collected and retransfused. Several techniques of varying levels of sophistication are available. The operative site must be free of bacteria, bowel contents and tumour cells.

The use of predeposit autologous transfusion was largely driven by concerns about transfusion-transmitted infection, particularly in the USA. It has been abandoned in the UK, except for those rare patients in whom it is not possible to identify compatible blood because of multiple antibodies. There is little evidence that this approach reduces blood requirements, and blood is perceived as being 'safe'. Blood salvage is increasingly being employed as a way of avoiding the use of donor blood. In developing countries, autologous blood and blood from relatives are commonly chosen because of a lack of donor blood.

BLOOD, BLOOD COMPONENTS AND BLOOD PRODUCTS

Most blood collected from donors is processed as follows:

- ***Blood components***, such as red cell and platelet concentrates, fresh frozen plasma (FFP) and cryoprecipitate, are prepared from a single donation of blood by simple separation methods such as centrifugation and are transfused without further processing. Platelet concentrates are also prepared by plateletpheresis (see below).
- ***Blood products***, such as coagulation factor concentrates, albumin and immunoglobulin solutions, are prepared by complex processes using the plasma from many donors as the starting material (UK donor plasma is not used; see above).

In most circumstances, it is preferable to transfuse only the blood component or product required by the patient ('***component therapy***') rather than using whole blood. This is the most effective way of using donor blood, which is a scarce resource, and reduces the risk of complications from transfusion of unnecessary components of the blood.

Patients should be provided with information about blood transfusion, wherever possible, and given the opportunity to ask questions: for example, about alternatives to transfusion. This discussion should be documented. Some patients, such as Jehovah's Witnesses, may refuse transfusion and need specialized management when they undergo surgery or receive medical treatments that usually require blood transfusion. The indications for transfusion have been summarized by the National Blood Transfusion Committee.

Whole blood

A unit of whole blood consists of 450 mL±10% of blood from a suitable donor plus 63 mL of anticoagulant, which is then leucocyte-depleted. Blood stored at 4°C is given a 'shelf-life' of 5 weeks in the UK (6 weeks in some other countries), when at least 70% of the transfused red cells should survive normally. Whole blood is now rarely used for transfusion; donated blood is processed into red cell concentrates and other blood components.

Red cell concentrates

Virtually all the plasma is removed and is replaced by about 100 mL of an optimal additive solution, such as SAG-M, which contains sodium chloride, adenine, glucose and mannitol. The mean volume is about 330 mL. The PCV is about 0.57 L/L but the viscosity is low, as there are no plasma proteins in the additive solution; this allows fast administration, if necessary.

Red cell concentrates are used to increase the oxygen-carrying capacity of patients with major haemorrhage ***(Fig. 16.29)***, and to treat non-bleeding patients with severe anaemia by maintaining the Hb above 70 g/L; a higher threshold – e.g. Hb of 9 g/L – is used for patients with severe cardiovascular disease. An algorithm for the management of major haemorrhage is available in the UK Blood Services *Handbook for Transfusion Medicine*.

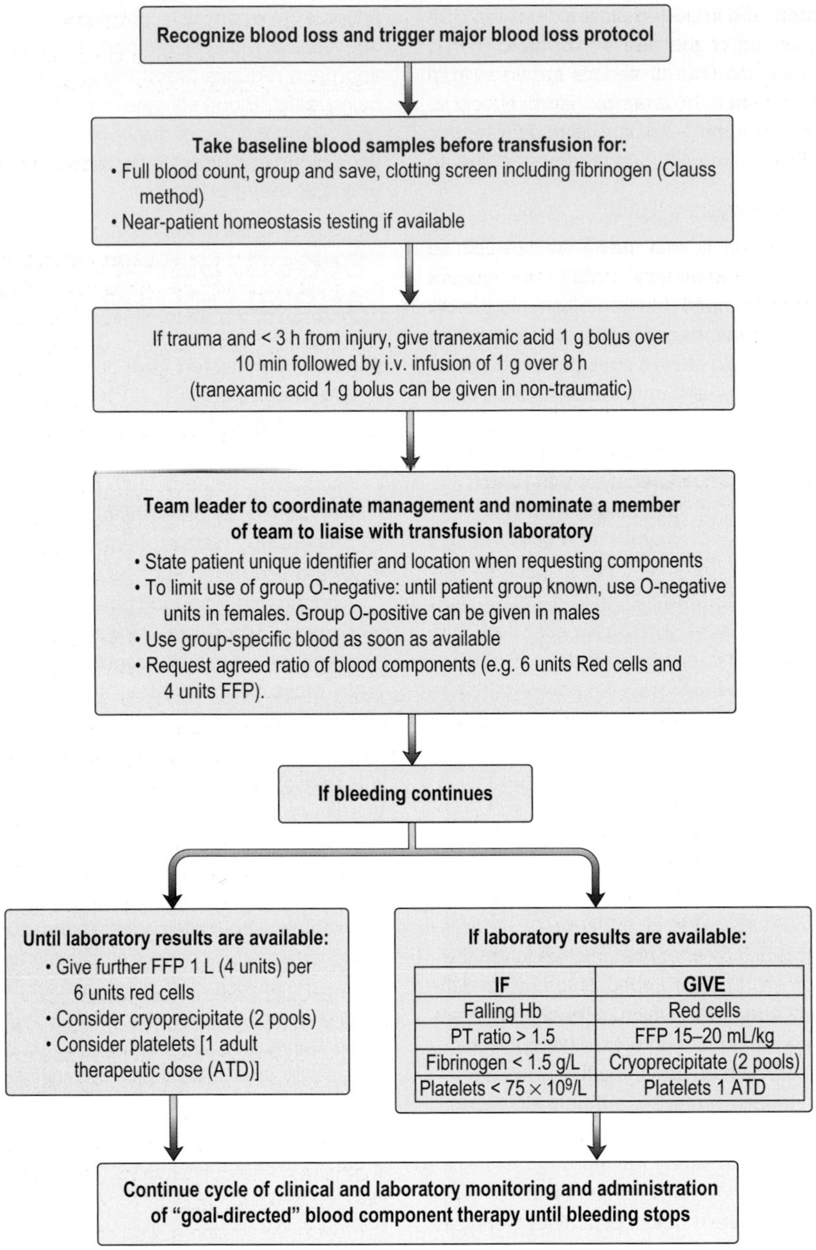

Figure 16.29 **Algorithm for the management of major haemorrhage.** ATD, adult therapeutic dose; FFP, fresh frozen plasma; PT, prothrombin time. *(From: Norfolk D 2013* Handbook of Transfusion Medicine. *The Stationery Office, with permission. Available at www.transfusionguidelines.com.)*

Washed red cell concentrates

These are preparations of red cells suspended in saline, produced by cell separators that remove all but traces of plasma proteins. They are used in patients who have had severe recurrent urticarial or anaphylactic reactions.

Platelet concentrates

These are prepared either by centrifugation of whole blood or by plateletpheresis of blood from single donors using cell separators. They may be stored for up to 5 days at 22°C with agitation. They are used to treat bleeding in patients with severe thrombocytopenia, and prophylactically to prevent bleeding in patients with bone marrow failure when the platelet count is $<10\times10^9$/L.

Granulocyte concentrates

These are prepared from whole blood as '***buffy coats***' or from blood from single donors using cell separators, and are used for patients with severe neutropenia when there is definite evidence of bacterial infection. The numbers of granulocytes collected may be increased by treating donors with G-CSF and steroids. The half-life of granulocytes is of the order of a few hours only and thus granulocytes need to be collected and transfused on a daily basis, making the practicalities of this treatment challenging.

Fresh frozen plasma

FFP is prepared by freezing the plasma from 1 unit of blood to –30°C to maintain the concentration of coagulation factors. The volume is approximately 200 mL. FFP contains all the coagulation factors present in fresh plasma and is used mostly for replacement of coagulation factors in acquired coagulation factor deficiencies, such as massive haemorrhage and DIC. It may be further treated by a pathogen-inactivation process – for example, methylene blue or solvent detergent – to minimize the risk of disease transmission. For children, see pages 558–559.

Prothrombin complex concentrates

These contain factors II, VII, IX and X, and have replaced FFP as the recommended treatment for rapid reversal of warfarin overdose in patients with an elevated INR and bleeding (see ***Box 16.38***) because of their superior efficacy and lower risk of allergic reactions and volume overload.

Cryoprecipitate

This is obtained by allowing the frozen plasma from a single donation to thaw at 4–8°C and removing the supernatant. The volume is about 20 mL and it is stored at −30°C. It contains factor VIII: C, von Willebrand factor (VWF) and fibrinogen, and may be useful in DIC and other conditions where the fibrinogen level is very low. It is no longer used for the treatment of haemophilia A and von Willebrand's disease because of the greater risk of virus transmission compared with virus-inactivated coagulation factor concentrates. Fibrinogen concentrates are now available, but are not yet approved for the treatment of patients with acquired disorders of haemostasis such as massive transfusion.

Specific coagulation factor concentrates

Specific factor concentrates are available for factors VII, VIII, IX, X, XI, XIII and VWF. These are freeze-dried preparations of the specific factor prepared from large pools of plasma. All products are produced from plasma sources at low risk of vCJD and are virus-inactivated during manufacture using either heat or chemicals. They are used for treating patients with inherited coagulation factor deficiencies, where recombinant coagulation factor concentrates are unavailable. If available, recombinant coagulation factor concentrates are the treatment of choice (see pp. 571–573).

Albumin

There are two preparations:

- ***Human albumin solution 4.5%*** contains 45 g/L albumin and 160 mmol/L sodium. It is available in 50, 100, 250 and 500 mL bottles.
- ***Human albumin solution 20%*** contains approximately 200 g/L albumin and 130 mmol/L sodium. It is available in 50 and 100 mL bottles.

Human albumin solutions are generally considered to be inappropriate fluids for acute volume replacement or for the treatment of shock because they are no more effective in these situations than synthetic colloid solutions, such as polygelatins (Gelofusine) or hydroxyethyl starch (Haemaccel). However, albumin solutions are indicated for treatment of acute severe hypoalbuminaemia and as the replacement fluid for plasma exchange. The 20% albumin solution is particularly useful for patients with nephrotic syndrome or liver disease who are fluid-overloaded and resistant to diuretics. Albumin solutions should not be used to treat patients with malnutrition or chronic renal or liver disease who have a low serum albumin.

Normal immunoglobulin

This is prepared from normal plasma. It is used in patients with hypogammaglobulinaemia, to prevent infections, and in patients with, for example, immune thrombocytopenic purpura (see pp. 569–570).

Specific immunoglobulins

These are obtained from donors with high titres of antibodies. Many preparations are available, such as anti-D, anti-hepatitis B and anti-varicella zoster.

Therapeutic use of haemopoietic stem cell transplantation

The use of haemopoietic stem cells to regenerate the bone marrow of patients whose own, usually diseased, marrow has been ablated by radiation and/or chemotherapy is the first and, to date, the only routine 'stem cell therapy' in clinical practice. Haemopoietic stem cell transplantation (HSCT) is used in a range of haematological malignancies, and occasionally in other cancers and non-malignant disorders, such as sickle cell disease. It relies on the regenerative potential of transfused haemopoietic stem cells to repopulate the marrow niche that has been rendered temporarily or permanently hypoplastic by chemotherapy with or without additional radiotherapy. Such procedures vary in the source of the stem cells and in the type and intensity of the preparatory conditioning regimen ***(Box 16.24)***.

Autologous stem cell transplantation

Most anticancer drugs have a sigmoid dose–response relationship, which suggests that, up to a point, a higher dose of a cytotoxic drug will induce a greater response. However, increasing a cytotoxic drug dose is often not possible, owing to toxicity. For those chemotherapeutic agents with a dose-limiting toxicity of bone marrow failure, infusion of previously harvested haemopoietic stem cells is able to 'rescue' the haemopoietic system and permits the use of higher doses to overcome tumour drug resistance. Haemopoietic stem cells are collected either from the patient's bone marrow or, more commonly, from the peripheral blood by leucopheresis, following stem cell mobilization from the marrow niche by the administration of the growth factor G-CSF (see p. 517), with or without chemotherapy. These stem cells are stored by cryopreservation and then re-infused intravenously after an intensive chemotherapy regimen. This approach has been particularly effective in relapsed lymphomas, myeloma and germ cell tumours, and the large majority of HSCT procedures are carried out to treat these conditions. However, tumour contamination of the re-infused stem cells remains a reality. The infused stem cells take a period of 2–4 weeks to regenerate normal blood cell production, and therefore patients undergoing autologous HSCT experience a prolonged period of severe cytopenias and immunosuppression, with a consequent treatment-related mortality in the region of 1–5%.

Allogeneic HSCT

Conventional myeloablative allogeneic HSCT

Conventional myeloablative allogeneic HSCT combines the cytotoxic effect of high-dose chemotherapy and/or radiotherapy with a potent immunotherapy effect. Historically, the transplantation of

Box 16.24 Sources of stem cells

Bone marrow or peripheral blood stem cells

- Autologous – from patient
- Syngeneic – from identical twin
- Allogeneic
  - related or unrelated donor
  - full (10/10) or partial (8 or 9/10) HLA match
  - umbilical cord blood

donor haemopoietic cells has been combined with myeloablative chemotherapy with or without radiotherapy, with the dual effects of treating the malignancy and causing temporary immunosuppression that allows the graft 'to take'. Donors are usually fully matched at the major HLA antigens. Thus siblings are more likely to be found to be potential donors (25% chance for each sibling) than unrelated volunteers, who have to be carefully selected by HLA-matching using large sample registries of potential donors. Allogeneic transplantation has been successfully used in a number of haemopoietic malignancies: most commonly, acute leukaemias. The engraftment of the donor immune system, with antitumour activity (graft-versus-tumour), is primarily responsible for the increased effectiveness of this approach. Complications include GvHD, an alloimmune reaction of the donor cells against normal host organs, which can affect 30–50% of transplant recipients and is potentially fatal in some cases. Immunosuppression, both from conditioning therapy and from the immunosuppressive drugs (ciclosporin or tacrolimus) given to prevent GvHD, results in a high incidence of opportunistic infection and viral reactivation, such as CMV. All patients receive prophylactic antibacterial, antifungal and antiviral drugs. Mortality from conventional allogeneic stem cell transplantation is therefore a major problem, with 15–40% at risk of dying from the procedure, depending on the age and status of the recipient and the degree of HLA compatibility of the donor. The use of donor lymphocyte infusions following allogeneic HSCT, while losing some of the specificity, has produced the strongest evidence for the efficacy of immunotherapy via graft-versus-tumour activity with clinical remissions observed, albeit with a risk of triggering GvHD.

Non-myeloablative allogeneic HSCT

The considerable toxicity associated with conventional myeloablative allogeneic HSCT limits use of the procedure to younger patients. This is problematic, as many haematological malignancies for which allogeneic HSCT is indicated primarily affect older patients. To address this problem, allogeneic HSCT approaches using 'reduced-intensity conditioning' have been developed since the turn of the century and are based on drugs such as fludarabine, which are primarily immunosuppressive rather than myelosuppressive. This maintains the anticancer 'graft-versus-leukaemia' effect of the transplant without the toxicity of conventional allogeneic stem cell transplantation. Treatment-related mortality is lower and the technique can be used successfully, particularly in the elderly and those with co-morbidities. GvHD remains an obstacle to success, however. Non-myeloablative allogeneic transplants are now more common than conventional myeloablative HSCT procedures.

Further reading

Bolton-Maggs PHB (ed), Poles D, Watt A et al on behalf of the Serious Hazards of Transfusion (SHOT) Steering Group. *The 2013 Annual SHOT Report*. Manchester: SHOT; 2014; http://www.shotuk.org.

Dodd RY, Stramer SL. Transfusion-transmitted emerging infectious diseases; 30 years of challenges and progress. *Transfusion* 2013; 53:2375–2383.

Goodnough LT, Levy JH, Murphy MF. Concepts of blood transfusion in adults. *Lancet* 2013; 381:1845–1854.

Goodnough LT, Murphy MF. Do liberal transfusions cause more harm than good? *Br Med J* 2014; 350:13–15.

Hewitt PE, Ijaz S, Brailsford SR et al. Hepatitis E virus in blood components: a prevalence and transmission study in southeast England. *Lancet* 2014; 384:1766–1773.

Jenq RR, van den Brink MR. Allogeneic haematopoietic stem cell transplantation: individualized stem cell and immune therapy of cancer. *Nat Rev Cancer* 2010; 10:213–221.

Murphy MF, Pamphilon D, Heddle N (eds). *Practical Transfusion Medicine*, 4th edn. Oxford: Wiley–Blackwell; 2013.

Norfolk D (ed). *Handbook of Transfusion Medicine*, 5th edn. Norwich: UK Blood Services/The Stationery Office; 2013; http://www.transfusionguidelines.org.

Padhi S, Kemmis-Betty S, Rajesh S et al. Blood transfusion: summary of NICE guideline. *BMJ* 2015;351:h5832.

Vlaar AP, Juffermans NP. Transfusion-related acute lung injury: a clinical review. *Lancet* 2013; 382:984–994.

THE WHITE CELL

The five types of leucocytes found in peripheral blood are: neutrophils, eosinophils and basophils (which are all called granulocytes), and lymphocytes and monocytes (see also pp. 124–125). The development of these cells is shown in ***Figure 16.1***.

Neutrophils

The earliest morphologically identifiable precursors of neutrophils in the bone marrow are myeloblasts, which are large cells constituting up to 3% of the nucleated cells in the marrow. The nucleus is large and contains 2–5 nucleoli. The cytoplasm is scanty and contains no granules. Promyelocytes are similar to myeloblasts but have some primary cytoplasmic granules, containing enzymes such as myeloperoxidase. Myelocytes are smaller cells without nucleoli but with more abundant cytoplasm and both primary and secondary granules. Indentation of the nucleus marks the change from myelocyte to metamyelocyte. The mature neutrophil is a smaller cell with a nucleus that has 2–5 lobes, with predominantly secondary granules in the cytoplasm, which contain lysozyme, collagenase and lactoferrin.

Peripheral blood neutrophils are equally distributed into a circulating pool and a marginating pool lying along the endothelium of blood vessels. In contrast to the prolonged maturation time of about 10 days for neutrophils in the bone marrow, their half-life in the peripheral blood is extremely short: only 6–8 hours. In response to stimuli (e.g. infection, corticosteroid therapy), neutrophils are released into the circulating pool from both the marginating pool and the marrow. Immature white cells are released from the marrow when a rapid response (within hours) occurs in acute infection (described as a 'shift to the left' on a blood film).

Function

The prime function of neutrophils is to ingest and kill bacteria, fungi and damaged cells. Neutrophils are attracted to sites of infection or inflammation by chemotaxins. Recognition of foreign or dead material is aided by the coating of particles with immunoglobulin and complement (opsonization), as neutrophils have Fc and C3b receptors (see pp. 124–125). The material is ingested into vacuoles, where it is subjected to enzymic destruction; this is either oxygen-dependent, with the generation of hydrogen peroxide (myeloperoxidase), or oxygen-independent (lysosomal enzymes and lactoferrin). Leucocyte alkaline phosphatase (LAP) is an enzyme found in leucocytes. It is raised when there is a neutrophilia due to an acute illness. It is also raised in polycythaemia and myelofibrosis, and reduced in chronic myeloid leukaemia.

Neutrophil leucocytosis

A rise in the number of circulating neutrophils to $>10\times10^9$/L occurs in bacterial infections or is a result of tissue damage. This may also be seen in pregnancy, during exercise and after corticosteroid administration ***(Box 16.25)***. With any tissue necrosis, there is a release of various soluble factors, causing a leucocytosis. Interleukin 1 is also released in tissue necrosis and causes a pyrexia. The pyrexia and leucocytosis that accompany a myocardial

Box 16.25 Causes of a neutrophil leucocytosis

- Bacterial infections
- Tissue necrosis, e.g. myocardial infarction, trauma
- Inflammation, e.g. gout, rheumatoid arthritis
- Drugs, e.g. corticosteroids, lithium, G-CSF
- Haematological:
  - Myeloproliferative disease
  - Leucoerythroblastosis (see text)
- Physiological, e.g. pregnancy, exercise
- Malignant disease, e.g. bronchial, breast, gastric
- Metabolic, e.g. renal failure, acidosis
- Congenital, e.g. leucocyte adhesion deficiency, hereditary neutrophilia
- Smoking
- Acute haemorrhage or haemolysis

G-CSF, granulocyte colony stimulating factor.

Box 16.26 Causes of neutropenia

Acquired
- Viral infection
- Severe bacterial infection, e.g. typhoid
- Felty syndrome (rheumatoid arthritis-associated)
- Immune neutropenia – autoimmune, autoimmune neonatal neutropenia
- Pancytopenia from any cause, including drug-induced marrow aplasia (see p. 530)
- Drug-induced agranulocytosis, e.g. carbimazole
- Pure white cell aplasia

Inherited
- Ethnic (neutropenia is common in black races)
- Kostmann syndrome (severe infantile agranulocytosis) due to mutation in the elastane 2 (*ELA2*) gene
- Cyclical (genetic mutation in *ELA2* gene with neutropenia every 2–3 weeks)
- Others, e.g. Schwachman–Diamond syndrome, dyskeratosis congenita, Chédiak–Higashi syndrome

infarction are a good example of this and may be wrongly attributed to infection.

A ***leucoerythroblastic blood film*** (an overproduction of white cells, with many immature cells and nucleated red cells) may occur in many types of severe acute illness (e.g. infection, haemorrhage), tuberculosis, malignant infiltration of the bone marrow, and occasionally after haemorrhage, haemolysis and severe haemolytic or megaloblastic anaemia.

Neutropenia and agranulocytosis

Neutropenia is defined as a circulatory neutrophil count of $<1.5\times10^9$/L. The causes are given in ***Box 16.26***. A virtual absence of neutrophils is called agranulocytosis. It is important to note that black patients may have somewhat lower neutrophil counts. Neutropenia caused by viruses is probably the most common type. Chemotherapy and radiotherapy predictably produce neutropenia; many other drugs have been known to produce an idiosyncratic cytopenia and a drug cause should always be considered.

Clinical features

Infections may be frequent, are often serious, and are more likely as the neutrophil count falls. An absolute neutrophil count

Box 16.27 Causes of eosinophilia

Parasitic infestations, such as:
- *Ascaris*
- Hookworm
- *Strongyloides*

Allergic disorders, such as:
- Hayfever (allergic rhinitis)
- Other hypersensitivity reactions, including drug reactions

Skin disorders, such as:
- Urticaria
- Pemphigus
- Eczema

Pulmonary disorders, such as:
- Bronchial asthma
- Tropical pulmonary eosinophilia
- Allergic bronchopulmonary aspergillosis
- Eosinophilic granulomatosis with polyangiitis

Malignant disorders, such as:
- Hodgkin's lymphoma
- T-cell non-Hodgkin's lymphoma
- Carcinoma
- Eosinophilic leukaemia
- Acute myeloid leukaemia
- Myeloproliferative diseases associated with PDGFR rearrangements

Miscellaneous disorders, such as:
- Hypereosinophilic syndrome
- Sarcoidosis
- Hypoadrenalism
- Eosinophilic gastroenteritis

of $<0.5\times10^9$/L is regarded as 'severe' neutropenia and may be associated with life-threatening infections, such as pneumonia and septicaemia. A characteristic glazed mucositis occurs in the mouth, and ulceration is common.

Investigations

The blood film shows marked neutropenia. The appearance of the bone marrow will indicate whether the neutropenia is due to depressed production or increased destruction of neutrophils. Neutrophil antibody studies are performed if an immune mechanism is suspected.

Management

Antibiotics should be given as necessary to patients with acute severe neutropenia (see pp. 604–605). Exposure to infections should be minimized. A neutropenic diet is instituted (see ***Box 17.21***).

If the neutropenia seems likely to have been caused by a drug, all current drug therapy should be stopped. Recovery of the neutrophil count usually occurs after about 10 days. G-CSF (see p. 517) is used to decrease the period of neutropenia after chemotherapy and haemopoietic transplantation. It is also employed successfully in the treatment of chronic neutropenia.

Steroids and high-dose intravenous immunoglobulin are used to treat patients with severe autoimmune neutropenia and recurrent infections, and G-CSF has produced responses in some cases.

Eosinophils

Eosinophils are slightly larger than neutrophils and are characterized by a nucleus, usually with two lobes, and large cytoplasmic granules that stain deeply red. The eosinophil plays a part in allergic responses (see p. 125) and in the defence against infections with helminths and protozoa.

Eosinophilia is defined as $>0.4\times10^9$/L eosinophils in the peripheral blood. The causes of eosinophilia are listed in ***Box 16.27***.

Basophils

The nucleus of basophils is similar to that of neutrophils but the cytoplasm is filled with large, black granules. The granules contain histamine, heparin, and enzymes such as myeloperoxidase. The physiological role of the basophil is not known. Binding of IgE causes the cells to degranulate and release histamine and other contents involved in acute hypersensitivity reactions (see p. 142).

Basophils are usually few in number ($<1\times10^9$/L) but are significantly increased in some myeloproliferative disorders, such as chronic myeloid leukaemia.

Monocytes

Monocytes are slightly larger than neutrophils. The nucleus has a variable shape and may be round, indented or lobulated. The cytoplasm contains fewer granules than neutrophils. Monocytes are precursors of tissue macrophages and dendritic cells; they spend only a few hours in the blood but can continue to proliferate in the tissues for many years.

A monocytosis ($>0.8\times10^9$/L) may be seen in chronic bacterial infections, such as tuberculosis or infective endocarditis, chronic neutropenia and myelodysplasia, particularly chronic myelomonocytic leukaemia.

Lymphocytes

Lymphocytes form nearly half of circulating white cells. They descend from pluripotential stem cells (see ***Fig. 16.1***). Circulating lymphocytes are small cells, a little larger than red cells, with a dark-staining central nucleus. There are two main types: T and B lymphocytes (see p. 121).

Lymphocytosis (lymphocyte count $>5\times10^9$/L) occurs in response to viral infections, particularly EBV, CMV and HIV, and chronic infections such as tuberculosis and toxoplasmosis. It is also found in chronic lymphocytic leukaemia and in some lymphomas.

HAEMOSTASIS AND THROMBOSIS

The integrity of the circulation is maintained by blood flowing through intact vessels lined by endothelial cells. Haemostasis is the host defence mechanism that protects this integrity after injury to the vessel wall and tissue injury.

HAEMOSTASIS

Haemostasis is a complex process that depends on interactions between the vessel wall, leucocytes, platelets, coagulation and fibrinolytic mechanisms. Haemostatic systems are normally quiescent but, following tissue injury, become rapidly activated. The formation of the haemostatic plug is shown in ***Figure 16.30***.

Vessel wall

The vessel wall is lined by endothelium, which, in normal conditions, prevents platelet adhesion and thrombus formation. This property is partly due to its negative charge but also to:

- thrombomodulin and heparan sulphate expression
- synthesis of prostacyclin (prostaglandin I_2, PGI_2) and nitric oxide (NO), which cause vasodilatation and inhibit platelet aggregation
- production of plasminogen activator.

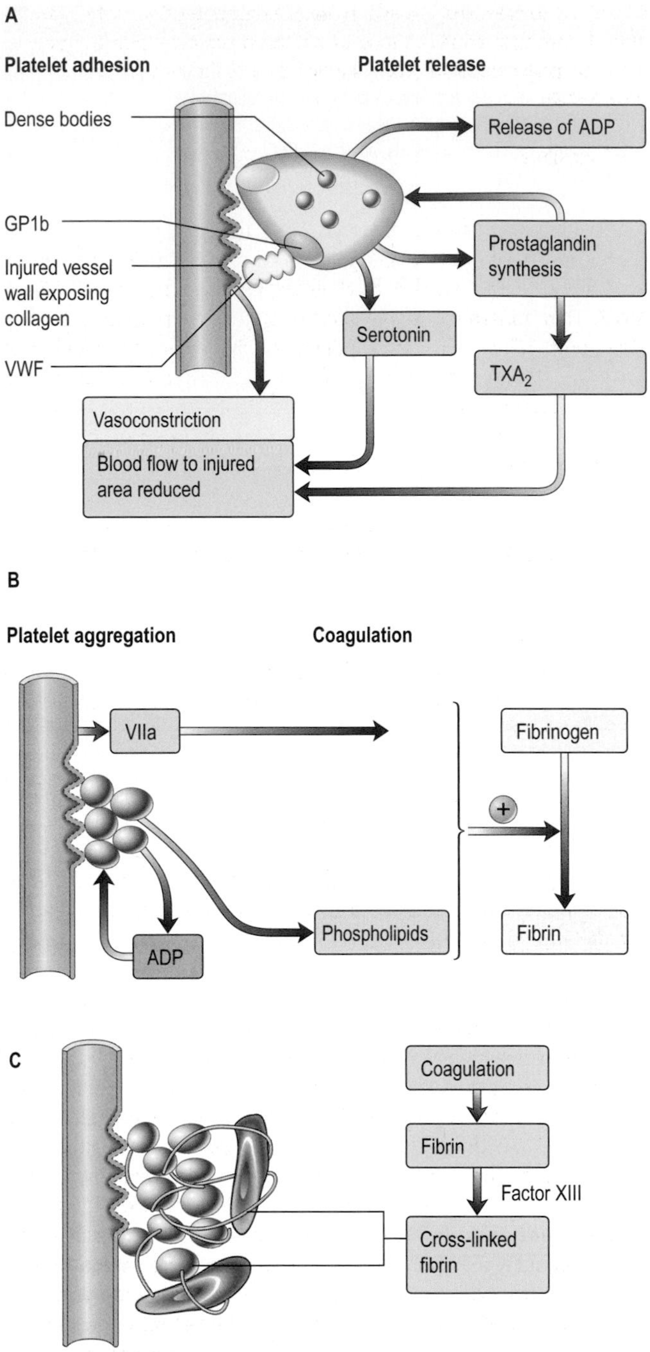

Figure 16.30 Formation of the haemostatic plug: sequential interactions between the vessel wall, platelets and coagulation factors.

A. ***Contact of platelets with collagen*** via the platelet receptor GP1b and factor von Willebrand factor (VWF) in plasma activates platelet prostaglandin synthesis, which stimulates release of adenosine diphosphate (ADP) from the dense bodies. Vasoconstriction of the vessel occurs as a reflex and by release of serotonin and thromboxane A_2 (TXA_2) from platelets.

B. ***Release of ADP from platelets*** induces platelet aggregation and formation of the platelet plug. The coagulation pathway is stimulated, leading to the formation of fibrin.

C. ***Fibrin strands are cross-linked by factor XIII*** and stabilize the haemostatic plug by binding platelets and red cells.

Injury to vessels causes reflex vasoconstriction, while endothelial damage results in loss of antithrombotic properties, activation of platelets and coagulation, and inhibition of fibrinolysis ***(Fig. 16.30)***.

Platelets

Platelet adhesion

When the vessel wall is damaged, the escaping platelets come into contact with and adhere to collagen and subendothelial bound VWF. This adherence is mediated through glycoprotein Ib (GPIb). Glycoprotein IIb–IIIa is then exposed, forming a second binding site for VWF. Within seconds of adhesion to the vessel wall, platelets begin to undergo a shape change, from a disc to a sphere, spread along the subendothelium and release the contents of their cytoplasmic granules. These are the dense bodies (containing adenosine diphosphate (ADP) and serotonin) and the α-granules (containing platelet-derived growth factor, platelet factor 4, β-thromboglobulin, fibrinogen, VWF, fibronectin, thrombospondin and other factors).

Platelet release

The release of ADP leads to a conformational change in the fibrinogen receptor, the glycoprotein IIb–IIIa complex (GPIIb–IIIa), on the surfaces of adherent platelets, allowing it to bind to fibrinogen (see also ***Fig. 16.39***).

Platelet aggregation

As fibrinogen is a dimer, it can form a direct bridge between platelets and so binds platelets into activated aggregates (platelet aggregation; ***Fig. 16.30B***), and further platelet release of ADP occurs. A self-perpetuating cycle of events is set up, leading to formation of a platelet plug at the site of the injury.

Coagulation

After platelet aggregation and release of ADP, the exposed platelet membrane phospholipids are available for the assembly of coagulation factor enzyme complexes (tenase and prothrombinase); this platelet phospholipid activity has been called platelet factor 3 (PF-3). The presence of thrombin encourages fusion of platelets, and fibrin formation reinforces the stability of the platelet plug. Central to normal platelet function is platelet ***prostaglandin synthesis***, which is induced by platelet activation and leads to the formation of thromboxane A_2 (TXA_2) in platelets ***(Fig. 16.31)***. TXA_2 is a powerful vasoconstrictor and also lowers cyclic adenosine monophosphate (AMP) levels and initiates the platelet release reaction. Prostacyclin (PGI_2) is synthesized in vascular endothelial cells and opposes the actions of TXA_2. It produces vasodilatation and increases the level of cyclic AMP, preventing platelet aggregation on the normal vessel wall, as well as limiting the extent of the initial platelet plug after injury.

Coagulation and fibrinolysis

Coagulation involves a series of enzymatic reactions that lead to the conversion of soluble plasma fibrinogen to fibrin-based clot ***(Fig. 16.33)***. Roman numerals are used for most of the factors, but I and II are referred to as fibrinogen and prothrombin, respectively; III, IV and VI are redundant. The active forms are denoted by 'a'. The coagulation factors are primarily synthesized in the liver and are either serine protease enzyme precursors (factors XI, X and IX, and thrombin) or co-factors (V and VIII), except for fibrinogen, which is polymerized to form fibrin.

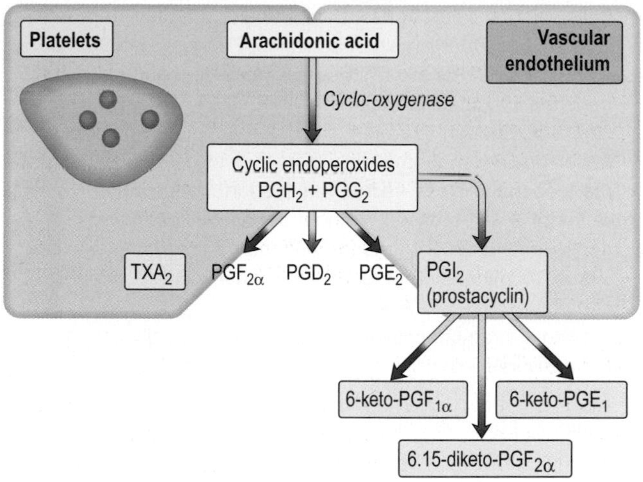

Figure 16.31 **Prostaglandin (PG) synthesis.**

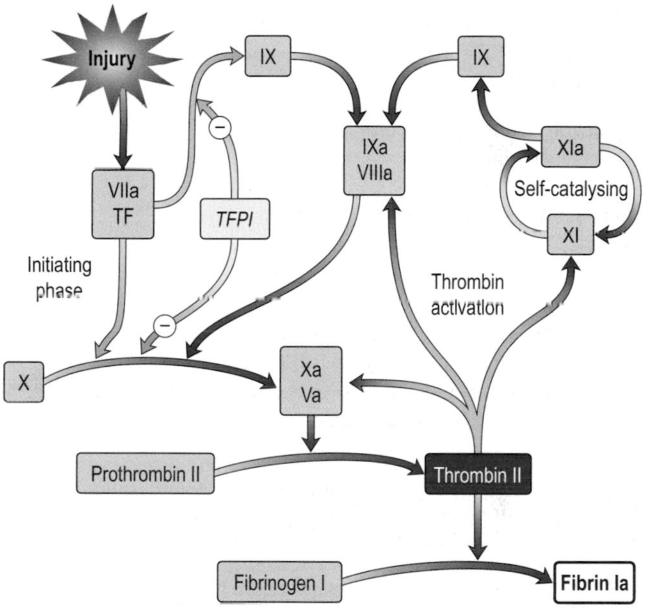

Figure 16.32 **Coagulation mechanism.** The *in vivo* pathway begins with tissue factor–factor VIIa (VIIa, TF) complex activating factor X (Xa) and amplifying factor IX (IXa). Thrombin activates factor XI (XIa), as well as factor IXa, VIIIa, and Va and Xa complexes. TFPI, tissue factor pathway inhibitor.

Coagulation pathway

This enzymatic amplification system was traditionally divided into 'extrinsic' and 'intrinsic' pathways. This concept is useful for the interpretation of clinical laboratory tests, such as the prothrombin time (PT) and activated partial thromboplastin time (APTT) (see ***Fig. 16.36***), but is unrepresentative and oversimplifies *in vivo* coagulation. Coagulation is initiated by tissue damage ***(Fig. 16.32)***:

- Tissue damage exposes tissue factor (TF), which binds to factor VII.
- The TF–factor VII complex directly converts factor X to active factor Xa, and some factor IX to factor IXa.
- In the presence of factor Xa, tissue factor pathway inhibitor (TFPI) inhibits further generation of factor Xa and factor IXa.

- Following inhibition by TFPI, the amount of factor Xa produced is insufficient to maintain coagulation. Further factor Xa, to allow haemostasis to progress to completion, can only be generated by the alternative factor IX/factor VIII pathway. However, enough thrombin exists at this point to activate factor VIII, which dramatically increases the activity of factor IXa (generated by TF–factor VIIa), so further activation of factor X can proceed. Without the amplification and consolidating action of factor VIII/factor IX, bleeding will ensue, as generation of factor Xa is insufficient to sustain haemostasis.
- Similarly, thrombin activates factor V, dramatically enhancing the conversion of prothrombin to thrombin by factor Xa.
- Thrombin hydrolyses the peptide bonds of fibrinogen, releasing fibrinopeptides A and B, and allowing polymerization between fibrinogen molecules to form fibrin. At the same time, thrombin, in the presence of calcium ions, activates factor XIII, which stabilizes the fibrin clot by cross-linking adjacent fibrin molecules.

Factor VIII

Factor VIII consists of a molecule with coagulant activity (VIII:C) associated with VWF. Factor VIII increases the activity of factor IXa by approximately 200 000 fold. VWF functions to prevent premature factor VIII:C breakdown and locate it to areas of vascular injury. Factor VIII:C has a molecular weight of about 350 000.

Von Willebrand factor

VWF is a glycoprotein with a molecular weight of about 200 000, which readily forms multimers in the circulation with molecular weights of up to 20×10^6. It is synthesized by endothelial cells and megakaryocytes, and stored in platelet granules as well as the endothelial cells. The high-molecular-weight multimeric forms of VWF are the most biologically active (see p. 573 and ***Fig. 16.37***).

Physiological limitation of coagulation

Without a physiological system to limit blood coagulation, dangerous thrombosis could ensue. The natural anticoagulant mechanism regulates and localizes thrombosis to the site of injury.

Antithrombin

Antithrombin (AT), a member of the serine protease inhibitor (serpin) superfamily, is a potent inhibitor of coagulation. It inactivates the serine proteases by forming stable complexes with them, and its action is greatly potentiated by heparin.

Activated protein C

This is generated from its vitamin K-dependent precursor, protein C, by thrombin; thrombin activation of protein C is greatly enhanced when thrombin is bound to thrombomodulin on endothelial cells ***(Fig. 16.33)***. Activated protein C inactivates factor V and factor VIII, reducing further thrombin generation.

Protein S

This is a co-factor for protein C, which acts by enhancing binding of activated protein C to the phospholipid surface. It circulates bound to C4b binding protein but some 30–40% remains unbound and active (free protein S).

Other inhibitors

Other natural inhibitors of coagulation include α_2-macroglobulin, α_1-antitrypsin and α_2-antiplasmin.

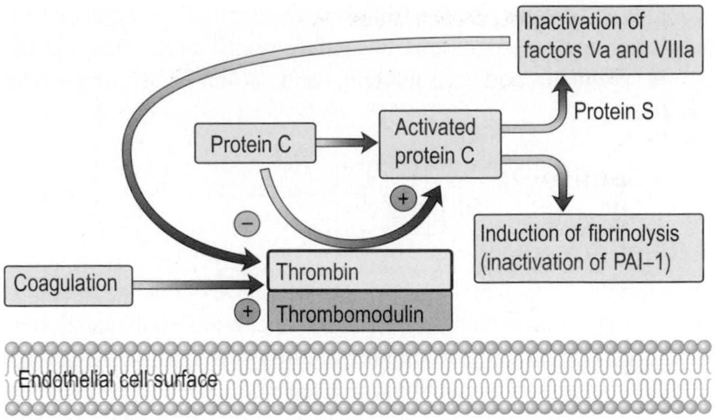

Figure 16.33 Activation of protein C. PAI-1, plasminogen activator inhibitor 1.

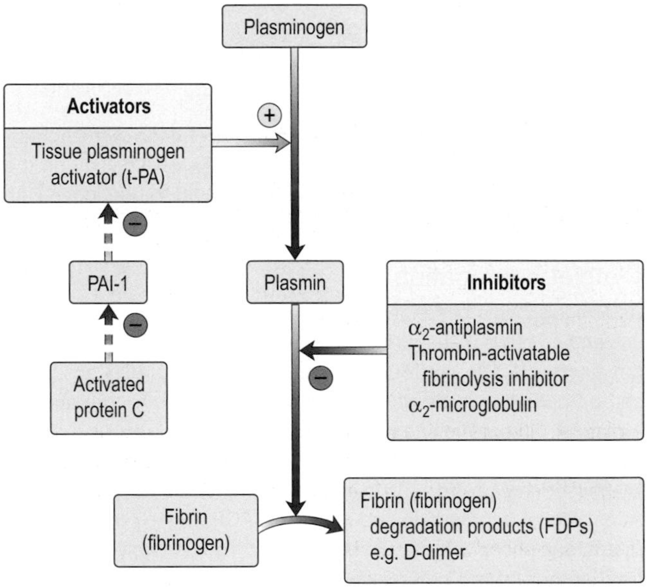

Figure 16.34 Fibrinolytic system. PAI-1, plasminogen activator inhibitor-1.

Fibrinolysis

Fibrinolysis is a normal haemostatic response that helps to restore vessel patency after vascular damage. The principal component is the enzyme plasmin, which is generated from its inactive precursor plasminogen ***(Fig. 16.34)***. This is achieved principally via tissue plasminogen activator (t-PA) released from endothelial cells. Some plasminogen activation may also be promoted by urokinase, produced in the kidneys. Other plasminogen activators (factor XII and prekallikrein) are of minor physiological importance.

Plasmin

Plasmin is a serine protease, which breaks down fibrinogen and fibrin into fragments X, Y, D and E, collectively known as fibrin (and fibrinogen) degradation products (FDPs). D-dimer is produced when cross-linked fibrin is degraded. Its presence in the plasma indicates that the coagulation mechanism has been activated.

Fibrinolytic system

This is activated by the presence of fibrin. Plasminogen is specifically adsorbed to fibrin and fibrinogen by lysine-binding sites.

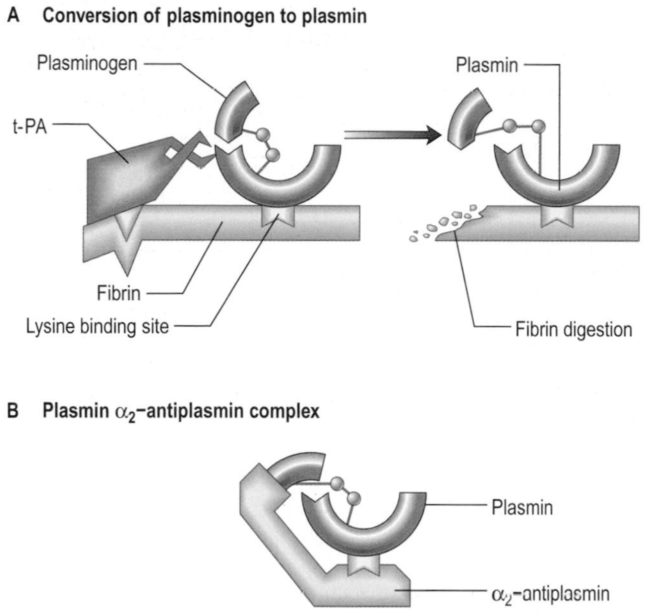

Figure 16.35 Fibrinolysis. A. ***The conversion of plasminogen to plasmin*** by tissue plasminogen activator (t-PA) occurs most efficiently on the surface of fibrin, which has binding sites for both plasminogen and t-PA. B. ***Free plasmin in the blood is rapidly inactivated by*** α_2***-antiplasmin.*** Plasmin generated on the fibrin surface is partially protected from inactivation. The lysine-binding sites on plasminogen are necessary for the interaction between plasmin(ogen) and fibrin, and between plasmin and α_2-antiplasmin.

However, little plasminogen activation occurs in the absence of polymerized fibrin, as fibrin also has a specific binding site for plasminogen activators, whereas fibrinogen does not ***(Fig. 16.35)***.

Tissue plasminogen activator

This is inactivated by plasminogen activator inhibitor-1 (PAI-1). Activated protein C inactivates PAI-1 and therefore induces fibrinolysis ***(Fig. 16.33)***. Inactivators of plasmin, such as α_2-antiplasmin ***(Fig. 16.35)*** and thrombin-activatable fibrinolysis inhibitor (TAFI), also contribute to the regulation of fibrinolysis.

Investigation of bleeding disorders

Although the precise diagnosis of a bleeding disorder will depend on laboratory tests, much information is obtained from the history and physical examination.

Is there a generalized haemostatic defect?

Supportive evidence for a generalized haemostatic defect includes bleeding from multiple sites, spontaneous bleeding, and excessive bleeding after injury.

Is the defect inherited or acquired?

A family history of a bleeding disorder should be sought. Severe inherited defects usually become apparent in infancy, sometimes at the time of birth with prolonged bleeding from the umbilical cord, while mild inherited defects may only come to attention later in life: for example, with excessive bleeding after surgery, childbirth, dental extractions or trauma. Some defects are revealed by routine coagulation screens that are performed before surgical procedures.

Is the bleeding suggestive of a vascular/platelet defect or a coagulation defect?

Vascular/platelet bleeding

This is characterized by easy bruising and spontaneous bleeding from small vessels. There is often bleeding into the skin. Purpura includes both petechiae, small skin haemorrhages varying from pinpoint size to a few millimetres in diameter and which do not blanch on pressure, and ecchymoses, larger areas of bleeding into the skin. Bleeding also occurs from mucous membranes, especially the nose and mouth.

Coagulation disorders

These are typically associated with bleeding after injury or surgery and, in more severe forms, haemarthroses and muscle haematomas. There is often a short delay between the precipitating event and overt haemorrhage or haematoma formation.

Laboratory investigations

Blood count and film

These show the number and morphology of platelets and any blood disorder, such as leukaemia or lymphoma. The normal range for the platelet count is 150–400 $\times 10^9$/L.

Coagulation tests

These are performed using blood collected into citrate, which neutralizes calcium ions and prevents clotting.

- ***The prothrombin time (PT)*** (also see p. 579) is measured by adding tissue factor (thromboplastin) and calcium to the patient's plasma and measuring the length of time taken for the blood to clot. The normal PT is 12–16 s. When used to measure warfarin-based oral anticoagulation, the PT is expressed as the international normalized ratio, or INR (see p. 579). The PT measures VII, X, V, prothrombin and fibrinogen (the classic 'extrinsic' pathway) ***(Fig. 16.36)***, and is prolonged in abnormalities of these factors. It may also be abnormal in liver disease, or if the patient is on oral anticoagulants, including warfarin and some of the new alternative oral anticoagulants.
- ***The activated partial thromboplastin time (APTT)*** is also sometimes known as the PTT with kaolin (PTTK). It is measured by adding a surface activator (such as kaolin, micronized silica or ellagic acid), phospholipid (to mimic platelet membrane) and calcium to the patient's plasma. The normal APTT is 26–37 s and depends on the exact methodology. The APTT measures XII, XI, IX, VIII, X, V, prothrombin and fibrinogen (the classic 'intrinsic' pathway), and is prolonged in deficiencies of one or more of these factors. It is not dependent on factor VII.
- ***The thrombin time (TT)*** is measured by adding thrombin to the patient's plasma. The normal TT is 12–14 s, and it is prolonged in fibrinogen deficiency, in qualitative defects of fibrinogen (dysfibrinogenaemia) or in the presence of inhibitors such as heparin or FDPs.
- ***Correction tests*** can be used to differentiate prolonged times in the PT, APTT and TT due to various coagulation factor deficiencies and inhibitors of coagulation. Prolonged PT, APTT or TT due to coagulation factor deficiencies can be corrected by addition of normal plasma to the patient's plasma. Failure to correct after addition of normal plasma is suggestive of the presence of an inhibitor of coagulation.

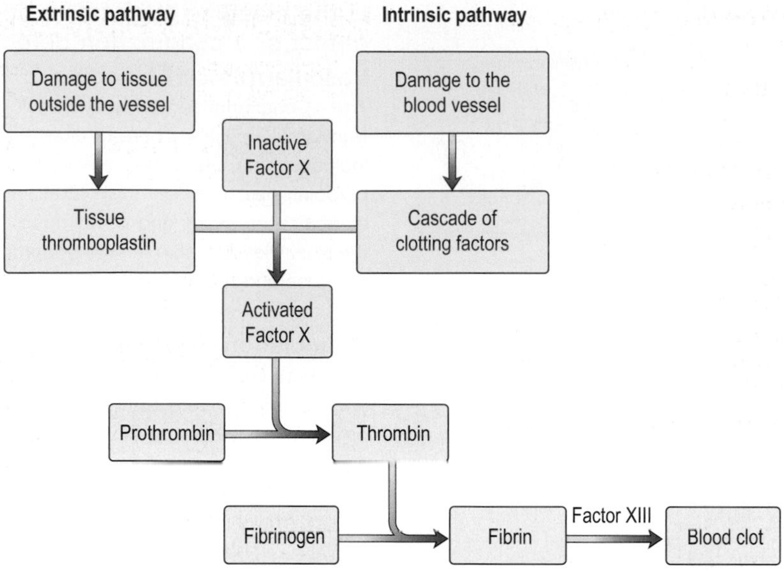

Figure 16.36 **The classic *in vitro* extrinsic and intrinsic coagulation cascade, as relevant to the prothrombin time (PT) and activated partial thromboplastin time (APTT).** See text and ***Fig. 16.32***. Initiation of coagulation differs significantly *in vitro* from *in vivo*.

- ***Factor assays*** are used to confirm coagulation defects, especially where a single inherited disorder is suspected.
- ***Special tests of coagulation*** will often be required to confirm the precise haemostatic defect. Such tests include estimation of fibrinogen and FDPs, platelet function tests such as platelet aggregation, and platelet granule contents.
- ***Bleeding time*** measures platelet plug formation *in vivo*. A sphygmomanometer cuff is inflated to 40 mmHg and incisions in the forearm 1 mm deep and 1 cm long are made with a template. Wounds are blotted every 30 s and the time taken for bleeding to stop is recorded (normally 3–10 min). Prolonged bleeding times are found in patients with platelet function defects, and when the platelet count is $<100 \times 10^9$/L. Nowadays, this test is very rarely done, as it can scar and is painful.

VASCULAR DISORDERS

The vascular disorders ***(Box 16.28)*** are characterized by easy bruising and bleeding into the skin. Bleeding from mucous membranes sometimes occurs but the bleeding is rarely severe. Laboratory investigations, including the bleeding time, are normal. The vascular disorders are described below.

Hereditary haemorrhagic telangiectasia

This is a rare disorder with autosomal dominant inheritance. In most cases, mutations occur in one of three genes – *ENG*, *ALK1* or *SMAD4* – that encode components of the TGF-β signalling pathway that is involved in blood vessel development. Dilatation of capillaries and small arterioles produces characteristic small, red spots that blanch on pressure in the skin and mucous membranes, particularly the nose and gastrointestinal tract. Recurrent epistaxis and chronic gastrointestinal bleeding are the major problems that cause chronic iron deficiency anaemia. Vascular malformations also occur in pulmonary, hepatic cerebral and spinal vasculature.

i Box 16.28 Vascular disorders

Congenital
- Hereditary haemorrhagic telangiectasia (Osler–Weber–Rendu disease)
- Connective tissue disorders (Ehlers–Danlos syndrome, osteogenesis imperfecta, pseudoxanthoma elasticum, Marfan syndrome)

Acquired

Severe infections
- Septicaemia
- Meningococcal infections
- Measles
- Typhoid

Allergic disorders
- Henoch–Schönlein purpura
- Autoimmune rheumatic disorders (systemic lupus erythematosus, rheumatoid arthritis)

Drug-induced disorders
- Steroids
- Sulphonamides

Others
- Senile purpura
- Easy bruising syndrome
- Scurvy
- Factitious purpura

Easy bruising syndrome

This is a common benign disorder occurring in otherwise healthy women. It is characterized by bruises on the arms, legs and trunk with minor trauma, possibly because of skin vessel fragility. It may give rise to the suspicion of a serious bleeding disorder.

Senile purpura and purpura due to steroids

These are both due to atrophy of the vascular supporting tissue.

Purpura due to infections

This is mainly caused by damage to the vascular endothelium. The rash of meningococcal septicaemia is particularly characteristic (see pp. 281–282).

Box 16.29 Clinical effects caused by different levels of platelet count

Platelet count ($\times 10^9$/L)	Clinical defect
>500	Haemorrhage or thrombosis
500–100	No clinical effect
100–50	Moderate haemorrhage after injury
50–20	Purpura may occur Haemorrhage after injury
<20	Purpura common Spontaneous haemorrhage from mucous membranes Intracranial haemorrhage (rare)

(From Colvin BT. Disorders of haemostasis. *Medicine* 2004; 32(5):27–33, with permission from Elsevier.)

Henoch–Schönlein purpura

This occurs mainly in children (see p. 748). It is a type III hypersensitivity (immune complex) reaction that is often preceded by an acute upper respiratory tract infection. Purpura is seen mainly on the legs and buttocks. Abdominal pain, arthritis, haematuria and glomerulonephritis also occur. Recovery is usually spontaneous but some patients develop renal failure.

Episodes of inexplicable bleeding or bruising

These may represent abuse, either self-inflicted or caused by others. These various forms of artificial or factitious purpura may be expressions of emotional or psychiatric disturbances.

PLATELET DISORDERS

Bleeding due to thrombocytopenia or abnormal platelet function is characterized by purpura and bleeding from mucous membranes. Bleeding is uncommon with platelet counts $>50\times10^9$/L, and severe spontaneous bleeding is unusual with platelet counts $>20\times10^9$/L ***(Box 16.29)***.

Thrombocytopenia

This is caused by reduced platelet production in the bone marrow, excessive peripheral destruction of platelets or sequestration in an enlarged spleen ***(Box 16.30)***. The underlying cause may be revealed by history and examination but a bone marrow examination will show whether the numbers of megakaryocytes are reduced, normal or increased, and will provide essential information on morphology. Specific laboratory tests may be useful to confirm the presence of such conditions as paroxysmal nocturnal haemoglobinuria (PNH) or SLE.

In patients with thrombocytopenia due to failure of production, no specific treatment may be necessary but the underlying condition should be treated if possible. Where the platelet count is very low or the risk of bleeding is very high, then platelet transfusion is indicated.

Immune thrombocytopenic purpura

In immune thrombocytopenic purpura (ITP), thrombocytopenia is due to immune destruction of platelets. The antibody-coated platelets are removed following binding to Fc receptors on macrophages.

Box 16.30 Causes of thrombocytopenia

Impaired production
- Selective megakaryocyte depression:
  - Rare congenital defects
  - Drugs, chemicals and viruses
- As part of a general bone marrow failure:
  - Cytotoxic drugs and chemicals
  - Radiation
  - Megaloblastic anaemia
  - Leukaemia
- Myelodysplastic syndromes
- Myeloma
- Myelofibrosis
- Solid tumour infiltration
- Aplastic anaemia
- HIV infection

Excessive destruction or increased consumption
- Immune
- Autoimmune – immune thrombocytopenic purpura
- Drug-induced, e.g. GP IIb/IIIa inhibitors, penicillins, thiazides
- Secondary immune (systemic lupus erythematosus, chronic lymphocytic leukaemia, viruses, drugs, e.g. heparin, bivalirudin)
- Alloimmune neonatal thrombocytopenia
- Post-transfusion purpura
- Disseminated intravascular coagulation
- Thrombotic thrombocytopenic purpura

Sequestration
- Splenomegaly
- Hypersplenism

Dilutional
- Massive transfusion

ITP in children

This occurs most commonly in the 2–6-year age group. ITP has an acute onset with mucocutaneous bleeding and there may be a history of a recent viral infection, including varicella zoster or measles. Although bleeding may be severe, life-threatening haemorrhage is rare (approximately 1%). Bone marrow examination is not usually performed unless treatment becomes necessary on clinical grounds.

ITP in adults

The presentation is usually less acute than in children. ITP is characteristically seen in women and may be associated with other autoimmune disorders such as SLE, thyroid disease and autoimmune haemolytic anaemia (*Evans syndrome*). It is also seen in patients with chronic lymphocytic leukaemia and solid tumours, and after infections with viruses such as HIV. Platelet autoantibodies are detected in about 60–70% of patients, and are presumed to be present, although not detectable, in the remaining patients; the antibodies often have specificity for platelet membrane glycoproteins IIb/IIIa and/or Ib.

Clinical features

Major haemorrhage is rare and is seen only in patients with severe thrombocytopenia. Easy bruising, purpura, epistaxis and menorrhagia are common. Physical examination is normal except for evidence of bleeding. Splenomegaly is rare.

Investigations

The only blood count abnormality is thrombocytopenia. Normal or increased numbers of megakaryocytes are found in the bone marrow (if examination is performed), which is otherwise normal. The detection of platelet autoantibodies is not essential for confirmation of the diagnosis, which often depends on exclusion of other causes of excessive destruction of platelets.

Management

Children

Children do not usually require treatment. Where treatment is necessary on clinical grounds, corticosteroids, intravenous immunoglobulin (i.v. IgG) and anti-D are effective; i.v. IgG is effective in more than 80% of children and raises the count more rapidly than steroids. Treatment should be reserved for very serious bleeding or urgent surgery. Chronic ITP is rare and requires specialist management.

Adults

Patients with platelet counts $>30\times10^9$/L generally require no treatment unless they are about to undergo a surgical procedure. Patients with even lower platelet counts may not require treatment unless they have spontaneous bruising or bleeding.

First-line therapy

This consists of oral corticosteroids 1 mg/kg body weight. Approximately 66% will respond to prednisolone but relapse is common when the dose is reduced. Only 33% of patients can expect a long-term response, and long-term remission is seen in only 10–20% of patients after stopping prednisolone. Patients who fail to respond to corticosteroids or require high doses to maintain a safe platelet count should be considered for splenectomy.

Intravenous immunoglobulin (i.v. IgG) is effective. It raises the platelet count in 75%, and in 50% the platelet count will normalize. Responses are only transient (3–4 weeks) with little evidence of any lasting effect. However, i.v. IgG is very useful where a rapid rise in platelet count is desired: for example, before surgery.

Second-line therapy

Therapies include:

- ***Splenectomy***, to which the majority of patients respond; two-thirds will achieve a normal platelet count. About 50% of patients who do not have a complete response can still expect some improvement in the platelet count.
- ***Rituximab (anti-CD20)***, to which about 60% of patients respond, although only 15–20% have longlasting responses.
- ***Thrombopoietin receptor agonists***, such as romiplostim and eltrombopag, which drive increased platelet production. They have been shown to increase platelet counts significantly in ITP on a long-term basis and are approved drugs for refractory ITP.
- ***Platelet transfusions***, reserved for intracranial or other extreme haemorrhage, where emergency splenectomy may be justified.

Other immune thrombocytopenias

Drugs

Drugs cause immune thrombocytopenia by the same mechanisms as those described for drug-induced immune haemolytic anaemia (see p. 546). The same drugs can be responsible for immune haemolytic anaemia, thrombocytopenia or neutropenia in different patients.

Heparin-induced thrombocytopenia

See pages 578–581.

Neonatal alloimmune thrombocytopenia

This condition is due to fetomaternal incompatibility for platelet-specific antigens, usually for human platelet alloantigen 1a (HPA-1a), and is the platelet equivalent of haemolytic disease of the newborn. The mother is HPA-1a-negative and produces antibodies that destroy the HPA-1a-positive fetal platelets. Thrombocytopenia is self-limiting after delivery, but platelet transfusions may be required initially to prevent or treat bleeding associated with severe thrombocytopenia; platelets are prepared from HPA-1a-negative volunteers or the mother herself. Severe bleeding, such as intracranial haemorrhage, may also occur *in utero*.

Antenatal treatment of the mother – usually with high-dose IgG and/or steroids – has been effective in preventing haemorrhage in severely affected cases.

Post-transfusion purpura

Post-transfusion purpura (PTP) is rare, occurring 7–10 days after a transfusion of platelet-containing blood components, usually red cells. PTP is associated with a platelet-specific alloantibody, usually anti-HPA-1a in an HPA-1a-negative individual. PTP always occurs in patients who have previously been immunized, either by blood transfusion or by pregnancy – hence it is more common in women. The cause of the destruction of the patient's own platelets is not well understood, but they may be destroyed as 'bystanders' during the acute immune response to HPA-1a. PTP is self-limiting, but intravenous IgG or plasma exchange may be required in severe bleeding.

Thrombotic thrombocytopenic purpura

Thrombotic thrombocytopenic purpura (TTP; see p. 750) is a rare but very serious condition, in which platelet consumption leads to profound thrombocytopenia. There is a characteristic symptom complex of florid purpura, fever, fluctuating cerebral dysfunction and microangiopathic haemolytic anaemia with red cell fragmentation, often accompanied by acute kidney injury. The coagulation screen is usually normal but lactate dehydrogenase (LDH) levels are markedly raised as a result of haemolysis. TTP arises due to endothelial damage and microvascular thrombosis. This occurs due to a reduction in ADAMTS-13 (*a d*isintegrin-like *a*nd *m*etalloproteinase domain with *t*hrombospondin-type motifs), a protease that is normally responsible for regulating the size of VWF. ADAMTS-13 is needed to break down ultra-large von Willebrand factor multimers (UL VWFMs) into smaller, haemostatically active fragments that interact with platelets. Reduction in ADAMTS-13 results in the adhesion and aggregation of platelets to UL VWFMs and multiorgan microthrombi. In most sporadic cases, there is a true deficiency of the ADAMTS-13, associated with antibodies to ADAMTS-13. In some congenital cases, the deficiency is due to mutations in the *ADAMTS-13* gene. Secondary causes of acute TTP include pregnancy, oral contraceptives, SLE, infection and drug treatment, including the use of ticlopidine and clopidogrel. Such cases may have a variable ADAMTS-13 activity at presentation, and may or may not have associated antibodies to ADAMTS-13.

Management

Plasma exchange is the mainstay of treatment. It provides a source of ADAMTS-13 and removes associated autoantibody in acute TTP. Cryoprecipitate and solvent-detergent FFP both contain ADAMTS-13. Pulsed intravenous methylprednisolone is given acutely; increasingly, rituximab is also a primary treatment of choice. Disease activity is monitored by measuring the platelet count and serum LDH. Platelet concentrates are contraindicated. The untreated condition has a mortality of up to 90% but modern management has reduced this figure to about 10%. Recurrent and relapsing TTP occurs, often associated with a persistent lack of ADAMTS-13. In secondary TTP cases, identifiable precipitating drugs should be stopped. Caplacizumab is a single-variable-domain immunoglobulin directed to the A1 region of the von Willebrand factor. It inhibits the VWF interaction with glycoprotein 1b and has shown short-term benefit in a phase 2 study.

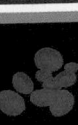

Platelet function disorders

Platelet function disorders ***(Box 16.31)*** are usually associated with excessive bruising and bleeding and, in some of the acquired forms, with thrombosis. The platelet count is often normal and the bleeding time is prolonged. The rare inherited defects of platelet function require more detailed investigations, such as platelet aggregation studies and factor VIII:C and VWF assays, if von Willebrand's disease is suspected.

If there is serious bleeding or if the patient is about to undergo surgery, drugs with antiplatelet activity should be withdrawn and any underlying condition should be corrected if possible.

Bleeding in renal disease is multifactorial, although platelet dysfunction is a major component. The degree of the defect of haemostasis is broadly proportional to the plasma urea concentration – platelet function is impaired by urea, guanidinosuccinic acid and other phenolic metabolites that accumulate in chronic kidney disease. Dialysis partially corrects platelet function. The haematocrit should be increased to >0.30 and the use of desmopressin may be helpful. Platelet transfusions may be required if these measures are unsuccessful or if the risk of bleeding is high.

Thrombocytosis

The platelet count may rise above 400×10^9/L as a result of:

- splenectomy
- malignant disease
- inflammatory disorders, such as rheumatoid arthritis and inflammatory bowel disease
- major surgery and post haemorrhage
- myeloproliferative disorders
- iron deficiency.

Thus, thrombocytosis is part of the acute-phase reaction, although platelet numbers are also elevated following splenectomy because of the loss of a major site of platelet destruction.

Essential thrombocythaemia, a myeloproliferative neoplasm that is described on page 550, and other myeloproliferative conditions such as polycythaemia vera, myelofibrosis and chronic myeloid leukaemia may also be associated with a high platelet count.

A persistently elevated platelet count can lead to arterial or venous thrombosis. It is usual to treat the underlying cause of the thrombocytosis but sometimes a small dose of aspirin (75 mg) is also given. In myeloproliferative diseases, the primary risk is thrombosis and specific action is often taken to reduce the platelet count, usually with hydroxycarbamide (hydroxyurea). Paradoxically, there is also a risk of abnormal bleeding if the platelet count is very high.

Box 16.31 Inherited and acquired types of platelet dysfunction

Inherited

- ***Glanzmann's thrombasthenia*** – lack of platelet membrane glycoprotein IIb–IIIa complex, resulting in defective fibrinogen binding and failure of platelet aggregation
- ***Bernard–Soulier syndrome*** – lack of platelet membrane glycoprotein Ib–IX–V complex (the binding site for VWF), causing failure of platelet adhesion and moderate thrombocytopenia
- ***Storage pool disease*** – lack of the storage pool of platelet dense bodies, causing poor platelet function

Acquired

- Myeloproliferative disorders
- Renal and liver disease
- Paraproteinaemias
- Drug-induced, such as with NSAIDs (aspirin) or other platelet inhibitory drugs

Further reading

British Committee for Standards in Haematology. Guideline for the investigation and management of adults and children presenting with a thrombocytosis. *Br J Haematol* 2010; 149:352–375.

National Institute for Health and Clinical Excellence. *NICE Technology Appraisal 221: Romiplostim for the Treatment of Chronic Immune (Idiopathic) Thrombocytopenic Purpura*. NICE 2011; http://www.nice.org.uk/guidance/TA221.

Neunert C, Lim W, Crowther M et al. The American Society of Hematology 2011 evidence-based practice guideline for immune thrombocytopenia. *Blood* 2011; 117:4190–4207.

Veyradier A. Von Willebrand factor – a new target for TTP treatment? *N Engl J Med* 2016; 374:583–585.

INHERITED COAGULATION DISORDERS

Inherited coagulation disorders are uncommon and usually involve deficiency of one factor only. Acquired coagulation disorders occur more frequently and almost always involve several coagulation factors (see pp. 573–575).

In inherited coagulation disorders, deficiencies of all factors have been described. Those leading to abnormal bleeding are rare, apart from haemophilia A (factor VIII deficiency), haemophilia B (factor IX deficiency) and von Willebrand's disease.

Haemophilia A

This is due to a lack of factor VIII. VWF is normal in haemophilia ***(Fig. 16.37)***. The prevalence of haemophilia A is about 1 in 5000 of the male population. It is inherited as an X-linked disorder. If a female carrier has a son, he has a 50% chance of having haemophilia; a daughter has a 50% chance of being a carrier. All daughters of men with haemophilia are carriers and the sons are normal.

Although a large number of different genetic defects have been found in the factor VIII gene, a common gene inversion in intron 22 is causative in approximately 50% of families with severe disease. There is a high mutation rate, one-third of cases being apparently sporadic with no family history of haemophilia.

Clinical features and investigations

The clinical features depend on the level of factor VIII. The normal level of factor VIII is 50–150 IU/dL.

- ***Levels of <1 IU/dL (severe haemophilia)*** are associated with frequent spontaneous bleeding from early life, typically into joints and muscles. Without adequate treatment, such recurrent bleeding into joints leads to crippling joint deformity.
- ***Levels of 1–5 IU/dL (moderate haemophilia)*** are associated with severe bleeding following injury and occasional spontaneous bleeds.
- ***Levels of >5 IU/dL (mild haemophilia)*** are usually associated with bleeding only after injury or surgery. Diagnosis in this group can often be delayed until quite late in life.

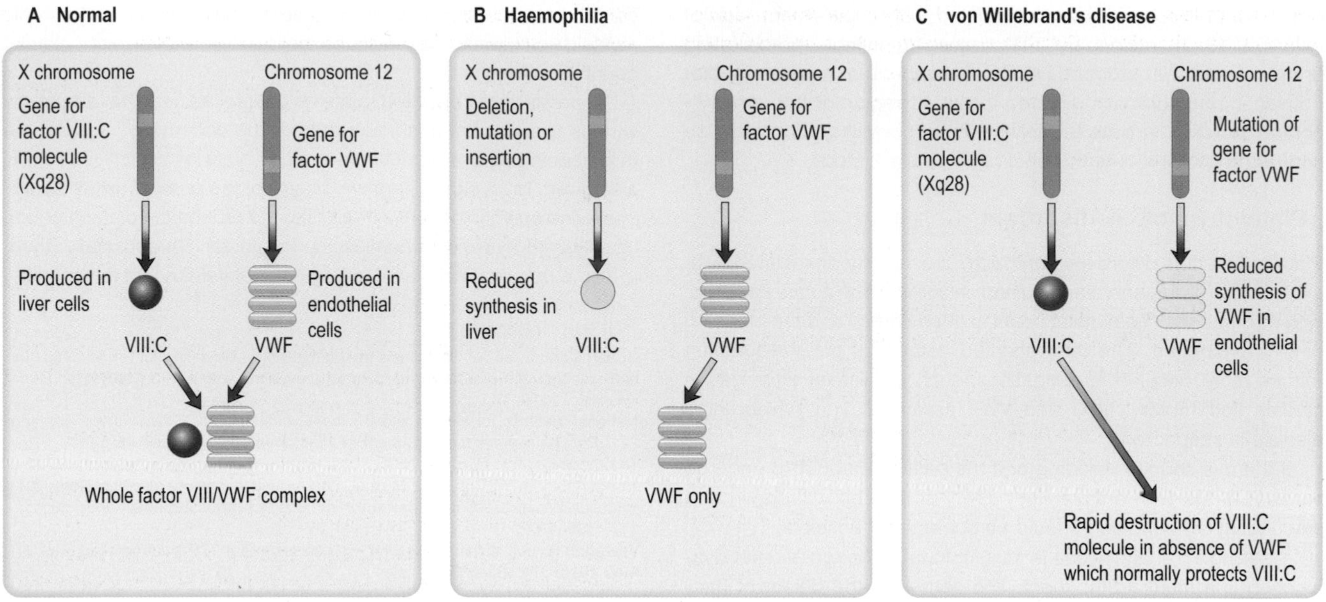

Figure 16.37 Synthesis of factor VIII and von Willebrand factor (VWF) in inherited coagulation disorders. A. Normal factor VIII synthesis. **B.** Haemophilia A, showing defective synthesis of factor VIIIc. **C.** Von Willebrand's disease, showing reduced synthesis of VWF.

Box 16.32 Blood changes in haemophilia A, von Willebrand's disease and vitamin K deficiency

	Haemophilia A	von Willebrand's disease	Vitamin K deficiency
Bleeding time	Normal	↑	Normal
PT	Normal	Normal	↑
APTT	↑+	↑±	↑
VIII:C	↓++	↓	Normal
VWF	Normal	↓	Normal

With treatment, life expectancy today is very good. The most common causes of death in people with haemophilia are cancer and heart disease, as for the general population, rather than bleeding, although cerebral haemorrhage is much more frequent than in the general population. The main laboratory features of haemophilia A are shown in ***Box 16.32***. The abnormal findings are a prolonged APTT and a reduced level of factor VIII. The PT, bleeding time and VWF level are normal.

Management

Bleeding is treated by administration of ***factor VIII concentrate*** by intravenous infusion to achieve normalization of levels. Factor VIII concentrate is available as plasma-derived and recombinant products. Recombinant products are the treatment of choice but economic constraints often limit availability, particularly in developing countries.

Many patients with severe haemophilia treat themselves at home with regular factor VIII infusions three or more times per week, to prevent recurrent bleeding into joints and subsequent joint damage. Such 'prophylaxis' is usually started in early childhood (around 2 years of age). Otherwise, patients at home may treat as and when they have a bleed: 'on-demand' treatment.

For surgery, levels should be kept to normal until healing has occurred; as factor VIII has a half-life of 12 hours, it is often administered twice daily to maintain the required level.

New bioengineered factor VIII products are now becoming available that have half lives approximately 1.5 times that of base factor VIII.

For those with milder haemophilia, ***synthetic vasopressin*** (desmopressin, an analogue of vasopressin) – intravenous, subcutaneous or intranasal – produces a 3–5-fold rise in factor VIII and VWF levels. It is very useful in patients with a baseline level of factor VIII >10 IU/dL. It avoids the complications associated with blood products and is useful for treating and preventing bleeding in mild haemophilia.

People with haemophilia should be registered at comprehensive care centres (CCC), which take responsibility for their full medical care, including social and psychological support.

Complications

Up to 30% of people with severe haemophilia will, during their lifetime, develop antibodies to factor VIII that inhibit its action. Such inhibitors usually develop after the first few treatment doses of factor VIII. Inhibitors are relatively rare in moderate and mild haemophilia, and are often associated with specific molecular defects.

Management of inhibitor patients is very difficult, as infused factor VIII is rapidly inactivated. Acute bleeding events require treatment with agents that can bypass factor VIII, such as recombinant factor VIIa or activated prothrombin complex concentrates.

In those recently identified as having developed an inhibitor, the long-term aim is to eradicate the inhibitory antibody. This is done using immune tolerance induction strategies, sometimes with additional immunosuppression. This is successful in around 80% of cases.

Although a historical legacy of plasma-derived concentrates, the risk of ***viral transmission*** has been virtually eliminated (see p. 558). Although many died as a consequence of HIV and hepatitis C infection, a considerable number of patients remain that have HIV and/or hepatitis C infection.

Carrier detection and antenatal diagnosis

Owing to Lyonization early in embryonic life (i.e. random inactivation of one chromosome; see p. 109), some female carriers may have low levels of factor VIII while others will have normal levels. Carrier detection is, therefore, definitively carried out using molecular genetic testing/mutation analysis. Antenatal diagnosis may be carried out by molecular analysis of chorionic villus biopsy at 11–12 weeks' gestation if selective termination is being considered, or by third trimester amniocentesis if not.

Haemophilia B (Christmas disease)

Haemophilia B is caused by a deficiency of factor IX. The inheritance and clinical features are identical to those of haemophilia A, but the incidence is only about 1 in 30 000 males. It has been identified as the type of haemophilia affecting the Russian royal family. The half-life of factor IX is longer at 18 hours. Haemophilia B is treated with factor IX concentrates, recombinant factor IX being generally available, and prophylactic doses are given twice a week. New bioengineered factor IX concentrates have half-lives 3–5 times that of regular factor IX. Desmopressin is ineffective. Gene therapy has shown promise in potential management of severe haemophilia B.

Von Willebrand's disease

In von Willebrand's disease (VWD), there is defective platelet function, as well as factor VIII deficiency. Both these defects are due to a deficiency or abnormality of VWF ***(Fig. 16.37)***. VWF plays a role in platelet adhesion to damaged subendothelium, as well as stabilizing factor VIII in plasma (see p. 565).

The VWF gene is located on chromosome 12 and numerous mutations of the gene have been identified. VWD has been classified into three types:

- ***Type 1*** is partial quantitative deficiency of VWF and significant type 1 VWD is usually inherited as an autosomal dominant.
- ***Type 2*** is due to a qualitative abnormality of VWF, and it too is usually inherited as an autosomal dominant.
- ***Type 3*** is recessively inherited and patients have virtually complete deficiency of VWF. Their parents are often phenotypically normal.

Many subtypes of VWD are described, particularly type 2 variants, which reflect the specific qualitative changes in the VWF protein.

Clinical features

These are very variable. Type 1 and type 2 patients usually have relatively mild clinical features. Bleeding follows minor trauma or surgery, and epistaxis and menorrhagia often occur. Haemarthroses are rare. Type 3 patients have more severe bleeding but rarely experience the joint and muscle bleeds seen in haemophilia A.

Characteristic laboratory findings are shown in ***Box 16.32***. These also include defective platelet aggregation with ristocetin.

Management

Management depends on the severity of the condition and may be similar to that of mild haemophilia, including the use of desmopressin where possible. Some plasma-derived factor VIII concentrates contain intact VWF and are the current mainstay of replacement therapy. Recombinant VWF is in late stage clinical trial. These specific products are used to treat bleeding or to cover surgery in patients who require replacement therapy, such as those with type 3 (severe) VWD and those who do not respond adequately to desmopressin. Cryoprecipitate can be used as a source of VWF but should be avoided if possible, since it is not virus-inactivated.

Further reading

Berntorp E, Shapiro AD. Modern haemophilia care. *Lancet* 2012; 379:1447–1456.
Nathwani AC, Reiss UM, Tuddenham GD et al. Long term safety and efficacy of factor IX gene therapy in hemophilia B. *N Engl J Med* 2014; 371:1994–2004.

ACQUIRED COAGULATION DISORDERS

Vitamin K deficiency

Vitamin K is necessary for the γ-carboxylation of glutamic acid residues on coagulation factors II, VII, IX and X, and on proteins C and S. Without it, these factors cannot bind calcium.

Deficiency of vitamin K (see also p. 197) may be due to:

- ***inadequate stores***, as in haemorrhagic disease of the newborn and severe malnutrition, especially when combined with antibiotic treatment (see p. 197)
- ***malabsorption of vitamin K***, a fat-soluble vitamin, which occurs in cholestatic jaundice owing to the lack of intraluminal bile salts
- ***oral anticoagulant drugs***, many of which are vitamin K antagonists.

The PT and APTT are prolonged ***(Box 16.32)*** and there may be bruising, haematuria and gastrointestinal or cerebral bleeding. Minor bleeding is treated with phytomenadione (vitamin K_1) 10 mg intravenously. Some correction of the PT is usual within 6 hours but it may not return to normal for 2 days.

Newborn babies have low levels of vitamin K and this may cause minor bleeding in the first week of life (***classical haemorrhagic disease of the newborn***). Vitamin K deficiency also causes *late* ***haemorrhagic disease of the newborn***, which occurs 2–26 weeks after birth and results in severe bleeding such as intracranial haemorrhage. Most infants with these syndromes have been exclusively breast-fed, and both conditions are prevented by administering 1 mg i.m. vitamin K to all neonates (see p. 197). Concerns about the safety of this are unfounded.

Liver disease

Liver disease may result in a number of defects in haemostasis:

- ***Vitamin K deficiency***. This occurs owing to intrahepatic or extrahepatic cholestasis.
- ***Reduced synthesis***. Reduced synthesis of coagulation factors may be the result of severe hepatocellular damage. The use of vitamin K does not improve the results of abnormal coagulation tests, but it is generally given to ensure that a treatable cause of failure of haemostasis has not been missed.
- ***Thrombocytopenia***. This results from hypersplenism due to splenomegaly associated with portal hypertension, or from folic acid deficiency.
- ***Functional abnormalities***. Functional abnormalities of platelets and fibrinogen are found in many patients with liver failure.
- ***Disseminated intravascular coagulation***. DIC (see below) occurs in acute hepatic failure.

Disseminated intravascular coagulation

Disseminated intravascular coagulation (DIC) never occurs in isolation. Recognition that the patient has a clinical disorder ***(Box 16.33)*** that may result in DIC is the key to investigation and management. DIC arises because of systemic activation of coagulation either by

Box 16.33 Causes of disseminated intravascular coagulation

- Malignant disease
- Septicaemia (e.g. Gram-negative, including meningococcal)
- Haemolytic transfusion reactions
- Obstetric causes (e.g. abruptio placentae, amniotic fluid embolism, pre-eclampsia)
- Trauma, burns, surgery
- Other infections (e.g. *falciparum* malaria)
- Liver disease
- Snake bite

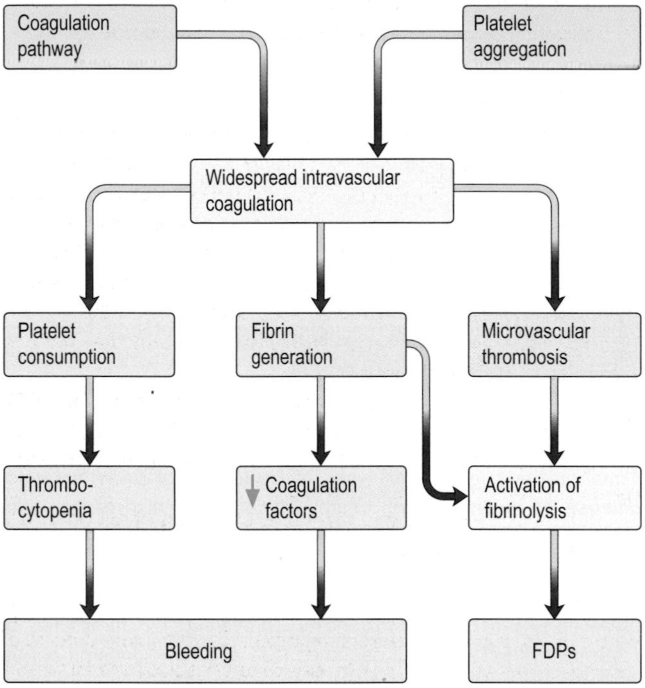

Figure 16.38 Disseminated intravascular coagulation. FDPs, fibrin degradation products.

release of procoagulant material, such as tissue factor, or via cytokine pathways as part of the inflammatory response. Such systemic activation leads to widespread generation of fibrin and deposition in blood vessels, leading to thrombosis and multiorgan failure. Due to the widespread coagulation activation there is consumption of platelets and coagulation factors and secondary activation of fibrinolysis, leading to production of fibrin degradation products (FDPs and D-dimer). These further contribute to the coagulation defect by inhibiting fibrin polymerization ***(Fig. 16.38)***. The consequences of these changes are a mixture of initial thrombosis, followed by a bleeding tendency due to consumption of coagulation factors and dysregulated fibrinolytic activation.

Clinical features

The underlying disorder is usually obvious. The patient is often acutely ill and shocked. The clinical presentation of DIC varies from no bleeding at all to profound haemostatic failure with widespread haemorrhage. Bleeding may occur from the mouth, nose and venepuncture sites, and there may be widespread ecchymoses.

Box 16.34 International Society on Thrombosis and Haemostasis (ISTH) Diagnostic Scoring System for DIC

Parameter	Score
Platelet count	$>100\times10^9$/L=0 $<100\times10^9$/L=1 $<50\times10^9$/L=2
Elevated fibrin marker (e.g. D-dimer, fibrin degradation products)	No increase=0 Moderate increase=2 Strong increase=3
Prolonged PT	<3 s=0 >3 s but <6 s=1 >6 s=2
Fibrinogen level	>1 g/L=0 <1 g/L=1

Calculate score:
>5 compatible with overt DIC: repeat score daily,
<5 suggestive of non-overt DIC: repeat next 1–2 days

Thrombotic events occur as a result of vessel occlusion by fibrin and platelets. Any organ may be involved but the skin, brain and kidneys are most often affected.

Investigations

The diagnosis needs to encompass both clinical and laboratory aspects. It is often suggested by the underlying condition of the patient. If the patient has an underlying disorder known to be compatible with overt DIC, the ISTH scoring system is a useful diagnostic tool. This scoring system provides an objective assessment ***(Box 16.34)***.

In severe cases with haemorrhage:

- The PT, APTT and TT are usually very prolonged and the fibrinogen level is markedly reduced.
- High levels of FDPs, including D-dimer, are found, owing to the intense fibrinolytic activity stimulated by the presence of fibrin in the circulation.
- There is severe thrombocytopenia.
- The blood film may show fragmented red blood cells.

Management

The cornerstone of management is treatment of the underlying condition and intensive support to manage hypoxia, acidosis and organ failure. In those that are not bleeding, this is often all that is necessary. Transfusions of platelet concentrates, FFP, cryoprecipitate and red cell concentrates is indicated in patients who are bleeding or to cover interventions. Transfusion of blood components on the basis of coagulation tests alone is not required. Inhibitors of fibrinolysis, such as tranexamic acid, should not be used in DIC, as dangerous fibrin deposition may result. In those cases with a dominant thrombotic component, the cautious use of unfractionated heparin should be considered. In critically ill, non-bleeding patients with DIC, thromboprophylactic doses of heparin are recommended.

Excessive fibrinolysis

Excessive fibrinolysis occurs in certain malignancies, such as acute promyelocytic leukaemia, and also during surgery involving tumours of the prostate, breast, pancreas and uterus owing to release of tissue plasminogen activators.

Primary hyperfibrinolysis is very rare but activation of fibrinolysis occurs in DIC as a secondary event in response to intravascular deposition of fibrin.

The clinical picture is similar to that of DIC, with widespread bleeding. Laboratory investigations are also similar, with a prolonged PT, APTT and TT, a low fibrinogen level and increased FDPs, although fragmented red cells and thrombocytopenia are not seen because disseminated coagulation with widespread fibrin deposition is not present.

If the diagnosis is certain, fibrinolytic inhibitors, such as tranexamic acid, can be given but evidence for efficacy is lacking.

Massive transfusion

Few platelets and reduced levels of clotting factors are found in stored blood, although there are adequate amounts of the other coagulation factors. During massive transfusion (defined as transfusion of a volume of blood equal to the patient's own blood volume within 24 hours, e.g. >10 units in an adult), the platelet count and PT and APTT should be checked at intervals.

Transfusion of platelet concentrates, FFP and cryoprecipitate should be given if thrombocytopenia or defective coagulation is thought to be contributing to continued blood loss. Other problems of massive transfusion are described on page 1157.

Inhibitors of coagulation

Factor VIII autoantibodies arise occasionally in patients without haemophilia but with autoimmune disorders such as SLE, in elderly patients, with malignant disease and sometimes after childbirth. There can be severe bleeding. Immediate bleeding problems are managed with concentrates that bypass factor VIII activity (e.g. recombinant factor VIIa or activated prothrombin complex concentrates; see p. 572). Longer-term therapy is to eliminate the autoantibody using immunosuppression, such as steroids, cyclophosphamide or rituximab.

Lupus anticoagulant antibodies (see p. 695) are autoantibodies directed against phospholipids (antiphospholipid antibodies) and lead to prolongation of phospholipid-dependent coagulation tests, particularly the APTT; they do not inhibit coagulation factor activity.

Further reading

George JN, Nester CM. Syndromes of thrombotic microangiopathy. *N Engl J Med* 2014; 371:654–666.
Hunt BJ. Bleeding and coagulopathies in critical care. *N Engl J Med* 2014; 370:847–859.
Lillicrap D. Von Willebrand disease: advances in pathogenetic understanding, diagnosis and therapy. *Blood* 2013; 122:3735–3740.
Tripodi A, Mannucci PM. The coagulopathy of chronic liver disease. *N Engl J Med* 2011; 365:147–156.

THROMBOSIS

A thrombus is defined as a solid mass formed in the circulation from the constituents of the blood during life. Fragments of thrombi (emboli) may break off and block vessels downstream. Thromboembolic disease is much more common than abnormal bleeding; nearly half of adult deaths in England and Wales are due to coronary artery thrombosis, cerebral artery thrombosis or pulmonary embolism.

A thrombus results from a complex series of events involving coagulation factors, platelets, red blood cells and the vessel wall.

Arterial thrombosis

This usually occurs in association with atheroma, which tends to form at areas of turbulent blood flow, such as the bifurcation of arteries. Platelets adhere to the damaged vascular endothelium and aggregate in response to ADP and TXA_2 to form a 'white thrombus'. The growth of the platelet thrombus is limited at its margins by PGI_2 and nitric oxide (NO). Plaque rupture leads to the exposure of blood containing factor VIIa to tissue factor within the plaque, which may trigger blood coagulation and lead to thrombus formation. This results in complete occlusion of the vessel or embolization that produces distal obstruction. The risk factors for arterial thrombosis are related to the development of atherosclerosis (see p. 992).

Arterial thrombi may also form in the heart, as mural thrombi in the left ventricle after myocardial infarction, in the left atrium in mitral valve disease, or on the surfaces of prosthetic valves.

Venous thrombosis

Unlike arterial thrombosis, venous thrombosis often occurs in normal vessels. Major causes are stasis and hypercoagulability. The majority of venous thrombi occur in the deep veins of the leg, originating around the valves as 'red thrombi' consisting mainly of red cells and fibrin. The propagating thrombus is formed of fibrin and platelets, and is particularly liable to embolize. Chronic venous obstruction following thrombosis in the deep veins of the leg frequently results in a permanently swollen limb and may lead to ulceration (post-phlebitic syndrome).

Risk factors for venous thrombosis are shown in ***Box 16.35***. Venous thrombosis may occur with changes in blood cells, such as polycythaemia and thrombocythaemia, and with coagulation abnormalities (thrombophilia; see below).

The clinical features and diagnosis of venous thrombosis are discussed on page 1055.

Thrombophilia

Thrombophilia is a term describing inherited or acquired defects of haemostasis leading to a predisposition to venous or arterial thrombosis. It occurs in people with:

- recurrent venous thrombosis
- venous thrombosis for the first time under the age of 40 years
- an unusual venous thrombosis, such as mesenteric or cerebral vein thrombosis
- unexplained neonatal thrombosis
- recurrent miscarriages
- arterial thrombosis in the absence of arterial disease.

Coagulation abnormalities

Factor V Leiden

Factor V Leiden differs from normal factor V by a single nucleotide substitution (Arg506Gln). This variation makes factor V less likely to be cleaved by activated protein C. As factor V is a co-factor for thrombin generation (see ***Fig. 16.32***), impaired inactivation by activated protein C (see ***Fig. 16.33***) results in a tendency to thrombosis. Factor V Leiden is found in 3–5% of healthy individuals in the Western world and in about 20–30% of patients with venous thrombosis. It is very rare in Chinese populations.

Factor V Leiden acts synergistically with other acquired thrombosis risk factors: for example, in those who are taking oral contraceptive pills or are pregnant. Thrombosis risk rises 35-fold in those on a combined oral contraceptive pill, although the absolute risk for thrombosis remains at significantly below 0.5% per year for any single individual.

Box 16.35 Risk factors for venous thromboembolism (VTE)

Patient factors
- Age
- Body mass index (BMI) >30 kg/m^2
- Varicose veins
- Continuous travel >3 h in preceding 4 weeks
- Immobility (bed rest ≥3 days)
- Pregnancy and puerperium
- Previous deep vein thrombosis or pulmonary embolism
- Thrombophilia
  - Antithrombin deficiency
  - Protein C or S deficiency
  - Factor V Leiden
  - Resistance to activated protein C (caused by factor V Leiden variant)
  - Prothrombin gene variant
  - Hyperhomocysteinaemia
  - Antiphospholipid antibody/lupus anticoagulant
- Oestrogen therapy, including hormone replacement therapy (HRT)
- Dysfibrinogenaemia
- Plasminogen deficiency

Disease or surgical procedure
- Trauma or surgery, especially of pelvis, hip or lower limb
- Malignancy
- Cardiac or respiratory failure
- Recent myocardial infarction or stroke
- Acute medical illness/severe infection
- Inflammatory bowel disease
- Behçet's disease
- Nephrotic syndrome
- Myeloproliferative disorders
- Paroxysmal nocturnal haemoglobinuria
- Paraproteinaemia
- Sickle cell anaemia
- Central venous catheter *in situ*

Prothrombin variant

A mutation in the 3′ untranslated region of the prothrombin gene has been described (G20210A). This variant is associated with elevated levels of prothrombin and a 2–3-fold increase in the risk of venous thrombosis. There is an interaction with factor V Leiden and contraceptive pill use or pregnancy. The prevalence is 2% in Caucasian populations, and 6% in unselected patients with thrombosis.

Antithrombin deficiency

This deficiency can be inherited as an autosomal dominant. Many variations have been described that lead to a conformational change in the protein. It can also be acquired following trauma, with major surgery and with the contraceptive pill. Low levels are also seen in severe proteinuria (e.g. the nephrotic syndrome). Recurrent thrombotic episodes occur, starting at a young age in the inherited variety. Patients may be relatively resistant to heparin, as antithrombin is required for its action. Antithrombin concentrates are available.

Protein C and S deficiencies

These autosomal dominant conditions result in an increased risk of venous thrombosis, often before the age of 40 years. Homozygous protein C or S deficiency causes neonatal purpura fulminans, which is fatal without immediate replacement therapy. Plasma-derived protein C concentrate is available.

Box 16.36 Drugs used in the treatment of thrombotic disorders

Antiplatelet
- Aspirin
- Thromboxane synthase, e.g. dipyridamole
- GP IIb/IIIa inhibitors, e.g. abciximab, eptifibatide, tirofiban
- ADP receptor antagonists/P2Y$_{12}$ inhibitors, e.g. clopidogrel, prasugrel, ticagrelor
- Epoprostenol
- Thromboxane prostaglandin receptor antagonists, e.g. terutroban

Thrombolytic
- Streptokinase
- Tissue-type plasminogen activator (t-PA or alteplase)
- Reteplase (r-PA)
- Tenecteplase (TNK-tPA)

Anticoagulant
- Heparin:
  - Unfractionated (or standard)
  - Low-molecular-weight
- Hirudin-like, e.g. bivalirudin
- Fondaparinux
- Warfarin
- Xa inhibitors, e.g. apixaban, rivaroxaban, otamixaban, edoxaban, betrixaban
- Direct thrombin inhibitors, e.g. dabigatran

Antiphospholipid antibody

See page 695.

Homocysteine

When elevated, this amino acid is associated with both arterial thrombosis and venous thromboembolism. The mechanism of vascular damage is unclear. Folate, vitamin B$_{12}$ and vitamin B$_6$ supplementation is often helpful in reducing levels.

Investigations

Haemostatic screening test

- ***Full blood count***, including platelet count.
- ***Coagulation screen***, including a fibrinogen level. These tests will detect erythrocytosis, thrombocytosis, dysfibrinogenaemia and the possible presence of a lupus anticoagulant.

Testing for specific causes of thrombophilia

- ***Assays*** for naturally occurring anticoagulants, such as antithrombin, protein C and protein S.
- ***Assay*** for activated protein C resistance and molecular testing for factor V Leiden and the prothrombin variant.
- ***Screening for a coagulation factor inhibitor***, including a lupus anticoagulant (and anticardiolipin antibodies) (see p. 695).

Prevention and treatment of arterial thrombosis

Attempts to prevent or reduce arterial thrombosis are directed mainly at minimizing factors predisposing to atherosclerosis. Treatment of established arterial thrombosis includes the use of antiplatelet drugs and thrombolytic therapy.

Antiplatelet drugs

Platelet activation at the site of vascular damage is crucial to the development of arterial thrombosis, and this can be altered by the following drugs ***(Box 16.36)***:

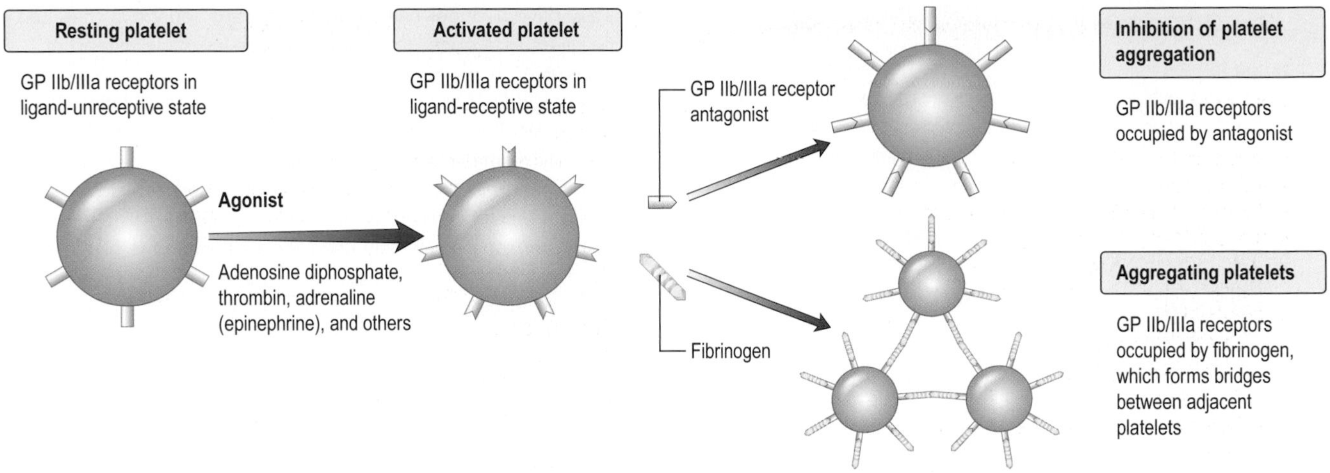

Figure 16.39 The role of glycoprotein IIb/IIIa in platelet aggregation and the inhibition of platelet aggregation by inhibitors of glycoprotein IIb/IIIa receptors.

- ***Aspirin*** irreversibly inhibits the enzyme cyclo-oxygenase (COX), resulting in reduced platelet production of TXA_2 (see ***Fig. 24.30***). At the low doses used in cardiovascular disease prevention or treatment, there is selective inhibition of the isoform COX-1, found within platelets. This inhibition cannot be repaired and is effective for the life of the circulating platelet, which is about 1 week. It has been suggested that there may be significant individual variability in the response to aspirin, although there is no clear reason for this. The term '***aspirin resistance***' has been loosely applied when the clinical effects of aspirin are less than expected. No large body of clinical trial data is specifically available to correlate clinical events and laboratory findings with respect to aspirin response and so it is difficult to determine whether the breakthrough events experienced by patients treated with aspirin represent aspirin resistance or are related to more mundane issues, such as aspirin dose, drug interactions or drug non-compliance.
- ***Dipyridamole***, which inhibits platelet phosphodiesterase, causing an increase in cyclic AMP with potentiation of the action of PGI_2, has been widely used as an antithrombotic agent but there is little evidence that it is effective.
- ***Clopidogrel*** irreversibly blockades the ADP ($P2Y_{12}$) receptor on platelet cell membranes, so affecting the ADP-dependent activation of the glycoprotein IIb/IIIa complex. It is similar to ticlopidine but has fewer side-effects. Trials support its use in acute coronary syndromes (see p. 999).
- ***Prasugrel***, a novel thienopyridine, is like clopidogrel and is licensed for use in acute coronary syndromes (see p. 999).
- ***Ticagrelor*** is also a P2Y12 platelet ADP receptor blocker but, unlike clopidogrel, is reversible and is not a prodrug, so having a faster onset of action than greater degree of platelet inhibition and consistency of effect. It is licensed for use in acute coronary syndromes.
- ***Glycoprotein IIb/IIIa receptor antagonists*** block the receptor on the platelet for fibrinogen and VWF (***Fig. 16.39***). Three classes have been described:
  - murine–human chimeric antibodies (e.g. abciximab)
  - synthetic peptides (e.g. eptifibatide)
  - synthetic non-peptides (e.g. tirofiban).

  They have been used as an adjunct in invasive coronary artery intervention and as primary medical therapy in coronary heart disease. Excessive bleeding has been a problem.
- ***Epoprostenol*** is a prostacyclin that is used to inhibit platelet aggregation during renal dialysis (with or without heparin), and also in primary pulmonary hypertension.
- ***Terutroban*** is a thromboxane prostaglandin receptor antagonist that is being trialled in secondary prevention of cerebrovascular and cardiovascular disease as an alternative to aspirin.

The indications for and results of antiplatelet therapy are discussed in the appropriate sections (see p. 999).

Thrombolytic therapy

Streptokinase

Streptokinase is a purified fraction of the filtrate obtained from cultures of haemolytic streptococci. It forms a complex with plasminogen, resulting in a conformational change, which activates other plasminogen molecules to form plasmin. Streptokinase is antigenic and the development of streptococcal antibodies precludes repeated use. Activation of plasminogen is indiscriminate, so that both fibrin in clots and free fibrinogen are lysed, leading to low fibrinogen levels and the risk of haemorrhage.

Plasminogen activators

Tissue-type plasminogen activators (alteplase (t-PA), tenecteplase (TNK-tPA)) are produced by recombinant technology. Reteplase (r-PA) is also a recombinant plasminogen activator. These agents are not antigenic and do not give allergic reactions. They are relatively fibrin-specific, and have relatively little systemic activity and short half-lives (around 5 min). The bleeding complications observed are similar in severity and frequency to those seen with streptokinase, suggesting that fibrin specificity does not confer protection against haemorrhage.

Indications

The use of thrombolytic therapy in myocardial infarction is discussed on page 1005. The combination of aspirin with thrombolytic therapy produces better results than thrombolytic therapy alone. The extent of the benefit depends on how quickly treatment is given. These agents are also used in cerebral infarction (see p. 836) and in massive pulmonary embolism where there is haemodynamic instability. The main risk of thrombolytic therapy is bleeding.

Box 16.37 Indications for warfarin and target INR

Target INR 2.5
- Pulmonary embolism
- Proximal and calf deep vein thrombosis
- Recurrence of venous thromboembolism when no longer on warfarin therapy
- Symptomatic inherited thrombophilia
- Atrial fibrillation
- Cardioversion
- Mural thrombus
- Cardiomyopathy
- Antiphospholipid syndrome
- Bioprosthetic heart valves

Target INR 3.5
- Recurrence of venous thromboembolism while on warfarin therapy
- Mechanical prosthetic heart valve

(Data from Keeling D, Baglin T, Tait C et al. and the British Committee for Standards in Haematology. Guidelines on oral anticoagulation with warfarin – fourth edn. Brit J Haematol *2011; 154(3):311–324.)*

Treatment should not be given to patients who have had recent bleeding, uncontrolled hypertension or a haemorrhagic stroke, or surgery or other invasive procedures within the previous 10 days.

Prevention and management of venous thromboembolism

Venous thromboembolism (VTE) is a common problem after surgery, particularly in high-risk patients such as the elderly, those with malignant disease and those with a history of previous thrombosis ***(Box 16.37)***. The incidence is also high in patients confined to bed following trauma, myocardial infarction or other illnesses. The prevention and treatment of venous thrombosis includes the use of anticoagulants.

Anticoagulants

Heparin (standard or unfractionated)

Heparin is not a single substance but rather a mixture of polysaccharides. Commercially available unfractionated heparin consists of components with molecular weights varying from 5000 to 35 000, with an average of about 13 000. It was initially extracted from liver (hence its name) but is now prepared from porcine gastric mucosa. Heparin acts immediately, binding to antithrombin. This induces a conformational change that increases the inhibitory activity of antithrombin (at least 5000-fold) towards activated serine protease coagulation factors (thrombin, XIIa, XIa, Xa, IXa and VIIa).

Low-molecular-weight heparins

Low-molecular-weight (LMW) heparins are produced by enzymatic or chemical degradation of standard heparin, producing fractions with molecular weights in the range of 2000–8000. Potentiation of thrombin inhibition (anti-IIa activity) requires a minimum length of the heparin molecule with an approximate molecular weight of 5400, whereas the inhibition of factor Xa requires only a smaller heparin molecule with a molecular weight of about 1700. LMW heparins have the following properties:

- Bioavailability is better than that of unfractionated heparin.
- They have greater activity against factor Xa than against factor IIa, suggesting that they may produce an equivalent anticoagulant effect to standard heparin but have a lower risk of bleeding, although this has not generally been confirmed. In addition, LMW heparins cause less inhibition of platelet function.
- They have a longer half-life than standard heparin and so can be given as a once-daily subcutaneous injection instead of every 8–12 h.
- They produce little effect on tests of overall coagulation, such as the APTT at doses recommended for prophylaxis. They are not fully neutralized by protamine.

LMW heparins are excreted renally and therefore dose reductions are required in those with renal impairment.

LMW heparins are widely used for antithrombotic prophylaxis: for example, in high-risk surgical patients and for the treatment of established thrombosis (see pp. 1055–1056).

The main complication of all heparin treatment is bleeding. This is managed by stopping heparin. Very occasionally, it is necessary to neutralize unfractionated heparin with protamine. Other complications include osteoporosis with prolonged therapy and thrombocytopenia.

Heparin-induced thrombocytopenia

Heparin-induced thrombocytopenia (HIT) is an uncommon complication of heparin therapy and usually occurs 5–14 days after first heparin exposure. It is due to an immune response directed against heparin/platelet factor 4 complexes. All forms of heparin have been implicated but the problem occurs less often with LMW heparins.

HIT is paradoxically associated with severe thrombosis; when it is diagnosed, all forms of heparin must be discontinued, including heparin flush. Unfortunately the diagnosis can be difficult to make because patients on heparin are often very sick and may be thrombocytopenic for many other reasons. Use of the '4Ts' pre-test probability score can help diagnosis (based on degree of thrombocytopenia, timing of thrombocytopenia, presence of new thrombosis, and likelihood of an alternative diagnosis for the thrombocytopenia). Those with an intermediate or high risk score should have the diagnosis confirmed or refuted using an anti-enzyme-linked immunosorbent assay (anti-ELISA).

It is always necessary to continue some form of anticoagulation in patients with HIT and the choice lies between the heparinoid danaparoid and the direct thrombin inhibitor argatroban. The introduction of warfarin should be covered by one of these agents, as warfarin alone may exacerbate thrombosis as protein C levels fall.

Fondaparinux

This is a synthetic pentasaccharide that inhibits activated factor X, similar to the LMW heparins. It is used in acute coronary syndrome (see pp. 999–1000). A long-acting version, idraparinux, is also available and only needs to be given weekly. Neither binds to platelet factor 4 and so has no capacity to cause HIT.

Direct thrombin inhibitors

Hirudins bind directly to thrombin and are, effectively, irreversible inhibitors. Recombinant hirudins are no longer available.

Bivalirudin is a 20 amino acid synthetic analogue of hirudin. Compared with hirudin, it appears to cause less bleeding, is a reversible thrombin inhibitor (as it is broken down by thrombin) and has a shorter half-life. It is used in percutaneous coronary interventions.

Argatroban is a small-molecule, direct thrombin inhibitor with a short half-life. It is licensed in the UK for treatment of HIT.

Oral anticoagulants

Coumarins and indanediones

These act by interfering with vitamin K metabolism. The coumarin warfarin is most commonly used because it has a low incidence of side-effects other than bleeding.

The dosage is controlled by prothrombin tests (PT). Thromboplastin reagents for PT testing are derived from a variety of sources and give different PT results for the same plasma.

It is standard practice to compare each thromboplastin with an international reference preparation so that it can be assigned an international sensitivity index (ISI). The ***international normalized ratio (INR)*** is the ratio of the patient's PT to a normal control when using the international reference preparation. Therapeutic ranges using the INR for warfarin in various conditions are shown in ***Box 16.37***.

Each laboratory can use a chart adapted to the ISI of their thromboplastin to convert the patient's PT to the INR. Suitably selected control plasmas can also be employed to achieve the same objective. Adoption of this system means that PT tests on a given plasma sample using different thromboplastins result in the same INR and that anticoagulant control is comparable in different hospitals across the world.

Contraindications Contraindications to the use of oral anticoagulants are seldom absolute and include:

- severe uncontrolled hypertension
- non-thromboembolic strokes
- peptic ulceration (unless cured by *Helicobacter pylori* eradication)
- severe liver and renal disease
- pre-existing haemostatic defects
- non-compliance.

Warfarin should be avoided in pregnancy because it is teratogenic in the first trimester and may be associated with fetal haemorrhage later in pregnancy. When anticoagulation is considered essential in pregnancy, self-administered subcutaneous heparin should be used as an alternative, although this may not be as effective for women with prosthetic cardiac valves. Specialist advice should be sought.

Many drugs interact with warfarin (see p. 24). More frequent PT testing should accompany changes in medication, which should be implemented with the full knowledge of the anticoagulant clinic.

Increased anticoagulant effect due to warfarin An increased anticoagulant effect caused by warfarin is usually produced by one of the following mechanisms:

- drugs causing a reduction in the metabolism of warfarin, including tricyclic antidepressants, cimetidine, sulphonamides, phenothiazines and amiodarone
- drugs such as clofibrate and quinidine, which increase the sensitivity of hepatic receptors to warfarin
- drugs interfering with vitamin K absorption (such as broad-spectrum antibiotics and colestyramine), which also potentiate the action of warfarin
- displacement of warfarin from its binding site on serum albumin by drugs such as sulphonamides (this is not usually responsible for clinically relevant interactions)
- drugs that inhibit platelet function (such as aspirin), which increase the risk of bleeding
- alcohol excess, cardiac failure, liver or renal disease, hyperthyroidism and febrile illnesses, which result in potentiation of the effect of warfarin.

Decreased anticoagulant effect due to warfarin A decreased anticoagulant effect due to warfarin is usually produced by drugs that increase the clearance of warfarin by induction of hepatic enzymes that metabolize warfarin, such as rifampicin and barbiturates.

Anticoagulant-related bleeding Bleeding is the most serious side-effect of warfarin. Bleeding occurs in up to 4% of patients on oral anticoagulants per year, requires hospital admission in 2% and has a 0.25% morbidity associated with it. The benefit of anticoagulants must therefore be notably more than the risk of bleeding. Management of warfarin-related bleeding ***(Box 16.38)*** is dependent upon the INR and the degree of bleeding. Minor bleeding may be treated with cessation of warfarin alone, while serious bleeding will require additional use of vitamin K and factor concentrates.

Box 16.38 Management of warfarin-related bleeding and excessive oral anticoagulation

INR/Bleeding	Actions
INR >3.0 <6.0 (target INR 2.5)	1. Reduce warfarin dose or stop
INR >4.0 <5.0 (target INR 3.5)	2. Restart warfarin dose or stop
INR >5.0 <8.0, no bleeding	1. Stop warfarin 2. Reduce maintenance warfarin dose and investigate cause of elevated INR
INR >8.0, no bleeding or minor bleeding	1. Stop warfarin 2. Reduce maintenance warfarin dose and investigate cause of elevated INR 3. If no bleeding, give 1–5 mg of oral vitamin K 4. If minor bleeding, give 1–3 mg intravenous vitamin K
Major bleeding	1. Stop warfarin 2. Give four-factor prothrombin complex concentrate 25–50 U/kg (FFP 15 mL/kg only if concentrate not available) 3. Give 5 mg of intravenous vitamin K

If unexpected bleeding occurs, investigate the possibility of a local anatomical cause.

(Data from Keeling D, Baglin T, Tait C et al. and the British Committee for Standards in Haematology. Guidelines on oral anticoagulation with warfarin – fourth edition. *Br J Haematol* 2011; 154:311–324.)

Direct oral anticoagulants (also called new/novel oral anticoagulants)

A number of orally active direct thrombin (e.g. dabigatran) and Xa inhibitor drugs (e.g. rivaroxaban, apixaban, edoxaban) have been introduced for the treatment and prevention of venous and arterial thrombosis. These new direct oral anticoagulants have a much broader therapeutic window than warfarin, have fewer drug interactions (aside from stronger inducers and inhibitors of P-glycoprotein and CYP3A4) and offer the prospect of fixed drug dosing without the need to monitor coagulation.

Monitoring The primary advantage of these drugs is that they do not require regular monitoring. Dose amendment is, however, recommended with some NOACs in relation to patient age, weight and renal/liver function. Although they may prolong routine clotting times, this is variable. In the rare event that any actual monitoring is required, specific drug levels must be measured.

Indications Dabigatran, apixaban and rivaroxaban are licensed for prevention of thrombosis in hip and knee replacement surgery, prevention of stroke in atrial fibrillation, and treatment of VTE. These drugs have proved at least as effective as warfarin in large-scale clinical trials, and in some regimes are more effective than warfarin. All have at least similar safety profiles in terms of clinically significant bleeding rates; they do have higher rates of gastrointestinal haemorrhage but lower rates of intracranial haemorrhage than warfarin. Large-scale studies for other indications in various aspects of thrombosis treatment and prevention are being undertaken using such drugs, which are replacing warfarin in a significant number of patients. However, patients with significant hepatic dysfunction or renal impairment may not be good candidates for these drugs due to their hepatic and renal excretion.

Bleeding and reversal Specific molecules (monoclonal antibody fragment against dabigatran or a factor Xa decoy for rivaroxaban and apixaban) are in clinical trials. Idarucizumab has recently obtained FDA approval as a reversal agent for dabigatran. If bleeding occurs with these new agents that requires anticoagulant reversal, this can be partially achieved using activated or traditional prothrombin complex concentrates. All agents have relatively short half-lives (<14 hours) and will leave the circulation relatively quickly. Care needs to be taken, however, in planning the timing of anticoagulant cessation prior to elective surgery.

Prophylaxis to prevent venous thromboembolism

Risk factors for VTE are well defined. Most hospitalized patients have one or more of these risk factors and VTE is common in hospitalized patients. The risk of developing deep vein thrombosis (DVT) after hip replacement surgery has been estimated to be as high as 50% when thromboprophylaxis is not used. Approximately 10% of hospital deaths may be due to pulmonary embolism (PE) and more people die from hospital-acquired venous thrombosis than the combined total of deaths from road traffic accidents, acquired immunodeficiency syndrome (AIDS) and breast cancer. PE is the most common preventable cause of hospital death.

Appropriate thromboprophylaxis is highly effective and cost-effective. Such prophylactic measures include early mobilization, elevation of the legs, and use of compression stockings, intermittent compression devices and anticoagulant drugs, such as LMW heparins and thrombin inhibitors. All patients, medical and surgical, admitted to hospital should be assessed for thrombotic risk and given appropriate thromboprophylaxis. National guidelines are available to guide appropriate management ***(Box 16.39)***.

- ***Low-risk patients (Box 16.39)*** require no specific measures other than early mobilization.
- ***High-risk patients*** based on risk assessment are most effectively managed using graduated compression stockings and LMW heparin subcutaneously daily.

The antithrombin agents dabigatran and rivaroxaban are routinely used after lower limb joint replacement surgery. They are as effective as LMW heparins and, as they are given orally, can be used for extended periods out of hospital.

Box 16.39 Risk assessment for deep vein thrombosis and pulmonary embolism for hospital patients (NICE CG92)

Patients who are at risk of VTE

Medical patients

- If mobility significantly reduced for ≥3 days *or*
- If expected to have ongoing reduced mobility due to normal state plus any VTE risk factor

Surgical patients and patients with trauma

- If total anaesthetic + surgical time >90 min *or*
- If surgery involves pelvis or lower limb and total anaesthetic + surgical time >60 min *or*
- If acute surgical admission with inflammatory or intra-abdominal condition *or*
- If expected to have significant reduction in mobility *or*
- If any VTE risk factor present

VTE risk factors[a]

- Active cancer or cancer treatment
- Age >60 years
- Critical care admission
- Dehydration (usually associated with surgery)
- Known thrombophilias
- Obesity (BMI >30 kg/m^2)
- One or more significant medical co-morbidities (e.g. heart disease, metabolic endocrine or respiratory pathologies, acute infectious diseases, inflammatory conditions)
- Personal history or first-degree relative with a history of VTE
- Use of HRT
- Use of oestrogen-containing contraceptive therapy
- Varicose veins with phlebitis

Patients who are at risk of bleeding

All patients who have any of the following:

- Active bleeding
- Acquired bleeding disorders (such as acute liver failure)
- Concurrent use of anticoagulants known to increase the risk of bleeding (such as warfarin with INR >2)
- Lumbar puncture/epidural/spinal anaesthesia within the previous 4 h or expected within the next 12 h
- Acute stroke
- Thrombocytopenia (platelets <75 × 10^9/L
- Uncontrolled systolic hypertension (≥230/120 mmHg)
- Untreated inherited bleeding disorders (such as haemophilia or von Willebrand's disease)

[a]*For women who are pregnant or have given birth within the previous 6 weeks, see recommendations 1.6.4–1.6.6 in NICE Clinical Guideline 92.*

Management of established venous thromboembolism

- ***The aim*** of anticoagulant treatment is to prevent further thrombosis and pulmonary embolization while resolution of venous thrombi occurs by natural fibrinolytic activity. Anticoagulation is started with heparin, as it produces an immediate anticoagulant effect. Heparin should be administered for approximately 5 days, the time taken for simultaneously administered warfarin to produce an anticoagulant effect (INR 2.5).
- ***LMW heparin*** (e.g. tinzaparin 175 U/kg daily, dalteparin 200 U/kg daily, enoxaparin 1.5 mg/kg daily) is equally effective and as safe as unfractionated heparin in the immediate treatment of DVT and PE. This creates the opportunity for treatment of VTE without admission to hospital, in compliant patients without coexisting risk factors for haemorrhage.
- ***Length of anticoagulation***. This is recommended for *at least* 6 weeks after precipitated isolated calf vein thrombosis and *at least* 3 months after precipitated proximal DVT or PE in patients who have temporary risk factors. For patients with idiopathic VTE or permanent risk factors, at least 3 months' anticoagulation is recommended and consideration should be given to indefinite anticoagulation.
- ***Use of longer-term anticoagulation*** in patients with previous thrombosis: it has been suggested that a lower INR might be safer and equally effective but the current view is that the target INR should be 2.0–3.0 where oral anticoagulation is used. Indefinite anticoagulation is considered appropriate for those with two or more episodes of VTE.
- ***Outpatient anticoagulation*** is best supervised in anticoagulant clinics. Patients are issued with national booklets for recording INR results and anticoagulant doses. Home monitoring is possible in well-motivated patients.

Inferior vena cava (IVC) filters are an important tool for preventing PE in patients who have a contraindication to anticoagulation. Most are now retrievable, allowing removal once a temporary contraindication to anticoagulation has passed. Long-term use of an IVC filter is associated with a risk of thrombosis at and below the site of the filter.

The role of thrombolytic therapy in the treatment of venous thrombosis is not established. It is used in patients with massive PE who are haemodynamically unstable and in patients with extensive deep venous thrombi.

Thrombolytic therapy should be followed by anticoagulation with heparin for a few days and then by oral anticoagulants to prevent rethrombosis.

Further reading

Heneghan C, Ward A, Perera R et al. Self-monitoring of oral anticoagulation: systematic review and meta-analysis of individual patient data. *Lancet* 2012; 379:322–324.

Bibliography

Baglin TP, Gray E, Greaves M et al. Guidelines for testing for heritable thrombophilia. *Br J Haematol* 2010; 149:209–220.

British Society for Haematology. Guidelines for the diagnosis and management of disseminated intravascular coagulation. *Br J Haematol* 2009; 145:24–33.

Kearon C, Elie AA, Comerota AJ et al. Antithrombotic therapy for VTE disease: antithrombotic therapy and prevention of thrombosis, 9th edition: American College of Chest Physicians evidence-based clinical practice guidelines. *Chest* 2012; 141(2 Suppl):e419S–494S.

Keeling D, Baglin T, Tait C et al. and the British Committee for Standards in Haematology. Guidelines on oral anticoagulation with warfarin – fourth edition. *Br J Haematol* 2011; 154:311–324.

Provan AB, Stasi R, Newland AC et al. International consensus report on the investigation and management of primary immune thrombocytopenia. *Blood* 2010; 115:168–186.

Watson H, Davidson S, Keeling D and the Haemostasis and Thrombosis Task Force of the British Committee for Standards in Haematology. Guidelines on the diagnosis and management of heparin-induced thrombocytopenia – second edition. *Br J Haematol* 2012; 159:528–540.

Significant websites

http://www.bcshguidelines.com *British Society for Haematology guidelines*
http://www.bloodline.net *General website on haematology*
http://www.hemophilia.org *US National Hemophilia Foundation*
http://www.isth.org/ *International Society on Thrombosis and Haemostasis (ISTH)*
http://www.shotuk.org *Serious Hazards of Transfusion (SHOT) scheme, covering UK and Ireland NHS and private hospitals, affiliated to the Royal College of Pathologists (based at the Manchester Blood Transfusion Centre)*
http://www.transfusionguidelines.org.uk *UK Blood Transfusion and Tissue Transplantation Services Professional Guidelines, including Handbook of Transfusion Medicine*
http://www.transfusion.org *Journal of the American Association of Blood Banks*
http://www.wfh.org *World Federation of Hemophilia*

17

Malignant disease

Christopher J Gallagher, Matthew Smith, Jonathan Shamash

See your e-book for key learning points, summaries, clinical tips, drug tips, extra tables, interactive Figures, learning challenges and MCQs.

INTRODUCTION

The term 'malignant disease' encompasses a wide range of illnesses, including common ones such as lung, breast and colorectal cancer (see ***Box 17.43***), as well as rare ones like the acute leukaemias. Malignant disease is widely prevalent and, in the West, almost one-third of the population will develop cancer at some time during their life. It is second only to cardiovascular disease as a cause of death. Although the mortality of cancer is high, many advances have been made, both in terms of treating the disease and in understanding its biology at the molecular level.

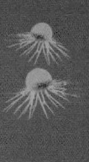

MALIGNANT DISEASE

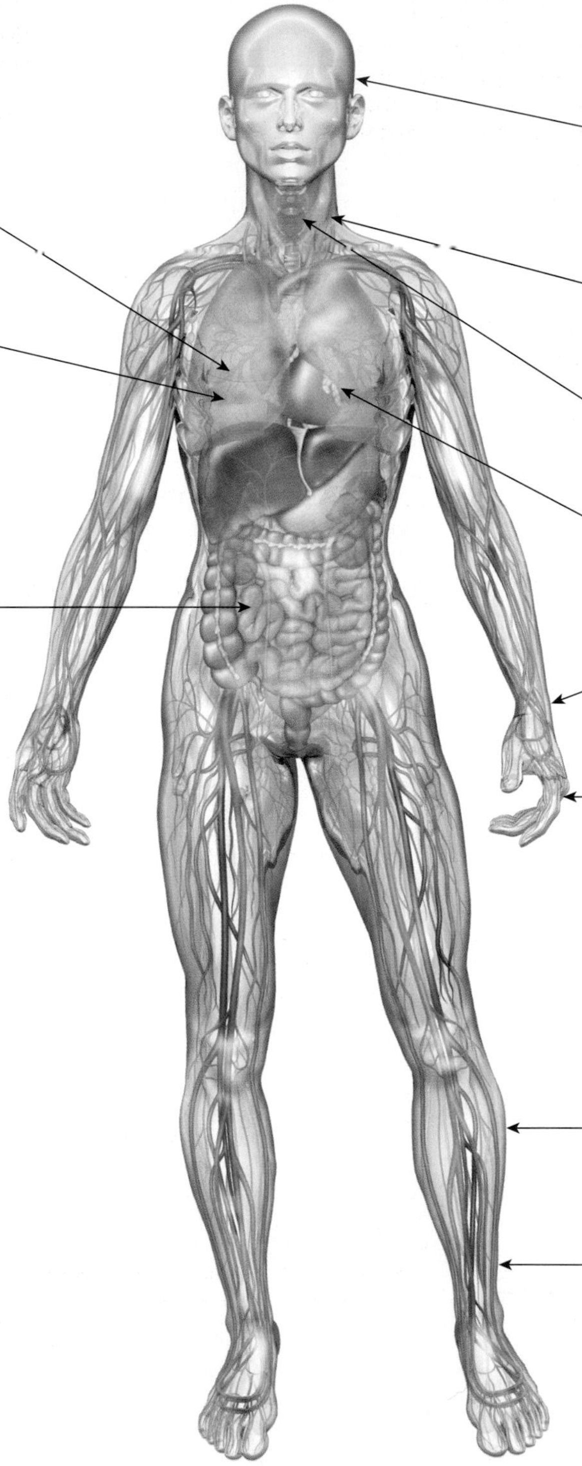

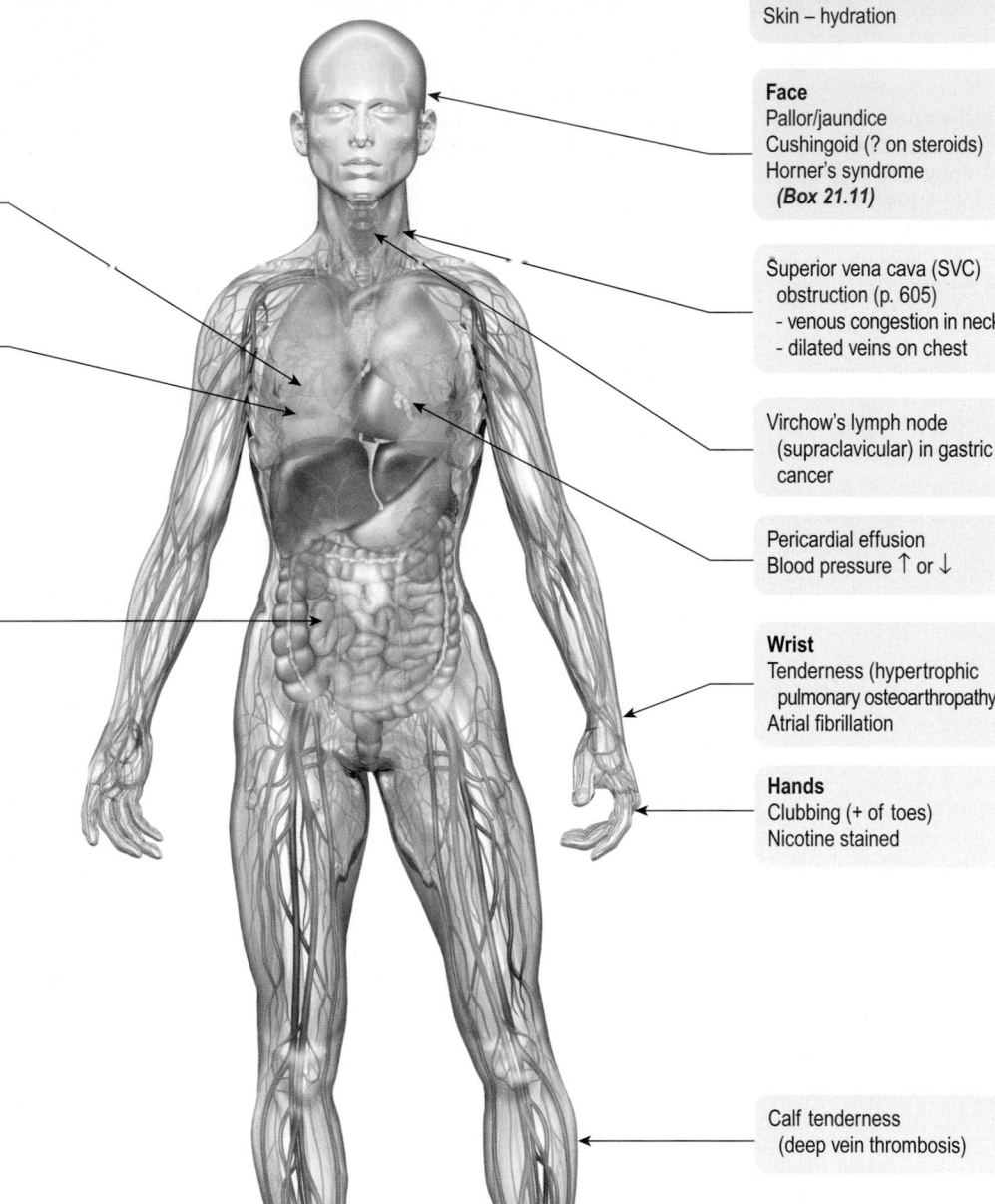

Neurological signs
Memory problems
Personality change (brain metastases)
Focal signs
Spinal cord compression (p. 872)

Breasts
Skin tethering

Respiratory
Consolidation (pneumonia)
Pleural effusion
Stridor (obstruction of trachea)

Abdomen
Surgical scars
Ascites
Masses, e.g. epigastric
Visible peristalsis (if intestinal obstruction)
Hepatomegaly
Splenomegaly
Renal mass
Mass in pelvis

Lymph nodes
Check:
- Neck (see opposite)
- Supraclavicular
- Axillary
- Inguinal
- Antecubital

Bones
Tenderness (long bones, spine, pelvis)

General
Cachexia
? Jaundiced
Skin – hydration

Face
Pallor/jaundice
Cushingoid (? on steroids)
Horner's syndrome *(**Box 21.11**)*

Superior vena cava (SVC) obstruction (p. 605)
- venous congestion in neck
- dilated veins on chest

Virchow's lymph node (supraclavicular) in gastric cancer

Pericardial effusion
Blood pressure ↑ or ↓

Wrist
Tenderness (hypertrophic pulmonary osteoarthropathy)
Atrial fibrillation

Hands
Clubbing (+ of toes)
Nicotine stained

Calf tenderness (deep vein thrombosis)

Peripheral oedema

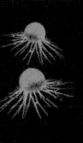

LYMPHADENOPATHY

Cervical lymph node enlargement – differential diagnosis

Infections	**Primary lymph node malignancies**
Acute	Hodgkin's lymphoma
Pyogenic infections	Non-Hodgkin's lymphoma
Epstein–Barr infection	Chronic lymphocytic leukaemia
Toxoplasmosis	Acute lymphoblastic leukaemia
Cytomegalovirus infection	**Secondary malignancies**
Infected eczema	Nasopharyngeal, oropharyngeal
Cat scratch fever	Thyroid
Acute childhood exanthema	Laryngeal
Chronic	Lung
Tuberculosis	Melanoma
Syphilis	Breast
HIV infection	Stomach
Autoimmune rheumatic disease	**Miscellaneous**
Rheumatoid arthritis	Sarcoidosis
Systemic lupus erythematous	Kawasaki's syndrome
Drug reactions	Kikuchi-Fujimoto disease (histiocytic necrotizing lymphadenitis)
Phenytoin	Castleman's disease (unicentric)

Abdominal examination:

Look for:
- Scars
- Distension (? ascites)
- Umbilicus – ? everted, ? nodule (Sister Mary Joseph's nodule – metastases from ovarian or gastric cancer)

Feel:
- Liver (enlarged from knobbly metastases)
- Spleen (haematological malignancy)
- Masses
- Inguinal nodes (e.g. ovarian, haematological)
- Ascites (shifting dullness)

Listen:
- Absent bowel sounds (paralytic ileus)

EXAMINATION OF LYMPH NODES IN THE HEAD AND NECK

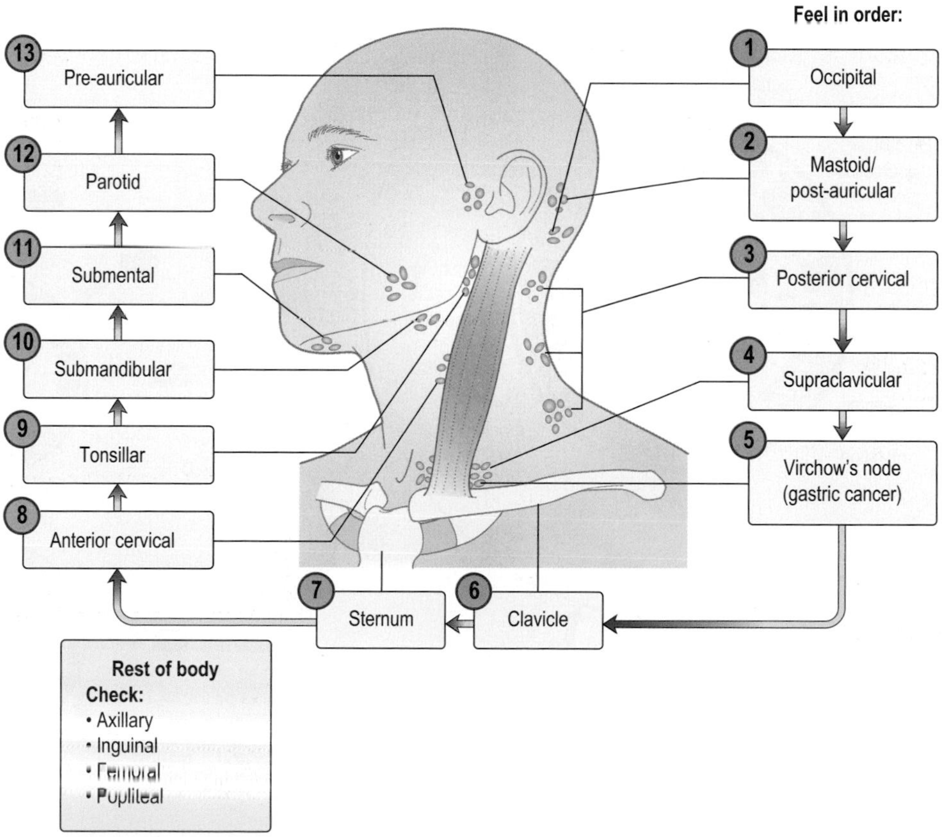

THE BIOLOGY OF CANCER

Most human neoplasms are clonal in origin: that is, they arise from a single population of precursor or cancer stem cells. This process is typically initiated by genetic aberrations within this precursor cell that may be inherited (germline) or acquired (somatic). Cancer becomes increasingly common as we get older, and can be related to a time-dependent accumulation of DNA damage that is not repaired by the normal mechanisms of genome maintenance, damage tolerance and checkpoint pathways. The hallmark areas of loss or gain in function in developing cancer are shown in ***Figure 17.1***. Whole-genome sequencing experiments are now identifying significant clonal genetic heterogeneity within tumours, including 'passenger' (inactive) and 'driver' (active) mutations. This heterogeneity is a potential source of treatment-resistant clones and is temporally variable, so that, at relapse, the predominant founder clone that has not been eradicated is seen to have acquired new mutations on its return; alternatively, a sub-clone, selected out by treatment pressure, has gained further mutations and led to a recurrence.

Sustaining proliferative signalling, enabling replicative immortality and resisting cell death

Malignant transformation may result from a gain in function as cellular proto-oncogenes become mutated (e.g. *ras*), amplified (e.g. *HER2*) or translocated (e.g. *BCR-ABL*). However, these mutations are insufficient to cause malignant transformation by themselves. Alternatively, there may be a loss of function of tumour suppressor genes, such as *p53*, that normally suppress growth. Loss or gain of function may also involve alterations in the genes controlling the transcription of the oncogenes or tumour suppressor genes (see p. 119). Over subsequent cell divisions, heterogeneity develops with the accumulation of further genetic abnormalities ***(Fig. 17.2)***. The genes most commonly affected can be characterized as those controlling cell cycle checkpoints, DNA repair and DNA damage recognition, apoptosis, differentiation, growth factor receptors, signalling pathways and tumour suppressor genes ***(Box 17.1)***. Recognition of critical genetic alterations has enabled extensive development of new targeted drugs, such as imatinib, which inhibits the growth signals of the abnormal tyrosine kinase *BCR/ABL*. Proliferation may continue at the expense of differentiation, which, together

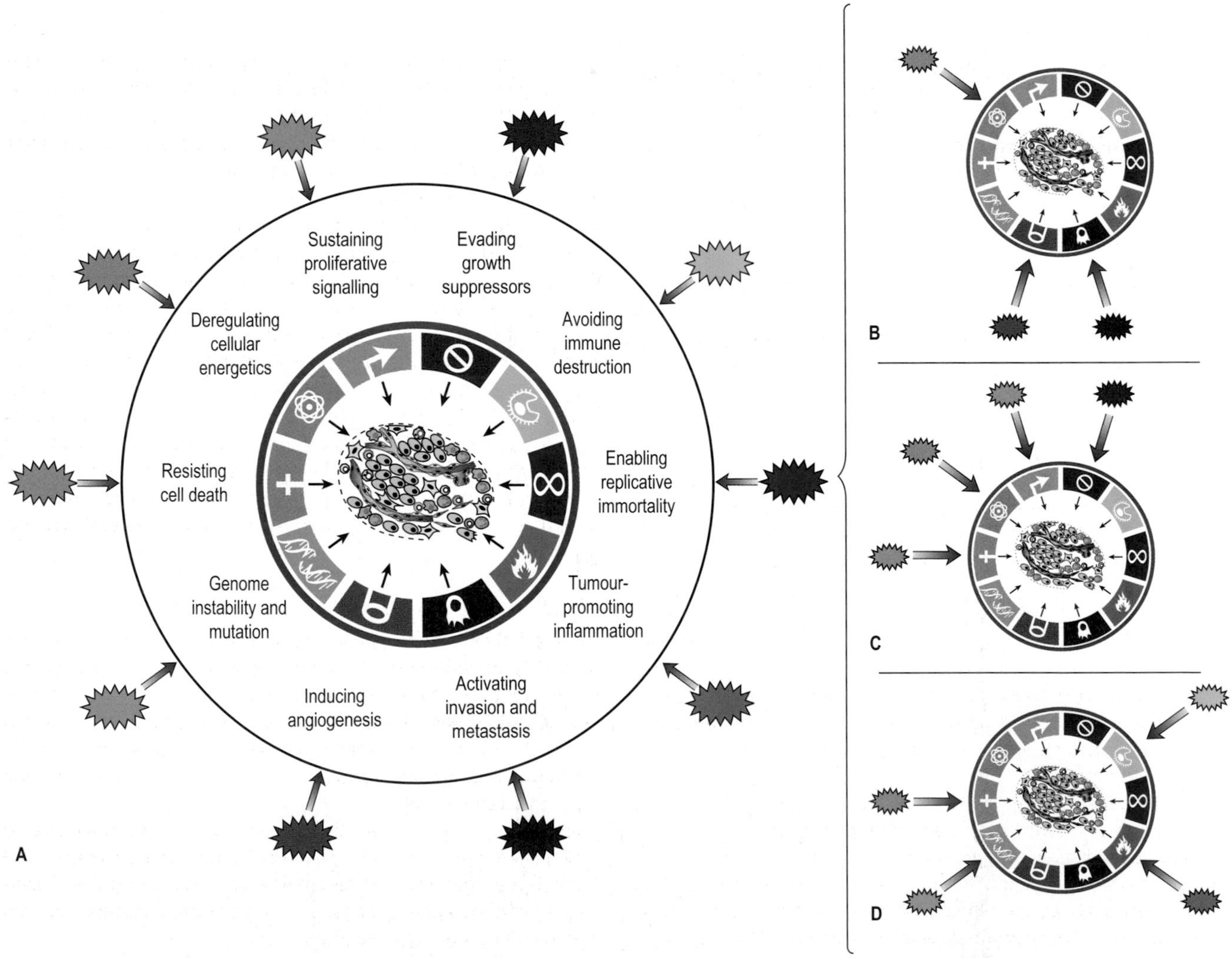

Figure 17.1 The hallmarks of cancer. Ten biologically damaging capabilities acquired during the multistep development of human tumours are shown. Each colour shows a different action as shown in the white circle. Each of these can be targeted as shown by the different-coloured 'explosion' shapes. **A.** In multi-targeting, toxicity to normal healthy tissue is a major challenge. **B–D.** These figures suggest possible selective targeting which would reduce toxicity to normal healthy tissue and optimize effectiveness on the specific target. *(From Hanahan D. The cancer wars 2: Rethinking the war on cancer.* Lancet *2014; 383:558–563, with permission. Adapted from Hanagan D, Weinberg PA. The hallmarks of cancer: the next generation.* Cell *2011; 144:646–474.)*

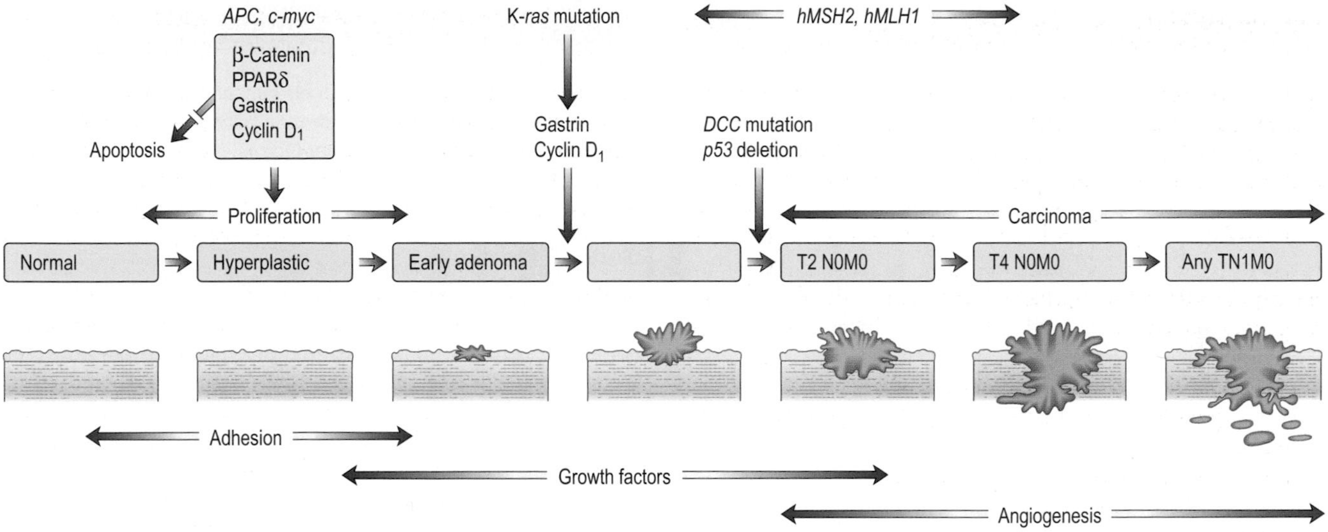

Figure 17.2 The adenoma–carcinoma progression sequence, showing genetic mutations at different stages. APC, adenomatous polyposis coli; PPARδ, peroxisome proliferator-activated receptor delta.

Box 17.1 Common genetic abnormalities in cancer

Gene	Examples
Control of cell cycle checkpoints	Cyclin D_1, *p15*, *p16*
DNA repair	*FANCA*, *ATM*
Apoptosis	*Bcl2*
Differentiation	*PML/RARA*
Growth factor receptors	*EGF*, *VEGF*, *FGF*, *BCR/ABL*, *TGF-B*, *KIT*, *L-FLT3*
Signalling pathways	*RAS*, *BRAF*, *JAK2*, *NF1*, *PTCH*
Hedgehog signalling pathway	See page 98
Tumour suppressor genes	*p53*, *Rb*, *WT1*, *VHL*

with failure of apoptosis, leads to tumour formation with the accumulation of morphologically abnormal cells varying in size, shape and cytoplasmic or nuclear maturity.

Evading growth suppression

Tumour cells are usually not recognized and killed by the immune system. There are two main reasons:

- There is a failure to express molecules such as human leucocyte antigen (HLA) and co-stimulatory B7 molecules that are required for activation of cytotoxic, or 'killer', T lymphocytes.
- Tumours may also actively secrete immunosuppressive cytokines and cause a generalized immunosuppression.

Successful strategies for tumour vaccines that overcome these obstacles are developing in renal cancer and prostate cancer. The monoclonal antibody ipilimumab, which works against the inhibitory cytotoxic T lymphocyte-associated antigen 4 (CTLA-4) molecule that is expressed after T-cell activation, is used in melanoma (see p. 601). There is increasing interest in the programmed death pathway (PD/PD-ligand). This checkpoint inhibitor (see p. 130) negatively affects the immune response. Recently, blocking either PD-1 (on T cells) or its ligand, PDL-1, which is present in some tumours, has been associated with an immune response that can produce tumour shrinkages that may be durable. Common tumours, such as squamous lung cancer and transitional cell carcinomas, have responded, in addition to those tumours expected to be susceptible to immunological therapies (melanoma and renal cancer).

Inducing angiogenesis

There is a progressive slowing of the rate of growth as many tumours become larger. This occurs for many reasons but outgrowing the blood supply is paramount. New vessel formation (angiogenesis) is stimulated by a variety of peptides produced both by tumour cells and by host inflammatory cells, such as basic fibroblast growth factor (bFGF), angiopoietin 2 and vascular endothelial growth factors (VEGFs), which are stimulated by hypoxia. The anti-VEGF-receptor monoclonal, bevacizumab, has had some success in colorectal and ovarian cancer. Alternatively, small molecules that target post-receptor response (tyrosine kinase inhibitors) may be used; examples include sunitinib and pazopanib.

Invasion and metastasis

Solid cancers spread by both local invasion and distant metastasis ***(Fig. 17.3)***, through the vessels of the blood and lymphatic systems. Infiltration into surrounding tissues is associated with loss of cell–cell cohesion, which is mediated by active homotypic cell adhesion molecules (CAMs). Epithelial cadherin (E-cadherin) is expressed by many carcinomas and mutated in some, such as familial gastric carcinoma (see p. 382).

Invasion is also determined by the balance of activators to inhibitors of proteolysis. The matrix metalloproteinases (MMPs) and their tissue inhibitors (TIMPs) are involved in tumour growth, invasion, metastasis and angiogenesis, and are being targeted by new therapeutic drugs for tumour treatment.

Dissemination of tumour cells occurs through intravasation into the vascular and lymphatic vessels and dissemination to distant sites, partly by chance, but also because of specific interactions between receptors and cytokines found on stromal and tumour cells, such as tumour necrosis factor (TNF), interleukin 6 (IL-6) and chemokines.

Further reading

Aparicio S, Caldas C. The implications of clonal genome evolution for cancer medicine. *N Engl J Med* 2013; 368:842–851.
Ding L, Ley TJ, Larson DE et al. Clonal evolution in relapsed acute myeloid leukaemia revealed by whole-genome sequencing. *Nature* 2012; 481:506–510.
Hanahan D. Rethinking war on cancer. *Lancet* 2014; 383:558–563.
Hodi FS, O'Day SJ, McDermott DF et al. Improved survival with ipilimumab in patients with metastatic melanoma. *N Engl J Med* 2010; 363:711–723.
Pritchard CC, Grady WM. Colorectal cancer molecular biology moves into clinical practice. *Gut* 2011; 60:116–129.

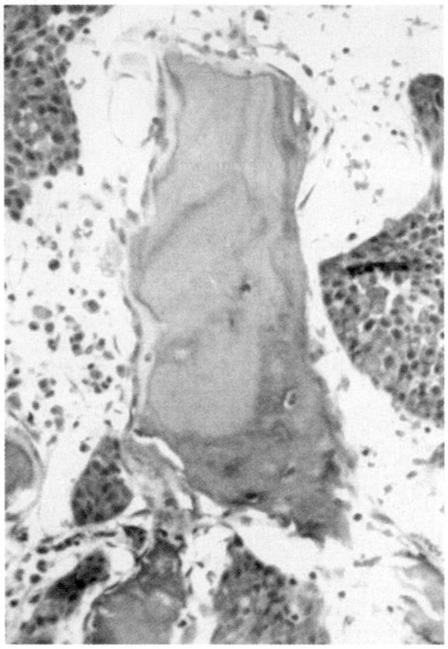

Figure 17.3 Bone metastasis with osteoclast and osteoblast activation.

AETIOLOGY AND EPIDEMIOLOGY

For most patients, the cause of their cancer is unknown, probably representing a multifactorial interaction between individual genetic predispositions and environmental factors.

Aetiology

Genetic factors

Rather than occurring by somatic mutation in response to mutagens, germline mutations in the genes that predispose to the development of cancer may be inherited and therefore present in all tissues. Examples of such cancer syndromes are given in **Box 17.2**. Expression of the mutation, and hence carcinogenesis, will depend on the penetrance (due to the level of expression and the presence of other genetic events) of the gene and whether the mutated allele has a dominant or recessive effect. There is a small group of autosomal dominant inherited mutations, such as RB (in retinoblastoma), and a small group of recessive mutations **(Box 17.2)**. Carriers of the recessive mutations are at risk of developing cancer if the second allele becomes mutated, leading to 'loss of heterozygosity' within the tumour, although this is seldom sufficient, as carcinogenesis is a multistep process.

Environmental factors

A wide range of environmental factors has been identified as being associated with the development of malignancy **(Box 17.3)** and may be amenable to preventative action, such as smoking cessation, dietary modification and antiviral immunization **(Box 17.4)**. Environmental factors interact with genetic predisposition. For example, subsequent generations of people moving from countries with a low incidence to those with a high incidence of breast or colon cancer

Box 17.2 Familial cancer syndromes

Syndrome	Gene	Neoplasms
Autosomal dominant		
Retinoblastoma	*RB1*	Eye
Wilms' tumour	*WT1*	Kidney
Li–Fraumeni	*p53*	Sarcoma/brain/leukaemia
Neurofibromatosis type 1	*NF1*	Neurofibromas/leukaemia
Familial adenomatous polyposis (FAP)	*APC*	Colon
Lynch syndrome (previously hereditary non-polyposis colon cancer, HNPCC)	*MLH1* and *MSH2*	Colon, endometrium
Hereditary diffuse gastric cancer syndrome	E-cadherin	Stomach
Breast/ovary families	*BRCA1* *BRCA2* *p53*	Breast/ovary
Melanoma	*p16*	Skin
Von Hippel–Lindau	*VHL*	Renal cell carcinoma and haemangioblastoma
Multiple endocrine neoplasia type 1	*MEN1*	Pituitary, pancreas, parathyroid
Multiple endocrine neoplasia type 2	*RET*	Thyroid, adrenal medulla
Autosomal recessive		
Xeroderma pigmentosa	*XP*	Skin
Ataxia telangiectasia	*AT*	Leukaemia, lymphoma
Fanconi's anaemia	*FA*	Leukaemia, lymphoma
Bloom syndrome	*BS*	Leukaemia, lymphoma

Box 17.3 Some causative factors associated with the development of cancer

Causative factors	Neoplasms
Smoking	Mouth, pharynx, oesophagus, larynx, lung, bladder, lip
Alcohol	Mouth, pharynx, larynx, oesophagus, colorectal
Iatrogenic	
Alkylating agents	Bladder, bone marrow
Oestrogens	Endometrium, vagina, breast, cervix
Androgens	Prostate
Radiotherapy (e.g. mantle radiotherapy)	Carcinoma of breast and bronchus
Diet	
High-fat diet	Colorectal
Environment/occupation	
Air pollution	Lung cancer
Vinyl chloride	Liver (angiosarcoma)
Polycyclic hydrocarbons	Skin, lung, bladder, myeloid leukaemia
Aromatic amines	Bladder
Asbestos	Lung, mesothelium
Ultraviolet light	Skin, lip
Radiation	e.g. Leukaemia, thyroid cancer
Aflatoxin	Liver
Biological agents	
Hepatitis B virus	Liver (hepatocellular carcinoma)
Hepatitis C virus	Liver (hepatocellular carcinoma)
Human T-cell leukaemia virus	Leukaemia/lymphoma
Epstein–Barr virus	Burkitt's lymphoma Hodgkin's lymphoma Nasopharyngeal carcinoma
Human papillomavirus types 16 and 18	Cervix Oral cancer (type 16)
Schistosoma japonicum	Bladder
Helicobacter pylori	Stomach

Box 17.4 Key messages for a healthy lifestyle for preventing cancer

- Stop smoking
- Moderate alcohol consumption
- Maintain a healthy weight
- Take moderate exercise
- Eat healthily (fruit and vegetables, high fibre, low fat/salt/sugar)
- Limit sun exposure
- Minimize occupational risk
- Minimize radiation exposure
- Vaccinate against hepatitis B and human papillomavirus

acquire the tumour incidence of the country to which they have moved, while Northern European people exposed to strong ultraviolet radiation have the highest risk of developing melanoma.

Tobacco

The incidence of lung cancer in both men and women increased dramatically in the last 25 years worldwide, but is now falling in many developed countries. The association of smoking with lung cancer is indisputable and causative mechanisms have been identified; cigarette tobacco is responsible for one-third of all deaths from cancer in the UK. Smoking not only causes lung cancer, but also is associated with cancer of the mouth, larynx, oesophagus and bladder. Smoking is discussed on pages 1074–1075.

Alcohol

Alcohol is associated with cancers of the upper respiratory and gastrointestinal tracts, and also interacts with tobacco in the aetiology of these tumours. It may be associated with an increased risk of breast cancer.

Diet

One-third of cancer deaths have been attributed to dietary factors, although it is often difficult to differentiate these from other epidemiological factors. For example, the incidence of stomach cancer is particularly high in the Far East, while breast and colon cancers are more common in Western, economically more developed countries. Many associations have been observed without a causative link being identified between the incidence of cancer and the consumption of dietary fibre, red meat, saturated fats, salted fish, vitamin E, vitamin A and many others. Food and its role in the causation of gastrointestinal cancer are discussed on page 183. Higher levels of obesity in the developed world have been associated with increases in cancers associated with oestrogenic stimulation of the breast and endometrium in women.

Environment/occupation

Environmental factors

Air pollution (see p. 56).

Ultraviolet (UV) light is known to increase the risk of skin cancer (basal cell, squamous cell and melanoma). The incidence of melanoma is therefore particularly high in the white Anglo-Celtic population of Australia, New Zealand and South Africa, where exposure to UV light is combined with a genetically predisposed population.

Arsenical contamination of water supplies has been linked to a high incidence of lung and colon cancers in South-east Asia, particularly where boreholes are the main water source.

Occupational factors

In 1775, Percival Pott described the association between carcinogenic hydrocarbons in soot and the development of scrotal epitheliomas in chimney sweeps. The principal causes now are ***asbestos*** (lung and mesothelial cancer) and ***polycyclic hydrocarbons*** from fossil fuel combustion (skin, lung and bladder cancers). ***Organic chemicals***, such as benzene, may cause the development of bone marrow conditions, such as myelodysplastic syndrome or acute myeloid leukaemia.

Infectious agents

The geographical distribution of a rare malignancy suggests that it might be caused by, or associated with, an infective agent. Chronic persistent infection provides growth stimulation, while many viruses contain transforming viral oncogenes.

T-cell leukaemia, seen almost exclusively in residents of the southern island of Japan and in the West Indies, is caused by infection with the locally endemic retrovirus human T-cell leukaemia virus (HTLV-1) and integration of the oncogene, *TAX*, into the cellular genome.

Hepatocellular carcinoma occurs in patients with hepatitis B and C virus infections, and Burkitt's lymphoma and nasopharyngeal carcinoma are associated with the Epstein–Barr virus (EBV). EBV is also linked with Hodgkin's lymphoma (see p. 616).

Patients with human immunodeficiency (HIV) infection or immunosuppression from organ transplantation have an increased incidence of EBV-related lymphoma and herpesvirus-8-associated Kaposi's sarcoma.

Human papillomavirus (HPV) infection types 16 and 18, for which an effective vaccine is now available, is an established cause of the rise in cervical cancer among sexually active women; more recently, it has also been associated with an increase in head and neck cancers. Bacterial infection with *Helicobacter pylori* predisposes to the development of gastric cancer and gastric lymphoma, while *Schistosoma japonicum* infection predisposes to the development of squamous cell carcinomas in the bladder.

Medication

Oestrogens have been implicated in the development of vaginal, endometrial and breast carcinoma. Certain cytotoxic drugs given, such as those for Hodgkin's lymphoma (see pp. 616–618) are themselves associated with an increased incidence of secondary acute myelogenous leukaemia (AML), and bladder and lung cancer. Androgens have been associated with both benign and malignant liver tumours.

Radiation

Accidental

The nuclear disasters of Hiroshima, Nagasaki and Chernobyl led to an increased incidence of leukaemia after 5–10 years in the exposed population, as well as increased incidences of thyroid and breast cancer. Radiation workers are at an increased risk of malignancy due to occupational exposure, unless precautions are taken to minimize the danger by using personal and environmental shielding, and to record and limit the amount of personal exposure.

Therapeutic

Long-term survivors following radiotherapy, such as that for Hodgkin's lymphoma, have an increased incidence of cancer, particularly at the radiation field margins.

Diagnostic

Imaging procedures involving radiation exposure are associated with an increased risk of cancer. This risk is cumulative, dose-dependent and time-dependent, and so children are at higher risk than adults. The cancer risk of various common investigations is shown in ***Box 17.5***. All doctors should strive to minimize diagnostic exposure to radiation where possible by using alternative modalities such as ultrasound or magnetic resonance imaging (MRI). Good documentation of radiation doses is required. This is particularly so in children and pregnant women.

Box 17.5 Radiation exposure from common diagnostic radiological procedures[a]

Procedure	mSv
Chest X-ray	0.02
Computed tomogram (CT) chest	7
CT abdomen	8–10
Whole-body CT	20
Percutaneous coronary intervention	15
Myocardial perfusion imaging	15.6

[a]UK background radiation is 2.6 mSv per year. 1 mSv carries a lifetime cancer risk of 1 in 17 500 and 5 mSv a risk of 1 in 3500.
(Modified from Smith-Bindman R, Lipson J, Marcus R et al. *Arch Intern Med* 2009; 169:2078–2086 and Fazel R, Krumholz HM, Wang Y et al. *N Engl J Med* 2009; 361:849–857.)

Epidemiology

The incidence and mortality from cancer vary by tumour type and geographical region across the world.

Geographical distribution

The incidence of cancer across the world is dependent on the local environmental factors, the diet and the genetics of the population (see above) (***Figs 17.4*** and ***17.5***). Age is also a factor, as most cancers occur in those over the age of 65, who comprise 3.3% of the population in Africa, compared with 15.2% in Europe. Reproductive patterns also influence breast cancer. Migrating individuals often take on the risks associated with the local environmental factors.

Other factors

Incidence and mortality are closely linked for those cancers for which treatment has yet to make significant improvements, such as lung, stomach and liver. However, in countries with effective screening programmes, there is an increasing incidence, but decreasing mortality, for breast, cervix, bowel and prostate cancers.

Further reading

Hoeijmakers JH. DNA damage, aging and cancer. *N Engl J Med* 2009; 361:1475–1485.
McDermott U, Downing JR, Stratton MR. Genomics and the continuum of cancer care. *N Engl J Med* 2011; 364:340–350.
Pearce MS, Salotti JA, Little MP et al. Radiation exposure from CT scans in childhood and subsequent risk of leukaemia and brain tumours: a retrospective cohort study. *Lancet* 2012; 380:499–505.

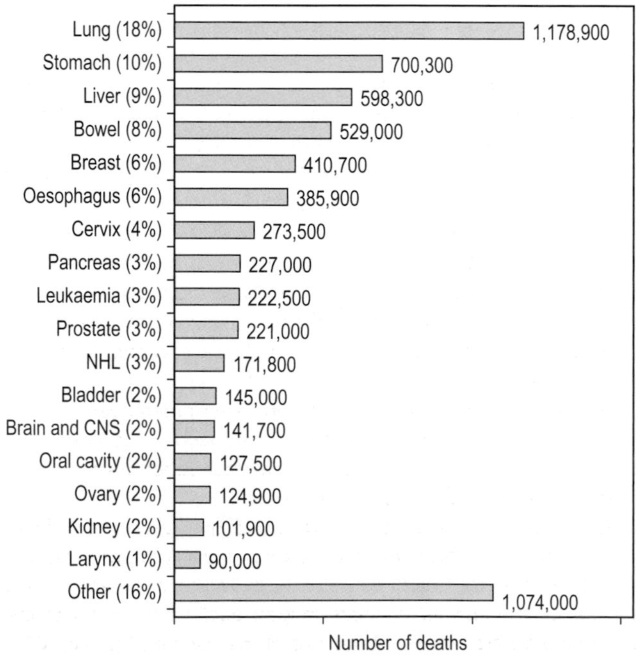

Figure 17.4 The most common causes of death from cancer worldwide, 2002 estimates. Non-melanoma skin cancers are excluded. CNS, central nervous system; NHL, non-Hodgkin's lymphoma. *(From* http://info.canceresearchuk.org/cancerstats/world/the-global-picture/*.)*

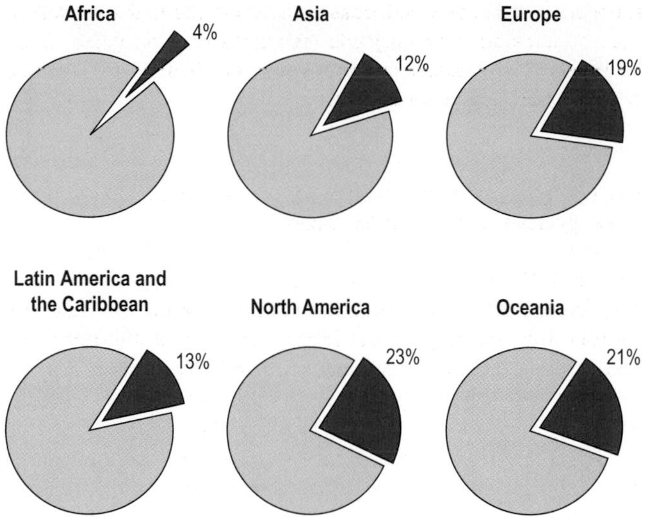

Figure 17.5 Percentage of all deaths due to cancer in the different regions of the world. *(From:* http://info.cancerresearchuk.org/cancerstats/world/the-global-picture/.*)*

CLINICAL APPROACH TO THE PATIENT WITH MALIGNANT DISEASE

Asymptomatic detection through screening

Most common cancers start as focal microscopic clones of transformed cells, and diagnosis only becomes likely once sufficient tumour bulk has accumulated to cause symptoms or signs. In order to try to make an earlier diagnosis and enhance the curative possibilities, an increasing number of screening programmes are being developed that either target the asymptomatic or pre-invasive stages of the cancer, as in cervix, breast and colon, or use serum tumour markers, as in prostate and ovarian cancers. Genetic screening can be used to target screening to those groups at most risk of developing cancer, such as *BRCA1*-positive individuals who may develop breast cancer (see ***Box 17.2***). The aim of screening programmes is to improve individual and/or population survival by detecting cancer in its very early stages, when the patient is asymptomatic. This strategy is dependent on finding tests that are sufficiently sensitive and specific, using detection methods that identify cancer before it has spread, and having curative treatments that are practical and consistent with maintenance of a normal lifestyle and quality of life.

Screening is provided to populations – for breast, cervical and colon cancer in the UK, for example – and also to individuals via annual check-ups; alternatively, it may be opportunistic, when patients see their doctor for other reasons.

Unfortunately, earlier diagnosis does not necessarily mean longer survival and randomized trials are necessary to prove benefit. With lead-time bias, the patient is merely treated at an earlier date and hence the survival appears longer; death still occurs at the same time from the point of genesis of the cancer ***(Fig. 17.6)***. With length-time bias, a greater number of slowly growing tumours are detected when asymptomatic individuals are screened, leading to a false impression of an improvement in survival.

The characteristics of effective screening programmes are shown in ***Box 17.6***.

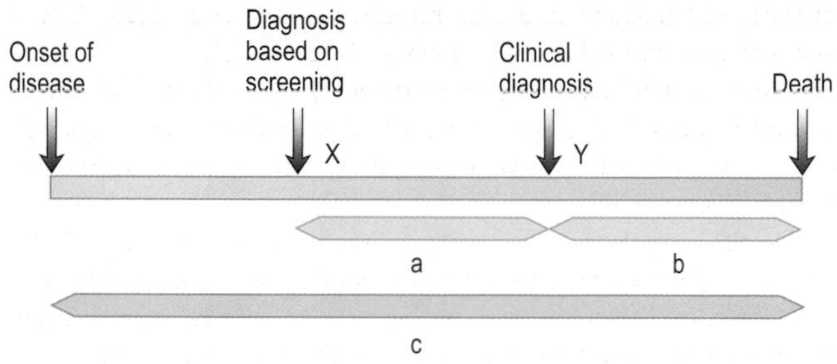

Figure 17.6 Lead-time bias. Earlier diagnosis, at X, made by screening tests before the clinical diagnosis, at Y, suggests an increased survival time of a+b. The actual survival time (c) remains unchanged.

i Box 17.6 Characteristics of an effective screening programme

- It must be affordable for the healthcare system
- It must be acceptable to all social groups so that they attend for screening
- It must have a good discriminatory index between benign and malignant lesions
- It must show a reduction in mortality from the cancer

Cervical cancer

The smear test is cheap and safe but requires a well-trained cytologist to identify the early changes (dyskaryosis and cervical intraepithelial neoplasia, CIN). However, developments in liquid cytology and co-testing for HPV DNA may overcome this. Effective treatment for high-risk, pre-invasive, malignant changes reduces the incidence and mortality from cervical cancer, although there are no randomized trials. Screening will continue to be required, despite the introduction of vaccination against HPV infection for women before they become sexually active, because the lag time between infection and the appearance of disease can be in the order of 40–50 years.

Breast cancer

The UK National Health Service Breast Screening Programme (i.e. biplanar mammography every 3 years) for women aged 50–70 years has been shown to reduce mortality from breast cancer in randomized controlled studies. The test is acceptable to most women, with 50–75% of individuals attending for screening when sufficiently educated about the benefits. In North America, there is continuing debate about whether annual mammography from a younger age is more effective.

The cost is estimated to be between £250 000 and £1.3 million per life saved, money which, according to critics, could be used more appropriately in better treatment.

Women from families with *BRCA1*, *BRCA2* and *p53* mutations require intensive screening starting at an earlier age, when mammography is inaccurate due to greater breast density and MRI scanning is preferred.

Colorectal cancer

Faecal occult blood is a cheap test for the detection of colorectal cancer. Large randomized studies have shown a reduction in cancer-related mortality of 15–33%. However, the false-positive rates are high, meaning many unnecessary colonoscopies (see

Box 17.7 Symptoms and signs of malignant disease

Degree of spread	Anatomical location	Examples of clinical problems
Local	Mass	Thyroid nodule, pigmented naevus, breast lump, abdominal mass, testicular mass
	Local infiltration of skin	Dermal nodules, peau d'orange, ulceration
	Local infiltration of nerve	Neuropathic pain and loss of function Horner syndrome, cord compression, Pancoast tumour, focal CNS deficit, hypopituitarism
	Local infiltration of vessel	Venous thrombosis, tumour emboli, haemorrhage, e.g. gastrointestinal
	Obstruction of viscera or duct	Small or large bowel obstruction, dysphagia, SVC obstruction Obstructive uropathy, acute kidney injury, urinary retention, stridor, lobar collapse, pneumonia, cholestatic jaundice
Nodal	Peripheral	Supraclavicular fossa, Virchow's node, lymphoedema
	Central	Mediastinum – SVC obstruction, porta hepatis – obstructive jaundice, para-aortic nodes and back pain
Metastatic	Lung	Pleuritic pain, cough, shortness of breath, lymphangitis and respiratory failure, recurrent pneumonia
	Liver	RUQ pain, anorexia, fever, raised serum liver enzymes, jaundice
	Brain	Headache and vomiting of raised intracranial pressure, focal deficit, coma, seizure
	Bone	Bone pain, cord compression, fracture, hypercalcaemia
	Pleura	Effusion, pain, shortness of breath
	Peritoneum	Ascites, Krukenberg tumours
	Adrenal	Addison's disease (hypoadrenalism)
	Umbilicus	Sister Mary Joseph's nodule

CNS, central nervous system; RUQ, right upper quadrant; SVC, superior vena cava.

p. 425). The UK has recently introduced a national screening programme using faecal occult blood in patients aged 60–64 years, in which positive tests have identified that 10% have cancer and 40% have adenomas. A randomized trial in Norway has found an increased number of early-stage cancers in the screened population but a high incidence of interval cancers between biennial screens.

Colonoscopy is the 'gold-standard' technique for the examination of the colon and rectum and is the investigation of choice for high-risk patients. Universal screening strategies have been recommended in the USA, but the shortage of skilled endoscopists, the expense, the need for full bowel preparation and the small risk of perforation make colonoscopy impractical as a population screening tool at present; computed tomographic (CT) colonography ('virtual colonoscopy') (see ***Fig. 13.5***) may become an alternative, along with genetic testing and stool DNA tests.

Prostate cancer

Serum prostate-specific antigen (PSA) can be used for the detection of this cancer, which is on the increase. Many men over 70 have evidence of prostate cancer at postmortem but had no symptoms of the disease, and it has been suggested that those over 75 should not have screening PSA tests. The test must be interpreted with caution due to the natural increase in PSA with age, benign prostatic hypertrophy and prostatitis. The early results of screening for prostate cancer have varied greatly, with any reductions in prostate cancer-specific mortality potentially not observed for 10 years or more. Currently, national screening programmes are not recommended but instead an informed choice programme is in existence in the UK. Screening may not be appropriate in those with a life expectancy of less than 10–15 years.

Epithelial ovarian cancer

Serum CA125 can be used for the early detection of this cancer and is the subject of ongoing trials. An improvement in survival of a screened population can be shown but at the cost of many unnecessary laparotomies, so that further enhancements are being investigated by serial testing and in combination with transvaginal ultrasound scans.

The symptomatic patient with cancer

Patients may offer information of predisposing conditions and family history that alerts the clinician to the likelihood of a cancer diagnosis. Many present with a history of tumour site-specific symptoms, such as pain, and physical signs, such as a mass, which readily identify the primary site of the cancer ***(Box 17.7)***. Cancer symptoms typically increase with time, and do not respond to measures such as antibiotics. However, some patients only seek medical attention when more systemic and non-specific symptoms occur, such as weight loss, night sweats, fever, fatigue, recurrent infections and anorexia. These usually indicate a more advanced stage of disease, except in some paraneoplastic and ectopic endocrine syndromes (see below). Other patients are only diagnosed on discovery of established metastases, such as the abdominal distension of ovarian cancer, the back pain of metastatic prostatic cancer, or the liver enlargement of metastatic gastrointestinal cancer

Paraneoplastic syndromes are indirect effects of cancer (***Box 17.8*** and ***Fig. 17.7***) that are often associated with specific types of cancer and may be reversible with treatment of the cancer. The effects and mechanisms can be very variable. For example, in the Lambert–Eaton syndrome (see p. 890), there is cross-reactivity between tumour antigens and the normal tissue acetylcholine receptors at neuromuscular junctions.

The ***coagulopathy of cancer*** may present with thrombophlebitis, deep venous thrombosis and pulmonary emboli, particularly in association with cancers of pancreas, stomach and breast. Some 18% of patients with recurrent pulmonary embolus will be found to have an underlying cancer and many cancer patients are at increased risk of venous thromboembolism (VTE) following diagnosis. Trousseau syndrome – superficial thrombophlebitis migrans – refers to this process in the superficial venous system. All patients with active cancer admitted to hospital are at high risk of VTE and should be given prophylaxis with, for example, subcutaneous low-molecular-weight heparin in the absence of any contraindications (see p. 578).

Other symptoms are related to peptide or hormone release, such as in carcinoid or Cushing syndrome.

Box 17.8 Paraneoplastic syndromes

Syndrome	Tumour	Serum antibodies
Neurological		
Lambert–Eaton syndrome	Lung (small-cell) carcinoma	Anti-VGCC
Peripheral sensory neuropathy	Lung (small-cell), breast and ovary lymphoma	Anti-Hu
Cerebellar degeneration	Lung (particularly small-cell) lymphoma	Anti-Yo
Opsoclonus/myoclonus	Breast, lung (small-cell)	Anti-Ri
Stiff person syndrome	Breast, lung (small-cell)	Anti-amphiphysin
Limbic, hypothalamic, brain stem encephalitis	Lung	Anti-Ma protein
	Testicular	Anti-NMDAR
Endocrine/metabolic		
SIADH	Lung (small-cell)	
Ectopic ACTH secretion	Lung (small-cell)	
Hypercalcaemia	Renal, breast, myeloma, lymphoma	
Fever	Lymphoma, renal	
Musculoskeletal		
Hypertrophic pulmonary osteoarthropathy	Lung (non-small-cell)	
Clubbing	Lung	
Skin		
Dermatomyositis/polymyositis	Lung and upper gastrointestinal	
Acanthosis nigricans	Mainly gastric	
Velvet palms	Gastric, lung (non-small cell)	
Hyperpigmentation	Lung (small-cell)	
Pemphigus	Non-Hodgkin's lymphoma, CLL	
Haematological		
Erythrocytosis	Renal cell carcinoma, hepatocellular carcinoma, cerebellar haemangioblastoma	
Thrombocytosis	Ovarian cancer	
Migratory thrombophlebitis	Pancreatic adenocarcinoma	
DVT	Adenocarcinoma	
DIC	Adenocarcinoma	
Renal		
Nephrotic syndrome	Myeloma, amyloidosis	
Membranous glomerulonephritis	Lymphoma	

ACTH, adrenocorticotrophic hormone; CLL, chronic lymphocytic leukaemia; DIC, disseminated intravascular coagulation; DVT, deep venous thrombosis; NMDAR, N-methyl-D-aspartate receptors; SIADH, syndrome of inappropriate antidiuretic hormone secretion; VGCC, voltage-gated calcium channels.

Cachexia of advanced cancer is thought to be due to release of chemokines such as tumour necrosis factor (TNF), as well as the fact that patients lose their appetite. The unexplained loss of >10% of body weight in a patient should always stimulate a search for an explanation.

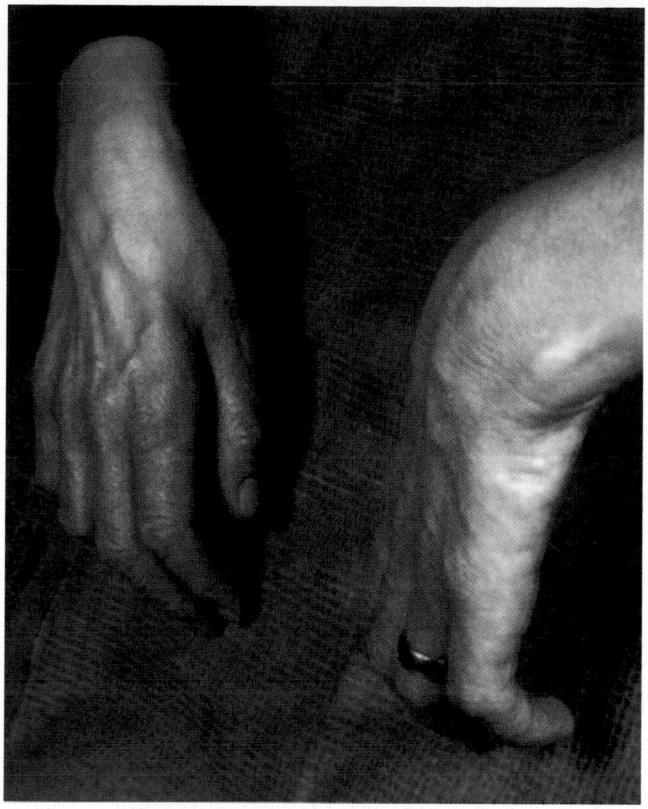

Figure 17.7 Paraneoplastic peripheral neuropathy. There is wasting of the small muscles of the hands.

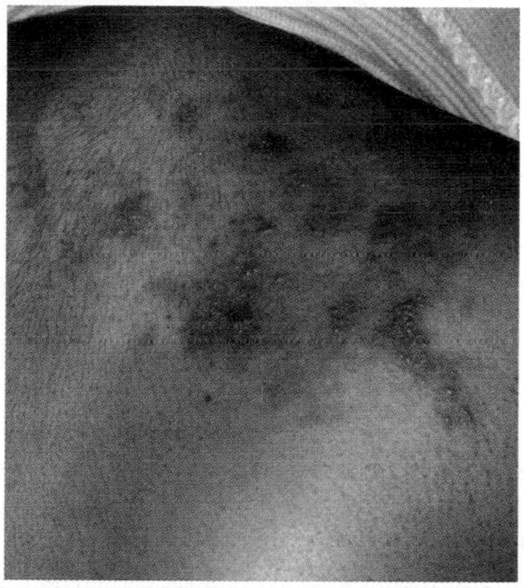

Figure 17.8 Reactivated herpes zoster (shingles).

Cancer-associated immunosuppression can lead to reactivation of latent infections such as herpes zoster ***(Fig. 17.8)*** and tuberculosis.

Serum tumour markers

Tumour markers are intracellular proteins or cell surface glycoproteins released into the circulation and detected by immunoassays. Examples are given in ***Box 17.9***. Values in the normal range do not necessarily equate with the absence of disease and a positive result must be corroborated by histology, as these markers can be seen in many benign conditions. They are most useful in the serial monitoring of response to treatment. As discussed in subsequent sections, a proportion of low-grade B-cell lymphomas and a majority

Box 17.9 Serum tumour markers

Serum tumour marker	Neoplasms
α-Fetoprotein	Hepatocellular carcinoma and non-seminomatous germ cell tumours of the gonads
β-Human chorionic gonadotrophin (β-hCG)	Choriocarcinomas, germ cell tumours (testicular) and lung cancers
β_2-microglobulin	Non-Hodgkin's lymphoma, myeloma
Prostate-specific antigen (PSA)	Carcinoma of the prostate
Carcinoma embryonic antigen (CEA)	Gastrointestinal cancers
CA125	Ovarian cancer
CA19–9	Gastrointestinal cancers, particularly pancreatic cancer
CA15–3	Breast cancer
Osteopontin	Many cancers, including mesothelioma
M-band (Ig or light chain)	Myeloma, chronic lymphocytic leukaemia, small lymphocytic lymphoma, lymphoplasmacytic lymphoma, amyloid
Calcitonin	Medullary carcinoma of thyroid
Thyroglobulin	Papillary and follicular thyroid cancer

of cases of myeloma will produce a monoclonal paraprotein of intact immunoglobulin molecule or light chains. This acts as a valuable tumour marker in the diagnosis and assessment of response.

Cancer imaging

Radiological investigation by experts is required at various stages: at initial diagnosis and staging of the disease, during the monitoring of treatment efficacy, at the detection of recurrence, and for the diagnosis and treatment of complications.

The choice of investigations needs to be guided by the patient's symptoms and signs, site and histology of the cancer, the curative or palliative potential of treatment, and the utility of the information in guiding treatment. Specific investigations are described under each tumour type.

Contrast agents are used for increased structural discrimination in cross-sectional imaging and can be further enhanced with functional specificity for metabolically active tissue with 19 fluorodeoxy-glucose uptake positron emission tomography-computed tomography (PET-CT) scan, as used extensively in head and neck cancer, lung cancer and lymphoma. ***Radionuclide imaging*** of sentinel lymph nodes is used to guide lymphatic surgery in breast cancer and melanoma. Tumour-targeted contrast agents can improve detection rates; examples include the radiolabelled monoclonal antibody (MAb) rituximab for lymphoma, or radiolabelled small molecules such as octreotide for neuroendocrine tumours. Research into the use of reporter agents that become visible only on activation within the tumour environment holds the promise of greater sensitivity and specificity in the future.

Biopsy and histological examination

The diagnosis of cancer may be suspected by both patient and doctor but advice about treatment can usually be given only on the basis of a tissue diagnosis. This may be obtained by endoscopic, radiologically guided or surgical biopsy, or by cytology (e.g. lung cancer may be diagnosed by sputum cytology). Malignant lesions can be distinguished morphologically from benign ones by the pleiomorphic nature of the cells, increased numbers of mitoses, nuclear abnormalities of size, chromatin pattern and nucleolar organization, and evidence of invasion into surrounding tissues, lymphatics or vessels. The degree of differentiation (or, conversely, of anaplasia) of the tumour has prognostic significance: generally speaking, more differentiated tumours have a better prognosis than poorly differentiated ones. In some tumours, the surgical procedure will vary depending on the presence of malignancy, and an intra-operative provisional histological opinion can be rapidly obtained with a tissue sample processed using 'frozen section' techniques, rather than having the sample paraffin embedded, which takes more than a day.

Immunocytochemistry, using monoclonal antibodies against tumour antigens, is very helpful in differentiating between lymphoid and epithelial tumours, and between some subsets of these (see ***Box 17.62***). However, there is much overlap in the expression of many of these ***tissue tumour markers*** and some adenocarcinomas and squamous carcinomas do not bear any distinctive immunohistochemical markers that are diagnostic of their primary site of origin.

Molecular markers of genetic abnormalities have long been available in the haematological cancers and are increasingly available in solid cancers. For example, ***fluorescence in situ hybridization*** (FISH; see p. 113) can be used to look for characteristic chromosomal translocations, as in lymphoma and leukaemia, as well as deletions or amplifications, as in breast cancer (see pp. 118–119). The development of the new targeted MAbs and tyrosine kinase inhibitors (TKis) has been guided by increasing use of mutation analysis of common oncogenes, such as RAS and RAF in colon cancer and melanoma. ***Tissue microarrays*** can identify patterns of multiple genomic alterations and single nucleotide polymorphisms (SNPs), as in breast cancer and lymphoma (see p. 107), and ***RNA assays*** with reverse transcriptase polymerase chain reaction (RT-PCR) can be used to identify tissue of origin with prognostic and predictive relevance.

Genomics and proteomics are being investigated in order to target new (and expensive) therapies, such as imatinib in chronic myeloid leukaemia (CML) and gastrointestinal stromal tumours (GIST); trastuzumab and lapatinib in breast cancer; erlotinib and crizotinib in lung cancer; and cetuximab and bevacizumab in colon cancer.

Further reading

Fearon KCH. Cancer cachexia and fat–muscle physiology. *N Engl J Med* 2011; 365:565–567.
Hugosson J, Carlsson S, Aus G et al. Mortality results from the Göteborg randomised population-based prostate-cancer screening trial. *Lancet Oncol* 2010; 11:725–732.
Ilic D, Neuberger MM, Djulbegovic M et al. *Screening for Prostate Cancer* (Cochrane Review). Chichester: Cochrane Library; 2013; issue 1.
Paimela H, Malila N, Palva T et al. Early detection of colorectal cancer with faecal occult blood test screening. *Br J Surg* 2010; 97:1567–1571.
Schröder FH, Hugosson J, Roobol MJ et al. Prostate cancer mortality at 11 years of follow-up. *N Engl J Med* 2012; 366:981–990.

CANCER TREATMENT

Aims of treatment

Optimal cancer treatment is delivered by a multidisciplinary team that coordinates the delivery of the appropriate anticancer treatment (surgery, chemotherapy, radiotherapy and biological/

endocrine therapy), supportive and symptomatic care, and psychosocial support.

Establishment of agreed patient pathways has enabled more effective and timely delivery of care and post-treatment rehabilitation. Central to this endeavour is the involvement of the patient, through education as to the nature of their disease and the treatment options available.

A curative approach

For most solid tumours, local control is necessary, but not sufficient, for cure because of the presence of systemic (microscopic) disease, while haematological cancers are usually disseminated from the outset. Improvement in the rate of cure of most cancers is thus dependent on earlier detection to increase the success of local treatment and effective systemic treatment. The likelihood of cure of the systemic disease rests on the type of cancer and its expression of appropriate treatment targets, its drug sensitivity and tumour bulk (microscopic or clinically detectable). A few rare cancers are so chemosensitive that even bulky metastases can be cured: for example, leukaemia, lymphoma, gonadal germ cell tumours and choriocarcinoma. For most common solid tumours, such as lung, breast and colorectal cancer, there is no current cure of bulky (clinically detectable) metastases, but micrometastatic disease treated by adjuvant systemic therapy (see below) after surgery can be cured in 10–20% of patients.

Adjuvant therapy for solid tumours

Micrometastatic spread by lymphatic or haematological dissemination often occurs early in the development of the primary tumour and can be demonstrated by molecular biological methods capable of detecting the small numbers (1 in 10^6) of circulating cells. Studies correlating prognosis with histological features of the primary cancer, such as differentiation, invasion of blood vessels or regional lymph nodes, and molecular markers like Her2 in breast cancer, enable risk stratification and increasing individualization of therapy. ***Adjuvant therapy*** is defined as treatment given, in the absence of macroscopic evidence of metastases, to patients at risk of recurrence from micrometastases, following treatment given for the primary lesion. ***'Neoadjuvant' therapy***, alternatively, is given before primary surgery, both to shrink the tumour in order to improve the local excision, and to treat any micrometastases as soon as possible.

The success of adjuvant treatment across many tumour types relies on careful selection of patients according to defined risk criteria, and reduction of treatment toxicity to reach a balanced risk/benefit ratio. However, the majority who receive such treatment do not benefit, either because they were already cured or because the cancer is resistant to the treatment. Better tests, such as gene arrays and circulating tumour cells, are being developed to identify those with micrometastases, who really benefit from treatment.

A palliative approach

When cure is no longer possible, palliation – that is, relief of tumour symptoms, preservation of quality of life and prolongation of life – is possible in many cancers in proportion to their drug and radiation sensitivity. There is, on average, a 2–18 month prolongation in median life expectancy with treatments for solid tumours (see specific tumour types for details) and up to 5–8 years for some leukaemias and lymphomas, those individuals with the most responsive tumours experiencing the greatest benefit. In addition, through early assessment during treatment, it is possible to stop if no evidence of benefit is demonstrable early on, so as to minimize exposure to toxic and unsuccessful treatment.

Assessment before treatment

Staging

Before a decision about treatment can be made, not only the type of tumour, but also its extent and distribution, need to be established. Various 'staging investigations' are therefore performed before a treatment decision is made. To be useful clinically, the staging system must sub-divide the patients into groups with different prognoses, which can guide treatment selection.

The staging systems vary according to the type of tumour and may be site-specific (see Hodgkin's lymphoma, p. 617). Alternatively, the TNM (tumour, node, metastases) classification is used (see ***Box 17.53***), and can be adapted for application to most common cancers.

Performance status

In addition to anatomical staging, the person's age and general state of health need to be taken into account when planning treatment. The latter has been called 'performance status' and is of great prognostic significance for all tumour types ***(Box 17.10)***. Performance status reflects the effects of the cancer on the patient's functional capacity. An alternative performance rating scale is provided by Karnofsky. With a performance status of 2, response to, and survival following, treatment are greatly reduced for most tumour types.

Assessment of the benefits of treatment

A measurable response to treatment can serve as a useful early surrogate marker when assessing whether to continue a given treatment for an individual patient. Trials to assess response to treatment in advanced disease have identified active agents for use in the more curative setting of adjuvant treatment of early-stage disease

Response to treatment can be subjective or objective.

A subjective response is one perceived by the patient in terms of, for example, relief of pain and dyspnoea, or improvement in appetite, weight gain or energy. Such a subjective response is a major aim of most palliative treatments. Quantitative measurements of these subjective symptoms (*p*atient *r*eported *o*utcome *m*easures, PROMs) form a part of the assessment of response to chemotherapy, especially in those situations where cure is not possible and where the aim of treatment is to provide prolongation of

Box 17.10 Eastern Cooperative Oncology Group (ECOG) performance status scale

Status	Description
0	Asymptomatic, fully active and able to carry out all pre-disease performance without restrictions
1	Symptomatic, fully ambulatory but restricted in physically strenuous activity and able to carry out performance of a light or sedentary nature, e.g. light housework, office work
2	Symptomatic, ambulatory and capable of all self-care but unable to carry out any work activities. Up and about >50% of waking hours; in bed <50% of day
3	Symptomatic, capable of only limited self-care, confined to bed or chair >50% of waking hours, but not bedridden
4	Completely disabled. Cannot carry out any self-care. Totally bedridden

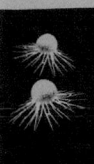

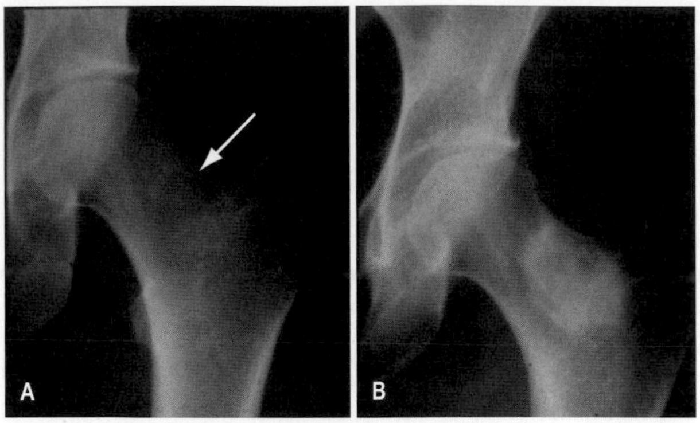

Figure 17.9 Chemotherapy: radiological response. X-rays showing response to chemotherapy and radiotherapy. **A** Bone metastasis responding to chemotherapy with sclerotic new bone formation. Tumour (arrowed). **B.** Following radiotherapy.

Box 17.11 RECIST criteria for assessing response to treatment in solid tumours

Criteria	Description
Complete response	Disappearance of all target lesions
Partial response	≥30% decrease in the baseline sum of the longest diameters of all target lesions
Progression	≥20% increase in the sum of the longest diameters of all target lesions compared with the smallest recorded sum since treatment started, or the appearance of any new lesions
Stable disease	All values between partial response and progressive disease
Target lesions	Measurable lesions up to 5 per organ and 10 in total, selected on size and replicable measurement
Non-target lesions	Non-measurable lesions recorded as present or absent at baseline and on follow-up
Measurable	Lesions with the longest diameter in one dimension ≥2.0 cm or ≥1.0 cm if assessed by spiral CT scan
Non-measurable	e.g. Bone, meningeal, ascites, pleural effusion, inflammatory breast cancer, lymphangitis cutis and pulmonis, cystic lesions

RECIST, Response Evaluation Criteria in Solid Tumours.

good-quality life. In these circumstances, measures of quality of life enable an estimate of the balance of benefit and side-effects to be made.

An objective response to treatment is assessed clinically and radiologically ***(Fig. 17.9)***. The term 'remission' is often used synonymously with 'response', which, if complete, means an absence of detectable disease without necessarily implying a cure of the cancer. The terms used to evaluate the responses of tumours are given in ***Box 17.11***. For a complete response, all previous clinical abnormalities should have resolved and this needs to be confirmed by clinical examination or sampling of the primary disease site, or by detection of serum tumour markers. Radiologically, a partial response, defined since 1999 by the *R*esponse *E*valuation *C*riteria *i*n *S*olid *T*umours (RECIST) convention, is a ≥30% reduction in the sum of all measurable lesion diameters.

The increasing use of PET-CT has meant that metabolic responses (reduction in tracer avidity with or without a reduction in the size of the mass) may predict long-term outcome more accurately; this is particularly the case in lymphoma, where a classification of metabolic response exists, as well as in gastrointestinal stromal tumour (GIST).

The final assessment of treatment outcome is the impact of the therapy on remission duration and survival: that is, the cure rate. Such survival figures are increasingly incorporating quality-of-life assessments and a health economic assessment to calculate the number of quality-adjusted life years (QALYs) gained for the cost of the treatment and judgements are made about health system affordability.

Further reading

Biggi A, Gallamini A, Chauvie S et al. International validation study for interim PET in ABVD-treated, advanced-stage Hodgkin lymphoma: interpretation criteria and concordance rate among reviewers. *J Nucl Med* 2013; 54:683–690.

PRINCIPLES OF CHEMOTHERAPY

Cytotoxic chemotherapy employs systemically administered drugs that directly damage cellular DNA (and RNA). It kills cells by promoting apoptosis and, sometimes, frank necrosis. Different cytotoxic drugs work at different stages in the cell cycle (***Fig. 17.10***; see also ***Fig. 7.16***).

There is a narrow therapeutic window between effective treatment of the cancer and normal tissue toxicity, because cytotoxic drugs are not cancer-specific (unlike some of the targeted biological agents) and the increased proliferation in cancers is not much greater than in normal tissues. The dose and schedule of the chemotherapy are limited by normal tissue tolerance, especially in those more proliferative tissues of the bone marrow and gastrointestinal tract mucosa. All tissues can be affected, however, depending on the pharmacokinetics of the drug and its affinity for particular tissues (e.g. heavy metal compounds for kidneys and nerves).

The therapeutic effect on the cancer is achieved by a variety of mechanisms that seek to exploit differences between normal and transformed cells. While most of the drugs have been derived in the past by empirical testing of many different compounds, such as alkylating agents, the new molecular biology is leading to targeting of particular genetic defects in the cancer (see p. 601).

Toxicity to normal tissue can be limited in some instances by supplying growth factors such as granulocyte colony-stimulating factor (G-CSF) or by infusing stem cell preparations to diminish bone marrow toxicity. The use of more specific targeted biological agents with relatively weak pro-apoptotic effects, in combination with the general cytotoxics, has also improved the therapeutic ratio (e.g. trastuzumab and breast cancer; see p. 634). Certain cytotoxic therapies may also be administered into the pleural space, peritoneum or cerebrospinal fluid (CSF), or into the arterial supply of a tumour.

Most tumours rapidly develop resistance to single agents given on their own through changes in membrane transport and DNA repair pathways. For this reason, the principle of intermittent combination chemotherapy was developed. Several drugs are combined, chosen on the basis of differing mechanisms of action and non-overlapping toxicities. These drugs are given over a period of a few days, followed by a rest of a few weeks, during which time the normal tissues have the opportunity for regrowth. If the normal tissues are more proficient at DNA repair than the cancer cells, it may be possible to deplete the tumour while allowing the restoration of normal tissues between chemotherapy cycles ***(Fig. 17.11)***.

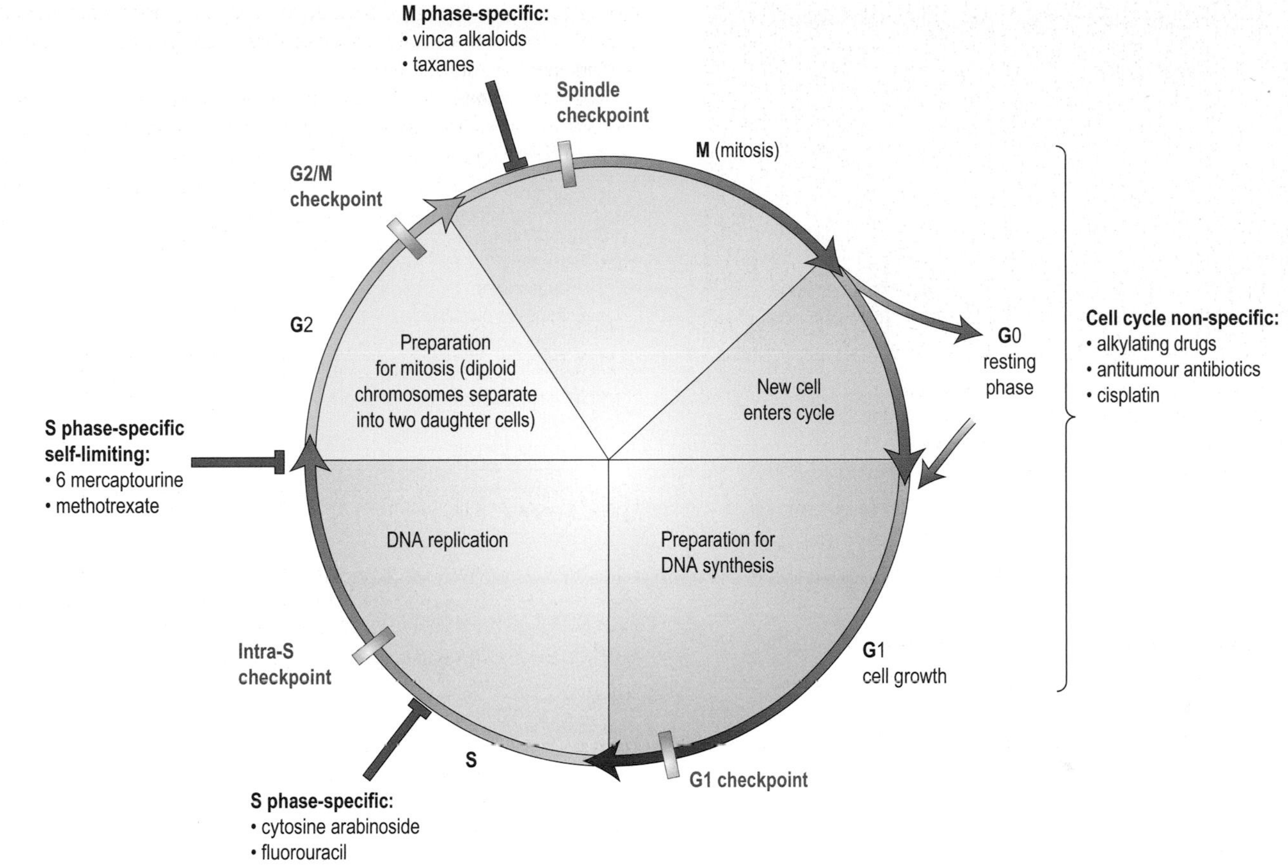

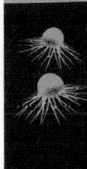

Figure 17.10 Cell cycle and chemotherapy drugs. (See also ***Fig. 7.16***.)

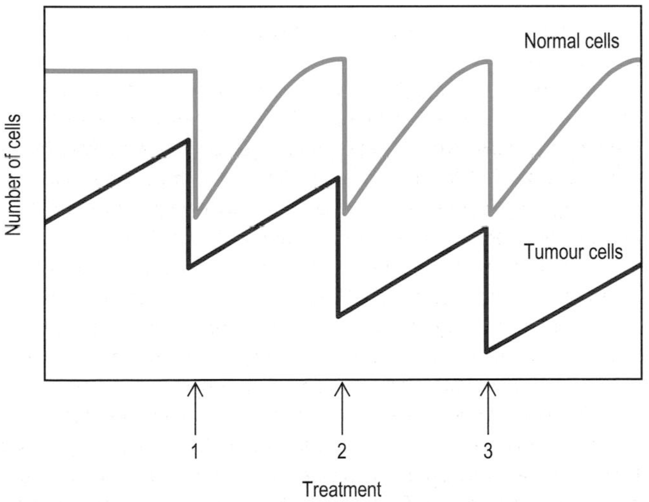

Figure 17.11 Effects of multiple courses of cytotoxic chemotherapy. The decrease in the number of cells with each course is shown.

In many experimental tumours, it has been shown that there is a log–linear relationship between drug dose and number of cancer cells killed, and that the maximum effective dose is very close to the maximum tolerated dose at which dose-limiting toxicity is reached. With a chemosensitive tumour, relatively small increases in dose may have a large effect on tumour cell kill. It is therefore apparent that, where cure is a realistic option, the dose administered is critical and may need to be maintained despite toxicity. In situations where cure is not a realistic possibility and palliation is the aim, a sufficient dose to exceed the therapeutic threshold, but not cause undue toxicity, is required, as the short-term quality of life becomes a major consideration.

Classification of cytotoxic drugs

See ***Box 17.12***.

DNA-damaging drugs

Alkylating agents

These act by covalently binding alkyl groups. Their major effect is to cross-link DNA strands, interfering with DNA synthesis and causing strand breaks.

Platinum compounds

Cisplatin, carboplatin and oxaliplatin cause interstrand cross-links of DNA and are often regarded as non-classical alkylating agents. They have transformed the treatment of testicular cancer (cisplatin) and have a major role against many other tumours.

Antimetabolites

Antimetabolites are usually structural analogues of naturally occurring metabolites that interfere with normal synthesis of nucleic acids by falsely substituting purines and pyrimidines in metabolic pathways.

Folic acid antagonists

This class includes methotrexate, which is structurally very similar to folic acid and binds preferentially to dihydrofolate reductase, the

Box 17.12 Chemotherapy: some cytotoxic drugs

DNA-damaging agents
- Free radicals:
  - Alkylators, e.g. cyclophosphamide, melphalan, chlorambucil, ifosfamide
  - Nitrosoureas, e.g. carmustine (BCNU), bendamustine, lomustine (CCNU), busulfan
  - Tetrazines, e.g. dacarbazine, temozolomide
- DNA cross-linking – platinum, e.g. cisplatin, carboplatin, oxaliplatin

Antimetabolites
- Pyrimidine synthesis, e.g. 5-fluorouracil, capecitabine, cytarabine, fludarabine, gemcitabine, cladribine, clofarabine, nelarabine, azacitidine
- Purine synthesis, e.g. mercaptopurine, tioguanine
- Antifolates, e.g. methotrexate, pemetrexed

DNA repair inhibitors
- Topoisomerase-I inhibitors, e.g. irinotecan
- Topoisomerase-II inhibitors, e.g. etoposide
- Anthracyclines, e.g. daunorubicin, doxorubicin, epirubicin, bleomycin, mitomycin

Antitubulin agents
- Tubulin-binding – alkaloids, e.g. vincristine, vinorelbine
- Taxanes, e.g. paclitaxel, docetaxel
- Eribulin, epothilones

enzyme responsible for the conversion of folic acid to folinic acid. It is used widely in the treatment of solid tumours and haematological malignancies. Folinic acid is often given to 'rescue' normal tissues from the effects of high doses of methotrexate. A related drug, pemetrexed, targets the enzyme thymidylate synthase, as well as glycinamide ribonucleotide formyltransferase (GARFT).

Pyrimidine antagonists

5-Fluorouracil (5-FU) consists of a uracil molecule with a substituted fluorine atom. It acts by blocking thymidylate synthase, which is essential for pyrimidine synthesis. Oral capecitabine is metabolized to 5-FU, as is tegafur with uracil.

Arabinosides

Arabinosides inhibit DNA synthesis by inhibiting DNA polymerase. Cytarabine is used almost exclusively in the treatment of acute myeloid leukaemia, where it remains the backbone of therapy.

Purine antagonists

This class includes 6-mercaptopurine and 6-tioguanine, which are both used almost exclusively in the treatment of acute leukaemia.

DNA repair inhibitors

Epipodophyllotoxins

These are semisynthetic derivatives of podophyllotoxin, which inhibit the topoisomerase enzymes that allow unwinding and uncoiling of supercoiled DNA, and maintain DNA strand breaks.

Cytotoxic antibiotics

The anthracyclines act by intercalating adjoining nucleotide pairs on the same strand of DNA and by inhibiting topoisomerase-II DNA repair. They have a wide spectrum of activity in haematological and solid tumours.

Antitubulin agents

Vinca alkaloids

Drugs such as vincristine, vinblastine and vinorelbine act by binding to tubulin and inhibiting microtubule formation during mitosis (see p. 92). They are associated with neurotoxicity due to their antimicrotubule effect and must never be given intrathecally, as this is lethal.

Box 17.13 Side-effects of chemotherapy

Common
- Nausea and vomiting
- Hair loss
- Myelosuppression
- Mucositis
- Fatigue

Drug-specific
- Cardiotoxicity, e.g. anthracyclines
- Progressive pulmonary fibrosis, e.g. bleomycin, busulfan
- Neurotoxicity, e.g. cisplatinum, vinca alkaloids, taxanes
- Nephrotoxicity, e.g. cisplatinum, TKis
- Skin, e.g. anti-EGFR TKis
- Skin plantar–palmar dermatitis, e.g. 5-fluorouracil liposomal doxorubicin
- Sterility, e.g. alkylating agents, anthracyclines, docetaxel
- Secondary malignancy, e.g. alkylating agents, epipodophyllotoxins
- CNS, e.g. TKis

CNS, central nervous system; EGFT, epidermal growth factor receptor; TKi, tyrosine kinase inhibitor.

Box 17.14 Some common chemotherapy regimens

Cancer	Abbreviation[a]	Regimen
Hodgkin's lymphoma	ABVD	Adriamycin (doxorubicin), bleomycin, vinblastine, dacarbazine
Non-Hodgkin's lymphoma	CHOP	Cyclophosphamide, hydroxy-doxorubicin, vincristine, prednisolone
Breast	AC	Adriamycin, cyclophosphamide
Lung	PE	Cisplatin, etoposide
Stomach	ECF	Epirubicin, cisplatin, 5-fluorouracil
Colorectal	FolFOX	Oxaliplatin, 5-fluorouracil, folinic acid

[a]Some abbreviations are related to trade names.

Taxanes

Paclitaxel and docetaxel bind to tubulin dimers and prevent their assembly into microtubules.

Side-effects of chemotherapy

Chemotherapy carries many potentially serious side-effects and should be used only by trained practitioners; however, an appreciation of its common potential side-effects is necessary for any general physician who is called to see a cancer patient on chemotherapy. The five most common side-effects are vomiting, hair loss, tiredness, myelosuppression and mucositis ***(Box 17.13)***. Side-effects are much more directly dose-related than anticancer effects and it has been the practice to give drugs at doses close to their maximum tolerated dose, although this is not always necessary to achieve their maximum anticancer effect. Common combination chemotherapeutic regimens are shown in ***Box 17.14***.

Common side-effects

Extravasation of intravenous drugs

Cytotoxic drugs should only be given by trained personnel. They cause severe local tissue necrosis if leakage occurs outside the vein. Stop the infusion immediately and institute local measures: for example, aspirate as much of the drug as possible from the cannula, infiltrate the area with 0.9% saline and apply warm compresses. Antihistamines and corticosteroids may give symptomatic relief.

Nausea and vomiting

The severity of these common side-effects varies with the cytotoxic and they can be eliminated in 75% of patients by using modern antiemetics. Nausea and vomiting are particular problems with platinum analogues. A stepped policy with antiemetics, such as metoclopramide and domperidone, followed by 5-HT_3 (serotonin) antagonists (e.g. ondansetron, granisetron) combined with dexamethasone, should be used to match the emetogenic potential of the chemotherapy. Aprepitant, a neurokinin receptor antagonist, is helpful in preventing acute and delayed nausea and vomiting. It is used with dexamethasone and a 5-HT_3 antagonist. Drugs such as cyclizine, olanzapine and levomepromazine, and benzodiazepines can be used to control persistent nausea.

Effects on hair, skin and nails

Many, but not all, cytotoxic drugs are capable of causing hair loss. Scalp cooling can sometimes be used to reduce hair loss but, in general, this side-effect can only be avoided by selection of drugs, where this is possible. Hair regrows on completion of chemotherapy. Nails will demonstrate banding, reflecting periods of cessation of growth during each chemotherapy cycle ***(Fig. 17.12)***, and skin toxicity may be particularly pronounced with 5-FU, capecitabine and docetaxel ***(Fig. 17.13)***.

Fatigue

This is often significant and may continue beyond completion of therapy. Other problems, such as anaemia or depression, may exacerbate fatigue. Attention should be paid to nutrition, hydration, sleep hygiene, gentle exercise, task prioritization, pacing, realistic target setting and scheduling rest within the day.

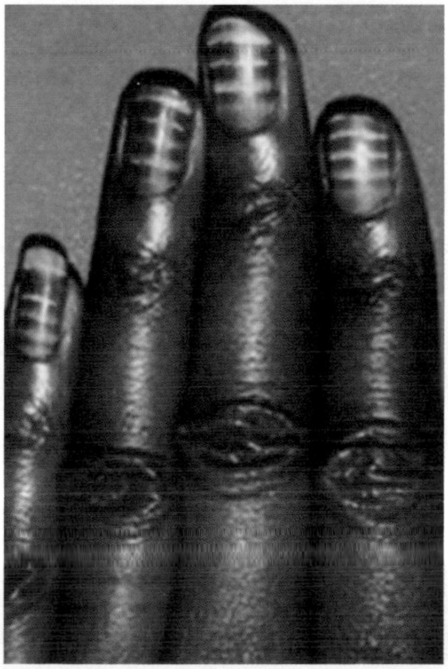

Figure 17.12 Nail growth cessation with each drug cycle (Beau's lines).

Bone marrow suppression and immunosuppression

Suppression of the production of red blood cells, white blood cells and platelets occurs with most cytotoxic drugs and is a dose-related phenomenon ***(Fig. 17.14)***. Severely myelosuppressive chemotherapy may be required if treatment is to be given with curative intent, despite the potential for rare but fatal infection or bleeding. Anaemia and thrombocytopenia are managed by red cell or platelet transfusions. (Neutropenic infection is discussed on pp. 604–605.) The risk of infective problems can be ameliorated by the use of prophylactic antimicrobials, such as ciprofloxacin, or the use of G-CSF as primary prophylaxis in those chemotherapy

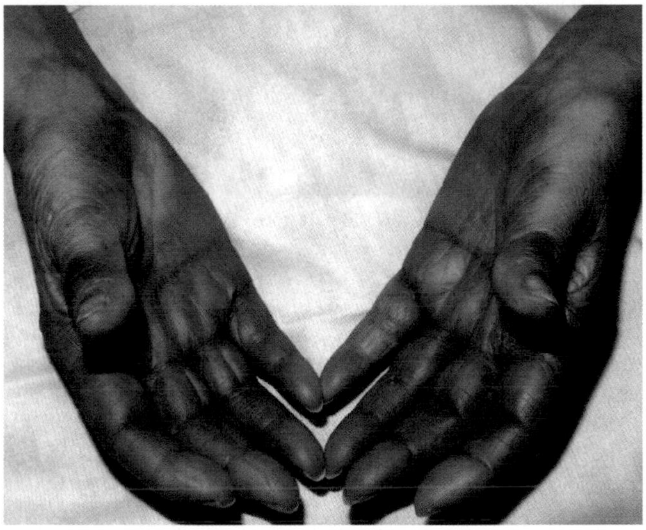

Figure 17.13 Hands showing palmar–plantar skin toxicity.

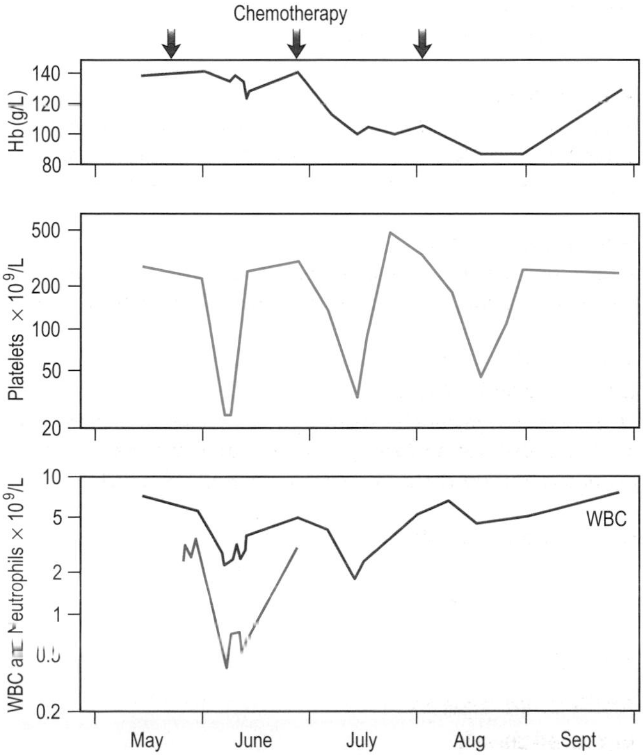

Figure 17.14 Cyclical myelosuppression from chemotherapy (arrowed). Hb, haemoglobin; WBC, white blood cells.

regimens that carry a significant risk of febrile neutropenia or in those patients on less intensive therapies who are at higher risk due to age or co-morbidity.

Mucositis

This common side-effect of chemotherapy reflects the sensitivity of the mucosa to antimitotic agents. Mucositis causes severe pain in the oropharyngeal region and problems with swallowing and nutrition. It can be generalized throughout the intestinal tract and can cause life-threatening diarrhoea. Treatment is with antiseptic and anti-candidal mouthwash; if mucositis is severe, fluid and antibiotic support is required, as the mucosa is a portal for entry of enteric organisms. Palifermin, a recombinant keratinocyte-derived growth factor, may ameliorate severe chemotherapy- and radiotherapy-induced mucositis.

Other toxicities

Cardiotoxicity

This is a rare side-effect of chemotherapy, and is usually associated with anthracyclines such as doxorubicin; effects can present as an acute arrhythmia during administration or cardiac failure due to cardiomyopathy after chronic exposure ***(Fig. 17.15)***. This effect is dose-related and can largely be prevented by restricting the cumulative total dose of anthracyclines within the safe range (equivalent to 450 mg/m^2 body surface area cumulative doxorubicin dose). The risk of anthracycline cardiomyopathy is also dependent on other treatments, such as trastuzumab or radiotherapy, as well as other cardiac risk factors, such as hypertension, smoking and hypercholesterolaemia. Cardiotoxicity can also be reduced by using the analogue, epirubicin, or by reducing peak drug concentrations through delayed-release preparations, such as liposomal doxorubicin. 5-Fluorouracil and its prodrug, capecitabine, can cause cardiac ischaemia.

Neurotoxicity

This occurs predominantly with the vinca alkaloids, taxanes and platinum analogues (but not carboplatin). It is dose-related and cumulative. Chemotherapy is usually stopped before the development of a significant polyneuropathy, which, once established, is only partially reversible. Vinca alkaloids, such as vincristine, must never be given intrathecally, as the neurological damage is progressive and fatal.

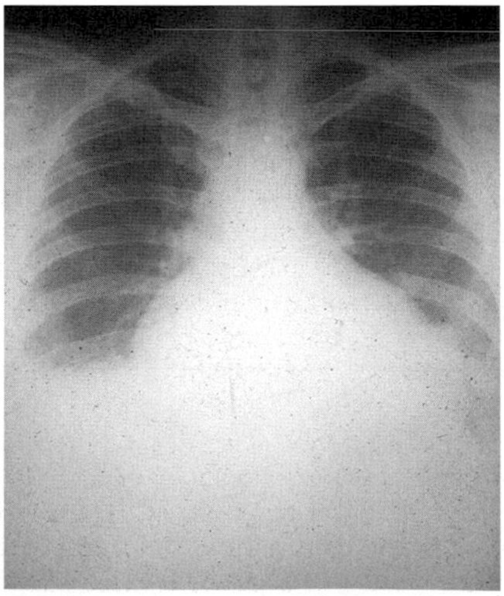

Figure 17.15 Anthracycline dilated cardiomyopathy with congestive heart failure.

Nephrotoxicity

Cisplatin (but not oxaliplatin or carboplatin), methotrexate and ifosfamide can potentially cause renal damage. This can usually be prevented by maintaining an adequate diuresis during treatment to reduce drug concentration in the renal tubules, and by monitoring of renal function.

Sterility and premature menopause

Some anticancer drugs, particularly alkylating agents, but also anthracyclines and docetaxel, may cause gonadal damage, resulting in sterility and, in women, the loss of ovarian oestrogen production, which may be irreversible.

In males, storage of sperm prior to chemotherapy should be offered to the patient when chemotherapy is given with curative intent.

In females, collection of oocytes to be fertilized *in vitro* and cryopreserved as embryos for subsequent implantation is most successful; however, it is also possible to collect and freeze by vitrification of unstimulated oocytes. Cryopreservation of ovarian tissue and retrieval of viable oocytes for subsequent fertilization are still experimental. The recovery of gonadal function is dependent on the status before treatment; in women, this is mostly related to age since menarche, with those under 40 years having significantly more ovarian reserve.

Secondary malignancies

Anticancer drugs have mutagenic potential and the development of secondary malignancies, predominantly acute leukaemia, is an uncommon but particularly unwelcome long-term side-effect in patients otherwise cured of their primary malignancies. The alkylating agents, anthracyclines and epipodophyllotoxins are particularly implicated in this complication.

PRINCIPLES OF HAEMATOPOIETIC STEM CELL TRANSPLANTATION

See pages 561–562.

PRINCIPLES OF ENDOCRINE THERAPY

Oestrogens are capable of stimulating the growth of breast and endometrial cancers, and androgens can stimulate the growth of prostate cancer. Removal of these growth factors by manipulation of the hormonal environment may result in apoptosis and regression of the cancer. Endocrine therapy can be curative in a proportion of patients treated for micrometastatic disease in the adjuvant setting for breast and prostate cancer, and provides a minimally toxic, non-curative (palliative) treatment in advanced/metastatic disease. The presence of detectable cellular receptors for the hormone is strongly predictive of response. However, this is also modified by the many molecular interactions between the activation pathways of, for example, epidermal growth factor receptor (EGFR), the androgen receptor (AR) and oestrogen receptor (ER) (see pp. 634 and 642).

PRINCIPLES OF BIOLOGICAL AND TARGETED THERAPY

Immunotherapy

The most dramatic evidence for the effectiveness of immunotherapy is seen in the response of the acute leukaemias to allogeneic haemopoietic stem cell transplantation (HSCT). Certain antigens that are specific to cancer cells, such as sequences of tumour immunoglobulin from B-cell lymphomas, or melanoma antigens, have been used as tumour vaccines, together with manipulation of the immune system to overcome tolerance. Engineered chimeric antigen receptors (CARs) that direct T cells to specific antigenic targets are emerging as a powerful potential tool in the treatment of a wide range of cancers.

Interferons

Interferons are naturally occurring cytokines that mediate the cellular immune response.

Interferon-alpha (IFN-α) has been used to treat advanced melanoma and renal cell carcinoma.

Treatment with IFN has side-effects (see p. 458): most commonly, influenza-like symptoms, which tend to diminish with time; and fatigue, which generally does not, and can be treatment-limiting. IFN used to be given as a daily subcutaneous injection, but conjugation with polyethylene glycol (PEG interferon) has led to a reduction in frequency of injection and severity of side-effects.

Interleukins

Interleukin 2 (IL-2), a recombinant protein, is used to activate T-cell responses, often in conjunction with IFN-stimulated B-cell activation. Anti-tumour activity has been observed in renal cell carcinoma and melanoma, with responses in 10–20% of patients, occasionally for prolonged periods. Toxicity is common; acutely, this includes the capillary leak syndrome with hypotension and pulmonary oedema, while autoimmune thyroiditis and vitiligo occur later.

Immune checkpoint inhibitors

These new agents directly interfere with the relationship between T cells and antigen-presenting cells or tumour cells to overcome the common problems of immune tolerance and anergy. Ipilimumab is a monoclonal antibody that blocks the CD152 (CTLA-4) receptor responsible for downregulating T-cell responses, and is active in the treatment of melanoma. The inhibitors of the programmed death (PD-1) receptor or its ligands, PD-L1 and L2, on activated T cells, further reactivate tumour-specific cytotoxic T cells, so that ipilimumab plus nivolumab doubled the response rate from 20% to 40% in metastatic melanoma. Many clinical trials are now examining these agents in the context of a variety of other cancers.

Immunomodulatory drugs: thalidomide, lenalidomide, pomalidomide

This family of immunomodulatory drugs (IMIDs) is increasingly being used in a range of malignancies, such as myeloma, chronic lymphocytic leukaemia (CLL) and myelodysplastic syndrome (MDS) as well some solid tumours. They have anti-angiogenic functions, as well as effects on cytokine production, tumour/stromal interactions and T-cell co-stimulatory functions. They are all considered teratogenic and should be avoided in women of reproductive potential, unless extra precaution is taken against conception. There is increasing evidence that IMIDs work through binding of the E3 ligase protein, cereblon, which acts to degrade two specific B-cell transcription factors, IKZF1 and IKZF3.

Box 17.15 Monoclonal antibodies (MAbs) in cancer

Antigen	Mutation/ amplification	Tumour type	MAb
CD20	+	NHL	**Rituximab**
EGFR	cERBB2/Her2 amplification	Breast, gastric	**Trastuzumab**
	cERBB2/Her2 amplification	Breast	**Pertuzumab**
	RAS/BRAF wt	Colorectal, oropharyngeal	**Cetuximab**
	RAS/BRAF wt	Colorectal	**Panitumumab**
	+	Melanoma	**Ipilumumab**
VEGFR	+	Colorectal, ovarian	**Bevacizumab**
PD-1	+	Melanoma, Hodgkin's lymphoma, NSCLC	**Nivolumab**
RANKL	+	Bone metastases	**Denosumab**

CD, cluster of differentiation; EGFR, epidermal growth factor receptor; NHL, non-Hodgkin's lymphoma; NSCLC, non-small cell lung cancer; PD-1, programmed cell death protein 1; RANKL, receptor activator of nuclear factor kappa-B ligand; VEGFR, vascular endothelial growth factor receptor.

Targeted therapies

The fast-developing field of targeted therapies includes monoclonal antibodies, receptor kinase inhibitors, and small molecule receptor blockers. Expression of the targeted molecule is not sufficient of itself to indicate that use of the corresponding drug will be therapeutic because it is also necessary for the drug to be able to interrupt a growth-critical pathway in that cancer.

Monoclonal antibodies

Monoclonal antibodies (MAbs; ***Box 17.15***) directed against tumour cell surface antigens are 'humanized' by being genetically engineered to have a range of functions:

- As direct treatment for B-cell lymphoid malignancy (e.g. rituximab anti-CD20 surface antigen). Tumour cell lysis occurs by both complement- and antibody-dependent cellular cytotoxicity
- As a carrier molecule to target toxins or radioisotopes to the tumour cells, e.g. anti-CD20 conjugated to radioactive yttrium for non-Hodgkin's lymphoma (NHL), and trastuzumab or trastuzumab emtansine for breast cancer.
- As anti-growth factor agents added to chemotherapy by inhibiting dimerization of the extracellular receptor molecules (see ***Box 17.14***). Side-effects are those of hypersensitivity to the foreign protein and specific cross-reactivities, e.g. trastuzumab for the myocardium, bevacizumab for the mucosa and renal tubule, and cetuximab for the skin follicles.

Intracellular signal inhibitors

Many cancer cells are transformed by the activity of the protein products of oncogenes that signal growth by phosphorylation of tyrosine residues on the intracellular portion of growth factor receptors. Small molecule inhibitors ***(Box 17.16)*** have many pharmacokinetic advantages over the MAb inhibitors. The first example was the TKi, imatinib, which specifically inhibits the BCR-ABL fusion

Box 17.16 Intracellular signal inhibitor therapies in cancer

Gene	Genetic alteration	Tumour type	Therapeutic agent
Receptor tyrosine kinase			
EGFR	Mutation, amplification	Lung	**Gefitinib, erlotinib, afatinib**
ERBB2	Amplification	Breast	**Lapatinib**
PDGFRA	Mutation	GIST	**Sunitinib, imatinib, nilotinib**
PDGFRB	Translocation	Chronic myelomonocytic leukaemia	**Sunitinib, sorafenib, imatinib**
ALK	Mutation or amplification	Lung, neuroblastoma, anaplastic large-cell lymphoma	**Crizotinib**
c-Met	Amplification	Gefitinib-resistant NSCLC, gastric	**Crizotinib**
c-Kit	Mutation	GIST	**Sunitinib, imatinib**
FLT3	Internal tandem duplication	AML	**Lestaurtinib, midostaurin**
RET	Mutation, translocation	Thyroid medullary carcinoma	**Vandetanib**
JAK2	Mutation	Myelofibrosis	**Ruxolitinib**
Non-receptor tyrosine kinase			
ABL	Translocation (BCR-ABL)	CML	**Imatinib** **Nilotinib, dasatinib** **Bosutinib, ponatinib**
BTK	Mutation in primary B-cell deficiency	CLL, mantle cell lymphoma	**Ibrutinib**
Serine–threonine–lipid kinase			
BRAF	Mutation (V600E)	Melanoma	**Vemurafenib**
mTOR	Increased activation	Renal cell carcinoma, breast	**Temsirolimus, everolimus**
PI3Kδ		CLL, mantle cell lymphoma	**Idelalisib**
DNA damage or repair			
BRCA1 and BRCA2	Mutation (synthetic lethal effect)	Breast, ovarian	**Olaparib (PARP inhibitors)**

AML, acute myeloid leukaemia; BCR, breakpoint cluster region; CLL, chronic lymphocytic leukaemia; CML, chronic myeloid leukaemia; GIST, gastrointestinal stromal tumour; NSCLC, non-small cell lung cancer; PARP, poly(adenosine diphosphate-ribose) polymerase.

oncoprotein and c-Kit. This compound is an extremely effective treatment for CML and GIST, which are characterized by the presence of the c-Kit target. Lapatinib, which inhibits Her2, has increased survival in breast cancer. The less specific TKis, sunitinib and pazopanib, which inhibit signalling by EGFR and vascular endothelial growth factor receptor (VEGFR), have proved effective in metastatic renal cancer, while afatinib, erlotinib and gefitinib have shown activity in lung cancer. Vemurafenib is a kinase inhibitor and has a specificity for BRAF-V600, as used in malignant melanoma (pp. 1373–1374). Many other similar molecules are in pre-clinical or early clinical development, but heterogeneity within a single tumour occurs and genomic anomalies may not all be represented in a single biopsy specimen. Vandetanib, a combined VEGF and C-RET inhibitor, is useful in the treatment of medullary thyroid cancer.

Proteasome inhibitors

The proteasome degrades redundant or damaged proteins that have been labelled by a process called ubiquitination. Such proteins include cyclins and cyclin-dependent kinases, as well as factors in the nuclear factor kappa-B (NFκB) pathway. Inhibition of the proteasome leads to apoptosis in cancer cells and is synergistic with other treatments such as steroids and chemotherapy. Bortezomib is the first of such inhibitors to reach clinical practice and is used in myeloma, as well as some types of NHL. There are also recent additions to this class, including carfilzomib and ixazomib.

Gene therapy

Antisense oligonucleotides are short sequences of DNA bases that specifically inhibit complementary sequences of either DNA or RNA. As a result, they can be generated against genetic sequences, which are specific for tumour cells. Their clinical development has been hampered by poor uptake by tumour cells and rapid degradation by natural endonucleases. However, one antisense sequence directed against the *Bcl-2* oncogene has been shown to have an anti-tumour effect in patients with NHL. Viral vectors for the transfection of tumour cells *in vivo* are being tested as a way of delivering specific replacement gene therapy in head and neck cancers.

Further reading

Longo DL. Tumor heterogeneity and personalized medicine. *N Engl J Med* 2010; 366:956–957.

Lu G, Middleton RE, Sun H et al. The myeloma drug lenalidomide promotes the cereblon-dependent destruction of Ikaros proteins. *Science* 2014; 343:305–309.

Maus MV, Grupp SA, Porter DL et al. Antibody-modifed T cells: CARS take the front seat for haematologic malignancies. *Blood* 2014; 123:2625–2635.

Touchefeu Y, Montassier E, Nieman K et al. Systematic review: the role of the gut microbiota in chemotherapy- or radiation-induced gastrointestinal mucositis. *Aliment Pharmacol Ther* 2014; 40:409–421.

Wolchok JD, Kluger H, Callahan MK et al. Nivolumab plus ipilimumab in advanced melanoma. *N Engl J Med* 2013; 369:122–133.

PRINCIPLES OF RADIATION THERAPY

Theoretical background

Radiation delivers energy to tissues, causing ionization and excitation of atoms and molecules. The biological effect is exerted through the generation of single- and double-strand DNA breaks, inducing apoptosis of cells as they progress through the cell cycle, and through the generation of short-lived free radicals, particularly from oxygen, which damage proteins and membranes. The generation of free radicals depends on the degree of oxygenation/hypoxia in the target tissues. This can affect the biological effect by up to threefold and is the subject of continuing research for hypoxic cell sensitizers to overcome the reduced efficacy of radiation for hypoxic tumours. Hypoxia, however, may also drive a more malignant potential further, so reduced efficacy is only part of the solution to the hypoxia problem.

The radiation effect will also depend on the intensity of the radiation source, measured as the linear energy transfer or frequency of ionizing events per unit of path, which is subject to the inverse square law as the energy diminishes with the distance from the source. The depth of penetration of biological tissues by the photons depends on the energy of the beam. Low-energy photons from an 85-kV source are suitable for superficial treatments, while high-energy 35-MV sources produce a beam with deeper penetration, less dose at the initial skin boundary (skin-sparing), sharper edges and less absorption by bone. Superficial radiation may be also delivered by electron beams from a linear accelerator that has had the target electrode that generates the X-rays removed.

The radiation dose is measured in Gray (Gy), where 1 Gray = 1 joule (J) absorbed per kilogram of absorbing tissue. The biological effect is dependent on the dose rate, duration, volume irradiated and tissue sensitivity. Sensitivity to photon damage is greatest during the G2–M phase of the cell cycle and is also dependent on the DNA repair capacity of the cell.

Types of radiation therapy

- ***External beam (or teletherapy)*** from a linear accelerator source produces X-rays. The energy is transmitted as photons and is the most commonly used form of radiotherapy. ^{60}Cobalt generators can also provide γ-rays and high-energy photons, but are being gradually phased out. Most external beam treatments that are given with curative intent are delivered in 1.5–2-Gy fractions daily for 5 days per week.
- ***Fractionation*** is the delivery of the radiation dose in increments separated by at least 4–6 h to try to exploit any advantage in DNA repair between normal and malignant cells.
- ***Hyperfractionation*** is when more than one fraction per day is given. This approach has been shown to improve outcome in head and neck, and lung cancer. The treatment can also be accelerated: that is, the total dose is given in a shorter overall time. For example, a standard curative treatment taking 6.5 weeks can be accelerated so that the same dose is delivered in 5.5 weeks. Radiation dose is thus described by three factors:
  - total dose in Gy
  - number of fractions
  - time for completion.
- ***Brachytherapy*** is the use of radiation sources in close contact with the tissue to provide intense exposure over a short distance to a restricted volume. Such techniques have been used to treat localized breast, prostatic and cervical carcinoma.
- ***Systemic radionuclides***, e.g. ^{131}Iodine or radioisotope-labelled MAbs (e.g. anti-CD20 for lymphoma) and hormones (e.g. somatostatin for carcinoid tumours), can be administered by intravenous or intracavitary routes to provide radiation targeted to particular tissue uptake via surface antigens or receptors.

Box 17.17 Curative radiotherapy treatment

Primary modality
- Retina
- Central nervous system
- Skin
- Pharynx and larynx
- Cervix and vagina
- Prostate
- Lymphoma

Adjuvant to primary surgery
- Lung
- Breast
- Uterus
- Bladder
- Rectum
- Testis – seminoma
- Sarcoma

Box 17.18 Palliative benefits of radiotherapy

- Pain relief, e.g. bone metastases
- Reduction of headache and vomiting in raised intracranial pressure from central nervous system metastases
- Relief of obstruction of bronchus, oesophagus, ureter and lymphatics
- Preservation of skeletal integrity from metastases in weight-bearing bones
- Reversal of neurological impairment from spinal cord or optic nerve compression by metastases

Clinical application of radiation therapy

Radiotherapy planning involves both detailed physics of the applied dose and knowledge of the biology of the cancer; it is also necessary to establish whether the intention is to treat the tumour site alone, or to include the likely loco-regional patterns of spread. Normal tissue tolerance will determine the extent of the side-effects and, therefore, the total achievable dose. A balanced decision is made according to the curative or palliative intent of the treatment and the likely early or late side-effects.

The cancers for which radiotherapy is usually employed in a primary curative approach, when the tumour is anatomically localized, are listed in ***Box 17.17***, along with those in which radiotherapy has curative potential when used in addition to surgery (adjuvant radiotherapy). Palliative treatments are frequently used to provide relief of symptoms and to improve quality, if not duration, of survival ***(Box 17.18)***. Palliative treatment is usually given in as few fractions as possible over as short a time as possible. Radiotherapy planning, by the use of CT scanning guidance, has been complemented by the introduction of three-dimensional planning and intensity modulated radiotherapy (IMRT), which can deliver curved dose distributions to enable an improved therapeutic ratio. This allows a greater differential in dose between the tumour and critical normal structures, in turn allowing dose escalation or a reduced risk of toxicity. Four-dimensional radiotherapy planning is also becoming widely used, and varies radiation dose over time: for example, the respiratory cycle during lung cancer treatment. Stereotactic focused irradiation (stereotactic body radiotherapy, SBRT), using the γ-knife or Cyberknife, can concentrate gamma radiation from multiple sources on to a small volume to generate an ablative dose for treating tumours of the central nervous system and isolated metastases.

Proton beam therapy is an alternative type of external beam radiotherapy using protons, which, due to their larger mass, have little side scatter and so offer a much more focused beam with less dose to surrounding structures. Electron beam therapy uses high-energy electrons that have a short range and so are preferable for superficial tumours, such as melanoma or cutaneous lymphoma.

Box 17.19 Side-effects of radiotherapy

Acute temporary side-effects/dependent on region being treated
- Anorexia, nausea, malaise
- Mucositis, oesophagitis, diarrhoea
- Alopecia
- Myelosuppression

Late side-effects
- Skin: ischaemia, ulceration
- Bone: necrosis, fracture, sarcoma
- Mouth: xerostomia, ulceration
- Bowel: stenosis, fistula, diarrhoea
- Bladder: fibrosis, frequency, incontinence
- Vagina: dyspareunia, stenosis
- Lung: fibrosis, breathlessness
- Heart: pericardial fibrosis, cardiomyopathy, vasculopathy
- Central nervous system: myelopathy
- Gonads: infertility, menopause
- Secondary malignancies: e.g. leukaemia, cancer (e.g. thyroid)
- Other: carotid artery stenosis

Combination chemoradiotherapy

The local efficacy of radiotherapy can be increased by the simultaneous but not serial addition of chemotherapy with agents such as cisplatin, mitomycin and 5-FU for cancers of the head and neck, lung, oesophagus, stomach, rectum, anus and cervix. Reduced local recurrence rates have translated into survival benefits and further research is investigating the concurrent use of biological agents (e.g. EGFR inhibitors) with radiation.

Side-effects of radiotherapy

Early radiotherapy side-effects may occur within days to weeks of treatment; at this point, they are usually self-limiting but associated with general systemic disturbance ***(Box 17.19)***. The side-effects will depend on tissue sensitivity, fraction size and treatment volume, and are managed with supportive measures until normal tissue repair occurs. The toxicity may also be enhanced by exposure to other radiation-sensitizing agents, especially some cytotoxics, such as bleomycin, actinomycin, anthracyclines, cisplatin and 5-FU.

Later side-effects occur months to years later, and are unrelated to the severity of the acute effects because of their different mechanism. Late effects reflect both the loss of slowly proliferating cells and a local endarteritis that produces ischaemia and proliferative fibrosis. The risks of late side-effects are related to the fraction size and total dose delivered to the tissue. Growth may be arrested if bony epiphyses are not yet fused and are irradiated, leading to distorted skeletal growth in later life.

Secondary malignancies following radiotherapy may appear 10–20 years after cure of the primary cancer. Haematological malignancies tend to occur sooner than solid tumours from the irradiated tissues. The latter are very dependent on the status of the tissue at the time of treatment; for example, the pubertal breast is up to 300 times more sensitive to malignant transformation than the breast tissues of a woman in her thirties. Patients who smoke are more liable to develop lung cancer. Treatment of these secondary cancers can be successful, providing there is normal bone marrow to reconstitute the haemopoietic system, or the whole tissue at risk can be resected (e.g. thyroid after mantle radiotherapy for lymphoma).

ACUTE ONCOLOGY

The acute care of all patients admitted to hospital with a cancer diagnosis has become known as acute oncology, in order to ensure a coordinated patient care, with access to all facets of the multidisciplinary team and thus the most efficient use of high-cost inpatient facilities. In addition, there are a number of common oncological emergencies for which urgent treatment is critical for success ***(Box 17.20)***.

Neutropenic sepsis

This is the most common cause of attendance in the accident and emergency department for any cancer patient and must be always considered in any patient who is unwell within a month of chemotherapy. Neutropenic patients are at high risk of bacterial and fungal infections, most often from enteric bowel flora; hence, many units will advocate a specific neutropenic diet that is low in bacterial and fungal contamination ***(Box 17.21)***. Patients must be warned of the possibility of neutropenic fever occurring. Non-specific symptoms are also common, such as nausea, diarrhoea, drowsiness and breathlessness. A fever may not always be present. The critical test is the full blood count. Patients with neutrophils $<1.0\times10^9$/L are managed by the immediate introduction of broad-spectrum antibiotics and fluid resuscitation. Signs of systemic illness, such as tachycardia, hypotension or oliguria, mandate urgent admission and resuscitation with intravenous treatment ***(Box 17.22)***. Initial empirical therapy should be reviewed following microbiological results.

All such patients need to be discussed with the appropriate specialist oncology team and hospitals should have clear protocols for the rapid institution of antibiotics in such patients within an hour

Box 17.20 Acute oncology: problems and common causes

Problem	Common causes
Fever	Neutropenic sepsis
Breathlessness	Pulmonary embolus, pleural effusion Neutropenic sepsis Bronchial obstruction and lobar collapse Tense ascites
Hypotension	Neutropenic sepsis Embolus, pericardial tamponade
Swollen facies	Superior vena caval obstruction
Leg weakness	Spinal cord compression
Mental deterioration	Hypercalcaemia Raised intracranial pressure
Renal failure	Obstructive uropathy, sepsis Drugs: NSAIDs, methotrexate, cisplatin Metabolic: calcium, uric acid, myeloma protein, tumour lysis
Haemorrhage	Tumour erosion, thrombocytopenia, DIC
Bone pain	Pathological fracture
Acute abdomen	Intestinal obstruction and perforation
Jaundice	Obstructing mass liver, parenchymal destruction by tumour or drugs

DIC, disseminated intravascular coagulation; NSAIDs, non-steroidal anti-inflammatory drugs.

Box 17.21 Neutropenic diet

Foods and drinks that should be avoided	Foods and drinks that are safe
• All uncooked vegetables and most fruits – peel off thick skin from foods like oranges and bananas • Raw or rare meat • Fish • Uncooked or undercooked eggs • Foods from salad bars and delicatessen counters • Soft blue/mould cheeses, e.g. brie, camembert, stilton • 'Well' water – or boil it for 1 min before drinking	• Cooked vegetables • Canned fruits and juices • Well-done meat • Hard-boiled eggs (no runny yolks) • Vacuum-packed lunch meats (not freshly sliced meats) • Pasteurized milk, cheese, yogurt and other dairy products only • Tap water if the source is known – or boil it; bottled water

Box 17.22 Management of febrile neutropenia

- Febrile neutropenia is classed as a one-off reading ≥38.5°C or a reading ≥38°C sustained for 1 h
- Patients on antipyretics/steroids and elderly patients may not mount a febrile response
- Hypothermia or clinical deterioration may be the first sign

Immediate intervention is essential

- Resuscitate with i.v. fluids to restore circulatory function; monitor urine output, Glasgow Coma Scale score and central venous pressure
- Take cultures of blood, urine, sputum and stool
- Give empirical antibiotics as per local policy and sensitivities
- Review intensive care and consider inotropic support at an early stage:
  - Commonly used antibiotics should include activity against enteric Gram-negative bacteria and *Pseudomonas*, e.g. co-amoxiclav, ceftazidime or piperacillin–tazobactam with gentamicin; meropenem monotherapy
  - Antibiotics against staphylococci may be needed, e.g. vancomycin, especially with indwelling venous access lines
  - Neutropenic diet should be started, low in bacteria and fungi
- Change antibiotics according to culture results, or empirically increase Gram-negative cover and consider adding Gram-positive cover, if the patient deteriorates clinically and/or temperature is still elevated after 48 h; discuss with the microbiology department
- Consider imaging, e.g. chest CT, if fever is not responding to broad-spectrum antibiotics, to detect an occult source of fever; consider adding treatment for opportunistic infections:
  - Liposomal amphotericin B or voriconazole – *Candida* and *Aspergillus*
  - High-dose co-trimoxazole – *Pneumocystis*
  - Clarithromycin – *Mycoplasma* and *Legionella*
  - Anti-tuberculous therapy – *Mycobacterium tuberculosis*

For further information, see Dellinger RP et al. Surviving sepsis campaign: international guidelines for management of severe sepsis and septic shock. Crit Care Med *2008; 36:296–327.*

of arrival in the accident and emergency department. In units practised in the assessment of febrile neutropenia, it is possible to follow a more risk-stratified antibiotic policy and to avoid or curtail admission with oral co-amoxiclav plus ciprofloxacin when low-risk features are present: that is, absence of tachycardia, hypotension, hypoxia and mucositis and an expected short duration of myelosuppression.

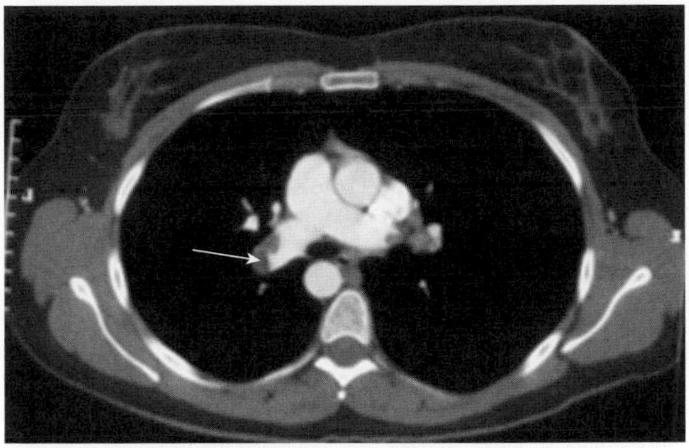

Figure 17.16 Pulmonary embolism (arrow).

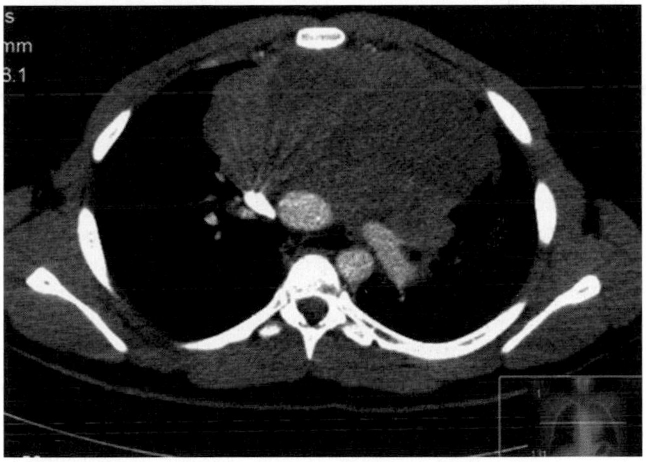

Figure 17.17 Bulky anterior mediastinal mass in a patient presenting with superior vena caval obstruction in T-lymphoblastic lymphoma.

Pulmonary embolus

This is a common complication of the coagulopathy of cancer and is a side-effect of chemotherapy ***(Fig. 17.16)***. It often presents with unexplained breathlessness and episodic exacerbations from multiple small emboli, rather than chest pain. A high level of suspicion should be maintained in any cancer patient with breathlessness, hypoxia or chest pain. CT pulmonary angiography is the investigation of choice. Prophylactic anticoagulation is given to all immobilized patients (see p. 580). Warfarin is ineffective in reversing the coagulopathy of cancer, and low-molecular-weight heparin is preferred.

Superior vena caval obstruction

Superior vena caval obstruction ***(Fig. 17.17)*** can arise from any upper mediastinal mass but is most commonly associated with lung cancer and lymphoma. The patient presents with difficulty breathing and/or swallowing; stridor; a swollen, oedematous facies and arms; venous congestion in the neck; and dilated veins in the upper chest and arms. Treatment is with immediate steroids, chemotherapy, where the tumour is expected to respond, and possibly mediastinal radiotherapy. Vascular stents and anticoagulation are also sometimes required. Some tumours, such as lymphomas, small cell lung cancers and germ cell tumours, are so sensitive to chemotherapy that this is preferred to radiotherapy, as the masses are likely to be both large and associated with more disseminated disease elsewhere. An early decision is necessary based on the patient's likely prognosis, as ventilatory support may be required until treatment has had time to relieve the obstruction.

Spinal cord compression

Spinal cord compression (see pp. 872–873) needs to be rapidly diagnosed and urgent treatment arranged within 24 hours of onset of paresis to salvage as much functional capacity as possible. Early neurological clinical features may be incomplete, more subjective than objective, and gradual in onset. MRI scanning is the investigation of choice. Treatment should begin with high-dose steroids and a joint neurosurgical and oncological consultation, with the neurosurgeons advising on spinal stability, the need for spinal precautions for movement, and the role of decompressive surgery and external bracing for limited-extent disease. In the absence of surgery, radiotherapy alone may be used.

Tumour lysis syndrome

This occurs if treatment triggers a massive breakdown of tumour cells, leading to increased serum levels of urate, potassium and phosphate, and a secondary hypocalcaemia. These biochemical changes can lead to cardiac arrhythmias and seizures. Urate deposition in the renal tubules can cause renal failure (hyperuricaemic nephropathy). Vigorous hydration, often with diuretics, is crucial to maintain high urine outputs in such patients; however, a proportion will require dialysis for uraemia, oliguria or severe electrolyte disturbances. The xanthine oxidase inhibitor, allopurinol, should be given before treatment is started in low-risk patients. Intravenous rasburicase, a recombinant urate oxidase, is used for prophylaxis in high-risk patients and in the treatment of tumour lysis syndrome.

Acute hypercalcaemia

This presents with vomiting, confusion, constipation and oliguria. Treatment is by resuscitation with intravenous fluids first, to establish a saline diuresis, and an intravenous bisphosphonate, such as pamidronate or the more potent zoledronic acid (see ***Box 26.48***). Treating the cause is crucial. Denosumab and calcitonin can be used in intractable cases.

Raised intracranial pressure

Raised intracranial pressure due to intracerebral metastases presents classically with headache, nausea and vomiting. There are often no localizing neurological signs and almost never papilloedema until very late in the disease. However, for many, there is a slower onset with non-specific symptoms such as drowsiness or mental deterioration. Treatment is by high-dose steroids and investigation by MRI. Surgery is appropriate if the condition is unifocal and/or threatening the fourth ventricle; otherwise, whole-brain or local stereotactic Cyberknife radiotherapy is required.

Hyperviscosity

This can affect patients with a very high haematocrit (haemoglobin >180 g/L), white cell count (>100×10^9/L) or platelet cell count (>1000×10^9/L) from untreated leukaemia or from a myeloproliferative disorder. Viscosity can also be increased by high levels of monoclonal immunoglobulin molecules, as seen in myeloma or Waldenström's macroglobulinaemia. IgA and IgM are more commonly implicated due to their respective dimeric and pentameric structures. Clinical features include hypoxia, pulmonary infiltrates, confusion, headache, visual disturbances, papilloedema and retinal venous dilatation; rarely, cardiac failure or priapism may be present. Treatment is by leucopheresis or plasmapheresis, followed by urgent treatment for the underlying malignancy.

Malignant bile duct obstruction

This will present with cholestatic jaundice. Lymphomatous obstruction will respond very well to prompt initiation of therapy. A small proportion of pancreatic and bile duct tumours are surgically resectable, more commonly those in the distal bile duct as compared to those in the hilar region. However, in the greater proportion of patients, treatment is palliative. In recent years, endoscopic techniques have allowed the insertion of stents into the biliary tree to re-establish bile flow. Self-expanding metal stents have long periods of patency but are at risk of ascending infection. In the small proportion of patients in whom bile duct drainage is not possible endoscopically, the percutaneous route offers an alternative. Endoscopic photodynamic laser therapy with a photoporphyrin sensitizer can also prolong patency.

Further reading

Howard SC, Jones DP, Pui CH. The tumor lysis syndrome. *N Engl J Med* 2011; 364:1844–1854.

HAEMATOLOGICAL MALIGNANCIES

The leukaemias, the lymphomas and multiple myeloma are an interrelated spectrum of malignancies of the myeloid and lymphoid systems. They are uncommon but not rare, the lymphomas alone being the fifth most common cancer in the UK. The aetiology of these diseases is unknown, for the most part, although viruses, irradiation, cytotoxic poisons and immune suppression have been implicated in a small proportion of cases (see pp. 589–590). The pathogenesis involves at least one molecular abnormality, or usually more, and non-random chromosomal abnormalities have been detected in several leukaemias and lymphomas. Classification has become increasingly complex, with the universally applied World Health Organization (WHO) scheme demanding morphological, cytogenetic and sometimes molecular criteria to be fulfilled. Transformation from low-grade to high-grade pathological sub-type may occur. Treatment options are multiple. Patients need to be supported through treatment involving prolonged myelosuppression and immunosuppression. These therapies are potentially life-threatening but can also be curative. These complexities have given rise to the need for highly skilled staff and specialist facilities; patients should be referred to these centres for treatment.

Haematological malignancies can be divided on the basis of speed of evolution of the disease and cell of origin, and according to whether there is primarily a marrow-based leukaemic presentation (with obvious circulating disease in the peripheral blood), or a nodal or extranodal lymphomatous presentation in which soft tissue masses predominate and there is little peripheral blood involvement. 'Acute' disorders are rapidly progressive and fatal within days to weeks if not treated, whereas 'chronic' disorders are typically indolent and slowly progressive, and patients can live with their disease for long periods. Myeloid disorders arise from the lineages within the marrow that produce granulocytes, red cells or platelets. Lymphoid disorders can arise from either B- or T-cell lineages. This classification is summarized in ***Box 17.23***. This is an arbitrary division

Box 17.23 Classification of leukaemia and lymphoma

Timeframe	Myeloid (bone marrow)	Lymphoid (bone marrow)	Lymphoid (node)
Acute Immature cells predominate	Acute myeloid leukaemia	Acute lymphocytic leukaemia	Lymphoma, 'high-grade', 'aggressive', e.g. Burkitt's lymphoma
	Myelodysplastic syndrome	Myeloma	
Chronic Mature cells predominate	Chronic myeloid leukaemia Other myeloproliferative disorder	Chronic lymphocytic leukaemia Others	Lymphoma, 'low-grade', 'indolent', e.g. follicular lymphoma

and there is movement across the divisions; for example, chronic myeloid leukaemia can transform to either acute myeloid leukaemia or acute lymphocytic leukaemia; myeloproliferative neoplasms and myelodysplastic syndrome (MDS; pp. 551–552) can transform to acute myeloid leukaemia; and chronic lymphocytic leukaemia and low-grade non-Hodgkin's lymphoma can transform to high-grade forms in 'Richter's transformation'. MDS and myeloma may both present with a range of clinical phenotypes, from indolent disease to very aggressive and rapidly progressive presentations that include MDS-refractory anaemia with excess of blasts or the plasma cell leukaemia variant of myeloma.

In the management of these diseases, it is critical for patients to be appraised of the natural history, its potential modification by treatment, and the risks of both severe morbidity and mortality. It must be made clear from the outset whether a curative or palliative strategy is most appropriate and the reasons for this decision should be explained. If cure is to be pursued, the patient must be informed of the approximate probability of success and its potential price. The possibility of failure needs to be addressed at the outset.

THE LEUKAEMIAS

There are four main subtypes, as discussed above:

1. acute myeloid leukaemia (AML)
2. acute lymphoblastic leukaemia (ALL)
3. chronic myeloid leukaemia (CML)
4. chronic lymphocytic leukaemia (CLL).

These are relatively uncommon diseases with an incidence of about 10/100 000 per year. They can occur at any age and the type of leukaemia varies with age; ALL is mainly seen in childhood and CLL is a disease of the elderly.

Leukaemia can be diagnosed by examination of a stained slide of peripheral blood and bone marrow, but immunophenotyping, cytogenetics and molecular genetics are essential for complete sub-classification and prognostication. The lineage and degree of maturity of the leukaemic clone can be assessed by the expression of cytosolic enzymes and surface antigens.

Aetiology

In the majority of patients, this is unknown but several factors have been associated:

- ***Radiation***. This can induce genetic damage to haemopoietic precursors and ALL, AML and CML have been seen in increased incidence in survivors of Hiroshima and Nagasaki, and in patients treated with ionizing radiation.
- ***Chemical and drugs***. Exposure to benzene, used in industry, may lead to marrow damage. AML occurs after treatment with alkylating agents (e.g. melphalan) and topoisomerase-II inhibitors (e.g. etoposide).
- ***Genetic factors***. Leukaemia risk is highly elevated in a number of germline conditions that result in genetic instability or bone marrow failure. These include Fanconi anaemia, ataxia telangiectasia and Li–Fraumeni syndrome. The risk is elevated some 30 times in people with trisomy 21. There is a high degree of concordance among monozygotic twins. Several genes have also been associated with familial AML, such as *CEBPA* and *RUNX1*.
- ***Viruses***. A type of leukaemia is associated with human T-cell lymphotropic retrovirus type 1 (HTLV-1), which is found particularly in Japan and the Caribbean.

Genetics

Leukaemic cells often have a somatically acquired cytogenetic abnormality, which may be of prognostic, as well as diagnostic, significance. These genetic alterations change the normal cell-regulating process by interfering with the control of normal proliferation, blocking differentiation, maintaining an unlimited capacity for self-renewal and, lastly, promoting resistance to death signals: that is, decreased apoptosis.

The first non-random chromosomal abnormality to be described was the Philadelphia (Ph) chromosome, which is associated with CML in 97% of cases (see ***Fig. 17.21A***, p. 612). The Ph chromosome is also found in ALL, the incidence in the latter illness increasing with age. The translocation is shown schematically in ***Figure 17.21A***. The Ph chromosome is an abnormal chromosome 22, resulting from a reciprocal translocation between part of the long arm of chromosome 22 and chromosome 9. The resulting karyotype is described as t(9; 22)(q34; q11). The molecular consequences of the translocation are that part of the Abelson proto-oncogene (*c-ABL*), normally present on chromosome 9, is translocated to chromosome 22, where it comes into juxtaposition with a region of chromosome 22 named the 'breakpoint cluster region' (BCR). The new 'fusion' gene, *BCR-ABL*, is capable of being expressed as a chimeric messenger RNA, which has been identified in cells from patients with CML. When translated, this produces a fusion protein that has tyrosine kinase activity and enhanced phosphorylating activity compared with the normal protein, resulting in altered cell growth, stromal attachment and apoptosis. The breakpoint differs in CML and Ph-positive ALL, leading to the production of two different tyrosine kinase proteins with molecular weights of 210 kDa and 190 kDa, respectively. It is unclear whether the presence of *BCR-ABL* is sufficient for development of the disease. It has been shown that normal subjects can carry low levels of the *BCR-ABL* fusion gene in their blood without developing leukaemia. Other genetic and cytogenetic abnormalities are often seen in leukaemic cells.

As well as cytogenetic and molecular aberrations, epigenetic modification via abnormal methylation patterns and chromatin modification due to histone acetylation is increasingly understood to be involved in oncogenesis and may represent potential therapeutic targets.

Acute leukaemias

The acute leukaemias increase in incidence with advancing age. Acute myeloid (myeloblastic, myelogenous) leukaemia has a median age at presentation of 65 years and may arise *de novo* or against a background of myelodysplasia or prior cytotoxic chemotherapy ('secondary'). Acute lymphoid (lymphoblastic) leukaemia has a substantially lower median age at presentation and, in addition, is the most common malignancy in childhood. The simplified WHO classification is shown in ***Box 17.24***.

Clinical features

The majority of patients with acute leukaemia, regardless of subtype, present with symptoms ***(Box 17.25)*** reflecting inadequate haemopoiesis secondary to infiltration of the bone marrow by leukaemic cells, symptoms due to tissue infiltration by leukaemic cells ***(Box 17.26)***, the consequences of a high white blood cell count, or substance release from the tumour cells.

Investigations

For confirming diagnosis

- ***Blood count***. Haemoglobin is low, the white blood cell count is usually raised (sometimes low) and platelets are low.
- ***Blood film***. Blast cells are almost invariably seen ***(Fig. 17.18A)***; lineage may be identified morphologically, e.g. the presence of Auer rods is consistent with a diagnosis of AML.
- ***Bone marrow aspirate***. Increased cellularity ***(Fig. 17.18B)***, reduced erythropoiesis and reduced megakaryocytes may be seen. Replacement by blast cells is >20% (often approaching 100%). Lineage is confirmed by immunophenotyping, e.g. AML – CD33 or CD13; B lineage ALL – CD10 and CD19; and T lineage – CD3. Cytogenetic and FISH analysis, as well as real-time PCR and molecular genetics, may be used for prognostication.
- ***Chest X-ray***. Mediastinal widening is often present in T-lymphoblastic leukaemia.
- ***Cerebrospinal fluid examination***. This is performed in all patients with ALL, as the risk of central nervous system involvement is high. It is less critical in AML.
- ***Coagulation profile***. This is performed to exclude the presence of disseminated intravascular coagulation (DIC): raised prothrombin time and activated partial thromboplastin time, reduced fibrinogen, and increased fibrinogen degradation products, e.g. D-dimers.

Box 17.24 World Health Organization classification of acute leukaemia

Acute myeloid leukaemia
- AML with recurrent genetic abnormalities
- AML with MDS-related changes
- Therapy-related myeloid neoplasm
- AML, not otherwise categorized[a]

Acute lymphoid leukaemia
- B-cell lymphoblastic leukaemia/lymphoma

[a]*These entities correspond with the French–American–British classification. MDS, myelodysplastic syndrome.*
(Modified from Jaffe ES, Harris NL, Stein H et al. (eds). World Health Organization Classification of Tumours. Pathology and Genetics of Tumours of Haematopoietic and Lymphoid Tissues. *Lyon: IARC Press; 2008, with permission from the World Health Organization.)*

Box 17.25 Symptoms and signs of leukaemia

	Symptoms	Signs	Type
Marrow failure			
Anaemia	Breathlessness Fatigue Angina Claudication	Pallor Cardiac flow murmur	ALL/AML
Neutropenia	Infections	Fever Mouth ulcers Septic focus	
Thrombocytopenia	Bleeding and bruising	Petechiae Gum bleeding Fundal haemorrhage	
High WBC			
Leucostasis	Breathlessness	Hypoxia, pulmonary infiltrates	ALL/AML
	Headache Confusion	Reduced GCS	
	Visual problems	Retinal vein dilatation, papilloedema, fundal haemorrhage	
Tissue infiltration			
Marrow	Bone pain		ALL/AML
Gums		Gum hypertrophy	AML
Skin		Violaceous skin deposits	AML
Liver/spleen		Hepatosplenomegaly	ALL/AML
Nodes		Lymphadenopathy	ALL/AML
CNS	Headache	Cranial nerve palsies	ALL/ (AML)
Testes		Testicular enlargement	ALL
Mediastinum		Mediastinal mass, SVCO	ALL
Substance release			
DIC	Bleeding and bruising	Ecchymoses Bleeding i.v. sites	AML
Hyperuricaemia	Acute gout Tumour lysis	Renal stones, tophi Acute kidney failure	ALL/AML

ALL, acute lymphoid leukaemia; AML, acute myeloid leukaemia; CNS, central nervous system; DIC, disseminated intravascular coagulation; GCS, Glasgow Coma Scale score; SVCO, superior vena caval obstruction; WBC, white blood cell count.

Box 17.26 Characteristics of blast cells

- A blast cell is an immature precursor of myeloid cells (myeloblasts) or lymphoid cells (lymphoblast)
- They are bigger than their normal counterparts
- There is an immature nucleus (nucleolus, open chromatin)
- Cytoplasmic appearances are often atypical
- They are rarely seen in normal individuals
- If present, they are highly suggestive of an acute leukaemia or a chronic disorder that is beginning to transform into an acute disease, e.g. transformed myeloproliferative neoplasms, MDS-RAEB, CML blast crisis.

CML, chronic myeloid leukaemia; MDS-RAEB, myelodysplastic syndrome-refractory anaemia with excess blasts.

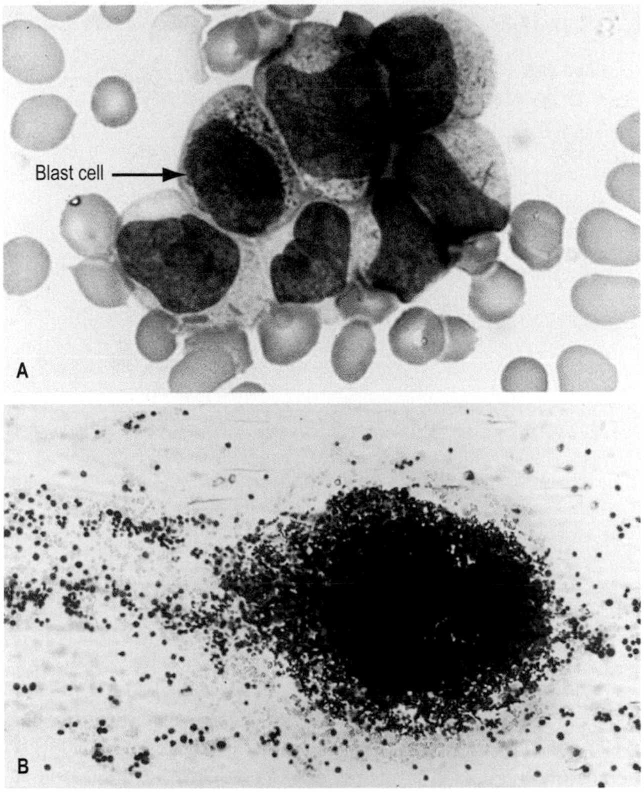

Figure 17.18 Acute leukaemia. A. Peripheral blood film showing characteristic blast cells. The arrow points to the abnormal blast cell. **B.** Bone marrow aspirate showing particle with increased cellularity. *(Courtesy of Dr Manzoor Mangi.)*

For planning therapy

- Biochemistry, serum urate, renal and liver biochemistry.
- Cardiac function: electrocardiography and direct tests of left ventricular function, e.g. echocardiogram (see pp. 944–948).
- HLA type.
- Check HBV status (p. 456).

Management

Untreated acute leukaemia is invariably fatal, most often within a few months, though with judicious palliative care it may be extended, perhaps to a year. Treatment with curative intent may be successful, or may fail, either because the leukaemia does not respond (i.e. refractory to treatment), because the disease returns after an initial favourable response (relapse), or because the patient succumbs to complications of the therapy (treatment-related mortality). At initial presentation, acute leukaemias range from being probably curable (e.g. childhood 'good-risk' ALL) through to probably incurable (e.g. AML with adverse cytogenetic features in the elderly). Since curative treatment carries considerable morbidity and potential mortality, it is essential for the 'risk/benefit' ratio to be clearly understood by physician and patient alike.

Palliative therapy

Every attempt should be made to ensure that the patients are at home as much as possible, while making available the full range of supportive care. Palliation may well include low-dose chemotherapy in addition to blood product support and antimicrobials.

Curative therapy

The decision to treat with curative intent, particularly if successful, implies severe disruption of normality for the patient and family for at least 6 months and often up to a year. In the short term, it may demand transfer to another hospital, as acute leukaemia should only be treated in units seeing a sufficient number of patients. It is highly likely to involve admission to hospital for up to a month in the first instance, with further, partly predictable, subsequent admissions of several days' to weeks' duration, requiring discussions and decisions about work or education.

The decision to treat with curative intent implies that the chance of cure justifies the risks of the therapy. It does not imply that cure is guaranteed or even expected.

Active therapy

Supportive care

This forms the basis of treatment, whether for cure or palliation:

- ***Avoidance of symptoms of anaemia*** (haemoglobin >80–100 g/L). Repeated transfusion of packed red cells is needed (sometimes, irradiation of cells is required)
- ***Prevention or control of bleeding*** (platelet count $<10\times10^9$/L in the stable patient and $<20\times10^9$/L in the septic patient, or $<50\times10^9$/L if a procedure is planned, e.g. lumbar puncture). The role of prophylactic platelet transfusion has been evaluated and remains superior to any alternative, certainly for patients with AML.
- ***Correction of coagulation abnormalities***. This is achieved with fresh frozen plasma (FFP) to keep the activated partial thromboplastin time ratio and INR <1.5 times normal, and with cryoprecipitate to keep the fibrinogen level >1.5 g/dL. Norethisterone is given to women of menstrual age to avoid menorrhagia during their thrombocytopenic phase.
- ***Leucopheresis***. This may be required to reduce the white cell count rapidly before the chemotherapy has started to be effective.
- ***Treatment of infection*** (see **Box 17.22**):
  - ***Prophylactic***. Education of patients, relatives and staff about diet, hand washing and isolation facilities is necessary. Selected antibiotics, antifungals, antivirals and *Pneumocystis jirovecii* prophylaxis may be required.
  - ***Therapeutic***. Fever is managed using local protocol/algorithm for antibiotic and antifungal combinations.
- ***Control of hyperuricaemia***. This should be achieved with hydration, prophylactic allopurinol and occasionally rasburicase (see p. 606).

Indwelling venous devices, such as a Hickman line, are required to allow easy access to the blood for tests and administration of therapy. Sperm banking is offered to postpubertal men and oocyte collection to women, if there is time before treatment.

Specific treatment

The initial requirement of therapy is to return the peripheral blood and bone marrow to normal (complete remission, CR). This 'induction chemotherapy' is tailored to the particular leukaemia and the individual patient's risk factors. Since this treatment is not leukaemia-specific but also impairs normal bone marrow function, it leads to a major risk of life-threatening infection, which increases the risk of early death in the short term.

Successful remission induction is always followed by further treatment (consolidation). Details are determined by the type of leukaemia and by the patient's risk factors and tolerance of

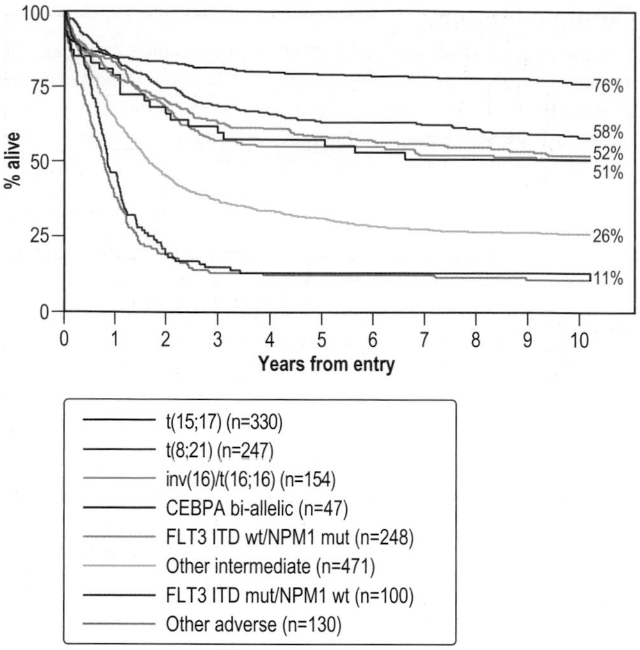

Figure 17.19 Prognosis related to cytogenetics and molecular data in acute myeloid leukaemia (AML). Outcome of younger adults with AML treated in the Medical Research Council AML10 and AML12 trials, stratified according to cytogenetic and molecular abnormalities. *(Reproduced with permission from Smith ML, Hills RK, Grimwade D. Independent prognostic variables in acute myeloid leukaemia.* Blood Reviews *2011; 25(1):39–51.)*

Box 17.27 Risk factors in acute myeloid leukaemia

Good risk
- *De novo* disease
- Favourable cytogenetics: t(15; 17) t(8; 21) or inv(16) or its variant t(16; 16)
- CEBPA bi-allelic mutation
- NPM1 mutation with FLT3 wild type

Poor risk
- Age >60
- Male gender
- Secondary disease, e.g. prior MDS or MPN
- High WBC
- Adverse cytogenetics: –5, del(5q), –7, abnormal 3q26 or a complex karyotype
- FLT3 internal tandem duplication mutation
- MRD positivity

CEBPA, transcription factor CCAAT/enhancer binding protein; FLT3, FMS-like tyrosine kinase 3; MDS, myelodysplastic syndrome, MPN, myeloproliferative neoplasm; MRD, minimal residual disease; NPM1, nucleophosmin; WBC, white blood cell count.

treatment. Recurrence is almost invariable if 'consolidation' therapy is not given. This reflects the lack of sensitivity of the definition of 'complete remission', which has been solely morphological. Cytogenetics and molecular genetic techniques can, however, identify residual leukaemic cells not detected morphologically ('minimal residual disease', MRD) and they are highly predictive of recurrence. Failure to achieve morphological CR with two cycles of therapy ('refractory') carries almost as bad a prognosis as the untreated leukaemia. If CR can be achieved – by new experimental approaches, for instance – cure may still be possible with stem cell transplantation (see pp. 561–562). A small proportion of patients with refractory disease may also be cured by a myeloablative allograft.

Acute myeloid leukaemia

In AML, the prognosis is dependent on a range of key variables, the two main ones being age and cytogenetics (***Fig. 17.19*** and ***Box 17.27***).

Management

Young patients: intensive therapy unless unfit

Treatment with curative intent is undertaken in the majority of adults below the age of 60 years, provided there is no significant co-morbidity. Treatment success reflects the cytogenetic pattern. Those with 'favourable risk' disease (e.g. inv(16) or t(8; 21) karyotypes, or solely NPM1-mutated AML, or AML with the bi-allelic transcription factor CCAAT/enhancer binding protein (CEBPA) mutation) are treated with moderately intensive combination chemotherapy. This always includes an anthracycline such as daunorubicin and cytarabine (cytosine arabinoside) and consolidation with a minimum of four cycles of treatment given at 3–4-week intervals.

Patients with favourable-risk disease do not benefit from allogeneic stem cell transplantation during their first complete remission because the risks outweigh the benefits. Those with 'intermediate-risk' cytogenetics (e.g. normal karyotype, +8, +21) are a heterogeneous and increasingly complex group. Where possible, they should be given consolidation chemotherapy after an initial remission has been achieved, followed by allogeneic transplantation in those deemed at increased risk of relapse because of risk factors, such as FLT3 internal tandem duplication. Patients with adverse cytogenetics (e.g. –7, –5, complex karyotype) should proceed to a stem cell transplant in first complete remission (CR1) because they respond poorly to conventional chemotherapy and have a high risk of relapse.

CR will be achieved in about 80% of patients under the age of 60. Failure is due to either resistant leukaemia (10%), or death due to infection or bleeding (10%). Approximately 50% of those entering complete remission will be cured (i.e. approximately 40% overall), although this varies from 60–70% in the favourable cytogenetic group to 10–20% in the adverse cytogenetic group.

Older patients: intensive versus non-intensive strategies

The initial treatment of the older patient (>60 years) is much more contentious. A decision needs to be taken initially as to whether the patient is 'fit' enough to tolerate intensive chemotherapy. This will require a full assessment of their co-morbidities and organ function. Older patients tolerate cytotoxic therapy less well than younger patients due to additional co-morbidities, and their disease is often more aggressive in its biology; for example, adverse cytogenetics are more common with increasing age. As a result, treatment-related morbidity and mortality are both higher and outcome is less successful. Reduced-intensity allogeneic transplantation is increasingly being used for this group but is limited by its toxicity. For those who are not fit for intensive chemotherapy, treatment will have a palliative aim to improve marrow function and to maximize quality of life. Choice of therapy will include low-dose cytarabine, azacitidine, oral cytotoxics (such as hydroxycarbamide) or enrolment into any one of a range of clinical trials of novel agents.

Relapsed AML

The management of recurrence is undertaken on an individual basis, since the overall prognosis is very poor, despite the fact that second remissions may be achieved. Long survival following recurrence is rarely achieved without allogeneic transplantation. New therapy should be considered. The use of minimal residual disease monitoring may allow the detection of a subgroup of patients during initial therapy who require treatment intensification, such as allograft, as well as patients in CR who are in the early stages of relapse and need pre-emptive therapy before frank marrow relapse occurs.

Newer agents that target the FLT3 mutation, present in a significant proportion of cases of AML, are in clinical trials in conjunction with conventional chemotherapy. Other novel therapies that are being considered in AML include chemotherapy-labelled monoclonal antibodies (gemtuzumab ozogamicin) and hypomethylating agents (e.g. azacitidine).

Acute promyelocytic leukaemia

Acute promyelocytic leukaemia (APML) is a variant of AML, occurring in 10–15% of cases; it is characterized by the translocation t(15; 17) and has particular morphological features. There is an almost invariable coagulopathy, which remains a major cause of early death. The empirical discovery that all-*trans*-retinoic acid (ATRA) causes differentiation of promyelocytes and rapid reversal of the bleeding tendency was a major breakthrough. APML is treated with ATRA combined with several courses of chemotherapy. Complete remission and molecular remission occur in at least 90% of younger adults with APML, and at least 70% will expect to be cured. Transplantation may be necessary either if the leukaemia is not eliminated at the molecular level, or following recurrence and re-induction therapy. Arsenic trioxide, which induces apoptosis via activation of the ***caspase cascade*** (see p. 105), is used in resistant or relapsed disease and is under investigation as first-line therapy.

Acute lymphoblastic leukaemia

This condition may present in leukaemic phase with significant marrow involvement (acute lymphoblastic leukaemia, ALL) or may present as localized disease, typically a mediastinal mass (lymphoblastic lymphoma). The tumour cells in each condition are indistinguishable and similar therapies are therefore used. The overall strategy for the treatment of ALL differs in detail from that for AML. Remission induction is undertaken with combination chemotherapy that includes vincristine, a glucocorticoid, an anthracycline and asparaginase. Once remission is achieved, the details of consolidation will be determined by the anticipated risk of relapse. Intensive consolidation of remission with variable numbers of chemotherapy cycles comprising cytotoxics with different mechanisms of action has been standard practice, including the administration of high-dose methotrexate. In those patients with high-risk features (see below) or an HLA-matched sibling donor, allogeneic transplantation is recommended on achieving CR1.

A major difference between therapy for ALL and AML is the need for central nervous system-directed therapy. Prophylaxis should be given with intrathecal chemotherapy under platelet cover if necessary, as soon as blasts are cleared from the blood. Depending on risk, this may be continued for up to 2 years and complemented by high doses of systemic cytarabine or methotrexate. Cranial irradiation was previously given to all patients to reduce the risk of relapse within the central nervous system; some risk-adapted strategies reserve this only for those patients at very high risk.

Additionally, after intensive induction and consolidation, maintenance therapy for 2 years is required to reduce the risk of disease recurrence. This typically comprises 2 years of treatment with methotrexate and mercaptopurine, although more intensive regimens are used by many groups.

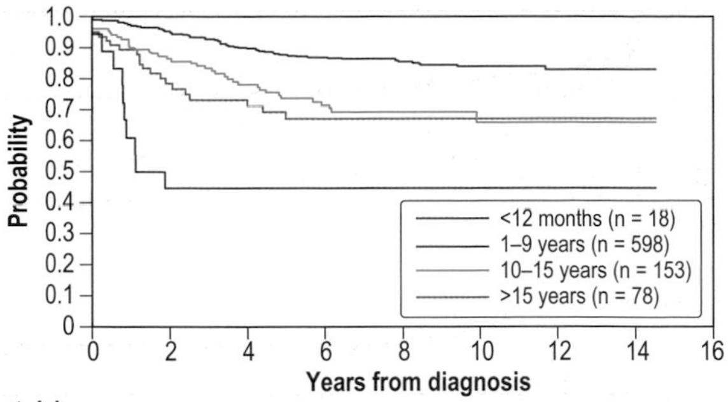

Number at risk

<12 months	18	11	8	8	6	1	1	0	0
1–9 years	598	528	378	295	213	149	85	31	4
10–15 years	153	130	100	77	50	26	11	6	1
>15 years	78	60	40	29	20	7	1	0	0

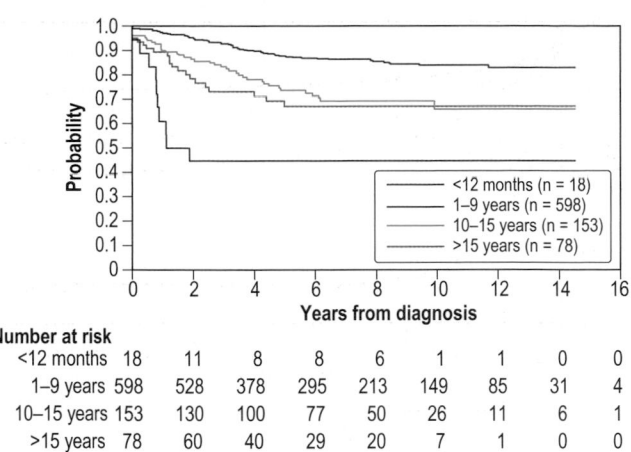

Figure 17.20 Overall survival in 2628 children of different ages with newly diagnosed acute lymphoblastic leukaemia. Outcome of participants in consecutive studies conducted at St Jude Children's Research Hospital from 1962 to 2005. *(From Pui C-M, Robinson LL, Lock T. Acute lymphoblastic leukaemia.* Lancet *2008; 371:1030–1043, Figure 3, with permission.)*

Box 17.28 Acute lymphoblastic leukaemia (ALL) risk factors

Risk factor	Good	Poor
Age	Younger	Older
WBC	$<50 \times 10^9$/L for B-lineage $<100 \times 10^9$/L for T-lineage	$>50 \times 10^9$/L for B-lineage $>100 \times 10^9$/L for T-lineage
Immunophenotype	CD10+ common ALL	Pro-B ALL
Cytogenetic aberrations	t(12; 21) hyperdiploidy	t(9; 22) or t(4; 11) hypodiploidy
Time to response	Early clearance of blasts	Failure to achieve a CR within 3–4 weeks
Minimal residual disease	MRD negative	MRD positive
Extramedullary disease	CSF clear	CSF positive

CR, complete remission; CSF, cerebrospinal fluid; MRD, minimal residual disease; WBC, white blood cell count.

Prognosis

A number of clinical and laboratory features are determinants of treatment response and survival in ALL ***(Box 17.28)***. Increasingly, therapeutic strategies based on prognostic risk are being used in management of the disease. Minimal residual disease (MRD) stratification is increasingly employed to select out patients who are at high risk (for treatment intensification) or low risk (for treatment de-escalation).

The prognosis ***(Fig. 17.20)*** of ALL in childhood is now excellent: complete remission is achieved in almost all, with up to 80% being alive without recurrence at 5 years. Failure occurs most frequently in those with high presentation blast counts or an 11q23 *MLL* translocation. Current treatment strategies lessen therapy for 'good-risk' children in order to avoid some of the long-term consequences of therapy, such as avascular necrosis of bone, infertility, neurotoxicity and cardiotoxicity.

The situation is far less satisfactory for adults, the prognosis getting worse with advancing years. Co-morbidity and t(9; 22) translocation increase in frequency with age. Overall, the CR rate is 70–80%. Disease that is refractory to first-line therapy carries a very poor prognosis. Between 30% and 40% of patients continue in durable first remissions, resulting in approximately 25–30% overall patient cure. Increasing numbers of patients are receiving transplants for this condition, including those with sibling donors and those high-risk individuals who have an available unrelated or alternative donor. Imatinib used in conjunction with chemotherapy increases the response rate and quality of response in patients with the t(9; 22) translocation and ALL. As with AML, most recurrences occur within the first 3 years and the outcome is extremely poor. Second remissions, though usually achieved, are rarely durable, except following allogeneic transplantation. Isolated extramedullary recurrences, however, may be cured. Novel cytotoxics drugs, including clofarabine and nelarabine, are increasingly used for relapsed/refractory cases. A range of monoclonals are currently under evaluation for use in B-ALL, including rituximab (anti-CD20), inotuzumab (calicheamicin-labelled anti-CD22) and blinatumomab (CD19/CD3 bi-specific T-cell engager antibody).

Chronic leukaemias

Chronic myeloid leukaemia

Chronic myeloid leukaemia (CML), which accounts for about 14% of all leukaemias, is a member of the family of myeloproliferative neoplasms (MPNs); it is almost exclusively a disease of adults, the peak of presentation being between 40 and 60 years. It is defined by the presence of the Philadelphia chromosome ***(Fig. 17.21)***, which is demonstrated either cytogenetically (95%) or molecularly (5%). Unlike the acute leukaemias, which are either rapidly reversed or rapidly fatal, CML has a more slowly progressive course; if not initially cured, it will be followed eventually by 'blast crisis' transformation to acute leukaemia (75% myeloid, 25% lymphoid) or myelofibrosis with death in a median of 3–4 years.

Clinical features

CML usually presents in the chronic phase and some patients have no symptoms.

Symptoms

When present, symptoms include:

- symptomatic anaemia (e.g. shortness of breath)
- abdominal discomfort due to splenomegaly
- weight loss
- fever and sweats in the absence of infection
- headache (occasionally) or priapism due to hyperleucocytosis
- bruising and bleeding (uncommon).

Signs

These include:

- pallor
- splenomegaly, often massive
- lymphadenopathy (uncommon; suggests blast crisis)
- extramedullary soft tissue leukaemic deposit – 'chloroma' (indicates blast crisis)
- retinal haemorrhage due to leucostasis.

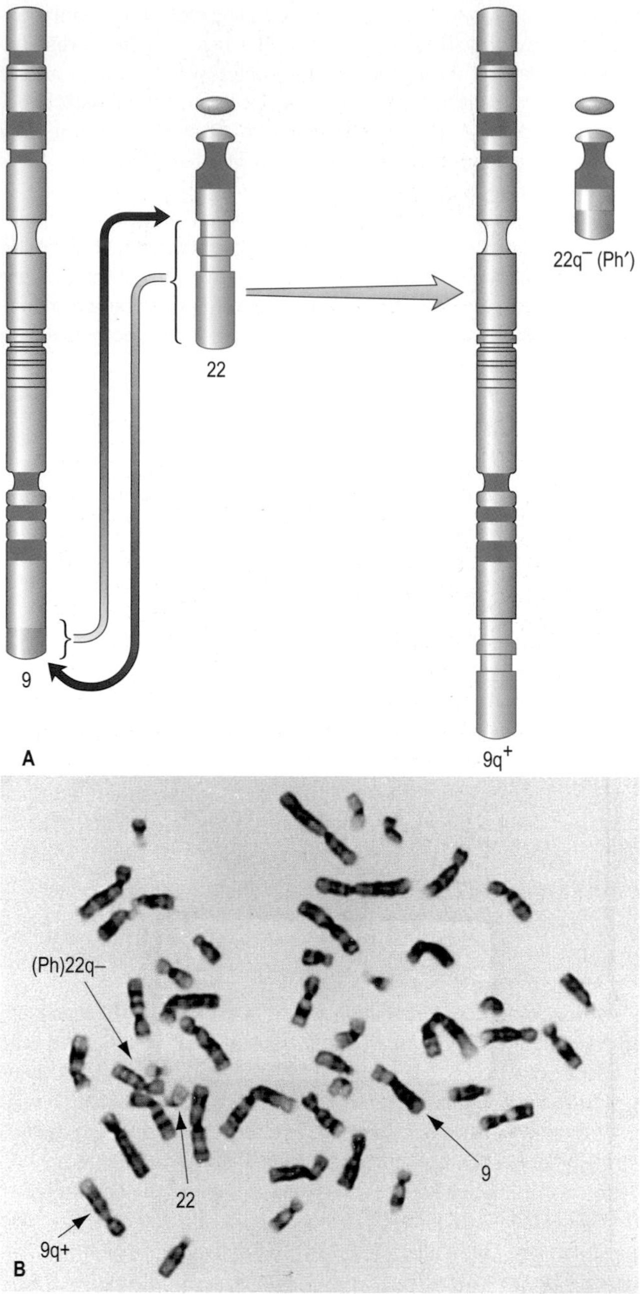

Figure 17.21 The Philadelphia chromosome (Ph). A. The long arm (q) of chromosome 22 has been shortened by the reciprocal translocation with chromosome 9. **B.** The Philadelphia chromosome is formed by a reciprocal translocation of part of the long arm (q) of chromosome 22 to chromosome 9. It is seen in 90–95% of patients with chronic myeloid leukaemia. The karyotype is expressed as 46XX, (9; 22)(q34; q11).

Investigations

- ***Blood count***. Haemoglobin is low (normochromic and normocytic) or normal; the white blood cell count is raised (usually >100× 10^9/L); and platelets are low, normal or raised.
- ***Blood film***. There is neutrophilia with the whole spectrum of mature myeloid precursors. Basophils and eosinophils are elevated. Increased numbers of blasts are suggestive of an accelerated phase or blast crisis ***(Fig. 17.22)***.

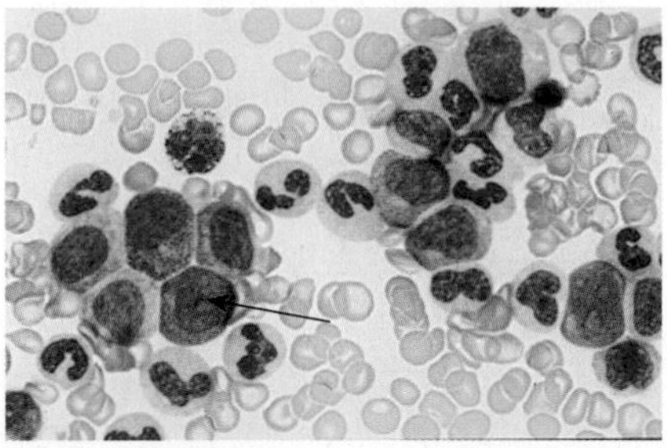

Figure 17.22 **Blood film showing blast cells (arrow) in chronic myeloid leukaemia.**

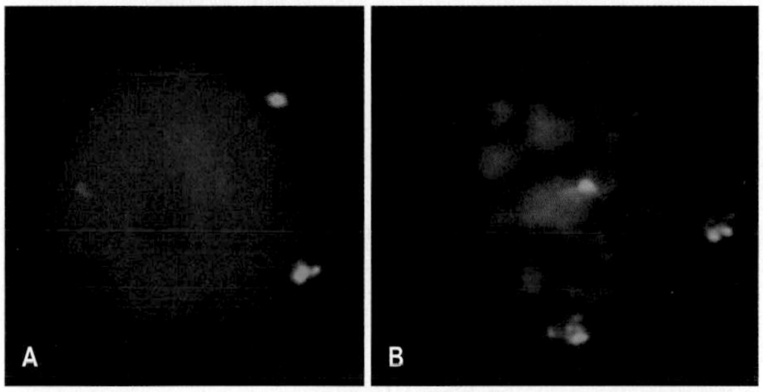

Figure 17.23 **Fluorescence *in situ* hybridization photomicrograph of a patient with chronic myeloid leukaemia. A.** 17p (green probe) and 11q (red probe) shows two green signals (TP53 deletion) with normal diploid complement of 11q. **B.** 12 centromere (green probe) and 13q14 (red probe) shows three green signals (trisomy 12) with normal diploid complement of 13q. *(Courtesy of Debra Lillington, Barts and the London NHS Trust.)*

- ***Bone marrow aspirate***. Increased cellularity is seen, with increased myeloid precursors. Cytogenetics reveals a t(9; 22) translocation (the Philadelphia chromosome; see ***Fig. 17.21B***).
- ***FISH (Fig. 17.23)*** or ***RT-PCR*** is used to demonstrate the cytogenetic/molecular abnormality. These tests are also used to monitor response to therapy quantitatively.

Management

Treatment has been transformed by the advent of imatinib, a tyrosine kinase inhibitor that specifically blocks the enzymatic action of the BCR-ABL fusion protein, and is now first-line treatment for the chronic phase. Imatinib produces a complete haematological response in over 95% of patients, and 70–80% of these have no cytogenetically detectable Ph^+ cells in the marrow (complete cytogenetic remission). A significant proportion will lose molecularly detectable BCR/ABL transcripts from the blood, achieving a molecular remission (MR) of varying depths: MR3 (a 3 log reduction; <0.1%), MR4 (<0.01%) or MR5 (<0.001%). Event-free and overall survival appears to be better than for other treatments. Side-effects of imatinib include nausea, headache, rashes and cytopenia. Imatinib can be continued indefinitely, although it should be stopped before attempts to conceive. Resistance to imatinib as a single agent may develop as a result of secondary BCR/ABL kinase mutations beyond t(9; 22). The use of second-generation TKis, dasatinib and nilotinib, may restore haematological or molecular remissions in those patients in the chronic phase that have primary or acquired resistance to imatinib, or are intolerant of imatinib. Both dasatinib and nilotinib have demonstrated promise in the first-line setting, although it remains to be seen whether their advantage over imatinib in speed and depth of response is sustained over time. Bosutinib and ponatinib are also available for intolerant or resistant patients.

In the acute phase (blast transformation), most patients have only a short-lived response to imatinib and other chemotherapy, as for acute leukaemia, and stem cell transplantation is used in the hope of achieving a durable remission.

Stem cell transplantation. Allogeneic haemopoietic stem cell transplantation (HSCT; pp. 561–562) can cure approximately 70% of chronic-phase CML patients. It is now used in those with an inadequate response to imatinib or disease progression on therapy.

Chronic lymphocytic leukaemia

Chronic lymphocytic leukaemia (CLL) is the most common leukaemia, occurring predominantly in later life and increasing in frequency with advancing years (median age of presentation is between 65 and 67 years). It results from the clonal expansion of small B lymphocytes. The majority of patients are asymptomatic, and are identified as a chance finding on a blood count performed for another indication. Others, however, present with the features of marrow failure or immunosuppression. The median survival is about 10 years and prognosis correlates with clinical stage at presentation ***(Box 17.29)***. A number of cytogenetic and molecular abnormalities are now recognized as being of prognostic significance (see below). This condition may present in leukaemic phase with significant marrow/blood involvement (CLL), or may present as localized disease (small lymphocytic lymphoma, SLL). The tumour cells in each condition are indistinguishable and a similar therapeutic approach is therefore used. A pre-malignant condition, monoclonal B cell lymphocytosis (MBL), exists where there are less than the 5×10^9/L B cells required for a diagnosis of CLL. Some of these have a CLL phenotype and may progress to CLL.

Clinical features

The majority of patients are asymptomatic at presentation. Common symptoms are:

- recurrent infection because of (functional) leucopenia and immune failure (reduced immunoglobulins)
- anaemia due to haemolysis or marrow infiltration
- painless lymphadenopathy
- left upper quadrant discomfort (from splenomegaly).

The most common findings on examination are:

- anaemia
- fever (due to infection)
- lymphadenopathy (may involve a single area or be generalized)
- hepatosplenomegaly, sometimes massive.

However, none of these may be present.

Investigations

- ***Blood count*** reveals a normal or low haemoglobin; a raised white blood cell count, which may be very high; lymphocytosis (criteria for diagnosis $>5 \times 10^9$/L); and normal or low platelets.
- ***Blood film*** demonstrates small or medium-sized mature and normal appearing lymphocytes. Smudge cells may be seen *in vitro*. No immature blasts are evident.
- ***Bone marrow*** reflects peripheral blood, often very heavily infiltrated with lymphocytes.
- ***Immunophenotyping*** shows mainly CD19+, CD5+ or CD23+ B cells with weak expression of CD20, CD79b and surface immunoglobulin (kappa and lambda light chains).

Box 17.29 The Rai and Binet staging systems for chronic lymphocytic leukaemia[a]

Stage	Risk	Manifestations	Patients (%)	Median survival (years)	Recommended treatment
Rai staging system					
0	Low	Lymphocytosis	31	>10	Watch and wait
I	Intermediate	Lymphadenopathy	35	9	Treat only with progression[b]
II	Intermediate	Splenomegaly, lymphadenopathy or both	26	7	Treat only with progression[b]
III	High	Anaemia, organomegaly	6	5	Treat in most cases
IV	High	One or more of the following: anaemia, thrombocytopenia and organomegaly	2	5	Treat in most cases
Binet staging system					
A	Low	Lymphocytosis, <3 lymphoid areas enlarged[c]	63[d]	>10	Watch and wait
B	Intermediate	≥3 lymphoid areas enlarged[c]	30	7	Treat in most cases
C	High	Anaemia, thrombocytopenia or both	7	5	Treat in most cases

[a]Lymphocytosis is present in all stages of the disease. [b]Progression is defined by weight loss, fatigue, fever, massive organomegaly and a rapidly increasing lymphocyte count. [c]Lymphoid areas include the cervical, axillary and inguinal lymph nodes, the spleen and the liver. [d]Stage A includes all patients with Rai stage 0 disease, two-thirds of patients with Rai stage I disease, and one-third of those with Rai stage II.
(From Dighiero G, Binet JL. When and how to treat chronic lymphocytic leukaemia. *N Engl J Med* 2000; 343:1800, with permission.)

- ***Cytogenetics/FISH analyses*** are not essential for diagnosis but help in the assessment of prognosis (see ***Fig. 17.23***).
- ***Direct Coombs' test*** may be positive if there is haemolysis.
- ***Immunoglobulins*** are low or normal.

Prognosis

The clinical course of CLL is variable. Several biomarkers are used to supplement clinical stage and have been shown to predict progression and survival. Cytogenetic abnormalities are detected in >90% of cases. Patients with an isolated deletion of 13q have an excellent prognosis, in contrast to those with either 11q deletion or 17p deletion (sites of the tumour suppressor genes *ATM* and *TP53*, respectively), who tend to have a rapidly evolving clinical course. In those tumours that demonstrate a high level of mutation within the variable region of the rearranged immunoglobulin heavy chain (IgVH) ('mutated'), the clinical course is more indolent than in those where the IgVH sequence more closely resembles that of the germline ('unmutated'). Expression of ZAP70, a 70-kDa tyrosine kinase protein, correlates well with mutational status. Patients with <20% expression of ZAP70 have median 10-year survival of >50%; in >20% expression, the median survival is <5 years. High expression of CD38 on leukaemic cells may also indicate adverse prognosis.

Management

In CLL, the major consideration is when to treat; indeed, 30% of patients will never require intervention. Treatment depends on the 'stage' ***(Box 17.29)*** of the disease. Early-stage disease is usually managed expectantly, advanced-stage disease is always treated immediately; and the approach to the intermediate stage is variable. Absolute indications for treatments are:

- marrow failure, manifest by worsening anaemia and/or thrombocytopenia
- recurrent infection
- massive or progressive splenomegaly or lymphadenopathy
- progressive disease manifest by doubling of the lymphocyte count in 6 months
- systemic symptoms (fever, night sweats or weight loss)
- presence of haemolysis or other immune-mediated cytopenias.

General/supportive treatment

Anaemia due to haemolysis is treated with steroids. Anaemia and thrombocytopenia caused by marrow infiltration is treated with chemotherapy and, when necessary, transfusion. Erythropoietin (see p. 519) may avoid the need for transfusions, particularly in patients receiving chemotherapy. Infection is treated as indicated, with prophylactic antibiotic, antiviral, anti-*Pneumocystis* and antifungal therapy potentially being given during periods of chemotherapy. Immunoglobulin replacement may be helpful, as well as pneumococcal and influenza vaccination. Allopurinol is given to prevent hyperuricaemia.

Specific treatment

Choice of therapy will depend on patient-related factors, such as age and co-morbidity, adverse prognostic features, and anticipated response and toxicities to therapy. Intervention, when indicated, usually causes improvement in symptoms and blood count. The effect on survival is unclear. There is a range of therapies available and these must be tailored to the patient's age, fitness, prior therapy exposure and concurrent co-morbidities. Those individuals with adverse cytogenetics are a particularly difficult group to treat.

- ***Purine analogues***, fludarabine alone or in combination with cyclophosphamide or mitoxantrone (with or without steroids), can induce complete remissions (and MRD-negative remissions), although they are not helpful in patients with 17p deletion or *TP53* mutation.
- ***Rituximab*** used as combination therapy shows a dramatic improvement in response rate, and ***FCR*** (fludarabine, cyclophosphamide, rituximab) has become the standard of care as first-line therapy.
- ***Chlorambucil*** usually reduces the white cell count in older patients and decreases lymphadenopathy and splenomegaly to palliate the disease successfully. Bendamustine is an alternative alkylator that may be appropriate for first-line therapy in older and less fit patients who cannot tolerate FCR.
- ***Alemtuzumab***, a humanized monoclonal antibody targeting CD52, which is highly expressed in B-CLL, is used in those

patients that progress after fludarabine or who have 17p deletion or *TP53* mutation.

- ***Ofatumumab*** is a new-generation anti-CD20 monoclonal antibody that binds to a different epitope to that of rituximab and is used for treatment of fludarabine- or alemtuzumab-refractory CLL. ***Obinutuzumab*** (GA101) is another novel anti-CD20 monoclonal antibody with type 2 binding, associated with increased direct cell death effects. In combination with chlorambucil, it has been shown to be superior to either chlorambucil alone or chlorambucil with rituximab.
- ***Allogeneic stem cell transplantation*** with non-myeloablative conditioning regimens is increasingly performed.

Novel drugs at varying stages of evaluation include lenalidomide and ABT-199 (a BCL-2 inhibitor), as well as three fascinating small molecules that work downstream of the B-cell receptor: ibrutinib (an inhibitor of the enzyme Bruton's tyrosine kinase, BTK), acalabrutinib (a selective inhibitor of BTK), and idelalisib (an inhibitor of phosphoinositide 3-kinase delta, PI3Kδ). These inhibit malignant B-cell survival signalling and disrupt B-cell localization in protective niches within lymph nodes. The consequence is a lymphocytosis, as tumour cells are displaced into the peripheral blood. Current trials are looking at combining these agents with conventional cytotoxics and monoclonals, and evaluating their place in current treatment algorithms.

Lymphomatous transformation

CLL may undergo lymphomatous (Richter's) transformation in 5–10% of cases, most typically to diffuse large B-cell lymphoma, although Hodgkin's-like transformation is recognized. In the main, response to cytotoxic chemotherapy is unsatisfactory and survival short.

Hairy cell leukaemia

Hairy cell leukaemia (HCL) is a clonal proliferation of abnormal B (or, very rarely, T) cells, which, as in CLL, accumulate in the bone marrow and spleen. It is a rare disease; median age at presentation is 52 years and the male to female ratio is 4:1. The bizarre name relates to the appearance of the cells on a blood film and in the bone marrow: they have an irregular outline owing to the presence of filament-like cytoplasmic projections. V600E *BRAF* mutations (see pp. 1373–1374) are seen in the majority of cases.

Clinical features

Clinical features include anaemia, fever and weight loss. Splenomegaly occurs in 80%; lymphadenopathy is uncommon. Anaemia, neutropenia, thrombocytopenia and low monocyte counts are found.

Management

The purine analogues 2-chloroadenosine acetate (2-CDA; cladribine) and pentostatin have specific activity in this condition; complete remission is achieved in 90% with just one cycle of treatment. The remissions can last for many years and patients can be successfully retreated. Rituximab is used in cases that do not respond to the above drugs.

Further reading

Diller L. Adult primary care after childhood acute lymphoblastic leukemia. *N Engl J Med* 2011; 365:1417–1424.

Ferarra F, Schiffe C. Acute myeloid leukaemia in adults. *Lancet* 2013; 381:484–495.

Godley LA. Profiles in leukaemia. *N Engl J Med* 2012; 366:1152–1153.

Inaba H, Greaves M, Mulligan CG. Acute lymphoblastic leukaemia. *Lancet* 2013; 381:1943–1955.

Jaffe ES, Harris NL, Stein H et al (eds). *World Health Organization Classification of Tumours. Pathology and Genetics of Tumours of Haematopoietic and Lymphoid Tissues*. Lyon: IARC Press; 2008.

Shannon K, Armstrong SA. Genetics, epigenetics and leukaemia. *N Engl J Med* 2010; 363:2460–2461.

Wilson WH. Progress in chronic lymphatic leukemia with targeted therapy. *N Engl J Med* 2016; 374:386–388.

THE LYMPHOMAS

The lymphomas are malignancies of the lymphoid system and hence may arise at any site where lymphoid tissue is present. Certain subtypes have increased in frequency over the past 50 years for reasons that are not clear, the overall incidence being 15–20 per 100 000 population, which makes them the fifth most common malignancy in the Western world. Most commonly, patients have peripheral lymphadenopathy or symptoms due to occult lymph nodes, although approximately 20% arise at primary extranodal sites. A relatively small proportion present with lymphoma-associated 'B' symptoms of weight loss, fever and sweats. The natural history and clinical course are determined by the pathological subtype, classified by histological, immunological and molecular criteria, the distribution of the disease ('stage'), non-specific prognostic features and general co-morbidity.

A significant proportion of patients are cured and many others are helped, in terms of both quality and length of life.

The increasingly complex WHO classification of tumours of haemopoietic and lymphoid tissues primarily distinguishes Hodgkin's lymphoma from non-Hodgkin's lymphoma, an umbrella term covering a multiply subclassified spectrum of B- and T-cell malignancies, reflecting the stage of lymphoid development at which they arise. Thus, lymphoblastic lymphoma and lymphoblastic leukaemia are considered as a single entity, as are small lymphocytic lymphoma and chronic lymphatic leukaemia, both discussed in the section above.

Overall management strategy common to all lymphomas

A suspected diagnosis of lymphoma should always be confirmed by an excision biopsy of the relevant tissue large enough to allow histological, immunological and molecular analysis. Cutting needle biopsy is an acceptable substitute for biopsy of impalpable, 'occult' disease but fine needle aspiration is inadequate. The opinion of an expert haemato-pathologist is essential.

Investigations

The diagnosis having been established, treatment strategy and details will depend on the outcome of investigations that are common to all the lymphomas. These investigations are conducted to provide a basis for prognostication and treatment decisions, against which the outcome of treatment may be assessed ***(Box 17.30)***, 'stage' being assigned notionally to the modification of the Ann Arbor classification for all nodal lymphomas, despite the fact that this was planned only for Hodgkin's disease.

The tests listed in ***Box 17.30*** are essential for planning specific therapy. Serum uric acid measurement is helpful, particularly in those lymphomas that carry a risk of tumour lysis syndrome (see p. 606); tests of cardiac function are valuable when potentially cardiotoxic chemotherapy is to be recommended, as is assessment of HIV and hepatitis B and C status.

Once a decision to 'treat' has been made, a course of treatment will begin, during which benefit will be assessed at appropriate

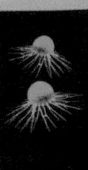

Box 17.30 Investigation of the patient with lymphoma

For diagnosis
- Clinical history and examination
- Chest X-ray for mediastinal widening (see ***Fig. 17.25***)
- CT scan of chest, abdomen, pelvis ± neck
- PET scan (see ***Fig. 17.26***)
- ± Bone marrow biopsy (for stage III or IV, or HIV-positive patients, or patients with B symptoms)
- Blood count, differential, film

For planning specific therapy
- Electrolytes and renal function, liver function tests and biochemistry
- Serum uric acid
- Virology: HIV, hepatitis B and C
- Cardiac function[a]
- Respiratory function[a]
- Fertility[a]

[a]*Depending on circumstances. CT, computed tomography; PET, positron emission tomography.*

Box 17.31 Hodgkin's lymphoma: pathological classification

Nodular lymphocyte-predominant Hodgkin's lymphoma	5%
Classical Hodgkin's lymphoma:	
Nodular sclerosis HL	70%
Lymphocyte-rich HL	5%
Mixed cellularity HL	20%
Lymphocyte-depleted HL	rare

(From Harris NL, Jaffe ES, Diebold J et al. World Health Organization classification of neoplastic diseases of the hematopoietic and lymphoid tissues: report of the clinical advisory committee meeting – Airlie House, Virginia, November 1997. J Clin Oncol *1999; 17:3835–3849, with permission.)*

intervals, and subsequent to which complete re-evaluation ('re-staging') will be performed. Depending on the outcome, future plans will be made. In the event of a decision to stop treatment, surveillance will, in the first instance, be close, the interval between attendances being extended with the passage of time. Beyond 5 years, the focus of attention is on the possible long-term consequences of therapy, rather than the disease itself. When initial therapy has been less successful than wished, management will be dictated by individual circumstances. As conventional treatment becomes exhausted, experimental therapy may be broached.

Hodgkin's lymphoma

Hodgkin's lymphoma (HL) has an incidence of approximately 3 per 100 000 in the Western world; there is a male predominance of approximately 1.3 : 1. The majority of cases occur between the ages of 16 and 65, with a peak in the third decade. The incidence is stable.

Aetiology

There is epidemiological evidence linking previous infectious mononucleosis with HL; up to 40% of patients with HL have increased Epstein–Barr virus (EBV) antibody titres at the time of diagnosis, and EBV DNA has been demonstrated in tissue from patients with HL. These data suggest a role for EBV in pathogenesis. Other viruses have not been detected. Other environmental and occupational exposures to pathogens have been postulated.

Diagnosis

Hodgkin's lymphoma is subclassified, according to the WHO classification ***(Box 17.31)***, into:

- ***Classical Hodgkin's lymphoma*** (***cHL***), the hallmark of which is the Reed–Sternberg cell ***(Fig. 17.24).*** cHL accounts for 90–95% of cases and is further subdivided into four distinct categories.
- ***Nodular lymphocyte predominant HL*** (***NLPHL***), characterized by the Reed–Sternberg cell variant, the 'popcorn cell'.

Clinical features

The most common presentation of HL is painless cervical lymphadenopathy, commonly described in examination as 'rubbery'. Other causes of cervical lymphadenopathy are shown on page 606. A smaller proportion of patients (often young women) present with

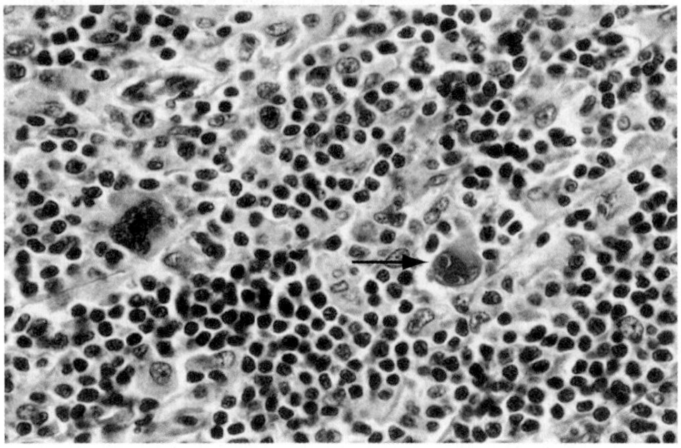

Figure 17.24 Histological appearance of Hodgkin's lymphoma. Scattered mononuclear Hodgkin's cells and a classical malignant binucleate Reed–Sternberg cell (arrowed) are seen to the right of centre on a background of benign small lymphocytes and histiocytes. *(Courtesy of Dr AJ Norton.)*

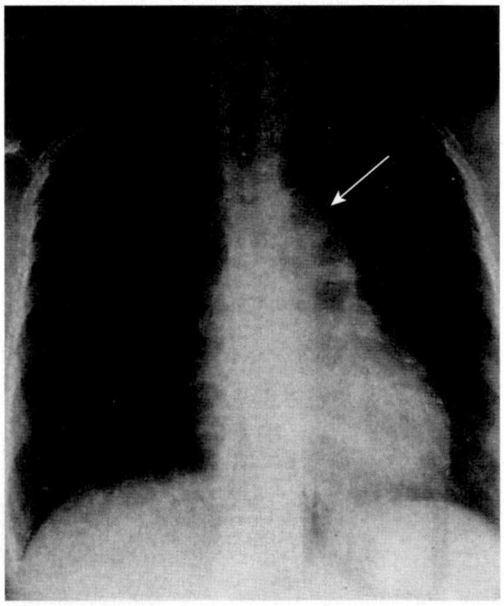

Figure 17.25 Chest X-ray of a mediastinal mass (arrowed) that is due to Hodgkin's lymphoma.

disease localized to the mediastinum, with cough due to mediastinal lymphadenopathy ***(Fig. 17.25)***; others present with 'generalized disease', including hepatosplenomegaly and constitutional 'B' symptoms. Other less common symptoms, undoubtedly associated with HL but not recognized in the staging classification, are pruritus and alcohol-related pain at the site of lymphadenopathy.

Investigations

These are summarized in ***Box 17.30***. Bone marrow biopsy is indicated only in patients with clinically advanced disease (stage III or IV), those with 'B' symptoms and those who are HIV-positive. The clinical utility of the PET scan is becoming established in the management of HL ***(Fig. 17.26)*** to stage a patient accurately and to establish sites of extranodal disease.

'Stage' is currently assigned according to the Cotswolds modification of the Ann Arbor classification, although this is under review ***(Box 17.32)***. The Hasenclever score is used for prognostication ***(Box 17.33)***; however, its relevance to treatment planning is limited because of the very small number of patients at high risk of standard treatment failure. On the basis of 'stage' and other prognostic factors, patients with HL are divided into three groups ***(Box 17.34)***.

Management

Principles of management

Management is aimed towards a curative intent with expectation of success. However, in patients with NLPHL, who usually present with stage I disease with longstanding lymphadenopathy, an expectant policy with close surveillance is followed. Older patients, with or without co-morbidity, require considerable modification of therapy and there is an expectation of success. Patients with HIV infection should be managed, in conjunction with their HIV clinicians, in the same way as those who are seronegative.

Treatment of early-stage, 'low-risk' disease

'Moderate' chemotherapy, comprising 2–4 cycles of doxorubicin, bleomycin, vinblastine and dacarbazine (ABVD), non-sterilizing and of a low second cancer risk, followed by involved field irradiation (20–30 Gy), has replaced large field irradiation (see p. 604), with 90% being cured. Current trials are evaluating the role of PET scanning to see if patients who become 'PET'-negative' after chemotherapy can be spared irradiation altogether. NLPHL is strongly CD20-positive and, as such, is often treated with retuximab-ABVD chemoimmunotherapy.

Box 17.32 Cotswolds modification of Ann Arbor staging of Hodgkin's lymphoma

Stage	Description
I	Involvement of a single lymph-node region or lymphoid structure (e.g. spleen, thymus, Waldeyer's ring) or involvement of a single extralymphatic site
II	Involvement of two or more lymph-node regions on the same side of the diaphragm (hilar nodes, when involved on both sides, constitute stage II disease); localized contiguous involvement of only one extranodal organ or site and lymph-node region(s) on the same side of the diaphragm (IIE). The number of anatomical regions involved should be indicated by a subscript (e.g. II_3)
III	Involvement of lymph-node regions on both sides of the diaphragm (III), which may also be accompanied by involvement of the spleen (IIIS) or by localized involvement of only one extranodal organ site (IIIE) or both (IIISE)
III1	With or without involvement of splenic, hilar, coeliac or portal nodes
III2	With involvement of para-aortic, iliac and mesenteric nodes
IV	Diffuse or disseminated involvement of one or more extranodal organs or tissues, with or without associated lymph-node involvement
Designations applicable to any disease state	
A	No symptoms
B	Fever (temperature >38°C), drenching night sweats, unexplained loss of >10% of body weight within the previous 6 months
X	Bulky disease (a widening of the mediastinum by more than one-third or the presence of a nodal mass with a maximal dimension >10 cm)
E	Involvement of a single extranodal site that is contiguous or proximal to the known nodal site

(From Diehl V, Thomas RK, Re D et al. Hodgkin's lymphoma – diagnosis and treatment. *Lancet Oncology* 2004; 5:19–26. with permission from Elsevier.)

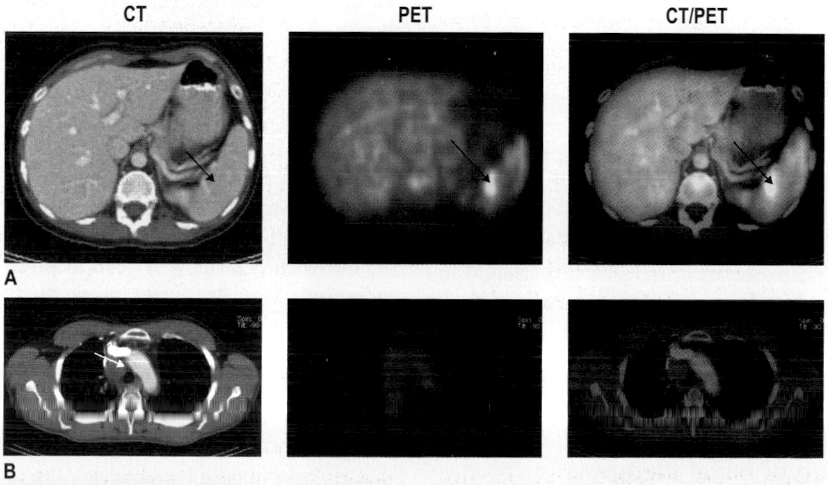

Figure 17.26 Positron emission tomography (PET) and computed tomography (CT) in the investigation of Hodgkin's lymphoma. **A.** Lymphoma in spleen (arrowed) detected on PET (centre) and CT/PET (right), but not on CT (left). **B.** Malignant lymphoma: mediastinal mass on CT scan (left), shown to be metabolically inactive on PET (centre) and PET/CT (right). *(Courtesy of Dr N Avril.)*

Box 17.33 Advanced stage Hodgkin's lymphoma (Hasenclever score)

Clinical prognostic factors	Score	
	0	*1*
Serum albumin	Normal	<40 g/L
Haemoglobin	>105 g/L	<105 g/L
Age	<45	>45
Sex	Female	Male
Stage	<IV	IV
Leucocytosis	<15 × 10^9/L	>15 × 10^9/L
Lymphopenia	>0.6 × 10^9/L	<0.6 × 10^9/L

Cumulative score

Score 0: 84% freedom from progression at 5 years; 7% (of all patients) frequency
Score 1: 77%; 22%
Score 2: 67%; 29%
Score 3: 60%; 28%
Score 4: 51%; 12%
Score 5: 42%; 7%

Box 17.34 Hodgkin's lymphoma: prognostic groups

Prognostic group	Description
Early favourable	Stage I+II without unfavourable prognostic factors
Early unfavourable	Stage I+II with unfavourable factors
Advanced	The remainder

Treatment of advanced disease (including locally advanced, unfavourable, early-stage)

This is also curable for a significant proportion of patients, having a median survival easily exceeding 5 years for 50–60%. Cyclical chemotherapy with 6–8 cycles of ABVD, with involved field irradiation to sites which were initially bulky, or at which there is 'persistent disease' after chemotherapy, is standard. Increasingly, the data from studies incorporating PET scanning, both part way through and after planned chemotherapy, have shown that PET-positive masses are likely to represent fibrous tissue; in this situation, irradiation may be omitted.

The major short-term toxicity relates to myelosuppression and mucositis, the mortality being no more than 1% and the long-term risks being to the heart and lungs. Infertility and second malignancy are uncommon.

The above approach fails for about 25% of patients. More intensive treatment programmes, e.g. BEACOPP with the addition of etoposide (E), procarbazine (P) and prednisolone (P) to the drugs in ABVD, have been tested, with an overall increase in efficacy but greater toxicity profiles (and expense). It remains a challenge to identify those who will be 'ABVD failures' at initial presentation. An alternative is to develop 'risk-adapted' therapy, based on response to the first two cycles of therapy, again with PET scanning, and then to escalate to more intensive therapy when the response is deemed inadequate, or de-escalate when response is superior.

Management of failure of initial therapy

Treatment failure has become a declining problem because of improvements in the outcome of first-line therapy. The median survival from first recurrence is more than 10 years, possibly influenced by the duration of the first remission; it may not be so good if failure occurs after very intensive therapy. Second and third remissions may be achieved with 'appropriate' re-induction therapy, consolidated, if possible, with an autograft. Registry data suggest this may be curative for up to 50%, but follow-up only extends to 15 years.

Experimental approaches

With such excellent results with first- and second-line conventional therapy, experimental treatment is seldom required. The antigen-targeted immunoconjugate, anti-CD-30–auristatin (SGN-35, brentuximab), has shown great efficacy in phase II trials; it is increasingly being used for relapsed patients and is in clinical trials for first line patients as ABrVD, in comparison to standard ABVD with bleomycin. Allogeneic HSCT following myeloablative conditioning has high treatment related mortality and morbidity. Reduced-intensity conditioning HSCT, followed, if necessary, by donor lymphocyte infusion, is being investigated.

Long-term follow-up

The risks of late effects of therapy, particularly second malignancy and cardiac and endocrine problems, require appropriate and indefinite surveillance of patients at 'high risk'.

Non-Hodgkin's lymphomas

As defined by the WHO classification ***(Box 17.35)***, approximately 80% of non-Hodgkin's lymphoma (NHL) is of B-cell origin and 20% of T-cell origin, there being considerable geographical variation. The incidence has increased, not necessarily for all subtypes, from 5 to 15 per 100 000 per year in the last half century.

Aetiology

A family history is associated with a minor increase in risk of lymphoma, and common genetic polymorphisms with only a small risk for an individual may be significant in population terms. Certain inherited syndromes, such as ataxia–telangiectasia and Wiskott–Aldrich syndrome, are associated with an increased risk of lymphoma. The human T-cell leukaemia virus type 1 (HTLV-1) is causally related to adult T-cell lymphoma/leukaemia. *Helicobacter pylori* is known to 'cause' extranodal marginal zone lymphoma in the stomach, and *Chlamydia psittaci* may be implicated in ocular MALT lymphoma. There is a very strong epidemiological relationship between EBV and endemic Burkitt's lymphoma, and a lesser one with sporadic Burkitt's lymphoma and Hodgkin's lymphoma.

Immune suppression, immunosuppressant drugs, particularly as used for solid organ transplantation, and HIV infection are all associated with an increased incidence of lymphoma. Agricultural work is associated with lymphoma, but no other data show any convincing evidence of a link with occupation or lifestyle. In the majority of individual cases, the cause is unknown.

Pathogenesis

Malignant clonal expansion of lymphocytes occurs at different stages of lymphocyte development, leading to the different subtypes of lymphoma ***(Fig. 17.27)***. In general, neoplasms of non-dividing mature lymphocytes are 'indolent', whereas those of proliferating cells (e.g. lymphoblastic) are much more 'aggressive'. Malignant transformation is usually due to errors in gene rearrangements, which occur during the class switch, or gene recombinations

Box 17.35 Modified WHO classification of lymphoid neoplasms other than ALL (2008)

B-cell lymphomas

Mature B-cell lymphoma

- Chronic lymphocytic leukaemia/small lymphocytic lymphoma
- B-cell prolymphocytic leukaemia
- Splenic marginal zone lymphoma
- Hairy cell leukaemia
- Lymphoplasmacytic lymphoma
- Extranodal marginal zone B-cell lymphoma of mucosa-associated lymphoid tissue (MALT-lymphoma)
- Nodal marginal zone B-cell lymphoma
- Follicular lymphoma (aggressive)
- Mantle cell lymphoma
- Diffuse large B-cell lymphoma (aggressive)
- Mediastinal (thymic) large B-cell lymphoma
- Intravascular large B-cell lymphoma
- Primary effusion lymphoma
- Burkitt's lymphoma/leukaemia (highly aggressive)

T/NK cell lymphomas

Mature T/NK cell lymphoma

- T-cell prolymphocytic leukaemia
- T-cell large granular lymphocytic leukaemia
- Chronic/lymphoproliferative disorder of NK cells
- Aggressive NK cell leukaemia
- Adult T-cell leukaemia/lymphoma (very aggressive)
- Extranodal NK/T-cell lymphoma, nasal type
- Enteropathy-type T-cell lymphoma
- Hepatosplenic T-cell lymphoma
- Subcutaneous panniculitis-like T-cell lymphoma
- Mycosis fungoides
- Sézary syndrome
- Primary cutaneous CD30+ peripheral T-cell lymphoproliferative disorders
- Peripheral T-cell lymphoma, unspecified (aggressive)
- Angioimmunoblastic T-cell lymphoma
- Anaplastic large cell lymphoma (aggressive) *ALK*-positive
- Anaplastic large cell lymphoma (aggressive) *ALK*-negative

ALK, anaplastic lymphoma kinase (gene); ALL, acute lymphoblastic leukaemia; NK, natural killer.

(Modified from Jaffe ES, Harris NL, Stein H et al. (eds). World Health Organization Classification of Tumours. Pathology and Genetics of Tumours of Haematopoietic and Lymphoid Tissues. *Lyon: IARC Press; 2008, with permission from the World Health Organization.)*

Box 17.36 Chromosome translocations in non-Hodgkin's lymphoma

Type	Translocation	Genes	Function
Follicular	t(14; 18)	*BCL2/IGH*	Suppressor of apoptosis
Lymphoplasmacytic	t(9; 14)	*PAX5/IGH*	Transcription factor
Mantle cell	t(11; 14)	*CCND1/IGH*	Cell cycle regulator
Diffuse large B cell	t(3; 4)	*BCL6*	Cell cycle regulator
Burkitt's	t(8; 14)	*MYC/IGH*	Transcription factor
Anaplastic	t(2; 5)	*NPM1/ALK*	Tyrosine kinase
MALT	t(11; 18)	*BIRC3/MALT1*	Suppressor of apoptosis

MALT, mucosa-associated lymphoid tissue.

for immunoglobulin and T-cell receptors. Thus, many of the errors occur within immunoglobulin loci or T-cell receptor loci. For example, an abnormal gene translocation may lead to the activation of a proto-oncogene, by moving it next to a promoter sequence for the immunoglobulin heavy chains (Ig-H).

The NHLs are subclassified according to the cell of origin (T or B lineage) and the stage of lymphocytic maturation at which they develop (precursor or mature).

Cytogenetic features

Burkitt's lymphoma was the first tumour in which a cytogenetic change was shown to involve the translocation of a specific gene (*Box 17.36*). The most frequent change is a translocation between chromosomes 8 and 14, in which the *MYC* oncogene is translocated from chromosome 8 to a position near the constant region of the immunoglobulin heavy chain gene on chromosome 14, resulting in upregulation of myc. Similar rearrangements involving the light chain loci are seen in the alternative Burkitt's lymphoma translocations between chromosome 8 and either chromosome 2 or 22. Other somatic cytogenetic abnormalities associated with human lymphoma are the t(14; 18) in follicular lymphoma, involving upregulation of BCL2, or the t(11; 14) in mantle cell lymphoma, involving upregulation of the cell cycle regulator cyclin D1. Gene expression profiling and other molecular techniques are identifying new molecular subclasses of lymphoma with prognostic significance.

Clinical features

The most common presentation overall is with painless lymphadenopathy or with symptoms caused by a lymph node mass. Primary extranodal lymphomas present with soft tissue masses and related symptoms at the relevant site.

The more common subtypes of NHL are described below.

B-cell lymphomas

See *Figure 17.28*.

Follicular lymphoma

This is the second most common NHL (comprising approximately 20% of lymphomas worldwide).

Clinical features and course

Follicular lymphoma occurs in middle to late life, being rare in childhood. The majority of patients will present with painless lymphadenopathy at more than one site, although a small proportion will be ill, some with 'B' symptoms. In the latter, there should be suspicion that the diagnostic biopsy was not representative. This may be the case when the presenting symptom relates to an abdominal mass but a peripheral node is biopsied. Percutaneous needle biopsy of the abdominal mass may reveal transformation to diffuse large B-cell lymphoma, with potentially different management. Bone marrow infiltration is common in certain subtypes.

There have been dramatic improvements in the outcome of therapy since the introduction of antibody therapy (rituximab), targeting the CD20 antigen expressed on almost all B-cell lymphomas, leading to the development of chemoimmunotherapy; to date,

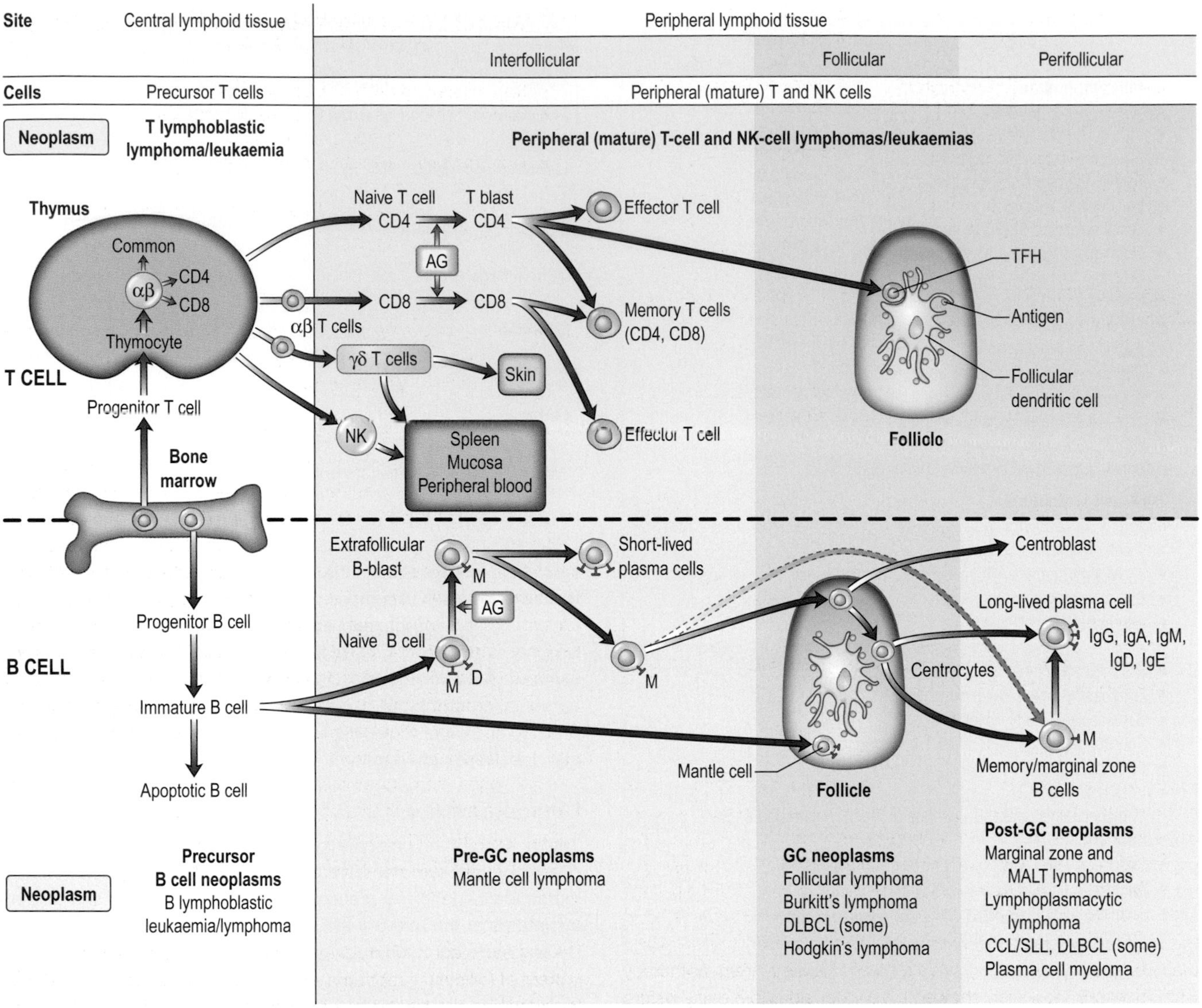

Figure 17.27 Differentiation of T and B lymphocytes and their relationship to neoplasms.
Top (above dotted line): ***T-cell differentiation.*** Progenitor T cells from the bone marrow enter the thymus and develop into different naive T cells. αβ T cells leave the thymus, are exposed to antigen (AG) and undergo blast transformation. They then develop into CD4+ and CD8+ effector and memory T cells. T regulatory cells are the major type of CD4+ effector cells. The other specific effector T cells are the follicular helper T cell (TFH) in the germinal centres (GC). Upon antigenic stimulation, T-cell responses to antigenic stimulation pathways of natural killer cells (NK) and γδ T cells are unknown.
Bottom: ***B-cell differentiation.*** Precursor B cells mature in the bone marrow and undergo apoptosis or mature to naive B cells. Following exposure to antigen and blast transformation, they develop into short-lived plasma cells or enter the GC. Somatic hypermutation and heavy chain class switching occur here (not shown). The transformed cells of the GC (centroblasts) undergo apoptosis or develop into centrocytes. Post-GC cells include long-lived plasma cells and memory/marginal cells.
DLBCL, diffuse large B-cell lymphoma; CLL/SLL, chronic lymphocytic leukaemia/small lymphocytic lymphoma; Ig, immunoglobulin; MALT, mucosa-associated lymphoid tissue; NOS, not otherwise specified. *(Redrawn from information in Swerdlow SH, Campo E, Harris NL et al.* WHO Classification of Tumours of Haematopoietic and Lymphoid Tissues*, 4th edn. Geneva: WHO; 2008.)*

however, the proportion of patients cured has been small. The illness has been shown to regress spontaneously in some cases, which has led to an expectant policy of treatment for many patients. The clinical course following initiation of treatment to date has been that of a remitting–recurring disease, often with several biopsy-proven episodes of lymphadenopathy that are responsive to therapy, albeit usually transiently. Transformation to diffuse large B-cell lymphoma occurs in up to 25% of patients over 15 years and usually heralds a grave prognosis, although this may be improving. Death occurs because of resistant disease, transformed or not, the complications of therapy, or unrelated causes. The median survival now exceeds 10 years. Prognostic factor comprising the FLIPI (follicular lymphoma international prognostic index) are shown in ***Box 17.37***.

Management

General management

Lymph node biopsy, accompanied by appropriate further investigation, should precede any treatment decision. The 'well' patient

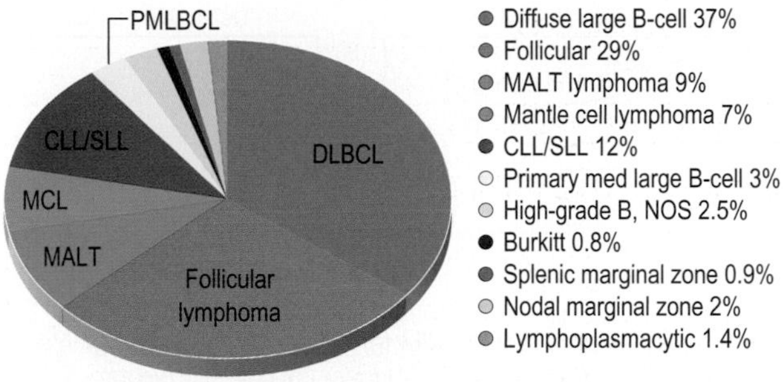

Figure 17.28 Relative frequencies of B-cell lymphoma subtypes in adults. CLL/SLL, chronic lymphocytic leukaemia/small lymphocytic lymphoma; MALT, mucosa-associated lymphoid tissue; NOS, not otherwise specified. *(From Swerdlow SH, Campo E, Harris NL et al. 2008* WHO Classification of Tumours of Haematopoietic and Lymphoid Tissues*, 4th edn. Geneva: WHO; 2008, with permission.)*

Box 17.37 Prognostic factors for survival in non-follicular lymphoma (FLIPI)

- Haemoglobin <120 g/L
- >4 nodal sites involved
- Age >60 years
- Stage III or IV disease
- Elevated serum LDH

FLIPI, Follicular Lymphoma International Prognostic Index; LDH, lactate dehydrogenase.

– variously defined, but certainly having no symptoms, organ impairment, 'bulky disease' or evidence of rapid progression or transformation – should be managed expectantly, after a careful explanation of the rationale. This approach is followed by progression mandating therapy in about 2.5 years for half of the patients, with 20% having had some spontaneous regression and 15% having had no treatment more than 10 years from diagnosis. A large trial comparing expectant management against immunotherapy with rituximab, however, showed a very considerable delay before having the first treatment in the rituximab group. The implications of this are unclear. Indications for treatment of low-grade NHL are shown in ***Box 17.38***.

Initial treatment: early disease

Stage I (possibly stage II) disease is treated with involved field megavoltage irradiation, which almost always induces complete remission, 50% of patients being disease-free after 10–15 years. In terms of overall survival, there are no randomized trials to show this is better than expectant management (i.e. observing and treating if progression occurs). Functional imaging – that is, PET scanning – may identify patients who are in 'surgical CR' post biopsy; no therapy is indicated for this group.

Initial treatment: advanced disease (stages II–IV)

Chemoimmunotherapy incorporating rituximab is the treatment of choice, having been shown in randomized trials to be superior to chemotherapy alone, in terms of disease-free, progression-free and overall survival. 'CHOP-R' (cyclophosphamide, doxorubicin, vincristine and prednisolone plus rituximab) and the less intensive 'R-CVP' (rituximab plus cyclophosphamide, vincristine and prednisolone) are both widely used and R-bendamustine is gaining popularity. Over the next few years, it will become clear which chemotherapy is the best for which group of patients. It has been shown that continuing rituximab 'maintenance' for 2 years has a dramatic effect on progression-free survival, although any benefits for overall survival remain unclear.

Box 17.38 Indications for treatment of low-grade NHL at presentation or progression

- Stage I disease; possibly limited stage II disease
- Advanced disease, i.e. stages II–IV with 'B' symptoms
- Organ impairment (i.e. bone marrow failure)
- Bulky disease (i.e. lymph node mass >10 cm)
- Histological transformation
- Progression of lymphadenopathy after expectant management
- Philosophy of physician and patient

Second therapy and beyond

Patients are managed expectantly in the first instance, provided full re-evaluation, including repeat biopsy, reveals no evidence of transformation. A number of options are available, including re-induction of remission with combined chemoimmunotherapy, followed by rituximab maintenance in those not 'rituximab-resistant'. Myeloablative autologous consolidation chemotherapy is used in younger patients, particularly those in whom the first remission was short. Reduced-intensity conditioning allogeneic HSCT has yielded very impressive results in selected patients and may be curative despite the toxicity of the treatment, due to the presence of a 'graft-versus-lymphoma effect' that can be enhanced by escalating doses of donor lymphocyte infusions.

The biggest challenges lie in patients with 'resistant disease' and in the treatment of 'transformation'. A number of experimental agents with new antibodies, immunomodulatory agents and drugs targeted to specific pathways are showing promise.

Prognosis

There has been a dramatic improvement in the overall survival pattern of follicular lymphoma as the result of introducing anti-CD20 (rituximab) in the treatment of advanced disease. The median survival has been extended, well beyond 10 years in several series, although these may possibly have involved selected patients. Improvements in disease-free survival, after both initial and second-line therapy, are encouraging. It is reasonable to anticipate that further improvement will be seen with the selective use of allogeneic stem cell transplantation and the new targeted therapies under investigation.

Diffuse large B-cell lymphoma

This is the most common adult lymphoma worldwide (increasing in incidence with age) and the second most common lymphoma in childhood, accounting for approximately 30% of all cases. There is a slight male preponderance. There is overlap between classical diffuse large B-cell lymphoma (DLBCL) and Burkitt's lymphoma, certain cases having a germinal centre phenotype and a high proliferative fraction but non-Burkitt morphology and variable occurrence of *MYC* and *BCL2* translocations detected by FISH. Gene expression profiling may, in the future, help place these tumours in the correct category to guide appropriate therapy.

Clinical features

The majority of patients present with painless lymphadenopathy, clinically at one or several sites. Intra-abdominal disease presents with bowel symptoms due to compression or infiltration of the gastrointestinal tract. In a small proportion, there is a primary mediastinal presentation, most often in men, with symptoms and signs akin to those of HL. There may be 'B' symptoms, which should not be confused with symptoms related to the site of involvement. Investigation will lead to the demonstration of either locally or systemically advanced disease in the majority of cases. The illness is itself rapidly progressive without intervention, death occurring within months rather than years. Approximately 30% of cases present at an extranodal site, as opposed to having nodal disease with extranodal spread.

Management

Initial treatment

Treatment should be initiated immediately after the diagnosis is confirmed. In younger patients without co-morbidity, there is a high expectation of cure. Treatment is assigned on the basis of the revised International Prognostic Index (R-IPI; ***Box 17.39*** and ***Fig. 17.29***). Further refinement using gene expression profiling has identified at least two distinct subtypes of DLBCL ***(Fig. 17.30)***: germinal centre cell (GC) and activated B-cell (AB).

Low-risk (IPI score 0–1) with anatomically localized disease

At present, 'CHOP-R' followed by involved field irradiation, or 'more CHOP-R' is used. Interim PET scanning may be used to inform individualization of therapy.

Two studies conducted in France suggest that the prognosis is better with chemotherapy alone, provided 'enough' is given, with more than 80% of younger patients being alive 10 years after therapy. A trial comparing chemotherapy with and without rituximab in all patients with low-risk disease showed a marked advantage for those receiving chemoimmunotherapy. Further studies are awaited ***(Fig. 17.31)***.

Intermediate and poor-risk (IPI score 2+)

The age of the patient and co-morbidity are critical for both the selection of treatment and the prognosis. Recognition of this fact has led to the use of an age-adjusted prognostic index for patients over the age of 60. Chemoimmunotherapy was established to be superior to chemotherapy alone for older patients in this category. 'CHOP-R', to a total of 6 or 8 cycles, has become standard care for the large majority of patients of all ages with DLBCL.

Many trials of increasing intensity of therapy for selected patients have yet to yield convincing results. However, there is an increasing consensus that the small group of patients having DLBCL with 'Burkitt-like features' should be treated as for Burkitt's lymphoma. The ability to distinguish between the molecularly distinct, 'germinal-centre' DLBCL and 'activated B-cell' DLBCL with immunohistochemistry has made it possible to explore different

Box 17.39 Adverse prognostic factors in diffuse large B-cell lymphoma (R-IPI)

- Age >60 years
- Stage III or IV, i.e. advanced disease
- High serum lactate dehydrogenase level
- More than one extranodal site involved
- ECOG performance status 2 or more (see ***Box 17.10***)

ECOG, Eastern Cooperative Oncology Group; R-IPI, revised International Prognostic Index.

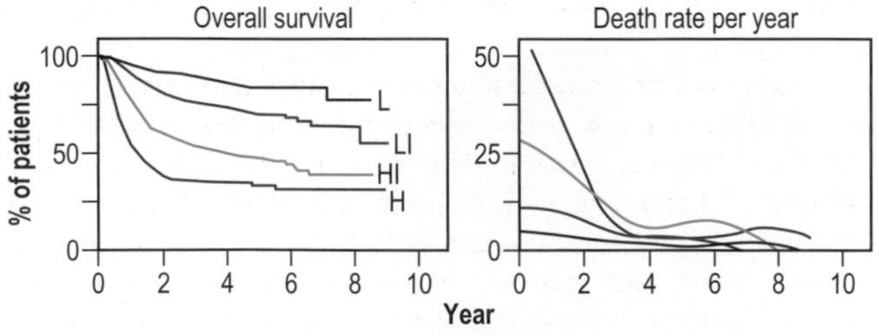

Figure 17.29 A predictive model for aggressive non-Hodgkin's lymphoma. Survival among 1274 younger patients (≤60 years), according to risk group defined by the age-adjusted international index. L, low risk; LI, low to intermediate risk; HI, high to intermediate risk; H, high risk. *(Reproduced with permission from The International Non-Hodgkin's Lymphoma Prognostic Factors Project. A predictive model for aggressive non-Hodgkin's lymphoma.* New Engl J Med *1993; 329(14):987–994.)*

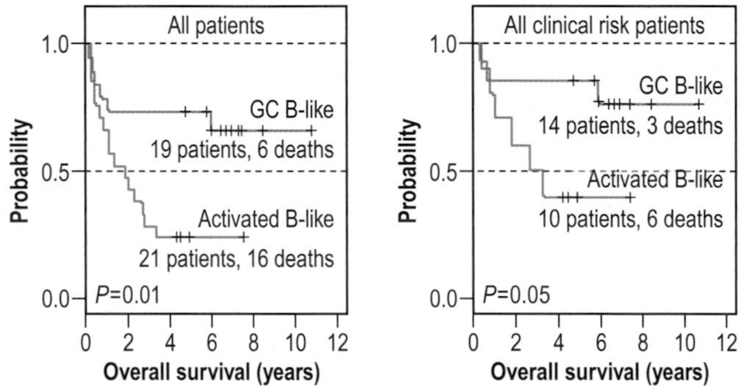

Figure 17.30 Kaplan–Meier plot of overall survival of DLBCL patients. Patients are grouped on the basis of gene expression profiling. GC, germinal centre cell. *(Reproduced with permission from Alizadeh AA. Distinct types of diffuse large B-cell lymphoma identified by gene expression profiling.* Nature *2000; 403(6769):503–511.)*

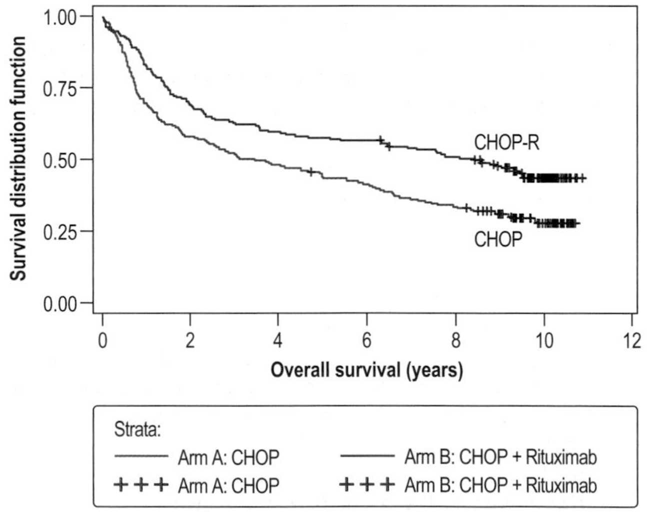

Figure 17.31 Overall survival in patients treated with CHOP and CHOP-R. Median overall survival (OS) was 3.5 years (95% confidence interval (CI): 2.2–5.5) in the CHOP arm and 8.4 years (95% CI: 5.4–not reached) in the CHOP-R arm ($p<0.0001$). DLBCL, diffuse large B-cell lymphoma. *(Reproduced with permission from Coiffier B, Thieblemont C, Van Den Neste E et al. Long-term outcome of patients in the LNH-98.5 trial, the first randomized study comparing rituximab-CHOP to standard CHOP chemotherapy in DLBCL patients: a study by the Groupe d'Etudes des Lymphomes de l'Adulte.* Blood *2010; 116(12):2040–2045.)*

therapeutic approaches in the two groups, with appropriate targeted agents.

Involvement of the central nervous system, most often meningeal, is an uncommon but devastating complication, confirming a very poor prognosis overall. Patients with a high IPI score, and particularly those with specific extranodal sites of involvement (breast, testis, paranasal sinuses, bone marrow) and those who are HIV-positive, should receive intrathecal methotrexate with each cycle of therapy. The management of overt leptomeningeal or parenchymal involvement, often in the context of generalized lymphoma, is difficult and usually unsuccessful in the long term. Most strategies involve high doses of systemic methotrexate and cytarabine (cytosine arabinoside), both of which cross the blood–brain barrier. Cranial or craniospinal irradiation may also be used.

Second (and subsequent) therapy

Although there may be responsiveness initially to alternative chemotherapy, after failure of initial therapy or subsequent progression, the prognosis is very poor. Patients entering a partial remission do better than those in whom disease recurs after they enter an initial complete remission.

The major issues to be addressed are whether treatment is to be undertaken with palliative or curative intent, and if the latter, what are the expectations of success. The ***palliative approach*** involves both chemotherapy and irradiation. The ***curative approach*** involves complete re-evaluation, followed by second-line chemotherapy; this has a proven response rate of approximately 50%. If at least a further partial remission is achieved, in the younger, fitter patient, peripheral blood stem cell harvest is undertaken, followed, if successful, by an autograft. Overwhelmingly, the best results are achieved in those entering an unequivocal second CR. Even so, the proportion of patients in a prolonged second remission does not exceed 25%.

Prognosis

The outlook for patients with DLBCL has improved by at least 15% in terms of cure, with the incorporation of rituximab into the initial therapy, the expectation of cure now being between 40% and 80% depending on the presenting features. The challenge of progressive disease following initial treatment is great, with less than 20% of patients overall staying alive in the long term. Options include palliation, clinical trial entry, lenalidomide, bortezomib combinations or the single agent pixantrone.

Burkitt's lymphoma

This is the most rapidly proliferating lymphoma, with a doubling time approaching 100% and a very rapid evolution. The most common childhood malignancy worldwide, it has a male to female preponderance of approximately 3 : 1 and occurs at all ages. There are three types:

- Endemic:
  - Always Epstein–Barr virus (EBV)-associated
  - Occurs in equatorial Africa
  - Corresponds to the distribution of malaria.
- Sporadic:
  - 30% EBV-related
- AIDS-related.

A similar picture to AIDS-related lymphoma may appear post transplant.

The most common presenting feature in the endemic type is a rapidly growing jaw tumour in a young child ***(Fig. 17.32)***. The next

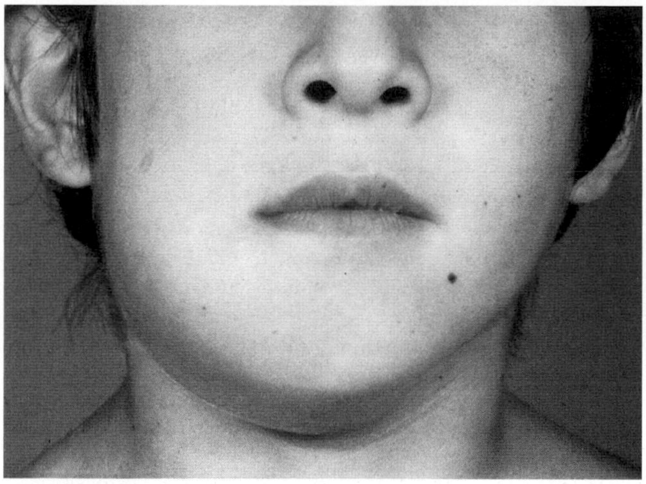

Figure 17.32 A child with Burkitt's lymphoma.

most common is an abdominal mass that is often associated with bone marrow involvement. Other common sites are the central nervous system, the kidney and the testis.

Investigation is along conventional lines for lymphoma, at least in the Western world, but must be conducted as a matter of urgency. A different staging classification is applied to children.

Management

Burkitt's lymphoma should be treated with curative intent whenever feasible, regardless of HIV status. Investigation having been completed, it is essential that the patient is haemodynamically and metabolically stable prior to the initiation of specific therapy. Particular attention must be paid to the risk of the tumour lysis syndrome so rasburicase prophylaxis should be given if available (see p. 606). If it is not, other standard measures based on fluids and allopurinol should be pursued to minimize the risk of tumour lysis syndrome. Very frequent monitoring of electrolyte balance is essential for at least 72 hours after treatment is commenced, with particular attention to potassium and phosphate levels.

Standard treatment comprises, if possible, intensive, cyclical combination chemotherapy, including cyclophosphamide, methotrexate and cytarabine in high doses. Rituximab is now included, although the evidence base for this is minimal. The details and number of cycles administered will be determined by the perceived level of 'risk'. Prophylactic central nervous system therapy is essential, intrathecal methotrexate or cytarabine often being given in addition to high-dose systemic administration.

Prognosis

In the Western world, the prognosis of Burkitt's lymphoma has improved markedly over the past 10 years. The chances of cure are very high for 'low-risk' patients and exceed 50% for 'poor-risk' patients, as well as the HIV-positive cases, provided all treatment can be administered.

Failure to achieve CR is a very poor prognostic factor, as is recurrence, which supervenes within the first year after completion of initial therapy if it does so at all. Although there may be further chemoresponsiveness, it is rare for second-line therapy to be more than transiently beneficial, regardless of whether it is followed by consolidation, with either myeloablative chemotherapy or allogeneic haemopoietic stem cell transplantation.

Mantle cell lymphoma

This is one of the less common B-cell lymphomas, usually presenting in later life, with a male to female preponderance of 3:1. The most frequent presentation is with painless lymphadenopathy, often generalized. There may be non-specific symptoms of tiredness, or ones related to the gastrointestinal tract. 'B' symptoms occur in <50%. Examination and standard investigation usually confirm generalized lymphadenopathy with or without hepatosplenomegaly ***(Fig. 17.33)***. Patients with bowel symptoms frequently have multiple lesions found on endoscopy. The bone marrow is usually involved and there may well be lymphoma cells in the peripheral blood. The t(11; 14) translocation with dysregulation of cyclin D1 is a classical feature of this lymphoma.

Management

In the majority of patients, therapy is started after investigation has been completed. It is usual for there to be regression of disease with chemotherapy, although it is not often that CR is achieved. A prognostic index is used to help determine whether more or less 'aggressive' treatment is best employed. In reality, the major determining factors are the age of the patient and the presence or absence of co-morbidities. The outcome is likely to be best when 'more' treatment is given. Hence, younger, fitter patients are now treated with relatively intensive chemoimmunotherapy, incorporating cycles of high-dose cytarabine as well as rituximab, followed by, in first remission, myeloablative chemotherapy with autologous stem cell rescue. Older, less fit patients are treated with less intensive therapy, such as CHOP-R or bendamustine. In general, the strategy is to stop treatment after the planned initial course of treatment, provided the patient is well and at least a partial remission has been achieved. Almost inevitable progression occurs in both older and younger patients, palliation being the expectation for most. Experimental approaches include reduced-intensity allogeneic HSCT and novel drugs targeting both the NFκB and mammalian target of rapamycin (mTOR) pathways, such as bortezomib and temsirolimus, respectively. In a recent study, replacement of vincristine with bortezomib in combination therapy has shown benefit.

Recently, two other drugs that inhibit malignant B-cell survival signalling and disrupt B-cell localization in their protective niches within lymph nodes have been successfully trialled in mantle cell lymphoma. These are ibrutinib (BTK inhibitor) and idelalisib (PI3Kδ inhibitor). Current trials are under way looking at combining these agents with current standards of care such as CHOP-R or R-bendamustine.

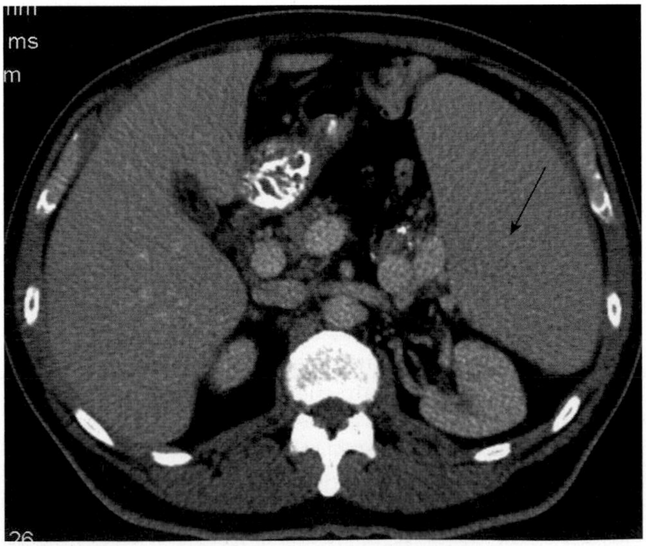

Figure 17.33 CT of the abdomen of a patient with mantle cell lymphoma (arrowed). Significant splenomegaly is also shown.

Prognosis

Untreated mantle cell lymphoma has a natural history that lies between that of DLBCL and follicular lymphoma. The prognosis has improved in recent years with the introduction of treatment strategies that have prolonged the period of remission without curing the patient, and with the discovery of new agents, bringing the overall median survival nearer 5 years.

Lymphoplasmacytic lymphoma

This is an uncommon B-cell malignancy, which is known as ***Waldenström's macroglobulinaemia*** when associated with an IgM paraprotein and bone marrow infiltration. It usually occurs in later life, the incidence being approximately the same in men and women. It may be preceded by a pre-lymphomatous phase, in which a small, monoclonal IgM band is present for many years; it is often an incidental finding. The presentation is with lymphadenopathy or, alternatively, symptoms of anaemia or hyperviscosity caused by the paraprotein (e.g. headaches, visual disturbance). Examination and investigation usually reveal little beyond minimal adenopathy and, commonly, splenomegaly.

Management

Following completion of investigation, the critical decision is whether to initiate specific therapy or not. In an emergency, with severe symptoms of hyperviscosity, it is most appropriate to lower the paraprotein by plasmapheresis. In some circumstances, particularly in the otherwise less fit, it may be best to use maintenance pheresis and blood transfusion as the primary therapy. Responses are seen in about 50% of cases, with a fall in the paraprotein to 50% of the baseline level with single-agent therapy and higher with combination chemotherapy and rituximab. Ibrutinib has shown promise in a recent study, particularly with *MYD88* and *CXCR4* mutations. Treatment, either repeating the initial therapy or changing it, is reinstated only when progression is clearly documented, most often by a fall in the haemoglobin or a significant rise in the M band. In the very small proportion of younger patients for whom CR is achieved, consolidation with a bone marrow transplant is used. Similarly, in the same group of patients who have recurrent disease, which is again responsive, allogeneic HSCT is also used.

Prognosis

Lymphoplasmacytic lymphoma is a relatively rare chemotherapy- and immunotherapy-sensitive disease, which may follow an indolent course for some years without therapy. Although the median survival is only 5 years, 10–20% of patients die of unrelated causes as it presents in later life.

Primary extranodal lymphoma

Lymphoma may arise anywhere in the body where there is lymphoid tissue and therefore the clinical presentation is that of a lesion or mass at the relevant site. In practice, the majority occur in the central nervous system, stomach or skin.

Primary central nervous system lymphoma

This diffuse, large B-cell lymphoma occurs in both the immunocompetent (predominantly the elderly) and the immunosuppressed, in the context of HIV infection or following solid organ transplant. It presents with symptoms relating to single or multiple parenchymal mass lesions. The diagnosis needs to be made on the basis of a biopsy, particularly in the immunocompromised, in whom an infectious aetiology of the symptoms is possible, such as toxoplasmosis. An MRI scan is the first choice of investigation; cerebrospinal fluid is usually normal. Further investigation is necessary to exclude the cerebral lesion being a manifestation of generalized disease.

Management

In some patients in the post-transplant setting, reduction of immunosuppression may be beneficial. Chemotherapy alone, with high-dose methotrexate and cytarabine, is used. The best 'disease-free' results have possibly been obtained by the use of chemotherapy and irradiation but toxicity is greater, with a risk of irreversible loss of cerebral function. The overall results are disappointing, only a small proportion of patients remaining alive in the long term without disability. The situation in the HIV-positive patient with cerebral lymphoma (fortunately, a declining problem) is much worse and palliative irradiation is the best option.

Primary gastric lymphoma

This B-cell lymphoma, either extranodal marginal-zone lymphoma of mucosa-associated lymphoid tissue (MALT) or DLBCL arising on a background of MALT lymphoma, is closely related to *Helicobacter* infection. It presents with symptoms of gastric ulceration or a mass, indigestion or bleeding; the diagnosis is made by endoscopic biopsy to include both the confirmation of lymphoma and *H. pylori* status. This is followed by investigation as for nodal lymphoma, which reveals local nodal involvement in a proportion of patients and distant spread in a small number only.

Management

Management is entirely dependent on whether or not there is any evidence of DLBCL. If only 'low-grade' gastric 'MALT' lymphoma is present, *Helicobacter* eradication therapy is the treatment of choice (see p. 380). This almost invariably alleviates the symptoms. Re-evaluation is carried out after 3 months with endoscopy, repeat biopsy and, in some circumstances, endoscopic ultrasound. In general, a conservative approach is followed, as responses may take many months to achieve and rapid progression is very unlikely. Regular endoscopy every 6 months should be continued for at least 2 years. Failure is not common. If it does occur, it is rarely rapid and the biopsy should be repeated. If the histology is unchanged after further *Helicobacter* eradication therapy (if necessary), either irradiation to the gastric bed or chemoimmunotherapy is likely to be effective or possibly curative. Overall, the prognosis is very good, the very large proportion of patients being alive 10 years after diagnosis.

Any evidence of DLBCL is an indication for chemoimmunotherapy. *Helicobacter* eradication therapy should also be given, but should not be considered definitive treatment. The potential risk of gastric perforation or haemorrhage because of therapy is not a contraindication to treatment. Surgery is rarely needed, but irradiation is used for persistent disease. The prognosis is approximately the same as for nodal DLBCL of equivalent extent.

Primary cutaneous (T- or B-cell) lymphoma

Lymphomas of both B- and T-cell types may arise singly and multiply in the skin and pursue a very long natural history, even though they may give rise to considerable discomfort.

Mycosis fungoides (Sézary syndrome)

This is the most common cutaneous lymphoma, predominantly arising in and confined to the skin, although spreading to other organs later in the disease. It has a long natural history, being sometimes preceded by a scaly 'pre-mycotic phase'. This T-cell lymphoma presents with multiple erythematous lesions, plaques and tumours, which, when associated with spread to the blood, become the Sézary syndrome. Generalized erythema may occur (erythroderma). The likelihood over time of disease extending beyond the skin is highest in patients with tumours.

Management

Treatment is palliative and there is little indication that the disease is ever eradicated. Many treatments result in regression of disease. Phototherapy (PUVA), topical steroids and topical chemotherapy all produce a response. Radiation is effective, and total skin electron beam therapy particularly so, although attention must be paid to potential side-effects, including erythroderma. Systemic chemotherapy, either at conventional or high doses, has been disappointing. Newer approaches include anti-T-cell antibodies and histone deacetylase inhibitors.

The median survival is approximately 10 years, there being a close correlation with the extent of disease at presentation. Interaction between oncologist and dermatologist is essential.

Cutaneous B-cell lymphoma

The two major subtypes have their origins in the extranodal marginal zone or follicle centre. Both usually present with either single or clustered cutaneous lesions, biopsy of which confirms the diagnosis. All conventional staging investigations are negative. Treatment is either expectant, surgical excision or irradiation, which may be used repeatedly over time. Antibiotics are used for marginal-zone lymphoma if there is evidence of *Borrelia burgdorferi* infection. Only if there are lesions at multiple sites should systemic chemotherapy be used. The long-term prognosis is excellent.

T-cell and natural killer cell lymphomas

These are much less common than their B-cell counterparts, although they are relatively more frequent in the East than the West. The most common presentations are nodal or cutaneous (see p. 1374) and specific subtypes involve the liver and subcutaneous tissue ***(Fig. 17.34)***. Peripheral T-cell lymphomas with nodal presentation have a poor prognosis. They are treated as for DLBCL without rituximab.

The two most common subtypes of nodal T-cell lymphoma are 'peripheral T-cell lymphoma, not otherwise specified (NOS)' and 'angioimmunoblastic T-cell lymphoma', which together account for about 50% of T-cell lymphomas. Both occur in the middle-aged to elderly population, the primary presentation being lymphadenopathy. In contrast to the B-cell lymphomas, 'B symptoms' are common. Patients with angioimmunoblastic T-cell lymphoma also present with features akin to inflammatory disease, with fevers, rashes and electrolyte abnormalities; in the first instance, these may be rapidly responsive to corticosteroids or low doses of alkylating agents.

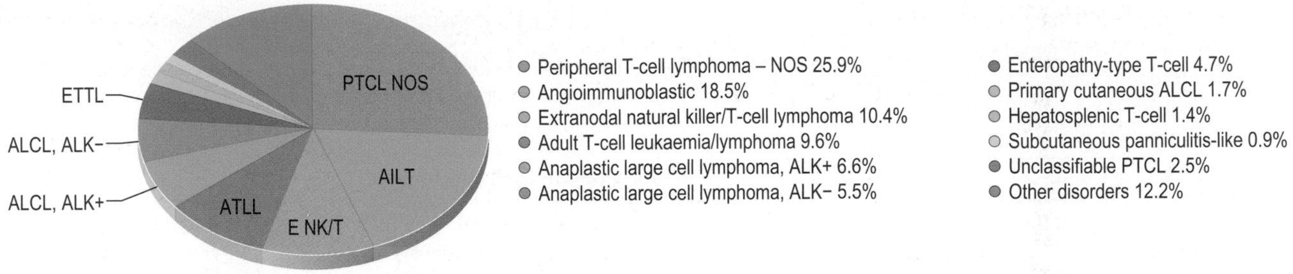

Figure 17.34 Relative frequencies of T-cell lymphoma subtypes in adults. NOS, not otherwise specified. *(Reproduced with permission from WHO. Swerdlow SH, Campo E, Harris NL et al.* WHO Classification of Tumours of Haematopoietic and Lymphoid Tissues, *4th edn. Geneva: WHO; 2008;* ***Fig 8.07****.)*

Management

Following standard investigation, which usually reveals widespread disease, patients are treated with cyclical combination chemotherapy as used for DLBCL. CD20 is not expressed on T cells so rituximab is not used and, as yet, there is no equivalent drug for T-cell lymphoma. Resolution of symptoms almost invariably occurs, although they may recur between cycles. Overall, the outcome of treatment is worse than for DLBCL, in terms of quality of response, duration of response and overall survival. Second-line therapy is rarely satisfactory, although a small proportion of patients may benefit from myeloablative therapy to consolidate a second response.

Further reading

Armitage JO. Early-stage Hodgkin's lymphoma. *N Engl J Med* 2010; 363:653–662.
Good DJ, Gascoyne RD. Classification of non-Hodgkin's lymphoma. *Hematol Oncol Clin North Am* 2008; 22:781–805.
Lister TA, Crowther D, Sutcliffe SB et al. Report of a committee convened to discuss the evaluation and staging of patients with Hodgkin's disease: Cotswolds meeting. *J Clin Oncol* 1989; 7:1630–1636.
Magrath IT, Boffetta P, Potter M (eds). *The Lymphoid Neoplasms*, 3rd edn. London: Hodder Arnold; 2010.
Mahadevan D, Fisher RI. Novel therapeutics for aggressive non-Hodgkin's lymphoma. *J Clin Oncol* 2011; 29:1876–1884.
Molyneux EM, Rochford R, Griffin B et al. Burkitt's lymphoma. *Lancet* 2012; 379:1234–1244.
Relander T, Johnson NA, Farinha P et al. Prognostic factors in follicular lymphoma. *J Clin Oncol* 2010; 28:2902–2913.
Robak T, Huang H, Jin J et al. Bortezomib-based therapy for newly diagnosed mantle cell lymphoma. *New Engl J Med* 2015; 372:944–953.
Salles G, Seymour JF, Offner F et al. Rituximab maintenance for 2 years in patients with high tumour burden follicular lymphoma responding to rituximab plus chemotherapy (PRIMA): a phase 3 randomised controlled trial. *Lancet* 2011; 377:42–51.
Shankland KR, Armitage JO, Hancock BW. Non-Hodgkin lymphoma. *Lancet* 2012; 380:848–857.
Swerdlow SH, Campo E, Harris NL et al. *WHO Classification of Tumours of Haematopoietic and Lymphoid Tissues*, 4th edn. Geneva: WHO; 2008.
Townsend W, Linch D. Hodgkin's lymphoma in adults. *Lancet* 2012; 380:836–847.
Viviani S, Zinzani PL, Rambaldi A et al. for the Michelangelo Foundation, the Gruppo Italiano di Terapie Innovative nei Linfomi and the Intergruppo Italiano Linfomi. ABVD versus BEACOPP for Hodgkin's lymphoma when high-dose salvage is planned. *N Engl J Med* 2011; 365:203–212.

MYELOMA

Myeloma is a malignant disease of bone marrow plasma cells, accounting for 1% of all malignant disease. There is a clonal expansion of abnormal, proliferating plasma cells producing a monoclonal paraprotein, mainly IgG (55%) or IgA (20%), and rarely IgM and IgD. The paraproteinaemia may be associated with excretion of light chains in the urine (Bence Jones protein), which are either kappa or lambda. In approximately 20%, there is no paraproteinaemia, only light chains in the urine. Rarely, patients produce no paraprotein or light chains – this is termed 'non-secretory myeloma' (<5%).

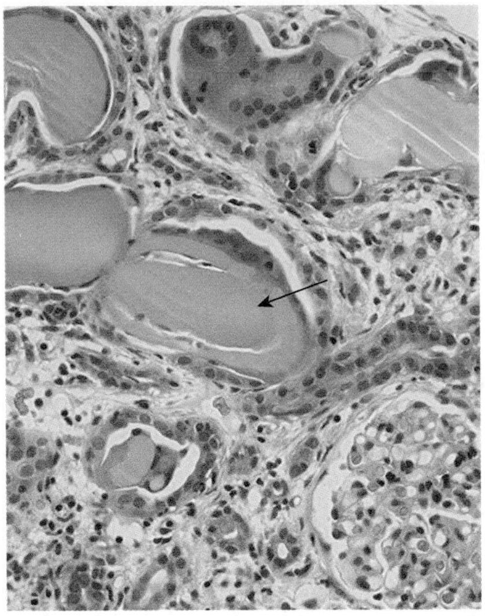

Figure 17.35 Kidney biopsy of a patient with myeloma and acute kidney injury due to light chain cast nephropathy. *(Courtesy of Professor Michael Sheaff, Barts and The London NHS Trust.)*

Clinicopathological features

Myeloma is a disease of the elderly, the median age at presentation being over 60 years. It is rare under 40 years of age. The annual incidence is 4 per 100 000 and it is more common in males and in black Africans, but less common in Asians. The clinical features include:

- ***Bone destruction***, often causing fractures of long bones or vertebral collapse (which can cause spinal cord compression) and hypercalcaemia. Soft tissue plasmacytomas also occur and they are the usual cause of spinal cord compression in myeloma.
- ***Bone marrow infiltration with plasma cells***, resulting in anaemia, neutropenia and thrombocytopenia, together with production of the paraprotein, which may (rarely) result in symptoms of hyperviscosity.
- ***Kidney injury*** (see p. 751) owing to a combination of factors: deposition of light chains in the renal tubules ***(Fig. 17.35)***, hypercalcaemia, hyperuricaemia, use of NSAIDs and, rarely, the deposition of AL amyloid (see p. 1288).

In addition, there is a reduction in the normal immunoglobulin levels (immune paresis), contributing to the tendency for patients with myeloma to have recurrent infections, particularly of the

Box 17.40 WHO (2008) classification of plasma cell neoplasms

- Monoclonal gammopathy of undetermined significance
- Plasma cell myeloma
- Solitary plasmacytoma of bone
- Extraosseous plasmacytoma
- Monoclonal immunoglobulin deposition diseases
- Heavy chain diseases:
  - Gamma (γ) heavy chain disease
  - Mu (μ) heavy chain disease
  - Alpha (α) heavy chain disease

Box 17.41 Life-threatening complications of myeloma

- ***Renal impairment*** – often a consequence of hypercalcaemia – requires urgent attention and patients may need to be referred for long-term peritoneal dialysis or haemodialysis
- ***Hypercalcaemia*** should be treated by rehydration and use of bisphosphonates, such as pamidronate
- ***Spinal cord compression*** due to myeloma is treated with dexamethasone, followed by radiotherapy to the lesion delineated by a magnetic resonance imaging scan
- ***Hyperviscosity*** due to high circulating levels of paraprotein may be corrected by plasmapheresis

respiratory tract. The WHO classification (2008) of plasma cell neoplasms is shown in ***Box 17.40***.

Cytogenetics

With FISH and microarray techniques, abnormalities are found in most cases of myeloma. Abnormalities of chromosome 13 and hypodiploidy (<45 chromosomes) have been shown to be associated with poor survival, as have t(4; 14), t(14; 16) and *p53* (17p) deletions. Conversely, t(11; 14) and hyperdiploidy (>50 chromosomes) are associated with a better prognosis.

Bone disease

There is dysregulation of bone remodelling, which leads to the typical lytic lesions, usually seen in the spine, skull, long bones and ribs. In myeloma, there is increased osteoclastic activity with no increased osteoblast formation of bone. Bisphosphonates that inhibit osteoclast activity are useful in myeloma but, surprisingly, there is no increase in bone deposition.

Adhesion of stromal cells to myeloma cells stimulates the production of receptor activator of nuclear factor kappa-B ligand (RANKL), IL-6 and also VEGF, which plays a role in angiogenesis. RANKL also stimulates osteoclast formation and the lytic lesions. Myeloma cells also produce dickkopf-1 (DKK1), which inhibits osteoblast activity and therefore production of new bone. This occurs because DKK1 binds to the Wnt co-receptor, lipoprotein receptor-related protein 5 (LRP5), inhibiting Wnt signalling (see p. 98) and osteoblast differentiation.

Symptoms

- Bone pain: most commonly backache, owing to vertebral involvement (60%).
- Symptoms of anaemia.
- Recurrent infections.
- Symptoms of renal failure (20–30%).
- Symptoms of hypercalcaemia.
- Rarely, symptoms of hyperviscosity and bleeding due to thrombocytopenia.

Patients can be asymptomatic, the diagnosis being suspected by abnormal 'routine' blood tests. Life-threatening complications are shown in ***Box 17.41***.

Investigations

General

- ***Full blood count***. Haemoglobin, white blood cell count and platelet count are normal or low.
- ***Erythrocyte sedimentation rate***. This is often high.
- ***Blood film***. There may be rouleaux formation as a consequence of the paraprotein and circulating plasma cells in the aggressive plasma cell leukaemia variant of myeloma.

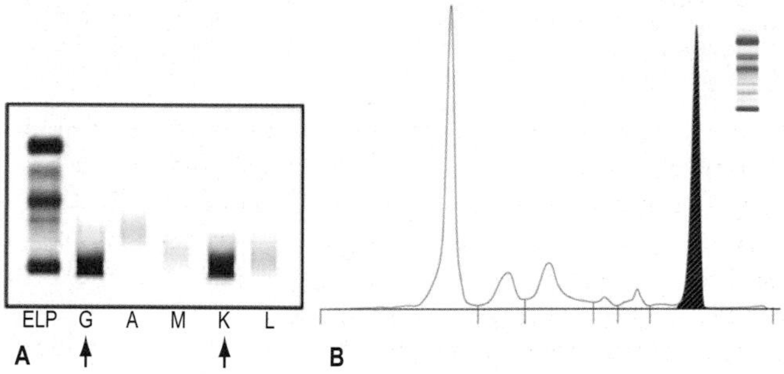

Figure 17.36 Serum protein electrophoresis and immunofixation. **A.** Immunofixation of immunoglobulin G (IgG) kappa monoclonal paraprotein. **B.** Quantitation and serum electrophoresis of IgG paraprotein. Serum electrophoresis and immunofixation of a patient with an IgG K paraprotein (left). The column on the far left is the total serum electrophoresis stained with anti-protein reagents. Albumin is at the top and the increased immunoglobulins at the bottom. These are shown to stain with anti-IgG and anti-kappa light chain reagents (arrows). The paraprotein is quantified (right) by calculating the area under the paraprotein spike and comparing it with the albumin concentration. A, immunoglobulin A; ELP, electrophoresis; G, immunoglobulin G; K, kappa; L, lambda; M, immunoglobulin M.

- ***Urea and electrolytes***. There may be evidence of kidney injury (see above).
- ***Serum calcium***. This is normal or raised. Serum alkaline phosphatase is usually normal.

Immunological

- ***Total protein*** is normal or raised.
- ***Serum protein electrophoresis and immunofixation*** characteristically shows a monoclonal band and immune paresis ***(Fig. 17.36)***. The serum free light chain assay, more sensitive than urine electrophoresis, may show an abnormal ratio and an increased total amount of free kappa or lambda chains, and is often abnormal earlier than routine electrophoresis.
- ***Twenty-four-hour urine electrophoresis and immunofixation*** is used for assessment of light-chain excretion.

Radiological

- ***Skeletal survey*** may show characteristic lytic lesions, most easily seen in the skull ***(Fig. 17.37)***. CT, MRI and PET are used in plasmacytomas (bone or soft tissue deposits).
- ***MRI spine*** is useful if there is back pain; it may show imminent compression/collapse.

Other

Bone marrow aspirate or trephine shows characteristic infiltration by plasma cells ***(Fig. 17.38)***. Amyloid may be found (see pp. 1288–1289).

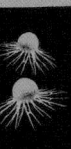

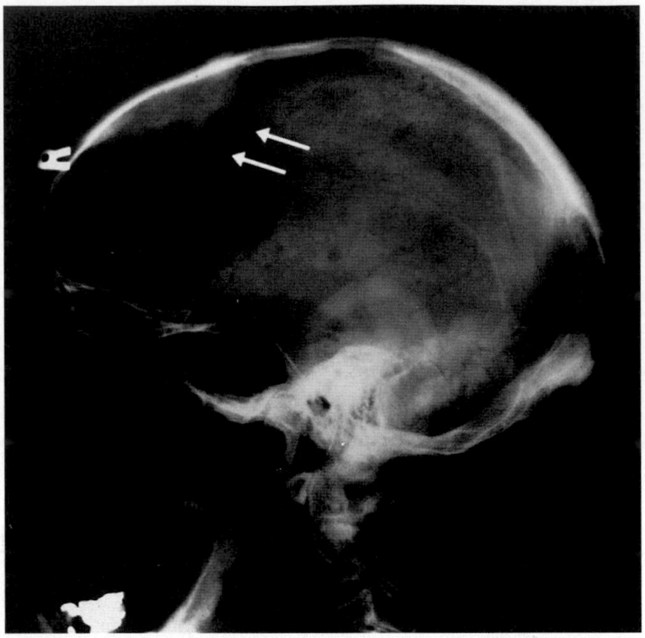

Figure 17.37 Myeloma affecting the skull. Note the rounded lytic translucencies produced by infiltration of the skull with myeloma cells (arrowed).

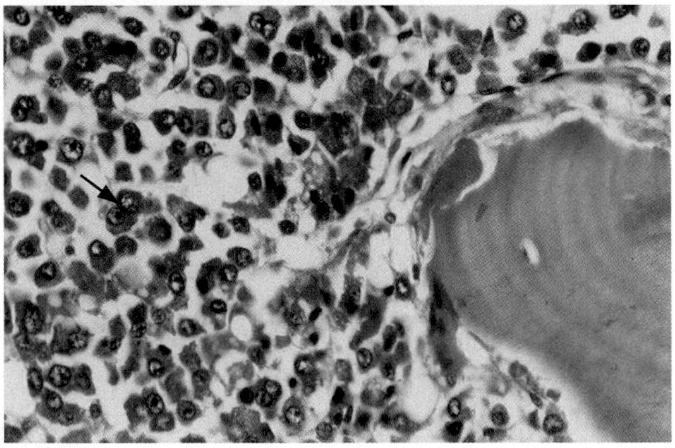

Figure 17.38 Multiple myeloma. Histology shows replacement of the medullary cavity by abnormal plasma cells with some binucleate forms (arrowed). A residual bony trabeculum is present towards the right. *(Courtesy of Dr AJ Norton.)*

Box 17.42 International prognostic index based on serum albumin and β_2-microglobulin (β_2M) for multiple myeloma

Stage	Median survival (months)
Stage 1 – β_2M <3.5 mg/L and serum albumin ≥35 g/L	62
Stage 2 – not stage 1 or 3	44
Stage 3 – β_2M >5.5 mg/L	29

Prognosis

Reduced serum albumin, increased serum β_2-microglobulin and increased serum lactate dehydrogenase (LDH) indicate a poor prognosis at diagnosis ***(Box 17.42)*** on an international prognostic index.

Diagnosis

Symptomatic myeloma (***SMM***) can be diagnosed if either of the following is present:

- significant paraproteinaemia (see ***Fig. 17.36***)
- increased bone marrow plasma cells (>10%); (see ***Fig 17.38***).

with evidence of end-organ failure: that is, hyper*c*alcaemia, *r*enal impairment, *a*naemia and lytic *b*one lesions (CRAB).

Asymptomatic myeloma (***AMM***; 10% of cases) has a significant paraprotein (IgG or IgA >30 g/dL or urinary light chain excretion >1 g/day) and/or a marrow plasmacytosis >10% but no end-organ damage. The median time to progression for these patients is 2–3 years. The risk is highest for those with IgA isotype and light chains in the urine.

Monoclonal gammopathy of unknown significance (***MGUS***) describes an isolated finding of a monoclonal paraprotein in the serum, usually in the elderly, that does not fulfil the diagnostic criteria for SMM or AMM. Between 20% and 30% go on to develop multiple myeloma over a 25-year period. Low-risk MGUS is characterized by an IgG subtype, a paraprotein <15 g/dL and a normal serum free light chain ratio.

Plasmacytoma is an isolated tumour of neoplastic plasma cells. Patients may present with a plasmacytoma and no evidence of multiple myeloma. This may be a 'solitary plasmacytoma of bone' within the skeleton or an 'extramedullary plasmacytoma' outside the marrow cavity, typically in the upper aerodigestive tract.

For paraprotein-associated neuropathy and POEMS syndrome, see page 884.

Management

With good supportive care and chemotherapy, median survival is now 5 years, some patients surviving to 10 years. Young patients receiving more intensive therapy may live longer.

Supportive therapy

- Anaemia should be corrected; blood transfusion may be required. Erythropoietin often helps. Transfusion should be undertaken slowly in patients with hyperviscosity.
- Hypercalcaemia, kidney injury and hyperviscosity should be treated as indicated (see pp. 606 and 772–773).
- Infection should be treated promptly with antibiotics. Give pneumococcal and yearly influenza vaccinations.
- Bone pain can be alleviated most rapidly by radiotherapy and systemic chemotherapy or high-dose dexamethasone. NSAIDs are usually avoided because of the risk of acute kidney injury. Bisphosphonates, such as zoledronate, which inhibit osteoclast activity, help ensure rapid normocalcaemia and, given long-term, reduce skeletal events such as pathological fracture, cord compression and bone pain.
- Pathological fractures may also be prevented by prompt orthopaedic surgery with pinning of lytic bone lesions at critical sites seen on the skeletal survey, such as the femoral shaft. Kyphoplasty and vertebroplasty may be useful in treating vertebral fractures (see p. 659).

Specific therapy

Myeloma remains incurable. Therapy is aimed at treatment or prevention of specific complications and prolongation of overall survival. There are a plethora of agents that can be used at first line or subsequent relapse in myeloma.

Initial treatment typically consists of an alkylator (cyclophosphamide or melphalan), steroid (prednisolone or dexamethasone) and novel agent (bortezomib or thalidomide). Melphalan is avoided in those who may require stem cell mobilization subsequently. Bortezomib is preferable in those with renal impairment. Thalidomide has activity as a single agent and is widely used in first-line and relapsed settings. It is teratogenic and associated with neuropathy, somnolence, constipation and an increased risk of venous thrombosis. Lenalidomide is a thalidomide analogue, which is also used for relapsed myeloma. It has greater potency than thalidomide with less toxicity.

In younger patients (<65–70 years), an orally active cyclophosphamide, thalidomide and dexamethasone-based induction (CTD), followed by a high-dose melphalan autograft, has a significantly higher response rate, with 40% of patients achieving a CR and median survival increasing to 6 years. A bortezomib-containing initial treatment schedule, such as bortezomib, thalidomide and dexamethasone, is also appropriate. The role of allogeneic transplantation is currently unclear but it should be considered in young patients, with a suitable donor and high-risk disease.

In older or less fit patients, melphalan and prednisolone was used, with a median survival of 29–37 months; complete remissions were rare. Recent phase III studies have suggested that these agents, combined with thalidomide as MPT, result in improved response rates and overall survival, albeit with increased toxicity. Additionally, a phase III study has shown that bortezomib plus melphalan and prednisolone (VMP) is superior to the latter two alone. Finally, the FIRST study showed superiority of lenalidomide/dexamethasone to MPT for older patients and this may come to be standard of care.

For relapsed patients, a second autograft may be considered if there was a favourable response duration to the first (>12–18 months). Choice of reinduction therapy will be tailored to the patient according to prior exposure and toxicities. New agents available or currently under evaluation include the proteasome inhibitors ixazomib and carfilzomib; pomalidomide, bendamustine, elotuzumab (monoclonal antibody to CS1), daratumumab (monoclonal antibody to CD38), panobinostat (histone deacetylase inhibitor) and plitidepsin are in clinical trials.

Further reading

Avigan D, Rosenblatt J. Current treatment for multiple myeloma. *N Engl J Med* 2014; 371:961–962.

Kyle RA, Durie BG, Rajkumar SV et al. Monoclonal gammopathy of undetermined significance (MGUS) and smoldering (asymptomatic) multiple myeloma: IMWG consensus perspectives risk factors for progression and guidelines for monitoring and management. *Leukemia* 2010; 24:1121–1127.

Ludwig H, Sonneveld P, Davies F et al. European perspective on multiple myeloma treatment strategies in 2014. *Oncologist* 2014; 19:829–844.

Rollig C, Knop S, Bornhauser M. Multiple myeloma. *Lancet* 2015; 385:2197–2208.

Stewart AK, Rajkvrar V, Dimopovids MA et al. Carfilzomib, lenalidomide, and dexamethasone for relapsed multiple myeloma. *N Engl J Med* 2015; 372:142–152.

COMMON SOLID TUMOUR TREATMENT

Common solid cancer mortality is listed in **Box 17.10**; the improvements in survival in recent years have come from advances in prevention, diagnosis and treatment. The presentation, diagnosis, natural history and systemic treatment of the common cancers are described in the relevant chapters. The decision to treat and the aim of that treatment, whether palliation or cure, require knowledge of the natural history of the disease, prognostic and predictive factors, the patient's performance status and the potential efficacy of treatment. Management should be carried out by multidisciplinary teams, usually led by an oncologist.

Box 17.43 Index of net survival of all cancers at 5 years after diagnosis

Cancer type	5-year survival (%)	
	Men	*Women*
Pancreas	3.6	3.1
Lung	8.4	11.6
Oesophagus	15.6	14.7
Stomach	19.5	17.7
Brain	17.8	19.5
Multiple myeloma	50	43.8
Ovary		46.4
Leukaemia	53.3	49.1
Kidney	56.7	55.6
Colon	59.2	57.3
Rectum	56.6	59.8
Non-Hodgkin's lymphoma	68.1	69.7
Prostate	84.8	
Larynx	67.9	
Bladder	56.5	45.3
Cervix		67.5
Melanoma	87.8	92.4
Breast		86.7
Hodgkin's lymphoma	84.1	86.3
Testis	98	
All cancers	49.2	59.2

(From Quaresma M, Coleman MP, Rachet B. 40-year trends in an index of survival for all cancers combined and survival adjusted for age and sex for each cancer in England and Wales, 1971–2011: a population-based study. Lancet 2015; 385:1206–1218, with permission.)

LUNG CANCER

The presentation and diagnosis of lung cancer ***(Fig. 17.39)*** are covered more fully on pages 1126–1127. Current treatment reflects the fact that the majority of patients are diagnosed at an advanced stage with a poor prognosis; there are therefore many trials assessing different screening strategies to try to achieve earlier diagnosis and more curative treatment.

Prognosis

Lung cancer histology is divided into two main types: small-cell (neuroendocrine) lung cancers (SCLC), which tend to disseminate early in their development, and non-small-cell lung cancers (NSCLC), which are more likely to be diagnosed in a localized form. As treatments have changed, it has become clear that what was simply called non-small-cell lung cancer needs to be separated into individual pathological entities, as the management varies and some therapies are effective only in particular subtypes. Tumour stage and patient performance status are used in selecting treatment and predicting response and prognosis. While overall 5-year

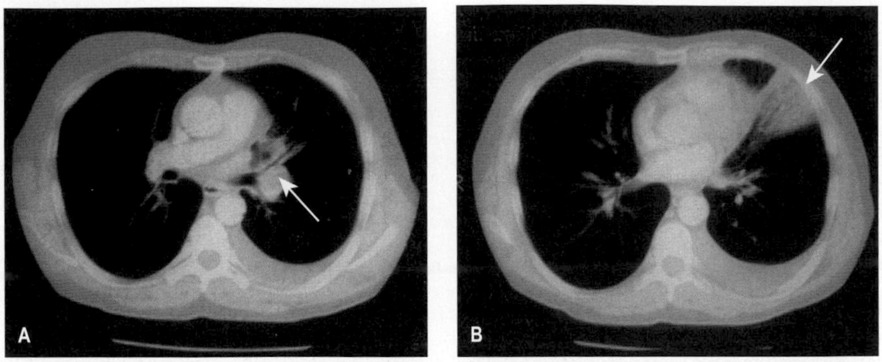

Figure 17.39 Computed tomography in lung cancer. A. Non-small-cell lung cancer of the left main bronchus (arrowed). **B.** Associated hilar lymphadenopathy and distal atelectasis of the lung (arrowed).

survival has remained approximately 10%, treatment is beginning to have an impact in selected groups and the multidisciplinary team can greatly aid in the appropriate application of treatment and the avoidance of nihilism.

Non-small-cell lung cancer

Staging of NSCLC has been improved by CT and PET scanning and is classified according to the TNM system (see ***Box 24.58*** and ***Fig. 24.44***); this system divides the disease into local, locally advanced and advanced stages, with 5-year survival varying from 55–67% to 23–40% and 1–3%, respectively.

Management

Surgery can be curative in NSCLC (T1, N0, M0) but only 5–10% of all cases are suitable for resection; about 70% of these survive for 5 years. Surgery is rarely appropriate in patients over 65 years, as the operative mortality rate exceeds the 5-year survival rate. Trial data suggest that neoadjuvant chemotherapy may downstage tumours to render them operable and may also improve 5-year survival in patients whose tumours are operable at presentation.

Preoperative assessment

Lung function tests, including walking oximetry, are used to predict postoperative potential. An active life after pneumonectomy is unlikely if the gas transfer is reduced below 50%.

In operable disease stages T1N0–T3N2 (stage I–IIIa), adjuvant radiotherapy and chemotherapy following surgery can improve prognosis in patients of good performance status, as shown by the international adjuvant lung cancer trial and a meta-analysis of 12 randomized controlled trials. Cisplatin-based combination chemotherapy induced a response in 60% and produced a relative risk reduction of 11% with an absolute improvement in 5-year survival for stage II and IIIa disease of 4%, from 40.4% to 44.5%. There appears to be no difference in survival if chemotherapy is given before (neo-adjuvant) or after surgery.

A practical molecular assay to predict survival in resected non-squamous lung cancer is still in development.

Radiation therapy for cure

In patients who are fit and who have a stage 1 NSCLC, high-dose radiotherapy (65 Gy or 6500 rads) can result in a 27-month median survival and a 22% 5-year survival. It is the treatment of choice if surgery is not appropriate; however, poor lung function can also be a relative contraindication to radiotherapy. Radiation pneumonitis (defined as an acute infiltrate precisely confined to the radiation area and occurring within 3 months of radiotherapy) develops in 10–15% of cases. Radiation fibrosis, a fibrotic change occurring within a year or so of radiotherapy and not precisely confined to the radiation area, occurs to some degree in all cases but is usually asymptomatic.

For unresectable disease, the combination of concurrent cisplatin with radiotherapy (chemoradiation), when compared with radiotherapy alone, has increased the resection rate and 3-year survival from 11% to 23%, at the expense of greater oesophageal toxicity.

Adenocarcinoma

Therapy depends on the presence or absence of activating mutations in the epidermal growth factor receptor (EGFR); these are much more likely to be present in non-smokers or light smokers and in those with an Asian background. In the most common mutation (del 19), the drug afatinib (EGFR tyrosine kinase inhibitor) has been associated with a survival advantage over first-line chemotherapy. In other activating mutations, while progression-free survival and quality of life with afatinib are improved over the use of chemotherapy, survival rates remain the same as when a tyrosine kinase inhibitor (TKi, e.g. erlotinib) is deferred until chemotherapy has failed. If mutations are found, the response to a TKi in the first-line setting is >60%, or 40% following chemotherapy. Other oncogenetic mutations include the anaplastic lymphoma kinase (ALK) which is seen in 57% of NSCLC adenocarcinoma, and these respond to crizotinib. Where chemotherapy is chosen, cisplatin plus either pemetrexed or vinorelbine is the most effective combination. Normally, four 3-weekly cycles are given. In patients who are fit at the end of chemotherapy (performance status 0–1), maintenance chemotherapy with pemetrexed until progression has been shown to prolong median survival by 3–5 months to around 14 months.

Squamous cell lung cancer

Unlike adenocarcinoma, this is usually smoking-associated and activating mutations are uncommon. Cisplatin (or carboplatin) plus gemcitabine remains the standard treatment (and is superior in this group to regimes based on cisplatin and pemetrexed). An alternative, particularly in older patients, is carboplatin and paclitaxel.

Second-line therapy in NSCLC

In all non-small-cell tumours where current targeted agents are not predicted to be beneficial, the single agent docetaxel may be offered as second-line therapy if patients are fit. A recent study has shown that nivolumab has a significantly better survival and response rate than docetaxel in advanced disease.

Small-cell lung cancer

Prognosis

SCLC is an aggressive neuroendocrine tumour. It is staged in the same way as NSCLC and stage 1 tumours may benefit from surgery. For non-operable cases, disease is split into limited- or extensive-stage disease.

Management

Limited-stage disease is confined to one anatomical area and is present in approximately 30% of patients. It is best treated with concurrent chemotherapy and radiotherapy using a combination of cisplatin and etoposide or irinotecan, which increases the survival at 5 years from 15% to 25%, compared with radiotherapy alone. A similar degree of improvement can also be achieved with hyperfractionated radiotherapy. Prophylactic whole-brain radiation to prevent cerebral metastases can reduce symptomatic central nervous system disease and improve overall survival by 5%.

Extensive disease can be palliated with the combination of carboplatin and etoposide or irinotecan; compared with best supportive care, this can increase median survival from 6 months to 9–13 months, and the 2-year survival to 20%. Second-line chemotherapy can provide further palliation for patients with good performance status.

Symptomatic care for lung cancer patients

The prognosis for the majority of patients remains poor because the disease is diagnosed at an advanced stage and the co-morbidity from other smoking-related diseases compromises treatment. Therefore, much of the treatment, whether symptomatic or anticancer, is delivered with palliative intent. (General palliative care is discussed in Chapter 3.) Specific issues for lung cancer are the relief of bronchial obstruction and breathlessness, and the alleviation of local pain, for which radiotherapy is often employed alongside appropriate opiate analgesia. Laser therapy, endobronchial irradiation and tracheobronchial stents are used (see p. 1132).

Metastases in the lung

Metastases are very common and usually present as round shadows (1.5–3.0 cm diameter). They are usually detected on chest X-ray in patients already diagnosed as having carcinoma, but may be the first presentation. Typical sites for the primary tumour include the kidney, prostate, breast, bone, gastrointestinal tract, cervix or ovary.

Metastases usually develop in the parenchyma or pleura and are often relatively asymptomatic, even when the chest X-ray shows extensive disease. Rarely, metastases may develop within the bronchi and present with haemoptysis.

Carcinoma, particularly of the stomach, pancreas and breast, can involve the mediastinal glands and spread along the lymphatics of both lungs (lymphangitis carcinomatosa), leading to progressive and severe breathlessness. Chest X-ray signs of hilar lymphadenopathy and basal shadowing are unreliable compared with the characteristic signs on CT scan of irregular thickening of the interlobular septa in a polygonal pattern around a thick-walled central vessel.

Occasionally, a pulmonary metastasis may be detected as a solitary round shadow on chest X-ray in an asymptomatic patient. The most common primary tumour to do this is a renal cell carcinoma.

The differential diagnosis includes:

- primary bronchial carcinoma
- tuberculoma
- benign tumour of the lung
- hydatid cyst.

Single pulmonary metastases can be removed surgically but, as CT scans usually show the presence of small metastases that remain undetected on chest X-ray, detailed imaging, including PET scanning and assessment, is essential before undertaking surgery.

Further reading

Ciuleanu T, Brodowicz T, Zielinski C et al. Maintenance pemetrexed plus best supportive care versus placebo plus best supportive care for non-small-cell lung cancer: a randomised, double-blind, phase 3 study. *Lancet* 2009; 374:1432–1440.
Kwak EL, Bang YJ, Camidge DR et al. Anaplastic lymphoma kinase inhibition in non-small-cell lung cancer. *N Engl J Med* 2010; 363:1693–1703.
Maemondo M, Inoue A, Kobayashi K et al. Gefitinib or chemotherapy for non-small-cell lung cancer with mutated EGFR. *N Engl J Med* 2010; 362:2380–2388.
Reck M, Heigener DF, Mok T et al. Management of non-small-cell lung cancer: recent developments. *Lancet* 2013; 382:709–719.
Rosell R, Bivona T, Karachaliou N. Genetics and biomarkers in personalisation of lung cancer treatment. *Lancet* 2013; 382:720–731.
Soloman BJ, Mok T, Kim DW, et al. First-line crizotinib versus chemotherapy in ALK-positive lung cancer. *N Engl J Med* 2014; 371:2167–2177.

BREAST CANCER

Breast cancer is the most common cancer in women who do not smoke. The screening programme in the UK, with biplanar digital mammography every 3 years in women aged 50–70, and improvements in multimodality treatment have increased overall survival and rates of cure, while breast-conserving surgery has greatly ameliorated the psychosexual impact of the disease.

Aetiology and pathology

The majority of breast cancers arise from the epithelial cells of the milk ducts and reproduce their histological features in a variety of patterns ***(Box 17.44)***, of which the most common is an infiltrating ductal carcinoma. Further biological typing ***(Box 17.45)*** has revealed that some triple negative cancers also resemble the *BRCA1* mutated cancers with an associated DNA repair deficiency that has been targeted with new drugs such as poly-ADP-ribose polymerase (PARP) inhibitors. For many cancers, it is thought that there is an identifiable precursor *in situ* stage, which is confined within the basement membrane and is still truly localized and detectable by its trademark microcalcification on a screening mammogram. For others, this stage may be non-existent or so brief as to be undetectable, and invasive disease is present from very early in development with a consequently worse prognosis. Approximately 10% of women have familial breast cancer ***(Box 17.46)*** and 3% have

Box 17.44 Breast cancer histology

Non-invasive
- Ductal cancer *in situ*
- Lobular cancer *in situ*

Invasive
- Infiltrating ductal cancer
- Infiltrating lobular cancer
- Metaplastic cancer
- Mucinous cancer
- Medullary cancer
- Papillary cancer
- Tubular cancer

Other
- Adenoid cystic, secretory, apocrine cancers
- Paget's disease of the nipple
- Phylloides tumour (sarcoma)

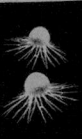

Box 17.45 Invasive breast cancer biological subtypes and treatment sensitivity

Subtype	Expression				Sensitivity		
	ER	*PR*	*Her2*	*Ki-67*	*ET*	*Anti-Her2*	*CT*
Luminal A	+	+	–	L	H	L	L
Luminal B	+	+	–	H	H	L	M
Basal	–	–	–	H	L	L	H
Her2	–/+	–/+	3+	H	L/H	H	H

+, present by immunohistochemistry; –, absent by immunohistochemistry; CT, chemotherapy; ER, oestrogen receptor; ET, endocrine therapy; H, high; HER2, human epidermal growth factor receptor 2; L, low; M, moderate; PR, progesterone receptor.

Box 17.46 Familial patterns of breast and ovarian cancer with increased risk of inherited *BRCA* mutations

- A mother or sister diagnosed with breast cancer before the age of 40
- Two close relatives from the same side of the family diagnosed with breast cancer; at least one must be a mother, sister or daughter
- Three close relatives diagnosed with breast cancer at any age
- A father or brother diagnosed with breast cancer at any age
- A mother or sister with breast cancer in both breasts, the first cancer diagnosed before the age of 50
- One close relative with ovarian cancer and one with breast cancer, diagnosed at any age; at least one must be a mother, sister or daughter
- A close relative of Ashkenazi Jewish origin with breast or ovarian cancer
- A close relative with pancreatic cancer and breast or ovarian cancer

detectable mutations in the *BRCA1* and *BRCA2* genes and *TP53*. The hormonal environment exerts a major effect on expression of the breast cancer potential and is related to reproductive behaviour, diet, exercise, weight and exogenous hormones from oral contraception and postmenopausal hormone replacement therapy.

Clinical features

Most women with symptomatic rather than screen-detected breast cancer present with a painless, increasing mass that may also be associated with nipple discharge, skin tethering, ulceration and, in inflammatory cancers, oedema and erythema. In developing countries, 80% are likely to present with advanced disease ***(Fig. 17.40)*** and metastases.

Investigations

The triple assessment of any symptomatic breast mass by palpation, radiology (mammography, ultrasound and MRI scan) and fine needle aspiration cytology is the most reliable way to differentiate breast cancer from the 15 times more common benign breast masses. Large-bore core needle biopsy should follow to provide histological confirmation and predictive factors, such as grade, Ki-67 (immunohistochemical test) proliferation index and oestrogen, progesterone and Her2 receptor status, to inform the subsequent decision-making process. Molecular profiling to assess risk of recurrence and benefit of chemotherapy with the Oncotype Dx assay (see below) of the expression of 21 genes is able to better identify good-prognosis patients who do not need chemotherapy. Assessment should be carried out in a dedicated one-stop clinic that is able to provide the appropriate support and referral. Staging is both surgical, with respect to tumour size and axillary lymph node

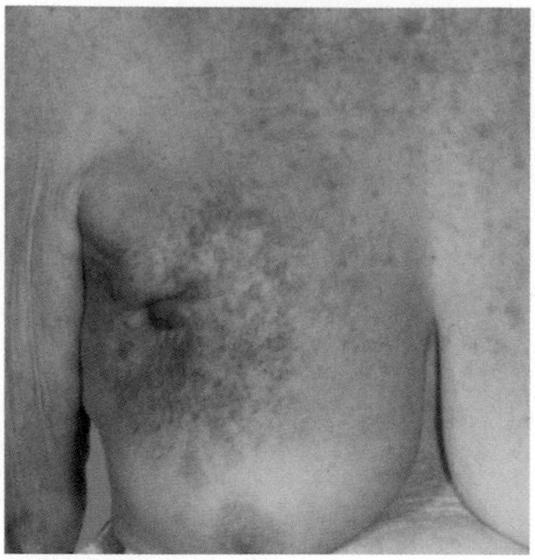

Figure 17.40 Locally advanced breast cancer invading skin and axillary lymph nodes.

Box 17.47 Risk of cancer associated with *BRCA1* or *BRCA2* germline mutation

Cancer	General population	*BRCA1* mutated	*BRCA2* mutated
Breast	12%	50–80%	40–70%
Breast second primary	3.5% at 5 years	27% at 5 years	12% at 5 years
Ovary	1–2%	24–40%	11–18%
Prostate	15% (North European) 18% (African American)	<30%	<39%
Pancreas	0.5%	1–3%	2–7%

(http://www.ncbi.nlm.nih.gov/books/NBK1247/)

status, and, in advanced disease, investigative, examining common sites of metastasis by chest X-ray and CT scan of lungs and liver, and by bone scan. At present, only 20% of patients are diagnosed with no evidence of microscopic nodal metastases.

Prognosis

The following are all significant independent predictors of a high risk of recurrence: large size of the primary tumour; metaplastic histological subtype that is high-grade/poorly differentiated; oestrogen and progesterone receptor (ER, PR)-negative; and young age and pre-menopausal status. Expression of Her2 is an adverse factor for small, otherwise good-prognosis tumours and, like ER and PR, is a predictor of treatment response.

Several gene expression profiles, such as the Oncotype Dx test score, have identified sets of between 20 and 70 genes, whose expression pattern can identify low- and high-risk subsets independently of clinical risk factors and predict treatment benefit. Clinical trials are in progress to test whether this leads to better decision-making and outcome than the traditional clinical factors. *BRCA* gene mutation testing, when there is a strong familial breast or ovarian cancer history, can inform the choice of local and contralateral breast treatment. ***Box 17.47*** shows the risk of cancer with *BRCA* genes in different cancers.

Management of early breast cancer

Survival probability and benefit from adjuvant treatment can be calculated using the website www.adjuvantonline.com, which is

Box 17.48 Worked example of risk and benefit calculation for adjuvant breast cancer treatment[a]

	Calculation	Result
Predicted 10-year risk of breast cancer mortality		40%
Tamoxifen RR reduction	25% relative mortality reduction	10%
Chemotherapy FEC-T RR reduction	30% =	13%
Trastuzumab RR reduction of post-chemotherapy risk	33% of residual 27% =	9%
Combined treatment mortality reduction		30%
Residual 10-year risk		10%

[a]Using www.adjuvantonline.com predictions. Example is for a 45-year-old, pre-menopausal woman with T1N1 grade 3 invasive ductal cancer, who is ER^+, PR^+ and $Her2^{3+}$. FEC-T, fluorouracil, epirubicin, cyclophosphamide, docetaxel; RR, relative risk.

Box 17.49 Indications for adjuvant radiotherapy in breast cancer

- Breast-conserving surgery
- Large, high-grade primary tumour
- Proximity to surgical margins
- Lymph node metastases

based on the American Surveillance Epidemiology and End Results (SEER) database and has been validated on independent datasets from British Columbia and Finland ***(Box 17.48)***.

Local treatment

Surgery may vary from wide local excision or segmental mastectomy and breast conservation for masses <3 cm in diameter, to simple mastectomy with or without reconstruction. The choice is dictated by the location and extent of the breast mass in relation to the breast size and patient preferences. In the absence of clinical or radiological (usually ultrasound) evidence of lymphadenopathy, surgery of the axilla can be minimized by sentinel lymph node-guided sampling (after dye or radioactive tracer injection); otherwise, dissection to level 3 is required if there are clinically involved nodes, in order to gain local control and provide prognostic information to guide adjuvant treatment. The greater the amount of axillary surgery, the greater is the risk of postoperative lymphoedema.

Radiotherapy is given to the conserved breast after wide local excision to reduce local recurrence, and to the chest wall after mastectomy if there are risk factors for local recurrence to complete the local control measures ***(Box 17.49)***.

Radiotherapy to the axilla is an equally effective alternative to axillary dissection following a positive sample but should not be added after full dissection of the axilla because the combination raises the risk of severe lymphoedema to 30%. Adjuvant radiotherapy reduces the risk of local recurrence by 75% and improves 10-year survival by 3%.

Data suggest that women over 70 years with oestrogen receptor (ER)-positive cancers of up to 2 cm diameter may be offered surgery and tamoxifen alone without radiotherapy, without compromising outcome.

Box 17.50 Side-effects of endocrine agents for breast cancer in order of frequency

Tamoxifen
- Hot flushes
- Weight gain
- Mood changes
- Vaginal discharge
- Thromboembolism
- Endometrial hyperplasia and neoplasia

Aromatase inhibitors
- Hot flushes
- Vaginal dryness
- Arthralgia
- Skin rash
- Osteoporosis
- Adverse lipid profile

Endocrine treatment

Anti-oestrogen drugs

In ***pre-menopausal women***, a reduction in oestrogens can be achieved via oophorectomy or via pituitary downregulation using a gonadotrophin-releasing hormone (GnRH) analogue, such as goserelin or leuprorelin.

Tamoxifen is a mixed agonist and antagonist of oestrogen action on the oestrogen receptor, while the more recent drug fulvestrant is a more selective oestrogen receptor modulator (SERM).

Synthetic progestogens, such as medroxyprogesterone acetate and megestrol acetate, have a direct effect on breast tumour cells through progesterone receptors, as well as effects on the pituitary/ovarian (pre-menopausal) and adrenal/pituitary axis (post-menopausal). They can be as effective as tamoxifen in metastatic breast cancer.

In ***post-menopausal women***, androgens are synthesized by the adrenal glands and converted in subcutaneous fat to oestrone by the enzyme aromatase. The aromatase inhibitors, anastrozole, letrozole and exemestane, reduce circulating oestrogen levels and oestrogen synthesis in tumour cells; they have shown greater efficacy than tamoxifen in the treatment of metastatic breast cancer and reduced distant recurrence rates in the adjuvant setting.

Side-effects (Box 17.50) are those of oestrogen deprivation, and women need support in managing them if they are to be able to complete the standard 5-year course.

Adjuvant systemic treatment

Endocrine therapy

In about one-third of patients, the breast cancer will express receptors for oestrogen and progesterone. For pre-menopausal women, tamoxifen adjuvant therapy for 5 years immediately following surgery for receptor-positive disease reduces the 10-year relative risk of women dying from breast cancer by about 25%, and the absolute 10-year death rate by an average of 12% for all stages. Recent trials have shown increased benefit from either continuing tamoxifen for a total of 10 years or, in those becoming post-menopausal on treatment, switching to an aromatase inhibitor (AI) for a further 5 years.

For post-menopausal women with ER- and/or PR-positive disease, adjuvant tamoxifen or an AI such as anastrozole, letrozole or exemestane, all given for 5 years, reduces the risk of death from breast cancer by a similar 25%. Extended AI treatment schedules are still under investigation.

AIs, however, are the treatment of choice for post-menopausal women because they avoid the adverse effects of tamoxifen on the uterus and venous thromboembolism, and achieve a greater reduction in contralateral breast cancers and in distant metastases, contributing to an overall improvement in relapse-free survival, though not an overall survival advantage. It is recommended that the choice should be discussed for each patient, taking the individual co-morbidities into account. The effects of endocrine therapy are additive to those of chemotherapy and are most effective when given after, not concurrently with, the chemotherapy.

Chemotherapy and targeted therapy

A meta-analysis of all randomized trials of adjuvant therapy in breast cancer has shown that, for women with high-risk features (**Box 17.51**), adjuvant chemotherapy with first-generation regimens, such as CMF (cyclophosphamide, 5-fluorouracil (5-FU) plus methotrexate) for 6 months, reduces the absolute 10-year death rate by about 10% and the relative risk of death (RR) by 20%. Ovarian ablation using a GnRH analogue for 2 years is equally effective as CMF chemotherapy in pre-menopausal women. More effective second-generation regimens that include an anthracycline, such as Epi-CMF (epirubicin) or FEC100 (5-FU, epirubicin 100 mg/m^2, cyclophosphamide), increase the RR to 25%. A third-generation regimen with a taxane, such as FEC-D (fluorouracil, epirubicin, cyclophosphamide followed by docetaxel) (see **Box 17.14**), gives a 33% RR reduction but with increased toxicity.

Chemotherapy is less effective in hormone receptor-positive disease, and although menopausal status does not affect the relative efficacy of chemotherapy, the risk of recurrence is lower after the menopause and thus the absolute improvement in survival is less. Toxicity may also be higher with increasing age, so that treatment decisions may need to be more individualized in discussion between the patient and her doctors. The combined effect of radiotherapy, chemotherapy and tamoxifen or AI approximately halves the risk of dying of breast cancer for appropriately selected patients.

Her2-/cERBB2-targeted therapy

The addition of adjuvant intravenous trastuzumab for a further year to chemotherapy for the treatment of the 15–20% of patients in whom the breast cancer overexpresses Her2 further reduces the risk of mortality by 25% when trastuzumab is used alone, and by 33% when it is administered concurrently with a taxane. Intravenous or, more recently, subcutaneous trastuzumab is the standard of care for these patients but has a direct toxic effect on the myocardium that is additive to pre-existing myocardial damage, especially that caused by anthracyclines, and should not be given concurrently. An alternative regimen with docetaxel, carboplatin and trastuzumab is equally as effective and can avoid much of the myocardial toxicity. Left ventricular ejection fraction must be monitored before and during treatment to avoid potentially severe congestive heart failure.

Her2 blockade is also clinically effective with the monoclonal antibody pertuzumab or the receptor tyrosine kinase inhibitor (TKi) lapatinib. The combination of pertuzumab and trastuzumab has doubled response rates in metastatic treatment and results of adjuvant trials are awaited.

Neoadjuvant and primary systemic treatment

There is no survival advantage for preoperative endocrine or chemotherapy treatment when compared with postoperative treatment; that is, the advantage over surgery alone is the same. However, there is a significant benefit from either rendering inoperable tumours operable (called primary systemic therapy) or making large tumours smaller and suitable for breast-conserving surgery in about two-thirds of such patients (called neoadjuvant therapy), in addition to the reduction in risk of death from distant metastases.

Management of advanced breast cancer

Patients with established metastatic disease may require endocrine therapy, chemotherapy and radiotherapy. The treatment is not curative but is of great palliative benefit and often consistent with many years of good-quality life. Little additional benefit has been gained by adding endocrine therapy and chemotherapy together, although the inclusion of anti-HER2 (antibodies) in chemotherapy has produced a survival advantage. Prolonging treatment can delay relapse but at the expense of treatment toxicity; therefore, the serial use of intermittent courses of the different endocrine and chemotherapies, starting with the least toxic and most effective treatment, is usually most consistent with maintaining a good quality of life for as long as possible. Median survival from diagnosis is 2 years with a wide 95% confidence interval of 6–54 months. Surgical resection of unifocal metastases in the liver, lung or chest wall may be appropriate for cancers with a long disease-free interval.

Endocrine treatment

Women who have high levels of ERs and PRs in their tumour have a greater chance of responding to endocrine treatments (i.e. 60% versus 10% for ER-negative disease; **Box 17.52**).

Endocrine therapy is usually tried first in those patients who have characteristics suggesting they are likely to respond and who do not have immediately life-threatening organ failure. Remission lasts 2 years on average and is consistent with an excellent quality of life. When relapse occurs, further treatment with different agents may produce another remission.

Chemotherapy

Chemotherapy is used for patients who lack the above features of hormone-responsive disease, those who fail to respond to endocrine therapy, or those who require a rapid response if at risk of, for example, liver or respiratory failure. Chemotherapy can provide good-quality palliation and prolongation of life. The drugs listed below are all able to induce objective responses in metastatic disease, and when the disease responds, patients are likely to experience further serial responses to subsequent treatment at relapse. Single-agent treatment is often as effective as combination therapy; there is no benefit with combining more than two drugs at a time, which has the advantage of preserving more options for future use. There is very little difference in efficacy between the different regimens for Her2-negative metastatic disease, with response rates varying from 40% to 60% for a median duration of 8–10 months. The most common regimens with either single agents or doublet combinations include:

Box 17.51 Poor prognostic factors for breast cancer

- Young age
- Pre-menopausal status
- Large tumour size
- High tumour grade
- Oestrogen/progesterone/Her2 receptor-negative
- Positive nodes

Box 17.52 Oestrogen-sensitive metastatic breast cancer characteristics

- Expression of oestrogen receptors and/or progesterone receptors
- Disease-free interval >1 year
- Skin, lymph node or bone disease
- Absence of life-threatening visceral disease

- MM: mitoxantrone and methotrexate
- AC/EC: doxorubicin or epirubicin and cyclophosphamide
- DC: docetaxel and capecitabine
- PG: paclitaxel and gemcitabine
- vinorelbine, carboplatin, mitomycin and eribulin.

The multiple regimens provide the possibility of avoiding drug resistance over several episodes of treatment interspersed with treatment-free periods so that the disease can be palliated, often for several years.

The addition of trastuzumab and pertuzumab or, to lesser degree, lapatinib to the cytotoxic drugs (except the anthracyclines; see above) has significantly improved survival for those women whose tumour overexpresses the *c-ERBB2/Her2* oncogene. Inhibition of VEGFR by bevacizumab may be effective in a small proportion of patients but as yet it lacks a predictive biomarker. Markers of DNA repair deficiency, such as *BRCA1* mutations, render the breast cancer potentially sensitive to the PARP inhibitors in development.

Anti-osteolytic therapy

Bone metastases are a common problem in the management of breast cancer. The bisphosphonates and the more potent anti-RANKL monoclonal antibody, denosumab, have a major role in reducing the incidence of new osteolytic deposits, bone pain and fracture when used preventatively, and in treating pain and hypercalcaemia from established metastases. While the second-generation bisphosphonate, pamidronate, may be sufficient, the more potent third-generation drugs, such as zoledronate or denosumab (the most effective), can be associated with hypocalcaemia and, in rare cases, impaired bone healing and osteonecrosis of the jaw (see p. 714).

Further reading

Baselga J, Cortés J, Kim SB et al. Pertuzumab plus trastuzumab plus docetaxel for metastatic breast cancer. *N Engl J Med* 2012; 366:109–119.

Burstein HJ, Morrow M. Nodal irradiation after breast cancer surgery in the era of effective adjuvant therapy. *N Engl J Med* 2015; 373:379–381.

Coudert B, Asselain B, Campone M et al. Extended benefit from sequential administration of docetaxel after standard fluorouracil, epirubicin, and cyclophosphamide regimen for node positive breast cancer: the 8-year follow-up results of the UNICANCER-PACS01 trial. *Oncologist* 2012; 17:900–909.

Donker M, van Teinhoven G, Straver ME et al. Radiotherapy or surgery of the axilla after a positive sentinel node in breast cancer (EORTC 10981-22023 AMROS): a randomized, multicenter, open-label, phase 3 non-inferiority trial. *Lancet Oncol* 2014; 15:1303–1310.

EBCTG (Early Breast Cancer Trialists Collaborative Group). Effect of radiotherapy after mastectomy and axillary surgery on 10-year recurrence and 20-year breast cancer mortality: meta-analysis of individual patient data for 8135 women in 22 randomised trials. *Lancet* 2014; 383:2127–2135.

Morrow M, Waters J, Morris E. MRI for breast cancer screening, diagnosis and treatment. *Lancet* 2011; 378:1804–1811.

Reis-Filho JS, Pusztai L. Gene expression profiling in breast cancer: classification, prognostication and prediction. *Lancet* 2011; 378:1812–1823.

Tutt A, Robson M, Garber JE et al. Oral poly(ADP-ribose) polymerase inhibitor olaparib in patients with BRCA1 or BRCA2 mutations and advanced breast cancer: a proof-of-concept trial. *Lancet* 2010; 376:235–244.

GASTROINTESTINAL CANCER

Upper gastrointestinal cancers

Oesophageal cancer

Presentation and diagnosis are described on page 374. Early diagnosis, as pioneered in Japan, where there is a particularly high incidence, has shown that it is possible to improve the prognosis of a disease that otherwise is typically diagnosed only when local metastases have already occurred.

Management and prognosis

Pre-treatment histology, stage, age and performance status are critical prognostic factors for treatment decisions, which should be made by a multidisciplinary team in designated units with the surgical expertise to avoid treatment mortality. The prognosis for the majority of symptomatic patients is poor, 50% have distant metastases at the time of diagnosis, and the majority of the remainder having loco-regional spread into adjacent mediastinal structures. Staging with endoscopic ultrasound, CT scan and PET-CT scan has improved the selection of patients of good performance status with truly localized disease, for whom curative treatment may be attempted.

Surgery provides the best chance of a cure and should be used as the primary modality only when imaging (see above) has shown that the tumour has not infiltrated outside the oesophageal wall (stage 1). The overall 5-year survival figures are poor (see p. 376), and only 4% for stage 4 cancers, because 70% of patients present late with stage ≥3 disease.

Response to neoadjuvant therapy is a further strong prognostic factor. Treatment of potentially resectable squamous carcinomas with cisplatin, 5-FU and concurrent radiotherapy, or postoperative chemotherapy with epirubicin, cisplatin and 5-FU for adenocarcinomas at the oesophagogastric junction in those of good performance status, achieves complete remission in 20–40%; there is a median survival of 19 months, and 25–35% of patients are alive 5 years after surgery.

Locally advanced or metastatic disease can be palliated with 5-FU or capecitabine chemotherapy in approximately 30%, increasing to 45–55% with the addition of oxaliplatin or irinotecan for a median duration of 6–8 months.

Distressing symptomatic problems with dysphagia can be partially relieved by endoscopic insertion of expanding metal stents or percutaneous endoscopic gastrostomy tubes to support liquid enteral feeding and endoscopic ablation to help control bleeding. The patient and family need considerable support and explanation to enable them to understand that feeding, including parenteral methods, does not improve survival beyond that dictated by the underlying cancer, and may introduce its own complications with adverse effects on quality of life.

Gastric cancer

The presentation and diagnosis of gastric cancer are described on pages 381–384.

Prognosis

The majority of patients are still diagnosed at an advanced stage, except in Japan, which has an active surveillance policy. Thus, in the West, the overall prognosis has not improved above 10% survival at 5 years. Selected groups may do much better and the histological grade and staging, with respect to the presence of serosal involvement (T3), nodal involvement (N1–2) and performance status, are the main factors in determining prognosis and selecting treatment.

Management

Early non-ulcerated, mucosal lesions can be removed endoscopically.

Surgery remains the most effective form of treatment if the patient is operable. Selection on operability has reduced the numbers undergoing surgery and has improved the overall surgical 5-year survival rates from 20% to 30%. Five-year survival rates in 'curative' operations are as high as 50%.

Adjuvant treatment trials of perioperative chemotherapy with regimens such as epirubicin, cisplatin and infusional 5-FU (ECF), or epirubicin, oxaliplatin and capecitabine (EOX), improved 5-year survival in operable gastric and lower oesophageal adenocarcinomas from 23% to 36–51%, depending on the preoperative stage. Adjuvant postoperative treatment with cisplatin, 5-FU and radiotherapy, compared with surgery alone, significantly increased median survival from 28 to 35 months, and 5-year survival from 41% to 47%.

Advanced disease may be palliated with chemotherapy, such as epirubicin or docetaxel combined with cisplatin and infusional 5-FU, or oxaliplatin and capecitabine, with a response in 40–50% of patients for a median of 8–12 months in those with good performance status (see p. 383). The addition of trastuzumab for tumours overexpressing Her2 has improved median survival from 11 to 16 months, but the addition of treatments targeting VEGFR (bevacizumab) or EGFR (cetuximab or panitumumab) have not proved successful.

Supportive care for patients with upper gastrointestinal cancers, more than cancers in any other site, must include attention to nutrition with the use of endoscopic stents to relieve obstruction, nasojejunal and percutaneous gastrostomy feeding tubes, and occasionally parenteral nutrition. When the disease progresses beyond active anticancer treatment, management of the distressing obstructive symptoms can include octreotide to reduce secretions and, if necessary, a venting gastrostomy.

Gastrointestinal stromal tumours

Gastrointestinal stromal tumours (GIST) are rare, slow-growing neoplasms that may arise in the stomach or small or large intestine. Prognosis depends on size, site, Ki-67 proliferation index (see p. 384), and association with neurofibromatosis type 1. Immunohistochemistry for CD117 and DOG-1 is usually positive. If it is negative, diagnosis can be reached by analysis of the known mutational sites in *cKIT* or *PDGFRA* oncogenes. These mutations are also predictive of dose requirements and treatment response to the receptor TKi, imatinib, or sensitivity to alternative TKis (see pp. 601–602). Surgery is potentially curative for localized disease, and imatinib adjuvant therapy for 3 years prolongs survival. In metastatic disease, imatinib treatment should continue until relapse and can induce remissions in 50–80% on PET-CT criteria for a median of 2 years; further responses are possible to alternative TKis, such as sunitinib and nilotinib.

Lower gastrointestinal cancers

Small intestine cancer

Predisposing factors for small intestinal cancer, and its presentation and treatment, are described on pages 402–403. The principles of treatment are determined by extrapolation from management of the more common colorectal cancers.

Colorectal cancer

Presentation and diagnosis of colorectal cancer are described on page 424.

Prevention

- ***A low-fat, high-fibre diet*** for the prevention of sporadic colorectal cancer, along with endoscopic screening, is recommended for at-risk patients with a strong family history and for inherited syndromes (e.g. familial adenomatous polyposis, Lynch syndrome).
- ***NSAIDs or aspirin*** may play a role in prevention. After 5 years' treatment with daily aspirin, there is a 35% reduction in all gastrointestinal cancers (used for those who are not at risk of gastric erosions).

Screening

See page 425.

Management

Management should be undertaken by multidisciplinary teams working in specialist units. About 80% of patients with colorectal cancer undergo surgery, though fewer than half of these survive more than 5 years. The operative procedure depends on the cancer site. Long-term survival is determined by the stage of the primary tumour, the achievement of clear surgical margins and the presence of metastatic disease ***(Box 17.53)***. There has been a gradual move from using Dukes' classification to the TNM system.

Prognostic factors

The site of the disease, above or below the pelvic peritoneal reflection, CT scan staging, surgical margins, TNM stage and performance status are the main clinical prognostic factors ***(Box 17.54)***. Gene expression profiling, using Oncotype Dx and Coloprint, for example, can identify prognostic subgroups but is not predictive of treatment benefit. High microsatellite instability (MSI) predicts for a better prognosis and can be used to identify low-risk patients for whom adjuvant therapy is unlikely to be of benefit. Mutations in *BRAF* occur in 6–8% and indicate a poor prognosis, as do mutations with predictive effect in *KRAS* in 40% and *NRAS* in 10–15% of cancers.

Surgery

Rectal cancer

Total mesorectal excision (TME) is used for careful removal of the entire package of mesorectal tissue surrounding the cancer. A low rectal anastomosis is then performed. Abdomino-perineal excision, which requires a permanent colostomy, is reserved for very low tumours within 5 cm of the anal margin. TME combined with preoperative chemo-radiotherapy reduces local recurrence rates in rectal cancer to around 8% and improves survival. Local transanal surgery is used very occasionally for early superficial rectal cancers.

Colon cancer

A segmental resection and restorative anastomosis, with removal of the draining lymph nodes as far as the root of the mesentery, is employed for cancer elsewhere in the colon. Surgery in patients with obstruction carries greater morbidity and mortality. Where technically possible, preoperative decompression by endoscopic stenting with a mesh-metal stent relieves obstruction; surgery can therefore be elective rather than emergency, and is probably associated with a decrease in morbidity and mortality.

Neoadjuvant chemotherapy and radiotherapy

Neoadjuvant chemo-radiation treatment of rectal cancers, using cisplatin and 5-FU with radiotherapy, has increased the proportion of locally advanced tumours that can be resected with clear surgical margins (long-course radiotherapy) and reduced local relapse rate (both short- and long-course radiotherapy), but has not improved distant metastatic relapse and overall survival. Preoperative rather than postoperative treatment has reduced toxicity to the other

Box 17.53 Staging and survival of colorectal cancers

TNM classification	Description	Notation	Modified Dukes' classification	5-year survival (%)
Stage I (N0, M0)	Tumours invade submucosa Tumours invade muscularis propria	T1 T2	A	90
Stage IIA (N0, M0) **Stage IIB**	Tumours invade into subserosa Tumours invade directly into other organs	T3 T4	B	70 65
Stage III (M0) **Stage IIIB**	T1, T2 + 1–3 regional lymph nodes involved T3, T4 + 1–3 regional lymph nodes involved	N1 N1	C	60 35
Stage IIIC	Any T + 4 or more regional lymph nodes	N2		25
Stage IV	Any T, any N + distant metastases	M1	D	7

Box 17.54 Prognostic and predictive factors for colorectal cancer

- Site above or below pelvic peritoneal reflection
- TNM stage and performance status
- Surgical margins
- Favourable mutational profile:
  - Low microsatellite instability
  - BRAF wild type
  - RAS wild type

pelvic structures due to preservation of the normal anatomical relations.

Adjuvant chemotherapy with 6 months of infusional 5-FU and folinic acid (leucovorin) or oral capecitabine for rectal and colonic adenocarcinoma reduces the risk of death by 30% and significantly increases 5-year survival for node-positive stage III disease (Dukes' C) by 10–15%, from 40% to 55%. A further 4% improvement in one trial was achieved by the addition of oxaliplatin but with additional toxicity. Less benefit is seen for stage II node-negative patients. The adjuvant use of anti-VEGF or EGFR-targeted treatments is still being investigated with respect to *RAS* gene status.

Follow-up

All patients who have surgery should have a total colonoscopy performed before surgery to look for additional lesions. If total colonoscopy cannot be achieved before surgery, a second 'clearance' colonoscopy within 6 months of surgery is essential. Patients with stage II or III disease should be followed up with regular colonoscopy and carcinoembryonic antigen (CEA) measurements; rising levels of CEA suggest recurrence. CT scanning to detect operable liver metastases should be performed for up to 5 years post surgery.

Metastatic colorectal cancer

Advanced colorectal cancer is successfully palliated with little toxicity by 5-FU and folinic acid regimens or oral capecitabine in approximately 30% of patients for a median of 12–14 months. The addition of irinotecan or oxaliplatin increases the proportion who benefit to 55%, and extends median survival to 18 months but with increased toxicity. Anti-EGFR and VEGFR agents ***(Box 17.55)*** increase the response rate with chemotherapy, such as 5-FU/folinic acid with oxaliplatin or irinotecan (FolFOX or FolFIRI), to 68% and the median survival from 19 to 24 months. Toxicity of the anti-VEGFR agents commonly leads to hypertension, proteinuria, arterial thrombus, mucosal bleeding and perforation, and delayed wound healing. The anti-EGFR agents cause acneiform rash, hypomagnesaemia, and hypersensitivity reactions.

Treatment can be intermittent or may comprise an intensive induction phase followed by maintenance with 5-FU and a relevant

Box 17.55 Benefit of adding targeted drugs to FolFOX or FolFIRI chemotherapy for metastatic colorectal cancer

Drug	Wild type	Mutated *KRAS/NRAS* and *BRAF*
Anti-EGFR		
Cetuximab	+	–
Panitumumab	+	–
Anti-VEGFR		
Bevacizumab	–	+
Aflibercept	–	+
Regorafenib	–	+

EGFR, endothelial growth factor receptor; FolFIRI, folinic acid (leucovorin), fluorouracil, ironotecan; FolFOX, folinic acid (leucovorin), fluorouracil, oxaliplatin; VEGFR, vascular endothelial growth factor receptor.

targeted agent which prolongs the progression-free survival but not the overall survival.

Liver and lung metastases are a common problem with colorectal cancers. With appropriate selection of patients who have a good performance status and in whom MRI and PET-CT scans do not demonstrate disease elsewhere, local treatment can prolong good-quality survival. This includes a variety of methods from surgical resection to gamma-knife irradiation, radiofrequency, cryoablation or hepatic artery embolization. Small lesions can be ablated, but larger lesions are best managed by partial hepatectomy or a combination approach, so that embolization is followed by hepatic regeneration before final resection. Patient selection is critical; long-term survival without recurrence is reported in up to 20% of patients at 5 years with a single <4-cm lesion amenable to resection presenting more than a year from initial diagnosis. More patients can be rendered suitable with perioperative chemotherapy, such as FolFOX or FolFIRI with cetuximab if *RAS* is wild-type.

Anal cancer

Management, where possible, is with surgery. If disease is locally advanced, downstaging is achieved by using chemoradiotherapy with mitomycin-C (MMC) and 5-FU, followed by surgery.

Further reading

Boland CR, Goel A. Prognostic subgroups among patients with stage II colon cancer. *N Engl J Med* 2016; 374:277–278.

Cunningham D, Atkin W, Lenz HJ et al. Colorectal cancer. *Lancet* 2010; 375:1030–1047.

Fiorica F, Cartei F, Licata A et al. Can chemotherapy concomitantly delivered with radiotherapy improve survival of patients with resectable rectal cancer? A meta-analysis of literature data. *Cancer Treat Rev* 2010; 36:539–549.

Northover J, Glynne-Jones R, Sebag-Montefiore D et al. Chemoradiation for the treatment of epidermoid anal cancer: 13-year follow-up of the first

randomised UKCCCR Anal Cancer Trial (ACT I). *Br J Cancer* 2010; 102:1123–1128.
O'Connell MJ, Lavery I, Yothers G et al. Relationship between tumor gene expression and recurrence in four independent studies of patients with stage II/III colon cancer treated with surgery alone or surgery plus adjuvant fluorouracil plus leucovorin. *J Clin Oncol* 2010; 28:3937–3944.
Rothwell PM, Fowkes FG, Belch JF et al. Effect of daily aspirin on long-term risk of death due to cancer: analysis of individual patient data from randomised trials. *Lancet* 2011; 377:31–41.
Rubenstein JH, Shaheen NJ. Epidemiology, diagnosis, and management of esophageal adenocarcinoma. *Gastroenterology* 2015; 149:642–643.

HEPATOBILIARY AND PANCREATIC CANCERS

Liver

Hepatocellular carcinoma

Hepatocellular carcinoma (HCC; see p. 485) arises in a cirrhotic liver in 95% of cases and can be screened and detected by cross-sectional imaging and a rise in serum α-fetoprotein.

Management and prognosis

Surgical resection of isolated lesions <5 cm in diameter or up to three lesions <3 cm in diameter is associated with a median survival of 5 years, although the remaining liver remains at risk of further recurrence. Liver transplantation offers the only opportunity for cure for patients with a small primary but is often limited by the underlying cause of the hepatitis and cirrhosis. Conventional chemotherapy and radiotherapy are unsuccessful; transarterial embolization or radiofrequency ablation in patients with small primaries as above and adequate liver function prolongs survival, though less successfully than surgery. Antiangiogenic compounds are being evaluated: sorafenib prolongs survival to 10 months in patients with non-resectable tumours.

Biliary tract

Cancer of the biliary tract may be intra- or extrahepatic. These malignancies represent approximately 1% of all cancers. A number of associations have been identified, such as choledochal cyst and chronic infection of the biliary tract with, for example, *Clonorchis sinensis*. There are also associations with autoimmune disease processes, such as primary sclerosing cholangitis, and inflammatory bowel disease.

Carcinoma of the gall bladder

(See pp. 497–498).

Cholangiocarcinoma

(See also p. 498.) This usually presents with jaundice and is detected by imaging: initially ultrasound and thereafter CT and, in particular, magnetic resonance cholangiopancreatography (MRCP). Spread is usually by local lymphatics or local extension. Cholangiocarcinoma of the common bile duct may be resectable at presentation but local extension precludes such management in the majority of more proximal lesions. Localized disease justifies an aggressive surgical approach, including partial hepatic resection. Hepatic transplantation for selected stage 1 and 2 disease has achieved 80% 5-year survival.

Palliative chemotherapy for patients with good performance status and advanced disease, using gemcitabine and cisplatin, achieves a response in 50% with a median survival of 12 months. Chemo-radiation has been used to treat localized small hilar cholangiocarcinoma, and radiotherapy can provide good analgesia.

Pancreas

Pancreatic adenocarcinoma

Prognosis

The 5-year survival rate for carcinoma of the pancreas is approximately 2–5%, with surgical intervention representing the only chance of long-term survival. Approximately 20% of all cases have a localized tumour suitable for resection and a median survival of 2 years, but in an elderly population, many of these individuals have co-morbid factors that preclude such major surgery.

Management

There is no proven adjuvant therapy for pancreatic cancer following surgery. To optimize the percentage of patients undergoing possible surgical resection, it is necessary to review each case in a multidisciplinary meeting. This approach also allows formulation of treatment strategies for those considered unsuitable for surgery.

In the majority of cases, management is palliative. Obstruction of the biliary tree and jaundice is a debilitating complication, often associated with severe pruritus but also the cause of non-specific malaise, lethargy and anorexia. Endoscopic placement of endoprostheses (stents) offers excellent palliation.

Palliative surgery has a role in duodenal obstruction (a complication seen in 10% of cases), but in advanced disease, self-expanding metal stents can be placed across the duodenal obstruction with excellent short-term results.

Chemo-radiotherapy with gemcitabine for small, locally advanced disease can achieve a response in 30% and a median survival of 17 months. Palliative chemotherapy for advanced disease with gemcitabine and cisplatin can achieve a response in approximately 20% of patients with advanced disease and an improvement in median survival from 6 to 12 months.

With disease progression, abdominal pain is a frequent complicating factor; it may prove extremely difficult to treat but can be sometimes helped by radiotherapy.

Neuroendocrine tumours of the pancreas

Treatment options for pancreatic neuroendocrine tumours (see also pp. 512–513) require a multidisciplinary approach and depend on the presence or absence of metastatic (usually hepatic) disease. Surgical resection of the pancreatic lesion is the only potential curative approach. Aggressive surgical intervention, including resection of the primary lesion, as well as liver resection for metastasis, has been used in selected cases. Somatostatin analogues, such as octreotide and lanreotide, have been used specifically for the control of symptoms secondary to the hormonal secretion. Radionuclide-labelled octreotide can also be used to induce responses in 23% for a median of 17 months.

The chemotherapeutic agents streptozotocin, 5-FU and cisplatin produce partial remission in 33% for a median of 9 months, while median survival is 31 months, reflecting the indolent natural history of these tumours. Everolimus and sunitinib can provide palliative benefit with prolongation of progression-free survival from 5.5 to 11 months and increased survival.

In patients with extensive liver metastasis, occlusion of the arterial blood flow by hepatic arterial embolization may control hormone-related symptoms. In most cases, the tumours are slowly progressive and may allow a reasonable quality of life for several years.

Further reading

Al-Rajabi R, Patel S, Ketchum NS et al. Comparative dosing and efficacy of sorafenib in hepatocellular cancer patients with varying liver dysfunction. *J Gastrointest Oncol* 2015; 6:259–267.
Caplin ME, Pavel M, Ćwikła JB et al. Lanreotide in metastatic enteropancreatic neuroendocrine tumors. *N Engl J Med* 2014; 371:224–233.
El-Serag HB. Hepatocellular carcinoma. *N Engl J Med* 2011; 365:1118–1127.
Gillmore R, Laurence V, Raouf S et al. Chemoradiotherapy with or without induction chemotherapy for locally advanced pancreatic cancer: a UK multi-institutional experience. *Clin Oncol* 2010; 22:564–569.
Grossman EJ, Millis JM. Liver transplantation for non-hepatocellular carcinoma malignancy: indications, limitations, and analysis of the current literature. *Liver Transpl* 2010; 16:930–942.
Raymond E, Dahan L, Raoul JL et al. Sunitinib malate for the treatment of pancreatic neuroendocrine tumors. *N Engl J Med* 2011; 364:501–513.
Turner NC, Strauss SJ, Sarker D et al. Chemotherapy with 5-fluorouracil, cisplatin and streptozocin for neuroendocrine tumours. *Br J Cancer* 2010; 102:1106–1112.
Valle J, Wasan H, Palmer DH et al. Cisplatin plus gemcitabine versus gemcitabine for biliary tract cancer. *N Engl J Med* 2010; 362:1273–1281.

EPITHELIAL OVARIAN CANCER

Aetiology and pathology

There is uncertainty over the tissue of origin that gives rise to the 80% of all ovarian cancers that are epithelial ***(Box 17.56)***. The ovarian surface epithelium of the serosal peritoneum or the epithelial lining of the fallopian tube fimbriae are the most likely candidates. There is a consistent relationship between the risk of epithelial ovarian cancer (EOC) and the frequency and duration of ovulation. While not mechanistically explained, this has provided a successful rationale for reducing the risk of EOC by up to one-third through early pregnancy and use of the oral contraceptive pill. The non-epithelial cancers are of germ cell or stromal origin, although molecular biological markers have shown that the category of mixed Müllerian carcino-sarcoma is an entirely epithelial tumour with metaplastic stromal elements.

BRCA1 or *BRCA2* germline mutations (see ***Box 17.47***) are present in 10% overall, except in those with a family history of breast or ovarian cancer. In high-grade serous histology, *BRCA* mutations are present in 23% of patients <50 years old, falling to 12% in those >50 years, despite a lack of family history in 40%.

Clinical features

Ovarian cancer typically causes few specific symptoms, often leading to late diagnosis; however, it is not silent ***(Box 17.57)***.

Sometimes, there is a sensation of a pelvic mass, which may become (acutely) painful; often, however, there is only vague abdominal distension and epigastric discomfort. Symptoms of irritable bowel syndrome can be confused with those of ovarian cancer but rarely present for the first time over the age of 50, when they should stimulate investigation for ovarian cancer.

On examination, the majority of patients present with a pelvic mass and advanced stage III (spread within the peritoneal cavity) or IV (extraperitoneal) disease. Screening (see p. 592) by serum CA125 tumour marker and transvaginal ultrasound scan does detect some early cancers with improved survival, but is being further refined with serial tests to avoid too many negative laparotomies and is thus still considered a research tool.

Investigations

Pelvic examination should be complemented by a serum CA125 tumour marker in primary care and transvaginal ultrasound. MRI is the definitive imaging technique for the pelvis, while CT-PET scans assist in staging the patient. A risk of malignancy index (RMI) of >250 ***(Box 17.58)*** should trigger investigation by a specialist gynaecological cancer team.

BRCA mutation status should be assessed in patients with a positive family history (see ***Box 17.46***), and in those with high-grade serous adenocarcinoma histology under the age of 50 to identify the potential for targeted treatment with PARP inhibitors.

Prognosis

Histological subtype (clear cell and mucinous are worse), grade/differentiation, stage, extent of residual disease following surgery (macroscopic versus microscopic or none) and performance status are all significant independent prognostic factors for survival ***(Box 17.59)***.

Five-year survival rates for stage III vary with *BRCA* mutational status: *BRCA1* 44% and *BRCA2* 61%, compared to *BRCA*-negative

Box 17.56 Ovarian cancer pathology

- Serous cystadenocarcinoma
- Papillary cystadenocarcinoma
- Endometrioid cancer
- Adenocarcinoma
- Mucinous cancer
- Clear cell cancer
- Mixed mesodermal Müllerian tumours
- Germ cell cancers:
  - Dysgerminoma
  - Embryonal cancer
  - Endodermal sinus tumour
  - Choriocarcinoma
  - Teratoma immature/mature
- Granulosa cell tumours
- Brenner, Sertoli–Leydig tumour, carcinoid tumours
- Other stromal cell tumours

Box 17.57 Symptoms associated with ovarian cancer that need investigation

- Persistent abdominal distension (women often refer to this as bloating)
- Feeling full when eating or early satiety and loss of appetite
- Pelvic or abdominal pain
- Increased urinary urgency or frequency

Box 17.58 Risk of ovarian malignancy index (RMI)

- RMI combines three pre-surgical features and is a product of the ultrasound scan score (U), the menopausal status (M) and the serum CA125 level (CA125):
  $RMI = U \times M \times CA125$
- The ultrasound result is scored as 1 point for each of the following characteristics: multilocular cysts, solid areas, metastases, ascites and bilateral lesions: U=0 (for an ultrasound score of 0), U=1 (for an ultrasound score of 1), U=3 (for an ultrasound score of 2–5).
- The menopausal status is scored as 1=pre-menopausal and 3=post-menopausal. The classification of 'post-menopausal' relates to women who have had no period for more than 1 year or women over the age of 50 who have had a hysterectomy.
- Serum CA125 is measured in IU/mL and can vary between 0 and hundreds or even thousands of units.
- If the RMI is >250, a strong suspicion of ovarian cancer should be maintained.

Box 17.59 Survival rates in invasive epithelial ovarian cancer

Stage	Relative 5-year survival rate	Stage	Relative 5-year survival rate
I	89%	IIC	57%
IA	94%	III	34%
IB	91%	IIIA	45%
IC	80%	IIIB	39%
II	66%	IIIC	35%
IIA	76%	IV	18%
IIB	67%		

(From Heintz AP, Odicino F, Maisonneuve P et al. Carcinoma of the ovary. FIGO 26th Annual Report on the Results of Treatment in Gynecological Cancer. *Int J Gynaecol Obstet* 2006; 95(Suppl 1):S161–192, with permission.)

25%. *BRCA* status is also a predictive marker for increased sensitivity to platinum and anthracycline cytotoxics, and to PARP inhibitors like olaparib.

Management

Debulking surgery (with total abdominal hysterectomy, bilateral salpingo-oophorectomy, omentectomy, and stripping of the subdiaphragmatic peritoneum) has a major role in the treatment of ovarian cancer. When disease is confined to the ovary – that is, stage I – surgery can be curative in 80–90% if the histology is well to moderately differentiated. For patients with poorly differentiated or more advanced disease, and spread throughout the peritoneal cavity, surgery still has a major role in staging and in improving survival when it is possible to debulk optimally to no visible residual disease. Primary chemotherapy and delayed surgery is an alternative approach when disease is too advanced to permit optimal primary debulking surgery and is able to render approximately one-third of inoperable patients fit for optimal debulking surgery. Survival of patients with such advanced disease is equal, whether chemotherapy is given before or after surgery, but preoperative downstaging can avoid much surgical morbidity.

Carboplatin, which is associated with fewer side-effects than cisplatin, has become the mainstay of EOC chemotherapy. Response is achieved in approximately two-thirds of patients. Paclitaxel has been shown to increase the response rate and improve the survival of many patients when added to a platinum-based treatment.

Adjuvant treatment with carboplatin and paclitaxel for stage I high-risk disease increases the absolute 5-year survival by 9%, from 70% to 79%, and for combined stages I–III completely debulked disease by 19%, from 60% to 79%, a relative risk reduction of 29%.

In more advanced disease, 75% of patients will respond to combination chemotherapy and the median survival is approximately 3 years. Treatment at recurrence may involve surgery for oligo-metastatic disease with a long treatment-free interval, but can also be delayed in advanced cases until the disease is symptomatic. Further palliative responses can be achieved with carboplatin and paclitaxel if the treatment-free interval is >6 months; liposomal doxorubicin, etoposide, gemcitabine and trabectedin are all active drugs for the palliation of recurrent disease. Up to 30% of those with metastatic disease may be alive after 5 years, although this falls to 5–10% if the cancer is not able to be debulked at operation or has spread outside the peritoneal cavity. It has proven difficult to develop more targeted biological agents for ovarian cancer, apart from olaparib for *BRCA*-mutated disease. Bevacizumab, when added to chemotherapy, has increased disease-free survival by 3–6 months without increasing overall survival, and has a limited role, except perhaps in platinum-resistant recurrent disease.

Stage III EOC tends to remain exclusively within the peritoneal cavity, which has led to new intraperitoneal routes of treatment administration with a 17% improved survival for those with minimal residual disease after surgery. However, at recurrence, bulk disease in the peritoneum commonly causes progressive bowel obstruction, which may require palliative operation or expert palliative care support to manage the terminal phases of the illness.

Further reading

Jayson GC, Kohn EC, Kitchener HC, Ledermann JA. Ovarian cancer. *Lancet* 2014; 384:1376–1388.

UROLOGICAL CANCERS

Renal cell carcinoma

Clinical features and diagnosis

See page 791.

Investigations and management

At diagnosis, renal cancers are staged using CT and/or MRI scans to assess operability and the presence of distant metastases.

A nephrectomy is performed unless bilateral tumours are present or the contralateral kidney functions poorly, in which case conservative surgery, such as partial nephrectomy, may be indicated.

For patients with metastatic disease, prognosis is predicted on the basis of the Heng criteria (Karnofsky performance status score <80, haemoglobin below the lower limit of normal, neutrophils and platelets above the upper limit of normal, raised calcium, <6 months from diagnosis). Those with no risk factors are considered as having a favourable prognosis and 75% will be alive at 2 years; those with 1–2 risk factors are considered intermediate-prognosis (53% alive at 2 years); and those with 3 or more risk factors are considered poor-prognosis (7% survival at 2 years). If metastases are present and the patient is in the favourable or intermediate group, nephrectomy may still be warranted when the primary tumour constitutes the main bulk of disease, since regression of metastases has been reported after removal of the main tumour mass. Adjuvant treatments are unproven and under investigation. The 5-year survival rate is 60–70% with tumours confined to the renal parenchyma, 15–35% with lymph node involvement, and only approximately 5% in those who have distant metastases.

TKis are the mainstay of treatment for metastatic renal cancer. Sunitinib has a 30–40% response rate and a median time to progression of 11 months. It is a toxic drug, with fatigue, diarrhoea, sore mouth and taste disturbance its main side-effects. It can also cause cardiac dysfunction with prolonged use. It is normally given for 28 days, followed by a 2-week break. Pazopanib, a related drug, is better tolerated and of similar efficacy. Patients who fall into the favourable-prognosis group may be treated with immunotherapy: for example, high-dose IL-2. Following failure of immunotherapy or a first-line TKi, the drug axitinib may be used; if that fails, some may respond to everolimus. Bevacizumab has activity and is sometimes combined with interferon. Isolated metastases – of brain or lung, for instance – may be suitable for excision.

Urothelial cancers

Clinical features and diagnosis

(See also pp. 791–792) Prognosis depends on the performance status of the patient, the TNM stage of the tumour (and whether it has penetrated the bladder muscle in bladder tumours, in particular), and its degree of differentiation. After surgery, the surgical margins, lymphovascular invasion and nodal involvement are further prognostic factors.

Management

Renal pelvis and ureteric tumours

Early-stage tumours are treated by nephro-ureterectomy. Adjuvant radiotherapy and chemotherapy appear to be of little or no value. The remainder of the urothelium is at risk of further primary transitional cell cancers (TCCs) in about half of patients and requires surveillance cystoscopy. Metastatic TCC is treated as for bladder tumours (see below).

Bladder tumours

Superficial bladder TCCs within the basement membrane are treated by transurethral resection or local diathermy. The risk of recurrence varies with the differentiation, and follow-up check cystoscopies and cytological examination of the urine are required. Recurrent superficial TCC can be treated with bladder instillation of BCG (bacille Calmette-Guérin) or, alternatively, with chemotherapy agents such as gemcitabine or mitomycin to delay further recurrence for 18 months on average.

Patients with muscle-invasive bladder tumours are treated with radical cystectomy if under 70 years, and radical radiotherapy if over 70 years, with salvage cystectomy for recurrences. In the absence of metastases and with adequate renal function (glomerular filtration rate >60 mL/min), surgery or radical radiotherapy should be preceded by neoadjuvant chemotherapy; this is cisplatin-based, with methotrexate, vinblastine and doxorubicin (MVAC) or cisplatin and gemcitabine. Neoadjuvant chemotherapy improves the absolute cure rate by 10%. The prognosis ranges from a 5-year survival rate of 80–90% for lesions not involving bladder muscle to 5% for those presenting with metastases.

Alternatively, those with T1 grade 3 to T4 tumours can be offered the chance of bladder preservation with chemo-radiotherapy using cisplatin and 5-FU. This can achieve complete response at subsequent transurethral resection in 66%, bladder preservation and a good quality of life in 67%, and a comparable long-term survival (30–50% at 5 years) to cystectomy. Cystectomy requires a new bladder to be made out of small bowel, joining this to the urethra if possible, or an ileal conduit.

Metastatic bladder cancer. This is a chemosensitive cancer; it is usually a TCC, although other variants may occur, such as squamous tumours where chemosensitivity is similar. Cisplatin-based treatment is the mainstay and response rates of 40–60% are seen. Approximately 5–10% are durable. Second-line chemotherapy often produces responses in previously responsive tumours; combinations include carboplatin and paclitaxel. Targeting the PD-1/PD-L1 axis (see p. 601) is producing encouraging results and is likely to be used increasingly in management of this disease.

Prostate cancer

Early prostate cancer

Clinical features and diagnosis

(See p. 792.) Diagnosis is usually made on a raised serum prostate-specific antigen (PSA), followed by a transrectal ultrasound-guided needle biopsy.

Prognosis

The histological appearances are graded and accorded a Gleason score; together with the height of the serum PSA, plus accurate staging of the local extent of disease with pelvic MRI (dynamic contrast) and transrectal ultrasound, this score can identify prognostic groups ***(Box 17.60)***. Treatment decisions must balance the age and performance status of the patient with the predicted behaviour of the cancer, which is becoming more objectively identifiable with advances in gene profiling. This allows the selection of patients with good prognosis for no active treatment; they may reasonably choose to be kept under surveillance and, like 75% of men over the age of 80, die with, but not because of, their prostate cancer.

Management

(See also p. 793.) Patients with disease localized to the prostate requiring treatment can be managed by curative surgery (radical prostatectomy), external beam radiotherapy, or brachytherapy implants, which can achieve equivalent survival rates but differ in the spectrum of unwanted side-effects with respect to incontinence and sexual dysfunction. Radiotherapy tends to be used more frequently in older patients who wish to avoid surgery. In appropriately selected series of patients, a 5-year survival of 85% can be achieved. Adjuvant radiotherapy after radical prostatectomy can reduce PSA relapse but has not increased overall survival. Discussion between patient and clinician is vital to enable a treatment choice that is most appropriate to the patient's circumstances; many of these individuals are elderly and the side-effects of treatment are significant, often not leading to an improvement in mortality. For many patients (those with combined Gleason scores of 6 or below), localized prostate cancer may be managed expectantly using the strategy of watchful waiting, in which regular PSA tests are supplemented with repeat prostatic biopsies to establish whether the cancer is becoming more aggressive and thus warrants active therapy. Alternatively, they may be managed through a strategy of simple surveillance using changes in symptoms and PSA alone to guide therapy.

Box 17.60 Prostate cancer: prognostic factors

At initial diagnosis
- Clinical stage
- Biopsy Gleason grade
- Serum PSA level

Post surgery
- Surgical/pathological stage
- Surgical margins
- Extracapsular spread, extension to seminal vesicles or lymph nodes

Metastatic hormone-resistant
- Performance status
- Serum PSA
- Haemoglobin, albumin, alkaline phosphatase and LDH level

LDH, lactate dehydrogenase; PSA, prostate-specific antigen.

Endocrine therapy

Prostate cancer is the most hormone-sensitive malignancy. The androgen receptor (AR) plays a critical role; prostate cancer tissue is able to trap circulating androgens so that tissue levels of androgens are maintained, despite very low (castration) levels of circulating androgens. Resistance may involve receptor super-sensitivity and altered ligand binding, allowing other steroids to act as agonists and eventually bypassing the androgen receptor.

Androgen deprivation

- ***GnRH agonists***, e.g. goserelin and leuprorelin, and orchidectomy are equally effective at lowering circulating androgens and inducing responses in prostate cancer. However, in the first week, GnRH agonists produce a rise in luteinizing hormone (LH) and testosterone, which can result in a tumour flare in metastatic disease; they must therefore be combined with an antiandrogen, e.g. flutamide, in the initial phases. An alternative is to use a gonadorelin antagonist, e.g. degarelix.
- ***Androgen receptor blockers*** include drugs such as bicalutamide and the more potent antagonist, enzalutamide.
- ***Androgen synthesis inhibitors*** such as abiraterone act by inhibiting *CYP17*.
- ***Corticosteroids and oestrogens*** may also be helpful in disease that has become refractory to castration.

Hormonal agents may also be used after chemotherapy for prostate cancer, and both enzalutamide and abiraterone have been shown to prolong life in this situation. Adjuvant androgen deprivation treatment, such as monthly depot goserelin, has not improved survival following surgery, but when given before and during radiotherapy, can improve the overall survival at 3 years for T1–T3 tumours from 62% to 78%.

Advanced prostate cancer

Management

Locally advanced prostate cancer (T3 N0) without distant metastases is best treated with combined androgen deprivation and radiotherapy, which improves 10-year survival, compared with endocrine treatment alone, from 61% to 71%.

Metastatic prostate cancer is normally treated initially with androgen deprivation to achieve castration and effectively palliated in 70% of patients for a median duration of response of 2 years. Once this fails, the disease is termed castration-resistant and further palliative options are more potent hormonal drugs or chemotherapy, such as docetaxel. If chemotherapy fails, a return to hormonal therapy may prolong disease control. The timing of chemotherapy remains unclear; rather like in breast cancer, it may be deferred until all available hormonal therapy has failed or it may be used earlier.

Other non-hormonal approaches are frequently used: bone-targeted drugs such as alpharadin (^{223}radium), zoledronic acid and denosumab, as well as palliative radiotherapy for painful metastases.

Germ cell tumours

Testicular and ovarian germ cell tumours

Germ cell tumours are the most common cancers in men aged 15–35 years but comprise only 1–2% of all cancers. They are much less common in women. There are two main histological types: seminoma (dysgerminoma in women) and non-seminoma. Non-seminomas may be comprised of varying proportions of mature and immature elements; the mature elements are now known as teratoma (previously, this term referred to all non-seminomas). Teratomas in women present as dermoid cysts with low malignant potential. Germ cell tumours may rarely occur in extragonadal sites in the midline from pituitary, mediastinum or retroperitoneum but should be treated in a similar manner ***(Box 17.61)***.

Clinical features

Most men present with a testicular mass, which is often painful; some have symptoms of metastases to the para-aortic lymph nodes with back pain and gynaecomastia if the tumour is hCG-secreting ***(Fig. 17.41)***. In women, the mass presents with vague pelvic symptoms but at a younger age than the more common epithelial ovarian cancers.

Investigations

- ***Ultrasound or MRI scanning*** of the testicle or ovary is required.
- ***Assay of serum tumour markers*** includes α-fetoprotein (AFP), β-human chorionic gonadotrophin (β-hCG) and lactate dehydrogenase (LDH). A urinary pregnancy test for hCG in the accident and emergency department has saved the lives of young men with metastatic germ cell cancer.
- ***CT or MRI scan*** is performed to seek distant metastases.

Treatment

- ***Surgery for men*** is by the inguinal approach to avoid spillage of highly metastatic tumour in the scrotum.
- ***Surgery in women*** for diagnosis and staging should always be conservative, compared to the approach in epithelial ovarian cancer, with preservation of fertility because of the efficacy of chemotherapy.

Management

Seminomas

Seminomas are very radiosensitive and chemosensitive. They are associated with a raised serum LDH but only rarely a mildly raised β-hCG and never a raised AFP. Stage I disease limited to the gonad

Box 17.61 Germ cell histology: WHO classification

- Seminoma
- Non-seminoma
  - Embryonal carcinoma
  - Choriocarcinoma
  - Yolk sac tumour
  - Teratoma

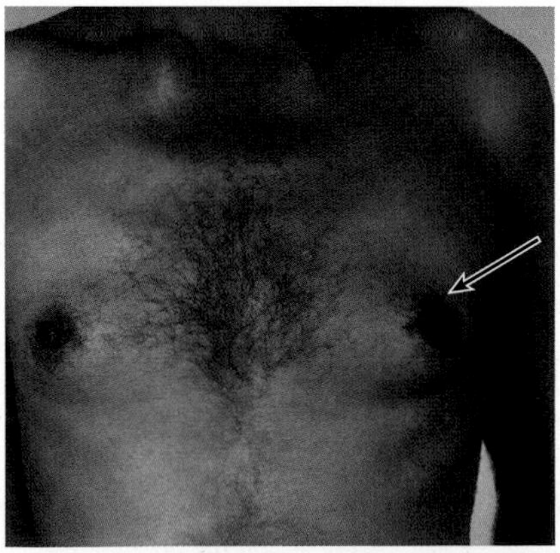

Figure 17.41 Gynaecomastia (arrowed) in a man with β-human chorionic gonadotrophin-secreting testicular cancer.

is associated with a 10–30% 5-year risk of recurrence with surgery alone. Adjuvant therapy, with either chemotherapy or radiotherapy to the para-aortic lymph nodes, is preferred as it leads to greater than 95% cure in early-stage disease. Carboplatin is the first choice because of convenience, reduced acute side-effects, and absence of the long-term risks of secondary malignancy that are associated with radiotherapy. Alternatively, intensive surveillance can be undertaken, with treatment reserved for those who relapse; this approach carries an equally high cure rate, since combination chemotherapy (e.g. cisplatin, etoposide and bleomycin, BEP) will cure 95% of those with visible metastatic disease.

Non-seminomas

The risk of relapse with stage I disease varies from 5% to 50%, depending on the prognostic factors of histological differentiation, presence of embryonal elements, and extent of local and vascular invasion.

For those at moderate to high risk, adjuvant chemotherapy with a single cycle of BEP leads to a 95% cure rate. The option of primary retroperitoneal lymph node dissection in high-risk non-seminoma is now rarely taken up, as it is less likely to reduce the risk of recurrence.

Metastatic disease commonly involves para-aortic lymph nodes and lungs but may spread rapidly (especially if there are trophoblastic (β-hCG-producing) elements present) and cause life-threatening respiratory or other organ failure. A rapid diagnosis can be made in the presence of gynaecomastia and a positive urinary pregnancy test before the institution of potentially life-saving treatment. About 80% of teratomas will express either β-hCG or AFP, and almost all metastatic disease will be associated with an elevation of the less specific serum marker, LDH.

The percentage cure rate depends on the height of the tumour markers (AFP >10000 and β-hCG >100000 IU/L) and the sites of metastases; it ranges from 50% to 95%. The most established regimen is BEP and 3–4 cycles are usually given.

Patients who relapse following initial chemotherapy may well be cured by subsequent chemotherapy with further cisplatin and ifosfamide, or high-dose chemotherapy with carboplatin and etoposide, and a stem cell transplant.

Although approximately 20% of men will be infertile due to azoospermia at the time of diagnosis, the majority of the remainder will retain their fertility after chemotherapy and be able to father normal children. Similarly, most women retain their fertility, although less is known about the association with infertility at presentation owing to the much lower frequency of germ cell tumours in women.

Further reading

Attard G, Parker C, Eeles RA et al. Prostate cancer. *Lancet* 2016; 387:70–82.

Beer TM, Armstrong AJ, Rathkopf DE et al. and PREVAIL Investigators. Enzalutamide in metastatic prostate cancer before chemotherapy. *N Engl J Med* 2014; 371:424–433.

Choueiri TK, Jacobus S, Bellmunt J et al. Neoadjuvant dose-dense methotrexate, vinblastine, doxorubicin, and cisplatin with pegfilgrastim support in muscle-invasive urothelial cancer: pathologic, radiologic, and biomarker correlates. *J Clin Oncol* 2014; 32:1889–1894.

Escudier B, Eisen T, Porta C and ESMO Guidelines Working Group. Renal cell carcinoma: ESMO Clinical Practice Guidelines for diagnosis, treatment and follow-up. *Ann Oncol* 2012; 23 Suppl 7:vii65–71.

James ND, Hussain SA, Hall E et al. Radiotherapy with or without chemotherapy in muscle-invasive bladder cancer. *N Engl J Med* 2012; 366:1477–1488.

Motzer RJ, Hutson TE, Cella D et al. Pazopanib versus sunitinib in metastatic renal-cell carcinoma. *N Engl J Med* 2013; 369:722–731.

Quinn DI, Lara PN Jr. Renal cell cancer - targeting an immune checkpoint or multiple kinases. *N Engl J Med* 2015; 373:1872–1874.

Ryan CJ, Smith MR, de Bono JS et al. and COU-AA-302 Investigators. Abiraterone in metastatic prostate cancer without previous chemotherapy. *N Engl J Med* 2013; 368:138–148.

METASTATIC CANCER OF UNKNOWN PRIMARY

Patients presenting with symptoms of their metastases, or with an incidental finding on imaging without a clinically obvious primary after investigation, represent a common clinical problem and comprise 5–10% of patients in a specialist oncological centre. As a result of several systematic studies, some with postmortem follow-up, the following guidance should aid the choice of appropriate investigation and treatment. On the other hand, poor-prognosis patients identified by performance status, histology, site and extent of disease can be spared the discomfort of intensive investigation and given more appropriate palliative care.

Diagnosis

Diagnosis requires histology first and foremost, as it will lead to the identification of several distinct groups.

- ***Squamous cancers*** mostly present in the lymph nodes of the cervical region; 80% will be associated with an occult head and neck primary, the remainder arising from the lung. Inguinal nodes usually point to a primary of the genital tract or anal canal. Treatment with radiotherapy and chemotherapy may have curative potential, especially in the head and neck area, and even in the absence of an identifiable primary on pan-endoscopy.
- ***Poorly differentiated or anaplastic cancers*** will include the majority of the curable cancers, such as high-grade lymphomas and germ cell tumours, and should be suspected in all young patients with midline masses. They are identifiable by their immunocytochemistry and tumour markers. Gene markers, such as ip12 for germ cell tumours and Bcl-2 for lymphomas, are increasingly available to aid this diagnosis. Treatment and prognosis are as outlined for lymphoma and germ cell tumours.
- ***Adenocarcinomas*** form the majority of cases. Their investigation should be guided by the desire to identify the most treatable options, and the knowledge that the largest proportion will have arisen from the lung or pancreas, with relatively poor treatment prospects.

Tissue tumour markers can be helpful ***(Box 17.62)*** and, increasingly, gene profiles are able to identify the primary site of origin by gene expression microarray and RT-PCR.

Mutation analysis is more easily available to identify potential targets for treatment, such as RAS, EGFR and RET; however, clinical trials are still necessary to identify whether specific pathway inhibitors have a therapeutic effect when so identified.

Investigations should therefore always start with a review of the histology, a chest X-ray and a CT scan of chest, abdomen and pelvis; in men, they should include serum PSA and rectal ultrasound to identify prostate cancers, and in women, mammography and breast MRI to identify occult breast cancer, and pelvic MRI to identify ovarian cancer.

For good-prognosis patients wishing to have palliative chemotherapy, investigations such as endoscopy to identify lung, colon or stomach primaries are indicated to guide the choice of chemotherapy agents, although the diagnostic yield of 4–5% must be set against the discomfort and risks. Serum tumour markers for other solid cancers, although highly sensitive, are too non-specific and unreliable to be useful as diagnostic aids in this situation.

Further investigation may require PET-CT for head and neck, lung and possibly other primaries, and radio-isotope scans for

Box 17.62 Carcinoma of unknown primary

Immunohistochemistry markers	Most probable (but not exclusive) tissue of origin
EMA (epithelial membrane antigen)	Epithelial
LCA (leucocyte common antigen)	Lymphoid
Cytokeratin 7+ 20+	Pancreas 65%, cholangiocarcinoma 65% Gastric 40%, transitional cell 65%, ovarian mucinous 90%
Cytokeratin 7+ 20–	Ovarian (except mucinous) 100%, breast 90%, lung adenocarcinoma 90%, uterus endometrioid 85%, transitional cell 35%, pancreas adenocarcinoma 30%, cholangiocarcinoma 30%, thyroid 100%, mesothelioma 65%
Cytokeratin 7– 20+	Colorectal adenocarcinoma 80%, gastric adenocarcinoma 35%, Merkel cell 70%
Cytokeratin 7– 20–	Hepatocellular 80%, carcinoid 80%, lung small cell and squamous 75%, prostate 85%, renal adenocarcinoma 80%, adrenal 100%, germ cell 95%, squamous cancer of head and neck, and oesophagus 70%, mesothelioma 35%
TTF-1 (thyroid transcription factor)	Lung and thyroid
Thyroglobulin	Thyroid
ER (oestrogen receptor), PR (progesterone receptor) and Her2 receptor	Breast
PSA (prostate specific antigen)	Prostate and breast
CEA (carcinoembryonic antigen)	Gastrointestinal
CDX2	Colorectal and small intestinal
Villin	Gastrointestinal
CA125 peritoneal antigen	Ovarian, fallopian tube and primary peritoneal and breast
WT1	Ovarian serous cancer, mesothelioma, desmoplastic tumours, Wilms' tumours
S100, melanin and HMB45	Melanoma
Myosin, desmin and factor VIII	Soft tissue sarcoma
Chromogranin and NSE (neurone specific enolase)	Neuroendocrine
AFP (α-fetoprotein)	Germ cell tumours and hepatocellular carcinoma
β-hCG (beta-human chorionic gonadotrophin)	Germ cell and trophoblastic tumours
CD117	Gastrointestinal stromal tumours

thyroid and carcinoid tumours. PET-CT may also be used to seek other metastatic sites if considering surgery for unifocal disease.

Prognosis

The histological type and extent of the disease and performance status of the patient are the key factors. Most large series report an overall median survival of 12 weeks but considerably better survival amongst the special subgroups, such as patients presenting with isolated nodal metastases who have a significantly better prognosis than the majority with visceral and/or bone metastases and may warrant more extensive investigation.

Management

If investigations have not identified a primary site, surgery may be considered for unifocal adenocarcinoma of unknown primary (ACUP) metastases in lymph nodes, lung, liver and brain, especially if due to melanoma and so having the potential for long-term survival.

In women, an isolated axillary lymph node metastasis should be treated as for lymph-node-positive breast cancer; this has a similar prospect for long-term cure, though without the need for breast surgery. Malignant ascites in women should be treated with a trial of chemotherapy, as for primary peritoneal, fallopian tube or epithelial ovarian cancer. The prognosis for those responding to the therapeutic trial is similar to that in the disease of known primary origin. Primary chemotherapy that achieves an excellent response by imaging and CA125 criteria should be followed by debulking surgery; if successful, it carries a median survival in excess of 4 years.

Box 17.63 Adenocarcinoma of unknown primary: where search for the primary is of therapeutic benefit

- Breast, e.g. isolated axillary lymphadenopathy
- Ovary, e.g. peritoneal carcinomatosis
- Prostate, e.g. pelvic lymphadenopathy
- Colon, e.g. liver metastases

For men, the occasional occult prostatic cancer found from a raised serum PSA offers some palliative treatment prospects ***(Box 17.63)***.

For the patient presenting with hepatic metastases, which are most commonly associated with an occult gastrointestinal primary, there is an increasing choice and efficacy of chemotherapy agents for gastrointestinal cancers that have the potential to improve their palliation.

If there is an excellent response, suitable patients may even be considered for hepatic ablation or resection. If, after all efforts, no primary has been identified, palliative chemotherapy treatment can achieve responses in 20–40% in highly selected series, with median survivals of 9–10 months, and 5–10% surviving to 5 years.

Further reading

Greco FA, Spigel DR, Yardley DA et al. Molecular profiling in unknown primary cancer: accuracy of tissue of origin prediction. *Oncologist* 2010; 15:500–506.

Varadhachary GR, Raber MN. Cancer of unknown primary site. *N Engl J Med* 2014; 371:757–763.

18

Rheumatic disease

Anisur Rahman, Ian Giles

See your e-book for key learning points, clinical tips, drug tips, extra tables, extra images, interactive Figures, videos, MCQs and Special Topics from the International Advisory Board.

INTRODUCTION

Musculoskeletal problems, particularly pain, are common. They represent 20–30% of the workload of the primary care physician. They can be divided into three types

- ***Pain arising from soft tissues around joints***, such as muscles and tendons. The joints themselves are normal. These are the most common locomotor problems, and are generally self-limiting or respond to simple analgesia, physiotherapy or exercise.
- ***Diseases of the joints themselves***. Osteoarthritis is more common than inflammatory arthritis, especially in the elderly.
- ***Autoimmune rheumatic diseases***. These include disorders such as systemic lupus erythematosus (SLE), where the locomotor symptoms are just one manifestation of a systemic disorder.

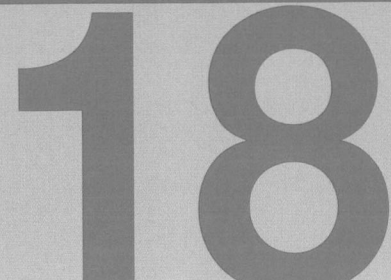

RHEUMATOLOGY

Clinical examination of joints

- **Ask patient to walk a few steps and come back**
- **Note gait**
- **Neck**

Ask patient to move head back and forward / Sideways moving ear to touch shoulder (testing cervical spine)

General
Look for walking aids
Ask patient to walk – note gait
Joint – swelling, redness, deformity
Rash
Weight loss
Depression

Head and neck
- ? Cushingoid
Face - Butterfly rash (malar) (SLE)
- Tight skin (scleroderma)
Eyes - Episcleritis
- Scleromalacia (RA)
- Red, painful eye
- Dry eyes
Mouth - Ulcers
- Small
Nose - Beaky
(Ulcers, Small, Beaky: Systemic sclerosis)

- **Arms**

Flex elbows to touch shoulders / Put hands behind head

Psoriatic rash

Rheumatoid nodules

- **Hands**

Inspect function / Make a fist / Open and close / Pain / Squeeze metacarpals / Turn palms up and down (supinate and pronate)

Hands and wrists
Rheumatoid arthritis
- Ulnar deviation
- Subluxation of MCPs
- PIP joints
- Fixed flexion (Boutonnière's)
- Fixed extension (swan neck deformity)
- Swellings and deformities
- SLE – Gottron's nodules

Osteoarthritis
- Heberden's and Bouchard's nodes

Raynaud's

- **Legs**

Flex hip / With hand on knee, move foot to left and right to rotate hips

- **Knee**

Touch for warmth and swelling / Test for effusion effusion

Knees
Effusion
Popliteal cyst (Baker's cyst)

- **Feet**

Look / Squeeze forefoot (checking for metatarsophalangeal inflammation, synovitis)

Feet
Deformities
Foot broader
Hammer toe deformities
Ulcers

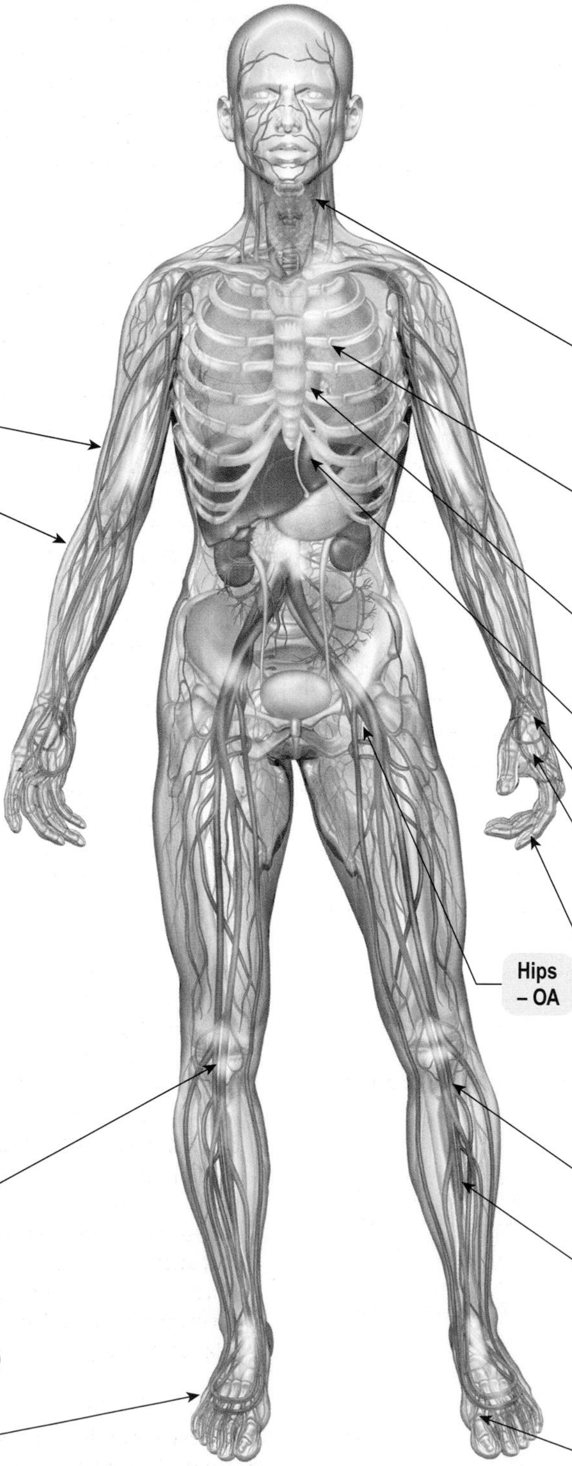

Hips – OA

Osteoarthritis
Large weight-bearing joints

Rheumatoid arthritis (RA)
Hands, feet, elbows, temporomandibular, sternoclavicular, acromioclavicular, cervical spine. Any synovial joint.

- **Spine**

Bend right and left by moving hands at side, to slide down leg towards knee / Look at spine for scoliosis, kyphosis, deformity / Bend forwards to try and touch toes (don't force to do this) / Standing – ask patient to turn from side to side

Lymphadenopathy (RA)

Lungs
Infections
Bronchiectasis
Pleural effusions

Heart
Murmurs
Pericardial sounds

Splenomegaly

Tenosynovitis

Carpal tunnel

Nails
Vasculitic lesions
Dystrophy and pitting in psoriasis

Bowed deformity in Paget's

Oedema

Sensory polyneuropathy

Acute gout

ANATOMY AND PHYSIOLOGY OF THE NORMAL JOINT

A joint can be defined as a place where two or more bones meet. There are three types of joints: fibrous, fibrocartilaginous and synovial.

Fibrous and fibrocartilaginous joints

These include the intervertebral discs, the sacroiliac joints, the pubic symphysis and the costochondral joints. Skull sutures are fibrous joints. Little movement occurs at such joints.

Synovial joints

Synovial joints ***(Fig. 18.1)*** include the ball-and-socket joints (e.g. hip) and the hinge joints (e.g. interphalangeal). They are designed to allow movement, which is restricted to a required range, and stability is maintained during use. The load is distributed across the surface, thus preventing damage by overloading or disuse. Each structural component of a synovial joint plays a key functional role, and different components are affected in different disease processes.

Juxta-articular bone

Bone structure and physiology are discussed on page 707. The bone that abuts a joint (juxta-articular bone) is highly vascular and comprises a light framework of mineralized collagen enclosed in a thin coating of tougher, cortical bone. It withstands pressure poorly if the normal intra-articular covering of hyaline cartilage is worn away, as in osteoarthritis (OA; see pp. 667–671). This process can lead to abnormalities of bone growth and remodelling (see p. 668).

Articular cartilage

The hyaline cartilage lining the bones within a joint is called articular cartilage. It is avascular and derives nourishment from synovial fluid. It is predominantly composed of type II collagen, encoded by the *COL2A1* gene, which forms a mesh-like network. Within the mesh are giant macromolecular aggregates of proteoglycan. These heterogeneous macromolecules comprise protein chains with side-chains of the carbohydrates keratan and chondroitin sulphate (aggrecans). These molecules have a negative charge and retain water in the structure by producing a dynamic tension between the retaining force of the collagen matrix and the expansive effect of osmotic pressure. Intermittent pressure from 'loading' of the joint is essential to normal cartilage function and encourages movement of water, minerals and nutrients between cartilage and synovial fluid. Chondrocytes secrete collagen and proteoglycans, and are embedded in the cartilage. They migrate towards the joint surface along with the matrix they produce. Defects in articular cartilage and underlying bone are features of ***osteoarthritis***.

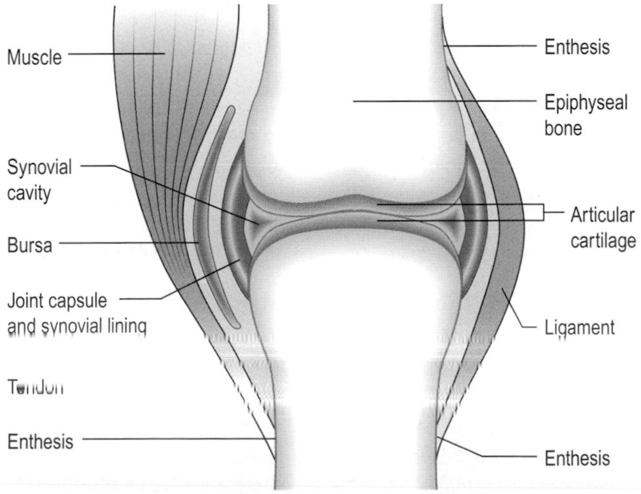

Figure 18.1 Normal synovial joint.

Synovium and synovial fluid

The joint capsule, which is connected to the periosteum, is lined with synovium, which is a few cells thick and vascular. Its surface is smooth and non-adherent, and is permeable to proteins and crystalloids. As there are no macroscopic gaps, it is able to retain normal joint fluid, even under pressure. Macrophages and fibroblast-like synoviocytes form the synovial layer by cell-to-cell interactions mediated by cadherin II. The synoviocytes release hyaluronan into the joint space, which helps to retain fluid in the joint. Synovial fluid is a highly viscous fluid secreted by the synovial cells and has a similar consistency to plasma. Glycoproteins ensure a low coefficient of friction between the cartilaginous surfaces. Tendon sheaths and bursae are also lined by synovium. Inflammation of the synovium is a feature of ***inflammatory arthritis***.

Ligaments and tendons

These structures stabilize joints. Ligaments are variably elastic and this contributes to the stiffness or laxity of joints (see pp. 666–667). Tendons are inelastic and transmit muscle power to bones. The joint capsule is formed by intermeshing tendons and ligaments. The point where a tendon or ligament joins a bone is called an ***enthesis*** and may be the site of inflammation. Whereas most ligaments and tendons run outside the joints, some, like the supraspinatus tendon in the shoulder and the cruciate ligaments in the knee, run through the joint. Inflammation or trauma to these joints can cause severe joint symptoms.

Blood vessels and nerves

The ligaments, periosteum, synovial tissue and capsule of the joint are richly supplied by blood vessels and nerves. Pain usually derives from inflammation of these sites because the synovial membrane is relatively insensitive.

Enzymes and cytokines

Connective tissue constantly undergoes repair and remodelling. Degradation is mediated by enzymes such as aggrecanase and matrix metalloproteinases (MMPs), which require zinc and act at a neutral pH. There are several MMPs that act on different collagens, such as the gelatinases (MMP-2 and 9), which degrade denatured collagen. MMPs also act on non-collagen proteins: for example, the stromelysins (MMP-3, 10 and 11), which degrade proteoglycans and fibronectin.

The turnover of normal collagen is initiated by cytokines: for example, interleukin-1 (IL-1) synthesized by chondrocytes. Activation of latent MMPs and tissue plasminogen activator then occurs.

Two inhibitors, TIMP (*t*issue *i*nhibitor of *m*etallo*p*roteinase) and plasminogen activator inhibitor 1 (PAI 1), inhibit degradation during matrix remodelling.

Skeletal muscle

This tissue consists of bundles of myocytes containing actin and myosin molecules. These molecules interdigitate and form myofibrils, which cause muscle contraction in a similar way to myocardial muscle (see p. 933). Bundles of myofibrils (fasciculi) are covered by connective tissue, the perimysium, which merges with the epimysium (covering the muscle) and forms the tendon, which attaches to the bone surface (enthesis).

Though not strictly a component of the joint itself, muscles are so closely related to joints that strain and tension in muscles are commonly interpreted by patients as joint pain. Pain in muscles and ligaments (myofascial pain) is a very common cause of locomotor symptoms. Primary inflammatory disease of muscle (myositis) is far less common.

CLINICAL APPROACH TO THE PATIENT WITH RHEUMATIC DISEASE

Taking a musculoskeletal history

In most rheumatological disorders, the diagnosis is ***clinical***: that is, made on the history and examination, and then supported by investigations. Taking a thorough history is therefore crucial, and the main points to consider are described below.

Who is the patient?

Age

Some diseases, such as OA, polymyalgia rheumatica and giant cell arteritis, present mainly in patients over the age of 50. Conversely, autoimmune rheumatic diseases and inflammatory arthritis frequently present in people under 50.

Gender

Most rheumatological diseases can occur in either gender, but rheumatoid arthritis (RA), SLE and systemic sclerosis are more common in women, whereas gout and ankylosing spondylitis are more common in men.

Ethnicity

SLE is more common in African–Caribbean people than in other ethnicities.

Job

Jobs that involve heavy use of one part of the body can lead to soft tissue pain and/or OA: for example, in the low back, hips and knees of people who do a lot of heavy lifting. Musculoskeletal pain may also affect people's ability to do their job, care for children or dependants, or enjoy social activities. It is important to assess these effects on quality of life.

Has something happened to the patient?

Physical trauma

Trauma to a particular region of the body may cause pain there and/or in related regions. Where an injury is associated with a legal or insurance claim, this process may affect longevity of symptoms.

Psychosocial stress and depression

The biopsychosocial model of disease holds that physical, psychological and social factors interact to contribute to symptoms. This model is used in musculoskeletal disorders, where pain may cause distress and poor sleep, which in turn build up muscle tension and worsen the pain (see pp. 663–665). Acute stressful events, such as bereavement, bullying, abuse and redundancy, may exacerbate these symptoms.

What are the symptoms?

Pain

- ***Where is it? Is it localized or generalized?*** The pattern of joint involvement is a useful clue to the diagnosis (e.g. distal interphalangeal joints in nodal OA).
- ***Is it arising from joints, spine, muscles or bone, with local tenderness?*** Soft tissue lesions and inflamed joints are locally tender.
- ***Could it be referred from another site?*** Joint pain is localized but may radiate distally – shoulder to upper arm; hip to thigh and knee.
- ***Is it constant, intermittent or episodic?*** How severe is it – aching or agonizing?
- ***Are there aggravating or precipitating factors?*** Is it made worse by activity and eased by rest (mechanical), or worse after rest (inflammatory).
- ***Are there any associated neurological features?*** Numbness, pins and needles and/or loss of power suggest 'nerve' involvement. The distribution of symptoms is a useful clue to the nerve or nerve root affected.

Stiffness

- ***Is it generalized or localized?*** Spine or joint stiffness is common after injury.
- ***Does it affect the limb girdles or periphery?***
- ***Is it worse in the morning and relieved by activity?***
  - Joint stiffness for more than 30 min each morning – think of inflammatory arthritis.
  - Morning spinal stiffness in younger adults – think of ankylosing spondylitis (see pp. 683–685).
  - Shoulder and pelvic girdle stiffness and pain in a patient over 55 years may be polymyalgia rheumatica (see p. 700).

Swelling

- ***Does it affect one joint or several?*** Look for symmetry or asymmetry, and/or a peripheral or proximal pattern. An acute monoarthritis may be due to trauma, gout, pseudogout or sepsis (fever or immunosuppression). A polyarthritis is more likely to be due to OA or RA.
- ***Is it constant or does it come in short-lived or longer episodes?***
- ***Is there associated inflammation*** (redness and warmth)?

Extra-articular symptoms

Osteoarthritis and soft tissue problems are not usually associated with symptoms outside the joints. The presence of features such as rash, breathlessness, neurological symptoms or blood disorders suggests that the locomotor problems may be one facet of a more systemic disorder, such as RA, psoriatic arthritis or SLE.

What medication is the patient taking?

- ***Could a drug be a cause?*** Diuretics may precipitate gout in men and older women. Steroids can cause avascular necrosis. Some drugs cause a lupus-like syndrome (see p. 692).
- ***Have the symptoms responded to medication?*** A good response to a trial of steroids suggests an inflammatory or autoimmune problem.

What is the family history?

Does anyone in the family have a similar problem or another related disorder?

Examination of the joints

Always observe patients, looking for disabilities, as they walk into the room and sit down. General and neurological examinations are often necessary. Guidelines for rapid examinations of the limbs and spine are shown in ***Box 18.1***.

Examining an individual joint involves three stages: looking, feeling and moving ***(Box 18.2)***. A screening examination of the locomotor system, known by the acronym GALS (*g*lobal *a*ssessment of the *l*ocomotor *s*ystem), has been devised. Video demonstrations are available (see 'Further reading'). GALS has been modified for examination of children.

Box 18.1 Rapid examinations of the limbs and spine

Upper limbs

- ***Raise the arms sideways to the ears*** (***abduction***). ***Reach behind the neck and back***. Difficulties with these movements indicate a shoulder or rotator cuff problem.
- ***Hold the arms forwards, with elbows straight and fingers apart, palm up and palm down***. Fixed flexion at the elbow indicates an elbow problem. Examine the hands for swelling, wasting and deformity.
- ***Place the hands in the 'prayer' position with the elbows apart***. Flexion deformities of the fingers may be due to arthritis, flexor tenosynovitis or skin disease. Painful restriction of the wrist limits the person's ability to move the elbows out with the hands held together.
- ***Make a tight fist***. Difficulty with this indicates a loss of flexion or grip. Grip strength can be measured.

Lower limbs

- ***Ask the patient to walk*** a short distance away from and towards you, and to stand still. Look for abnormal posture or stance.
- ***Ask the patient to stand on each leg***. Severe hip disease causes the pelvis on the non-weight-bearing side to sag (positive Trendelenburg test).
- ***Watch the patient stand and sit***, looking for hip and/or knee problems.
- ***Ask the patient to straighten and flex each knee***.
- ***Ask the patient to place each foot in turn on the opposite knee with the hip externally rotated***. This tests for painful restriction of the hip or knee. Abnormal hips or knees must be examined with the patient lying down.
- ***Move each ankle up and down***. Examine the ankle joint and tendons, medial arch and toes while the patient is standing.

Spine

Stand behind the patient.

- ***Ask the patient to (a) bend forwards to touch the toes with straight knees, (b) extend backwards, (c) flex sideways, and (d) look over each shoulder, flexing and extending and side-flexing the neck***. Observe abnormal spinal curves – scoliosis (lateral curve), kyphosis (forward bending) or lordosis (backward bending). A cervical and lumbar lordosis and a thoracic kyphosis are normal. Muscle spasm is worse whilst standing and bending. Leg length inequality leads to a scoliosis that decreases on sitting or lying (the lengths are measured with the patient lying down).
- ***Ask the patient to lie supine***. Examine any restriction of straight-leg raising (see disc prolapse, below).
- ***Ask the patient to lie prone***. Examine for anterior thigh pain during a femoral stretch test (flexing knee whilst prone), which indicates a high lumbar disc problem.
- ***Palpate the spine and buttocks for tender areas***.

Investigation of rheumatic disease

Investigations are unnecessary in many of the common musculoskeletal problems; the diagnosis is clear from the history and examination findings. Tests help to exclude another condition and to reassure the patient or their primary care physician.

Useful blood screening tests

- Full blood count:
  - ***Haemoglobin***. Normochromic, normocytic anaemia suggests chronic inflammatory and autoimmune diseases. Hypochromic, microcytic anaemia indicates iron deficiency, sometimes due to non-steroidal anti-inflammatory drug (NSAID)-induced gastrointestinal bleeding.
  - ***White cell count***. Neutrophilia is seen in bacterial infection (e.g. septic arthritis). It also occurs with corticosteroid treatment. Lymphopenia is found in viral illnesses or SLE. Neutropenia may reflect drug-induced bone marrow suppression. Eosinophilia is seen in eosinophilic granulomatosis with polyangiitis (see p. 1121).

Box 18.2 Examination of the joint

Look at the appearance of the joint

- Swelling – could be bony, fluid or synovial
- Deformity:
  - ***Valgus***, where the distal bone is deviated laterally (e.g. knock-knees or genu valgum)
  - ***Varus***, where the distal bone is deviated medially (bow-legs or genu varum)
  - Fixed flexion or hyperextension
- Rash – especially psoriasis
- Muscle wasting – easier to see in large muscles like the quadriceps
- Scars – from surgery or trauma
- Signs of inflammation
- Symmetry:
  - Are the right and left joints (e.g. hips, knees, any other paired joint) the same?
  - If not, which do you think is abnormal?

Feel

- Swelling:
  - ***Fluid swelling*** (effusion) usually represents increased synovial fluid in inflammatory arthritis, but can be due to blood or pus
  - ***Synovial swelling*** is rubbery or boggy and usually occurs in inflammatory arthritis
  - ***Bony swelling***, such as Heberden's nodes in the fingers, is usually seen in osteoarthritis
- Warmth – a warm joint may be inflamed or infected
- Tenderness – may represent joint inflammation, but many people have chronic tenderness all over the body (e.g. in fibromyalgia)

Move

- Active movement:
  - Is the range full and pain-free?
  - Is the movement fluid?
  - In the hands, can the patient perform fine movements?
  - In the legs, can the patient walk properly?
- Compare movements on the right and left sides – are they symmetrical?
- Is there crepitus when the joint is moved?
- If active movement is limited, try passive movement:
  - In a joint problem both will usually be affected.
  - In a muscle or nerve problem, passive movement may remain full.

- *Platelets*. Raised platelets occur with any chronic inflammation. Thrombocytopenia is seen in drug-induced bone marrow suppression and may be a feature of SLE.
- ***Erythrocyte sedimentation rate (ESR) and C-reactive protein (CRP)***. An increase in these reflects inflammation. Plasma viscosity is also raised in inflammatory disease.
- ***Bone and liver biochemistry***. A raised serum alkaline phosphatase may indicate liver or bone disease. A rise in liver enzymes is seen with drug-induced toxicity. For other investigations of bone, see pages 708–711.

Other blood and urine tests

- Protein electrophoretic strip (and/or immunofixation), serum free light chain testing and urinary Bence Jones protein – to exclude myeloma as a cause of a raised ESR.
- Serum uric acid – for gout.
- Antistreptolysin O titre – in rheumatic fever.

Serum autoantibody studies

- ***Rheumatoid factors (RFs)*** (see also pp. 674–675). Rheumatoid factors are detected by enzyme-linked immunosorbent assay (ELISA). RFs are antibodies (usually immunoglobulin (Ig) M, but also IgG or IgA) against the Fc portion of IgG. They are detected in 70% of people with RA, but are not diagnostic. RFs are detected in many autoimmune rheumatic disorders (e.g. SLE), in chronic infections, and in asymptomatic older people ***(Box 18.3)***.
- ***Anti-citrullinated peptide antibodies (ACPA)***. These antibodies are directed against citrullinated antigens, vimentin, fibrinogen, alpha enolase and type II collagen. They are measured by an ELISA technique and are present in up to 80% of people with RA. They have a high specificity for RA (90%, with a sensitivity of 60%). They are helpful in early disease when the RF is negative, to distinguish it from acute transient synovitis (see ***Box 18.26***). Positivity for RF and/or ACPA is associated with a worse prognosis and an increase in the likelihood of bony erosions in people with RA.
- ***Antinuclear antibodies (ANAs)***. These are detected by indirect immunofluorescent staining of fresh frozen sections of rat liver or kidney or Hep-2 cell lines. Different patterns reflect a variety of antigenic specificities that occur with different clinical pictures (see ***Box 18.36***). ANA is used as a screening test for SLE and systemic sclerosis – a negative ANA makes either condition highly unlikely – but low titres occur in RA and chronic infections and in normal individuals, especially the elderly ***(Box 18.4)***.
- ***Anti-double-stranded DNA (dsDNA) antibodies***. These are usually detected by a precipitation test (Farr assay), ELISA or an immunofluorescent test using *Crithidia luciliae* (which contains dsDNA). Raised anti-dsDNA is highly specific for SLE; the levels usually rise and fall in parallel with disease activity so can be used to monitor the level of treatment required.
- ***Anti-extractable nuclear antigen (ENA) antibodies*** (see ***Box 18.36***). These produce a speckled ANA fluorescent pattern, and can be identified by ELISA. The most commonly measured ENAs are:
  - ***anti-Ro and anti-La***, which occur in Sjögren syndrome and SLE
  - ***anti-Sm***, which is highly specific for SLE
  - ***anti-Jo-1***, which is the most common of the anti-tRNA synthetase enzymes that occur in some people with dermatomyositis or polymyositis
  - ***anti-topoisomerase I (anti-Scl 70)***, which is specific for systemic sclerosis
  - ***anti-RNA polymerase I and III***, which occur in systemic sclerosis and are associated with pulmonary fibrosis.
- ***Anti-neutrophil cytoplasmic antibodies (ANCAs)*** (see p. 702). These are predominantly IgG autoantibodies directed against the primary granules of neutrophil and macrophage lysosomes. They are strongly associated with small-vessel vasculitis. Two major clinically relevant ANCA patterns are recognized on ***immunofluorescence***:
  - ***proteinase 3 (PR3-ANCA)***, also called cytoplasmic or cANCA, producing a granular immunofluorescence and seen in granulomatosis with polyangiitis (GPA)

Box 18.3 Conditions in which rheumatoid factor (RF) is found in the serum

Condition	RF (IgM) %
Autoimmune rheumatic diseases	
Rheumatoid arthritis	70
Systemic lupus erythematosus	25
Sjögren syndrome	90
Systemic sclerosis	30
Polymyositis/dermatomyositis	50
Juvenile idiopathic arthritis	Variable
Viral infections	**Hyperglobulinaemias**
Hepatitis	Chronic liver disease
Infectious mononucleosis	Sarcoidosis
Cryoglobulinaemia	
Chronic infections	**Normal population**
Tuberculosis	Elderly
Leprosy	Relatives of people with rheumatoid arthritis
Infective endocarditis	
Syphilis	

Box 18.4 Conditions in which serum antinuclear antibodies are found

Condition	%
Systemic lupus erythematosus	95
Systemic sclerosis	70
Sjögren syndrome	80
Polymyositis and dermatomyositis	40
Rheumatoid arthritis	30
Juvenile idiopathic arthritis	Variable
Other diseases	
Autoimmune hepatitis	100
Drug-induced lupus	>95
Myasthenia gravis	50
Idiopathic pulmonary fibrosis	30
Diabetes mellitus	25
Infectious mononucleosis	5–10
Normal population	8

   - ***myeloperoxidase*** (***MPO-ANCA***), also called perinuclear or pANCA, producing a perinuclear stain and seen in microscopic polyarteritis (polyangiitis) and eosinophilic (E)GPA.
- ***Antiphospholipid antibodies*** (see p. 695). These are detected in the antiphospholipid syndrome (see p. 695).
- ***Immune complexes***. Immune complexes are infrequently measured, largely because of variability between assays and difficulty in interpreting their meaning. Assays based on the polyethylene glycol (PEG) precipitation method or C1q binding are available commercially.
- ***Complement***. Low complement levels indicate consumption and suggest an active disease process in SLE.

Joint aspiration and examination of synovial fluid

Examination of joint (or bursa) fluid is used mainly to diagnose septic, reactive or crystal arthritis. The appearance of the fluid is an indicator of the level of inflammation. The procedure is often undertaken in combination with injection of a corticosteroid. Aspiration alone is therapeutic in crystal arthritis ***(Box 18.5)***.

Aspiration and analysis of synovial fluid are always indicated when septic or crystal-induced arthritis is suspected, particularly a monoarthritis. Normal fluid is clear and straw-coloured, and contains <3000 white blood cells (WBC)/mm^3. Inflammatory fluid is cloudy and contains >3000 WBC/mm^3. Septic fluid is opaque and less viscous, and contains up to 75 000 WBC/mm^3. There is much overlap.

Polarized light microscopy is performed for crystals:

- ***gout***: negatively bi-refringent, needle-shaped crystals of sodium urate
- ***calcium pyrophosphate deposition arthropathy***: rhomboidal, weakly positively bi-refringent crystals of calcium pyrophosphate.

Gram staining is essential if septic arthritis is suspected and may identify the organism immediately. Joint fluid should be cultured and antibiotic sensitivities requested.

Diagnostic imaging and visualization

- ***X-rays*** can be diagnostic in certain conditions (e.g. established RA) and are the first investigation in many cases of trauma. X-rays can detect joint space narrowing, erosions in RA, calcification in soft tissue, new bone formation, e.g. osteophytes, and decreased bone density (osteopenia) or increased bone density (osteosclerosis):
   - In acute low back pain (see pp. 656–657), X-rays are indicated only if the pain is persistent, recurrent, associated with neurological symptoms or signs, or worse at night or associated with symptoms such as fever or weight loss.
   - Radiological changes are common in older people and may not indicate symptomatic OA or spondylosis.
   - X-rays are of little diagnostic value in early inflammatory arthritis but are useful as a baseline from which to judge later change.
- ***Ultrasound*** is particularly useful for periarticular structures, soft tissue swellings and tendons, and for detecting active synovitis in inflammatory arthritis. It is increasingly used to examine the shoulder and other structures during movement, e.g. shoulder impingement syndrome (see pp. 653–654). Doppler ultrasound measures blood flow and hence inflammation. Ultrasound may be used to guide local injections.
- ***Magnetic resonance imaging*** (***MRI***) shows bone changes and intra-articular structures in striking detail. Visualization of particular structures can be enhanced with different resonance sequences. T_1-weighted MRI is used for anatomical detail, T_2-weighted for fluid detection and short tau inversion recovery (STIR) for the presence of bone marrow oedema. MRI is more sensitive than X-rays in the early detection of articular and periarticular disease. Gadolinium injection enhances inflamed tissue. MRI is especially useful for detection of damage to non-bony tissues in or near joints, e.g. meniscal tears in the knee and torn rotator cuff muscles in the shoulder; detection of nerve root compression in the spine; detection of inflamed muscle in myositis; and early detection of synovitis in inflammatory arthritis.
- ***Computerized axial tomography*** (***CT***) is useful for detecting changes in calcified structures but the dose of irradiation is high.
- ***Bone scintigraphy*** utilizes radionuclides, usually ^{99m}Tc, and detects abnormal bone turnover and blood circulation; although non-specific, it helps in detecting areas of inflammation, infection or malignancy. It is best used in combination with other anatomical imaging techniques.
- ***Dual-energy X-ray absorptiometry (DXA) scanning*** uses very low doses of X-irradiation to measure bone density and is used in the screening and monitoring of osteoporosis.
- ***Positron emission tomography*** (***PET***) ***scanning*** uses radionuclides, which decay by emission of positrons. ^{18}F-Fluorodeoxyglucose uptake indicates areas of increased glucose metabolism. PET is used to locate tumours and demonstrate large-vessel vasculitis, e.g. Takayasu's arteritis (see pp. 1054–1055). PET scans are combined with CT to improve anatomical details.
- ***Arthroscopy*** is a direct means of visualizing a joint, particularly the knee or shoulder. Biopsies can be taken, surgery performed in certain conditions (e.g. repair or trimming of meniscal tears), and loose bodies removed.
- ***Nerve conduction studies and electromyography*** are used to diagnose nerve entrapment syndromes (such as carpal or tarsal tunnel) and to distinguish myositis from neuropathies.

Box 18.5 Joint aspiration

This is a sterile procedure that should be carried out in a clean environment.

Explain the procedure to the patient; obtain consent.

1. Decide on the site to insert the needle and mark it.
2. Clean the skin and your hands scrupulously. Remove rings and wristwatch. Put on gloves.
3. Draw up local anaesthetic (and corticosteroid if it is being used) and then use a new needle.
4. Warn the patient. Insert the needle, injecting local anaesthetic as it advances; if a joint effusion is suspected, attempt to aspirate as you advance it.
5. If fluid is obtained, change syringes and aspirate fully.
6. Examine the fluid in the syringe and decide whether or not to proceed with a corticosteroid injection (if fluid is clear or slightly cloudy) or send for microbiological tests.
7. Cover the injection site and advise the patient to rest the affected area for a few days. Warn the patient that the pain may increase initially but to report urgently if this persists beyond a few days, if the swelling worsens or if they become febrile, since this might indicate an infected joint.

Further reading

Foster HE, Kay LJ, May CR et al. Pediatric regional examination of the musculoskeletal system: a practice and consensus-based approach. *Arthritis Care Res* 2011; 63:1503–1510.
Male D, Brostoff J, Roth DB et al. *Immunology*, 8th edn. St Louis: Elsevier; 2012.
http://www.arthritisresearchuk.org/ *Musculoskeletal screening examination: GALS video*.

COMMON REGIONAL MUSCULOSKELETAL PROBLEMS

See ***Figure 18.2***.

Pain in the neck and shoulder

See ***Box 18.6***.

Mechanical or muscular neck pain (shoulder girdle pain)

Unilateral or bilateral muscular-pattern neck pain is common and usually self-limiting. It can follow injury, falling asleep in an awkward position, or prolonged keyboard working. Chronic burning neck pain occurs because of muscle tension from anxiety and stress.

Spondylosis seen on X-ray increases after the age of 40 years but it is not always related to pain. Spondylosis can, however, cause stiffness and increases the risk of mechanical or muscular neck pain. Muscle spasm is palpable and tender, and may lead to abnormal neck posture (e.g. acute torticollis). Muscular-pattern neck pain is not localized but affects the trapezius muscle, the C7 spinous process and the paracervical musculature (shoulder girdle pain). Pain often radiates upwards to the occiput and is commonly associated with tension headaches. These features are also seen in chronic widespread pain (see pp. 664–665).

Management

Patients are given short courses of analgesic therapy, along with reassurance and explanation. Physiotherapists can help to relieve spasm and pain, teach exercises and relaxation techniques, and improve posture. An occupational therapist can advise about the ergonomics of the workplace if the problem is work-related (see p. 665).

Nerve root entrapment

This is caused by an acute cervical disc prolapse or pressure on the root from spondylotic osteophytes narrowing the root canal.

Acute cervical disc prolapse presents with unilateral pain in the neck, radiating to the interscapular and shoulder regions. This diffuse, aching, dural pain is followed by sharp, electric shock-like pain down the arm, in a nerve root distribution, often with pins and needles, numbness, weakness and loss of reflexes ***(Box 18.7)***.

Cervical spondylosis occurs in the older patient with postero-lateral osteophytes compressing the nerve root and causing root pain (see ***Fig. 21.64***), commonly at C5/C6 or C6/C7; it is seen on oblique radiographs of the neck. An MRI scan clearly distinguishes facet joint OA, root canal narrowing and disc prolapse.

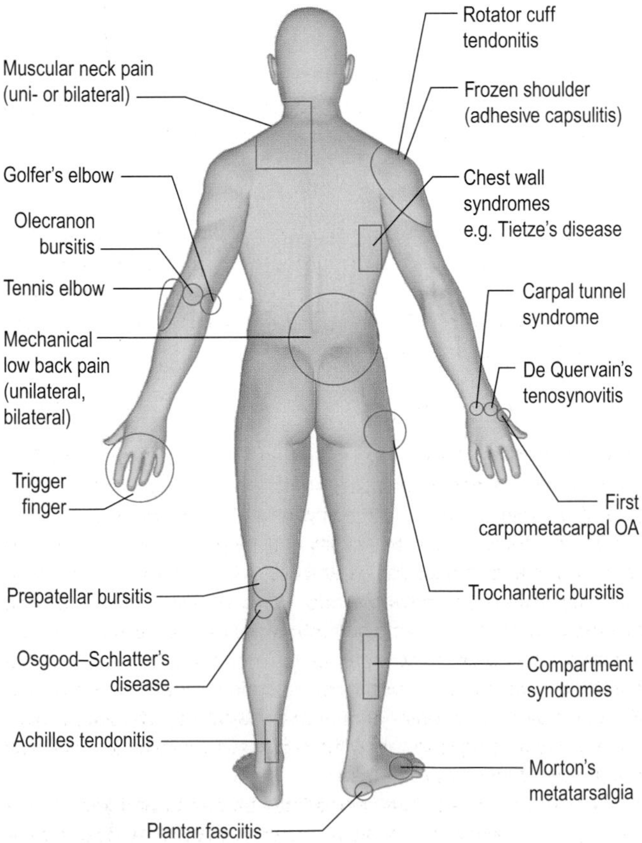

Figure 18.2 Common regional musculoskeletal problems. OA, osteoarthritis.

Box 18.6 Pain in the neck and shoulder

- Trauma (e.g. a fall)
- Mechanical or muscular neck pain
- Whiplash injury
- Disc prolapse – nerve root entrapment
- Ankylosing spondylitis
- Shoulder lesions:
  - Rotator cuff tendonitis
  - Calcific tendonitis or bursitis
  - Impingement syndrome or rotator cuff tear
  - Adhesive capsulitis (true 'frozen' shoulder)
  - Inflammatory arthritis or osteoarthritis
- Polymyalgia rheumatica
- Fibromyalgia (chronic widespread pain)
- Chronic (work-related) upper limb pain syndrome
- Tumour

Box 18.7 Cervical nerve root entrapment: symptoms and signs

Nerve root	Sensory changes	Reflex loss	Weakness
C5	Lateral arm	Biceps	Shoulder abduction Elbow flexion
C6	Lateral forearm Thumb and index finger	Biceps Supinator	Elbow flexion Wrist extension
C7	Middle finger	Triceps	Elbow extension
C8	Medial forearm Little and ring fingers	None	Finger flexion
T1	Medial upper arm	None	Finger abduction and adduction

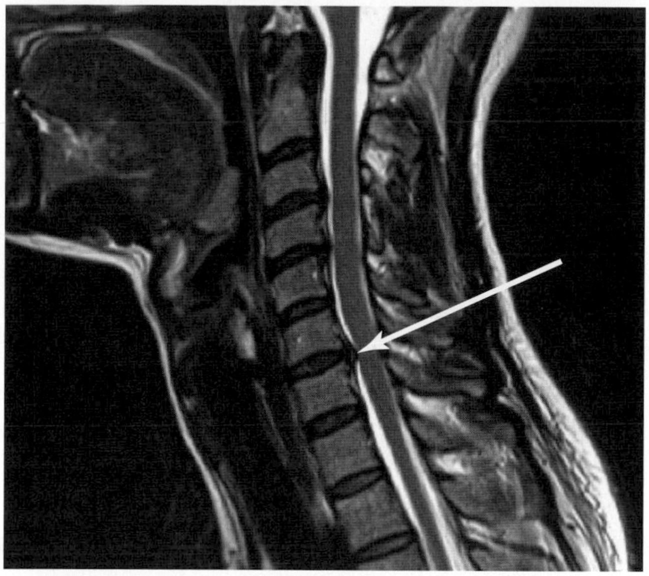

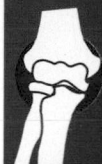

Figure 18.3 Magnetic resonance image of the cervical spine. A large central disc prolapse (arrowed) is shown at the C6/7 level, and smaller disc bulges at C3/4 and C4/5.

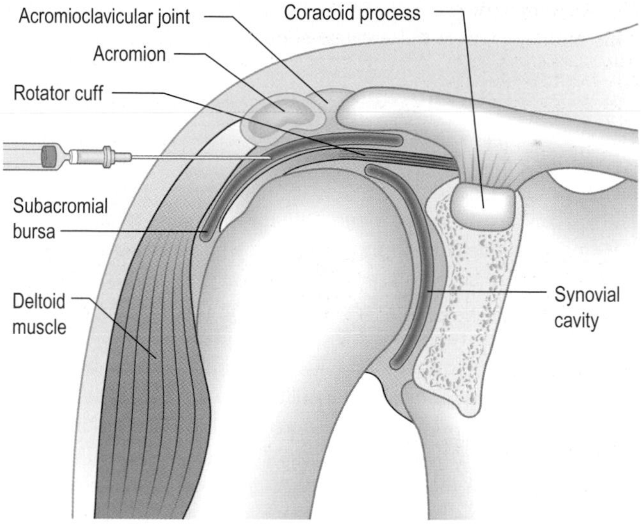

Figure 18.4 The shoulder region, showing site of injection and subacromial space.

Management

A support collar, rest, analgesia and sedation are used initially as necessary. Patients should be advised not to carry heavy items. They usually recover in 6–12 weeks. MRI is the investigation of choice if surgery is being considered or the diagnosis is uncertain ***(Fig. 18.3)***. A cervical root block, administered under direct vision by an experienced pain specialist, may relieve pain while the disc recovers. Neurosurgical referral is recommended if the pain persists or if the neurological signs of weakness or numbness are severe or bilateral. Bilateral root pain, with or without long track symptoms or signs, is a neurosurgical emergency because a central disc prolapse may compress the cervical spinal cord. Posterior osteophytes may cause spinal claudication and cervical myelopathy.

Whiplash injury

Whiplash injury results from acceleration–deceleration forces applied to the neck, usually in a road traffic accident when the car of a person wearing a seat belt is struck from behind. A simple decision plan based on clinical criteria helps to distinguish those most at risk and who warrant radiography. There is a low probability of serious bony injury if there is:

- no midline cervical tenderness
- no focal neurological deficit
- normal alertness
- no intoxication
- no other painful distracting injury.

CT scans are reserved for those with bony injury. MRI scans occasionally show severe soft tissue injury. Whiplash injuries may lead to litigation or insurance claims.

Whiplash injury is a common cause of chronic neck pain, although most people recover within a few weeks or months. Delayed recovery depends, in part, on the severity of the initial injury. The pattern of chronic neck pain is often complex, involving pain in the neck, shoulder and arm. It may be accompanied by subjective symptoms, such as headache, dizziness and poor concentration. The subjective nature of these symptoms has led to controversy about their cause. The problem is more commonly seen in industrialized countries, where the conflictive nature of the compensation process may actually delay recovery. Non-conflictive means of compensation may lead to a better prognosis.

Box 18.8 Differential diagnosis of 'shoulder' pain

- Rotator cuff tendonitis pain is worse at night and radiates to the upper arm.
- Painful shoulders produce secondary muscular neck pain.
- Muscular neck pain (also known as shoulder girdle pain) does not radiate to the upper arm.
- Cervical nerve root pain is usually associated with pins and needles or neurological signs in the arm.

Management

Management is with reassurance (the patient is often distressed and anxious), analgesia, a short-term support collar and physiotherapy. Pain may take a few weeks or months to settle and the patient should be warned of this. Clinical trial evidence shows no benefit with prolonged physiotherapy.

Pain in the shoulder

The shoulder is a shallow joint with a large range of movement. The humeral head is held in place by the rotator cuff ***(Fig. 18.4)***, which is part of the joint capsule. It is comprised of the tendons of infraspinatus and teres minor posteriorly, supraspinatus superiorly, and teres major and subscapularis anteriorly. The rotator cuff (particularly supraspinatus) prevents the humeral head from blocking against the acromion during abduction; the deltoid pulls up and the supraspinatus pulls in to produce a turning movement, and the greater tuberosity glides under the acromion without impingement. Shoulder pathology restricts or is made worse by shoulder movement. Specific diagnoses are difficult to make clinically but that may not matter for pain management.

Pain in the shoulder can sometimes be due to problems in the neck; the differential diagnosis is shown in ***Box 18.8***. Adhesive capsulitis (true frozen shoulder) is uncommon (see below). Early inflammatory arthritis and polymyalgia rheumatica in the elderly may present with shoulder pain. Shoulder pain is more common in diabetic patients than in the general population.

Rotator cuff (supraspinatus) tendonosis

This condition is a common cause of shoulder pain at all ages. It follows trauma in 30% of cases and is bilateral in under 5%. The pain radiates to the upper arm and is made worse by arm abduction and elevation, which are often limited. The pain is often worse during the middle of the range of abduction, reducing as the arm is raised fully; a so-called 'painful arc syndrome'. When examined from behind, the scapula rotates earlier than usual during elevation. Passive elevation reduces impingement and is less painful. Severe pain virtually immobilizes the joint, although some rotation is retained (compare adhesive capsulitis; see below). There is also painful spasm of the trapezius. There may be an associated subacromial bursitis. Isolated subacromial bursitis occurs after direct trauma, falling on to the outstretched arm or elbow. Acromioclavicular osteophytes increase the risk of impingement and may need to be removed surgically.

X-ray or ultrasound is necessary only when rotator cuff tendonosis is persistent or the diagnosis is uncertain.

Management

Analgesics, NSAIDs and/or physiotherapy may suffice, but severe pain responds to an injection of corticosteroid into the subacromial bursa ***(Fig. 18.4)***. Patients should be warned that 10% will develop worse pain for 24–48 hours after injection. Some 70% improve over 5–20 days and mobilize the joint themselves. Physiotherapy helps persistent stiffness. Further ultrasound-guided corticosteroid injections may be needed but the long-term benefit is unclear.

Torn rotator cuff

This condition is caused by trauma but also occurs spontaneously in the elderly and in RA. It prevents active abduction of the arm but patients learn to initiate elevation using the unaffected arm. Once elevated, the arm can be held in place by the deltoid muscle. In younger people, the tear is repaired surgically but this is rarely possible in the elderly or in RA. Some patients require arthroscopic surgery.

Calcific tendonosis and bursitis

Calcium pyrophosphate deposits in the tendon are visible on X-ray but they are not always symptomatic. The pathogenesis is unclear, although ischaemia may play a part. The deposit is usually just proximal to the greater tuberosity. It may lead to acute or chronic recurrent shoulder pain and restriction of movement. A local corticosteroid injection may relieve the pain. The calcification may persist or resolve. Aspiration or breaking up of the deposit under ultrasound control may be required for persistent pain. Rarely, arthroscopic removal is necessary.

Shedding of crystals into the subacromial bursa causes a bursitis with severe pain and shoulder restriction. The shoulder feels hot and is swollen, and an X-ray shows a diffuse opacity in the bursa. The differential diagnosis of calcific bursitis is gout, pseudogout or septic arthritis. Aspiration and injection with corticosteroid can help.

Adhesive capsulitis (true 'frozen' shoulder)

This condition is uncommon but can develop with rotator cuff lesions, or following hemiplegia, chest or breast surgery, or myocardial infarction. Initially, it causes severe shoulder pain and a gradually reducing range of movement, leading to a 'frozen' phase where there is loss of all shoulder movements but little pain. NSAIDs and intra-articular injections of local anaesthetic and corticosteroids are helpful in the painful phase. Subsequently, there is usually a gradual improvement in function over weeks to months. Therapeutic exercises and physiotherapy help in later phases. Once the pain settles, arthroscopic release speeds functional recovery.

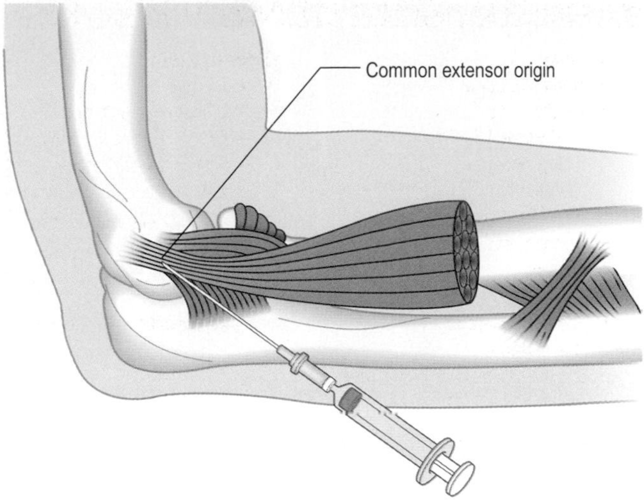

Figure 18.5 Injection for tennis elbow.

Pain in the elbow

Pain in the elbow can be due to epicondylitis, inflammatory arthritis or, occasionally, OA.

Epicondylitis

Two common sites where the insertions of tendons into bone become inflamed (enthesitis) are the common wrist extensor origin at the lateral humeral epicondyle ('tennis elbow') and the common wrist flexor origin at the medial epicondyle ('golfer's elbow'). Despite the names, both conditions are usually unrelated to either sport!

There is local tenderness. Pain radiates into the forearm on using the affected muscles – typically, gripping or holding a heavy bag in tennis elbow or carrying a tray in golfer's elbow. Pain at rest also occurs.

Management

Advise rest and arrange review by a physiotherapist. A local injection of corticosteroid at the point of maximum tenderness is helpful when the pain is severe but needs physiotherapy follow-up to prevent recurrences ***(Fig. 18.5)***. Avoid the ulnar nerve when injecting golfer's elbow. Both conditions settle spontaneously eventually, but occasionally persist and require surgical release.

Pain in the hand and wrist

(See ***Box 18.9***.) Hand pain is commonly caused by injury or repetitive, work-related activities. When associated with pins and needles or numbness, it suggests a neurological cause arising at the wrist, elbow or neck. Pain and stiffness that are worse in the morning are due to tenosynovitis or inflammatory arthritis. The distribution of hand pain often indicates the diagnosis.

Box 18.9 Causes of pain in the hand and wrist

All ages
- Trauma/fractures
- Tenosynovitis:
  - Flexor with/without triggering
  - Dorsal
  - De Quervain's
- Carpal tunnel syndrome
- Ganglion
- Inflammatory arthritis
- Raynaud syndrome (see p. 1054)
- Chronic regional pain syndrome type I (see p. 665)

Older patients
- Nodal OA:
  - DIPs (Heberden's nodes)
  - PIPs (Bouchard's nodes)
  - First carpometacarpal joint
- Trauma – scaphoid fracture
- Pseudogout
- Gout:
  - Acute
  - Tophaceous

DIPs/PIPs, distal/proximal interphalangeal joints.

Tenosynovitis

The finger flexor tendons run through synovial sheaths and under loops that hold them in place. Inflammation occurs with repeated or unaccustomed use, or in inflammatory arthritis. The thickened sheaths are often palpable.

Flexor tenosynovitis causes finger pain when gripping and stiffness of the fingers in the morning. Occasionally, a tendon causes a trigger finger, when the finger remains flexed in the morning or after gripping, and has to be pulled straight. A tender tendon nodule is palpable, usually in the distal palm. Trigger finger or thumb is more common in diabetic patients.

Dorsal tenosynovitis is less common, except in RA. The hourglass swelling extends from the back of the hand and under the extensor retinaculum.

De Quervain's tenosynovitis causes pain and swelling around the radial styloid, where the abductor pollicis longus tendon is held in place by a retaining band. There is local tenderness, and the pain at the styloid is worsened by flexing the thumb into the palm.

Management

Resting, splinting and NSAIDs may help. Local corticosteroids injected alongside the tendon under low pressure (not into the tendon itself) are helpful. Occasionally, surgery is needed if symptoms persist.

Carpal tunnel syndrome

This condition arises due to median nerve compression in the limited space of the carpal tunnel. Thickened ligaments, tendon sheaths or bone enlargement can cause it, but it is usually idiopathic. (Causes are discussed on p. 882.) The history is usually typical and diagnostic, the patient waking with numbness, tingling and pain in a median nerve distribution. The pain may radiate to the forearm. The fingers feel swollen but usually are not. Wasting of the abductor pollicis brevis develops with sensory loss in the radial three and a half fingers. The pain may be produced by tapping the nerve in the carpal tunnel (Tinel's sign) or by holding the wrist in flexion (Phalen's test).

Management

Management is with a splint to hold the wrist in dorsiflexion overnight, which relieves the symptoms and is diagnostic; used nightly for several weeks, it may produce full recovery. If it does not, a corticosteroid injection into the carpal tunnel (avoid the nerve!) helps in about 70% of cases, although it may recur. Persistent symptoms or nerve damage produce prolonged latency across the carpal tunnel on nerve conduction studies and require surgical decompression.

Other conditions causing pain

Inflammatory arthritis

This may present with pain, swelling and stiffness of the hands. In RA, the wrists, proximal interphalangeal (PIP) joints and metacarpophalangeal (MCP) joints are affected symmetrically. In psoriatic arthritis and reactive arthritis, a finger may be swollen (dactylitis), or the distal interphalangeal (DIP) joints and nails are affected asymmetrically.

Nodal osteoarthritis

This affects the DIP and less commonly PIP joints, which are initially swollen and red. The inflammation and pain settle but bony swellings remain (see pp. 669–670).

First carpometacarpal osteoarthritis

This causes pain at the base of the thumb when gripping, or painless stiffness at the base of the thumb, often in people with nodal OA.

Scaphoid fractures

These cause pain in the anatomical snuffbox. They are not seen immediately on X-ray; if there is clinical suspicion, a cast is necessary. Untreated scaphoid fractures can eventually cause pain because of failed union.

Ganglion

A ganglion is a jelly-filled, often painless swelling caused by a partial tear of the joint capsule or tendon sheath. The wrist is a common site. Treatment is not essential, as many resolve or cause little trouble; otherwise, surgical excision is the best option.

Dupuytren's contracture

This condition is a painless, palpable fibrosis of the palmar aponeurosis, with fibroblasts invading the dermis. It causes puckering of the skin and gradual fixed flexion, usually of the ring and little fingers. It is more common in males, Caucasians, individuals with diabetes mellitus, and those who overuse alcohol. A similar fibrosis occurs in the feet and is often more aggressive. It is also associated with Peyronie's disease of the penis – a painful inflammatory disorder of the corpora cavernosa, leading eventually to painless fibrosis and angulation of the penis during erection. Intralesional steroid injections may help in early disease and some advocate transcutaneous needle aponeurotomy. Percutaneous collagenase injection into the lesion has been shown to be effective in several studies and is now first-line treatment used before surgery. Surgical release of the contracture is restricted to those with severe deformity of the fingers.

Pain in the lower back

Low back pain is a common symptom. It is often traumatic and work-related, although lifting apparatus, other mechanical devices and improved office seating help to avoid it. Episodes are generally short-lived and self-limiting, and patients attend a physiotherapist or osteopath more often than a doctor. Chronic back pain is the cause of 14% of long-term disability in the UK. The causes are listed in ***Box 18.10***.

Box 18.10 Causes of pain in the back (lumbar region)

Mechanical
- Trauma
- Muscular and ligamentous pain
- Fibrositic nodulosis
- Postural back pain (sway back)
- Lumbar spondylosis
- Facet joint syndrome
- Lumbar disc prolapse
- Spinal and root canal stenosis
- Spondylolisthesis
- Disseminated idiopathic skeletal hyperostosis (DISH)
- Fibromyalgia, chronic widespread pain (see pp. 664–665)

Inflammatory
- Infective lesions of the spine
- Ankylosing spondylitis/sacroiliitis (see pp. 683–685)

Metabolic
- Osteoporotic spinal fractures (see pp. 711–715)
- Osteomalacia (see pp. 717–718)
- Paget's disease (see pp. 715–717)

Neoplastic (see p. 749)
- Metastases
- Multiple myeloma
- Primary tumours of bone

Referred pain

Box 18.11 Management of back pain

- Most back pain presenting to a primary care physician needs no investigation
- Pain between the ages of 20 and 55 years is likely to be mechanical and is managed with analgesia, brief rest if necessary and physiotherapy
- Patients should stay active within the limits of their pain
- Early treatment of the acute episode, advice and exercise programmes reduce long-term problems and prevent chronic pain syndromes
- Physical manipulation of uncomplicated back pain produces short-term relief and enjoys high patient satisfaction ratings
- Psychological and social factors may influence the time of presentation
- Appropriate early management reduces long-term disability

The majority of cases of low back pain are uncomplicated and arise from mechanical causes. Management of this type of back pain is summarized in ***Box 18.11***.

One should be alert to clues in the history and examination that could suggest more serious causes of low back pain, as summarized in ***Figure 18.6***.

Investigations

- ***Spinal X-rays (Fig. 18.7)*** are required only if the pain is associated with certain 'red flag' symptoms or signs, which indicate a high risk of more serious underlying problems:
  - starts before the age of 20 years or after 50
  - is persistent and a serious cause is suspected
  - is worse at night or in the morning, when an inflammatory arthritis (e.g. ankylosing spondylitis), infection or a spinal tumour may be the cause
  - is associated with a systemic illness, fever or weight loss
  - is associated with neurological symptoms or signs.
- ***MRI (Fig. 18.8)*** is preferable to CT scanning when neurological signs and symptoms are present. CT scans demonstrate bony pathology better. Interpretation of the relevance of the findings may require a specialist opinion.
- ***Bone scans*** are useful in infective and malignant lesions but are also positive in degenerative lesions.
- ***Full blood count, ESR and biochemical tests*** are required only when the pain is likely to be due to malignancy, infection or a metabolic cause. Normal ESR and CRP distinguish mechanical back pain from polymyalgia rheumatica, a likely differential in the elderly.

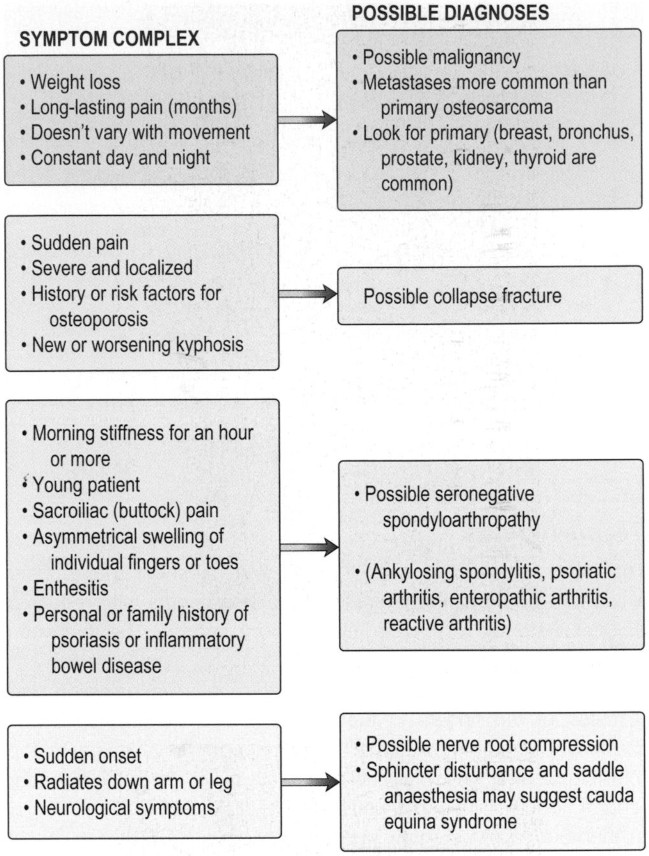

Figure 18.6 Diagnoses for serious causes of back pain.

Mechanical low back pain

Mechanical low back pain starts suddenly, may be recurrent and is helped by rest. It is often precipitated by an injury and may be unilateral or bilateral. It is usually short-lived.

Examination

The back is stiff and a scoliosis may be present when the patient is standing. Muscular spasm is visible and palpable, and causes local pain and tenderness. It lessens when sitting or lying. Excessive rest should be avoided. Once a patient develops low back pain, although the episode itself is usually self-limiting, there is a significantly increased risk of further back pain episodes. Risk factors for recurrent back pain include:

- female sex
- increasing age
- pre-existing chronic widespread pain (fibromyalgia)
- psychosocial factors, such as high levels of psychological distress, poor self-rated health and dissatisfaction with employment.

Chronic low back pain is a major cause of disability and time off work and is reduced by appropriate early management.

Spinal movement occurs at the disc and the posterior facet joints, and stability is normally achieved by a complex mechanism of spinal ligaments and muscles. Any of these structures may be a source of pain. An exact anatomical diagnosis is difficult but some typical syndromes are recognized (see below). They are often

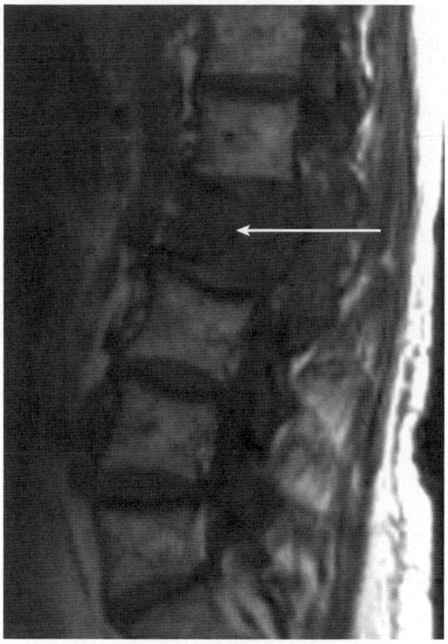

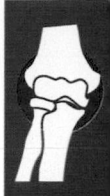

Figure 18.7 Spinal metastasis in L2. The patient had severe back pain and weight loss, and prior carcinoma of the breast.

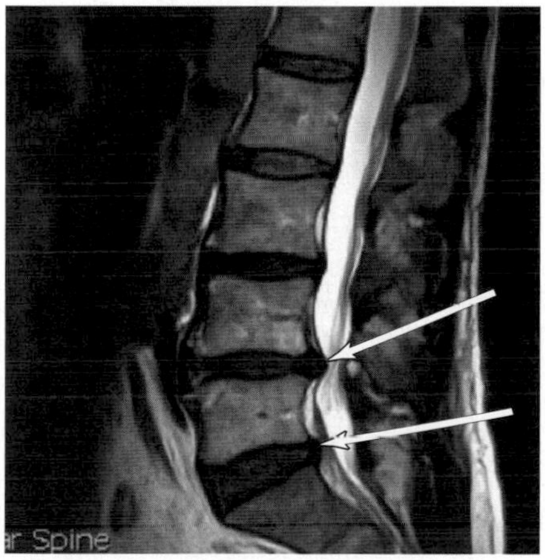

Figure 18.8 Magnetic resonance image of the lumbar spine. A large disc prolapse is shown at the L4/L5 level and a smaller prolapse at L5/S1 (arrowed). The signal from all the lumbar discs indicates dehydration.

associated with, but not necessarily caused, by radiological spondylosis (see pp. 886–888).

Postural back pain develops in individuals who sit in poorly designed, unsupportive chairs.

Lumbar spondylosis

The fundamental lesion in spondylosis occurs in an intervertebral disc, a fibrous structure whose tough capsule inserts into the rim of the adjacent vertebrae. This capsule encloses a fibrous outer zone and a gel-like inner zone. The disc allows rotation and bending.

Changes in the discs occasionally start in teenage years or early twenties and often increase with age. The gel changes chemically, breaks up, shrinks and loses its compliance. The surrounding fibrous zones develop circumferential or radial fissures. In the majority, this is initially asymptomatic but visible on MRI as decreased hydration. Later, the discs become thinner and less compliant. These changes cause circumferential bulging of the intervertebral ligaments.

Reactive changes develop in adjacent vertebrae; the bone becomes sclerotic and osteophytes form around the rim of the vertebra ***(Fig. 18.8)***. The most common sites of lumbar spondylosis are L5/S1 and L4/L5.

In young people, disc prolapse through an adjacent vertebral end-plate produces a Schmorl's node on X-ray. This process is painless but may accelerate disc degeneration.

Spondylosis may be symptomless but can cause:

- episodic mechanical spinal pain
- progressive spinal stiffening
- facet joint pain
- acute disc prolapse, with or without nerve root irritation
- spinal stenosis
- spondylolisthesis.

Facet joint syndrome

Lumbar spondylosis also causes secondary OA of the misaligned facet joints. Pain is typically worse on bending backwards and when straightening from flexion. It is lumbar in site, unilateral or bilateral, and radiates to the buttock. The facet joints are well seen on MRI and may show OA, an effusion or a ganglion cyst. Direct corticosteroid injections into the joints under imaging may help but their long-term value is unclear. Physiotherapy to reduce hyperlordosis and weight reduction are helpful.

Fibrositic nodulosis

This condition causes unilateral or bilateral low back and buttock pain. There are tender nodules in the upper buttock and along the iliac crest. Such nodules are relevant only if they are tender. They are probably traumatic. Local, intralesional corticosteroid injections may help. No imaging is required.

Postural back pain and sway back of pregnancy

Low back pain is common in pregnancy and reflects altered spinal posture and increased ligamentous laxity. There is usually a hyperlordosis on examining the patient standing. Weight control and pre- and postnatal exercises are helpful, and the pain usually settles after delivery. Analgesics and NSAIDs are best avoided during pregnancy and breast-feeding. Epidurals during delivery are not associated with an increased incidence of subsequent back pain. Poor posture causes a similar syndrome in the non-pregnant, owing to obesity or muscular weakness. Poor sitting posture at work is a frequent cause of chronic low back pain.

Management of mechanical back pain

Adequate analgesia to allow normal mobility and avoidance of bed rest is best, combined with physical treatments such as physiotherapy, back muscle training regimens and manipulation. Manipulation produces more rapid pain relief in some patients. Acupuncture may help. [illegible] lifting and exercises help to prevent recurrent attacks of pain. Most episodes recover, irrespective of the treatment given. A positive approach probably reduces the development of chronic pain. A comfortable sleeping position should be adopted using a mattress of medium (not hard) firmness.

Acute lumbar disc prolapse

The central disc gel may extrude into a fissure in the surrounding fibrous zone and cause acute pain and muscle spasm. These

Box 18.12 Lumbar nerve root entrapment: symptoms and signs

Nerve root	Sensory changes	Reflex loss	Weakness	Usual disc prolapse
L2	Front of thigh	None	Hip flexion/ adduction	L1/2
L3	Inner thigh and knee	Knee	Knee extension	L2/3
L4	Inner calf	Knee	Knee extension	L3/4
L5	Outer calf Upper, inner foot	None	Inversion of foot Dorsiflexion of toes	L4/5
S1	Posterior calf Lateral border of foot	Ankle	Plantar flexion of foot	L5/S1

events are often self-limiting. A disc prolapse occurs when the extrusion extends beyond the limits of the fibrous zone ***(Fig. 18.8)***. The weakest point is posterolateral, where the disc may impinge on emerging spinal nerve roots in the root canal.

The episode often starts dramatically during lifting, twisting or bending, and produces a typical combination of low back pain and muscle spasm, and severe, lancinating pains, paraesthesia, numbness and neurological signs in one leg (rarely both). The back pain is diffuse and usually unilateral, and radiates into the buttock. The muscle spasm leads to a scoliosis that reduces when lying down. The nerve root pain develops with, or soon after, the onset. The site of the pain and other symptoms are determined by the root affected ***(Box 18.12)***. A central high lumbar disc prolapse may cause spinal cord compression and long tract signs (i.e. upper motor neurone). Below L2/L3, it produces lower motor neurone lesions.

Examination

On examination, the back often shows a marked scoliosis and muscle spasm. The straight-leg-raising test, whilst the patient is lying, is positive in a lower lumbar disc prolapse – raising the straight leg beyond 30° produces pain radiating down the leg further than the knee. Slight limitation or pain in the back limiting this movement is seen with mechanical back pain. Pain in the affected leg produced by a straight raise of the other leg suggests a large or central disc prolapse. Look for perianal sensory loss and urinary retention or incontinence, which indicate a cauda equina lesion – a neurosurgical emergency (see p. 888). An upper lumbar disc prolapse produces a positive femoral stretch test: pain in the anterior thigh when the knee is flexed in the prone position.

Management

Advise a short period (2–3 days) of bed rest, lying flat for a lower disc but semi-reclining for a high lumbar disc, and prescribe analgesia and muscle relaxants. Once the pain is tolerable, encourage the patient to mobilize and refer them to a physiotherapist for exercises and preventative advice. The investigation of choice is MRI, which identifies the abnormal disc and any compressed nerves. An imaging-guided epidural or nerve root canal injection reduces pain rapidly, although the evidence that it speeds resolution or prevents surgery is unclear. Caudal epidural injections are less effective than lumbar ones. Resuscitation equipment must be available for these procedures. Referral to a surgeon for possible microdiscectomy or hemi-laminectomy is necessary if the neurological signs are severe, if the pain persists and is severe for more than 6–10 weeks, or if the disc is central. If bladder or anal sphincter tone is affected, it becomes a neurosurgical emergency.

Spinal and root canal stenosis

Progressive loss of disc height, OA of the facet joints, posterolateral osteophytes and buckling of the ligamentum flavum all contribute to root canal stenosis. These changes cause nerve root pain or spinal root claudication – pain and paraesthesiae in a root distribution brought on by walking and relieved slowly by rest. The associated sensory symptoms, slower recovery when the patient rests, and presence of normal foot pulses distinguish this from peripheral arterial claudication. Severe cervical spondylosis may also produce spinal claudication, often with arm symptoms and signs.

The investigation of choice to identify the location and extent of stenosis is MRI. Spinal canal stenosis at more than one level is often associated with severe spondylosis and/or a congenitally narrow spinal canal. It causes buttock and bilateral leg pain, ‘heaviness’, paraesthesiae and numbness when walking. Rest helps, as does bending forwards, a manœuvre that opens the spinal canal. Specialist surgical advice is necessary.

Spondylolisthesis

This condition occurs in adolescents and young adults when bilateral congenital pars interarticularis defects cause instability and permit a vertebra to slip, with or without preceding injury. Rarely, a cauda equina syndrome develops, with loss of bladder and anal sphincter control, and saddle-distribution anaesthesia. It is diagnosed radiologically and can be seen on plain radiographs, though MRI may be necessary if entrapment of nerve roots or cauda equina syndrome is suspected. Low back pain in adolescents warrants investigation, and spondylolisthesis requires orthopaedic assessment. It needs careful monitoring during the growth spurt.

A degenerative spondylolisthesis may also develop in older people with lumbar spondylosis and OA of the facet joints.

Diffuse idiopathic skeletal hyperostosis

Diffuse idiopathic skeletal hyperostosis (DISH, or Forestier's disease) affects the spine and extraspinal locations. It causes bony overgrowths and ligamentous ossification, and is characterized by flowing calcification over the anterolateral aspects of the vertebrae. The spine is stiff but not always painful, despite the dramatic changes seen on plain radiographs, which are the imaging investigation of choice. Ossification at muscle insertions around the pelvis produces radiological ‘whiskering’. Similar changes occur at the patella and in the feet. It is more common in people with metabolic syndrome (high body mass index (BMI), diabetes mellitus, hypertension and dyslipidaemia; see p. 209).

Management is with analgesics or NSAIDs for pain, and exercise to retain movement and muscle strength.

Osteoporotic crush fracture of the spine

Osteoporosis is asymptomatic but leads to an increased risk of fracture of peripheral bones, particularly neck of femur and wrist, and thoracic or lumbar vertebral crush fractures. Such vertebral fractures develop without trauma, after minimal trauma, or as part of a major accident. They may develop painlessly or cause agonizing localized pain that radiates around the ribs and abdomen. Multiple fractures lead to an increased thoracic kyphosis. They cause disability and reduced quality of life. The diagnosis is confirmed by

X-rays, showing loss of anterior vertebral body height and wedging, with sparing of the vertebral end-plates and pedicles. Bone oedema on MRI indicates that a fracture is recent. An underlying tumour and pathological fracture need to be excluded.

Management

Advise bed rest and analgesia until the severe pain subsides over a few weeks, then gradual mobilization. It may warrant hospitalization, and the prescription of intravenous bisphosphonates or subcutaneous or nasal calcitonin to relieve pain. There may be some residual pain and deformity.

The role of percutaneous vertebroplasty and balloon kyphoplasty remains unclear; there are no randomized controlled trials (RCTs) showing any benefit. Both involve inserting a needle through a pedicle into the affected vertebral body under CT guidance with the aim of stabilizing the fracture. Kyphoplasty involves inflating a balloon filled with methyl methacrylate cement in order to restore vertebral shape. Vertebroplasty is the injection of cement alone, without restoring vertebral shape. Pain relief is usual with both but the risks are higher with vertebroplasty. Deciding when to intervene is complicated by the spontaneous recovery that many experience.

Bone density measurement and preventative treatment of osteoporosis are essential (see pp. 713–715).

Septic discitis

Septic discitis may cause severe pain and rapid adjacent vertebral destruction. It is seen on MRI and requires urgent neurosurgical referral.

Ankylosing spondylitis

Buttock pain and low back stiffness in a young adult suggest ankylosing spondylitis (see pp. 683–685), especially if they are worse at night and in the morning.

Pain in the hip

'Hip' refers to a wide area between the upper buttock, trochanter and groin. It is useful to ask the patient to point to the site of pain and its field of radiation. Pain arising from the hip joint itself is felt in the groin, lower buttock and anterior thigh, and may radiate to the knee. Occasionally and inexplicably, hip arthritis causes pain only in the knee ***(Box 18.13)***.

? Box 18.13 Pain in the hip: causes

Hip region problems	Main sites of pain
Osteoarthritis of hip	Groin, buttock, front of thigh to knee
Trochanteric bursitis (or gluteus medius tendonopathy)	Lateral thigh to knee
Meralgia paraesthetica	Anterolateral thigh to knee
Referred from back	Buttock
Facet joint pain	Buttock and posterior thigh
Fracture of neck of femur	Groin and buttock
Inflammatory arthritis	Groin, buttock, front of thigh to knee
Sacroiliitis (ankylosing spondylitis)	Buttock(s)
Avascular necrosis	Groin and buttocks
Polymyalgia rheumatica	Lumbar spine, buttocks and thighs

Osteoarthritis of the hip

OA (see pp. 667–671) is the most common cause of hip joint pain in a person over the age of 50 years. It gives rise to pain in the buttock and groin on standing and walking. Stiff hip movements cause difficulty in putting on a sock and may produce a limp. Sudden-onset pain may be associated with an effusion on MRI and can be treated by an ultrasound-guided steroid injection. Severe hip OA is characterized by pain and limitation even at rest and abnormal gait. In severe cases, total hip replacement is the only successful therapy.

Lateral hip pain syndrome: trochanteric bursitis and gluteus medius tendonopathy

This syndrome may be due to trochanteric bursitis and caused by trauma or unaccustomed exercise. It also occurs in inflammatory arthritis. The pain over the trochanter is worse on going up stairs, lying on that side in bed and crossing the legs. The best management is unclear but exercises help, as may a local corticosteroid injection, although the evidence base for treatment is poor. Surgery is rarely necessary. Lateral hip pain may be referred from the upper lumbar spine. A tear of the gluteus medius tendon at its insertion into the trochanter causes a similar syndrome but does not respond to injection. MRI scans have demonstrated this new syndrome.

Meralgia paraesthetica

This condition causes numbness and burning dysaesthesia (increased sensitivity to light touch) over the anterolateral thigh, and may be precipitated by a sudden increase in weight, an injury or pelvic surgery. It is usually self-limiting but can be helped by amitriptyline or gabapentin at night.

Fracture of the femoral neck

This fracture usually occurs after a fall, occasionally spontaneously. There is pain in the groin and thigh, weight-bearing is painful or impossible, and the leg is shortened and externally rotated. Occasionally, a fracture is not displaced and remains undetected. X-rays are diagnostic. Anyone with a hip fracture, especially after minimal trauma, should be reviewed for osteoporosis (see pp. 711–715).

Avascular necrosis (osteonecrosis) of the femoral head

This condition is uncommon but occurs at any age. (Risk factors are discussed on p. 715.) There is severe hip pain. X-rays are diagnostic after a few weeks, when a well-demarcated area of increased bone density is visible at the upper pole of the femoral head. The affected bone may collapse. Early, the X-ray is normal but bone scintigraphy or MRI demonstrates the lesion and shows bone marrow oedema.

Inflammatory arthritis of the hip

Inflammatory arthritis produces pain in the groin and stiffness, which is worse in the morning. RA rarely presents with hip pain, although the hip is involved eventually in severe RA. Ankylosing spondylitis and other seronegative spondyloarthropathies cause inflammatory hip arthritis in younger people.

Polymyalgia rheumatica

Bilateral hip, buttock and thigh pain and stiffness that are worse in the morning in an elderly patient may be attributable to polymyalgia rheumatica (see p. 700). Neck and shoulder pain and stiffness are usually also present.

Box 18.14 Pain in the knee

Trauma and overuse

Problems arising within the joint
- Osteoarthritis
- Inflammatory arthritis
- Meniscal tear
- Cruciate ligament tear
- Chrondromalacia
- Osteochondritis dissecans
- Spontaneous osteonecrosis of the knee

Problems arising in tissues around the joint

Medial
- Medial ligament strain
- Anserine bursitis

Anterior
- Pre-patellar bursitis
- Infrapatellar bursitis
- Quadriceps tendon enthesitis
- Osgood–Schlatter disease

Posterior
- Popliteal (Baker's) cyst

Other
- Hypermobility syndrome
- Referred from hip joint

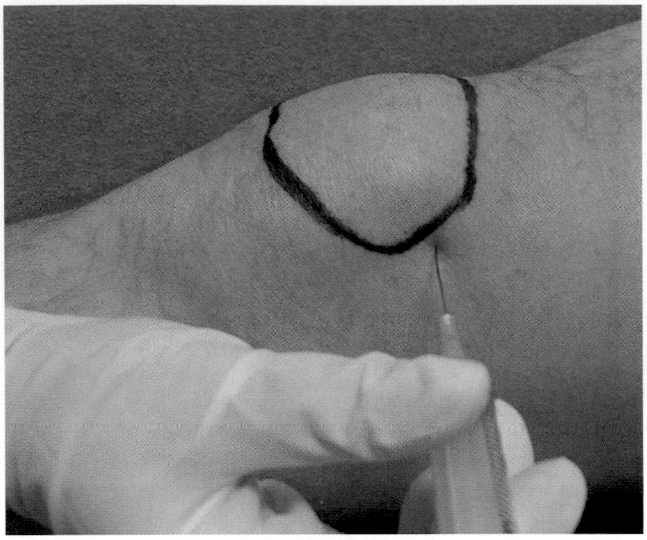

Figure 18.9 Aspiration of the knee.

Pain in the knee

The knee depends on ligaments and quadriceps muscle strength for stability. It is frequently injured, particularly during sports. Trauma or overuse of the knee leads to a variety of peri- and intra-articular problems. Some are self-limiting; others require physiotherapy, local corticosteroid injections or surgery.

Painful knee problems can be divided into those that arise within the joint and those that arise in the soft tissues around the joint ***(Box 18.14)***. Only problems arising within the joint are likely to cause accumulation of fluid (effusion). Identification and aspiration of fluid from effusions are important diagnostic procedures.

Knee joint effusions

An effusion of the knee causes swelling, stiffness and pain. The pain is more severe with an acute onset and with increasing inflammation because the capsule that contains the pain receptors is stretched. A full clinical history must include a past medical, family and drug history.

Examination

A large and tense effusion is easily seen and felt on each side of the patella and in the suprapatellar pouch, and is fluctuant. The effusion delays the patella tapping against the femur when it is pressed firmly and quickly with the knee held straight and relaxed (the 'patellar tap' sign). Small effusions also demonstrate the 'bulge' sign when the patient is lying with the quadriceps relaxed. For this test, apply a gentle sweeping pressure, first to the medial side of the joint and then, watching the medial dimple, to the lateral side. Slightly delayed bulging of the medial dimple indicates fluid in the joint.

Investigations

These are:
- blood tests (urate, blood cultures)
- aspiration ***(Fig. 18.9)*** and examination of the knee effusion.

The basic technique of aspiration is described in ***Box 18.5***. If the fluid obtained is very cloudy, septic arthritis (or occasionally gout) is the likeliest diagnosis. Slightly cloudy or blood-stained fluid that does not clot is likely to indicate pseudogout. Frank blood that clots suggests a haemarthrosis. Fluid should be sent for Gram stain and culture if sepsis is suspected. It should be sent for polarized light microscopy if looking for crystals (see p. 651).

Pain arising from within the knee

Osteoarthritis of the knee

Minor radiographic changes of OA (see ***Fig. 18.16***) are very common in the over-fifties and do not usually cause pain, which is more likely to arise from surrounding soft tissues. X-ray appearances and the degree of pain felt in OA of the knee are not closely correlated. Marked valgus, varus or fixed flexion deformities suggest severe OA. For severe cases, surgery, usually total knee replacement, is the treatment of choice. In milder cases, pain relief, physiotherapy and, sometimes, intra-articular corticosteroid injections may help.

Inflammatory arthritis of the knee

Monoarthritis of the knee, associated with severe pain and marked redness, may be due to septic arthritis, gout or pseudogout. A cool, clear, viscous effusion is seen in elderly people with moderate or severe symptomatic OA (see pp. 667–671). RA rarely presents with knee involvement alone, though seronegative spondyloarthritis may do so.

Haemarthrosis of the knee

This condition is caused by:
- trauma: meniscal, cruciate or synovial lining tear
- clotting or bleeding disorders, e.g. haemophilia, sickle cell disease or von Willebrand's disease.

Torn meniscus

The menisci are partially attached fibrocartilages that stabilize the rounded femoral condyles on the flat tibial plateaux. In the young, they are resilient, but this decreases with age. They can be torn by an injury, commonly in sports that involve twisting and bending. The history is usually diagnostic. There is immediate medial or lateral knee pain and swelling within a few hours. The affected side is tender. If the tear is large, the knee may lock flexed. The immediate treatment is to apply ice. MRI demonstrates the tear ***(Fig. 18.10)***. In most circumstances, especially in active sportsmen and sportswomen, early arthroscopic repair or trimming of the torn meniscus is essential. Surgical intervention reduces recurrent pain, swelling and locking but not the risk of secondary OA. In older patients with OA plus meniscal tear, surgery is no more effective than physiotherapy alone. The long-term benefit of early repair of tears is not

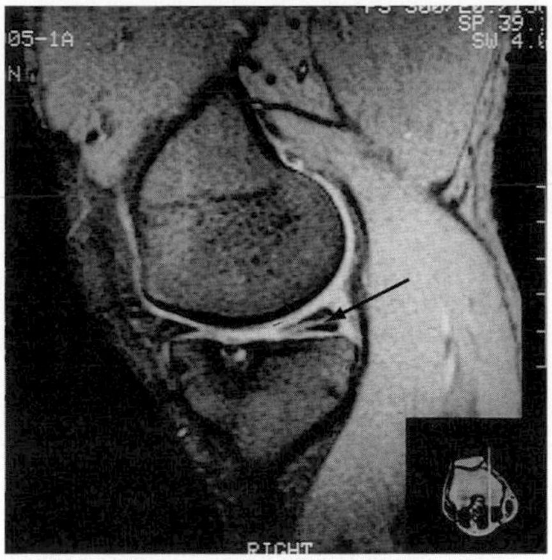

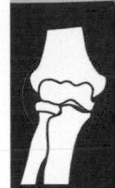

Figure 18.10 Magnetic resonance image of a knee. A complete tear of the posterior horn of the medial meniscus is shown, extending to its lower surface (arrowed).

yet known. Post-surgical quadriceps exercises aid a return to sport and other activities.

Torn cruciate ligaments

Torn cruciate ligaments account for around 70% of knee haemarthroses in young people. They often coexist with a meniscal tear. Partial cruciate tears are difficult to diagnose clinically. On flexing the knee to 90°, a torn anterior cruciate allows the tibia to be pulled forwards on the femur. MRI is the investigation of choice. Such injuries need urgent orthopaedic referral, reconstructive surgery usually being necessary in young active adults. There is a significant incidence of secondary OA.

Chondromalacia patellae

This diagnosis is made arthroscopically. The retropatellar cartilage is fibrillated. In most cases, the pain settles eventually. When there is patellar misalignment, it may need surgery, as does recurrent patellar dislocation in adolescent girls.

Osteochondritis dissecans

This condition occasionally causes knee pain and swelling in adolescents and young adults, more commonly males. It is probably traumatic, possibly with hereditary predisposing factors. A fragment of bone and its attached cartilage detach by shearing, most commonly from the lateral aspect of the medial femoral condyle.

There is aching pain after activity and, if the fragment becomes loose, locking or 'giving way' occurs. The lesion is seen on a tunnel-view X-ray but MRI is more sensitive, especially if the fragment is undisplaced. Undisplaced lesions are treated with rest, then isometric quadriceps exercises. Loose fragments can be fixed arthroscopically or removed. A similar lesion affecting the lateral femoral condyle occurs in older people.

Spontaneous osteonecrosis of the knee

Osteonecrosis may occur spontaneously or after injury. There is local pain and there are marked bone marrow changes on MRI ***(Fig. 18.11A)*** or single-photon emission computed tomography (SPECT; ***Fig. 18.11B***). In particular, weight-bearing must be avoided. Pamidronate by infusion is sometimes used. Spontaneous osteonecrosis of the knee (SONK) may progress to bone infarction and require replacement surgery.

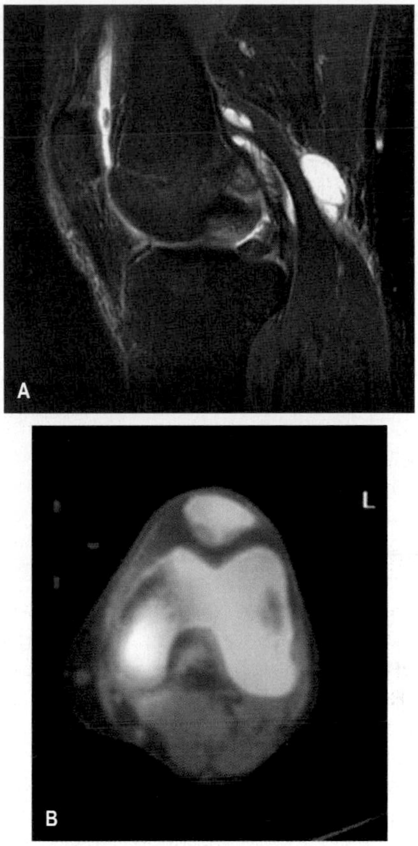

Figure 18.11 Spontaneous osteonecrosis of the knee. A. Magnetic resonance image showing a high signal in the posterior aspect of the femoral condyle, a small effusion and a popliteal cyst. **B.** Single-photon emission computed tomography (SPECT) image showing a high signal in the posterior medial femoral condyle.

Pain from structures around the knee

Medial knee pain

There may be medial or lateral ligament strain but the medial ligament is more commonly affected. There is pain at the ligament's insertion into the upper medial tibia, which is worsened by standing or stressing the affected ligament.

Anserine bursitis causes pain and localized tenderness 2–3 cm below the posteromedial joint line in the upper part of the tibia at the site of the bursa. It occurs in obese women, often with valgus deformities, and in breast-stroke swimmers.

Management is with physiotherapy and a local corticosteroid injection.

Anterior knee pain

Anterior knee pain is common in adolescence. In many cases, no specific cause is found, despite investigation. This is called 'anterior knee pain syndrome' and settles with time. Isometric quadriceps exercises and avoidance of high heels both help the condition. Patients and parents often need firm reassurance. Abnormal patellar tracking may be a cause and may need surgical treatment. Hypermobility of joints causes joint pain, maltracking and, rarely, recurrent patellar dislocation (see also p. 704).

Pre- and infrapatellar bursitis

This can occur in patients whose jobs involve frequent kneeling ('housemaid's knee', 'clergyman's knee', 'carpet-layer's knee').

There is local pain, tenderness and sometimes swelling. Avoidance of kneeling and a local corticosteroid injection are helpful. Septic bursitis can occur.

Osgood–Schlatter disease

Osgood–Schlatter disease (see p. 704) causes pain and swelling over the tibial tubercle. It is a traction apophysitis of the patellar tendon and occurs particularly in teenage sports players.

Enthesitis

This may occur at the patellar end of the quadriceps tendon (jumper's knee).

Posterior knee pain

Popliteal cyst (Baker's cyst)

In approximately 5% of people with a knee effusion, a swollen, painful popliteal cyst develops. The semi-membranosus bursa in some individuals has a valve-like connection to the knee, allowing the effusion to flow into the bursa but not back. The cyst is best seen and felt in the popliteal fossa with the patient standing.

Ruptured popliteal cyst

Fluid escapes into the soft tissue of the popliteal fossa and upper calf, causing sudden and severe pain, swelling and tenderness of the upper calf. Dependent oedema of the ankle develops, and the knee effusion reduces dramatically in size and may be undetectable.

A history of previous knee problems and the sudden onset of pain and tenderness high in the calf suggest a ruptured cyst rather than a deep vein thrombosis (DVT). However, the diagnosis is often missed and treated inappropriately with anticoagulants. A diagnostic ultrasound examination distinguishes a ruptured cyst from a DVT (see p. 1055). Analgesics or NSAIDs, rest with the leg elevated, and aspiration and injection with corticosteroids into the knee joint are required.

Pain in the shin, calf and ankle

Sever's disease

This is a traction apophysitis of the Achilles tendon in young people (compare Osgood–Schlatter disease, p. 704).

Pain at the insertion of the Achilles tendon into the calcaneum is an enthesitis. This is traumatic or it can complicate spondyloarthritis. Raising the shoe heel reduces pain. Occasionally, a low-pressure corticosteroid injection near the enthesis is necessary.

Achilles tendonosis

This causes a painful, tender swelling a few centimetres above the tendon's insertion. Advise against walking barefoot and jumping. Tendon damage or rupture can occur with quinolone, e.g. ciprofloxacin therapy. Therapeutic ultrasound is helpful. (*Caution*: a local injection may cause the tendon to rupture.) Autologous platelet concentrates are used but evidence of efficacy is poor.

Achilles bursitis

This lies clearly anterior to the tendon and can be safely injected with corticosteroid.

Compartment syndromes

The muscles of the lower leg are enclosed in fascial compartments, with little room for expansion to occur. Compartment syndromes can be acute and severe, such as following exercise.

In the ***anterior tibial syndrome***, there is severe pain in the front of the shin, occasionally with foot drop. Immediate surgical decompression to prevent muscle necrosis is sometimes required.

Chronic compartment syndrome produces pain in the lower leg that is aggravated by exercise and may therefore be mistaken for a vascular or neurological disorder.

Pain in the foot

(See ***Box 18.15***). The feet are subjected to extreme pressures by weight-bearing and inappropriate shoes. They are commonly painful. Broad, deep, thick-soled shoes are essential for sporting activities, prolonged walking or standing, and in people with congenitally flat or arthritic feet.

There are two common types of foot deformity:

- ***Flat feet***. These stress the ankle and throw the hindfoot into a valgus (everted) position. A flat foot is rigid and inflexible.
- ***High-arched feet***. These place pressure on the lateral border and ball of the foot.

The foot is affected by a variety of inflammatory arthritic conditions. After the hand, the foot joints are the most commonly affected by RA. The diagnosis depends on careful assessment of the distribution of the joints affected, the pattern of other joint problems or the finding of an associated condition (e.g. psoriasis; see pp. 1353–1356).

Hallux valgus

The big toe migrates laterally. In the congenital form, the first metatarsal bone is displaced medially (metatarsus primus varus). The shape of modern shoes causes later onset of hallux valgus. It is a common complication of RA.

Hallux rigidus

OA of the first metatarsophalangeal (MTP) joint in a normally aligned or valgus joint causes hallux rigidus: a stiff, dorsiflexed and painful big toe. Careful choice of footwear and the help of a podiatrist suffice for most cases but some require surgery.

Metatarsalgia

This is common, especially in women who wear high heels, after trauma and in those with hammer toes. The ball of the foot is painful to walk and stand on. Callosities and pressure-induced bursae develop under the metatarsal heads. RA causes misalignment of the metatarsal bones and severe metatarsalgia.

Management is with podiatry and the wearing of appropriate shoes. Surgery is occasionally needed, particularly in the rheumatoid forefoot.

? Box 18.15 Pain in the foot and heel: causes

- Structural – flat (pronated) or high-arched (supinated)
- Hallux valgus/rigidus (± osteoarthritis)
- Metatarsalgia
- Morton's neuroma
- Stress fracture
- Inflammatory arthritis
- Acute, monoarticular – gout
- Chronic, polyarticular – rheumatoid arthritis
- Chronic, pauciarticular – spondyloarthritis
- Tarsal tunnel syndrome
- Heel pain
- Plantar fasciitis: below heel
- Plantar spur: below heel
- Achilles tendonitis/bursitis: behind heel
- Sever's disease: behind heel
- Arthritis of ankle/subtaloid joints

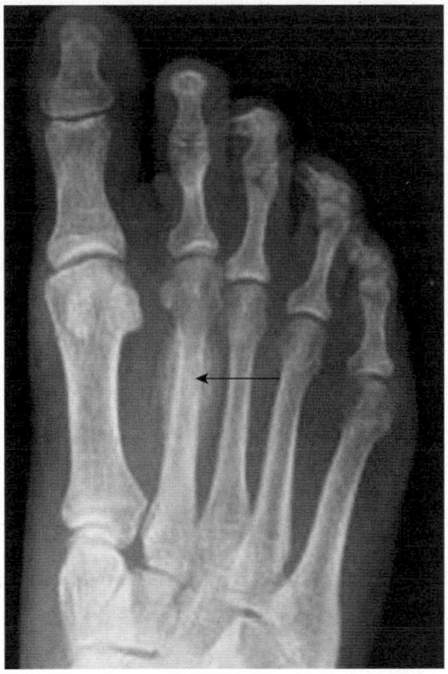

Figure 18.12 Callus forming around a stress fracture. The image shows a stress fracture of the second metatarsal at 4 weeks. X-rays initially were normal.

Morton's neuroma

This usually occurs between the third and fourth metatarsal heads. It causes pain, burning and numbness in the adjacent surfaces of the affected toes when walking. It is helped by wearing wider, cushion-soled shoes. Occasionally, a steroid injection or excision is necessary.

Stress fractures of the metatarsals

These cause sudden, severe, weight-bearing pain in the distal shaft of the fractured metatarsal bone. They occur after unaccustomed walking or with new shoes. There is local tenderness and swelling, but initially X-rays are normal and diagnosis delayed ***(Fig. 18.12)***. A radioisotope bone scan or MRI reveals the fracture earlier than X-rays. Reduced weight-bearing for a few weeks usually suffices. Underlying osteoporosis may be a cause.

Tarsal tunnel syndrome

This is an entrapment neuropathy of the posterior tibial nerve at the medial malleolus. It produces burning, tingling and numbness of the toes, sole and medial arch. The nerve is tender below the malleolus and, when tapped, produces a shock-like pain (Tinel's sign). A local steroid injection under the retinaculum, between the medial malleolus and calcaneum, is helpful.

Pain under the heel

See ***Box 18.15***.

Plantar fasciitis

This is an enthesitis at the insertion of the plantar fascia into the calcaneum. It produces localized pain under the heel when standing and walking, and local tenderness. It occurs alone or in spondyloarthritis. Obesity, particularly in flat-footed people who walk a lot, can predispose to plantar fasciitis.

Plantar spurs

These are traction lesions at the insertion of the plantar fascia in older people and are usually asymptomatic. They become painful after trauma.

Calcaneal bursitis

This is a pressure-induced (adventitious) bursa that produces diffuse pain and tenderness under the heel. Compression of the heel pad from the sides is painful, which distinguishes it from plantar fascia pain.

Clinical features and management of heel pain

Whatever the cause, heel pain is always worse in the morning as soon as weight is placed on the foot.

All of these lesions are treated with heel pads, and reduced walking; they are often self-limiting. A dorsiflexion splint at night to stretch the plantar fascia is worth trying. When an injection is necessary, a medial approach is used, rather than advancing through the heel pad, often under ultrasound guidance.

Pain in the chest

Musculoskeletal conditions are sometimes a cause of chest pain. An example is Tietze's disease. In this condition, pain arises from the costosternal junctions. It is usually unilateral and affects one, two or three ribs. There is local tenderness, which helps to make the diagnosis. The condition is benign and self-limiting. It often responds well to anti-inflammatory drugs. Other causes of chest wall pain include rib fractures due to trauma, osteoporosis or a malignant deposit. Costochondral pain occurs in ankylosing spondylitis (see pp. 683–685). In people with heart disease, costochondral pain may cause severe anxiety but it is not like angina and the patient should be reassured.

Pain associated with sport and the performing arts

Pain in muscles and soft tissues is common after sport or associated with performing arts, such as dancing or playing musical instruments. General advice, such as warming up properly and using appropriate supportive footwear for running, can help. However, in cases of prolonged pain or where the person suffering pain is a professional sportsperson or performer, referral to a sports medicine specialist is advisable.

Further reading

Balagué F, Mannion A, Pellise F et al. Non-specific low back pain. *Lancet* 2012; 379:482–491.

Coombes BK, Bisset L, Vicenzino B. Efficacy and safety of corticosteroid injections and other injections for management of tendinopathy: a systematic review of randomised controlled trials. *Lancet* 2010; 376:1751–1767.

Ensrud KE, Schousboe JT. Clinical practice. Vertebral fractures. *N Engl J Med* 2011; 364:1634–1642.

Klazan CA, Lohle PN, de Vries J et al. Vertebroplasty versus conservative treatment in acute osteoporotic vertebral compression fractures: an open-labelled study. *Lancet* 2010; 376:1085–1092.

Lamb SE, Hansen Z, Lall R et al. Group cognitive behavioural therapy for low back pain in primary care. *Lancet* 2010; 375:916–923.

Ropper AH, Zafonte RD. Sciatica. *New Engl J Med* 2015; 372:1240–1248.

CHRONIC PAIN SYNDROMES

Chronic pain is defined as pain lasting more than 3 months (the natural tissue-healing time). Many rheumatological illnesses (e.g.

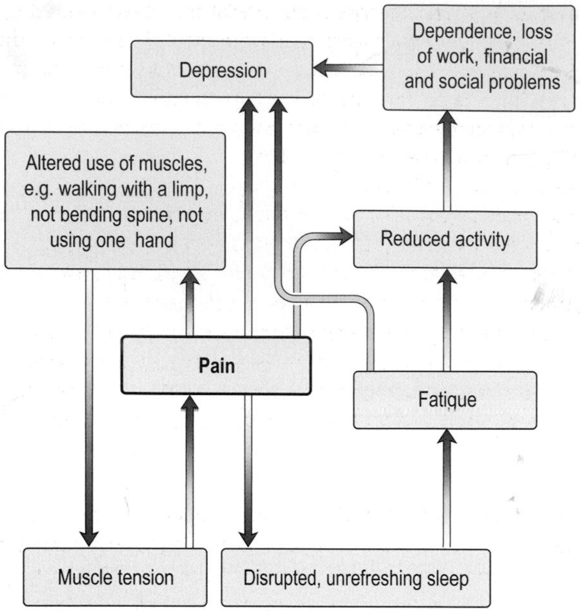

Figure 18.13 **Interaction of physical and psychological factors in chronic widespread pain.**

RA and OA) cause pain of such duration but are not considered as chronic pain syndromes. In chronic pain syndromes, the pain generally has no clear structural cause or curative treatment and is often combined with psychological distress, poor sleep and altered use of the muscles due to the pain (called fear-avoidance behaviour or abnormal pain behaviour). This altered behaviour can lead to more stress and tension in the muscles, exacerbating the pain ***(Fig. 18.13)***.

The pain suffered by these patients is neither imaginary nor artefactual, even though there may be no structural abnormality in the painful area. There is a problem with the pain processing system in the nervous system, leading to amplification of pain signals. Psychological factors often contribute to this amplification, and the pain can make psychological distress worse in a vicious circle. The combination of physical pain and psychological distress makes these syndromes difficult to manage.

Living with chronic pain is difficult. Patients may become anxious, depressed or socially isolated, and their quality of life is reduced. There are often adverse effects on employment, personal relationships and dependence on others. Consultations need to address these issues, as well as the pain itself, to be effective. In chronic pain syndromes, patients need help to lead a more normal life despite their pain, and are best referred to a specialist, multidisciplinary pain service. Medications alone are not the answer.

These syndromes can be conveniently subdivided into chronic widespread pain (above and below the waist and on both sides of the body) and chronic regional pain (any other distribution). Both are very common. Epidemiological studies show that the prevalence of chronic widespread pain is 10–11% and that of chronic regional pain 20–30%.

Chronic widespread pain

Pain that starts in a single area can spread to other areas of the body, as more muscles become tense and tender. Conversely, patients with chronic widespread pain can develop new, localized causes of pain (e.g. appendicitis, OA) that can be treated

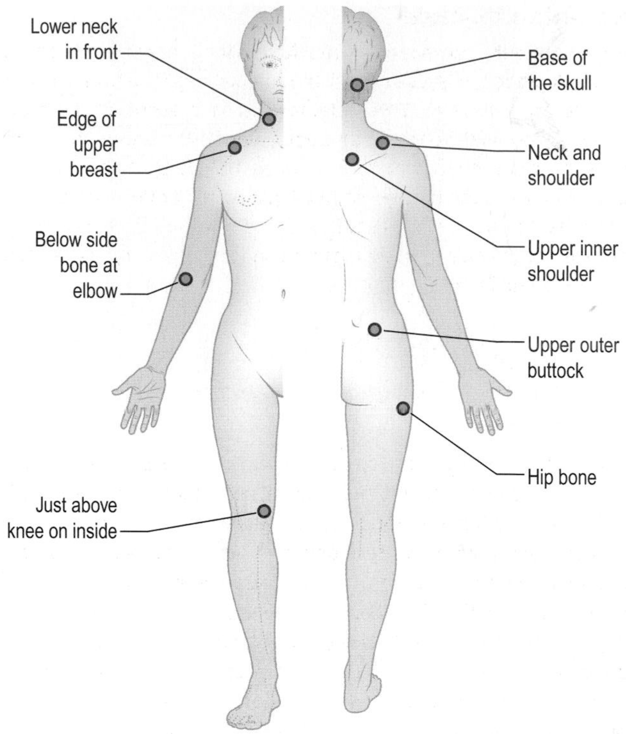

Figure 18.14 **Trigger points in fibromyalgia.**

successfully. It should not be assumed that every pain in these patients is always due to the same chronic problem.

Two of the main causes of chronic widespread pain are fibromyalgia and joint hypermobility syndrome (see pp. 666–667).

Fibromyalgia

Fibromyalgia is not a diagnosis of exclusion. It can occur in patients who have other illnesses like RA and SLE. Individuals suffer chronic widespread pain with disrupted and unrefreshing sleep, constant tiredness, and tender points detectable on pressing their muscles ***(Fig. 18.14)***. Multiple other symptoms, such as irritable bowel syndrome (IBS), tension headaches, dysmenorrhoea, atypical facial or chest pain and forgetfulness, often coexist. It occurs in about 1 in 50 people, can develop at any age and affects women more than men (2 : 1). The diagnosis is clinical, and blood tests and imaging are normal. These tests may be requested to exclude other causes of pain.

Management

(See p. 901.) A clear explanation of the diagnosis is critically important. While being honest about the fact that there is no cure for fibromyalgia, it is also necessary to reassure the patient that it is not arthritis and that the pain is not causing damage to joints or muscles. Many patients have never had an explanation of the cause of their symptoms, which leads to fear and doubt. Treatment options that can be offered to help (not cure) are described below.

Drugs

There is evidence from clinical trials for use of analgesics, anticonvulsants and antidepressants. Commonly used drugs include amitriptyline (which may also improve sleep), pregabalin, paracetamol, tramadol and gabapentin. Benefits, however, are often short-term and adverse effects common.

Non-drug therapies

A sympathetic, psychosocial, multidisciplinary approach is appropriate. A graded, supervised aerobic exercise regimen over 3 months is safe and effective. When depression is present, it should be treated. Cognitive behavioural therapy can help the person to pace their life more effectively and to cope better. Pain management programmes, combining psychology with physiotherapy, are designed to improve physical function and quality of life but do not reduce pain intensity. Acupuncture can lessen pain in some cases but the effect is usually transient.

Chronic regional pain

Chronic (work-related) upper-limb pain syndrome

This name is preferred to 'repetitive strain injury' (RSI). The predominant symptoms are pain in all or part of one or both arms. A specific lesion, such as tennis elbow or carpal tunnel syndrome, or muscular-pattern neck pain often develops first, and early recognition and treatment may prevent chronicity. After a variable period, the pain becomes more diffuse and no longer simply work-related, and there is often severe distress. It is seen in keyboard workers and in musicians. When it arises at work, it is often at a time of changing work practices, shortage of staff or disharmony. Middle managers find it difficult to deal with and this compounds the stress.

Management

If possible, there should be a brief period off work and a gradual return to activity as the pain settles. Use of analgesia and NSAIDs, with physiotherapy, is helpful during the initial phase to prevent a vicious circle developing. Amitriptyline or pregabalin is helpful for some patients.

A review of working practices and the positioning of screen, keyboard and chair are essential, as is support of the patient by their manager. Musicians are helped by expert advice on playing technique and should reduce playing times temporarily, but not stop completely.

Temporomandibular pain dysfunction syndrome

This pain syndrome is a disorder of the temporomandibular joint that is associated with nocturnal tooth grinding or abnormalities of bite. It occurs in anxious people. It gives rise to pain in one or both temporomandibular joints.

Dental correction of the bite helps a few, but when no dental cause is found, low-dose tricyclic antidepressant therapy is used. Many patients are made worse by unnecessary dental treatment.

Complex regional pain syndrome

Complex regional pain syndrome (CRPS) is a rare condition (prevalence 20 : 100 000), in which regional neuropathic pain is associated with abnormal sensory, autonomic, motor and/or trophic changes. There are two types. In CRPS type I, there is no identifiable overt nerve lesion, whereas such a lesion is identifiable in CRPS type II. CRPS usually occurs after trauma but the pain is disproportionate in time or intensity to that usually caused by such an injury. It may also develop after central nervous system lesions (e.g. strokes) or without cause.

Its features are pain and other sensory abnormalities, including hyperaesthesia; and autonomic vasomotor dysfunction, leading to abnormal blood flow and sweating; and motor system abnormalities, leading to structural changes of superficial and deep tissues (trophic changes). Not all components need be present. The sensory, motor and sympathetic nerve changes are not restricted to the distribution of a single nerve and may be remote from the site of injury. The early phase, with pain, swelling and increased skin temperature, is difficult to diagnose but potentially reversible.

After a period of weeks or months, a second, still painful, dystrophic phase develops, characterized by articular stiffness, cold skin and trophic changes, often with localized osteoporosis.

A late phase involves continued pain, skin and muscle atrophy, and muscle contractures, and is extremely disabling.

Diagnosis is clinical – a high index of suspicion and recognition of the unusual distribution of the pain. There are no specific or sensitive investigations, though demineralization may be seen on X-ray. Bone scan and MRI are not required to make the diagnosis.

Management

Management is difficult and the problem often very disabling. The evidence base for treatment is poor. Early diagnosis, effective pain relief and general care of the patient are essential. NSAIDs, tricyclic antidepressants, serotonin–norepinephrine reuptake inhibitors, and pregabalin or gabapentin are used in the early phase, together with active exercise of the limb, encouraged by a physiotherapist. Intravenous bisphosphonates can also be effective. Referral to a specialist pain clinic is essential. Nerve blocks were used in the past but are less common now. Intravenous immunoglobulins have been used in clinical trials but are not yet an accepted therapy.

Further reading

Fukushima FB, Bezerra DM, Vilas Boas PJF et al. Complex regional pain syndrome. *Br Med J* 2014; 348:g3683.
Rahman A, Underwood, M, Carnes D. Fibromyalgia. *Br Med J* 2014; 348:g1224.

ANALGESIC AND ANTI-INFLAMMATORY DRUGS FOR MUSCULOSKELETAL PROBLEMS

The key to using drugs, particularly in chronic disorders and the elderly, is to balance risk and benefit and to review their appropriateness constantly. ***Box 18.16*** shows the main drugs available.

Simple and compound analgesic agents

Simple agents, such as paracetamol, aspirin or codeine compounds (or combination preparations), used when necessary or regularly, relieve pain and improve function. Sleep may also be improved. Side-effects are relatively infrequent, although drowsiness and constipation occur with codeine preparations, especially in the elderly.

Stronger analgesics, such as dihydrocodeine, tramadol or morphine derivatives, should be used only with severe pain.

Non-steroidal anti-inflammatory drugs

Non-steroidal anti-inflammatory drugs (NSAIDs) have anti-inflammatory and centrally acting analgesic properties. They inhibit cyclo-oxygenase (COX), a key enzyme in the formation of prostaglandins, prostacyclins and thromboxanes (see ***Fig. 24.30***). There are two specific cyclo-oxygenase enzymes:

- ***COX-1*** is the constitutive form present in many normal tissues.
- ***COX-2*** is the form mainly induced in response to pro-inflammatory cytokines and is not found in most normal

Box 18.16 Analgesics and NSAIDs

Drug	Dose	Frequency
Analgesics[a] *To be taken only if needed. Maximum doses are indicated.*		
Paracetamol	500–1000 mg	6-hourly
Paracetamol (500 mg) and codeine (8–30 mg)	1–2 tablets	6-hourly
Dihydrocodeine	30–60 mg	Every 6–8 h
Paracetamol with dihydrocodeine	1–2 tablets	Every 6–8 h
Non-steroidal anti-inflammatory drugs (NSAIDs) *Always to be taken with food. Slow-release preparations are used in inflammatory conditions or if more regular pain control is needed. Examples are shown.*		
Ibuprofen	200–400 mg	Every 6–8 h
Ibuprofen slow-release	600–800 mg	12-hourly
Diclofenac	25–50 mg	8-hourly
Diclofenac slow-release	75–100 mg	×1–2 daily
Naproxen	250 mg	×3–4 daily
Naproxen slow-release	550 mg	×2 daily
Celecoxib[b]	100–200 mg	×2 daily

[a]In order of potency. [b]COX-2-specific NSAID (coxib).

tissues (except the kidney). It is associated with oedema and the nociceptive and pyretic effects of inflammation.

Effects and side-effects

Most of the older NSAIDs are non-specific and block both enzymes but with variable specificity ('non-specific NSAIDs', or nsNSAIDs). Their therapeutic effect depends on blocking COX-2 and their side-effects mainly on blocking COX-1. COX-1 protects the gastric mucosa and blocking it accounts for the majority of upper gastrointestinal side-effects.

The most common side-effects with non-specific NSAIDs are indigestion or skin rashes. More serious upper gastrointestinal side-effects are gastric erosions and peptic ulceration with perforation and bleeding. These occur more frequently in the elderly, in whom mortality is higher, in long-term use, and in those with high risk factors: a history of ulcers, *Helicobacter pylori*, and concurrent corticosteroid or anticoagulant therapy. Ibuprofen, in combination with low-dose aspirin, significantly increases the risk of severe gastrointestinal bleeding. Practice guidelines recommend proton pump inhibitors in high-gastrointestinal-risk patients on non-specific NSAIDs. H_2 blockers are less effective as gastroprotective agents. Prostaglandin E_2 analogues, such as misoprostol, reduce ulcer complications and are popular, but may cause nausea and diarrhoea. Lower gastrointestinal side-effects of non-specific NSAIDs are becoming more common.

COX-2 inhibitors ('coxibs') produce fewer gastrointestinal side-effects but these still occur. Coxibs are used in patients who have a high risk of gastrointestinal disease but no cardiovascular risk. People with a high risk of both may be better off taking an NSAID (ibuprofen or naproxen) or a coxib with a proton pump inhibitor.

Coxibs and NSAIDs may reduce renal function, especially in the elderly (see ***Box 20.20***). Coxibs and all NSAIDs except naproxen, if used in high dose for long periods, cause a small increase in risk of vascular events, such as myocardial infarction or stroke. All these drugs, including naproxen, increase the risk of heart failure.

Uses

- ***In musculoskeletal pain and in OA and spondylosis***, short courses of NSAIDs or coxibs are used but simple analgesia is often more appropriate.
- ***In crystal synovitis***, NSAIDs and coxibs have a true anti-inflammatory effect.
- ***In chronic inflammatory synovitis***, NSAIDs and coxibs do not alter the chronic inflammatory process or decrease the risk of joint damage, but they do reduce pain and stiffness.
- ***In inflammatory arthritis and situations where more constant pain control is needed***, slow-release preparations are useful.
- ***In chronic arthritis***, NSAID gels have some value.

The standard advice is to use NSAID in the lowest dose possible for the shortest time necessary to control pain. Be aware of the patient's gastrointestinal and cardiac risks before prescribing NSAIDs or coxibs.

DISORDERS OF COLLAGEN

Collagen is responsible for many of the structural, tensile and load-bearing properties in the various tissues where it is found. The structure of collagen is discussed on page 647. Thirty or more dispersed genes encode for more than 19 different types of collagen ***(Box 18.17)***.

Joint hypermobility syndrome (Ehlers–Danlos syndrome type III)

These two terms describe the same syndrome. Inheritance appears to be autosomal dominant but the underlying genetic abnormality is unknown. Hypermobility itself is very common (15–20% of adults); it may be demonstrated by showing increased flexibility in the thumbs, little fingers, elbows, knees and lumbar spine, and quantified using the Beighton score ***(Box 18.18)***. The majority of hypermobile people suffer no adverse effects from the hypermobility but in some it can cause recurrent subluxations of individual joints and/or persistent widespread musculoskeletal pains. These people are said to have joint hypermobility syndrome. Other symptoms, such

Box 18.17 The major types of collagen

Collagen structure	Type number	Encoding gene	Associated conditions
Fibrillar	I, II, III, V, XI	*COL1A1–2, COL2A2, COL3, COL5, COL11*	Osteogenesis imperfecta, Ehlers–Danlos syndrome (subtypes)
Basement membrane	IV	*COL4A1–5*	Alport syndrome (see p. 743)
Fibril-associated collagen with interrupted triple helix (FACIT)	IX, XII, XIV	*COL9, 12, 14*	
Filament-producing	VI	*COL6A1–3*	
Network-forming	VIII, X	*COL8A1, 10A1*	
Anchoring fibril	VII	*COL7A1*	Epidermolysis bullosa (see p. 1371)

Box 18.18 The Beighton hypermobility score[a] and diagnostic criteria for joint hypermobility syndrome

Joint	Finding	Score
Little (fifth) finger	Passive dorsiflexion >90°	1 for each side
Thumb	Passive dorsiflexion to the flexor aspect of the forearm	1 for each side
Elbow	Hyperextends >10°, extends ≤10°	1 for each side
Knee	Hyperextends >10°, extends ≤10°	1 for each side
Forward flexion of trunk with the knees fully extended	Palms can rest flat on the floor	1

Diagnostic criteria for joint hypermobility syndrome: Beighton score ≥4; arthralgia for ≥3 months in ≥4 joints.

[a]In this 9-point system, the higher the score, the higher the laxity. Young adults can score 4–6.

as bowel disturbance, easy scarring and faintness on standing (postural orthostatic tachycardia syndrome, or POTS), can also occur and the combination can be very disruptive to normal life. Treatment of the musculoskeletal symptoms relies on specialist physiotherapy to advise on exercises that take the patient's hypermobility into account. Pain management programmes can be helpful in more severe cases. It is usually better to avoid surgery due to difficulties in healing.

Other forms of Ehlers–Danlos syndrome

Ehlers–Danlos syndrome (EDS) is a heterogeneous group of disorders of collagen. Ten different types have been recognized with varying degrees of skin fragility, skin hyper-extensibility and joint hypermobility.

- ***Types I and II*** (classic EDS) are inherited in an autosomal dominant fashion. Mutations in *COL5A1* and *COL5A2* result in abnormal type V collagen.
- ***Type IV*** (vascular type) is also autosomal dominant and involves arteries, bowel and uterus, as well as skin. Mutations in the *COL3A1* gene produce abnormalities in structure, synthesis or secretion of type III collagen.
- ***Type VI*** is a recessively inherited disorder and results from a mutation in the gene that encodes lysyl hydroxylase.
- ***Type VII*** is an autosomal dominant disorder in which there is a defect in the conversion of procollagen to collagen; *COL1A1* and *COL1A2* mutations delete the N-proteinase cleavage sites.

Type III EDS was described above. The other forms of EDS are very rare and their defects have not been elucidated here. The clinical features are described on page 1378.

Marfan syndrome

This condition is described on pages 1028–1029.

Osteogenesis imperfecta

This is a heterogeneous group of disorders inherited mainly in autosomal dominant fashion with mutations in *COL1A1* and *COL1A2* genes. There are four main types of osteogenesis imperfecta and clinical subtypes are also described (V, VI and VII). The major clinical feature is bone fragility but other collagen-containing tissues are also involved, such as tendons, skin and eyes.

- ***Type I***: mild bony deformities, blue sclerae, defective dentine, early-onset deafness, hypermobility of joints and heart valve disorders
- ***Type II***: death in the perinatal period
- ***Type III***: severe bone deformity and blue sclerae
- ***Type IV***: fewer fractures, normal sclerae, normal lifespan but can also be severe, as in type III.

Management with daily oral risedronate in children improves BMD and reduces fracture risk. Intravenous pamidronate is another option. Prognosis is variable, depending on the severity of the disease. Stem cell therapy is being used.

Achondroplasia

Achondroplasia ('dwarfism') is diagnosed in the first years of life. The disease is inherited in an autosomal dominant manner and is caused by a defect in the fibroblast growth factor receptor-3 gene. The trunk is of normal length but the limbs are very short and broad due to abnormal endochondral ossification. The vault of the skull is enlarged, the face is small and the nose bridge is flat. Intelligence is normal.

Further reading

Coxib and Traditional NSAID Trialists Collaboration. Vascular and upper gastrointestinal effects of non-steroidal anti-inflammatory drugs: meta-analyses of individual participant data from randomized trials. *Lancet* 2013; 382:769–779.

Grahame R, Bird H A, Child A. The revised (Brighton 1998) criteria for the diagnosis of benign joint hypermobility syndrome. *J Rheumatol* 2000; 27:1777–1779.

OSTEOARTHRITIS

Osteoarthritis (OA) is the most common type of arthritis and is no longer viewed as a simple degenerative process due to ageing. It is now recognized to occur as a result of damage to articular cartilage induced by a complex interaction of genetic, metabolic, biochemical and biomechanical factors, leading to an inflammatory response affecting cartilage, subchondral bone, ligaments, menisci, synovium and capsule. It is the subject of intense investigation to develop disease-modifying therapies, with limited success so far.

Epidemiology

The prevalence of OA rises with age, being uncommon before 50 years of age and increasing, so that most people over 60 years will have some radiological evidence of it, although only a quarter of these are symptomatic. It occurs worldwide with a variable distribution. For instance, hip OA is less common and knee OA more common in Asians than in Europeans. Beyond 55 years of age, women are affected more commonly than men, with a familial pattern of inheritance in nodal and primary generalized forms of OA. It has a variable distribution ***(Fig. 18.15)*** and resulting disabilities have major socioeconomic resource implications, particularly in the developed world. OA is the most common cause of disability in the Western world in older adults.

Aetiology and pathogenesis

Cartilage is a matrix of collagen fibres, enclosing a mixture of proteoglycans and water (see p. 647); it has a smooth surface and is shock-absorbing. Under normal circumstances, there is a dynamic balance between cartilage degradation by wear and its production by chondrocytes. Early in the development of OA, this balance is lost and, despite increased synthesis of extracellular matrix, the cartilage becomes oedematous. Subsequently, focal erosion of

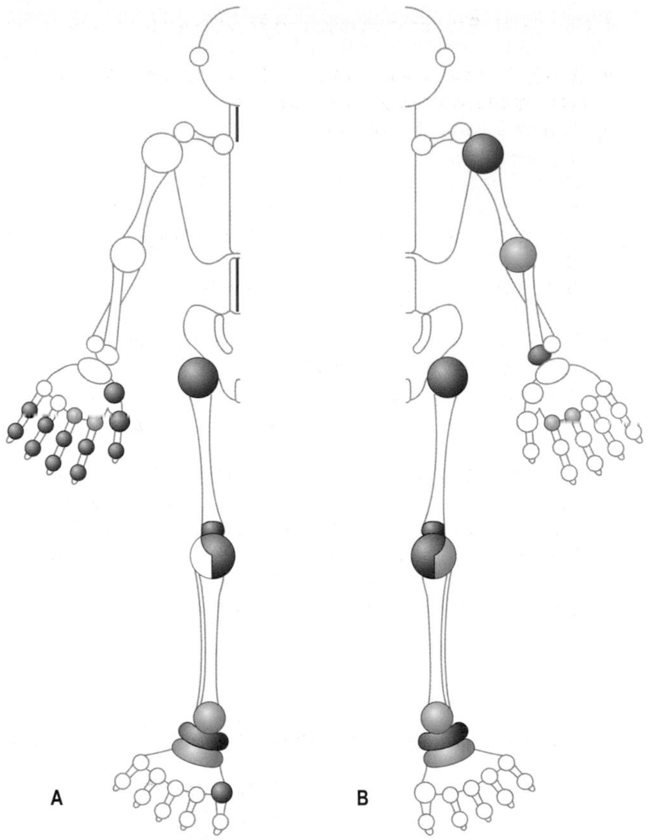

Figure 18.15 Typical distribution of affected joints in arthritis. **A.** Primary generalized osteoarthritis. **B.** Pyrophosphate arthropathy. Red circles indicate the more commonly affected sites, and blue the less commonly affected sites.

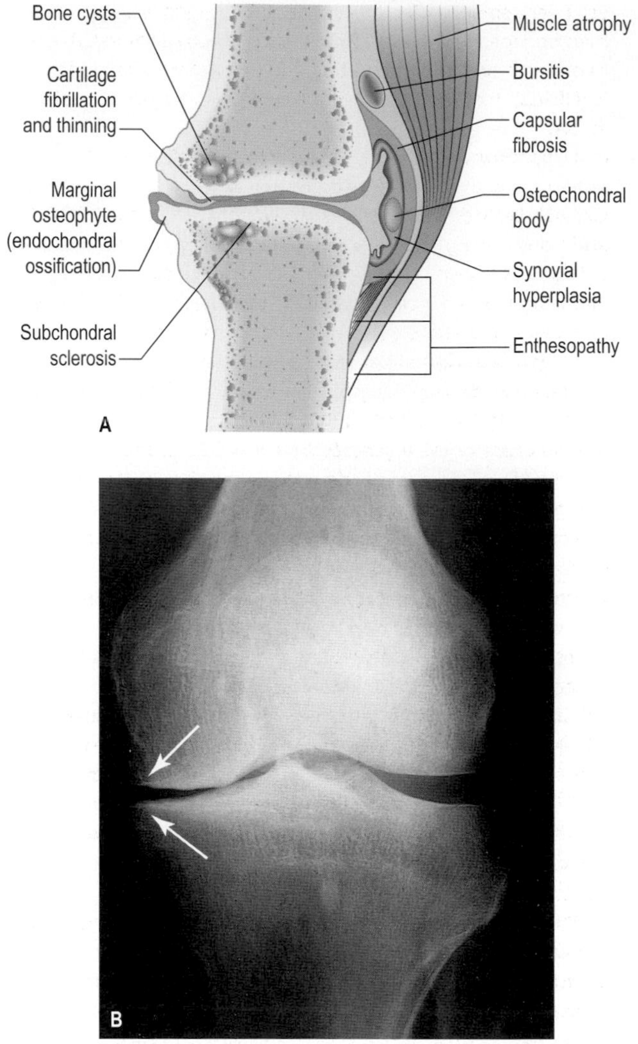

Figure 18.16 Early osteoarthritis of a knee. A. Pathology. **B.** On the X-ray, there is medial compartment narrowing owing to cartilage thinning with subarticular sclerosis and marginal osteophyte formation (arrowed).

cartilage develops, chondrocytes die and, although repair is attempted from adjacent cartilage, the process is disordered, leading to a failure of synthesis of extracellular matrix so that the surface becomes fibrillated and fissured. Cartilage ulceration exposes underlying bone to increased stress, producing microfractures and cysts. The bone attempts repair but produces abnormal sclerotic subchondral bone and overgrowths at the joint margins, called osteophytes ***(Fig. 18.16)***. There is some secondary inflammation. This process produces a spectrum of OA, ranging from atrophic disease in which cartilage destruction occurs without any subchondral bone response, to hypertrophic disease in which there is massive new bone formation at the joint margins.

Joint specific genetic factors are involved in the pathogenesis of OA. Polymorphisms in the gene for human aggrecan have been correlated with OA of the hand in older men, and familial concordance for hip and knee OA is greater in surgically defined than in radiographically defined disease. There is no single gene, however, that associates with all patterns of OA, and several other mechanisms have been suggested:

- ***Abnormal stress and loading***, leading to mechanical cartilage damage, play a role in secondary OA.
- ***Obesity*** is a risk factor for developing OA of the hand and knee, but not the hip, in later life. Increased skeletal mass increases cartilage volume.
- ***Collagenases*** (MMP-1 and MMP-13) cleave collagen, and other metalloproteinases, such as stromelysin (MMP-3) and gelatinases (MMP-2 and MMP-9), are also present in the extracellular matrix. MMPs are secreted by chondrocytes in an inactive form. Extracellular activation then leads to the degradation of both collagen and proteoglycans around chondrocytes.
- ***Tissue inhibitors of metalloproteinases*** (TIMPs) regulate the MMPs. Disturbance of this regulation may lead to an increase in cartilage degradation over synthesis and contribute to the development of OA. TIMPs have not yet proven to be of therapeutic value.
- ***Osteoprotegerin (OPG), RANK and RANK ligand*** (RANKL) control subchondral bone remodelling. Their levels are significantly different in OA chondrocytes. Inhibition of RANKL is being investigated as a new therapeutic approach in OA.
- ***Aggrecanase*** production is stimulated by pro-inflammatory cytokines, and aggrecan (the major proteoglycan) levels fall.
- ***Synovial inflammation*** is present in OA, and CRP in the serum may be raised. Interleukin-1 (IL-1) and tumour necrosis factor alpha (TNF-α) release stimulates metalloproteinase production, and IL-1 inhibits type II collagen production. IL-6 and IL-8 may also be involved. Anti-cytokine therapy has not

yet been tested in OA. The production of cytokines by macrophages and that of MMPs by chondrocytes in OA are dependent on the transcription factor nuclear factor kappa B (NF-κB). Inhibition of NF-κB may have a therapeutic role in OA.

- ***IL-1 receptor antagonist*** genes are associated with radiographic severity of knee OA.
- ***Growth factors***, including insulin-like growth factor 1 (IGF-1) and transforming growth factor beta (TGF-β), are involved in collagen synthesis, and their deficiency may play a role in impairing matrix repair. Paradoxically, increased TGF-β may also cause increased subchondral bone density.
- ***Cartilage breakdown products*** lead to macrophage infiltration and vascular hyperplasia, and IL1-β and TNF-α may contribute to further cartilage degradation.
- ***Vascular endothelial growth factor*** (VEGF) from macrophages is a potent stimulator of angiogenesis and may contribute to inflammation and neovascularization in OA. Innervation can accompany vascularization of the articular cartilage.
- ***A strong hereditary element*** underlying OA is suggested by twin studies. The influence of genetic factors is estimated at 35–65%. Mutations in the gene for type II collagen (*COL2A1*) have been associated with early polyarticular OA. Large genome-wide association studies (GWAS) of subjects undergoing total knee replacement have identified the strongest association on chromosome 3 with rs6076, which is in perfect linkage disequilibrium with rs11177. This single nucleotide polymorphism (SNP) encodes a missense polymorphism within the nucleostemin encoding gene, *GNL3*.
- ***In the Caucasian population***, there is an inverse relationship between the risk of developing OA and osteoporosis.
- ***Gender***. In women, weight-bearing sports produce a two- to threefold increase in risk of OA of the hip and knee. In men, there is an association between hip OA and certain occupations: farming and labouring. OA may flare after the female menopause or after cessation of hormone replacement therapy.
- ***Periarticular enthesitis*** has been proposed as a factor in the pathogenesis of nodal generalized OA (NGOA) and is the subject of investigation.

The term ***primary OA*** is sometimes used when there is no obvious known predisposing factor.

Box 18.19 shows some of the predisposing factors for the development of OA, and ***Box 18.20*** lists other conditions that sometimes cause secondary arthritis.

Clinical features

OA affects many joints, in diverse clinical patterns, typically causing mechanical pain with movement and/or loss of function. Hip and knee OA are major causes of disability. Early OA is rarely symptomatic, however, unless accompanied by a joint effusion, whilst advanced radiological and pathological OA is not always symptomatic.

Symptoms are usually gradual in onset and progressive. Episodic disease flare-ups may be inflammatory in nature, with an associated slight rise in ESR or CRP. Focal synovitis is caused by fragments of shed bone or cartilage. Radiological OA is usually, but not inevitably, progressive. This progression may be stepwise or continual. Radiological improvement is uncommon but has been observed, suggesting that repair is possible.

Box 18.19 Factors predisposing to osteoarthritis (OA)

- ***Obesity***: This predicts a later risk of radiological and symptomatic OA of the hip and hand in population studies
- ***Heredity***: There is a familial tendency to develop nodal and generalized OA
- ***Gender***: Polyarticular OA is more common in women; a higher prevalence after the menopause suggests a role for sex hormones
- ***Hypermobility*** (see p. 704): Increased range of joint motion and reduced stability lead to OA
- ***Osteoporosis***: There is a reduced risk of OA
- ***Diseases***: See Box 18.20
- ***Trauma***: A fracture through any joint predisposes. Meniscal and cruciate ligament tears cause OA of the knee
- ***Congenital joint dysplasia***: This alters joint biomechanics and leads to OA. Mild acetabular dysplasia is common and leads to earlier onset of hip OA
- ***Joint congruity***: Congenital dislocation of the hip or a slipped femoral epiphysis or Perthes' disease predispose; osteonecrosis of the femoral head (see p. 659) in children and adolescents causes early-onset OA
- ***Occupation***: Miners develop OA of the hip, knee and shoulder, cotton workers OA of the hand, and farmers OA of the hip
- ***Sport***: Repetitive use and injury in some sports cause a high incidence of lower-limb OA

Box 18.20 Causes of osteoarthritis

Primary OA
- No known cause

Secondary OA

Pre-existing joint damage
- Rheumatoid arthritis
- Gout
- Spondyloarthritis
- Septic arthritis
- Paget's disease
- Avascular necrosis, e.g. corticosteroid therapy

Metabolic disease
- Cartilage calcification
- Hereditary haemochromatosis
- Acromegaly

Systemic disease
- Haemophilia – recurrent haemarthrosis
- Haemoglobinopathies, e.g. sickle cell disease
- Neuropathies

Symptoms

- Joint pain with movement and/or weight-bearing.
- Short-lived morning joint stiffness.
- Functional limitation.

Signs

- Crepitus.
- Restricted movement.
- Bony enlargement.
- Joint effusion and variable levels of inflammation.
- Bony instability and muscle wasting.

Clinical subsets

Localized OA

Nodal OA

In nodal OA (***Box 18.21***), joints of the hand are usually affected one at a time over several years, with the DIPs more frequently involved than the PIPs. Nodal OA often begins around the female menopause, with inflammation causing painful, tender, swollen interphalangeal joints and impairment of hand function. At this stage, enthesitis can be seen on MRI. Intra-articular corticosteroid injections may be helpful at this stage. The inflammatory phase settles

Box 18.21 Features of nodal osteoarthritis

- Demonstrates a familial nature
- Has a higher incidence in women
- Shows a typical pattern of polyarticular involvement of the hand joints
- Develops in late middle age and around female menopause
- Has a generally good long-term functional outcome
- Is associated with osteoarthritis of the knee, hip and spine (nodal generalized osteoarthritis)

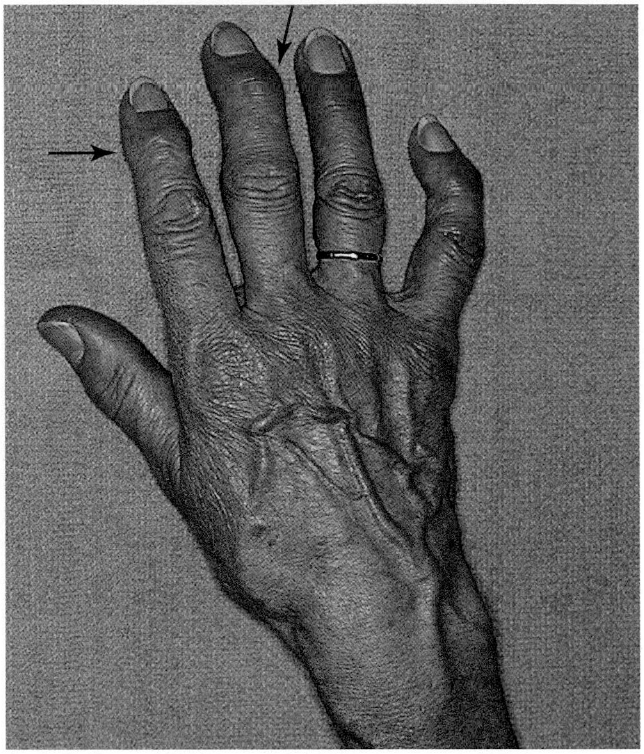

Figure 18.17 Severe nodal osteoarthritis. The distal interphalangeal joints (DIPs) demonstrate Heberden's nodes (arrowed). The middle finger DIP joint is deformed and unstable. The thumb is adducted and the bony swelling of the first carpometacarpal joint is clearly shown – 'the squared hand of nodal osteoarthritis'.

after some months or years, leaving painless bony swellings posterolaterally: ***Heberden's nodes (DIPs)*** and ***Bouchard's nodes (PIPs)***, along with stiffness and deformity ***(Fig. 18.17)***. Functional impairment is usually limited, although PIP OA restricts grip more than DIP involvement. On X-ray, the nodes are marginal osteophytes and there is joint space loss.

Thumb-base OA coexists with nodal OA and causes pain and disability, which decrease as the joint stiffens. The 'squared' hand in OA ***(Fig. 18.17)*** is caused by bony swelling of the first carpometacarpal joint and fixed adduction of the thumb. Function is rarely severely compromised.

Polyarticular hand OA is associated with a slightly increased frequency of OA at other sites.

Hip OA

Hip OA affects 7–25% of adult Caucasians but is significantly less common in black African and Asian populations. There are two major subgroups defined by the radiological appearance. The most common is ***superior-pole hip OA***, where joint space narrowing and sclerosis predominantly affect the weight-bearing upper surface of the femoral head and adjacent acetabulum. This finding is most common in men and unilateral at presentation, although both hips may become involved in progressive disease. Early onset of hip OA is associated with acetabular dysplasia or labral tears. Less commonly, ***medial cartilage loss*** occurs. This appearance is seen most commonly in women and is associated with hand involvement (NGOA), and is usually bilateral. It is more rapidly disabling.

Knee OA

The prevalence of symptomatic knee OA is 40% in individuals over 75 years of age and is more common in women. There is a strong relationship with obesity. The disease is generally bilateral and strongly associated with nodal OA of the hand in elderly women, or is seen as part of generalized OA. The medial compartment is most commonly affected, leading to a varus (bow-legged) deformity. Often, retropatellar OA is also present. Previous trauma and meniscal and cruciate ligament tears are risk factors for developing knee OA. Bone marrow lesions seen on MRI predict disease progression and eventual joint replacement.

Primary generalized OA

This condition is rare and usually seen in combination with NGOA. Other affected areas include the knees, first MTP, hip and intervertebral (spondylosis) joints. Its onset is often sudden and severe. There is a female preponderance and a strong familial tendency. Periarticular ligamentous pathology may have an important role in the phenotypic expression of NGOA.

Erosive OA

In this rare subgroup, the DIPs and PIPs are inflamed and equally affected, with a poor functional outcome. Radiologically, there is marked osteolysis. Destructive phases are followed by phases of remodelling.

Crystal-associated OA

This condition most commonly occurs with calcium pyrophosphate deposition (CPPD) in the cartilage. It increases in frequency with age and causes cartilage calcification (CC) on over 40% of knee X-rays in the over-eighties, but is usually asymptomatic. The joints most frequently affected are the knees (hyaline cartilage and fibrocartilage) and wrists (triangular fibrocartilage; see ***Fig. 18.15***). There is patchy linear CC on X-ray ***(Fig. 18.18)***.

A chronic arthropathy (pseudo-OA) occurs, predominantly in elderly women with severe CC. There is a florid inflammatory component and marked osteophyte and cyst formation visible on X-rays. The joints affected differ from those in NGOA, being predominantly the knees, then wrists and shoulders. CC is associated with CPPD crystal-induced arthritis (see p. 689).

A rare, rapidly destructive arthritis in elderly women, affecting shoulders, hips and knees, is associated with the finding of crystals of calcium apatite in a bloody joint effusion. The outlook is poor and joints require early surgical replacement.

Investigations

- ***Blood tests***. There is no specific test; the ESR is usually normal, although high-sensitivity CRP may be slightly raised. Rheumatoid factor and antinuclear antibodies are negative.
- ***X-rays***. These are abnormal only when the damage is advanced. They are useful in preoperative assessments.

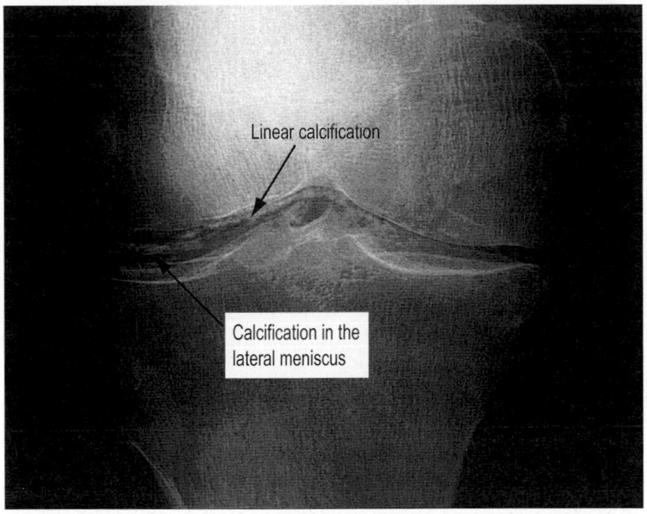

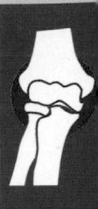

Figure 18.18 Cartilage calcification of the knee. Note the linear calcification in the hyaline cartilage and calcification of the lateral meniscus (plus mild secondary osteoarthritis).

For knees, a standing X-ray (stressed) is used to assess cartilage loss, and 'skyline' views in flexion are used for patello-femoral OA.

- ***MRI***. This demonstrates meniscal tears, early cartilage injury and subchondral bone marrow changes (osteochondral lesions).
- ***Arthroscopy***. This reveals early fissuring and surface erosion of the cartilage.
- ***Aspiration of synovial fluid*** (if there is a painful effusion). This shows a viscous fluid with few leucocytes (see p. 651).

Management

The guiding principle is to treat the symptoms and disability, not the radiological appearances; depression and poor quadriceps strength are better predictors of pain than radiological severity in OA of the knee. Patient education about the disease and its effects reduces pain, distress and disability, and increases compliance with treatment. Psychological or social factors alter the impact of the disease.

Physical measures

Weight loss and exercises for strength and stability are useful. Hydrotherapy helps, especially in lower-limb OA. Local heat, ice packs, massage, and rubefacients or local NSAID gels are all used. Insoles for flat feet and a walking stick held on the contralateral side to the affected lower limb joint are useful.

There is increasing evidence that acupuncture helps knee OA. Other forms of complementary medicine are commonly used, despite lack of scientific evidence that they have any effect.

Medication

Potential benefit must be balanced against potential side-effects, especially in the elderly. Paracetamol is used but its value has been questioned (see ***Box 18.16***). NSAIDs or coxibs should be used intermittently when possible. Opioids are a last resort and should be used cautiously in older patients.

Intra-articular corticosteroid injections produce short-term improvement when there is a painful joint effusion. Frequent injections into the same joint should be avoided. Heterogeneity of relevant studies means that the potential role of intra-articular hyaluronan preparations is not effective in general.

Glucosamine and chondroitin (sold as food supplements) have no clinically relevant effect on joint pain or joint space narrowing.

There are no proven agents that halt or reverse OA, although they are greatly needed. The role of bisphosphonates in reducing bone changes is unclear. The role of drugs that block tissue metalloproteinases or cytokines (see pathogenesis, above) is also unclear.

Surgery

Arthroscopy for knee OA is rarely beneficial. Replacement arthroplasty, however, has transformed the management of severe OA. More than 1 million hip arthroplasties are being performed worldwide each year, predominantly for OA, and this number is projected to double in the next two decades. Furthermore, there has been a significant fall in 90-day mortality from 0.56% in 2003 to 0.29% in 2018. The safety of hip and knee replacements is now equal, with a complication rate of about 1%, loosening and late blood-borne infection being the most serious. These slight but definite risks make it essential for the patient to be certain that surgery is necessary. Resurfacing hip surgery has become popular but may have higher complication rates in women, particularly with metal on metal resurfacing. Uni-compartmental knee replacement is a less major procedure and may be appropriate in some cases. For most patients, a total hip or knee replacement reduces pain and stiffness, and greatly increases function, mobility and – particularly significant for the elderly – independence.

Other surgical procedures include re-alignment osteotomy of the knee or hip, excision arthroplasty of the first MTP and base of the thumb, and fusion of a first MTP joint.

Further reading

Brandt KD. *Diagnosis and Nonsurgical Management of Osteoarthritis*, 5th edn. New York: Professional Communications; 2010.
Haseeb A, Haqqi TM. Immunopathogenesis of osteoarthritis. *Clin Immunol* 2013; 146:185–196.
Hunter DJ. Viscosupplementation for osteoarthritis of the knee. *New Engl J Med* 2015; 372:1040–1047.
Pivec R. Hip arthroplasty. *Lancet* 2012; 380:1768–1777.

INFLAMMATORY ARTHRITIS

Inflammatory arthritis includes a large number of diseases in which the predominant feature is synovial inflammation. The three main subgroups of inflammatory arthritis are rheumatoid arthritis (RA), spondyloarthritis and crystal arthritis ***(Box 18.22)***. The diagnosis of these conditions is helped by distinguishing:

- the pattern of joint involvement (symmetrical or asymmetrical, large or small) ***(Box 18.23)***
- presence of any non-articular disease
- a past and family history
- periodicity of the arthritis (single acute, relapsing, chronic and progressive).

Box 18.22 The three main subgroups of inflammatory arthritis

1. Rheumatoid arthritis (associated with antibodies)
2. Spondyloarthritis (associated with human leucocyte antigen (HLA)-B27)
3. Metabolic arthritis (e.g. associated with crystals)

Box 18.23 Pattern of joint involvement in inflammatory arthritis

Diseases presenting as an inflammatory monoarthritis
- Crystal arthritis, e.g. gout, CPPD
- Septic arthritis
- Palindromic rheumatism
- Traumatic ± haemarthrosis
- Arthritis due to juxta-articular bone tumour
- Occasionally, psoriatic, reactive, rheumatoid may present as monoarthritis

Diseases presenting as an inflammatory polyarthritis
- Rheumatoid arthritis
- Reactive arthritis
- Spondyloarthritis associated with psoriasis or ankylosing spondylitis
- Postviral arthritis
- Lyme arthritis
- Enteropathic arthritis
- Arthritis associated with erythema nodosum

CPPD, calcium pyrophosphate deposition arthropathy.

Certain non-articular diseases, such as psoriasis, iritis, IBS, non-specific urethritis or recent dysentery, suggest spondyloarthritis. There may be evidence of recent viral illness (rubella, hepatitis B or erythrovirus), rheumatic fever, or a tick bite and skin rash (Lyme disease). In early arthritis, it may not be possible to make a specific diagnosis until the disease has evolved from an undifferentiated arthritis into a chronic form.

There is a distinct genetic separation of rheumatoid-pattern synovitis and spondyloarthritis; RA (see below) is associated with a genetic marker in the class II major histocompatibility complex (MHC) genes, whilst spondyloarthritis shares certain alleles in the B locus of class I MHC genes, usually B27 (see p. 683).

In general, the pain and stiffness of inflammatory arthritis are worse in the morning, often lasting for several hours and improving with activity, in contrast with the much shorter morning stiffness and mechanical pain with activity of OA. Inflammatory markers (ESR and CRP) are often raised in inflammatory arthritis, and there is often a normochromic, normocytic anaemia. Specific types of arthritis are discussed below.

Early inflammatory polyarthritis

Undifferentiated polyarthritis requires urgent referral to a rheumatologist for diagnosis and treatment, including the early introduction of disease-modifying agents when indicated (see p. 680). In persistent inflammatory arthritis, sustained remission depends on rapid diagnosis and intensive treatment. Poor prognostic features for undifferentiated polyarthritis are:

- polyarticular onset
- positive anti-citrullinated peptide antibodies (ACPA)
- positive rheumatoid factor
- joint erosion on X-ray at presentation
- disease >3–6 months.

RHEUMATOID ARTHRITIS

RA is an autoimmune disease associated with autoantibodies to the Fc portion of immunoglobulin G (rheumatoid factor) and to citrullinated cyclic peptide. There is persistent synovitis, causing chronic symmetrical polyarthritis with systemic inflammation. Genetically, RA is a heterogeneous group of diseases.

Epidemiology

RA has a worldwide distribution affecting 0.5–1% of the population (with a female preponderance of 3:1). The prevalence is low in black Africans and Chinese people. The incidence is falling. RA remains a significant cause of disability and mortality and carries a high socioeconomic cost. It presents from early childhood (when it is rare) to late old age. The most common age of onset is between 30 and 50 years.

Aetiology and pathogenesis

There has been a greater understanding of genetic and environmental factors in the last two decades.

- ***Gender***. Women, before the menopause, are affected three times more often than men. Post-menopause, the frequency of onset is similar between the sexes; thus sex hormones may be important in the pathogenesis. A meta-analysis of the use of the oral contraceptive pill has shown no effect on RA overall, but it may delay the onset of disease.
- ***Genetic factors***. There is an increased incidence in first-degree relatives and a high concordance amongst monozygotic twins (up to 15%) and dizygotic twins (3.5%). Overall, genetic factors account for about 60% of disease susceptibility. There is a strong association between susceptibility to RA and certain human leucocyte antigen (HLA) haplotypes: HLA-DR4, which occurs in 50–75% of patients and correlates with a poor prognosis, as does possession of certain shared alleles of HLA-DRB1*04. The possession of these shared epitope alleles in HLA-DRB1 (S2 and S3P) increases susceptibility to RA and may predispose to ACPA directed against citrullinated antigens. Citrullination is a process that modifies antigens, allowing them to fit into the shared epitope on HLA alleles. In a genome-wide association study in ACPA-positive RA, an association was found with loci near HLA-DRB1 and PTPN22 in people of European descent. These genes affect the presentation of autoantigens (*HLA-DRB1*), T-cell receptor signal transduction (*PTPN22*) and targets of ACPA (*PAD14*).
- ***Environment***. Smoking and other forms of bronchial stress increase the risk of RA with HLA-DR4 and acts synergistically with HLA-DRB1 to increase the risk of having ACPA. Environmental stress, such as smoking, is thought to promote post-translational modifications, leading to citrullination of mucosal proteins in pulmonary tissue. A loss of tolerance at other mucosal sites is suggested by the association of periodontal disease and alterations in the gut microbiome with RA.

Immunology

RA is primarily a synovial disease, and synovitis occurs when chemoattractants produced in the joint recruit circulating inflammatory cells. Over-production of tumour necrosis factor alpha (TNF-α) leads to synovitis and joint destruction. Interaction of macrophages and T and B lymphocytes drives this over-production. TNF-α stimulates over-production of IL-6, as well as other cytokines. The increased understanding of the immunopathogenesis of this disease has informed the development of targeted biological therapies ***(Fig. 18.19)***. Blockade of TNF-α and IL-6 has produced marked improvement in synovitis and systemic malaise, indicating the pivotal role of these cytokines in the chronic synovitis (see pp. 680–682).

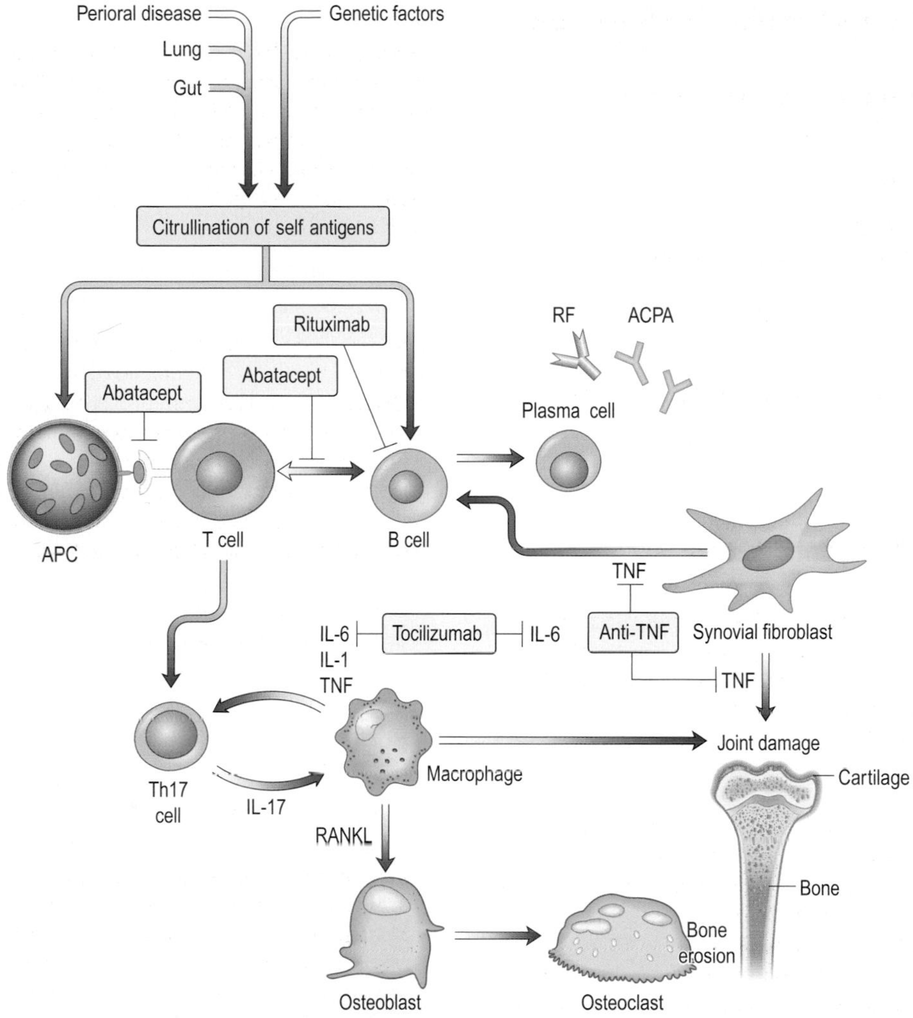

Figure 18.19 Pathogenesis of rheumatoid arthritis. Environment–gene interactions promote citrullination of self proteins, which can then be detected by T and B cells; this leads to a loss of tolerance and promotion of the inflammatory response, resulting in joint damage. Targeted therapy is also shown. **ACPA**, anti-citrullinated peptide antibody; **APC**, antigen-presenting cell; **IL**, interleukin; **RANKL**, receptor activator of nuclear factor kappa B ligand; **RF**, rheumatoid factor; **Th**, T helper; **TNF**, tumour necrosis factor.

An imbalance in the number of certain cell types appears to be central to immune regulation and its dysfunction.

- ***Synovial cells*** in chronic rheumatoid synovitis are predominantly fibroblast-like synoviocytes, and macrophage-like synoviocytes that produce pro-inflammatory cytokines. Abnormal fibroblast-like synoviocytes circulate between joints and may be the trigger for polyarthritis.
- ***Osteoclasts*** cause bone and cartilage destruction.
- ***Synovial B cells***, activated by cytokine-activated macrophages and T cells, produce autoantibodies, of which IgM and IgA RF are the most typical in RA. As RFs bind the Fc portion of IgG, they have the potential for self-aggregation and immune complex formation in the synovium. These may then trigger macrophages via IgG Fc receptors to produce even more cytokines, including IL-1, IL-8, TNF-α and granulocyte macrophage colony stimulating factor, and fibroblasts to produce IL-6.
- ***CD20-positive B-cell ablation*** (a technique used for treating B-cell lymphomas) induces temporary remission, reinforcing the central role of B cells in the chronic inflammation of RA. As the B cells return, the CRP rises and the disease flares again.
- ***Synovial fibroblasts*** have high levels of the adhesion molecule, vascular cell adhesion molecule (VCAM-1, a molecule that supports B-lymphocyte survival and differentiation), decay accelerating factor (DAF, a factor that prevents complement-induced cell lysis) and cadherin II (which mediates cell-to-cell interactions). These molecules may facilitate the formation of ectopic lymphoid tissue in synovium. Mice deficient in cadherin II are resistant to a form of inflammatory arthritis.
- ***T cells*** can be a part of the destructive process. T cell-associated cytokines, such as IL-2 and IL-4, however, are not present in high amounts. Th17 helper cells (see pp. 131–132), which produce IL-17A, 17F, 21 and 22, and TNF-α, may cause inflammation. The normal regulatory T cells are suppressed by TGF-β and interleukins (produced by macrophages and dendritic cells), allowing the Th17 helper cells to increase.

The role of innate immunity in RA pathogenesis and in predisposing the joint to inflammation is still unknown (see pp. 123–128).

The ***triggering antigen***, which leads to self-maintained inflammation in RA, remains unclear. Triggers for ACPA production include filaggrin, type II collagen and vimentin. There is little evidence that type II collagen is the triggering antigen, although it is a cause of arthritis in animal models of RA. Smoking is a potential trigger, particularly in ACPA-positive RA (see p. 675).

Pathology

RA is typified by widespread, persistent synovitis of joints, tendon sheaths or bursae. Normal synovium is thin, comprising a lining layer a few cells thick that contains fibroblast-like synoviocytes and macrophages overlying loose connective tissue. The synoviocytes play a central role in synovial inflammation. In RA, the synovium becomes greatly thickened, causing 'boggy' swelling around joints and tendons, with proliferation of the synovium into folds and fronds, and infiltration by a variety of inflammatory cells, including polymorphs, which transit through the tissue into the joint fluid, and lymphocytes and plasma cells. There are disorganized lymphoid follicles. The normally sparse surface layer of lining cells becomes hyperplastic and thickened ***(Fig. 18.20)***. There is marked vascular proliferation. Increased permeability of blood vessels and the synovial lining layer leads to joint effusions that contain lymphocytes and dying polymorphs.

The hyperplastic synovium spreads from the joint margins on to the cartilage surface. This 'pannus' of inflamed synovium damages the underlying cartilage by blocking its normal route for nutrition and by the direct effects of cytokines on the chondrocytes. The cartilage becomes thinned and the underlying bone exposed. Local cytokine production and joint disuse combine to cause juxta-articular osteoporosis during active synovitis.

Fibroblasts from the proliferating synovium also grow along the course of blood vessels between the synovial margins and the epiphyseal bone cavity, and damage the bone. This process is shown by MRI to occur in the first 3–6 months following onset of the arthritis before the diagnostic, ill-defined, juxta-articular bony 'erosions' appear on X-ray ***(Fig. 18.21)***. This early damage justifies the use of disease-modifying anti-rheumatic drugs (DMARDs; see p. 680) within 3 months of onset of the arthritis to try to induce disease remission. Low-dose steroids delay, and anti-TNF-α agents halt and occasionally reverse, erosion formation. Erosions lead to a variety of deformities and contribute to long-term disability.

Rheumatoid factors and anti-citrullinated peptide antibodies (ACPA)

Transient production of RF (see pp. 650–651) is an essential part of the body's normal mechanism for removing immune complexes, but in RA they show a much higher affinity and their production is persistent and occurs in the joints. They are of any immunoglobulin class (IgM, IgG or IgA), but the most common tests employed clinically detect IgM RF. Around 70% of people with polyarticular RA have IgM rheumatoid factor in the serum. Positive titres can predate the onset of RA.

The term 'seronegative RA' is used when the standard tests for IgM RF are persistently negative. These patients tend to have a more limited pattern of synovitis.

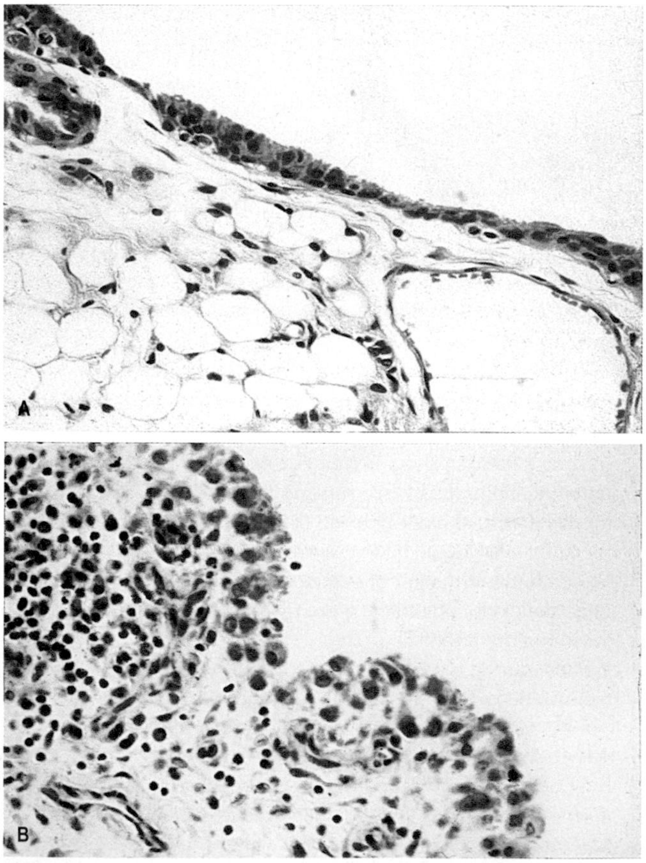

Figure 18.20 Histological appearance of synovium in rheumatoid arthritis (RA). A. Normal synovium. **B.** Synovial appearances in established RA, showing marked hypertrophy of the tissues with infiltration by lymphocytes and plasma cells. *(From Shipley M.* Colour Atlas of Rheumatology, *3rd edn. London: Mosby–Wolfe; 1993, with permission.)*

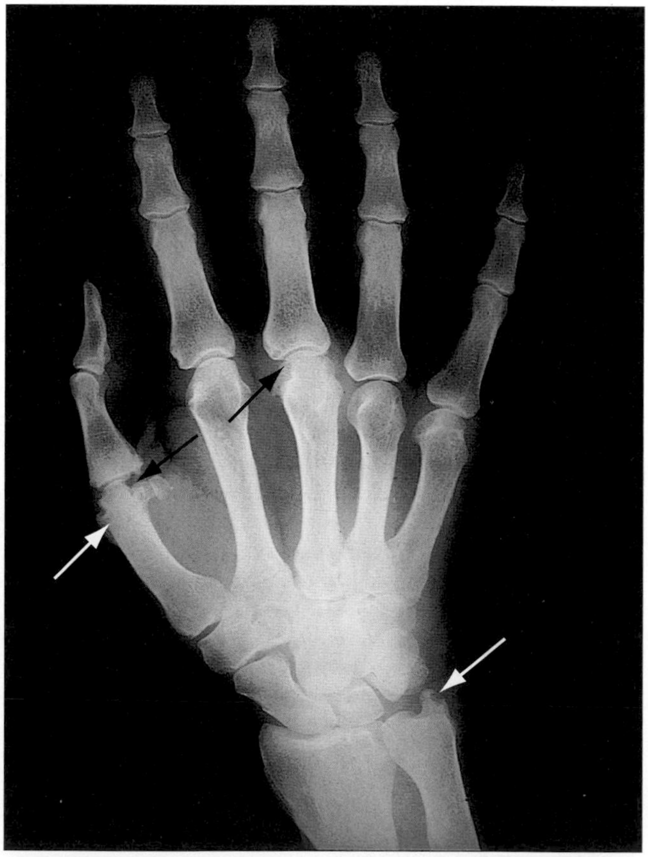

Figure 18.21 X-ray of early rheumatoid arthritis. Typical erosions may be seen at the thumb (black and white arrows on the left), middle metacarpophalangeal joints (central black arrow) and ulnar styloid (white arrow on the right).

Box 18.24 Factors predicting a poor prognosis for progression in early rheumatoid arthritis

- Older age
- Female sex
- Symmetrical small joint involvement
- Morning stiffness >30 min
- >4 swollen joints
- Cigarette smoking
- Co-morbidity
- C-reactive protein >20 g/dL
- Positive rheumatoid factor and anti-citrullinated peptide antibodies

Box 18.25 Differential diagnosis of early rheumatoid arthritis

- Postviral arthritis: rubella, hepatitis B or erythrovirus
- Seronegative spondyloarthropathies
- Polymyalgia rheumatica
- Acute nodal osteoarthritis (proximal and distal interphalangeal joints involved)

IgM RF is not diagnostic of RA and its absence does not rule the disease out; however, it is a useful predictor of prognosis. A persistently high titre in early disease implies more persistently active synovitis, more joint damage and greater disability eventually, and justifies earlier use of DMARDs.

ACPAs (see p. 650) are usually present with RF in RA. They are better predictors of a transition from early transient inflammatory arthritis to persistent synovitis and early RA. RF and ACPA together are even more specific.

Box 18.26 ACR/EULAR 2010 criteria for rheumatoid arthritis[a]

Criteria	Points
1. Joint involvement	**0–5**
1 medium to large joint	0
2–10 medium to large joints	1
1–3 small joints (large joints not counted)	2
4–10 small joints (large joints not counted)	3
>10 joints; at least one small joint	5
2. Serology	**0–3**
Negative RF and negative ACPA	0
Low positive RF or low positive ACPA	2
High positive RF or high positive ACPA	3
3. Acute-phase reactants	**0–1**
Normal CRP and normal ESR	0
Abnormal CRP or abnormal ESR	1
4. Duration of symptoms	**0–1**
<6 weeks	0
≥6 weeks	1

[a]The cut-off point for RA is at ≥6 points. Patients can also be classified as having RA if they have both typical erosions and longstanding disease previously satisfying the classification criteria. **ACPA**, anti-citrullinated peptide antibody; **ACR**, American College of Rheumatology; **CRP**, C-reactive protein; **EULAR**, European League Against Rheumatism; **ESR**, erythrocyte sedimentation rate; **RF**, rheumatoid factor.
(Adapted from Scott DL, Wolfe F, Huizinga TW. Rheumatoid arthritis. *Lancet* 2010; 376:1094–1108.)

Clinical features

Typical presentation

RA typically presents (approximately 70% of cases) as a progressive, symmetrical, peripheral polyarthritis, evolving over a period of a few weeks or months in patients between 30 and 50 years of age, although the disease can occur at any age. Less commonly (15%), a rapid onset can occur over a few days (or explosively overnight), with a severe symmetrical, polyarticular involvement, especially in the elderly. Factors indicating a poor prognosis are listed in ***Box 18.24***. The differential diagnosis of early RA is shown in ***Box 18.25***.

Revised classification (American College of Rheumatology, ACR) criteria from 2010 are more suitable for assessing and diagnosing early arthritis than previous versions because they do not rely on later changes, such as erosions and extra-articular disease to distinguish RA ***(Box 18.26)***.

In early RA, the combination of at least one swollen joint for more than 6 weeks with no prior injury, no associated history or family history of spondyloarthritis or associated conditions such as psoriasis (see pp. 1353–1356), and a positive ACPA test is the best way to select patients for earlier treatment to avoid joint damage. This benefit of earlier treatment is evidence-based and has been shown to reduce the risk of the development of damage and permanent joint deformities.

Symptoms and signs of early RA

The majority of patients complain of pain and stiffness of the small joints of the hands (MCPs, PIPs) and feet (MTPs). The DIPs are usually spared. The wrists, elbows, shoulders, knees and ankles are also affected. In most cases, many joints are involved, but 10% of patients present with a monoarthritis of the knee or shoulder or with carpal tunnel syndrome.

Fatigue is a common complaint. The pain and stiffness are significantly worse in the morning. Sleep is disturbed.

The joints are usually warm and tender with some joint swelling. There is limitation of movement and muscle wasting. Deformities and non-articular features develop if the disease cannot be controlled (see below).

RA in the older patient may mimic polymyalgia rheumatica; the synovitis becomes apparent as the corticosteroid dose is reduced.

Other presentations

The presentation and progression of RA are variable. Presentations are shown in ***Box 18.27***. Relapses and remissions occur either spontaneously or on drug therapy. In some patients, the disease remains active, producing progressive joint damage. Rarely, the process may cease ('burnt-out RA').

Seronegative RA initially affects the wrists more often than the fingers and has a less symmetrical joint involvement. It has a better long-term prognosis but some cases progress to severe disability. This form can be confused with psoriatic arthropathy, which has a similar distribution (see pp. 685–686).

Palindromic rheumatism is unusual (5%) and consists of short-lived (24–48-hour) episodes of acute monoarthritis. The joint becomes acutely painful, swollen and red, but resolves completely. Further attacks occur in the same or other joints. About 50% of patients go on to develop typical chronic rheumatoid synovitis after a delay of months or years. The rest remit or continue to have acute episodic arthritis. The detection of RF or ACPA predicts conversion to chronic, destructive synovitis.

Box 18.27 Presentations of rheumatoid arthritis

- ***Palindromic.*** Palindromic monoarticular attacks last 24–48 h; 50% progress to other types of RA.
- ***Transient.*** Disease is self-limiting, lasting <12 months and leaving no permanent joint damage. It is usually seronegative for IgM RF and ACPA. Some of these patients may have undetected postviral arthritis.
- ***Remitting.*** There is a period of several years during which the arthritis is active but then remits, leaving minimal damage.
- ***Chronic, persistent.*** This is the most typical form; it may be seropositive or seronegative for IgM RF. The disease follows a relapsing and remitting course over many years. Seropositive (plus ACPA) patients tend to develop greater joint damage and long-term disability. They warrant earlier and more aggressive treatment with disease-modifying agents.
- ***Rapidly progressive.*** The disease progresses remorselessly over a few years and leads rapidly to severe joint damage and disability. It is usually seropositive (plus ACPA), has a high incidence of systemic complications and is difficult to treat.

ACPA, anti-citrullinated peptide antibody; RF, rheumatoid factor.

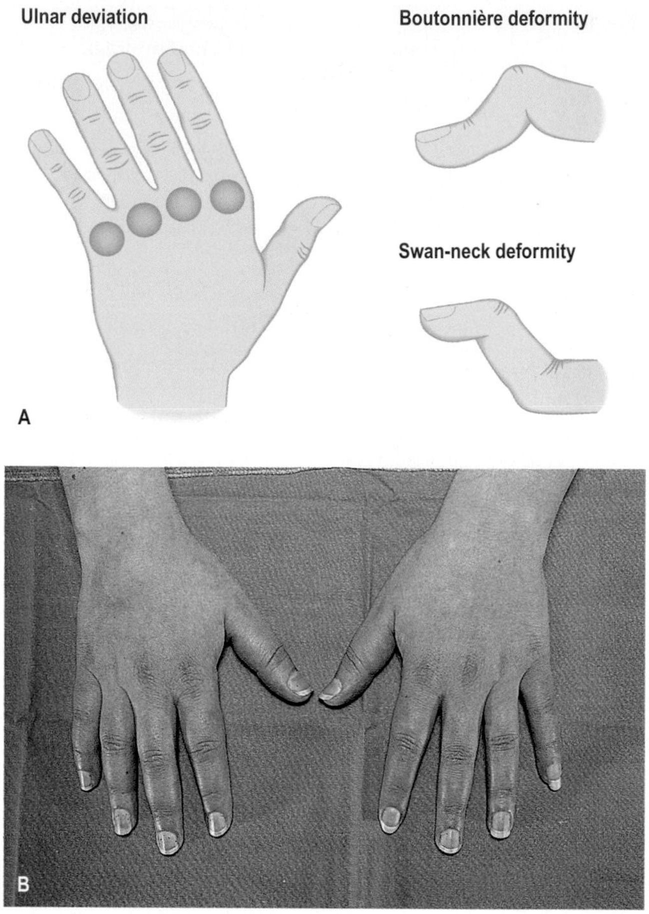

Figure 18.22 Rheumatoid arthritis. A. Characteristic hand deformities. **B.** Early rheumatoid arthritis – dorsal tenosynovitis of the right wrist and small joints of both hands with spindling of the fingers.

Complications

Septic arthritis

This complication is serious and has significant morbidity and mortality. In immunosuppressed patients, the affected joints may not display the typical signs of inflammation with accompanying fever found in patients with an intact immune system. There is usually a neutrophil leucocytosis. Any effusion, particularly of sudden onset, should be aspirated. *Staphylococcus aureus* is the most common organism. Blood cultures are often positive. Treatment is with systemic antibiotics (see p. 690) and drainage.

Amyloidosis

Amyloidosis (see pp. 1288–1289) is found in a very small number of people with uncontrolled RA. RA is the most common cause of secondary AA amyloidosis. AL amyloidosis causes a polyarthritis that resembles RA in distribution and is also often associated with carpal tunnel syndrome and subcutaneous nodules.

Joint involvement in RA

The changes described below are seen in established disease or when early drug treatment has been ineffective.

Hands and wrists

The impact of RA on the hands is severe. In early disease, the fingers are swollen, painful and stiff. Inflamed flexor tendon sheaths increase functional impairment and may cause a carpal tunnel syndrome. Joint damage causes:

- ***A combination of ulnar drift and palmar subluxation of the MCPs (Fig. 18.22).*** This change leads to unsightly deformity, but function may be preserved once the patient has learned to adapt and pain is controlled.
- ***Fixed flexion*** (buttonhole or boutonnière deformity) or ***fixed hyperextension*** (swan-neck deformity) of the PIP joints, which impairs hand function.
- ***Swelling and dorsal subluxation of the ulnar styloid***, which causes wrist pain and may cause rupture of the finger extensor tendons, leading in turn to a sudden onset of finger drop of the little and ring fingers predominantly; this needs urgent surgical repair.

Shoulders

RA commonly affects the shoulders. Initially, the symptoms mimic rotator cuff tendonosis (see p. 654) with a painful arc syndrome and pain in the upper arms at night. Further joint damage leads to global stiffening; rotator cuff tears become more common (see p. 654) and interfere with dressing, feeding and personal toilet.

Elbows

Synovitis of the elbows causes swelling and a painful fixed flexion deformity. In late disease, flexion may be lost and severe difficulties with feeding result, especially combined with shoulder, hand and wrist deformities.

Feet

One of the earliest manifestations of RA is painful swelling of the MTP joints.

- The foot becomes broader and a hammer-toe deformity develops.
- Exposure of the metatarsal heads to pressure by the forward migration of the protective fibrofatty pad ***(Fig. 18.23)*** causes pain.
- Ulcers or calluses may develop under the metatarsal heads and over the dorsum of the toes.
- Mid- and hindfoot RA causes a flat medial arch and loss of flexibility of the foot.
- The ankle often assumes a valgus position.

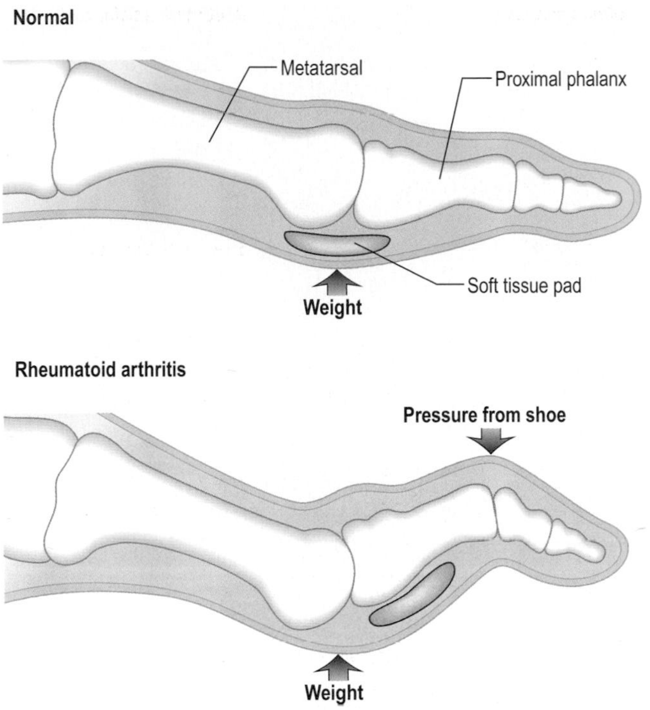

Figure 18.23 **The toes in rheumatoid arthritis.** There is exposure of the metatarsal heads with forward migration of the soft tissue pad.

Appropriate broad, deep, cushioned shoes are essential but rarely wholly adequate, and walking is often painful and limited. Podiatry helps and surgery may be required.

Knees

Massive synovitis and knee effusions occur but respond well to aspiration and steroid injection (see p. 660). A persistent effusion increases the risk of popliteal cyst formation and rupture (see p. 662). In later disease, erosion of cartilage and bone causes loss of joint space on X-ray and damage to the medial and/or lateral and/or retropatellar compartments of the knees. Depending on the pattern of involvement, the knees may develop a varus or valgus deformity. Secondary OA follows. Total knee replacement is often the only way to restore mobility and relieve pain.

Hips

The hips are occasionally affected in early RA but less commonly so than the knees at all stages of the disease. Pain and stiffness are accompanied by radiological loss of joint space and juxta-articular osteoporosis. The latter may permit medial migration of the acetabulum (protrusio acetabulae). Later, secondary OA develops. Hip replacement is usually necessary.

Cervical spine

Painful stiffness of the neck in RA is often muscular, but it may be due to rheumatoid synovitis affecting the synovial joints of the upper cervical spine and the bursae, which separate the odontoid peg from the anterior arch of the atlas and its retaining ligaments. This synovitis leads to bone destruction, damages the ligaments and causes atlantoaxial or upper cervical vertebral instability. Subluxation and local synovial swelling may damage the spinal cord, producing pyramidal and sensory signs. MRI is the imaging of choice, but lateral flexed and extended neck X-rays can demonstrate instability. In late RA, difficulty walking that cannot be explained by articular disease, weakness of the legs or loss of control of bowel or bladder may be due to spinal cord compression and is a neurosurgical emergency.

Imaging of the cervical spine in flexion and extension is recommended in patients with RA before surgery or upper gastrointestinal endoscopy to check for instability and reduce the risk of cord injury during intubation.

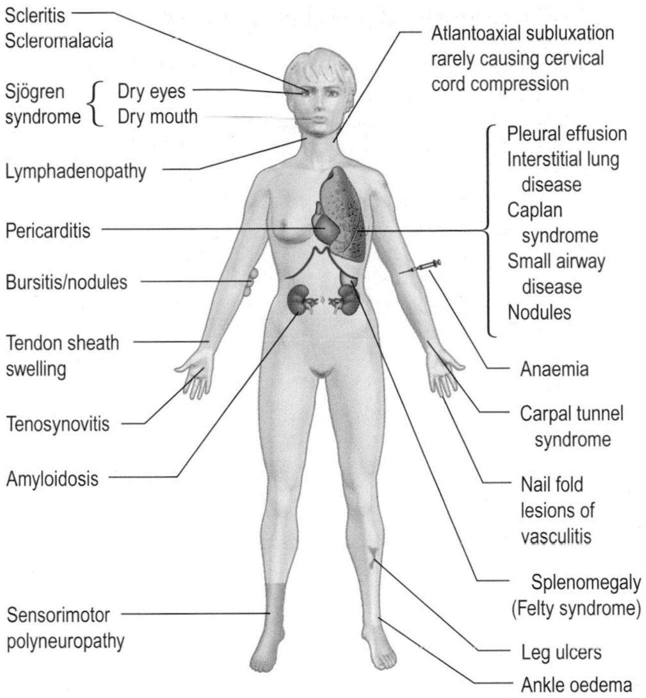

Figure 18.24 **Non-articular manifestations of rheumatoid arthritis.**

Other joints

The temporomandibular, acromioclavicular, sternoclavicular, crico-arytenoid and any other synovial joint can be affected.

Non-articular manifestations

See ***Figure 18.24***.

Soft tissue surrounding joints

Subcutaneous nodules are firm and intradermal, generally occurring over pressure points: typically, the elbows, the finger joints and the Achilles tendon in patients with seropositive erosive disease. They can be removed surgically but they tend to recur.

The olecranon and other bursae may be swollen (bursitis).

Tenosynovitis of flexor tendons in the hand can cause stiffness and occasionally a trigger finger. Swelling of the extensor tendon sheath over the dorsum of the wrist is common.

Muscle wasting around joints is common. Corticosteroid-induced myopathy occurs. Osteoporosis is more common in poorly controlled RA.

Less common non-articular manifestations

Non-articular complications are becoming less common, probably because of more effective disease control.

Lungs

Findings in the lungs (see pp. 1121–1122) include:

- airways disease: a spectrum from predominant bronchiectasis (cough and daily sputum) to predominant obliterative bronchiolitis (progressive breathlessness)

- disease of the pleura: pleural effusion (asymptomatic to mildly breathless) and thickening
- interstitial lung disease: a combination of inflammation and basal lung fibrosis
- peripheral, intrapulmonary nodules: asymptomatic but may cavitate, especially with pneumoconiosis (Caplan syndrome)
- infective lesions, e.g. tuberculosis in patients on biological DMARDs.

Vasculitis

Vasculitis (see pp. 699–702) caused by immune complex deposition in arterial walls is uncommon. Smoking is a risk factor. Findings include:

- nail-fold infarcts due to cutaneous vasculitis
- widespread cutaneous vasculitis with necrosis of the skin (seen in people with very active, strongly seropositive disease)
- mononeuritis multiplex (see p. 883).

Heart and peripheral vessels

Poorly controlled RA with a persistently raised CRP and high cholesterol is a cardiovascular risk factor, independent of traditional risk factors (i.e. high cholesterol and hypertension). Other cardiovascular problems include:

- pericarditis, which is rarely symptomatic
- endocarditis and myocardial disease, rarely symptomatic, found at postmortem in approximately 20% of cases
- Raynaud syndrome, rarely (see p. 1054).

Nervous system

- Peripheral sensory neuropathies: mononeuritis multiplex or symmetrical, peripheral – due to vasculitis of the vasa nervorum.
- Compression neuropathies: carpal or tarsal tunnel syndrome – due to synovitis.
- Cord compression: due to atlantoaxial subluxation (see above).

Eyes

- Sicca syndrome causes dry mouth and eyes (see Sjögren syndrome, p. 698).
- Scleritis and episcleritis occur in severe, seropositive disease, resulting in painful red eye.
- Scleromalacia perforans is a rare feature.

Kidneys

Amyloidosis causes proteinuria, nephrotic syndrome and chronic kidney disease. It occurs rarely in severe, longstanding rheumatoid disease and is due to the deposition of highly stable serum amyloid A protein (SAP) in the intercellular matrix of a variety of organs. SAP is an acute-phase reactant, produced normally in the liver.

Spleen, lymph nodes and blood

Felty syndrome is splenomegaly and neutropenia in a patient with RA. Leg ulcers and sepsis are complications. HLA-DR4 is found in 95% of patients, compared with 50–75% of people with RA alone.

Lymph nodes may be palpable, usually proximal to affected joints. There may be peripheral lymphoedema of the arm or leg.

Anaemia is almost universal and is usually normochromic and normocytic. It may be iron-deficient owing to gastrointestinal blood loss from NSAID ingestion, or rarely haemolytic (Coombs-positive). There may be a pancytopenia due to hypersplenism in Felty syndrome or as a complication of DMARD treatment. A high platelet count occurs with active disease.

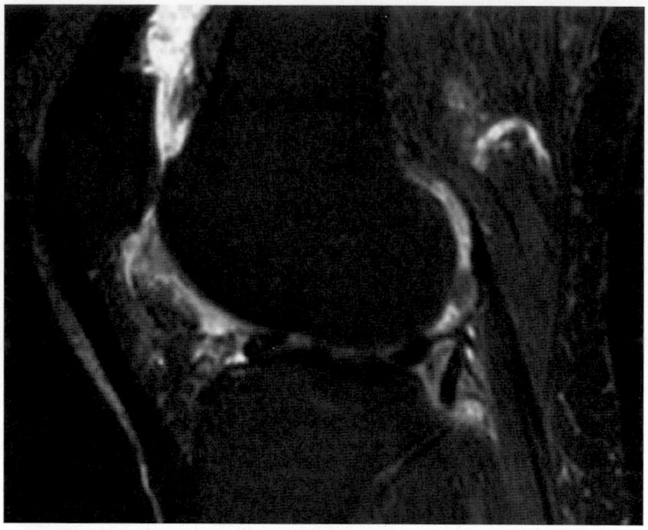

Figure 18.25 MRI of chronic rheumatoid arthritis of the knee. There is inflamed synovium throughout joint and spreading into the popliteal bursa.

Diagnosis and investigations

Diagnosis relies on the clinical features described above. The predictors of poor prognosis arthritis are listed in ***Box 18.24***. Initial investigations include:

- ***Blood count*** may show a normochromic, normocytic anaemia.
- ***ESR and/or CRP*** are raised in proportion to the activity of the inflammatory process and are useful in monitoring treatment.
- ***Serology*** reveals ACPA positivity (see p. 650). This is present earlier in the disease (and may predate it by many years), and in early inflammatory arthritis indicates the likelihood of progressing to RA. RF is present in approximately 70% of cases and ANA at low titre in 30%.
- ***X-rays*** show soft tissue swelling in early disease, but ultrasound and MRI ***(Fig. 18.25)*** are useful to demonstrate synovitis and early erosions.
- ***Aspiration of the joint*** may be needed if an effusion is present. The aspirate looks cloudy owing to white cells. In a suddenly painful joint, septic arthritis should be suspected (see p. 690).
- ***Doppler ultrasound*** is a very effective way of demonstrating persistent synovitis when deciding on the need for DMARDs or assessing their efficacy.

Other investigations will depend on the clinical picture, as outlined above. In severe disease, extensive imaging of joints may be required. MRI is the technique of choice, especially for the knee and cervical spine.

Management

(See ***Box 18.28***.) The diagnosis of RA inevitably causes concern and fear in the patient and requires explanation and reassurance. Anyone with early inflammatory arthritis should be referred to a specialist arthritis clinic within 3 months of onset.

The doctor should have a positive approach and remind the patient that, with the help of drugs, most people continue to lead a more or less normal life, as the aim of therapy is disease remission; 25% will recover completely. The earliest years are often the most difficult and people should be helped and encouraged to stay at work, as 30% lose their job within 2 years of diagnosis.

> **Box 18.28 Management of rheumatoid arthritis**
>
> - Establish the diagnosis clinically.
> - Use NSAIDs and analgesics to control symptoms.
> - Try to induce remission with i.m. depot methylprednisolone 80–120 mg if synovitis persists beyond 6 weeks.
> - If synovitis recurs, refer to a rheumatologist to start DMARDs and consider combinations of sulfasalazine, methotrexate and hydroxychloroquine. Give a second dose of i.m. depot methylprednisolone or oral steroids.
> - Refer for physiotherapy and general advice through a specialist team.
> - As improvement occurs, as measured by less pain, less morning stiffness and reduced acute-phase response, tail off steroids and possibly reduce drugs.
> - If no better, use anti-TNF-α therapy or other biological agent.
>
> *DMARDs, disease-modifying anti-rheumatic drugs; TNF-α, tumour necrosis factor alpha.*

Patients adjust and cope remarkably with time and support from the specialist team in a rheumatology unit (including doctors, nurses, physiotherapists, podiatrists and psychologists) and from leaflets, websites and local patient groups.

Patients from socially deprived backgrounds and smokers have a worse prognosis. Consideration must also be given to reducing the increased prevalence of cardiovascular risk that occurs in RA; statins are thought to be beneficial in this respect, although more clinical studies are required.

Drug therapy

There is no curative agent available for RA but early recognition and intensified treatment, with regular review until remission occurs, reduces disability. Less frequent review is then continued to assess disease activity, damage, function and co-morbidities.

The disease activity score DAS28 is widely used to measure disease activity in RA by counting the number of tender and swollen joints in 28 joints in the upper limbs and knees, combining these values with the ESR and the patient's assessment of their general health on a visual analogue scale to generate a numerical score ***(Fig. 18.26)***. A DAS28 score of greater than 5.1 implies active disease, less than 3.2 low disease activity and less than 2.6 remission. Data now support the use of multiple traditional DMARDs (started sequentially as 'step-up' or together) as combination therapy early in the disease to prevent the long-term irreversible damaging effects of joint inflammation. Biological therapies (known as biologics) are recombinant proteins: most commonly, monoclonal IgG1 antibodies directed against specific immunological targets or fusion proteins containing the Fc portion of IgG1 joined to receptor-blocking proteins. These drugs are increasingly used earlier in disease to reduce disease activity and damage. Searching for persistent synovitis in patients in apparent remission using Doppler ultrasound leads to more intensive therapeutic regimes to reduce longer-term disability.

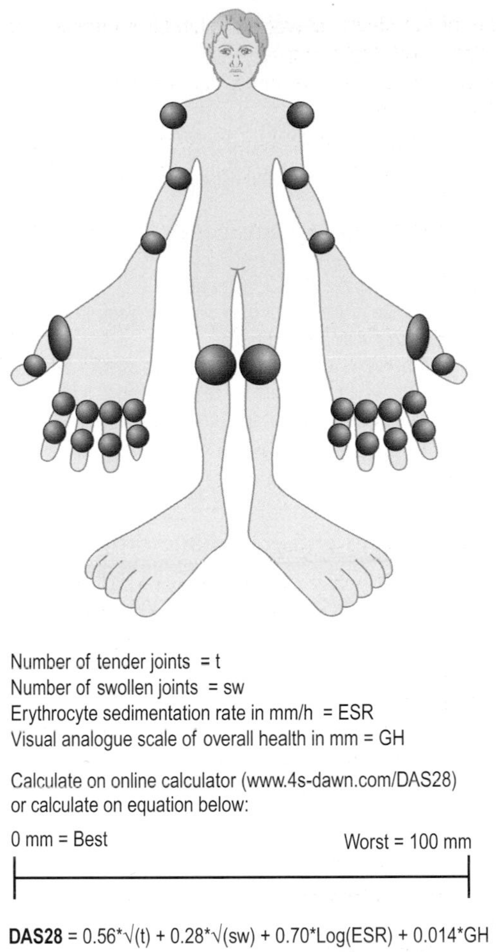
Number of tender joints = t
Number of swollen joints = sw
Erythrocyte sedimentation rate in mm/h = ESR
Visual analogue scale of overall health in mm = GH
Calculate on online calculator (www.4s-dawn.com/DAS28)
or calculate on equation below:
0 mm = Best
Worst = 100 mm
DAS28 = 0.56*√(t) + 0.28*√(sw) + 0.70*Log(ESR) + 0.014*GH

Figure 18.26 Calculation of disease activity score from 28 joints (DAS28).

Non-steroidal anti-inflammatory drugs and coxibs

Most people with RA are unable to cope without an NSAID to relieve night pain and morning stiffness. In addition to disease-modifying drugs. The individual response to NSAIDs varies greatly, so several different drugs may have to be tried for at least a week for a particular patient to find the most effective (see ***Box 18.16***), starting with an inexpensive NSAID with few side-effects. The major side-effects of NSAIDs and the use of coxibs are discussed on page 666. If gastrointestinal side-effects are prominent, or the patient is over 65 years of age, add a proton pump inhibitor. For additional relief, a simple analgesic is taken as required (e.g. paracetamol or a combination of codeine or dihydrocodeine and paracetamol).

Corticosteroids

The early use of corticosteroids slows down the course of the disease but intensive short courses in very early arthritis do not appear to stop progressive disease. Corticosteroids are the most common cause of secondary osteoporosis and the risk of fracture is increased by as much as 75% within the first 3 months of treatment. Therefore, concomitant vitamin D and bisphosphonates are necessary to reduce fracture risk in patients expected to be on corticosteroid therapy for more than 3 months' duration.

Intra-articular injections with semi-crystalline steroid preparations have a powerful but sometimes only short-lived effect.

Intramuscular depot injections (40–120 mg depot methylprednisolone) are used to help induce remission whilst waiting for DMARDs to work and to control severe disease flares.

Oral corticosteroids are powerful disease-controlling drugs but cause a number of problems (***Box 18.30***; see also ***Box [illegible]***), they are best avoided in the long term because side-effects are inevitable. Early intensive short-term regimens are often used to help induce remission. Doses of 5–7.5 mg daily as maintenance therapy are used in some centres. Corticosteroids are invaluable to people with severe disease who have extra-articular manifestations such as vasculitis.

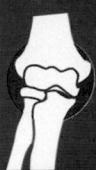

Box 18.29 Problems associated with the use of corticosteroids

- Patients are increasingly anxious about the use of corticosteroids because of adverse publicity about their potential side-effects. This must be discussed frankly and the risks of not using corticosteroids in treatment should be described and balanced against the risks posed by the drugs themselves.
- Patients must be warned to avoid sugars and saturated fats, and to eat less because of the risk of weight gain.
- The skin becomes thin and easily damaged.
- Patients should be monitored for diabetes and hypertension.
- Cataract formation may be accelerated.
- Osteoporosis develops within 3 months on doses above 7.5 mg daily. Monitor with DXA scan and treat with calcium, vitamin D and bisphosphonate (see pp. 713–715).

DXA, dual-energy absorptiometry.

Disease-modifying anti-rheumatic drugs

Traditional disease-modifying anti-rheumatic drugs (DMARDs) are synthetic small-molecule drugs; they are listed in ***Box 18.30***. Despite their mechanism of action being incompletely understood, they have been shown to reduce inflammation, joint swelling and plasma acute-phase reactants, and to slow the development of joint erosions as well as irreversible damage. Their beneficial effect is not immediate, taking 2–3 months to become apparent. As monotherapy, traditional DMARDs often have only a partial effect, achieving between 20% and 50% improvement by ACR criteria for disease remission ***(Box 18.31)***, and are more effective used in combination.

Early intervention with traditional DMARDs within 6 weeks to 6 months of disease onset improves the outcome. Combinations of three or four drugs (steroids, sulfasalazine, methotrexate and hydroxychloroquine) in early RA are increasingly common; the number of agents is reduced once remission has been achieved. Several DMARDs are contraindicated in pregnancy (see ***Box 29.10***). Effective treatment with DMARDs including TNF-α blockers reduces the increased cardiovascular risk in RA.

Methotrexate

Methotrexate remains the anchor drug in RA therapy, although it should not be used in pregnancy and conception should be delayed until women have been off the drug for 6 weeks. A screening history, chest X-ray and an interferon gamma release assay (IGRA) in high-risk patients are performed to exclude tuberculosis. Initial pneumococcal and annual influenza vaccinations are given. The starting *weekly* dose of 7.5–10 mg orally is increased up to 15–25 mg as necessary to reduce disease activity. It is well tolerated, although nausea or poor absorption may limit its efficacy, in which case it is given by subcutaneous injection. Oral folic acid reduces side-effects but may also lessen efficacy. Full blood counts and liver biochemistry should be monitored. Methotrexate usually works within 1–2 months. More patients remain on this agent than on most other DMARDs, indicating that it is effective and has relatively few side-effects.

Sulfasalazine

Sulfasalazine is a combination of sulfapyridine and 5-amino-salicylic acid. Sulfapyridine is probably the active component. It is well tolerated and can be used during pregnancy. The usual starting dose of 500 mg per day is increased to a maintenance dose of 2–3 g per day. Around 50% of patients respond in the first 3–6 months, but efficacy can be lost. Blood monitoring is obligatory because of the risk of leucopenia and thrombocytopenia.

Hydroxychloroquine

A dose of 200–400 g daily is well tolerated. It is used alone in mild disease or commonly as an adjunct to other DMARDs. Retinopathy is extremely rare (about 1 in 2000 patients). Some rheumatologists arrange an initial check of macular function with an Amsler chart and further reviews annually, as retinopathy is irreversible.

Leflunomide

This DMARD exerts an immunomodulatory effect by preventing pyrimidine production in proliferating lymphocytes through blockade of the enzyme dihydro-orotate dehydrogenase, thus blocking clonal expansion of T cells. Most other cells are able to bypass this blockade. It has a long half-life of 4–28 days. A dose of 20 mg daily (10 mg if diarrhoea is a problem) is used. Diarrhoea diminishes with time. Blood monitoring is obligatory (full blood count, platelets, liver biochemistry). The onset of action is 4 weeks with some further improvement sustained at 2 years. Leflunomide works in some patients who have failed to respond to methotrexate. Its long half-life means that it is best avoided in women planning a family.

Biological therapies

TNF-α blockers

These agents are more expensive than traditional DMARDs so they are used after at least two DMARDs (usually sulfasalazine and methotrexate) have failed. They represent a major therapeutic advance, particularly in the number of combination therapies that are now available to treat RA, although not all patients respond and there is loss of efficacy in some responders. They are usually given in combination with methotrexate to reduce loss of efficacy due to anti-drug antibody formation.

- ***Etanercept*** is a fully humanized p75 TNF-α receptor IgG1 fusion protein given by self-administered subcutaneous injection. Around 65% of patients respond well. Some develop an injection reaction.
- ***Adalimumab*** is a fully human monoclonal antibody against TNF-α, given along with methotrexate.
- ***Infliximab*** is a monoclonal antibody against TNF-α, given intravenously and co-prescribed with methotrexate to prevent loss of efficacy because of antibody formation.
- ***Certolizumab pegol*** is an Fab fragment of a humanized TNF-α inhibitor monoclonal antibody. It is pegylated: that is, polyethylene glycol groups are added to reduce its immunogenicity and prolong its half-life. The lack of an Fc portion on the antibody aims to reduce the risk of complement-dependent, as well as antibody-dependent, cytotoxicity and may reduce placental transfer. It is useful with or without methotrexate for severe active RA.
- ***Golimumab*** is a human IgG1-κ monoclonal antibody against TNF, which is given by subcutaneous injection once monthly for severe RA.

These products slow or halt erosion formation in up to 70% of people with RA and produce healing in a few. Malaise and tiredness improve in a manner that is not seen with other DMARDs. Secondary failure may occur with all in the first year; changing to another anti-TNF agent is justified and often regains control of the disease. Potential biomarkers for responsiveness are being studied. Failure to respond to one does not predict failure to others.

Safety data. To answer questions regarding rare or delayed onset of adverse events, as well as long-term outcomes and problems arising from biological therapies, national registers have been set up in different countries. These longitudinal, observational

Box 18.30 Disease-modifying anti-rheumatic drugs (DMARDs)

Drug	Dose	Side-effects	Monitoring
Sulfasalazine (enteric coated)	500 mg daily after food, increasing to 2–3 g daily	Nausea Skin rashes and mouth ulcers Neutropenia and/or thrombocytopenia Abnormal liver biochemistry	Baseline FBC, U&Es, LFTs, then at 2, 4 and 8 weeks, then 4-monthly
Methotrexate (give pneumococcal and annual influenza vaccinations)	7.5–10 mg increasing to max. 25 mg weekly, orally or s.c.	Nausea, mouth ulcers and diarrhoea Abnormal liver biochemistry Neutropenia and/or thrombocytopenia Renal impairment Rare – pulmonary fibrosis	Baseline CXR, FBC, U&Es, LFTs, then repeat blood tests at 2, 4 and 8 weeks, then 8-weekly
Leflunomide	10–20 mg daily, occasionally with initial loading dose	Diarrhoea Neutropenia and/or thrombocytopenia Abnormal liver biochemistry Alopecia Hypertension	Baseline FBC, U&Es, LFTs, then repeat at 2, 4 and 8 weeks, then 2-monthly
Cytokine modulators			
TNF-α blockers			
Etanercept (alone or with methotrexate)	s.c. 25 mg × 2-weekly or 50 mg weekly	Injection site reactions Infections, e.g. tuberculosis and septicaemia Hypersensitivity reactions Heart failure Rare – demyelination and autoimmune syndromes Reversible lupus-like syndrome Infections Hypersensitivity reactions	Baseline CXR, hepatitis B and C, HIV, FBC, U&Es, LFTs Exclude TB and CMV with QuantiFERON-TB or -CMV, if indicated Monitor as per concomitant DMARD; if monotherapy, repeat FBC, U&Es and LFTs 6-monthly
Adalimumab (with methotrexate)	s.c. 40 mg alternate weeks		As per etanercept
Infliximab (with methotrexate)	i.v. 3–10 mg/kg every 4–8 weeks		As per etanercept; see p. 680
Certolizumab pegol (alone or with methotrexate)	s.c. 400 mg in weeks 0, 2, 4, then 200 mg fortnightly		As per etanercept; see p. 680
Golimumab	s.c. monthly 50 mg		
Other biological agents (used with methotrexate)			
Rituximab	i.v. 500–1000 mg	Hypo-/hypertension Skin rash Nausea Pruritus Back pain Rare – toxic epidermal necrolysis	Baseline CXR, hepatitis B and C, HIV, Igs, CD19, FBC, U&Es, LFTs Quantiferon if indicated Monitor as per concomitant DMARD; if monotherapy, repeat FBC, U&Es, LFTs, Igs and CD19 6-monthly
Abatacept	i.v. 10 mg/kg on days 1, 15, 30 and then monthly s.c. preparations available	Nausea, vomiting Headache Rare – hypersensitivity	Baseline CXR, hepatitis B and C, HIV, FBC, U&Es, LFTs Quantiferon if indicated Monitor as per concomitant DMARD; if monotherapy, repeat FBC, U&Es and LFTs 6-monthly
Tocilizumab	i.v. 8 mg/kg infusion	Headache Skin eruption Stomatitis Fever Anaphylactic reactions	As per abatacept plus baseline and 6-monthly lipids

CD19, cluster of differentiation 19; CXR, chest X-ray; FBC, full blood count; HIV, human immunodeficiency virus; Igs, immunoglobulins; i.v., intravenous; LFTs, liver function tests; NICE, National Institute for Health and Care Excellence; s.c., subcutaneous; TNF-α, tumour necrosis factor alpha: U&Es, urea and electrolytes.

Box 18.31 The 2011 ACR/EULAR definitions for disease remission in rheumatoid arthritis clinical trials

- Tender joint count (including feet and ankles) ≥1
- Swollen joint count (including feet and ankles) ≥1
- C-reactive protein ≥1 mg/L
- Patient global assessment ≥1 (on a 10-cm visual analogue scale)

ACR, American College of Rheumatology; EULAR, European League Against Rheumatism.

cohort studies are mostly focused on TNF-α blockers but are expanding to include other biological therapies.

To date, the results are reassuring. Infection rates are increased with TNF-α blockers, particularly in the first few months of treatment, but the rate then declines. There is a known association between RA and non-Hodgkin's lymphoma (NHL) but, overall, registers have not shown an increased risk of NHL in patients with RA treated with TNF-α blockers, although mean follow-up is relatively short at 5 years. There is no convincing evidence of any increased risk of other cancers. Reactivation of old tuberculosis may occur but is probably less common with etanercept. A pre-treatment chest X-ray is recommended, with a specialist review for high-risk groups. Tuberculosis should be treated before these agents are prescribed, and a course of prophylaxis is used in latent disease. Hepatitis B and C infection requires careful risk analysis and regular aminotransferase monitoring if anti-TNF agents are prescribed. They should not be used in patients who have severe cardiac failure.

These agents are extremely expensive when compared with traditional DMARDs but they may save costs in the longer term by reducing disability and the need for hospitalization. To date, there is no evidence of an adverse effect on pregnancy outcome but care is essential (see **Box 29.10**).

Other biological agents

- ***Rituximab*** is a chimeric monoclonal antibody (see pp. 146–147), directed against the CD20 receptor expressed on pre-B and mature B cells that is not present on stem cells and is lost before differentiation into plasma cells. Rituximab produces significant improvement in RF-positive RA for 8 months to several years when used alone or in combination with corticosteroids and/or methotrexate. This clinical improvement is associated with a 6–9-month B-cell lymphopenia and little change in circulating immunoglobulins. A re-flare is often accompanied by a return of peripheral B lymphocytes and rise in CRP. Rituximab can be re-used as the disease flares. Repeated courses are well tolerated and around 80% of RF-positive patients respond, with 50–60% showing persistent disease control; however, immunoglobulin levels should be monitored, as they may fall with repeated treatments. Rituximab is mainly used in patients who have failed to respond to anti-TNF agents.
- ***Abatacept*** is a recombinant fusion protein of CTLA4 and the Fc portion of IgG1, which selectively modulates T-cell activation by co-stimulation blockade. It may be used in patients who do not respond to anti-TNF regimens.
- ***Tocilizumab*** is a humanized monoclonal anti-IL-6 receptor antibody; it is used with methotrexate for moderate to severe RA, usually after at least one other biologic has failed, but it may also be considered as a first-line biological therapy.
- ***Anakinra*** is a human recombinant IL-1 receptor antagonist; it is recommended for use in combination with methotrexate but is not often given in RA, as it is less efficacious than other biologics.
- ***Tofacitinib*** is oral Janus kinase (JAK) inhibitor, which selectively blocks JAK3/1 receptors that inhibit cytokine (IL-2, 4, 7, 9, 15 and 21) signalling. Three phase 3 studies have shown improvements with tofacitinib compared with placebo, methotrexate and adalimumab. There remain concerns, however, regarding infection and cardiovascular risk (due to raised lipids), as well as abnormal liver biochemistry. Therefore, the drug has not been approved in Europe, although it has been approved by the Food and Drug Administration (FDA) in the United States.

Drugs used less commonly
Gold, azathioprine, cyclophosphamide and ciclosporin

These drugs are very rarely used to treat RA because of the availability of other agents with more favourable risk–benefit profiles. Gold (sodium aurothiomalate) is given by deep intramuscular injection and can induce remission. Due to side-effects or lack of effect, however, few patients remain on it beyond 2 years. Azathioprine and cyclophosphamide may be given when extra-articular features, particularly vasculitis, are severe. Ciclosporin is only used when conventional therapy has been ineffective and may cause a rise in creatinine level and hypertension.

Physical measures

Input is required from the multidisciplinary team. Physiotherapists advise a combination of rest for active arthritis and exercises to maintain joint range and muscle power. Exercise in a hydrotherapy pool is popular and effective. Occupational therapists help to manage activities of daily living despite the arthritis and provide functional adaptations in the home or at work. Family and friends should be involved. Podiatry, footwear advice and psychological support should also be offered to all people with RA.

Surgery

Surgery has a useful role in the long-term approach to patient management but is less frequently needed as therapeutic disease control becomes more effective. Its main objectives are prophylactic, to prevent joint destruction and deformity, and reconstructive, to restore function.

Single-joint disease can be treated by surgical synovectomy to reduce the bulk of inflamed tissue and prevent damage. Excision arthroplasty of the ulnar styloid reduces pain and the risk of extensor tendon damage. Excision arthroplasties of the metatarsal heads reduce metatarsal pain and relieve pressure points. The major surgical advance has been the development of total replacement arthroplasty of the hip, knee, finger joints, elbow and shoulder. Such procedures need careful planning and the expected outcomes and risks should be explained to the patient.

Prognosis

A poor prognosis is indicated by:

- ***a clinical picture*** of an insidious rather than an explosive onset of RA, female sex, increasing number of peripheral joints involved and the level of disability at the onset
- ***blood tests*** showing a high CRP/ESR, normochromic normocytic anaemia, and high titres of ACPA and of RF
- ***X-rays*** with early erosive damage (*note*: ultrasound and MRI can show cartilage and bone damage prior to conventional X-rays).

Prognosis can be altered dramatically with early DMARD therapy under expert supervision.

Spondyloarthritis

Spondyloarthritis (SpA) is an umbrella term for a group of conditions that affects the spine and peripheral joints with familial clustering and a link to certain type 1 HLA antigens ***(Box 18.32)***. Joint

Box 18.32 Spondyloarthritis

- Axial spondyloarthritis, including ankylosing spondylitis
- Psoriatic arthritis
- Reactive arthritis (sexually acquired)
- Post-dysenteric reactive arthritis
- Enteropathic arthritis (ulcerative colitis/Crohn's disease)

involvement is different from that seen in RA, as it is usually more limited and has a different distribution and associated extra-articular features. These diseases occasionally present in childhood.

They may also be categorized according to their predominant clinical manifestation of axial (sacroiliac and/or spine) or peripheral (arthritis, enthesitis and/or dactylitis) disease with possible overlap. The Assessment of Spondyloarthritis International Society has developed classification criteria for both axial and peripheral SpA, which were developed to enhance diagnosis, treatment and design of clinical trials. Despite this, distinct SpA conditions exist, as shown in ***Box 18.32***.

Histologically, the synovitis itself is similar to that of RA, but there is no production of rheumatoid factor (RF) or anti-citrullinated peptide antibody (ACPA). Inflammation of the enthesis (junction of ligament or tendon and bone) and joint ankylosis develop more commonly than in RA. All are associated with an increased frequency of sacroiliitis and HLA-B27.

Aetiology

The common aetiological thread linking these disorders is their striking association with HLA-B27, particularly ankylosing spondylitis (AS). HLA type B27 is present in >90% of Caucasians with AS but only 8% of controls. HLA-B27 exhibits a number of unusual characteristics, including a high tendency to misfold. The role of class I HLA antigens in pathogenesis is supported by the fact that HLA-B27 transgenic mice spontaneously develop arthritis and skin, gut and genitourinary lesions.

Infections have been postulated to be involved, possibly by molecular mimicry, with parts of the organism that are structurally similar to the HLA molecule triggering cross-reactive antibody formation, although this hypothesis is unproven. The acquired immunodeficiency syndrome (AIDS) is increasing the prevalence of reactive arthritis and spondylitis in sub-Saharan Africa, even in the absence of HLA-B27. The explanation for this changing epidemiology is unclear.

The types of arthritis that follow a precipitating infection are called reactive arthritis (see p. 686).

The specialized immune systems of the gut and genitourinary mucous membranes may also play a causal role, perhaps reacting to local infections or to antigens, which cross the damaged mucosa.

Axial spondyloarthritis

Axial spondyloarthritis occurs in 1% of the general population. It is an inflammatory disorder primarily affecting fibrous and synovial joints of the spine. Sacroiliac joint changes are seen only on MRI. When radiographic changes at the sacroiliac joints are present, the term ankylosing spondylitis (AS) is used.

Ankylosing spondylitis

It is now recognized that AS forms part of the spectrum of axial spondyloarthritis. It presents with inflammatory back pain and sacroiliac inflammation. It is seen in 0.2–0.5% of the population in Northern Europe and approximately 0.5% in the USA, affecting mainly young adults (late teens to early thirties) and occurring worldwide, with a male to female ratio of 3 : 1. Women present later and are under-diagnosed. The frequency of axial spondyloarthritis in different populations is roughly paralleled by the incidence of HLA-B27; Africans and Japanese have a low incidence of both HLA-B27 and AS, while the North American Haida Indians have a high incidence of both.

Aetiology

This is probably a combination of genetic and environmental features:

- There are at least 24 subtypes of HLA-B27 (B*2701 to B*2724). Some appear to increase risk; others have a protective role. Twin studies indicate a much higher disease concordance in HLA-B27-positive monozygotic twins (up to 70%) than in dizygotic twins (about 20–25%).
- Other genes lying within the major histocompatibility complex (the *IL-1* gene cluster and *CYP2D6*) also influence susceptibility to AS but the disease is polygenic and genome-wide association studies have identified significant associations with the endoplasmic reticulum aminopeptidase (*ERAP*)-1 and *IL-23* genes.
- The association of *ERAP-1* with axial spondyloarthritis may support the arthritogenic peptide hypothesis, whereby disease is triggered by presentation of peptide by HLA-B27 to cytotoxic CD8-positive T cells. Furthermore, misfolding of HLA-B27 leads to the production of IL-23, and T cells resident in entheses promote inflammation characteristic of spondyloarthritis in response to IL-23.
- The interaction of environmental factors has been proposed, but although Gram-negative organisms, such as *Yersinia*, *Klebsiella*, *Salmonella* and *Shigella*, can cause a reactive arthropathy, there is no conclusive evidence for their involvement in the pathogenesis of axial spondyloarthritis.
- Lymphocyte and plasma cell infiltration occurs with local erosion of bone at the attachments of the intervertebral and other ligaments (enthesitis), which heals with new bone (syndesmophyte) formation.

Clinical features

Initially, the diagnosis is often missed because the patient is asymptomatic between episodes and radiological abnormalities are absent.

- ***Back pain*** with episodic inflammation of the sacroiliac joints in the late teenage years or early twenties is the first manifestation of axial spondyloarthritis.
- ***Pain in one or both buttocks*** and low back pain and stiffness are typically worse in the morning and relieved by exercise.
- ***Retention of the lumbar lordosis during spinal flexion*** is an early sign. Later, paraspinal muscle wasting develops.

Criteria for classifying inflammatory back pain as axial spondyloarthritis are shown in ***Box 18.33***. These criteria encompass the whole spectrum of disease, with evidence of sacroiliitis being based on radiographic or MRI evidence of disease. Spinal stiffness can be measured by Schober's test; the skin over the midline of the spine is marked 5 cm below and 10 cm above the dimples of Venus and the increase in distance between those marks during flexion is recorded. An increase of <5 cm implies spinal stiffness.

Box 18.33 Back pain criteria for diagnosing axial/ankylosing spondylitis

- ***Age of onset*** <45 years
- ***Insidious onset***
- ***Improvement of back pain with exercise***
- ***No improvement of back pain with rest***
- ***Pain at night*** with improvement on getting up

The presence of **four of the five criteria suggests ankylosing spondylitis with 80% sensitivity**. All criteria have high sensitivity.

Box 18.34 Non-articular problems in spondyloarthritis

- Uveitis, in all types
- Cutaneous lesions in reactive arthritis (keratoderma blennorrhagica), histologically identical to pustular psoriasis
- Nail dystrophy, in psoriasis and reactive arthritis
- Aortitis, occasionally in ankylosing spondylitis and reactive arthritis

Non-spinal complications (uveitis or costochondritis) suggest the diagnosis of spondyloarthritis ***(Box 18.34)***:

- ***Costochondral junction inflammation*** causes anterior chest pain. Measurable reduction of chest expansion is due to costovertebral joint involvement.
- ***Peripheral joint involvement*** is asymmetrical and affects a few, predominantly large, joints. Hip involvement leads to fixed flexion deformities of the hips and further deterioration of posture. Young teenage boys occasionally present with a lower-limb monoarthritis (see p. 704), which later develops into AS.
- ***Acute anterior uveitis*** occurs in approximately 30% of patients with axial spondyloarthritis and related diseases, and is occasionally the presenting complaint. Severe eye pain, photophobia and blurred vision are an emergency (see pp. 1332–1333).
- ***Other extra-articular features*** include:
  - cardiovascular disease – aortic incompetence occurs in up to 1% of patients with established AS and cardiac conduction abnormalities in around 5%
  - respiratory disease – rarely, chest wall rigidity is associated with interstitial lung disease
  - renal impairment – reported in 10–35% of patients with AS and most commonly linked to chronic NSAID use
  - axial osteoporosis – occurs in approximately 25%. with vertebral fracture in 10%.

Overall clinical assessment of disease activity is based on a 1–10 score for levels of fatigue, spinal pain, arthralgia, swelling, localized tenderness, inflammation of tendons/enthesis, and duration and severity of morning stiffness. This can be measured using the Bath Ankylosing Spondylitis Disease Activity Index (see Further reading).

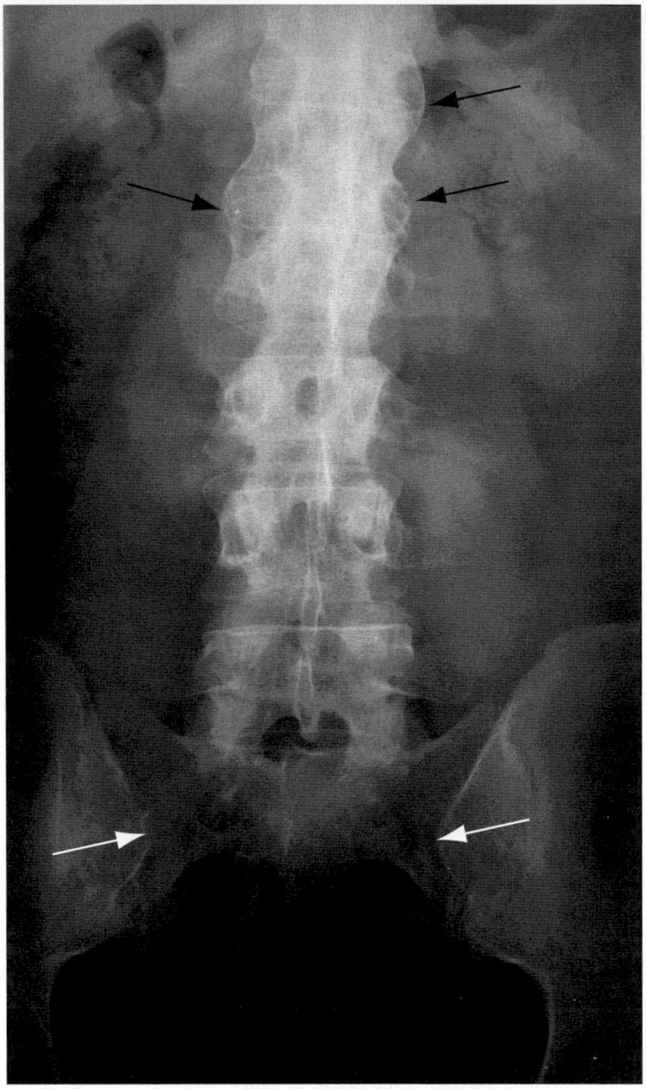

Figure 18.27 X-ray of ankylosing spondylitis. The sacroiliac joints are eroded and show marginal sclerosis (white arrows). There is bridging syndesmophyte formation at the thoracolumbar junction (black arrows).

Investigations

- ***Blood***. ESR and CRP are usually raised.
- ***HLA testing***. This is rarely of value because of the high frequency of HLA-B27 in the population, but may give supporting evidence in a difficult case.
- ***X-rays***. The medial and lateral cortical margins of both sacroiliac joints lose definition owing to erosions and eventually become sclerotic ***(Fig. 18.27)***. Radiological appearances in the spine of blurring of the upper or lower vertebral rims at the thoracolumbar junction are caused by an enthesitis at the insertion of the intervertebral ligaments and may eventually affect the whole spine. Persistent inflammatory enthesitis causes bony spurs (syndesmophytes), which lead to bony ankylosis and permanent stiffening. The sacroiliac joints eventually fuse, as may the costovertebral joints, reducing chest expansion. Calcification of the intervertebral ligaments and fusion of the spinal facet joints and syndesmophytes leads to what is often called a 'bamboo' spine ***(Fig. 18.28)***.
- ***MRI***. MRI with gadolinium demonstrates sacroiliitis before it is seen on X-rays, as well as persistent enthesitis.

Management

- The key to effective management of AS is early diagnosis so that a regimen of preventative exercises is started before syndesmophytes have formed. Morning exercises aim to maintain spinal mobility, posture and chest expansion; regular NSAIDs to improve symptoms and signs of spondyloarthritis are often required to achieve this goal.
- Failure to control pain and to encourage regular spinal and chest exercises leads to an irreversible dorsal kyphosis and wasted paraspinal muscles, which, along with stiffening of the cervical spine, makes forward vision difficult.
- When the inflammation is active and the morning pain and stiffness are too severe to permit effective exercise, an evening dose of a long-acting or slow-release NSAID or an NSAID suppository improves sleep, pain control and exercise compliance.
- Sulfasalazine, methotrexate and leflunomide may help peripheral arthritis but not spinal disease.

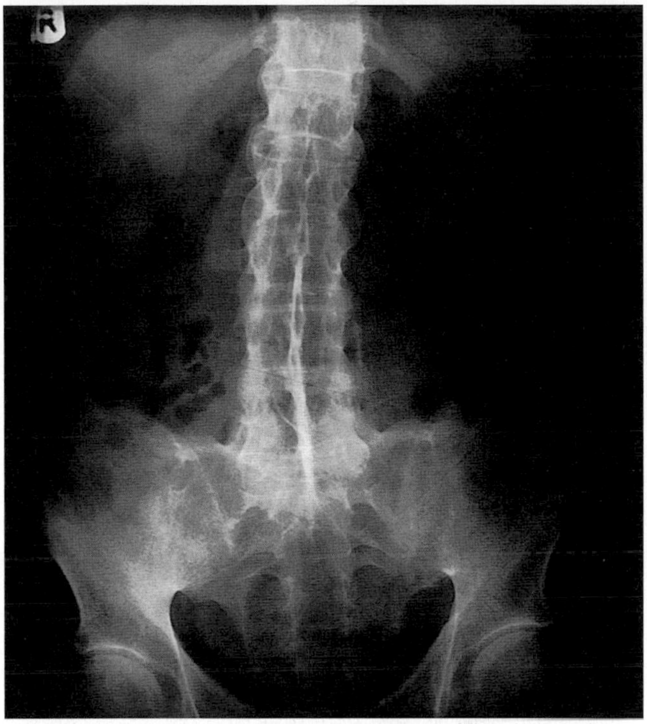

Figure 18.28 X-ray of bamboo spine in ankylosing spondylitis. In advanced disease, there is calcification of the interspinous ligaments and fusion of the facet joints, as well as syndesmophytes at all levels. The sacroiliac joints fuse.

- When NSAIDs have failed, the TNF-α-blocking drugs adalimumab, etanercept, golimumab, certolizumab and infliximab (see ***Box 18.30***) have all been shown to reduce symptoms of spinal and peripheral joint inflammation substantially and to improve function, as well as quality of life. Evidence of reduction of bony progression, however, has not been found. Relapse occurs on stopping therapy but may be delayed by several months making intermittent treatment feasible. Other biologics do not help spondyloarthritis.
- Early clinical studies have shown apremilast, a phosphodiesterase type 4 (PDE4) inhibitor, and secukinumab, an anti-IL-17, to be effective in spondyloarthritis.

Prognosis

With exercise and pain relief, the prognosis is excellent and over 80% of patients are fully employed. Anti-TNF therapies are likely to reduce the morbidity of severe disease, lowering the risk of permanent spinal stiffness and progressive peripheral joint disease.

Psoriatic arthritis

The prevalence of psoriasis is 2–3% worldwide; in this population, around 10% have arthritis, which precedes skin disease in around 15% of cases. A family history of psoriasis may be a clue to the diagnosis. The aetiology and pathogenesis are described on page 1333.

Clinical features

Patterns of psoriatic arthritis include:

- ***Mono- or oligoarthritis***.
- ***Polyarthritis***: often begins with an asymmetrical pattern and progresses to be virtually indistinguishable from RA.

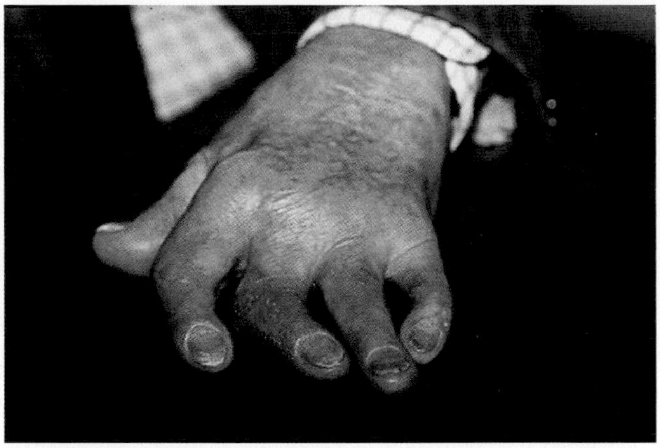

Figure 18.29 Hand showing psoriatic arthritis mutilans. All the fingers are shortened and the joints unstable, owing to underlying osteolysis.

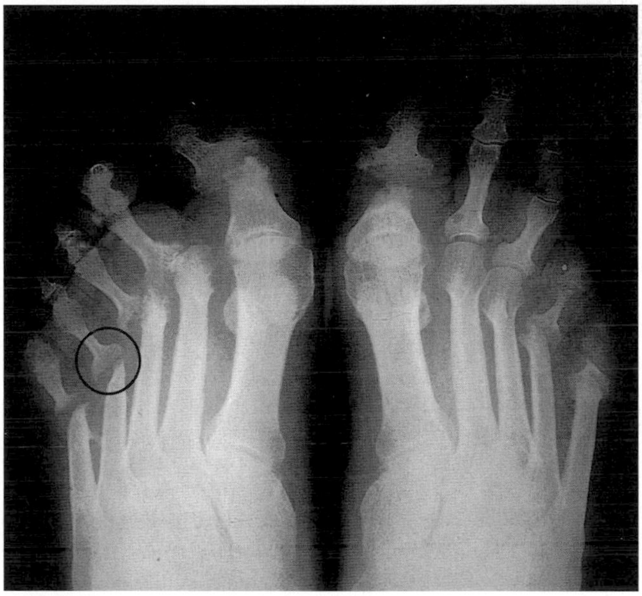

Figure 18.30 X-ray of psoriatic arthritis. There is osteolysis of the metatarsal heads and central erosion of the proximal phalanges to produce the 'pencil in cup' appearance (circle). All the lesser toes are subluxed.

- ***Spondylitis***: unilateral or bilateral sacroiliitis and early cervical spine involvement; only 50% are HLA-B27-positive.
- ***Distal interphalangeal arthritis***: the most typical pattern of joint involvement in psoriasis, often with adjacent nail dystrophy (see p. 1355) reflecting enthesitis extending into the nail root. Dactylitis, in which an entire finger or toe is swollen, with joint and tendon sheath involvement, is characteristic of this condition.
- ***Arthritis mutilans***: affects about 5% of patients who have psoriatic arthritis and causes marked periarticular osteolysis and bone shortening ('telescopic' fingers) ***(Fig. 18.29)***.

Radiologically, psoriatic arthritis is erosive but the erosions are central in the joint, not juxta-articular, and produce a 'pencil in cup' appearance ***(Fig. 18.30)***. The skin and nail disease can be mild and may develop after the arthritis.

Management and prognosis

NSAIDs and/or analgesics help the pain but can occasionally worsen the skin lesions. Local synovitis responds to intra-articular corticosteroid injections. Sulfasalazine, methotrexate and leflunomide are commonly used in patients with persistent peripheral joint synovitis, although none has a proven effect on slowing the development of joint damage. Ciclosporin may also be considered in severe disease. Hydroxychloroquine is best avoided because it may rarely cause acute psoriatic skin reactions. Similarly, oral corticosteroids may destabilize skin disease; they are best avoided but are valuable when injected into a single inflamed joint.

Anti-TNF-α agents, such as etanercept and golimumab (see pp. 680–682), and ustekinumab (an anti-IL-12/23 inhibitor), are highly effective and safe for severe skin and joint disease. They should be used when methotrexate has failed. An anti-IL-17 inhibitor has shown promise in late-phase clinical trials, and apremilast, a PDE4 inhibitor given orally, has been approved by the FDA for psoriatic arthritis. Rituximab has no role in treating psoriatic arthritis.

The prognosis for the joint involvement is generally better than in RA.

Reactive arthritis

Reactive arthritis is a sterile synovitis, which occurs following an infection.

Spondyloarthritis develops in 1–2% of patients after an acute attack of dysentery, or after a sexually acquired infection – non-specific urethritis (NSU) in the male, non-specific cervicitis in the female. In males, positivity for HLA-B27 increases the risk of developing reactive arthritis after such an infection by 30–50-fold but not all patients are HLA-B27-positive. Women are less commonly affected.

Aetiology

A variety of organisms can be the trigger, including strains of *Salmonella* or *Shigella* spp. in bacillary dysentery. *Yersinia enterocolitica* causes diarrhoea and a reactive arthritis. In NSU, the organisms are *Chlamydia trachomatis* or *Ureaplasma urealyticum*.

People with reactive arthritis are not more susceptible to infection but appear to respond differently. Bacterial antigens or bacterial DNA have been found in the inflamed synovium of affected joints, suggesting that this persistent antigenic material is driving the inflammatory process. The methods by which HLA-B27 increases susceptibility to reactive arthritis include:

- T-cell receptor repertoire selection
- molecular mimicry causing autoimmunity against HLA-B27 and/or other self antigens
- mode of presentation of bacteria-derived peptides to T lymphocytes.

There are other organisms that also trigger reactive arthritis but have a different genetic basis; see post-streptococcal arthritis (pp. 703–704), gonococcal arthritis (pp. 690–691) and brucellosis (p. 691). In these conditions, the borderline between reactive arthritis and septic arthritis is more indistinct and they can cause both.

Clinical features

The arthritis is typically an acute, asymmetrical, lower-limb arthritis, occurring a few days to a couple of weeks after the infection. The arthritis may be the presenting complaint if the infection is mild or asymptomatic. Enthesitis is common, causing plantar fasciitis or Achilles tendon enthesitis (see p. 662), and dactylitis may also occur ***(Fig. 18.31)***. Seventy per cent of patients recover fully within 6 months but many have a relapse.

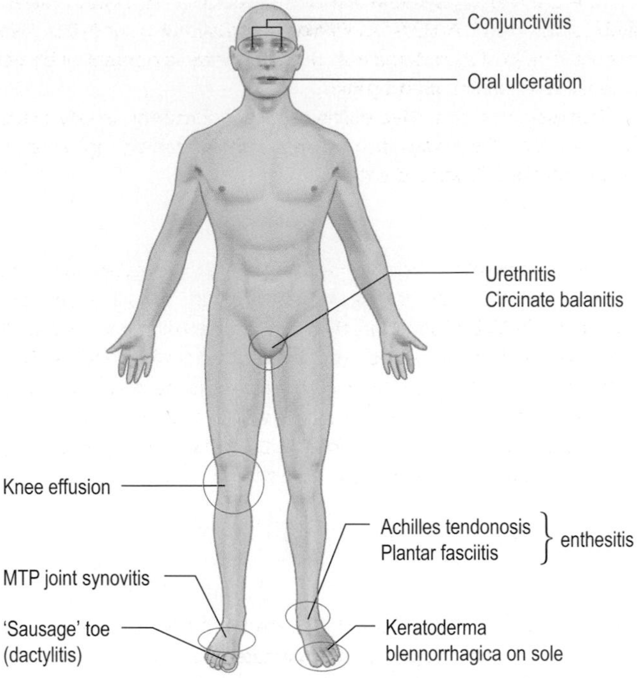

Figure 18.31 Clinical features of reactive arthritis. MTP, metatarsophalangeal.

In susceptible individuals with reactive arthritis, sacroiliitis and spondylitis may also develop. Sterile conjunctivitis occurs in 30%. Acute anterior uveitis complicates more severe or relapsing disease but is not synchronous with the arthritis.

The skin lesions resemble psoriasis:

- ***Circinate balanitis*** in the uncircumcised male causes painless superficial ulceration of the glans penis. In the circumcised male, the lesion is raised, red and scaly. Both heal without scarring.
- ***Keratoderma blennorrhagica*** involves the skin of the feet and hands, which develops painless, red and often confluent raised plaques and pustules that are histologically similar to pustular psoriasis.
- ***Nail dystrophy*** occurs.

Management

Treating persisting infection with antibiotics alters the course of the arthritis, once it has developed. Cultures should be taken and any infection treated. Sexual partners must be screened.

Pain responds well to NSAIDs and locally injected or oral corticosteroids. The majority of individuals with reactive arthritis have a single attack that settles, but a few develop a disabling relapsing and remitting arthritis. Relapsing cases are sometimes treated with sulfasalazine or methotrexate (see ***Box 18.30***). TNF-α-blocking agents remain the drugs of next choice in severe and persistent disease but are rarely necessary.

Enteropathic arthritis associated with inflammatory bowel disease

Enteropathic synovitis occurs in up to 10–15% of patients who have ulcerative colitis or Crohn's disease (see pp. 408–411). The link between the bowel disease and the inflammatory arthritis is not clear. Selective mucosal leakiness may expose the individual to antigens that trigger synovitis.

The arthritis is asymmetrical and predominantly affects lower-limb joints. An HLA-B27-associated sacroiliitis or spondylitis also occurs. The joint symptoms may predate the development of bowel disease and lead to its diagnosis.

Remission of ulcerative colitis or total colectomy usually leads to remission of the joint disease, but arthritis can persist even in well-controlled Crohn's disease.

Management

The inflammatory bowel disease should be treated (see pp. 409–411). In all cases of enteropathic arthritis, the symptoms are helped by NSAIDs, although they may make diarrhoea worse. A monoarthritis is best treated by intra-articular corticosteroids. Sulfasalazine is more frequently prescribed than mesalazine, as it may help both bowel and joint disease. The TNF-α-blocking drugs infliximab, adalimumab and certolizumab are used in inflammatory bowel disease and can help the arthritis.

Crystal arthritis

Aetiology

The two main types of crystal-induced arthritis are caused by sodium urate and calcium pyrophosphate crystals, which are distinguished by their different shapes and refringence properties under polarized light with a red filter ***(Fig. 18.32)***. Rarely, crystals of calcium apatite (see p. 670) or cholesterol cause acute synovitis.

Gout and hyperuricaemia

Gout is an inflammatory arthritis associated with hyperuricaemia and intra-articular sodium urate crystals.

Epidemiology

The prevalence of gout has increased substantially in the last two decades to 2.5% in the UK and 3.9% in the USA. Asian populations are also increasingly at risk as their diet becomes more Western. This rising prevalence is due to changing diets with purine-rich foods, high saturated fats and fructose-containing drinks; alcohol misuse; increasing co-morbidities that promote hyperuricaemia; and suboptimal management. Gout is more common in men than women (5 : 1); it rarely occurs before young adulthood (when it suggests a specific genetic defect), and seldom in pre-menopausal females. Some 85–90% of cases are idiopathic. Hyperuricaemia is common in certain ethnic groups (e.g. Maoris).

The last two steps of purine metabolism in humans are the conversion of hypoxanthine to xanthine, and of xanthine to uric acid, catalysed by the enzyme xanthine oxidase. Primates lost the gene for uricase, which degrades uric acid, during evolution 10–20 million years ago, so hyperuricaemia possibly offered an evolutionary advantage.

Serum uric acid (SUA) levels are higher in men than in women. Hyperuricaemia is defined as a serum uric acid level greater than two standard deviations from the mean, of 420 μmol/L in males and 360 μmol/L in females. The limit of solubility when crystal formation may occur is 360 μmol/L at 35°C and 300 μmol/L at 30°C. Hyperuricaemia is mostly asymptomatic, although OA joints are more prone to attacks of gout. The range of SUA for individuals with gout is higher than in healthy controls. SUA levels increase with age, obesity, a 'Western' diet (see above) and combined hyperlipidaemia, diabetes mellitus, ischaemic heart disease and hypertension (metabolic syndrome; see p. 209). Gout is often familial.

Pathogenesis of hyperuricaemia and gout

Uric acid is the final product of endogenous and dietary purine metabolism in humans, and SUA depends on the balance between purine synthesis, ingestion of dietary purines and the elimination of urate by the kidney (66%) and intestine (33%).

Some 90% of people with gout have impaired excretion of uric acid (10% have increased production due to high cell turnover and <1% due to an inborn error of metabolism). Renal excretion is coordinated by a group of renal tubular urate transport molecules and a complex process of glomerular filtration, proximal tubule reabsorption via the urate transporter-1 (URAT1) and active re-secretion ***(Fig. 18.33)***. GLUT9 (a product of the *SLC2A9* gene) transports uric acid, along with glucose and fructose, into the cell from the tubule and back into the circulation. Genetic variations in both URAT1 and SLC2A9 have been linked to the development of hyperuricaemia in humans. Both the entry of uric acid via the URAT1 mechanism and the exit into circulation by SLC2A9 can be blocked by uricosuric drugs, such as probenecid. The body pool is about 1000 mg and 60% is turned over daily. Low-dose aspirin blocks uric acid secretion. Insulin resistance enhances uric acid resorption. Causes of hyperuricaemia are shown in ***Box 18.35***.

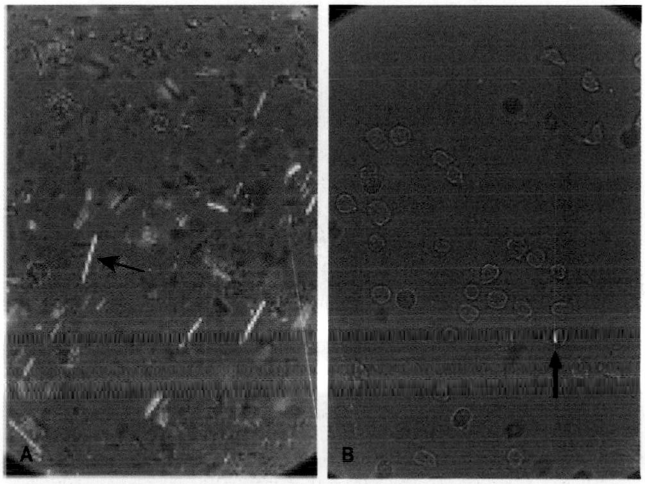

Figure 18.32 Crystal arthritis. A. Needle-shaped urate crystals (arrowed). **B.** A small, intracellular pyrophosphate crystal (arrowed). Both are viewed under polarized light with a red filter.

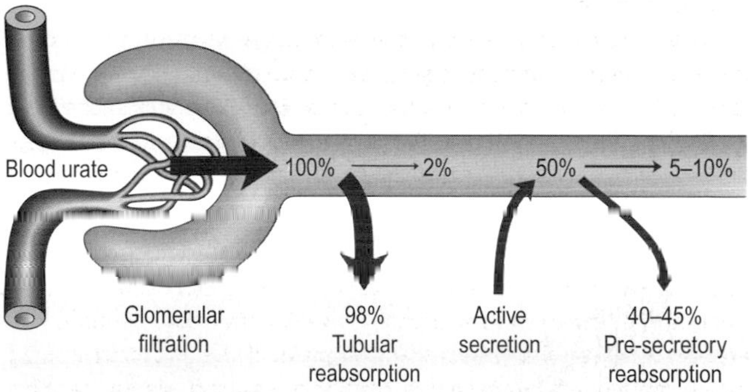

Figure 18.33 Urate renal transport. The net result is that about 5–10% of the glomerular load is excreted in the urine under normal circumstances.

Box 18.35 Causes of hyperuricaemia

Impaired excretion of uric acid
- Chronic renal disease (clinical gout unusual)
- Drug therapy, e.g. thiazide diuretics, low-dose aspirin
- Hypertension
- Lead toxicity
- Primary hyperparathyroidism or hypothyroidism
- Increased lactic acid production from alcohol, exercise, starvation
- Glucose-6-phosphatase deficiency (interferes with renal excretion)

Increased production of uric acid
Increased purine synthesis de novo *due to:*
- Hypoxanthine–guanine–phosphoribosyl transferase (HGPRT) reduction (an X-linked inborn error causing the Lesch–Nyhan syndrome)
- Phosphoribosyl-pyrophosphate synthase overactivity
- Glucose-6-phosphatase deficiency with glycogen storage disease type 1

Increased turnover of purines due to:
- Myeloproliferative disorders, e.g. polycythaemia vera
- Lymphoproliferative disorders, e.g. leukaemia
- Others, e.g. carcinoma, severe psoriasis

Gout as an autoinflammatory disease

The involvement of the innate immune system and inflammasomes indicates that gout is an autoinflammatory disease, similar to the hereditary periodic fevers (see pp. 705–706). A series of receptors recognize bacteria and viruses as 'foreign' and eliminate them by activating the cytokine cascade. One such receptor (NLRP3) has been implicated in crystal-triggered inflammation. Activation of the inflammasome (see p. 126) activates IL-1β, leading to cellular activation, which triggers an IL-8-mediated influx of neutrophils. Ingestion by polymorphonuclear leucocytes of sodium urate crystals causes the release of pro-inflammatory cytokines, particularly IL-1β and complement. Colchicine inhibits the microtubule formation that is necessary for this process to occur.

Clinical features

Hyperuricaemia may be asymptomatic or may cause:
- ***Acute gout***, followed by an asymptomatic intercritical phase; a second acute attack is likely within 2 years.
- ***Chronic interval gout***, with acute attacks superimposed on low-grade inflammation and potential joint damage.
- ***Chronic polyarticular gout***, which is rare, except in elderly people on longstanding diuretic treatment, in renal failure, or when allopurinol is started too soon after an acute attack.
- ***Tophaceous gout***.
- ***Urate renal stone*** formation (see pp. 754–757).

Acute gout presents typically in a middle-aged male with a sudden onset of agonizing pain, swelling and redness of the first MTP joint. The attack may be precipitated by excess food, alcohol, dehydration or diuretic therapy. Untreated attacks last about 7 days. Recovery is typically associated with desquamation of the overlying skin. In 25% of attacks, a joint other than the great toe is affected.

In severe attacks, overlying crystal cellulitis makes gout difficult to distinguish clinically from infective cellulitis. A family or personal history of gout and the finding of a raised SUA suggest the diagnosis but, if in doubt, blood and joint fluid cultures should be taken to exclude sepsis.

Chronic tophaceous gout is described below.

Investigations

The clinical picture is often diagnostic, as is the rapid response to NSAIDs or colchicine.
- ***Joint fluid microscopy*** is the most specific and diagnostic test but is technically difficult.
- ***Serum uric acid*** is usually raised (>600 μmol/L). If it is not, it should be rechecked several weeks after the attack, as levels fall immediately after an acute episode. Acute gout rarely occurs with a serum uric acid in the lower half of the normal range below the saturation point of 360 μmol/L.
- ***Serum urea, creatinine*** and estimated glomerular filtration rate (eGFR) are monitored for signs of renal impairment.

Management

The use of NSAIDs or coxibs in high doses rapidly reduces the pain and swelling. The first dose should be taken at the first indication of an attack:
- ***naproxen***: 750 mg immediately, then 500 mg every 8–12 h
- ***diclofenac***: 75–100 mg immediately, then 50 mg every 6–8 h

After 24–48 hours, reduced doses are given for a further week. *Caution*: NSAIDs may cause renal impairment. In individuals with renal impairment or a history of peptic ulceration, alternative treatments include:
- ***Colchicine***: loading doses will cause diarrhoea or colicky abdominal pain, so 500 μg 2–3 times per day is usually sufficient to terminate attacks without side-effects.
- ***Corticosteroids***: oral prednisolone or intramuscular or intra-articular depot methylprednisolone is used.

Dietary advice

The first attacks may be separated by up to 2 years and are managed symptomatically. Recognition and prompt treatment, including lifestyle modifications, are paramount. Advice to reduce alcohol intake, especially beer, which is high in purines and fructose, and consumption of non-diet carbonated soft drinks, which are also high in fructose, is essential; other dietary change include reduction of total calorie and cholesterol intake, and avoidance of purine-rich foods, such as offal, red meat, shellfish and spinach. These modifications can reduce serum urate by 15% and delay the need for drugs that reduce serum urate levels. Dietary advice is readily available on the Internet.

Treatment with agents that reduce serum uric acid levels

The aim of treatment is to reduce the uric acid level below the 360 μmol/L level; some guidelines recommend a level below 300 μmol/L.

Allopurinol

Allopurinol should only be used when the attacks are frequent and severe (despite dietary changes), or associated with renal impairment or tophi, or when the patient finds NSAIDs or colchicine difficult to tolerate. Allopurinol is a xanthine oxidase inhibitor, which reduces serum uric acid levels rapidly; it is relatively non-toxic but should be used at low doses (50–100 mg) in renal impairment. It should never be started within a month of an acute attack and always under cover of NSAIDs or colchicine for the first 2–4 weeks before and 4 weeks after starting allopurinol, as it may induce acute gout. The dose can be increased gradually from 100 mg every few weeks until the uric acid level is below the 360 μmol/L level. Skin rashes and gastrointestinal intolerance are the most common side-effects. A hypersensitivity reaction is the most serious but rare adverse event, as is bone marrow suppression.

Febuxostat

Febuxostat (80–120 mg) is a non-purine analogue inhibitor of xanthine oxidase that is well tolerated and as effective as allopurinol. It is safer in renal impairment, as it undergoes hepatic metabolism rather than renal excretion, and is helpful in patients who cannot tolerate allopurinol; however, there is evidence that it may increase cardiovascular risks, and this is being monitored in ongoing observational studies. Allopurinol remains the drug of first choice, unless there are strong contraindications to its use.

Pegloticase

Pegloticase, a pegylated recombinant uricase given intravenously, lowers urate levels dramatically but its place in therapy is unclear.

Uricosuric agents

These also lower the serum uric acid but their use is restricted throughout Europe by the very rare occurrence of serious hepatotoxicity. ***Benzbromarone*** acts on the URAT1 transporter and is well tolerated. ***Sulfinpyrazone*** and ***probenecid*** are best avoided in renal impairment. Availability of these drugs varies between countries – in the UK, benzbromarone and probenecid can be obtained for treating named patients.

Losartan

Losartan is an angiotensin I receptor antagonist and is uricosuric in hypertensive patients with gout. It may reduce the risk of gout in patients with the metabolic syndrome.

Anakinra and canakinumb

Anakinra blocks IL-1β and canakinumab is a human monoclonal antibody with specific cross-reactivity for IL-1β but not for other members of the IL-1 family. Their cost-effectiveness in managing gout resistant to conventional agents is still subject to trials. Increased knowledge of the mechanisms of urate transport and the inflammatory response it induces is likely to provide new therapeutic targets in the future.

Chronic tophaceous gout

Individuals with persistently high levels of uric acid can present with chronic tophaceous gout, as sodium urate forms smooth white deposits (tophi) in skin and around joints, on the ear, fingers ***(Fig. 18.34)*** or the Achilles tendon. Large deposits are unsightly and ulcerate. There is chronic joint pain and sometimes superimposed acute gouty attacks.

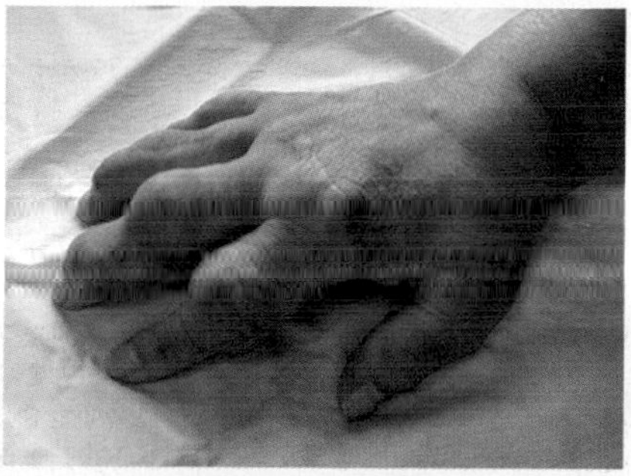

Figure 18.34 Gout with tophi. *(Courtesy of Dr Varkey Alexander, Al-Sabah Hospital, Kuwait.)*

Periarticular deposits lead to a halo of radio-opacity and clearly defined ('punched out') bone cysts on X-ray.

Tophaceous gout is often associated with renal impairment and/or the long-term use of diuretics. There may be acute or chronic urate nephropathy or renal stone formation. Whenever possible, diuretics should be stopped or changed to less urate-retaining ones, such as bumetanide. Treat with allopurinol and/or uricosuric agents (see above). Pegloticase is used preventatively in people undergoing chemotherapy for malignancies (tumour lysis syndrome), and in those rare individuals who have refractory tophaceous gout.

Calcium pyrophosphate dihydrate deposition arthropathy (DPPD)

There has been a complex evolution of descriptive terminology for this condition over time and previous terms, including pseudogout, have been unified into calcium pyrophosphate dihydrate deposition (CPPD) arthropathy. This condition occurs in hyaline and fibrocartilage, and is the most common cause of cartilage calcification. CPPD-associated arthritis is the third most common inflammatory arthritis, which increases with age, OA, joint trauma/injury and metabolic disease (hyperparathyroidism, haemochromatosis, hypomagnesaemia), and has a familial predisposition. Shedding of crystals into a joint precipitates acute synovitis that resembles gout, except that it is more common in elderly women and usually affects the knee or wrist.

Diagnosis

The diagnosis is made by detecting rhomboidal, weakly positively bi-refringent crystals in joint fluid (see ***Fig. 18.32***), or deduced from the presence of cartilage calcification on X-ray. Joint fluid looks purulent so should be sent for culture to exclude septic arthritis, as the attacks may also be associated with fever and a raised white blood cell count.

Management

Unlike in gout, there is no specific treatment to eliminate calcium pyrophosphate crystals. Therefore, management is focused on symptom control and treatments overlap with those for gout and OA. An evidence base is lacking in this condition, however, and there have been no randomized controlled clinical trials of acute management. Aspiration of the joint reduces the pain dramatically but it is usually necessary to use an NSAID or colchicine, as for gout. If infection can be excluded, an intra-articular injection of a corticosteroid helps. Studies of blockade of the NLRP3 inflammasome-IL-1 pathway (see p. 688) are under way.

Basic calcium phosphate deposition disease

Basic calcium phosphate (BCP) crystals, including hydroxyapatite, tricalcium phosphate and octacalcium phosphate, can be deposited in any tissues, particularly at intra-articular and periarticular locations. Crystal formation is thought to be partly regulated by the effects of extracellular inorganic phosphate on chondrocytes and is linked with the development of OA. BCP crystals cause joint damage through induction of fibroblast proliferation, inflammatory cytokines (IL-1β and TNF-α), nitric oxide and metalloproteinases.

BCP crystal deposits in periarticular soft tissue may be asymptomatic or can cause acute calcific periarthritis (particularly in the supraspinatus tendon), tendonitis, bursitis and enthesitis. Less frequently, they can cause arthritis. In acute attacks, periarticular tissues or joints can be swollen, tender and hot. This presentation may mimic cellulitis, gout, CPPD disease and septic arthritis. Periarticular or articular BCP crystal deposits are also found in an extremely destructive chronic arthropathy of the elderly that occurs most often in shoulders (Milwaukee shoulder) or other large joints, such as the hips and knees, and in erosive OA of the fingers.

Diagnosis

The diagnosis is made clinically and septic arthritis should be excluded. A neutrophilia with elevation of ESR and CRP may occur during an acute attack. Intra- and/or periarticular calcifications, with or without erosive, destructive or hypertrophic changes, may be seen on X-ray. Alizarin red S staining is not specific for BCP crystals in synovial fluid and other calcium-containing particulates are also stained by this method.

Management

Management of acute attacks is similar to that of CPPD disease with NSAIDs, oral colchicine, aspiration of effusions and/or intra-/periarticular injection of steroids to try to shorten the duration of symptoms. In patients with underlying progressive articular changes, the response to medical therapy is usually less rewarding. Total joint replacement may be required for patients with severe destructive arthropathy in large joints.

Further reading

Burns CM, Wortmann RL. Gout therapeutics: new drugs for old disease. *Lancet* 2011; 377:165–177.
Dougados M, Baeten D. Spondyloarthritis. *Lancet* 2011; 377:2127–2137.
Guidelli GM, Barskova T, Brizi MG et al. One year in review: novelties in the treatment of rheumatoid arthritis. *Clin Exp Rheumatol* 2015; 33:102–108.
Neogi T. Gout. *N Engl J Med* 2011; 364:443–452.
Richette P, Bardin T. Gout. *Lancet* 2010; 375:318–328.
Sieper J, Rudwaleit M, Baraliakos X et al. The Assessment of SpondyloArthritis international Society (ASAS) handbook: a guide to assess spondyloarthritis. *Ann Rheum Dis* 2009; 68 Suppl 2:i1–44.
Taylor PC. Aetiopathology of rheumatoid arthritis. *Medicine* 2014; 42:227–230.
Zhang W, Doherty M, Bardin T et al. European League Against Rheumatism recommendations for calcium pyrophosphate deposition. Part I: terminology and diagnosis, Part II: management. *Ann Rheum Dis* 2011; 70:563–575.
http://basdai.com Bath Ankylosing Spondylitis Disease Activity Index.

INFECTIONS OF JOINTS

Joints become infected by direct injury or by blood-borne infection from an infected skin lesion or other site. The incidence of definite and probable septic arthritis in Western Europe is 4–10 per 100 000 patient-years per year. The rising global incidence of this condition has been linked with an ageing population, increased immunosuppressive use, musculoskeletal prostheses and surgical procedures. It is a medical emergency that requires prompt treatment to prevent irreversible joint destruction and has a significant mortality of up to 11%, reaching 50% in polyarticular sepsis.

Chronically inflamed joints (e.g. in RA) are more prone to infection than are normal joints. Individuals who are immunosuppressed, by AIDS or by immunosuppressive agents, are particularly at risk, as are infants, the elderly and those who use excess alcohol. Artificial joints are also potential sites for infection.

Septic arthritis

The organism that most commonly causes septic arthritis is *Staphylococcus aureus*. Other organisms include streptococci, other species of staphylococcus, *Neisseria gonorrhoeae*, *Haemophilus influenzae* in children, and these and other Gram-negative organisms in the elderly or complicating RA.

Clinical features

Suspected septic arthritis is a medical emergency. In young and previously fit people, the joint is hot, red, swollen and agonizingly painful; it is held immobile by muscle spasm. In contrast, the onset may be insidious with a lack of systemic symptoms; in the elderly, immunosuppressed and patients with RA, a high index of suspicion is needed.

In 20% of patients, the sepsis affects more than one joint. Chronic destructive arthritis due to tuberculosis is rare.

Investigations

- ***Aspirate*** the joint and send the fluid for urgent Gram-staining and culture. The fluid is usually frankly purulent. The culture techniques should include those for gonococci and anaerobes.
- ***Blood cultures*** are often positive.
- ***Leucocytosis*** is usual, unless the person is severely immunosuppressed.
- ***X-rays*** are of no value in diagnosis in acute septic arthritis.
- ***Skin wound swabs, sputum and throat swab or urine*** may be positive and indicate the source of infection.

Management

There are no RCTs to guide management in adults. The prognosis is similar for patients with a proven microbiological diagnosis to those with a suspected but not proven diagnosis; therefore it is vital to treat on the basis of clinical suspicion, probability (with subsequent confirmed identity) of organism, local pattern of antibiotic sensitivity and microbiological advice.

Therapy should be started immediately before culture results are available because joint destruction may occur within weeks.

- The joint should be immobilized initially, followed by early physiotherapy to prevent stiffness and muscle wasting.
- Intravenous antibiotics should be given for 1–2 weeks. It is usual to give two antibiotics to which the organism is sensitive for 6 weeks, then one for a further 6 weeks, orally. Response is monitored clinically and with ESR and CRP.

Empirical treatment in septic arthritis

Empirical regimens include intravenous flucloxacillin 2 g given 6-hourly, plus sodium fusidate 500 mg orally 8-hourly. If the patient is allergic to penicillin, replace flucloxacillin with erythromycin 1 g i.v. 6-hourly or clindamycin 600 mg i.v. 8-hourly. In immunosuppressed patients, flucloxacillin 1–2 g i.v. 6-hourly plus gentamicin (to cover Gram-negative organisms) should be used. Teicoplanin i.v. should replace flucloxacillin if meticillin-resistant *Staphylococcus aureus* (MRSA) is likely. Change the antibiotics if the organism is not sensitive. Drainage of the joint and arthroscopic joint washouts are helpful in relieving pain.

Management of infected prostheses

If chronically infected, the prosthesis is removed and the joint space filled with an antibiotic-impregnated spacer for 3–6 weeks before a new prosthesis is inserted. The whole process is covered by antibiotics, such as teicoplanin i.v. and oral sodium fusidate.

Specific types of bacterial arthritis

Gonococcal arthritis

This is the most common cause of a septic arthritis in previously fit young adults, more commonly affecting women, and men who have sex with men.

Patients present with a fever and characteristic pustules on the distal limbs, often in association with polyarthralgia and tenosynovitis, when about 40% have a gonococcaemia. This phase settles and blood cultures usually become negative. Nucleic acid amplification tests may be positive even when cultures are negative. Later, large-joint mono- or pauciarticular arthritis may follow. Culture is usually positive from the genital tract, although the joint fluid may be sterile. It is not clear whether this joint inflammation is simply a septic arthritis (which responds rapidly to antibiotics), or whether there is also a reactive element to bacterial lipopolysaccharide.

Management consists of oral penicillin, ciprofloxacin or doxycycline for 2 weeks, and joint rest. Resistance to antibiotics is increasing (see pp. 234–235).

Tuberculous arthritis

Around 1% of people with tuberculosis develop joint and/or bone involvement. It occurs as the primary disease in children. In adults, it is usually due to haematogenous spread from secondary pulmonary or renal lesions. The onset is insidious and diagnosis often delayed.

The organism invades the synovium or intervertebral disc. There are caseating granulomas and rapid destruction of cartilage and adjacent bone. Some patients develop a reactive polyarthritis (Poncet's disease).

The hip or knee (30%) is quite commonly affected but around 50% develop spinal disease. Patients become febrile with night sweats, anorexia and weight loss. The usual risk factors for tuberculosis apply – debility, excess alcohol use or immunosuppression. HIV-positive/AIDS patients are at particular risk.

Investigations should include culture of fluid, and culture and biopsy of the synovium. *Mycobacterium tuberculosis* is the usual organism but atypical mycobacteria are occasionally implicated. A chest X-ray should be performed. Initially, joint or spinal X-rays may be normal but joint-space reduction and bone destruction develop rapidly if treatment is delayed. MRI shows the abnormality earlier in the spine and CT-guided biopsy from the affected disc is often necessary to obtain cultures.

Management is as for pulmonary tuberculosis with therapy for 9 months. The joint should be rested and the spine immobilized in the acute phase.

Meningococcal arthritis

Joint inflammation may complicate meningococcal septicaemia, presenting as a migratory polyarthritis. Organisms are rarely cultured from the joint and most cases are due to immune complex deposition. Treatment is urgent with immediate penicillin therapy.

Infective endocarditis

This condition may present with arthralgia, polymyalgia rheumatica-like symptoms or an infective arthritis. It is discussed on pages 1017–1021.

Lyme arthritis

About 80% of people with Lyme disease develop arthralgia, less commonly an acute pauciarticular arthritis (see p. 284); this usually resolves but 10% of untreated cases go on to develop a chronic arthritis. There are no positive markers in these patients of an ongoing infection (see p. 284).

Diagnosis is by the detection of IgM antibodies against the spirochaete *Borrelia burgdorferi*.

Treatment with antibiotics (amoxicillin or doxycycline) is highly effective in early disease. The response of chronic arthritis to antibiotic treatment is discussed below.

Brucellosis

Brucellosis (see p. 283) has a worldwide distribution. The most common cause of chronic brucellosis and of arthritis is *Brucella melitensis*. There is usually a migratory large joint mono- or oligoarticular arthritis, which is septic or reactive. Arthritis is more common in chronic infections of more than 6 months.

Syphilitic arthritis

Congenital syphilis (see p. 329) can cause an acute painful epiphysitis or osteochondritis sometimes associated with para-articular swelling in the first few weeks of life. Later, at age 8–16 years, painless effusion of the knees may occur (Clutton's joints).

In acquired syphilis, arthralgia and arthritis occur in the secondary stage. Charcot's (neuropathic) joints usually involve the knees in tabes dorsalis (see p. 866).

Leprosy

Acute or chronic symmetrical polyarthritis resembling RA, swollen hands and feet due to lepra reactions, tenosynovitis and thickened nerves with or without cutaneous manifestations are seen in leprosy (see pp. 285–286).

Actinomycetes infection

Actinomycetes can affect the mandible or vertebrae.

Arthritis in viral disease

A transient polyarthritis or arthralgia can occur before, during or after many viral illnesses. These include infectious mononucleosis, chickenpox, mumps, adenovirus, rubella, erythrovirus B19, hepatitis B and C, arboviral infections and HIV. In most of these, it is due to a direct toxic effect or immune complex deposition.

Rubella

In rubella (see p. 252), the virus can occasionally be isolated from the joint. This arthritis is rare in countries where rubella vaccination is routine. It occurs most commonly in up to 50% of young adult females a few days after rubella infection (6% of men). It is a symmetrical polyarthritis involving the MCP or PIP joints most commonly, but many joints can be affected. It closely resembles RA. IgM rubella antibodies are present. It resolves within a few weeks in most cases. A mild arthritis occurs rarely 2–4 weeks after rubella vaccination.

Erythrovirus B19

Erythrovirus B19 (see p. 252) causes an acute, self-limiting arthritis and is associated with erythema infectiosum ('slapped cheek disease').

Hepatitis

In hepatitis B infection (see pp. 454–457), a sudden, symmetrical polyarticular arthritis of the small joints of the hands occurs in approximately one third of patients, often in the prodromal phase, and mostly resolves before the onset of jaundice. Hepatitis C infection causes type II mixed cryoglobulinaemia (see p. 748).

Arbovirus

Arbovirus infections (see p. 257), which are endemic in many parts of the world, give rise to an arthralgia and/or arthritis. For example, the Ross River virus causes an epidemic polyarthritis in Australia and the South Pacific; it involves the small joints of the hands and clears in 2–4 weeks. Other viral infections causing epidemic arthritis include chikungunya (see p. 257) and o'nyong-nyong.

Musculoskeletal aspects of infection with HIV and AIDS

Musculoskeletal manifestations are common in these patients and are often caused by triggers such as opportunistic infections and drug therapy rather than HIV itself. Infective arthritis seen in these immunosuppressed patients often has minimal symptoms and signs. Certain of the antiviral agents cause an acute arthritis, possibly because of crystallization in the joint.

Arthralgia is common in AIDS. There is a ***seronegative, predominantly lower-limb arthritis***, similar to psoriasis or Reiter's disease. ***Spondylitis*** also occurs but is not associated with HLA-B27. ***Avascular necrosis***, possibly associated with corticosteroids or alcohol, is seen.

Non-articular diseases, such as Sjögren- and lupus-like syndromes, systemic vasculitis of the necrotizing and hypersensitivity types and myositis, also occur.

Fungal infections

Fungal infections of joints occur rarely. Bone abscesses may be seen. Destructive joint lesions can also occur with blastomycosis. A benign polyarthritis accompanied by erythema nodosum occasionally occurs in coccidioidomycosis and histoplasmosis. Culture of purulent synovial fluid and skin tests for fungi may help the diagnosis.

Further reading

Mathews CJ, Weston VC, Jones A et al. Bacterial septic arthritis in adults. *Lancet* 2010; 375:846–855.

AUTOIMMUNE RHEUMATIC DISEASES

Autoimmunity and autoantibodies

Autoimmune diseases are conditions in which the immune system attacks tissues of the body. The antigens can be present in multiple organs so the clinical manifestations are systemic and diverse. In some diseases, such as Graves' disease, Hashimoto's thyroiditis and type 1 diabetes mellitus, only a single organ is affected. Each individual autoimmune rheumatic disease (ARD) has a characteristic pattern of symptoms and signs, which are used to make the diagnosis. In some ARDs, there are also characteristic autoantibodies (i.e. antibodies that recognize antigens that are normal constituents of the body, such as DNA and phospholipids). Positive blood tests for autoantibodies are useful but not essential in the diagnosis of ARDs (see ***Box 18.4***).

Systemic lupus erythematosus

Systemic lupus erythematosus (SLE) is an inflammatory, multisystem autoimmune disorder with arthralgia and rashes as the most common clinical features, and cerebral and renal disease as the most serious problems.

Epidemiology

SLE occurs worldwide and is about nine times as common in women as in men, with a peak age of onset between 20 and 40 years. The prevalence varies between ethnic groups, being highest (at 1:250) in African/Caribbean women. In other populations, the prevalence varies between 1:1000 and 1:10 000.

Aetiology

The cause is unknown but there are several predisposing factors:

- ***Heredity***. There is a higher concordance rate in monozygotic twins (up to 25%) compared with dizygotic twins (3%). First-degree relatives have a 3% chance of developing the disease but approximately 20% have autoantibodies.
- ***Genetics***. Three whole-genome analyses have led to the identification of approximately 20 genes linked to the development of SLE. These include some HLA genes, as well as genes involved in T- and B-lymphocyte function. Homozygous deficiencies of the complement genes C1q, C2 or C4 are very rare but convey a high risk of developing SLE.
- ***Sex hormone status***. Pre-menopausal women are most frequently affected.
- ***Drugs***. Drugs such as hydralazine, isoniazid, procainamide and penicillamine can induce a form of SLE that is usually mild, in that the kidneys and central nervous system are not affected.
- ***Ultraviolet light***. This can trigger flares of SLE, especially in the skin.
- ***Exposure to Epstein–Barr virus***. This has been suggested as a trigger for SLE.

Pathogenesis

When cells die by apoptosis, the cellular remnants appear on the cell surface as small blebs that carry self antigens. These antigens include nuclear constituents (e.g. DNA and histones), which are normally hidden from the immune system. In people with SLE, removal of these blebs by phagocytes is inefficient, so that they are transferred to lymphoid tissues, where they can be taken up by antigen-presenting cells. The self antigens from these blebs can then be presented to T cells, which in turn stimulate B cells to produce autoantibodies directed against these antigens (see pp. 144–146). It has been shown that, in some patients, the autoantibodies are present in stored blood samples that were taken years before the patient developed clinical features of SLE. The combination of availability of self antigens and failure of the immune system to inactivate B cells and T cells that recognize these self antigens (i.e. a breakdown of *tolerance*; see pp. 144–146) leads to the following immunological consequences.

- Development of autoantibodies that either form circulating complexes or deposit by binding directly to tissues.
- Activation of complement and influx of neutrophils, causing inflammation in those tissues.
- Abnormal cytokine production: increased blood levels of IL-10 and interferon-alpha are particularly closely linked to high activity of inflammation in SLE. However, no form of anticytokine biological therapy has yet been adopted routinely in the treatment of SLE.

More recently, other cells have been implicated in the pathogenesis of SLE. These include dendritic cells, which are activated by immune complexes containing nucleic acids to produce interferon, and invariant natural killer T cells (iNKT cells), which are reduced in number and function in patients with SLE.

Pathology

SLE of the skin and kidneys is characterized by deposition of complement and IgG antibodies, and by influx of neutrophils and

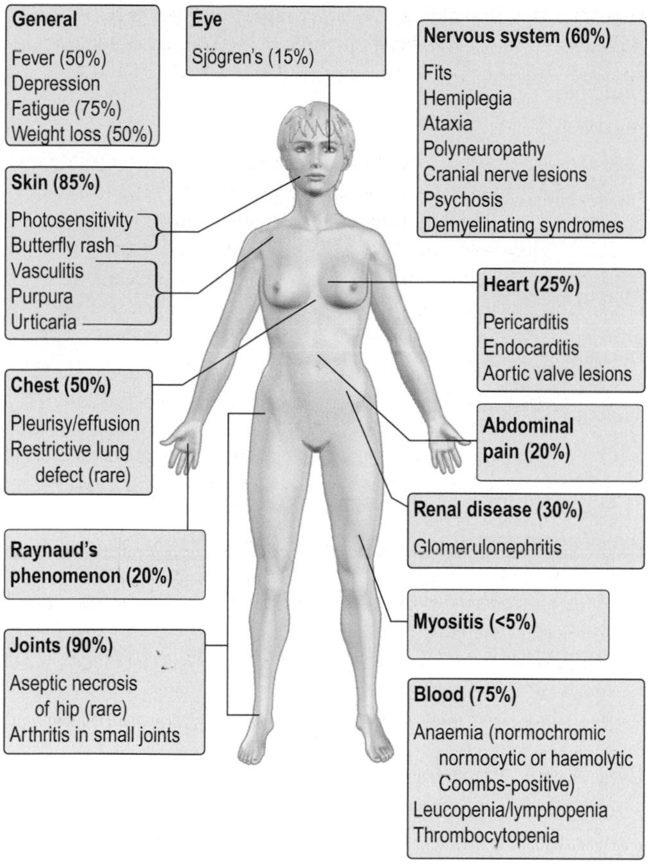

Figure 18.35 Clinical features of systemic lupus erythematosus.

lymphocytes. Biopsies of other tissues are carried out less frequently but can show vasculitis affecting capillaries, arterioles and venules. The synovium of joints can be oedematous and may contain immune complexes. Haematoxylin bodies (rounded, blue, homogeneous haematoxylin-stained deposits) are seen in inflammatory infiltrates and are thought to result from the interaction of antinuclear antibodies and cell nuclei.

The pathology of lesions in other organs is described in the appropriate chapters.

Clinical features

The manifestations of SLE vary greatly between patients. Most patients suffer fatigue, arthralgia and/or skin problems. Involvement of major organs is less common but more serious ***(Fig. 18.35)***.

General features

Fever is common in exacerbations. Patients complain of marked malaise and tiredness, and these symptoms do not correlate with disease activity or severity of organ-based complications.

The joints and muscles

Joint involvement is the most common clinical feature (>90%). Patients often present with symptoms resembling RA with symmetrical small joint arthralgia. Joints are painful but characteristically appear clinically normal, although sometimes there is slight soft tissue swelling surrounding the joint. Deformity because of joint capsule and tendon contraction is rare, as are bony erosions. Rarely, major joint deformity resembling RA (known as *Jaccoud's arthropathy*) is seen. Avascular necrosis affecting the hip or knee is a rare complication of the disease or of treatment with corticosteroids.

Myalgia is present in up to 50% of patients but a true myositis is seen in only <5%. If myositis is prominent, the patient may well have an overlap ARD with both polymyositis and SLE.

The skin

The skin (see p. 1367) is affected in 85% of cases. Erythema, in a 'butterfly' distribution on the cheeks of the face and across the bridge of the nose (see ***Fig. 31.33***), is characteristic. Vasculitic lesions on the fingertips and around the nail folds, purpura and urticaria occur. In 40–50% of cases, there is photosensitivity (especially in patients positive for anti-Ro antibodies). Prolonged exposure to sunlight can lead to exacerbations of the disease. Livedo reticularis, palmar and plantar rashes, pigmentation and alopecia are seen. Scarring alopecia can lead to irreversible bald patches, which are especially upsetting for women, who form the majority of people with SLE. Raynaud's phenomenon (see p. 1054) is common and may precede the development of other clinical problems by years.

Discoid lupus is a benign variant of lupus in which only the skin is involved. The rash is characteristic and appears on the face as well-defined erythematous plaques that progress to scarring and pigmentation (see p. 1366). Subacute cutaneous lupus erythematosus, a rare variant, is described on page 1367.

The lungs

Up to 50% of patients will have lung involvement at some time during the course of the disease (see p. 1122). Recurrent pleurisy and pleural effusions (exudates) are the most common manifestations and are often bilateral. Pneumonitis and atelectasis are seen; eventually, a restrictive lung defect develops, with loss of lung volumes and raised hemidiaphragms. This 'shrinking lung syndrome' is poorly understood but may have a neuromuscular basis. Rarely, pulmonary fibrosis occurs, more commonly in overlap syndromes (see p. 699). Intrapulmonary haemorrhage associated with vasculitis is a rare but potentially life-threatening complication.

The heart and cardiovascular system

The heart is involved in 25% of cases. Pericarditis, with small pericardial effusions detected by echocardiography, is common. A mild myocarditis also occurs, giving rise to arrhythmias. Aortic valve lesions and a cardiomyopathy can rarely be present. A non-infective endocarditis involving the mitral valve (Libman–Sacks syndrome) is very rare. Raynaud's, vasculitis, and arterial and venous thromboses can occur, especially in association with the antiphospholipid syndrome (see below). There is an increased frequency of ischaemic heart disease and stroke in people with SLE, which is partly due to altered levels of common risk factors such as hypertension and lipid levels, but the presence of chronic inflammation over many years may also be contributory. It is not known whether intensive treatment of cardiovascular risk factors in SLE will alter the risk of developing coronary disease or stroke. The benefit of statin therapy in the absence of significant hypercholesterolaemia remains to be proved.

The kidneys

A classification of types of nephritis is given on pages 733–734. Postmortem studies suggest that histological changes are very frequent, but clinical renal involvement occurs in only approximately 30% of cases. All patients should have regular screening of urine for blood and protein. An asymptomatic patient with proteinuria may be in the early stages of lupus nephritis, and treatment may prevent progression to renal impairment. Proteinuria should be quantified and haematuria should prompt examination for urinary casts or fragmented red cells that suggest glomerulonephritis. Renal biopsy is important to define the type and severity of nephritis. Renal vein thrombosis can occur in nephrotic syndrome or in association with antiphospholipid antibodies.

The nervous system

Involvement of the nervous system occurs in up to 60% of cases and symptoms often fluctuate. There may be a mild depression, but occasionally, more severe psychiatric disturbances occur. Epilepsy, migraines, cerebellar ataxia, aseptic meningitis, cranial nerve lesions, cerebrovascular disease or a polyneuropathy may be seen. The pathogenic mechanism for cerebral lupus is complex. Lesions may be due to vasculitis or immune-complex deposition, thrombosis or non-inflammatory microvasculopathy. In people with cerebral lupus, infection should be excluded, or treated in parallel with administration of corticosteroids and immunosuppression.

The eyes

Retinal vasculitis can cause infarcts (cytoid bodies), which appear as hard exudates, and haemorrhages. There may be episcleritis, conjunctivitis or optic neuritis, but blindness is uncommon. Secondary Sjögren syndrome is seen in about 15% of cases.

The gastrointestinal system

Mouth ulcers are common and may be a presenting feature. These may be painless or become secondarily infected and painful. Mesenteric vasculitis can produce inflammatory lesions involving the small bowel (infarction or perforation). Liver involvement and pancreatitis are uncommon.

Investigations

Blood

- ***A full blood count*** may show a leucopenia, lymphopenia and/or thrombocytopenia. Anaemia of chronic disease or autoimmune haemolytic anaemia also occurs. The ESR is raised in proportion to the disease activity. In contrast, the CRP is usually normal but may be high when the patient has lupus pleuritis, arthritis or a coexistent infection.
- ***Urea and creatinine*** only rise when renal disease is advanced. Low serum albumin or high urine albumin/creatinine ratio are earlier indicators of lupus nephritis.
- ***Autoantibodies*** of many different types may be present in SLE but the most significant are ANA, anti-dsDNA, anti-Ro, anti-Sm and anti-La ***(Box 18.36)***. Antiphospholipid antibodies are present in 25–40% of cases but not all of these patients develop antiphospholipid syndrome (see below).
- ***Serum complement*** C3 and C4 levels are often reduced during active disease. The combination of high ESR, high anti-dsDNA and low C3 may herald a flare of disease. All these markers tend to return towards normal as the flare improves, but in some patients, anti-dsDNA levels remain high even during clinical remission.

Histology

- Characteristic histological and immunofluorescent abnormalities (deposition of IgG and complement) are seen in biopsies from the kidney and skin.

Box 18.36 Antinuclear autoantibodies and disease associations

Antibody	Disease	Prevalence
ds-DNA	SLE	70%
Anti-histone	Drug-induced lupus	–
Anti-centromeric	Limited scleroderma	70%
Anti-Ro (SS-A)	SLE Primary Sjögren's	40–60% 60–90%
Anti-La (SS-B)	SLE Primary Sjögren's	15% 35–85%
Anti-Sm	SLE	10–25% (Caucasian) 30–50% (Black African)
Anti-UI-RNP	SLE Overlap syndrome	30%
Anti-Jo-1 (antisynthetase)	Polymyositis Dermatomyositis	30%
Anti-topoisomerase-1 (Scl-70)	Diffuse cutaneous SSc	30%

ds-DNA, double-stranded DNA; RNP, ribonucleoprotein; Ro, La, first two letters of name of patients; Sm, Smith, patient's name; SS-A, SS-B, Sjögren syndrome A and B; SSc, systemic scleroderma; SLE, systemic lupus erythematosus.

Diagnostic imaging

- CT scans of the brain sometimes show infarcts or haemorrhage with evidence of cerebral atrophy. MRI can detect lesions in white matter that are not seen on CT. However, it can be very difficult to distinguish true vasculitis from small thrombi.

Management

General measures

The disease and its management should be discussed with the patient, particularly the effect upon the patient's lifestyle: for example, appearance and debility due to fatigue. Patients are advised to avoid excessive exposure to sunlight and it is also necessary to reduce cardiovascular risk factors.

Symptomatic treatment

Many patients do not need treatment with corticosteroid tablets or immunosuppressive agents. Arthralgia, arthritis, fever and serositis all respond well to standard doses of NSAIDs (see pp. 665–666). Topical corticosteroids are effective and widely used in cutaneous lupus. Antimalarial drugs (chloroquine or hydroxychloroquine) help mild skin disease, fatigue and arthralgias that cannot be controlled with NSAIDs but patients require regular eye checks because of rare retinal toxicity (1 in 2000).

Corticosteroids and immunosuppressive drugs

Single intramuscular injections of long-acting corticosteroids or short courses of oral corticosteroids are useful in treating severe flares of arthritis, pleuritis or pericarditis. In some cases, these symptoms can only be kept under control using long-term oral corticosteroids.

Renal or cerebral disease and severe haemolytic anaemia or thrombocytopenia must be treated with high-dose oral corticosteroids, and the first two of these require immunosuppressive drugs in addition. Cyclophosphamide was most commonly used to achieve remission in these severe forms of lupus but is being replaced by mycophenolate mofetil, which has fewer side-effects. Azathioprine is also used to maintain remission. Newer agents, which specifically target cells or cytokines in the immune system, are coming into use, especially in refractory cases. These include rituximab (anti-CD20) and belimumab, which are both monoclonal antibodies acting against B lymphocytes.

Prognosis

An episodic course is characteristic, with exacerbations and complete remissions that may last for long periods. However, SLE can also be a chronic persistent condition. The mortality rate in SLE has fallen dramatically over the last 50 years; the 10-year survival rate is about 90%, but this is lower if major organ-based complications are present. Deaths early in the course of disease are mainly due to renal or cerebral disease or infection. Later, coronary artery disease and stroke become more prevalent. Chronic progressive destruction of joints, as seen in RA and OA, occurs rarely, but a few patients develop deformities such as ulnar deviation. People with SLE have an increased long-term risk of developing some cancers, especially lymphoma.

Pregnancy and SLE

Fertility is usually normal, except in severe disease, and there is no major contraindication to pregnancy. Recurrent miscarriages can occur, especially in women with antiphospholipid antibodies. Exacerbations can arise during pregnancy and are frequent postpartum. The patient's medications should be reviewed. Mycophenolate should be stopped, whereas azathioprine, hydroxychloroquine and low-dose oral corticosteroids are safe. Hypertension must be controlled. People with anti-Ro or anti-La antibodies have a 2% risk of giving birth to babies with neonatal lupus syndrome (rash, hepatitis and fetal heart block).

Antiphospholipid syndrome

Patients who have thrombosis (arterial or venous) and/or recurrent miscarriages (see p. 1299), and who also have persistently positive blood tests for antiphospholipid antibodies (aPL), have the antiphospholipid syndrome (APS). Antiphospholipid antibodies can be detected by several different tests:

- The ***anticardiolipin test***, which detects antibodies (IgG or IgM) that bind the negatively charged phospholipid, cardiolipin.
- The ***lupus anticoagulant test***, which detects changes in the ability of blood to clot in a test tube. Despite the name, it is not a test for lupus. It is a test for APS. The ***anticoagulant*** effect caused by aPL in the test tube causes an opposite ***procoagulant*** effect inside the body because the balance of factors stimulating thrombosis is different there.
- The ***anti-β_2-glycoprotein I test***, which detects antibodies that bind β_2-glycoprotein I, a molecule that interacts closely with phospholipids.

A persistently positive test (i.e. positive on at least two occasions ≤12 weeks apart) in one or more of these assays is needed to diagnose APS. However, some people who test positive for aPL will never develop APS; that is, not all aPLs are harmful. APS can present in patients who already have another ARD, especially SLE. APS can also occur on its own (primary APS).

New diagnostic tests for APS are being developed and include anti-prothrombin assays, tests for IgA aPL and tests for antibodies to the N-terminal domain of β_2-glycoprotein I. Although not currently used in clinical practice, these tests may soon be helpful for assessing the overall thrombosis risk of a patient with APS, or for diagnosing patients with 'seronegative' APS who have typical clinical features but test negative for anti-cardiolipin, lupus anticoagulant and anti-β_2-glycoprotein I.

Pathogenesis

Negatively charged phospholipids and β_2-glycoprotein I are present on the outer surface of apoptotic blebs, and so aPLs are believed to arise by a similar mechanism to the lupus autoantibodies described above. Pathogenic aPLs bind to the N-terminal domain of β_2-glycoprotein I. Changes in the oxidation state of β_2-glycoprotein I in patients with APS enhance the availability of this domain to bind aPLs, and this interaction is facilitated when the protein is bound to phospholipid on the surface of cells such as endothelial cells, platelets, monocytes and trophoblasts. This change alters the functioning of those cells, leading to thrombosis and/or miscarriage.

Clinical features

Since APS is defined by the presence of thrombosis and/or pregnancy loss, it is not surprising that these are the most common features. Ischaemic strokes occur in about 20% of patients and deep vein thrombosis in about 40%. Unlike most causes of thrombophilia, APS can cause either arterial or venous thrombosis (though rarely both in the same patient). Some 27% of women who have had two or more spontaneous miscarriages have APS.

Large studies, however, show that people with APS can also have many other features, including:

- thrombocytopenia
- chorea, migraine and epilepsy
- valvular heart disease
- cutaneous manifestations (e.g. livedo reticularis)
- positive Coombs test
- renal impairment due to ischaemia in the small renal vessels.

Occasionally, APS is catastrophic. Catastrophic APS is a rare variant (about 1% of cases) in which multiple infarcts in different organs of the body cause failure of multiple organs simultaneously. There is a high mortality from catastrophic APS.

Management

In people with APS who have had one thrombosis or more, the recommended treatment to prevent further thrombosis is long-term anticoagulation with warfarin. The optimal target INR is unclear and many patients are managed with a lower target INR. Pregnant women with APS are given oral aspirin and subcutaneous low-molecular-weight heparin from early in gestation. This therapy reduces the chance of a miscarriage but pre-eclampsia and poor fetal growth remain common. There are no definite guidelines for managing people with aPL who have never had thrombosis. Aspirin or clopidogrel is sometimes given prophylactically, especially in those with high-IgG aPL. Warfarin is given much more rarely in these circumstances, but may be indicated in patients at particularly high risk: for example, those who test positive for all three of anti-cardiolipin, lupus anticoagulant and anti-β_2-glycoprotein I. Newer anticoagulants that act against specific clotting factors are replacing warfarin in some clinical situations and may come into use in APS. An example is the factor X inhibitor rivaroxaban, which is currently being assessed in a clinical trial in APS.

Systemic sclerosis (scleroderma)

Systemic sclerosis (SSc, or scleroderma; see p. 1366) is a multisystem disease and is distinct from localized scleroderma syndromes, such as morphea, that do not involve internal organ disease and are rarely associated with vasospasm (Raynaud's phenomenon). SSc has the highest case-specific mortality of any of the autoimmune rheumatic diseases. It occurs worldwide but there may be racial or ethnic differences in clinical features. For example, renal involvement is less frequent in Japanese cases.

The incidence of SSc is 10/million population per year with a 3:1 female to male ratio. The peak incidence is between 30 and 50 years of age. It is rare in children.

Environmental risk factors for scleroderma-like disorders include exposure to vinyl chloride, silica dust, adulterated rapeseed oil and trichloroethylene. Drugs such as bleomycin also produce a similar picture. Although unusual, familial cases are reported and twin cohorts suggest higher concordance in monozygotic pairs, consistent with genetic determinants of aetiology.

Pathology and pathogenesis

Vascular features

Widespread vascular damage involving small arteries, arterioles and capillaries is an early lesion. There is initial endothelial cell damage with release of cytokines, including endothelin-1, which causes vasoconstriction. There is continued intimal damage with increasing vascular permeability, leading to cellular activation and activation of adhesion molecules (E-selectin, VCAM, intercellular adhesion molecule 1 (ICAM-1)), with migration of cells into the extracellular matrix. Migrating lymphocytes are IL-2-producing cells, expressing surface antigens such as CD3, CD4 and CD5. All these factors cause release of other mediators (e.g. IL-1, 4, 6 and 8, TGF-β and platelet-derived growth factor) with activation of fibroblasts. Plasma levels of the chemokine CXCL4 are elevated in SSc and correlate with skin and lung fibrosis.

The damage to small blood vessels also produces widespread obliterative arterial lesions and subsequent chronic ischaemia.

Fibrotic features

Fibroblasts synthesize increased quantities of collagen types I and III, as well as fibronectin and glycosaminoglycans, producing fibrosis in the lower dermis of the skin as well as the internal organs. It is possible that antibodies to platelet-derived growth factor receptor, which have been found in blood of people with SSc, stimulate fibroblasts to cause fibrosis.

Clinical features (Fig. 18.36)

Raynaud's phenomenon

Raynaud's phenomenon is seen in almost 100% of cases and can precede the onset of the full-blown disease by many years.

Limited cutaneous scleroderma (LcSSc): 70% of cases

This condition usually starts with Raynaud's phenomenon many years (up to 15) before any skin changes. The skin involvement is limited to the hands, face, feet and forearms. The skin is tight over the fingers and often produces flexion deformities of the fingers. Involvement of the skin of the face produces a characteristic 'beak'-like nose and a small mouth (microstomia). Painful digital ulcers and telangiectasia with dilated nail-fold capillary loops are seen. Digital ischaemia may lead to gangrene. Gastrointestinal tract involvement is common. Pulmonary hypertension develops in 21% of people with LcSSc and pulmonary interstitial disease also occurs.

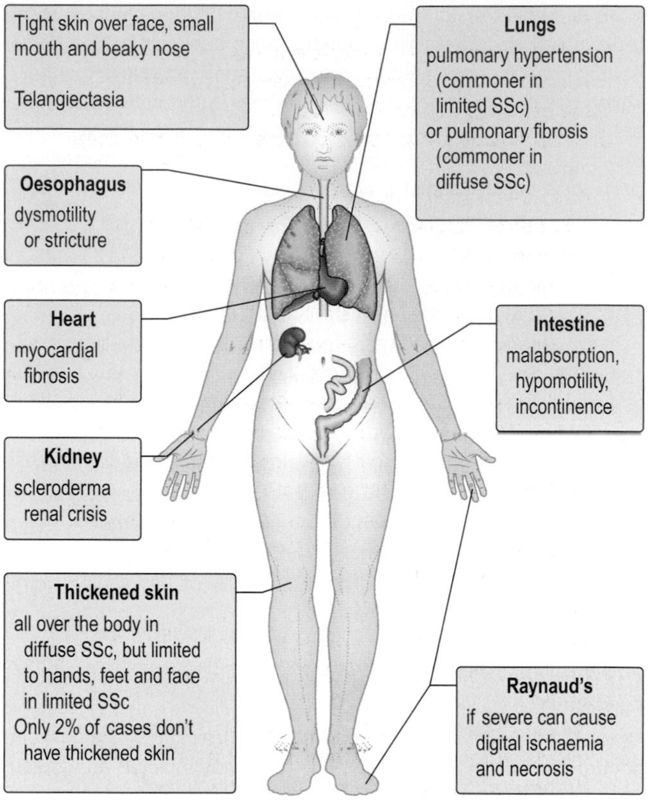

Figure 18.36 Clinical features of systemic sclerosis (SSc).

Diffuse cutaneous scleroderma (DcSSc): 30% of cases

Initially oedematous in onset, skin sclerosis rapidly follows. Raynaud's phenomenon usually starts just before or concomitant with the oedema.

Diffuse swelling and stiffness of the fingers is rapidly followed by more extensive skin thickening, which can involve most of the body in the severest cases. Later, the skin becomes atrophic. Early involvement of other organs occurs with general symptoms of lethargy, anorexia and weight loss.

- ***Gastrointestinal involvement*** includes heartburn, reflux or dysphagia due to oesophageal involvement (see p. 372), which is almost invariable, and anal incontinence occurs in many patients. Malabsorption from bacterial overgrowth due to dilatation and atony of the small bowel is not infrequent; more rarely, dilatation and atony of the colon occurs. Pseudo-obstruction is a known complication.
- ***Renal involvement*** is acute or chronic (see pp. 749–750). Acute hypertensive renal crisis used to be the most common cause of death in systemic sclerosis. Angiotensin-converting enzyme (ACE) inhibitors and better care, along with dialysis and renal transplantation, have changed this.
- ***Lung disease***, both fibrosis (in 41% of cases) and pulmonary hypertension (17% of cases), contributes significantly to mortality in SSc. Pulmonary hypertension can be isolated or secondary to fibrosis, and high plasma levels of endothelin-1 are seen.
- ***Myocardial fibrosis*** leads to arrhythmias and conduction defects. Pericarditis is found occasionally.

Sometimes, these systemic features occur without skin involvement (SSc *sine* scleroderma).

Investigations

- ***Full blood count***. A normochromic, normocytic anaemia occurs and a microangiopathic haemolytic anaemia is seen in some people with renal disease.
- ***Urea and electrolytes***. Urea and creatinine rise in acute kidney injury.
- ***Autoantibodies (Box 18.36)***:
  - ***In LcSSc***: speckled, nucleolar or anti-centromere antibodies (ACAs) occur in 70% of cases. Anti-Th/To antibodies target small nuclear ribonucleoproteins and are found in up to 7% of cases of LcSSC.
  - ***In DcSSc***: there are anti-topoisomerase-1 antibodies (called anti-Scl-70) in 30% of cases, and anti-RNA polymerase (I, II and III) antibodies in 20–25%. Anti-Scl-70 is highly specific for DcSSC. Anti-RNA polymerase positivity is associated with an increased risk of renal involvement. Anti-U3RNP antibodies bind a small nuclear ribonucleoprotein called fibrillarin and are present in up to 6% of patients with SSc – more commonly in DcSSc than LcSSc.
  - ***RF*** is positive in 30%.
  - ***ANA*** is positive in 95%.
- ***Urine*** microscopy and, if there is proteinuria, the urine albumin/creatinine ratio should be measured.
- ***Imaging***:
  - ***Chest X-ray***: to exclude other pathology, for changes in cardiac size and established lung disease.
  - ***Hands***: deposits of calcium around the fingers (in severe cases, erosion and absorption of the tufts of the distal phalanges, termed 'acro-osteolysis').
  - ***Barium swallow***: generally confirms impaired oesophageal motility. Scintigraphy, manometry, impedance and upper gastrointestinal endoscopy are also valuable.
  - ***High-resolution CT***: to demonstrate fibrotic lung involvement.
- ***Other investigations*** of gastrointestinal tract (e.g. see ***Fig. 13.5***), lung, renal and cardiac as appropriate.

Management

Treatment should be organ-based in order to try to control the disease. Currently, there is no cure. In contrast to many other ARDs, corticosteroids and immunosuppressants are rarely used in SSc, with the exception of SSc-related pulmonary fibrosis.

- ***Education***, counselling and family support are essential.
- ***Regular exercises*** and skin lubricants may limit contractures but no treatment has proven efficacy in reducing skin fibrosis.
- ***Raynaud's phenomenon*** may be improved by hand warmers and oral vasodilators (calcium-channel blockers, ACE inhibitors, angiotensin receptor blockers). In severe cases, parenteral vasodilators (prostacyclin analogues and calcitonin gene-related peptide) are used. Lumbar sympathectomy can help foot symptoms. Radical micro-arteriolysis (digital sympathectomy) can be used where individual fingers or toes are severely ischaemic, and thoracic sympathectomy under video-assisted thoracic surgery is now performed.
- ***Oesophageal symptoms*** can almost always be improved by proton pump inhibitors but prokinetic drugs are rarely helpful.
- ***Symptomatic malabsorption*** requires nutritional supplements and rotational antibiotics to treat small intestinal bacterial overgrowth.
- ***Renal involvement*** requires intensive control of hypertension. The first drug of choice is an ACE inhibitor. Vigilance for hypertensive scleroderma renal crisis (SRC) is critical, especially in early-stage dcSSc with rapidly progressive skin and tendon friction rubs. High-dose corticosteroids (above 10 mg prednisolone daily) may increase the risk of SRC.
- ***Pulmonary hypertension*** is treated with oral vasodilators, oxygen and warfarin. Advanced cases should receive prostacyclin therapy (inhaled, subcutaneous or intravenous) or the oral endothelin-receptor antagonists (bosentan and sitaxentan). Right heart failure is treated conventionally and transplantation (heart–lung or single lung) is used in eligible cases.
- ***Pulmonary fibrosis*** is currently treated with immunosuppression, most often with cyclophosphamide or azathioprine combined with low-dose oral prednisolone.

Prognosis

In limited cutaneous scleroderma, the disease is often milder, with much less severe internal organ involvement and a 70% 10-year survival. Pulmonary hypertension is a significant later cause of death. Lung fibrosis and severe gut involvement also determine mortality. In diffuse disease, where organ involvement is often severe at an earlier stage, many patients die of pulmonary, cardiac or renal involvement. Overall, pulmonary involvement (vascular or interstitial) accounts for around 50% of scleroderma-related deaths.

Localized forms of scleroderma occur either in patches (morphea; see p. 1366) or linear forms. These are more commonly seen in children and adolescents, and do not convert into systemic forms, although ANA may occur in localized scleroderma and, very occasionally, localized and systemic forms coexist.

Polymyositis and dermatomyositis

Polymyositis (PM) is a rare disorder of unknown cause, in which the clinical picture is dominated by inflammation of striated muscle, causing proximal muscle weakness. When the skin is involved, it is called 'dermatomyositis' (DM). The incidence is about 2–10/million population *per annum* and it occurs in all races and at all ages. The aetiology is unknown, although viruses (e.g. *Coxsackie*, rubella, influenza) have been implicated and persons with HLA-B8/DR3 appear to be genetically predisposed.

Clinical features

Adult polymyositis

Women are affected three times more commonly than men.

The onset can be insidious, over months, or acute. General malaise, weight loss and fever can develop during the acute phase, but the cardinal symptom is proximal muscle weakness. The shoulder and pelvic girdle muscles become wasted but are not usually tender. Face and distal limb muscles are not usually affected. Movements such as squatting and climbing stairs become difficult. As the disease progresses, involvement of pharyngeal, laryngeal and respiratory muscles can lead to dysphonia and respiratory failure. These severe complications are rare if the disease is treated early.

Adult dermatomyositis

This condition is also more common in women. Apart from muscle weakness, these patients often suffer from myalgia, polyarthritis and Raynaud's phenomenon, but DM is primarily distinguished from PM by the characteristic rash. This typically affects the eyelids,

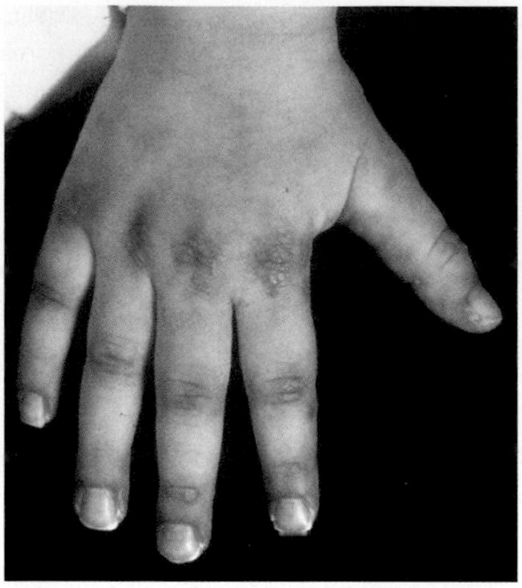

Figure 18.37 **Purplish Gottron's papules over the knuckles (dermatomyositis).** *(Courtesy of David Paige, London.)*

where heliotrope (purple) discoloration is accompanied by periorbital oedema, and the fingers, where purple–red, raised vasculitic patches are seen. These patches occur over the knuckles (Gottron's papules; ***Fig. 18.37***) in 70% of patients, and this appearance is highly specific for DM. Ulcerative vasculitis and calcinosis of the subcutaneous tissue are seen in 25% of cases. In the long term, muscle fibrosis and contractures of joints occur.

Antisynthetase syndrome

Some 20–30% of people with PM or DM have antibodies to tRNA synthetase enzymes. These people are more likely to develop pulmonary interstitial fibrosis, Raynaud's phenomenon, arthritis, and hardening and fissuring of skin over the pulp surface of the fingers (mechanic's hands). This variant of PM/DM is sometimes called anti-synthetase syndrome and often has a poor outcome. Respiratory muscles are affected in PM/DM and this compounds the effects of interstitial fibrosis. Dysphagia is seen in about 50% of patients owing to oesophageal muscle involvement.

Association with other ARDs

There is an association with other ARDs (e.g. SLE, RA and SSc) and their associated clinical features, such as deforming arthritis, malar rash and skin sclerosis.

Association with malignancies

The relative risk of cancer is 2.4 for male and 3.4 for female patients, and a wide variety of cancers have been reported. The onset and clinical picture do not differ from those of typical DM/PM. The associated cancer may not become apparent for 2–3 years, and recurrent, refractory or ANA-negative DM should prompt a search for occult malignancy.

Malignancy (e.g. lung, ovary, breast, stomach) can also predate the onset of myositis, particularly in males with DM.

Childhood dermatomyositis

This variant most commonly affects children between the ages of 4 and 10 years. The typical rash of DM is usually accompanied by muscle weakness. Muscle atrophy, subcutaneous calcification and contractures may be widespread and severe. Ulcerative skin vasculitis is common and recurrent abdominal pain due to vasculitis is also a feature.

Investigations

- ***Serum creatine kinase*** **(*CK*)**, aminotransferases, lactate dehydrogenase (LDH) and aldolase are usually raised and are useful guides to muscle damage, but may not reflect activity.
- ***ESR*** and ***CRP*** may be raised.
- ***Serum autoantibody studies*** include antinuclear antibody testing, which is usually positive in people with DM. RF is present in up to 50%, and many ***myositis-specific antibodies*** (MSAs) have been recognized and correlate with certain subsets. Anti-synthetase antibodies have been described above.
- ***Electromyography*** **(*EMG*)** shows a typical triad of changes with myositis: spontaneous fibrillation potentials at rest, polyphasic or short-duration potentials on voluntary contraction, and salvos of repetitive potentials on mechanical stimulation of the nerve.
- ***MRI*** can be used to detect abnormally inflamed muscle.
- ***Needle muscle biopsy*** shows fibre necrosis and regeneration in association with an inflammatory cell infiltrate with lymphocytes around the blood vessels and between muscle fibres. Open biopsy allows more thorough assessment.
- ***Screening for malignancy*** is usually limited to relatively non-invasive investigations such as chest X-ray, mammography, pelvic/abdominal ultrasound, urine microscopy and a search for circulating tumour markers.
- ***PET*** scanning can detect malignancy.

Management

Bed rest may be helpful but must be combined with an exercise programme. Prednisolone is the mainstay of treatment: 0.5–1.0 mg/kg body weight as initial therapy, continued until at least 1 month after myositis has become clinically and enzymatically inactive. Tapering of steroids must be slow. Early intervention with steroid-sparing agents, such as methotrexate, azathioprine, ciclosporin, cyclophosphamide and mycophenolate mofetil, is common, especially where there is clinical relapse or a rise in CK as the dose of steroids is reduced. Intravenous immunoglobulin therapy (IVIG) is helpful in some recalcitrant cases. Treatment of childhood DM tends to be more intensive, with earlier use of immunosuppressive agents. Use of biological agents such as rituximab has been described. Rituximab is more likely to be effective in autoantibody-positive cases.

Inclusion body myositis

Inclusion body myositis is an idiopathic inflammatory myopathy usually occurring in men over 50 years. Weakness of the pharyngeal muscles causes difficulty in swallowing in over 50%. It is a slowly progressive weakness of mainly distal muscles. In contrast to polymyositis, the CK is only slightly elevated; the EMG shows both myopathic and neuropathic changes. On MRI, the changes are often more distal but can be similar to those of polymyositis. A muscle biopsy shows inflammation and basophilic rimmed vacuoles with diagnostic filamentous inclusions and vacuoles on electron microscopy. A trial of corticosteroids is worthwhile but generally the response is poor.

Sjögren syndrome

The syndrome of dry eyes (keratoconjunctivitis sicca) in the absence of RA or any of the autoimmune diseases is known as 'primary Sjögren syndrome'. There is an association with HLA-B8/DR3.

Dryness of the mouth, skin or vagina may also be a problem. Salivary and parotid gland enlargement is seen. In the majority of cases, dryness and fatigue are the only symptoms, and Sjögren syndrome is irritating and inconvenient rather than dangerous. However, in a minority there may be systemic symptoms such as:

- arthralgia and occasional non-progressive polyarthritis, like that seen in SLE (but much less common)
- Raynaud's phenomenon
- dysphagia and abnormal oesophageal motility, as seen in systemic sclerosis (but less common)
- other organ-specific autoimmune disease, including thyroid disease, myasthenia gravis, primary biliary cirrhosis, autoimmune hepatitis and pancreatitis
- renal tubular defects (uncommon) causing nephrogenic diabetes insipidus and renal tubular acidosis
- pulmonary diffusion defects and fibrosis
- polyneuropathy, fits and depression
- vasculitis
- increased incidence of non-Hodgkin's B-cell lymphoma.

Pathology and investigations

Biopsies of the salivary gland or of the lip show a focal infiltration of lymphocytes and plasma cells.

- ***Schirmer tear test***. A standard strip of filter paper is placed on the inside of the lower eyelid; wetting of <10 mm in 5 min indicates defective tear production.
- ***Rose Bengal staining***. Staining of the eyes shows punctate or filamentary keratitis.
- ***Laboratory abnormalities***. These include raised immunoglobulin levels, circulating immune complexes and autoantibodies. RF is usually positive. Antinuclear antibodies are found in 80% of cases and anti-mitochondrial antibodies in 10%. Anti-Ro (SSA) antibodies are found in 60–90%, compared with 10% of cases of RA and secondary Sjögren syndrome. This antibody is of particular interest because it can cross the placenta and cause congenital heart block.

Management

Symptomatic treatment is with artificial tears and saliva replacement solutions. Hydroxychloroquine may help fatigue and arthralgia. Corticosteroids are rarely needed but are used to treat persistent salivary gland swelling or neuropathy. A trial of rituximab in Sjögren syndrome is under way but it is not yet standard therapy.

'Overlap' syndromes and undifferentiated autoimmune rheumatic disease

An ***overlap syndrome*** is one where the patient shows the characteristic clinical features of more than one ARD. Treatment of each ARD is usually the same as when they occur separately.

Undifferentiated ARD is a term used for the condition of patients who have evidence of autoimmunity (e.g. positive autoantibody test) and some clinical features of such diseases (commonly, Raynaud's phenomenon and/or arthralgia) but not enough to make a clear diagnosis of any individual ARD. These patients sometimes develop a clearer ARD over time, but some always remain undifferentiated and tend to have relatively mild disease without major organ problems.

Further reading

Giannokopoulos B, Krilis S. The pathogenesis of the antiphospholipid syndrome. *New Engl J Med* 2013; 368:1033–1044.

Rahman A, Isenberg DA. Systemic lupus erythematosus. *N Engl J Med* 2008; 358:929–939.

Ruiz-Irastorza G, Crowther M, Branch W et al. Antiphospholipid syndrome. *Lancet* 2011; 376:1498–1509.

Tsokos G. Systemic lupus erythematosus. *N Engl J Med* 2011; 378:1949–1961.

SYSTEMIC INFLAMMATORY VASCULITIS

Vasculitis is a histological term describing inflammation of the vessel wall. Vasculitis can be seen in many diseases ***(Boxes 18.37–18.38)***. The group of diseases described in this section (systemic inflammatory vasculitides) is characterized by widespread vasculitis leading to systemic symptoms and signs, generally requiring treatment with corticosteroids and/or immunosuppressive drugs. Two main features are helpful in classifying these vasculitides: the ***size of the blood vessels involved*** and the ***presence or absence of anti-neutrophil cytoplasmic antibodies*** (***ANCA***) in the blood. Revisions in the commonly used terms for various vasculitides have been proposed to reflect increased pathophysiological understanding of these conditions (***Fig. 18.38*** and ***Box 18.38***).

- ***Large-vessel vasculitis*** refers to the aorta and its major tributaries.
- ***Medium-vessel vasculitis*** refers to medium- and small-sized arteries and arterioles.
- ***Small-vessel vasculitis*** refers to small arteries, arterioles, venules and capillaries.

Box 18.37 Types of systemic vasculitis

Large-vessel
- Giant cell arteritis/polymyalgia rheumatica
- Takayasu's arteritis

Medium-vessel
- Classical polyarteritis nodosa (PAN)
- Kawasaki's disease

Small-vessel

• Microscopic polyangiitis • Granulomatosis with polyangiitis • Eosinophilic granulomatosis with polyangiitis (30–50% ANCA-positive) • Immunoglobulin A (Henoch–Schönlein) vasculitis	ANCA-associated
• Cutaneous leucocytoclastic vasculitis • Essential cryoglobulinaemia	ANCA-negative

ANCA, anti-neutrophil cytoplasmic antibodies.

Box 18.38 Other conditions associated with vasculitis[a]

Infective
- e.g. Subacute infective endocarditis

Non-infective
- Vasculitis with rheumatoid arthritis
- Systemic lupus erythematosus
- Scleroderma
- Polymyositis/dermatomyositis
- Drug-induced Behçet's disease
- Goodpasture syndrome
- Hypocomplementaemia
- Serum sickness
- Paraneoplastic syndromes
- Inflammatory bowel disease

[a]*See also* ***Box 18.37***.

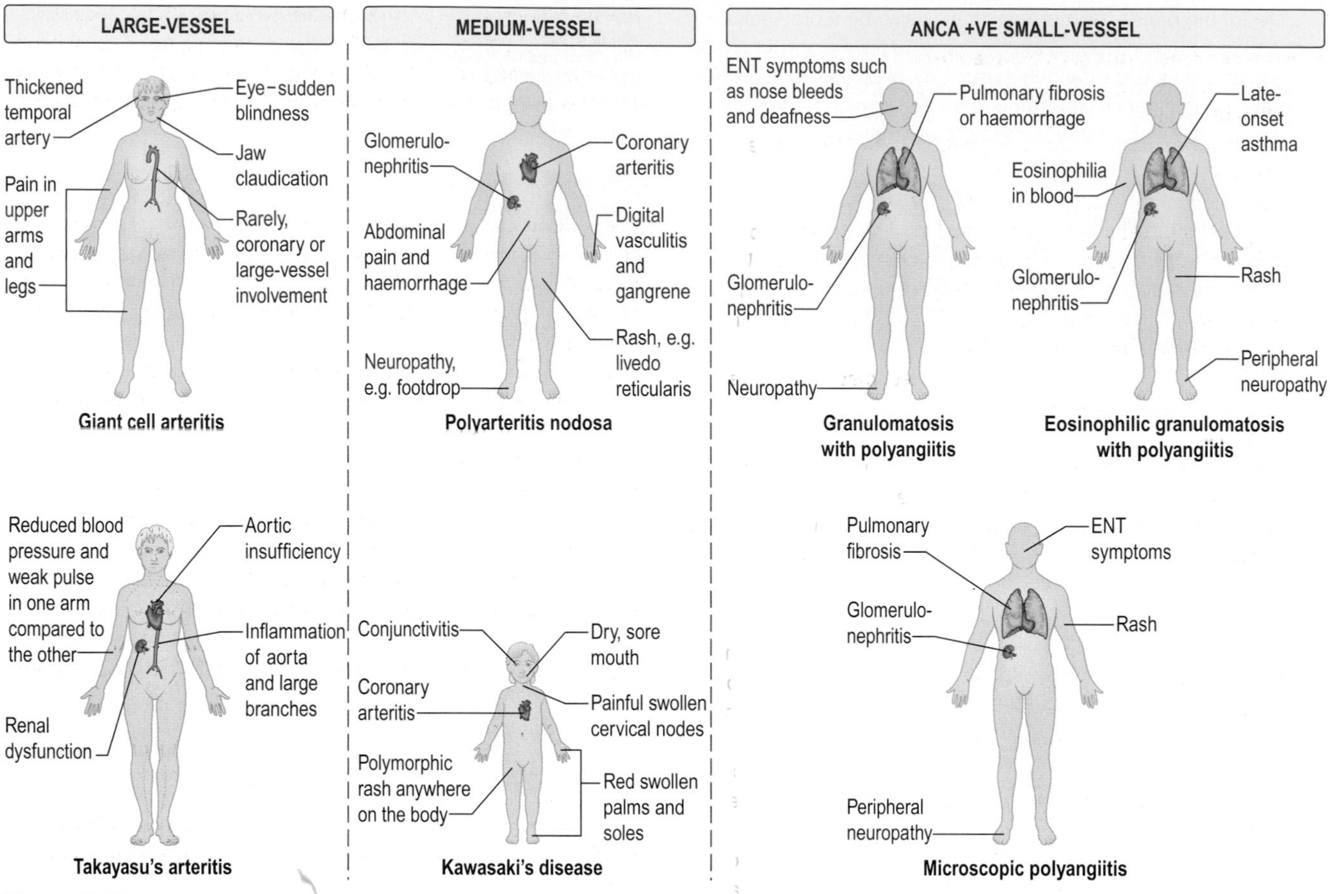

Figure 18.38 Clinical features of systemic inflammatory vasculitides. These illnesses all frequently present with joint pain, as well as systemic symptoms such as fatigue, malaise and weight loss. The most common organ-specific manifestations are shown. Giant cell arteritis is usually seen in people over 50, whereas Takayasu's disease is seen in people under 50. Kawasaki's disease is usually seen in children under 5. ANCA, anti-neutrophil cytoplasmic antibodies; ENT, ear, nose and throat.

Box 18.39 Symptom patterns in some muscle disorders

- ***Polymyositis*** – proximal muscle ache and weakness
- ***Polymyalgia rheumatica*** – proximal morning stiffness and pain
- ***Myopathy*** – weakness, but no pain or stiffness

Large-vessel vasculitis

Polymyalgia rheumatica and giant cell (temporal) arteritis are systemic illnesses of the elderly. Both are associated with the finding of a giant cell arteritis on temporal artery biopsy.

Polymyalgia rheumatica

Polymyalgia rheumatica (PMR) causes a sudden onset of severe pain and stiffness of the shoulders and neck, and of the hips and lumbar spine: a limb girdle pattern. These symptoms are worse in the morning, lasting from 30 minutes to several hours. The clinical history is usually diagnostic and the patient is always over 50 years old. Up to 25% of patients may have some inflammation of peripheral joints.

Approximately one-third of patients develop systemic features of tiredness, fever, weight loss, depression and occasionally nocturnal sweats, especially if PMR is not diagnosed and treated early. A differential diagnosis is shown in ***Box 18.39***.

Investigation of PMR

- ***A raised ESR and/or CRP*** is a hallmark of this condition. It is rare to see PMR without an acute-phase response. If it is absent, the diagnosis should be questioned and the tests repeated a few weeks later before treatment is started.
- ***Serum alkaline phosphatase and γ-glutamyl-transpeptidase*** may be raised as markers of the acute inflammation.
- ***Anaemia*** (mild normochromic, normocytic) is often present.
- ***Temporal artery biopsy*** shows giant cell arteritis in 10–30% of cases, but is rarely performed unless giant cell arteritis is also suspected.

Giant cell arteritis

Giant cell arteritis (GCA) is inflammatory granulomatous arteritis of large cerebral arteries, which occurs in association with PMR. The patient may have current PMR or a history of recent PMR, or may be on treatment for PMR. It is extremely rare under 50 years of age. Presenting symptoms of GCA include severe headaches, tenderness of the scalp (combing the hair may be painful) or of the temple, claudication of the jaw when eating, and tenderness and swelling of one or more temporal or occipital arteries. The most feared manifestation is sudden, painless, temporary or permanent loss of vision in one eye due to involvement of the ophthalmic artery (see pp. 845–846). Systemic manifestations of severe malaise, tiredness and fever occur.

Investigation of GCA

- ***Normochromic, normocytic anaemia***.
- ***ESR*** is usually raised (in the region of 50–120 mm/h) and the CRP very high.
- ***Liver biochemistry*** may be abnormal, as in PMR. The albumin may be low.
- A ***temporal artery biopsy*** from the affected side is the definitive diagnostic test. This should be taken before, or within 7 days of starting, high doses of corticosteroids. The lesions are patchy and the whole length of the biopsy (>1 cm long) must be examined; even so, negative biopsies occur.

The ***histological features*** of GCA are:

- Cellular infiltrates of CD4+ T lymphocytes, macrophages and giant cells in the vessel wall. Note that giant cells are not visible in all cases.
- Granulomatous inflammation of the intima and media.
- Breaking up of the internal elastic lamina.
- Giant cells, lymphocytes and plasma cells in the internal elastic lamina.

Management of PMR or GCA

Corticosteroids produce a dramatic reduction of symptoms of PMR within 24–48 hours of starting treatment, provided the dose is adequate. If this improvement does not occur, the diagnosis should be questioned and an alternative cause sought, such as RA, vasculitis, infection or malignancy. This treatment should reduce the risk of patients who have PMR developing GCA. NSAIDs are less effective and should not be used.

In GCA, corticosteroids are obligatory because they significantly reduce the risk of irreversible visual loss and other focal ischaemic lesions, but much higher doses are needed than in PMR. If GCA is suspected, it may not be possible to arrange a temporal artery biopsy rapidly. In these circumstances, treatment should not be delayed, especially if there have already been episodes of visual loss or stroke.

Starting daily doses of prednisolone are:

- ***PMR***: 10–15 mg prednisolone as a single dose in the morning
- ***GCA***: 60–100 mg prednisolone, usually in divided doses.

The dose should then be reduced gradually in weekly or monthly steps. While the dose is above 20 mg, the step reductions are 5 mg, reducing the evening doses first. Between 20 mg and 10 mg, the reduction can be in 2.5 mg steps, but below 10 mg the rate should be slower and the steps of 1 mg each. Most patients will eventually be able to stop corticosteroids after 12–18 months but up to 25% may need low doses long-term. Steroid-sparing immunosuppressive agents are used in refractory cases where it is hard to reduce the corticosteroid dose without causing a flare of disease or a rise in ESR or CRP.

Calcium and vitamin D supplements, and sometimes bisphosphonates, are necessary to prevent osteoporosis while high-dose steroids are being used (see pp. 713–715).

Takayasu's arteritis

Takayasu's is a granulomatous inflammation of the aorta and its major branches; it is discussed on pages 1054–1055.

Medium-sized vessel vasculitis

Polyarteritis nodosa

Classical polyarteritis nodosa (PAN) is a rare condition that usually occurs in middle-aged men. It is accompanied by severe systemic manifestations, and its occasional association with hepatitis B antigenaemia suggests a vasculitis secondary to the deposition of immune complexes. Pathologically, there is fibrinoid necrosis of vessel walls with microaneurysm formation, thrombosis and infarction.

Clinical features

These include fever, malaise, weight loss and myalgia. These initial symptoms are followed by dramatic acute features that are due to organ infarction.

- ***Neurological***. Mononeuritis multiplex is due to arteritis of the vasa nervorum.
- ***Abdominal***. Pain is due to arterial involvement of the abdominal viscera, mimicking acute cholecystitis, pancreatitis or appendicitis. Gastrointestinal haemorrhage occurs because of mucosal ulceration.
- ***Renal***. Presentation is with haematuria and proteinuria. Hypertension and acute/chronic kidney disease occur.
- ***Cardiac***. Coronary arteritis causes myocardial infarction and heart failure. Pericarditis also occurs.
- ***Skin***. Subcutaneous haemorrhage and gangrene occur. A persistent livedo reticularis is seen in chronic cases. Cutaneous and subcutaneous palpable nodules occur but are uncommon.
- ***Lung***. Involvement is rare.

Investigations and management

- ***Blood count***. Anaemia, leucocytosis and a raised ESR occur.
- ***Biopsy***. Material from an affected organ shows features listed above.
- ***Angiography***. Microaneurysms in hepatic, intestinal or renal vessels can be demonstrated if necessary.
- ***Other investigations***. These are performed as appropriate (e.g. electrocardiogram and abdominal ultrasound), depending on the clinical problem. ANCA is positive only rarely in classic PAN.

Treatment is with corticosteroids, usually in combination with immunosuppressive drugs such as azathioprine.

Kawasaki's disease

Kawasaki's disease is an acute systemic vasculitis involving medium-sized vessels, affecting mainly children under 5 years of age. It is very frequent in Japan and an infective trigger is suspected. It occurs worldwide and is also seen in adults.

Clinical features and management

The clinical features are:

- fever lasting 5 days or more
- bilateral conjunctival congestion 2–4 days after onset
- dryness and redness of the lips and oral cavity 3 days after onset
- acute cervical lymphadenopathy accompanying the fever
- polymorphic rash involving any part of the body
- redness and oedema of the palms and soles 2–5 days after onset

The persistent fever plus at least four of the other five features should be present to make the diagnosis, or fewer than four if coronary aneurysms can be seen on two-dimensional echocardiography, MRI or angiography.

Cardiovascular changes in the acute stage include pancarditis and coronary arteritis, leading to aneurysms or dilatation.

Other features include diarrhoea, albuminuria, aseptic meningitis and arthralgia; in most, there is a leucocytosis, thrombocytosis and a raised CRP. Anti-endothelial cell autoantibodies are often detectable.

Treatment is with a single dose of high-dose intravenous immunoglobulin (2 g/kg), which prevents the coronary artery disease, followed after the acute phase by aspirin 200–300 mg daily. There is no evidence that steroid treatment improves the outcome.

Small-vessel vasculitis

The two revised categories of small-vessel vasculitis (SVV) are characterized by a ***paucity of vessel wall immunoglobulin*** and presence (in many but not all patients) of ANCA in one, and a ***prominence of vessel wall immunoglobulin*** in the other (see pp. 1120–1121).

ANCA-associated vasculitis (AAV) includes:

- granulomatosis with polyangiitis (GPA; see p. 1121)
- eosinophilic granulomatosis with polyangiitis (EGPA; see p. 1121)
- microscopic polyangiitis (MPA; see p. 1121).

Immune complex (ANCA-negative) small-vessel vasculitis includes:

- anti-glomerular basement membrane (anti-GBM) disease (see p. 1121)
- IgA vasculitis (IgAV, Henoch–Schönlein) (see p. 748)
- cryoglobulinaemic vasculitis (CV) (see p. 748)
- hypocomplementaemic urticarial vasculitis (HUV, anti-C1q vasculitis)
- cutaneous leucocytoclastic vasculitis (see p. 1377).

Cutaneous leucocytoclastic vasculitis is the characteristic acute purpuric lesion that histologically involves the dermal post-capillary venules. This lesion affects only the skin and should be differentiated from similar lesions produced in systemic vasculitis. The purpura may be accompanied by arthralgia and glomerulonephritis. Hepatitis C infection is common and may be an aetiological agent. The condition can also be caused by drugs such as sulphonamides and penicillin.

Primary central nervous system vasculitis is a very rare condition (incidence 2–4 cases per million person years) characterized by clinical features confined to the central nervous system and characteristic appearances on angiography or cerebral biopsy. The most common clinical features are headache, altered cognition, focal weakness and stroke. Blood tests, including inflammatory markers and autoantibodies, are usually normal but a normal cerebral MRI essentially excludes the diagnosis.

Management of small-cell vasculitis

The treatment depends on the organs involved. Vasculitis confined to the skin may not require systemic treatment, whereas involvement of major organs (e.g. lungs or kidneys in GPA) requires high-dose corticosteroids, immunosuppression and, sometimes, plasma exchange. Clinical trials have shown that depletion of B cells with rituximab is as effective as cyclophosphamide in treating AAV and can help reduce the dose of corticosteroids required to maintain remission.

Behçet's disease

Behçet's disease is an inflammatory disorder of unknown cause. There is a striking geographical distribution, it being most common in Turkey, Iran and Japan. The prevalence per 100 000 is 10–15 in Japan and 80–300 in Turkey. There is a link to the HLA-B51 allele, with a relative risk of 5–10; this association is not seen in patients in the USA and Europe.

Clinical features

The cardinal clinical feature is recurrent oral ulceration. The ***international criteria for diagnosis*** require oral ulceration and any two of the following:

- genital ulcers
- defined eye lesions, including an anterior or posterior uveitis or retinal vascular lesions
- defined skin lesions – erythema nodosum, pseudofolliculitis and papulopustular lesions
- positive skin pathergy test (see below)
- oral ulcers – aphthous or herpetiform.

Other manifestations include a self-limiting peripheral mono- or oligoarthritis affecting knees, ankles, wrists and elbows; gastrointestinal symptoms of diarrhoea, abdominal pain and anorexia; pulmonary and renal lesions; thrombophlebitis (especially in the legs); vasculitis; and a brainstem syndrome, organic confusional states and a meningoencephalitis. All the common manifestations are self-limiting except for the ocular attacks. Repeated attacks of uveitis can cause blindness.

The ***pathergy reaction*** is highly specific to Behçet's disease. Skin injury – by a needle prick, for example – leads to papule or pustule formation within 24–48 hours. Blood tests usually show raised ESR and CRP but not autoantibodies.

Management

Corticosteroids, immunosuppressive agents and ciclosporin are used for chronic uveitis and the rare neurological complications. Colchicine helps erythema nodosum and joint pain. Thalidomide may be useful in some cases, although side-effects of drowsiness and peripheral neuropathy are common. It should not be used in pregnant women because of phocomelia (limb abnormalities). Anti-TNF agents can be used to control severe uveitis and serious manifestations such as neurological and gastrointestinal Behçet's disease.

Further reading

Jennette JC, Falk RJ, Bacon PA et al. 2012 revised International Chapel Hill Consensus Conference nomenclature of vasculitides. *Arthritis Rheum* 2013; 65:1–11.

Kermani TA, Warrington KJ. Polymyalgia rheumatica. *Lancet* 2013; 381:63–72.

Warrell DA, Cox TM, Firth JD (eds). *Oxford Textbook of Medicine*, 5th edn. Oxford: Oxford University Press; 2010. Section 19.11 Autoimmune rheumatic disorders and vasculitides; Section 21.10.2 The kidney in systemic vasculitis.

ARTHRITIS IN CHILDREN

Joint and limb pains are common in children but arthritis is, fortunately, rare. Babies and young children may present with immobility of a joint or a limp, but the diagnosis can be extremely difficult. ***Figure 18.39*** summarizes the differential diagnosis.

For chronic conditions, the child and family often need a great deal of support from physiotherapists, occupational therapists, psychologists, teachers, social workers and orthopaedic surgeons. These are best obtained in specialist paediatric centres.

Juvenile idiopathic arthritis

Systemic-onset juvenile idiopathic arthritis

Still's disease (which accounts for 10% of cases of juvenile idiopathic arthritis (JIA)) affects boys and girls equally up to 5 years of age; after this, girls are more commonly affected. Adult-onset Still's disease is rare.

Juvenile idiopathic arthritis

Systemic arthritis
Oligoarthritis (persistent)
Oligoarthritis (extended)
Polyarthritis (rheumatoid-factor positive)
Polyarthritis (rheumatoid-factor negative)
Enthesitis-related arthritis
Psoriatic arthritis
Unclassified

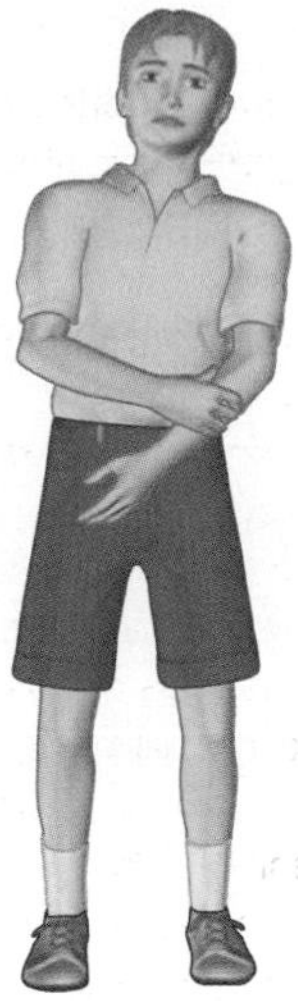

Other conditions

Henoch–Schönlein purpura
Infections, e.g. tuberculosis, septic arthritis, viral arthritis
Rheumatic fever
Hypermobility syndrome
Leukaemia
Sickle cell disease
SLE and other autoimmune rheumatic disease
Transient synovitis of the hip
Perthes' disease

Figure 18.39 **The differential diagnosis of arthritis in children.** SLE, systemic lupus erythematosus.

Clinical features include a high (>39°) fever with an evanescent pink maculopapular rash and arthralgia, arthritis, myalgia and generalized lymphadenopathy. Hepatosplenomegaly, pericarditis and pleurisy occur. The differential diagnoses include malignancy – in particular, leukaemia and neuroblastoma – and infection. Laboratory tests show a high ESR and CRP, neutrophilia and thrombocytosis. Autoantibodies are negative. Macrophage activation syndrome (an excessive proliferation of T cells and macrophages) is a rare but potentially fatal complication, which can follow infection (often viral) or a change in medication.

Oligoarthritis (persistent)

This variant is the most common form of JIA (50–60%) but is still a relatively uncommon condition. It affects, by definition, four or fewer joints, especially knees, ankles and wrists, often in an asymmetrical pattern. It affects mainly girls, with a peak age of 3 years. The prognosis is generally good, with most going into remission. Uveitis (often with a positive ANA) occurs and requires regular screening by slit-lamp examination. Blindness can occur if it is untreated. Prognosis is generally good, with remission occurring eventually in most patients.

Oligoarthritis (extended)

In approximately 25% of patients, oligoarthritis extends to affect many more joints after around 6 months. This form of arthritis can be very destructive.

Polyarthritis JIA

The ***RF-positive*** form (usually also ACPA-positive) occurs in older girls, usually over 8 years. It is a systemic disease; the arthritis commonly involves the small joints of the hands, wrists, ankles and feet initially, and eventually larger joints. It can be a very destructive arthritis and needs aggressive treatment.

The ***RF-negative*** form is more common. It usually affects girls under 12 years but can occur at any age. The arthritis is often asymmetrical, with a distribution similar to that seen in the RF-positive form. It may also affect the cervical spine, temporomandibular joints and elbows. Patients may be ANA-positive, with a risk of chronic uveitis. All children must have regular ophthalmological examination.

Enthesitis-related arthritis

This form affects teenage and younger boys mainly, often those with a family history of HLA-B27 disorders. It produces an asymmetrical arthritis of lower-limb joints and enthesitis. It is associated with HLA-B27 and a risk of iritis. It is the childhood equivalent of adult ankylosing spondylitis but spinal involvement is rare in childhood. Approximately 1 in 3 develops spinal disease in adulthood.

Psoriatic arthritis

This arthritis occurs in children and is similar in pattern to the adult form. The arthritis can be very destructive. Psoriasis may develop long after the arthritis but is found commonly in a first-degree relative.

Management of JIA

Early recognition and aggressive treatment prevent joint damage and allow normal growth and development. There is no cure but clinical remission is an achievable goal. JIA should always be referred to a specialist paediatric rheumatology unit with facilities to assess and design treatment plans that aim to prevent long-term disability. These units also need facilities for rehabilitation, education and surgical intervention. NSAIDs reduce pain and stiffness, but disease-modifying agents such as methotrexate are used to control moderate and severe disease. Corticosteroids are often required in systemic disease: intravenous pulsed methylprednisolone is used, followed by methotrexate (10–15 mg/m^2) weekly to control disease and prevent growth suppression.

Cytokine modulators (see ***Box 18.30***) are used if methotrexate fails; they are highly effective in all types except systemic-onset JIA, where the results are variable. Etanercept and adalimumab are the most common drugs used but anakinra, tocilizumab and abatacept are being used in systemic-onset JIA. Anakinra (see p. 682), an IL-1β receptor antagonist, helps in methotrexate-resistant systemic-onset disease. Sulfasalazine is used only in enthesitis-related JIA. Aspirin may be a cause of Reye syndrome and should not be used under the age of 12 years.

Prognosis

Before cytokine modulators, up to 50% of children developed long-term disability; 25% continued to have active arthritis into adult years. Death was due to infection or systemic disease with pericarditis or amyloidosis. The prognosis is much improved but long-term studies, particularly on safety, are awaited.

Childhood rheumatic diseases other than juvenile idiopathic arthritis

IgA vasculitis (Henoch–Schönlein purpura)

This condition is the most common systemic vasculitis seen in children. It is described on page 748.

Rheumatic fever

Rheumatic fever still occurs occasionally in developed countries but is more common in developing countries. It is described on page 282.

The arthritis affects large joints and migrates between joints, each being affected for a few days at a time. This pattern is unlike systemic-onset JIA, where arthritis is usually much more persistent in each affected joint. The fever is persistent but rarely as high as in systemic-onset JIA, and the temperature often remains above normal. A child may not volunteer a history of sore throat and the carditis may be silent. Isolated arthritis is the presenting symptom in 14–42%. The disease is easily missed if not included in the differential diagnosis of acute childhood arthritis.

Treatment is described on page 282.

Hypermobility and hypermobility syndrome

A large proportion of children are hypermobile in at least one joint. Though in most cases it is asymptomatic and causes no problems, a proportion of them will develop various musculoskeletal complaints in early childhood, such as late walking, flat feet or nocturnal leg pains, probably due to hypermobile ankles and knees suffering recurrent sprains and strains after exercise. Joint effusions, subluxation, dislocation and ligamentous injuries may occur throughout childhood. Low back pain may develop in affected adolescents. These symptoms in hypermobile children may lead to a diagnosis of joint hypermobility syndrome (Ehlers–Danlos syndrome type III; see pp. 666–667).

More severe hypermobility is also seen in the other, rarer forms of Ehlers–Danlos syndrome and Marfan syndrome (see pp. 667 and 1028–1029).

Management is with exercise directed at improving the strength of muscles that cross affected joints, as well as overall fitness and endurance. It may be necessary to reduce or change sporting and other activities. Cognitive behavioural therapy helps in teenagers.

Idiopathic musculoskeletal pain

This can become chronic in children. Management requires exclusion of the causes shown in ***Figure 18.39***, but without performing unnecessary laboratory investigations. Nocturnal musculoskeletal pains are episodic and may be associated with hypermobility. They are called ‘growing pains’. They often last 15–30 minutes and awaken the child from sleep, and may require physiotherapy and analgesics, together with advice and support for the parents.

Low back pain in children may reflect psychosocial problems at home or school as much as any obvious musculoskeletal pathology.

Osteochondritis

Osteochondritis can affect the ossification centre of the ends of bones. A typical condition is ***Osgood–Schlatter disease***, which is characterized by localized pain and swelling over the tibial tubercle or at the patellar tendon insertion. It is usually seen in athletic teenagers and responds to local treatment and changes of sporting activities. ***Sever’s disease*** is an osteochondritis of the insertion of the Achilles tendon into the calcaneum.

Perthes’ disease

This is an idiopathic, possibly avascular, necrosis of the proximal femoral epiphysis, of unknown aetiology. It presents as a painless limp, usually in boys aged 3–12 years, and is occasionally bilateral. If severe, it may require surgical correction.

Transient synovitis of the hip (irritable hip)

This causes painful limitation of movement, usually of one hip, after an upper respiratory infection in young children (usually boys). Symptoms usually resolve within a few weeks (2–3% develop Perthes’ disease) but other more serious causes of hip pain should be excluded. Management is with rest and analgesia until the pain resolves.

Further reading

Prakken B, Albani S, Martini A. Juvenile idiopathic arthritis. *Lancet* 2011; 377:2138–2149.

Prince FH, Otten MH, van Suijlekom-Smit WA. Diagnosis and management of juvenile idiopathic arthritis. *BMJ* 2011; 342:95–102.

RHEUMATOLOGICAL PROBLEMS SEEN IN OTHER DISEASES

Gastrointestinal and liver disease

- ***Enteropathic synovitis*** (see pp. 686–687).
- ***Autoimmune hepatitis*** (see pp. 463–464) may be accompanied by an arthralgia similar to that seen in SLE. Joint pain occurs in a bilateral, symmetrical distribution, predominantly affecting the small joints of the hands. Joints usually look normal but sometimes there is a slight soft tissue swelling. These patients often have positive tests for antinuclear antibodies.
- ***Primary biliary cholangitis*** patients occasionally have a symmetrical arthropathy.
- ***Hereditary haemochromatosis*** is associated with arthritis in 50% of cases, which is often the first sign of the disease and cartilage calcification is common.
- ***Whipple’s disease*** (see p. 400) is accompanied by fever and arthralgia.

Malignant disease

It is not uncommon for malignant diseases to present with musculoskeletal symptoms. Gout occurs in conditions such as chronic myeloid leukaemia. Neoplastic disease of bone is described on pages 718–719.

Hypertrophic pulmonary osteoarthropathy

Hypertrophic pulmonary osteoarthropathy (HPO) is a paraneoplastic, non-metastatic complication, frequently associated with carcinoma of the bronchus. It may be the presenting feature of the disease. It rarely occurs with other conditions that also cause clubbing, presenting most often in middle-aged men with pain and swelling of the wrists and ankles. Other joints are occasionally involved. The mechanism is unclear. One suggestion is the release of VEGF into the circulation. Primary HPO is a hereditary condition involving a mutation in the *HPGD* gene that degrades prostaglandin E_2 (PGE_2). The mutation therefore allows over-production of PGE_2, which may cause clubbing.

The diagnosis is made on the presence of clubbing of the fingers (usually gross in primary) and periosteal new bone formation along the shafts of the distal ends of the radius, ulna, tibia and fibula on X-ray. A chest X-ray usually shows the malignancy.

Management should be directed at the underlying carcinoma; if this can be removed, the arthropathy disappears. NSAIDs relieve the symptoms.

Sarcoidosis

Sarcoidosis (see pp. 1118–1120) is a multisystem granulomatous disease and is associated with erythema nodosum, which occurs in 20% of cases at or soon after the onset of the disease. The most useful diagnostic test is a chest X-ray, which shows hilar lymphadenopathy in 80% of cases. The serum ACE may be raised.

Other patterns of arthritis occur later in the disease. These include a transient rheumatoid-like polyarthritis and an acute monoarthritis that can be mistaken for gout. Bone cysts can also develop.

Treatment is with NSAIDs; if these fail to control the symptoms, corticosteroids are usually very effective.

Paraneoplastic polyarthritis

This condition is seen with carcinoma of the breast in women and of the lung in men, and also with renal cell carcinoma. The neoplasm may be occult at onset and the diagnosis is then difficult to make.

Skin disease

Psoriatic arthritis

This disease is discussed on pages 685–686.

Erythema nodosum

Erythema nodosum (see p. 1363) is accompanied by arthritis in over 50% of cases. The knees and ankles are particularly affected, being swollen, red and tender. The arthritis subsides, along with the skin lesions, within a few months. Treatment is with NSAIDs or occasionally steroids.

Neurological disease

Neuropathic (Charcot's) joints

These are damaged by trauma as a result of the loss of the protective pain sensation. They were first described by Charcot in relation to tabes dorsalis. They also occur in syringomyelia, diabetes mellitus and leprosy. The site of the neuropathic joint depends on the localization of the pain loss:

- In tabes dorsalis, the knees and ankles are most often affected.
- In diabetes mellitus, the joints of the tarsus are involved.
- In syringomyelia, the shoulder is involved.

Neuropathic joints are not painful, although there may be painful episodes associated with crystal deposition. Presentation is usually with swelling and instability. Eventually, severe deformities develop.

The characteristic finding is a swollen joint with abnormal but painless movement, in association with neurological findings that depend on the underlying disease (e.g. dissociated sensory loss in syringomyelia or polyneuropathy in diabetes). X-ray changes are characteristic, with gross joint disorganization and bony distortion.

Treatment is symptomatic. Surgery may be required in advanced cases.

Blood disease

Arthritis due to haemarthrosis is a common presenting feature of people with ***haemophilia*** (see pp. 571–573). Attacks begin in early childhood in most cases and are recurrent. The knee is the most commonly affected joint but the elbows and ankles are sometimes involved. The arthritis can lead to bone destruction and disorganization of joints. Apart from replacement of factor VIII, affected joints require initial immobilization followed by physiotherapy to restore movement and measures to prevent and correct deformities.

Sickle cell crises (see p. 539) are often accompanied by joint pain that particularly affects the hands and feet in a bilateral, symmetrical distribution. Affected joints usually look normal but are occasionally swollen. This condition may also be complicated by avascular necrosis (see p. 715) and by osteomyelitis.

Arthritis can also occur in ***acute leukaemia*** (see pp. 608–612); it may be the presenting feature in childhood. The knee is particularly affected and is very painful, warm and swollen. Treatment is directed at the underlying leukaemia. Arthritis may also occur in chronic leukaemia, with leukaemic deposits in and around the joints.

Individuals with ***thalassaemia major*** (see pp. 536–537) are living longer and are presenting with back pain due to premature disc degeneration, secondary spondylosis and crush fractures caused by osteoporosis. There is marked discal calcification.

Endocrine and metabolic disorders

Hypothyroid patients may complain of pain and stiffness of proximal muscles, resembling polymyalgia rheumatica. They may also have carpal tunnel syndrome. Less often, there is an arthritis accompanied by joint effusions, particularly in the knees, wrist and small joints of the hands and feet. These problems respond rapidly to thyroxine.

Hyperparathyroidism may be complicated by cartilage calcification and acute CPPD.

In ***acromegaly***, arthralgia occurs in about 50% of patients. It particularly affects the small joints of the hands and knees. There may be a carpal tunnel syndrome.

In ***Cushing's disease***, back pain is common.

Joint disorders related to ***diabetes mellitus*** are described on page 1273.

Familial hypercholesterolaemia is associated with oligo- or polyarthritis, usually with tendon xanthomata. Arthritis also occurs in combined hyperlipidaemia.

MISCELLANEOUS ARTHROPATHIES

Familial Mediterranean fever

Systemic autoinflammatory syndromes (SAIDs) are rare genetic and acquired disorders which present with recurrent attacks of fever in childhood and adult life.

Familial Mediterranean fever (FMF) is inherited as an autosomal recessive condition and occurs in certain ethnic groups, particularly Arabs, Turks, Armenians and Sephardic Jews. The gene, called *MEFV*, has been localized to chromosome 16. It encodes for pyrin (or marenostrin), a suppressor of the activation of caspase 1, which stimulates the biosynthesis of IL-1β, which drives inflammation. Failure of suppression leads to FMF attacks.

These are characterized by recurrent episodes of fever, arthritis and serositis. Abdominal or chest pain due to peritonitis or pleurisy occurs. The arthritis is usually monoarticular and episodes last up to 1 week. The CRP is markedly raised during the attacks. The condition may be mistaken for palindromic rheumatism (see p. 675), but such attacks are not usually accompanied by fever.

The diagnosis can be made by PCR, if available, but is based on the clinical picture and exclusion of other conditions.

Treatment involves regular colchicine 1000–1500 μg daily, which can usually prevent the attacks. In resistant patients, thalidomide (see p. 601) and anakinra can be tried. In general, the disorder is benign, but in 25% of cases, renal amyloidosis develops.

Other systemic autoinflammatory syndromes (SAIDs) are being increasingly recognized. These include tumour necrosis factor receptor-associated periodic syndrome (TRAPS), mevalonate kinase deficiency (MKD), cryopyrin-associated periodic syndrome (CAPS), and periodic fever, aphthous stomatitis, pharyngitis and adenitis (PFAPA).

SAPHO (synovitis, acne, palmoplantar pustulosis, hyperostosis, osteitis)

This rare syndrome appears to be a reaction to chronic *Propionibacterium acnes* infection. It produces chronic multifocal osteitis with anterior chest wall pain and peripheral synovitis. There is inflammatory cytokine release and global neutrophil activation. Etanercept (see p. 680) may help.

Osteochondromatosis

In this condition, foci of cartilage form within the synovial membrane. These foci become calcified and then ossified (osteochondromas). They may give rise to loose bodies within the joint. The condition occurs in a single joint of a young adult and X-rays are usually diagnostic.

Management involves removal of loose bodies and synovectomy.

Pigmented villonodular synovitis

This is characterized by exuberant synovial proliferation that occurs either in joints or in tendon sheaths. The main manifestation in joints is recurrent haemarthrosis. It may produce progressive local bone destruction. A malignant form is seen occasionally.

Management is synovectomy or radiotherapy. In tendon sheaths, the condition gives rise to a nodular mass that requires excision.

Relapsing polychondritis

Relapsing polychondritis is a rare inflammatory condition of cartilage. It occurs equally in males and females, usually the elderly. Tenderness, inflammation and eventual destruction of cartilage occur, mainly in the ear, nose, larynx or trachea. A seronegative polyarthritis occurs, as well as episcleritis and evidence of a vasculitis (e.g. glomerulonephritis). The diagnosis is clinical with laboratory evidence of acute inflammation.

Treatment involves corticosteroids and immunosuppressive agents.

Further reading

Lachmann HJ. Autoinflammatory syndromes as causes of fever of unknown origin. *Clin Med* 2015; 15:295–298.

19 Bone disease

Donncha O'Gradaigh, Richard Conway

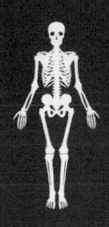

See your e-book for key learning points, clinical tips, drug tips, extra tables, extra images and MCQs.

ANATOMY AND PHYSIOLOGY OF BONE

Bone is a specialized connective tissue serving three major functions:

- ***mechanical*** – supplying structure and muscle attachment for movement
- ***metabolic*** – providing the body's primary store of calcium and phosphate
- ***protective*** – enclosing the marrow and other vital organs.

Bone structure

Bone is comprised of cells and a matrix of organic protein and inorganic mineral. Long bones (femur, tibia, humerus) and flat bones (skull, scapula) have different embryological templates, with varying proportions of cortical and trabecular bone.

- ***Cortical (compact or lamellar) bone*** forms the shaft of long bones and the outer shell of flat bones. Formed of concentric rings of bone, it is particularly adapted to withstand bending strain.
- ***Trabecular (cancellous) bone*** is found at the ends of long bones and inside flat bones. Comprised of a network of interconnecting rods and plates of bone, it offers resistance to compressive loads. It is also the main site of bone turnover for mineral homeostasis.
- ***Woven bone*** lacks an organized structure. It appears in the first few years of life, at sites of fracture repair and in high-turnover bone disorders such as Paget's disease.

Matrix components

- ***Type I collagen*** is the main protein, forming parallel lamellae of differing density (which impairs spreading of cracks). In cortical bone, concentric lamellae form around a central blood supply (Haversian system), which communicates via transverse (Volkmann's) canals.
- ***Non-collagen proteins*** include osteopontin, osteocalcin and fibronectin.
- ***Bone mineral*** largely consists of calcium and phosphate in the form of hydroxyapatite.

Bone cells

Osteoblasts

Derived from local mesenchymal stem cells, these cells synthesize matrix (osteoid) and regulate its mineralization. After bone formation, the majority of osteoblasts are removed by apoptosis (see p. 105), others remaining at the bone/marrow interface as lining cells or within the bone as osteocytes. Osteoblasts regulate bone resorption through the balance in expression of the stimulatory receptor activator of nuclear factor kappa B ligand (RANKL) and its antagonist, osteoprotegerin (OPG). Osteoblasts are rich in alkaline phosphatase and express receptors for parathyroid hormone (PTH), oestrogen, glucocorticoids, vitamin D, inflammatory cytokines and the transforming growth factor-beta (TGF-β) family, all of which may therefore influence bone remodelling.

Osteocytes

These small cells, derived from osteoblasts, are embedded in bone and interconnected with each other and with bone lining cells through cytoplasmic processes. They respond to mechanical strain by undergoing apoptosis or through altered cell signalling, which in turn activates bone formation with or without prior resorption. As osteocytes also express RANKL and OPG, the relative importance of osteocytes and osteoblasts in bone resorption function continues to be explored.

Osteoclasts

These cells have the unique capacity to resorb bone and are derived from haemopoietic precursors of the macrophage lineage. In response to RANKL, macrophage colony stimulating factor (M-CSF) and local adhesion factors (integrins), osteoclasts attach to bone, creating a ruffled border that forms a number of extracellular lysosomal compartments. Hydrogen ions are actively secreted into these spaces and the acid environment removes the mineral phase before specialized cysteine proteases (e.g. cathepsin K) resorb the collagen matrix.

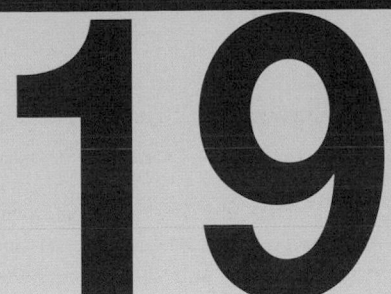

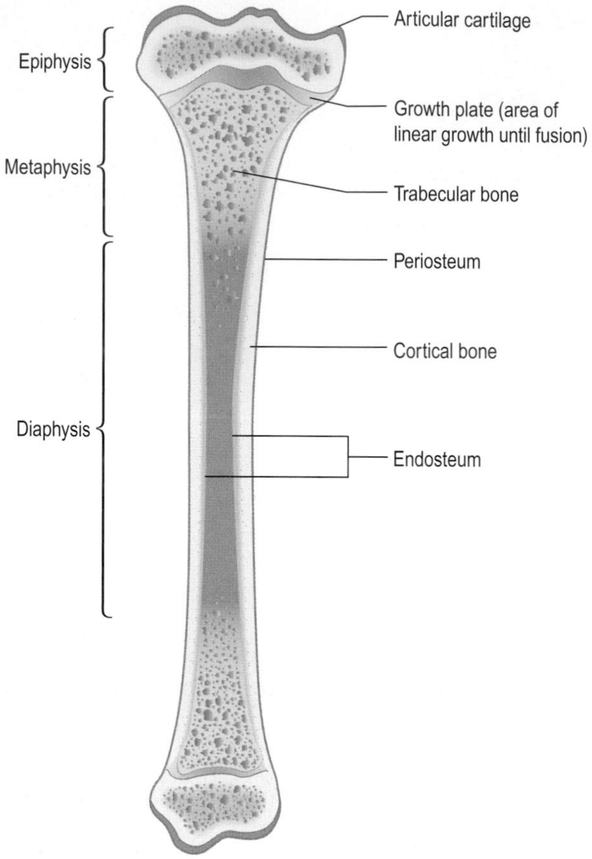

Figure 19.1 **A longitudinal section of a growing long bone.** *(From NICE guidelines: Osteoporosis – primary prevention. http://www.nice.org.uk/Guidance/TA160 (23 July 2012).)*

Bone growth and remodelling

Longitudinal growth occurs at the epiphyseal growth plate, a cartilage structure between the epiphysis and metaphysis ***(Fig. 19.1)***. Cartilage production is tightly regulated, with subsequent mineralization and growth finally arrested at 18–21 years, when the epiphysis and metaphysis fuse.

In adults, bone is regularly remodelled to ensure repair of microdamage and turnover of calcium and phosphate for homeostasis. This remodelling cycle is carried out by the basic multicellular unit (BMU; ***Fig. 19.2***). Signals initiating resorption include osteocyte apoptosis and altered signalling (sclerostin, prostaglandins, RANKL and other molecules), resulting in localized retraction of bone-lining cells and binding of multinucleate osteoclasts to the bone surface, followed by bone resorption. Bone formation involves reciprocal effects of *wnt* versus *dickkopf* (*Dkk*) and sclerostin on the LRP5/6-β-catenin pathway. The switch from resorption to formation may rely on osteocyte signalling or on release of signals from the bone matrix, such as TGF-β. Bone remodelling is said to be coupled when formation follows resorption, but may be unbalanced when the amount of bone removed is not replaced with an equal amount.

Examples of bone remodelling include:

- Myeloma cells have dual lytic effects, with enhanced expression of RANKL and expression of *Dkk*
- In rheumatioid arthritis, RANKL and *Dkk* are increased
- In spondyloarthritis (characterized by new bone formation alongside erosion) *Dkk* is inhibited, with the increased *wnt* activity also increasing OPG relative to RANKL
- Corticosteroids may increase osteocyte SOST expression, and stimulate expression of *Dkk*.

Calcium homeostasis and its regulation

Calcium homeostasis is regulated by the effects of PTH and 1,25-dihydroxyvitamin D (1,25$(OH)_2D_3$) on gut, kidney and bone. Calcium-sensing receptors are present in the parathyroid glands, kidney and brain.

Calcium absorption and distribution

Daily calcium consumption ***(Fig. 19.3)***, primarily from dairy foods, is 20–25 mmol (800–1000 mg). The combined effect of calcium and vitamin D deficiency contributes to the bone fragility seen in some older persons. Intestinal absorption of calcium is reduced by vitamin D deficiency and in malabsorption states (see p. 204).

Vitamin D metabolism

The primary source of vitamin D ***(Fig. 19.4)*** in humans is photoactivation in the skin of 7-dehydrocholesterol to cholecalciferol, which is then converted first in the liver to 25-hydroxyvitamin D (25$(OH)D_3$) and subsequently in the kidney (by the enzyme 1α-hydroxylase) to 1,25$(OH)_2D_3$. (This step can occur in lymphomatous and sarcoid tissue, resulting in hypercalcaemia.) Regulation of the latter step is by PTH, phosphate and feedback inhibition by 1,25$(OH)_2D_3$.

Parathyroid hormone

Parathyroid hormone (PTH), an 84-amino-acid hormone, is secreted from the chief cells of the parathyroid gland, which have calcium-sensing and vitamin D receptors. PTH increases renal phosphate excretion and increases plasma calcium by:

- increasing osteoclastic activity in bone (a rapid response)
- increasing intestinal absorption of calcium (a slower response)
- increasing 1α-hydroxylation of vitamin D (the rate-limiting step)
- increasing renal tubular reabsorption of calcium.

Hypomagnesaemia can suppress the normal PTH response to hypocalcaemia.

Calcitonin

Calcitonin is produced by thyroid C cells. Although calcitonin inhibits osteoclastic bone resorption and increases the renal excretion of calcium and phosphate, neither excess calcitonin (seen in medullary carcinoma of the thyroid) nor its deficiency following thyroidectomy has significant skeletal effects in humans.

Further reading

Rosen CJ. Vitamin D insufficiency. *N Engl J Med* 2011; 364:248–254.
Xiong J, Onal M, Jilka RL et al. Matrix-embedded cells control osteoclast formation. *Nat Med* 2011; 17:1235–1241.
Zebaze RM, Ghasem-Zadeh A, Bohte A et al. Intracortical remodelling and porosity in the distal radius and post-mortem femurs of women: a cross-sectional study. *Lancet* 2010; 375:1729–1736.
http://courses.washington.edu/bonephys/ *Bone physiology*.

CLINICAL APPROACH TO THE PATIENT WITH BONE DISEASE

Investigation of bone and calcium disorders

(See ***Box 19.1***.)

Total plasma calcium

Normal range 2.2–2.6 mmol/L. About 40% is ionized and physiologically active; the remainder is complexed or protein-bound. As

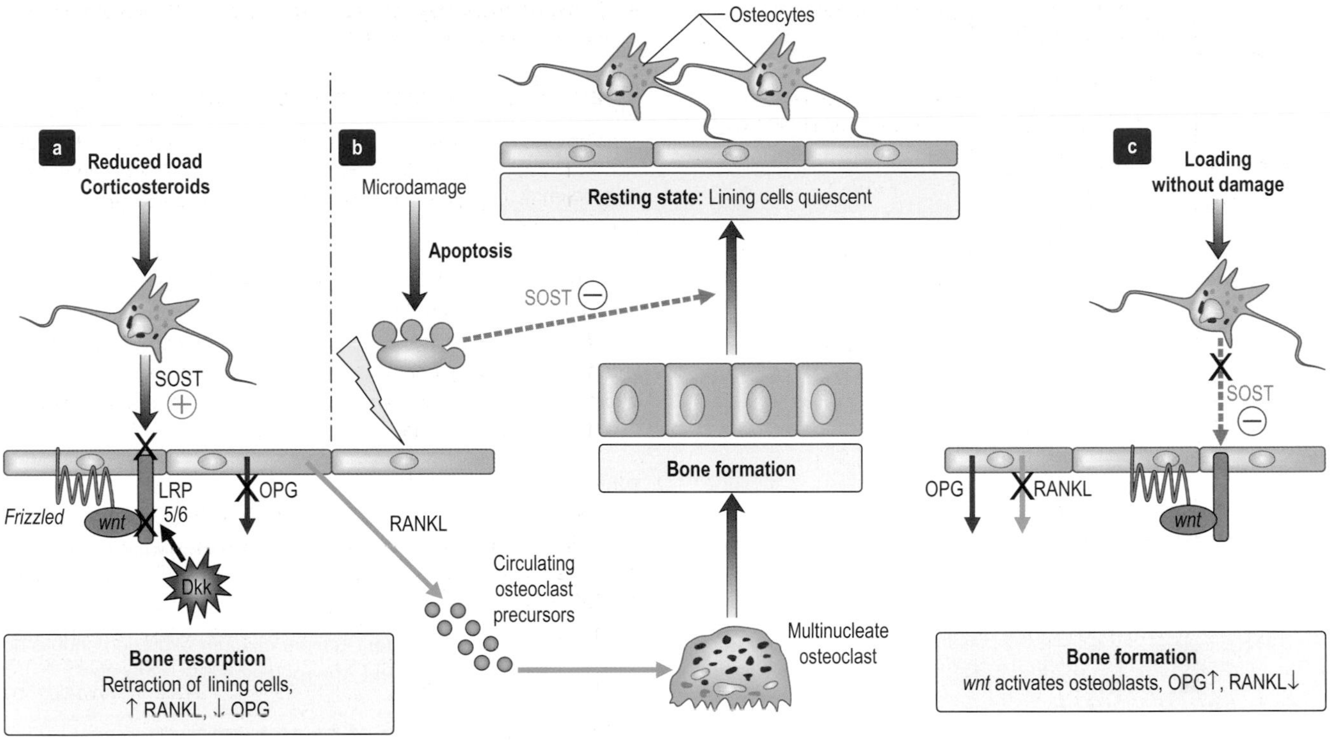

Figure 19.2 Bone is remodelled in response to alterations in two reciprocal systems.
(a) ***Quiescent bone (centre)*** may experience *reduced load* in response, the osteocyte increases expression of ***sclerostin (SOST+)***, inhibiting the response to *wnt* via the ***LRP5/frizzled co-receptor complex*** (orange).
(b) ***Microdamage*** causes osteocyte apoptosis, with direct osteoclast-generating effects via receptor activator of nuclear factor kappa B ligand (RANKL), and loss of the inhibitory effect of SOST on later bone formation (dashed line, SOST–). The osteoblastic lining cells retract from an area of bone, forming a bone remodelling unit, while increased expression of RANKL and reduced osteoprotegerin (OPG) activates the formation of bone-resorbing multinucleate osteoclasts from circulating precursors; the resorbed area is then replaced by new osteoid, formed by cuboidal osteoblasts. As new osteocytes are formed, SOST levels rise and the osteoblasts cease formation, the majority undergoing apoptosis.
(c) If bone experiences *loading without damage*, ***sclerostin expression*** is reduced (SOST–), increasing signal response to *wnt*, activation of osteoblast bone formation, and increased OPG expression.

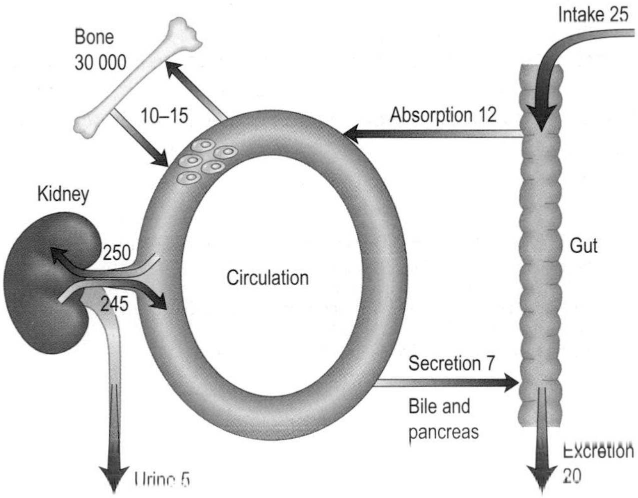

Figure 19.3 Calcium exchange in the normal human. The amounts are shown in mmol per day.

Box 19.1 Common blood test patterns in bone disorders

Test results (serum)	Probable diagnosis	Confirmatory test
A patient with fragility fracture		
Ca, Phosphate, ALP normal	Osteoporosis	Check vitamin D, PTH, DXA
Ca high	Paget's disease of bone	Review imaging to rule out tumour
Ca normal, Phosphate low	Hyperparathyroidism	
Vitamin D low	Secondary hyperparathyroidism	
Vitamin D normal	Primary hyperparathyroidism	Check calcium – may be raised
A patient with bone pain		
Ca, Phosphate normal, ALP high	Paget's disease of bone	Check PTH, vitamin D for osteomalacia
Phosphate high, ALP high, PTH high	MBD-CKD	

ALP, alkaline phosphatase; Ca, calcium; DXA, dual energy X-ray absorptiometry; MBD-CKD, metabolic bone disorder of chronic kidney disease; PTH, parathyroid hormone.

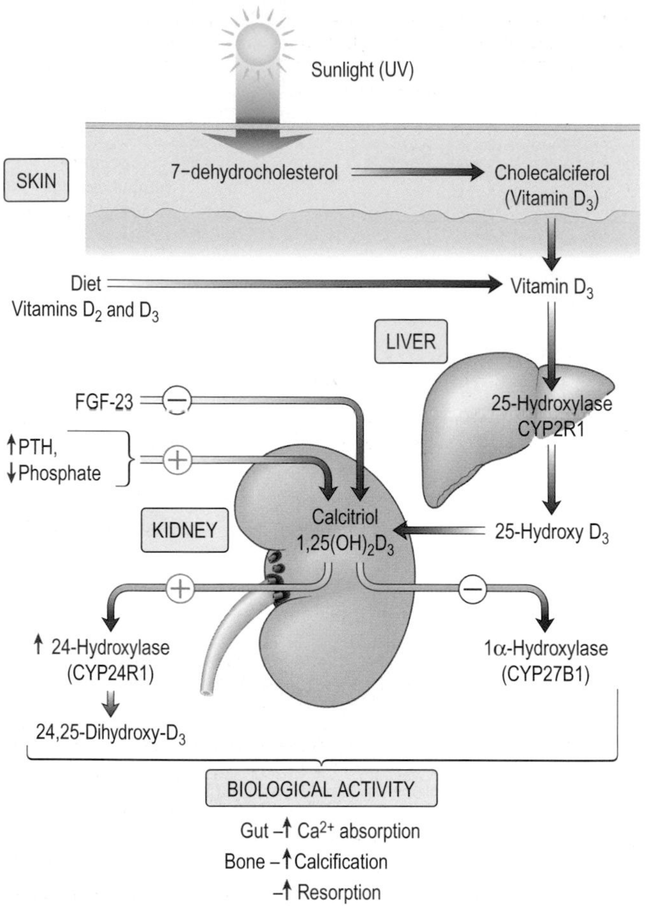

Figure 19.4 The metabolism and actions of vitamin D. 1,25-Dihydroxycholecalciferol (calcitriol) is the biologically active agent. It inhibits 1α-hydroxylase and stimulates 24-hydroxylase to produce 24,25-dihydroxy-D_3, which is not biologically active. CYP, cytochrome P enzyme; FGF, fibroblast growth factor secreted mainly by osteocytes (see p. 171).

ionized calcium is difficult to measure, normal practice is to measure total calcium, correcting the value to allow for protein binding according to the following formula: add or subtract 0.02 mmol/L for each gram per litre of a simultaneous albumin level below or above 40 g/L. For critical measurements, samples should be taken in the fasting state and without a tourniquet (the latter may increase local plasma calcium concentration).

Plasma phosphate

Normal range 0.8–1.4 mmol/L. Phosphate is essential to most biological systems. High levels are found in chronic kidney disease (CKD) and hypoparathyroidism, while low levels are associated with primary hyperparathyroidism, hypophosphataemic rickets and osteomalacia, and other disorders associated with reduced renal tubular phosphate reabsorption.

Plasma PTH

Normal range 10–65 ng/mL. The PTH assay measures the intact hormone. In hypercalcaemia not due to hyperparathyroidism, serum PTH levels are suppressed. Lithium toxicity may be associated with raised PTH levels; in familial hypocalciuric hypercalcaemia (FHH), serum PTH may be normal or marginally elevated.

Serum 25-hydroxyvitamin D

Vitamin D status is best assessed using serum 25-$(OH)D_3$, as $1,25(OH)_2D_3$ has a short half-life and does not accurately reflect true vitamin D status. ***Vitamin D deficiency*** is defined as <25 nmol/L (10 ng/mL) and ***vitamin D insufficiency*** as <75 nmol/L (30 ng/mL). Rickets and osteomalacia occur with prolonged vitamin D deficiency.

The significance of vitamin D insufficiency is uncertain but it has been linked to a wide range of conditions, including ischaemic heart disease, multiple sclerosis and a variety of cancers. Recent evidence suggests that racial differences are present in the assessment of vitamin D status. Black Americans have consistently lower levels of 25-$(OH)D_3$ than white Americans but also lower levels of ***vitamin D-binding protein***, resulting in equivalent bioavailable 25-$(OH)D_3$.

24-hour urinary calcium

Normal range 2.5–6.25 (female) and 7.5 (male) mmol/24 h. This is increased where renal tubular reabsorption of calcium is decreased, and in hypercalcaemia. One exception is FHH, where the genetic defect leads to inappropriately reduced calcium excretion. Measurement of 24-hour urinary calcium excretion should be performed in the assessment of hypercalcaemic patients.

Biochemical markers of bone formation and resorption

The clinical use of these biochemical markers is limited by large biovariability and measurement variance. Serial measurements at the same time of day in individual patients are useful in assessing response to treatment of metabolic bone diseases.

- ***Bone-specific alkaline phosphatase***. Circulating alkaline phosphatase is derived from bone, liver and placenta. The bone-specific isoenzyme can be measured as a marker of formation, although there is some overlap with the liver isoenzyme. Elevated serum levels occur during bone growth: for example, in adolescents, fracture repair, and high-bone-turnover states.
- ***Type 1 collagen pro-peptides***. These are by-products of collagen synthesis. Serum levels of both the carboxyterminal (P1CP) and aminoterminal (P1NP) pro-peptides reflect bone formation.
- ***Serum osteocalcin***. This is another bone formation marker.
- ***Serum or urine levels of N-terminal (NTX) and C-terminal (CTX) cross-linked telopeptides***. These reflect bone resorption. They may change rapidly in response to anti-resorptive drugs or in disease states, and have been used to assess fracture risk.

Diagnostic imaging

- ***Plain radiographs***. These identify fractures, tumours and infections. Other specific features may be seen (see following sections).
- ***Radionucleotide imaging***. The uptake of a ^{99m}technetium-labelled bisphosphonate in bone reflects bone turnover and blood flow. Increased uptake is therefore seen in fractures, tumour and metastatic deposits, infection and Paget's disease of bone.
- ***Magnetic resonance imaging (MRI)***. This is the most sensitive and specific test for the diagnosis of osteomyelitis. It is also useful in the detection of stress fractures, which may

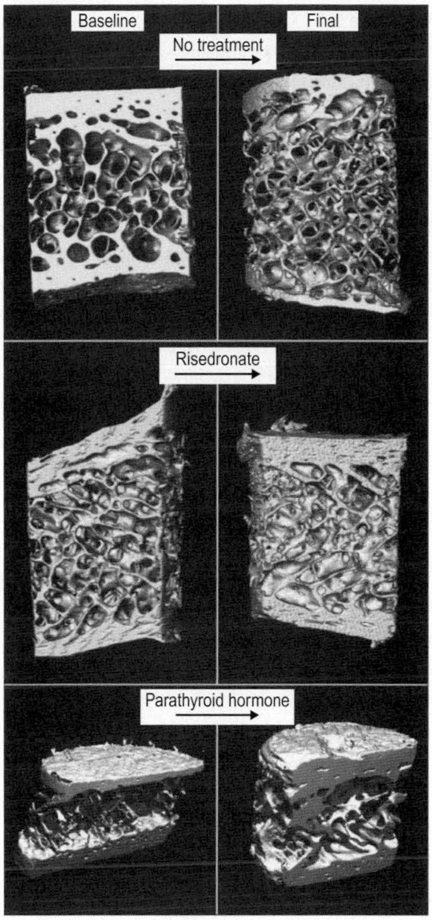

Figure 19.5 Computerized images of bone biopsies in osteoporosis. These images demonstrate changes in bone architecture over time. ***Upper pair***: Without treatment, the bone cortex becomes thinner and numerous trabecular rods and plates are lost. ***Centre pair***: In response to bisphosphonate treatment, resorption is reduced, with preservation of bone mineral and structure. ***Lower pair***: In response to anabolic therapy, bone is increased at both trabecular and cortical sites. *(From Jiang Y, Zhao JJ, Mitlak BH et al. Recombinant human parathyroid hormone (1–34) improves both cortical and cancellous bone structure.* Journal of Bone and Mineral Research *2003; 18:1932–1941, with permission of the American Society for Bone and Mineral Research.)*

not be demonstrated on plain radiographs. A technique to suppress the high signal associated with bone marrow (such as STIR sequences; see p. 651) allows highly sensitive recognition of 'bone marrow oedema', a non-specific feature of a number of bone disorders, including osteonecrosis.

- ***Bone biopsy (Fig. 19.5)***. A core of bone is removed, including both cortices of the iliac crest using a trephine. The non-decalcified specimen is examined for static and dynamic (bone turnover) indices. An oral tetracycline is given to the patient prior to the biopsy, for 2 days on two occasions 10 days apart, allowing assessment of the rate of bone turnover and mineralization. Biopsy is most commonly used in the assessment of suspected renal bone disease and osteomalacia.
- ***Bone densitometry measurements*** (see p. 712).

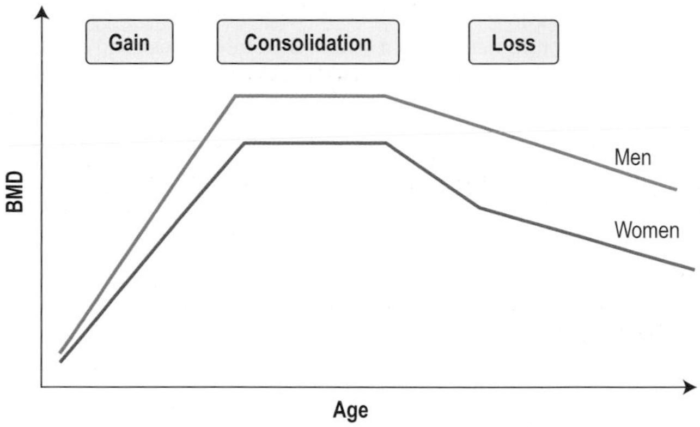

Figure 19.6 Lifetime changes in bone mineral density (BMD). Peak bone mass is achieved between 20 and 30 years of age (gain), and consolidated up to around the age of 40 years. Then, age-related bone loss occurs in both men and women, with an accelerated loss in women starting around the time of menopause, which lasts between 5 and 10 years.

OSTEOPOROSIS

Osteoporosis is defined as 'a disease characterized by low bone mass and micro-architectural deterioration of bone tissue, leading to enhanced bone fragility and an increase in fracture risk'.

Using bone densitometry at the hip or spine measured by dual X-ray absorptiometry (DXA), the World Health Organization (WHO) also defines osteoporosis as a bone density of 2.5 standard deviations (SDs) below the young healthy adult mean value (T-score ≤–2.5) or lower. Values between –1 and –2.5 SDs below the young adult mean are termed 'osteopenia'. The rationale for this definition is the inverse relationship between bone mineral density (BMD) and fracture risk in postmenopausal women and older men. However, this definition should not be applied to younger populations.

Fractures due to osteoporosis are a major cause of morbidity and mortality in elderly populations, with osteoporotic fractures of the spine causing acute pain or deformity and postural back pain. One in two women and one in five men aged 50 years will have an osteoporotic fracture during their remaining lifetime. Caucasian and Asian races are particularly at risk. As the risk of fracture increases exponentially with age, changing population demographics will increase the burden of disease.

Pathogenesis

Osteoporosis results from increased bone breakdown by osteoclasts and decreased bone formation by osteoblasts, leading to loss of bone mass.

Bone mass decreases with age ***(Fig. 19.6)*** but will depend on the 'peak' mass attained in adult life and on the rate of loss in later life. Genetic factors are the single most significant influence on peak bone mass. Multiple genes are involved, including collagen type 1A1, vitamin D receptor and oestrogen receptor genes. Nutritional factors, sex hormone status and physical activity also affect peak mass. Not all causes of osteoporosis affect bone remodelling and architecture in the same way.

Oestrogen deficiency results in increased numbers of remodelling units, premature arrest of osteoblastic synthetic activity and perforation of trabeculae, with a loss of resistance to fracture that is not fully reflected in the bone density measurement.

Glucocorticoids induce a high-turnover state initially, with increased fracture risk evident within 3 months of starting therapy. More prolonged use leads to a reduced-turnover state but with a net loss due to reduced synthesis (through increased inhibition of the *wnt*-LRP5/6 axis).

Ageing results in increased turnover at the bone/vascular interface within cortical bone, resulting in a weak structure for the stresses occurring in this area of long bones (trabecularization of cortical bone).

Risk factors

Risk factors for fracture may exert their effect through reducing BMD, or they may increase risk over that attributable to BMD, meaning that they are BMD-independent ***(Box 19.2)***. Oestrogen deficiency is a major factor in the pathogenesis of accelerated bone loss due to a normal or premature menopause or amenorrhoea in anorexia and in athletes. In the elderly, vitamin D insufficiency and consequent hyperparathyroidism reduce BMD. However, previous fracture, increasing age, glucocorticoid therapy, smoking and falls increase the risk of fracture at any given BMD. For instance, 10% of women who are 65 years old and have a T-score of –2 at the hip would be expected to sustain a fracture over the next 10 years; if similar women had a Colles' fracture, smoked and had prolonged exposure to steroids, their risk would be closer to 26% in the same period.

Treatment depends on the type of risk factors: if they are recognized as 'BMD-dependent', they respond to bone-directed treatment; if classed as 'BMD-independent', they require additional intervention (e.g. reduction of falls risk).

Box 19.2 Risk factors for fragility fractures

BMD-dependent
Female sex
Caucasian/Asian
Gastrointestinal disease
Hypogonadism
Immobilization
Chronic liver disease
Chronic kidney disease
Low dietary calcium intake
Vitamin D insufficiency
Chronic obstructive pulmonary disease
Cushing syndrome
Hyperthyroidism
Hyperparathyroidism
Diabetes mellitus
Mastocytosis
Multiple myeloma
Osteogenesis imperfecta

Drugs
Heparin
Calcineurin inhibitors, e.g. ciclosporin
Anticonvulsants
Thiazolidinediones
Aromatase inhibitors
Anti-androgens
GnRH analogues
Proton pump inhibitors
?Selective serotonin reuptake inhibitors

BMD-independent
Increasing age
Previous fragility fracture
Family history of hip fracture
Low body mass index
Smoking
Excess alcohol use
Glucocorticoid therapy
High bone turnover
Increased risk of falling
Rheumatoid arthritis

Clinical features

Fracture is the only cause of symptoms in osteoporosis. ***Vertebral crush fracture*** is suggested by the sudden onset of severe pain in the spine, often radiating around to the front. However, only about 1 in 3 vertebral fractures is symptomatic. Pain from mechanical derangement, increasing kyphosis, height loss and abdominal protuberance follow crushed vertebrae. ***Colles' fractures*** typically follow a fall on an outstretched arm. ***Fractures of the proximal femur*** usually occur in older individuals falling on their side or back.

Other causes of low-trauma fractures must not be overlooked, including metastatic disease and myeloma.

Investigations

Plain radiographs (Fig. 19.7) usually show a fracture and may reveal previously asymptomatic vertebral deformities. Such clinically silent fractures may also be detected during DXA scanning with an additional analysis (called ***lateral vertebral assessment***, carried out with a much lower radiation dose than conventional imaging).

Bone density

DXA measures areal bone density (mineral per surface area rather than a true volumetric density), usually of the lumbar spine and proximal femur. It is precise and accurate, uses low doses of radiation and is the 'gold standard' in diagnosis of osteoporosis ***(Fig. 19.8)***. Because of osteophytes, spinal deformity and vertebral fractures, spinal values may be artefactually elevated and should be interpreted with caution in the elderly.

Associated disease and risk factors

Investigations to exclude other diseases or identify contributory factors associated with osteoporosis should be performed and are particularly necessary in men, in whom secondary causes are more common ***(Box 19.2)***.

Selection of individuals for treatment: risk assessment

The purpose of treatment in osteoporosis is to reduce the risk of fractures ***(Box 19.3)***. Thus, assessment of absolute fracture risk

Box 19.3 Management of osteoporosis: summary

Treatment is guided by risk of fracture, not BMD alone.

If there is an intermediate risk from clinical factors, request a DXA scan (see http://www.shef.ac.uk/FRAX or other risk calculator until familiar with assessments).

Do not under-estimate the risk from steroids or previous fracture.

Many guidelines (e.g. NICE) recommend bisphosphonate as first-line drugs in most cases. Other options include:

- **denosumab:**
  - in the young (to defer bisphosphonate use)
  - for a new fracture on a bisphosphonate *or* a fall in BMD *or* bisphosphonate use for 5–10 years
  - after hip fracture
- **teriparatide** if there are multiple vertebral fractures or a high risk
- **i.v. zoledronate** after hip fracture
- **strontium ranelate** if the patient is at high risk and there is no possible alternative.

BMD monitoring is required in:

- selected high-risk cases
- low-risk cases not treated.

BMD, bone mineral density; DXA, dual-energy X-ray absorptiometry; NICE, National Institute for Health and Care Excellence.

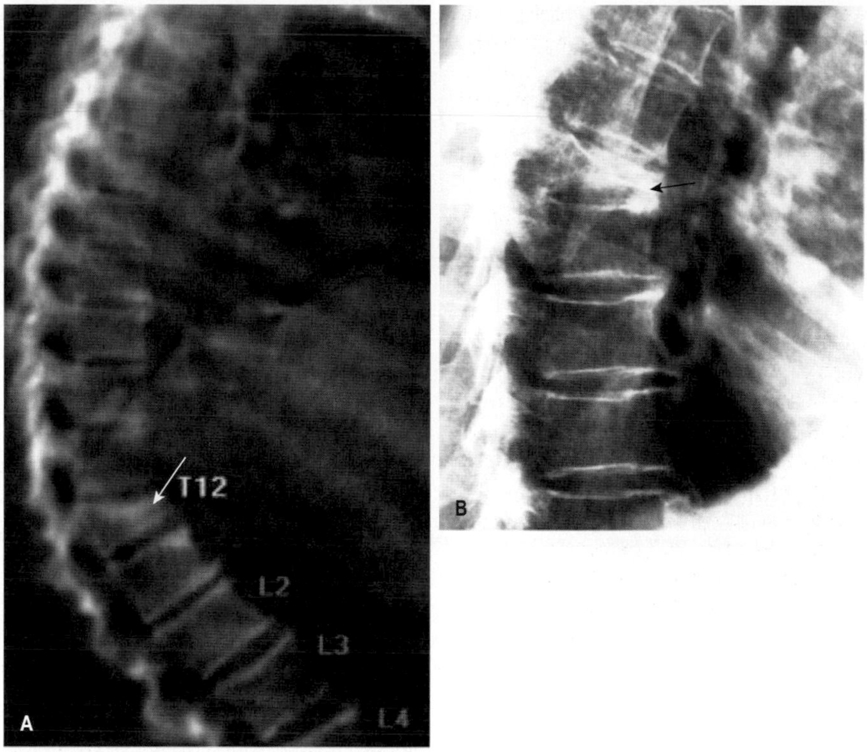

Figure 19.7 Vertebral fracture as seen on lateral vertebral assessment (LVA) and plain radiograph. A. The LVA image shows a vertebra with reduced height at T12 (arrow). **B.** The radiograph shows a typical wedge compression fracture.

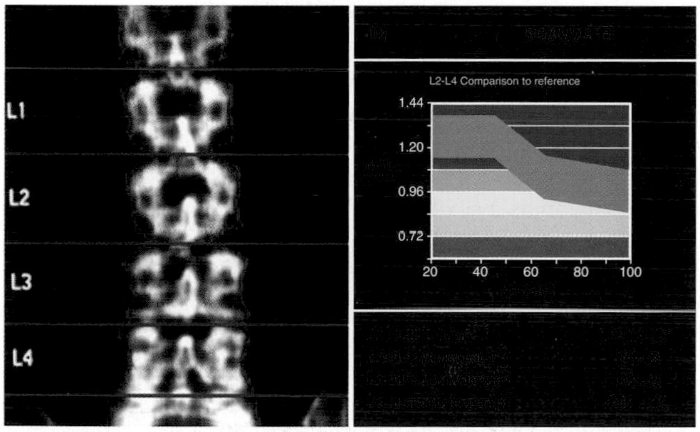

A B

Figure 19.8 Dual energy X-ray absorptiometry of the lumbar spine. **A.** Anteroposterior image of the lumbar spine. **B.** The patient's value is expressed in relation to the reference range.

should be made in every case. All patients with a history of fragility fracture should be reviewed for treatment. In those aged over 75 years, DXA is often not necessary prior to treatment, but in those under 75 years of age, DXA is useful in guiding treatment decisions (***Box 19.4*** and ***Fig. 19.9***). Although age and BMD measurements in the spine and proximal femur are the most useful data for assessing fracture risk, it is vital to recognize that the majority of fragility fractures occur in women with a T-score better than –2.5. Therefore, factors that are known to increase fracture risk independently of BMD should be taken into account when assessing an individual's risk of fracture, for example, using risk calculators such as FRAX®. The threshold for recommending treatment will be determined by the cost-effectiveness of treatment in a particular healthcare setting and by clinical judgement.

Box 19.4 Indications for DXA scanning

- Radiographic osteopenia
- Previous fragility fracture (in those aged <75 years)
- Glucocorticoid therapy (in those aged <65 years)
- Body mass index <19 kg/m^2
- Maternal history of hip fracture
- BMD-dependent risk factors (see ***Box 19.2***)

In patients presenting with height loss and/or kyphosis, lateral thoracic spine X-ray should be the initial investigation.

BMD, bone mineral density; DXA, dual-energy X-ray absorptiometry.

Prevention and management

- ***Symptomatic management***. New vertebral fractures may require bed rest for 1–2 weeks with strong analgesia, muscle relaxants (e.g. diazepam 2 mg 3 times daily) and gradual physiotherapy to restore confident mobilization (see p. 659). Non-spinal fractures should be treated by conventional orthopaedic means.
- ***Calcium and vitamin D***. Daily intakes of 800–1200 mg of calcium and 400–800 IU of vitamin D are recommended throughout life for optimum bone health. Dietary intake of calcium, and vitamin D from sunshine and diet, are preferable. For those not meeting calcium intake targets, or those with low serum 25-(OH)D$_3$ levels, supplements are recommended, e.g. colecalciferol 20 μg and calcium 2 g daily.
- ***Lifestyle measures***. Weight-bearing exercise for 30 min 3 times a week may increase BMD, while gentle exercise in the elderly may reduce the risk of falls and improve the protective responses to falling. Smoking and excess alcohol use should be avoided.

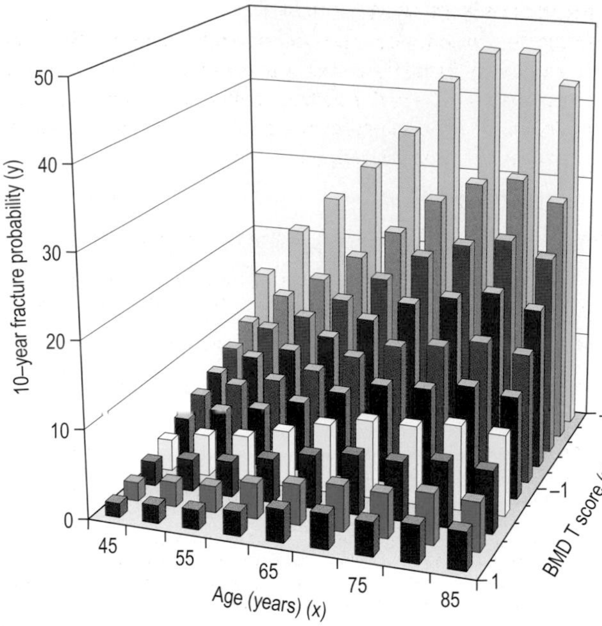

Figure 19.9 Graph illustrating the combined effects of age (x-axis) and reduced bone mass (expressed as T-scores on the z-axis) on the 10-year probability of fracture (y-axis) in a population of women. Reduced bone mass osteopenia, T-scores between −1 and −2.5. Osteoporotic bone (T-scores <−2.5) is shown in pale green. Note that the risk of fracture may be greater in an older woman with osteopenia than in a young woman with osteoporosis. *(Data from Kanis JA. Diagnosis of osteoporosis and assessment of fracture risk.* Lancet *359:1929–1936.)*

- ***Reduction of falls***. Physiotherapy and assessment of home safety are helpful. Hip protectors do reduce fractures in the elderly in residential care when worn correctly, but compliance is poor.

Pharmacological intervention

Most interventions (see ***Fig. 19.5***) act by inhibiting bone resorption (anti-resorptives), the exception being PTH peptides, which stimulate bone formation. The impression from bone turnover markers that strontium ranelate may have both anti-resorptive and stimulatory effects remains poorly understood.

The evidence base for the ***anti-fracture efficacy*** of interventions varies. Some interventions have been shown to reduce fracture at vertebral and non-vertebral sites, including the hip, whereas others have not been demonstrated to be effective at all sites ***(Box 19.5)***. Since a fracture at one site increases the risk of subsequent fracture at any site, treatments with efficacy at all major fracture sites (particularly spine and hip) are preferable. Hence, **the bisphosphonates and denosumab are generally regarded as first-line options in the majority of postmenopausal women with osteoporosis**.

Bisphosphonates

Synthetic analogues of bone pyrophosphate, bisphosphonates adhere to hydroxyapatite and inhibit osteoclasts. Alendronate and risedronate are given as once-weekly doses, zoledronate as a once-yearly infusion, and ibandronate usually as a once-monthly oral therapy (a 3-monthly intravenous injection is rarely used).

Oral bisphosphonates should be taken fasting, with a large drink of water, while standing or sitting upright. The patient should then remain upright and avoid food and drink for at least 30 minutes.

Box 19.5 Medications to reduce fracture risk in postmenopausal women

Intervention	Vertebral fracture	Non-vertebral fracture	Hip fracture
Alendronate	+	+	+
Risedronate	+	+	+
Ibandronate	+	+[a]	ND
Zoledronate	+	+	+
Bazedoxifene	+	ND	ND
Raloxifene	+	ND	ND
Strontium ranelate	+	+	+[a]
Denosumab	+	+	+[a]
Teriparatide	+	+	ND

[a]Demonstrated only in high-risk subgroup. ND, not demonstrated.

Bisphosphonates are generally well tolerated but may be associated with upper gastrointestinal side-effects such as oesophagitis, particularly if the dosing instructions are not closely followed. Bisphosphonates should be used with careful monitoring in patients who have chronic kidney disease (stage 4 or 5). Osteonecrosis of the jaw is rarely seen following high-dose intravenous bisphosphonates in patients who have malignant disease. It is associated with poor dental hygiene. As prolonged suppression of bone turnover is linked with atypical femoral fractures, it is currently advised to reassess bisphosphonate treatment after 5 years. Only those with vertebral fractures and a T-score at the neck of femur of <−2.5 at this 5-year scan appear to have a reduced risk of fracture with continued treatment.

Denosumab

Denosumab is a fully human monoclonal antibody to RANKL and is administered as a single subcutaneous injection every 6 months. It is an anti-resorptive agent that increases BMD and reduces fractures at the spine, hip and other non-vertebral sites. Fracture risk reduction at the spine is equivalent to that with most bisphosphonates, and risk reduction at the hip is superior (with the exception of zoledronic acid). Adverse effects are infrequent: most commonly dysuria, rarely cellulitis. Osteonecrosis of the jaw and atypical femoral fractures have also occurred but estimating the true frequency of these rare adverse events is not possible with current data.

Strontium ranelate

This is used only when no alternative exists because of its adverse cardiovascular effects. It has weak anti-resorptive activity whilst maintaining bone formation. It reduces the risk of vertebral fractures in postmenopausal women with osteoporosis, and the risk of hip and other non-vertebral fractures in high-risk subgroups (women with previous fracture and T-scores at the hip of −2.4 or less). Nausea, diarrhoea and headaches are infrequent side-effects.

Selective oestrogen-receptor modulators

Selective oestrogen-receptor modulators (SERMs) include raloxifene and bazedoxifene. They have no stimulatory effect on the endometrium but activate oestrogen receptors in bone. Both prevent BMD loss at the spine and hip in postmenopausal women, but have been found to reduce only vertebral fracture rates. Leg cramps and flushing may occur and the risk of thromboembolic complications is also increased to a degree similar to that seen with hormone replacement therapy (HRT; see pp. 1296–1297 and ***Box 29.1***). The use of SERMs is associated with a small increase in the risk of stroke.

Recombinant human parathyroid hormone

Recombinant human PTH peptide 1–34 (teriparatide) and recombinant human PTH 1–84 are anabolic agents that stimulate bone formation. Teriparatide reduces vertebral and non-vertebral fractures in postmenopausal women with established osteoporosis, although data on hip fracture are not available. It is given by daily subcutaneous injection for 24 months. Recombinant human PTH 1–84 is also administered by once-daily subcutaneous injection but has been shown to reduce only vertebral fractures. An anti-resorptive drug, such as denosumab, should be given on completion of PTH peptide therapy to maintain the increase in BMD. Non-osteoporotic bone diseases, such as osteomalacia, should be excluded prior to treatment. PTH peptide therapy is indicated mainly in severe cases of vertebral osteoporosis or in women who fail to respond to other therapies. Teriparatide may cause mild transient hypercalcaemia but routine monitoring is not required. Nausea and headache may occur. Recombinant human PTH 1–84 is associated with a higher incidence of hypercalcaemia and hypercalciuria, and routine monitoring is advised. Neither agent should be used in people with skeletal metastases or osteosarcoma.

Hormone replacement therapy

Because of its adverse effects on breast cancer and cardiovascular disease risk, HRT is not indicated for osteoporosis except in early postmenopausal women who also have significant perimenopausal symptoms.

Calcitriol ($1,25\text{-}(OH)_2D_3$) and calcitonin

These may reduce vertebral fracture rate, although the data are inconsistent.

Combination therapies

Combination therapies, either with two anti-resorptive agents, or an anti-resorptive and an anabolic agent, often produce larger increases in BMD than monotherapy but have not been shown to result in greater fracture reduction.

Surgery

This is required to stabilize vertebral fractures. Percutaneous vertebroplasty and balloon kyphoplasty are discussed on page 659. Hip fractures are dealt with by hip replacements or stabilization with pins.

Treatment of specific conditions

Glucocorticoid-induced osteoporosis

Individuals requiring continuous oral glucocorticoid therapy for 3 months or more (at any dose) should be assessed for coexisting risk factors (age, previous fracture, hormone status). Postmenopausal women and men aged over [illegible] years and any individuals who have sustained a fragility fracture should receive treatment without waiting for DXA scanning. DXA results and fracture risk assessment guide treatment for other patients (see ***Box 19.4***). For these individuals, bisphosphonates and teriparatide are the approved agents. Denosumab is likely to be equally effective; though it is not yet formally approved for this indication, its mode of delivery may be advantageous in some settings.

Osteoporosis in men

Alendronate, risedronate and denosumab increase BMD and reduce vertebral fractures in men with osteoporosis. Teriparatide is also approved for use in this setting. In men with osteoporosis who have clinical and biochemical evidence of hypogonadism, testosterone replacement is also used.

Further reading

Coughlan T, Dockery F. Osteoporosis and fracture risk in older people. *Clin Med* 2014; 14:187–191.

Cummings SR, Martin J, McClung MR et al. Denosumab for prevention of fractures in postmenopausal women with osteoporosis. *N Engl J Med* 2009; 361:756–757.

Favus MJ. Bisphosphonates for osteoporosis. *N Engl J Med* 2010; 363:2027–2035.

Gourley ML, Fine JP, Preisser JS et al. Bone-density testing interval and transition to osteoporosis in older women. *N Engl J Med* 2012; 366:225–233.

Rachner TD, Khosla S, Hofbauer LC. Osteoporosis: now and the future. *Lancet* 2011; 377:1276–1287.

Weinstein RS. Glucocorticoid-induced bone disease. *N Engl J Med* 2011; 365:62–70.

http://www.nhsgrampian.org *Sample calcium intake questionnaire.*

http://www.nof.org/ *National Osteoporosis Foundation clinical guidelines.*

http://www.shef.ac.uk/FRAX *FRAX tool for 10-year probability of hip fracture and 10-year probability of major osteoporotic fracture.*

OSTEONECROSIS

This is also known as aseptic, avascular or ischaemic necrosis of bone. There are a multitude of risk factors but over 80% of cases are attributed to glucocorticoid treatment or alcohol excess. Less frequent causes include sickle cell disease, systemic lupus erythematosus (SLE), deep-sea diving (Caisson's disease), endocrine disorders (e.g. Cushing's, diabetes mellitus), trauma, human immunodeficiency virus (HIV) infection and irradiation.

Osteonecrosis usually presents with joint pain, the shoulder or hip being most commonly affected, but can be asymptomatic, particularly on the opposite side in the same person. It may only be recognized when it results in collapse of the articular bone.

MRI best confirms the diagnosis by showing bone marrow oedema. If advanced, it can be seen on plain X-rays.

Management is mainly symptomatic. Surgical options include drilling through the bone cortex (decompression), vascularized bone grafts, or rotation of the affected bone away from the load-bearing area; however, joint replacement is often required. Bisphosphonates may reduce pain, and progression has been reduced with statin therapy in steroid-associated osteonecrosis.

PAGET'S DISEASE OF BONE

Paget's disease of bone is a focal disorder of bone remodelling. Increased osteoclastic bone resorption is followed by a compensatory increase in new bone formation, increased local bone blood flow and fibrous tissue in adjacent bone marrow. Ultimately, formation [illegible] resorption but the new woven bone is weaker than normal bone, which leads to deformity and increased fracture risk. Paget's disease does not spread, but can become symptomatic at previously silent sites.

Epidemiological studies are difficult because most affected individuals are asymptomatic. Paget's disease is most often seen in Europe and particularly in northern England. It affects men and women (2:3) over the age of 40 years. The incidence approximately doubles per decade thereafter, with up to 10% of individuals radiologically affected by the age of 90. For unknown reasons, the incidence and severity of Paget's disease have decreased in recent years.

Aetiology and pathogenesis

Genetic factors are implicated in Paget's disease. A positive family history is noted in about 15%. Mutations in *SQSTM1*, which encodes the osteoclast mediator protein p62, have been reported in up to 10% of cases. Intracellular inclusions in the osteoclasts in pagetic lesions are believed to be paramyxovirus nucleocapsid (e.g. canine distemper virus, measles or respiratory syncytial virus). However, similar inclusions are seen in other bone disorders, and theories of a viral aetiology in Paget's remain contentious. Altered expression of *c-fos* (an oncogene) is one suggested mechanism linking viral infection with the pathogenic changes in osteoclasts, which are more numerous and contain an increased number of nuclei (up to 100).

Clinical features (see *Fig. 19.10A*)

Between 60% and 80% of people with radiologically identified Paget's disease are asymptomatic. Diagnosis often follows the finding of an asymptomatic elevation of serum alkaline phosphatase, or a plain X-ray performed for other indications. The disease may involve one bone (monostotic, in 15%) or many (polyostotic). The most common sites, in order of frequency, are pelvis, femur, lumbar spine, skull and tibia (see ***Fig. 19.10C***). Small bones of the feet and hands are rarely involved.

Symptoms and complications include:

- **bone pain**
- **joint pain** when an involved bone is close to a joint, leading to cartilage damage and osteoarthritis
- **deformities,** in particular bowed tibia and skull changes
- **neurological complications** – nerve compression (deafness from VIIIth cranial nerve involvement; cranial nerves II, V and VII may also be involved); spinal stenosis; hydrocephalus due to blockage of the aqueduct of Sylvius
- **high-output cardiac failure** and myocardial hypertrophy due to increased bone blood flow
- **hypercalcaemia** – rarely seen outside the setting of fracture
- **pathological fractures**
- **osteosarcoma** – occurs in fewer than 1% of cases of Paget's and may be heralded by an increase in bone pain or swelling in a previous pagetic bone area.

Investigations

- ***Increased serum alkaline phosphatase*** with normal serum calcium and phosphate reflects increased bone turnover. Levels may be normal with limited or monostotic Paget's disease. Levels are reduced with treatment and increased during relapse.
- ***Vitamin D*** should be measured, as deficiency is frequent in the age group affected by Paget's disease and should be corrected (see p. 718) to avoid hypocalcaemia following bisphosphonate treatment
- ***X-ray*** features ***(Fig. 19.10B)*** vary from predominantly lytic lesions (osteoporosis circumscripta in the skull is characteristic), through a mixed phase, to a mainly sclerotic phase of bone expansion, cortical thickening and coarsening of the trabecular pattern.
- ***Isotope bone scans*** are useful to determine the extent of skeletal involvement, but are unable to distinguish between Paget's disease and sclerotic metastatic carcinoma (especially breast and prostate).

Management

Bisphosphonates are the mainstay of treatment. New bone formed after treatment is lamellar, not woven (reflecting normalization of bone turnover rather than a direct effect on osteoblasts). Treatment is interrupted and repeat courses are guided by symptoms and by recurrence in elevation of alkaline phosphatase. In addition to treatment of symptomatic patients, treatment of asymptomatic lesions is appropriate if there is a significant risk of potential

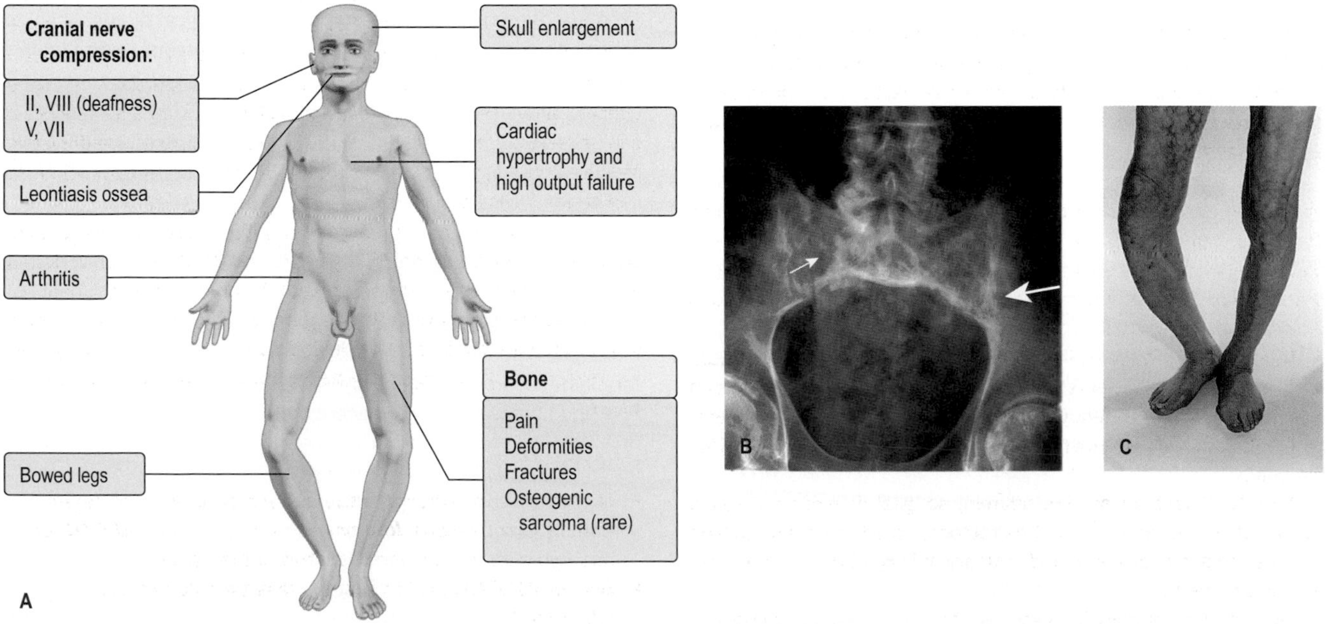

Figure 19.10 **Paget's disease. A.** Clinical features. **B.** X-ray appearance of the pelvis, showing osteolytic (thin arrow) and osteosclerotic (thick arrow) lesions. **C.** Legs showing bowing of the tibia caused by increased bone growth. Note the erythema ab igne on the medial aspect of the thigh.

complications, such as fracture in weight-bearing long bones or the spine, nerve entrapment or deafness with skull involvement, and before orthopaedic procedures in involved bone (to reduce vascularity).

Intravenous bisphosphonates

Zoledronate is the most commonly used agent for Paget's disease, administered as a single infusion over 15 min. **Pamidronate** is an alternative but takes longer to infuse and is less potent; some patients develop drug resistance for unknown reasons. Both drugs can be associated with a first-dose reaction characterized by 'flu-like' symptoms, including transient pyrexia over 24–48 hours, which can be ameliorated with paracetamol.

Oral bisphosphonates

Oral bisphosphonates are used at doses higher than those for osteoporosis (e.g. 30 mg risedronate daily for 2 months, or 40 mg alendronate daily for 6 months) and are less effective than intravenous zoledronic acid.

Surgery

Joint replacement or osteotomy is sometimes necessary to correct deformity or pain due to associated degenerative joint disease. Neurosurgery may be needed where there is spinal disease. Osteosarcoma usually requires amputation, though wide excision and limb salvage can be successful at distal sites.

Further reading

Ralston SH. Paget's disease of bone. *N Engl J Med* 2013; 368:644–650.

RICKETS AND OSTEOMALACIA

Osteomalacia is defective mineralization of newly formed bone matrix or osteoid. Rickets is defective mineralization at the epiphyseal growth plate and is found in association with osteomalacia in children.

Aetiology

Many factors can result in defective mineralization of the osteoid. For normal mineralization, adequate levels of vitamin D, calcium and phosphate, adequate activity of alkaline phosphatase, a normal pH at the osteoid surface and normal osteoid composition are all necessary ***(Box 19.6)***.

The most common cause of osteomalacia is hypophosphataemia due to hyperparathyroidism secondary to vitamin D deficiency. The most common cause of vitamin D deficiency worldwide is dietary deficiency. Bread, milk and cereals in high-income countries are now fortified with vitamin D. This has led to a much-reduced incidence of osteomalacia and rickets.

Vitamin D is produced in the skin through the action of sunlight on 7-dehydrocholesterol (see ***Fig. 19.4***). Lack of sun exposure can lead to vitamin D deficiency, especially in individuals living in temperate regions who keep large parts of the skin covered throughout the year.

Vitamin D is a fat-soluble vitamin, so gastrointestinal disease can result in malabsorption. Gastrectomy, cystic fibrosis, coeliac disease, Crohn's disease and primary biliary cirrhosis are well-recognized causes.

Due to the intimate involvement of the kidney in phosphate balance, a number of causes of osteomalacia are mediated by the kidney (see p. 779). Primary renal phosphate wasting occurs in tumour-induced osteomalacia, multiple myeloma and Fanconi syndrome. Proximal (type 2) renal tubular acidosis can cause osteomalacia due to both renal phosphate wasting and abnormal osteoid pH secondary to metabolic acidosis.

Box 19.6 Causes of rickets/osteomalacia

Deficient intake or absorption of vitamin D
- Inadequate sun exposure or deficient synthesis in skin
- Low dietary intake
- Malabsorption: coeliac disease, Crohn's disease, gastrectomy, primary biliary cirrhosis

Defective 1α-hydroxylation
- Chronic kidney disease
- Vitamin D-dependent rickets type I – due to deficiency of 1α-hydroxylase

Primary renal phosphate wasting
- Renal tubular acidosis (also by causing metabolic acidosis)
- Hereditary hypophosphataemic rickets (vitamin D-resistant rickets)
- Dent's disease
- Fanconi syndrome
- Multiple myeloma
- Tumour-induced osteomalacia

Inhibitors of mineralization
- Fluoride, aluminium, bisphosphonates
- Metabolic acidosis

Defective vitamin D receptors
- Hereditary vitamin D-resistant rickets (previously known as vitamin D-dependent rickets type II)

Clinical features

Osteomalacia may be asymptomatic and identified incidentally on routine investigations following a fragility fracture. When symptomatic, it characteristically causes muscle weakness and widespread bone pain. Muscle weakness is due to a multifactorial proximal myopathy, with low vitamin D, hypophosphataemia and high PTH levels all contributing. It results in a characteristic waddling gait with difficulty climbing stairs and getting out of a chair. Generalized bone pain and tenderness are thought to be caused by hydration of the demineralized matrix, resulting in periosteal distension. The pain is typically a dull ache that is worse on weight-bearing and walking. It can be reproduced by pressure on the sternum or tibia. Insufficiency fractures can occur when the quality of the bone is insufficient to handle the stress of weight-bearing.

At birth, neonatal rickets may present as craniotabes (a thin, deformed skull). In the first few years of life, there may be widened epiphyses at the wrists and beading at the costochondral junctions, producing the 'rickety rosary', or a groove in the rib cage (Harrison's sulcus). In older children, lower limb deformities are seen. A myopathy may also occur. Hypocalcaemic tetany may occur in severe cases.

Investigations

- ***Serum alkaline phosphatase*** is elevated in 90% of cases.
- ***Low serum calcium***, ***low phosphate*** and ***elevated PTH*** are each present in approximately half of the cases.
- ***Serum 25-(OH)D_3*** is low, usually less than 25 nmol/L (10 ng/mL).
- ***Serum FGF-23*** is elevated in many people with tumour-induced osteomalacia and in hypophosphataemic rickets.

- ***Plain radiographs*** demonstrate decreased bone mineralization. The characteristic finding in osteomalacia is Looser's pseudofractures. These are narrow radiolucent lines with sclerotic borders running perpendicular to the cortex. They can be found at any site but are most commonly seen in the femur and pelvis.
- ***Tetracycline-labelled bone biopsy*** is the gold standard diagnostic test. This is not practical in most clinical settings and is used mainly in research studies.

Management

Vitamin D replacement is the cornerstone of treatment. Treatment involves two stages: an initial loading stage to replenish body stores of vitamin D, and a subsequent maintenance phase to avoid repeat deficiency. All patients should also receive supplementary calcium of 1000–1200 mg/day. In nutritional deficiency, recommended initial replacement is with vitamin D 50 000 units per week orally. The initial replacement dose should be continued for 8 weeks. Vitamin D is also available as an intramuscular injection; two doses of 300 000 units are usually enough to replenish body stores. Adequacy of vitamin D replacement should be evaluated by re-assaying vitamin D levels, or PTH levels if initially abnormal. This should be followed by regular supplementation with 800–1000 units of vitamin D per day.

Doses for children are lower and are age-dependent. People with gastrointestinal disease and vitamin D deficiency due to malabsorption need higher doses of 10 000–50 000 units per day of vitamin D.

Tumour-induced osteomalacia is best treated by removal of the causative neoplasm, which is usually occult and frequently benign. This leads to rapid resolution of symptoms.

Further reading

Elder C J, Bishop NJ. Rickets. *Lancet* 2014; 383:1665–1676.
Pearce SH, Cheetham TD. Diagnosis and management of vitamin D deficiency. *BMJ* 2010; 340:b5664.

BONE INFECTIONS

Acute and chronic osteomyelitis

Osteomyelitis predominantly occurs in children and chronicity is common. In children, it commonly arises due to haematogenous spread to the vascular metaphysis. In high-income countries, it occurs in around 8 per 100 000 children per year, but it is considerably more common in low-income countries, with boys affected twice as often as girls. Malnutrition, debilitating disease and decreased immunity play a role in the pathogenesis. Without prompt recognition, it has devastating consequences.

Staphylococcus is the organism responsible for 90% of cases of acute osteomyelitis. Other organisms include *Haemophilus influenzae* and *Salmonella*; infection with the latter may occur as a complication of sickle cell anaemia. The classic presentation is with fever and localized bone pain with overlying tenderness and erythema, although it is rare in adults and often hard to diagnose, requiring a bone biopsy.

Diagnosis

- ***Imaging***:
  - Plain X-ray is not sensitive in early infection but osteopenia may be present.
  - MRI is highly sensitive, showing marrow oedema in 3 days.
  - Bone scans are also helpful.
- ***Blood cultures*** are often positive with staphylococcal infection.
- ***Bone biopsy and culture*** identifies the organism and sensitivities.

Management

Treatment of osteomyelitis centres on immobilization and antibiotic therapy with intravenous teicoplanin or intravenous flucloxacillin 1–2 g every 6 hours and oral sodium fusidate. Switch to oral antibiotics after 2 weeks and continue for a further 4 weeks. Surgical drainage and removal of dead bone (sequestrum) may be necessary but recurrence is common.

Delayed treatment leads to chronic osteomyelitis. In chronic osteomyelitis, sinus formation is usual. Subacute osteomyelitis is associated with a chronic abscess within the bone (Brodie's abscess). Symptoms may be limited to local pain.

Tuberculous osteomyelitis

This is usually due to haematogenous spread from a reactivated primary focus in the lungs or gastrointestinal tract. The disease starts in intra-articular bone. The spine is commonly involved **(Pott's disease)**, with damage to the bodies of two neighbouring vertebrae leading to vertebral collapse and acute angulation of the spine (gibbus). Later, an abscess forms ('cold abscess'). Pus can track along tissue planes and discharge at a point far from the affected vertebrae. Symptoms consist of local pain and later swelling if pus has collected. Systemic symptoms of malaise, fever and night sweats occur.

Management is as for pulmonary tuberculosis but extended to 9 months (see pp. 1110–1113), together with initial immobilization.

NEOPLASTIC DISEASE OF BONE

Bone pain may be due to multiple myeloma, lymphoma, a primary tumour of bone or secondary deposits. The pain is typically unremitting and worse at night, and there are other clinical clues such as weight loss or ill-health.

Malignant tumours of bone are shown in ***Box 19.7.*** The most common tumours are metastases from the bronchus, breast and prostate. Metastases from kidney and thyroid are less common. Primary bone tumours are rare and usually seen only in children and young adults.

Symptoms are usually related to the anatomical position of the tumour, with local bone pain. Systemic symptoms (e.g. malaise and pyrexia) and aches and pains occur and are occasionally related to hypercalcaemia. The diagnosis of metastases can often be made from the history and examination, particularly if the primary tumour has already been diagnosed. Symptoms from bony metastases may, however, be the first presenting feature.

Box 19.7 Malignant neoplasms of bone

- Metastases (osteolytic):
  - Bronchus
  - Breast
  - Prostate (often osteosclerotic as well)
  - Thyroid
  - Kidney
- Multiple myeloma
- Primary bone tumours (rare; seen in the young), e.g.:
  - Osteosarcomas
  - Fibrosarcomas
  - Chondromas
  - Ewing's tumour

Investigations

- ***Skeletal isotope scans*** show bony metastases as 'hot' areas before radiological changes occur.
- ***X-rays*** may show metastases as osteolytic areas with bony destruction. Osteosclerotic metastases are characteristic of prostatic carcinoma.
- ***MRI*** is used extensively, particularly for vertebral lesions.
- ***CT and computed tomography-positron emission tomography (CT-PET)*** are useful.
- ***Serum alkaline phosphatase*** (from bone) is usually raised.
- ***Hypercalcaemia*** occurs in 10–20% of patients who have metastatic malignancies, or is due to ectopic parathormone or PTH-related protein secretion.
- ***Prostate-specific antigen*** (PSA) and serum acid phosphatase are raised in the presence of prostatic metastases.

Management

Treatment is usually with analgesics and anti-inflammatory drugs. Local radiotherapy to bone metastases relieves pain and reduces the risk of pathological fracture. Some tumours respond to chemotherapy; others are hormone-dependent and respond to hormonal therapy. Bisphosphonates (see p. 714) can help symptomatically. Occasionally, pathological fractures require internal fixation.

OTHER BONE DISORDERS

Osteopetrosis (marble bone disease)

This condition may be inherited in either an autosomal dominant or a typically severe, autosomal recessive pattern. Another recessive form associated with renal tubular acidosis is due to carbonic anhydrase II deficiency.

The severe form is caused by a mutation in the gene encoding a chloride channel necessary for osteoclast activity. Bone density is increased throughout the skeleton but bones tend to fracture easily. Encroachment on the marrow space leads to a leucoerythroblastic anaemia. There is mental retardation and early death. In the mild form, there may be only X-ray changes, but fractures and infection can occur. The acid phosphatase level may be raised. Stem cell transplantation has been successful.

Scheuermann's disease

This disease predominantly occurs in adolescent boys. The main feature is a progressive dorsal kyphosis of the thoracic spine. Pain may or may not be present. The cause is unknown. A genetic predisposition, exacerbated by excessive exercise prior to epiphyseal fusion, is one suggested explanation. Older patients with kyphosis may be referred with suspected osteoporotic fractures but found to have long-standing kyphosis due to Scheuermann's. Management is focused on postural exercises and avoidance of precipitants. Surgery may be undertaken to correct kyphosis in severe cases.

Bibliography

Rosen CJ, ed. *Primer on the Metabolic Bone Diseases and Disorders of Mineral Metabolism*, 8th edn. Hoboken, New Jersey: Wiley–Blackwell, American Society for Bone and Mineral Research; 2013.

Significant websites

http://nof.org *National Osteoporosis Foundation – useful clinicians' guide.*
http://www.iscd.org *International Society for Clinical Densitometry – guidelines on DXA scanning.*
http://www.nos.org.uk/ *UK National Osteoporosis Society – useful information and reviews of ongoing research.*

20 Kidney and urinary tract disease

M Magdi Yaqoob, Neil Ashman

See your e-book for key learning points, summaries, clinical tips, drug tips, extra tables, extra images, interactive Figures, videos, MCQs and Special Topics from the International Advisory Board.

KIDNEYS AND URINARY TRACT

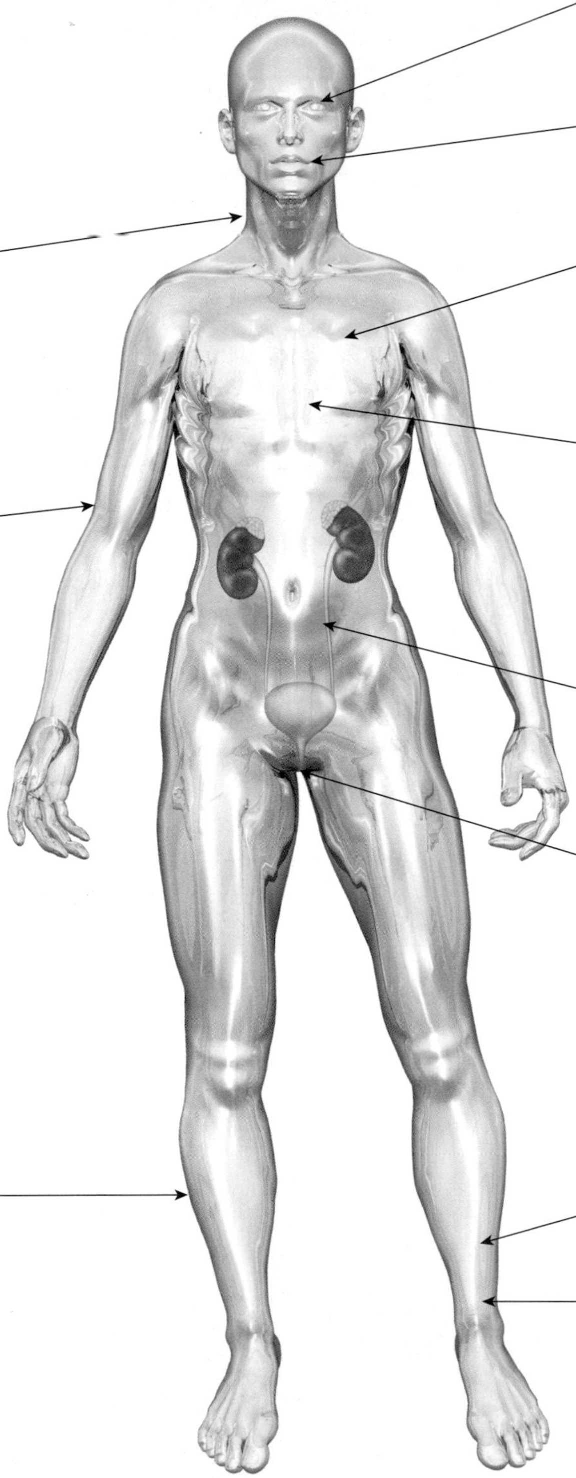
General
Looks tired
Pale (anaemia with high urea/creatinine)
Tachypnoea (metabolic acidosis)
Yellowish complexion
? confused (e.g. elderly with urinary tract infection)
↑ Jugular venous pressure (fluid overload)
Blood pressure
(? raised)
Skin
Pruritus (with high urea)
Vasculitic rash
Fundoscopy
- may show hypertensive changes
Dry mouth if fluid depletion
Lungs
- basal crackles in fluid overload
Heart
- pericardial friction rub (in uraemia)
- Extra heart sound (fluid overload)
- Arrhythmias from hyperkalaemia
Abdomen
+/– enlarged kidneys
Tender
Arterial bruits (renal vascular disease)
Suprapubic tenderness (infection)
Rectal examination
? enlarged prostate
Urine analysis
- Blood and protein
- Microscopy
- Bacteriology
Ankle (or sacral) oedema
Peripheral sensorimotor neuropathy

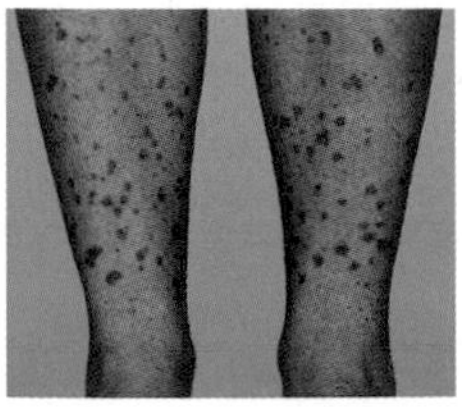

ANATOMY AND PHYSIOLOGY OF THE KIDNEY AND URINARY TRACT

Functional anatomy

The ***kidneys*** are paired organs, 11–14 cm in length in adults, 5–6 cm in width and 3–4 cm in depth. They lie in the retroperitoneum, on either side of the vertebral column at the level of T12–L3 (the right kidney lies lower than the left, pushed down by the liver). Each kidney is enclosed in a fibrous capsule, and has an outer cortex and an inner medulla ***(Fig. 20.1)***. There are about 1 million ***nephrons*** in each kidney. Each nephron contains a glomerulus, proximal tubule, loop of Henle, distal tubule and collecting duct. All glomeruli lie in the cortex, and tubules dip in and out of the medulla, where the collecting ducts merge to form the ducts of Bellini, emptying at a papilla at the apex of renal pyramid into a calyx. Urine then flows through merging calyces into the renal pelvis, ureters and bladder.

The renal arteries branch off the abdominal aorta, dividing into smaller branches until arterial blood reaches the glomerulus. About 25% of people have dual or multiple renal arteries on one or both sides. ***Afferent glomerular arterioles*** arise from interlobular branch arteries to supply the glomerular capillary tuft, which drains into ***efferent glomerular arterioles***. Efferent arterioles from (outer) cortical glomeruli drain into a peritubular capillary network within the renal cortex and then into increasingly large and more proximal branches of the renal vein. By contrast, blood from the (inner) juxtamedullary glomeruli passes via vasa recta in the medulla and returns via the cortex to renal veins that drain into the inferior vena cava.

The renal capsule and ureters are innervated via T10–12 and L1 nerve roots, and renal pain is felt over the corresponding dermatomes.

The nephron

A ball of capillaries makes up the glomerular tuft, enclosed by Bowman's capsule, a chamber lined with specialized ***parietal epithelial cells*** that marks the origin of the tubule ***(Fig. 20.2)***. The tuft, held together and regulated by ***mesangial cells***, then serves as the filtration barrier, allowing filtrate from plasma to move into the urinary (Bowman's) space. The rate of glomerular filtration is influenced by changes in the contractile tone in either the afferent or the efferent arterioles; for example, efferent vasoconstriction will increase the transglomerular capillary pressure, and increase filtration.

Glomerular capillaries are lined with ***endothelial cells***, fenestrated with 60–80-nm pores, and covered with charged glycocalyx. The glomerular basement membrane (GBM), about 300 nm thick

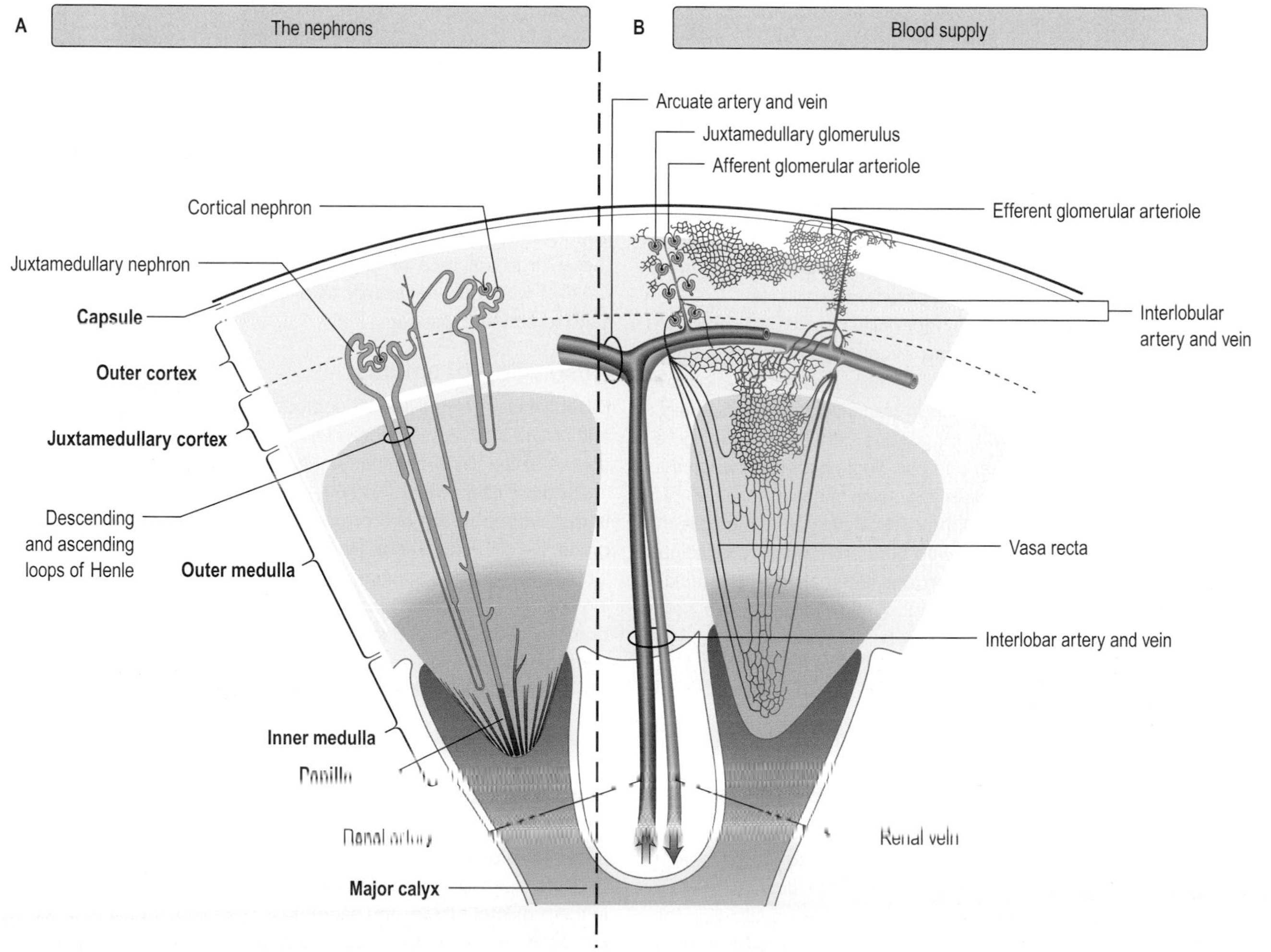

Figure 20.1 Functional anatomy of the kidney. A. The nephrons. **B.** Arterial and venous supply. *(After Standring S (ed.).* Gray's Anatomy, *40th edn. Edinburgh: Churchill Livingstone; 2008.)*

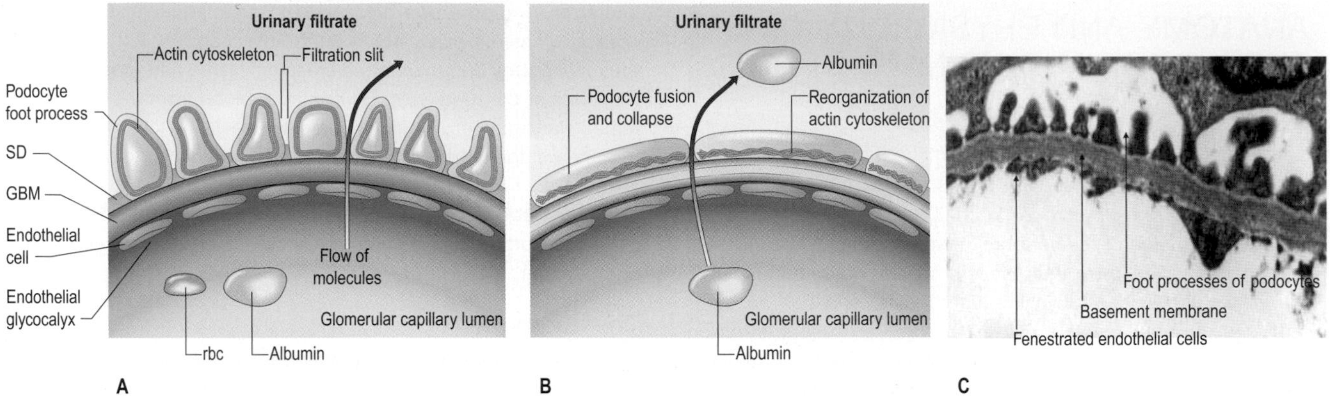

Figure 20.2 The glomerular filtration barrier. A. Blood enters the glomerular capillaries and is filtered across the endothelium and the glomerular basement membrane (GBM), and through the filtration slits between podocyte foot processes to produce the primary urine filtrate. In healthy glomeruli, this barrier restricts the passage of macromolecules. The proteins that form the slit diaphragm (SD) are essential for the normal functioning of the filtration barrier. **B.** Loss of these proteins, either genetically or by acquired means, leads to foot process effacement, breakdown of the barrier and leakage of albumin. **C.** Electron micrograph of the normal filtration barrier. rbc, red blood cell. *(A, B. Adapted from Quaggin S. Sizing up sialic acid in glomerular disease.* Journal of Clinical Investigation *2007; 117:1480–1483.)*

and made of type IV collagen, laminin and heparin sulphate, separates endothelium from podocytes (or visceral epithelial cells). Podocytes anchor on to the GBM by means of an extensive trabecular network of foot processes, and hang into Bowman's space. The interdigitating foot processes of podocytes then form the 40-nm filtration slit, a narrow potential space traversed by a protein 'zipper' that may prevent the passage of larger molecules (such as albumin) into the urinary space, and regulates the architecture and function of podocytes.

Mesangial cells (thought to be related to macrophages) sit within the tuft, able to contract and relax to control blood flow and the filtration surface area along the glomerular capillaries in response to a host of mediators. They also secrete the ***mesangial matrix***, which provides the scaffolding for glomerular capillaries.

The ***renal tubules*** are lined by epithelial cells, which alter the composition of filtrate to form urine eventually. Proximal tubular cells have a luminal brush border to increase (by 30-fold) the surface area exposed to filtrate, rich in transporters and channels. The loop of Henle is lined with squamous cells, which are more permeable to water than solute, and cuboidal epithelium, when the reverse is true. The distal tubule regulates electrolytes and pH through cuboidal epithelium, and the cortical portion of the collecting ducts contains two cell types with different functions: principal cells (sodium, potassium and water) and intercalated cells (acid–base; see p. 153). Finally, resident interstitial fibroblast-like cells in the renal cortex produce erythropoietin in response to hypoxia (see p. 728).

The juxtaglomerular apparatus

The juxtaglomerular apparatus regulates flow and filtration in each individual nephron. Columnar epithelium in the macula densa ***(Fig. 20.3)*** senses the concentration of tubular fluid sodium (higher filtrate flow means more delivered sodium), triggering adenosine-mediated vasoconstriction of the afferent arteriole to drop glomerular filtration (so-called tubule–glomerular feedback). Juxtaglomerular cells secrete renin, able to induce aldosterone release, allowing the apparatus to monitor flow, and respond when necessary to drop glomerular filtration rate (GFR) and retain salt to maintain fluid balance.

Physiology

A ***hydrostatic pressure gradient*** of approximately 10 mmHg (a capillary pressure of 45 mmHg minus 10 mmHg of pressure within Bowman's space and 25 mmHg of plasma oncotic pressure) provides the driving force for ultrafiltration of virtually protein-free and fat-free fluid across the glomerular filter into Bowman's space and so into the renal tubule ***(Fig. 20.4)***.

The ***ultrafiltration rate*** (GFR) varies with age and sex but is approximately 120–130 mL/min per 1.73 m^2 surface area in adults. This means that, each day, ultrafiltration of 170–180 L of water and unbound small-molecular-weight constituents of blood occurs. If these large volumes of ultrafiltrate were excreted unchanged as urine, it would be necessary to drink huge amounts of water and salts to stay in balance.

Absorption of solutes

Essential electrolytes and other blood constituents, such as glucose and amino acids, are absorbed from filtrate in transit along the long course of the nephron (see ***Fig. 20.3***).

Sodium filters freely, and 60–80% of filtered sodium (and water) is reabsorbed in the late proximal tubule, where the apical membrane Na^+/H^+ exchanger (NHE3) trades hydrogen ions into the lumen for absorbed sodium, with anionic chloride (Cl^-) accompanying sodium to maintain electric neutrality. Secreted H^+ allows bicarbonate (HCO_3^-), formed from water and CO_2 by cellular and luminal carbonic anhydrase, to exit the basolateral membrane with absorbed Na^+. Around 25% is then absorbed in the thick ascending limb of the loop of Henle, as NaCl by the $Na^+/K^+/2Cl^-$ co-transporter (NKCC). The remaining 5% is absorbed by the thiazide-sensitive NaCl co-transporter and the epithelial sodium channel (ENaC), in the principal cell of the collecting duct. Of the recommended allowance of <6 g/day of ***salt*** (equivalent to around 2 g Na^+), around 5–10% will be excreted in urine, stool and sweat.

Potassium is freely filtered at the glomerulus, largely reabsorbed in the proximal tubule, and secreted in the distal tubule and collecting ducts. A clinical consequence of this is that the ability to eliminate unwanted potassium is less dependent on GFR than is the elimination of urea or creatinine. Virtually all bicarbonate, glucose

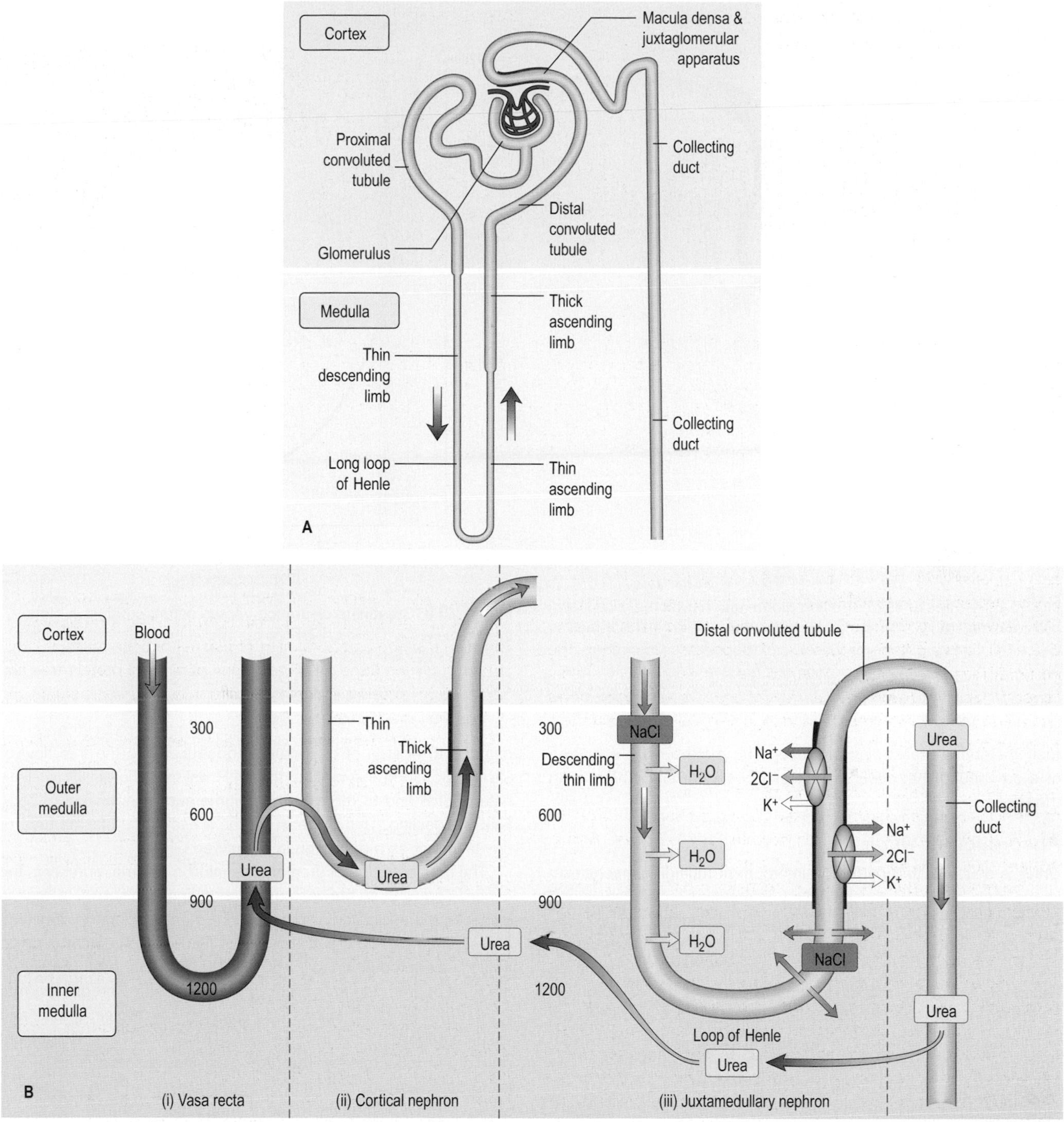

Figure 20.3 Functional anatomy of the nephron. A. Principal parts of the nephron. The point where the distal tubule is in close proximity to its own glomerulus is called the juxtaglomerular apparatus. This contains the macula densa. **B.** The countercurrent system. (i) *Vasa recta*: these vessels descend from the cortex into the medulla and then turn back towards the cortex. (ii) *Cortical nephron*: these have short descending limbs extending into the outer medulla. (iii) *Juxtamedullary nephron*: the descending limb dips deeply into the hypertonic inner medulla. Numbers indicate approximate osmolalities.

and amino acids (**Fig. 20.3B**) are absorbed in the proximal tubule, making use of the large surface area of this segment of the nephron.

The proximal tubule has a maximal absorptive capacity for many compounds. For instance, if blood glucose levels are elevated above the normal range, the amount filtered (filtered load = GFR × plasma concentration) may exceed the maximal absorptive capacity of the proximal tubule and glucose will 'spill over' into the urine as glycosuria. Inherited or acquired defects in tubular function may also lead to incomplete absorption of a *normal* filtered load, and substances such as glucose (renal glycosuria), amino acids, phosphate, sodium, potassium and calcium will appear in the urine, either singly or in combination. Examples include cystinuria (a defect of a specific amino acid transporter) or Fanconi syndrome (see pp. 1286–1287).

Other compounds filtered and reabsorbed or secreted to a variable extent include urate, many organic acids and many drugs or

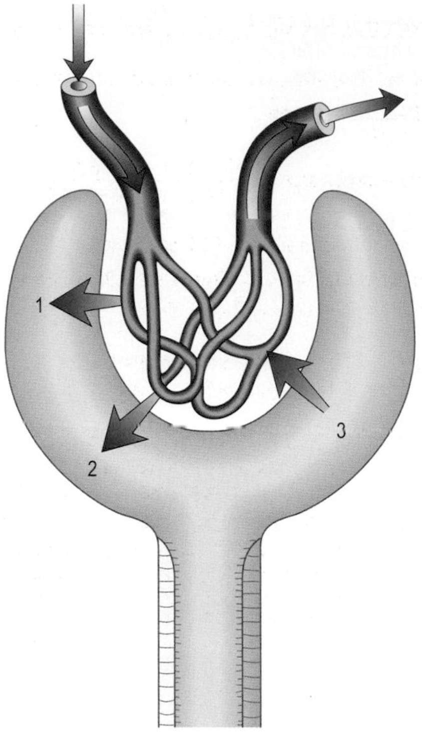

Figure 20.4 Pressures controlling glomerular filtration. (1) Capillary hydrostatic pressure (45 mmHg). **(2)** Hydrostatic pressure in Bowman's space (10 mmHg). **(3)** Plasma protein oncotic pressure (25 mmHg). Arrows (1, 2, 3) indicate the direction of a pressure gradient.

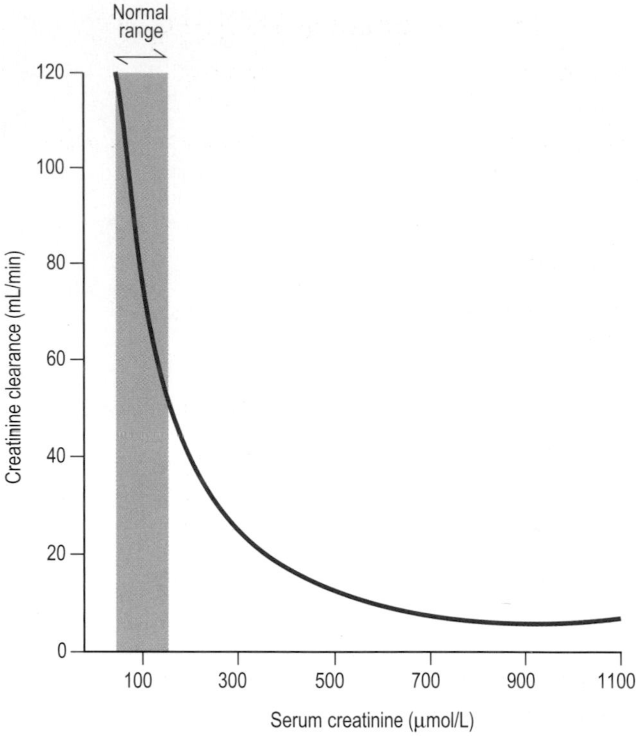

Figure 20.5 Creatinine clearance versus serum creatinine. Note that the serum creatinine does not rise above the normal range until there is a reduction of 50–60% in the glomerular filtration rate (creatinine clearance).

their metabolic breakdown products. The more tubular secretion of a compound that occurs, the less dependent elimination is on the GFR.

Absorption of water

Urine is concentrated by the countercurrent multiplier mechanism in the loop of Henle, the medullary interstitium, medullary blood vessels (vasa recta) and, finally, the collecting ducts (see pp. 153–154). Sodium and urea in water flow as filtrate into the descending loop, permeable to water and impermeable to sodium. In the thick ascending limb (impermeable to water), active absorption of sodium by the $Na^+/K^+/2Cl^-$ co-transporter into the interstitium increases the tissue osmolarity. Because of the hairpin nature of the loop, water from the permeable descending limb enters the interstitium by osmosis, where the vasa recta return fluid to the circulation. Constant active absorption of sodium in the ascending loop multiplies this process over time, and the solute concentration at the tip of the loop is fourfold that of extracellular fluid. By this mechanism, salt and water are returned to the circulation. Filtrate entering the collecting duct is increasingly concentrated by the action of antidiuretic hormone (ADH, or vasopressin), leading to the release of intracellular aquaporin water channels, which insert themselves across the apical membrane. Water then enters the cell along an osmotic gradient. When the effect of ADH wears off, water channels return to the cell cytoplasm (see ***Fig. 9.5***). The final urine volume is 1–2 L daily.

Glomerular filtration rate

In health, the GFR remains constant owing to intrarenal regulatory mechanisms. In disease (e.g. a reduction in intrarenal blood flow, damage to or loss of glomeruli or obstruction to the free flow of ultrafiltrate along the tubule), the GFR will fall. The ability to eliminate wastes and to regulate the volume and composition of body fluid will decline. This is measured as a rise in the plasma urea or creatinine, or as a reduction in measured GFR.

The concentration of urea or creatinine in plasma represents the dynamic equilibrium between production and elimination. In healthy subjects, there is an enormous reserve of renal excretory function, and serum urea and creatinine do not rise above the normal range until there is a reduction of 50–60% in the GFR ***(Fig. 20.5)***. Thereafter, the level of urea depends on both the GFR and its production rate ***(Box 20.1)***. The latter is heavily influenced by protein intake and tissue catabolism. The level of creatinine is much less dependent on diet but is more related to age, sex and muscle mass. Once it is elevated, serum creatinine is a better guide to GFR than urea and is widely used to monitor further deterioration in the GFR.

Measuring or estimating the GFR

If a substance is filtered, and then unmodified by the tubules as it passes along the nephron, the concentration of that substance per mL will be the same in blood and urine. Accurate calculations of the GFR, particularly in cases where the urea and creatinine may be in the normal range or near normal, can be assessed by cystatin C and creatinine clearance. Alternatives for quantifying the true GFR include measuring ***iohexol*** or ***inulin clearance***, or radio-isotope (^{51}Cr-EDTA) GFR. Neither is practical for daily clinical practice.

Cystatin C

This is a freely filtered, low-molecular-weight protein that appears to be a more accurate marker of kidney function than creatinine.

Box 20.1 Factors influencing serum urea levels

Production	Elimination
Increased by	
High-protein diet	Elevated GFR, e.g. pregnancy
Increased catabolism	
Surgery	
Infection	
Trauma	
Corticosteroid therapy	
Tetracyclines	
Gastrointestinal bleeding	
Cancer	
Decreased by	
Low-protein diet	Glomerular disease
Reduced catabolism, e.g. old age	Reduced renal blood flow
Liver failure	Hypotension
	Dehydration
	Urinary obstruction
	Tubulointerstitial nephritis

GFR, glomerular filtration rate.

Box 20.2 Estimation of glomerular filtration rate (GFR)

To convert creatinine values in μmol/L to mg/dL, multiply by 0.0113.

Cockcroft–Gault equation

$$\text{Creatinine clearance} = \frac{(140 - \text{age}) \times \text{weight (kg)} \times \text{constant}}{\text{Serum creatinine } [\mu\text{mol/L}]}$$

Constant = 1.23 for males and 1.04 for women.

Modification of diet in renal disease (MDRD) equation

Calculation of estimated GFR by four variables:

$$\text{Estimated GFR (mL/min/1.73 m}^2) = 32788 \times (S_{Cr})^{-1.154} \times (\text{age})^{-0203} \times \text{constant (0.742 if female)} \times (1.210 \text{ if black African})$$

CKD Epidemiology (CKD-EPI) Collaboration equation

GFR (mL/min/1.73 m^2) = 141 × min (serum creatinine/κ, 1)$^{\alpha}$ × max (serum creatinine/κ, 1)$^{-1.209}$ × 0.993^{Age} × 1.018 [if female] × 1.159 [if black] where κ is 0.7 for females and 0.9 for males, α is −0.329 for females and −0.411 for males, min indicates the minimum or serum creatinine/κ or 1, and max indicates the maximum of serum creatinine/κ or 1.

(Adapted from MacGregor MS, Boag DE, Innes A. Chronic kidney disease. Quarterly Journal of Medicine *2006; 99:365–375.)*

Blood concentrations are less affected by muscle mass, age and gender, but measurement of cystatin C has not widely entered clinical practice as yet.

Creatinine clearance

Daily production of creatinine (principally from muscle cells) is fairly constant and little affected by protein intake. Serum creatinine and excreted (urinary) creatinine vary little throughout the day. Small quantities of creatinine are secreted into the tubule but this does not usually affect the assay. Urine is collected over 24 hours for measurement of urinary creatinine. A single plasma level of creatinine is measured some time during the 24-hour period, and a creatinine clearance calculated as $U \times VP$, where U = urine concentration of creatinine, V = rate of urine flow in mL/min, and P = plasma concentration of creatinine. Normal ranges are 90–140 mL/min in men and 80–125 mL/min in women.

Estimated or calculated GFR – the eGFR

Measurement of GFR is cumbersome and time-consuming, and may be inaccurate if 24-hour urine collections are incomplete. Several formulae have been developed that predict creatinine clearance or GFR from serum creatinine and patient characteristics, often derived from large trials. Variables might include age, weight, gender and ethnicity. Commonly used equations are displayed in ***Box 20.2***. All have their shortcomings, and are less accurate the closer a GFR is to normal (so patients with seemingly abnormal calculated GFRs may have normal kidney function). Of the equations, the CKD-EPI equation is more accurate than the modification of diet in renal disease (MDRD) study equation overall and is most reliable for predicting eGFR >60 mL/min/1.73 m^2.

All these equations have not, however, been fully validated across all ranges of renal impairment, weights or body mass index (BMI), or in all ethnic groups. However, for monitoring patients with gouts or chronic kidney disease, the convenience and ease of the eGFR has led to its widespread adoption.

Drugs, toxins, proteins and the kidney

A substantial fraction of prescription drugs is handled and eliminated by the kidney. Many of these medications (e.g. penicillins, cephalosporins, diuretics, non-steroidal anti-inflammatory drugs (NSAIDs) and antivirals) circulate in the plasma as small organic anions, and are actively eliminated in the proximal tubule by a specific organic anion transporter (OAT) system.

The kidney is also a major site for the catabolism (and so elimination) of many small-molecular-weight proteins and polypeptides, including many hormones such as insulin, parathyroid hormone (PTH) and calcitonin, by endocytosis carried out by the megalin–cubilin complex in the brush border of proximal tubular cells. In chronic kidney disease (CKD), the metabolic clearance of these substances is reduced and their half-life is prolonged. This accounts, for example, for the reduced insulin requirements of patients with diabetes as their renal function declines.

Endocrine function

Renin–angiotensin system

(See ***Fig. 20.6***.) The ***juxtaglomerular apparatus*** (JGA) regulates flow and filtration in each individual nephron. Columnar epithelium in the macula densa (see ***Fig. 20.3***) senses the concentration of tubular fluid sodium (higher filtrate flow means more delivered sodium), triggering adenosine-mediated vasoconstriction of the afferent arteriole to drop glomerular filtration (tubuloglomerular feedback). Juxtaglomerular cells secrete renin, able to induce aldosterone release, allowing the apparatus to monitor flow, and respond when necessary to drop GFR and retain salt to maintain fluid balance.

Pro-renin, synthesized by specialized arteriolar smooth muscle cells in the JGA, is cleaved into the active proteolytic enzyme, renin. Active renin is stored in the JGA, and released in response to triggers related to a falling intravascular volume, pressure or increased fluid losses via the kidney. Specifically, these are:

- pressure changes in the afferent arteriole
- changes in sympathetic tone
- chloride and osmotic concentration in the distal tubule via the macula densa (see ***Fig. 20.3A***) – ***tubuloglomerular feedback***
- local prostaglandin and nitric oxide release.

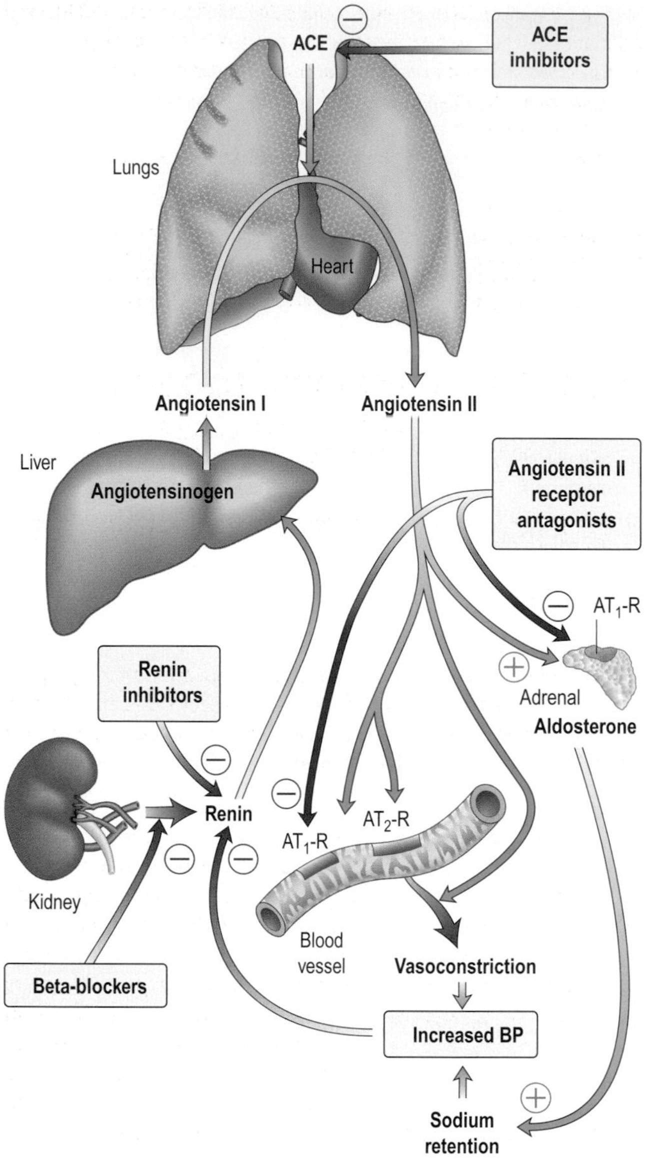

Figure 20.6 The renin–angiotensin–aldosterone system. Angiotensin-converting enzyme (ACE) inhibitors and angiotensin II antagonists can inhibit this system. BP, blood pressure.

In the blood, renin converts angiotensinogen, an α_2-globulin of hepatic origin, to inactive angiotensin I. Angiotensin I is further cleaved by angiotensin-converting enzyme (ACE, present in lung and vascular endothelium) into active ***angiotensin II*** (***AII***), which has two major actions (mediated by two types of receptor, AT_1 and AT_2). When AII binds the AT_1 subtype (found in the heart, blood vessels, kidney, adrenal cortex, lung and brain), this binding mediates vasoconstriction. AII binding AT_2 is probably involved in vascular growth.

AII:
- causes rapid, powerful vasoconstriction
- stimulates the adrenal zona glomerulosa to increase aldosterone production (over hours or days), leading to sodium (and water) absorption in the collecting duct
- causes vasoconstriction of efferent (but also, to a lesser extent, afferent) renal arterioles, resulting in increase of glomerular capillary pressure to maintain GFR.

The net result is that AII has opposing effects on the regulation of GFR:
- an increase in glomerular pressure and consequent rise in GFR
- reduction in renal blood flow and mesangial cell contraction, reducing filtration (see ***Fig. 20.44***).

In renal artery stenosis with resultant low perfusion pressure, AII maintains GFR.

The renin–angiotensin system can be blocked at several points with renin inhibitors, ACE inhibitors and angiotensin II receptor antagonists (AII-RAs). These are useful agents in the treatment of hypertension and heart failure (see pp. 1047 and 985) but have differences in action: ACE inhibitors also block kinin production while AII-RAs are specific for AT_1 receptors.

Erythropoietin

Erythropoietin (see also p. 519) is the major stimulus for erythropoiesis, the synthesis of red cells. It is a glycoprotein produced principally by fibroblast-like cells in the renal interstitium.
- Under ***hypoxic*** conditions, both the α and β subunits of hypoxia inducible factor 2 (HIF-2) are expressed, forming a heterodimer and causing erythropoietin gene transcription. Erythropoietin, once formed, binds to its receptors on erythroid precursor cells, to maintain normal red cell synthesis.
- Under ***normal oxygen*** conditions, only the HIF-2-β subunit is constitutively expressed. The α subunit undergoes proline hydroxylation in the presence of iron and oxygen.
- The hydroxylated HIF-2-α subunit binds to von Hippel–Lindau protein, with the activating ubiquitination (see p. 104) and subsequent degradation of HIF-2-α via proteosomes so that no erythropoietin is transcribed.

This and other hydroxylation steps have an absolute requirement for molecular oxygen; this forms the basis of oxygen sensing.

Loss of renal substance, with decreased erythropoietin production, results in a normochromic, normocytic anaemia. Conversely, erythropoietin secretion may be increased, with resultant polycythaemia, in people with polycystic renal disease, benign renal cysts or renal cell carcinoma.

Recombinant human erythropoietin has been biosynthesized and is available for clinical use, particularly in people with CKD (see p. 778).

Vitamin D metabolism

Naturally occurring vitamin D (see also p. 708; cholecalciferol) requires hydroxylation in the liver at position 25 and again by a renal 1α-hydroxylase enzyme to produce the metabolically active 1,25-dihydroxycholecalciferol (1,25-$(OH)_2D_3$).

Activity of 1α-hydroxylase is increased by:
- high plasma levels of PTH
- low serum phosphate
- low 1,25-$(OH)_2D_3$.

Both 1,25-dihydroxycholecalciferol and 25-hydroxycholecalciferol are degraded in part by being hydroxylated at position 24 by 24-hydroxylase. The activity of this enzyme is reduced by PTH and increased by 1,25-$(OH)_2D_3$ (which therefore promotes its own inactivation).

Reduced 1α-hydroxylase activity in diseased kidneys leads to relative deficiency of 1,25-$(OH)_2D_3$. As a result, gastrointestinal calcium and, to a lesser extent, phosphate absorption is reduced and bone mineralization impaired. Reduced gut calcium absorption leads to hypocalcaemia, which is sensed by a specific calcium-sensing receptor (CaSR) on parathyroid glands, and in turn induces release of PTH. Receptors for 1,25-$(OH)_2D_3$ are also found on parathyroid glands, and reduced receptor binding alters the set-point for release of PTH when plasma calcium falls. This combination contributes to the (common) secondary hyperparathyroidism seen in patients with CKD, even of modest degree.

Autocrine function

Endothelins

The endothelins (ETs) are a family of potent vasoactive peptides that also influence cell proliferation, tissue fibrosis and epithelial solute transport. They do not circulate but act locally. ETs are produced by most types of cell in the kidney. When binding ET-type A receptor, ET mediates vasoconstriction. When binding to ET-type B receptor, ETs cause vasodilatation. Through vasoconstriction by ETA and salt and water retention via ETB receptors, ETs cause hypertension.

Prostaglandins

Prostaglandins are unsaturated, oxygenated fatty acids, derived from the enzymatic metabolism of arachidonic acid, mainly by constitutively expressed cyclo-oxygenase-1 (COX-1) or inducible COX-2 (see ***Fig. 24.30***). COX-1 is highly expressed in the collecting duct, while COX-2 expression is restricted to the macula densa. Both COX isoforms convert arachidonic acid to unstable prostaglandin H_2 (PGH_2). PGH_2 is then converted to:

- PGE_2 in the collecting duct, responsible for natriuretic and diuretic effects
- PGD_2, which is of undetermined significance, produced in the proximal tubule
- prostacyclin (PGI_2), synthesized in the interstitium and vessels
- thromboxane A_2, a vasoconstrictor, mainly synthesized in the glomerulus.

They all maintain renal blood flow and GFR in the face of vasoconstrictors such as angiotensin II, catecholamines and α-adrenergic stimulation. Inhibition of prostaglandin synthesis by NSAIDs results in a further reduction in GFR, which is sometimes sufficiently severe as to cause acute kidney injury (AKI), particularly in the elderly, with volume depletion, or where ACE inhibitors or AII-RAs are used.

Natriuretic peptides

Atrial natriuretic peptides (ANPs) are secreted from granules in the cardiac atria in response to atrial stretch (as might be caused by increased venous return or by volume overload). They produce marked sodium and water excretion and increase GFR rate. ANP is also a direct vasodilator, lowering blood pressure; it reduces renin release and aldosterone secretion, and consequently inhibits AII synthesis. Their effects are to reverse salt and water retention. ***Brain natriuretic peptide*** (BNP) is found in the ventricle as well as the brain and has sequence homology with ANP. Normally, its circulating level is 25% less than for ANP but may exceed it in congestive cardiac failure (see p. 983).

Nitric oxide and the kidney

Nitric oxide (see ***Fig.*** [illegible]), a molecular gas, is formed by the action of three isoforms of nitric oxide synthase (NOS), all of which are expressed in the kidney: eNOS is found in vessels, nNOS mainly in the macula densa and inner medullary collecting duct, and iNOS in several tubule segments. Nitric oxide binds soluble guanylate cyclase, enhancing the synthesis of cyclic guanosine monophosphate (cGMP) from guanosine triphosphate (GTP), and mediates the following physiological actions in the kidney:

- regulation of renal perfusion and glomerular pressure
- natriuresis, by inhibiting Na^+/K^+-ATPase and NHE3
- antagonism of ADH
- modulation of tubule–glomerular feedback (see p. 724).

Further reading

Kapitsinou PP, Liu Q, Unger TL et al. Hepatic HIF-2 regulates erythropoietic responses to hypoxia in renal anemia. *Blood* 2010; 116:3039–3048.
Stevens LA, Schmid CH, Zhang Y et al. Development and validation of GFR-estimating equations. *Nephrol Dial Transplant* 2010; 25:449–457.

CLINICAL APPROACH TO THE PATIENT WITH KIDNEY AND URINARY TRACT DISEASE

Investigation of kidney and urinary tract disease

Examination of the urine

Appearance

Unless urine is visibly bloody (or cola-coloured, in cases of myoglobinuria or haemoglobinuria), inspection of the urine is not helpful. Cloudy, offensive-smelling urine may denote infection, but this should be further tested by dipsticks.

Volume

In temperate climates, healthy adults will pass between 800–2500 mL per 24 hours (roughly 1 mL/kg/h). Usually, the minimum urine output capable of maintaining solute excretion for health (without accumulation in the body) is around 650 mL. If the kidney loses concentrating capacity (as occurs in CKD or diabetes insipidus), higher urine volumes are needed for the same daily solute output, and urine outputs may rise well above 2500 mL. ***Nocturia*** is a symptom of kidney disease, as patients without the ability to concentrate solute into a small urine volume will waken, needing to pass urine during the night. High daily volumes are also seen with glycosuria or increased protein catabolism following surgery, as the solute load requiring excretion is higher.

Specific gravity and osmolality

Urine specific gravity (SG, where <1.008 is dilute and >1.020 is concentrated) is a measure of the weight of dissolved particles in urine, whereas urine osmolality reflects the number of such particles. Usually, the relationship between the two is close. Measurement of urine SG or osmolality can be helpful in confirming loss of concentrating ability (as might be seen when tubular function fails in acute tubular necrosis or CKD). It can also be helpful in oliguric patients, when a high SG might suggest pre-renal AKI, as opposed to established acute tubular necrosis (see pp. 771–772).

Urinary pH

Measurement of urinary pH (usually 5.5–6.5) is helpful only in the investigation and treatment of renal tubular acidosis (see pp. 177–178).

Dipsticks (chemical testing) and urine microscopy

Dipsticks are cheap and hugely helpful in investigating suspected kidney disease, using reagents fixed on pads that change colour on reacting with specific elements in urine. Microscopy on a midstream sample spun at 2000 rpm is essential to understand dipstick findings fully.

Blood

Haematuria may originate from anywhere in the urinary tract. Once found on dipstick, a mid-stream sample should be examined for red cells or casts. Red cells (usually 1–2 per high-power field) are described as dysmorphic if they originate from the early nephron (glomerular bleeding), and may be accompanied by red-cell casts. Casts are cylindrical bodies, moulded in the shape of the distal tubular lumen. Red-cell casts – even if only single – always indicate renal disease. A dipstick that is strongly positive for haematuria with no red cells seen on microscopy might suggest haemoglobinuria or myoglobinuria. Bleeding may come from any site within the urinary tract ***(Fig. 20.7)***:

- ***Overt bleeding from the urethra*** is suggested when blood is seen at the start of voiding and then the urine becomes clear.
- ***Blood diffusely present*** throughout the urine comes from the bladder or above.
- ***Blood only at the end of micturition*** suggests bleeding from the prostate or bladder base.

Women will commonly have dipstick-positive haematuria during a period; it is usually worth repeating testing after menstruation.

Protein

Proteinuria is one of the most common signs of renal disease. Dipsticks will detect proteinuria from around 50–150 mg/L, and may be designed to test for either albuminuria or proteinuria. They will not detect light chains or immunoglobulins (Bence Jones proteins). Normal individuals excrete less than 20 μg of albumin per minute (30 mg in 24 h). Dipsticks, however, detect albumin only in a concentration above 200 μg/min (300 mg per 24 h if urine volume is normal). If two separate urine samples find proteinuria on dipstick testing, a random urine protein : creatinine ratio (uPCR) should be measured. This convenient test has largely replaced formal (timed) 24-hour urine collections for proteinuria; an alternative is the albumin : creatinine ratio (ACR). As albumin is usually the dominant

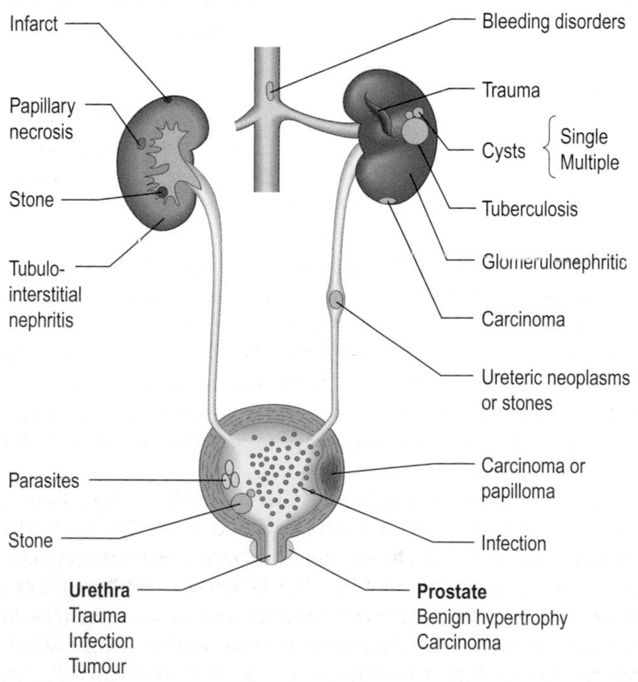

Figure 20.7 Sites and causes of bleeding from the urinary tract.

protein lost in the urine, patients who have albuminuria always have proteinuria (and the urine PCR will be higher than the urine ACR). Confusingly, the terms are often used interchangeably. For people with diabetes, the urine ACR has particular prognostic significance, and is usually the preferred screening test (see p. 1269) for the ***microalbuminuria*** found in early diabetic kidney disease.

Both tests are expressed as mg (protein)/mmol creatinine. Generally, an ACR of 2.5–20 mg/mmol corresponds to albuminuria of 30–300 mg daily (crudely, multiply the result by a factor of 15 – so an ACR of 50 mg/mmol = 750 mg/day albuminuria). Similarly, a uPCR of 3–30 mg/mmol corresponds to 30–300 mg daily (multiplying by a factor of 10 for this test – so a PCR of 50 mg/mmol = 500 mg proteinuria per day). The uPCR assay is relatively cheap and identifies patients whose proteinuria is of tubular and glomerular origin. ACR or PCR levels independently predict all-cause and cardiovascular mortality in the general population in addition to better risk stratifications of patients with CKD for future renal outcomes. Pyrexia, exercise and adoption of the upright posture (***postural proteinuria***) all increase urinary protein output but are benign. Proteinuria may associate with coarse granular casts seen on urine microscopy.

Glucose

Renal glycosuria is uncommon, so that a positive test for glucose might prompt consideration of diabetes mellitus. Dipsticks for glucose are very sensitive, however.

Bacteria and pus cells

Dipstick tests for bacteriuria are based on the detection of ***nitrite*** produced from the reduction of urinary nitrate by bacteria, and also on the detection of leucocyte esterase, an enzyme specific for neutrophils. Although each test on its own has limitations, a positive reaction with both tests has a high predictive value for urinary tract infection (see pp. 763–764). Where positive, a mid-stream sample should be sent for microscopy, culture and sensitivities (MC&S). White blood (pus) cells (WBCs) may be seen on microscopy, as may bacteria. A measurement of ≥10 WBCs/mL in fresh mid-stream urine samples is abnormal and suggests urinary tract infection (UTI). Not all pyuria is UTI, though; pus cells are seen with renal stones, tubule-interstitial nephritis, papillary necrosis, tuberculosis and interstitial cystitis. White cell casts may be seen with (and are more characteristic of) acute pyelonephritis.

Blood and quantitative tests

The use of serum urea, creatinine and GFR as measures of renal function is discussed on pages 726–727. Other quantitative tests of disturbed renal function are described under the relevant disorders, as are diagnostic tests, such as anti-neutrophil cytoplasmic antibody (ANCA), immunofluorescence and complement.

Imaging techniques

Ultrasonography

Ultrasound of the kidneys and bladder is safe and non-invasive, avoiding ionizing radiation and intravascular contrast medium. In renal diagnosis, it is the imaging method of choice for:

- Assessing renal size and symmetry (normal-sized kidneys with abnormal function suggest an acute cause, as kidneys scar as they fail, and may shrink in length and volume), and allowing directed renal biopsy.
- Ruling out obstruction, either of the bladder and ureters (with unilateral or bilateral hydronephrosis), or of the kidney itself (where pelvicalyceal dilatation may suggest high ureteric or pelvic disease).

- Characterizing renal masses as cystic (either simple cysts or polycystic kidneys) or complex and solid (benign and malignant renal tumours, or infected collections).
- Guiding intervention aimed at relieving obstruction (percutaneous nephrostomy).
- Confirming renal vein patency, and suggesting (but not proving) renal artery disease, in the case of ***Doppler ultrasonography*** (***duplex***).
- Looking for bladder tumours or stones. A scan obtained after voiding (post-micturition) allows bladder emptying to be assessed.

Computed tomography

Unenhanced computed tomography (CT) is the first-line investigation for cases of ***ureteric colic*** and suspected renal calculi. It has superseded excretion urography (also known as intravenous urography (IVU) or intravenous pyelography (IVP)).

Multislice detector CT has both improved image resolution and allowed reconstruction of the imaging data in a variety of planes. CT is also used to:

- characterize renal masses that are indeterminate at ultrasonography
- stage renal and bladder tumours
- evaluate the retroperitoneum for tumours, retroperitoneal fibrosis (peri-aortitis) and other causes of ureteric obstruction
- assess severe renal trauma
- visualize the renal arteries and veins by CT angiography.

Disadvantages include radiation and contrast nephrotoxicity (see p. 774).

Positron emission tomography (***PET***), using 18-F-fluorodeoxyglucose (FDG), is useful for detection of infection (e.g. in a cyst), inflammation or tumours, and is often used with CT (PET/CT).

Magnetic resonance imaging

Magnetic resonance imaging (MRI) is used as an alternative to CT with no irradiation:

- To stage prostate (but also renal and bladder) cancer.
- To reconstruct the anatomy of the renal arteries using magnetic resonance ***angiography*** with gadolinium as contrast medium. In experienced hands, its sensitivity and specificity approach that of renal angiography.

The Food and Drug Administration (FDA) advises not using gadolinium in patients with renal insufficiency because of the development of nephrogenic systemic fibrosis (see pp. 1365 and 781).

Plain X-ray

A plain radiograph of the abdomen may be useful to identify renal calcification or radiodense calculi in the kidney, renal pelvis, and the line of the ureters or bladder ***(Fig. 20.8)***.

Antegrade pyelography

Antegrade pyelography ***(Fig. 20.9)*** involves percutaneous puncture of a pelvicalyceal system with a needle and the injection of contrast medium to outline the pelvicalyceal system and ureter to the level of obstruction. Drains can be sited and stents placed during the procedure. Retrograde pyelography under screening control allows a contrast study of the ureter from the bladder. It is invasive, commonly requires a general anaesthetic, and may result in the introduction of infection.

Micturating cystourethrography

After bladder catheterization, contrast is instilled into the bladder. The catheter is then removed and the patient screened during voiding to check for vesicoureteric reflux and to study the urethra and bladder emptying. Micturating cystourethrography (MCUG) is used in children with recurrent infection (see p. 764). It is rarely appropriate in adults, as with bladder wall hypertrophy in adulthood, vesicoureteric reflux tends to disappear.

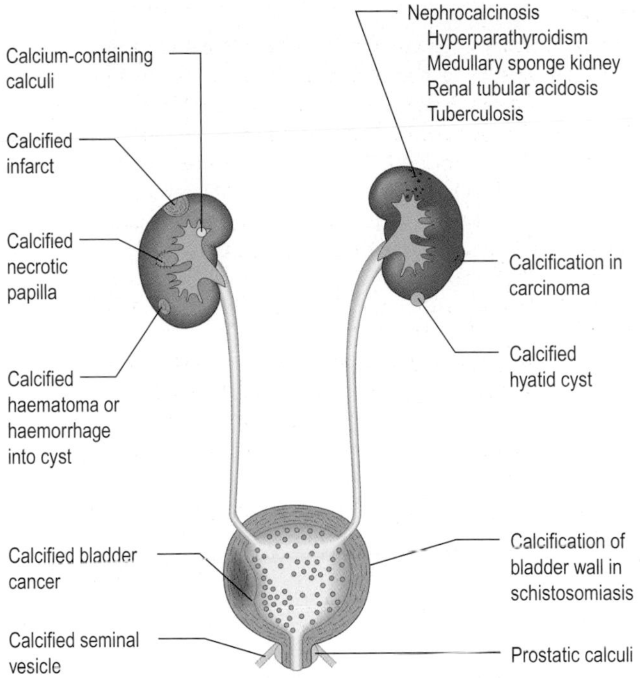

Figure 20.8 **Calcification in the renal tract.** Calculi can occur at any site.

Aortography or renal arteriography

Conventional or digital subtraction angiography (DSA) is used both diagnostically, and in cases of suspected renal artery stenosis, to allow therapeutic renal artery balloon angioplasty and stenting. Complications include cholesterol embolization (see pp. 753–754) and contrast-induced kidney damage (contrast nephropathy).

Renal scintigraphy

Isotope studies are helpful for dynamic or static studies of perfusion or excretion. Following venous injection of a bolus of tracer, emissions from the kidney can be recorded by gamma camera. Technetium-labelled diethylenetriaminepenta-acetic acid (^{99m}Tc-DTPA) is excreted by glomerular filtration and can be used to confirm renal perfusion. In patients with unilateral renal artery stenosis, there is, typically, a slowed and reduced uptake of tracer with a delay in reaching a peak. Studies carried out before and after administration of an ACE inhibitor may demonstrate a fall in uptake that is suggestive of functional arterial stenosis. Both false-positive and false-negative results are common, particularly in patients with CKD, and renal arteriography remains the 'gold standard' in the diagnosis of renal artery stenosis.

Dimercaptosuccinic acid labelled with technetium (^{99m}Tc-DMSA) is filtered by the glomerulus and then binds to proximal tubular cells. Static studies are useful to assess the relative contribution in function of asymmetric kidneys. ^{99m}Tc-DMSA is also useful in highlighting 'photon-deficient' areas (where isotope is not seen), suggestive of scars or infarction, when compared to healthy tissue uptake. Mercapto-acetyltriglycine (MAG3) labelled with technetium (^{99m}Tc) is excreted by renal tubular secretion, so resistance to flow in the

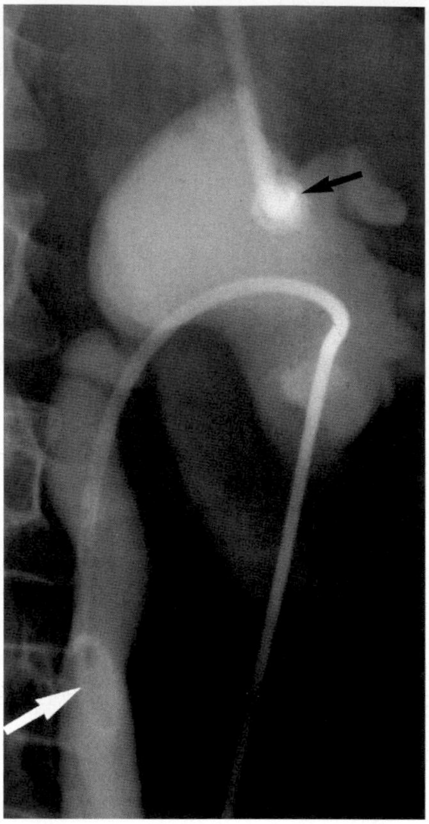

Figure 20.9 Antegrade pyelography via percutaneous catheter (black arrow) of obstructed system. A percutaneous drainage catheter (white arrow) has been inserted.

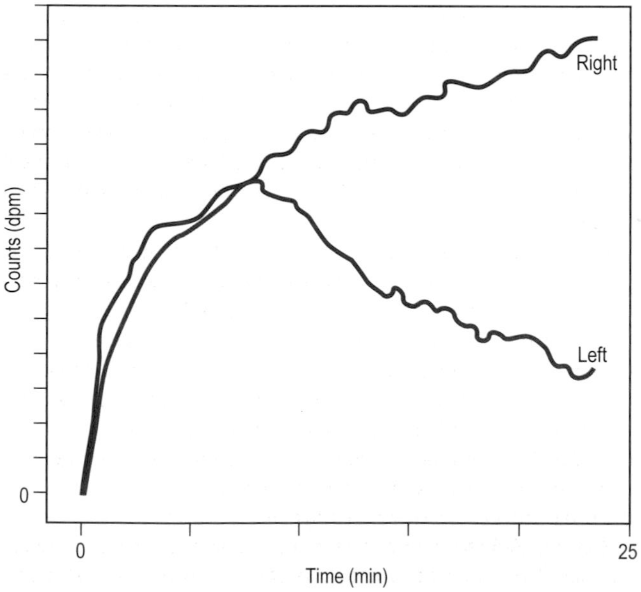

Figure 20.10 Dynamic scintigram. Note the progressive rise of the right kidney curve to a plateau (in contrast to the normal left kidney curve), owing to urinary tract obstruction on the right side.

pelvis or ureter (with obstruction) prolongs the parenchymal transit of tracer with a delay in emptying the pelvis. On whole-kidney renograms, the time–activity curve fails to fall after an initial peak, or continues to rise ***(Fig. 20.10)***, confirming hold-up to flow. Furosemide may be given to exaggerate urine output and emphasize the delay, in order to aid diagnosis.

Transcutaneous renal biopsy

Renal biopsy ***(Box 20.3)*** is carried out under ultrasound control in specialized centres and requires interpretation by an experienced pathologist. It is helpful in the investigation of the nephritic and nephrotic syndromes, acute and chronic kidney disease, haematuria after urological investigations and renal graft dysfunction. Native renal biopsy material must be examined by conventional histochemical staining, by electron microscopy, and by immunoperoxidase or immunofluorescence. Techniques like *in situ* hybridization and polymerase chain reaction (PCR) analysis are also widely used in renal biopsy specimens.

The complications of transcutaneous renal biopsy are shown in ***Box 20.4***.

Glomerular disease is usually described by kidney biopsy findings. Commonly used terms are shown in ***Box 20.5***.

Box 20.3 Transcutaneous renal biopsy

Before biopsy

1. Perform a coagulation screen; it must be normal.
2. Group and save the serum for cross-matching.
3. Give the patient a full explanation of what is involved and obtain consent.

During biopsy

1. Ask the patient to lie prone with a hard pillow under the abdomen.
2. Localize the kidney by ultrasound.
3. Inject local anaesthetic along the biopsy track.
4. Instruct the patient to hold a breath when the biopsy is performed.

After biopsy

1. Apply pressure dressing to the biopsy site and ask the patient to rest in bed for 8–24 h.
2. Maximize fluid intake to prevent clot colic.
3. Check the pulse and blood pressure regularly.
4. Advise the patient to avoid heavy lifting or gardening for 2 weeks.

Box 20.4 Complications of transcutaneous renal biopsy

- Macroscopic haematuria – up to 10%
- Pain in the flank, sometimes referred to the shoulder tip
- Perirenal haematoma
- Arteriovenous aneurysm formation – about 20%, almost always of no clinical significance
- Profuse haematuria demanding blood transfusion – 1–3%
- Profuse haematuria demanding occlusion of the bleeding vessel at angiography or nephrectomy – approximately 1 in 400
- Introduction of infection
- Mortality rate of about 0.1%

Box 20.5 Glomerular disease: commonly used terms

- ***Focal***: some, but not all, glomeruli show the lesion
- ***Diffuse*** (global): most of the glomeruli (>75%) contain the lesion
- ***Segmental***: only a part of the glomerulus is affected (most focal lesions are also segmental, e.g. focal segmental glomerulosclerosis)
- ***Global***: all of the glomerulus is symmetrically involved
- ***Proliferative***: an increase in cell numbers due to hyperplasia of one or more of the resident glomerular cells with or without inflammation
- ***Membrane alterations***: capillary wall thickening due to deposition of immune deposits or alterations in basement membrane
- ***Crescent formation***: epithelial cell proliferation with mononuclear cell infiltration in Bowman's space

THE GLOMERULUS AND GLOMERULAR DISEASE

A glomerulus consists of a collection of capillaries seated within Bowman's capsule in the urinary space. Blood flows in via the afferent arteriole, and exits via the efferent arteriole. Filtrate leaves Bowman's space into the proximal tubule. The capillary tuft is supported by mesangial cells and mesangial matrix. Filtrate moves from the capillary lumen into the urinary space across the glomerular filter (see p. 724). Three elements are involved in allowing or preventing filtration: endothelium, the glomerular basement membrane (GBM) and podocytes ***(Fig. 20.11)***.

Filtration barrier (slit diaphragm)

The glomerular filtration barrier (see ***Fig. 20.2***) consists of the fenestrated endothelium, the GBM and the terminally differentiated visceral epithelial cells known as podocytes. Podocytes attach to the GBM by foot processes via adhesion molecules, such as $\alpha_3\beta_1$ and dystroglycans. Adjacent podocytes are joined laterally via their foot process by slit diaphragms, which bridge across the filtration slits. The various proteins comprising the slit diaphragm include nephrin, CD2-associated protein (CD2AP), canonical transient receptor potential channel 6 (TRPC6), podocin, P-cadherin, α- and β-catenin, and zonula occludens-1 (ZO-1). These co-localize within the subcellular domain to function as a molecular sieve. These proteins, in addition to providing structural support to the cytoskeletal proteins like filamentous actin, also have signalling functions in order to maintain the normal function of podocytes. Abnormalities in any of these proteins result in the breakdown of the filtration barrier with consequent torrential leak of macromolecules.

Podocyte changes

The podocyte structure (see above) is maintained by actin, which supports the cytoskeleton (see ***Fig. 20.2***). A rearrangement of the fluid actin cytoskeleton leads to foot process effacement (flattening). As the architecture of the filtration slit is now disrupted, albumin leaks into the urine, and recovery of the cytoskeleton reverses proteinuria. The cytoskeleton can be altered by:

- abnormalities of cytoskeletal proteins like α-actinin-4, which causes hereditary focal segmental glomerular sclerosis
- injury to or abnormalities of slit diaphragm proteins
- changes in the GBM itself
- direct injury to podocytes by viral infection, drugs, toxins or the local activation of the renin–angiotensin system.

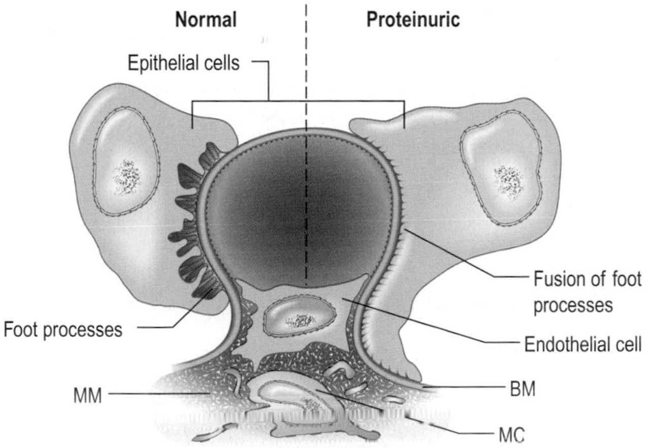

Figure 20.11 **A normal (left) and a proteinuric (right) glomerulus.** A capillary loop shows normal glomerular morphology on the left with an epithelial cell with pseudopodia (foot processes). In the proteinuric diagram (right), there is fusion of the foot processes, which is characteristic of many diseases. BM, basement membrane; MC, mesangial cell; MM, mesangial matrix.

Glomerular disease

Glomerular disease is the third most common cause (after diabetes and hypertension) of end-stage kidney disease (ESKD) in Europe and the USA, accounting for some 10–15% of such patients. These are diseases in which:

- there may be an immunologically mediated inflammatory injury to glomeruli, or structural or functional glomerular damage without inflammation
- renal interstitial damage is a regular accompaniment
- the kidneys are involved symmetrically
- secondary mechanisms of glomerular injury may come into play following an initial immune insult, such as fibrin deposition, platelet aggregation, neutrophil infiltration and free radical-induced damage
- haemodynamic consequences of a primary injury may further disturb glomerular function
- renal lesions may be part of a generalized disease (e.g. systemic lupus erythematosus, SLE).

Describing glomerular disease

The nomenclature for glomerular disease can be confusing, as descriptive terms (as seen on histology) overlap with clinical syndromes and more recent molecular insights into the pathogenesis of disease. If there is predominant inflammation on histology, glomerular disease may be described as a ***glomerulonephritis***. If inflammation is absent, ***glomerulopathy*** is more correct. There remains much overlap between the two, and the terms are often (wrongly) used interchangeably. It may be better to think about glomerular disease in terms of the predominant compartment involved, where the GBM separates podocytes from mesangial and endothelial cells.

- Podocytes (in the urinary compartment) are principally involved in glomerular diseases (usually glomerulopathies) that present as the nephrotic syndrome, where proteinuria is often heavy.
- Endothelial and mesangial cells (in the endocapillary compartment) are principally involved in glomerular disease presenting as nephritis (glomerulonephritis), where haematuria, proteinuria and often hypertension are equally evident.
- Podocytes, endothelial and mesangial cells may be equally involved where a glomerulonephritis presents with heavy proteinuria and the nephrotic syndrome as well.

Clinical classification of glomerular disease is also often used, although there is no complete correlation between histopathological types and clinical features. Four major glomerular syndromes are often described:

- ***Nephrotic syndrome***: massive proteinuria (>3.5 g/day), hypoalbuminaemia, oedema, lipiduria and hyperlipidaemia. Podocyte malfunction or injury is often causative.
- ***Glomerulonephritis (nephritic syndrome)***:
  - ***Acute glomerulonephritis***: abrupt onset of glomerular haematuria (red blood cell casts or dysmorphic red blood cells), non-nephrotic-range proteinuria, oedema, hypertension and transient renal impairment, *or*

Box 20.6 Investigation of glomerular diseases

Investigations	Positive findings
Urine microscopy	Red cells, red-cell casts
Urinary protein	Nephrotic or sub-nephrotic-range proteinuria
Serum urea	May be elevated
Serum creatinine	May be elevated
Culture (throat swab, discharge from ear, swab from inflamed skin)	Nephritogenic organism (not always)
Antistreptolysin-O titre	Elevated in post-streptococcal nephritis
C3 and C4 levels	May be reduced
Antinuclear antibody (ANA)	Present in significant titre in systemic lupus erythematosus
Antinuclear cytoplasmic antibody (ANCA)	Positive in some vasculitides
Anti-glomerular basement membrane (anti-GBM)	Positive in Goodpasture syndrome
Cryoglobulins	Increased in cryoglobulinaemia
Chest X-ray	Cardiomegaly, pulmonary oedema (not always)
Renal imaging	Usually normal
Renal biopsy	Any glomerulopathy

  - ***Rapidly progressive glomerulonephritis***: features of acute nephritis, focal necrosis with or without crescents, and rapidly progressive renal failure over weeks.
- ***Mixed nephritic/nephrotic presentations***: where glomerulonephritis is part of a systemic disease (e.g. lupus nephritis, cryoglobulinaemia and Henoch–Schönlein purpura), a nephritic syndrome is often associated with the nephrotic syndrome.
- ***Asymptomatic haematuria, proteinuria*** or both.

Investigation of glomerular diseases is shown in ***Box 20.6***.

Nephrotic syndrome

Nephrotic syndrome is characterized by:

- hypoalbuminaemia
- >3.5 g proteinuria/day
- dyslipidaemia
- salt and water retention, leading to oedema.

Pathophysiology

Hypoalbuminaemia

Loss of urinary protein (largely albumin) of the order ≥3.5 g daily in an adult may lead to hypoalbuminaemia. Normal dietary protein intake in the UK is around 70 g daily and the normal liver can synthesize albumin at a rate of 10–12 g daily. How, then, does a daily urinary protein loss of 3.5 g result in hypoalbuminaemia? This can be partly explained by increased catabolism of reabsorbed protein, largely albumin, in the proximal tubules, even though the rate of albumin synthesis is increased.

Proteinuria

Proteinuria occurs partly because structural damage to the glomerular barrier (podocytes, basement membrane, fenestrated endothelium and endothelial charge) allows the passage of more and larger molecules. The filtration slit between podocytes and normal podocyte architecture, and interdigitating podocyte foot processes are critical to maintaining a barrier to protein loss into the urinary space, as is a functional GBM and healthy capillary endothelium (and its charge).

Hyperlipidaemia

This is a consequence of increased synthesis of lipoproteins (such as apolipoprotein B, C-III lipoprotein (a)), as a direct consequence of a low plasma albumin. Low-density lipoprotein (LDL) increases, partly due to upregulation of a liver serine protease, ***pro-protein convertase subtilisin kexin-9*** (***PCSK9***), which causes internalization of LDL receptors. Very-low-density lipoprotein (VLDL) and/or intermediate-density lipoprotein (IDL) fractions increase, with no change (or a decrease) in HDL (the LDL/HDL cholesterol ratio increases). There is also reduced clearance of the principal triglycerides bearing lipoprotein (chylomicrons and VLDL), as high plasma levels of free fatty acid (FFA) trigger release of appropriately sialylated angiopoietin-like 4 (Angptl4) protein from adipose tissue, heart and skeletal muscles, inhibiting lipoprotein lipase and resulting in hypertriglyceridaemia.

Oedema in hypoalbuminaemia

See page 155.

Management

General measures

- ***Initial management*** should be with dietary sodium restriction and a thiazide diuretic (e.g. bendroflumethiazide 5 mg daily). Unresponsive patients require furosemide 40–120 mg daily with the addition of amiloride (5 mg daily; monitor serum potassium concentration regularly). Nephrotic patients may malabsorb diuretics (as well as other drugs) owing to gut mucosal oedema, and intravenous administration may be needed initially. Patients are sometimes hypovolaemic, and moderate oedema may have to be accepted in order to avoid postural hypotension.
- ***Normal protein intake*** is advisable. A high-protein diet (80–90 g protein daily) increases proteinuria and can be harmful in the long term.
- ***Albumin infusion*** produces only a transient effect. It is only given to patients who are diuretic-resistant and those with oliguria and uraemia in the absence of severe glomerular damage: for example, in minimal-change nephropathy. Albumin infusion is combined with diuretic therapy, and diuresis often continues with diuretic treatment alone.
- ***Hypercoagulable states*** predispose to venous thrombosis. The hypercoagulable state is due to loss of clotting factors (e.g. antithrombin) in the urine and an increase in hepatic production of fibrinogen. Prolonged bed rest should be avoided, as thromboembolism is very common (particularly in membranous nephropathy). Long-term prophylactic anticoagulation may be indicated, and if renal vein thrombosis occurs, permanent anticoagulation is required.
- ***Sepsis*** is a major cause of death in nephrotic patients. The increased susceptibility to infection is partly due to loss of immunoglobulin in the urine. Pneumococcal infections are particularly common and pneumococcal vaccine should be given. Early detection and aggressive treatment of infections,

rather than long-term antibiotic prophylaxis, constitute the best approach.

- ***Lipid abnormalities*** are responsible for an increase in the risk of cardiovascular disease in patients with proteinuria. Treatment of hypercholesterolaemia starts with an HMG-CoA reductase inhibitor (a statin).
- Lastly, ***ACE inhibitors and/or angiotensin II receptor antagonists*** (AII-RAs) are indicated for their antiproteinuric properties in all types of glomerulonephropathy, but most especially the nephrotic syndrome. These drugs reduce proteinuria by lowering glomerular capillary filtration pressure (a fall in efferent tone drops the transglomerular capillary pressure, and so protein loss into the urinary space); blood pressure and renal function should be monitored regularly.

Specific measures

Treat the underlying cause of any urinary protein leak. ***Box 20.7*** shows the glomerular lesions commonly associated with the nephrotic syndrome.

Causes of nephrotic syndrome

Minimal-change nephropathy (minimal-change disease)

In minimal-change nephropathy (MCN; also called minimal-change disease, MCD), glomeruli appear normal on light microscopy ***(Fig. 20.12)***. On electron microscopy, fusion of the foot processes of podocytes is seen, consistent with a disrupted podocyte actin cytoskeleton (see ***Fig. 20.2B***). Neither immune complexes nor anti-GBM antibody can be demonstrated by immunofluorescence on glomerular staining for antibody.

Immature differentiating CD34 stem cells (rather than mature T lymphocytes) appear to be responsible for the pathogenesis of MCN. Podocyte function is also affected by interleukin 13 (IL-13), the production of vascular endothelial growth factor (VEGF), or the upregulation of vascular hyposialylated-angiopoietin-like 4 (ANGPTL4), secreted by the podocytes.

Many drugs have been implicated in MCN, including NSAIDs, lithium, antibiotics (cephalosporins, rifampicin, ampicillin), bisphosphonates and sulfasalazine. Atopy is present in 30% of cases of MCN, and allergic reactions can trigger the nephrotic syndrome. Infections, such as hepatitis C virus (HCV), the human immunodeficiency virus (HIV) and tuberculosis, are rarer causes.

Clinical features

MCN is most common in children, particularly boys, and is responsible for the large majority of cases of nephrotic syndrome in childhood. Proteinuria is usually 'highly selective', where albumin, but not higher-molecular-weight proteins such as immunoglobulins, is lost in the urine. Oedema is usual and in children this may present predominantly around the face. The condition accounts for 20–25% of cases of adult nephrotic syndrome. It is often regarded as a condition that does not lead to CKD (but see focal segmental glomerulosclerosis below).

Management

- Manage symptoms with general measures (above).
- High-dose corticosteroid therapy with prednisolone 60 mg/m^2 daily (up to a maximum of 80 mg/day) for a maximum of 4–6 weeks, followed by 40 mg/m^2 every other day for a further 4–6 weeks, reverses proteinuria in more than 95% of children. Response rates in adults are significantly lower and response may occur only after many months (12 weeks with daily steroid therapy and 12 weeks of maintenance with alternate-day therapy). Spontaneous remission also occurs and steroid therapy should, in general, be withheld if urinary protein loss is insufficient to cause hypoalbuminaemia or oedema. In both children and adults, if remission lasts for 4 years after steroid therapy, further relapse is very rare.
- In children, two-thirds relapse after steroid therapy and further courses of corticosteroids are required. One-third of these children regularly relapse on steroid withdrawal, so that a second-line agent should be added after repeat induction with steroids.
- Cyclophosphamide 1.5–2.0 mg/kg daily is given for 8–12 weeks with prednisolone 7.5–15 mg/day. This increases the likelihood of long-term remission. Steroid-unresponsive patients may also respond to cyclophosphamide. No more than two courses of cyclophosphamide should be prescribed in children because of the risk of side-effects, which include future infertility (azoospermia and premature ovarian failure).
- An alternative to cyclophosphamide is ciclosporin 3–5 mg/kg per day, which is effective but must be continued long-term to prevent relapse on stopping treatment. The antiproteinuric effect of ciclosporin is normally attributed to its immunosuppressive action but may result from the stabilization of the actin cytoskeleton in kidney podocytes.

Box 20.7 Glomerulopathies associated with the nephrotic syndrome

Primary glomerular disease	Secondary glomerular disease
Nephrotic syndrome	
Minimal-change nephropathy Congenital nephrotic syndrome Focal segmental glomerular sclerosis Membranous nephropathy	Amyloidosis Diabetic nephropathy
Mixed nephrotic/nephritic	
Mesangiocapillary glomerulonephritis Mesangial proliferative glomerulonephritis	Systemic lupus erythematosus Cryoglobulinaemic disease Henoch–Schönlein syndrome Idiopathic fibrillary glomerulopathy Immunotactoid glomerulopathy Fibronectin glomerulonephropathy

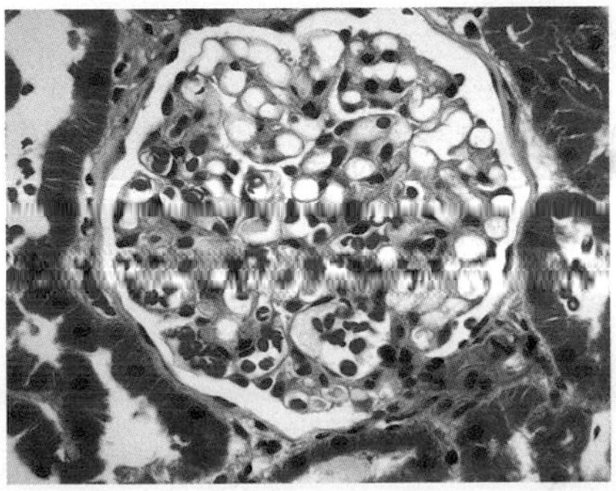

Figure 20.12 Normal glomerulus on light microscopy in minimal-change nephropathy.

Ciclosporin inhibits the calcineurin-mediated dephosphorylation of synaptopodin (a regulator of actin cytoskeleton) and protects it from cathepsin L-mediated degradation. These results have shed new light on the role of calcineurin signalling in proteinuric kidney diseases. Excretory function and ciclosporin blood levels (recommended trough levels 80–150 ng/mL) must be monitored regularly, as ciclosporin is potentially nephrotoxic.

- Rituximab, a depleting monoclonal antibody directed against CD20, present on B lymphocytes, is showing promise in reducing the number of relapses in frequently relapsing disease, and also in minimizing the immunosuppressant burden in corticosteroid-dependent disease.
- In corticosteroid-dependent children, the anthelminthic agent levamisole 2.5 mg/kg to a maximum of 150 mg on alternate days is also useful in maintenance of remission but its mode of action is unexplained.

Congenital nephrotic syndrome

Congenital nephrotic syndrome (Finnish type) is an autosomal recessively inherited disorder due to mutations in the gene coding for a transmembrane protein, nephrin; it occurs at a frequency of 1 per 8200 live births in Finland. Nephrin is a critical element of the filtration slit, and its loss of function results in massive proteinuria shortly after birth. The disorder can be diagnosed *in utero*, as increased α-fetoprotein in amniotic fluid is a common feature. Histologically, some glomeruli are small and infantile, whereas others are enlarged and more mature, and have diffuse mesangial hypercellularity. Because of the massive proteinuria, some tubules develop microcysts and are dilated. On electron microscopy, complete effacement of the foot processes of visceral epithelial cells is observed. This condition is characterized by relentless progression to ESKD.

Other inherited nephrotic syndromes involve mutations in other genes that encode other podocyte proteins, such as podocin, α-actinin 4 and Wilms' tumour suppressor gene.

Focal segmental glomerulosclerosis

Focal segmental glomerulosclerosis (FSGS) describes a sclerotic glomerular lesion that affects some (but not all) glomeruli, and some (but not all) segments of each tuft.

- ***Primary FSGS*** is an unusual primary cause of the nephrotic syndrome.
- ***Secondary FSGS*** looks similar on light microscopy. Although proteinuria may be heavy, hypoalbuminaemia is *unusual*.

Primary focal segmental glomerulosclerosis

Clinical features of primary FSGS

This disease of unknown aetiology usually presents as massive proteinuria (usually non-selective), haematuria, hypertension and renal impairment. The associated nephrotic syndrome is often resistant to steroid therapy. All age groups are affected. It usually recurs in transplanted kidneys, sometimes within days of transplantation, and particularly in patients with aggressive primary renal disease.

Aetiology of primary FSGS

A circulating permeability factor causes the increased protein leak; plasma from patients increases membrane permeability in isolated glomeruli. Kidneys transplanted into murine models of FSGS develop the lesion, but kidneys from FSGS-prone mice transplanted to a normal strain are protected. Removal of this factor by plasmapheresis results in transient amelioration of proteinuria. The identity of the permeability factor remains unknown but recent findings suggest that cardiotrophin-like cytokine 1 is likely a candidate in FSGS. Soluble urokinase-like plasminogen activator receptor (SuPAR) was initially thought to be involved but now appears less likely to be causative, based on recent experimental and clinical evidence. Mutations in the *MYO1E* gene, which encodes for myosin 1E, found in podocytes, has been described in families with FSGS.

Pathology

Segmental glomerulosclerosis is seen on light microscopy, which later progresses to global sclerosis. The deep glomeruli at the corticomedullary junction are affected first. These may be missed on transcutaneous biopsy, leading to a mistaken diagnosis of MCN (pp. 735–736). A pathogenetic link may exist between MCN and FSGS, as a proportion of cases classified as having the former condition develop progressive CKD, which is unusual. Immunofluorescence shows deposits of C3 and immunoglobulin M (IgM) in affected portions of the glomerulus. The other glomeruli are usually enlarged but may be of normal size. Focal tubular atrophy and interstitial fibrosis are invariably present. Electron microscopy demonstrates primarily foot process effacement, occasionally in a patchy distribution. The degree of podocyte foot process effacement on electron microscopy can help distinguish between 'primary' and 'secondary' FSGS. If severe foot process effacement is present in normal and sclerosed glomeruli on electron microscopy, primary FSGS is more likely (this is not the case if foot process effacement is largely localized to sclerosed glomeruli alone).

Five histological variants of FSGS exist:

- In ***classic FSGS*** ***(Fig. 20.13A)***, the involved glomeruli show sclerotic segments in any location of the glomerulus.
- The ***glomerular tip lesion*** is characterized by segmental sclerosis, at the tubular pole of all the affected glomeruli at a very early stage (tip FSGS; ***Fig. 20.13B***). These patients have a more favourable response to steroids and disease runs a more benign course.
- In ***collapsing FSGS*** ***(Fig. 20.13C)***, podocytes are usually enlarged and coarsely vacuolated with wrinkled and collapsed capillary walls. Collapsing FSGS is commonly seen in young blacks with HIV infection or disease, and is known as HIV-associated nephropathy (HIVAN; see below).
- The ***perihilar variant*** ***(Fig. 20.13D)*** consists of perihilar sclerosis and hyalinosis in more than 50% of segmentally sclerotic glomeruli. It is frequently observed with secondary FSGS.
- The ***cellular variant*** ***(Fig. 20.13E)*** is characterized by at least one glomerulus with segmental hypercellularity (proliferation) that occludes the capillary lumen.

Management

- ***Prednisolone*** 0.5–2 mg/kg per day is used in most patients and continued for 6 months before the patient is considered resistant to therapy, which is common.
- ***Ciclosporin*** at doses to maintain serum trough levels at 150–300 ng/mL may be effective in reducing or stopping urinary protein excretion (tacrolimus is an alternative). Relapse after reducing or stopping ciclosporin is very common so that long-term use is required.

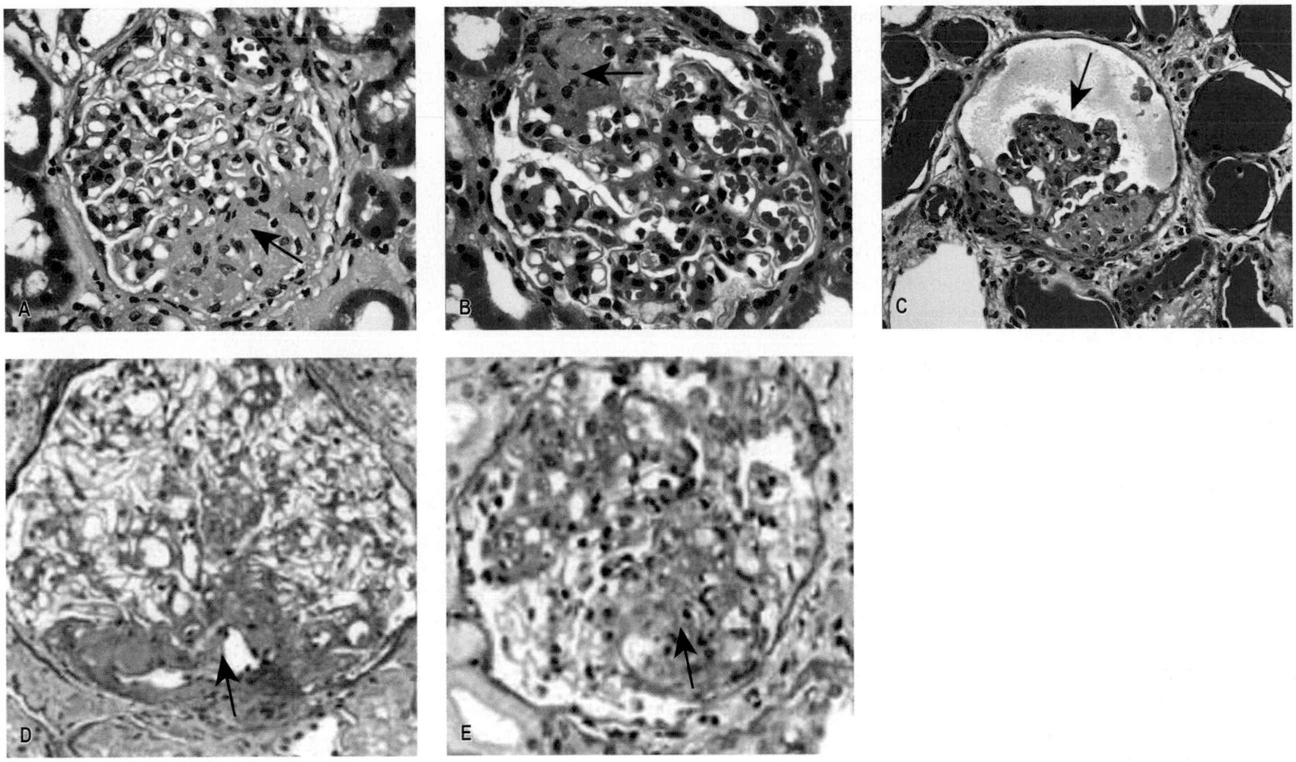

Figure 20.13 **Focal segmental glomerulosclerosis (FSGS). A.** Classic FSGS showing sclerotic segments (arrow) in glomerulus. **B.** Glomerular tip lesions showing segmental sclerosis (arrow) at pole of glomerulus. **C.** Collapsing FSGS (arrow). **D.** FSGS perihilar variant. **E.** FSGS cellular variant.

- ***Cyclophosphamide***, ***chlorambucil*** or ***azathioprine*** is used for second-line therapy in adults. In patients with FSGS with mesangial hypercellularity and tip lesion, cyclophosphamide 1–1.5 mg/kg per day with 60 mg of prednisolone for 3–6 months, followed by prednisolone and azathioprine, can be used as maintenance therapy.

About 50% of patients progress to ESKD within 10 years of diagnosis, particularly those who are resistant to therapy. The recurrence of this renal lesion following renal transplantation is very high with a poor renal prognosis. Plasmapheresis or immunoabsorption has been the mainstay of treatment in patients with post-transplant recurrence but has had modest results. Anti-CD80 antibodies (abatacept), used in rheumatology, have been tried with success in this condition.

Secondary FSGS

Secondary FSGS with similar glomerular changes is seen as a ***secondary phenomenon*** when the number of functioning nephrons is reduced for any reason. Here, FSGS represents the common final glomerular lesion seen in response to subsequent haemodynamic glomerular strain. As nephrons fail, increased flow through the remaining nephrons leads to glomerular hypertrophy and hyperfiltration and hydraulic injury, with the secondary changes of FSGS. It is also described as remnant nephropathy (see p. 776). Associations include:

- ***reduced nephron number*** (e.g. nephrectomy, hypertension, gross obesity, ischaemia, sickle nephropathy, reflux nephropathy, chronic allograft nephropathy, IgA nephropathy, and scarring following renal vasculitis)
- ***mutations*** in specific podocyte genes
- ***viruses***, e.g. HIV type 1, erythrovirus B19, cytomegalovirus, Epstein–Barr virus and simian virus 40
- ***drugs*** such as heroin, all interferons, anabolic steroids, lithium, sirolimus, pamidronate and calcineurin inhibitors, e.g. ciclosporin, which can also cause FSGS
- ***APOL1 gene mutations*** in patients of African ancestry, which makes them susceptible to FSGS in response to insults such as hypertension, SLE and HIV.

HIV-associated nephropathy

In HIV-associated nephropathy (HIVAN), glomeruli are characteristically 'collapsed' on light microscopy ***(Fig. 20.13C)***; podocytes are enlarged, hyperplastic and coarsely vacuolated, containing protein absorption droplets and overlying capillaries with varying degrees of wrinkling and collapse of the walls. Direct podocyte HIV-1 infection is associated with loss of podocyte-specific markers such as Wilms' tumour factor and synaptopodin in HIVAN. HIVAN presents with nephrotic-range proteinuria, oedema and CKD, which can be rapid in progression. Antiretroviral therapy (ART) may reverse the renal lesions seen, and restores renal function if treatment is commenced early.

Membranous glomerulopathy

Idiopathic membranous glomerulopathy is an autoimmune disease that occurs mainly in adults, and predominantly in men. It presents with asymptomatic proteinuria or frank nephrotic syndrome. Microscopic haematuria, hypertension and/or renal impairment may accompany the nephrotic syndrome. As in other glomerular disease, hypertension and a greater degree of renal impairment are poor prognostic signs. In membranous glomerulopathy, almost half of the patients undergo spontaneous or therapy-related remission. Eventually, however, about 40% develop CKD, usually in association with persistent nephrotic-range proteinuria. Younger people, females and those with asymptomatic proteinuria of modest degree at the time of presentation do best.

Pathogenesis

In the primary or idiopathic form (which comprises 75% of the cases), glomerular histology is identical to that seen when membranous glomerulopathy is secondary to another insult. These include:

- drugs (e.g. penicillamine, gold, NSAIDs, probenecid, mercury, captopril)
- autoimmune disease (e.g. SLE, thyroiditis)
- infections (e.g. hepatitis B, hepatitis C, schistosomiasis, *Plasmodium malariae*)
- cancers (e.g. carcinoma of the lung, colon, stomach, breast and lymphoma)
- other causes (e.g. sarcoidosis, kidney transplantation, sickle cell disease).

A majority of patients (70%) with idiopathic membranous nephropathy have been found to have IgG4-type autoantibodies against phospholipase A_2 receptor (PLA_2R), a glycoprotein constituent of normal glomeruli. PLA_2R is present in normal human podocytes and in immune deposits in patients with idiopathic membranous nephropathy, indicating that it could be a major autoantigen in this disease; it is linked to human leucocyte antigen (HLA)-DQA1. Specific IgG4 autoantibodies to anti-aldose reductase (AR) and anti-manganese superoxide dismutase (SOD2) have also been found in the sera and glomeruli of patients with membranous nephropathy but not in other renal pathologies or normal kidney. Recently, antibodies against a novel antigen, thrombospondin type 1 domain-containing 7A (THSD7A), have been identified in anti-PLA_2R-negative patients with membranous nephropathy. This suggests that AR, THSD7A and SOD2 could be additional renal autoantigens of human membranous nephropathy under certain clinical circumstances.

On light microscopy, capillary loops appear thick. Using a periodic acid–Schiff, or silver, stain (which highlights basement membrane), 'spikes' of basement membrane are visible. On electron microscopy, small, electron-dense deposits in the sub-epithelial aspects of the capillary walls are seen, encircled by perpendicular basement membrane spikes. Uniform granular capillary wall deposits of PLA_2R antigen and IgG subclasses (IgG4 is predominant in idiopathic membranous nephropathy), as well as complement C3, are seen on immunofluorescence. Late in the disease, deposits are completely surrounded by basement membrane and are undergoing resorption, which appears as uniform thickening of the capillary basement membrane on light microscopy ***(Fig. 20.14)***.

Management

As many as a third or more of patients will undergo spontaneous remission if watched for at least 6–12 months, particularly if kidney function is normal and proteinuria modest. In general, patients with heavier proteinuria, progressive renal dysfunction and a high titre of anti-PLA_2R antibodies are considered for early treatment.

- All patients should receive ACE inhibition at the maximum tolerated dose.
- The alkylating agents, cyclophosphamide (1.5–2.5 mg/kg per day for 6–12 months with 1 mg/kg per day of oral prednisolone on alternate days for the first 2 months) and chlorambucil (0.2 mg/kg per day in months 2, 4 and 6, alternating with oral prednisolone 0.4 mg/kg per day in months 1, 3 and 5), are both effective.

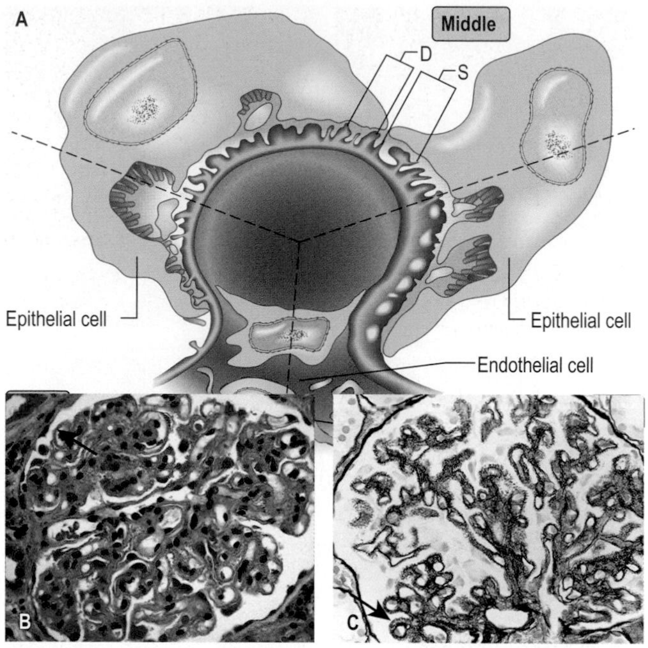

Figure 20.14 Membranous glomerulopathy. A. Membranous nephropathy showing the early, middle and late stages. D, subepithelial deposits; MC, mesangial cell; MM, mesangial matrix; S, spikes.
B. Light microscopy of membranous nephropathy showing thickened basement membrane (arrow).
C. Silver stain showing spikes (arrow) in membranous nephropathy.
(A, After Marsh FP. Postgraduate Nephrology. *Oxford: Butterworth Heinemann; 1985.)*

- Ciclosporin or tacrolimus is also of use, though remission is less well sustained and treatment courses are longer.
- Mycophenolate mofetil has demonstrated benefit in smaller studies with short follow-up.
- Anti-CD20 antibodies (rituximab, which ablates B lymphocytes) have been shown to improve renal function, reduce proteinuria and increase the serum albumin; no significant adverse affects have been shown in the short term.
- Oral corticosteroids are of no benefit alone but may be additive. A pilot study has shown promise with subcutaneous administration of adrenocorticotrophic hormone (tetracosactide) twice weekly, demonstrating an improvement in proteinuria. It is believed that it acts directly on podocytes by binding to melanocortin receptors. It is licensed by the FDA for use in nephrotic syndrome of any cause.

Amyloidosis

Amyloidosis (see pp. 1288–1289) is a systemic acquired or inherited disorder of protein folding, in which normally soluble proteins or fragments are deposited extracellularly as abnormal insoluble fibrils, causing progressive organ dysfunction and death.

The abnormal protein may be derived from light chains or immunoglobulin (AL amyloid), or from serum amyloid A protein (AA amyloid). The renal consequences are similar, even if systemic features differ.

Pathology

On light microscopy, widespread eosinophilic deposits are seen in the mesangium, capillary loops and arteriolar walls. Deposits stain pink, with green bi-refringence under polarized light with Congo red

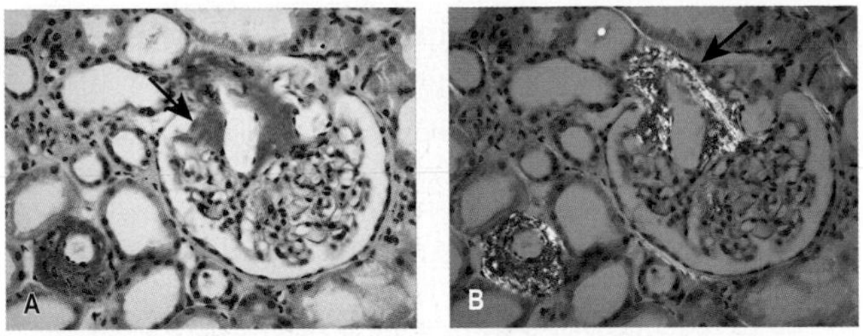

Figure 20.15 **Amyloid. A.** Light microscopy of eosinophilic amyloid deposits (arrow). **B.** Congo red stain under polarized light showing apple green refringence.

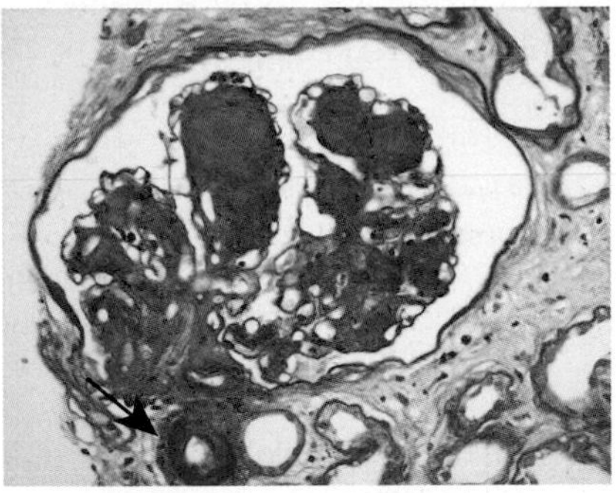

Figure 20.16 **Diabetes mellitus.** Advanced diabetic glomerulopathy and arteriolar sclerosis (arrow).

(Fig. 20.15). On electron microscopy, the characteristic fibrils of amyloid can be seen. Amyloid consisting of immunoglobulin light chains (AL amyloid) can be identified by immunohistochemistry in only 40% of cases, as compared to almost 100% of patients with protein found in secondary amyloid (AA amyloid).

Diagnosis

The diagnosis can often be made clinically when features of amyloidosis are present elsewhere (see p. 1289). On imaging, the kidneys are often large. Scintigraphy with radiolabelled serum amyloid P (SAP), a technique for quantitatively imaging amyloid deposits *in vivo*, is used to detect the rate of regression or progression of amyloidosis over a period of time (see p. 1289). Renal biopsy is necessary in all suspected cases of renal involvement.

Management

Treatments that reduce production of the amyloidogenic protein can improve organ function and survival in immunoglobulin-light-chain-related (AL) amyloidosis and hereditary transthyretin-associated (ATTR) amyloidosis (see p. 1288). In AA amyloidosis, production of serum amyloid A can sometimes be decreased by treatment of the underlying inflammatory condition but cannot be completely suppressed.

Renoprotective measures should be started (see ***(Box 20.9)***). The success of dialysis and kidney transplantation depends on the extent of amyloid deposition in extrarenal sites, especially the heart.

Diabetic nephropathy

Diabetic renal disease is the leading cause of ESKD in the Western world, arising largely as a complication of type 2 diabetes mellitus. Diabetic kidney disease occurs in about 20–30% of both type 1 and type 2 diabetics (see pp. 1269–1270); the natural history is similar from the onset of proteinuria, and the histological lesion is the same. Risk factors for nephropathy include poor glycaemic control, hypertension, male gender, ethnicity and social deprivation.

Pathology

Glomerular hyperfiltration (the GFR increases to >150 mL/min/m^2) and initial enlargement of kidney volume occur as local vasoactive factors increase flow. The GBM thickens and the mesangium expands. Progressive depletion of podocytes (see p. 733) from the filtration barrier (through apoptosis or detachment) results in podocyturia early in the disease. Proteinuria evolves as filtration pressures rise and the filter is compromised. Later, glomerulosclerosis develops with nodules (Kimmelstiel–Wilson lesion) and hyaline deposits in the glomerular arterioles ***(Fig. 20.16)***. Mesangial expansion and hyalinosis are partly due to amylin (β-islet-specific amyloid protein) deposits, with increasingly heavy proteinuria.

The Renal Pathology Society has developed a consensus classification combining type 1 and type 2 diabetic nephropathies ***(Box 20.8)***. This discriminates lesions by various degrees of severity for use in international clinical practice.

The pathophysiology is discussed on page 1269.

Box 20.8 Renal Pathology Society classification of types 1 and 2 diabetic nephropathy

Class	Name
I	Isolated glomerular basement membrane thickening (>395 nm in females, >430 nm in males). No evidence of mesangial expansion, mesangial matrix increase, or global glomerulosclerosis involving >50% of glomeruli
IIa	Mild mesangial expansion
IIb	Severe mesangial expansion (in a severe lesion, >25% of the total mesangium contains areas of expansion larger than the mean area of a capillary lumen)
III	Nodular intercapillary glomerulosclerosis (≥1 Kimmelstiel–Wilson lesion(s)) and <50% global glomerulosclerosis
IV	Advanced diabetic glomerulosclerosis and >50% global glomerulosclerosis

Management

Lifestyle changes (cessation of smoking, attention to salt intake, weight loss and increased exercise) are necessary in preventing progression of any diabetic complication.

- ***Aim for good (intensive) glycaemic control***. If achieved for even a limited period, this reduces the incidence of ESKD and other microvascular complications in the long term (the so-called 'legacy effect' in both type 1 and type 2 diabetes mellitus).
- ***Control dyslipidaemia***.
- ***Control blood pressure*** to <120/80 mmHg with ACE inhibitors or AII-RA; these should be used once microalbuminuria develops, even if blood pressure control is good. Combined use of ACE inhibitors and AII-RA (dual blockade) does not provide additional benefit but is associated with an increased risk of AKI and hyperkalaemia; it is no longer recommended in recent trials.

As in other kidney diseases, however, nearly the entire course of renal injury in diabetes is clinically silent. The aim of medical intervention during this silent phase is renoprotection ***(Box 20.9)***, as judged by a slowed loss of glomerular filtration over time. Despite intensified metabolic control and antihypertension treatment in

Box 20.9 Renoprotection

Goals of treatment
- Blood pressure <120/80 mmHg
- Proteinuria <0.3 g/24 h

Treatment measures
Patients with chronic kidney disease and proteinuria >1 g/24 h:
- Angiotensin-converting enzyme inhibitor increasing to maximum dose
  Angiotensin receptor antagonist if goals are not achieved[a]
- Addition of diuretic to prevent hyperkalaemia and help to control blood pressure
  Addition of calcium-channel blocker (verapamil or diltiazem) if goals are not achieved

Additional management
- Statins to lower cholesterol to <4.5 mmol/L
- Smoking cessation (threefold higher rate of deterioration in chronic kidney disease)
- Treatment of diabetes (HbA_{1c} <7%, 53 mmol/mol)
- Normal protein diet (0.8–1 g/kg body weight)

[a]*In type 2 diabetes start with angiotensin receptor antagonist.*

patients with diabetes, a substantial number still go on to develop ESKD.

Other interventions with a less robust evidence base include:
- ***Paricalcitol*** (a selective activator of the vitamin D receptor), added to treatment with ACE inhibitors, reduced albuminuria (a surrogate marker of progressive renal disease) in patients with type 2 diabetes in a randomized controlled trial. Paricalcitol worked best in patients with a high sodium intake in their diet, who are known to respond poorly to ACE inhibitor and angiotensin receptor blocker therapy.
- ***Bardoxolone methyl*** is a nuclear 1 factor (erythroid-derived 2)-related factor 2 (NRF-2) activator, an anti-inflammatory known to reduce oxidative stress. A large study failed to demonstrate benefit in patients with type 2 diabetes mellitus and CKD.
- ***Pentoxyphylline*** (previously used for peripheral vascular disease) slows the rate of GFR decline and proteinuria (by putatively reducing the production of tumour necrosis factor-alpha, TNF-α). This interesting observation requires external validation.
- ***Atrasentan*** (a selective endothelin A receptor (ET_AR) antagonist when used with renin–angiotensin system inhibitors) is similarly generally safe and effective in reducing residual albuminuria. This could ultimately translate into improved renal outcomes in patients with type 2 diabetic nephropathy, but needs confimation in long-term follow-up studies.

Isolated proteinuria without haematuria

In asymptomatic patients, this is often an incidental finding. It is usually found at <1 g/day) with normal renal function. Over 50% of these patients have postural proteinuria. The outcome of isolated proteinuria (postural or non-postural) is excellent in the majority of patients, with a gradual decline in proteinuria over time. Occasionally, it may be an early sign of a serious glomerular lesion such as membranous glomerulopathy, IgA nephropathy, FSGS, diabetic nephropathy or amyloidosis (see above). Mild proteinuria may also accompany a febrile illness, congestive heart failure or infectious diseases with no clinical renal significance.

Glomerulonephritis (asymptomatic, acute and rapidly progressive)

Glomerulonephritis (GN) is immunologically mediated, with involvement of cellular immunity (T lymphocytes, macrophages/dendritic cells), humoral immunity (antibodies, immune complexes, complement) and other inflammatory mediators (including cytokines, chemokines and the coagulation cascade). The immune response can be directed against known target antigens, particularly when GN complicates infections, cancers or drugs. The underlying antigenic target is more often unknown. Primary GN may occur in genetically susceptible individuals (usually determined by major histocompatibility complex (MHC) genes like *HLA-A1*, *B8*, *DR2* and *DR3*), following environmental insults. Circulating autoantibodies and/or abnormalities in serum complement, and glomerular deposition of antibodies, immune complexes, complement and fibrin characterize the condition. Glomerulonephritis may present as:
- asymptomatic urinary abnormalities
- acute nephritis (nephritic syndrome)
- rapidly progressive glomerulonephritis.

The same underlying histology may often present in any of the above ways, and these should be seen as clinical syndromes on a spectrum rather than as distinct diseases.

Asymptomatic urinary abnormalities

Haematuria with or without sub-nephrotic-range proteinuria in an asymptomatic patient may lead to the early discovery of potentially serious glomerular disease such as SLE, Henoch–Schönlein purpura, post-infectious GN or idiopathic hypercalciuria in children. Asymptomatic haematuria is also the primary presenting manifestation of a number of specific glomerular diseases discussed below.

Acute nephritis (nephritic syndrome)

This classically presents as:
- haematuria (macroscopic or microscopic) – with red-cell casts on urine microscopy
- proteinuria
- hypertension
- oedema (periorbital, leg or sacral)
- temporary oliguria and uraemia.

Nephritis can present indolently or incidentally, and is usually distinguished from rapidly progressive glomerulonephritis (see below) by the lack of cellular necrosis (and crescent formation) in the glomeruli seen on biopsy, and the rate at which renal decline evolves. These syndromes should be seen as a continuum.

Rapidly progressive glomerulonephritis

Rapidly progressive glomerulonephritis (RPGN) is a syndrome with glomerular haematuria (red blood cell casts or dysmorphic red blood cells), rapidly developing acute kidney failure over weeks to months and focal glomerular necrosis ***(Fig. 20.17)*** with or without glomerular crescent development on renal biopsy. The 'crescent' is an aggregate of macrophages and epithelial cells in Bowman's space ***(Fig. 20.17)***. RPGN can develop with immune deposits (anti-GBM or immune complex type, e.g. SLE) or without immune deposits (pauci-immune, e.g. anti-PR3 and or anti-MPO-ANCA-positive vasculitides). It can also develop as an idiopathic primary glomerular disease, or can be superimposed on secondary glomerular diseases such as IgA nephropathy, membranous GN and post-infective GN. It can be classified based on the pattern of immune complex deposition in glomeruli (seen on immunofluorescence):

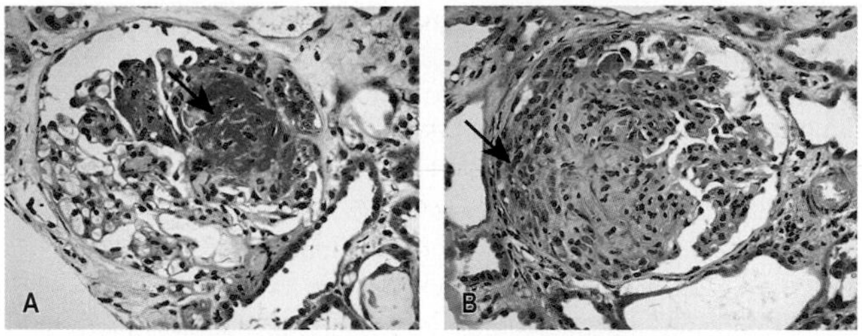

Figure 20.17 **Rapidly progressive glomerulonephritis (RPGN).** Arrows show 'crescents' with aggregates of macrophages and epithelial cells in Bowman's space. **A.** Focal necrotizing glomerulonephritis. **B.** Crescentic glomerulonephritis.

Box 20.10 Types of rapidly progressive glomerulonephritis (RPGN)

Linear immunofluorescent pattern *(Fig. 20.20A)*
- Idiopathic anti-GBM antibody-mediated RPGN
- Goodpasture syndrome

Granular immunofluorescent pattern (immune complex-mediated RPGN; see *Fig. 20.20B*)
- Idiopathic immune complex-mediated RPGN
- Associated with other primary GN:
  - Mesangiocapillary GN (type II > type I)
  - IgA nephropathy
  - Membranous glomerulopathy
- Associated with secondary GN:
  - Post-infectious GN
  - Systemic lupus erythematosus
  - Henoch–Schönlein syndrome
  - Cryoglobulinaemia

Negative immunofluorescent pattern (pauci-immune RPGN)
- ANCA-associated systemic vasculitides

ANCA, anti-neutrophil cytoplasmic antibody; GBM, glomerular basement membrane; IgA, immunoglobulin A.

that is, linear, granular and negative immunofluorescent patterns ***(Box 20.10)***.

Post-streptococcal glomerulonephritis

Post-streptococcal glomerulonephritis (PSGN) occurs in childhood. An acute nephritis follows 1–3 weeks after a streptococcal infection. Streptococcal throat infection, otitis media or cellulitis can all be responsible. The infecting organism is a Lancefield group A β-haemolytic streptococcus of a nephritogenic type. The latent interval between infection and the development of symptoms and signs of renal involvement reflects the time taken for immune complex formation and deposition and glomerular injury to occur. PSGN is now rare in developed countries. Renal biopsy shows diffuse, florid, acute inflammation in the glomerulus (without necrosis but occasionally cellular crescents), with neutrophils and deposition of IgG and complement ***(Fig. 20.18)***. Ultrastructural findings are those of electron-dense deposits, characteristically but not solely in the sub-epithelial aspects of the capillary walls. Endothelial cells often are swollen. Similar biopsy findings may be seen in ***non-streptococcal post-infectious glomerulonephritis (Box 20.11)***.

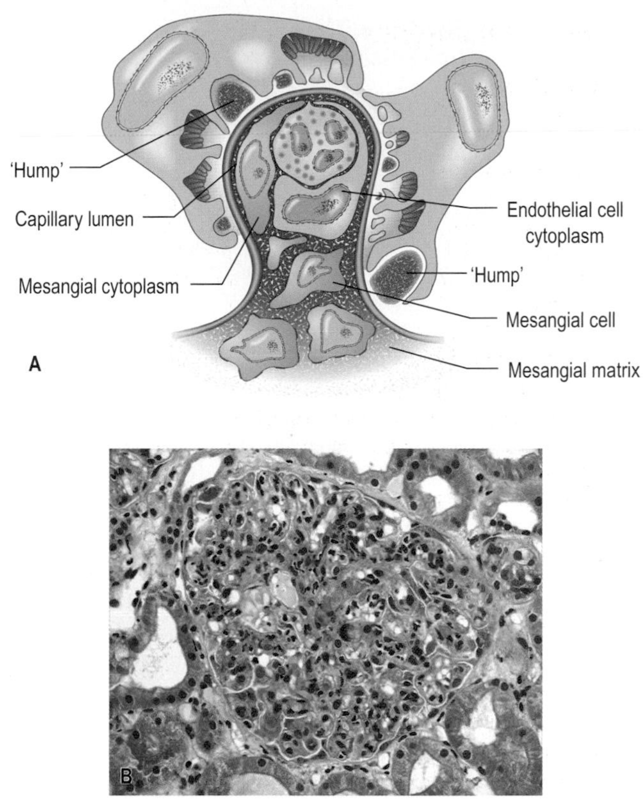

Figure 20.18 **Post-streptococcal glomerulonephritis. A.** Large aggregates of immune material (humps) in the extracapillary area. There is an increase in mesangial matrix and mesangial cells with occlusion of the capillary lumen by endothelial cell cytoplasm, leucocytes and mesangial cell cytoplasm. **B.** Light microscopy showing acute inflammation of the glomerulus with neutrophils. *(After Marsh FP.* Postgraduate Nephrology. *Oxford: Butterworth Heinemann; 1985.)*

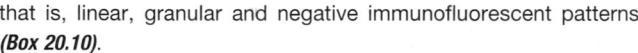

Box 20.11 Diseases commonly associated with the acute nephritic syndrome

- Post-streptococcal glomerulonephritis
- Non-streptococcal post-infectious glomerulonephritis, e.g. *Staphylococcus*, pneumococcus, *Legionella*, syphilis, mumps, varicella, hepatitis B and C, echovirus, Epstein–Barr virus, toxoplasmosis, malaria, schistosomiasis, trichinosis
- Infective endocarditis
- Shunt nephritis
- Visceral abscess
- Systemic lupus erythematosus (see pp. 692–695)
- Henoch–Schönlein syndrome (see p. 748)
- Cryoglobulinaemia (see p. 748)

Management

The acute phase should be treated with good blood pressure control, diuretics and salt restriction for oedema, and dialysis as necessary. If recovery is slow, corticosteroids may be helpful. The prognosis is usually good in children. A small number of adults develop hypertension and/or CKD later in life. Therefore, in older patients, an annual blood pressure check and measurement of serum creatinine are required. Evidence in support of long-term penicillin prophylaxis after the development of glomerulonephritis is lacking. In non-streptococcal post-infectious glomerulonephritis, prognosis is equally good if the underlying infection is eradicated.

Glomerulonephritis with infective endocarditis

GN occurs rarely in patients with infective endocarditis (usually intravenous drug users), or in patients with infected ventriculoperitoneal shunts (***shunt nephritis***). Histology appearances resemble post-infectious GN but lesions are usually focal and segmental. Crescentic GN with AKI has been described, particularly with *Staphylococcus aureus* infection. Appropriate antibiotic therapy or surgical eradication of infection in fulminant cases usually results in a return of normal renal function.

GN also occurs associated with ***visceral abscesses*** (mainly pulmonary) and is indistinguishable from post-infectious GN. Complement levels are normal and immune deposits are absent on biopsy. Antibiotic therapy and surgical drainage of the abscess result in complete recovery of renal function in approximately 50% of patients.

IgA nephropathy

IgA nephropathy ***(Fig. 20.19)*** has replaced post-streptococcal glomerulonephritis as the most common form of GN worldwide. Demographic and family studies support the existence of a genetic contribution to the pathogenesis of IgA nephropathy, but results from genetic association studies of candidate genes are inconsistent. A genome-wide analysis study conducted in European patients showed a strong association on chromosome 6p in the region of the MHC/DQ and HLA-B loci, suggesting that the HLA region contains the strongest common susceptibility alleles that predispose to IgA nephropathy.

Histology

There is a focal and segmental proliferative glomerulonephritis with mesangial deposits of polymeric IgA1. In some cases, IgG, IgM and C3 are also seen in the glomerular mesangium. Superimposed crescent formation is frequent, particularly following macroscopic haematuria associated with upper respiratory tract infection.

An Oxford histological classification for IgA nephropathy is shown in ***Box 20.12***. The features have prognostic significance and it is recommended that they be taken into account for predicting outcome independent of the clinical features, both at the time of presentation and during follow-up.

Pathogenesis

The disease may be a result of a number of events, including:

- exaggerated bone marrow and tonsillar IgA1 immune response to viral or other antigens
- an association with an abnormality in O-linked galactosylation in the hinge region of the IgA1 molecule
- functional abnormalities of two IgA receptors – CD89 expressed on blood myeloid cells and the transferring receptor (CD71) on mesangial cells
- circulating immune complexes composed of a glycan-specific IgG and a galactose-deficient IgA1 antibody.

IgA-rich immune complexes deposit in the glomerular mesangium, inducing mesangial cell activation and proliferation, and matrix synthesis and deposition. Removal of these complexes by bacterial proteases attenuates injury, and it is thought that glycan-specific autoantibodies, rather than IgA1 itself, play a key role in the pathogenesis. Up to 50% of patients exhibit elevated serum IgA (polyclonal).

Several diseases are associated with IgA deposits, including Henoch–Schönlein purpura, chronic liver disease, malignancies (especially carcinoma of bronchus), seronegative spondyloarthritis, coeliac disease, mycosis fungoides and psoriasis.

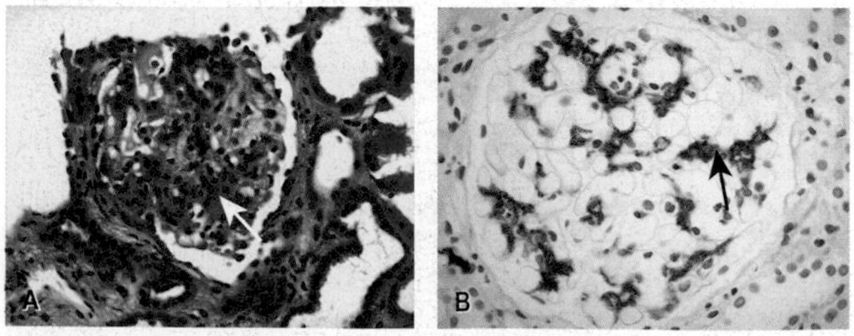

Figure 20.19 **IgA nephropathy. A.** Light microscopy showing mesangial cell proliferation (arrow) and increased matrix. **B.** IgA deposits (arrow) on immunoperoxidase staining.

Clinical features

IgA nephropathy tends to occur in children and young males, presenting with asymptomatic microscopic haematuria or recurrent macroscopic haematuria following an upper respiratory or gastrointestinal viral infection. Proteinuria occurs and 5% of cases can be nephrotic. The prognosis is usually good, especially in those with normal blood pressure, normal renal function and absence of proteinuria at presentation. Surprisingly, recurrent macroscopic haematuria is a good prognostic sign, although this may be due to 'lead-time bias' (see p. 591), as patients with overt haematuria come to medical attention at an earlier stage of their illness. The risk of eventual development of ESKD is about 25% in those with proteinuria of more than 1 g per day, elevated serum creatinine, hypertension, *ACE* gene polymorphism (DD isoform) and tubulointerstitial fibrosis on renal biopsy.

Box 20.12 Oxford histological classification of IgA nephropathy

Histological variable	Description	Class
Mesangial hypercellularity	Average mesangial hypercellularity[a] >0.5	M1
	Average mesangial hypercellularity <0.5	M0
Segmental glomerulosclerosis	Part of the glomerular tuft is involved in sclerosis	S1
	No segmental glomerulosclerosis	S0
Endocapillary hypercellularity	Hypercellularity present and results in luminal narrowing	E1
	No hypercellularity	E0
Tubular atrophy/ interstitial fibrosis	Percentage of cortical area involved:	
	>50	T2
	26–50	T1
	0–25	T0

[a]Mesangial hypercellularity is scored 0 for glomeruli with <4 mesangial cells per mesangial area; 1 for those with 4–5 cells; 2 for 6–7 cells; and 3 for ≥8 cells. Scores obtained for all glomeruli are then averaged.

Management

- All patients, with or without hypertension and proteinuria, should receive an ACE inhibitor or an AII-RA, to reduce proteinuria and preserve renal function.
- Patients with proteinuria of over 1–3 g/day, mild glomerular changes only and preserved renal function should be treated with steroids. Steroids reduce proteinuria and stabilize renal function.
- Addition of azathioprine to steroids does not confer additional benefits. The combination of cyclophosphamide, dipyridamole and warfarin should not be used; nor should ciclosporin.
- In patients with progressive disease (falling to eGFR <60 mL/min), fish oils or prednisolone with cyclophosphamide for 3 months, followed by maintenance with prednisolone and azathioprine, may be tried.
- A tonsillectomy can reduce proteinuria and haematuria in those patients with recurrent tonsillitis.
- Mesangial IgA deposits are commonly found in the allografts of transplanted patients but loss of graft function as a result is uncommon.

Alport syndrome

Alport syndrome is a rare hereditary nephritis with haematuria, proteinuria (<1–2 g/day), progressive kidney disease and high-frequency nerve deafness. Approximately 15% of cases may have ocular abnormalities, such as bilateral anterior lenticonus, and macular and perimacular retinal flecks. In about 85% of patients with Alport syndrome there is an X-linked inherited mutation in the *COL4α5* gene encoding the COL4α5 collagen chain, a critical component of the glomerular basement membrane. In female carriers, penetrance is variable and depends on the type of mutation or degree of mosaicism following hybridization of the X chromosome. Patients with autosomal recessive or dominant modes of inheritance have also been described with mutations in *COL4α3* or *COL4α4* gene. In families with stromal cell tumours, there is an additional mutation in the *COL4α6* gene.

These mutations present as post-translational defects in α3, α4 and α5 chains, and result in incorrect assembly or folding of monomers; defective monomers are rapidly degraded. Over time, the basement membrane undergoes selective proteolysis, and glomerular membranes thicken unevenly, split and ultimately deteriorate.

Although the basement membrane is abnormal, podocyte function and the slit diaphragm are unaffected. Proteinuria in Alport syndrome is often mild and is the result of glomerular sclerosis, rather than primary loss of slit pores.

In some patients with Alport syndrome and carriers, a thin basement membrane, as seen in benign familial haematuria, is the only abnormality detected on histology. For this reason, the boundary between Alport's and benign familial haematuria has become increasingly vague.

Management

The disease is progressive and accounts for some 5% of cases of ESKD in childhood or adolescence. Patients with mild CKD can be treated with ACE inhibitors to attenuate proteinuria. Exciting experimental evidence suggests that mesenchymal stem cells can transdifferentiate into podocytes and repair basement abnormalities and slow the rate of progression. Anti-GBM antibody does not adhere normally to the glomerular basement membrane of affected individuals but development of crescentic glomerulonephritis in the transplanted kidney due to anti-GBM alloantibody is a well-recognized complication.

Thin glomerular basement membrane disease

This condition is inherited as an autosomal dominant and typically presents with persistent microscopic glomerular haematuria (red blood cell casts or dysmorphic red blood cells). The diagnosis is made on renal biopsy, which shows thinning of the glomerular capillary basement membrane on electron microscopy. The condition was under-diagnosed and is much more common than previously believed. The prognosis for renal function is usually very good but some patients develop renal insufficiency over decades. The cause of renal impairment in this condition is not known but may be due to secondary FSGS or concomitant IgA nephropathy. Misdiagnosis occurs with Alport syndrome, which shares similar histological features. No treatment is of known benefit.

Anti-GBM glomerulonephritis

Anti-GBM glomerulonephritis ***(Fig. 20.20A)***, characterized by linear capillary loop staining with IgG and C3 and extensive crescent formation, accounts for 15–20% of all cases of RPGN, although overall represents less than 5% of all forms of glomerulonephritis.

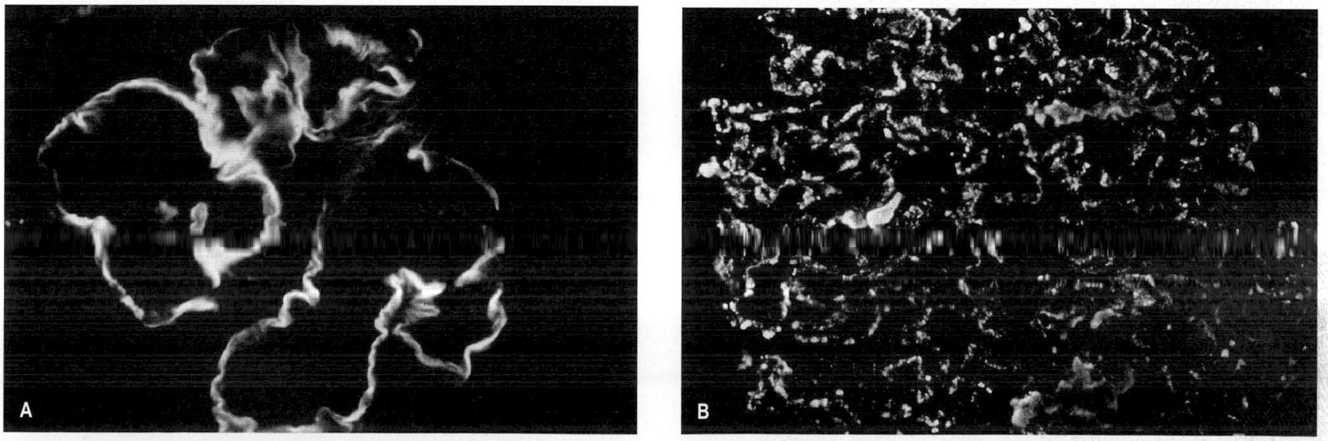

Figure 20.20 **Immunofluorescence. A.** Anti-glomerular basement membrane antibody (anti-GBM) deposition in a linear pattern typical of Goodpasture syndrome. **B.** Showing immune complex deposition in a diffuse granular pattern.

This condition is rare, with an incidence of 1 per 2 million in the general population. About two-thirds of these patients have ***Goodpasture syndrome*** with associated lung haemorrhage (see p. 1121). The remainder have a renal restricted anti-GBM RPGN, which is seen in patients over 50 years and affects both genders equally.

Anti-GBM antibodies (detected by enzyme-linked immunosorbent assay, or ELISA) are present in serum and are directed against the ***non-collagenous (NCI) component*** of $\alpha 3$ (IV) collagen of the basement membrane. This target antigen must be present as a component of the native $\alpha 3$, $\alpha 4$, $\alpha 5$ (IV) network of selected basement membrane in order for pulmonary and renal disease to develop. Anti-GBM glomerulonephritis never occurs in patients with Alport syndrome; although it can develop after patients with Alport's receive a kidney transplant, anti-GBM alloantibodies evolve in response to the 'foreign' $\alpha 3$, $\alpha 4$, $\alpha 5$ (IV) collagen network absent in a patient's own kidneys.

Anti-GBM RPGN is restricted by the major histocompatibility complex; HLA-DRB1*1501 and HLA-DRB1*1502 alleles increase susceptibility, whereas HLA-DR7 and HLA-DR1 are protective. The thymus expresses $\alpha 3$ (IV) NCI peptides that can eliminate autoreactive $CD4^+$ helper T cells, but a few such cells escape deletion and are kept in check by circulating regulatory cells (Treg). Breakdown of this peripheral tolerance (the mechanism of which is unknown) results in these autoreactive $CD4^+$ cells producing anti-GBM antibodies. These antibodies are very specific: antibodies against $\alpha 1$, $\alpha 2$ and $\alpha 3$ NCI domains do not cause RPGN. Since the $\alpha 3$ (IV) NCI epitope is hidden within the $\alpha 3$, $\alpha 4$ and $\alpha 5$ (IV) promoter, it is presumed that an environmental factor, such as exposure to hydrocarbons or tobacco smoke, is required in order to reveal cryptic epitopes to the immune system.

The mechanism of renal injury is complex. When anti-GBM antibody binds basement membrane, it activates complement and proteases, and results in disruption of the filtration barrier and Bowman's capsule, causing proteinuria and the formation of crescents. Crescent formation is facilitated by IL-12 and γ-interferon, which are produced by resident and infiltrating inflammatory cells.

Management involves:

- ***plasma exchange*** to remove circulating anti-GBM antibodies
- ***steroids*** to suppress inflammation from antibody already deposited in the tissue
- ***cyclophosphamide*** to suppress further antibody synthesis.

The ***prognosis*** is directly related to the extent of glomerular damage (measured by percentage of glomeruli containing crescents, serum creatinine and need for dialysis) at the initiation of treatment. When oliguria occurs or serum creatinine rises above 600–700 μmol/L, renal failure is usually irreversible. Once the active disease is treated, this condition, unlike other autoimmune diseases, does not follow a remitting/relapsing course. If left untreated, autoantibodies diminish spontaneously within 3 years and autoreactive T cells cannot be detected in the convalescent patients. This is suggestive of re-establishment of peripheral tolerance, which coincides with re-emergence of regulatory $CD25^+$ cells in the peripheral blood; these play a key role in inhibiting the autoimmune response. The emergence and persistence of these regulatory cells may underlie the 'single hit' nature of this condition.

ANCA-positive small-vessel vasculitis

(See also p. 702.) Inflammation and necrosis of the blood vessel wall occurs in many primary vasculitic disorders. The small-vessel vasculitides affecting the kidney include:

- granulomatosis with polyangiitis (GPA)
- microscopic polyangiitis (MPA)
- renal-limited vasculitis (without systemic features)
- eosinophilic granulomatosis with polyangiitis (which is frequently ANCA-negative).

The anti-neutrophil cytoplasmic antibody (ANCA)-associated small-vessel vasculitides are GPA, MPA and renal-limited vasculitis. GPA and MPA share a common pathology with focal necrotizing lesions, which affect many different vessels and organs:

- in the lungs, a capillaritis may cause lung haemorrhage
- within the glomerulus of the kidney, crescentic GN and/or focal necrotizing lesions (FNGN) may cause AKI (see ***Fig. 20.17***)
- in the dermis, a purpuric rash or vasculitic ***(Fig. 20.21)*** ulceration.

Renal histology is regarded as a 'gold standard' for the diagnosis and prognostication of ANCA-associated GN. A consensus group proposed a new classification around four general categories of lesions:

- ***focal*** (≥50% normal glomeruli that are not affected by the disease process)
- ***crescentic*** (≥50% of glomeruli with cellular crescents)
- ***mixed*** (a heterogeneous glomerular phenotype in which no glomerular feature predominates)
- ***sclerotic*** (≥50% of glomeruli with global sclerosis).

This system has been shown to have a prognostic value for 1- and 5-year renal outcomes, and may guide therapy.

Pathogenesis

There are two forms of ANCA (see p. 650; ***Fig. 20.22***):

- PR3-ANCA (cANCA)
- MPO-ANCA (pANCA).

If ELISA and indirect immunofluorescence techniques are combined, diagnostic specificity is 99%. ANCA and anti-GBM antibodies do occur together; such patients tend to follow the natural history of Goodpasture syndrome.

- ***PR3-ANCA positivity*** is found in the large majority (>90%) of patients with active GPA and in up to 50% of patients with MPA.
- ***Anti-MPO positivity*** is present in the majority of patients with renal-limited vasculitis and in a variable number of cases of MPA. There is some evidence to suggest that ANCAs are pathogenic and not just markers of disease; for example, development of drug-induced ANCA is associated with

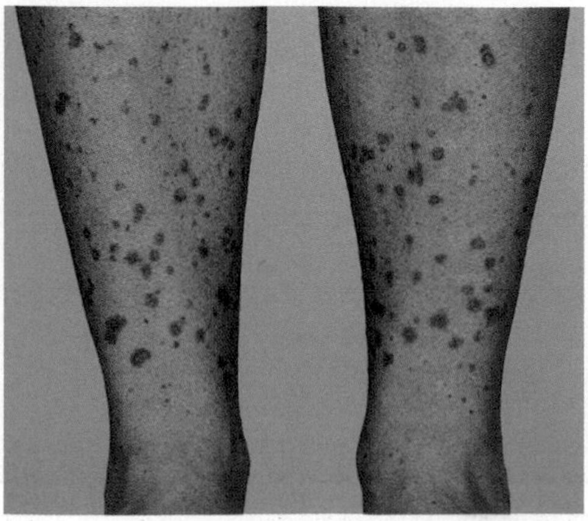

Figure 20.21 Vasculitic rash.

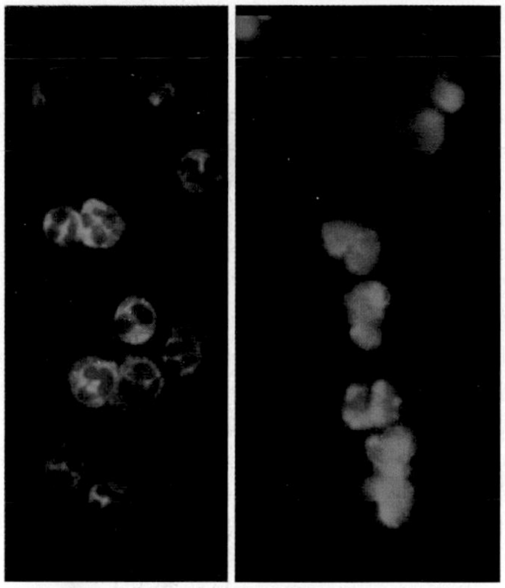

A cANCA. B pANCA.

Figure 20.22 ANCA-positive glomerulonephritis – immunofluorescence. A. cANCA. **B.** pANCA. *(From Schrier RW 1999.* The Schrier Atlas of Diseases of the Kidney, Vol. IV: Systemic Diseases and the Kidney. *Wiley–Blackwell, with permission.)*

vasculitic lesions in humans. Eosinophilic GPA may have either anti-MPO or anti-PR3 ANCA.

- ***Positivity for both types of ANCA*** antibodies occurs in up to 10% of patients, who have a variable clinical course but a worse renal outcome.
- ***Drugs*** (e.g. propylthiouracil, hydralazine, minocycline, penicillamine) may induce vasculitis associated (most commonly) with MPO-ANCA, often in very high titres. Many cases of drug-induced ANCA-associated vasculitis present with constitutional symptoms, arthralgias/arthritis and cutaneous vasculitis. Crescentic GN and lung haemorrhage can also occur.

Both ANCA autoantigens are present in immature neutrophil granules. In contrast to the normally silenced state of these two genes in mature neutrophils of healthy subjects, *PR3* and *MPO* are aberrantly expressed in mature neutrophils of patients with ANCA vasculitis due to unsilencing of both antigens because of epigenetic modifications.

- It is unclear how and why ***autoimmunity*** causes the formation of ANCA antibodies. Patients with anti-PR3 also have autoantibodies to a peptide translated from the antisense DNA strand of PR3 (complementary PR3; cPR3) or to a mimetic of this peptide. This suggests that autoimmunity can be initiated through an immune response against a peptide that is antisense or complementary to the autoantigen, which then induces anti-idiotypic antibodies (autoantibodies) that cross-react with the autoantigen.
- A recent study has shown that infection by fimbriated bacteria (Gram-negative pathogens such as *Escherichia coli*, *Klebsiella pneumoniae* and *Proteus mirabilis*) can trigger, due to molecular mimicry, a cross-reactive autoimmunity to lysosomal membrane protein 2 (LAMP-2), a glycosylated membrane protein that is co-localized with PR3 and MPO in the intracellular vesicles of neutrophils.

Other factors that contribute to the initiation of an ANCA autoimmune response and the induction of injury by ANCA include genetic predisposition (α_1-antitrypsin deficiency, Pi-Z allele) and environmental factors (e.g. silica exposure, viral infection, *Staph. aureus* infection).

Management

The sooner treatment is instituted, the greater chance there is of recovery of renal function.

- ***High-dose oral corticosteroids*** and ***intravenous pulsed cyclophosphamide*** are of benefit in inducing remission. The best indicators of prognosis are pulmonary haemorrhage and severity of renal failure at presentation.
- ***Rituximab*** has been shown in two studies to be equally effective as cyclophosphamide for inducing remission in ANCA-associated vasculitides in the short term (6–12 months), with similar adverse event rates. Rituximab may be a therapeutic option in patients who cannot tolerate cyclophosphamide, and in those whose disease is poorly controlled and who relapse while on cyclophosphamide.
- ***Fulminant disease*** requires intensification of immunosuppression with adjuvant plasma exchanges or intravenous pulsed methylprednisolone (1 g/day for 3 consecutive days). Plasma exchange appeared to have a better outcome than pulsed methylprednisolone in one study.
- Once remission has been achieved, mycophenolate mofetil or azathioprine should be substituted for cyclophosphamide. Use of rituximab every 3 months in fixed dose has recently been shown to be superior to azathioprine in the maintenance of remission.
- Colonization of the upper respiratory tract with *Staph. aureus* increases the risk of relapse, and treatment with sulfamethoxazole/trimethoprim reduces the relapse rate.
- Relapse after complete cessation of immunosuppressive therapy has been observed relatively frequently, and therefore long-term, albeit relatively low-dose, immunosuppression is necessary.
- Intravenous immunoglobulin (anti-thymocyte globulin (ATG) directed against activated T lymphocytes causes lymphopenia), lymphocyte-depleting anti-CD52 (campath-IH) antibodies and anti-TNF therapy have shown promise in the treatment of severe and drug-resistant cases as induction therapy. However, an anti-TNF agent, etanercept, has been ineffective as a sole agent for maintenance.
- Up to 25% of patients with PR3-ANCA harbour antibodies against human plasminogen and/or tissue plasminogen activator. Their presence has been correlated with venous thromboembolic events and fibrinoid necrotic glomerular lesions, suggesting functional interference with fibrinolysis. However, a formal role for anticoagulation in patients with ANCA-associated GN remains uncertain.

Mixed nephritic and nephrotic syndrome

Injury involves mesangial cells, endothelium, the basement membrane and podocytes in this heterogenous group of conditions.

Mesangiocapillary (membranoproliferative) glomerulonephritis

Mesangiocapillary (membranoproliferative) glomerulonephritis (MCGN) is an uncommon descriptive lesion that has three subtypes with similar clinical presentations: the nephrotic syndrome, haematuria, hypertension and renal impairment. They also produce similar microscopic findings, although the pathogenesis may be different. Electron microscopy defines:

- ***Type 1 MCGN*** involves mesangial cell proliferation, with mainly sub-endothelial immune deposition and apparent splitting of the capillary basement membrane, giving a 'tramline' effect. It can be associated with persistently reduced plasma levels of C3 and normal levels of C4, and activation of the classical complement cascade. It is often idiopathic but occurs with chronic infection (abscesses, infective endocarditis, infected ventriculoperitoneal shunt) or cryoglobulinaemia secondary to hepatitis C infections ***(Fig. 20.23A)***.

- ***Type 2 MCGN*** demonstrates mesangial cell proliferation with electron-dense, linear (ribbon-like) intramembranous deposits that usually stain for C3 only ***(Fig. 20.23B)***. This ***dense deposit disease*** may be idiopathic or may be associated with factor H deficiency and partial lipodystrophy (loss of subcutaneous fat on the face and upper trunk). Alternatively, ***C3 nephropathy*** presents with low C3 levels (as in type 1 MCGN), due in this case to activation of the alternative pathway of the complement cascade, where loss-of-function mutations in complement factor H allow uncontrolled alternative pathway activation. Autoantibodies to the C3 convertase enzyme (C3 nephritic factor) are present. In patients of Cypriot origin, an autosomal dominant inherited heterozygous duplication in the *CFHR5* gene (CFHR5 nephropathy) leads to a similar presentation.
- ***Type 3 MCGN*** has features of both type 1 and type 2 disease. Complement activation appears to be via the final common pathway of the cascade.

Most patients eventually go on to develop ESKD over several years. Type 2 MCGN recurs in virtually 100% of renal transplant patients but recurrence is less common in type 1 (25%).

Management

In idiopathic MCGN (***all age groups***) with normal renal function and non-nephrotic-range proteinuria, no specific therapy is required. Good blood pressure control, ideally with an ACE inhibitor, is of benefit.

In ***children*** with the nephritic syndrome and/or impaired renal function, a trial of steroids is warranted (alternate-day prednisolone 40 mg/m^2 for a period of 6–12 months). If no benefit is seen, this treatment is discontinued. Regular follow-up, with control of blood pressure, use of agents to reduce proteinuria and correction of lipid abnormalities, is necessary.

In ***adults*** with the nephritic syndrome and/or renal impairment, aspirin (325 mg) or dipyridamole (75–100 mg) daily, or a combination of the two, should be given for 6–12 months. Again, if no benefits are seen, the treatment should be stopped. Treatment to slow the rate of progression of CKD is instituted (see p. 782). In C3 nephropathy due to loss-of-function mutation in complement factor H, anti-C5 antibody (eculizumab) has been used successfully in several patients.

IgM nephropathy

This disorder is characterized by increased mesangial cellularity in most of the glomeruli, associated with granular immune deposits of IgM and complement. People present with episodic or persistent haematuria and the nephrotic syndrome. Unlike in minimal-change disease, the prognosis is not uniformly good, as steroid response is only 50%. Between 10% and 30% develop progressive renal insufficiency with evidence of secondary FSGS (see p. 737) on repeat biopsy. A trial of cyclophosphamide with prednisolone is used with persistent nephrotic syndrome, particularly when there is a rising plasma creatinine concentration.

C1q nephropathy

C1q nephropathy is very similar to IgM nephropathy in presenting features and microscopic appearance, with the exception of C1q deposits in the mesangium. Sometimes it is misdiagnosed as lupus nephritis, particularly in people with negative serology (so-called 'seronegative lupus'). The distinguishing features are intense C1q staining and absence of tubuloreticular inclusions (attributable to high circulating α-interferon) on electron microscopy. Only some people are steroid-dependent. Progression to CKD is, as in most glomerular diseases, most likely to occur in people with heavy proteinuria and renal insufficiency.

Idiopathic fibrillary glomerulopathy

In this rare condition, microfibrillary structures are seen in the mesangium and glomerular capillary wall on electron microscopy that are clearly different from those seen in amyloidosis; the fibrils are larger than in amyloidosis (20–30 nm versus 10 nm in diameter) and do not stain with Congo red. The median age at presentation is approximately 45 years (range 10–80 years). People present with proteinuria, mostly in the nephrotic range (60%), and microscopic

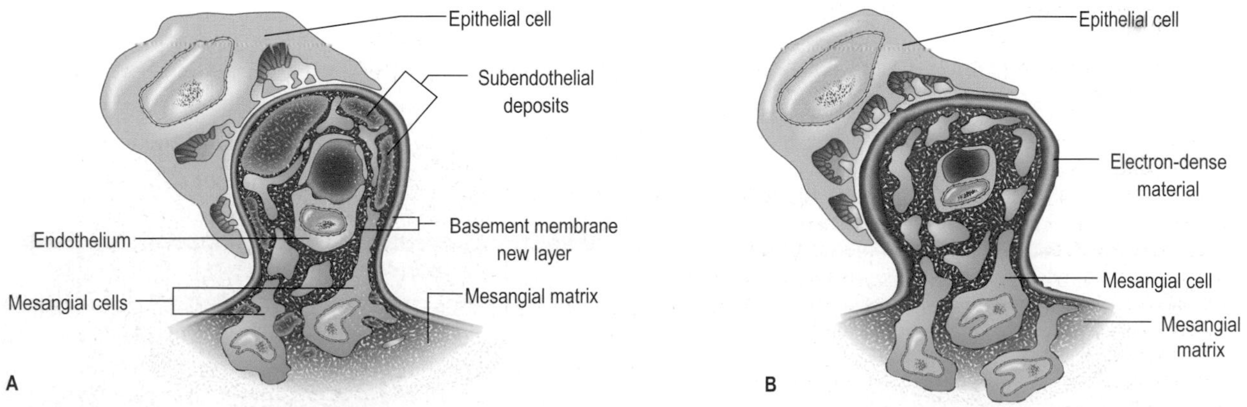

Figure 20.23 Mesangiocapillary glomerulonephritis (MCGN). A. Type 1 MCGN showing expanded mesangial matrix and mesangial cells, thickened capillary wall, large subendothelial deposits and formation of a new layer of basement membrane (tramline effect). **B.** Type 2 MCGN. This shows a variable glomerular appearance; very electron-dense material has replaced Bowman's capsule, tubular basement membrane and part of the capillary. There is some proliferation of mesangial cells. *(After Marsh FP.* Postgraduate Nephrology. *Oxford: Butterworth–Heinemann; 1985.)*

haematuria (70%), hypertension and CKD (50%) that may progress rapidly; 40–50% of patients develop ESKD within 2–6 years. No treatment is known to be of benefit.

Immunotactoid glomerulopathy

In this disorder, microtubules that are much larger (30–40 nm in diameter) than the fibrils in fibrillary glomerulopathy are seen on electron microscopy. The majority of patients have circulating paraproteins, or monoclonal immunoglobulin deposition is seen in the glomeruli on immunofluorescence microscopy. A lymphoproliferative disease is the underlying cause in over 50% of cases. The clinical presentation and course are similar to those of fibrillary glomerulopathy. Complete or partial remission of the nephrotic syndrome can be achieved with chemotherapy in 80% of patients.

Fibronectin glomerulopathy

This is also a form of glomerulonephritis due to fibrillar deposits, which, unlike amyloidosis but like fibrillary glomerulonephritis and immunotactoid glomerulopathy, is negative for Congo red staining. It is inherited as an autosomal dominant disorder and is associated with the massive deposition of fibronectin, a large dimeric glycoprotein consisting of two similar subunits (approximately 250 kDa in weight). The possible genetic abnormality in this disorder is a loss-of-function mutation in uteroglobin.

Fibronectin glomerulopathy is extremely rare and was originally described only in Caucasians of European descent. An Asian family with this disease has since been reported. There are as yet no known cases in black or Hispanic people. It presents with varying degrees of proteinuria seen first between the ages of 20 and 40, followed by hypertension, microscopic haematuria, and slow progression to ESKD in most patients.

Systemic lupus erythematosus (lupus nephritis)

Overt renal disease occurs in at least one-third of systemic lupus erythematosus (SLE) patients and, of these, 25% reach end-stage CKD within 10 years (see also pp. 693–694). Histologically, almost all patients will have changes. ***Box 20.13*** shows the progression of the histological findings and the clinical picture from classes I to VI.

Serial renal biopsies show that in approximately 25% of patients, histological appearances change from one class to another during the inter-biopsy interval. Immune deposits in the glomeruli and mesangium are characteristic of SLE (tubuloreticular structure in glomerular endothelial cells) and stain positive for IgG, IgM, IgA and the complement components C3, C1q and C4 on immunofluorescence.

Box 20.13 Classification of lupus nephritis

- ***Class I – Minimal mesangial lupus nephritis*** (***LN***), with immune deposits but normal on light microscopy. Asymptomatic.
- ***Class II – Mesangial proliferative LN*** with mesangial hypercellularity and matrix expansion. Clinically, there is mild renal disease.
- ***Class III – Focal LN*** (involving <50% of glomeruli) with subdivisions for active or chronic lesions. Subepithelial deposits seen. Clinically, there is haematuria and proteinuria; 10–20% of all LN.
- ***Class IV – Diffuse LN*** (involving >50% of glomeruli; ***Fig. 20.24***) classified by the presence of segmental and global lesions as well as active and chronic lesions. Subendothelial deposits are present. Clinically, there is progression to the nephrotic syndrome, hypertension and renal insufficiency. Most common and most severe form of LN.
- ***Class V – Membranous LN*** affects 10–20% of patients. Can occur in combination with class III or IV. Good prognosis.
- ***Class VI – Advanced sclerosing LN*** (≥90% globally sclerosed glomeruli without residual activity). This represents the advanced stages of the above, as well as healing. Immunosuppressive therapy is unlikely to help, as it is 'inactive'. Progressive CKD.

(Modified from International Society of Nephrology/Renal Pathological Society 2004.)

Pathophysiology

SLE is known to be a multifactorial autoantigen-driven, T-cell-dependent and B-cell-mediated autoimmune disorder (see pp. 692–695).

- Lupus nephritis typically associates with multiple circulating autoantibodies to cellular antigens (particularly anti-dsDNA, anti-Ro), and with complement activation, which leads to reduced serum levels of C3, C4 and (particularly) C1q.
- C1q is the first component of the classical pathway of the complement cascade (see p. 124) and is involved in the activation of complement and clearance of self-antigens generated during apoptosis.
- Although self DNA was thought to be the inciting autoantigen, nucleosomes (structures comprising DNA and histone, generated during apoptosis) are more likely to be antigenic.
- Nucleosome-specific T cells, antinucleosome antibodies and nephritogenic immune complexes are generated.
- T-helper 2 (Th2) cells, with basophils and B-cell survival factors (such as BLyS), enhance B-cell differentiation and survival, and stimulated nucleic acid-binding receptors promote the production of autoreactive antibodies.
- Positively charged histone components of the nucleosome bind to the negatively charged heparan sulphate of the GBM, targeting an inflammatory reaction to the kidney.
- Inflammation stimulates complement activation, mesangial cell proliferation, mesangial matrix expansion and recruitment of inflammatory leucocytes.

The extraglomerular renal features of lupus nephritis include tubulointerstitial nephritis (75% of patients), renal vein thrombosis and renal artery stenosis. Thrombotic manifestations are associated with autoantibodies to phospholipids (anticardiolipin or lupus anticoagulant) (see p. 695), and may present as infarction of glomerular segments, thrombotic microangiopathy or vasculitis.

Management

Initial treatment depends on the clinical presentation but hypertension and oedema should always be treated. Disease activity, kidney

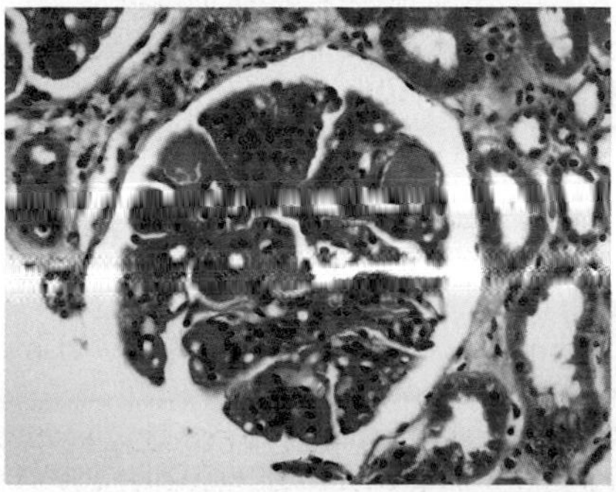

Figure 20.24 Lupus nephritis type IV – a diffuse proliferative nephritis. There is proliferation of endothelial and mesangial cells.

biopsy and histology, as well as the presence or absence of extra-renal manifestations of lupus, guide therapy. ***Type I lupus nephritis*** requires no specific treatment. ***Type II*** usually runs a benign course but some patients are treated with hydroxychloroquine and/or steroids alone.

- There have been a number of clinical trials with immunosuppressive agents in ***types III, IV and V*** lupus nephritis. Outcomes are affected by ethnicity, clinical characteristics, irreversible damage (on renal biopsy), initial response to treatment and the future frequency of renal flares.
- Steroids and high-dose intravenous cyclophosphamide or mycophenolate mofetil (MMF) are usually used for induction. In white populations, low-dose cyclophosphamide is a good alternative to high-dose cyclophosphamide, as it is similarly effective and associated with less toxicity.
- MMF is as effective as high-dose intravenous cyclophosphamide in the induction phase with a similar safety profile, but cyclophosphamide may be inferior to MMF in black and Hispanic people.
- Most patients respond to induction therapy. Remission is maintained with MMF (superior to azathioprine) or azathioprine, which is similar in effectiveness to ciclosporin in reducing the risk of relapse.
- B-cell depletion with rituximab (anti-CD20) has been used in some patients, with favourable results over the short term. However, controlled trials have not shown consistent results. It might be useful in severe, refractory lupus nephritis.

Prognosis

Treatment leading to the normalization of proteinuria, hypertension and renal dysfunction indicates a good prognosis. The prognosis is better in patients with types I, II and V disease. Glomerulosclerosis (type VI) usually predicts ESKD.

Cryoglobulinaemic renal disease

Cryoglobulins (CGs) are individual or mixed immunoglobulins and complement components, which precipitate reversibly in the cold. Three types are recognized:

- ***Type I*** is characterized by a cryoprecipitable immunoglobulin of a single monoclonal type, as is found in multiple myeloma and lymphoproliferative disorders.
- ***Types II and III*** cryoglobulinaemias are mixed types. In each, an antiglobulin is bound to the *Fc* portion of polyclonal IgG. In type II, the antiglobulin is usually monoclonal IgM with rheumatoid factor activity, often associated with hepatitis C virus infection, but also with other causes listed below. In type III, the antiglobulin is polyclonal IgM. Type II CGs account for 40–60% cases, while 40–50% of all CG cases are of type III.

Glomerular disease is more common in type II than in type III cryoglobulinaemia. In approximately 30% of these 'mixed' cryoglobulinaemias, no underlying or associated disease is found (essential cryoglobulinaemia). Recognized associations include viral infections (hepatitis B and C, HIV, cytomegalovirus, Epstein–Barr infection), fungal and spirochaetal infections, malaria and infective endocarditis, and autoimmune rheumatic diseases (SLE, rheumatoid arthritis and Sjögren syndrome). Glomerular pathological changes resemble those of MCGN (see ***Fig. 20.23***).

Presentation is usually in the fourth or fifth decades of life, and women are more frequently affected than men. Systemic features include purpura, arthralgia, leg ulcers, Raynaud's phenomenon, evidence of systemic vasculitis, a polyneuropathy and hepatic involvement. The glomerular disease presents typically as asymptomatic proteinuria, microscopic haematuria or both, but presentation with an acute nephritic and nephrotic syndrome (the most common presentation) or features of CKD also occurs.

Complement is consumed, cryoglobulins can be detected, and protein electrophoresis, rheumatoid factor, autoantibodies and antiviral antibodies or mRNA of hepatitis C, depending on the associated disorder, should be sought.

The underlying cause should be treated; as hepatitis C virus infection is the most common cause, antivirals, such as proteases, are highly efficacious. Intensive plasma exchange or cryofiltration has been used in selected cases where vasculitis is limb-, organ- or life-threatening to achieve rapid removal of cryoglobulins. Uncontrolled studies of the anti-CD20 chimeric monoclonal antibody rituximab, which depletes B cells, appear promising.

Henoch–Schönlein syndrome (purpura)

This clinical syndrome comprises a characteristic skin rash, abdominal colic, joint pain and glomerulonephritis. Approximately 30–70% have clinical evidence of renal disease with haematuria and/or proteinuria. The renal disease is usually mild but the nephrotic syndrome and AKI can occur. The renal lesion is a focal segmental proliferative glomerulonephritis, sometimes with mesangial hypercellularity. In the more severe cases, epithelial crescents may be present. Immunoglobulin deposition is mainly IgA in the glomerular mesangium distribution, similar to IgA nephropathy. There is no treatment of proven benefit; steroid therapy is ineffective. Treatment is usually supportive; in crescentic GN, aggressive immunosuppression has been tried but with variable outcome.

Other glomerular disorders

Fabry's disease

This is an X-linked lysosomal storage disease resulting from a deficiency of the enzyme α-galactosidase. Glycosphingolipids accumulate in many cells; in the kidney, podocytes are affected. Systemic features include angiokeratomas in the skin, cardiovascular disease, neuropathies and proteinuric progressive CKD. Enzyme replacement with agalsidase (α-galactosidase) slows progression and injury to the heart, kidney and skin (see pp. 1287–1288).

Sickle nephropathy

Sickle disease or trait is complicated relatively commonly by papillary sclerosis or necrosis, nephrogenic diabetes insipidus and incomplete renal tubular acidosis. Glomerular lesions are rare and can sometimes be traced to hepatitis B or C infection acquired through repeated blood transfusions. Occasionally, proteinuria or nephrotic syndrome with progressive renal insufficiency is seen without prior infection. Rarely, membranous GN or mesangiocapillary GN with IgG deposits occurs in association. No form of effective therapy is known.

Glomerulopathy associated with pre-eclampsia

Patients with pre-eclampsia present with hypertension and proteinuria, often of rapid onset, which usually disappears after delivery. The glomerular lesion is characterized by marked endothelial swelling and obliteration of capillary lumina. Fibrinogen–fibrin deposits may be found in the mesangium. The renal lesion may not be reversible and 30% of patients have changes for ≥6 months. In severe cases, associated with cortical necrosis, there may be a microangiopathic haemolytic anaemia. Normal placental development, regulated by angiogenic factors like vascular endothelial growth factor (VEGF) and by placental growth factors, does not occur in pre-eclampsia. Implantation is abnormal, in part due to a soluble fms-like tyrosine kinase (sFlt1) receptor, an antagonist of placental growth factor and specifically of VEGF, which is upregulated in the placenta of patients with pre-eclampsia. High circulating levels of these receptors antagonize angiopoietic factors and cause endothelial dysfunction. Excessive free radical generation in the placenta of pre-eclamptic patients is due to upregulation of NADPH oxidase activity, caused by generation of an angiotensin II receptor agonist antibody in some patients.

Paraneoplastic glomerulonephritis

A rare complication of malignancy, paraneoplastic glomerulonephritis is usually misdiagnosed as idiopathic glomerulonephritis. A number of cancers involve the kidney:

- ***Thymoma or Hodgkin's lymphoma***: polarization of the immune response towards a Th2 profile and possibly excessive production of IL-13 leads to the development of minimal change disease, mesangiocapillary glomerulonephritis or membranous nephropathy.
- ***B-cell lymphoma and leukaemia***: these may induce injury through the presence of monoclonal immunoglobulin, cryoglobulin, and possibly hepatitis C virus infection.
- ***Polycythaemia vera, essential thrombocythaemia or primary myelofibrosis***: severe thrombocytosis may induce focal segmental glomerulosclerosis, possibly due to elevated levels of platelet-derived growth factor.
- ***Myelodysplastic syndromes***: autoimmunity causes a variety of glomerulonephritides.
- ***Epithelial carcinoma***: glomerular inflammatory cells and sub-epithelial immune IgG1- and IgG2-containing complexes are usually present and may aid in the diagnosis of paraneoplastic membranous nephropathy.

Further reading

ACCORD Study Group. Long-term effects of intensive glucose lowering on cardiovascular outcomes. *N Engl J Med* 2011; 364:818–828.
Berden AE, Ferrario F, Hagen EC et al. Histopathologic classification of ANCA-associated glomerulonephritis. *J Am Soc Nephrol* 2010; 21:1628–1636.
D'Agali VD, Kaskel FJ, Falk RJ. Focal segmental glomerulosclerosis. *N Engl J Med* 2011; 365:2398–2411.
Deegens JK, Wetzels JF. Glomerular disease: the search goes on: suPAR is not the elusive FSGS factor. *Nat Rev Nephrol* 2014; 10:431–432.
Devuyst O, Knoers NV, Remuzzi G et al. Rare inherited kidney diseases: challenges, opportunities, and perspectives. *Lancet* 2014; 383:1844–1859.
de Zeeuw D. The end of dual therapy with renin-angiotensin-aldosterone system blockade? *N Engl J Med* 2013; 369:1960–1962.
de Zeeuw D, Agarwal R, Amdahl M et al. Selective vitamin D receptor activation with paricalcitol for reduction of albuminuria in patients with type 2 diabetes (VITAL study): a randomised controlled trial. *Lancet* 2010; 376:1543–1551.
Fogo AB. Milk and membranous nephropathy. *N Engl J Med* 2011; 364:2154–2159.
Gale DP, de Jorge EG, Cook HT et al. Identification of a mutation in complement factor H-related protein 5 in patients of Cypriot origin with glomerulonephritis. *Lancet* 2010; 376:794–801.
Ingelfinger J. MYO1E, [illegible] *N Engl J Med* 2011; 365:368–369.
Parving HH, Brenner BM, McMurray JJ et al. Cardiorenal end points in a trial of aliskiren for type 2 diabetes. *N Engl J Med* [illegible].
Pickering MC, D'Agati VD, Nester CM et al. C3 glomerulopathy: consensus report. *Kidney Int* 2013; 84:1079–1089.
Prunotto M, Carnevali ML, Candiano G et al. Autoimmunity in membranous nephropathy targets aldose reductase and SOD2. *J Am Soc Nephrol* 2010; 21:507–519.
Ramos-Casals M, Stone JH, Cid MC et al. The cryoglobulinaemias. *Lancet* 2012; 379: 348–360.
Runco P, Debies H. Pathophysiological advances in membranous nephropathy: time for a shift in patients' care. *Lancet* 2015; 385:1983–1992.
Schwartz N, Goilav B, Putterman C. The pathogenesis, diagnosis and treatment of lupus nephritis. *Curr Opin Rheumatol* 2014; 26:502–509.
Sethi S, Fervenza FC. Membranoproliferative glomerulonephritis. *N Engl J Med* 2012; 366:1119–1131.
Stone JH, Zen Y, Deshpande V. Mechanisms of disease: IgG4-related disease. *N Engl J Med* 2012; 366:539–551.
Tervaert TW, Mooyaart AL, Amann K et al. Pathologic classification of diabetic nephropathy. *J Am Soc Nephrol* 2010; 21:556–563.
Tian SY, Feldman BM, Beyene J et al. Immunosuppressive therapies for the induction treatment of proliferative lupus nephritis: a systematic review and network metaanalysis. *J Rheumatol* 2014; 41:1998–2007.
Zoungas S, Chalmers J, Neal B et al. ADVANCE-ON Collaborative Group. Follow-up of blood-pressure lowering and glucose control in type 2 diabetes. *N Engl J Med* 2014; 371:1392–1406.

KIDNEY INVOLVEMENT IN OTHER DISEASES

Polyarteritis nodosa

Classical polyarteritis nodosa (PAN) is a multisystem disorder (see also p. 701). Aneurysmal dilatation of medium-sized arteries presents as hypertension, polyneuropathy and ischaemic infarction of a number of organs (including skin, gut, heart and brain). Aneurysms may be seen on renal arteriography. The condition is more common in men and in the elderly; typically, patients are ANCA-negative. It may be associated with drug use and hepatitis B infection. This form of polyangiitis is linked with slowly progressive CKD, often accompanied by severe hypertension. Rapidly progressive kidney failure is rare. Treatment with immunosuppression is less effective than it is for microscopic polyangiitis.

Systemic sclerosis (scleroderma)

Systemic sclerosis (scleroderma, SSc; see pp. 695–697) is a chronic, multisystem disease characterized by fibrosis and vasculopathy of the skin and visceral organs. Plasmacytoid dendritic cells appear to produce high plasma levels of CXCL4, which associate with both skin and lung fibrosis, as well as with pulmonary arterial hypertension in patients with SSc.

Some 10% of SSc patients develop scleroderma renal crisis, characterized by accelerated hypertension, rapidly progressive kidney failure and proteinuria. On kidney biopsy, 'onion skinning' in arcuate and interlobular arteries results from vessel intimal proliferation, fibrin thrombi and fibrinoid necrosis. The treatment of choice is ACE inhibitors, which have led to a remarkable improvement in outcomes in scleroderma renal crisis. Death is now rarely due to renal failure, though <30% of patients progress to ESKD.

Haemolytic uraemic syndrome

Haemolytic uraemic syndrome (HUS) is characterized by intravascular haemolysis with red cell fragmentation (microangiopathic haemolysis), thrombocytopenia and AKI due to thrombosis in small arteries and arterioles ***(Fig. 20.25)***. These features are also seen in disseminated intravascular coagulation, but coagulation tests are typically normal in HUS.

Diarrhoea-associated HUS

Diarrhoea-associated HUS (D+ HUS) often follows a febrile illness, particularly gastroenteritis associated with *Escherichia coli*, notably strain O157. This strain of *E. coli* produces verocytotoxin (or shiga toxin), with a pathogenic A unit that inhibits protein synthesis and initiates endothelial damage. B units facilitate entry of the A unit into the endothelial cells by binding to a receptor (Gb3) on the endothelial cell. Toxins are transported to and into endothelial cells from the gut on neutrophils. Most patients with D+ HUS recover renal

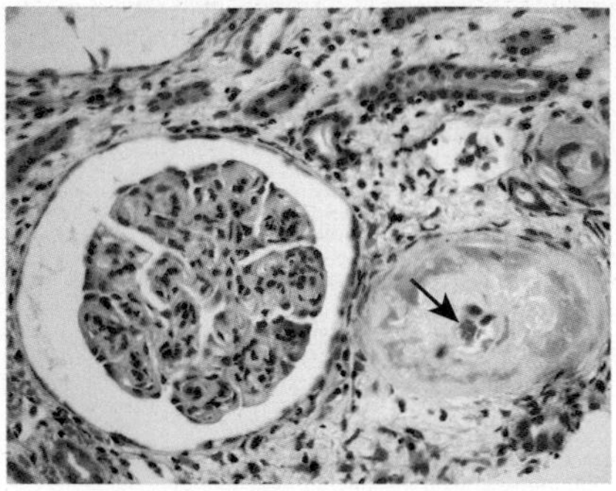

Figure 20.25 Typical haemolytic uraemic syndrome (HUS) renal lesion – light microscopy. Arrow shows microthrombi.

function but supportive care, including fluid and electrolyte balance, antihypertensives, nutritional support and dialysis, is commonly required. Plasmapheresis is not beneficial. About 5% die during the acute episode, 5% develop ESKD and 30% exhibit evidence of long-term damage with persistent proteinuria. Antibiotic and anti-motility agents for diarrhoea increase the risk of HUS and its complications.

In 2011, an outbreak caused by shiga toxin-producing *E. coli* O104:H4 was reported in Germany and other European countries. In this outbreak, HUS occurred far more than might usually be expected, and was associated with significant morbidity and mortality (see p. 276). Severe neurological complications were seen; immunoadsorption was successful in many cases.

Recurrent episodes of HUS have been described in the same individual, and familial forms of the disease (with both recessive and dominant inheritance) exist.

Atypical HUS

Atypical HUS (aHUS) is a complement-driven illness, often related to a deficiency of complement factor H (CFH) or complement factor I (CFI). Factor H is a soluble protein produced by the liver, which regulates the activity of the alternative complement activation pathway; in particular, it protects host cell surfaces from complement-mediated damage. In some families with aHUS, a mutation has been traced to another complement regulatory protein, CD46 (previously known as membrane co-factor protein, MCP). This protein is highly expressed in the kidney and normally prevents glomerular C3 activation. A loss-of-function mutation in CD46 results in unopposed complement activation and development of HUS. Functional deficiency of these factors can be acquired due to autoantibody formation, either as an isolated phenomenon or as part of an autoimmune disease such as SLE. A loss-of-function mutation in thrombomodulin (a membrane-bound anti-coagulant glycoprotein) has been identified as an alternative complement pathway. Rarely, gain-of-function mutations can affect genes encoding the alternative pathway C3 convertase components, CFB and C3. CFB mutations, which lead to chronic alternative pathway activation, occur in only 1–2% of patients with D+ HUS. About 4–10% of patients have heterozygous mutations in C3, usually with low C3 levels. Most mutations reduce C3b binding to CFH and CD46, which severely impairs degradation of mutant C3b.

Management of atypical HUS

Treatment is often difficult, and severe hypertension and recurrence are frequent. The course of the disease is often indolent and progressive.

- Plasmapheresis or plasma infusion is used at initiation of therapy in the majority of patients, often until diagnosis is clear.
- C5 activation is one of the critical steps in the activation of complement cascade. ***Eculizumab***, a monoclonal humanized anti-C5 antibody, has transformed outcomes, both at acute presentation and in prevention of recurrence (in native kidneys and in transplants).
- Liver transplantation is a potentially curative treatment in patients harbouring CFH and CFI mutations.

Sporadic cases of aHUS

These can be associated with pregnancy, SLE, scleroderma, malignant hypertension, metastatic cancer, HIV infection and various drugs, including oral contraceptives, ciclosporin, tacrolimus, chemotherapeutic agents (e.g. cisplatin, mitomycin C, bleomycin) and heparin. Treatment is supportive, with removal of the offending agent or specific treatment of the underlying cause. There is no evidence in favour of plasma infusion or plasmapheresis in these sporadic cases but it is tried, usually as a last resort.

Streptococcus pneumoniae produces an enzyme (possibly neuroaminidase) that can expose an antigen (Thomsen antigen) present on red blood cells, platelets and glomeruli. Antibodies to the Thomsen antigen result in an antigen–antibody reaction and can lead to HUS and anaemia. The improved outcome is due to increasing awareness of this complication, judicious use of blood products (washed blood products) and avoidance of plasma infusion or plasmapheresis.

Metabolism-associated HUS

Cobalamin C disease is a hereditary disorder of vitamin B_{12} metabolism that may cause HUS and multiple organ damage in infants and, rarely, adults. It is caused by mutations in a gene encoding the methylmalonic aciduria and homocystinuria type C protein (*MMACHC*). The resulting deficiency in methylcobalamin causes hyperhomocysteinaemia, decreased plasma methionine levels, and methylmalonic aciduria.

Abnormal cobalamin C metabolism is associated with platelet activation, generation of reactive oxygen species, endothelial dysfunction, increased tissue factor expression, coagulation activation and HUS.

Parenteral hydroxocobalamin is the principal treatment for infants.

Thrombotic thrombocytopenic purpura

Thrombotic thrombocytopenic purpura (TTP; see pp. 570–571) is characterized by microangiopathic haemolysis, renal failure and evidence of neurological disturbance. Young adults are most commonly affected.

Antiphospholipid syndrome

In the antiphospholipid syndrome (APS; see p. 695), the binding of antiphospholipid antibodies (aPL) to beta 2 glycoprotein I (β2GPI) induces endothelial cell–leucocyte adhesion and thrombus formation through the inhibition of endothelial nitric oxide synthase (eNOS).

The central feature of APS is recurrent thrombosis (both venous and arterial) and early pregnancy loss in the presence of antiphospholipid antibodies. Antibodies may be primary or secondary to

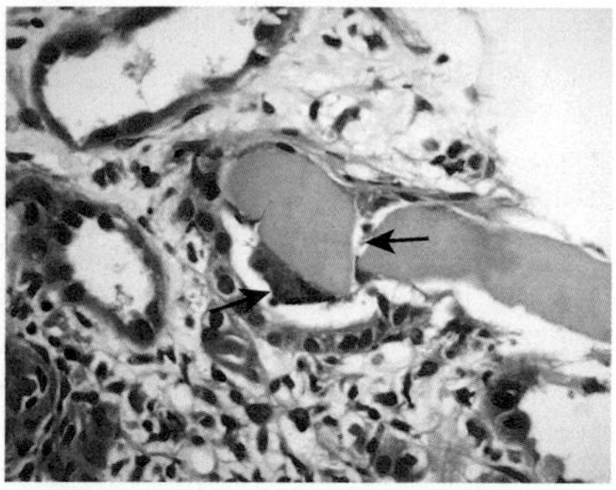

Figure 20.26 Cast nephropathy in a patient with multiple myeloma. Light microscopy showing a characteristic fractured cast and giant cell reaction (arrows).

infections (HIV, hepatitis C) or autoimmune disease (SLE). Some 50% have renal involvement with proteinuria. Thrombotic microangiopathy is a rare but well-recognized presentation. In some cases, a lupus nephritis-like (usually mesangiocapillary GN) lesion is seen. The only proven treatment for APS is systemic anticoagulation. Use of steroids or plasmapheresis is reserved for patients with APS and life-threatening renal involvement with thrombotic microangiopathy. Treatment is variably successful (30–70%).

Multiple myeloma

AKI is relatively common in myeloma, occurring in 20–30% of affected individuals at the time of diagnosis, and is mainly due to the nephrotoxic effects of the abnormal immunoglobulins. It is often irreversible and may present as:

- ***light chain cast nephropathy*** – intratubular deposition of light chains, particularly kappa chains, which characteristically appear on renal histology as fractured casts with a giant cell reaction ***(Fig. 20.26)***
- ***AL amyloidosis*** – deposition of amyloid fibrils of light chains (Congo red-positive)
- ***light chain deposition disease*** – nodular glomerulosclerosis with granular deposits of usually lambda light chains (Congo red-negative)
- ***plasma cell infiltration*** – often an incidental finding at postmortem
- ***Fanconi syndrome*** – tubular toxicity due to light chains
- ***hypercalcaemic nephropathy*** – bone resorption causing hypercalcaemia
- ***hyperuricaemic nephropathy*** – tumour lysis causing tubular crystallization of uric acid
- ***radiocontrast nephropathy*** – interaction between light chains and radiocontrast.

Treatment of the underlying myeloma is key to recovery (see pp. 628–629). If a patient with cast nephropathy and severe AKI remains dialysis-dependent, the prognosis is poor. Commencement of effective bortezomib-based chemotherapy, which decreases light chain production, and a high-cut-off haemodialysis have shown some promise in relapsed myeloma.

Further reading

Kömhoff M, Roofthooft MT, Spronsen F. Syndromes of thrombotic microangiopathy. *N Engl J Med* 2014; 371:1846–1847.

Salvadori M, Bertoni E. Update on hemolytic uremic syndrome: diagnostic and therapeutic recommendations. *World J Nephrol* 2013; 2:56–76.

HYPERTENSION AND THE KIDNEY

Hypertension can be the cause or the result of renal disease. It is often difficult to differentiate between the two on clinical grounds. Routine tests (as described on p. 1046) should be performed on all hypertensive patients, though renal imaging is usually unnecessary.

The ***mechanisms*** responsible for the normal regulation of arterial blood pressure and the development of essential primary hypertension are unclear (see pp. 1046–1049). One basic concept is that the long-term regulation of arterial pressure is closely linked to the ability of the kidneys to excrete sufficient salt to maintain normal sodium balance, extracellular fluid volume and normal blood volume at normotensive arterial pressures. Cross-transplantation experiments suggest that hypertension travels with the kidney, as hypertension develops in the normotensive recipient of a kidney genetically programmed for hypertension. Similarly, patients with ESKD due to hypertension become normotensive after receiving a kidney transplant from normotensive donors, provided the new kidney functions well.

One renal factor contributing to future hypertension is the total number of nephrons per kidney ('nephron dose'). People with hypertension and normal renal function have a significantly reduced number of nephrons in each kidney, and individual nephrons are enlarged as a result of glomerular hyperfiltration (see p. 739). Where hypertension is more common (as it is in black or Hispanic men and women), increased glomerular volume is found (a surrogate marker for reduced nephron number).

Whether reduced nephron number is genetic or environmental in origin is unclear. Changes in the intrauterine environment may lead to poor renal growth (and reduced renal volume suggesting lower nephron number) before birth, low birth weight, and hypertension in adult life.

Excess renal sympathetic activity may also contribute. Strategies to achieve bilateral renal sympathetic denervation were hugely effective in patients with refractory hypertension in uncontrolled studies; to date, this benefit has not been borne out by a recent well-controlled trial.

Essential hypertension

In essential hypertension, arteriosclerosis of major renal arteries and changes in the intrarenal vasculature (nephrosclerosis) occur. Arterial pressure is a product of cardiac output and systemic vascular resistance (SVR). The compliance of systemic arteries is, then, a critical component; 'stiff' (sclerotic) arteries cannot modulate pressure surges in systole, and systolic pressures rise. Over time, vessels (and the kidney) remodel:

- In small vessels and arterioles, intimal thickening with reduplication of the internal elastic lamina occurs and the vessel wall becomes hyalinized.
- In large vessels, concentric reduplication of the internal elastic lamina and endothelial proliferation produce an 'onion skin' appearance.
- Reduction in size of both kidneys occurs; this may be asymmetrical if one major renal artery is more affected than the other.
- The proportion of sclerotic (scarred) glomeruli is increased compared with age-matched controls.

Renal function does deteriorate with these changes but severe CKD is unusual in whites (1 in 10 000). In black Africans, by contrast, hypertension much more often results in the development of CKD, with a fourfold higher incidence of ESKD in blacks compared to whites. This difference in incidence of hypertensive renal disease may be due to overestimation of diagnosis on clinical grounds, a higher incidence of hypertension (usually salt-sensitive), reduced nephron number and a higher frequency of susceptibility alleles for ESKD in the (West) African than the European gene pool.

A genome-wide study found statistically stronger associations between two independent sequence variants in the apolipoprotein L1 gene (*APOL1*) and non-diabetic nephropathy in African–Americans, in hypertension-attributed ESKD. These kidney disease risk variants most likely arose due to the positive selection for evolutionary advantage that these variants in *APOL1* conferred against trypanosomal infection and protection from African sleeping sickness. These observations provide some evidence, similar to findings with sickle cell anaemia, that natural selection might protect from one disease but allow another one to develop.

In accelerated or malignant-phase hypertension:

- Arteriolar fibrinoid necrosis occurs, probably as a result of plasma entering the media of the vessel through splits in the intima. It is prominent in afferent glomerular arterioles.
- Fibrin deposition within small vessels is often associated with thrombocytopenia and red cell fragmentation seen in the peripheral blood film (microangiopathic haemolytic anaemia).

Microscopic haematuria, proteinuria, usually of modest degree (1–3 g daily), and progressive CKD occur. If disease is untreated, fewer than 10% of patients survive 2 years.

Management

The management of benign essential and malignant hypertension is described on page 1048. If treatment is begun before CKD has developed, the prognosis for renal function is good. Stabilization or improvement in renal function, with healing of intrarenal arteriolar lesions and resolution of microangiopathic haemolysis, occurs with effective treatment of malignant-phase hypertension.

Renal hypertension

Hypertension commonly complicates bilateral renal disease such as chronic glomerulonephritis, bilateral reflux nephropathy, polycystic disease and analgesic nephropathy. Two main mechanisms are responsible:

- activation of the renin–angiotensin–aldosterone system
- retention of salt and water as excretory function declines, leading to an increase in blood volume and blood pressure.

As CKD progresses, salt and water overload becomes ever more involved in driving high blood pressure.

Hypertension occurs earlier, is more common and tends to be more severe in patients with glomerular disease (glomerulonephritis) than in those with tubulointerstitial diseases such as reflux or analgesic nephropathy.

Management is described on pages 1047–1048. Meticulous control of the blood pressure may prevent ongoing or new vascular or parenchymal changes, and further deterioration of renal function. There is good evidence that ACE inhibitors offer additional renoprotective benefits for the same degree of blood pressure control than other agents. In a study of African–Americans with hypertension, intensive blood pressure control (130/78 mmHg) was not superior to standard control (141/86 mmHg) in the prevention of ESKD. However, in the same study, patients with proteinuria benefited more from intensive blood pressure control. However, presence of the *APOL1* risk allele was associated with rapid decline of GFR irrespective of achieved blood pressure or baseline proteinuria.

Renovascular disease

Renal ischaemia, or a fall in perfusion pressures in the afferent glomerular arterioles, leads to increased production and release of renin from the juxtaglomerular apparatus (see p. 727). This, in turn, causes a consequent increase in angiotensin II, a potent vasoconstrictor, which also triggers aldosterone secretion, stimulates thirst and leads to vascular smooth muscle hypertrophy and fibrosis in the kidney.

In renal artery stenosis, narrowing of the renal artery or arteries causes a fall in renal perfusion pressure on the distal side of the stenosis; in each affected kidney, angiotensin release occurs, and local salt and water reabsorption is increased. Urine from the ischaemic kidney is more concentrated, with a lower sodium concentration than urine from an unaffected kidney. GFR is decreased on the ischaemic side as well.

Narrowing of the renal arteries (renal artery stenosis) is caused by one of two pathologies: ***atherosclerotic renovascular disease*** or ***fibromuscular dysplasia***.

Atherosclerotic renovascular disease

Atherosclerotic renovascular disease (ARVD) is a common cause of hypertension and CKD due to ischaemic nephropathy. Its incidence increases with age:

- 5% in those under 60 years of age
- 16% in those over 60 years of age.

In most patients, the atherosclerotic lesion is ostial (within 1 cm of the origin of the renal artery) and usually associated with symptomatic atherosclerotic vascular disease elsewhere. Patients with peripheral vascular disease (39%), coronary artery disease (10–29%), congestive cardiac failure (34%) and aortic aneurysm (38%) are at high risk of developing significant renal artery stenosis.

Many patients are asymptomatic and are discovered incidentally during investigation for other conditions. Aortography experience from the USA shows that 11% of asymptomatic patients have significant unilateral stenosis and 4% have bilateral disease. ARVD results in hypertension (present in 50%), sodium retention (ankle and flash pulmonary oedema), proteinuria (usually in the sub-nephrotic range) and decreased GFR. Beyond the stenosis, affected kidneys demonstrate changes histologically, with vascular sclerosis, tubular atrophy, interstitial fibrosis with inflammatory cellular infiltrate, atubular glomeruli, cholesterol emboli and secondary FSGS changes. These changes are often described as 'ischaemic nephropathy'. The affected kidney loses volume (as fibrosis replaces normal tissue), and becomes smaller on ultrasound measurement. These morphological changes are responsible for the associated fall in GFR; the arterial stenosis itself drives hypertension.

Renovascular disease should be considered in:

- patients with hypertension and/or CKD with abdominal or other audible bruits
- patients with renal asymmetry – particularly where ultrasound suggests >1.5 cm difference in length
- recurrent flash pulmonary oedema without cardiopulmonary disease
- progressive CKD in patients with evidence of generalized atherosclerosis.

Management

The ***aim of treatment*** is to prevent decline in renal function and to reverse salt and water overload. Most patients with ARVD will die a cardiovascular death, and modifiable risk factors should be addressed. All patients with ARVD should be managed with a combination of aspirin, statins and optimal control of blood pressure as prophylaxis against progression of atherosclerosis. Hypertension should be controlled, ideally with an ACE inhibitor. This is the paradox of ARVD: angiotensin drives the renal and cardiac events, so ACE inhibition is ideal medical therapy. However, because ACE inhibitors will cause a fall (often significant) in renal perfusion beyond the stenosis, ACE inhibitors can cause AKI in patients with bilateral, haemodynamically significant ARVD.

Renal artery stenosis can also progress to occlusion, particularly in patients with stenosis of >75%, as shown by serial angiography. Revascularization offers definitive treatment of stenotic lesions in ARVD:

- ***Options in renal artery stenosis***. These include transluminal angioplasty to dilate the stenotic region, insertion of stents across the stenosis (sometimes the only endoscopic option when the stenosis occurs close to the origin of the renal artery from the aorta, making angioplasty technically difficult or impossible), reconstructive vascular surgery and nephrectomy.
- ***Indications for revascularization***. Vessels with stenosis of >75% and recurrent flash pulmonary oedema, drug-resistant severe hypertension, ARVD affecting solitary functioning kidney, patients with cardiac failure needing ACE inhibitors, unexplained progressive CKD and dialysis-dependent renal failure.

In a number of recent trials, renal artery stenting did not confer a significant benefit with respect to the prevention of clinical events (cardiovascular events, progressive renal insufficiency or the need for renal replacement therapy) when added to comprehensive, multifactorial medical therapy in people with atherosclerotic renal artery stenosis and hypertension or CKD. Up to 30% of renal artery interventions will be complicated by atheroembolism, which may lead to further functional deterioration.

Prognosis

Mortality is high because of other associated co-morbidities, and ARVD patients have generalized endothelial dysfunction. ARVD patients with ESKD have higher death rates than those with other causes of ESKD. Five-year survival is only 18% in patients with ESKD due to ARVD.

Fibromuscular dysplasia of the renal arteries

Fibromuscular dysplasia (FMD) is often asymptomatic, occurring in younger women with hypertension. It is far less common than ARVD. FMD affects many arterial beds, including the carotid and coronary arteries. Renal function is often normal.

Magnetic resonance angiography (MRA; gadolinium-enhanced) reveals a characteristic string of beads appearance in the mid-renal artery (rather than affecting the ostium, as occurs in ARVD)

Angioplasty (occasionally with stent insertion) or, rarely, surgery was offered to affected individuals. Cure rates were only 36% and 54% after angioplasty and surgery, respectively, in a recent study of over 2000 patients (defining cure as blood pressure <140/90 mmHg without treatment), and the blood pressure outcome was strongly age-related. Procedural complications were common: 12% after angioplasty and 17% after surgery. Current medical antihypertensive therapy is very effective in this group, and angioplasty is now not usually performed.

Screening for renovascular disease

- ***Radionuclide studies*** (see pp. 731–732) can demonstrate decreased renal perfusion on the affected side. In unilateral renal artery stenosis, a disproportionate fall in isotope uptake occurs on the affected side after administration of captopril. A completely normal result makes renovascular disease unlikely.
- ***Doppler ultrasound*** is sensitive but highly operator-dependent and time-consuming. Higher renal artery velocity on Doppler may mean a higher pressure differential across a stenosis. Doppler also describes the intrarenal vascular resistance, which can be valuable in predicting the success of revascularization procedures. A resistive index of >80 is a predictor of poor response following intervention.
- ***MRA*** can be used to visualize the renal arteries and there is a good – though not perfect – correlation between MRA findings and those of renal arteriography.
- ***CT scanning*** permits non-invasive imaging of the renal arteries. It is much less expensive than MRA but does expose the patient to ionizing radiation and to contrast injection, and is less reliable than MRA.
- ***Renal arteriography*** (see p. 731) is used to confirm the diagnosis of renal arterial disease. It also allows therapeutic intervention if needed at diagnosis.

Further reading

Appel LJ, Wright JT Jr, Greene T et al. Intensive blood pressure control in hypertensive chronic kidney disease. *N Engl J Med* 2010; 363:918–929.

Cooper CJ, Murphy TP, Cutlip DE et al and CORAL Investigators. Stenting and medical therapy for atherosclerotic renal-artery stenosis. *N Engl J Med* 2014; 370:13–22.

Genovese G, Friedman DJ, Ross MD et al. Association of trypanolytic ApoL1 variants with kidney disease in African Americans. *Science* 2010; 329:841–845.

Parsa A, Kao WH, Xie D et al and AASK Study Investigators; CRIC Study Investigators. APOL1 risk variants, race, and progression of chronic kidney disease. *N Engl J Med* 2013; 369:2183–2196.

OTHER VASCULAR DISORDERS OF THE KIDNEY

Renal artery occlusion

This occurs from thrombosis *in situ*, usually in a severely damaged atherosclerotic vessel, or more commonly from embolization, such as in atrial fibrillation. Both lead to renal infarction, either of a wedge of kidney or of the whole kidney. Occlusion of a small branch artery may produce no effect, but occlusion of larger vessels results in dull flank pain, macroscopic haematuria and varying degrees of CKD. Intra-arterial thrombolytic therapy has been tried with mixed results.

Cholesterol embolization (atheroembolic renal disease)

Showers of cholesterol-rich atheromatous material from ulcerated plaques reach the kidney from the aorta and/or renal arteries, particularly after catheterization of the abdominal aorta or attempts at renal artery angioplasty. Anticoagulants and thrombolytic agents also precipitate non-traumatic cholesterol embolization. Renal failure from cholesterol emboli may be acute or slowly progressive.

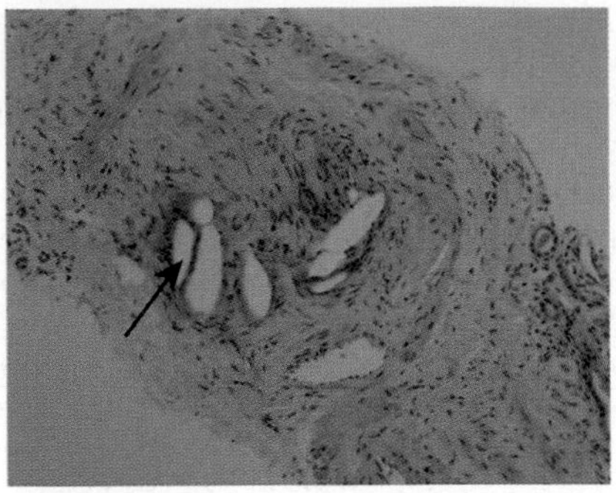

Figure 20.27 Renal cholesterol emboli showing the characteristic cholesterol biconvex clefts.

Clinical features include fever, eosinophilia, back and abdominal pain, and evidence of embolization elsewhere, such as to the retina or digits. The diagnosis can be confirmed by renal biopsy ***(Fig. 20.27)***. It is more common in males, the elderly (>70 years) and patients with cardiovascular disease. Over 80% have abnormal renal function at baseline. Atheroembolic renal disease (AERD) occurs spontaneously in 25% of the cases. The 2-year mortality is 30% and a similar percentage of patients develop CKD. Baseline co-morbidities – that is, reduced renal function, presence of diabetes, history of heart failure, acute/subacute presentation, and gastrointestinal tract involvement – are significant predictors of event occurrence. The risk of dialysis and death is 50% lower among those receiving statins.

Renal vein thrombosis

This is usually of insidious onset, occurring in patients with the nephrotic syndrome, with a renal cell carcinoma, and in thrombophilia (see p. 575) with an increased risk of venous thrombosis. Anticoagulation is indicated.

RENAL CALCULI AND NEPHROCALCINOSIS

Renal and vesical calculi

Nephrolithiasis, or renal stones, usually occurs in the upper urinary tract. It is very common worldwide, with a lifetime risk of about 10%.

Most stones are composed of calcium oxalate and phosphate; these are more common in men ***(Box 20.14)***. Mixed infective stones, which account for about 15% of all calculi, are twice as common in women as in men. The overall male to female ratio of stone disease is 2:1.

Stone disease is frequently recurrent, and more than 50% of patients will experience a second stone within 10 years of their first. The risk of recurrence increases if a metabolic or structural abnormality predisposing to stone formation is present and is not modified by treatment. Nephrolithiasis is not a benign condition; observational studies show an association with an increased risk of ESKD, bone diseases, hypertension and myocardial infarction.

Aetiology

Stones form because solute concentrations exceed saturation, often in the context of a trigger or nidus to crystallize around. Inhibitors of crystal formation prevent stone formation in normal urine, despite the concentrations of stone-forming substances exceeding maximum solubility in water. Factors predisposing to stone formation in these so-called 'idiopathic stone-formers' are:

- ***Chemical composition of urine*** that favours stone crystallization.
- ***A concentrated urine*** resulting from dehydration (particularly in those living or working in a hot climate or environment).
- ***Impairment of inhibitors that prevent crystallization*** in normal urine. These inhibitors include inorganic magnesium, pyrophosphate and citrate. Organic inhibitors include glycosaminoglycans and nephrocalcin (an acidic protein of tubular origin). Tamm–Horsfall protein may have a dual role in both inhibiting and promoting stone formation. Tamm–Horsfall protein usually inhibits crystallization of urinary oxalate but in an undersialylated form promotes stone formation.

Recognized risk factors for stone formation are listed in ***Box 20.15***.

Stones may be single or multiple and vary enormously in size from minute, sand-like particles to staghorn calculi or large stone concretions in the bladder. They may be located within the renal parenchyma or within the collecting system. Stones regularly cause obstruction, leading to hydronephrosis; a combination of obstruction and infection often causes lasting damage to the kidney.

Hypercalcaemia

If the GFR is normal, hypercalcaemia almost invariably leads to hypercalciuria. Common causes of hypercalcaemia leading to stone formation are:

- primary hyperparathyroidism (see p. 1236)
- vitamin D ingestion
- sarcoidosis.

Hypercalciuria

This is by far the most common metabolic abnormality detected in calcium stone-formers. Approximately 8% of men excrete more than 7.5 mmol of calcium per day. Calcium stone formation is more common in this group, although the cutoff is entirely arbitrary. In women, a 24-hour calcium excretion of >6.25 mmol tends to make stone formation more likely.

Box 20.14 Type and frequency of renal stones in the UK

Type of renal stone	Percentage of stones
Calcium oxalate usually with calcium phosphate	65
Calcium phosphate alone	15
Magnesium ammonium phosphate (struvite)	10–15
Uric acid	3–5
Cystine	1–2

Box 20.15 Causes of urinary tract stones

- Dehydration
- Hypercalcaemia
- Hypercalciuria
- Hyperoxaluria
- Hyperuricaemia and hyperuricosuria
- Infection
- Cystinuria
- Primary renal disease (polycystic kidneys, medullary sponge kidneys, renal tubular acidosis)
- Drugs (see text)

About 90% of ionized calcium filtered by the kidney is reabsorbed in the tubule, controlled largely by PTH. Causes of hypercalciuria include:

- hypercalcaemia
- high dietary intake of calcium
- excessive resorption of calcium from the skeleton, such as occurs with prolonged immobilization or weightlessness
- idiopathic hypercalciuria.

Idiopathic hypercalciuria is a common risk factor for the formation of stones, and can be thought of as accelerated calcium transport, with enhanced gut uptake, and increased urine excretion of calcium.

Hyperoxaluria

There are two inborn errors of glyoxylate metabolism that cause increased endogenous oxalate biosynthesis and are inherited in an autosomal recessive manner:

- ***type 1***: alanine–glyoxylate aminotransferase deficiency
- ***type 2***: glyoxylate reductase hydroxypyruvate reductase deficiency.

In both types, calcium oxalate stone formation occurs. The prognosis is poor, as widespread calcium oxalate crystal deposition in the kidneys leads to CKD in the late teens or early twenties. Successful liver transplantation has been shown to cure the metabolic defect.

Much more common causes of mild hyperoxaluria are:

- excess ingestion of foodstuffs high in oxalate, such as spinach, rhubarb and tea
- dietary calcium restriction, with compensatory increased absorption of oxalate
- gastrointestinal disease (e.g. Crohn's), usually with an intestinal resection, associated with increased absorption of oxalate from the colon.

Dehydration secondary to fluid loss from the gut also plays a part in stone formation.

Hyperuricaemia and hyperuricosuria

Uric acid stones account for 3–5% of all stones in the UK, but in Israel the proportion is as high as 40%. Uric acid is the endpoint of purine metabolism. Hyperuricaemia (see pp. 687–689) can occur as a primary defect in idiopathic gout, and as a secondary consequence of increased cell turnover: for example, in myeloproliferative disorders. Increased uric acid excretion occurs in these conditions, and stones will develop in some patients. Some uric acid stone-formers have hyperuricosuria (>4 mmol/24 h on a low-purine diet), without hyperuricaemia.

Dehydration alone may also cause uric acid stones to form. Patients with ileostomies are at particular risk, both from dehydration and from the fact that loss of bicarbonate from gastrointestinal secretions results in the production of an acid urine (uric acid is more soluble in an alkaline medium than in an acid one).

Some patients with calcium stones also have hyperuricaemia and/or hyperuricosuria; it is believed that the calcium salts precipitate on an initial nidus of uric acid in such patients.

Urinary tract infection

Mixed infective stones are composed of magnesium ammonium phosphate together with variable amounts of calcium. Such struvite stones are often large, forming a cast of the collecting system (staghorn calculus). These stones are usually due to urinary tract infection with organisms such as *Proteus mirabilis* that hydrolyse urea, with formation of the strong base ammonium hydroxide. The availability of ammonium ions and the alkalinity of the urine favour stone formation. An increased production of mucoprotein from infection also creates an organic matrix on which stone formation can occur.

Cystinuria

Cystinuria (see also pp. 1286–1287) results in the formation of cystine stones (about 1–2% of all stones).

Primary renal disease

- ***Polycystic renal disease*** (see pp. 789–790) shows a high prevalence of stone disease.
- ***Medullary sponge kidney*** involves dilatation of the collecting ducts that leads to urinary stasis and calcification ***(Fig. 20.28)***. Approximately 20% of these patients have hypercalciuria and a similar proportion have a renal tubular acidification defect.
- ***Renal tubular acidosis***, either inherited and acquired, is associated with nephrocalcinosis and stone formation. Persistently alkaline urine and reduced urinary citrate excretion leads to stone formation, as calcium and citrate form a *soluble* complex in urine.

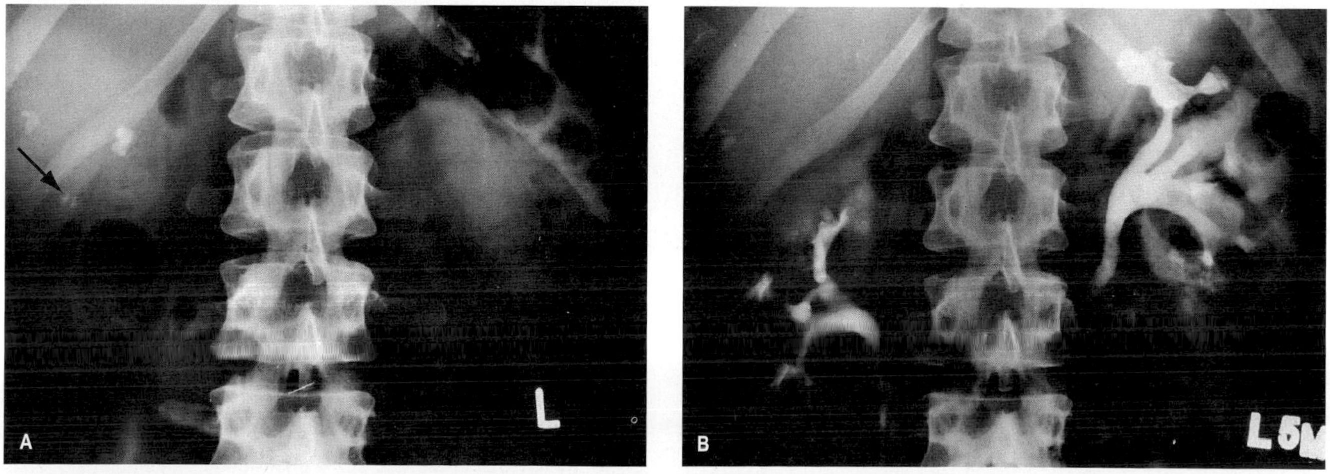

Figure 20.28 Medullary sponge kidney. A. Plain film showing 'spotty' calcification in the renal areas (arrow). **B.** After injection of contrast, the calcification is shown to be small calculi in the papillary zones.

Drugs

Some drugs promote calcium stone formation (e.g. loop diuretics, antacids, glucocorticoids, theophylline, vitamins D and C, acetazolamide); some promote uric acid stones (e.g. thiazides, salicylates); and some precipitate into stones (e.g. indinavir, triamterene, sulfadiazine).

Clinical features

Most people with urinary tract calculi are asymptomatic.

- Pain is the most common symptom and may be sharp or dull, constant, intermittent or colicky ***(Box 20.16)***.
- If the urinary tract is obstructed, fluids or diuretics (including alcohol) make the pain worse as peristaltic flow increases.
- Exertion may cause mobile calculi to move, precipitating pain and, occasionally, haematuria.
- Ureteric colic occurs when a stone enters the ureter and either obstructs it or causes spasm during its passage down the ureter. Classically, pain radiates from the flank to the iliac fossa, testis or labia (in the distribution of the first lumbar nerve root). Pallor, sweating and vomiting often occur and the patient is restless, trying to obtain relief from the pain. Haematuria often occurs. Untreated, the pain of ureteric colic typically subsides after a few hours.

When urinary tract obstruction and infection are present, the features of acute pyelonephritis or of a Gram-negative septicaemia may dominate the clinical picture.

Calcified papillae may mimic ordinary calculi, so that causes of papillary necrosis such as analgesic abuse should be considered (see p. 768).

Bladder stones

Bladder stones ***(Box 20.17)*** are usually associated with bacteriuria and present with frequency, dysuria and haematuria; severe introital or perineal pain may occur if trigonitis is present.

A calculus at the bladder neck or an obstruction in the urethra may cause bladder outflow obstruction, resulting in anuria and painful bladder distension.

Investigations

- ***Dipsticks*** for red cells, protein, glucose
- ***Chemical analysis*** should be employed for passed stones.
- ***A mid-stream specimen of urine*** should be taken for microscopy (crystals) and culture.
- ***Serum urea, electrolyte, creatinine (eGFR) and calcium levels.***
- ***Ultrasonography*** shows kidney stones and renal pelvis dilatation well but ureteric stones can be missed.
- ***Computed tomography of kidneys, ureters and bladder (CT-KUB)*** is the best diagnostic test available with a sensitivity of >95%. It involves radiation and in young patients many physicians perform ultrasonographs as the first investigation.

A normal CT excludes the diagnosis of pain due to calculous disease. The CT-KUB appearances in a patient with acute left ureteric obstruction are shown in ***Figure 20.29***.

Pure uric acid stones are radiolucent and show as a filling defect after injection of contrast medium if excretion urography is performed. Uric acid stones are readily seen on CT scanning ***(Fig. 20.30)***. Mixed infective stones in which organic matrix predominates are barely radio-opaque.

Management

Renal colic is painful. Analgesia with an NSAID, such as diclofenac 75 mg i.m. compares favourably with opiates such as diamorphine or pethidine. Stones of <0.5 cm diameter usually pass spontaneously, particularly if hydration is maintained (patients that can drink should aim for >2.5 L intake). Alpha-blockers (e.g. tamsulosin)

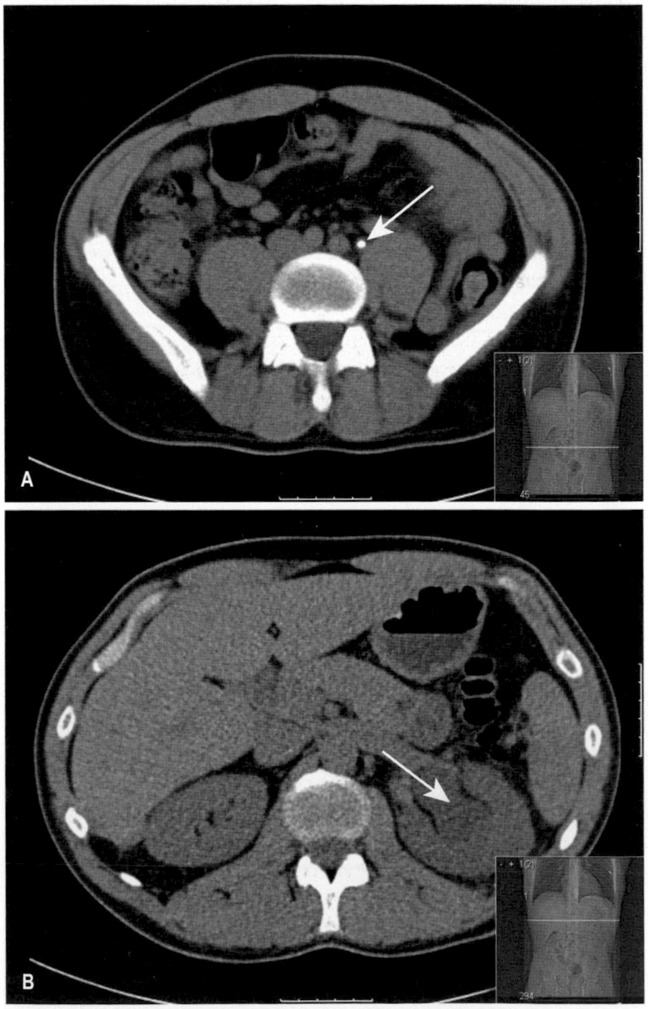

Figure 20.29 Computed tomography of kidneys, ureters and bladder (CT-KUB) in ureteric stone obstruction. A. Left ureteric calculus (arrow). **B.** A dilated renal pelvis (arrow) proximal to the ureteric stone in **A.**

Box 20.16 Clinical features of urinary tract stones

- Asymptomatic
- Pain: renal colic
- Haematuria
- Urinary tract infection
- Urinary tract obstruction

Box 20.17 Bladder stones

Occur where stasis, infection and a nidus for stone formation come together:

- Bladder outflow obstruction (e.g. urethral stricture, neuropathic bladder, prostatic obstruction)
- Presence of a foreign body (e.g. catheters, non-absorbable sutures)

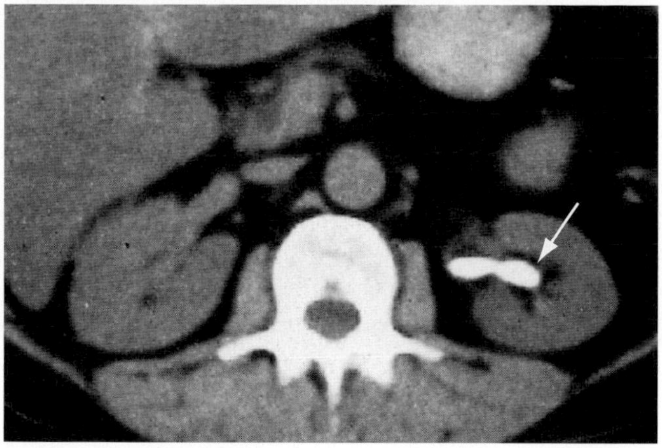

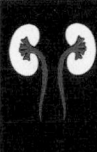

Figure 20.30 CT scan showing a uric acid stone. The stone appears as a bright lesion in the left kidney (arrow).

were thought to help expulsion of distal ureteral stones of <6 mm size (alpha receptors are predominantly present in the distal ureter and detrusor) but a recent RCT has shown no benefit.

Stones of >1 cm diameter usually need urological or radiological intervention. Extracorporeal shock-wave lithotripsy (ESWL) will fragment most stones, which then pass spontaneously. Ureteroscopy with a YAG laser can be used for larger stones. Percutaneous nephrolithotomy is also used. Open surgery is rarely needed.

Investigation of the cause of stone formation

In an elderly patient who has had a single episode with one stone, only limited investigation is required. Younger patients and those with recurrent stone formation need detailed investigation.

- ***Renal imaging*** excludes structural abnormalities of the urinary tract.
- ***Urine culture*** excludes significant bacteriuria.
- ***Chemical analysis*** is performed on any stone passed (required in the diagnosis of cystinuria or uric acid stone formation).
- ***Serum calcium*** is investigated if hypercalcaemia is present (see p. 754).
- ***Serum urate concentration*** is often, but not invariably, elevated in uric acid stone-formers.
- ***A screening test for cystinuria*** should be carried out by adding sodium nitroprusside to a random unacidified urine sample; a purple colour indicates that cystinuria may be present. Urine chromatography is required to define the diagnosis precisely.
- ***Urinary calcium, oxalate and uric acid output*** should be measured in two consecutive, carefully collected 24-h urine samples. After aliquots are withdrawn for estimation of uric acid, the urine is acidified to prevent crystallization of calcium salts on the walls of the container, which would give falsely low results for urinary calcium and oxalate.
- ***Plasma bicarbonate*** is low in renal tubular acidosis. The finding of a urine pH that does not fall below 5.5 in the face of metabolic acidosis is diagnostic of this condition (see pp. 177–178).

Prevention of recurrent stones

- In all idiopathic stone-formers, where no metabolic abnormality is present, maintain a high intake of fluid throughout the day and night to ensure a daily urine volume of 2–2.5 L. This reduces saturation of solute.
- With idiopathic hypercalciuria, dietary calcium restriction is inappropriate, as restriction results in hyperabsorption of oxalate. Foods rich in oxalate should be avoided (nuts, spinach, chocolate, rhubarb). Patients who live in a hard-water area may benefit from drinking softened water.
- Salt intake should be limited to 50 mmol/day (calcium excretion increases by 0.6 mmol/day for every 100 mmol Na^+ in the urine).
- If hypercalciuria stone formation persists, a thiazide diuretic (e.g. bendroflumethiazide 2.5 or 5 mg each morning) reduces urinary calcium excretion. This indirect effect is due to mild volume contraction resulting in increased calcium absorption in the proximal renal tubule.
- Reduction of animal proteins to 50 g/day is also advisable.
- Where mixed infective stones recur, long-term, low-dose prophylactic antibiotics may prevent bacteriuria.
- Uric acid stones can be prevented by the long-term use of allopurinol to maintain the serum urate and urinary uric acid excretion in the normal range. Uric acid is more soluble at alkaline pH, and long-term sodium bicarbonate supplementation to maintain an alkaline urine is an alternative approach in those few patients unable to take allopurinol (see p. 769). However, alkalinization of the urine facilitates precipitation of calcium oxalate and phosphate.

Cystine stones can be prevented and indeed will dissolve slowly with a high fluid intake. To achieve this, up to 5 L of water is drunk in each 24 hours. Patients need to wake twice during the night to drink 500 mL or more of water. Understandably, many patients cannot tolerate this regimen. Alkalinization to a pH of 7 requires high doses of potassium citrate or bicarbonate. An alternative option is the long-term use of the chelating agent penicillamine; this causes cystine to be converted to the more soluble penicillamine–cysteine complex. Side-effects include drug rashes, blood dyscrasias and immune complex-mediated glomerulonephritis. However, it is especially effective in promoting dissolution of cystine stones already present. Other cystine-binding drugs include captopril and tiopronin.

Monogenic hyperoxaluria can be managed with oral high-dose pyridoxine if type 1 (though no response will occur with type 2). Unfortunately, there is currently no proven pharmacotherapy for effective treatment of the more common form of 'idiopathic' hyperoxaluria present in up to 40% of stone-formers. Probiotic *Oxalobacter formigenes* has shown some promise.

Nephrocalcinosis

The term 'nephrocalcinosis' means diffuse renal parenchymal calcification that is detectable radiologically ***(Fig. 20.31)***. The condition is typically painless. Hypertension and CKD commonly occur. The main causes of nephrocalcinosis are listed in ***Box 20.18***.

Dystrophic calcification occurs following renal cortical necrosis. In ***hypercalcaemia and hyperoxaluria***, deposition of calcium oxalate results from the high concentration of calcium and oxalate within the kidney.

In ***renal tubular acidosis*** (see pp. 177–178), failure of urinary acidification and a reduction in urinary citrate excretion both favour calcium phosphate and oxalate precipitation, since precipitation occurs more readily in an alkaline medium and the calcium-chelating action of urinary citrate is reduced.

Management and prevention of nephrocalcinosis consist of treating the cause.

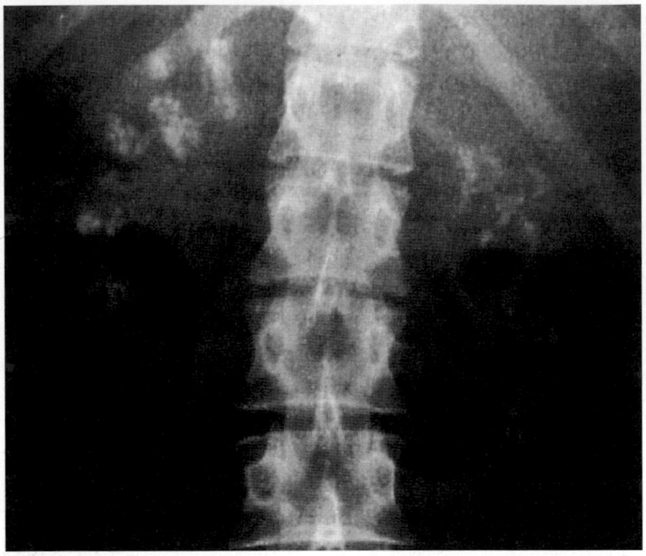

Figure 20.31 X-ray showing nephrocalcinosis.

Box 20.18 Causes of nephrocalcinosis

Mainly cortical (rare)
- Renal cortical necrosis (tramline calcification)

Mainly medullary
- Hypercalcaemia (primary hyperparathyroidism, hypervitaminosis D, sarcoidosis)
- Renal tubular acidosis (inherited and acquired)
- Primary hyperoxaluria
- Medullary sponge kidney
- Tuberculosis

Further reading

Moe OW, Pearle MS, Sakhaee K. Pharmacotherapy of urolithiasis: evidence from clinical trials. *Kidney Int* 2011; 79:385–392.
Pickard R, Starr K, MacLennan G et al. Medical expulsive therapy in adults with ureteric colic: a multicentre, randomised, placebo-controlled trial. *Lancet* 2015; 386:341–349.
Worcester EM, Coe FL. Calcium kidney stones. *N Engl J Med* 2010; 363:954–963.

URINARY TRACT OBSTRUCTION

Urinary tract obstruction can occur at any point between the kidney and the urethral meatus. Obstruction can be partial or complete, and leads to delayed transit of urine, rising urinary tract (and intra-renal) pressure, and – if obstructing both kidneys – eventual renal impairment.

Aetiology

Obstructing lesions may lie within the lumen, or in the wall of the urinary tract, or outside the wall, causing obstruction by external pressure. Obstruction causing dilatation of the renal pelvis and/or ureter is known as hydronephrosis. The major causes of obstruction are shown in ***Box 20.19***. In children, obstruction usually results from congenital abnormalities or urethral valves. In young women, pelvic tumours, pregnancy or stones cause obstruction. In younger men, stones are the dominant cause, but bladder outflow obstruction (prostatic disease) dominates later in life.

Box 20.19 Causes of urinary tract obstruction

Within the lumen
- Calculus
- Blood clot
- Sloughed papilla (diabetes; analgesia misuse; sickle cell disease or trait)
- Tumour of renal pelvis, ureter or bladder

Within the wall
- Pelviureteric neuromuscular dysfunction (congenital, 10% bilateral)
- Ureteric stricture (tuberculosis, especially after treatment; calculus; after surgery)
- Ureterovesical stricture (congenital; ureterocele; calculus; schistosomiasis)
- Congenital megaureter
- Congenital bladder neck obstruction
- Neuropathic bladder
- Urethral stricture (calculus; gonococcal; after instrumentation)
- Congenital urethral valve
- Pin-hole meatus

Pressure from outside
- Pelviureteric compression (bands; aberrant vessels)
- Tumours (e.g. retroperitoneal tumour or glands; carcinoma of colon; tumours in pelvis, e.g. carcinoma of cervix)
- Diverticulitis
- Aortic aneurysm
- Retroperitoneal fibrosis (peri-aortitis)
- Accidental ligation of ureter
- Retrocaval ureter (right-sided obstruction)
- Prostatic obstruction
- Phimosis

Pathophysiology

Urine continues to be formed despite obstruction to flow. This leads to:

- progressive rise in intraluminal pressure
- dilatation proximal to the site of obstruction
- compression and thinning of the renal parenchyma, eventually reducing it to a thin rim and resulting in a decrease in the size of the kidney.

Acute obstruction is followed by transient renal arterial vasodilatation succeeded by vasoconstriction, probably mediated mainly by angiotensin II and thromboxane A_2. Ischaemic interstitial damage mediated by free oxygen radicals and inflammatory cytokines compounds the damage induced by compression of the renal substance.

Clinical features

Symptoms

Loin pain occurs, which can be dull or sharp, and constant or intermittent. Pain is made worse if urine flow and volume increase, as the collecting system distends. A high fluid intake or diuretics, including alcohol and coffee, may provoke pain.

Complete anuria is strongly suggestive of complete bilateral obstruction or complete obstruction of a single kidney.

Polyuria may occur in partial obstruction, as rising pressures impair renal tubular concentrating capacity; intermittent anuria and polyuria indicate intermittent complete obstruction.

Infection is a major complication, and may give rise to malaise, fever and septicaemia.

Bladder outflow obstruction may occur with few symptoms. Hesitancy, narrowing and diminished force of the urinary stream, terminal dribbling (lower urinary tract symptoms, or LUTS) and a sense of incomplete bladder emptying are typical features (see p. 792). Infection is common (and may precipitate acute retention) with frequency, urgency, urge incontinence, dysuria and the passage of cloudy, smelly urine. Acute bladder retention causes significant discomfort and distress, though in the elderly may present as confusion and agitation alone.

Signs

On abdominal palpation, loin tenderness may be present, and occasionally an enlarged hydronephrotic kidney is palpable. In acute or chronic retention, the enlarged bladder can be felt or percussed. Examination of the genitalia, rectum and vagina is performed, since prostatic obstruction and pelvic malignancy are common causes of urinary tract obstruction. However, the apparent size of the prostate on digital examination is a poor guide to the presence of prostatic obstruction.

Investigations

- ***Urinalysis*** is performed for haematuria.
- ***A mid-stream sample of urine for MC&S*** to exclude infection.
- ***Routine biochemical investigations*** may show a raised serum urea or creatinine (or a reduced eGFR), hyperkalaemia, or anaemia of chronic disease. Prostate-specific antigen may be abnormal (see p. 592).
- ***Ultrasonography*** (see pp. 730–731) is the investigation of choice to confirm or rule out upper urinary tract dilatation. Ultrasound cannot distinguish a baggy, low-pressure, unobstructed system from a tense, high-pressure, obstructed one, so that false-positive scans are seen. Stones in the ureter can be missed.
- ***Plain abdominal X-ray*** may detect radiolucent stones/ calcification but can miss stones lying over the bone.
- ***CT scanning*** has a high sensitivity and can visualize uric acid (radiolucent) stones as small as 1 mm, as well as details of the obstruction. CT also allows detection of local mass lesions or lymphadenopathy.
- ***Excretion urography*** is now seldom used. A characteristic delayed nephrogram is seen on the obstructed side (owing to a reduction in the GFR). With time, the nephrogram on the affected side becomes denser than normal, owing to the prolonged nephron transit time, and the site of obstruction with proximal dilatation is seen ***(Fig. 20.32)***.
- ***Radionuclide studies*** (see pp. 731–732) have a role in longstanding obstruction to differentiate true obstructive nephropathy from retention of tracer in a baggy, low-pressure, unobstructed pelvicalyceal system.
- ***Antegrade pyelography and ureterography*** (see p. 731) define the site and cause of obstruction. This technique can be combined with drainage of the collecting system by percutaneous needle nephrostomy.
- ***Retrograde ureterography*** (see p. 731) offers the option of relieving ureteric obstruction from below at the time of examination. In obstruction due to neuromuscular dysfunction at the pelviureteric junction or retroperitoneal fibrosis, the collecting system may fill normally from below.
- ***Cystoscopy, urethroscopy and urethrography*** can visualize obstructing lesions within the bladder and urethra directly. Urethrography involves introducing contrast medium into the bladder by catheterization or suprapubic bladder puncture, and taking X-ray films during voiding to show obstructing lesions in the urethra. It is of particular value in the diagnosis of urethral valves and strictures.

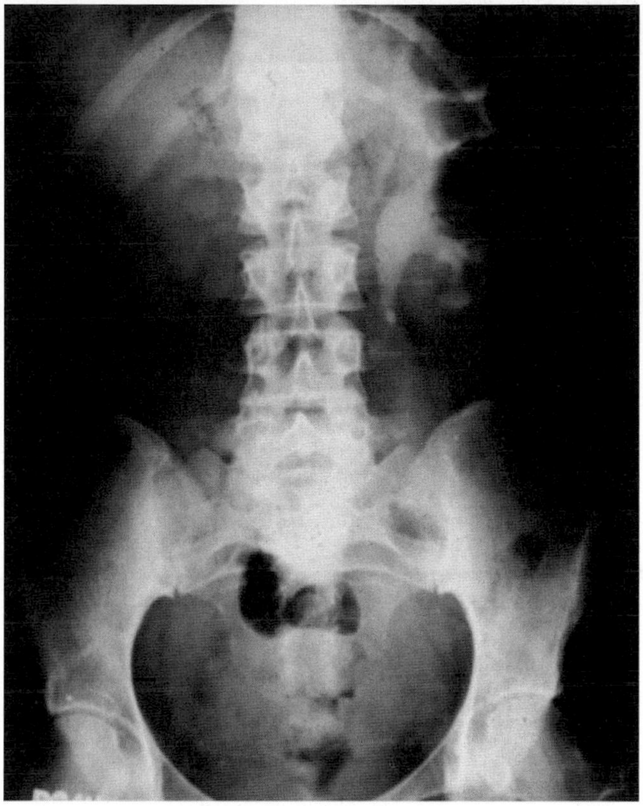

Figure 20.32 Intravenous urographic X-ray taken 24 hours after injection of contrast. A delayed nephrogram and pyelogram are shown on the left side, with dilatation of the system to the level of the block. By this time, contrast medium has disappeared from the normal right side.

Management

Treatment aims to:

- relieve the obstruction
- treat the underlying cause
- prevent and treat infection
- preserve renal function.

An obstructed and infected urinary tract is a medical emergency; delay can lead to septicaemia.

- Bladder catheterization offers rapid relief of outflow tract obstruction. If a urinary catheter cannot be passed urethrally, a suprapubic catheter should be placed.
- Obstructed and hydronephrotic kidneys can be relieved by placing a percutaneous nephrostomy under ultrasound guidance.
- It is also possible to relieve obstructed ureters by cystoscopic (retrograde) stenting.

In contrast, with partial urinary tract obstruction, particularly if spontaneous relief is expected – such as by passage of a calculus there is no immediate urgency. ***Surgical management*** depends on the cause of the obstruction (see below) and local expertise. Dialysis may be required in the ill patient prior to surgery.

Post-obstructive diuresis

This occurs after the relief of obstruction at any site in the urinary tract. Massive diuresis may occur following relief of bilateral obstruction, as prior sodium and water retention, the osmotic effect of retained solutes and defective renal tubular reabsorptive capacity correct. This diuresis is associated with increased blood volume and high levels of atrial natriuretic peptide (ANP). The diuresis is usually self-limiting, but a minority of patients develop severe sodium, water and potassium depletion needing intravenous replacement. In milder cases, oral salt and potassium supplements, together with a high water intake, are sufficient.

Specific causes of obstruction

Calculi

These are discussed on pages 754–757.

Pelviureteric junction obstruction

A functional disturbance in peristalsis of the collecting system, without any mechanical obstruction, causes pelvic hydronephrosis ***(Fig. 20.33)***. In patients with recurrent loin pain or progressive kidney damage, surgical correction by open or percutaneous pyeloplasty is indicated. If longstanding obstruction has destroyed kidney function, nephrectomy prevents future pyonephrosis.

Obstructive megaureter

This childhood condition may become evident only in adult life. It results from the presence of a region of defective peristalsis at the lower end of the ureter adjacent to the ureterovesical junction. The condition is more common in males. It presents with urinary tract infection, flank pain or haematuria. The diagnosis is made on imaging with ultrasound, CT or, if necessary, ascending ureterography.

Excision of the abnormal portion of ureter with re-implantation into the bladder is always indicated in children and in adults when the condition is associated with evidence of progressive deterioration in renal function, bacteriuria that cannot be controlled by medical means, or recurrent stone formation.

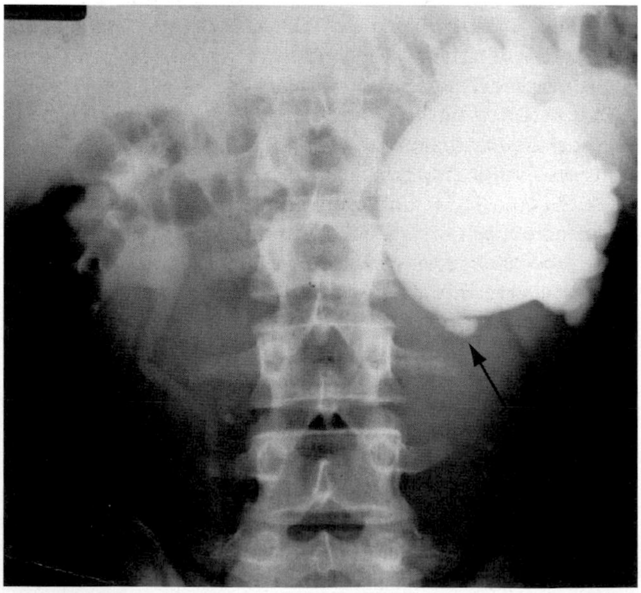

Figure 20.33 X-ray showing left pelviureteric junction obstruction (arrow).

Retroperitoneal fibrosis (chronic peri-aortitis)

Retroperitoneal fibrosis (RPF) is a descriptive term used when inflammatory fibrotic tissue encases the aorta and ureters; it has a number of underlying causes. RPF is three times more common in men than in women, and is an IgG4-related disease (see p. 145).

Extraluminal ureteric obstruction leads to unilateral or bilateral obstruction. The condition may extend from the level of the second lumbar vertebra to the pelvic brim. In up to 15% of patients, the fibrotic process can extend outside the retroperitoneum, consistent with it being a systemic condition. Mediastinal fibrosis, Riedel fibrosing thyroiditis, sclerosing cholangitis, fibrotic orbital pseudotumour, fibrotic arthropathy, and pleural, pericardial and lung fibrosis have been reported with increasing frequency.

RPF is thought to be either an autoallergic response to leakage of material, probably ceroid, from atheromatous plaques, producing an inflammatory reaction, or a systemic autoimmune disease. There is an association with HLA-DRB1*03, an allele linked to various autoimmune diseases. RPF is possibly initiated as a vasa vasorum vasculitis in the aortic wall, which is often seen in chronic peri-aortitis. This inflammatory process can cause medial wall thinning and promote atherosclerosis, and also extends into the surrounding retroperitoneum with a fibro-inflammatory reaction typical of chronic peri-aortitis. The autoimmune reaction to plaque antigens could be an epiphenomenon of this immune-mediated process. Activating antibodies against fibroblasts (detectable in one-third of patients) have also been implicated in the pathogenesis, as has the presence of ***IgG4-bearing plasma cells***; the latter is a common finding in autoimmune chronic pancreatitis, a disorder sometimes associated with idiopathic retroperitoneal fibrosis. In addition, several infiltrating B cells show clonal or oligoclonal immunoglobulin heavy chain rearrangement. These findings raise the possibility of RPF being a primary B-cell disorder.

Aetiology of RPF

Causes are many:

- ***Idiopathic*** (in 60–70%).
- ***Secondary*** causes include:
  - drugs (methysergide, lysergic acid, ergot-derived dopamine receptor agonists (cabergoline, bromocriptine, pergolide), ergotamine, methyldopa, hydralazine, beta-blockers)
  - malignancy (carcinomas of the colon, prostate, breast, stomach, carcinoid, Hodgkin's and non-Hodgkin's lymphomas, sarcomas)
  - infection (tuberculosis, syphilis, histoplasmosis, actinomycosis, fungal infections)
  - surgery/radiotherapy (lymph node resection, colectomy, hysterectomy, aortic aneurysm repair).

Recognized associations include untreated abdominal aortic aneurysm, smoking and asbestosis.

Clinical features and investigation of RPF

RPF may present with malaise, low back pain, weight loss, testicular pain, claudication and haematuria.

Laboratory tests show normochromic anaemia, CKD, a raised erythrocyte sedimentation rate (ESR) and C-reactive protein (CRP), and increased serum IgG4 levels. ***Imaging*** with ultrasound will show a poorly circumscribed peri-aortic mass. The test of choice is contrast-enhanced CT, which will show the mass, lymph nodes and tumour ***(Fig. 20.34)***. MRI will show similar findings but does not require contrast. Fluorodeoxyglucose-PET (FDG-PET), a functional

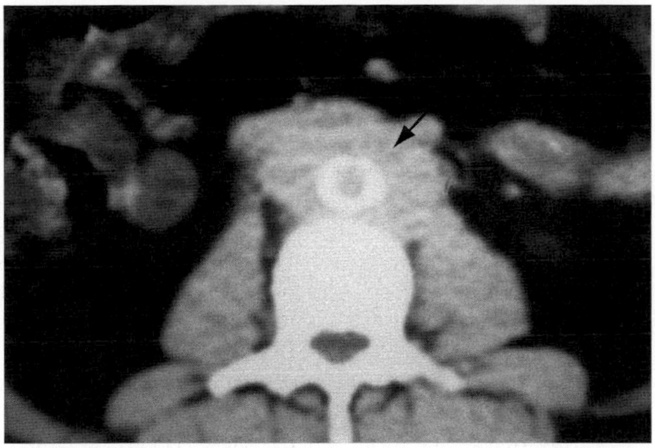

Figure 20.34 Retroperitoneal fibrosis (peri-aortitis). Note the large mass surrounding the abdominal aorta on this CT scan (arrow).

imaging modality, assesses the metabolic activity of the retroperitoneal mass. FDG-PET also allows whole-body imaging and can detect occult malignant or infectious foci, particularly in secondary retroperitoneal fibrosis.

Management of RPF

A biopsy is performed to exclude an underlying infection, lymphoma or carcinoma. Initial management may involve decompressing obstructed ureters by stenting (anterograde or retrograde). Corticosteroids may reverse the obstructing inflammatory tissue, if only as a holding measure before definitive treatment of the underlying cause. Response to treatment and disease activity are assessed by serial measurements of ESR and eGFR, and repeat FDG-PET scans can also monitor disease.

Obstruction is relieved surgically by ureterolysis. A long-term ureteric stent or stents can be used with chronic corticosteroid therapy, but regular (usually 6-monthly) changes of the stent(s) are required if the peri-aortic mass does not regress.

Relapse after withdrawal of steroid therapy may occur and treatment may need to be continued for years. Mycophenolate or tamoxifen is also effective. Long-term follow-up is mandatory.

Benign prostatic hypertrophy

Benign prostatic hypertrophy is a common cause of urinary tract obstruction. It is described on page 792.

Prognosis of urinary tract obstruction

The prognosis depends on the cause and the stage at which obstruction is relieved. Four factors influence the rate at which kidney damage occurs, its extent, and the degree and rapidity of recovery of renal function after relief of obstruction:

- whether obstruction is partial or complete
- the duration of obstruction
- the presence or absence of infection
- the site of obstruction.

Complete obstruction for several weeks will lead to irreversible or only partially reversible kidney damage. If complete obstruction lasts several months, irreversible destruction of the affected kidney occurs. Partial obstruction carries a better prognosis, depending on its severity. Bacterial infection with obstruction rapidly increases kidney damage. Obstruction at or below the bladder neck leads to hypertrophy and trabeculation of the bladder without a rise in pressure within the upper urinary tract, in which case the kidneys are protected from the effects of back-pressure.

Box 20.20 Non-steroidal anti-inflammatory drugs and the kidney

Problem	Cause
Sodium and water retention	Reduction of prostaglandin production
Acute tubulointerstitial nephritis	Hypersensitivity reaction
Nephrotic syndrome	Membranous glomerulopathy
Analgesic nephropathy	Papillary necrosis after chronic use
Acute kidney injury	Acute tubular necrosis
Hyperkalaemia	Decreased renal excretion of K^+

Further reading

Stone JH, Zen Y, Deshpande V. IgG4-related disease. *N Engl J Med* 2012; 366:539–551.

Yaqoob M, Junaid I. Urinary tract obstruction. In: Warrell DA, Cox TM, Firth JD (eds). *Oxford Textbook of Medicine*, 5th edn. Oxford: Oxford University Press; 2010.

DRUGS AND THE KIDNEY

The kidney eliminates many drugs, as well as the (often active) products of drug metabolism in the liver. Dosing requires some thought with CKD, particularly in the elderly. Many drugs can further impair renal function, either over time, or acutely if hypovolaemia occurs (with vomiting or diarrhoea, for example), where a prescribed drug (such as an ACE inhibitor) prevents an appropriate response.

Drug-induced impairment of renal function

Renal perfusion falls with drugs that cause:

- hypovolaemia, e.g.:
  - loop diuretics such as furosemide, especially in elderly patients
  - renal salt and water loss, such as from hypercalcaemia induced by vitamin D therapy (since hypercalcaemia adversely affects renal tubular salt and water conservation)
- decrease in cardiac output, which impairs renal perfusion (e.g. beta-blockers)
- decrease in renal blood flow (e.g. ACE inhibitors, particularly in the presence of renovascular disease).

Drugs may directly damage the kidney:

- ***Acute tubular necrosis produced by direct nephrotoxicity*** from prolonged or high-dose treatment with aminoglycosides (e.g. gentamicin, amikacin), amphotericin B, tenofovir, cisplatin or calcineurin inhibitors. The combination of aminoglycosides with furosemide is particularly nephrotoxic.
- ***Crystal nephropathies*** caused by antivirals such as aciclovir and indinavir.
- ***Acute tubulointerstitial nephritis*** (see pp. 767–768), a cell-mediated hypersensitivity nephritis occurring with many drugs, including penicillins, cephalosporins, proton pump inhibitors, diuretics, sulphonamides and NSAIDs (which have many other effects on the kidney; ***Box 20.20***).
- ***Chronic tubulointerstitial nephritis*** due to drugs (see pp. 768–769).
- ***Membranous glomerulonephritis***, e.g. penicillamine, gold, anti-TNF (see pp. 737–738).

- ***Retroperitoneal fibrosis with urinary tract obstruction*** – can result from the use of drugs (see pp. 760–761).

Using drugs in patients with impaired renal function

See ***Box 20.21***.

Absorption

Absorption can be unpredictable in uraemia, as gastric emptying may be delayed, and nausea and vomiting are frequent.

Metabolism

The rate of drug metabolism by the kidney is reduced as a result of:

- ***Reduced drug catabolism***. Insulin, for example, is in part catabolized by the normal kidney. In renal disease, insulin catabolism is reduced. The insulin requirements of diabetics decline as renal function deteriorates, for this reason.
- ***Reduced conversion of a precursor to a more active metabolite***. An example is the conversion of 25-hydroxycholecalciferol to the more active 1,25-$(OH)_2D_3$. The 1α-hydroxylase enzyme responsible for this conversion is located in the kidney. In renal disease, production of the enzyme declines and deficiency of 1,25-$(OH)_2D_3$ results.

Box 20.21 Safe prescribing in kidney disease

Safe prescribing in CKD demands knowledge of the clinical pharmacology of the drug and its metabolites in normal individuals and in uraemia. The clinician should ask the following questions when prescribing, and discuss them with the patient:

1. ***Is treatment mandatory?*** Unless it is, it should be withheld.
2. ***Can the drug reach its site of action?*** For example, there is little point in prescribing the urinary antiseptic, nitrofurantoin, in severe CKD since bacteriostatic concentrations will not be attained in the urine.
3. ***Is the drug's metabolism altered in uraemia?***
4. ***Will accumulation of the drug or metabolites occur?*** Even if accumulation is a potential problem, owing to the drug or its metabolites being excreted by the kidneys, it is not necessarily an indication to change the drug given. The size of the loading dose will depend on the size of the patient and is unrelated to renal function. Avoidance of toxic levels of drug in blood and tissues subsequently requires the administration of normal doses of the drug at longer time intervals than usual, or in smaller doses at the usual time intervals.
5. ***Is the drug toxic to the kidney?***
6. ***Are the effective concentrations*** of the drug in biological tissues similar to the toxic concentrations? Should blood levels of the drug be measured?
7. ***Will the drug worsen the uraemic state*** by means other than nephrotoxicity, e.g. steroids, tetracycline?
8. ***Is the drug a sodium or potassium salt?*** These are potentially hazardous in uraemia.

Not surprisingly, adverse drug reactions are more than twice as common in patients with CKD as in normal individuals. Elderly patients, in whom unsuspected CKD is common, are particularly at risk. Attention to the above and titration of the dose of drugs employed should reduce the problem.

The dose may be titrated by:

- observation of its clinical effect, e.g. hypotensive agents
- early detection of toxic effects
- measurement of drug levels in the blood, e.g. gentamicin levels.

Protein binding

Reduced protein binding of a drug potentiates its activity and increases the potential for toxic side-effects. Hypoalbuminaemia (in the nephrotic syndrome) leads to increased free drug, as does uraemic toxins binding to albumin (occupying drug-binding sites). Measuring total plasma concentration (albumin-bound and free drug) of such drugs can give misleading results. For example, more free phenytoin than albumin-bound phenytoin is present in CKD, for the same total plasma concentration seen in healthy individuals – and lower levels will control seizures in patients with CKD.

Volume of distribution

Salt and water overload or depletion may occur in patients with renal disease. This affects the concentration of drug obtained from a given dose.

End-organ sensitivity

The renal response to drug treatment may be reduced in renal disease. For example, mild thiazide diuretics have little diuretic effect in patients with severe CKD.

Renal elimination

In CKD, drugs eliminated by the kidneys are no longer excreted normally. Water-soluble drugs, such as gentamicin, which are poorly absorbed from the gut, typically given by injection and not metabolized by the liver, give rise to far more problems than lipid-soluble drugs such as propranolol, which are well absorbed and principally metabolized by the liver.

Drugs affecting protein anabolism and catabolism

Tetracyclines, with the exception of doxycycline, have a catabolic effect. Increased nitrogenous waste products are not well cleared, and uraemia may be more marked. Corticosteroids also have a catabolic effect and may lead to a disproportionate increase in urea compared to creatinine when used in high doses in CKD.

Problem patients

Particular problems are presented by patients with rapidly changing renal function, such as those with evolving AKI or recovering acute tubular necrosis. In addition, drugs may be removed by dialysis and haemofiltration, which will affect the dosage required.

URINARY TRACT INFECTION

Urinary tract infection (UTI) is common, particularly in women, most often occurring in a normal urinary tract and usually as cystitis; half of all women will experience a UTI in their lifetime. Most UTIs occur in isolation (***Fig. 20.35***). It is uncommon in men and children; when diagnosed, it often occurs in an abnormal urinary tract. Between 1% and 2% of patients presenting in primary care will have a UTI.

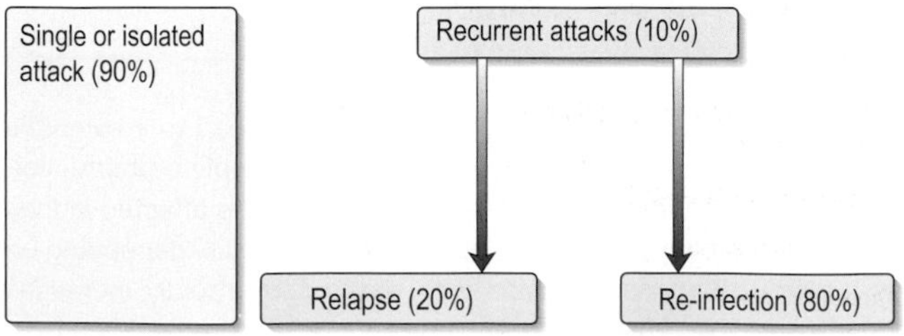

Figure 20.35 The natural history of urinary tract infection.

UTI is not always uncomplicated; recurrent infection causes considerable morbidity, and infection can lead to life-threatening Gram-negative septicaemia and kidney failure.

Aetiology and pathogenesis

Infection is most often caused by bacteria from a patient's own bowel flora ***(Box 20.22)***, and infection usually ascends up the urethra. In women, the short urethra makes ascending infection more likely. Rarely, infection may arise from the bloodstream or lymphatics, or by direct extension (e.g. from a vesicocolic fistula).

Bacterial virulence

How well an organism adheres to urothelium determines its virulence. The presence of flagella (for motility), aerobactin (used to acquire iron), haemolysin (to form pores) and, above all, the presence of fimbriae (adhesins that attach organisms to the perineum and urothelium) on the bacterial cell surface make *E. coli* such a common pathogen.

Innate host defence

Innate host defence prevents UTI in the following ways:

- ***Neutrophils***. Bacterial adhesins activate receptors, e.g. Toll receptor 4, on the mucosal surface, resulting in IL-8 production and expression of its receptor, CXCR1, on neutrophil surfaces. Activation of neutrophils is essential for bacterial killing.
- ***Urine osmolality and pH***. Urinary osmolality >800 mOsm/kg and low or high pH reduce bacterial survival.
- ***Complement***. Complement activation with mucosal IgA production by uroepithelium (acquired immunity) plays a major role in defence against UTI.
- ***Commensal organisms***. Eradication of commensal organisms such as lactobacilli, corynebacteria, streptococci and bacteroides by spermicidal jelly or antibiotics results in overgrowth of *E. coli*.
- ***Urine flow***. Good urine flow and normal micturition wash out bacteria. Urine stasis promotes UTI.
- ***Uroepithelium***. Mannosylated Tamm–Horsfall proteins (THPs), present in the mucus and glycocalyx covering uroepithelium, have antibacterial properties and interfere with bacterial binding to uroepithelium. Cranberry juice and blueberry juice contain a large-molecular-weight factor (pro-anthrocyanidins) that prevents binding of *E. coli* to the uroepithelium.
- ***Blood group antigens***. Women who are non-secretors of ABH blood group antigens are 3–4 times more likely to have recurrent UTIs.

Box 20.22 Organisms causing urinary tract infection in domiciliary practice

Organism	Approximate frequency (%)
Escherichia coli and other 'coliforms'	70
Proteus spp.	12
Staphylococcus saprophyticus or *epidermidis*[a]	10
Enterococcus faecalis[b]	6
Pseudomonas spp.	5
Klebsiella spp.	4

[a]More common in young women (20–30%). [b]More common in hospital practice.

Risk factors

- Female gender, especially postmenopausal women.
- New sexual activity, particularly in young women.
- Indwelling urinary catheter or instrumentation of the urinary tract.
- Urinary tract stones.
- Urinary tract stasis (incomplete bladder emptying).
- Diabetes mellitus or immunosuppression.
- Dementia.

Clinical features

The most typical symptoms of (lower) UTI are:

- frequency of micturition by day and night
- dysuria (painful voiding)
- suprapubic pain and tenderness
- haematuria
- smelly urine.

These are the symptoms of bladder and urethral inflammation, or 'cystitis'. Loin pain and tenderness, with fever, chills, night sweats and rigors, suggest extension of infection to the pelvis and kidney, known as pyelitis or pyelonephritis. Localization of the site of infection on the basis of symptoms alone is unreliable.

UTI can also present with few or no symptoms (particularly in the immunocompromised), or even with abdominal pain, fever or haematuria in the absence of frequency or dysuria. In the elderly, new confusion may be the only symptom of UTI. In small children, who cannot complain of dysuria, symptoms are often 'atypical'. The possibility of UTI must always be considered in the fretful, febrile, sick child who fails to thrive.

Diagnosis

Uncomplicated UTIs in younger women (age ≤65) can be diagnosed in those without known urinary tract abnormalities, recent urinary tract instrumentation, or systemic illness if they exhibit at least two of three cardinal symptoms – dysuria, urgency or frequency – along with absence of vaginal discharge. Neither urine dipstick testing for leucocyte esterase nor urine culture enhances diagnostic sensitivity. Telephone-based protocols have outcomes similar to those of surgery-based diagnosis and treatment, and such methods are often preferred by patients. Patients with histories of uncomplicated UTIs can be taught to self-diagnose and initiate therapy.

Otherwise, diagnosis is based on culture of a clean-catch mid-stream specimen of urine and the presence or absence of pyuria. The criteria for the diagnosis of UTI, particularly in symptomatic women, are shown in ***Box 20.23***. Most Gram-negative organisms

Box 20.23 Criteria for the diagnosis of bacteriuria

Symptomatic young women

- $\geq 10^2$ coliform organisms/mL urine plus pyuria (>10 white blood cells/mm^3)

  or

- $\geq 10^5$ any pathogenic organisms/mL urine

  or

- Any growth of pathogenic organisms in urine by suprapubic aspiration

Symptomatic men

- $\geq 10^3$ pathogenic organisms/mL urine

Asymptomatic patients

- $\geq 10^5$ pathogenic organisms/mL urine on two occasions reduce nitrates to nitrites and produce a red colour in the reagent square. False-negative results are common. Dipsticks that detect significant pyuria depend on the release of esterases from leucocytes. Dipstick tests positive for both nitrite and leucocyte esterase are highly predictive of acute infection (sensitivity of 75% and specificity of 82%).

Re-infection versus relapsing infection may be distinguished as follows:

- ***Relapse*** is diagnosed by recurrence of bacteriuria with the same organism within 7 days of completion of antibacterial treatment. Treatment failure may suggest ***(Fig. 20.36)*** associated stones, scarred kidneys, polycystic disease or bacterial prostatitis.
- ***Re-infection*** is when bacteriuria is absent after treatment for at least 14 days, usually longer, followed by recurrence of infection with the same or different organisms. This is not due to failure to eradicate infection, but is the result of re-invasion of a susceptible tract with new organisms. Approximately 80% of recurrent infections are due to re-infection.

Where culture is negative and symptoms persist, consider:

- ***Abacteriuric frequency or dysuria ('urethral syndrome')***. This is caused by bladder trauma after intercourse; vaginitis, atrophic vaginitis or urethritis in the elderly; and *Chlamydia* infection and tuberculosis in symptomatic young women with 'sterile pyuria'.
- ***Interstitial cystitis***. This is uncommon but distressing, affecting women over the age of 40. Patients present with frequency, dysuria and often severe suprapubic pain but cultures are sterile. Cystoscopy shows typical inflammatory changes with ulceration of the bladder base. It is now thought to be an autoimmune disorder. Treatments include oral prednisolone, bladder instillation of sodium cromoglicate or dimethyl sulphoxide, and bladder stretching under anaesthesia. Unfortunately, relief of symptoms can be difficult to achieve.
- ***Predominant frequency*** and passage of small volumes of urine ('irritable bladder'). These may occur after previous UTI.

Natural history

Serious morbidity is unusual. However, renal scarring can result from recurrent UTI and dissemination of infection as septicaemia can be fatal. In patients with a ***normal urinary tract (with normal renal imaging)***, outcomes are very good, and persistent or recurrent infection seldom results in serious kidney damage (uncomplicated UTI). In those with ***abnormal urinary tracts*** (stones or stasis), recurrence is more common and outcomes are less good. The combination of infection and obstruction results in severe, sometimes rapid, kidney damage (obstructive pyonephrosis) and is a major cause of Gram-negative septicaemia from *Pseudomonas* and *Enterobacter* spp. Complicated and uncomplicated infection is compared in ***Figure 20.37***.

Acute pyelonephritis

Fever, loin pain with tenderness and significant bacteriuria usually imply infection of the kidney (acute pyelonephritis). Small renal cortical abscesses and streaks of pus in the renal medulla are often present. Histologically, there is focal infiltration by polymorphonuclear leucocytes and many polymorphs in tubular lumina.

Although, with antibiotics, significant permanent kidney damage in adults with normal urinary tracts is rare, CT scanning can show wedge-shaped areas of inflammation in the renal cortex ***(Fig. 20.38)***, where renal function will be impaired.

Reflux nephropathy

This was called chronic pyelonephritis or atrophic pyelonephritis, resulting from a combination of:

- vesicoureteric reflux
- infection acquired in infancy or early childhood.

Normally, the vesicoureteric junction acts as a one-way valve ***(Fig. 20.39)***, urine entering the bladder from above; the ureter is shut off during bladder contraction, thus preventing reflux of urine. In some infants and children – possibly even *in utero* – this valve mechanism is incompetent, bladder voiding being associated with variable reflux of a jet of urine up the ureter. A secondary consequence is incomplete bladder emptying, as refluxed urine returns

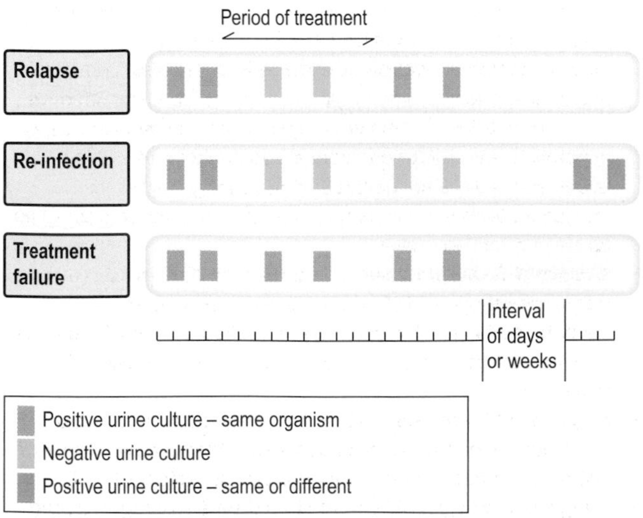

Figure 20.36 A comparison of re-infection, relapse and treatment failure in urinary tract infection.

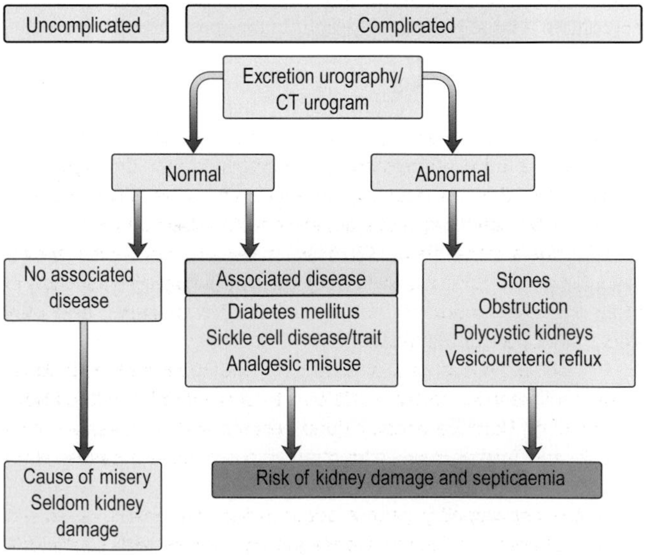

Figure 20.37 Complicated versus uncomplicated urinary tract infection.

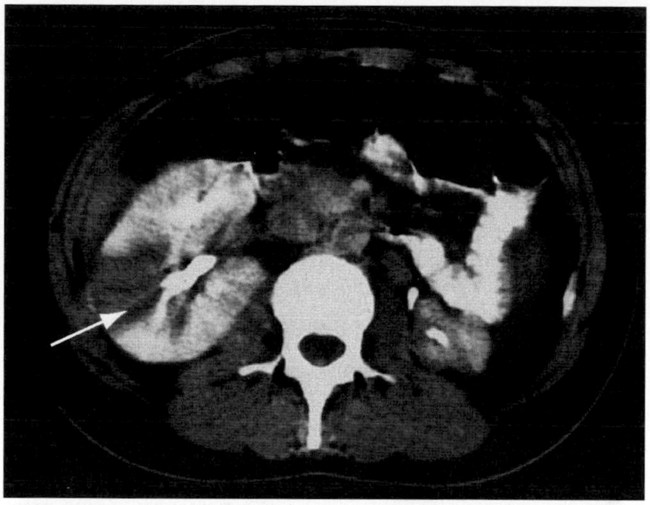

Figure 20.38 Computed tomogram showing a wedge-shaped area of renal cortical loss (arrow) following acute pyelonephritis.

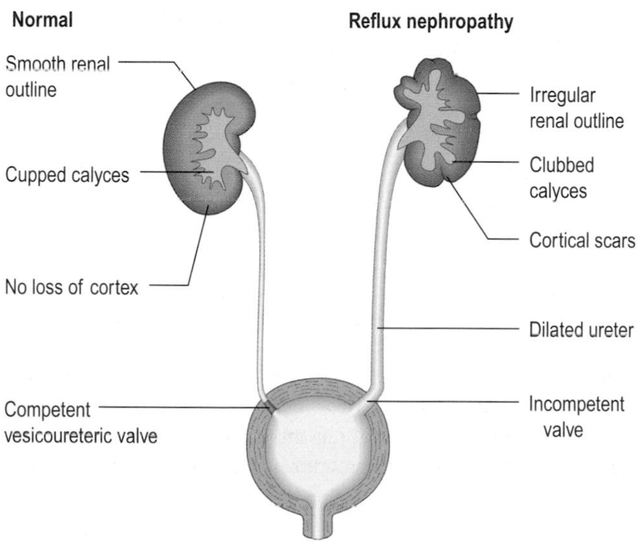

Figure 20.39 Findings in patients with reflux nephropathy compared with normal individuals.

to the bladder after voiding. This latter event predisposes to infection, and the reflux of infected urine leads to kidney damage.

Typically, there is papillary damage, tubulointerstitial nephritis and cortical scarring in areas adjacent to 'clubbed calyces'.

Diagnosis is based on CT scan of the kidneys, which shows irregular renal outlines, clubbed calyces and a variable reduction in renal size. The condition may be unilateral or bilateral, and may affect all or part of the kidney.

Reflux usually ceases around puberty with growth of the bladder base (a thickened bladder wall is able to prevent reflux with bladder contraction). Damage already done persists and progressive renal fibrosis and further loss of function occur in severe cases, even though there is no further infection.

Reflux nephropathy cannot occur in the absence of reflux – it does not begin in adult life. Consequently, women with bacteriuria and a normal urogram can be reassured that kidney damage will not develop.

Chronic reflux nephropathy acquired in infancy predisposes to hypertension in later life and, if severe, is a relatively common cause of ESKD in childhood or adult life. Meticulous early detection and control of infection, with or without ureteral re-implantation to create a competent valve, can prevent further scarring and allow normal growth of the kidneys. No proof exists, however, that re-implantation surgery confers long-term benefit.

Continuous antibiotic prophylaxis (CAP), compared with no treatment, significantly reduces the risk of symptomatic UTI in children with chronic reflux nephropathy but at the expense of increased risk for developing antimicrobial-resistant bacterial strains. CAP does not have a significant impact on the occurrence of new renal scarring.

Special investigations

Uncomplicated UTI usually does not require imaging. If infection is recurrent or affects men or children, or if there are unusually severe symptoms, it should be investigated further. Patients with diabetes mellitus and those on immunosuppression benefit from early imaging.

- ***Ultrasound*** allows the detection of calculi, obstruction, abnormal urinary anatomy and incomplete bladder emptying (post-micturition scan). It is helpful in the assessment of suspected pyelonephritis or an obstructed, infected kidney that may require drainage.
- ***CT*** is more sensitive for diagnosis and follow-up of complicated renal tract infection. Contrast-enhanced CT allows different phases of excretion to be studied, and can define the extent of disease and identify significant complications or obstruction.
- ***MRI*** is particularly useful in those with iodinated contrast allergies, offering an ionizing radiation-free alternative in the diagnosis of both medical and surgical diseases of the kidney.
- ***Nuclear medicine*** has a limited role in the evaluation of UTI in adults. Its main role is in the assessment of renal function and detection of scars by DMSA scan, often prior to surgery.

Management

Management of a single isolated attack

- ***The most appropriate antibiotic choices*** are trimethoprim–sulfamethoxazole (160/800 mg twice daily for 3–7 days) or nitrofurantoin (100 mg twice daily for 5–7 days). Fluoroquinolones offer no advantage in cure rates; β-lactam antibiotics, such as amoxicillin–clavulanate, are less effective than the first-line recommendations. Most patients who delay antibiotic treatment to encourage spontaneous resolution eventually receive antibiotics and have longer times to resolution. Men with uncomplicated UTIs should be treated as above but for 7–14 days.
- ***Shorter 3–5-day courses*** with amoxicillin (250 mg three times daily), trimethoprim (200 mg twice daily) or an oral cephalosporin are also used, and modified in light of the result of urine culture and sensitivity testing, and/or the clinical response.
- ***Single-shot treatment*** with 3 g of amoxicillin or 1.92 g of co-trimoxazole is used for patients with bladder symptoms of <36 hours' duration who have no previous history of UTI.
- ***A high (2 L daily) fluid intake*** should be encouraged during treatment and for some subsequent weeks. Urine culture should be repeated 5 days after treatment.

- ***If the patient is acutely ill with high fever, loin pain and tenderness*** (acute pyelonephritis), antibiotics are given intravenously, e.g. aztreonam, cefuroxime, ciprofloxacin or gentamicin, switching to a further 7 days' treatment with oral therapy as symptoms improve. Intravenous fluids may be required to achieve a good urine output.
- ***In patients presenting for the first time with high fever, loin pain and tenderness***, urgent renal ultrasound examination is required to exclude an obstructed pyonephrosis. If this is present, it should be drained by percutaneous nephrostomy (see p. 731).

Management of recurrent infection

Pre-treatment and post-treatment urine cultures are necessary to confirm the diagnosis and to establish whether recurrent infection is due to relapse or re-infection.

Relapse. A search should be made for a cause (e.g. stones or scarred kidneys), and treatment modified if possible. Intense or prolonged treatment may be required. If this fails, long-term antibiotics are necessary.

Re-infection. This implies that the patient has a predisposition to periurethral colonization or poor bladder defence mechanisms. Contraceptive advice should be offered and the use of a diaphragm or spermicidal jelly discouraged. Atrophic vaginitis should be identified in postmenopausal women, who should be treated (see below). Preventative measures may help:

- a 2 L daily fluid intake
- voiding at 2–3-h intervals, with double micturition if reflux is present
- voiding before bedtime and after intercourse
- avoidance of spermicidal jellies and of bubble baths and other chemicals in bath water
- avoidance of constipation, which may impair bladder emptying.

Evidence of impaired bladder emptying on excretion urography/ultrasound requires urological assessment. If UTI continues to recur, treatment for 6–12 months with low-dose alternating monthly prophylaxis (trimethoprim 100 mg, co-trimoxazole 480 mg, cefalexin 125 mg at night or macrocrystalline nitrofurantoin) is required; it should be taken last thing at night when urine flow is low. Intravaginal oestrogen therapy has been shown to produce a reduction in the number of episodes of UTI in postmenopausal women. Cranberry juice is said to reduce the risk of symptoms and re-infection by 12–20% but studies are limited.

Urinary infections in the presence of an indwelling catheter

Colonization of the bladder by a pathogen is common after a urinary catheter has been *in situ* for more than a few days, partly due to organisms forming biofilms. So long as the bladder catheter is in place, antibiotics are likely to be ineffective and will encourage the development of resistant organisms. The patient should be treated only if there are symptoms or evidence of infection. The catheter should always be replaced. When changing catheters, a single dose of antibiotic (e.g. gentamicin) is recommended.

Infection by *Candida* is a frequent complication of prolonged bladder catheterization. Treatment should be reserved for patients with evidence of invasive infection and those who are immunosuppressed. The catheter should be removed or replaced. In severe infections, continuous bladder irrigation with amphotericin 50 μg/mL is useful.

Bacteriuria in pregnancy

Pregnant women should have their urine cultured, as 2–6% have asymptomatic bacteriuria (see p. 1308). Usually harmless in non-pregnant women, bacteriuria in pregnancy can lead to acute pyelonephritis, and in late pregnancy may trigger pre-term labour. Ureteric dilatation in response to hormonal changes may allow ascending infection. *Bacteriuria must always be treated and shown to be eradicated.* Re-infection may require prophylactic therapy. Tetracycline, trimethoprim, sulphonamides and 4-quinolones are contraindicated in pregnancy. Amoxicillin and ampicillin, nitrofurantoin and oral cephalosporins may be used safely in pregnancy.

Bacterial prostatitis

Bacterial prostatitis is a relapsing infection that presents as perineal pain, recurrent epididymo-orchitis and prostatic tenderness, with pus in expressed prostatic secretions. Treatment is for 4–6 weeks with drugs that penetrate into the prostate, such as trimethoprim or ciprofloxacin. Long-term, low-dose treatment may be required. Prostadynia (prostatic pain in the absence of active infection) may persist long after the infection. Amitriptyline and carbamazepine may alleviate the symptoms.

Renal carbuncle

Renal carbuncle is an abscess in the renal cortex caused by a blood-borne staphylococcus, usually from a boil or carbuncle of the skin. It presents with a high, swinging fever, loin pain and tenderness, and fullness in the loin. The urine shows no abnormality, as the abscess does not communicate with the renal pelvis, more often extending into the perirenal tissue. Staphylococcal septicaemia is common. Diagnosis is by ultrasound or CT scanning. Treatment involves antibacterial therapy with flucloxacillin and surgical drainage.

Tuberculosis of the urinary tract

Tuberculous infection is on the increase worldwide, partly due to the reservoir of infection in susceptible HIV-infected individuals and the emergence of drug-resistant strains. Tuberculosis of the urinary tract presents with frequency, dysuria or haematuria. In the UK, it is seen mainly in the Asian immigrant population. Cortical lesions result from haematogenous spread in the primary phase of infection. Most heal, but in some, infection persists and spreads to the papillae, with the formation of cavitating lesions and the discharge of mycobacteria into the urine. Infection of the ureters and bladder commonly follows, with the potential for development of ureteral strictures and a contracted bladder. Rarely, cold abscesses may form in the loin. In males, the disease may present with testicular or epididymal discomfort and thickening.

Diagnosis depends on constant awareness, especially in patients with sterile pyuria. Imaging may show cavitating lesions in the renal papillary areas, commonly with calcification. There may also be evidence of ureteral obstruction with hydronephrosis. Culture of mycobacteria from early-morning urine samples is not straightforward. Imaging may be normal in diffuse interstitial renal tuberculosis, when diagnosis is made instead by renal biopsy, which demonstrates caseating granulomata with multinucleate giant cells and acid-fast bacilli on Ziehl–Neelsen staining ***(Fig. 20.40)***. Some patients present late with small, unobstructed kidneys, when the diagnosis is easy to miss.

Treatment is as for pulmonary tuberculosis (see pp. 1110–1113). Renal ultrasonography and/or CT scanning should be carried

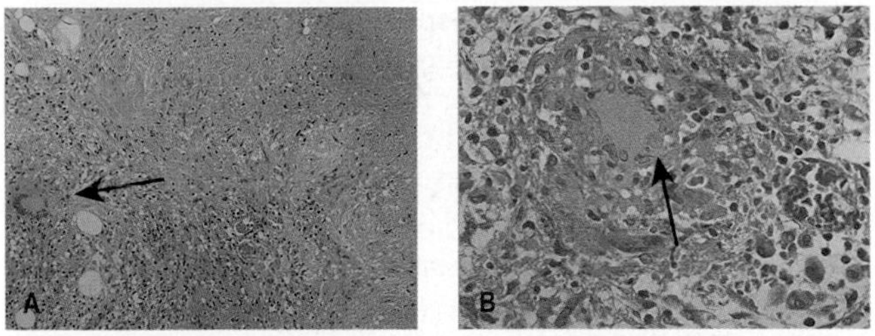

Figure 20.40 **Renal tuberculosis. A.** Caseating granulomatous interstitial nephritis showing multinuclear giant cell (arrow). **B.** Ziehl–Neelsen staining showing mycobacteria (arrow).

out 2–3 months after initiation of treatment, as ureteric strictures may first develop in the healing phase.

Xanthogranulomatous pyelonephritis

This is an uncommon chronic interstitial infection of the kidney, most often due to *Proteus*, in which there is fever, weight loss, loin pain and a palpable enlarged kidney. It is usually unilateral and associated with staghorn calculi and UTI. CT scanning shows up intrarenal abscesses as lucent areas within the kidney. Nephrectomy is the treatment of choice; antibacterial treatment rarely, if ever, eradicates the infection.

Further reading

Chapagain A, Dobbie H, Sheaff M et al. Presentation, diagnosis, and treatment outcome of tuberculous-mediated tubulointerstitial nephritis. *Kidney Int* 2011; 79:671–677.
Hooton TM. Uncomplicated urinary tract infection. *N Engl J Med* 2012; 366:1028–1037.
Wise GJ, Schlegel PN. Sterile pyuria. *New Engl J Med* 2015; 372:1048–1054.

TUBULOINTERSTITIAL NEPHRITIS

Diseases of the kidney primarily affect the glomeruli, vasculature, or the substance of the renal parenchyma, made up of tubules and the interstitium. Tubular and interstitial injury and recovery tend to go hand in hand.

Acute tubulointerstitial nephritis

In approximately 70% of the cases, acute tubulointerstitial nephritis (TIN) is a hypersensitivity reaction to drugs ***(Box 20.24)***, most commonly penicillins, NSAIDs or proton-pump inhibitors.

Drug-induced acute TIN

Patients may be wholly asymptomatic (with impaired renal function found incidentally), or present with fever, arthralgia, skin rashes and acute oliguric or non-oliguric kidney injury. Many have eosinophilia and eosinophiluria. Renal histology shows an intense interstitial cellular infiltrate, often including eosinophils, with variable tubular necrosis ***(Fig. 20.41)***. Rarely, NSAIDs can cause a glomerular minimal-change lesion [illegible] TIN and [illegible] the nephrotic syndrome. Treatment involves stopping the offending drug. High-dose prednisolone (60 mg daily) is given but efficacy has not been proven. Patients may require dialysis for management of the AKI. Most patients make a good recovery in terms of kidney function, but some may be left with significant interstitial fibrosis and CKD.

Box 20.24 Common causes of acute tubulointerstitial nephritis

- Drugs (70%):
  - Antibiotics:
    Cephalosporins
    Ciprofloxacin
    Erythromycin
    Penicillin
    Rifampicin
    Sulphonamides
  - Analgesics:
    Non-steroidal anti-inflammatory drugs
  - Diuretics:
    Furosemide
    Thiazides
  - Miscellaneous:
    Allopurinol
    Carbamazepine
    Cimetidine
    Phenytoin
    Proton pump inhibitors
    Valproate
- Infection (15%):
  - Viruses, e.g. hantavirus
  - Bacteria, e.g. streptococci
- Idiopathic (8%)
- Tubulointerstitial nephritis with uveitis (TINU) (5%)
- Systemic inflammatory disorders, e.g.:
  - Systemic lupus erythematosus (2%)
  - IgG4-related disorder

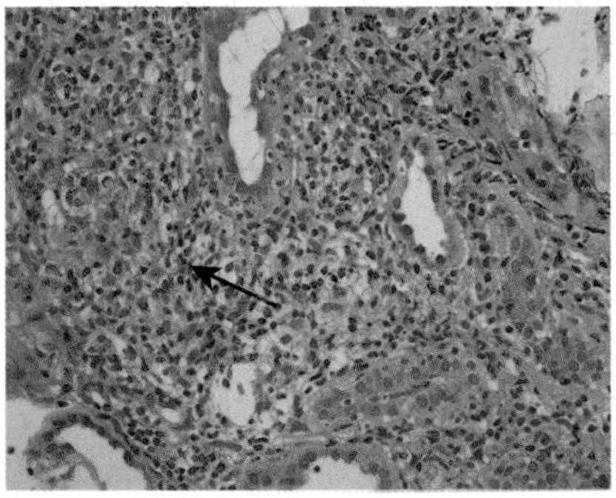

Figure 20.41 **Tubulointerstitial nephritis showing diffuse interstitial infiltrate with red staining (arrow).**

Infection causing acute TIN

Acute pyelonephritis leads to inflammation of the tubules, producing a neutrophilic cellular infiltrate. TIN can complicate systemic infections with viruses (Hantavirus, Epstein–Barr virus, HIV, measles, adenovirus), bacteria (*Legionella*, *Leptospira*, streptococci, *Mycoplasma*, *Brucella*, *Chlamydia*) and others (*Leishmania*, *Toxoplasma*). Hantavirus causes haemorrhagic fever with TIN and can be fatal. Epstein–Barr virus DNA has been found in renal biopsy tissue of cases of idiopathic TIN. In immunocompromised patients, such as those who have had renal transplantation, cytomegalovirus, polyoma (BK) and herpes simplex virus can cause acute TIN in the renal graft. Treatment involves eradication of infection with appropriate antibiotics or antiviral agents; in renal transplantation, the immunosuppressive regimen is modified.

Acute TIN as part of multisystem inflammatory diseases

Several non-infectious inflammatory disorders, such as Sjögren syndrome, SLE and granulomatosis, can cause acute or chronic TIN rather than glomerulonephritis. Sjögren syndrome may additionally present as renal tubular acidosis. Sarcoidosis presents as granulomatous TIN in up to 20% of patients. Associated hypercalcaemia causes AKI. These heterogeneous conditions with TIN generally respond to steroids.

Tubulointerstitial nephritis with uveitis syndrome

Patients with tubulointerstitial nephritis with uveitis (TINU) syndrome present with uveitis, an acute TIN, weight loss, anaemia and a raised ESR of unknown cause. It is common in childhood but has been reported in adulthood, and is more frequently found in women. It may be associated with autoantibodies directed against modified CRP. A prolonged course of steroids leads to improvement in both renal function and uveitis.

Chronic tubulointerstitial nephritis

The major causes of chronic TIN are given in ***Box 20.25***. Patients present with any of polyuria, nocturia, proteinuria (usually slight, <1 g daily) or uraemia. Chronic TIN may be linked with papillary necrosis (ischaemic damage to the papillae, which then slough into the calyces and urine) when associated with longstanding analgesic use, diabetes mellitus, sickle cell disease or trait. Microscopic or overt haematuria or sterile pyuria also occurs, and occasionally a sloughed papilla may cause ureteric colic or produce acute ureteric obstruction. Histologically, a generalized chronic inflammatory cellular infiltration of the interstitium with tubular atrophy and generalized interstitial oedema or fibrosis is present, and in many cases no cause is found.

IgG4-related tubulointerstitial nephritis is distinguished by very low concentrations of complement and increased serum IgG4. This may lead to immune complex formation.

The radiological appearances must be distinguished from those of reflux nephropathy ***(Fig. 20.42)*** or obstructive uropathy.

Tubular damage to the medullary area of the kidney leads to defects in urine concentration and sodium conservation with polyuria and salt wasting. Fibrosis progressing into the cortex leads to loss of excretory function and urea.

Analgesic nephropathy

The chronic consumption of large amounts of analgesics (classically, phenacetin but now NSAIDs) leads to chronic TIN and papillary necrosis. Analgesic nephropathy is more common in women and typically presents in middle age. Presentation may be with anaemia, CKD, UTIs, haematuria or urinary tract obstruction (owing to sloughing of a renal papilla). Salt- and water-wasting renal disease may occur. Chronic analgesic use also predisposes to the development of uroepithelial tumours. Diagnosis is usually made on clinical grounds combined with the non-pathognomonic appearance on imaging (such as ultrasonography or CT scan), which demonstrates smallish, irregularly outlined kidneys.

Box 20.25 Causes of chronic tubulointerstitial nephritis

Drugs and toxins, e.g.
- All causes of acute tubulointerstitial nephritis, e.g. analgesics
- Ciclosporin
- 5-aminosalicylates
- Cadmium, lead, titanium
- Irradiation

Systemic disease, e.g.
- Diabetes mellitus
- Sickle cell disease or trait
- Systemic lupus erythematosus/vasculitis
- Sarcoidosis
- IgG4-related disease

Metabolic, e.g.
- Hyperuricaemia
- Nephrocalcinosis
- Hyperoxaluria

Infection, e.g.
- Human immunodeficiency virus
- Epstein–Barr virus

Miscellaneous
- Hypertension
- Balkan nephropathy
- Herbal nephropathy
- Alport syndrome

Patients should be encouraged to avoid NSAIDs, and if necessary, dihydrocodeine or paracetamol may be offered as a reasonable alternative (this may stop further damage and even achieve an improvement). The development of flank pain or an unexpectedly rapid deterioration in renal function should prompt ultrasonography to screen for urinary tract obstruction due to a sloughed papilla.

Balkan nephropathy

Balkan nephropathy (BN) is a chronic TIN endemic in areas along the tributaries of the River Danube. Inhabitants of the low-lying plains, which are subjected to frequent flooding and where the water supply comes from shallow wells, are affected, whereas the disease does not occur in hillside villages where surface water provides the supply. Chronic dietary poisoning by aristolochic acid (AA) is thought to be responsible for BN and the urothelial cancers that accompany the diagnosis. The disease is insidious in onset, with mild proteinuria progressing to ESKD in 3 months to 10 years. There is no treatment.

Chinese herb nephropathy

Chinese herbal medicines may contain AA, produced as a result of fungal contamination of the product. Histology is similar to that of BN but the clinical course is aggressive, with relentless progression to ESKD and a high incidence of uroepithelial tumours.

Other forms of chronic TIN

These are rare ***(Box 20.25)***. Diagnosis of all forms depends on a history of drug ingestion or industrial exposure to nephrotoxins. In patients with unexplained renal impairment with normal-sized

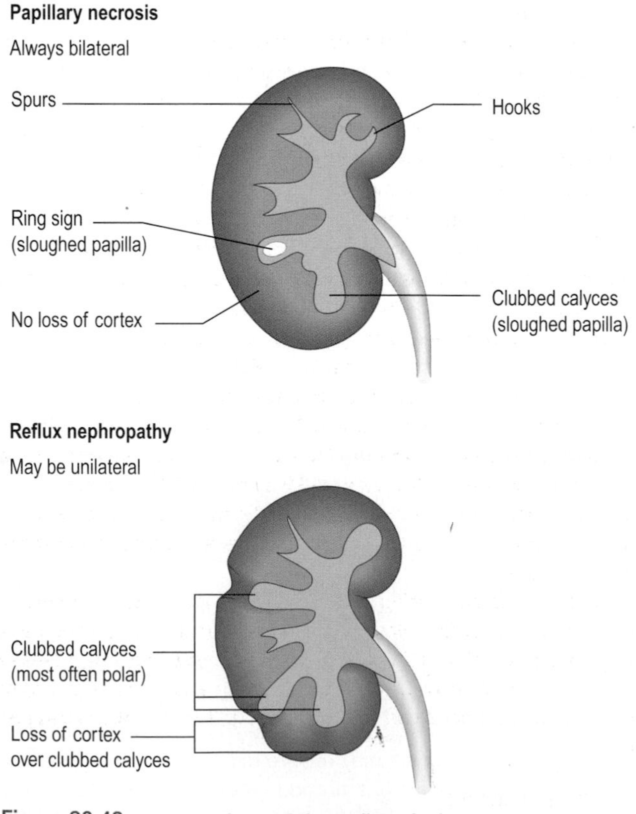

Figure 20.42 A comparison of the radiological appearances of papillary necrosis and reflux nephropathy.

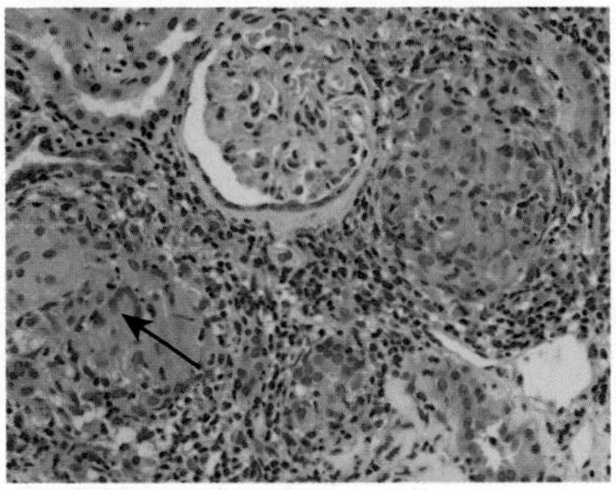

Figure 20.43 Granulomatous tubulointerstitial nephritis. The granuloma consists of both giant cells (arrow) and epithelioid cells. These findings are characteristic of renal sarcoid but can be seen with any cause (drug or infection) of interstitial nephritis.

kidneys, renal biopsy must always be undertaken to exclude a treatable TIN, such as granulomatous TIN due to ***renal sarcoidosis (Fig. 20.43)***, which may be the first presentation of sarcoidosis (see pp. 1118–1120). Renal sarcoidosis generally responds rapidly to steroids.

Hyperuricaemic nephropathy

Acute hyperuricaemic nephropathy (see p. 606), as part of tumour lysis syndrome, causes AKI in patients with very high serum urate concentrations. It may occur prior to treatment of haematological malignancies, but more often supervenes after treatment. As the abundant tumour cells lyse in response to chemotherapy, large amounts of nucleoprotein are released with increased uric acid production. Renal failure is due to intrarenal and extrarenal obstruction caused by deposition of uric acid crystals in the collecting ducts, pelvis and ureters.

There may be flank pain or colic, and oliguria or anuria with increasing uraemia. Plasma urate levels are >0.75 mmol/L and may be as high as 4.5 mmol/L. ***Diagnosis*** is based on the hyperuricaemia and the clinical setting. Ultrasound may demonstrate extrarenal obstruction due to stones but may be unremarkable.

Allopurinol 100–200 mg three times daily for 5 days is given prior to and throughout treatment with radiotherapy or cytotoxic drugs. A high rate of urine flow must be maintained by oral or parenteral fluid, and the urine kept alkaline by the administration of sodium bicarbonate 600 mg four times daily and acetazolamide 250 mg three times daily, since uric acid is more soluble in an alkaline than an acid medium. Febuxostat, a non-purine-analogue inhibitor of xanthine oxidase, can be used if allopurinol cannot be tolerated and eGFR is >30 mL/min. ***Rasburicase***, a recombinant urate oxidase (see p. 774), and ***pegloticase***, a pegylated uricase, are successfully used to lower serum urate concentrations rapidly for both treatment and prevention. In severely oliguric or anuric patients, dialysis is required to lower the plasma urate.

There is no convincing direct evidence for ***chronic hyperuricaemia nephropathy***. However, a few observational studies have suggested that elevated levels of uric acid independently increase the risk for new-onset CKD, and that plasma urate reduction with allopurinol has a beneficial effect in slowing the rate of progression of CKD.

Further reading

Kamisawa T, Zen Y, Pillais S et al. IgG4-related disease. *Lancet* 2015; 385:1460–1471.

ACUTE KIDNEY INJURY

Acute kidney injury (AKI) is defined as follows:

- There is an abrupt deterioration in renal function, usually over hours or days.
- It is usually (but not always) reversible over days or weeks.

AKI may cause sudden, life-threatening biochemical disturbances as a medical emergency. Oliguria is often a feature. The distinction between AKI and CKD, or even acute-on-chronic kidney disease, is not always obvious. AKI is usually recognized by a falling urine output and rising serum urea and creatinine, or both. In some situations, urea and creatinine are less accurate predictors of deteriorating renal function ***(Box 20.26)***.

AKI may result from:

- ***pre-renal*** causes (reduced kidney perfusion leads to a falling GFR)
- ***renal*** parenchymal disorders (injury to glomerulus, tubule or vessels)
- ***post-renal*** causes (urinary tract obstruction – functioning kidneys cannot excrete urine with back-pressure affecting function).

The Acute Dialysis Quality Initiative group proposed the **RIFLE classification** (**r**isk, **i**njury, **f**ailure, **l**oss, **e**nd-stage renal disease) to define AKI better, using either an increase in serum creatinine or a decrease in urine output. RIFLE describes three levels of renal dysfunction (R, I, F) and two outcome measures (L, E). These criteria indicate an increasing degree of renal damage and have a predictive value for mortality.

The Acute Kidney Injury Network (AKIN) proposed a modification of the original RIFLE criteria to include less severe AKI and a time constraint of 48 hours, and gives a correction for volume status before classification.

'R' in RIFLE is ***stage 1*** (a serum creatinine rise of ≥26.4 μmol/L – that is, a 1.5-fold increase within 48 hours).

'I' is ***stage 2*** – that is, a 2–3-fold increase in serum creatinine.

'F' is ***stage 3*** – that is, an increase in serum creatinine of >300% (equal to ≥354 μmol/L).

Urine output data are the same.

Using the same criteria of serum creatinine and urine output, a more recent classification (The Kidney Diseases: Improving Global Outcomes (KDIGO) classification) is shown in ***Box 20.27***.

Epidemiology

Incidence varies widely, depending on the population studied and the definition of AKI used, e.g.:

Box 20.26 Causes of altered serum urea and creatinine concentration other than altered renal function

Decreased concentration	Increased concentration
Urea	
Low protein intake	Corticosteroid treatment
Liver failure	Tetracycline treatment
Sodium valproate treatment	Gastrointestinal bleeding
Creatinine	
Low muscle mass	High muscle mass
	Red meat ingestion
	Muscle damage (rhabdomyolysis)
	Decreased tubular secretion (e.g. therapy with cimetidine or trimethoprim)

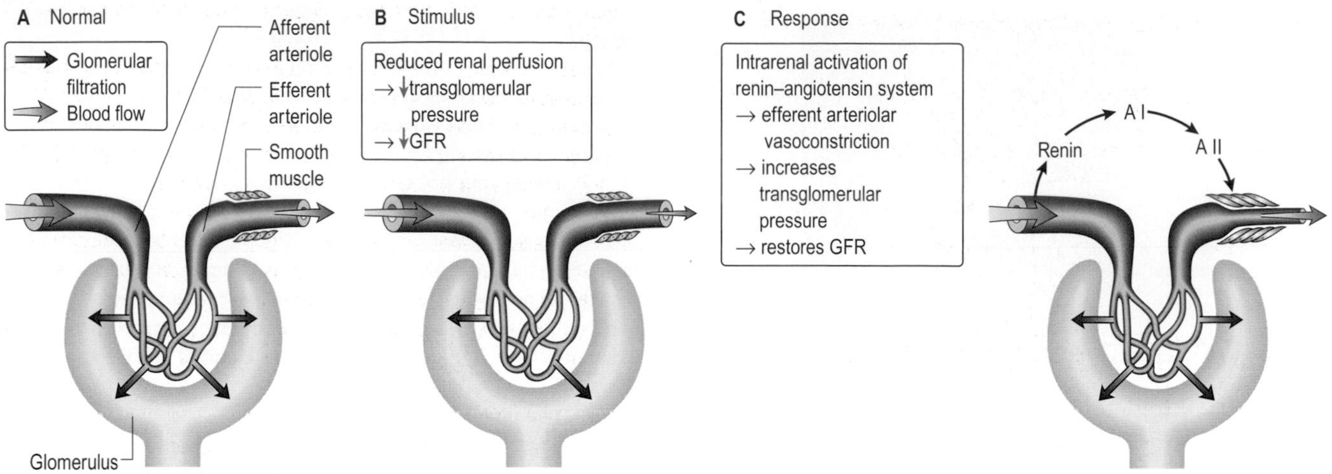

Figure 20.44 Glomerular dynamics. Effect of the renin–angiotensin system. AI, angiotensin I; AII, angiotensin II; GFR, glomerular filtration rate.

Box 20.27 KDIGO[a] classification of acute kidney injury

Stage	Serum creatinine concentration (SCr)	Urine output criteria
1	SCr 1.5–1.9 times baseline OR ≥26.5 μmol/L (0.3 mg/dL) increase	<0.5 mL/kg/h for 6–12 h
2	SCr 2–2.9 times baseline	<0.5 mL/kg/h for 6–12 h
3	SCr 3 times baseline OR Initiation of renal replacement therapy OR In patients <18 years, decrease in eGFR to <35 mL/min/1.73 m^2	Anuria for ≥12 h

[a]Kidney Diseases: Improving Global Outcomes.

- Community-acquired AKI on admission to hospital affects approximately 5% in the UK (superimposed on CKD in half of these patients).
- Severe AKI (creatinine >500 μmol/L, often requiring dialysis) affects about 130–140 per million population per year.
- About 25% of patients with sepsis and 50% of patients with septic shock will have AKI.

Outcomes vary: uncomplicated AKI carries a good prognosis, with mortality rates <5–10%. In contrast, AKI complicating non-renal organ system failure (in the intensive treatment unit (ITU) setting) is associated with mortality rates of 50–70%, which have not changed for several decades. Sepsis-related AKI has a significantly worse prognosis than AKI in the absence of sepsis.

Clinical approach to the patient with AKI

Pre-renal AKI

Falling renal blood flow leads to a falling GFR. This might be due either to changes in the circulation, or to intrarenal vasomotor changes that drop glomerular perfusion pressures. Common causes of a falling effective circulating volume include ***(Box 20.28)***:

- hypovolaemia of any cause, including dehydration or haemorrhage
- hypotension without hypovolaemia, including cirrhosis or septic shock
- low cardiac output, including cardiac failure or cardiogenic shock

Box 20.28 Causes of hypovolaemia

- Dehydration
- Reduced intake (nil by mouth, confusion)
- Gut losses (vomiting, nasogastric tube losses, diarrhoea)
- Renal losses (diuretics, hyperglycaemia)
- Burns, sweating
- Haemorrhage
- Third space losses (pancreatitis, peritonitis, bowel obstruction)
- Systemic vasodilatation (septic shock, cirrhosis)
- Cardiac failure or shock (myocardial infarction, arrhythmias, cardiomyopathy, tamponade)

Box 20.29 Criteria for distinction between pre-renal and intrinsic causes of renal dysfunction

Criteria	Pre-renal	Intrinsic
Urine specific gravity	>1.020	<1.010
Urine osmolality (mOsm/kg)	>500	<350
Urine sodium (mmol/L)	<10	>20
$Fe_{Na} = \frac{U_{Na}}{P_{Na}} + \frac{U_{Cr}}{P_{Cr}} \div 100$	<1%	>1%

Cr, creatinine; FE, fractional excretion; Na, sodium; P, plasma; U, urine.

- combinations of the above.

Common intra-renal causes include:

- NSAIDs, ACE inhibitors ***(Fig 20.44)***, amphotericin B and calcineurin inhibitors, often in the context of added changes in renal blood flow.

Usually, the kidney maintains glomerular filtration close to normal, despite wide variations in renal perfusion pressure and volume status – so-called ‘autoregulation’ (prostaglandins, nitric oxide and angiotensin acting on afferent and efferent arterioles). Once autoregulation fails, GFR drops and AKI develops. Over time, reduced blood flow may lead to established parenchymal injury, but if renal perfusion is corrected early, AKI will resolve fully.

A few simple biochemical measures have long been used to prove pre-renal AKI ***(Box 20.29)***. Urine specific gravity or osmolality will rise, as solutes are concentrated into smaller urine volumes (the kidney is retaining fluid to improve renal blood flow). Urine sodium will be low, as salt is retained for the same reason. The fractional

Box 20.30 Distinguishing causes of shock on clinical examination

	Hypovolaemia	Low cardiac output	Vasodilatation
Hypotension	Postural hypotension	Hypotension	Hypotension
Peripheries	Cool	Cool	Warm
Jugular venous pressure (JVP)	Low	Raised	Low

Box 20.31 Some causes of acute tubular necrosis

- Haemorrhage
- Burns
- Diarrhoea and vomiting, fluid loss from fistulae
- Pancreatitis
- Diuretics
- Myocardial infarction
- Congestive cardiac failure
- Endotoxic shock
- Snake bite
- Myoglobinaemia
- Haemoglobinaemia (due to haemolysis, e.g. in falciparum malaria, 'blackwater fever')
- Hepatorenal syndrome
- Radiological contrast agents (see p. 774)
- Drugs, e.g. aminoglycosides, non-steroidal anti-inflammatory drugs, angiotensin-converting enzyme inhibitors, platinum derivatives
- Abruptio placentae
- Pre-eclampsia and eclampsia

excretion of sodium (FE_{Na}) is a more reliable measure of sodium retention. None of these measures is reliable on its own and laboratory tests are no substitute for clinical assessment ***(Box 20.30)***.

Management of pre-renal AKI

This largely depends on the underlying cause. Most cases of AKI have an element of hypovolaemia, so prompt fluid resuscitation is most often indicated. When there is uncertainty as to the volume status of a patient, a fluid challenge of 250 mL crystalloid will often prove whether hypotension is fluid-responsive. Heart rate, blood pressure and urine output will all guide response to resuscitation. For cardiogenic shock and septic shock, see pages 1154 and 1150–1161, respectively.

Post-renal AKI

Obstruction of the urinary tract may occur at any point from the calyces to the external urethral orifice but commonly takes the form of bladder outflow obstruction (prostate disease in men) or bilateral ureteric obstruction (stones or tumours). The causes and presentation of urinary tract obstruction are dealt with on pages 758–761. Almost every case of unexplained AKI should result in an ultrasound to exclude obstruction, as, once this is relieved (and if acute), renal function will return to baseline.

Renal parenchymal AKI

This is most commonly (80–90%) due to ***acute tubular necrosis*** (ATN; see below and ***Box 20.31***). Almost any cause of pre-renal AKI, if prolonged to the point at which renal autoregulation fails (see above), will lead to ischaemic ATN. If not ischaemic, then ATN usually results from direct tubular toxins ***(Box 20.31)***. As a result, ATN is common in hospital practice. Other causes of parenchymal AKI include:

- Disease affecting the intrarenal arteries and arterioles, as well as glomerular capillaries, such as a vasculitis (see pp. 744–745), accelerated hypertension, cholesterol embolism, haemolytic uraemic syndrome, thrombotic thrombocytopenic purpura (TTP), pre-eclampsia and crescentic glomerulonephritis.
- Acute tubulointerstitial nephritis (see pp. 767–768). This also occurs when renal tubules are acutely obstructed by crystals, e.g. after rapid lysis of certain malignant tumours following chemotherapy (acute hyperuricaemic nephropathy).
- Acute bilateral suppurative pyelonephritis or pyelonephritis of a single kidney, which can cause acute uraemia.

Acute tubular necrosis

Acute tubular necrosis (ATN) ***(Box 20.31)*** occurs due to:

- sustained under-perfusion and reduced renal blood flow of renal tubules leads to tubular cell death (hence the name), or
- nephrotoxins causing direct injury and cell death in renal tubules.

Factors involved in the development of ATN include:

- ***Intrarenal microvascular vasoconstriction with falling delivery of O_2 and increasing tubular hypoxia***:
  - vasoconstriction in response to endothelin, adenosine, thromboxane A_2, leukotrienes and sympathetic nerve activity
  - impaired vasodilatation due to reduced sensitivity to nitric oxide, prostaglandins (PGE_2), acetylcholine and bradykinin
- ***Increased endothelial and vascular smooth muscle cell structural damage***:
  - increased leucocyte–endothelial adhesion, vascular congestion and obstruction, leucocyte activation and inflammation.
- ***Tubular cell injury***. Ischaemic injury results in rapid depletion of intracellular ATP stores resulting in cell death either by necrosis or apoptosis, with:
  - increased cytosolic cell calcium concentration
  - induction of nitric oxide synthases with increased production of nitric oxide, causing cell death
  - increased production of intracellular proteases such as calpain, which cause proteolysis of cytoskeletal proteins and cell wall collapse
  - tubular obstruction by desquamated viable or necrotic cells and casts
  - loss of cell polarity, i.e. integrins located on the basolateral side of the cell are translocated to the apical surface, which, when combined with other desquamated cells, forms casts, with tubular obstruction and back-leak of tubular fluid.
- ***Tubular cellular recovery***. Tubular cells have the capacity to regenerate rapidly and to reform the disrupted tubular basement membrane, which explains the reversibility of ATN. Multiple growth factors, including insulin-like growth factor 1, epidermal growth factor and hepatocyte growth factor, and their receptors are upregulated during the regenerative process after injury.

Once established, renal blood flow is much reduced in ATN, particularly blood flow to the renal cortex. Ischaemic tubular damage contributes to a reduction in glomerular filtration as glomeruli contract through afferent arteriolar spasm, filtrate leaks back towards the glomerulus, and tubular obstruction evolves ***(Fig. 20.45)***.

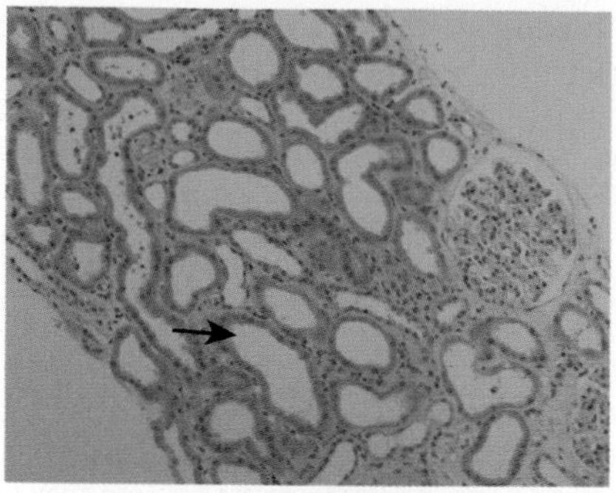

Figure 20.45 Acute tubular necrosis. Effacement and loss of the proximal tubule brush border, patchy loss of tubular cells and focal areas of proximal tubule dilatation (arrow).

Oliguria is common in the early stages; non-oliguric AKI is usually the result of a less severe renal insult. Recovery of renal function typically occurs after 7–21 days, although recovery is delayed by continuing sepsis. The use of intravenous mannitol, furosemide or 'renal-dose' dopamine is not supported by controlled trial evidence, and none of these treatments is without risk.

Clinical features of AKI

Symptoms of uraemia, such as anorexia, nausea, vomiting and pruritus, develop, followed by intellectual clouding, drowsiness, fits, coma and haemorrhagic episodes. Epistaxis and gastrointestinal haemorrhage are relatively common. ***Signs*** of the underlying insult are often obvious and infection, in particular, must be sought and excluded. Severe infection may have initiated AKI or have complicated it, owing to impaired immune defences in uraemic patients, or insertion and retention of an unnecessary bladder catheter with complicating UTI and bacteraemia.

- ***Hyperkalaemia*** is common, particularly with sepsis or muscle trauma.
- ***Metabolic acidosis*** is usual, unless hydrogen ion loss by vomiting or aspiration of gastric contents is a feature.
- ***Hyponatraemia*** may be present owing to water overload if patients have continued to drink in the face of oliguria, or if over-enthusiastic fluid replacement with 5% glucose has been carried out.
- ***Pulmonary oedema*** owing to salt and water retention is not uncommon, particularly after inappropriate attempts to initiate a diuresis by infusion of crystalloid without adequate monitoring of the patient's volume status.

Investigation of AKI

Emergency investigation

The aim is to define the AKI syndrome – pre-renal, renal or post-renal – and decide if the deterioration in function is all acute or acute-on-chronic kidney disease.

Pre-renal, renal or post-renal AKI?

Pre-renal AKI is diagnosed largely on clinical examination, and assessing the volume status is vital; it can be difficult to distinguish pre-renal and renal AKI (particularly since prolonged renal hypoperfusion will lead to ATN). Bladder outflow obstruction is ruled out by clinical examination (a large palpable bladder suggests long-standing outflow obstruction), after inserting a urethral catheter (or flushing of an existing catheter) and draining large urine volumes, or on ultrasound of the kidneys and bladder. Absence of upper tract dilatation on renal ultrasonography will, with very rare exceptions, rule out urinary tract obstruction.

Other investigations are as follows:

- Urinalysis, urine microscopy, particularly for red cells and red-cell casts (indicative of glomerulonephritis), and urine culture. Urine should be tested for free haemoglobin and myoglobin, where appropriate. Urine protein : creatinine ratio is helpful if parenchymal disease is possible.
- In AKI, it takes 48–72 h before creatinine rises in the plasma; by that time, cell injury is well established and irreversible. Urinary and plasma biomarkers (e.g. kidney injury molecule 1, neutrophil gelatinase-associated lipocalin) rise within few hours of AKI and may allow earlier treatment.
- Blood tests include measurement of serum urea, electrolytes, creatinine, calcium, phosphate, albumin, alkaline phosphatase and urate concentrations, as well as a full blood count and examination of the peripheral blood film where necessary. Coagulation studies, blood cultures and measurements of nephrotoxic drug blood levels should be carried out.

Acute or chronic uraemia?

The distinction between AKI and longstanding CKD depends on the history and duration of symptoms (a long history of nocturia suggests progressive tubular failure). Previous urinalysis or measurement of renal function is often vital in understanding the length of renal injury. Rapid changes in creatinine or GFR over days or weeks suggest an acute process.

Ultrasound is key; renal size (measured as the pole-to-pole length) and reflectivity (or echogenicity) are helpful, as small, scarred (increased echogenicity) kidneys suggest a longstanding process. The reverse is not true; the kidney may remain normal in size in diabetes and amyloidosis, for instance.

An anaemia of chronic disorder, hyperparathyroidism or renal osteodystrophy also suggests CKD.

Management of AKI

Early specialist review is advisable. Often unwell, patients with AKI should be monitored in a high-dependency setting.

General measures

Good nursing, infection control and physiotherapy are vital. Fluid balance, as intake and output (particularly urine output), will be key to recovery. Daily measurements of weight, lying and standing blood pressure, medication review to withhold nephrotoxins, collateral history and past results will all form part of the management plan.

Specific issues are described below.

Hyperkalaemia

This may be life-threatening, leading to cardiac dysrhythmias, particularly ventricular fibrillation. Treatment is outlined in ***Box 9.18***.

Intravenous sodium bicarbonate reduces potassium as it corrects acidosis but should not be used in volume-overloaded patients, as the sodium content may trigger or exacerbate pulmonary oedema. Rapid correction of acidosis in a hypocalcaemic patient may also trigger tetany (the ionized calcium fraction falls as albumin binding increases with a normalizing pH). Ion exchange resins can be used to prevent chronic hyperkalaemia, but in many patients, hyperkalaemia will be controlled only by dialysis or haemofiltration.

Pulmonary oedema

Unless a diuresis can be induced with intravenous furosemide, dialysis or haemofiltration will be required.

Sepsis

Infection needs to be treated promptly, avoiding nephrotoxic antibiotics. Use of prophylactic antibiotics or barrier nursing is not usually recommended.

Use of drugs

Nephrotoxins must be avoided and all drug dosing requires thought; GFR may be changing on a day-by-day basis and dose modification needs to follow. There is a particular risk with anticoagulants (oral and heparins; see p. 579).

Fluid and electrolyte balance

Twice-daily clinical assessment is needed. In general, once the patient is euvolaemic, daily fluid intake should equal urine output plus losses from the gut (including nasogastric loss) plus an allowance of 500 mL daily for insensible loss. Febrile patients will require an additional allowance.

Replacement fluid may be a balanced replacement solution, 0.9% saline (e.g. burns, pancreatitis) or colloids such as 4% albumin. There are no significant differences between them with respect to death rates, organ failure, the need for renal replacement therapy (RRT) or the duration of hospitalization.

Large-volume fluid infusion or changes in daily weight (reflecting changes in fluid balance) make more regular review necessary. When overload is present, loop diuretics may be useful. Non-oliguric patients with AKI fare better than oliguric patients. However, conversion of oliguria to non-oliguria has not been shown to decrease mortality, and diuretics have not been demonstrated to prevent AKI or improve outcomes.

Nutrition

Salt and potassium should be restricted. Protein intake is sometimes limited to approximately 40 g daily (0.5 g/kg/day) to avoid the need for RRT, but this poses the risk of a negative nitrogen balance. Patients on RRT are managed on a 70 g protein (and not >1.5 g/kg/day) diet, with hypercatabolic individuals requiring a greater nitrogen intake. Ideally, nutrition should be by mouth or nasogastric tube, or, as a last resort, by parenteral feeding (with sustained bowel dysfunction >14 days).

Renal replacement therapy – haemodialysis and haemofiltration

The main indications for blood purification and/or fluid removal are:

- symptomatic uraemia (including pericarditis or tamponade)
- hyperkalaemia not controlled by conservative measures
- pulmonary oedema unresponsive to diuresis
- severe acidosis
- for removal of drugs causing the AKI, e.g. gentamicin, lithium, severe aspirin overdose.

Contemporary RRT options include intermittent haemodialysis or haemodiafiltration (HDF), continuous venovenous haemofiltration (CVVHF) or peritoneal dialysis. It is not clear when to start RRT; there is some evidence that early initiation (urea <27 mmol/L) may be associated with better outcomes.

There are no data to favour haemodialysis or CVVHF as a superior mode of therapy in AKI. However, there is a consensus that in haemodynamically unstable patients, particularly those on the ITU, continuous treatments like CVVHF are more widely used for systemically unwell patients with AKI. Fluids (including nutrition, blood products or antibiotics) can be administered as volume is ultrafiltered off, preventing swings in volume and delivering more cardiovascular stability. More RRT is not necessarily better; two large trials have failed to show a survival benefit with augmented doses of RRT in critically ill patients.

Haemodialysis is explained on pages 783–784. CVVHF achieves blood flow using a blood pump to draw and return blood (hence, venovenous) from the lumen of a dual-lumen catheter placed in the jugular, subclavian or femoral vein. Ultrafiltrate (plasma in this case) is continually removed from the patient, usually at rates of up to 1000 mL/h, combined with simultaneous infusion of replacement solution. For instance, in a fluid-overloaded patient, one might remove filtrate at 1000 mL/h and replace at a rate of 900 mL/h, achieving a net fluid removal of 100 mL/h.

Peritoneal dialysis is used infrequently in the management of AKI. Peritoneal dialysis has low efficiency in AKI (removing solutes slowly and less completely), and is not appropriate for patients with intra-abdominal causes or complications of their AKI. Increasing intra-abdominal pressure as peritoneal dialysis fluid is instilled can compromise lung function as well.

Management of the recovery phase

Usually, after 1–3 weeks, renal function improves, with an increase in urine output and better kidney function. Dialysis or haemofiltration, if it has been required, can be discontinued. A characteristic recovery phase, with a large-volume diuresis, develops as GFR recovers ahead of renal tubular reabsorptive capacity for sodium, potassium and water. Intravenous fluids are often needed to support patients, with replacement sodium chloride and potassium. Typically, the diuretic phase lasts for only a few days.

Other causes of AKI

Rhabdomyolysis

Rhabdomyolysis, or 'crush syndrome', occurs when skeletal muscle injury provokes the release of intracellular myoglobin, a direct tubular toxin leading to ATN. Causes include trauma, compartment syndrome, excessive exertion (marathon runners), status epilepticus and muscle toxins (statins, malaria and antimalarials, and snake and insect venom). Rapid rises in potassium, phosphate and lactate accompany elevated muscle enzymes (aspartate aminotransferase (AST)); characteristically, creatine phosphokinase (CK) is massively elevated. Early and vigorous fluid resuscitation is vital (injured muscle sequesters large amounts of fluid, causing hypovolaemic shock). Inflamed, injured muscle may become ischaemic in compartments, and a careful examination for typical 'woody-hard' muscle compartments may suggest a need for fasciotomies to release at-risk muscle. Sodium bicarbonate used to alkalinize the urine may limit myoglobin-induced injury.

A similar syndrome can arise with massive haemolysis, where the tubular toxin is haemoglobin rather than myoglobin. As cell breakdown is on a far smaller scale, the biochemical derangements seen with muscle injury may be absent.

Acute cortical necrosis

Renal hypoperfusion results in diversion of blood flow from the cortex to the medulla, with a drop in GFR. Medullary ischaemic damage is largely reversible because tubular cells have the capacity for regeneration. In contrast, glomerular ischaemic injury does not heal with regeneration but with scarring – glomerulosclerosis.

Prolonged cortical ischaemia may lead to irreversible loss of renal function termed 'cortical necrosis'. This may be patchy or complete. Any cause of ATN, if sufficiently severe or prolonged, may lead to cortical necrosis. Cortical necrosis occurs more commonly where the vasculature and endothelium have been damaged (with or without coagulopathy), such as haemolytic uraemic syndrome and with complications of pregnancy.

Contrast nephropathy

In patients with impaired renal function, iodinated radiological contrast media may be nephrotoxic, possibly by causing renal vasoconstriction and by exerting a direct toxic effect on renal tubules. The effect is dose-dependent and more commonly seen in procedures that require large amounts of contrast, such as angiography with or without angioplasty. In many patients, the effect is mild, transient and fully reversible. However, it is not benign; even a transient elevation of creatinine following contrast administration is associated with long-term consequences (an increased risk of cardiac events, ESKD and mortality). Risk factors include:

- associated hypovolaemia
- more advanced CKD
- cardiac failure
- diabetic nephropathy
- nephrotoxins (ACE inhibitors and NSAIDs in particular).

Diabetes *per se* is not a risk factor. However, metformin can precipitate a lactic acidosis and should be stopped if creatinine is >130 μmol/L and not restarted until renal function returns to the baseline level.

Prevention is key: minimize the dose of contrast administered, use an iso-osmolar or low-osmolality contrast medium, and ensure patients are pre-hydrated with 1 L of 0.9% saline or 1 L of sodium bicarbonate 1.4% peri-procedure and up to 8–12 h post-procedure, avoiding volume overload in susceptible patients. A recently completed trial confirmed that fluid administration guided by left end-diastolic pressure was safe and more effective in the prevention of contrast-induced AKI among high-risk patients undergoing cardiac catheterization.

N-acetylcysteine (a potent antioxidant) given 48 h prior to radiological intervention may be of borderline benefit at best. Dopamine, theophylline (an adenosine antagonist) and prophylactic haemodialysis (removing contrast agent from the circulation) are of no benefit.

Acute phosphate nephropathy

Administration of oral sodium phosphate solution as bowel preparation for gastrointestinal investigations is a cause of AKI. Oral phosphate solution is contraindicated in patients with CKD, congestive heart failure, gastrointestinal obstruction, and pre-existing electrolyte disorders like hypercalcaemia. Renal biopsy shows abundant calcium phosphate deposits. Treatment is usually supportive and dialysis is carried out if necessary, with good renal recovery.

Tumour lysis syndrome

Tumour lysis syndrome (TLS; see p. 606) complicates the first treatment of lymphoproliferative tumours; it can occur spontaneously, and can be found with other cancers. Chemotherapy (or even steroids), causing rapid death of malignant cells, sees the release of intracellular and membrane products, including uric acid, potassium and phosphate. A high filtered uric acid load leads to an obstructive crystal uropathy; serum urate may be 4- or 5-fold the upper limit of normal. The danger is hyperkalaemia; at-risk patients should be pre-hydrated to maintain a good urine output (allowing large urinary potassium losses), and xanthine oxidase inhibitors such as allopurinol may prevent uric acid formation. Rasburicase, a recombinant urase oxidase that does not occur in primates, oxidizes uric acid to soluble allantoin; urate levels can be undetectable after administration.

Hepatorenal syndrome

The renal failure observed in hepatorenal syndrome (HRS) results from profound renal vasoconstriction with histologically normal kidneys (see p. 475). HRS only occurs once portal hypertension and ascites have complicated liver disease. Patients are not hypovolaemic, and renal recovery is usually observed after successful liver transplantation.

Further reading

Bellomo R, Kellum JA, Ronco C. Acute kidney injury. *Lancet* 2012; 380:756–766.
Bosch X, Esteban Poch E, Grau JM. Rhabdomyolysis and acute kidney injury. *N Engl J Med* 2009; 361:62–72.
Palevsky PM. Renal support in acute kidney injury – how much is enough? *N Engl J Med* 2009; 361:1699–1701.

CHRONIC KIDNEY DISEASE

The term 'chronic kidney disease' (CKD) has replaced terms like chronic renal failure or insufficiency. CKD is a descriptive term and is used for deteriorating kidney function of any underlying cause. CKD implies longstanding (>3 months), potentially progressive, impairment in renal function. However, in most cases of stage 1–3 CKD, kidney function does not continue to decline over time, and patients do not die as a direct result of kidney disease.

In many cases, there is no effective means to reverse the underlying disease process. There are exceptions where reversal is likely:

- relief of urinary tract obstruction
- immunosuppressive therapy for glomerulonephritis or systemic vasculitis
- treatment of accelerated hypertension
- correction of critical narrowing of renal arteries.

In many other cases of CKD, even if the underlying diagnosis cannot be fully treated, the rate of deterioration in renal function can be slowed (see p. 782). A list of causes of CKD is given in ***Box 20.32***.

Staging and prevalence

CKD is staged according to the National Kidney Foundation's Kidney Disease Outcomes Quality Initiative (K/DOQI), and endorsed by International Kidney Disease: Improving Global Outcomes (KDIGO). Staging is intended to reflect patient prognosis and outcomes ***(Fig. 20.46)***. Using this MDRD-GFR-based system (see p. 727), high prevalences of CKD are now found in population-based surveys, particularly in elderly patients ***(Box 20.33)***.

There is increasing complexity in staging:

- Stage 3 CKD may be divided into two stages, to recognize the increased disease and cardiovascular complications seen with more advanced stage 3 CKD.
- It has been advocated that cystatin C (see pp. 726–727), a more accurate marker of GFR, be used in patients with stage 3 CKD to stratify risk better in this group.
- Some bodies recommend adding measured proteinuria to the staging system, by adding the suffix 'p' to any stage if a urine protein : creatinine ratio (PCR) of >45 mg/mmol (see p. 730) or

Box 20.32 Causes of chronic kidney disease

Congenital and inherited disease
- Polycystic kidney disease (adult and infantile forms)
- Medullary cystic disease
- Tuberous sclerosis
- Oxalosis
- Cystinosis
- Congenital obstructive uropathy

Glomerular disease

Primary glomerulonephritides
- Including focal glomerulosclerosis

Secondary glomerular disease
- (Systemic lupus, polyangiitis, granulomatosis with polyangiitis, amyloidosis, diabetic glomerulosclerosis, accelerated hypertension, haemolytic uraemic syndrome, thrombotic thrombocytopenic purpura, systemic sclerosis, sickle cell disease)

Vascular disease
- Hypertensive nephrosclerosis (common in black Africans)
- Renovascular disease
- Small- and medium-sized-vessel vasculitis

Tubulointerstitial disease
- Tubulointerstitial nephritis – idiopathic, due to drugs (especially nephrotoxic analgesics), immunologically mediated
- Reflux nephropathy
- Tuberculosis
- Schistosomiasis
- Nephrocalcinosis
- Multiple myeloma (myeloma kidney)
- Balkan nephropathy
- Renal papillary necrosis (diabetes, sickle cell disease and trait, analgesic nephropathy)
- Chinese herb nephropathy

Urinary tract obstruction
- Calculus disease
- Prostatic disease
- Pelvic tumours
- Retroperitoneal fibrosis
- Schistosomiasis

albumin:creatinine ratio (ACR) of >30 mg/mmol is found – so proteinuric kidney disease with a GFR of 42 mL/min would be classed as stage 3Bp. By adding proteinuria into the classification, a more at-risk population is identified.

- Confusingly, people with stage 2 CKD are not thought to have a disease unless they have other evidence of kidney damage; this might include haematuria, proteinuria, structurally abnormal kidneys, inherited kidney diseases or biopsy changes consistent with kidney disease.

Between 6% and 11% of people can be defined as having CKD, diagnosis becoming more likely as people live longer. There is wide geographical variation in the incidence, prevalence and causes of CKD across the globe. For instance, the most common cause of glomerulonephritis in sub-Saharan Africa is malaria. Schistosomiasis is a common cause of CKD due to urinary tract obstruction in parts of the Middle East, including southern Iraq.

The incidence of ESKD varies between ethnic groups, being 3–4 times as common in black Africans in the UK and USA as it is in whites, and hypertensive nephropathy is a much more frequent cause of ESKD in this group. The prevalence of diabetes mellitus, and hence of diabetic nephropathy, is higher in some Asian groups than in whites. Age is also of relevance; CKD due to atherosclerotic renal vascular disease is much more common in the elderly than in the young. Over 70% of all cases with CKD are due to diabetes mellitus, hypertension and atherosclerosis.

Box 20.33 Prevalence of CKD

CKD stage	Age in years (% of population affected)			
	<65	*65–74*	*75–84*	*≥85*
3	1.4	15.4	29.4	30.9
4	0.04	0.4	1.3	2.4
5	0.03	0.2	0.1	0.1
Total	**1.5**	**15.9**	**30.9**	**33.4**

GFR and ACR categories and risk of adverse outcomes			Description	ACR (mg/mmol) / description		
				<3	3–30	>30
				A1	A2	A3
GFR (mL/min/1.73 m²)	≥90	G1	Normal or increased GFR with other evidence of kidney damage	No CKD markers of kidney damage		
	60–89	G2	Slight decrease in GFR with other evidence of kidney damage			
	45–59	G3a	Moderate decrease in GFR with or without other evidence of kidney damage			
	30–44	G3b	Moderate to severe increase in GFR			
	15–29	4	Severe decrease in GFR with or without other evidence of kidney damage			
	<15	5	End-stage renal disease			

Increasing risk (down the GFR categories)

Increasing risk (across the ACR categories)

Figure 20.46 Classification of chronic kidney disease using glomerular filtration rate (GFR) and albumin:creatinine (ACR) categories. CKD, chronic kidney disease. *(Adapted with permission from Kidney Disease: Improving Global Outcomes (KDIGO) CKD Work Group. KDIGO 2012 clinical practice guideline for the evaluation and management of chronic kidney disease. Kidney International 2013; (Suppl. 3):1–150.)*

Progression

CKD tends to progress to ESKD, although the rate of progression may be slow. The speed of decline tends to depend on the underlying nephropathy and on control of blood pressure. Patients with chronic glomerular diseases tend to deteriorate more quickly than those with chronic tubulointerstitial nephropathies. Regardless of cause, there may be common pathways to progression in CKD:

- Each kidney has roughly a million nephrons. In CKD, where many nephrons have failed, and scarred, the burden of filtration falls to fewer functioning nephrons.
- Functioning ('remnant') nephrons experience increased flow per nephron (hyperfiltration), as renal blood flow has not changed, and adapt with glomerular hypertrophy and reduced arteriolar resistance.
- Increased flow, increased pressure and increased shear stress set in motion a vicious circle of raised intraglomerular capillary pressure and strain, which accelerates remnant nephron failure.
- Increased flow and strain may be detected as new or increasing proteinuria.

Angiotensin II produced locally modulates intraglomerular capillary pressure and GFR, causing vasoconstriction of postglomerular arterioles, and increasing the glomerular hydraulic pressure and filtration fraction (see ***Fig. 20.44***). In addition, by its effect on mesangial cells and podocytes, it increases the pore sizes and impairs the size-selective function of basement membrane for macromolecules.

Angiotensin II also modulates cell growth directly and indirectly by upregulating transforming growth factor-beta (TGF-β), a potent fibrogenic cytokine, increasing collagen synthesis and epithelial cell transdifferentiation to myofibroblasts that contribute to excessive matrix formation. Angiotensin II also upregulates plasminogen activator inhibitor-1 (PAI-1), which inhibits matrix proteolysis by plasmin, with accumulation of excessive matrix and scarring in both the glomeruli and interstitium.

Proteinuria itself may be harmful in the tubulointerstitium. Albumin, in disease, may appear in the urinary space carrying bound fatty acids, growth factors and cytokines. When reabsorbed in the proximal tubule and degraded, these carried molecules may themselves then cause proximal tubular cell activation and interstitial scarring.

The prognosis of CKD correlates with:

- hypertension, particularly if poorly controlled
- proteinuria
- on histology, the degree of scarring in the interstitium (but not the changes seen in glomeruli).

Therapy (see ***Box 20.9***) aimed at inhibiting angiotensin II and reducing proteinuria mainly with ACE inhibitors or angiotensin-receptor antagonists offers benefit in slowing the rate of progression of CKD in both diabetic and non-diabetic renal diseases in humans.

Clinical approach to the patient with CKD and renal disease

History

- ***Duration of symptoms***.
- ***Drug ingestion***, including NSAIDs, analgesic and other medications, and unorthodox treatments such as herbal remedies.
- ***Previous medical and surgical history***, e.g. previous chemotherapy, multisystem diseases such as SLE, malaria.
- ***Previous occasions on which urinalysis or measurement of urea and creatinine might have been performed***, e.g. pre-employment or insurance medical examinations, new patient checks.
- ***Family history of renal disease***.

Clinical features

The kidneys have a great deal of reserve; as a result, the early stages of CKD are often completely asymptomatic, even as renally cleared metabolites begin to accumulate. It is not clear which metabolites lead to specific symptoms, but they are thought to be products of protein catabolism (nitrogenous waste products). These metabolites, also called uraemic toxins, must be of relatively small molecular size (since haemodialysis, which clears only relatively small molecules, improves symptoms). Little else is known with certainty.

Serum urea and creatinine concentrations are measured in CKD as surrogates of accumulating metabolites (uraemic toxins) because their measurement is easy, and there is a rough correlation between urea and creatinine concentrations and symptoms. These substances are not, however, particularly toxic in themselves.

Symptoms are common when the serum urea concentration exceeds 40 mmol/L but many patients develop uraemic symptoms at lower levels of serum urea. Symptoms include:

- malaise, loss of energy
- loss of appetite, loss of weight
- insomnia
- nocturia and polyuria due to impaired concentrating ability
- itching
- nausea, vomiting and diarrhoea
- paraesthesiae due to polyneuropathy
- 'restless legs' syndrome (the overwhelming need to alter the position of the lower limbs frequently)
- bone pain due to metabolic bone disease
- paraesthesiae and tetany due to hypocalcaemia
- symptoms due to salt and water retention – peripheral or pulmonary oedema
- symptoms due to anaemia
- amenorrhoea in women; erectile dysfunction in men.

In more advanced uraemia CKD stage 5, these symptoms become more severe and central nervous system symptoms are common:

- mental slowing, clouding of consciousness and seizures
- myoclonic twitching.

Urine volume is not a good symptom of advancing CKD. Oliguria is a powerful symptom of sudden kidney injury, but slowly progressive kidney disease can see urine volume actually increase, as failing tubular function leads to a salt- and water-wasting state. As concentrating ability in the tubules fails, urine volume increases through day and night, and so polyuria and nocturia are useful symptoms to suggest the length of time for which CKD has been present.

Examination

There are few physical signs specific to uraemia. Findings include short stature (in patients who have had CKD in childhood); pallor (due to anaemia); increased photosensitive pigmentation (which may make the patient look misleadingly healthy); brown discoloration of the nails; scratch marks due to uraemic pruritus; signs of fluid overload (see p. 773); pericardial friction rub; flow murmurs (mitral regurgitation due to mitral annular calcification; aortic and pulmonary regurgitant murmurs due to volume overload); and glove and stocking peripheral sensory loss (rare).

The kidneys themselves are usually impalpable unless grossly enlarged as a result of polycystic disease, obstruction or tumour. Rectal and vaginal examination may disclose evidence of an underlying cause of CKD, particularly urinary obstruction, and should always be performed.

In addition to these findings, there may be physical signs of any underlying disease that may have caused the CKD, for instance:

- cutaneous vasculitic lesions in systemic vasculitides
- retinopathy in diabetes and hypertensive retinopathy in hypertension
- evidence of peripheral vascular disease and associated renal artery stenosis
- evidence of spina bifida or other causes of neurogenic bladder.

An assessment of the central venous pressure, skin turgor, blood pressure both lying and standing and peripheral circulation should also be made. The major symptoms and signs of CKD are shown in ***Figure 20.47***.

Investigations

The following investigations are common to all renal patients. This includes individuals with glomerular or non-glomerular disease, renal involvement in systemic diseases, AKI and CKD, as renal symptoms and signs are non-specific.

Urinalysis

- ***Haematuria*** may indicate glomerulonephritis but other sources must be excluded. Haematuria should not be assumed to be due to the presence of an indwelling catheter.

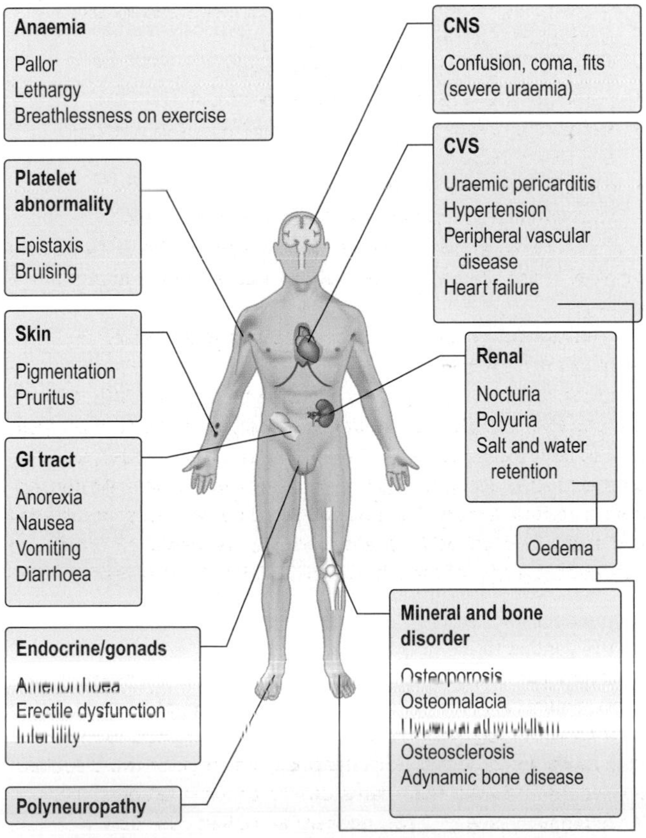

Figure 20.47 Symptoms and signs of chronic kidney disease. Oedema may be due to a combination of primary renal salt and water retention and heart failure.

- ***Proteinuria***, if heavy, is strongly suggestive of glomerular disease. Urinary infection may also cause proteinuria. ***Glycosuria*** with normal blood glucose is common in CKD.
- ***Leucocytes or nitrites***, if present, might suggest infection.

Urine microscopy

(See pp. 729–730.)

- ***White cells*** in the urine usually indicate active bacterial urinary infection but this is an uncommon cause of CKD; sterile pyuria suggests papillary necrosis or renal tuberculosis.
- ***Eosinophiluria*** is strongly suggestive of allergic tubulointerstitial nephritis or cholesterol emboli.
- ***Granular casts*** are formed from abnormal cells within the tubular lumen and indicate active renal disease. ***Red-cell casts*** are highly suggestive of glomerulonephritis.
- ***Red cells in the urine*** may be from anywhere between the glomerulus and the urethral meatus (see ***Fig. 20.7***).

Urine biochemistry

- ***Proteinuria*** is a key finding, and urine PCR or ACR should be performed on an early morning sample (see p. 730).
- ***Urinary electrolytes*** are unhelpful in CKD. The use of urinary sodium concentration in the distinction between pre-renal and intrinsic renal disease is discussed on pages 770–771.
- ***Urine osmolality*** is a measure of concentrating ability. A low urine osmolality is normal in the presence of a high fluid intake but indicates renal disease when the kidney should be concentrating urine, such as in hypovolaemia or hypotension.
- ***Urine electrophoresis and immunofixation*** is necessary for the detection of light chains, which can be present in myeloma without a detectable serum paraprotein.

Serum biochemistry

- ***Urea, electrolytes, bicarbonate and creatinine*** are measured.
- ***Calculation of eGFR*** is performed.
- ***Electrophoresis and immunofixation*** are carried out, and ***free light chains*** for myeloma.
- ***Elevations of creatine kinase and a disproportionate elevation in serum creatinine and potassium*** compared with urea suggest rhabdomyolysis.
- ***Blood glucose and HbA1C*** estimate chronic diabetic control.

Haematology

- ***Eosinophilia*** suggests vasculitis, allergic tubulointerstitial nephritis or cholesterol embolism.
- ***Markedly raised viscosity*** or ESR suggests myeloma or vasculitis.
- ***Fragmented red cells and/or thrombocytopenia*** suggest intravascular haemolysis due to accelerated hypertension, haemolytic uraemic syndrome or thrombotic thrombocytopenic purpura.
- ***Tests for sickle cell disease*** should be performed when relevant.

Immunology

- ***Complement components*** may be low in active renal disease due to SLE, mesangiocapillary glomerulonephritis, post-streptococcal glomerulonephritis, and cryoglobulinaemia.
- ***Autoantibody screening*** is useful in detection of SLE (see pp. 692–695), scleroderma (p. 695–697), granulomatosis with

polyangiitis and microscopic polyangiitis (p. 1121), and Goodpasture syndrome (p. 1121).
- ***Cryoglobulins*** are measured in unexplained glomerular disease, particularly mesangiocapillary glomerulonephritis.
- ***Antibodies to streptococcal antigens*** (antistreptolysin O titre (ASOT), anti-DNAse B) are sought if post-streptococcal glomerulonephritis is possible.
- ***Antibodies to hepatitis B and C*** may point to polyarteritis or membranous nephropathy (hepatitis B) or to cryoglobulinaemic renal disease (hepatitis C).
- ***Antibodies to HIV*** raise the possibility of HIV-associated renal disease.

Radiological investigation

- ***Ultrasound*** should be performed in every patient (to establish renal size and exclude hydronephrosis).
- ***CT*** is useful for the diagnosis of calculi, retroperitoneal fibrosis and some other causes of urinary obstruction, and may also demonstrate cortical scarring.
- ***Magnetic resonance angiography*** is carried out in renovascular disease.

Renal biopsy

(See p. 732.) This should be performed in every person with unexplained CKD and normal-sized kidneys, unless there are strong contraindications. If rapidly progressive glomerulonephritis is possible, this investigation must be performed within 24 hours of presentation, if at all possible.

Complications of CKD

Anaemia

Anaemia in CKD impairs quality of life and well-being. A normochromic, normocytic anaemia develops by a number of mechanisms:
- ***Erythropoietin deficiency*** – this is the most significant mechanism.
- ***Increased blood loss*** – there may be occult gastrointestinal bleeding, repeated blood sampling, blood loss during haemodialysis, or platelet dysfunction.
- ***Bone marrow toxins*** – these are retained in CKD, or there is fibrosis secondary to hyperparathyroidism.
- ***Haematinic deficiency*** – there may be decreased iron, vitamin B_{12} or folate.
- ***Increased red-cell destruction*** – red cells have a shortened lifespan in uraemia, and haemodialysis itself may cause a degree of haemolysis.
- ***ACE inhibitors*** – these may cause anaemia in CKD, probably by interfering with the control of endogenous erythropoietin release.

Management

Synthetic (recombinant) human erythropoiesis stimulating agents (ESAs; epoetin-α or β, or the longer-acting darbepoetin-α) have transformed the management of renal anaemia. ESAs can be given subcutaneously or by intravenous injection, at a starting dose of 50 U/kg of epoetin-α three times weekly, or darbepoetin 30 μg weekly. Supplemental intravenous iron may promote a response to erythropoietin and can be given prior to starting ESAs. Haemoglobin is then measured every 2 weeks, and the dose adjusted to maintain a target haemoglobin of 100–120 g/L (see below). As hypertension can be a significant side-effect in 30% of patients new to ESAs, blood pressure should be monitored in the first 6 months, and treated if rising. Peripheral resistance increases in all patients, owing to loss of hypoxic vasodilatation and to an increase in blood viscosity. The rare complication of encephalopathy with fits, transient cortical blindness and hypertension can complicate treatment.

Targets and treatment are as follows:
- ***Target haemoglobin*** is between 100 and 120 g/L. Studies in pre-dialysis CKD patients have not shown any outcome benefits in patients who were treated to achieve higher haemoglobin targets (>120 g/L).
- Patients who ***fail to respond*** to 300 U/kg weekly of epoetin-α should be screened to exclude associated iron deficiency, bleeding, malignancy, infection, inflammation, or formation of anti-erythropoietin neutralizing antibodies.
- The increased demand for iron by the bone marrow is enormous when an ESA is started. Functional iron deficiency (poor mobilization of iron, despite adequate iron stores with ferritin >500 μg/L) is a common finding in patients with chronic inflammation. Hepcidin synthesis, as an acute phase reactant produced by the liver in response to cytokines (particularly IL-6), inhibits gastrointestinal iron absorption (see p. 524) and sequesters iron in the liver, preventing its release. Intravenous (rather than oral) iron supplements optimize the response to ESAs in CKD.
- Correcting anaemia with ESAs improves quality of life, exercise tolerance, and sexual and cognitive function in dialysis patients, and leads to regression of left ventricular hypertrophy. By avoiding blood transfusion, the risk is minimized of sensitization to HLA antigens, which may complicate future renal transplantation.
- Several reports of anti-erythropoietin antibody-mediated pure red-cell aplasia in patients receiving subcutaneous ESA therapy (particularly epoetin-α) have been described. Changes in the manufacturing process of the pre-filled syringes used to deliver ESAs have reduced the number of cases; the rubber stoppers interacted with the drug vehicle to act as an immunological adjuvant, stimulating anti-erythropoietin antibody production in hosts.

Several novel erythropoiesis-stimulating agents are in clinical trials. An engineered peptide that stimulates the erythropoietin receptor has been withdrawn because of anaphylaxis in a few patients. Oral agents that inhibit prolyl hydroxylase and prolong the life of hypoxia inducible factors (HIF) 1α, a transcription factor for endogenous production of erythropoietin, have shown promise in phase 2 trials.

CKD mineral and bone disorder

Once called 'renal osteodystrophy' but now more appropriately described as a mineral and bone disorder, CKD-MBD describes:
- changes in calcium, phosphorus, PTH and vitamin D metabolism
- the various forms of bone disease that may develop alone or in combination in CKD
- the vascular consequences that accompany it.

Altered bone morphology might be described in CKD ***(Fig. 20.48)*** as:
- hyperparathyroid bone disease
- osteomalacia
- osteoporosis
- osteosclerosis
- adynamic bone disease.

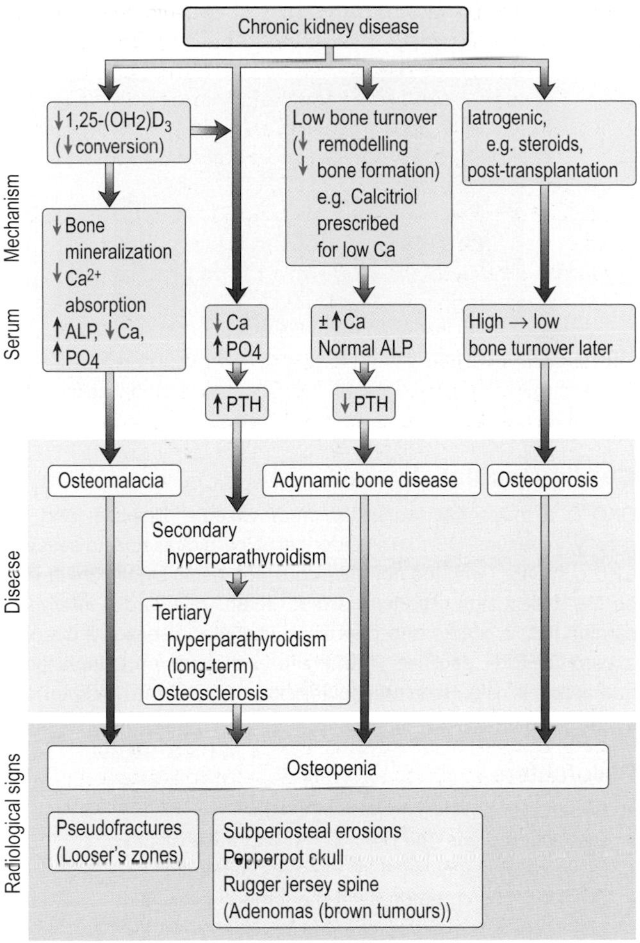

Figure 20.48 Chronic kidney disease mineral and bone disorder (CKD-MB). Pathogenesis and radiological features of renal bone disease. ALP, alkaline phosphatase; PTH, parathyroid hormone.

Most patients with CKD are found on bone biopsy to have mixed bone disease. CKD-MBD is almost universal by late stage 3 CKD. Vascular calcification is common in CKD patients; it is speculated that vascular smooth muscle cells, modulated by uraemia and/or phosphate, differentiate to an osteoblast-like phenotype, able to synthesize and deposit matrix, which is then mineralized. Calcified vessel walls become increasingly stiff and non-compliant (leading to left ventricular hypertrophy over time), cardiac valves calcify, and soft-tissue calcium is deposited widely. There is an association between vascular calcification and mortality in CKD but a causal link has not yet been proved.

Pathogenesis of CKD-MBD

Phosphate excretion falls in the very early stages of CKD. Retained phosphate then results in the release of fibroblast growth factor 23 (FGF23) and other phosphaturic agents by osteoblasts as a compensatory mechanism (see p. 171). FGF23 causes phosphaturia to bring the plasma phosphate level to within the normal range. FGF23 also downregulates renal 1α-hydroxylase, reducing the action of activated vitamin D in increasing intestinal absorption of phosphate. Despite consistently elevated levels of FGF23, phosphate levels in blood will once again rise as CKD progresses. Elevated FGF23 levels are the strongest independent predictor of mortality in patients with CKD. This underscores the necessity of controlling phosphate levels during the very early stages of CKD.

As CKD progresses, *secondary hyperparathyroidism* develops:

- Decreased renal production of 1α-hydroxylase results in reduced conversion of 25-$(OH)_2D_3$ to the more metabolically active 1,25-$(OH)_2D_3$ (1,25-dihydroxycholecalciferol).
- 1,25-$(OH)_2D_3$ deficiency results in reduced gut calcium absorption and a fall in calcium.
- Reduced activation of vitamin D receptors in the parathyroid glands by 1,25-$(OH)_2D_3$ increases the release of PTH.
- Calcium-sensing receptors, expressed in the parathyroid glands, react rapidly to acute changes in extracellular calcium concentrations, and a low calcium triggers increased PTH release.
- Retained phosphate also indirectly lowers ionized calcium (and probably directly via a putative but unrecognized phosphate receptor), resulting in increased PTH synthesis and release.
- PTH promotes reabsorption of calcium from bone and increased proximal renal tubular reabsorption of calcium. This mechanism attempts to reverse the hypocalcaemia caused by 1,25-$(OH)_2D_3$ deficiency and phosphate retention.

This 'secondary' hyperparathyroidism leads to increased osteoclastic activity, cyst formation and bone marrow fibrosis (osteitis fibrosa cystica). The typical biochemical findings are hypocalcaemia, hyperphosphataemia, an elevated PTH and a raised serum alkaline phosphatase (as a marker of increased bone turnover). Radiologically, digital subperiosteal erosions and a 'pepperpot skull' are seen. Longstanding secondary hyperparathyroidism ultimately leads to hyperplasia of the glands with autonomous or ***tertiary hyperparathyroidism***. PTH release now occurs independently of calcium or 1,25-$(OH)_2D_3$ control, and high turnover in bone leads to hypercalcaemia.

Longstanding hyperparathyroidism causes increased bone density (***osteosclerosis***), seen particularly in the spine, where alternating bands of sclerotic and porotic bone give rise to a characteristic 'rugger jersey' appearance on X-ray.

Deficiency of 1,25-$(OH)_2D_3$ and hypocalcaemia can also result in impaired mineralization of osteoid (***osteomalacia***).

'***Adynamic bone disease***' describes a state in which both bone formation and resorption are depressed and the skeleton becomes inert. Bone turnover is reduced, usually where there is overtreatment with active vitamin D, low PTH (after surgical parathyroidectomy), accumulation of aluminium used as a phosphate binder, or diabetes. There may be hypercalcaemia, particularly if calcium intake is high (excess calcium cannot be laid down in bone); the serum alkaline phosphatase is normal and the PTH is low. X-rays and dual X-ray absorptiometry (DXA) scans show osteopenia. No treatment is of proven benefit.

Osteoporosis is commonly found in CKD, often after transplantation and the use of corticosteroids. Monitoring is with yearly DXA scanning.

Management of CKD-MBD

The aim is to keep serum calcium and phosphate in the normal range as CKD progresses, and once dialysis is needed, to control PTH within 2- to 9-fold the upper limit of normal. This is to ensure that bone turnover continues and adynamic bone does not develop (see above). The less well-understood goal is to limit vascular calcification as well, by maintaining good bone health and avoiding calcium exposure.

Calcium, phosphate and PTH should be measured 3-monthly, and some would define the extent of vascular calcification (e.g. by X-ray of the lumbar spine or of the abdomen). Treatment and targets, then, aim to reduce phosphate (and preferably limit calcium load), and to control PTH and achieve a normal calcium.

Reduction of phosphate and limiting of calcium load

- ***Dietary restriction***. This is seldom effective alone because so many foods are phosphate-rich
- ***Gut phosphate binders***. Sevelamer carbonate, lanthanum carbonate, calcium carbonate and calcium acetate all reduce phosphate absorption and serum phosphate levels when taken with meals. Sevelamer (unlike calcium-containing binders) attenuates vascular calcification and lowers cholesterol levels by 10%; it has not been shown to reduce mortality.
- ***Aluminium-containing gut phosphate binders***. These are very effective but absorption of aluminium poses the risk of aluminium bone disease and development of cognitive impairment. They are rarely used in the developed countries but are still employed in developing countries because they are extremely cheap.
- ***Nicotinamide***. An alternative to phosphate binders, nicotinamide blocks the intestinal sodium/inorganic phosphate (Na/Pi) co-transporter. It reduces phosphate levels and PTH levels alongside improvement in the lipid profile in dialysis patients.

Control of PTH and achievement of normal calcium

- ***Calcitriol (1,25-dihydroxycholecalciferol), vitamin D analogues*** such as alfacalcidol, or novel vitamin D metabolites (22-oxacalcitriol, paricalcitol, doxercalciferol). These are given orally to suppress PTH once the level is three times or more above the upper limit of normal. Newer vitamin D analogues, such as paricalcitol (19-nor-1,25 dihydroxyvitamin D_2), may be less likely to lead to hypercalcaemia, but their usefulness over the conventional but less expensive calcitriol or alfacalcidol remains to be established.
- ***Calcimimetic agents*** (e.g. cinacalcet, a calcium-sensing receptor agonist; see p. 1237). These have also been tried in established secondary hyperparathyroidism with successful suppression of PTH levels and lowering of calcium × phosphate product. Calcimimetics act by activating the calcium-sensing receptor, leading the parathyroid to respond as though serum calcium levels were high, reducing PTH synthesis and release. The long-term safety and efficacy of these agents have been confirmed; however, a recent controlled trial to assess potential survival benefits on treatment was non-conclusive.

Calciphylaxis

Also known as calcific uraemic arteriolopathy, this is a rare but serious life-threatening complication in CKD patients. It presents as painful skin patches, plaques and ulcers, with non-healing eschars, panniculitis and dermal necrosis. The characteristic feature on histology is vascular calcification and superimposed small-vessel thrombosis ***(Fig. 20.49)***. Risk factors include hyperparathyroidism, elevated serum phosphate, morbid obesity and warfarin use. Control of hyperparathyroidism is either with surgical intervention or with a calcimimetic agent, aiming to drop both calcium and phosphate to low–normal ranges. Despite treatment, subsequent infection escalates the risk, as patients are often already frail, and many die within a year of diagnosis.

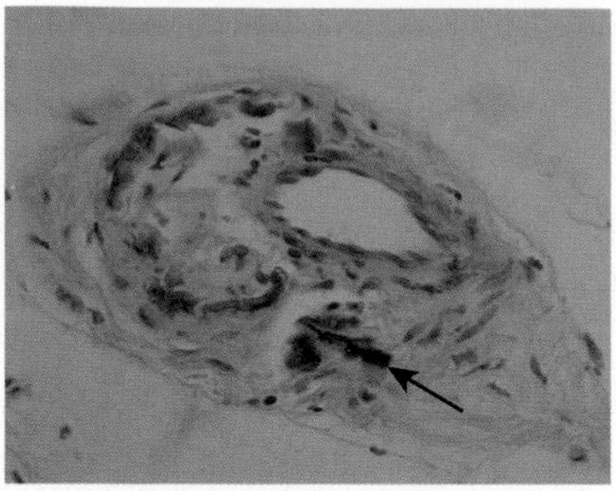

Figure 20.49 Calciphylaxis. Characteristic arterial calcification of the skin microvasculature in the absence of vasculitic change (arrow).

Cardiovascular disease

CKD is a major risk factor for cardiovascular disease, and the greatly increased (16-fold) incidence of cardiovascular disease in CKD compared with the normal population has a significant impact on life expectancy. Sudden cardiac death, myocardial infarction, cardiac failure, stroke and peripheral vascular disease all occur in excess as GFR declines (and the presence of proteinuria adds further to this risk). Renal transplantation reverses the risk seen with stage 5 CKD.

Risk factors

- Hypertension (very common in CKD).
- Diabetes mellitus (the most common cause of CKD).
- Dyslipidaemia (universal in uraemic patients).
- Smoking – as common as in the general population.
- Male gender – over-represented in patients with CKD.

Also clustering with CKD, ventricular hypertrophy is common, as is systolic and diastolic dysfunction. Left ventricular hypertrophy is a risk factor for early death in CKD, as in the general population. Systolic dysfunction is also a marker for early death. Myocardial fibrosis, abnormal myocyte function, calcium overload and hyperparathyroidism, and carnitine and selenium deficiencies all contribute to the systolic dysfunction seen with the uraemic cardiomyopathy.

Coronary artery and generalized vascular calcification

Traditional risk factors (e.g. smoking, diabetes) only partly explain the increased cardiovascular risk in patients with CKD. Coronary artery calcification is more common in patients with ESKD than in normal individuals and it is likely that this contributes to cardiovascular mortality. Peripheral vessel calcification ***increases vascular stiffness*** (***reduced compliance***), which manifests as increased pulse pressure, increased pulse wave velocity, and an increased afterload with advancing left ventricular hypertrophy. Risk factors related to calcification include the following:

- ***A raised (calcium × phosphate) product*** promotes calcification.
- ***Hyperparathyroidism*** increases intracellular calcium.
- ***Uraemia leads to loss of constitutive inhibitors of calcification***, with vascular smooth muscle cells acquiring osteoblast-like characteristics.
- ***Inflammation*** further inhibits fetuin (a glycoprotein synthesized by liver, and a potent inhibitor of vascular calcification).

Plain abdominal X-ray (demonstrating 'pipe-stem' calcification of large arteries), electron beam or multislice CT of the coronaries, and vascular Doppler can all identify and quantify vascular calcification.

Risk factor modification is similar to that undertaken in patients without CKD, although clear evidence of benefit is less obvious.

Other cardiovascular risk factors

Hyperhomocysteinaemia, *Chlamydophila pneumoniae* infection, malnutrition, inflammation, insulin resistance, oxidative stress and elevated endogenous inhibitor of nitric oxide synthase and asymmetric dimethyl arginine (ADMA) all contribute to increased cardiovascular events. High ADMA levels in uraemia are caused, in part, by oxidative stress and can possibly explain the 52% increase in the risk of death and 34% increase in the risk of cardiovascular events in uraemic patients. The use of antioxidants, vitamin E or acetylcysteine has been associated with a significant reduction in all-cause and cardiovascular mortality. However, trials to reduce levels of homocysteine with folic acid, B_6 and B_{12} supplementation have been unsuccessful.

The conclusion from a study of heart and renal protection (SHARP) in over 9500 CKD patients was that around one-quarter of all heart attacks, strokes and revascularizations could be avoided in CKD by using a combination of ezetimibe and simvastatin to lower blood cholesterol. This combination did not, however, confer any survival advantage or prevent the development of ESKD.

Pericarditis

This is common and occurs in two clinical settings:

- Uraemic pericarditis is a feature of severe, pre-terminal uraemia or of under-dialysis. Haemorrhagic pericardial effusion and atrial arrhythmias are often associated. There is a danger of pericardial tamponade, and anticoagulants should be used with caution. Pericarditis usually resolves with intensive dialysis.
- Dialysis pericarditis occurs as a result of an intercurrent illness or surgery in a patient receiving apparently adequate dialysis.

Skin disease

Pruritus (itching) is common, and is caused by:

- accumulating nitrogenous waste products of protein catabolism (and itching improves following dialysis)
- hypercalcaemia and hyperphosphataemia
- an elevated calcium × phosphate product
- hyperparathyroidism (even if calcium and phosphate levels are normal)
- iron deficiency.

In dialysis patients, inadequate dialysis is a treatable cause of pruritus. However, for many, the cause of itching is unknown and no effective treatment exists.

Many patients with CKD suffer from dry skin, for which simple aqueous creams are helpful. CKD may also cause porphyria cutanea tarda (PCT), a blistering, photosensitive skin rash. This results from a decrease in hepatic uroporphyrinogen decarboxylase combined with a decreased clearance of porphyrins in the urine or by dialysis. Pseudoporphyria, a condition similar to PCT but without enzyme deficiency, is also seen in CKD with increased frequency.

Nephrogenic systemic fibrosis

See ***Box 20.34***.

> **Box 20.34 Nephrogenic systemic fibrosis (NSF)**
>
> NSF is a systemic fibrosing skin disorder seen only in patients with moderate to severe CKD (eGFR <30 mL/min), particularly those on dialysis. Gadolinium-containing contrast agents, which are excreted exclusively by the kidney, have been implicated in the causation of over 95% cases of NSF (see p. 1365).
>
> The ***diagnosis*** is based on biopsy of an involved site, showing proliferation of dermal fibrocytes with excessive collagen deposition. Special testing may show gadolinium.
>
> NSF is chronic and unremitting, with 30% having no improvement, 20% having modest improvement and 30% dying. No single or combination therapy offers benefit, except for improving renal function following transplantation. ***Prevention*** is key, so gadolinium-based contrast agents should be avoided in patents with eGFR <30 mL/min or those on dialysis.

Gastrointestinal complications

Decreased gastric emptying, and an increased risk of reflux oesophagitis, gastritis and peptic ulceration are all common (hypergastrinaemia increases as GFR declines); gastrointestinal tract bleeding is more frequently seen as a result. Constipation is particularly common in patients on continuous ambulatory peritoneal dialysis (CAPD).

Acute pancreatitis occurs more frequently, though elevations of serum amylase of up to three times normal may be found in CKD without any evidence of pancreatic disease, owing to retention of high-molecular-weight forms of amylase normally excreted in the urine.

Metabolic abnormalities

Gout

Urate is retained as GFR declines, and many drugs used to manage CKD increase the risk of gout. Nephrotoxic NSAIDs are less useful in treatment, though colchicine is useful for the acute attack. Reduced-dose allopurinol is effective in the prevention of further attacks.

Insulin

Insulin is catabolized by, and to some extent excreted via, the kidneys. Moreover, renal glucose production is diminished with progressive CKD. For these reasons, insulin requirements in diabetic patients decrease as CKD progresses. By contrast, end-organ resistance to insulin is a feature of advanced CKD, resulting in modestly impaired glucose tolerance. Insulin resistance may contribute to hypertension and lipid abnormalities.

Lipid metabolism

Abnormalities in lipid metabolism are common in CKD and include:

- impaired clearance of triglyceride-rich particles
- hypercholesterolaemia (particularly in advanced CKD).

The situation is further complicated in ESKD, when regular heparinization (in haemodialysis), excessive glucose absorption (in CAPD) and immunosuppressive drugs (in transplantation) may all contribute to lipid abnormalities.

Endocrine abnormalities

These include:

- Hyperprolactinaemia, which may present with galactorrhoea in men as well as women.
- Decreased serum testosterone levels (only seldom below the normal level). Loss of libido, erectile dysfunction and decreased spermatogenesis are common.

- Menstrual irregularities, oligomenorrhoea or amenorrhoea (very few women on dialysis will have periods), which are common, as is loss of libido (see p. 1175).
- Complex abnormalities of growth hormone secretion and action, resulting in impaired growth in uraemic children (pharmacological treatment with recombinant growth hormone and insulin-like growth factor is used)
- Altered protein binding (and increased thyroid-binding globulin loss with proteinuria). These make thyroid function tests difficult to interpret. Thyroid-stimulating hormone (TSH) is the best test of thyroid function. True hypothyroidism occurs with increased frequency in CKD.

Posterior pituitary gland function is normal in CKD.

Muscle dysfunction

Uraemia appears to interfere with muscle energy metabolism but the mechanism is uncertain. Decreased physical fitness (cardiovascular deconditioning) also contributes.

Nervous system abnormalities

Uraemia affects the ***central nervous system*** as depressed cerebral function, a decreased seizure threshold, asterixis, tremor and myoclonus. Anxiety, depression and impaired cognition also occur. In people with profound uraemia, and high blood urea prior to their first dialysis, the sudden correction of urea can cause ***dialysis disequilibrium*** (urea does not equilibrate rapidly across the blood–brain barrier and, as blood urea falls on dialysis in advance of central nervous system urea, rapid movement of water into the higher-urea environment within the central nervous system leads to osmotic cerebral swelling and even fits). This can be avoided by correcting uraemia gradually by short, repeated haemodialysis treatments or by the use of peritoneal dialysis.

Increased circulating catecholamines lead to downregulation of α-receptors, impaired baroreceptor sensitivity and impaired efferent vagal function in the ***autonomic nervous system***. Overactivity of the sympathetic nervous system may contribute to the hypertension seen in CKD. These abnormalities correct to some extent with regular dialysis, and resolve after successful renal transplantation.

Peripherally, median nerve compression in the carpal tunnel is common, usually due to β_2-microglobulin-related amyloidosis (see p. 1289). Advanced uraemia leads to a symmetrical polyneuropathy (which may recur in inadequately dialysed patients).

Management of CKD

General measures

- As always, make a diagnosis, and treat any modifiable underlying cause.
- Address cardiovascular risk factors – in particular, smoking cessation, exercise and weight loss.
- Avoid nephrotoxic drugs (see below).
- Arrange systematic follow-up, depending on the stage of CKD, to identify those most likely to progress ***early***.

As stage 3 CKD progresses to stage 4 CKD, attention should be paid to correcting the complications described above: anaemia, CKD-MDB and metabolic abnormalities. Primary prevention of cardiovascular disease is a major part of CKD management at this stage.

Renoprotection

The multidrug approach to chronic nephropathies has been formalized in an international protocol (see ***Box 20.9***).

Correction of specific complications

Hyperkalaemia often responds to dietary restriction of potassium intake. Drugs that cause potassium retention (see p. 168) should be stopped. Occasionally, it may be necessary to prescribe ion-exchange resins to remove potassium in the gastrointestinal tract. Two new orally active drugs, patiromer and sodium zirconium cyclosilicate, have been successful in controlling hyperkalaemia in phase 3 trials and will be available soon for use in clinical practice. Emergency treatment of severe hyperkalaemia is described on page 168.

Correction of acidosis helps to address hyperkalaemia in CKD and may also decrease muscle catabolism. Sodium bicarbonate supplements are effective (4.8 g (57 mmol) of Na^+ and HCO_3^- daily), without significant risk of oedema or hypertension. Correcting metabolic acidosis with sodium bicarbonate at a mean dose of 1.8 g/day also reduces the rate of decline of GFR (slowing progression) in advanced (stage 4 and 5) CKD. Calcium carbonate, also used as a calcium supplement and phosphate binder, has a beneficial effect on acidosis.

Drug therapy should be reviewed and nephrotoxins avoided in patients with CKD. These include:

- Tetracyclines (with the possible exception of doxycycline).
- Drugs excreted by the kidneys, such as gentamicin. These should be prescribed only in the absence of any alternative, and drug levels monitored if feasible.
- NSAIDs.
- Potassium-sparing agents, such as spironolactone and amiloride. These pose particular dangers, as do artificial salt substitutes, all of which contain potassium.

Antibiotics, anticoagulants (particularly anti-thrombin oral anticoagulants, which currently lack a practical monitoring measurement of effect), beta-blockers, oral hypoglycaemics, insulin, antidepressants and analgesics (particularly opioids, which can accumulate, leading to an opiate narcosis) often need dose adjustment when prescribed for patients with CKD.

Early referral

Patients need time to adjust to the demands of CKD and its treatment, and to absorb information. Those who share in the decisions about their care, who are able to understand and choose treatments, make the best transition to dialysis or transplantation. As GFR declines below 20 mL/min/1.73 m^2, a dedicated team should counsel patients as to their diet, review medication, encourage risk factor modification, and support men and women to RRT (or the choice not to undertake dialysis).

If the patient opts for regular haemodialysis, an arteriovenous fistula should be fashioned well in advance of the need for dialysis (when serum creatinine is in the order of 400–500 μmol/L in non-diabetics, and at an even earlier stage in diabetics with poorer vasculature). Such fistulae require several weeks to mature and become usable for vascular access. Veins required for future arteriovenous fistulae should not be rendered useless by cannulation ***(Fig. 20.50)***. Patients choosing peritoneal dialysis might have a buried catheter placed and left subcutaneously for some time, able to be externalized on the day dialysis starts.

Where suitable, patients should be offered and prepared for ***pre-emptive living donor transplantation*** as the best option for RRT.

Renal replacement therapy

About 3 million people across the globe either are treated by haemodialysis or peritoneal dialysis, or live with a functioning renal

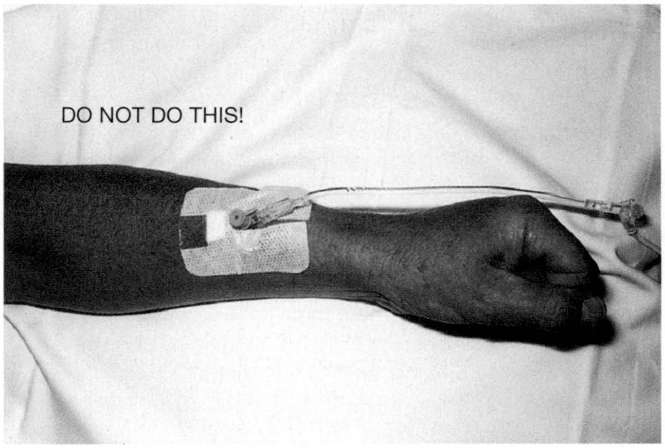

Figure 20.50 Intravenous cannula in exactly the WRONG place. The cannula is shown in a right-handed patient with CKD, who will, in future, need a left (non-dominant arm) radiocephalic fistula.

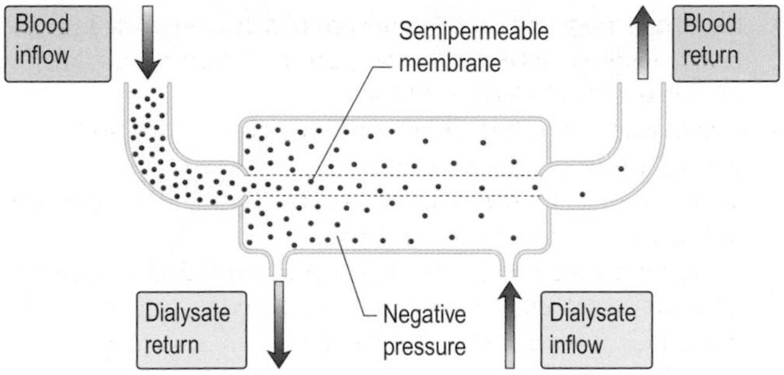

Figure 20.51 Changes across a semipermeable dialysis membrane.

transplant. In the UK, around 53 000 people receive treatment for ESKD; around 50% have been transplanted, 42% are on haemodialysis and 8% are on peritoneal dialysis. Dialysis aims to mimic the excretory function of normal kidneys by:

- eliminating (nitrogenous and small molecular) wastes
- maintaining normal electrolyte concentrations
- preventing systemic acidosis
- maintaining a normal extracellular volume.

Box 20.35 Range of concentrations in routinely available final dialysates used for haemodialysis

Dialysate	Range of concentration (mmol/L)
Sodium	130–145
Potassium	0.0–4.0
Calcium	1.0–1.6
Magnesium	0.25–0.85
Chloride	99–108
Bicarbonate	35–40
Glucose	0–10

Initiation of dialysis

It is not widely agreed *when* to start dialysis in patients with stage 5 CKD, and trials have suggested that early initiation of dialysis is not associated with improved survival or clinical outcomes. There is a general tendency to start dialysis at an eGFR closer to 15 mL/min rather then below 10 mL/min, but this decision is best shared with an individual patient, taking into account symptoms and life plans.

An informed choice

Many people, particularly if they are frail or living with other co-morbidities, will choose not to undergo RRT if able to make a shared, informed decision with their physician and families. For some, the *quantity* of extended life offered by dialysis is not matched by the perceived impact on the *quality* of their lives. For others, events and complications of dialysis can make the daily experience of treatment difficult to endure, and they may choose to withdraw from dialysis. Support through their last illness, good symptom control, and respect for the individual's informed choices can allow patients a comfortable end of life after a period of long illness.

A difficult choice

Across the globe, RRT (like other treatments) can be an expensive option. For many societies, health resources may be allocated to other pressing priorities, or may be available for a defined time period only, or one form of RRT may be preferred over others. The drive for more cost-effective and low-technology solutions to treat renal failure is a pressing need for the specialty worldwide.

Haemodialysis

Basic principles

Anticoagulated blood from a patient is pumped around an extracorporeal circuit and through a biocompatible, semipermeable membrane (the dialyser, or 'artificial kidney') before being returned to the circulation. In the dialyser, ultrapure dialysate flowing in the opposite direction is in close contact with blood. Small solutes (but not cells and larger-molecular-weight proteins) can cross the membrane, and move by diffusion down a concentration gradient ***(Fig. 20.51)***. A transmembrane pressure allows controlled fluid removal by ultrafiltration (and with fluid, more solute removal by convection). Over a standard 4-hour session, up to 80 L of blood (at around 300 mL/min) is circulated through the dialyser; even so, this only provides an equivalent GFR of 10–12 mL/min/m^2. ***Box 20.35*** describes a typical dialysate; dialysis is individually prescribed for any particular patient to obtain optimal results.

Access

Effective dialysis needs blood flows of between 250 and 450 mL/min. In order to achieve this, a surgically fashioned arteriovenous fistula (AVF; ***Fig. 20.52***) is formed, using the radial or brachial artery and the cephalic vein. Large-bore needles are inserted into the arterialized vein of the AVF to take blood to and from the dialysis machine. In patients with poor-quality veins or arterial disease (e.g. diabetes mellitus), synthetic arteriovenous grafts offer an alternative.

For many, an AVF is not an immediate or appropriate solution, and a ***semipermanent dual-lumen venous catheter*** can be inserted under a skin tunnel into the jugular or femoral vein. Although easy to place and offering immediate use, there is a significant risk of bloodstream infection (with a foreign body directly accessing the circulation), catheter malfunction (thrombosis), or venous stenosis or occlusion.

For urgent dialysis, a temporary (and untunnelled) large-bore, double-lumen dialysis catheter may be inserted into a central vein – usually the subclavian, jugular or femoral vein.

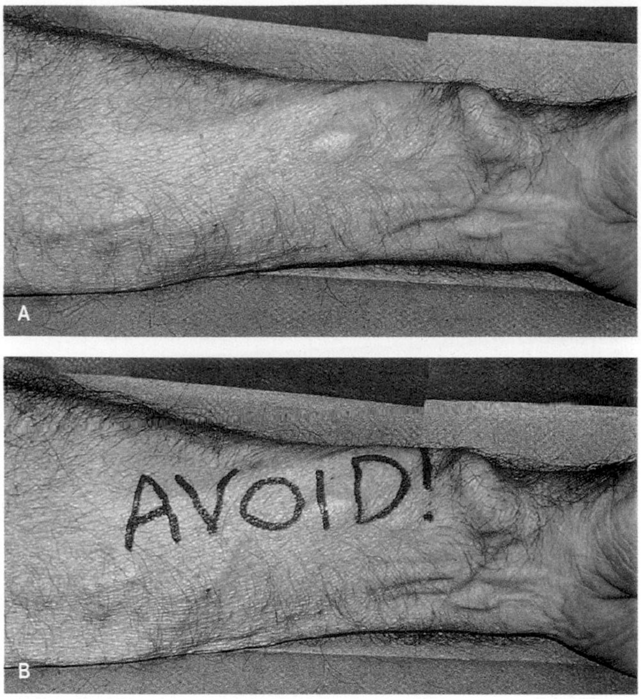

Figure 20.52 **Arteriovenous (radiocephalic) fistula. A.** In the left forearm. **B.** One way of reminding the anaesthetic, nursing and surgical teams about the presence of an existing arteriovenous fistula in a haemodialysis patient about to undergo surgery. In particular, the fistula should not be compressed during surgery to avoid thrombosis within it.

Aims

- ***Maintain euvolaemia*** – the ideal (or 'dry') weight. Fluid gains (in kilograms) between each dialysis session are the sum of fluid intake less fluid losses over a 48-h interdialytic interval. A patient who is anuric (with no urine output) who drinks 2 L/day will gain 4 kg if no insensible or stool losses occur. If a patient is weighed before and after each session (with the post-dialysis weight described as the 'dry' weight), dialysis can deliver long-term volume and blood pressure control.
- ***Maintain electrolytes*** in balance. A low dialysate potassium (of 1–3 mmol/L) allows rapid control of hyperkalaemia and a negative potassium balance (of 1–2 mmol/kg/session) over a treatment. Dialysate sodium is carefully controlled to prevent large fluid shifts (at 137–141 mmol/L, although this can be individualized), and calcium fixed to mimic the ionized fraction (and prevent net calcium gain during dialysis).
- ***Prevent acidosis***. Dialysate is buffered with bicarbonate at (for example) 36 mmol/L. This will diffuse into blood to correct acidosis during treatment.
- ***Balance frequency and duration with quality of life***. Between 4 and 5 h of treatment three times a week is considered 'adequate' to maintain volume and solute balance over time. Shorter or less frequent dialysis is usually only sufficient if a patient has considerable ***residual renal function*** (usually assessed by measuring 24- or 48-h urine volumes and clearances, then adding this to the dialysis clearance). Recent evidence is pointing towards more frequent dialysis (up to 5–6 dialysis sessions per week) or longer treatment duration (6–8 h three times weekly) as offering more benefit in terms of quality of life, solute clearance and cardiovascular health.
- ***Deliver enough dialysis*** (adequacy). The size, number and nature of 'uraemic toxins' are not clear, and the only true measure of adequacy is patient mortality and morbidity. Symptoms of under-dialysis are non-specific and include insomnia, itching and fatigue (despite adequate correction of anaemia), restless legs and a peripheral sensory neuropathy. Formal measures using urea as a surrogate calculate the urea reduction ratio (URR, targeting >65% per session) or the eKt/V (where K is the dialyser clearance, t is the duration of dialysis in minutes, and V is the urea distribution volume estimated as total body water) as minimum thresholds required for well-nourished dialysis patients dialysed three times per week. It is unclear whether a higher eKt/V (more dialysis than is thought of as adequate) associates with better outcomes; initial trial data suggest not.

Specific complications

- Access (either AVF or catheter) malfunction, thrombosis or bleeding
- Bloodstream infections, which may disseminate to soft tissue (septic arthritis), cardiac valves (endocarditis) or spinal column (vertebritis).
- Dialysis disequilibrium, when dialysis is initiated with too rapid early urea removal. Subsequent movement of fluid towards the higher urea seen across the blood–brain barrier can cause cerebral oedema and fitting.
- Intradialytic hypotension (where too rapid fluid removal exceeds refill of the circulation from the extravascular space).
- Dialysis-related amyloidosis, where failure of clearance of β_2-microglobulin, a molecule of 11.8 kDa, leads to amyloid deposits, median nerve compression in the carpal tunnel, a dialysis arthropathy, bone cysts and fractures, pseudotumours and gastrointestinal bleeding.

Haemofiltration

Haemofiltration differs from haemodialysis in that there is no dialysate; rather, plasma water (and suspended solutes) is removed by convection across a high-flux semipermeable membrane. Substitution fluid (with the desired biochemical composition) is then infused to replace (large) fluid losses ***(Fig. 20.53)***. Haemofiltration may be preferred in the acute setting, where haemodynamic instability is common (particularly on ITUs). Modern dialysis machines have built-in facilities to generate online ultra-pure water, which has minimized the cost of the procedure. It has also given the clinician the option to use this technique either as haemofiltration or in combination with dialysis as ***haemodiafiltration*** to increase middle

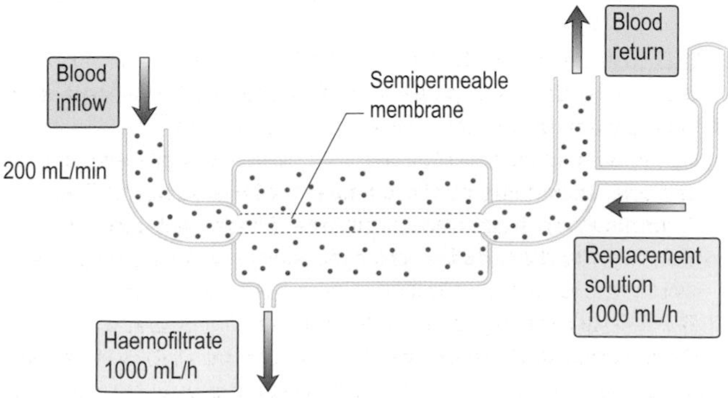

Figure 20.53 **Principles of haemofiltration.**

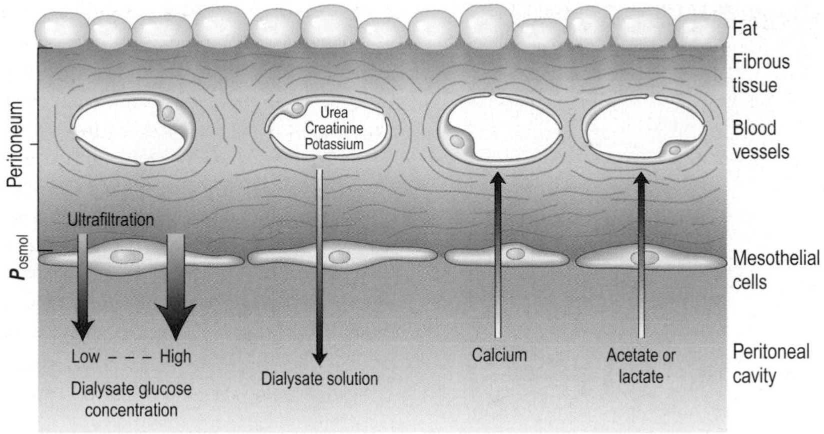

Figure 20.54 Principles of peritoneal dialysis. Water is attracted into the peritoneal cavity, depending on the osmolarity of the dialysate.

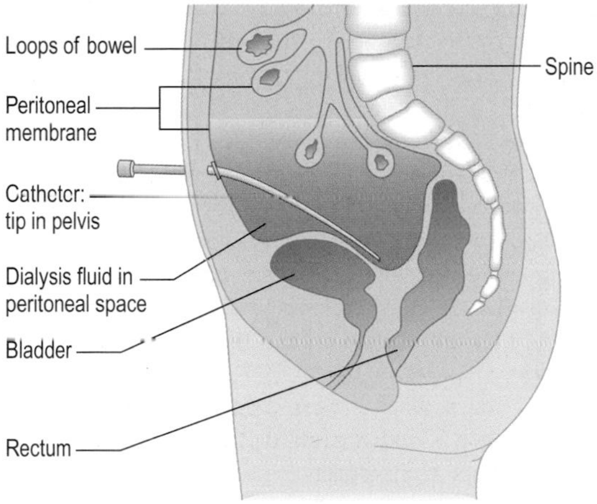

Figure 20.55 The siting of a Tenckhoff peritoneal dialysis catheter.

Box 20.36 Range of concentrations in routinely available CAPD dialysates

Dialysate	Range of concentration (mmol/L)
Sodium	130–134
Potassium	0
Calcium	1.0–1.75
Magnesium	0.25–0.75
Chloride	95–104
Lactate	35–40
Glucose[a]	77–236
Total osmolality	356–511 mOsm/kg

[a]Glucose content is often expressed as g/dL of anhydrous glucose (e.g. 1.36% = 77 mmol/L). An even more hypertonic dialysate (6.36%) is available for acute (intermittent) peritoneal dialysis. CAPD, continuous ambulatory peritoneal dialysis.

molecule clearance (e.g. β_2-microglobulin) and prevent long-term dialysis complications such as dialysis-related amyloidosis, particularly in young, highly sensitized, non-transplantable patients.

Peritoneal dialysis

Peritoneal dialysis uses the peritoneal membrane as a semipermeable membrane, avoiding the need for extracorporeal circulation of blood. It is a very simple, low-technology (and effective) treatment compared to haemodialysis ***(Fig. 20.54)***.

- A soft catheter is placed through a skin tunnel into the peritoneal cavity through the midline of the anterior abdominal wall ***(Fig. 20.55)***.
- Dialysate is run into the peritoneal cavity, usually under gravity.
- Urea, creatinine, phosphate and other uraemic toxins pass into the dialysate down their concentration gradients.
- Water (with solutes) is attracted into the peritoneal cavity by osmosis, depending on the osmolarity of the dialysate. This is determined by the glucose or polymer (icodextrin) content of the dialysate ***(Box 20.36)***. More hypertonic solutions (rising from around 1.5% to 4% glucose) will improve fluid removal.
- The fluid is exchanged regularly to repeat the process.

Continuous ambulatory peritoneal dialysis (***CAPD***) has dialysate present within the peritoneal cavity continuously, except during an exchange (done 3–5 times a day using a sterile no-touch technique to connect 1.5–3-L bags of dialysate to the peritoneal catheter; each exchange takes 20–40 min.

Automated peritoneal dialysis (***or nightly intermittent peritoneal dialysis***) has a simple exchange machine performing continuous low-volume exchanges each night while the patient is asleep. Sometimes dialysate is left in the peritoneal cavity during the day in addition, to increase the time during which biochemical exchange is taking place.

Specific complications

- Bacterial peritonitis, presenting as fever, abdominal pain, and a cloudy peritoneal dialysate effluent (>100 cells/mm^3 on microscopy is suggestive) progressing to frank peritonitis, occurs at the rate of about one episode for every 2 patient-years. Once peritoneal effluent is sent for culture, empirical antibiotic treatment is started. Common causative organisms are listed in ***Box 20.37***.
- Catheter exit-site infections may progress to skin tunnel infections and peritonitis.
- Constipation may impair flow of dialysate in and out of the pelvis.
- Hernias are caused by raised intra-abdominal pressure, and dialysate 'leaks' into the pleural cavity or scrotum (down a patent processus vaginalis).

Box 22.37 Some causes of CAPD peritonitis[a]

Cause	Approximate % of cases
Staphylococcus epidermidis	40–50
Escherichia coli, *Pseudomonas* and other Gram-negative organisms	25
Staphylococcus aureus	15
Mycobacterium tuberculosis	2
Candida and other fungal species	2

[a]In approximately 20%, no bacteria are found. CAPD, continuous ambulatory peritoneal dialysis.

- Sclerosing peritonitis is a potentially fatal complication of CAPD, where long-term patients develop progressive thickening of the peritoneal membrane. This occurs in association with adhesions and strictures, turning the small bowel into a mass of matted loops and causing repeated episodes of small bowel obstruction.

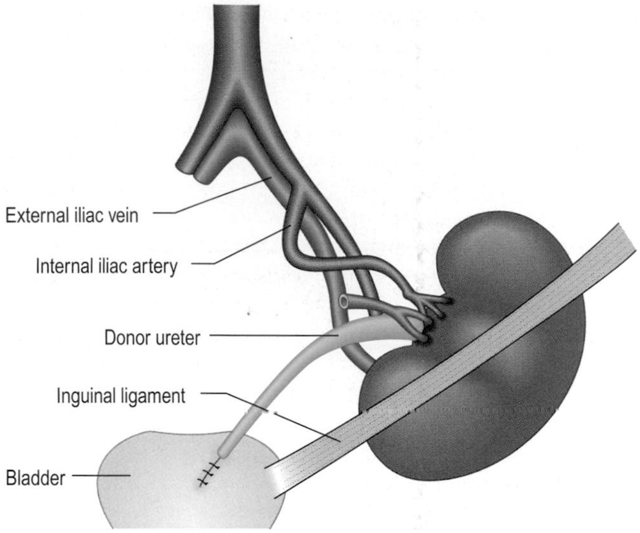

Figure 20.56 Anatomy of a renal transplant operation.

Adequacy

Most clinicians aim for a weekly *Kt/V* of 2.0 (see above), coupled with a creatinine clearance of 60 L per week. Once patients stop passing urine (and have no residual renal function), peritoneal dialysis inadequacy becomes common, and a switch in technique to haemodialysis may be required.

Dialysis in the frail

Dialysis can prolong life, but the benefit to any individual, and particularly to frail patients, varies widely. Outcomes in frail elderly people who are undergoing dialysis are poor. Small studies suggest that mortality or quality-of-life outcomes do not differ significantly among selected patients who elect to undergo dialysis, compared to those who decide against dialysis. In one study, over 50% died within the first year of initiating dialysis and around 30% had a decrease in functional status.

Renal transplantation

Successful renal transplantation offers the potential for almost complete rehabilitation in ESKD.

- Survival is significantly better compared to dialysis patients on transplant waiting lists.
- Transplantation allows freedom from dietary and fluid restrictions.
- Anaemia and infertility are corrected.
- Any need for parathyroidectomy is reduced.

It is the treatment of choice for any *appropriate* patients with ESKD. However, the supply of donor organs (in the UK, 44 per million population per year) is exceeded by demand. Donor organs are a scarce and valuable resource that must be used optimally.

Kidney transplantation involves the anastomosis of an explanted human kidney, usually either from a deceased donor or from a living related or unrelated donor, on to the iliac vessels of the recipient ***(Fig. 20.56)***. The donor ureter is placed into the recipient's bladder. Unless the donor is genetically identical (i.e. an identical twin), immunosuppressive treatment is needed, for as long as the transplant remains in place, to prevent rejection. Patient and graft survival has steadily improved with:

- more appropriate patient selection and assessment
- better donor–recipient compatibility
- improvements in surgical techniques
- more efficient immunosuppressive regimens.

Some 80% of grafts now survive for 5–10 years in the best centres, and 50% for 10–30 years. However, the half-life of renal allografts is still 13–16 years. The three most common causes of late graft loss are death of patients with a functioning graft, recurrence of the original (or new) renal disease, and chronic allograft nephropathy.

Considerations in successful kidney transplantation

ABO (blood group) compatibility between donor and recipient is preferred. ABO-incompatible renal transplants (where donor and recipient have different blood groups) are successful with directed immunosuppression (including immunoadsorption to remove preformed antibodies, splenectomy, anti-CD20 antibodies to remove B lymphocytes, and intravenous pooled immunoglobulins for immunomodulation or anti-idiotypic antibodies).

Donor and recipient HLA mismatches should ideally be minimized. Nationwide matching schemes for kidneys retrieved from deceased donors form the basis for kidney transplant offers. Complete compatibility at A, B and DR loci offers the best long-term outcomes when compared to multiply mismatched organs (i.e. antigens possessed by the donor and not possessed by the recipient). However, transplanting completely mismatched kidneys, particularly with living donation, is routine and results are as good as, if not better than, properly matched deceased donor kidneys.

Pre-formed (historical) anti-HLA antibodies in recipients, resulting from either sensitization from prior blood transfusions, kidney transplants or past pregnancy in women, tend to predict less good outcomes. This is particularly true if these existing antibodies are donor-specific (or recipient anti-HLA antibodies against donor antigens). Transplantation can still be successful but pre-transplant strategies to minimize these antibodies (with plasmapheresis, intravenous immunoglobulin and/or the anti-B cell monoclonal antibody, rituximab) are necessary.

Organs may be retrieved from donors who have sustained brainstem death or even cardiac arrest. Most countries allow the removal of kidneys and other organs from patients who have suffered irretrievable brain damage ('brainstem death') while the heart is still beating (donation after brainstem death, DBD; see pp. 1172–1173).

Due to the shortage of solid organs and increasing numbers of patients waiting for them, several countries now allow the retrieval of organs after cardiac death (donation after cardiac death, DCD), with comparable results to 'heart-beating' donations. Expanded criteria donors (ECD), aged >60 years, or those between the ages of 55 and 59 years but with co-morbidity such as hypertension, diabetes, pre-retrieval AKI and intracranial haemorrhage as a cause of death, are also increasingly used.

Living related or unrelated donation offers the best kidney outcomes. Potential living donors undergo comprehensive preoperative evaluation to ensure that they will come to no harm through donating a kidney to another person. Recent evidence suggests that live donors carry a statistically increased risk of CKD/ESKD post donation but the inherent risk is too low for it to be of clinical significance. Young women donors are at increased risk of gestational hypertension or pre-eclampsia in subsequent pregnancies, though without any ill-effects on their children. As a result, all living donors should be monitored regularly.

Timing transplantation so that it takes place prior to dialysis initiation (pre-emptive transplantation) offers benefits to both the recipient and the graft.

Immunosuppression for transplantation

Long-term inhibition of the recipient immune system is needed to prevent immune-mediated injury to grafts recognized as non-self. This is almost universally the case, except where living related donation from an identical twin occurs. Some degree of immunological tolerance does develop, and the risk of rejection is highest in the first 3 months after transplantation. In the early months, rejection episodes occur in less than 20% of cadaver kidney recipients on current immunosuppression protocols, and most cases are reversible. A combination of immunosuppressive drugs is usually used ***(Box 20.38)***. Individualizing immunosuppression to a specific recipient remains an inexact science, and preventing the complications of over-immunosuppression is as necessary as preventing rejection. Therapeutic drug monitoring is useful in delivering the most intense immunosuppression in the early post-transplant phase, and allows lower target ranges further out.

Early complications

Early (technical) failure

Occlusion or stenosis of the arterial anastomosis, occlusion of the venous anastomosis, and urinary leaks owing to damage to the lower ureter or to defects in the anastomosis between ureter and recipient bladder can occur despite best surgical technique.

Acute tubular necrosis

Delayed graft function resulting from ATN is the most common cause of deceased donor graft dysfunction (up to 40–50%), particularly in kidneys from DCD or ECD donors (see above). Hypotension or loss of cardiac output will have an understandable impact on the retrieved organ. A prolonged 'cold ischaemia time' (the period during which the retrieved organ is cooled on ice in transit and awaits implantation) also leads to delayed graft function due to ATN. Finally, calcineurin inhibitors used to prevent rejection are themselves nephrotoxic where high peak and trough concentrations cause tubular injury.

Acute rejection

Acute rejection is seen in between 10% and 30% of transplant recipients and usually presents with declining renal function within the first 3 months. Renal biopsy ***(Fig. 20.57A)*** can confirm the diagnosis and also assesses the severity and type of rejection, but sampling errors do occur. Urinary measurement of RNA is also being used to detect acute cellular rejection (T-cell or antibody-mediated, with or without endothelial injury – so-called 'vascular rejection').

Cellular rejection may respond to high-dose intravenous corticosteroids, increased or switched calcineurin inhibition, or the use of T-cell-depleting agents such as anti-thymocyte globulin (ATG) or anti-lymphocyte globulin (ALG). Antibody-mediated rejection (diagnosed by the presence of circulating donor-specific anti-HLA antibodies and evidence of complement activation on renal biopsy by C4 staining; ***Fig. 20.57B***) is usually treated empirically by a combination of intravenous immunoglobulin (to neutralize and promote the clearance of anti-HLA antibodies), plasmapheresis (to remove antibodies) and anti-CD20 antibody administration (to deplete B lymphocytes), with variable success.

More than one rejection within the first 3 months, vascular and/or antibody-mediated rejection, delayed rejection (requirement of dialysis within the first week after transplantation), and failure of serum creatinine to return to baseline (<130 μmol/L) after a rejection episode are associated with worse long-term outcome.

Infection

- Bacterial infections occur early (<1 month postoperatively), as urinary tract, wound and chest infections.
- Cytomegalovirus (CMV) infection develops weeks or months after transplantation in 70% of CMV-seronegative recipients receiving grafts from a seropositive donor, and in patients receiving biological agents (antibodies) as induction or therapy for rejection, unless prophylaxis with valganciclovir is given.

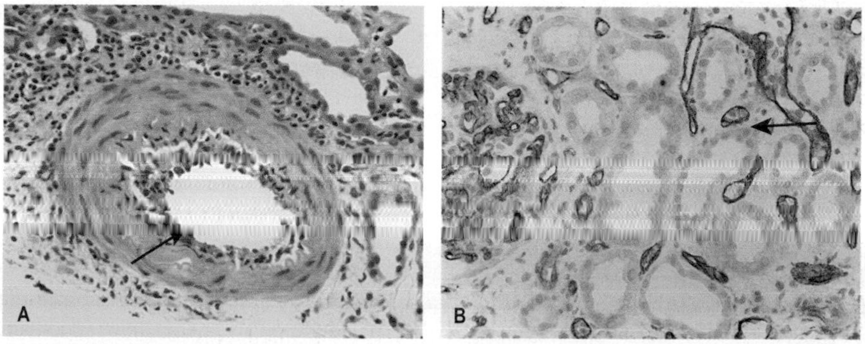

Figure 20.57 Histology of kidney in rejection. A. Acute vascular rejection: the mononuclear inflammatory cell infiltrate is limited to the expanded intima and does not involve the entire vascular wall as in systemic vasculitis. **B.** Antibody-mediated rejection: an acute tubular necrosis with capillary glomerulitis and peritubular and glomerular capillary C4d positivity.

Box 20.38 Immunosuppressive drugs used in renal transplantation

Class	Mechanism of action	Examples	Clinical role	Side-effects
Calcineurin inhibitors	Disrupt T-cell signalling	Ciclosporin Tacrolimus	Mainstay of most regimens	Nephrotoxicity (monitor levels), hypertension, diabetes, hirsutism, virilization
Inhibitors of purine synthesis	Inhibit purine synthesis and hence active proliferation of cells (especially lymphocytes)	Azathioprine Mycophenolate mofetil (MMF)	Used in most regimens	Neutropenia, pancytopenia, deranged LFTs (azathioprine), diarrhoea (MMF) Interaction with allopurinol (azathioprine)
Steroids	Inhibit cytokine- regulated T-cell signalling	Prednisolone (oral) Methylprednisolone (i.v.)	Used in most regimens. Dose tapers over first few weeks I.v. methylprednisolone used on induction and to treat acute rejection	Multiple, including osteoporosis, hypertension, diabetes, weight gain, poor wound healing, lipid abnormalities
Rapamycin (Sirolimus)	Inhibits cytokine-dependent cell proliferation		Role still being explored Alternative to calcineurin inhibitors	Delayed graft function, myelosuppression, impaired wound healing, thrombocytopenia Levels should be monitored
Anti-CD25 antibodies	Monoclonal antibody, blocking the IL-2 receptor	Daclizumab Basiliximab	Given on induction Usually used in patients with medium to high risk of rejection	Well tolerated
Antibodies causing T-cell depletion	Target and destroy T cells	Anti-thymocyte globulin (ATG)=polyclonal OKT3=monoclonal anti-CD3 antibody	For steroid-resistant rejection (7–10-day course) May be used as induction agent for patients at high risk of rejection	Severe T-cell depletion (risk of sepsis) Late development of malignancy, esp. lymphoma
Anti-CD52 antibody	Depletes both T and B cells	Alemtuzumab	Used as induction agent	Over-immunosuppression, risk of sepsis and malignancy in longer term Long-term outcome data awaited
Anti-B7 antibody	Prevents engagement of B7 and CD28 Blocks co-stimulatory signal	Belatacept	Has been tried with success in maintenance regimens instead of calcineurin inhibitors	Relatively high but mild rejection High incidence of post-transplant lymphoma in EBV-negative patients
Anti-C5a antibody	Inhibits complement activation by blocking activated C5	Eculizumab	Success in acute antibody-mediated rejections Atypical HUS post transplant	Infections, particularly meningococcal meningitis. Patients should be vaccinated against meningitis prior to its use

EBV, Epstein–Barr virus; HUS, haemolytic uraemic syndrome; IL-2, interleukin 2; LFTs, liver function tests.

Opportunist infections, such as those with *Pneumocystis jiroveci*, occur and prophylactic co-trimoxazole is given in the early months. These infections also occur in the months after transplantation and associate with heavier immunosuppressant burdens.

- Polyomavirus infection (***BK nephropathy***) causes an often aggressive tubulointerstitial nephritis that may lead to graft loss. The only existing therapy is minimization of immunosuppression in the hope of spontaneous viral clearance.

Late complications

- ***Post-transplantation lymphoproliferative disorders*** (PTLD), often associated with Epstein–Barr virus, are malignancies more frequent in patients who received profound immunosuppression. Immunization is minimized and standard chemotherapy offered, with mixed outcomes.
- ***Immunosuppressive therapy*** increases the risk of skin tumours, including basal and squamous cell carcinoma. Other cancers that occur at increased frequency include renal, cervical and vaginal malignancies.
- ***Cardiovascular disease*** causes 50% of patient deaths after transplantation. Increased hypertension, obesity, diabetes and insulin resistance, and lipid disorders all play a role, as does an often long history of CKD.
- ***Post-transplant osteoporosis*** may occur as a result of steroid use.
- ***Recurrent renal disease*** is surprisingly common. Primary FSGS often recurs and causes early graft loss. Mesangiocapillary GN, diabetic nephropathy and IgA nephropathy also commonly recur, with variable effects on long-term graft survival.

Most grafts fail eventually through lasting immunological injury, the toxicities of immunosuppressant drugs, or even both.

A common histological finding is interstitial fibrosis and tubular atrophy, a lesion once called chronic allograft nephropathy. There is a growing understanding of the role of subclinical chronic antibody-mediated rejection due to existing or *de novo* donor-specific antibodies, but non-immunological factors play an important part as well. Progressive irreversible decline in graft function is associated with mild to modest proteinuria (<3 g/day), and interventions to change this trajectory currently lack evidence of benefit.

Renal transplantation in HIV patients

Modern antiretroviral therapy (ART) offers patients with HIV infection a near-normal life expectancy. However, an increasing number develop ESKD, and HIV was considered to be a contraindication to renal transplantation. However, a study of outcomes for 150 HIV-infected patients undergoing renal transplantation has shown that kidney transplantation is safe and effective in these individuals, at least in the short term. The patients in the study had $CD4^+$ T-cell counts of ≥200 cells/mm^3 and undetectable plasma levels of HIV type 1 RNA while on stable ART during the 16 weeks before renal transplantation. Median follow-up was 1.7 years. Survival rates at 1 year (95%) and 3 years (88%) were worse in HIV-infected patients than in the general population of kidney transplant recipients, but better than those in patients aged ≥65 years. Many rejection episodes were glucocorticoid-resistant, suggesting an aggressive response to donor antigens.

Further reading

EVOLVE Trial Investigators, Chertow GM, Block GA, Correa-Rotter R et al. Effect of cinacalcet on cardiovascular disease in patients undergoing dialysis. *N Engl J Med* 2012; 367:2482–2494.

Kurella Tamura M, Covinsky KE, Chertow GM et al. Functional status of elderly adults before and after initiation of dialysis. *N Engl J Med* 2009; 361:1539–1547.

Levey AS, Coresh J. Chronic kidney disease. *Lancet* 2012; 379:165–180.

Levey AS, de Jong PE, Cooper BA et al and IDEAL Study. A randomized, controlled trial of early versus late initiation of dialysis. *N Engl J Med* 2010; 363:609–619.

Levey AS, de Jong PE, Coresh J et al. The definition, classification, and prognosis of chronic kidney disease: a KDIGO Controversies Conference report. *Kidney Int* 2011; 80:17–28.

Nankivell BJ, Alexander SI. Mechanisms of disease: rejection of the kidney allograft. *N Engl J Med* 2010; 363:1451–1462.

Ortiz A, Covic A, Fliser D et al and Board of the EURECA-m Working Group of ERA-EDTA. Epidemiology, contributors to, and clinical trials of mortality risk in chronic kidney failure. *Lancet* 2014; 383:1831–1843.

Steiner RW. The risks of living kidney donation. *N Engl J Med* 2016; 374:479–481.

Tonelli M, Muntner P, Lloyd A et al. Using proteinuria and estimated glomerular filtration rate to classify risk in patients with chronic kidney disease: a cohort study. *Ann Intern Med* 2011; 154:12–21.

Vincenti F, Charpentier B, Vanrenterghem Y et al. A phase III study of belatacept-based immunosuppression regimens versus cyclosporine in renal transplant recipients (BENEFIT study). *Am J Transplant* 2010; 10:536–546.

http://www.ctsu.ox.ac.uk/~sharp/ *The SHARP study.*

CYSTIC RENAL DISEASE

Solitary or multiple renal cysts are common, especially with advancing age; 50% of those over 50 years of age have one or more such cysts. They have no special significance except in the differential diagnosis of renal tumours (see pp. 791–792). These cysts are often asymptomatic and are found on ultrasound examination performed for some other reason. Occasionally, they may cause pain and/or haematuria if large, or bleeding may occur into the cyst. Cystic degeneration (the formation of multiple cysts that enlarge with time) occurs regularly in the non-functioning kidneys of patients with ESKD treated by dialysis and/or transplantation. These acquired cysts have malignant potential.

Autosomal dominant polycystic kidney disease

Autosomal dominant polycystic kidney disease (ADPKD) is an inherited disorder that usually presents in adulthood. It is characterized by the development of multiple renal cysts, variably associated with extrarenal (mainly hepatic and cardiovascular) abnormalities. ADPKD is by far the most common inherited nephropathy, with a prevalence rate ranging from 1 : 400 to 1 : 1000 in white populations. It accounts for 3–10% of all patients commencing regular dialysis in the West (see ciliopathies, pp. 92–93).

Mutations in *PKD1* (on chromosome 16) are responsible for 85% of cases, with mutations on *PKD2* (on chromosome 4) accounting for the remainder. These genetic abnormalities are distinct from the autosomal recessive form of polycystic disease (due to mutations in the *PKHD1* gene on chromosome 6p21.1-p12), which is often lethal in early life.

PKD1 encodes polycystin 1, involved in cell–cell and/or cell–matrix interactions. *PKD2* encodes polycystin 2, which functions as a calcium ion channel. The polycystin complex occurs in cilia, responsible for sensing flow in the tubule. Disruption of the polycystin pathway results in reduced cytoplasmic calcium, which, in principal cells (see p. 175) of the collecting duct, causes defective ciliary signalling and disoriented cell division, resulting in cyst formation. Progressive loss of renal function is usually attributed to mechanical compression, apoptosis of the healthy tissue and reactive fibrosis. Renal function declines at a variable rate, depending on the growth and size of cysts; patients with rapidly growing cysts on MRI lose renal function more rapidly. Strategies to slow the growth rate of cysts have been very effective in preserving renal function in animal models. These therapies include the vasopressin V_2 receptor inhibitors (vaptans, to reduce cyclic adenosine monophosphate (cAMP) in the principal cells), roscovitine (a cyclin-dependent kinase inhibitor) and antiproliferative therapy with sirolimus (mammalian target of rapamycin (mTOR) inhibitor).

Clinical features

Presenting symptoms occur from any point in the second decade onwards:

- loin pain and/or haematuria from haemorrhage into a cyst, cyst infection or urinary tract stone formation
- loin or abdominal discomfort as the size of the kidneys increases
- subarachnoid haemorrhage associated with berry aneurysm rupture
- complications of hypertension
- complications of associated liver cysts (occurs in around 50%)
- symptoms of uraemia and/or anaemia associated with CKD.

Complications and associations

- Pain from large cysts can be difficult to manage, with surgical decompression of some benefit in about two-thirds of affected patients.
- Cyst infection is most effectively treated with lipophilic antibiotics that penetrate into infected cysts and are active against Gram-negative bacteria, such as co-trimoxazole and fluoroquinolones.
- Renal calculi occur in 10–20% and are often composed of uric acid and are radiolucent (see ***Fig. 20.30***).
- Hypertension is an early and very common feature of ADPKD. Intrarenal activation of the renin–angiotensin system is thought to be contributory, so ACE inhibitors are logical first-line

agents in treatment. Early control of blood pressure is essential as left ventricular hypertrophy is common, and cardiovascular complications are a major cause of death in ADPKD.
- Progressive CKD is the most serious complication of ADPKD. At glomerular filtration rates below 50 mL/min, the rate of decline in GFR averages 5 mL/min each year, which is more rapid than in other primary renal disorders. The probability of being alive without requiring dialysis or transplantation by the age of 70 years is in the order of 30%. Survival rates on regular haemodialysis and after renal transplantation in ADPKD are better than those in patients with other primary renal diseases.
- Approximately 30% of patients have hepatic cysts, occasionally massive enlargement of the polycystic liver with pain, infection and, more rarely, compression of the bile duct, portal vein or hepatic venous outflow.
- Some 10% of ADPKD patients have an asymptomatic intracranial aneurysm (see p. 839). The prevalence is twice as high if a family history of aneurysms or intracranial haemorrhage is present. Screening for intracranial aneurysm in ADPKD is recommended for patients aged 18–40 years who have a positive family history.
- Mitral valve prolapse is found in 20% of individuals with ADPKD.

Diagnosis and screening

Physical examination commonly reveals large, irregular kidneys and possibly hepatomegaly. Definitive diagnosis is established by ultrasound examination (***Fig. 20.58*** and ***Box 20.39***). However, such renal imaging techniques may be equivocal, especially in subjects under the age of 15 years. A number of conditions can mimic the clinical and radiological appearance of ADPKD (***Box 20.40***).

The children and siblings of patients with established ADPKD should, in general, be offered screening. Affected individuals should have regular blood pressure checks and should be offered genetic counselling. Gene linkage analysis can be utilized in many families.

Management

No definitive therapy is yet available. Potential strategies include:
- ***Vasopressin receptor antagonists***, which act by inhibiting cAMP in principal cells, reduce cyst growth and slow the rate of progression of renal failure. Liver toxicity has limited widespread use.
- ***Octreotide***, a long-acting somatostatin analogue (which also inhibits cAMP), has been beneficial in halting the growth of both liver and renal cysts.
- In the HALT-PKD study A, patients with early PKD and eGFR >60 mL/min, when randomized to a low blood pressure group (95/60–110/75 mmHg), had slower annualized increase in total kidney volume, lower albuminuria and left ventricular mass index compared to the standard blood pressure group (120/70–130/80 mmHg). In late-stage PKD (with eGFR of 25–60 mL/min), adding an angiotensin receptor blocker to an ACE inhibitor (dual blockade) did not confer additional benefit at 5–8-year follow-up.
- Two studies of mTOR inhibitors, e.g. rapamycin, in PKD were essentially negative for the primary end-point of cyst growth and preservation of renal function, but studies of patients with early disease are in progress.

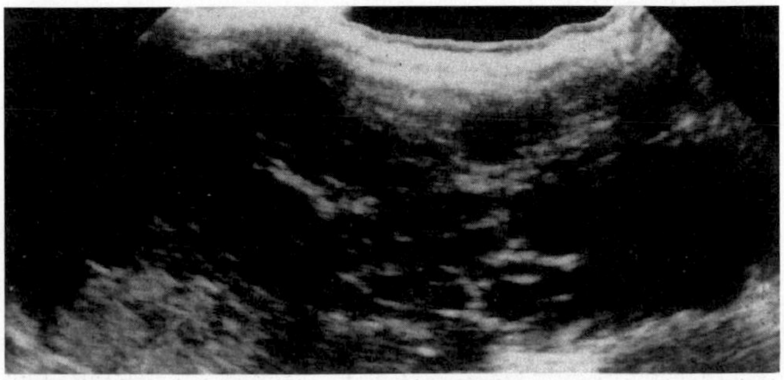

Figure 20.58 Ultrasound scan of a polycystic kidney. An enlarged kidney is shown, with many cysts of varying size.

Medullary cystic disease ('juvenile nephronophthisis')

Juvenile nephronophthisis develops early in childhood and is inherited in an autosomal recessive manner. Mutations in the genes *NPHP1–4*, encoding nephrocystin and inversin (both co-localized in the cilia of the renal tubules) leads to multiple cyst formation. Polyuria, polydipsia and growth retardation result from impaired tubular function. A similar condition developing later in childhood (medullary cystic disease) is inherited as an autosomal dominant trait, but sporadic cases occur in both conditions. The dominant

Box 20.39 Ultrasonographic diagnostic criteria for testing individuals at risk of autosomal dominant polycystic kidney disease (ADPKD)

In at-risk individuals, a diagnosis of ADPKD is established if patients meet the following criteria:
- 15–39 years: $\geq$3 cysts (unilateral or bilateral)
- 40–59 years: $\geq$2 cysts in each kidney
- $\geq$60 years: $\geq$4 cysts in each kidney

ADPKD is excluded in patients meeting the following criteria:
- $\geq$40 years: <2 cysts
- 30–39 years: 0 cysts (this excludes ADPKD in 98% of cases).

At <30 years, a negative renal ultrasound scan does not exclude a diagnosis of ADPKD; other imaging techniques, such as CT and MRI, may be useful and molecular genetic testing might be needed.

Box 20.40 Conditions that clinically and radiologically mimic polycystic kidney disease

- ***Tuberous sclerosis***: includes lymphangiomyomatosis and lymphangioleiomyomatosis, and can be associated with the *TSC2–PKD1* contiguous gene syndrome
- ***von Hippel–Lindau syndrome***
- ***Multicystic dysplastic kidney***: a non-heritable unilateral syndrome or a systemic syndrome (e.g. prune belly syndrome)
- ***Juvenile nephronophthisis*** and medullary cystic kidney disease: can be autosomal recessive (presenting in the second decade of life) or autosomal dominant (presenting in the third to fourth decades)
- ***Glomerulocystic kidney disease***: involves the expansion of Bowman's space and is autosomal dominant
- ***Acquired cystic disease***: involves end-stage kidney disease and hypokalaemia
- ***Renal-cell carcinoma***: involves cystic changes

histological findings are interstitial inflammation and tubular atrophy, with later development of medullary cysts.

Diagnosis is based on family history and renal biopsy, the cysts rarely being visible on imaging.

Medullary sponge kidney

Medullary sponge kidney is an uncommon cystic condition presenting as intermittent renal colic, the passage of small stones and haematuria. Although it is most often sporadic, a few affected families have been reported. Dilatation of the collecting ducts in the papillae occurs, sometimes with cystic change. In severe cases, the medullary area has a sponge-like appearance. The condition may affect one or both kidneys, or only part of one kidney. Cyst formation is commonly associated with the development of small calculi within the cyst. In about 20% of patients, there is associated hypercalciuria or renal tubular acidosis (see pp. 177–178). Hemihypertrophy of the skeleton has been described in this condition.

CT or IVU (see ***Fig. 20.28***) is diagnostic. Renal function is usually well maintained and CKD is unusual, except where obstructive nephropathy develops owing to the presence of stones in the pelvis or ureters.

Further reading

Caroli A, Perico N, Perna A et al and ALADIN study group. Effect of long acting somatostatin analogue on kidney and cyst growth in autosomal dominant polycystic kidney disease (ALADIN): a randomised, placebo-controlled, multicentre trial. *Lancet* 2013; 382:1485–1495.
Ellison DH, Ingelfinger JR. A quest – halting the progression of autosomal dominant polycystic kidney disease. *N Engl J Med* 2014; 371:2329–2331.
Hildebrandt F, Benzing T, Katsanis N. Ciliopathies. *N Engl J Med* 2011; 364:1533–1543.
Ong ACM, Devuyst O, Knebelmann B et al. Autosomal dominant polycystic kidney disease: the changing face of clinical management. *Lancet* 2015; 385:1993–2002.
Simms RJ. Autosomal dominant polycystic kidney disease. *BMJ* 2016; 352:i679.
Torres VE, Chapman AB, Devuyst O et al and TEMPO 3:4 Trial Investigators. Tolvaptan in patients with autosomal dominant polycystic kidney disease. *N Engl J Med* 2012; 367:2407–2418.

TUMOURS OF THE KIDNEY AND GENITOURINARY TRACT

Renal cell carcinoma

Renal cell carcinomas (RCCs) arise from proximal tubular epithelium. They are the most common renal tumour in adults (accounting for 1–2% of all malignancies), and affect men more often than women (2:1). They usually present after 50 years of age (and rarely before the age of 40).

RCCs are highly vascular tumours; microscopically, most tumours are composed of large cells containing clear cytoplasm.

Clinical features

- RCCs are often asymptomatic and discovered incidentally.
- Haematuria, loin pain and a mass in the flank occur.
- Malaise, anorexia and weight loss may be present (30%).
- Some 5% of patients have polycythaemia (see pp. 548–550).
- Around 30% of patients have hypertension (due to secretion of renin by the tumour) and anaemia, due to depression of erythropoietin in approximately the same number.
- Pyrexia occurs in about 20% of patients.
- Approximately one-third present with metastases.
- Rarely, a left-sided varicocele may be associated with left-sided tumours that have invaded the renal vein and caused obstruction to drainage of the left testicular vein.

Diagnosis

Ultrasound may demonstrate a solid lesion. CT scanning is used to identify the renal lesion and involvement of the renal vein or inferior vena cava. MRI is better than CT for tumour staging. Urine cytology for malignant cells is of no value. The ESR is usually raised. Liver biochemistry may be abnormal, returning to normal after surgery.

Management

Medical management of RCC is discussed on pages 640–641. A nephrectomy is performed unless bilateral tumours are present or the contralateral kidney functions poorly, in which case conservative surgery, such as partial nephrectomy, may be indicated. If metastases are present, nephrectomy may still be warranted, since regression of metastases has been reported after removal of the main tumour mass.

Von Hippel–Lindau (VHL) disease is an autosomal dominant disorder presenting with bilateral RCCs, retinal and cerebellar haemangioblastomas, phaeochromocytomas, pancreatic neuroendocrine tumours and renal cysts. VHL protein acts as a tumour suppressor by tagging hypoxia-inducible gene products (VEGF, TGF) for degradation. Inactivating mutations of the *VHL* gene lead to uncontrolled angiogenesis and neoplasia. Mutations of the same tumour suppressor gene are responsible for RCC and VHL.

Nephroblastoma (Wilms' tumour)

Seen within the first 3 years of life, Wilms' tumour presents as an (occasionally bilateral) abdominal mass, rarely with haematuria. Diagnosis is established by ultrasound, CT and MRI. A combination of nephrectomy, radiotherapy and chemotherapy has much improved survival rates, even in children with metastatic disease. Overall, the 5-year survival rate is 90%.

Urothelial tumours

The calyces, renal pelvis, ureter, bladder and urethra are lined by transitional cell epithelium. Transitional cell cancers account for about 3% of deaths from all forms of malignancy. These tumours are uncommon below the age of 40 years, and more common in men (the male:female ratio is 4:1). Bladder tumours are about 50 times as common as those of the ureter or renal pelvis. Predisposing factors include:

- cigarette smoking
- exposure to industrial carcinogens such as β-naphthylamine and benzidine (workers in the petroleum, chemical, cable and rubber industries are at particular risk) or ingestion of aristolochic acid found in some herbal weight-loss preparations
- exposure to drugs (e.g. phenacetin, cyclophosphamide)
- chronic inflammation (e.g. schistosomiasis, usually associated with squamous carcinoma).

Clinical features

Painless haematuria is the most common presenting symptom (80%) of bladder malignancy, although pain may occur owing to clot retention. Symptoms suggestive of UTI develop in the absence of significant bacteriuria. In patients with bladder cancer, pain also results from local nerve involvement. Presenting symptoms may result from local metastases. Flank pain may occur with urinary tract obstruction in ureteric lesions.

Investigations

- Urine cytology for malignant cells.
- Urinary tumour markers.
- Cystoscopy to assess the tumour burden and for biopsy.
- CT or MRI of the pelvis.

Management

Medical management of urothelial and testicular tumours is discussed on pages 641 and 642–643, respectively.

DISEASES OF THE PROSTATE GLAND

Benign enlargement of the prostate gland

Benign prostatic enlargement occurs most often in men over the age of 60 years. The aetiology is not established, but the condition is unknown with hypogonadism, confirming the androgen dependency of the condition. Microscopically, hyperplasia affects the glandular and connective tissue elements of the prostate. Enlargement of the gland stretches and distorts the urethra, obstructing bladder outflow.

Clinical features

Frequency of urination, usually first noted as nocturia, is a common early symptom. Difficulty or delay in initiating urination, with variability and reduced forcefulness of the urinary stream and post-void dribbling, are often present (so-called 'LUTS', or lower urinary tract symptoms). Acute retention of urine (see below) or retention with overflow incontinence may occur. Occasionally, severe haematuria results from rupture of prostatic veins or is a consequence of bacteriuria or stone disease.

Examination and investigations

Abdominal examination for bladder enlargement, together with digital rectal examination, is performed (a benign prostate characteristically feels smooth). Investigations should include urine culture, a serum prostate-specific antigen (PSA), renal function, ultrasound and pressure flow studies of bladder emptying.

Management and prognosis

Patients with mild to moderate symptoms are managed by lifestyle change alone, as symptoms following therapy are sometimes greater than those with no therapy at all.

Individuals with moderate prostatic symptoms can be treated with:

- alpha-blockers (such as tamsulosin, which relaxes prostate and bladder smooth muscle tone)
- 5α-reductase inhibitors (e.g. finasteride, which blocks the conversion of testosterone to dihydrotestosterone, the androgen primarily responsible for prostatic growth and enlargement)
- combination therapy.

Surgical treatment includes:

- laser therapy (enucleation or vaporization)
- trans-urethral needle ablation (TUNA)
- trans-urethral resection of the prostate (TURP)
- open prostatectomy.

Deterioration in renal function or the development of upper tract dilatation usually requires surgery.

In acute retention or retention with overflow, the priorities are to relieve pain and catheterize (and drain) the bladder. If urethral catheterization is impossible, a suprapubic catheter can be placed.

Prostatic carcinoma

Prostatic carcinoma accounts for 7% of all cancers in men and is the sixth most common cancer in the world. Malignant change within the prostate becomes increasingly common with advancing age. By the age of 80 years, 80% of men have malignant foci within the gland but most of these appear to lie dormant. Histologically, the tumour is an adenocarcinoma.

Pathogenesis

Risk factors for prostate cancer include advancing age, race (common in the black population in the USA and rare in China and Japan) and a family history. The first degree relatives of men with prostate cancer have twice the risk compared to the general population. This is higher in those diagnosed below the age of 60 years and 50% higher in monozygotic twins. Genetic studies have shown that the homeobox gene *HOXB13* is a predisposition gene. Genome-wide association studies have identified about 77 SNPs associated with prostate cancer. *BRCA2* confers a 5–7 times higher risk.

Hormonal factors also play a role in aetiology.

Clinical features

Presentation is usually with LUTS if there is local disease, or back and skeletal pain, weight loss or anaemia if metastatic. The diagnosis is also made by the incidental finding of a hard, irregular gland on digital rectal examination, or as an unexpected histological result after prostatectomy for what was believed to be benign prostatic enlargement.

In developed countries, patients now present as a result of screening for prostate cancer by measurement of serum PSA. However, on the evidence available, national screening programmes are not justified. Treatment of well people carries a high morbidity of urinary incontinence and sexual dysfunction, with no evidence as yet of increased overall survival. In future, screening of 'at-risk' groups may be useful:

- PSA >4 ng/mL: this is abnormal but a measurement of between 4 and 10 ng/mL can be due to benign hypertrophy and cancer.
- PSA >10 ng/mL: a prostatic biopsy will show cancer in >50% of cases.

Investigations

These include trans-rectal ultrasound (TRUS) of the prostate and extended sampling prostatic biopsy. A histological diagnosis is essential before treatment. The Gleason scoring system is based on the histological appearances. If metastases are present, serum PSA levels usually are markedly elevated (>16 ng/mL) but can be normal; it is a myth that elevated levels occur as a result of rectal examination.

Ultrasonography and TRUS are also of value in defining the size of the gland and staging any tumour present. Endorectal coil MRI helps to detect extraprostatic extension. The upper renal tracts can be examined by ultrasonography for evidence of dilatation. Bone metastases appear as osteosclerotic lesions on X-ray and are also detected by isotopic bone scans.

Management

Non-surgical treatment of prostatic carcinoma is discussed on pages 641–642. Microscopic, impalpable tumours can sometimes be managed expectantly. Treatment for disease confined to the gland is radical prostatectomy (provided the patient is fit for the procedure), now performed by robotic surgery or radiotherapy. Metastatic disease can be treated with orchidectomy but many men refuse.

Further reading

Attard G, Parker C, Eeles RA et al. Prostate cancer. *Lancet* 2016; 387:70–82.
Richter HE, Albo ME, Zyczynski HM et al. Retropubic versus transobturator midurethral slings for stress incontinence. *N Engl J Med* 2010; 362:2066–2076.

THE URINARY TRACT IN THE ELDERLY

Progressive sclerosis of glomeruli occurs with ageing and this, together with the development of atheromatous renal vascular disease, accounts for the progressive reduction in GFR seen as people age. A GFR of 50–60 mL/min (about half the normal value for a young adult) may be regarded as 'normal' in patients over 80 years of age. The reduction in muscle mass often seen with ageing may mask this deterioration in renal function as creatinine falls despite a falling GFR. Accurate estimation of GFR in the elderly is necessary, particularly when prescribing drugs wholly or partly excreted by the kidney.

Urinary tract infections

UTIs are common in the elderly, where impaired bladder emptying (due to prostatic disease in men) or a neuropathic bladder (especially common in women) is frequently found. Symptoms may be atypical, with confusion, incontinence, nocturia, smelly urine or a vague change in well-being with little in the way of dysuria more common (see p. 763).

Urinary incontinence

This is defined as involuntary passage of urine sufficient to be a health or social problem; 25% of women and 15% of men over 65 describe the problem.

- ***Urge incontinence*** is usually due to detrusor muscle overactivity with leakage of urine because the bladder is sensed as full. It may occur as an isolated event, secondary to local factors (e.g. bladder infection or stones) or to central factors (e.g. stroke, dementia or Parkinson's disease).
- ***Stress incontinence*** occurs when the intra-abdominal pressure is increased, e.g. after a cough or sneeze, with a weak pelvic floor musculature or urethral sphincter. It is more common in women after childbirth.
- ***Overflow incontinence*** occurs with leakage of urine from a full, distended bladder. It occurs commonly in men with prostatic obstruction, following spinal cord injury, or in women with cystoceles or after gynaecological surgery.
- ***Functional incontinence*** involves the passage of urine that occurs owing to inability to get to a toilet because of disability, e.g. stroke, trauma, the unavailability of toilet facilities or dementia.

Management

Examine for local problems, such as prostatic enlargement in men and gynaecological disorders in women, and for central problems, such as neurological disorders or dementia. Urine analysis (note glycosuria) and culture should be carried out to exclude UTI. Treat contributing causes, such as constipation, drug therapy and other co-existing disease.

- ***Urge incontinence*** – bladder training, antimuscarinics, e.g. oxybutynin, tolterodine, solifenacin and darifenacin.
- ***Stress incontinence*** – pelvic floor exercises. Trans-urethral injections of autologous myoblasts can aid in regeneration of the rhabdosphincter, and fibroblasts in reconstruction of the urethral submucosa. Mid-urethral slings are increasingly used for the treatment of stress incontinence; either the retropubic or the trans-obturator approach is used, with comparable efficiency.
- ***Overflow incontinence*** – removal of the obstruction.
- ***Functional incontinence*** – improvement facilities, regular urine voiding, absorbent padding.

In patients who do not respond to simple measures, pressure flow studies (urodynamics) should be performed. Incontinence is distressing, and an expert and committed incontinence advisory and treatment service combining nursing and medical skills can be of real benefit. For established incontinence, catheterization may be necessary, but should be avoided if at all possible.

Further reading

Tonelli M, Riella M. Chronic kidney disease and the ageing population. *Lancet* 2014; 383:1278–1279.
Schaeffer AJ, Nicolle LE. Urinary tract infections in older men. *New Engl J Med* 2016; 374:562-571.

Bibliography

Cameron JS, Davison AM, Grunfeld JP et al. (eds). *Oxford Textbook of Clinical Nephrology*. Oxford: Oxford University Press; 2004.
Current Opinion in Nephrology and Hypertension A monthly journal with review articles, each issue devoted to one or two topics.
Journal of the American Society of Nephrology The highest-impact journal in nephrology with bi-monthly self-assessment programme (SAP) supplements.
Kidney International The major journal associated with the International Society of Nephrology – monthly with original and review articles.
Nephrology, Dialysis, Transplantation The major European journal devoted to the subject, with review articles, editorial comments and original papers.

Significant websites

http://www.kidney.org.uk *UK charity run by and for patients.*
http://www.tinkershop.net/nephro.htm *Nephrology calculator.*

21 Neurological disease

Paul Jarman

NEUROLOGICAL DISEASE

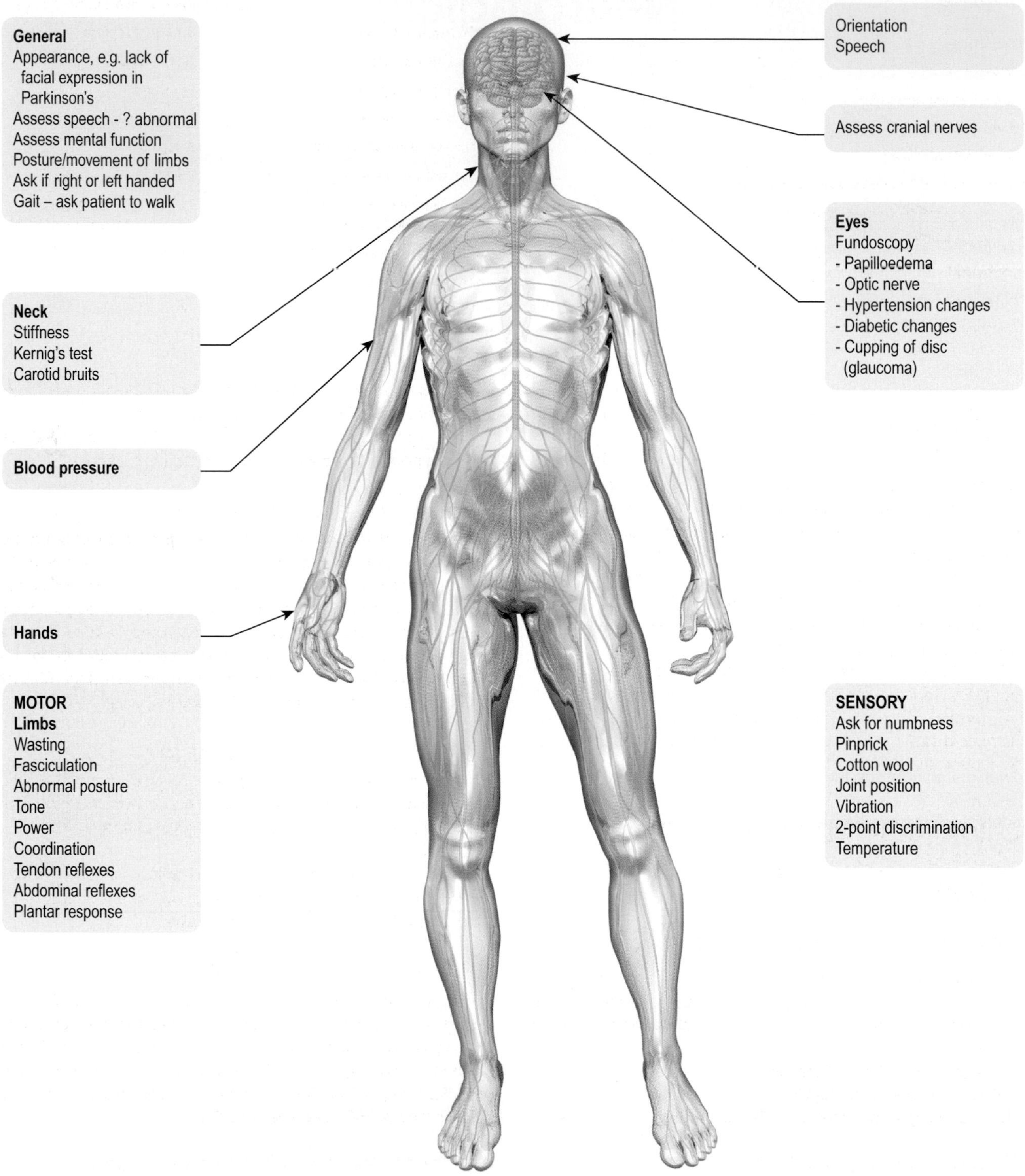
General
Appearance, e.g. lack of facial expression in Parkinson's
Assess speech - ? abnormal
Assess mental function
Posture/movement of limbs
Ask if right or left handed
Gait – ask patient to walk
Neck
Stiffness
Kernig's test
Carotid bruits
Blood pressure
Hands
MOTOR
Limbs
Wasting
Fasciculation
Abnormal posture
Tone
Power
Coordination
Tendon reflexes
Abdominal reflexes
Plantar response
Orientation
Speech
Assess cranial nerves
Eyes
Fundoscopy
- Papilloedema
- Optic nerve
- Hypertension changes
- Diabetic changes
- Cupping of disc (glaucoma)
SENSORY
Ask for numbness
Pinprick
Cotton wool
Joint position
Vibration
2-point discrimination
Temperature

Box 21.1 UK incidence of common neurological conditions

Conditions	Events per 100 000/year
Migraine	400
Stroke	240
Dementia over age of 85	68
Epilepsy	50
Parkinson's disease	19
Severe brain injury and subdural haematoma	13
All central nervous system tumours	9
Trigeminal neuralgia	8
Meningitis	7
Multiple sclerosis	7
Myasthenia, all muscle and motor neurone disease	5

Box 21.2 Common gait abnormalities

Cause	Gait abnormality
Stroke	Spastic/hemiparetic
Parkinson's disease	Shuffling/festinant
Cerebellar ataxia	Broad-based
Sensory neuropathy	Stamping
Position sensory loss	High-stepping
Distal weakness/foot drop	Slapping
Proximal weakness, e.g. myopathy	Waddling
Apraxia of gait, e.g. diffuse cerebrovascular disease	Incoordinated/gait initiation failure; marche à petits pas
Normal-pressure hydrocephalus	Hesitant
Arthritis and muscle pain	Antalgic

INTRODUCTION

Neurology is a large and diverse subject that covers many conditions requiring long-term coordinated care and having serious effects on the daily lives of patients and their families. Neurology includes conditions as diverse as cognitive disorders involving higher-level mental functioning and disorders of peripheral nerve and skeletal muscle. It is a specialty requiring good clinical skills and examination technique, which cannot be replaced with investigations or imaging techniques alone.

Some 17% of general practitioner consultations and 10% of Emergency Department visits are for neurological symptoms; 19% of all hospital admissions are for neurological disorders and 25% of chronic disability in adults below the age of 64 is due to neurological disorders ***(Box 21.1)***.

CLINICAL APPROACH TO THE PATIENT WITH NEUROLOGICAL DISEASE

Clinical features of neurological disease

Pattern recognition in neurology – interpretation of history, symptoms and examination – is very reliable. Practical experience is vital. There are three critical questions in formulating a clinical diagnosis:

- What is/are the site(s) of the lesion(s)?
- What is the likely pathology?
- Does a recognizable disease fit this pattern?

Difficulty walking and falls

Change in walking pattern is a common complaint ***(Box 21.2)***. Arthritis and muscle pain make walking painful and slow (antalgic gait). The ***pattern*** of gait is valuable diagnostically.

Spasticity and hemiparesis

Spasticity (see pp. 812–813), more pronounced in extensor muscles and with or without weakness, causes stiff, effortful and slow walking. Toes of shoes become scuffed, catching level ground. Pace shortens; a narrow base is maintained. Clonus – involuntary extensor rhythmic leg jerking – may occur.

In a hemiparesis, when spasticity is unilateral and weakness marked, the stiff, weak leg is circumducted and drags.

Parkinson's disease: shuffling gait

Stride length shortens and, in advanced forms, the gait slows to a shuffle. Posture is stooped and arm swing reduced (initially, unilateral). Gait becomes festinant (hurried) with short, rapid steps. There is difficulty turning quickly (count the number of steps to turn around). Eventually, gait initiation difficulty and freezing episodes (sudden involuntary halts, such as when passing through a doorway) may develop. Falls are uncommon, except in late-stage disease, and may indicate a 'Parkinson's plus' syndrome.

Cerebellar ataxia: broad-based gait

In lateral cerebellar lobe disease (see p. 814), stance becomes broad-based, unstable and tremulous. Ataxia describes this incoordination. When walking, the person tends to veer to the side of the affected cerebellar lobe.

In disease of midline structures (cerebellar vermis), the trunk becomes unsteady without limb ataxia, and there is a tendency to fall backwards or sideways – truncal ataxia.

Sensory ataxia: stamping gait

Peripheral sensory loss (e.g. polyneuropathy; see pp. 883–886) causes ataxia because of loss of ***proprioception*** (position sense). A broad-based, high-stepping, 'stamping' gait develops as feet are placed clumsily, relying in part on vision, so balance is worse in the dark. Romberg's test, first described in sensory ataxia of tabes dorsalis (see p. 866), becomes positive.

Lower limb weakness: high-stepping and waddling gaits

When weakness is distal, affecting ankle dorsiflexors, such as in a common peroneal nerve palsy (see p. 883), gait becomes high-stepping to avoid tripping. The sole returns to the ground with an audible ***slap***.

Weakness of proximal leg muscles (e.g. polymyositis, muscular dystrophy) causes difficulty rising from sitting. Walking becomes a ***waddle***, the pelvis being poorly supported by each leg.

Box 21.3 Medical risk factors for falls in the elderly

- Cognitive impairment (dementia and delirium)
- Arthritis, muscle weakness
- Disorders of balance and gait, e.g. Parkinsonism, ataxia, stroke
- Visual impairment
- Postural hypotension and syncope
- Vestibular disorders
- Polypharmacy, especially with sedative drugs, neuroleptics, antihypertensives and anticonvulsants
- Alcohol excess
- Peripheral neuropathy
- Effects of ageing on strength, postural stability and reaction time
- Use of walking aid

Box 21.4 Five-part short neurological examination

1. Look at patient
- General demeanour
- Speech
- Gait
- Arm swinging

2. Head
- Fundi
- Pupils
- Eye movements
- Facial movements
- Tongue

3. Upper limbs
- Posture of outstretched arms
- Wasting, fasciculation
- Power, tone
- Coordination
- Reflexes

4. Lower limbs
- Power
- Tone
- Reflexes
- Plantar responses

5. Sensation
- Ask the patient

Gait apraxia

With frontal lobe disease (e.g. diffuse cerebrovascular disease, normal-pressure hydrocephalus), ***walking skills*** become disorganized, despite normal motor and sensory function when examined on the couch. The gait is shuffling with small steps (***marche à petits pas***), gait ignition failure and hesitancy with fear of falling. Unlike in the gait of Parkinson's disease, arm swing and posture are normal. Urinary incontinence and dementia are often present.

Falls

Falls are a major health problem in elderly people, often leading to hospital admission; they are frequently a reason for requiring residential care. A third of people over the age of 65 will fall each year and 10% sustain serious injury, such as hip fracture or head injury. Falls are the leading cause of injury-related death in elderly people.

The cause of falls is usually multifactorial and a multidisciplinary approach to assessment and prevention is essential, taking into account both intrinsic medical risk factors and external environmental factors, such as rugs, stairs, footwear, poor lighting and so on. Medical risk factors for falls ***(Box 21.3)*** are additive, with multiple factors substantially increasing the risk of falling. Prevention of falls relies on identification of those at risk, treatment of medical risk factors where possible (e.g. rationalization of medications, treatment of postural hypotension), modification of environmental hazards in the home, patient education and training, and mitigation of the consequences of falls: for example, treating osteoporosis to reduce risk of fracture, and use of hip protectors, aids such as walking frames, and personal alarms. Involvement of physiotherapy and occupational therapy colleagues is a part of the assessment and management of falls.

Dizziness, vertigo and blackouts

Dizziness covers many complaints, from a vague feeling of unsteadiness to severe, acute vertigo. It is frequently used to describe light-headedness (e.g. due to hypotension), panic, anxiety, palpitations and chronic ill-health. The real nature of this symptom must be determined.

Vertigo (see p. 809) means the illusion of movement, a sensation of rotation or tipping. The patient feels the surroundings are spinning or moving. This is distressing and often accompanied by nausea or vomiting.

Blackout, like dizziness, is simply descriptive, implying either altered consciousness (see epilepsy, pp. 846–850, and syncope, p. 851), transient visual disturbance as part of pre-syncope or falling, or hypoglycaemia in a diabetic patient. A good history is essential.

Collapse is a vague term but often used. It should be avoided.

Fatigue is common. When it is an isolated symptom, it rarely indicates neurological disease, although it may be a symptom of many neurological disorders. General medical causes, such as anaemia and endocrine disorders, should be excluded. No serious disease is found in many (>20%) patients referred with symptoms suggestive of possible neurological conditions.

Examination and formulation

Following a short or detailed examination, relevant findings are summarized in a brief formulation, which becomes the basis for investigation, transfer of information and management ***(Boxes 21.4–21.6)***.

Further reading

Clarke C. The language of neurology – symptoms, signs and basic investigations. In: Clarke C, Howard R, Rossor M et al. (eds). *Neurology: A Queen Square Textbook*. Oxford: Blackwell; 2009.

Dykes PC, Carroll DL, Hurley A et al. Fall prevention in acute care hospitals. *JAMA* 2010; 304:1912–1918.

Keall MD, Pierse N, Howeden-Chapman P et al. Home modifications to reduce injuries from falls in the home injury prevention (HIPI) study: a cluster-randomised controlled trial. *Lancet* 2015; 385:231–238.

FUNCTIONAL NEUROANATOMY

The neurone and synapse

The neurone is the functional unit of the entire nervous system ***(Fig. 21.1)***. Its cell body and axon terminate in a synapse. The size and type of each group of neurones vary. A thoracic spinal cord α-motor neurone has an axonal length of >1 metre and innervates between several hundred and 2000 muscle fibres in one leg – a motor unit. By contrast, some spinal or intracerebral interneurones have axons <100 μm long, terminating on one neuronal cell body.

Neurotransmitters

Neurotransmitters are excitatory (acetylcholine, noradrenaline (norepinephrine), adrenaline (epinephrine), 5-hydroxytryptamine (5-HT, serotonin), dopamine, glutamate and aspartate) or inhibitory (γ-aminobutyric acid (GABA), histamine and glycine). Neuropeptides, such as vasopressin, adrenocorticotrophic hormone (ACTH), substance P and opioid peptides, as well as the purines adenosine triphosphate (ATP) and adenosine monophosphate (AMP) are both excitatory and inhibitory.

Box 21.5 Ten-part neurological examination

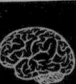

1. ***State of consciousness, arousal, appearance***
2. ***Mental state, attitude, insight***
3. ***Cognitive function*** – orientation, recall, level of intellect, language, other cortical problems, e.g. apraxia
4. ***Gait and balance tests***, including tandem walking and Romberg's test
5. ***Neck*** – stiffness, palpation and auscultation of carotids
6. ***Cranial nerves*** (see ***Box 21.8***)
7. ***Motor system***
   Upper limbs:
   - Wasting and fasciculation
   - Posture of arms: drift, rebound, tremor
   - Tone: spasticity, clonus, extrapyramidal rigidity
   - Power: 0–5 scale (see ***Box 21.6***)
   - Tendon reflexes: + or ++ normal; +++ pathological; 0=absent with reinforcement

   Thorax and abdomen:
   - Respiration
   - Thoracic and abdominal muscles
   - Abdominal reflexes

   Lower limbs:
   - Wasting and fasciculation
   - Tone, power and tendon reflexes
   - Plantar responses
8. ***Coordination and fine movements***
9. ***Sensory system***
   - Chart area of sensory loss; start in area with abnormal sensation and move stimulus towards normal area to demarcate boundaries

   Posterior columns:
   - Vibration (128 Hz tuning fork)
   - Joint position – small movements of distal interphalangeal joints in toes and fingers
   - Light touch – use cotton wool
   - Two-point discrimination (normal: 2–4 mm fingertips, 2 cm soles)

   Spinothalamic tracts:
   - Pain: use a split orange-stick or a sterile pin (never a hypodermic needle)
   - Temperature: warm and cold objects

   Cortical sensory loss – dysgraphaesthesia and astereognosis
10. ***Specialized tests*** as required e.g. Hallpike for vertigo, Phalen's test and so on

Box 21.6 Muscle power – the Medical Research Council (MRC) scale

Grade	Definition
5	Normal power
4	Active movement against gravity and resistance
3	Active movement against gravity only
2	Active movement with gravity eliminated
1	Flicker of contraction
0	No contraction

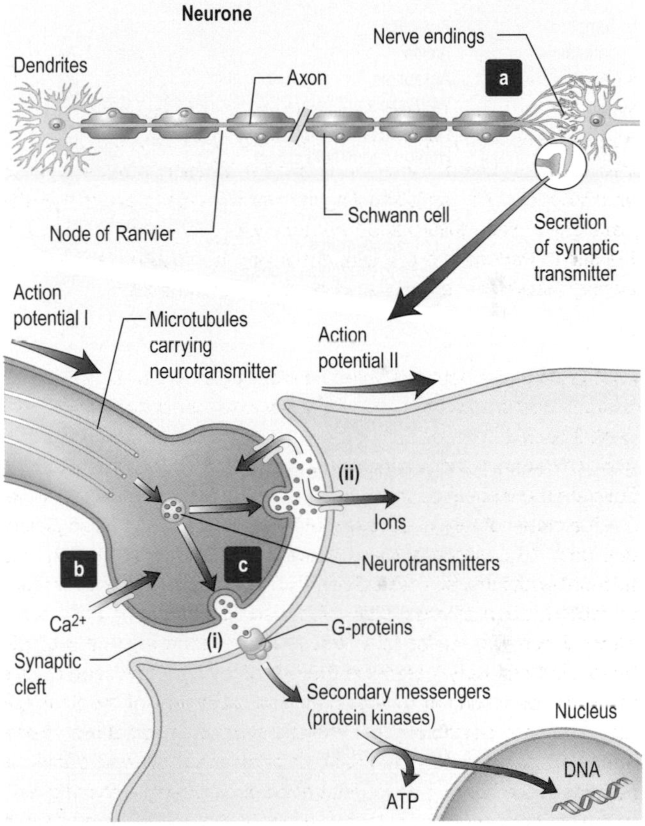

Figure 21.1 The functional unit: neurone and neurotransmitters. **(a)** ***The action potential*** – that is, the nerve impulse – travels down the axon. Microtubules carry neurotransmitters to nerve endings. **(b)** ***Action potential I*** depolarizes the synaptic membrane, opening voltage-gated calcium channels. **(c)** Influx of calcium ions causes vesicles to fuse with the membrane, allowing neurotransmitter binding to receptors **(i)** and activation of secondary messengers that modulate gene transcription and also open ligand-gated channels **(ii)**. This allows ions to enter, depolarize the membrane and ***initiate action potential II.***

Synaptic transmission is mediated by neurotransmitters released by action potentials passing down an axon. Neurotransmitters activate postsynaptic receptors and are removed by transporter proteins. The neurotransmitter–receptor reaction increases ionic permeability and propagates a further action potential. Axonal electrical activity and synaptic chemical release are the basis of neurological function.

Clinical features of focal brain lesions: general mechanisms

The symptoms and signs suggest the area of the brain that is malfunctioning (e.g. aphasia – the left frontal lobe; hemiparesis – the internal capsule, or a Bell's palsy – VIIth cranial (facial) nerve).

Focal lesions of the cortex, and lesions throughout the nervous system, cause symptoms and signs by two processes:

- ***Suppression or destruction of neurones*** and surrounding structures ***(Fig. 21.2)***. This is the most common process: part of the system simply fails to work.
- ***Synchronous discharge of neurones*** by *irritative* lesions ***(Fig. 21.3)***, e.g. cortical lesions, causes epilepsy, either partial or generalized.

Localization within the cerebral cortex

This subject causes unnecessary difficulty. Work on neuronal networks, functional imaging and plasticity questions the traditional views of highly specific localization of cortical function. The following paragraphs summarize areas of clinical relevance.

Site of lesion	Disorder	R L
Frontal, either	Intellectual impairment Personality change Urinary incontinence Monoparesis or hemiparesis	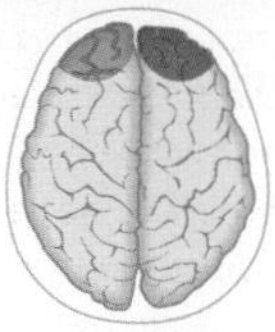
Frontal, left	Broca's aphasia	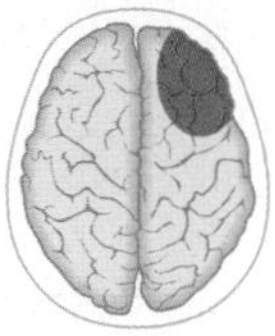
Temporo-parietal, left	Acalculia Alexia Agraphia Wernicke's aphasia Right-left disorientation Homonymous field defect	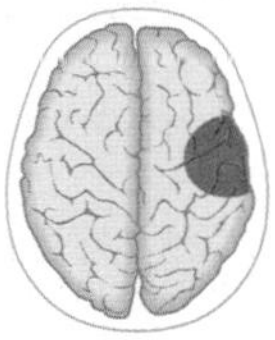
Temporal, right	Confusional states Failure to recognize faces Homonymous field defect	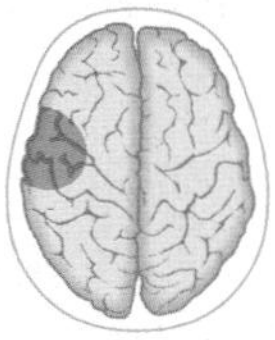
Parietal, either	Contralateral sensory loss or neglect Agraphaesthesia Homonymous field defect	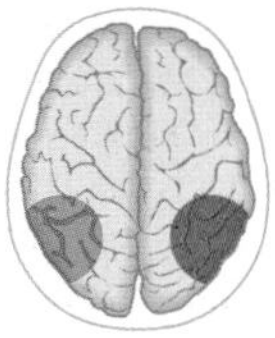
Parietal, right	Dressing apraxia Failure to recognize faces	
Parietal, left	Limb apraxia	
Occipital/ occipitoparietal	Visual field defects Visuospatial defects Disturbances of visual recognition	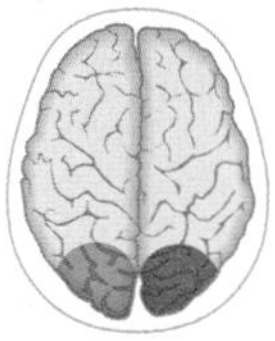

Figure 21.2 Principal features of destructive cortical lesions in a right-handed individual.

Site of lesion	Effects	R L
Frontal	Partial seizures–focal motor seizures of contralateral limbs Conjugate deviation of head and eyes away from the lesion	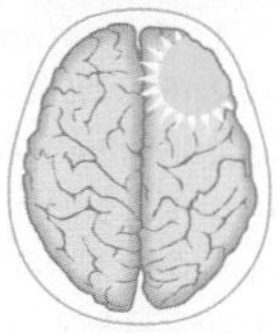
Temporal	Formed visual hallucinations Complex partial seizures Memory disturbances (e.g. *déjà vu*)	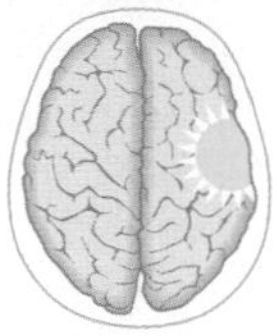
Parietal Parieto-occipital	Partial seizures–focal sensory seizures of contralateral limbs Crude visual hallucinations (e.g. shapes in one part of the field)	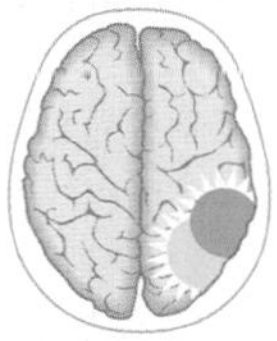
Occipital	Visual disturbances (e.g. flashes)	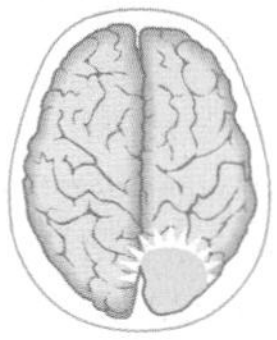

Figure 21.3 Effects of irritative cortical lesions.

The dominant hemisphere (usually left)

The concept of cerebral dominance arose from a simple observation: right-handed stroke patients with acquired language disorders had destructive lesions within the left hemisphere. Right-handed (and 70% of left-handed) people have language function on the left.

More specifically, destructive lesions within the left fronto-temporo-parietal region cause disorders of communication:

- spoken language – ***aphasia***, also called ***dysphasia***
- writing – ***agraphia***
- reading – acquired ***alexia***.

Developmental dyslexia describes delayed, disorganized reading and writing ability in children, usually with normal intelligence.

Aphasia

Aphasia is loss of, or defective language from damage to, the speech centres within the left hemisphere. Numerous varieties have been described.

Broca's (expressive, anterior) aphasia

Damage in the left frontal lobe causes reduced speech fluency with relatively preserved comprehension. The patient makes great efforts to initiate language, which becomes reduced to a few disjointed words with failure to construct sentences (sometimes described as ***telegrammatic***). Patients who recover say they knew what they wanted to say but could not get the words out.

Wernicke's (receptive, posterior) aphasia

Left temporo-parietal damage leaves fluency of language but words are muddled. This varies from insertion of a few incorrect or non-existent words into speech to a profuse outpouring of jargon (non-existent words). Severe jargon aphasia is bizarre and often mistaken for psychotic behaviour.

Patients who recover from Wernicke's aphasia say that they found speech, both their own and others', like an unintelligible foreign language – that is, incomprehensible – but they could neither stop speaking nor understand speech.

Nominal (anomic) aphasia

This means difficulty in naming objects. Naming difficulty is an early feature in all types of aphasia. This is often tested in practice by asking patient to name parts of a watch; a more sensitive test utilizes pictures to test low-frequency words, such as rhinoceros, violin, tricycle or ladybird.

Global (central) aphasia

This means the combination of the expressive problems of Broca's aphasia and the loss of comprehension of Wernicke's, with loss of both language production and understanding. It is due to widespread damage to speech areas and is the most common aphasia after a severe left hemisphere infarct. Writing and reading are also affected.

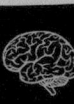

Dysarthria

Dysarthria is disordered articulation – slurred speech. Language is intact. Paralysis, slowing or incoordination of the muscles of articulation causes various patterns of dysarthria. Examples are the ***gravelly*** speech of pseudobulbar palsy (see p. 811), the ***jerky***, ataxic speech of cerebellar lesions, the hypophonic ***monotone*** of Parkinson's, and speech in myasthenia that ***fatigues*** and dies away. Many aphasic patients are also dysarthric.

The non-dominant hemisphere

Disorders in right-handed patients with right hemisphere lesions are often difficult to recognize. There are abnormalities of perception of internal and external space. Examples are loss of the way in familiar surroundings, failure to put on clothing correctly (dressing apraxia), or inability to draw simple shapes – constructional apraxia.

Memory and its disorders

Like most brain functions, memory has a modular organization, with different aspects of memory dependent on functionally and anatomically distinct brain networks. Three distinct processes are required: learning, storage and subsequent retrieval of learned information. There is a fundamental distinction between ***explicit*** memory, which can be consciously accessed, such as long-term memory for events (***episodic*** memory) and knowledge of word meaning (***semantic*** memory) on the one hand, and ***implicit*** memory, which is not conscious: for example, how to ride a bike ***(Fig. 21.4)***. Short-term memory is frequently misunderstood and refers to ***working*** memory lasting seconds only: for example, phone numbers.

Disorders of memory can result from damage to the medial structures of the temporal lobes and their brainstem connections – the hippocampi, fornices and mammillary bodies, as well as from damage to the thalamus and frontal lobe. The distributed anatomical basis of memory means that bilateral lesions are necessary to cause ***amnesia***. Impairment of episodic memory usually results in a temporal memory gradient: recent and new memories are mainly affected, with relative preservation of distant memories.

Memory loss (the amnestic syndrome) is frequently a symptom of dementia, especially Alzheimer's disease (see pp. 876–878), but also occurs as an isolated entity ***(Box 21.7)***.

Essential elements of neuroanatomy

For clinical purposes, the complexity of neuroanatomy must be reduced to its core elements:

- cranial nerves
- three systems of motor control:
  - corticospinal or pyramidal system
  - extrapyramidal system
  - cerebellum

Box 21.7 Causes of an amnestic syndrome[a]

- Dementia (note: multiple cognitive domains affected, not memory in isolation)
- Amnestic mild cognitive impairment (see p. 876)
- Alcohol – thiamine deficiency (Wernicke–Korsakoff syndrome)
- Head injury (severe)
- Anoxic brain damage and that following carbon monoxide poisoning
- Stroke, including bilateral thalamic infarction, subarachnoid haemorrhage, diffuse small-vessel disease, and post cardiac surgery
- Viral, paraneoplastic and autoimmune encephalitis
- Drugs – psychotropics, anticholinergics and solvent abuse
- Bilateral invasive tumours
- Temporal lobe epilepsy and temporal lobectomy
- Following hypoglycaemia
- Temporary amnesia: transient global amnesia, transient epileptic amnesia, post-traumatic amnesia
- Dissociative (functional/psychogenic)

[a] *Amnesia must be distinguished from delirium.*

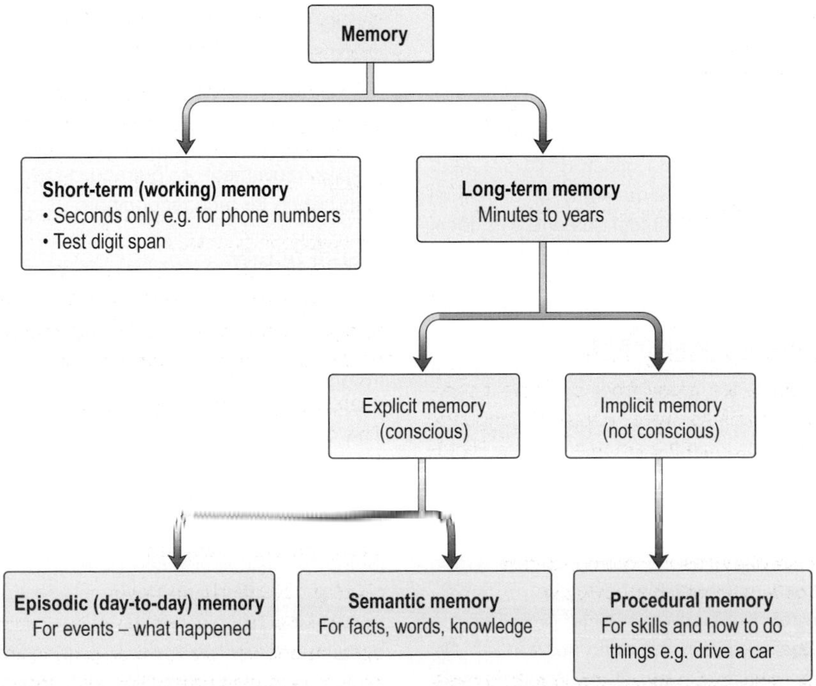

Figure 21.4 Types of memory.

Box 21.8 Cranial nerves

Number	Name	Main clinical action
I	Olfactory	Smell
II	Optic	Vision, fields, afferent light reflex
III	Oculomotor	Eyelid elevation, eye elevation, **ad**duction, depression in **ab**duction, efferent pupil – light reflex
IV	Trochlear	Eye intorsion, depression in **ad**duction
V	Trigeminal	Facial (and corneal) sensation, mastication muscles
VI	Abducens	Eye **ab**duction
VII	Facial	Facial movement, taste fibres
VIII	Vestibulo-cochlear Cochlear	Balance and hearing
IX	Glossopharyngeal	Sensation – soft palate, taste fibres
X	Vagus	Cough, palatal and vocal cord movements
XI	Accessory	Head turning, shoulder shrugging
XII	Hypoglossal	Tongue movement

- motor unit
- reflex arc
- sensory pathways and pain
- control of the bladder and sexual function.

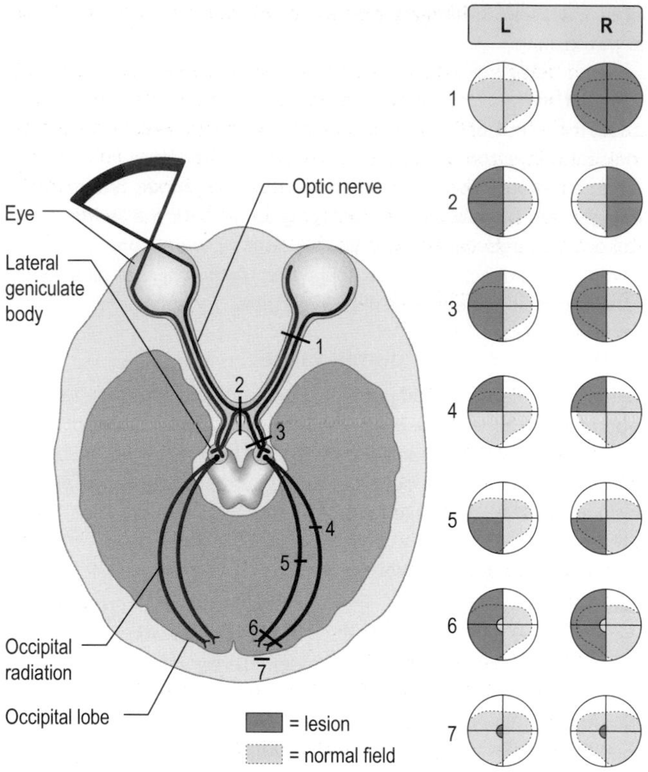

Figure 21.5 The visual pathway. (1) Mononuclear field loss – complete optic nerve lesion. **(2)** Bitemporal hemianopia – chiasmal lesion. **(3)** Homonymous hemianopia – optic tract lesion. **(4)** Homonymous quadrantanopia – temporal lesion. **(5)** Homonymous quadrantanopia – parietal lesion. **(6)** Homonymous hemianopia with macular sparing – occipital cortex or optic radiation. **(7)** Homonymous hemianopia (hemiscotoma) – occipital pole lesion.

CRANIAL NERVES

See ***Box 21.8***.

I: Olfactory nerve

This sensory nerve arises from olfactory (smell) receptors within nasal mucosa. Branches pierce the cribriform plate and synapse in the olfactory bulb. The olfactory tract passes to the olfactory cortex.

Anosmia (loss of the sense of smell) is caused by head injury (shearing of olfactory neurones as they pass through the cribriform plate at the skull base) or tumours of the olfactory groove (e.g. meningioma). Olfaction is temporarily (or permanently, on occasion) lost or diminished after upper respiratory infections and with local disorders of the nose. Many patients with gradual-onset anosmia over many years may be unaware of the deficit: for example, in Parkinson's disease, where anosmia precedes motor symptoms by many years but is often not noticed by the patient.

Detailed smell testing is difficult in routine clinical practice and rarely performed. Adequate testing requires use of commercially available kits, such as scratch and sniff cards or odour-filled pens with forced multiple choice identification.

II: Optic nerve and visual system

Light regulated by the pupillary aperture is converted into action potentials by retinal rod, cone and ganglion cells (see pp. 1323–1324). The lens, under control of the ciliary muscle, produces the image (inverted) on the retina. Axons in the optic nerve (1 on ***Fig. 21.5***) decussate at the optic chiasm (2), and fibres from the nasal retina cross and join with uncrossed fibres originating in the temporal retina to form the optic tract (3). Each optic tract thus carries information from the contralateral visual hemifield.

From the lateral geniculate body, fibres pass in the optic radiation through the parietal and temporal lobes (4 and 5) to reach the visual cortex of the occipital lobe (6 and 7), which is somatotopically organized with macular vision located at the occipital pole.

Beyond the visual cortex, visual information is further processed by neighbouring visual association areas to detect lines, orientation, shapes, movement, colour and depth; there is even a distinct area responsible for face recognition.

Visual acuity

Visual acuity (see p. 1324) is assessed in each eye with a Snellen chart and/or Near Vision Reading Types, corrected for refractive errors with lenses or a pinhole. The patient should stand 6 metres from a well-lit chart. Acuity is recorded as distance in metres from the chart over distance at which the line should be legible, e.g. 6/6 indicates 'normal' acuity and 6/60 very poor acuity.

Visual field defects

Visual fields are assessed at the bedside by confrontation – comparing the examiner's and patient's fields, one eye at a time and quadrant by quadrant. Patience and good technique are required to produce reliable results. White and red targets (traditionally, hatpins) are used to assess peripheral and central fields, respectively, although in practice a fingertip is often substituted as a cruder screening test. More detailed quantification of fields may be obtained using Goldmann (manual) or Humphrey (automated) perimetry testing.

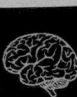

Field defects are described as hemianopic when half the field is affected and quadrantanopic when a quadrant is affected. Lesions posterior to the optic chiasm produce ***homonymous*** field defects, indicating involvement of the same part of the visual field in both eyes, as information from the two visual hemifields is separated beyond this point. Lesions damaging decussating nasal fibres at the optic chiasm cause bitemporal defects.

Retinal and local eye lesions

See pages 1333–1334.

Optic nerve lesions

Unilateral visual loss, commencing with a central or paracentral (off-centre) scotoma, is the hallmark of an optic nerve lesion. Because most fibres in the optic nerve subserve macular vision, lesions within the nerve disproportionately affect central vision and colour vision. A total optic nerve lesion causes unilateral blindness with loss of pupillary light reflex. Examination findings in optic neuropathy are:

- reduced acuity in the affected eye
- a scotoma (usually central)
- impaired colour vision (assess with Ishihara plates)
- an afferent pupillary defect (see below)
- optic atrophy – pale disc (develops late).

Causes are listed in ***Box 21.9***.

Papilloedema

Papilloedema means swelling of the optic disc. Causes are shown in ***Box 21.10***. The earliest signs of swelling are disc pinkness, with blurring and heaping up of disc margins, nasal first. There is loss of spontaneous pulsation of retinal veins within the disc. The physiological cup becomes obliterated, and the disc is engorged with dilated vessels. Small haemorrhages often surround the disc.

Various conditions simulate true disc swelling. Marked hypermetropic (long-sighted) refractive errors make a disc appear pink, distant and ill defined. Myelinated nerve fibres at disc margins and hyaline bodies (drusen; see p. 1334) can be mistaken for disc swelling.

Disc infiltration also causes a swollen disc with raised margins (e.g. in leukaemia).

When there is doubt about disc oedema, intravenous fluorescein angiography is diagnostic; retinal leakage is seen with papilloedema.

Papilloedema produces few, if any, visual symptoms other than momentary visual obscurations with changes in posture. The underlying disease is the source of the patient's symptoms. The blind spot is enlarged but this is not noticed by the patient. However, over time, progressive and permanent constriction of visual fields occurs, ultimately culminating in optic atrophy.

Inflammatory optic neuropathy (optic neuritis)

Optic neuritis is one of the most common causes of subacute visual loss. Symptoms may vary from a mild fogging of central vision with colour desaturation to a dense central scotoma, but very rarely complete blindness. Pain on eye movements is almost universal. The optic disc usually appears normal, despite severe visual loss (unless the inflammation is at the optic nerve head, in which case the disc may appear swollen in the acute phase).

A plaque of demyelination within the optic nerve is the most common cause in Western populations. Dedicated magnetic resonance imaging (MRI) of the optic nerves may show the inflammatory plaque, and imaging of the brain may show additional inflammatory lesions, which confer a higher risk of developing multiple sclerosis (MS). Approximately 50% of patients go on to develop MS with prolonged follow-up (see pp. 858–862). Recovery of visual acuity to 6/9 or better occurs in 95% of cases over months; recovery time is improved by high-dose intravenous steroids given acutely.

Optic neuritis may be caused by infective or other inflammatory disorders, such as sarcoidosis or vasculitides (see ***Box 21.9***).

Anterior ischaemic optic neuropathy

The anterior part of the optic nerve is supplied by the posterior ciliary arteries, occlusion or hypoperfusion of which leads to infarction of all or part of the optic nerve head. There is sudden or stuttering altitudinal visual loss (typically, the lower half of the visual field) with disc swelling, later replaced by optic atrophy. The other eye is affected later in one-third of cases.

Individuals with small hypermetropic discs seem to be predisposed, and often there are relatively few vascular risk factors. Less commonly, arteritis is the cause (see p. 694).

Optic atrophy

Optic atrophy means disc pallor, from loss of axons, glial proliferation and decreased vascularity. This may eventually develop following any type of optic neuropathy of sufficient severity to damage axons extensively within the nerve, including chronic papilloedema.

Box 21.9 Causes of optic neuropathy

- Inflammatory (optic neuritis), e.g. demyelination, sarcoidosis, vasculitis
- Optic nerve trauma or compression, e.g. glioma, meningioma, aneurysm, bone disorders affecting orbit
- Toxic, e.g. tobacco/alcohol, ethambutol, methyl alcohol, quinine, hydroxychloroquine, radiation
- Ischaemic optic neuropathy, e.g. giant cell arteritis
- Hereditary optic neuropathies, e.g. Leber's
- Nutritional deficiency, e.g. vitamins B_1 and B_{12}
- Infection, e.g. orbital cellulitis, syphilis, tuberculosis
- Neurodegenerative disorders, e.g. leucodystrophies
- Papilloedema and its causes (see ***Box 21.10***)

Box 21.10 Causes of optic disc swelling

- Raised intracranial pressure (papilloedema)
- Brain tumour, abscess or haemorrhage
- Idiopathic intracranial hypertension, hydrocephalus
- Optic nerve disease
- Optic neuritis, e.g. multiple sclerosis
- Ischaemic optic neuropathy, e.g. giant cell arteritis
- Toxic optic neuropathy, e.g. methanol
- Venous occlusion
- Venous sinus thrombosis
- Central retinal vein thrombosis
- Orbital mass lesions
- Retinal vascular disease
- Malignant hypertension
- Vasculitis, e.g. systemic lupus erythematosus
- Metabolic causes
- Hypercapnia, chronic hypoxia, hypocalcaemia
- Disc infiltration
- Leukaemia, sarcoidosis, optic nerve glioma

Optic chiasm

Bitemporal hemianopia or quadrantanopia occurs with compression of the chiasm from above or below. Common causes are:
- pituitary tumours (see pp. 1182–1183)
- meningioma
- craniopharyngioma.

Optic tract and optic radiation

Optic tract lesions (rare) cause a homonymous hemianopia (loss of the contralateral visual field in both eyes). Optic radiation lesions cause homonymous quadrantanopic defects. Temporal lobe lesions (e.g. tumour, infarction) cause upper quadrantic defects, and parietal lobe lesions cause lower quadrantic defects.

Occipital cortex

Homonymous hemianopic defects are produced by unilateral posterior cerebral artery infarction (see p. 834). The macular cortex (at each occipital pole) may be spared.

Widespread bilateral occipital lobe damage by infarction (‘***top of the basilar***’ syndrome, occlusion of the rostral basilar artery), trauma or coning causes ***cortical blindness*** (Anton syndrome). The patient cannot see but characteristically lacks insight into this; he or she may even deny it. Pupillary responses remain normal (see p. 834).

The pupils

A slight difference between the size of each pupil (up to 1 mm) is common (***physiological anisocoria***) and does not vary with differing light levels. The pupil tends to become smaller and irregular in old age (senile miosis); anisocoria is more pronounced. ***Convergence*** becomes sluggish with ageing.

Pupillary reactions to light and accommodation may be tested ***(Fig. 21.6)***. A bright torch (not an ophthalmoscope light!) should be used to test the pupillary light reaction.

Afferent pupillary defect (APD). A complete optic nerve lesion causes a dilated pupil and an APD. For a left APD:
- The pupil is unreactive to light (i.e. the direct reflex is absent).
- The consensual reflex (constriction of the right pupil when the left is illuminated) is absent. Conversely, the left pupil constricts when light is shone in the intact right eye: that is, the consensual reflex of the right eye remains intact.

Relative afferent pupillary defect (RAPD). This occurs with incomplete damage to one optic nerve relative to the other. An RAPD is a sensitive sign of optic nerve pathology and can provide evidence of an optic nerve lesion, even after recovery of vision. For a left RAPD:
- Direct and indirect reflexes are intact in each eye but differ in relative strength.
- When the light is swung from one eye to the other, the left pupil ***dilates*** slightly when illuminated and ***constricts*** slightly when the right eye is illuminated (the consensual reflex is stronger than the direct).

Horner syndrome

The sympathetic nervous supply to the eye is a three-neurone pathway originating in the hypothalamus and descending by way of the brainstem and cervical cord to the T1 nerve root, paravertebral sympathetic chain and, on via the carotid artery wall, to the eye. Damage to any part of the pathway results in Horner syndrome ***(Box 21.11)***. This is significant not only because it affects vision but also because it may indicate serious underlying pathology.

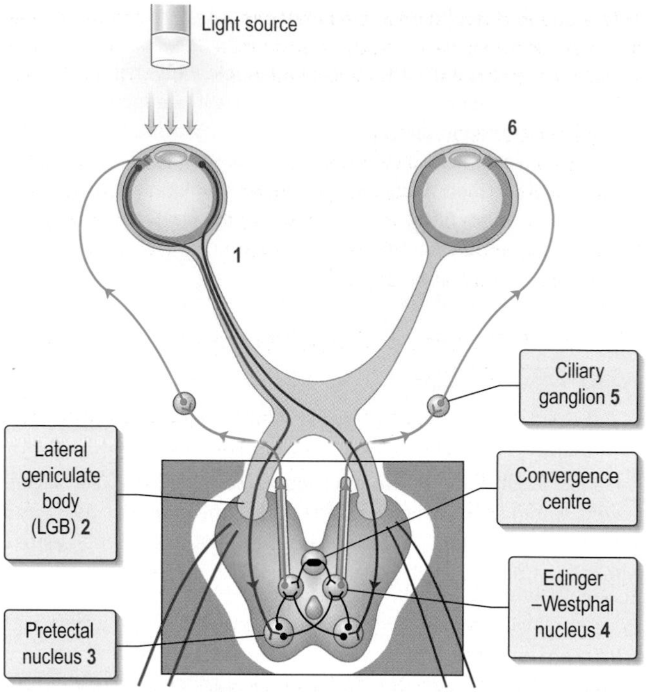

Figure 21.6 Pupillary light reflex. *Afferent pathway*: **(1)** Light activates optic nerve axons. **(2)** Axons (some decussating at the chiasm) pass through each lateral geniculate body, and **(3)** synapse at pretectal nuclei. *Efferent pathway*: **(4)** Action potentials pass to Edinger–Westphal nuclei of the IIIrd nerve, then, **(5)** via parasympathetic neurones in IIIrd nerves to cause **(6)** pupil constriction.

Box 21.11 Causes of Horner syndrome

Hypothalamic, hemisphere and brainstem lesions
- Massive cerebral infarction
- Brainstem demyelination or lateral medullary infarction

Cervical cord
- Syringomyelia and cord tumours

T1 root
- Apical lung tumour or tuberculosis
- Cervical rib
- Brachial plexus trauma

Sympathetic chain and carotid artery in neck
- Following thyroid/laryngeal/carotid surgery
- Carotid artery dissection
- Neoplastic infiltration
- Cervical sympathectomy

Miscellaneous
- Congenital
- Cluster headache, usually transient
- Idiopathic

The clinical features of Horner syndrome are:
- unilateral miosis (constricted pupil)
- partial ptosis
- loss of sweating on the same side (extent depending on the level of the lesion)
- possible subtle conjunctival injection and enophthalmos.

The miosis is most easily seen in low light, as the pupil cannot dilate, and may not be apparent in bright light.

Myotonic pupil (Holmes–Adie pupil)

This is a dilated, often irregular, pupil and more frequent in women; it is common and usually unilateral. There is no (or very slow) reaction to bright light and also incomplete constriction to convergence.

This is due to denervation in the ciliary ganglion, of unknown cause, and has no other pathological significance. A myotonic pupil is sometimes associated with diminished or absent tendon reflexes.

Argyll Robertson pupil

Now rarely seen in clinical practice, an Argyll Robertson pupil is small and irregular; it is fixed to light but constricts on convergence. The lesion is in the brainstem surrounding the aqueduct of Sylvius. Once considered diagnostic of neurosyphilis, it is now only occasionally seen in diabetes or MS.

III, IV, VI: Oculomotor, trochlear and abducens nerves

These cranial nerves supply the extraocular muscles and disorders commonly result in abnormal eye movements and diplopia (double vision) due to breakdown of conjugate (yoked) eye movements. Diplopia may also occur with local orbital lesions or myasthenia gravis.

Examination of eye movements

Pursuit (slow) eye movements and saccadic (fast) eye movements are tested separately. The examiner assesses the range of eye movements in all directions and asks the patient to report double vision. Jerky pursuit movements with saccadic intrusion (i.e. brief, fast saccades interspersed with slower pursuit movements) overshoot on saccadic movements, and nystagmus may indicate cerebellar or brainstem pathology.

Control of eye movements

Fast voluntary eye movements originate in the frontal lobes. Fibres descend and cross in the pons to end in the centre for lateral gaze (paramedian pontine reticular formation, PPRF), close to the VIth nerve nucleus. Each PPRF also receives input from:

- the ipsilateral occipital cortex – pathway concerned with tracking objects
- the vestibular nuclei – pathways linking eye movements with position of the head and neck (vestibulo-ocular reflex)

Conjugate lateral eye movements are coordinated from each PPRF via the medial longitudinal fasciculus (MLF; ***Fig. 21.7***). Fibres from the PPRF pass both to the ipsilateral VIth nerve nucleus (lateral rectus) and, having crossed the midline, to the opposite IIIrd nerve nucleus (medial rectus and other muscles) via the MLF, thus linking the eyes for lateral gaze.

Abnormalities of conjugate lateral gaze

A destructive lesion on one side allows the eyes to be driven by the intact opposite pathway. A left frontal destructive lesion (e.g. an infarct) leads to failure of conjugate lateral gaze to the right. In an acute lesion, the eyes are often deviated to the side of the lesion, past the midline, and therefore look towards the left (normal) limbs; there is usually a contralateral (i.e. right) hemiparesis.

In the brainstem, a unilateral destructive lesion involving the PPRF leads to failure of conjugate lateral gaze towards that side. There is usually a contralateral hemiparesis, and lateral gaze is deviated towards the side of the paralysed limbs.

Internuclear ophthalmoplegia

Damage to one MLF causes internuclear ophthalmoplegia (INO), a common complex brainstem eye movement disorder seen frequently in MS. In a right INO, there is a lesion of the right MLF ***(Fig. 21.7)***. On attempted left lateral gaze, the right eye fails to **ad**duct or does so slowly as compared to the **ab**ducting eye. The left eye develops nystagmus in **ab**duction. The side of the lesion is on the side of impaired **ad**duction, not on the side of the (obvious, unilateral) nystagmus. Bilateral INO is almost pathognomonic of MS.

One and a half syndrome

Pontine infarction involving the PPRF, VIth nerve nucleus and MLF on one side results in an ipsilateral horizontal gaze palsy and an INO, so that abduction of the opposite eye (with nystagmus) is the only horizontal eye movement possible. Vertical gaze and convergence are preserved, as they have distinct neural control mechanisms.

Vestibulo-ocular (doll's eye) reflexes

Examination is of diagnostic value in coma (see p. 1172) and assessment of vertigo (see p. 809).

Abnormalities of vertical gaze

Failure of up-gaze may be caused by dorsal midbrain lesions, such as pinealoma or infarct. When the pupillary light reflex fails in addition, this is called Parinaud syndrome. Defective up-gaze also develops in certain degenerative disorders (e.g. progressive supranuclear palsy). Some impairment of up-gaze occurs as part of normal ageing.

Principal output from PPRF

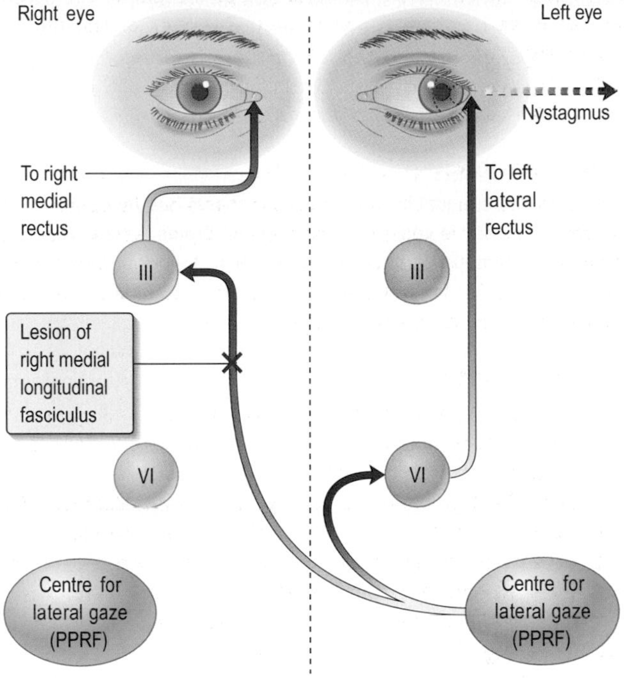

Figure 21.7 Paramedian pontine reticular formation (PPRF) and internuclear ophthalmoplegia. Impulses from the PPRF pass via the ipsilateral VIth nerve nucleus to the lateral rectus muscle (**ab**duction), and via the medial longitudinal fasciculus to the opposite third nerve nucleus and thus to the opposite medial rectus muscle (**ad**duction). A lesion of the medial longitudinal fasciculus (X) causes failure of or slow **ad**duction in the right eye, and nystagmus in the left eye with left lateral gaze.

Nystagmus

Nystagmus is rhythmic oscillation of eye movement; it is a sign of disease of the retina, cerebellum and/or vestibular systems and their connections. Nystagmus is either ***jerk*** or ***pendular***. Nystagmus must be sustained within binocular gaze to be of diagnostic value; a few beats at the extremes of gaze are normal.

Jerk nystagmus

Jerk nystagmus (usual in neurological disease) is a fast/slow oscillation. This is seen in vestibular, VIIIth nerve, brainstem and cerebellar lesions. The direction of nystagmus is decided by the fast component, a reflex attempt to correct the slower, primary movement.

- ***Horizontal or rotary jerk nystagmus*** may be either of peripheral (vestibular) or central origin (VIIIth nerve, brainstem, cerebellum and connections).
  - In peripheral lesions, nystagmus is usually acute and transient (minutes or hours) and associated with severe prostrating vertigo.
  - In central lesions, nystagmus tends to be long-lasting (weeks, months or more). Vertigo caused by central lesions tends to wane after days or weeks, the nystagmus outlasting it.
- ***Vertical jerk nystagmus*** is typically caused by central lesions.
- ***Down-beat jerk nystagmus*** is a rarity caused by lesions around the foramen magnum (e.g. meningioma, cerebellar ectopia).

Pendular nystagmus

Pendular describes movements to and fro, similar in velocity and amplitude. Pendular nystagmus is usually vertical and present in all directions of gaze. The causes are generally ocular (e.g. poor visual fixation from longstanding, severe visual impairment) or congenital.

III: Oculomotor nerve lesions

The nucleus of the IIIrd nerve lies ventral to the aqueduct in the midbrain. It supplies four external ocular muscles (superior, inferior and medial recti, and inferior oblique) and levator palpebrae superioris (which lifts the eyelid), and effects parasympathetic constriction of the pupil. Causes of a IIIrd nerve lesion are listed in ***Box 21.12***.

Signs of a complete IIIrd nerve palsy include:

- unilateral complete ptosis (levator weakness)
- deviation of the eye down and out (unopposed lateral rectus and superior oblique)
- a fixed and dilated pupil.

Patients do not complain of diplopia as the ptosis effectively covers the eye. ***Sparing of the pupil*** indicates that parasympathetic fibres are undamaged; these run in a discrete bundle on the surface of the nerve, and so the pupil is of normal size and reacts normally. Diabetic IIIrd nerve infarction is usually painless and pupil-sparing, unlike compression by a posterior communicating artery aneurysm.

? Box 21.12 Some causes of a IIIrd nerve lesion

- Aneurysm of the posterior communicating artery
- Infarction of IIIrd nerve, e.g. diabetes, atheroma
- Coning of the temporal lobe
- Midbrain infarction
- Midbrain tumour (primary or secondary)

IV: Trochlear nerve lesions

The trochlear nerve supplies the superior oblique muscle. The patient complains of torsional diplopia (two objects at an angle) when attempting to look down (e.g. descending stairs); the head is tilted away from that side. The most common cause is head injury, often with bilateral trochlear nerve palsies occurring.

VI: Abducens nerve lesions

The abducens nerve supplies the lateral rectus muscle (**ab**duction). Lesions cause horizontal diplopia when looking into the distance, which is maximal when looking to the side of the lesion. The eye cannot be fully abducted and an esotropia (inward eye deviation) may be visible in the primary position.

The VIth nerve has a long intracranial course. It can be damaged in the brainstem (e.g. by MS or infarction). In raised intracranial pressure, it is compressed against the tip of the petrous temporal bone (this may be bilateral). The nerve sheath may be infiltrated by tumours, particularly nasopharyngeal carcinoma. Microvascular ischaemia of the nerve may occur in diabetes with acute onset, followed by recovery within 3 months in most cases.

Complete external ophthalmoplegia

Complete external ophthalmoplegia describes an immobile eye when IIIrd, IVth and VIth nerves are paralysed at the orbital apex (e.g. by metastasis) or within the cavernous sinus (e.g. by sinus thrombosis or meningioma).

Wernicke's encephalopathy due to thiamine deficiency (see p. 885) may cause a complex eye movement disorder or complete ophthalmoplegia, as may neuromuscular junction disorders such as myasthenia, botulism and some myopathies or metabolic disorders.

V: Trigeminal nerve

The trigeminal is the largest cranial nerve; it is mainly sensory with a motor component to the muscles of mastication.

Sensory fibres (***Fig. 21.8***; see also ***Figs 21.13*** and ***21.14***) of the three divisions – ophthalmic (V_1), maxillary (V_2) and mandibular (V_3) – pass to the trigeminal (Gasserian) ganglion at the apex of the petrous temporal bone. Ascending fibres transmitting light touch enter the fifth nucleus in the pons. Descending central fibres carrying pain and temperature form the spinal tract of V, to end in the spinal fifth nucleus that extends from the medulla into the cervical cord.

Clinical features of a Vth nerve lesion

A complete Vth nerve lesion causes unilateral sensory loss on the face, scalp anterior to the vertex, and the anterior two-thirds of the tongue and buccal mucosa; the jaw deviates to that side as the mouth opens (motor fibres). Diminution of the corneal reflex is an early and sometimes isolated sign of a Vth nerve lesion.

Aetiology

- ***Brainstem pathology*** (infarction, demyelination or tumour) may damage the nucleus, with light touch and spinothalamic pathways sometimes being differentially involved.

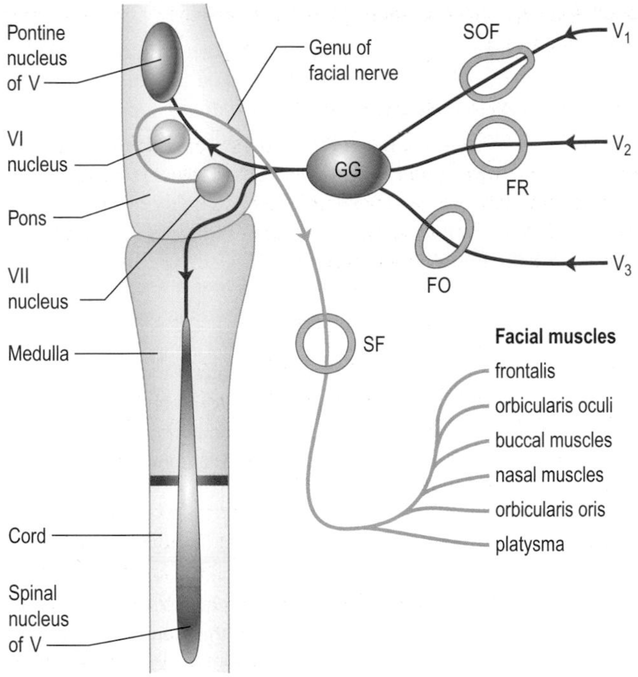

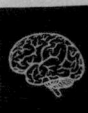

Figure 21.8 Sensory input of fifth nerve (red) and motor output of the VIIth nerve (blue). FO, foramen ovale; FR, foramen rotundum; GG, Gasserian ganglion; SF, stylomastoid foramen; SOF, superior orbital fissure.

- ***Cerebellopontine angle tumours*** (acoustic neuroma or meningioma) may compress the nerve and also affect the VIIth and VIIIth nerves, producing facial weakness and deafness.
- ***Cavernous sinus and skull base pathology*** (tumour or infection) may affect the ganglion and proximal branches.
- ***Peripheral branches*** may be picked off individually, e.g. the 'numb chin syndrome' seen with a breast cancer metastasis in the mandible.

Trigeminal neuralgia

Trigeminal neuralgia is discussed with facial pain (see p. 845).

Trigeminal sensory neuropathy

This causes gradually progressive, unilateral, facial sensory loss and tingling with normal imaging. The condition is probably heterogeneous in aetiology but may have an autoimmune basis, with inflammation of the trigeminal ganglion, occurring mainly in association with mixed and undifferentiated connective tissue disease and primary Sjögren syndrome.

VII: Facial nerve

The VIIth nerve is largely motor, supplying muscles of facial expression. It carries sensory taste fibres from the anterior two-thirds of the tongue via the chorda tympani and supplies motor fibres to the stapedius muscle. The VIIth nerve ***(Fig. 21.8)*** arises from its nucleus in the pons and leaves the skull through the stylomastoid foramen. Neurones in each VIIth nucleus supplying the upper face (principally frontalis) receive bilateral supranuclear innervation.

Unilateral facial weakness

Upper motor neurone (UMN) lesions. These cause weakness of the lower part of the face on the opposite side. Frontalis is spared: normal furrowing of the brow is preserved; eye closure and blinking are largely unaffected. The earliest sign is slowing of one side of the face: for example, on baring the teeth. There is sometimes relative preservation of spontaneous emotional movement (e.g. smiling) compared with voluntary movement.

Lower motor neurone (LMN) lesions. A complete unilateral LMN VIIth lesion causes weakness (ipsilateral) of all facial expression muscles. The angle of the mouth falls; unilateral dribbling develops. Frowning (frontalis) and eye closure are weak. Corneal exposure and ulceration occur if the eye does not close during sleep. Taste sensation is frequently also impaired.

Causes of facial weakness

The most common cause of a UMN lesion is hemispheric stroke with hemiparesis on the opposite side. At lower levels, lesion sites are recognized by LMN weakness with additional signs.

Pons. Here the VIIth nerve loops around the VIth (abducens) nucleus ***(Fig. 21.8)***, leading to a lateral rectus palsy (see p. 806) with unilateral LMN facial weakness. When the neighbouring PPRF and corticospinal tract are involved, there is the combination of:

- LMN facial weakness
- failure of conjugate lateral gaze (towards lesion)
- contralateral hemiparesis.

Causes include pontine tumours (e.g. glioma), MS and infarction.

Cerebellopontine angle (***CPA***). The neighbouring Vth, VIth and VIIIth nerves are compressed with VII in the CPA: for example, by acoustic neuroma, meningioma or metastasis.

Petrous temporal bone. The nerve may be damaged within the bony facial canal, within which lies the sensory geniculate ganglion (receiving taste fibres from the anterior two-thirds of the tongue via the chorda tympani). As well as LMN facial weakness, lesions in this region cause:

- loss of taste on the anterior two-thirds of the tongue
- hyperacusis (loud noise distortion – paralysis of stapedius).

Causes include:

- Bell's palsy
- trauma
- middle ear infection
- herpes zoster (Ramsay Hunt syndrome; see p. 808)

Skull base, parotid gland and within the face. The facial nerve can be compressed by skull base tumours and in Paget's disease of bone. Branches of VII may be damaged by parotid gland tumours as the nerve traverses the parotid, and by sarcoidosis (see pp. 1118–1120) and trauma.

Bell's palsy

This common (37 per 100 000 incidence), acute facial palsy is thought to be due to viral infection/reactivation (often herpes simplex) causing swelling of nerve within the tight petrous bone facial canal. Unilateral LMN facial weakness develops over 24–48 hours, sometimes with lost or altered taste on the tongue, and hyperacusis. Pain behind the ear is common at onset. Patients often suspect a stroke and may be very distressed. Vague altered facial sensation is often reported, although examination of facial sensation is normal.

Diagnosis is made on clinical grounds and tests are usually not required. The ear (and palate) should be examined for vesicles (see Ramsay Hunt syndrome below), hearing loss or evidence of local pathology such as cholesteatoma or malignant otitis externa; parotid tumours should be excluded. Involvement of other cranial nerves means facial weakness is not due to Bell's palsy. Lyme disease may account for one-quarter of cases of facial palsy in endemic areas and HIV seroconversion is the most common cause in parts of Africa.

(***Bell's phenomenon*** is the upward conjugate eye movement that occurs normally when the eyes are closed but is accentuated when the orbicularis oculi muscle is weak.)

Management and prognosis

Complete, or almost complete, recovery over 4–12 weeks occurs in at least 85% of patients, even without specific treatment. Patients should be reassured that the prognosis is good and that the condition is unlikely to recur.

Inability to blink in severe facial weakness may lead to exposure keratitis. Use of lubricating eye ointment is often required and patients should be advised to tape the eye closed carefully at night. For more severe facial weakness with complete inability to close the eye, early ophthalmological assessment is necessary and lateral tarsorrhaphy and/or insertion of a gold weight into the upper lid may be required until recovery occurs.

Early treatment with corticosteroids (prednisolone 50 mg for 10 days) improves outcome if started within 72 hours of onset. The latest evidence does not support use of antiviral agents.

Recovery sometimes takes up to a year if axons have to regrow rather than just remyelinate, in which case aberrant re-innervation of facial muscles (e.g. mouth twitching with blinking) is a frequent late complication. Plastic surgery may be helpful where recovery is not complete. Bell's palsy rarely recurs; if it does, this should prompt a search for an alternative cause.

Ramsay Hunt syndrome

This is herpes zoster (shingles) of the geniculate ganglion. There is a facial palsy (identical to Bell's) with vesicles around the external auditory meatus and/or the soft palate (sensory twigs from VII). Deafness and vertigo/unsteadiness may occur. Complete recovery is less likely than in Bell's. Antiviral treatment (aciclovir/valaciclovir) is usually given with steroids.

Bilateral facial weakness

Bilateral facial palsy is rare, accounting for less than 1% of cases of facial palsy, but is more likely than unilateral palsies to have an identifiable underlying cause. Paradoxically, bilateral weakness is often less obviously apparent than unilateral weakness, as there is no facial asymmetry.

Causes include:

- infections:
  - Lyme disease (bilateral in 25% – Bannwarth syndrome)
  - viral: human immunodeficiency virus (HIV) seroconversion, Epstein–Barr virus
  - mastoiditis (bilateral)
  - diphtheria and botulism (rare)
- sarcoidosis
- skull-base trauma and tumours
- pontine lesions, e.g. gliomas
- neuromuscular disorders as part of more generalized weakness:
  - Guillain–Barré syndrome
  - myasthenia
  - myotonic dystrophy and facioscapulohumeral dystrophy
- congenital and genetic causes (Gelsolin gene mutations).

Hemifacial spasm

Hemifacial spasm (HFS) is an irregular, painless unilateral spasm of facial muscles, usually occurring after middle age. It starts in the orbicularis oculi and usually progresses gradually over the years to involve other facial muscles on the same side. It varies from a mild to a severe, disfiguring spasm.

HFS is usually caused by compression of the root entry zone of the facial nerve, generally by vascular structures such as the vertebral or basilar arteries or their branches (a mechanism similar to that of trigeminal neuralgia; see p. 845). Other mass lesions in the cerebellopontine angle, including tumours, are the cause in approximately 1% of cases.

Occasionally, HFS may occur with ipsilateral trigeminal neuralgia, one symptom usually preceding the other: a combination called ***tic convulsif***. The paroxysms of pain and spasm occur independently. A compressive cause, such as a vascular loop or other structural lesion, is usually identified.

Management

Mild cases require no treatment. Botulinum toxin injection into affected muscles every 3–4 months is now the standard treatment. Drugs (e.g. carbamazepine) are of little value. Decompression of the VIIth nerve in the CPA is sometimes helpful. Surgical decompression of the facial nerve in the posterior fossa involves interposing a non-resorbable sponge between the nerve and any adjacent vascular loop identified at operation. The procedure results in complete resolution of symptoms in up to 90% of cases but is associated with a risk of facial weakness or deafness.

Other involuntary facial movements

Myokymia of orbicularis oculi is an irritating twitch, usually of the lower eyelid. It is a normal phenomenon but sometimes a cause of anxiety. More extensive facial myokymia may result from intrinsic brainstem pathology.

Tics and tardive dyskinesia frequently involve facial or perioral muscles (see pp. 856–857).

Blepharospasm is a form of focal dystonia affecting orbicularis oculi (see p. 857).

VIII: Vestibulo-cochlear nerve and cochlear nerve

Auditory fibres from the spiral organ of Corti within the cochlea pass to the cochlear nuclei in the pons. Fibres from these nuclei cross the midline and pass upwards via the medial lemnisci to the medial geniculate bodies and then to the temporal cortex.

Symptoms of a cochlear nerve lesion are deafness and tinnitus (see p. 1317). Sensorineural and conductive deafness can be distinguished with tuning fork tests, e.g. Rinne's and Weber's (using a 256 Hz, not 128 Hz, tuning fork; see p. 1313).

Basic investigations of cochlear lesions

- Pure tone audiometry and auditory thresholds.
- Auditory evoked potentials (recording responses from repetitive clicks via scalp electrodes; lesion levels are determined from the response pattern).

Causes of deafness

These are listed in ***Box 21.13*** and ***Box 30.2***.

Box 21.13 Some causes of vertigo and hearing loss

Conditions	Symptom(s)
Benign paroxysmal positional vertigo	V
Vestibular neuritis	V
Ménière's disease	V, D
Alcohol, antiepileptic drug intoxication	V
Cerebellar lesions	V
Partial (temporal lobe) seizures	V
Migraine	V+ phonophobia
Brainstem ischaemia	V, occasionally D
Multiple sclerosis	V, occasionally D
Mumps, intrauterine rubella and congenital syphilis	D
Advancing age (presbyacusis) and otosclerosis	D
Acoustic trauma	D
Congenital, e.g. Pendred syndrome	D
Gentamicin, furosemide	V, D
Middle and external ear disease	V, D
Cerebellopontine angle lesions, e.g. acoustic neuroma	V, D
Carcinomatous meningitis, sarcoidosis and tuberculous meningitis	V, D

D, hearing loss; V, vertigo.

Vertigo and the vestibular system

The vestibular system of the inner ear detects head movements and has three primary functions:

- to stabilize gaze during head movements, e.g. looking ahead while running (the vestibulo-ocular reflex)
- to control posture and balance
- to facilitate perception of orientation and motion.

Nerve impulses generated by movement of hair cells within the three semicircular canals detect head motion in the three planes (yaw/pitch/roll). Balance is maintained by integrating information from:

- the vestibular system
- the visual system
- the somatosensory system – proprioception from limbs, trunk and neck.

The ***main symptoms*** of vestibular lesions are vertigo and loss of balance.

Vertigo

Vertigo is the illusion of movement of the subject or surroundings, typically rotatory, and should be distinguished from other causes of non-specific dizziness. It can be described to patients as being similar to the sensation one feels after getting off a child's roundabout or after spinning on the spot and suddenly stopping.

Vomiting frequently accompanies acute vertigo of any cause. Vertigo is always made worse by head movements and patients prefer to remain still and maintain visual fixation. Walking is unsteady. Nystagmus (see p. 806) is the principal sign.

The dizzy patient

Complaints of 'dizziness' require careful history taking and may be caused by:

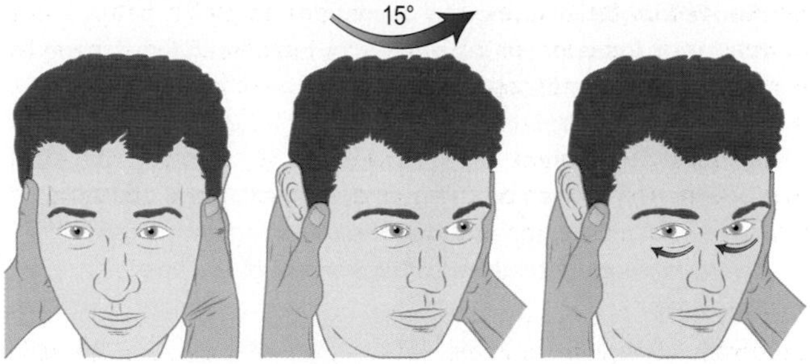

Figure 21.9 The head impulse test. When tested on the normal side, a patient can maintain fixation on a distant object as the examiner rapidly turns the patient's head sideways through about 15°. If there is unilateral vestibulopathy, the patient cannot maintain fixation on the target and can be observed to make a voluntary eye movement (a saccade) back to the target after the head impulse, as shown on the right. It is essential for the head to be turned as rapidly as possible; otherwise, smooth pursuit eye movements will compensate for the head turn.

- vertigo
- pre-syncopal sensations due to transient cerebral hypoperfusion, e.g. orthostatic light-headedness
- unsteadiness or disequilibrium, e.g. cerebellar or postural stability disorders
- non-specific 'dizziness', e.g. due to medication or anxiety and hyperventilation.

Causes of vertigo

Vertigo indicates a disturbance of the vestibular apparatus or brainstem and associated neural pathways ***(Box 21.13)***. Causes:

- ***Peripheral causes*** (vestibular system) are common. Deafness and tinnitus accompanying vertigo indicate involvement of the ear or cochlear nerve (see pp. 1313–1317).
- ***Central causes*** (brainstem and connections) are rarer. Other clinical features, such as diplopia, weakness, cerebellar signs or cranial nerve palsies, may help localize the lesion.

Peripheral (vestibular) disorders

Vestibular disorders are fully discussed elsewhere (see pp. 1316–1317). Attack duration and frequency, as well as trigger factors, help the clinician distinguish on history between different pathological causes. The ability to perform a Hallpike test (see pp. 1316–1317), head impulse test and Epley particle repositioning manœuvre are invaluable skills for all clinicians (see pp. 1316–1317; ***Fig. 21.9*** and see ***Fig. 30.8***).

The most commonly encountered vestibular disorders presenting with vertigo are:

- ***benign paroxysmal positional vertigo*** (BPPV) – frequent attacks lasting seconds only (see pp. 1316–1317).
- ***vestibular neuronitis*** – acute onset lasting days or weeks; non-recurrent
- ***Ménière's disease*** – recurrent attacks lasting minutes or hours, usually accompanied by hearing loss, tinnitus and a feeling of fullness in the ear
- ***trauma*** – vestibular disruption following head injury.

Central causes of vertigo

Vertigo may be a manifestation of brainstem pathology, including:

- ***infarcts involving the vestibular nuclei*** in the medulla (e.g. the lateral medullary syndrome)

- ***demyelination*** involving the brainstem
- ***posterior fossa mass lesions*** – e.g. tumours, haemorrhage or vascular malformations
- ***migrainous vertigo*** (see p. 843) – lasts hours, occurring every few weeks or months
- ***CPA mass lesions*** and tumours compressing the vestibular nerve (technically, these should be classified as 'peripheral' disorders, but are distinct from disorders of the vestibular apparatus)
- ***drugs*** – e.g. anticonvulsant toxicity and alcohol.

Although vertigo occasionally occurs in isolation with brainstem pathology, it is more typically a single component of a more complex clinical picture, associated with other symptoms or examination findings. The brainstem nuclei and tracts are tightly packed into a small space and most pathological processes affect multiple contiguous neural pathways, resulting, for example, in diplopia, eye movement disorders, cranial nerve palsies, cerebellar signs or hemiparesis.

Slowly growing CPA tumours, such as vestibular nerve schwannomas, may cause vertigo but rarely do so in the absence of unilateral deafness and tinnitus.

Basic investigations for vestibular problems

Bedside assessment is usually sufficient to make a diagnosis in the majority of patients:

- examination of eye movements for nystagmus (see p. 806)
- assessment of hearing and otoscopic examination of the ear (see p. 808)
- head impulse (thrust) test – to assess the vestibulo-ocular reflex (VOR) and identify a unilateral vestibulopathy
- Hallpike manœuvre – a positioning test to stimulate the posterior semicircular canal and trigger an attack in BPPV (see ***Fig. 30.8***).

Specialist testing is occasionally required to assess vestibular function and hearing. This includes:

- caloric testing – irrigation of the external auditory meatus with cold and then warm water to stimulate the horizontal semicircular canal and induce nystagmus; labyrinthine function is tested in each ear separately
- electro-nystagmography – to quantify and characterize nystagmus under different conditions, e.g. in a rotating chair
- posturography – assesses body sway on a moving platform
- pure-tone audiograms
- high-definition MRI – provides the best structural imaging of the brainstem and CPA, and is useful where a central cause of vertigo is suspected.

Vestibular neuronitis

Vestibular neuronitis is a common but poorly understood problem. It is an acute attack of isolated vertigo with nystagmus, often with vomiting, and is believed to follow viral infections. The disturbance lasts for several days or weeks, is self-limiting and rarely recurs. Vestibular neuronitis is sometimes followed by BPPV (see pp. 1316–1317). Deafness is absent. Acute treatment is with vestibular sedatives. Similar symptoms can be caused by MS or brainstem vascular lesions. Other signs are usually apparent.

Lower cranial nerves IX, X, XI, XII

The glossopharyngeal (IX), vagus (X) and accessory (XI) nerves arise in the medulla and leave the skull through the jugular foramen. The hypoglossal (XII) arises in the medulla, to leave the skull base via the hypoglossal foramen. Outside the skull, the four cranial nerves lie together, close to the carotid artery and sympathetic trunk.

Glossopharyngeal (IX)

This nerve is largely sensory, supplying sensation and taste from the posterior third of the tongue and the pharynx (afferent pathway of gag reflex). Motor fibres supply some pharyngeal muscles, and parasympathetic fibres supply the parotid.

Vagus (X)

The vagus is a mixed nerve, largely motor, which supplies striated muscle of the pharynx (efferent gag reflex pathway), larynx (including vocal cords via recurrent laryngeal nerves) and upper oesophagus. There are sensory fibres from the larynx. Parasympathetic fibres supply the heart and abdominal viscera.

Accessory (XI)

The accessory nerve, a complex motor nerve, supplies the trapezius and sternomastoid muscles.

Hypoglossal (XII)

The hypoglossal nerve is a motor nerve to tongue muscles.

IXth and Xth nerve lesions

Principal causes of IXth, Xth, XIth and XIIth nerve lesions are listed in ***Box 21.14***.

Isolated lesions of IXth and Xth nerves are unusual, since disease at the jugular foramen affects both nerves and sometimes XI.

A unilateral IXth nerve lesion causes diminished sensation on the same side of the pharynx and is hard to recognize in isolation. A Xth nerve palsy produces ipsilateral failure of voluntary and reflex elevation of the soft palate (which is drawn to the opposite side) and ipsilateral vocal cords.

Bilateral lesions of IXth and Xth nerves cause palatal weakness, reduced palatal sensation, an absent gag reflex, dysphonia and choking with nasal regurgitation. ***Bulbar palsy*** is a general term describing palatal, pharyngeal and tongue weakness of LMN or muscle origin.

Recurrent laryngeal nerve lesions. Paralysis of this branch of each vagus causes hoarseness (dysphonia) and failure of the forceful, explosive part of coughing ('bovine cough'). There is no visible palatal weakness; vocal cord paralysis is seen endoscopically. Bilateral acute lesions (e.g. postoperatively) cause respiratory obstruction – an emergency.

Box 21.14 Principal causes of IXth, Xth, XIth and XIIth nerve lesions

Within brainstem
- Infarction
- Syringobulbia
- Motor neurone disease (motor fibres)

Around skull base
- Nasopharyngeal carcinoma
- Glomus tumour
- Neurofibroma
- Jugular venous thrombosis
- Trauma

Within neck and nasopharynx
- Nasopharyngeal carcinoma
- Metastases
- Carotid artery dissection (XII)
- Trauma
- Lymph node biopsy in posterior triangle (XI)

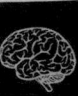

The left recurrent laryngeal nerve (looping beneath the aorta) is damaged more commonly than the right.

Causes of recurrent laryngeal nerve lesions include:

- mediastinal primary tumours (e.g. thymoma)
- secondary spread from bronchial carcinoma
- aortic aneurysm
- trauma or surgery of neck or thorax.

XIth nerve lesions

XIth nerve lesions cause weakness of sternomastoid (rotation of the head and neck to the opposite side) and trapezius (shoulder shrugging). Nerve section (e.g. following lymph node biopsy in the neck posterior triangle) is followed by persistent neuralgic pain.

XIIth nerve lesions

LMN lesions of XII lead to unilateral tongue weakness, wasting and fasciculation. The protruded tongue deviates towards the weaker side. Bilateral supranuclear (UMN) lesions produce slow, limited tongue movements and a stiff tongue that cannot be protruded far. Fasciculation is absent.

Bulbar and pseudobulbar palsy

Bulbar palsy

This is LMN weakness of muscles whose cranial nerve nuclei lie in the medulla (the bulb). Paralysis of bulbar muscles is caused by disease of lower cranial nerve nuclei, lesions of IXth, Xth and XIIth nerves ***(Box 21.14)***, malfunction of their neuromuscular junctions (e.g. myasthenia gravis, botulism) or disease of muscles themselves (e.g. dystrophies).

Pseudobulbar palsy

Describes bilateral supranuclear (UMN) lesions of lower cranial nerves producing weakness of the tongue and pharyngeal muscles. This resembles, superficially, a bulbar palsy: hence pseudobulbar. Findings are a stiff, slow, spastic tongue (not wasted), dysarthria and dysphagia. Gag and palatal reflexes are preserved and the jaw jerk exaggerated. Emotional lability (inappropriate laughing or crying) often accompanies pseudobulbar palsy. Principal causes are:

- motor neurone disease, often both UMN and LMN lesions (i.e. elements of both pseudobulbar and bulbar palsy)
- cerebrovascular disease, typically following multiple infarcts
- neurodegenerative disorders such as progressive supranuclear palsy (see p. 855)
- severe traumatic brain injury
- MS, mainly as a late event.

Difficulty swallowing, dysarthria and drooling also develop in later stages of Parkinson's disease.

Dropped head syndrome

As the name suggests, weakness of neck extensors causes neck flexion and inability to hold the head up. Seen mainly in the elderly, it is often due to isolated neck extensor myopathy of uncertain cause but may be a presenting feature of motor neurone disease, myasthenia or various myopathic disorders.

Further reading

Biousse V, Newman NJ. Ischemic optic neuropathies. *N Engl J Med* 2015; 372:2428–2436.

MOTOR CONTROL SYSTEMS

There are three systems, each of which interacts by feedback loops with the other two, with sensory input from the reticular formation:

- ***The corticospinal*** (or ***pyramidal***) ***system*** enables purposive, skilled, intricate, strong and organized movements. Defective function is recognized by a distinct pattern of signs – loss of skilled voluntary movement, spasticity and reflex change – seen, for example, in a hemiparesis, hemiplegia or paraparesis.
- ***The extrapyramidal system*** facilitates fast, fluid movements that the corticospinal system has generated. Defective function produces slowness (bradykinesia), stiffness (rigidity) and/or disorders of movement (rest tremor, chorea and other dyskinesias). One feature (e.g. stiffness, tremor or chorea) will often predominate.
- ***The cerebellum*** and its connections have a role coordinating smooth and learned movement, initiated by the pyramidal system, and in posture and balance control. Cerebellar disease leads to unsteady and jerky movements (ataxia), with characteristic limb signs of past-pointing, action tremor and incoordination, gait ataxia and/or truncal ataxia.

Corticospinal (pyramidal) system

The corticospinal tracts originate in neurones of the cortex and terminate at motor nuclei of cranial nerves and spinal cord anterior horn cells. The pathways of particular clinical significance ***(Fig. 21.10)*** congregate in the internal capsule and cross in the medulla (decussation of the pyramids), passing to the contralateral cord as the lateral corticospinal tracts. This is the pyramidal system, disease of which causes UMN lesions. 'Pyramidal' is simply a descriptive term that draws together anatomy and characteristic physical signs; it is used interchangeably with the term UMN.

A proportion of the corticospinal outflow is uncrossed (anterior corticospinal tracts). This is of no relevance in practice.

Characteristics of pyramidal lesions

Signs of an early pyramidal lesion may be minimal ***(Box 21.15)***. Weakness, spasticity or changes in reflexes can predominate, or be present in isolation.

Pyramidal drift of an upper limb

Normally, the outstretched upper limbs are held symmetrically, when the eyes are closed. With a pyramidal lesion, when both upper limbs are held outstretched, palms uppermost, the affected limb drifts downwards and pronates. This sign, with slowing of fast finger movements, is an early one, sometimes occurring before weakness and/or reflex changes become apparent.

Weakness and loss of skilled movement

A unilateral pyramidal lesion above the decussation in the medulla causes weakness of the opposite limbs. When acute and complete, this weakness will be immediate and total: a hemiplegia – for example, following an internal capsule infarct. With slowly progressive lesions (e.g. a hemisphere glioma), a characteristic pattern of weakness emerges: a hemiparesis.

In the upper limb, flexors remain stronger than extensors, whereas in the lower limb, extensors remain stronger than flexors. In the upper arm, weaker movements are thus shoulder abduction and elbow extension; in the forearm and hand, wrist and finger

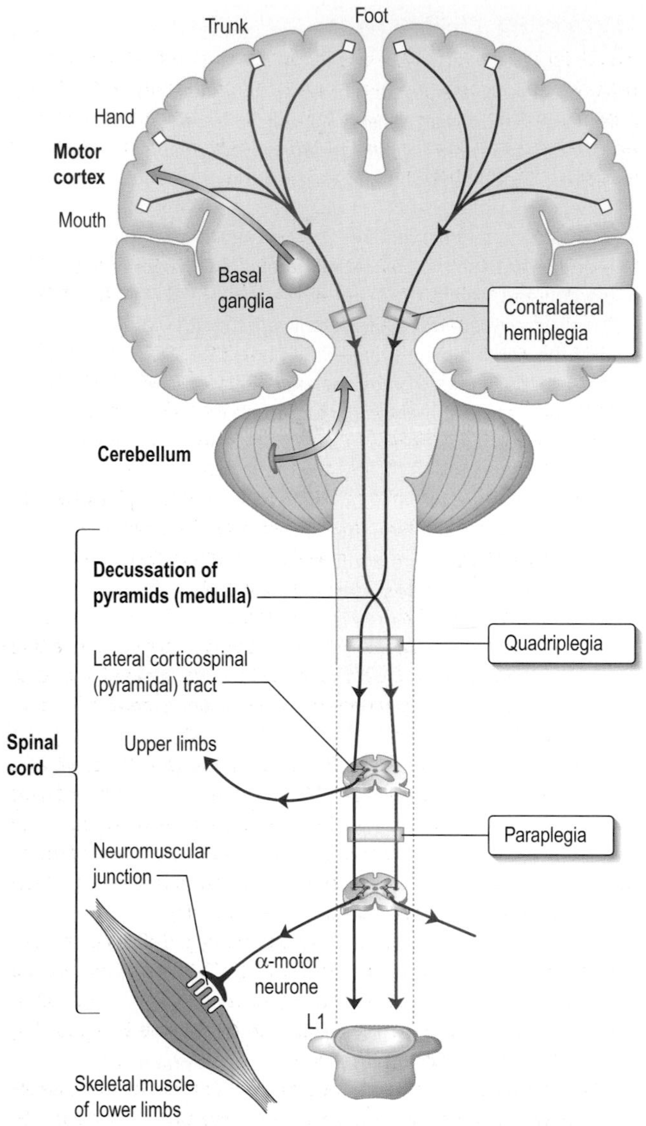

Figure 21.10 The motor (corticospinal, pyramidal) system.

Box 21.15 Features of upper motor neurone lesions

- Drift of upper limb
- Weakness with characteristic distribution
- Changes in tone: flaccid–spastic
- Exaggerated tendon reflexes
- Extensor plantar response
- Loss of skilled finger/toe movements
- Loss of abdominal reflexes
- No muscle wasting
- Normal electrical excitability of muscle

extensors and abductors are weaker than their antagonists. In the lower limb, weaker movements are hip flexion, knee flexion, ankle dorsiflexion and eversion. There is also loss of skilled movement; fine finger and toe control diminishes. Wasting (except from disuse) is not a feature. When a UMN lesion is below the decussation of the pyramids – in the cervical cord, for example – hemiparesis is on the same side as the lesion; this is an unusual situation.

Changes in tone and tendon reflexes

An acute lesion of one pyramidal tract (e.g. internal capsule stroke) causes initially flaccid paralysis with loss of tendon reflexes. Increase in tone follows, usually within several days, due to loss of inhibitory effects of the corticospinal pathways and an increase in spinal reflex activity. This increase in tone (spasticity) is most easily detectable in stronger muscles. Spasticity is characterized by sudden ***changing resistance*** to rapid passive movement – the clasp-knife effect. Relevant tendon reflexes become exaggerated; clonus may emerge.

Changes in superficial reflexes

The normal flexor plantar response becomes extensor. In a severe acute lesion, this extensor response can be elicited from a wide area of the foot. As recovery progresses, the receptive area diminishes until the lateral posterior third of the sole remains receptive to an orange-stick stimulus (the appropriate instrument). An extensor plantar response is certain when great toe dorsiflexion is accompanied by abduction of adjacent toes. Abdominal reflexes are abolished on the affected side.

Patterns of UMN disorders

There are three main patterns:

- ***Hemiparesis*** means weakness of the limbs on one side; it is usually caused by a lesion in the brain and occasionally in the cord.
- ***Paraparesis*** means weakness of both lower limbs and is usually diagnostic of a cord lesion; bilateral medial brain lesions (e.g. parasagittal meningioma) occasionally cause paraparesis.
- ***Tetraparesis*** (also called ***quadriparesis***) means weakness of four limbs.

Hemiplegia, paraplegia and tetraplegia (strictly) indicate *total* paralysis but are often used to describe severe weakness.

Hemiparesis

The level within the corticospinal system is recognized from particular features.

Motor cortex. Weakness and/or loss of skilled movement confined to one contralateral limb (an arm or a leg – monoparesis) or part of a limb (e.g. a clumsy hand) is typical of an isolated motor cortex lesion (e.g. an infarct or secondary neoplasm). A defect in cognitive function (e.g. aphasia) and focal epilepsy may occur.

Internal capsule. Corticospinal fibres are tightly packed in the internal capsule (about 1 cm^2); thus a small lesion causes a large deficit. A middle cerebral artery branch infarction (see p. 833) produces a sudden, dense, contralateral hemiplegia.

Pons. A pontine lesion (e.g. an MS plaque) is rarely confined to the corticospinal tract. Adjacent structures, e.g. VIth and VIIth nuclei, MLF and PPRF (see p. 805) are involved. Diplopia, facial weakness, internuclear ophthalmoplegia (INO) and/or a lateral gaze palsy occur with contralateral hemiparesis.

Spinal cord. An isolated lesion of one lateral corticospinal tract (e.g. a cervical cord injury) causes an ipsilateral UMN lesion, the level being indicated by changes in reflexes (e.g. absent biceps, C5/6), features of a Brown–Séquard syndrome (see p. 817) and muscle wasting at the level of the lesion (p. 818).

Spastic paraparesis

Paraparesis indicates bilateral damage to corticospinal pathways, causing weakness and spasticity (or flaccid weakness in the initial phase of spinal shock after an acute cord insult). Cord compression (see pp. 872–873) or cord diseases are the usual causes; cerebral lesions occasionally produce paraparesis. Paraparesis is a feature of many neurological conditions; finding the cause is crucial (see p. 872).

Extrapyramidal system

The extrapyramidal system is a general term for basal ganglia motor systems: that is, corpus striatum (caudate nucleus + globus pallidus + putamen), subthalamic nucleus, substantia nigra and parts of the thalamus. In basal ganglia/extrapyramidal disorders, two features (either or both) become apparent, in limbs and axial muscles:

- reduction in speed of movement (***bradykinesia***) or akinesia (no movement), with muscle rigidity
- involuntary ***hyperkinetic*** movements (tremor, chorea, dystonia, tics, myoclonus).

Extrapyramidal disorders are classified broadly into ***akinetic–rigid syndromes*** (see p. 855) where poverty of movement predominates, and ***hyperkinetic*** movement disorders where there are abnormal involuntary movements (see pp. 855–857).

The most common extrapyramidal disorder is Parkinson's disease.

Essential anatomy

The corpus striatum lies close to the substantia nigra, thalami and sub-thalamic nuclei, lateral to the internal capsule (***Fig. 21.11***; see ***Fig. 21.10***).

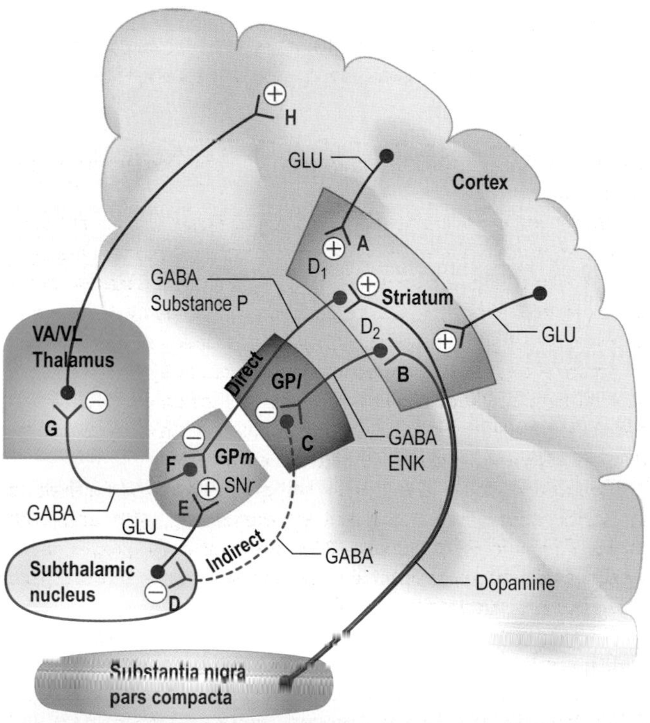

Figure 21.11 Extrapyramidal system: connections and neurotransmitters. The ***inhibitory pathways*** are in blue (B, C, D, F, G) and the ***excitatory pathways*** are in red (A, E, H). ENK, enkephalin; GABA, γ-aminobutyric acid; GLU, glutamate; GP*l*, lateral globus pallidus; GP*m*, medial globus pallidus; SN*r*, substantia nigra pars reticulate; VA/VL, ventral anterior and ventrolateral thalamic nuclei.

Function and dysfunction

Overall function of this system is modulation of cortical motor activity by a series of loops between cortex and basal ganglia ***(Fig. 21.11)***. In involuntary movement disorders, there are specific changes in neurotransmitters ***(Box 21.16)*** rather than focal lesions seen on imaging or at postmortem.

Proposed model of principal pathways

1. Direct pathway from striatum to medial globus pallidus (GP*m*) and substantia nigra pars reticulata (SN*r*). Inhibitory ***synapse F***, GABA and substance P.
2. Indirect pathway from striatum to globus pallidus, via lateral globus pallidus (GP*l*; inhibitory ***synapse C***, GABA, enkephalin) and subthalamic nucleus (inhibitory ***synapse D***, GABA). Terminates in GP*m*-SN*r* (in excitatory ***synapse E***, glutamate).
3. Direct pathways, both inhibitory and excitatory, from substantia nigra pars compacta (SNc) to striatum. ***Synapse A***, dopamine, D_1, excitatory; and ***synapse B***, D_2, inhibitory.
4. GP*m* and SN*r* to thalamus. Inhibitory ***synapse G***, GABA.
5. Thalamus to cortex. Excitatory, ***synapse H***.
6. Cortex to striatum. Excitatory, glutamate.

The model helps explain how basal ganglia disease can either reduce excitatory thalamo-cortical activity at synapse H – that is, movement – causing bradykinesia, or increase it, causing hyperkinetic disorders.

Parkinson's disease (***PD***). This is characterized by slowness, stiffness and rest tremor (see p. 853). Degeneration in SNc causes loss of dopamine activity in the striatum. Dopamine is excitatory for synapse A and inhibitory for synapse B. Through the direct pathway there is reduced activity at synapse F, leading to increased inhibitory output (G) and decreased cortical activity (H).

Also in PD, in the indirect pathway, dopamine deficiency results in disinhibition of neurones synapsing at C. This leads to reduced activity at D, and to increased activity of neurones in the subthalamic nucleus. There is excess stimulation at synapse E, enhancing further inhibitory output of GP*m*–SN*r*.

The net effect via both pathways is to inhibit the ventral anterior (VA) and ventrolateral (VL) nuclei of the thalamus at synapse G. Cortical (motor) activity at H is thus reduced.

Levodopa helps slowness and tremor in PD (see p. 854) but induces unwanted dyskinesias by increasing dopamine activity at

Box 21.16 Changes in neurotransmitters in Parkinson's and Huntington's diseases

Site	Neurotransmitter
Parkinson's	
Putamen	Dopamine ↓ 90% Noradrenaline (norepinephrine) ↓ 60% 5-HT ↓ 60%
Substantia nigra	Dopamine ↓ 90% GAD + GABA ↓↓
Cerebral cortex	GAD + GABA ↓↓
Huntington's	
Corpus striatum	Acetylcholine ↓↓ GABA ↓↓ Dopamine: normal GAD + GABA ↓↓

5-HT, 5-hydroxytryptamine; GABA, γ-aminobutyric acid; GAD, glutamic acid decarboxylase, the enzyme responsible for synthesizing GABA.

synapses A and B; it is thought to do this by reversing sequences in both direct and indirect pathways.

Hemiballismus (see p. 856). Wild, flinging (ballistic) limb movements are caused by a lesion in the subthalamic nucleus, typically an infarct. This reduces excitatory activity at synapse E, reduces inhibition at G, with increased thalamo-cortical neuronal activity, and increases activity at H.

Cerebellum

The third system of motor control modulates coordination and learned movement patterns, rather than speed. Ataxia, i.e. unsteadiness, is characteristic.

The cerebellum receives afferents from:

- proprioceptive receptors (joints and muscles)
- vestibular nuclei
- basal ganglia
- the corticospinal system
- olivary nuclei.

Efferents pass from the cerebellum to:

- each red nucleus
- vestibular nuclei
- basal ganglia
- the corticospinal system.

Each lateral cerebellar lobe coordinates movement of the ipsilateral limbs. The vermis (a midline structure) is concerned with maintenance of axial (midline) posture and balance.

Cerebellar lesions

Box 21.17 summarizes the main causes of cerebellar disease. Expanding lesions obstruct the aqueduct to cause hydrocephalus, with severe pressure headaches, vomiting and papilloedema. Coning of the cerebellar tonsils (see p. 869) through the foramen magnum leads to respiratory arrest, sometimes within minutes/hours. Rarely, tonic seizures (attacks of limb stiffness) occur.

Lateral cerebellar hemisphere lesions

A lesion within one cerebellar lobe (e.g. tumour or infarction) causes disruption of the normal sequence of movements (dyssynergia) on the same side.

Box 21.17 Principal causes of cerebellar syndromes

Tumours
- Haemangioblastoma
- Medulloblastoma
- Secondary neoplasm
- Compression by acoustic neuroma

Vascular
- Haemorrhage
- Infarction
- Arteriovenous malformation

Infection
- Abscess
- HIV
- Prion diseases
- Encephalitis

Developmental
- Arnold–Chiari malformation
- Cerebral palsy

Toxic and metabolic
- Antiepileptic drugs
- Chronic alcohol use
- Carbon monoxide poisoning
- Lead poisoning
- Solvent misuse

Inherited
- Friedreich's and other spinocerebellar ataxias
- Ataxia telangiectasia

Miscellaneous
- Multiple sclerosis (common in MS)
- Hydrocephalus
- Hypothyroidism
- Paraneoplastic syndromes (rapidly progressive)
- Multiple system atrophy
- Superficial siderosis

Posture and gait. The outstretched arm is held still in the early stages of a cerebellar lobar lesion (cf. the drift of pyramidal lesions) but there is rebound upward overshoot when the limb is pressed downwards and released. Gait becomes broad and ataxic, faltering towards the side of the lesion.

Tremor and ataxia. Movement is imprecise in direction, force and distance (dysmetria). Rapid alternating movements (tapping, clapping or rotary hand movements) become disorganized (dysdiadochokinesia). Intention tremor (action tremor with past-pointing) is seen, but speed of fine movement is preserved (cf. extrapyramidal and pyramidal lesions).

Nystagmus. Coarse horizontal nystagmus (see p. 806) develops with a lateral cerebellar lobe lesion. The fast component is always towards the side of the lesion.

Dysarthria. Halting, jerking speech (scanning speech) develops.

Other signs. Titubation – rhythmic head tremor as either forward and back (yes–yes) movements or rotary (no–no) movements – can occur, mainly when cerebellar connections are involved (e.g. in essential tremor and MS; see pp. 856 and 858–862). Hypotonia (floppy limbs) and depression of reflexes (with slow, pendular reflexes) are also sometimes seen.

Midline cerebellar lesions

Cerebellar vermis lesions have dramatic effects on trunk and axial muscles. There is difficulty standing and sitting unsupported (truncal ataxia), with a broad-based, ataxic gait. Lesions of the flocculonodular region cause vertigo and vomiting with gait ataxia if they extend to the roof of the IVth ventricle.

Tremor

Tremor means a regular and sinusoidal oscillation of the limbs, head or trunk.

Postural tremor

Everyone has a physiological tremor (often barely perceptible) of the outstretched hands at 8–12 Hz. This is increased with anxiety, caffeine, hyperthyroidism and drugs (e.g. sympathomimetics, sodium valproate, lamotrigine, lithium) and occurs in mercury poisoning. A higher-amplitude, postural tremor is seen in benign essential tremor (usually quite fast at 5–12 Hz).

Intention tremor

Tremor exacerbated by action, with past-pointing and accompanying incoordination of rapid alternating movement (dysdiadochokinesia), occurs in cerebellar lobe disease and with lesions of cerebellar connections. Titubation (head tremor) and nystagmus may be present.

Rest tremor

Seen typically in Parkinson's disease, this tremor is noticeably worse at rest, usually 4–7 Hz (often pill-rolling, between thumb and forefinger). Unlike essential tremor, Parkinsonian tremor is generally unilateral for the first few years.

Other tremors

Dystonic tremor occurs after the age of 50 and is a manifestation of dystonia that is often seen without dystonic posturing. It is generally unilateral (or asymmetric), affecting hand/arm or head, and worse with posture and certain tasks such as drinking, pouring

Box 21.18 Features of lower motor neurone lesions

- Weakness
- Wasting
- Hypotonia
- Reflex loss
- Fasciculation
- Fibrillation potentials (electromyography)
- Muscle contractures
- Trophic changes in skin and nails

liquids, or using cutlery or a pen. It is often mistaken for parkinsonian tremor. Holmes tremor (present at rest, action and posture) is seen following lesions of the red nucleus (e.g. infarction, multiple sclerosis).

LOWER MOTOR NEURONE LESIONS

The lower motor neurone (LMN) is the pathway from anterior horn cell (or cranial nerve nucleus) via a peripheral nerve to muscle motor end-plates. The motor unit consists of one anterior horn cell, its single fast-conducting axon that leaves the cord via the anterior root, and the group of muscle fibres (100–2000) supplied via the nerve. Anterior horn cell activity is modulated by impulses from:

- corticospinal tracts
- the extrapyramidal system
- the cerebellum
- afferents via posterior roots.

Clinical features of lower motor neurone lesions

These are seen in voluntary muscles that depend on an intact nerve supply for both contraction and metabolic integrity. Signs follow rapidly if the LMN is interrupted ***(Box 21.18)***.

Aetiology

Examples of LMN lesions at various levels include:

- cranial nerve nuclei (Bell's palsy) and anterior horn cell (motor neurone disease)
- spinal root – ***radiculopathy***, e.g. cervical and lumbar disc protrusion (see p. 887)
- peripheral (or cranial) nerve – trauma, entrapment (see pp. 882–883) and polyneuropathy (pp. 883–886).

Spinal reflex arc

Components are illustrated in ***Figure 21.12***. The stretch reflex is the physiological basis for all tendon reflexes. In the knee jerk, a tap on the patellar tendon activates stretch receptors in the quadriceps. Impulses in first-order sensory neurones pass directly to LMNs (L3 and L4) that contract quadriceps. Loss of a tendon reflex is caused by a lesion anywhere along the spinal reflex path. The reflex lost indicates its level ***(Box 21.19)***.

Reinforcement. Distraction of the patient's attention, clenching teeth or pulling interlocked fingers enhances reflex activity (Jendrassik manœuvre). Such reinforcement manœuvres should be done before a reflex is recorded as absent.

SENSORY PATHWAYS AND PAIN

Peripheral nerves and spinal roots

Peripheral nerves carry all modalities of sensation from either free or specialized nerve endings to dorsal roots and thence to the cord. Sensory distribution of spinal roots (dermatomes) is shown in ***Figure 21.13***.

Box 21.19 Spinal levels: recording/interpretation of tendon reflexes

Level	Reflex	Symbol	Meaning
C5–6	Supinator	0	Absent
C5–6	Biceps	±	Present with reinforcement
C7	Triceps	+	Normal
L3–4	Knee	++	Brisk, normal
S1	Ankle	+++ CL	Exaggerated (abnormal) Clonus

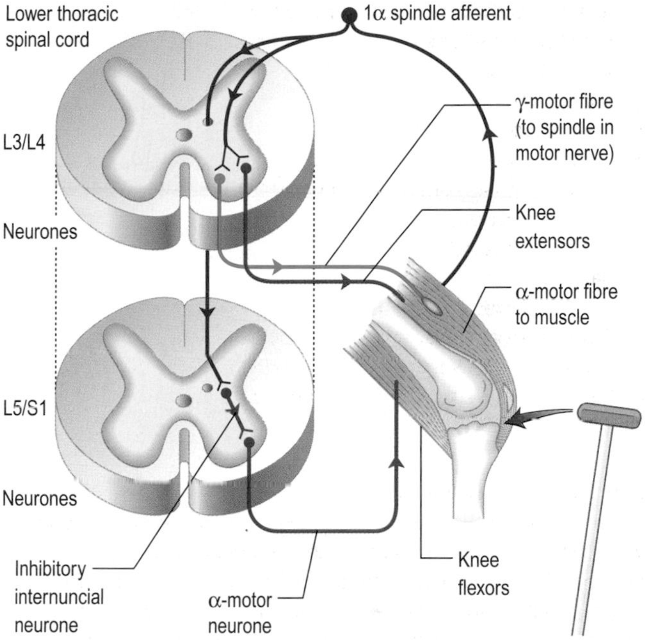

Figure 21.12 Knee jerk: a spinal reflex arc. Sudden patellar tendon stretching generates sensory action potentials in 1α-muscle spindle afferents that synapse with γ motor fibres to spindles and α-motor fibres. Motor action potentials cause brisk extensor muscle contraction; there is also inhibition of knee flexors.

Spinal cord

Posterior columns

Axons in the posterior columns whose cell bodies are in the ipsilateral gracile and cuneate nuclei in the medulla carry sensory modalities of vibration, joint position (proprioception), light touch and two-point discrimination. Axons from second-order neurones then cross in the brainstem to form the medial lemniscus, passing to the thalamus ***(Fig. 21.14)***.

Spinothalamic tracts

Axons carrying pain and temperature sensation synapse in the dorsal horn of the cord, cross within the cord, and pass in the spinothalamic tracts to the thalamus and reticular formation.

Sensory cortex

Fibres from the thalamus pass to the parietal region sensory cortex ***(Fig. 21.14)***. Connections exist between the thalamus, sensory cortex and motor cortex.

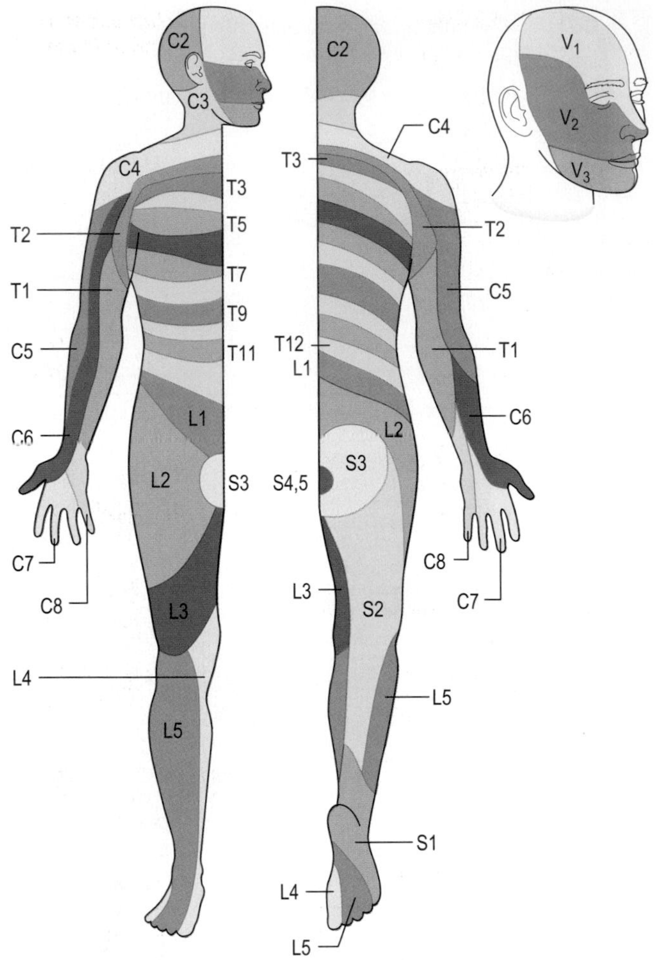

Figure 21.13 **Dermatomes of spinal roots and Vth nerve.**

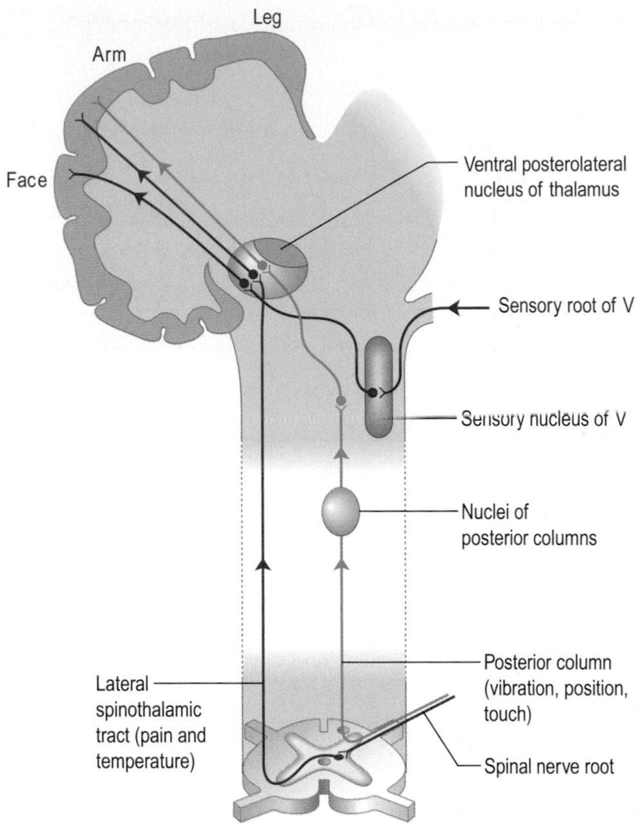

Figure 21.14 **Principal sensory pathways.** Posterior columns remain uncrossed until the medulla. Spinothalamic tracts cross close to their entry into the cord.

Lesions of the sensory pathways

Altered sensation, tingling (paraesthesia), clumsiness, numbness and pain are the principal symptoms of sensory lesions. The pattern and distribution point to the site of pathology ***(Fig. 21.15)***.

Peripheral nerve lesions

Symptoms are felt within the distribution of a peripheral nerve (see pp. 881–888). Section of a sensory nerve is followed by complete sensory loss. Nerve entrapment (see pp. 882–883) causes numbness, pain and tingling. Tapping the site of compression sometimes causes a sharp, electric shock-like pain in the distribution of the nerve, known as Tinel's sign, such as in carpal tunnel syndrome (see p. 882).

Neuralgia

Neuralgia refers to pain, usually of great severity, in the distribution of a damaged nerve. Examples are:

- trigeminal neuralgia (see p. 845)
- postherpetic neuralgia (see p. 866)
- complex regional pain syndrome type II (causalgia) – chronic burning pain that occasionally follows peripheral nerve damage.

Spinal root lesions

Root pain

Pain of root compression is felt in the myotome supplied by the root, and there is also a tingling discomfort in the dermatome. The pain is worsened by manœuvres that either stretch the root (e.g. straight leg raising in lumbar disc prolapse) or increase pressure in the spinal subarachnoid space (coughing and straining). Cervical and lumbar disc protrusions (see p. 887) are common causes of root lesions.

Dorsal spinal root lesions

Section of a dorsal root causes loss of all modalities of sensation within a dermatome ***(Fig. 21.13)***. However, overlap between adjacent dermatomes makes it difficult to detect anaesthesia when a single root is destroyed.

Spinal cord lesions

Posterior column lesions

These cause:

- tingling
- electric shock-like sensations
- clumsiness
- numbness
- tight band-like sensations.

These symptoms, though lateralized, are often felt vaguely without a clear sensory level. Position sense, vibration sense, light touch and two-point discrimination are diminished below the lesion.

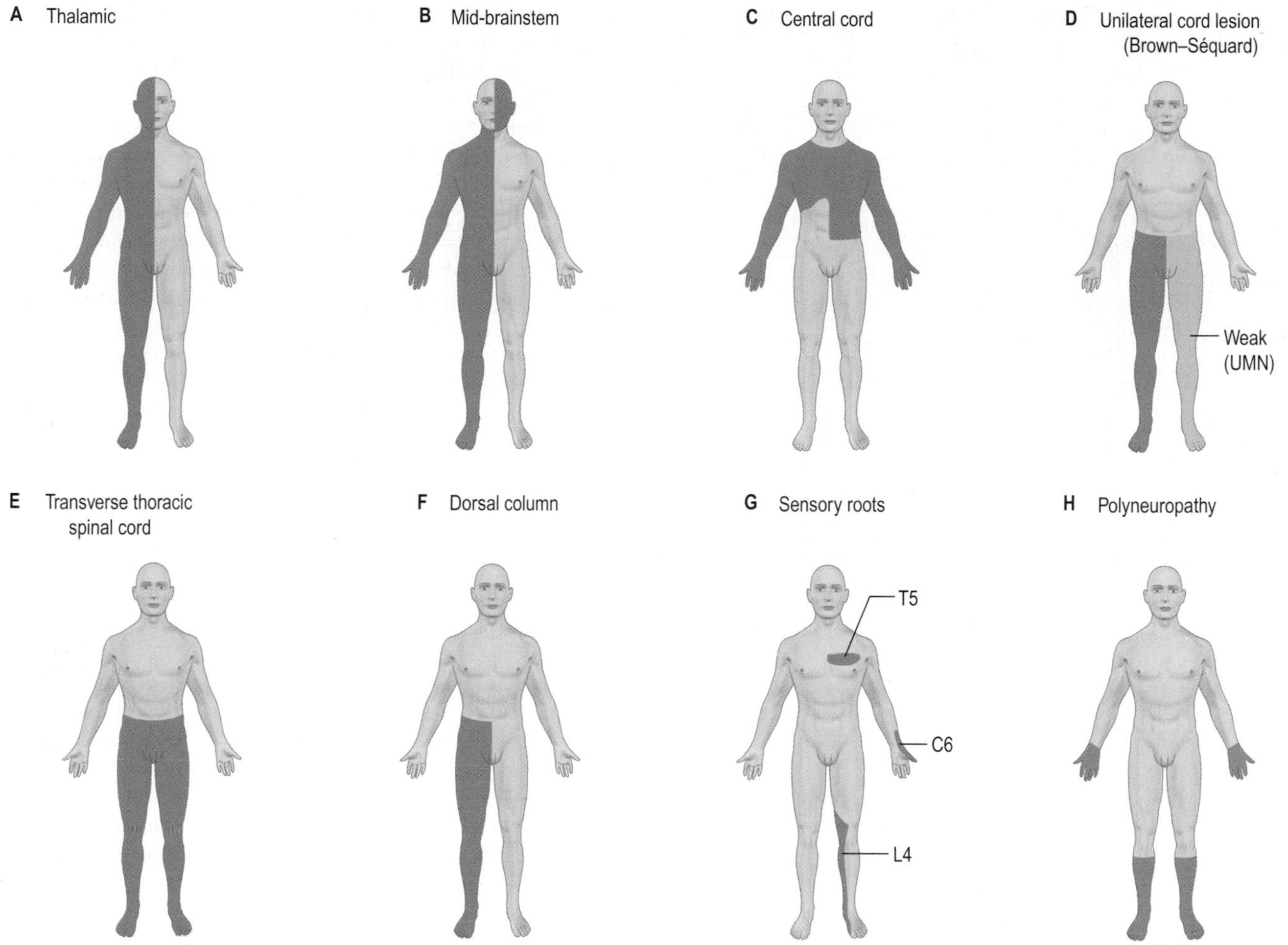

Figure 21.15 Principal patterns of loss of sensation. A. ***Thalamic lesion:*** sensory loss throughout opposite side (rare). **B.** ***Brainstem lesion:*** contralateral sensory loss below face and ipsilateral loss on face. **C.** ***Central cord lesion,*** e.g. syrinx: 'suspended' areas of loss, often asymmetrical and 'dissociated': i.e. pain and temperature lost but light touch intact. **D.** ***Hemisection of cord/unilateral cord lesion*** – Brown–Séquard syndrome: contralateral spinothalamic (pain and temperature) loss with ipsilateral weakness and dorsal column loss below lesion. **E.** ***Transverse cord lesion:*** loss of all modalities, including motor, below lesion. **F.** ***Dorsal column lesion,*** e.g. multiple sclerosis: loss of proprioception, vibration and light touch. **G.** ***Individual sensory root lesions,*** e.g. C6, T5, L4. **H.** ***Polyneuropathy:*** distal sensory loss. UMN, upper motor neurone.

Position sense loss produces a stamping gait (sensory ataxia; see p. 797).

Lhermitte's phenomenon

Electric shock-like sensations radiate down the trunk and limbs on neck flexion. This points to a cervical cord lesion. Lhermitte's is common in acute exacerbations of MS (see p. 859), and also occurs in cervical myelopathy (pp. 887–888), subacute combined degeneration of the cord (p. 886), radiation myelopathy (p. 888) and cord compression.

Spinothalamic tract lesions

Pure spinothalamic spinal lesions cause contralateral loss of pain and temperature sensation with a clear level below the lesion. This is called ***dissociated*** sensory loss – pain and temperature are dissociated from light touch, which remains preserved. This is seen typically in syringomyelia where a cavity occupies the central cord (see p. 874).

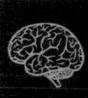

The spinal level is modified by lamination of fibres within the spinothalamic tracts. Fibres from lower spinal roots lie superficially and are damaged first by compressive lesions from outside the cord. As an external compressive lesion (e.g. a mid-thoracic extradural meningioma; ***Fig. 21.16***) enlarges, the spinal sensory level ascends as deeper fibres become involved. Conversely, a central cord lesion (e.g. a syrinx; see p. 874) affects deeper fibres first. Spinothalamic tract lesions cause loss of pain and temperature perception (e.g. painless burns). Perforating ulcers and neuropathic (Charcot) joints develop.

Spinal cord compression

Cord compression ***(Fig. 21.16)*** causes progressive spastic paraparesis (or tetraparesis/quadriparesis) with sensory loss below the level of compression. Sphincter disturbance is common. Root pain is frequent but not invariable, felt characteristically at the level of compression. With thoracic cord compression (e.g. an extradural meningioma), pain radiates around the chest and is exacerbated by coughing and straining, as meningeal root sheaths are stretched.

Damage to one spinothalamic tract (contralateral loss of pain and temperature) with the ipsilateral corticospinal tract is known as the ***Brown–Séquard syndrome*** (originally, cord hemisection). The patient complains of numbness on one side and weakness on the other. Paraparesis/spinal cord lesions are discussed on page 859.

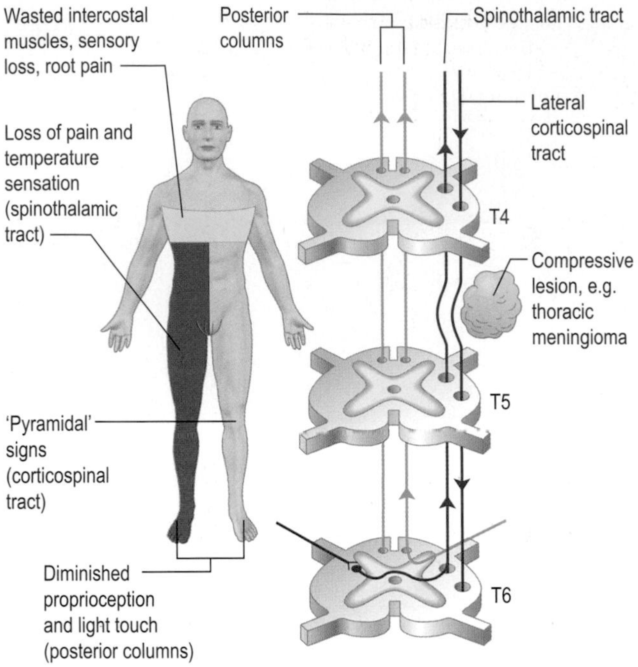

Figure 21.16 Spinal cord compression: features and anatomy.

Pontine lesions

Since lesions (e.g. an MS plaque) lie above the decussation of the posterior columns, and both medial lemniscus and spinothalamic tracts are close together, there is loss of all forms of sensation on the side opposite the lesion. Combinations of IIIrd, IVth, Vth, VIth and VIIth cranial nerve nuclei are seen, and may indicate a level ***(Fig. 21.14)***.

Thalamic lesions

Thalamic pain (also called ***central post-stroke pain*** or ***thalamic syndrome***) follows a small thalamic infarct. The patient has a stroke (hemiparesis and sensory loss). Weakness improves but deep-seated constant pain in the paretic limbs develops. Choreo-athetotic movements occur. Secondary depression may lead to self-harm. Thalamic lesions can also cause diminished sensation alone, on the opposite side; this is less usual.

Parietal cortex lesions

Sensory loss, neglect of one side, apraxia (see p. 798) and subtle disorders of sensation occur. Pain is not a feature of destructive cortical lesions. Irritative phenomena (e.g. focal sensory seizures from a parietal cortex glioma) cause tingling sensations in a limb or elsewhere.

Pain

Pain is an unpleasant, complex sensory and emotional experience. Acute pain serves a biological purpose (e.g. withdrawal) and is typically self-limiting, ceasing as healing ensues. Some forms of chronic pain (e.g. causalgia) outlast the period required for healing and may be permanent.

Essential physiology of pain

Pain perception is mediated by small-diameter myelinated A-delta and non-myelinated C fibres. Chemicals released following injury produce pain either by direct stimulation or by sensitization of nerve endings. A-delta fibres give rise to perception of sharp, immediate pain; slower-onset, more diffuse and prolonged pain is mediated by slower-conducting C fibres.

Nociceptive (pain) impulses enter the cord via dorsal spinal roots forming synapses in the spinal cord dorsal horn (substance P and glutamate neurotransmitters). Second-order neurones then decussate to the contralateral side and ascend in the spinal cord via two main pathways: the spinothalamic tract (for pain localization) and the spinoreticular tract (mediation of the emotional component of pain; ***Fig. 21.17***). Both pathways project via synapses in the thalamus to the sensory cortex and limbic system. There are projections to brainstem structures: the reticular formation (spinoreticular tract) and periaqueductal grey matter (spinothalamic tract), which modulates pain transmission via descending monoaminergic pathways to the spinal cord dorsal horn. The emotional and affective components of pain, mediated through cortical and limbic networks, are now recognized to be fundamental to pain perception.

Gate theory of pain

Gate theory proposes that transmission of afferent nociceptive (pain) impulses is regulated ('gated') in the spinal cord dorsal horn synapses by afferent impulses from non-nociceptive, large-diameter sensory fibres and descending pathways from the periaqueductal grey (PAG) and other brainstem structures. It explains the phenomenon of rubbing a painful area to ease the pain and is also the basis of transcutaneous electrical nerve stimulation (TENS) therapy. Similar gating and modulation of afferent pain signals occur in the brainstem under the influence of connections from the thalamus and limbic system.

Peripheral and central sensitization

Sensitization is an increase in the excitability of peripheral nociceptors and central pain pathways, causing normal sensory inputs such as light touch to produce abnormal responses: that is, pain (termed ***allodynia***). For example, warm water in a shower feels painfully burning on sunburnt skin and touching the scalp is painful during a migraine. This is an adaptive protective response to ensure that contact with an injured area is minimized. However, maladaptive responses to pain via this mechanism at the central or peripheral level may be the basis for chronic pain when it becomes permanent and out of proportion to the initial painful stimulus.

Plasticity and receptor changes

Pain results in neural plasticity changes and reorganization in pain pathways at spinal cord and cortical/brainstem level. These modulate pain and may be maladaptive in some cases, leading to maintenance of chronic pain. Molecular changes also occur in response to painful stimuli, including upregulation of sodium channels and receptor changes.

Neuropathic pain

Pain results directly from damage to, or dysfunction of, the pain/sensory pathways, such as in peripheral nerve damage, radiculopathy, post-stroke pain and post-herpetic neuralgia ***(Box 21.20)***. It is common, affecting 6–8% of people. Clinically, the pain usually has an unpleasant burning, electrical or stabbing quality, with allodynia being a frequent feature. It often becomes chronic due to peripheral and central sensitization processes.

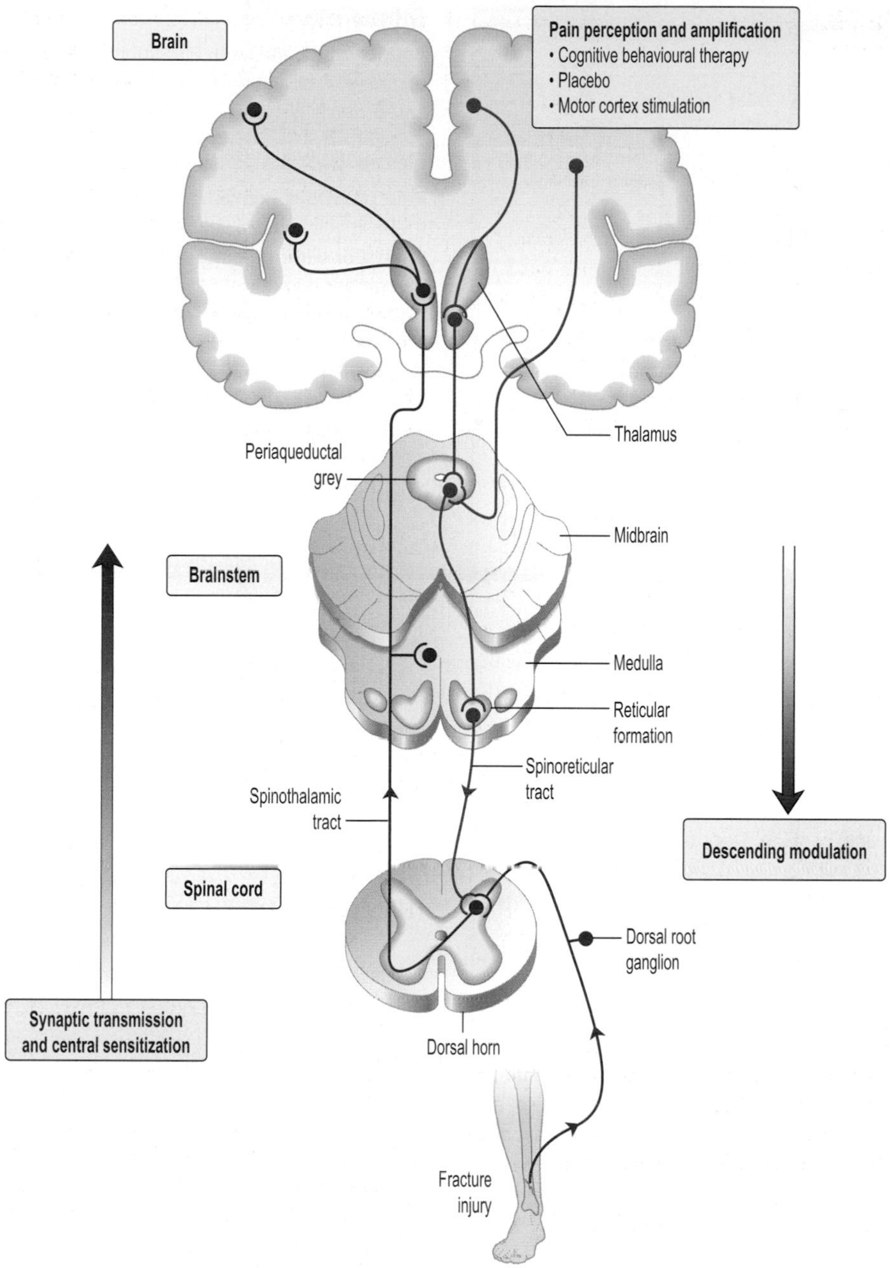

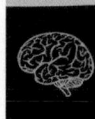

Figure 21.17 The spinothalamic and spinoreticular tracts in pain perception.

Neurotransmitters and receptors involved in pain

These are involved in pain processing, explaining why a wide range of drug classes are helpful in treating pain.

- ***Excitatory neurotransmitters*** include substance P, glutamate and calcitonin gene-related peptide (CGRP) in the dorsal horn of the spinal cord and peripherally.
- ***Gamma-aminobutyric acid*** (***GABA***) is a key inhibitory neurotransmitter.
- ***Opioid receptors***, activated by endogenous endorphins or opiate medications, are widely distributed in pain pathways, including in the spinal cord, PAG and other brainstem structures.
- ***Noradrenaline*** (***norepinephrine***) and 5-HT (serotonin) are distributed in descending regulatory pathways.
- ***The vanilloid receptor*** (TRPV1 – transient receptor potential cation channel VI) on peripheral nociceptors is activated by capsaicin, the active constituent of chilli peppers.

Management of chronic pain

Chronic pain is gravely disabling, distressing and difficult to treat (see pp. 663–665). Multidisciplinary pain clinics provide the best setting for long-term management.

Management plans for intractable pain have seven components.

Diagnostic

Rigorous attention must be paid to the diagnosis, reviewing the entire history and investigations. A specific surgical approach may

Box 21. 20 Causes of neuropathic pain

Peripheral nerve injury
- Peripheral neuropathy – especially if small (pain) fibres are affected, e.g. diabetes, AL amyloid, HIV, chemotherapy (e.g. carboplatin neuropathy), vitamin deficiency, alcohol, Fabry's
- Vasculitic nerve lesions – e.g. diabetic femoral neuropathy (neuralgic amyotrophy)
- Nerve compression – carpal tunnel syndrome, meralgia paraesthetica
- Post-herpetic neuralgia
- Nerve trauma or section – e.g. phantom limb pain
- Trigeminal neuralgia

Nerve root and plexus
- Radiculopathy due to intervertebral disc prolapse
- Plexopathy – e.g. inflammatory (brachial neuritis) or neoplastic infiltrative (e.g. breast cancer)

Central nervous system disorders
- Multiple sclerosis (pain is common in progressive forms)
- Post-stroke pain – e.g. thalamic strokes
- Spinal cord lesions – intrinsic cord lesions, inflammatory or vascular (infarcts) especially
- Parkinson's disease

become apparent (e.g. nerve root or peripheral nerve compression or trigeminal neuralgia).

Psychological

Chronic pain influences quality of life. Depression (see pp. 907–908) is commonly associated with pain; antidepressants can help. Psychology-based pain management programmes and cognitive behavioural therapy are now a cornerstone of chronic pain management, helping people to control symptoms and the response to pain.

Analgesics

These include aspirin, paracetamol, non-steroidal anti-inflammatory drugs (NSAIDs) and opiates. Some opiates, such as tramadol and tapentadol, also have a monoamine reuptake inhibition mechanism of action. The World Health Organization (WHO) analgesic ladder (see pp. 32–33) is useful.

Co-analgesics

Co-analgesics have a primary use other than for pain, and help when used alone or added to analgesics. They may have a synergistic effect when used in combination. Examples are:
- ***tricyclic antidepressants***, e.g. amitriptyline
- ***duloxetine*** – a serotonin (5-HT)–noradrenaline (norepinephrine) reuptake blocker (SNRI)
- ***anticonvulsants***, e.g. carbamazepine, gabapentin, pregabalin and lamotrigine (see ***Box 3.3***)
- ***calcium-channel blockers***, e.g. ziconotide used intrathecally
- ***muscle relaxants***, e.g. baclofen
- ***capsaicin*** topical preparations – extracts from capsicum plants (chilli peppers), which bind to vanilloid receptors (see above)
- ***N-methyl-D-aspartate*** (***NMDA***) antagonists, e.g. ketamine
- ***cannabinoids*** – administered via oral spray in MS and resistant cancer pain
- ***botulinum*** toxin – licensed for chronic migraine; increasing evidence supports a role in modulating pain neurotransmitters.

Stimulation

Acupuncture, ice, heat, ultrasound, massage, TENS and spinal cord stimulation all achieve analgesia by gating effects on large myelinated nerve fibres.

Nerve blocks

Pain pathways can be blocked, either temporarily by local anaesthetic (by injection or with topical patches) or permanently with phenol or with radiofrequency lesions:
- somatic blocks:
  - peripheral nerve and plexus injections
  - epidural and spinal analgesia
- sympathetic blocks:
  - sympathetic ganglia injections
  - central epidural and spinal sympathetic blockade.

Neurosurgery

Highly specialized techniques have a place alongside drugs. Examples are dorsal rhizotomy, sympathectomy, cordotomy and neurostimulation.

Further reading

Cohen SP, Mao J. Neuropathic pain: mechanisms and their clinical implications. *BMJ* 2014; 348:f7656.
Magrinelli R, Zanette G, Tamburin S. Neuropathic pain: diagnosis and treatment. *Prac Neurol* 2013; 13:292–307.
Turk DC, Wilson HD, Cahana A. Treatment of chronic non-cancer pain. *Lancet* 2011; 377:2226–2235.

BLADDER CONTROL AND SEXUAL DYSFUNCTION

Changes in micturition and failure of normal sexual activity due to neurological conditions are seen in sacral, spinal cord and cortical disease.

Essential functions and anatomy

The bladder has two functions: storage and voiding. Afferent pathways (T12–S4) respond to pressure within the bladder and sensation from the genitalia. As the bladder distends, continence is maintained by suppression of parasympathetic outflow and reciprocal activation of sympathetic outflow. Both are under some voluntary control. Voiding takes place by parasympathetic activation of the detrusor, and relaxation of the internal sphincter ***(Box 21.21)***.

Cortical awareness of bladder fullness is located in the post-central gyrus, parasagittally, while initiation of micturition is in the pre-central gyrus. Voluntary control of micturition is located in the frontal cortex, parasagittally.

Box 21.21 Efferents to the bladder and genitalia

Nerve supply	Function
Parasympathetic S2–4	Bladder wall: contraction Internal sphincter: relaxation Penis/clitoris: engorgement
Sympathetic T12–L2	Bladder wall: relaxation Internal sphincter: contraction Orgasm, ejaculation
Pudendal nerves	External sphincter (skeletal muscle)

Neurological disorders of micturition

Urogenital tract disease is dealt with largely by urologists. Incontinence is common and easy to recognize; neurological causes are sometimes not obvious. These are:

Cortical:

- Post-central lesions cause loss of the sense of bladder fullness.
- Pre-central lesions cause difficulty in initiating micturition.
- Frontal lesions cause socially inappropriate micturition.

Spinal cord. Bilateral UMN lesions (pyramidal tracts) cause urinary frequency and incontinence. The bladder is small and hypertonic: that is, sensitive to small changes in intravesical pressure. Frontal lesions can also cause a hypertonic bladder.

LMN. Sacral lesions (conus medullaris, sacral root and pelvic nerve – *bilateral*) cause a flaccid, atonic bladder that overflows (cauda equina; see p. 888), often unexpectedly.

Management. Assessment of both urological causes (e.g. calculi, prostatism, gynaecological problems) and potential neurological causes of incontinence is necessary. Intermittent self-catheterization is used by many patients who have, for example, spinal cord lesions.

Male erectile dysfunction

Failure of penile erection often has mixed organic and psychological causes. Depression is common. Erectile dysfunction is described on page 1217.

INVESTIGATION OF NEUROLOGICAL DISEASE

Neurological investigations, such as brain scans, should not be a substitute for clinical evaluation through history-taking and examination. An experienced clinician will be able to make an accurate diagnosis in most patients without recourse to investigations: for example, in most individuals presenting with headache. However, cross-sectional imaging will allow confirmation of the anatomical localization of lesions and may reveal the presence of other clinically 'silent' lesions. Imaging does not always indicate the pathological nature of a visualized lesion (careful history-taking is essential in this regard) and therefore needs to be carefully interpreted in the clinical context. Neurophysiological investigations provide information about nervous system *function* and are more diagnostically helpful than imaging in some situations: for example, in patients with primary generalized epilepsies or peripheral nerve disorders.

Unnecessary or inappropriate use of investigations, particularly brain imaging, exposes patients to risk, such as radiation, is an inefficient use of resources, and may lead to identification of incidental findings that cause considerable anxiety (3% incidental abnormality rate for brain MRI scans). Clinicians should also be familiar with the range of normal in the population: for example the high prevalence of white-matter hyperintensities on brain MRI in older people and the range of common non-specific electroencephalogram (EEG) changes.

Neuroimaging

Skull and spinal X-rays

Skull X-rays have now been largely superseded by computed tomography (CT) and MRI. They show fractures, bone metastases, osteomyelitis, Paget's disease, sinus disease and intracranial calcification.

Spinal X-rays show fractures, congenital and destructive lesions (bone cysts, infection, metastases), and degenerative spondylosis.

Brain computed tomography

In brain CT, an X-ray beam and detectors revolve rapidly as the patient is moved slowly through the scanner, producing a spiral set of 'slices'. The digital data are converted to cross-sectional images.

Differences in attenuation (density, expressed as Hounsfield units) between different tissues allow accurate recognition of, for example, fresh blood, bone or calcification ***(Fig. 21.18)***. Enhancement with intravenous iodinated contrast delineates areas of vascular leak, such as with tumours and inflammation ***(Box 21.22)***.

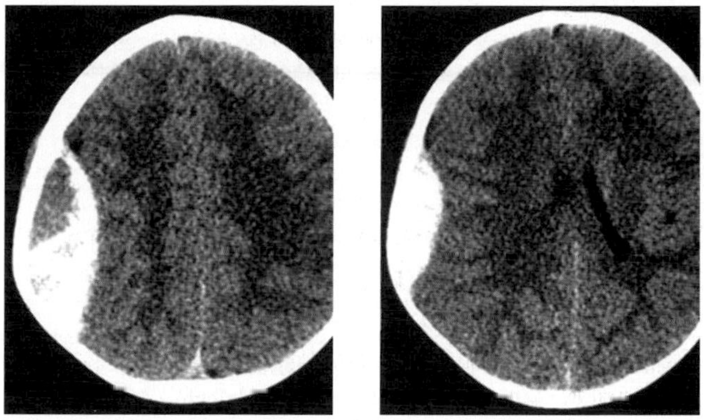

Figure 21.18 Extradural haematoma.

Box 21.22 Comparison of magnetic resonance imaging and computed tomography

Advantages of CT over MRI

- Speed – brain imaging takes seconds, an advantage in restless or critically ill patients; CT is also less sensitive to artefact due to patient motion
- Patient access – critically ill patients can be monitored more easily than in an MRI scanner
- Method of choice to detect acute haemorrhage
- Detailed evaluation of bone, e.g. spinal vertebrae and fractures
- Easier identification of calcification and metal foreign bodies
- Toleration by claustrophobic patients
- Safety with implanted devices, e.g. pacemakers
- Wider availability than MRI
- Imaging modality of choice in trauma and acute stroke for these reasons

Advantages of MRI over CT

- Superior spatial resolution and soft tissue contrast for imaging of brain parenchyma, spinal cord and nerve roots, e.g. white-matter disease such as multiple sclerosis plaques and spinal cord, which are not visible on CT
- No bone artefact, so superior visualization of posterior fossa and spinal cord
- Availability of numerous special sequences, e.g. diffusion-weighted sequence sensitive to early infarction; multiple sequences increase diagnostic utility
- No ionizing radiation
- MR angiography may be performed without contrast
- Viewing of images in axial, sagittal and coronal planes

CT angiography

Spiral CT after intravenous injection of contrast produces high-quality arterial angiograms (or venograms), which are now considered the gold standard for non-invasive angiography.

Spinal CT and CT myelography

Spinal CT is useful for assessing the bone architecture of the spine but provides little information about soft tissues, such as nerve roots and spinal cord (MRI is required). CT myelography (spinal CT after intrathecal injection of contrast) is used for identification of spinal fluid leaks/blockage or for situations where MRI is contraindicated.

Magnetic resonance imaging

A hydrogen nucleus is a proton whose electrical charge creates a local electrical field. In MRI, protons are aligned by sudden, strong magnetic impulses and then imaged with radiofrequency waves at right angles to their alignment. The protons resonate and spin, then revert to their normal alignment. As they do so, images are made at different phases of relaxation, known as T_1, T_2, T_2 STIR, FLAIR, diffusion-weighted imaging (DWI) and other sequences. The combination of these sequences increases the diagnostic sensitivity and specificity of MRI. Gadolinium is used as intravenous contrast to show areas of increased vascularity.

The superior spatial resolution and soft tissue contrast of MRI, as compared to CT, makes MRI of the brain and spine generally preferable in the non-emergency situation. It can image pathology not easily visualized on CT, such as small lesions, white-matter disease such as MS plaques and spinal cord lesions or compression, and demonstrate anatomy more accurately.

Doppler studies

Ultrasound is a safe, low-cost and rapid method for detecting and quantifying carotid stenosis and assessing carotid plaque burden. It is operator-dependent and less reproducible than other imaging modalities.

Catheter angiography

Contrast is injected intra-arterially in selected vessels via a catheter inserted in the femoral artery. Angiography carries a mortality and stroke risk (<1%). Images of aorta, carotid, vertebral and brain arteries demonstrate occlusion, stenoses, aneurysms and arteriovenous malformations (AVMs). Spinal angiography is complex and is used to identify spinal AVMs and dural fistulas. Aneurysms and AVMs may be treated by endovascular means (embolization with glue or platinum coils) during the procedure.

Positron emission tomography, single proton emission computed tomography, dopamine transporter imaging and functional MRI

These functional imaging techniques track uptake of radioisotopes and/or metabolites. Fluorodeoxyglucose positron emission tomography (FDG-PET) is used principally to detect occult neoplasms or tumour recurrence, outside the central nervous system (CNS), or to identify large-vessel vasculitis. Dopamine transporter imaging (DAT) is used to identify reduced nigrostriatal dopaminergic terminals in parkinsonian disorders, mainly in patients with atypical tremor where the clinical diagnosis is uncertain. Functional MRI (fMRI) is largely a research tool for mapping brain function, in health and disease. New techniques using radionuclide tracers to image brain amyloid deposits in Alzheimer's disease are in development and will soon be available for clinical use.

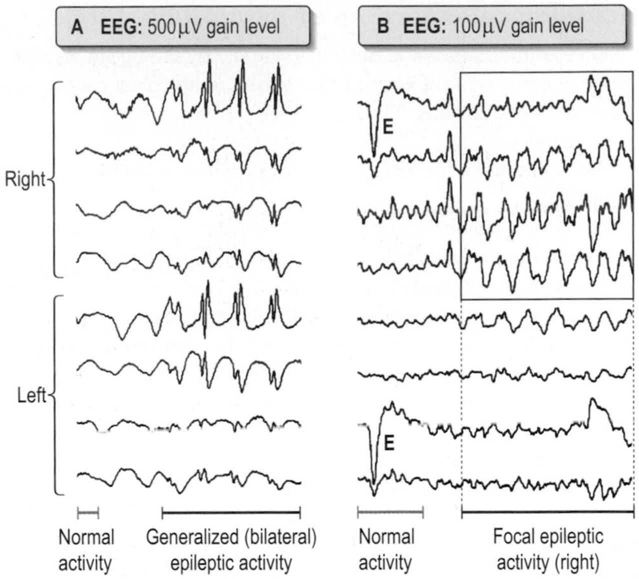

Figure 21.19 Examples of EEG traces. A. Normal activity followed by generalized epileptic spikes in all leads. **B.** Normal activity followed by focal spikes in right leads. E, eye-movement artefact.

Isotope bone scanning

The radioisotope [^{99m}Tc]-pertechnetate is given intravenously. The technique is used principally in detection of vertebral, skull and bone metastases.

Neurophysiological investigations

Electroencephalography

Brain electrical activity ***(Fig. 21.19)*** is recorded from scalp electrodes (20 channels simultaneously). Its main use is to characterize epilepsy syndromes. Recordings are usually made between seizures (inter-ictal). Sleep-deprived EEG and 24-hour ambulatory EEG increase diagnostic sensitivity. Videotelemetry (VT) combines continuous EEG with video over several days to record the semiology and electrical characteristics of seizures. VT is invaluable diagnostically to identify seizure type where there is clinical uncertainty, and to pinpoint the seizure focus in focal epilepsies.

Epilepsy

Spikes, or spike-and-wave abnormalities, are hallmarks of epilepsy, but it is important to emphasize that patients with epilepsy often have a normal EEG between seizures (see p. 849).

Diffuse brain disorders

Slow-wave EEG abnormalities appear in encephalopathy (e.g. hepatic coma), encephalitis and prion (Creutzfeldt–Jakob) diseases.

Brain death

The EEG is isoelectric (flat); EEG is not necessary to confirm brain death in many countries (see p. 1172).

Electromyography and nerve conduction studies

Electromyography (EMG) and nerve conduction studies (NCS) are skilled investigations of nerve function that are essential for investigation of peripheral nerve, anterior horn cell, neuromuscular junction (NMJ) and, to a lesser extent, muscle disorders. NCS are highly sensitive in identification of peripheral neuropathy, and assessment

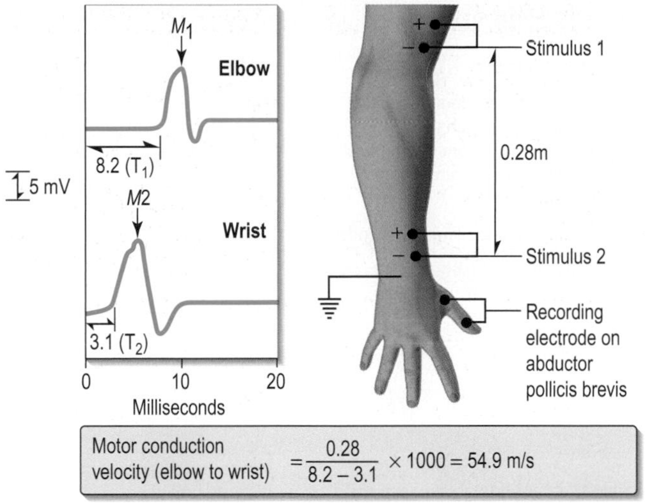

Figure 21.20 Measurement of motor conduction velocity (MCV) in ulnar nerve. The recording electrode on abductor pollicis brevis measures the muscle action potential (M) from ulnar nerve stimulation at the elbow (stimulus 1) and wrist (stimulus 2). MCV calculation:
M_1 = muscle action potential (MAP) from stimulus 1
M_2 = MAP from stimulus 2
T_1 = time from elbow to recording electrode
T_2 = time from wrist to recording electrode
$\text{MCV} = \dfrac{\text{distance (metres)} \times 1000}{T_1 - T_2} = \text{m/s}$

of the nerves affected and the type of pathology (axonal loss versus demyelinating). In mononeuropathies, the anatomical site of the lesion may be identified with considerable accuracy and prognostic information obtained.

Electromyography

A concentric needle electrode is inserted into voluntary muscle. Amplified recordings, on an oscilloscope, are also heard through a speaker. The main EMG features include:

- normal interference pattern
- denervation and re-innervation changes
- myopathic and myotonic features (see p. 889).

Single-fibre EMG is used for disorders of NMJ transmission.

Peripheral nerve conduction

Electrical stimulation of a peripheral nerve generates a nerve impulse that may be recorded ***(Fig. 21.20)***. Four measurements are of principal value in neuropathies and nerve entrapment:

- nerve conduction velocity
- distal motor latency
- sensory action potentials (SAPs)
- compound muscle action potentials (CMAPs).

Small action potential size (SAP and CMAP) indicates loss of axons. Conduction block and slowing of conduction velocity indicate demyelinating neuropathy, as salutatory conduction is lost with damage to the myelin sheath. Repetitive nerve stimulation is used to identify NMJ conduction disorders (myasthenia).

Cerebral-evoked potentials

Visual-evoked potentials (VEPs) record the interval visual stimuli take to reach the occipital cortex, and the amplitude of response. VEPs are used to confirm previous optic neuritis (see p. 803); this leaves a delayed latency despite clinical recovery.

Box 21.23 The normal cerebrospinal fluid (CSF)

Appearance	Crystal clear, colourless
Pressure	60–150 mm of CSF, recumbent
Cell count	<5/mm^3 No polymorphs Mononuclear cells only
Protein	0.2–0.4 g/L
Glucose	2/3–1/2 of blood glucose
Immunoglobulin G	<15% of total CSF protein
Oligoclonal bands	Absent

Similar techniques for auditory and somatosensory potentials (from a limb) are also used.

Lumbar puncture and cerebrospinal fluid examination

See ***Boxes 21.23*** and ***21.24***. Indications for lumbar puncture (LP) include:

- diagnosis of meningitis and encephalitis
- diagnosis of subarachnoid haemorrhage (in a patient with a normal CT)
- measurement of CSF pressure, e.g. idiopathic intracranial hypertension (see p. 845)
- removal of CSF therapeutically, e.g. idiopathic intracranial hypertension
- diagnosis of various conditions, e.g. MS, neurosyphilis, sarcoidosis, Behçet's, malignant meningitis, polyneuropathies
- intrathecal injection/drugs.

In suspected CNS infection, close liaison between clinician and microbiologist is essential. Specific techniques (e.g. polymerase chain reaction to identify specific pathogens) are invaluable. Repeated CSF examination is often necessary in chronic infection such as tuberculosis. Post-LP headaches, worse on standing, are a common complaint for several days (or more). Prolonged headaches can be treated by an 'autologous intrathecal blood patch': injection of 20 mL of the patient's venous blood into the lumbar epidural space.

Biopsy

Interpretation of brain, tonsillar, muscle and nerve histology requires specialist neuropathology services.

Brain and meninges

Brain biopsy (e.g. of a non-dominant frontal lobe) is rarely used to diagnose inflammatory and degenerative brain diseases. CT and MR stereotactic biopsies of intracranial lesions are standard procedures.

Muscle

Muscle biopsy (usually quadriceps), with light/electron microscopy and immunohistochemical analysis, is performed routinely for diagnosis of inflammatory, metabolic and dystrophic disorders (see p. 889).

Peripheral nerve

Nerve biopsy, usually of the (sensory) sural nerve or superficial sensory branch of the radial nerve, can be of value in the diagnosis of peripheral neuropathy: for example, if vasculitis, amyloid

Box 21.24 Lumbar puncture (LP)

Explain the procedure to the patient and obtain consent. LP should not be performed in the presence of raised intracranial pressure or when an intracranial mass lesion is a possibility.

Technique

- Place the patient on the edge of the bed in the left lateral position, with knees and chin as close together as possible.
- Mark the third and fourth lumbar spines. The fourth lumbar spine usually lies on a line joining the iliac crests.
- Using sterile precautions, inject 2% lidocaine into the dermis by raising a bleb in either the third or fourth lumbar interspace.
- Push the LP needle through the skin in the midline, steadily forwards and slightly towards the head, with the head and spine bolstered horizontally with pillows.
- When you feel the needle penetrate the dura, withdraw the stylet and allow a few drops of CSF to escape.
- You can then measure CSF pressure with a manometer connected to the needle. The patient's head must be on the same level as the sacrum. Normal CSF pressure is 60–150 mm of CSF. The level rises and falls with respiration and heartbeat, and rises on coughing.
- Collect CSF specimens in three sterile bottles and take a sample for CSF glucose, together with a simultaneous blood glucose sample.
- Record CSF naked-eye appearance: clear, cloudy, yellow (xanthochromic) or red.
- Ask the patient to lie flat after the procedure to avoid subsequent headaches; this manœuvre is probably of little value, however.
- Analgesics may be required for post-LP headaches.

Contraindications

- Suspicion of a mass lesion in the brain or cord. Caudal herniation of the cerebellar tonsils (coning) may occur if an intracranial mass is present and the pressure below is reduced by removal of CSF
- Any cause of raised intracranial pressure
- Local infection near the LP site
- Congenital lesions in the lumbosacral region (e.g. meningomyelocele)
- Platelet count $<40 \times 10^9$/L and other clotting abnormalities, including anticoagulant drugs
- Unconscious patients and those with papilloedema must have a CT scan before LP.

Notes

- Contraindications are relative; there are circumstances when LP is carried out despite them.
- Composition of normal CSF is shown in Box 21.23.

deposition or malignant infiltration is suspected. There may be significant complications (wound healing and pain), so it should be undertaken only where all other investigations are non-diagnostic and where there is clinical evidence of a severe or progressive neuropathy.

Psychometric assessment

Psychometric testing, performed by neuropsychologists, assesses cognitive function in more detail than bedside testing during clinical examination. Decline in intellectual function, as compared to estimated pre-morbid IQ, is seen following brain injury or in dementia, for example. Individual cognitive domains, such as various types of memory, language, visuospatial function and frontal executive function, are tested separately, as they may be differentially involved in different disorders, the pattern of involvement often being of considerable diagnostic value. Serial testing at intervals of 6–12 months may be needed to show clear evidence of progression in neurodegenerative disorders such as dementias.

Box 21.25 Neurological autoantibody tests[a]

Clinical disorder	Antibody (Ab) test
Paraneoplastic disorders: cerebellar ataxia, limbic encephalitis, opsoclonus–myoclonus, progressive encephalomyelitis with rigidity and myoclonus	Anti-Hu, Yo, Ma2/Ma1, CV2, Ri, Tr, amphiphysin
Teratoma-associated limbic encephalitis	NMDA Abs
Limbic encephalitis (non-paraneoplastic)	Anti-potassium channel, glycine Abs
Myasthenia gravis[b]	Acetylcholine receptor, MUSK Abs
Lambert–Eaton myasthenic syndrome[b]	Voltage-gated calcium channel Abs
Neuromyelitis optica	Aquaporin 4 Abs
Stiff person syndrome	Anti-GAD Abs
Transverse myelitis	Anti-MOG Abs
Peripheral neuropathy	Anti-ganglioside and MAG Abs
Hashimoto's encephalopathy	Anti-TPO Abs
Dermatomyositis/polymyositis[b]	Anti-Jo-1 and other tRNA synthetases, SRP, Mi-2 and other Abs

[a]See also Box 17.8. [b]May be paraneoplastic.

Routine tests

Standard blood tests, such as full blood count, erythrocyte sedimentation rate (ESR), biochemistry, glucose/HbA_{1c}, C-reactive protein, creatine kinase and protein electrophoresis, are helpful to identify underlying disorders such as diabetes, metabolic disorders and other systemic disorders that may underlie neurological presentations (e.g. coma or peripheral neuropathy). Relevant tests are covered in disease-specific sub-sections.

Specialized tests in specific diseases

An increasing number of highly specialized tests are employed to diagnose individual (sometimes rare) diseases ***(Box 21.25)***.

Genetic tests

Several hundred neurogenetic disorders are now recognized and, for many of these, specific molecular genetic investigations are available for diagnostic and predictive testing (see pp. 880–881). As genetic testing is complex and expensive, it should only be undertaken after senior specialist advice. It is likely that there will be gene chip-based testing of panels of disease genes (e.g. for dementias or muscular dystrophies) in the near future. Informed patient consent is required, as a positive test may have implications for other family members. Predictive testing in non-affected, at-risk individuals should only be undertaken after detailed genetic counselling by a specialist.

Immunological tests

An increasing number of autoimmune neurological disorders are recognized, many of which are associated with specific antibody tests ***(Box 21.25)***. Many of these are paraneoplastic syndromes but an increasing number of non-cancer-related autoimmune syndromes have been identified, such as forms of encephalitis or myasthenia gravis. In addition, monoclonal paraproteins associated with plasma cell dyscrasias may cause immune-mediated peripheral neuropathy.

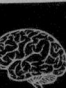

Further reading

Morris Z, Whiteley WM, Longstreth Jr WT et al. Incidental findings on brain magnetic resonance imaging: systematic review and meta-analysis. *BMJ* 2009; 339:b3016.

Whittaker RG. SNAPs, CMAPs and F-waves: nerve conduction studies for the uninitiated. *Prac Neurol* 2012; 12:108–115.

UNCONSCIOUSNESS AND COMA

Consciousness is dependent on the functioning of two separate anatomical and physiological systems:

- The ascending reticular activating system (ARAS), projecting from brainstem to thalamus. This determines arousal (the level of consciousness).
- The cerebral cortex, which determines the content of consciousness.

Impaired functioning of either anatomical system may cause coma.

Disturbed consciousness: definitions

- ***Coma***: a state of unrousable unresponsiveness. Level of consciousness represents a continuum between being alert and deeply comatose. It may be quantified using the Glasgow Coma Scale (GCS) with a score between 3 and 15 ***(Box 21.26)***. Coma may be conveniently defined as a GCS score of 8 or lower. Terms such as stupor and obtundation have been superseded by the GCS score and are no longer used.
- ***Delirium***: a confusional state in which reduced attention is a cardinal feature, usually with altered behaviour, cognition, orientation and a fluctuating level of consciousness (from agitation to hypoarousal; see pp. 926–927).

Box 21.26 Glasgow Coma Scale (GCS)[a]

Parameter	Score
Eye opening (*E*)	
Spontaneous	4
To speech	3
To pain	2
No response	1
Motor response (*M*)	
Obeys	6
Localizes	5
Withdraws	4
Flexion	3
Extension	2
No response	1
Verbal response (*V*)	
Orientated	5
Confused conversation	4
Inappropriate words	3
Incomprehensible sounds	2
No response	1

[a]GCS score = $E+M+V$ (GCS minimum = 3; maximum = 15).

Mechanisms and causes of coma

Altered consciousness is produced by four mechanisms affecting the ARAS in the brainstem or thalamus, and/or widespread impairment of cortical function (***Box 21.27*** and ***Fig. 21.21***).

- ***Brainstem lesion***. A discrete brainstem or thalamic lesion, e.g. stroke, may damage the ARAS.

Box 21.27 Principal causes of coma: examples of mechanisms

Diffuse brain dysfunction

- Drug overdose (accidental or deliberate), including alcohol
- CO poisoning
- Traumatic brain injury
- Hypoglycaemia, hyperglycaemia
- Severe uraemia (see p. 772)
- Hepatic encephalopathy (see p. 474)
- Respiratory failure with CO_2 retention (see p. 1081)
- Hypercalcaemia, hypocalcaemia
- Hypoadrenalism, hypopituitarism and hypothyroidism
- Hyponatraemia, hypernatraemia
- Metabolic acidosis
- Hypothermia, hyperpyrexia
- Seizures – post-ictal state and non-convulsive status
- Metabolic rarities, e.g. porphyria
- Extensive cortical damage
- Hypoxic–ischaemic brain injury, e.g. cardiac arrest
- Encephalitis, meningitis, cerebral malaria
- Subarachnoid haemorrhage

Direct effect within brainstem

- Brainstem haemorrhage, infarction or demyelination
- Brainstem neoplasm, e.g. glioma
- Wernicke–Korsakoff syndrome

Pressure effect on brainstem

- Tumour, massive hemisphere infarction with oedema, haematoma, abscess
- Cerebellar mass

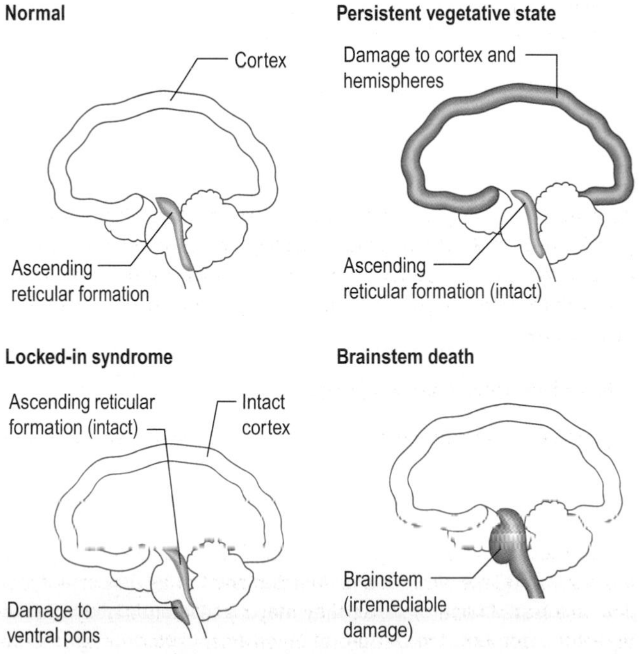

Figure 21.21 Anatomy of vegetative state, locked-in syndrome and brainstem death. *(Adapted from Bates D. Coma and brainstem death.* Medicine *2004; 32.)*

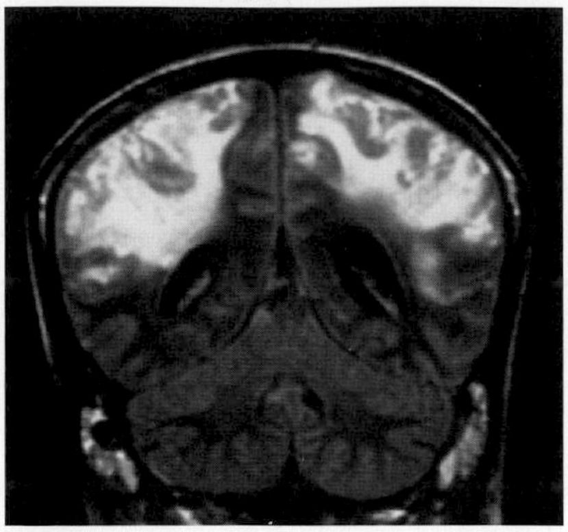

Figure 21.22 **Magnetic resonance image showing extensive cortical damage following meningitis.** A permanent vegetative state resulted.

- ***Brainstem compression***. A supratentorial mass lesion within the brain compresses the brainstem, inhibiting the ARAS, e.g. 'coning' from a brain tumour or haemorrhage. Mass lesions within the posterior fossa are particularly prone to causing brainstem compression and hydrocephalus.
- ***Diffuse brain dysfunction***. Generalized severe metabolic or toxic disorders (e.g. alcohol, sedatives, uraemia, hypercapnia) depress cortical and ARAS function.
- ***Massive cortical damage***. Unlike brainstem lesions, extensive damage of the cerebral cortex and cortical connections is required to cause coma, e.g. meningitis or hypoxic–ischaemic damage after cardiac arrest ***(Fig. 21.22)***.

A single focal hemisphere (or cerebellar) lesion does not produce coma, unless it compresses the brainstem. Cerebral oedema frequently surrounds masses, increasing their pressure effects.

The most common causes of coma are:

- metabolic disorders – 35%
- drugs and toxins – 25%
- mass lesions – 20%
- other – including trauma, stroke and CNS infections.

The unconscious patient

Immediate assessment and management

- Check the ***a***irway, ***b***reathing, ***c***irculation, ***d***isability and ***e***xposure/***e***xamination.
- Use Stix to measure blood glucose; if the patient is hypoglycaemic, give glucose (25 mL 50%).
- Treat seizures with buccal midazolam; if not terminated, use intravenous phenytoin.
- If there is fever and meningism, give intravenous antibiotics.
- Give intravenous naloxone or flumazenil (for overdose) and thiamine (in Wernicke's encephalopathy) in people who use excess alcohol.

Obtain as much history as possible. A limited history is one of the problems in assessing the unconscious patient. What were the circumstances? Ask paramedics, police and witnesses. Contact the patient's relatives, friends and GP, and obtain past hospital notes. Look for drug details/bottles and identification data.

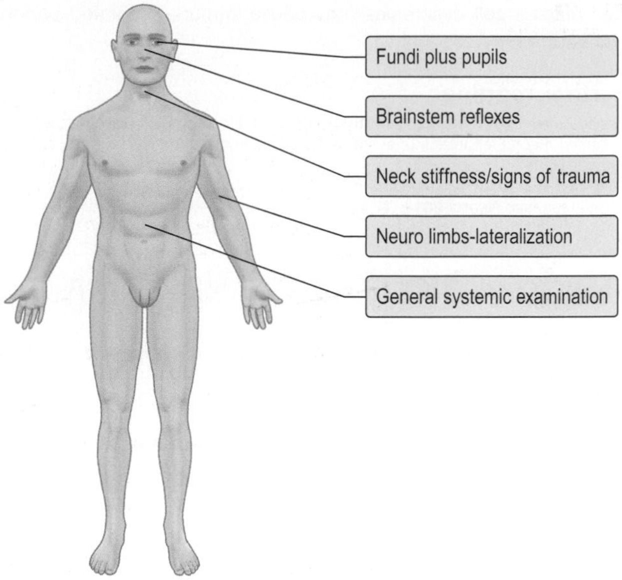

Figure 21.23 **Assessing the level of consciousness.**

General and neurological examination

General examination

(See ***Fig. 21.23***.)

- Measure the patient's temperature (with a low-reading rectal thermometer if hypothermic). Check for meningism.
- Sniff the patient's breath for ketones, alcohol and hepatic fetor.
- Survey the skin for signs of trauma or spinal injury, rash (meningococcal sepsis), jaundice or stigmata of chronic liver disease, cyanosis and injection marks.
- Assess the respiratory pattern, e.g. Cheyne–Stokes (alternating hyperpnoea and periods of apnoea indicating bilateral cerebral or upper brainstem dysfunction) or acidotic (Kussmaul) respiration (deep, sighing hyperventilation seen in diabetic ketoacidosis and uraemia).

Neurological examination

Neurological examination aims to determine:

- depth of coma (GCS)
- brainstem function
- lateralization of pathology.

Depth of coma

GCS. Assessment of the GCS score is repeated regularly to determine whether the patient's level of consciousness is progressively declining. Use a painful stimulus (e.g. nail-bed pressure) to each limb and central area (sternal rub or pressure over the supraorbital nerve), and record the *best* response. Shout commands.

Fundi. Look for papilloedema and subhyaloid retinal haemorrhage (seen in subarachnoid haemorrhage).

Brainstem function

Pupils

Record their size and reaction to light ***(Fig. 21.24)***:

- ***Dilatation of one pupil*** that then becomes fixed to light indicates compression of the IIIrd nerve. This is a potential neurosurgical emergency ***(Fig. 21.25)***.

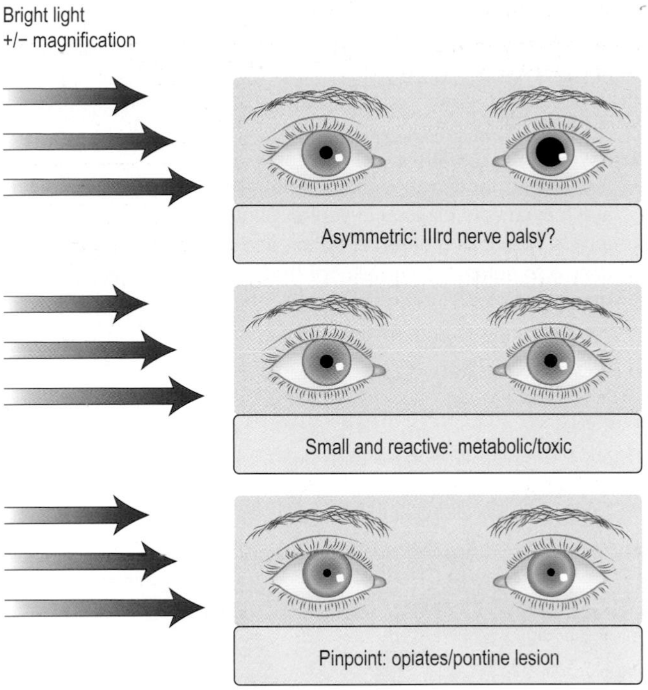

Figure 21.24 Examination of the pupils.

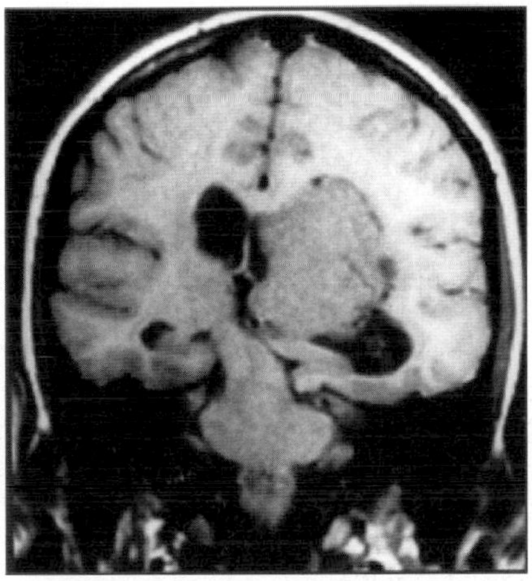

Figure 21.25 Medial temporal lobe (uncal) herniation causing compression.

- ***Bilateral mid-point reactive pupils*** (i.e. normal pupils) are characteristic of metabolic comas and follow coma due to sedative drugs (except opiates).
- ***Bilateral light-fixed, dilated pupils*** are one cardinal sign of brain death. They can occur in deep coma of any cause, but particularly in barbiturate intoxication and hypothermia.
- ***Bilateral pinpoint, light-fixed pupils*** occur with pontine lesions (e.g. haemorrhage) and with opiates.

Mydriatic drugs and previous pupillary surgery can cause diagnostic difficulty.

Eye movements and position

- Disconjugate eyes (divergent ocular axes) indicate a brainstem lesion, e.g. ***skew deviation*** (one eye up, one eye down; ***Fig. 21.26***).
- Conjugate gaze deviation means the eyes deviate towards the lesion in the frontal lobe and the normal limbs (unopposed activity of the intact frontal eye fields drives eyes to the opposite side); and away from the lesion in the brainstem and towards the weak limbs (the PPRF in the pons controls lateral gaze to the ipsilateral side; see p. 805) ***(Fig. 21.27)***.
- Vestibulo-ocular reflex means that passive head-turning produces conjugate ocular deviation away from the direction of rotation (doll's eye reflex). This reflex disappears in deep coma, brainstem lesions and brain death ***(Fig. 21.28)***.
- In light coma, slow, side-to-side eye movements are seen ('windscreen wiper' eyes; ***Fig. 21.29***). This is also seen with extensive cortical damage in deep coma.

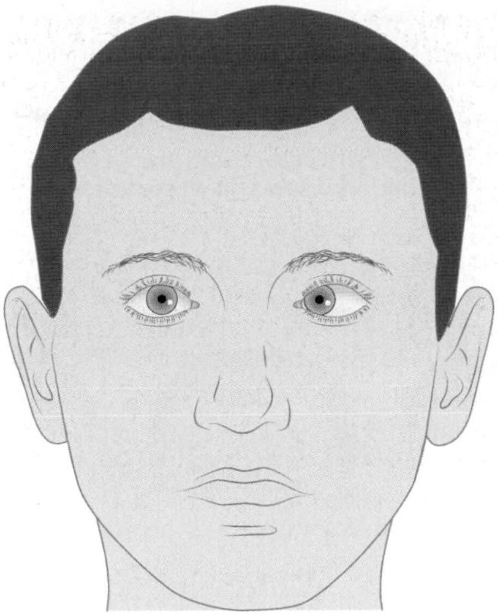

Figure 21.26 Disconjugate eye position. This usually indicates brainstem lesion (the eyes may be mildly disconjugate in metabolic coma).

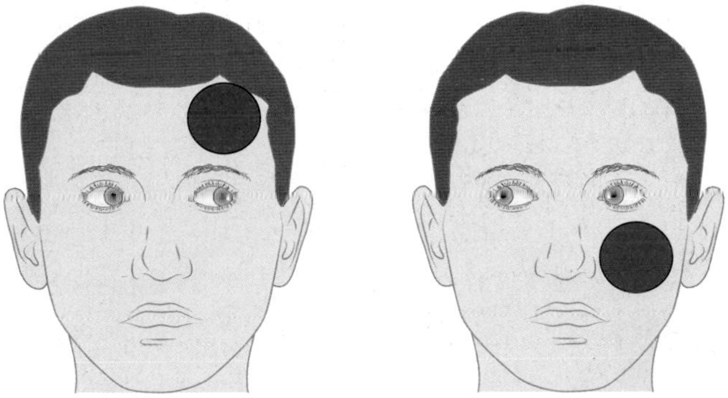

A B

Figure 21.27 Conjugate gaze deviation. A. Frontal lesion. **B.** Brainstem lesion.

Other brainstem reflexes

- Corneal reflex.
- Gag/cough reflex (via endotracheal tube if intubated).
- Respiratory drive (see p. 1081).

Lateralizing signs

Coma makes it difficult to recognize lateralizing signs. These are helpful:

- ***Asymmetry of response to visual threat*** in a stuporose patient: suggests hemianopia.

- ***Asymmetry of face***: drooping or dribbling on one side; blowing in and out of mouth when the paralysed cheek does not move.
- ***Asymmetry of tone***: unilateral flaccidity or spasticity – may be the only sign of hemiparesis.
- ***Asymmetry of decerebrate and decorticate posturing***.

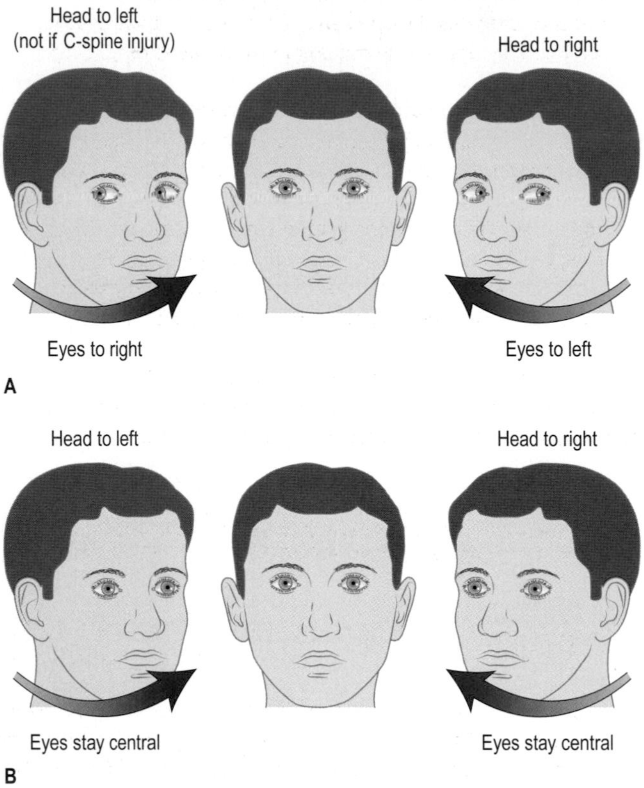

Figure 21.28 **Doll's eye movements. A.** Normal. **B.** Abnormal.

- ***Asymmetrical response*** to painful stimuli.
- ***Asymmetry of tendon reflexes and plantar responses***: both plantars are often extensor in deep coma.

Coma 'look-alikes'

- Psychogenic coma.
- 'Locked-in' syndrome – complete paralysis, except for vertical eye movements/blinking in ventral pontine infarction. Patients have a functioning cerebral cortex and are fully aware but unable to communicate, except through eye movements ***(Box 21.28)***.
- Severe paralysis, e.g. myaesthenic crisis or severe Guillain–Barré syndrome.

Diagnosis and investigations in coma

Often, the cause is evident (e.g. head injury, metabolic disorder, overdose). Where lateralizing signs or brainstem pathology are

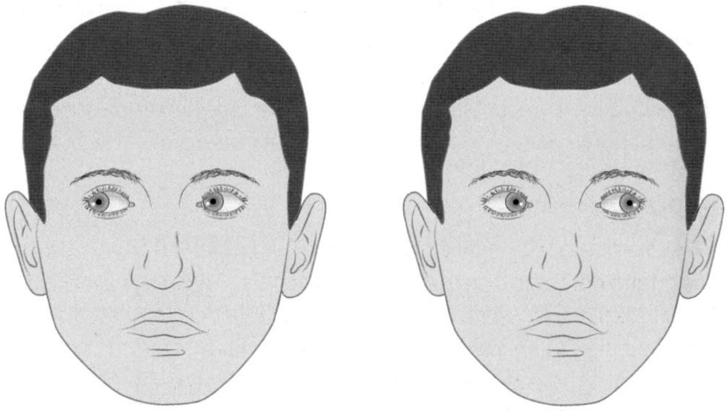

Figure 21.29 **'Windscreen wiper' eyes ('ping pong' eyes).** Slow, side-to-side movements demonstrate diffuse cortical dysfunction. This is common in light coma and implies normal brainstem function. In deep coma it indicates extensive cortical damage.

Box 21.28 Differential diagnosis of prolonged disorders of consciousness

Condition	Vegetative state	Minimally conscious state	Locked-in syndrome	Coma	Death confirmed by brainstem tests
Awareness	Absent	Present	Present	Absent	Absent
Sleep–wake cycles	Present	Present	Present	Absent	Absent
Response to noxious stimuli	±	Present	Present (in eyes only)	±	Absent
Glasgow Coma Scale	E4, M1–4, V1–2	E4, M1–5, V1–4	E4, M1, V1	E1–2, M1–4, V1–2	E1, M1–3, V1
Motor function	No purposeful movement	Some consistent verbal or purposeful behaviour	Volitional vertical eye movements or eye blink typically preserved	No purposeful movement	None or only reflex spinal movement
Respiratory function	Typically preserved	Typically preserved	Typically preserved	Variable	Absent
EEG activity	Typically slow-wave activity	Insufficient data	Typically normal	Typically slow-wave activity	Typically absent
Cerebral metabolism (PET)	Severely reduced	Intermediate reduction	Mildly reduced	Moderately to severely reduced	Severely reduced or absent
Prognosis	Variable: if permanent, continued VS or death	Variable: if permanent, continued MCS or death	Depends on cause but full recovery unlikely	Recovery, vegetative state or death within weeks	Organ function can be sustained only temporarily with life support

EEG, electroencephalography; MCS, minimally conscious state; PET, positron emission tomography; vegetative state.
(Reproduced from Royal College of Physicians. *Prolonged Disorders of Consciousness: National Clinical Guidelines*. London: RCP, 2013; with permission.)

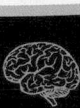

found on examination, a mass lesion or infarction/haemorrhage is likely (note that hypoglycaemia may also cause focal signs). If no cause is obvious after clinical assessment, further investigations are essential.

Blood and urine

- ***Drug screen*** – blood alcohol and salicylates, urine toxicology including screening for benzodiazepines, narcotics, amfetamines.
- ***Biochemistry*** – urea, electrolytes, glucose, calcium, liver biochemistry.
- ***Metabolic and endocrine studies*** – thyroid stimulating hormone, cortisol.
- ***Arterial blood gases*** – for acidosis or high CO_2 levels.
- ***Other*** – e.g. cerebral malaria (request *thick* blood film; see pp. 299–300) and porphyria (pp. 1289–1291).

Brain imaging

CT brain imaging is the most readily available and safest modality in the unconscious patient (MRI is useful where CT is normal but presents greater monitoring challenges in the unconscious patient). CT is quick and effective in demonstrating all types of brain haemorrhage and most mass lesions; infarcts may be missed in the early stages and where only the brainstem is affected.

CSF examination

LP should be performed in coma only after careful risk assessment. It is contraindicated when an intracranial mass lesion is a possibility; CT is essential to exclude this. CSF examination is likely to alter therapy only if undiagnosed meningoencephalitis or other infection is present, or in subarachnoid haemorrhage where CT may give a false negative result, particularly after 24 hours.

Electroencephalography

EEG is of some value in the diagnosis of metabolic coma, encephalitis and non-convulsive status epilepticus.

General management

Comatose patients need careful nursing, meticulous attention to the airway, and frequent monitoring of vital functions.

Longer-term essentials are:

- skin care – turning (to avoid pressure ulcers and pressure palsies)
- oral hygiene – mouthwashes, suction
- eye care – prevention of corneal damage (lid taping, irrigation)
- fluids – nasogastric or intravenous
- feeding – via a fine-bore nasogastric tube or via PEG
- sphincters – catheterization when essential (use a penile urinary sheath if possible in men); rectal evacuation.

Prognosis in coma and the vegetative state

Prognosis depends on the cause of coma and the extent of brain damage sustained. Metabolic and toxic causes of coma have the best prognosis when the underlying problem can be corrected. Following hypoxic–ischaemic brain injury, such as after cardiac arrest, only 11% make a good recovery; after stroke, the prognosis is worse still, with only 7% recovering. Of those patients who do not recover consciousness, a substantial proportion will remain in a vegetative or minimally responsive state.

- ***The vegetative state*** (VS) is usually a consequence of extensive cortical damage. Brainstem function is intact and so breathing is normal without the need for mechanical ventilation, and the patient appears awake with eye-opening and sleep–wake cycles. However, there is no sign of awareness or response to environmental stimuli, except reflex movements. Feeding is via gastrostomy. Patients may remain in this state for years. It is considered permanent (PVS) if there is no recovery after 12 months where trauma is the cause, and after 6 months for all other causes. Prolonged support of patients after this time presents a number of ethical issues; families may apply to the courts for withdrawal of feeding in PVS.
- ***Minimally conscious state*** (MCS) describes patients with some, often fluctuating, limited awareness, with inconsistent but reproducible responses, e.g. movements in response to voice; crying or laughing in response to emotional stimuli; and vocalization in response to questions. A patient may emerge from VS into MCS. Distinguishing VS from MCS requires careful specialist assessment over a long period. Functional brain imaging has recently been used for this purpose.
- ***Brainstem death*** is discussed on pages 1172–1173.

Distinction between these states is essential before addressing issues of prognosis and cessation of supportive care.

Further reading

Royal College of Physicians of London. *Prolonged Disorders of Consciousness: National Clinical Guidelines*. London: RCP; 2013.

STROKE

Stroke is the third most common cause of death in high-income countries (11% of all deaths in the UK) and the leading cause of adult disability worldwide. Approximately two-thirds of the global burden of stroke is in middle- and low-income countries. Stroke rates are higher in Asian and black African populations than in Caucasians. Stroke risk increases with age but one-quarter of all strokes occur before the age of 65. The death rate following stroke is 20–25%, and 40% of surviving patients are dependent at 6 months.

Definitions

- ***Stroke***. To the public, stroke means weakness, usually permanent on one side, often with loss of speech. Stroke is *defined* as a syndrome of rapid onset of neurological deficit caused by focal, cerebral, spinal or retinal infarction. Tissue injury is confirmed by neuroimaging. Hemiplegia following middle cerebral arterial thromboembolism is the typical example.
- ***Transient ischaemic attack*** (***TIA***) means a brief episode of neurological dysfunction due to temporary focal cerebral or retinal ischaemia without infarction, e.g. a weak limb, aphasia or loss of vision, usually lasting seconds or minutes with complete recovery. TIAs may herald a stroke. The arbitrary time of <24 hours is no longer used.

'Cerebrovascular accident' is a vague term and should be avoided.

Pathophysiology

The underlying pathology responsible for stroke is either infarction or haemorrhage. Stroke mechanism and pathophysiology

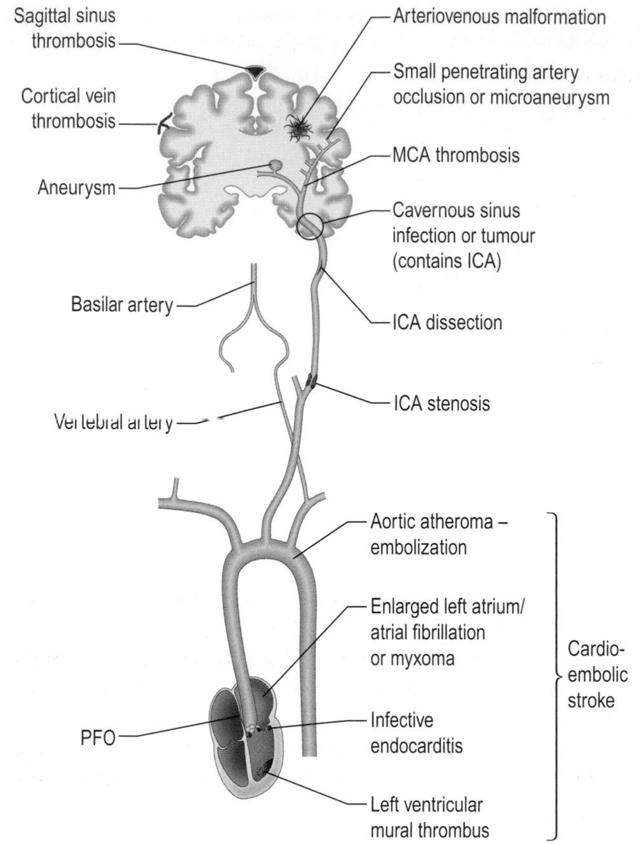

Figure 21.30 **Pathophysiology of ischaemic stroke.** ICA, internal carotid artery; MCA, middle cerebral artery; PFO, patent foramen ovale.

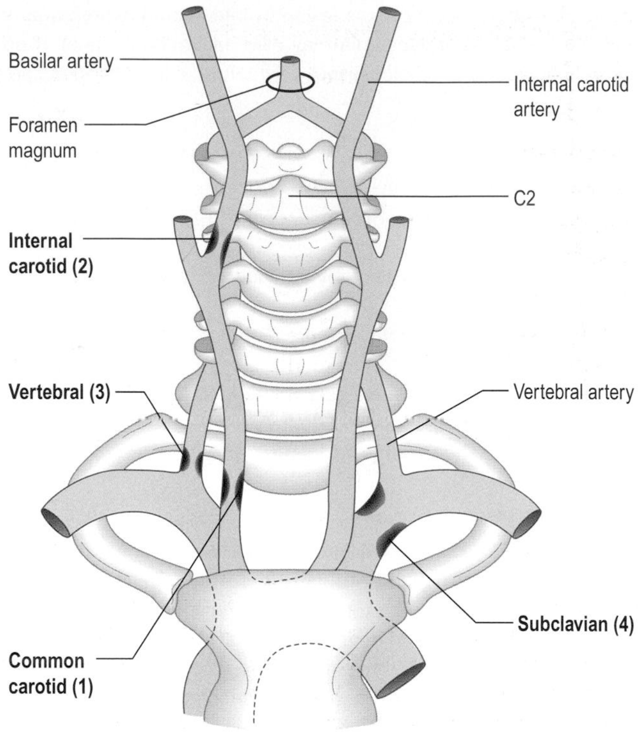

Figure 21.31 **Principal sites of stenoses in extracerebral arteries.** (These are shown in bold, 1–4.)

depend on the population studied but are broadly as follows ***(Fig. 21.30)***:

- ischaemic stroke/infarction (85%)
  - thrombotic
  - large-artery stenosis
  - small-vessel disease
  - cardio-embolic
  - hypoperfusion
- haemorrhagic stroke (10%) (see pp. 838–839)
  - intracerebral haemorrhage (12%) (see pp. 838–839)
  - subarachnoid haemorrhage (5%) (see pp. 839–841)
- other (5%), e.g. arterial dissection, venous sinus thrombosis, vasculitis (see p. 699).

Ischaemic stroke

Arterial disease and atherosclerosis are the main pathological processes causing stroke. Arterial branch points, such as the origin of the great vessels arising from the aorta, the proximal internal carotid artery and its distal intracranial branches, are particularly affected ***(Fig. 21.31)***. Non-Caucasian populations tend to have more intracranial narrowing and white populations more extracranial disease (which is strongly correlated with co-morbid coronary artery and peripheral vascular disease).

Thrombosis. Thrombosis at the site of ruptured mural plaque leads to artery-to-artery embolism or vessel occlusion.

Large-artery stenosis. This usually causes stroke by acting as an embolic source rather than by occluding the vessel (which may not in itself cause stroke if it occurs gradually and collateral circulation is adequate).

Small-vessel disease. Small penetrating arterial branches supply the deep brain parenchyma and are affected by a different pathological process: an occlusive vasculopathy – lipohyalinosis – that is a consequence of hypertension. This leads to small infarcts called 'lacunes' and/or gradual accumulation of diffuse ischaemic change in deep white matter.

Cardio-embolic stroke. The heart is a common source of embolic material. Atrial fibrillation (and other arrhythmias) leading to thrombosis in a dilated left atrium is the most common cause. Cardiac valve disease, including congenital valve disorders, infective vegetations, and rheumatic and degenerative calcific changes, may cause embolization. Mural thrombosis may occur in a damaged or akinetic segment of the ventricle. A patent foramen ovale (PFO), which is a common variant, may occasionally allow passage of fragments of thrombus (e.g. from a lower limb deep vein thrombosis) from the right atrium to the left when Valsalva causes shunting of blood across the PFO. Pulmonary arteriovenous fistulas may also act as a conduit for paradoxical embolization. Rarer causes include fat emboli after long bone fracture, atrial myxomas and iatrogenic causes, such as cardiac bypass and air embolism. Simultaneous infarcts in different vascular territories are very suggestive of a proximal source of emboli in the heart or aorta.

Hypoperfusion. Severe hypotension, such as in cardiac arrest, may lead to border-zone infarction in the watershed areas between vascular territories, particularly if there is severe stenosis of proximal carotid vessels. The parieto-occipital area between the middle and posterior cerebral artery territories is particularly vulnerable.

Carotid and vertebral artery dissection

Dissection accounts for around 1 in 5 strokes below the age of 40 and is sometimes a sequel of trivial neck trauma or hyperextension: for example, after whiplash, osteopathic manipulation, hairwashing

Box 21.29 Factors reducing stroke risk

Risk factor	Action	Reduction in stroke risk		
		Infarction	*Haemorrhage*	*Relative risk reduction in secondary prevention*
Hypertension	Treatment and monitoring	++	++	28%
Smoking	Cessation	++	+	33%
Lifestyle	Greater activity	+	0	
Alcohol	Moderate intake	+	+	
High cholesterol	Statins, diet	+	0	24%
Atrial fibrillation	Anticoagulation	++	*Increases* risk slightly	67%
Obesity	Weight reduction	Probable	Probable	
Diabetes	Good control	+	0	
Severe carotid stenosis	Surgery	++	0	44%
Sleep apnoea	Treatment	+	0	

++, major correlation with reduced stroke risk; +, moderate correlation; SAH, subarachnoid haemorrhage.

in a salon or exercise. Subtle collagen disorders, such as partial forms of Marfan syndrome, may be a predisposing factor.

Most dissections are in large extracranial neck vessels. Blood penetrates the subintimal vessel wall, forming a false lumen, but it is thrombosis within the true lumen due to tissue thromboplastin release that leads to embolization from the site of dissection and stroke, sometimes days after the initial event.

Pain in the neck or face is often the clue leading to diagnosis. Horner syndrome or lower cranial nerve palsies may occur with carotid dissection, as these structures are intimately associated with the carotid artery in the neck.

Venous stroke

Only 1% of strokes are venous. Thrombosis within intracranial venous sinuses, such as the superior sagittal sinus, or in cortical veins, may occur in pregnancy, hypercoagulable states and thrombotic disorders, or with dehydration or malignancy. Cortical infarction, seizures and raised intracranial pressure result.

Haemorrhagic stroke

See page 838.

Transient ischaemic attacks

TIAs are usually the result of microemboli but different mechanisms produce similar clinical events. For example, TIAs may be caused by a fall in cerebral perfusion (e.g. a cardiac dysrhythmia, postural hypotension or decreased flow through atheromatous arteries). Infarction is usually averted by autoregulation. Rarely, tumours and subdural haematomas cause episodes that are indistinguishable from thromboembolic TIAs. Principal sources of emboli to the brain are cardiac thrombus and atheromatous plaques/thrombus within the aortic arch and carotid and vertebral systems. Cardiac thrombus often results from atrial fibrillation (which can be paroxysmal) or myocardial infarction. Cardiac valve disease may be a source of emboli: for example, calcific material or vegetations in infective endocarditis. Polycythaemia is also a cause.

Risk factors for stroke

The principal risk factors are those for atherosclerosis: age, smoking, dyslipidaemia, diabetes, obesity, inactivity and genetic/ethnic factors.

Hypertension is overall the most modifiable stroke risk factor in the population; stroke is decreasing in the 40–60 age group partly because hypertension is now more effectively identified and treated ***(Box 21.29)***. There is a linear relationship between blood pressure and stroke risk.

On an individual rather than population basis, anticoagulation for atrial fibrillation is the intervention resulting in the greatest stroke risk reduction.

Other risk factors and rarer causes of stroke

- Thrombocythaemia, polycythaemia and hyperviscosity states – thrombophilia (e.g. protein C deficiency, factor V Leiden) is weakly associated with arterial stroke but predisposes to cerebral venous thrombosis.
- Anti-cardiolipin and lupus anticoagulant antibodies (anti-phospholipid syndrome; see p. 695) predispose to arterial thrombotic strokes in young patients.
- Low-dose, oestrogen-containing oral contraceptives do not increase stroke risk significantly in healthy women but probably do so in combination with other risk factors, e.g. uncontrolled hypertension or smoking.
- Migraine is a rare cause of cerebral infarction.
- Vasculitis (systemic lupus erythematosus (SLE), polyarteritis, giant cell arteritis, granulomatous CNS angiitis) is a rare cause of stroke.
- Amyloidosis can present as recurrent cerebral haemorrhage (see p. 1288).
- Hyperhomocysteinaemia predisposes to thrombotic strokes. Folic acid therapy does not reduce the incidence.
- Neurosyphilis, mitochondrial disease, Fabry's disease (see pp. 1287–1288).
- Sympathomimetic drugs such as cocaine, and possibly over-the-counter cold remedies containing vasoconstrictors; neuroleptics in older patients.
- CADASIL (cerebral dominant arteriopathy with subcortical infarcts and leucoencephalopathy) is a rare inherited cause of stroke/vascular dementia.

Vascular anatomy

Knowledge of normal arterial anatomy and likely sites of atheromatous plaques and stenoses helps understanding of the main stroke syndromes.

The circle of Willis is supplied by the two internal carotid arteries (the anterior cerebral circulation) and by the vertebro-basilar posterior cerebral circulation. The distribution of the anterior, middle and posterior cerebral arteries that supply the cerebrum is shown in ***Figures 21.32*** and ***21.33*** (see also ***Figs 21.30*** and ***21.31***).

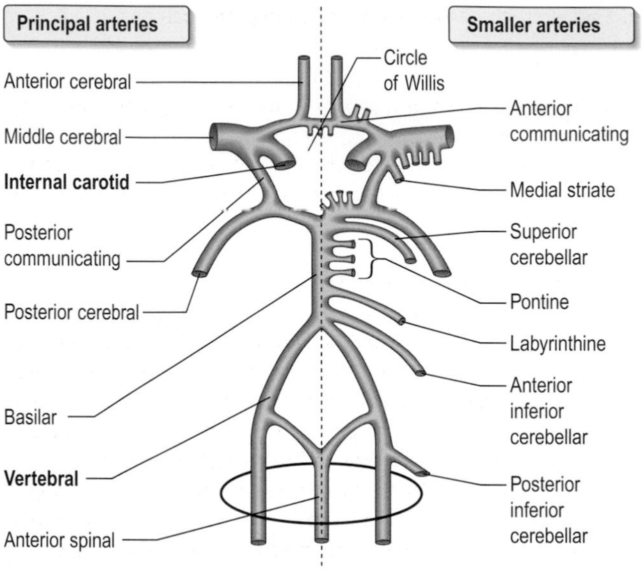

Figure 21.32 **Arteries supplying the brain and cord.**

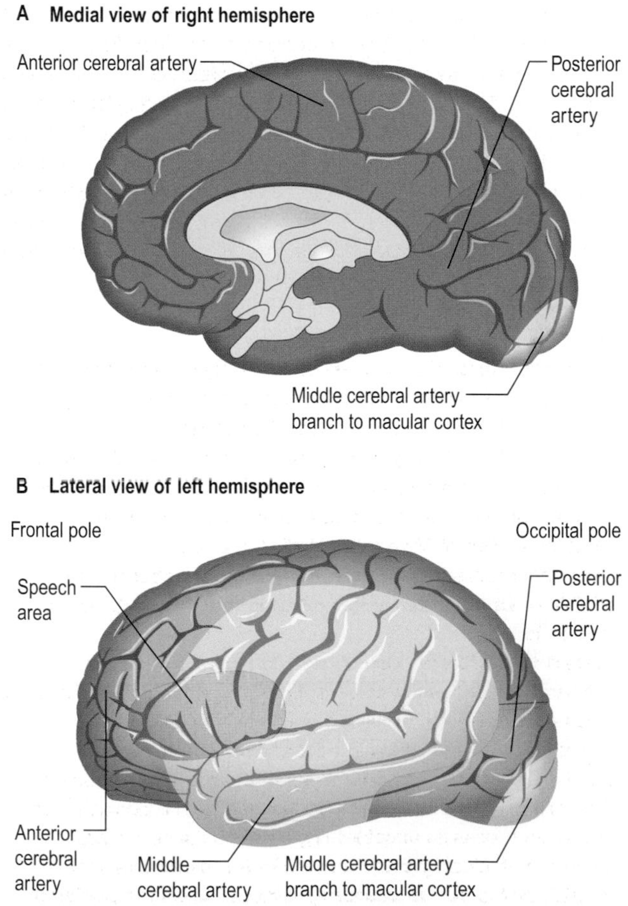

Figure 21.33 **The three major cerebral arteries. A.** Medial view of right hemisphere. **B.** Lateral view of left hemisphere.

Box 21.30 Features of transient ischaemic attacks

Anterior circulation	Posterior circulation
Carotid system	*Vertebrobasilar system*
• Amaurosis fugax	• Diplopia, vertigo, vomiting
• Aphasia	• Choking and dysarthria
• Hemiparesis	• Ataxia
• Hemisensory loss	• Hemisensory loss
• Hemianopic visual loss	• Hemianopic visual loss
	• Bilateral visual loss
	• Tetraparesis
	• Loss of consciousness (rare)
	• Transient global amnesia (possibly)

Clinical syndromes

Transient ischaemic attacks

Clinical features

TIAs cause sudden loss of function, usually lasting for minutes only, with complete recovery and no evidence of infarction on imaging. The previous classical definition of a duration of <24 hours is no longer used. Clinical features of the principal forms of TIA are given in ***Box 21.30***. Hemiparesis and aphasia are the most common.

Amaurosis fugax

This is a sudden transient loss of vision in one eye. When it is due to the passage of emboli through the retinal arteries, the embolus is sometimes visible through an ophthalmoscope during an attack (Hollenhorst plaque). A TIA causing an episode of amaurosis fugax is often the first clinical evidence of internal carotid artery (ICA) stenosis – a warning sign of incipient ICA territory stroke.

Diagnosis

Diagnosis of TIA is often based solely on its description. It is unusual to witness an attack, as it is so brief. Consciousness is usually preserved in TIA. There may be clinical evidence of a source of embolus, such as:

- carotid arterial bruit (stenosis)
- atrial fibrillation or other dysrhythmia
- valvular heart disease/endocarditis
- recent myocardial infarction.

An underlying condition may be evident:

- atheroma
- hypertension
- postural hypotension
- bradycardia or low cardiac output
- diabetes mellitus
- rarely, arteritis, polycythaemia, neurosyphilis, HIV
- antiphospholipid syndrome (see p. 695).

Differential diagnosis

TIAs can be distinguished, usually on clinical grounds, from other transient episodes (see p. 851). Occasionally, events identical to TIAs are produced by mass lesions. Focal epilepsy is usually recognized by its positive features (e.g. limb jerking and loss of consciousness) and progression over minutes. In a TIA, involuntary limb movements do occur occasionally – ***limb-shaking TIA*** – and are pathognomonic of severe carotid stenosis causing transient focal cerebral hypoperfusion. Cerebral amyloid angiopathy can cause TIA-like events; identification on imaging is necessary, as antiplatelet therapy is contraindicated.

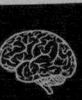

Migraine aura causing visual loss or dysphasia, particularly when it occurs without subsequent headache in elderly people, often causes diagnostic difficulty. Headache, common but not invariable in migraine, is rare in TIA. Positive visual phenomena such as shimmering, which are typical of migraine, are not seen in TIA. The onset and evolution of symptoms is usually slower with migraine aura than TIA (minutes rather than seconds). Limb weakness is rarely due to migraine.

Prognosis

Prospective studies show that 5 years after a single thromboembolic TIA:

- 30% have had a stroke, a third of these in the first year
- 15% have suffered a myocardial infarct.

TIAs in the anterior cerebral circulation carry a more serious prognosis than those in the posterior circulation (see ***Box 21.30***).

The ***ABCD² score (Box 21.31)*** can help to stratify stroke risk in the first 2 days. If patients are considered to have had a high-risk TIA – that is, ABCD² score of >4, or have had two recent TIAs, especially within the same vascular territory, then they should have urgent investigation and commencement of secondary prevention. *All* patients should be referred to a TIA clinic and ideally should be seen within 24 hours. Investigation and treatment should be regarded as urgent and completed within 2 weeks.

Investigations should include Doppler of the internal carotid arteries, cardiac echo, ECG and 24-hour tape, MRI brain and MR or CT angiography. Treat with medical therapy (see pp. 836–837) and surgery if appropriate (pp. 837–838). Surgery or stenting of high-grade symptomatic carotid stenosis should take place within 1 week of TIA (pp. 837–838).

Cerebral infarction

Major thromboembolic cerebral infarction usually causes an obvious stroke. The clinical picture is thus very variable, depending on the infarct site and extent.

Following vessel occlusion, brain ischaemia occurs, with electrical neuronal failure causing symptoms, followed by infarction and cell death. The infarcted region is surrounded by a swollen ischaemic area that does not function but is structurally intact. This is the ***ischaemic penumbra***, which is detected on MRI and can regain function following revascularization.

Within the ischaemic area, hypoxia leads to neuronal damage. There is a fall in ATP with release of glutamate, which opens calcium channels with release of free radicals. These alterations lead to inflammatory damage, necrosis and apoptotic cell death.

Clinical features

An acute onset (over minutes) of 'negative' symptoms indicating focal deficits in brain function, such as weakness, sensory loss, dysphasia and visual loss, are the characteristic defining features of ischaemic stroke. The exact clinical picture depends on the vascular territory affected.

Anterior circulation infarcts

This includes infarcts in the territory of the internal carotid, middle cerebral (MCA), anterior cerebral (ACA) and ophthalmic arteries. Complete MCA occlusion results in devastating stroke with contralateral hemiplegia and facial weakness, hemisensory loss and neglect syndromes (parietal lobe – severe if the non-dominant side is affected), eye deviation towards the affected side (frontal eye fields), aphasia (dominant hemisphere lesions) and hemianopia. Brain swelling of infarcted tissue leads to a high risk of death due to coning – ***malignant MCA infarction***. Decompressive craniectomy ***(Fig. 21.34)*** within the first 48 hours has been shown to reduce mortality and slightly improve the long-term severe disability.

A similar picture to MCA stroke is caused by ***internal carotid occlusion***, although collateral circulation may reduce the infarct size (see ***Fig. 21.31***). MCA branch occlusions produce fragments of the picture described above, such as hemiparesis, monoparesis and aphasia. Occlusion of lenticulostriate perforating arteries (or MCA occlusion with collateral circulation protecting the cortex) causes infarction of deep sub-cortical structures such as the internal capsule, resulting in hemiplegia and hemisensory deficits. ACA infarcts are significantly less common than MCA infarcts and typically produce hemiparesis affecting the leg more than arm, and frontal lobe deficits such as apathy or apraxia.

Posterior circulation infarcts

- ***Brainstem infarction*** causes complex signs, depending on the relationship of the infarct to cranial nerve nuclei, long tracts and brainstem connections ***(Box 21.32)***.
- ***The lateral medullary syndrome*** (Wallenberg syndrome) is a common brainstem vascular syndrome presenting as acute vertigo with cerebellar and other signs, including Horner syndrome (***Box 21.33*** and ***Fig. 21.35***). It follows thromboembolism in the posterior inferior cerebellar artery (PICA) or its branches, vertebral artery thromboembolism or dissection.
- ***Cerebellar infarcts*** occur in isolation or as part of a more extensive brainstem syndrome. Swelling of the cerebellum may cause brainstem compression and coma or obstructive hydrocephalus necessitating decompressive surgery.
- ***Basilar artery thrombosis*** is more common than embolism. The clinical picture depends on the level of the occlusion and the branch vessels affected. High lesions cause midbrain infarction, including coma and ***locked-in syndrome*** (see p. 828) or ***top of the basilar syndrome***, when the posterior cerebral artery (PCA) is also affected, causing devastating midbrain, occipital lobe and thalamic infarction.

Box 21.31 ABCD² score in the stratification of stroke risk

Parameter	Score
Age >60 years	1
BP >140 mmHg systolic and/or diastolic >90 mmHg	1
Clinical features	
Unilateral weakness	2
Isolated speech disturbance	1
Other	0
Duration of symptoms (min)	
>60	2
10–59	1
<10	0
Diabetes	
Present	1
Absent	1

A score of <4 is associated with a minimal risk whereas >6 is high-risk for a stroke within 7 days of a TIA.

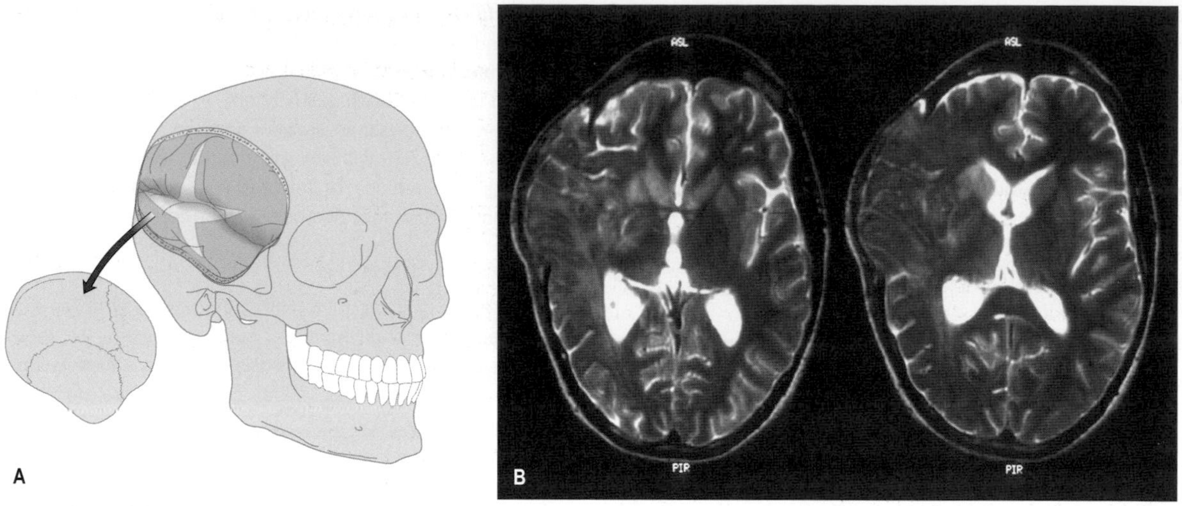

Figure 21.34 Decompressive craniectomy for stroke.

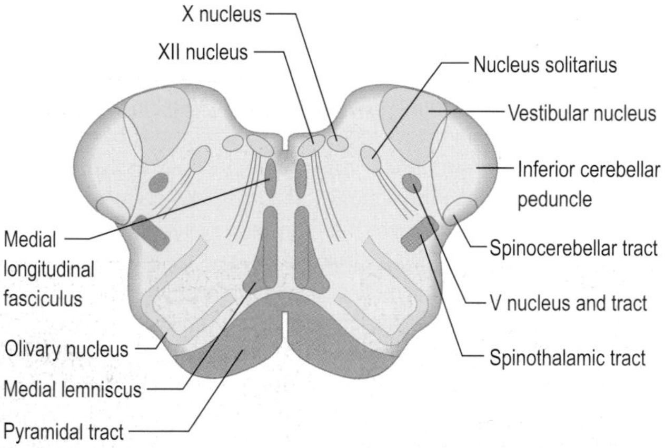

Figure 21.35 Medulla (cross-section). Structures at risk after brainstem infarction.

Box 21.32 Features of brainstem infarction

Clinical feature	Structure involved
Hemiparesis or tetraparesis	Corticospinal tracts
Sensory loss	Medial lemniscus and spinothalamic tracts
Diplopia	Oculomotor system
Facial numbness	Vth nerve nuclei
Facial weakness	VIIth nerve nucleus
Nystagmus, vertigo	Vestibular connections
Dysphagia, dysarthria	IXth and Xth nerve nuclei
Dysarthria, ataxia, hiccups, vomiting	Brainstem and cerebellar connections
Horner syndrome	Sympathetic fibres
Coma, altered consciousness	Reticular formation

Posterior cerebral artery infarcts are typically embolic. Homonymous hemianopia results from unilateral lesions, cortical blindness (***Anton syndrome***) from bilateral lesions (see ***Fig. 21.33*** and p. 804). Neglect syndromes and visual agnosias are associated with involvement of more anterior visual association areas. The PCA supplies the thalamus, and postero-medial temporal lobe and infarction of these structures causes confusion or memory impairment.

Box 21.33 Some clinical stroke syndromes

Vascular supply/ region affected	Neurological deficits
Left middle cerebral artery	Right-sided weakness involving face and arm > leg Dysphasia
Right middle cerebral artery	Left-sided weakness involving face and arm > leg Visual and/or sensory neglect Denial of disability
Lateral medulla (posterior inferior cerebellar artery or vertebral artery)	Ipsilateral Horner syndrome Xth nerve palsy Facial sensory loss Limb ataxia with contralateral spinothalamic sensory loss Vertigo Dysphagia
Posterior cerebral artery	Homonymous hemianopia Varied deficits due to thalamic, occipito-parietal and/or temporal lobe involvement
Internal capsule	Motor, sensory or sensorimotor loss Face = arm = leg Possible profound dysarthria from involvement of corticobulbar fibres No dysphasia or other cortical deficits
Bilateral paramedian thalamus and midbrain	Coma or reduced alertness Ophthalmoplegia Ataxia Memory impairment Thalamic pain
Carotid artery dissection	Neck/face pain Ipsilateral Horner syndrome from compression of sympathetic plexus around the carotid artery Lower cranial nerves (Xth and XIIth most clinically obvious) Embolic infarcts in anterior circulation territory

Lacunar infarction

Lacunes are small (<1.5 cm^3) infarcts seen on MRI or at postmortem. Hypertension is the major risk factor. Strokes without cortical features, such as pure motor stroke, pure sensory stroke, sudden unilateral ataxia and sudden dysarthria with a clumsy hand, are typical lacunar syndromes. Lacunar infarction is often symptomless.

Multi-infarct dementia (vascular dementia)

Multiple lacunes or larger infarcts cause generalized intellectual loss seen with advanced cerebrovascular disease. In the late stages, there is dementia (see pp. 874–879), pseudobulbar palsy and a shuffling gait – ***marche à petits pas*** (small steps), sometimes called atherosclerotic parkinsonism. ***Binswanger's disease*** is a term for widespread low attenuation in cerebral white matter, usually with dementia, TIAs and stroke episodes in hypertensive patients (the changes being seen on imaging/autopsy).

Watershed (border-zone) infarction

Severe cerebral hypoperfusion, such as hypotension after cardiac arrest or bypass surgery, causes ischaemia in the border zones between areas supplied by the anterior, middle and posterior cerebral arteries (affecting the occipito-parietal cortex, hippocampi and motor pathways). Complex patterns of visual loss (e.g. ***Balint syndrome***), memory loss, intellectual impairment and sometimes motor deficits are typical. A vegetative state or minimally conscious state may result from severe hypoxic–ischaemic encephalopathy after prolonged cerebral hypoperfusion (see p. 829).

Investigations in stroke

The purpose of investigations in stroke is to:

- confirm the clinical diagnosis, distinguish between haemorrhage and thromboembolic infarction, and exclude stroke mimics, e.g. tumour
- identify an underlying cause for the purposes of secondary prevention and identification of stroke mimics.

Investigations in thromboembolic stroke and TIA are listed in ***Box 21.34***.

Neuroimaging

- ***CT*** will demonstrate haemorrhage immediately but cerebral infarction is often not detected in the acute phase or only subtle changes are seen ***(Fig. 21.36A)***. Repeat CT at 24–48 h may be helpful.
- ***MRI*** is more sensitive than CT for early changes of infarction (diffusion-weighted sequences, DWI; ***Fig. 21.36B***) and for small infarcts ***(Fig. 21.37)***. MRI also clearly demonstrates the extent and anatomy of an infarct and shows evidence of clinically silent simultaneous infarcts that indicate an embolic cause. MRI can also help identify the underlying cause, e.g. arterial dissection using specific sequences to show the false lumen (***crescent sign***) or venous cortical infarcts. Many stroke mimics, such as demyelination, are shown with MRI but not CT. For these reasons, MRI is increasingly used in routine assessment of stroke and is essential in younger patients or in those where the cause is uncertain.
- ***Vascular imaging*** by carotid Doppler within 24 h is essential to identify high-grade symptomatic carotid stenosis requiring surgery. CT or MR angiography is now widely used to corroborate the results of Doppler, to identify arterial stenosis in the posterior circulation or intracranial vessels that are not visible on Doppler, and also to identify arterial dissection and venous sinus thrombosis. Catheter angiography is rarely needed following ischaemic stroke.

Box 21.34 Stroke investigations

Immediate urgent investigations

(Within 1 h if considering thrombolysis or patient is on anticoagulants or has reduced conscious level; otherwise within 24 h)

- CT brain scan
- Blood count and glucose (and clotting studies if anticoagulated)

Further investigations

(Within 24 h)

- Routine blood tests – blood count, erythrocyte sedimentation rate, glucose, clotting studies, lipids
- Electrocardiography (ECG) and later 24-h ECG for atrial fibrillation
- Carotid Doppler studies (in patients with anterior circulation stroke fit for surgery)

In addition

In selected patients, e.g. young stroke or no cause identified

- CT or MR angiography
- MRI brain scan with dissection protocol
- Echocardiogram (consider transoesophageal echocardiography)
- Prolonged cardiac monitoring for paroxysmal atrial fibrillation in cryptogenic stroke, e.g. implantable loop recorder
- Vasculitis screen
- Antiphospholipid antibodies
- Thrombophilia screen
- Other: genetics for CADASIL and mitochondrial disorders; alpha-galactosidase for Fabry's disease; drugs of abuse screen, e.g. cocaine

CADASIL, cerebral dominant arteriopathy with subcortical infarcts and leucoencephalopathy.

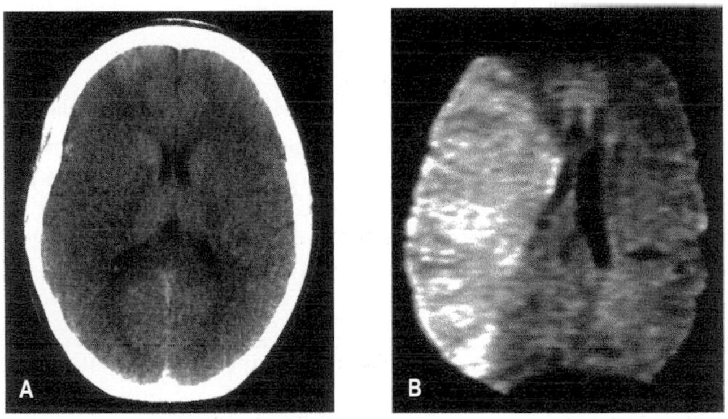

Figure 21.36 **Middle cerebral artery (MCA) infarction. A.** ***CT*** performed initially shows only very subtle low-density changes in the right MCA territory. **B. *Diffusion-weighted magnetic resonance imaging*** done at the same time shows the full extent of the area of ischaemia. *(Courtesy of Dr Paul Jarman.)*

Cardiac investigations

Identification of a cardioembolic source of stroke, principally atrial fibrillation, is achieved with electrocardiography (ECG) or 24-hour ECG. Other causes, such as valve disease, patent foramen ovale or mural thrombus, require transthoracic echocardiography, or transoesophageal echo in selected patients. Recent research has shown that prolonged cardiac monitoring (e.g. with an implantable loop recorder) demonstrates paroxysmal atrial fibrillation in a significant minority of people with stroke of unknown cause.

Other investigations

In young patients with stroke or in those individuals where there is no evidence of atherosclerosis or an embolic source, more specialist investigations may be required to look for an underlying

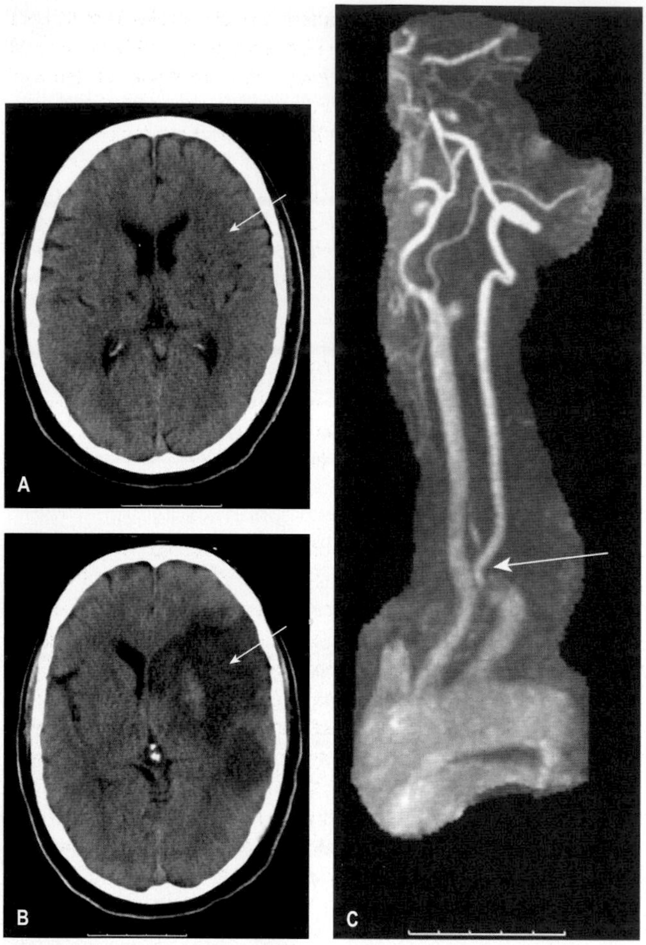

Figure 21.37 Magnetic resonance imaging of cerebral infarction and subsequent magnetic resonance angiography performed in the same patient. A. Early changes (arrowed). **B.** Changes after 5 days (arrowed). **C.** Magnetic resonance angiography showing internal carotid artery occlusion (arrowed). *(Courtesy of Dr Paul Jarman.)*

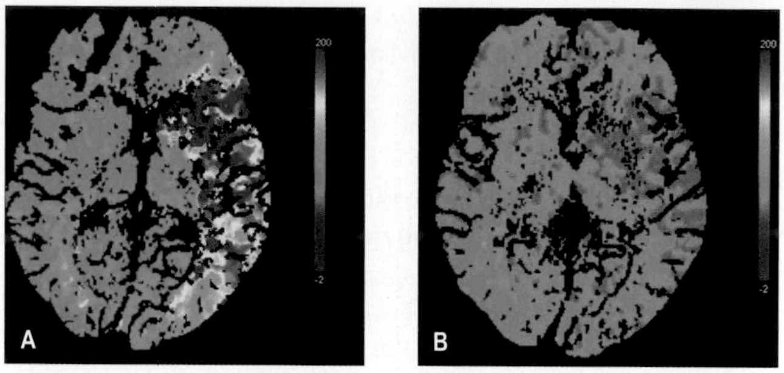

Figure 21.38 CT perfusion scans. A. Pre-thrombolysis; **B.** Post-thrombolysis showing reperfusion of the ischaemic site. *(Courtesy of Professor Adrian Dixon, Cambridge Radiology Department, UK.)*

vasculitic, inflammatory, infective, metabolic or genetic cause (see ***Box 21.34*** and p. 831).

Acute stroke: immediate care and thrombolysis

(See ***Box 21.35***.) Stroke is a medical emergency. Paramedics and members of the public are encouraged to make the diagnosis of stroke on a simple history and examination – ***FAST***:

- ***F***ace – sudden weakness of the face
- ***A***rm – sudden weakness of one or both arms
- ***S***peech – difficulty speaking, slurred speech
- ***T***ime – the sooner treatment can be started, the better.

During initial assessment, immediate, continued and meticulous attention to the airway, blood pressure and swallowing is essential. Management of unconscious or stuporose patients is outlined on page 826.

Box 21.35 Stroke management outline

1. Immediate general medical measures:
   - Airway: confirm patency and monitor
   - Continue care of the unconscious or stuporose patient
   - Give oxygen by mask
   - Monitor blood pressure
2. Is thrombolysis appropriate?
   - If so (see ***Box 21.36***), *immediate* brain imaging is essential
3. Brain imaging:
   - CT should always be available; this will indicate haemorrhage, other pathology and sometimes infarction
4. Cerebral infarction
   - If CT excludes haemorrhage, give immediate thrombolytic therapy. Give aspirin 300 mg/day if thrombolytic therapy is contraindicated
5. Cerebral haemorrhage:
   - If CT shows haemorrhage, give no drugs that could interfere with clotting; neurosurgery may occasionally be needed
6. Admit to multidisciplinary stroke unit:
   - Assess swallowing
   - Start thromboembolism prophylaxis
   - Treat medical complications, e.g. infection, hyperglycaemia, atrial fibrillation and so on
   - Investigate for cause and risk factors (see ***Box 21.34***)
   - Arrange early therapy input (physiotherapy, occupational therapy, speech and language therapy)
   - Initiate secondary prevention measures initiated
   - Give lifestyle advice – smoking cessation, weight reduction, diet and so on
7. Rehabilitation – specialized unit or community

Thrombolysis

Thrombolysis significantly increases the chances of having no disability or minimal disability after stroke, by reducing infarct size (***Figs 21.38*** and ***21.39***; ***Box 21.36***). Earlier treatment within the 4.5-hour time window significantly improves outcome, *so every minute counts*. Approximately 10% of patients are potential candidates for thrombolysis, most being excluded due to late presentation outside the time window for treatment. Two recent studies have shown benefit, with a low complication rate, from endovascular therapy (usually performed with retrievable stents) following alteplase therapy. In both studies, patients with proximal vessel occlusion and salvageable brain tissue were selected, with improved function and reduced mortality after treatment.

In a recent meta-analysis of five trials, endovascular thrombectomy has been shown to benefit most patients with an acute stroke caused by occlusion of the proximal anterior circulation. This treatment may become the accepted standard of care.

Antiplatelet therapy and anticoagulation

High-dose aspirin (300 mg) is started 24 hours after thrombolysis, or immediately haemorrhage is excluded if thrombolysis is contraindicated, and continued for 2 weeks before switching to clopidogrel. The number needed to treat (NNT) to prevent one stroke is 100.

Anticoagulants are started for atrial fibrillation-associated cardioembolic stroke only after 2 weeks to reduce the risk of acute haemorrhagic transformation of infarcts (NNT=12). However, for

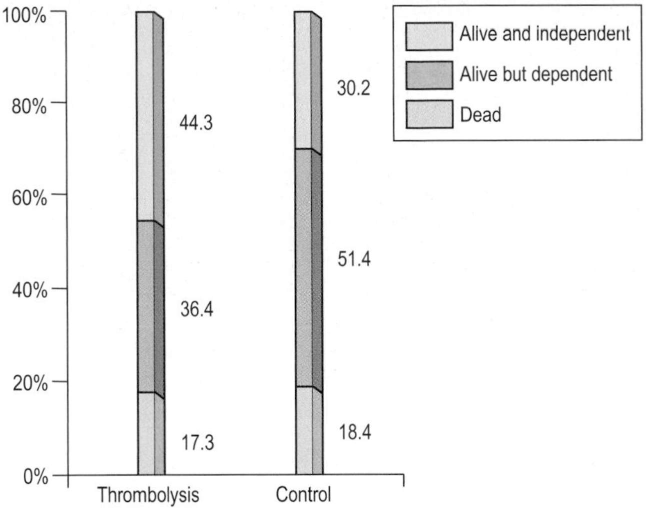

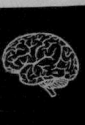

Figure 21.39 Risk of death, dependency and good functional outcome in randomized trials of tissue plasminogen activator rt-PA given within 3 hours of acute stroke. *(Data from Stroke Module,* Cochrane Database of Systematic Reviews. *Cochrane Collaboration issue 4, 1999.)*

Box 21.36 Thrombolysis in acute ischaemic stroke[a]

Eligibility
- Clinical diagnosis of acute ischaemic stroke
- Assessment by experienced team
- Persisting neurological deficit
- Imaging excludes haemorrhage
- Timing of onset well established
- Thrombolysis should commence as soon as possible and up to 4.5 h after acute stroke

Exclusion criteria

Historical
- Stroke or head trauma within the prior 3 months
- Any prior history of intracranial haemorrhage
- Major surgery within 14 days
- Gastrointestinal or genitourinary bleeding within the previous 21 days
- Arterial puncture at a non-compressible site within 7 days
- Lumbar puncture within 7 days

Clinical
- Rapidly improving stroke syndrome
- Minor and isolated neurological signs
- Seizure at the onset of stroke if the residual impairments are due to post-ictal phenomena
- Symptoms suggestive of subarachnoid haemorrhage, even if the CT is normal
- Persistent systolic blood pressure (BP) >185, diastolic BP >110 mmHg, or requiring aggressive therapy to control BP
- Pregnancy
- Active bleeding or acute trauma (fracture)

Laboratory
- Platelets <100 000/mm^3
- Serum glucose <2.8 mmol/L or >22.2 mmol/L
- International Normalized Ratio (INR) >1.7 if on warfarin
- Elevated partial thromboplastin time if on heparin

Dose of i.v. alteplase (tissue plasminogen activator)
- Total dose 0.9 mg/kg (max. 90 mg)
- 10% of total dose by initial i.v. bolus over 1 min
- Remainder infused intravenously over 60 min

[a]*See* ***Figure 21.38***.

arterial dissection, the risk of recurrent embolic stroke from the site of dissection is considered to be high enough to justify immediate anticoagulation, although controlled trial evidence is lacking. Venous sinus or cortical vein thrombosis causing stroke is also treated with anticoagulation. In addition to warfarin for oral anticoagulation, other oral anticoagulants (OACs; see p. 972) that inhibit factor Xa or thrombin are now available. They have the advantage over warfarin of a wider therapeutic index with a lower rate of haemorrhage, no need for monitoring and few drug interactions. Idarucizumab has FDA approval for intravenous use, fully reversing dabigatran in 4 hours.

Decompressive craniectomy

This should be performed within 48 hours in MCA strokes causing infarction of more than 50% of the MCA territory to prevent coning and improve long-term outcome (see p. 833).

Stroke units

Direct admission to a stroke unit has been demonstrated to be one of the most effective interventions in acute stroke, saving lives and reducing long-term disability. Specialized multidisciplinary teams and clear protocols for aspects of care, such as swallowing assessment, thromboembolism prevention, treatment of infections, management of hyperglycaemia and other medical complications, improve quality and consistency of care, and thus outcomes. Early mobilization and access to physiotherapy, occupational therapy and speech therapy, as well as initiation of secondary prevention and patient education, are equally necessary. Early supported discharge and assessment of rehabilitation needs are also better coordinated on a stroke unit than a general ward.

Secondary prevention interventions

Antihypertensive therapy

Recognition and good control of high blood pressure are the major factors in primary and secondary stroke prevention. Transient hypertension, often seen following stroke, usually does not require treatment, provided diastolic pressure does not rise above 100 mmHg. Sustained severe hypertension needs treatment after 72 hours (see p. 1048); blood pressure should be lowered slowly to avoid any sudden fall in perfusion.

Lipid-lowering therapy

Statins, typically simvastatin 40 mg, should be offered to all patients unless there is a contraindication, aiming for a target total cholesterol <4 mmol/L (low-density lipoprotein <2 mmol/L).

Lifestyle modification and education

Education of patient and family is an essential aspect of secondary prevention. Smoking cessation and advice about diet, exercise, weight reduction and alcohol consumption should be started on the stroke unit and continued after discharge.

Surgery and stenting for carotid stenosis

High grade symptomatic carotid stenosis is associated with a significant risk of recurrent stroke during the weeks after TIA or stroke. Carotid endarterectomy should be performed within 2 weeks in patients with 70–99% stenosis on the affected side, provided the initial stroke was not severely disabling. A second imaging modality, such as CT angiography, should be performed to confirm the results of Doppler studies. For patients with moderate symptomatic stenosis (50–69%), there is a modest benefit with intervention over the 3% stroke risk associated with the procedure itself. Carotid stenting is an alternative to surgery in some patients (major stroke risk is the same for surgery and stenting but the chance of minor non-disabling stroke is higher for stenting).

The case for intervention in asymptomatic stenosis is debatable. Patients with 70–99% stenosis may have a modest stroke risk reduction at 5 years, but moderate stenosis should be treated conservatively. Screening asymptomatic individuals for carotid stenosis is not helpful. Carotid occlusion is always treated conservatively (there is no risk of distal embolization).

Stroke in the elderly

Thrombolysis is not contraindicated. Age is no barrier to recovery; elderly patients benefit from good rehabilitation. Consider social isolation, pre-existing cognitive impairment, nutrition, and skin and sphincter care, and reassess swallowing. Carotid endarterectomy over 75 years of age confers greater risk reduction than in younger patients.

Rehabilitation: multidisciplinary approach

Physiotherapy has particular value in the first few weeks after stroke to relieve spasticity, prevent contractures and teach patients to use walking aids. The benefits of physiotherapy for longer-term outcome are still inadequately researched. Baclofen and/or botulinum toxin are sometimes helpful in the management of severe spasticity.

Speech and language therapists have a vital understanding of aphasic patients' problems and frustration. Return of speech is hastened by conversation generally. If swallowing is unsafe because of the risk of aspiration, either nasogastric feeding or percutaneous gastrostomy will be needed. Video-fluoroscopy while attempting to swallow is helpful.

Physiotherapy, occupational and speech therapy have a vital role in assessing and facilitating the future care pathway. Stroke is frequently devastating and, particularly during working life, radically alters the patient's remaining years. Many become unemployable, lose independence and are financially embarrassed. Loss of self-esteem makes depression common.

At home, aids and alterations may be needed: stair and bath rails, portable lavatories, hoists, sliding boards, wheelchairs, tripods, stair lifts, electric blinds and modified sleeping arrangements, kitchen, steps, flooring and doorways. Liaison between hospital-based and community care teams, and primary care physician, is essential.

Prognosis

About 25% of patients die within 2 years of a stroke, nearly 10% within the first month ***(Fig. 21.39)***. This early mortality is higher following intracranial haemorrhage than ischaemic stroke. Poor outcome is likely when there is coma, a defect in conjugate gaze and hemiplegia. Many complications, such as aspiration or pressure ulcers, are preventable, particularly in the elderly. Coordinated care reduces deaths.

Recurrent strokes are, however, common (10% in the first year) and many patients die subsequently from myocardial infarction. Of initial stroke survivors, some 30–40% remain alive at 3 years.

Gradual improvement usually follows stroke, with recovery plateauing after 12 months. One-third of survivors return to independent mobility and one-third have disability requiring institutional care.

Further reading

Bonati LH, Dobson J, Featherstone RL et al. Long-term outcomes after stenting versus endarterectomy for treatment of symptomatic carotid stenosis: the International Carotid Stenting Study (ICSS) randomised trial. *Lancet* 2015; 385:529–538.
Campbell BCV. Endovascular therapy for ischaemic stroke with perfusion imaging selection. *N Engl J Med* 2015; 372:1009–1018.
Furlan AJ. Endovascular therapy for stroke – it's about time. *N Engl J Med* 2015; 372:2347–2349.
Goyal M, Demchuk AM, Menon BK et al. Randomised assessment of rapid endovascular treatment of ischaemic stroke. *N Engl J Med* 2015; 372:1019–1030.
Goyal M, Menon BK, van Zwam WH et al. Endovascular thrombectomy of large vessel ischaemic stroke: a meta-analysis of individual patient data from five randomised trials. *Lancet* 2016; 387:1723–31.
IST-3 Collaborative Group. The benefits and harms of intravenous thrombolysis with recombinant tissue plasminogen activator within 6 h of acute ischaemic stroke (the third International Stroke Trial [IST-3]): a randomised controlled trial. *Lancet* 2012; 379:2352–2363.
Jüttler E, Unterberg A, Woitzik J et al. Hemicraniectomy in older patients with extensive middle-cerebral-artery stroke. *N Engl J Med* 2014; 370:1091–1100.
Langhorne P, Bernhardt J, Kwakkel G. Stroke rehabilitation. *Lancet* 2011; 377:1693–1702.
Qureshi AI, Caplan LR. Intracranial atherosclerosis. *Lancet* 2014; 383:984–998.
Rothwell PM, Algra A, Amarenco P. Medical treatment in acute and long-term secondary prevention after transient ischaemic attack and ischaemic stroke. *Lancet* 2011; 377:1681–1692.
Wechsler LR. Intravenous thrombolytic therapy for acute ischemic stroke. *N Engl J Med* 2011; 364:2138–2146.

Intracranial haemorrhage

This comprises:

- intracerebral and cerebellar haemorrhage
- subarachnoid haemorrhage
- subdural and extradural haemorrhage/haematoma.

Intracerebral haemorrhage

Aetiology

Intracerebral haemorrhage causes approximately 10% of strokes. It is associated with a higher mortality than ischaemic stroke (up to 50%). A large haematoma may act as a space-occupying lesion, causing raised intracranial pressure with brain displacement and herniation.

- ***Hypertensive***. Rupture of microaneurysms (Charcot–Bouchard aneurysms, 0.8–1.0 mm in diameter) and degeneration of small, deep, penetrating arteries are the principal pathologies. Such haemorrhage is usually massive, often fatal, and occurs in chronic hypertension and at well-defined sites: basal ganglia, pons, cerebellum and sub-cortical white matter. Vasopressor drugs, such as cocaine, may cause haemorrhage. Alcohol is also a risk factor (probably as a result of impaired coagulation/platelet function).
- ***Cerebral amyloid angiopathy*** (***CAA***). Deposition of amyloid-β in the walls of small and medium-sized arteries in normotensive patients, particularly over 60 years, causes *lobar* intracerebral haemorrhage (especially posterior, i.e. occipital/parietal lobes), which is often recurrent. CAA is associated with particular apolipoprotein E genotypes (E2) and is more common in patients with Alzheimer's disease. Cerebral microbleeds are usually seen on MRI sequences sensitive to haemosiderin deposition. CAA may occasionally cause TIA-like, transient neurological symptoms.
- ***Secondary***. Arteriovenous malformations, cavernomas, aneurysms and dural venous thrombosis cause around 20% of intracerebral haemorrhages. Coagulopathies, anticoagulants and thrombolysis may cause haemorrhage. Haemorrhagic transformation of a large ischaemic infarct may sometimes present as a haemorrhage.

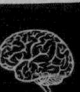

Clinical features and investigations

At the bedside, there is no entirely reliable way of distinguishing between haemorrhage and ischaemic infarcts. Intracerebral haemorrhage is more often associated with severe headache or coma. Patients on oral anticoagulants should be assumed to have had a haemorrhage unless it is proved otherwise.

Brain haemorrhage is seen on CT imaging immediately (compare infarction; see pp. 821–822) as intraparenchymal, intraventricular or subarachnoid blood. Routine MRI may not identify an acute small haemorrhage reliably in the first few hours. MRI and MR angiography are necessary to identify underlying vascular malformations such as AVMs or aneurysms. Catheter angiography may be required in selected patients with no obvious risk factors or no underlying cause identified on imaging.

Management of haemorrhagic stroke

Medical

Treatment should be on a stroke unit or a neuroscience intensive care unit. Frequent monitoring of GCS and neurological signs is essential, as neurosurgery may be required. Antiplatelet drugs are, of course, contraindicated. Anticoagulation should be rapidly reversed where possible (for patients on warfarin give intravenous vitamin K and clotting factor concentrates). Control of hypertension is vital with intravenous drugs in an intensive care unit setting for systolic blood pressure >160–180 mmHg. Measures to reduce intracranial pressure may be required, including mechanical ventilation and mannitol. Recombinant activated factor VII administration may prevent haematoma expansion but has not yet been shown to improve outcome.

Surgical

Cerebellar haematomas may cause obstructive hydrocephalus or coma due to brainstem compression; urgent neurosurgical clot evacuation is life-saving (and is required where the haematoma is >3 cm or the patient is drowsy or deteriorating). The role of surgical decompression for non-cerebellar bleeds is less clear-cut and liaison with neurosurgeons is vital. Use of minimally invasive surgical techniques to evacuate haematomas is an area of active research. Placement of an external ventricular drain is needed if obstructive hydrocephalus develops: for example, with extension of the haemorrhage into the ventricular system.

Subarachnoid haemorrhage

Subarachnoid haemorrhage (SAH) means spontaneous arterial bleeding into the subarachnoid space, and is usually clearly recognizable clinically from its dramatic onset. SAH accounts for some 5% of strokes and has an annual incidence of 6 per 100 000.

Aetiology

The causes of SAH are shown in ***Box 21.37***; it is unusual to find any contributing disease.

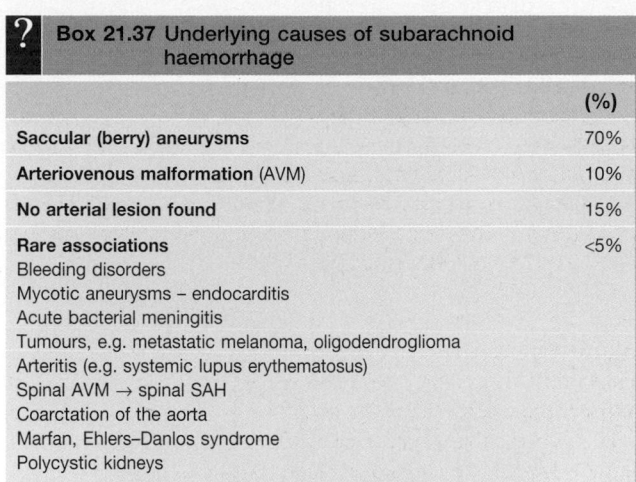

Box 21.37 Underlying causes of subarachnoid haemorrhage

	(%)
Saccular (berry) aneurysms	70%
Arteriovenous malformation (AVM)	10%
No arterial lesion found	15%
Rare associations	<5%
Bleeding disorders	
Mycotic aneurysms – endocarditis	
Acute bacterial meningitis	
Tumours, e.g. metastatic melanoma, oligodendroglioma	
Arteritis (e.g. systemic lupus erythematosus)	
Spinal AVM → spinal SAH	
Coarctation of the aorta	
Marfan, Ehlers–Danlos syndrome	
Polycystic kidneys	

Saccular (berry) aneurysms

Saccular aneurysms ***(Fig. 21.40)*** develop within the circle of Willis and adjacent arteries. Common sites are at arterial junctions:

- between posterior communicating and internal carotid artery – posterior communicating artery aneurysm
- between anterior communicating and anterior cerebral artery – anterior communicating and anterior cerebral artery aneurysm

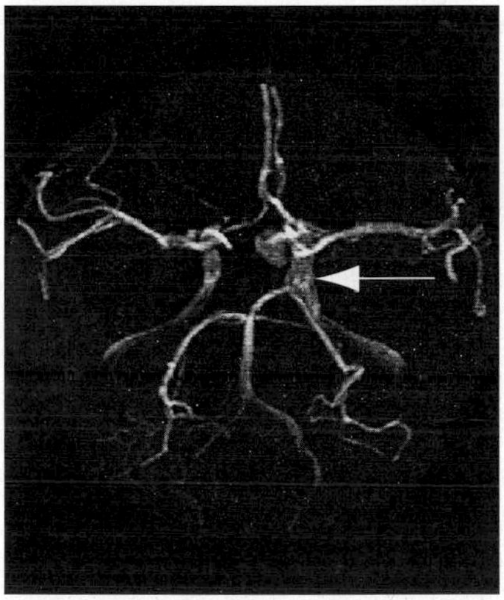

Figure 21.40 Digital subtraction angiogram: posterior communicating artery aneurysm.

- at the trifurcation or a bifurcation of the middle cerebral artery – middle cerebral artery aneurysm.

Other aneurysm sites are on the basilar, posterior inferior cerebellar, intracavernous internal carotid and ophthalmic arteries. Saccular aneurysms are an incidental finding in 1% of autopsies and can be multiple.

Aneurysms cause symptoms either by spontaneous rupture, when there is usually no preceding history, or by direct pressure on surrounding structures; for example, an enlarging unruptured posterior communicating artery aneurysm is the most common cause of a painful IIIrd nerve palsy (see p. 806).

Arteriovenous malformation

Arteriovenous malformation (AVM) is a vascular developmental malformation, often with a fistula between arterial and venous systems, causing high flow through the AVM and high-pressure arterialization of draining veins. An AVM usually presents following a spontaneous intracerebral haemorrhage or with a seizure, often focal in onset. The risk of a first haemorrhage in unruptured AVMs (20% fatal and 30% resulting in permanent disability) is approximately 2–3% per year. Once an AVM has caused a haemorrhage, the risk of rebleeds is increased to approximately 10% per year. AVMs may be ablated with endovascular treatment (catheter injection of glue into the

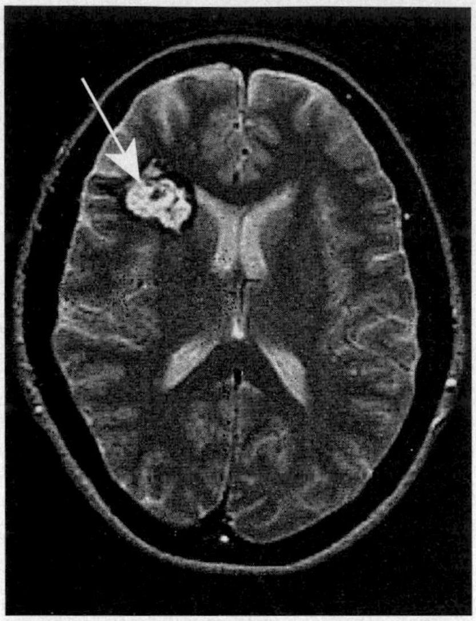

Figure 21.41 Magnetic resonance T2-weighted image: symptomless frontal cavernoma (arrowed).

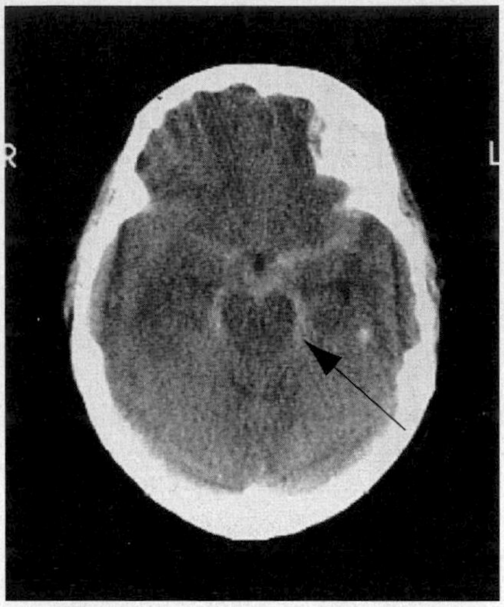

Figure 21.42 Subarachnoid haemorrhage CT showing blood around the brainstem (arrowed).

nidus, usually), microsurgery or stereotactic radiotherapy. A multidisciplinary team approach with neurologist, interventional neuroradiologist and neurosurgeon is required in deciding on treatment options. There is no clear consensus on the best treatment modality or, indeed, whether the considerable risk of intervention is lower than with a conservative approach.

Cavernous haemangiomas (cavernomas) are common (0.1–0.5% prevalence) and consist of a tangle of low-pressure dilated vessels without a major feeding artery; they are frequently symptomless ***(Fig. 21.41)*** and seen incidentally on imaging. Multiple cavernomas often have a genetic basis. Cavernomas may cause seizures. Small haemorrhages may occur but are usually low-pressure bleeds and rarely cause severe deficits. Surgical resection is rarely needed, except where the cavernoma is gradually enlarging or causing significant neurological symptoms.

Clinical features of subarachnoid haemorrhage

There is a sudden, very severe headache, often occipital (mean time to peak headache 3 min). Headache is usually followed by vomiting and often by coma and death. Survivors of SAH may remain comatose or drowsy for hours, days or longer. SAH is a *possible* diagnosis in any sudden headache.

Following major SAH, there is neck stiffness and a positive Kernig's sign. Papilloedema is sometimes present, with retinal and/or subhyaloid haemorrhage (tracking beneath the retinal hyaloid membrane). Minor bleeds cause few signs but almost invariably do cause headache (approximately 17% of patients have small 'sentinel bleeds' in the weeks before presenting with SAH).

Investigations

CT imaging is the immediate investigation ***(Fig. 21.42)***. Subarachnoid and/or intraventricular blood is usually seen (sensitivity of CT to detect subarachnoid blood is 95% within 24 hours of onset but much lower over subsequent days). Lumbar puncture is not necessary if SAH is confirmed by CT, but should be performed if doubt remains. CSF becomes yellow (xanthochromic) within 12 hours of SAH and remains detectable for 2 weeks. Visual inspection of supernatant CSF is usually sufficiently reliable for diagnosis. Spectrophotometry to estimate bilirubin in the CSF released from lysed cells is used to define SAH with certainty. CT angiography or catheter angiography to identify the aneurysm or other source of bleeding is performed in patients potentially fit for surgery. In some, no aneurysm or source of bleeding is found, despite a definite SAH.

Differential diagnosis

SAH must be differentiated from migraine. This is sometimes difficult but a short time to maximal headache intensity and the presence of neck stiffness usually indicate SAH. ***Thunderclap headache*** is used (confusingly) to describe either SAH or a sudden (benign) headache for which no cause is ever found. The syndrome of reversible cerebral vasoconstriction (Call–Fleming syndrome) presents with thunderclap headache. Acute bacterial meningitis occasionally causes a very abrupt headache, when a meningeal microabscess ruptures; SAH also occasionally occurs at the onset of acute bacterial meningitis. Cervical arterial dissection can present with a sudden headache.

Complications

Blood in the subarachnoid space can lead to obstructive hydrocephalus, seen on CT. Hydrocephalus can be asymptomatic but may cause deteriorating consciousness following SAH. Shunting may be necessary. Arterial spasm (visible on angiography and a cause of coma or hemiparesis) is a serious complication of SAH and a poor prognostic feature.

Management

Immediate treatment of SAH involves bed rest and supportive measures. Hypertension should be controlled. Nimodipine, a calcium-channel blocker given for 3 weeks, reduces mortality.

All SAH cases should be discussed urgently with a neurosurgical centre. Nearly half of SAH cases are either dead or moribund before reaching hospital. Of the remainder, a further 10–20% rebleed and die within weeks. Failure to diagnose SAH – for example, mistaking SAH for migraine – contributes to this mortality.

Where angiography demonstrates an aneurysm (the cause of the vast majority of SAHs), endovascular treatment by placing platinum coils via a catheter in the aneurysm sac, to promote thrombosis and ablation of the aneurysm, is now the first-line treatment.

Endovascular coiling has a lower complication rate than surgery but direct surgical clipping of the aneurysm neck is still required in some selected cases. For asymptomatic (unruptured) aneurysms over 8 mm in diameter, the risk of treatment is less than the risk of haemorrhage if not treated. Patients who remain comatose or who have persistent severe deficits after SAH have a poor outlook.

Subdural and extradural bleeding

These conditions can cause death following head injuries unless treated promptly.

Subdural haematoma

Subdural haematoma (SDH) means accumulation of blood in the subdural space following rupture of a vein. This usually follows a head injury, sometimes a trivial one. The interval between injury and symptoms can be days, or may extend to weeks or months. Chronic, apparently spontaneous, SDH is common in the elderly, and also occurs with anticoagulants.

Headache, drowsiness and confusion are common; symptoms are indolent and can fluctuate. Focal deficits, such as hemiparesis or sensory loss, develop. Epilepsy occasionally occurs. Stupor, coma and coning may follow.

Extradural haemorrhage

Extradural haemorrhage (EDH) typically follows a linear skull vault fracture tearing a branch of the middle meningeal artery. Extradural blood accumulates rapidly over minutes or hours. A characteristic picture is that of a head injury with a brief duration of unconsciousness, followed by improvement (the lucid interval). The patient then becomes stuporose; there is an ipsilateral dilated pupil and contralateral hemiparesis, with rapid transtentorial coning. Bilateral fixed, dilated pupils, tetraplegia and respiratory arrest follow. An acute progressive SDH presents similarly.

Management

Possible extradural or subdural bleeding needs immediate imaging. CT ***(Fig. 21.43A)*** is the most widely used investigation because of its immediate availability. MRI is more sensitive for the detection of small haematomas. T1-weighted MRI ***(Fig. 21.43B)*** shows bright images due to the presence of methaemoglobin.

EDHs *require urgent neurosurgery*; if it is performed early, the outlook is excellent. When the patient is far from a neurosurgeon, such as in wartime or at sea, drainage through skull burr-holes has been life-saving when an EDH has been diagnosed clinically.

Subdural bleeding usually needs less immediate attention but close neurosurgical liaison is necessary. Even large collections can resolve spontaneously without drainage. Serial imaging is required to assess progress.

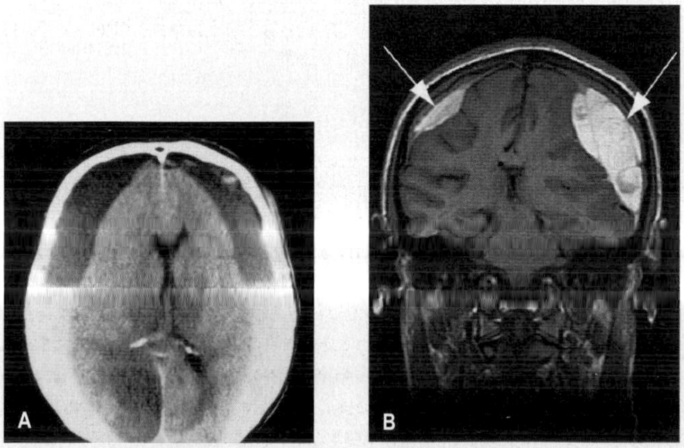

Figure 21.43 Bilateral subdural haematomas. A. CT scan. **B.** Magnetic resonance T1-weighted image.

Cortical venous thrombosis and dural venous sinus thrombosis

Intracranial venous thromboses are usually (>50%) associated with a pro-thrombotic risk factor, such as oral contraceptives, pregnancy, genetic or acquired pro-thrombotic states, and dehydration. Head injury is also a cause. Infection, such as from a paranasal sinus, may be present. Venous thromboses can also arise spontaneously.

Cortical venous thrombosis

The venous infarct leads to headache, focal signs (e.g. hemiparesis) and/or seizures. Cortical haemorrhagic infarction is shown on MRI.

Dural venous sinus thromboses

Cavernous sinus thrombosis causes eye pain, fever, proptosis and chemosis. External and internal ophthalmoplegia with papilloedema develops.

Thrombosis of the dural venous sinuses, such as when the sagittal sinus causes raised intracranial pressure with headache, papilloedema and frequently seizures, may progress to coma.

Management

MRI and MR venography (MRV) show occluded sinuses and/or veins. Treatment is with heparin initially, followed by warfarin or other oral anticoagulants for 6 months. Anticonvulsants are given if necessary.

Further reading

Knopman J, Stieg PE. Management of unruptured brain arteriovenous malformations. *Lancet* 2014; 383:581–583.

Molyneaux AJ, Birks J, Clarke A et al. The durability of endovascular coiling versus neurosurgical clipping of ruptured cerebral aneurysms: 18-year follow-up. *Lancet* 2015; 385:691–697.

Mendelow AD, Gregson BA, Rowan EN et al; STICH II Investigators. Early surgery versus initial conservative treatment in patients with spontaneous supratentorial lobar intracerebral haematomas (STICH II): a randomised trial. *Lancet* 2013; 382:397–408.

http://www.bestpractice.bmj.com *BMJ best practice guidelines for haemorrhagic stroke.*

HEADACHE, MIGRAINE AND FACIAL PAIN

Headache is an almost universal experience and one of the most common symptoms in medical practice. It varies from an infrequent and trivial nuisance to a pointer to serious disease. Headache symptoms are unpleasant, disabling and common worldwide, and have a substantial economic impact because of time lost from work.

Mechanisms

Pain receptors are located at the base of the brain in arteries and veins, and throughout meninges, extracranial vessels, scalp, neck and facial muscles, paranasal sinuses, eyes and teeth. Curiously, brain substance is almost devoid of pain receptors. Head pain is mediated by the Vth and IXth cranial nerves and upper cervical sensory roots.

Box 21.38 Some causes of secondary headache

- Raised intracranial pressure, e.g. idiopathic intracranial hypertension
- Infections, e.g. meningitis, sinusitis
- Giant cell arteritis
- Intracranial haemorrhage, esp. subarachnoid haemorrhage or subdural haematoma
- Low cerebrospinal fluid volume (low-pressure) headache
- Post-traumatic headache
- Cervicogenic headache
- Acute glaucoma

A clinical approach to the patient with headache

In assessing patients with headache, the aim should be to make a confident diagnosis based on the history. Examination is helpful in excluding underlying medical disorders as a cause of headache but will not distinguish between different types of primary headache.

There is an internationally agreed classification for headaches that defines all headache patterns. Headache is divided into primary headache disorders such as migraine, and secondary headaches due to underlying pathology such as raised intracranial pressure or meningitis ***(Box 21.38)***. It is also useful to distinguish between episodic (recurrent) headache, single first headache episodes and patients with chronic headache.

In an outpatient clinic setting, most headaches will be benign. Fewer than 1% of outpatients with non-acute headache have a serious underlying cause but in the Emergency Department there will be a much higher prevalence of serious underlying pathology presenting with headache. New-onset severe headache in those without a previous headache history, especially in older patients (>50), requires exclusion of underlying pathology causing secondary headache.

There are some widely believed 'headache myths'. Headaches are not caused by hypertension, except rarely with malignant hypertension (see p. 1048). Eye strain from refractive error does not cause headache and sinusitis is rarely the explanation for recurrent or chronic headache.

Taking a history for 'headaches'

Ask about:

- Headache location (e.g. hemicranial), severity and character (e.g. throbbing versus non-throbbing).
- Associated symptoms, e.g. nausea, photophonia, phonophobia and motion sensitivity.
- Presence of autonomic symptoms, e.g. tearing or ptosis.
- Relieving or exacerbating features, e.g. effect of posture.
- Headache pattern: Is headache episodic and part of a pattern of previous similar headaches? Age at onset and headache frequency.
- Duration of headache episodes (helpful in distinguishing between different primary headache types).
- Triggers.
- Pattern of analgesic use.
- Family history of headache.
- 'Red flag' symptoms: fever (meningitis, sinusitis).
- Sudden onset in less than 1 minute (SAH).
- Features of raised intracranial pressure.
- Jaw claudication (giant cell arteritis).

Examination

Examination should include fundoscopy to look for papilloedema. In older patients, temporal arteries should be palpated for loss of pulsatility and tenderness that may be features of giant cell arteritis (GCA). Fever and neck stiffness suggest meningitis. Examination is generally normal in patients with primary headache disorders.

Investigations

Investigations, including brain imaging, do not contribute to the diagnosis of primary headache disorders. Neuroimaging is indicated only where history or examination suggests an underlying secondary cause. Older patients with new-onset headache and those with 'red flag' symptoms should have brain CT. In patients over 50 with new headache, the ESR should be checked to exclude GCA.

Primary headache disorders

Migraine

Migraine is the most common cause of episodic headache (15–20% of women and 5–10% of men); in 90%, onset is before 40 years of age. Episodes of headache are associated with sensory sensitivity such as to light, sound or movement, and sometimes with nausea and vomiting. There is a spectrum of severity between individuals and from one attack to another. Migraine is usually high-impact, with inability to function normally during episodes. Headache frequency in migraine varies from an occasional inconvenience to frequent headaches severely impacting on quality of life, and may transform into chronic daily headache.

Mechanisms

Genetic factors play a part in causing the neuronal hyper-excitability that is probably the biological basis of migraine. Migraine is polygenic but a rare form of familial migraine is associated with mutations in the α-1 subunit of the P/Q-type voltage-gated calcium channel or neuronal sodium channel (*SCN1A*), and a dominant loss-of-function mutation in a potassium channel gene (*TRESK*) has been identified in some patients with migraine with aura.

The pathophysiology of migraine is now thought to have a primarily neurogenic rather than vascular basis. Spreading cortical depression – a wave of neuronal depolarization followed by depressed activity slowly spreading anteriorly across the cerebral cortex from the occipital region – is thought to be the basis of the migraine aura. Activation of trigeminal pain neurones is the basis of the headache. The innervation of the large intracranial vessels and dura by the first division of the trigeminal nerve is known as the trigeminovascular system. Release of calcitonin gene-related peptide (CGRP), substance P and other vasoactive peptides, including 5-HT, by activated trigeminovascular neurones causes painful meningeal inflammation and vasodilatation. Peripheral and central sensitization of trigeminal neurones and brainstem pain pathways makes otherwise innocuous sensory stimuli (such as CSF pulsation and head movement) painful, and light and sound are perceived as uncomfortable.

Clinical features

Migraine without aura

Migraine typically starts around puberty with increasing prevalence into the fourth decade. There is a spectrum of severity and associated features, but attacks have recognizable core features ***(Box 21.39)***. Most migraine attacks are usually of sufficient severity to

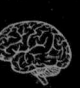

> **Box 21.39 Migraine: simplified diagnostic criteria**
>
> Headache lasting 4 hours to 3 days (untreated)
>
> **At least two of:**
> - Unilateral pain (may become holocranial later in attack)
> - Throbbing-type pain
> - Moderate to severe intensity
> - Motion sensitivity (headache made worse with head movement or physical activity)
>
> **At least one of:**
> - Nausea/vomiting
> - Photophobia/phonophobia
> - Normal examination and no other cause of headache

prevent sufferers continuing with normal activities; sleep usually helps. A washed-out feeling follows the attack. The scalp may be tender to touch during episodes (allodynia) and the preference is to be still in a dark, quiet environment.

Some patients recognize changes in routine as trigger factors:

- Sleep (too little or too much).
- Stress (including letdown after a period of stress).
- Hormonal factors for women – changes in oestrogen levels, e.g. menstrual migraine (usually just before menses) and worsening with the oral contraceptive pill and menopause.
- Eating – skipping meals and alcohol. Contrary to popular belief, individual foods are rarely a trigger.
- Other – sensory stimuli, such as bright lights or loud sounds; physical exertion; and changes in weather patterns, e.g. stormy weather. Minor head injuries may trigger a worsening of migraine frequency and severity.

Migraine with aura

Approximately 25% of migraine sufferers experience focal neurological symptoms immediately preceding the headache phase in some or all attacks; this is termed migraine aura. Most never experience aura, and the presence of aura is therefore not required for a diagnosis of migraine. Aura usually evolves over 5–20 minutes, with symptoms changing as the wave of spreading neuronal depression moves across the surface of the cortex. It rarely lasts longer than 60 minutes and is followed immediately by the headache phase.

Visual aura is the most common type, with positive visual symptoms such as shimmering, teichopsia (zigzag lines, also called fortification spectra) and fragmentation of the image (like looking through a pane of broken glass) often accompanied by patches of loss of vision, which may move across the visual field (scotomas) and even evolve into hemianopia or tunnel vision. Positive sensory symptoms (mainly tingling), dysphasia and, rarely, loss of motor function may also occur, and may occur successively within the same episode of aura following the visual symptoms.

Migraine aura usually presents no diagnostic difficulty, but problems with diagnosis may sometimes arise in men over the age of 50 who develop migraine aura for the first time without subsequent headache (sometimes referred to as acephalic migrainous aura). This is frequently misdiagnosed as a TIA (see p. 833). Distinguishing the two conditions is often difficult and relies on the characteristic evolution of symptoms over minutes and the presence of positive symptoms in aura, in contrast to TIA where symptom onset is acute and negative symptoms (visual loss as opposed to visual distortion and teichopsia) are the norm. There may also be a history of previous typical migraine aura in early adult life to help distinguish the conditions.

Migraine-related dizziness

Vertigo is now recognized as being a migrainous symptom in some individuals, with attacks lasting for hours in the context of migraine attacks. There is an overlap with what is sometimes described as basilar migraine, a poorly defined migraine subtype associated with brainstem aura-type symptoms before or during attacks, including perioral paraesthesiae, diplopia, unsteadiness and, rarely, reduced level of consciousness.

Hemiplegic migraine

This rare autosomal dominant disorder causes a hemiparesis and/or coma and headache, with recovery within 24 hours. Some patients have permanent cerebellar signs, as it is allelic with episodic ataxia. It is distinct from more common forms of migraine.

Management

General measures include:

- explanation
- avoidance of trigger factors and lifestyle modification where possible.

Acute treatment of attacks

Analgesics, such as high-dose dispersible aspirin (900 mg), paracetamol 1 g or an NSAID (e.g. naproxen 250–500 mg), are often effective, with an antiemetic such as metoclopramide if necessary. Acute treatment should be taken as soon as possible after onset of headache. Patients should be aware that repeated use of analgesics leads to further headaches (see medication overuse headache, p. 844).

Triptans (5-$HT_{1B/1D}$ agonists) are specific for migraine and may be effective where simple analgesics are insufficient. Sumatriptan was the first marketed; almotriptan, eletriptan, frovatriptan, naratriptan, rizatriptan and zolmitriptan are now available, with various routes of administration. Subcutaneous sumatriptan injection may be effective where vomiting prevents absorption of oral medication (note that nasal triptan sprays rely on gastrointestinal rather than nasal absorption). Triptans should be avoided when there is vascular disease, and like analgesics, they should not be overused. CGRP antagonists, e.g. telcagepant, are proving to be very effective for acute treatment of migraine.

Migraine suppression medication

When migraine episodes are frequent – >1–2 per month, for example – and impacting on quality of life, migraine suppression medication should be offered. The key principles are that a period of 3–6 months' treatment is usually sufficient to reduce headache frequency and severity by approximately 50%, with the effect of 'resetting' migraine frequency beyond the treatment period. However, these medications will not be effective where ongoing analgesic overuse is an issue. Treatment options include:

- ***Anticonvulsants***. Valproate (800 mg) or topiramate (100–200 mg daily) is generally the most effective option.
- ***Beta-blockers***, e.g. propranolol slow-release 80–160 mg daily.
- ***Tricyclics***, e.g. amitriptyline 10 mg, increasing weekly in 10 mg steps to 50–60 mg.
- ***Botulinum toxin***. This was recommended as a treatment for chronic migraine (see p. 844). The technique involves 31 injections over the scalp and neck repeated every 3 months. Its effect is inconsistent.
- ***Pizotifen***. This is rarely used. Flunarizine (a calcium antagonist) and methysergide are used in refractory patients.

Tension-type headache

The exact pathogenesis of tension-type headache (TTH) remains unclear. There is overlap with migraine, and many headaches traditionally subsumed under this category probably, in fact, represent mild migraine. Since there are no diagnostic tests to separate TTH from mild migraine it is difficult to know if the conditions are biologically distinct. In contrast to migraine, pain is usually of mild to moderate severity, bilateral and relatively featureless, with tight band sensations, pressure behind the eyes, and bursting sensations being described.

Depression is also a frequent co-morbid feature. TTH is often attributed to cervical spondylosis, refractive errors or high blood pressure; evidence for such associations is poor.

Simple analgesics are often effective but overuse should be avoided. Physical treatments, such as massage, ice packs and relaxation, are often recommended. Frequent or chronic TTH may respond to migraine suppression medications as above, with tricyclics often being used first-line.

Trigeminal autonomic cephalalgias

The trigeminal autonomic cephalalgias are a group of primary headache disorders characterized by unilateral trigeminal distribution pain (usually in the ophthalmic division of the nerve) and prominent ipsilateral autonomic features.

Cluster headache

Cluster headache is distinct from migraine and much rarer (1 per 1000). It affects adults, mostly males aged between 20 and 40. Patients describe recurrent bouts (clusters) of excruciating unilateral retro-orbital pain with parasympathetic autonomic activation in the same eye, causing redness or tearing of the eye, nasal congestion or even a transient Horner syndrome. The pain is reputed to be the worst known to humans, and patients often contemplate, and sometimes commit, suicide, such is the severity of the pain. Unlike with migraine attacks, patients prefer to move about or rock rather than remain still.

Attacks are shorter than migraine, usually 30–90 minutes, and may occur several times per day, especially during sleep. Clusters last 1–2 months, with attacks most nights, before stopping completely and typically recurring a year or more later, often at the same time of year. Although the cause is not known, hypothalamic activation is seen on functional imaging studies during an attack.

Management. Analgesics are unhelpful. Subcutaneous sumatriptan is the drug of choice for acute treatment, as no other drug works quickly enough. High-flow oxygen is also used. Most prophylactic migraine drugs are unhelpful. Verapamil, lithium and/or a short course of steroids help terminate a bout of cluster headaches.

Paroxysmal hemicrania and SUNCT

Paroxysmal hemicrania is a rare condition with similarities to cluster headache, differing mainly in that attacks are briefer (10–30 min) and more frequent (>5 per day, at any time of day) and do not occur in clusters. Women are more often affected than men. There is a rapid and complete response to indometacin.

Short-lasting unilateral neuralgiform headache with conjunctival injection and tearing (***SUNCT***) is very rare. Attacks are short, 5 seconds to 2 minutes, and very frequently occur in bouts. Distinguishing SUNCT from trigeminal neuralgia can be difficult.

Other primary headache disorders

- ***Primary stabbing headache*** (***'ice pick headache'***) involves momentary jabs or stabs of localized pain occurring either in the same spot or moving about the head. Symptoms wax and wane, and are more common in patients with other primary headache disorders, particularly migraine. Treatment is usually not needed but this type of headache responds well to indometacin.
- ***Primary cough headache*** is a sudden, sharp head pain on coughing. No underlying cause is found but intracranial pathology should be excluded. The problem often resolves spontaneously. Indometacin is the treatment of choice; LP with removal of CSF can help.
- ***Primary sex headache*** is characterized by explosive headache at or before orgasm. It often resolves spontaneously after several attacks. Investigation to exclude SAH is required after the first episode.
- ***Other varieties*** of primary headache include hemicrania continua, primary exertional headache, hypnic headache (headache triggered by sleep), and primary thunderclap headache.

Chronic daily headache

This is defined as headache on ≥15 days per month for at least 3 months. Up to 4% of the population are affected by daily or near-daily headache. Although there are many possible causes, including secondary headache disorders, in practice, primary headache disorders, particularly migraine, are responsible for the majority. Where migraine is the cause, the term chronic migraine is now preferred.

Overuse of analgesic medication or triptans (termed ***medication overuse headache***) is often a major factor leading to and maintaining chronicity, particularly in those with migrainous biology. Use of ≥10 doses per month of any analgesic or triptan, particularly codeine or opiate-containing drugs such as co-codamol, or numerous over-the-counter analgesics, may eventually lead to transformation of episodic headache into chronic daily headache.

Explanation that medication overuse is part of the problem is essential to help patients withdraw from or substantially reduce analgesic intake. This is a difficult process for many patients, especially as there may be a period of transient rebound worsening of headache after withdrawal. Concurrent introduction of migraine suppression medication (see above) may help withdrawal but will not be effective if patients cannot withdraw from frequent analgesic use. Occasionally, hospital admission for analgesic withdrawal with parenteral administration of dihydroergotamine is required.

Secondary headache disorders

Raised intracranial pressure headache

Any headache present on waking and made worse by coughing, straining or sneezing may be due to raised intracranial pressure (ICP) caused by a mass lesion. Vomiting often accompanies pressure headaches. Visual obscurations (momentary bilateral visual loss with bending or coughing) are characteristic and seen in the presence of papilloedema. Occasionally, where ICP rises quickly, papilloedema may not be present.

Neuroimaging is mandatory if raised ICP is suspected. Where no mass lesion, venous sinus thrombosis or hydrocephalus is detected on imaging in the presence of papilloedema, idiopathic intracranial hypertension may be the cause and LP is performed to measure CSF opening pressure.

Idiopathic intracranial hypertension

Idiopathic intracranial hypertension (IIH) probably results from reduced CSF resorption. IIH typically develops in younger, overweight female patients, many of whom have polycystic ovaries. Headaches and transient visual obscurations due to the florid papilloedema are the presenting features. A VIth nerve palsy may develop – a false localizing sign (see p. 806). CSF pressure is very elevated, with normal constituents. Brain imaging is normal, although ventricles may be small and appear 'slit-like'.

Various drugs, such as tetracyclines, and vitamin A supplements have been implicated. Other causes of papilloedema should be excluded. Sagittal sinus thrombosis can cause a similar picture and should always be looked for on MR venography.

IIH is usually self-limiting. However, optic nerve damage can result from longstanding severe papilloedema with progressive loss of peripheral visual fields. Regular monitoring of visual fields with perimetry is essential. Repeated LP, acetazolamide and thiazide diuretics are used to reduce CSF production. Weight reduction is helpful. Ventriculoperitoneal shunt insertion or optic nerve sheath fenestration to protect vision is sometimes necessary.

Low-CSF-volume (low-pressure) headache

Although most often seen following LP, CSF leaks may occur spontaneously, leading to postural headache, worse on standing or sitting and relieved completely by lying flat. The patient may give a history of vigorous Valsalva, straining or coughing just prior to onset. Leptomeningeal enhancement may be seen on MRI but is not reliably present. LP is generally avoided for obvious reasons but may reveal low opening pressure. The site of the leak is usually within the spine; thus treatment consists of injection of autologous blood into the spinal epidural space to seal the leak (a 'blood patch'), or occasionally surgical repair of the dural tear. Intravenous caffeine infusion and bed rest are sometimes effective.

Post-traumatic headache

Pre-existing migraine may worsen following head injury. *De novo* headache sometimes follows a minor head injury but post-traumatic headache is an ill-defined entity. Improvement over a few weeks is the norm, but where litigation is ongoing, symptoms can persist for long periods. Subdural haematoma and low-pressure headache need to be considered as a possible cause.

Facial pain

The face has many pain-sensitive structures: teeth, gums, sinuses, temporomandibular joints, jaw and eyes. Dental causes are common and should always be considered. Facial pain is also caused by specific neurological conditions.

Trigeminal neuralgia

Trigeminal neuralgia typically starts in the sixth and seventh decades; hypertension is the main risk factor. Compression of the trigeminal nerve at or near the pons by an ectatic vascular loop is the usual cause. High-resolution MRI studies may demonstrate the vascular loop in contact with the nerve in a high proportion of cases. In younger patients, multiple sclerosis or a cerebellopontine angle tumour (acoustic schwannomas, meningiomas, epidermoids) is more likely to be the cause.

Clinical features

Paroxysms of knife-like or electric shock-like pain, lasting seconds, occur in the distribution of the Vth nerve. Pain tends to commence in the mandibular division (V_3) but may spread over time to involve the maxillary (V_2) and, occasionally, the ophthalmic divisions (V_1). Bilateral trigeminal neuralgia is rare (3%) and usually due to intrinsic brainstem pathology, such as demyelination. Episodes occur many times a day with a refractory period after each. They may be brought on by stimulation of one or more trigger zones in the face. Washing, shaving, a cold wind and chewing are examples of trivial stimuli that provoke pain. The face may be screwed up in agony. Spontaneous remissions last months or years before (almost invariable) recurrence. There are no signs of Vth nerve dysfunction on examination.

Management

Carbamazepine (600–1200 mg daily) reduces the severity of attacks in the majority. Oxcarbazepine, lamotrigine and gabapentin are also used. If drugs fail or are not tolerated, a number of surgical options are available that, in general, are more effective than medical treatments. Percutaneous radiofrequency selective ablation of the trigeminal ganglion is performed as a day-case procedure; recurrence may occur after an average of 2 years. Microvascular decompression of the nerve in the posterior fossa has a high long-term success rate (approximately 90%).

Atypical facial pain

Facial pain differs from trigeminal neuralgia in quality and distribution, and trigger points are absent. The condition is probably heterogeneous in aetiology but is believed by some (on little evidence) to be a somatic manifestation of depression. Tricyclic antidepressants and drugs used in neuropathic pain are sometimes helpful.

Other causes of facial pain

Facial pain occurs in the trigeminal autonomic cephalgias (see above), occasionally in migraine and in carotid dissection.

Giant cell arteritis (temporal arteritis)

A granulomatous large-vessel arteritis is seen almost exclusively in people over 50 (see p. 842).

Clinical features

- ***Headache***. This is almost invariable in giant cell arteritis (GCA). Pain develops over inflamed superficial temporal and/or occipital arteries. Touching the skin over an inflamed vessel (e.g. when combing the hair) causes pain. Arterial pulsation is soon lost; the artery becomes hard, tortuous and thickened. The scalp over inflamed vessels may become red. Rarely, gangrenous patches appear.
- ***Facial pain***. Pain in the face, jaw and mouth is caused by inflammation of facial, maxillary and lingual branches of the external carotid artery in GCA. Pain is characteristically worse on eating (jaw claudication). Mouth opening and protruding the tongue become difficult. A painful, ischaemic tongue occurs rarely.
- ***Visual problems***. Visual loss from arterial inflammation and occlusion occurs in 25% of untreated cases. Posterior ciliary artery occlusion causes anterior ischaemic optic neuropathy in three-quarters of these. Other mechanisms are central retinal artery occlusion, cilioretinal artery occlusion and posterior

ischaemic optic neuropathy. There is sudden monocular visual loss (partial or complete), usually painless. Amaurosis fugax (see p. 832) may precede permanent blindness.

When the posterior ciliary vessels are affected, ischaemic optic neuropathy causes the disc to become swollen and pale; retinal branch vessels usually remain normal. When the central retinal artery is occluded, there is sudden permanent unilateral blindness, disc pallor and visible retinal ischaemia. Bilateral blindness may develop, with the second eye being affected 1–2 weeks after the first.

Diagnosis and management

See page 701.

Further reading

Headache Classification Committee of the International Headache Society. The International Classification of Headache Disorders, 3rd edn (beta version). *Cephalgia* 2013; 33:629–808.

Wessman M. Migraine: a complex genetic disorder. *Lancet Neurol* 2007; 6:521–532.

http://www.bash.org.uk *British Association for the Study of Headache guidelines on headache diagnosis and management.*

EPILEPSY AND LOSS OF CONSCIOUSNESS

Epilepsy

An epileptic seizure can be defined as a sudden synchronous discharge of cerebral neurones causing symptoms or signs that are apparent either to the patient or to an observer. For example, a limited discharge affecting only part of the cortex may cause a subjective aura apparent only to the patient, or a generalized seizure may cause a convulsion witnessed by an observer of which the patient may be unaware. This definition excludes disorders such as migrainous aura that are more gradual in onset and usually more prolonged, and EEG discharges that do not have a clinical correlate. Epilepsy is an ongoing liability to recurrent epileptic seizures.

Epidemiology

Epilepsy is common. Its population prevalence is 0.7–0.8% (higher in developing countries). Approximately 440 000 people in the UK have epilepsy. The incidence of epilepsy is age-dependent; it is highest at the extremes of life, most cases starting before the age of 20 or after the age of 60. The cumulative incidence (lifetime risk) of epilepsy is over 3% and the lifetime risk of having a single seizure is 5%. The fact that the prevalence is much lower than the cumulative incidence in part reflects the fact that epilepsy often goes into remission.

Classification

Seizures are divided by clinical pattern into two main groups (***Box 21.40*** and ***Fig. 21.44***): ***focal*** seizures and ***generalized*** seizures.

- ***A focal seizure*** is caused by electrical discharge restricted to a limited part of the cortex of one cerebral hemisphere. Partial seizures are further characterized according to whether or not there is:
  - aura, e.g. smell or auditory hallucination, déjà vu, fear, visual distortion, sensory symptoms such as tingling, abdominal rising sensation
  - motor features, e.g. one limb jerking (a Jacksonian seizure)
  - loss of awareness or responsiveness, e.g. in many temporal lobe seizures.
- ***In a generalized seizure***, there is simultaneous involvement of both hemispheres, always associated with loss of consciousness or awareness.

Focal seizures with electrical activity confined to one part of the brain may spread after a few seconds, due to failure of inhibitory mechanisms, to involve the whole of both hemispheres, causing a ***secondary generalized seizure***. The patient may remember the initial focal seizure before losing consciousness, in which case this is called an ***aura***; sometimes, however, the spread of electrical

Box 21.40 Classification of seizures

1. Generalized seizures
   A. Tonic–clonic seizures (grand mal)
   B. Absence seizures with 3 Hz spike-and-wave discharge (petit mal)
   C. Myoclonic seizures
   D. Tonic, clonic and atonic seizures
2. Focal seizures (originating within one hemisphere)
   Characterized according to one or more features:
   A. Aura
   B. Motor (without impaired awareness, e.g. Jacksonian seizures)
   C. Awareness and responsiveness altered or retained (e.g. with impaired awareness, in temporal lobe seizures)
   A focal seizure can evolve into bilateral convulsive seizure – secondary generalization
3. Unknown (insufficient evidence to characterize as focal, generalized or both)

(Abridged from algorithm in Berg AT, Berkovic SF, Brodie MJ et al. Revised terminology and concepts for organization of seizures and epilepsies: report of the ILAE Commission on Classification and Terminology 2005–2009. Epilepsia 2010; 51:676–685.)

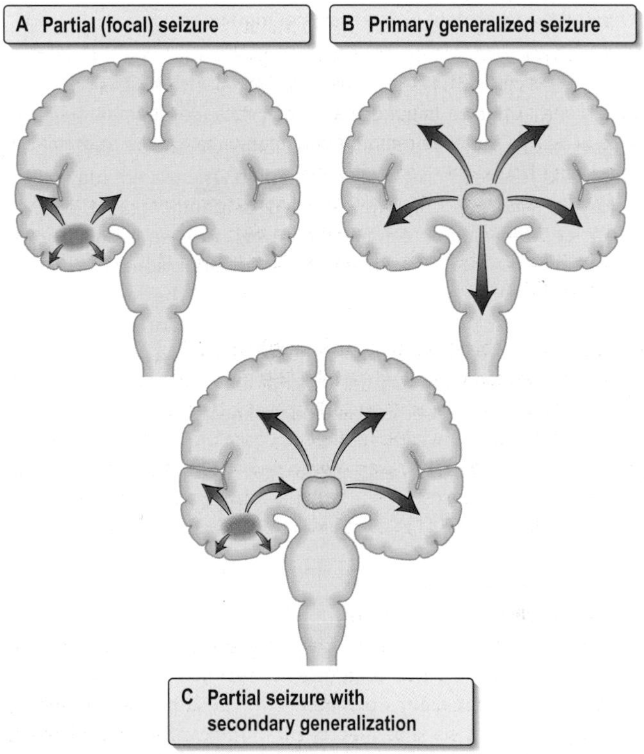

Figure 21.44 Seizure types.

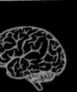

activity is so rapid that the patient does not experience any warning before a secondary generalized seizure.

Generalized seizure types

Typical absence seizures (petit mal)

This generalized epilepsy almost invariably begins in childhood. Each attack is accompanied by 3 Hz spike-and-wave EEG activity (see ***Fig. 21.19***). There is loss of awareness and a vacant expression for <10 seconds before returning abruptly to normal and continuing as though nothing had happened. Apart from slight fluttering of the eyelids, there are no motor manifestations. Patients often do not realize they have had an attack but may have many per day. Typical absence attacks are never due to acquired lesions such as tumours; they are a manifestation of primary generalized epilepsy. Children with absence seizures may go on to develop generalized convulsive seizures. Absence seizures are often confused with temporal lobe seizures causing transient alteration of awareness.

Generalized tonic–clonic seizures (grand mal seizures)

Prodrome. There is often no warning before generalized tonic–clonic seizures (GTCS), or there may be an aura prior to a secondary generalized seizure.

Tonic–clonic phase. An initial tonic stiffening is followed by the clonic phase with synchronous jerking of the limbs, reducing in frequency over about 2 minutes until the convulsion stops. The patient may utter an initial cry and then falls, sometimes suffering serious injury. The eyes remain open and the tongue is often bitten. There may be incontinence of urine or faeces.

Post-ictal phase. A period of flaccid unresponsiveness is followed by gradual return of awareness with confusion and drowsiness lasting 15 minutes to an hour or longer. Headache is common after a GTCS.

Myoclonic, tonic and atonic seizures

Myoclonic seizures or 'jerks' take the form of momentary brief contractions of a muscle or muscle groups: for example, causing a sudden involuntary twitch of a finger or hand. They are common in primary generalized epilepsies. ***Tonic seizures*** consist of stiffening of the body, not followed by jerking. ***Atonic seizures*** involve a sudden collapse with loss of muscle tone and consciousness.

Focal seizure types

Focal seizures with aura

The nature of the aura helps to localize the seizure focus. Temporal lobe auras include déjà vu or jamais vu; fear (may be mistaken for panic attacks); olfactory, gustatory or auditory hallucinations; altered perception, such as macropsia or micropsia; an abdominal rising sensation; nausea; and vertigo. With some frontal seizures, conjugate gaze (see p. 827) deviates away from the epileptic focus and the head turns; this is known as an adversive seizure. Occipital lobe auras include visual phenomena such as zigzag lines and coloured scotomas. Some auras are vague or hard for patients to describe but they are generally stereotyped: that is, the same on each occasion.

Focal motor seizures

These originate within the motor cortex. Jerking typically begins on one side of the mouth or in one hand, sometimes spreading to involve the entire side. This visible spread of activity is called the ***Jacksonian march*** of a seizure. Local temporary paralysis of the limbs affected sometimes follows: Todd's paralysis.

Box 21.41 Causes of epilepsy

- Primary generalized epilepsy, e.g. juvenile myoclonic epilepsy
- Developmental, e.g. neuronal migration abnormalities, cortical dysplasia
- Hippocampal sclerosis
- Brain trauma and surgery
- Intracranial mass lesions, e.g. tumour
- Vascular, e.g. cerebral infarction, arteriovenous malformation, venous sinus thrombosis
- Infectious, e.g. viral encephalitis, meningitis, cerebral tuberculosis, HIV, cerebral toxoplasmosis, neurocysticercosis
- Immune, e.g. NMDA receptor antibody and potassium channel antibody encephalitis
- Genetic, e.g. channelopathies
- Metabolic abnormalities, e.g. hyponatraemia, hypocalcaemia
- Neurodegenerative disorders, e.g. Alzheimer's
- Drugs, e.g. ciclosporin, lidocaine, quinolones, tricyclic antidepressants, antipsychotics, lithium, stimulant drugs such as cocaine
- Alcohol withdrawal

Focal seizures with altered awareness or responsiveness

These usually arise from the temporal lobe (60%) or the frontal lobe. There is often a preceding aura followed by a period of complete or partial loss of awareness of surroundings, lasting for 1–2 minutes on average (as opposed to 10 seconds in absence seizures), which the patient generally does not remember subsequently. This stage is accompanied by speech arrest and often by ***automatisms***: semi-purposeful stereotyped motions such as lip smacking or dystonic limb posturing, or more complex motor behaviours such as walking in a circle or undressing. The attacks may be followed by a short period of post-ictal confusion or may develop into a secondary generalized convulsive seizure.

Epilepsy syndromes and aetiology of epilepsy

The range of causes of epilepsy (***Box 21.41***) is different at different ages and in different countries.

- ***Children and teenagers***: genetic, perinatal and congenital disorders predominate.
- ***Younger adults***: trauma, drugs and alcohol are common.
- ***Older ages (>60 years)***: vascular disease and mass lesions such as neoplasms are important.

Primary generalized epilepsies

Presenting in childhood and early adult life, primary generalized epilepsies (PGEs) account for up to 20% of all patients with epilepsy. The cause is thought to be polygenic with complex inheritance. The brain is structurally normal but abnormalities of ion channels influencing neuronal firing, abnormalities of neurotransmitter release and synaptic connections are probably the underlying molecular pathological substrates. They include:

- ***Childhood absence epilepsy***: absence seizures. Spontaneous remission by age 18 is usual.
- ***Juvenile myoclonic epilepsy*** (JME, ***Box 21.42***). This accounts for 10% of all epilepsy patients. Typically, myoclonic jerks start in the teenage years (and are usually ignored by the patient; ask about jerks when taking an epilepsy history – ***Box 21.42***), followed by generalized tonic–clonic seizures that bring the patient to medical attention. One-third of patients also have absences. Seizures and jerks often occur in the morning after waking. Lack of sleep, alcohol and strobe or flickering lights are seizure triggers in JME. JME usually responds well

Box 21.42 Juvenile myoclonic epilepsy

- 10% of all epilepsy patients
- Starts in teenage years
- Clinical features:
  - Myoclonic jerks
  - Generalized tonic–clonic seizures
  - Absence in one-third
  - Triggers: sleep deprivation, alcohol, strobe lighting
- Abnormal EEG
- Good response to treatment
- Requires life-long treatment

to treatment, is usually associated with EEG abnormalities and requires life-long treatment.

- ***Monogenic disorders***: research has identified a number of single-gene epilepsy disorders, e.g. autosomal dominant nocturnal frontal lobe epilepsy (caused by mutations in the nicotinic acetylcholine receptor gene). Many are due to mutations of neuronal voltage-gated channels, e.g. potassium and sodium channels, or ligand-gated channels and receptors (channelopathies).

Focal epilepsy

Almost any process disrupting the cortical grey matter can cause epilepsy. Seizures arise from the affected area of cortex, with or without secondary generalized seizures (these may obscure the focal onset). A focal seizure onset often indicates a structural cause and detailed imaging is required to identify this. In general, the response to treatment is less good than with PGE.

Hippocampal sclerosis

This is a major cause of epilepsy. Hippocampal sclerosis (damage with scarring and atrophy of the hippocampus and surrounding cortex) is the main pathological substrate causing temporal lobe epilepsy and the leading cause of localization-related epilepsy. Childhood febrile convulsions are the main risk factor. Hippocampal sclerosis is usually visible on MRI. It is one of the more common causes of refractory epilepsy, in which case it may be amenable to surgical resection of the damaged temporal lobe.

Genetic and developmental disorders

Over 200 genetic disorders, such as tuberous sclerosis, include epilepsy among their features. These account for less than 2% of epilepsy cases. Neuronal migration defects during brain development, dysplastic areas of cerebral cortex and hamartomas contribute to seizures in both infancy and adult life.

Trauma, hypoxia and neurosurgery

Traumatic brain injury. This may cause epilepsy, sometimes years after the event. The risk is not increased after mild injury (loss of consciousness or post-traumatic amnesia <30 min). Depressed skull fracture, penetrating injury and intracranial haemorrhage increase risk significantly.

Perinatal brain injury and cerebral palsy. Periventricular leukomalacia and brain haemorrhage associated with prematurity and fetal hypoxia, may cause early-onset epilepsy. One-third of children with cerebral palsy have epilepsy.

Brain surgery. This is followed by seizures in up to 17% of cases. Prophylactic anticonvulsant use after surgery is not recommended.

Brain tumours and other mass lesions

Mass lesions involving the cortex cause epilepsy. Seizures are one of the most common presenting features of brain tumours. Brain tumours cause 6% of cases of adult-onset epilepsy.

Vascular disorders

Stroke and small-vessel cerebrovascular disease is the most common cause of epilepsy after the age of 60.

Cortical venous thrombosis or venous sinus thrombosis

Arteriovenous malformations commonly cause epilepsy.

Cavernous haemangiomas (***cavernomas***) usually present with epilepsy (see ***Fig. 21.41***).

Neurodegenerative disorders

Neurodegenerative disorders involving the cerebral cortex, such as Alzheimer's disease, are associated with an increased risk of epilepsy.

Infection

Seizures are often the presenting feature of encephalitis, cerebral abscess and tuberculomas. They also occur in chronic meningitis (e.g. tuberculosis) and may rarely be the first sign of acute bacterial meningitis. Neurocysticercosis is a major cause of seizures in countries where the pork tapeworm is endemic, such as India and South America. HIV and complications of immunosuppression, such as cerebral toxoplasmosis, may also lead to seizures.

Immunological disorders

Autoimmune antibody-mediated encephalitis, such as that due to antibodies against potassium channels or NMDA or glycine receptors, typically present with seizures, as may autoimmune limbic encephalitis.

Alcohol and drugs

Chronic alcohol use is a common cause of seizures. These occur either during heavy drinking bouts or during periods of withdrawal. Alcohol-induced hypoglycaemia and head injury also lead to seizures.

Several drugs, including antipsychotics, tricyclic antidepressants, selective serotonin reuptake inhibitors (SSRIs), lithium, class Ib anti-arrhythmics such as lidocaine, ciclosporin and mefloquine, sometimes provoke fits, either in overdose or at therapeutic doses in individuals with a low seizure threshold. Stimulant drugs such as cocaine also cause seizures.

Withdrawal of antiepileptic drugs (especially barbiturates) and benzodiazepines may provoke seizures.

Metabolic abnormalities

Seizures can be caused by:

- hypocalcaemia, hypoglycaemia, hyponatraemia
- acute hypoxia
- uraemia, hepatic encephalopathy
- porphyria.

Diagnosis of the first fit and investigations

The diagnosis of a seizure is essentially a clinical one, based on taking a history from the patient and any witnesses (***Boxes 21.43*** and ***21.44***). Investigations have a limited role in distinguishing between a seizure and other causes of a blackout or attack (see p. 851).

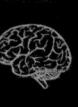

Box 21.43 Diagnosis of a seizure: taking a history after an episode of loss of consciousness

Witness account is crucial
- What happened:
  - Before: aura versus pre-syncopal prodrome
  - During: convulsion, automatisms versus brief syncopal blackout and pallor
  - After: post-ictal confusion and headache versus rapid recovery in syncope
- Circumstances:
  - Seizure triggers? Sleep deprivation, alcohol binge or drugs
  - Syncope triggers? Pain, heat, prolonged standing and so on
- Epilepsy risk factors?
  - Childhood febrile convulsions
  - Significant head injury
  - Meningitis or encephalitis
  - Family history of epilepsy
- Previous unrecognized seizures?
  - Myoclonic jerks
  - Absences
  - Auras (focal seizures)
- Alcohol excess?
- Medication lowering seizure threshold?
- Hold a driving licence?

Box 21.44 Useful points when diagnosing epilepsy

Diagnosis is a clinical one. Tests such as EEG have little role in distinguishing between epilepsy and other attack types:
- Poor clinical discriminators between types of blackout:
  - Urinary incontinence – may occur in both seizure and syncope
  - Presence of injury
- Good discriminators between types of blackout:
  - Prolonged recovery period (seizure)
  - Bitten tongue – side usually (seizure)
  - Colour change – pallor (syncope), cyanosis (seizure)
- Stereotyped attacks are usually due to epilepsy
- If in doubt, do not diagnose epilepsy – best to wait and see rather than label and treat as epilepsy
- There is no role for a 'trial of anticonvulsant treatment' in uncertain cases

Box 21.45 Checklist after a first seizure

- Perform tests:
  - Blood tests and ECG
  - EEG
  - MRI brain (most patients – see text)
- Avoid or remove precipitants: drugs, alcohol, sleep deprivation
- Give advice on safety: e.g. avoid swimming, baths, working at heights
- Stop driving and ask the patient to inform the Driver and Vehicle Licensing Authority (DVLA; in the UK)
- Discuss recurrence risk and treatment

The majority of patients referred to a first fit clinic have not had a seizure. The most common error is to misdiagnose a syncopal blackout for a seizure.

Which investigations are needed?

Blood tests, including serum calcium, and an ECG (rhythm, conduction abnormalities, QT interval) are necessary in most patients following an episode of loss of consciousness ***(Box 21.45)***.

Electroencephalography

EEG is most useful to categorize epilepsy and understand its cause, rather than as a means of confirming a doubtful diagnosis of epilepsy. EEG has a high false-negative rate in epilepsy (>20% even with awake and sleep recordings) and a low false-positive rate (1% of people without epilepsy have epileptiform changes on EEG).

- ***EEG abnormalities in epilepsy***: focal cortical spikes (e.g. over a temporal lobe) or generalized spike-and-wave activity (in PGE). Epileptic activity is continuous in status epilepticus.
- ***Sleep recordings or 24h ambulatory EEG*** increase sensitivity when routine EEG is normal.
- ***Inpatient EEG videotelemetry*** is helpful for diagnosis in attacks of uncertain cause.

Brain imaging

MRI is indicated in most patients after a first seizure, particularly in focal-onset seizures and in older patients where the chance of a focal brain lesion is greatest. In patients below the age of 30 with a definite electroclinical diagnosis of PGE, brain imaging is not essential.

Recurrence risk after a first fit

Some 70–80% of people will have a second seizure, the risk being highest in the first 6 months after the initial seizure. The vast majority of those who have a second seizure will have further seizures if not started on treatment. The risk of seizure recurrence is significantly increased by features of PGE on EEG, focal seizures and the presence of structural brain lesions.

Management

Emergency measures

Most seizures last only minutes and end spontaneously. A prolonged seizure (>5 min) or repeated seizures may be terminated with rectal diazepam, intravenous lorazepam or buccal midazolam. Oxygen should be given and the airway monitored in the post-ictal phase.

Status epilepticus

This medical emergency ***(Box 21.46)*** means continuous seizures for 30 minutes or longer (or two or more seizures without recovery of consciousness between them over a similar period). Status epilepticus has a mortality of 10–15%. The longer the duration of status, the greater the risk of permanent cerebral damage. Rhabdomyolysis may lead to acute kidney injury in convulsive status epilepticus.

Over 50% of cases occur without a previous history of epilepsy. Some 25% with apparent refractory status have ***pseudostatus*** (non-epileptic attack disorder).

Not all status is convulsive. In ***absence status***, for example, status is non-convulsive; the patient is in a continuous, distant, stuporose state. ***Focal status*** also occurs. ***Epilepsia partialis continua*** is continuous seizure activity in one part of the body, such as a finger or a limb, without loss of consciousness. This is often due to a cortical neoplasm or, in the elderly, a cortical infarct.

Antiepileptic drugs

Antiepileptic drugs (AEDs; ***Box 21.47***) are indicated when there is a firm clinical diagnosis of epilepsy and a substantial risk of recurrent seizures. Some general principles apply:
- Introduce AEDs at low dose and slowly titrate upwards until the seizures are controlled or side-effects become unacceptable.
- Aim for monotherapy; 70% of patients will have good seizure control with a single AED.

Box 21.46 Status epilepticus: management

Early status (up to 30 min)
- Administer oxygen, monitor ECG and blood pressure, perform routine blood tests (include glucose, calcium, drug screen, anticonvulsant levels urgently)
- Give lorazepam i.v. 4 mg bolus. Repeat once if necessary. Buccal midazolam is an alternative

Established status (30–90 min)
- Phenytoin: give 15 mg/kg i.v. diluted to 10 mg/mL in saline into a large vein at 50 mg/min (ECG monitoring required)
  or
- Fosphenytoin: this is a prodrug of phenytoin and can be given faster than phenytoin. Doses are expressed in phenytoin equivalents (PE): fosphenytoin 1.5 mg = 1 mg phenytoin. Give 15 mg/kg (PE) fosphenytoin (15 mg × 1.5 = 21.5 mg) diluted to 10 mg/mL in saline at 50–100 mg (PE)/min

If ongoing seizures
- Phenobarbital 10 mg/kg i.v. diluted 1 in 10 in water for injection at <100 mg/min
- Valproate i.v. (25 mg/kg) is an alternative

Refractory status (>90 min) – general anaesthesia
- Only in intensive care setting; intubation and ventilation usually required
- Propofol bolus 2 mg/kg, repeat, followed by continuous infusion of 5–10 mg/kg per hour
- Thiopental and midazolam infusions may also be used
- Use continuous EEG monitoring to assess efficacy of treatment – aim for EEG burst suppression pattern
- Reinstate previous AED medication via nasogastric tube
- Establish diagnosis: CT or MRI may reveal an underlying cause
- Remember: 25% of apparent status cases turn out to be pseudostatus

Box 21.47 Antiepileptic drugs and common seizure types

	Generalized tonic–clonic seizures (grand mal)	Focal seizures with or without secondary generalization	Myoclonic seizures
First-line	Sodium valproate Levetiracetam Lamotrigine Carbamazepine Oxcarbazepine Topiramate	Carbamazepine Lamotrigine Levetiracetam Sodium valproate Oxcarbazepine Topiramate	Sodium valproate Levetiracetam Topiramate
Second-line and/or add-ons	Phenobarbital Clobazam Clonazepam Phenytoin	Clobazam Gabapentin Pregabalin Zonisamide Lacosamide Tiagabine	Clonazepam Clobazam Lamotrigine Piracetam
May worsen attacks			Carbamazepine Oxcarbazepine

- If seizures are not controlled with the first AED, gradually introduce a second agent and then slowly withdraw the first AED. If the patient is still not seizure-free, then combination therapy is required.
- Epilepsy is one of the few disorders where non-generic ('brand name') prescribing is justified to ensure consistent drug levels.
- Routine monitoring of AED levels is not needed and should be reserved for assessing compliance and toxicity. Measuring sodium valproate levels is rarely useful, as levels fluctuate widely.
- There are interactions between AEDs (and with other medications), e.g. between sodium valproate and lamotrigine. New-generation AEDs have fewer interactions.
- Phenytoin is no longer considered a first-line AED; it is now principally used in emergency control of seizures (see status epilepticus above). Levetiracetam is increasingly used in most types of epilepsy.

Unwanted effects of drugs

Intoxication with most AEDs causes unsteadiness, nystagmus and drowsiness. Side-effects are more common with multiple AED usage. Skin rashes are seen particularly with lamotrigine, carbamazepine and phenytoin. A wide variety of idiosyncratic drug reactions may occur, such as blood dyscrasias with carbamazepine.

Epilepsy in women

See page 1306.

Epilepsy and driving

Patients should be asked to stop driving after a seizure and to inform the regulatory authorities if they hold a driving licence. After a seizure, a temporary driving ban until seizure-free is usual but regulations vary from country to country. Many driving regulatory bodies also suggest refraining from driving while withdrawing from AEDs.

Lifestyle and safety

People with epilepsy (the term 'epileptic' is no longer used) should be encouraged to lead lives as unrestricted as reasonably possible, though observing simple safety measures such as avoiding swimming and dangerous sports like rock-climbing. Advice at home includes leaving bathroom and lavatory doors unlocked and taking showers rather than baths. Epilepsy triggers, such as sleep deprivation, excess alcohol and drugs, should be avoided, as should strobe lighting where there is EEG evidence of a photo-paroxysmal response.

Drug withdrawal

Withdrawal of AEDs should be considered after a seizure-free period of at least 2–3 years. There is a 50% seizure recurrence rate after withdrawal so detailed discussion and explanation are essential.

Refractory epilepsy

- Seizures may persist despite treatment, especially with temporal lobe epilepsy.
- Re-evaluate the diagnosis.
- Consider concordance (compliance).
- Combine AEDs and use the maximum tolerated dose.
- Refer to a specialist unit for consideration of epilepsy surgery.
- Other non-pharmacological treatments, such as vagal nerve stimulation and the ketogenic low-carbohydrate diet, may sometimes be useful.

Epilepsy surgery

Temporal lobectomy will result in seizure freedom in 50–70% of selected patients with uncontrolled seizures caused by hippocampal sclerosis (defined by imaging and confirmed by EEG).

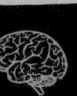

Box 21.48 Causes of blackouts and 'funny turns'

- Epilepsy
- Syncope:
  - Neurocardiogenic syncope (vasovagal)
  - Cardiac syncope (Stokes–Adams attacks)
  - Micturition syncope
  - Cough syncope
  - Postural hypotension
  - Carotid sinus syncope
- Non-epileptic attacks (pseudoseizures)
- Panic attacks and hyperventilation
- Hypoglycaemia
- Drop attacks
- Hydrocephalic attacks
- Basilar migraine
- Severe vertigo
- Cataplexy, narcolepsy, sleep paralysis

Other causes of blackouts

The distinction between a fit (seizure), a faint (syncope) or another type of attack is primarily a clinical one, dependent on the history and an eyewitness account ***(Box 21.48)***. Mistaking a syncopal loss of consciousness for a seizure is the most frequent error made in differential diagnosis.

Syncope or faints

The simple faint that over half the population experiences at some time (particularly in childhood, youth or pregnancy) is due to sudden reflex bradycardia with vasodilatation of both peripheral and splanchnic vasculature (***neurocardiogenic or vasovagal syncope***).

- ***Precipitants***: a common response to prolonged standing, fear, venesection or pain. Syncope almost never occurs in the recumbent posture.
- ***Prodrome***: usually brief. There is dizziness and a light-headed feeling, often with nausea, sweating, a feeling of heat and visual grey-out.
- ***Blackout*** (see p. 798): patients usually lie still but jerking and twitching movements can occur and are sometimes mistaken for a convulsion. Their appearance is pale. Incontinence of urine or faeces can occur and is not a good discriminator between seizure and syncope.
- ***Recovery***: rapid, usually taking place over seconds, but may be followed by a feeling of general fatigue (as opposed to post-ictal drowsiness and confusion following a seizure).

Other types of syncope

Cardiac syncope (Stokes–Adams attacks) is potentially serious and often treatable. Typically, there is little or no warning. Cardiac arrhythmias, such as those due to heart block, or left ventricular outflow tract obstruction may be the cause. Syncope during exercise is often cardiac in origin.

Micturition syncope occurs during micturition in men, particularly at night.

Cough syncope occurs when venous return to the heart is obstructed by bouts of severe coughing; it is also seen with laughter occasionally.

Postural hypotension (see p. 939) can cause syncope and occurs in the elderly, in autonomic neuropathy, and with some drugs, such as antihypertensives.

Carotid sinus syncope (see p. 940) is due to a vagal response caused by pressure over the carotid sinus baroreceptors in the neck: for example, due to a tight collar.

Convulsive syncope is when collapsing in a propped-up position following a syncope results in delayed restoration of cerebral blood flow and may lead to a secondary anoxic seizure following syncope.

Investigations

A 12-lead ECG should always be performed after a syncope to identify heart block, pre-excitation or long QT syndrome. Cardiac ECG holter monitoring and echocardiography are required where cardiac syncope is suspected. An implantable loop recorder is occasionally needed for infrequent events with a possible cardiac origin. Tilt-table testing (see p. 948) is sometimes diagnostic but has low sensitivity.

Other conditions

Non-epileptic attack disorder (***pseudoseizures***) regularly causes difficulty in diagnosis. Attacks may look like grand mal fits. Usually, there are bizarre thrashing, non-synchronous limb movements, but there can be extreme difficulty in separating these attacks from seizures. EEG videotelemetry is valuable. Apparent status epilepticus can occur. The serum prolactin level is of some value; this rises during a grand mal seizure but not during a pseudoseizure (or a partial seizure).

Panic attacks (see p. 916) trigger sudden sympathetic activation and often hyperventilation, leading to respiratory alkalosis. They cause some or all of the following symptoms: dizziness, chest pains or tightness, a feeling of choking or shortness of breath, tingling in face and extremities, palpitations, trembling and a feeling of dissociation or of impending doom. Consciousness is usually preserved and attacks are easily recognized. Blood gases should be measured.

Hypoglycaemia (see p. 1258) causes confusion followed by loss of consciousness, sometimes with a convulsion, dysphasia or hemiparesis. There is often a warning, with hunger, malaise, shaking and sweating. Prompt recovery occurs with intravenous (or oral) glucose. Prolonged hypoglycaemia causes widespread cerebral damage. Hypoglycaemic attacks unrelated to diabetes are rare (see pp. 1275–1276). Feeling faint after fasting does not indicate anything serious.

Vertigo, when acute, can be sufficiently severe as to cause prostration; a few seconds' unresponsiveness sometimes follows.

Migraine, in the form of severe basilar migraine and familial hemiplegic migraine, may occasionally lead to loss of consciousness.

Drop attacks are instant, unexpected episodes of lower limb weakness with falling, largely in women over 60 years. Awareness is preserved. They are due to sudden change in lower limb tone, presumably of brainstem origin. Sudden attacks of leg weakness also occur in hydrocephalus.

TIAs are almost never a cause of loss of consciousness.

Sleep disorders

Sleep architecture and insomnia are discussed on pages 904–905. Myoclonic jerks when falling asleep are a normal phenomenon (see p. 856). Seizures may occur predominantly or solely during sleep.

Narcolepsy and cataplexy

Narcolepsy is caused by abnormalities of the brain neurotransmitter hypocretin (orexin), which is a regulator of sleep. CSF levels are usually low, thought in most cases to be due to autoimmune damage to the hypothalamic cells secreting the neurotransmitter. Narcolepsy is strongly associated with human leucocyte antigen (HLA)-DR2 and HLA-DQBI*0602 antigens. The prevalence is estimated at 30–50/100 000.

There are four main clinical features but not all patients have the full tetrad:

- ***Excessive daytime sleepiness*** (***EDS***). This is the usual presenting symptom and the main cause of disability. Patients have frequent irresistible sleep attacks during the day, often in inappropriate circumstances, e.g. during meals or conversations or while driving. EDS may be quantified with the Epworth Sleepiness Scale. Night-time sleep may be disrupted and, paradoxically, insomnia may occur.
- ***Cataplexy***. This is sudden loss of muscle tone leading to head droop or even falling with intact awareness. Attacks are often set off by sudden surprise or emotion, e.g. laughter.
- ***Hypnagogic/hypnopompic hallucinations***. These terms refer to dream-like hallucinations occurring while falling asleep or waking from sleep; these are often frightening.
- ***Sleep paralysis***. A brief paralysis on waking or while falling asleep is due to intrusion of rapid eye movement (REM) atonia into wakefulness. This occasionally occurs in people without narcolepsy.

Diagnosis and management

Multiple sleep latency testing demonstrating a rapid transition from wakefulness to sleep and a short time to onset of REM sleep confirms the diagnosis. HLA testing may also be useful.

Good sleep hygiene advice is necessary. Modafinil dexamfetamine and methylphenidate are used to treat EDS, often with only partial response. Tricyclic antidepressants, particularly clomipramine, or SSRIs can improve cataplexy. Sodium oxybate is also used.

Parasomnias

Disruptive motor or verbal behaviours occurring during sleep are divided into REM and non-REM parasomnias, depending on which stage of sleep they arise in. They include sleepwalking, night terrors, confusional arousals and REM sleep behaviour disorder (which may be an early feature of Parkinson's disease).

Obstructive sleep apnoea

See pages 1085–1086.

Restless leg syndrome (Willis–Ekbom disease)

This affects about 10% of adults, both women and men, and is also seen in children. Most people do not seek medical advice but it can be quite severe in 2–3%. The syndrome is characterized by an unpleasant sensation of 'wanting to move' the legs with throbbing or pulling, and usually occurs when the person is resting, sitting or lying; it can be totally or partially relieved by stretching or walking. It often occurs in the evenings or night-time and appears to be more frequent in the elderly. The condition is usually idiopathic and there is a familial tendency. It has been associated with pregnancy, Parkinson's disease, uraemia or a haematinic deficiency. Some drugs have been implicated.

There is no specific treatment. Dopamine agonist drugs and benzodiazepines may help. Some suggest a decreased use of alcohol or caffeine.

Further reading

Kwan P, Schachter SC, Brodie MJ. Drug resistant epilepsy. *N Engl J Med* 2011; 365:919–926.

Leach JP, Abassi H. Modern management of epilepsy. *Clin Med* 2013; 13:84–86.

Moshé SL, Perucca E, Ryvlin P et al. Epilepsy: new advances. *Lancet* 2015; 385:884–898.

Scammell TE. Narcolepsy. *N Engl J Med* 2015; 373:2054–2662.

Shorvon SD. Epilepsy and related disorders. In: Clarke C, Howard R, Rossor M et al (eds). *Neurology: A Queen Square Textbook*. Oxford: Blackwell; 2009.

http://www.epilepsysociety.org.uk *National Society for Epilepsy, UK patient support group*.

http://www.narcolepsy.org.uk *Narcolepsy UK*.

MOVEMENT DISORDERS

Disorders of movement divide broadly into two categories:

- hypokinesias – characterized by slowed movements with increased tone (parkinsonism)
- hyperkinesias – excessive involuntary movements.

Both types may coexist: for example, in Parkinson's disease, where there are both slowed movements and tremor. Many of these disorders (not all) relate to dysfunction of the basal ganglia.

Parkinsonian disorders

Idiopathic Parkinson's disease

In 1817, James Parkinson, a physician in Hoxton, London, published *The Shaking Palsy*, describing this common worldwide condition that has a prevalence of 150/100 000. Parkinson's disease (PD) is clinically and pathologically distinct from other parkinsonian syndromes.

Aetiology

The causes of idiopathic PD are still not fully understood. The relatively uniform worldwide prevalence suggests that a single environmental agent is not responsible. There may be multiple interacting risk factors, including genetic susceptibility.

Age and gender

Prevalence increases sharply with age, particularly over 70 years, with prevalence of 1 in 200 over age 80. Ageing changes are likely to be a factor in causation. Prevalence is higher in men (1.5 : 1 male to female).

Environmental factors

Epidemiological studies consistently show a small increased risk with rural living and drinking well water. Pesticide exposure has been implicated and pesticide-induced rodent models of PD exist, which increases biological plausibility of a link. The chemical compound methyl-phenyl tetrahydropyridine (MPTP), a potent mitochondrial toxin, causes severe parkinsonism, leading to suggestions that oxidative stress may be a factor leading to neuronal cell death in idiopathic PD. Studies consistently show that non-smokers have a higher risk of PD than smokers (even after controlling for shorter life expectancy in smokers), an observation that is difficult to explain.

Genetic factors

Idiopathic PD is not usually familial but twin studies show there is a significant genetic component in early-onset PD (onset before 40). Several genetic loci for Mendelian inherited monogenic forms of PD have now been identified ***(Box 21.49)***, designated *PARK* 1–11. Most of these are rare but together they account for a large proportion of early-onset and familial PD, and a small proportion (perhaps 1–2%), of sporadic late-onset cases. The main significance of the *PARK* genes is that they provide insights into the

Box 21.49 Selected Parkinson's disease (PD) genes

Locus	Protein	Inheritance	Comments
PARK1	α-synuclein	AD	Rare but a major protein in Lewy bodies
PARK2	Parkin	AR	Responsible for most cases of juvenile PD and 20% of early-onset PD cases
PARK6	Pink-1	AR	Rare. Protein involved in mitochondrial function
PARK8	LRRK2 (a kinase of unknown function)	AD	Phenotype almost identical to sporadic PD. Found in 1% of apparently sporadic PD patients. High frequency in Jewish and North African Arab patients

AD, autosomal dominant; AR, autosomal recessive.

pathophysiological mechanisms underlying PD that may be relevant to sporadic cases. Polymorphisms in these and other genes may, in combination, constitute a susceptibility to PD that can be triggered by environmental factors or the ageing process.

Pathology

The pathological hallmarks of PD are the presence of neuronal inclusions called Lewy bodies (see pp. 877–878) and loss of the dopaminergic neurones from the pars compacta of the substantia nigra in the midbrain that project to the striatum of the basal ganglia (see ***Fig. 21.11***). Lewy bodies contain tangles of α-synuclein and ubiquitin, and become gradually more widespread as the condition progresses, spreading from the lower brainstem to the midbrain and then into the cortex. Degeneration also occurs in other basal ganglia nuclei. The extent of nigrostriatal dopaminergic cell loss correlates with the degree of akinesia.

Clinical features

PD almost always presents with the typical motor symptoms of tremor and slowness of movement but it is likely that the pathological process starts many years before these symptoms develop. By the time of first presentation, on average 70% of dopaminergic nigrostriatal cells have already been lost.

Prodromal pre-motor symptoms

Patients develop a variety of non-specific non-motor symptoms during the approximately 7 years, sometimes longer, before the motor symptoms become manifest. These include:

- anosmia (present in 90%) – the olfactory bulb is one of the first structures to be affected
- depression/anxiety (50%)
- aches and pains
- REM sleep behaviour disorder
- autonomic features – urinary urgency, hypotension
- constipation
- restless legs syndrome.

Motor symptoms

These develop slowly and insidiously, and are often initially attributed to 'old age' by patients. The core motor features of PD are:

- akinesia
- tremor
- rigidity
- postural and gait disturbance.

Slowness causes difficulty rising from a chair or getting into or out of bed. Writing becomes small (micrographia) and spidery, tending to tail off. Relatives often notice other features: slowness and an impassive face. Idiopathic PD is almost always more prominent initially on one side. The diagnosis is usually evident from the overall appearance.

Akinesia

Poverty/slowing of movement (also called bradykinesia) is the cardinal clinical feature of Parkinsonism and the main cause of disability. What distinguishes it from slowness of movement from other causes is a progressive ***fatiguing*** and ***decrement*** in amplitude and speed of repetitive movements, such as opening and closing the hand or finger tapping.

There is difficulty initiating movement. The upper limb is usually affected first and is almost always unilateral for the first years. Rapid dexterous movements are impaired, causing difficulty writing (micrographia) and doing up buttons and zips, for example. Facial immobility gives a mask-like semblance of depression. Frequency of spontaneous blinking diminishes, producing a ***serpentine stare***.

Tremor

Tremor is the presenting symptom in 70% of patients. It typically starts in the fingers or hand (3–6 Hz) and is unilateral initially, spreading later to the leg on the same side and, after some years, to the opposite side. The tremor is present at rest, and reduces or stops completely when the hand is in motion. It is often described as ***pill-rolling*** because the patient appears to be rolling something between thumb and forefinger. As with most tremors, it is made worse by emotion or stress.

Rigidity

This is a sign rather than a symptom. Stiffness on passive limb movement is described as 'lead pipe', as it is present throughout the range of movement and, unlike spasticity, is not dependent on speed of movement. When stiffness occurs with tremor (not always visible), a ratchet-like jerkiness is felt, described as 'cogwheel' rigidity.

Postural and gait changes

A stooped posture is characteristic. Gait gradually becomes shuffling with small stride length, slow turns, freezing and reduced arm swing. Postural stability eventually deteriorates, leading to falls, but this is a late-stage feature that should arouse suspicion of an alternative diagnosis if present during the first 5 years.

Speech and swallowing

Speech becomes quiet, indistinct and flat. Drooling may be an embarrassing problem and swallowing difficulty is a late feature that may eventually lead to aspiration pneumonia as a terminal event.

Cognitive and psychiatric changes

Cognitive impairment is now recognized to be common in late-stage PD (80%) and may develop into dementia. Visual hallucinations on treatment, and psychosis are not uncommon, and may herald evolving cognitive decline. Cholinesterase inhibitors (see p. 879) may be helpful.

Depression is common, probably due to involvement of serotonergic and adrenergic systems, and is a cause of reduced quality of life in PD. Anxiety is also co-morbid with PD.

The clinical evolution of PD

Most patients respond well to treatment and there is generally a period of several years in which symptoms are well controlled with relatively little disability. Response to dopaminergic drugs is never lost but treatment-related fluctuations may develop (see below), which can be limiting, especially for patients with early age at onset. Eventually, usually by the mid-seventies, late-stage, treatment-unresponsive features, such as cognitive impairment, swallowing difficulty, loss of postural stability and falls, start to emerge.

The rate of progression is very variable, with a benign form running over several decades. Usually, the course is over 10–20 years, death resulting from bronchopneumonia and immobility.

Diagnosis

There is no laboratory test; diagnosis is made by recognizing physical signs and distinguishing idiopathic PD from other Parkinsonian syndromes. Patients with suspected PD should be referred to a specialist without initiation of treatment.

MRI is normal and not necessary in typical cases. Dopamine transporter (DAT) imaging using SPECT or PET makes use of a radio-labelled ligand binding to dopaminergic terminals to assess the extent of nigrostriatal cell loss. It may occasionally be needed to distinguish PD from other causes of tremor or from drug-induced parkinsonism, but it cannot discriminate between PD and other akinetic-rigid syndromes.

Management

Education about the condition is necessary and physical activity is beneficial and should be encouraged. Dopamine replacement with levodopa or a dopamine agonist improves motor symptoms and is the basis of pharmacological therapy. Treatment of non-motor symptoms, such as depression, constipation, pain and sleep disorders, is also necessary and significantly improves quality of life.

Dopamine replacement may not always be needed in early-stage PD and is only started when symptoms begin to cause disability. The mechanism of action of drugs in PD is shown in ***Figure 21.45***.

Levodopa

Levodopa remains the most effective form of treatment and all patients with PD will eventually need it. It is combined with a dopa decarboxylase inhibitor – benserazide (co-beneldopa) or carbidopa (co-careldopa) – to reduce the peripheral adverse effects (e.g. nausea and hypotension); 50 mg of levodopa (e.g. co-careldopa 62.5 mg) three times daily, increasing after 1 week to 100 mg three times daily, is a typical starting dose. The response is often dramatic.

Dopamine agonists

Dopamine agonists (DAs) may be used in combination with levodopa or as initial monotherapy in younger patients (below age 65–70) with mild to moderate impairment. Although less efficacious in symptom control than levodopa and generally less well tolerated, DAs are associated with fewer motor complications over a 5-year

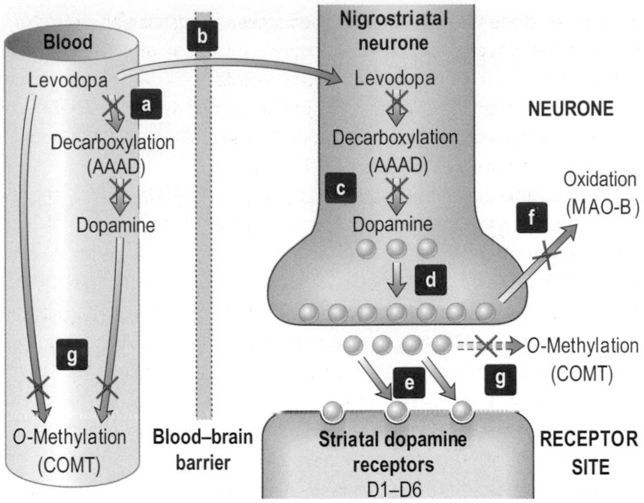

Figure 21.45 Drugs in Parkinson's disease. Levodopa crosses the blood–brain barrier, enters the nigrostriatal neurone and is converted to dopamine. **(a)** Carbidopa and benserazide reduce peripheral conversion of levodopa to dopamine, thus reducing the side-effects of circulating dopamine. **(b)** Dietary amino acids from high-protein meals can inhibit active transport across the blood–brain barrier by competing with levodopa. **(c)** Levodopa is converted (aromatic amino acid decarboxylase, AAAD) to dopamine. **(d)** Amantadine enhances dopamine release. **(e)** Dopamine agonists react with dopamine receptors. **(f)** Monoamine oxidase (MAO)-B inhibitors block dopamine breakdown. **(g)** Catechol-O-methyl transferase (COMT) inhibitors prolong dopamine activity by blocking breakdown.

period. Non-ergot DAs (pramipexole and ropinirole or rotigotine via transdermal patch) are used in preference to ergot-derived drugs, which may be associated with fibrotic reactions, including cardiac valvular fibrosis. Domperidone is used as an antiemetic when initiating DA therapy (other antiemetics should not be used, as they may worsen symptoms by blocking central dopamine receptors).

Other drugs used in PD

- ***Selegiline*** 5–10 mg once daily (a monoamine oxidase (MAO)-B inhibitor) reduces catabolism of dopamine in brain. It has a mild symptomatic effect. ***Rasagiline*** is another MAO-B inhibitor.
- ***Amantadine*** has a modest anti-parkinsonian effect but is used mainly to improve dyskinesias in advanced disease.
- ***Antimuscarinics*** (e.g. ***orphenadrine***, ***procyclidine***, ***trihexyphenidyl***) may help tremor but are rarely used in PD except in younger patients. They have a high propensity to cause confusion and cognitive impairment in older patients.
- ***Apomorphine*** is a potent, short-acting DA administered subcutaneously by an autoinjector pen as intermittent 'rescue' injection for off periods or by continuous infusion pump. It is used in advanced PD.

Long-term response to treatment

As the disease progresses, medical therapy for PD becomes more difficult as higher doses of dopamine replacement therapy are required and response becomes more unpredictable with the development of motor fluctuations and dyskinesias; response to dopaminergic drugs is never lost, however.

Approximately 10% of patients per year develop motor complications in the form of 'wearing off' (the duration of effect of individual doses of levodopa becomes progressively shorter), dyskinesias (involuntary choreiform movements) and, eventually, 'on/off' phenomena (sudden, unpredictable transitions from mobile to immobile). Eventually, patients may alternate between the 'on' state with dopamine-induced dyskinesias and periods of complete immobility ('off').

Management of the motor complications of treatment represents one of the greatest challenges in the management of PD. Strategies include:

- dose fractionation of levodopa – increasing dose frequency
- addition of the catechol-O-methyl transferase (COMT) inhibitor ***entacapone*** (200 mg with each levodopa dose) to prolong duration of action; this is also available as a combined preparation with levodopa and carbidopa
- slow-release levodopa – mostly used for overnight symptoms, as absorption is erratic and difficult to predict, so limiting effectiveness in control of daytime symptoms
- avoidance of protein-rich meals (which impair levodopa absorption) and taking doses at least 40 minutes prior to meals
- apomorphine continuous subcutaneous infusion (see above)
- deep brain stimulation and levodopa intestinal gel (see below).

Deep brain stimulation

Stereotactic insertion of electrodes into the brain has proved to be a major therapeutic advance in selected patients (usually under age 70) with disabling dyskinesias and motor fluctuations not adequately controlled with medical therapy. Targets include:

- the subthalamic nucleus – response similar to levodopa with reduction in dyskinesia
- the globus pallidus – improves dyskinesia but levodopa is still required for motor symptoms
- the thalamus – for tremor only.

Dopaminergic drugs can be reduced (but not withdrawn) after deep brain stimulation (DBS). Approximately 10% of patients will be candidates at some point, usually patients with younger onset, as they have a higher rate of motor complications such as dyskinesia. There is a trend towards earlier use of DBS before motor complications become severe.

Levodopa intestinal gel infusion

Continuous infusion of this gel into the small intestine via a jejunostomy using a patient-operated pump is effective for selected patients with severe motor complications. At present, it is used only where apomorphine and DBS are contraindicated, partly because of high costs.

Tissue transplantation

Transplantation of embryonic mesencephalic dopaminergic cells directly into the putamen has produced mixed results but is potentially promising; research is ongoing to refine the technique. Stem cells and gene therapy approaches are in development.

Physiotherapy, occupational therapy and physical aids

Physiotherapy, occupational therapy and speech therapy all have a role to play in managing PD and reducing disability, speech and swallowing problems, and falls. Walking aids are often a hindrance early on, but later a frame or a tripod may help. A variety of external cueing techniques may help with freezing.

Other akinetic–rigid syndromes

Drug-induced parkinsonism

Dopamine-blocking or depleting drugs, particularly neuroleptics (with the exception of clozapine), induce parkinsonism or worsen symptoms in affected patients, and may precipitate symptoms in elderly patients in the pre-symptomatic phase. Antimuscarinic drugs reduce these symptoms, although tardive dyskinesia may be made worse.

Atypical parkinsonism

A number of neurodegenerative disorders affect the basal ganglia, causing prominent parkinsonism as part of the clinical picture; they may be mistaken for idiopathic PD in the early stages. These include:

- ***Progressive supranuclear palsy*** (Steele–Richardson–Olszewski syndrome). This causes parkinsonism, postural instability with early falls, vertical supranuclear gaze palsy, pseudobulbar palsy and dementia. Tau deposition is seen pathologically in the substantia nigra, subthalamic nucleus and midbrain.
- ***Multiple system atrophy*** (***MSA***). Autonomic and cerebellar symptoms occur in addition to parkinsonism. Either parkinsonism or cerebellar symptoms predominate. Pathologically, α-synuclein-positive glial cytoplasmic inclusions are found in the basal ganglion, cerebellum and motor cortex. Patients do not respond to levodopa therapy. Management is symptomatic and they have a poorer prognosis than patients with Parkinson's disease.
- ***Corticobasal degeneration***. Alien limb phenomena, myoclonus and dementia occur.

These disorders are relentlessly progressive; although they sometimes respond to levodopa, they usually cause death within a decade. 'Red flag' symptoms suggesting one of these disorders include:

- symmetrical presentation and absence of tremor
- levodopa unresponsiveness (or poor response)
- early falls (within first year)
- additional neurological features.

Wilson's disease

This rare and treatable disorder of copper metabolism is inherited as an autosomal recessive trait. Copper deposition occurs in the basal ganglia, cornea and liver (see p. 479), where it can cause cirrhosis. All young patients (below age 50) with any hyperkinetic movement disorder or with liver cirrhosis should be screened for Wilson's disease (serum copper and caeruloplasmin should be checked). Intellectual impairment develops. Neurological damage is reversible with early treatment. Diagnosis and treatment with the chelating agent penicillamine are discussed on page 479.

Hyperkinetic movement disorders

There are five hyperkinetic movement disorders, which can sometimes be difficult to separate from one another and may occur in combination.

- ***tremor*** – rhythmic sinusoidal oscillation of a body part
- ***chorea*** – excessive, irregular movements flitting from one body part to another ('dance-like')
- ***myoclonus*** – brief, electric shock-like jerks

- ***tics*** – stereotyped movements or vocalizations (may be temporarily suppressed)
- ***dystonia*** – sustained muscle spasms causing twisting movements and abnormal postures.

Essential tremor

This common condition, often inherited as an autosomal dominant trait, causes a bilateral, fast, low-amplitude tremor, mainly in the upper limbs. The head and voice are occasionally involved. Tremor is postural, such as when holding a glass or cutlery. Essential tremor occurs at any age but usually starts in early life. Tremor is slowly progressive but rarely produces severe disability. There may be a cerebellar-type action tremor component. Anxiety exacerbates the tremor.

Treatment is often unnecessary or unsatisfactory. Many patients are reassured to find they do not have PD, with which essential tremor is often confused. Small amounts of alcohol, beta-blockers (propranolol), primidone or gabapentin may help. Sympathomimetics (e.g. salbutamol) make all tremors worse. Stereotactic thalamotomy and thalamic DBS are used in severe cases.

Chorea

There are a wide variety of possible causes of chorea. These include:

- systemic disease – thyrotoxicosis, SLE, antiphospholipid syndrome, polycythaemia vera
- genetic disorders – Huntington's disease and genetic phenocopies, neuroacanthocytosis, benign hereditary chorea
- structural and vascular disorders affecting the basal ganglia
- drugs (e.g. levodopa and the oral contraceptive pill)
- post-infectious (Sydenham's chorea) – following months after streptococcal infection or as part of acute rheumatic fever
- pregnancy.

Treatment is of the underlying cause but dopamine-blocking drugs, such as phenothiazines (e.g. sulpiride) and dopamine-depleting drugs (tetrabenazine), reduce chorea (as the prototypical *excessive* movement condition the treatment is the *opposite* of PD).

Huntington's disease

Huntington's disease is a cause of chorea, usually presenting in middle life, initially with subtle 'fidgetiness' followed by development of progressive psychiatric and cognitive symptoms.

Prevalence worldwide is about 5/100 000. HD is due to a CAG trinucleotide repeat expansion, which forms the basis of the diagnostic test (see p. 115). This results in translation of an expanded polyglutamine repeat sequence in huntingtin, the protein gene product, the function of which is unclear. The expansion is thought to be a toxic 'gain-of-function' mutation. Most adult-onset patients have 36–55 repeats and there is an inverse relationship between repeat length and age at onset, with juvenile-onset patients having over 60 repeats. Expansion of the unstable CAG repeat during meiosis, particularly spermatogenesis, is the molecular basis for the phenomenon of anticipation (a tendency for successive generations to have earlier onset and more severe disease), particularly when inherited from the father.

HD is inherited in an autosomal dominant manner with complete penetrance (all gene carriers will develop the disease eventually). Previous family history is often not known. There is no disease-modifying treatment at present, although chorea can improve with treatment, such as risperidone or sulpiride, but progressive neurodegeneration leads to dementia and ultimately death after 10–20 years. Patients with small or intermediate-range expansions may present in old age with isolated chorea.

Absence of treatment results in a low take-up rate for presymptomatic testing in at-risk individuals. Test centres have protocols for counselling families and addressing ethical issues.

Hemiballismus

Hemiballismus (see ***Fig. 21.11***) describes violent swinging movements of one side, usually caused by infarction or haemorrhage in the contralateral subthalamic nucleus.

Acute chorea–hemiballismus also occurs after diabetic hyperosmolar hyperglycaemia, with signal change seen in the basal ganglia on CT or MRI; it is thought to be due to osmotic shifts causing myelinolysis.

Myoclonus

Cortical myoclonus is usually distal (hands and fingers especially) and stimulus-sensitive (spontaneous but also triggered by touch or loud noises). It is caused by a wide variety of pathologies affecting the cerebral cortex; spinal and brainstem myoclonus are caused by localized lesions affecting these structures.

Primary myoclonus

Physiological myoclonus. Nocturnal myoclonus consisting of sudden jerks (often with a feeling of falling) on dropping off to sleep or waking; it is common and not pathological. The startle response is also a form of brainstem myoclonus.

Myoclonic dystonia (***DYT11***). Myoclonic 'lightning jerks', often with dystonia, are inherited as a rare autosomal dominant disorder due to mutations in the ε-sarcoglycan gene. The condition is thought to be allelic with benign essential myoclonus (caused by disruption of the same gene).

Myoclonus in epilepsy

Myoclonic jerks occurs in several forms of epilepsy (see p. 847). An antiepileptic drug, such as valproate, may be helpful.

Progressive myoclonic epilepsy–ataxia syndromes

These rare conditions include genetic and metabolic disorders in which myoclonus accompanies progressive epilepsy, cognitive decline and/or ataxia. ***Lafora body disease***, ***neuronal ceroid lipofuscinosis*** and ***Unverricht–Lundborg*** disease are examples.

Secondary myoclonus

Myoclonus may be seen in a wide variety of metabolic disorders, including hepatic and renal failure (asterixis), as part of several dementias and neurodegenerative disorders (e.g. Alzheimer's disease) and encephalitis.

Post-anoxic myoclonus sometimes follows severe cerebral anoxia.

Tics

Tics are common (15% lifetime prevalence), brief, stereotyped movements usually affecting the face or neck but which may involve any body part; they include vocal tics. Unlike other movement disorders, they may be transiently suppressed, leading to a build-up of anxiety and overflow after release.

Simple transient tics (e.g. blinking, sniffing or facial grimacing) are common in childhood but may persist. Adult-onset tics are rare and usually have a secondary cause. The borderland between normal and pathological is vague.

Tourette syndrome

The most common cause of tics, characterized by multiple motor tics and at least one vocal tic, starts in childhood and persists longer than a year. Boys are affected more often than girls in a 3 : 1 ratio. Behavioural problems, including attention deficit hyperactivity disorder (ADHD) and obsessive–compulsive disorder (OCD), are common and may sometimes be the major cause of disability. There is sometimes explosive barking and grunting of obscenities (coprolalia) and gestures (copropraxia) or echolalia (copying what other people say). Many affected individuals never come to medical attention. The cause is not known but it may be a complex problem with histaminergic neurotransmission.

Dystonias

Dystonia ***(Box 21.50)*** is most usefully classified by aetiology into:

- ***primary dystonias*** – where dystonia is the only, or main, clinical manifestation (usually genetic)
- ***secondary dystonia*** – due to brain injury, cerebral palsy or drugs, for example
- ***heredo-degenerative dystonia*** – part of a wider neurodegenerative disorder
- ***paroxysmal dystonias*** – rare, mostly genetic, attacks of sudden involuntary movements with elements of dystonia and chorea.

Primary dystonias

Young onset. Mutations in the *DYT1* gene locus, seen particularly in the Ashkenazi Jewish population, cause limb-onset dystonia (usually foot), before the age of 28. Most patients have a three base-pair GAG deletion in the torsinA endoplasmic reticulum ATPase protein encoded by the *DYT1* gene. Penetrance is low (autosomal dominant) and phenotype very variable, but the disorder often spreads over years to become generalized dystonia, and can result in severe disability. Cognitive function remains normal. The condition is rare and the definitive form of treatment for severe cases is DBS (electrodes inserted into the globus pallidus).

Adult onset. This is much the most common type of primary dystonia. Onset is usually around 55 and dystonia is usually focal (restricted to one body part), particularly affecting the head and neck, unlike *DYT1* dystonia. Various patterns are recognized.

Torticollis

Dystonic spasms gradually develop in neck muscles, causing the head to turn (torticollis) or to be drawn backwards (retrocollis). There may also be a jerky head tremor. A gentle touch with a fingertip at a specific site may relieve the spasm temporarily (sensory trick or 'geste').

Box 21.50 A classification of dystonias

- Generalized dystonia
- Primary torsion dystonia (PTD)
- Dopamine-responsive dystonia (DRD)
- Drug-induced dystonia (e.g. metoclopramide)
- Symptomatic dystonia (e.g. after encephalitis lethargica or in Wilson's disease)
- Paroxysmal dystonia (very rare, familial, with marked fluctuation)
- Local dystonia
- Spasmodic torticollis
- Writer's cramp
- Oromandibular dystonia
- Blepharospasm
- Hemiplegic dystonia, e.g. following stroke
- Multiple sclerosis – rare

Writer's cramp and task-specific dystonias

There is a specific inability to perform a previously highly developed, repetitive, skilled movement, such as writing. The movement provokes dystonic posturing. Other functions of the hand remain normal. Overuse may lead to task-specific dystonias in certain occupations, such as musicians, typists and even golfers.

Blepharospasm and oromandibular dystonia

These consist of spasms of forced blinking or involuntary movement of the mouth and tongue (e.g. lip-smacking and protrusion of the tongue and jaw). Speech may be affected.

Dopa-responsive dystonia

In this rare disorder, dystonia is completely abolished by small doses of levodopa. Typically, dystonic walking begins in childhood and may resemble a spastic paraparesis or even present as cerebral palsy. Dominantly inherited mutations in the *GTP* cyclohydrolase gene on chromosome 14q21.3 (necessary for synthesis of a co-factor – tetrahydrobiopterin – needed for dopamine synthesis) lead to brain dopamine deficiency. Patients with dystonic gaits are sometimes given test doses of levodopa.

Neuroleptics and movement disorders

Neuroleptics (antipsychotic drugs used to treat schizophrenia) and related drugs used as antiemetics (e.g. metoclopramide) can cause a variety of movement disorders:

- ***Akathisia***. This is a restless, repetitive and irresistible need to move.
- ***Parkinsonism***. This is due to D_1 and D_2 dopamine receptor blockade (see above).
- ***Acute dystonic reactions***. Spasmodic torticollis, trismus and oculogyric crises (episodes of sustained upward gaze) develop, dramatically and unpredictably, after single doses.
- ***Tardive dyskinesia***. These mouthing and lip-smacking grimaces occur after several years of neuroleptic use. They often become temporarily worse when the drug is stopped or the dose reduced. Even if treatment ceases, resolution seldom follows. Atypical neuroleptics are less prone to cause this complication.

Management

Targeted injection of botulinum toxin into affected muscles is now the principal form of treatment for all focal dystonias. Antimuscarinics (e.g. trihexyphenidyl) are sometimes helpful.

Further reading

Kalia LV, Lang AE. Parkinson's disease. *Lancet* 2015; 386:896–912.
Obeso JA, Rodriguez-Oroz MC, Stamelou M et al. Expanding the universe of disorders of basal ganglion. *Lancet* 2014; 384:523–531.
Schapira AH, Olanow CW, Greenamyre JT et al. Slowing of neurodegeneration in Parkinson's disease and Huntington's disease: future therapeutic perspectives. *Lancet* 2014; 384:545–555.
Stoessi AJ, Leherly S, Strafella AD. Imaging insights into basal ganglion function, Parkinson's disease and dystonia. *Lancet* 2014; 384:532–544.

NEUROINFLAMMATORY DISORDERS

Multiple sclerosis is by far the most common neuroinflammatory disorder in Western populations. Other CNS inflammatory conditions include post-infectious disorders such as acute disseminated encephalomyelitis (ADEM) and transverse myelitis, distinct autoimmune disorders such as neuromyelitis optica (NMO), and multisystem inflammatory disorders such as sarcoidosis and Behçet's disease.

Multiple sclerosis

Multiple sclerosis (MS) is a chronic autoimmune, T-cell-mediated, inflammatory disorder of the CNS. Multiple plaques of demyelination are found throughout the brain and spinal cord, occurring sporadically over years (dissemination in space and time is crucial for diagnosis).

MS is a major cause of disability in young adults but several disease-modifying therapies are now available.

Epidemiology

Prevalence. MS is a common neurological disorder with over 2500000 cases worldwide. In the UK, the prevalence is 1.2/1000. Approximately 80000 people in the UK have MS.

Gender. Women outnumber men by 2 : 1. There is evidence that this ratio is widening, with an increasing proportion of women being affected.

Age. Presentation is typically between 20 and 40 years of age. Presentation after age 60 is rare, although diagnosis may sometimes be much delayed, occurring years after the initial symptoms.

Prevalence varies widely in different geographical regions and ethnic groups. This probably reflects both genetic (see below) and environmental influences in pathogenesis. MS is much more common in white populations and with increasing distance from the equator. Even within the UK, there is a north–south divide, prevalence being higher in Scotland than southern England. Migration studies show that children moving from a low-risk to a high-risk area (e.g. the UK) develop a higher risk of MS, similar to the population of the country to which they migrate, indicating that environmental factors are a factor in pathogenesis.

Other autoimmune disorders occur with increased frequency in patients with MS and their relatives, indicating a genetic predisposition to autoimmunity.

Aetiology and pathogenesis

MS is a T-cell-mediated autoimmune disease that causes an inflammatory process mainly within the white matter of the brain and spinal cord. The aetiology of MS is complex and not yet fully understood.

Genetic susceptibility

Multiple genes interact to confer an increased risk of MS, giving a complex polygenic inheritance pattern. Genetic differences between different populations probably account for part of the observed variation in MS incidence around the world.

Family studies show that there is a much-increased risk of MS in first-degree relatives of affected patients (approximately 5% lifetime risk of developing MS). Twin studies confirm a major genetic component to susceptibility, with 30% of monozygotic twins being concordant for MS versus 5% of dizygotic twins.

Genes. Variations in some 60 different genes have been identified as conferring an increased risk of MS; 80% of these are genes relating to immune system function and regulation, including HLA and major histocompatibility complex (MHC) polymorphisms. HLA-associated genes include haplotypes HLA-DRB1*1501, DQA1*102 and DQB1*0602. HLA-DR15 appears to be associated with an earlier disease onset.

Environmental factors

Migration studies (see above) and twin studies indicate that environmental factors play a role in the development of MS but these factors are still largely unknown. Viral infections can precipitate MS relapses, and exposure to infectious agents at critical times in development may trigger MS in genetically susceptible individuals. There is evidence that exposure to Epstein–Barr virus (EBV) may be linked to MS; EBV seropositivity is higher in patients with MS than in the general population. Human herpesvirus 6 (HHV-6) has also been implicated. Exposure to infectious agents in childhood may reduce the risk of developing MS and other autoimmune disorders (the 'hygiene hypothesis'). There is also some evidence that low levels of vitamin D and lack of sunlight exposure may be a risk factor for MS.

Pathology

Plaques of demyelination, 2–10 mm in size, are the cardinal features ***(Fig. 21.46)***. Plaques occur anywhere in CNS white matter but have a predilection for distinct CNS sites: optic nerves, the periventricular region, the corpus callosum, the brainstem and its cerebellar connections, and the cervical cord (corticospinal tracts and posterior columns). MRI studies show that most inflammatory plaques are asymptomatic. Recent advances in pathology and MRI techniques show that the grey matter of the cortex and the sub-pial meninges is also affected from an early stage in MS. Peripheral myelinated nerves are not directly affected in MS.

Acute relapses are caused by focal inflammation causing myelin damage and conduction block. Recovery follows as inflammation subsides and remyelination occurs. When damage is severe, secondary permanent axonal destruction occurs. Progressive axonal damage is the pathological basis of the progressive disability seen in progressive forms of MS. The extent of grey matter damage correlates with the severity of disability and cognitive involvement. The exact relationship between the inflammatory lesions seen in early relapsing–remitting forms of MS and the progressive axonal loss of chronic forms of MS is disputed.

Clinical features

No single group of signs or symptoms is diagnostic. A wide variety of possible symptoms may occur, depending on the anatomical site of the lesions; MS has been described as the modern 'great imitator'. The clinical time course of attacks and tempo of evolution of

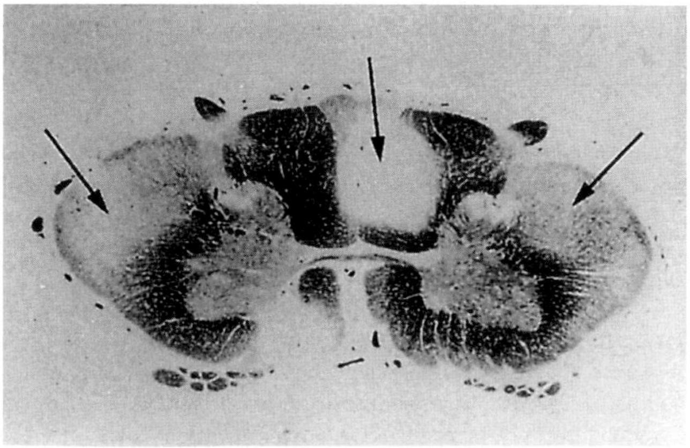

Figure 21.46 Multiple sclerosis (MS). Cross-section of spinal cord showing MS plaques in posterior column and lateral corticospinal tracts (arrowed). *(Courtesy of the late Professor Ian Macdonald.)*

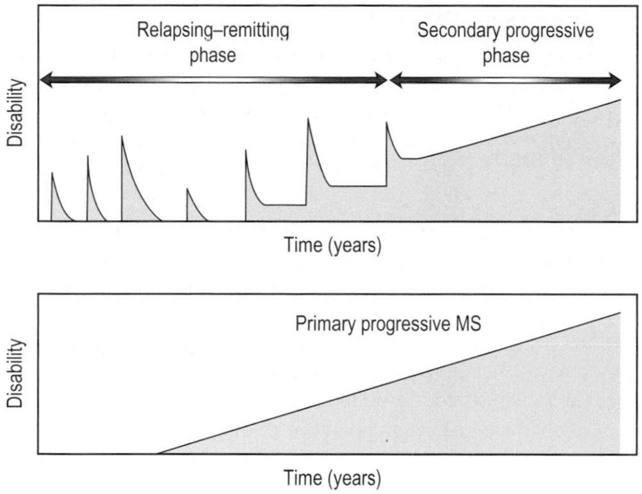

Figure 21.47 **Clinical patterns of multiple sclerosis.**

symptoms are as helpful as the symptoms themselves in making the diagnosis of MS.

Types of MS

There are four main clinical patterns ***(Fig. 21.47)***:

- ***Relapsing–remitting MS*** (***RRMS***) (85–90%). This is the most common pattern of MS. Symptoms occur in attacks (relapses) with a characteristic time course: onset over days and typically recovery, either partial or complete, over weeks. On average, patients have one relapse per year but occasionally many years may separate relapses (benign MS – 10% of patients). Patients may accumulate disability over time if they do not recover fully after relapses.
- ***Secondary progressive MS***. This late stage of MS consists of gradually worsening disability progressing slowly over years. Some 75% of patients with relapsing–remitting MS will eventually evolve into a secondary progressive phase by 35 years after onset. Relapses may sometimes occur in this progressive phase (relapsing–progressive MS).
- ***Primary progressive MS*** (***PPMS***) (10–15%). This pattern is characterized by gradually worsening disability without relapses or remissions. It typically presents later and is associated with fewer inflammatory changes on MRI.
- ***Relapsing–progressive MS*** (<5%). This is the least common form of MS. It is similar to PPMS but with occasional supra-added relapses on a background of progressive disability from the outset.

Clinical presentations

Three characteristic common presentations of MS are optic neuropathy (neuritis), brainstem demyelination and spinal cord lesions.

Optic neuritis

See page 803.

Brainstem demyelination

A relapse affecting the brainstem causes combinations of diplopia, vertigo, facial numbness/weakness, dysarthria or dysphagia. Pyramidal signs in the limbs occur when the corticospinal tracts are involved. A typical picture is sudden diplopia, and vertigo with nystagmus, but without tinnitus or deafness. Bilateral internuclear ophthalmoplegia (see p. 805) is pathognomonic of MS.

Spinal cord lesions

Paraparesis developing over days or weeks (see ***Box 21.60***) is a typical result of a plaque in the cervical or thoracic cord, causing difficulty in walking and limb numbness with tingling, often asymmetric. Lhermitte's sign may be present (see p. 817). Sometimes the arms are also involved in high cervical cord lesions. A tight band sensation around the abdomen or chest is common with thoracic cord lesions.

Common symptoms in MS

Disability and neurological impairments accumulate gradually over the years. Several symptoms are common and many can be improved with symptomatic treatments.

- Visual changes (see p. 803).
- Sensory symptoms – often unusual, e.g. a sensation of water trickling down the skin. Sensory symptoms are the presenting feature in 40% of patients. Reduced vibration sensation and proprioception in the feet are among the most common abnormalities on examination, but examination may be normal despite significant sensory symptoms.
- Clumsy/useless hand or limb – due to loss of proprioception (often a dorsal column spinal plaque).
- Unsteadiness or ataxia.
- Urinary symptoms – bladder hyper-reflexia causing urinary urgency and frequency. Treatment is with antimuscarinics or intravesical botulinum toxin injections.
- Pain – neuropathic pain is common.
- Fatigue – a common and often debilitating symptom, which can occur in patients with otherwise mild disease. This sometimes responds to amantadine or a fatigue management programme.
- Spasticity – may require baclofen or other muscle relaxants. Occasionally, botulinum toxin injections are used for focal spasticity.
- Depression.
- Sexual dysfunction.
- Temperature sensitivity – temporary worsening of pre-existing symptoms with increases in body temperature, e.g. after exercise or a hot bath, is known as Uhthoff's phenomenon.

Unusual presentations

Epilepsy and trigeminal neuralgia (see p. 845) occur more commonly in MS patients than in the general population. Tonic spasms (frequent brief spasms of one limb) are rare but pathognomonic of MS.

Late-stage MS

Late MS causes severe disability with spastic tetraparesis, ataxia, optic atrophy, nystagmus, brainstem signs (e.g. bilateral internuclear ophthalmoplegia), pseudobulbar palsy and urinary incontinence. Cognitive impairment, often with frontal lobe features, may occur in late-stage disease. In a proportion of patients, disability eventually becomes severe, with median time to requiring walking aids of 15 years and time to wheelchair use 25 years from onset.

Diagnosis

Few other neurological diseases have a similar relapsing and remitting course. The diagnosis of MS requires two or more attacks affecting different parts of the CNS: that is, dissemination in time and space, and exclusion of other possible causes. History and support from investigations, particularly MRI, make the diagnosis. The McDonald criteria formalize the diagnostic features but are

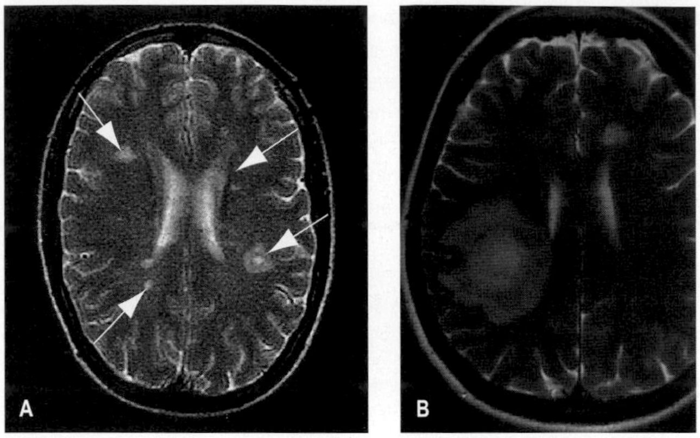

Figure 21.48 Multiple sclerosis. A. T2-weighted magnetic resonance image. Brain plaques are shown (arrowed). Typical lesions are oval in shape, up to 2 cm in diameter, and often orientated perpendicular to the lateral ventricles. **B.** Tumefactive multiple sclerosis lesion.

designed mainly for research purposes and rarely used in clinical practice.

When taking a history at the time of initial presentation, it is essential to ask about previous episodes of neurological symptoms, often years previously, that may represent episodes of unrecognized demyelination: for example, a severe episode of vertigo lasting weeks or loss of vision in one eye that gradually recovered.

Investigations

The purpose of investigations is to provide supportive evidence of dissemination in time and space (i.e. to show scattered demyelinating lesions that evolve over time), to exclude other diseases and to provide evidence of immunological disturbance.

- MRI of brain and cord is the definitive investigation, as it demonstrates areas of demyelination with high sensitivity. Multiple scattered plaques are usually seen ***(Fig. 21.48A)***, demonstrating dissemination in space. Typical lesions are oval in shape, up to 2 cm in diameter, and often orientated perpendicular to the lateral ventricles. Occasionally, large 'tumefactive' (swelling) lesions are seen ***(Fig. 21.48B)***. Acute lesions show gadolinium enhancement for 6–8 weeks. Although a sensitive technique to demonstrate plaques (normal MRI in MS is possible but distinctly rare), it is limited by lower specificity. Over the age of 50, small ischaemic lesions may be difficult to distinguish from demyelination, and in younger patients other neuroinflammatory disorders such as sarcoidosis, Behçet syndrome and vasculitis may produce similar imaging appearances. The presence of spinal cord lesions is quite specific for inflammatory disorders such as MS rather than ischaemic lesions, so cord imaging is often useful where there is diagnostic difficulty.
- Plaques are rarely visible on CT.
- CSF examination is often unnecessary with suggestive MRI imaging and a compatible clinical picture. CSF analysis shows oligoclonal IgG bands in over 90% of cases but these are not specific for MS. The CSF cell count may be raised (5–60 mononuclear cells/mm^3).
- Evoked responses, e.g. visual evoked responses in optic nerve lesions, may demonstrate clinically silent lesions. However, since the advent of MRI, they are less used in diagnosis.
- Blood tests are used to exclude other inflammatory disorders such as sarcoidosis or SLE, or other causes of paraparesis, e.g. adrenoleucodystrophy, HIV, human T-cell lymphotropic virus 1 (HTLV-1) and vitamin B_{12} deficiency.

The clinically isolated syndrome (CIS)

In patients presenting with a first ever episode of neurological symptoms suggestive of neuroinflammation, termed a 'clinically isolated syndrome' (CIS), a diagnosis of MS cannot be made by definition. In up to 70% of such patients, MRI shows multiple clinically silent lesions. An abnormal brain MRI at presentation, with multiple inflammatory-type lesions, confers an 85% chance of developing MS over subsequent years (50% if presenting with optic neuritis). Patients need to be made aware of this possibility.

A second clinical event indicative of a new lesion in a different anatomical location allows the diagnosis of MS to be confirmed. Alternatively, a repeat MRI brain scan at least 1 month later showing either a new lesion or a gadolinium-enhancing lesion is sufficient to demonstrate dissemination in time and space and confirm the diagnosis, even in the absence of new symptoms.

Management

There is no cure for MS but, in recent years, several immunomodulatory treatments have been introduced that have dramatically altered the ability to modify the course of the inflammatory relapsing–remitting phase of MS. It is hoped that these will translate into reduced long-term disability but this has yet to be proven.

General measures

Education, provision of appropriate written materials and support from a multidisciplinary team, including an MS nurse specialist, are essentials. Treatments are available for various symptoms, e.g. pain, spasticity and urinary features ***(Box 21.51)***. Physiotherapy and occupational therapy are helpful where there is persisting impairment between relapses. Infections should be treated early, as they may precipitate relapses or lead to worsening of existing symptoms. Immunizations are safe (but not live vaccines if on disease-modifying drugs).

Acute relapses

Short courses of steroids, such as i.v. methylprednisolone 1 g/day for 3 days or high-dose oral steroids, are used for severe relapses. They speed recovery but do not influence long-term outcome.

Disease-modifying drugs

Immunomodulatory disease-modifying drugs (DMDs; ***Box 21.52***), such as β-interferon (both IFN-β1b and 1a, and pegylated β1a) and glatiramer acetate, reduce relapse rate by one-third and serious relapses by up to half in RRMS. They also significantly reduce development of new MRI lesions and may reduce accumulation of disability over the short term. They are self-administered by subcutaneous or intramuscular injection and are generally well tolerated, apart from influenza-like side-effects and injection site irritation. From a health economics point of view, cost is an issue, as these drugs are very expensive. IFN-β and glatiramer acetate are considered first-line DMDs. ***Current recommendations*** in the UK are that DMDs are offered to ambulant patients with RRMS where there have been two or more *significant* relapses over a 2-year period or after one major disabling relapse. When used after CIS, the conversion rate to definite MS is reduced from 50% to 30% over 3 years, but in the UK treatment with DMDs after CIS is rarely

Box 21.51 Symptomatic treatments in multiple sclerosis

Urinary symptoms
- Antimuscarinics, e.g. oxybutynin, tolterodine, solifenacin, trospium
- Desmopressin spray ± antimuscarinic
- Intermittent self-catheterization (ISC)
- Botulinum toxin type A intravesical injections (usually also require ISC)
- Bladder training exercises
- Indwelling catheter

Spasticity
- Self-management, including stretching, physiotherapy, splinting
- Skeletal muscle relaxants: baclofen, tizanidine, clonazepam
- Gabapentin
- Botulinum toxin type A (electromyelography-guided injections) for focal spasticity
- Cannabis: oromucosal spray
- Intrathecal baclofen pump
- Intrathecal phenol destructive procedure in advanced disease with paraplegia

Pain
- As for treatment of neuropathic pain (see pp. 819–820)
- Trigeminal neuralgia – carbamazepine, lamotrigine
- Lhermitte's – carbamazepine

Depression
- Cognitive behavioural therapy
- Antidepressants (see p. 901)

Impaired mobility
- Physiotherapy ± walking aids
- Treat spasticity
- Fampridine – selected patients

Erectile dysfunction
- Sildenafil, tadalafil or vardenafil

Tremor
- Beta-adrenoceptor-blocking drugs
- Botulinum toxin type A injections (head or arms)
- Deep brain stimulation for severe Holmes tremor

Fatigue
- Fatigue management programme, treat depression
- Amantadine (often ineffective)

recommended. DMDs are not effective in primary progressive or secondary progressive MS.

Oral DMDs

Three oral agents, ***fingolimod***, ***teriflunomide*** and ***dimethyl fumarate***, have been licensed for treatment of RRMS. They all reduce relapse rate significantly and, in the case of fingolimod and dimethyl fumarate, are superior to interferons. In general, they seem well tolerated but have more serious adverse events than interferons. Their exact place in MS treatment is not yet established (cost is an issue); in some countries, they are used as first-line DMDs but in the UK are likely to be used where first-line drugs are not tolerated or not sufficiently effective.

Treatment of aggressive RRMS

Immunomodulatory drugs and biological agents (monoclonal antibodies), such as ***natalizumab*** and ***alemtuzumab***, have shown high efficacy in preventing relapses and may reduce accumulation of disability significantly ***(Box 21.52)***. They have the potential to cause serious adverse effects and are generally used only in very aggressive disease or where relapses are not reduced by β-IFN or glatiramer acetate.

Other drugs and symptomatic therapies

- ***Vitamin D***. There is some evidence that vitamin D supplementation may be beneficial in MS but this is still controversial. Some specialists advocate treatment with up to 2000 IU daily.
- ***Fampridine*** (4-aminopyridine, an oral potassium-channel blocker). This has been shown to improve walking significantly in selected patients with significant MS-related disability.
- ***Other symptomatic treatments***. Symptomatic treatments are available for most complications of MS and significantly improve quality of life ***(Box 21.51)***. Urinary urgency and frequency, pain, spasticity and depression are all common and treatable.

Box 21.52 Disease-modifying drugs used in relapsing–remitting multiple sclerosis

Drug	Mode of action	Administration	Reduction in relapse rate	Effect on disability	Adverse effects/ comments
β-interferon (IFN-β1b and 1a)	Immunomodulatory	s.c. alternate days or i.m. weekly	33%	?	Few
Glatiramer acetate	Unknown	s.c. daily	33%	?	Few
Natalizumab	MCA blocks α-4 integrin vascular adhesion molecule. Prevents T cells entering CNS	i.v. monthly	68%	+	Rarely, PML (fatal) Hypersensitivity reactions
Alemtuzumab	MCA. Anti-CD52. Depletes T > B cells	i.v. once and repeat at 1 year	65% relapse-free at 4 years	++	Autoimmune disorders: Graves' disease and ITP
Fingolimod	Sphingosine-1-phosphate receptor (S1-PR) ligand. Prevents T cells leaving lymph nodes	Oral daily	60%	?+	Bradycardia and increased infection rate
Dimethyl fumarate	Unknown	Oral twice daily	50–60%	?	Good safety record in psoriasis; well tolerated but one case of PML
Teriflunomide	Blocks proliferation of activated lymphocytes	Oral daily	30%	+	Abnormal liver enzymes
Mitoxantrone	Cytotoxic agent	i.v. every 3 months	?>60%	?	Cardiotoxicity and secondary malignancy. Sometimes used in relapsing–progressive MS

ITP, immune thrombocytopenic purpura; MCA, monoclonal antibody; PML, progressive multifocal leucoencephalopathy.

Prognosis

The clinical course of MS is unpredictable; a high MR lesion load at initial presentation, high relapse rate, male gender and late presentation are poor prognostic features but not invariably so. There is wide variation in severity. Many patients continue to live independent, productive lives; a minority become severely disabled. Life expectancy is reduced by 7 years on average.

Transverse myelitis

Transverse myelitis is an acute inflammatory disorder affecting the spinal cord with cord swelling and loss of function. Typically, one or two spinal segments are affected with part or all of the cord area at that level involved (*transverse* indicates involvement of the whole cross-section of the cord at the affected level). Clinically, a myelopathy evolves over days, and recovery (often partial) follows over weeks or months. MRI is sensitive and shows cord swelling and oedema with gadolinium enhancement at the affected level(s). Usually, images are also taken of the brain to look for evidence of demyelination. CSF may be inflammatory with an excess of lymphocytes. Causes include:

- ***Para-infectious autoimmune inflammatory response***. This is the most common cause and may follow viral infection or immunization, for example.
- ***Systemic inflammatory disorders***, e.g. SLE, Sjögren's, sarcoidosis.
- ***Infection***. This may be caused by viruses – e.g. herpesviruses, such as varicella zoster or EBV, HIV, HTLV-1 and 2 (tropical spastic paraparesis); mycobacteria, e.g. tuberculosis; bacteria – e.g. syphilis and Lyme disease; or flatworms – e.g. schistosomiasis.
- ***Multiple sclerosis***. Transverse myelitis may occur as part of a relapse or be a presenting feature of MS. If the brain MRI is normal, the risk of later development of MS is around 20%; in those that do develop MS with a normal brain MRI, prognosis is better than average.
- ***Neuromyelitis optica*** – see below.

Treatment is usually with high-dose steroids or other immunosuppression, or antimicrobial therapy in the case of specific infections.

Neuromyelitis optica

This is a distinct inflammatory relapsing demyelinating disorder, previously thought to be a variant of MS. It is characterized by longitudinally extensive transverse myelitis (>3 segments) and bilateral or recurrent optic neuritis. Limited forms occur, such as recurrent myelitis only. Serum antibodies to aquaporin-4 water channels on astrocytes are diagnostic. It is rarer than MS but there is a higher incidence in Asians and Afro-Caribbeans.

Treatment with steroids and immunosuppressive drugs is essential from the time of diagnosis, as the relapse rate is high and relapses are much more disabling than in MS. A similar syndrome that follows a monophasic course occurs with myelin oligodendrocyte (MOG) antibodies.

Acute disseminated encephalomyelitis

Acute disseminated encephalomyelitis (ADEM) is usually post-infectious, following infections such as measles, mycoplasma, mumps and rubella, and occasionally following 1–2 weeks after immunization. There is a monophasic illness with multifocal brain, brainstem and often spinal cord inflammatory lesions in white matter, with demyelination. ADEM is caused by an immune-mediated host response to infection and occurs principally in children and young adults. Mild cases recover completely. Survivors often have permanent brain damage. Treatment is supportive, with steroids and anticonvulsants.

Other neuroinflammatory conditions

Neurosarcoidosis

Neurosarcoid with or without systemic sarcoid causes chronic meningoencephalitis, cord lesions, cranial nerve palsies – particularly bilateral VIIth nerve lesions, polyneuropathy and myopathy (see pp. 1118–1120). Diagnosis can be difficult if disease is confined to the CNS.

Behçet's disease

Behçet's principal features (see p. 702) are recurrent oral and/or genital ulceration, inflammatory ocular disease (uveitis; see pp. 1332–1333) and neurological syndromes. Brainstem and cord lesions, aseptic meningitis, encephalitis and cerebral venous thrombosis occur. There is a predilection for ethnic groups along the ancient 'Silk Road' – Turkey, the Middle East and Asia. Behçet's is associated with the HLA-B51 allele.

Further reading

Frohman EM, Wingerchuk DM. Clinical practice. Transverse myelitis. *N Engl J Med* 2010; 363:564–572.
Perry M, Swain S, Kemmis-Betty S et al. Multiple sclerosis: summary of NICE guidance. *BMJ* 2014; 349:g5701.
Polman CH, Reingold SC, Banwell B et al. Diagnostic criteria for multiple sclerosis: 2010 revisions to the McDonald criteria. *Ann Neurol* 2011; 69:292–302.
Scolding N, Barnes D, Cader S et al. Association of British Neurologists: revised (2015) guidelines for prescribing disease-modifying treatments in multiple sclerosis. *Pract Neurol* 2015; 15:273–279.
http://www.mssociety.org.uk *MS Society (UK National Charity).*

NERVOUS SYSTEM INFECTION

Meningitis

Meningitis usually implies serious *infection* of the meninges ***(Box 21.53)***. Bacterial meningitis is fatal unless treated. Microorganisms

Box 21.53 Infective causes of meningitis in the UK

Bacteria
- *Neisseria meningitidis*
- *Streptococcus pneumoniae*[a]
- *Staphylococcus aureus*
- *Streptococcus* group B
- *Listeria monocytogenes*
- Gram-negative bacilli, e.g. *Escherichia coli*
- *Mycobacterium tuberculosis*
- *Treponema pallidum*

Viruses
- Enteroviruses:
  - ECHO
  - Coxsackie
- (Poliomyelitis – mainly eradicated worldwide)
- Mumps
- Herpes simplex
- HIV
- Epstein–Barr

Fungi
- *Cryptococcus neoformans*
- *Candida albicans*
- *Coccidioides immitis, Histoplasma capsulatum, Blastomyces dermatitidis* (USA)

[a]*These organisms account for 70% of acute bacterial meningitis outside the neonatal period. A wide variety of infective agents are responsible for the remaining 30% of cases.* Haemophilus influenzae b *(Hib) has been eliminated as a cause in many countries by immunization. Malaria often presents with cerebral symptoms and a fever.*

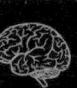

reach the meninges either by direct extension from the ears, nasopharynx, cranial injury or congenital meningeal defect, or by bloodstream spread. Immunocompromised patients are at risk of infection with unusual organisms. Non-infective causes of meningeal inflammation include malignant meningitis, intrathecal drugs and blood following subarachnoid haemorrhage.

Pathology

In acute bacterial meningitis, the pia-arachnoid is congested with polymorphs. A layer of pus forms. This may organize to form adhesions, causing cranial nerve palsies and hydrocephalus.

In chronic infection (e.g. tuberculosis), the brain is covered in a viscous grey–green exudate with numerous meningeal tubercles. Adhesions are invariable. Cerebral oedema occurs in any bacterial meningitis.

In viral meningitis there is a predominantly lymphocytic inflammatory CSF reaction without pus formation, polymorphs or adhesions; there is little or no cerebral oedema unless encephalitis develops.

Clinical features

The meningitic syndrome

This is a simple triad: headache, neck stiffness and fever. Photophobia and vomiting are often present. In acute bacterial infection, there is usually intense malaise, fever, rigors, severe headache, photophobia and vomiting, developing within hours or minutes. The patient is irritable and often prefers to lie still. Neck stiffness and a positive Kernig's sign usually appear within hours.

In less severe cases (e.g. many viral meningitides), there are less prominent meningitic signs. However, bacterial infection may also be indolent, with a deceptively mild onset.

In uncomplicated meningitis, consciousness remains intact, although anyone with a high fever may be delirious. Progressive drowsiness, lateralizing signs and cranial nerve lesions indicate complications such as venous sinus thrombosis (see p. 848), severe cerebral oedema or hydrocephalus, or an alternative diagnosis such as cerebral abscess (see p. 867) or encephalitis (see pp. 865–866).

Specific varieties of meningitis

Clinical clues point to the diagnosis ***(Box 21.54)***. If there is access to the subarachnoid space via skull fracture (recent or old) or occult spina bifida, bacterial meningitis can be recurrent, and the infecting organism is usually pneumococcus.

Box 21.54 Clinical clues in meningitis

Clinical feature	Possible cause
Petechial rash	Meningococcal infection
Skull fracture **Ear disease** **Congenital CNS lesion**	Pneumococcal infection
Immunocompromised patients	HIV with opportunistic infection
Rash or pleuritic pain	Enterovirus infection
International travel	Malaria
Occupational (work in drains, canals, polluted water, recreational swimming) **Clinical:** myalgia, conjunctivitis, jaundice	Leptospirosis

Acute bacterial meningitis

Onset is typically sudden, with rigors and high fever. Meningococcal septicaemia is associated with a petechial rash, sometimes sparse (***Box 21.55*** and ***Fig. 21.49***). The meningitis may be part of a generalized meningococcal septicaemia with septic shock and peripheral vascular infarcts (see pp. 281–282). Acute septicaemic shock may develop in any bacterial meningitis.

Viral meningitis

This is almost always a benign, self-limiting condition lasting 4–10 days. Headache may follow for some months. There are no serious sequelae, unless an encephalitis is present (see pp. 865–866).

Chronic meningitis (see below)

For further discussion on chronic meningitis, see below.

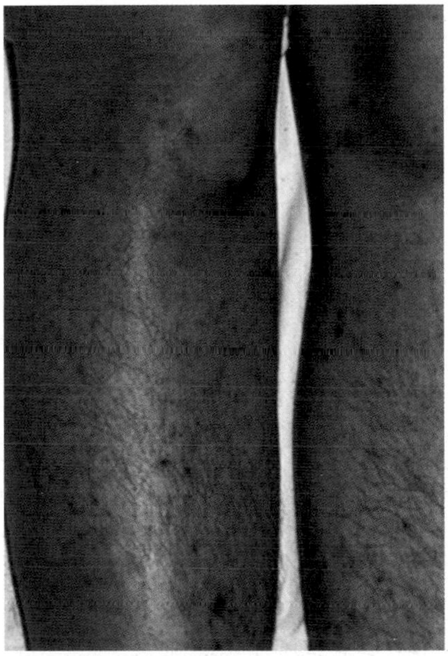

Figure 21.49 Rash of meningococcal septicaemia with meningitis.

Box 21.55 Meningococcal meningitis and meningococcaemia: emergency treatment

Suspicion of meningococcal infection is a medical emergency requiring treatment immediately.

Clinical features

- Petechial or non-specific blotchy, red rash
- Fever, headache, neck stiffness.

All these features may not be present – and meningococcal infection may sometimes begin like any apparently non-serious infection.

Immediate treatment for suspected meningococcal meningitis at first contact before investigation

- Third-generation cephalosporin, e.g. cefotaxime, as empirical therapy (increasing rates of penicillin resistance)
- Switch to benzylpenicillin if sensitivity confirmed
- Dexamethasone 0.6 mg/kg i.v. with or before first dose of antibiotic

In meningitis, minutes count – delay is unacceptable.

On arrival in hospital

- Blood tests, including blood cultures, immediately
- Monitoring for septic shock.

For further management and prophylaxis, see text.

Box 21.56 Typical changes in cerebrospinal fluid in viral, pyogenic and tuberculous meningitis

	Normal	Viral	Pyogenic	Tuberculous
Appearance	Crystal clear	Clear/turbid	Turbid/purulent	Turbid/viscous
Mononuclear cells	<5/mm³	10–100/mm³	<50/mm³	100–300/mm³
Polymorph cells	Nil	Nil[a]	200–300/mm³	0–200/mm³
Protein	0.2–0.4 g/L	0.4–0.8 g/L	0.5–2.0 g/L	0.5–3.0 g/L
Glucose	⅔–½ blood glucose	>½ blood glucose	<½ blood glucose	<½ blood glucose

[a]Some CSF polymorphs may be seen in the early stages of viral meningitis and encephalitis.

Differential diagnosis

It may be difficult to distinguish between the sudden headache of subarachnoid haemorrhage, migraine and acute meningitis. Meningitis should be considered seriously in anyone with headache and fever, and in any sudden headache. Neck stiffness should be looked for; it may not be obvious.

Chronic meningitis sometimes resembles an intracranial mass lesion, with headache, epilepsy and focal signs. Cerebral malaria can mimic bacterial meningitis.

Management

Recognition and immediate treatment of acute bacterial meningitis ***(Box 21.55)*** are vital. Minutes save lives. Bacterial meningitis has a high mortality and morbidity. Even with optimal care, mortality is around 15%. The following applies to adult patients; management is similar in children.

When meningococcal meningitis is diagnosed clinically by the petechial rash, immediate intravenous antibiotics should be given and blood cultures taken; lumbar puncture is unnecessary. In other causes of meningitis, an LP is performed if there is no clinical suspicion of a mass lesion (see p. 823). If the latter is suspected, an immediate CT scan must be performed because coning of the cerebellar tonsils may follow LP, but normal brain imaging does not exclude raised intracranial pressure and clinical features of raised pressure contraindicate LP. Typical CSF changes are shown in ***Box 21.56***. CSF pressure is characteristically elevated.

Immediate ***antibiotic*** treatment in acute bacterial meningitis is shown in ***Box 21.57***. Treatment with antibiotics should be continued for at least 5 days.

Adjunctive immediate high-dose ***steroid*** (dexamethasone 0.6 mg/kg i.v. for 4 days), given with or before the first dose of antibiotics, has been shown to reduce neurological complications in bacterial meningitis (e.g. deafness), and some studies also show reduced mortality in Western populations.

Blood should be taken for cultures, glucose and routine tests. Chest and skull films should be obtained if appropriate.

CSF stains demonstrate organisms (e.g. Gram-positive intracellular diplococci – pneumococcus; Gram-negative cocci – meningococcus). Ziehl–Neelsen stain demonstrates acid-fast bacilli (tuberculosis), though TB organisms are rarely numerous. Indian ink stains fungi.

Meticulous attention should focus on microbiological studies in suspected CNS infection with close liaison between clinician and microbiologist. Specific techniques, such as polymerase chain reaction for meningococci and viruses, or CSF bacterial antigen testing, are invaluable. Syphilis serology should always be carried out.

Local infection (e.g. paranasal sinus) should be treated surgically if necessary. Repair of a depressed skull fracture or meningeal tear may be required.

Box 21.57 Antibiotics in acute bacterial meningitis

Organism	Antibiotic	Alternative (e.g. allergy)
Unknown pyogenic	Third-generation cephalosporin, e.g. cefotaxime (+ vancomycin in areas of high pneumococcal penicillin/cephalosporin resistance)	Benzylpenicillin and chloramphenicol
Age >50 or immunocompromised	As above but add ampicillin to cover *Listeria*	Co-trimoxazole for *Listeria*
Meningococcus	Third-generation cephalosporin initially Switch to benzylpenicillin if confirmed sensitive	Cefotaxime
Pneumococcus	Third-generation cephalosporin, e.g. cefotaxime	Penicillin
Haemophilus	Third-generation cephalosporin, e.g. cefotaxime	Chloramphenicol

Prophylaxis

Meningococcal infection should be notified to the public health authorities, and advice sought about immunization and prophylaxis of contacts. Chemoprophylaxis with rifampicin or ciprofloxacin should be offered to all close contacts. MenC vaccine is given in the UK and MenB, a meningococcal B vaccine, is now available for population immunization of infants and for use in outbreaks. A combined A and C meningococcal vaccine is sometimes used prior to travel from the UK to endemic regions, such as Africa or Asia, and there is a quadrivalent ACWY vaccine for specific events, such as the Hajj and Umrah in Mecca.

Pneumococcal conjugated vaccine is now given to infants in many countries and pneumococcal polysaccharide vaccine is offered to older adults and those with, for example, immunodeficiency or splenectomy. Pneumococcal immunization has reduced the incidence of pneumococcal meningitis.

Hib (*Haemophilus influenzae*) vaccine is given routinely in childhood in the UK and many other countries, virtually eliminating a common cause of fatal meningitis.

Chronic meningitis

Tuberculous meningitis (TBM) and ***cryptococcal meningitis*** typically commence with vague headache, lassitude, anorexia and vomiting. Acute meningitis can occur but is unusual. Meningitic signs often take some weeks to develop. Drowsiness, focal signs (e.g. diplopia, papilloedema, hemiparesis) and seizures are common.

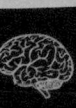

Syphilis, sarcoidosis and Behçet's also cause chronic meningitis. In some cases of chronic meningitis, an organism is never identified.

Investigation and management of tuberculous meningitis

TBM is a common and serious disease worldwide. Brain imaging, usually with MRI, may show meningeal enhancement, hydrocephalus and tuberculomas (see pp. 870–871 and 867), although it may remain normal (see **Box 21.56** for CSF changes). In many cases, the sparse tuberculous organisms cannot be seen on staining and PCR testing should be performed, although results may be negative. Repeated CSF examination is often necessary and it will be some weeks before cultures are confirmatory. Treatment with antituberculosis drugs (see p. 1111) – rifampicin, isoniazid and pyrazinamide – must commence on a presumptive basis and continue for at least 9 months. Ethambutol should be avoided because of its eye complications. Adjuvant corticosteroids, such as prednisolone 60 mg for 3 weeks, are now recommended (often tapered off). Relapses and complications (e.g. seizures, hydrocephalus) are common in TBM. The mortality remains over 60%, even with early treatment.

Malignant meningitis

Malignant cells can cause a subacute or chronic, non-infective, meningitic process. A meningitic syndrome, cranial nerve lesions, paraparesis and root lesions are seen, often in confusing and fluctuating patterns. CSF cytology may demonstrate malignant cells but yield is low so multiple LPs may be required to confirm the diagnosis. Treatment with intrathecal cytotoxic agents is sometimes helpful.

Cells in a sterile CSF (pleocytosis)

A raised CSF cell count is present without an evident infecting organism. CSF pleocytosis, i.e. a mixture of lymphocytes and polymorphs, is the usual situation **(Box 21.58)**.

Encephalitis

Encephalitis means acute inflammation of brain parenchyma, usually viral. In viral encephalitis, fever (90%) and meningism are usual; in contrast to meningitis, however, the clinical picture is dominated by brain parenchyma inflammation. Personality and behavioural change is a common early manifestation, which progresses to a reduced level of consciousness and even coma. Seizures (focal and generalized) are very common and focal neurological deficits, such as speech disturbance, often occur (especially in herpes simplex encephalitis).

Box 21.58 Causes of sterile CSF pleocytosis

- Partially treated bacterial meningitis
- Viral meningitis
- Tuberculous or fungal meningitis
- Intracranial abscess
- Neoplastic meningitis
- Parameningeal foci, e.g. paranasal sinus
- Syphilis
- Cerebral venous thrombosis
- Cerebral malaria
- Cerebral infarction
- Following subarachnoid haemorrhage
- Encephalitis, including HIV
- Rarities, e.g. cerebral malaria, sarcoidosis, Behçet syndrome, Lyme disease, endocarditis, cerebral vasculitis

Viral encephalitis

(See p. 260.) The viruses isolated from adult UK cases are usually herpes simplex (HSV), varicella zoster (VZV) and other herpes group viruses, HHV-6, 7, enteroviruses and adenovirus. HSV encephalitis typically affects the temporal lobes initially, and is often asymmetric. Frequently, the virus is never identified. Outside the UK, in endemic regions, different pathogens cause encephalitis, including flaviviruses (Japanese encephalitis, West Nile virus, tick-borne encephalitis) and rabies.

Local epidemics can occur. For example, in New York in the 1990s, West Nile virus caused an epidemic and Venezuelan equine virus was isolated from encephalitis cases in South America.

Investigations

- MRI shows areas of inflammation and swelling, generally in the temporal lobes in HSV encephalitis. Raised intracranial pressure and midline shift may occur, leading to coning.
- EEG shows periodic sharp and slow-wave complexes.
- CSF shows an elevated lymphocyte count (95%).
- Viral detection by CSF PCR is highly sensitive for several viruses, such as HSV and VZV. However, a false-negative result may occur within the first 48 hours of symptom onset. Serology (blood and CSF) is also helpful.
- Brain biopsy is rarely required since the advent of MRI and PCR.

Management

Suspected HSV and VZV encephalitis is treated immediately with intravenous aciclovir (10 mg/kg 3 times a day for 14–21 days), even before investigation results are available. Early treatment significantly reduces both mortality and long-term neurological damage in survivors. Seizures are treated with anticonvulsants. Occasionally, decompressive craniectomy is required to prevent coning but coma confers a poor prognosis.

Long-term complications are common and include memory impairment, personality change and epilepsy.

Autoimmune encephalitis

This group of disorders are increasingly being recognized. Autoantibodies directed against neuronal epitopes cause a subacute encephalitic illness: limbic encephalitis or panencephalitis. Limbic encephalitis presents over weeks or months with memory impairment, confusion, psychiatric disturbance, and seizures – usually temporal lobe seizures, reflecting involvement of the hippocampus and mesial temporal lobes.

Paraneoplastic limbic encephalitis **(*PLE*)**. PLE is seen particularly with small-cell lung cancer and testicular tumours, and is associated with a variety of antibodies, including anti-Hu and anti-Ma2. Antibodies can be detected in 60% of cases. MRI usually shows a hippocampal high signal. PLE precedes the diagnosis of cancer in most cases and should prompt investigation to identify the tumour.

Voltage-gated potassium channel (VGKC) limbic encephalitis. VGKC antibodies (which can be tested for) produce a variety of disorders, including limbic encephalitis with characteristic faciobrachial dystonic seizures, in combination with confusion, agitation and hyponatraemia. This usually occurs in patients over 50 years of age but is rarely associated with cancer (thymoma). Treatment is with high-dose steroids. Neuromyotonia and peripheral nerve hyperexcitability syndromes may also be seen with antibodies to VGKC.

Anti-NMDA receptor antibody encephalitis. This presents as limbic encephalitis followed by coma and often status epilepticus. Orofacial dyskinesias are characteristic. Patients are usually younger and most have teratomas, such as ovarian.

Patients may respond to immunotherapy: intravenous immunoglobulin or plasma exchange initially, followed by steroids, rituximab or cyclophosphamide. PLE responds less well to treatment.

HIV and neurology

HIV-infected individuals frequently present with or develop neurological conditions. The human immunodeficiency virus itself is directly neuroinvasive and neurovirulent. Immunosuppression leads to indolent, atypical clinical patterns (see p. 337). HIV patients also have a high incidence of stroke. The pattern of disease is changing with anti-retroviral (ART) therapy.

CNS and peripheral nerve disease in HIV

HIV seroconversion can cause meningitis, encephalitis, Guillain–Barré syndrome and Bell's palsy (the most common cause of Bell's palsy in South Africa).

Chronic meningitis occurs with fungi (e.g. *Cryptococcus neoformans* or *Aspergillus*), tuberculosis, *Listeria*, coliforms or other organisms. Raised CSF pressure is common in cryptococcal meningitis.

AIDS–dementia complex (***ADC***). A progressive, HIV-related dementia, sometimes with cerebellar signs, is still seen where ART is unavailable.

Encephalitis and brain abscess. *Toxoplasma*, cytomegalovirus, herpes simplex and other organisms cause severe encephalitis. Multiple brain abscesses develop in HIV infection, usually due to toxoplasmosis.

CNS lymphoma. This is typically fatal (see p. 625).

Progressive multi-focal leucoencephalopathy (***PML***) is due to JC virus and occurs with very low CD4 counts (see p. 263).

Spinal vacuolar myelopathy. This occurs in advanced disease.

Peripheral nerve disease. HIV-related peripheral neuropathy is common (70%) and can be difficult to distinguish from the effects of ART, which is also toxic to peripheral nerves.

Other infections and post-infectious inflammatory conditions

Many other infections involve the CNS and are discussed in Chapter 11: for example, rabies, tetanus, botulism, Lyme disease and leprosy.

Herpes zoster (shingles)

This is caused by reactivation of varicella zoster virus (VZV), usually within dorsal root ganglia. Primary infection with VZV causes chickenpox, following which the virus remains latent in sensory ganglia. Development of shingles may indicate a decline in cell-mediated immunity, such as that due to age or malignancy.

Clinical patterns and complications

Dermatomal shingles. See pages 249–250 and 1344.

Postherpetic neuralgia. This is defined as pain lasting for more than 4 months after developing shingles; it occurs in 10% of patients (often elderly). Burning, intractable pain responds poorly to analgesics. Response to treatment is unsatisfactory but there is a trend towards gradual recovery over 2 years. Amitriptyline or gabapentin is commonly used and topical lidocaine patches may help.

Cranial nerve involvement. Only cranial nerves with sensory fibres are affected, particularly the trigeminal and facial nerves. Ophthalmic herpes is due to involvement of V_1. This can lead to corneal scarring and secondary panophthalmitis. Involvement of the geniculate ganglion of the facial nerve is also called Ramsay Hunt syndrome (see p. 808).

Myelitis. This may occur in the context of shingles, when the inflammatory process spreads from the dorsal root ganglion to the adjacent spinal cord.

Immunization. Older adults (p. 250) can be vaccinated against herpes zoster (even those who have had shingles previously), as it boosts immunity against VZV and reduces the incidence of shingles by about 50%.

Neurosyphilis

Many neurological symptoms occur, sometimes mixed (see also syphilis; pp. 328–330).

Asymptomatic neurosyphilis

This means positive CSF serology without signs.

Meningovascular syphilis

This causes:

- subacute meningitis with cranial nerve palsies and papilloedema
- a gumma – a chronic expanding intracranial mass
- paraparesis – a spinal meningovasculitis.

Tabes dorsalis

Demyelination in dorsal roots causes a complex deafferentation syndrome. The elements of tabes are:

- lightning pains
- ataxia, stamping gait, reflex/sensory loss, wasting
- neuropathic (Charcot) joints
- Argyll Robertson pupils (see p. 805)
- ptosis and optic atrophy.

General paralysis of the insane

The grandiose title describes dementia and weakness. The dementia of general paralysis of the insane (GPI) is typically similar to that of Alzheimer's (see pp. 876–878). Progressive cognitive decline, seizures, brisk reflexes, extensor plantar reflexes and tremor develop. Death follows within 3 years. Argyll Robertson pupils are a usual finding. GPI and tabes are rarities in the UK.

Other forms of neurosyphilis

In ***congenital*** neurosyphilis (acquired *in utero*), features of combined tabes and GPI develop in childhood: taboparesis.

Secondary syphilis can be symptomless or may cause a self-limiting subacute meningitis.

Management

Benzylpenicillin 1 g daily i.m. for 10 days in primary infection eliminates any risk of neurosyphilis. Allergic (Jarisch–Herxheimer) reactions can occur; steroid cover is usually given with penicillin (see pp. 329–330). Established neurological disease is arrested but not reversed by penicillin.

Neurocysticercosis

The pork tapeworm, *Taenia solium*, is endemic in Latin America, Africa, India and much of South-east Asia (see p. 315). Epilepsy is the most common clinical manifestation of neurocysticercosis and one of the most common causes of epilepsy in endemic countries. Most infected people remain asymptomatic.

Brain CT and MRI show ring-enhancing lesions with surrounding oedema when the cyst dies, and later calcification. Multiple cysts are often seen in both brain and skeletal muscle. Serological tests indicate infection but not activity. Biopsy of a lesion is rarely necessary. Management is primarily the control of seizures, and the anthelminthic agent, albendazole, is often given too (usually with steroid cover).

Subacute sclerosing panencephalitis

Persistence of measles antigen in the CNS is associated with this rare late sequel of measles. Progressive mental deterioration, fits, myoclonus and pyramidal signs develop, typically in a child. Diagnosis is made by high measles antibody titre in blood and CSF. Measles immunization protects against subacute sclerosing panencephalitis (SSPE), which has now been almost eliminated in the UK.

Progressive rubella encephalitis

Some 10 years after primary rubella infection, this causes progressive cognitive impairment, fits, optic atrophy, cerebellar and pyramidal signs. Antibody to rubella viral antigen is produced locally within the CNS. It is even rarer than SSPE.

Mollaret's meningitis

Recurrent, self-limiting episodes of aseptic meningitis (i.e. no bacterial cause is found) occur over many years. Herpes simplex has been shown to be the cause in most cases.

Whipple's disease

CNS Whipple's disease, due to *Tropheryma whipplei* infection, is characterized by neurological symptoms, e.g. myoclonus, dementia and supranuclear ophthalmoplegia (see p. 400). Diagnosis of CNS involvement is made by CSF PCR (only 50% sensitivity) or brain biopsy.

Brain and spinal abscesses

Brain abscess

Focal bacterial infection behaves as any expanding mass. The typical bacteria found are *Streptococcus anginosus* and *Bacteroides* species (paranasal sinuses and teeth), and staphylococci (penetrating trauma). Mixed infections are common. Multiple abscesses develop, particularly in HIV infection. Fungi also cause brain abscesses. A parameningeal infective focus (e.g. ear, nose, paranasal sinus, skull fracture) or a distant source of infection (e.g. lung, heart, abdomen) may be present. Frequently, no underlying cause is found. An abscess is more than 10 times rarer than a brain tumour in the UK.

Clinical features and management

Headache, focal signs (e.g. hemiparesis, aphasia, hemianopia), epilepsy and raised intracranial pressure develop. Fever, leucocytosis and raised ESR are usual, although not invariable.

Urgent imaging is essential. MRI shows a ring-enhancing mass, usually with considerable surrounding oedema ***(Fig. 21.50)***. The search for a focus of infection should include a detailed examination of the skull, ears, paranasal sinuses and teeth, and distant sites such as heart and abdomen. LP is dangerous and should not be performed. Neurosurgical aspiration with stereotactic guidance

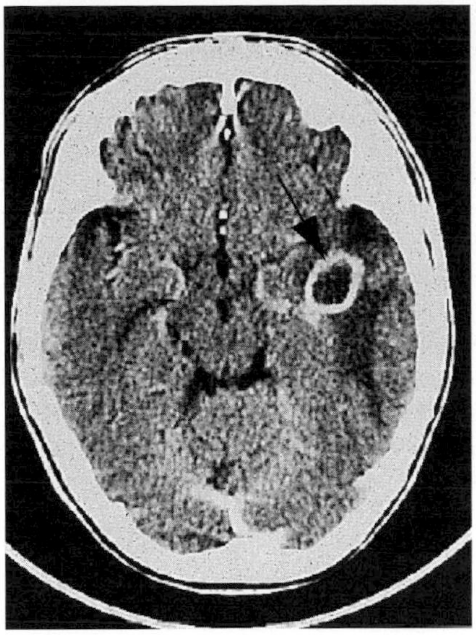

Figure 21.50 Pyogenic cerebral abscess: CT. There is a ring-enhancing lesion with adjacent oedema.

allows the infective organism to be identified. Treatment is with high-dose antibiotics and, sometimes, surgical resection/decompression. Despite treatment, mortality remains high at approximately 25%. Epilepsy is common in survivors.

Brain tuberculoma

Tuberculosis causes chronic caseating intracranial granulomatous masses: tuberculomas. These are the most common intracranial masses in countries where tuberculosis is common, such as India. Brain tuberculomas either present as mass lesions *de novo* or develop during tuberculous meningitis; they are also found as symptomless intracranial calcification on imaging. Spinal cord tuberculomas also occur. Treatment is described on pages 1110–1113.

Subdural empyema and intracranial epidural abscess

Intracranial subdural empyema is a collection of subdural pus, usually secondary to local skull or middle ear infection. Features are similar to those of a cerebral abscess. Imaging is diagnostic.

In ***intracranial epidural abscess***, a layer of pus, 1–3 mm thick, tracks along the epidural space, causing sequential cranial nerve palsies. There is usually local infection: in the middle ear, for example. MRI shows the collection; CT is typically normal. Drainage is required, as are antibiotics.

Spinal epidural abscess

Staphylococcus aureus is the usual organism, reaching the spine via the bloodstream: for example, from a boil. Fever and back pain are followed by paraparesis and/or root lesions. Emergency imaging and antibiotics are essential and surgical decompression is often necessary.

Further reading

Brouwer MC, Tunkel GM, McKhann HGM. Brain abscess. *New Engl J Med* 2014; 371:447–456.

van de Beek D, Brouwer MC, Thwaites GE et al. Advances in treatment of bacterial meningitis. *Lancet* 2012; 380:1693–1702.

http://www.meningitisnow.org/ *Formed in 2013 by merger of Meningitis UK and the Meningitis Trust.*

BRAIN TUMOURS

Primary intracranial tumours account for some 10% of neoplasms. The most common tumours are outlined in ***Box 21.59***. ***Cerebral metastases*** are the most common intracranial tumours ***(Fig. 21.51)***. Symptomless meningiomas (benign) are found quite commonly on imaging or at autopsy.

Gliomas

These malignant tumours of neuroepithelial origin are usually seen within the hemispheres, but occasionally in the cerebellum, brainstem or cord ***(Fig. 21.52)***. Their cause is unknown. Gliomas are occasionally associated with neurofibromatosis. They tend to spread by direct extension, virtually never metastasizing outside the CNS.

- ***Astrocytomas*** are gliomas that arise from astrocytes. They are classified histologically into grades I–IV. Grade I astrocytomas grow slowly over many years, while grade IV tumours (glioblastoma multiforme) cause death within several months. Cystic astrocytomas of childhood are relatively benign and usually cerebellar.
- ***Oligodendrogliomas*** arise from oligodendrocytes. They grow slowly, usually over several decades. Calcification is common.

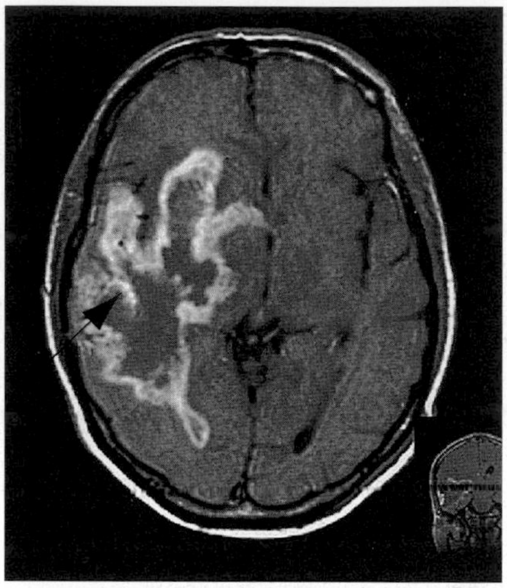

Figure 21.52 Cerebral glioblastoma multiforme: T1-weighted MRI.

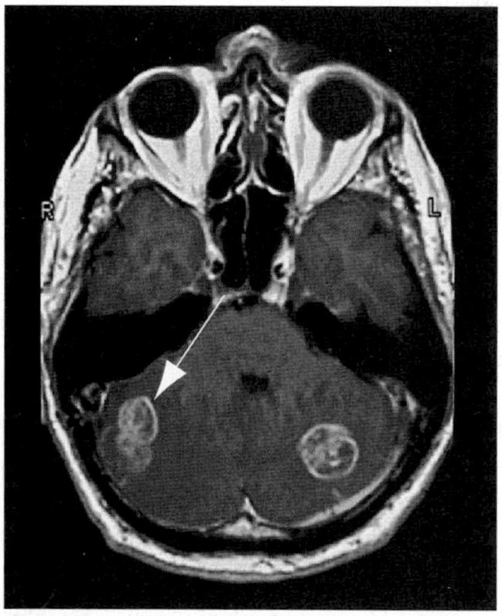

Figure 21.51 Bilateral cerebellar metastases (arrowed): T1-weighted MRI.

Box 21.59 Common brain tumours

Tumour	Approximate frequency
Metastases	50%
Bronchus	
Breast	
Stomach	
Prostate	
Thyroid	
Kidney	
Primary malignant tumours of neuroepithelial tissues	35%
Astrocytoma	
Oligodendroglioma	
Mixed (oligoastrocytoma) glioma	
Ependymoma	
Primary cerebral	
Lymphoma	
Medulloblastoma	
Benign tumours	15%
Meningioma	
Neurofibroma	

Meningiomas

These benign tumours ***(Fig. 21.53)*** arise from the arachnoid and may grow to a large size, usually over years. Those close to the skull erode bone or cause local hyperostosis. They often occur along the intracranial venous sinuses, which they may invade. They are unusual below the tentorium. Common sites are the parasagittal region, sphenoidal ridge, subfrontal region, pituitary fossa and skull base.

Neurofibromas (schwannomas)

These solid benign tumours arise from Schwann cells and occur principally in the cerebellopontine angle, where they arise from the VIIIth nerve sheath (acoustic neuroma; see p. 807). They may be bilateral in neurofibromatosis type 2 (see p. 881).

Other neoplasms

Other less common neoplasms include cerebellar haemangioblastomas, ependymomas of the IVth ventricle, colloid cysts of the IIIrd ventricle, pinealomas, chordomas of the skull base, glomus tumours of the jugular bulb, medulloblastomas (a cerebellar childhood tumour), craniopharyngiomas (see p. 1187) and primary CNS lymphomas (p. 625). For pituitary tumours, see pages 1185–1188.

Clinical features

Mass lesions within the brain produce symptoms and signs by three mechanisms:

- direct effect – brain is infiltrated and local function impaired
- secondary effects of raised intracranial pressure and shift of intracranial contents (e.g. papilloedema, vomiting, headache)
- provocation of generalized and/or partial seizures.

Although neoplasms, either secondary or primary, are the most common mass lesions in the UK, cerebral abscess, tuberculoma, neurocysticercosis, and subdural and intracranial haematomas can also produce features that are clinically similar.

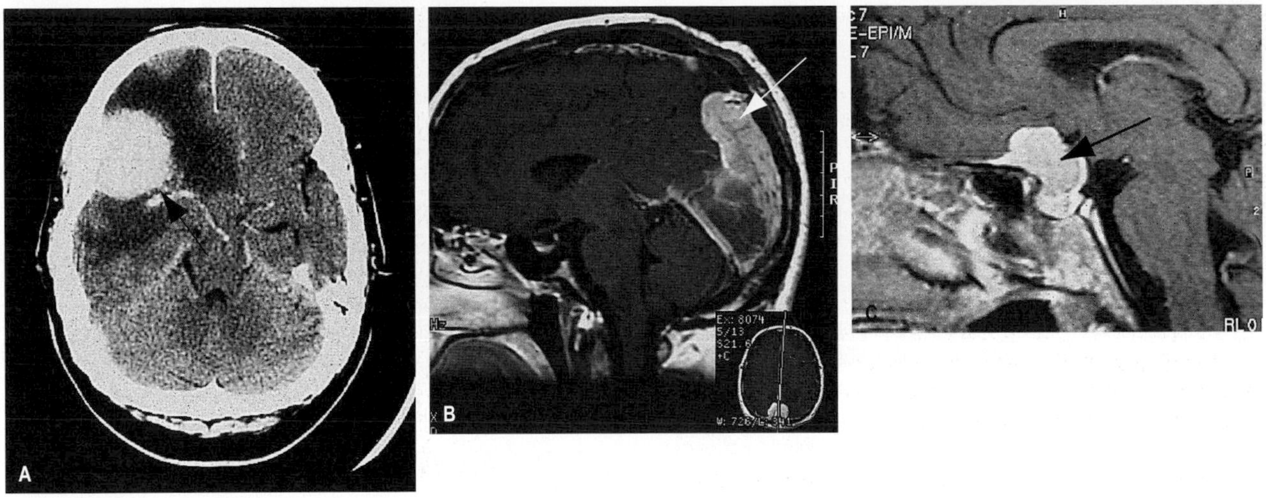

Figure 21.53 **Meningiomas (arrowed). A.** Frontal: CT. **B.** Falx meningioma (occipital): T1-weighted MRI. **C.** Within sella and suprasellar extension: T1-weighted MRI.

Direct effects of mass lesions

The hallmark of a direct effect of a mass is local progressive deterioration of function. Tumours can occur anywhere within the brain. Three examples are given:

- ***A left frontal meningioma*** caused a frontal lobe syndrome over several years with vague disturbance of personality, apathy and impaired intellect. Expressive aphasia developed, followed by progressive right hemiparesis as the corticospinal pathways became involved. As the mass enlarged further, pressure headaches and papilloedema occurred.
- ***A right parietal lobe glioma*** caused a left homonymous field defect (optic radiation). Cortical sensory loss in the left limbs and left hemiparesis followed over 3 months. Partial seizures (episodes of tingling of the left limbs) developed.
- ***A left VIIIth nerve sheath neurofibroma (acoustic neuroma, schwannoma)*** in the cerebellopontine angle caused, over 3 years, progressive deafness (VIII), left facial numbness (V) and weakness (VII), followed by cerebellar ataxia on the same side.

With a hemisphere tumour, epilepsy and the direct effects commonly draw attention to the problem. The rate of progression varies greatly, from a few days or weeks in a highly malignant glioma, to several years with a slowly enlarging mass such as a meningioma. Cerebral oedema surrounds mass lesions; its effect is difficult to distinguish from that of the tumour itself.

Raised intracranial pressure

Raised intracranial pressure causing headache, vomiting and papilloedema is a relatively unusual presentation of a mass lesion in the brain. These symptoms often imply hydrocephalus: obstruction to CSF pathways. Typically, this is produced early by posterior fossa masses that obstruct the aqueduct and IVth ventricle, but only later by lesions above the tentorium. Shift of the intracranial contents produces features that coexist with the direct effects of any expanding mass:

- ***Distortion of the upper brainstem*** as midline structures are displaced either caudally or laterally by a hemisphere mass (see ***Fig. 21.52***). This causes impairment of consciousness, progressing to coning and death as the medulla and cerebellar tonsils are forced into the foramen magnum.
- ***False localizing signs***, termed false only because they do not point *directly* to the site of the mass.
  Three examples of false localizing signs are:
- ***A VIth nerve lesion***, first on the side of a mass and later bilaterally as the VIth nerve is compressed or stretched during its long intracranial course.
- ***A IIIrd nerve lesion*** developing as the temporal lobe uncus herniates caudally, compressing the IIIrd nerve against the petroclinoid ligament. The first sign is ipsilateral pupil dilatation as parasympathetic fibres are compressed.
- ***Hemiparesis*** on the same side as a hemisphere tumour – that is, the side that might not be expected – from compression of the contralateral cerebral peduncle on the edge of the tentorium.

Seizures

Seizures are a common presenting feature of malignant brain tumours. Partial seizures, simple or complex, that may evolve into generalized tonic–clonic seizures, are characteristic of many hemisphere masses, whether malignant or benign. The pattern of partial seizure is that of localizing value (see p. 847).

Investigations

Imaging

Both CT and MRI are useful in detecting brain tumours; MRI is superior for posterior fossa lesions. Benign and malignant tumours, brain abscess, tuberculosis, neurocysticercosis and infarction have characteristic, but not entirely reliable, appearances, and refined imaging techniques and biopsy are often necessary. MR angiography is used occasionally to define blood supply and MR spectroscopy to identify patterns typical of certain gliomas. PET is sometimes helpful to locate an occult primary tumour with brain metastases.

Routine tests

Since metastases are more common than primary tumours, routine tests, such as chest X-ray, should be performed.

Lumbar puncture

This is contraindicated when there is any possibility of a mass lesion, as withdrawing CSF may provoke immediate coning.

CSF examination is rarely helpful and has been superseded by imaging.

Biopsy and tumour removal

Stereotactic biopsy via a skull burr-hole is carried out to ascertain the histology of most suspected malignancies. With a benign tumour, such as a symptomatic, accessible meningioma, craniotomy and removal are usual.

Management

Cerebral oedema surrounding a tumour responds rapidly to steroids: intravenous or oral dexamethasone. Epilepsy is treated with anticonvulsants.

While complete surgical removal of a tumour is an objective, it is often not possible; nor is surgery always necessary. Follow-up with serial imaging is sometimes preferable in low-grade gliomas. At exploration, some benign tumours can be entirely removed (e.g. acoustic neuromas, some parasagittal meningiomas). With a malignant tumour, it is not possible to remove an infiltrating mass entirely. Biopsy and debulking are performed.

Within the posterior fossa, tumour removal is often necessary because of raised pressure and danger of coning. Overall mortality for posterior fossa exploration remains around 10%.

For gliomas and metastases, radiotherapy is usually given and improves survival, if only slightly. Solitary metastases can often be excised successfully. Chemotherapy has little real value in the majority of primary or secondary brain tumours. Vincristine, procarbazine and temozolomide (an oral alkylating agent) can be used. Bevacizumab has been shown to have some benefit, although no effect on overall survival. Most malignant gliomas have a poor prognosis despite advances in imaging, surgery, chemotherapy and radiotherapy: survival for grade IV gliomas at 2 years is less than 50%. Surgical debulking and radiotherapy improve survival by 4–5 months.

Stereotactic radiotherapy (gamma knife)

Only available in selected centres, a collimated radiotherapy beam can deliver high doses of radiation to small targets up to 3 cm in diameter with precision. It may be used to target small metastases, and inaccessible skull-base tumours such as meningiomas or schwannomas. It may also be used to treat intracerebral AVMs.

Further reading

Bredel M, Scholtens DM, Yadav AK et al. NFKBIA deletion in glioblastomas. *N Engl J Med* 2011; 364:627–637.

HYDROCEPHALUS

Hydrocephalus is an excessive accumulation of CSF within the head, caused by a disturbance of formation, flow or absorption. High pressure and ventricular dilatation result ***(Fig. 21.54)***.

Infantile hydrocephalus

Head enlargement in infancy occurs in 1 in 2000 live births. There are several causes:

- ***Arnold–Chiari malformations***. The cerebellar tonsils descend into the cervical canal ***(Fig. 21.55)***. Associated spina bifida is common. Syringomyelia may develop (see p. 874).
- ***Stenosis of the aqueduct of Sylvius***. Aqueduct stenosis is either congenital (genetic), or acquired following neonatal meningitis/haemorrhage.
- ***Dandy–Walker syndrome***. There is cerebellar hypoplasia and obstruction to IVth ventricle outflow foramina.

Hydrocephalus in adults

Hydrocephalus is sometimes an unsuspected finding on imaging. Stable childhood hydrocephalus can become apparent in adult life ('arrested hydrocephalus') but can suddenly decompensate. Combinations of headache, cognitive impairment, features of raised

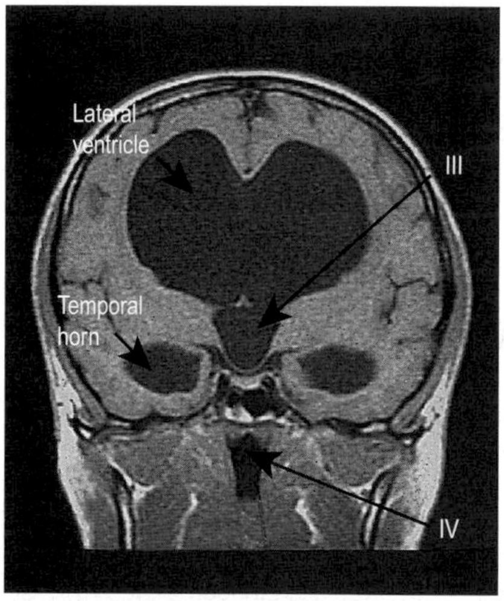

Figure 21.54 Hydrocephalus with gross IIIrd, IVth and lateral ventricle enlargement (arrowed): T1-weighted MRI.

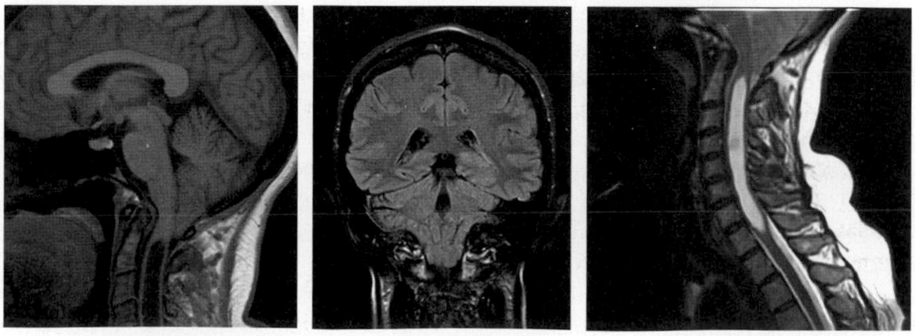

Figure 21.55 Arnold–Chiari malformation with spinal cord syrinx.

intracranial pressure, and ataxia develop, depending on how high the CSF pressure rises and how rapid the onset is. Elderly patients with more compliant brains may present with gradual-onset gait apraxia and subtle cognitive slowing.

Hydrocephalus may be caused by:

- ***posterior fossa and brainstem tumours*** obstructing the aqueduct or IVth ventricular outflow
- ***subarachnoid haemorrhage***, head injury or meningitis (particularly tuberculous), causing obstruction of CSF flow and reabsorption
- ***a IIIrd ventricle colloid cyst*** causing intermittent hydrocephalus – recurrent prostrating headaches with episodes of lower limb weakness
- ***choroid plexus papilloma*** (rare) secreting CSF.

Frequently, the underlying cause of hydrocephalus remains obscure.

Management

Ventriculoperitoneal shunting is necessary when progressive hydrocephalus causes symptoms. Removal of tumours is carried out when appropriate. Endoscopic IIIrd ventriculostomy may be performed.

Normal-pressure hydrocephalus

This describes a syndrome of enlarged lateral ventricles in elderly patients with the clinical triad of:

- a gait disorder – gait apraxia
- dementia
- urinary incontinence.

The term is a misnomer, as it is a low-grade hydrocephalus with intermittently raised ICP. Ventriculoperitoneal shunting may be required. A trial of prolonged drainage of lumbar CSF over several days predicts response to shunt insertion.

TRAUMATIC BRAIN INJURY

In most Western countries, head injury accounts for about 250 hospital admissions per 100 000 population annually. Traumatic brain injury (TBI) describes injuries with potentially permanent consequences. For each 100 000 people, 10 die annually following TBI; 10–15 are transferred to a neurosurgical unit, the majority of these requiring rehabilitation for a prolonged period of 1–9 months. The prevalence of survivors with a major persisting handicap is around 100/100 000. Road traffic accidents and excessive alcohol use are the principal aetiological factors in this major cause of morbidity and mortality, in many countries.

Skull fractures

Linear skull fracture of the vault or base is one indication of the severity of a blow, but in itself is not necessarily associated with any brain injury. Healing of linear fractures takes place spontaneously. ***Depressed*** skull fracture is followed by a high incidence of post-traumatic epilepsy. Surgical elevation and debridement are usually necessary.

Principal local complications of skull fracture are:

- ***meningeal artery rupture*** causing extradural haematoma (see p. 841)
- ***dural vein tears*** causing subdural haematoma (see p. 841)
- ***CSF rhinorrhoea/otorrhoea*** and consequent meningitis.

Mechanisms of brain damage

Older classifications attempted to separate ***concussion***, transient coma for hours followed by apparent complete clinical recovery, from brain ***contusion*** – that is, bruising – with prolonged coma, focal signs and lasting damage. Pathological support for this division is poor. Mechanisms of TBI are complex and interrelated:

- diffuse axonal injury – shearing and rotational stresses on decelerating brain, sometimes at the site opposite impact (the *contrecoup* effect)
- neuronal and axonal damage from direct trauma
- brain oedema and raised intracranial pressure
- brain hypoxia
- brain ischaemia.

Clinical course

In a mild TBI, a patient is stunned or dazed for a few seconds or minutes. Following this, the patient remains alert without post-traumatic amnesia. Headache can follow; complete recovery is usual. In more serious injuries, duration of unconsciousness, and particularly of post-traumatic amnesia (PTA), helps grade severity. PTA lasting more than 24 hours defines severe TBI. The Glasgow Coma Scale (GCS; see p. 825) is used to record the degree of coma; this has prognostic value. A GCS below 5/15 at 24 hours implies a serious injury; 50% of such patients die or remain in a vegetative or minimal conscious state (see p. 829). However, prolonged coma of up to some weeks is occasionally followed by good recovery.

Recovery after severe TBI takes many weeks or months. During the first few weeks, patients are often intermittently restless or lethargic, and have focal deficits such as hemiparesis or aphasia. Gradually, they become more aware, though they may remain in PTA, being unable to lay down any continuous memory despite being awake. This amnesia may last some weeks or more, and may not be obvious clinically. PTA is one predictor of outcome. PTA of over a week implies that persistent organic cognitive deficit is almost inevitable, although return to unsupported paid work may be possible.

Late sequelae

Sequelae of TBI are major causes of morbidity and can have serious social and medicolegal consequences. They include:

- ***Incomplete recovery***, e.g. cognitive impairment, hemiparesis.
- ***Post-traumatic epilepsy*** (see p. 848).
- ***The post-traumatic (post-concussional) syndrome***. This describes the vague complaints of headache, dizziness and malaise that follow even minor head injuries. Litigation is frequently an issue. Depression is prominent. Symptoms may be prolonged.
- ***Benign paroxysmal positional vertigo*** (see pp. 1316–1317).
- ***Chronic subdural haematoma*** (see p. 841).
- ***Hydrocephalus*** (see pp. 870–871).
- ***Chronic traumatic encephalopathy***. This follows repeated and often minor injuries. It is known as the '***punch-drunk syndrome***' and consists of cognitive impairment and extrapyramidal and pyramidal signs, seen typically in professional boxers.

Management

Immediate management

Attention to the airway is vital. If there is coma, depressed fracture or suspicion of intracranial haematoma, CT imaging and discussion with a neurosurgical unit are essential. Indications for CT vary from imaging all minor head injuries in some US centres to more stringent criteria elsewhere.

In many severe TBI cases, assisted ventilation will be needed. Intracranial pressure monitoring is valuable. Hypothermia lowers intracranial pressure when used early after a TBI; an effect on outcome has been seen only in specialized neurotrauma centres. Care of the unconscious patient is described on pages 826–829. Prophylactic antiepileptic drugs have been shown to be of no value in prevention of late post-traumatic epilepsy. Trials using progesterone have shown no benefit.

Rehabilitation

TBI cases require skilled, prolonged and energetic support. Survivors with severe physical and cognitive deficits require rehabilitation in specialized units. Rehabilitation includes care from a multidisciplinary team with physiotherapeutical, psychological and practical skills. Many survivors are left with cognitive problems (amnesia, neglect, disordered attention and motivation) and behavioural/emotional problems (temper dyscontrol, depression and grief reactions). Long-term support for both patients and families is necessary.

Further reading

Stocchetti N, Maas AI. Traumatic intracranial hypertension. *N Engl J Med* 2014; 370:2121–2130.

SPINAL CORD DISEASE

The cord extends from C1, the junction with the medulla, to the lower vertebral body of L1, where it becomes the conus medullaris. Blood supply is from the anterior spinal artery and a plexus on the posterior cord. This network is supplied by the vertebral arteries and by several branches from lumbar and intercostal vessels, including the artery of Adamkiewicz.

Spinal cord compression

The principal features of chronic and subacute cord compression are spastic paraparesis or tetraparesis, radicular pain at the level of compression, and sensory loss below the compression ***(Box 21.60)***.

For example, in compression at T4 (see ***Fig. 21.16***), a band of pain radiates around the thorax, characteristically worse on coughing or straining. Spastic paraparesis develops over months, days or hours, depending on underlying pathology. Numbness commencing in the feet rises to the level of compression. This is called the ***sensory level*** and is usually 2–3 dermatome levels below the level of anatomical compression. Retention of urine and constipation develop.

Aetiology

Disc and vertebral lesions. Central cervical disc and thoracic disc protrusion causes cord compression (see p. 887). Chronic compression due to cervical spondylotic myelopathy is frequently seen in clinical practice and is the most common cause of a spastic paraparesis in an elderly person.

Trauma. Stabilize the neck and back, and move patient with extreme caution in trauma. Any trauma to the back is potentially serious and the patient should be immobilized until the extent of the injury can be determined.

Spinal cord tumours. Extramedullary tumours, such as meningiomas and neurofibromas, cause cord compression (***Fig. 21.56*** and ***Box 21.61***) gradually over weeks to months, often with root pain and a sensory level (see p. 817). Vertebral body destruction by bony metastases, such as in prostate or breast cancer, is a common cause of spinal cord compression.

Intramedullary tumours (e.g. ependymomas) are less common and typically progress slowly, sometimes over many years. Sensory disturbances similar to syringomyelia may develop (see p. 874).

Tuberculosis. Spinal tuberculosis is the most common cause of cord compression in countries where the disease is common. There is destruction of vertebral bodies and disc spaces, with local spread of infection. Cord compression and paraparesis follow, culminating in paralysis: Pott's paraplegia.

Spinal epidural abscess. This is described on page 867.

Epidural haemorrhage and haematoma. These are rare sequelae of anticoagulant therapy, bleeding disorders or trauma, and can follow LP when clotting is abnormal. A rapidly progressive cord or cauda equina lesion develops.

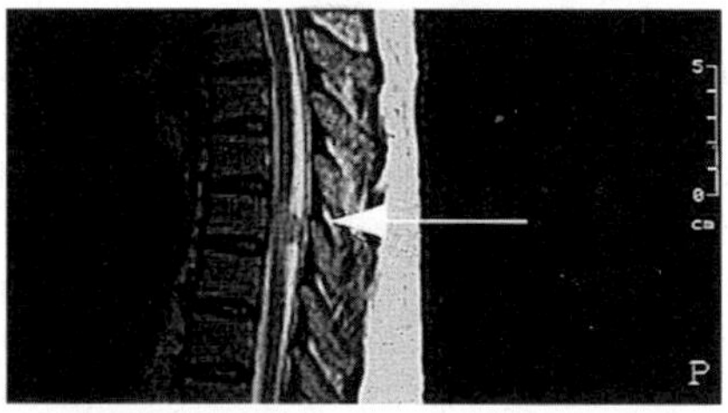

Figure 21.56 Thoracic meningioma (arrowed) compressing the spinal cord: T2-weighted MRI.

? Box 21.60 Causes of spinal cord compression

- Spinal cord tumours
- Extramedullary, e.g. meningioma or neurofibroma
- Intramedullary, e.g. ependymoma or glioma
- Vertebral body destruction by bone metastases, e.g. prostate primary
- Disc and vertebral lesions:
  - Chronic degenerative and acute central disc prolapse
  - Trauma
- Inflammatory:
  - Epidural abscess
  - Tuberculosis
  - Granulomatous
- Epidural haemorrhage/haematoma

i Box 21.61 Principal spinal cord neoplasms

Extradural
- Metastases:
  - Bronchus
  - Breast
  - Prostate
  - Lymphoma
  - Thyroid
  - Melanoma

Extramedullary
- Meningioma
- Neurofibroma
- Ependymoma

Intramedullary
- Glioma
- Ependymoma
- Haemangioblastoma
- Lipoma
- Arteriovenous malformation
- Teratoma

Management

Acute spinal cord compression is a medical emergency. Early diagnosis and treatment is vital. MRI is the imaging technique of choice.

Routine tests (e.g. chest X-ray) may indicate a primary neoplasm or infection. Surgical exploration is frequently necessary; if decompression is not performed promptly, irreversible cord damage ensues. Results are excellent if benign tumours and haematomas are removed early. Radiotherapy is used to treat cord malignancies, or compression due to inoperable malignant vertebral body disease causing cord compression.

Other spinal cord disorders

Inflammatory cord lesions (transverse myelitis)

See page 862.

Anterior spinal artery occlusion

There is acute paraplegia and loss of spinothalamic (pain and temperature) sensation, with infarction of the anterior two-thirds of the spinal cord. This may result from aortic atherosclerosis, dissection, trauma or cross-clamping in surgery. Vasculitis, emboli, haematological disorders causing thrombosis and severe hypotension are other causes. Occlusion of the artery of Adamkiewicz, which supplies the thoracic anterior spinal artery, causes watershed infarction of the cord, typically at the T8 level where perfusion is relatively poor.

Arteriovenous malformations of the cord

Although rare, spinal arteriovenous malformations (AVMs) may be difficult to diagnose but are potentially curable. The two main types seen are dural arteriovenous fistulas (acquired) and true intramedullary AVMs (probably congenital but gradually enlarging). Dural arteriovenous fistulas occur mainly in middle-aged men due to formation of a direct connection between an artery and vein in a dural nerve root sleeve. This causes arterialization of veins with venous hypertension, and thus oedema and congestion of the spinal cord at and below the affected level. Presentation is with a gradually progressive myelopathy over months or a few years, often with thoracic back pain. MRI usually shows cord swelling ***(Fig. 21.57)*** and may show the enlarged arterialized veins over the surface of the cord. Spinal angiography demonstrates the fistula and allows endovascular ablation with glue, often with complete resolution of symptoms if permanent neuronal damage has not already occurred.

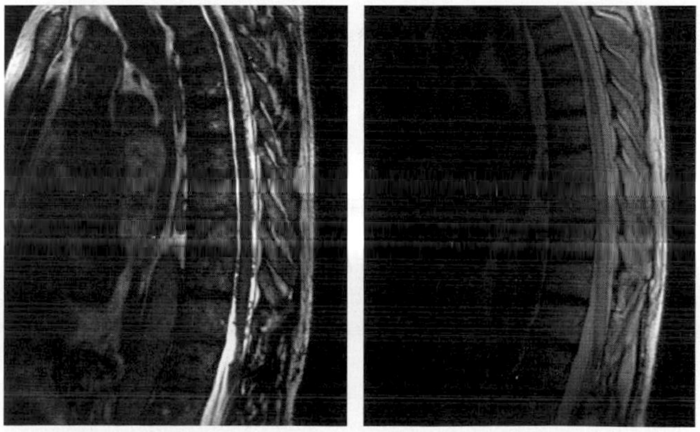

Figure 21.57 Dural arteriovenous fistulas.

Genetic disorders – hereditary spastic paraparesis (HSP)

Several genetic disorders may present with a gradually evolving upper motor neurone syndrome resembling a myelopathy. Typically, spasticity and stiffness dominate the clinical picture rather than weakness, especially in hereditary spastic paraparesis (HSP). Muscle relaxants, such as baclofen, improve gait. There are 28 known genes associated with HSP, some causing 'pure' spasticity and others with associated neurological features, such as thinning of the corpus callosum.

Other genetic disorders such as adrenoleucodystrophy may cause a slowly progressive spastic paraparesis (including in manifesting female carriers), as can the spinocerebellar ataxias (see p. 881) or presenilin-1 mutations (see p. 877).

Vitamin B_{12} deficiency

Subacute combined degeneration of the cord resulting from vitamin B_{12} deficiency (see p. 886) is the most common example of metabolic disease causing spinal cord damage. Abuse of nitrous oxide may precipitate functional B_{12} deficiency with normal serum B_{12} levels.

Other causes of a spastic paraparesis

Motor neurone disease may present initially with a spastic paraparesis before lower motor neurone features develop (see pp. 879–880). Paraneoplastic disorders, radiotherapy, copper deficiency, liver failure and rare toxins (e.g. lathyrism) may cause spinal cord damage. Not all causes of paraparesis relate to spinal cord pathology; beware a parasagittal cerebral meningioma presenting with a paraparesis due to bilateral compression of the leg area of the motor cortex.

Care of the patient with paraplegia

Where patients are left with a severe paraplegia, there are several issues in long-term care, and specialist nursing is vital.

Bladder management. The bladder does not empty and urinary retention results. Patients self-catheterize or develop reflex bladder emptying, helped by abdominal pressure. Early treatment of urine infections is essential. Chronic kidney disease is a common cause of death.

Bowel function. Constipation and impaction must be avoided. Following acute paraplegia, manual evacuation is necessary; reflex emptying develops later.

Skin care. Risks of pressure ulcers and their sequelae are serious. Meticulous attention must be paid to cleanliness and regular turning. The sacrum, iliac crests, greater trochanters, heels and malleoli should be inspected frequently (see p. 1376). Pressure-relieving mattresses are useful initially until patients can turn themselves. If pressure ulcers develop, plastic surgical repair may be required. Pressure palsies, such as those of ulnar nerves, can occur.

Lower limbs. Passive physiotherapy helps to prevent contractures. Severe spasticity, with flexor or extensor spasms, may be helped by muscle relaxants such as baclofen or by botulinum toxin injections.

Rehabilitation. Many patients with traumatic paraplegia or tetraplegia return to self-sufficiency (especially if the level is at C7 or below). A specialist spinal rehabilitation unit is necessary. Lightweight, specially adapted wheelchairs provide independence. Tendon transfer operations may allow functional grip if hands are weak. Autonomic dysreflexia may be a problem. Patients with paraplegia have substantial practical, psychological and sexual needs.

Syringomyelia and syringobulbia

A syrinx is a fluid-filled cavity within the spinal cord. Syringobulbia means a cavity in the brainstem. Syringomyelia is frequently associated with the Arnold–Chiari malformation (see p. 870). The abnormality at the foramen magnum probably allows normal pulsatile CSF pressure waves to be transmitted to fragile tissues of the cervical cord and brainstem, causing secondary cavity formation. The syrinx is in continuity with the central canal of the cord. Syrinx formation may also follow spinal cord trauma and lead to secondary damage years later, and can also be caused by intrinsic cord tumours.

Pathophysiology

The expanding cavity in the cord gradually destroys spinothalamic neurones, anterior horn cells and lateral corticospinal tracts. In the medulla (syringobulbia), lower cranial nerve nuclei are affected.

Clinical features

Cases associated with the Arnold–Chiari malformation usually develop symptoms around the age of 20–30. Upper limb pain exacerbated by exertion or coughing is typical. Spinothalamic sensory loss – pain and temperature – leads to painless upper limb burns and trophic changes. Paraparesis develops. The following are typical signs of a substantial cervical syrinx ***(Fig. 21.58)***:

- ***a 'suspended' area of dissociated sensory loss*** – i.e. spinothalamic loss in the arms and hands without loss of light touch.
- ***loss of upper limb reflexes***.
- ***muscle wasting*** in the hand and forearm.
- ***spastic paraparesis*** – initially mild.
- ***brainstem signs*** – as the syrinx extends into the brainstem (syringobulbia) there may be tongue atrophy and fasciculation, bulbar palsy, a Horner syndrome and impairment of facial sensation.

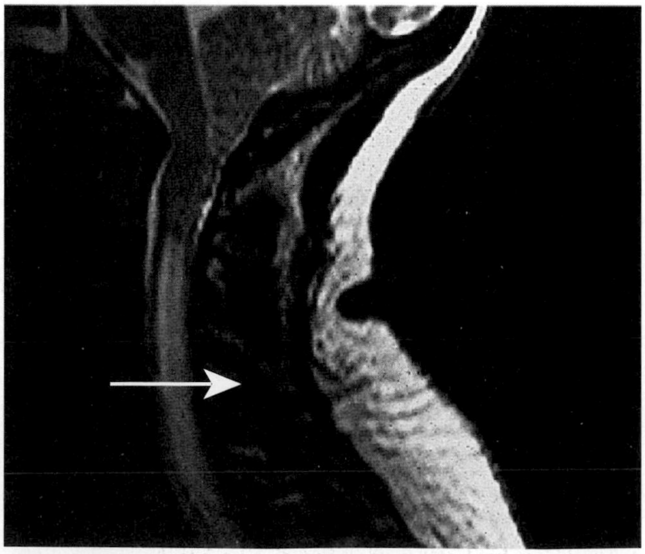

Figure 21.58 Cervical syrinx – cavity within cord (arrowed): T2-weighted MRI.

Investigations and management

MRI demonstrates the cavity and herniation of cerebellar tonsils. Syringomyelia is gradually progressive over several decades. Sudden deterioration sometimes follows minor trauma or occurs spontaneously. Surgical decompression of the foramen magnum often causes the syrinx to collapse.

Further reading

Ginsberg L. Disorders of the spinal cord and roots. *Pract Neurol* 2011; 11:259–267.

NEURODEGENERATIVE DISEASES

Neurodegenerative disease is an umbrella term for disorders characterized by progressive neuronal cell loss with distinct patterns in different disorders. These disorders are increasing in an ageing population.

Dementia

Dementia is a clinical syndrome with multiple causes, defined by:

- an acquired loss of higher mental function, affecting two or more cognitive domains, including:
  - episodic memory (acquisition of new information) – usually (but not always) involved
  - language function
  - frontal executive function
  - visuospatial function
  - apraxia
- being of sufficient severity to cause significant social or occupational impairment
- being chronic and stable (which distinguishes it from delirium, which is acute and fluctuating).

Although dementia is usually progressive, it is not invariably so, and may even be reversible in some cases. Dementia robs patients of their independence, and is a serious burden on carers and a major socioeconomic challenge for society as a whole.

Epidemiology

Dementia is common and becoming even more so as a result of an ageing population and better case ascertainment. Age is the main risk factor, followed by family history. Over the age of 65, there is a 6% prevalence; over the age of 85, the prevalence increases to 20%.

Clinical assessment

There are two main considerations:

- Does the patient have dementia?
- Are the pattern of cognitive deficits, tempo of progression or associated features suggestive of a distinct cause? Cognitive problems need to be interpreted in the context of estimated premorbid abilities (e.g. based on educational attainments or occupation).

Taking a history from a spouse or relative is essential. Patients may tend to downplay or deny symptoms (anosognosia) or constantly look to the relative for answers (the 'head-turning sign'). See ***Box 21.62*** for the key elements in history-taking.

Box 21.62 Taking a dementia history

- Memory:
  - Is (s)he repetitive, e.g. with questions?
  - Is there a temporal gradient of amnesia – preservation of more distant memories with amnesia for recent events?
  - Is there difficulty learning to use new devices, e.g. computer, mobile phone?
- Functional ability:
  - Has work performance or ability to cook and do domestic tasks declined?
  - Has responsibility for finances and administration shifted to the spouse?
  - Does (s)he get easily muddled?
- Personality and frontal lobe function:
  - Has personality altered?
  - More aggressive/apathetic/lacking initiative
  - Disinhibition
  - Change in food preference or religiosity
- Language:
  - Difficulty with word finding or remembering names
- Visuospatial ability:
  - Does (s)he get lost in familiar places?
  - Difficulty dressing, e.g. putting jacket on the wrong way round
- Psychiatric features:
  - Features of depression
- Tempo of progression
- Family history of dementia
- Alcohol and drug use
- Medication
- Any other neurological problems, e.g. parkinsonism, gait disorder, strokes

Examination

Conversation with the patient during history-taking may be as revealing as formal cognitive assessment but many patients hide deficits well behind an intact social façade.

Bedside cognitive assessment

The mini-mental state examination (MMSE; see pp. 893–897) is commonly used to assess cognitive function but has its limitations, such as relative insensitivity to milder cognitive impairment and to frontal lobe dysfunction, especially in those with premorbid abilities. The Addenbrooke's Cognitive Examination (ACE) is a tool developed to address the deficiencies of the MMSE but is short enough to use in clinical practice.

It is useful to ask patients to give an account of recent news events to assess episodic memory.

Individual cognitive domains can be tested separately in detail: for example, clock drawing for visuospatial (parietal lobe) function, naming and reading tasks for language function, verbal fluency, conceptual similarity to test abstract thinking, and stop–go tasks, which are components of the Frontal Assessment Battery (FAB).

Check for primitive reflexes (frontal release signs), such as grasp, palmo-mental and pout reflexes, and perseveration or utilization behaviour with frontal lobe involvement.

Test:

- limb praxis – copying hand gestures and miming tasks, e.g. 'Show me how you brush your teeth',
- oro-buccal praxis, e.g. 'Show me how you would blow out a candle'.

Complete neurological examination to look for evidence of papilloedema, parkinsonism, myoclonus and gait disorders, for example, is also necessary, in addition to is general examination and assessment of mental state.

Box 21.63 Tests in dementia

Blood tests
- Full blood count, erythrocyte sedimentation rate, vitamin B_{12}
- Urea and electrolytes
- Glucose
- Liver biochemistry
- Serum calcium
- Thyroid stimulating hormone, T_3, T_4
- HIV serology

Imaging
- CT or MRI brain scan

Other – selected patients only
- Cerebrospinal fluid
  – including tau and Aβ42 measurement
- Genetic studies, e.g. for AD and FTD genes, HD, prion mutations
- Electroencephalography
- Brain biopsy

AD, Alzheimer's disease; FTD, fronto-temporal dementia; HD, Huntington's disease.

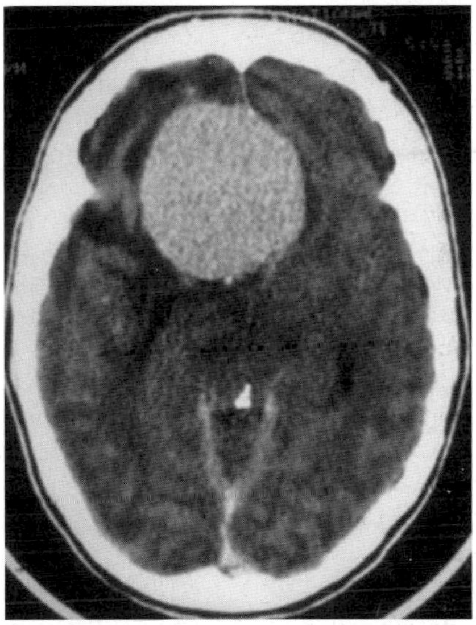

Figure 21.59 CT scan showing a large frontal meningioma presenting with apathy and frontal dementia.

Investigations

Investigations ***(Box 21.63)*** are aimed at identifying treatable causes and helping support a clinical diagnosis of dementia type. For most patients, this should include the elements listed below.

Blood tests. These should include a full blood count and measurement of vitamin B_{12}, thyroid function, urea and electrolytes, liver function, glucose and ESR.

Brain imaging. CT is adequate to exclude structural lesions ***(Fig. 21.59)***, such as tumours or hydrocephalus. The superior anatomical resolution of MRI helps identify patterns of regional brain atrophy and so distinguish between different types of degenerative dementia (e.g. hippocampal atrophy in Alzheimer's disease (AD) versus temporal lobe and frontal atrophy in frontotemporal dementia). Imaging also allows assessment of brain 'vascular load'. MRI is always preferable to CT in patients with cognitive disorders.

Detailed neuropsychometric assessment (see p. 924). Appropriate in most patients, this allows quantification of the relative involvement of different cognitive domains and may be helpful if performed serially over time to assess progression.

Younger patients (<65 years). More intensive investigation may be necessary. This may include EEG, genetic tests (e.g. for

Huntington's, familial AD and FTD genes), voltage-gated potassium channel antibodies, antineuronal antibodies (for paraneoplastic limbic encephalitis), HIV serology and metabolic tests; on rare occasions, brain biopsy may be appropriate.

CSF examination. Measurement of CSF protein biomarkers has been shown to be useful in distinguishing between different types of dementia; for example, in Alzheimer's disease, CSF tau is raised and Aβ42 reduced. In Creutzfeldt–Jakob disease (CJD) and other rapidly progressive dementias, protein 14–3–3 is increased. A new CSF assay for abnormal prion protein, real-time quaking induced conversion (rt-QUIC), has proved to be highly sensitive and specific for CJD.

New imaging modalities. Radionuclide scans using radioactively labelled ligands that bind directly to amyloid allow amyloid deposition in the brain to be directly visualized and have great potential for earlier and more accurate diagnosis of AD. Amyloid imaging is now beginning to enter clinical practice in some specialist centres.

Mild cognitive impairment

Mild cognitive impairment (MCI) is an intermediate state between normal cognition and dementia. Often mild memory impairment, greater than expected for age but not sufficient to classify as dementia, is the only symptom ('amnestic MCI'). MCI may be a pre-dementia state, with 10–15% of patients per year developing overt AD.

Causes of dementia

There are many causes of dementia ***(Box 21.64)***, by far the most common being AD. Cause varies according to age ***(Fig. 21.60)***.

Alzheimer's disease

Although technically a definitive diagnosis can only be made by histopathology, in practice the clinical features are sufficiently characteristic that a diagnosis can usually be made with considerable accuracy in life, supported by diagnostic investigations. The key clinical features are:

- ***Memory impairment***. Episodic (day-to-day) memory is affected. There is progressive loss of ability to learn, retain and process new information. There is a characteristic temporal gradient, with relative preservation of distant memory and amnesia for more recent events. Patients often refer to this as 'short-term memory loss', which technically refers to loss of working memory: for example, digit span, which is preserved in AD.
- ***Language***. This usually becomes impaired as the disease advances. Difficulty with word finding is characteristic.
- ***Apraxia***. Ability to carry out skilled motor activities is impaired (see p. 798).
- ***Agnosia***. There is a failure to recognize objects such as clothing, and places or people.
- ***Frontal executive function***. Organizing, planning and sequencing are impaired.
- ***Parietal presentation***. Presentation with visuospatial difficulties and difficulty with orientation in space and navigation may occur. Parietal lobe involvement is also seen as a later feature in more typical presentations.

Box 21.64 Causes of dementia

Degenerative
- Alzheimer's disease
- Dementia with Lewy bodies
- Frontotemporal dementia
- Huntington's disease
- Parkinson's disease
- Prion diseases, e.g. Creutzfeldt–Jakob

Vascular
- Vascular dementia
- Cerebral vasculitis (rare)

Metabolic
- Uraemia
- Liver failure

Toxic
- Alcohol
- Solvent misuse
- Heavy metals

Vitamin deficiency
- B_{12} and thiamine

Traumatic
- Severe or repeated brain injury

Intracranial lesions
- Subdural haematoma
- Tumours
- Hydrocephalus

Infections
- HIV
- Neurosyphilis
- Whipple's disease
- Tuberculosis

Endocrine
- Hypothyroidism
- Hypoparathyroidism

Psychiatric
- Depression causing 'pseudo-dementia'

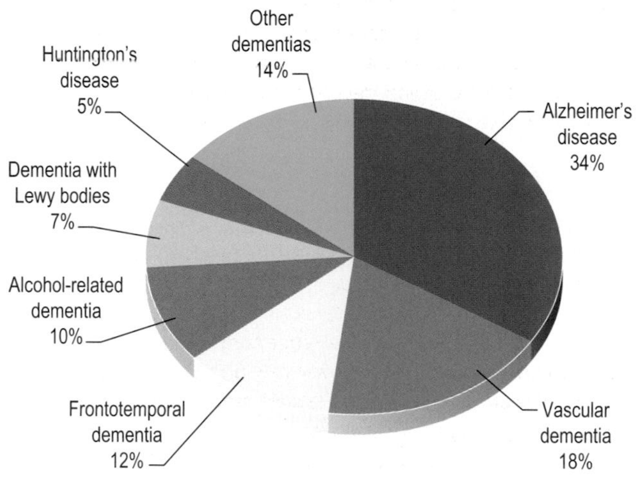

A

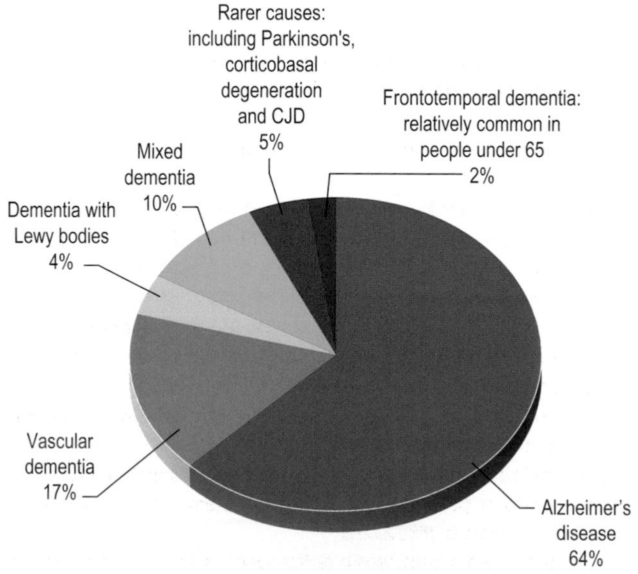

B

Figure 21.60 Causes of dementia at different ages. A. Under 65 years. **B.** At 65 years or more. CJD, Creutzfeldt–Jakob disease. *(Data from Prince M, Knapp M, Guerchet M et al.* Alzheimer's Society Dementia UK Update. *London: Alzheimer's Society; 2014.)*

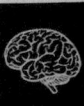

- ***Posterior cortical atrophy*** (***PCA***). This is the least common presentation of AD with visual disorientation due to initial involvement of the occipital lobes and occipito-parietal regions. Patients have complex visual symptoms that may be difficult to describe; they often say that it is easier to see distant than close-up objects. Memory is initially well preserved.
- ***Personality***. In contrast to other dementias such as frontotemporal dementia, basic personality and social behaviour remain intact until late AD.
- ***Anosognosia***. Lack of insight by the patient into their difficulties is common; they may be reluctant to seek medical attention but be brought to clinic by a family member.
- ***Tempo***. Onset is insidious and often not noticed by family members initially. Progression is gradual but inexorable over a decade or longer, with eventual severe deficits in multiple cognitive domains.
- ***Late non-cognitive features***. Myoclonus may develop, sometimes followed by seizures (the cortex is the main site of pathology). Sleep–wake cycle reversal and incontinence may place a great strain on carers. Motor function is usually strikingly preserved so patients are capable of wandering and getting lost. Swallowing may become impaired, leading to aspiration pneumonia – often a terminal event.

Investigations

MRI typically shows characteristic atrophy of mesial temporal lobe structures, including hippocampi, progressing eventually to generalized cerebral atrophy. Imaging may be normal in the early stages and selective regional atrophy is seen in AD variants such as 'posterior presentations', such as posterior cortical atrophy (PCA) with occipital lobe atrophy. Characteristic MRI and psychometric testing abnormalities are sufficient to make a diagnosis if the clinical picture is suggestive (a progressive amnestic cognitive disorder in an older person). CSF tau and β-amyloid measurement is helpful in cases of diagnostic difficulty but not yet widely available (see above).

Molecular pathology and aetiology

Although the cause of AD is still not known, a great deal is now understood about the molecular pathology. The pathological hallmarks are:

- The deposition of β-amyloid (Aβ) in amyloid plaques in the cortex.
- Structural and conformational changes in tau protein, i.e. hyperphosphorylation and formation of paired helical filaments, which are the binding blocks of neurofibrillary tangles. These protein aggregates damage synapses and ultimately lead to neuronal death. Early pathological changes in the brain, including Aβ deposition, pre-date clinical symptoms and diagnosis by up to 25 years.

Amyloid may also be laid down in cerebral blood vessels, leading to amyloid angiopathy.

The amyloid precursor protein (APP) is processed by secretase enzymes to form pathogenic $A\beta_{1-42}$ monomers, which polymerize into amyloid plaques ***(Fig. 21.61)***.

A basal forebrain cholinergic deficit occurs and may explain the therapeutic response to cholinesterase inhibitor drugs.

Genetics of AD

A first-degree relative with AD confers a doubled lifetime risk of AD. There are rare autosomal dominant monogenic early-onset forms of familial AD with high penetrance, caused by mutations in specific genes; taken together, these account for only 1% of cases of AD.

Other genes. The E4 allele of the apolipoprotein E gene confers an increased risk of AD (2–3 times lifetime risk), especially if two copies of the E4 allele are inherited (6–8 times risk). Several other candidate genes have been identified as risk factors for AD in large genome-wide association studies.

Amyloid precursor protein (***APP***). Point mutations in the *APP* gene can cause AD, and the presence of three copies of the *APP* gene on chromosome 21 in Down syndrome patients is responsible for the high incidence of AD in that condition.

Presenilin (PS)-1 and 2. Mutations in these genes affect the γ-secretase enzyme function ***(Fig. 21.61)***. *PS1* mutations account for 50% of monogenic forms of AD. The *PS1/2* and *APP* genes may be sequenced for mutations in selected early-onset cases with a family history.

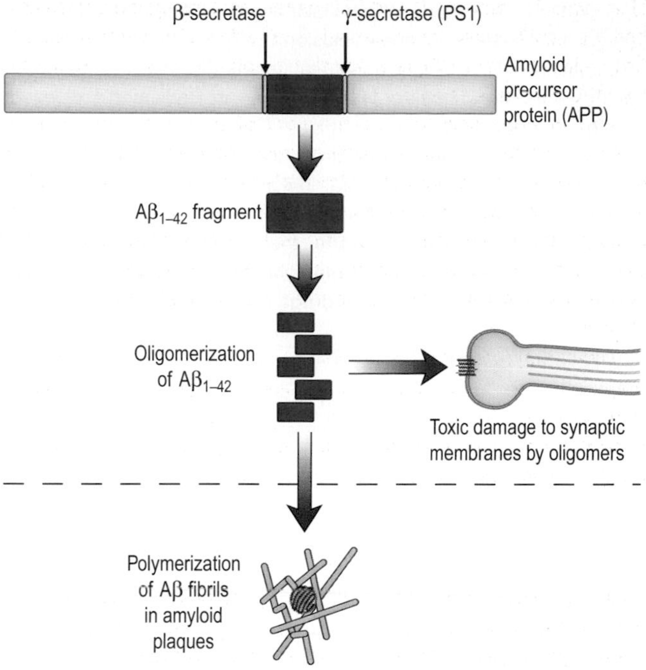

Figure 21.61 Molecular pathogenesis of Alzheimer's disease. Processing of the amyloid precursor protein (APP) molecule by secretase enzymes releases $A\beta_{1-42}$ monomers, which are the building block of amyloid plaques. Aβ oligomers may damage synaptic membranes. Mutations in APP or γ-secretase (presenilin-1) cause genetic forms of Alzheimer's. Disruption of the balance between formation and degradation of $A\beta_{1-42}$ is thought to be a major problem.

Environmental risk factors

Age is the main risk factor for AD, as incidence increases exponentially with age. Head trauma and vascular risk factors also increase AD risk. Epidemiological studies show that taking anti-inflammatory drugs over a long period may confer some protection.

Dementia with Lewy bodies and Parkinson's disease dementia

Dementia with Lewy bodies (DLB) is characterized by the early feature of visual hallucinations, fluctuating cognition with variation in attention and alertness, sleep disorders (especially REM sleep behaviour disorder), dysautonomia and parkinsonism. The visual hallucinations often take the form of people or animals, or the sense of a presence ('extracampine hallucinations'). Memory loss may be absent in the early stages. Delusions and transient loss of consciousness occur. Lewy bodies, inclusions containing aggregates of the protein α-synuclein first described in Parkinson's disease, are found in the cortex.

In DLB, the cognitive features dominate; parkinsonism may evolve later and is typically mild. In Parkinson's disease dementia (PDD), cognitive problems are a late feature, occurring at least 1 year after onset and usually after the age of 75. Both conditions may respond to cholinesterase inhibitors. Patients with DLB may be very sensitive to neuroleptic drugs with dramatic worsening.

Vascular dementia

This common cause of dementia is due to different mechanisms, including multi-infarct dementia, cerebral small-vessel disease and post-stroke dementia. Most vascular dementias are of mixed cause. Vascular dementia is distinguished from AD by its clinical features and imaging. Dementia can be progressive and similar to AD. There is sometimes a history of TIAs or the dementia follows a succession of cerebrovascular events or has a stepwise course. Apraxic gait disorder, pyramidal signs and urinary incontinence are common additional features. Widespread small-vessel disease seen on MRI is the typical finding and may produce a variety of cognitive deficits, reflecting the site of ischaemic damage.

Frontotemporal dementia

Frontotemporal dementia (FTD) is the term used to describe a group of neurodegenerative disorders characterized by asymmetric frontal lobe and temporal lobe atrophy on MRI and at postmortem (also called ***Pick's disease***). Onset is usually below the age of 65 and there is often a family history. FTD is considerably less common than AD, prevalence being approximately 10 per 100 000 before the age of 65. There are three distinct presentations, depending on which anatomical region is affected first.

Frontal presentation. This ***behavioural variant*** is characterized by personality change, emotional blunting, apathy, disinhibition, carelessness and behavioural change with striking preservation of episodic memory.

Temporal presentations. ***Primary progressive aphasia*** is characterized by progressive impairment of language function. Involvement of the left temporal lobe produces 'semantic dementia', with fluent speech relatively lacking in meaningful content and progressive difficulty with comprehension of the meaning of words (e.g. a patient may respond to the MMSE question 'What season is it?' by asking 'What is a season?'). The second temporal lobe presentation is ***progressive non-fluent aphasia*** due to peri-Sylvian atrophy, with loss of verbal fluency and increasingly telegrammatic speech.

The frontal and temporal presentations eventually merge as cognitive decline becomes more widespread.

Pathology

About 25% of cases are familial, associated with mutations in the tau and progranulin genes or hexanucleotide repeat expansion in the *C9ORF72* gene. The characteristic pathology consists of deposition of abnormally aggregated proteins: phosphorylated tau, transactive response DNA-binding protein 43 (TDP-43) or fused in sarcoma (FUS). 10% of patients have overlap syndromes with motor neurone disease or parkinsonian disorders such as progressive supranuclear palsy. There is no cure or specific treatment at present.

Prion diseases, including Creutzfeldt–Jakob disease

Prion diseases (see pp. 267–268) are transmissible neurodegenerative disorders with a long incubation period, caused by accumulation of misfolded native prion protein (PrP^c). Misfolding and conformational change in PrP^c is caused either by exposure to the abnormal misfolded isoform of the protein (PrP^{sc}) or by mutations in the PrP gene (*PRNP*), leading to toxic accumulation of PrP^{sc} as amyloid in beta-pleated sheets. Neuronal cell damage and 'spongiform' change in the brain result (see pp. 267–268), the clinical correlate being a rapidly progressive dementia in most cases.

Creutzfeldt–Jakob disease

Creutzfeldt–Jakob disease (CJD) is the most common prion disease in humans, the animal equivalents being bovine spongiform encephalopathy (BSE) in cattle and scrapie in sheep. CJD may be sporadic, iatrogenic or familial.

Sporadic CJD is the most common form, occurring over the age of 50, with an incidence of approximately 1 per million. It is thought to be due to spontaneous somatic mutations in the *PRNP* gene or stochastic conformational change in PrP^c to PrP^{sc} with a subsequent 'domino effect' inducing misfolding in other PrP molecules. A rapidly progressive dementia leads to death within 6 months of onset. Rapidly progressive cognitive decline should always lead to suspicion of CJD. The presence of myoclonus is also a clinical clue (present in 90%). New forms of monoclonal antibody treatment are being studied.

Iatrogenic CJD is transmitted from neurosurgical instruments (prions are resistant to sterilization), transplant material (e.g. corneal grafts) and cadaveric pituitary-derived growth hormone taken from patients with CJD or pre-symptomatic CJD. Iatrogenic CJD has a long incubation period of several years.

Familial CJD (rare) is associated with *PRNP* gene mutations. Other clinical phenotypes, such as ***familial fatal insomnia***, also occur.

Variant CJD

Variant CJD (vCJD) was first seen in the UK in 1995. vCJD patients are younger than sporadic cases with a mean age of 29. Early symptoms are neuropsychiatric, followed by ataxia and dementia with myoclonus or chorea. The diagnosis can be confirmed by tonsillar biopsy but a sensitive blood test has been developed. vCJD has a longer course than sporadic CJD – up to several years. vCJD and BSE are caused by the same prion strain, giving rise to speculation that transmission from animal to human food chain took place: that is, infection from BSE-infected cattle to humans (see p. 267). Transmission via blood transfusion may also occur. Most patients with vCJD and sporadic CJD have a specific polymorphism at codon 129 of the *PRNP* gene that leads to susceptibility.

Other dementias

Other neurodegenerative disorders may include dementia as one of their clinical manifestations. For example, corticobasal degeneration (CBD), progressive supranuclear palsy (PSP) and dementia may be a feature of a number of genetic and metabolic disorders, such as Huntington's disease (see p. 856) and the leucodystrophies.

Management of dementia

It is rare for a reversible cause for dementia to be found, such as normal pressure hydrocephalus or frontal meningioma. Other disorders, such as limbic encephalitis or severe depression, may present as dementia mimics and every effort should be made to distinguish these treatable conditions from degenerative dementias.

Management is supportive, to preserve dignity and to provide care for as long as possible in the familiar home environment. The burden of illness frequently falls on relatives. Dementia clinical nurse specialists form a central part of the multidisciplinary team.

General measures. Some evidence suggests that participation in cognitively demanding activities in later life may protect against or delay the onset of dementia. High-dose B vitamins may possibly slow conversion from MCI to AD in patients with above-average levels of the amino acid homocysteine. There is some recent evidence supporting use of vitamin E to slow progression.

Cognitive enhancing drugs. These have a modest symptomatic benefit in AD, equivalent to an increase in 1–2 points on the MMSE. They are not disease-modifying, so do not slow or prevent progression. Whilst there has been some dispute about the place for these drugs, they contribute to patients being able to prolong independence and remain at home for longer than might otherwise be the case.

Cholinesterase inhibitors (donepezil, rivastigmine and galantamine) increase brain acetylcholine levels by inhibiting CNS acetylcholinesterase. Patients with AD have a central cholinergic deficit. There is usually a small but significant improvement in memory, cognition and function. Cholinesterase inhibitors are also effective in DLB and Parkinson's dementia but not in FTD or vascular dementia. Side-effects, particularly cholinergic gastrointestinal symptoms, may be a problem. An ECG should be performed to exclude cardiac conduction deficits before starting therapy.

Memantine is an NMDA receptor antagonist. It is used in moderate or severe AD or where cholinesterase inhibitors are not tolerated. There is some evidence that combination of memantine and cholinesterase inhibitors is better than either used alone. It is generally well tolerated.

Psychiatric and behavioural problems. Depression is common in dementia and may be difficult to distinguish from dementia symptoms, such as apathy and worsening cognitive function. A trial of an antidepressant is appropriate where depression is suspected. Distinguishing depressive pseudo-dementia from organic dementia can be difficult but is crucial. Behavioural disturbance (e.g. due to agitation or delusions) and hallucinations may occur in late-stage disease. Use of antipsychotic medications is associated with significantly increased stroke risk in patients with dementia and should be used only as a last resort.

Drugs in development. The greatest need is for disease-modifying therapies that halt or slow progression in early-stage disease before significant irreversible neuronal damage has accumulated. Potential treatments in development include anti-amyloid therapies, such as monoclonal antibodies directed against Aβ and inhibitors of secretase enzymes that process APP into Aβ fragments. Solanuzemab is a monoclonal antibody targeting Aβ that has shown efficacy in slowing progression in early-stage AD in phase III clinical trials.

Financial and legal issues. Patients may want to set up a Lasting Power of Attorney (if they retain mental capacity to do so in legal terms) to allow a spouse or relative to deal with their financial affairs on their behalf when they lose the capacity to do so. Patients and carers may be entitled to state financial benefits.

Driving. After a diagnosis of dementia, patients in the UK have a duty to inform the Driver and Vehicle Licensing Authority (DVLA), who may request a driving safety assessment.

Further reading

Bang J, Spina S, Miller BL. Frontotemporal dementia. *Lancet* 2015; 386:1672–1682.
Mitchell SL. Advanced dementia. *N Engl J Med* 2015; 372:2533–2540.
O'Brien JT, Thomas A. Vascular dementia. *Lancet* 2015; 386:1698–1706.
Walker Z, Possin KL, Boeve BF, Aarsland D. Lewy body dementias. *Lancet* 2015; 386:1683–1697.

Motor neurone disease

Motor neurone disease (MND) is a devastating condition causing progressive weakness and eventually death, usually as a result of respiratory failure or aspiration. It is relatively uncommon, with an annual incidence of 2/100 000. Presentation is usually between the ages of 50 and 75. Below age 70, men are affected more often than women. Amyotrophic lateral sclerosis (ALS) is the term more commonly used for MND in some countries.

Pathogenesis

MND predominantly affects upper and lower motor neurones in the spinal cord, cranial nerve motor nuclei and cortex. However, other neuronal systems may also be affected; 5% of patients also develop FTD (see p. 878) and up to 40% have some measurable frontal lobe cognitive impairment. MND is usually sporadic and of unknown cause, with no established environmental risk factors. Ubiquinated cytoplasmic inclusions containing the RNA processing proteins TDP-43 and FUS are the pathological hallmarks found in axons, indicating that protein aggregation may be involved in pathogenesis, as with other neurodegenerative disorders. Oxidative neuronal damage and glutamate-mediated excitotoxicity have also been implicated in pathogenesis.

Between 5% and 10% of cases of MND are familial, and mutations in the free radical scavenging enzyme superoxide dismutase (SOD-1) and in a number of other genes, including *TDP-43* and *FUS*, have been identified. A hexanucleotide GGGGCC repeat expansion in the *C9ORF72* gene on chromosome 9 accounts for a significant proportion of familial cases of MND–FTD overlap.

Clinical features

Four main clinical patterns are seen. These different presentations usually merge as MND progresses. The sensory system is not involved and so sensory symptoms such as numbness, tingling and pain do not occur.

- ***Amyotrophic lateral sclerosis*** (***ALS***). This is the classic paraneoplastic presentation with simultaneous involvement of upper and lower motor neurones, usually in one limb, spreading gradually to other limbs and trunk muscles. The typical picture is one of progressive focal muscle weakness and wasting (e.g. in one hand), with muscle fasciculations due to spontaneous firing of abnormally large motor units formed by surviving axons branching to innervate muscle fibres that have lost their nerve supply. Cramps are a common but non-specific symptom. Examination often reveals upper motor neurone signs, such as brisk reflexes (a brisk reflex in a wasted muscle is a classic sign), extensor plantar responses and spasticity. Sometimes, an asymmetric spastic paraparesis is the presenting feature, with lower motor neurone features developing months later. Relentless progression of signs and symptoms over months allows confirmation of a diagnosis that may initially be suspected.
- ***Progressive muscular atrophy***. This is a pure lower motor neurone presentation with weakness, muscle wasting and fasciculations, usually starting in one limb and gradually spreading to involve other adjacent spinal segments.

- ***Progressive bulbar and pseudobulbar palsy*** (20%). The lower cranial nerve nuclei and their supranuclear connections are initially involved. Dysarthria, dysphagia, nasal regurgitation of fluids and choking are the presenting symptoms. A fasciculating tongue with slow, stiff tongue movements is the classic finding in a mixed bulbar palsy. Emotional incontinence with pathological laughter and crying may occur in pseudobulbar palsy.
- ***Primary lateral sclerosis*** (rare, 1–2%). This is the least common form of MND and is confined to upper motor neurones, causing a slowly progressive tetraparesis and pseudobulbar palsy.

Diagnosis

Diagnosis is largely clinical. There are no diagnostic tests but investigations allow exclusion of other disorders and may confirm subclinical involvement of muscle groups, such as paraspinal muscles. Denervation of muscles due to degeneration of lower motor neurones is confirmed by EMG.

Cervical spondylosis causing radiculopathy with myelopathy (upper and lower motor neurone signs) can cause diagnostic difficulty. Motor neuropathies, such as multifocal motor neuropathy, can also appear like MND (see p. 884).

Prognosis and management

Survival for more than 3 years is unusual, although there are rare MND cases who survive for a decade or longer.

No treatment has been shown to influence outcome substantially. Riluzole, a sodium-channel blocker that inhibits glutamate release, slows progression slightly, increasing life expectancy by 3–4 months on average. Non-invasive ventilatory support and feeding via a gastrostomy help prolong survival. Patients should be supported by a specialist multidisciplinary team with access to palliative care and a clinical nurse specialist.

Further reading

Atarashi R, Satoh K, Sano K et al. Ultrasensitive human prion detection in cerebrospinal fluid by real-time quaking-induced conversion. *Nat Med* 2011; 17:175–178.
Dubois B, Lirvan I. The FAB A frontal assessment battery at the bedside. *Neurology* 2000; 55:1621–1626.
Howard R, McShane R, Lindesay J et al. Donepezil and memantine for moderate-to-severe Alzheimer's disease. *N Engl J Med* 2012; 366:893–903.
National Institute for Health and Care Excellence. NICE Dementia guideline and technology appraisal; NICE 2011; http://www.nice.org.uk.
Petersen RC. Mild cognitive impairment. *N Engl J Med* 2011; 364:2227–2234.
Prince M, Knapp M, Guerchet M et al. *Dementia UK: Update*. London: Alzheimer's Society; 2014.
Querfurth HW, LaFerla FM. Alzheimer's disease. *N Engl J Med* 2010; 362:329–344.
Warren JD, Rohrer JD, Rossor MN. Frontotemporal dementia. *BMJ* 2013; 347:f4827.
White AR, Enever P, Tayebi M et al. Monoclonal antibodies inhibit prion replication and delay the development of prion disease. *Nature* 2003; 422:80–83.

CONGENITAL DISORDERS

Cerebral palsy

Cerebral palsy (CP) is an umbrella term encompassing disparate disorders that are apparent at birth or in childhood and are characterized by non-progressive motor deficits. It is the most common form of physical disability in childhood and most affected children survive into adulthood. A variety of intrauterine and neonatal cerebral insults may cause CP, including prematurity and its complications, hypoxia, intrauterine infections and kernicterus. In many cases, no specific cause can be identified.

Clinical features

Failure to achieve normal milestones is usually the earliest feature. Specific motor syndromes become apparent later in childhood or, rarely, in adult life.

- ***Spastic diplegia*** – lower limb spasticity, with scissoring of gait.
- ***Athetoid cerebral palsy*** (see p. 856).
- ***Infantile hemiparesis*** – may be noted at birth or later. One hemisphere is hypotrophic and the contralateral, hemiparetic limbs small (hemiatrophy).
- ***Ataxic and dystonic CP***.
- ***Co-morbidity*** – particularly epilepsy and learning difficulty, which are common and at least as disabling as the motor deficit.

Dysraphism

Failure of normal fusion of the fetal neural tube leads to a group of congenital anomalies. Folate deficiency during pregnancy is contributory and supplements should always be given (see p. 201). Antiepileptic drugs, such as valproate, are also implicated (see pp. 849–850). If there is access from the skin, such as from a sinus connecting to the subarachnoid space, bacterial meningitis may follow.

- ***Meningoencephalocele*** involves extrusion of brain and meninges through a midline skull defect; protrusion can be minor or massive.
- ***Spina bifida*** is failure of lumbosacral neural tube fusion. Several varieties occur.
- ***Spina bifida occulta*** is isolated failure of vertebral arch fusion (usually lumbar), often seen incidentally on X-rays (3% of the population). A dimple or a tuft of hair may overlie the anomaly; clinical abnormalities are unusual.
- ***Meningomyelocele*** may occur with spina bifida.

Meningomyelocele consists of elements of spinal cord and lumbosacral roots within a meningeal sac. This herniates through a vertebral defect. In severe cases, both lower limbs and sphincters are paralysed. Meningocele is a meningeal defect alone. The defect should be closed in the first 24 hours after birth.

Further reading

Colver A, Fairhurst C, Pharoah POD. Cerebral palsy. *Lancet* 2014; 383:1240–1249.
Kiernan MC, Vucic S, Cheah BC et al. Amyotrophic lateral sclerosis. *Lancet* 2011; 377:942–955.
Renton AE, Majounie E, Waite A et al. A hexanucleotide repeat expansion in C9ORF72 is the cause of chromosome 9p21-linked ALS-FTD. *Neuron* 2011; 72:257–268.

NEUROGENETIC DISORDERS

Approximately 80% of the 20 000–30 000 human genes are expressed in the brain. It is therefore not surprising that of the 5000 or so Mendelian disorders of humans, a high proportion are neurological disorders. Several hundred neurological disease genes have been identified and molecular genetic testing is now part of the neurological diagnostic process. Many of these disorders are covered in largely individual disease sections of this chapter.

Neurocutaneous syndromes

Neurofibromatosis type 1 (von Recklinghausen's disease)

One of the most common neurogenetic disorders, neurofibromatosis type 1 (NF-1) has a prevalence of 1 in 3000. Inheritance is

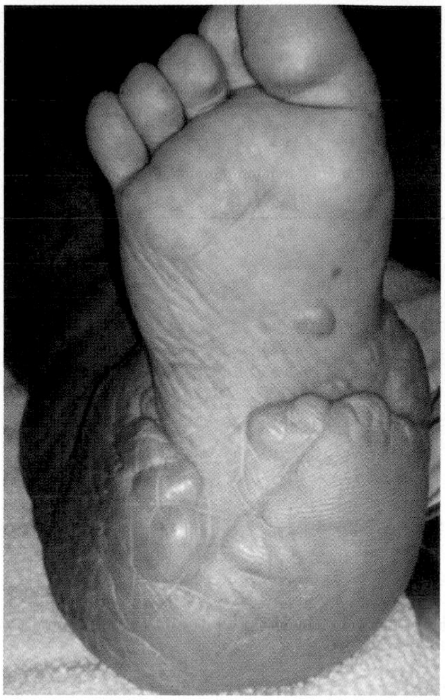

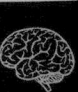

Figure 21.62 Plexiform neurofibroma.

autosomal dominant but 50% of cases are due to new mutations with no family history. The protein is called neurofibromin 1. NF-1 is characterized by multiple skin neurofibromas and pigmentation (*café-au-lait* patches – see p. 1367, axillary freckling and Lisch nodules of the iris). The neurofibromas arise from the neurilemmal sheath.

Skin neurofibromas present as soft subcutaneous, sometimes pedunculated, lumps (see p. 1367). They increase in number throughout life. Plexiform neurofibromas ***(Fig. 21.62)*** may develop on major nerves and proximal nerve roots, sometimes involving the spinal cord. Treatment is surgical removal if pressure symptoms develop. Associated features include learning difficulties, malignant transformation of neurofibromas, and bone abnormalities including scoliosis and fibrous dysplasia.

Neurofibromatosis type 2

Neurofibromatosis type 2 (NF-2) is much less common than NF-1. It is also autosomal dominant; the gene product, merlin or schwannomin, is a cytoskeletal protein. Many neural tumours occur:

- acoustic neuromas (usually bilateral) in 90%
- meningiomas
- gliomas (including optic nerve glioma)
- cutaneous neurofibromas (30%).

Tuberous sclerosis (epiloia)

Features of this rare multisystem, autosomal dominant condition include adenoma sebaceum, renal tumours and glial overgrowth in the brain (cortical tubers and sub-ependymal nodules). Epilepsy (70%) and learning difficulties (50%) are common complications.

Von Hippel–Lindau disease

This rare condition is dominantly inherited. Cerebellar, spinal and retinal haemangioblastomas develop and can be surgically removed. Tumours – renal cell carcinoma and phaeochromocytomas – may also occur. Polycythaemia sometimes develops.

Spinocerebellar ataxias

A wide variety of genetic disorders cause cerebellar ataxia as the sole or predominant clinical feature. Many are due to trinucleotide repeat insertions (see p. 115).

Early-onset ataxia

Most early (<20 years of age) childhood-onset inherited ataxias are autosomal recessive. Friedreich's ataxia is by far the most common, caused by a GAA trinucleotide repeat expansion in the frataxin gene (involved in mitochondrial iron metabolism). Onset is in the early teens with progressive difficulty in walking due to cerebellar ataxia and sensory neuropathy. Associated features include scoliosis, cardiomyopathy, optic atrophy, areflexia and diabetes.

Ataxia telangiectasia and ataxia with vitamin E deficiency are other rarer forms of autosomal recessive inherited ataxia.

Late-onset ataxia

Adult-onset (>20 years of age) inherited ataxias are usually dominantly inherited and there are some 30 different genetic forms, many caused by CAG trinucleotide repeats. There are three main categories of autosomal dominant cerebellar ataxia (ADCA):

- ***ADCA-1***: progressive ataxia with variable additional features, including peripheral neuropathy, pyramidal and extrapyramidal signs, and cognitive impairment. ADCA-1 is caused by mutations in loci *SCA1–3*.
- ***ADCA-2***: progressive ataxia with macular dystrophy. ADCA-2 is rare and involves the *SCA7* gene.
- ***ADCA-3***: late adult-onset 'pure' ataxia. ADCA-3 is associated with the *SCA6* gene in 50%. Non-genetic phenocopies must be excluded.

PARANEOPLASTIC SYNDROMES

Neurological disease may accompany malignancy in the absence of metastases. These paraneoplastic syndromes are associated with anti-neuronal antibodies, believed to be involved in the generation of signs and symptoms. Numerous anti-neuronal antibodies have been described.

Clinical pictures include:

- sensorimotor neuropathy (see p. 884)
- Lambert–Eaton myasthenic–myopathic syndrome (LEMS; see p. 890) and myasthenia gravis with thymoma
- motor neurone disease variants (see pp. 879–880)
- spastic paraparesis (see p. 873)
- cerebellar syndrome (see p. 814)
- limbic encephalitis (see pp. 865–866)
- paraneoplastic stiff person syndrome (see p. 892).

The neurological syndrome usually precedes evidence of the neoplasm: often a small-cell bronchial carcinoma, or breast or ovarian cancer. Diagnosis is based on the clinical pattern and antibody profile. Neuroimaging is typically normal. Treatment is often unsatisfactory.

PERIPHERAL NERVE DISEASE

Mechanisms of damage to peripheral nerves

Peripheral nerves consist of two principal cellular structures: the nerve nucleus with its axon, and the myelin sheath, which is produced by Schwann cells between each node of Ranvier (see ***Fig. 21.1***). Blood supply is via vasa nervorum. Several mechanisms, some coexisting, cause nerve damage.

Demyelination

Schwann cell damage leads to myelin sheath disruption. This causes marked slowing of conduction, seen, for example, in Guillain–Barré syndrome and many genetic neuropathies.

Axonal degeneration

Axon damage causes the nerve fibre to die back from the periphery. Conduction velocity initially remains normal (compare demyelination) because axonal continuity is maintained in surviving fibres. Axonal degeneration typically occurs in toxic neuropathies. A wide range of toxic and metabolic disorders damage peripheral nerves, as their long axons (requiring cellular transport of proteins from cell body to nerve terminals) make them uniquely vulnerable. This explains the concept of length-dependent neuropathy with the longest, most vulnerable axons (to the toes) being affected first.

Compression

Focal demyelination at the point of compression causes disruption of conduction. This typically occurs in entrapment neuropathies, such as carpal tunnel syndrome.

Infarction

Microinfarction of vasa nervorum occurs in diabetes and arteritis, such as polyarteritis nodosa and eosinophilic granulomatosis with polyangiitis (see p. 1121). Wallerian degeneration occurs distal to the infarct.

Infiltration

Infiltration of peripheral nerves occurs by inflammatory cells in leprosy and granulomas, such as sarcoid, and by neoplastic cells.

Nerve regeneration

Regeneration occurs either by remyelination – Schwann cells produce new myelin sheaths around an axon – or by axonal growth down the nerve sheath with sprouting from the axonal stump. Axonal growth takes place at up to 1 mm/day.

Types of peripheral nerve disease

(See ***Fig. 21.63***.)

- ***Neuropathy*** simply means a pathological process affecting a peripheral nerve or nerves.
- ***Mononeuropathy*** means a process affecting a single nerve.
- ***Mononeuritis multiplex*** means that several individual nerves are affected.
- ***Polyneuropathy*** describes diffuse, symmetrical disease, usually commencing peripherally. The course may be acute, chronic, static, progressive, relapsing or towards recovery. Polyneuropathies are motor, sensory, sensorimotor and autonomic. They are classified broadly into demyelinating and axonal types, depending on which principal pathological process predominates. It is often impossible to separate these clinically. Many systemic diseases cause neuropathies. Widespread loss of tendon reflexes is typical, with distal weakness and distal sensory loss.
- ***Radiculopathy*** means disease affecting nerve roots and ***plexopathy***, the brachial or lumbosacral plexus.

Diagnosis is made by clinical pattern, nerve conduction studies/EMG, nerve biopsy, usually sural or radial, and identification of systemic or genetic disease.

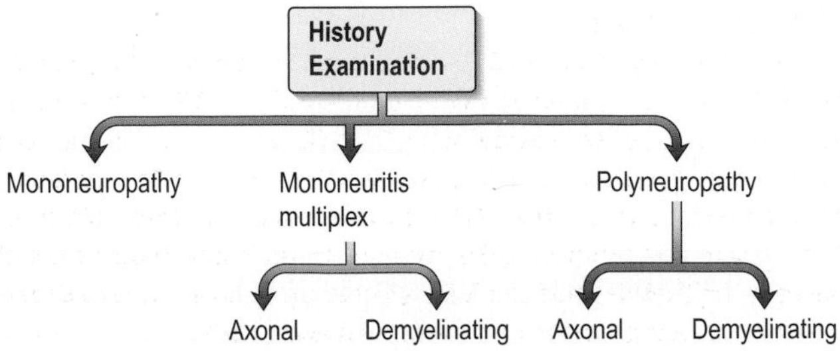

Figure 21.63 Peripheral neuropathies. The type of neuropathy (axonal or demyelinating) can be assessed by electrical nerve studies (see pp. 822–823).

Mononeuropathies

Peripheral nerve compression and entrapment

Nerves are vulnerable to mechanical compression at a few key sites ***(Box 21.65)***, such as the common peroneal nerve at the head of the fibula, or the ulnar nerve at the elbow. Entrapment develops in relatively tight anatomical passages, such as the carpal tunnel. Focal demyelination predominates at the compression site, and some distal axonal degeneration occurs.

These neuropathies are recognized largely by their clinical features. Diagnosis is confirmed by nerve conduction studies.

The most common are mentioned here. All are seen more frequently in people with diabetes.

Carpal tunnel syndrome

This common mononeuropathy, median nerve entrapment at the wrist, is usually known as carpal tunnel syndrome (CTS; see p. 655). CTS is typically not associated with any underlying disease. It is, however, seen in:

- hypothyroidism
- pregnancy (third trimester)
- rheumatoid disease
- acromegaly
- amyloidosis, including in dialysis patients.

Symptoms, signs and management are discussed on page 655.

Ulnar nerve compression

The nerve is compressed in the cubital tunnel at the elbow. This follows prolonged or recurrent pressure and elbow fracture ('tardy ulnar palsy', as onset is very delayed).

Box 21.65 Nerve compression and entrapment

Nerve	Entrapment/compression site
Median	Carpal tunnel (wrist)
Ulnar	Cubital tunnel (elbow)
Radial	Spiral groove (of humerus)
Posterior interosseous	Supinator muscle (forearm)
Lateral cutaneous of thigh	Inguinal ligament
Common peroneal	Neck of fibula
Posterior tibial	Tarsal tunnel (flexor retinaculum – foot)

There is clawing of the hand, wasting of interossei and hypothenar muscles, and weakness of interossei and medial two lumbricals with sensory loss in the little finger and splitting of the ring finger. Decompression and transposition of the nerve at the elbow is sometimes helpful but often disappointing.

The deep, solely motor branch of the ulnar nerve can be damaged in the palm by repeated trauma, such as from a crutch, screwdriver handle or cycle handlebars.

Radial nerve compression

The radial nerve is compressed acutely against the humerus: for example, when the arm is draped over a hard chair for several hours, known as Saturday night palsy. Wrist drop and weakness of brachioradialis and finger extension follow. Recovery is usual, though not invariable, within 1–3 months. Posterior interosseous nerve compression in the forearm also leads to wrist drop, without weakness of brachioradialis.

Lateral cutaneous nerve of the thigh compression

This is also known as meralgia paraesthetica and is described on page 659.

Common peroneal nerve palsy

The common peroneal nerve is compressed against the head of the fibula following prolonged squatting, yoga, pressure from a cast, prolonged bed rest or coma, or for no apparent reason. There is foot drop and weakness of ankle eversion. The ankle jerk (S1) is preserved. A patch of numbness develops on the anterolateral border of the dorsum of the foot and/or lateral calf. Confusion with an L5 motor radiculopathy may occur. Recovery is usual, though not invariable, within several months.

Hereditary neuropathy with pressure palsies

The genetic converse of Charcot–Marie–Tooth disease 1A (see p. 886), this dominantly inherited disorder is due to deletion (as opposed to duplication) of the *PMP-22* gene. Patients are susceptible to pressure palsies after minor compression episodes; even the brachial plexus may be involved. There is also a mild background neuropathy that develops gradually. Genetic testing can be performed.

Mononeuritis multiplex

This occurs in:

- diabetes mellitus
- leprosy
- vasculitis, including eosinophilic granulomatosis with polyangiitis
- amyloidosis
- malignancy
- neurofibromatosis
- HIV and hepatitis C infection
- multifocal motor neuropathy with conduction block.

Several nerves, such as the ulnar, median, radial and lateral popliteal, become affected sequentially or simultaneously. When multifocal neuropathy is symmetrical, there is difficulty distinguishing it from polyneuropathy.

Polyneuropathies (peripheral neuropathy)

Many diseases cause polyneuropathy. The diagnosis should not stop with identification of the polyneuropathy, but should involve a full diagnostic work-up to identify the underlying cause ***(Box 21.66)***.

Box 21.66 Varieties of polyneuropathy

- Guillain–Barré syndrome
- Chronic inflammatory demyelinating polyradiculoneuropathy
- Idiopathic sensorimotor neuropathy
- Metabolic, toxic and vitamin deficiency neuropathies (see ***Box 21.68***)

Box 21.67 Investigations in peripheral neuropathy

Initial investigations

- Blood tests:
  - Full blood count, erythrocyte sedimentation rate, vitamin B_{12}
  - Renal, liver, thyroid function
  - Glucose
  - Protein electrophoresis, immunoglobulins/immunofixation
  - Antinuclear antibody
- Chest X-ray
- Urine: Bence Jones proteins, casts

Selected patients

- Nerve biopsy
- Blood tests:
  - Anti-ganglioside antibodies
  - Anti-myelin-associated glycoprotein (anti-MAG) antibodies
  - HIV, Lyme disease, hepatitis C
  - Cryoglobulins, vasculitis screen
  - Anti-Ro and anti-La
  - Porphyrins
  - Genetic tests (e.g. Friedreich's ataxia)
  - Angiotensin-converting enzyme
  - Serum free light chains
  - Anti-neuronal antibodies
- Search for malignancy
- CSF analysis for protein
- Labial salivary gland biopsy for Sjögren's
- Slit-skin smear for leprosy
- Nerve conduction studies: to differentiate axonal from demyelinating forms

However, despite thorough investigation, the aetiology remains unknown in 50% of cases.

Clinical features. Duration, distribution and pattern of the different types of polyneuropathy vary considerably.

Neurophysiological features. Nerve conduction studies allow separation into axonal and demyelinating forms.

Diagnostic investigations (in addition to neurophysiology). A stepped approach can be taken ***(Box 21.67)***.

Immune-mediated neuropathies

Guillain–Barré syndrome (GBS)

Clinical features

Guillain–Barré syndrome (GBS) is also called acute inflammatory demyelinating polyradiculoneuropathy (AIDP). GBS is the most common acute polyneuropathy (3/100 000 per year); it is usually demyelinating or occasionally axonal, and has an immune-mediated, often post-infectious, basis. GBS is monophasic – it does not recur. The clinical spectrum of GBS extends to an acute motor axonal neuropathy (AMAN) and the Miller–Fisher syndrome – a rare proximal form causing ocular muscle palsies and ataxia.

Paralysis follows 1–3 weeks after an infection that is often trivial and seldom identified. *Campylobacter jejuni* and cytomegalovirus infections are well-recognized causes of severe GBS. Infecting organisms induce antibody responses against peripheral nerves. Molecular mimicry – that is, sharing of homologous epitopes between microorganism liposaccharides and nerve gangliosides (e.g. GM1) – is the possible mechanism.

The patient complains of weakness of the distal limb muscles and/or distal numbness. Low back pain is a frequent early feature. The weakness and sensory loss progress proximally, over several days to 6 weeks. Predominant proximal muscle involvement may occur and, rarely, pure sensory forms. Loss of tendon reflexes is almost invariable. In mild cases, there is mild disability before spontaneous recovery begins, but in some 20% respiratory and facial muscles become weak, sometimes progressing to complete paralysis. Autonomic features sometimes develop.

Diagnosis

This is established on clinical grounds and confirmed by nerve conduction studies; these show slowing of conduction in the common demyelinating form, prolonged distal motor latency and/or conduction block. CSF protein is often raised to 1–3 g/L; cell count and glucose level remain normal.

In the Miller–Fisher syndrome, antibodies against GQ1b (ganglioside) have a sensitivity of 90%.

The differential diagnosis includes other acute paralytic illnesses, such as botulism, cord compression, muscle disease and myasthenia.

Course and management

Paralysis may progress rapidly (hours/days) to require ventilatory support. It is essential for ventilation (vital capacity) to be monitored repeatedly to recognize emerging respiratory muscle weakness. Low-molecular-weight heparin (see p. 578) and compression stockings should be used to reduce the risk of venous thrombosis.

Immunoglobulin given intravenously within the first 2 weeks reduces duration and severity of paralysis. Patients should be screened for IgA deficiency before immunoglobulin is given, as severe allergic reactions due to IgG antibodies may occur when congenital IgA deficiency is present. Plasma exchange is an alternative. Prolonged ventilation may be necessary. Improvement towards independent mobility is gradual over many months or even years but may be incomplete. Some 5–8% die and 30% are left disabled.

Chronic inflammatory demyelinating polyradiculoneuropathy

Chronic inflammatory demyelinating polyradiculoneuropathy (CIDP) develops over months, causing progressive or relapsing proximal and distal limb weakness with sensory loss. Variants, such as the sensory ataxic form and multifocal motor neuropathy, occur. In some cases, cranial nerves may be involved.

There is no single diagnostic test but CSF protein is raised and patchy demyelination is usually seen on nerve conduction studies. Some cases are associated with a serum paraprotein. Nerve biopsy is sometimes required. CIDP responds to long-term immunosuppression with steroids or to intravenous immunoglobulin in the acute stages.

Multifocal motor neuropathy with conduction block

A distal immune-mediated focal demyelinating motor neuropathy (often asymmetrical and predominantly in the hands) develops gradually over months with profuse fasciculation; hence there is confusion with motor neurone disease (see pp. 879–880). Conduction block and denervation are seen electrically. Antibodies to the ganglioside GM_1 are found in over 50% of cases; this is non-specific, as antibodies are sometimes seen in other neuropathies, such as GBS.

Treatment is usually with regular intravenous immunoglobulin infusions that produce immediate improvement. Steroids may cause the condition to worsen and should be avoided.

Paraproteinaemic neuropathies

Up to 70% of patients with a serum paraprotein have a neuropathy and some 10% of patients with no other identifiable cause for their neuropathy have a paraprotein. Most are associated with monoclonal gammopathy of unknown signification (MGUS; see p. 628) but they are also seen in myeloma (see pp. 626–629). The antibody may be pathogenic for the neuropathy (e.g. anti-MAG) or coincidental in some cases.

IgM paraproteins: usually a demyelinating neuropathy. The paraproteins are often directed against myelin-associated glycoprotein (anti-MAG). The anti-MAG phenotype is a slowly progressive distal neuropathy with ataxia and prominent tremor.

POEMS syndrome (**P**olyneuropathy (demyelinating), **O**rganomegaly (hepatomegaly 50%), **E**ndocrinopathy (reduced testosterone usually), an ***M*** (para)protein band, and **S**kin changes): probably caused by vascular endothelial growth factor (VEGF) release from a plasmacytoma. Treatment is of the plasmacytoma/plasma cell dyscrasia.

Chronic sensorimotor neuropathy: no cause found

This situation is common. Progressive symmetrical numbness and tingling occur in hands and feet, spreading proximally in a glove and stocking distribution. Distal weakness also ascends. Tendon reflexes are lost. Symptoms may progress, remain static or occasionally remit. Autonomic features are sometimes seen.

Nerve conduction studies usually show axonal degeneration. Nerve biopsy helps to classify some cases: for example, diagnosing CIDP or unsuspected vasculitis.

Metabolic, toxic and vitamin deficiency neuropathies

Causes of the most common neuropathies are shown in ***Box 21.68***.

Metabolic neuropathies

Diabetes mellitus

This is the most common cause of neuropathy in developed countries; 50% of patients with diabetes have neuropathy after 25 years. Good glycaemic control is protective against this microvascular complication of diabetes. Several varieties of neuropathy occur (see pp. 1270–1272):

- ***distal symmetrical sensory neuropathy***: usually mild and asymptomatic; related to diabetes duration and glycaemic control
- ***acute painful sensory neuropathy*** (reversible with improved glycaemic control)
- ***mononeuropathy and multiple mononeuropathy (mononeuritis multiplex)***:
  - cranial nerve lesions
  - individual mononeuropathies (e.g. carpal tunnel syndrome) or mononeuritis multiplex
- ***diabetic amyotrophy***: a reversible vasculitic plexopathy or femoral neuropathy
- ***autonomic neuropathy***.

Box 21.68 Metabolic, toxic and vitamin deficiency neuropathies

Metabolic
- Diabetes mellitus
- Uraemia
- Hepatic disease
- Thyroid disease
- Porphyria
- Amyloid disease
- Malignancy
- Refsum's disease
- Critical illness

Toxic
- Drugs (see ***Box 21.70***)
- Alcohol
- Industrial toxins, e.g. lead, organophosphates

Vitamin deficiency
- B_1 (thiamine)
- B_6 (pyridoxine)
- Nicotinic acid
- B_{12}

Other
- Hereditary sensorimotor neuropathies, e.g. Charcot–Marie–Tooth
- Other polyneuropathies:
  - Neuropathy in cancer
  - Neuropathy in systemic diseases
  - Autonomic neuropathy
  - HIV-associated neuropathy
  - Critical illness neuropathy

Uraemia

Progressive sensorimotor neuropathy develops in chronic uraemia. Response to dialysis is variable; the neuropathy usually improves after transplantation.

Thyroid disease

A mild chronic sensorimotor neuropathy is sometimes seen in both hyperthyroidism and hypothyroidism. Myopathy also occurs in hyperthyroidism (see pp. 1205–1206).

Porphyria

In acute intermittent porphyria (see p. 1290), there are episodes of a severe, mainly proximal neuropathy in the limbs, sometimes with abdominal pain, confusion and coma. Alcohol, barbiturates and intercurrent infection can precipitate attacks.

Amyloidosis

Polyneuropathy or multifocal neuropathy develops (see pp. 1288–1289).

Toxic neuropathies

Alcohol

Polyneuropathy, mainly in the lower limbs, occurs with chronic alcohol use. It is a common cause of neuropathy. A myopathy may accompany it. For other neurological consequences of alcohol, see ***Box 21.69***.

Drugs and industrial toxins

Many drugs ***(Box 21.70)*** and a wide variety of industrial toxins cause polyneuropathy. Toxins include:
- lead – motor neuropathy
- acrylamide (plastics industry), trichlorethylene, hexane, fat-soluble hydrocarbons, e.g. solvent abuse; see p. 923
- arsenic, thallium and heavy metals.

Vitamin deficiency neuropathies

Vitamin deficiencies cause nervous system damage that is potentially reversible if treated early, and progressive if not. Deficiencies, often of multiple vitamins, develop in malnutrition.

Box 21.69 Neurological effects of ethyl alcohol

- Acute intoxication:
  - Disturbance of balance, gait and speech
  - Coma
  - Head injury and sequelae
- Alcohol withdrawal:
  - Morning shakes
  - Tremor
  - Delirium tremens
- Thiamine deficiency:
  - Polyneuropathy
  - Wernicke–Korsakoff syndrome
- Epilepsy
- Acute intoxication
- Alcohol withdrawal
- Hypoglycaemia
- Cerebellar degeneration
- Cerebral infarction
- Cerebral atrophy, dementia
- Osmotic demyelination syndrome (ODS)
- Marchiafava–Bignami syndrome (corpus callosum degeneration, rare)

Box 21.70 Drug-related neuropathies

Drug	Neuropathy	Mode/site of action
Phenytoin	M	A
Chloramphenicol	S, M	A
Metronidazole	S, S/M	A
Isoniazid	S, S/M	A
Dapsone	M	A
Anti-retroviral drugs	S > M	A
Nitrofurantoin	S/M	A
Vincristine	S > M	A
Paclitaxel	S > M	A
Disulfiram	S, M	A
Cisplatin	S	A
Amiodarone	S, M	D, A
Chloroquine	S, M	A, D
Suramin	M > S	D, A

A, axonal; D, demyelinating; M, motor; S, sensory.

Thiamine (vitamin B_1)

Dietary deficiency causes ***beriberi*** (see p. 198). Its principal features are polyneuropathy and cardiac failure. Thiamine deficiency also leads to Wernicke's encephalopathy and Korsakoff psychosis. Alcohol is the most common cause in Western countries and, rarely, anorexia nervosa or vomiting of pregnancy.

Wernicke–Korsakoff syndrome. This thiamine-responsive encephalopathy is due to damage in the brainstem and its connections. It consists of:
- ***eye signs –*** nystagmus, bilateral lateral rectus palsies, conjugate gaze palsies
- ***ataxia –*** broad-based gait, cerebellar signs and vestibular paralysis
- ***cognitive change –*** acutely, stupor and coma, later, an amnestic syndrome with confabulation.

Wernicke–Korsakoff syndrome is under-diagnosed. Thiamine should be given parenterally if the diagnosis is a possibility. Untreated Wernicke–Korsakoff syndrome commonly leads to an irreversible amnestic state. Erythrocyte transketolase activity is reduced but the test is rarely available.

Pyridoxine (vitamin B_6)

Deficiency causes a mainly sensory neuropathy. In practical terms, this is seen as limb numbness developing during anti-tuberculosis therapy in slow isoniazid acetylators (see p. 1111). Prophylactic pyridoxine 10 mg daily is given with isoniazid.

Vitamin B_{12} (cobalamin)

Deficiency causes damage to the spinal cord, peripheral nerves and brain.

Subacute combined degeneration of the cord (***SACD***). Combined cord and peripheral nerve damage is a sequel of addisonian pernicious anaemia and, rarely, other causes of vitamin B_{12} deficiency (see p. 528). Initially, there is numbness and tingling of fingers and toes; distal sensory loss, particularly of the posterior column, absent ankle jerks, and, with cord involvement, exaggerated knee jerks and extensor plantars. Optic atrophy and retinal haemorrhage may occur. In later stages, sphincter disturbance, severe generalized weakness and dementia develop. Exceptionally, dementia develops in the early stages.

Activated vitamin B_{12}, methylmalonic acid and homocysteine levels should be checked. Macrocytosis with megaloblastic marrow is usual, though not invariable, in SACD. Parenteral B_{12} reverses nerve damage but has little effect on the cord and brain. Copper deficiency is a very rare cause of a similar picture. Nitrous oxide abuse may cause functional B_{12} deficiency.

Genetic neuropathies

Inherited neuropathy may occur as 'pure' neuropathy disorders (e.g. Charcot–Marie–Tooth disease) or as part of a neurological multisystem disorder (e.g. spinocerebellar ataxias; see p. 881).

Charcot–Marie–Tooth disease

Charcot–Marie–Tooth (CMT) disease is a complex group of heterogeneous hereditary motor and sensory neuropathies (HMSNs) with multiple causative genes. Distal limb wasting and weakness typically progress slowly over many years, mostly in the legs, with variable loss of sensation and reflexes. In advanced disease, severe foot drop results but patients usually remain ambulant. Mild cases have pes cavus and toe clawing that can pass unnoticed.

- ***HSMN Ia (CMT 1A)*** – the most common (70% of CMT; 1:2500 births) autosomal dominant demyelinating neuropathy, caused by duplication (or point mutation) of a 1.5 megabase portion p11.2 of chromosome 17 encompassing the peripheral myelin protein 22 gene (*PMP-22*, 17p11.2)
- ***HSMN Ib (CMT 1B)*** – the second most common autosomal dominant demyelinating neuropathy due to mutations in the myelin protein zero gene (*MPZ*) on chromosome 1 (1q22)
- ***HSMN II (CMT 2)*** – rare axonal polyneuropathies also caused by *MFN2* or *KIFIB* on chromosome 1p36 and other mutations; there is prominent sensory involvement with pain and paraesthesias.
- ***distal spinal muscular atrophy*** – a rare cause of the CMT phenotype
- ***CMT with optic atrophy***, deafness, retinitis pigmentosa and spastic paraparesis
- ***CMTX*** – an X-linked dominant HSMN on chromosome Xq13.1; the gene product is a gap junction B1 protein (GJB1) or connexin 32 (see pp. 94–95).

Hereditary motor and sensory neuropathy type III

HSMN III is a rare childhood demyelinating sensory neuropathy (Déjérine–Sottas disease) leading to severe incapacity during adolescence. Nerve roots become hypertrophied. CSF protein is greatly elevated to ≥10 g/L. Point mutations, either of *PMP-22* gene or of *P0*, can generate this phenotype.

Other polyneuropathies

Neuropathy in cancer

Polyneuropathy is seen as a paraneoplastic syndrome (non-metastatic manifestation of malignancy). Polyneuropathy occurs in myeloma and other plasma cell dyscrasias via several mechanisms, including direct effects of paraproteins, amyloidosis and nerve infiltration, POEMS and effects of chemotherapy. Individual nerves may be infiltrated with malignant cells, such as lymphoma.

Neuropathies in systemic diseases

Vasculitic neuropathy occurs in SLE (see pp. 692–695), polyarteritis nodosa (p. 701), granulomatosis with eosinophilia (p. 1121) and rheumatoid disease (p. 678). Both multifocal neuropathy and symmetrical sensorimotor polyneuropathy occur.

Autonomic neuropathy

Autonomic neuropathy causes postural hypotension, urinary retention, erectile dysfunction, nocturnal diarrhoea, diminished sweating, impaired pupillary responses and cardiac arrhythmias. This can develop in diabetes and amyloidosis, and may complicate GBS and Parkinson's disease. Many varieties of neuropathy cause autonomic problems in a mild form. Occasionally, such as with amyloidosis, a severe autonomic neuropathy may occur.

Neuromuscular weakness complicating critical illness

Some 50% of critically ill intensive care unit patients with multiple organ failure and/or sepsis develop an axonal polyneuropathy (see p. 1167). Typically, distal weakness and absent reflexes are seen during recovery from critical illness. Resolution is usual.

Plexus and nerve root lesions

The common conditions that cause these are summarized in ***Box 21.71***.

Cervical and lumbar degeneration

Spondylosis ***(Box 18.10)*** describes vertebral and ligamentous degenerative changes occurring during ageing or following trauma. Several factors produce neurological signs and symptoms:

- osteophytes – local overgrowth of bony spurs or bars
- thickening of spinal ligaments
- congenital narrowing of the spinal canal

Box 21.71 Common root and plexus problems

Nerve root	Plexus
• Cervical and lumbar spondylosis • Trauma • Herpes zoster • Tumours, e.g. neurofibroma, metastases • Meningeal inflammation, e.g. syphilis, arachnoiditis	• Trauma • Malignant infiltration • Neuralgic amyotrophy • Thoracic outlet syndrome (cervical rib)

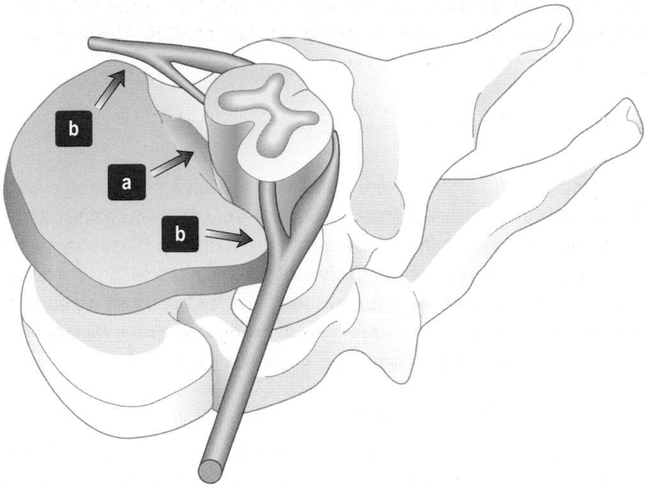

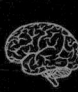

Figure 21.64 **Central and lateral disc protrusions. (a)** Central disc protrusion compressing the cord. **(b)** Lateral disc protrusion compressing nerve roots.

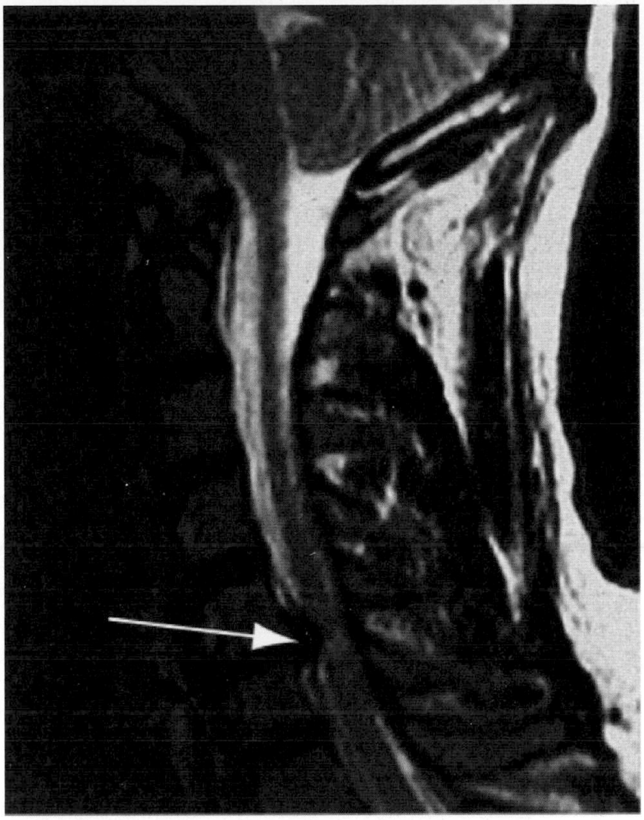

Figure 21.65 **C5/6 disc (arrowed) compressing the cord: T2-weighted MRI.**

- disc degeneration and protrusion (posterior and lateral protrusion: cord and root compression)
- vertebral collapse (osteoporosis, infection)
- rheumatoid synovitis (see p. 677)
- ischaemic changes within cord and nerve roots.

Narrowing of disc spaces, osteophytes, narrowing of exit foramina and narrowing of the spinal canal are also seen on X-rays and MRI in the *symptomless* population, commonly in the mid- and lower cervical and lower lumbar region, and so imaging must not be over-interpreted.

Lateral cervical disc protrusion

The patient complains of pain in the arm. A C7 protrusion is the most common problem ***(Fig. 21.64)***. There is root pain that radiates to the C7 myotome (triceps, deep to scapula and extensor aspect of forearm), with a sensory disturbance, tingling and numbness in the C7 dermatome.

In an established C7 root lesion there is:

- weakness/wasting – triceps, wrist and finger extensors
- loss of the triceps jerk (C7 reflex arc)
- C7 dermatome sensory loss.

Although the initial pain can be very severe, most cases recover with rest and analgesics. It is usual to immobilize the neck. Disc protrusion with root compression is seen on MRI. Root decompression is sometimes helpful.

Lateral lumbar disc protrusion

The L5 and S1 roots are commonly compressed by lateral prolapse of L4–L5 and L5–S1 discs; the root number below a disc interspace is compressed. There is low back pain and ***sciatica***: pain radiating from the back to buttock and leg. Onset is typically acute. This can follow lifting, bending or minor injury. When pain follows such an event, it is tempting to ascribe the disc protrusion to it. However, commonly, lateral lumbar disc protrusion is apparently spontaneous; lifting or injury is usually only bringing forward an inevitable disc prolapse.

Straight-leg raising is limited. There is reflex loss, such as ankle jerk in an S1 root lesion, and weakness of plantar flexion (S1) or great toe extension (L5). Sensory loss is found in the affected dermatome.

Most sciatica resolves with initial rest and analgesia, followed by early mobilization. MRI is sometimes appropriate. Surgery is indicated when a substantial persistent symptomatic disc lesion is shown.

Acute low back pain

Acute low back pain is extremely common. Often, pain is of disc or facet joint origin. Significant nerve root compression is unusual. Maintenance of activity and a trial of gentle manipulation are recommended (see also p. 657).

Cervical spondylotic myelopathy

This is a relatively common disorder of older adults. Posterior disc protrusion ***(Fig. 21.65)***, common at C4–5, C5–6 and C6–7 levels, causes spinal cord compression. Congenital spinal canal narrowing, osteophytic bars, ligamentous thickening and ischaemia are contributory. Usually, there are no or few neck symptoms. The patient complains of slowly progressive difficulty walking as a spastic paraparesis develops. A reflex level in the upper limbs and evidence of cervical radiculopathy may coexist. MRI demonstrates the level and extent of cord compression and T2 signal change is usually evident in the cervical cord at the point of maximal compression. Neck manipulation should be avoided.

Decompression by anterior cervical discectomy may be necessary when cord compression is severe or progressive. Complete recovery of the pyramidal signs may occur; progression is generally halted.

Central thoracic disc protrusion

Central protrusion of a thoracic disc is an unusual cause of paraparesis, as the thoracic spine is relatively non-mobile and disc degeneration and protrusion, other than that due to trauma, is rare.

The cauda equina syndrome

A central lumbosacral disc protrusion causes a cauda equina syndrome: that is, bilateral flaccid (compare spasticity in higher lesions) lower limb weakness, sacral numbness, retention of urine, erectile dysfunction and areflexia, usually with back pain. Multiple lumbosacral nerve roots are involved. Onset is either acute – an acute flaccid paraparesis – or chronic, sometimes with intermittent claudication. A central lumbosacral protrusion should be suspected if a patient with back pain develops retention of urine or sacral numbness. Urgent imaging and surgical decompression are indicated for this emergency. Neoplasms in the lumbosacral region can present with similar features.

Spinal stenosis

A narrow spinal canal is developmental and frequently symptomless, but a congenital narrowing of the cervical canal predisposes the cervical cord to damage from minor disc protrusion later.

In the lumbosacral region, further narrowing of the canal by disc protrusion causes root pain and/or buttock and lower limb claudication. As the patient walks, nerve roots become hyperaemic and swell, producing buttock and lower limb pain with numbness (claudication). Surgical decompression is required.

Neuralgic amyotrophy

Severe pain in the muscles around one shoulder is followed by wasting, usually of infraspinatus, supraspinatus, deltoid and serratus anterior. A demyelinating brachial plexopathy develops over several days. The cause is unknown; an allergic or viral basis is postulated. Rarely, a similar condition develops in distal upper limb muscles or in a lower limb. Recovery of wasted muscles is usual, but not invariable, over several months.

Thoracic outlet syndrome

A fibrous band or cervical rib extending from the tip of the C7 transverse process towards the first rib compresses the lower brachial plexus roots, C8 and T1. There is forearm pain (ulnar border), T1 sensory loss and thenar muscle wasting, principally of abductor pollicis brevis. A Horner syndrome may develop. The rib or band can be excised. Frequency of this diagnosis varies widely; thoracic outlet problems are sometimes invoked to explain ill-defined arm symptoms, typically on poor evidence.

A rib or band can also produce subclavian artery or venous occlusion. Neurological and vascular problems rarely occur together.

Malignant infiltration and radiation plexopathy

Metastatic disease of nerve roots or the brachial or lumbosacral plexus causes a painful radiculopathy and/or plexopathy. An example is apical bronchial carcinoma (Pancoast's tumour) causing a T1 and sympathetic outflow lesion: wasting of small hand muscles, pain and T1 sensory loss with an ipsilateral Horner syndrome. This also occurs in apical tuberculosis. In the upper limb, radiotherapy following breast cancer can produce a plexopathy.

MUSCLE DISEASES

Definitions

- ***Myopathy*** means a disease of voluntary muscle.
- ***Myositis*** indicates inflammation.
- ***Muscular dystrophies*** are inherited disorders of muscle cells.
- ***Myasthenia*** means fatiguable (worse on exercise) weakness – seen in neuromuscular junction diseases.
- ***Myotonia*** is sustained contraction/slow relaxation.
- ***Channelopathies*** are ion channel disorders of muscle cells.

Weakness is the predominant feature of muscle disease. A selection of these conditions is given in ***Box 21.72***.

Pathophysiology

Muscle fibres are affected by:

- acute inflammation and fibre necrosis (e.g. polymyositis, infection)
- genetically determined metabolic failure (e.g. Duchenne muscular dystrophy)
- infiltration by inflammatory tissue (e.g. sarcoidosis)
- fibre hypertrophy and regeneration
- mitochondrial diseases
- immunological damage, e.g. myasthenia gravis and Lambert–Eaton myasthenic syndrome
- ion channel disorders, e.g. chloride channel mutations in hereditary myotonias.

Diagnosis

Clinical features, including the distribution of weakness, wasting or hypertrophy, and the tempo of progression and presence of family history contribute to a clinical diagnosis. Several investigations help make a definitive diagnosis.

Serum muscle enzymes

Serum creatine kinase (CK) is a marker of muscle fibre damage and is greatly elevated in many dystrophies, such as Duchenne, and in inflammatory muscle disorders, such as polymyositis.

Box 21.72 Muscle disease: classification

- Acquired
  - Inflammatory
  - Polymyositis
  - Dermatomyositis
  - Inclusion body myositis
  - Viral, bacterial and parasitic infection
  - Sarcoidosis
- Endocrine and toxic
  - Corticosteroids/Cushing's
  - Thyroid disease
  - Calcium disorders
  - Alcohol misuse
  - Drugs, e.g. statins
- Myasthenic
  - Myasthenia gravis
  - Lambert–Eaton myasthenic–myopathic syndrome (LEMS)
- Genetic dystrophies
  - Duchenne
  - Facioscapulohumeral
  - Limb girdle and others
- Myotonic
  - Myotonic dystrophy
  - Myotonia congenita
- Channelopathies
  - Hypokalaemic periodic paralysis
  - Hyperkalaemic periodic paralysis
- Metabolic
  - Myophosphorylase deficiency (McArdle syndrome)
  - Other defects of glycogen and fatty acid metabolism
- Mitochondrial disease

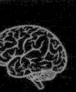

Neurogenetic tests

These are essential in muscular dystrophies and mitochondrial disease.

Electromyography

Characteristic EMG patterns are as follows:

- ***Myopathy***. Short-duration spiky polyphasic muscle action potentials are seen. Spontaneous fibrillation is occasionally recorded.
- ***Myotonic discharges***. A characteristic high-frequency whine is heard.
- ***Decrement and increment***. In myasthenia gravis, a characteristic decrement in evoked muscle action potential follows repetitive motor nerve stimulation. The reverse occurs, i.e. increment, following repetitive stimulation in LEMS (see p. 890).
- In ***denervation***, profuse fibrillation potentials are seen.

Muscle biopsy

Unlike neural tissue skeletal muscle can be easily biopsied to provide a definitive diagnosis using powerful molecular immunohistochemical techniques. Histology and muscle histochemistry of fibre types demonstrate denervation, inflammation and dystrophic changes. Electron microscopy is often valuable. In dystrophies, immunohistochemistry in specialist laboratories allows identification of the abnormal muscle protein and a precise molecular diagnosis.

Imaging

MRI shows ***signal changes*** within muscles in some cases of myositis, and fatty replacement of muscle in chronically damaged muscles.

Inflammatory myopathies

Inflammatory myopathies, including polymyositis, dermatomyositis and inclusion body myositis, are described on pages 697 and 698. Granulomatous muscle infiltration and inflammation may occur in sarcoidosis and other disorders such as rheumatoid arthritis, causing a mild myopathy. Viral myositis may also occur and muscles may be involved in other infections such as neurocysticercosis (see pp. 866–867).

Metabolic and endocrine myopathies

Corticosteroids and Cushing syndrome

Proximal weakness occurs with prolonged high-dose steroid therapy and in Cushing syndrome (see pp. 1197–1199). Selective type-2 fibre atrophy is seen on biopsy.

Thyroid disease

Several myopathies occur (see also p. 1207). Thyrotoxicosis can be accompanied by severe proximal myopathy. There is also an association between thyrotoxicosis and myasthenia gravis, and between thyrotoxicosis and hypokalaemic periodic paralysis (see p. 891). Both associations are seen more frequently in South-east Asia. In ophthalmic Graves' disease, there is swelling and lymphocytic infiltration of extraocular muscles (see p. 1208).

Hypothyroidism is sometimes associated with muscle pain and stiffness, resembling myotonia. A proximal myopathy also occurs.

Disorders of calcium and vitamin D metabolism

Proximal myopathy develops in hypocalcaemia, rickets and osteomalacia (see p. 717).

Hypokalaemia

Acute hypokalaemia (e.g. with diuretics) causes flaccid paralysis reversed by potassium, given slowly (see p. 167). Chronic hypokalaemia leads to mild, mainly proximal, weakness. (See also periodic paralysis; p. 891).

Alcohol and drugs

Severe myopathy with muscle pain, necrosis and myoglobinuria occurs in acute excess. A subacute proximal myopathy occurs with chronic alcohol use. A similar syndrome occurs in diamorphine and amfetamine addicts.

Drugs

Drug-induced muscle disorders include proximal myopathy (steroids), muscle weakness (lithium), painful muscles (fibrates), rhabdomyolysis (a fibrate combined with a statin, or interaction between statins and other drugs such as certain antibiotics) and malignant hyperpyrexia. Most respond to drug withdrawal.

Myophosphorylase deficiency (McArdle syndrome)

McArdle syndrome is a muscle only glycogenosis where there is a deficiency of muscle glycogen phosphorylase (PYGM). It presents with muscle cramps, fatigue, anaesthetic problems and myoglobinuria after exercise in adults. Diagnosis is made on a muscle biopsy with analysis of PYGM at 11q13. Patients have a normal life span. Sucrose should be given before exercise.

Malignant hyperpyrexia

Widespread skeletal muscle rigidity with hyperpyrexia as a sequel of general anaesthesia or neuroleptic drugs, such as haloperidol, is due to a genetic defect in the sarcoplasmic reticulum calcium-release channel of the muscle ryanodine receptor, RyR1. Death during or following anaesthesia can occur in this rarity, sometimes inherited as an autosomal dominant trait. Dantrolene is of some help for rigidity.

Neuromuscular junction disorders

Myasthenia gravis

Myasthenia gravis (MG) is an autoimmune disorder of neuromuscular junction (NMJ) transmission, characterized by weakness and fatiguability of proximal limb, bulbar and ocular muscles, the latter sometimes in isolation. The prevalence is about 4 in 100 000. MG is twice as common in women as in men, with a peak age incidence around 30 and a second smaller peak in incidence in older men.

Antibodies to acetylcholine receptor protein (anti-AChR antibodies) are pathogenic. Immune complexes of anti-AChR IgG and complement are deposited at the postsynaptic membranes, causing destruction of AChRs. Antibodies against muscle-specific receptor tyrosine kinase (anti-MuSK antibodies) have been identified in anti-AChR antibody-negative cases.

Thymic hyperplasia is found in 70% of MG patients below the age of 40. In some 10%, a thymic tumour is found (paraneoplastic myasthenia), the incidence increasing with age; antibodies to striated muscle can be demonstrated in some of these patients.

There is an association between MG and other autoimmune disorders: thyroid disease, rheumatoid disease, pernicious anaemia and SLE. Transient MG is sometimes caused by D-penicillamine treatment.

Clinical features

Weakness and fatiguability are typical. Limb muscles (proximal), extraocular muscles, speech, facial expression and mastication muscles are commonly affected. Symptoms are worse towards the end of the day. Fluctuating diplopia and ptosis (often asymmetric) are frequently early symptoms and symptoms may be confined to the eyes: ocular myasthenia. Respiratory difficulties can occur in generalized myasthenia. Early complaints of fatigue are frequently dismissed.

Complex extraocular palsies, ptosis and fatiguable proximal weakness are found on examination (prolonged upgaze should be checked and limb power tested after repetitive contractions). The reflexes are initially preserved but may be fatiguable: that is, they disappear following repetitive activity. Wasting is sometimes seen after many years.

Investigations

- ***Serum anti-AChR and anti-MuSK antibodies***. Anti-AChR antibodies are present in some 80–90% of cases of generalized MG. In pure ocular MG, anti-AChR antibodies are detectable in less than 30% of cases. These antibodies are highly specific for MG and confirm the diagnosis. Anti-MuSK antibodies define a subgroup of MG patients characterized by weakness predominantly in bulbar, facial and neck muscles.
- ***Repetitive nerve stimulation and single-fibre EMG***. A characteristic decrement occurs in the evoked muscle action potential during repetitive stimulation. Single-fibre EMG of orbicularis oculi is more sensitive than repetitive stimulation and shows block and jitter.
- ***Imaging and other tests***. Mediastinal MRI or CT is needed to look for thymoma in all cases. Antibodies to striated muscle suggest a thymoma.
- ***Tensilon (edrophonium) test***. This is seldom required and the drug is not available worldwide. Edrophonium 10 mg is given intravenously following a 1–2 mg test dose from the 10 mg vial. When the test is positive, there is substantial improvement in weakness within seconds and this lasts for up to 5 minutes. A control test using saline is performed. The sensitivity of the test is 80% but there are false-negative and false-positive tests. Occasionally, edrophonium (an anticholinesterase) causes bronchospasm and syncope. Resuscitation facilities must be available.

Course and management

MG fluctuates in severity; most cases have a protracted, life-long course. Respiratory impairment, nasal regurgitation and dysphagia occur; emergency ventilation may be required. Simple monitoring tests, such as the duration for which an arm can be held outstretched, and the vital capacity are useful.

Exacerbations are usually unpredictable and unprovoked but may be brought on by infections and by aminoglycosides and other drugs.

Drug treatment

Oral anticholinesterases

Pyridostigmine (60 mg tablet) is widely used. The duration of action is 3–4 hours, the dose (usually 3–16 tablets daily) determined by response. Pyridostigmine prolongs acetylcholine action by inhibiting cholinesterase. Overdose of anticholinesterases causes severe weakness (cholinergic crisis). Muscarinic side-effects, such as colic and diarrhoea, are common; oral atropine (antimuscarinic) 0.5 mg helps to reduce this. Anticholinesterases help weakness but do not alter the natural history of myasthenia.

Immunosuppressant drugs

These drugs are used in patients who do not respond to pyridostigmine or who have severe weakness. Steroids are usually used. There is improvement in 70%, although this may be preceded by an initial relapse; steroid dose should be increased slowly. Azathioprine, mycophenolate and other immunosuppressants are also used as steroid-sparing agents.

Thymectomy

Thymectomy improves myasthenia in patients with thymic hyperplasia and positive AChR antibodies (approximately one-third improve, one-third enter remission and one-third do not benefit). When a thymoma is present, the potential for malignancy makes surgery necessary but the myasthenia may not improve.

Plasmapheresis and intravenous immunoglobulin

These produce a rapid dramatic response and are used in exacerbations and severe myasthenic crisis.

Other rare myasthenic syndromes exist, such as congenital myasthenia.

Lambert–Eaton myasthenic–myopathic syndrome

Lambert–Eaton myasthenic–myopathic syndrome (LEMS) is a paraneoplastic manifestation of small-cell bronchial carcinoma due to defective acetylcholine release at the neuromuscular junction. A smaller proportion of cases are autoimmune without underlying malignancy. Proximal limb muscle weakness, sometimes with ocular/bulbar muscles, develops, with some absent tendon reflexes: a cardinal sign. Weakness tends to improve after a few minutes of muscular contraction, and absent reflexes return (compare myasthenia). Diagnosis is confirmed by repetitive nerve stimulation (increment; see above). Antibodies to voltage-gated calcium channels are found in most cases (90%). Treatment with 3,4-diaminopyridine (DAP) is reasonably safe and effective.

Muscular dystrophies

These progressive, genetically determined disorders of skeletal and sometimes cardiac muscle have a complex clinical and neurogenetic classification.

Duchenne muscular dystrophy and Becker's muscular dystrophy

These are inherited as X-linked recessive disorders, though one-third of cases are spontaneous mutations. Duchenne muscular dystrophy (DMD) occurs in 1 in 3000 male infants. There is absence of the gene product *dystrophin*, a rod-shaped cytoskeletal muscle protein in DMD. In Becker's dystrophy, dystrophin is present but levels are low. DMD is usually obvious by the fourth year, and often causes death by the age of 20.

Dystrophin is essential for cell membrane stability. Deficiency leads to reduction in three glycoproteins (α-, β- and γ-sarcoglycans) in the dystrophin-associated protein complex (DAP complex) that links dystrophin to laminin within cell membranes.

Becker's muscular dystrophy is less severe than Duchenne and weakness only becomes apparent in young adults.

Clinical features

A boy with DMD is noticed to have difficulty running and rising to his feet; he uses his hands to climb up his legs (Gowers' sign). There is initially a proximal limb weakness with calf pseudohypertrophy. The myocardium is affected. Severe disability is typical by the age of 10.

Investigations

The diagnosis is often suspected clinically. CK is grossly elevated (100–200 times normal). Biopsy shows variation in muscle fibre size, necrosis, regeneration and replacement by fat, and on immunochemical staining, absence of dystrophin.

Management

There is no curative treatment but new gene-editing therapies are in development. Steroids may delay progression. Physiotherapy helps prevent contractures in the later stages. Non-invasive respiratory support and multidisciplinary care improve life expectancy.

Carrier detection. Females with an affected brother have a 50% chance of carrying the *DMD* gene. In carriers, 70% have a raised CK, and usually EMG abnormalities and/or changes on biopsy. Carrier and prenatal diagnosis is available with genetic counselling.

Limb-girdle and facioscapulohumeral dystrophy

These less severe but disabling dystrophies are summarized in ***Box 21.73***. There are many other varieties of dystrophy; facioscapulohumeral dystrophy is one of the most common. Genes for numerous forms of limb-girdle muscular dystrophy have been identified. CK is usually moderately elevated.

Box 21.73 Limb-girdle and facioscapulohumeral dystrophies

	Limb-girdle	Facioscapulohumeral
Inheritance	Recessive, dominant or X-linked	Dominant, new mutations common
Onset	10–20 years	10–40 years
Muscles affected	Proximal: shoulders, pelvic girdle	Face, shoulders, scapular winging, upper arms, foot drop. Typically asymmetric
Progression	Severe disability <25 years	Life expectancy normal, slow progression
Associated features	Very variable. Contractures in Emery Dreifuss dystrophy	Occasionally, deafness and retinal abnormalities
Diagnosis	Multiple genetic types Diagnosis on muscle biopsy immunohistochemistry and genetic testing	Genetic testing (muscle biopsy usually not required but may show inflammatory changes)

Myotonias

Myotonias are characterized by continued, involuntary muscle contraction after cessation of voluntary effort: that is, failure of muscle relaxation. EMG is characteristic (see p. 823). The two most common myotonias are described below. Patients with myotonia tolerate general anaesthetics poorly.

Myotonic dystrophy

This autosomal dominant condition is a genetic disorder with two different triple repeat mutations: most commonly, an expanded CTG repeat in a protein-kinase (*DMPK*) gene (DM1). The less common variety (DM2) is caused by an expanded CCTG repeat in a zinc finger protein gene. There is a correlation between disease severity, age at onset and approximate size of triplet repeat mutations. There is progressive distal muscle weakness, with ptosis, weakness and thinning of the face and sternomastoids. Myotonia is typically present. Muscle disease is part of a syndrome comprising:

- cataracts
- frontal baldness
- cognitive impairment (mild)
- oesophageal dysfunction (and aspiration)
- cardiomyopathy and conduction defects (sudden death can occur in type 1)
- small pituitary fossa and hypogonadism
- glucose intolerance
- low serum IgG.

This gradually progressive condition usually becomes evident between 20 and 50 years. Phenytoin or procainamide helps.

Myotonia congenita

Autosomal dominant myotonia, usually mild, becomes evident in childhood. The gene, *CLC1*, codes for a muscle chloride channel. The myotonia, which persists, is accentuated by rest and by cold. Diffuse muscle hypertrophy occurs; the patient has bulky muscles.

Channelopathies

Hypokalaemic periodic paralysis

This disorder is characterized by generalized weakness, including that of bulbar muscles, which often starts after a heavy carbohydrate meal or following exertion. Attacks last for several hours. The disorder often first comes to light in the teenage years and tends to remit after the age of 35. Serum potassium is usually below 3.0 mmol/L in an attack. The weakness responds to (slow) intravenous potassium chloride. It is usually inherited as an autosomal dominant trait caused by mutation in a muscle voltage-gated calcium channel gene (*CACLN1A3*). Other mutations in the sodium channels (*SCNA4*) and potassium channels (*KCNE3*) also occur. Acetazolamide sometimes helps prevent attacks. Weakness can be caused by diuretics. A similar condition can also occur with thyrotoxicosis.

Hyperkalaemic periodic paralysis

This condition, also autosomal dominant, is characterized by attacks of weakness, sometimes with exercise. Attacks start in childhood and tend to remit after the age of 20; they last about 30–120 minutes. Myotonia may occur. Serum potassium is elevated. An attack can be terminated by intravenous calcium gluconate or chloride. There are point mutations in a muscle voltage-gated sodium channel gene (*SCN4A*). Acetazolamide or a thiazide diuretic can be helpful.

A very rare normokalaemic, sodium-responsive periodic paralysis also occurs.

Stiff person syndrome

Stiff person syndrome (SPS) is a rare autoimmune disease, more common in females, causing axial muscle stiffness with abnormal posture, spasms and falls. Attacks of stiffness are sometimes provoked by noise or emotion, but sometimes occur spontaneously. Between attacks, which last from hours to days or even weeks, the patient may appear normal.

Widespread muscle stiffness is typical during an attack; there are no other neurological signs. SPS has been mistaken for Parkinson's, dystonia and non-organic conditions. Anti-glutamic acid decarboxylase antibodies (anti-GAD) are found in very high titre in >50% of cases and are believed to be involved in the generation of muscle stiffness. Continuous motor activity in paraspinal muscles is seen on EMG.

Treatment with diazepam, other muscle relaxants and intravenous immunoglobulin can be helpful during attacks.

A form of SPS is also seen occasionally as a paraneoplastic condition associated with antibodies to the synaptic protein amphiphysin (see ***Box 17.8***).

Mitochondrial diseases

These comprise a complex group of rare disorders involving muscle, peripheral nerves and CNS, characterized by morphological and biochemical abnormalities in mitochondria. Mitochondrial DNA is inherited maternally (see p. 109). The spectrum is wide, ranging from optic atrophy (see Leber's; p. 112) to myopathies, neuropathies and encephalopathy.

- *MELAS* (*m*itochondrial *e*ncephalomyopathy, *l*actic *a*cidosis, *s*troke-like episodes) is one well-recognized form.
- Chronic progressive ophthalmoplegia (CPEO) is another.
- *MERRF* describes *m*yoclonic epilepsy with abnormal muscle histology, the muscle appearance being described as *r*agged *r*ed *f*ibres.

Further reading

Ryan A, Matthews E, Hanna MG. Skeletal muscle channelopathies. *Curr Opin Neurol* 2007; 20:558–563.
Shapira AHV. Mitochondrial disease. *Lancet* 2006; 368:70–82.

Bibliography

Clarke C, Howard R, Rossor M et al. (eds). *Neurology: A Queen Square Textbook*. Oxford: Blackwell; 2009.

Significant websites

http://jnnp.bmjjournals.com *Journal of Neurology, Neurosurgery and Psychiatry*.
http://www.patient.co.uk/selfhelp.asp *UK Patient Support Group*.
http://www.theabn.org *Association of British Neurologists information service*.

22 Psychological medicine

Julius Bourke, Peter D White

See your e-book for key learning points, clinical tips, drug tips, extra images, extra tables, case studies, MCQs and Special Topics from the International Advisory Board.

INTRODUCTION

Psychiatry is concerned with the study and management of disorders of mental function: primarily, thoughts, perceptions, emotions and purposeful behaviours. Psychological medicine, or liaison psychiatry, is concerned primarily with psychiatric disorders in patients who have physical complaints or conditions. This chapter will mainly address this branch of psychiatry.

The long-held belief that diseases are either physical or mental has been replaced by the accumulated evidence that the brain is functionally or anatomically abnormal in psychiatric disorders. Physical, psychological and social factors, and their interactions, must be looked into, in order to understand psychiatric conditions – replacing the mind/body ***biomedical model*** with an integrated ***biopsychosocial*** one.

Epidemiology

The point prevalence of psychiatric disorders in adults in the UK is about 20%, mostly composed of depressive and anxiety disorders and substance misuse (mainly alcohol) ***(Box 22.1)***. The prevalence is about twice as high in patients attending the general hospital, with the highest rates in the accident and emergency department and medical wards.

Culture and ethnicity

These can alter either the presentation or the prevalence of psychiatric ill-health. Biological factors in mental illness are similar across cultural boundaries but may vary by ethnic groups, whereas psychological and social factors will vary across culture. For example, the prevalence and presentation of schizophrenia vary little between countries, suggesting that biological factors operate independently of cultural ones. In contrast, disorders in which social factors play a greater role vary between cultures, so that anorexia nervosa is found more often in Western-influenced cultures. Culture can also influence the presentation of illnesses, such that physical symptoms are more common presentations of depressive illness in Asia than in Europe. Similarly, culture will influence the healthcare that is both sought and provided for the same condition.

CLINICAL APPROACH TO THE PATIENT WITH A PSYCHIATRIC DISORDER

The psychiatric history

The history is essential in making a diagnosis. The method is similar to that used in all specialties, but tailored to help to make a psychiatric diagnosis, determine possible aetiology and estimate prognosis. The history may be taken from the patient, or a friend or relative (usually with the patient's permission), or from relevant healthcare professionals. The patient interview also enables a doctor to establish a therapeutic relationship with the patient. ***Box 22.2*** gives essential guidance on how to conduct such an interview safely, although it is rare for a patient to harm a healthcare professional. When interviewing a patient for the first time, follow the guidance outlined on page 10.

Components of the history are summarized in ***Box 22.3***.

The mental state examination

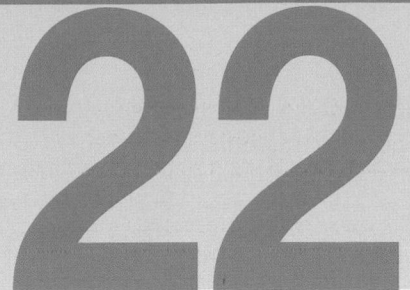

The history will already have assessed several aspects of the mental state examination (MSE), but several of these will need to be expanded on and specific areas, such as cognition, tested. The MSE is typically followed by a physical examination, and concluded with an assessment of insight and risk, and a formulation that takes into account a differential diagnosis and aetiology. Each domain of the MSE is given below; abnormalities that might be detected and the disorders in which they are found are summarized in ***Box 22.4***.

Box 22.1 The approximate prevalence of psychiatric disorders in different UK populations

Population/disorder	Approximate percentage
Community	20[a]
Neuroses	16
Psychoses	0.5
Alcohol misuse	5
Drug misuse	2[b]
Primary care	25
General hospital outpatients	30
General hospital inpatients	40

[a]Total in the community (general population) is 20% due to co-morbidity.
[b]An under-estimate.

Box 22.2 The essentials of a safe psychiatric interview

- ***Beforehand***: Ask someone with experience who knows the patient whether it is safe to interview the patient alone.
- ***Access to others***: If in doubt, interview in the view or hearing of others, or accompanied by another member of staff.
- ***Setting***: If safe, conduct the interview in a quiet room alone for confidentiality, not by the bed.
- ***Seating***: Place yourself between the door and the patient.
- ***Alarm***: If one is available, find out where the alarm is and how to use it.

Aspects of the MSE

Appearance and general behaviour

The state and colour of the clothes, facial appearance, eye contact, posture and movement provide information about a patient's affect. Agitation and anxiety cause an easy startle response, sweating, tremor, restlessness, fidgeting and visual scanning (for danger).

Speech

The rate, rhythm, volume and content of the patient's speech should be examined for abnormalities. Note that speech is the only way that you can examine thoughts and, as such, disorders of thought form are typically observed in this section. Thought content (literally, the content of the patient's thoughts) is dealt with separately (see below). Abnormalities that may reflect neurological lesions, such as dysarthria and dysphasia, should also be assessed.

Mood and affect

The patient has an ***emotion*** or ***feeling***, tells you about their ***mood***, and what you observe is the patient's ***affect***. Mood may be altered in three ways: persistent change in mood, fluctuation and incongruity.

Thoughts

Abnormalities of thought content and thought possession are recorded here. Delusions (see ***Box 22.4***) can be further categorized as primary or secondary, depending on whether they arise *de novo* or secondary to other abnormalities of the mental state.

Abnormal perceptions

Assessing perceptions will involve you observing the patient as well as asking questions of them. For example, patients experiencing auditory hallucinations may appear startled by sounds or voices that you cannot hear, or may interact with them: for example, appearing to be engaged in conversation when nobody else is in the room. Hallucinations can affect any sensory modality and

Box 22.3 Summary of the components of the psychiatric history

Component	Description
Reason for referral	Why and how the patient came to the attention of the doctor
Present illness	How the illness progressed, from the earliest time at which a change was noted until the patient came to the attention of the doctor
Past psychiatric history	Prior episodes of illness, and where and how they were treated. Prior self-harm
Past medical history	This should include emotional reactions to illness and procedures
Family history	History of psychiatric illnesses and relationships within the family
Personal (biographical) history	*Childhood*: mother's pregnancy and patient's birth (complications, nature of delivery), early development and attainment of developmental milestones (e.g. learning to crawl, walk, talk). School history: age started and finished; truancy, bullying, reprimands; qualifications *Adulthood*: employment (age at first job, total number of jobs, reasons for leaving, problems at work), relationships (sexual orientation, age at first relationship, total number of relationships, reasons for ending them), children and dependants
Reproductive history	*Women*: menstrual problems, pregnancies, terminations, miscarriages, contraception and menopause
Social history	Current employment, benefits, housing, current stressors
Personality	This may help to determine prognosis. How do they normally cope with stress? Do they trust others and make friends easily? Irritable? Moody? A loner? This list is not exhaustive
Drug history	Prescribed and over-the-counter medication, units and type of alcohol/week, tobacco, caffeine and illicit drugs
Forensic history	Explain that you need to ask about this, since ill-health can sometimes lead to problems with the law. Note any violent or sexual offences. This is part of a *risk assessment*. Worst harm they have ever inflicted on someone else? Under what circumstances? Would they do the same again, were the situation to recur?
Systematic review	Psychiatric illness is not exclusive of physical illness! The two may not only coexist but also have a common aetiology

Box 22.4 The mental state examination and the psychopathology it is used to detect

Type of disorder	Abnormality	Description	Typical of which disorder(s)?
Appearance and behaviour			
		Colour and state of clothes, facial appearance, eye contact, posture, movement, agitation. Startle response, sweating, tremor, restlessness, fidgeting, visual scanning (for danger), distractibility	
Speech			
Disorders of stream of thought	Pressured speech	Rapid rate, increased volume, difficult to interrupt	Mania
	Poverty of speech	Lengthy pauses between brief utterances	Depressive illness Schizophrenia
	Thought block	A sentence is suddenly stopped for no obvious reason	Schizophrenia
Disorders of thought form	Flight of ideas	Thoughts rapidly jump from one topic to another	Mania
	Word salad or schizophasia	The connection between themes, sentences and even words is lost, resulting in unintelligible speech, although words are still identifiable	Schizophrenia Receptive (Wernicke's) aphasia
	Perseveration	Persistent, inappropriate repetition of the same thought or action	Schizophrenia, Obsessive–compulsive disorder Frontal lobe lesions
Mood			
Persistent change	Depression	Low mood, tearfulness, low spirits	Depression
	Anxiety	Constant, inappropriate or excessive worry, fear, apprehension, tension or inner restlessness	Anxiety disorders (±depressive illnesses) Drug intoxication and withdrawal
	Elation	A feeling of high spirits, exuberant happiness, vitality	Mania, drug intoxication
	Irritability	Either expressed (as in a temper or impatience) or an internal feeling of exasperation or anger	Depression (especially men) Mania
	Blunted affect	A total absence of emotion	Schizophrenia (in chronic illness)
Fluctuating change		Different emotions rapidly follow one another. Alternatively, excessive emotion over events	Mixed affective states Pseudobulbar palsy
Incongruity		Mood and context do not reflect one another, e.g. laughing whilst describing the death of a loved one	Schizophrenia Mania
Thoughts			
Disorders of content	Delusions	A false belief held with absolute conviction, and out of keeping with the patient's cultural, social and religious beliefs	Psychosis
	Overvalued ideas	Deeply held personal convictions that are understandable when the individual's background is known	–
	Obsessions	Recurrent, persistent thought, impulse, image or musical theme occurring despite the patient's effort to resist it. May be accompanied by compulsions (repetitive, seemingly purposeful action performed stereotypically)	Obsessive–compulsive disorder
Disorders of thought possession	Thought broadcast	The patient experiences their thoughts as being understood by others without talking	Schizophrenia
	Thought insertion	The patient's thought is perceived as being planted in their mind by someone else	Schizophrenia
	Thought withdrawal	The patient experiences their thoughts being taken away from them, without their control	Schizophrenia
Perceptions			
	Hallucinations	Perception in the absence of a stimulus, perceived in objective space with the qualities of normal perceptions	Psychosis Organic brain states, e.g. delirium
	Pseudo-hallucinations	Usually auditory: true externally sited hallucinations, but with insight into their imaginary nature, or internally sited (e.g. 'I heard a voice in my head speaking to me')	Depressive illness Personality disorders Not indicative of psychotic disorder
	Illusions	Misperceptions of external stimuli, most likely when the general level of sensory stimulation is reduced	Normal experience Some neurological disorders
	Depersonalization	A change in self-awareness such that the patient feels unreal or detached from their body. The patient is aware, however, of the subjective nature of this alteration	Anxiety disorders Schizophrenia Temporal lobe epilepsy, in healthy people when tired
	Derealization	The unpleasant feeling that the external environment has become unreal and/or remote; patients may describe themselves as though they are in a dream-like state	As in depersonalization
	Heightened sensitivity	Photosensitivity and phonosensitivity	Anxiety disorders Drug intoxication and withdrawal Migraine Epilepsy

Box 22.5 Cognitive examination[a]

Cognitive domain	Assessment
Diffuse functions	
Premorbid intelligence	An estimate is helpful in assessing changes in cognitive abilities: Ask the patient about the final year and level of their education, and the highest qualifications or skills they achieved
Orientation	Assess orientation to time, place and person. Consciousness can be defined as the awareness of the self and the environment. Clouding of consciousness is more accurately a fluctuating level of awareness and is commonly seen in delirium
Attention	Ask the patient to say the months of the year or days of the week backwards
Verbal memory	*Immediate recall or registration*: ask the patient to repeat a name and address with 10 or so items, noting how many times it takes to recall it with 100% accuracy (normal is 1 or 2). *Short-term memory*: ask the patient to try to remember the address and then ask it of them again after 5 min (0 or 1 error is normal).
Long-term memory	Ask the patient to recall the news from that morning or recently. If they are not interested in the news, find out their interests (football team, favourite soap opera) and ask relevant questions. *Amnesia* is literally an absence of memory; *dysmnesia* indicates a dysfunctioning memory
Focal functions	
Frontal, temporal and parietal lobe function	These are covered in detail on pages 798–802
Behaviour	Disinhibited behaviour that cannot be explained by a psychiatric illness is suggestive of frontal lobe lesions
Sequential tasks	Ask the patient to alternate making a fist with one hand at the same time as a flat hand with the other Ask the patient to tap a table once if you tap twice, and vice versa Note any motor perseveration whereby the patient cannot change the movement once established Observe for verbal perseveration, in which the patient repeats the same answer as given previously for a different question
Abstract thinking	Ask the patient the meaning of common proverbs: a literal meaning may suggest frontal lobe dysfunction, assuming reasonable premorbid intelligence

[a]This correlates well with more time-consuming intelligence quotient (IQ) tests, but it will not pick up cognitive problems caused by focal brain lesions as easily.

specific types of hallucination will be addressed later in the chapter along with the disorders in which they most commonly occur.

Cognitive state

Examination of the cognitive state is necessary to diagnose organic brain disorders, such as delirium and dementia. Poor concentration, confusion and memory problems are the most common subjective complaints. Clinical testing involves the screening of cognitive functions, which may suggest the need for more formal psychometry. Simple questioning will detect about 90% of people who have cognitive impairments, with about 10% false positives. Testing can be divided into tests of diffuse and focal brain functions, and the means of assessment are set out in ***Box 22.5***.

Insight and illness beliefs

Insight is the degree to which a person recognizes that he or she is unwell, and is minimal in people with a psychosis. ***Illness beliefs*** are the patient's own explanations of their ill-health, including diagnosis and causes. These beliefs should be elicited because they can help to determine prognosis and adherence to treatment.

Defence mechanisms

Although not strictly part of the mental state examination, it is useful to be able to identify psychological defences in ourselves and our patients. Defence mechanisms are unconscious mental processes. Some of the most commonly used defence mechanisms are described in ***Box 22.6*** and are useful in understanding many aspects of behaviour.

Box 22.6 Common defence mechanisms

Defence mechanism	Description
Repression	Exclusion from awareness of memories, emotions and/or impulses that would cause anxiety or distress if allowed to enter consciousness
Denial	Similar to repression and occurs when patients behave as though unaware of something that they might be expected to know, e.g. a patient who, despite being told that a close relative has died, continues to behave as though the relative were still alive
Displacement	Transferring of emotion from a situation or object with which it is properly associated to another that gives less distress
Identification	Unconscious process of taking on some of the characteristics or behaviours of another person, often to reduce the pain of separation or loss
Projection	Attribution to another person of thoughts or feelings that are in fact one's own
Regression	Adoption of primitive patterns of behaviour appropriate to an earlier stage of development. It can be seen in ill people who become child-like and highly dependent
Sublimation	Unconscious diversion of unacceptable behaviours into acceptable ones

Risk assessment

The assessment of risk may sound daunting but it is common to all clinical practice: for instance, when determining whether a patient with chest pain should be reviewed in the resuscitation room of the emergency department rather than a normal cubicle. Risk must be assessed in people with a psychiatric diagnosis, although the nature of 'risk' is different.

Risk can be broken down into two parts: the risk that the patient poses to themselves and that which they pose to others ***(Box 22.7)***.

Box 22.7 The assessment of risk

	Risk to self	Risk to others
Active	Acts of self-harm or suicide attempts Look for prior history of self-harm and what may have precipitated or prevented it	Aggression towards others – this may be actual violence or threatening behaviour A past history of aggression is a good predictor of its recurrence. Look at the severity and quality of, and remorse for, prior violent acts, as well as identifiable precipitants that might be avoided in the future (e.g. alcohol)
Passive	Self-neglect Manipulation by others	Neglect of others – always find out whether there are children or other dependants at home

Box 22.8 The main causes of disturbed behaviour

- Drug intoxication (especially alcohol)
- Delirium (acute confusional state)
- Acute psychosis
- Personality disorder

An appraisal of risk will already have been made in the initial preparations for seeing a patient (see ***Box 22.2***) and in checking 'forensic history' (see ***Box 22.3***). Additional information from family, friends or professionals who know the patient may prove invaluable.

Severe behavioural disturbance

Patients who are aggressive or violent cause understandable apprehension in all staff, and are most commonly seen in the accident and emergency department. Information from anyone accompanying the patient, including police or carers, can help considerably. ***Box 22.8*** lists the main causes of disturbed behaviour.

Management of the severely disturbed patient

The primary aims of management are the control of dangerous behaviour and the establishment of a provisional diagnosis. Four specific strategies may be necessary when dealing with the violent patient:

- reassurance and explanation
- medication
- physical restraint
- monitoring.

These are explained in ***Box 22.9***. Remember that the behaviour exhibited is normally a reflection of an underlying disorder and, as such, portrays suffering and often fear. The approach to the agitated or even the violent patient must therefore take this into account and the steps listed are used with the intention of alleviating this suffering whilst maintaining the safety of the individual, and of other patients and staff. Management begins at the point of an initial assessment that takes into account prior episodes of disturbed behaviour and its precipitants. Armed with this knowledge, it may be possible to prevent a recurrence.

Box 22.9 The management of the severely disturbed patient

Method	Description
'Verbal de-escalation'	First step – try to defuse the situation by talking to the patient. The disturbed behaviour may be simple to correct, e.g. if staff explain their intentions on approaching the patient
Medication	Where possible, use oral medication first. Start with a short-acting benzodiazepine unless the patient is elderly or delirious (can worsen confusion and agitation). Give medications sequentially, rather than together, allowing 30 min to 1 h for them to take effect: Lorazepam (oral/i.m.) 0.5–1 mg Haloperidol (oral) 2.5–5 mg Promethazine (i.m.) 50 mg Haloperidol (i.m.) 5–10 mg Olanzapine (i.m.) 10 mg
Physical restraint	Use only to maintain safety and to administer intramuscular medications. It should be performed by adequately trained psychiatric nurses and security staff. In the UK, doctors will never be involved in restraining the patient. Restraint is a potentially dangerous intervention, even more so when mixed with psychotropic medication, and deaths have occurred as a direct consequence
Monitoring	Where medications are used, monitor blood pressure, pulse, respiratory rate and oxygen saturation frequently, dictated by the level of ongoing agitation and consciousness

The relevant physical examination

This should be guided by the history and mental state examination. Particular attention should be paid to the neurological and endocrinological examinations when organic brain syndromes and affective illnesses are suspected.

Summary or formulation

When the full history and mental state have been assessed, you should make a concise assessment or 'formulation' of the case. In addition to summarizing the essential features of the history and examination, the formulation includes a differential diagnosis, possible causal factors, and any further investigations or interviews that are needed. It concludes with a concise plan of treatment and a statement of the likely prognosis.

Further reading

Dudas RB, Berrios GE, Hodges JR. The Addenbrooke's Cognitive Examination (ACE) in the differential diagnosis of early dementias versus affective disorder. *Am J Geriatr Psychiatry* 2005; 13:218–226.

McAllister-Williams RH, Cousins D, Lunn B. Clinical assessment and investigation in psychiatry. *Medicine* 2012; 40:568–573.

CLASSIFICATION OF PSYCHIATRIC DISORDERS

The classification of psychiatric disorders into categories is mainly based on symptoms and behaviours, since there are few diagnostic tests for psychiatric disorders. There currently exists an unhelpful dualistic division of psychiatric disorders from neurological diseases into separate chapters in the main classification system. Since the brain or nervous system is the organ affected in both groups of conditions, some have argued that neurological and

Box 22.10 International Classification of Psychiatric Disorders (ICD-10)

- Organic disorders
- Mental and behavioural disorders due to psychoactive substance use
- Schizophrenia and delusional disorders
- Mood (affective) disorders
- Neurotic, stress-related and somatoform disorders
- Behavioural syndromes
- Disorders of adult personality and behaviour
- Mental retardation

psychiatric disorders should be classified in future in one chapter as disorders of the nervous system.

Psychiatric classifications have traditionally divided up disorders into neuroses and psychoses:

- ***Neuroses*** are illnesses in which symptoms vary only in severity from normal experiences, such as depressive illness.
- ***Psychoses*** are illnesses in which symptoms are qualitatively different from normal experience, with little insight into their nature, such as schizophrenia.

There are several problems with a neurotic–psychotic dichotomy. First, neuroses may be as severe in their effects as psychoses. Second, neuroses may cause symptoms that fulfil the definition of psychotic symptoms. For instance, someone with anorexia nervosa may be convinced that they are fat when they are thin, and this belief would meet all the criteria for a delusional belief, yet we would traditionally classify the illness as a neurosis.

The ***ICD-10 Classification of Mental and Behavioural Disorders***, published by the World Health Organization, has largely abandoned the traditional division between neurosis and psychosis, although the terms are still used. The disorders are now arranged in groups according to major common themes (e.g. mood disorders and delusional disorders). A classification of psychiatric disorders derived from ICD-10 is shown in ***Box 22.10***, and this is the classification mainly used in this chapter (ICD-11 will be available in 2017).

The Diagnostic and Statistical Manual of the American Psychiatric Association (DSM-5) is an alternative classification system.

Further reading

American Psychiatric Association. *Diagnostic and Statistical Manual of Mental Disorders*, 5th edn. Text Revision (DSM-5). Washington, DC: APA; 2013.
Jacob KS, Patel V. Classification of mental disorders: a global mental health perspective. *Lancet* 2014; 383:1433–1435.
White PD, Rickards H, Zeman AZJ. Time to end the distinction between mental and neurological illnesses. *BMJ* 2012; 344:e3454.
World Health Organization. *The ICD-10 Classification of Mental and Behavioural Disorders: Clinical Descriptions and Diagnostic Guidelines*. Geneva: World Health Organization; 1992.

AETIOLOGY OF PSYCHIATRIC DISORDERS

A psychiatric disorder may result from several causes, which may interact. It can be helpful to divide causes into the three 'Ps', as having predisposing, precipitating and perpetuating factors:

- ***Predisposing factors*** often stem from early life and include genetic factors, pregnancy- and delivery-related factors, previous emotional traumas and personality factors.
- ***Precipitating factors*** are 'triggers' that may be physical, psychological or social. Whether or not they produce a disorder depends on their nature and severity, and the presence of predisposing factors.

Box 22.11 Psychiatric conditions sometimes caused by physical diseases

Depressive illness
- Hypothyroidism
- Cushing syndrome
- Steroid treatment
- Brain tumour

Anxiety disorder
- Thyrotoxicosis
- Hypoglycaemia (transient)
- Phaeochromocytoma
- Complex partial seizures (transient)
- Alcohol withdrawal

Irritability
- Post-concussion syndrome
- Frontal lobe syndrome
- Hypoglycaemia (transient)

Memory problem
- Brain tumour
- Hypothyroidism

Altered behaviour
- Acute drug intoxication
- Post-ictal state
- Acute delirium
- Dementia

Brain tumour

- ***Perpetuating factors*** maintain the disorder once it has been triggered and may be physical, psychological or social. There may be more than one and these may interact.

PSYCHIATRIC ASPECTS OF PHYSICAL DISEASES

People with non-psychiatric, 'physical' diseases are more likely to suffer from psychiatric disorders than those who are well. The most common psychiatric disorders in such patients are mood and acute organic brain disorders (delirium). The relationship between mental and physical conditions may be understood in one of four ways:

- Psychological distress and disorders can precipitate physical diseases (e.g. the cardiac risk associated with depressive disorders, or hypokalaemia causing arrhythmias in anorexia nervosa).
- Physical diseases and their treatments can cause mental symptoms or ill-health ***(Box 22.11)***.
- Both the mental and physical symptoms are caused by a common disease process (e.g. Huntington's chorea, Parkinson's disease).
- Physical and mental symptoms and disorders may be independently co-morbid, particularly in the elderly.

Factors that increase the risk of a psychiatric disorder in someone with a physical disease are shown in ***Box 22.12***.

Differences in management

Although the basic principles are the same as in treating psychiatric illnesses in the physically healthy, there are some differences:

- ***A physical disease or treatment*** may be exacerbating the psychiatric condition and may be revealed in the history (see ***Box 22.11***); this should then be addressed. For example, dopamine agonists may precipitate a psychosis.
- ***Disorders affecting pharmacokinetics*** entail a reduction in dosage when psychotropic drugs are prescribed, e.g. fluoxetine in acute kidney injury or hepatic failure.
- ***Drug interactions*** should be of particular concern, e.g. lithium and non-steroidal anti-inflammatory drugs (NSAIDs).
- ***Women who might become pregnant*** need to avoid certain drugs, such as sodium valproate, which can cause fetal malformations.
- ***A planned physical treatment*** may sometimes exacerbate the psychiatric condition. An example would be high-dose

Box 22.12 Factors increasing the risk of psychiatric disorders in the general hospital

Patient factors
- Previous psychiatric history
- Current social or interpersonal stresses
- Homelessness
- Recent alcohol misuse

Setting
- Accident and emergency department
- Neurology, oncology and endocrinology wards
- Intensive care unit
- Renal dialysis unit

Physical conditions
- Chronic ill health
- Chronic pain
- Life-threatening illness
- Recent bad prognostic news
- Disabling condition
- Brain disease
- Recent live birth, stillbirth or miscarriage
- Functional illness

Treatment
- Certain drugs (e.g. dopamine agonists)
- Second postoperative day
- Surgery affecting body image (e.g. emergency stomata)

steroids as part of chemotherapy in a patient with leukaemia and depressive illness.

- ***The risk of suicide*** should always be remembered in an inpatient with a mood disorder and steps should be taken to reduce that risk, e.g. by moving the patient to a room on the ground floor and/or having a registered mental health nurse attend the patient while at risk.

Further reading

Becker AE, Kleinman A. Mental health and the global agenda. *N Engl J Med* 2013; 369:66–73.

THE SICK ROLE AND ILLNESS BEHAVIOUR

The ***sick role*** describes the behaviour usually adopted by ill people. Such people are not expected to fulfil their normal social obligations. They are treated with sympathy by others and are only obliged to see their doctor and take medical advice or treatments.

Illness behaviour is the way in which given symptoms may be differentially perceived, evaluated and acted (or not acted) upon. We all have illness behaviour when we choose what to do about a symptom. Going to see a doctor is generally more likely with more severe, disabling and numerous symptoms. It is also more likely in introspective individuals who focus on their health.

Abnormal illness behaviour occurs when there is a discrepancy between the objective pathology present and the patient's response to it, in spite of adequate medical investigation and explanation.

FUNCTIONAL SOMATIC SYNDROMES

So-called ***functional*** (in contrast to 'organic') somatic syndromes are illnesses in which no obvious pathology is found and there is an assumed dysfunction of an organ or system. Examples are given

Box 22.13 'Functional' somatic syndromes

- 'Tension' headaches
- Atypical facial pain
- Atypical chest pain
- Fibromyalgia (chronic widespread pain)
- Other chronic regional pain syndromes
- Chronic fatigue syndrome
- Multiple chemical sensitivity
- Premenstrual syndrome
- Irritable or functional bowel syndrome
- Irritable bladder

in ***Box 22.13***. The psychiatric classification of these disorders might be ***somatoform disorders***, if there are clear psychological precipitating or perpetuating factors, but they do not fit easily within either medical or psychiatric classification systems, since they occupy the borderland between them. This classification also implies a dualistic 'mind or body' dichotomy, which is not backed up by evidence. Since current classifications still support this outmoded understanding, this chapter will address these conditions in this way.

The word ***psychosomatic*** has had several colloquial meanings, including 'all in the mind' and imaginary, but the modern concept is that psychosomatic disorders are syndromes in which both physical and psychological factors are likely to be causative. So-called medically unexplained symptoms and syndromes are very common in both primary care and the general hospital (over half the outpatients in gastroenterology and neurology clinics have these syndromes). Because orthodox medicine has not been particularly effective in treating or understanding these disorders, many patients perceive their doctors as unsympathetic and seek out complementary or even alternative treatments of uncertain efficacy.

Because epidemiological studies suggest that having one of these syndromes significantly increases the risk of having another, some doctors believe that these conditions represent different manifestations of a single 'functional syndrome', indicating a global somatization process, particularly since they are also associated with depressive and anxiety disorders. Against this view is the evidence that the majority of primary care patients with one of these disorders do not have a mood or other functional disorder. It also seems that it requires a major stress or the development of a co-morbid psychiatric disorder in order for such sufferers to see their doctor, which might explain why doctors are overly impressed with the associations with both stress and psychiatric disorders. Doctors have historically tended to diagnose 'stress' or 'psychosomatic disorders' in people with symptoms that they cannot explain. History is full of such disorders being reclassified as research clarifies the pathology. An example is writer's cramp (see p. 857), which most neurologists agree is a dystonia rather than a neurosis.

The likelihood is that these functional disorders will be reclassified as their causes and pathophysiology are revealed. Functional brain scans and peripheral sensory testing suggest that central nervous system sensitization is found in a number of these disorders, which might help to explain their clustering together.

Chronic fatigue syndrome

There has probably been more controversy over the existence and causes of chronic fatigue syndrome (CFS) than any other functional somatic syndrome in recent decades. This is reflected in its uncertain classification as ***neurasthenia*** in the psychiatric classification and as ***myalgic encephalomyelitis*** (***ME***) under neurological diseases. There is good evidence for the independent existence of this syndrome, although the diagnosis is made clinically and by exclusion of other fatiguing disorders. Its prevalence is 0.5–2.5%

Box 22.14 Aetiological factors commonly seen in 'functional' disorders

Predisposing
- Perfectionist and introspective personality traits
- Childhood traumas (physical and sexual abuse)
- Similar illnesses in first-degree relatives

Precipitating (triggering)
- Infections (CFS, irritable bowel syndrome)
- Traumatic events (especially accidents)
- Acute painful conditions ('fibromyalgia' and other chronic pain syndromes)
- Life events that precipitate changed behaviours (e.g. taking time off sick)
- Incidents where the patient believes others are responsible

Perpetuating (maintaining)
- Inactivity with consequent physiological adaptation (CFS, 'fibromyalgia')
- Avoidant behaviours (MCS, CFS)
- Maladaptive illness beliefs (that maintain maladaptive behaviours) (CFS, MCS)
- Excessive dietary restrictions ('food allergies')
- Stimulant drugs (e.g. caffeine)
- Sleep disturbance
- Mood disorders
- Somatization disorder
- Unresolved anger or guilt
- Disputed compensation claim

CFS, chronic fatigue syndrome; MCS, multiple chemical sensitivities.

worldwide, mainly depending on how it is defined. It occurs most commonly in women between the ages of 20 and 50 years.

Clinical features

The cardinal symptom is chronic fatigue made worse by minimal exertion. The fatigue is usually both physical and mental, and is most commonly associated with:

- poor concentration
- impaired registration of memory
- alteration in sleep pattern (either insomnia or hypersomnia)
- muscular pain.

Mood disorders are present in a significant minority of patients, and can cause problems in diagnosis because of the overlap in symptoms. These mood disorders may be secondary, independent (co-morbid) or primary (with a misdiagnosis of CFS).

Aetiology

Functional disorders often have some aetiological factors in common with each other ***(Box 22.14)***, as well as more specific aetiologies. For instance, CFS can be triggered by certain infections, such as infectious mononucleosis and viral hepatitis. About 12% of patients who have infectious mononucleosis have CFS 6 months after the onset of infection, yet there is no evidence of persistent infection in these patients. Those fatigue states that clearly do follow on from a viral infection can also be classified as ***post-viral fatigue syndromes***.

Other aetiological factors are uncertain. Immune and endocrine abnormalities noted in CFS may be secondary to the inactivity or sleep disturbance commonly seen. The role of stress is uncertain, with some indication that the influence of stress is mediated through consequent psychiatric disorders exacerbating fatigue, rather than any direct effect.

Box 22.15 Management of functional somatic syndromes

- The first principle is the identification and treatment of maintaining factors (e.g. dysfunctional beliefs and behaviours, mood and sleep disorders).

Communication
- Explanation of ill-health, including diagnosis and causes
- Education about management (including self-help leaflets)

Stopping drugs
- e.g. Caffeine causing insomnia, analgesics causing dependence

Rehabilitative therapies
- Cognitive behaviour therapy (to challenge unhelpful beliefs and change coping strategies)
- Supervised and graded exercise therapy for approximately 3 months (to reduce inactivity and improve fitness)

Pharmacotherapies
- Specific antidepressants for mood disorders, analgesia and sleep disturbance (e.g. 10–50 mg of amitriptyline at night for sleep and pain)
- Symptomatic medicines (e.g. appropriate analgesia, taken only when necessary)

Management

The general principles of the management of functional disorders are given in ***Box 22.15***. Specific management of CFS should include a mutually agreed and supervised programme of gradually increasing activity. However, only about a quarter of patients recover after treatment. It is sometimes difficult to persuade a patient to accept what are inappropriately perceived as 'psychological therapies' for such a physically manifested condition. Antidepressants do not work in the absence of a mood disorder or insomnia.

Prognosis

Prognosis is poor without treatment, with less than 10% of hospital attenders recovered after 1 year. Outcomes are worse with greater severity, increasing age, co-morbid mood disorders, and the conviction that the illness is entirely physical. A large trial showed that about 60% improve with active rehabilitative treatments, such as graded exercise therapy and cognitive behaviour therapy, when added to specialist medical care.

Fibromyalgia (chronic widespread pain)

This controversial condition of unknown aetiology overlaps with chronic fatigue syndrome, both conditions causing fatigue and sleep disturbance. Diffuse muscle and joint pains are more constant and severe in chronic widespread pain (CWP); the 'tender points', previously thought to be pathognomonic (see pp. 664–665), are now known to be of no diagnostic importance, but this is disputed by some.

CWP occurs most commonly in women aged 40–65 years, and has a prevalence in the community of 1–11%, varying by definition. There are associations with depressive and anxiety disorders, other functional disorders, physical deconditioning and a possibly characteristic sleep disturbance (see ***Box 22.14***). Functional brain scans suggest that patients perceive greater pain, supporting the idea of abnormal sensory processing that may be related to abnormal regulation of central opioidergic mechanisms.

Management

Apart from the general principles set out in ***Box 22.15***, management consists of:

- centrally acting analgesia
- reversal of the sleep disturbance
- a physically orientated rehabilitation programme.

A meta-analysis suggests that tricyclic antidepressants such as amitriptyline and dosulepin that inhibit reuptake of both serotonin (5-hydroxytryptamine, 5-HT) and noradrenaline (norepinephrine) have the greatest effect on sleep, fatigue and pain. The doses used are too low to exert an antidepressant effect and the drugs may work primarily through their hypnotic effects. Other centrally acting anti-nociceptive agents that are also antidepressants include duloxetine and milnacipran (not available in the UK), used at full doses, or anticonvulsants, such as pregabalin and gabapentin.

Other chronic pain syndromes

A chronic pain syndrome is a condition of chronic disabling pain for which no medical cause can be found. The psychiatric classification would be a persistent ***somatoform pain disorder***; this is unsatisfactory since the criteria include the stipulation that emotional factors must be the main cause, and it is clinically difficult to be that certain.

The main sites affected in chronic pain syndromes are the head, face, neck, lower back, abdomen, genitalia or all over (fibromyalgia). 'Functional' low back pain is the most common 'physical' reason for being off sick long-term in the UK (see pp. 655–659). Quite often, a minor abnormality will be found on investigation (such as mild cervical spondylosis on the neck X-ray), but this will not be severe enough to explain the severity of the pain and resultant disability. These pains are often unremitting and respond poorly to analgesics. Sleep disturbance is almost universal and co-morbid psychiatric disorders are commonly found.

Aetiology

The perception of pain involves sensory (nociceptive), emotional and cognitive processing in the brain. Functional brain scans suggest that the brain responds abnormally to pain in these conditions, with increased activation in response to chronic pain. This could be related to conditioned physiological and behavioural responses to an initial acute pain. The brain may then adapt to the prolonged stimulus of the pain by changing its central processing. The insula, striatum, thalamus and cingulate gyrus seem to be particularly affected, all of which are involved in the experience of pain in general. Thus, it is possible to start to understand how cognitions, emotions and behaviour might influence the perception of chronic pain (see ***Box 22.14***).

Management

Management involves the same principles as are applied in other functional syndromes ***(Box 22.15)***. Since analgesics are rarely effective and can cause long-term harm, patients should be encouraged to reduce their use gradually. It is often helpful to involve the patient's immediate family or partner, to ensure that the partner is also supported and not unconsciously discouraging progress.

Specific drug treatments are few:

- ***Nerve blocks*** are not usually effective.
- ***Anticonvulsants*** include gabapentin and pregabalin (see p. 820).
- ***Antidepressants*** may be dual-acting drugs (serotonin and noradrenaline reuptake inhibitors, SNRIs) that affect both serotonin and noradrenaline (norepinephrine) reuptake; these demonstrate the greatest efficacy (e.g. duloxetine). Low-dose tricyclic antidepressants that affect both of these neurotransmitters (e.g. amitriptyline, dosulepin) are also effective, although this may be primarily through an improvement in sleep. Serotonergic antidepressants (selective serotonin reuptake inhibitors, SSRIs) tend to be less effective, except in the presence of comorbid anxiety and depressive disorders.

Irritable bowel syndrome

This is one of the most common functional somatic syndromes, affecting some 10–30% of the population worldwide. The clinical features and management of the irritable bowel syndrome (IBS) and the related functional bowel disorders are described in more detail in on pages 430–431. Although the majority of people with IBS do not have a psychiatric disorder, depressive illness should be excluded in those with constipation and a poor appetite. Anxiety disorders should be excluded in individuals with nausea and diarrhoea. Persistent abdominal pain or a feeling of emptiness may occasionally be the presenting symptom of a severe depressive illness, particularly in the elderly, with a ***nihilistic delusion*** that the body is empty or dead inside (see pp. 906–913).

Management

This is dealt with in more detail in ***Box 22.15***. Seeing a physician who provides specific education that addresses individual illness beliefs and concerns can provide lasting benefit.

Antidepressants are frequently indicated in moderate to severe cases and the choice of agent will depend on the presence of pain, sleep disturbance and psychiatric comorbidity, as well as the effect of drug families on bowel transit times (e.g. this is reduced with SSRIs). Milder cases will often respond well to low doses of amitriptyline, although this may be poorly tolerated if constipation is predominant. Non-pharmacological treatments are also effective, and these include:

- cognitive behaviour therapy
- hypnotherapy
- brief interpersonal psychotherapy.

Multiple chemical sensitivity, *Candida* hypersensitivity and food allergies

Some complementary health practitioners, doctors and patients themselves make diagnoses of multiple chemical sensitivities (MCS) (e.g. to foods, smoking, perfumes, petrol), *Candida* hypersensitivity and allergies (to food, tap water and even electricity). Symptoms and syndromes attributed to these putative disorders are numerous and variable, and include all the functional disorders, ***mood disorders*** and ***arthritis***. Scientific support for the existence of these disorders is weak, particularly when double-blind methodologies have been used.

Type 1 hypersensitivities to foods such as nuts certainly exist, although they are fortunately uncommon (approximately 3/1000) (see p. 142). Direct ***specific food intolerances*** also occur (e.g. chocolate with migraine, caffeine with IBS).

Candidiasis can occur in the gastrointestinal tract in immunocompromised individuals, such as those with the acquired immunodeficiency syndrome (AIDS). Vaginal candidiasis can follow antibiotic treatment in otherwise healthy women. A double-blind and controlled study of nystatin in women diagnosed as having candidiasis hypersensitivity syndrome showed that vaginitis was the only condition relieved more by nystatin than placebo. There is little evidence of *Candida* having a systemic role in other symptoms. In spite of this evidence, the patient is often convinced of the legitimacy and usefulness of these diagnoses and their treatments.

Aetiology

Surveys of patients diagnosed with MCS or food allergies have shown high rates of current and previous mood and anxiety disorders (see **Box 22.14**). Eating disorders (see pp. 927–928) should be excluded in people with food intolerances. Some patients taking very-low-carbohydrate diets as putative treatments may develop reactive hypoglycaemia after a high carbohydrate meal, which they then interpret as a food allergy.

Classical conditioning can produce intolerance to foods and smells in healthy people and this may be a causative mechanism in some individuals with intolerances. This supports the existence of these intolerance conditions, but suggests they may be conditioned responses with attendant physiological consequences. This might explain why double-blinding sometimes abolishes the reaction to the stimulus.

Management

The general principles in **Box 22.15** apply. If one assumes a phobic or conditioned response is responsible, graded exposure (systematic desensitization) to the conditioned stimulus may be worthwhile. Preliminary studies do suggest that this approach may successfully treat such intolerances, in the context of cognitive behaviour therapy.

Premenstrual syndrome

The premenstrual syndrome (PMS) consists of both physical and psychological symptoms that regularly occur during the premenstrual phase and substantially diminish or disappear soon after the period starts.

- ***Physical symptoms*** include headache, fatigue, breast tenderness, abdominal distension and fluid retention.
- ***Psychological symptoms*** can include irritability, emotional lability or low mood, and tension.

The ***premenstrual*** (***late luteal***) ***dysphoric disorder*** (***PMDD***) is a severe form of PMS with marked mood swings, irritability, depression and anxiety accompanying the physical symptoms. Women who generally suffer from mood disorders may be more prone to experience this. The prevalence of PMS does not vary between cultures and is reported by the majority (75%) of women at some time in their lives. Severely disabling PMS (PMDD) occurs in about 3–8% of women.

The cause of PMS remains unclear, although exacerbating factors include some of those outlined in **Box 22.14**. Abnormalities of reproductive hormone receptors may also play a role.

Management

The general principles in **Box 22.15** apply. Treatments with vitamin B_6 (see p. 200), diuretics, progesterone, oral contraceptives, oil of evening primrose, and oestrogen implants or patches (balanced by cyclical norethisterone) remain empirical. Psychotherapies aimed at enhancing the patient's coping skills can reduce disability. Two trials suggest that graded exercise therapy improves symptoms. Several studies have demonstrated that SSRIs (see p. 910) are effective treatments for PMDD.

The menopause

The clinical features and management of the menopause are described on pages 1296–1297. A prospective study has shown that there is no increased incidence of depressive disorders at this time. Such a significant bodily change, sometimes occurring at the same time as children leave home, is naturally accompanied by an emotional adjustment that does not normally amount to a pathological state.

Further reading

Bass C, Hallingan P. Factitious disorders and malingering: challenges for clinical assessment and management. *Lancet* 2014; 383:1422–1432.

Ford AC, Talley NJ, Schoenfeld PS et al. Efficacy of antidepressants and psychological therapies in irritable bowel syndrome: systematic review and meta-analysis. *Gut* 2009; 58:367–378.

White PD, Goldsmith KA, Johnson AL et al. Comparison of adaptive pacing therapy, cognitive behaviour therapy, graded exercise therapy, and specialist medical care for chronic fatigue syndrome (PACE): a randomised trial. *Lancet* 2011; 377:823–836.

Yonkers KA, O'Brien PM, Eriksson E. Premenstrual syndrome. *Lancet* 2008; 371:1200–1210.

SOMATOFORM DISORDERS

As explained in the section on functional disorders (see pp. 899–902), the classification of somatoform disorders is unsatisfactory because of the uncertain nature and aetiology of these disorders. However, there are certain disorders, beyond those described in 'functional somatic syndromes', that present frequently and coherently enough to be usefully recognized.

Somatization disorder

One in 10 patients presenting with a functional disorder will fulfil the criteria of a chronic somatization disorder. The condition is composed of multiple, recurrent, medically unexplained physical symptoms, usually starting early in adult life. Symptoms may be referred to almost any part or bodily system. The patient has often had multiple medical opinions and repeated negative investigations. Medical reassurance that the symptoms do not have a demonstrable physical cause fails to reassure the patient, who will continue to 'doctor-shop'. The patient is usually reluctant to accept that psychological and/or social factors may play a role. Abnormal illness behaviour is evident and patients can be attention-seeking and dependent on doctors.

The aetiology is unknown, but both mood and personality disorders are often also present. Somatization disorder is frequently associated with dependence upon or overuse of prescribed medication, usually sedatives and analgesics. There is often a history of significant childhood traumas, or chronic ill-health in the child or parent, which may play an aetiological role or help to explain difficult therapeutic relationships (see **Box 22.14**). The condition is probably the somatic presentation of psychological distress, although iatrogenic damage (from postoperative and drug-related problems) soon complicates the clinical picture. The course of the disorder is chronic and disabling, with longstanding family, marital and/or occupational problems.

Hypochondriasis

The conspicuous feature is a preoccupation with an assumed serious disease and its consequences. Patients commonly believe that they suffer from cancer, AIDS or some other serious condition. Characteristically, such patients repeatedly request investigations either to prove they are ill or to reassure themselves that they are well. Such reassurance rarely lasts long before another cycle of worry and requests begins. The symptom of hypochondriasis may be secondary to or associated with a variety of psychiatric disorders, particularly depressive and anxiety disorders. Occasionally, the hypochondriasis is delusional, secondary to schizophrenia or a depressive psychosis. Hypochondriasis may coexist with physical disease but the diagnostic point is that the patient's concern is disproportionate and unjustified.

Management of somatoform disorders

The principles outlined in ***Box 22.15*** apply to these disorders. Since they have a poor prognosis, the aim is to minimize disability. Furthermore, it is vital that all members of staff and close family members adopt the same approach to the patient's problems. The patients often, consciously or unconsciously, split both medical staff and family members into 'good' and 'bad' (or caring and uncaring) people, as a way of projecting their distress.

Patients appreciate a discussion and explanation of their symptoms. You should sensitively explore possible psychological and social difficulties, if possible by asking about or demonstrating links between symptoms and stresses. Such discussion usually gives information that can be used to formulate an agreed plan of management. A contract of mutually agreed care, involving the appropriate professionals (general practitioner, and a choice of psychotherapist, health psychologist, complementary health professional, physician or psychiatrist), with agreed frequency of visits and a review date, can be helpful in managing the condition. Management also includes cessation of reassurance that no serious disease has been uncovered, since this simply reinforces dependence on the doctor. Repeated investigations should be discouraged. Cognitive behaviour therapy has been shown to provide effective rehabilitation in significant numbers of patients suffering from a somatoform disorder.

DISSOCIATIVE/CONVERSION DISORDERS

A ***dissociative disorder*** is a condition in which there is a profound loss of awareness or cognitive ability without medical explanation. The term dissociative indicates the disintegration of different mental activities, and covers such phenomena as amnesia, fugues and pseudoseizures (non-epileptic attacks).

Conversion disorder occurs when an unresolved conflict is converted into, usually symbolic, physical symptoms as a defence against it. Such symptoms commonly include paralysis, abnormal movements, sensory loss, aphonia, disorders of gait and pseudocyesis (false pregnancy). The lifetime prevalence has been estimated at 3–6 per 1000 in women, with a lower prevalence in men. Most cases begin before the age of 35 years. Conversion is unusual in the elderly.

Clinical features

The various symptoms are usually divided into dissociative and conversion categories ***(Box 22.16)***. Dissociative disorders have the following three characteristics that are necessary in order to make the diagnosis:

- They occur in the absence of physical pathology that would fully explain the symptoms.
- They are produced unconsciously.
- Symptoms are not caused by over-activity of the sympathetic nervous system.

Box 22.16 Common dissociative/conversion symptoms

Dissociative (mental)	Conversion (physical)
• Amnesia	• Paralysis
• Fugue	• Disorders of gait
• Pseudodementia	• Tremor
• Dissociative identity disorder	• Aphonia
	• Mutism
	• Sensory symptoms
	• Globus
	• Pseudoseizures
	• Blindness

Other characteristics include:

- Symptoms and signs often reflect a patient's ideas about illness.
- There is usually abnormal illness behaviour, with exaggeration of disability.
- There may have been significant childhood traumas.
- ***Primary gain*** is the immediate relief from the emotional conflict.
- ***Secondary gain*** refers to the social advantage gained by the patient by being ill and disabled (sympathy of family and friends, time off work, disability pension).
- Physical disease is, not uncommonly, also present (e.g. pseudoseizures are more common in someone with epilepsy).

Dissociative amnesia commences suddenly. Patients are unable to recall long periods of their lives and may even deny any knowledge of their previous life or personal identity. In a ***dissociative fugue***, patients not only lose their memory but also wander away from their usual surroundings; when found, they have no memory of their whereabouts during this wandering. The differential diagnosis of a fugue state includes post-epileptic automatism, depressive illness and alcohol misuse.

Multiple personality disorder is rare but dramatic, and may be triggered by suggestion on the part of a psychotherapist. There are rapid alterations between two or more 'personalities' in the same person, each of which is repressed and dissociated from the other 'personalities'. A differential diagnosis is rapid-cycling manic depressive disorder which would explain sudden apparent changes in personality.

Differential diagnosis

Dissociation is usually a stable and reliable diagnosis over time, although high rates of co-morbid mood and personality disorders are found in chronic sufferers. Particular care should be taken to make the diagnosis on positive grounds, and not simply on the basis of an absence of a medical diagnosis. Care should also be taken to exclude or treat co-morbid psychiatric disorders.

Aetiology

Functional brain scans differ between healthy controls feigning a motor abnormality and people with a similar conversion motor symptom, which suggests that dissociation involves different areas of the brain from simulation ***(Fig. 22.1)***. Functional brain scanning of a patient with conversion paralysis has shown that recalling a past trauma not only activated the emotional areas, such as the amygdala, but also reduced motor cortex activity. This would suggest that conversion involves a disinhibition of voluntary will at an unconscious level, so that the patient can no longer *will* something to happen.

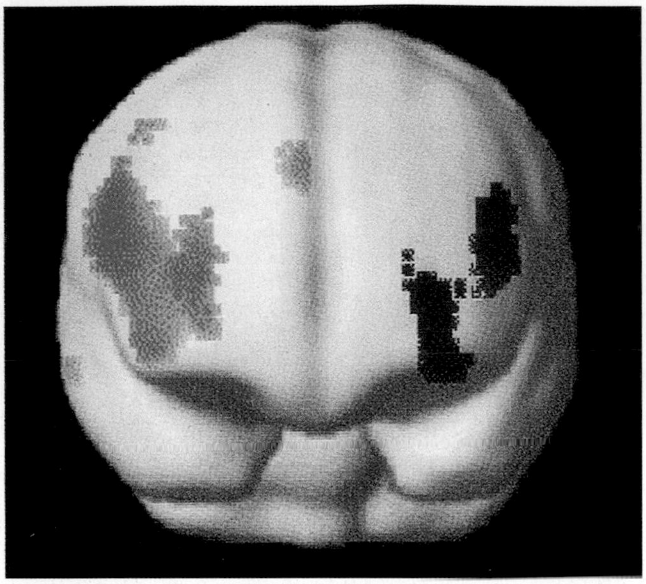

Figure 22.1 Statistical parametric maps superimposed on a magnetic resonance imaging scan of the anterior surface of the brain, orientated as though looking at a person head on. The red region shows hypofunction of people with conversion motor symptoms. The green region shows hypofunction of healthy controls feigning the same motor abnormality. *(From Spence SA, Crimlisk HL, Cope H et al. Discrete neurophysiological correlates in prefrontal cortex during hysterical and feigned disorders of movement.* Lancet *2000; 355:1243–1244, with permission.)*

The psychoanalytical theory of dissociation is that it is the result of emotionally charged memories that are repressed into the unconscious at some point in the past. Symptoms are explained as the combined effects of repression and the symbolic conversion of this emotional energy into physical symptoms. This hypothesis is difficult to test, although there is some evidence that people with dissociative disorders are more likely to have suffered childhood abuse, particularly when the abuse was both sexual and physical, and started early in childhood. Caution should be taken with such a history obtained by therapies that 'recover' childhood memories that were previously completely unknown to the patient.

Management

The treatment of dissociation is similar to the treatment of somatoform disorders in general, outlined above and in **Box 22.15**. The first task is to engage the patient and their family with an explanation of the illness that makes sense to them, is acceptable, and leads to the appropriate management. An invented example of a suitable explanation is given in **Box 22.17**. Such an explanation would be modified by mutual discussion until an agreed understanding was achieved, which would serve as a working model for the illness. Provision of a rehabilitation programme that addresses both the physical and the psychological needs and problems of the patient would then be planned.

- ***A graded and mutually agreed plan for a return to normal function*** can usually be led by the appropriate therapist (e.g. speech therapist for dysphonia, physiotherapist for paralysis).
- ***A psychotherapeutic assessment*** should be made at the same time, in order to determine the appropriate form of psychotherapy. For instance, couple therapy will address a significant relationship difficulty; individual psychotherapy could ease an unresolved conflict from childhood (see management of post-traumatic stress disorder, p. 918).

Box 22.17 An example of an explanation that might be given for a dissociative disorder

'You told me about the tremendous shock you felt when your mother suddenly died. This was particularly the case since you hadn't spoken to her for so long beforehand, after that big disagreement with her over your wedding to John. You weren't able to say good-bye before she died. Your brain was overloaded with grief, guilt and anger all at once. I wonder whether that is why you aren't able to speak now. I wonder whether it's difficult to think of anything to say that would make things right, particularly since you can't speak with your mother now.'

Abreaction brought about by ***hypnosis*** or by intravenous injections of small amounts of midazolam may produce a dramatic, if sometimes short-lived, recovery. In the abreactive state, the patient is encouraged to relive the stressful events that provoked the disorder and to express the accompanying emotions: that is, to abreact. Such an approach has been useful in the treatment of acute dissociative states in wartime but appears to be of less value in civilian life. It should only be contemplated in the presence of an anaesthetist with suitable resuscitation equipment to hand.

Hypnotherapy is psychotherapy applied while the patient is in a hypnotic trance, the idea being that therapy is more easily possible because the patient is relaxed and not using repression. This may allow the therapist access to the previously unconscious emotional conflicts or memories. There are no published trials of this technique in dissociation, which Freud gave up as unsuccessful in order to found psychoanalysis, but some hypnotherapists claim good results. Care should be taken to avoid a catastrophic emotional reaction when the patient is suddenly faced with the previously repressed memories.

Prognosis

Most cases of recent onset recover quickly with treatment, which is why a positive diagnosis should be made early. Those cases that last longer than a year are likely to persist, with entrenched abnormal illness behaviour patterns. One study found that 83% were still unwell at 12 years' follow-up.

SLEEP DIFFICULTIES

Sleep is divided into rapid eye movement (REM) and non-REM sleep:

- As drowsiness begins, the alpha rhythm on an electroencephalogram (EEG) disappears and is replaced by deepening ***slow-wave*** activity (***non-REM***).
- After 60–90 minutes, this slow-wave pattern is replaced by low-amplitude waves, on which are superimposed ***rapid eye movements*** lasting a few minutes.
- This cycle is repeated during the duration of sleep, with the REM periods becoming longer and the slow-wave periods shorter and less deep ***(Fig. 22.2)***.

REM sleep is accompanied by dreaming and physiological arousal. ***Slow-wave sleep*** is associated with release of anabolic hormones and cytokines, with an increased cellular mitotic rate. It helps to maintain host defences, metabolism and repair of cells. For this reason, slow-wave sleep is increased in those conditions where

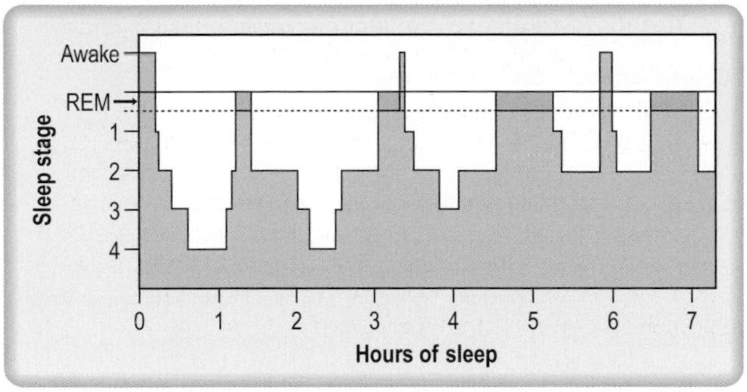

Figure 22.2 Sleep architecture. Cycles of slow-wave sleep are interspersed with rapid eye movement (REM) sleep. Sleep is 'staged' by the electroencephalogram (EEG). Deeper sleep (stages 3 and 4) is demonstrated by slow waves on the EEG. Sleep occurs in cycles, light sleep (accompanied by REM sleep and dreaming) to deep sleep and back again, and these cycles last about 90 minutes.

growth or conservation is required (e.g. adolescence, pregnancy, thyrotoxicosis).

Insomnia

Insomnia is difficulty in sleeping; a third of adults complain of insomnia, and in a third of these it can be severe.

Primary sleep disorders

These include sleep apnoea (see pp. 1085–1086), narcolepsy (pp. 851–852), the ***restless legs syndrome*** (Ekbom syndrome; see p. 852) and the related ***periodic leg movement disorder***, in which the legs (and sometimes the arms) jerk while asleep.

Delayed sleep phase syndrome

This occurs when the circadian pattern of sleep is delayed, so that the patient sleeps from the early hours until midday or later; it is most common in young people. ***Night terrors***, ***sleep-walking*** and ***sleep-talking*** are non-REM phenomena, called parasomnias; they are most commonly found in children, but can recur in adults when under stress or suffering from a mood disorder. Sleep disorders secondary to another medical diagnosis will not be discussed here.

Psychophysiological insomnia

This is commonly secondary to functional, mood and substance misuse disorders, and is frequently present in individuals under stress ***(Box 22.18)***. It can often be triggered by one of these factors, but then becomes a habit on its own, driven by anticipation of insomnia and daytime naps.

Insomnia causes daytime sleepiness and fatigue, with consequences such as road traffic accidents. Assessment should pay particular attention to mood, life difficulties and drug intake (especially alcohol, nicotine and caffeine), and the timing of the insomnia should be ascertained:

- ***Initial insomnia*** (trouble going off to sleep) is common in mania, anxiety, depressive disorders and substance misuse.
- ***Middle insomnia*** (waking up in the middle of the night) occurs with medical conditions such as sleep apnoea and prostatism.
- ***Late insomnia*** (early morning waking) is caused by depressive illness and malnutrition (anorexia nervosa).

Habitual ***alcohol*** consumption should be carefully estimated, since even a small excess can be a potent cause of insomnia, as well as recent withdrawal. ***Caffeine*** is perhaps the most commonly taken drug in the UK, and its effects are easily under-estimated. Six cups of coffee a day are likely to cause insomnia in the average healthy adult. Caffeine is found not only in tea and coffee, but also in chocolate, cola drinks and some analgesics. Prescription drugs that can either disturb sleep or cause vivid dreams include most appetite suppressants, glucocorticoids, dopamine agonists, lipid-soluble beta-blockers (e.g. propranolol) and certain psychotropic drugs (especially when first prescribed, e.g. fluoxetine, reboxetine, risperidone).

? Box 22.18 Common causes of insomnia

Primary sleep disorders
- Periodic leg movements
- Restless legs syndrome

Secondary sleep disorders
- Psychiatric disorders:
  - Mood disorders (mania, depressive and anxiety disorders)
  - Delirium and dementia
- Drug use or misuse:
  - Addictive drug withdrawal (alcohol, benzodiazepines)
  - Stimulant drugs (caffeine, amfetamines)
  - Prescribed drugs (steroids, dopamine agonists)
- Physical conditions:
  - Pain (classically with carpal tunnel syndrome)
  - Nocturia (e.g. from prostatism)
  - Malnutrition

Hypersomnia

This is not uncommon in adolescents with depressive illness. It occurs in narcolepsy, and may temporarily follow infections such as infectious mononucleosis.

Management of insomnia

This is determined by diagnosis. Where none is immediately apparent, it is worth educating the patient about sleep hygiene. In addition:

- ***Simple measures***, such as decreasing alcohol intake, having supper earlier, exercising daily, having a hot bath prior to going to bed and establishing a routine of going to bed at the same time, should all be tried.
- ***Relaxation techniques and cognitive behaviour therapy*** have a role in those with intractable insomnia.
- ***Short-half-life benzodiazepines*** can be useful for acute insomnia, but should not be used for more than 2 weeks continuously to avoid dependence.
- ***Non-benzodiazepine hypnotics*** (zaleplon, zopiclone, zolpidem) act at γ-aminobutyric acid type A (GABA-A) receptors and occasional dependence has been reported.
- ***Certain antihistamines*** (e.g. diphenhydramine and promethazine) ***and antidepressants*** (e.g. amitriptyline, trimipramine, trazodone, mirtazapine) are not addictive and can be used as hypnotics in low dose, with the added advantage of improving slow-wave sleep. The most common adverse effects are morning sedation and weight gain.

Further reading

Falloon K, Arroll B, Elley CR et al. The assessment and management of insomnia in primary care. *BMJ* 2011; 342:d2899.
Morin CM, Benca R. Chronic insomnia. *Lancet* 2012; 379:1129–1141.

MOOD (AFFECTIVE) DISORDERS

The central feature of these disorders is an abnormality of mood. Mood is best described in terms of a continuum ranging from severe depression at one extreme to severe mania at the other, with the normal, stable mood in the middle. Mood disorders are divided into unipolar and bipolar affective disorders.

Unipolar affective disorders

Patients suffer from depressive episodes alone, although they are commonly recurrent.

Bipolar affective disorder

Patients suffer bouts of both depression and mania. Although mania can rarely occur by itself without depressive mood swings (thus being 'unipolar'), it is far more commonly found in association with depressive swings, even if sometimes it takes several years for the first depressive illness to appear.

- ***Bipolar I*** disorder is defined as one or more manic or mixed (signs of mania and depression) episodes.
- ***Bipolar II*** is defined as a depressive episode with at least one episode of hypomania (this is shorter-lived than mania and is not accompanied by psychotic symptoms). Hypomania is noticeably abnormal but does not result in functional impairment or hospitalization.
- ***Bipolar III*** disorder is less well established and describes depressive episodes, with hypomania occurring only when taking an antidepressant.

About 10% of patients who have depressive illness are eventually found to have a bipolar illness.

Depressive disorders

Depressive disorders or 'episodes' are classified by the ICD-10 as mild, moderate or severe, with or without somatic symptoms. Severe depressive episodes are divided according to the presence or absence of psychotic symptoms.

Clinical features of depressive disorder

Whereas everyone will, at some time or other, feel 'fed up' or 'down in the dumps', it is when such symptoms become qualitatively different and pervasive or interfere with normal functioning that a depressive illness has occurred. Depressive disorder, clinical or 'major' depression, is characterized by disturbances of mood, speech, energy and ideas ***(Box 22.19)***. Patients often describe their symptoms in physical terms. Marked fatigue and headache are the two most common physical symptoms in depressive illness and may be the first symptoms to appear. Patients describe the world as looking grey, and themselves as lacking a zest for living, and being devoid of pleasure and interest in life (anhedonia). Anxiety and panic attacks are common; secondary obsessional and phobic symptoms may emerge. Symptoms should last for at least 2 weeks and cause significant incapacity (e.g. trouble working or relating to others) in order to be considered an illness.

In the more severe forms, diurnal variation in mood can occur, patients feeling worse in the morning, after waking in the early hours with apprehension. Suicidal ideas are more frequent, intrusive and prolonged. Delusions of guilt, persecution and bodily disease are not uncommon, along with second-person auditory hallucinations insulting the patient or suggesting suicide. In severe depressive illness, particularly in the elderly, concentration and memory can be so badly affected that the patient appears to have dementia (pseudodementia). Delusions of poverty and non-existence (nihilism) occur particularly in this age group. Suicide is a real risk; lifetime risk is approximately 6% in all patients, but higher in those with depressive illness severe enough to warrant admission to hospital, those with bipolar affective disorder and those with co-morbid substance misuse. Screening questions for depressive illness are shown in ***Box 22.20***.

Box 22.19 Characteristic features of depressive illness

Characteristic	Clinical features
Mood	Depressed, miserable or irritable
Talk	Impoverished, slow, monotonous
Energy	Reduced, lethargic, lacking motivation
Ideas	Feelings of futility, guilt, self-reproach, unworthiness, hypochondriacal preoccupations, worrying, suicidal thoughts, delusions of guilt, nihilism and persecution
Cognition	Impaired learning, pseudodementia in elderly patients
Physical	Insomnia (especially early waking), poor appetite and weight loss, constipation, loss of libido, erectile dysfunction, bodily pains
Behaviour	Retardation or agitation, poverty of movement and expression
Hallucinations	Auditory – often hostile, critical

Box 22.20 Screening questions for depressive illness

- During the last month, have you often been bothered by feeling down, depressed or hopeless?
- During the last month, have you often been bothered by having little interest or pleasure in doing things?

If the answer to one or both of these questions is 'yes', assess further for depressive illness.

Epidemiology

About a third of the population will feel unhappy at any one time but this is not the same as depressive illness; the middle-aged feel least happy compared to the young and elderly. The point prevalence of depressive illness is 5% in the community, with a further 3% having dysthymia (see below). It is more common in women, but there is no increase with age, and no difference by ethnic group or socioeconomic class (apart from a clear association with unemployment). Married and never-married people have similar prevalence rates, with separated and divorced people having two to three times the prevalence. Depressive illnesses are becoming more common.

Depressive illnesses are more frequently found in the presence of:

- physical diseases, particularly if chronic, stigmatizing or painful
- excessive and chronic alcohol use
- social stresses, particularly loss events, such as separation, redundancy and bereavement
- interpersonal difficulties with those close to the patient, especially when socially humiliated
- lack of social support, with no confiding relationship.

Depressed people with another physical disorder view themselves as more sick and disabled, visit their doctors almost four times as often as the non-depressed physically ill, stay in hospital longer, adhere less to medical advice and medication, and undergo more medical and surgical procedures. Depressive illness may be associated with increased mortality (excluding suicide) in people with physical illness, such as myocardial infarct.

Dysthymia

Dysthymia is a mild or moderate depressive illness that lasts intermittently for 2 years or more and is characterized by tiredness and low mood, lack of pleasure, low self-esteem and feelings of discouragement. The mood relapses and remits, with several weeks of feeling well, soon followed by longer periods of being unwell. It can be punctuated by depressive episodes of greater severity, so-called 'double depression'.

Seasonal affective disorder

Seasonal affective disorder is characterized by recurrent episodes of depressive illness occurring during the winter months in the northern hemisphere. Symptoms are similar to those found with atypical depressive illness, in that patients complain of hypersomnia, increased appetite (with carbohydrate craving) and weight gain, with profound fatigue. Such patients have a higher prevalence of bipolar affective disorder, and some doctors are uncertain whether the condition is different from normal depressive illness, with the accentuation of mood that naturally occurs by season. However, there is evidence that seasonal depressive illness can be successfully treated with bright light therapy given in the early morning, which causes a phase advance in the circadian rhythm of melatonin. In contrast, the same treatment given in the early evening, with consequent phase delay of melatonin secretion, is less antidepressant. Selective serotonin reuptake inhibitors (SSRIs) are alternative treatments.

Puerperal affective disorders

Affective illnesses and distress are common in women soon after they have given birth.

'Maternity blues' describe the brief episodes of emotional lability, irritability and tearfulness that occur in about 50% of women 2–3 days postpartum and resolve spontaneously in a few days.

Postpartum psychosis occurs once in every 500–1000 births. Over 80% of cases are 'affective' in type and the onset is usually within the first 2 weeks following delivery. In addition to the classical features of an affective psychosis, disorientation and confusion are often noted. Severely depressed patients may have delusional ideas that the child is deformed, evil or otherwise affected in some way, and such false ideas may lead to either attempts to kill the child or suicide. The response to speedy treatment is generally good. The recurrence rate for a psychosis in a subsequent puerperium is 20–30%.

Non-psychotic postnatal depressive disorders occur during the first postpartum year in 10% of mothers, especially in the first 3 months, with a higher prevalence in developing countries. Risk factors are first pregnancy, poor relationship with the partner, ambivalence about the pregnancy, and emotional personality traits. The Edinburgh Postnatal Depression Scale (EPDS) is a ten-item questionnaire that can be used as an effective screening tool. Depressive illness after childbirth is clinically similar to other depressive illnesses, but lack of emotional bonding with the baby is common.

Differential diagnosis of depressive disorders

The differential diagnoses of depressive illness are shown in ***Box 22.21***. Other psychiatric disorders are the most common misdiagnoses. Some 90% of patients presenting with a depressive illness while misusing alcohol will no longer be depressed 2 weeks after their last drink.

Pathological (abnormal) grief and normal grief are described on page 918. Pathological grief is closely associated with depressive illness.

? Box 22.21 Common differential diagnoses of depressive illness

Other psychiatric disorders
- Alcohol misuse
- Amfetamine (and derivatives) misuse and withdrawal
- Borderline personality disorder
- Dementia
- Delirium
- Schizophrenia
- Normal and pathological grief

Organic (secondary) affective illness

Physical causes that are both necessary and sufficient as a cause
- Cushing syndrome
- Thyroid disease (although sometimes depression persists after treatment)
- Hyperparathyroidism
- Corticosteroid treatment
- Brain tumour (rarely without other neurological signs)

Investigation of depressive disorders

A corroborative history can be valuable in helping to exclude differential diagnoses such as alcohol misuse, and in elucidating maintaining factors such as a poor relationship with a partner. Investigations should be guided by the history and examination but those commonly performed are:

- full blood count, urea and electrolytes, serum creatinine, estimated glomerular filtration rate (eGFR)
- liver biochemistry (including glutamyl transpeptidase)
- serum calcium
- erythrocyte sedimentation rate/C-reactive protein (ESR/CRP)
- thyroid function tests (free T_4, thyroid-stimulating hormone (TSH))

Other tests include:

- serum cortisol (morning and evening)
- antinuclear antibody
- chest X-ray
- EEG or brain scan, as indicated

Aetiology of unipolar depressive disorders

The aetiology of unipolar depressive disorders is multifactorial and is composed of a mixture of genetic and environmental factors.

Genetic factors

Unipolar depression is probably polygenic but no linkage has been firmly identified. The risk of unipolar depression in a first-degree relative of a patient is approximately three times that in the non-affected. The concordance of unipolar depression in monozygotic twins is between 30% and 60%, increasing with more recurrent illnesses. Polymorphisms that increase the risk of depression involve monoamines and their receptors, but studies are inconclusive. Recent research suggests a possible role for epigenetic changes. The issue is complicated by the genetic influence on sleep habits, emotional personality and even life events, which are all involved in the genesis of depressive illness.

Biochemical changes

Monoamines

The monoamine deficiency theory of depressive illness is supported by the efficacy of monoamine reuptake inhibitors and the depressive effect of dietary tryptophan depletion, but the timing of changes in neurotransmitter metabolism and clinical improvement is discrepant.

Neuroimaging studies have revealed a raised density of monoamine oxidase A (MAO-A) receptors. Depression is proposed to be related to a chronic and ongoing depletion of these neurotransmitters as a result of this enzyme's increased activity and its interaction with region-specific monoamine transporter densities. The relative transporter densities in particular regions and how they are affected by the global reduction in monoamine levels are then thought to determine the particular expression of the depressive illness and the predominance of particular symptoms.

Neuroendocrine tests also suggest that the serotonin neurotransmitter system is downregulated. 5-HT_{1a} and 5-HT_2 receptor subtypes are thought most likely to be involved. Receptor-labelled functional brain scans suggest that dopamine under-activity is related to psychomotor retardation.

Hypothalamo–pituitary–adrenal axis

The administration of exogenous steroids is associated with the onset of depressive symptoms and people with Cushing syndrome often demonstrate depressive episodes. Acute stress, whether physical or psychological, is associated with a rise in serum glucocorticoids. Severe depressive episodes have been linked with hypercortisolaemia (of note is the fact that cortisol is low in 'atypical' depression), but whether this is aetiological or secondary to sleep disturbance and weight loss is unknown. This cortisol dysregulation has been associated with impaired glucocorticoid negative feedback, adrenal hyper-responsiveness to adrenocorticotrophic hormone (ACTH) and hypersecretion of cortisol-releasing hormone (CRH).

Exposure to the high levels of cortisol is thought to have a direct effect on neuronal plasticity and to lower resistance to neuronal damage. The hippocampus seems especially susceptible, resulting in atrophic changes. This, in turn, has further deleterious effects on wider neuroendocrine function, leading to a self-perpetuating dysregulation that may serve to maintain and/or worsen the illness.

The interplay at this level becomes more complicated, with reduced central and peripheral glucocorticoid receptor sensitivity, hypothalamo–pituitary–adrenal (HPA) axis upregulation, and the release of pro-inflammatory cytokines that may, in turn, explain changes in mood, fatigue, appetite, sensitivity to pain and reduced libido (note that depression is a side-effect of interferon treatment). Additionally, at the cellular level, this affects monoamine transport and causes neuronal apoptosis and dysfunction of glial cells, normally responsible for maintaining neuronal homeostasis.

Brain-derived neurotrophic factor

Healthy interactions between neurones and glial cells are maintained by brain-derived neurotrophic factor (BDNF), which is found in its greatest concentration in the hippocampus and cerebral cortex. It promotes cell growth and long-term potentiation (the enhancement of synchronous firing between two neurones). Pro-BDNF, its precursor, promotes the reduction of dendritic spines and apoptosis. BDNF is then involved in the growth and activity of neural networks.

- Animal studies show BDNF is reduced under stressful conditions.
- Adult humans with untreated depressive illness have lower serum concentrations of BDNF when compared with both healthy controls and those that have received antidepressant treatment.
- Low levels normalize with antidepressant treatment.

BDNF therefore has potential as an objective marker of depression and its response to treatment, as well as being a potential target for treatment of the disorder itself.

Neuroimaging changes

The use of functional magnetic resonance imaging (fMRI) and positron emission tomography (PET) has revealed a number of abnormalities in the brains of people with major depression. These changes are non-specific but involve regions that are associated with both the emotional and the cognitive abnormalities seen in depression. Increased brain ventricle volume, and orbitofrontal, dorsolateral frontal and anterior cingulate cortex altered activation have been implicated. The hippocampus is smaller in several stress-related neuropsychiatric disorders, including recurrent depression.

Sleep

A reduced time between onset of sleep and REM sleep (shortened REM latency), and reduced slow-wave sleep both occur in depressive illness. These abnormalities persist in some patients when they are not depressed. Families with several sufferers of depressive illness can share these traits, suggesting that sleep patterns may be inherited and may predispose to depression.

Childhood traumas and personality

Physical, sexual and emotional abuse and neglect in childhood all predispose adults to depressive illness but the effect is non-specific. Both 'neurotic' (emotional) and perfectionist personality traits are risks for depressive illness, and these may be determined as much by genetic factors as childhood environment.

Social factors

Some 30% of women will develop a depressive illness after a severe life event or difficulty, such as a divorce, and this is compounded by low self-esteem and a lack of a confiding relationship. Unemployment is a significant risk factor in men.

An integrated model of aetiology

Stress is more likely to trigger depressive illness in a person predisposed by lack of social support and/or certain personality traits. Stress, in turn, triggers various brain changes in both stress hormones (such as the release of CRH) and neurotransmitters (e.g. serotonin), which are both known to be altered in depressive illness. This suggests an integrated biopsychosocial model of depressive illness and challenges dualistic ideas that depressive illnesses are either psychological or physical. Depressive illnesses involve both the mind and the body, which are themselves indivisible.

Management of depressive illness

The patient needs to know the diagnosis to provide understanding and rationalization of the overwhelming distress inherent in depressive illness. Knowing that self-loathing, guilt and suicidal thoughts are caused by the illness may have an 'antidepressant' effect. The further treatment of depressive disorders involves physical, psychological and social interventions ***(Box 22.22)***.

Patients who are actively suicidal or severely depressed (with or without psychotic symptoms) should be admitted to hospital. Admission is necessary for perhaps 1 in 1000 people with clinical depression in primary care. This provides the patient with a break

Box 22.22 Management of depressive illness

Physical
- Cessation of depressing drugs (alcohol, steroids)
- Regular exercise (good for mild to moderate depression)
- Antidepressants (choice determined by adverse effects, co-morbid illnesses and interactions)
- Adjunctive drugs (e.g. lithium; if no response to two different antidepressants)
- Electroconvulsive therapy (ECT; if depression is life-threatening or non-responsive)

Psychological
- Education and regular follow-up by same professional
- Cognitive behaviour therapy (CBT)
- Other indicated psychotherapies (couple, family, interpersonal)

Social
- Financial: eligible benefits, debt counselling
- Employment: acquiring or changing a job or career
- Housing: adequate, secure tenancy, safe, social neighbours
- Young children: child-care support

Treatments combined
- The most effective treatment is a mixture of CBT and an antidepressant

from self-care, and allows support, listening, observation, the close monitoring of treatments and the prevention of suicide. The pitfall of not treating a depressive illness just because it seems an 'understandable' reaction to serious illness or difficult circumstances should be avoided. This is particularly likely to happen if the patient is elderly, or severely or even terminally ill.

Psychological treatments

There is good evidence that mild to moderate depressive episodes respond well to 'talking therapies'.

Cognitive behaviour therapy

Beck developed cognitive behaviour therapy (CBT) to reverse the negative cognitive triad with which patients regard themselves, their situation and their futures. It involves the identification of the negative automatic thoughts that maintain the negative perceptions that feed depression. These commonly include catastrophizing (e.g. making a 'mountain out of a mole-hill'), over-generalizing (e.g. 'I failed an exam; therefore I am a failure as a person') and categorical ('all-or-none') thinking (e.g. 'My work is either perfect or abysmal'). CBT then involves identifying the links between these thoughts, consequent behaviour and feeling low, and then testing their logic. This is done by looking at the evidence either in the therapy sessions (e.g. Q: 'Did you pass the other exams you took?'; A: 'Yes; I guess I did') or in behavioural 'experiments' (e.g. showing the 'abysmal' work to a colleague and asking their opinion).

There is good evidence that individual CBT is as effective as antidepressant drugs for mild and moderate depressive illness, and should be offered as first-choice treatment. It is also effective in preventing a relapse of clinical depression after therapy has ceased. Individual CBT is more effective than group-delivered therapy, and computer-delivered CBT programs are also helpful when used to supplement therapist involvement. Third-wave CBT therapies, such as mindfulness-based CBT, centred on the use of meditation, can prevent recurrence. Acceptance and commitment therapy (accepting the things that cannot be changed, and committing oneself to things that can be) shows promise.

Interpersonal psychotherapy

This psychotherapy is probably as effective as both antidepressants and CBT in mild and moderate clinical depression. The therapist focuses on those interpersonal relationships involved in, or affected by, the patient's illness (especially relationship changes or deficiencies), using problem-solving techniques to help the individual to find solutions.

Other psychotherapies

Couple therapy is particularly effective when a patient is in a problematic relationship that may be contributing to the depressive illness; both the patient and partner attend therapy.

Family therapy is effective not only to treat a family with problems, but also to assist the family to help a patient get better. It may involve understanding one family member's 'depression' as a systemic 'solution' for a wider problem within the family.

Physical treatments

Exercise and other self-help

There is good evidence that regular exercise, particularly involving other people, can help relieve depressive illness of mild severity. The benefit is independent of a physical training effect. The role of exercise is unclear but recent evidence suggests that kynurenine is prevented from crossing the blood–brain barrier, thereby reducing neuroactive metabolites. Other self-help and psycho-educational advice (e.g. reduction of alcohol consumption, regular meals and sleep–wake cycle) may be helpful, particularly if supported by bibliotherapy.

Use of drugs in the treatment of clinical depression

Moderate and severe episodes of depression can be effectively treated using medication. Antidepressants are designed to provide an acute increase in monoamine activity. They do this through either prevention of reuptake or enzymatic degradation. This occurs acutely and, although an equally rapid ***depletion*** of monoamines has an acute mood-lowering effect, the mood-elevating benefits of these drugs require weeks of continuous administration. The benefits are therefore unlikely to be due to this mechanism alone.

The effects of chronic administration of monoamine reuptake inhibitors are various. Examples include an increase in the synthesis of binding proteins necessary for serotonin receptor activity and increases in cyclic adenine monophosphate activation, which, in turn, increases BDNF synthesis, enhances glucocorticoid receptor sensitivity and inhibits cytokine signalling. These effects may be secondary to the acute restoration of monoamine levels but rely upon transcriptional and translational changes that alter neuronal plasticity. It is this protein synthesis-dependent process that is thought to be the final pathway responsible for the clinical effect of the drugs.

As the neurobiology for depressive illness becomes clearer, so too are novel approaches to its treatment; some of the novel targets under active investigation are listed in ***Box 22.23***.

A general approach to the prescription of antidepressants is outlined in ***Box 22.24***.

Drug choices in specific circumstances

- ***Recurrent episodes***. Maintenance treatment with the antidepressant at the dose that obtained remission should be continued for at least 2 years. Maintenance treatment beyond this point should be re-evaluated, taking into account age, co-morbidities and risk factors.

Box 22.23 Potential targets for novel antidepressant agents

- Brain-derived neurotrophic factor (BDNF)
- Tumour necrosis factor-alpha (TNF-α)
- Interleukin-1 beta (IL-1β)
- Glucocorticoid receptors
- Corticotrophin-releasing hormone
- Melatonin-concentrating hormone
- Alpha-melanocyte stimulating hormone
- Ghrelin
- Leptin
- Orexins
- Neuropeptide Y
- Nesfatin-1

Box 22.24 A general approach to the prescription of antidepressants

- Any drugs that may contribute to or exacerbate depression, e.g. corticosteroids, should be stopped
- An ECG should be performed prior to institution of antidepressants
- Patient education should be provided (e.g. 80% of the UK public wrongly believe that antidepressants are addictive)
- Regular follow-up (especially weeks 1–6) should accompany the prescription of antidepressants to increase adherence
- All antidepressants have similar efficacy and speed of onset
- Selective serotonin reuptake inhibitors (SSRIs) are considered first-line agents
- Choice of agent will depend on safety and adverse effects, which can be used to positive effect (sedating drugs given at night to enhance sleep)
- The rate of improvement is greatest in weeks 1–2
- An alternative agent should be considered at week 4 in the absence of any response
- With resolution of symptoms, antidepressants should be continued for 6–9 months after a single episode but for at least 2 years in the case of multiple prior episodes
- Some 50% of patients who stop antidepressants immediately on recovery relapse in the next 6 months

- ***Refractory depressive illness***. Whilst 50% may show a response, as few as 30% of individuals (outpatients) experience complete remission with the first choice of antidepressant agent. Strategies available at this point are switching drug classes or augmenting with other agents. This should be overseen by a specialist.
- ***Psychotic depression***. This needs either a combination of an antidepressant and an antipsychotic drug, or electroconvulsive therapy.
- ***Depressive episodes in bipolar affective disorder***. Monotherapy with quetiapine has been proposed as the treatment of choice. Other drugs include mood stabilizers or olanzapine, either alone or in combination with an SSRI antidepressant (see p. 914).

Selective serotonin reuptake inhibitors

Selective serotonin reuptake inhibitors (SSRIs) selectively inhibit the reuptake of the monoamine serotonin (5-HT) within the synapse ***(Fig. 22.3)***. Citalopram and its laevo-isomer, escitalopram, fluvoxamine, fluoxetine, paroxetine and sertraline have the advantage of causing less serious adverse effects than tricyclic antidepressants. For instance, SSRIs do not usually lead to significant weight gain. Because of their long half-lives, they can also be given just once a day, normally in the morning after breakfast. For these reasons, patients adhere better to treatment and therefore SSRIs are now first-line treatments for depressive disorders.

The most common adverse effects of SSRIs resemble a 'hangover' and include nausea, vomiting, headache, diarrhoea and dry mouth. Insomnia and paradoxical agitation can occur when first starting the drugs. Adolescents, in particular, may develop suicidal thoughts with SSRIs; for this reason, only fluoxetine is licensed in the UK for adolescents. Further studies suggest that this is a small risk, if present, and no study has shown a significant increased risk of suicide itself. One in five patients also has sexual adverse effects, such as erectile dysfunction and loss of libido. Uncommon adverse effects include restless legs syndrome (see p. 852) and hyponatraemia.

A ***risk of bleeding*** is associated with SSRIs and is thought to be due to the inhibition of serotonin uptake by platelets as part of normal aggregation in response to vascular injury. To date, much of the reported incidence relates to gastrointestinal bleeding, and any patient with one or more risk factors for upper gastrointestinal bleeding, such as taking an NSAID, should be given gastroprotection with a proton pump inhibitor or advised to stop the NSAID. A risk of intra- and postoperative bleeding has also been reported. Whilst antidepressants are certainly not a reason to withhold a surgical intervention, there is certainly an added risk, of which the surgeon and anaesthetist should be aware.

'***Serotonin syndrome***' is a toxic hyper-serotonergic state, which can be caused by the ingestion of two or more drugs that increase serotonin levels, e.g. an SSRI combined with a monoamine oxidase inhibitor, a dopaminergic drug (e.g. selegiline) or a tricyclic antidepressant. Symptoms include agitation, confusion, tremor, diarrhoea, tachycardia and hypertension; hyperthermia is characteristic. This is a medical emergency and treatment may require admission to hospital.

Discontinuation syndrome, a specific withdrawal syndrome, has also been reported with SSRIs, and may occur with any antidepressant if stopped suddenly. The syndrome is characterized by shivering, anxiety, dizziness, 'electric shocks', headache and nausea. Patients should be warned not to omit a dose and to reduce SSRIs gradually when stopping them.

A ***prolonged QTc interval*** has been noted, particularly with high doses of citalopram and escitalopram.

Tricyclic antidepressants

Tricyclic antidepressants (TCAs) potentiate the action of the monoamines, noradrenaline (norepinephrine) and serotonin, by inhibiting their reuptake into nerve terminals ***(Fig. 22.3)***. Other tricyclics in common use include nortriptyline, doxepin and clomipramine. Dosulepin, imipramine and amitriptyline are the three most commonly used TCAs in the UK, but many related compounds have been introduced, some having fewer autonomic and cardiotoxic effects (e.g. lofepramine).

TCAs have a number of adverse effects ***(Box 22.25)***. In long-term treatment or prophylaxis, weight gain is most troublesome. Because of their toxicity in overdose, it is wisest not to prescribe them to outpatients who have suicidal thoughts without monitoring or giving the drugs to a reliable family member to look after.

Serotonergic and noradrenergic antidepressants

These antidepressants block a number of different neurotransmitter receptors both at the synapse and elsewhere. Their different receptor profiles cause different adverse effects.

- ***Dual-acting agents*** (***serotonin and noradrenaline reuptake inhibitors, SNRIs***). Venlafaxine is a potent blocker of both

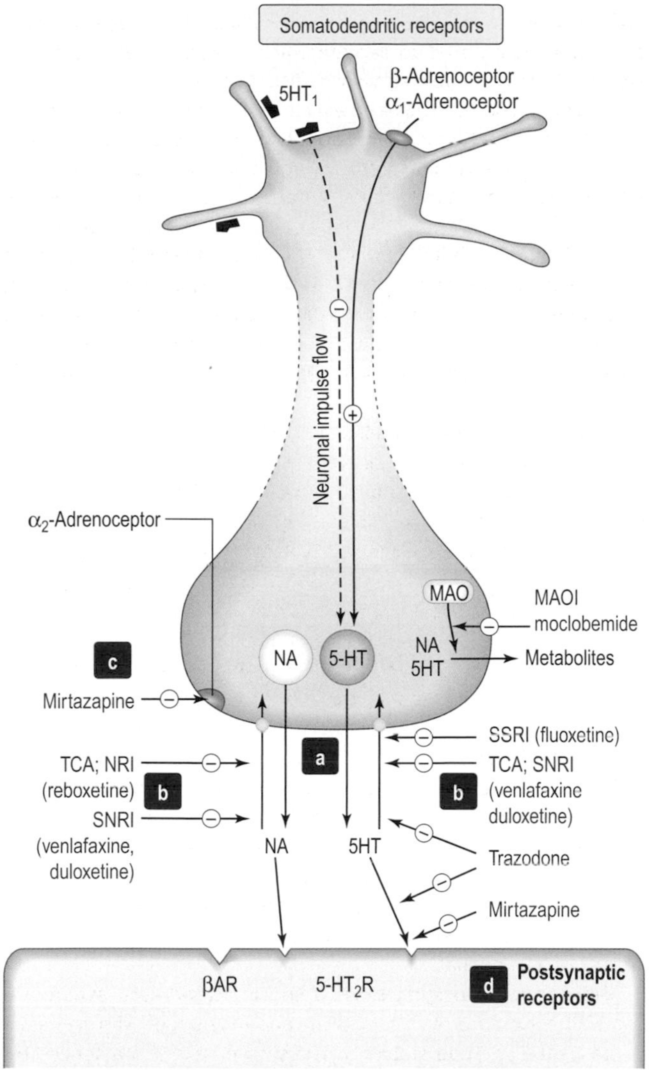

Figure 22.3 The effect of drugs used in the treatment of depression on central nervous system serotonergic and adrenergic functioning.
(a) The majority of released serotonin 5-HT and noradrenaline (NA; norepinephrine) is rapidly removed from the synapse by reuptake into the neurone (yellow circles).
(b) There is a range of antidepressants, which vary in their abilities to inhibit the reuptake of serotonin or noradrenaline, thus enhancing the synapse concentrations of these transmitters.
(c) Stimulation of presynaptic α_2-adrenoceptors reduces monoamine release; mirtazapine blocks these presynaptic autoreceptors, and increases the release and transmission of noradrenaline and serotonin.
(d) Other drugs act by significantly blocking postsynaptic receptors that are upregulated in depression. βAR, β-adrenoceptor; MAO, monoamine oxidase; MAOI, monoamine oxidase inhibitor; NA, noradrenaline; NRI, (selective) noradrenaline reuptake inhibitor; SNRI, serotonin and noradrenaline reuptake inhibitor; SSRI, selective serotonin reuptake inhibitor; TCA, 'classic' tricyclic antidepressant. *(From Waller DG, Sampson AP, Renwick A, Hillier K. Medical Pharmacology and Therapeutics. Edinburgh: Saunders; 2014, with permission.)*

serotonin and noradrenaline (norepinephrine) reuptake. At higher doses, it also affects dopamine transmission. It has negligible affinity for other neurotransmitter receptor sites and so produces less sedation and fewer antimuscarinic effects. It can be given in slow-release form with the advantage of once-daily dosage. Nausea is the most common side-effect

Box 22.25 Adverse effects of tricyclic antidepressants

Antimuscarinic effects
- Dry mouth
- Constipation
- Tremor
- Blurred vision
- Urinary retention

Cardiovascular effects
- QT prolongation
- Arrhythmias
- Postural hypotension

Convulsant activity
- Lowered seizure threshold

Other effects
- Weight gain
- Sedation
- Mania (rarely)

and patients should be monitored for hypertension. It should not be prescribed in those with uncontrolled hypertension or cardiac arrhythmias. Duloxetine works in a similar way to venlafaxine and has been found to be especially helpful with chronic pain.

- ***Tetracyclics***. Trazodone is a tetracyclic compound that acts as a serotonin antagonist (except at 5-HT_1A receptors, where it acts as a partial agonist) and reuptake inhibitor. It is used in the treatment of anxiety and depressive disorders, and also for insomnia due to its sedative effects. It has low cardiotoxic and antimuscarinic effects. However, dizziness and postural hypotension can be problems for some patients, and blood pressure should be monitored during the initial titration.
- ***Mirtazapine*** is a 5-HT_2 and 5-HT_3 receptor antagonist and a potent α_2-adrenergic blocker. The consequent effect is to increase both noradrenaline and selective serotonin transmission: an NSSA. It can be given at night to aid sleep and rarely causes sexual adverse effects. Mirtazapine can be sedating in low dose and can cause weight gain. An uncommon adverse effect is agranulocytosis.
- ***Noradrenaline (norepinephrine) reuptake inhibitors*** (***NRIs***). Reboxetine is an NRI that is an effective antidepressant but has also demonstrated benefit in the treatment of panic disorder and attention deficit disorder. It can cause insomnia in some patients in addition to antimuscarinic adverse effects.

Monoamine oxidase inhibitors

Monoamine oxidase inhibitors (MAOIs) act by irreversibly inhibiting the intracellular enzymes monoamine oxidase A and B, leading to an increase of noradrenaline (norepinephrine), dopamine and 5-HT in the brain (see ***Fig. 22.3***). Because of their adverse effects and restrictions placed on patients taking them, they are rarely used by non-psychiatrists. MAOIs also produce a dangerous hypertensive reaction with foods containing tyramine or dopamine and therefore a restricted diet is prescribed. Tyramine is present in cheese, pickled herrings, yeast extracts, certain red wines, and any food, such as game, that has undergone partial decomposition. Dopamine is present in broad beans. MAOIs interact with drugs such as pethidine and can also cause liver damage occasionally.

Reversible inhibitors of monoamine oxidase A

An example of a reversible inhibitor of monoamine oxidase A (RIMA) is moclobemide; the usual dose is 300 mg daily. These drugs appear to have fewer adverse effects than the MAOIs (insomnia and headache, but some sexual problems) and constitute a low risk in overdose. Patients prescribed such antidepressants should be told that they can eat a normal diet, but should be careful to avoid excessive amounts of food rich in tyramine (see above).

Selective irreversible inhibitors of monoamine oxidase B

Selegiline is a selective irreversible inhibitor of MAO-B. At higher doses, it loses its specificity and also inhibits MAO-A. It is more frequently used in the treatment of Parkinson's disease (see p. 854) than in depression, as it prolongs the activity of levodopa because dopamine is a substrate of MAO-B.

Melatonin receptor agonist and serotonin receptor antagonist (see *Box 22.23*)

Agomelatine is the only drug in this class. It is an agonist at both the melatonin MT_1 and MT_2 receptors. It is a weak antagonist at 5-HT_{2C} receptors. It does not affect the uptake of serotonin, noradrenaline (norepinephrine) or dopamine. Agomelatine has the same antidepressant efficacy as the SSRIs.

Antidepressant augmentation

If two trials of antidepressants have failed, adding a second concomitant drug, such as lithium, an atypical antipsychotic or triiodothyronine, can be helpful.

Antidepressant use in general medicine

- ***Cardiac disease***. In people with cardiac disease, SSRIs, lofepramine and trazodone are preferred over more quinidine-like compounds.
- ***Epilepsy***. MAOIs and mirtazapine do not affect epileptic thresholds.
- ***Drug interactions***. SSRIs are metabolized by the cytochrome P450 system, unlike venlafaxine, mirtazapine and reboxetine; the latter therefore have fewer drug interactions.
- ***Herbal medicine***. Care should be taken not to prescribe antidepressants while a patient is taking the herbal antidepressant St John's wort, which interacts with serotonergic drugs in particular.
- ***Elderly***. Doses of antidepressants should initially be halved in the elderly and in people with renal or hepatic failure.
- ***Pregnancy***. Antidepressants should be avoided if possible in pregnancy and breast-feeding. If other treatments are ineffective, the risks of drug therapy should be balanced against those of taking no treatment, since depression can affect fetal progress and future mother–child bonding. TCAs are generally believed to be safe in pregnancy, with no significant increase in congenital malformations in fetuses exposed to them. However, occasionally, their antimuscarinic adverse effects produce jitteriness, sucking problems and hyperexcitability in the newborn. Postpartum plasma levels of babies breast-fed by treated mothers are negligible. SSRIs do not seem to be teratogenic but manufacturers advise against their use in pregnancy until more data are available. Pulmonary hypertension in the newborn is a rare complication. MAOIs should be avoided during pregnancy because of the possibility of a hypertensive reaction in the mother.

Combining antidepressants with psychotherapy

Historically, the understanding has been that combining psychotherapy with antidepressants provided no additive benefit. Recently, however, a well-designed randomized controlled trial has suggested that an additive effect can be achieved with this approach (specifically, with CBT). However, this is both a modest and a specific effect. Patients with more severe and non-chronic episodes attain this benefit, whilst those with milder forms of the disorder, chronic depression and co-morbid personality disorders do not, when compared to antidepressants alone. Individuals who obtained benefit from the combined treatment also experienced fewer adverse effects from the antidepressants prescribed.

Electroconvulsive therapy

Electroconvulsive therapy (ECT) is the treatment of choice in severe, life-threatening depressive illness, particularly when psychotic symptoms are present. It is sometimes essential treatment when the patient is dangerously suicidal or refusing to eat and drink, and when a rapid resolution is required, such as in postpartum depressive illness, when returning baby to mother as soon as it is safe to do so forms part of the treatment.

The treatment is performed under general anaesthetic and involves the passage of an electric current across two electrodes applied to the anterior temporal areas of the scalp, in order to induce a seizure. The motoric seizure is less significant than its electrophysiological evidence (spike-and-wave activity on an EEG), without which benefit is unlikely to be seen. Treatments are normally given twice a week for 3–6 weeks.

ECT is a controversial treatment, yet it is free of serious adverse effects. Most adverse effects are due to the general anaesthetic. Post-ictal confusion and headache are not uncommon, while transient and short-term retrograde amnesia and a temporary defect in new learning can occur during the weeks of treatment, but these are typically short-lived effects. The frequency with which defects in autobiographical memory occur during the time of treatment should be noted. These are discrete and, in most instances, not recognized by the patient, unless the particular memory is actively sought. It is necessary to warn patients of its possibility beforehand.

Uncommonly used physical treatments

Transcranial magnetic stimulation* (*TMS*)** shows moderate efficacy, but is uncommonly used. ***Psychosurgery is very occasionally considered in people with severe intractable depressive illness, when all other treatments have failed (see p. 920). A third of them improve remarkably, while a further third improve somewhat.

Vagal nerve and deep brain stimulation may represent major advances in the management of chronic and treatment-refractory depressive disorders, but definitive trials are not available.

Social treatments

Many people with clinical depression have associated social problems (see *Box 22.22*). Assistance with these can make a significant contribution to clinical recovery. Other social interventions include the provision of group support, social clubs, occupational therapy and referral to a social worker. Educational programmes, self-help groups, and informed and supportive family members can help improve outcome.

Prognosis

Depression is one of the leading causes of disease burden worldwide. People with major depressive illness are between 1.5 and 2 times more likely to die than non-depressed people in the next 16 years, and the risks encompass not only suicide, but also cardiovascular disorders. Depression produces greater disability than angina, arthritis, asthma and diabetes, which makes effective treatment and prevention imperative.

The majority of patients have recovered by 6 months in primary care and 12 months in secondary care. About a quarter of patients attending hospital with depressive illnesses will have a recurrence within 1 year, and three-quarters will have a recurrence within

Box 22.26 Clinical features of mania

Characteristic	Clinical feature
Mood	Elevated or irritable
Talk	Fast, pressurized, flight of ideas
Energy	Excessive
Ideas	Grandiose, self-confident, delusions of wealth, power, influence or of religious significance, sometimes persecutory
Cognition	Disturbance of registration of memories
Physical	Insomnia, mild to moderate weight loss, increased libido
Behaviour	Disinhibition, increased sexual activity, excessive drinking or spending
Hallucinations	Fleeting auditory

10 years. People with recurrent depressive illnesses should be offered prevention. This may involve CBT that concentrates on relapse prevention, other forms of psychotherapy, prolonged antidepressant use, and advice on lifestyle activities such as regular exercise. Full-dose antidepressants are the most effective prophylaxis in recurrent depressive disorders.

Mania, hypomania and bipolar disorder

Mania and hypomania almost always occur as part of a bipolar disorder. The clinical features of mania include a marked elevation of mood, characterized by euphoria, over-activity and disinhibition ***(Box 22.26)***. Hypomania lasts a shorter time and is less severe, with no psychotic features and less disability. Hypomania can be distinguished from normal happiness by its persistence, non-reactivity (not provoked by good news and not affected by bad news) and social disability.

The social disability of mania can be severe, with disinhibited behaviour leading to significant debts (from overspending), lost relationships (from promiscuity or irritability), social ostracism and lost employment (from reckless or disinhibited behaviour).

Some patients have a ***rapid-cycling*** illness, with frequent swings from one mood state to another. A ***mixed affective state*** occurs when features of mania and depressive illness are seen in the same episode. ***Cyclothymia*** is a personality trait with spontaneous swings in mood that are not sufficiently severe or persistent to warrant another diagnosis.

Differential diagnosis

Acute intoxication with recreational drugs such as amfetamines, amfetamine derivatives (MDMA: ecstasy), and cocaine can mimic mania. Up to a quarter of people with Cushing syndrome develop mania. Similarly, corticosteroids can induce mania less commonly than depressive illness. Dopamine agonists (e.g. bromocriptine) are also known to induce mania sometimes.

Epidemiology

The lifetime prevalence of bipolar affective disorder is 1% across the world. Unlike unipolar depressive illness, it is equally common in men and women, supporting its different aetiology. There is no variation by socioeconomic class or race. The mean age of onset is 21, earlier than unipolar depression. The higher prevalence found in divorced people is probably a consequence of the condition.

Box 22.27 Treatment options in acute mania or hypomania

Choice of agent is determined largely by clinical judgement, contraindications and prior response

- Stop antidepressant medication

If the patient is NOT on antimanic medication, then start

- Antipsychotic, e.g. aripiprazole 15 mg daily
- *Or* Valproate 750 mg daily
- *Or* Lithium 0.4 mg daily to serum lithium of 0.4–1.0 mmol/L

If response is inadequate:

- Antipsychotic + valproate or lithium

If the patient is already ON antimanic medication

- If taking an antipsychotic: check dose and compliance; increase if possible, or add valproate or lithium
- If taking valproate: check plasma levels and increase dose, aiming for a serum concentration of 125 mg/L as tolerated and/or add an antipsychotic (this should be done if mania is severe)
- If taking lithium: check plasma levels and increase dose to gain a level of 1.0–1.2 mmol/L if necessary (*Note*: higher than usual reference range) or add an antipsychotic (this should be done if mania is severe)
- If taking carbamazepine: add an antipsychotic if appropriate

A short-acting benzodiazepine may be added to assist with agitation in all patients

Aetiology

Genetic factors

There is strong evidence for a genetic aetiology in this disorder. There is a 60–80% concordance rate in monozygotic twins, compared to 15% in dizygotic twins, suggesting a high rate of heritability. Studies in adoptive twins show similar rates, so this high rate is probably genetic and not due to the family environment. Linkage studies have so far proved disappointing, with several polymorphism associations being found, similar to polymorphisms associated with schizophrenia.

Biochemical changes

Brain monoamines, such as serotonin, are increased in mania. Dexamethasone tends not to suppress cortisol levels in people with mania, suggesting a similar pattern of non-suppression to that seen in severe depressive illness.

Psychological factors

The effect of life events is weaker in bipolar compared with unipolar illnesses, most effects being apparent at first onset. Similarly, personality does not seem to be a major influence, in contrast to unipolar depression, although there is some evidence of a link with the creativity and divergent thinking that is an advantage in the right occupation.

Management

Acute mania or hypomania

Treatment is summarized in ***Box 22.27***. Acute mania is treated with an atypical antipsychotic (neuroleptic), sodium valproate or lithium.

- The atypical antipsychotics aripiprazole, olanzapine, quetiapine and risperidone are particularly recommended, especially with behavioural disturbance. Doses are similar to those used in schizophrenia. The behavioural excitement and overactivity are usually reduced within days, but elation, grandiosity and associated delusions often take longer to respond.

- Lithium may be used in instances where compliance is likely to be good; however, the screening necessary prior to its prescription (see below) may prohibit its use in these circumstances as a first-line agent.
- Valproic acid is also helpful in hypomania or in rapid-cycling illnesses (see below).

Prevention in bipolar disorders

Since bipolar illnesses tend to be relapsing and remitting, prevention of recurrence is the major therapeutic challenge in management. A patient who has experienced more than two episodes of affective disorder within a 5-year period is likely to benefit from preventive treatments. Recommendations include lithium, olanzapine and valproic acid (so long as the patient is not a woman at risk of pregnancy).

Lithium

Lithium (carbonate or citrate) is one of the two main agents used for prophylaxis in people with repeated episodes of bipolar illness (the other being valproic acid). It is rapidly absorbed from the gastrointestinal tract and more than 95% is excreted by the kidneys; small amounts are found in the saliva, sweat and breast milk. Renal clearance of lithium correlates with renal creatinine clearance. Lithium is a mood-stabilizing drug that prevents mania more than depression. It lowers the frequency and severity of relapses by half and significantly reduces the likelihood of suicide. Its mode of action is unknown, but lithium is known to act on the serotonergic system. Poor response to lithium is associated with a negative family history, an unstable premorbid personality and a rapid-cycling illness. Pharmacogenetic work suggests that certain polymorphisms may predict response.

Plasma levels

These should be monitored weekly, with blood drawn 12 h after the last dose (a 'trough' level) until a steady state is reached and at 3-monthly intervals thereafter. The minimum level for prophylaxis is 0.4 mmol/L, with an optimum range of between 0.6 and 0.75 mmol/L. Levels higher than this may afford further protection against manic episodes but the relationship with depression is less clear. For this reason, the therapeutic range is typically quoted as 0.5–1.0 mmol/L. Fluctuations in plasma levels increase the risk of relapse.

Screening prior to starting lithium and at 6-monthly intervals thereafter includes:

- ***Thyroid function*** (free T_4, TSH and thyroid autoantibodies). Lithium interferes with thyroid function and can produce frank hypothyroidism. The presence of thyroid autoantibodies increases the risk.
- ***Parathyroid function***. Serum calcium and parathyroid hormone levels are higher in 10% of patients.
- ***Renal function*** (serum urea and creatinine, eGFR and 24-h urinary volume). Long-term treatment with lithium causes two renal problems: nephrogenic diabetes insipidus (p. 1234) and reduced glomerular function. The best screen for diabetes insipidus is to ask the patient about polyuria and polydipsia.

Toxicity

Patients should carry a lithium card with them at all times, be advised to avoid dehydration, and be warned of drug interactions, such as with NSAIDs and diuretics. As with all medications, it is vital to discuss adverse effects and signs of toxicity (these are listed in ***Box. 22.28***).

Box 22.28 Lithium

Adverse effects

- Nausea
- Diarrhoea
- Fine tremor
- Weight gain, mainly through increased appetite
- Polyuria } due to nephrogenic diabetes insipidus
- Polydipsia } due to nephrogenic diabetes insipidus

Toxicity (>1.5 mmol/L, more likely with dehydration and drug interactions)

- Drowsiness
- Nausea
- Vomiting
- Blurred vision
- Coarse tremor
- Ataxia
- Dysarthria
- Delirium
- Convulsions
- Coma
- Death

Pregnancy

As a rule, lithium is not advised during pregnancy, particularly in the first trimester, because of an increased risk of fetal malformation (Ebstein's anomaly). About 25% of women with a history of bipolar disorder relapse within 2 weeks of delivery. Restarting lithium within 24 h of delivery (if the mother is prepared to forgo breast-feeding) markedly reduces the risk of relapse.

Other mood stabilizers

Valproic acid (as the semisodium salt) is recommended in both prophylaxis and treatment of manic states. Second-line treatments include ***carbamazepine*** and ***lamotrigine***. Some patients who do not respond to lithium may respond to these anticonvulsants or a combination of both. People with rapid-cycling illnesses show a better response to anticonvulsants than to lithium. For antimanic treatment, dosage in the initial stage of treatment will be 200 mg twice daily of carbamazepine, increasing to a normal dose of 800–1000 mg.

Other drugs that appear to exert a prophylactic mood-stabilizing effect include ***olanzapine*** and ***risperidone***.

Both carbamazepine and valproate can be teratogenic (neural tube defects) and should be avoided in pregnancy. Other adverse effects of these drugs are given on page 850.

Prognosis

The mean duration of a manic episode is 2 months, with 95% making a full recovery in time. Recurrence is the rule in bipolar disorders, up to 90% relapsing within 10 years.

Further reading

BALANCE Investigators. Lithium plus valproate combination versus monotherapy for relapse prevention in bipolar disorders (BALANCE). *Lancet* 2010; 375:365–375.

Cipriani A, Barbui C, Salanti G et al. Comparative efficacy and acceptability of antimanic drugs in acute mania. *Lancet* 2011; 378:1306–1315.

Craddock N, Sklar P. Genetics of bipolar disorder. *Lancet* 2013; 381:1654–1662.

Geddes JR, Miklowitz DJ. Treatment of bipolar disorder. *Lancet* 2013; 381:1672–1682.

Grande I, Berk M, Birmaher B et al. Bipolar disorders. *Lancet* 2016;387:1561–1572.

Krishnan V, Nestler EJ. The molecular neurobiology of depression. *Nature* 2008; 455:894–902.

Kupfer DJ, Frank E, Phillips ML. Major depressive disorder: new clinical, neurobiological, and treatment perspectives. *Lancet* 2012; 379:1045–1055.

McKnight RF, Adida M, Budge K et al. Lithium toxicity profile: a systematic review and meta-analysis. *Lancet* 2012; 379:721–728.

Phillips ML, Kupfer DJ. Bipolar disorder diagnosis: challenges and future directions. *Lancet* 2013; 381:1663–1671.

Stewart DE. Depression during pregnancy. *N Engl J Med* 2011; 365:1605–1611.

SUICIDE AND SELF-HARM

(See also p. 63.) Suicide accounts for 2% of male deaths and 1% of female deaths in England and Wales each year, equivalent to a rate of 8 per 100 000. The rate increases with age, peaking for women in their sixties and for men in their seventies. Suicide is the second most common cause of mortality in 15- to 34-year-olds. Meta-analyses of relevant studies suggest that the lifetime risk of suicide is 7% in alcohol dependence, 6% in affective disorders and 4% in schizophrenia.

The highest rates of suicide have been reported in rural southern India (148/100 000 in young women and 58/100 000 in young men) and in Eastern Europe (30–40/100 000), while the lowest are found in Spain (4/100 000) and Greece (3/100 000), but such variations may reflect differences in reporting, which may be related to religion, as much as genuine differences. The provision of mental health care to suicidal individuals varies greatly around the world; a World Health Organization (WHO) study suggests that most receive no treatment at all. Factors that increase the risk of suicide are indicated in ***Box 22.29***.

A distinction must be drawn between those who attempt suicide – self-harm (SH) – and those who succeed (suicide):

- The majority of cases of SH occur in people under 35 years of age.
- The majority of suicides occur in people aged over 60.
- Suicides are more common in men, while SH is more common in women.
- Suicides are more common in older men, although rates are falling. Rates in young men are rising fast throughout the UK and Europe.
- Suicides in women are slowly falling in the UK.
- Approximately 90% of cases of SH involve self-poisoning.
- A formal psychiatric diagnosis can be made retrospectively in 90% of suicides but is unusual in SH.

There is, however, an overlap between SH and suicide. Between 1% and 2% of people who attempt suicide will kill themselves in the year following SH. The risk of suicide stays elevated in those with SH, with 0.5% per annum committing suicide in the following 20 years. Following the guidelines for the assessment of such patients ***(Box 22.30)*** will help ensure that the risk factors relating to suicide are assessed. Indications for referral to a psychiatrist before discharge from hospital are also given.

In general, it is worth trying to interview a family member or close friend and checking these points with them. Requests for immediate re-prescription on discharge should be denied, except in cases of essential medication. In such cases, however, only 3 days' supply of medication should be given, and the patient should be requested to report to their general practitioner or to their psychiatric outpatient clinic for further supplies. Occasionally, involuntary admission to hospital may be required (see pp. 929–930).

Box 22.29 Factors that increase the risk of suicide

- Male sex
- Older age
- Living alone
- Immigrant status
- Recent bereavement, separation or divorce
- Unemployment or retirement
- Living in a socially disorganized area
- Family history of affective disorder, suicide or alcohol misuse
- Previous history of affective disorder, alcohol or drug misuse
- Previous suicide attempt
- Addiction to alcohol or drugs
- Severe depression or early dementia
- Incapacitating painful physical illness

Box 22.30 Guidelines for the assessment of patients who harm themselves

Questions to ask: of concern if positive answer

- Was there a clear precipitant/cause for the attempt?
- Was the act premeditated or impulsive?
- Did the patient leave a suicide note?
- Had the patient taken pains not to be discovered?
- Did the patient make the attempt in strange surroundings (i.e. away from home)?
- Would the patient do it again?

Other relevant factors

- Has the precipitant or crisis resolved?
- Is there a continuing suicidal intent?
- Does the patient have any psychiatric symptoms?
- What is the patient's social support system?
- Has the patient inflicted self-harm before?
- Has anyone in the family ever taken their life?
- Does the patient have a physical illness?

Indications for referral to a psychiatrist

Absolute indications

- Clinical depression
- Psychotic illness of any kind
- Clearly pre-planned suicidal attempt that was not intended to be discovered
- Persistent suicidal intent (the more detailed the plans, the more serious the risk)
- A violent method used

Other common indications

- Alcohol and drug misuse
- Patients over 45 years, especially if male, and young adolescents
- Those with a family history of suicide in first-degree relatives
- Those with serious (especially incurable) physical disease
- Those living alone or otherwise unsupported
- Those in whom there is a major unresolved crisis
- Persistent suicide attempts
- Any patients who give you cause for concern

Further reading

Bruffaerts R, Demyttenaere K, Hwang I et al. Treatment of suicidal people around the world. *Br J Psychiatry* 2011; 199:64–70.
Moran P, Coffey C, Romaniuk H et al. The natural history of self-harm from adolescence to young adulthood. *Lancet* 2012; 379:236–243.
van Heeringen K, Mann JJ. The neurobiology of suicide. *Lancet Psychiatry* 2014; 1:63–72.

ANXIETY DISORDERS

These are conditions in which anxiety dominates the clinical symptoms. They are classified according to whether the anxiety is persistent (general anxiety) or episodic, with the episodic conditions classified according to whether the episodes are regularly triggered by a cue (phobia) or not (panic disorder). The differential diagnoses of anxiety disorders are given in ***Box 22.31***. A patient with one anxiety disorder may well develop others in time.

Box 22.31 Anxiety disorders: the differential diagnosis

Psychiatric disorders
- Depressive illness
- Obsessive–compulsive disorder
- Pre-senile dementia
- Alcohol dependence
- Drug dependence
- Benzodiazepine withdrawal

Endocrine disorders
- Hyperthyroidism
- Hypoglycaemia
- Phaeochromocytoma

Box 22.32 Physical and psychological symptoms of anxiety

Physical symptoms

Gastrointestinal
- Dry mouth
- Difficulty in swallowing
- Epigastric discomfort
- Aerophagy (swallowing air)
- 'Diarrhoea' (usually frequency)

Respiratory
- Feeling of chest constriction
- Difficulty in inhaling
- Over-breathing
- Choking

Cardiovascular
- Palpitations
- Awareness of missed beats
- Chest pain

Genitourinary
- Increased frequency
- Failure of erection
- Lack of libido

Nervous system
- Fatigue
- Blurred vision
- Dizziness
- Sensitivity to noise and/or light
- Headache
- Sleep disturbance
- Trembling

Psychological symptoms
- Apprehension and fear
- Irritability
- Difficulty in concentrating
- Distractibility
- Restlessness
- Depersonalization
- Derealization

General anxiety disorder

General anxiety disorder (GAD) occurs in 4–6% of the population and is more common in women. Symptoms are persistent and often chronic. GAD and the related panic disorder are differential diagnoses for functional somatic syndromes, owing to the many physical symptoms that are caused by these conditions.

Clinical features

The physical and psychological symptoms are outlined in ***Box 22.32***. The patient looks worried, and has a tense posture, restless behaviour, a pale and sweaty skin, or neck and chest intermittent flushing. The patient takes time to go to sleep; once asleep, they wake intermittently with worry dreams. Associated conditions include hyperventilation, which is even more common in panic disorders ***(Box 22.33)***. The patient will either breathe rapidly and shallowly or sigh deeply, particularly when talking about the stresses in their life.

Mixed anxiety and depressive disorder

This disorder is the most common mood disorder in primary care (7% point prevalence), in which there are equal elements of both anxiety and depression, showing how closely associated these two abnormal mood states are.

Box 22.33 The hyperventilation syndrome

Clinical features
- Panic attacks – fear, terror and impending doom – accompanied by some or all of the following:
  - Dyspnoea (trouble getting a good breath in)
  - Palpitations
  - Chest pain or discomfort
  - Suffocating sensation
  - Dizziness
  - Paraesthesiae in hands and feet
  - Perioral paraesthesiae
  - Sweating
  - Carpopedal spasms

Aetiology
- Over-breathing leading to a decrease in P_aCO_2 and an increase in arterial pH, causing relative hypocalcaemia

Diagnosis
- A provocation test – voluntary overbreathing for 1 minute – provokes similar symptoms; rebreathing from a large paper bag relieves them

Management
- Explanation and reassurance is given
- The patient is trained in relaxation techniques and slow, controlled breathing
- The patient is asked to breathe into a closed paper bag

Panic disorder

Panic disorder is diagnosed when the patient has repeated, sudden attacks of overwhelming anxiety, accompanied by severe physical symptoms, usually related to both hyperventilation (see ***Box 22.33***) and sympathetic nervous system overactivity (palpitations, tremor, restlessness and sweating). The lifetime prevalence is 5%. People with a panic disorder often have catastrophic illness beliefs during the panic attack, such as the conviction that they are about to die from a stroke or heart attack. The fear of a stroke is related to dizziness and headache. Fear of a heart attack accompanies chest pain (atypical chest pain). The occasional patient with longstanding attacks may no longer feel anxious and simply notices the physical symptoms.

Aetiology

General anxiety and panic disorders occur four times more commonly in first-degree relatives of affected patients. Sympathetic nervous system overactivity, increased muscle tension and hyperventilation are the common pathophysiological associations. Anxiety is the emotional response to the threat of a loss, whereas depression is the response to the loss itself. There is some evidence that being bullied, with the explicit threats involved, leads to anxiety disorders in adolescents.

Phobic (anxiety) disorders

Phobias are common conditions in which intense fear is triggered by a stimulus, or group of stimuli, that are predictable and normally cause no particular concern to others (e.g. agoraphobia, claustrophobia, social phobia). This leads to avoidance of the stimulus ***(Box 22.34)***. The patient knows that the fear is irrational but cannot control

Box 22.34 Phobias
- A phobia is an abnormal fear and avoidance of an object or situation
- Phobias are common (the incidence varies from 3.5% to 12.8% worldwide), disabling and treatable with behaviour therapy

it. The prevalence of all phobias is 8%, with many patients having more than one. Many phobias of 'medical' stimuli exist (e.g. of doctors, dentists, hospitals, vomit, blood and injections), which affect the patient's ability to receive adequate healthcare.

Aetiology

Phobias may be caused by classical conditioning, in which a response (fear and avoidance) becomes conditioned to a previously benign stimulus (e.g. a lift), often after an initiating emotional shock (e.g. being stuck in a lift). In children, phobias can arise through imagined threats (e.g. stories of ghosts told in the playground). Women have twice the prevalence of phobias than men. Phobias aggregate in families, with increasing evidence of the importance of genetic factors being published.

Agoraphobia

Translated as 'fear of the marketplace', this common phobia (4% prevalence) presents as a fear of being away from home, with travelling, walking down a road and going to supermarkets being common cues. This can be a very disabling condition, since the patient often avoids leaving home, particularly when unaccompanied. It is often associated with ***claustrophobia***, a fear of enclosed spaces.

Social phobia

This is the fear and avoidance of social situations: crowds, strangers, parties and meetings. Public speaking would be the sufferer's worst nightmare. It is suffered by 2% of the population.

Simple phobias

The most common is the phobia of spiders (arachnophobia), particularly in women. The prevalence of simple phobias is 7% in the general population. Other common phobias include insects, moths, bats, dogs, snakes, heights, thunderstorms and the dark. Children are particularly phobic about the dark, ghosts and burglars, but the large majority grow out of these fears.

Management of anxiety disorders

Psychological management

For many people with brief episodes, discussion with a doctor concerning the nature of anxiety and its precipitants is sufficient.

- ***Relaxation techniques*** can be effective in mild/moderate anxiety. Relaxation can be achieved in many ways, including complementary techniques such as meditation and yoga. Conventional relaxation training involves a slowing down of the rate of breathing, muscle relaxation and mental imagery.
- ***Anxiety management*** training involves two stages. In the first stage, verbal cues and mental imagery are used to arouse anxiety to demonstrate the link with symptoms. In the second stage, the patient is trained to reduce this anxiety by relaxation, distraction and reassuring self-statements.
- ***Biofeedback*** is useful for showing patients that they are not relaxed, even when they fail to recognize it, having become so used to anxiety. Biofeedback involves feeding back to the patient a physiological measure that is abnormal in anxiety. These measures may include electrical resistance of the skin of the palm, heart rate, muscle electromyography or breathing pattern. The effect tends not to generalize to everyday life away from the feedback.
- ***Behaviour therapies*** are treatments that are intended to change behaviour and thus symptoms. The most common and successful behaviour therapy (with 80% success in some phobias) is graded exposure, otherwise known as systematic desensitization. First, the patient rates the phobia into a hierarchy or 'ladder' of worsening fears (e.g. in agoraphobia: walking to the front door with a coat on; walking out into the garden; walking to the end of the road). Second, the patient practises exposure to the least fearful stimulus until no fear is felt. The patient then moves 'up the ladder' of fears until they are cured.
- ***Cognitive behaviour therapy*** (CBT; see p. 909) is the treatment of choice for panic disorder and general anxiety disorder because the therapist and patient need to identify the mental cues (thoughts and memories) that may subtly provoke exacerbations of anxiety or panic attacks. CBT also allows identification and alteration of the patient's 'schema', or way of looking at themselves and their situation, which feeds anxiety.

Drug treatments

Initial 'drug' treatment should involve advice for gradual cessation of anxiogenic recreational drugs such as caffeine and alcohol (which can cause a rebound anxiety and withdrawal). Prescribed drugs used in the treatment of anxiety can be divided into two groups: those that act primarily on the central nervous system, and those that block peripheral autonomic receptors.

- ***Benzodiazepines*** are centrally acting anxiolytic drugs. They are agonists of the inhibitory transmitter γ-aminobutyric acid (GABA). Diazepam (5 mg twice daily, up to 10 mg three times daily in severe cases), alprazolam (250–500 μg three times daily) and chlordiazepoxide have relatively long half-lives (20–40 h) and are used as anti-anxiety drugs in the short term. Adverse effects include sedation and memory problems, and patients should be advised not to drive while on treatment. They can cause dependence and tolerance within 4–6 weeks, particularly in those with dependent personalities. A withdrawal syndrome ***(Box 22.35)*** can occur after just 3 weeks of continuous use and is particularly severe when high doses have been given for a longer time. Thus, if a benzodiazepine drug is prescribed for anxiety, it should be given in as low a dose as possible, preferably on an 'as necessary' basis, and for not more than 2–4 weeks. A withdrawal programme from chronic use includes changing the drug to the long-acting diazepam, followed by a very gradual reduction in dosage.
- ***Most SSRIs*** (e.g. fluoxetine, paroxetine, sertraline, escitalopram, citalopram) are useful symptomatic treatments for general anxiety and panic disorders, as well as some phobias (social phobia), although doses higher than those used in depression are often required. Duloxetine, mirtazapine, venlafaxine and pregabalin are alternative treatments for GADs, with the added benefit of possibly preventing the subsequent development of depression. Treatment response is often delayed several weeks; a trial of treatment should last 3 months.

Box 22.35 Withdrawal syndrome with benzodiazepines

- Insomnia
- Anxiety
- Tremulousness
- Muscle twitching
- Perceptual distortions
- Hallucinations (which may be visual)
- Hypersensitivities (light, sound, touch)
- Convulsions

- ***Antipsychotics***, such as aripiprazole or olanzapine, can be effective for more severe or refractory cases.
- ***Beta-blockers*** are effective in reducing peripheral symptoms, as many of the symptoms of anxiety are due to an increased or sustained release of adrenaline (epinephrine) and noradrenaline (norepinephrine) from the adrenal medulla and sympathetic nerves. Beta-blockers, such as propranolol (20–40 mg two or three times daily), can reduce peripheral symptoms such as palpitations, tremor and tachycardia, but they do not help central symptoms such as anxiety.

Acute stress reactions and adjustment disorders

Acute stress reaction

This occurs in individuals in response to exceptional physical and/or psychological stress. While severe, such a reaction usually subsides within days. The stress may be an overwhelming traumatic experience (e.g. accident, battle, physical assault, rape) or a sudden change in the social circumstances of the individual, such as a bereavement. Individual vulnerability and coping capacity play a role in the occurrence and severity of an acute stress reaction, as evidenced by the fact that not all people exposed to exceptional stress develop symptoms. Symptoms usually include an initial state of feeling 'dazed' or numb, with inability to comprehend the situation. This may be followed either by further withdrawal from the situation, or by anxiety and overactivity. No treatments beyond reassurance and support are normally necessary.

Adjustment disorder

This disorder can follow an acute stress reaction and is common in the general hospital. This is a more prolonged (up to 6 months) emotional reaction to a significant life event, with low mood joining the initial shock and consequent anxiety, but not of sufficient severity or persistence to fulfil a diagnosis of a depressive or anxiety disorder. Supportive counselling is usually a successful treatment, allowing facilitation of unexpressed feelings, elucidation of unspoken fears, and education about the likely future.

Normal grief

Normal grief immediately follows bereavement, is expressed openly, and allows a person to go through the social ceremonies and personal processes of bereavement. The three stages are, first, shock and disbelief; second, the emotional phase (anger, guilt and sadness); and, third, acceptance and resolution. This normal process of adjustment may take up to a year, with movement between all three stages occurring in a sometimes haphazard fashion.

Pathological (abnormal) grief

This is a particular kind of adjustment disorder. It can be characterized as excessive and/or prolonged grief, or even absent grieving with abnormal denial of the bereavement. Usually, a relative will be stuck in grief, with insomnia and repeated dreams of the dead person, anger at doctors or even the patient for dying, consequent guilt in equal measure, and an inability to 'say good-bye' to the loved person by dealing with their effects. ***Guided mourning*** uses cognitive and behavioural techniques to allow the relative to stop grieving and move on in life.

Post-traumatic stress disorder

Post-traumatic stress disorder (PTSD) is a protracted response to a stressful event or situation of an exceptionally threatening nature, likely to cause pervasive distress in almost anyone. Causes include natural or human disasters, war, serious accidents, witnessing the violent death of others, and being the victim of sexual abuse, rape, torture, terrorism or hostage-taking. Predisposing factors, such as personality, previously unresolved traumas or a history of psychiatric illness, may prolong the course of the syndrome. These factors are neither necessary nor sufficient to explain its occurrence, which is mostly related to the intensity of the trauma, the proximity of the patient to the traumatic event, and its prolonged or repeated nature. Functional brain scan research suggests a possible neurophysiological relationship with obsessive–compulsive disorder (see pp. 919–920).

Clinical features

The typical symptoms of PTSD include:

- '***flashbacks***', repeated vivid reliving of the trauma in the form of intrusive memories, often triggered by a reminder of the trauma
- ***insomnia***, usually accompanied by nightmares, the nocturnal equivalent of flashbacks
- ***emotional blunting***, emptiness or 'numbness', alternating with ***intense anxiety*** on exposure to events that resemble an aspect of the traumatic event, including anniversaries of the trauma
- ***avoidance*** of activities and situations reminiscent of the trauma
- ***emotional detachment*** from other people
- ***hypervigilance***, with autonomic hyperarousal and an enhanced startle reaction.

This clinical picture represents the severe end of a spectrum of emotional reactions to trauma, which might alternatively take the form of an adjustment or mood disorder. The course is often fluctuating but recovery can be expected in two-thirds of cases at the end of the first year. Complications include depressive illness and alcohol misuse. In a small proportion of cases, the condition may follow a chronic course over many years and a transition to an enduring personality change.

Management and prevention

Compulsory ***psychological debriefing*** immediately after a trauma does not prevent PTSD and may be harmful. Prevention is better achieved by the support offered by others who were also involved. Trauma-focused CBT is often effective. ***Eye movement desensitization and reprocessing*** (EMDR) is an equally effective treatment and may require fewer sessions. SSRIs and venlafaxine have a place in the management of chronic PTSD but dropout from pharmacotherapy is common.

The adult consequences of childhood abuse

Estimates of the prevalence of childhood sexual abuse vary, depending on definition, but there is reasonable evidence that 20% of women and 10% of men suffered significant, coercive and inappropriate sexual activity in childhood. The abuser is usually a member of the family or known to the child in social care homes. The likelihood of long-term consequences is determined by:

- an earlier age of onset
- the severity of the abuse
- the repeated nature and duration of the period of abuse
- the association with physical abuse.

Consequent adult psychiatric disorders include depressive illness, substance misuse, eating disorders, borderline personality disorder and deliberate self-harm. Other negative outcomes include a decline in socioeconomic status, sexual problems, prostitution and difficulties in forming adult relationships.

Repeated childhood physical and emotional abuse or neglect may also affect emotional and personality development, predisposing the adult to similar psychiatric disorders. Those who have undergone repeated abuse are more likely to have long-term physical stress related consequences, such as hypothalamic–pituitary–adrenal axis downregulation and smaller brain hippocampal sizes.

Management

Psychodynamic psychotherapy

Psychodynamic psychotherapy is derived from psychoanalysis and is based on a number of key analytical concepts. These include Freud's ideas about psychosexual development, defence mechanisms, free association as the method of recall, and the therapeutic techniques of interpretation, including that of transference, defences and dreams. Such therapy usually involves once-weekly sessions, the length of treatment varying between 3 months and 2 years. The long-term aim of such therapy is twofold: symptom relief and personality change. Psychodynamic psychotherapy is classically indicated in the treatment of unresolved conflicts in early life, as might be found in non-psychotic and personality disorders, but there is no convincing evidence concerning its superiority over alternative forms of treatment.

Cognitive analytical therapy

Cognitive analytical therapy is an integration of CBT and psychodynamic therapy. It is a short-term therapy that involves the patient and therapist recognizing the origins of a recurrent problem, reformulating how it continues to occur, and revising other ways of coping and internalizing it, using both the transference of the patient–therapist relationship and behavioural experiments.

Obsessive–compulsive disorder

Obsessive–compulsive disorder (OCD) is characterized by obsessional ruminations and compulsive rituals. It is particularly associated with, and/or secondary to, both depressive illness and ***Tourette syndrome*** (see p. 857). The prevalence is between 1% and 2% in the general population, and patients uncommonly seek help. There is an equal distribution by gender, and the mean age of onset ranges from 20 to 40 years.

Clinical features

The obsessions and compulsions are time-consuming and intrusive, so that they affect functioning and cause considerable distress. Ruminations are often unpleasant repetitive thoughts, out of character, such as being dirty or violent. This can lead to a constant need to check that everything and everyone is all right and that things have been done correctly, and reassurance cannot remove the doubt that persists. Some rituals are derived from superstitions, such as actions repeated a fixed number of times, with the need to start again if interrupted. When severe and primary, OCD can last for many years and may be resistant to treatment. However, obsessional symptoms commonly occur in other disorders, most notably depressive illness, and remit with the resolution of the primary disorder.

Minor degrees of obsessional symptoms and compulsive rituals or superstitions are common in people who are not ill or in need of treatment, particularly in times of stress and in children, who usually grow out of it. The mildest grade is that of obsessional personality traits, such as over-conscientiousness, tidiness, punctuality, and other attitudes and behaviours indicating a strong tendency towards conformity and inflexibility. Such individuals are *perfectionists* who are intolerant of shortcomings in themselves and others, and take pride in their high standards. When such traits are so marked that they dominate other aspects of the personality, in the absence of clear-cut OCD, the diagnosis is obsessional (anankastic) personality (see p. 929).

Aetiology

Genetic factors

OCD is found in 5–7% of the first-degree relatives. Twin studies showed 80–90% concordance in monozygotic twins and about 50% in dizygotic twins. Genetic factors account for more of the variance in childhood-onset cases than in those who develop it as an adult.

Biological model

Neuroimaging studies suggest dysfunction in the orbito-striatal area (including the caudate nucleus) and dorsolateral prefrontal cortex, combined with abnormalities in serotonergic (underactive) and glutamatergic (overactive) neurotransmission. Further support for this model comes from an association with a number of neurological disorders involving dysfunction of the striatum, including Parkinson's disease, Huntington's disease, Tourette syndrome and Sydenham's chorea. The latter has also been associated with OCD and tic disorders in the *p*aediatric *a*utoimmune *n*europsychiatric *d*isorder *a*ssociated with *s*treptococcal infection (PANDAS). This is a rare condition in children that follows group A haemolytic streptococcal infection. OCD also can follow head trauma.

Cognitive behavioural model

Most people have the occasional intrusive thoughts, but would ordinarily dismiss these as meaningless and not focus upon them further. These develop into an obsession when they assume great significance to the individual, causing greater anxiety. This anxiety motivates suppression of these thoughts, and ritual behaviours are developed to reduce anxiety further.

Management

Psychological management

CBT focusing on exposure and response prevention is reasonably effective. This involves confronting the anxiety-provoking stimulus in a controlled environment and not performing the associated ritual. The aim is for the individual to habituate to the stimulus, thus reducing anxiety. Since it provokes anxiety, the dropout rate is often high.

Physical management

Tricyclic antidepressants (TCAs) and serotonin reuptake inhibitors (SSRIs)

Clomipramine (a TCA) and the SSRIs are the mainstay of drug treatment. Their efficacy is independent of their antidepressant action but the doses required are usually some 50–100% higher than those effective in depression. Although many sufferers respond, relapse rates on discontinuation are high. Three months' treatment with maximum tolerated doses may be necessary for a positive response; in those who fail to respond, the addition of an antipsychotic significantly improves outcome, especially when tics occur co-morbidly. Positive correlations between reduced severity

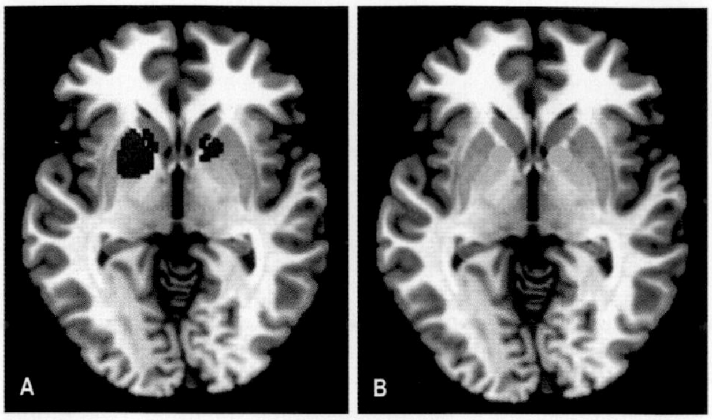

Figure 22.4 Grey matter increase and deep brain stimulation targets in obsessive–compulsive disorder. A. Main areas of increased grey matter regions (lenticular nuclei and caudate) in individuals with obsessive–compulsive disorder (red). **B.** The usual targets for deep brain stimulation in the treatment of obsessive compulsive disorder (green). *(From Radua J, Mataix-Cols D. Voxel-wise meta-analysis of grey matter changes in obsessive compulsive disorder.* British Journal of Psychiatry *2009; 195:393–402, with permission.)*

Box 22.36 Behavioural effects of alcohol

Blood alcohol concentration (BAC) (mg/dL)	Expected effect
20–99	Impaired coordination, euphoria
100–199	Ataxia, poor judgement, labile mood
200–299	Marked ataxia and slurred speech; poor judgement, labile mood, nausea and vomiting
300–399	Stage 1 anaesthesia, memory lapse, labile mood
400+	Respiratory failure, coma, death

of OCD and decreased orbitofrontal and caudate metabolism following behavioural and SSRI treatments have been demonstrated in a number of studies.

Deep brain stimulation

This is a non-ablative, and therefore potentially reversible, surgical technique that involves the electrical stimulation of the basal ganglia by implanted electrodes, creating a 'functional lesion' ***(Fig. 22.4)***. Although this has had success, often impressively so in intractable cases, issues still remain regarding subject selection and the optimum anatomical targets.

Psychosurgery

This is very occasionally recommended in cases of chronic and severe OCD that has not responded to other treatments. The development of stereotactic techniques has led to the replacement of the earlier, crude leucotomies with more precise surgical interventions such as subcaudate tractotomy and cingulotomy, with small yttrium radioactive implants, which induce lesions in the cingulate area or the ventromedial quadrant of the frontal lobe.

Prognosis

Two-thirds of cases improve within a year. The remainder run a fluctuating or persistent course. The prognosis is worse when the personality is obsessional or anankastic and the OCD is primary and severe.

Further reading

Grant JE. Obsessive-compulsive disorder. *N Engl J Med* 2014; 371:646–653.
National Institute for Health and Clinical Excellence. *Nice Clinical Guideline 113: Generalised Anxiety Disorder and Panic Disorder (with or without Agoraphobia) in Adults: Management in Primary, Secondary and Community Care.* NICE 2011; http://www.nice.org.uk/CG113/.
Shear MK. Complicated grief. *N Engl J Med* 2015; 372:153–160.

ALCOHOL MISUSE AND DEPENDENCE

A wide range of physical, social and psychiatric problems are associated with excessive drinking. Alcohol misuse occurs when a patient is drinking in a way that regularly causes problems to the patient or others.

- ***The problem drinker*** is one who causes or experiences physical, psychological and/or social harm as a consequence of drinking alcohol. Many problem drinkers, while heavy drinkers, are not physically addicted to alcohol.
- ***Heavy drinkers*** are those who drink significantly more in terms of quantity and/or frequency than is safe in the long term.
- ***Binge drinkers*** are those who drink excessively in short bouts, usually 24–48 h long, separated by often quite lengthy periods of abstinence. Their overall monthly or weekly alcohol intake may be relatively modest.
- ***Alcohol dependence*** is defined by a physical dependence on or addiction to alcohol. The term 'alcoholism' is a confusing one and has off-putting connotations of vagrancy, 'meths' drinking and social disintegration. It has been replaced by the term 'alcohol dependence syndrome'.

Epidemiology

A total of 20% of men and 10% of women drink more than double the recommended limits of 3 units a day of alcohol for men, and 2 units for women in the UK. The amount of alcohol consumed in the UK has doubled over the last 50 years. Some 4% of men and 2% of women report alcohol withdrawal symptoms, suggesting dependence. Approximately 1 in 5 male admissions to acute medical wards is directly or indirectly due to alcohol. People with serious drinking problems have a two to three times increased risk of dying compared with members of the general population of the same age and sex.

Box 22.36 provides an approximate estimate of what can be expected in an average individual in the way of behavioural impairment resulting from a particular blood alcohol level. The amount of alcohol is measured for convenience in units that contain about 8 g of absolute alcohol and raise the blood alcohol concentration by about 15–20 mg/dL, the amount that is metabolized in 1 h. One unit of alcohol is found in half a pint of ordinary beer (3.5% alcohol by volume, ABV) and 125 mL of 9% wine. However, some beers and most lagers are now 5% ABV (3 units per pint). Wine is often 13% ABV and sold in 175 mL glasses (2–3 units per glass).

Diagnosis

Alcohol misuse should be suspected in any patient presenting with one or more of the physical problems commonly associated with excessive drinking (see pp. 217–218). Alcohol misuse may also be associated with a number of psychiatric symptoms/disorders and social problems ***(Box 22.37)***.

Box 22.37 Common alcohol-related psychological and social problems

Psychological
- Depression
- Anxiety
- Memory problems
- Delirium tremens
- Attempted suicide
- Suicide
- Pathological jealousy

Social
- Domestic violence
- Marital and sexual difficulties
- Child abuse
- Employment problems
- Financial difficulties
- Accidents at home, on the roads, at work
- Delinquency and crime
- Homelessness

Box 22.38 Symptoms of alcohol dependence

- Inability to keep to a drink limit
- Difficulty in avoiding getting drunk
- Spending a considerable time drinking
- Missing meals
- Memory lapses, blackouts
- Restlessness without drink
- Organizing the day around drink
- Trembling after drinking the day before
- Morning retching and vomiting
- Sweating excessively at night
- Withdrawal fits
- Morning drinking
- Increased tolerance
- Hallucinations, frank delirium tremens

Guidelines

The patient's frequency of drinking and the quantity drunk during a typical week should be established:

- Up to 21 units of alcohol a week for men and 14 units for women: this carries no long-term health risk.
- 21–35 units a week for men and 14–24 units for women: there is unlikely to be any long-term health damage, provided the drinking is spread throughout the week.
- Over 36 units a week for men and 24 for women: damage to health becomes increasingly likely.
- Above 50 units a week for men and 35 for women: this is a definite health hazard.

Diagnostic markers of alcohol misuse

Laboratory parameters indicating alcohol misuse in recent weeks include elevated γ-glutamyl transpeptidase (γ-GT) and mean corpuscular volume (MCV). Blood or breath alcohol tests are useful in anyone suspected of very recent drinking.

Alcohol dependence syndrome

Dependence is a pattern of repeated self-administration that causes tolerance, withdrawal and compulsive drug-taking, the essential element of which is the continued use of the substance despite significant substance-related problems. Symptoms of alcohol dependence in a typical order of occurrence are shown in ***Box 22.38***. Diagnostic criteria for alcohol withdrawal syndrome are shown in ***Box 22.39***.

Course

About 25% of all cases of alcohol misuse will lead to chronic alcohol dependence. This most commonly ends in social incapacity, death or abstinence. Alcohol dependence syndrome usually develops after 10 years of heavy drinking (3–4 years in women). In some individuals who use alcohol to alter consciousness, obliterate conscience and defy social mores, dependence and loss of control may appear in only a few months or years.

Box 22.39 Diagnostic criteria for alcohol withdrawal syndrome

Any three of the following:
- Tremor of outstretched hands, tongue or eyelids
- Sweating
- Nausea, retching or vomiting
- Tachycardia or hypertension
- Anxiety
- Psychomotor agitation
- Headache
- Insomnia
- Malaise or weakness
- Transient visual, tactile or auditory hallucinations or illusions
- Grand mal convulsions

Delirium tremens

Delirium tremens (DTs) is the most serious withdrawal state and occurs 1–3 days after alcohol cessation, so is commonly seen 1–2 days after admission to hospital. Patients are disorientated and agitated, and have a marked tremor and visual hallucinations (e.g. insects or small animals coming menacingly towards them). Signs include sweating, tachycardia, tachypnoea and pyrexia. Complications include dehydration, infection, hepatic disease or the Wernicke–Korsakoff syndrome (see p. 885).

Aetiology of alcohol dependence

Genetic factors

Sons of alcohol-dependent people who are adopted by other families are four times more likely to develop drinking problems than are the adopted sons of non-alcohol misusers. Genetic markers include the serotonin transported gene, dopamine-2 receptor allele A1, alcohol dehydrogenase subtypes and monoamine oxidase B activity, but they are not specific.

Environmental factors

Childhood maltreatment increases the risk of subsequent alcohol dependence and this rises if there is also a history of parental alcohol dependence or other substance misuse.

Biochemical factors

Several factors have been suggested, including abnormalities in alcohol dehydrogenase, neurotransmitter substances and brain amino acids, such as GABA. There is no conclusive evidence that these or other biochemical factors play a causal role.

Psychiatric illness

This is an uncommon cause of addictive drinking but it is a treatable one. Some depressed patients drink excessively in the hope of raising their mood. People with anxiety states or phobias are also at risk.

Excess consumption in society

The prevalence of alcohol dependence and problems correlates with the general level (*per capita* consumption) of alcohol use in a society. This, in turn, is determined by factors that may control overall consumption, including price, licensing laws, availability, and the societal norms concerning the use and misuse of alcohol.

Management

Psychological management of problem drinking

Successful identification at an early stage can be a helpful intervention in its own right. It should lead to:

- the provision of information concerning safe drinking levels
- a recommendation to cut down where indicated
- simple support and advice concerning associated problems.

Such a brief intervention is effective in its own right. Successful alcohol misuse treatment involves ***motivational enhancement*** (***motivational therapy***), feedback, education about the adverse effects of alcohol, and agreed drinking goals. A motivational approach is based on five stages of change: pre-contemplation, contemplation, determination, action and maintenance. The therapist uses motivational interviewing and reflective listening to allow the patient to persuade himself along the five stages to change.

This technique, CBT and 12-step facilitation (as used by Alcoholics Anonymous, AA) have all been shown to reduce harmful drinking. With addictive drinking, self-help group therapy, which involves long-term support by fellow members of the group (e.g. AA), is helpful in maintaining abstinence. Family and marital therapy involving both the alcohol misuser and spouse may also be helpful. Families of drinkers find meeting others in a similar situation helpful (Al-Anon).

Drug treatments for problem drinking

Alcohol withdrawal and DTs

Addicted drinkers often experience considerable difficulty when they attempt to reduce or stop their drinking. Withdrawal symptoms are a particular problem and delirium tremens needs urgent treatment ***(Box 22.40)***. In the absence of DTs, alcohol withdrawal can be treated on an outpatient basis, using one of the fixed schedules in ***Box 22.40***, so long as the patient attends daily for medication and monitoring, and has good social support. Outpatient schedules are sometimes given over 5 days. Long-term treatment with benzodiazepines should not be prescribed in those patients who continue to misuse alcohol. Some alcohol misusers add dependence on diazepam to their problems.

Drugs for prevention of alcohol dependence

Naltrexone, the opioid antagonist (50 mg per day), reduces the risk of relapse into heavy drinking and the frequency of drinking. ***Acamprosate*** (1–2 g/day) acts on several receptors, including those for GABA, noradrenaline (norepinephrine) and serotonin. There is reasonable evidence that it reduces drinking frequency. Neither drug seems particularly helpful in maintaining abstinence. The effects of both drugs are enhanced by combining them with counselling, but their moderate efficacy precludes regular use.

Drugs such as ***disulfiram*** react with alcohol to cause unpleasant acetaldehyde intoxication and histamine release. A daily maintenance dose means that the patient must wait until the disulfiram is eliminated from the body before drinking safely. There is mixed evidence of efficacy.

Oral thiamine (300 mg/day) can prevent Wernicke–Korsakoff syndrome (see p. 885) in heavy drinkers.

Prognosis

Research suggests that 30–50% of alcohol-dependent drinkers are abstinent or drinking very much less up to 2 years following traditional intervention. The long-term outcome of patients treated with the latest psychological and pharmacological therapies remains uncertain.

Further reading

Friedmann PD. Alcohol use in adults. *N Engl J Med* 2013; 368:365–373.
Schuckit MA. Recognition and management of withdrawal delerium (delerium tremens). *N Engl J Med* 2014; 371:2100–2113.

DRUG MISUSE AND DEPENDENCE

In addition to alcohol and nicotine, there are a number of psychotropic substances that are taken for their effects on mood and other mental functions ***(Box 22.41)***.

Aetiology of drug misuse

There is no single cause of drug misuse and/or dependence. Three factors appear commonly, in a similar way to alcohol problems:

- the availability of drugs
- a vulnerable personality
- social pressures, particularly from peers.

Box 22.40 Management of delirium tremens (DTs)

General measures

- Admit the patient to a medical bed.
- Correct electrolyte abnormalities and dehydration.
- Treat any co-morbid disorder (e.g. infection).
- Give parenteral thiamine slowly (250 mg daily for 3–5 days) in the absence of Wernicke–Korsakoff syndrome.
- Give parenteral thiamine slowly (500 mg daily for 3–5 days) with Wernicke–Korsakoff encephalopathy. *Note*: Beware anaphylaxis.
- Give prophylactic phenytoin or carbamazepine, if there is a previous history of withdrawal fits.

Specific drug treatment

- Give one of the following orally:
  - Diazepam 10–20 mg
  - Chlordiazepoxide 30–60 mg
- Repeat 1 h after the last dose, depending on response.

Fixed-schedule regimens

- Diazepam 10 mg every 6 h for 4 doses, then 5 mg 6-hourly for 8 doses ***OR***
- Chlordiazepoxide 30 mg every 6 h for 4 doses, then 15 mg 6-hourly for 8 doses.
- Provide additional benzodiazepine when symptoms and signs are not controlled.

Box 22.41 Commonly used drugs of misuse and dependence

Stimulants

- Methylphenidate
- Phenmetrazine
- Phencyclidine ('angel dust')
- Cocaine
- Amfetamine derivatives
- Ecstasy (MDMA)

Hallucinogens

- Cannabis preparations
- Solvents
- Lysergic acid diethylamide (LSD)
- Mescaline

Narcotics

- Morphine
- Heroin
- Codeine
- Pethidine
- Methadone

Tranquillizers

- Barbiturates
- Benzodiazepines

Once regular drug-taking is established, pharmacological factors determine dependence.

Drugs of misuse and their effects

Inhaled substances

Some 1% of adolescents in the UK sniff solvents such as glue for their intoxicating effects. Tolerance develops over weeks or months. Intoxication is characterized by euphoria, excitement, a floating sensation, dizziness, slurred speech and ataxia. Acute intoxication can cause amnesia and visual hallucinations.

Nitric oxide (laughing gas) is also popular in the UK.

Amfetamines and related substances

These have temporary stimulant and euphoriant effects that are followed by fatigue and depression, the latter sometimes prolonged for weeks. Psychological rather than true physical dependence occurs with amfetamine sulphate ('speed'). Methyl amfetamine, also known as 'methamphetamine' or 'crystal meth', is another amfetamine psychostimulant. The particularly high potential for abuse is associated with the activation of neural reward mechanisms involving nucleus accumbens dopamine release.

In addition to a manic-like presentation, amfetamines can produce a paranoid psychosis indistinguishable from schizophrenia.

'Ecstasy' (also known as E, white burger or white dove) is the street name for 3,4-methylenedioxy-metamfetamine (MDMA), a psychoactive phenylisopropylamine, synthesized as an amfetamine derivative. It is a psychedelic drug, which is often used as a 'dance drug'. It has a brief duration of action (4–6 h). Deaths have been reported from malignant hyperpyrexia and dehydration. Acute renal and liver failure can occur.

Cocaine

Cocaine (see pp. 73–74) is a central nervous system stimulant (with similar effects to amfetamines), derived from *Erythroxylon coca* trees grown in the Andes. In purified form, it may be taken by mouth, or snorted or injected. If cocaine hydrochloride is converted to its base ('crack'), it can be smoked. This causes an intense stimulating effect, and 'free-basing' is common. Compulsive use and dependence occur more frequently among users who are free-basing. Dependent users take large doses and alternate between withdrawal phenomena of depression, tremor and muscle pains, and the hyper-arousal produced by increasing doses. Prolonged use of high doses produces irritability, restlessness, paranoid ideation and, occasionally, convulsions. Persistent sniffing of the drug can cause perforation of the nasal septum. Overdoses cause death through myocardial infarction, cerebrovascular disease, hyperthermia and arrhythmias (see pp. 73–74).

Hallucinogenic drugs

Hallucinogenic drugs, such as lysergic acid diethylamide (LSD) and mescaline, produce distortions and intensifications of sensory perceptions, as well as frank hallucinations in acute intoxication. Psychosis is a long-term complication.

Cannabis

Cannabis (also known as grass, pot, skunk, spliff or marijuana) is a widely used drug in some sub-cultures. It is derived from the dried leaves and flowers of the plant *Cannabis sativa*. It can cause tolerance and dependence. Hashish is the dried resin from the flower tops, whilst marijuana refers to any part of the plant. The drug, when smoked, seems to exaggerate the pre-existing mood, be it depression, euphoria or anxiety. It has specific analgesic properties. Cannabis use, especially of the more potent 'skunk', has increased in the UK. An amotivational syndrome with apathy and memory problems has been reported with chronic daily use. Cannabis may, of itself, sometimes cause psychosis in the right circumstances (see below).

Tranquillizers

Drugs that cause dependence include barbiturates and benzodiazepines. Benzodiazepine dependence is common and may be iatrogenic, when the drugs are prescribed and not discontinued. Discontinuing treatment with benzodiazepines may cause withdrawal symptoms (see ***Box 22.35***). For this reason, withdrawal should be supervised and gradual.

Opiates

Physical dependence occurs with morphine, heroin and codeine, as well as with synthetic and semi-synthetic opiates such as methadone, pethidine and fentanyl. These substances display cross-tolerance – the withdrawal effects of one are reduced by administration of another. The psychological effects of opiates are a calm, slightly euphoric mood associated with freedom from physical discomfort and a flattening of emotional response. This is believed to be due to the attachment of morphine and its analogues to endorphin receptors in the central nervous system. Tolerance to this group of drugs is rapidly developed and marked, but is quickly lost following abstinence. The ***opiate withdrawal syndrome*** consists of a constellation of signs and symptoms ***(Box 22.42)*** that reaches peak intensity on the second or third day after the last dose of the opiate. These rapidly subside over the next 7 days. Withdrawal is dangerous in people with heart disease or other chronic debilitating conditions.

Opiate addicts have a relatively high mortality rate, owing to both the ease of accidental overdose and the blood-borne infections associated with shared needles. Heart disease (including infective endocarditis), tuberculosis and AIDS are common causes of death, while the complications of hepatitis B and C are also common.

Management of chronic misuse

Blood and urine screening for drugs is required in circumstances where drug misuse is suspected (see ***Box 22.41***). When a patient with an opiate addiction is admitted to hospital for another health problem, advice should be sought from a psychiatrist or drug misuse clinic regarding management of their addiction while an inpatient.

Box 22.42 Opiate withdrawal syndrome

12–16 h after last dose of opiate

- Yawning
- Rhinorrhoea
- Lacrimation
- Pupillary dilatation
- Sweating
- Piloerection
- Restlessness

24–72 h after last dose of opiate

- Muscular twitches
- Aches and pains
- Abdominal cramps
- Vomiting
- Diarrhoea
- Hypertension
- Insomnia
- Anorexia
- Agitation
- Profuse sweating

The treatment of chronic dependence is directed towards helping the patient either to live without drugs, or to regularize and control use, and to prevent secondary ill-health. Patients need help and advice in order to avoid a withdrawal syndrome. Some people with opiate addiction who cannot manage abstinence may be maintained on oral methadone. In the UK, only specially licensed doctors may legally prescribe heroin and cocaine to an addict for maintenance treatment of addiction. An overdose should be treated immediately with the opioid antagonist naloxone. Injectable diacetylmorphine, the active ingredient in heroin, has been proposed as a more effective alternative to methadone but adverse effects (accidental overdose and seizures) remain a potential concern.

Drug-induced psychosis

Drug-induced psychosis has been reported with amfetamine and its derivatives, and with cocaine and hallucinogens. It can occur acutely after drug use but is more usually associated with chronic misuse. Psychoses are characterized by vivid hallucinations (usually auditory, but often occurring in more than one sensory modality), misidentifications, delusions and/or ideas of reference (often of a persecutory nature), psychomotor disturbances (excitement or stupor) and an abnormal affect. For diagnosis, ICD-10 requires the condition to occur within 2 weeks and usually within 48 h of drug use, and to persist for more than 48 h but not more than 6 months.

Cannabis use can result in anxiety, depression or hallucinations. Manic-like psychoses occurring after long-term cannabis use have been described but seem more likely to be related to the toxic effects of heavy ingestion. Evidence suggests that the risk of psychosis is significantly raised in those using cannabis at an early age (before, as compared to after, 15 years) and on a daily basis. High-potency cannabis ('skunk') is associated with an increased risk. A meta-analysis suggests that daily cannabis use doubles the risk of psychosis, and that 14% of schizophrenia in the UK would be prevented if cannabis use ceased.

Further reading

Degenhardt L, Hall W. Extent of illicit drug use and dependence, and their contribution to the global burden of disease. *Lancet* 2012; 379:55–70.

Kuepper R, van Os J, Lieb R et al. Continued cannabis use and risk of incidence and persistence of psychotic symptoms: 10 year follow-up cohort study. *BMJ* 2011; 342:d738.

Room R, Reuter P. How well do international drug conventions protect public health? *Lancet* 2012; 379:84–91.

Strang J, Babor T, Caulkins J et al. Drug policy and the public good: evidence for effective interventions. *Lancet* 2012; 379:71–83.

Strang J, Metrebian N, Lintzeris N et al. Supervised injectable heroin or injectable methadone versus optimised oral methadone as treatment for chronic heroin addicts in England after persistent failure in orthodox treatment (RIOTT): a randomised trial. *Lancet* 2010; 375:1885–1895.

Volkow ND, Baler RD, Compton WM et al. Adverse health effects of marijuana use. *New Engl J Med* 2014; 370:2219–2227.

Volkow ND, Koob GF, McLellan AT. Neurobiologic advances from the brain disease model of addiction. *N Engl J Med* 2016; 374:363–371.

SCHIZOPHRENIA

The group of illnesses conventionally referred to as 'schizophrenia' is diverse in nature and covers a broad range of perceptual, cognitive and behavioural disturbances. The point prevalence of the condition is 0.5% throughout the world, with equal gender distribution. A non-psychiatrist primarily needs to know how to recognize schizophrenia, what problems it might present with in the general hospital, and how it is treated.

Aetiology

No single cause has been identified. Schizophrenia is likely to be a disease of neurodevelopmental disconnection caused by an interaction of genetic and multiple environmental factors that affect brain development. It is likely that daily cannabis use is a risk factor. The genetic aetiology is likely to be polygenic and non-mendelian; a recent very large study suggests there are about 100 single nucleotide polymorphisms that are associated. Schizophrenia has a heritability of about 60%. Functional neuroimaging studies and histology point towards alterations in prefrontal and, less consistently, temporal lobe function, with enlarged lateral ventricles and disorganized cytoarchitecture in the hippocampus, supporting the neurodevelopmental theory of aetiology. Dopamine excess (D_2) is the oldest and most widely accepted neurochemical hypothesis, although this may explain only one group of symptoms (the positive ones). The cognitive impairments in schizophrenia may be related to dopamine D_1 abnormalities. The interaction between serotonergic and dopaminergic systems is likely to play a role, although direct evidence is lacking. Additional hypotheses involving glutamate (NMDA) and GABA systems are under scrutiny.

Clinical features

The illness can begin at any age but is rare before puberty. The peak age of onset is the early twenties. The symptoms that are diagnostic of the condition have been termed ***first-rank symptoms*** and were described by the German psychiatrist Kurt Schneider. They consist of:

- ***auditory hallucinations*** in the third person and/or voices commenting on the patient's behaviour
- ***thought withdrawal***, insertion and broadcast
- ***primary delusion*** (arising out of nothing)
- ***delusional perception***
- ***somatic passivity and feelings*** – patients believe that their thoughts, feelings or acts are controlled by others.

The more of these symptoms a patient has, the more likely it is that the diagnosis is schizophrenia, but these symptoms may also occur in other psychoses.

Other symptoms of ***acute schizophrenia*** include behavioural disturbances, other hallucinations, secondary (usually persecutory) delusions and blunting of mood. Schizophrenia is sometimes divided into 'positive' (type 1) and 'negative' (type 2) types:

- ***Positive schizophrenia*** is characterized by acute onset, prominent delusions and hallucinations, normal brain structure, a biochemical disorder involving dopaminergic transmission, a good response to neuroleptics, and a better outcome.
- ***Negative schizophrenia*** is characterized by a slow, insidious onset, a relative absence of acute symptoms, the presence of apathy, social withdrawal, lack of motivation, underlying brain structure abnormalities and poor neuroleptic response.

Chronic schizophrenia is characterized by its long duration and by the 'negative' symptoms of underactivity, lack of drive, social withdrawal and emotional emptiness.

Differential diagnosis

Schizophrenia should be distinguished from:

- organic mental disorders (e.g. partial complex epilepsy)
- mood (affective) disorders (e.g. mania)
- drug psychoses (e.g. amfetamine psychosis)
- personality disorders (schizotypal).

In older patients, any acute or chronic brain syndrome can present in a schizophrenia-like manner. A helpful diagnostic point

Box 22.43 Unwanted effects of antipsychotic drugs[a]

Motor
- Acute dystonia
- Parkinsonism
- Akathisia (motor restlessness)
- Tardive dyskinesia

Autonomic
- Hypotension
- Failure of ejaculation

Antimuscarinic
- Dry mouth
- Urinary retention
- Constipation
- Blurred vision

Metabolic
- Weight gain

Others
- Precipitation of glaucoma
- Galactorrhoea (due to hyperprolactinaemia)
- Amenorrhoea
- Cardiac arrhythmias
- QTc interval prolongation
- Seizures
- Leucopenia
- Cholestatic jaundice
- Skin reactions
- Hypersensitivity

[a]*The frequency and type of side effects will depend upon the choice of antipsychotic agent and its dose.*

is the fact that altered consciousness and disturbances of memory do not occur in schizophrenia, and visual hallucinations are unusual.

A ***schizoaffective psychosis*** describes a clinical presentation in which clear-cut affective and schizophrenic symptoms coexist in the same episode.

Management

The best results are obtained by combining drug and social treatments.

Antipsychotic (neuroleptic) drugs

These act by blocking the D_1 and D_2 groups of dopamine receptors. Such drugs are most effective against acute, positive symptoms and are least effective in the management of chronic, negative symptoms. Complete control of positive symptoms can take up to 3 months, and premature discontinuation of treatment can result in relapse.

As antipsychotic drugs block both D_1 and D_2 dopamine receptors, they usually produce extrapyramidal adverse effects. This limits their use in the maintenance therapy of many patients. They also block adrenergic and muscarinic receptors and thereby cause a number of unwanted effects ***(Box 22.43)***.

Neuroleptic malignant syndrome

This is an infrequent but potentially dangerous adverse effect. Neuroleptic malignant syndrome is a medical emergency and should be managed by medical admission. It occurs in 0.2% of patients on neuroleptic drugs, particularly the potent dopaminergic antagonists, such as haloperidol. Symptoms occur a few days to a few weeks after starting treatment and consist of hyperthermia, muscle rigidity, autonomic instability (tachycardia, labile blood pressure, pallor) and a fluctuating level of consciousness. Investigations show a raised creatine kinase, raised white cell count and abnormal liver biochemistry. The more severe consequences include acute kidney injury, pulmonary embolus and death. Treatment consists of stopping the drug and general resuscitation measures, such as temperature reduction. Bromocriptine enhances dopaminergic activity and dantrolene will reduce muscle tone but no treatment has proven benefit.

Pregnancy

Data on the potential teratogenicity of antipsychotic (neuroleptic) medications are still limited. The disadvantages of not treating during pregnancy have to be balanced against possible developmental risks to the fetus. The butyrophenones (e.g. haloperidol) are probably safer than the phenothiazines, such as chlorpromazine. Subsequent management decisions relating to dosage will depend primarily on the ability to avoid adverse effects, since the antiparkinsonian agents are still believed to be teratogenic and should be avoided.

Typical or first-generation antipsychotics

Phenothiazines were the first group of antipsychotics to be developed but are used less frequently now. Chlorpromazine (100–1000 mg daily) is the drug of choice when a more sedating drug is required. Trifluoperazine is used when sedation is undesirable. Fluphenazine decanoate is used as a long-term prophylactic to prevent relapse, as a depot injection (25–100 mg i.m. every 1–4 weeks). ***Butyrophenones*** (e.g. haloperidol 2–15 mg daily) are also powerful antipsychotics, and are used in the treatment of acute schizophrenia and mania. They are likely to cause a dystonia and/or extrapyramidal adverse effects, but are much less sedating than the phenothiazines.

Atypical antipsychotics or serotonin dopamine antagonists

Atypical antipsychotics or serotonin dopamine antagonists (SDAs), also referred to as the 'second-generation antipsychotics', are 'atypical' in that they block D_2 receptors less than D_1, and thus cause fewer extrapyramidal adverse effects and less tardive dyskinesia. They are now recommended as first-line drugs for newly diagnosed schizophrenia and for patients taking typical antipsychotics who are experiencing significant adverse effects.

Risperidone is a benzisoxazole derivative with combined dopamine D_2 receptor and 5-HT_{2A}-receptor blocking properties. Dosage ranges from 6 to 10 mg/day. The drug is not markedly sedative and the overall incidence and severity of extrapyramidal adverse effects is lower than with more conventional antipsychotics. Hyperprolactinaemia can be problematic and prolactin levels should be monitored. Paliperidone is an active metabolite of risperidone, available in oral and depot (4-weekly) preparations.

Olanzapine has affinity for 5-HT_2, D_1, D_2, D_4 and muscarinic receptor sites. Clinical studies indicate that it has a lower incidence of extrapyramidal adverse effects. The apparent better compliance with the drug may be related to its lower side-effect profile and its once-daily dosage of 5–15 mg. Weight gain is a problem with long-term treatment and there is an increased risk of type 1 diabetes mellitus with this and other atypical drugs.

Other atypical antipsychotics include amisulpride, lurasidone, sulpiride, zotepine, ziprasidone and quetiapine, the latter causing less hyperprolactinaemia. Those taking atypical antipsychotics should have regular monitoring of their body mass index, cholesterol levels, blood sugar and QTc interval on ECG. No more than one antipsychotic should be prescribed routinely. Neither risperidone nor olanzapine seems as specific a treatment for intractable chronic schizophrenia as clozapine.

Clozapine is used in patients who have intractable schizophrenia and have failed to respond to at least two conventional antipsychotic drugs; alternatively, it may be used as first-line therapy. This drug is a dibenzodiazepine with a relative high affinity for D_4 dopamine receptors, as compared with D_1, D_2, D_3 and D_5. In addition to muscarinic and α-adrenergic receptors. It acts additionally as a partial agonist at 5-HT_{1A} receptors, which may be of benefit in treating the 'negative' symptoms of psychosis. Functional brain scans have shown that clozapine selectively blocks limbic dopamine receptors more than striatal ones, which is probably why it causes considerably fewer extrapyramidal adverse effects. Clozapine exercises a strong therapeutic effect on both intractable positive and negative symptoms. However, it is expensive and produces severe agranulocytosis in 1–2% of patients. Therefore, in the UK, for example, it can only be prescribed to registered patients by doctors and pharmacists registered with a patient-monitoring service. The starting dose is 25 mg per day with a maintenance dose of 150–300 mg daily. White cell counts should be monitored weekly for 18 weeks and then 2-weekly for the length of treatment. In addition to its antipsychotic actions, clozapine may also help reduce aggressive and hostile behaviour and the risk of suicide. It can cause considerable weight gain and sialorrhoea. There is an increased risk of diabetes mellitus, and gastrointestinal hypomotility resulting in a functional obstruction has also been reported.

Psychological management

This consists of reassurance, support and a good doctor–patient relationship. Psychotherapy of an intensive or exploratory kind is contraindicated. In contrast, individual CBT may have some efficacy, particularly in those who decline drug treatment.

Social management

Social treatment involves attention being paid to the patient's environment and social functioning. Family education can help relatives and partners to provide the optimal amount of emotional and social stimulation, so that not too much emotion is expressed (a risk for relapse). Over 90% of patients are unemployed but sheltered employment can be helpful. Assertive outreach mental health teams will follow up those adhering poorly to treatment.

Medical presentations related to treatment

The motor adverse effects of neuroleptics are the most common reason for a patient with schizophrenia to present to a physician, followed by self-harm. ***Acute dystonia*** normally arises in patients newly started on neuroleptics, causing torticollis. ***Extrapyramidal adverse effects*** are common and present in the same way as Parkinson's disease. They remit once the drug is stopped and on use of antimuscarinic drugs, such as procyclidine. ***Akathisia*** is motor restlessness, most commonly affecting the legs. It is similar to the restless legs syndrome but is apparent during the day. ***Amenorrhoea*** and ***galactorrhoea*** can be caused by dopamine antagonists. Postural hypotension can affect the elderly, and neuroleptics can be the cause of delirium in this age group, if their antimuscarinic effects are prominent.

Long-term benefits outweigh the risks in most cases, and long-term treatment is associated with a lower mortality rate when compared with no treatment. In this respect, the atypical antipsychotics are preferable to the typical antipsychotics and clozapine is the class leader.

Prognosis

The prognosis of schizophrenia is variable: 15–25% of people with schizophrenia recover completely, about 70% will have relapses and may develop mild to moderate negative symptoms, and about 20% will remain seriously disabled. There is some evidence that early drug treatment improves prognosis.

Further reading

Howes OD, Murray RM. Schizophrenia: an integrated sociodevelopmental-cognitive model. *Lancet* 2014; 383:1677–1687.

Leucht S, Cipriani A, Spineli L et al. Comparative efficacy and tolerability of 15 antipsychotic drugs in schizophrenia: a multiple-treatments meta-analysis. *Lancet* 2013; 382:951–962.

ORGANIC MENTAL DISORDERS

Organic brain disorders result from structural pathology, as in dementia (see pp. 874–879), or from disturbed central nervous system function, as in fever-induced delirium.

Delirium

Delirium, also termed ***toxic confusional state*** and ***acute organic psychosis***, is an acute or subacute brain failure in which impairment of attention is accompanied by abnormalities of perception and mood. It is the most common psychosis seen in the general hospital setting, where it occurs in 14–24% of patients. This figure rises in specialist populations such as intensive care patients. Agitation is usually worse at night, with consequent sleep reversal, so that the patient is asleep in the day and awake all night. In addition to an agitated, 'hyperactive' presentation, a hypoactive variant is also recognized and is thought to represent a worse prognosis in the elderly. Most cases will demonstrate a fluctuation between these two psychomotor forms. During the acute phase, thought and speech are incoherent, memory is impaired and misperceptions occur. Episodic visual hallucinations (or illusions) and persecutory delusions occur. As a consequence, the patient may be frightened, suspicious, restless and uncooperative.

A developing, deteriorating or damaged brain predisposes a patient to develop delirium ***(Box 22.44)***. A large number of diseases may cause delirium, particularly in elderly patients, such that it is wise to assess for delirium in patients over 65 years who are admitted to hospital. Some causes of delirium are listed in ***Box 22.45***.

Box 22.44 Predisposing factors in delirium

- Extremes of age (developing or deteriorating brain)
- Damaged brain:
  - Any dementia (most common predisposition)
  - Previous head injury
  - Alcohol brain damage
  - Previous stroke
- Dislocation to an unfamiliar environment (e.g. hospital admission)
- Sleep deprivation
- Sensory extremes (overload or deprivation)
- Immobilization
- Visual or hearing impairment

Box 22.45 Some common causes of delirium

- Systemic infection:
  - Any infection, particularly with high fever (e.g. malaria, septicaemia)
- Metabolic disturbance:
  - Hepatic failure
  - Chronic kidney disease
  - Disorders of electrolyte balance, dehydration
  - Hypoxia
- Vitamin deficiency:
  - Thiamine (Wernicke–Korsakoff syndrome, beriberi)
  - Nicotinic acid (pellagra)
  - Vitamin B_{12}
- Endocrine disease:
  - Hypothyroidism
  - Cushing syndrome
- Intracranial causes:
  - Trauma
  - Tumour
  - Abscess
  - Subarachnoid haemorrhage
  - Epilepsy
- Drug intoxication:
  - Anticonvulsants
  - Antimuscarinics
  - Anxiolytics/hypnotics
  - Tricyclic antidepressants
  - Dopamine agonists
  - Digoxin
- Drug/alcohol withdrawal
- Postoperative states

Box 22.46 Delirium: diagnostic criteria[a]

- Disturbance of consciousness:
  - ↓Clarity of awareness of environment
  - ↓Ability to focus, sustain or shift attention
- Change in cognition:
  - Memory deficit, disorientation, language disturbance, perceptual disturbance
- Disturbance develops over a short period (hours or days)
- Fluctuation over the course of a day

[a]*Derived from* Diagnostic and Statistical Manual *of the American Psychiatric Association, 5th edn: text revision (DSM-5).*

Delirium tremens should be considered in the differential diagnosis (see p. 921), as well as Lewy body dementia (pp. 877–878). Diagnostic criteria are given in ***Box 22.46***.

Management

History should be taken from a witness. Examination may reveal the cause. Investigation and treatment of the underlying physical disease should be undertaken (see ***Box 22.45***). The patient should be carefully nursed and rehydrated in a quiet single room with a window that does not allow exits. If a high fever is present, the patient's temperature should be reduced. All current drug therapy should be reviewed and, where possible, stopped. If they are needed, ensure that patients have hearing aids, glasses and dentures. Psychoactive drugs should be avoided if possible (because of their own risk of exacerbating delirium). In severe delirium, haloperidol is an effective choice, the daily dose usually ranging between 1.5 mg (in the elderly) and 20 mg per day. Benzodiazepines should not be used as first-line medication and may prolong confusion. If necessary, the first dose can be administered intramuscularly. Olanzapine is an effective alternative, especially if given at night for insomnia.

Prognosis

Delirium usually clears within a week or two, but brain recovery usually lags behind recovery from the causative physical illness. The prognosis depends not only on the successful treatment of the causative disease, but also on the underlying state of the brain. Some 25% of the elderly with delirium will have an underlying dementia; 15% of patients do not survive their underlying illness; 40% are in institutional care at 6 months. Mortality rates are raised in patients with delirium in the 18 months after admission and this is greatest in those who present to emergency departments with the diagnosis.

Further reading

Inouye SK, Westendorp RGJ, Saczynski JS. Delirium in elderly people. *Lancet* 2014; 383:911–922.

van Munster BC, de Rooij S. Delirium: a synthesis of current knowledge. *Clin Med* 2014; 14:192–195.

Witlox J, Eurelings LS, de Jonghe JF et al. Delirium in elderly patients and the risk of postdischarge mortality, institutionalization, and dementia: a meta-analysis. *JAMA* 2010; 304:443–451.

EATING DISORDERS

Obesity

Obesity is the most common eating disorder (see pp. 206–212) and has become epidemic in many developed countries. It is usually caused by a combination of constitutional and social factors, but a binge eating disorder and psychological determinants of 'comfort eating' should be excluded.

Anorexia nervosa

Case register data suggest an incidence rate of 19/100 000 females aged between 15 and 34 years. Surveys have suggested a prevalence rate of approximately 1% among schoolgirls and university students. However, many more young women have amenorrhoea accompanied by less weight loss than the 15% required for the diagnosis of anorexia nervosa. The condition is much less common among men (ratio of 1:10).

Clinical features

The main clinical criteria for diagnosis are shown in ***Box 22.47***. Clinical features include the following:

- Onset is usually in adolescence.
- There is a previous history of faddish eating.
- The patient generally eats little, yet is obsessed by food.
- Exercising is excessive.

The physical consequences of anorexia include sensitivity to cold, constipation, hypotension and bradycardia. In most cases, amenorrhoea is secondary to the weight loss. In those who also binge and vomit or abuse purgatives, there may be hypokalaemia and alkalosis.

Aetiology

Biological factors

Genetic

Some 6–10% of female siblings of affected women suffer from anorexia nervosa. There is an increased concordance amongst monozygotic twins, suggesting a genetic predisposition.

Hormonal

The reductions in sex hormones and downregulation of the hypothalamic–pituitary–adrenal axis are secondary to malnutrition and usually reversed by refeeding.

Psychological factors

Individual

Anorexia nervosa has often been seen as an escape from the emotional problems of adolescence and a regression into childhood. Patients will often have had dietary problems in early life. Perfectionism and low self-esteem are common antecedents. Studies suggest that survivors of childhood sexual or other abuse are at greater risk of developing an eating disorder, usually anorexia nervosa, in adolescence.

Box 22.47 Clinical criteria for anorexia nervosa

- Body weight >15% below the standard weight or a body mass index <17.5 kg/m^2 (ICD-10)
- Self induced weight loss: avoidance of fattening foods, vomiting, purging, exercise or appetite suppressants
- Distortion of body image, i.e. patients regard themselves as fat when they are thin
- Morbid fear of fatness
- Amenorrhoea in women

ICD-10, Classification of Mental and Behavioural Disorders, *10th edn.*

Family

Family problems are most commonly secondary to the stress of coping with a family member with the illness.

Social and cultural factors

There is a higher prevalence in higher social classes, Westernized families, certain occupational groups (e.g. ballet dancers and nurses) and societies where cultural value is placed on thinness.

Management

Treatment can be conducted on an outpatient basis, unless the weight loss is severe and accompanied by marked cardiovascular signs and/or electrolyte and vitamin disturbances. Hospital admission may then be unavoidable and may need to be on a medical ward initially. Uncommonly, the patient's weight loss may be so severe as to be life-threatening. If the patient cannot be persuaded to enter hospital, compulsory admission may have to be used. Inpatient treatment goals include:

- establishing a therapeutic relationship with both the patient and her family
- restoring the weight to a level between the ideal body weight and the patient's ideal weight
- providing a balanced diet, aimed at gaining 0.5–1 kg weight per week
- eliminating purgative and/or laxative use and vomiting.

Outpatient treatment should include cognitive behavioural or interpersonal psychotherapies. Setting up a therapeutic alliance is vital. Family therapy is more effective than individual psychotherapy in adolescents and those still at home, and less effective in those who have left home. Motivational enhancement techniques are being used with some success.

Drug treatment has met with limited success, and those drugs that increase the QTc interval should be avoided. Vitamins and minerals may need replacement.

Prognosis

The condition runs a fluctuating course, with exacerbations and partial remissions. Long-term follow-up suggests that about two-thirds of patients maintain normal weight and that the remaining one-third are split between those who are moderately underweight and those who are seriously underweight. Indicators of a poor outcome include:

- a long initial illness
- severe weight loss
- older age at onset
- bingeing and purging
- personality difficulties
- difficulties in relationships.

Suicide has been reported in 2–5% of people with chronic anorexia nervosa. The mortality rate per year is 0.5% from all causes. The illness can quickly cause osteopenia, and later osteoporosis. More than one-third have recurrent affective illness, and various family, genetic and endocrine studies have found associations between eating disorders and depression.

Bulimia nervosa

This refers to episodes of uncontrolled excessive eating, which are also termed 'binges', accompanied by means to lose weight. There is a preoccupation with food and habitual behaviours to avoid the fattening effects of periodic binges. These behaviours include:

- self-induced vomiting
- misuse of drugs – laxatives, diuretics, thyroid extract or anorectics.

Box 22.48 Clinical features of bulimia nervosa

- Physical complications of vomiting:
  - Cardiac arrhythmias
  - Renal impairment
  - Muscular paralysis
  - Tetany – from hypokalaemic alkalosis
  - Swollen salivary glands – from vomiting
  - Eroded dental enamel
- Associated psychiatric disorders:
  - Depressive illness
  - Alcohol misuse
- Fluctuations in body weight within normal limits
- Menstrual function – periods irregular but amenorrhoea is rare
- Personality – perfectionism and/or low self-esteem present premorbidly

Additional clinical features are shown in ***Box 22.48***.

The lifetime prevalence of bulimia ranges between 3% and 7% for women. Bulimia is sometimes associated with anorexia nervosa. A premorbid history of dieting is common. The prognosis for bulimia nervosa is better than that for anorexia nervosa.

Management

Individual CBT is more effective than both interpersonal psychotherapy and drug treatments. SSRIs (e.g. fluoxetine) are also an effective treatment, even in the absence of a depressive illness, but may require high doses.

Atypical eating disorders

These include eating disorders that do not conform clinically to the diagnostic criteria for anorexia nervosa or bulimia nervosa. ***Binge eating disorders*** (BEDs) consist of bulimia without the vomiting and other weight-reducing strategies. The new DSM-5 considers binge eating disorder as a separate diagnosis, characterized by discrete episodes of significant over-eating combined with a sense of having no control over eating during these episodes. Periods of binging need to be present at least once a week over a period of 3 months or more. ICD-10 continues to consider the diagnosis as an otherwise undefined eating disorder. Management strategies include self-help programmes and CBT, which are often combined with an SSRI.

Further reading

Bulik CM. The challenges of treating anorexia nervosa. *Lancet* 2014; 383:105–106.

Royal College of Psychiatrists. *College Report 130. Guidelines for the Nutritional Management of Anorexia Nervosa.* Royal College of Psychiatrists 2005; http://www.rcpsych.ac.uk.

Treasure J, Claudino AM, Zucker N. Eating disorders. *Lancet* 2010; 375:583–593.

SEXUAL DISORDERS

Sexual disorders can be divided into sexual dysfunctions and deviations, and gender role disorders ***(Box 22.49)***.

Sexual dysfunction

Sexual dysfunction in men refers to the repeated inability to achieve normal sexual intercourse, whereas in women it refers to a repeatedly unsatisfactory quality of sexual satisfaction. Problems of sexual dysfunction can usefully be classified into those affecting sexual desire, arousal and orgasm.

Among men presenting for treatment of sexual dysfunction, erectile dysfunction is the most frequent complaint. The prevalence

Box 22.49 Classification of sexual disorders

Sexual dysfunction

Affecting sexual desire
- Low libido

Impaired sexual arousal
- Erectile dysfunction
- Failure of arousal in women

Affecting orgasm
- Premature ejaculation
- Retarded ejaculation
- Orgasmic dysfunction in women

Sexual deviations

Variations of the sexual 'object'
- Fetishism
- Transvestism
- Paedophilia
- Bestiality
- Necrophilia

Variations of the sexual act
- Exhibitionism
- Voyeurism
- Sadism
- Masochism
- Frotteurism

Disorders of the gender role
- Transsexualism

Box 22.51 Drugs affecting sexual arousal

Male arousal
- Alcohol[a]
- Benzodiazepines
- Neuroleptics
- Cimetidine
- Opiate analgesics
- Methyldopa
- Clonidine
- Spironolactone
- Antihistamines
- Metoclopramide
- Diuretics
- Beta-blockers
- Cannabis

Female arousal
- Alcohol[a]
- Central nervous system depressants
- Antidepressants (SSRIs)
- Oral combined contraceptives
- Methyldopa
- Clonidine

[a]Alcohol increases the desire but diminishes the performance. SSRIs, selective serotonin reuptake inhibitors.

Box 22.50 Medical conditions affecting sexual performance

Endocrine
- Diabetes mellitus
- Hyperthyroidism
- Hypothyroidism

Cardiovascular
- Angina pectoris
- Previous myocardial infarction
- Disorders of peripheral circulation

Hepatic
- Cirrhosis, particularly alcohol-related

Renal
- Chronic kidney disease

Neurological
- Neuropathy
- Spinal cord lesions

Respiratory
- Asthma
- Chronic obstructive pulmonary disease

Psychiatric
- Depressive illness
- Substance misuse

of premature ejaculation is low, except in young men, while ejaculatory failure is rare.

Common female problems include reduced libido, vaginismus and anorgasmia.

Sexual drive is affected by constitutional factors, ignorance of sexual technique, anxiety about sexual performance, medical and psychiatric conditions, and certain drugs (***Boxes 22.50*** and ***22.51***).

The treatment of sexual dysfunction involves careful assessment of both physical and psychosocial factors, the participation (where appropriate) of the patient's partner, sex education, and specific therapeutic techniques, including relaxation, behavioural therapy and couple therapy. The introduction of phosphodiesterase type 5 inhibitors (e.g. sildenafil) has provided an effective therapy for the treatment of erectile dysfunction (see p. 1217).

Sexual deviation

Sexual deviations are regarded as unusual forms of behaviour rather than as an illness. Doctors are only likely to be involved when the behaviour involves breaking the law (e.g. paedophilia) and when there is a question of an associated mental or physical disorder. Men are more likely than women to have sexual deviations.

Gender role disorders

Transsexualism involves a disturbance in gender identity in which the patient is convinced that their body is the wrong gender. A person's gender identity refers to the individual's sense of masculinity or femininity, as distinct from sex. There is increasing evidence that transsexualism is biologically determined, perhaps by prenatal endocrine influences, and functional brain imaging shows specific differences from normal controls.

For males, treatment includes oestrogen administration and, if surgery is to be recommended, a period of living as a woman as a trial beforehand. In the case of female transsexuals, treatment involves surgery and the use of methyltestosterone.

PERSONALITY DISORDERS

These disorders comprise enduring patterns of behaviour that manifest themselves as inflexible responses to a broad range of personal and social situations. Personality disorders are developmental conditions that appear in childhood or adolescence and continue into adult life. Their prevalence is about 15% in the population. They are not secondary to another psychiatric disorder or brain disease, although they may precede or coexist with other disorders. In contrast, personality change is acquired, usually in adult life, following severe or prolonged stress, extreme environmental deprivation, serious psychiatric disorder or brain injury or disease.

Personality disorders are usually subdivided according to clusters of traits that correspond to the most frequent or obvious behavioural manifestations, but many will show the characteristics of more than one category. The main categories of personality disorder are described in ***Box 22.52***.

Further reading

Bateman AW, Gunderson J, Mulder R. Treatment of personality disorder. *Lancet* 2015; 385:735–743.

Gunderson JG. Borderline personality disorder. *N Engl J Med* 2011; 364:2037–2042.

Leichsenring F, Leibing E, Kruse J et al. Borderline personality disorder. *Lancet* 2011; 377:74–84.

Newton-Howes G, Clark LA, Chanen A. Personality disorder across the life course. *Lancet* 2015; 385:727–734.

Tyrer P, Reed GM, Crawford MJ. Classification, assessment, prevalence, and effect of personality disorder. *Lancet* 2015; 385:717–726.

INVOLUNTARY DETENTION OR COMMITMENT

Involuntary detention in hospital is typically used as a last resort and treatment on an outpatient basis is preferable in most cases.

Box 22.52 The main categories of personality disorder

Category	Description
Borderline (emotionally unstable)	Impulsive actions Intense, short-lived emotional attachments Chronic internal emptiness Frequent self-harm Transient 'pseudo'-psychotic features Strong family history of mood disorders
Paranoid	Extreme sensitivity Suspicion Litigiousness Self-importance Preoccupation with conspiracy theories
Schizoid	Emotional coldness and detachment Limited capacity to express emotions Indifference to praise or criticism Preference for solitary activities Lack of close friendships Marked insensitivity to social norms
Antisocial	Callous unconcern for the feelings of others Incapacity to maintain enduring relationships Very low tolerance of frustration Incapacity to experience guilt and to learn from experience Tendency to blame others
Histrionic	Self-dramatization, theatricality, suggestibility Shallow and labile emotions Continual seeking for excitement and appreciation Inappropriately seductive appearance and behaviour
Narcissistic	Inflated sense of self-importance Need to be admired Self-referential nature Arrogance
Anankastic (obsessional)	Feelings of excessive doubt and caution Preoccupation with details, rules and order Perfectionism Excessive conscientiousness, scrupulousness, pedantry and rigidity
Dependent	Encouragement of others to make their personal decisions Subordination of their needs to others Unwillingness to make demands on others Feelings of inability to care for themselves Preoccupation with fears of being abandoned

The term describes the practice of ***admitting or keeping a patient in hospital against their will***. This is done in compliance with the mental health legislation relevant to a particular country. Application for such a course of action may be made by a doctor (typically, but not always, a psychiatrist), social worker, psychologist or, in some instances, a police officer.

Mental health laws differ between countries and, in the case of the USA, also between states. However, in broad terms, the principles remain the same and are summarized in ***Box 22.53***.

The potential for abuse of such 'powers' is a constant focal point for the review of such legislation. Although this is thankfully uncommon, the detention of individuals as a means to suppress dissent against regimes is well known.

Box 22.53 The basis of mental health laws for detention or commitment

1. The individual to be detained must be suffering from a defined mental disorder.
2. Detention is for the purposes of observation and refinement of the diagnosis and/or to actively treat the disorder (i.e. detention is a means to an end).
3. Attempts to treat the individual on an outpatient basis have failed.
4. The offer of a voluntary admission to hospital has been refused or is impractical.
5. Treatment in hospital is necessary:
   - because it will benefit the outcome of the illness
   - to protect the patient from harm (in terms of physical health, mental health, and abuse or manipulation at the hands of others)
   - to protect others from harm that the patient might cause them passively (neglect) or actively.

Box 22.54 Assessment of mental capacity to make a decision

The patient has a demonstrated impairment or disturbance of their mind/brain and a demonstrated inability to do any of the following:

- Understand relevant information
- Retain that information for sufficient time to make the decision
- Use or weigh that information
- Communicate their decision

MENTAL CAPACITY ACT

Mental capacity is the ability to make decisions about all aspects of one's life, including, but not exclusively, healthcare. All doctors need to be able to assess mental capacity. In England and Wales, a new act was passed in 2005, which, for the first time, formally protects patients who lack capacity (see ***Boxes 1.4*** and ***22.54***). Some 3% of people in the UK are thought to lack capacity due to conditions affecting brain function, such as dementia. However, the assessment of capacity is specific to an individual decision, so it is possible to have capacity to make one decision but not another. The assessment of capacity is outlined in ***Box 22.54***. Capacity is assumed unless there is evidence to the contrary. In the absence of capacity, it is best to act in the best interests of the patient and provide the least restrictive management, after consulting the nearest relative or an independent advocate.

Further reading

Nicholson TR, Cutter W, Hotopf M. Assessing mental capacity: the Mental Capacity Act. *BMJ* 2008; 336:322–325.

http://www.legislation.gov.uk *Mental Capacity Act 2005. Code of Practice 2013.*

Significant websites

http://psych.org *American Psychiatric Association.*
http://www.b-eat.co.uk *Beating Eating Disorders (formerly the Eating Disorders Association).*
http://www.cebmh.com *Centre for Evidence-Based Mental Health.*
http://www.mentalhealth.org.uk *Mental Health Foundation – charity.*
http://www.rcpsych.ac.uk *UK Royal College of Psychiatrists.*
http://www.sleepfoundation.org *National Sleep Foundation.*

23 Cardiovascular disease

Nicholas H Bunce, Robin Ray

See your e-book for section summaries, clinical tips, drug tips, videos, audio, extra images, interactive Figures, MCQs and Special Topics from the International Advisory Board.

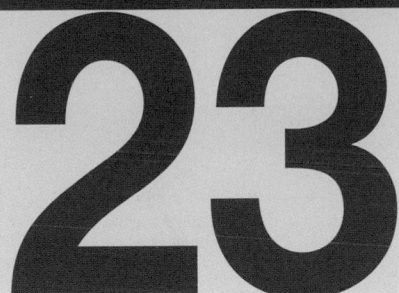

CARDIOVASCULAR

General
- Breathless
- Position - sitting up?
- Colour - cyanosed (central)
  - pale
  - malar flush (mitral stenosis)
- Pain
- Obesity/cachexia
- Signs of other conditions, e.g. Marfan
- Temperature
- Sweating

Jugular venous pulsation
- Height
- Character

Carotid pulse
- Character
- Bruits

Blood pressure

Tendon xanthoma

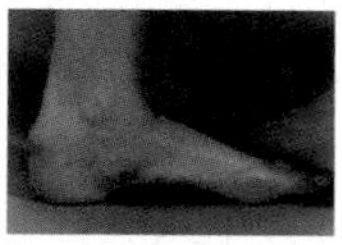

(From Gaw A 2013 Clinical Biochemistry, An Illustrated Colour Text, 5th Edn. Elsevier, with permission)

Radial pulse
- Rate
- Rhythm
- Volume

Hands
Splinter haemorrhoids
Clubbing
Peripheral cyanosis
Tendon xanthomata (hyperlipidaemia)

Splinter haemorrhages

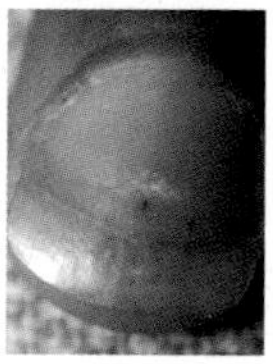

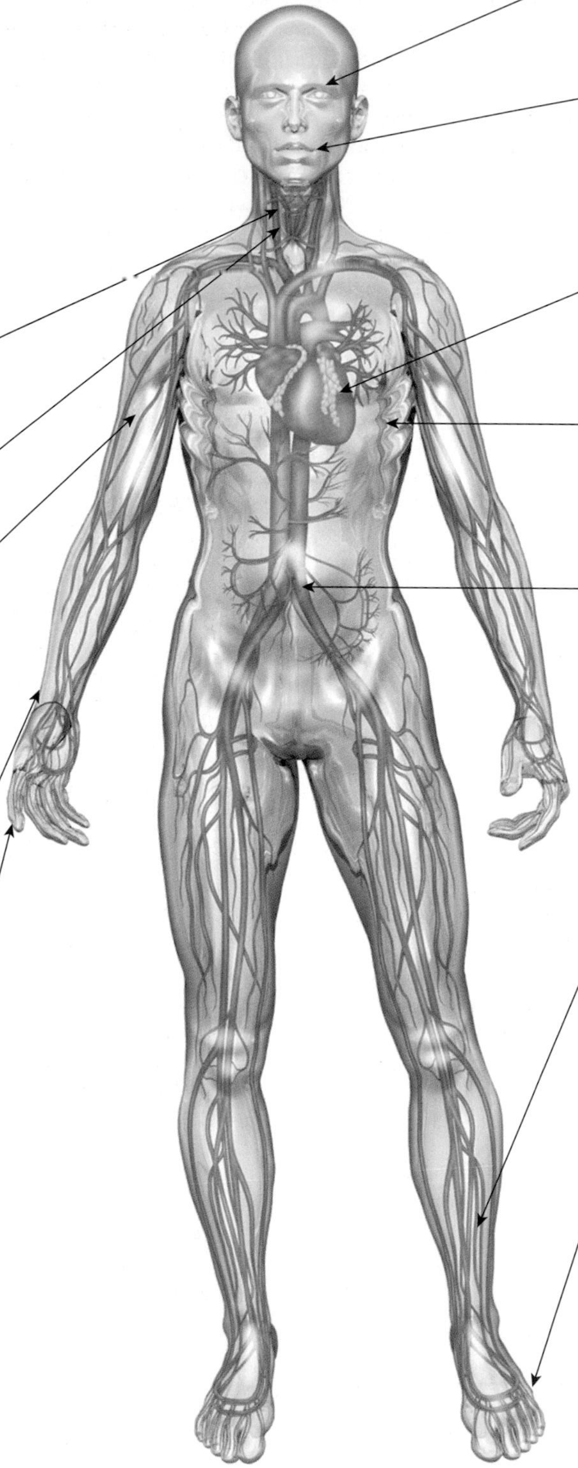

Xanthelasma

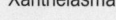

Mouth
Oral hygiene
Poor dentition

Precordium
Inspect - look for scars
Palpate - apex beat
- thrills
- ventricular heaves

Respiratory
- Basal crackles

Abdomen
- Hepatomegaly (pulsatile in tricuspid incompetence)
- Ascites
- Aortic aneurysm

Legs
Oedema
Feel for peripheral pulses

Feet
Look for ischaemia
- Feel for pulses
- Temperature
Vasculitis rash

Infective endocarditis, septic embolization

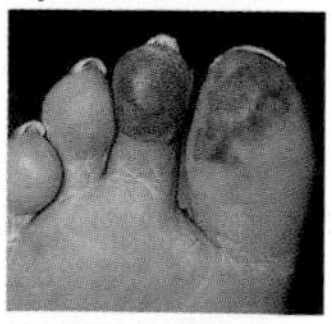

(From Johnson RJ, Feehally J 2000 Comprehensive Clinical Nephrology, 2nd ed. St. Louis, Mosby, 2000, with permission)

ANATOMY, PHYSIOLOGY AND EMBRYOLOGY OF THE HEART

Myocardial cells constitute 75% of the heart mass but only about 25% of the cell number. They are designed to perform two fundamental functions: initiation and conduction of electrical impulses and contraction. Although most myocardial cells are able to perform both these functions, the vast majority are predominantly contractile cells (myocytes) and a small number are specifically designed as electrical cells. The latter, collectively known as the conducting system of the heart, are not nervous tissue but modified myocytes lacking in myofibril components. They have the ability to generate electrical impulses, which are then conducted to the myocytes, leading to contraction by a process known as excitation–contraction coupling. The rate of electrical impulse generation and the force of myocardial contraction are modified by numerous factors, including autonomic input and stretch.

Three epicardial coronary arteries supply blood to the myocardium, and a more complex network of veins is responsible for drainage. In the face of continuous arterial pressure fluctuations, blood vessels, especially in the cerebral circulation, maintain constant tissue perfusion by a process known as '***autoregulation***'; blood vessel control is, however, complex, involving additional local and central mechanisms.

The conduction system of the heart

The sinus node (sinoatrial node)

The sinus node is a complex, spindle-shaped structure that lies in the lateral and epicardial aspects of the junction between the superior vena cava and the right atrium ***(Fig. 23.1)***. Physiologically, it generates impulses automatically by spontaneous depolarization of its membrane at a rate quicker than any other cardiac cell type. It is therefore the natural pacemaker of the heart.

A number of factors are responsible for the spontaneous decay of the sinus node cell membrane potential ('the pacemaker potential'), the most significant of which is a small influx of sodium ions into the cells. This small sodium current has two components: the background inward (I_b) current and the 'funny' (I_f) current (or pacemaker current) ***(Fig. 23.2)***. The term 'funny' current denotes ionic flow through channels activated in ***hyperpolarized*** cells (−60 mV or greater), unlike other time- and voltage-dependent channels activated by ***depolarization***. The rate of depolarization of the sinus node membrane potential is modulated by autonomic tone (i.e. sympathetic and parasympathetic input), stretch, temperature, hypoxia and blood pH and responds to other hormonal influences (e.g. tri-iodothyronine and serotonin).

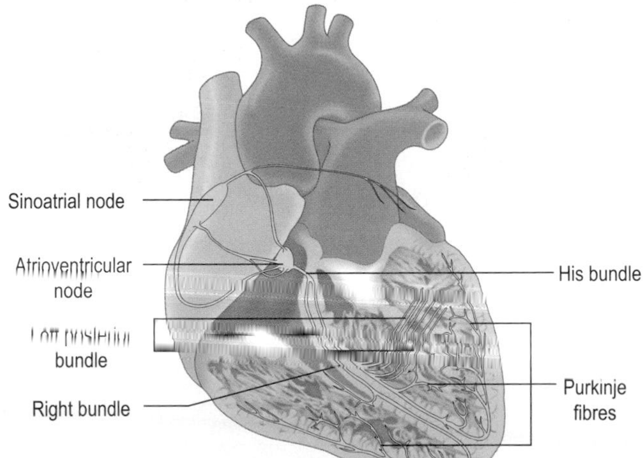

Figure 23.1 **The conducting system of the heart.**

Atrial and ventricular myocyte action potentials

Action potentials in the sinus node trigger depolarization of the atrial, and subsequently the ventricular, myocytes. These cells have a different action potential from that of sinus node cells ***(Fig. 23.2)***. Their resting membrane potential is a consequence of a small flow of potassium ions into the cells through open 'inward rectifier' channels (I_{Ki}); at this stage, sodium and calcium channels are closed. The arrival of adjacent action potentials triggers the opening of voltage-gated, fast, self-inactivating sodium channels, resulting in a sharp depolarization spike. This is followed by a partial repolarization of the membrane due to activation of 'transient outward' potassium channels.

The plateau phase that follows is unique to myocytes and results from a small, but sustained, inward calcium current through L-type calcium channels (I_{CaL}) lasting 200–400 ms. This calcium influx is caused by a combined increase in permeability of the cell, especially the sarcolemmal membranes to calcium ***(Fig. 23.3)***. This plateau (or refractory) phase in myocyte action potential prevents early reactivation of the myocytes and directly determines the strength of contraction. The gradual inactivation of the calcium channels activates delayed rectifier potassium channels (I_K), repolarizing the membrane. Atrial tissue is activated like a 'forest fire', but the activation peters out when the insulating layer between the atrium and the ventricle – the annulus fibrosus – is reached. Controversy exists about whether impulses from the sinoatrial (SA) node travel over specialized conducting 'pathways' or over ordinary atrial myocardium.

The atrioventricular node, His bundle and Purkinje fibres

The depolarization continues to conduct slowly through the atrioventricular (AV) node. This is a small, bean-shaped structure that lies beneath the right atrial endocardium within the lower interatrial septum. The AV node continues as the His bundle, which penetrates the annulus fibrosus and conducts the cardiac impulse rapidly towards the ventricle. The His bundle reaches the crest of the interventricular septum and divides into the right bundle branch and the main left bundle branch.

The ***right bundle branch*** continues down the right side of the interventricular septum to the apex; from here, it radiates and

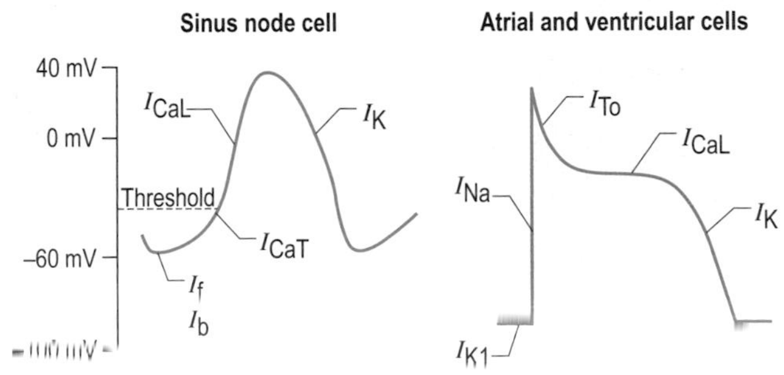

Figure 23.2 **Myocardial action potentials.** I_b, background inward sodium current; I_{CaL}, long-lasting (or 'L' type) calcium channel; I_{CaT}, transient (or 'T' type) calcium channel; I_f, 'funny' current; I_K, delayed rectifier potassium current; I_{K1}, inward rectifier potassium current; I_{Na}, inward sodium current; I_{To}, transient outward potassium current.

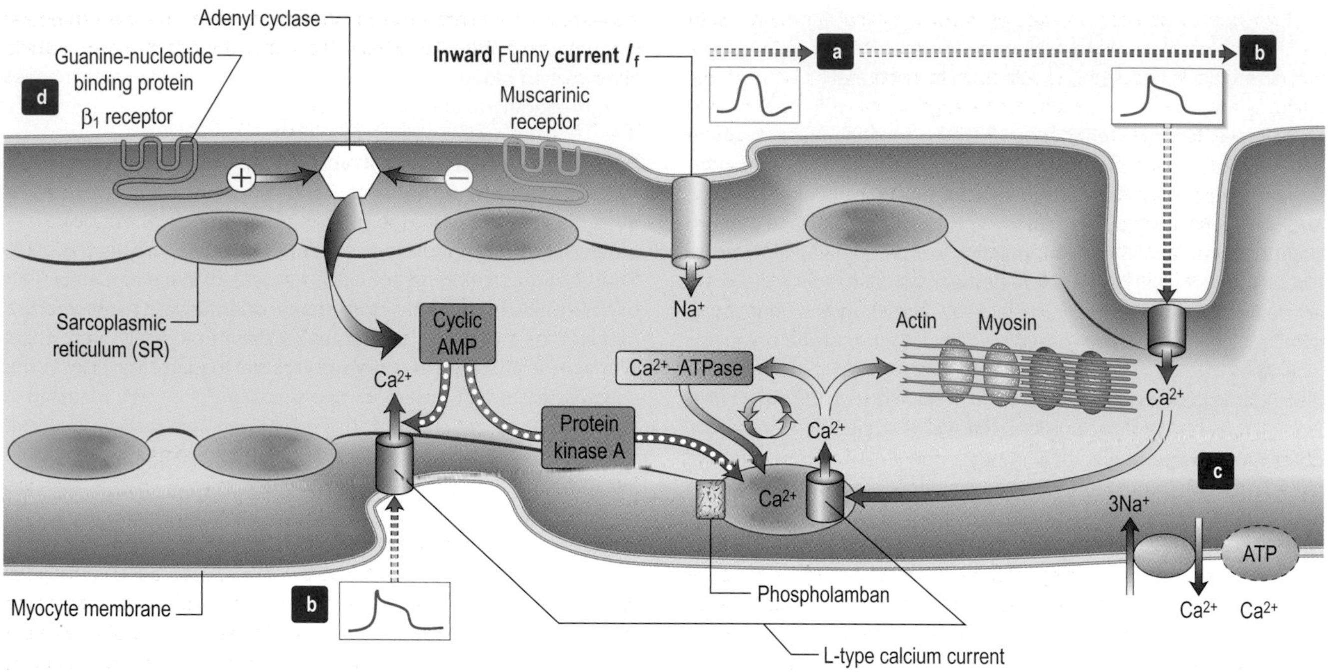

Figure 23.3 The 'complete' cardiac cell. (a) *Spontaneous depolarization* in sinus node cells, due to sodium (Na) influx through the 'funny' current, generates the 'pacemaker' potential. **(b)** This activates other atrial and ventricular myocytes, triggering *action potentials* and activating L-type calcium (Ca) channels in the surface and transverse tubule membranes (at the top and bottom of the figure). **(c)** The resulting *Ca influx* acts on Ca-induced Ca release channels (RyR2) on the sarcoplasmic reticulum (SR); this causes the release of stored Ca, which acts on actin and myosin fibrils, leading to contraction. Ca reuptake pumps in the SR, regulated by phospholamban, replenish the stores; various exchange pumps also expel Ca from the cell. **(d)** *Autonomic input* has either a positive chronotropic/inotropic effect (β_1 receptors) or a negative chronotropic/inotropic effect (muscarinic receptors). AMP, adenosine monophosphate; ATPase, adenosine triphosphatase.

divides to form the Purkinje network, which spreads throughout the sub-endocardial surface of the right ventricle. The ***main left bundle branch*** is a short structure, which fans out into many strands on the left side of the interventricular septum. These strands can be grouped into an anterior superior division (the anterior hemi-bundle) and a posterior inferior division (the posterior hemi-bundle). The anterior hemi-bundle supplies the sub-endocardial Purkinje network of the anterior and superior surfaces of the left ventricle, and the inferior hemi-bundle supplies the inferior and posterior surfaces. Impulse conduction through the AV node is slow and depends on action potentials largely produced by slow transmembrane calcium flux. In the atria, ventricles and His–Purkinje system, conduction is rapid and is due to action potentials generated by rapid transmembrane sodium diffusion.

The cellular basis of myocardial contraction – excitation–contraction coupling

Each myocyte, approximately 100 μm long, branches and interdigitates with adjacent cells. An intercalated disc permits electrical conduction to adjacent cells. Myocytes contain bundles of parallel myofibrils. Each myofibril is made up of a series of sarcomeres ***(Fig. 23.4)***. A sarcomere (which is the basic unit of contraction) is bound by two transverse Z lines, to each of which is attached a perpendicular filament of the protein actin. The actin filaments from each of the two Z bands overlap with thicker parallel protein filaments known as myosin. Actin and myosin filaments are attached to each other by cross-bridges that contain adenosine triphosphatase (ATPase), which breaks down adenosine triphosphate (ATP) to provide the energy for contraction.

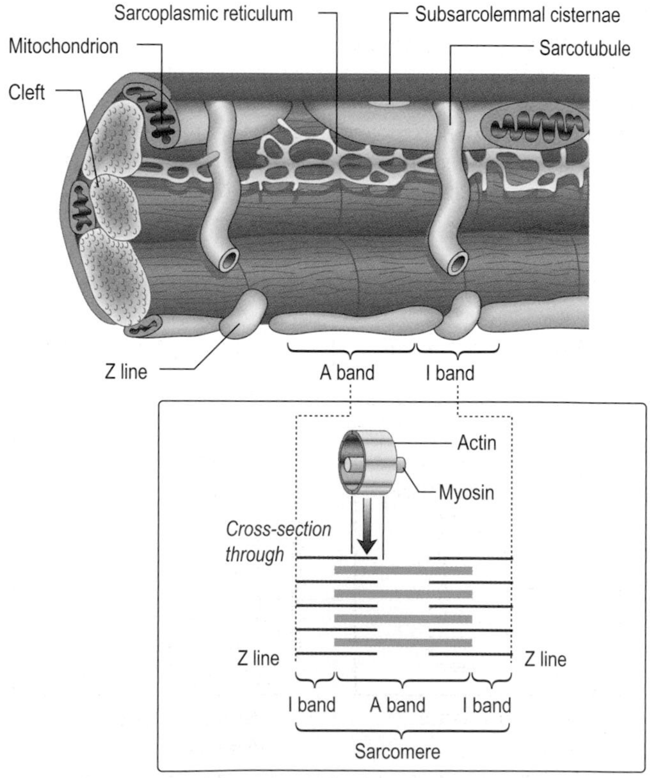

Figure 23.4 The structure of a myofibril within a myocyte. The myofibrils are made up of a series of sarcomeres joined at the Z line.

Two chains of actin molecules form a helical structure, with another molecule, tropomyosin, in the grooves of the actin helix; a further molecule, troponin, is attached to every seven actin molecules. During cardiac contraction, the length of the actin and myosin monofilaments does not change. Rather, the actin filaments slide between the myosin filaments when ATPase splits a high-energy bond of ATP. To supply the ATP, the myocyte (which cannot stop for a rest) has a very high mitochondrial density (35% of the cell volume). As calcium ions bind to troponin C, the activity of troponin I is inhibited, which induces a conformational change in tropomyosin. This event unlocks the active site between actin and myosin, enabling contraction to proceed.

Calcium is made available during the plateau phase of the action potential when calcium ions enter the cell and are mobilized from the sarcoplasmic reticulum (SR) through the ryanodine receptor (RyR2) calcium-release channel (see p. 1039). RyR2 activity is regulated by the protein calstabin 2 and nitric oxide. The force of cardiac muscle contraction ('inotropic state') is thus regulated by the influx of calcium ions into the cell through calcium channels ***(Fig. 23.3)***. T (transient) calcium channels open when the muscle is more depolarized, whereas L (long-lasting) calcium channels require less depolarization. The extent to which the sarcomere can shorten determines the stroke volume of the ventricle. It is maximally shortened in response to powerful inotropic drugs or severe exercise.

Starling's law of the heart

The contractile function of an isolated strip of cardiac tissue can be described by the relationship between the velocity of muscle contraction, the load that is moved by the contracting muscle, and the extent to which the muscle is stretched before contracting. As with all other types of muscle, the velocity of contraction of myocardial tissue is reduced by increasing the load against which the tissue must contract. However, in the non-failing heart, pre-stretching of cardiac muscle improves the relationship between the force and velocity of contraction ***(Fig. 23.5)***.

This phenomenon was described in the intact heart as an increase of stroke volume (ventricular performance) with an enlargement of the diastolic volume (preload), and is known as 'Starling's law of the heart' or the 'Frank–Starling relationship'. It has been transcribed into more clinically relevant indices. Thus, stroke work (aortic pressure × stroke volume) is increased as ventricular end-diastolic volume is raised. Alternatively, within certain limits, cardiac output rises as pulmonary capillary wedge pressure increases. This clinical relationship is described by the ventricular function curve ***(Fig. 23.5)***, which also shows the effect of sympathetic stimulation.

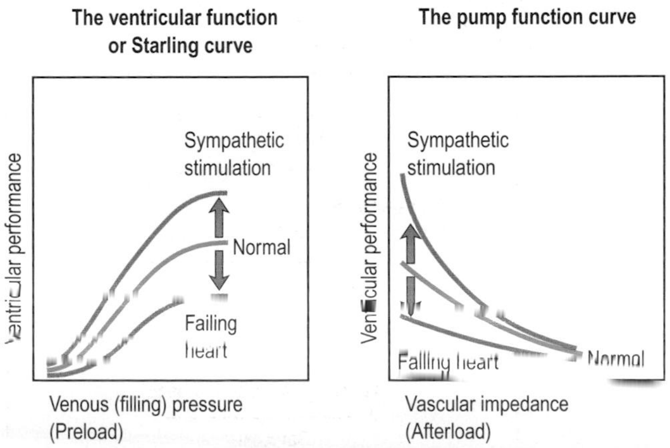

Figure 23.5 The Frank–Starling mechanism. The effect on ventricular contraction of alteration in filling pressures and outflow impedance in the normal, failing and sympathetically stimulated ventricle is shown.

Nerve supply of the myocardium

Adrenergic nerves supply atrial and ventricular muscle fibres, as well as the conduction system. Beta$_1$-receptors predominate in the heart with both adrenaline (epinephrine) and noradrenaline (norepinephrine) having positive inotropic and chronotropic effects. Cholinergic nerves from the vagus supply mainly the SA and AV nodes via M_2 muscarinic receptors. The ventricular myocardium is sparsely innervated by the vagus. Under basal conditions, vagal inhibitory effects predominate over the sympathetic excitatory effects, resulting in a slow heart rate.

Adrenergic stimulation and cellular signalling

Beta$_1$-adrenergic stimulation enhances Ca^{2+} flux in the myocyte and thereby strengthens the force of contraction (see ***Fig. 23.3***). Binding of catecholamines, such as noradrenaline, to the myocyte β_1-adrenergic receptor stimulates membrane-bound adenylate kinases. These enzymes enhance production of cyclic adenosine monophosphate (cAMP), which activates intracellular protein kinases; these, in turn, phosphorylate cellular proteins, including L-type calcium channels within the cell membrane. Beta$_1$-adrenergic stimulation of the myocyte also enhances myocyte relaxation.

The return of calcium from the cytosol to the SR is regulated by phospholamban (PL), a low-molecular-weight protein in the SR membrane. In its dephosphorylated state, PL inhibits Ca^{2+} uptake by the SR ATPase pump (see ***Fig. 23.3***). However, β_1-adrenergic activation of protein kinase phosphorylates PL and blunts its inhibitory effect. The subsequently greater uptake of Ca^{2+} ions by the SR hastens Ca^{2+} removal from the cytosol and promotes myocyte relaxation.

The increased cAMP activity also results in phosphorylation of troponin I, an action that inhibits actin–myosin interaction and further enhances myocyte relaxation.

The cardiac cycle

The cardiac cycle ***(Fig. 23.6)*** consists of precisely timed rhythmic electrical and mechanical events that propel blood into the systemic and pulmonary circulations. The first event in the cardiac cycle is atrial depolarization (a P wave on the surface electrocardiogram (ECG)), followed by right atrial and then left atrial contraction. Ventricular activation (the QRS complex on the ECG) follows after a short interval (the PR interval). Left ventricular contraction starts and, shortly thereafter, right ventricular contraction begins. The increased ventricular pressures exceed the atrial pressures, and close first the mitral and then the tricuspid valves.

Until the aortic and pulmonary valves open, the ventricles contract with no change of volume (isovolumetric contraction). When ventricular pressures rise above the aortic and pulmonary artery pressures, the pulmonary valve and then the aortic valve open and ventricular ejection occurs. As the ventricles begin to relax, their pressures fall below the aortic and pulmonary arterial pressures, and aortic valve closure is followed by pulmonary valve closure. Isovolumetric relaxation then occurs. After the ventricular pressures have fallen below the right atrial and left atrial pressures, the tricuspid and mitral valves open. The cardiac cycle can be depicted graphically as the relationship between the pressure and volume of the ventricle. This is shown in ***Figure 23.7***, which illustrates the changing pressure–volume relationships in response to increased contractility and to exercise.

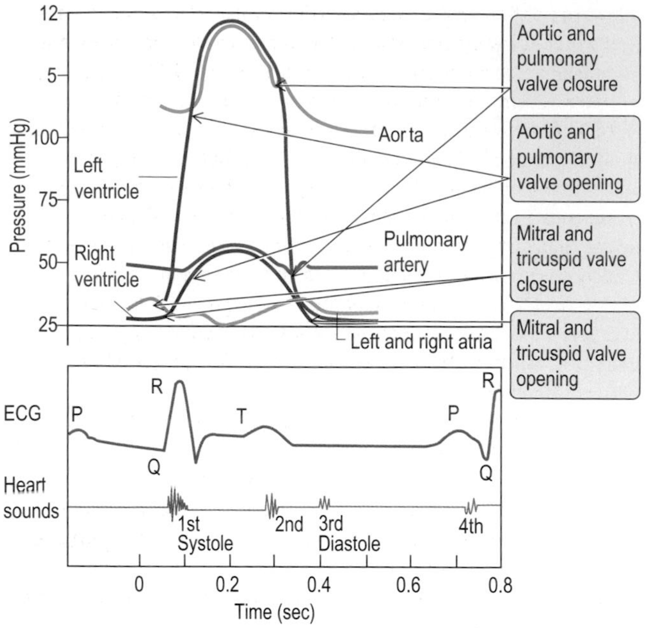

Figure 23.6 **The cardiac cycle.**

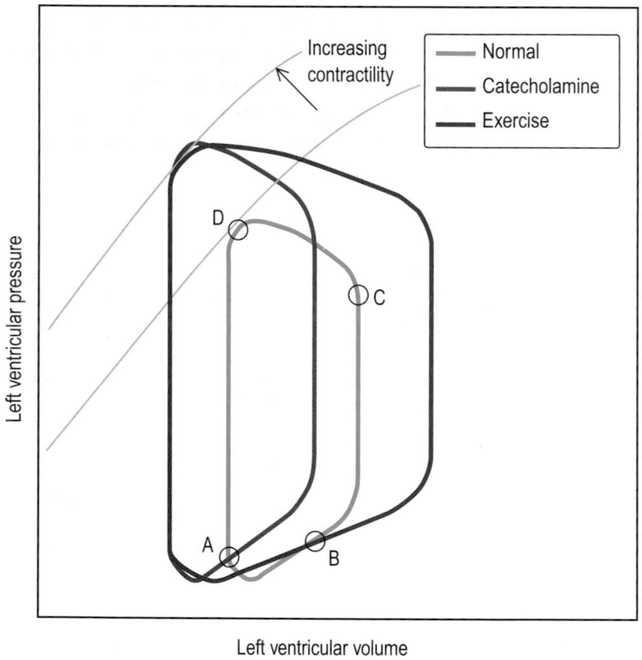

Figure 23.7 **Pressure–volume loop.** AB, diastole: ventricular filling; BC systole: isovolumetric ventricular contraction; CD, systole: ventricular emptying; DA, diastole: isovolumetric ventricular relaxation.

The coronary circulation

The coronary arterial system *(Fig. 23.8)* consists of the right and left coronary arteries. These arteries branch from the aorta, arising immediately above two cusps of the aortic valve. The right and left coronary arteries are unique in that they fill during diastole, when

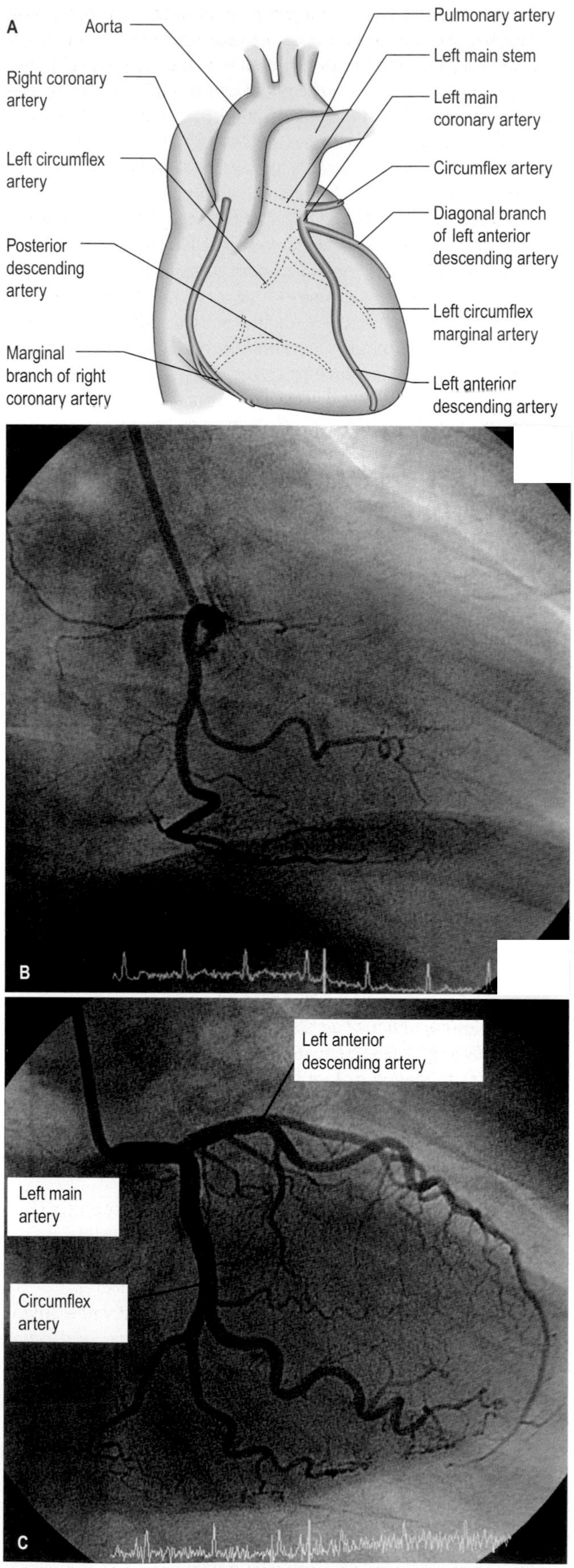

Figure 23.8 **The coronary circulation. A.** The normal coronary arterial anatomy. **B.** Angiogram of the dominant right coronary system. **C.** Angiogram of the left coronary system from the same patient (right anterior oblique projection).

not occluded by valve cusps and when not squeezed by myocardial contraction. The right coronary artery arises from the right coronary sinus and courses through the right side of the AV groove, giving off vessels that supply the right atrium and the right ventricle. The vessel usually continues as the posterior descending coronary artery, which runs in the posterior interventricular groove and supplies the posterior part of the interventricular septum and the posterior left ventricular wall.

Within 2.5 cm of its origin from the left coronary sinus, the left main coronary divides into the left anterior descending artery and the circumflex artery. The left anterior descending artery runs in the anterior interventricular groove and supplies the anterior septum and the anterior left ventricular wall. The left circumflex artery travels along the left AV groove and gives off branches to the left atrium and the left ventricle (marginal branches).

The sinus node and the AV node are supplied by the right coronary artery in about 60% and 90% of people, respectively. Therefore, disease in this artery may cause sinus bradycardia and AV nodal block. The majority of the left ventricle is supplied by the left coronary artery and disease in this vessel can cause significant myocardial dysfunction.

Some blood from the capillary beds in the wall of the heart drains directly into the cavities of the heart via tiny veins, but the majority returns by veins that accompany the arteries, to empty into the right atrium via the coronary sinus. An extensive lymphatic system drains into vessels that travel along the coronary vessels and then into the thoracic duct.

Blood vessel control and functions of the vascular endothelium

In functional terms, the tunica intima with the vascular endothelium and the smooth-muscle-cell-containing tunica media are the main constituents of blood vessels. These two structures are closely interlinked by a variety of mechanisms to regulate vascular tone. The central control of blood vessels is achieved via the neuroendocrine system. Sympathetic vasoconstrictor and parasympathetic vasodilator nerves regulate vascular tone in response to daily activity. Where neural control is impaired or in various pathological states, such as haemorrhage, endocrine control of blood vessels, mediated through adrenaline (epinephrine), angiotensin and vasopressin, takes over.

At a local level, tissue perfusion is maintained automatically and by the effect of various factors synthesized and/or released in the immediate vicinity. In the face of fluctuating arterial pressures, blood vessels vasoconstrict independently of nervous input when blood pressure drops and vice versa. This process of ***autoregulation*** is a consequence of:

- the ***Bayliss myogenic*** response – the ability of blood vessels to constrict when distended
- the ***vasodilator washout*** effect – the vasoconstriction triggered by a decrease in the concentration of tissue metabolites.

The vascular endothelium is a cardiovascular endocrine organ, which occupies a strategic interface between blood and other tissues. It produces various compounds (e.g. nitric oxide (NO), prostacyclin (PGI_2), endothelin, endothelial-derived hyperpolarizing factor (EDHF), adhesion molecules, vascular endothelial growth factor (VEGF)) and has enzymes located on the surface, controlling the levels of circulating compounds such as angiotensin, bradykinin and serotonin. It has many regulatory roles:

Vasomotor control

- ***Nitric oxide*** is a diffusible gas with a very short half-life; it is produced in endothelial cells from the amino acid L-arginine via the action of the enzyme NO synthase (NOS), which is controlled by cytoplasmic calcium/calmodulin ***(Fig. 23.9)***. It is produced in response to various stimuli ***(Box 23.1)***, triggering vascular smooth muscle relaxation through activation of guanylate cyclase; this leads to an increase in the intracellular levels of cyclic 3,5-guanine monophosphate (cGMP). Its cardiovascular effects protect against atherosclerosis, high blood pressure, heart failure and thrombosis. NO is also the neurotransmitter in various 'nitrergic' nerves in the central and peripheral nervous systems and may play a role in the central regulation of vascular tone. The class of drugs used to treat erectile dysfunction, the phosphodiesterase (PDE_5) inhibitors, prevent the breakdown of cGMP and promote vasodilatation.
- ***PGI_2*** is synergistic to NO and also plays a role in the local regulation of vasomotor tone.
- ***Endothelin*** is a 21-amino-acid peptide that counteracts the effects of NO. Its production is inhibited by shear stress – that is, the stress exerted on the vessel wall by the flowing blood – and it causes profound vasoconstriction and vascular smooth muscle hypertrophy. It is thought to play a role in the genesis of hypertension and atheroma.
- ***Angiotensin-converting enzyme***, located on the endothelial cell membrane, converts circulating angiotensin I (synthesized by the action of renin on angiotensinogen) to angiotensin II, which has vasoconstrictor properties and leads to aldosterone release (see ***Fig. 20.6***). Aldosterone promotes sodium absorption from the kidney and, together with the angiotensin-induced vasoconstriction, provides haemodynamic stability.

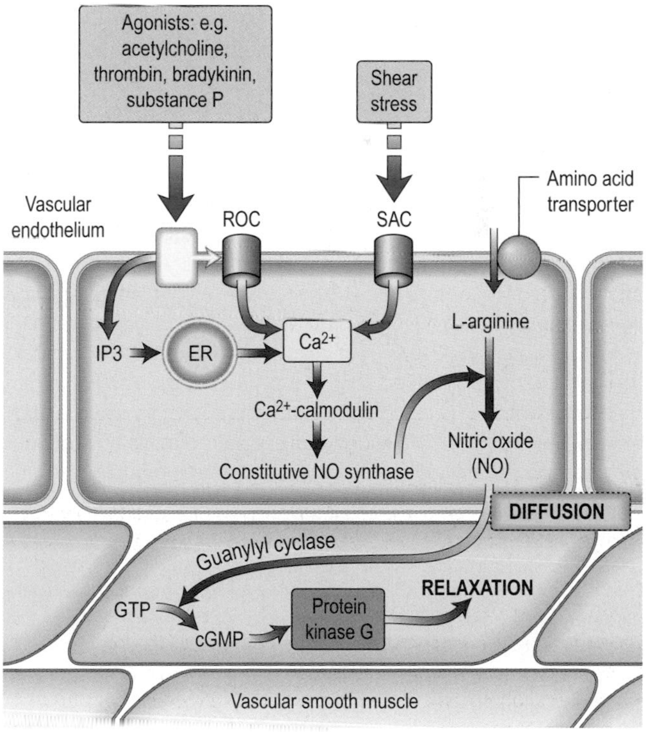

Figure 23.9 The stimulus for production and function of nitric oxide (NO). Various stimuli lead to the production of NO via cytoplasmic calcium/calmodulin. NO triggers smooth muscle relaxation via the activation of guanylyl cyclase. cGMP, cyclic guanine monophosphate; ER, endoplasmic reticulum; GTP, guanine triphosphate; IP3, inositol triphosphate; ROC, receptor-operated Ca^{2+} channel; SAC, stretch-activated Ca^{2+} channel.

Box 23.1 Some of the products and functions of the vascular endothelium

Endothelial product	Function(s)	Stimulus
Nitric oxide	Vasodilatation Inhibition of platelet aggregation Inhibition of transcription of adhesion molecules Inhibition of vascular smooth muscle proliferation	Shear stress, e.g. induced by exercise Agonists: thrombin, acetylcholine, endothelin, bradykinin, serotonin, substance P Inflammation/endotoxin shock
Prostacyclin (PGI_2)	Vasodilation Inhibition of platelet aggregation	Agonist: thrombin Inflammation
Prostanoids	Vasoconstriction	Hypoxia
Endothelin	Vasoconstriction	Thrombin, angiotensin II, vasopressin Hypoxia *Note*: Inhibited by shear stress
Endothelial-derived hyperpolarizing factor	Vasodilatation	Agonists: bradykinin, acetylcholine
Angiotensin-converting enzyme	Vasoconstriction	Expressed naturally
von Willebrand factor	Promotion of platelet aggregation Stabilization of factor VIII	Agonists: thrombin, adrenaline (epinephrine)
Adhesion molecules		
P, L, E selectins ICAM, VCAM, PECAM	Margination of white blood cells Binding and diapedesis of WBCs into vessel wall	Inflammatory mediators: histamine, thrombin, TNF, IL-6
Vascular endothelial growth factor (VEGF)	Angiogenesis Vasodilatation Increase in vascular permeability	Pregnancy Hypoxia Inflammation, e.g. rheumatoid arthritis Trauma Tumours

ICAM, intracellular adhesion molecule; IL, interleukin; PECAM, platelet/endothelial cell adhesion molecule; TNF, tumour necrosis factor; VCAM, vascular cell adhesion molecule; WBC, white blood cell.

- ***Other factors*** that influence vasomotor tone include histamine (released by mast cells), bradykinin (synthesized from kininogen by the action of coagulation factor XIIa) and serotonin (released by platelets).

Anti- and prothrombotic mechanisms

PGI_2, produced from arachidonic acid in the endothelial cell membrane by the action of the enzyme cyclo-oxygenase, inhibits platelet aggregation. Low-dose aspirin prevents activation of the cyclo-oxygenase pathway in platelets but only to a degree that does not affect PGI_2 synthesis, unlike higher doses. Other antithrombotic agents, such as clopidogrel (an adenosine diphosphate (ADP) receptor antagonist) and glycoprotein IIb/IIIa inhibitors, achieve their effects by acting directly on platelet receptors. The antithrombotic effect of PGI_2 is aided by NO, affecting platelets via activation of guanylate cyclase. The endothelial cell membrane also produces other anticoagulant molecules, such as thrombomodulin, heparin sulphate and various fibrinolytic factors. Clinically used, fast-acting heparin preparations are identical to this naturally occurring molecule.

In addition to their ability to prevent clotting, endothelial cells also aid thrombosis. They are responsible for the production of von Willebrand factor through a unique organelle called the Weibel–Palade body, which not only acts as a carrier for factor VIII but also promotes platelet adhesion by binding to exposed collagen (see p. 565).

Modulation of immune responses

In response to various inflammatory mediators, the vascular endothelium expresses various so-called 'adhesion molecules', which promote leucocyte attraction, adhesion and infiltration into the blood vessel wall (see p. 133).

Regulation of vascular cell growth

The endothelial cells are also responsible for the development of new blood vessels ('angiogenesis') in the placenta, wound healing, tissue repair and tumour growth. This process is facilitated by VEGF.

Further reading

Levick JR. *An Introduction to Cardiovascular Physiology*, 5th edn. London: Arnold; 2009.

CLINICAL APPROACH TO THE PATIENT WITH HEART DISEASE

Clinical features of heart disease

The following symptoms occur with heart disease:

- chest pain
- dyspnoea (breathlessness)
- palpitations
- syncope
- fatigue
- peripheral oedema.

The severity of cardiac symptoms or fatigue is classified according to the New York Heart Association (NYHA) grading of cardiac status (see ***Box 23.21***). The differential diagnosis of chest pain is given in ***Box 23.2***.

Central chest pain

This is the most common symptom associated with heart disease. The pain of angina pectoris and myocardial infarction is due to myocardial hypoxia.

Box 23.2 Differential diagnosis of chest pain

Central

Cardiac
- Ischaemic heart disease (infarction or angina)
- Coronary artery spasm
- Pericarditis/myocarditis
- Mitral valve prolapse
- Aortic aneurysm/dissection

Non-cardiac
- Pulmonary embolism
- Oesophageal disease (see ***Box 13.11***)
- Mediastinitis
- Costochondritis (Tietze disease)
- Trauma (soft tissue, rib)

Lateral/peripheral

Pulmonary
- Infarction
- Pneumonia
- Pneumothorax
- Lung cancer
- Mesothelioma

Non-pulmonary
- Bornholm disease (epidemic myalgia)
- Herpes zoster
- Trauma (ribs/muscular)

Types of pain include:
- retrosternal heavy or gripping sensation with radiation to the left arm or neck that is provoked by exertion and eased with rest or nitrates – ***angina*** (see pp. 993–997)
- similar pain at rest – ***acute coronary syndrome*** (see pp. 997–1006)
- severe, tearing chest pain radiating through to the back – ***aortic dissection*** (see pp. 1053–1054)
- sharp, central chest pain that is worse with movement or respiration but relieved with sitting forward – ***pericarditis pain*** (see pp. 1043–1044)
- sharp, stabbing, left sub-mammary pain associated with anxiety – ***da Costa syndrome***.

Dyspnoea

Left ventricular failure causes dyspnoea due to oedema of the pulmonary interstitium and alveoli. This makes the lungs stiff (less compliant), thus increasing the respiratory effort required to ventilate them. ***Tachypnoea*** (increased respiratory rate) is often present owing to stimulation of pulmonary stretch receptors.

Orthopnoea refers to breathlessness on lying flat. Blood is redistributed from the legs to the torso, leading to an increase in central and pulmonary blood volume. The patient uses an increasing number of pillows to sleep.

Paroxysmal nocturnal dyspnoea (PND) is when a patient is woken from sleep fighting for breath. It is caused by the same mechanisms as orthopnoea. However, as sensory awareness is reduced whilst asleep, the pulmonary oedema can become quite severe before the patient is awoken.

Hyperventilation with alternating episodes of apnoea (***Cheyne–Stokes respiration***) occurs in severe heart failure.

If hypopnoea occurs rather than apnoea, the phenomenon is termed 'periodic breathing', but the two variations are known together as ***central sleep apnoea syndrome (CSAS)***. This occurs due to malfunctioning of the respiratory centre in the brain, caused by poor cardiac output with concurrent cerebrovascular disease. The symptoms of CSAS, such as daytime somnolence and fatigue, are similar to those of obstructive sleep apnoea syndrome (OSAS; see pp. 1085–1086) and there is considerable overlap with the symptoms of heart failure. CSAS is believed to lead to myocardial hypertrophy and fibrosis, deterioration in cardiac function and complex arrhythmias, including non-sustained ventricular tachycardia, hypertension and stroke. Patients with CSAS have a worse prognosis than similar patients without CSAS.

Box 23.3 Cardiovascular causes of syncope

Vascular
- Neurocardiogenic (vasovagal)
- Postural hypotension
- Postprandial hypotension
- Micturition syncope
- Carotid sinus syncope

Obstructive
- Aortic stenosis
- Hypertrophic cardiomyopathy
- Pulmonary stenosis
- Tetralogy of Fallot
- Pulmonary hypertension/ embolism
- Atrial myxoma/thrombus
- Defective prosthetic valve

Arrhythmias
- Rapid tachycardias
- Profound bradycardias (Stokes–Adams)
- Significant pauses (in rhythm)
- Artificial pacemaker failure

Palpitations

These represent an increased awareness of the normal heart beat or the sensation of slow, rapid or irregular heart rhythms. The most common arrhythmias felt as palpitations are premature ectopic beats and paroxysmal tachycardias. A useful trick is to ask patients to tap out the rate and rhythm of their palpitations, as the different arrhythmias have different characteristics:
- ***Premature beats (ectopics)*** are felt by the patient as a pause followed by a forceful beat. This is because premature beats are usually followed by a pause before the next normal beat, as the heart resets itself. The next beat is more forceful, as the heart has had a longer diastolic period and therefore is filled with more blood before this beat.
- ***Paroxysmal tachycardias*** (see pp. 963–964) are felt as a sudden, racing heart beat.
- ***Bradycardias*** (see p. 964) may be appreciated as slow, regular, heavy or forceful beats. Most often, however, they are simply not sensed. All palpitations can be graded by the NYHA cardiac status (see ***Box 23.21***).

Syncope

Syncope is a transient loss of consciousness due to inadequate cerebral blood flow. The cardiovascular causes are listed in ***Box 23.3***.

Vascular

- ***A vasovagal attack*** is a simple faint and is the most common cause of syncope. The mechanism begins with peripheral vasodilatation and venous pooling of blood, leading to a reduction in the amount of blood returned to the heart. The near-empty heart responds by contracting vigorously, which, in turn, stimulates mechanoreceptors (stretch receptors) in the inferoposterior wall of the left ventricle. These, in turn, trigger reflexes via the central nervous system, which act to reduce ventricular stretch (i.e. further vasodilatation and sometimes profound bradycardia), but this causes a drop in blood pressure and therefore syncope. These episodes are usually associated with a prodrome of dizziness, nausea, sweating, tinnitus, yawning and a sinking feeling. Recovery occurs within a few seconds, especially if the patient lies down.
- ***Postural (orthostatic) hypotension*** is a drop in systolic blood pressure of ≥20 mmHg or more on standing from a sitting or lying position. Usually, reflex vasoconstriction prevents a drop in pressure, but if this is absent or the patient is fluid-depleted or on vasodilating or diuretic drugs, hypotension occurs.

- ***Postprandial hypotension*** is a drop in systolic blood pressure of ≥20 mmHg, or the systolic blood pressure drops from >100 mmHg to <90 mmHg within 2 hours of eating. The mechanism is unknown but may be due to pooling of blood in the splanchnic vessels. In normal subjects, this elicits a homeostatic response via activation of baroreceptors and the sympathetic system, peripheral vasoconstriction and an increase in cardiac output.
- ***Micturition syncope*** refers to loss of consciousness whilst passing urine.
- ***Carotid sinus syncope*** occurs when there is an exaggerated vagal response to carotid sinus stimulation, provoked by wearing a tight collar, looking upwards or turning the head.

Obstructive

The obstructive cardiac causes listed in ***Box 23.3*** all lead to syncope due to restriction of blood flow from the heart into the rest of the circulation, or between the different chambers of the heart.

Arrhythmias

Stokes–Adams attacks (see p. 966) are a sudden loss of consciousness unrelated to posture and caused by intermittent high-grade AV block, profound bradycardia or ventricular standstill. The patient falls to the ground without warning, and is pale and deeply unconscious. The pulse is usually very slow or absent. After a few seconds, the patient flushes brightly and recovers consciousness as the pulse quickens. Often there are no sequelae, but patients may injure themselves during falls. Occasionally, a generalized convulsion may occur if the period of cerebral hypoxia is prolonged, leading to a misdiagnosis of epilepsy.

Fatigue

Fatigue may be a symptom of inadequate systemic perfusion in heart failure. It is due to poor sleep; is a direct side-effect of medication, particularly beta-blockers; is due to electrolyte imbalance caused by diuretic therapy; or is a systemic manifestation of infection, such as endocarditis.

Peripheral oedema

Heart failure results in salt and water retention due to renal underperfusion and consequent activation of the renin–angiotensin–aldosterone system (see pp. 727–728). This leads to dependent pitting oedema.

Further reading

Freeman R. Neurogenic orthostatic hypotension. *N Engl J Med* 2008; 358:615–624.

Moya A, Sutton R, Ammirati F et al. Task Force for the Diagnosis and Management of Syncope; European Society of Cardiology (ESC); European Heart Rhythm Association (EHRA); Heart Failure Association (HFA); Heart Rhythm Society (HRS). Guidelines for the diagnosis and management of syncope (version 2009). *Eur Heart J* 2009; 30:2631–2671.

National Institute for Health and Care Excellence. *NICE Clinical Guideline 109: Transient Loss of Consciousness ('Blackouts') Management in Adults and Young People*. NICE 2010; https://www.nice.org.uk/guidance/cg109.

Examination of the cardiovascular system

General examination

General features of the patient's wellbeing should be noted, as well as the presence of conjunctival pallor, obesity, jaundice and cachexia.

- ***Clubbing*** (see p. 1067) is seen in congenital cyanotic heart disease, particularly Fallot's tetralogy, and also in 10% of patients with sub-acute infective endocarditis.
- ***Splinter haemorrhages*** are small, sub-ungual linear haemorrhages that are frequently due to trauma, but also seen in infective endocarditis.
- ***Cyanosis*** is a dusky blue discoloration of the skin (particularly at the extremities) or of the mucous membranes when the capillary oxygen saturation is <85%. ***Central cyanosis*** (see p. 1067) is seen with shunting of deoxygenated venous blood into the systemic circulation, as in the presence of a right-to-left heart shunt. ***Peripheral cyanosis*** is seen in the hands and feet, which are cold. It occurs in conditions associated with peripheral vasoconstriction and stasis of blood in the extremities, leading to increased peripheral oxygen extraction. Such conditions include congestive heart failure, circulatory shock, exposure to cold temperatures and abnormalities of the peripheral circulation, such as Raynaud's (see p. 1054).

The arterial pulse

The first pulse to be examined is the right radial pulse. A delayed femoral pulsation occurs because of a proximal stenosis, particularly of the aorta (coarctation).

Rate

The pulse rate should be between 60 and 80 beats per minute (b.p.m.) when an adult patient is lying quietly in bed.

Rhythm

The rhythm is regular, except for a slight quickening in early inspiration and a slowing in expiration (sinus arrhythmia).

- ***Premature beats*** occur as occasional or repeated irregularities superimposed on a regular pulse rhythm. Similarly, intermittent heart block is revealed by occasional beats dropped from an otherwise regular rhythm.
- ***Atrial fibrillation*** produces an 'irregularly irregular' pulse. This irregular pattern persists when the pulse quickens in response to exercise, in contrast to pulse irregularity due to ectopic beats, which usually disappears on exercise.

Character

- ***Carotid pulsations*** are not normally apparent on inspection of the neck but may be visible (Corrigan's sign) in conditions associated with a large-volume pulse, including high-output states (such as thyrotoxicosis, anaemia or fever), and in aortic regurgitation.
- ***A 'collapsing' or 'water hammer' pulse (Fig. 23.10)*** is a large-volume pulse characterized by a short duration with a brisk rise and fall. This is best appreciated by palpating the radial artery with the palmar aspect of four fingers while elevating the patient's arm above the level of the heart. A collapsing pulse is characteristic of aortic valvular regurgitation or a persistent ductus arteriosus.
- ***A small-volume pulse*** is seen in cardiac failure, shock, and obstructive valvular or vascular disease. It may also be present during tachyarrhythmias.
- ***A plateau pulse (Fig. 23.10)*** is small in volume and slow in rising to a peak; it is due to aortic stenosis.
- ***An alternating pulse (pulsus alternans) (Fig. 23.10)*** is characterized by regular alternate beats that are weak and strong. It is a feature of severe myocardial failure and is due to the prolonged recovery time of damaged myocardium; it indicates a very poor prognosis. It is easily noticed when taking the blood pressure because the systolic pressure may vary from beat to beat by as much as 50 mmHg.

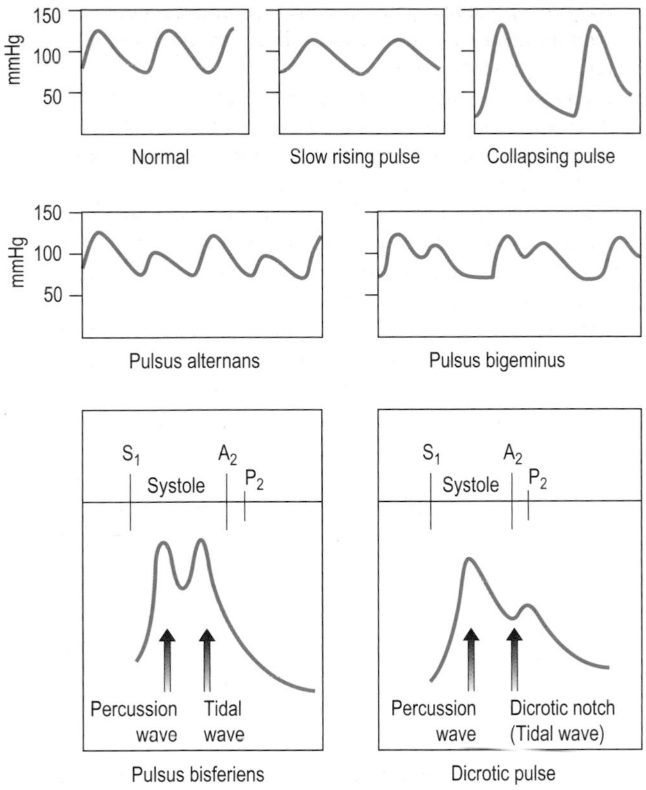

Figure 23.10 Arterial waveforms. A_2, aortic component of the second heart sound; P_2, pulmonary component of the second heart sound; S_1, first heart sound.

- ***A bigeminal pulse* (*pulsus bigeminus*) *(Fig. 23.10)*** is caused by a premature ectopic beat following every sinus beat. The rhythm is not regular because every weak pulse is premature.
- ***Pulsus bisferiens (Fig. 23.10)*** is found in hypertrophic cardiomyopathy and in mixed aortic valve disease (regurgitation combined with stenosis). The first systolic wave is the 'percussion' wave, produced by the transmission of the left ventricular pressure in early systole. The second peak is the 'tidal' wave, caused by recoil of the vascular bed. This normally happens in diastole (the dicrotic wave), but when the left ventricle empties slowly or is obstructed and cannot empty completely, the tidal wave occurs in late systole. The result is a palpable double pulse.
- ***A dicrotic pulse (Fig. 23.10)*** results from an accentuated dicrotic wave. It occurs in sepsis and hypovolaemic shock, and after aortic valve replacement.
- ***Paradoxical pulse*** is a misnomer, as it is actually an exaggeration of the normal pattern. In normal subjects, the systolic pressure and the pulse pressure (the difference between the systolic and diastolic blood pressures) fall during inspiration. The normal fall of systolic pressure is <10 mmHg, and this can be measured using a sphygmomanometer. It is due to increased pulmonary intravascular volume during inspiration. In severe airflow limitation (especially severe asthma), there is an increased negative intrathoracic pressure on inspiration, which enhances the normal fall in blood pressure. In patients with cardiac tamponade, the fluid in the pericardium increases the intrapericardial pressure, thereby impeding diastolic filling of the heart. The normal inspiratory increase in venous return to the right ventricle is at the expense of the left ventricle, as both ventricles are confined by the accumulated pericardial fluid within the pericardial space. Paradox can occur via a similar mechanism in constrictive pericarditis but is less common.

Box 23.4 Taking the blood pressure

Use a properly calibrated machine.

1. Take the blood pressure in the (right) arm with the patient relaxed and comfortable.
2. Wrap the sphygmomanometer cuff around the upper arm and place the inflation bag over the brachial artery.
3. Inflate the cuff until the pressure exceeds the arterial pressure – when the radial pulse is no longer palpable.
4. Position the diaphragm of the stethoscope over the brachial artery just below the cuff.
5. Slowly reduce the cuff pressure until sounds (Korotkoff sounds) can be heard (***phase 1***). This is the systolic pressure.
6. Allow the pressure to fall further until the Korotkoff sounds suddenly become muffled (***phase 4***).
7. Allow the pressure to fall still further until the sounds disappear (***phase 5***).
8. The diastolic pressure is usually taken as ***phase 5*** because this phase is more reproducible and nearer to the intravascular diastolic pressure. The Korotkoff sounds may disappear (***phase 2***) and reappear (***phase 3***) between the systolic and diastolic pressures. Do not mistake ***phase 2*** for the diastolic pressure or ***phase 3*** for the systolic pressure.

Box 23.5 Measurement of jugular venous pressure (JVP)

- The patient is positioned at about 45° to the horizontal (between 30° and 60°), wherever the top of the venous pulsation can be seen in a good light.
- The JVP is measured as the vertical distance between the manubriosternal angle and the top of the venous column.
- The normal JVP is usually <3 cmH_2O, which is equivalent to a right atrial pressure of 8 cmH_2O when measured with reference to a point midway between the anterior and posterior surfaces of the chest.
- The venous pulsations are not usually palpable (except for the forceful venous distension associated with tricuspid regurgitation).
- Compression of the right upper abdomen causes a temporary increase in venous pressure and makes the jugular venous pulse more visible (hepatojugular reflux).

Blood pressure

The peak systemic arterial blood pressure is produced by transmission of left ventricular systolic pressure. Vascular tone and an intact aortic valve maintain the diastolic blood pressure. Instructions for taking the blood pressure are outlined in ***Box 23.4***.

Jugular venous pressure

There are no valves between the internal jugular vein and the right atrium. Observation of the column of blood in the internal jugular system is therefore a good measure of right atrial pressure. The external jugular cannot be relied upon because of its valves and because it may be obstructed by the fascial and muscular layers through which it passes; it can only be used if typical venous pulsation is seen, indicating no obstruction to flow.

Measurement of jugular venous pressure

See ***Box 23.5***.

Elevation of the jugular venous pressure (JVP) occurs in ***heart failure***. An elevated JVP also occurs in constrictive pericarditis and cardiac tamponade (increases in inspiration – ***Kussmaul's sign***), renal disease with salt and water retention, over-transfusion or excessive infusion of fluids, congestive cardiac failure and superior vena cava obstruction.

A reduced JVP occurs in hypovolaemia.

The jugular venous pressure wave

This consists of three peaks and two troughs ***(Fig. 23.11)***. The peaks are described as **a**, **c** and ***v*** waves and the troughs are known as ***x*** and ***y*** descents:

- ***The a wave*** is produced by atrial systole and is increased with right ventricular hypertrophy secondary to pulmonary hypertension or pulmonary stenosis. Giant cannon waves occur in complete heart block and ventricular tachycardia.
- ***The x descent*** occurs when atrial contraction finishes.
- ***The c wave*** occurs during the ***x*** descent and is due to transmission of right ventricular systolic pressure before the tricuspid valve closes.
- ***The v wave*** occurs with venous return filling the right atrium. Giant ***v*** waves occur in tricuspid regurgitation.
- ***The y descent*** follows the ***v*** wave when the tricuspid valve opens. A steep ***y*** descent is seen in constrictive pericarditis and tricuspid incompetence.

The precordium

- With the patient at 45°, the cardiac apex is located in the fifth intercostal space mid-clavicular line. Left ventricular dilatation will displace the apex downwards and laterally. It may be impalpable in patients with emphysema, obesity, or pericardial or pleural effusions.
- ***A tapping apex*** is a palpable first sound and occurs in mitral stenosis.
- ***A vigorous apex*** may be present in diseases with volume overload, e.g. aortic regurgitation.
- ***A heaving apex*** may occur with left ventricular hypertrophy – aortic stenosis, systemic hypertension and hypertrophic cardiomyopathy.
- ***A double pulsation*** may occur in hypertrophic cardiomyopathy.
- ***A sustained left parasternal heave*** occurs with right ventricular hypertrophy or left atrial enlargement.
- ***A palpable thrill*** may be felt overlying an abnormal cardiac valve, e.g. systolic thrill with aortic stenosis.

Auscultation

The ***bell*** of the stethoscope is used for low-pitched sounds (heart sounds and mid-diastolic murmur in mitral stenosis). The ***diaphragm*** is used for high-pitched sounds (systolic murmurs, aortic regurgitation, ejection clicks and opening snaps). The areas of auscultation are shown in ***Figure 23.12***. Left-sided valve murmurs may be more prominent in expiration and right-sided in inspiration. Mitral murmurs may be more audible with the patient reclining to the left.

First heart sound (S1)

This is due to mitral and tricuspid valve closure. A loud S1 occurs in thin people, hyperdynamic circulation, tachycardias and mild to moderate mitral stenosis. A soft S1 occurs in obesity, emphysema, pericardial effusion, severe calcific mitral stenosis, mitral or tricuspid regurgitation, heart failure, shock, bradycardias and first-degree block.

Second heart sound (S2)

This is due to aortic and pulmonary valve closure. Physiological splitting of S2 occurs during inspiration in children and young adults.

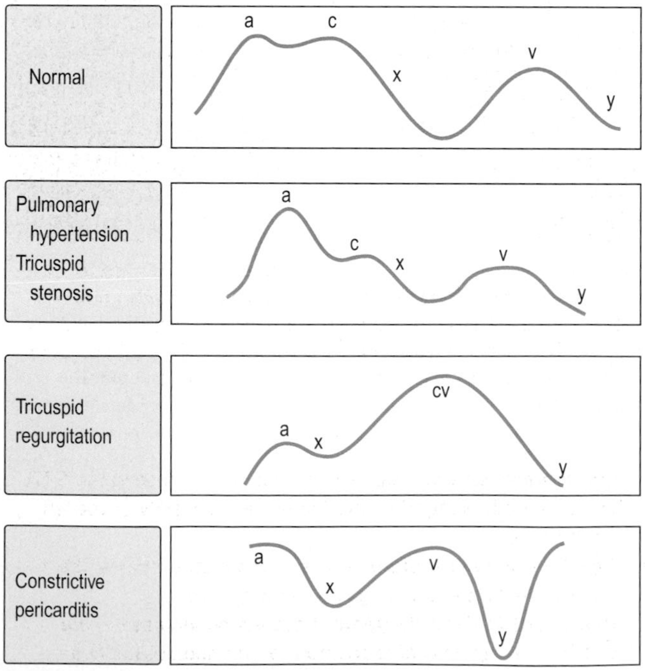

Figure 23.11 **Jugular venous waveforms.**

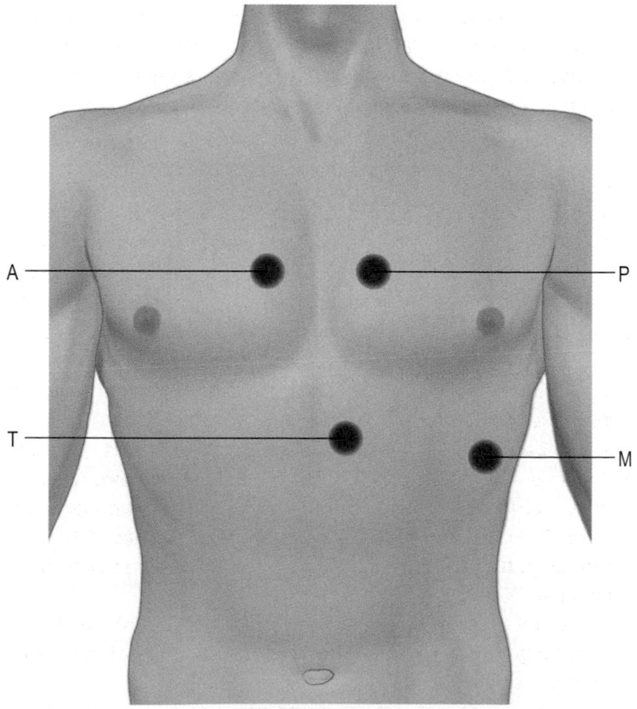

Figure 23.12 **Heart auscultation.** Aortic area second intercostal space (ICS) right sternal edge (**A**). Pulmonary area second ICS left sternal edge (**P**). Mitral area fifth ICS, mid-clavicular line (**M**). Tricuspid area third to fifth ICS, left sternal edge (**T**).

Third and fourth heart sounds

These are pathological:

- ***A third heart sound*** is due to rapid ventricular filling and is present in heart failure.
- ***A fourth heart sound*** occurs in late diastole and is associated with atrial contraction.

Singly or together, they will produce a gallop rhythm.

Heart murmurs

These are due to turbulent blood flow and occur in hyperdynamic states or with abnormal valves. (Listen online on Student Consult.) Innocent or flow murmurs are soft, early systolic, short and non-radiating. They are heard frequently in children and young adults. Heart murmurs can be graded on the following scale:

- 1/6 very faint; not always heard in all positions
- 2/6 quiet but not difficult to hear
- 3/6 moderately loud
- 4/6 loud ± thrills
- 5/6 very loud ± thrills; heard with the stethoscope partly off the chest
- 6/6 ± thrills; heard with the stethoscope completely off the chest.

The individual murmurs are discussed under valve disease (see pp. 1006–1017).

CARDIAC INVESTIGATIONS

Blood tests

These include routine haematology, urea/creatinine and electrolytes, liver biochemistry, cardiac enzymes, thyroid function and brain natriuretic peptides (BNP).

Chest X-ray

Ideally, this is taken in the postero-anterior (PA) direction at maximum inspiration with the heart close to the X-ray film to minimize magnification with respect to the thorax. A lateral view may give additional information if the PA film is abnormal. The cardiac structures and great vessels that can be seen on these X-rays are indicated in ***Figure 23.13***. An antero-posterior (AP) view is taken only in an emergency.

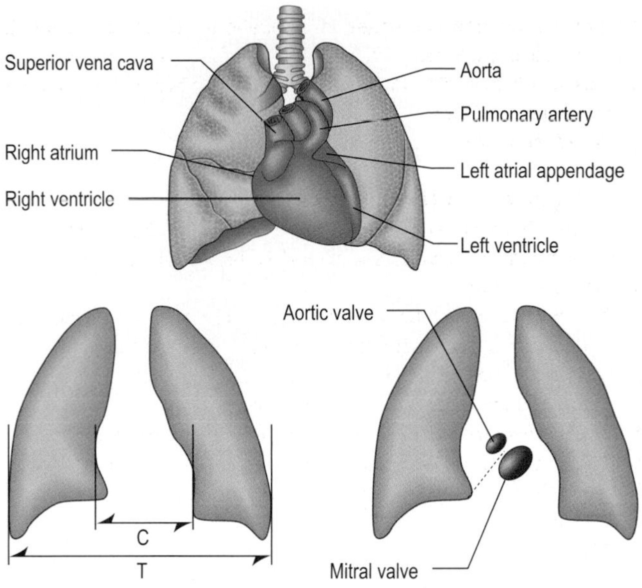

Figure 23.13 The heart silhouette as it is seen on the chest X-ray. Measurements of the cardiothoracic ratio (CTR) and the location of the cardiac valves are also shown. The dotted line is an arbitrary line from the left hilum to the right cardiophrenic angle; a calcified aortic valve is seen above this line. CTR=(C/T)×100%; normal CTR <50%.

Heart size

Heart size can be reliably assessed only from the PA chest film. The maximum transverse diameter of the heart is compared with the maximum transverse diameter of the thorax measured from the inside of the ribs (the cardiothoracic ratio, CTR). The CTR is usually <50%, except in neonates, infants, athletes, and patients with skeletal abnormalities such as scoliosis and funnel chest. A transverse cardiac diameter >15.5 cm is abnormal. Pericardial effusion or cardiac dilatation causes an increase in the ratio.

A ***pericardial effusion*** produces a globular heart (see ***Fig. 23.121***). This enlargement may occur quite suddenly and, unlike in heart failure, there is no associated change in the pulmonary vasculature. The echocardiogram is more specific (see ***Fig. 23.122***).

Certain patterns of specific chamber enlargement may be seen on the chest X-ray:

- ***Left atrial dilatation*** leads to prominence of the left atrial appendage and a straightening or convex bulging of the upper left heart border, a double atrial shadow to the right of the sternum, and splaying of the carina because a large left atrium elevates the left main bronchus ***(Fig. 23.14)***. On a lateral chest X-ray, an enlarged left atrium bulges backwards, impinging on the oesophagus.

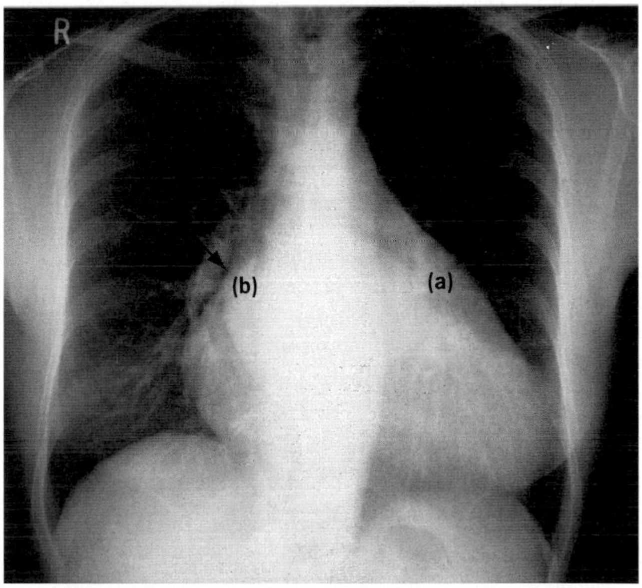

Figure 23.14 A plain postero-anterior chest X-ray of a patient with mixed mitral valve disease. The left atrium (**a**) is markedly enlarged. Note the large bulge on the left heart border (left atrium). The 'double shadow' (border of the right and left atria, (**b**)) is on the right side of the heart. There is cardiac (left ventricular) enlargement due to mitral regurgitation.

- ***Left ventricular enlargement*** causes an increase in the CTR and a smooth elongation and increased convexity of the left heart border.
- ***Right atrial enlargement*** results in the right border of the heart projecting into the right lower lung field.
- ***Right ventricular enlargement*** causes an increase in the CTR and an upward displacement of the apex of the heart because the enlarging right ventricle pushes the left ventricle

leftwards, upwards and eventually backwards. Differentiation of left from right ventricular enlargement may be difficult using the shape of the left heart border alone, but the lateral view shows enlargement anteriorly for the right ventricle and posteriorly for the left ventricle.

- ***Ascending aortic dilatation or enlargement*** is seen as a prominence of the aortic shadow to the right of the mediastinum between the right atrium and superior vena cava.
- ***Dissection of the ascending aorta*** is seen as a widening of the mediastinum on chest X-ray but an ultrasound/magnetic resonance imaging (MRI) should be performed.
- ***Enlargement of the pulmonary artery*** in pulmonary hypertension, pulmonary artery stenosis and left-to-right shunts produces a prominent bulge on the left-hand border of the mediastinum below the aortic knuckle.

Calcification

Calcification in the cardiovascular system occurs because of tissue degeneration. Calcification is visible on a lateral or a penetrated PA film, but is best studied with computed tomography (CT) scanning.

Lung fields

- ***Pulmonary plethora*** results from left-to-right shunts (e.g. atrial or ventricular septal defects). It is seen as a general increase in the vascularity of the lung fields and as an increase in the size of hilar vessels (e.g. in the right lower lobe artery), which normally should not exceed 16 mm diameter.
- ***Pulmonary oligaemia*** is a paucity of vascular markings and a reduction in the width of the arteries. It occurs in situations where there is reduced pulmonary blood flow, such as pulmonary embolism, severe pulmonary stenosis and Fallot's tetralogy.
- ***Pulmonary hypertension*** may result from pulmonary embolism, chronic lung disease or chronic left heart disease, e.g. left ventricular failure or mitral valve disease such as shunts due to a ventricular septal defect or mitral valve stenosis. In addition to the X-ray features of these conditions, the pulmonary arteries are prominent close to the hila but are reduced in size (pruned) in the peripheral lung fields. This pattern is usually symmetrical. Normal pulmonary capillary pressure is 5–14 mmHg at rest. Mild pulmonary capillary hypertension (15–20 mmHg) produces isolated dilatation of the upper zone vessels.
- ***Interstitial oedema*** occurs when the pressure is between 21 and 30 mmHg. This manifests as fluid collections in the interlobar fissures, interlobular septa (Kerley B lines) and pleural spaces. This gives rise to indistinctness of the hilar regions and haziness of the lung fields.
- ***Alveolar oedema*** occurs when the pressure exceeds 30 mmHg, appearing as areas of consolidation and mottling of the lung fields ***(Fig. 23.15)*** and pleural effusions. Patients with longstanding elevation of the pulmonary capillary pressure have reactive thickening of the pulmonary arteriolar intima, which protects the alveoli from pulmonary oedema. Thus, in these patients, the pulmonary venous pressure may increase to well above 30 mmHg before frank pulmonary oedema develops.

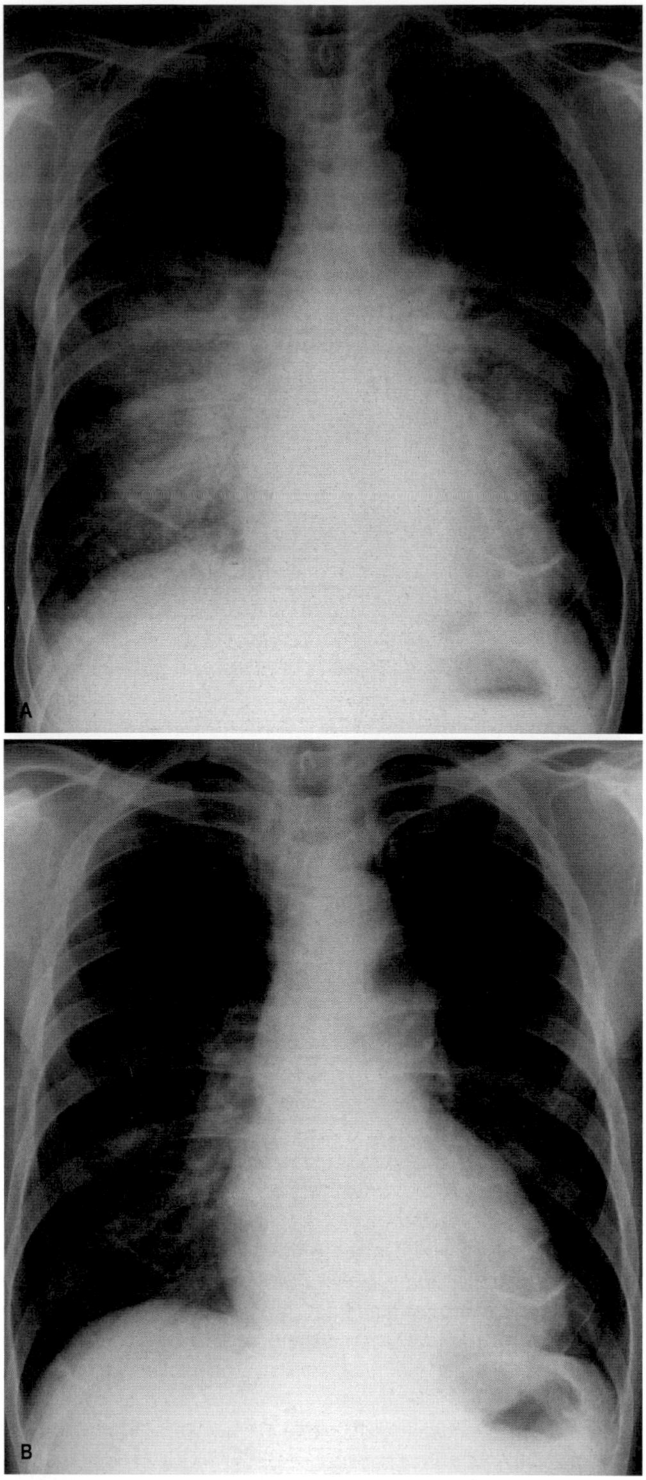

Figure 23.15 Acute pulmonary oedema: chest X-rays taken before and after treatment. A. The X-ray taken when the oedema was present demonstrates hilar haziness, Kerley B lines, upper lobe venous engorgement, and fluid in the right horizontal interlobar fissure. **B.** These abnormalities are resolved on the film taken after successful treatment.

Electrocardiography

The electrocardiogram (ECG) is a recording of the electrical activity of the heart. It is the vector sum of the depolarization and repolarization potentials of all myocardial cells (see ***Fig. 23.2***). At the body surface, these generate potential differences of about 1 mV, and the fluctuations of these potentials create the familiar P-QRS-T pattern. At rest, the intracellular voltage of the myocardium is polarized at −90 mV compared with that of the extracellular space. This

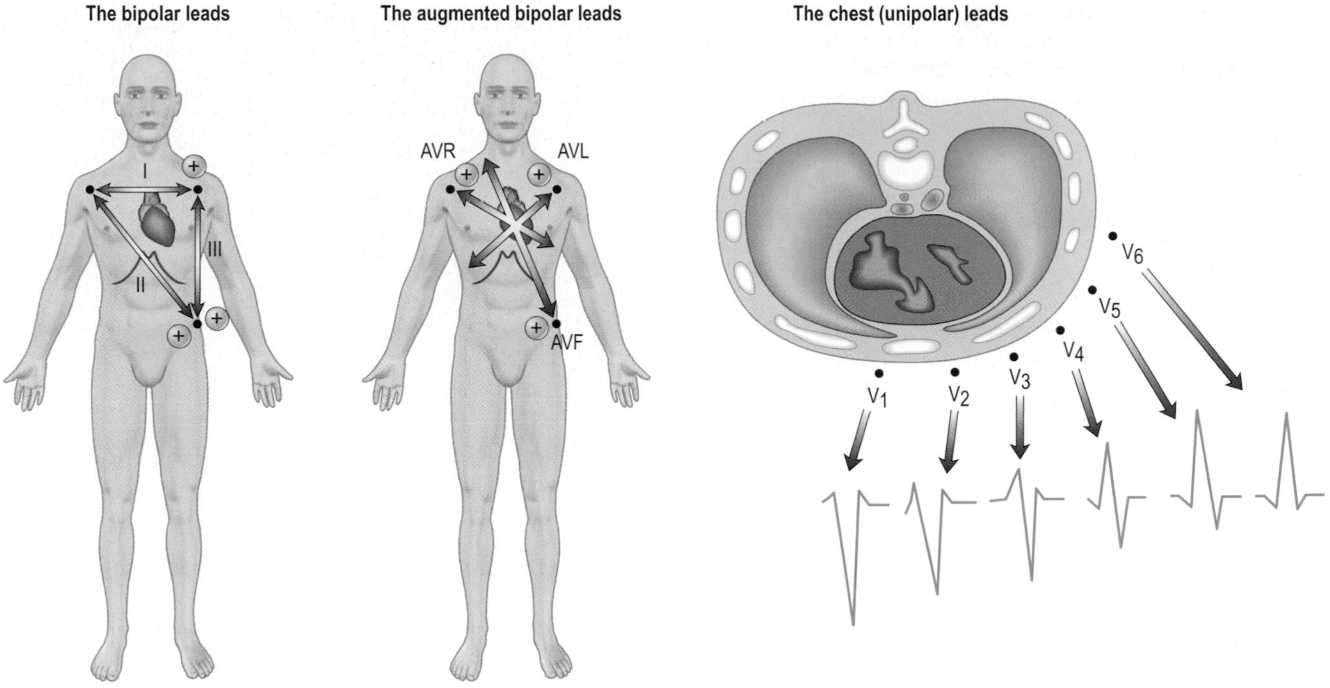

Figure 23.16 The connections or directions that comprise the 12-lead electrocardiogram.

diastolic voltage difference occurs because of the high intracellular potassium concentration, which is maintained by the sodium potassium pump despite the free membrane permeability to potassium. Depolarization of cardiac cells occurs when there is a sudden increase in the permeability of the membrane to sodium. Sodium rushes into the cell and the negative resting voltage is lost (phase 0 on ***Fig. 23.39***). The depolarization of a myocardial cell causes the depolarization of adjacent cells and, in the healthy heart, the entire myocardium is depolarized in a coordinated fashion. During repolarization, cellular electrolyte balance is slowly restored (phases 1, 2 and 3). Slow diastolic depolarization (phase 4) follows until the threshold potential is reached. Another action potential then follows.

The ECG is recorded from two or more simultaneous points of skin contact (electrodes). When cardiac activation proceeds towards the positive contact, an upward deflection is produced on the ECG. Correct representation of a three-dimensional spatial vector requires recordings from three mutually perpendicular (orthogonal) axes. The shape of the human torso does not make this easy, so the practical ECG records 12 projections of the vector, called 'leads' ***(Fig. 23.16)***.

Six of the leads are obtained by recording voltages from the limbs (I, II, III, AVR, AVL and AVF). The other six leads record potentials between points on the chest surface and an average of the three limbs: RA, LA and LL. These are designated V_1–V_6 and aim to select activity from the right ventricle (V_1–V_2), interventricular septum (V_3–V_4) and left ventricle (V_5–V_6). Note that leads AVR and V_1 are oriented towards the cavity of the heart, leads II, III and AVF face the inferior surface, and leads I, AVL and V_6 face the lateral wall of the left ventricle. A V_4 on the right side of the chest (V_4R) is occasionally useful (e.g. for the diagnosis of right ventricular infarction).

Most ECG machines are simultaneous three-channel recorders with output given either as a continuous strip or with automatic channel switching. Many ECG machines also analyse the recordings and print the analysis on the record. Usually, the machine interpretation is correct but many arrhythmias still defy automatic analysis.

The ECG waveform

The shape of the normal ECG waveform ***(Fig. 23.17)*** has similarities, whatever the orientation. The first deflection is caused by atrial depolarization; it is a low-amplitude, slow deflection called a ***P wave***. The ***QRS complex*** reflects ventricular activation or depolarization, and is sharper and larger in amplitude than the P wave. An initial downward deflection is called the ***Q wave***. An initial upward deflection is called an ***R wave***. The ***S wave*** is the last part of ventricular activation. The ***T wave*** is another slow and low-amplitude deflection that results from ventricular repolarization.

The ***PR interval*** is the length of time from the start of the P wave to the start of the QRS complex. It is the time taken for activation to pass from the sinus node, through the atrium, AV node and His–Purkinje system, to the ventricle.

The ***QT interval*** extends from the start of the QRS complex to the end of the T wave. This interval represents the time taken to depolarize and repolarize the ventricular myocardium. The QT interval varies greatly with heart rate and is often represented as a corrected QT interval (or QTc) for a given heart rate. There are a number of formulae for derivation of QTc, but the most widely accepted are Bazett's formula and Fridericia's correction ***(Box 23.6)***.

An abnormally prolonged QTc can predispose to a risk of dangerous ventricular arrhythmias. Prolongation of the QT interval may be congenital or can occur in many acquired conditions (see ***Box 23.15***).

The ***ST segment*** is the period between the end of the QRS complex and the start of the T wave. In the normal heart, all cells are depolarized by this phase of the ECG; that is, the ST segment represents ventricular repolarization.

Box 23.6 Normal ECG intervals

Parameter	Interval
P wave duration	≤0.12 s
PR interval	0.12–0.22 s
QRS complex duration	≤0.10 s
Corrected QT (QTc)	≤0.44 s in males
	≤0.46 s in females
QT_{cB}=QT√^{2} (R–R)	Bazett's square root formula
QT_{cF}=QT√^{3} (R–R)	Fridericia's cube root formula

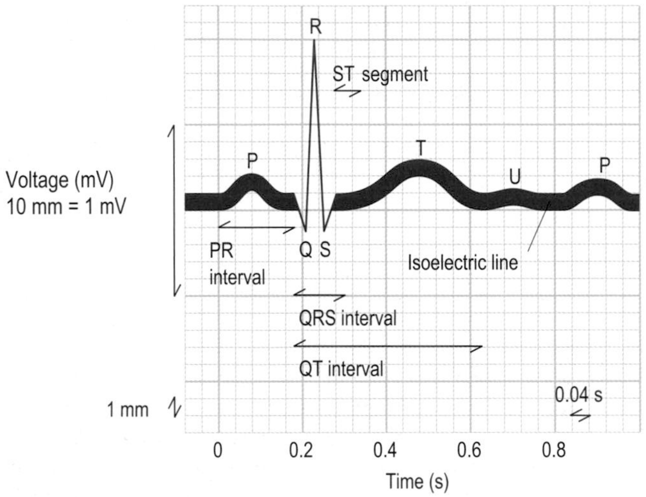

Figure 23.17 **The waves and elaboration of the normal electrocardiogram.**

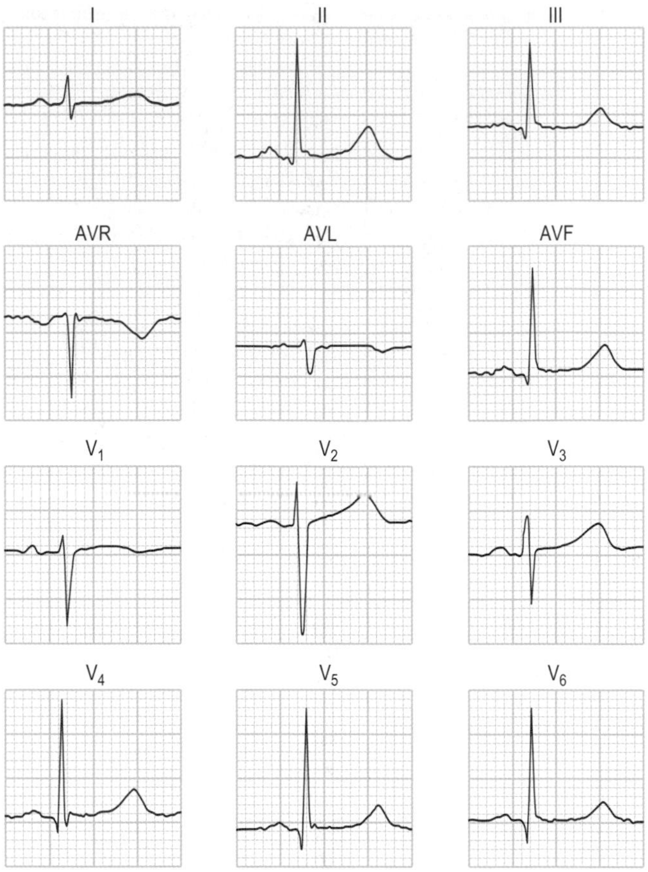

Figure 23.18 **A normal 12-lead electrocardiogram.**

A normal 12-lead ECG is shown in ***Figure 23.18***, and the normal values for the electrocardiographic intervals are indicated in ***Box 23.6***. Leads that face the lateral wall of the left ventricle have predominantly positive deflections, and leads looking into the ventricular cavity are usually negative. Detailed patterns depend on the size, shape and rhythm of the heart and the characteristics of the torso.

Cardiac vectors

At any point in time during depolarization and repolarization, electrical potentials are being propagated in different directions. Most of these cancel each other out and only the net force is recorded. This net force in the frontal plane is known as the cardiac vector.

The mean QRS vector can be calculated from the six standard leads ***(Fig. 23.19)***:

- Normal between –30° and +90°
- Left axis deviation between –30° and –90°
- Right axis deviation between +90° and +150°.

Calculation of this vector is useful in the diagnosis of some cardiac disorders.

Exercise electrocardiography

This is less used than previously (see p. 995) because of its low sensitivity. The ECG is recorded while the patient walks or runs on a motorized treadmill. The test is based on the principle that exercise increases myocardial demand on coronary blood supply, which may be inadequate during exercise, and at peak stress can result in relative myocardial ischaemia. Most exercise tests are performed according to a standardized method, such as the Bruce protocol. Recording an ECG after exercise is not an adequate form of stress test. Normally, there is little change in the T wave or ST segment during exercise.

The patient's exercise capacity (the total time achieved) will depend on many factors; however, patients who can only exercise for <6 min generally have a poorer prognosis.

Myocardial ischaemia provoked by exertion results in ST segment depression (>1 mm) in leads facing the affected area. The form of ST segment depression provoked by ischaemia is characteristic: it is either planar or shows down-sloping depression ***(Fig. 23.20)***. Up-sloping depression is a non-specific finding. The degree of ST segment depression is positively correlated to the degree of myocardial ischaemia.

ST segment elevation during an exercise test is induced much less frequently than ST depression. When it occurs, it reflects transmural ischaemia caused by coronary spasm or critical stenosis.

Although most abnormalities are detected in lead V_5 (anterior and lateral ischaemia) or AVF (inferior ischaemia), it is best to record a full 12-lead ECG. During an exercise test, the blood pressure and rhythm responses to exercise are also assessed. Exercise normally causes an increase in heart rate and blood pressure. A sustained fall in blood pressure usually indicates severe coronary artery disease. A slow recovery of the heart rate to basal levels has also been reported to be a predictor of mortality.

Frequent premature ventricular depolarizations during the test are associated with a long-term increase in the risk of death from

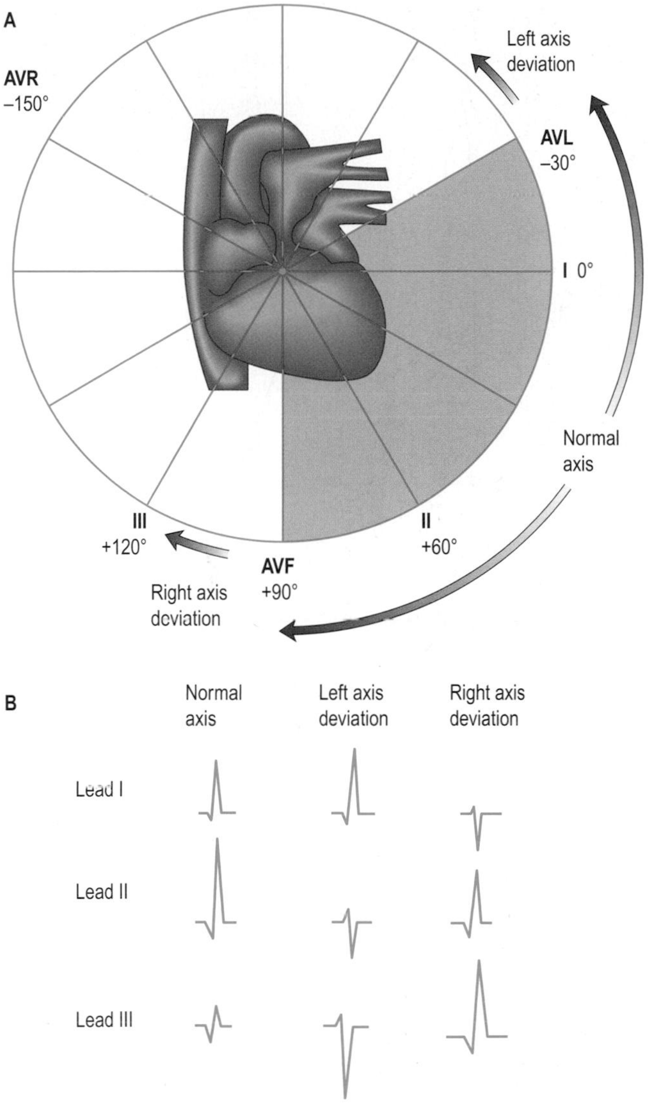

Figure 23.19 Cardiac vectors. A. *The hexaxial reference system*, illustrating the six leads in the frontal plane; for example, lead I is 0°, lead II is +60° and lead III is +120°. **B.** *Calculating the direction of the cardiac vector*. In the first column, the QRS complex with zero net amplitude (i.e. when the positive and negative deflections are equal) is seen in lead III. The mean QRS vector is therefore perpendicular to lead III and is either −150° or +30°. Lead I is positive, so the axis must be +30°, which is normal. In left axis deviation (second column), the main deflection is positive (R wave) in lead I and negative (S wave) in lead III. In right axis deviation (third column), the main deflection is negative (S wave) in lead I and positive (R wave) in lead III. The frontal plane QRS axis is normal only if the QRS complexes in leads I and II are predominantly positive.

cardiovascular causes, and further testing is required in these patients.

Twenty-four-hour ambulatory taped electrocardiography

This records transient changes such as a brief paroxysm of tachycardia, an occasional pause in the rhythm, or intermittent ST segment shifts ***(Fig. 23.21)***. A conventional 12-lead ECG is recorded in less than a minute and usually samples fewer than 20 complexes. In a 24-hour period, over 100 000 complexes are recorded. Such a

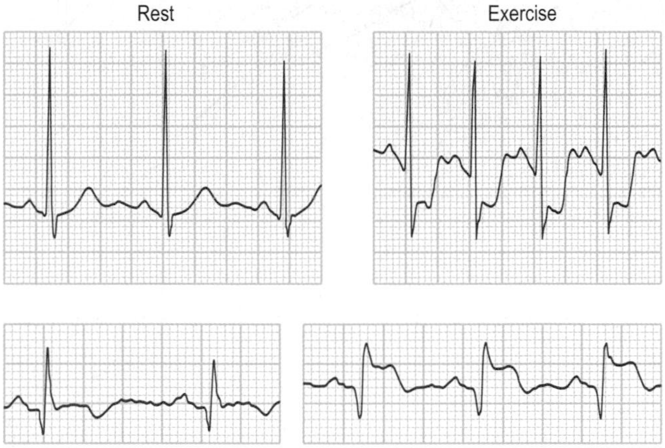

Figure 23.20 Electrocardiographic changes during exercise testing. The upper traces show significant horizontal ST segment depression during exercise. The lower traces show ST elevation during exercise.

large amount of data must be analysed by automatic or semi-automatic methods. This technique is called ***Holter electrocardiography*** after its inventor.

Event recording is another technique that is used to record less frequent arrhythmias. The patient is provided with a pocket-sized device that can record and store a short segment of the ECG. The device may be kept for several days or weeks until the arrhythmia is recorded. Most units of this kind will also allow transtelephonic ECG transmission so that the physician can determine the need for treatment or the continued need for monitoring.

A very small event recorder, known as an implantable loop recorder (ILR), can also be implanted subcutaneously, triggered by events or a magnet, and interrogated by the physician.

Other tests

Non-invasive methods that make use of digitalized Holter recordings to identify increased risk of ventricular arrhythmias include assessment of heart rate variability, signal-averaged ECG and T wave alternans.

- ***Heart rate variability* (*HRV*)** can be assessed from a 24-hour ECG. HRV is decreased in some patients following myocardial infarction and represents an abnormality of autonomic tone or cardiac responsiveness. Low HRV is a major risk factor for sudden death and ventricular arrhythmias in patients discharged from hospital following myocardial infarction.
- ***Signal-averaged ECG* (*SAECG*)** is a technique that requires amplification and averaging of abnormal low-amplitude signals that occur beyond the end of the QRS complex and extend well into the ST segment. These signals are therefore also known as late potentials and are too small to be detected on a surface ECG. They arise in areas of slow conduction in the myocardium, such as the border zone of an infarct, where re-entrant ventricular arrhythmias can originate.
- ***T wave alternans* (*TWA*)** is a valuable technique used as a non-invasive marker of susceptibility to ventricular arrhythmias and sudden cardiac death. TWA represents microvolt level changes in the morphology of the T waves in every other beat and can be detected during acute myocardial ischaemia using

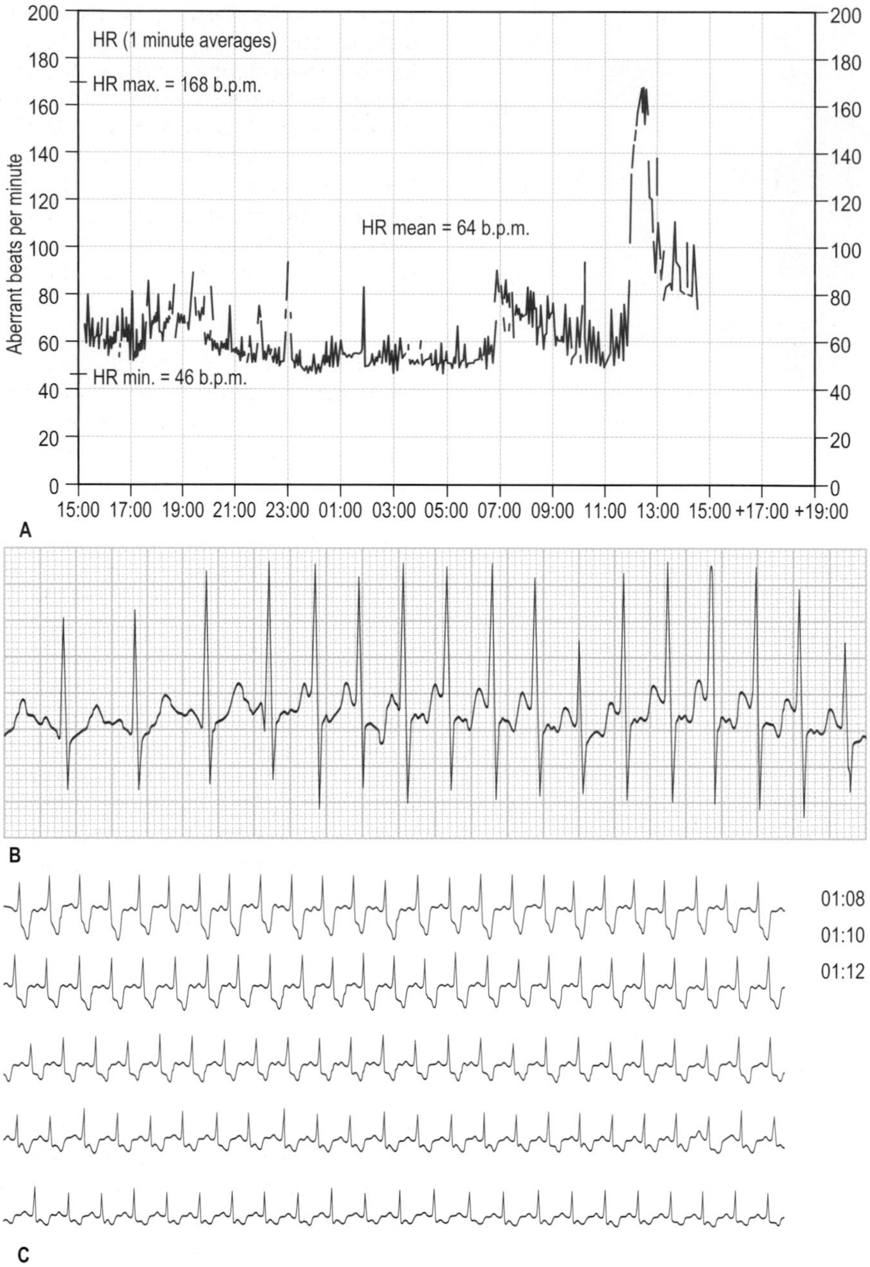

Figure 23.21 Examples of Holter recordings. A. A tachograph showing a sudden increase in heart rate (HR) between 11:00 and 13:00h. **B.** An ambulatory ECG record of the same patient, revealing supraventricular tachycardia. **C.** An ambulatory ECG showing ST depression in a patient with silent myocardial ischaemia.

amplification techniques. Visible TWA on an ordinary surface ECG is quite a rare phenomenon, except in patients with long QT syndromes, particularly during emotion or exercise.

Tilt testing

Patients with suspected neurocardiogenic (vasovagal) syncope should be investigated by upright tilt testing. The patient is secured to a table which is tilted to +60° to the vertical for ≥45 minutes. The ECG and blood pressure are monitored throughout. If neither symptoms nor signs develop, isoprenaline may be slowly infused or glyceryl trinitrate inhaled and the tilt repeated. A positive test results in hypotension, sometimes bradycardia ***(Fig. 23.22)*** and pre-syncope/syncope, and supports the diagnosis of neurocardiogenic syncope. If symptoms and signs appear, placing the patient flat can quickly reverse them. The effect of treatment can be evaluated by repeating the tilt test, but it is not always reproducible. The overall sensitivity, specificity and reproducibility are low.

Carotid sinus massage

Carotid sinus massage ***(Box 23.7)*** may lead to asystole (>3 s) and/or a fall in systolic blood pressure (>50 mmHg). This hypersensitive response occurs in many of the normal (especially elderly) population, but may also be responsible for loss of consciousness in some patients with carotid sinus syndrome (see p. 940). In one-third of cases, carotid sinus massage is only positive when the patient is standing. Atherosclerosis can cause narrowing and stenosis of

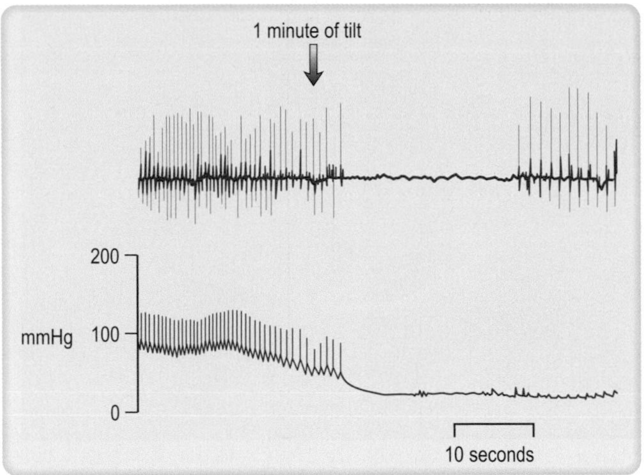

Figure 23.22 **Tilt test.** The ECG (top trace) and arterial blood pressure (bottom trace) recorded during a tilt test. After 1 min of tilt, hypotension, bradycardia and syncope occur.

Box 23.7 Carotid sinus massage

- Explanation and informed consent.
- Ensure there is no significant carotid artery disease (carotid bruits).
- Provide continuous electrocardiographic monitoring.
- Place the patient in the supine position with the head slightly extended.
- Start with right carotid sinus massage.
- Apply firm rotary pressure to the carotid artery at the level of the third cervical vertebra for 5 s.
- Alternatively, apply steady pressure.
- If there is no response, massage the left carotid sinus.
- Generally, right carotid sinus massage decreases the sinus node discharge, and left carotid sinus massage slows atrioventricular conduction.
- Do not massage both carotid sinuses at the same time.
- Single application of carotid sinus pressure may be effective in about 20–30% of patients with paroxysmal supraventricular tachycardias; multiple applications can terminate tachycardia in about 50% of patients.
- Asystole is a potential but rare complication.

carotid arteries. Carotid sinus massage should thus be avoided in patients with carotid bruits.

Echocardiography

Echocardiography is a non-invasive diagnostic technique that is widely employed in clinical cardiology. It involves the use of ultrasound (either alone or with contrast agent) to assess cardiac structure and function. A physician or technician performs the studies and a comprehensive examination takes 15–45 minutes. The ultrasound machines are either mobile on wheels, or handheld.

Physics

Echocardiography uses transmitted ultrasound wavelengths of ≤1 mm, which correspond to frequencies of approximately ≥2 MHz (≥2 million cycles per second). At such high frequencies, the ultrasound waves can be focused into a 'beam' and aimed at a particular region of the heart. The waves are generated in very short bursts or pulses a few microseconds long by a crystal transducer, which also detects returning echoes and converts them into electrical signals.

When the handheld crystal transducer is placed on the body surface, the emitted ultrasound pulses encounter interfaces between various body tissues as they pass through the body. In crossing each interface, some of the wave energy is reflected, and if the beam path is approximately at right angles to the plane of the interface, the reflected waves return to the transducer as an echo. Since the velocity of sound in body tissues is almost constant (1550 m/s), the time delay for the echo to return measures the distance of the reflecting interface. Thus, if a single ultrasound pulse is transmitted, a series of echoes return, the first of which is from the closest interface.

Echocardiographic modalities

M-mode and two-dimensional echocardiography

M-mode echocardiography is a technique that details the changing motion of structures along the ultrasound beam with time. Thus, the motion of the interventricular septum during the cardiac cycle (either towards or away from the transducer placed on the chest wall) can be assessed and quantified. Stationary structures thus generate horizontal straight lines; the distances of these lines from the top of the screen indicate the depth of the structures, and movements, such as those of heart valves, are indicated by zigzag lines ***(Fig. 23.23C)***. Alternatively, a series of views from different positions can be obtained in the form of a two-dimensional image (cross-sectional 2-D echocardiography; ***Fig. 23.23A,B***). This method is useful for delineating anatomical structures and for quantifying volumes of the cardiac chambers. M mode can be used to estimate left ventricular (LV) systolic function by comparing end-diastolic and end-systolic dimensions. For example, the percentage reduction in the left ventricular cavity size ('shortening fraction', SF) is given by:

$$SF = \frac{LVDD - LVSD}{LVDD} \times 100\%$$

where LVDD is left ventricular diastolic diameter and LVSD is left ventricular systolic diameter, at the base of the heart. The normal range is 30–45%.

This method is easy to perform, but is an inaccurate measure of ***ejection fraction*** (***EF***) because it does not take account of reduced regional function of the mid or apical myocardium – due to infarction, for example. For this reason, estimation of EF based on the difference in LV volumes from systole to diastole, derived from planimetered measurements of LV area in at least two planes, is more accurate. A normal EF is >55%. This method is helpful in assessing the response of the patient with heart failure to therapy. It also permits estimation of LV mass.

Three-dimensional echocardiography

Three-dimensional echocardiography is a novel development in cardiac imaging in which a volumetric dataset is acquired using a multiplane probe rotating around a fixed axis. Clinical uses include accurate volumetric assessment of ventricular function and mass, assessment of mitral and aortic valve disease, and assessment of adult congenital heart disease ***(Fig. 23.24)***.

Doppler echocardiography

Echocardiography imaging utilizes echoes from tissue interfaces. Using high amplification, it is also possible to detect weak echoes scattered by small targets, including those from red blood cells. Blood velocity in the heart chambers is typically much more rapid (>1 m/s) than the movement of myocardial tissue. If the blood is moving in the same direction as the direction of the ultrasound beam, the frequency of the returning echoes will be changed according to the Doppler phenomenon. The Doppler shift frequency

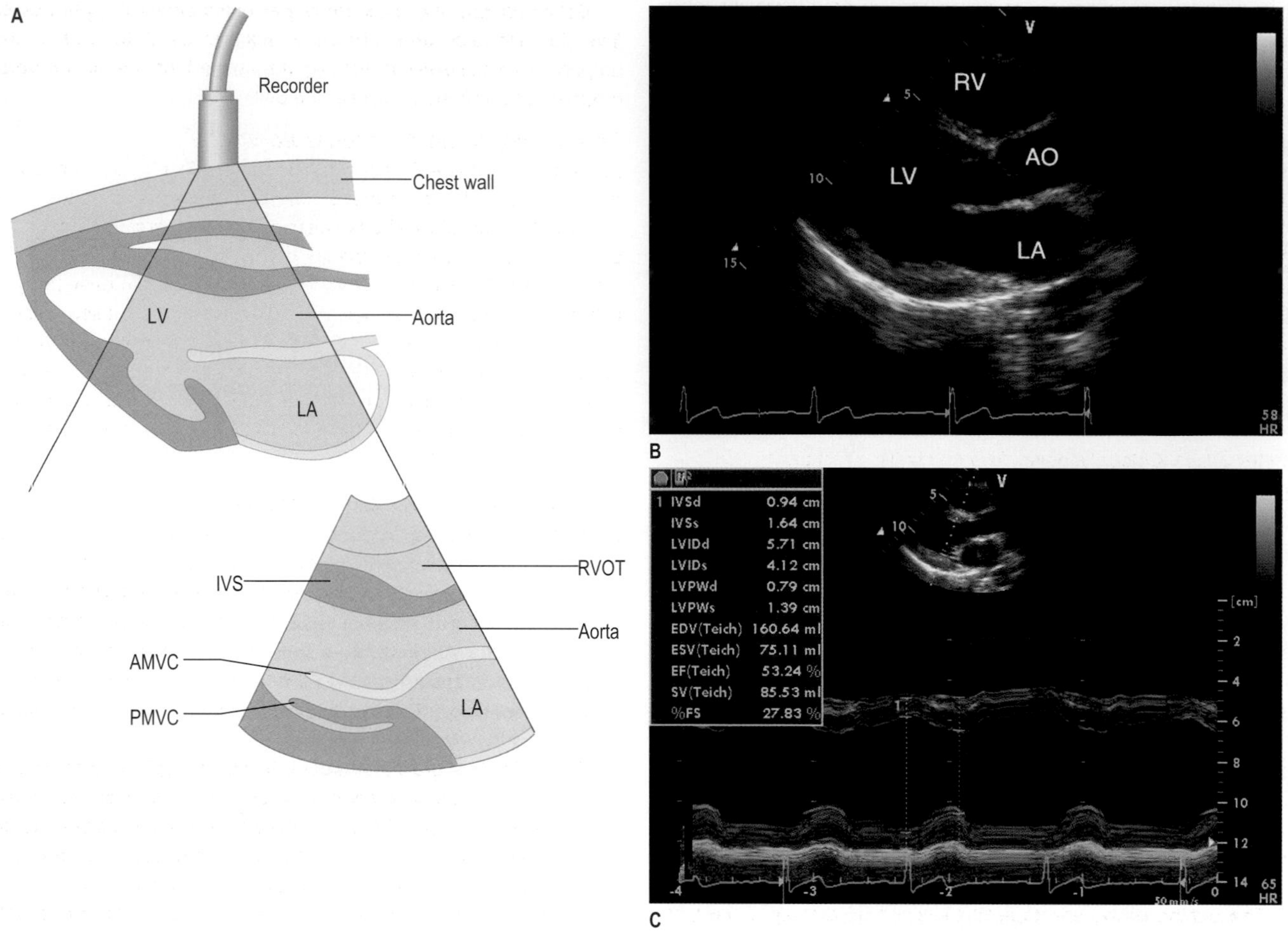

Figure 23.23 Echocardiograms. A. ***Diagrammatic representations*** of the anatomy of the area scanned and of the echocardiogram. **B. *Two-dimensional long-axis view*** from a normal subject. **C. *M-mode recording*** from a normal subject with the ultrasound beam directed across the left ventricle, just below the mitral valve. AMVC, anterior mitral valve cusp; AO, aorta; IVS, interventricular septum; LA, left atrium; LV, left ventricle; LV(d)/LV(s), left ventricular end-diastolic/end-systolic dimensions; MV, mitral valve; PM, papillary muscle; PMVC, posterior mitral valve cusp; PVW, posterior ventricular wall; RA, right atrium; RV, right ventricle; RVOT, right ventricular outflow tract.

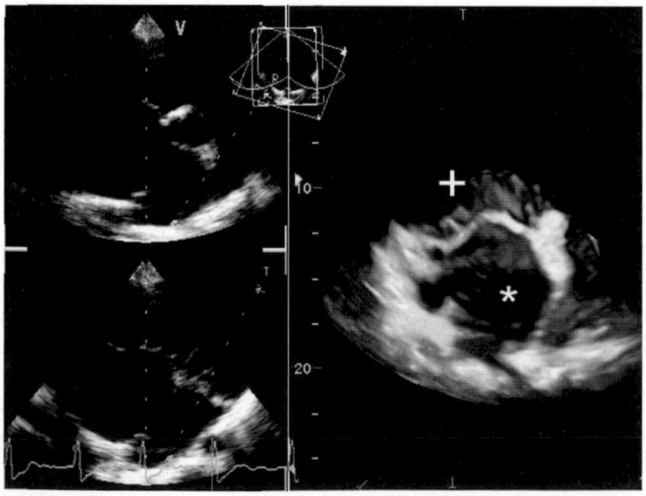

Figure 23.24 Three-dimensional echocardiograph in a patient with an atrial septal defect (*). The mitral valve (+) and the left atrial anatomy are well delineated.

is directly proportional to the blood velocity. Blood velocity data can be acquired and displayed in several ways.

Pulsed-wave Doppler Pulsed-wave (PW) Doppler extracts velocity data from the pulse echoes used to form a 2-D image and gives useful qualitative information. PW echoes can be specified from locations within an image identified by a sample volume cursor placed on the screen. Such information from the left ventricular outflow tract (LVOT) and right ventricular outflow tract provides the stroke distance, and is used to estimate cardiac output (CO) and also to quantify intracardiac shunts.

Cardiac output can then be derived using the formula:

$$CO = \text{stroke volume} \times \text{heart rate}$$

Stroke volume is the stroke distance multiplied by the area of the LVOT, which can also be measured echocardiographically. PW Doppler of the flow across the mitral valve and into the left atrium through the pulmonary veins can be used as an element of the estimation of left ventricular filling pressure.

Colour flow Doppler Doppler colour flow imaging uses one colour for blood flowing towards the transducer and another colour for blood flowing away. This technique allows the direction, velocity and timing of the flow to be measured with a simultaneous view of

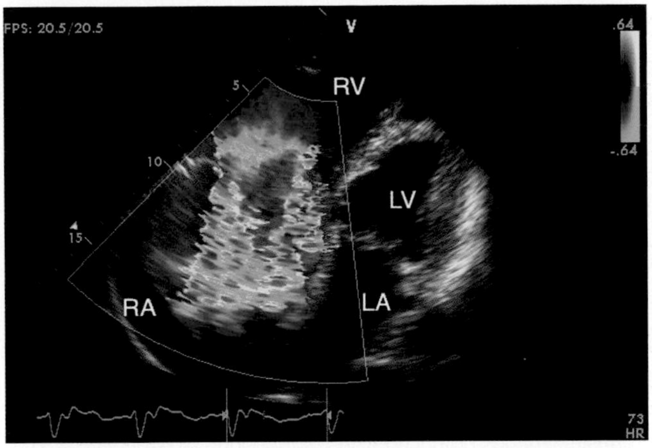

Figure 23.25 Colour Doppler. Blood is shown flowing away from the echocardiography probe as a blue signal and towards the probe as a red signal. In this patient with tricuspid regurgitation, blood leaks from the right ventricle (RV) to the right atrium (RA) during cardiac systole. LA, left atrium; LV, left ventricle.

cardiac structure and function. Colour flow Doppler is used to help assess valvular regurgitation ***(Fig. 23.25)*** and may be helpful in the assessment of coronary blood flow.

Continuous-wave Doppler Continuous-wave (CW) Doppler collects all the velocity data from the path of the beam and analyses it to generate a spectral display. This is unlike PW Doppler, which provides information from a particular sample volume at one location along a line. Thus, CW Doppler does not provide any depth information.

The outline of the envelope of the spectral display is used to estimate the value of peak velocity throughout the cardiac cycle. CW Doppler is typically used to assess valvular obstruction, which then causes increased velocities. For example, normal flow velocities are of the order of 1 m/s across the normal aortic valve, but if there is a severe obstructive lesion, such as a severely stenotic aortic valve, velocities of 4 m/s or more can occur. These velocities are generated by the pressure gradient that exists across the lesion.

According to the Bernoulli equation, the pressure difference between two chambers is calculated as: 4 multiplied by the square of the CW Doppler velocity between chambers. Thus a velocity of 5 m/s across the aortic valve suggests a peak gradient of $4 \times 5 \times 5 = 100$ mmHg between the ascending aorta and the left ventricle. This equation has been validated in a wide variety of clinical situations, including valve stenoses, ventricular septal defects and intraventricular obstruction (as in hypertrophic cardiomyopathy). It is often clinically unnecessary to resort to invasive methods such as cardiac catheterization to measure intracardiac pressure gradients.

Similarly, pulmonary artery (PA) systolic pressure and right ventricular diastolic pressure can be calculated using the Bernoulli equation. In this case, CW Doppler tracing of the tricuspid regurgitant jet is used to estimate the pressure gradient between the right ventricle and the right atrium. The PA systolic pressure is then calculated by adding the estimated right atrial pressure to the pressure gradient between the right ventricle and the right atrium.

Tissue Doppler Tissue Doppler is similar to PW Doppler. It measures myocardial tissue velocities within a particular sample volume placed on the image. Such velocities are of the order of 1 cm/s. Currently, tissue Doppler of the mitral annulus is used as part of the estimation of left ventricular filling pressure.

Other ultrasound modalities Harmonic power Doppler, pulse inversion Doppler and ultraharmonics are used to detect and amplify microsphere-specific signals as part of the echocardiographic assessment of myocardial perfusion.

Transoesophageal echocardiography

In transoesophageal echocardiography (TOE), a transducer mounted on a flexible tube is placed into the oesophagus. This involves the use of local anaesthesia and, sometimes, intravenous sedation. High-resolution images can be obtained because of the close proximity of the heart to the transducer in the oesophagus, and also because of the higher frequencies that are used relative to transthoracic imaging. TOE is most commonly used to assess valve structure and function (for reparability of mitral valve prolapse), the features and complications of infective endocarditis, and the aorta (for aortic dissection); and to seek a cardiac source of embolus.

Wall motion stress echocardiography

Echocardiography can be used clinically to evaluate the patient for the presence of myocardial scars and reversible ischaemia. Since ultrasound cannot directly detect red blood cells in capillaries, myocardial wall motion is used as a surrogate for perfusion. Myocardial segments that demonstrate a change in function (defined as a change or reduction in thickening) from rest to stress can be assumed to be supplied by a flow-limiting stenosis in the epicardial artery or graft.

Stress for this indication needs to be inotropic to induce true ischaemia. Physiological stress includes treadmill exercise, which is complicated by the difficulty in obtaining reliable images rapidly as the patient comes off the treadmill, before heart rate reduces back to sub-maximal levels. Alternatively, pharmacological stress can be induced with dobutamine at graded doses. This is relatively safe but complications such as ventricular arrhythmia have been reported. This technique can also be used to assess viability of the myocardium, and hibernating or stunned myocardium (see p. 987).

Myocardial perfusion echocardiography

In order to assess myocardial perfusion by echocardiography (MPE), microspheres of similar size to red blood cells are used as an intravenous contrast agent. Microsphere-specific ultrasound modes, such as harmonic power Doppler, can be used for detection. MPE involves the use of intravenous infusion of contrast to fill the myocardium. A pulse of ultrasound destroys microspheres within the capillaries (and not the left ventricular cavity), and the time taken to replenish the capillaries is a measure of myocardial blood flow. The time taken to fill should be significantly shorter at stress than at rest.

Contrast echo for left ventricular opacification

Intravenous contrast agents opacify the left ventricle and can define the endocardial border. Their clinical utility has reduced with the advent of harmonic imaging, which has improved image quality in patients who were previously 'difficult to image'.

Intravascular (coronary) ultrasound

Intravascular (coronary) ultrasound probes can be used to obtain images of proximal coronary arteries as part of a percutaneous transluminal coronary angioplasty (PTCA) procedure: for example, to assess adequacy of deployment of intracoronary stents.

Nuclear imaging

Nuclear imaging is used to detect myocardial infarction or to measure myocardial function, perfusion or viability, depending on the radiopharmaceutical and the imaging technique chosen. These data are particularly valuable when used in combination. All involve a significant radiation dose (see p. 953).

Image type

Gamma cameras produce a planar image in which structures are superimposed, as in a standard radiograph. Single-photon-emission computed tomography (SPECT) imaging uses similar raw data to construct tomographic images, just as a CT image is reconstructed from X-rays. This gives finer anatomical resolution, but is technically demanding. These methods may be used with any of the radiopharmaceuticals.

Myocardial perfusion and viability

Thallium-201 is rapidly taken up by the myocardium, so an image taken immediately after injection reflects the distribution of blood flow to the myocardium. Areas of ischaemia or infarction receive less ^{201}Tl and appear dark. Between 2 and 24 hours after injection, ^{201}Tl is redistributed so that all cardiac myocytes contain a comparable concentration. Images obtained at this time show dark areas where the myocardium has infarcted, but normal density in ischaemic areas. Comparison of the early and late images is one method of predicting whether an ischaemic area of myocardium contains enough viable tissue to justify coronary bypass or angioplasty. Technetium-99-labelled tetrofosmin ***(Fig. 23.26)*** is also taken up rapidly by cardiac myocytes but does not undergo redistribution. When this substance is injected during exercise, its distribution in the myocardium reflects the distribution of blood at the time of the exercise, even if the image is taken several hours later. This is a sensitive method of detecting myocardial viability. Images produced following injection of [^{99m}Tc]tetrofosmin during exercise can be compared to images produced following injection at rest to decide which areas of ischaemia are reversible (see p. 987). In patients unable to exercise, the heart can be stressed with drugs, e.g. dipyridamole or dobutamine.

Infarct imaging

Perfusion images produced using compounds labelled with ^{201}Tl or [^{99m}Tc]sestamibi show a myocardial infarction as a perfusion defect or 'cold spot'. These methods are sensitive for detecting and localizing the infarct, but give no information about its age. [^{99m}Tc] Pyrophosphate is preferentially taken up by myocardium that has undergone infarction within the previous few days. Images are difficult to interpret because the isotope is also concentrated by bone and cartilage.

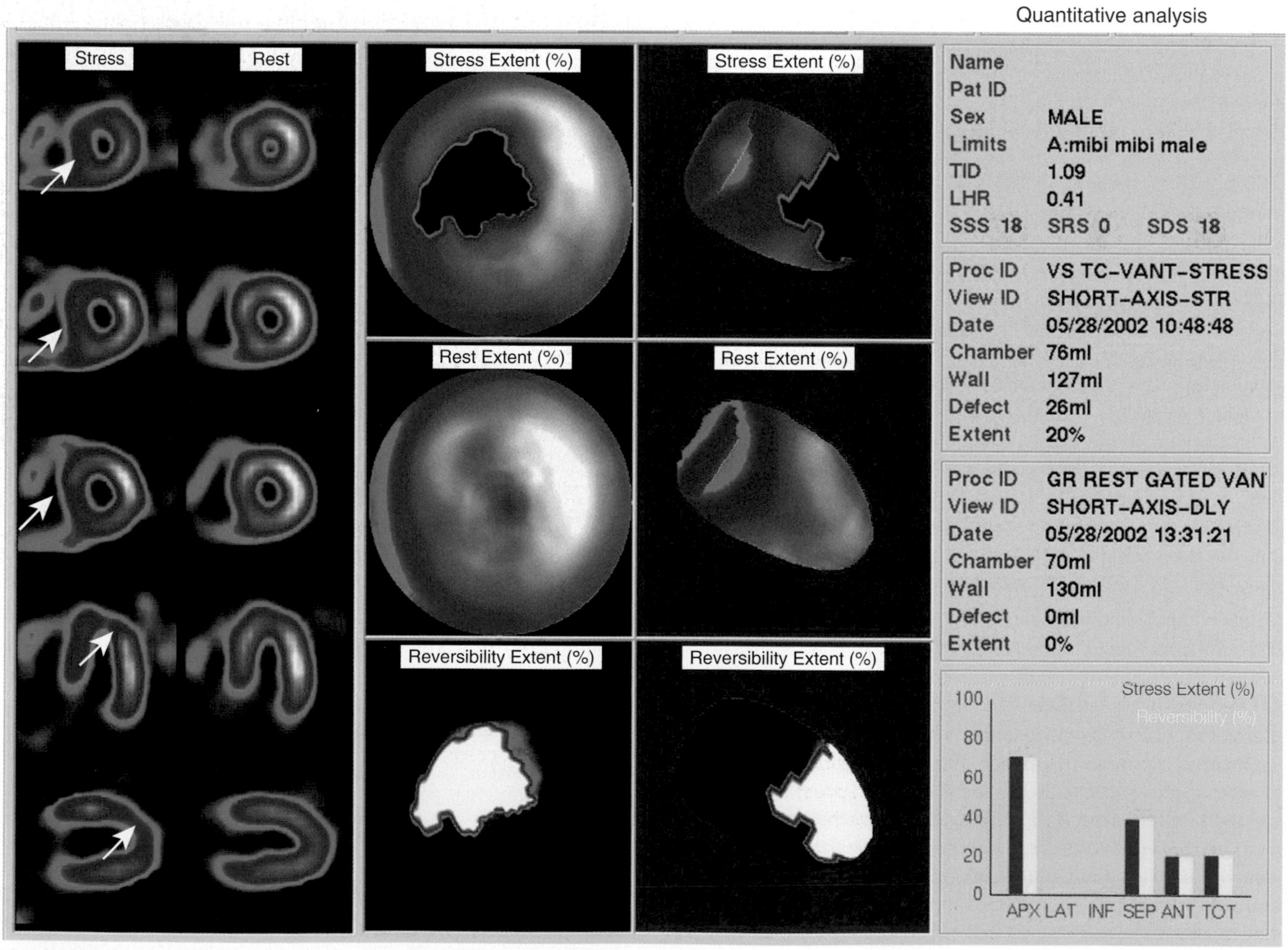

Figure 23.26 Myocardial SPECT study acquired with [^{99m}Tc]tetrofosmin tracer. *Left panel*: Three short-axis slices and a horizontal and a vertical axis plane of the left ventricle after stress and following a resting re-injection of tracer. The rest images demonstrate normal tracer uptake (orange signal) in the whole of the left ventricle. The stress images demonstrate reduced tracer uptake (arrows; purple-blue signal) in the anterior and septal walls, consistent with a significant stenosis in the left anterior descending artery. *Middle panel*: Polar maps of the whole myocardium can localize the ischaemic territory. *Right panel*: Quantitative analysis can help define the extent and reversibility of the ischaemia.

Cardiac computed tomography

Computed tomography (CT) is useful for the assessment of the thoracic aorta and mediastinum. The development of 64-slice multidetector CT (MDCT) scanners has enabled accurate non-invasive imaging of the coronary arteries.

Coronary artery calcification

Calcium is absent in normal coronary arteries, but is present in atherosclerosis and increases with age. Studies have demonstrated a positive correlation between calcification and the presence of coronary artery stenoses, although the relationship is non-linear. Electron beam CT (EBT) and MDCT scanners are used to obtain multiple thin axial slices through the heart and then the calcium score is calculated. The calcium score is based on the X-ray attenuation coefficient or CT number measured in Hounsfield units. Meta-analyses have demonstrated that a higher calcium score is associated with a higher event rate and higher relative risk ratios, although currently no study has shown a net effect on health outcomes of calcium scoring. The current National Institute for Health and Care Excellence (NICE) chest pain guidelines recommend the use of CT calcium scoring in patients with chest pain and a 10–29% likelihood of coronary artery disease (see p. 995).

CT coronary angiography

CT coronary angiography (CTCA) is performed with a supine patient connected to a three-lead ECG for cardiac synchronization. The 64-slice MDCT scanners have a temporal resolution of 165–210 ms; image quality is optimal with a slow and steady heart rate (<65–70 b.p.m.), which can be obtained with the use of oral or intravenous beta-blockers. Sublingual nitroglycerin (0.4–0.8 mg dose) may improve visualization of the coronary artery lumen. A volume dataset containing the whole heart is acquired during a single breath-hold with the injection of 60–80 mL of iodinated contrast agent at 4–6 mL/s. The radiation dose during the scan is 11–22 mSv but this can be reduced to 7–11 mSv with ECG-controlled dose modulation; this compares with 2.5–5.0 mSv for diagnostic coronary angiography and 15–20 mSv for SPECT. The volume dataset is then analysed with multiplanar reformatting for the presence of coronary artery stenoses ***(Fig. 23.27)***. Studies have reported high sensitivity (>85%) and specificity (>90%) for the detection of coronary artery disease, with a very high negative predictive value (>95%). CTCA may become part of an acute chest pain service in the emergency medicine department to exclude aortic dissection, pulmonary embolism and coronary artery disease. However, this technique does expose the patient to ionizing radiation.

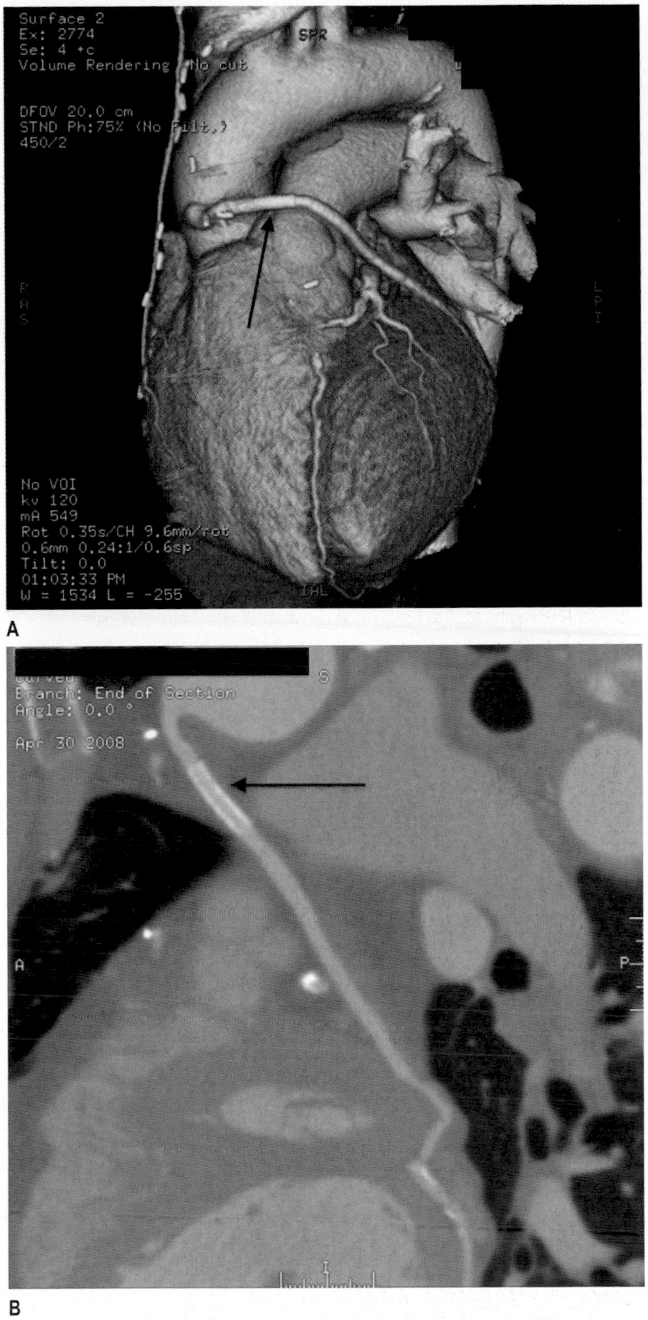

Figure 23.27 Coronary artery stent: multislice computed tomography. A. A volume-rendered image in a patient with coronary artery stent insertion (arrow) in a saphenous vein graft to the native circumflex coronary artery. **B.** The multiplanar reformatted image demonstrates stent patency (arrow) and insertion of the graft to the circumflex coronary artery.

Cardiovascular magnetic resonance

Cardiovascular magnetic resonance (CMR), a non-invasive imaging technique that does not involve harmful radiation, is increasingly used in the investigation of patients with cardiovascular disease.

CMR is usually performed with multiple breath-holds to minimize respiratory motion artefacts and cardiac gating to reduce blurring during the cardiac cycle. Several different sequences are used to provide anatomical and functional information. Most sequences do not require a contrast agent but intravenous gadolinium may be needed for magnetic resonance angiography, myocardial perfusion, infarct and fibrosis imaging. The major contraindications are permanent pacemaker or defibrillator, intracerebral clips and significant claustrophobia. Patients with coronary stents and prosthetic valves can be safely scanned.

Clinical use of CMR

The current indications for CMR are summarized in ***Box 23.8***.

Congenital heart disease

CMR provides additional and complementary information to echocardiography in patients with congenital heart disease. Cine-imaging can accurately assess systemic and non-systemic ventricular function and mass. Extracardiac conduits, anomalous pulmonary venous return and aortic coarctations before and after repair can be studied by CMR, and the studies repeated for long-term follow-up without the risk of ionizing radiation.

Cardiomyopathies, pericardial disease and cardiac masses

In hypertrophic cardiomyopathy, CMR accurately defines the extent and distribution of myocardial hypertrophy and can be used in patients with sub-optimal echocardiograms. Intravenous gadolinium can be utilized to demonstrate regional myocardial fibrosis, which is associated with an adverse prognosis. In patients with suspected arrhythmogenic right ventricular cardiomyopathy, CMR is the imaging investigation of choice to detect global and regional wall motion abnormalities of the right ventricle and right ventricular outflow tract, and to detect fatty or fibro-fatty infiltration of the right and left ventricles. In constrictive pericarditis and restrictive cardiomyopathy, CMR can demonstrate the effects of the impaired ventricular filling common to both conditions (dilated right atrium and inferior vena cava), and can also determine the thickness of the pericardium (usually 4 mm in normal individuals) ***(Fig. 23.28)***. In patients with dilated cardiomyopathy, CMR can accurately quantify biventricular function and, with gadolinium, can demonstrate myocardial fibrosis. In inflammatory and infiltrative conditions of the myocardium, such as myocarditis, sarcoidosis and amyloidosis, CMR is increasingly used as a diagnostic investigation due to different patterns of signal enhancement seen with gadolinium. In patients with thalassaemia, CMR can detect iron deposition within the myocardium and guide chelation therapy. CMR can be useful in patients with cardiac masses to differentiate benign from malignant tumours and to identify thrombus not visualized on echocardiography.

Box 23.8 Indications for cardiovascular magnetic resonance (CMR)

- Congenital heart disease (CHD):
  - Anatomical assessment following echocardiography, particularly in patients with complex CHD or following surgical intervention
  - Follow-up/surveillance studies
  - Anomalous pulmonary or systemic venous return
  - Assessment of right or left ventricular function/dilatation
- Cardiomyopathies/cardiac infiltration/pericardial disease
- Disease of the aorta, including aortic dissection, aneurysm, coarctation
- Valvular heart disease:
  - Quantification of stenosis and regurgitation
  - Accurate ventricular dimensions/function
  - Planimetry of valvular stenosis
- Coronary artery disease:
  - Left and right ventricular function
  - Wall motion assessment during dobutamine stress
  - Myocardial perfusion during adenosine stress
  - Coronary artery and coronary artery bypass graft imaging
  - Myocardial infarct imaging and viability assessment with dobutamine CMR or delayed enhancement
- Pulmonary vessels

Diseases of the aorta

CMR is an excellent technique for assessing patients with aortic dissection and can detect the clinical features of an aortic dissection: the intimal flap, thrombosis in a false lumen, aortic regurgitation, pericardial effusion and aortic dilatation. As it does not involve radiation or need contrast, CMR is an ideal method of surveillance of patients with dilated thoracic aortas or repaired coarctation.

Valvular heart disease

Valvular stenosis produces signal void on gradient-echo CMR. CMR can quantify the velocity across a stenosed valve using phase-contrast velocity mapping. Valvular regurgitation can be accurately quantified using phase-contrast velocity mapping across the valve, or by calculating the stroke volumes of the left and right ventricles, which are equal in the absence of significant regurgitation. However, in most patients, transthoracic and transoesophageal echocardiography should provide sufficient information.

Coronary artery disease

CMR can be used to assess coronary artery anatomy, left ventricular function, myocardial perfusion and viability in a 'one-stop' approach to the assessment of patients with coronary artery disease. Coronary artery anatomy and stenoses can be identified with ultra-fast breath-hold or respiratory-gated sequences with high accuracies. Global left ventricular function and wall motion abnormalities can be detected with cine-imaging performed at rest and during dobutamine stress. Myocardial perfusion can be assessed with gadolinium and first-pass imaging; ischaemia can be demonstrated with adenosine for coronary vasodilatation. Myocardial viability can be determined using gadolinium and 'delayed enhancement' images. With these techniques, CMR is increasingly used to assess both ischaemia in patients with suspected coronary disease, and myocardial viability prior to revascularization in patients with impaired cardiac function (***Figs 23.29*** and ***23.30***).

Pulmonary vessels

Magnetic resonance angiography (MRA) with gadolinium can provide high-quality images of the pulmonary veins, which can be

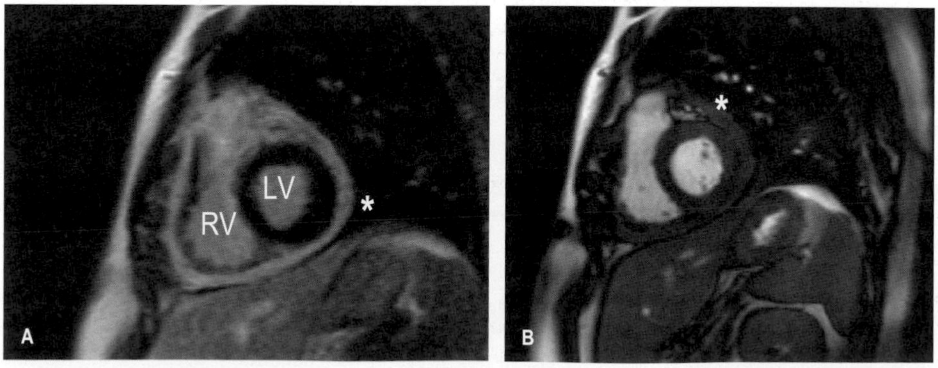

Figure 23.28 Short-axis cardiac magnetic resonance (CMR) in a patient with constrictive pericarditis. A and **B** show thickening of the pericardium (*). LV, left ventricle; RV, right ventricle.

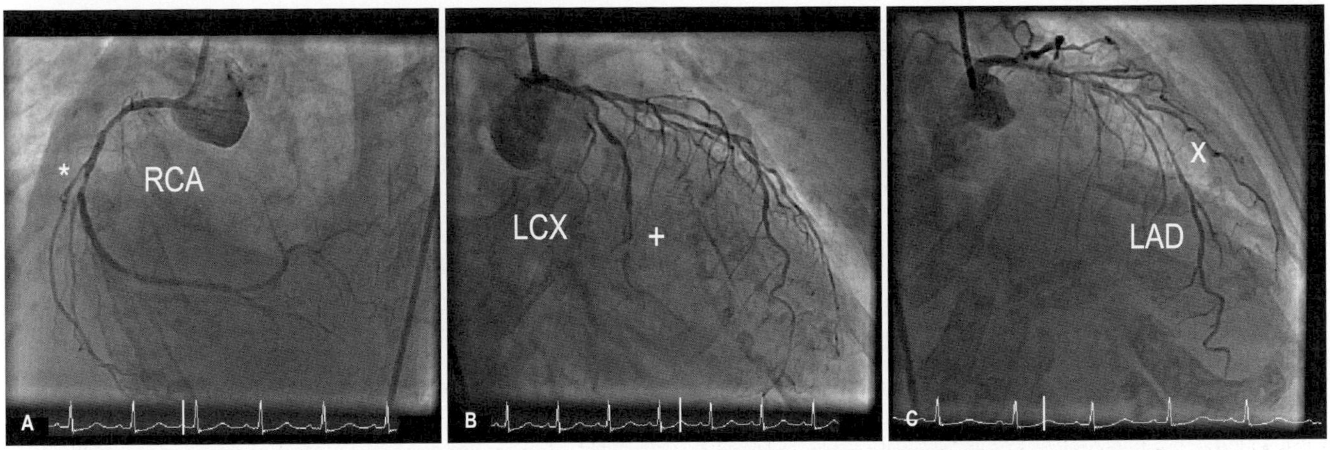

Figure 23.29 Cardiac magnetic resonance (CMR) in a patient with type 2 diabetes mellitus and exertional breathlessness. A. Diagnostic coronary angiography demonstrates a severe stenosis (*) in the right coronary artery (RCA). **B.** There is a sub-totally occluded (+) circumflex coronary artery (LCX). **C.** A long diseased segment (X) is also seen in the left anterior descending coronary artery (LAD).

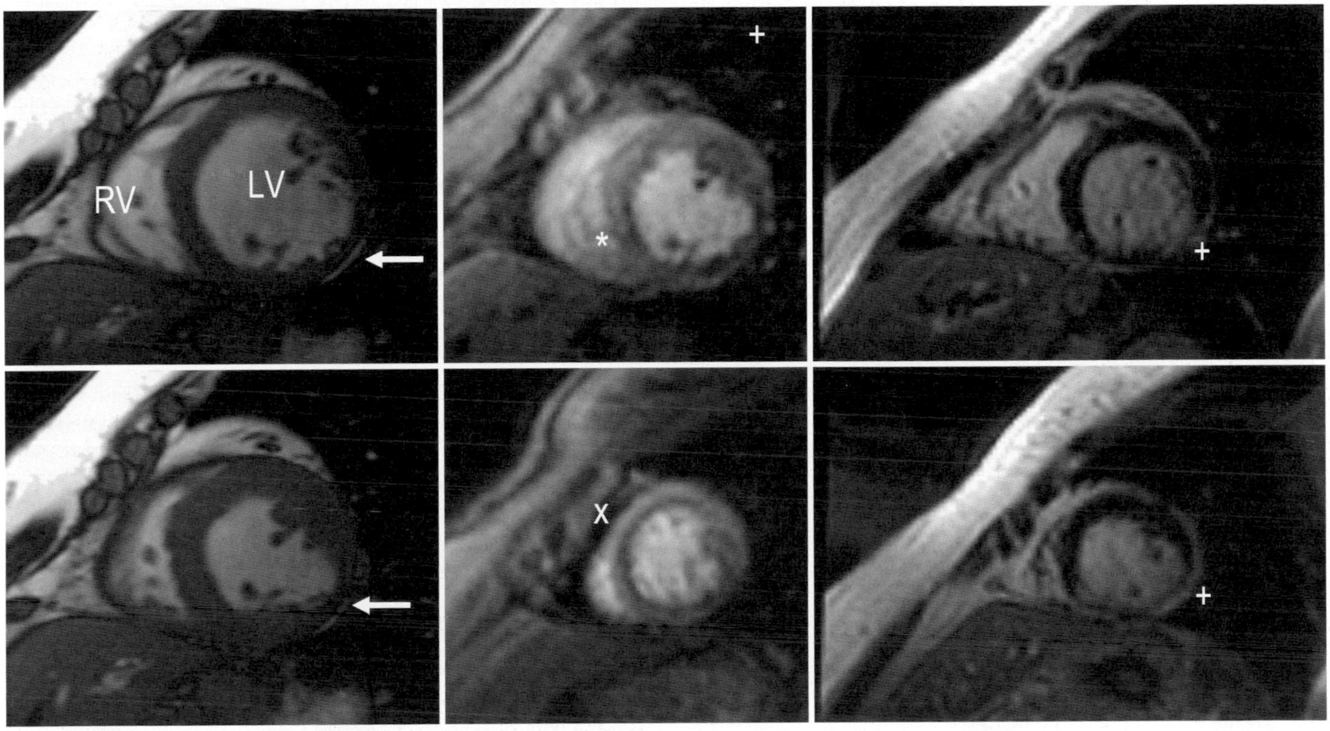

A B C

Figure 23.30 Cardiac magnetic resonance (CMR). A. *Short-axis CMR FIESTA cine-imaging* (diastole top, systole bottom) demonstrates thinning and hypokinesia of the inferolateral wall (arrowed) but preserved function of the rest of the myocardium. **B.** *First-pass perfusion CMR* (mid top, apex bottom) demonstrates sub-endocardial perfusion defects in the inferolateral wall (+), infero-septum (*) and apical segments (X). **C.** *Delayed-enhancement CMR* confirms a transmural myocardial infarction of the mid-apical infero-lateral wall (+) secondary to a previous infarction from the circumflex coronary artery, and confirms inducible ischaemia in the right and left coronary territories. LV, left ventricle; RV, right ventricle.

fused with electrical data during pulmonary vein isolation for the treatment of atrial fibrillation.

Positron emission tomography

Positron emission tomography (PET) is based on detection of high-energy emissions caused by annihilation of positrons released from unstable isotopes. PET has several advantages over other techniques, such as improved spatial resolution, accurate quantification, and use of biological isotopes of carbon, nitrogen and oxygen. However, it is expensive and requires a cyclotron to produce the short-lived tracers. PET/CT has become a useful investigation in the detection of viable myocardium in patients who are suitable for revascularization.

Myocardial perfusion and ischaemia can be determined using PET with ^{13}N-ammonia or ^{15}oxygen with greater sensitivity than SPECT. Myocardial metabolism and viability can be detected with the use of ^{18}F-fluorodeoxyglucose (FDG), which the cardiac myocyte utilizes for energy production in the presence of reduced oxygen supply and blood flow. There may be reduced perfusion to infarcted or fibrotic myocardium, but also reduced FDG uptake. In hibernating myocardium, with viable but dysfunctional myocardium, PET can demonstrate reduced myocardial perfusion but with preserved or increased FDG uptake.

Cardiac catheterization

Cardiac catheterization is the introduction of a thin radio-opaque tube (catheter) into the circulation. The right heart is catheterized by introducing the catheter into a peripheral vein (usually the right femoral or internal jugular vein) and advancing it through the right atrium and ventricle into the pulmonary artery. The pressures in the right heart chambers and in the pulmonary artery can be measured directly. An indirect measure of left atrial pressure can be obtained by 'wedging' a catheter into the distal pulmonary artery (see p. 1147). In this position, the pressure from the right ventricle is obstructed by the catheter, and only the pulmonary venous and left atrial pressures are recorded. Left heart catheterization is usually performed via the right femoral or radial artery. A pigtail catheter is advanced up the aorta and manipulated through the aortic valve into the left ventricle. Pressure tracings are taken from the left ventricular cavity. The end-diastolic pressure is invariably elevated in patients with left ventricular dysfunction. A power injection of radio-opaque contrast material is used to opacify the left ventricular cavity (left ventriculography) and thereby assesses left ventricular systolic function. The catheter is then withdrawn across the aortic valve into the aorta and the 'pullback' gradient across the valve is measured. Aortography (a power injection into the aortic root) can be performed to assess the aortic root and the presence and severity of aortic regurgitation. Specially designed catheters are then used to engage the left and right coronary arteries selectively, and contrast cine-angiograms are taken in order to define the coronary circulation and identify the presence and severity of any coronary artery disease. During the procedure, intracoronary nitrate or adenosine may be used to dilate the coronary arteries. During cardiac catheterization, blood samples may be withdrawn to measure the oxygen content. These estimations are used to quantify intracardiac shunts and measure cardiac output.

Further reading

Budoff MJ, Ashenbach S, Blumenthal RS et al. Assessment of coronary artery disease by cardiac computed tomography: a scientific statement from the American Heart Association Committee on Cardiovascular Imaging and Intervention, Council on Cardiovascular Radiology and Intervention, and Committee on Cardiac Imaging, Council on Clinical Cardiology. *Circulation* 2006; 114:1761–1791.

Grayburn PA. Interpreting the coronary-artery calcium score. *N Engl J Med* 2012; 366:294–296.

Hundley WG, Bluemke DA, Finn JP et al. and the American College of Cardiology Foundation Task Force on Expert Consensus Documents. ACCF/ACR/AHA/NASCI/SCMR 2010 expert consensus document on cardiovascular magnetic resonance: a report of the American College of Cardiology Foundation Task Force on Expert Consensus Documents. *Circulation* 2010; 121:2462–2508.

Hung J, Lang R, Flachskampf F et al. 3D echocardiography: a review of the current status and future directions. *J Am Soc Echocardiogr* 2007; 20:213–233.

Quinones MA, Otto CM, Stoddard M et al. Recommendations for quantification of Doppler echocardiography: a report from the Doppler Quantification Task Force of the Nomenclature and Standards Committee of the American Society of Echocardiography. *J Am Soc Echocardiogr* 2002; 15:167–184.

http://bsecho.org/toe-minimum-dataset/ *Minimum dataset for a standard transoesphageal echocardiogram; British Society of Echocardiography Education Committee.*

THERAPEUTIC PROCEDURES

Cardiac resuscitation

Each year in the UK, there are approximately 100 000 unexpected deaths occurring within 24 hours of the development of cardiac symptoms. About half of these deaths are almost instantaneous. Most deaths are due to ventricular fibrillation or rapid ventricular tachycardia; a small proportion are caused by severe bradyarrhythmias. Coronary artery disease accounts for approximately 80% of sudden cardiac deaths in Western society. Transient ischaemia is suspected of being the major trigger factor; however, only a small proportion of survivors have clinical evidence of acute myocardial infarction.

When cardiac arrest occurs, basic life support must be started immediately. The longer the period of respiratory and circulatory arrest, the lower is the chance of restoring healthy life. The chain of survival ***(Fig. 23.31)*** includes early recognition of cardiac arrest; early activation of emergency services; early cardiopulmonary

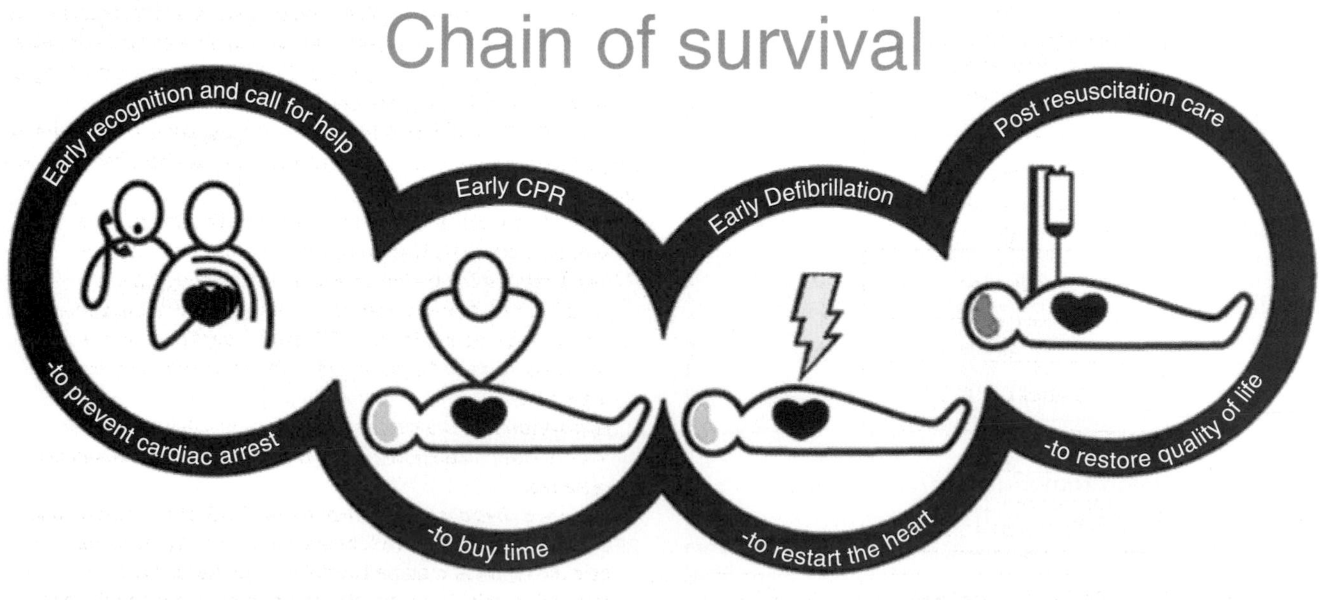

Figure 23.31 Cardiopulmonary resuscitation chain of survival.

resuscitation (CPR); early defibrillation and early advanced life support; and high-quality post-resuscitation care.

Basic life support

The first step in basic life support (BLS) is to ensure the safety of the victim and rescuer. The next is to ascertain that the victim is unresponsive by shaking him/her and shouting into one ear. If no response is obtained, help should be sought immediately prior to commencement of BLS. If the victim has absent or abnormal breathing, then cardiac arrest is confirmed and BLS should be started ***(Box 23.9)***.

Airway

Debris (e.g. blood and mucus) in the mouth and pharynx should be removed. Loose or ill-fitting dentures should be removed. The airway should be opened gently by flexing the neck and extending the head ('sniffing the morning air' position). This manœuvre is not recommended if a cervical spine injury is suspected. Any obstruction deep in the oral cavity or upper respiratory tract may need to be removed using abdominal and/or chest thrusts (Heimlich manœuvre; see p. 1078).

Circulation

Most adult cardiac arrest is due to a primary cardiac disorder, such as acute coronary syndrome, and results in circulatory collapse. Pulse detection can be difficult, and if the victim is unresponsive, with absent or abnormal breathing, external chest compression should be started immediately. The heel of one hand is placed over the centre of the patient's chest and the heel of the second hand is placed over the first with the fingers interlocked. The arms are kept straight and the sternum is rhythmically depressed by 5–6 cm at a rate of approximately 100–120 per minute, allowing for complete recoil between compressions. Chest compressions do not massage the heart. The thorax acts as a pump and the heart provides a system of one-way valves to ensure forward circulation. Respiratory and circulatory support is continued by providing two effective breaths for every 30 cardiac compressions (30 : 2 for one or two persons, 15 : 2 in paediatric patients). It is easier for the lay public to give compressions without interruption (hands only). This maintains adequate cerebral and coronary perfusion pressures. The initiation of CPR by the lay public at the site of the arrest saves lives. There is evidence to suggest that if the person performing compressions tires, the quality of resuscitation deteriorates. Mechanical CPR devices are available but not yet widely used.

Box 23.9 Adult basic life support (out of hospital)

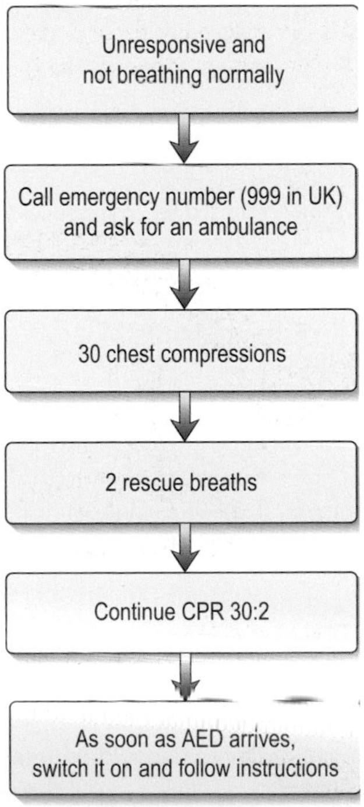
Unresponsive and
not breathing normally
Call emergency number (999 in UK)
and ask for an ambulance
30 chest compressions
2 rescue breaths
Continue CPR 30:2
As soon as AED arrives,
switch it on and follow instructions

(AED, automated external defibrillator; CPR, cardiopulmonary resuscitation. With permission from Resuscitation Council UK; http://www.resus.org.uk.)

Breathing

After 30 compressions, the rescuer opens the victim's airway by tilting the head backwards (***head tilt***) and pulling the chin forwards (***chin lift*** or ***jaw thrust***). The rescuer then pinches the victim's nostrils firmly, takes a deep breath, and seals his/her lips around the mouth of the victim. Two effective breaths are given, each over 1 second. In paediatric patients, respiratory arrests are more common and patients should be given rescue breaths and a minute of CPR before a sole rescuer leaves the victim to seek help. CPR should not be interrupted to re-assess the victim unless he/she starts to show signs of life and starts to breathe normally.

Advanced cardiac life support

By the time effective life support has been established, more help should have arrived and advanced cardiac life support (ACLS) can begin. This consists of ECG monitoring, advanced airway management (endotracheal intubation or supraglottic airway tube) and establishment of an intravenous infusion in a large peripheral or central vein (an intra-osseous needle may be used if intravenous access is not possible). As soon as possible, the cardiac rhythm should be established, as this determines which pathway of the European Resuscitation Council and the Resuscitation Council UK ACLS algorithm is followed ***(Fig. 23.32)***. This can be determined with an automated external defibrillator (AED), or the paddles or limb leads of a standard defibrillator.

If the ECG shows a shockable rhythm – ventricular fibrillation or pulseless ventricular tachycardia, then an unsynchronized shock of 150–200 J biphasic (360 J monophasic) is delivered without delay via paddles or self-adhesive pads, followed immediately by 2 minutes of CPR. For a non-shockable rhythm – asystole or pulseless electrical activity, 2 minutes of CPR is delivered with 1 mg of intravenous adrenaline (epinephrine).

For both sides of the algorithm, it is vital to maintain CPR, ensure oxygenation and exclude or treat reversible causes: the 'four Hs and four Ts':

- ***Hypoxia*** should be minimized by ventilating the patient with oxygen and a bag-valve mask or advanced airway (endotracheal intubation or supraglottic airway tube), ensuring that there is bilateral air entry and chest expansion. With an advanced airway, CPR should continue, with a ventilation rate of 10 per minute without interrupting cardiac massage.
- ***Hypovolaemia*** is a frequent cause of pulseless electrical activity due to haemorrhage. Intravenous volume should be replaced.
- ***Hyper- or hypokalaemia*** may cause ECG abnormalities and should be detected by biochemical testing. Intravenous calcium chloride may be helpful in hyperkalaemia or hypocalcaemia. Acidosis should be managed with effective ventilation.

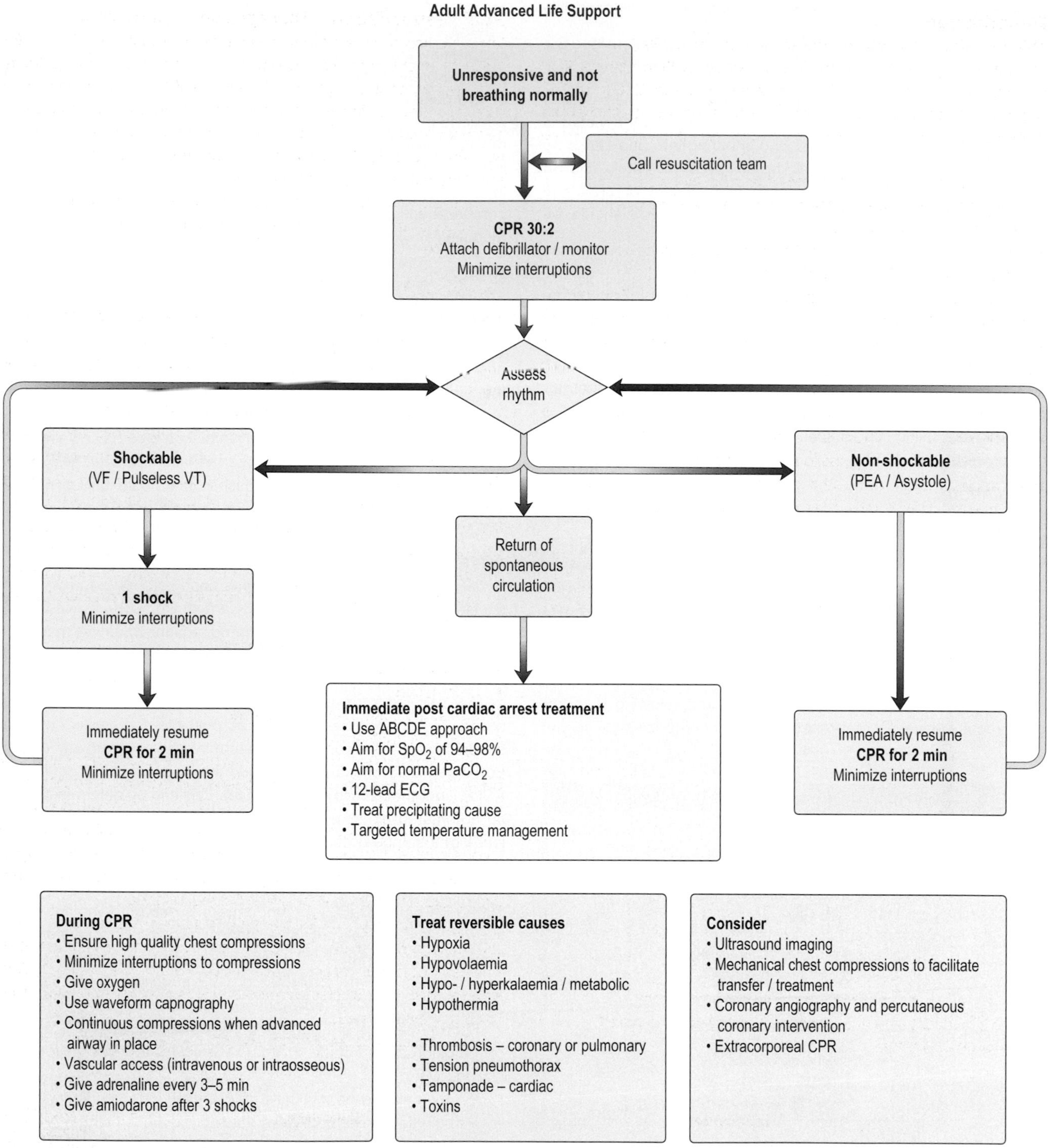

Figure 23.32 Adult advanced life support algorithm. ABCDE, Airway, Breathing, Circulation, Disability, Exposure; CPR, cardiopulmonary resuscitation; PEA, pulseless electrical activity; VF, ventricular fibrillation; VT, ventricular tachycardia. *(Reproduced with permission from the Resuscitation Council;* http://www.resus.org.uk.*)*

- ***Hypothermia*** should be excluded with a low-reading thermometer and treated with external or internal warming.
- ***Thromboembolism*** and massive pulmonary embolism may cause pulseless electrical activity and patients should be considered for intravenous thrombolysis.
- ***Tension pneumothorax*** may occur during central venous cannulation or following chest trauma. Clinical diagnosis (deviated trachea, hyper-resonant chest, absent breath sounds, ultrasound) and needle thoracocentesis or thoracostomy may be required.
- ***Tamponade*** should be excluded with echocardiography; if present, it should be treated with pericardiocentesis.
- ***Toxins*** may have been ingested by accident or deliberate self-harm, and specific antidotes should be used in appropriate patients.

Defibrillation

This technique is used to convert ventricular fibrillation to sinus rhythm. When the defibrillator is discharged, a high-voltage field envelops the heart, depolarizing the myocardium and allowing an organized heart rhythm to emerge. Electrical energy is discharged through two paddles with gel pads or adhesive pads placed on the chest wall.

The paddles are placed in one of two positions:

- One paddle is placed to the right of the upper sternum and the other over the cardiac apex.
- One paddle is placed under the tip of the left scapula and the other is over the anterior wall of the left chest.

All personnel should stand clear of the patient. The person performing defibrillation has the responsibility for ensuring the safety of the patient and of the other people present. Conventional defibrillators employ a damped monophasic waveform. Biphasic defibrillators, which require less energy, are increasingly common. AEDs, which recognize ventricular fibrillation automatically, deliver a shock if indicated. These are available in some public places (in the UK, their location is signalled by a specific sign; ***Fig. 23.33***). It is the responsibility of all healthcare practitioners to be familiar with the range of defibrillators they may be called on to use in their workplace.

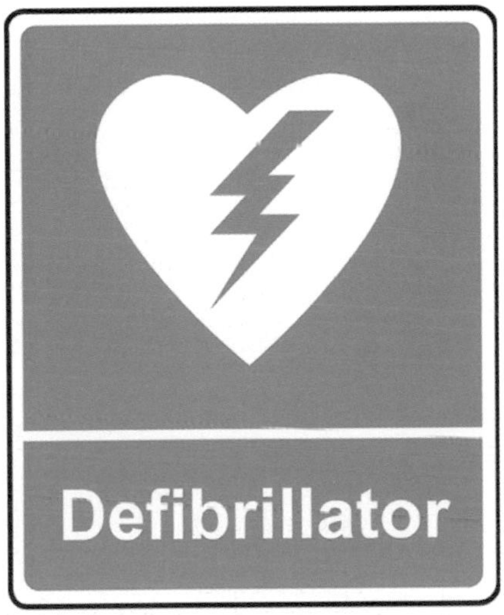

Figure 23.33 **UK sign indicating the location of automated external defibrillators.**

Post resuscitation – therapeutic hypothermia

Initial studies suggested that therapeutic hypothermia (32–34°C for 12–24h) might improve outcomes in unconscious adult patients with spontaneous circulation after an out-of-hospital cardiac arrest due to ventricular fibrillation. However a recent multinational study demonstrated a similar improvement in outcome with therapeutic hypothermia at 33°C, compared to a targeted temperature of 36°C; thus, the value of hypothermia is unclear.

Neurological recovery appears to be more favourable in patients with purposeful movements and EEG activity within 3days of a cardiac arrest.

Direct current cardioversion

Tachyarrhythmias that do not respond to medical treatment or that are associated with haemodynamic compromise (e.g. hypotension, worsening heart failure) may be converted to sinus rhythm by the use of a transthoracic electric shock. A short-acting general anaesthetic is used. Muscle relaxants are not usually given.

When the arrhythmia has definite QRS complexes, the delivery of the shock should be timed to coincide with the downstroke of the QRS complex (synchronization) ***(Fig. 23.34)***. The machine being used to perform the direct current cardioversion (DCC) will do this automatically if the appropriate button is pressed. There is a crucial difference between defibrillation and cardioversion: a non-synchronized shock is used to defibrillate. Accidental defibrillation of a patient who does not require it may itself precipitate ventricular fibrillation.

Typical indications for DCC include:

- atrial fibrillation
- atrial flutter
- sustained ventricular tachycardia
- junctional tachyarrhythmias.

If atrial fibrillation or flutter has been present for more than a few days, it is necessary to anticoagulate the patient adequately for 3weeks before elective cardioversion to reduce the risk of embolization. The duration of anticoagulation after successful cardioversion for atrial fibrillation is a complex issue and depends on a number of factors: it should be given for at least 4weeks after the procedure and may well be given for much longer.

Digoxin toxicity may lead to ventricular arrhythmias or asystole following cardioversion. Therapeutic digitalization does not increase the risks of cardioversion, but it is conventional to omit digoxin several days prior to elective cardioversion in order to be sure that toxicity is not present.

Cardiac enzyme levels may rise after a cardioversion.

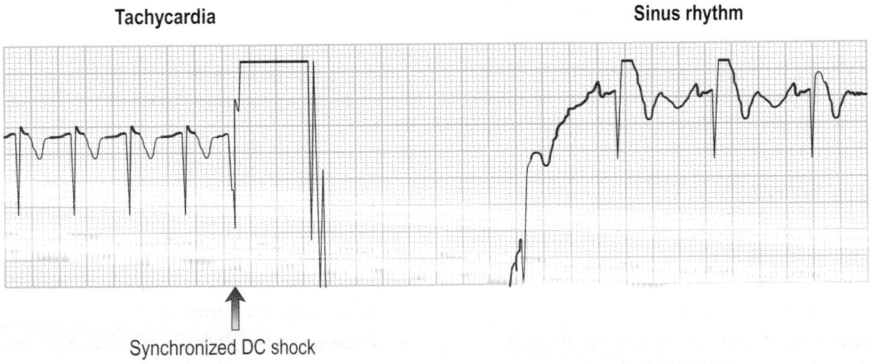

Figure 23.34 **Direct current (DC) cardioversion of a supraventricular tachycardia to sinus rhythm.** The direct current shock is delivered synchronously with the QRS complex.

Temporary pacing

Therapeutic cardiac pacing is employed in any patient with sustained symptomatic or haemodynamically compromising bradycardia. Bradycardias may be due to either a slow intrinsic heart rate (e.g. sinus node dysfunction) or AV block. Prophylactic cardiac pacing is employed in asymptomatic patients with either bradycardia or conduction abnormalities, in whom the risk of progression to symptomatic bradycardia justifies such a strategy.

Transvenous pacing is the preferred method in patients with symptomatic bradycardias. In summary, a thin (French gauge 5 or 6), bipolar pacing electrode wire is inserted via an internal jugular vein, a femoral vein or a subclavian vein and is positioned at the right ventricular apex using cardiac fluoroscopy. The energy needed for successful pacing (the pacing threshold) is assessed by reducing the energy until the pacemaker fails to stimulate the tissue (loss of capture). The output energy is then set at three times the threshold value to prevent inadvertent loss of capture. If the threshold increases above 5V, the pacemaker wire should be resited. A temporary pacemaker unit ***(Fig. 23.35A)*** is almost always set to work 'on demand' – to fire only when a spontaneous beat has not occurred. The rate of temporary pacing is usually 60–80 per minute.

Transcutaneous pacing is the preferred method in selected patients with asymptomatic bradycardia or conduction abnormalities, and may be life-saving when a cardiac arrest is precipitated by bradycardia. In this method, the myocardium is depolarized by current flow between two large adhesive electrodes positioned anteriorly and posteriorly on the chest wall. Transcutaneous pacing is uncomfortable for the conscious patient. However, it can usually be tolerated until a temporary transvenous pacemaker is inserted.

Permanent pacing

Permanent pacemakers are fully implanted in the body and connected to the heart by one or two electrode leads (***Fig. 23.35B***). The pacemaker is powered by solid-state lithium batteries, which usually last 5–10 years. Pacemakers are 'programmable', in that their operating characteristics (e.g. the pacing rate) can be changed by a programmer that transmits specific electromagnetic signals through the skin. The pacemaker leads are passed transvenously to the right heart chambers. Leadless pacemakers are in trials.

Pacemakers are designed both to pace and to sense either the ventricles, the atria or, more commonly, both chambers. A single-chamber ventricular pacemaker is described as a 'VVI' unit because it paces the ventricle (V), senses the ventricle (V) and is inhibited (I) by a spontaneous ventricular signal. Occasionally (e.g. in symptomatic sinus bradycardia), an atrial pacemaker (AAI) may be implanted. Pacemakers that are connected to both the right atrium and ventricle ('dual-chamber' pacemakers) are used to simulate the natural pacemaker and activation sequence of the heart. This form of pacemaker is called DDD because it paces the two (dual) chambers, senses both (D) and reacts in two (D) ways: pacing in the same chamber is inhibited by spontaneous atrial and ventricular signals, and ventricular pacing is triggered by spontaneous atrial events ***(Fig. 23.35C)***.

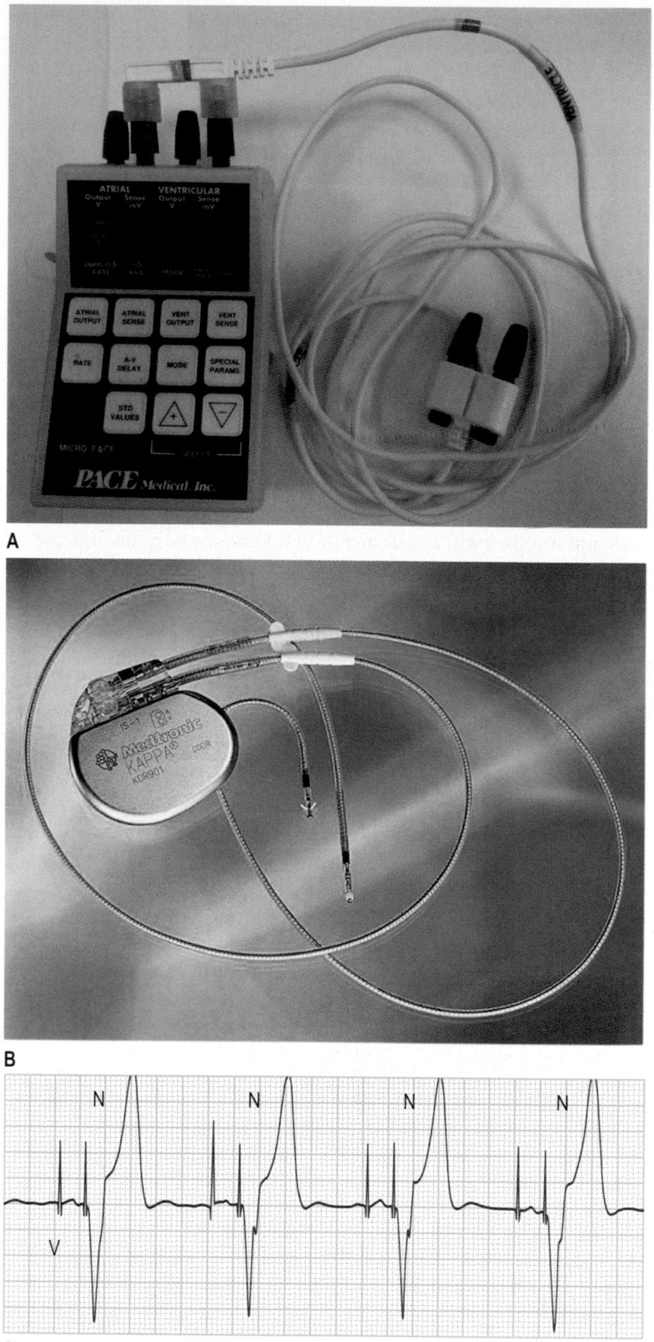

A

B

C

Figure 23.35 Pacemakers. A. A temporary pacemaker unit. **B.** A permanent pacemaker with atrial (placed in the right atrium, usually in its high lateral wall) and ventricular (placed in the right ventricular apex) leads. **C.** An electrocardiogram showing dual (atrial and ventricular) chamber pacing. A wide QRS complex results from abnormal activation of the ventricles from the right ventricular apex.

In addition, pacemakers may be 'rate-responsive' (R). A rate-responsive pacemaker detects motion (level of vibration or acceleration), respiration or changes in QT interval; by employing one or more biosensors, it changes its rate of pacing so that it is appropriate to the level of exertion.

The choice of pacemaker mostly depends on the underlying rhythm abnormality and the general condition of the patient. For example, complete heart block in patients with sinus rhythm should be treated with a dual-chamber device in order to maintain AV synchrony, whereas inactive or infirm patients may not benefit from the most sophisticated units. Specialized biventricular pacemakers are used for the treatment of severe heart failure.

Permanent pacemakers are inserted under local anaesthetic using fluoroscopy to guide the insertion of the electrode leads via the cephalic or subclavian veins. Perioperative prophylactic antibiotics are routinely prescribed. The pacemaker is usually positioned subcutaneously in front of the pectoral muscle. Following surgery, which usually takes 60–90 minutes, the patient rests in bed for 6–12 hours before being discharged. Patients may not drive for at least 1 week after implantation, and must inform the licensing authorities and their motor insurers.

Complications are few but can prove to be very difficult to manage, and patients should be referred to the pacemaker clinic. They include the following:

- infection
- erosion
- pocket haematoma
- lead displacement
- electromagnetic interference.

Pericardiocentesis

A pericardial effusion is an accumulation of fluid between the parietal and visceral layers of pericardium. Fluid is removed for relief of symptoms that are due to haemodynamic embarrassment or for diagnostic purposes. This can be a technically difficult procedure, particularly in the acute setting, and should be performed in a cardiac laboratory. In an emergency, it can be performed at the bedside.

Pericardial aspiration or pericardiocentesis ***(Fig. 23.36)*** is performed by inserting a needle into the pericardial space, usually via a sub-xiphisternal route under ultrasound guidance. Certain effusions, particularly posterior ones, require surgical drainage under a general anaesthetic. If a large volume of fluid is to be removed, a wide-bore needle and cannula are inserted. The needle may be removed and the cannula left *in situ* to drain the fluid. Fluid that is removed is sent for chemical analysis, microscopy, including cytology, Gram stain and culture. If a re-accumulation of pericardial fluid is anticipated, the cannula may be left in place for several days, or an operation can be performed to cut a window in the parietal pericardium (fenestration) or to remove a large section of the pericardium.

Right-heart bedside catheterization

Bedside catheterization (see ***Fig. 25.14***) of the pulmonary artery with a pulmonary artery balloon flotation catheter (Swan–Ganz catheter) is performed in patients with:

- cardiac failure
- cardiogenic shock
- doubtful fluid status.

Intra-aortic balloon pumping

This technique is used to assist the failing left ventricle temporarily. A catheter with a long sausage-shaped balloon at its tip is introduced percutaneously into the femoral artery and manipulated under X-ray control so that the balloon lies in the descending aorta just below the aortic arch ***(Fig. 23.37)***. The balloon is rhythmically deflated and inflated with carbon dioxide gas. Using the ECG or intra-aortic pressure changes, the inflation is timed to occur during ventricular diastole to increase diastolic aortic pressure and, consequently, to improve coronary and cerebral blood flow. During systole, the balloon is deflated, resulting in a reduction in the

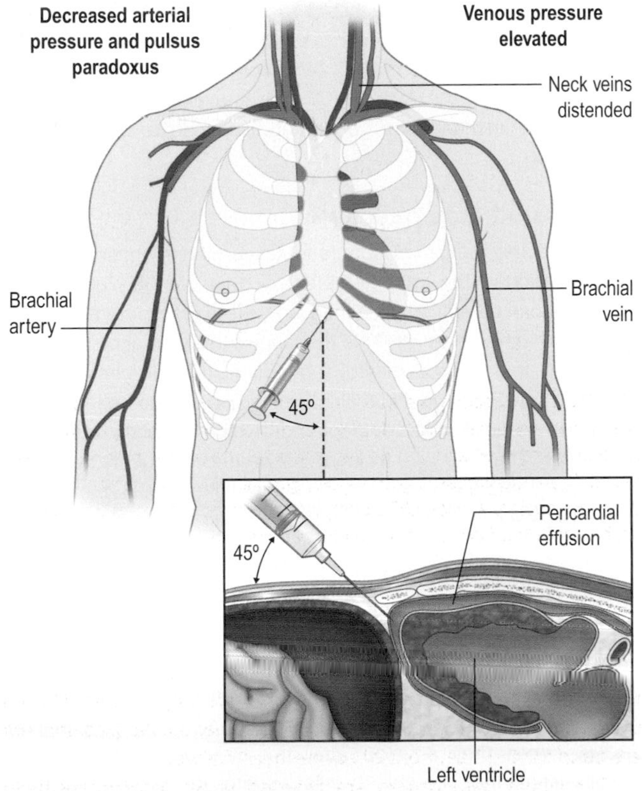

Figure 23.36 **Pericardiocentesis.**

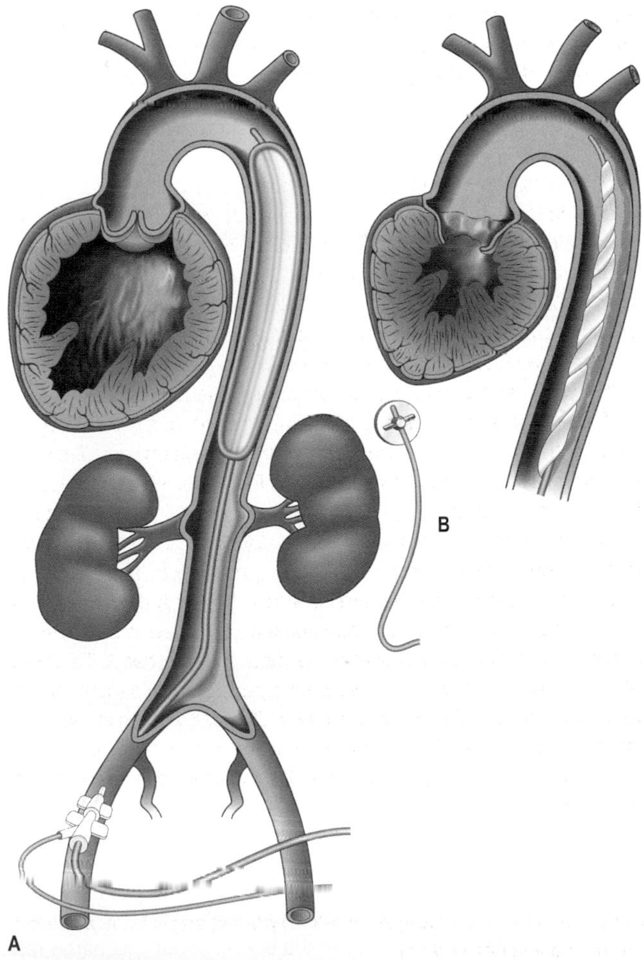

Figure 23.37 **Intra-aortic balloon pump. A.** The pump is inflated in the aorta. **B.** The balloon is deflated.

resistance to left ventricular emptying. Intra-aortic balloon pumping is used for circulatory support in the following acute situations:

- ***Acute heart failure***. Balloon pumping is employed to improve cardiac output when there is a transient or reversible depression of left ventricular function, such as in a patient with severe mitral valve regurgitation who is awaiting surgical replacement of the mitral valve, or in a patient with a ventricular septal defect that is due to septal infarction. It may also be used to support patients awaiting heart transplantation.
- ***Unstable angina pectoris***. Balloon pumping is utilized to treat unstable angina pectoris by improving coronary flow and decreasing myocardial oxygen consumption by reducing the 'afterload'. This technique may be successful, even when medical therapy has failed. It is followed by early angiography and appropriate definitive therapy, such as surgery or coronary angioplasty.

Balloon pumping should not be used when there is no remediable cause of cardiac dysfunction. It is also unsuitable in patients with severe aortic regurgitation, aortic dissection and severe peripheral vascular disease.

Complications of balloon pumping occur in about 20% of patients and include aortic dissection, leg ischaemia, emboli from the balloon, and balloon rupture. Embolic complications are reduced by anticoagulation with heparin.

Further reading

Nielsen N, Wettersley J, Cronberg T et al. Targeted temperature management at 33°C versus 36°C after cardiac arrest. *N Engl J Med* 2013; 369:2197–2206.

Various authors. American Heart Association guidelines for cardiopulmonary resuscitation and emergency cardiovascular care. *Circulation* 2010; 122(Suppl 3):S640–933.

http://www.resus.org.uk *Resuscitation Council (UK) Resuscitation Guidelines 2010.*

CARDIAC ARRHYTHMIAS

An abnormality of the cardiac rhythm is called a cardiac arrhythmia. Arrhythmias may cause sudden death, syncope, heart failure, chest pain, dizziness, palpitations or no symptoms at all. There are two main types of arrhythmia:

- ***Bradycardia***: the heart rate is slow (<60 b.p.m. during the day or <50 b.p.m. at night).
- ***Tachycardia***: the heart rate is fast (>100 b.p.m.).

Tachycardias are more symptomatic when the arrhythmia is fast and sustained. Tachycardias are subdivided into supraventricular tachycardias, which arise from the atrium or the AV junction, and ventricular tachycardias, which arise from the ventricles.

Some arrhythmias occur in patients with apparently normal hearts; in others, arrhythmias originate from diseased tissue, such as scar, as a result of underlying structural heart disease. When myocardial function is poor, arrhythmias are more symptomatic and are potentially life-threatening.

Sinus node function

The normal cardiac pacemaker is the sinus node (see p. 933) and, like most cardiac tissue, it depolarizes spontaneously.

The rate of sinus node discharge is modulated by the autonomic nervous system. Normally, the parasympathetic system predominates, resulting in slowing of the spontaneous discharge rate from approximately 100 to 70 b.p.m. A reduction of parasympathetic tone or an increase in sympathetic stimulation leads to tachycardia; conversely, increased parasympathetic tone or decreased sympathetic stimulation produces bradycardia. The sinus rate in women is slightly faster than in men. Normal sinus rhythm is characterized by P waves that are upright in leads I and II of the ECG (see ***Fig. 23.18***), but inverted in the cavity leads AVR and V_1 ***(Fig. 23.38)***.

Sinus arrhythmia

Fluctuations of autonomic tone result in phasic changes of the sinus discharge rate. During inspiration, parasympathetic tone falls and the heart rate quickens; on expiration, the heart rate falls. This variation is normal, particularly in children and young adults. Typically, sinus arrhythmia results in predictable irregularities of the pulse.

Sinus bradycardia

A sinus rate of <60 b.p.m. during the day or <50 b.p.m. at night is known as sinus bradycardia. It is usually asymptomatic unless the rate is very slow. Sinus bradycardia is normal in athletes owing to increased vagal tone. Other causes may be divided into systemic or cardiac, and are discussed below in the section entitled 'Bradycardias and heart block' (see pp. 964–968).

Sinus tachycardia

Sinus rate acceleration to >100 b.p.m. is known as sinus tachycardia. Again, causes may be divided into systemic or cardiac, and are discussed below in the section entitled 'Supraventricular tachycardias' (see pp. 968–973).

Mechanisms of arrhythmia production

Abnormalities of automaticity, which could arise from a single cell, and abnormalities of conduction, which require abnormal interaction between cells, account for both bradycardia and tachycardia. Sinus bradycardia is a result of abnormally slow automaticity while bradycardia due to AV block is caused by abnormal conduction within the AV node or the intraventricular conduction system. The mechanisms generating tachycardia are shown in ***Figure 23.39***.

Accelerated automaticity

The normal mechanism of spontaneous cardiac rhythmicity is slow depolarization of the transmembrane voltage during diastole until the threshold potential is reached and the action potential of the pacemaker cells takes off. This mechanism may be accelerated by increasing the rate of diastolic depolarization or changing the threshold potential ***(Fig. 23.39A)***. For example, sympathetic stimulation releases adrenaline (epinephrine), which enhances automaticity. Such changes are thought to produce sinus tachycardia, escape rhythms and accelerated AV nodal (junctional) rhythms.

Triggered activity

Myocardial damage can result in oscillations of the transmembrane potential at the end of the action potential. These oscillations, which are called 'after-depolarizations', may reach threshold potential and produce an arrhythmia. If they occur before the transmembrane potential reaches its threshold (at the end of phase 3 of the action potential), they are called 'early after-depolarizations' (E in ***Fig. 23.39B***). When they develop after the transmembrane potential is completed, they are called 'delayed after-depolarizations' (D in ***Fig. 23.39B***).

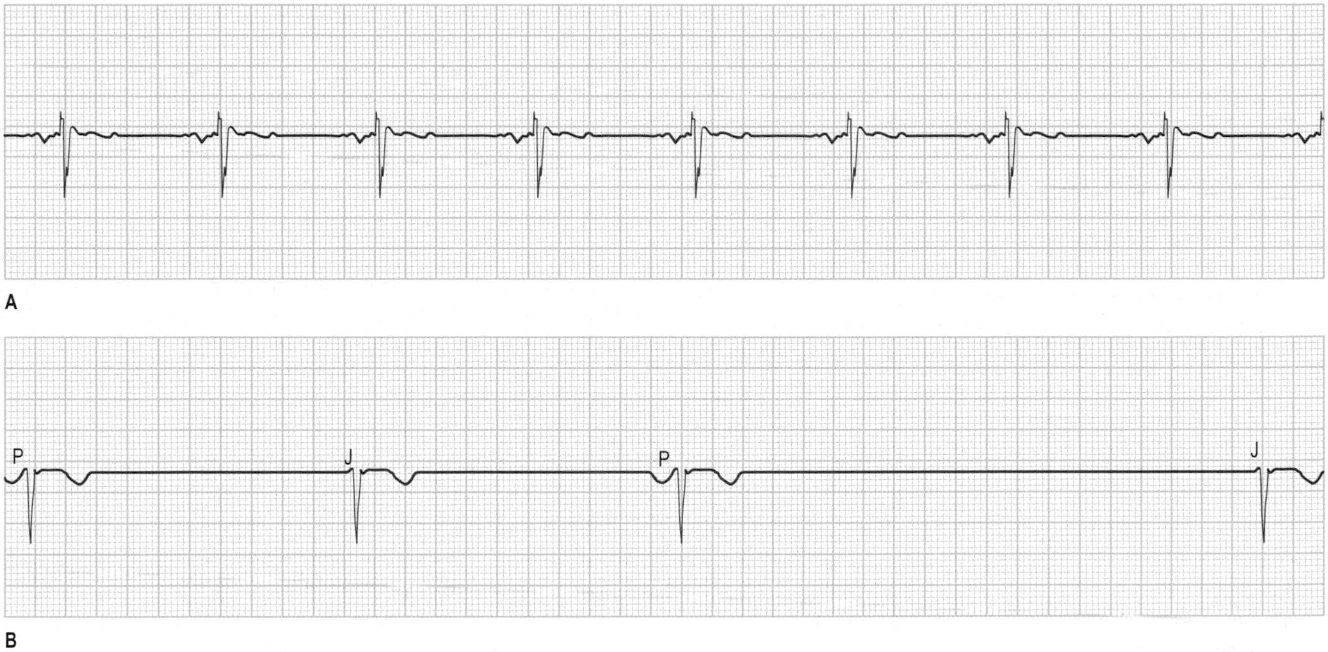

Figure 23.38 **Sinus node. A.** An ECG showing *normal sinus rhythm* (PR interval <0.2 s). A P wave precedes each QRS complex. **B.** A patient with *sick sinus syndrome*. The ECG shows sinus arrest (only occasional sinus P waves) and junctional escape beats (J). P waves are inverted in the cavity loads that are shown here.

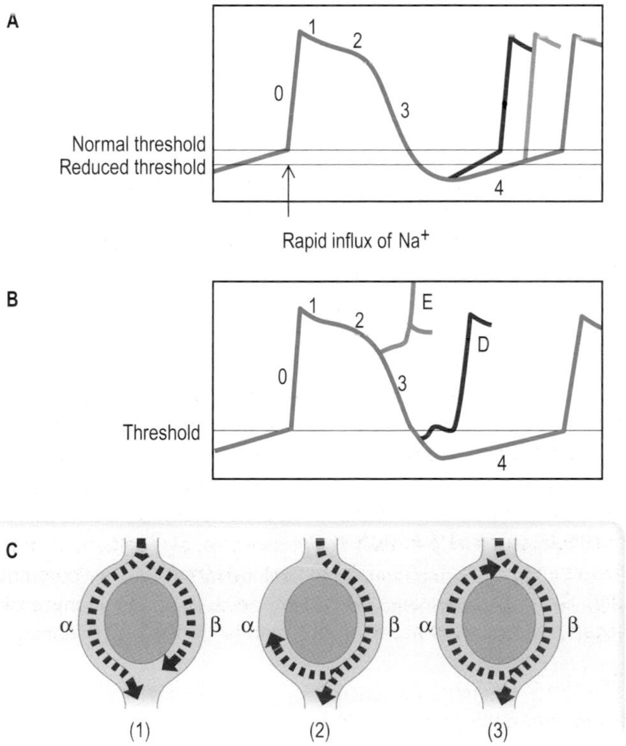

Figure 23.39 **Mechanisms of arrhythmogenesis. A–B.** *Action potentials* (i.e. the potential difference between intracellular and extracellular fluid) of ventricular myocardium after stimulation. **A.** Increased (accelerated) automaticity due to reduced threshold potential or an increased slope of phase 4 depolarization (see pp. 944–945). **B.** Triggered activity due to early (E) or delayed (D) 'after-depolarizations' reaching threshold potential. **C.** *Mechanism of circus movement or re-entry*. In panel (**1**) the impulse passes down both limbs of the potential tachycardia circuit. In panel (**2**) the impulse is blocked in one pathway (α) but proceeds slowly down pathway β, returning along pathway α until it collides with refractory tissue. In panel (**3**) the impulse travels so slowly along pathway β that it can return along pathway α and complete the re-entry circuit, producing a circus movement tachycardia.

The abnormal oscillations can be exaggerated by pacing, catecholamines, electrolyte disturbances, hypoxia, acidosis and some medications, which may then trigger an arrhythmia. The atrial tachycardias produced by digoxin toxicity are due to triggered activity. The initiation of ventricular arrhythmia in the long QT syndrome (see p. 975) may be caused by this mechanism.

Re-entry (or circus movements)

The mechanism of re-entry (***Fig. 23.39C***) occurs when a 'ring' of cardiac tissue surrounds an inexcitable core (e.g. in a region of scarred myocardium). Tachycardia is initiated if an ectopic beat finds one limb refractory (α), resulting in unidirectional block, and the other limb excitable. Provided conduction through the excitable limb (β) is slow enough, the other limb (α) will have recovered and will allow retrograde activation to complete the re-entry loop. If the time to conduct around the ring is longer than the recovery times (refractory periods) of the tissue within the ring, circus movement will be maintained, producing a run of tachycardia. The majority of regular paroxysmal tachycardias are produced by this mechanism.

BRADYCARDIAS AND HEART BLOCK

Bradycardias may be due to failure of impulse formation (sinus bradycardia) or failure of impulse conduction from the atria to the ventricles (atrioventricular block).

Bradycardia

Sinus bradycardia

Sinus bradycardia is due to extrinsic factors that influence a relatively normal sinus node, or due to intrinsic sinus node disease. The mechanism can be acute and reversible, or chronic and degenerative.

Common ***extrinsic causes*** of sinus bradycardia include:

- hypothermia, hypothyroidism, cholestatic jaundice and raised intracranial pressure
- drug therapy with beta-blockers, digitalis and other antiarrhythmic drugs
- neurally mediated syndromes (see below).

Common ***intrinsic causes*** include:

- acute ischaemia and infarction of the sinus node (as a complication of acute myocardial infarction)
- chronic degenerative changes, such as fibrosis of the atrium and sinus node (sick sinus syndrome).

Sick sinus syndrome or ***sinoatrial disease*** is usually caused by idiopathic fibrosis of the sinus node. Other causes of fibrosis, such as ischaemic heart disease, cardiomyopathy or myocarditis, can also cause the syndrome. Patients develop episodes of sinus bradycardia or sinus arrest (see ***Fig. 23.38B***), and commonly experience paroxysmal atrial tachyarrhythmias (tachy–brady syndrome) owing to diffuse atrial disease.

Neurally mediated syndromes

Neurally mediated syndromes are due to a reflex (called Bezold–Jarisch) that may result in both bradycardia (sinus bradycardia, sinus arrest and AV block) and reflex peripheral vasodilatation. These syndromes usually present as syncope or pre-syncope (dizzy spells).

- ***Carotid sinus syndrome*** occurs in the elderly and mainly leads to bradycardia. Syncope occurs (see p. 940).
- ***Neurocardiogenic (vasovagal) syncope (syndrome)*** usually presents in young adults but may present for the first time in elderly patients (see pp. 939–940). It results from a variety of situations (physical and emotional) that affect the autonomic nervous system. The efferent output may be predominantly bradycardic, predominantly vasodilatory or mixed.
- ***Postural orthostatic tachycardia syndrome (POTS)*** is a sudden and significant increase in heart rate associated with normal or mildly reduced blood pressure and produced by standing. The underlying mechanism is a failure of the peripheral vasculature to constrict appropriately in response to orthostatic stress, which is compensated by an excessive increase in heart rate.

Many medications, such as antihypertensives, tricyclic antidepressants and neuroleptics, can be the cause of syncope, particularly in the elderly. Careful dose titration and avoidance of combining two agents with the potential to cause syncope help to prevent iatrogenic syncope.

Management

The management of sinus bradycardia is first to identify and then, if possible, to remove any extrinsic causes. Temporary pacing may be employed in patients with reversible causes until a normal sinus rate is restored, and in patients with chronic degenerative conditions until a permanent pacemaker is implanted.

Chronic symptomatic sick sinus syndrome requires permanent pacing (DDD), with additional antiarrhythmic drugs (or ablation therapy) to manage any tachycardic element. Thromboembolism is common in tachy–brady syndrome and patients should be anticoagulated unless there is a contraindication.

Patients with carotid sinus hypersensitivity (asystole >3 s), especially if symptoms are reproduced by carotid sinus massage, and in whom life-threatening causes of syncope have been excluded, benefit from pacemaker implantation.

Treatment options in vasovagal attacks include avoidance, if possible, of situations known to cause syncope in a particular patient, and sitting/lying down and applying counter-pressure manœuvres (pushing the palms together or crossing the legs) if an attack threatens. Increased salt intake, compression of the lower legs with hose, and drugs such as beta-blockers, alpha-agonists (e.g. midodrine) or myocardial negative inotropes (e.g. disopyramide) may be helpful.

In selected patients with 'malignant' neurocardiogenic syncope (syncope associated with injuries and demonstrated asystole), permanent pacemaker therapy is helpful. These patients benefit from dual-chamber pacemakers with a feature called 'rate drop response', which, once activated, paces the heart at a fast rate for a set period of time in order to prevent syncope.

Heart block

Heart block or conduction block may occur at any level in the conducting system. Block in either the AV node or the His bundle results in AV block, whereas block lower in the conduction system produces bundle branch block.

Atrioventricular block

There are three forms.

First-degree AV block

This is simple prolongation of the PR interval to >0.22 s. Every atrial depolarization is followed by conduction to the ventricles but with delay ***(Fig. 23.40)***.

Second-degree AV block

This occurs when some P waves conduct and others do not. There are several forms ***(Fig. 23.41)***:

- ***Mobitz I block*** (Wenckebach block phenomenon) is progressive PR interval prolongation until a P wave fails to conduct. The PR interval before the blocked P wave is much longer than the PR interval after the blocked P wave.
- ***Mobitz II block*** occurs when a dropped QRS complex is not preceded by progressive PR interval prolongation. Usually, the QRS complex is wide (>0.12 s).

- ***2:1 or 3:1 (advanced) block*** occurs when every second or third P wave conducts to the ventricles. This form of second-degree block is neither Mobitz I nor II.

Wenckebach AV block in general is due to block in the AV node, whereas Mobitz II block signifies block at an infra-nodal level, such as the His bundle. The risk of progression to complete heart block is greater and the reliability of the resultant escape rhythm is less with Mobitz II block. Therefore, pacing is usually indicated in Mobitz II block, whereas patients with Wenckebach AV block are usually monitored.

Acute myocardial infarction may produce ***second-degree heart block***. In inferior myocardial infarction, close monitoring and transcutaneous temporary back-up pacing are all that is required. In anterior myocardial infarction, second-degree heart block is associated with a high risk of progression to complete heart block, and temporary pacing followed by permanent pacemaker implantation is usually indicated. Block either in the AV node or at an infra-nodal level may cause 2:1 heart block. Management depends on the clinical setting in which it occurs.

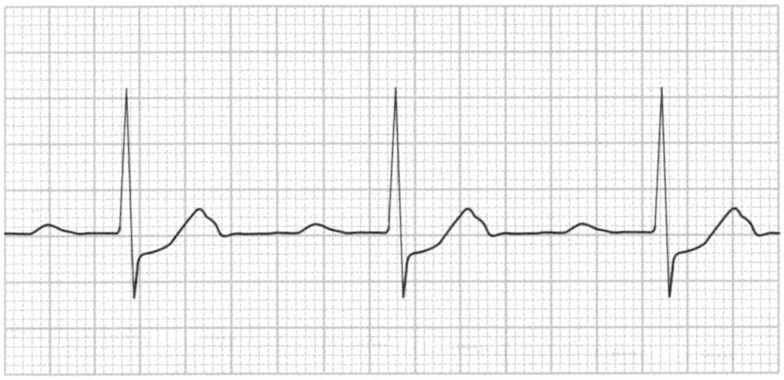

Figure 23.40 An ECG showing first-degree atrioventricular block with a prolonged PR interval. In this trace, coincidental ST depression is also present.

Third-degree (complete) AV block

Complete heart block occurs when all atrial activity fails to conduct to the ventricles ***(Fig. 23.42)***. In patients with complete heart block, the aetiology needs to be established ***(Box 23.10)***. In this situation, life is maintained by a spontaneous escape rhythm.

Narrow-complex escape rhythm (<0.12 s QRS complex) implies that it originates in the His bundle and therefore that the region of block lies more proximally in the AV node. The escape rhythm occurs with an adequate rate (50–60 b.p.m.) and is relatively reliable. Treatment depends on the aetiology. Recent-onset, narrow-complex AV block that has transient causes may respond to intravenous atropine, but temporary pacing facilities should be

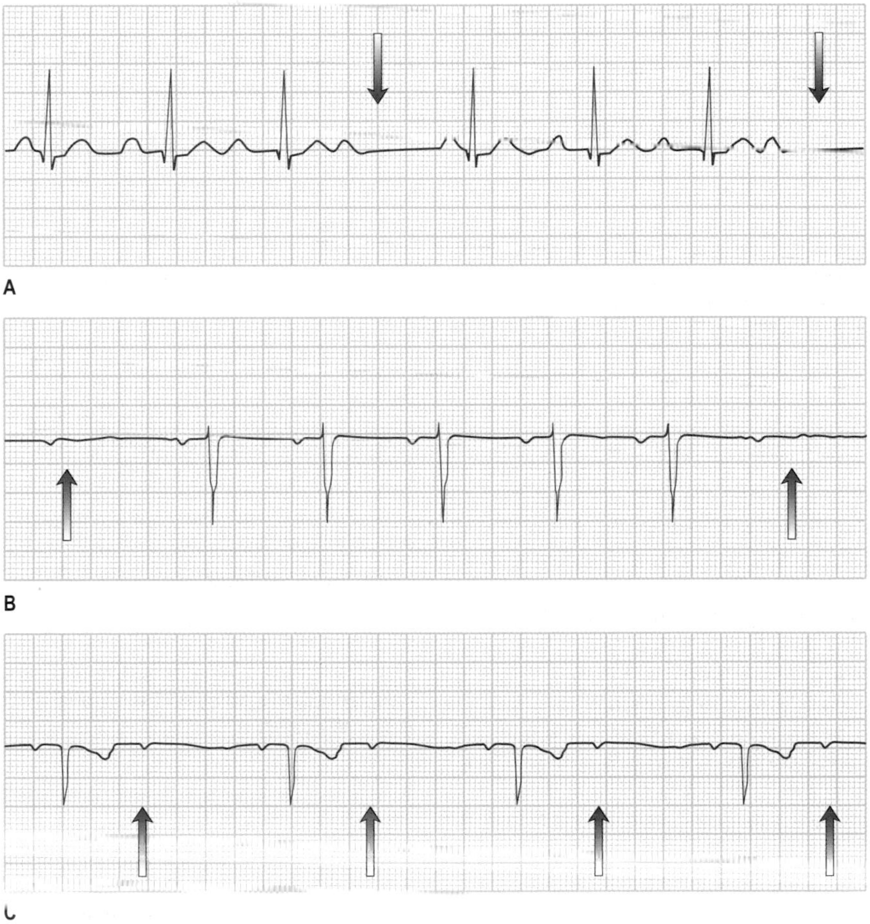

Figure 23.41 Three varieties of second-degree atrioventricular (AV) block. A. *Wenckebach (Mobitz type I) AV block*. The PR interval gradually prolongs until the P wave does not conduct to the ventricles (arrowed). **B.** *Mobitz type II AV block*. The P waves that do not conduct to the ventricles (arrowed) are not preceded by gradual PR interval prolongation. **C.** *Two P waves to each QRS complex*. The PR interval prior to the dropped P wave is always the same. It is not possible to define this type of AV block as type I or type II Mobitz block and it is, therefore, a third variety of second-degree AV block (arrows show P waves).

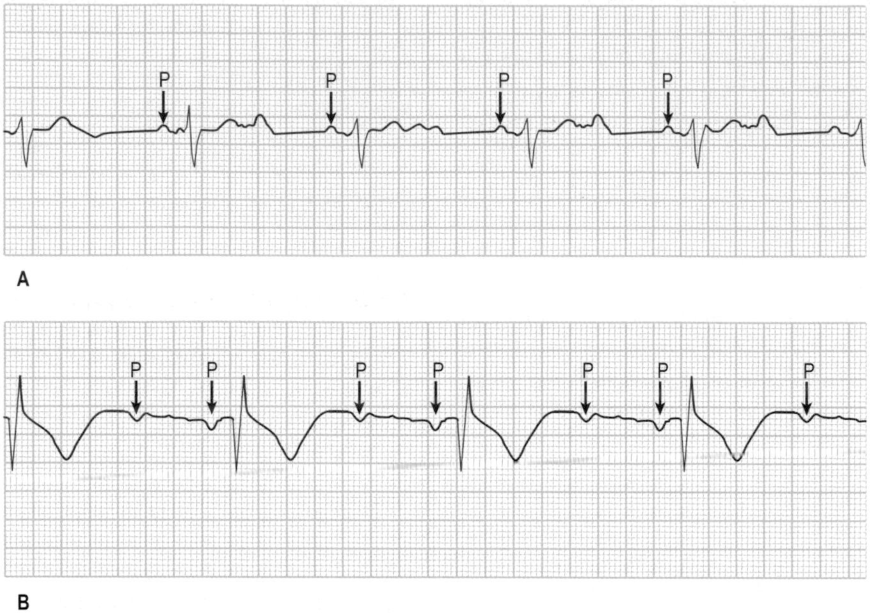

Figure 23.42 Two examples of complete heart block. **A.** *Congenital complete heart block.* The QRS complex is narrow (0.08 s) and the QRS rate is relatively rapid (52/min). **B.** *Acquired complete heart block.* The QRS complex is broad (0.13 s) and the QRS rate is relatively slow (38/min).

Box 23.10 Causes of complete heart block

Congenital
- Autoimmune (e.g. maternal SLE)
- Structural heart disease (e.g. transposition of great vessels)

Idiopathic fibrosis
- Lev's disease (progressive fibrosis of distal His–Purkinje system in elderly patients)
- Lenegre's disease (proximal His–Purkinje fibrosis in younger patients)

Ischaemic heart disease
- Acute myocardial infarct
- Ischaemic cardiomyopathy

Non-ischaemic heart disease
- Calcific aortic stenosis
- Idiopathic dilated cardiomyopathy
- Infiltrations (e.g. amyloidosis, sarcoidosis, neoplasia)

Cardiac surgery
- e.g. Following aortic valve replacement, CABG, VSD repair

Iatrogenic
- Radiofrequency AV node ablation and pacemaker implantation

Drug-induced
- e.g. Digoxin, beta-blockers, non-dihydropyridine calcium-channel blockers, amiodarone

Infections
- Endocarditis
- Lyme disease
- Chagas' disease

Autoimmune rheumatic disease
- e.g. SLE, rheumatoid arthritis

Neuromuscular diseases
- e.g. Duchenne muscular dystrophy

AV, atrioventricular; CABG, coronary artery bypass graft surgery; SLE, systemic lupus erythematosus; VSD, ventricular septal defect.

available for the management of these patients. Chronic narrow-complex AV block requires permanent pacing (dual-chamber; see p. 960) if it is symptomatic or associated with heart disease. Pacing is also advocated for isolated, congenital AV block, even if asymptomatic.

Broad-complex escape rhythm (>0.12 s) implies that the escape rhythm originates below the His bundle and therefore that the region of block lies more distally in the His–Purkinje system. The resulting rhythm is slow (15–40 b.p.m.) and relatively unreliable. Dizziness and blackouts (***Stokes–Adams attacks***) often occur. In the elderly, it is usually caused by degenerative fibrosis and calcification of the distal conduction system (***Lev's disease***). In younger individuals, a proximal progressive cardiac conduction disease due to the inflammatory process is known as ***Lenegre's disease***. Sodium channel abnormalities have been identified in both syndromes. Broad-complex AV block may also be caused by ischaemic heart disease, myocarditis or cardiomyopathy. Permanent pacemaker implantation (see pp. 960–961) is indicated, as pacing considerably reduces the mortality. Because ventricular arrhythmias are not uncommon, an implantable cardioverter–defibrillator (ICD) may be indicated in those with severe left ventricular dysfunction (>0.30 s duration).

Bundle branch block

The His bundle gives rise to the right and left bundle branches. The left bundle subdivides into the anterior and posterior divisions of the left bundle. Various conduction disturbances can occur.

Bundle branch conduction delay

This produces slight widening of the QRS complex (up to 0.11 s). It is known as incomplete bundle branch block.

Complete block of a bundle branch

This is associated with a wider QRS complex (≥0.12 s). The shape of the QRS depends on whether the right or the left bundle is blocked.

Right bundle branch block (Fig. 23.43A) produces late activation of the right ventricle. This is seen as deep S waves in leads I and V_6, and as a tall late R wave in lead V_1 (late activation moving towards right-sided leads and away from left-sided leads).

Left bundle branch block (Fig. 23.44) produces the opposite: a deep S wave in lead V_1 and a tall late R wave in leads I and V_6. Because left bundle branch conduction is normally responsible for the initial ventricular activation, left bundle branch block also produces abnormal Q waves.

Hemiblock

Delay or block in the divisions of the left bundle branch produces a swing in the direction of depolarization (electrical axis) of the heart. When the anterior division is blocked (left anterior hemiblock), the left ventricle is activated from inferior to superior. This produces a superior and leftward movement of the axis (left axis deviation).

Delay or block in the postero-inferior division swings the QRS axis inferiorly to the right (right axis deviation).

Bifascicular block

Bifascicular block (see ***Fig. 23.43B***) is a combination of a block of any two of the following: the right bundle branch, the left antero-superior division and the left postero-inferior division. Block of the remaining fascicle will result in complete AV block.

Clinical features of heart blocks

Bundle branch blocks are usually asymptomatic. Right bundle branch block causes wide but physiological splitting of the second heart sound. Left bundle branch block may cause reverse splitting of the second sound. Patients with intraventricular conduction disturbances may complain of syncope. This is due to intermittent complete heart block or to ventricular tachyarrhythmias. ECG monitoring and electrophysiological studies are needed to determine the cause of syncope in these patients.

Aetiology

Right bundle branch block occurs as an isolated congenital anomaly or is associated with cardiac or pulmonary conditions. Right bundle branch block can be a normal finding in about 5% of individuals. Conditions commonly associated with right bundle branch block include congenital cardiac disorders, such atrial and ventricular septal defects, pulmonary stenosis and Fallot's tetralogy, pulmonary embolism, pulmonary hypertension, myocardial infarction, fibrosis of conduction tissue and Chagas' disease. Block in the right bundle alone does not tend to alter the electrical axis of the heart unless accompanied by right ventricular hypertrophy (RV overload) or coexistent fascicular block. The combination of right bundle branch block with left axis deviation is seen in patients with ostium primum atrial septal defects, but more often signifies diffuse conduction tissue disease affecting the right bundle and the left anterior fascicle. Complete left bundle branch block is often associated with

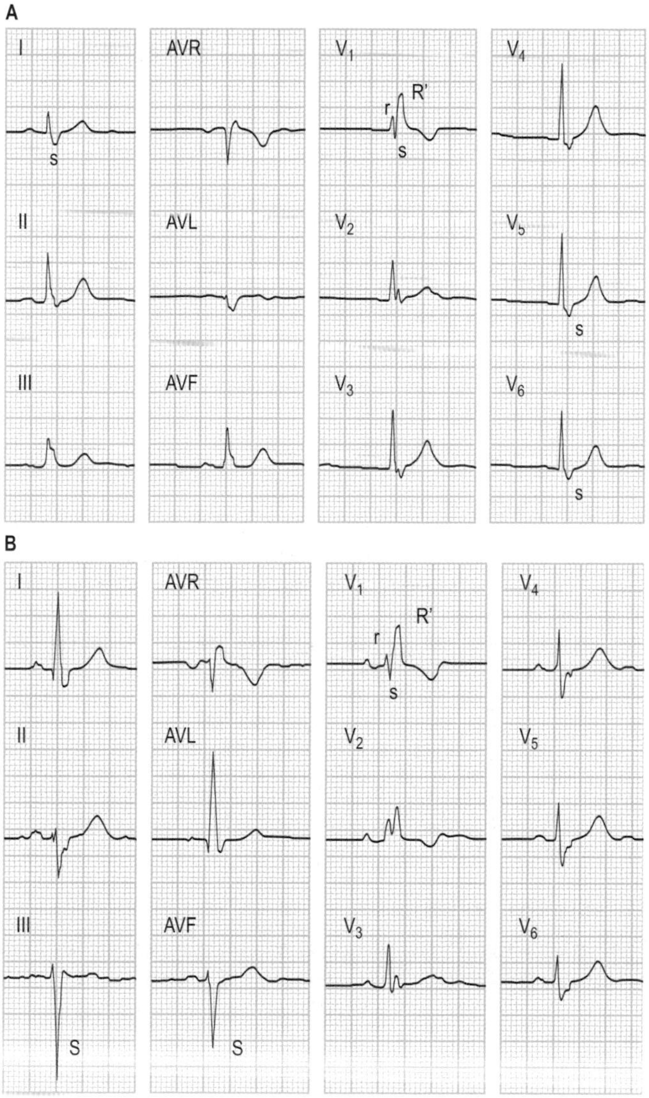

Figure 23.43 Right bundle branch block versus bifascicular block. **A.** A 12-lead ECG showing *right bundle branch block*. Note an rsR′ pattern with the tall R′ in lead V_1–V_2 and the broad S waves in leads I and V_5–V_6. **B.** Compare this ECG showing *bifascicular block*. In addition to right bundle branch block, note the left axis deviation and deep S waves in leads III and AVF, which are typical of left anterior hemiblock.

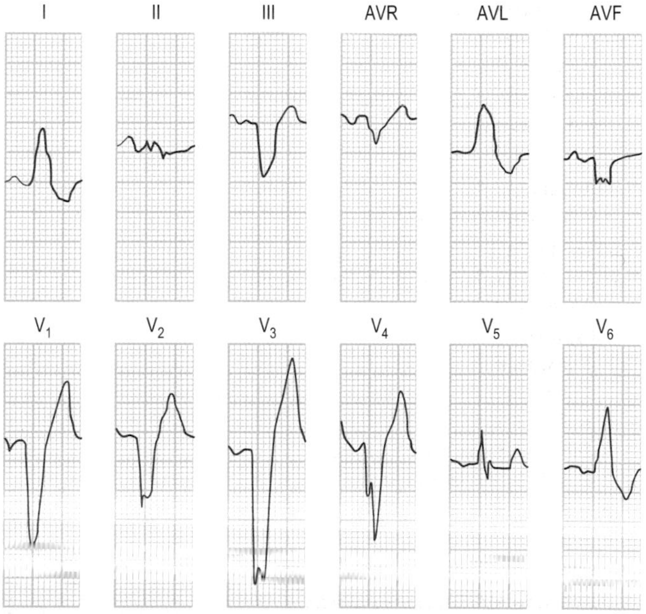

Figure 23.44 A 12-lead ECG showing left bundle branch block. The QRS duration is >0.12 s. Note the broad, notched R waves with ST depression in leads I, AVL and V_6, and the broad QS waves in V_1–V_3.

extensive left ventricular disease. The most common causes include aortic stenosis, hypertension, myocardial infarction and severe coronary disease, and are similar to those of complete heart block.

SUPRAVENTRICULAR TACHYCARDIAS

Supraventricular tachycardias (SVTs) arise from the atrium or the atrioventricular junction. Conduction is via the His–Purkinje system; therefore, the QRS shape during tachycardia is usually similar to that seen in the same patient during baseline rhythm. A classification of supraventricular tachycardia is given in ***Box 23.11***. Some of these tachycardias are discussed in more detail below.

Inappropriate sinus tachycardia

Inappropriate sinus tachycardia is a persistent increase in resting heart rate unrelated to, or out of proportion with, the level of physical or emotional stress. It is found predominantly in young women and is not uncommon in health professionals. Sinus tachycardia due to intrinsic sinus node abnormalities, such as enhanced automaticity, or abnormal autonomic regulation of the heart with excess sympathetic and reduced parasympathetic input, is extremely rare.

In general, sinus tachycardia is a secondary phenomenon and the underlying causes need to be actively investigated. Depending on the clinical setting, acute causes include exercise, emotion, pain, fever, infection, acute heart failure, acute pulmonary embolism and hypovolaemia. Chronic causes include pregnancy, anaemia, hyperthyroidism and catecholamine excess. The underlying cause should be found and treated, rather than treating the compensatory physiological response. If necessary, beta-blockers may be used to slow the sinus rate, in hyperthyroidism, for example (see p. 1206); ivabradine, an I_F (pacemaker current) blocker, may be useful when beta-blockade cannot be tolerated.

Box 23.11 Causes of supraventricular tachycardia (SVT)

Tachycardia	ECG features	Comment
Sinus tachycardia	P wave morphology similar to sinus rhythm preceding QRS	Need to determine underlying cause
Atrioventricular nodal re-entrant tachycardia (AVNRT)	No visible P wave, or inverted P wave immediately before or after QRS complex	Most common cause of palpitations in patients with normal hearts
Atrioventricular re-entrant tachycardia (AVRT) complexes	P wave visible between QRS and T wave	Due to an accessory pathway. If pathway conducts in both directions, ECG during sinus rhythm may be pre-excited
Atrial fibrillation	'Irregularly irregular' RR intervals and absence of organized atrial activity	Most common tachycardia in patients >65 years
Atrial flutter	Visible flutter waves at 300 b.p.m. (sawtooth appearance), usually with 2:1 AV conduction	Suspect in any patient with regular SVT at 150 b.p.m.
Atrial tachycardia	Organized atrial activity with P wave morphology different from sinus rhythm preceding QRS	Usually occurs in patients with structural heart disease or following extensive ablation within atria
Multifocal atrial tachycardia	Multiple P wave morphologies (≥3) and irregular RR intervals	Rare arrhythmia; most commonly associated with significant chronic lung disease
Accelerated junctional tachycardia	ECG similar to that in AVNRT	Rare in adults

Atrioventricular junctional tachycardias

AV nodal re-entrant and AV re-entrant tachycardias are usually referred to as paroxysmal SVTs and are often seen in young patients with no or little structural heart disease, although congenital heart abnormalities (e.g. Ebstein's anomaly, atrial septal defect, Fallot's tetralogy) can coexist in a small proportion of patients with these arrhythmias. The first presentation is commonly between ages 12 and 30, and the prevalence is approximately 2.5/1000.

In these tachycardias the AV node is an essential component of the re-entry circuit.

Atrioventricular nodal re-entrant tachycardia

Atrioventricular nodal re-entrant tachycardia (***AVNRT***) is twice as common in women. Clinically, the tachycardia often strikes suddenly without obvious provocation, but exertion, emotional stress, coffee, tea and alcohol may aggravate or induce the arrhythmia. An attack may stop spontaneously or may continue indefinitely until medical intervention.

In AVNRT, there are two functionally and anatomically different pathways predominantly within the AV node: one is characterized by a short effective refractory period and slow conduction, and the other has a longer effective refractory period and conducts faster. In sinus rhythm, the atrial impulse that depolarizes the ventricles usually conducts through the fast pathway. If the atrial impulse (e.g. an atrial premature beat) occurs early when the fast pathway is still refractory, the slow pathway takes over in propagating the atrial impulse to the ventricles. It then travels back through the fast pathway, which has already recovered its excitability, thus initiating the most common 'slow–fast', or typical, AVNRT.

The rhythm is recognized on ECG from normal regular QRS complexes, usually at a rate of 140–240/min ***(Fig. 23.45A)***. Sometimes, the QRS complexes will show typical bundle branch block. P waves either are not visible or are seen immediately before or after the QRS complex because of simultaneous atrial and ventricular activation. It is less common (5–10%) to observe a tachycardia when the atrial impulse conducts anterogradely through the fast pathway and returns through the slow pathway, producing a long RP′ interval ('fast–slow' or long RP′ tachycardia).

Atrioventricular re-entrant tachycardia

This large circuit comprises the AV node, the His bundle, the ventricle and an abnormal connection of myocardial fibres from the ventricle back to the atrium. It is called an accessory pathway or bypass tract and results from an incomplete separation of the atria and the ventricles during fetal development.

In contrast to AVNRT, atrioventricular re-entrant tachycardia (***AVRT***) is due to a macro re-entry circuit and each part of the circuit

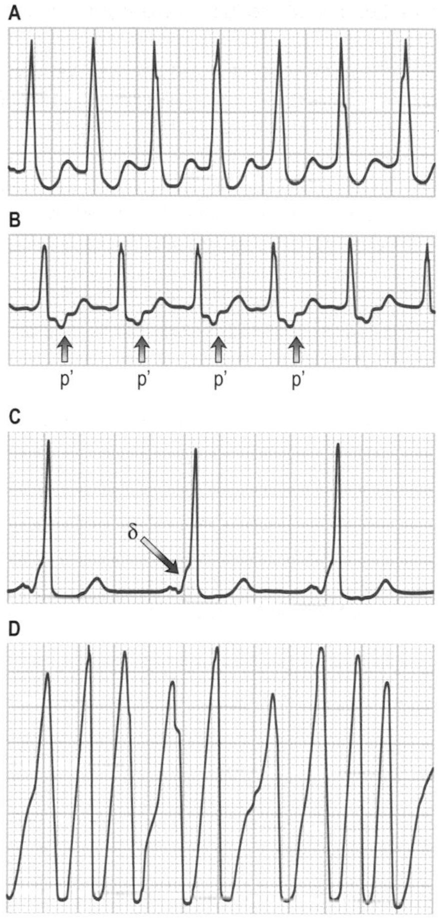

Figure 23.45 **Atrioventricular junctional tachycardia.** **A.** ***Atrioventricular nodal re-entrant tachycardia (AVNRT)***. The QRS complexes are narrow and the P waves cannot be seen. **B.** ***Atrioventricular re-entrant tachycardia (AVRT)*** *(Wolff–Parkinson–White syndrome, WPW)*. The tachycardia P waves (arrowed) are clearly seen after narrow QRS complexes. **C.** An ECG taken in a patient with ***WPW syndrome during sinus rhythm***. Note the short PR interval and the δ wave (arrowed). **D.** ***Atrial fibrillation in the WPW syndrome***. Note the tachycardia with broad QRS complexes and the fast and irregular ventricular rate.

is activated sequentially. As a result, atrial activation occurs after ventricular activation and the P wave is usually seen clearly between the QRS and T waves ***(Fig. 23.45B)***.

Accessory pathways are most commonly situated on the left but may occur anywhere around the AV groove. The most common accessory pathways, known as ***Kent bundles***, are in the free wall or septum. In about 10% of cases, multiple pathways occur. ***Mahaim fibres*** are atrio-fascicular or nodo-fascicular fibres that enter the ventricular myocardium in the region of the right bundle branch. Accessory pathways that conduct from the ventricles to the atria only are not visible on the surface ECG during sinus rhythm and are therefore 'concealed'. Accessory pathways that conduct bidirectionally usually are manifest on the surface ECG. If the accessory pathway conducts from the atrium to the ventricle during sinus rhythm, the electrical impulse can conduct quickly over this abnormal connection to depolarize part of the ventricles abnormally (pre-excitation). A pre-excited ECG is characterized by a short PR interval and a wide QRS complex that begins as a slurred part known as the ***delta*** wave ***(Fig. 23.45C)***. Patients with a history of palpitations and a pre-excited ECG have a syndrome known as Wolff–Parkinson–White (WPW) syndrome.

During AVRT, the AV node and ventricles are activated normally (***orthodromic AVRT***), usually resulting in a narrow QRS complex. Less commonly, the tachycardia circuit can be reversed, with activation of the ventricles via the accessory pathway, and atrial activation via retrograde conduction through the AV node (***antidromic AVRT***). This results in a broad-complex tachycardia. These patients are also prone to atrial fibrillation.

During atrial fibrillation, the ventricles may be depolarized by impulses travelling over both the abnormal and the normal pathways. This results in pre-excited atrial fibrillation, a characteristic tachycardia that is characterized by irregularly irregular broad QRS complexes ***(Fig. 23.45D)***. If an accessory pathway has a short antegrade effective refractory period (<250 ms), it may conduct to the ventricles at an extremely high rate and may cause ventricular fibrillation. The incidence of sudden death is 0.15–0.39% per patient-year and it may be a first manifestation of the disease in younger individuals. Verapamil and digoxin may allow a higher rate of conduction over the abnormal pathway and precipitate ventricular fibrillation. Therefore, neither verapamil nor digoxin should be used to treat atrial fibrillation associated with the WPW syndrome.

Clinical features of AVNRT and AVRT

The leading symptom of most SVTs, in particular AVNRT and AVRT, is rapid regular palpitations, usually with abrupt onset and sudden termination, which can occur spontaneously or be precipitated by simple movements. A common feature is termination by Valsalva manœuvres. In younger individuals with no structural heart disease, the rapid heart rate can be the main pathological finding.

Irregular palpitations may be due to atrial premature beats, atrial flutter with varying AV conduction block, atrial fibrillation or multifocal atrial tachycardia. In patients with depressed ventricular function, uncontrolled atrial fibrillation can reduce cardiac output and cause hypotension and congestive heart failure.

Other symptoms may include anxiety, dizziness, dyspnoea, neck pulsation, central chest pain and weakness. Polyuria may occur because of the release of atrial natriuretic peptide in response to increased atrial pressures during the tachycardia, especially during AVNRT and atrial fibrillation. Prominent jugular venous pulsations due to atrial contractions against closed AV valves may be observed during AVNRT.

Syncope has been reported in 10–15% of patients, usually just after initiation of the arrhythmia or in association with a prolonged pause following its termination. It is more common if the patient is standing. However, in older patients with concomitant heart disease, such as aortic stenosis, hypertrophic cardiomyopathy and cerebrovascular disease, significant hypotension and syncope may result from moderately fast ventricular rates.

Management of AVNRT and AVRT

Acute management

In an emergency, distinguishing between AVNRT and AVRT may be difficult, but it is usually not critical as both tachycardias respond to the same treatment. Patients presenting with SVTs and haemodynamic instability (e.g. hypotension, pulmonary oedema) require emergency cardioversion. If the patient is haemodynamically stable, vagal manœuvres, including right carotid massage (see ***Box 23.7***), the Valsalva manœuvre and facial immersion in cold water, can be successfully employed.

The Valsalva manœuvre is the best of these techniques and is often easier for the patient to perform successfully. It should be undertaken when the patient is resting in the supine position (thus avoiding elevated background sympathetic tone) and involves abrupt voluntary increase in intra-abdominal and intrathoracic pressure by straining. Patient should not take a deep inspiration before straining. Several seconds after the release of the strain, the resulting intense vagal effect may terminate AVNRT or AVRT, or may produce sufficient AV block to reveal an underlying atrial tachyarrhythmia.

If physical manœuvres have not been successful, intravenous adenosine (initially 6 mg by i.v. push, followed by 12 mg if needed) should be tried. Adenosine is a very short-acting (half-life <10 s), naturally occurring purine nucleoside that causes complete heart block for a fraction of a second following intravenous administration. It is highly effective at terminating AVNRT and AVRT or unmasking underlying atrial activity, but rarely affects ventricular tachycardia. The side-effects of adenosine are very brief but include:

- bronchospasm
- flushing
- chest pain
- heaviness of the limbs
- sense of impending doom.

Adenosine is contraindicated in patients with a history of asthma. In some patients, it can induce atrial fibrillation.

An alternative treatment is verapamil 5–10 mg i.v. over 5–10 min, i.v. diltiazem, or beta-blockers (esmolol, propranolol, metoprolol). Verapamil (or diltiazem) must not be given after beta-blockers *or* if the tachycardia presents with broad (>0.12 s) QRS complexes.

Long-term management

Patients with suspected cardiac arrhythmias should always be referred to the cardiologist for electrophysiological evaluation and long-term management, as both pharmacological and non-pharmacological treatments, including ablation of an accessory pathway, are readily available. Verapamil, diltiazem and beta-blockers have proven efficacy in 60–80% of patients. Sodium-channel blockers (flecainide and propafenone), potassium repolarization current blockers (sotalol, dofetilide, azimilide) and the multichannel blocker amiodarone may also prevent the occurrence of tachycardia.

Refinement of catheter ablation techniques has rendered many AV junctional tachycardias entirely curable. Modification of the slow pathway is successful in 96% of patients with AVNRT, although a 1% risk of AV block is present. In AVRT, the target for catheter ablation is the accessory pathway(s). The success rate of ablation of a single accessory pathway is approximately 95%, with a recurrence rate of 5%, requiring a repeat procedure.

Atrial tachyarrhythmias

Atrial tachyarrhythmias, including atrial fibrillation, atrial flutter, atrial tachycardia and atrial ectopic beats, all arise from the atrial myocardium ***(Fig. 23.46)***. They share similar aetiologies, of which the most commonly encountered in clinical practice are increasing age, myocardial infarction, hypertension, obesity, diabetes mellitus, hypertrophic cardiomyopathy, heart failure, valvular heart disease, myocarditis, pericarditis, cardiothoracic surgery, electrolyte imbalance, alcohol use, obstructive airway disease, chest infections and hyperthyroidism.

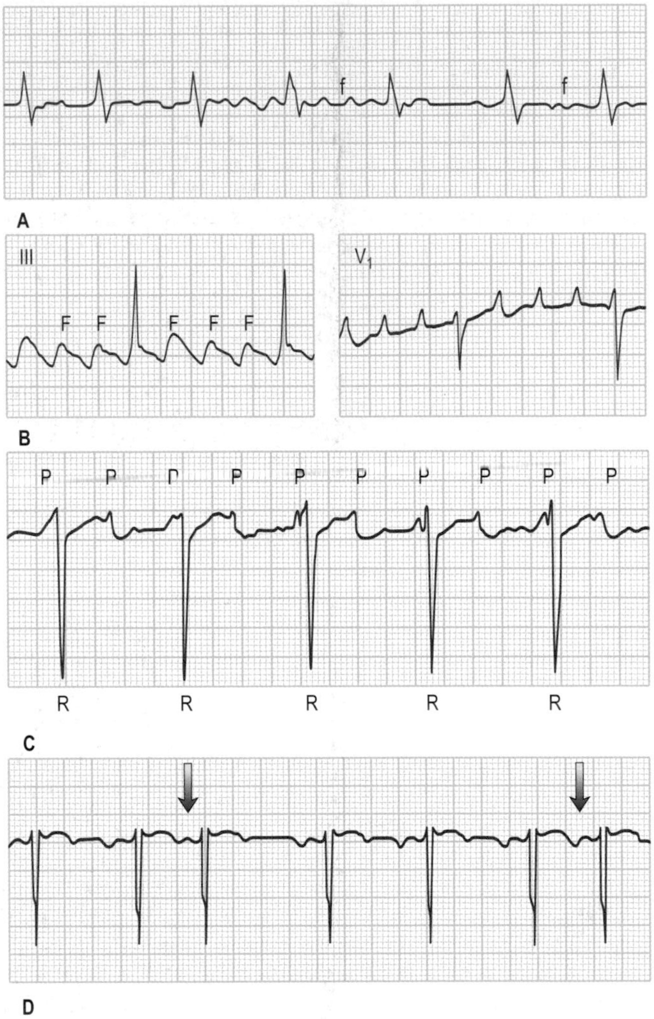

Figure 23.46 **ECGs showing a variety of atrial arrhythmias. A.** *Atrial fibrillation*. Note the absolute rhythm irregularity and baseline undulations (*f* waves). **B.** *Atrial flutter*. Some flutter waves are marked with an F. In this case, the flutter frequency is 240/min. Every fourth flutter wave is transmitted to the ventricles and the ventricular rate is therefore 60/min. **C.** *Atrial tachycardia* with second-degree atrioventricular block. Note the fast atrial (P wave) rate of 150/min and the slower ventricular (R wave) rate of 75/min. **D.** *Atrial premature beats* (arrowed). The premature P wave is different from the sinus P wave and conducts to the ventricle with a slightly prolonged PR interval.

Atrial fibrillation

This is a common arrhythmia, occurring in 1–2% of the general population and 5–15% of patients over 75 years of age. It also occurs, particularly in a paroxysmal form, in younger patients. Any condition resulting in raised atrial pressure, increased atrial muscle mass, atrial fibrosis, or inflammation and infiltration of the atrium may cause atrial fibrillation.

Although rheumatic heart disease, alcohol intoxication and thyrotoxicosis are the 'classic' causes of atrial fibrillation, hypertension and heart failure are the most common causes in the developed world. Hyperthyroidism may provoke atrial fibrillation, sometimes as virtually the only feature of the disease, and thyroid function tests are mandatory in any patient with atrial fibrillation that is unaccounted for. Atrial fibrillation occurs in one-third of patients after cardiac surgery. It usually manifests during the first 4 days and is associated with increased morbidity and mortality, largely due to stroke and circulatory failure, a longer hospital stay and later recurrences.

In some patients, no cause can be found, and this group is labelled as having 'lone' atrial fibrillation. The pathogenesis of 'lone', or 'idiopathic', atrial fibrillation is unknown but genetic predisposition or even specific genetically predetermined forms of the arrhythmia have been proposed. About 30–40% of those with atrial fibrillation, especially those who present at a young age, have at least one parent with the arrhythmia, and genes associated with the sodium channel, the potassium channel, gap junction proteins and right–left isomerism have been implicated. Gene defects linked to chromosomes 10, 6, 5 and 4 have been associated with familial atrial fibrillation.

Atrial fibrillation is maintained by continuous, rapid (300–600/min) activation of the atria by multiple meandering re-entry wavelets, often driven by rapidly depolarizing automatic foci, located predominantly within the pulmonary veins. The atria respond electrically at this rate but there is no coordinated mechanical action and only a proportion of the impulses are conducted to the ventricles. The ventricular response depends on the rate and regularity of atrial activity, particularly at the entry to the AV node, the refractory properties of the AV node itself, and the balance between sympathetic and parasympathetic tone.

Clinical features

Symptoms attributable to atrial fibrillation are highly variable. In some patients (about 30%), it is an incidental finding, while others attend hospital as an emergency with rapid palpitations, dyspnoea and/or chest pain following the onset of atrial fibrillation. Most patients with on-going atrial fibrillation experience some deterioration of exercise capacity or wellbeing, but this may be appreciated only once sinus rhythm is restored. When caused by rheumatic mitral stenosis, the onset of atrial fibrillation results in considerable worsening of cardiac failure.

The patient has an 'irregularly irregular' pulse, as opposed to a basically regular pulse with an occasional irregularity (e.g. extrasystoles) or recurring irregular patterns (e.g. Wenckebach block). The irregular nature of the pulse in atrial fibrillation is maintained during exercise.

The ECG shows fine oscillations of the baseline (so-called fibrillation or *f* waves) and no clear P waves ***(Fig. 23.46A)***. The QRS rhythm is rapid and irregular. Untreated, the ventricular rate is usually 120–180/min but it slows with treatment.

The clinical classification of atrial fibrillation includes:

- first detected – irrespective of duration or severity of symptoms
- paroxysmal – stops spontaneously within 7 days
- persistent – continuous >7 days
- longstanding persistent – continuous >1 year
- permanent – continuous, with a joint decision between the patient and the physician to cease further attempts to regain sinus rhythm.

The classification is helpful in choosing between rhythm restoration and rate control. Atrial fibrillation may be asymptomatic and the 'first detected episode' should not be regarded as necessarily the true onset.

Management

Acute management

When atrial fibrillation is due to an acute precipitating event, such as alcohol toxicity, chest infection or hyperthyroidism, the provoking cause should be treated. Strategies for the acute management of atrial fibrillation are:

- ***Ventricular rate control***. This is achieved by drugs that block the AV node (see below).
- ***Cardioversion***. This is achieved electrically by DC shock (see p. 959), or medically by intravenous infusion of an antiarrhythmic drug such as flecainide, propafenone, vernakalant or amiodarone. Cardioversion can also be achieved by giving an oral agent (flecainide or propafenone) previously tested in hospital and found to be safe in a particular patient ('pill-in-pocket' approach).

The choice depends on:

- how well the arrhythmia is tolerated (is cardioversion urgent?)
- whether anticoagulation is required before considering elective cardioversion
- whether spontaneous cardioversion is likely (previous history? reversible cause?).

Conversion to sinus rhythm can be achieved by electrical DC cardioversion (see p. 959) in about 80% of patients. Biphasic waveform defibrillation is more effective than conventional (monophasic) defibrillation, and biphasic defibrillators are now standard. To minimize the risk of thromboembolism associated with cardioversion, patients are fully anticoagulated with warfarin (International Normalized Ratio (INR) 2.0–3.0) or with dabigatran 150 mg twice daily for 3 weeks before cardioversion (unless atrial fibrillation is of <48 h duration) and at least 4 weeks after the procedure. The patient is then assessed for the necessity for long-term anticoagulation based on their thromboembolic risk score (see below). If cardioversion is urgent and the patient is not on any anticoagulation, transoesophageal echocardiography is used to exclude the presence of atrial thrombus.

Long-term management

Two strategies are available:

- 'rate control' (AV nodal slowing agents ***plus oral anticoagulation***)
- 'rhythm control' (antiarrhythmic drugs plus DC cardioversion ***plus oral anticoagulation***).

Major randomized studies in patients predominantly over the age of 65 years (AFFIRM) or in patients with heart failure (AF-CHF) have shown that there is no net mortality or symptom benefit to be gained from one strategy compared with the other. Which strategy to adopt needs to be assessed for each individual patient. Factors to consider include the likelihood of maintaining sinus rhythm and the safety/tolerability of antiarrhythmic drugs in a particular patient.

Rhythm control

This is advocated for younger, symptomatic and physically active patients. ***Recurrent paroxysms*** may be prevented with oral medication. In general, patients with no significant heart disease can be treated with any class Ia, Ic or III antiarrhythmic drug, although it is recommended that amiodarone (because of its substantial extracardiac adverse effect profile) should be reserved until other drugs have failed. For patients with ***heart failure*** or ***left ventricular hypertrophy*** only amiodarone is recommended. Patients with ***coronary artery disease*** may be treated with sotalol or amiodarone. Patients with ***paroxysmal atrial fibrillation*** or with early ***persistent atrial fibrillation*** (little left atrial dilatation) may be treated with left atrial ablation. The ectopic triggers for atrial fibrillation are generally found in the pulmonary veins, which can be isolated from the atria using radiofrequency or cryothermal energy. Occasionally, more extensive ablation within the left atrium is needed. These techniques are more successful than antiarrhythmic drugs and may represent a 'cure' in some patients. However, the procedure is invasive and carries some hazard of serious complications such as stroke, and bleeding in about 2% of cases. In the long term, recurrence is not uncommon and an apparently successful ablation does not remove the obligation for appropriate anticoagulation. Ablation has not been shown to improve long-term cardiovascular outcome but it does successfully treat symptoms due to atrial fibrillation.

Rate control

As a primary strategy, this is appropriate in patients who:

- have the permanent form of the arrhythmia associated with symptoms that can be further improved by slowing heart rate, or are older than 65 years with recurrent atrial tachyarrhythmias ('accepted' atrial fibrillation)
- have persistent tachyarrhythmias and have failed cardioversion(s) and serial prophylactic antiarrhythmic drug therapy, and in whom the risk/benefit ratio from using specific antiarrhythmic agents is shifted towards increased risk.

Rate control is usually achieved with a combination of ***digoxin***, ***beta-blockers*** or ***non-dihydropyridine calcium-channel blockers*** (***verapamil*** or ***diltiazem***). Digoxin monotherapy may be sufficient for elderly, non-ambulant patients. In younger patients, the effect of catecholamines easily overwhelms the vagotonic effect of digoxin and additional AV nodal slowing agents are needed. The ventricular rate response is generally considered to be controlled if the resting heart rate is <110 b.p.m. but stricter control, between 60 and 80 b.p.m. at rest and <110 b.p.m. during moderate exercise, may be needed if symptoms persist. To assess the adequacy of rate control, an ECG rhythm strip may be sufficient in an elderly patient but ambulatory 24-hour Holter monitoring and an exercise stress test (treadmill) are needed in younger individuals. Older patients with poor rate control despite optimal medical therapy should be considered for AV node ablation and pacemaker implantation ('***ablate and pace***' ***strategy***). These patients usually experience a marked symptomatic improvement but require life-long anticoagulation because of the on-going risk of thromboembolism.

Anticoagulation

This is indicated in patients with atrial fibrillation related to rheumatic mitral stenosis or in the presence of a mechanical prosthetic heart valve. In patients with non-valvular atrial fibrillation (in the absence of mitral stenosis, artificial heart valves or mitral valve repair), a scoring system known as CHA_2DS_2VASc is used ***(Box 23.12)*** as the first step in determining the need for anticoagulation.

Long-term prophylaxis against ischaemic stroke with oral anticoagulation must be balanced against the risk of haemorrhage. The HAS-BLED score is recommended by European, Canadian and UK (NICE) guidelines. A high HAS-BLED score identifies patients with a high risk of bleeding (***Box 23.13*** and ***Fig. 23.47***).

When oral anticoagulation is required, either warfarin (dose adjusted to maintain an INR between 2.0 and 3.0) or one of the new oral anticoagulant agents (NOACs) can be used. These latter agents fall into two classes: direct thrombin inhibitors (e.g. dabigatran) and oral direct factor Xa inhibitors (e.g. rivaroxaban and apixaban). NOACs specifically block a single step in the coagulation cascade, in contrast to warfarin, which blocks several vitamin K-dependent factors (II, VII, IX and X). Unlike warfarin, the NOACs have a rapid onset of action, shorter half-life and fewer food and drug interactions, and do not require INR testing. Trial data have shown them to be equally effective as, and safer than, warfarin. However, these agents require dose reduction or avoidance in patients with renal impairment, the elderly or those with low body weight.

Atrial flutter

Atrial flutter is often associated with atrial fibrillation and frequently requires a similar initial therapeutic approach. Atrial flutter is usually an organized atrial rhythm with an atrial rate typically between 250 and 350 b.p.m. Typical, or isthmus-dependent, atrial flutter involves a macro re-entrant right atrial circuit around the tricuspid annulus. The wavefront circulates down the lateral wall of the right atrium, through the Eustachian ridge between the tricuspid annulus and the inferior vena cava, and up the interatrial septum, giving rise to the most frequent pattern, referred to as counter-clockwise flutter.

Box 23.12 CHA_2DS_2-VASc scoring system for non-valvular atrial fibrillation

	Risk factors	Score/points
C	Congestive heart failure	1
H	Hypertension	1
A_2	Age ≥75	2
D	Diabetes mellitus	1
S_2	Stroke/TIA/thromboembolism	2
V	Vascular disease (aorta, coronary or peripheral arteries)	1
A	Age 65–74	1
Sc	Sex category: female	1

Annual risk of stroke

0 points = 0% risk: No prophylaxis
1 point = 1.3% risk: Anticoagulant (oral) or aspirin
2+ points = 2.2% risk: Oral anticoagulant

TIA, transient ischaemic attack.

Box 23.13 HAS-BLED score for bleeding risk on oral anticoagulation in atrial fibrillation

Clinical characteristic	Score/points
Hypertension (systolic ≥160≥mmHg)	1
Abnormal renal function	1
Abnormal liver function	1
Stroke in past	1
Bleeding	1
Labile INRs	1
Elderly: age ≥65 years	1
Drugs as well	1
Alcohol intake at same time	1

INR, International Normalized Ratio.
(Adapted from European Society of Cardiology Clinical Practice Guidelines. *Eur Heart J* 2012; 33:2719–2747.)

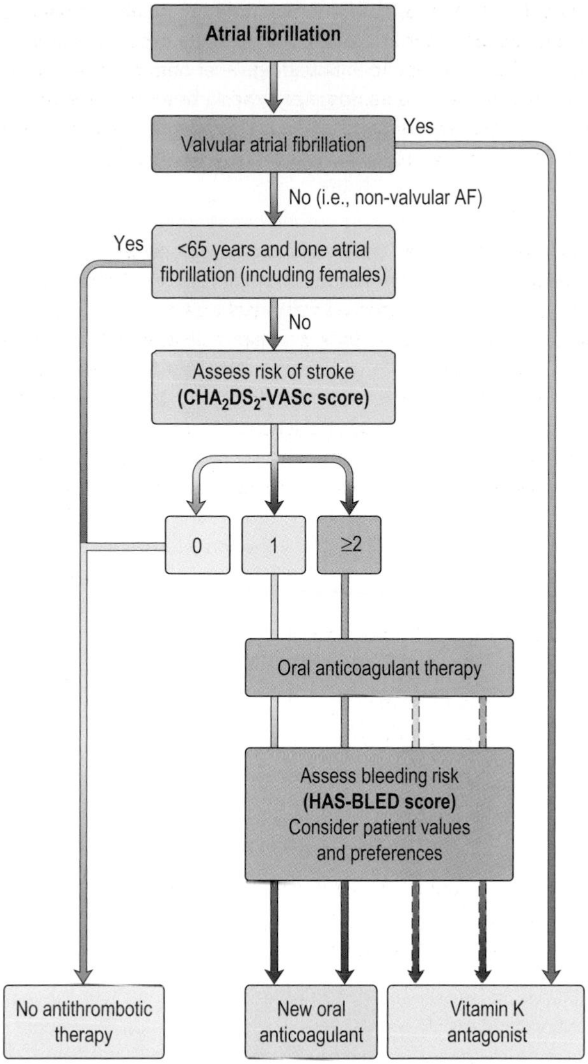

Figure 23.47 Choice of anticoagulant. Antiplatelet therapy with aspirin plus clopidogrel (or, less effectively, aspirin only) should be considered in patients who refuse any oral anticoagulant therapy or cannot tolerate anticoagulants for reasons unrelated to bleeding. *(Adapted from European Society of Cardiology Clinical Practice Guidelines.* Eur Heart J *2012; 33:2719–2747, with permission.)*

Re-entry can also occur in the opposite direction (clockwise or reverse flutter).

The ECG shows regular sawtooth-like atrial flutter waves (F waves) between QRS complexes ***(Fig. 23.46B)***. In typical counter-clockwise atrial flutter, the F waves are negative in the inferior leads and positive in leads V_1 and V_2. In clockwise atrial flutter, the deflection of the F waves is the opposite. If F waves are not clearly visible, it is worth trying to reveal them by slowing AV conduction by carotid sinus massage or by the administration of AV nodal blocking drugs such as adenosine or verapamil.

Symptoms are largely related to the degree of AV block. Most often, every second flutter beat conducts, giving a ventricular rate of 150 b.p.m. Occasionally, every beat conducts, producing a heart rate of 300 b.p.m. More often, especially when patients are receiving treatment, AV conduction block reduces the heart rate to approximately 75 b.p.m.

Management

Management of a symptomatic acute paroxysm is by electrical ***cardioversion***. Patients who have been in atrial flutter for more than 1–2 days should be treated in a similar manner to patients with atrial fibrillation and ***anticoagulated*** for 3 weeks prior to cardioversion. Acute pharmacological cardioversion can be achieved using class Ic (flecainide, propafenone) or certain class III antiarrhythmic agents (dofetilide, ibutilide; these have better efficacy than in atrial fibrillation but are not available in many countries).

Recurrent paroxysms may be prevented by ***class III*** antiarrhythmic agents (sotalol, amiodarone). ***AV nodal blocking agents*** may be used to control the ventricular rate if the arrhythmia persists. However, the treatment of choice for patients with recurrent atrial flutter is catheter ***ablation*** (see p. 979), which permanently interrupts re-entry by creating a line of conduction block within the isthmus between the inferior vena cava and the tricuspid valve ring. This technique offers patients whose only arrhythmia is typical atrial flutter an almost certain chance of a cure, although the later occurrence of atrial fibrillation is not uncommon.

Atrial tachycardia

This is an uncommon arrhythmia. Its prevalence is believed to be <1% in patients with arrhythmias. It is usually associated with structural heart disease but, in many cases, it is referred to as idiopathic. Macro re-entrant tachycardia often occurs after surgery for congenital heart disease. Atrial tachycardia with block is often a result of digitalis poisoning.

The mechanisms of atrial tachycardia are attributed to enhanced automaticity, triggered activity or intra-atrial re-entry. Atrial re-entrant tachycardia is usually relatively slow (125–150 b.p.m.) and can be initiated and terminated by atrial premature beats. The P′P′ intervals are regular. The PR interval depends on the rate of tachycardia and is longer than in sinus rhythm at the same rate.

Automatic tachycardia usually presents with higher rates (125–250 b.p.m.) and is often characterized by a progressive increase in the atrial rate with onset of the tachycardia ('warm-up') and progressive decrease prior to termination ('cool-down'). Atrial tachycardia is typically caused by a focus that is frequently located along the crista terminalis in the right atrium, adjacent to a pulmonary vein in the left atrium, or around one of the atrial appendages. Automatic atrial tachycardia may also present as an incessant variety leading to tachycardia-induced cardiomyopathy. Short runs of atrial tachycardia may provoke more sustained episodes of atrial fibrillation.

Figure 23.46C demonstrates an atrial tachycardia at an atrial rate of 150/min. The P waves are abnormally shaped and occur in front of the QRS complexes. Carotid sinus massage may increase AV block during tachycardia, thereby facilitating the diagnosis, but does not usually terminate the arrhythmia. Management options include ***cardioversion***, ***antiarrhythmic drug therapy*** to maintain sinus rhythm, ***AV nodal slowing agents*** to control rate and, in selected cases, radiofrequency catheter ***ablation***.

Atrial ectopic beats

These often cause no symptoms, although they may be sensed as an irregularity or heaviness of the heart beat. On the ECG, they appear as early and abnormal P waves and are usually, but not always, followed by normal QRS complexes ***(Fig. 23.46D)***. Treatment is not normally required unless the ectopic beats provoke more significant arrhythmias, when ***beta-blockers*** may be effective.

VENTRICULAR TACHYARRHYTHMIAS

Ventricular tachyarrhythmias can be discussed under the following headings:

- life-threatening ventricular tachyarrhythmias (sustained ventricular tachycardia, ventricular fibrillation, torsades de pointes)
- normal heart ventricular tachycardia
- non-sustained ventricular tachycardia
- ventricular premature beats (ectopics).

Some of these conditions are cardiac channelopathies. These are congenital disorders that are caused by mutations that affect the function of cardiac ion channels and hence the electrical activity of the heart. They include Brugada syndrome, congenital long QT syndrome, short QT syndrome, catecholaminergic polymorphic ventricular tachycardia (CPVT) and idiopathic ventricular fibrillation.

Sustained ventricular tachycardia

Sustained ventricular tachycardia (>30 s) often results in ***pre-syncope*** (dizziness), ***syncope***, ***hypotension*** and ***cardiac arrest***, although it may be remarkably well tolerated in some patients. Examination reveals a pulse rate typically between 120 and 220 b.p.m. Usually, there are clinical signs of atrioventricular dissociation (i.e. intermittent cannon 'a' waves in the neck) and variable intensity of the first heart sound).

The ECG shows a rapid ventricular rhythm with broad (often ≥0.14 s), abnormal QRS complexes. AV dissociation may result in visible P waves, which appear to march through the tachycardia, capture beats (an intermittent narrow QRS complex owing to normal ventricular activation via the AV node and conducting system) and fusion beats (intermediate between ventricular tachycardia beat and capture beat).

Supraventricular tachycardia with bundle branch block may resemble ventricular tachycardia on the ECG. However, if a broad-complex tachycardia is due to SVT with either right or left bundle branch block, then the QRS morphology should resemble a typical right bundle branch block or left bundle branch block pattern (see ***Figs 23.43A*** and ***23.44***). Other ECG criteria to differentiate VT from SVT with aberrancy are indicated in ***Box 23.14***. Some 80% of all broad-complex tachycardias are due to ventricular tachycardia, and the proportion is even higher in patients with structural heart disease. Therefore, in all cases of doubt, ventricular tachycardia should be diagnosed.

Management

Treatment may be urgent, depending on the haemodynamic situation. If the patient is haemodynamically compromised (e.g. hypotensive or pulmonary oedema), emergency DC cardioversion may be required. On the other hand, if the blood pressure and cardiac output are well maintained, intravenous therapy with beta-blockers (esmolol), class I drugs or amiodarone is usually used. DC cardioversion is necessary if medical therapy is unsuccessful.

Box 23.14 ECG distinction between SVT with bundle branch block and VT

VT is more likely than SVT with bundle branch block where there is:

- a very broad QRS (>0.14 s)
- atrioventricular dissociation
- a bifid, upright QRS with a taller first peak in V_1
- a deep S wave in V_6
- a concordant (same polarity) QRS direction in all chest leads (V_1–V_6)

SVT, supraventricular tachycardia; VT, ventricular tachycardia.

Ventricular fibrillation

This involves very rapid and irregular ventricular activation with no mechanical effect. The patient is pulseless and becomes rapidly unconscious; respiration ceases (cardiac arrest). The ECG shows shapeless, rapid oscillations and there is no hint of organized complexes ***(Fig. 23.48)***. It is usually provoked by a ventricular ectopic beat. Ventricular fibrillation rarely reverses spontaneously. The only effective treatment is electrical defibrillation. Basic and advanced cardiac life support is needed (see p. 957).

If the attack of ventricular fibrillation occurs during the first day or two of an acute myocardial infarction, it is probable that prophylactic therapy will be unnecessary. If the ventricular fibrillation was not related to an acute infarction, the long-term risk of recurrent cardiac arrest and sudden death is high.

Survivors of these ventricular tachyarrhythmias are, in the absence of an identifiable reversible cause (e.g. acute myocardial infarction, severe metabolic disturbance), at high risk of sudden death. Implantable cardioverter–defibrillators are first-line therapy in the management of these patients (see pp. 979–980).

Brugada syndrome

This inheritable condition accounts for part of a group of patients with idiopathic ventricular fibrillation who have no evidence of causative structural cardiac disease. It is more common in young male adults and in South-east Asia. The diagnosis is made by identifying the classic ECG changes that may be present spontaneously or may be provoked by the administration of a class I antiarrhythmic (flecainide or ajmaline): right bundle branch block with coved ST elevation in leads V_1–V_3 ***(Fig. 23.49)***. Atrial fibrillation may occur.

In 20% of cases, this is a monogenic inheritable condition associated with loss of sodium-channel function due to a mutation in the *SCN5A* gene. Recently, other mutations in the *SCN1B* gene, glycerol-3-phosphate dehydrogenase-1-like gene (*GPD1L*-type) and genes related to calcium-channel sub-units *CACNA1C* and *CACNB2* have also been implicated in the genesis of this syndrome. It can present with sudden death during sleep, resuscitated cardiac arrest and syncope, or the patient may be asymptomatic and diagnosed incidentally or during familial assessment. There is a high risk of sudden death, particularly in the symptomatic patient or those with spontaneous ECG changes. The only successful treatment is

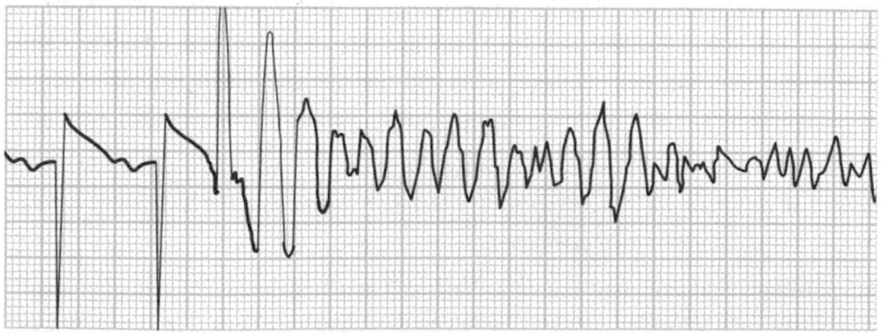

Figure 23.48 Ventricular fibrillation. Two beats of sinus rhythm are followed by a ventricular ectopic beat that initiates ventricular fibrillation. The ST segment during sinus rhythm is elevated owing to acute myocardial infarction in this case.

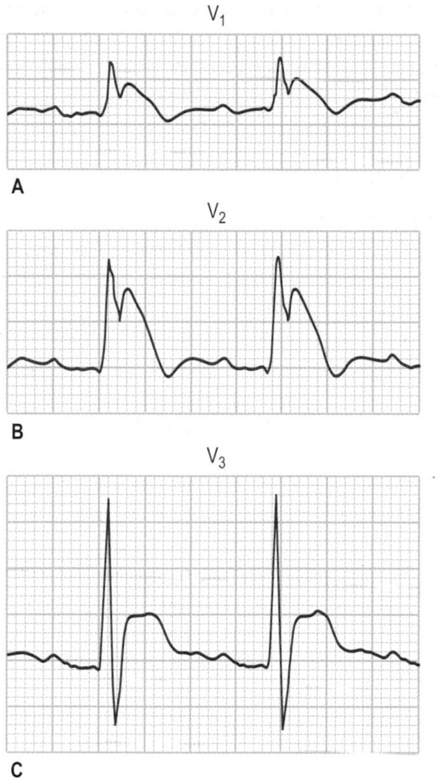

Figure 23.49 **The Brugada ECG.** ST elevation with right bundle branch block. **A.** V_1. **B.** V_2. **C.** V_3.

an ICD. Beta-blockade is not helpful and may be harmful in this syndrome.

Long QT syndrome

This describes an ECG where the ventricular repolarization (QT interval) is greatly prolonged. The causes of long QT syndrome are listed in ***Box 23.15***.

Congenital long QT syndrome

Two major syndromes have been described, which may (Jervell–Lange-Nielsen syndrome) or may not (Romano–Ward syndrome) be associated with congenital deafness.

The molecular biology of the congenital long QT syndromes has been shown to be heterogeneous. It is usually a monogenic disorder and has been associated with mutations in cardiac potassium and sodium-channel genes. The different genes involved appear to correlate with different phenotypes ***(Fig. 23.50A)*** that can exhibit such variable penetrance that carriers may have completely normal ECGs. To date, thirteen long QT (LQT) sub-types have been identified but three major sub-types account for the majority of cases. These are: LQT1 (*KCNQ1* gene mutation affecting the $I_{ks}\alpha$ sub-unit), in which the arrhythmia is usually provoked by exercise, particularly swimming; LQT2 (*KCNH2* gene mutation affecting the $I_{Kr}\alpha$ sub-unit), in which arrhythmia provocation is associated with emotion and acoustic stimuli; and LQT3 (*SCN5A* gene mutation affecting the $I_{Na}\alpha$ sub-unit), in which the arrhythmias occur during rest or when asleep. It is likely that identification of the mutation involved will not only improve diagnostic accuracy, particularly with cascade screening in affected families, but also guide future therapy for the congenital long QT syndrome.

Box 23.15 Causes of long QT syndrome

Congenital
- Jervell–Lange-Nielsen syndrome (autosomal recessive)
- Romano–Ward syndrome (autosomal dominant)

Acquired

Electrolyte abnormalities
- Hypokalaemia
- Hypomagnesaemia
- Hypocalcaemia

Drugs
- Quinidine, disopyramide
- Sotalol, amiodarone
- Tricyclic antidepressants, e.g. amitriptyline
- Phenothiazine drugs, e.g. chlorpromazine
- Antipsychotics, e.g. haloperidol, olanzapine
- Macrolides, e.g. erythromycin
- Quinolones, e.g. ciprofloxacin
- Methadone

Poisons
- Organophosphate insecticides

Miscellaneous
- Bradycardia
- Mitral valve prolapse
- Acute myocardial infarction
- Diabetes
- Prolonged fasting and liquid protein diets (long-term)
- Central nervous system diseases, e.g. dystrophia myotonica

Acquired long QT syndrome

QT prolongation and torsades de pointes are usually provoked by bradycardia.

Clinical features

Patients with a long QT develop syncope and palpitations as a result of polymorphic ventricular tachycardia (torsades de pointes). They usually terminate spontaneously but may degenerate to ventricular fibrillation, resulting in sudden death.

Torsades de pointes is characterized on the ECG by rapid, irregular, sharp complexes that continuously change from an upright to an inverted position ***(Fig. 23.50B)***.

Between spells of tachycardia, or immediately preceding the onset of tachycardia, the ECG shows a prolonged QT interval; the corrected QT (see ***Box 23.6***) is usually >0.50 s.

Management

Acute (acquired) long QT syndrome is treated as follows:
- Any electrolyte disturbance is corrected.
- Causative drugs are stopped.
- The heart rate is maintained with atrial or ventricular pacing.
- Magnesium sulphate 8 mmol (Mg^{2+}) is given over 10–15 min for acquired long QT.
- Intravenous isoprenaline may be effective when QT prolongation is acquired (isoprenaline is contraindicated for congenital long QT syndrome).

Long-term, congenital long QT syndrome is generally treated by beta-blockade, pacemaker therapy and, occasionally, left cardiac sympathetic denervation. LQT1 patients seem to respond well to beta-blockade while LQT3 patients are better treated with sodium-channel blockers. All long QT patients should avoid drugs known to prolong the QT interval. Patients who remain symptomatic despite conventional therapy, and those with marked QT prolongation or a strong family history of sudden death, usually need ICD therapy.

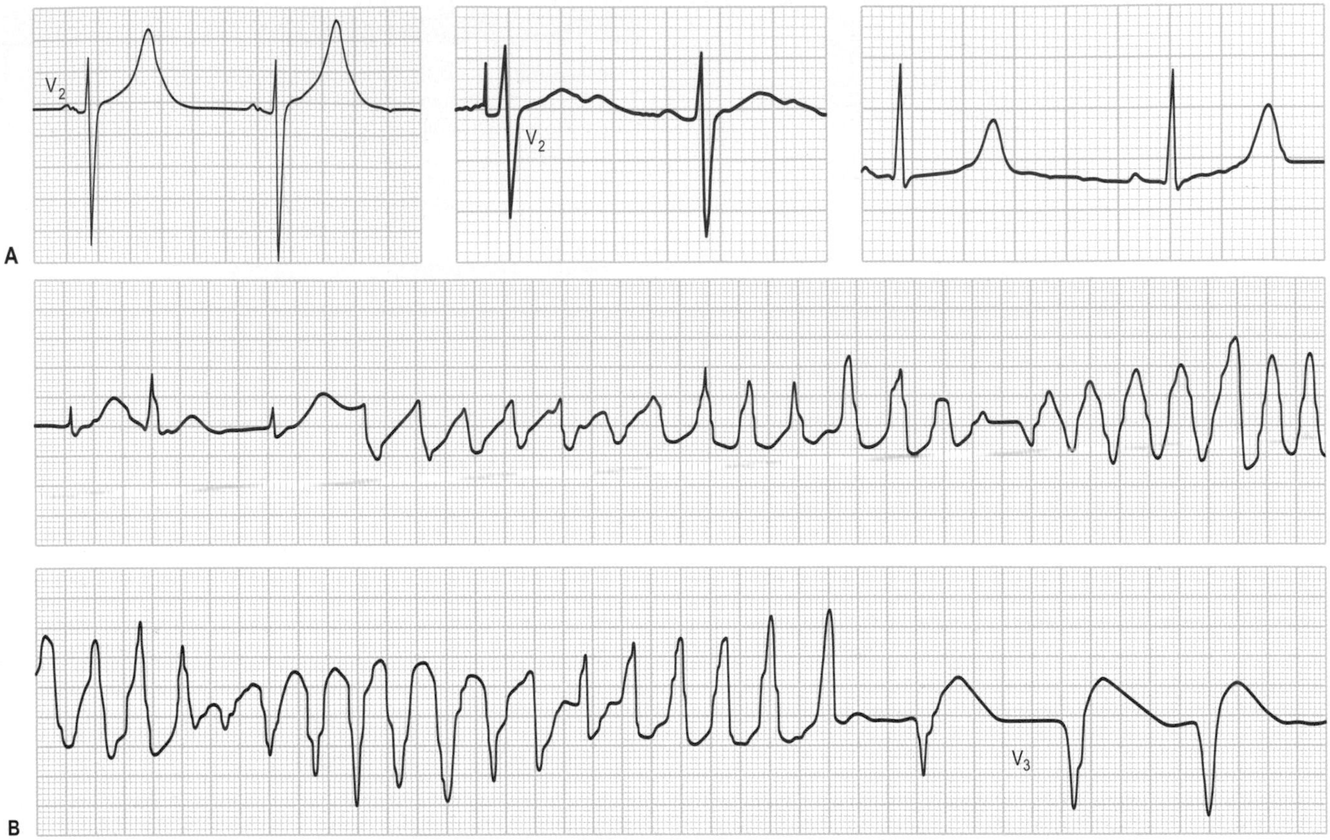

Figure 23.50 Prolonged QT syndrome. A. Three examples of a *prolonged QT interval* corresponding to three different types of long QT syndrome. **B.** An ECG demonstrating a supraventricular rhythm with a long QT interval giving way to atypical ventricular tachycardia (*torsades de pointes*). The tachycardia is short-lived and is followed by a brief period of idioventricular rhythm.

Short QT syndrome

Five types have been described; they are caused by genetic abnormalities that lead to faster repolarization. Ventricular arrhythmias and sudden death may occur and an ICD is the best treatment.

Normal heart ventricular tachycardia

Monomorphic ventricular tachycardia in patients with structurally normal hearts (idiopathic ventricular tachycardia) is usually a benign condition with an excellent long-term prognosis. Occasionally, it is incessant (so called Gallavardin's tachycardia) and, if untreated, may lead to cardiomyopathy.

Normal heart ventricular tachycardia arises from a focus either in the right ventricular outflow tract or in the left ventricular septum. Treatment of symptoms is usually with beta-blockers. There is a special form of verapamil-sensitive tachycardia that responds well to non-dihydropyridine calcium antagonists. In symptomatic patients, radiofrequency catheter ablation is highly effective, resulting in a cure in >90% of cases. It is sometimes difficult to distinguish arrhythmogenic right ventricular hypertrophy (see pp. 1038–1040) from this seemingly benign disorder.

Non-sustained ventricular tachycardia

Non-sustained ventricular tachycardia (NSVT) is defined as ventricular tachycardia that is ≥5 consecutive beats but lasts <30 s ***(Fig. 23.51A)***. NSVT can be found in 6% of patients with normal hearts and usually does not require treatment. It is documented in up to 60–80% of patients with heart disease. There is insufficient evidence on prognosis, but an ICD has been shown to improve survival of patients with particularly poor left ventricular function (ejection fraction ≤30%) by preventing arrhythmic death. Antiarrhythmic suppression of NSVT is not usually advocated but beta-blockers may improve quality of life in symptomatic individuals.

Ventricular premature beats (ectopics)

These may be uncomfortable, especially when frequent. The patient complains of extra beats, missed beats or heavy beats because it may be the premature beat, the post-ectopic pause or the next sinus beat that is noticed by the patient. The pulse is irregular owing to the premature beats. Some early beats may not be felt at the wrist. When a premature beat occurs regularly after every normal beat, 'pulsus bigeminus' may occur. If premature ventricular beats are highly symptomatic, treatment with beta-blockade may be helpful. If the ectopics are very frequent, left ventricular dysfunction may develop; if the ectopics stem from a single focus, especially when in the right ventricle, catheter ablation can be very effective.

These premature beats ***(Fig. 23.51B–D)*** have a broad (>0.12 s) and bizarre QRS complex because they arise from an abnormal (ectopic) site in the ventricular myocardium. Following a premature beat, there is usually a complete compensatory pause because the AV node or ventricle is refractory to the next sinus impulse. Early 'R-on-T' ventricular premature beats (occurring simultaneously with the upstroke or peak of the T wave of the previous beat) may induce ventricular fibrillation in patients with heart disease, particularly following myocardial infarction.

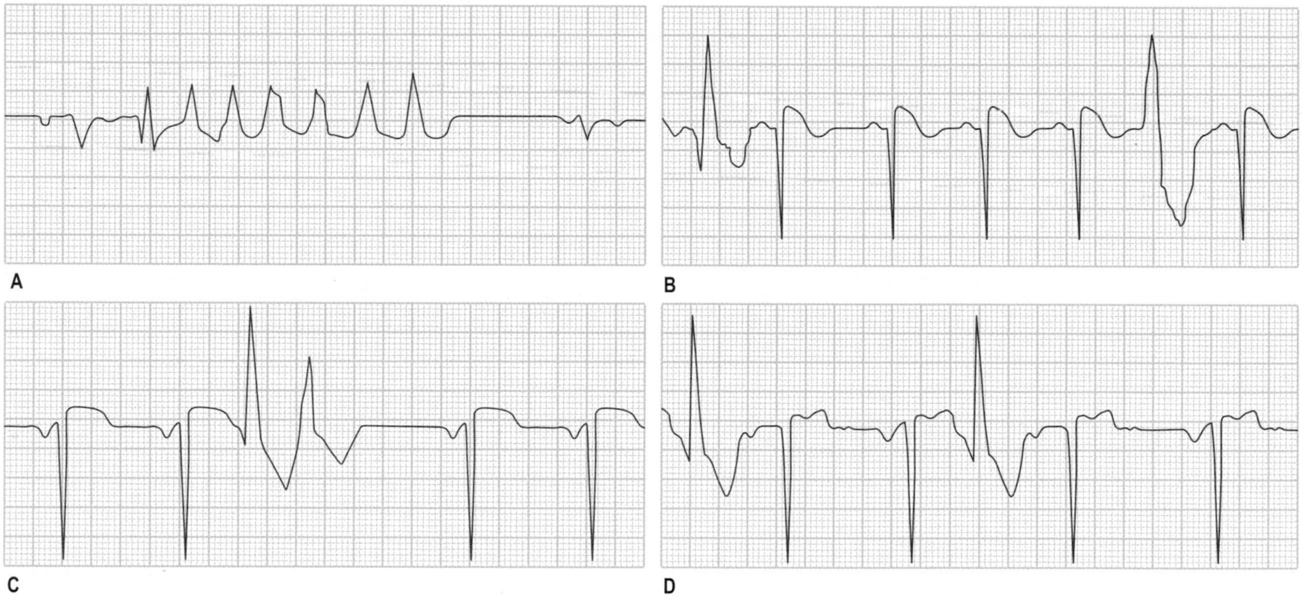

Figure 23.51 Varieties of ventricular ectopic activity. A. A brief run of ventricular tachycardia (*non-sustained ventricular tachycardia*) that follows previous ectopic activity. **B.** Two ventricular ectopic beats of different morphology (multimorphological). **C.** Two ventricular premature beats (VPBs) occurring one after the other (a pair or couplet of VPBs). **D.** Frequently repetitive ventricular ectopic activity of a single morphology.

Ventricular premature beats are usually treated only if symptomatic. Simple measures, such as reassurance and beta-blocker therapy, are normally all that is required.

Long-term management of cardiac tachyarrhythmias

Options for the long-term management of cardiac tachyarrhythmias include:

- antiarrhythmic drug therapy
- ablation therapy
- device therapy.

To determine the optimal strategy for a given patient, the following questions must be addressed:

- Is the principal aim of treatment symptom relief or prevention of sudden death?
- Is maintaining sinus rhythm or controlling ventricular rates the treatment goal?

Commonly employed treatment strategies for the management of specific tachyarrhythmias are outlined in ***Box 23.16***.

Antiarrhythmic drugs

Drugs that modify the rhythm and conduction of the heart are used to treat cardiac arrhythmias. Antiarrhythmic drugs may aggravate or produce arrhythmias (proarrhythmia) and they may also depress ventricular contractility and must therefore be used with caution. They are classified according to their effect on the action potential (Vaughan Williams' classification; ***Box 23.17*** and ***Fig. 23.52***).

Class I drugs

These are membrane-depressant drugs that reduce the rate of entry of sodium into the cell (sodium-channel blockers). They may slow conduction, delay recovery or reduce the spontaneous discharge rate of myocardial cells. Class I agents have been found to increase mortality compared to placebo in post-myocardial infarction patients with ventricular ectopy (Cardiac Arrhythmia Suppression

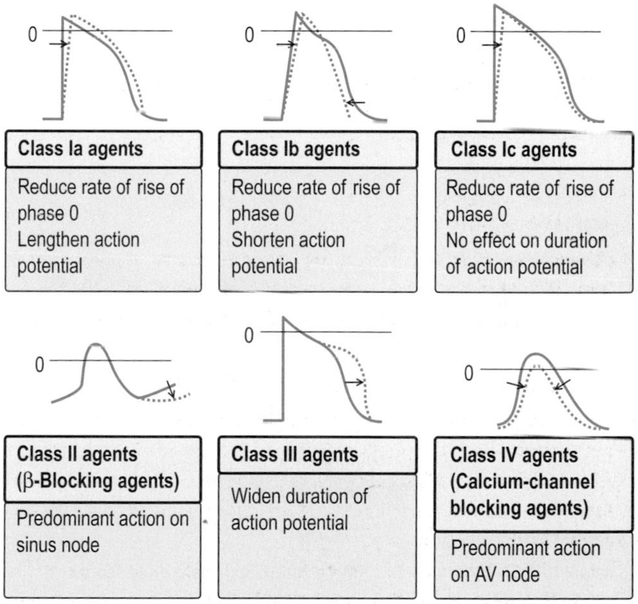

Figure 23.52 Vaughan Williams' classification of antiarrhythmic drugs based on their effect on cardiac action potentials (see also *Fig. 23.39*). *(0=0 mV. The dotted curves indicate the effects of the drugs. AV, atrioventricular.)*

Trial (CAST) trials – class Ic agents) and in patients treated for atrial fibrillation (class Ia agent, quinidine). In view of this, class Ic agents, such as flecainide, and all other class I drugs should be reserved for patients who do not have significant coronary artery disease, left ventricular dysfunction, or other forms of significant structural heart disease.

Class II drugs

These antisympathetic drugs prevent the effects of catecholamines on the action potential. Most are β-adrenoceptor antagonists.

Box 23.16 Long-term management of tachyarrhythmias

Tachycardia	Management aims	Management strategies
AV node re-entrant tachycardia (AVNRT)	Relieve symptoms	Beta-blockers, calcium-channel blockers, digoxin Class Ic or class III drugs Catheter ablation
AV re-entrant tachycardia (AVRT)	Relieve symptoms	Beta-blockers, calcium-channel blockers, digoxin Class Ic or class III drugs Catheter ablation
Wolff–Parkinson–White (WPW) syndrome	Relieve symptoms Prevent sudden death (esp. if documented pre-excited atrial fibrillation)	Class Ic or class III drugs Catheter ablation
Atrial fibrillation	Relieve symptoms Prevent worsening heart failure due to poor rate control Prevent thromboembolic complications	Maintenance of sinus rhythm: Class Ic or class III drugs ± cardioversion Catheter ablation Rate control: Beta-blockers, calcium-channel blockers, digoxin AV node ablation plus pacemaker Anticoagulation: Warfarin, novel oral anticoagulant (e.g. dabigatran, rivaroxaban, apixaban)
Atrial flutter	Relieve symptoms Prevent worsening heart failure due to poor rate control Prevent thromboembolic complications	Class Ic or class III drugs Catheter ablation Beta-blockers, calcium-channel blockers, digoxin Anticoagulation
Atrial tachycardia	Relieve symptoms Prevent worsening heart failure due to poor rate control Prevent thromboembolic complications	Class Ic or class III drugs Catheter ablation Beta-blockers, calcium-channel blockers, digoxin Anticoagulation
Life-threatening ventricular tachyarrhythmias	Prevent sudden death	ICD Beta-blockers, amiodarone
Congenital long QT	Prevent sudden death	Beta-blockers ± pacemaker, ICD Correction of bradycardia Correction of electrolytes
Acquired long QT	Prevent sudden death	Avoidance of all QT-prolonging drugs
Normal heart ventricular tachycardias	Relieve symptoms	Beta-blockers, calcium-channel blockers Catheter ablation
Non-sustained VT (NSVT)	Relieve symptoms Prevent sudden death in certain situations	Beta-blockers Class Ic and class III drugs (amiodarone, sotalol) ICD in clearly defined subgroups

AV, atrioventricular; ICD, implantable cardioverter–defibrillator.

Box 23.17 Vaughan Williams' classification of antiarrhythmic drugs

Class/action	Drugs
Class I	Membrane-depressant drugs (sodium-channel blockers)
Ia Lengthen action potential	Disopyramide
Ib Shorten action potential	Lidocaine, mexiletine
Ic No effect on action potential	Flecainide, propafenone
Class II Block β-adrenoceptors	Atenolol, acebutolol, bisoprolol, propranolol, esmolol
Class III Lengthen action potential	Amiodarone, dronedarone, sotalol, dofetilide, ibutilide, vernakalant
Class IV Reduce plateau phase of action potential	Calcium-channel blockers, e.g. verapamil, diltiazem
Other	Adenosine, digoxin

Cardioselective beta-blockers (β_1) include metoprolol, bisoprolol, atenolol and acebutolol. Beta-blockers suppress AV node conduction, which may be effective in preventing attacks of junctional tachycardia, and may help to control the ventricular rate during paroxysms of other forms of SVT (e.g. atrial fibrillation). In general, beta-blockers are anti-ischaemic and anti-adrenergic, and have proven beneficial effects in patients post myocardial infarction (by preventing ventricular fibrillation) and in patients with congestive heart failure. It is therefore advisable to use beta-blocker therapy either alone or in combination with other antiarrhythmic drugs in patients with symptomatic tachyarrhythmias, particularly in those with coronary artery disease.

Class III drugs

These prolong the action potential, usually by blocking the rapid component of the delayed rectifier potassium current (IKr), and do not affect sodium transport through the membrane. The drugs in this class are amiodarone and sotalol. Sotalol is also a beta-blocker.

Sotalol may result in acquired long QT syndrome and torsades de pointes. The risk of torsades is increased in the setting of hypokalaemia, and particular care should be taken in patients taking diuretic therapy. Amiodarone therapy, in contrast to most other antiarrhythmic drugs, carries a low risk of proarrhythmia in patients with significant structural heart disease, but its use may be limited due to toxic and potentially serious side-effects. Dronedarone is a multichannel blocking drug that suppresses the recurrence of atrial fibrillation and reduces hospital admissions in patients with cardiovascular risk. However, it has proven harmful in patients with left ventricular dysfunction and is contraindicated in heart failure.

Vernakalant is a multichannel blocker that is approved for the rapid intravenous medical cardioversion of new-onset atrial fibrillation.

Class IV drugs

The non-dihydropyridine calcium-channel blockers are particularly effective at slowing conduction in nodal tissue. These drugs can prevent attacks of junctional tachycardia (AVNRT and AVRT) and may help to control ventricular rates during paroxysms of other forms of SVT (e.g. atrial fibrillation).

Antiarrhythmic drugs have not been shown to prolong life. Patient safety is the main factor in determining the choice of antiarrhythmic therapy, and proarrhythmic risks need to be carefully assessed prior to initiating therapy. As a generalization, class Ic agents are employed in patients with structurally normal hearts, and class III agents are used in patients with structural heart disease, although exceptions exist.

Patients with structurally normal hearts and normal QT intervals, or those with implantable defibrillators, either are at very low risk of proarrhythmia or are protected from any life-threatening consequences; in these individuals, it is possible to persevere with drug therapy.

Catheter ablation

Catheter ablation (radiofrequency or cryoablation) is frequently employed in the management of symptomatic tachyarrhythmias. Ablations are performed percutaneously by placing electrode catheters into the heart chambers, usually via femoral vessels. Successful ablation depends on accurate identification of either the site of origin of a focal tachycardia or a critical component of a macro re-entry tachycardia. Catheter ablation has been found to be highly effective in the following tachyarrhythmias:

- AV node re-entrant tachycardia (AVNRT)
- AV re-entrant tachycardia (AVRT) with an accessory pathway, including Wolff–Parkinson–White (WPW) syndrome
- normal heart ventricular tachycardia
- atrial flutter
- atrial tachycardia
- paroxysmal atrial fibrillation (pulmonary vein isolation).

Symptomatic patients with a ***pre-excited*** ECG because of accessory pathway conduction (WPW syndrome) are advised to undergo catheter ablation as first-line therapy, owing to the risk of sudden death associated with this condition. This is especially the case in patients with pre-excited atrial fibrillation. Patients with accessory pathways that only conduct retrogradely from the ventricles to the atrium are not at increased risk of sudden death but experience symptoms due to AVRT. These patients are commonly offered an ablation procedure if simple measures, such as AV nodal slowing agents, fail to suppress tachycardia. Asymptomatic patients with the WPW ECG pattern are now frequently offered an ablation procedure for prophylactic reasons. The main risk associated with accessory pathway ablation is thromboembolism in patients with left-sided accessory pathways. The success rate for catheter ablation of AVNRT and accessory pathways is >95%.

Patients with ***normal hearts and documented ventricular tachycardia*** should be referred for specialist evaluation. Unlike VT in patients with structural heart disease, normal heart VT is not associated with increased risk of sudden death and is easily cured by catheter ablation.

Catheter ablation is recommended in patients with ***atrial flutter*** that is not easily managed medically. Ablation of typical flutter is effective in 90–95% of cases. In the direct comparison of catheter ablation and antiarrhythmic therapy, the rate of recurrence was significantly lower following ablation. ***Atrial tachycardia***, especially in patients with structurally normal hearts, may also be cured by catheter ablation. In atrial fibrillation, adequate control of ventricular rates is sometimes not possible, despite optimal medical therapy. These patients experience a marked symptomatic improvement following AV node ablation (which leads to complete heart block) and pacemaker implantation.

In ***younger patients*** with structurally normal hearts, ***atrial ectopic beats***, which commonly arise from a focus situated in the pulmonary veins, may trigger atrial fibrillation. Catheter ablation of this ectopic focus includes the application of radiofrequency energy around the pulmonary veins in order to abolish the connection between the sleeves of arrhythmogenic atrial myocardium surrounding or extending into the veins from the atrium (pulmonary vein isolation). The trigger is therefore eliminated and the arrhythmia does not recur. These techniques appear to be highly effective, especially in young patients with paroxysmal atrial fibrillation, normal atrial size and no underlying heart disease (70–80% long-term success), but are presently time-consuming procedures (4 h or more) and carry a risk of serious complications such as stroke, pericardial haemorrhage, pulmonary vein stenosis and atrio-oesophageal fistula in a small minority of patients (in experienced centres <2% altogether).

Implantable cardioverter–defibrillator

Life-threatening ventricular arrhythmias (ventricular fibrillation or rapid ventricular tachycardia with hypotension) result in death in up to 40% within 1 year of diagnosis. Large multicentre prospective trials, such as the Antiarrhythmics (amiodarone) Versus Implantable Defibrillator (AVID) trial, have proven that implantable defibrillators improve overall survival in patients who have experienced an episode of life-threatening ventricular tachyarrhythmia.

The implantable cardioverter–defibrillator (ICD) recognizes ventricular tachycardia or fibrillation and automatically delivers pacing or a shock to the heart to cause cardioversion to sinus rhythm. Modern ICDs are only a little larger than a pacemaker and are implanted in a pectoral position ***(Fig. 23.53)***. The device may have leads to sense and pace both the right atrium and ventricle, and the lithium batteries employed are able to provide energy for over 100 shocks, each of around 30 J. ICD discharges are painful if the patient is conscious. However, ventricular tachycardia may often be terminated by overdrive pacing the heart, which is painless. The ICD is superior to all other treatment options at preventing sudden cardiac death. The use of this device has cut the sudden death rate in patients with a history of serious ventricular arrhythmias to approximately 2% per year. However, the majority of these patients have significant structural heart disease and overall cardiac mortality due to progressive heart failure remains high. As a result, the ICD is now first-line therapy in the secondary prevention of sudden death.

ICDs are also employed in the primary prevention of sudden cardiac death. The chances of surviving an out-of-hospital cardiac

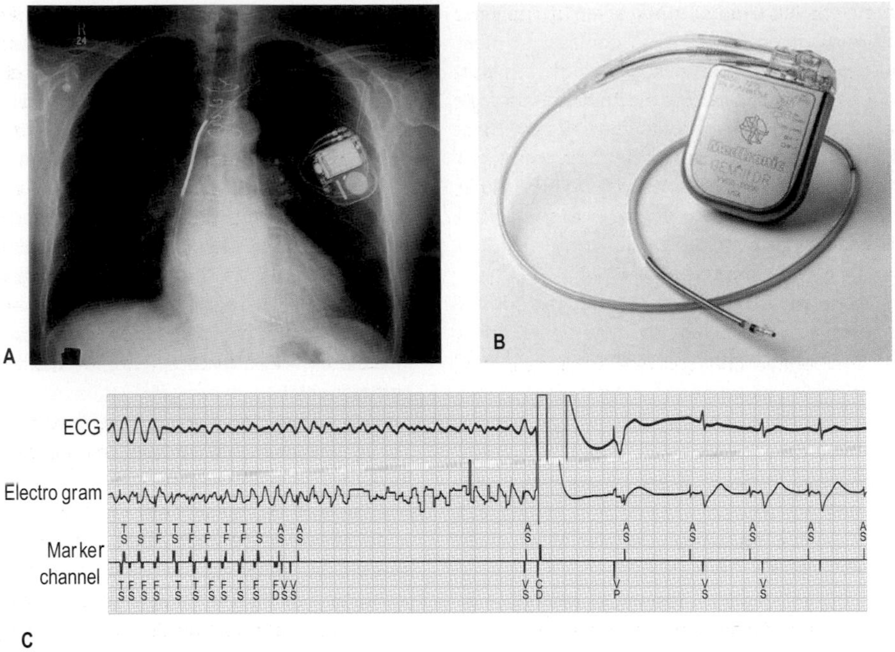

Figure 23.53 Implantable cardioverter–defibrillator. A. *X-ray of a 'dual-chamber' defibrillator* in a left pectoral position with atrial and ventricular leads. **B.** *Medtronic GEM® III DR defibrillator.* **C.** *ECG showing the termination of ventricular fibrillation by a direct current shock at 20 J.* The electrogram, recorded internally from the ventricular lead of an ICD, reveals chaotic ventricular activity consistent with ventricular fibrillation. This is confirmed by an electrocardiogram (lead V_2). The marker channel demonstrates that the device detects ventricular fibrillation correctly (FS, fibrillation sensing, lower line) and delivers an appropriate shock (CD) that terminates the arrhythmia and restores normal sinus rhythm (VS, ventricular sensing, lower line). Incidentally, atrial fibrillation is also detected before shock delivery (upper line on the marker channel).

arrest are as low as 10%. Therefore, selected patients who have never experienced a spontaneous episode of life-threatening ventricular tachyarrhythmia but who are assessed to be at high risk of sudden death are advised to undergo ICD implantation. In two large primary prevention ICD trials, Multicenter Automated Defibrillator Implantation Trial (MADIT II) and Sudden Cardiac Death in Heart Failure Trial (SCD-HeFT), therapy with an ICD reduced mortality by 23–31% on top of conventional treatment, which included revascularization, beta-blockers and angiotensin-converting enzyme (ACE) inhibitors. ICD combined with cardiac resynchronization therapy may improve both symptoms and life expectancy of patients with any degree of heart failure (COMPANION, CARE-HF and MADIT-CRT).

The following groups of patients may merit prophylactic ICD placement for primary prevention:

- Patients with heart failure with a left ventricular ejection fraction of ≤35% and NYHA functional class <IV (see ***Box 23.21***). In such patients who also have left bundle branch block (QRS >120 ms), there is additional benefit in combining ICD with cardiac resynchronization therapy (CRT-D; see p. 988).
- Those with a familial condition and high risk of sudden death, such as dilated and hypertrophic cardiomyopathy, long QT syndrome, Brugada syndrome or other channelopathies, who have a strong family history of sudden cardiac death and arrhythmogenic right ventricular dysplasia.

Further reading

Ackerman MJ, Mohler PJ. Defining a new paradigm for human arrhythmia syndromes: phenotypic manifestations of gene mutations in ion channel- and transporter-associated proteins. *Circul Res* 2010; 107:457–465.

Brignole M, Arruchio A, Baron-Esquivias G et al. 2013 ESC Guidelines on cardiac pacing and cardiac resynchronization therapy. The Task Force on Cardiac Pacing and Resynchronization Therapy of the European Society of Cardiology (ESC). Developed in collaboration with the European Heart Rhythm Association (EHRA). *Eur Heart J* 2013; 34:2281–2329.

Camm AJ, Kirchhof P, Lip GY et al. and European Heart Rhythm Association; European Association for Cardio-Thoracic Surgery. Guidelines for the management of atrial fibrillation. The Task Force for the Management of Atrial Fibrillation of the European Society of Cardiology (ESC). *Europace* 2010; 12:1360–1420. [Focused update: *Eur Heart J* 2012; 33:2719–2747.]

Heist EK, Ruskin JN. Drug-induced arrhythmia. *Circulation* 2010; 122:1426–1435.

Lip GYH. Atrial fibrillation. *Lancet* 2012; 379:648–661.

National Institute for Health and Care Excellence. *NICE Clinical Guideline 180: Atrial Fibrillation: The Management of Atrial Fibrillation*. NICE 2014; http://www.nice.org.uk/CG180.

National Institute for Health and Care Excellence. *NICE Technology Appraisal 314: Implantable Cardioverter Defibrillators and Cardiac Resynchronisation Therapy for Arrhythmias and Heart Failure*. NICE 2014; https://www.nice.org.uk/guidance/ta314.

Priori SG, Wilde AA, Horie M et al. Executive summary: HRS/EHRA/APHRS expert consensus statement on the diagnosis and management of patients with inherited primary arrhythmia syndromes. *Europace* 2013; 15:1389–1406.

Schwartz PJ, Ackerman MJ. The long QT syndrome: a transatlantic clinical approach to diagnosis and therapy. *Eur Heart J* 2013; 34:3109–3116.

Verheugt FWA, Granger CB. Novel antithrombotic agents. Oral anticoagulants for stroke prevention in atrial fibrillation: current status, special situations and unmet needs. *Lancet* 2015; 386:303–310.

Wazri O, Wilkoff B, Saliba W. Catheter ablation for atrial fibrillation. *N Engl J Med* 2011; 365:2296–2304.

HEART FAILURE

Heart failure is a complex syndrome that can result from any structural or functional cardiac disorder that impairs the ability of the heart to function as a pump to support a physiological circulation.

Worldwide, the incidence of heart failure is variable but increases with advancing age. For example, in Scotland, the prevalence of heart failure is high at 7.1 in 1000, increasing with age to 90.1 in 1000 among people over 85 years. In the UK, overall incidence is about 2 in 1000. Approximately 26 million people worldwide have heart failure.

The prognosis of heart failure has improved over the past 10 years with evidence-based therapy, but the mortality rate remains high and approximately 50% of patients are dead at 5 years. Heart failure accounts for 5% of admissions to hospital medical wards. The cost of managing heart failure in the UK exceeds £1 billion per year. Coronary artery disease is the most common cause of heart failure in Western countries.

The causes of heart failure are shown in ***Box 23.18***.

Pathophysiology

When the heart fails, considerable changes affect the heart and peripheral vascular system in response to the haemodynamic changes associated with heart failure ***(Box 23.19)***. These physiological changes are compensatory and maintain cardiac output and peripheral perfusion. However, as heart failure progresses, these mechanisms are overwhelmed and become pathophysiological. The development of pathological peripheral vasoconstriction and sodium retention in heart failure by activation of the renin–angiotensin–aldosterone system entails a loss of beneficial compensatory mechanisms and represents cardiac decompensation. Factors involved are venous return, outflow resistance, contractility of the myocardium, and salt and water retention.

Venous return (preload)

In the intact heart, myocardial failure leads to a reduction of the volume of blood ejected with each heart beat, and an increase in the volume of blood remaining after systole. This increased diastolic volume stretches the myocardial fibres and, as Starling's law of the heart (see p. 935) would suggest, myocardial contraction is restored. However, the failing myocardium results in depression of the ventricular function curve (cardiac output plotted against the ventricular diastolic volume) ***(Fig. 25.7)***.

Mild myocardial depression is not associated with a reduction in cardiac output because it is maintained by an increase in venous pressure (and hence diastolic volume). However, the proportion of blood ejected with each heart beat (ejection fraction) is reduced early in heart failure. Sinus tachycardia also ensures that any reduction of stroke volume is compensated for by the increase in heart rate; cardiac output (stroke volume × heart rate) is therefore maintained.

When there is more severe myocardial dysfunction, cardiac output can be maintained only by a large increase in venous pressure and/or marked sinus tachycardia. The increased venous pressure contributes to the development of dyspnoea, owing to the accumulation of interstitial and alveolar fluid, and to the occurrence of hepatic enlargement, ascites and dependent oedema due to increased systemic venous pressure. However, the cardiac output at rest may not be much depressed, but myocardial and haemodynamic reserve is so compromised that a normal increase in cardiac output cannot be produced by exercise.

In very severe heart failure, the cardiac output at rest is depressed, despite high venous pressures. The inadequate cardiac output is redistributed to maintain perfusion of vital organs, such as the heart, brain and kidneys, at the expense of the skin and muscle.

Box 23.18 Causes of heart failure

Main causes

- Ischaemic heart disease (35–40%)
- Cardiomyopathy (dilated) (30–34%)
- Hypertension (15–20%)

Other causes

- Cardiomyopathy (undilated): hypertrophic, restrictive (amyloidosis, sarcoidosis)
- Valvular heart disease (mitral, aortic, tricuspid)
- Congenital heart disease (ASD, VSD)
- Alcohol and drugs (chemotherapy – trastuzumab, imatinib)
- Hyperdynamic circulation (anaemia, thyrotoxicosis, haemochromatosis, Paget's disease)
- Right heart failure (right ventricular infarct, pulmonary hypertension, pulmonary embolism, COPD)
- Tricuspid incompetence
- Arrhythmias (atrial fibrillation, bradycardia (complete heart block, sick sinus syndrome)
- Pericardial disease (constrictive pericarditis, pericardial effusion)
- Infections (Chagas' disease), e.g. myocarditis

ASD, atrial septal defect; COPD, chronic obstructive pulmonary disease; VSD, ventricular septal defect.

Box 23.19 Pathophysiological changes in heart failure

- Ventricular dilatation
- Myocyte hypertrophy
- Increased collagen synthesis
- Altered myosin gene expression
- Altered sarcoplasmic Ca^{2+} ATPase density
- Increased ANP secretion
- Salt and water retention
- Sympathetic stimulation
- Peripheral vasoconstriction

ANP, atrial natriuretic peptide; ATPase, adenosine triphosphatase.

Outflow resistance (afterload)

Outflow resistance (afterload) (see ***Fig. 23.5***) is the load or resistance against which the ventricle contracts. It is formed by:

- pulmonary and systemic resistance
- physical characteristics of the vessel walls
- the volume of blood that is ejected.

An increase in afterload decreases the cardiac output. This results in a further increase of end-diastolic volume and dilatation of the ventricle itself, which further exacerbates the problem of afterload. This is expressed by Laplace's law: the tension of the myocardium (T) is proportional to the intraventricular pressure (P) multiplied by the radius of the ventricular chamber (R) – that is, $T \propto PR$.

Myocardial contractility (inotropic state)

The state of the myocardium also influences performance. The sympathetic nervous system is activated in heart failure via baroreceptors as an early compensatory mechanism, which provides inotropic support and maintains cardiac output. Chronic sympathetic activation, however, has deleterious effects by further increasing neurohormonal activation and myocyte apoptosis. This is compensated by a downregulation of β-receptors. Increased contractility (positive inotropism) can result from increased sympathetic drive, and this is a normal part of the Frank–Starling relationship (see ***Fig. 23.5***). Conversely, myocardial depressants (e.g. hypoxia) decrease myocardial contractility (negative inotropism).

Neurohormonal and sympathetic system activation: salt and water retention

The increase in venous pressure that occurs when the ventricles fail leads to retention of salt and water and their accumulation in the interstitium, producing many of the physical signs of heart failure. Reduced cardiac output also leads to diminished renal perfusion, activating the renin–angiotensin system and enhancing salt and water retention (see ***Fig. 20.6***), which further increases venous pressure ***(Fig. 23.54)***. The retention of sodium is, in part, compensated by the action of circulating atrial natriuretic peptides and antidiuretic hormone (see pp. 150–153).

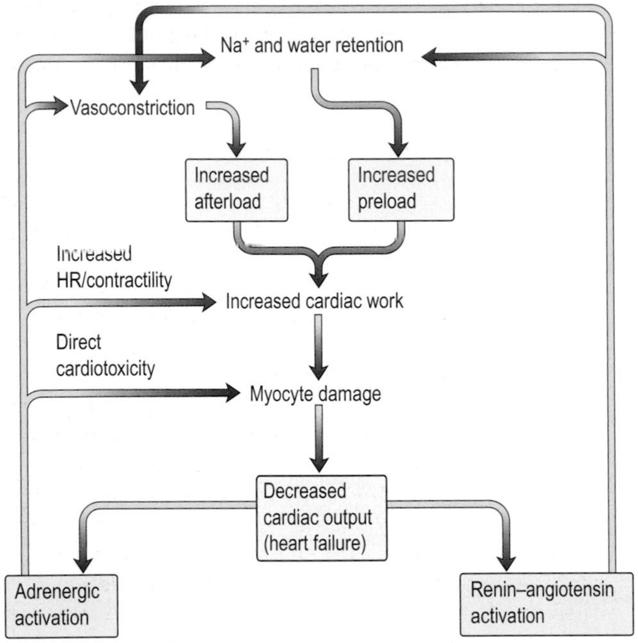

Figure 23.54 The compensatory physiological response to heart failure. Chronic activation of the renin–angiotensin and adrenergic systems results in a 'vicious circle' of cardiac deterioration that further exacerbates the physiological response. HR, heart rate.

The interaction of haemodynamic and neurohumoral factors in the progression of heart failure remains unclear. Increased ventricular wall stress promotes ventricular dilatation and further worsens contractile efficiency. In addition, prolonged activation of the sympathetic nervous and renin–angiotensin–aldosterone systems exerts direct toxic effects on myocardial cells.

Myocardial remodelling in heart failure

Left ventricular remodelling is a process of progressive alteration of ventricular size, shape and function owing to the influence of mechanical, neurohumoral and possibly genetic factors in several clinical conditions, including myocardial infarction, cardiomyopathy, hypertension and valvular heart disease. Its hallmarks include hypertrophy, loss of myocytes and increased interstitial fibrosis. Remodelling continues for months after the initial insult, and the eventual change in the shape of the ventricle becomes responsible for significant impairment of overall function of the heart as a pump ***(Fig. 23.55A)***. In cardiomyopathy, the process of progressive ventricular dilatation or hypertrophy takes place without ischaemic myocardial injury or infarction ***(Fig. 23.55B)***.

Changes in myocardial gene expression

Haemodynamic overload of the ventricle stimulates changes in cardiac contractile protein gene expression. The overall effect is to increase protein synthesis, but many proteins also switch to fetal and neonatal isoforms. Human myosin is composed of a pair of heavy chains and two pairs of light chains. Myosin heavy chains (MHCs) exist in two isoforms, α and β, that have different contractile properties and ATPase activity; $\alpha\alpha$-MHC predominates in the atria and $\beta\beta$-MHC in the ventricles. In animal models, pressure overload results in a shift from $\alpha\alpha$- to $\beta\beta$-MHC in the atria, in parallel with atrial size. This results in a reduction in atrial contractility but lower energy demands. This shift is less significant in the human ventricle, as the $\beta\beta$-MHC isoform already predominates. Other genes affected

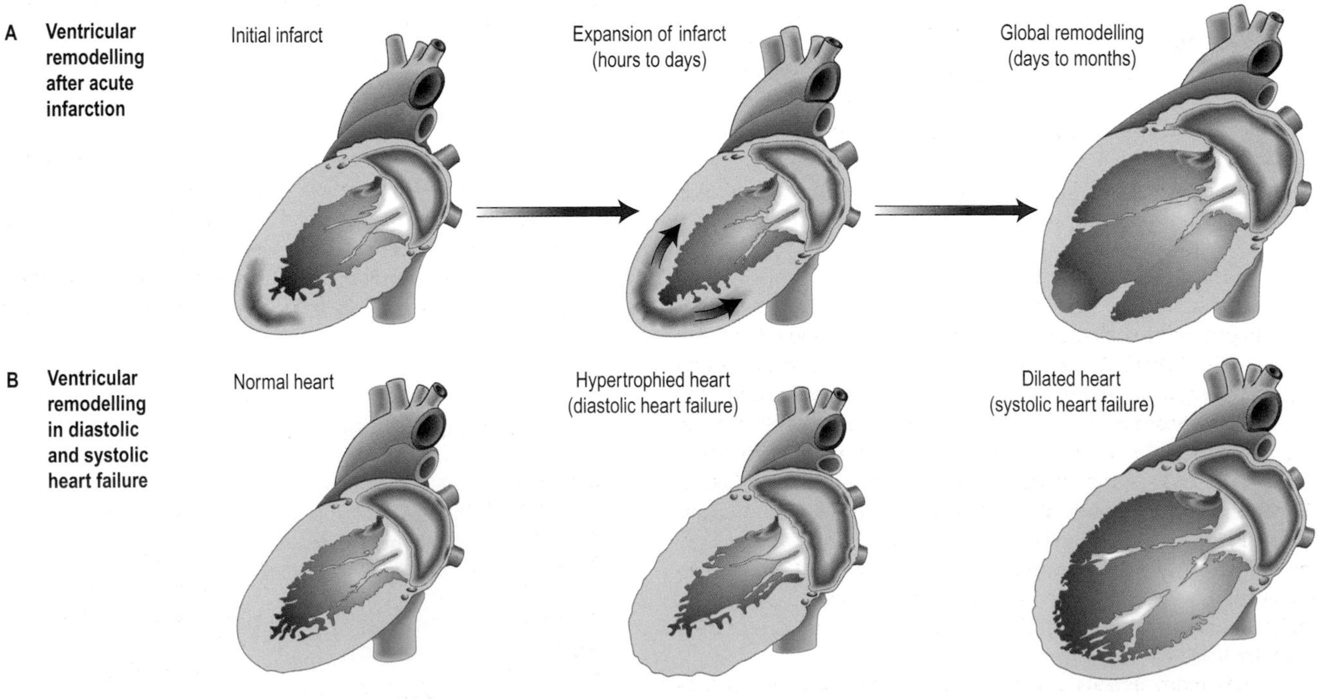

Figure 23.55 Ventricular remodelling. A. In ischaemic (myocardial infarction) heart failure. **B.** In non-ischaemic heart failure (e.g. in cardiomyopathy).

in heart failure include those encoding Na^+/K^+-ATPase, Ca^{2+}-ATPase and β_1-adrenoceptors.

Abnormal calcium homeostasis

Calcium ion flux within myocytes plays a pivotal role in the regulation of contractile function. Excitation of the myocyte cell membrane causes the rapid entry of calcium into myocytes from the extracellular space via calcium channels. This triggers the release of intracellular calcium from the sarcoplasmic reticulum and initiates contraction (see ***Fig. 23.3***). Relaxation results from the uptake and storage of calcium by the sarcoplasmic reticulum (see ***Fig. 23.9***), controlled by changes in nitric oxide. In heart failure, there is a prolongation of the calcium current in association with prolongation of contraction and relaxation.

Apoptosis

Apoptosis (or 'programmed cell death'; see p. 105) of myocytes has been demonstrated in animal models of ischaemic reperfusion, rapid ventricular pacing, mechanical stretch and pressure overload. Apoptosis is associated with irreversible congestive heart failure, and the spiral of ventricular dysfunction, characteristic of heart failure, results from the initiation of apoptosis by cytokines, free radicals and other triggers.

Natriuretic peptides (ANP, BNP and C-type)

- ***Atrial natriuretic peptide*** (***ANP***) is released from atrial myocytes in response to stretch. ANP induces diuresis, natriuresis, vasodilatation and suppression of the renin–angiotensin system. Levels of circulating ANP are increased in congestive cardiac failure and correlate with functional class, prognosis and haemodynamic state.
- ***Brain natriuretic peptide*** (***BNP***) (so called because it was first discovered in the brain) is predominantly secreted by the ventricles in response to increased myocardial wall stress. N-terminal (NT)-proBNP is an inactive protein that is cleaved from proBNP to release BNP. Both BNP and NT-proBNP are increased in patients with heart failure, and levels correlate with ventricular wall stress and the severity of heart failure. BNP and NT-proBNP are good predictors of cardiovascular events and mortality, and there is increasing interest in monitoring levels to help guide heart failure therapy.
- ***C-type peptide***, which is limited to vascular endothelium and the central nervous system, has similar effects to those of ANP and BNP.

Endothelial function in heart failure

The endothelium has a central role in the regulation of vasomotor tone. In patients with heart failure, endothelium-dependent vasodilatation in peripheral blood vessels is impaired and may be one mechanism of exercise limitation. The cause of abnormal endothelial responsiveness relates to abnormal release of both nitric oxide and vasoconstrictor substances, such as endothelin (ET). The activity of nitric oxide, a potent vasodilator, is blunted in heart failure. ET secretion from a variety of tissues is stimulated by many factors, including hypoxia, catecholamines and angiotensin II. The plasma concentration of ET is elevated in patients with heart failure, and levels correlate with the severity of haemodynamic disturbance. The major source of circulating ET in heart failure is the pulmonary vascular bed.

ET has many actions that potentially contribute to the pathophysiology of heart failure: vasoconstriction, sympathetic stimulation, renin–angiotensin system activation and left ventricular hypertrophy. Acute intravenous administration of ET antagonists improves haemodynamic abnormalities in patients with congestive cardiac failure, and oral ET antagonists are being developed. Plasma concentrations of some cytokines, in particular tumour necrosis factor (TNF), are increased in patients with heart failure.

Antidiuretic hormone (vasopressin)

Antidiuretic hormone (ADH) is raised in severe chronic heart failure, particularly in patients on diuretic treatment. A high ADH concentration precipitates hyponatraemia, which is an ominous prognostic indicator.

Clinical syndromes of heart failure

There are many causes of heart failure (see ***Box 23.18***) that can present suddenly, with acute heart failure (AHF), or more insidiously, with chronic heart failure (CHF).

- ***Left ventricular systolic dysfunction*** (***LVSD***) or ***heart failure and a reduced (R) ejection fraction*** (***HFREF***) is commonly caused by ischaemic heart disease but can also occur with valvular heart disease and hypertension.
- ***Diastolic heart failure*** is a syndrome consisting of symptoms and signs of ***heart failure with preserved (P) left ventricular ejection fraction*** (***HFPEF***) >45–50%. There is increased stiffness in the ventricular wall and decreased left ventricular compliance, leading to impairment of diastolic ventricular filling and hence decreased cardiac output. Echocardiography may demonstrate an increase in left ventricular wall thickness, increased left atrial size and abnormal left ventricular relaxation with normal or near-normal left ventricular volume. Diastolic heart failure is more common in elderly hypertensive patients but may occur with primary cardiomyopathies (hypertrophic, restrictive, infiltrative).
- ***Right ventricular systolic dysfunction*** (***RVSD***) may be secondary to chronic LVSD but can occur with primary and secondary pulmonary hypertension, right ventricular infarction, arrhythmogenic right ventricular cardiomyopathy and adult congenital heart disease.

Clinical features of heart failure

The symptoms and signs of heart failure are shown in ***Box 23.20***.

The New York Heart Association (NYHA) classification of heart failure ***(Box 23.21)*** can be used to describe the symptoms of heart failure and limitation of exercise capacity, and is useful for assessing response to therapy. It does not include left ventricular ejection fraction as a means of determining severity of heart failure.

Box 23.20 Clinical features of heart failure

Symptoms
- Exertional dyspnoea
- Orthopnoea
- Paroxysmal nocturnal dyspnoea
- Fatigue

Signs
- Tachycardia
- Elevated jugular venous pressure
- Cardiomegaly
- Third and fourth heart sounds
- Bi-basal crackles
- Pleural effusion
- Peripheral ankle oedema
- Ascites
- Tender hepatomegaly

Box 23.21 New York Heart Association (NYHA) classification of heart failure

Class	Features
Class I	No limitation. Normal physical exercise does not cause fatigue, dyspnoea or palpitations
Class II	Mild limitation. Comfortable at rest but normal physical activity produces fatigue, dyspnoea or palpitations
Class III	Marked limitation. Comfortable at rest but gentle physical activity produces marked symptoms of heart failure
Class IV	Symptoms of heart failure occur at rest and are exacerbated by any physical activity

Box 23.22 Diagnosis of heart failure (European Society of Cardiology guidelines)

Diagnosis of HF-REF requires three conditions to be satisfied

1. Symptoms typical of heart failure
2. Signs typical of heart failure
3. Reduced LV ejection fraction

Diagnosis of HF-PEF requires four conditions to be satisfied

1. Symptoms typical of heart failure
2. Signs typical of heart failure
3. Normal or only mildly reduced LV ejection fraction and LV not dilated
4. Relevant structural heart disease (LV hypertrophy/left atrial enlargement) and/or diastolic dysfunction

HF-REF = heart failure and a reduced ejection fraction; HF-PEF = heart failure with 'preserved' ejection fraction; LV = left ventricular.

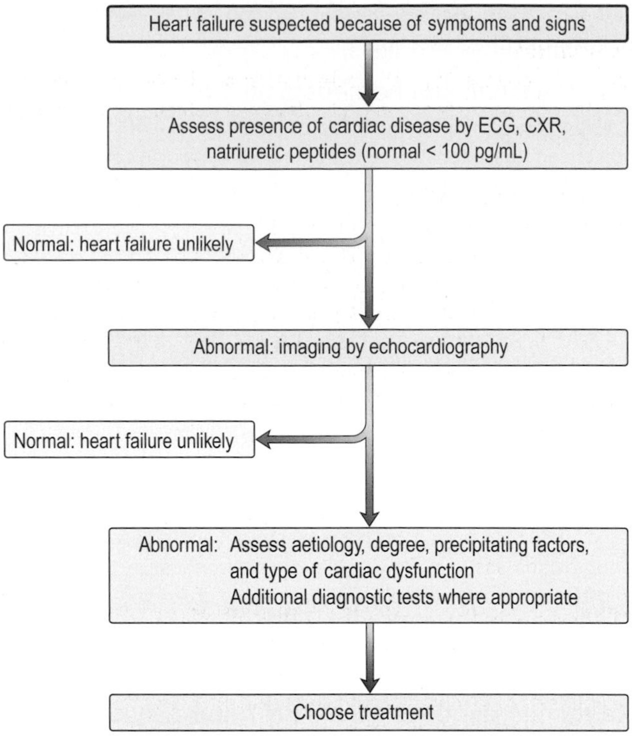

Figure 23.56 Algorithm for the diagnosis of heart failure. *(Based on the European Society of Cardiology and NICE guidelines.)*

Diagnosis of heart failure

The diagnosis of heart failure should not be based on history and clinical findings alone; it requires evidence of cardiac dysfunction using objective measures of left ventricular structure and function (usually echocardiography). Similarly, the underlying cause of heart failure should be established in all patients (***Box 23.22*** and ***Fig. 23.56***).

Investigations in heart failure

- ***Blood tests***. Full blood count, urea and electrolytes, liver biochemistry, cardiac enzymes in acute heart failure, BNP or NT-proBNP, and thyroid function should be tested.
- ***Chest X-ray***. Look for cardiomegaly, pulmonary congestion with upper lobe diversion, fluid in fissures, Kerley B lines and pulmonary oedema.
- ***Electrocardiogram***. Identify ischaemia, hypertension or arrhythmia.
- ***Echocardiography***. Assess cardiac chamber dimension, systolic and diastolic function, regional wall motion abnormalities, valvular disease and cardiomyopathies.
- ***Stress echocardiography***. Assess viability in dysfunctional myocardium – dobutamine identifies contractile reserve in stunned or hibernating myocardium.
- ***Nuclear cardiology***. Radionucleotide angiography (RNA) can quantify ventricular ejection fraction; SPECT or PET can demonstrate myocardial ischaemia and viability in dysfunctional myocardium.
- ***Cardiac MRI*** (***CMR***). Assess cardiac structure and function and viability in dysfunctional myocardium with the use of dobutamine for contractile reserve or with gadolinium for delayed enhancement ('infarct imaging').
- ***Cardiac catheterization***. This technique is employed for the diagnosis of ischaemic heart failure (and suitability for revascularization) and for measurement of pulmonary artery pressure, left atrial (wedge) pressure, left ventricular end-diastolic pressure.
- ***Cardiac biopsy***. This is used for diagnosis of cardiomyopathies, such as amyloid, and for follow-up of transplanted patients to assess rejection.
- ***Cardiopulmonary exercise testing***. Peak oxygen consumption (VO_2) is predictive of hospital admission and death in heart failure. A 6-minute exercise walk is an alternative.
- ***Ambulatory 24-hour ECG monitoring*** (***Holter***). This is used in patients with suspected arrhythmia, and may be used in those with severe heart failure or inherited cardiomyopathy to determine whether a defibrillator is appropriate (non-sustained ventricular tachycardia).

Management of heart failure

Management is aimed at relieving symptoms, prevention and control of disease leading to cardiac dysfunction and heart failure, retarding disease progression and improving quality and length of life.

Measures to prevent heart failure include cessation of smoking, alcohol and illicit drugs, effective treatment of hypertension, diabetes and hypercholesterolaemia, and pharmacological therapy following myocardial infarction.

The management of heart failure requires any factor aggravating the failure to be identified and treated. Similarly, the cause of heart failure must be elucidated and, where possible, corrected. Community nursing programmes to help with drug compliance and to detect early deterioration may prevent acute hospitalization.

General lifestyle advice

Education

Effective counselling of patients and family, emphasizing weight monitoring and dose adjustment of diuretics, may prevent hospitalization.

Dietary modification

Large meals should be avoided and, if necessary, weight reduction instituted. Salt restriction is required and foods rich in salt or added salt in cooking and at the table should be avoided. In severe heart failure, fluid restriction is necessary and patients may need to weigh themselves daily. Alcohol has a negative inotropic effect and heart failure patients should moderate consumption. Omega-3 polyunsaturated fatty acids (see p. 187) reduce mortality and hospital admission.

Smoking

Smoking should be stopped, with help from anti-smoking clinics if necessary (see p. 1075).

Physical activity, exercise training and rehabilitation

For patients with exacerbations of congestive cardiac failure, bed rest reduces the demands on the heart and is useful for a few days. Migration of fluid from the interstitium promotes a diuresis, reducing heart failure. Prolonged bed rest may lead to the development of deep vein thrombosis (DVT); this can be avoided by daily leg exercises, low-dose subcutaneous heparin and elastic support stockings. Low-level endurance exercise (e.g. 20–30 min walking three or five times per week or 20 min cycling at 70–80% of peak heart rate five times per week) is actively encouraged in patients with compensated heart failure in order to reverse 'deconditioning' of peripheral muscle metabolism. Strenuous isometric activity should be avoided.

Vaccination

While prospective clinical trials are lacking, it is recommended that patients with heart failure be vaccinated against pneumococcal disease and influenza (see p. 1078)

Air travel

This is possible for most patients, subject to clinical circumstances. Check with the airline – most have guidelines on who should travel.

Sexual activity

Tell patients on nitrates not to take phosphodiesterase type 5 inhibitors (e.g. sildenafil), as they may induce profound hypotension.

Driving

Driving cars and motorcycles may continue, provided there are no symptoms that distract the driver's attention. The Driver and Vehicle Licensing Authority (DVLA) in the UK does not need to be notified. Symptomatic heart failure disqualifies patients from driving large lorries and buses. Re/licensing may be permitted, as long as the left ventricular ejection fraction is good (i.e. >40%), the exercise test requirements can be met and there are no other disqualifying conditions.

Monitoring

The clinical condition of a person with heart failure fluctuates; lengthy and repeated hospital admissions are common, with an average inpatient stay of between 5 and 10 days. Monitoring of clinical status is necessary and this responsibility should be shared between primary and secondary healthcare professionals.

Essential monitoring includes assessment of:

- functional capacity (e.g. NYHA functional class, exercise tolerance test, echocardiography, maximum VO_2)
- fluid status (body weight, clinical assessment and urea and electrolytes)
- cardiac rhythm (ECG, 24-h tape).

Multidisciplinary team approach

Heart failure care should be delivered by a multidisciplinary team with an integrated approach across the healthcare community. The multidisciplinary team should involve specialist healthcare professionals: cardiologist or physician with a specialist interest in heart failure, heart failure nurse, dietician, pharmacist, occupational therapist, physiotherapist and palliative care adviser.

Understanding the information needs of patients and carers is vital. Good communication is essential for best clinical management, which should include advice on anxiety, depression and 'end-of-life' issues.

Drug management

Box 23.23 lists the drugs used in heart failure. ***Figure 23.57*** shows the stages of heart failure and the treatment options.

Diuretics

These act by promoting the renal excretion of salt and water by blocking tubular reabsorption of sodium and chloride (see p. 156). Loop diuretics (e.g. furosemide and bumetanide) and thiazide diuretics (e.g. bendroflumethiazide, hydrochlorothiazide) should be given in patients with fluid overload. Although diuretics provide symptomatic relief of dyspnoea and improve exercise tolerance, there is limited evidence that they affect survival. In severe heart failure patients, the combination of a loop and thiazide diuretic may be required. Serum electrolytes and renal function must be monitored regularly (risk of hypokalaemia and hypomagnesaemia).

Angiotensin-converting enzyme inhibitors

The use of angiotensin-converting enzyme (ACE) inhibitors in patients with heart failure has been demonstrated in multiple large randomized controlled trials (CONSENSUS, SOLVD) to improve symptoms and significantly reduce mortality. ACE inhibitors also benefit patients with asymptomatic heart failure following myocardial infarction. Thus, ACE inhibitors improve survival in patients in all functional classes (NYHA I–IV) and are recommended in all patients at risk of developing heart failure. The main adverse effects of ACE inhibitors are cough, hypotension, hyperkalaemia and renal dysfunction. Contraindications to their use include renal artery stenosis, pregnancy and previous angio-oedema. In patients with heart failure, ACE inhibitors should be introduced at a low initial dose and gradually titrated, with regular monitoring of blood pressure and renal function.

Angiotensin II receptor antagonists

The angiotensin II receptor antagonists (ARBs, candesartan and valsartan) are indicated as second-line therapy in patients intolerant of ACE inhibitors. Unlike ACE inhibitors, they do not affect bradykinin metabolism and do not produce a cough. The CHARM Alternative Trial showed that candesartan reduced the risk of heart failure hospitalization compared to placebo in patients intolerant of ACE inhibitors. Other trials (Val HeFT and ELITE II) have assessed other

Box 23.23 Drugs used in heart failure

Drug	Dose (initial/maximum)	Precautions
ACE inhibitors/ARAs		
Ramipril	1.25–2.5 mg daily/2.5–5 mg ×2 daily	Monitor renal function and use with caution if baseline serum creatinine >250 µmol/L or baseline blood pressure <90 mmHg
Enalapril	2.5 mg daily/10 mg ×2 daily	
Captopril	6.25 mg ×3 daily/25–50 mg ×3 daily	
Candesartan	4 mg daily/32 mg daily	
Valsartan	80 mg daily/320 mg daily	
Losartan	50 mg daily/100 mg daily	
Beta-adrenoceptor-blocking drugs		
Bisoprolol	1.25 mg daily/10 mg daily	Use with caution in obstructive airways disease, bradyarrhythmias
Carvedilol	3.125 mg daily/50 mg daily	Avoid in acute heart failure until patient is cardiovascularly stable
Nebivolol	1.25 mg daily/10 mg daily	
Diuretics		
Furosemide	20–40 mg daily/250–500 mg daily	Monitor renal function and check for hypokalaemia and hypomagnesaemia
Bumetanide	0.5–1.0 mg daily/5–10 mg daily	
Bendroflumethiazide	2.5 mg daily/10 mg daily	
Metolazone	2.5 mg daily/10 mg daily	Use in severe heart failure
Aldosterone antagonists		
Spironolactone	12.5–25 mg daily/50–200 mg daily (lower if on ACE inhibitor)	Monitor renal function, check for hyperkalaemia, gynaecomastia with spironolactone
Eplerenone	25 mg daily/50 mg daily	
Cardiac glycosides		
Digoxin	0.125–0.25 mg daily (reduce dose in elderly or in renal impairment)	Use with caution in renal impairment or conduction disease, and with amiodarone
Vasodilators		
Isosorbide dinitrate	20–40 mg ×3 daily	
Hydralazine	37.5–75 mg ×3 daily	
Ivabradine	5 mg daily/7.5 mg ×2 daily	Use with caution in sick sinus syndrome; AV block

ACE, angiotensin-converting enzyme; ARA, angiotensin II receptor antagonist; AV, atrioventricular.

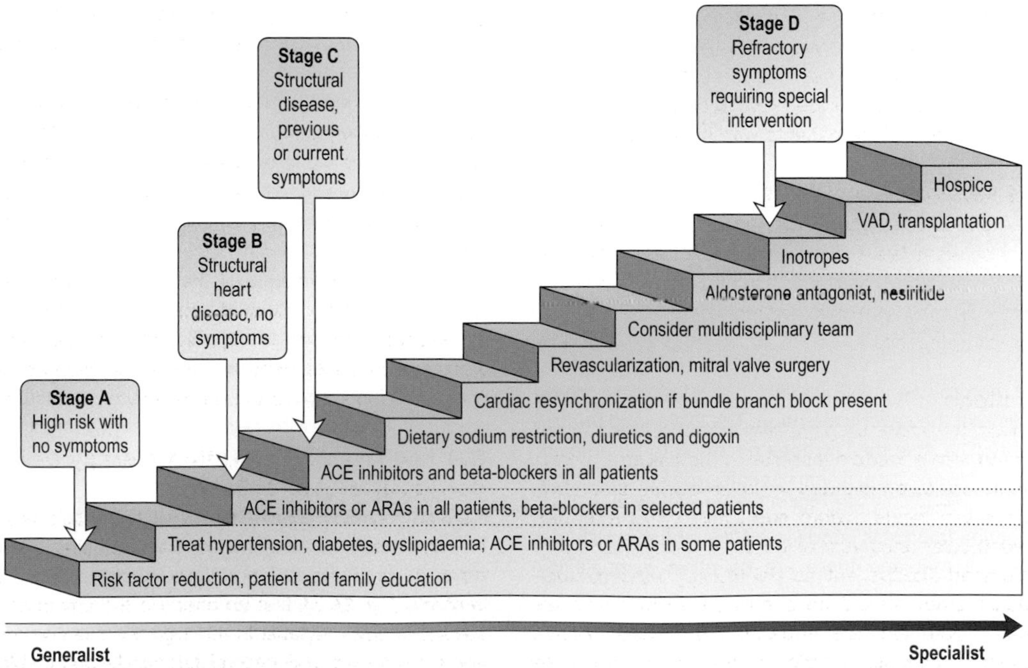

Figure 23.57 Stages of heart failure and treatment options for systolic heart failure. ACE, angiotensin-converting enzyme; ARA, angiotensin II receptor antagonist; VAD, ventricular assisted device.

ARAs. A recent study using the ARA valsartan and a neprilysin inhibitor sacubitril has shown promise in the treatment of heart failure.

Beta-blockers

Beta-blockers have been shown to improve functional status and reduce cardiovascular morbidity and mortality in patients with heart failure. Several trials (CIBIS, CIBIS II, MERIT-HF, COMET) have assessed the effects of beta-blockers in varying degrees of heart failure. Bisoprolol and carvedilol reduce mortality in any grade of heart failure. Nebivolol is used in the treatment of stable mild to moderate heart failure in patients over 70 years old (SENIORS). In patients with significant heart failure, beta-blockers are started at a low dose and gradually increased, with monitoring of heart rate and blood pressure.

Aldosterone antagonists

The aldosterone antagonists spironolactone and eplerenone have been shown to improve survival in patients with heart failure. In RALES, spironolactone reduced total mortality by 30% in patients with severe heart failure. However, gynaecomastia or breast pain occurred in 1 in 10 men taking spironolactone. In EPHESUS, eplerenone given to patients with an acute myocardial infarction and heart failure reduced total mortality by 15% and sudden cardiac death by 21%, with no gynaecomastia.

Cardiac glycosides

Digoxin is a cardiac glycoside that is indicated in patients in atrial fibrillation with heart failure. It is used as add-on therapy in symptomatic heart failure patients already receiving ACE inhibitors and beta-blockers. Although the DIG study demonstrated that digoxin reduced hospital admissions in patients with heart failure, a subanalysis in the ROCKET AF trial suggested that mortality may, in fact, be increased.

Vasodilators and nitrates

The combination of hydralazine and nitrates reduces preload and afterload, and is used in patients intolerant of ACE inhibitors or ARAs. The Veterans Administration Cooperative Study demonstrated that the combination of hydralazine (with nitrates) improved survival in patients with chronic heart failure. The A-HeFT trial showed that the same combination reduced mortality and hospitalization for heart failure in black patients with heart failure.

Inotropic and vasopressor agents

Intravenous inotropes and vasopressor agents (see ***Box 23.27***) are used in patients with acute heart failure and severe haemodynamic compromise. Although they produce haemodynamic improvements, they have not been shown to improve long-term mortality when compared with placebo.

Other medications

In hospital, all patients require prophylactic anticoagulation. Heart failure is associated with a fourfold increase in the risk of a stroke. Oral anticoagulants are recommended in patients with atrial fibrillation and in those with sinus rhythm and a history of thromboembolism, left ventricular aneurysm or thrombus. In patients with known ischaemic heart disease, antiplatelet therapy (aspirin, clopidogrel) and statin therapy should be continued. Arrhythmias are common in heart failure and are implicated in sudden death. Although treatment of complex ventricular arrhythmias might be expected to improve survival, there is no evidence to support this and it may increase mortality. In the Sudden Cardiac Death Heart Failure Trial (SCD-HeFT), amiodarone showed no benefit compared to placebo in patients with impaired left ventricular function and mild to moderate heart failure (whereas an ICD reduced mortality by 23% compared to placebo). Patients with heart failure and symptomatic ventricular arrhythmias should be assessed for suitability for an ICD.

Ivabradine selectively decreases heart rate without affecting blood pressure by inhibiting the I_F channels in the sinoatrial node (see pp. 933–935). An elevated heart rate in patients with heart failure is associated with worse cardiovascular outcomes. The SHIFT study reported a reduction in cardiovascular death and heart failure hospitalization in patients in sinus rhythm with chronic heart failure and left ventricular dysfunction (LVEF ≤35%). Ivabradine can be used in patients in sinus rhythm with an elevated heart rate despite beta-blocker treatment or in those who are unable to tolerate beta-blockers.

Non-pharmacological treatment

Revascularization

While coronary artery disease is the most common cause of heart failure, the role of revascularization in patients with heart failure is unclear. Patients with angina and left ventricular dysfunction have a higher mortality from surgery (10–20%), but have the most to gain in terms of improved symptoms and prognosis. Factors that must be considered before recommending surgery include age, symptoms and evidence of reversible myocardial ischaemia.

Hibernating myocardium and myocardial stunning

'Hibernating' myocardium can be defined as reversible left ventricular dysfunction due to chronic coronary artery disease that responds positively to inotropic stress and indicates the presence of viable heart muscle that may recover after revascularization. It is due to reduced myocardial perfusion, which is just sufficient to maintain viability of the heart muscle. Myocardial hibernation results from repetitive episodes of cardiac stunning that occur: for example, with repeated exercise in a patient with coronary artery disease.

Myocardial stunning is reversible ventricular dysfunction that persists following an episode of ischaemia when the blood flow has returned to normal: that is, there is a mismatch between flow and function.

The prevalence of hibernating myocardium in patients with coronary artery disease can be estimated from the frequency of improvement in regional abnormalities in wall motion after revascularization; it is thought to be 33% of such patients. Techniques to try to identify hibernating myocardium include stress echocardiography, nuclear imaging, CMR and PET.

The clinical relevance of the hibernating and stunned myocardium is that ventricular dysfunction due to these mechanisms may be wrongly ascribed to myocardial necrosis and scarring, which seems untreatable, whereas reversible hibernating and stunning myocardium responds to coronary revascularization.

Cardiac resynchronization therapy or implantable cardioverter–defibrillator

Cardiac resynchronization therapy (CRT) entails simultaneous pacing of both ventricles (biventricular pacing) using a lead placed in the right ventricle and another in the coronary sinus to pace the left ventricle ***(Fig. 23.58)***. It is an effective therapy in addition to optimal medical therapy in patients with significant left ventricular impairment and a prolonged QRS interval (left bundle branch block). Resynchronization may reverse the process of ventricular remodelling, reduce functional mitral regurgitation and improve left ventricular function.

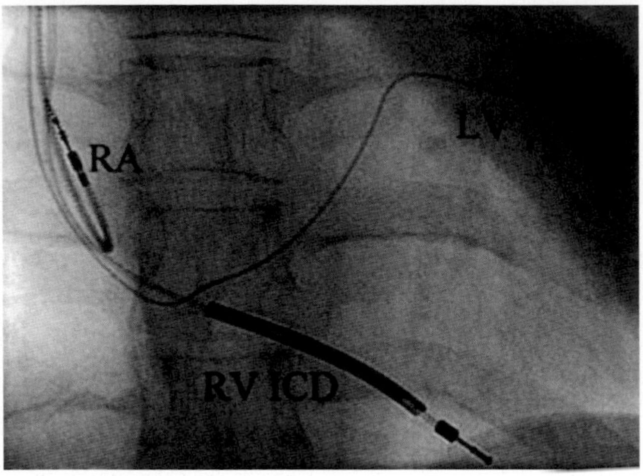

Figure 23.58 Implanted biventricular pacemaker with implantable cardioverter–defibrillator device (CRT-D). LV, left ventricle; RA, right atrium; RV, right ventricle.

The CARE-HF and COMPANION trials reported symptomatic benefit and a reduction in heart failure events and mortality following CRT implantation in patients with heart failure in NYHA classes III and IV. Similar findings have been noted in more recent trials in patients with mild heart failure or no symptoms.

Most patients with heart failure who receive CRT also meet the criteria for use of an implantable cardioverter–defibrillator (ICD) and should receive a combined device (CRT-D). Patients with end-stage heart failure (NYHA IV) or other co-morbidities that may significantly reduce lifespan are generally not candidates for an ICD.

Cardiac transplantation

Cardiac transplantation has become the treatment of choice for younger patients with severe intractable heart failure, whose life expectancy is less than 6 months. With careful recipient selection, the expected 1-year survival for patients following transplantation is over 90%, and is 75% at 5 years. Irrespective of survival, quality of life is dramatically improved for the majority of patients. The availability of heart transplantation is limited.

Heart allografts do not function normally. Cardiac denervation results in a high resting heart rate, loss of diurnal blood pressure variation and impaired renin–angiotensin–aldosterone regulation. Some patients develop a 'stiff heart' syndrome, caused by rejection, denervation and ischaemic injury during organ harvest and implantation. Transplantation of an inappropriately small donor heart can also result in elevated right and left heart pressure.

The complications of heart transplantation are summarized in ***Box 23.24***. Many (infection, malignancy, hypertension and hyperlipidaemia) are related to immunosuppression. Allograft coronary atherosclerosis is the major cause of long-term graft failure and is present in 30–50% of patients at 5 years. It is due to a 'vascular' rejection process in conjunction with hypertension and hyperlipidaemia.

There are specific contraindications to cardiac transplantation ***(Box 23.25)***; notably, high pulmonary vascular resistance and active malignancy are absolute contraindications. Several options to transplantation are available: cardiomyoplasty (augmentation of left ventricular contraction by wrapping a latissimus dorsi muscle flap around the ventricle) and the Batista procedure (surgical ventricular size reduction and remodelling of the geometry of the left ventricle). Both procedures have a high mortality and there is limited evidence of substantial benefit in the medium term.

Box 23.24 Complications of cardiac transplantation

- Allograft rejection:
  - 'Humoral'
  - 'Vascular'
  - 'Cell-mediated'
- Infections:
  - Early: hospital-acquired organisms – staphylococci; Gram-negative bacteria
  - Late (2–6 months): opportunistic (toxoplasmosis, cytomegalovirus, fungi, *Pneumocystis*)
- Allograft vascular disease
- Hypertension
- Hypercholesterolaemia
- Malignancy

Box 23.25 Contraindications to cardiac transplantation

- Age >60 years (some variations between centres)
- Alcohol/drug misuse
- Uncontrolled psychiatric illness
- Uncontrolled infection
- Severe renal/liver failure
- High pulmonary vascular resistance
- Systemic disease with multiorgan involvement
- Treated cancer in remission but with <5 years' follow-up
- Recent thromboembolism
- Other disease with a poor prognosis

Acute heart failure

Acute heart failure (AHF) occurs with the rapid onset of symptoms and signs of heart failure secondary to abnormal cardiac function, causing elevated cardiac filling pressures. This leads to severe dyspnoea, and fluid accumulates in the interstitium and alveolar spaces of the lung (pulmonary oedema). AHF is the leading cause of hospital admission in people above the age of 65 years; it has a poor prognosis, with a 60-day mortality rate of nearly 10% and a rate of death or rehospitalization of 35% within 60 days. In patients with ***acute pulmonary oedema***, the in-hospital mortality rate is 12% and by 12 months this rises to 30%. Poor prognostic indicators include a high (>16 mmHg) pulmonary capillary wedge pressure (PCWP), low serum sodium concentration, increased left ventricular end-diastolic dimension on echo and low oxygen consumption.

The aetiology of AHF is similar to that of chronic heart failure:

- ***Ischaemic heart disease*** patients present with an acute coronary syndrome or develop a complication of a myocardial infarction, such as papillary muscle rupture or ventricular septal defect requiring surgical intervention.
- ***Valvular heart disease*** patients also present with AHF due to valvular regurgitation in endocarditis or prosthetic valve thrombosis. A thoracic aortic dissection may produce severe aortic regurgitation.
- ***Hypertension*** patients present with episodes of 'flash' pulmonary oedema despite preserved left ventricular systolic function.
- ***Acute and chronic kidney disease*** both involve fluid overload and reduced renal excretion, which will produce pulmonary oedema.
- ***Atrial fibrillation*** is frequently associated with AHF and may require emergency cardioversion.

Several clinical syndromes of AHF can be defined ***(Box 23.26)***. In a clinical environment, both the Killip score (see p. 1004, based on a cardiorespiratory clinical assessment) and Forrester classification (based on right catheterization findings) are used to provide therapeutic and prognostic information.

Box 23.26 Clinical syndromes of acute heart failure (AHF)

Type	Clinical features
Acute decompensated heart failure	Mild features of heart failure, e.g. dyspnoea
Hypertensive AHF	High blood pressure, preserved left ventricular function, pulmonary oedema on chest X-ray
Acute pulmonary oedema	Tachypnoea, orthopnoea, pulmonary crackles, oxygen saturation <90% on air, pulmonary oedema on chest X-ray
Cardiogenic shock	Systolic blood pressure <90 mmHg, mean arterial pressure drop >30 mmHg, urine output <0.5 mL/kg per hour, heart rate >60 b.p.m.
High-output heart failure	Warm peripheries, pulmonary congestion, blood pressure may be low, e.g. septic shock
Right heart failure	Low cardiac output, elevated jugular venous pressure, hepatomegaly, hypotension

(Modified from the European Society of Cardiology.)

Pathophysiology

The pathophysiology of AHF is similar to that of chronic heart failure with activation of the renin–angiotensin–aldosterone axis and sympathetic nervous system. In addition, prolonged ischaemia (e.g. in acute coronary syndromes) results in myocardial stunning (see p. 987), which exacerbates myocardial dysfunction but may respond to inotropic support. If myocardial ischaemia persists, the myocardium may exhibit hibernation (persistently impaired function due to reduced coronary blood flow), which may recover with successful revascularization.

Diagnosis

In a person presenting with symptoms and signs of heart failure, a structured assessment should result in the clinical diagnosis of AHF and direct initial treatment to stabilize the patient. Initial investigations performed in the emergency room should include the following:

- ***A 12-lead ECG*** will identify acute coronary syndromes, left ventricular hypertrophy, atrial fibrillation, valvular heart disease and left bundle branch block.
- ***A chest X-ray*** may demonstrate cardiomegaly, pulmonary oedema, pleural effusion or non-cardiac disease.
- ***Blood investigations*** should include serum creatinine and electrolytes, full blood count, blood glucose, cardiac enzymes and troponin, C-reactive protein (CRP) and D-dimer.
- ***Plasma BNP*** or ***NT-proBNP*** (BNP >100 pg/mL or NT-proBNP >300 pg/mL) is suggestive of heart failure.
- ***Transthoracic echocardiography*** should be performed without delay to confirm the diagnosis of heart failure (see pp. 949–951) and possibly identify the cause.

If the baseline investigations confirm AHF, then treatment should be commenced.

Management

The goals of treatment in a patient with AHF include:

- immediate relief of symptoms and stabilization of haemodynamics (short-term benefits)

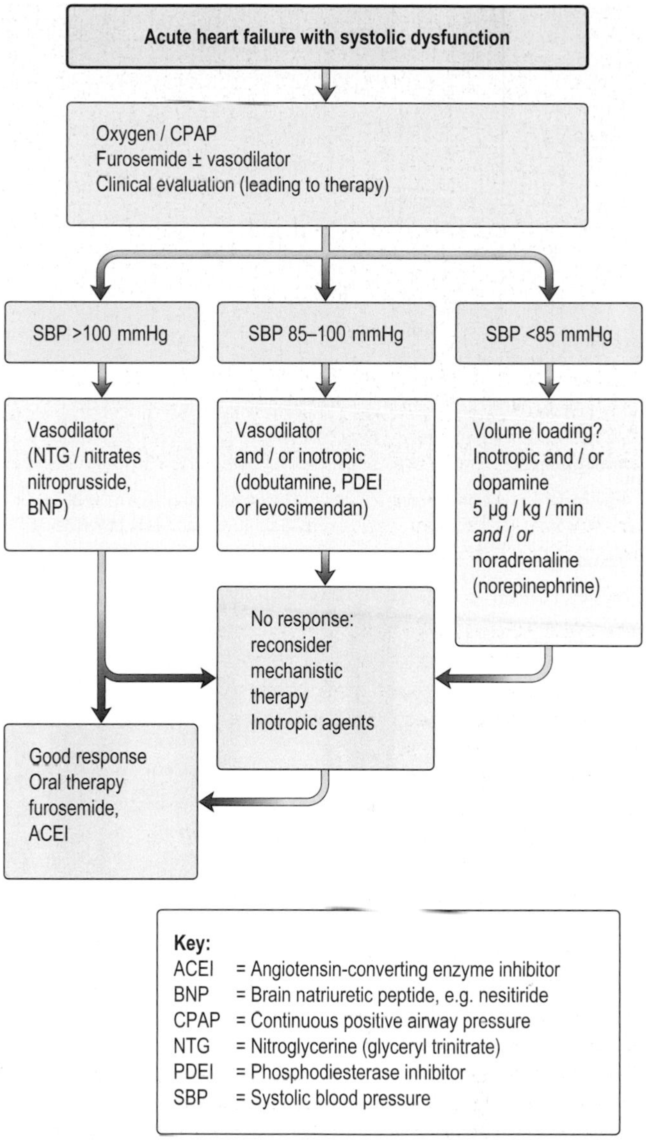

Figure 23.59 Algorithm for the management of acute heart failure with systolic dysfunction. *(From Nieminen MS, Böhm M, Cowie MR et al. Executive summary of the guidelines on the diagnosis and treatment of acute heart failure: the Task Force on Acute Heart Failure of the European Society of Cardiology.* Eur Heart J *2005; 26:384–416, Figure 6, with permission from Oxford University Press and the European Society of Cardiology.)*

- reduction in length of hospital stay and hospital re-admissions
- reduction in mortality from heart failure.

Patients with AHF should be managed in a high-dependency area with regular measurement of temperature, heart rate, blood pressure and cardiac monitoring. All require prophylactic anticoagulation with low-molecular-weight heparin.

Individuals with haemodynamic compromise may need arterial lines for invasive blood pressure monitoring and arterial gas sampling, central venous cannulation (intravenous medication, inotropic support, monitoring of central venous pressure) and pulmonary artery cannulation (calculation of cardiac output/index, peripheral vasoconstriction and pulmonary wedge pressure).

Initial therapy (***Fig. 23.59*** and ***Box 23.27***) includes oxygen and diuretics (e.g. i.v. furosemide 50 mg). If intravenous nitrates (e.g.

Box 23.27 Pharmacological therapy in acute heart failure

Drug	Dose	Indications/mechanism of action
Myocardial oxygenation		
Oxygen	35–50% inspired oxygen concentration	Ensure airway is patent and maintain arterial saturation at 95–98%
Non-invasive positive pressure ventilation (NIPPV), e.g. CPAP		Use if failing to maintain arterial saturation Increases pulmonary recruitment and functional residual capacity – reduces work of breathing
Intubation/mechanical ventilation		Use if patient is failing to maintain arterial saturation and is fatigued (reduced respiratory rate, increased arterial CO_2, confusion)
Opiate		
Morphine	2.5–5.0 mg i.v. (with antiemetic metoclopramide 10 mg i.v.)	Use in agitated patient Relieves dyspnoea, venous and arterial dilatation
Antithrombin		
Low-molecular-weight heparin	e.g. Enoxaparin 1 mg/kg s.c. ×2 daily ACS or 40 mg s.c. daily prophylaxis	Use in patients with AHF, ACS or atrial fibrillation, or for DVT prophylaxis Caution if creatinine clearance <30 mL/min
Vasodilators		
Glyceryl trinitrate	10–200 μg/min i.v. infusion	Reduces pulmonary congestion; at low doses causes venodilatation, reducing preload; at high doses causes arterial vasodilatation, reducing afterload Ensure BP >85–90 mmHg
Sodium nitroprusside	0.3–5 μg/kg per min i.v. infusion	Use in severe AHF where there is predominantly high afterload, e.g. hypertensive AHF Needs arterial BP monitoring for profound hypotension
Diuretic		
Furosemide	Bolus 40–100 mg i.v. or infusion 5–40 mg/h	Low doses produce vasodilatation and reduce right atrial pressure and PCWP; promote diuresis Need to monitor sodium, potassium and creatinine
Inotropes		
Dopamine	Low dose <2 μg/kg per min	Low dose acts on peripheral dopamine receptors to produce vasodilatation (renal, splanchnic, coronary, cerebrovascular) and may improve diuresis
	Medium dose >2 μg/kg per min	Medium dose acts on β-receptors to increase myocardial contractility and cardiac output
	High dose >5 μg/kg per min	High dose acts on α-receptors, causing vasoconstriction and increasing total peripheral resistance (increases afterload, PAP)
Dobutamine	2–20 μg/kg per min (patients on beta-blockers may need high dose)	Stimulates β_1 and β_2-receptors, producing vasodilatation. Increases heart rate and cardiac output, and also diuresis as haemodynamics are improved
Milrinone	Bolus 25–75 μg/kg over 10–20 min then 0.375–0.75 μg/kg per min	Inhibits phosphodiesterase and maintains cAMP Increases cardiac output and stroke volume, reduces PAP/PCWP/total peripheral resistance/BP
Levosimendan	Bolus 12–24 μg/kg over 10 min then 0.05–2 μg/kg per min	Positive inotropic drug with vasodilator effects by increasing sensitivity of contractile proteins to calcium and opening potassium channels Increases cardiac output and reduces PCWP
Vasopressors		
Noradrenaline (norepinephrine)	0.2–1.0 μg/kg per min	Stimulates α-receptors Increases total peripheral resistance and BP
Adrenaline (epinephrine)	Bolus 1 mg at resuscitation then 0.05–0.5 μg/kg per min	Stimulates α, β_1- and β_2-receptors Increases cardiac output, heart rate, total peripheral resistance and BP
Cardiac glycoside		
Digoxin	0.5 mg i.v. repeated after 2–6 h	Inhibits myocardial sodium/potassium ATPase, leading to increased calcium and sodium exchange Increases cardiac output and slows AV conduction Use in AF; avoid in ACS

ACS, acute coronary syndrome; AF, atrial fibrillation; AHF, acute heart failure; ATPase, adenosine triphosphatase; AV, atrioventricular; BP, blood pressure; cAMP, cyclic adenosine monophosphate; CPAP, continuous positive airway pressure; i.v., intravenous; NIPPV, non-invasive positive pressure ventilation; PAP, positive airway pressure; PCWP, pulmonary capillary wedge pressure; s.c., subcutaneous.

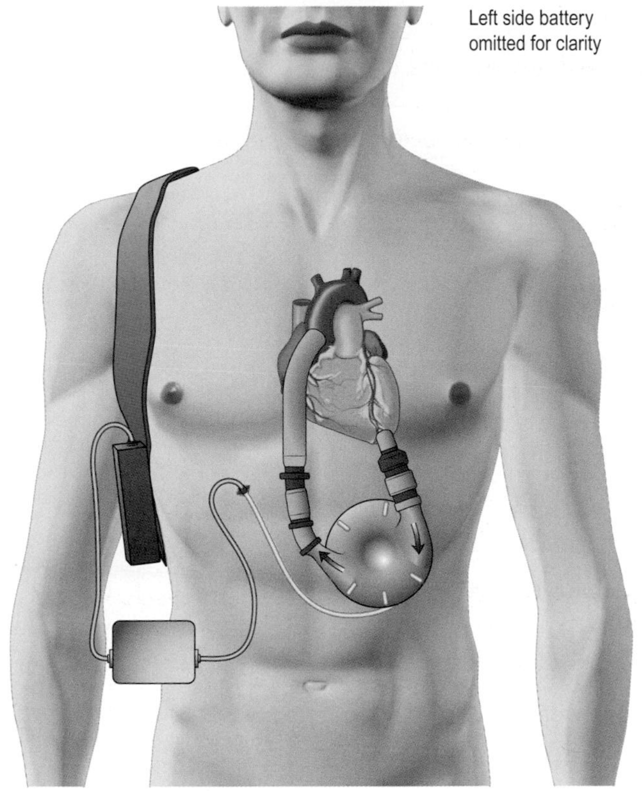

Figure 23.60 **Left ventricular assist device.** *(From Moser DK, Riegel B. Cardiac Nursing. Philadelphia: Saunders; 2007, p. 981, with permission of Elsevier.)*

glyceryl trinitrate infusion 10–200 μg/min) are required (e.g. concomitant myocardial ischaemia, severe hypertension), careful monitoring of the blood pressure is mandatory. Inotropic support (see pp. 1158–1160) with dobutamine, phosphodiesterase inhibitors or levosimendan can be added in patients who do not respond to the initial therapy ***(Fig. 23.59)***. A BNP (nesiritide) can also be used in AHF as a bolus injection followed by an infusion.

Patients with profound hypotension may require inotropes and vasopressors to improve the haemodynamic status and alleviate symptoms, but these have not been shown to improve mortality. Non-invasive continuous positive airway pressure/positive pressure ventilation (CPAP/NIPPV; see pp. 1165–1166) has been shown to provide earlier improvement in dyspnoea and respiratory distress than standard oxygen via mask; mortality is, however, unaffected.

Mechanical assist devices

Mechanical assist devices can be used in patients who fail to respond to standard medical therapy but in whom there is either transient myocardial dysfunction with likelihood of recovery (e.g. post anterior myocardial infarction treated with coronary angioplasty) or as a bridge to cardiac surgery, including transplantation.

Ventricular assist devices

Ventricular assist devices (VADs, ***Fig. 23.60***) are mechanical devices that replace or help the failing ventricles in delivering blood around the body. A left ventricular assist device (LVAD) receives blood from the left ventricle and delivers it to the aorta; a right ventricular assist device (RVAD) receives blood from the right ventricle and delivers it to the pulmonary artery. The devices can be extracorporeal (suitable for short-term support) or intracorporeal (suitable for long-term support as a bridge to transplantation or as destination therapy in patients with end-stage heart failure not candidates for transplantation). The main problems with VADs include thromboembolism, bleeding, infection and device malfunction.

Further reading

Armstrong PW. Aldosterone antagonists – last man standing? *N Engl J Med* 2011; 364:79–80.

Bonow RO, Maurer G, Lee KL et al. for the STICH Trial Investigators. Myocardial viability and survival in ischemic left ventricular dysfunction. *N Engl J Med* 2011; 364:1617–1625.

Braunwald E. Biomarkers in heart failure. *N Engl J Med* 2008; 358:2148–2158.

Braunwald E. The war against heart failure. *Lancet* 2015; 385:812–824.

Dworzynski K, Roberts E, Ludman A et al. Diagnosing and managing acute heart failure in adults: summary of NICE guidance. *BMJ* 2014; 349:g5695.

Fang JC. Underestimating medical therapy for coronary disease ... again [Editorial]. *N Engl J Med* 2011; 364:1671–1673.

Holzmeister J, Leclercq C. Implantable cardioverter defibrillators and cardiac resynchronisation therapy. *Lancet* 2011; 378:722–730.

Krum H, Teerlink JR. Medical therapy for chronic heart failure. *Lancet* 2011; 378:713–772.

McMurray JJ. Clinical practice. Systolic heart failure. *New Engl J Med* 2010; 362:228–238.

McMurray JJ, Adamopoulos S, Anker SD et al. ESC Guidelines for the Diagnosis and Treatment of Acute and Chronic Heart Failure 2012: The Task Force for the Diagnosis and Treatment of Acute and Chronic Heart Failure 2012 of the European Society of Cardiology. Developed in collaboration with the Heart Failure Association (HFA) of the ESC. *Eur J Heart Fail* 2012; 14:803–869.

National Institute for Health and Care Excellence. *NICE Clinical Guideline 108: Chronic Heart Failure: Management of Chronic Heart Failure in Adults in Primary and Secondary Care*. NICE 2010; https://www.nice.org.uk/guidance/cg108.

National Institute for Health and Care Excellence. *NICE Clinical Guideline 187: Acute Heart Failure: Diagnosing and Managing Acute Heart Failure in Adults*. NICE 2014; https://www.nice.org.uk/guidance/cg187.

Swedberg K, Komajda M, Böhm M et al. on behalf of the SHIFT Investigators. Ivabradine and outcomes in chronic heart failure (SHIFT): a randomised placebo-controlled study. *Lancet* 2010; 376:875–885.

Velazquez EJ, Lee KL, Deja MA et al. for the STICH Investigators. Coronary-artery bypass surgery in patients with left ventricular dysfunction. *N Engl J Med* 2011; 364:1607–1616.

Zannad F, McMurray JJ, Krum H et al. for the EMPHASIS-HF Study Group. Eplerenone in patients with systolic heart failure and mild symptoms. *N Engl J Med* 2011; 364:11–21.

CORONARY ARTERY DISEASE

Myocardial ischaemia occurs when there is an imbalance between the supply of oxygen (and other essential myocardial nutrients) and the myocardial demand for these substances.

Coronary blood flow to a region of the myocardium may be reduced by a mechanical obstruction that is due to:

- atheroma
- thrombosis
- spasm
- embolus
- coronary ostial stenosis
- coronary arteritis (e.g. in systemic lupus erythematosus).

There can be a decrease in the flow of oxygenated blood to the myocardium that is due to:

- anaemia
- carboxyhaemoglobulinaemia
- hypotension, causing decreased coronary perfusion pressure.

An increased demand for oxygen may occur owing to an increase in cardiac output (e.g. thyrotoxicosis) or myocardial hypertrophy (e.g. from aortic stenosis or hypertension).

Myocardial ischaemia most commonly arises as a result of obstructive coronary artery disease (CAD) in the form of coronary atherosclerosis. In addition to this fixed obstruction, variations in the tone of smooth muscle in the wall of a coronary artery may add another element of dynamic or variable obstruction.

CAD is the largest single cause of death in the UK and many parts of the world. In 2010, cardiovascular diseases were the UK's biggest killer, accounting for nearly 180000 deaths. CAD was responsible for 1 in 5 male deaths and 1 in 10 female deaths (approximately 80000 deaths). Sudden cardiac death is a prominent feature of CAD, 1 in every 6 coronary attacks presenting with sudden death as the first, last and only symptom.

Pathophysiology of coronary atherosclerosis

Coronary atherosclerosis is a complex inflammatory process characterized by the accumulation of lipid, macrophages and smooth muscle cells in intimal plaques in the large and medium-sized epicardial coronary arteries. The vascular endothelium plays a critical role in maintaining vascular integrity and homeostasis. Mechanical shear stresses (e.g. from morbid hypertension), biochemical abnormalities (e.g. elevated low-density lipoprotein (LDL), diabetes mellitus), immunological factors (e.g. free radicals from smoking), inflammation (e.g. infection such as *Chlamydophila pneumoniae*) and genetic alteration may contribute to the initial endothelial 'injury' or dysfunction, which is believed to trigger atherogenesis.

The ***development of atherosclerosis*** follows the endothelial dysfunction, with increased permeability to and accumulation of oxidized lipoproteins, which are taken up by macrophages at focal sites within the endothelium to produce lipid-laden foam cells. Macroscopically, these lesions are seen as flat, yellow dots or lines on the endothelium of the artery and are known as '***fatty streaks***'. The 'fatty streak' progresses with the appearance of extracellular lipid within the endothelium ('***transitional plaque***'). Release of cytokines, such as platelet-derived growth factor and transforming growth factor beta (TGF-β), by monocytes, macrophages or the damaged endothelium promotes further accumulation of macrophages, as well as smooth muscle cell migration and proliferation. The proliferation of smooth muscle with the formation of a layer of cells covering the extracellular lipid separates it from the adaptive smooth muscle thickening in the endothelium. Collagen is produced in larger and larger quantities by the smooth muscle and the whole sequence of events cumulates as an '***advanced*** or ***raised fibrolipid plaque***'. The 'advanced plaque' may grow slowly and encroach on the lumen, or become unstable, undergo thrombosis and produce an obstruction ('***complicated plaque***').

Two different mechanisms are responsible for thrombosis on the plaques ***(Fig. 23.61)***:

- ***The first process*** is superficial endothelial injury, which involves denudation of the endothelial covering over the plaque. Sub-endocardial connective tissue matrix is then exposed and platelet adhesion occurs because of reaction with collagen. The thrombus is adherent to the surface of the plaque.
- ***The second process*** is deep endothelial fissuring, which involves an advanced plaque with a lipid core. The plaque cap tears (ulcerates, fissures or ruptures), allowing blood from the lumen to enter the inside of the plaque itself. The core with lamellar lipid surfaces, tissue factor (which triggers platelet adhesion and activation) produced by macrophages and exposed collagen, is highly thrombogenic. Thrombus forms within the plaque, expanding its volume and distorting its shape. Thrombosis may then extend into the lumen.

A 50% reduction in luminal diameter (producing a reduction in luminal cross-sectional area of approximately 70%) causes a haemodynamically significant stenosis. At this point, the smaller distal intramyocardial arteries and arterioles are maximally dilated (coronary flow reserve is near zero), and any increase in myocardial oxygen demand provokes ischaemia.

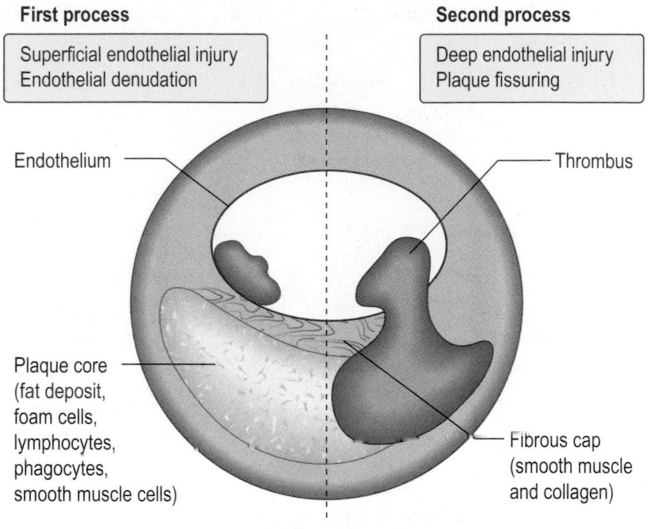

Figure 23.61 The mechanisms for the development of thrombosis on plaques.

Box 23.28 Risk factors for coronary disease

Fixed
- Age
- Male sex
- Positive family history
- Deletion polymorphism in the angiotensin-converting enzyme (*ACE*) gene (DD)

Potentially changeable
- Hyperlipidaemia
- Cigarette smoking
- Hypertension
- Diabetes mellitus
- Lack of exercise
- Blood coagulation factors – high fibrinogen, factor VII
- Elevated C-reactive protein
- Homocysteinaemia
- Obesity
- Gout
- Soft water
- Drugs, e.g. contraceptive pill, nucleoside analogues, COX-2 inhibitors, rosiglitazone
- Heavy alcohol consumption

CAD gives rise to a wide variety of clinical presentations, ranging from relatively stable angina through to the acute coronary syndromes of unstable angina and myocardial infarction ***(Fig. 23.62)***. ***Figure 23.63*** shows a plaque rupture.

Risk factors for coronary artery disease

CAD is an atherosclerotic disease that is multifactorial in origin, giving rise to the risk factor concept. Certain living habits promote atherogenic traits in genetically susceptible persons. A number of 'risk' factors are known to predispose to the condition ***(Box 23.28)***. Some of these, such as age, gender, race and family history, cannot be changed, whereas other major risk factors, such as serum cholesterol, smoking habits, diabetes and hypertension, can be modified.

Atherosclerotic disease manifest in one vascular bed is often advanced in other territories. Patients with intermittent claudication have a two- to fourfold increased risk of CAD, stroke or heart failure. Following initial myocardial infarction (MI), there is a three- to sixfold increase in the risk of heart failure and stroke. After stroke, the risk of heart failure and MI is increased twofold.

The disease can be asymptomatic in its most severe form, with 1 in 3 myocardial infarctions going unrecognized. Some 30–40% of

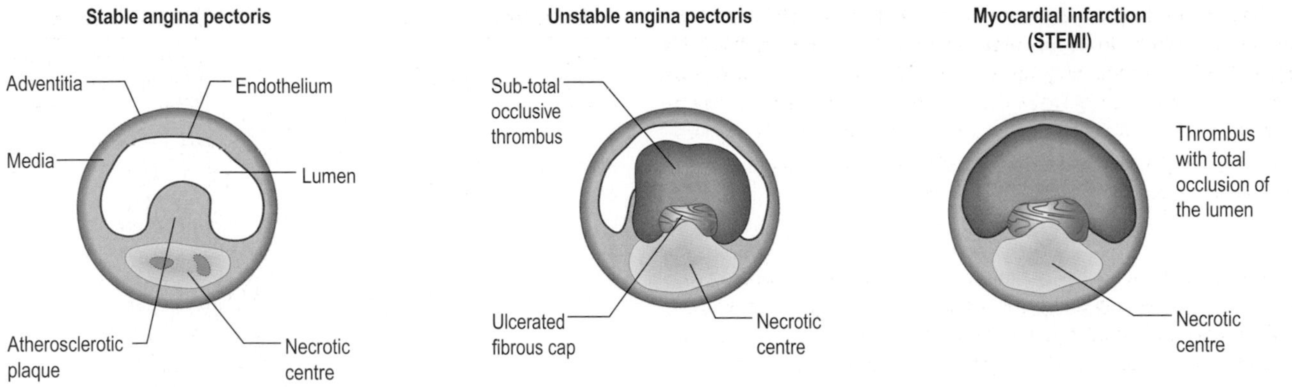

Figure 23.62 The mechanisms for the development of thrombosis on plaques in various clinical syndromes. Relationship between the state of coronary artery vessel wall and the various syndromes.

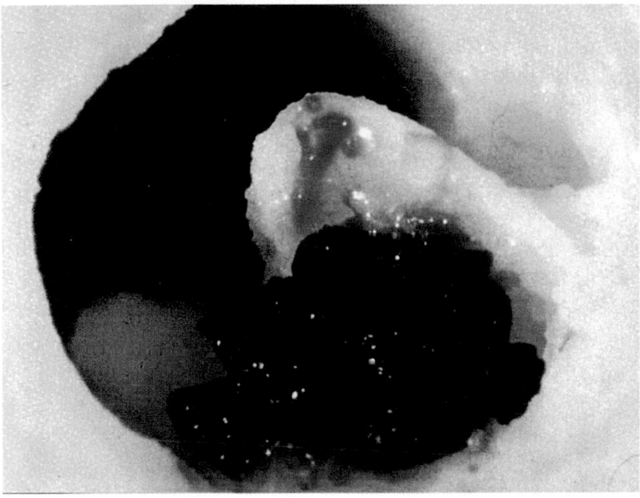

Figure 23.63 Acute coronary thrombus. Cross-section (×30) of the epicardial coronary artery, demonstrating a rupture of the shoulder region of the plaque with a luminal thrombus.

individuals who present with an acute coronary syndrome have had no prior warning symptom to suggest the presence of underlying disease.

Diagnosis

Cardiovascular risk assessment for primary and secondary prevention of cardiovascular disease

Primary prevention can be defined as the prevention of the atherosclerotic disease process and ***secondary prevention*** as the treatment of the atherosclerotic disease process (i.e. treatment of the disease or its complications). The objective of prevention is to reduce the incidence of first or recurrent clinical events due to CAD, ischaemic stroke and peripheral artery disease.

In the UK, NICE guidelines recommend that primary care should use the QRISK®2 risk assessment tool (see 'Further reading') to identify people who are likely to be at high risk (10-year risk of cardiovascular disease ≥10%).

Lipids

A full lipid profile should be obtained, including total cholesterol, high-density lipoprotein (HDL) cholesterol, non-HDL cholesterol, and triglyceride concentrations. Patients with a total cholesterol concentration >7.5 mmol/L and a family history of premature coronary heart disease may have ***familial hypercholesterolaemia***.

Lifestyle modifications

Patients should eat a diet with a reduced fat intake (≤30% of total energy intake, saturated fats ≤7% total energy intake) and a dietary cholesterol intake <300 mg/day. Saturated fats should be replaced by monounsaturated and polyunsaturated fats (rapeseed and olive oils). People should aim to reduce their intake of sugar and food products that contain refined sugars (e.g. fructose), and to eat at least five portions of fruit and vegetables per day, two portions of fish per week, and four to five portions of unsalted nuts, seeds and legumes per week. The weekly exercise recommendations are ≥150 minutes of moderate-intensity aerobic activity or 75 minutes of vigorous-intensity aerobic activity. Weight/body mass index should be <25 kg/m^2 (see p. 208). Daily alcohol intake should not exceed 3–4 units for men and 2–3 units for women, and smoking should be discontinued. Blood pressure and diabetes should be managed according to NICE guidelines in the UK.

Statin treatment

Atorvastatin 20 mg is recommended for the primary prevention of cardiovascular disease in people with a 10-year risk of cardiovascular disease of ≥10%. In patients with established cardiovascular disease, NICE recommends atorvastatin 80 mg, unless there are potential drug interactions, a high risk of adverse effects, or a different patient preference.

ANGINA

Myocardial ischaemia in patients with stable CAD occurs when there is a mismatch between blood supply and metabolic demand. This results in regional wall motion abnormalities, ST-T changes on the 12-lead ECG and cardiac ischaemic pain – angina. Ischaemic metabolites, including adenosine, stimulate nerve endings and produce pain.

Epidemiology

The prevalence of angina increases with age in both sexes; in women it is 5–7% at 45–64 years as opposed to 10–12% at 65–84 years, while in men it is 4–7% at 45–64 years as opposed to 12–14% at 65–84 years. The annual mortality rate ranges from 1.2% to 2.4% and there is an annual incidence of cardiac death of 0.6–1.4%. Risk factors include hypertension, hyperlipidaemia, diabetes mellitus, sedentary lifestyle, obesity, smoking and family history.

Diagnosis

The diagnosis of angina is largely based on the clinical history.

- ***Classical angina*** is characterized by chest pain that is described as 'heavy', 'tight' or 'gripping'. Typically, the pain is central/retrosternal and may radiate to the jaw and/or arms. The pain tends to occur with exercise or emotional stress, or when walking up slopes in cold weather, and eases rapidly with rest.
- ***Stable angina*** can be classified according to the Canadian Cardiovascular Society guidelines ***(Box 23.29)***.
- ***Unstable angina*** refers to angina of recent onset (<24 h) or deterioration in previous stable angina, with symptoms frequently occurring at rest: that is, **acute coronary syndrome**.
- ***Refractory angina*** refers to patients with severe coronary disease in whom revascularization is not possible and angina is not controlled by medical therapy.
- ***Vasospastic*** or ***variant (Prinzmetal's) angina*** refers to angina that occurs without provocation, usually at rest, as a result of coronary artery spasm. It occurs more frequently in women. Characteristically, there is ST segment elevation on the ECG during the pain.
- ***Microvascular angina*** patients have exercise-induced angina but normal or unobstructed coronary arteries (on coronary angiography, CTCA). Intracoronary acetylcholine may cause coronary spasm. Whilst they have a good prognosis, they are often highly symptomatic and can be difficult to treat. In women with this syndrome, the myocardium shows an abnormal metabolic response to stress, consistent with the suggestion that the myocardial ischaemia results from abnormal dilator responses of the coronary microvasculature to stress.

Box 23.29 Canadian Cardiovascular Society functional classification of angina

Class	Description
Class I	No angina with ordinary activity. Angina with strenuous activity
Class II	Angina during ordinary activity, e.g. walking up hills, walking rapidly upstairs, with mild limitation of activities
Class III	Angina with low levels of activity, e.g. walking 50–100 metres on the flat, walking up one flight of stairs, with marked restriction of activities
Class IV	Angina at rest or with any level of exercise

Examination

There are usually no abnormal findings in angina, although occasionally a fourth heart sound may be heard. Signs to suggest anaemia, thyrotoxicosis or hyperlipidaemia (e.g. lipid arcus, xanthelasma, tendon xanthoma) should be sought. It is essential to exclude aortic stenosis (i.e. slow-rising carotid impulse and ejection systolic murmur radiating to the neck) as a possible cause of the angina. The blood pressure should be taken to identify coexistent hypertension.

Investigations

Patients with suspected angina should have initial investigations ***(Box 23.30)***. The diagnosis of stable angina can be made on clinical assessment alone *or* by clinical assessment combined with anatomical (cardiac catheterization or CTCA) or functional imaging (SPECT, stress echocardiography, stress MRI).

UK NICE guidance recommends assessing the likelihood of CAD in patients without known CAD who present with typical angina, atypical angina or non-anginal chest pain ***(Box 23.31)***.

- Patients with ***non-anginal chest pain*** (more likely if the pain is continuous, unrelated to exertion, exacerbated by respiration, or associated with dizziness, palpitations or difficulty in swallowing) should be considered for alternative diagnoses and investigated appropriately.

Box 23.30 Investigations in stable angina

Laboratory tests
- Full blood count
- Thyroid function tests
- Fasting glucose
- HbA_{1c} (see p. 1251)
- Fasting lipid profile
- Glomerular filtration rate
- Troponin if unstable

12-lead ECG
- Exclude: ACS, pathological Q waves, left ventricular hypertrophy, left bundle branch block

Echocardiography
- Regional wall motion abnormalities
- Left ventricular ejection fraction
- Diastolic function
- Alternative causes of chest pain

Ambulatory ECG
- Paroxysmal arrhythmia
- Vasospastic angina

Chest X-ray
- Atypical presentation
- Pulmonary disease
- Heart failure

ACS, acute coronary syndrome.

Box 23.31 Likelihood of coronary artery disease in relation to type of presentation, age and risk[a]

Age	Non-anginal chest pain				Atypical angina				Typical angina			
	Men		*Women*		*Men*		*Women*		*Men*		*Women*	
	Lo	*Hi*	*Lo*	*Hi*	*Lo*	*Hi*	*Lo*	*Hi*	*Lo*	*Hi*	*Lo*	*Hi*
35	3	35	1	19	8	59	2	39	30	88	10	78
45	9	47	2	22	21	70	5	43	51	92	20	79
55	23	59	4	25	45	79	10	47	80	95	38	82
65	49	69	9	29	71	86	20	51	93	97	56	84

[a]Data are percentage of people at each mid-decade age with significant coronary artery disease. Hi, high risk – diabetes, smoking, hyperlipidaemia (total cholesterol >6.47 mmol/L); Lo, low risk – none of the above. Men >70 years with atypical or typical angina: assume risk >90%. Women >70 years: assume risk 61–90% unless high risk and typical angina (risk >90%). Resting ECG abnormalities (ST-T changes, Q waves, left bundle branch block) increase likelihood.

- Patients with ***typical angina and a risk of disease of >90%*** do not need further diagnostic investigation and should be managed for stable angina.
- Patients with ***typical or atypical angina and a risk of disease of 61–90%*** should have cardiac catheterization *if appropriate*.
- Patients with ***typical or atypical angina and a risk of disease of 30–60%*** should be referred for functional testing (SPECT, stress echocardiography, stress MRI).
- Patients with ***typical or atypical angina and a risk of disease of 10–29%*** should be referred for CTCA:
  - If the CT calcium score is 0, then angina is unlikely and other causes of chest pain should be sought (although young patients may have non-calcified plaque and CT angiography may be appropriate if they are symptomatic).
  - If the CT calcium score is 1–400, proceed to CT angiography.
  - If the CT calcium score is >400, invasive coronary angiography or functional imaging would be appropriate.
- If stable angina cannot be diagnosed in patients with known coronary artery disease, then functional assessment would be appropriate.

NICE does *not* recommend exercise ECG as a diagnostic test.

Management of stable angina

Patients should be informed as to the nature of their condition and reassured that the prognosis is good (annual mortality <2%). Lifestyle management should be instigated, as for prevention of CAD. The stable angina algorithm in ***Figure 23.64*** should be used to guide initial patient management, while ***Box 23.32*** outlines pharmacological therapy.

Revascularization

Percutaneous coronary intervention

Percutaneous coronary intervention (PCI) is the process of dilating a coronary artery stenosis by introducing an inflatable balloon and metallic stent ***(Fig. 23.65)*** into the arterial circulation via the femoral, radial or brachial artery ***(Fig. 23.66)***; the radial artery is the best (see below). Fractional flow reserve (FFR) measurement can be used to assess the severity of a stenosis prior to PCI. An FFR of >0.80 treated medically (i.e. no stent) is associated with improved patient outcomes. Complications of PCI include bleeding, haematoma, dissection and pseudoaneurysm from the arterial puncture site, although use of the radial artery reduces these risks and is the standard technique in the UK. Serious complications include acute myocardial infarction (2%), stroke (0.4%) and death (1%). ***Bare metal stents*** (BMS) are associated with a 20–30% risk of coronary artery re-stenosis within 6–9 months of implantation. First-generation ***drug-eluting stents*** (DES) with ***sirolimus*** and ***paclitaxel*** reduced re-stenosis but suffered from late and very late stent thrombosis. Second-generation DES (with thinner struts and biodegradable or biocompatible polymers) demonstrated better safety and efficacy, and are recommended for most patients (BMS may be preferred in patients requiring anticoagulation and early surgery). Dual antiplatelet therapy (aspirin and a P2Y12 inhibitor, e.g. prasugrel) should continue for 6–12 months.

PCI versus medical therapy

The Courage Trial, published in April 2007, randomized patients with stable but significant CAD and inducible ischaemia to PCI with stenting or optimal medical therapy. The primary composite outcome (all-cause death and non-fatal MI) occurred in 18.3% of the PCI patients and 17.8% of the medically treated patients. This supports an initial strategy of optimal medical therapy in patients

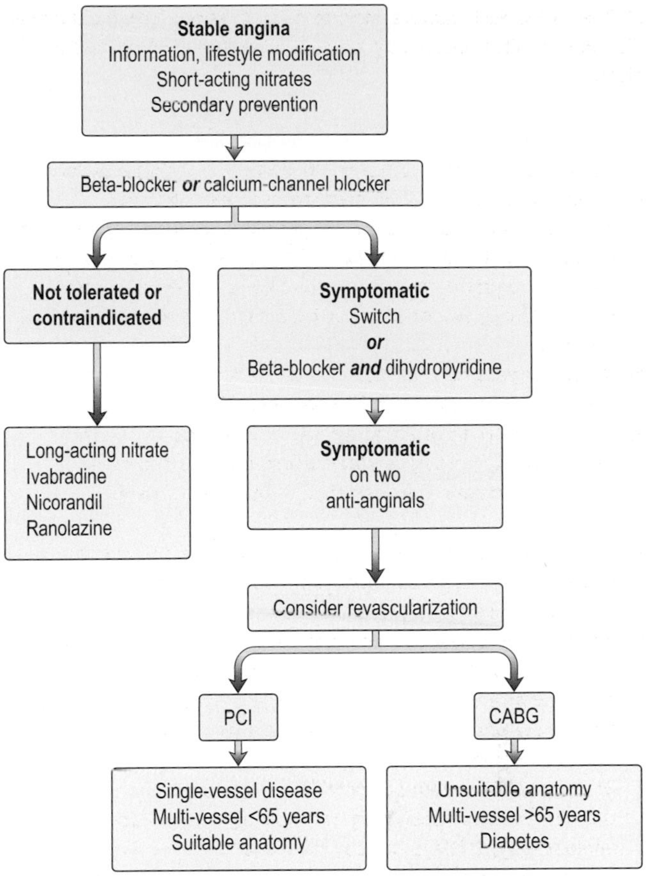

Figure 23.64 Algorithm for management of patients with stable angina. CABG, coronary artery bypass grafting; PCI, percutaneous coronary intervention. *(From NICE Guideline CG126.* Management of Stable Angina. *July 2011 (guidance under review), with permission.)*

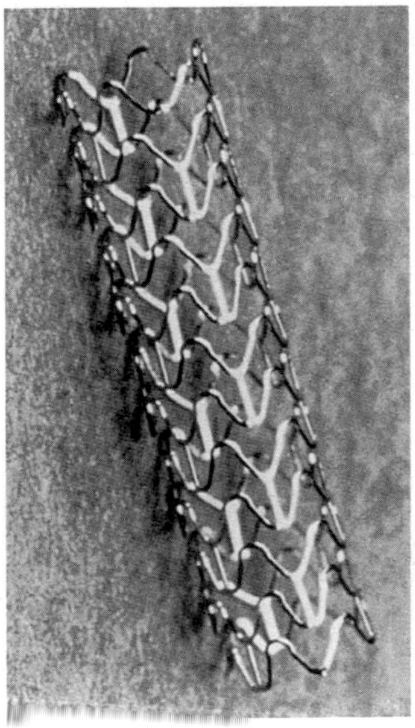

Figure 23.65 An intracoronary stent.

Box 23.32 Pharmacological therapy in stable angina

Drug	Dose	Indications/mechanism of action/cautions
Vasodilators		
Glyceryl trinitrate	0.3–1.0 mg sublingual 2.0–3.0 mg buccal	Prophylaxis and treatment of angina – rapid onset Repeat after 5 min if symptomatic Vasodilatation (causes headache and flushing)
Isosorbide mononitrate	10–60 mg ×2 daily (slow-release preparations available)	Prophylaxis of angina Side-effects – headache and flushing Contraindicated with phosphodiesterase type 5 inhibitors
Beta-blocker		
Bisoprolol	2.5–10 mg daily	Inhibits β-adrenoceptors, reduces heart rate and BP, reduces myocardial oxygen consumption Caution – COPD, acute heart failure, AV conduction Side-effects – fatigue, peripheral vasoconstriction (cold peripheries), sexual dysfunction, bronchospasm
Calcium-channel blockers		
Verapamil (*phenylalkylamines*)	80–120 mg ×3 daily (or 240–480 mg daily slow-release)	Inhibit calcium channels in myocardium, cardiac conductive tissue and vascular smooth muscle Diltiazem and verapamil – contraindicated in severe bradycardia, left ventricular failure with pulmonary congestion, second- or third-degree AV block Side-effects – constipation (verapamil), ankle oedema (amlodipine, diltiazem), reflex tachycardia (amlodipine)
Diltiazem (*benzothiapines*)	60–120 mg ×3 daily (longer-acting preparations available)	
Amlodipine (*dihydropyridines*)	5–10 mg daily	
Other anti-anginal drugs		
Ivabradine	2.5–7.5 mg ×2 daily	Inhibits pacemaker I_f current in SA node Use in sinus rhythm ± beta-blocker Side-effects – bradycardia, phosphenes Contraindications – sick sinus syndrome, AV block
Nicorandil	5–30 mg ×2 daily	Activates ATP-sensitive potassium channels and has nitrate properties – peripheral and coronary vasodilatation Use as adjunctive therapy Side-effects – headache, flushing, oral ulceration
Ranolazine	375–750 mg ×2 daily	Inhibits late sodium channels into cardiac cells Use as adjunctive therapy Metabolized by cytochrome P450 3A4 Side-effects – constipation, dizziness, lengthened QT
Event-reducing drugs		
Antiplatelet	Aspirin 75 mg daily	Reversible inhibition of platelet COX-1 and thromboxane production
	Clopidogrel 75 mg daily	Thienopyridine that antagonizes platelet ADP receptor P2Y12. Use if aspirin-intolerant
ACE inhibitor or ARB	Enalapril 10 mg daily	Indicated if treating other condition, e.g. hypertension, heart failure, chronic kidney disease
Statins	Atorvastatin 80 mg daily	Use to reduce LDL cholesterol to <1.8 mmol/L

ACE, angiotensin-converting enzyme; ADP, adenosine diphosphate; ARB, angiotensin receptor blocker; ATP, adenosine triphosphate; AV, atrioventricular; BP, blood pressure; COPD, chronic obstructive pulmonary disease; COX-1, cyclo-oxygenase-1; LDL, low-density lipoprotein; SA, sinoatrial.

with stable angina symptoms, although revascularization should be considered in those who remain symptomatic despite taking two anti-anginals.

Coronary artery bypass grafting

With coronary artery bypass grafting (CABG), autologous veins or arteries are anastomosed to the ascending aorta and to the native coronary arteries distal to the area of stenosis (see ***Fig. 23.67***). Improved graft survival can be obtained with *in situ* internal mammary and gastroepiploic arteries grafted on to the stenosed coronary artery, compared to vein grafts. Off-pump surgery is very comparable to standard CABG surgery in all outcomes, except that there are possibly more repeat vascularizations in the first year with off-pump surgery.

CABG versus medical therapy

Three major randomized controlled trials compared CABG with medical therapy: the Coronary Artery Surgery Study (CASS), the Veterans Administration (VA) Cooperative Study and the European Coronary Surgery Study (ECSS). A meta-analysis has been performed and demonstrated that, compared to medical therapy, CABG significantly improved angina symptoms and exercise capacity, and reduced the need for anti-anginal therapy. Operative mortality is well below 1% in patients with normal left ventricular function. Perioperative strokes occur in up to 2% of cases and more subtle neurological deficits are common. CABG is recommended for patients with triple-vessel CAD and impaired left ventricular function (LVEF 35–49%). Left stem disease with a stenosis of ≥50% is a class I indication for revascularization.

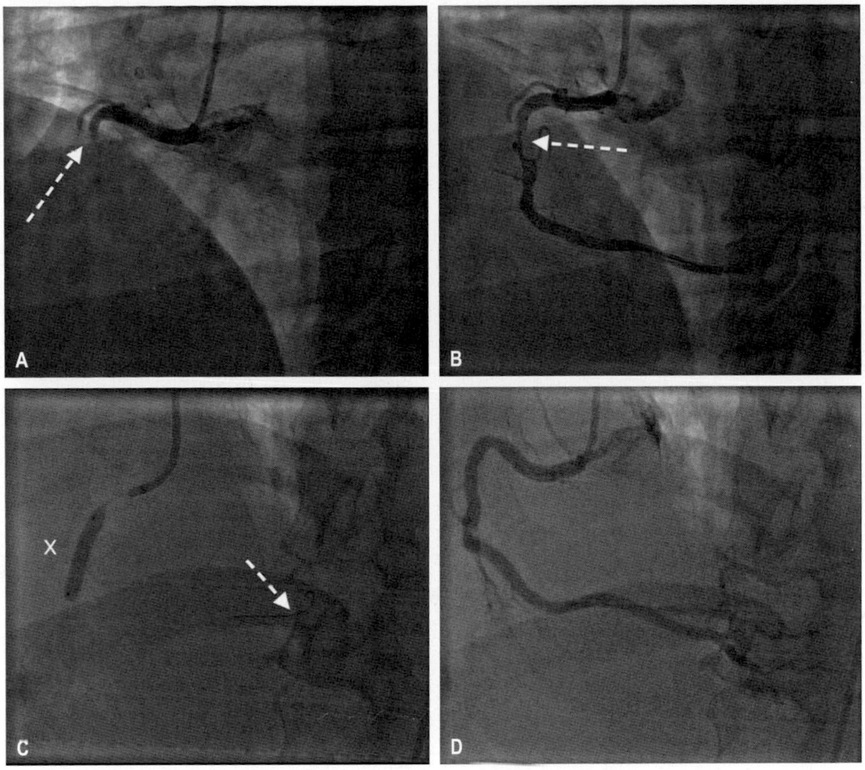

Figure 23.66 Percutaneous transluminal coronary angioplasty (PTCA). A. Coronary angiography demonstrates an occluded right coronary artery (arrowed). **B.** A soft wire passed through the guide catheter reopens the artery but a severe stenosis remains (arrowed). **C.** A balloon (X) is inflated to dilate the stenosis. The soft guidewire can be seen in the distal posterior descending artery (arrowed). **D.** The right coronary artery has now been successfully reopened with good antegrade flow.

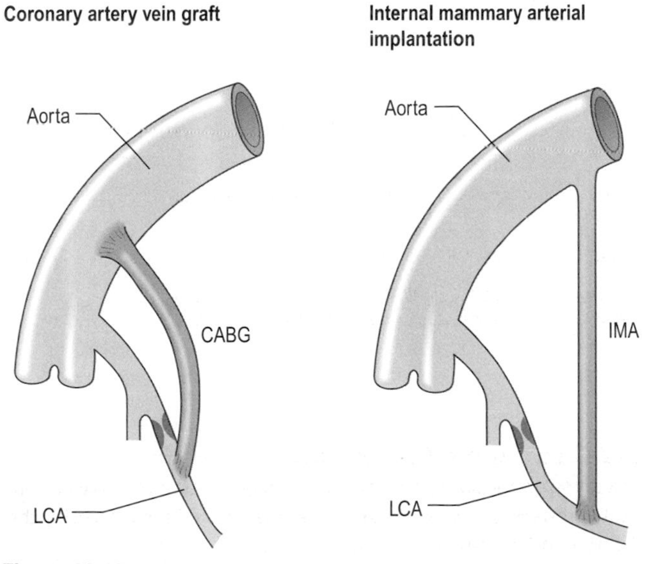

Figure 23.67 Relief of coronary obstruction by surgical techniques. Coronary artery bypass grafting (CABG) and internal mammary arterial implantation (IMA) are shown. In both of these examples, the graft bypasses a coronary obstruction in the left coronary artery (LCA).

PCI versus CABG

Comparative trials between CABG and PCI all demonstrate a higher need for repeat revascularization with PCI than with CABG. In the ERACI II study, PCI patients had fewer major adverse events initially and better 18-month survival than the CABG group. The Stent or Surgery (SoS) Trial reported a 2-year incidence of death or Q wave MI of 9% in PCI versus 10% in CABG patients, but fewer deaths with CABG (2% versus 5%). The SYNTAX study compared PCI with DES against CABG in patients with three-vessel disease and/or left main stem disease. The primary end-point (all-cause death, stroke, MI or repeat revascularization) occurred in more PCI patients. Although the draft NICE guidance for stable angina recommends PCI for young patients with single or multivessel disease (and no diabetes), the European Society of Cardiology (ESC) has recommended PCI *only* in cases of single- or double-vessel disease that does *not* involve the proximal left anterior descending artery.

Patients with intractable angina

Some patients remain symptomatic despite medication and are not suitable for (further) revascularization. These patients need a pain management programme.

ACUTE CORONARY SYNDROMES

Acute coronary syndromes (ACS) include:

- ***ST-elevation myocardial infarction (STEMI)***
- ***non-ST-elevation myocardial infarction (NSTEMI)***
- ***unstable angina (UA).***

Box 23.33 Definition of myocardial infarction

Criteria for acute myocardial infarction

The term acute myocardial infarction (MI) should be used when there is evidence of myocardial necrosis in a clinical setting consistent with acute myocardial ischaemia. Under these conditions, any one of the following criteria meets the diagnosis for MI:

- Detection of a rise and/or fall of cardiac biomarker values (preferably cardiac troponin, cTn), with at least one value above the 99th percentile upper reference limit (URL) and with at least one of the following:
  - symptoms of ischaemia
  - new, or presumed new, and significant ST-segment–T wave (ST–T) changes or new left bundle branch block (LBBB)
  - development of pathological Q waves on the ECG
  - imaging evidence of new loss of viable myocardium or new regional wall motion abnormality; identification of an intracoronary thrombus by angiography or autopsy.
- Cardiac death with symptoms suggestive of myocardial ischaemia and presumed new ischaemic ECG changes or new LBBB, but death occurred before cardiac biomarkers were obtained, or before cardiac biomarker values would be increased.
- Percutaneous coronary intervention (PCI)-related MI is arbitrarily defined by elevation of cTn values (>5×99th percentile URL) in patients with normal baseline values (≤99th percentile URL), or a rise of cTn values of >20% if the baseline values are elevated and are stable or falling. In addition, one of the following is required:
  - symptoms suggestive of myocardial ischaemia
  - new ischaemic ECG changes
  - angiographic findings consistent with a procedural complication *or*
  - imaging demonstration of new loss of viable myocardium or new regional wall motion abnormality.
- Stent thrombosis associated with MI when detected by coronary angiography or autopsy in the setting of myocardial ischaemia and with a rise and/or fall of cardiac biomarker values with at least one value above the 99th percentile URL.
- Coronary artery bypass grafting (CABG)-related MI is arbitrarily defined by elevation of cardiac biomarker values (>10×99th percentile URL) in patients with normal baseline cTn values (≤99th percentile URL). In addition, either:
  - new pathological Q waves or new LBBB
  - angiographically documented new graft or new native coronary artery occlusion *or*
  - imaging evidence of new loss of viable myocardium or new regional wall motion abnormality.

Criteria for prior myocardial infarction

Any one of the following criteria meets the diagnosis for prior MI:

- pathological Q waves with or without symptoms in the absence of non-ischaemic causes
- imaging evidence of a region of loss of viable myocardium that is thinned and fails to contract, in the absence of a non-ischaemic cause
- pathological findings of a prior MI.

(From Thygesen K, Alpert JS, Jaffe AS et al. Third universal definition of myocardial infarction. Eur Heart J *2012; 33:2251–2267.)*

The difference between UA and NSTEMI is that, in the latter, there is occluding thrombus, which leads to myocardial necrosis and a rise in serum troponins or creatine kinase-MB (CK-MB). Myocardial infarction (MI) occurs when cardiac myocytes die due to myocardial ischaemia, and can be diagnosed on the basis of appropriate clinical history, 12-lead ECG and elevated biochemical markers – troponin I and T, and CK-MB. The definition of MI is shown in ***Box 23.33***.

There are five types of MI:

- ***Type 1 – spontaneous MI with ischaemia*** due to a primary coronary event, e.g. plaque erosion/rupture, fissuring or dissection
- ***Type 2 – MI secondary to ischaemia*** due to increased oxygen demand or decreased supply, such as in coronary spasm, coronary embolism, anaemia, arrhythmias, hypertension or hypotension
- ***Type 3 – diagnosis of MI in sudden cardiac death***
- ***Type 4a – MI related to PCI***
- ***Type 4b – MI related to stent thrombosis***
- ***Type 5 – MI related to CABG***.

Pathophysiology

The mechanism that is common to all ACS is rupture or erosion of the fibrous cap of a coronary artery plaque. This leads to platelet aggregation and adhesion, localized thrombosis, vasoconstriction and distal thrombus embolization. The presence of a rich lipid pool within the plaque and a thin, fibrous cap is associated with an increased risk of rupture. Thrombus formation and the vasoconstriction produced by platelet release of serotonin and thromboxane A_2 result in myocardial ischaemia due to reduction of coronary blood flow.

Diagnosis and investigations

Clinical features

Patients with an ACS may complain of a new onset of ***chest pain***, chest pain at rest, or a deterioration of pre-existing angina. However, some present with atypical features, including indigestion, pleuritic chest pain or dyspnoea. Physical examination can detect alternative diagnoses, such as aortic dissection, pulmonary embolism or peptic ulceration. In addition, it can also identify adverse clinical signs, such as hypotension, basal crackles, fourth heart sounds and cardiac murmurs.

Electrocardiogram

Although the 12-lead ECG may be normal in patients, ST depression and T-wave inversion are highly suggestive of an ACS, particularly if associated with anginal chest pain. The ECG should be repeated when the patient is in pain, and continuous ST-segment monitoring is recommended. With a STEMI, complete occlusion of a coronary vessel will result in a persistent ST-elevation or left bundle branch block pattern, although transient ST elevation is seen with coronary vasospasm or Prinzmetal's angina.

Biochemical markers

- ***The cardiac troponin complex*** is made up of three distinct proteins (I, T and C), which are situated with tropomyosin on the thin actin filament that forms the skeleton of the cardiac myofilament. Troponin T attaches the complex to tropomyosin, troponin C binds calcium during excitation–contraction coupling, and troponin I inhibits the myosin binding site on the actin. 'Highly sensitive' troponin assays can now detect troponins in normal people. There are many different assays and results should be interpreted in the context of the clinical picture and the ECG. A negative predictive value of 99.4% has been shown for a serum troponin of <5 ng/L; this has been shown to be consistent across a wide group of patients. If the initial troponin assay is negative, then it should be repeated 4–12 h later. The troponin assay has prognostic information: that is, a high serum troponin level has an increased mortality

Box 23.34 Relationship between troponin I and risk of death in acute coronary syndrome

Serum troponin levels (ng/mL)	Mortality at 42 days (% of patients)
0 to <0.4	1.0
0.4 to <1.0	1.7
1.0 to <2.0	3.4
2.0 to <5.0	3.7
5.0 to <9.0	6.0
>9.0	7.5

(Adapted from Antman EM, Tanasijevic MJ, Thompson B et al. Cardiac-specific troponin I levels to predict the risk of mortality in patients with acute coronary syndromes. *New Engl J M* 1996; 335:1342–1349.)

risk in ACS **(*Box 23.34*)**, and defines which patients may benefit from aggressive medical therapy and early coronary revascularization.

- ***CK-MB*** level was the standard marker for myocyte death used in ACS. However, the presence of low levels of CK-MB in the serum of normal individuals and in patients with significant skeletal muscle damage has limited its accuracy. It can, however, be used to determine re-infarction, as levels drop back to normal after 36–72 h.
- ***Myoglobin*** becomes elevated very early in MI but the test has poor specificity for ACS, as myoglobin is present in skeletal muscle.

NSTEMI and unstable angina

Risk stratification

Initial risk in ACS is determined by complications of the acute thrombosis. This may produce recurrent myocardial ischaemia, marked ST depression, dynamic ST changes and a raised troponin level, and may be demonstrated with coronary angiography.

Long-term risks are defined by clinical risk factors: age, prior MI or bypass surgery, diabetes or heart failure. Biological markers, such as CRP, fibrinogen, BNP, modified albumin and serum creatinine, can be used to further stratify patient risk. Left ventricular dysfunction and the presence of left main or triple vessel disease significantly increase the future cardiovascular risk. Both the Thrombolysis in Myocardial Infarction (TIMI) score **(*Box 23.35*)** and the Global Registry of Acute Coronary Events (GRACE) prediction score can be used in patients with ACS to define risk. The GRACE score is based on age, heart rate, systolic blood pressure, serum creatinine and the Killip score (***Boxes 23.36*** and ***23.37***; see also p. 1004).

Investigation and treatment

All patients require immediate management of their chest pain, as outlined on pages 1002–1004 and in ***Box 23.30***.

High-risk patients for progression to MI or death require urgent coronary angiography (<24 h). This includes those individuals with persistent or recurrent angina with ST changes ≥2 mm or deep negative T-wave changes, clinical signs of heart failure or haemodynamic instability, or life-threatening arrhythmias (ventricular fibrillation, ventricular tachycardia).

Box 23.35 TIMI risk score in acute coronary syndrome (NSTEMI/UA)

Risk factor	Score
Age >65 years	1
>3 CAD risk factors – hypertension, hyperlipidaemia, family history, diabetes, smoking	1
Known CAD (coronary angiography stenosis >50%)	1
Aspirin use in the last 7 days	1
Severe angina (>2 episodes of rest pain in 24 h)	1
ST deviation on ECG (horizontal ST depression or transient ST elevation >1 mm)	1
Elevated cardiac markers (CK-MB or troponin)	1
Total score	

0–1: rate of death/MI in 14 days 3%; rate of death/MI/urgent revascularization 4.75%
2: 3%; 8.3%
3: 5%; 13.2%
4: 7%; 19.9%
5: 12%; 26.2%
6–7: 19%; 40.9%

CAD, coronary artery disease; CK-MB, creatine kinase MB; MI, myocardial infarction; NSTEMI, non-ST-elevation myocardial infarction; TIMI, Thrombolysis in Myocardial Infarction; UA, unstable angina.

Patients with ***intermediate or high-risk*** TIMI or GRACE scores should be referred for coronary angiography within <72 hours.

Low-risk patients can be managed with oral aspirin, ADP-receptor antagonists, beta-blockers and nitrates. These include patients with no recurrence of chest pain during observation, no signs of heart failure, normal ECG or minor T-wave changes on arrival and at 6–12 hours, and normal troponins on the initial assays and at 6–12 hours after admission. An exercise test should be performed; a negative result has a good prognosis but an early positive test should direct the patient to an invasive strategy. If the patient is unable to exercise satisfactorily, or if the baseline ECG is abnormal (e.g. left ventricular hypertrophy or left bundle branch block), then dobutamine stress echocardiography or myocardial perfusion scintigraphy is recommended. These tests are often used as the first-line investigation.

Antiplatelet drugs

The platelet is a key part of the thrombosis cascade involved in ACS. Rupture of the atheromatous plaque exposes the circulating platelets to adenosine diphosphate (ADP), thromboxane A_2 (TxA_2), adrenaline (epinephrine), thrombin and collagen tissue factor. This causes platelet activation, with thrombin as an especially potent stimulant of such activity. Platelet activation stimulates the expression of glycoprotein (GP) IIb/IIIa receptors on the platelet surface. These receptors bridge fibrinogen between adjacent platelets, causing platelet aggregates (see ***Fig. 16.39***). ACS patients should be treated with dual antiplatelet agents: ***aspirin 300 mg*** loading dose then 75 mg daily and an ADP-receptor antagonist (***clopidogrel 300–600 mg*** loading then 75 mg daily *or* ***prasugrel 60 mg*** loading then 10 mg daily *or* ***ticagrelor 180 mg*** loading then 90 mg twice daily).

Antithrombin drugs

An antithrombin should be added to dual antiplatelets in patients with ACS. ***Unfractionated heparin*** (***UFH***) requires frequent monitoring; the low-molecular-weight heparin ***enoxaparin*** appears to be

Box 23.36 Risk calculator for 6-month post-discharge mortality after hospitalization for acute coronary syndrome (GRACE score)

Medical history		Findings at initial hospital presentation		Findings during hospitalization		History of CCF	History of MI	Systolic BP		Elevated cardiac enzymes	ST segment depression	No in-hospital PCI
Age (years)	*Points*	*Resting heart rate (b.p.m.)*	*Points*	*Initial serum creatinine (mg/dL)*	*Points*	*Points*	*Points*	*(mmHg)*	*Points*	*Points*	*Points*	*Points*
≤29	0	≤49.9	0	0–0.39	1	24	12	≤79.9	24	15	11	14
30–39	0	50–69.9	3	0.4–0.79	3			80–99.9	22			
40–49	18	70–89.9	9	0.8–1.19	5			100–119.9	18			
50–59	36	90–109.9	14	1.2–1.59	7			120–139.9	14			
60–69	55	110–149.9	23	1.6–1.99	9			140–159.9	10			
70–79	73	150–199.9	35	2–3.99	15			160–199.9	4			
80–89	91	≥200	43	≥4	20			≥200	0			
≥90	100											

BP, blood pressure; CCF, congestive cardiac failure; GRACE, Global Registry of Acute Coronary Events; MI, myocardial infarction; PCI, percutaneous coronary intervention.

Box 23.37 Mortality in low-, intermediate- and high-risk categories according to the GRACE risk score

Syndrome type/timeframe	Risk category (tertiles)	GRACE risk score	Deaths (%)
NSTEMI-ACS			
In hospital	Low	≤108	<1
	Intermediate	109–140	1–3
	High	>140	>3
Post discharge to 6 months	Low	≤88	<3
	Intermediate	89–118	3–8
	High	>118	>8
STEMI-ACS			
In hospital	Low	49–125	<2
	Intermediate	126–154	2–5
	High	155–319	>5
Post discharge to 6 months	Low	27–99	<3
	Intermediate	100–127	3–8
	High	128–263	>8

ACS, acute coronary syndrome; GRACE, Global Registry of Acute Coronary Events; NSTEMI, non-ST-elevation myocardial infarction; STEMI, ST-elevation myocardial infarction.
(http://www.outcomes-umassmed.org/grace/grace_risk_table.aspx)

superior and can be given subcutaneously twice daily. ***Bivalirudin*** is a direct thrombin inhibitor that reversibly binds to thrombin and inhibits clot-bound thrombin. In the ACUITY trial, bivalirudin appeared as effective as heparin plus GPIIb/IIIa inhibitors in reducing ischaemic events in patients pre-treated with a thienopyridine and undergoing diagnostic angiography or percutaneous intervention, but with less bleeding. ***Fondaparinux*** is a synthetic pentasaccharide that selectively binds to antithrombin; this inactivates factor Xa, resulting in a strong inhibition of thrombin generation and clot formation. It does not inactivate thrombin and has no effect on platelets.

Activated glycoprotein (GP) IIb/IIIa receptors on platelets bind to fibrinogen, initiating platelet aggregation. Receptor antagonists have been developed that are powerful inhibitors of platelet aggregation. Abciximab is a monoclonal antibody that binds tightly and has a long half-life. Eptifibatide is a cyclic peptide that selectively inhibits GPIIb/IIIa receptors, but has a short half-life and wears off in 2–4 hours. Tirofiban is a small non-peptide that rapidly blocks the GPIIb/IIIa receptors and is reversible in 4–6 hours. In the GUSTO-IV ACS study of 7800 patients, abciximab was administered but coronary intervention discouraged. At 30 days, 8.2% of abciximab patients and 8.0% of placebo patients had reached the composite end-point of death or MI. In the PRISM study of 3232 patients with angina, tirofiban reduced the 30-day death or MI rate from 7.1% with placebo to 5.8%. Troponin-positive patients with diabetes scheduled to have coronary intervention benefit most from GPIIb/IIIa receptor antagonists. However, GPIIb/IIIa receptor antagonists may provide no extra benefit in patients who have already received clopidogrel and aspirin.

Anti-ischaemia agents

In patients with no contraindications (asthma, AV block, acute pulmonary oedema), beta-blockers are administered orally, to reduce myocardial ischaemia by blocking circulating catecholamines. This will lower the heart rate and blood pressure, reducing myocardial oxygen consumption. The dose can be titrated to produce a resting heart rate of 50–60 b.p.m. In patients with on-going angina, nitrates should be given either sublingually or intravenously. They effectively reduce preload and produce coronary vasodilatation. However, tolerance can become a problem and patients should be weaned off intravenous administration if symptoms resolve.

Plaque stabilization/remodelling

HMG-CoA reductase inhibitor drugs (statins) and ACE inhibitors are routinely administered to patients with ACS. These agents may produce plaque stabilization, improve vascular and myocardial remodelling, and reduce future cardiovascular events. Starting the drugs whilst the patient is still in hospital increases the likelihood of these individuals receiving secondary drug therapy.

Box 23.38 Pharmacological therapy in acute coronary syndrome

Drug	Dose	Notes
Myocardial oxygenation		
Oxygen	35–50%	Check ABG in severe COPD
Antiplatelet drugs		
Aspirin	150–300 mg chewable or soluble aspirin, then 75 mg orally daily	Caution if active peptic ulceration
Clopidogrel	300 mg orally loading dose, then 75 mg orally daily	Caution: increased risk of bleeding; avoid if CABG planned
Prasugrel	60 mg oral loading dose, then 10 mg orally daily (5 mg daily if <60 kg or >75 years old)	
Ticagrelor	Initially 180 mg, then 90 mg ×2 daily	Risk of bleeding
Antithrombin drugs		
Heparin	5000 units i.v. bolus, then 0.25 units/kg per hour	Measure anticoagulant effect with APTT at 6 h
Low-molecular-weight heparins, e.g. enoxaparin	1 mg/kg s.c. ×2 daily	
Bivalirudin	750 µg/kg i.v. bolus, then 1.75 mg/kg per hour for 4 h post PCI	
Fondaparinux	2.5 mg s.c. daily, for up to 8 days	
Rivaroxaban	Oral 2.5–10 mg daily	Risk of bleeding
Glycoprotein IIB/IIIA inhibitors*		
Abciximab	0.25 mg/kg i.v. bolus, then 0.125 µg/kg per min up to 10 µg/min i.v. ×12 h	Indicated if coronary intervention likely within 24 h
Eptifibatide	180 µg/kg i.v. bolus, then 2 µg/kg per min ×72 h	Indicated in high-risk patients managed without coronary intervention or during PCI
Tirofiban	0.4 µg/kg per min for 30 min, then 0.1 µg/kg per min ×48–108 h	Indicated in high-risk patients managed without coronary intervention or during PCI
Analgesia		
Diamorphine or morphine	2.5–5.0 mg i.v.	Prescribe with antiemetic, e.g. metoclopramide 10 mg i.v.
Myocardial energy consumption		
Atenolol	5 mg i.v. repeated after 15 min, then 25–50 mg orally daily	Avoid in asthma, heart failure, hypotension, bradyarrhythmias
Metoprolol	5 mg i.v. repeated to a maximum of 15 mg, then 25–50 mg orally ×2 daily	Avoid in asthma, heart failure, hypotension, bradyarrhythmias
Coronary vasodilatation		
Glyceryl trinitrate	2–10 mg/h i.v./buccal/sublingual	Maintain systolic BP >90 mmHg
Plaque stabilization/ventricular remodelling		
HMG-CoA reductase inhibitors (statins)		
Simvastatin	20–40 mg orally	Combine with dietary advice and modification
Pravastatin	20–40 mg orally	
Atorvastatin	80 mg orally	
ACE inhibitors		
Ramipril	2.5–10 mg orally	Monitor renal function
Lisinopril	5–10 mg orally	

*Not now used in patients pretreated with clopidogrel and aspirin prior to coronary intervention.

ABG, arterial blood gases; ACE, angiotensin-converting enzyme; APTT, activated partial thromboplastin time; BP, blood pressure; CABG, coronary artery bypass graft; COPD, chronic obstructive pulmonary disease; i.v., intravenous; PCI, percutaneous coronary intervention; s.c., subcutaneous.

Coronary intervention

Coronary revascularization is recommended in high-risk patients with ACS. Coronary stenting may stabilize the disrupted coronary plaque. The mortality rates with CABG are greater in the high-risk group patients, particularly those with a recent MI. Single-vessel lesions are usually treated with PCI, unless the anatomy is unfavourable. Conversely, patients with left main stem or triple-vessel disease with impaired left ventricular function are best managed with surgery.

ST elevation myocardial infarction (STEMI)

Myocardial infarction occurs when cardiac myocytes die due to prolonged myocardial ischaemia. The diagnosis can be made in patients with an appropriate clinical history together with findings

Box 23.39 TIMI risk score in ST elevation myocardial infarction (STEMI)

Risk factor	Score
Age >65 years	2
Age >75 years	3
History of angina	1
History of hypertension	1
History of diabetes	1
Systolic BP <100	3
Heart rate >100	2
Killip score II–IV	2
Weight >67 kg	1
Anterior MI or LBBB	1
Delay to treatment >4 h	1
Total score	

0: risk of death at 30 days 0.8%
1: 1.6%
2: 2.2%
3: 4.4%
4: 7.3%
5: 12.4%
6: 16.1%
7: 23.4%
8: 26.8%
9–16: 35.9%

BP, blood pressure; LBBB, left bundle branch block; MI, myocardial infarction.

from repeated 12-lead ECGs and elevated biochemical markers – troponin I and T, and CK-MB.

Pathophysiology

Rupture or erosion of a vulnerable coronary artery plaque can produce prolonged occlusion of a coronary artery, leading to myocardial necrosis within 15–30 minutes. The sub-endocardial myocardium is initially affected but, with continued ischaemia, the infarct zone extends through to the sub-epicardial myocardium, producing a transmural Q wave MI. Early reperfusion may salvage regions of the myocardium, reducing future mortality and morbidity.

The in-hospital mortality rate is between 6% and 14%. Several risk factors can be identified that predict death rate at 30 days (TIMI STEMI score; ***Box 23.39***).

Diagnosis

Clinical features

Any patient presenting with severe chest pain lasting more than 20 minutes may be suffering from an MI. The pain does not usually respond to sublingual glyceryl trinitrate, and opiate analgesia is required. The pain may radiate to the left arm, neck or jaw. However, in some patients, particularly elderly or diabetic ones, the symptoms may be atypical and include dyspnoea, fatigue, pre-syncope or syncope. Autonomic symptoms are common and on examination the patient is pale and clammy, with marked sweating. In addition, the pulse is thready with significant hypotension, bradycardia or tachycardia.

Box 23.40 Typical ECG changes in myocardial infarction (STEMI)

Infarct site	Leads showing ST elevation
Anterior	
Small	V_3–V_4
Extensive	V_2–V_5
Anteroseptal	V_1–V_3
Anterolateral	V_4–V_6, I, AVL
Lateral	I, AVL
Inferior	II, III, AVF
Posterior	V_1, V_2 (reciprocal)
Sub-endocardial	Any lead
Right ventricle	VR_4

Electrocardiography

An ECG in patients with chest pain should be performed on admission to the accident and emergency department. The baseline ECG is rarely normal, but if it is, it should be repeated every 15 minutes, while the patient remains in pain. Continuous cardiac monitoring is required because of the high likelihood of significant cardiac arrhythmias. ECG changes ***(Box 23.40)*** are usually confined to the ECG leads that 'face' the infarction. The presence of new ST elevation (due to opening of the K^+ channels) of ≥0.2 mV at the J-point in leads V_1–V_3, and ≥0.1 mV in other leads, suggests anterior MI ***(Fig. 23.68)***. An inferior wall MI is diagnosed when ST elevation is seen in leads II, III and AVF ***(Fig. 23.69)***. Lateral MI produces changes in leads I, AVL and V_5/V_6. In patients with a posterior MI, there may be ST depression in leads V_1–V_3 with a dominant R wave, and ST elevation in lead V_5/V_6. New, or presumed new, left bundle branch block is compatible with coronary artery occlusion requiring urgent reperfusion therapy. The evolution of the ECG during the course of STEMI is illustrated in ***Figure 23.70***.

Investigations

Blood samples should be taken for cardiac troponin I or T levels, although treatment should not be deferred until the results are available. Full blood count, serum electrolytes, glucose and lipid profile should be obtained. Transthoracic echocardiography (TTE) may be helpful to confirm an MI, as wall-motion abnormalities are detectable early in STEMI. TTE may detect alternative diagnoses, such as aortic dissection, pericarditis or pulmonary embolism.

Management

Early medical management

Initial assessment involves rapid triage for chest pain (*Note*: time is muscle) and referral for reperfusion therapy (primary PCI or thrombolysis). Initial medical therapy includes oxygen, intravenous opioids (morphine) and aspirin (300 mg) (see ***Box 23.38***).

Percutaneous coronary intervention

PCI performed within 90 minutes is the preferred reperfusion therapy in interventional cardiology centres that have the expertise available. Current recommendations are to treat the target vessel only, unless the patient is in cardiogenic shock or there is ongoing ischaemia. Data from the RIVAL and RIFLE STEACS studies

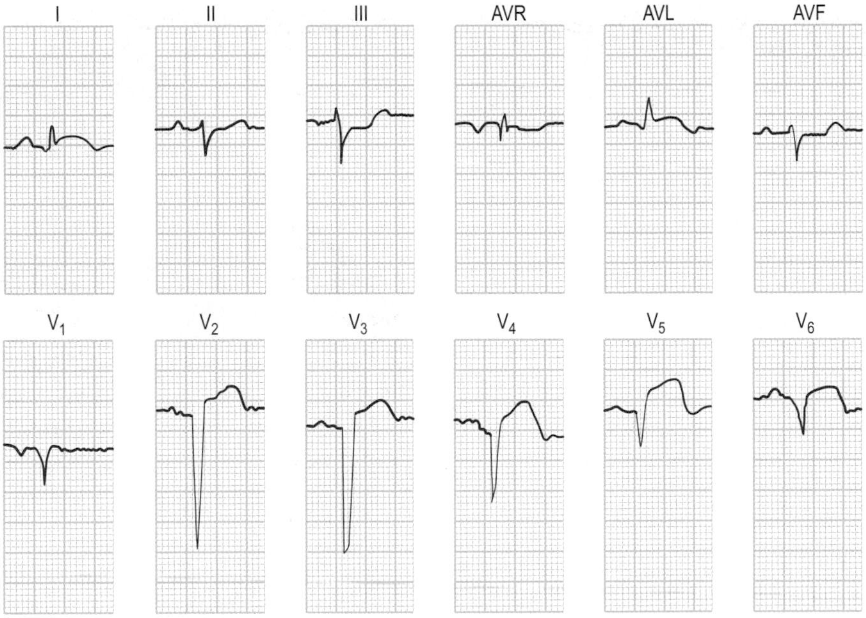

Figure 23.68 An acute anterolateral myocardial infarction, shown by a 12-lead ECG. Note the ST segment elevation in leads I, AVL and V_2–V_6. The T wave is inverted in leads I, AVL and V_3–V_6. Pathological Q waves are seen in leads V_2–V_6.

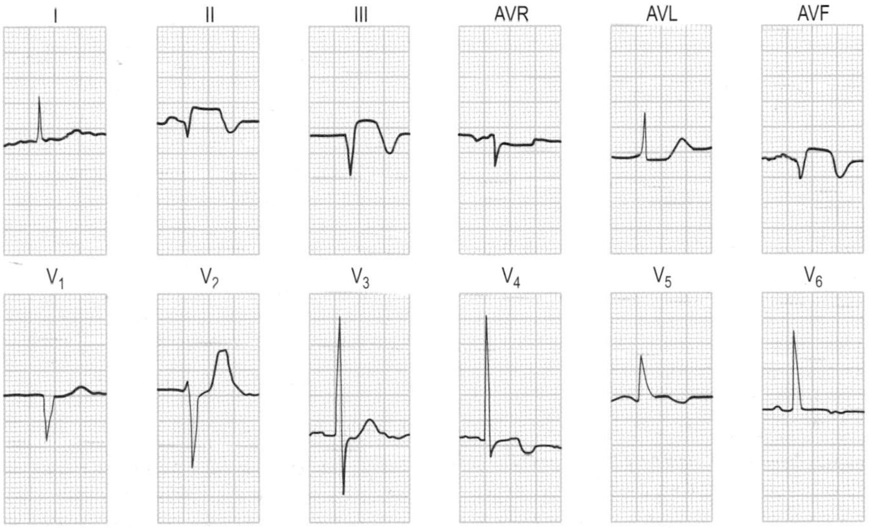

Figure 23.69 An acute inferior wall myocardial infarction, shown by a 12-lead ECG. Note the raised ST segment and Q waves in the inferior leads (II, III and AVF). The additional T-wave inversion in V_4 and V_5 probably represents anterior wall ischaemia.

demonstrate that radial PCI reduces bleeding complications at the arterial puncture site. The TAPAS study showed some benefit from thrombus aspiration, although this did not reduce infarct size when combined with intracoronary abciximab (INFUSE-AMI study). Patients undergoing primary PCI should be given dual antiplatelet therapy with aspirin and an ADP-receptor blocker, such as prasugrel or ticagrelor. Anticoagulant options include unfractionated heparin, enoxaparin or bivalirudin. The routine use of GP IIb/IIIa inhibitors is no longer recommended.

Fibrinolysis

Fibrinolytic agents (see pp. 566–567) enhance the breakdown of occlusive thromboses by the activation of plasminogen to form plasmin. Fibrinolysis is still used if PCI is unavailable. A meta-analysis of fibrinolytics (FTT), fibrinolysis within 6 hours of STEMI or left bundle branch block MI, prevented 30 deaths in every 1000 patients treated. Between 7 and 12 hours, 20 in every 1000 deaths were prevented. After 12 hours, the benefits are limited, and there is evidence to suggest less benefit for older patients, possibly because of the increased risk of strokes. Prompt reperfusion therapy (door to needle time <30 min) will reduce the death rate following MI. Double-bolus reteplase (r-PA) and single-bolus tenecteplase (TNK-t-PA) facilitate rapid administration of fibrinolytic therapy and can be used for pre-hospital thrombolysis. For patients who fail to reperfuse by 60–90 minutes, as demonstrated by <50% resolution of the ST-segment elevation, re-thrombolysis or referral for rescue coronary angioplasty is recommended. The contraindications to thrombolysis are provided in ***Box 23.41***. Aspirin and clopidogrel are recommended in patients undergoing fibrinolysis. Anticoagulant options include unfractionated heparin, enoxaparin or fondaparinux.

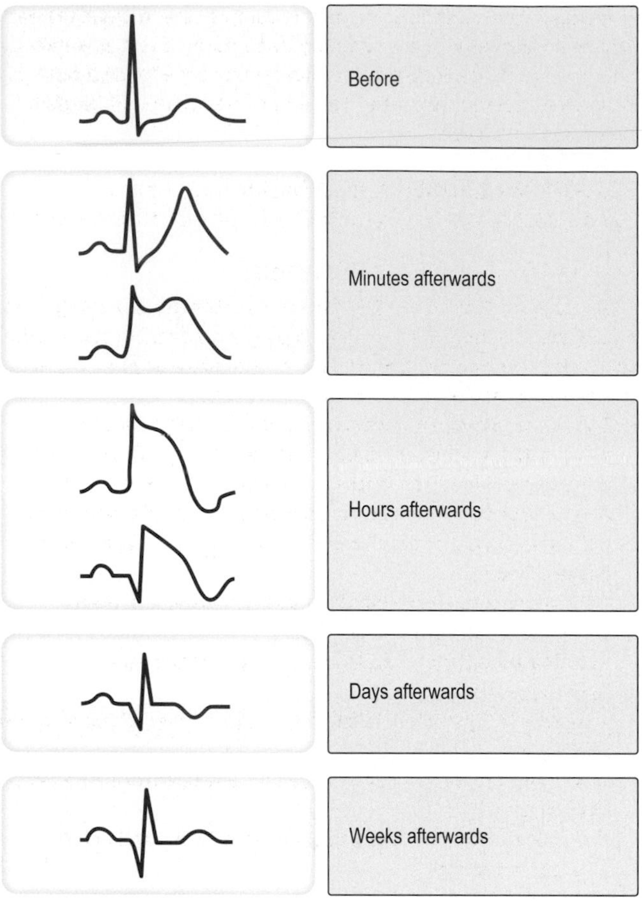

Figure 23.70 Electrocardiographic evolution of myocardial infarction (STEMI). After the first few minutes, the T waves become tall, pointed and upright, and there is ST segment elevation. After the first few hours, the T waves invert, the R-wave voltage is decreased and Q waves develop. After a few days, the ST segment returns to normal. After weeks or months, the T wave may return to upright but the Q wave remains.

Box 23.41 Contraindications to thrombolysis

Absolute contraindications
- Haemorrhagic stroke or stroke of unknown origin at any time
- Ischaemic stroke in preceding 3 months
- Central nervous system damage/neoplasm/vascular malformation
- Recent major trauma/surgery/head injury (within preceding 3 weeks)
- Gastrointestinal bleeding within the last month
- Known bleeding disorder
- Aortic dissection

Relative contraindications
- Ischaemic stroke in preceding 3 months
- Oral anticoagulant therapy
- Pregnancy or within 1 week postpartum
- Non-compressible vascular punctures
- Traumatic resuscitation
- Refractory hypertension (systolic blood pressure >180 mmHg)
- Advanced liver disease
- Internal bleeding, e.g. active peptic ulcer
- Dementia

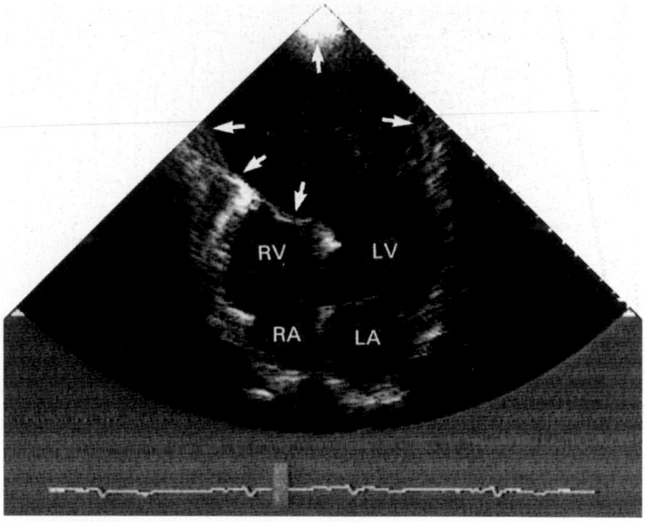

Figure 23.71 Two-dimensional echocardiogram (apical four-chamber view) showing a very large apical left ventricular aneurysm (arrowed). The relatively static blood in the aneurysm produces a swirling 'smoke' effect. This aneurysm was successfully resected surgically. LA, left atrium; LV, left ventricle; RA, right atrium; RV, right ventricle.

Coronary artery bypass surgery

Cardiac surgery is usually reserved for the complications of MI, such as ventricular septal defect or mitral regurgitation.

Complications of myocardial infarction

Heart failure

Cardiac failure post STEMI is a poor prognostic feature that necessitates medical and invasive therapy to reduce the death rate. The Killip classification is used to assess patients with heart failure post-MI:

- ***Killip I*** – no crackles and no third heart sound
- ***Killip II*** – crackles in <50% of the lung fields or a third heart sound
- ***Killip III*** – crackles in >50% of the lung fields
- ***Killip IV*** – cardiogenic shock.

Mild heart failure may respond to intravenous furosemide 40–80 mg i.v., with glyceryl trinitrate administration if the blood pressure is satisfactory. Oxygen is required, with regular oxygen monitoring. ACE inhibitors can be given in <24–48 hours if the blood pressure is satisfactory. Patients with severe heart failure may require Swan–Ganz catheterization to determine the pulmonary wedge pressure. Intravenous inotropes, such as dopamine or dobutamine, are used in patients with severe heart failure. If the patient is in cardiogenic shock, then revascularization with or without intra-aortic balloon pump insertion may be required.

Myocardial rupture and aneurysmal dilatation

Rupture of the free wall of the left ventricle is usually an early, catastrophic and fatal event. The patient will have a haemodynamic collapse, then an electromechanical cardiac arrest. A sub-acute rupture may allow for pericardiocentesis followed by surgical repair of the rupture. Aneurysmal dilatation of the infarcted myocardium ***(Fig. 23.71)*** is a late complication that may require surgical repair.

Ventricular septal defect

A ventricular septal defect (VSD) may occur in 1–2.0% of patients with STEMI, and may be associated with delayed or failed

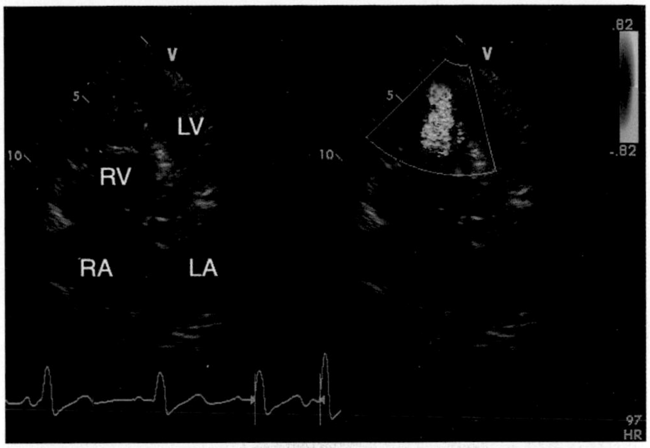

Figure 23.72 **Post-infarct ventricular septal defect.** LA, left atrium; LV, left ventricle; RA, right atrium; RV, right ventricle.

fibrinolysis. However, mortality is very high and there is a 12-month inoperative mortality of 92%. An intra-aortic balloon pump (IABP) and coronary angiography may allow patient optimization prior to surgery. A post-infarct VSD is demonstrated in ***Figure 23.72***.

Mitral regurgitation

Severe mitral regurgitation can occur early in the course of STEMI. Three mechanisms may be responsible for the mitral regurgitation, and a transoesophageal echocardiogram (TOE) may be necessary to confirm the aetiology:

- severe left ventricular dysfunction and dilatation, causing annular dilatation of the valve and subsequent regurgitation
- myocardial infarction of the inferior wall, producing dysfunction of the papillary muscle that may respond to coronary intervention
- myocardial infarction of the papillary muscles, producing sudden severe pulmonary oedema and cardiogenic shock (IABP, coronary angiography and early surgery may improve patient survival).

Cardiac arrhythmias

Ventricular tachycardia and ventricular fibrillation are common in STEMI, particularly with reperfusion. Cardiac arrest requires defibrillation. Ventricular tachycardia should be treated with intravenous beta-blockers (metoprolol 5 mg, esmolol 50–200 μg/kg per min), lidocaine 50–100 mg, or amiodarone 900–1200 mg/24 h. If the patient is hypotensive, synchronized cardioversion may be performed. Ensure that the serum potassium is >4.5 mmol/L. Refractory ventricular tachycardia or fibrillation may respond to magnesium 8 mmol/L over 15 min i.v.

Atrial fibrillation occurs frequently, and treatment with beta-blockers and digoxin may be required. Cardioversion is possible but relapse is common.

Bradyarrhythmias can be treated initially with i.v. atropine 0.5 mg repeated up to six times in 4 h. Temporary transcutaneous or transvenous pacemaker insertion may be necessary in patients with symptomatic heart block.

Conduction disturbances

These are common following MI. AV block may occur during acute MI, especially of the inferior wall (the right coronary artery usually supplies the sinoatrial and atrioventricular nodes). Heart block, when associated with haemodynamic compromise, may need treatment with atropine or a temporary pacemaker. Such blocks may last for only a few minutes, but frequently continue for several days. Permanent pacing may need to be considered if heart block persists for over 2 weeks.

Post-MI pericarditis and Dressler syndrome

See the section entitled 'Pericardial disease' (pp. 1042–1046).

Post-ACS lifestyle modification

After recovery from an ACS, patients should be encouraged to participate in a cardiac rehabilitation programme that provides education and information appropriate to their requirements. An exercise programme forms part of the rehabilitation.

- Dietary recommendations include calorie control of obesity, increased fruit and vegetables, reduced *trans* and saturated fats, and reduced salt intake in patients with hypertension.
- Alcohol consumption should be maintained within safe limits (≤21 units/week for men or <14 units for women) and avoid binge drinking.
- Patients should be physically active (30 min of moderate aerobic exercise 5 times per week).
- Patients should stop smoking (nicotine patches and buprenorphine are safe).
- A healthy weight (body mass index (BMI) <25 kg/m^2) should be maintained.
- Blood pressure should be reduced to a systolic measurement <140 mmHg.
- Patients with diabetes should be treated to maintain HbA_{1c} <7% (53 mmol/mol).

Post-ACS drug therapy and assessment

Extensive clinical trial evidence has been gathered in post-MI patients, demonstrating that a range of pharmaceuticals are advantageous in reducing mortality over the following years. Therefore, after MI, most patients should be taking most of the following medications:

- aspirin 75 mg daily
- an ADP-receptor blocker
- an oral beta-blocker to maintain heart rate <60 b.p.m.
- ACE inhibitors or angiotensin receptor blockers, particularly if LVEF is <40%
- high-intensity statins with target LDL cholesterol <1.8 mmol/L
- aldosterone antagonist, if there is clinical evidence of heart failure and LVEF is <40%; the serum creatinine is ≤221 μmol/L (men) or <177 μmol/L (women); and the serum potassium is <5.0 mEq/L.

Further reading

Anderson JL, Adams CD, Antman EM et al. 2012 ACCF/AHA focused update incorporated into the ACCF/AHA 2007 guidelines for the management of patients with unstable angina/non-ST-elevation myocardial infarction. *Circulation* 2013; 127:e663–e828.

Berry JD, Dyer A, Cal X et al. Lifetime risks of cardiovascular disease. *N Engl J Med* 2012; 366:321–329.

Blaha MJ, Budoff MJ, DeFilippis AP et al. Associations between C-reactive protein, coronary artery calcium, and cardiovascular events: implications for the JUPITER population from MESA, a population based cohort study. *Lancet* 2011; [illegible]

Bonaca MP, Bhatt DL, Cohen M et al; PEGASUS-TIMI 54 Steering Committee and Investigators. Long-term use of ticagrelor in patients with prior myocardial infarction. *N Engl J Med* 2015; 372:1791–1800.

Borissoff JI, Spronk HM, ten Cate H. The hemostatic system as a modulator of atherosclerosis. *N Engl J Med* 2011; 364:1746–1760.

De Bruyne B, Pijls NH, Kalesan B et al. Fractional flow reserve-guided PCI versus medical therapy in stable coronary disease. *N Engl J Med* 2012; 367:991–1001.

Diegeler A. Off-pump versus on-pump coronary-artery bypass grafting in elderly patients. *N Engl J Med* 2013; 368:1189–1198.
Gottlieb I, Miller JM, Arbab-Zadeh A et al. The absence of coronary calcification does not exclude obstructive coronary artery disease or the need for revascularization in patients referred for conventional coronary angiography. *J Am Coll Cardiol* 2010; 55:627–634.
Greenwood JD. Cardiovascular magnetic resonance and single photon computed tomography for the diagnosis of coronary artery disease (CE-MARC): a prospective study. *Lancet* 2012; 379:453–460.
Harrington RA. Selecting revascularization strategies in patients with coronary disease. *N Engl J Med* 2015; 372:1261–1263.
Head SJ, Börgermann J, Osnabrugge RL et al. Coronary artery bypass grafting: Part 2–optimizing outcomes and future prospects. *Eur Heart J* 2013; 34:2873–2886.
McCaul M, Lourens A, Kredo T. Pre-hospital versus in-hospital thrombolysis for ST-elevation myocardial infarction. *Cochrane Database Syst Rev (Online)* 2014; 9:CD010191.
Mehta SR, Jolly SS, Cairns J et al. Effects of radial versus femoral artery access in patients with acute coronary syndromes with or without ST-segment elevation. *J Am Coll Cardiol* 2012; 60:2490–2499.
Montalescot G, Sechtem U, Achenbach S et al. 2013 ESC guidelines on the management of stable coronary artery disease. *Eur Heart J* 2013; 34:2949–3003.
Montalescot G, Zeymer U, Silvain J et al. for the ATOLL Investigators. Intravenous enoxaparin or unfractionated heparin in primary percutaneous coronary intervention for ST-elevation myocardial infarction: the international randomised open-label ATOLL trial. *Lancet* 2011; 378:693–703.
Ong P, Athanasiadis A, Borgulya G et al. High prevalence of a pathological response to acetylcholine testing in patients with stable angina pectoris and unobstructed coronary arteries: the ACOVA study (Abnormal COronary VAsomotion in patients with stable angina and unobstructed coronary arteries). *J Am Coll Cardiol* 2012; 59:655–662.
Prasad A, Herrmann J. Myocardial infarction due to percutaneous coronary intervention. *N Engl J Med* 2011; 364:453–464.
Romagnoli E, Biondi-Zoccai G, Sciahbasi A et al. Radial versus femoral randomized investigation in ST-segment elevation acute coronary syndrome. *J Am Coll Cardiol* 2012; 60:2481–2489.
Schmermund A, Voigtländer T. Predictive ability of coronary artery calcium and CRP. *Lancet* 2011; 378:641–643.
Shah AS, Anand A, Sandoval Y et al. High-sensitivity cardiac troponin I at presentation in patients with suspected acute coronary syndrome: a cohort study. *Lancet* 2015;386:2481–2488.
Shahian DM, Meyer GS, Yeh RW et al. Percutaneous coronary interventions without on-site cardiac surgical backup. *N Engl J Med* 2012; 366:1814–1823.
Silber S, Windecker S, Vranckx P et al. on behalf of the RESOLUTE All Comers investigators. Unrestricted randomised use of two new generation drug-eluting coronary stents: 2-year patient-related versus stent-related outcomes from the RESOLUTE All Comers trial. *Lancet* 2011; 377:1241–1247.
Steg PG, James SK, Atar D et al. ESC Guidelines for the management of acute myocardial infarction in patients presenting with ST-segment elevation. *Eur Heart J* 2012; 33:2569–2619.
Stone GW, Maehara A, Lansky AJ et al. for the PROSPECT Investigators. A prospective natural-history study of coronary atherosclerosis. *N Engl J Med* 2011; 364:226–235.
Stone GW, Maehara A, Witzenbichler B et al. Intracoronary abciximab and aspiration thrombectomy in patients with large anterior myocardial infarction: the INFUSE-AMI randomized trial. *JAMA* 2012; 307:1817–1826.
Wijns W, Kolh P, Danchin N et al. and Task Force on Myocardial Revascularization of the European Society of Cardiology (ESC) and the European Association for Cardio-Thoracic Surgery (EACTS). Guidelines on myocardial revascularization. *Eur Heart J* 2010; 31:2501–2555.
Wiviott SD, Steg PG. Clinical evidence for oral antiplatelet therapy in acute coronary syndromes. *Lancet* 2015; 386:292–302.
http://www.qrisk.org *QRISK®2-2015 Cardiovascular disease risk assessment tool.*

VALVULAR HEART DISEASE

MITRAL VALVE

The mitral valve consists of the fibrous annulus, anterior and posterior leaflets, chordae tendineae and the papillary muscles ***(Fig. 23.73)***.

Mitral stenosis

The most common cause of mitral stenosis is rheumatic heart disease secondary to previous rheumatic fever due to infection with group A β-haemolytic streptococcus; in the developing world, this affects nearly 20 million people. The condition is more common in women than men. Inflammation leads to commissural fusion and a reduction in mitral valve orifice area, causing the characteristic doming pattern seen on echocardiography. Over many years, the condition progresses to valve thickening, cusp fusion, calcium deposition, a severely narrowed (stenotic) valve orifice and progressive immobility of the valve cusps.

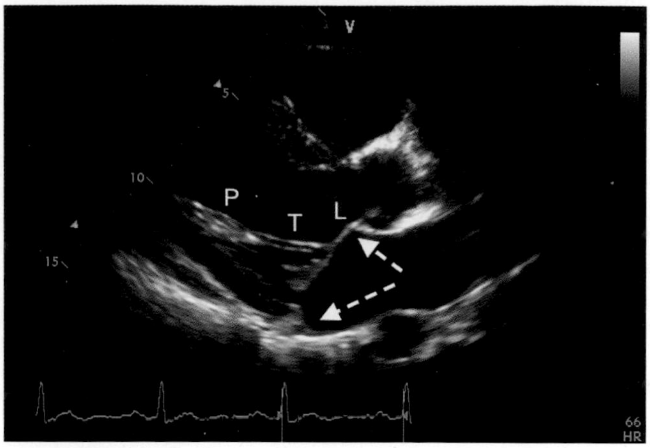

Figure 23.73 Mitral valve apparatus – parasternal long axis. Arrows, annulus; L, leaflets; P, papillary muscle; T, chordae tendineae.

Other causes of mitral stenosis include:

- congenital mitral stenosis
- Lutembacher syndrome (the combination of acquired mitral stenosis and an atrial septal defect)
- mitral annular calcification, rarely; this may lead to mitral stenosis if extensive, particularly in elderly patients and those with end-stage renal disease
- carcinoid tumours metastasizing to the lung, or primary bronchial carcinoid.

Pathophysiology

When the normal valve orifice area of 4–6 cm^2 is reduced to <1 cm^2, severe mitral stenosis is present. In order for sufficient cardiac output to be maintained, the left atrial pressure increases and left atrial hypertrophy and dilatation occur. Consequently, pulmonary venous, pulmonary arterial and right heart pressures also increase. The increase in pulmonary capillary pressure is followed by the development of pulmonary oedema, particularly when the rhythm deteriorates to atrial fibrillation with tachycardia and loss of coordinated atrial contraction. This is partially prevented by alveolar and capillary thickening and pulmonary arterial vasoconstriction (reactive pulmonary hypertension). Pulmonary hypertension leads to right ventricular hypertrophy, dilatation and failure with subsequent tricuspid regurgitation.

Clinical features

Symptoms

Usually, there are no symptoms until the valve orifice is moderately stenosed (area <2 cm^2). In Europe, this does not usually occur until several decades after the first attack of rheumatic fever, but in developing countries, children of 10–20 years of age may have severe mitral stenosis.

Progressively ***severe dyspnoea*** develops from the elevation in left atrial pressure, vascular congestion and interstitial pulmonary oedema. A cough productive of blood-tinged, frothy sputum or frank haemoptysis may occur. The development of pulmonary hypertension eventually leads to ***right heart failure*** and its symptoms of weakness, fatigue, and abdominal or lower limb swelling.

The large left atrium predisposes to ***atrial fibrillation***, giving rise to symptoms such as palpitations. Atrial fibrillation may result in ***systemic emboli***, most commonly to the cerebral vessels, producing neurological sequelae, but mesenteric, renal and peripheral emboli are also seen.

Signs

See the 'Clinical memo' in ***Figure 23.74***.

Face

Severe mitral stenosis with pulmonary hypertension is associated with the so-called mitral facies or malar flush. This is a bilateral, cyanotic or dusky pink discoloration over the upper cheeks, which is due to arteriovenous anastomoses and vascular stasis.

Pulse

Mitral stenosis may be associated with a small-volume pulse, which is usually regular early on in the disease process, when most patients are in sinus rhythm. However, as the severity of the disease progresses, many patients develop atrial fibrillation, resulting in an 'irregularly irregular' pulse. The development of atrial fibrillation in these patients often causes a dramatic clinical deterioration.

Jugular veins

If right heart failure develops, there is obvious distension of the jugular veins. If pulmonary hypertension or tricuspid stenosis is present, the 'a'-wave will be prominent, provided that atrial fibrillation has not supervened.

Palpation

There is a tapping impulse felt parasternally on the left side. This is the result of a palpable first heart sound combined with left ventricular backward displacement produced by an enlarging right ventricle. A sustained parasternal impulse due to right ventricular hypertrophy may also be felt.

Auscultation

Auscultation (***Fig. 23.74***) reveals a loud first heart sound if the mitral valve is pliable, but this will not occur in calcific mitral stenosis. As the valve suddenly opens with the force of the increased left atrial pressure, an 'opening snap' will be heard. This is followed by a low-pitched, 'rumbling', mid-diastolic murmur, best heard with the bell of the stethoscope held lightly at the apex and the patient lying on the left side in expiration. If the patient is in sinus rhythm, the murmur becomes louder at the end of diastole as a result of atrial contraction (pre-systolic accentuation).

The severity of mitral stenosis is judged clinically on the basis of several criteria:

- The presence of pulmonary hypertension implies that mitral stenosis is severe. Pulmonary hypertension is recognized by a right ventricular heave, a loud pulmonary component to the second heart sound and, eventually, signs of right-sided heart failure, such as oedema and hepatomegaly. Pulmonary hypertension results in pulmonary valvular regurgitation, which causes an early diastolic murmur in the pulmonary area, known as a Graham Steell murmur.
- The time between the opening snap and second heart sound (S2–OS interval) shortens with more severe degrees of mitral stenosis.
- The length of the mid-diastolic murmur is proportional to the severity.
- As the valve cusps become immobile, the loud first heart sound softens and the opening snap disappears. (For recordings of heart sounds, see online at Student Consult.) When pulmonary hypertension occurs, the pulmonary component of the second sound is increased in intensity and the mitral diastolic murmur may become quieter because of the reduction of cardiac output.

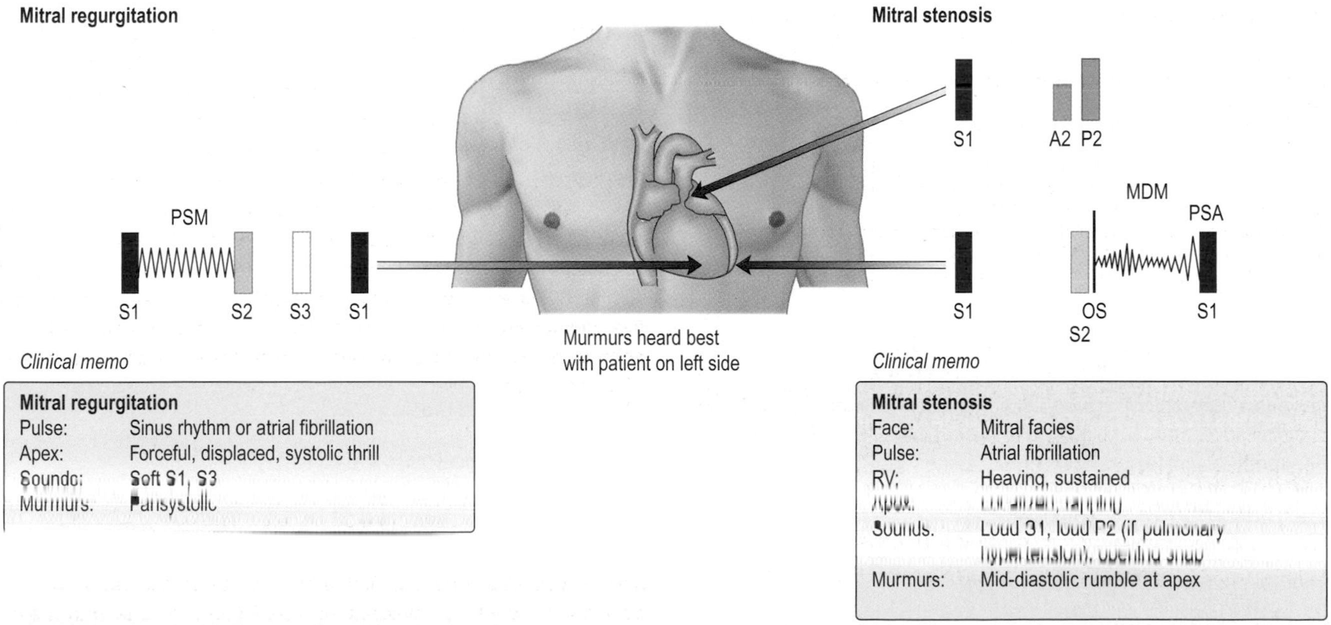

Figure 23.74 Features associated with mitral regurgitation and mitral stenosis. A2, aortic component of the second heart sound; MDM, mid-diastolic murmur; OS, opening snap; P2, pulmonary component of the second heart sound (loud with pulmonary hypertension); PSA, pre-systolic accentuation; PSM, pansystolic murmur; RV, right ventricle; S1, first heart sound; S2, second heart sound; S3, third heart sound.

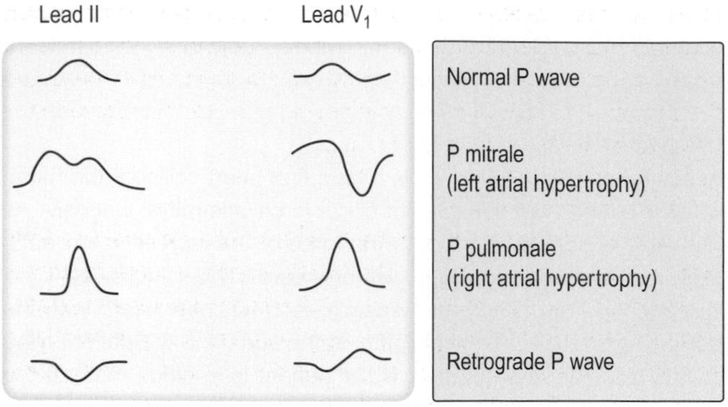

Figure 23.75 A bifid P wave, as seen on the ECG in mitral stenosis (P mitrale). Other P wave abnormalities are also shown for comparison.

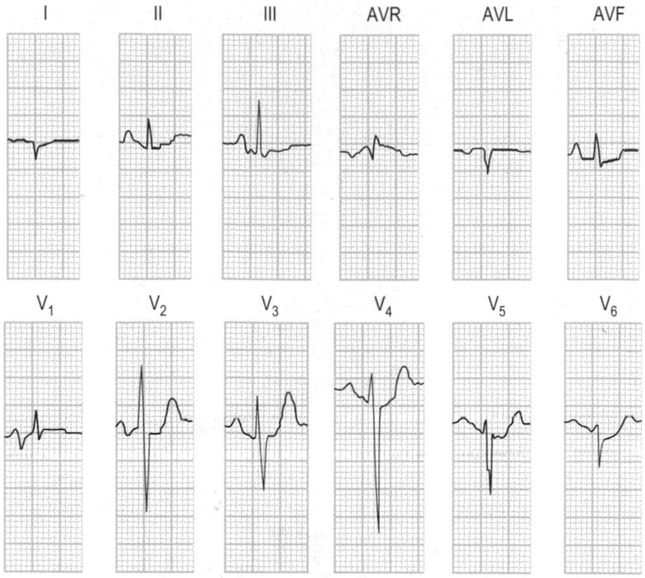

Figure 23.76 Severe mitral stenosis, shown by a 12-lead ECG. Note the right axis deviation (frontal plane axis=+120°), the left atrial conduction abnormality (large terminal negative component of the P wave in V_1) and the right ventricular hypertrophy (R wave in V_1 and right axis deviation).

Investigations

Chest X-ray

The chest X-ray may show left atrial enlargement with straightening of the left heart border and a 'double shadow' on the border of the right and left atria (see ***Fig. 23.14***). Late in the course of the disease, a calcified mitral valve may be seen on a penetrated or lateral view. Pulmonary vascular congestion and enlargement of the main pulmonary arteries may also be apparent in severe disease.

Electrocardiogram

In sinus rhythm, the ECG shows a bifid P wave owing to delayed left atrial activation ***(Fig. 23.75)***. However, atrial fibrillation is frequently present. As the disease progresses, the ECG features of right ventricular hypertrophy (right axis deviation and, perhaps, tall R waves in lead V_1) may develop ***(Fig. 23.76)***.

Echocardiogram

Transthoracic echocardiography is able to determine left atrial size and the degree of thickening, calcification and mobility of the mitral leaflets, as well as the degree of commissural fusion ***(Fig. 23.77)***. The severity of the mitral stenosis ***(Box 23.42)*** can be defined by mitral valve area on two-dimensional echocardiography, with continuous wave (CW) Doppler to measure the pressure half-time (the time taken for the pressure to halve from the peak value) and mean pressure drop across the valve. CW Doppler may also be used to estimate pulmonary artery pressure through measurement of the degree of tricuspid regurgitation.

Transoesophageal echocardiography **(*TOE*)** is performed to detect the presence of left atrial thrombus (see p. 951) or to carry out a detailed assessment prior to consideration of surgical or percutaneous intervention. The Wilkins score can be used to determine whether the valve is suitable for percutaneous valvotomy. The Wilkins score is an echocardiographic assessment of the mitral valve (leaflet mobility, valve thickening, valve calcification and subvalvular apparatus) and is used to determine suitability for percutaneous mitral valvuloplasty.

Cardiac magnetic resonance

CMR (see pp. 953–955) can show mitral valve anatomy accurately, although it is rarely used in mitral stenosis.

Cardiac catheterization

This is seldom required and is only used if coexisting cardiac problems (e.g. mitral regurgitation or CAD) are suspected. Right heart catheterization may be needed to determine pulmonary artery pressure in patients referred for valve intervention.

Box 23.42 Echocardiographic severity of mitral stenosis

Parameter	Normal	Mild	Moderate	Severe
Pressure half-time (ms)	40–70	71–139	140–219	>219
Mean pressure drop (mmHg)		<5.0	5–10	>10
Valve area (cm^2)	4.0–6.0	1.5–2.0	1.0–1.5	<1.0

(Source: British Society of Echocardiography.)

Management

Mild mitral stenosis may need no treatment other than prompt therapy for attacks of bronchitis. Infective endocarditis in pure mitral stenosis is uncommon. Early symptoms of mitral stenosis, such as mild dyspnoea, can usually be treated with low doses of diuretics. The onset of atrial fibrillation requires treatment with beta-blockers or DC cardioversion and anticoagulation to prevent atrial thrombus and systemic embolization. If pulmonary hypertension develops or the symptoms of pulmonary congestion persist despite therapy, surgical relief of the mitral stenosis is advised. There are four operative measures.

Trans-septal balloon valvotomy

A catheter is introduced into the right atrium via the femoral vein under local anaesthesia in the cardiac catheter laboratory. The interatrial septum is then punctured and the catheter advanced into the left atrium and across the mitral valve. A balloon is passed over the catheter to lie across the valve, and then inflated briefly to split the valve commissures. As with other valvotomy techniques, significant regurgitation may result, necessitating valve replacement (see below). This procedure is ideal for patients with pliable valves

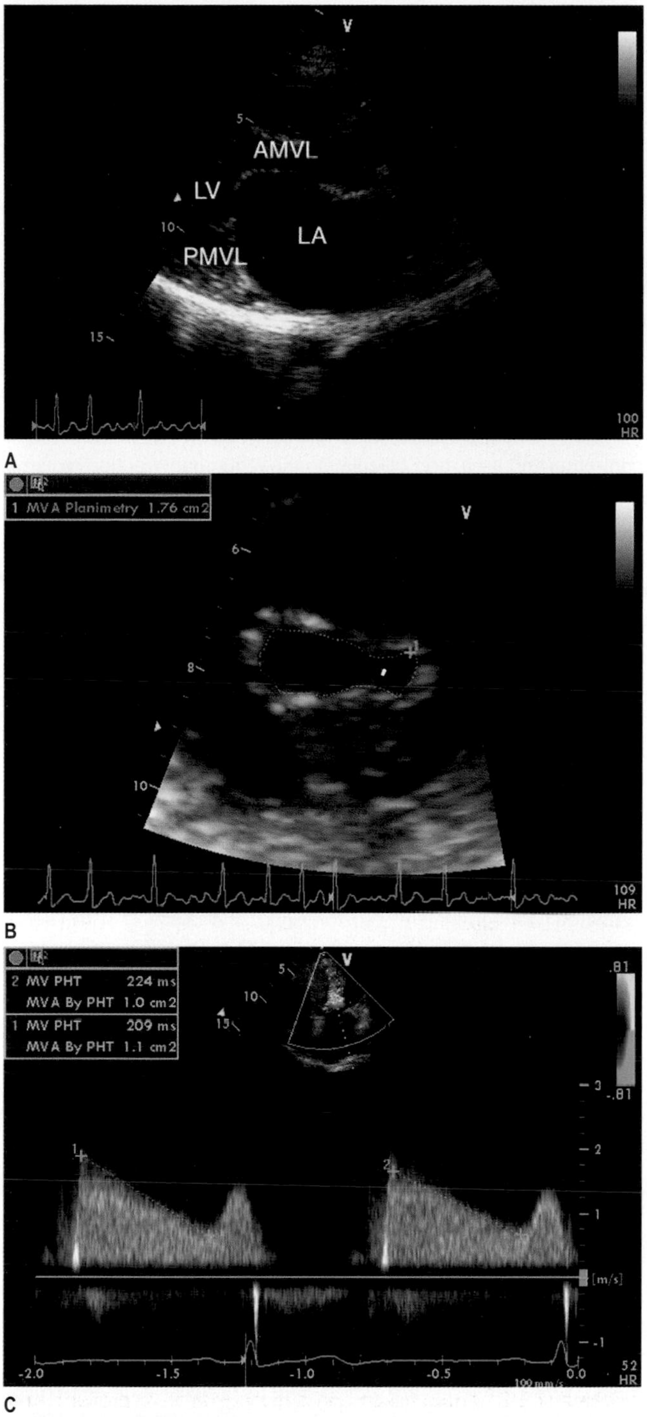

Figure 23.77 Echocardiograms in rheumatic mitral valve disease. **A.** *A two-dimensional long-axis view*, showing an enlarged left atrium and the 'hooked' appearance of the mitral valve leaflets, resulting from commissural fusion. **B.** *A magnified short-axis view*, showing the mitral valve orifice as seen from the left atrium. The orifice area can be planimetered to assess the severity; in this case, it is 1.5 cm^2, indicating moderately severe disease. **C.** *A continuous-wave (CW) Doppler recording*, showing the slow rate of decay of flow velocity from the left atrium to the left ventricle during diastole. It is also possible to derive the valve orifice area from the velocity decay rate. AMVL, anterior mitral valve leaflet; LA, left atrium; LV, left ventricle; PMVL, posterior mitral valve leaflet.

in whom there is little involvement of the sub-valvular apparatus and minimal mitral regurgitation. Contraindications include heavy calcification or more than mild mitral regurgitation and thrombus in the left atrium. TOE must be performed prior to this technique in order to exclude left atrial thrombus.

Closed valvotomy

This operation is advised for patients with mobile, non-calcified and non-regurgitant mitral valves. The fused cusps are forced apart by a dilator introduced through the apex of the left ventricle and guided into position by the surgeon's finger inserted via the left atrial appendage. Cardiopulmonary bypass is not needed for this operation. Closed valvotomy may produce a good result for 10 years or more. The valve cusps often re-fuse and, eventually, another operation may be necessary.

Open valvotomy

This operation is often preferred to closed valvotomy. The cusps are carefully dissected apart under direct vision. Cardiopulmonary bypass is required. Open dissection reduces the likelihood of causing traumatic mitral regurgitation.

Mitral valve replacement

Replacement of the mitral valve is necessary if:

- mitral regurgitation is also present
- there is a badly diseased or calcified stenotic valve that cannot be re-opened without producing significant regurgitation
- there is moderate or severe mitral stenosis and thrombus in the left atrium despite anticoagulation.

Artificial valves (see pp. 1016–1017) may work successfully for >20 years. Anticoagulants are generally necessary to prevent the formation of thrombus, which might obstruct the valve or embolize.

Mitral regurgitation

Mitral regurgitation can occur due to abnormalities of the valve leaflets, the annulus, the chordae tendineae or papillary muscles, or the left ventricle. The most frequent causes of mitral regurgitation are degenerative (myxomatous) disease, ischaemic heart disease, rheumatic heart disease and infectious endocarditis. Mitral regurgitation is also seen in diseases of the myocardium (dilated and hypertrophic cardiomyopathy), rheumatic autoimmune diseases (e.g. systemic lupus erythematosus), collagen diseases (e.g. Marfan and Ehlers–Danlos syndromes) and disorders caused by drugs, including centrally acting appetite suppressants (fenfluramine) and dopamine agonists (cabergoline).

Pathophysiology

Regurgitation into the left atrium produces left atrial dilatation but little increase in left atrial pressure if the regurgitation is longstanding, as the regurgitant flow is accommodated by the large left atrium. With acute mitral regurgitation, the normal compliance of the left atrium does not allow much dilatation and the left atrial pressure rises. Thus, in acute mitral regurgitation, the left atrial *v*-wave is greatly increased and pulmonary venous pressure rises, leading to pulmonary oedema. Since a proportion of the stroke volume is regurgitated, the stroke volume increases to maintain the forward cardiac output and the left ventricle therefore enlarges.

The Carpentier classification ***(Fig. 23.78)*** uses mitral leaflet motion to divide patients into different classes according to the mechanism of regurgitation, which can be useful when considering surgical intervention.

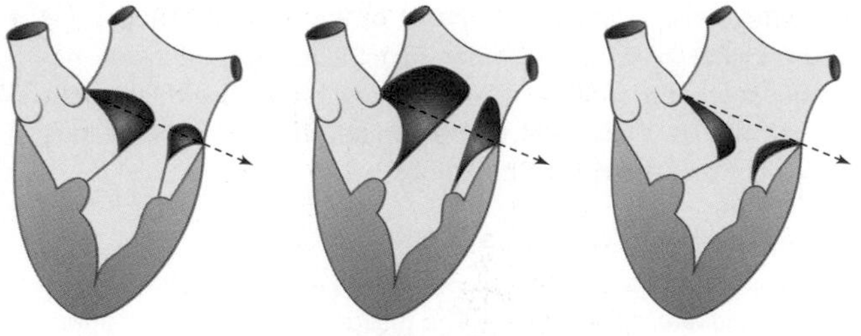

Figure 23.78 **Carpentier classification of mitral regurgitation and its causes. A.** Normal leaflet motion. **B.** Increased leaflet motion/ prolapse. **C.** Restricted leaflet motion. *(Reproduced from Tuladhar SM, Punjabi PP. Surgical reconstruction of the mitral valve.* Heart *2006; 92(10):1373–1377, with permission.)*

Clinical features

Symptoms

Mitral regurgitation can be present for many years and the cardiac dimensions greatly increased before any symptoms occur. The increased stroke volume is sensed as a 'palpitation'. ***Dyspnoea*** and ***orthopnoea*** develop because of pulmonary venous hypertension that arises as a direct result of the mitral regurgitation and secondarily as a consequence of left ventricular failure. ***Fatigue*** and ***lethargy*** develop because of the reduced cardiac output. In the late stages of the disease, the symptoms of ***right heart failure*** also occur and eventually lead to congestive cardiac failure. ***Cardiac cachexia*** may develop. Thromboembolism is less common than in mitral stenosis but ***subacute infective endocarditis*** is much more common.

Signs

See the 'Clinical memo' in ***Figure 23.74***.

The physical signs of uncomplicated mitral regurgitation are:

- ***Laterally displaced (forceful) diffuse apex beat*** and a ***systolic thrill*** (if severe).
- ***Soft first heart sound***, owing to the incomplete apposition of the valve cusps and their partial closure by the time ventricular systole begins.
- ***Pansystolic murmur***, due to the occurrence of regurgitation throughout the whole of systole, being loudest at the apex but radiating widely over the precordium and into the axilla.
- ***Mid-systolic click***, which may be present with a floppy mitral valve (see below); it is produced by the sudden prolapse of the valve and the tensing of the chordae tendineae that occurs during systole. This may be followed by a late systolic murmur owing to some regurgitation.
- ***Prominent third heart sound*** (S3), owing to the sudden rush of blood back into the dilated left ventricle in early diastole (sometimes a short mid-diastolic flow murmur may follow the third heart sound).

The signs related to atrial fibrillation, pulmonary hypertension, and left and right heart failure develop later in the disease. The onset of atrial fibrillation has a much less dramatic effect on symptoms than in mitral stenosis.

Investigations

Chest X-ray

The chest X-ray may show left atrial and left ventricular enlargement. There is an increase in the cardiothoracic ratio and valve calcification may be present.

Electrocardiogram

The ECG shows the features of left atrial delay (bifid P waves) and left ventricular hypertrophy ***(Fig. 23.79)***, as manifested by tall R waves in the left lateral leads (e.g. leads I and V_6) and deep S waves in the right-sided precordial leads (e.g. leads V_1 and V_2). (Note that S in V_1 plus R in V_5 or R in V_6 >35 mm indicates left ventricular hypertrophy.) Left ventricular hypertrophy occurs in about 50% of patients with mitral regurgitation. Atrial fibrillation may be present.

Echocardiogram

The echocardiogram ***(Fig. 23.80)*** shows a dilated left atrium and left ventricle. There may be specific features of chordal or papillary muscle rupture. The severity of regurgitation can be assessed with the use of colour Doppler, looking at the narrowest jet width (vena contracta) and area, and calculating the regurgitant fraction, volume or orifice area. Useful information regarding the severity of the condition can be obtained indirectly by observing the dynamics of ventricular function. ***Transoesophageal echocardiography*** can be helpful to identify structural valve abnormalities before surgery ***(Fig. 23.80)*** and intraoperative TOE can aid assessment of the efficacy of valve repair.

Cardiac catheterization

This demonstrates a prominent left atrial systolic pressure wave; when contrast is injected into the left ventricle, it is seen regurgitating into an enlarged left atrium during systole.

Management

Mild mitral regurgitation in the absence of symptoms can be managed conservatively by following the patient with serial echocardiograms. Prophylaxis against endocarditis is discussed on pages 236–237. Any evidence of progressive cardiac enlargement generally warrants early surgical intervention by either mitral valve repair or replacement. The current ESC guidelines recommend surgical intervention in patients with symptomatic severe mitral regurgitation, left ventricular ejection fraction >30% and end-diastolic dimension of <55 mm, and in asymptomatic patients with left ventricular dysfunction (end-systolic dimension >45 mm and/or ejection fraction of <60%). Surgery should also be considered in patients with asymptomatic severe mitral regurgitation with preserved left ventricular function and atrial fibrillation and/or pulmonary hypertension. The advantages of surgical intervention are diminished in more advanced disease. (*Sudden torrential mitral regurgitation, as seen with chordal or papillary muscle rupture or infective endocarditis, necessitates emergency mitral valve replacement.*) When patients are not suited to surgical intervention, or when surgery will be performed at a later date, management involves treatment with diuretics, ACE inhibitors and possibly anticoagulants. A percutaneous mitral valve repair (MitraClip) has been compared to cardiac surgery in the EVEREST II trial and appears effective in the short term at reducing the severity of mitral regurgitation and providing symptomatic relief. It is appropriate in selected patients unsuitable for cardiac surgery.

Prolapsing (billowing) mitral valve

This is also known as Barlow syndrome or floppy mitral valve. It is due to excessively large mitral valve leaflets, an enlarged mitral annulus, abnormally long chordae or disordered papillary muscle contraction. Histology may demonstrate myxomatous degeneration of the mitral valve leaflets. Prolapsing mitral valve is

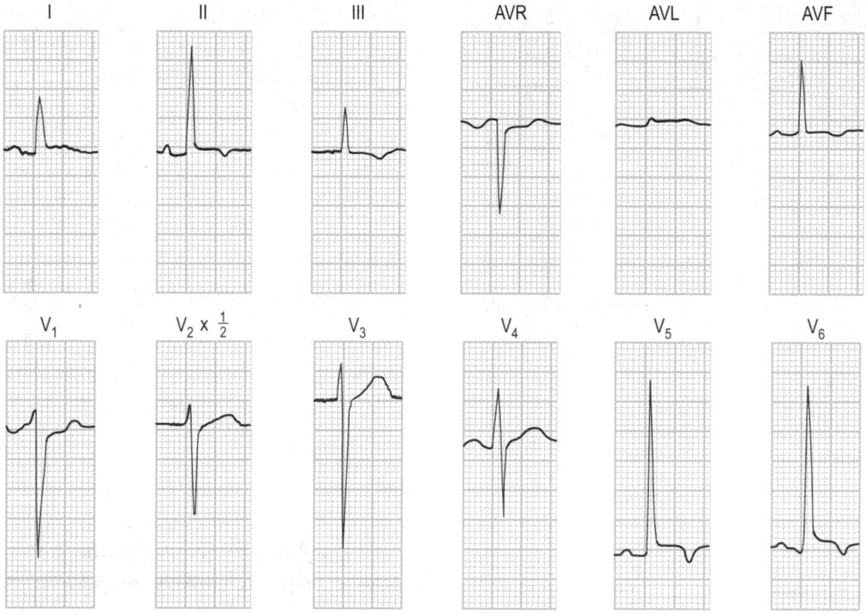

Figure 23.79 Left ventricular hypertrophy, shown in a 12-lead ECG. Note the size of the S wave seen in V_1 (21 mm); S in V_1+R in V_6=>35 mm.

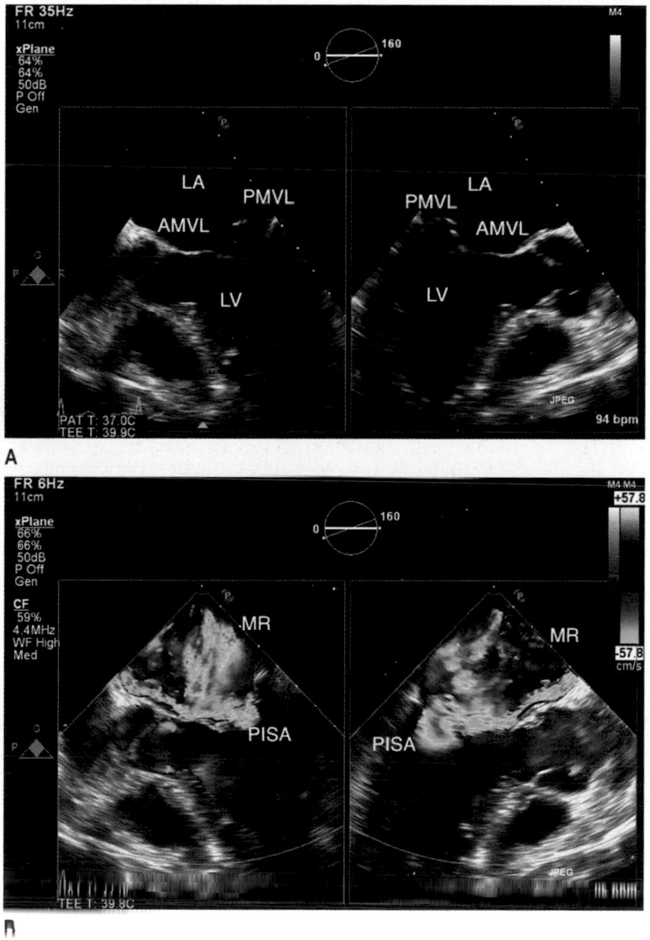

Figure 23.80 Mitral regurgitation. A. Transoesophageal echocardiography with *marked prolapse of part of the posterior mitral valve leaflet* (PMVL). **B.** Transoesophageal echocardiography with colour Doppler demonstrates *severe mitral regurgitation* (MR) into the left atrium (LA). AMVL, aortic mitral valve leaflet; LV, left ventricle; PISA, proximal isovelocity surface area.

more commonly seen in young women than in men or older women, and has a familial incidence. Its cause is unknown but it is associated with connective tissue disorders (Marfan syndrome, Ehlers–Danlos syndrome and pseudoxanthoma elasticum). It also occurs in association with an atrial septal defect and Ebstein's anomaly (see p. 1016).

AORTIC VALVE

Aortic stenosis

Aortic stenosis is a chronic progressive disease that produces obstruction to the left ventricular stroke volume, leading to symptoms of chest pain, breathlessness, syncope and pre-syncope, and fatigue.

Aortic valve stenosis includes calcific stenosis of a trileaflet aortic valve, stenosis of a congenitally bicuspid valve, and rheumatic aortic stenosis.

Calcific aortic valvular disease (***CAVD***) is the most common cause of aortic stenosis and mainly occurs in the elderly. This is an inflammatory process involving macrophages and T lymphocytes, initially with thickening of the sub-endothelium and adjacent fibrosis. The lesions contain lipoproteins, which calcify, increasing leaflet stiffness and reducing systolic opening. This can occur in a tri- or bileaflet aortic valve. Risk factors for CAVD include old age, male gender, elevated lipoprotein(a) and LDL, hypertension, diabetes and smoking.

Bicuspid aortic valve (***BAV***) ***(Fig. 23.81)*** is the most common form of congenital heart disease, occurring in 1–2% of live births; in about [illegible] of cases, it is [illegible] BAV [illegible] valve tend to present at an earlier age. BAV is associated with aortic coarctation, root dilatation and, potentially, aortic dissection, and patients should have regular follow-up echocardiography.

Rheumatic fever can produce progressive fusion, thickening and calcification of the aortic valve. In rheumatic heart disease, the aortic valve is affected in about 30–40% of cases and there is usually associated mitral valve disease.

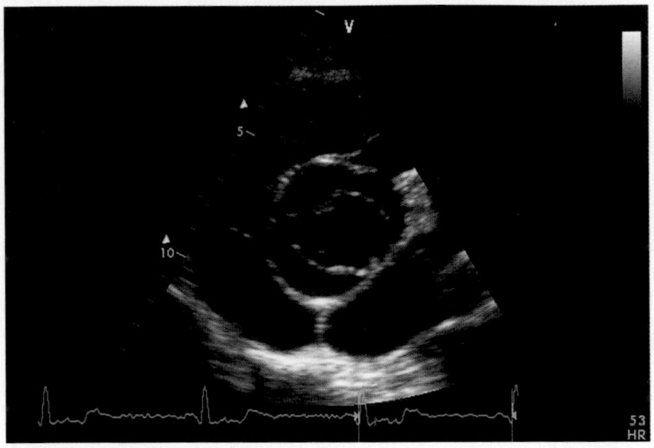

Figure 23.81 Bicuspid aortic valve.

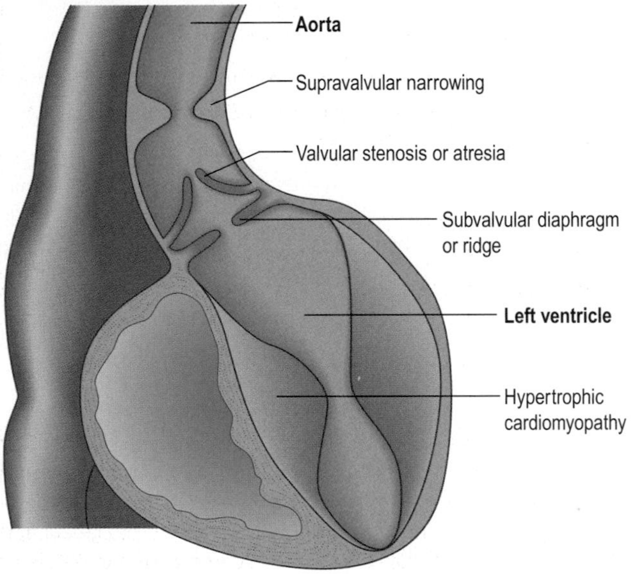

Figure 23.82 Several forms of left ventricular outflow tract obstruction.

Other causes of valvular stenosis include chronic kidney disease, Paget's disease of bone, previous radiation exposure and systemic lupus erythematosus. ***Valvular aortic stenosis*** should be distinguished from other causes of obstruction to left ventricular emptying ***(Fig. 23.82)***, which include:

- supravalvular obstruction – a congenital fibrous diaphragm above the aortic valve, often associated with mental retardation and hypercalcaemia (Williams syndrome)
- subvalvular aortic stenosis – a congenital condition in which a fibrous ridge or diaphragm is situated immediately below the aortic valve.
- hypertrophic cardiomyopathy – septal muscle hypertrophy obstructing left ventricular outflow.

Pathophysiology

Obstructed left ventricular emptying leads to increased left ventricular pressure and compensatory left ventricular hypertrophy. In turn, this results in relative ischaemia of the left ventricular myocardium, and consequent angina, arrhythmias and left ventricular failure. The obstruction to left ventricular emptying is relatively more severe on exercise. Normally, exercise causes a many-fold increase in cardiac output, but when there is severe narrowing of the aortic valve orifice, the cardiac output can hardly increase. Thus, the blood pressure falls, coronary ischaemia worsens, the myocardium fails and cardiac arrhythmias develop. Left ventricular systolic function is typically preserved in patients with aortic stenosis (compare this with aortic regurgitation).

Clinical features

Symptoms

There are usually no symptoms until aortic stenosis is moderately severe (when the aortic orifice is reduced to one-third of its normal size). At this stage, ***exercise-induced syncope***, ***angina*** and ***dyspnoea*** develop. When symptoms occur, the prognosis is poor – on average, death occurs within 2–3 years, if there has been no surgical intervention.

Signs

See the 'Clinical memo' in ***Figure 23.83***.

Pulse

The carotid pulse is of small volume and is slow-rising or plateau in nature (see pp. 940–941).

Precordial palpation

The apex beat is not usually displaced because hypertrophy (as opposed to dilatation) does not produce noticeable cardiomegaly. However, the pulsation is sustained and obvious. A double impulse is sometimes felt because the fourth heart sound or atrial contraction ('kick') may be palpable. A systolic thrill may be felt in the aortic area.

Auscultation

The most obvious auscultatory finding in aortic stenosis is an ejection systolic murmur that is usually 'diamond-shaped' (crescendo–decrescendo). The murmur is usually longer when the disease is more severe, as a longer ejection time is needed. The murmur is usually rough in quality and best heard in the aortic area. It radiates into the carotid arteries and also the precordium. The intensity of the murmur is not a good guide to the severity of the condition because it is lessened by a reduced cardiac output. In severe cases, the murmur may be inaudible.

Other findings include:

- ***systolic ejection click***, unless the valve has become immobile and calcified
- ***soft or inaudible aortic second heart sound*** when the aortic valve becomes immobile
- ***reversed splitting of the second heart sound*** (splitting on expiration) (see p. 942)
- ***prominent fourth heart sound***, caused by atrial contraction, and heard unless coexisting mitral stenosis prevents this.

Investigations

Chest X-ray

The chest X-ray usually reveals a relatively small heart with a prominent, dilated, ascending aorta. This occurs because turbulent blood flow above the stenosed aortic valve produces so-called 'post-stenotic dilatation'. The aortic valve may be calcified. The cardiothoracic ratio increases when heart failure occurs.

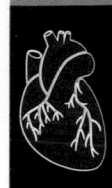

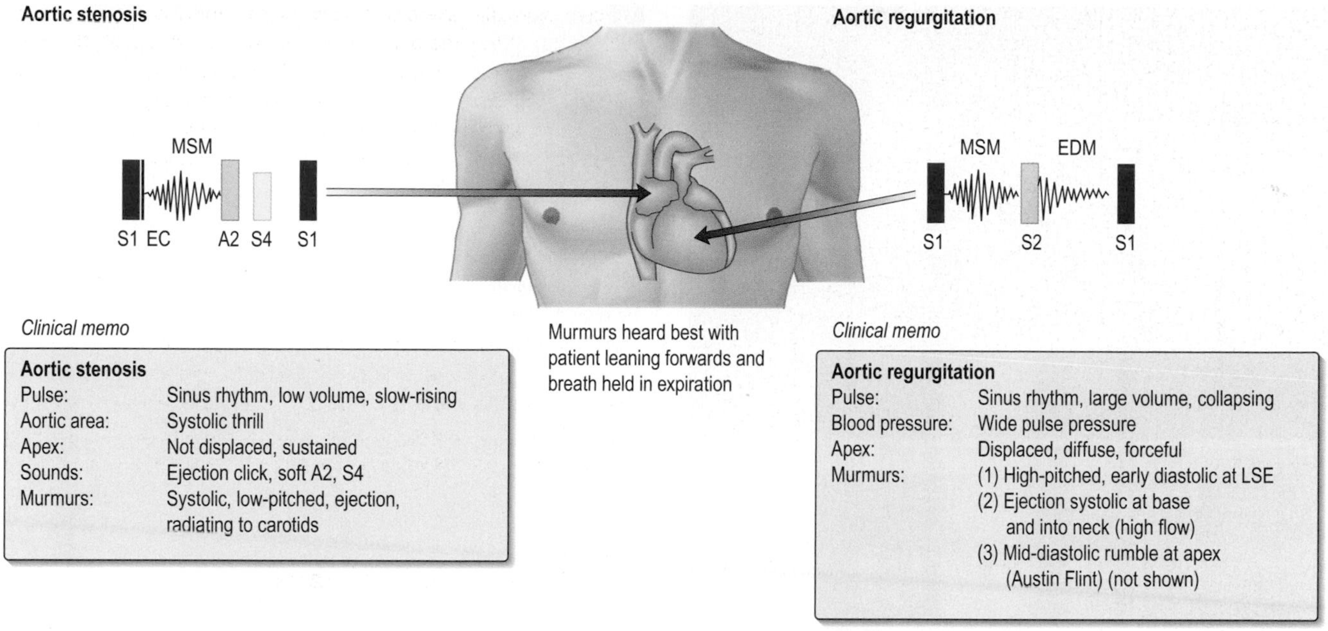
Aortic stenosis
MSM
S1 EC A2 S4 S1
Aortic regurgitation
MSM EDM
S1 S2 S1
Murmurs heard best with patient leaning forwards and breath held in expiration
Clinical memo
Aortic stenosis
Pulse: Sinus rhythm, low volume, slow-rising
Aortic area: Systolic thrill
Apex: Not displaced, sustained
Sounds: Ejection click, soft A2, S4
Murmurs: Systolic, low-pitched, ejection, radiating to carotids
Clinical memo
Aortic regurgitation
Pulse: Sinus rhythm, large volume, collapsing
Blood pressure: Wide pulse pressure
Apex: Displaced, diffuse, forceful
Murmurs: (1) High-pitched, early diastolic at LSE
(2) Ejection systolic at base and into neck (high flow)
(3) Mid-diastolic rumble at apex (Austin Flint) (not shown)

Figure 23.83 Features of aortic stenosis and aortic regurgitation. EC, ejection click; EDM, early diastolic murmur; LSE, left sternal edge; MSM, mid-systolic murmur; A2, aortic component of the second heart sound; S1, first heart sound; S4, fourth heart sound.

Box 23.43 Echocardiographic severity of aortic stenosis

Parameter	Normal	Mild	Moderate	Severe
Peak velocity (m/s)	<1.7	1.7–2.9	3.0–4.0	>4.0
Peak pressure drop (mmHg)		<36	36–64	>64
Mean pressure drop (mmHg)		<25	25–40	>40
Valve area (cm^2)	>2.0	1.5–2.0	1.0–1.4	<1.0

(Source: British Society of Echocardiography.)

Electrocardiogram

The ECG shows left ventricular hypertrophy and left atrial delay. A left ventricular 'strain' pattern due to 'pressure overload' (depressed ST segments and T-wave inversion in leads orientated towards the left ventricle, i.e. leads I, AVL, V_5 and V_6) is common when disease is severe. Usually, sinus rhythm is present, but ventricular arrhythmias may be recorded.

Echocardiogram

Echocardiography readily demonstrates the thickened, calcified and immobile aortic valve cusps, and the presence of left ventricular hypertrophy; it can be used to determine the severity of aortic stenosis (Box 23.43 and Fig. 23.84). Transoesophageal echocardiography is rarely indicated.

Cardiac catheterization

Cardiac catheterization is rarely necessary since all of this information can be gained non-invasively with echocardiography and CMR. Coronary angiography is required before surgery is recommended.

Cardiac magnetic resonance and cardiac computed tomography

These techniques are indicated for assessing the thoracic aorta for the presence of aneurysm, dissection or coarctation but are rarely needed.

Management

In patients with aortic stenosis, symptoms are a good index of severity and all symptomatic patients should have ***aortic valve replacement***. Patients with a BAV and ascending aorta >50 mm or expanding at >5 mm/year should be considered for surgical intervention. Asymptomatic patients should be under regular review for assessment of symptoms and echocardiography. Surgical intervention for asymptomatic people with severe aortic stenosis is recommended in those with:

- symptoms during an exercise test or with a drop in blood pressure
- an LVEF of <50%
- moderate to severe stenosis undergoing CABG, surgery of the ascending aorta or other cardiac valve.

Antibiotic prophylaxis against infective endocarditis is discussed on pages 236–237. Provided that the valve is not severely deformed or heavily calcified, critical aortic stenosis in childhood or adolescence can be treated by valvotomy (performed under direct vision by the surgeon or by balloon dilatation using X-ray visualization). This produces temporary relief from the obstruction. Aortic valve replacement will usually be needed a few years later. Balloon dilatation (valvuloplasty) has been tried in adults, especially in the elderly, as an alternative to surgery. Generally results are poor and such treatment is reserved for patients unfit for surgery or as a 'bridge' to surgery (as systolic function will often improve).

Percutaneous valve replacement

A novel treatment for patients unsuitable for surgical aortic valve replacement is transcatheter implantation with a balloon

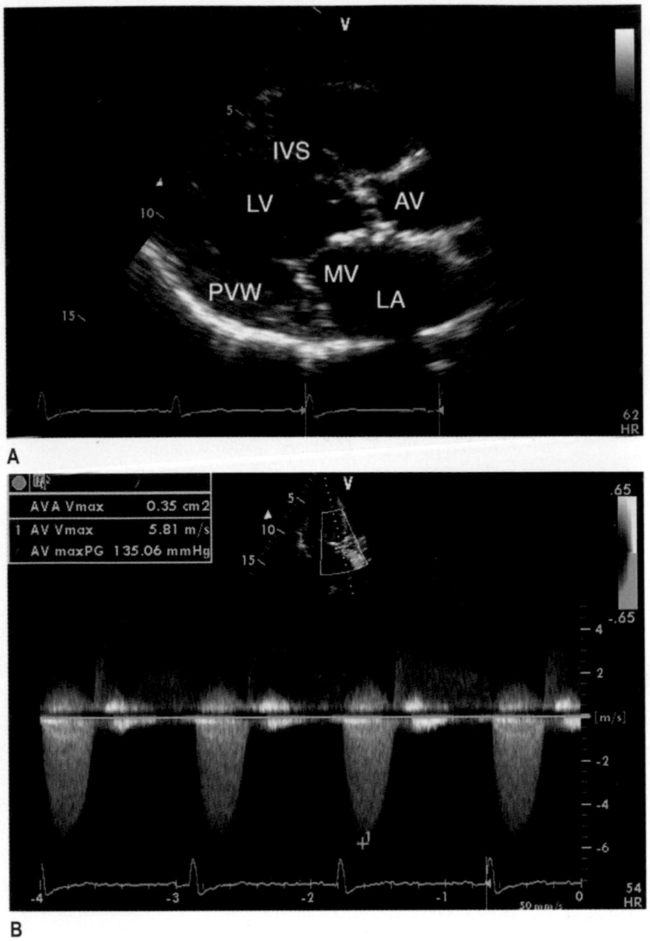

Figure 23.84 **Cardiac echograms. A.** *Two-dimensional echocardiogram (long-axis view)* in a patient with ***calcific aortic stenosis***. The calcium in the valve generates abnormally intense echoes. There is some evidence of associated left ventricular hypertrophy. **B.** *Continuous-wave (CW) Doppler* signals obtained from the right upper parasternal edge, where the high-velocity jet from the ***stenotic valve*** is coming towards the transducer. AV, aortic valve; IVS, interventricular septum; LA, left atrium; LV, left ventricle; MV, mitral valve; PVW, posterior ventricular wall.

expandable stent valve. Valve implantation has been shown to be successful (86%) with a procedural mortality of 2% and 30-day mortality of 12%. Good results have been reported in 5-year follow-up studies but further larger and randomized studies with long-term follow-up are required.

Aortic regurgitation

Aortic regurgitation can occur in diseases affecting the aortic valve, such as endocarditis, and diseases affecting the aortic root, such as Marfan syndrome ***(Box 23.44)***.

Pathophysiology

Aortic regurgitation is reflux of blood from the aorta through the aortic valve into the left ventricle during diastole. If net cardiac output is to be maintained, the total volume of blood pumped into the aorta must increase and, consequently, the left ventricular size must enlarge. Because of the aortic runoff during diastole, diastolic blood pressure falls and coronary perfusion is decreased. In addition, the larger left ventricular size is mechanically less efficient, so that the demand for oxygen is greater and cardiac ischaemia develops.

Box 23.44 Causes and associations of aortic regurgitation

Acute aortic regurgitation
- Acute rheumatic fever
- Infective endocarditis
- Dissection of the aorta
- Ruptured sinus of Valsalva aneurysm
- Failure of prosthetic valve

Chronic aortic regurgitation
- Rheumatic heart disease
- Syphilis
- Arthritides:
  - Reactive arthritis
  - Ankylosing spondylitis
  - Rheumatoid arthritis
- Hypertension (severe)
- Bicuspid aortic valve
- Aortic endocarditis
- Marfan syndrome
- Osteogenesis imperfecta

Clinical features

Symptoms

In aortic regurgitation, significant symptoms occur late and do not develop until ***left ventricular failure*** occurs. As with mitral regurgitation, a common symptom is ***pounding of the heart*** because of the increased left ventricular size and its vigorous pulsation. ***Angina pectoris*** is a frequent complaint. Varying grades of ***dyspnoea*** occur, depending on the extent of left ventricular dilatation and dysfunction. ***Arrhythmias*** are relatively uncommon.

Signs

See the 'Clinical memo' in Figure 23.83. The signs of aortic regurgitation are many and are due to the hyperdynamic circulation, reflux of blood into the left ventricle and the increased left ventricular size.

The pulse is bounding or collapsing (see p. 940). The following signs, which are rare, also indicate a hyperdynamic circulation:
- ***Quincke's sign*** – capillary pulsation in the nail beds
- ***de Musset's sign*** – head nodding with each heart beat
- ***Duroziez's sign*** – a to-and-fro murmur heard when the femoral artery is auscultated with pressure applied distally (if found, it is a sign of severe aortic regurgitation)
- ***pistol shot femorals*** – a sharp bang heard on auscultation over the femoral arteries in time with each heart beat.

The apex beat is displaced laterally and downwards, and is forceful in quality. On auscultation, there is a high-pitched early diastolic murmur best heard at the left sternal edge in the fourth intercostal space with the patient leaning forwards and the breath held in expiration. Because of the volume overload there is commonly an ejection systolic flow murmur. The regurgitant jet can impinge on the anterior mitral valve cusp, causing a mid-diastolic murmur (Austin Flint rumble).

Investigations

Chest X-ray

The chest X-ray features are those of left ventricular enlargement and, possibly, of dilatation of the ascending aorta. The ascending aortic wall may be calcified in syphilis, and the aortic valve calcified if valvular disease is responsible for the regurgitation.

Electrocardiogram

The ECG appearances are those of left ventricular hypertrophy due to 'volume overload' – tall R waves and deeply inverted T waves in

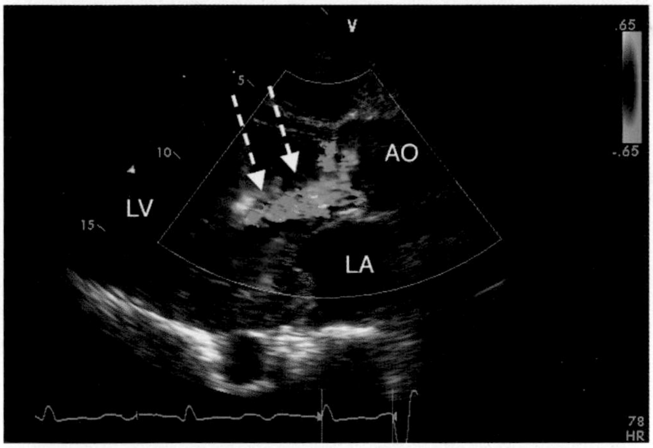

Figure 23.85 **Aortic regurgitation: colour Doppler.** AO, aorta; LA, left atrium; LV, left ventricle.

the left-sided chest leads, and deep S waves in the right-sided leads. Normally, sinus rhythm is present.

Echocardiogram

The echocardiogram ***(Fig. 23.85)*** demonstrates vigorous cardiac contraction and a dilated left ventricle. The aortic root may also be enlarged. Diastolic fluttering of the mitral leaflets or septum occurs in severe aortic regurgitation (producing the Austin Flint rumble). The severity of aortic regurgitation is assessed with a combination of colour Doppler (extent of the regurgitant jet, width of the vena contracta; ***Fig. 23.85***) and CW Doppler (diastolic flow reversal in the descending thoracic aorta, pressure half-time). Transoesophageal echocardiography may provide additional information about the valves and aortic root.

Cardiac catheterization

Cardiac catheterization is required to assess CAD in patients requiring surgery. During cardiac catheterization, injection of contrast medium into the aorta (aortography) will outline aortic valvular abnormalities and allow assessment of the degree of regurgitation.

Cardiac magnetic resonance and cardiac computed tomography

These techniques may be indicated for assessing the thoracic aorta in cases of aortic dilatation or dissection. CMR can be used to quantify regurgitant volume.

Management

The underlying cause of aortic regurgitation (e.g. syphilitic aortitis or infective endocarditis) may require specific treatment. Patients with acute aortic regurgitation may need treatment with vasodilators and inotropes. ACE inhibitors are useful in patients with left ventricular dysfunction and beta-blockers may slow aortic dilatation in Marfan patients. Because symptoms do not develop until the myocardium fails and because the myocardium does not recover fully after surgery, operative valve replacement may be performed before significant symptoms occur.

Aortic surgery is indicated in:

- acute severe aortic regurgitation, e.g. endocarditis
- symptomatic patients (dyspnoea, NYHA class II–IV, angina) with chronic severe aortic regurgitation
- in asymptomatic patients with an LVEF of ≤50%
- in asymptomatic patients with an LVEF of >50% but with a dilated left ventricle (end-diastolic dimension >70 mm or systolic dimension >50 mm)
- in those undergoing CABG or surgery of the ascending aorta or other cardiac valve.

Both mechanical prostheses and tissue valves are used. Tissue valves are preferred in the elderly and when anticoagulants must be avoided, but are contraindicated in children and young adults because of the rapid calcification and degeneration of the valves.

Antibiotic prophylaxis against infective endocarditis (see pp. 236–237) is not recommended.

TRICUSPID VALVE

Tricuspid stenosis

This uncommon valve lesion, which is seen much more often in women than in men, is usually due to rheumatic heart disease and is frequently associated with mitral and/or aortic valve disease. Tricuspid stenosis is also seen in the carcinoid syndrome.

Pathophysiology

Tricuspid valve stenosis results in a reduced cardiac output, which is restored towards normal when the right atrial pressure increases. The resulting systemic venous congestion produces hepatomegaly, ascites and dependent oedema.

Clinical features

Symptoms

Usually, patients with tricuspid stenosis complain of symptoms due to associated left-sided rheumatic valve lesions. The ***abdominal pain*** (due to hepatomegaly) and swelling (due to ascites), and ***peripheral oedema*** that occur are relatively severe when compared with the degree of ***dyspnoea***.

Signs

If the patient remains in sinus rhythm, which is unusual, there is a prominent jugular venous *a*-wave. This pre-systolic pulsation may also be felt over the liver. There is usually a rumbling mid-diastolic murmur, which is heard best at the lower left sternal edge and is louder on inspiration. It may be missed because of the murmur of coexisting mitral stenosis. A tricuspid opening snap may occasionally be heard.

Hepatomegaly, abdominal ascites and dependent oedema may be present.

Investigations

On the chest X-ray, there may be a prominent right atrial bulge. On the ECG, the enlarged right atrium is shown by peaked, tall P waves (>3 mm) in lead II. The echocardiogram may show a thickened and immobile tricuspid valve, but this is not so clearly seen as an abnormal mitral valve.

Management

Medical management consists of diuretic therapy and salt restriction. Tricuspid valvotomy is occasionally possible but tricuspid valve replacement is often necessary. Usually, other valves also need replacement because tricuspid valve stenosis is rarely an isolated lesion.

Tricuspid regurgitation

Functional tricuspid regurgitation (see ***Fig. 23.25***) may occur whenever the right ventricle dilates: for example, in cor pulmonale, MI or pulmonary hypertension.

Organic tricuspid regurgitation may occur with rheumatic heart disease, infective endocarditis, carcinoid syndrome, Ebstein's anomaly (a congenitally malpositioned tricuspid valve) and other congenital abnormalities of the AV valves.

Clinical features

The valvular regurgitation gives rise to high right atrial and systemic venous pressures. Patients may complain of the symptoms of ***right heart failure*** (see pp. 1006–1007).

Physical signs include a large jugular venous '*cv*'-wave and a palpable liver that pulsates in systole. Usually, a right ventricular impulse may be felt at the left sternal edge, and there is a blowing pansystolic murmur, best heard on inspiration at the lower left sternal edge. Atrial fibrillation is common.

Investigations

An ***echocardiogram*** shows dilatation of the right ventricle with thickening of the valve.

Management

Functional tricuspid regurgitation usually disappears with medical management. Severe organic tricuspid regurgitation may require operative repair of the tricuspid valve (annuloplasty or annuloplication). Very occasionally, tricuspid valve replacement may be necessary. In drug addicts with infective endocarditis of the tricuspid valve, surgical removal of the valve is recommended to eradicate the infection. This is usually well tolerated in the short term. The insertion of a prosthetic valve for this condition is sometimes necessary.

PULMONARY VALVE

Pulmonary stenosis

This is usually a congenital lesion but may rarely result from rheumatic fever or from the carcinoid syndrome. Congenital pulmonary stenosis may be associated with Fallot's tetralogy, Noonan syndrome or congenital rubella syndrome.

Pulmonary stenosis may be valvular, sub-valvular or supra-valvular.

Clinical features

The obstruction to right ventricular emptying results in right ventricular hypertrophy, which, in turn, leads to right atrial hypertrophy. Severe ***pulmonary obstruction*** may be incompatible with life, but lesser degrees of obstruction give rise to ***fatigue***, ***syncope*** and the symptoms of ***right heart failure***. Mild pulmonary stenosis may be asymptomatic.

The physical signs are characterized by a harsh mid-systolic ejection murmur, best heard on inspiration, to the left of the sternum in the second intercostal space. This murmur is often associated with a thrill. The pulmonary closure sound is usually delayed and soft. There may be a pulmonary ejection sound if the obstruction is valvular. A right ventricular fourth sound and a prominent jugular venous *a*-wave are present when the stenosis is moderately severe. A right ventricular heave (sustained impulse) may be felt.

Investigations

The chest X-ray usually shows a prominent pulmonary artery owing to post-stenotic dilatation. The ECG demonstrates both right atrial and right ventricular hypertrophy, although it may sometimes be normal, even in severe pulmonary stenosis. A Doppler echocardiogram is the investigation of choice.

Management

Management of severe pulmonary stenosis requires pulmonary valvotomy (balloon valvotomy or direct surgery).

Pulmonary regurgitation

This is the most common acquired lesion of the pulmonary valve. It results from dilatation of the pulmonary valve ring, which occurs with pulmonary hypertension (Graham Steell murmur). It may also occur following tetralogy of Fallot repair. It is characterized by a decrescendo diastolic murmur, beginning with the pulmonary component of the second heart sound that is difficult to distinguish from the murmur of aortic regurgitation. Pulmonary regurgitation usually causes no symptoms and treatment is rarely necessary.

PROSTHETIC VALVES

There is no ideal replacement for our own normally functioning, native heart valves. There are two options for valve prostheses: mechanical or tissue (bioprosthetic) ***(Fig. 23.86)***.

The valves consist of two basic components: an opening to allow blood to flow through and an occluding mechanism to regulate the flow. Mechanical prostheses rely on artificial concluders: a ball and cage (Starr–Edwards), tilting disc (Bjork–Shiley) or double tilting disc (St Jude). Tissue prostheses are derived from human (homograft) or from porcine or bovine (xenograft) sources. A valve replacement from within the same patient (i.e. pulmonary to aortic valve position) is termed an autograft.

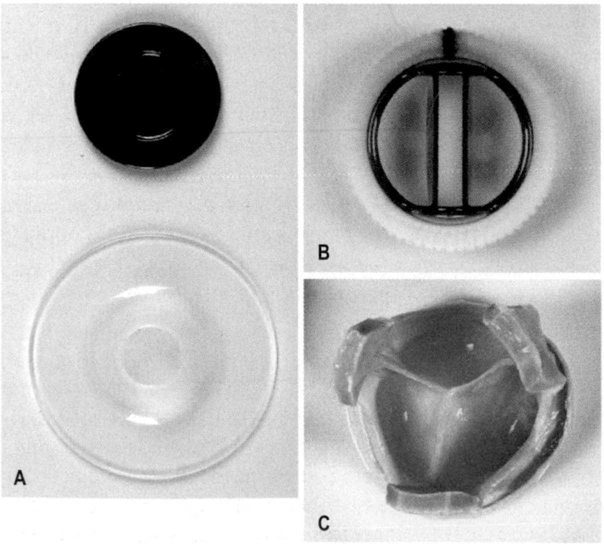

Figure 23.86 Prosthetic valves. A. Bjork–Shiley mechanical prosthetic valve. **B.** St Jude double tilting disc. **C.** Aortic valve tissue prosthesis (aortic view).

Mechanical versus tissue valves

Mechanical valves, being artificial structures, are more durable than their tissue counterparts, which tend to degenerate after 10 years. However, artificial structures are more thrombogenic. Mechanical valves require formal anticoagulation for the lifetime of the prosthesis. The target INR is determined by what type of valve is inserted, where it is positioned, and whether the patient has additional risk factors for thromboembolism (mitral, tricuspid, pulmonary valve disease; previous thromboembolism; atrial fibrillation; left atrial diameter >50 mm; mitral stenosis; LVEF <35%; hypercoagulable state) (see p. 575):

- low thrombogenicity valve (Carbomedics (aortic position), Medtronic Hall, St Jude Medical (without silzone)): INR 2.5 without and 3.0 with additional risk factors
- medium thrombogenicity valve (Bjork–Shiley, other bileaflet valves): INR 3.0 without and 3.5 with additional risk factors
- high thrombogenicity valve (Lillehei–Kaster, Omniscience, Starr–Edwards): INR 3.5 without and 4.0 with additional risk factors.

Tissue valves require anticoagulation for a limited postoperative period only, while the suture lines endothelialize (the ESC recommends 3 months with a target INR of 2.5, although some centres use low-dose aspirin 75–100 mg daily); it can then be discontinued unless another risk factor for thromboembolism (e.g. atrial fibrillation) persists. There is currently no role for the non-vitamin K antagonist oral anticoagulants (NOACs).

On auscultation, tissue valve heart sounds are comparable to those of a native valve. Mechanical valve heart sounds are generally louder and both opening and closing sounds can be heard.

Complications

All prostheses carry a risk of infection. Prosthetic valve endocarditis is associated with significant morbidity and mortality; prevention is the cornerstone of management. Patient education about antibiotic prophylaxis is vital and this should be reinforced at clinic visits. Any procedure that results in a breach of the body's innate defences (i.e. dental treatment, catheter insertion) increases the risk of exposing the prosthesis to a bacteraemia. This must be borne in mind when managing a patient with a prosthetic heart valve and steps should be taken to minimize the risk involved. The prosthetic valve occluding mechanism can be interrupted by vegetations, but also by thrombosis and calcification, resulting in either stenosis or regurgitation. The prosthesis can become detached from the valve ring, resulting in a ***para-prosthetic leak***. Evidence of structural failure can be detected by simple auscultation, with echocardiography as the initial investigation of choice. Transthoracic echocardiography is non-invasive, but scattering of echoes by mechanical valves makes assessment difficult. Transoesophageal echocardiography provides alternative views and higher image resolution, making it the investigation of choice when prosthetic valve endocarditis is suspected.

Interruption of anticoagulant therapy

For minor surgical procedures, including dental extraction and diagnostic endoscopy, anticoagulation should not be interrupted, although the INR should be reduced to a target of 2.0. Percutaneous arterial puncture is safe with an INR <2.0, although radial catheterization may be possible at higher INR levels. For major surgical procedures, anticoagulation should be discontinued 5 days before the procedure and intravenous unfractionated heparin or subcutaneous low-molecular-weight heparin commenced when the INR is <2.0.

Pregnancy and prosthetic heart valves

The types of valve prosthesis in women of childbearing age are as follows:

- ***Bioprosthetic valves*** are preferable during pregnancy, as they are less thrombogenic and do not require anticoagulation. However, valve degradation in women of childbearing age has been shown to be as high as 50% at 10 years and 90% at 15 years; women with a bioprosthetic valve may require redo valve surgery.
- ***Mechanical heart valves*** have excellent durability but are thrombogenic and require life-long anticoagulation with warfarin. Pregnancy is a hypercoagulable state due to increased levels of fibrinogen and factors VII, VIII and X, decreased levels of protein S activity, venous hypertension and stasis.

Pregnancy in women with a mechanical heart valve is associated with increased maternal mortality (1–4%) due to valve thrombosis because safe anticoagulation in these patients is complex. Warfarin crosses the placenta and is associated with a 5–12% risk of embryopathy during the first trimester. Warfarin also has an anticoagulant effect in the fetus, which may lead to spontaneous fetal intracranial haemorrhage. Many women will chose unfractionated heparin or low-molecular-weight heparin, as they do not cross the placenta and do not cause fetal embryopathy. However, unfractionated heparin may not provide consistent therapeutic anticoagulation during pregnancy and there is a high incidence (25%) of valve thrombosis. Low-molecular-weight heparin provides a more consistent anticoagulant effect when given twice daily, with dose adjustment to maintain anti-Xa levels of 0.8–1.2 U/mL 4 h after administration.

Further reading

Feldman T, Foster E, Glower DD et al. for the EVEREST II Investigators. Percutaneous repair or surgery for mitral regurgitation. *N Engl J Med* 2011; 364:1395–1406.

Joint Task Force on the Management of Valvular Heart Disease of the European Society of Cardiology (ESC); European Association for Cardio-Thoracic Surgery (EACTS). Guidelines on the management of valvular heart disease. *Eur Heart J* 2012; 33:2451–2496.

Lancet series 1, 2, 3. Valvular heart disease. *Lancet* 2016; 387:1312–1323, 1324–1334, 1335–1346

Mack MJ, Leon MB, Smith CR et al; PARTNER 1 trial investigators. 5-year outcomes of transcatheter aortic valve replacement or surgical aortic valve replacement for high surgical risk patients with aortic stenosis (PARTNER 1): a randomised controlled trial. *Lancet* 2015; 385:2477–2484.

Marijon E, Mirabel M, Celermajer DS et al. Rheumatic heart disease. *Lancet* 2012; 379:953–964.

INFECTIVE ENDOCARDITIS

Infective endocarditis is an endovascular infection of cardiovascular structures, including cardiac valves, atrial and ventricular endocardium, large intrathoracic vessels and intracardiac foreign bodies, such as prosthetic valves, pacemaker leads and surgical conduits. The annual incidence in the UK is 6–7/100 000, but it is more common in developing countries. Without treatment, the mortality approaches 100%; even with treatment, there is a significant morbidity and mortality.

Aetiology

Endocarditis is usually the consequence of two factors: the presence of organisms in the bloodstream, and abnormal cardiac endothelium that facilitates their adherence and growth.

Bacteraemia may arise for patient-specific reasons (poor dental hygiene, intravenous drug use, soft tissue infections) or may be associated with diagnostic or therapeutic procedures (dental treatment, intravascular cannulae, cardiac surgery or permanent pacemakers). Although bacteraemia may occur, there is no good evidence that it leads to infective endocarditis (see pp. 236–237).

Damaged endocardium promotes platelet and fibrin deposition, which allows organisms to adhere and grow, leading to an infected vegetation. Valvular lesions may create non-laminar flow, and jet lesions from septal defects or a patent ductus arteriosus result in abnormal vascular endothelium. Aortic and mitral valves are most commonly involved in infective endocarditis; intravenous drug users are the exception, as right-sided lesions are more common in them.

Organisms

Common organisms and the sources of infection are shown in ***Figure 23.87***.

Rare causes

These include the HACEK group of organisms, which tend to run a more insidious course ***(Box 23.45)***.

Culture-negative endocarditis

This accounts for 5–10% of endocarditis cases. The usual cause is prior antibiotic therapy (good history-taking is vital) but some cases are due to a variety of fastidious organisms that fail to grow in normal blood cultures. These include *Coxiella burnetii* (the cause of Q fever), *Chlamydia* species, *Bartonella* species (organisms that cause trench fever and cat scratch disease) and *Legionella*.

Clinical features

The clinical presentation of infective endocarditis ***(Box 23.46)*** is dependent on the organism and the presence of predisposing cardiac conditions. Infective endocarditis may occur as an acute, fulminating infection but also as a chronic or subacute illness with low-grade fever and non-specific symptoms. A high index of clinical suspicion is required to identify patients with infective endocarditis and certain criteria should alert the physician.

High clinical suspicion

- New valve lesion/(regurgitant) murmur.
- Embolic event(s) of unknown origin.
- Sepsis of unknown origin.
- Haematuria, glomerulonephritis and suspected renal infarction.
- 'Fever' plus:
  - Prosthetic material inside the heart
  - Other high predisposition for infective endocarditis, e.g. intravenous drug use
  - Newly developed ventricular arrhythmias or conduction disturbances
  - First manifestation of congestive cardiac failure
  - Positive blood cultures (with typical organism)
  - Cutaneous (Osler, Janeway) or ophthalmic (Roth) lesions ***(Fig. 23.88)***
  - Peripheral abscesses (renal, splenic, spine) of unknown origin
  - Predisposition and recent diagnostic/therapeutic interventions known to result in significant bacteraemia.

Low clinical suspicion

- Fever plus none of the above.

Diagnosis

The criteria for the clinical diagnosis of endocarditis have been established – the modified Duke criteria (see ***Box 23.45***).

Investigations

Investigations are required to confirm the diagnosis of infective endocarditis, to identify the organism in order to ensure appropriate

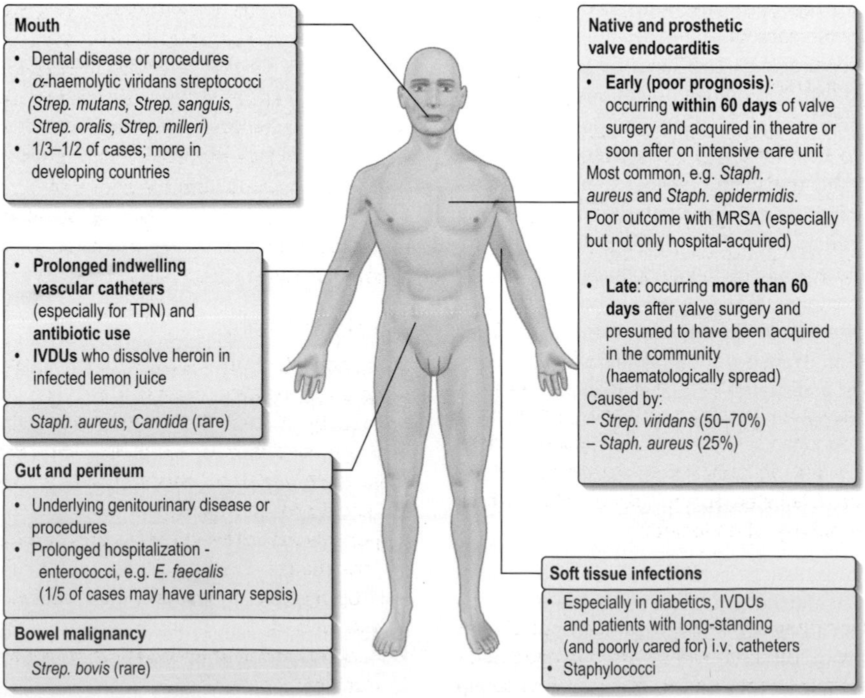

Figure 23.87 Infective endocarditis: aetiology and sources of infection. IVDU, intravenous drug user; MRSA, meticillin-resistant *Staphylococcus aureus*; TPN, total parenteral nutrition.

Box 23.45 Modified Duke criteria for endocarditis[a]

Major criteria

- A positive blood culture for infective endocarditis, as defined by the recovery of a typical microorganism from two separate blood cultures in the absence of a primary focus (viridans streptococci, *Abiotrophia* species and *Granulicatella* species; *Streptococcus bovis*, HACEK group[b], or community-acquired *Staphylococcus aureus* or enterococcus species) *or*
- A persistently positive blood culture, defined as the recovery of a microorganism consistent with endocarditis from either blood samples obtained more than 12 h apart or all three or a majority of four or more separate blood samples, with the first and last obtained at least 1 h apart *or*
- A positive serological test for Q fever, with an immunofluorescence assay showing phase 1 IgG antibodies at a titre >1 : 800 *or*
- Echocardiographic evidence of endocardial involvement:
  - an oscillating intracardiac mass on the valve or supporting structures, in the path or regurgitant jets, or on implanted material in the absence of an alternative anatomical explanation; *or*
  - an abscess; *or*
- New partial dehiscence of a prosthetic valve; *or*
- New valvular regurgitation.

Minor criteria

- Predisposition: predisposing heart condition or intravenous drug use
- Fever: temperature ≥38°C (100.4°F)
- Vascular phenomena: major arterial emboli, septic pulmonary infarcts, mycotic aneurysm, intracranial haemorrhage, conjunctival haemorrhages, Janeway lesion
- Immunological phenomena: glomerulonephritis, Osler nodes, Roth spots, rheumatoid factor
- Microbiological evidence: a positive blood culture but not meeting a major criterion as noted above, or serological evidence of an active infection with an organism that can cause infective endocarditis[c]
- Echocardiogram: findings consistent with infective endocarditis but not meeting a major criterion as noted above.

[a]*The diagnosis of infective endocarditis is definite when: (1) a microorganism is demonstrated by culture of a specimen from a vegetation, an embolism or an intracardiac abscess; (2) active endocarditis is confirmed by histological examination of the vegetation or intracardiac abscess; (3) two major clinical criteria, one major and three minor criteria, or five minor criteria are met.*
[b]*HACEK denotes* Haemophilus *species,* Actinobacillus actinomycetemcomitans, Cardiobacterium hominis, Eikenella corrodens *and* Kingella kingae.
[c]*Excluded from this criterion is a single positive blood culture for coagulase-negative staphylococci or other organisms that do not cause endocarditis. Serological tests for organisms that cause endocarditis include tests for* Brucella, Coxiella burnetii, Chlamydia, Legionella *and* Bartonella *species.*
(After Raoult D, Abbara S, Jassal DS et al. Case records of the Massachusetts General Hospital. Case 5–2007. A 53-year-old man with a prosthetic aortic valve and recent onset of fatigue, dyspnea, weight loss, and sweats. New Engl J Med *2007; 356:715. ©2007 Massachusetts Medical Society. All rights reserved.)*

Box 23.46 Clinical features of infective endocarditis

Clinical feature	Approximate %
General	
Malaise	95
Clubbing	10
Cardiac	
Murmurs	90
Cardiac failure	50
Arthralgia	25
Pyrexia	90
Skin lesions	
Osler nodes	15
Splinter haemorrhages	10
Janeway lesions	5
Petechiae	50
Eyes	
Roth spots	5
Conjunctival splinter haemorrhages	Rare
Splenomegaly	40
Neurological	
Cerebral emboli	20
Mycotic aneurysm	10
Renal	
Haematuria	70

therapy, and to monitor the patient's response to therapy ***(Box 23.47)***. Echocardiography is an extremely useful tool if used appropriately. A negative echocardiogram does not exclude a diagnosis of endocarditis. It is not an appropriate screening test for patients with just a fever or an isolated positive blood culture, where there is a low pre-test probability of endocarditis.

Management

The location of the infection means that prolonged courses of antibiotics are usually required in the treatment of infective endocarditis. The combination of antibiotics may be synergistic in eradicating microbial infection and minimizing resistance. Blood cultures should be taken prior to empirical antibiotic therapy (but this should not delay therapy in unstable patients). Antibiotic treatment should continue for 4–6 weeks. Typical therapeutic regimens are shown in ***Box 23.48*** but advice on specific therapy should be sought from the local microbiology department, according to the organism identified and current sensitivities. Serum levels of gentamicin and vancomycin need to be monitored to ensure adequate therapy and prevent toxicity. In patients with penicillin allergy, one of the glycopeptide antibiotics, vancomycin or teicoplanin, can be used. Penicillins, however, are fundamental to the therapy of bacterial endocarditis; allergies therefore seriously compromise the choice of antibiotics. It is essential to confirm the nature of a patient's allergy to ensure that the appropriate treatment is not withheld needlessly. Anaphylaxis would be much more influential on antibiotic choice than a simple gastrointestinal disturbance.

Persistent fever

Most patients with infective endocarditis should respond within 48 hours of initiation of appropriate antibiotic therapy. This is evidenced by a resolution of fever, reduction in serum markers of infection, and relief of systemic symptoms of infection. Failure of these factors to occur needs to be taken very seriously. The following should be considered:

- perivalvular extension of infection and possible abscess formation
- drug reaction (the fever should resolve promptly after drug withdrawal)
- hospital-acquired infection (i.e. venous access site, urinary tract infection)
- pulmonary embolism (secondary right-sided endocarditis or prolonged hospitalization).

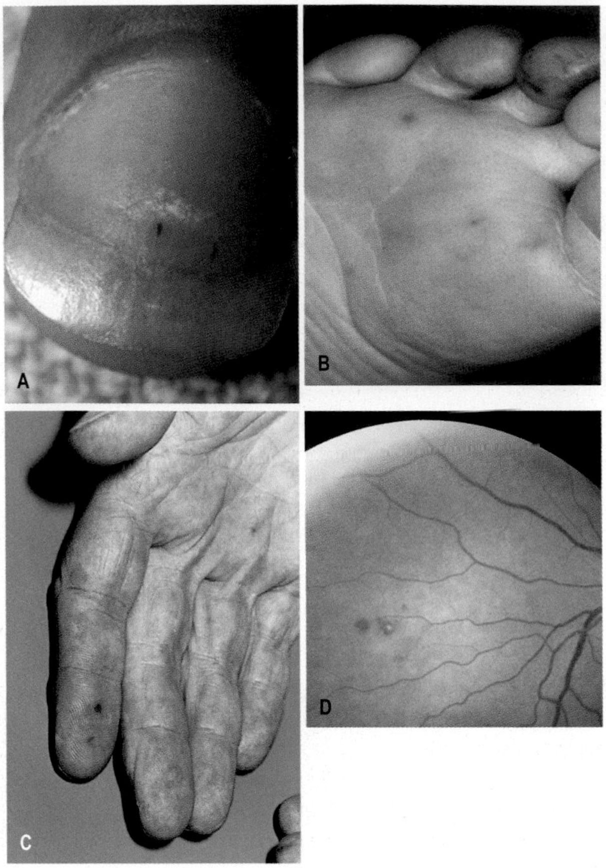

Figure 23.88 **Infective endocarditis. A.** Splinter haemorrhages. **B.** Janeway lesions. **C.** Osler nodes. **D.** Roth spots. *(A, B From Moser DK, Riegel B.* Cardiac Nursing. *Philadelphia: Saunders; 2007, p. 1127, with permission from Elsevier. C. From Forbes CD, Jackson WF.* Color Atlas and Text of Clinical Medicine, *3rd edn. St Louis: Mosby; 2003, p. 232; ©Elsevier. D. Courtesy of Professor Ian Constable.)*

In such cases, samples for culture should be taken from all possible sites and evidence sought of the above causes. A change of antibiotic dosage or regimen should be avoided unless there are positive cultures or a drug reaction is suspected. Emergence of bacterial resistance is uncommon. Close liaison with the microbiology department is recommended and a cardiothoracic surgical opinion should be sought.

Surgery

Decisions about surgical intervention in patients with infective endocarditis should be made after joint consultation between the cardiologist and cardiothoracic surgeon, taking into account patient-specific features (age, non-cardiac morbidities, presence of prosthetic material or cardiac failure) and infective endocarditis features (infective organism, vegetation size, presence of perivalvular infection, systemic embolization).

Prevention

Evidence suggested that antibiotic prophylactic therapy is not required (see pp. 236–237) but a recent study has disputed this. Another study shows no increase in the number of new cases following implementation of the NICE guidelines.

Box 23.47 Investigations and findings in endocarditis

Investigation	Findings and notes
Blood cultures	Three sets from different venepuncture sites
Serological tests	Consider in culture-negative cases for *Coxiella*, *Bartonella*, *Legionella*, *Chlamydia*
Full blood count	Reduced haemoglobin, increased white cells, increased or reduced platelets
Urea and electrolytes	Increased urea and creatinine
Liver biochemistry	Increased serum alkaline phosphatase
Inflammatory markers	Increased erythrocyte sedimentation rate and C-reactive protein (CRP reduces in response to therapy and increases with relapse)
Urine	Proteinuria and haematuria
Electrocardiogram	PR prolongation/heart block is associated with aortic root abscess
Chest X-ray	Pulmonary oedema in left-sided disease, pulmonary emboli/abscess in right-sided disease
Transthoracic echocardiography	First-line non-invasive imaging test with sensitivity of 60–75%; demonstrates vegetations, valvular dysfunction, ventricular function, abscesses
Transoesophageal echocardiography	Second-line invasive imaging test with greater sensitivity (>90%) and specificity; useful in suspected aortic root abscess and essential in prosthetic valve endocarditis

Box 23.48 Antibiotics in endocarditis (adapted from British Society for Antimicrobial Chemotherapy (BSAC) guidelines)

Clinical situation	Suggested antibiotic regimen to start
Clinical endocarditis, culture results awaited, no suspicion of staphylococci	Penicillin 1.2 g 4-hourly, gentamicin 80 mg 12-hourly
Suspected staphylococcal endocarditis (IVDU, recent intravascular devices or cardiac surgery, acute infection)	Vancomycin 1 g 12-hourly, gentamicin 80–120 mg 8-hourly
Streptococcal endocarditis (penicillin-sensitive)	Penicillin 1.2 g 4-hourly, gentamicin 80 mg 12-hourly
Enterococcal endocarditis (no high-level gentamicin resistance)	Ampicillin/amoxicillin 2 g 4-hourly, gentamicin 80 mg 12-hourly
Staphylococcal endocarditis[a]	Vancomycin 1 g 12-hourly, *or*
	Flucloxacillin 2 g 4-hourly, *or*
	Benzylpenicillin 1.2 g 4-hourly
	plus gentamicin 80–120 mg 8-hourly

Notes: (1) Monitor vancomycin and gentamicin levels, and adjust if necessary. (2) Choice of antibiotic for staphylococci depends on sensitivities. (3) Optimum choice of therapy needs close liaison with microbiology/infectious diseases departments. All antibiotics given i.v. IVDU, intravenous drug user. [a]MRSA can affect valves.

Further reading

Duval Z, Hoen B. Prophylaxis for infective endocarditis: let's end the debate. *Lancet* 2015; 385:1164–1165.
Habib G, Hown B, Tornos P et al. Guidelines on the prevention, diagnosis, and treatment of infective endocarditis (new version 2009): the Task Force on the Prevention, Diagnosis, and Treatment of Infective Endocarditis of the European Society of Cardiology (ESC). Endorsed by the European Society of Clinical Microbiology and Infectious Diseases (ESCMID) and the International Society of Chemotherapy (ISC) for Infection and Cancer. *Eur Heart J* 2009; 30:2369–2413.
Hoen B, Duval X. Infective endocarditis. *N Engl J Med* 2013; 368:1425–1433.
Thornhill MH. Impact of the NICE guidelines recommending cessation of antibiotic prophylaxis for prevention of infective endocarditis: before and after study. *BMJ* 2011; 342:2392.
Thuny F, Grisoli D, Collart F et al. Management of infective endocarditis. *Lancet* 2012; 379:965–975.
Werdan K, Dietz S, Löffler B et al. Mechanisms of infective endocarditis: pathogen–host interaction and risk states. *Nat Rev Cardiol* 2014; 11:35–50.

CONGENITAL HEART DISEASE

A congenital cardiac malformation occurs in about 1% of live births. There is an overall male predominance, although some individual lesions (e.g. atrial septal defect and persistent ductus arteriosus) occur more commonly in females. As a result of improved medical and surgical management, more children with congenital cardiac disease are surviving into adolescence and adulthood. Thus, there is a need for an increased awareness, among general physicians and cardiologists, of the problems posed by these individuals.

Fetal circulation

In the developing fetus, oxygenated blood and nutrients are supplied to the fetus via the placenta and the umbilical vein ***(Fig. 23.89)***. Half of that blood is directed to the fetal ductus venosus and carried to the inferior vena cava (IVC); the other half enters the liver.

Blood moves from the IVC to the right atrium of the heart. In the fetus, there is an opening between the right and left atrium (the foramen ovale), and most of the blood (which is a mixture of oxygenated and deoxygenated blood) flows from the right into the left atrium, bypassing the pulmonary circulation. This blood goes into the left ventricle and is pumped through the aorta into the fetal body. Some of the blood flows from the aorta through the internal iliac arteries to the umbilical arteries and re-enters the placenta, where carbon dioxide and other waste products from the fetus are taken up and enter the woman's circulation.

Some of the blood from the right atrium does not enter the left atrium, but enters the right ventricle and is pumped into the pulmonary artery. In the fetus, there is a connection between the pulmonary artery and the aorta, the ductus arteriosus, which directs most of this blood away from the lungs. With the first breath after delivery, the vascular resistance in the pulmonary arteries falls and more blood moves from the right atrium to right ventricle and pulmonary arteries, and oxygenated blood travels back to the left atrium through the pulmonary veins. The decrease in right atrial pressure and relative increase in left atrial pressure results in closure of the foramen ovale.

The ductus arteriosus usually closes off within 1 or 2 days of birth, completely separating the left and right systems. The umbilical vein and the ductus venosus closes off within 2–5 days of birth, leaving behind the ligamentum teres and the ligamentum venosus of the liver, respectively.

Aetiology

The aetiology of congenital cardiac disease is often unknown but recognized associations include:

- maternal prenatal rubella infection (persistent ductus arteriosus, and pulmonary valvular and arterial stenosis)
- maternal alcohol misuse (septal defects)

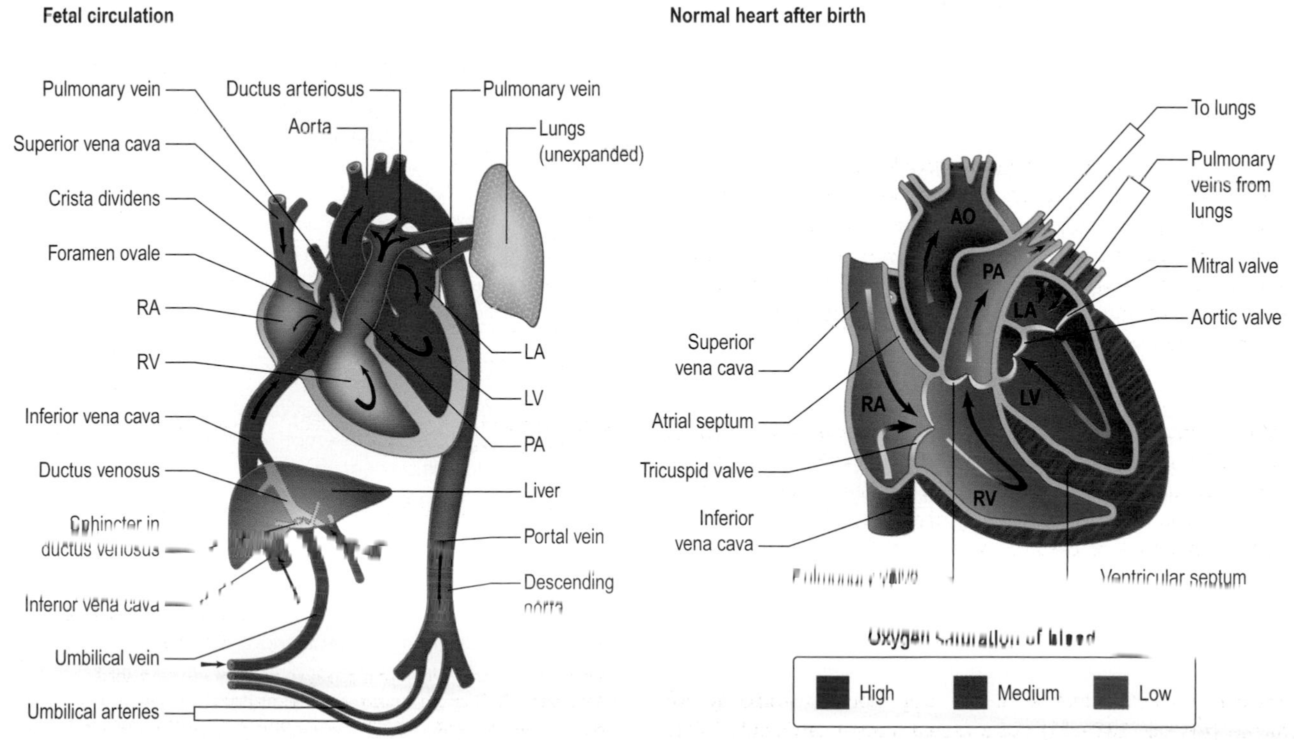

Figure 23.89 **Anatomy showing the circulation.** AO, aorta; LA, left atrium; LV, left ventricle; PA, pulmonary artery; RA, right atrium; RV, right ventricle.

Box 23.49 Classification of congenital heart disease

Acyanotic	Cyanotic
With shunts	**With shunts**
Atrial septal defect Ventricular septal defect Patent ductus arteriosus Partial anomalous venous drainage	Fallot's tetralogy Transposition of the great vessels Severe Ebstein's anomaly
Without shunts	**Without shunts**
Coarctation of the aorta Congenital aortic stenosis	Severe pulmonary stenosis Tricuspid atresia Pulmonary atresia Hypoplastic left heart

- maternal drug treatment and radiation
- genetic abnormalities (e.g. the familial form of atrial septal defect and congenital heart block)
- chromosomal abnormalities (e.g. septal defects and mitral and tricuspid valve defects, which are associated with Down syndrome (trisomy 21), or coarctation of the aorta in Turner syndrome (45, XO).

Classification

See ***Box 23.49***.

Clinical features

Symptoms and signs

Congenital heart disease should be recognized as early as possible, as the response is usually better the earlier the treatment is initiated. Some symptoms, signs and clinical problems are common in congenital heart disease:

- ***Central cyanosis*** occurs because of right-to-left shunting of blood or because of complete mixing of systemic and pulmonary blood flow. In the latter case, such as in Fallot's tetralogy, the abnormality is described as cyanotic congenital heart disease.
- ***Pulmonary hypertension*** results from large left-to-right shunts. The persistently raised pulmonary flow leads to the development of increased pulmonary artery vascular resistance and consequent pulmonary hypertension. This is known as Eisenmenger's reaction (or Eisenmenger's complex when due specifically to a ventricular septal defect). The development of pulmonary hypertension significantly worsens the prognosis.
- ***Clubbing of the fingers*** occurs in congenital cardiac conditions associated with prolonged cyanosis.
- ***Paradoxical embolism*** of thrombus from the systemic veins to the systemic arterial system may occur when a communication exists between the right and left heart. There is therefore an increased risk of cerebrovascular emboli and also abscesses (as with endocarditis).
- ***Polycythaemia*** can develop secondary to chronic hypoxaemia, leading to a hyperviscosity syndrome and an increased thrombotic risk, such as in strokes.
- ***Growth retardation*** is common in children with cyanotic heart disease.
- ***Syncope*** is common when severe right or left ventricular outflow tract obstruction is present. Exertional syncope, associated with deepening central cyanosis, may occur in Fallot's tetralogy. Exercise increases resistance to pulmonary blood flow but reduces systemic vascular resistance. Thus, the right-to-left shunt increases and cerebral oxygenation falls.
- ***Squatting*** is the posture adopted by children with Fallot's tetralogy. It results in obstruction of venous return of desaturated blood and an increase in the peripheral systemic vascular resistance. This leads to a reduced right-to-left shunt and improved cerebral oxygenation.

Box 23.50 Common congenital lesions

	Percentage of congenital lesions	Occurrence in first-degree relatives (%)
Ventricular septal defect	39	4
Atrial septal defect	10	2
Persistent ductus arteriosus	10	4
Pulmonary stenosis	7	
Coarctation of the aorta	7	2
Aortic stenosis	6	4
Fallot's tetralogy	6	4
Others	15	

Presentation

Adolescents and adults with congenital heart disease present with specific common problems related to the longstanding structural nature of these conditions and any surgical treatment:

- endocarditis (particularly in association with otherwise innocuous lesions, such as a small ventricular septal defect or a bicuspid aortic valve that can give up to 10% lifetime risk)
- progression of valvular lesions (calcification and stenosis of congenitally deformed valves, e.g. bicuspid aortic valve)
- atrial and ventricular arrhythmias (often quite resistant to treatment)
- sudden cardiac death
- right heart failure (especially when surgical palliation results in the right ventricle providing the systemic supply)
- end-stage heart failure (rarely managed by heart or heart–lung transplantation).

Genetic counselling

These conditions necessitate active follow-up of adult patients. Pregnancy is normally safe, except when pulmonary hypertension or vascular disease is present, in which case the prognosis for both mother and fetus is poor.

Box 23.50 lists the most common congenital lesions and their occurrence in first-degree relatives.

Genetic factors should be considered in all patients presenting with congenital heart disease. For example, parents with a child suffering from Fallot's tetralogy stand a 4% chance of conceiving another child with the disease, and so fetal ultrasound screening of the mother during pregnancy is essential. Parents with congenital heart disease are also more likely to have affected offspring. Fathers have a 2% risk, while mothers have a higher risk (around 5%). Individual families can exhibit even higher risks of recurrence.

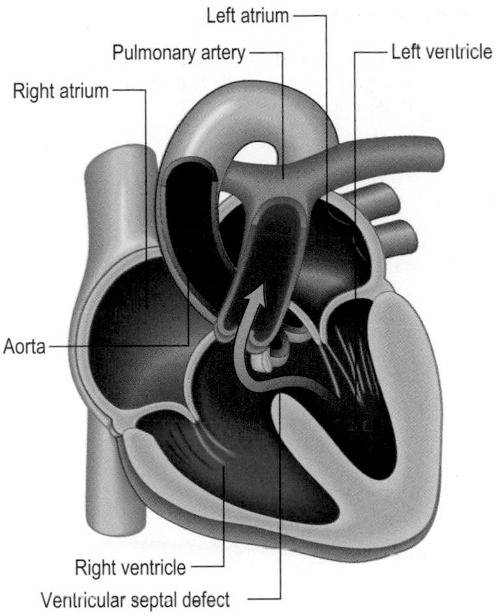

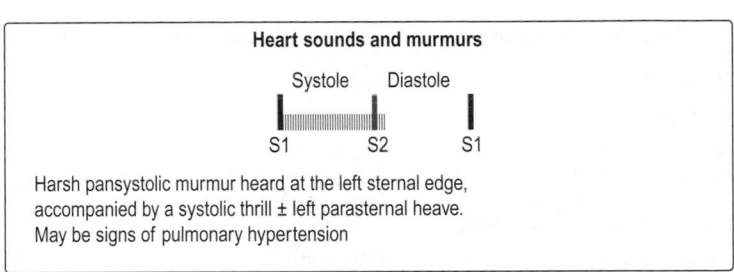

Heart sounds and murmurs

Systole Diastole

S1 S2 S1

Harsh pansystolic murmur heard at the left sternal edge, accompanied by a systolic thrill ± left parasternal heave. May be signs of pulmonary hypertension

Pathophysiology

- Left-to-right shunt
- When the left ventricle contracts, it ejects some blood into the aorta and some across the ventricular septal defect into the right ventricle and pulmonary artery
- **Small** VSDs ('maladie de Roger'): loud and sometimes long systolic murmur
- **Moderate** VSDs: loud 'tearing' pansystolic murmur
- **Large** VSDs: cause pulmonary hypertension and soft murmur Eisenmenger's complex may result

Figure 23.90 Ventricular septal defect (VSD). Pathophysiology and auscultatory findings.

Ventricular septal defect

Ventricular septal defect (VSD; ***Fig. 23.90***) is the most common congenital cardiac malformation (1:500 live births). The haemodynamic consequences are dependent on the shunt size. Left ventricular pressure is higher than right; blood therefore moves from left to right and pulmonary blood flow increases. In large defects, the large volumes of blood flow through the pulmonary vasculature leads to pulmonary hypertension and eventual Eisenmenger's complex, when right ventricular pressure becomes higher than left; as a result, blood starts to shunt from right to left, causing cyanosis.

- ***Small restrictive VSDs*** ('maladie de Roger') are often found incidentally, as patients are asymptomatic. They are associated with a loud pansystolic murmur. The majority close spontaneously by the age of 10 years.
- ***Large (non-restrictive) VSDs*** result in significant left atrial and left ventricular dilatation (due to left ventricular volume overload). Large defects usually present with heart failure symptoms in childhood and eventually lead to pulmonary hypertension and Eisenmenger's complex. As pressures equalize, the murmur becomes softer.

Investigations and treatment

A small VSD produces no abnormal X-ray or ECG findings. In larger defects, the chest X-ray may demonstrate prominent pulmonary arteries owing to increased pulmonary blood flow, but with pulmonary hypertension there may be 'pruned' pulmonary arteries. Cardiomegaly occurs when a moderate or large VSD is present and the ECG may show both left and right ventricular hypertrophy. Echocardiography can assess the size and location of the VSD and its haemodynamic consequences. Interventional options are either surgical patch repair or device closure, if it is an isolated muscular VSD. Indications for intervention include left atrial and ventricular enlargement, with or without early left ventricular dysfunction; reversible pulmonary hypertension (mild) where there is a residual left-to-right shunt and no significant desaturation with exercise; and infective endocarditis. Patients with a restrictive VSD and those who have had a successful closure have an excellent long-term outcome. Prophylaxis of endocarditis is discussed on pages 236–237.

Atrial septal defect

Atrial septal defect (ASD) is often first diagnosed in adulthood and represents one-third of congenital heart disease. It is 2–3 times more common in women than in men. There are three main types of ASD ***(Fig. 23.91)***:

- ***Sinus venosus defects*** – located in the superior part of the septum near the superior vena cava (superior sinus venosus defect), or the inferior part of the septum near the IVC (inferior sinus venosus defect) entry point.
- ***Ostium secundum defects*** (75%) – located in the mid-septum (fossa ovalis). This should not be confused with a patent foramen ovale (PFO), which is a normal variant and not a true septal defect. PFO is usually asymptomatic but is associated with paradoxical emboli and an increased incidence of embolic stroke.
- ***Ostium primum (atrioventricular septal) defects*** (15%) – located in the lower part of atrial septum.

Adult patients with an unrepaired ASD with a significant left-to-right shunt develop right heart overload and dilatation. These patients develop symptoms of dyspnoea and exercise intolerance, and may develop atrial arrhythmias from right atrial dilatation. There is also increased pulmonary vascular flow, but significant pulmonary hypertension develops in <5% of patients and it is thought that these individuals have additional factors, including genetic predisposition to pulmonary hypertension. The physical signs of ASD reflect the volume overloading of the right ventricle ***(Fig. 23.91)***. A right ventricular heave can usually be felt.

Investigations and treatment

The chest X-ray may demonstrate prominent pulmonary arteries with pulmonary plethora. Right bundle branch block and right axis deviation may be present on the ECG (because of dilatation of the right ventricle). Ostium primum defects may have left axis deviation on the ECG. Echocardiography may demonstrate hypertrophy and dilatation of the right heart and pulmonary arteries. Subcostal views with two-dimensional and colour Doppler demonstrate the ASD ***(Fig. 23.92)*** and allow calculation of the left-to-right shunt (QP:QS ratio). CMR and CT are helpful for assessing anomalous pulmonary

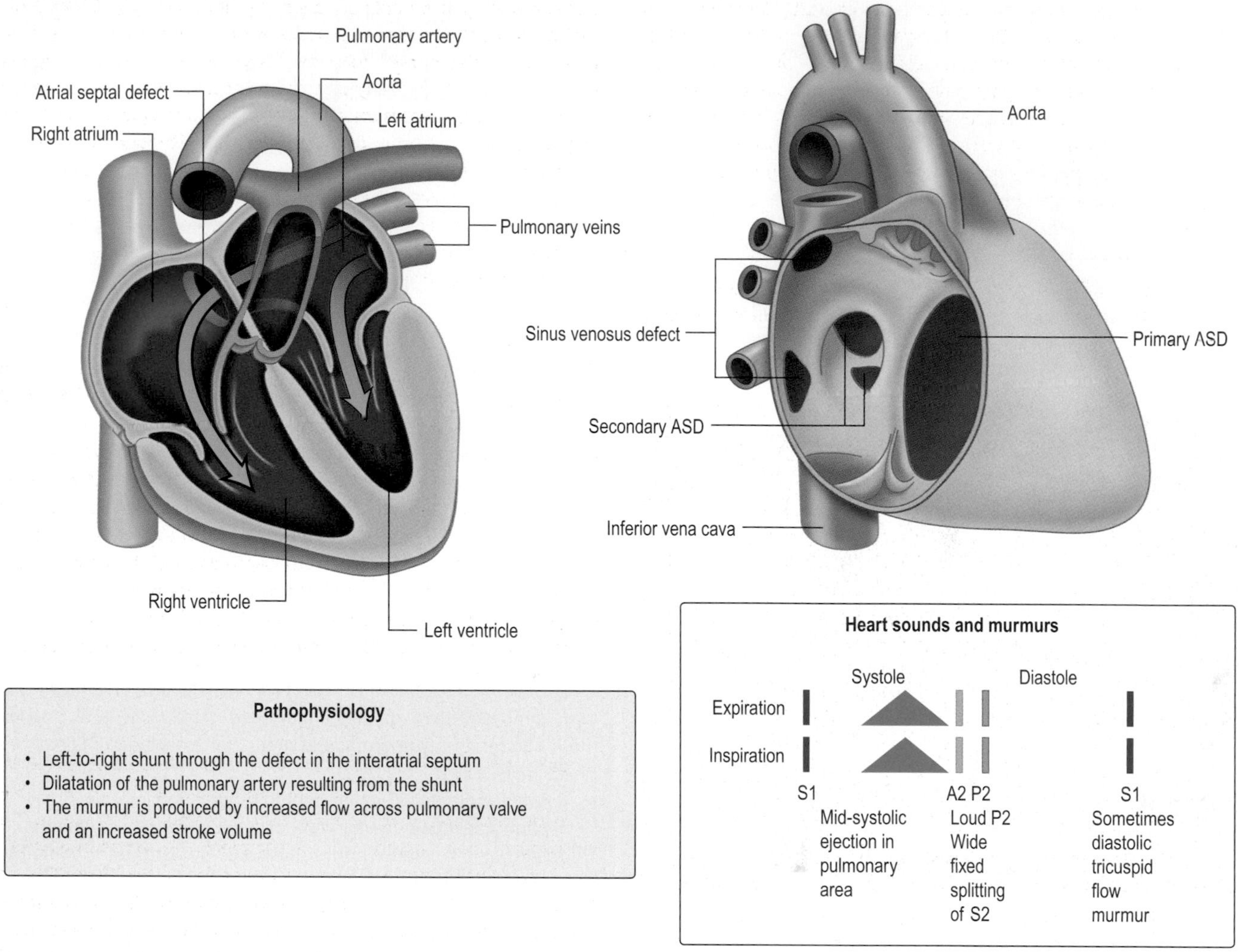

Figure 23.91 **Atrial septal defect (ASD).** Pathophysiology and auscultatory findings.

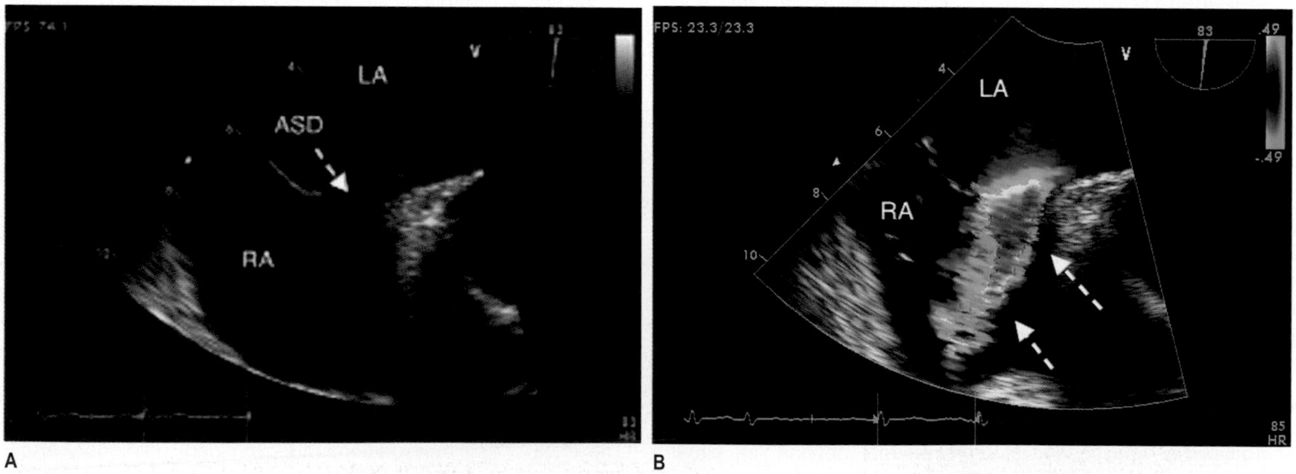

Figure 23.92 **Ostium secundum atrial septal defect (arrowed) in a young girl. A.** The defect is shown by a two-dimensional echocardiogram subcostal four-chamber view. **B.** Colour Doppler can demonstrate the left-to-right shunt. LA, left atrium; RA, right atrium.

venous drainage, which may accompany an ASD. Indications for intervention include: an ASD with significant left-to-right shunting, resulting in right atrial/ventricular enlargement, which should be closed irrespective of symptoms; and thromboembolic events, including a patent foramen ovale in certain patients. The options for intervention include device closure using a transcatheter clamshell device ***(Fig. 23.93)*** for most secundum ASDs (if they are of a suitable size), and surgical closure for all other ASD types.

Patent ductus arteriosus

A patent ductus arteriosus (PDA) is a persistent communication between the proximal left pulmonary artery and the descending aorta, resulting in a continuous left-to-right shunt ***(Fig. 23.94)***. Normally, the ductus arteriosus closes within a few hours of birth in response to decreased pulmonary resistance; however, in some cases (particularly in premature babies and in cases with maternal rubella), the ductus persists. Indometacin (a prostaglandin inhibitor) is given to stimulate duct closure. If the shunt is moderate to large, it will result in left heart volume overload and, in some cases, pulmonary hypertension and Eisenmenger syndrome. The characteristic clinical signs are a bounding pulse and continuous 'machinery murmur'; however, as pulmonary hypertension develops in a large PDA, the murmur becomes softer.

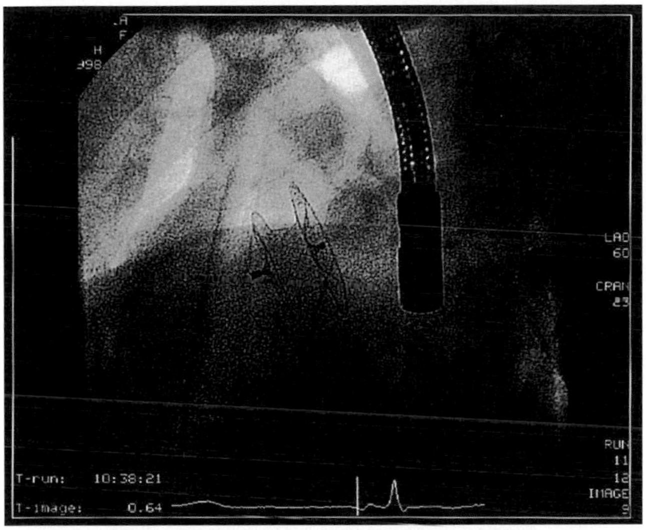

Figure 23.93 Angiographic appearance of a fully deployed atrial septal defect (ASD) closure device. The device bridges the ASD and wedges against the surfaces of the right and left atrial septa, occluding flow. The metal object in frame is the distal end of a transoesophageal echocardiography probe. *(Courtesy of Dr D Ward, St George's, University of London.)*

Investigations and treatment

With a large shunt, the aorta and pulmonary arterial system may be prominent on chest X-ray. The ECG may demonstrate left atrial abnormality and left ventricular hypertrophy. The development of an Eisenmenger reaction will produce right ventricular hypertrophy. Echocardiography may show a dilated left atrium and left ventricle, with right heart changes occurring late. Colour Doppler imaging of the proximal pulmonary arteries may demonstrate the shunt. Indications for intervention (usually with percutaneous devices) include left ventricular dilatation, and mild to moderate pulmonary arterial hypertension (not Eisenmenger's). Small defects may predispose to endarteritis and should be considered for device closure unless clinically silent.

Coarctation of the aorta

A coarctation of the aorta is a narrowing of the aorta at, or just distal to, the insertion of the ductus arteriosus (distal to the origin of the left subclavian artery; ***Fig. 23.95***). Rarely, it can occur proximal to the left subclavian. It occurs twice as commonly in men as in women. It is also associated with Turner syndrome (see p. 1220). In 80% of cases, the aortic valve is bicuspid (and potentially stenotic or endocarditic). Other associations include patent ductus arteriosus, ventricular septal defect, mitral stenosis or regurgitation, and circle of Willis aneurysms. Severe narrowing of the aorta encourages the formation of a collateral arterial circulation involving the periscapular and intercostal arteries. Decreased renal perfusion can lead to

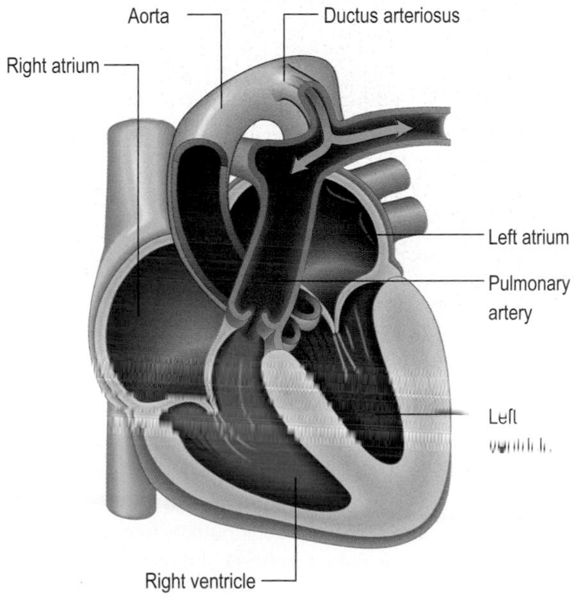

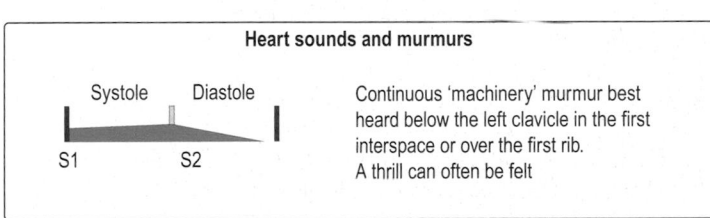

Heart sounds and murmurs

Systole Diastole
S1 S2

Continuous 'machinery' murmur best heard below the left clavicle in the first interspace or over the first rib.
A thrill can often be felt

Pathophysiology

- Left-to-right shunt
- Some of the blood from the aorta crosses the ductus arteriosus and flows into the pulmonary artery
- Murmur is produced by the turbulent aortic-to-pulmonary artery shunting in both systole and diastole
- Dilatation of the pulmonary artery, left atrium and left ventricle
- As pulmonary hypertension (Eisenmenger's reaction) develops, the murmur becomes quieter, may be confined to systole or may even disappear causing central cyanosis

Figure 23.94 Patent ductus arteriosus. Pathophysiology and auscultatory findings.

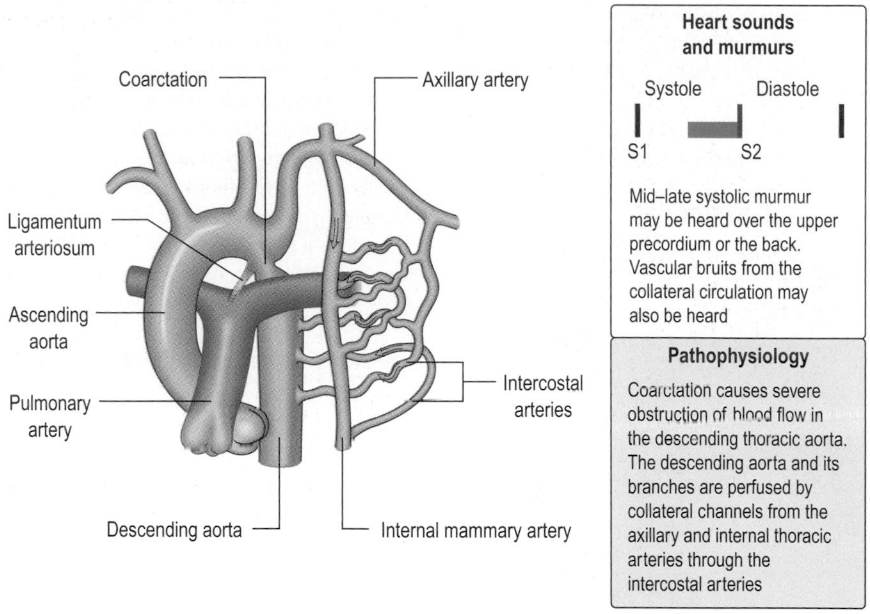
Coarctation
Axillary artery
Ligamentum arteriosum
Ascending aorta
Pulmonary artery
Intercostal arteries
Descending aorta
Internal mammary artery
Heart sounds and murmurs
Systole
Diastole
S1
S2
Mid–late systolic murmur may be heard over the upper precordium or the back. Vascular bruits from the collateral circulation may also be heard
Pathophysiology
Coarctation causes severe obstruction of blood flow in the descending thoracic aorta. The descending aorta and its branches are perfused by collateral channels from the axillary and internal thoracic arteries through the intercostal arteries

Figure 23.95 Coarctation of the aorta. Pathophysiology and auscultatory findings.

the development of systemic hypertension that persists even after surgical correction.

Coarctation of the aorta is often asymptomatic for many years. ***Headaches*** and ***nose bleeds*** (due to hypertension), and ***claudication*** and cold legs (due to poor blood flow in the lower limbs) may be present. Physical examination reveals hypertension in the upper limbs, and weak, delayed (radiofemoral delay) pulses in the legs. If coarctation is present in the aorta, proximal to the left subclavian artery, there will be asynchronous radial pulses in right and left arms. Poor peripheral pulses are seen in severe cases. For heart sounds and murmurs in coarctation of aorta, see ***Figure 23.95***.

Investigations and treatment

Chest X-ray may reveal a dilated aorta indented at the site of the coarctation. This is manifested by an aorta (seen in the upper right mediastinum) shaped like a 'number 3'. In adults, tortuous and dilated collateral intercostal arteries may erode the under-surfaces of the ribs ('rib notching'). The ECG demonstrates left ventricular hypertrophy. Echocardiography sometimes shows the coarctation and other associated anomalies. CT and CMR ***(Fig. 23.96)*** scanning can accurately demonstrate the coarctation and quantify flow.

Intervention is required if there is a peak–peak gradient across the coarctation of >20 mmHg and/or proximal hypertension. In neonates, coarctation is treated with surgical repair. In older children and adults, balloon dilatation and stenting is an option, although many centres still prefer surgery. Balloon dilatation is preferred for re-coarctation.

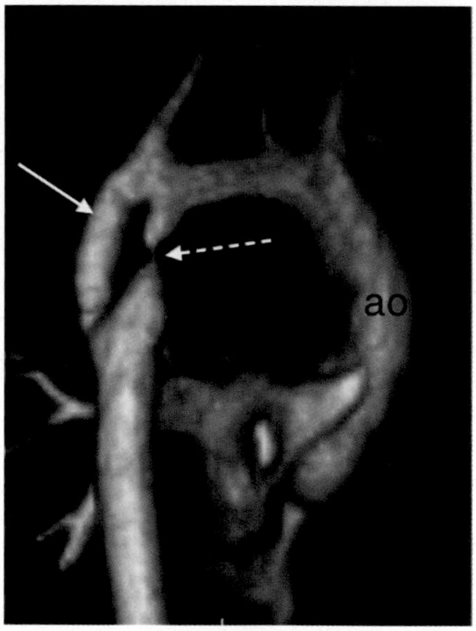

Figure 23.96 Severe aortic coarctation in an adult. The coarctation is shown on cardiac magnetic resonance angiography. The solid arrow indicates the jump bypass graft; the dotted arrow indicates severe aortic coarctation. ao, aorta.

Fallot's tetralogy

Tetralogy of Fallot ***(Fig. 23.97)*** consists of:

- a large, malaligned VSD
- an overriding aorta
- right ventricular outflow tract obstruction
- right ventricular hypertrophy.

Symptoms depend on the degree of pulmonary stenosis. Often, this is progressive in the first year of life and cyanosis develops due to increased right-sided pressures, resulting in a right-to-left shunt. Fallot's spells are episodes of severe cyanosis noted in children due to spasm of the subpulmonary muscle; these can be relieved by increasing systemic resistance using postural manœuvres, such as squatting. In babies with severe pulmonary stenosis, systemic-to-pulmonary artery shunts (i.e. a Blalock–Taussig, or subclavian-to-pulmonary artery shunt) may be used initially to increase pulmonary blood flow in severe cases of pulmonary stenosis. The majority of adults with tetralogy of Fallot will have undergone complete repair, which involves relief of the right ventricular outflow tract obstruction and closure of the VSD. The overall survival of those who have had operative repair is excellent. DiGeorge syndrome is found in 15% of those with tetralogy of Fallot.

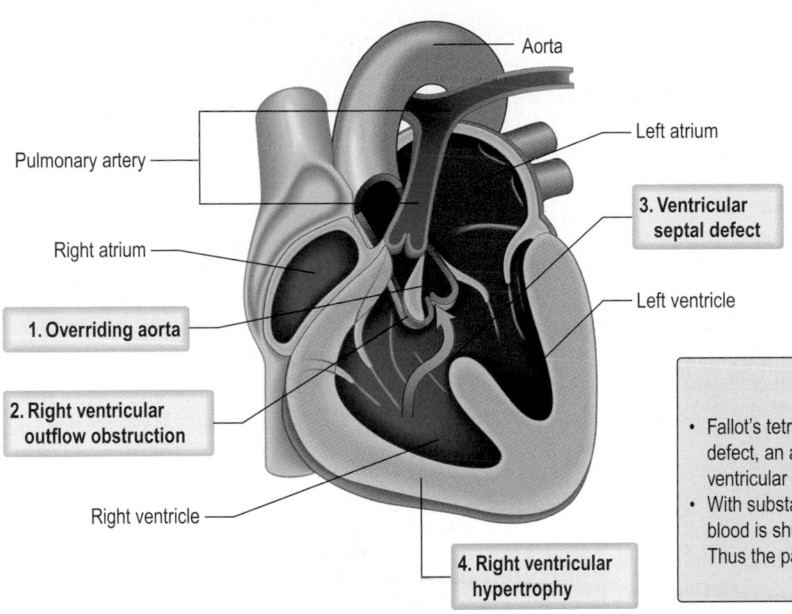

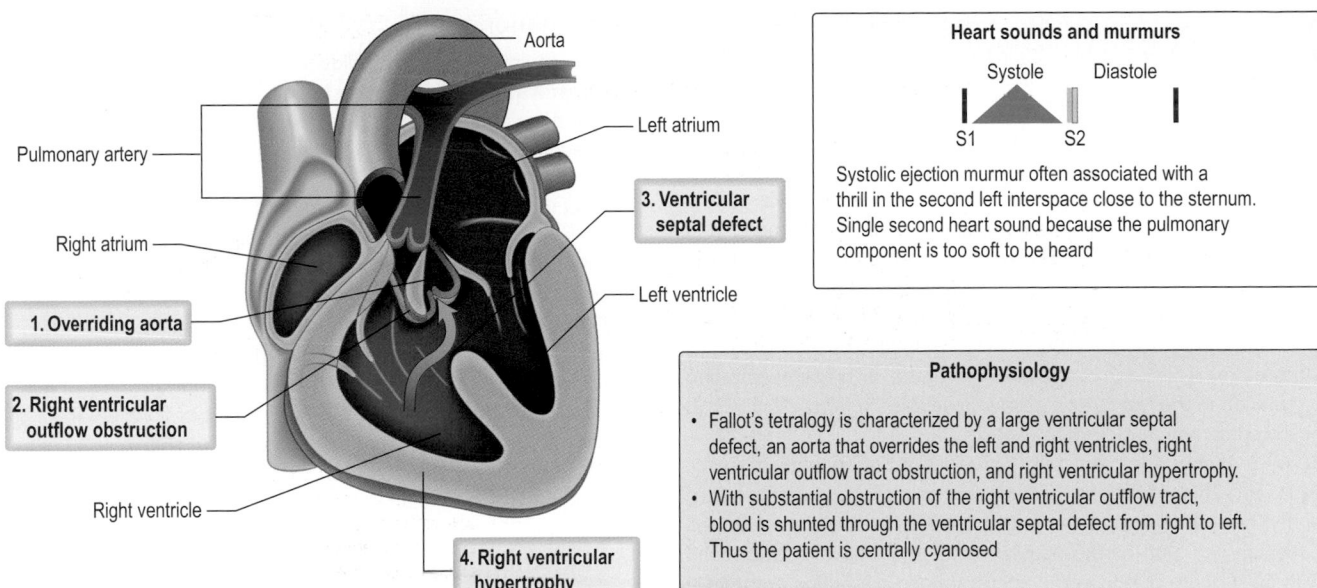

Heart sounds and murmurs

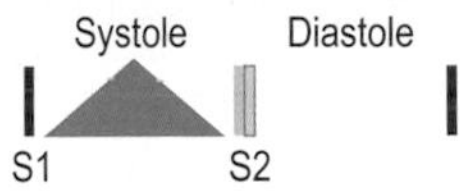

Systolic ejection murmur often associated with a thrill in the second left interspace close to the sternum. Single second heart sound because the pulmonary component is too soft to be heard

Pathophysiology

- Fallot's tetralogy is characterized by a large ventricular septal defect, an aorta that overrides the left and right ventricles, right ventricular outflow tract obstruction, and right ventricular hypertrophy.
- With substantial obstruction of the right ventricular outflow tract, blood is shunted through the ventricular septal defect from right to left. Thus the patient is centrally cyanosed

Figure 23.97 **Fallot's tetralogy.** Pathophysiology and auscultatory findings.

Transposition of the great arteries

Complete transposition of the great arteries

In complete transposition of the great arteries (TGA), the right atrium connects to the morphological right ventricle, which gives rise to the aorta, and the left atrium connects to the morphological left ventricle, which gives rise to the pulmonary artery ***(Fig. 23.98)***. This is incompatible with life, as blood circulates in two parallel circuits: that is, deoxygenated blood from the systemic veins passes into the right heart and then via the aorta back to the systemic circulation. Oxygenated blood from the pulmonary veins passes through the left heart and back to the lungs. Babies with transposition are usually born cyanosed; if there is a significant ASD, VSD or PDA allowing a shunt (i.e. mixing of oxygenated and deoxygenated blood), the diagnosis might be delayed. In those without a shunt, an atrial septostomy is performed. A Rashkind's balloon is deployed to dilate the foramen ovale and is used to maintain saturations at 50–80% until a definitive procedure can be performed. The arterial switch procedure is now performed in the first 2 weeks of life; the aorta is reconnected to the left ventricle and the pulmonary artery is connected to the right ventricle. The coronary arteries are re-implanted.

Currently, the majority of adult patients with transposition of the great arteries will have had an 'atrial switch' operation. The right ventricle remains the systemic ventricle in this situation. Although most of these patients do well for many years, life expectancy is clearly limited by eventual failure of the systemic right ventricle.

Congenitally corrected transposition of the great arteries

In congenitally corrected transposition of the great arteries (ccTGA), systemic venous return to the right atrium enters a morphological left ventricle, which pumps into the pulmonary artery. Pulmonary venous blood returns to the left atrium and then, via the morphological right ventricle, to the aorta. The circulation is physiologically corrected but the systemic circulation is supported by a morphological right ventricle. ccTGA is often associated with cardiac lesions; systemic (tricuspid) AV valve abnormalities with valve insufficiency; VSD; subpulmonary stenosis; complete heart block; Wolff–Parkinson–White syndrome; and dextrocardia. Many patients with ccTGA live a normal life, although others require pacemaker insertion (the AV node is abnormal, leading to heart block), or surgery for a regurgitant tricuspid valve, or they develop heart failure from the systemic (right) ventricle.

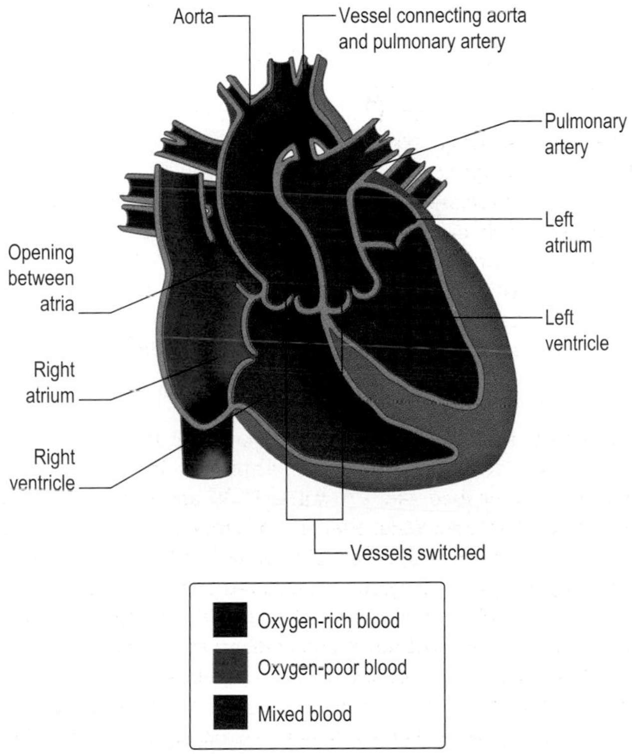

Figure 23.98 **Transposition of the great arteries.**

Further reading

Furlan AJ, Reisman M, Massaro J et al. Closure or medical therapy for cryptogenic stroke in patent foramen ovale. *N Engl J Med* 2012; 366:991–999.
Lindsey J, Hillis LD. Clinical update: atrial septal defects in adults. *Lancet* 2007; 369:1244–1246.

MARFAN SYNDROME

Clinical features

Marfan syndrome (MFS) is one of the most common autosomal dominant inherited disorders of connective tissue, affecting the heart and blood vessels (aortic aneurysm and dissection, mitral valve prolapse), eye (dislocated lenses, retinal detachment) and skeleton (tall, thin body build with long arms, legs and fingers; scoliosis and pectus deformity) (***Figs 23.99*** and ***23.100***).

Clinically, two of three major systems must be affected, to avoid over-diagnosing the condition. Diagnosis may be confirmed by studying family linkage to the causative gene, or by demonstrating a mutation in the Marfan syndrome gene (*MFS1*) for fibrillin (*FBN1*) on chromosome 15q21.

MFS affects approximately 1 in 5000 of the population worldwide, and 25% of patients are affected as a result of a new mutation. This group includes many of the more severely affected patients, with high cardiovascular risk. Other known associations with early death due to aortic aneurysm and dissection are: family history of early cardiac involvement; family history of dissection with an aortic root diameter of >5 cm; male sex; and extreme physical characteristics, including markedly excessive stature and widespread striae. Histological examination of aortas often shows widespread medial degeneration, described as 'cystic medial necrosis'.

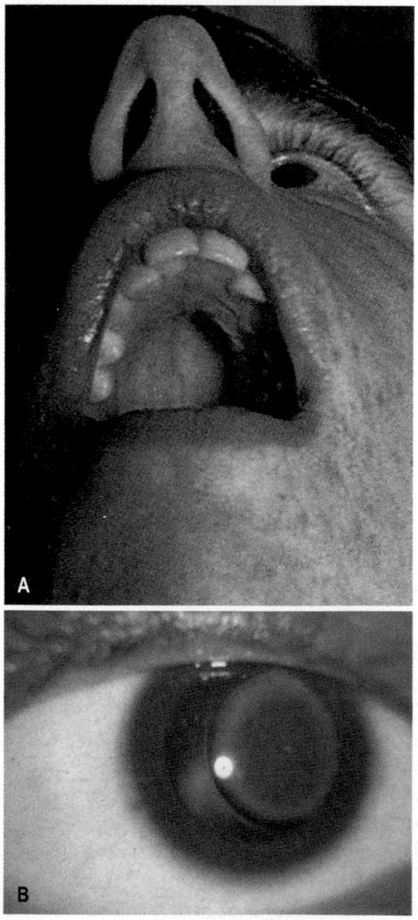

Figure 23.99 Marfan syndrome. A. High arched palate. **B.** Eye lens dislocation. *(From Forbes CD, Jackson WF.* Color Atlas and Text of Clinical Medicine, *3rd edn. St Louis: Mosby; 2003, p. 134, ©Elsevier.)*

Investigations

Cardiac investations are as follows:

- ***Chest X-ray*** is often normal but may show signs of aortic aneurysm and unfolding, or of widened mediastinum. Pneumothorax affects 11% and scoliosis is present in 70% of patients.
- ***ECG*** may be misleadingly normal with an acute dissection. In conjunction with mitral valve prolapse, 40% of patients usually have an arrhythmia, with premature ventricular and atrial arrhythmias.
- ***Echocardiography*** shows mitral valve prolapse, and mitral regurgitation in the majority of patients. High-quality serial echocardiogram measurements of aortic root diameter in the sinuses of Valsalva, at 90° to the direction of flow, are the basis for medical and surgical management ***(Fig. 23.100B)***.
- ***CT or CMR*** can detect aortic dilatation and both are useful in monitoring.

Management

- ***Beta-blocker therapy*** slows the rate of dilatation of the aortic root and atenolol is now standard therapy.
- ***Angiotensin receptor blockers*** specifically inhibit TNF-β, which is upregulated in Marfan. A trial of losartan compared with atenolol has shown no difference in aortic root dilatation at 3 years.
- ***Lifestyle alterations*** are required because of ocular, cardiac or skeletal involvement. Sports that necessitate prolonged exertion at maximum cardiac output, such as cross-country running, are to be avoided. Sedentary occupations are usually best, as patients tend to suffer from easy fatigability and hypermobile, painful joints.
- ***Monitoring*** should be carried out, with yearly echocardiograms up to aortic root diameter of 4.5 cm, and 6-monthly with diameters of 4.5–5 cm; the patient is then referred directly for elective surgery to a surgeon who is experienced in aortic root replacement in Marfan syndrome.

Pregnancy is generally well tolerated if no serious cardiac problems are present, but is preferably avoided if the aortic root diameter is >4 cm, with aortic regurgitation. Echocardiography should be performed every 6–8 weeks throughout pregnancy and during the initial 6 months postpartum. Blood pressure should be regularly monitored and hypertension treated actively. Delivery should be by the least stressful method, ideally vaginal. Caesarean section should not be routinely performed. However, if the aortic root is >4.5 cm, delivery at 39 weeks by induction or caesarean section is recommended. Beta-blocker therapy may be safely instituted or continued throughout pregnancy, to help prevent aortic dissection.

Medical and surgical management have increased the overall survival rate. On average, 13 years of life are added when surgical survival is compared to that reported in the natural history of MFS.

Genetic counselling

The condition is inherited in an autosomal dominant mode, with each child of one affected parent having a 50 : 50 chance of inheriting the condition. Males and females are affected equally often. In 25% of all cases, the condition arises as the result of a ***spontaneous mutation in gene 5*** of one of the parents. *FBN1* gene mutations can be identified in 80% of those affected, confirming diagnosis and aiding prognosis. The mutation can also be used to screen at-risk family members, including postnatal or prenatal offspring.

A

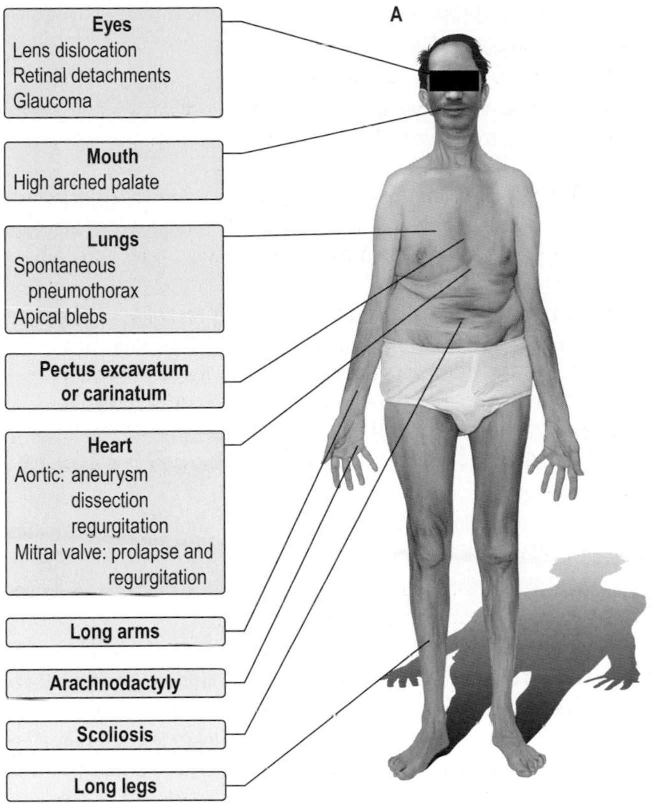

B

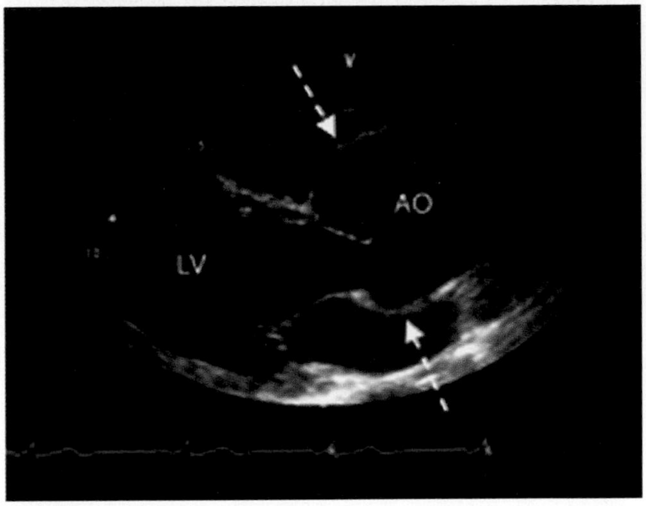

C

	Aortic size			
Yearly risk	> 3.5cm	> 4cm	> 5cm	> 6cm
Rupture	0.0%	0.3%	1.7%	3.6%
Dissection	2.2%	1.5%	2.5%	3.7%
Death	5.9%	4.6%	4.8%	10.8%
Any of the above	7.2%	5.3%	6.5%	14.1%

Figure 23.100 **Marfan syndrome. A.** Photograph of a 63-year-old man. **B.** Two-dimensional longitudinal echocardiogram of the aortic root. **C.** Yearly risk of complications based on aortic size.

Further reading

Brooke BS, Habashi JP, Judge DP et al. Angiotensin II blockade and aortic root dilation in Marfan's syndrome. *N Engl J Med* 2008; 358:2787–2795.

PULMONARY HEART DISEASE

The normal mean pulmonary artery pressure (mPAP) at rest is 14±3 mmHg with an upper limit of normal of 20 mmHg. The normal values for mPAP, mean capillary wedge pressure (mPCWP) and cardiac output (CO) are 12±2 mmHg, 6±2 mmHg and 5 L/min, respectively. The fall in pressure across the lung circulation is known as the transpulmonary gradient and reflects the difference between mPAP and mPCWP. The normal transpulmonary gradient is 6±2 mmHg.

The *pulmonary vascular resistance* (PVR) is calculated by the formula:

$$\frac{\text{mPAP} - \text{mPCWP}}{\text{CO}}$$

It is normally about 1.5 mmHg/L per min (1.5 Wood units). Approximately 60% of the body's endothelial surface is in the lungs and the lungs normally offer a low resistance to blood flow. This is because the media of the pre-capillary pulmonary arterioles is thin, as compared with their more muscular systemic counterparts that have to respond constantly to postural changes under the influence of gravity. The fact that the lung circulation normally offers a low resistance to flow explains the preferential passage of blood through the lungs in specific forms of congenital heart disease, which may eventually lead to remodelling of the lung circulation and pulmonary hypertension.

Pulmonary hypertension

Pulmonary hypertension (PH) is defined as an mPAP of >25 mmHg at rest, as measured on right heart catheterization. The clinical classification of PH is provided in ***Box 23.51***.

Pathophysiology

The different groups are characterized by variable amounts of hypertrophy, proliferation and fibrotic changes in distal pulmonary arteries (pulmonary arterial hypertension, PAH; pulmonary veno-occlusive disease, PVOD; pulmonary hypertension, PH, due to left heart disease; PH due to lung disease and/or hypoxia). Pulmonary venous changes are seen in PVOD and PH groups due to left heart disease, and the vascular bed may be destroyed in emphysematous or fibrotic areas seen in lung disease. In chronic thromboembolic pulmonary hypertension (CTEPH), organized thrombi are seen in the elastic pulmonary arteries. Patients with PH with unclear and/or multifactorial mechanisms have variable pathological findings.

Box 23.51 Updated clinical classification of pulmonary hypertension[a]

Group	Aetiological classification	Subtypes
1	Pulmonary arterial hypertension (PAH)	1.1. Idiopathic 1.2. Heritable 1.2.1. *BMPR2* 1.2.2. *ALK1, ENG, SMAD9, CAV1, KCNK3* 1.2.3. Unknown 1.3. Drugs and toxins 1.4. Associated with 1.4.1. Connective tissue disease[b] 1.4.2. HIV infection 1.4.3. Portal hypertension 1.4.4. Congenital heart disease 1.4.5. Schistosomiasis
1′	Pulmonary veno-occlusive disease (PVOD) and / or pulmonary capillary haemangiomatosis	
1″	Persistent pulmonary hypertension of the newborn (PPHN)	
2	Pulmonary hypertension due to left heart disease	2.1. Systolic dysfunction 2.2. Diastolic dysfunction 2.3. Valvular disease 2.4. Congenital/acquired left heart inflow/outflow tract obstruction and congenital cardiomyopathies
3	Pulmonary hypertension due to lung diseases and/ or hypoxia	3.1. Chronic obstructive pulmonary disease 3.2. Interstitial lung disease 3.3. Other pulmonary disease with mixed restrictive and obstructive pattern 3.4. Sleep-disordered breathing 3.5. Alveolar hypoventilation disorders 3.6. Chronic exposure to high altitude 3.7. Developmental abnormalities
4	Chronic thromboembolic pulmonary hypertension (CTEPH)	
5	Pulmonary hypertension with unclear and/or multifactorial mechanisms	5.1. Haematological disorders: chronic haemolytic anaemia, myeloproliferative disorders, splenectomy 5.2. Systemic disorders: sarcoidosis, pulmonary histiocytosis, lymphangioleiomyomatosis 5.3. Metabolic disorders: glycogen storage disease, Gaucher disease, thyroid disorders 5.4. Others: tumoral obstruction, fibrosing mediastinitis, chronic renal failure on dialysis, segmental pulmonary hypertension

[a]5th World Symposium on Pulmonary Hypertension, Nice, 2013.
[b]Now called 'autoimmune rheumatic disease'.
ALK1, activin-like receptor kinase-1; BMPR, bone morphogenetic protein receptor type II; CAV1, caveolin-1; ENG, endoglin; HIV = human immunodeficiency virus; KCNK3, potassium channel super-family K member-3; SMAD9, mothers against decapentaplegic 9.
(From: Simonneau G, Gatzoulis MA, Adatia I et al. Updated clinical classification of pulmonary hypertension. *J Am Coll Cardiol* 2013; 62:D34–41.)

Patients with progressive PH develop right ventricular hypertrophy, dilatation, heart failure and death.

Pulmonary artery hypertension

Epidemiology

A French registry of 674 patients with PAH identified 39.2% with idiopathic pulmonary artery hypertension (IPAH), 3.9% with familial (or heritable) disease, 9.5% with drug and toxin (anorexigens) causes, 15.3% with autoimmune rheumatic disease, 11.3% with congenital heart disease, 10.4% with portal hypertension and 6.2% with HIV-associated disease. In familial or heritable PAH, mutations in the bone morphogenetic protein receptor type 2 (*BMPR2*) gene, are detected in over 70% of cases; other mutations are seen in patients with hereditary haemorrhagic telangiectasia (Osler–Weber–Rendu syndrome).

Drugs and toxins known to cause PAH include fenfluramine, dexfenfluramine, toxic rapeseed oil and the anorectic agents aminorex and benfluorex.

Clinical features of PAH

Patients with PAH may present with symptoms of dyspnoea, fatigue, weakness, angina, syncope or abdominal distension. Clinical signs of PAH and right heart hypertrophy include a left parasternal heave, a loud P2 heart sound, a soft pansystolic murmur with tricuspid regurgitation or early diastolic murmur with pulmonary regurgitation. Right heart failure leads to jugular venous distension, ascites, peripheral oedema and hepatomegaly. Clinical signs of associated diseases, such as systemic sclerosis or chronic liver disease, should be sought.

Investigation of PAH

- ***Routine blood tests*** include full blood count, renal and liver biochemistry, thyroid function tests, and serological assays for underlying autoimmune rheumatic diseases, HIV and hepatitis.
- ***Chest X-ray*** shows enlargement of the pulmonary arteries and the major branches, with marked tapering (pruning) of peripheral arteries. The lung fields are usually lucent and there may be right atrial and right ventricular enlargement. The chest X-ray may facilitate the diagnosis of PH due to left heart or chronic lung disease.
- ***ECG*** shows right ventricular hypertrophy and right atrial enlargement (P pulmonale).
- ***Echocardiography (Fig. 23.101)*** with tricuspid regurgitation can be used for determination of PAP using the simplified Bernoulli equation (PAP $= 4\times$ (tricuspid regurgitation velocity)$^2 +$ estimated right atrial pressure). Right atrial pressure can be assumed at 5–10 mmHg unless there is significant dilatation of the inferior vena cava with reduced respiratory variation. Mean PAP $= 0.61 \times$ PA systolic pressure $+ 2$ mmHg (although the Bernoulli equation may not be accurate in cases of severe tricuspid regurgitation).
- ***CMR*** may be useful in adult congenital heart disease and in assessing right ventricular function on serial assessment.
- ***Abdominal liver ultrasound*** is useful to exclude liver cirrhosis and portal hypertension.
- ***Right heart catheterization*** may be indicated as part of the clinical assessment to confirm the diagnosis (elevated PAP), determine the pulmonary wedge pressure (PWP), calculate the cardiac output, and assess for pulmonary vascular resistance

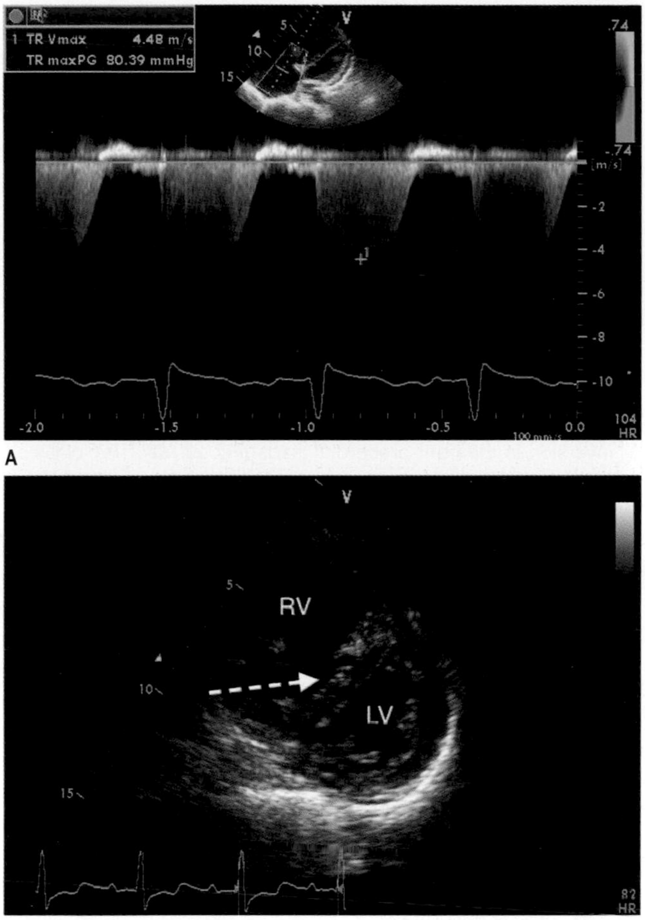

A

B

Figure 23.101 **Pulmonary hypertension. A.** Continuous wave Doppler echocardiography demonstrates markedly elevated tricuspid regurgitation velocity consistent with pulmonary hypertension. **B.** Parasternal short-axis echocardiogram with a dilated right ventricle (RV) and septal flattening (arrowed) in a patient with pulmonary hypertension. LV, left ventricle.

and reactivity. In PAH, a vasodilator challenge (inhaled nitric oxide, intravenous adenosine or epoprostenol) should be performed to identify patients who may benefit from vasodilator therapies. A responder is defined as a reduction in mean PAP of >10 mmHg to reach an absolute mean PAP of ≤40 mmHg with increased or unchanged cardiac output. These vasodilator challenges are not recommended in patients with other types of PH (types 2–5).

Management of PAH

- ***Physical activity***. Patients should be encouraged to remain physically active but avoid exertion that precipitates severe dyspnoea, chest pain or pre-syncope.
- ***Pregnancy***. Patients with PAH have a very high mortality rate during pregnancy (30–50%) and should be counselled against conception. Contraception may include barrier methods, progesterone-only pill or the Mirena coil.
- ***Travel***. During plane travel, supplementary oxygen at 2 L/min may be appropriate for patients with reduced functional class and with resting hypoxia of <8 kPa.
- ***Vaccination***. Vaccination should be given for influenza and pneumococcal pneumonia.
- ***Elective surgery***. Epidural anaesthesia may be preferable to a general anaesthetic.
- ***Oral anticoagulation***. There is evidence to support the use of oral anticoagulation in patients with IPAH, heritable PAH, and PAH due to anorexigens. The European target INR is 2.0–3.0.
- ***Diuretics***. These are used in patients with right heart failure and fluid overload.
- ***Digoxin***. This may be helpful in patients with tachyarrhythmias.
- ***Calcium channel blockers***. These can be effective in high doses in selected patients with IPAH who demonstrate a response to a vasodilator challenge. Right heart catheterization should be repeated in 3–4 months to assess response to therapy.
- ***Prostanoids***. Prostacyclin is a potent vasodilator that also inhibits platelet aggregation and cell proliferation. Synthetic prostacyclins are generally short-acting compounds requiring continuous intravenous or subcutaneous infusion or regular aerosol inhalation. They provide symptomatic relief and can improve exercise capacity; ***epoprostenol*** can improve survival in patients with both IPAH and APAH. Oral ***selexipag*** has been approved by the FDA for PAH treatment.
- ***Endothelin receptor antagonists***. Endothelin-1 is a potent vasoconstrictor and mitogen that binds to endothelin A and B receptors in the pulmonary vasculature. Both dual antagonists (***bosentan***) and selective A receptor antagonists (***sitaxentan***, ***ambrisentan***) can improve symptoms, exercise capacity and haemodynamics in patients with IPAH.
- ***Phosphodiesterase type 5 inhibitors***. These produce vasodilatation in the pulmonary vasculature and reduce cellular proliferation. ***Sildenafil*** and ***tadalafil*** have been demonstrated to provide symptomatic relief and improve exercise capacity in patients with IPAH.
- ***Balloon atrial septostomy***. This technique may be considered as palliative therapy in severe cases of PH.
- ***Cardiac transplantation***. This is used in patients with an adverse prognosis, although the 5-year survival following transplantation may be only 40–50%.

Other pulmonary hypertension groups

Left-sided heart disease (systolic and diastolic heart failure) and valvular heart disease is frequently associated with PH, as is advanced chronic obstructive pulmonary disease (see pp. 1079–1085), pulmonary fibrosis and emphysema. Following acute pulmonary embolism, 0.5–2.0% of patients will develop chronic thromboembolic pulmonary hypertension (CTEPH).

Pulmonary embolism

Thrombus, usually formed in the systemic veins or rarely in the right heart (<10% of cases), may dislodge and embolize into the pulmonary arterial system. Postmortem studies indicate that this is a very common condition (microemboli are found in up to 60% of autopsies) but it is not usually diagnosed this frequently in life. Ten per cent of clinical pulmonary emboli are fatal.

Most clots that cause clinically relevant pulmonary emboli actually come from the pelvic and abdominal veins, but femoral DVT and even occasionally axillary thrombosis can be the origin of the clot. Clot forms as a result of a combination of sluggish blood flow, local injury or compression of the vein and a hypercoagulable state. Emboli can also occur from tumour, fat (long bone fractures), amniotic fluid and foreign material during intravenous drug misuse. Risk factors are shown in ***Box 16.35*** and discussed on pages 575–578.

After pulmonary embolism, lung tissue is ventilated but not perfused, producing an intrapulmonary dead space and resulting in impaired gas exchange. After some hours, the non-perfused lung no longer produces surfactant. Alveolar collapse occurs and exacerbates hypoxaemia. The primary haemodynamic consequence of pulmonary embolism is a reduction in the cross-sectional area of the pulmonary arterial bed, which causes an elevation of pulmonary arterial pressure and a reduction in cardiac output. Right ventricular ischaemia can be detected with elevations of troponin and creatine kinase and is associated with adverse outcomes. Distal embolization leads to alveolar haemorrhage with haemoptysis, pleural inflammation and effusion (pulmonary infarction).

Clinical features

Sudden onset of ***unexplained dyspnoea*** is the most common, and often the only, symptom of pulmonary embolism. ***Pleuritic chest pain*** and ***haemoptysis*** are present only when infarction has occurred.

On examination, the patient may be tachypnoeic with a localized pleural rub and, often, coarse crackles over the area involved. An exudative pleural effusion (occasionally blood-stained) can develop. The patient may have a fever, and cardiovascular examination is typically normal.

Massive pulmonary embolism

Sudden collapse may occur with acute obstruction of the right ventricular outflow tract. The patient has severe central chest pain (cardiac ischaemia due to lack of coronary blood flow) and becomes shocked, pale and sweaty. Syncope may result if the cardiac output is transiently but dramatically reduced, and death may occur. On examination, the patient is tachypnoeic, and has a tachycardia with hypotension and peripheral shutdown. The JVP is raised with a prominent *a*-wave. There is a right ventricular heave, a gallop rhythm and a widely split second heart sound.

Chronic recurrent pulmonary embolism

This may present with dyspnoea, weakness, syncope on exertion and, occasionally, angina. Examination may reveal signs of right ventricular overload with a right ventricular heave and loud pulmonary second sound.

Investigations

- ***Chest X-ray*** is often normal, but linear atelectasis or blunting of a costophrenic angle (due to a small effusion) is not uncommon. Occasionally, a wedge-shaped pulmonary infarct, the abrupt cut-off of a pulmonary artery or a translucency of an under-perfused distal zone is seen. Patients with massive pulmonary embolism may have pulmonary oligaemia. Those with recurrent pulmonary emboli may have enlarged pulmonary arterioles with oligaemic lung fields.
- ***ECG*** findings include sinus tachycardia, right atrial dilatation with tall peaked P waves in lead II, right ventricular strain with right axis deviation and right bundle branch block, and T-wave inversion in the right precordial leads ***(Fig. 23.102)***. The 'classic' ECG pattern with an S wave in lead I, and a Q wave and inverted T waves in lead III (S1, Q3, T3), is rare.
- ***Blood gases*** may be normal, but with significant pulmonary embolism there will be arterial hypoxaemia with a low arterial CO_2 level, i.e. a type I respiratory failure pattern.
- ***Cardiac troponins and BNP*** may be elevated and are associated with an adverse outcome.
- ***Plasma D-dimer*** (see p. 566) is elevated in patients with thromboembolism and a negative test excludes a diagnosis of pulmonary embolism. However, elevated levels may be detected in patients with cancer, those who are pregnant, and in hospitalized and elderly patients.
- ***Radionuclide ventilation/perfusion scanning ($\dot{V}/\dot{Q}$ scan)*** is a good diagnostic investigation that is widely available. Pulmonary ^{99m}Tc scintigraphy demonstrates under-perfused areas ***(Fig. 23.103)***, which, if not accompanied by a ventilation defect on a ventilation scintigram performed after inhalation of radioactive xenon gas (see p. 1070), is highly suggestive of a pulmonary embolus. There are limitations to the test, however. For example, a matched defect may arise with a pulmonary embolus that causes an infarct, or with emphysematous bullae. This test is therefore conventionally reported as a

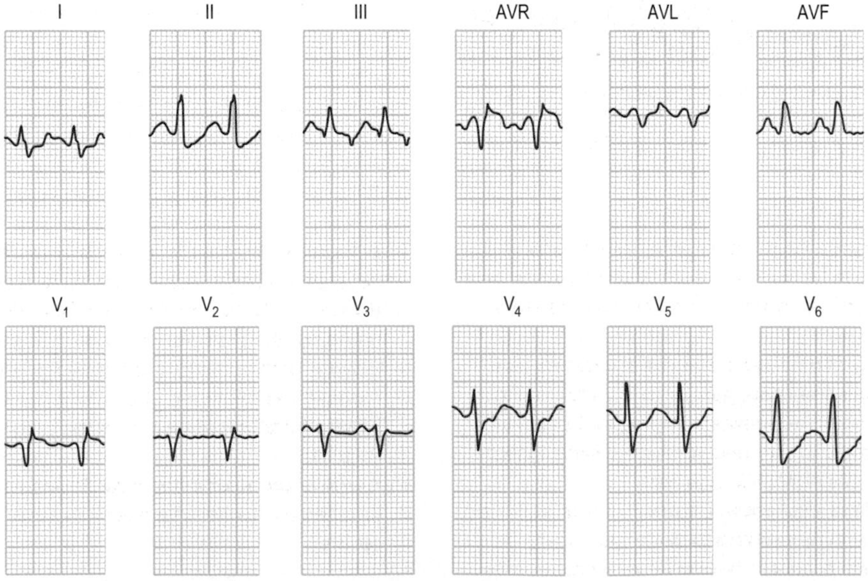

Figure 23.102 Acute pulmonary embolism shown on a 12-lead ECG. There is an S wave in lead I, a Q wave in lead III and an inverted T wave in lead III (the S1, Q3, T3 pattern). There is sinus tachycardia (160 b.p.m.) and an incomplete right bundle branch block pattern (an R wave in AVR and V_1 and an S wave in V_6).

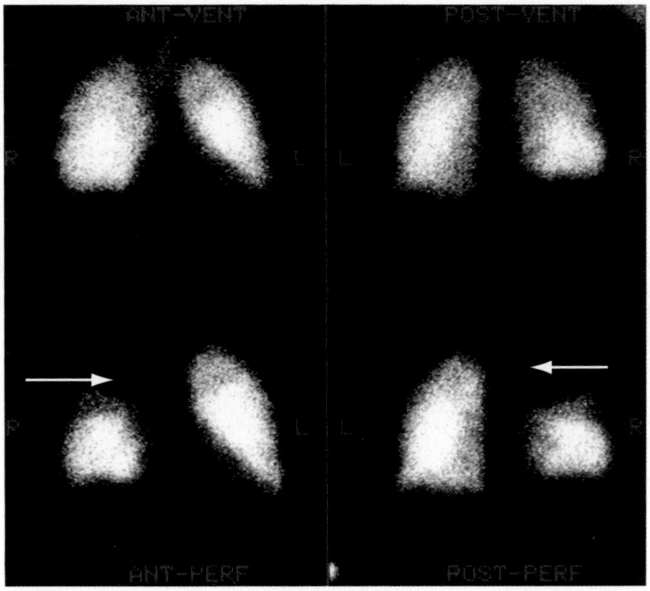

Figure 23.103 **Radionuclide ventilation/perfusion scanning.** Ventilation (top) and perfusion (bottom) lung scans demonstrate an absence of perfusion in the right upper lobe, i.e. probable pulmonary embolism (arrowed).

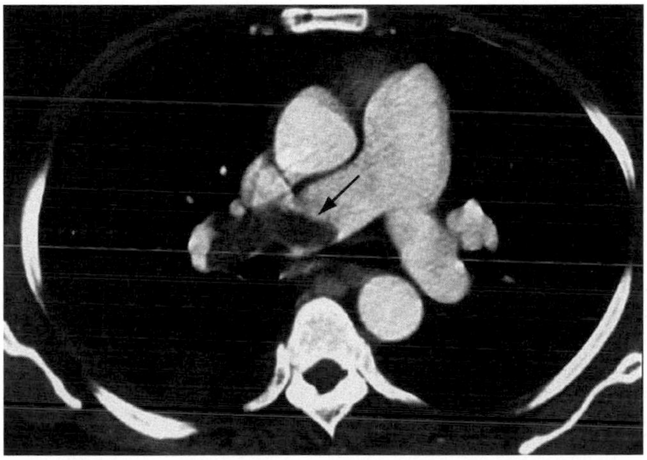

Figure 23.104 **CT pulmonary angiography in pulmonary embolism.** The image is taken at the level of the main right and left pulmonary arteries, and shows a large thrombus (arrowed) in the right pulmonary artery.

probability (low, medium or high) of pulmonary embolus and should be interpreted in the context of the history, examination and other investigations. A normal V̇/Q̇ scan has a negative predictive value of 97%.

- ***Ultrasound scanning*** can be performed for the detection of clots in pelvic or iliofemoral veins (see p. 1055). This may be very useful as a screening assessment in pregnant patients; a positive scan may preclude the need for further investigation with CT angiography (CTA) or V̇/Q̇ scanning.
- ***Contrast-enhanced multidetector CT angiograms*** (CTA; ***Fig. 23.104***) can accurately diagnose and exclude pulmonary embolism, and modern scanners have a negative predictive value of 95–97%. In pregnancy, CTA exposes the mother to a greater radiation risk than a V̇/Q̇ scan but delivers a lower radiation dose to the fetus.
- ***MRI*** can provide similar results and may be appropriate if CTA is contraindicated.
- ***Echocardiography*** can be useful in acute pulmonary embolism to assess for evidence of right ventricular dysfunction and, in some cases, may demonstrate thrombus. In chronic recurrent pulmonary emboli, there may be right ventricular dilatation and hypertrophy with pulmonary arterial hypertension.

Classification and investigation of acute pulmonary embolism

Clinical status at presentation can be used to divide patients into 'high-risk' and 'not high-risk', based on the presence of shock or hypotension ***(Fig. 23.105A)***.

High-risk patients should proceed to CTA; a positive test confirms the diagnosis. A negative test should lead to investigations for other causes of haemodynamic instability. Echocardiography may be useful if patients are too unstable for CTA. Right ventricular dysfunction or visible thrombi are consistent with pulmonary embolism; normal right ventricular function should suggest an alternative diagnosis.

In ***not high-risk*** patients, the clinical probability of pulmonary embolus should be determined using the Wells rule ***(Box 23.52)***.

- High-clinical-probability or PE-likely patients should proceed to multidetector contrast-enhanced CTA (see ***Fig. 23.104***). A positive test confirms the diagnosis. A negative test that has high probability may require further investigation. (Patients with renal failure or contrast allergy can have V̇/Q̇ scanning).
- Low- or intermediate-probability or PE-unlikely patients should have a D-dimer assay performed. A negative D-dimer rules out a pulmonary embolism. A positive D-dimer requires further investigation with CTA ***(Fig. 23.105B)***.

Management

Acute management

- ***High-flow oxygen*** (60–100%) should be given to all patients, unless they have significant chronic lung disease. Patients with pulmonary infarcts require bed rest and analgesia.
- ***Initial anticoagulation*** with subcutaneous low-molecular-weight heparin or fondaparinux or intravenous unfractionated heparin should be given.
- ***Intravenous fluids and even inotropic agents*** to improve the pumping of the right heart are sometimes required in severe cases, and very ill patients will require care on the intensive therapy unit (see pp. 1157–1158).
- ***Thrombolysis therapy*** can improve pulmonary perfusion quicker than anticoagulation. It should be used in unstable patients and should be considered in stable patients with adverse features, such as right ventricular dysfunction. The Pulmonary Embolism Thrombolysis (PEITHO) trial compared tenecteplase and heparin versus placebo and heparin in 1006 patients with acute pulmonary embolism. Thrombolysis reduced the primary end-point (all-cause death or haemodynamic collapse or compromise) (2.6% versus 5.6%, $P = 0.015$).
- ***Surgical embolectomy*** is rarely necessary, but there may be no alternative when the haemodynamic circumstances are very severe.

Prevention of further emboli

Patients should be anticoagulated with vitamin K antagonists (e.g. warfarin) for a period of 3–6 months with a target INR of 2.0–3.0.

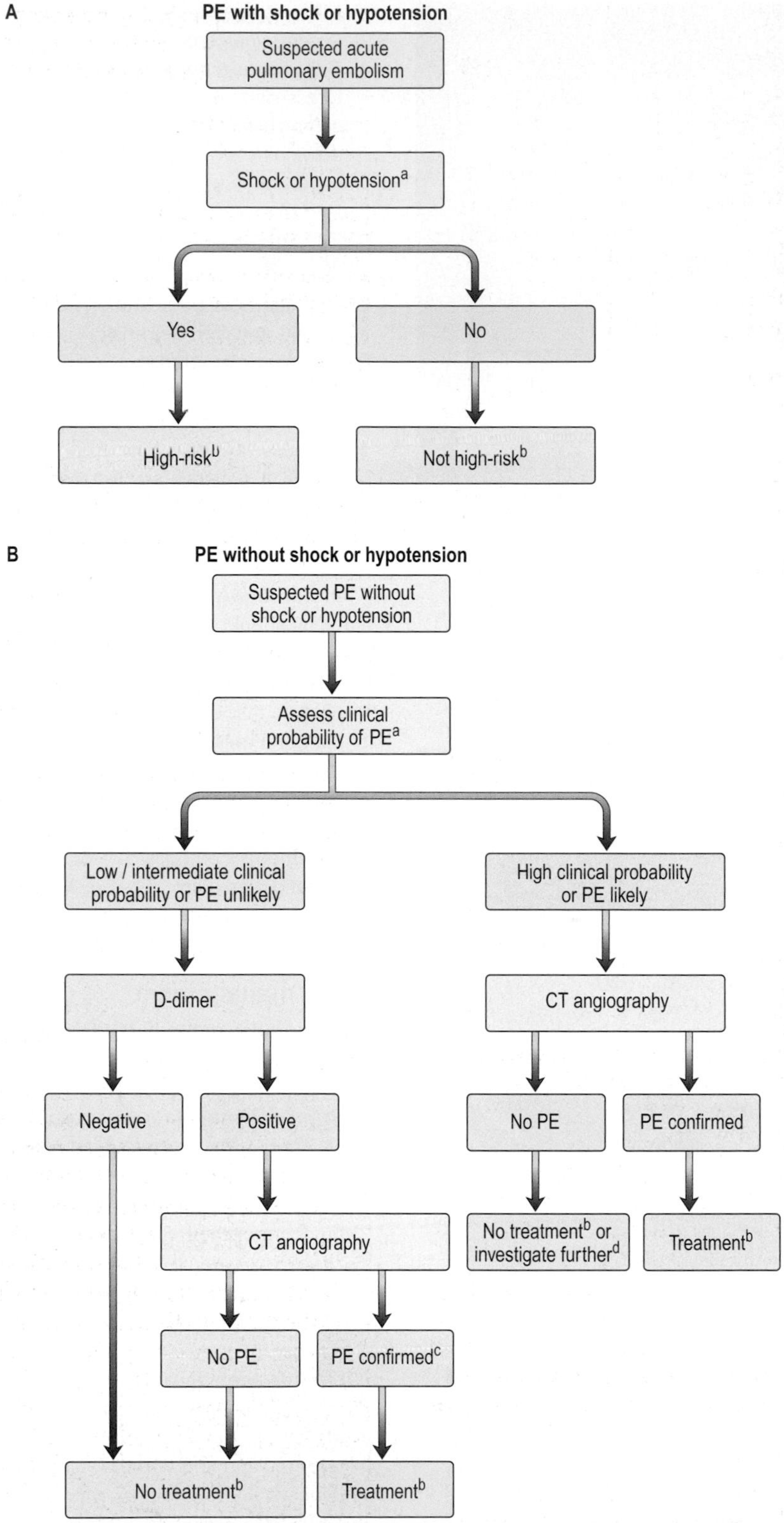

Figure 23.105 **Initial stratification of acute pulmonary embolism (PE). A.** *With shock or hypotension.* **B.** *Without shock or hypotension.*
[a]Systolic blood pressure <90 mmHg, or a systolic pressure drop of ≥40 mmHg for >15 min, if not caused by new-onset arrhythmia, hypovolaemia or sepsis.
[b]Based on the estimated PE-related in-hospital or 30-day mortality.
[c]Treatment refers to anticoagulation for PE.
[d]In case of a negative CT angiogram in patients with a high clinical probability, further investigation may be considered before withholding PE-specific treatment. *(From European Society of Cardiology Clinical Practice Guidelines 2014 Acute Pulmonary Embolism (Diagnosis and Management of), with permission.)*

Box 23.52 Wells rule

Rule	Points
Simplified Wells rule[a]	
Previous PE or DVT	1
Heart rate ≥100 b.p.m.	1
Surgery or immobilization <4 weeks	1
Haemoptysis	1
Active cancer	1
Clinical signs of DVT	1
Alternative diagnosis less likely than PE	1
2-level score	
PE unlikely	0–1
PE likely	≥2
Original Wells rule[b]	
Previous PE or DVT	1.5
Heart rate ≥100 b.p.m.	1.5
Surgery or immobilization < 4 weeks	1.5
Haemoptysis	1
Active cancer	1
Clinical signs of DVT	3
Alternative diagnosis less likely than PE	3
3-level score	
Low	0–1
Intermediate	2–6
High	≥7
2-level score	
PE unlikely	0–4
PE likely	≥5

DVT, deep venous thrombosis; PE, pulmonary embolism.
([a]Gibson NS, Sohne M, Kruip MJ et al. Further validation and simplification of the Wells clinical decision rule in pulmonary embolism. *Thromb Haemost* 2008; 99:229–234. [b]Wells PS, Anderson DR, Rodger M et al. Derivation of a simple clinical model to categorize patients probability of pulmonary embolism: increasing the models utility with the SimpliRED D-dimer. *Thromb Haemost* 2000; 83:416–420.)

More recently, non-vitamin-K-antagonist oral anticoagulants (NOACs; dabigatran, rivaroxaban and apixaban) have been used in patients with venous thromboembolism; they appear to be effective and possibly safer than standard vitamin K antagonists. Patients with cancer or pregnant women should be treated with long-term low-molecular-weight heparin. In high-risk patients in whom anticoagulation is absolutely contraindicated, a vena cava filter may be inserted via the femoral vein to above the level of the renal veins.

Chronic thromboembolic pulmonary hypertension

Chronic thromboembolic obstruction of the major pulmonary arteries has an incidence of 5 per million population in the UK. The mean age is 63 years, and males and females are equally affected. Patients may present with dyspnoea, haemoptysis and/or ankle oedema.

The clinical diagnosis of chronic thromboembolic pulmonary hypertension (CTEPH) is made following 3 months of adequate anticoagulation with an elevated PAP ≥25 mmHg, wedge pressure ≥15 mmHg associated with a segmental defect on $\dot{V}/\dot{Q}$ scan, or pulmonary artery obstruction on CT or pulmonary angiography. Pulmonary endarterectomy is the treatment of choice. Medical treatment includes anticoagulation, oxygen and diuretics. If the patient is inoperable, riociguat (a vasodilator) is used under specialist care.

Further reading

Agnelli G. Current concepts. Acute pulmonary embolism. *N Engl J Med* 2010; 363:266–284.
Bourjeily G. Pulmonary embolism in pregnancy. *Lancet* 2010; 375:500–512.
Humbert M, Sitbon O, Chaouat A et al. Pulmonary arterial hypertension in France: results from a national registry. *Am J Respir Crit Care Med* 2006; 173:1023–1030.
Konstantinides S, Torbicki A, Agnelli G et al. 2014 ESC Guidelines on the diagnosis and management of acute pulmonary embolism. *Eur Heart J* 2014; 35:3033–3080.
Suntharalingam J, Ross RM, Easaw J et al. Who should be referred to a specialist pulmonary hypertension centre – a referrer's guide. *Clin Med* 2016; 16:135–141.

MYOCARDIAL AND ENDOCARDIAL DISEASE

CARDIAC TUMOURS

Atrial myxoma

This is the most common primary cardiac tumour. It occurs at all ages and shows no sex preference. Although most myxomas are sporadic, some are familial or are part of a multiple system syndrome. Histologically, they are benign. The majority of myxomas are solitary, usually develop in the left atrium, and are polypoid, gelatinous structures attached by a pedicle to the atrial septum. The tumour may obstruct the mitral valve or may be a site of thrombi, which then embolize. It is also associated with constitutional symptoms: the patient may present with dyspnoea, syncope or a mild fever. The physical signs are a loud first heart sound, a tumour 'plop' (a loud third heart sound produced as the pedunculated tumour comes to an abrupt halt), a mid-diastolic murmur and signs due to embolization. A raised erythrocyte sedimentation rate (ESR) is usually present.

The diagnosis is easily made by echocardiography because the tumour is demonstrated as a dense, space-occupying lesion ***(Fig. 23.106)***. Surgical removal usually results in a complete cure.

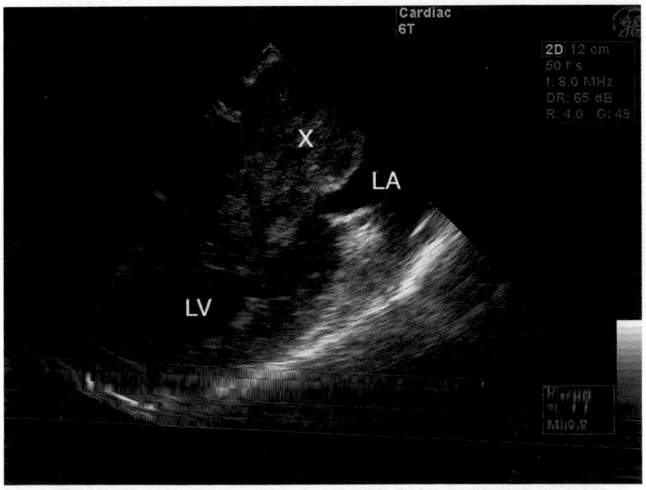

Figure 23.106 Atrial myxoma shown by a two-dimensional echocardiogram (long-axis view). The myxoma (X) is an echo-dense mass obstructing the mitral valve orifice. It was removed surgically. LV, left ventricle; LA, left atrium.

Myxomas may also occur in the right atrium or in the ventricles. Other primary cardiac tumours include rhabdomyomas and sarcomas.

MYOCARDIAL DISEASE

Myocardial disease that is not due to ischaemic, valvular or hypertensive heart disease, or a known infiltrative, metabolic/toxic or neuromuscular disorder, may be caused by:

- an acute or chronic inflammatory pathology (myocarditis)
- idiopathic myocardial disease (cardiomyopathy).

Myocarditis

Acute inflammation of the myocardium has many causes ***(Box 23.53)***. Establishment of a definitive aetiology, with isolation of viruses or bacteria, is difficult in routine clinical practice.

In Western societies, the most common cause of infective myocarditis is Coxsackie or adenoviral infection. Myocarditis in association with HIV infection is seen at postmortem in up to 20% of cases but causes clinical problems in less than 10% of cases. Chagas' disease, due to *Trypanosoma cruzi*, which is endemic in South America, is one of the most common causes of myocarditis worldwide. Additionally, toxins (including prescribed drugs), physical agents, hypersensitivity reactions and autoimmune conditions may also cause myocardial inflammation.

Pathology

In the acute phase, myocarditic hearts are flabby with focal haemorrhages; in chronic cases, they are enlarged and hypertrophied. Histologically ***(Fig. 23.107)***, an inflammatory infiltrate is present – lymphocytes predominating with viral causes, polymorphonuclear cells with bacterial causes, and eosinophils with allergic and hypersensitivity causes.

Clinical features

Myocarditis may be an acute or chronic process; its clinical presentations range from an asymptomatic state associated with limited and focal inflammation, to ***fatigue***, ***palpitations***, ***chest pain***, ***dyspnoea*** and ***fulminant congestive cardiac failure*** due to diffuse myocardial involvement. An episode of viral myocarditis, perhaps unrecognized and forgotten, may be the initial event that eventually culminates in an 'idiopathic' dilated cardiomyopathy. Physical examination includes soft heart sounds, a prominent third sound and often a tachycardia. A pericardial friction rub may be heard.

Investigations

- ***Chest X-ray***. This may show some cardiac enlargement, depending on the stage and virulence of the disease.
- ***ECG***. The ECG demonstrates ST- and T-wave abnormalities and arrhythmias. Heart block may be seen with diphtheritic myocarditis, Lyme disease and Chagas' disease (see below).
- ***Cardiac enzymes***. These are elevated.
- ***Viral antibody titres***. These may be increased. However, since enteroviral infection is common in the general population, the diagnosis depends on the demonstration of acutely rising titres.
- ***Endomyocardial biopsy***. Biopsy may show acute inflammation but false negatives are common by conventional criteria. Biopsy is of limited value outside specialized units.
- ***Viral RNA***. DNA can be measured from biopsy material using polymerase chain reaction (PCR). Specific diagnosis requires demonstration of active viral replication within myocardial tissue.

Management

The underlying cause must be identified, treated, eliminated or avoided. Bed rest is recommended in the acute phase of the illness and athletic activities should be avoided for 6 months. Heart failure should be treated conventionally with the use of diuretics, ACE inhibitors/angiotensin II receptor antagonists, beta-blockers or spironolactone with or without digoxin. ***Antibiotics*** should be administered immediately where appropriate. Non-steroidal anti-inflammatory drugs (***NSAIDs***) are contraindicated in the acute phase of the illness but may be used in the late phase. The use of ***corticosteroids*** is controversial and no studies have demonstrated

Box 23.53 Causes of myocarditis

- Idiopathic
- Infective
  - Viral: Coxsackievirus, adenovirus, cytomegalovirus, echovirus, influenza, polio, hepatitis, HIV
  - Parasitic: *Trypanosoma cruzi*, *Toxoplasma gondii* (a cause of myocarditis in the newborn or immunocompromised)
  - Bacterial: streptococcus (most commonly, rheumatic carditis), diphtheria (toxin-mediated heart block common)
  - Spirochaetal: Lyme disease (heart block common), leptospirosis
  - Fungal
  - Rickettsial
- Toxic
  - Drugs: those causing hypersensitivity reactions, e.g. methyldopa, penicillin, sulphonamides, antituberculous, modafinil
  - Radiation: may cause myocarditis but pericarditis is more common
- Autoimmune
  - An autoimmune form with autoactivated T cells and organ-specific antibodies may occur
  - Giant cell myocarditis
- Alcohol
- Hydrocarbons

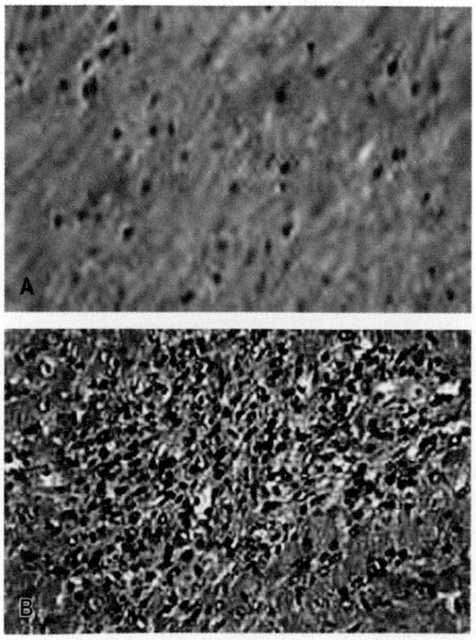

Figure 23.107 Myocardial biopsies. A. Normal myocardium. **B.** Myocarditis, with increased interstitial inflammatory cells.

an improvement in left ventricular ejection fraction or survival following their use. The administration of high-dose intravenous ***immunoglobulin***, on the other hand, appears to be associated with a more rapid resolution of the left ventricular dysfunction and improved survival. Effective antiviral, immunosuppressive (e.g. interferon-gamma) and ***immunomodulating*** (e.g. interleukin-10) agents are available to treat viral myocarditis.

Giant cell myocarditis

This is a severe form of myocarditis characterized by the presence of multinucleated giant cells within the myocardium. The cause is unknown but it may be associated with sarcoidosis, thymomas and autoimmune disease. It has a rapidly progressive course and a poor prognosis. Immunosuppression is recommended.

Chagas' disease

Chagas' disease is caused by the protozoan *Trypanosoma cruzi* and is endemic in South America, where upwards of 20 million people are infected. Acutely, features of myocarditis are present with fever and congestive heart failure. Chronically, there is progression to a dilated cardiomyopathy with a propensity towards heart block and ventricular arrhythmias. Treatment is discussed on page 303. Amiodarone is helpful for the control of ventricular arrhythmias; heart failure is treated in the usual way (see pp. 985–987).

CARDIOMYOPATHY

Cardiomyopathies are a group of diseases of the myocardium that affect the mechanical or electrical function of the heart. They are frequently genetic and a reclassification through the World Health Federation has endorsed the MOGE(S) nomenclature. This classification incorporates *m*orphological phenotype, *o*rgan or system involvement, *g*enetics, *a*etiological annotation and *s*tage of clinical function. This will aid understanding of the complexity of the inherited cardiomyopathies with the hope of integrating genotype assessment to individualize therapy. Clinically, these diseases can be divided into hypertrophic cardiomyopathy (HCM), arrhythmogenic cardiomyopathies (ACs) and dilated cardiomyopathy (DCM).

Secondary cardiomyopathies cover a wide range of aetiologies: infiltrative (e.g. amyloidosis, Gaucher's disease); storage-related (e.g. haemochromatosis); drugs (e.g. alcohol); inflammatory (e.g. sarcoidosis); neuromuscular (e.g. Friedreich's ataxia); nutritional (e.g. beriberi); autoimmune (e.g. systemic lupus erythematosus); and cancer therapy (e.g. anthracyclines – doxorubicin).

Inherited cardiomyopathies

Hypertrophic cardiomyopathy

Hypertrophic cardiomyopathy (HCM) includes a group of inherited conditions that produce hypertrophy of the myocardium in the absence of an alternative cause (e.g. aortic stenosis or hypertension). It is the most common cause of sudden cardiac death in young people and affects 1 in 500 of the population. The majority of cases are familial autosomal dominant, due to mutations in the genes encoding sarcomeric proteins (*Fig. 23.108*). The most common causes of HCM are mutations of the β-myosin heavy chain MYH7 and myosin-binding protein C MYBPC3. Other mutations include troponin T and I, regulatory and essential myosin light chains, titin, α-tropomyosin, α-actin, α-myosin heavy chain and muscle LIM protein (although over 400 mutations have been identified.) There are non-sarcomeric protein mutations in genes that control cardiac

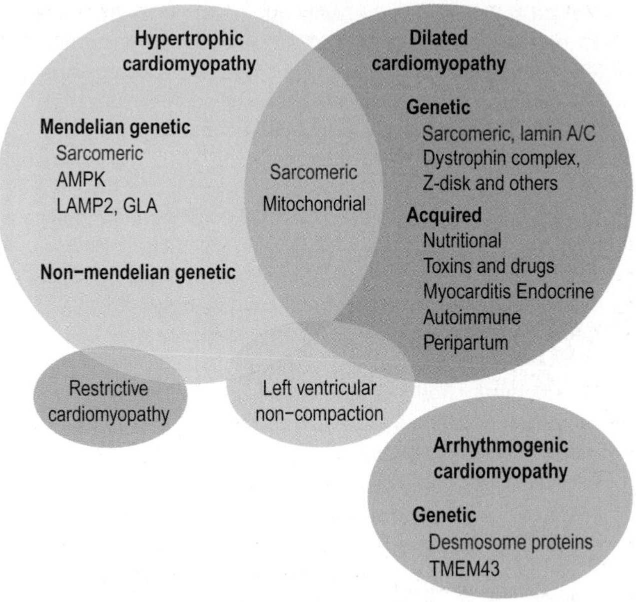

Figure 23.108 Cardiomyopathy: clinical categories and genetic basis. Hypertrophic and dilated cardiomyopathies share the same genes, as do the less common restrictive cardiomyopathy and left ventricular non-compaction. Arrhythmogenic cardiomyopathy (ACM) is genetically different. AMPK, adenosine monophosphate-activated kinase; GLA, galactosidase A; LAMP2, lysosomal assisted membrane protein 2; TMEM43, transmembrane protein 43. *(From Watkins H, Ashrafian H, Redwood C. Inherited cardiomyopathies.* N Engl J Med *2011; 364:1643–1656, with permission.)*

metabolism, which result in glycogen storage diseases (Danon's, Pompe's and Fabry's diseases) that are indistinguishable from HCM.

Clinical features

HCM is characterized by variable myocardial hypertrophy that frequently involves the interventricular septum, and by disorganization ('disarray') of cardiac myocytes and myofibrils. Some 25% of patients have dynamic left ventricular outflow tract obstruction due to the combined effects of hypertrophy, systolic anterior motion (SAM) of the anterior mitral valve leaflet and rapid ventricular ejection. The salient clinical and morphological features of the disease vary according to the underlying genetic mutation. For example, marked hypertrophy is common with β-myosin heavy chain mutations, whereas mutations in troponin T may be associated with mild hypertrophy but a high risk of sudden death. The hypertrophy may not manifest before completion of the adolescent growth spurt, making the diagnosis difficult in children. HCM due to myosin-binding protein may not manifest until the sixth decade of life or later.

Symptoms

- Many cases are asymptomatic and are detected by family screening of an affected individual or by a routine ECG examination.
- Chest pain, dyspnoea, syncope or pre-syncope (typically with exertion), cardiac arrhythmias and sudden death are seen
- Sudden death occurs at any age but the highest rates (up to 6% per annum) occur in adolescents or young adults. Risk factors for sudden death are discussed below.
- Dyspnoea occurs due to impaired relaxation of the heart muscle or the left ventricular outflow tract obstruction that occurs in some patients. The systolic cavity remains small until

the late stages of disease, when progressive dilatation may occur. If a patient develops atrial fibrillation, there is often a rapid deterioration in clinical status due to the loss of atrial contraction and the tachycardia – resulting in elevated left atrial pressure and acute pulmonary oedema.

Signs

- Double apical pulsation (forceful atrial contraction producing a fourth heart sound).
- Jerky carotid pulse because of rapid ejection and sudden obstruction to left ventricular outflow during systole.
- Ejection systolic murmur due to left ventricular outflow obstruction late in systole; it can be increased by manœuvres that decrease afterload, such as standing or Valsalva, and decreased by manœuvres that increase afterload and venous return, such as squatting.
- Pansystolic murmur due to mitral regurgitation (secondary to SAM).
- Fourth heart sound (if not in atrial fibrillation).

Investigations

- ***ECG*** abnormalities in HCM include left ventricular hypertrophy (see ***Fig. 23.79***), ST- and T-wave changes, and abnormal Q waves, especially in the inferolateral leads.
- ***Echocardiography*** is usually diagnostic. In classical HCM, there is asymmetric left ventricular hypertrophy (involving the septum more than the posterior wall), systolic anterior motion of the mitral valve, and a vigorously contracting ventricle ***(Fig. 23.109)***. However, any pattern of hypertrophy may be seen, including concentric and apical hypertrophy.
- ***CMR*** can detect both the hypertrophy and abnormal myocardial fibrosis ***(Fig. 23.110)***.
- ***Genetic analysis***, where available, may confirm the diagnosis and provide prognostic information for the patient and relatives.

Management

The management of HCM includes treatment of symptoms and prevention of sudden cardiac death in the patient and relatives.

Risk factors for sudden death are as follows:

- massive left ventricular hypertrophy (>30 mm on echocardiography)
- family history of sudden cardiac death (<50 years old)
- non-sustained ventricular tachycardia on 24-hour Holter monitoring
- prior unexplained syncope
- abnormal blood pressure response on exercise (flat or hypotensive response).

The presence of these cardiac risk factors is associated with an increased risk of sudden death ***(Box 23.54)***, and patients with two or more should be assessed for ICD insertion. When the risk is less, amiodarone is an appropriate alternative.

Chest pain and dyspnoea are treated with beta-blockers and verapamil, either alone or in combination. An alternative agent is disopyramide if patients have left ventricular outflow tract obstruction. In some individuals with significant left outflow obstruction and symptoms, dual-chamber pacing is necessary. Alcohol (non-surgical) ablation of the septum has been investigated and appears to give good results in reduction of outflow tract obstruction and subsequent improvement in exercise capacity. This procedure carries risks, including the development of complete heart block and MI. Occasionally, surgical resection of septal myocardium may be indicated. Vasodilators should be avoided because they may aggravate left ventricular outflow obstruction or cause refractory hypotension.

Arrhythmogenic cardiomyopathy/ arrhythmogenic right ventricular cardiomyopathy

Arrhythmogenic cardiomyopathy (ACM) is an uncommon (1 in 1000–5000 population) inherited condition that predominantly affects the right ventricle with fatty or fibro-fatty replacement of

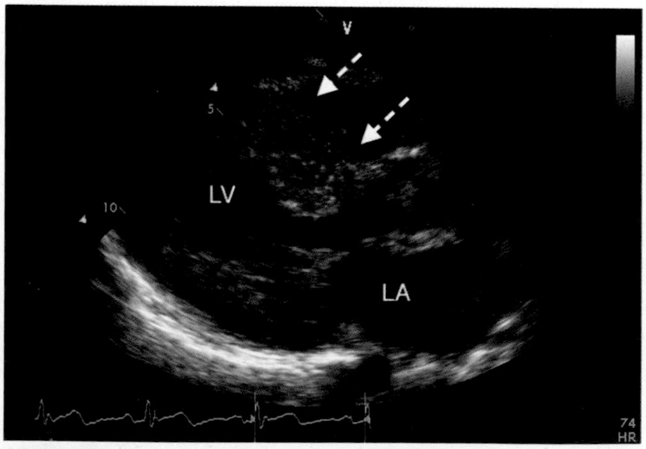

Figure 23.109 Hypertrophic cardiomyopathy. A two-dimensional echocardiogram (short-axis view). The grossly thickened interventricular septum is shown, resulting in a small left ventricular cavity. This condition is associated with an abnormal anterior motion of the mitral valve during systole (arrows). LA, left atrium; LV, left ventricle.

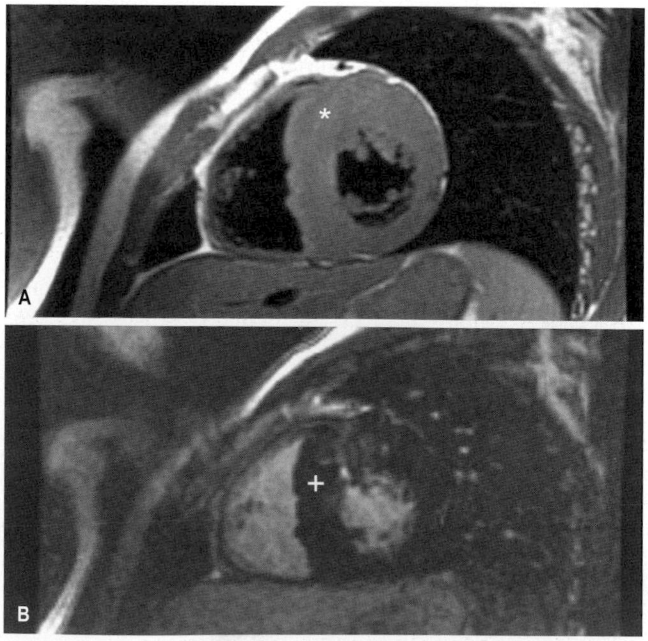

Figure 23.110 Cardiac magnetic resonance imaging in a patient with hypertrophic cardiomyopathy. A. Turbo spin-echo demonstrates marked thickening of the basal to mid-anterior wall and septum (*). **B.** Inversion recovery image post gadolinium demonstrates regional fibrosis with enhancement (+).

Box 23.54 Causes of sudden cardiac death

Coronary artery disease
- Acute myocardial infarction – STEMI
- Chronic ischaemic heart disease
- Following coronary artery bypass surgery
- After successful resuscitation for cardiac arrest
- Congenital anomaly of coronary arteries
- Coronary artery embolism
- Coronary arteritis

Non-coronary artery disease
- Hypertrophic cardiomyopathy
- Dilated cardiomyopathy (ischaemic or idiopathic)
- Arrhythmogenic right ventricular cardiomyopathy
- Congenital long QT syndrome
- Brugada syndrome
- Valvular heart disease (aortic stenosis, mitral valve prolapse) ± infective endocarditis
- Cyanotic heart disease (tetralogy of Fallot, transposition)
- Acyanotic heart disease (ventricular septal defect, patent ductus arteriosus)

STEMI, ST elevation myocardial infarction.

myocytes, leading to segmental or global dilatation ***(Fig. 23.111)***. Left ventricular involvement has been reported in up to 75% of cases. The fibro-fatty replacement leads to ventricular arrhythmia and risk of sudden death in its early stages, and right ventricular or biventricular failure in its later stages.

Autosomal dominant ACM has been mapped to mutations in genes coding for desmosomal proteins. These are the cardiac ryanodine receptor RyR2 (also responsible for familial catecholaminergic polymorphic ventricular tachycardia, CPVT), desmoplakin, plakophillin-2 and mutations altering the regulatory sequences of the transforming growth factor-β gene.

There are two recessive forms: ***Naxos disease*** (associated with palmoplantar keratoderma and woolly hair), which is due to a mutation in junctional plakoglobin, and ***Carvajal syndrome***, due to a mutation in desmoplakin.

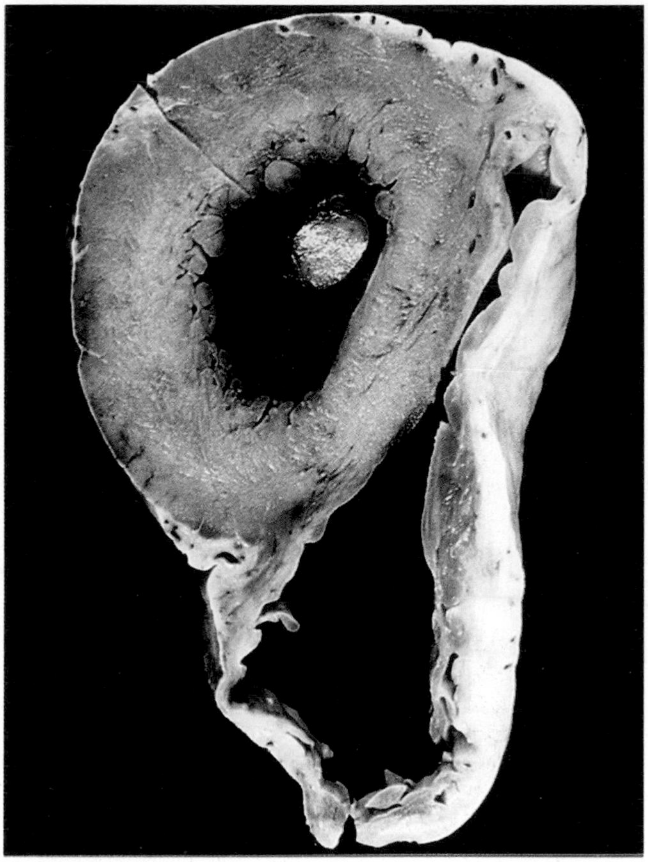

Figure 23.111 Gross pathological specimen demonstrating thinning and fibro-fatty replacement of the right ventricular free wall. *(From Basso C, Thiene G, Corrado D et al. Arrhythmogenic right ventricular cardiomyopathy. Dysplasia, dystrophy, or myocarditis?* Circulation *1996; 94:983–991, with permission.)*

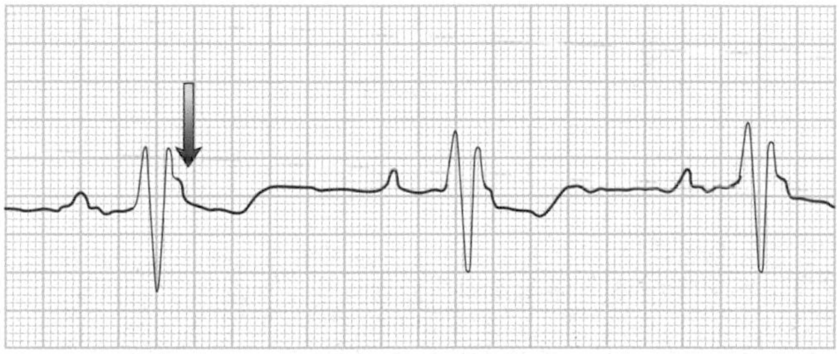

Figure 23.112 Electrocardiogram from an adult with arrhythmogenic cardiomyopathy. The ECG demonstrates right bundle branch block and precordial T-wave insertion, with epsilon waves visible at the terminal of the QRS complex (arrowed).

Clinical features

Most patients are asymptomatic. Symptomatic ventricular arrhythmia, syncope or sudden death occurs. Occasionally, presentation is with symptoms and signs of right heart failure, although this is more common in the later stages of the disease. Some patients may be detected through family screening, although frequently the morphological appearance of the right ventricle is normal, despite significant cardiac arrhythmias.

Investigations and diagnosis

- ***ECG*** is usually normal but may demonstrate T-wave inversion in the precordial leads related to the right ventricle (V_1–V_3). Small amplitude potentials occurring at the end of the QRS complex (epsilon waves) may be present ***(Fig. 23.112)***, and incomplete or complete right bundle branch block is sometimes seen. Signal-averaged ECG may indicate the presence of late potentials, and the delayed depolarization of individual muscle cells; 24-hour Holter monitoring may demonstrate frequent extrasystoles of right ventricular origin or runs of non-sustained ventricular tachycardia.
- ***Echocardiography*** is frequently normal but with more advanced cases may demonstrate right ventricular dilatation and aneurysm formation; there may be left ventricular dilatation.
- ***CMR*** can assess the right ventricle more accurately and in some cases can demonstrate fibro-fatty infiltration ***(Fig. 23.110)***.
- ***Genetic testing*** may soon be the diagnostic 'gold standard'.

Clinical diagnosis is made using Task Force Criteria, which include structural abnormalities of the right ventricle and right ventricular outflow tract (dilatation and abnormal wall motion on echocardiography or MRI), fibro-fatty replacement of myocytes on tissue biopsy, repolarization and conduction abnormalities on ECG

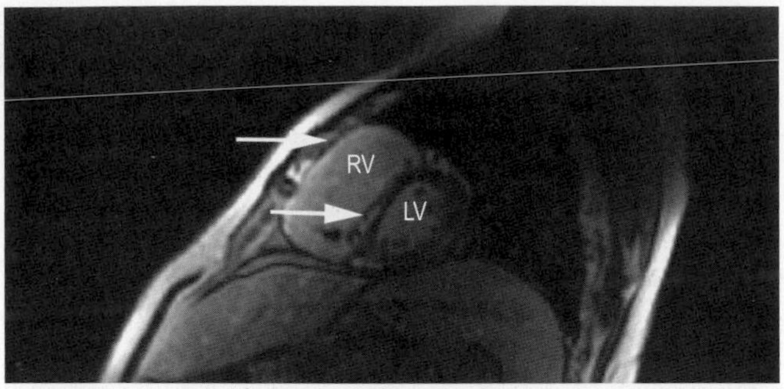

Figure 23.113 **Arrhythmogenic cardiomyopathy (ACM).** Inversion recovery magnetic resonance image post gadolinium demonstrates marked hyper-enhancement (arrowed) in the right ventricular free wall and infero-septum consistent with fibro-fatty replacement in right ventricle (RV) and left ventricle (LV)

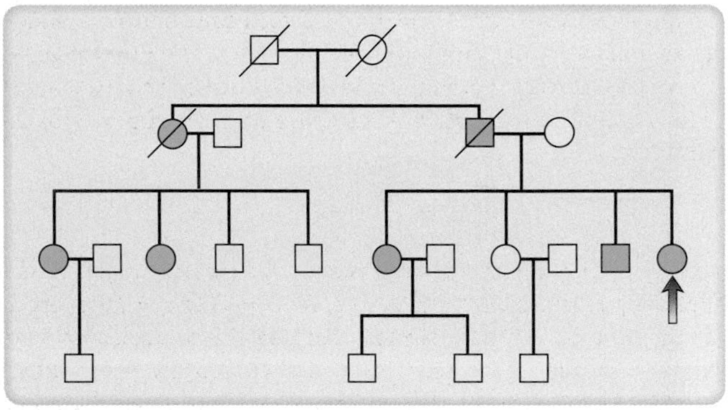

Figure 23.114 **Pedigree of a family with dilated cardiomyopathy.** Blue symbols are affected family members. The arrow indicates the index case.

or signal-averaged ECG, ventricular tachycardia or frequent ventricular extrasystoles on Holter monitoring, family history of ACM in a first- or second-degree relative, or premature sudden death (<35 years) due to ACM.

Management

Beta-blockers are first-line treatment for patients with non-life-threatening arrhythmias. Amiodarone or sotalol is used for symptomatic arrhythmias but for refractory or life-threatening arrhythmias an ICD is required. Occasionally, cardiac transplantation is indicated for either intractable arrhythmia or cardiac failure.

Dilated cardiomyopathy

Dilated cardiomyopathy (DCM) has a prevalence of 7–12 in 100 000 and is characterized by dilatation of the ventricular chambers and systolic dysfunction with preserved wall thickness.

Familial DCM is predominantly autosomal dominant and can be associated with over 20 abnormal loci and genes ***(Fig. 23.114)***. Many of these are genes encoding cytoskeletal or associated myocyte proteins (dystrophin in X-linked cardiomyopathy; actin, desmin, troponin T, β-myosin heavy chain, sarcoglycans, vinculin and lamin a/c in autosomal dominant DCM; ***Fig. 23.115***). Many of these have prominent associated features, such as skeletal myopathy or conduction system disease, and therefore differ from the majority of cases of DCM.

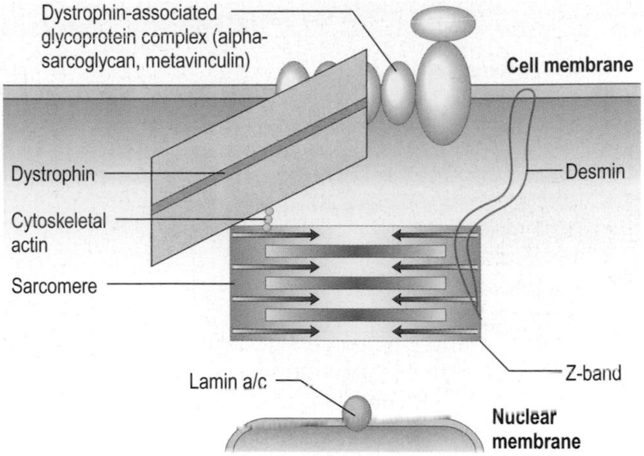

Figure 23.115 **Myocyte proteins implicated in dilated cardiomyopathy.**

Sporadic DCM can be caused by multiple conditions:

- myocarditis – Coxsackievirus, adenoviruses, erythroviruses, HIV, bacteria, fungi, mycobacteria, parasitic (Chagas' disease)
- toxins – alcohol, chemotherapy, metals (cobalt, lead, mercury, arsenic)
- autoimmune disorders
- endocrine disorders
- neuromuscular disorders.

Clinical features

DCM can present with heart failure, cardiac arrhythmias, conduction defects, thromboembolism or sudden death. Increasingly, evaluation of relatives of DCM patients is allowing identification of early asymptomatic disease, prior to the onset of these complications. Clinical evaluation should include a family history and construction of a pedigree where appropriate.

Investigations

- ***Chest X-ray*** demonstrates generalized cardiac enlargement.
- ***ECG*** may demonstrate diffuse non-specific ST-segment and T-wave changes. Sinus tachycardia, conduction abnormalities and arrhythmias (i.e. atrial fibrillation, ventricular premature contractions or ventricular tachycardia) are also seen.
- ***Echocardiogram*** reveals dilatation of the left and/or right ventricle with poor global contraction function ***(Fig. 23.116)***.
- ***CMR*** may demonstrate other aetiologies of left ventricular dysfunction (e.g. previous MI) or show abnormal myocardial fibrosis ***(Fig. 23.117)***.
- ***Coronary angiography*** should be performed to exclude coronary artery disease in all individuals at risk (generally, patients >40 years, or younger if symptoms or risk factors are present).
- ***Biopsy*** is not normally indicated outside specialist care.

Management

Treatment consists of the conventional management of heart failure with the option of cardiac resynchronization therapy and ICDs in patients with NYHA III/IV grading. Cardiac transplantation is appropriate for certain patients.

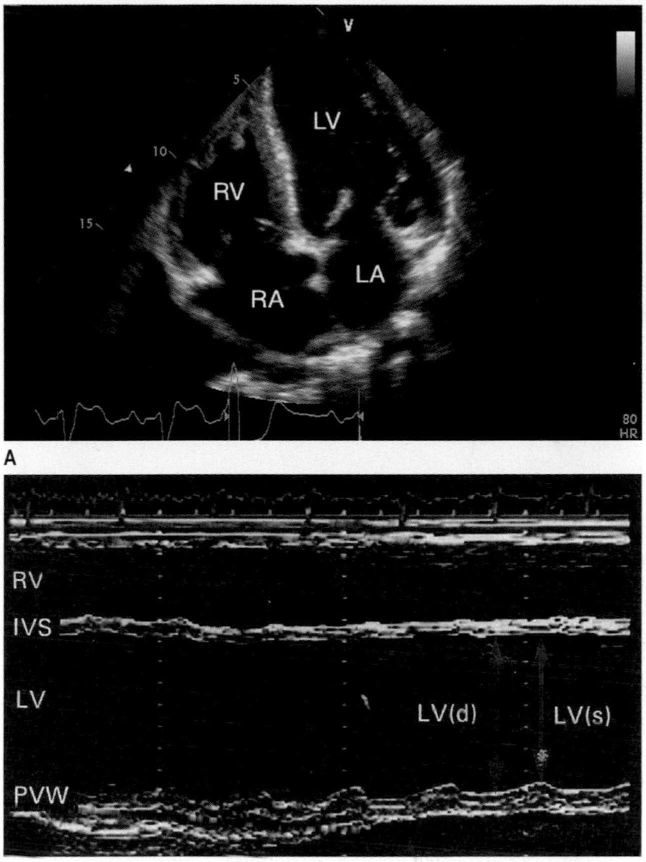

Figure 23.116 **Dilated cardiomyopathy. A.** *Two-dimensional (apical four-chamber view) echocardiogram.* **B.** *M-mode echocardiogram.* The heart has a 'globular' appearance with all four chambers dilated. The extremely impaired left ventricular function can be appreciated from the M-mode recording. Compare the systolic shortening fraction with that of Figure 23.23. IVS, interventricular septum; LA, left atrium; LV, left ventricle; LV(d), left ventricle (diastole); LV(s), left ventricle (systole); PVW, posterior ventricular wall; RA, right atrium.

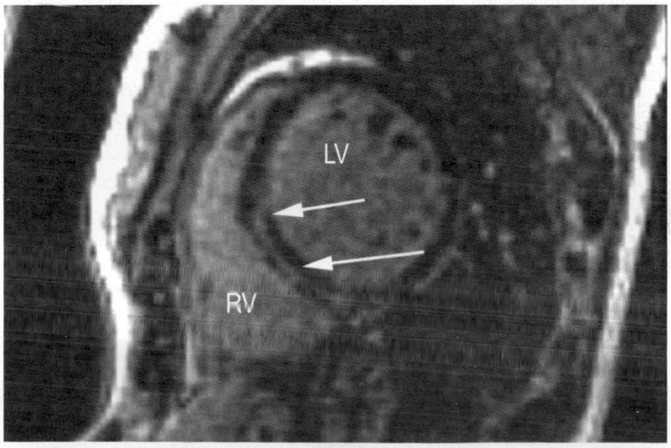

Figure 23.117 **Dilated cardiomyopathy.** Inversion recovery magnetic resonance scan post gadolinium demonstrates septal mid-wall hyper-enhancement (arrowed) consistent with fibrosis in a patient with dilated cardiomyopathy.

Left ventricular non-compaction

Left ventricular non-compaction (LVNC) is associated with a sponge-like appearance of the left ventricle. The condition predominantly affects the apical portion of the left ventricle and may be associated with congenital heart abnormalities. LVNC is diagnosed by echocardiography, CMR or left ventricular angiography. The natural history of the condition is unresolved but includes congestive cardiac failure, thromboembolism, cardiac arrhythmias and sudden death. Familial and spontaneous cases have been described.

Primary restrictive non-hypertrophic cardiomyopathy

This is a rare condition in which there is normal or decreased volume of both ventricles with bi-atrial enlargement, normal wall thickness, normal cardiac valves and impaired ventricular filling with restrictive physiology but near-normal systolic function. The restrictive physiology produces symptoms and signs of heart failure. Conditions associated with this form of cardiomyopathy include amyloidosis (most common), sarcoidosis, Loeffler's endocarditis and endomyocardial fibrosis; in the latter two conditions, there is myocardial and endocardial fibrosis, associated with eosinophilia. The idiopathic form of restrictive cardiomyopathy may be familial.

Clinical features

Patients with restrictive cardiomyopathy may present with dyspnoea, fatigue and embolic symptoms. On clinical examination, there will be elevated JVP with diastolic collapse (Friedreich's sign) and elevation of venous pressure with inspiration (Kussmaul's sign), hepatic enlargement, ascites and dependent oedema. Third and fourth heart sounds may be present.

Investigations

- ***Chest X-ray*** may show pulmonary venous congestion. The cardiac silhouette can be normal or show cardiomegaly and/or atrial enlargement.
- ***ECG*** may demonstrate low-voltage QRS and ST-segment and T-wave abnormalities.
- ***Echocardiography*** shows symmetrical myocardial thickening and often a normal systolic ejection fraction, but impaired ventricular filling. In amyloid patients, the myocardium typically appears speckled with absent radial thickening, as demonstrated by 'tramlines' on M-mode echocardiography ***(Fig. 23.118)***.
- ***CMR*** may demonstrate abnormal myocardial fibrosis in amyloidosis or sarcoidosis.
- ***Cardiac catheterization*** and haemodynamic studies may help distinguish between restrictive cardiomyopathy and constrictive pericarditis, although volume loading may be required.
- ***Endomyocardial biopsy*** in this condition is often useful, in contrast to other cardiomyopathies, and may permit a specific diagnosis, such as amyloidosis, to be made.

Management

There is no specific treatment. Cardiac failure and embolic manifestations should be treated. Cardiac transplantation is necessary in some severe cases, especially the idiopathic variety. In primary amyloidosis, combination therapy with melphalan plus prednisolone, with or without colchicine, may improve survival. However,

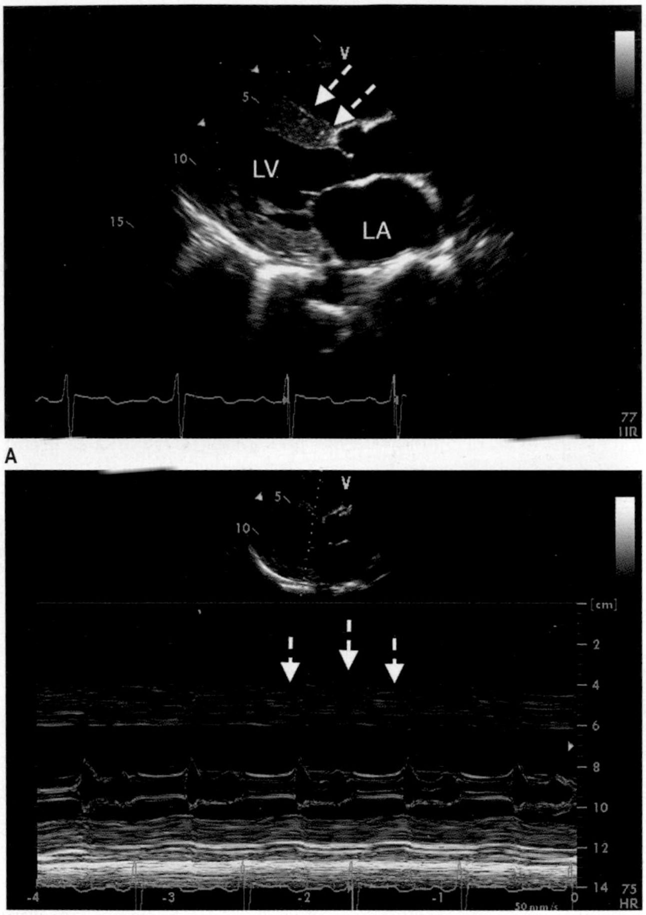

A

B

Figure 23.118 **Amyloid. A.** Parasternal long-axis echocardiogram demonstrating *left ventricular hypertrophy with reduced systolic function*. The septum has a speckled appearance (arrowed). **B.** M-mode echocardiogram demonstrates *reduced septal thickening with a 'tramline' appearance* (arrowed). These features are suggestive of cardiac amyloid – confirmed on cardiac biopsy. LA, left atrium; LV, left ventricle.

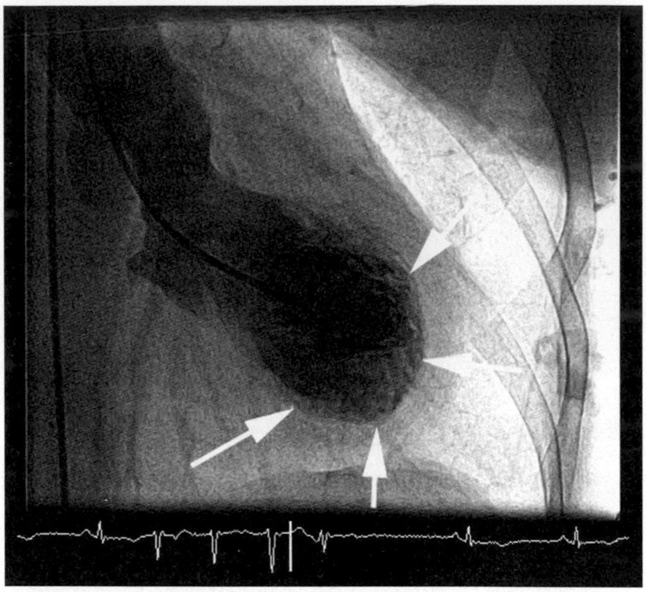

Figure 23.119 **Tako-tsubo cardiomyopathy.** Left ventricular angiography in a patient admitted with chest pain following emotional stress demonstrates apical ballooning (arrowed) consistent with Tako-tsubo cardiomyopathy. Diagnostic coronary angiography showed normal coronary arteries.

patients with cardiac amyloidosis have a worse prognosis than those with other forms of the disease, and the disease often recurs after transplantation. Liver transplantation may be effective in familial amyloidosis (due to production of mutant pre-albumin) and may lead to reversal of the cardiac abnormalities.

Acquired cardiomyopathies

Stress (Tako-tsubo/octopus pot/apical ballooning syndrome) cardiomyopathy

Patients with this condition present acutely with chest pain and breathlessness associated with ECG changes and elevated cardiac biomarkers consistent with acute MI. Diagnostic coronary angiography typically demonstrates unobstructed coronary arteries, with characteristic akinesia of the mid-apical segments of the left ventricle on ventriculography or echocardiography, and preserved basal function ***(Fig. 23.119)***. The pathophysiology is uncertain but disease may be due to transient catecholamine excess, coronary vasospasm, abnormalities of the coronary microcirculation and hypertrophy of the basal septum. The syndrome is more common in middle-aged to elderly women. Severe cases may have cardiogenic shock and pulmonary oedema. Patients with a significant left ventricular gradient may respond to cautious beta-blockade. Complete recovery of function is usual within 4–6 weeks but recurrences occur.

Peripartum cardiomyopathy

This rare condition affects women in the last trimester of pregnancy or within 5 months of delivery. It presents as a dilated cardiomyopathy, is more common in obese, multiparous women over 30 years old, and is associated with pre-eclampsia. Nearly half of patients will recover to normal function within 6 months but in some it can cause progressive heart failure and sudden death.

Tachycardia cardiomyopathy

Prolonged periods of supraventricular or ventricular tachycardia will lead to dilated cardiomyopathy. Cardioversion and ablation may be necessary to restore sinus rhythm and allow for recovery of cardiac function.

Further reading

Arbustini E, Narula N, Dec OW et al. The MOGE(S) classification for a phenotype-genotype nomenclature of cardiomyopathy. *J Am Coll Cardiol* 2013; 62:2046–2072.

Watkins H, Ashrafian H, Redwood C. Inherited cardiomyopathies. *N Engl J Med* 2011; 364:1643–1656.

PERICARDIAL DISEASE

The pericardium acts as a protective covering for the heart. It consists of an outer fibrous pericardial sac and an inner serous pericardium; the latter is made up of the inner visceral epicardium that lines the heart and great vessels, and its reflection, the outer parietal pericardium that lines the fibrous sac. The normal amount of

Box 23.55 Aetiology of pericarditis

I. Infectious pericarditis
  - Viral (Coxsackievirus, echovirus, mumps, herpes, HIV)
  - Bacterial (staphylococcal, streptococcal, pneumococcal and meningococcal infections, *Haemophilus influenzae*, mycoplasmosis, borreliosis, chlamydia)
  - Tuberculous
  - Fungal (histoplasmosis, coccidioidomycosis, candida)

II. Post-myocardial infarction pericarditis
  - Acute myocardial infarction (early)
  - Dressler syndrome (late)

III. Malignant pericarditis
  - Primary tumours of the heart (mesothelioma)
  - Metastatic pericarditis (breast and lung carcinoma, lymphoma, leukaemia, melanoma)

IV. Uraemic pericarditis

V. Myxoedematous pericarditis

VI. Chylopericardium

VII. Autoimmune pericarditis
  - Collagen-vascular (rheumatoid arthritis, rheumatic fever, systemic lupus erythematosus, scleroderma)
  - Drug-induced (procainamide, hydralazine, isoniazid, doxorubicin, cyclophosphamides)

VIII. Post-radiation pericarditis

IX. Post-surgical pericarditis
  - Post-pericardiotomy syndrome

X. Post-traumatic pericarditis

XI. Familial and idiopathic pericarditis

pericardial fluid is 20–49 mL and this fluid lubricates the surface of the heart. Presentations of pericardial disease include:

- acute and relapsing pericarditis
- pericardial effusion and cardiac tamponade
- constrictive pericarditis.

Acute pericarditis

This term refers to inflammation of the pericardium. Classically, fibrinous material is deposited into the pericardial space and pericardial effusion often occurs. Acute pericarditis has numerous aetiologies ***(Box 23.55)***, although, in most cases, a cause is not identified (idiopathic).

Viral pericarditis

The most common viral causes are Coxsackie B virus and echovirus. Viral pericarditis is usually painful but follows a short time course and rarely has long-term effects. Increasingly, HIV is implicated in the aetiology of pericarditis, both directly and via immunosuppression, which predisposes the subject to infective causes.

Bacterial pericarditis

This may rarely occur with septicaemia or pneumonia, may stem from an early postoperative infection after thoracic surgery or trauma, or may complicate endocarditis. *Staphylococcus aureus* is a frequent cause of purulent pericarditis in HIV patients. This form of pericarditis, especially staphylococcal, is fulminant and often fatal.

Other ***endemic infectious types of pericarditis*** include mycoplasmosis and Lyme pericarditis, which are often effusive and require pericardial drainage. The diagnosis is based on serological tests of pericardial fluid and identification of organisms in pericardial or myocardial biopsies.

Tuberculous pericarditis

This usually presents with chronic low-grade fever, particularly in the evening, associated with features of acute pericarditis, dyspnoea, malaise, night sweats and weight loss. Pericardial aspiration is often required to make the diagnosis. Constrictive pericarditis is a frequent outcome. Treatment is as for pulmonary tuberculosis (see pp. 1110–1113) with added prednisolone 60 mg daily for 2–6 weeks.

Fungal pericarditis

Pericarditis is a common complication of endemic fungal infections, such as histoplasmosis and coccidioidomycosis, but may be also caused by *Candida albicans*, especially in immunocompromised patients and drug addicts, or after cardiac surgery.

Post-myocardial infarction pericarditis

This occurs in about 20% of patients in the first few days following MI. It is more common with anterior MI and STEMI with high serum cardiac enzymes, but its incidence is reduced to 5–6% with thrombolysis. It may be difficult to differentiate this pain from recurrent angina when it occurs early (day 1–2 post infarct) but a good history of the pain and serial ECG monitoring are helpful. Pericarditis may also be present later on in the recovery phase after infarction. It is usually a feature of ***Dressler syndrome***, an autoimmune response to cardiac damage occurring 2–10 weeks' post infarct. Autoimmune reaction to myocardial damage is the main aetiology, and antimyocardial antibodies can often be found. Recurrences are common. Differential diagnosis includes new MI or unstable angina.

Malignant pericarditis

Carcinoma of the bronchus, ***carcinoma of the breast*** and ***Hodgkin's lymphoma*** are the most common causes of malignant pericarditis. Leukaemia and malignant melanoma are also associated with pericarditis. A substantial pericardial effusion is very typical and is due to obstruction of the lymphatic drainage from the heart. The effusion is often haemorrhagic. Radiation and therapy for thoracic tumours may cause radiation injury to the pericardium, resulting in serous or haemorrhagic pericardial effusion and pericardial fibrosis. Absence of neoplastic cells in the pericardial fluid in these conditions often helps diagnosis.

Uraemic pericarditis

This is due to irritation of the pericardium by accumulating toxins. It can occur in 6–10% of patients with advanced kidney disease if dialysis is delayed. It is an indication for urgent dialysis, as it continues to be associated with significant morbidity and mortality.

Clinical features

Pericardial inflammation produces sharp central ***chest pain*** that is exacerbated by movement, respiration and lying down. It is typically relieved by sitting forwards. It may be referred to the neck or shoulders. The main differential diagnoses are angina and pleurisy. The classical clinical sign is a pericardial friction rub occurring in three phases that correspond to atrial systole, ventricular systole and ventricular diastole. It may also be heard as a biphasic 'to-and-fro' rub. The rub is heard best with the diaphragm of the stethoscope at the lower left sternal edge at the end of expiration with the patient leaning forwards. There is usually a ***fever***, ***leucocytosis*** or ***lymphocytosis*** when pericarditis is due to viral or bacterial infection, rheumatic fever or MI. Features of a pericardial effusion may also be present. Large ***pericardial effusion*** can compress adjacent bronchi and lung tissue and may cause ***dyspnoea***.

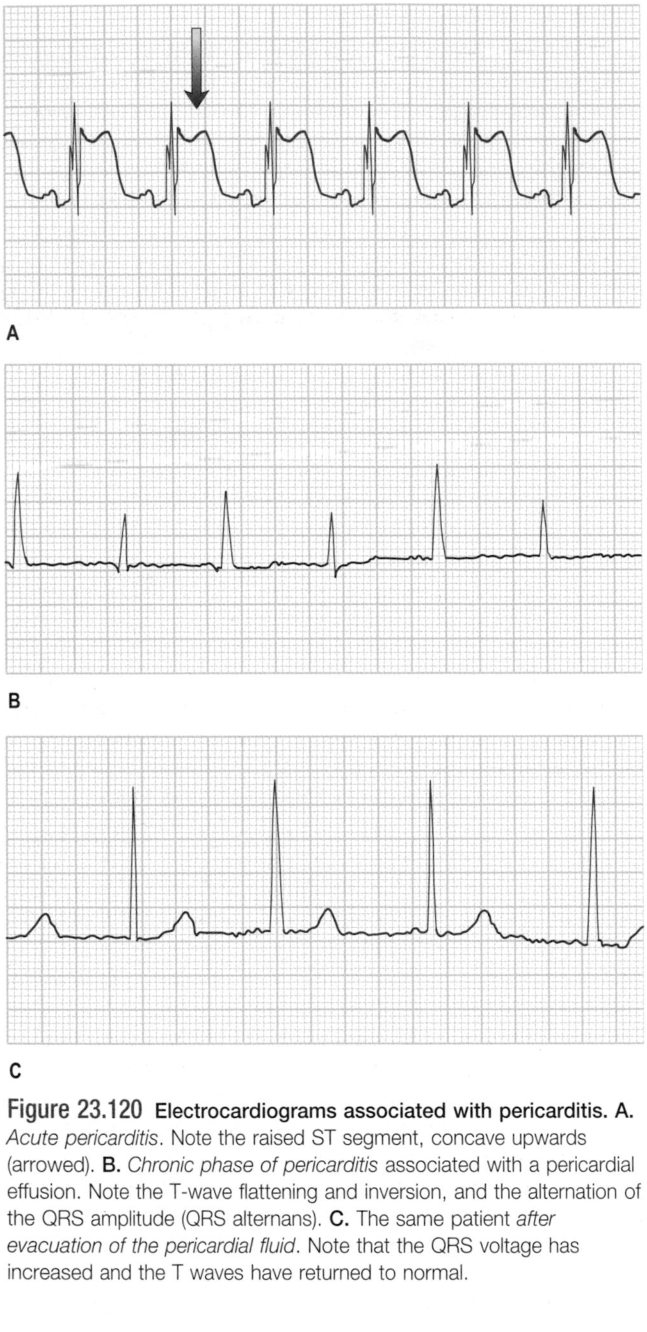

Figure 23.120 Electrocardiograms associated with pericarditis. A. *Acute pericarditis*. Note the raised ST segment, concave upwards (arrowed). **B.** *Chronic phase of pericarditis* associated with a pericardial effusion. Note the T-wave flattening and inversion, and the alternation of the QRS amplitude (QRS alternans). **C.** The same patient *after evacuation of the pericardial fluid*. Note that the QRS voltage has increased and the T waves have returned to normal.

Investigations

ECG is diagnostic. There is widespread concave-upwards (saddle-shaped) ST elevation ***(Fig. 23.120)***, reciprocal ST depression in leads AVR and V_1, and PR segment depression. These changes evolve over time, with resolution of the ST elevation, T-wave flattening/inversion and, finally, T-wave normalization. The early ECG changes must be differentiated from the ST elevation found in MI, which is limited to the infarcted area: for example, anterior or inferior. Sinus tachycardia may result from fever or haemodynamic embarrassment, and rhythm and conduction abnormalities may be present if myocardium is involved. Cardiac enzymes may be elevated if there is associated myocarditis (see pp. 1036–1037). Chest X-ray may demonstrate cardiomegaly (in cases with an effusion), which should be confirmed with echocardiography. CT and CMR may be helpful in cases with thickened (>4 mm) or inflamed (abnormal delayed enhancement) pericardium.

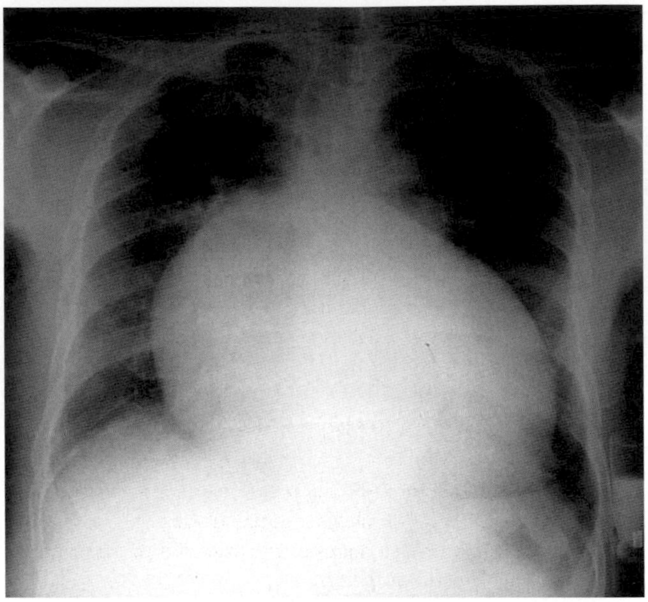

Figure 23.121 Chest X-ray showing a pericardial effusion. The heart appears globular.

Management

If a cause is found, this should be treated. Bed rest and oral NSAIDs (high-dose aspirin, indometacin or ibuprofen) are effective in most patients. Aspirin is the drug of choice for patients with a recent MI. Colchicine is also effective in combination with conventional therapy, as demonstrated in the COPE trial. Corticosteroids should be reserved for patients with a known immune cause, as their use is associated with an increased rate of recurrence.

Recurrent or relapsing pericarditis

About 20% of cases of acute pericarditis go on to develop idiopathic relapsing pericarditis, which may be incessant (recurring within 6 weeks during weaning off NSAIDs) or intermittent (recurs >6 weeks after the initial presentation). The first-line treatment is, again, oral NSAIDs. The trial of colchicine as first-choice therapy for recurrent pericarditis demonstrated that prolonged colchicine (for 6 months) was more effective than aspirin alone in reducing recurrence. In resistant cases, oral corticosteroids may be effective, and in some patients, pericardiectomy may be appropriate.

Pericardial effusion and cardiac tamponade

A pericardial effusion is a collection of fluid within the potential space of the serous pericardial sac ***(Fig. 23.121)***; it commonly accompanies an episode of acute pericarditis. When a large volume collects in this space, ventricular filling is compromised, leading to embarrassment of the circulation. This is known as cardiac tamponade.

Clinical features

Symptoms of a pericardial effusion commonly reflect the underlying pericarditis. On examination:

- Heart sounds are soft and distant.
- Apex beat is commonly obscured.
- A friction rub may be evident due to pericarditis in the early stages, but this becomes quieter as fluid accumulates and pushes the layers of the pericardium apart.

- Rarely, the effusion may compress the base of the left lung, producing an area of dullness to percussion below the angle of the left scapula (Ewart's sign).
- As the effusion worsens, signs of cardiac tamponade may become evident:
  - Raised JVP with sharp rise and y descent (Friedreich's sign)
  - Kussmaul's sign (rise in JVP/increased neck vein distension during inspiration)
  - Pulsus paradoxus (an exaggeration in the normal variation in pulse pressure seen with inspiration, such that there is a drop in systolic blood pressure of ≥10 mmHg)
  - Reduced cardiac output.

Investigations

- ***ECG*** reveals low-voltage QRS complexes (<0.5 mV in limb leads) with sinus tachycardia and there may be electric alternans (alteration of QRS amplitude or axis between beats).
- ***Chest X-ray (Fig. 23.121)*** shows a large, globular or pear-shaped heart with sharp outlines. Typically, the pulmonary veins are not distended.
- ***Echocardiography (Fig. 23.122)*** is the most useful technique for demonstrating the effusion and looking for evidence of tamponade – late diastolic collapse of the right atrium, early diastolic collapse of the right ventricle, ventricular septum displacement into the left ventricle during inspiration, diastolic flow reversal in the hepatic veins during expiration, dilated inferior vena cava with <50% reduction during inspiration.
- ***Cardiac CT or MRI*** is helpful if loculated pericardial effusions are suspected (post cardiac surgery).
- ***Pericardiocentesis*** is the removal of pericardial fluid with an aseptic technique under echocardiographic guidance (see ***Fig. 23.26***). It is indicated when a tuberculous, malignant or purulent effusion is suspected.
- ***Pericardial biopsy*** may be needed if tuberculosis is suspected and pericardiocentesis is not diagnostic.

Other tests may be needed to identify underlying causes: for example, blood cultures or autoantibody screen.

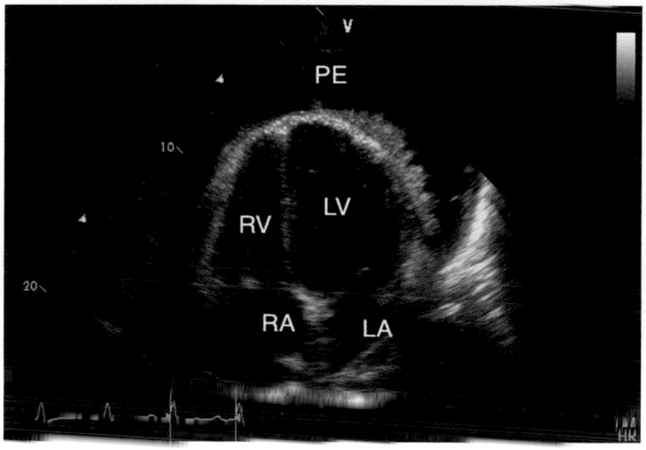

Figure 23.122 Two-dimensional echocardiogram (short-axis view) from a patient with a large pericardial effusion associated with pulmonary tuberculosis. The exudate is seen between the visceral and parietal layers of the pericardium and would give a false impression of cardiomegaly on a chest X-ray. Note the multiple fibrous strands within the effusion, showing that it is consolidating and will probably lead to constriction of cardiac function. LA, left atrium; LV, left ventricle; PE, pericardial effusion; RA, right atrium; RV, right ventricle.

Management

An underlying cause should be sought and treated if possible. Most pericardial effusions resolve spontaneously. However, when the effusion collects rapidly, tamponade may result. Pericardiocentesis is then indicated to relieve the pressure; a drain may be left in place temporarily to allow sufficient release of fluid. Pericardial effusions may re-accumulate, most commonly due to malignancy (in the UK). This may require pericardial fenestration: that is, creation of a window in the pericardium to allow the slow release of fluid into the surrounding tissues. This procedure may be performed either transcutaneously under local anaesthetic or using a conventional surgical approach.

Constrictive pericarditis

Certain causes of pericarditis, such as tuberculosis, haemopericardium, bacterial infection and rheumatic heart disease, result in the pericardium becoming thick, fibrous and calcified. This may also develop late after open heart surgery, and fibrosis also occurs with the use of dopamine agonists, such as cabergoline and pergolide. In many cases, these pericardial changes do not cause any symptoms. If, however, the pericardium becomes so inelastic as to interfere with diastolic filling of the heart, constrictive pericarditis is said to have developed. As these changes are chronic, allowing the body time to compensate, this condition is not as immediately life-threatening as cardiac tamponade, in which the circulation is more acutely embarrassed.

Constrictive pericarditis should be distinguished from restrictive cardiomyopathy (see pp. 1041–1042). The two conditions are very similar in their presentation, but the former is fully treatable, whereas most cases of the latter are not. In the later stages of constrictive pericarditis, the sub-epicardial layers of myocardium may undergo fibrosis, atrophy and calcification.

Clinical features

The symptoms and signs of constrictive pericarditis occur due to:

- reduced ventricular filling (similar to cardiac tamponade, i.e. Kussmaul's sign, Friedreich's sign, pulsus paradoxus)
- systemic venous congestion (ascites, dependent oedema, hepatomegaly and raised JVP)
- pulmonary venous congestion (dyspnoea, cough, orthopnoea, paroxysmal nocturnal dyspnoea), less commonly
- reduced cardiac output (fatigue, hypotension, reflex tachycardia)
- rapid ventricular filling ('pericardial knock' heard in early diastole at the lower left sternal border)
- atrial dilatation (30% of cases have atrial fibrillation).

Investigations

- ***Chest X-ray*** shows a relatively small heart in view of the symptoms of heart failure. Pericardial calcification may be present in up to 50%. A lateral chest film may be useful for detecting calcification that is missed on a postero-anterior film. However, a calcified pericardium is not necessarily a constricted one.
- ***ECG*** reveals low-voltage QRS complexes with generalized T-wave flattening or inversion.
- ***Echocardiography*** shows thickened, calcified pericardium, and small ventricular cavities with normal wall thickness. Doppler studies may be useful.
- ***CT and CMR*** are used to assess pericardial anatomy and thickness (≥4 mm) (see ***Fig. 23.28***).

- ***Endomyocardial biopsy*** may be helpful in distinguishing constrictive pericarditis from restrictive cardiomyopathy in difficult cases.
- ***Cardiac catheterization*** will usually reveal equal end-diastolic pressures in the left and right ventricles, owing to pericardial constriction.

Restrictive cardiomyopathy is a close mimic of constrictive pericarditis and all the above tests may help to distinguish the two conditions.

Management

The treatment for chronic constrictive pericarditis is complete resection of the pericardium. This is a risky procedure with a high complication rate due to the presence of myocardial atrophy in many cases at the time of surgery. Thus, early pericardiectomy is suggested in non-tuberculous cases, before severe constriction and myocardial atrophy have developed.

In cases of tuberculous constriction, the presence of pericardial calcification implies chronic disease. Early pericardiectomy with antituberculous drug cover is used in these cases. If there is no calcification, a course of antituberculous therapy should be attempted first. If the patient's haemodynamic state remains static or deteriorates after 4–6 weeks of therapy, pericardiectomy is recommended.

Further reading

Khandaker MH, Espinosa RE, Nishimura RA et al. Pericardial disease: diagnosis and management. *Mayo Clin Proc* 2010; 85:572–593.
Syed FF, Schaff HV, Oh JK. Constrictive pericarditis – a curable diastolic heart failure. *Nat Rev Cardiol* 2014; 11:530–544.
Yusuf S, Cairns JA, Camm AJ et al (eds). Pericardial disease. In: *Evidence-Based Cardiology*, 3rd edn. London: BMJ Books; 2011.

SYSTEMIC HYPERTENSION

High blood pressure (hypertension) is a major cause of premature vascular disease, leading to cerebrovascular events, ischaemic heart disease and peripheral vascular disease. Blood pressure (BP) is normally distributed in the population and mortality rises with increasing BP. The prevalence of hypertension may be 30–45% of the general population.

Diagnosis

BP should be measured in a quiet room; the patient should be seated, with an outstretched and supported arm. An automated machine with an appropriate cuff size is recommended. If postural hypotension (reduction in systolic BP of ≥20 mmHg) is suspected, then BP should be repeated after 1 minute of standing. In the UK, NICE recommends that ambulatory blood pressure monitoring (ABPM) is offered to patients with a clinic BP of ≥140/90 mmHg to confirm the diagnosis of hypertension. Home blood pressure monitoring (HBPM) can also be used.

- ***Stage 1 hypertension*** – clinic BP ≥140/90 mmHg and daytime average ABPM or HBPM ≥135/85 mmHg.
- ***Stage 2 hypertension*** – clinic BP ≥160/100 mmHg and daytime average ABPM or HBPM ≥150/95 mmHg.
- ***Severe hypertension*** – clinic systolic BP ≥180 mmHg and/or diastolic BP ≥110 mmHg.

Patients with a diagnosis of hypertension should have their cardiovascular risk assessed using an appropriate calculator. NICE recommends QRISK®2-2015 but the European Society of Cardiology/European Association for Cardiovascular Prevention and Rehabilitation's 'Heartscore' is an alternative.

Investigations

- ***Urinalysis*** for protein, albumin : creatinine ratio and haematuria.
- ***Blood tests*** for glucose, electrolytes, creatinine, estimated glomerular filtration rate (eGFR), and total and HDL cholesterol.
- ***Fundoscopy*** to detect hypertensive retinopathy:
  - Grade 1 – tortuosity of the retinal arteries with increased reflectiveness (silver wiring)
  - Grade 2 – grade 1 plus the appearance of arteriovenous nipping, produced when thickened retinal arteries pass over the retinal veins
  - Grade 3 – grade 2 plus flame-shaped haemorrhages and soft ('cotton wool') exudates due to small infarcts
  - Grade 4 – grade 3 plus papilloedema (blurring of the optic disc; ***Fig. 23.123***).
- ***A 12-lead ECG*** to detect left ventricular hypertrophy (see ***Fig. 23.79***).

The clinical history and examination may suggest a secondary cause of hypertension ***(Box 23.56)***, and referral to a specialist for specific investigations is recommended.

Management

Lifestyle intervention

The following lifestyle changes are recommended in patients with hypertension:

- ***diet***: high consumption of vegetables and fruits and low-fat diet
- ***regular physical exercise*** (30 min of moderate-intensity aerobic exercise 5–7 days/week)
- ***reduction of alcohol intake*** (<140 g/week men, <80 g/week women)
- ***reduction of dietary sodium intake*** (5–6 g/day) and use of low-sodium salt

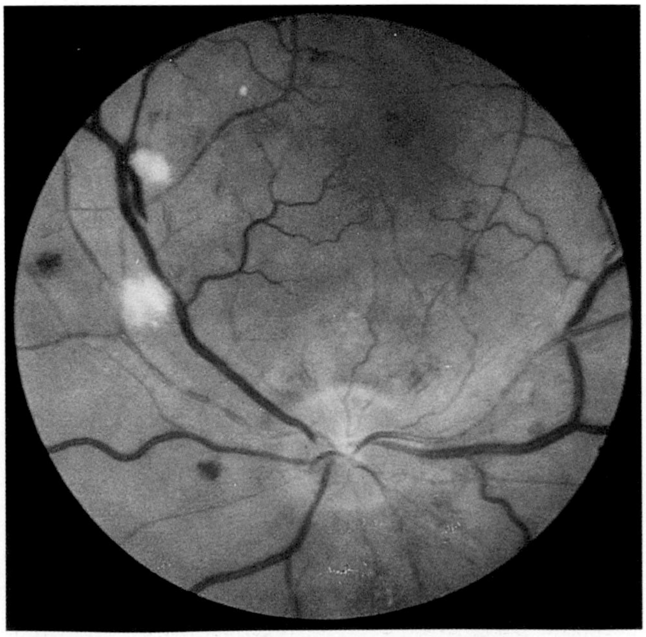

Figure 23.123 Fundus showing hypertensive changes. There is grade 4 retinopathy with papilloedema, haemorrhages and exudates.

Box 23.56 European Society of Cardiology clinical indications and diagnostics of secondary hypertension

Cause	Clinical history	Physical examination	Laboratory investigations	First-line tests	Additional tests
Common causes					
Renal parenchymal disease	History of urinary tract infection or obstruction, haematuria, analgesic abuse, family history of polycystic kidney disease	Abdominal masses (polycystic kidney disease)	Protein, erythrocytes or leucocytes in urine, decreased GFR	Renal ultrasound	Detailed work-up for kidney disease
Renal artery stenosis	Fibromuscular dysplasia: early-onset hypertension (especially in women) Atherosclerotic stenosis: abrupt-onset hypertension, worsening or difficult to treat; flash pulmonary oedema	Abdominal bruit	Difference of >1.5 cm in length between the two kidneys (renal ultrasound), rapid deterioration in renal function (spontaneous or in response to RAA blockers)	Renal duplex Doppler ultrasonography	MR angiography, spiral CT, intra-arterial digital subtraction angiography
Primary aldosteronism	Muscle weakness; family history of early-onset hypertension and cerebrovascular events age <40 years	Arrhythmias (if severe hypokalaemia)	Hypokalaemia (spontaneous or diuretic-induced); incidental discovery of adrenal masses	Aldosterone : renin ratio under standardized conditions (correction of hypokalaemia and withdrawal of drugs affecting RAA system)	Confirmatory tests (oral sodium loading, saline infusion, fludrocortisone suppression, or captopril test); adrenal CT scan; adrenal vein sampling
Uncommon causes					
Phaeochromocytoma	Paroxysmal hypertension; headache, sweating, palpitations, pallor; positive family history	Skin stigmata of neurofibromatosis (café-au-lait spots, neurofibromas)	Incidental discovery of adrenal (or in some cases, extra-adrenal) masses	Measurement of urinary fractionated metanephrines or plasma-free metanephrines	CT or MRI of abdomen and pelvis; ^{123}I-labelled meta-iodobenzyl guanidine scanning; genetic screening for pathogenic mutations
Cushing's syndrome	Weight gain, polyuria, polydipsia, psychological disturbances	Typical body habitus (central obesity, moon face, buffalo hump, red striae, hirsutism)	Hyperglycaemia	24-h urinary cortisol excretion	Dexamethasone suppression tests

CT, computed tomography; GFR, glomerular filtration rate; MRI, magnetic resonance imaging; RAA, renin–angiotensin–aldosterone.
(From The Task Force for the management of arterial hypertension of the European Society of Hypertension (ESH) and of the European Society of Cardiology (ESC). 2013 ESH/ESC Guidelines for the management of arterial hypertension. *Eur Heart J* 2013; 34:2159–2219 (Table 13), with permission. http://eurheartj.oxfordjournals.org/content/ehj/34/28/2159.full.pdf.)

- ***smoking cessation***
- ***weight reduction*** (BMI 25 kg/m^2, waist circumference <102 cm men, <88 cm women).

Pharmacological therapy

NICE guidance ***(Fig. 23.124)*** recommends that treatment should be offered to all people under 80 years of age with stage 1 hypertension and at least one of the following risk factors:

- target organ damage ***(Fig. 23.125)***
- cardiovascular disease
- renal disease
- diabetes
- 10-year cardiovascular risk ≥20%.

Patients under 40 years old with no risk factors should be referred to a specialist to exclude secondary causes of hypertension. All patients with stage 2 hypertension should be offered treatment. Using clinic BP, the target for treated patients is <140/90 mmHg in patients below 80 years of age, and <150/90 mmHg in patients of 80 years and above. In patients with 'white-coat' hypertension ***(Fig. 23.126)***, ABPM or HBPM may be more appropriate, with targets of <135/85 mmHg (below 80 years) and <145/85 mmHg (80 years and above). A recent study (SPRINT) found that in patients with hypertension but without diabetes, reducing systolic BP to a target of <120 mmHg reduced the rates of fatal and non-fatal cardiovascular events and death from any cause. A more recent study suggests a systolic BP of <130 mmHg is optimal in people with co-morbidities of renal, cardiovascular diseases and diabetes.

Step 1

First-line therapy for patients under 55 years is an ACE inhibitor such as enalapril or a low-cost ARB, such as candesartan. In young women of childbearing potential, treatment with beta-blockers may be preferred ***(Box 23.57)***. Patients aged 55 years and above, and black African or Caribbean patients, should be treated with a calcium-channel blocker, such as amlodipine (a thiazide-like diuretic should be used in patients with heart failure or those who develop troublesome ankle oedema).

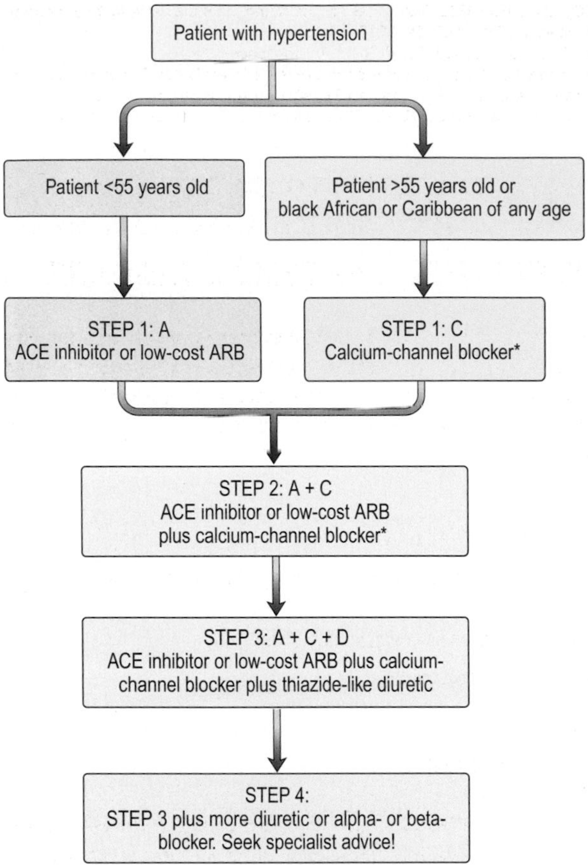

Figure 23.124 Hypertension treatment algorithm. *Thiazide-like diuretic if a calcium-channel blocker is not tolerated or is contraindicated. ACE, angiotensin-converting enzyme; ARB, angiotensin receptor blocker. *(From National Institute for Health and Care Excellence 2011 CG127* Hypertension: The Clinical Management of Primary Hypertension in Adults. *London: NICE, with permission.)*

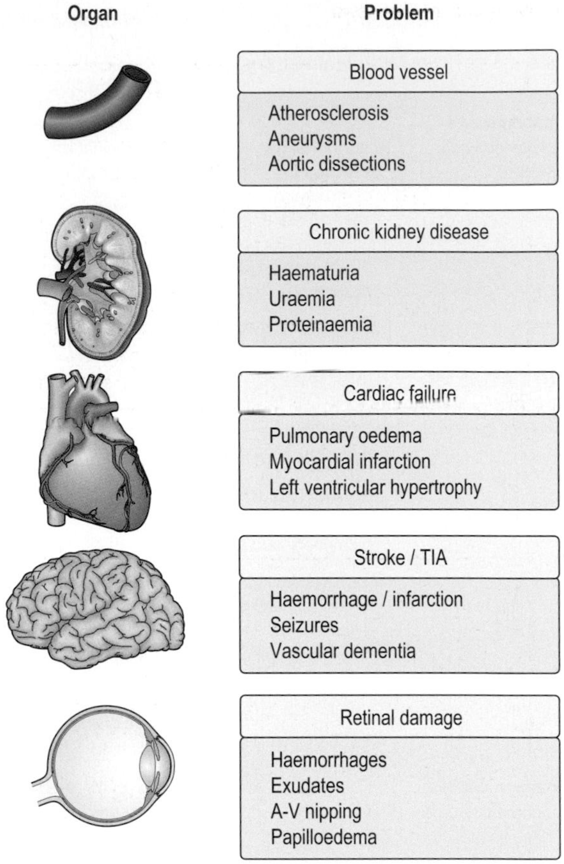

Figure 23.125 Target organ damage in hypertension. A-V, arteriovenous; TIA, transient ischaemic attack.

Step 2

If BP control is inadequate, then the combination of an ACE-inhibitor or ARB with a calcium-channel blocker is recommended (or a thiazide-like diuretic as above).

Step 3

At this point, therapy should be reviewed (including compliance and optimal dosage). Triple therapy of an ACE inhibitor or ARB with a calcium-channel blocker and a thiazide-like diuretic is recommended.

Step 4

If BP remains >140/90 mmHg on three agents, then the patient should be referred for specialist advice. In those with preserved renal function and resistant hypertension, spironolactone 25 mg daily can be added if the serum potassium is ≤4.5 mmol/L. If the potassium is >4.5 mmol/L, an increased dose of thiazide-like diuretic can be used with monitoring of electrolytes. Alpha- or beta-blockers can be used if these measures are not effective.

Management of severe or malignant hypertension

Patients with severe hypertension (diastolic pressure >140 mmHg), malignant hypertension (grade 3 or 4 retinopathy) and hypertensive encephalopathy or those with severe hypertensive complications, such as cardiac failure, should be admitted to hospital for immediate initiation of treatment. However, it is unwise to reduce the BP too rapidly, since this may lead to cerebral, renal and retinal ischaemia or MI, and the BP response to therapy must be carefully monitored, preferably in a high-dependency unit. In most cases, the aim is to reduce the diastolic BP to 100–110 mmHg over 24–48 hours. This is usually achieved with oral medication, such as amlodipine. The BP can then be normalized over the next 2–3 days. When rapid control of BP is required (e.g. in an aortic dissection), the agent of choice is intravenous sodium nitroprusside. Alternatively, an infusion of labetalol can be used. The infusion dosage must be titrated against the BP response.

Management of resistant hypertension

A patient with resistant hypertension is defined as having inadequate BP control on three or more antihypertensive drugs. Following investigations for any underlying cause, endovascular renal denervation of the sympathetic nerves, performed with a single electrode radio-frequency catheter, has shown to be effective in further reduction of BP, although results are variable.

Hypertension in pregnancy

See page 1302.

Further reading

Ettehad D, Emdin CA, Kiran A et al. Blood pressure lowering for prevention of cardiovascular disease and death: a systematic review and meta-analysis. *Lancet* 2016; 387:957–967.

Haller H, Ito S, Izzo JL Jr et al and ROADMAP Trial Investigators. Olmesartan for the delay or prevention of microalbuminuria in type 2 diabetes. *N Engl J Med* 2011; 364:907–917.

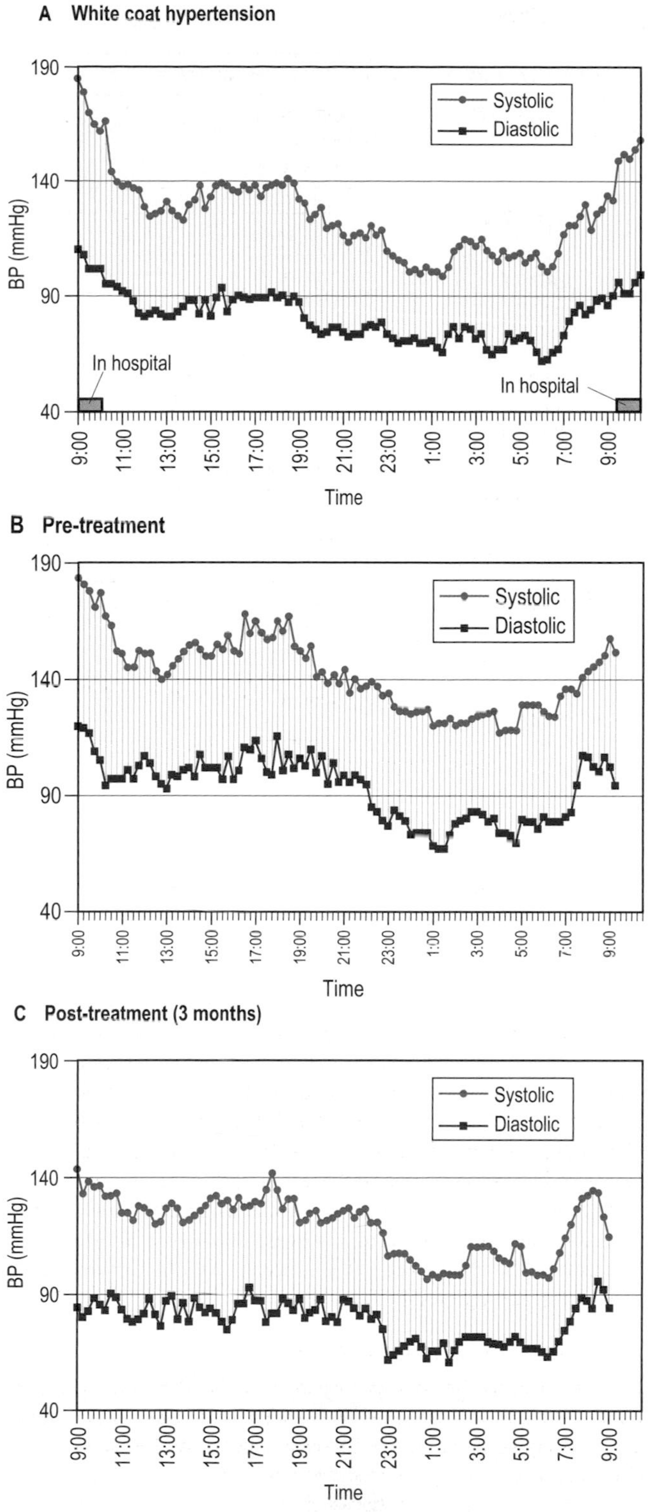

Figure 23.126 Twenty-four-hour ambulatory blood pressure monitoring. A, White-coat hypertension. B, Before treatment. C, After 3 months' treatment.

National Institute for Health and Care Excellence. *NICE Clinical Guideline 127. Hypertension: Clinical Management of Primary Hypertension in Adults*. NICE 2011; https://www.nice.org.uk/guidance/cg127.

Perkovic V, Rodgers A. Redefining blood-pressure targets--SPRINT starts the marathon. *N Engl J Med* 2015; 373:2175–2178.

Poulter NR, Prabhakaran D, Caulfield M. Hypertension. *Lancet* 2015; 386:801–812.

Task Force for the Management of Arterial Hypertension of the European Society of Hypertension (ESH) and of the European Society of Cardiology (ESC). 2013 ESH/ESC Guidelines for the management of arterial hypertension. *Eur Heart J* 2013; 34:2159–2219.

http://www.bhsoc.org/ *British Hypertension Society.*

http://www.heartscore.org *European Society of Cardiology/European Association for Cardiovascular Prevention and Rehabilitation's 'Heartscore' tool.*

http://www.qrisk.org *QRISK®2-2015 cardiovascular disease risk calculator.*

PERIPHERAL VASCULAR DISEASE

PERIPHERAL ARTERIAL DISEASE

Peripheral vascular disease (PVD) is commonly caused by atherosclerosis and usually affects the aorto-iliac or infra-inguinal arteries. It is present in 7% of middle-aged men and 4.5% of middle-aged women, but these patients are more likely to die of MI or stroke than lose their leg.

Limb ischaemia

Limb ischaemia may be classified as chronic or acute.

Chronic lower limb ischaemia

Common risk factors are:

- smoking
- diabetes
- hypercholesterolaemia
- hypertension.

Premature atherosclerosis in patients aged <45 years may be associated with thrombophilia and hyperhomocysteinaemia.

Clinical features

Symptoms

Peripheral arterial disease can be described using the Fontaine classification:

- Stage I – asymptomatic
- Stage II – intermittent claudication
- Stage III – rest pain/nocturnal pain
- Stage IV – necrosis/gangrene.

Patients with ***intermittent claudication*** complain of exertional discomfort, most commonly in the calf, which is relieved by rest. Patients with aorto-iliac disease may experience pain in the buttock, hip or thigh and may notice erectile dysfunction. The 'claudication distance' may be reproducible.

Patients with ***rest pain*** experience severe, unremitting pain in the foot, which stops a patient from sleeping. It is partially relieved by dangling the foot over the edge of the bed or standing on a cold floor.

Patients with severe PVD or critical lower limb ischaemia may have ulceration or ***necrosis*** of the tissue (***gangrene***).

Signs

The lower limbs are cold with dry skin and lack of hair. Pulses may be diminished or absent. Ulceration may occur in association with dark discoloration of the toes or gangrene. The abdomen should be examined for a possible aneurysm.

Differential diagnosis

Symptoms may be confused with those of:

- spinal canal claudication (but all pulses are present)
- osteoarthritis hip/knee (knee pain often at rest)

Box 23.57 Pharmacological therapy in hypertension

Drug	Dose	Conditions favouring use	Cautions/contraindications
Alpha-blockers			
Doxazosin	1.0–16 mg daily	Benign prostatic hypertrophy	Postural hypotension, urinary incontinence
Indoramin	25–100 mg ×2 daily		
Phenoxybenzamine	1 mg/kg i.v. over >2 h	Phaeochromocytoma crisis	Profound hypotension
Phentolamine	2.0–5.0 mg i.v.		
Aldosterone antagonists			
Spironolactone	50–400 mg daily	Primary hyperaldosteronism, heart failure	Hyperkalaemia
Eplerenone	50–100 mg daily		
Angiotensin-converting enzyme inhibitors			
Enalapril	5.0–40 mg daily	<55 years old, Caucasian, heart failure or left ventricular dysfunction, myocardial infarction or cardiovascular disease, diabetic nephropathy, chronic kidney disease, stroke secondary prevention	Renal failure (monitor electrolytes), peripheral vascular disease (if renovascular disease), pregnancy
Lisinopril	2.5–40 mg daily		
Perindopril	2.0–8.0 mg daily		
Ramipril	1.25–10 mg daily		
Angiotensin II receptor blockers			
Losartan	50–100 mg daily	ACE inhibitor-intolerant, <55 years old, Caucasian, hypertension with left ventricular hypertrophy, heart failure or left ventricular dysfunction, myocardial infarction, diabetic nephropathy, chronic kidney disease	Renal failure (monitor electrolytes), peripheral vascular disease (if renovascular disease), pregnancy
Candesartan	2.0–32 mg daily		
Valsartan	40–320 mg daily		
Olmesartan	10–40 mg daily		
Telmisartan	40 mg daily		
Beta-blockers			
Atenolol	25–100 mg daily	Coronary heart disease (post myocardial infarction or angina), heart failure (bisoprolol and carvedilol)	Diabetes, peripheral vascular disease, asthma/chronic obstructive pulmonary disease, heart block, unstable heart failure
Bisoprolol	1.25–20 mg daily		
Carvedilol	12.5–50 mg daily		
Labetalol	100–200 mg ×2 daily (max. 2.4 g/day)	Hypertension in pregnancy	
Calcium-channel blockers			
Amlodipine	5.0–10 mg daily	>55 years, black patients, angina	
Nifedipine (long-acting)	20–90 mg daily		
Diltiazem (long-acting)	90–180 mg ×2 daily		Bradycardia, heart block, heart failure, beta-blockers (verapamil)
Verapamil	120–240 mg ×2 daily		
Centrally acting drugs			
Methyldopa	250 mg–1 g ×3 daily	Hypertension in pregnancy, breastfeeding	Monitor blood counts and liver function tests
Moxonidine	200–600 μg daily	Resistant hypertension, insulin resistance	Renal or heart failure, glaucoma, angio-oedema, bradycardia
Diuretics			
Bendroflumethiazide	2.5 mg daily	>55 years, black patients, heart failure, stroke secondary prevention	Gout, diabetes, hypokalaemia
Chlortalidone	25 mg daily		
Furosemide	40–80 mg daily	Heart failure, renal dysfunction	Hypokalaemia
Renin inhibitors			
Aliskiren	150–300 mg daily	Resistant hypertension	Renal failure, pregnancy
Vasodilators			
Hydralazine	25–50 mg ×2 daily	Black patients, heart failure (when combined with nitrates)	Systemic lupus erythematosus
Minoxidil	5.0–50 mg daily	Severe hypertension (with a diuretic and beta-blocker)	Pregnancy
Sodium nitroprusside	0.3–5 μg/kg per min i.v.	Hypertensive crisis	Needs intra-arterial blood pressure monitoring, avoid prolonged use

- peripheral neuropathy (associated with numbness and tingling)
- popliteal artery entrapment (young patients who may have normal pulses)
- venous claudication (bursting pain on walking with a previous history of a DVT)
- fibromuscular dysplasia
- Buerger's disease (young males, heavy smokers).

Investigations

An estimation of the anatomical level of disease may be possible with the examination of pulses. The severity of disease is indicated by the ***ankle/brachial pressure index*** (ABPI). This is a measurement of the cuff pressure at which blood flow is detectable by Doppler in the posterior tibial or anterior tibial arteries compared to the brachial artery (ankle/brachial pressure). Intermittent claudication is associated with an ABPI of 0.5–0.9. Values of <0.5 are associated with critical limb ischaemia. The sensitivity of the test may be improved by a fall in ABPI after exercise. If the arteries are heavily calcified and incompressible – that is, in renal or diabetic disease, the ABPI will be falsely elevated. In these patients, toe pressure values are more sensitive. Diagnostic imaging includes the following options:

- ***Digital subtraction angiography*** (DSA) provides an arterial map ***(Fig. 23.127)*** but requires peripheral arterial cannulation and exposes the individual to iodinated contrast; it should be reserved for use in patients immediately prior to intervention.
- ***Duplex ultrasound using B-mode ultrasound and colour Doppler*** can provide an accurate anatomical map of the lower limbs with sensitivity of 87% and specificity of 94% compared to angiography, although it is operator-dependent.
- ***Three-dimensional contrast-enhanced MR angiography*** provides excellent imaging of both legs with a single contrast injection without exposure to ionizing radiation. Sensitivity of 97% and specificity of 96% are reported.

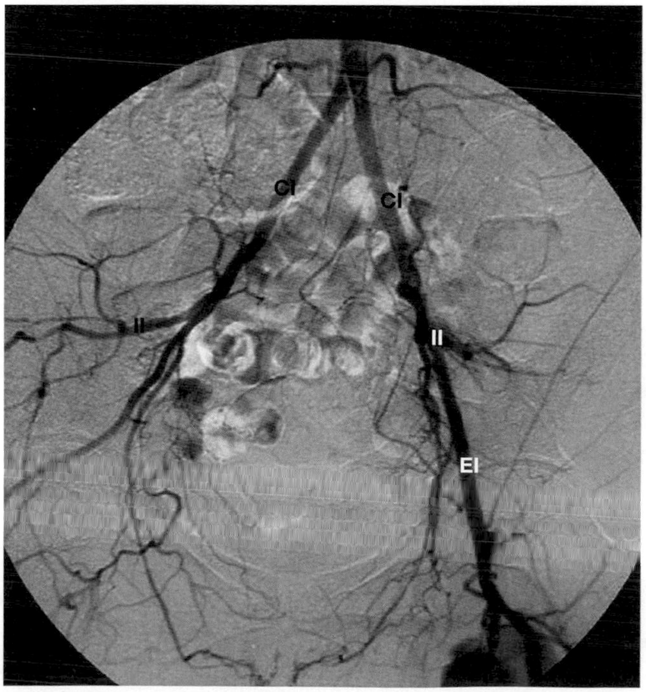

Figure 23.127 Angiogram showing occlusion of the right external iliac artery. CI, common iliac; EI, external iliac; II, internal iliac.

- ***CT angiography*** is an effective alternative to MRA, although extensive calcification may obscure stenoses. CTA requires ionizing radiation and iodinated contrast media.

Management

Medical

All patients with PVD need aggressive risk factor management. They should be encouraged to stop smoking and require smoking cessation advice. Individuals with diabetes mellitus need regular chiropody care and diabetic management. Hypercholesterolaemia should be treated, as this reduces disease progression. The Heart Protection Study showed that even the reduction of a normal cholesterol level reduces mortality from cardiovascular disease. Patients with peripheral arterial disease and a total cholesterol >3.5 mmol/L should receive statin therapy. Low-dose aspirin reduces the risk of MI and stroke in patients with PVD. Patients should be encouraged to exercise and to avoid obesity.

Pharmacological

- ***Cilostazol*** is a phosphodiesterase III inhibitor that increases levels of cAMP, produces vasodilatation and reversibly inhibits platelet aggregation. At a dose of 100 mg twice daily, it can increase walking distance in patients with short-distance claudication.
- ***Naftidrofuryl*** is a vasodilator agent that inhibits vascular and platelet 5-hydroxytryptamine$_2$ (5-HT$_2$) receptors and can reduce lactic acid levels. At a dose of 1–200 mg three times a day, it may increase walking distance and improve quality of life.
- ***Oxpentifylline, inositol nicotinate and cinnarizine*** are not recommended for patients with claudication.

Surgical/radiological

Vascular intervention for stable claudication is not generally recommended except in patients with severe or disabling symptoms. ***Percutaneous transluminal angioplasty*** is the first option and is carried out via a catheter inserted into the femoral artery. The long-term patency rates decrease as the angioplasty becomes more distal. The long-term results of angioplasty appear to be similar to those of a continued exercise programme. Arterial stents may be deployed in recurrent iliac disease, and drug-eluting stents allowing long-term patency are being used – with paclitaxel, for example. ***Bypass procedures*** may be performed using Dacron, polytetrafluoroethylene (PTFE) or autologous veins. Bypasses to distal vessels have poorer long-term patencies. Prosthetic grafts have equal patencies in above-knee bypasses but are inferior to grafts to veins below the knee. In severe ischaemia with unreconstructable arterial disease, an ***amputation*** may be necessary. An amputation may lead to loss of independence, only 70% of below-knee and 30% of above-knee amputees achieving full mobility.

Acute lower limb ischaemia

Clinical features

Symptoms

Patients complain of the 'five Ps': ***pain***, the fact that the leg looks white (***pallor***), ***paraesthesia***, ***paralysis*** and the sensation that it is ***perishingly*** cold. The pain is unbearable and normally requires opioids for relief.

Signs

The limb is cold, with mottling or marbling of the skin. Pulses are diminished or absent. The sensation and movement of the leg are reduced in severe ischaemia. Patients may develop a compartment syndrome with pain in the calf on compression.

Aetiology

Acute limb ischaemia (ALI) may occur because of embolic or thrombotic disease. ***Embolic disease*** is commonly due to cardiac thrombus and cardiac arrhythmias. Rheumatic fever is now an uncommon cause and the frequency of cardiac embolic ALI is also on the decline. Emboli may also occur secondary to aneurysm thrombus or thrombus on atherosclerotic plaques. Emboli from atrial myxomas are rare.

ALI is now often due to ***thrombotic disease***. Acute thrombus usually forms on a chronic atherosclerotic stenosis in a patient who has previously reported symptoms of claudication. Thrombus may also form in normal vessels in individuals who are hypercoagulable because of malignancy or thrombophilia defects. Prosthetic or venous grafts may also thrombose either *de novo* or secondary to a developing stenosis, which may be in the graft or in the native vessels. Popliteal aneurysms may thrombose or embolize distally. ***Acute upper limb ischaemia*** may be caused by similar processes or occur secondary to external compression with a cervical rib/band.

Investigations

Investigations are similar to those described for chronic lower limb disease.

Management

Medical

Management is dependent on the degree of ischaemia. Patients showing improvement may be treatable with heparin and appropriate treatment of the underlying cause. Patients with emboli following MI or atrial fibrillation need long-term warfarin.

Surgical/radiological

Patients with mild to moderate ischaemic symptoms who have an occluded graft may need graft thrombolysis. Intra-arterial thrombolysis may reveal an underlying stenosis within a graft or native vessel that could be treated with angioplasty. Patients with an embolus may benefit from its surgical removal (embolectomy). A bypass graft may be required after occlusion of a popliteal aneurysm or acute-on-chronic lower limb arterial disease. When an ischaemic limb is revascularized, the sudden improvement in blood flow can cause reperfusion injury, with release of toxic metabolites into the circulation. In muscle compartments, the consequent oedema may lead to a 'compartment syndrome', which requires fasciotomies (release of the fascia to prevent muscle damage). An amputation may be warranted in unreconstructable or severe ischaemia. In patients dying from other causes, acute limb ischaemia may occur and intervention may then be inappropriate.

Aneurysmal disease

Aneurysms are classified as true and false. An aneurysm is defined if there is a permanent dilatation of the artery to twice the normal diameter. In true aneurysms, the arterial wall forms the wall of the aneurysm. The arteries most frequently involved are the abdominal aorta, the iliac, popliteal and femoral arteries, and the thoracic aorta (in decreasing frequency). In false aneurysms (pseudoaneurysms), the surrounding tissues form the wall of the aneurysm. False aneurysms can occur following femoral artery puncture. A haematoma is formed because of inadequate compression of the entry site and continued bleeding into the surrounding compressed soft tissue forms the wall of this aneurysm.

Abdominal aortic aneurysm

Abdominal aortic aneurysms (AAAs) occur most commonly below the renal arteries (infra-renal). The incidence increases with age, AAAs being present in 5% of the population >60 years. They arise five times more frequently in men, and in 1 in 4 male children of an affected individual. Aneurysms may occur secondary to atherosclerosis, infection (syphilis, *Escherichia coli*, *Salmonella*) and trauma, or may be genetic (Marfan syndrome, Ehlers–Danlos syndrome).

Screening

In England and Wales, the prevalence of AAA is 3–4% of men ≥65 years old, and approximately 6000 deaths occur each year from a ruptured aortic aneurysm. The mortality rate for elective surgery is ≤3.5%, compared to 50% for an emergency repair. There are fixed risk factors – age, male gender, strong family history – and modifiable risk factors – smoking, hypertension, hypercholesterolaemia.

The UK recommendation is that screening should be offered to men aged 65–74 years, who will receive an abdominal ultrasound.

- ***Normal*** or ***<3 cm*** aorta will not require treatment or further scans.
- ***Small*** (***3–4.4 cm***) aorta will require annual ultrasound surveillance and a GP review to optimize lifestyle.
- ***Medium*** (***4.5–5.4 cm***) aorta requires quarterly ultrasound surveillance and cardiovascular secondary prevention therapy.
- ***Large*** (***≥5.5 cm***) aorta will be referred for assessment and possible elective repair.

Screening of female patients is *not* recommended, as the prevalence is much lower.

Clinical features

Symptoms

Most aneurysms are asymptomatic and are found on routine abdominal examination or plain X-ray, or during urological investigations. Rapid expansion or rupture of an AAA may cause ***severe pain*** (epigastric pain radiating to the back). A ruptured AAA causes ***hypotension***, ***tachycardia***, ***profound anaemia*** and ***sudden death***. The symptoms of rupture may mimic renal colic, diverticulitis and severe lower abdominal or testicular pain. Gradual erosion of the vertebral bodies may cause non-specific back pain. The aneurysm may embolize distally. Inflammatory aneurysms can obstruct adjacent structures, such as the ureter, duodenum and vena cava. Rarely, patients with aneurysms can present with severe haematemesis secondary to an aortoduodenal fistula.

Signs

The aorta is retroperitoneal and in overweight patients there may be no overt signs. An aneurysm is suspected if a pulsatile, expansile abdominal mass is felt. The presence of an AAA should alert a clinician to the possibility of popliteal aneurysms. Patients may present with 'trash feet', dusky discoloration of the digits secondary to emboli from the aortic thrombus.

Management

As with any operation, the management of an asymptomatic aneurysm depends on the balance of operative risk and conservative management. The UK Small Aneurysm Trial showed that patients with infra-renal AAAs did best with an operation if the aneurysm was:

- ≥5.5 cm diameter
- expanding at a rate of >1 cm/year
- symptomatic.

Medical

Patients with aneurysmal disease need careful control of hypertension, smoking cessation and lipid-lowering medication. Patients with AAAs <5.5 cm are followed up by regular ultrasound surveillance.

Surgical repair

Standard therapy is open surgical repair with insertion of a Dacron or Gore-Tex graft.

Endovascular stent

Endovascular stent insertion (via the femoral or iliac arteries) is a non-surgical approach to AAA repair. The Endovascular Aneurysm Repair (EVAR) studies (stent versus open surgical repair) and EVAR 2 (stent versus medical therapy in patients unsuitable for open repair) investigated the role of endovascular stents in patients with an AAA ≥5.5 cm on CT. In EVAR, the 30-day mortality rate was 1.7% with stenting versus 4.7% with surgery ($p = 0.009$) but the long-term mortality rate was similar in both groups at 4 years. In EVAR 2, the 30-day mortality rate with stenting was 9%. Long-term mortality rate was similar in both stent and medical therapy groups. A meta-analysis of three randomized control trials demonstrated a 30-day mortality rate of 2% for stent-graft repair versus 5% for open surgical repair; there were also reductions in intensive treatment unit and in-hospital stays with stent-graft repair.

Laparoscopic surgery

An alternative to open surgical repair or endovascular stenting is laparoscopic repair, which is performed with hand-assisted laparoscopic surgery (HALS, requiring a midline mini-laparotomy) or total laparoscopic surgery (TLS). In non-randomized controlled trials, both methods were associated with reduced length of stay, although the operating times were longer.

Prognosis

After repair, patients with an AAA should return to normal activity within a few months.

Thoraco-abdominal aneurysm

The ascending, arch or descending thoracic aorta may become aneurysmal. Ascending thoraco-abdominal aneurysms (TAAs) occur most commonly in patients with Marfan syndrome or hypertension. Descending or arch TAAs occur secondary to atherosclerosis and are now rarely due to syphilis.

Clinical features

Most aneurysms are asymptomatic and are found on routine chest X-ray or cardiological investigation. Rapid expansion may cause severe pain (chest pain radiating to the upper back) and rupture is associated with hypotension, tachycardia and death. Chest symptoms from expansion may include stridor (compressed bronchial tree), haemoptysis (aortobronchial fistula) and hoarseness (compression of the recurrent laryngeal nerve). Aorto-oesophageal fistula uncommonly causes haematemesis.

Investigations

- ***CT or MRI scan*** is used for assessment of a TAA.
- ***Aortography*** may be helpful for assessing the position of the key branches in relation to the aneurysm.
- ***Transoesophageal echocardiography*** can be useful for identifying an aortic dissection.

Management

If the aneurysm is >6 cm, then operative repair or stenting may be appropriate, but these can be technically difficult and carry a high risk of mortality and paraplegia. EVAR is, at present, the procedure of choice for isolated descending thoracic aneurysms.

Acute aortic syndromes

Acute aortic syndromes include aortic dissection, intramural haematoma (IMH) and penetrating aortic ulcers. Aortic dissection usually begins with a tear in the intima. Blood penetrates the diseased medial layer and then cleaves the intimal laminal plain, leading to dissection. IMH is considered a precursor of dissection, in which there is rupture of the vasa vasorum in the aortic media with aortic wall infarction. IMH is typically in the descending thoracic aorta. Deep penetrating aortic plaques may lead to IMH, dissection or ulceration/perforation. There is a predisposition to aortic dissection in patients with autoimmune rheumatic disorders and Marfan and Ehlers–Danlos syndromes.

Aortic dissection can be classified according to the timing of diagnosis from the origin of symptoms: acute <2 weeks, subacute 2–8 weeks and chronic >8 weeks, with mortality and extension decreasing with time. It can also be classified anatomically:

- ***Type A*** involves the aortic arch and aortic valve proximal to the left subclavian artery origin. This category includes De Bakey type I (extends to the abdominal aorta) and De Bakey type II (localized to the ascending aorta).
- ***Type B*** involves the descending thoracic aorta distal to the left subclavian artery origin. This category includes De Bakey type III ***(Fig. 23.128)***.

Clinical features

Symptoms

Most patients present with a sudden onset of severe and central ***chest pain*** that often radiates to the back and down the arms, mimicking MI. The pain is often described as tearing in nature and may be migratory.

Signs

Patients may be shocked and may have neurological symptoms secondary to loss of blood supply to the spinal cord. They may develop aortic regurgitation, coronary ischaemia and cardiac tamponade. Distal extension may produce acute kidney failure, acute lower limb ischaemia or visceral ischaemia. Peripheral pulses may be absent.

Investigations

The mediastinum may be widened on chest X-ray; urgent CT scan, transoesophageal echocardiography or MRI will confirm the diagnosis (see ***Fig. 23.100***).

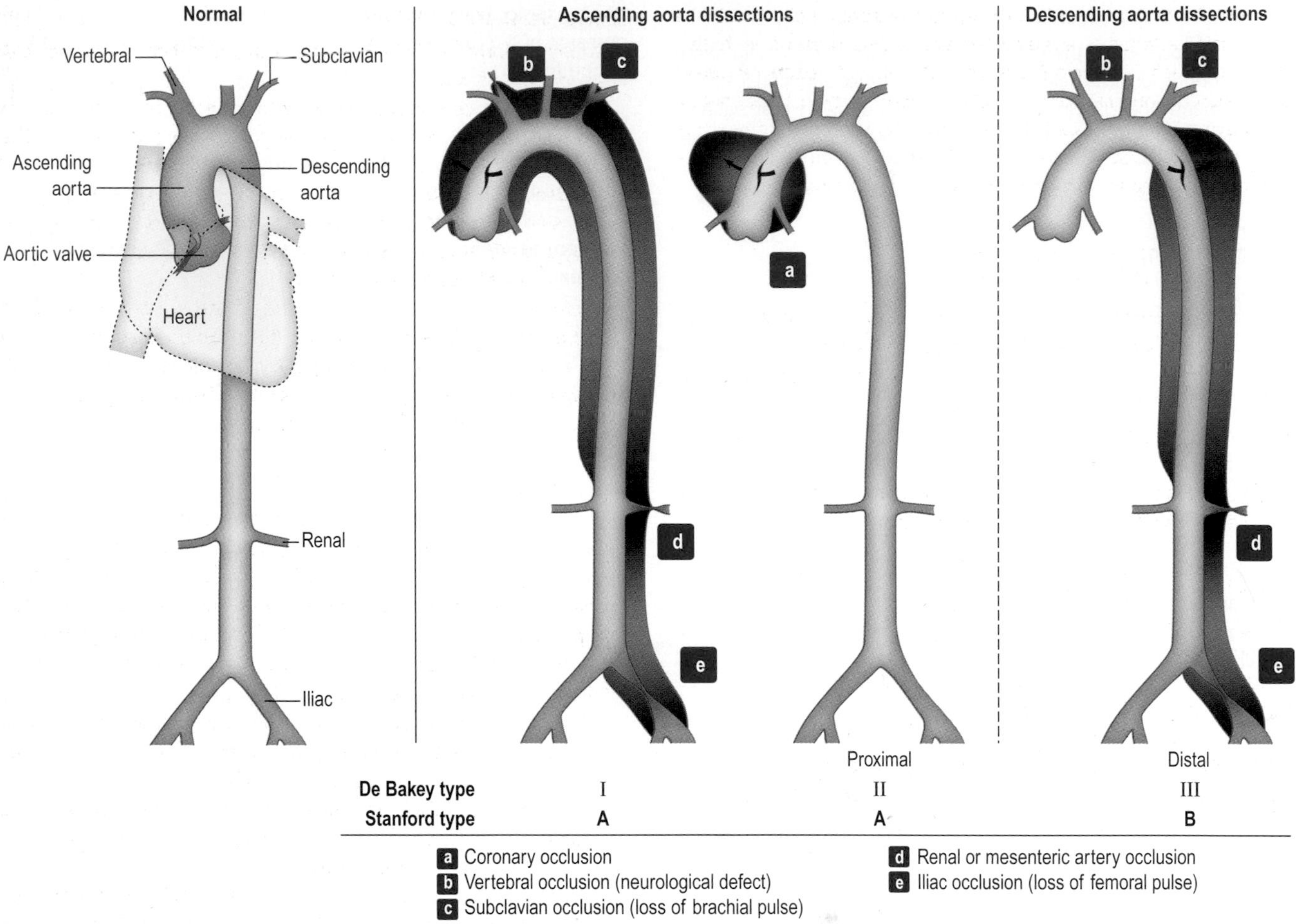

Figure 23.128 Classification of aortic aneurysms.

Management

At least 50% of patients are hypertensive and may require urgent antihypertensive medication to reduce blood pressure to <120 mmHg; intravenous beta-blockers (labetalol, metoprolol) and vasodilators (GTN) are used. Type A dissections should undergo surgery (arch replacement) if the patient is fit enough, as medical management carries a high mortality (50% within 2 weeks). Type B dissections carry a better prognosis and have a survival rate of 89% at 1 month; initially, these patients should be managed medically unless they develop complications. Endovascular intervention with stents may be indicated in individuals with rapidly expanding dissections (>1 cm/year), critical diameter (>5.5 cm), refractory pain or malperfusion syndrome, blunt chest trauma, penetrating aortic ulcers or IMH. Patients will require long-term follow-up with CT or MRI.

Other types of peripheral arterial disease

Raynaud's phenomenon or Raynaud's disease

Raynaud's phenomenon consists of spasm of the digital arteries, usually precipitated by cold and relieved by heat. If there is no underlying cause, it is known as Raynaud's disease. This affects 5% of the population, mostly women. The disorder is usually bilateral and fingers are affected more commonly than toes.

Clinical features

Vasoconstriction causes skin ***pallor*** followed by ***cyanosis*** due to sluggish blood flow, then redness secondary to hyperaemia. The duration of the attacks is variable but they can sometimes last for hours. Numbness, a burning sensation and severe pain occur as the fingers warm up. In chronic, severe disease tissue, ***infarction*** and ***digital loss*** can occur.

Diagnosis

Primary Raynaud's disease needs to be differentiated from secondary treatable causes leading to Raynaud's phenomenon. These are the rheumatic autoimmune disorders, such as systemic sclerosis. It can be associated with atherosclerosis or occupations that involve the use of vibrating tools. Ergot-containing drugs and beta-blockers, as well as smoking, can aggravate symptoms.

Management

Patients should avoid cold provocation by wearing gloves and warm clothes, and stop smoking. Vasodilators can be prescribed but are often unacceptable, as cerebral vasodilatation causes severe headaches. Sympathectomy or prostacyclin infusion can be helpful in severe disease.

Takayasu's disease

This is rare, except in Japan. It is known as the pulseless disease or aortic arch syndrome. It is of unknown aetiology and occurs in females. There is a vasculitis involving the aortic arch, as well as other major arteries. A systemic illness is also present, with pain and tenderness over the affected arteries. Absent peripheral pulses and hypertension are common. Corticosteroids help the constitutional symptoms. Eventually, heart failure and strokes may occur but most patients survive for at least 5 years. Treatment may involve a surgical bypass to improve perfusion of the affected areas.

Thromboangiitis obliterans (Buerger's disease)

This disease, involving the small vessels of the lower limbs, occurs in young men who smoke. It is thought by some workers to be indistinguishable from atheromatous disease. However, pathologically, there is inflammation of the arteries, and sometimes veins, which may indicate a separate disease entity. Clinically, it presents with severe claudication and rest pain, leading to gangrene. A thrombophlebitis is sometimes present. Treatment is as for all peripheral vascular disease, but patients must stop smoking.

Cardiovascular syphilis

This gives rise to:

- uncomplicated aortitis
- aortic aneurysms, usually in the ascending part
- aortic valvulitis with regurgitation
- stenosis of the coronary ostia.

The diagnosis is confirmed by serology. Treatment is with penicillin. Aneurysms and valvular disease are treated as necessary by the usual methods.

PERIPHERAL VENOUS DISEASE

Varicose veins

Varicose veins are a common problem, sometimes giving rise to pain. They are treated by injection with ultrasound-guided foam sclerotherapy or thermal ablation with, for example, endovenous lasers or surgery.

Venous thrombosis

Thrombosis can occur in any vein but the veins of the leg and the pelvis are the most common sites.

Superficial thrombophlebitis

This commonly involves the saphenous veins and is often associated with varicosities. Occasionally, the axillary vein is involved, usually as a result of trauma. There is local superficial inflammation of the vein wall, with secondary thrombosis.

The clinical picture is of a painful, tender, cord-like structure with associated redness and swelling.

The condition usually responds to symptomatic treatment with rest, elevation of the limb and analgesics (e.g. NSAIDs). The Comparison of Arixtra in Lower Limb Superficial Vein Thrombosis with Placebo (CALISTO) trial demonstrated that a 45 day course of subcutaneous fondaparinux 2.5 mg daily, compared with placebo, significantly reduced the rate of thromboembolic events (pulmonary embolism and deep vein thrombosis) from 1.3% to 0.2%, and limited the extension of superficial vein thrombosis to the saphenofemoral junction from 3.4% to 0.3% with no increased risk of bleeding.

Deep vein thrombosis

A thrombus forms in the vein, and any inflammation of the vein wall is secondary to this.

Thrombosis commonly occurs after periods of immobilization but it can occur in normal individuals for no obvious reasons. The precipitating factors are discussed on pages 992–993.

A deep vein thrombosis (DVT) in the legs occurs in 50% of patients after prostatectomy (without prophylactic heparin) or following a cerebral vascular event. In addition, 10% of patients with an MI have a clinically detected DVT.

Thrombosis can occur in any vein of the leg or pelvis, but is found particularly in veins of the calf. It is often undetected; autopsy figures give an incidence of over 60% in hospitalized patients. Axillary vein thrombosis occasionally occurs, sometimes related to trauma, but usually for no obvious reason.

Clinical features

The individual may be asymptomatic, presenting with clinical features of pulmonary embolism (see pp. 1031–1035).

A major presenting feature is ***pain*** in the calf, often with swelling, redness and ***engorged superficial veins***. The affected calf is often warmer and there may be ankle oedema. ***Homan's sign*** (pain in the calf on dorsiflexion of the foot) is often present, but is not diagnostic and occurs with all lesions of the calf.

Thrombosis in the iliofemoral region can present with severe pain, but there are often few physical signs apart from occasional swelling of the thigh and/or ankle oedema.

Complete occlusion, particularly of a large vein, can lead to a ***cyanotic discoloration*** of the limb and severe oedema, which can, very rarely, lead to venous gangrene.

Pulmonary embolism can occur with any DVT but is more frequent from an iliofemoral thrombosis and is rare with thrombosis confined to veins below the knee. In 20–30% of patients, spread of thrombosis can occur proximally without clinical evidence, so careful monitoring of the leg, usually by ultrasound, is required.

Investigations

Clinical diagnosis is unreliable, but combined with D-dimer level, it has a sensitivity of 80%. Confirmation of an iliofemoral thrombosis can usually be made with ***B mode venous compression***, ***ultrasonography*** or ***Doppler ultrasound*** with a sensitivity and specificity over 90%.

Below-knee thromboses can be detected reliably only by venography with non-invasive techniques, ultrasound, fibrinogen scanning and impedance plethysmography, having a sensitivity of only 70%. A venogram is performed by injecting a vein in the foot with contrast, which will detect virtually all thrombi that are present.

Management

The main aim of therapy is to prevent pulmonary embolism, and all patients with thrombi above the knee must be anticoagulated. Anticoagulation of below-knee thrombi is now recommended for 3 months, as 30% of patients will have an extension of the clot proximally. Bed rest is advised until the patient is fully anticoagulated. The patient should then be mobilized, with an elastic stocking giving graduated pressure over the leg.

Low-molecular-weight heparins (see p. 578) have replaced unfractionated heparin, as they are more effective and do not require monitoring; there is also less risk of bleeding. DVTs are being treated at home with low-molecular-weight heparin. Warfarin is started immediately and the heparin stopped when the INR is in

Box 23.58 Risk factors for venous thromboembolism (VTE)

- Active cancer or cancer treatment
- Age >60 years
- Critical care admission
- Long distance flight ± dehydration
- Known thrombophilias
- Obesity (BMI >30 kg/m^2)
- Significant medical co-morbidities (e.g. heart disease; metabolic, endocrine or respiratory pathologies; acute infectious diseases; inflammatory conditions)
- Personal history or first-degree relative with a history of VTE
- Use of hormone replacement therapy or oestrogen-containing contraceptive therapy
- Varicose veins with phlebitis
- Pregnancy/childbirth

BMI, body mass index.
(From http://guidance.nice.org.uk/CG92/QuickRefGuide/pdf/English.)

the target range. The duration of ***warfarin*** treatment is debatable: 3 months is the period usually recommended, but 4 weeks is long enough if a definite risk factor (e.g. bed rest) has been present. Recurrent DVTs need permanent anticoagulants. The target INR should be 2.5. Anticoagulants do not lyse the thrombus that is already present. Unfractionated heparin should only be used if LMWH is unavailable.

Thrombolytic therapy (see pp. 577–578) is occasionally used for patients with a large iliofemoral thrombosis.

Prognosis

Destruction of the deep vein valves produces a clinically painful, swollen limb that is made worse by standing and is accompanied by oedema and, sometimes, venous eczema. It occurs in approximately half of the patients with clinically symptomatic DVT, and it means that elastic support stockings are then required for life.

Prevention

An estimated 25 000 people in the UK die every year from a preventable hospital-acquired venous thromboembolism (VTE). In January 2010, NICE provided guidelines on the assessment and prevention of VTE in patients admitted to hospital (see p. 580):

- All patients should be assessed on admission to hospital (and again within 24 h or when a change occurs in the patient's clinical condition).
- Medical patients are at risk if they have reduced mobility for ≥3 days or if their mobility is reduced and they have one or more risk factors for VTE ***(Box 23.58)***.
- Surgical and trauma patients are at risk if they:
  - undergo a surgical procedure with a combined anaesthetic and surgery of >90 min (60 min if surgery is to the pelvis or lower limb)
  - are admitted with an acute inflammatory or intra-abdominal condition
  - have significantly reduced mobility
  - have one or more risk factors for VTE.

Box 23.59 Risk factors for bleeding

- Active bleeding
- Acquired bleeding disorders (e.g. acute liver failure)
- Concurrent use of anticoagulants (e.g. warfarin with INR >2)
- Lumbar puncture/epidural/spinal anaesthesia within the previous 4 h or expected within 12 h
- Acute stroke
- Thrombocytopenia (platelets <75 × 10^9/L)
- Uncontrolled systolic hypertension (≥230/120 mmHg)
- Untreated inherited bleeding disorders (haemophilia and von Willebrand's disease)

INR, International Normalized Ratio.

Patients at risk should be considered for pharmacological prophylaxis (fondaparinux or low-molecular-weight heparin or unfractionated heparin if there is renal impairment), unless they have a risk factor for bleeding ***(Box 23.59)*** that outweighs the benefits of VTE prophylaxis. Patients should also be encouraged to mobilize where possible and mechanical VTE (anti-embolism) stockings (thigh or knee length), foot impulse devices, and intermittent pneumatic compression devices (thigh or knee length) may be appropriate in certain patients. On discharge, patients should be provided with advice on the signs and symptoms of VTE; if pharmacological or mechanical prophylaxis has been prescribed, advice should be given on its usage. (Antithrombins are now being used in orthopaedic surgery; see p. 580.)

Further reading

Decousus H, Prandoni P, Mismetti P et al. for the CALISTO study group. Fondaparinux for the treatment of superficial-vein thrombosis in the legs. *N Engl J Med* 2010; 363:1222–1232.
House of Commons Health Committee. *The Prevention of Venous Thromboembolism in Hospitalised Patients*. London: The Stationery Office; 2005.
Johnston SL, Lock RJ, Gompels MM. Takayasu arteritis: a review. *J Clin Pathol* 2002; 55:481–486.
Kullo IJ, Rooke TW. Peripheral artery disease. *N Engl J Med* 2016; 374:861–871.
Kyrle PA, Eichinger S. Deep venous thrombosis. *Lancet* 2005; 365:1163–1174.
National Institute for Health and Care Excellence. *NICE Clinical Guideline 92: Venous Thromboembolism in Adults Admitted to Hospital: Reducing the Risk*. NICE 2010; https://www.nice.org.uk/guidance/cg92.
National Institute for Health and Care Excellence. *NICE Interventional Procedure Guidance 163: Stent-graft Placement in Abdominal Aortic Aneurysm.* NICE 2006; http://www.nice.org.uk/guidance/ipg163.
National Institute for Health and Care Excellence. *NICE Interventional Procedure Guidance 229: Laparoscopic Repair of Abdominal Aortic Aneurysm* NICE 2007; http://www.nice.org.uk/guidance/ipg229.
Nienaber CA, Clough RE. Management of acute aortic dissection. *Lancet* 2015; 385:800–811.
Schermerhorn ML, Buck DB, O'Malley AJ et al. Long term outcomes of aortic aneurysms in the Medicare Population. *N Engl J Med* 2015; 373:328–338.
United Kingdom EVAR Trial Investigators. Endovascular versus open repair of abdominal aortic aneurysm. *N Engl J Med* 2010; 362:1863–1871.
http://aaa.screening.nhs.uk UK *National Health Service population screening programme for abdominal aortic aneurysm.*

Significant websites

http://www.achd-library.com *Nevil Thomas Adult Congenital Heart Library.*
http://www.americanheart.org *American Heart Association.*
http://www.dh.gov.uk *UK National Service Framework: Coronary Heart Disease (2000).*
http://www.ecglibrary.com/ecghome.html *ECG tracings library.*
http://www.erc.edu *European Resuscitation Council.*
http://www.resus.org.uk *Resuscitation Council (UK).*

24

Respiratory disease

Anthony J Frew, Sarah R Doffman, Katharine Hurt, Rachel Buxton-Thomas

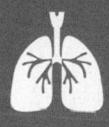

See your e-book for key learning points, clinical tips, drug tips, extra tables, extra images, interactive Figures, audio, videos, learning challenges and MCQs.

INTRODUCTION

The main role of the respiratory system is to extract oxygen from the external environment and to dispose of waste gases, principally carbon dioxide. This requires the lungs to function as efficient bellows, bringing in fresh air and delivering it to the alveoli, and expelling used air at an appropriate rate. Gas exchange is achieved by exposing thin-walled capillaries to the alveolar gas and matching ventilation to blood flow through the pulmonary capillary bed. In doing this, the lungs expose a large area of tissue, which can be damaged by dusts, gases and infective agents. Host defence is therefore a key priority for the lung and is achieved by a combination of structural and immunological defences.

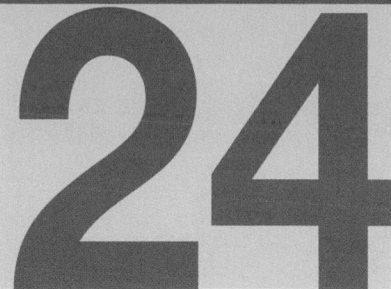

RESPIRATORY

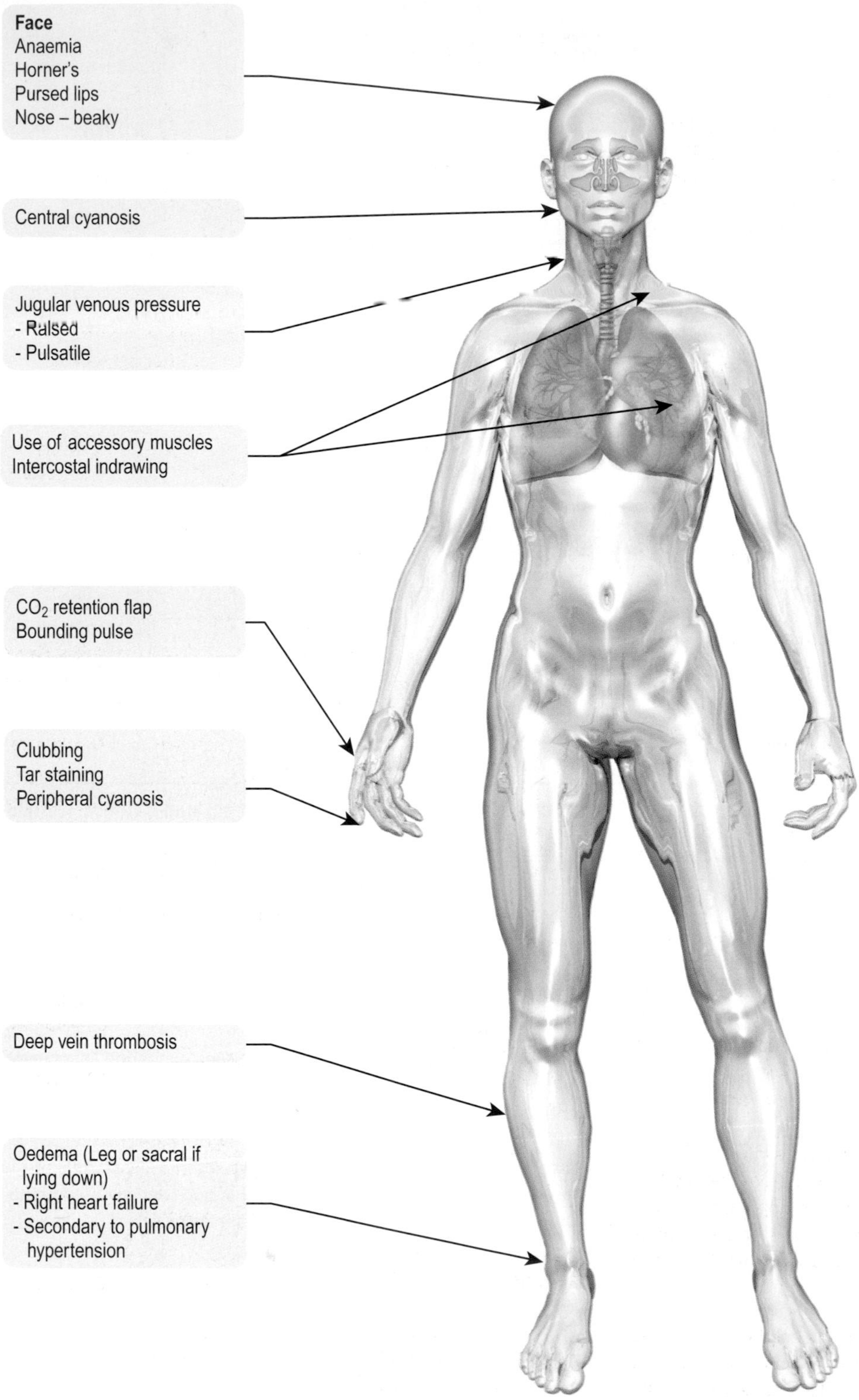

INSPECTION
- Colour
- Breathlessness
- Deformity
- Scars
- Symmetry of movement
- Abdominal paradox (diaphragm weakening)
- Hyperinflation
- Prominent veins (SVC obstruction)
- Intercostal indrawing
- Scoliosis

Observe
- Posture – lying flat or raised
- Colour – cyanosed?
- Respiratory rate
- Pain on breathing (pleuritic)?
- Sputum – colour/amount
- Fever
- Cachexia

Palpation
Tracheal position / Crico-sternal distance / Supraclavicular fossa nodes / Apex beat / Tenderness – Costochondritis – Rib fracture / Liver – Position (low lying) – Enlargement

Percussion
Dull (consolidation / collapse) / Stony dull (fluid) / Hyperresonance (pneumothorax)

Auscultation
Normal vesicular / Bronchial breathing / Wheeze – Monophonic (single large airway obstruction) – Polyphonic (narrowing of small airways) / Crackles – Early, diffuse (airflow limitation) – Late, pulmonary oedema, lung fibrosis – Bronchiectasis / Pleural rub / Vocal resonance / Whispered pectriloquy

Sputum
Volume (↑↑ bronchiectasis)
Mucopurulent (infection)
Purulent (green = infection)
Blood-stained (cancer, pulmonary embolism, tuberculosis, bronchiectasis)

Additional tests
Sputum
Chest X-ray
Spirometry (see p. 1070)
Pulmonary function tests

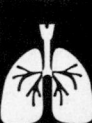

ANATOMY OF THE RESPIRATORY SYSTEM

The nose, pharynx and larynx

See pages 1317 and 1319.

The trachea, bronchi and bronchioles

The trachea is 10–12 cm in length. It lies slightly to the right of the midline and divides at the carina into right and left main bronchi. The carina lies under the junction of the manubrium sterni and the second right costal cartilage. The right main bronchus is more vertical than the left and, hence, inhaled material is more likely to end up in the right lung.

The right main bronchus divides into the upper lobe bronchus and the intermediate bronchus, which further subdivides into the middle and lower lobe bronchi. On the left, the main bronchus divides into upper and lower lobe bronchi only. Each lobar bronchus further divides into segmental and sub-segmental bronchi. There are about 25 divisions in all between the trachea and the alveoli.

The first seven divisions are bronchi that have:

- walls consisting of cartilage and smooth muscle
- an epithelial lining with cilia and goblet cells
- submucosal mucus-secreting glands
- endocrine cells – Kulchitsky or amine precursor and uptake decarboxylation (APUD) cells containing 5-hydroxytryptamine (5-HT, serotonin).

The next 16–18 divisions are bronchioles that have:

- no cartilage and a muscular layer that progressively becomes thinner
- a single layer of ciliated cells but very few goblet cells
- granulated Clara cells that produce a surfactant-like substance.

The ciliated epithelium is a key defence mechanism. Each cell bears approximately 200 cilia beating at 1000 beats per minute (b.p.m.) in organized waves of contraction. Each cilium consists of nine peripheral parts and two inner longitudinal fibrils in a cytoplasmic matrix ***(Fig. 24.1)***. Nexin links join the peripheral pairs. Dynein arms consisting of adenosine triphosphatase (ATPase) protein project towards the adjacent pairs. Bending of the cilia results from a sliding movement between adjacent fibrils powered by an ATP-dependent shearing force developed by the dynein arms (see also pp. 92–93). Absence of dynein arms leads to immotile cilia. Mucus, which contains macrophages, cell debris, inhaled particles and bacteria, is moved by the cilia towards the larynx at about 1.5 cm/min (the 'mucociliary escalator'; see below).

The bronchioles finally divide within the acinus into smaller respiratory bronchioles that have alveoli arising from the surface ***(Fig. 24.2)***. Each respiratory bronchiole supplies approximately 200 alveoli via alveolar ducts. The term 'small airways' refers to bronchioles of <2 mm; the average lung contains about 30 000 of these.

The alveoli

There are approximately 300 million alveoli in each lung. Their total surface area is 40–80 m^2. The epithelial lining consists mainly of ***type I pneumocytes (Fig. 24.3)***. These cells have an extremely thin layer of cytoplasm, which only offers a thin barrier to gas exchange. Type I cells are connected to each other by tight junctions that limit the movements of fluid in and out of the alveoli. Alveoli are not completely airtight; many have holes in the alveolar wall, allowing communication between alveoli of adjoining lobules (pores of Kohn).

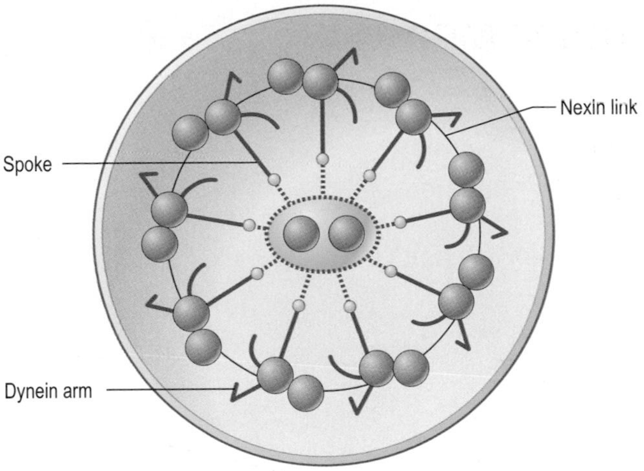

Figure 24.1 Cross-section of a cilium. Nine outer microtubular doublets and two central single microtubules are linked by spokes, nexin links and dynein arms.

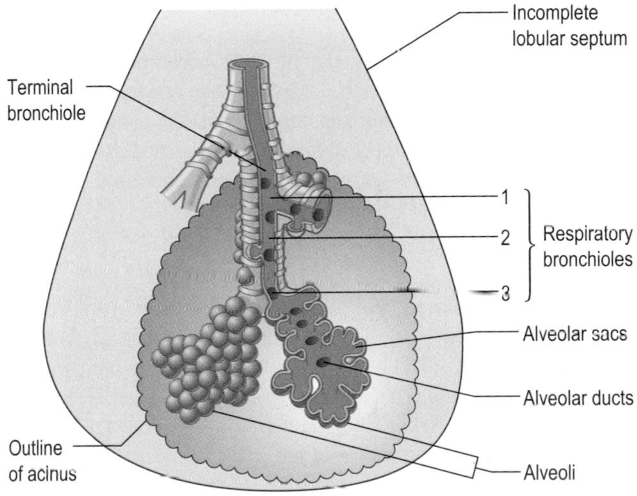

Figure 24.2 Branches of a terminal bronchiole ending in the alveolar sacs.

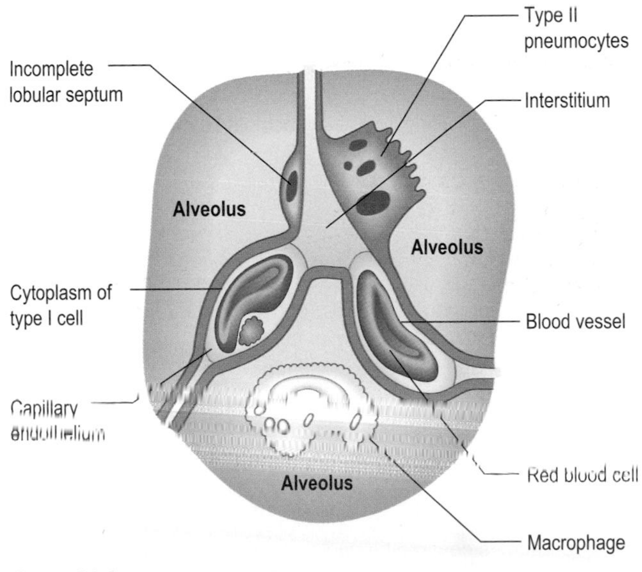

Figure 24.3 The structure of alveoli, showing the pneumocytes and capillaries.

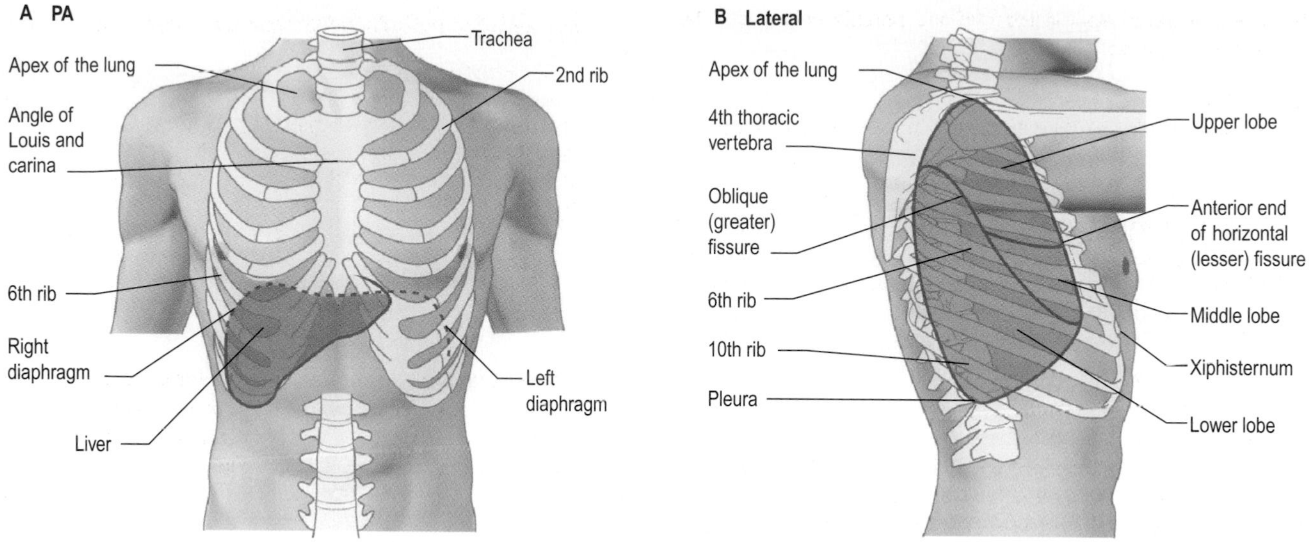

Figure 24.4 Surface anatomy of the chest. A. Anterior. **B.** Lateral.

Type II pneumocytes are slightly more numerous than type I cells but cover less of the epithelial lining. They are found generally in the borders of the alveolus and contain distinctive lamellar vacuoles, which are the source of surfactant. Type I pneumocytes are derived from type II cells. Large alveolar macrophages are present within the alveoli and assist in defending the lung.

The lungs

The lungs are separated into lobes by invaginations of the pleura, which are often incomplete. The right lung has three lobes, whereas the left lung has two. The positions of the oblique fissures and the right horizontal fissure are shown in ***Figure 24.4***. The upper lobe lies mainly in front of the lower lobe and therefore physical signs on the right side in the front of the chest are due to lesions of the upper lobe or the middle lobe.

Each lobe is further subdivided into bronchopulmonary segments by fibrous septa that extend inwards from the pleural surface. Each segment receives its own segmental bronchus.

The bronchopulmonary segment is further divided into individual lobules approximately 1 cm in diameter and generally pyramidal in shape, the apex lying towards the bronchiole that supplies it. Within each lobule, a terminal bronchus supplies an acinus; within this structure, further divisions of the bronchioles eventually give rise to the alveoli.

The pleura

The pleura is a layer of connective tissue covered by a simple squamous epithelium. The visceral pleura covers the surface of the lung, lines the interlobar fissures, and is continuous at the hilum with the parietal pleura, which lines the inside of the hemithorax. At the hilum, the visceral pleura continues alongside the branching bronchial tree for some distance before reflecting back to join the parietal pleura. In health, the pleurae are in apposition, apart from a small quantity of lubricating fluid.

The diaphragm

The diaphragm is covered by parietal pleura above and peritoneum below. Its muscle fibres arise from the lower ribs and insert into the central tendon. Motor and sensory nerve fibres go separately to each half of the diaphragm via the phrenic nerves. Fifty per cent of the muscle fibres are of the slow-twitch type with a low glycolytic capacity; they are relatively resistant to fatigue.

Pulmonary vasculature and lymphatics

The lung has a dual blood supply, receiving deoxygenated blood from the right ventricle via the pulmonary artery and oxygenated blood via the bronchial circulation.

The pulmonary artery divides to accompany the bronchi. The arterioles accompanying the respiratory bronchioles are thin-walled and contain little smooth muscle. The pulmonary venules drain laterally to the periphery of the lobules, pass centrally in the interlobular and intersegmental septa, and eventually join to form the four main pulmonary veins.

The bronchial circulation arises from the descending aorta. These bronchial arteries supply tissues down to the level of the respiratory bronchiole. The bronchial veins drain into the pulmonary veins, forming part of the normal physiological shunt.

Lymphatic channels lie in the interstitial space between the alveolar cells and the capillary endothelium of the pulmonary arterioles.

The tracheobronchial lymph nodes are arranged in five main groups: pulmonary, bronchopulmonary, subcarinal, superior tracheobronchial and paratracheal. For practical purposes, these form a continuous network of nodes from the lung substance up to the trachea.

Nerve supply to the lung

The innervation of the lung remains incompletely understood. Parasympathetic and sympathetic fibres (from the vagus and sympathetic chain, respectively) accompany the pulmonary arteries and the airways. Airway smooth muscle is innervated by vagal afferents, postganglionic muscarinic vagal efferents and vagally derived non-adrenergic non-cholinergic (NANC) fibres, which use a range of neurotransmitters including substance P, neurokinins A and B, calcitonin gene-related peptide, vasoactive intestinal polypeptide, and various adenine and guanine phosphates. Three muscarinic receptor subtypes have been identified: M_1 receptors on parasympathetic ganglia, a smaller number of M_2 receptors on muscarinic nerve terminals, and M_3 receptors on airway smooth muscle. The parietal pleura is innervated from intercostal and phrenic nerves but the visceral pleura has no innervation.

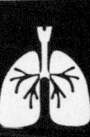

Further reading

Albert RK, Spiro SG, Jett JR. *Clinical Respiratory Medicine*, 4th edn. Chicago: Mosby; 2012.

PHYSIOLOGY OF THE RESPIRATORY SYSTEM

The nose

The major functions of nasal breathing are:

- to heat and moisten the air
- to remove particulate matter.

About 10 000 L of air are inhaled daily. The relatively low flow rates and turbulence of inspired air in the nose mean that few particles >10 microns (μm) in diameter pass through the nose. Particles deposited on the nasal mucosa are removed within 15 minutes, compared with 60–120 days for particles that reach the alveoli. Nasal secretion contains immunoglobulin A (IgA) antibodies, lysozyme and interferons. In addition, the cilia of the nasal epithelium move the mucous gel layer rapidly back to the oropharynx, where it is swallowed. Bacteria have little chance of settling in the nose. Mucociliary protection is less effective against viral infections because viruses bind to receptors on epithelial cells. The majority of rhinoviruses bind to an adhesion molecule, intercellular adhesion molecule 1 (ICAM-1), which is shared by neutrophils and eosinophils. Many noxious gases, such as SO_2, are almost completely removed by nasal breathing.

Breathing

Lung ventilation can be considered in two parts:

- the mechanical process of inspiration and expiration
- the control of respiration to a level appropriate for metabolic needs.

The mechanical process

The lungs have an inherent elastic property that causes them to tend to collapse away from the thoracic wall, generating a negative pressure within the pleural space. The strength of this retractive force relates to the volume of the lung: at higher lung volumes the lung is stretched more, and a greater negative intrapleural pressure is generated. ***Lung compliance*** is a measure of the relationship between this retractive force and lung volume. At the end of a quiet expiration, the retractive force exerted by the lungs is balanced by the tendency of the thoracic wall to spring outwards. At this point, respiratory muscles are resting. The volume of air remaining in the lung after a quiet expiration is called the ***functional residual capacity*** (***FRC***).

Inspiration from FRC is an active process: a negative intrapleural pressure is created by descent of the diaphragm and movement of the ribs upwards and outwards through contraction of the intercostal muscles. During tidal breathing in healthy individuals, inspiration is almost entirely due to contraction of the diaphragm. More vigorous inspiration requires the use of accessory muscles of ventilation (sternomastoid and scalene muscles). Respiratory muscles are similar to other skeletal muscles but are less prone to fatigue. However, inspiratory muscle fatigue contributes to respiratory failure in patients with severe chronic airflow limitation and in those with primary neurological and muscle disorders.

Box 24.1 Normal values for respiratory physiology

In a typical normal adult at rest:

- Pulmonary blood flow is about 5 L/min
- This carries 11 mmol/min (250 mL/min) of O_2 to tissues
- Ventilation is about 6 L/min
- This removes 9 mmol/min (200 mL/min) of CO_2 from the body
- Normal pressure of oxygen in arterial blood (P_aO_2) is 11–13 kPa
- Normal pressure of carbon dioxide in arterial blood (P_aCO_2) is 4.8–6.0 kPa

At rest or during low-level exercise, expiration is passive and results from the natural tendency of the lung to collapse.

Forced expiration involves activation of accessory muscles, chiefly those of the abdominal wall, which help to push up the diaphragm.

The control of respiration

Coordinated respiratory movements result from rhythmical discharges arising in an anatomically ill-defined group of interconnected neurones in the reticular substance of the brainstem, known as the respiratory centre. Motor discharges from the respiratory centre travel via the phrenic and intercostal nerves to the respiratory musculature.

Ventilation is controlled by a combination of neurogenic and chemical factors ***(Fig. 24.5)***. In healthy individuals, the main driver for respiration is the arterial pH, which is closely related to the partial pressure of carbon dioxide in arterial blood. Oxygen levels in arterial blood are usually above the level that triggers respiratory drive. Typical normal values are shown in ***Box 24.1***.

Breathlessness on physical exertion is normal and not considered a symptom unless the level of exertion is very light, such as when walking slowly. Surveys of healthy Western populations reveal that over 20% of the general population report themselves as breathless on relatively minor exertion. Although breathlessness is a very common symptom, the sensory and neural mechanisms underlying it remain obscure. The sensation of breathlessness is derived from at least three sources:

- ***Changes in lung volume***. These are sensed by receptors in thoracic wall muscles signalling changes in their length.
- ***Tension developed by contracting muscles***. This is sensed by Golgi tendon organs.
- ***Central perception of the sense of effort***.

The airways of the lungs

From the trachea to the periphery, the airways decrease in size but increase in number. Overall, the cross-sectional area available for airflow increases as the total number of airways increases. The airflow rate is greatest in the trachea and slows progressively towards the periphery (since the velocity of airflow depends on the cross-sectional area). In the terminal airways, gas flow occurs solely by diffusion. The resistance to airflow is very low (0.1–0.2 kPa/L in a normal tracheobronchial tree), steadily increasing from the small to the large airways.

Airways expand as the lung volume increases. At full inspiration (***total lung capacity***, TLC) they are 30–40% larger in calibre than at full expiration (***residual volume***, RV). In chronic obstructive pulmonary disease (COPD), the small airways are narrowed but this can be partially compensated by breathing closer to TLC.

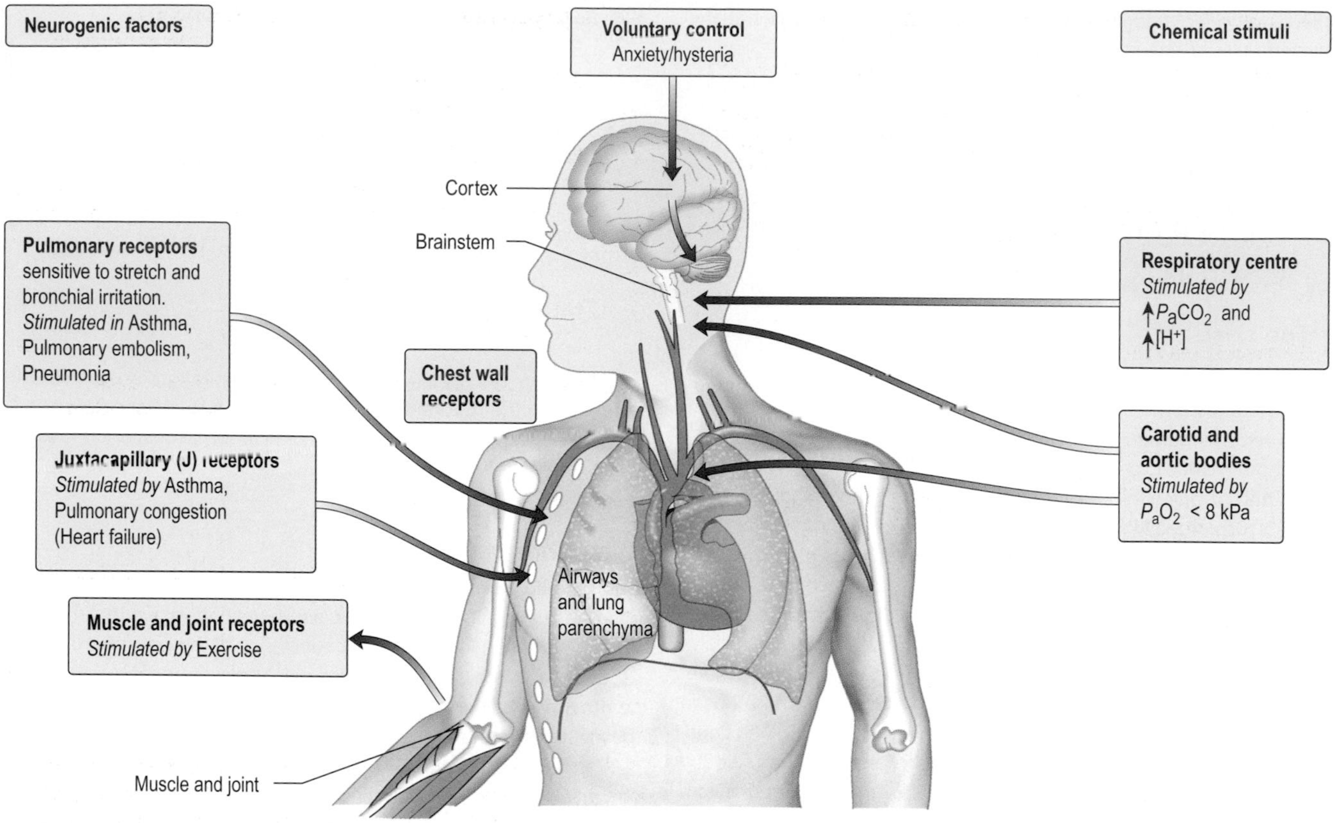

Figure 24.5 Chemical and neurogenic factors in the control of ventilation. The strongest stimulant to ventilation is a rise in P_aCO_2, which increases $[H^+]$ in cerebrospinal fluid. ***Sensitivity*** to this may be lost in ***chronic obstructive pulmonary disease***. In these patients, hypoxaemia is the chief stimulus to respiratory drive; oxygen treatment may therefore reduce respiratory drive and lead to a further rise in P_aCO_2. An increase in $[H^+]$ due to metabolic acidosis, as in diabetic ketoacidosis, will increase ventilation with a fall in P_aCO_2 causing deep sighing (Kussmaul) respiration. The respiratory centre is depressed by severe hypoxaemia and sedatives (e.g. opiates).

Control of airway tone

Bronchomotor tone is maintained by vagal efferent nerves and can be reduced by atropine or β-adrenoceptor agonists. Adrenoceptors on the surface of bronchial muscles respond to circulating catecholamines; there is no direct sympathetic innervation. Airway tone shows a ***circadian rhythm***, which is greatest at 04.00 and lowest in the mid-afternoon. Tone can be increased transiently by inhaled stimuli acting on epithelial nerve endings, which trigger reflex bronchoconstriction via the vagus. These stimuli include cigarette smoke, solvents, inert dust and cold air. Airway responsiveness to these stimuli increases following respiratory tract infections, even in healthy subjects. In asthma, the airways are very irritable and as the circadian rhythm remains the same, asthmatic symptoms are usually worse in the early morning.

Airflow

Movement of air through the airways results from a difference between atmospheric pressure and the pressure in the alveoli; alveolar pressure is negative in inspiration and positive in expiration. During quiet breathing, the pleural pressure is negative throughout the breathing cycle. With vigorous expiratory efforts (e.g. cough), the pleural pressure becomes positive (up to 10 kPa). This compresses the central airways, but the smaller airways do not close off because the driving pressure for expiratory flow (alveolar pressure) is also increased.

Alveolar pressure (P_{ALV}) is equal to the pleural pressure (P_{PL}) plus the elastic recoil pressure (P_{EL}) of the lung.

When there is no airflow (i.e. during a pause in breathing), the tendency of the lungs to collapse (the positive recoil pressure) is exactly balanced by an equivalent negative pleural pressure.

As air flows from the alveoli towards the mouth, there is a gradual drop of pressure owing to flow resistance ***(Fig. 24.6A)***.

In forced expiration, as mentioned above, the driving pressure raises both the alveolar pressure and the intrapleural pressure. Between the alveolus and the mouth, there is a point (C in ***Fig. 24.6B***) where the airway pressure equals the intrapleural pressure, and the airway collapses. However, this collapse is temporary, as the transient occlusion of the airway results in an increase in pressure behind it (i.e. upstream), and this raises the intra-airway pressure so that the airways open and flow is restored. The airways thus tend to vibrate at this point of 'dynamic collapse'.

As lung volume decreases during expiration, the elastic recoil pressure of the lungs decreases and the 'collapse point' moves upstream (i.e. towards the smaller airways; see ***Fig. 24.6C***). Where there is pathological loss of recoil pressure (as in COPD), the 'collapse point' is located even further upstream and causes expiratory flow limitation. The measurement of the forced expiratory volume in 1 second (FEV_1) is a useful clinical index of this phenomenon. To compensate, patients with COPD often 'purse their lips' in order to increase airway pressure so that their peripheral airways do not collapse. During inspiration, the intrapleural pressure is always less than the intraluminal pressure within the intrathoracic airways, so increasing effort does not limit airflow. Inspiratory flow is limited only by the power of the inspiratory muscles.

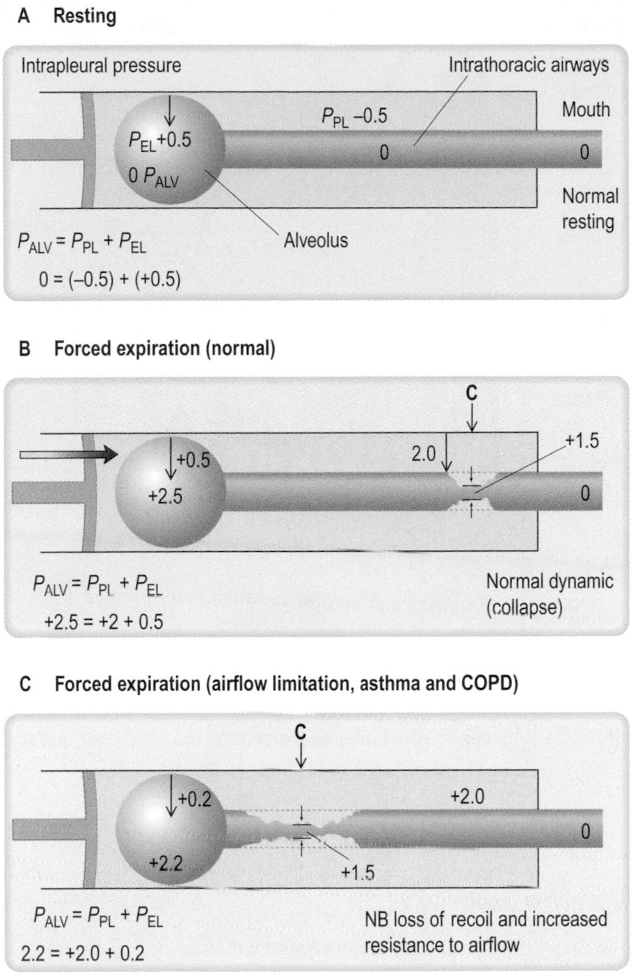

Figure 24.6 **Ventilatory forces. A.** During ***resting*** at functional residual capacity. **B.** During ***forced expiration*** in normal subjects. **C.** ***During forced expiration in a patient with chronic obstructive pulmonary disease*** (COPD). The respiratory system is represented as a piston with a single alveolus and the collapsible part of the airways within the piston (see text). C, collapse point; P_{ALV}, alveolar pressure; P_{EL}, elastic recoil pressure; P_{PL}, pleural pressure.

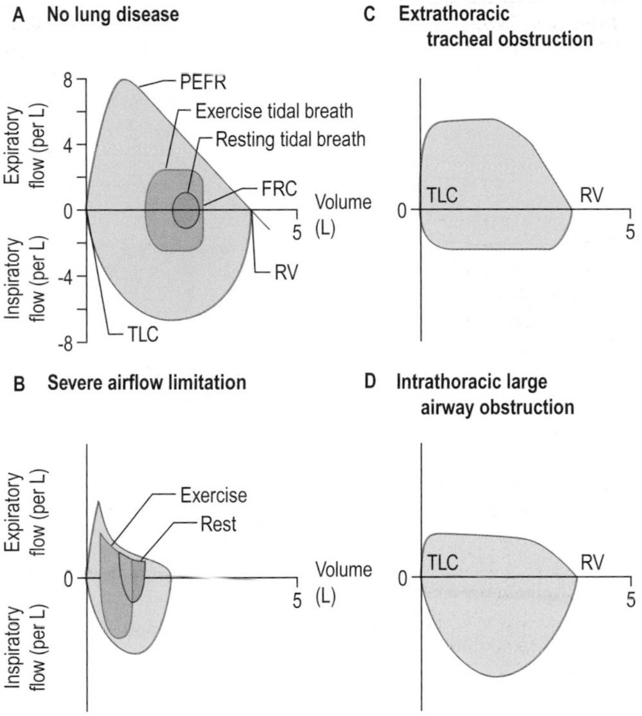

Figure 24.7 **Flow–volume loops.**
A, B. ***Maximal flow–volume loops,*** *showing the relationship between maximal flow rates on expiration and inspiration*. **A. *Normal subject.*** **B. *Severe airflow limitation.*** Flow–volume loops during tidal breathing at rest (starting from the functional residual capacity, FRC) and during exercise are also shown. The highest flow rates are achieved when forced expiration begins at total lung capacity (TLC) and represent the peak expiratory flow rate (PEFR). As air is blown out of the lung, so the flow rate decreases until no more air can be forced out, a point known as the residual volume (RV). Because inspiratory airflow is only dependent on effort, the shape of the maximal inspiratory flow–volume loop is quite different, and inspiratory flow remains at a high rate throughout the manœuvre.
C, D. ***Flow–volume loops in large airway (tracheal) obstruction,*** *showing plateauing of maximal expiratory flow*. **C. *Extrathoracic tracheal obstruction*** with a proportionally greater reduction of maximal inspiratory (as opposed to expiratory) flow rate. **D. *Intrathoracic large airway obstruction***; the expiratory plateau is more pronounced and inspiratory flow rate is less reduced than in **(C)**. In ***severe airflow limitation***, the ventilatory demands of exercise cannot be met (compare **A, B**), greatly reducing effort tolerance.

Flow–volume loops

The relationship between maximal flow rates and lung volume is demonstrated by the maximal flow–volume (MFV) loop ***(Fig. 24.7A)***.

In subjects with healthy lungs, maximal flow rates are rarely achieved even during vigorous exercise. However, in patients with severe COPD, limitation of expiratory flow occurs even during tidal breathing at rest ***(Fig. 24.7B)***. To increase ventilation, these patients have to breathe at higher lung volumes and allow more time for expiration, both of which reduce the tendency for airway collapse. To compensate, they increase flow rates during inspiration, where there is relatively less flow limitation.

The volume that can be forced in from the residual volume in 1 second (FIV_1) will always be greater than that which can be forced out from TLC in 1 second (FEV_1). Thus, the ratio of FEV_1 to FIV_1 is <1. The only exception to this occurs when there is significant obstruction to the airways outside the thorax, such as tracheal tumour or retrosternal goitre. Expiratory airway narrowing is prevented by tracheal resistance and expiratory airflow becomes more effort-dependent. During forced inspiration, this same resistance causes such negative intraluminal pressure that the trachea is compressed by the surrounding atmospheric pressure. Inspiratory flow thus becomes less effort-dependent, and the ratio of FEV_1 to FIV_1 is >1. This phenomenon, and the characteristic flow–volume loop, is diagnostic of extrathoracic airways obstruction ***(Fig. 24.7C)***.

Ventilation and perfusion relationships

For optimum gas exchange there must be a match between ventilation of the alveoli ($\dot{V}$) and their perfusion ($\dot{Q}$). However, in reality there is variation in the ($\dot{V}_A/\dot{Q}$) ratio in both normal and diseased lungs ***(Fig. 24.8)***. In the normal lung, both ventilation and perfusion are greater at the bases than at the apices, but the gradient for perfusion is steeper, so the net effect is that ventilation exceeds perfusion towards the apices, while perfusion exceeds ventilation at the bases. Other causes of $\dot{V}_A/\dot{Q}$ mismatch include direct shunting of deoxygenated blood through the lung without passing through alveoli (e.g. the bronchial circulation) and areas of lung that

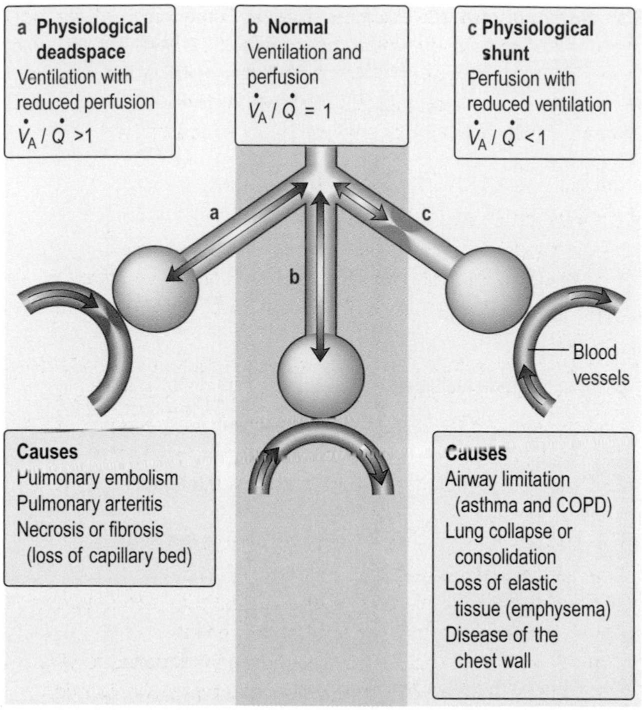

Figure 24.8 Relationships between ventilation and perfusion: the alveolar–capillary interface. ***The centre*** **(b)** shows ***normal ventilation*** and perfusion. On the left **(a)** there is a ***block in perfusion (physiological deadspace)***, while on the right **(c)** there is ***reduced ventilation (physiological shunting)***. COPD, chronic obstructive pulmonary disease.

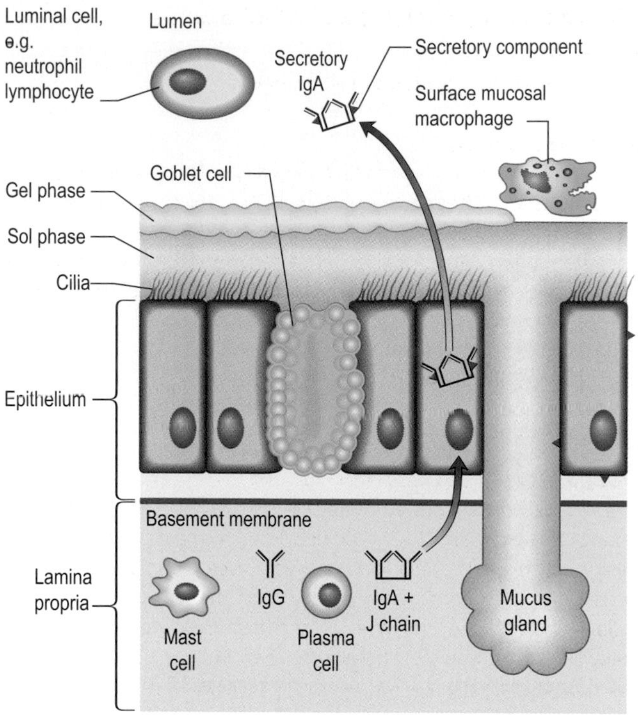

Figure 24.9 Defence mechanisms present at the epithelial surface.

receive no blood (e.g. anatomical deadspace, bullae and areas of under-perfusion during acceleration and deceleration, e.g. in aircraft and high-performance cars).

An increased physiological shunt results in arterial hypoxaemia since it is not possible to compensate for some of the blood being under-oxygenated by increasing ventilation of the well-perfused areas. An increased physiological deadspace just increases the work of breathing and has less impact on blood gases since the normally perfused alveoli are well ventilated. In more advanced disease this compensation cannot occur, leading to increased alveolar and arterial PCO_2 (P_aCO_2), together with hypoxaemia, which cannot be compensated for by increasing ventilation.

Hypoxaemia occurs more readily than hypercapnia because of the different ways in which oxygen and carbon dioxide are carried in the blood. Carbon dioxide is carried in three forms (in bicarbonate, in carbamino compounds and in simple solution), but the volume carried is proportional to the partial pressure of CO_2. Oxygen is carried in chemical combination with haemoglobin in the red blood cells, with a non-linear relationship between the volume carried and the partial pressure (see ***Fig. 24.5***). Alveolar hyperventilation reduces the alveolar PCO_2 (P_ACO_2) and diffusion leads to a proportional fall in the carbon dioxide content of the blood (P_aCO_2). However, as the haemoglobin is already saturated with oxygen, increasing the alveolar PO_2 through hyperventilation will not increase blood oxygen content. This means that hypoxaemia due to physiological shunting cannot be compensated for by hyperventilation.

In individuals who have mild degrees of $\dot{V}_A/\dot{Q}$ mismatch, the P_aO_2 and P_aCO_2 will still be normal at rest. Increasing the requirements for gas exchange by exercise will widen the $\dot{V}_A/\dot{Q}$ mismatch and the P_aO_2 will fall. $\dot{V}_A/\dot{Q}$ mismatch is by far the most common cause of arterial hypoxaemia.

Alveolar stability

Pulmonary alveoli are polygonal spaces within a sponge-like matrix. Surface tension acting at the curved internal surface tends to cause the alveoli to decrease in size. The surface tension within the alveoli would make the lungs extremely difficult to distend were it not for the presence of surfactant, an insoluble lipoprotein largely consisting of dipalmitoyl lecithin, which forms a thin monomolecular layer at the air–fluid interface. Surfactant is secreted by type II pneumocytes within the alveolus and reduces surface tension so that alveoli remain stable.

Fluid surfaces covered with surfactant exhibit a phenomenon known as hysteresis; that is, the surface-tension-lowering effect of the surfactant can be improved by a transient increase in the size of the surface area of the alveoli. During quiet breathing, small areas of the lung undergo collapse, but it is possible to re-expand these rapidly by a deep breath: hence the importance of sighs or deep breaths as a feature of normal breathing. Failure of this mechanism, such as in patients with fractured ribs, gives rise to patchy basal lung collapse. Surfactant levels may be reduced in a number of lung diseases (e.g. pneumonia). Lack of surfactant plays a central role in the respiratory distress syndrome of the newborn. Severe reduction in perfusion of the lung impairs surfactant activity and this may explain the characteristic areas of collapse associated with pulmonary embolism.

Defence mechanisms of the respiratory tract

Pulmonary disease often results from a failure of the normal host defence mechanisms of the healthy lung (***Fig. 24.9***). These can be divided into physical, physiological, humoral and cellular mechanisms.

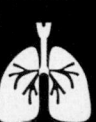

Physical and physiological mechanisms

Humidification

This prevents dehydration of the epithelium.

Particle removal

Over 90% of particles >10 μm in diameter are removed in the nostril or nasopharynx. This includes most pollen grains, which are typically >20 μm in diameter. Particles between 5 and 10 μm become impacted at the carina. Particles of <1 μm tend to remain airborne, thus the particles capable of reaching the deep lung are those in the 1–5 μm range.

Particle expulsion

This is effected by coughing, sneezing or gagging.

Respiratory tract secretions

The mucus of the respiratory tract is a gelatinous substance consisting of water and highly glycosylated proteins (mucins). The mucus forms a thick gel that is relatively impermeable to water and floats on a liquid or sol layer found around the cilia of the epithelial cells ***(Fig. 24.9)***. The gel layer is secreted from goblet cells and mucous glands as distinct globules that coalesce increasingly in the central airways to form a more or less continuous mucus blanket. In addition to the mucins, the gel contains various antimicrobial molecules (lysozyme, defensins), specific antibodies (IgA) and cytokines, which are secreted by cells in airways and are incorporated into the mucus gel. Bacteria, viruses and other particles become trapped in the mucus and are either inactivated or simply expelled before they can do any damage. Under normal conditions, the tips of the cilia engage with the undersurface of the gel phase and by coordinated movement they push the mucus blanket upwards and outwards to the pharynx, where it is either swallowed or coughed up. While it only takes 30–60 minutes for mucus to be cleared from the large bronchi, it can be several days before mucus is cleared from respiratory bronchioles. One of the major long-term effects of cigarette smoking is a reduction in mucociliary transport. This contributes to recurrent infection and prolongs contact with carcinogenic material. Air pollutants, local and general anaesthetics, and products of bacterial and viral infection also reduce mucociliary clearance.

Congenital defects in mucociliary transport lead to recurrent infections and eventually to bronchiectasis. For example, in the 'immotile cilia' syndrome there is an absence of the dynein arms in the cilia themselves, while in cystic fibrosis there is ciliary dyskinesia and abnormally thick mucus.

The respiratory microbiome

It has always been thought that the lower respiratory tract is sterile. Recent evidence has shown that there is a resident bacterial flora that is very similar to that of the mouth. The composition of the respiratory microbiome is determined by three factors:

- ***microbial immigration***, e.g. by inhalation, or microaspiration from the gastrointestinal tract
- ***the local growth conditions*** for the bacteria, e.g. temperature, pH, nutrients, concentration and activation of local inflammatory cells, and epithelial cell interactions
- ***microbial elimination*** by the usual mechanisms, i.e. the mucociliary escalator, coughing, and the innate and adaptive humoral mechanisms.

All of these factors will change in both acute and chronic lung conditions when there is an increase in pathological bacteria. This respiratory tract dysbiosis causes a disregulation of the local immune response and favours the growth of bacteria: for example, in the exacerbation of chronic diseases in which inflammation is perpetuated. The background composition of the bacterial microbiome in different conditions might favour exacerbations.

Humoral and cellular mechanisms

Non-specific soluble factors

- ***α-Antitrypsin*** (α_1-antiprotease; see p. 479) in lung secretions is derived from plasma. It inhibits chymotrypsin and trypsin, and neutralizes proteases including neutrophil elastase.
- ***Antioxidant defences*** include enzymes such as superoxide dismutase and low-molecular-weight antioxidant molecules (ascorbate, urate) in the epithelial lining fluid. In addition, lung cells are protected by an extensive range of intracellular defences, especially members of the glutathione S-transferase superfamily.
- ***Lysozyme*** is an enzyme found in granulocytes that has bactericidal properties.
- ***Lactoferrin*** is synthesized from epithelial cells and neutrophil granulocytes, and has bactericidal properties.
- ***Interferons*** are produced by most cells in response to viral infection and are potent modulators of lymphocyte function.
- ***Complement*** in secretions is also derived from plasma. In association with antibodies, it plays a major role in cytotoxicity.
- ***Surfactant protein A*** (SPA) is one of four species of surfactant proteins that opsonize bacteria/particles, enhancing phagocytosis by macrophages.
- ***Defensins*** are bactericidal peptides present in the azurophil granules of neutrophils.
- ***Dimeric secretory IgA*** targets specific antigens (see p. 392).

Innate and adaptive immunity

These mechanisms act as a defence against microbes, inorganic substances such as asbestos, particulate matter such as dust, and other antigens. They act by aiding opsonization so that macrophages can better ingest foreign material.

With infection, neutrophils migrate out of pulmonary capillaries into the air spaces and phagocytose and kill microbes with, for example, antimicrobial proteins (lactoferrin), degradative enzymes (elastase) and oxidant radicals. In addition, neutrophil extracellular traps ensnare and kill extracellular bacteria. Neutrophils also generate a variety of mediators, e.g. tumour necrosis factor alpha (TNF-α), interleukin 1 (IL-1), and chemokines that activate dendritic cells and B cells, and produce the T-cell-activating cytokine IL-12, which enhances neutrophil-mediated defence during pneumonia. Dendritic cells are antigen-presenting cells and are key to the adaptive immune response (see pp. 128–132).

Microbes are detected by host cells by pattern recognition receptors, such as toll-like receptors. These act via nuclear factor kappa B (NF-κB) transcription factors in the epithelial cells to produce adhesion molecules, chemokines and colony stimulating factors to initiate inflammation. Inflammation is necessary for innate immunity and host defence but can lead to lung damage; there is a fine line between defence and injury.

Further reading

Dickson RP, Martinez FJ, Huffnagle GB. The role of the microbiome in exacerbations of chronic lung diseases. *Lancet* 2014; 384:691–702.

Fahy JV, Dickey BF. Airway mucus function and dysfunction. *N Engl J Med* 2010; 363:2233–2247.

CLINICAL APPROACH TO THE PATIENT WITH RESPIRATORY DISEASE

Clinical features of respiratory disease

Runny, blocked nose and sneezing

Nasal symptoms are extremely common; 'runny nose' (rhinorrhoea), nasal blockage and attacks of sneezing can be caused by allergic rhinitis (see p. 1075) and by common colds (pp. 1075–1076).

Nasal secretions are usually thin and runny in allergic rhinitis but thicker and discoloured with viral infections. Nose bleeds and blood-stained nasal discharge are common and rarely indicate serious pathology. However, a blood-stained nasal discharge associated with nasal obstruction and pain may be the presenting feature of a nasal tumour (see p. 1318). Nasal polyps typically present with nasal blockage and loss of smell.

Cough

Cough (see also pp. 1089–1090) is the most common symptom of lower respiratory tract disease. It is caused by mechanical or chemical stimulation of cough receptors in the epithelium of the pharynx, larynx, trachea, bronchi and diaphragm. Afferent receptors go to the cough centre in the medulla, where efferent signals are generated to the expiratory musculature. Smokers often have a morning cough with a little sputum. A productive cough is the cardinal feature of chronic bronchitis, while dry coughing, particularly at night, can be a symptom of asthma or acid reflux. Cough also occurs in asthmatics after mild exertion or following forced expiration. Cough can occur without any definable pathology; psychological causes may be blamed but there is only limited evidence.

A worsening cough is the most common presenting symptom of lung cancer. The normal explosive character of the cough is lost when a vocal cord is paralysed, usually as a result of lung cancer infiltrating the left recurrent laryngeal nerve – sometimes termed a bovine cough. Cough can be accompanied by stridor in whooping cough or in laryngeal or tracheal obstruction.

Sputum

Approximately 100 mL of mucus is produced daily in a healthy, non-smoking individual. This flows gradually up the airways, through the larynx, and is then swallowed. Excess mucus is expectorated as sputum. Cigarette smoking is the most common cause of excess mucus production.

Mucoid sputum is clear and white but can contain black specks resulting from the inhalation of carbon. Yellow or green sputum is due to the presence of cellular material, including bronchial epithelial cells, or neutrophil or eosinophil granulocytes. Yellow sputum is not necessarily due to infection, as eosinophils in the sputum, as seen in asthma, can give the same appearance. The production of large quantities of yellow or green sputum is characteristic of bronchiectasis.

Haemoptysis (blood-stained sputum) varies from small streaks of blood to massive bleeding.

- The most common cause of mild haemoptysis is acute infection, particularly in exacerbations of COPD, but it should not be attributed to this without investigation.
- Other common causes are pulmonary infarction, bronchial carcinoma and tuberculosis.
- In lobar pneumonia, the sputum is usually rusty in appearance rather than frankly blood-stained.
- Pink, frothy sputum is seen in pulmonary oedema.
- In bronchiectasis, the blood is often mixed with purulent sputum.
- Massive haemoptysis (>200 mL of blood in 24 h) is usually due to bronchiectasis or tuberculosis.
- Uncommon causes of haemoptysis include idiopathic pulmonary haemosiderosis, Goodpasture syndrome, microscopic polyangiitis, trauma, blood disorders and benign tumours.

Haemoptysis should always be investigated. Although a diagnosis can often be made from a chest X-ray, a normal chest X-ray does not exclude disease. However, if the chest X-ray is normal, CT scanning and bronchoscopy are diagnostic in only about 5% of patients with haemoptysis.

Firm plugs of sputum may be coughed up by patients suffering from an exacerbation of allergic bronchopulmonary aspergillosis. Sometimes such sputum looks like casts of inflamed bronchi.

Breathlessness

Dyspnoea is a sense of awareness of increased respiratory effort that is unpleasant and that is recognized by the patient as being inappropriate. Patients often complain of tightness in the chest; this must be differentiated from angina.

Breathlessness should be assessed in relation to the patient's lifestyle. For example, a moderate degree of breathlessness will be totally disabling if the patient has to climb many flights of stairs to reach home.

Orthopnoea (see p. 939) is breathlessness on lying down. While it is classically linked to heart failure, it is partly due to the weight of the abdominal contents pushing the diaphragm up into the thorax. Such patients may also become breathless on bending over.

Tachypnoea and ***hyperpnoea*** are, respectively, an increased rate of breathing and an increased level of ventilation. These may be appropriate responses (e.g. during exercise).

Hyperventilation is inappropriate overbreathing. This may occur at rest or on exertion, and results in a lowering of the alveolar and arterial PCO_2 (see p. 916).

Paroxysmal nocturnal dyspnoea (see p. 939) is acute episodes of breathlessness at night, typically due to heart failure.

Wheezing

Wheezing is a common complaint and results from airflow limitation due to any cause. The symptom of wheezing is not diagnostic of asthma; other causes include vocal chord dysfunction, bronchiolitis and COPD. Conversely, wheeze may be absent in the early stages of asthma.

Chest pain

The most common type of chest pain reported in respiratory disease is a localized sharp pain, often termed pleuritic. It is made worse by deep breathing or coughing and the patient can usually localize it. Localized anterior chest pain with tenderness of a costochondral junction is caused by costochondritis. Shoulder tip pain suggests irritation of the diaphragmatic pleura, while central chest pain radiating to the neck and arms is likely to be cardiac. Retrosternal soreness is associated with tracheitis, while malignant invasion of the chest wall causes a constant, severe, dull pain.

Examination of the respiratory system

The nose

See page 1318.

The chest

Inspection

Assessment should be made of mental alertness, cyanosis, breathlessness at rest, use of accessory muscles, any deformity or scars on the chest and movement on both sides. CO_2 intoxication causes coarse tremor or flap of the outstretched hands. Prominent veins on the chest may imply obstruction of the superior vena cava.

Cyanosis (see p. 940) is a dusky colour of the skin and mucous membranes, due to the presence of >50 g/L of desaturated haemoglobin. When it has a central cause, cyanosis is visible on the tongue (especially the underside) and lips. Patients with central cyanosis will also be cyanosed peripherally. Peripheral cyanosis without central cyanosis is caused by a reduced peripheral circulation and is noted on the fingernails and skin of the extremities with associated coolness of the skin.

Finger clubbing is present when the normal angle between the base of the nail and the nail fold is lost. The base of the nail is fluctuant owing to increased vascularity, and there is an increased curvature of the nail in all directions, with expansion of the end of the digit. Some causes of clubbing are given in ***Box 24.2***. Clubbing is not a feature of uncomplicated COPD.

Palpation and percussion

The position of the trachea and apex beat should be checked. The supraclavicular fossa is examined for enlarged lymph nodes. The distance between the sternal notch and the cricoid cartilage (3–4 finger-breadths in full expiration) is reduced in patients with severe airflow limitation. Chest expansion should be checked; a tape measure may be used if precise or serial measurements are needed, such as in ***ankylosing spondylitis***. Local discomfort over the sternochondral joints suggests costochondritis. In rib fractures, compression of the chest laterally and anteroposteriorly produces localized pain. On percussion, liver dullness is usually detected anteriorly at the level of the sixth rib. Liver and cardiac dullness disappear when the lungs are over-inflated ***(Box 24.3)***.

Auscultation

The patient is asked to take deep breaths through the mouth. Inspiration should be more prolonged than expiration. Normal breath sounds are caused by turbulent flow in the larynx and sound harsher anteriorly over the upper lobes (particularly on the right). Healthy lungs filter out most of the high-frequency component, and the resulting sounds are called vesicular.

If the lung is consolidated or collapsed, the high-frequency hissing components of breath are not attenuated, and can be heard as 'bronchial breathing'. Similar sounds may be heard over areas of localized fibrosis or bronchiectasis. Bronchial breathing is accompanied by whispering pectoriloquy (whispered, high-pitched sounds can be heard distinctly through a stethoscope).

Box 24.2 Some causes of finger clubbing

Respiratory
- Bronchial carcinoma, especially epidermoid (squamous cell) type (major cause)
- Chronic suppurative lung disease:
  - Bronchiectasis
  - Lung abscess
  - Empyema
- Idiopathic lung fibrosis
- Pleural and mediastinal tumours (e.g. mesothelioma)
- Cryptogenic organizing pneumonia

Cardiovascular
- Cyanotic heart disease
- Subacute infective endocarditis
- Atrial myxoma

Miscellaneous
- Congenital – no disease
- Cirrhosis
- Inflammatory bowel disease

Box 24.3 Physical signs of respiratory disease

Pathological process	Mediastinal displacement	Percussion note	Breath sounds	Vocal resonance	Added sounds
Consolidation (i.e. lobar pneumonia)	None	Dull	Bronchial	Increased	Fine crackles
Collapse					
Major bronchus	Towards lesion	Dull	Diminished or absent	Reduced or absent	None
Peripheral bronchus	Towards lesion	Dull	Bronchial	Increased	Fine crackles
Fibrosis					
Localized	Towards lesion	Dull	Bronchial	Increased	Coarse crackles
Generalized (e.g. idiopathic lung fibrosis)	None	Normal	Vesicular	Increased	Fine crackles
Pleural effusion (>500 mL)	Away from lesion (in massive effusion)	Stony dull	Vesicular reduced or absent	Reduced or absent	None
Large pneumothorax	Away from lesion	Normal or hyper-resonant	Reduced or absent	Reduced or absent	None
Asthma	None	Normal	Vesicular Prolonged expiration	Normal	Expiratory polyphonic wheeze
Chronic obstructive pulmonary disease	None	Normal	Vesicular Prolonged expiration	Normal	Expiratory polyphonic wheeze and coarse crackles

Added sounds

Wheeze. Wheeze results from vibrations in the collapsible part of the airways when apposition occurs as a result of the flow-limiting mechanisms. Wheeze is usually heard during expiration and is commonly but not invariably present in asthma and COPD. In acute severe asthma, wheeze may not be heard, as airflow may be insufficient to generate the sound. Wheezes may be monophonic (single large airway obstruction) or polyphonic (narrowing of many small airways). An end-inspiratory wheeze or 'squeak' may be heard in obliterative bronchiolitis.

Crackles. These brief crackling sounds are probably produced by opening of previously closed bronchioles; early inspiratory crackles are associated with diffuse airflow limitation, while late inspiratory crackles are characteristically heard in pulmonary oedema, lung fibrosis and bronchiectasis.

Pleural rub. This creaking or groaning sound is usually well localized. It indicates inflammation and roughening of the pleural surfaces, which normally glide silently over one another.

Vocal resonance. Healthy lung attenuates high-frequency notes, as compared to the lower-pitched components of speech. Consolidated lung has the reverse effect, transmitting high frequencies well; the spoken word then takes on a bleating quality. Whispered (and therefore high-pitched) speech can be clearly heard over consolidated areas, as compared to healthy lung. Low-frequency sounds such as 'ninety-nine' are well transmitted across healthy lung to produce vibration that can be felt over the chest wall. Consolidated lung transmits these low-frequency noises less well, and pleural fluid severely dampens or obliterates the vibrations altogether. Tactile vocal fremitus is the palpation of this vibration, usually by placing the edge of the hand on the chest wall. For all practical purposes, this duplicates the assessment of vocal resonance and is not routinely performed as part of the chest examination.

Cardiovascular system examination

This gives additional information about the lungs (see pp. 940–943).

Additional bedside tests

Since so many patients with respiratory disease have airflow limitation, airflow should be routinely measured using a peak flow meter or spirometer. This is a much more useful assessment of airflow limitation than any physical sign.

Investigation of respiratory disease

Imaging

Imaging is essential in the investigation of most chest symptoms. Some diseases, such as tuberculosis or lung cancer, may be undetectable on clinical examination but are obvious on the chest X-ray. Conversely, asthma or chronic bronchitis may be associated with a normal chest X-ray. Always try to obtain previous images for comparison.

Chest X-ray

See ***Box 24.4***.

Collapse and consolidation

Simple pneumonia is easy to recognize (see ***Fig. 24.33***) but a careful search should be made for any evidence of collapse (***Fig. 24.10***; ***Box 24.5***). Loss of volume or crowding of the ribs is the best indicator of lobar collapse. The lung lobes collapse in characteristic directions. The lower lobes collapse downwards and towards the mediastinum; the left upper lobe collapses forwards against the anterior chest wall; and the right upper lobe collapses upwards and inwards, giving the appearance of an arch over the remaining lung. The right middle lobe collapses anteriorly and inwards, obscuring the right heart border. If a whole lung collapses, the mediastinum

Box 24.4 The chest X-ray

Check

- ***Centring of the image***. The distance between each clavicular head and the spinal processes should be equal.
- ***Penetration***. Check the image is not too dark and adjust the contrast.
- ***View:***
  - *Postero-anterior (PA) views* are used for routine images; the X-ray source is behind the patient.
  - *Anteroposterior (AP) views* are used only in patients who are unable to stand or cannot be taken to the radiology department; the cardiac outline appears bigger and the scapulae cannot be moved out of the way.
  - *Lateral views* were used to localize pathology but have been replaced by CT scans.

Look at

- Shape and bony structure of the chest wall
- Centrality of the trachea
- Elevation/flatness of the diaphragm
- Shape, size and position of the heart
- Shape and size of the hilar shadows
- Shape and size of any lung abnormalities
- Vascular shadowing

Box 24.5 Causes of lung collapse

- Enlarged tracheobronchial lymph nodes due to malignant disease or tuberculosis
- Inhaled foreign bodies (e.g. peanuts) in children, usually in the right main bronchus
- Bronchial casts or plugs (e.g. allergic bronchopulmonary aspergillosis)
- Retained secretions – postoperatively and in debilitated patients

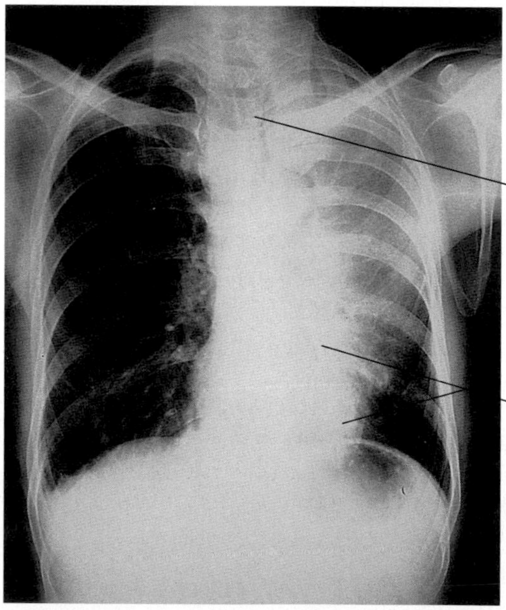

Figure 24.10 Collapse of the left upper lobe. Chest X-ray showing a triangular shadow in the left upper zone, next to the mediastinum.

Box 24.6 Causes of round shadows (>3cm) in the lung

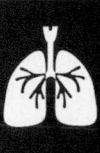

- Carcinoma
- Metastatic tumours (usually multiple shadows)
- Lung abscess (usually with fluid level)
- Encysted interlobar effusion (usually in horizontal fissure)
- Hydatid cysts (often with a fluid level)
- Arteriovenous malformations (usually adjacent to a vascular shadow)
- Aspergilloma
- Rheumatoid nodules
- Tuberculoma (may be calcification within the lesion)

Rare causes

Bronchial carcinoid

- Cylindroma
- Chondroma
- Lipoma

Other shadows related to mediastinum

- Pericardium
- Oesophagus
- Spinal cord

} Seen on lateral chest X-ray

will shift towards the side of the collapse. Uncomplicated consolidation does not cause mediastinal shift or loss of lung volume, so any of these features should raise the suspicion of an endobronchial obstruction.

Pleural effusion

Pleural effusions (see ***Fig. 24.45***) need to be larger than 500mL to cause much more than blunting of the costophrenic angle. On an erect film, they produce a characteristic shadow with a curved upper edge rising into the axilla. If they are very large, the whole of one hemithorax may be opaque, with mediastinal shift away from the effusion.

Fibrosis

Localized fibrosis produces streaky shadowing, and the accompanying loss of lung volume causes mediastinal structures to move to the same side. More generalized fibrosis can lead to a honeycomb appearance (see p. 1115), seen as diffuse shadows containing multiple circular translucencies a few millimetres in diameter.

Round shadows

Lung cancer is the most common cause of large round shadows but many other causes are recognized ***(Box 24.6)***.

Miliary mottling

This term, derived from the Latin for millet, describes numerous minute opacities, 1–3mm in size. The most common causes are tuberculosis, pneumoconiosis, sarcoidosis, idiopathic pulmonary fibrosis and pulmonary oedema (see Fig. 23.15), although pulmonary oedema is usually perihilar and accompanied by larger, fluffy shadows. Pulmonary microlithiasis is a rare but striking cause of miliary mottling.

Computed tomography

Computed tomography (CT) provides excellent images of the lungs and mediastinal structures ***(Fig. 24.11)***. It is essential in staging bronchial carcinoma by demonstrating tumour size, nodal involvement, metastases and invasion of mediastinum, pleura or chest wall. CT-guided needle biopsy allows samples to be obtained from peripheral masses. Staging scans should assess liver and adrenals, which are common sites for metastatic disease. Mediastinal structures are shown more clearly after injecting intravenous contrast medium.

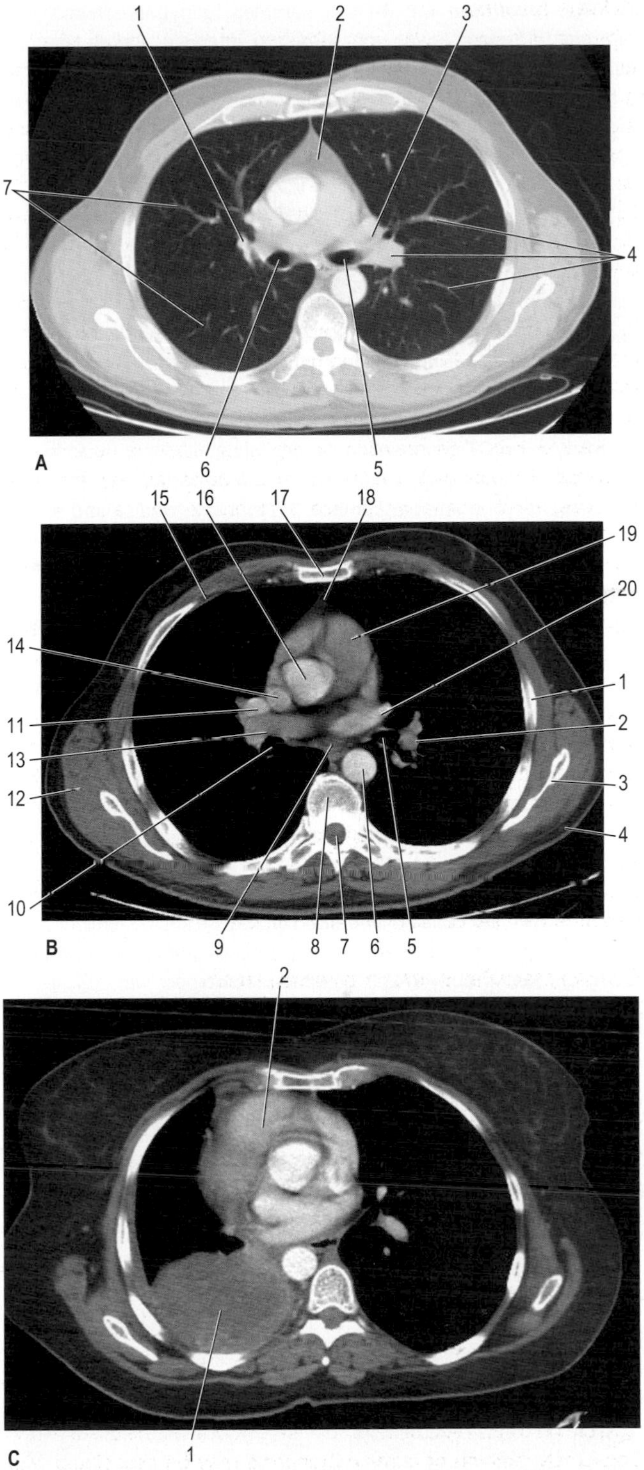

Figure 24.11 Computed tomography scans of the lung. A. *Lung setting* – showing normal lung markings. 1, right hilum; 2, mediastinum; 3, left hilum; 4, lung vessels; 5, left main bronchus; 6, right main bronchus; 7, peripheral lung vessels. **B. *Mediastinal (soft tissue) setting*** – showing normal mediastinal structures following intravenous contrast enhancement. 1, rib; 2, descending left pulmonary artery; 3, scapula; 4, subcutaneous fat; 5, left main bronchus; 6, descending aorta; 7, spinal canal; 8, vertebral body; 9, oesophagus; 10, right main bronchus; 11, right pulmonary artery; 12, muscle; 13, right superior pulmonary vein; 14, superior vena cava; 15, costal cartilage; 16, ascending aorta; 17, sternum; 18, thymic remnant; 19, pulmonary trunk; 20, left superior pulmonary vein. **C. *Post-contrast scan*** – showing large right upper zone carcinoma (1) with enlarged lymph nodes (2) in the mediastinum surrounding the trachea.

High-resolution CT (HRCT) samples lung parenchyma with 1–2 mm thickness scans at 10–20 mm intervals and is used to assess diffuse inflammatory and infective parenchymal processes. It is valuable in:

- evaluation of diffuse disease of the lung parenchyma, including sarcoidosis, hypersensitivity pneumonitis, occupational lung disease, and any other form of interstitial pulmonary fibrosis
- diagnosis of bronchiectasis; HRCT has a sensitivity and specificity of >90%
- distinction of emphysema from diffuse parenchymal lung disease or pulmonary vascular disease as a cause of a low gas transfer factor with otherwise normal lung function
- suspected opportunistic lung infection in immunocompromised patients
- diagnosis of lymphangitis carcinomatosa.

Multi-slice CT scanners can produce detailed images in two or three dimensions in any plane. This detail is particularly useful for the detection of pulmonary emboli. Pulmonary nodules and airway disease are more easily defined, reducing the need for HRCT.

Magnetic resonance imaging

Magnetic resonance imaging (MRI) with electrocardiography (ECG) gating allows accurate imaging of the heart and aortic aneurysms, and MRI has been used in staging lung cancer, for assessing tumour invasion in the mediastinum, chest wall and at the lung apex, because it produces good images in the sagittal and coronal planes. Vascular structures can be clearly differentiated, as flowing blood produces a signal void on MRI. MRI is less valuable than CT in assessing the lung parenchyma.

Positron emission tomography

Tumours take up labelled fluorodeoxyglucose (FDG), which emits positrons that can be imaged. In bronchial carcinoma, positron emission tomography (PET) scanning combined with CT is the investigation of choice for assessing lymph nodes and metastatic disease, and helps to differentiate benign from malignant tumours.

Scintigraphic imaging

Isotopic lung scans were used widely for the detection of pulmonary emboli but are now performed less often owing to widespread use of CT pulmonary angiography.

Perfusion scan

Macro-aggregated human albumin labelled with technetium-99m (^{99m}Tc) is injected intravenously. The particles impact in pulmonary capillaries, where they remain for a few hours. A gamma camera is then used to detect the deposition of the particles. The resultant pattern indicates the distribution of pulmonary blood flow; cold areas occur where there is defective blood flow (e.g. in pulmonary emboli).

Ventilation–perfusion scan

Xenon-133 gas is inhaled and its distribution is detected at the same time as the perfusion scan. Areas affected by pulmonary embolism will have reduced perfusion relative to ventilation (see pp. 1032–1033). Other lung diseases (e.g. asthma or pneumonia) impair both ventilation and perfusion. Unfortunately, a pulmonary embolus can affect the lung substance (e.g. atelectasis), leading to reduced ventilation. Nevertheless, this is a better technique than perfusion scanning alone.

Ultrasound

Ultrasound (USS) is useful for diagnosing and aspirating small pleural effusions, and for placing intercostal drains safely. USS-guided biopsy is used for lung masses that abut the pleura. Endobronchial USS is increasingly being used to assess mediastinal lymphadenopathy and to stage lung cancer.

Respiratory function tests

In clinical practice, airflow limitation can be assessed by relatively simple tests that have good intra-subject repeatability ***(Box 24.7)***. Results must be compared with predicted values for healthy subjects, as normal ranges vary with sex, age and height. Moreover, there is considerable variation between healthy individuals of the same size and age; the standard deviation for the peak expiratory flow rate is approximately 50 L/min, and for the FEV_1 it is approximately 0.4 L. Repeated measurements of lung function are useful for assessing the progression of disease in individual patients.

Tests of ventilatory function

These tests are used mainly to assess the degree of airflow limitation during expiration.

Spirometry

The patient takes a maximum inspiration followed by a forced expiration (for as long as possible) into the spirometer. The spirometer measures the 1-second forced expiratory volume (FEV_1) and the total volume of exhaled gas (forced vital capacity, FVC). Both FEV_1 and FVC are related to height, age and sex ***(Fig. 24.12)***.

In airflow limitation, the FEV_1 is reduced as a percentage of FVC. In normal health, the FEV_1/FVC ratio is around 75%. With increasing airflow limitation, FEV_1 falls proportionately more than FVC, so the FEV_1/FVC ratio is reduced. With restrictive lung disease, FEV_1 and FVC are reduced proportionately and the FEV_1/FVC ratio remains normal or may even increase because of enhanced elastic recoil.

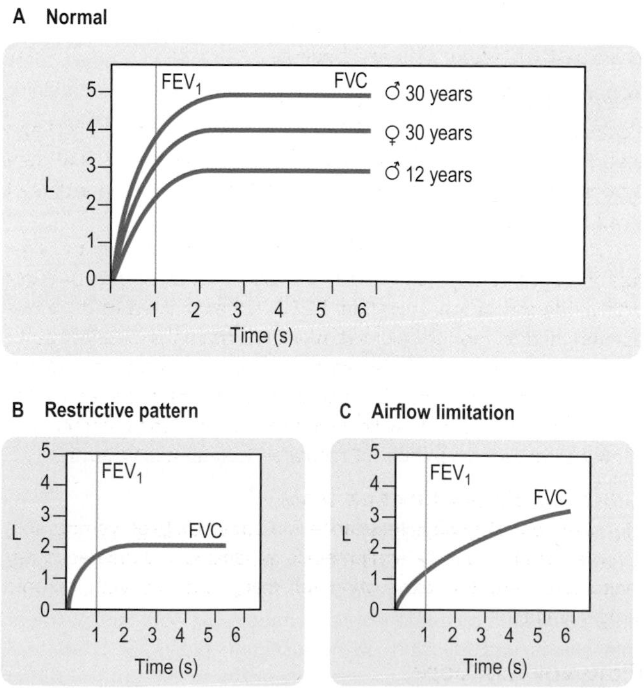

Figure 24.12 Spirometry: volume–time curves. A. Normal patterns for age and sex. **B.** Restrictive pattern (FEV_1 and FVC reduced). **C.** Airflow limitation (FEV_1 only reduced). FEV_1, forced expiratory volume in 1 s; FVC, forced vital capacity.

Box 24.7 Respiratory function and exercise tests

Test	Use	Advantages	Disadvantages
PEFR	Monitoring changes in airflow limitation in asthma	Portable Can be used at the bedside	Effort-dependent Poor measure of chronic airflow limitation
FEV, FVC, FEV_1/FVC	Assessment of airflow limitation The best single test	Reproducible Relatively effort-independent	Bulky equipment but smaller portable machines available
Flow–volume curves	Assessment of flow at lower lung volumes Detection of large-airway obstruction, both intra- and extrathoracic (e.g. tracheal stenosis, tumour)	Recognizes patterns of flow–volume curves for different diseases	Sophisticated equipment needed for full test but expiratory loop possible with compact spirometry
Airways resistance	Assessment of airflow limitation	Sensitive	Technique difficult to perform
Lung volumes	Differentiation between restrictive and obstructive lung disease	Effort-independent, complements FEV_1	Sophisticated equipment needed
Gas transfer	Assessment and monitoring of extent of interstitial lung disease and emphysema	Non-invasive (compared with lung biopsy or radiation from repeated chest X-rays and CT)	Sophisticated equipment needed
Blood gases	Assessment of respiratory failure	Can detect early lung disease when measured during exercise	Invasive
Pulse oximetry	Postoperative, sleep studies and respiratory failure	Continuous monitoring Non-invasive	Measures saturation only
Exercise tests (6-min walk)	Practical assessment for disability and effects of therapy	No equipment required	Time-consuming Learning effect At least two walks required
Cardiorespiratory assessment	Early detection of lung/heart disease Fitness assessment	Differentiates breathlessness due to lung or heart disease	Expensive and complicated equipment required

CT, computed tomography; FEV, forced expiratory volume; FEV_1, forced expiratory volume in 1 s; FVC, forced vital capacity; PEFR, peak expiratory flow rate.

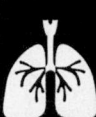

In chronic airflow limitation (particularly in COPD and asthma), the total lung capacity (TLC) is usually increased, yet there is nearly always some reduction in the FVC. This is because collapse of small airways causes obstruction to airflow before the normal residual volume (RV) is reached. This trapping of air within the lung is a characteristic feature of these diseases.

Peak expiratory flow rate

Peak expiratory flow rate (PEFR) is an extremely simple and cheap test. Subjects take a full inspiration to total lung capacity and then blow out forcefully into the peak flow meter ***(Fig. 24.13)***. The best of three attempts is recorded.

Although reproducible, PEFR is mainly dependent on the flow rate in larger airways and it may be falsely reassuring in patients with moderate airflow limitation. PEFR is mainly used to diagnose asthma, and to monitor exacerbations of asthma and response to treatment. Regular measurements of peak flow rates on waking, during the afternoon, and before going to bed demonstrate the wide diurnal variations in airflow limitation that characterize asthma and allow objective assessment of response to treatment ***(Fig. 24.14)***.

Other ventilatory function tests

Measurement of airways resistance in a body box (plethysmograph) is more sensitive but the equipment is expensive and the manoeuvres are too exhausting for many patients with chronic airflow limitation.

Flow–volume loops

Plotting flow rates against expired volume (flow–volume loops; see ***Fig. 24.7***) shows the site of airflow limitation within the lung. At the start of expiration from TLC, maximum resistance is from the large airways, and this affects the flow rate for the first 25% of the curve. As air is exhaled, lung volume reduces and the flow rate becomes dependent on the resistance of smaller airways. In COPD, where the disease mainly affects the smaller airways, expiratory flow rates at 50% or 25% of the vital capacity are disproportionately reduced when compared with flow rates at larger lung volumes. Flow–volume loops will also show obstruction of large airways: for example, tracheal narrowing due to tumour or retrosternal goitre.

Lung volumes

The subdivisions of lung volume are shown in ***Figure 24.15***. Tidal volume and vital capacity can be measured using a simple spirometer, but alternative techniques are needed to measure TLC and RV. TLC is measured by inhaling air containing a known concentration of helium and measuring its dilution in the exhaled air. RV can be calculated by subtracting the vital capacity from the TLC.

TLC measurements using this technique are inaccurate if there are large cystic spaces in the lung because helium cannot diffuse into them. Under these circumstances, the thoracic gas volume can be measured more accurately using a body plethysmograph (see above). The difference between measurements made by these two methods shows the extent of non-communicating air space within the lungs.

Transfer factor

To measure the efficiency of gas transfer across the alveolar–capillary membrane, carbon monoxide is used as a surrogate, since its diffusion rate is similar to oxygen. A low concentration of carbon monoxide is inhaled and the rate of absorption calculated. In normal lungs, the transfer factor accurately reflects the diffusing capacity of the lungs for oxygen and depends on the thickness of the alveolar–capillary membrane. In lung disease, the diffusing capacity

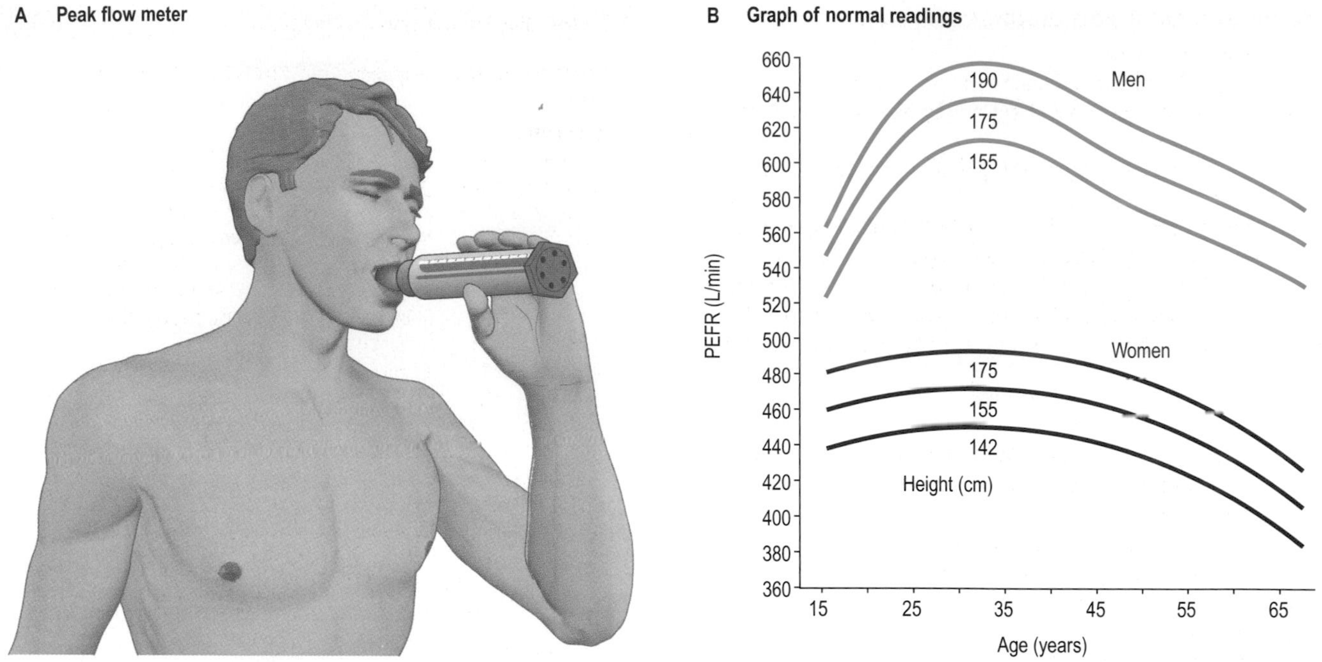

Figure 24.13 **Peak flow measurements. A.** Peak flow meter; the lips should be tight around the mouthpiece. **B.** Normal readings. PEFR, peak expiratory flow rate.

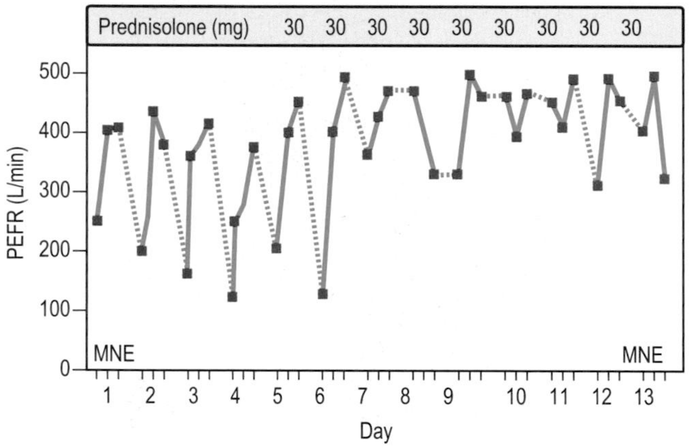

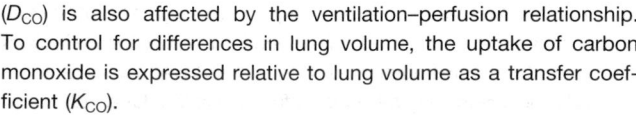

Figure 24.14 **Diurnal variability in peak expiratory flow rate (PEFR) in asthma, showing the effect of steroids.** M, morning; N, noon; E, evening.

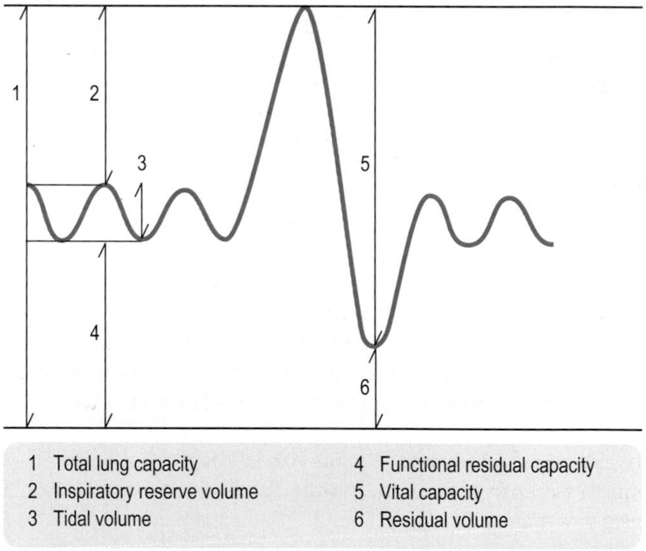

Figure 24.15 **The subdivisions of the lung volume.**

(D_{CO}) is also affected by the ventilation–perfusion relationship. To control for differences in lung volume, the uptake of carbon monoxide is expressed relative to lung volume as a transfer coefficient (K_{CO}).

Gas transfer is reduced in patients with severe degrees of emphysema and fibrosis, but also in heart failure and anaemia. Although relatively non-specific, gas transfer is particularly useful in the detection and monitoring of diseases affecting the lung parenchyma (e.g. idiopathic pulmonary fibrosis, sarcoidosis and asbestosis).

Measurement of blood gases

This technique is described on pages 1161–1162.

Measurement of the partial pressures of oxygen and carbon dioxide in arterial blood is essential in managing respiratory failure and severe asthma, when repeated measurements are often the best guide to therapy.

Peripheral oxygen saturation (S_pO_2) can be continuously measured using an oximeter with either ear or finger probes. Pulse oximetry has become an essential part of the routine monitoring of patients in hospital and clinics. It is also useful in exercise testing and reduces the need to measure arterial blood gases.

Exhaled nitric oxide

Nitric oxide (NO) is produced by the bronchial epithelium and increases in asthma and other forms of airway inflammation. Measuring exhaled NO can guide therapy in asthma that is difficult to control.

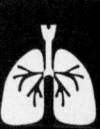

Haematological and biochemical tests

It is useful to measure:

- haemoglobin, to detect anaemia or polycythaemia
- packed cell volume (secondary polycythaemia occurs with chronic hypoxia)
- routine biochemistry (often disturbed in carcinoma and infection)
- D-dimer to detect intravascular coagulation; a negative test makes pulmonary embolism very unlikely.

Other blood investigations sometimes required include α_1-antitrypsin levels, *Aspergillus* antibodies, viral and mycoplasma serology, autoantibody profiles and specific IgE measurements.

Sputum

Sputum should be inspected for colour:

- Yellowish-green indicates inflammation (infection or allergy).
- Blood suggests a neoplasm or pulmonary infarct (see 'Haemoptysis', p. 1066).

Microbiological studies (e.g. Gram stain and culture) are rarely helpful in upper respiratory tract infections or in acute or chronic bronchitis. They are of value in:

- pneumonia
- tuberculosis
- unusual clinical problems
- *Aspergillus* lung disease.

Sputum cytology

This is useful in the diagnosis of bronchial carcinoma and asthma. Its advantages are speed, cheapness and its non-invasive nature.

However, not everyone can produce sputum and a reliable cytologist is needed. Sputum can be induced by inhalation of nebulized hypertonic saline (5%). Better samples can be obtained by bronchoscopy and bronchial washings (see p. 1074).

Exercise tests

The predominant symptom in respiratory medicine is breathlessness. The degree of disability produced by breathlessness can be assessed by asking the patient to walk for 6 minutes along a measured track. This has been shown to be a reproducible and useful test once the patient has undergone an initial training walk to overcome the learning effect. Additional information can be obtained by using pulse oximetry during exercise to assess desaturation.

More sophisticated cardiopulmonary exercise tests are useful in investigating unexplained breathlessness. These involve measurement of oxygen uptake ($\dot{V}O_2$), work performed, heart rate, blood pressure and serial ECGs.

Pleural aspiration

Diagnostic aspiration is necessary for all but very small effusions. Nowadays, this is usually done under ultrasound guidance, using full aseptic precautions. A needle is inserted under local anaesthesia through an intercostal space towards the top of the area identified on ultrasound. Fluid is withdrawn and the presence of any blood is noted. Samples are sent for cytology, protein estimation, lactate dehydrogenase (LDH) and bacteriological examination, including culture and Ziehl–Neelsen/auramine staining for tuberculosis. Large amounts of fluid can be aspirated through a large-bore needle to help relieve extreme breathlessness.

Pleural biopsy

Pleural biopsy used to be performed at the bedside but is now generally done under direct vision using video-assisted thoracoscopy (VATS).

Box 24.8 Intercostal drainage

Explain the nature of the procedure to the patient and obtain written consent.

Technique

1. Identify the site for aspiration (using ultrasound in most cases).
2. Carefully sterilize the skin over the aspiration site.
3. Anaesthetize the skin, muscle and pleura with 2% lidocaine.
4. Make a small incision and insert an 8–12 French gauge drain, using the Seldinger technique. A needle is used to enter the pleural space, and then withdrawn over a guide wire over which the catheter is then inserted. (A larger-calibre catheter is needed for drainage of empyema, or a 28 French gauge Argyle catheter.)
5. Attach to a three-way tap and 50 mL syringe, and aspirate up to 1000 mL. Stop aspiration if the patient becomes uncomfortable; shock may ensue if too much fluid is withdrawn too quickly.
6. If the drain is to stay in, secure it to skin with suture and sterile dressing.
7. Attach the drain to an underwater seal drainage bottle and allow fluid to drain. Clamp the drain and release periodically, especially if patient becomes uncomfortable (usually up to 1000 mL at a time before clamping for a few hours).
8. Perform a chest X-ray to check the position of the rain.

Pleurodesis

- Instil lidocaine 3 mg/kg and then talc 4–5 g in 50 ml sodium chloride 0.9% solution into the pleural cavity to achieve pleurodesis in recurrent/malignant effusion.

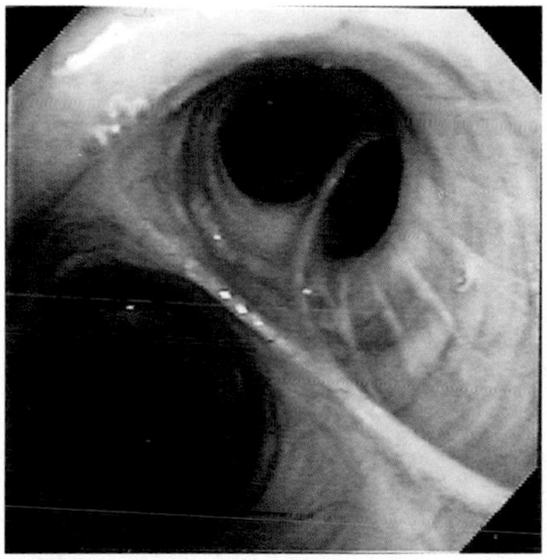

Figure 24.16 Normal endobronchial appearances as seen at fibreoptic bronchoscopy.

Intercostal drainage

This is carried out when large effusions are present, producing severe breathlessness, or for drainage of an empyema ***(Box 24.8)***. Drains should be inserted with ultrasound guidance. Pleurodesis is performed for recurrent/malignant effusion. Occasionally, a ***long-term pleural drain*** may be needed for recurrent effusions.

Mediastinoscopy

Mediastinoscopy is used in the diagnosis of mediastinal masses and in the staging of nodal disease in carcinoma of the bronchus. An incision is made just above the sternum and a mediastinoscope inserted by blunt dissection. Mediastinoscopy is needed much less often now, since the introduction of endobronchial ultrasound (EBUS).

Fibreoptic bronchoscopy

See ***Box 24.9*** and ***Figure 24.16***.

Box 24.9 Fibreoptic bronchoscopy

This enables the direct visualization of the bronchial tree as far as the sub-segmental bronchi under a local anaesthetic. Obtain informed written consent after explaining the nature of the procedure.

Indications
- Lesions requiring biopsy seen on chest X-ray
- Haemoptysis
- Stridor
- Positive sputum cytology for malignant cells with no chest X-ray abnormality
- Collection of bronchial secretions for bacteriology, especially tuberculosis
- Recurrent laryngeal nerve paralysis of unknown aetiology
- Infiltrative lung disease (to obtain a transbronchial biopsy)
- Investigation of collapsed lobes or segments and aspiration of mucus plugs

Disadvantages
- All patients require sedation to tolerate the procedure
- Minor and transient cardiac dysrhythmias occur in up to 40% of patients on passage of the bronchoscope through the larynx. Monitoring is required
- Oxygen supplementation is required in patients with P_aO_2 <8 kPa
- Fibreoptic bronchoscopy should be performed with care in the very sick, and transbronchial biopsies avoided in ventilated patients owing to the increased risk of pneumothorax
- Massive bleeding may occur after biopsy of vascular lesions or carcinoid tumours. Rigid bronchoscopy may be required to allow adequate access to the bleeding point for haemostasis

Under local anaesthesia and sedation, the central airways can be visualized down to sub-segmental level and biopsies taken for histology. More distal lesions may be sampled by washing or blind brushing. Diffuse inflammatory and infective lung processes may be sampled by bronchoalveolar lavage and transbronchial biopsy. The yield is best in sarcoidosis, lymphangitis carcinomatosa and hypersensitivity pneumonitis. Other fibrotic lung diseases rarely yield diagnostic samples so it may be preferable to perform open or thoracoscopic lung biopsy. EBUS enables direct sampling of lymph nodes for diagnostic staging of lung cancer.

Video-assisted thoracoscopic lung biopsy

Video-assisted thoracoscopic (VATS) lung biopsy has largely replaced open thoracotomy when a lung biopsy is required (see p. 1115).

Skin-prick tests

Allergen solutions are placed on the skin (usually the volar surface of the forearm) and the epidermis is broken using a 1 mm tipped lancet. A separate lancet should be used for each allergen. If the patient is sensitive to the allergen, a weal develops. The weal diameter is measured after 10 minutes. A weal of at least 3 mm diameter is regarded as positive, provided that the control test is negative. The results should always be interpreted in the light of the history. Skin tests are not affected by bronchodilators or corticosteroids but antihistamines should be discontinued at least 48 hours before testing.

Further reading

Bohadana A, Izbicki G, Kraman SS. Fundamentals of lung auscultation. *N Engl J Med* 2014; 370:744–751.

Hansell DM, Lynch DA, Page McAdams H et al. *Imaging of Diseases of the Chest*, 5th edn. Chicago: Elsevier Mosby; 2010.

Box 24.10 The dangers of cigarette smoking

General
- Lung cancer
- Chronic obstructive pulmonary disease (COPD)
- Carcinoma of the oesophagus
- Ischaemic heart disease
- Peripheral vascular disease
- Bladder cancer
- An increase in abnormal spermatozoa
- Memory problems

Maternal smoking
- A decrease in birth weight of the infant
- An increase in fetal and neonatal mortality
- An increase in asthma

Passive smoking
- Risk of asthma, pneumonia and bronchitis in infants of smoking parents
- An increase in cough and breathlessness in smokers and non-smokers with COPD and asthma
- An increase in cancer risk

SMOKING

Prevalence

Cigarette smoking is declining in the Western world. In 1974 in the UK, 51% of men and 41% of women smoked cigarettes – nearly half the adult population. Now, about 21% of men and 19% of women aged 16 years and over smoke. The highest rates are in people aged 20–24 (28% of women and 30% of men in this age group smoke). The highest rates of cigarette consumption per capita are in Serbia, Bulgaria, Greece and Russia. In global terms, the USA ranks 51st and the UK ranks 73rd, close to the rates in Sweden, Canada and the Netherlands. Smoking continues to increase in many developing countries, particularly among women.

Toxic effects

Cigarette smoke contains polycyclic aromatic hydrocarbons and nitrosamines, which are potent carcinogens. It causes release of enzymes from neutrophil granulocytes and macrophages that are capable of destroying elastin and leading to lung damage. Pulmonary epithelial permeability increases, even in symptomless cigarette smokers, and correlates with the concentration of carboxyhaemoglobin in blood. This altered permeability may allow easier access for carcinogens.

The dangers

Cigarette smoking is addictive and harmful to health ***(Box 24.10)***. People usually start smoking in adolescence for psychosocial reasons and, once they smoke regularly, the pharmacological properties of nicotine encourage persistence, by their effect on the smoker's mood. Very few cigarette smokers (<2%) can limit themselves to occasional or intermittent smoking.

Significant dose–response relationships exist between cigarette consumption, airway inflammation and lung cancer mortality ***(Box 24.11)***. Sputum production and airflow limitation increase with daily cigarette consumption, and effort tolerance decreases. Smoking 20 cigarettes daily for 20 years increases the lifetime risk of lung cancer by about 10 times compared to a lifelong non-smoker. Smoking and asbestos exposure are synergistic risk factors for lung cancer, with a combined risk of about 90 times that of unexposed non-smokers.

Cigarette smokers who change to cigars or pipe-smoking can reduce their risk of lung cancer. However, pipe- and cigar-smokers remain at greater risk of lung cancer than lifelong non-smokers or former smokers.

Box 24.11 Effects of smoking on the lung

Large airways
- Increase in submucosal gland volume
- Increase in number of goblet cells
- Chronic inflammation
- Metaplasia and dysplasia of the surface epithelium

Small airways
- Increase in number and distribution of goblet cells
- Airway inflammation and fibrosis
- Epithelial metaplasia/dysplasia
- Carcinoma

Parenchyma
- Proximal acinar scarring
- Increase in alveolar macrophage numbers
- Emphysema (centri-acinar, pan-acinar)

Environmental tobacco smoke ('passive smoking') has been shown to increase the frequency and severity of asthma attacks in children and may also increase the incidence of asthma. It is also associated with a small but definite increase in lung cancer. Worldwide, second-hand smoke was estimated to affect 40% of children, 33% of non-smoking males and 35% of non-smoking females in 2004. This caused a 1% worldwide mortality and 0.7% of the total worldwide burden of disease in disability-adjusted life years (DALYs).

Stopping smoking

If the entire population could be persuaded to stop smoking, the effect on healthcare use would be enormous. National campaigns, bans on advertising and a substantial increase in the cost of cigarettes are the best ways of achieving this at the population level. Smoking bans in the workplace and public spaces have also helped. Meanwhile, active encouragement to stop smoking remains a useful approach for individuals. Smokers who want to stop should have access to smoking cessation clinics to provide behavioural support. Nicotine replacement therapy (NRT) and bupropion are effective aids to smoking cessation in those smoking more than 10 cigarettes/day. Both should be used only in smokers who commit to a target stop date, and the initial prescription should be for 2 weeks beyond the target stop date. NRT is the preferred choice; there is no evidence that combined therapy offers any advantage. Therapy should be changed after 3 months if abstinence is not achieved.

Varenicline is an oral partial agonist on the $\alpha_4\beta_2$ subtype of the nicotinic acetylcholine receptor. It stimulates the nicotine receptor and reduces withdrawal symptoms and also the craving for cigarettes. A 12-week course quadruples the chance of stopping smoking; its main side-effects are nausea and sometimes severe depression. Cytisine, which has high affinity for the same receptor, also aids smoking cessation. Electronic cigarettes (battery-operated vaporizer) are a useful alternative for ex-smokers who miss the physical process of handling cigarettes and inhaling nicotine. While E-cigarettes are not harmless, they are much less harmful than ordinary cigarettes.

Further reading

Colditz GA. Smoke alarm – tobacco control remains paramount. *N Engl J Med* 2015; 372:665–666.

Gu Dongfeng, Kelly TN, Wu Xigui et al. Mortality attributable to smoking in China. *N Engl J Med* 2009; 360:150–159.

Oberg M, Jaakkola MS, Woodward A et al. Worldwide burden of disease from exposure to second-hand smoke: a retrospective analysis of data from 192 countries. *Lancet* 2008; 372:139–146.

Oncken C. Nicotine replacement for smoking cessation during pregnancy. *N Engl J Med* 2012; 366:846–847.

DISEASES OF THE UPPER RESPIRATORY TRACT

Rhinitis

The common cold (acute coryza)

This highly infectious illness (see p. 253) is due to a variety of respiratory viruses: for example, the rhinoviruses (most common), coronaviruses and adenoviruses. Infectivity from close personal contact (nasal mucus on hands) or droplets is high in the early stages of the infection, and spread is facilitated by overcrowding and poor ventilation. There are at least 100 different antigenic strains of rhinovirus, making it difficult for the immune system to confer protection. The incubation period varies from 12 hours to 5 days.

The clinical features are tiredness, slight pyrexia, malaise, and a sore nose and pharynx. Sneezing and profuse, watery nasal discharge are followed by thick mucopurulent secretions that may persist for up to a week. Secondary bacterial infection occurs in only a minority of cases.

Other forms of rhinitis

Rhinitis is defined clinically as sneezing attacks, nasal discharge or blockage occurring for more than an hour on most days:

- for a limited period of the year (seasonal or intermittent rhinitis)
- throughout the whole year (perennial or persistent rhinitis).

Seasonal rhinitis

This is the most common allergic disorder. It is often called 'hayfever', but as this implies that only grass pollen is responsible, it is better described as seasonal (or intermittent) allergic rhinitis. Worldwide prevalence rates vary from 2% to 20%. Prevalence is maximal in the second decade, and up to 30% of UK teenagers and young adults are affected each June and July.

Nasal irritation, sneezing and watery rhinorrhoea occur, but many also suffer from itching of the eyes and soft palate, and occasionally even itching of the ears because of the common innervation of the pharyngeal mucosa and the ear. In addition, approximately 20% suffer from seasonal wheezing. The common seasonal allergens are shown in ***Figure 24.17***.

Since pollination of plants that give rise to high pollen counts varies from country to country, seasonal rhinoconjunctivitis and accompanying wheeze may occur at different times of year in different regions.

Perennial rhinitis

In about 50% of patients with perennial rhinitis, symptoms of sneezing and watery rhinorrhoea predominate, whilst the other half complain mostly of nasal blockage. The patient may lose the senses of smell and taste but rarely has eye or throat symptoms. Sinusitis occurs in about 50% of cases, due to mucosal swelling that obstructs drainage from the sinuses. Perennial rhinitis is most frequent in the second and third decades, decreasing with age, and can be divided into four main types.

Perennial allergic rhinitis

The most common cause is allergy to the faecal particles of the house-dust mite, *Dermatophagoides pteronyssinus* or *D. farinae*; these are under 0.5 mm in size, invisible to the naked eye ***(Fig. 24.18)***, and found in dust throughout the house, particularly in older, damp dwellings. Mites live off desquamated human skin scales and the highest concentrations (4000 mites/g of surface dust) are found in human bedding. Their faecal particles are approximately 20 μm in

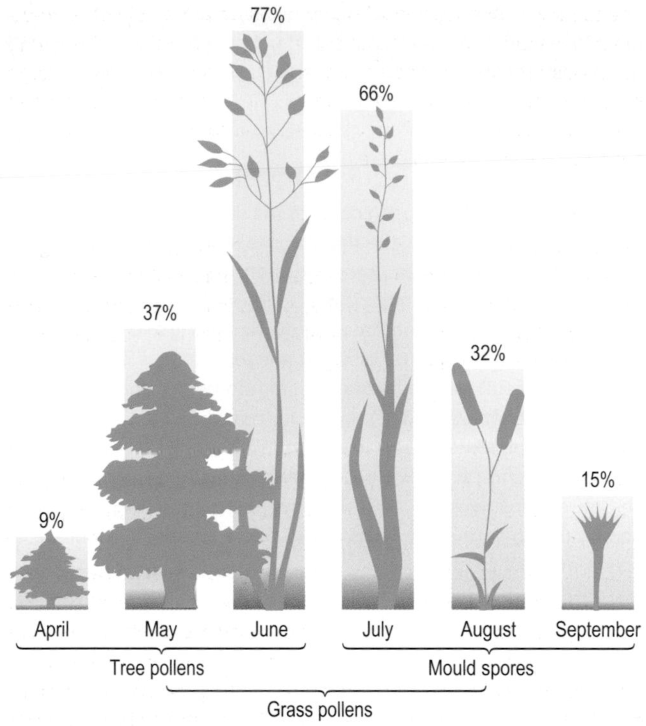

Figure 24.17 Seasonal allergic rhinitis. Bar graph showing the proportion of patients whose symptoms are worst in the month or months indicated. The causative agents are also shown.

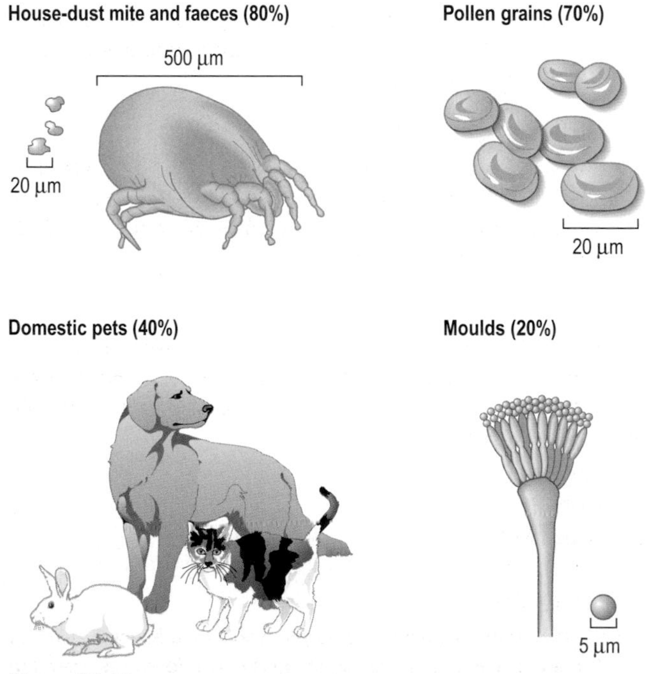

Figure 24.18 Common allergens causing allergic rhinitis and asthma. These include the house-dust mite, faeces of house-dust mites, pollen grains, domestic pets and moulds. Percentages indicate the proportion of positive skin-prick tests to these allergens in patients with allergic rhinitis.

diameter ***(Fig. 24.18)***, and impact in the nose rather than the lungs, unless the patient breathes through the mouth.

The next most common allergens come from domestic pets (especially cats) and are proteins derived from urine or saliva spread over the surface of the animal, as well as skin protein. Allergy to urinary protein from small mammals is a major cause of morbidity among laboratory workers.

Industrial dust, vapours and fumes cause occupationally related perennial rhinitis more often than asthma.

The presence of perennial rhinitis makes the nose more reactive to non-specific stimuli, such as cigarette smoke, washing powders, household detergents, strong perfumes and traffic fumes. Although patients often think they are allergic to these stimuli, these are irritant responses and do not involve antibodies.

Perennial non-allergic rhinitis with eosinophilia

No extrinsic allergic cause can be identified, either from the history or on skin testing, but eosinophilic granulocytes are present in nasal secretions. Most of these patients are intolerant of aspirin/non-steroidal anti-inflammatory drugs (NSAIDs).

Vasomotor rhinitis

These patients with perennial rhinitis have no demonstrable allergy or nasal eosinophilia. Watery secretions and nasal congestion are triggered by, for example, cold air, smoke, perfume or newsprint, possibly because of an imbalance of the autonomic nerves controlling the erectile tissue (sinusoids) in the nasal mucosa.

Nasal polyps

These are round, smooth, soft, semi-translucent, pale or yellow, glistening structures attached to the sinus mucosa by a relatively narrow stalk or pedicle, occurring in patients with allergic or vasomotor rhinitis. The mechanism(s) of their formation is not known. They contain mast cells, eosinophils and mononuclear cells in large numbers and cause nasal obstruction, loss of smell and taste, and mouth breathing, but rarely sneezing, since the mucosa of the polyp is largely denervated.

Pathogenesis of rhinitis

Sneezing, increased secretion and changes in mucosal blood flow are mediated both by efferent nerve fibres and by released mediators (see p. 1094). Mucus production results largely from parasympathetic stimulation. Blood vessels are under both sympathetic and parasympathetic control. Sympathetic fibres maintain tonic contraction of blood vessels, keeping the sinusoids of the nose partially constricted and aiding nasal patency. Stimulation of the parasympathetic system dilates these blood vessels. This stimulation varies spontaneously in a cyclical fashion so that air intake alternates slowly over several hours from one nostril to the other. The erectile cavernous nasal sinusoids can be influenced by emotion and hence affect nasal patency.

B cells produce IgE antibody against allergens. IgE binds to mast cells via high-affinity cell surface receptors, whose crosslinking causes degranulation and release of histamine, proteases (tryptase, chymase), prostaglandins (PGDs), cysteinyl leukotrienes (LTC_4, LTD_4, LTE_4) and cytokines. These mediators cause the acute symptoms of sneezing, itch, rhinorrhoea and nasal congestion. Sneezing results from stimulation of afferent nerve endings (mostly via histamine) and begins within minutes of an allergen entering the nose. This is followed by nasal exudation and secretion, and eventually nasal blockage, peaking 15–20 minutes after allergen exposure. These latter symptoms are driven by increased epithelial permeability, mostly due to histamine.

Additionally, allergens are presented to T cells via antigen-presenting cells (dendritic cells). This causes release of IL-4 and IL-13, which further stimulate the B cells, and also IL-5, IL-9 and granulocyte macrophage colony stimulating factor (GM-CSF), switching from a Th1 to a Th2 response to activate and recruit eosinophils, basophils, neutrophils and T lymphocytes. These cause chronic swelling and irritation, leading to nasal obstruction, hyper-reactivity and anosmia.

Investigations and diagnosis

The allergic factors causing rhinitis can usually be identified from the history. Skin-prick testing is used to support the history. A positive test does not necessarily mean that an allergen causes the respiratory disease. However, if there is a compatible clinical history, it is more likely to be relevant. Allergen-specific IgE antibodies can be measured in blood but such tests are much more expensive than skin tests and should be used only in patients who cannot be skin-tested for some reason (e.g. dermatographism, active eczema or inability to stop antihistamines for 3 days before skin tests).

Management

Allergen avoidance

Removal of a household pet or total enclosure of industrial processes releasing sensitizing agents can lead to cure of rhinitis and, indeed, asthma. However, pollen avoidance is impossible. Contact may be diminished by wearing sunglasses, driving with the car windows shut, avoiding walks in the countryside (particularly in the late afternoon, when the number of pollen grains is highest at ground level), and keeping bedroom windows shut at night. These measures are rarely sufficient in themselves to control symptoms. Exposure to pollen is generally lower in coastal regions, where sea breezes carry pollen grains inland.

The house-dust mite infests most areas of the house, but particularly the bedroom. Mite allergen exposure can be reduced by enclosing bedding in fabric specifically designed to prevent the passage of mite allergen, while allowing water vapour through. This is comfortable and also reduces symptoms. Acaricides are less effective and cannot be recommended. Increased room ventilation and reduced soft furnishings, including carpets, curtains and soft toys, can all help to reduce the mite load. However, the value of house-dust mite control measures in asthma has been challenged (see pp. 1096–1097).

H_1 antihistamines

Antihistamines remain the most common therapy for rhinitis; most can be purchased directly over the counter in the UK. They are particularly effective against sneezing and itching of the eyes and palate, but are less effective against rhinorrhoea and have little influence on nasal blockage. First-generation antihistamines (chlorphenamine, hydroxyzine) cause sedation and loss of concentration in all patients (including those who are not aware of the problem) and should no longer be used. Second-generation drugs, such as loratadine (10 mg once daily), desloratadine (5 mg daily), cetirizine (10 mg daily) and fexofenadine (120 mg daily), are at least as potent and do not cause sedation.

Decongestants

Drugs with sympathomimetic activity (α-adrenergic agents) are widely used to treat nasal obstruction. They may be taken orally or, more commonly, as nasal drops or sprays (e.g. ephedrine nasal drops). Xylometazoline and oxymetazoline are widely used because they have a prolonged action and tachyphylaxis does not develop. Secondary nasal hyperaemia can occur some hours later as a rebound effect and rhinitis medicamentosa can develop if patients take increasing quantities of decongestant to overcome this phenomenon. Although local decongestants are an effective treatment for vasomotor rhinitis, patients must be warned about rebound nasal obstruction and should use the drugs carefully. Ideally, such preparations should be prescribed for only a limited period to open the nasal airways and allow better access for other local therapy, such as topical corticosteroids.

Anti-inflammatory drugs

Sodium cromoglicate and nedocromil sodium act by blocking an intracellular chloride channel and influence mast cell and eosinophil activation and nerve function. Topical sodium cromoglicate and nedocromil sodium can be very effective in allergic conjunctivitis but are of limited value in allergic rhinitis.

Corticosteroids

The most effective treatment for rhinitis is a topical corticosteroid preparation (e.g. beclometasone, fluticasone propionate, fluticasone furoate or mometasone furoate spray). Topical steroids should be started before the beginning of seasonal symptoms. The combination of a topical corticosteroid with a non-sedating antihistamine taken regularly is particularly effective. Patients should be carefully instructed in how to use the nasal steroid device to achieve optimal drug deposition. In selected cases, an α-adrenergic agonist may help to decongest the nose prior to taking the topical corticosteroid. Patients often worry about possible side-effects; nasal steroids can cause epistaxis, but the amount used is insufficient to cause systemic effects.

If other therapy has failed, seasonal and perennial rhinitis respond readily to a short course (maximum 2 weeks) of treatment with oral prednisolone 5–10 mg daily. Nasal polyps may respond to oral corticosteroids and their recurrence may be prevented by continuous use of topical corticosteroids.

Leukotriene antagonists

In patients who do not respond to antihistamines or topical steroids, a leukotriene antagonist (e.g. montelukast 10 mg daily in the evening) may be helpful, especially in those with a history of NSAID sensitivity or concomitant asthma.

Immunotherapy

This is used for patients with seasonal allergic rhinitis who have not responded to standard drugs. Both oral and injectable vaccines are available (see p. 143). Other forms of desensitizing vaccines are under development.

Sinusitis

See page 1319.

Pharyngitis

The most common viruses causing pharyngitis are adenoviruses, of which there are about 32 serotypes. Endemic adenovirus infection causes the common sore throat, in which the oropharynx and soft palate are reddened and the tonsils are inflamed and swollen. Within 1–2 days, the tonsillar lymph nodes enlarge. Occasionally, localized epidemics occur due to adenovirus serotype 8, particularly in schools during summer, with episodes of fever, conjunctivitis, pharyngitis and lymphadenitis of the neck glands. The disease is self-limiting and requires only symptomatic treatment without antibiotics.

Over several decades, the proportion of sore throats due to bacterial infections, such as haemolytic streptococcus, has fallen. Many different pathogens have been implicated in pharyngitis but most do not require specific treatment. Persistent and severe tonsillitis should be treated with phenoxymethylpenicillin 500 mg four times a day or cefaclor 250 mg three times daily. Amoxicillin and ampicillin should be avoided if there is a possibility of infectious mononucleosis (see p. 258), as they are likely to cause drug rashes in this context.

Acute laryngotracheobronchitis

Acute laryngitis is an occasional but striking complication of upper respiratory tract infections, particularly those caused by parainfluenza viruses and measles. The condition is most severe in children under the age of 3 years. Inflammatory oedema extends to the vocal cords and the epiglottis, causing narrowing of the airway; there may be associated ***tracheitis*** or ***tracheobronchitis***. The voice becomes hoarse, with a barking cough (croup), and there is audible stridor. Progressive airways obstruction may occur, with recession of the soft tissue of the neck and abdomen during inspiration and, in severe cases, central cyanosis. Steam inhalations are not helpful. Nebulized adrenaline (epinephrine) gives short-term relief. Oral or intramuscular corticosteroids (e.g. dexamethasone) should be given with oxygen and adequate fluids. If steroids are used, endotracheal intubation is rarely necessary. Rarely, a tracheostomy is required.

Acute epiglottitis

H. influenzae type b (Hib) can cause life-threatening infection of the epiglottis, usually in children under 5 years of age. The child becomes extremely ill with a high fever, and severe airflow obstruction may rapidly occur. This is a life-threatening emergency and requires urgent endotracheal intubation and intravenous antibiotics (e.g. ceftazidime 25–150 mg/kg). Chloramphenicol (50–100 mg/kg) is also used in some countries. The epiglottis, which is red and swollen, should not be inspected until facilities to maintain the airways are available.

Other manifestations of Hib infection are meningitis, septic arthritis and osteomyelitis. A highly effective vaccine is now available, which is given to infants at 2, 3 and 4 months, with their primary immunizations against diphtheria, tetanus and pertussis (DTP). In many countries, this programme has reduced death rates from Hib infections virtually to zero.

Influenza

The influenza virus belongs to the orthomyxovirus group and exists in two main forms, A and B. Influenza B is associated with localized outbreaks of mild disease, whereas influenza A causes worldwide pandemics (see p. 254).

Clinical features

The incubation period of influenza is usually 1–3 days. The illness starts abruptly with a fever, shivering and generalized aching in the limbs. This is associated with severe headache, soreness of the throat and a dry cough that can persist for several weeks. Diarrhoea occurs in 70% of cases of H5N1 ('bird flu'). Influenza infection can be followed by a prolonged period of debility and depression that may take weeks or months to clear.

Complications

Secondary bacterial infection is common following influenza virus infection, particularly with *Streptococcus pneumoniae* and *Haemophilus influenzae*. Secondary pneumonia caused by *Staphylococcus aureus* is rarer, but more serious, and carries a mortality of up to 20%. Post-infectious encephalomyelitis is rare after influenza infection.

Diagnosis and management

Laboratory diagnosis is not usually necessary, but a definitive diagnosis can be established by demonstrating a four-fold increase in complement-fixing antibody or haemagglutinin antibody measured at onset and after 1–2 weeks, or by demonstrating the virus in throat or nasal secretions.

Management is by bed rest and paracetamol, with antibiotics to prevent secondary infection in those with chronic bronchitis, or cardiac or renal disease.

Neuraminidase inhibitors help to shorten the duration of symptoms in patients with influenza, if given within 48 hours of the first symptom. The cost–benefit of zanamivir and oseltamivir remains unproven but these are currently recommended in the UK for patients with suspected influenza over the age of 65 and 'at-risk' adults, as part of a strategy to reduce admissions to hospital when influenza is circulating in the community.

Prophylaxis

Protection by influenza vaccines is effective in only about 70% of people and lasts only for about a year. New vaccines have to be prepared to cover each change in viral antigenicity and are therefore in limited supply at the start of an epidemic. Nevertheless, routine vaccination is recommended for all individuals over 65 years of age and also for younger people with chronic heart disease, chronic lung disease (including asthma), chronic kidney disease or diabetes mellitus and for those who are immunosuppressed. During pandemics, key hospital and health service personnel should also be vaccinated. Influenza vaccine should not be given to individuals who are allergic to egg protein, as some are manufactured in chick embryos.

Inhalation of foreign bodies

Children inhale foreign bodies, such as peanuts, more commonly than do adults. In adults, inhalation may occur after excess alcohol or under general anaesthesia (loose teeth or dentures).

When the foreign body is large, it may impact in the trachea. The person chokes and then becomes silent; death ensues unless the material is quickly removed ***(Box 24.12)***.

More often, impaction occurs in the right main bronchus and produces:

- choking
- persistent monophonic wheeze
- persistent suppurative pneumonia
- lung abscess (common).

Box 24.12 Treatment of inhaled foreign bodies (Heimlich manœuvre)

Emergency

The Heimlich manœuvre is used to expel the obstructing object:

1. Stand behind the patient.
2. Encircle the upper part of the patient's abdomen just below the rib cage with your arms.
3. Give a sharp, forceful squeeze, forcing the diaphragm sharply into the thorax. This should expel sufficient air from the lungs to force the foreign body out of the trachea.

Non-emergency

Rigid bronchoscopy should be performed.

Further reading

Bjornson CL, Russell K, Foisy M et al. Treatment of croup in children: an overview of reviews. *Evid-based Child Health* 2010; 5:1555–1565.
Greiner AN, Hellings PW, Rotiroti G et al. Allergic rhinitis. *Lancet* 2011; 378:2112–2122.
Wessels MR. Streptococcal pharyngitis. *N Engl J Med* 2011; 364:648–655.
Zimmer SM, Burke DS. Historical perspective – emergence of influenza A (H1N1) viruses. *N Engl J Med* 2009; 361:279–285.

DISEASES OF THE LOWER RESPIRATORY TRACT

Lower respiratory tract infection accounts for approximately 10% of the worldwide burden of morbidity and mortality. Some 75% of all antibiotic usage is for these diseases, despite the fact that they are mainly due to viruses.

Acute bronchitis

Acute bronchitis in previously healthy subjects is often viral. Bacterial infection with *Strep. pneumoniae* or *H. influenzae* is a common sequel to viral infections, and is more likely to occur in cigarette smokers or people with COPD.

The illness begins with an irritating, non-productive cough, together with discomfort behind the sternum. There may be associated chest tightness, wheezing and shortness of breath. Later, the cough becomes productive, with yellow or green sputum. There is a mild fever and a neutrophil leucocytosis; wheeze with occasional crackles can be heard on auscultation. In otherwise healthy adults, the disease improves spontaneously in 4–8 days without them becoming seriously ill.

Antibiotics are often given (e.g. amoxicillin 250 mg three times daily), but it is not known whether this hastens recovery in otherwise healthy individuals and they should not be given in most cases.

Chronic obstructive pulmonary disease

Chronic obstructive pulmonary disease (COPD) is predicted to become the third most common cause of death and fifth most common cause of disability worldwide by 2020.

COPD is an overarching diagnosis that brings together a variety of clinical syndromes associated with airflow limitation and destruction of the lung parenchyma.

COPD is associated with a number of co-morbidities, e.g. ischaemic heart disease, hypertension, diabetes, heart failure and cancer, suggesting that it may be part of a generalized systemic inflammatory process.

Definition

COPD has been described as 'a disease state characterized by airflow limitation that is not fully reversible. The airflow limitation is usually both progressive and associated with an abnormal inflammatory response of the lungs to noxious particles or gases.'

Epidemiology and aetiology

COPD is caused by long-term exposure to toxic particles and gases. In developed countries, cigarette smoking accounts for over 90% of cases. In developing countries, other factors are also implicated, such as inhalation of smoke from biomass heating fuels and cooking in poorly ventilated areas. However, only 10–20% of heavy smokers develop COPD, indicating individual susceptibility. The development of COPD is proportional to the number of cigarettes smoked per day; the risk of death from COPD in patients smoking 30 cigarettes daily is 20 times that of a non-smoker. Autopsy studies have shown substantial numbers of centri-acinar emphysematous spaces in the lungs of 50% of British smokers over the age of 60 years, independently of whether significant respiratory disease was diagnosed before death.

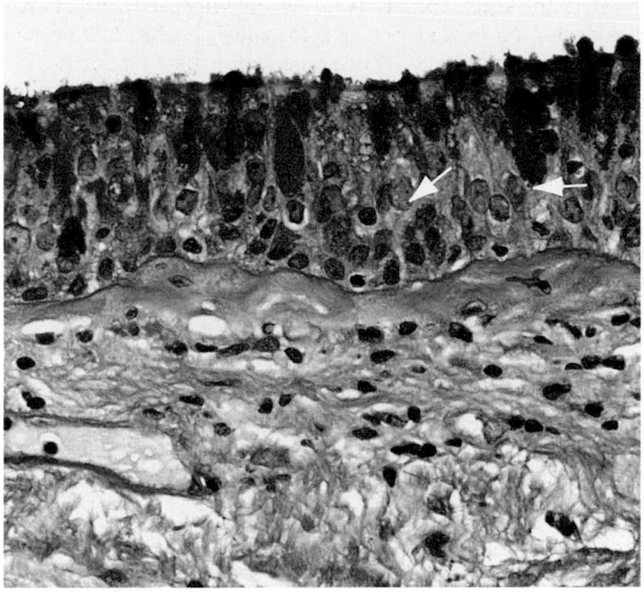

Figure 24.19 Chronic obstructive pulmonary disease (COPD). Section of bronchial mucosa stained for mucus glands by periodic acid–Schiff (PAS) showing an increase in mucus-secreting goblet cells (arrowed). *(Courtesy of Dr J Wilson and Dr S Wilson, University of Southampton.)*

Climate and air pollution are lesser causes of COPD, but mortality from COPD increases dramatically during periods of heavy atmospheric pollution (see pp. 56–57). Urbanization, social class and occupation may also play a part in the aetiology but these effects are difficult to separate from that of smoking. Some animal studies suggest that diet could be a risk factor for COPD but this has not been proven in humans.

The socioeconomic burden of COPD is considerable. In the UK, COPD causes approximately 18 million lost working days annually for men and 2.1 million lost working days for women, accounting for approximately 7% of all days of absence from work due to sickness. Nevertheless, the number of COPD admissions to UK hospitals has been falling steadily over the last 30 years.

Pathophysiology

The most consistent pathological finding in COPD is increased numbers of mucus-secreting goblet cells in the bronchial mucosa, especially in the larger bronchi ***(Fig. 24.19)***. In more advanced cases, the bronchi become overtly inflamed and pus is seen in the lumen. The role of the resident microbiome (see p. 1065) in exacerbations of COPD is as yet unknown.

Microscopically, there is infiltration of the walls of the bronchi and bronchioles with acute and chronic inflammatory cells; lymphoid follicles may develop in severe disease. In contrast to asthma, the lymphocytic infiltrate is predominantly $CD8^+$. The epithelial layer may become ulcerated and, with time, squamous epithelium replaces the columnar cells. The inflammation is followed by scarring and thickening of the walls, which narrows the small airways ***(Fig. 24.20)***.

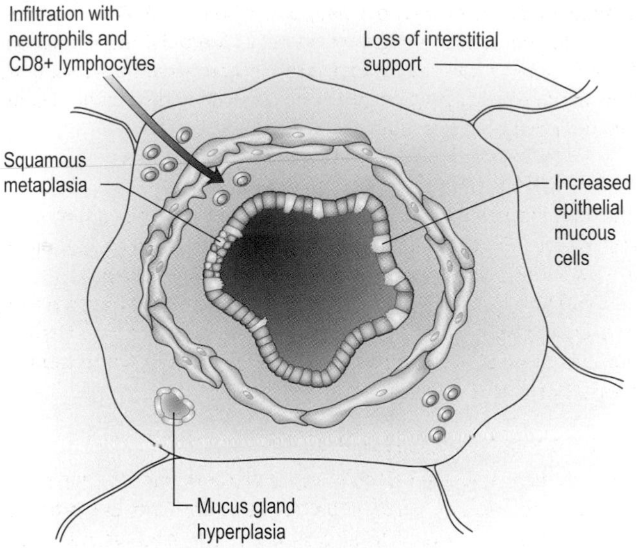

Figure 24.20 Pathological changes in the airways in COPD.

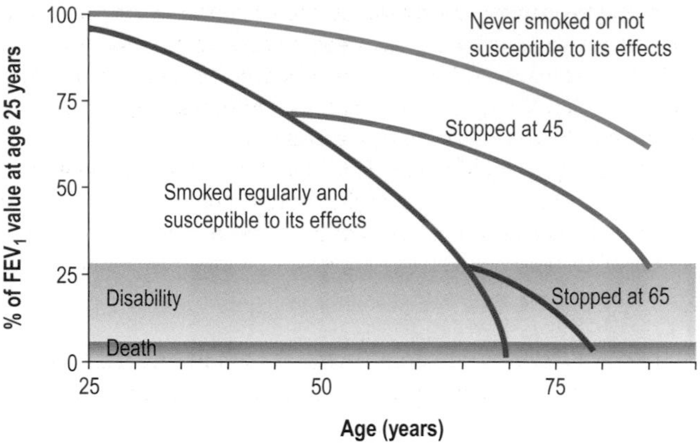

Figure 24.21 Influence of smoking on airflow limitation. *(From Fletcher CM, Peto R. The natural history of chronic airflow obstruction.* British Medical Journal *1977; 1:1645.)*

The small airways are particularly affected early in the disease, initially without the development of any significant breathlessness. This initial inflammation of the small airways is reversible and accounts for the improvement in airway function if smoking is stopped early. In later stages, the inflammation continues, even if smoking is stopped.

Further progression of the airways disease leads to progressive squamous cell metaplasia and fibrosis of the bronchial walls. The physiological consequence of these changes is the development of airflow limitation. If the airway narrowing is combined with emphysema (causing loss of the elastic recoil of the lung with collapse of small airways during expiration), the resulting airflow limitation is even more severe.

Emphysema is defined as abnormal, permanent enlargement of air spaces distal to the terminal bronchiole, accompanied by destruction of their walls and without obvious fibrosis. Enlargement of the distal air spaces (i.e. emphysema) is thought to be a secondary result of small airway inflammation and destruction. It is classified according to the site of damage:

- ***Centri-acinar emphysema***. Distension and damage of lung tissue is concentrated around the respiratory bronchioles, whilst the more distal alveolar ducts and alveoli tend to be well preserved. This form of emphysema is extremely common; when of modest extent, it is not necessarily associated with disability. Severe centri-acinar emphysema is associated with substantial airflow limitation.
- ***Pan-acinar emphysema***. This is less common but is the type associated with α_1-antitrypsin deficiency (see p. 1081). Distension and destruction affect the whole acinus, and in severe cases the lung is just a collection of bullae. Severe airflow limitation and $\dot{V}_A/\dot{Q}$ mismatch occur.
- ***Irregular emphysema***. There is scarring and damage that affect the lung parenchyma patchily, independent of acinar structure.

Emphysema leads to expiratory airflow limitation and air trapping. The loss of lung elastic recoil results in an increase in total lung capacity (TLC). Premature closure of airways limits expiratory flow while the loss of alveoli decreases capacity for gas transfer.

$\dot{V}_A/\dot{Q}$ mismatch is partly due to damage and mucus plugging of smaller airways from chronic inflammation, and partly due to rapid closure of smaller airways in expiration owing to loss of elastic support. The mismatch leads to a fall in P_aO_2 and increased work of respiration.

CO_2 excretion is less affected by $\dot{V}_A/\dot{Q}$ mismatch and many patients have low-normal P_aCO_2 values due to increasing alveolar ventilation in an attempt to correct their hypoxia ('pink puffers'). Other patients fail to maintain their respiratory effort and then their P_aCO_2 levels increase. In the short term, this rise in CO_2 leads to stimulation of respiration, but in the longer term, these patients often become insensitive to CO_2 and come to depend on hypoxaemia to drive ventilation. Such patients appear less breathless and, because of renal hypoxia, they start to retain fluid and increase erythrocyte production (leading eventually to polycythaemia). In consequence, they become bloated, plethoric and cyanosed, the typical appearance of the 'blue bloater'. Attempts to abolish hypoxaemia by administering oxygen can make the situation much worse by decreasing respiratory drive in these patients who depend on hypoxia to drive their ventilation.

The *classic Fletcher and Peto studies* ***(Fig. 24.21)*** showed a loss of 50 mL per year in FEV_1 in patients with COPD compared with 20 mL per year in healthy people. A more recent study has shown a 40 mL loss per year but only in 38% of the patients studied. Biomarkers to predict the rate of decline have been unhelpful, although serum levels of Clara cell secretory protein 16 (CC16) has been proposed as a possible indicator; it is an indication of acute or chronic bronchial epithelium injury.

Three mechanisms have been suggested to explain airflow limitation in small airways (<2 mm in diameter).

- ***Loss of elasticity*** and alveolar attachments of airways due to emphysema. This reduces the elastic recoil and the airways collapse during expiration.
- ***Inflammation and scarring***, which cause the small airways to narrow.
- ***Mucus secretion***, which blocks the airways.

Each of these narrows the small airways and causes air trapping, leading to hyperinflation of the lungs, $\dot{V}_A/\dot{Q}$ mismatch, increased work of breathing and breathlessness.

Pathogenesis

Cigarette smoking

Bronchoalveolar lavage and biopsies of the airways of smokers show increased numbers of neutrophil granulocytes. These granulocytes can release elastases and proteases, which may help to produce emphysema. It has been suggested that an imbalance between protease and antiprotease activity causes the damage. Alpha$_1$-antitrypsin is a major serum antiprotease, which can be inactivated by cigarette smoke (see below).

Mucous gland hypertrophy in the larger airways is thought to be a direct response to persistent irritation resulting from the inhalation of cigarette smoke. The smoke has an adverse effect on surfactant, favouring over-distension of the lungs.

Infections

Patients with COPD cope badly with respiratory infections, which are often the precipitating cause of acute exacerbations of the disease. However, it is less clear whether infection is responsible for the progressive airflow limitation that characterizes disabling COPD. Prompt use of antibiotics and routine vaccinations against influenza and pneumococci are appropriate.

Alpha$_1$-antitrypsin deficiency

Alpha$_1$-antitrypsin (see also pp. 479–480) is a proteinase inhibitor that is produced in the liver; it is secreted into the blood and diffuses into the lung. Here it inhibits proteolytic enzymes such as neutrophil elastase, which are capable of destroying alveolar wall connective tissue. In α_1-antitrypsin deficiency, the protein accumulates in the liver, leading to low levels in the lung.

More than 75 alleles of the α_1-antitrypsin gene have been described. The three main phenotypes are MM (normal), MZ (heterozygous deficiency) and ZZ (homozygous deficiency). About 1 child in 5000 in the UK is born with the homozygous deficiency, but not all develop chest disease. Those who do develop breathlessness under the age of 40 years have radiographic evidence of basal emphysema and are usually, but not always, cigarette smokers. Hereditary deficiency of α_1-antitrypsin accounts for about 2% of UK emphysema cases. A small minority develop liver disease (see p. 480).

Clinical features

Symptoms

The characteristic symptoms of COPD are productive cough with white or clear sputum, wheeze and breathlessness, usually following many years of a smoker's cough. Colds seem to 'settle on the chest' and frequent infective exacerbations occur, with purulent sputum. Symptoms can be worsened by cold or damp weather and atmospheric pollution. With advanced disease, breathlessness is severe, even after mild exercise such as getting dressed. Systemic effects include hypertension, osteoporosis, depression, weight loss and reduced muscle mass with general weakness.

Signs

In mild COPD, there may be no signs or just quiet wheezes throughout the chest. In severe disease, the patient is tachypnoeic, with prolonged expiration. The accessory muscles of respiration are used and there may be intercostal indrawing on inspiration and pursing of the lips on expiration (see p. 1061). Chest expansion is poor, the lungs are hyperinflated, and there is loss of the normal cardiac and liver dullness.

Patients who remain responsive to CO_2 are usually breathless and rarely cyanosed. Heart failure and oedema are rare features, except as terminal events. In contrast, patients who become insensitive to CO_2 are often oedematous and cyanosed but not particularly breathless. Those with hypercapnia may have peripheral vasodilatation, a bounding pulse, and when the P_aCO_2 is above about 10 kPa, a coarse flapping tremor of the outstretched hands. Severe hypercapnia causes confusion and progressive drowsiness. Papilloedema may be present but this is neither specific nor sensitive as a diagnostic feature.

Respiratory failure

The later stages of COPD are characterized by the development of respiratory failure. For practical purposes, this is defined as either a P_aO_2 <8 kPa (60 mmHg) or a P_aCO_2 >7 kPa (53 mmHg).

Chronic alveolar hypoxia and hypercapnia lead to constriction of the pulmonary arterioles and pulmonary hypertension. Cardiac output is normal or increased but salt and fluid retention occurs as a result of renal hypoxia.

Pulmonary hypertension

Patients with advanced COPD may develop pulmonary hypertension (cor pulmonale), which is defined as symptoms and signs of fluid overload secondary to lung disease. The fluid retention and peripheral oedema are due to failure of excretion of sodium and water by the hypoxic kidney rather than heart failure. It is characterized by pulmonary hypertension and right ventricular hypertrophy. On examination, the patient is centrally cyanosed (owing to the lung disease), and later becomes more breathless and develops ankle oedema. Initially, there may be a prominent parasternal heave, due to right ventricular hypertrophy, and a loud pulmonary second sound. In very severe pulmonary hypertension, the pulmonary valve becomes incompetent. With severe fluid overload, tricuspid incompetence may develop with a greatly elevated jugular venous pressure (JVP), ascites and upper abdominal discomfort due to liver swelling.

Diagnosis

This is usually clinical ***(Box 24.13)*** and based on a history of breathlessness and sputum production in a chronic smoker. In the absence of a history of cigarette smoking, asthma is a more likely explanation, unless there is a family history suggesting α_1-antitrypsin deficiency.

No individual clinical feature is diagnostic. The patient may have signs of hyperinflation and typical pursed lip respiration. There may be signs of overinflation of the lungs (e.g. loss of liver dullness on percussion), but this also occurs in other diseases such as asthma. Conversely, centri-acinar emphysema may be present without signs of overinflation. The chest may become 'barrel-shaped' but this can also result from osteoporosis of the spine in older men without emphysema.

Box 24.13 Classification of severity of airflow limitation in COPD (2016)

GOLD stage	FEV_1 / FVC	FEV_1% predicted[a]
1. **Mild**	<70%	>80%
2. **Moderate**	<70%	<80%
3. **Severe**	<70%	<50%
4. **Very severe**	<70%	<30%

[a]FEV_1 levels post bronchodilator therapy.

(Modified from Global Initiative for Chronic Obstructive Lung Disease (GOLD), 2016. www.goldcopd.com.)

Investigations

- ***Lung function tests*** show evidence of airflow limitation (see ***Figs 24.7*** and ***24.12***). The FEV_1:FVC ratio is reduced and the PEFR is low. In many patients, the airflow limitation is partly reversible (usually a change in FEV_1 of <15%), and it can be difficult to distinguish between COPD and asthma. Lung volumes may be normal or increased; carbon monoxide gas transfer factor is low when significant emphysema is present.
- ***Chest X-ray*** is often normal, even when the disease is advanced. The classic features are overinflation of the lungs with low, flattened diaphragms, and sometimes the presence of large bullae. Blood vessels may be 'pruned', with large proximal vessels and relatively little blood visible in the peripheral lung fields.
- ***High resolution CT (HRCT) scans*** are useful, particularly when the plain chest X-ray is normal.
- ***Haemoglobin level and packed cell volume*** can be elevated as a result of persistent hypoxaemia (secondary polycythaemia; see p. 550).
- ***Blood gases*** are often normal at rest but patients desaturate on exercise. In more advanced cases, there is resting hypoxaemia and there may also be hypercapnia.
- ***Sputum examination*** is not useful in ordinary cases. *Strep. pneumoniae* and *H. influenzae* are the only bacterial common organisms to produce acute exacerbations. Occasionally, *Moraxella catarrhalis* may cause infective exacerbations. Many acute episodes are viral in origin.
- ***ECG*** is often normal. In advanced pulmonary hypotension, the P wave is tall (P pulmonale) and there may be right bundle branch block and evidence of right ventricular hypertrophy (see p. 1030).
- ***Echocardiogram*** is useful to assess cardiac function where there is disproportionate dyspnoea.
- ***α_1-Antitrypsin*** levels and genotype are worth measuring in premature disease or lifelong non-smokers.

Management

See ***Figure 24.22*** for management strategies.

Smoking cessation

The single most useful measure is to persuade the patient to stop smoking. Even in advanced disease, this may slow down the rate of deterioration and prolong the time before disability and death occur (see ***Fig. 24.22***). Smoke from burning biomass fuels in poorly ventilated homes should also be reduced.

Drug therapy

This is used both for the short-term management of exacerbations and for the long-term relief of symptoms. Many of the drugs used are similar to those employed in asthma (see pp. 1097–1099).

Bronchodilators

- ***β-Adrenoceptor agonists.*** Many patients with mild COPD feel less breathless after inhaling a β-adrenergic agonist such as salbutamol (200 µg every 4–6 h). In more severe airway limitation (moderate and severe COPD), a long-acting β_2

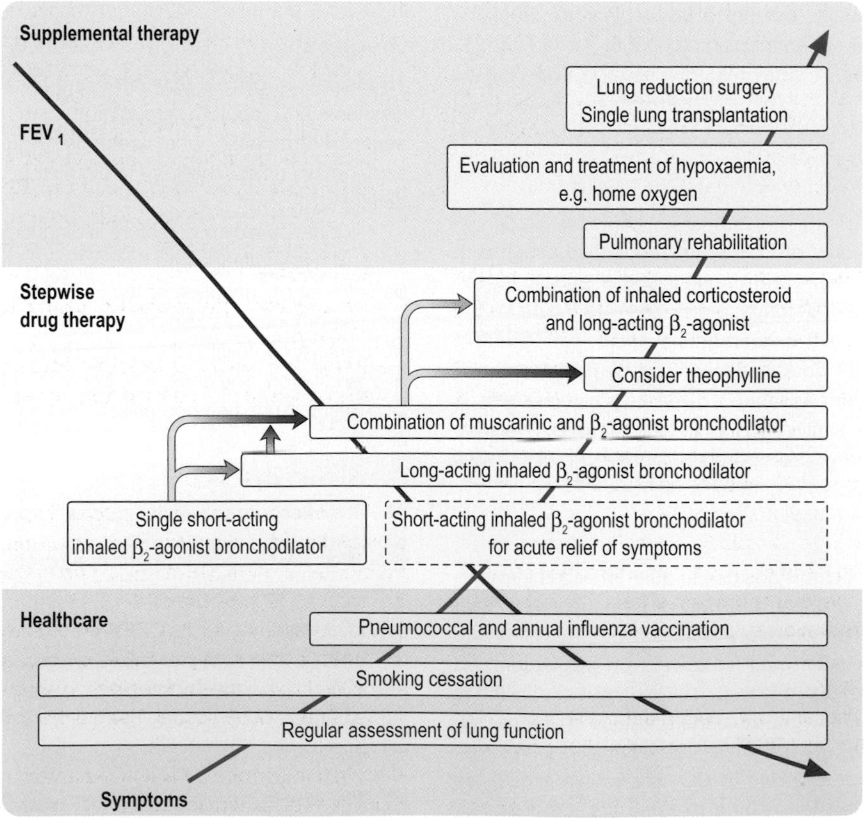

Figure 24.22 Algorithm for the treatment of COPD. The various components of management are shown as the FEV_1 decreases and the symptoms become more severe. *(After Sutherland ER, Cherniack RM. Management of chronic obstructive pulmonary disease.* New England Journal of Medicine *2004; 350:2689–2697.*

agonist should be used, e.g. formoterol 12 μg powder inhaled twice daily, salmeterol 50 μg twice daily or indacaterol 150–300 μg once daily.

- ***Antimuscarinic drugs***. More prolonged and greater bronchodilatation is achieved with antimuscarinic agents; the long-acting agents tiotropium (18 μg daily) and aclidinium (375 μg daily) are preferred to ipratropium or oxitropium. Tiotropium improves function and quality of life but does not affect the decline in FEV_1. If patients find inhalers difficult to use, spacer devices improve delivery. Objective evidence of improvement in peak flow rate or FEV_1 may be small, and decisions to continue or stop therapy are based mainly on the patient's reported symptoms.
- ***Theophyllines***. Long-acting preparations of theophylline are of little benefit in COPD.

Phosphodiesterase type 4 inhibitors

Roflumilast is a phosphodiesterase inhibitor with anti-inflammatory properties. It is used as an adjunct to bronchodilators for the maintenance treatment of COPD patients.

Corticosteroids

In symptomatic patients with moderate/severe COPD, a trial of corticosteroids is always indicated, since a proportion of individuals have an unsuspected reversible element to their disease and airway function may improve considerably. Prednisolone 30 mg daily should be given for 2 weeks, with measurements of lung function before and after the treatment period. If there is objective evidence of a substantial degree of improvement in airflow limitation (FEV_1 increase of >15%), prednisolone should be discontinued and replaced by inhaled corticosteroids (beclometasone 40 μg twice daily in the first instance, adjusted according to response). The value of long-term regular inhaled corticosteroids in all patients with COPD has not been proven.

Combinations of corticosteroids with long-acting β_2 agonists may protect against lung function decline but do not improve overall mortality. High-dose inhaled steroids are not advised, as their use is linked to increased rates of pneumonia.

Antibiotics

Prompt antibiotic treatment shortens exacerbations and should always be given in acute episodes, as it may prevent hospital admission and further lung damage. Patients can be given antibiotics to keep at home, starting them as soon as their sputum turns yellow or green. Although amoxicillin-resistant *H. influenzae* is increasing worldwide (occurring in about 20% of isolates from sputum), it is not a serious clinical problem. Resistance to cefaclor (500 mg 8-hourly) or cefixime (400 mg once daily) is significantly less frequent; co-amoxiclav is a useful alternative.

Long-term treatment with antibiotics remains controversial. They were once thought to be of no value, but eradication of infection and maintenance of the lower respiratory tract free of bacteria may help to prevent deterioration in lung function.

Antimucolytic agents

These reduce sputum viscosity and can reduce the number of acute exacerbations. A 4-week trial of carbocisteine 2.25 g daily can be tried.

Diuretic therapy

Diuretic therapy (see p. 156) is necessary for all oedematous patients. Daily weights should be recorded during acute inpatient episodes.

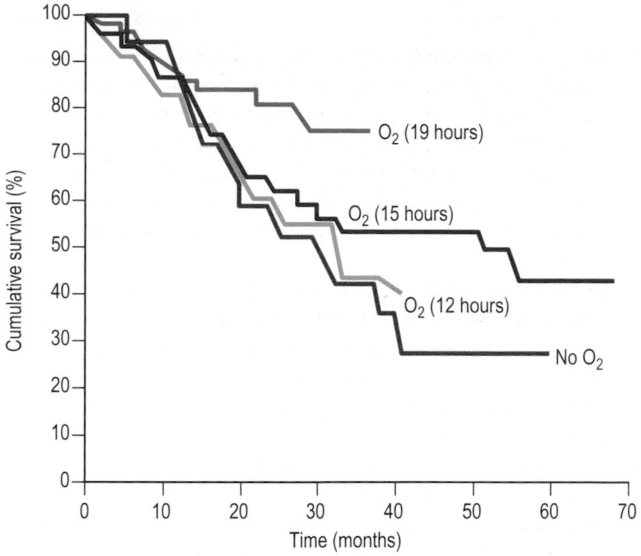

Figure 24.23 Cumulative survival curves for patients receiving oxygen. Oxygen doses are in hours per day.

Oxygen therapy

Two controlled trials (chiefly in males) have shown improved survival with the continuous administration of oxygen at 2 L/min via nasal prongs to achieve an oxygen saturation of >90% for large proportions of the day and night. Survival curves from these two studies are shown in ***Figure 24.23***. Only 30% of those not receiving long-term oxygen therapy survived for more than 5 years. A fall in pulmonary artery pressure was achieved if oxygen was given for 15 hours daily, but substantial improvement in mortality was achieved only by the administration of oxygen for 19 hours daily. These results suggest that long-term continuous domiciliary oxygen therapy will benefit patients who have:

- P_aO_2 of <7.3 kPa (55 mmHg) when breathing air. Measurements should be taken on two occasions at least 3 weeks apart after appropriate bronchodilator therapy ***(Box 24.14)***.
- P_aO_2 7.3–8 kPa with secondary polycythaemia, nocturnal hypoxaemia, peripheral oedema or evidence of pulmonary hypertension.
- Carboxyhaemoglobin of <3% (i.e. patients who have stopped smoking).

Domiciliary oxygen is best provided by using an oxygen concentrator, which is considerably cheaper than using oxygen cylinders.

Nocturnal hypoxia

COPD patients with severe arterial hypoxaemia may experience profound nocturnal hypoxaemia, which may cause the P_aO_2 to drop as low as 2.5 kPa (19 mmHg), particularly during the rapid eye movement (REM) phase of sleep.

Because patients with COPD are already hypoxic, the fall in P_aO_2 produces a much larger fall in oxygen saturation (owing to the shape of the oxygen–haemoglobin dissociation curve) and desaturation at up to 80% occurs. The mechanism is alveolar hypoventilation due to:

- inhibition of intercostal and accessory muscles in REM sleep
- shallow breathing in REM sleep, which reduces ventilation, particularly in severe COPD
- an increase in upper airway resistance because of a reduction in muscle tone.

Box 24.14 Guidelines for domiciliary oxygen (Royal College of Physicians, 1999)

- Chronic obstructive pulmonary disease with P_aO_2 <7.3 kPa when breathing air during a period of clinical stability
- Chronic obstructive pulmonary disease with P_aO_2 7.3–8 kPa in the presence of secondary polycythaemia, nocturnal hypoxaemia, peripheral oedema or evidence of pulmonary hypertension
- Severe chronic asthma with a P_aCO_2 <7.3 kPa or persistent disabling breathlessness
- Diffuse lung disease with P_aO_2 <8 kPa and in patients with P_aO_2 >8 kPa with disabling dyspnoea
- Cystic fibrosis when P_aO_2 <7.3 kPa or if P_aO_2 7.3–8 kPa in the presence of secondary polycythaemia, nocturnal hypoxaemia, pulmonary hypertension or peripheral oedema
- Pulmonary hypertension without parenchymal lung involvement when P_aO_2 <8 kPa
- Neuromuscular or skeletal disorders, after specialist assessment
- Obstructive sleep apnoea despite continuous positive airways pressure therapy, after specialist assessment
- Pulmonary malignancy or other terminal disease with disabling dyspnoea
- Heart failure with daytime P_aO_2 <7.3 kPa (on air) or with nocturnal hypoxaemia

These nocturnal hypoxaemic episodes are associated with a further rise in pulmonary arterial pressure owing to vasoconstriction. Most deaths in patients with COPD occur at night, possibly from cardiac arrhythmias due to hypoxaemia. Secondary polycythaemia may be exacerbated by the severe nocturnal hypoxaemia.

Each episode of desaturation is usually terminated by arousal from sleep, so the amount of normal sleep is reduced and patients suffer from daytime sleepiness.

Management is with nocturnal administration of oxygen and ventilatory support. Patients with arterial hypoxaemia should not be given sleeping tablets, as these will further depress respiratory drive.

Non-invasive positive-pressure ventilation can be administered with a tightly fitting nasal mask and bilevel positive airway pressure (BiPAP) – inspiratory to provide inspiratory assistance and expiratory to prevent alveolar closure, each adjusted independently. This improves ventilation during sleep and allows respiratory muscles to rest at night. BiPAP helps prevent hypoxaemic damage at night in COPD but it does not improve daytime respiratory function, respiratory muscle strength, exercise tolerance or breathlessness.

Pulmonary rehabilitation

Exercise training can modestly increase exercise capacity, with a diminished sense of breathlessness and improved general well-being. Regular training periods can be instituted at home; climbing stairs or walking fixed distances can be combined with regular clinic visits for encouragement. Breathing exercises are probably of less value. Quality of life can be improved by a multidisciplinary approach involving physiotherapy, exercise and education, although this does not alter life expectancy or the rate of decline in lung function; stopping smoking is still the most useful thing patients can do to help themselves. Nutritional advice and psychological, social and behavioural interventions are also helpful.

Additional measures

- ***Vaccines***. Patients with COPD should receive a single dose of the polyvalent pneumococcal polysaccharide vaccine and yearly influenza vaccinations.
- ***α_1-Antitrypsin replacement***. Weekly or monthly infusions of α_1-antitrypsin have been recommended for patients with serum levels <310 mg/L and abnormal lung function. Whether this modifies the long-term progression of the disease remains to be determined.
- ***Heart failure***. This should be treated (see pp. 948–988).
- ***Secondary polycythaemia***. This requires venesection if the PCV is >55%.
- ***Pulmonary hypertension***. This can be partially relieved by the use of oral β-adrenergic agonists, such as salbutamol (4 mg three times daily), but the long-term value is unknown.
- ***Sensation of breathlessness***. This can be reduced by either promethazine 125 mg daily or dihydrocodeine 1 mg/kg by mouth. Although opiates are the most effective treatment for intractable breathlessness, they depress ventilation and carry the risk of increasing respiratory failure.
- ***Leukotriene receptor antagonists***. Although these have been tried, they are rarely effective (see p. 1099).
- ***Air travel***. Commercial aircraft are pressurized to the equivalent of 2000–2400 m altitude. In healthy people, this causes P_aO_2 to fall from 13.5 to 10 kPa, leading to a trivial 3% drop in oxygen saturation, but patients with moderate COPD may desaturate significantly. The desaturation associated with air travel can be simulated by breathing 15% oxygen at sea level. Patients whose saturation drops below 85% within 15 minutes should be advised to contact their airline to request supplemental oxygen during their flight.
- ***Surgery***. Some patients have large emphysematous bullae that reduce lung capacity. Surgical bullectomy can enable adjacent areas of collapsed lung to re-expand and start functioning again. In addition, carefully selected patients with severe COPD (FEV_1 <1 L) have been treated with lung volume reduction surgery. This increases elastic recoil, which reduces the expiratory collapse of the airway and decreases expiratory airflow limitation. It also enables the diaphragm to work at a mechanical advantage. Initial studies suggested that ventilation was improved and patients felt less breathless, although mortality was unchanged. However, a controlled trial in severe emphysema found increased mortality and no improvement in the patients' condition. ***Single lung transplantation*** (see p. 1090) is used for end-stage emphysema, with 3-year survival rates of 75%. The principal benefit is improved quality of life but it does not extend survival.

Acute respiratory failure in COPD

- ***Oxygen therapy***. COPD is by far the most common cause of respiratory failure. In managing respiratory failure, the main goal is to improve the P_aO_2 by continuous oxygen therapy ***(Fig. 24.24)***. In type II respiratory failure, the P_aCO_2 is elevated and the patient is dependent on hypoxic drive. In this setting, giving additional oxygen will nearly always cause a further rise in P_aCO_2. Small increases in P_aCO_2 can be tolerated but the pH should not be allowed to fall below 7.25; if it does, non-invasive ventilation is required. In COPD exacerbations, a fixed-percentage mask (Venturi mask; ***Fig. 24.25***) is used to deliver controlled concentrations of oxygen. Initially, 24% oxygen is given, and the concentration of inspired oxygen can be gradually increased, provided the P_aCO_2 does not rise unacceptably.
- ***Removal of retained secretions***. Patients should be encouraged to cough up secretions. Physiotherapy is helpful.

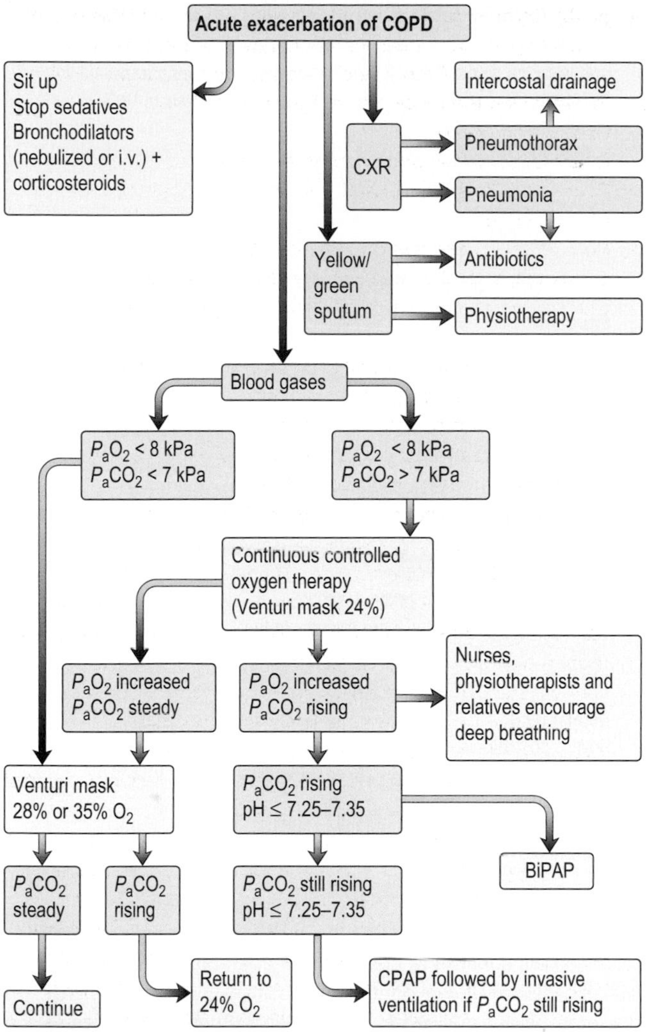

Figure 24.24 Algorithm for the treatment of respiratory failure in COPD. BiPAP, bilevel positive airway pressure; CPAP, continuous positive airway pressure; CXR, chest X-ray.

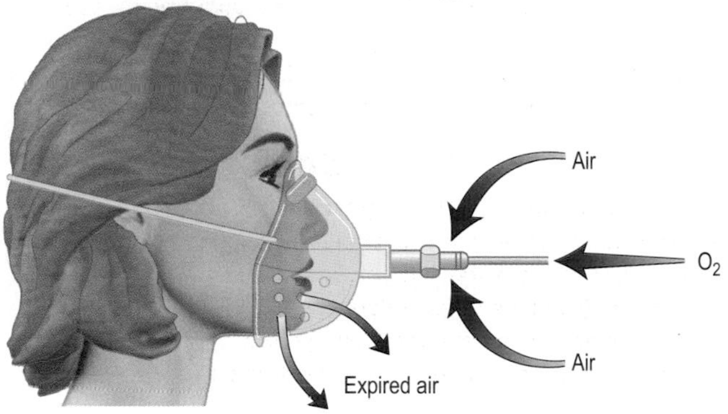

Figure 24.25 'Fixed-performance' device for administration of oxygen in spontaneously breathing patients (Venturi mask). Oxygen is delivered through the injector of the Venturi mask at a given flow rate. A proportionate amount of air is entrained and the inspired oxygen can be predicted accurately. Masks are available to deliver 24%, 28% and 35% oxygen.

Box 24.15 BODE index[a]

Variable	Points on BODE index			
	0	*1*	*2*	*3*
FEV$_1$ (% of predicted)	≥65	50–64	36–49	≤35
Distance walked in 6 min (metres)	≥350	250–349	150–249	≤149
MMRC dyspnoea scale[b]	0–1	2	3	4
Body mass index	>21	≤21		

[a]Body mass index, degree of airflow obstruction, dyspnoea and exercise capacity. [b]Scores on the modified Medical Research Council (MMRC) dyspnoea scale range from 0 to 4, with a score of 4 indicating that the patient is breathless when dressing.

If this fails, secretions can be aspirated by bronchoscopy or via an endotracheal tube.

- ***Respiratory support*** (see pp. 1163–1167). Non-invasive ventilatory techniques can be very helpful in avoiding the need for endotracheal intubation. The best current technique uses tight-fitting facial masks to deliver BiPAP. Assisted ventilation with an endotracheal tube is occasionally used for patients with COPD who have severe respiratory failure but only when there is a clear precipitating factor and the overall prognosis is reasonable. Assessing the likelihood of reversibility in an acute setting can present a difficult ethical problem.
- ***Respiratory stimulants***. Respiratory stimulants such as doxapram were used, but are now rarely chosen due to improvements in non-invasive ventilation.
- ***Corticosteroids, antibiotics and bronchodilators***. These should be administered in the acute phase of respiratory failure but decisions on long-term use should wait until the patient has recovered (see above).

Prognosis of COPD

Predictors of a poor prognosis are increasing age and worsening airflow limitation: that is, decreasing FEV$_1$. A predictive index (BODE: *b*ody mass index (BMI), degree of airflow *o*bstruction, *d*yspnoea and *e*xercise capacity) is shown in ***Box 24.15***. A patient with a BODE index of 0–2 has a 4-year mortality rate of 10%, compared with an 80% rate in someone with a BODE index of 7–10.

Obstructive sleep apnoea

Obstructive sleep apnoea (OSA) affects 1–2% of the population and occurs most often in overweight, middle-aged men. It can occur in children, particularly those with enlarged tonsils. The major symptoms and their frequency are listed in ***Box 24.16***. During sleep, activity of the respiratory muscles is reduced, especially during REM sleep when the diaphragm is virtually the only active muscle.

Box 24.16 Symptoms (%) of obstructive sleep apnoea

Loud snoring	95	**Nocturnal choking**	30
Daytime sleepiness	90	**Reduced libido**	20
Unrefreshed sleep	40	**Morning drunkenness**	5
Restless sleep	40	**Ankle swelling**	5
Morning headache	30		

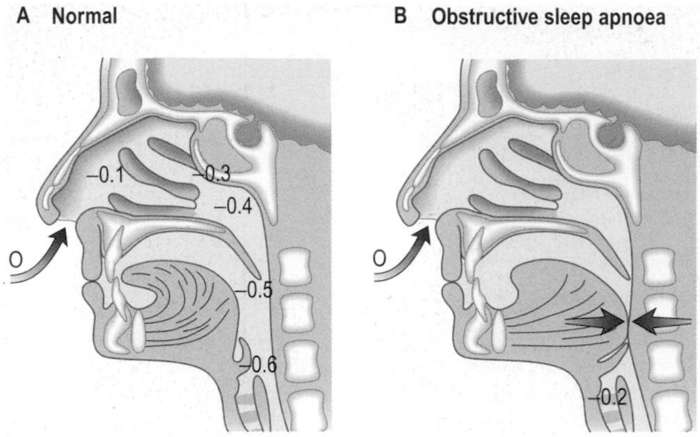

Figure 24.26 Section through head, showing pressure changes. Changes are shown in kPa. There is a pressure drop during inspiration as air is sucked through the turbinates. In patients with obstructive sleep apnoea, this is sufficient to collapse the pharynx (B – arrows on right), obstructing inspiration.

Apnoeas occur when the airway at the back of the throat is sucked closed when breathing in during sleep. When awake, this tendency is overcome by the action of opening muscles of the upper airway, the genioglossus and palatal muscles, but these become hypotonic during sleep ***(Fig. 24.26)***. Partial narrowing results in snoring, complete occlusion causes apnoea and critical narrowing causes hypopnoeas. Apnoea leads to hypoxia and increasingly strenuous respiratory efforts until the patient overcomes the resistance. The combination of the central hypoxic stimulation and the effort to overcome obstruction wakes the patient from sleep. These awakenings are so brief that patients remain unaware of them but may be woken hundreds of times per night, leading to sleep deprivation, especially a reduction in REM sleep, with consequent daytime sleepiness and impaired intellectual performance. Contributory factors are obesity, narrow pharyngeal opening and coexistent COPD.

Correctable factors occur in about one-third of cases and include:

- ***encroachment on pharynx*** – obesity, acromegaly, enlarged tonsils
- ***nasal obstruction*** – nasal deformities, rhinitis, polyps, adenoids
- ***respiratory depressant drugs*** – alcohol, sedatives, strong analgesics.

Diagnosis

Relatives often provide a good history of the snore–silence–snore cycle. The Epworth Sleepiness Scale ***(Box 24.17)*** helps discriminate OSA from simple snoring. The diagnosis is supported by overnight pulse oximetry performed at home. Characteristically, oxygen saturation falls in a cyclical manner, giving a sawtooth appearance to the tracing. If oximetry is negative or equivocal, inpatient assessment with oximetry and video-recording is indicated, preferably in a room specifically adapted for sleep studies. Full polysomnographic studies are rarely needed for clinical diagnosis but are useful in research laboratories. These involve oximetry, direct measurements of thoracic and abdominal movement to assess breathing, and electroencephalography to record patterns of sleep and arousal.

The diagnosis of sleep apnoea/hypopnoea is confirmed if there are more than 10–15 apnoeas or hypopnoeas in any 1 hour of sleep. There is, however, overlap with ***central sleep apnoea*** (see p. 939).

Box 24.17 Epworth sleepiness scale

How likely are you to doze off or fall asleep in the following situations, in contrast to just feeling tired? This refers to your usual way of life in recent times. Even if you have not done some of these things recently, try to work out how they would have affected you. Use the following scale to choose the most appropriate number for each situation.

0 = would never doze
1 = slight chance of dozing
2 = moderate chance of dozing
3 = high chance of dozing

Situation	**Chance of dozing**
Sitting and reading	______
Watching TV	______
Sitting and inactive in a public place (theatre or meeting)	______
As a passenger in a car for an hour without a break	______
Lying down to rest in the afternoon when circumstances permit	______
Sitting and talking to someone	______
Sitting quietly after lunch (without alcohol)	______
In a car, while stopped for a few minutes in the traffic	______
TOTAL	______

Normal 5±4
Severe obstructive sleep apnoea 16 (±4)
Narcolepsy 17

Management

Management consists of correction of treatable factors (see above) with, if necessary, nasal continuous positive airway pressure (CPAP) delivered by a nasal mask during sleep. Such systems raise the pressure in the pharynx by about 1 kPa, keeping the walls apart. Nasal CPAP improves symptoms, quality of life, daytime alertness and survival. However, up to 50% of OSA patients cannot tolerate CPAP. Modafinil (a central nervous system (CNS) stimulant) is a useful short-term alternative.

Bronchiectasis

Bronchiectasis describes abnormal and permanently dilated airways. The disease is characterized by a vicious circle of neutrophilic inflammation, recurrent infection and damage to the airway. This further impairs mucociliary clearance, and persistent inflammation leads to impairment of immunity.

Bronchiectasis is associated with a number of diseases but a cause will only be found in around 50% of cases. Little is known about the epidemiology of bronchiectasis and there is a wide variation in reported incidence. Bronchiectasis related to cystic fibrosis (see p. 1088) is generally considered a separate entity.

Aetiology

The causes of bronchiectasis are listed in ***Box 24.18***. Globally, tuberculosis is the leading cause. Bronchiectasis associated with other lung diseases – in particular, COPD – is becoming increasingly recognized.

Clinical features

See ***Box 24.19***.

Box 24.18 Causes of bronchiectasis

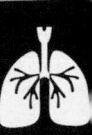

Congenital
- Deficiency of bronchial wall elements
- Pulmonary sequestration

Mechanical bronchial obstruction

Intrinsic
- Foreign body
- Inspissated mucus
- Post-tuberculous stenosis
- Tumour

Extrinsic
- Lymph node
- Tumour

Postinfective bronchial damage
- Bacterial and viral pneumonia, including pertussis, measles and aspiration pneumonia

Granuloma
- Tuberculosis, sarcoidosis

Diffuse diseases of the lung parenchyma
- e.g. Idiopathic pulmonary fibrosis

Immunological over-response
- Allergic bronchopulmonary aspergillosis
- Post-lung transplant

Immune deficiency

Primary
- Panhypogammaglobulinaemia
- Selective immunoglobulin deficiencies (IgA and IgG_2)

Secondary
- Human immunodeficiency virus (HIV) and malignancy

Mucociliary clearance defects

Genetic
- Primary ciliary dyskinesia (Kartagener syndrome with dextrocardia and situs inversus)
- Cystic fibrosis

Acquired
- Young syndrome – azoospermia, sinusitis

Box 24.19 Symptoms and signs in bronchiectasis

- Cough, usually persistent
- Sputum production, large amounts and purulent
- Breathlessness occurs as disease progresses
- Haemoptysis is usually a sign of infection; streaking is common but massive haemoptysis is a rare medical emergency
- Infection, usually characterized by increased sputum volume and increased purulence
- Pleuritic chest pain can be a feature of infection, as well as fever and systemic upset
- Coarse crackles heard on auscultation but examination can be normal
- Clubbing can occur, especially in cystic fibrosis

Investigations

The aims of investigation are to confirm the diagnosis, rule out an underlying cause, look for reversible factors and exclude complications.

- ***HRCT scanning*** is the investigation of choice. Characteristically, non-tapering 'tram track' airways and an increased bronchoarterial ratio 'signet ring' sign can be seen *(Fig. 24.27)*.
- ***Chest X-ray*** may often be normal but tram track airways, ring shadows and cysts may be seen.
- ***Sputum examination*** is useful for a focused antibiotic treatment plan, as well as the exclusion of non-tuberculous mycobacterial disease.
- ***Immune assessment*** would include immunoglobulins and responses to Hib, tetanus and pneumococcal vaccines as baseline tests. Second-line immunological investigation by an immunologist may be necessary.

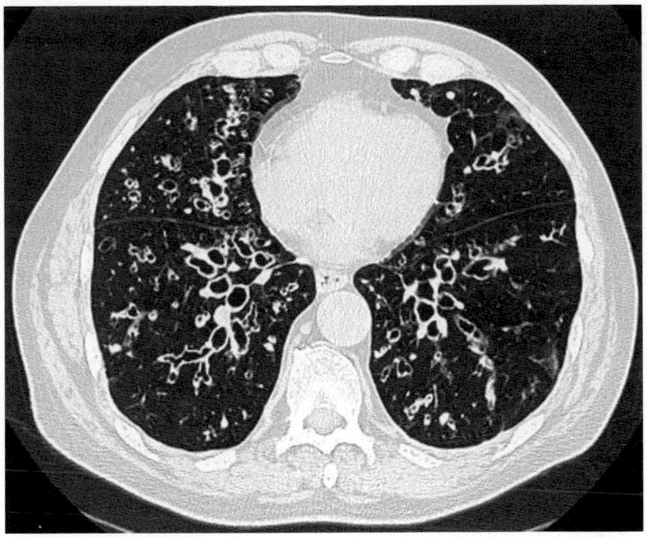

Figure 24.27 CT scan showing bronchiectasis. Note the dilated bronchi with thickened wall, which are larger than adjacent arteries, giving a signet ring appearance.

- ***Sweat test (pp. 1089) and cystic fibrosis genetic assessment (pp. 1088)*** should be carried out for all patients under 40, but also for patients at any age where there is a high index of suspicion.
- ***Nasal nitric oxide*** is a useful test for screening for primary ciliary dyskinesia (PCD). It is very low in PCD. Further ciliary investigation in a specialist centre may be required.
- ***Total IgE and* Aspergillus*-specific IgE or* Aspergillus *skin-prick testing*** should be done to exclude allergic bronchopulmonary aspergillosis.

Management

There is a distinct lack of trials in bronchiectasis to guide therapies, and therapeutic options often have been extrapolated from trials in cystic fibrosis and COPD. Therapy can broadly be divided into airway clearance, anti-inflammatories, and treatment of infection and complications.

Airway clearance

Daily airway clearance therapies are advised. The activated cycle of breathing technique, ***autogenic (self-)drainage*** and postural drainage are popular modalities. A number of devices are available to assist this, such as the 'Flutter' or 'Acapella', which provide positive expiratory pressure with or without airway oscillation

Nebulized hypertonic saline is also approved for use in bronchiectasis; it works as a mucoactive agent.

Anti-inflammatories

Long-term azithromycin has an immunomodulatory effect and has been demonstrated to reduce exacerbation frequency. Inhaled corticosteroids are beneficial to some patients.

Treatment of infection

Treatment of exacerbations usually lasts 2 weeks and is based on previously obtained microbiological information. When *Pseudomonas aeruginosa* is being treated, dual therapy is often used where there are multi-resistant pathogens and where multiple antibiotic courses would be expected. High-dose ciprofloxacin (750 mg twice daily) is a useful oral drug for treatment of *Pseudomonas*. *Haemophilus influenzae* infection is common in bronchiectasis and usually responds to oral antibiotics such as amoxicillin, co-amoxiclav or doxycycline. Some multi-resistant species need intravenous cephalosporin treatment.

Experience in cystic fibrosis has promoted the use of aggressive antibiotic strategies in bronchiectasis, with eradication therapy and chronic suppressive nebulized therapy with colistimethate or an aminoglycoside for *Pseudomonas aeruginosa* (see p. 1089).

Rotating oral antibiotic regimes are no longer recommended routinely. Long-term quinolones should be avoided.

Treatment of complications

- Pulmonary rehabilitation should be offered to patients with a reduced exercise capacity and breathlessness.
- Massive haemoptysis is a life-threatening medical emergency; treatment is resuscitation with airway protection until a bronchial artery embolization can be performed to control the bleeding. If this is not successful, surgery may be required.
- Treatment of *Aspergillus* lung disease and non-tuberculous mycobacteria is covered on pages 1113 and 1122–1123.
- Respiratory failure should be treated with oxygen and non-invasive ventilation. Suitable patients should be referred to a transplant centre.
- Surgery is used for localized disease.

Prognosis

Prognosis is undefined and obviously quite variable, depending on disease severity. A lower FEV_1 and infection with *Pseudomonas aeruginosa* are associated with a poorer outcome.

Cystic fibrosis

Cystic fibrosis (CF) is an autosomal recessive condition. In the UK, the birth prevalence is 1 in 2415 and the carrier rate is 1 in 25. Prevalence is a little lower in North America, rates being much lower in the non-Caucasian population. CF is no longer a disease that causes most patients to die in childhood: survival is improving dramatically. The current expected median survival is now around 36 years. CF is a multisystem disease, although respiratory problems are usually the most prominent. A vicious circle of mucus stasis, inflammation and infection leads to respiratory failure and death in the majority of patients. Most individuals with CF also have pancreatic insufficiency.

Pathogenesis

The CF gene is located on the long arm of chromosome 7 at position 31.2 (see pp. 117–118). Mutations lead to abnormalities in the production of the cystic fibrosis transmembrane conductance regulator (CFTR) protein. This protein is expressed in the apical membrane of epithelial cells and acts as a chloride channel. Over 1000 mutations have been identified, most of them rare. The F508del mutation is the most common, accounting for around 70% of cases. Mutations have been divided into different classes, depending on their effect on CFTR ***(Box 24.20)***. This classification is used therapeutically, with new CF treatments aimed at improving CFTR function. Ivacaftor is the first drug available for CF that improves CFTR function. Previous therapeutic strategies have been based on managing downstream complications only. Ivacaftor is available for patients with the G551D mutation (class III gating defect).

In the lungs, CFTR dysfunction leads to dehydrated airway surface liquid, mucus stasis, airway inflammation and recurrent infection. This process originates in the small airways, leading to progressive airway obstruction and bronchiectasis ***(Fig. 24.28)***.

Box 24.20 CFTR abnormalities in CF

Class	CFTR effect	Mutation example
I	Protein synthesis defect. No functional CFTR	G542X, R553X, R1162X
II	Folding/trafficking defect. Does not reach apical membrane	F508del
III	Gating defect	G551D
IV	Conductance impairment due to narrow channel	R117H
V	Splicing defect	3849+10kbC>T
VI	Reduced stability	4326delTC

Box 24.21 Clinical features and complications of cystic fibrosis (CF)

Respiratory
- Recurrent respiratory infection
- Chronic daily cough and sputum production
- Breathlessness
- Nasal polyps
- Haemoptysis (sometimes massive)
- Pneumothorax
- Respiratory failure and cor pulmonale
- Recurrent sinusitis

Gastrointestinal
- Failure to thrive in infancy and low body mass index in adults
- Meconium ileus in infancy
- Distal intestinal obstruction syndrome
- Steatorrhoea secondary to pancreatic insufficiency
- CF-related liver disease and cirrhosis
- Increased risk of gastrointestinal malignancy

Other
- CF-related diabetes
- Male infertility
- Osteoporosis
- Arthropathy

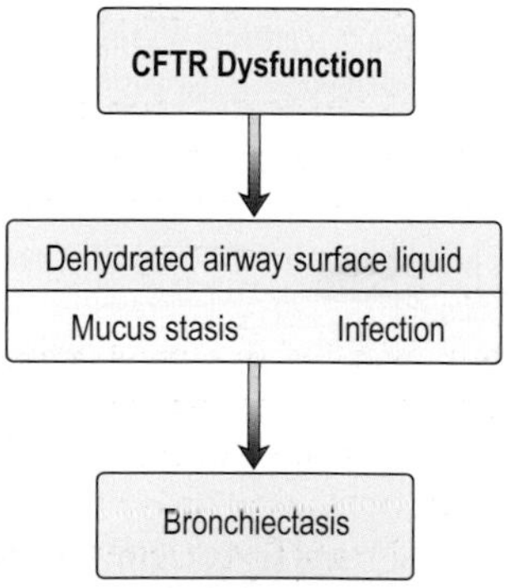

Figure 24.28 **Cystic fibrosis: pathogenesis of lung disease.**

Clinical features and complications

CF is a multisystem disease but in 90% of cases the eventual cause of death is related to respiratory disease. Pancreatic insufficiency occurs in the majority of patients and CF-related diabetes is becoming increasingly common as survival improves, occurring in up to 40–50% of older adults with CF. Liver disease occurs in around 20% of the CF population and can lead to cirrhosis in around 2%. Clinical manifestations and complications are summarized in ***Box 24.21***.

Diagnosis

Most new CF diagnoses are currently made at newborn screening. The test involves measuring immunoreactive trypsinogen at the time of the neonatal heel prick test. If the concentration is raised, formal testing is performed.

Aside from neonatal screening, diagnosis for children and adults is based on a combination of:

- Common clinical features **(Box 24.21)**.
- CFTR functional testing. The ***sweat test (pilocarpine iontophoresis)*** measures chloride concentration and is the test routinely performed. The normal range is <30 mmol/L, with borderline cases at 30–60 mmol/L. These cases often represent patients with a milder 'atypical' phenotype. In difficult cases, nasal potential difference can be measured.
- Confirmatory genetic testing.

Management

Patients with CF should be managed in a specialist centre by a multidisciplinary group of experienced healthcare professionals. Patients should be seen at least every 3 months and have an annual review. Lung function (FEV_1) and BMI should be recorded at every appointment, as they have prognostic importance.

Pulmonary disease

The aim of chronic pulmonary therapies is to reduce FEV_1 decline, daily symptoms and exacerbation frequency.

- ***Airway clearance techniques*** are a vital part of CF treatment regimens. There is no consensus on the best type and patient choice is the main factor.
- ***Nebulized therapy***:
  - Recombinant human DNase (rhDNase) is advised for routine treatment from early childhood (regardless of disease status). There is clear evidence of improvement in lung disease and therapy may influence survival.
  - Hypertonic saline works as an osmotic agent to draw water to the cell surface.
  - Inhaled mannitol also increases mucociliary clearance.
- ***Anti-inflammatory treatment*** with long-term azithromycin is widely used in CF and has an immunomodulatory effect.

Respiratory infection

Spread of respiratory infection is a great threat to CF patients. Clinics are microbiologically cohorted, patients are managed in single rooms and no patient social events are organized.

Pseudomonas aeruginosa infection is common in patients with CF and is associated with accelerated lung function decline. Eradication is the treatment aim. A combination of nebulized colistimethate and oral ciprofloxacin, or inhaled tobramycin, can be given. Long-term nebulized suppression therapy with these medications is also used to improve respiratory health.

Other organisms, such as *Burkholderia cepacia*, meticillin-resistant *Staph. aureus* (MRSA) and *Stenotrophomonas maltophilia*, have been associated with worsening respiratory outcomes, so eradication regimes for these bacteria are being used. Non-tuberculous mycobacterial disease, in particular *Mycobacterium abscessus*, can be associated with a rapid decline and active infection may preclude transplantation.

In exacerbations, intravenous antibiotic therapy is based on previous infection history. For *Pseudomonas*, a combination of a β-lactam antibiotic such as ceftazidime with an aminoglycoside such as tobramycin would be the first-line choice. *In vitro* sensitivities are less useful in CF. Many CF patients have a permanently implanted venous access device for delivery of intravenous therapy.

Advanced disease

Respiratory failure should be treated with oxygen and non-invasive ventilation. Patients should be referred for consideration of lung transplantation when FEV_1 falls to around 30% predicted. In end-stage disease, palliative care is an essential part of management. This can be challenging when patients are on an active waiting list for a lung transplant.

Non-respiratory complications

Pancreatic enzymes and vitamin supplements are used to treat those patients with pancreatic insufficiency. Close attention is paid to diet and calorie supplementation. Overnight gastric feeding may be required to maintain BMI in some patients.

CF-related diabetes will often require treatment with insulin and is screened for at annual review. It is distinct from type 1 and type 2 diabetes. Osteoporosis is screened for and treated. Fertility treatment is available for men with CF who are infertile.

The future

CFTR modulation has proved to be a major therapeutic advance. Chemical libraries have been screened and a number of compounds have been developed. Studies for therapies for the F508Del mutation are ongoing. Recently, lumacaftor (a CFTR corrector) in combination with ivacaftor has been shown to be beneficial in patients with p.Phe508del CFTR mutation. Other trials continue.

Chronic cough

Pathological coughing (see p. 1066) results from two mechanisms:

- stimulation of sensory nerves in the epithelium (by secretions, foreign bodies, cigarette smoke and tumours)
- sensitization of the cough reflex with abnormal increase in the sensitivity of the cough receptors.

Sensitization of the cough reflex can be demonstrated by inhalation of capsaicin or saline solution; it presents clinically as a persistent tickling sensation in the throat with paroxysms of coughing induced by changes in air temperature, aerosol sprays, perfumes and cigarette smoke. It is found in association with viral infections, oesophageal reflux, postnasal drip, cough-variant asthma, and in 15% of patients taking angiotensin-converting enzyme (ACE) inhibitors. The association with ACE inhibitors implicates neuropeptides, prostaglandins E_2 and F_2, and bradykinin as causes of cough. In some patients, no cause can be found (idiopathic cough). In the absence of chest X-ray abnormalities, possible investigations include:

- ENT examination (see p. 1318) and sinus CT for postnasal drip
- lung function tests and bronchial provocation testing (see p. 1092) for cough-variant asthma
- ambulatory oesophageal pH monitoring and manometry for oesophageal reflux
- fibreoptic bronchoscopy for inhaled foreign body or tumour
- ECG, echocardiography and exercise testing and impedance for cardiac causes
- hyperventilation testing
- psychiatric appraisal.

Symptomatic management of unexplained cough can be difficult. Morphine depresses the sensitized cough reflex but its unwanted effects limit its long-term use. Dihydrocodeine linctus may help some patients. Demulcent preparations and cough sweets provide only temporary relief. Patients who cough while taking ACE inhibitors should switch to an angiotensin II receptor antagonist, such as losartan (see pp. 985–987), which does not block bradykinin breakdown.

Lung and heart–lung transplantation

Indications and donor selection

The main diseases treated by transplantation are:

- pulmonary fibrosis
- primary pulmonary hypertension
- cystic fibrosis
- bronchiectasis
- emphysema – particularly α_1-antitrypsin inhibitor deficiency
- Eisenmenger syndrome.

Patients selected for transplantation are usually under 60 years with a life expectancy of less than 18 months, no underlying cancer and no serious systemic disease.

Organs are taken from donors under 40 years, with good cardiac and lung function, and chest measurements slightly smaller than those of the recipient. Matching for ABO blood group is essential, but rhesus blood group compatibility is not essential. Since donor material is limited, single-lung transplantation is preferred to double-lung or heart–lung transplantation; this can be successfully undertaken in pulmonary fibrosis, pulmonary hypertension and emphysema. Bilateral lung transplantation is required in infective conditions to prevent spillover of bacteria from the diseased lung to a single transplanted lung. Eisenmenger syndrome requires heart–lung transplant.

Complications and their treatment

- ***Early post-transplant pulmonary oedema*** requires diuretics and ventilatory support.
- ***Infections***, particularly within the first 3 months, are treated as follows:
  - bacterial pneumonia – antibiotics
  - cytomegalovirus – ganciclovir
  - herpes simplex – aciclovir.
  - *Pneumocystis jiroveci* – prophylactic co-trimoxazole.
- ***Immunosuppression*** is with ciclosporin (inhaled formulation has shown benefit) or tacrolimus, azathioprine or mycophenolate mofetil and prednisolone.
- ***Rejection***:
  - Early (first few weeks) – high-dose intravenous corticosteroids
  - Late (after 3 months) – high-dose intravenous corticosteroids are sometimes effective in obliterative bronchiolitis. Post-transplant lymphoproliferative disease may respond to rituximab, an anti-B-cell monoclonal antibody.

Prognosis

Several studies show a major improvement in overall quality of life. One-year survival rates have improved, with a yearly mortality rate of about 10%. Death is due mainly to bronchiolitis. Overall survival varies with the original diagnosis but the median survival is approximately 4 years.

Further reading

Barnes PJ. Small airways in COPD. *N Engl J Med* 2004; 350:2635–2637.
Davis PB. Another beginning for cystic fibrosis therapy. *N Engl J Med* 2015; 373:274–276.
Martinez FJ, Donohue JF, Rennard SI et al. The future of COPD treatment – difficulties of and barriers to drug development. *Lancet* 2011; 378:1027–1037.
Mitzner W. Emphysema – a disease of small airways or lung parenchyma? *N Engl J Med* 2011; 365:1637–1639.
Niewoehner DE. Outpatient management of severe COPD. *N Engl J Med* 2012; 362:1407–1416.
Postma DS, Bush A, van den Berge M. Risk factors and early origins of chronic obstructive pulmonary disease. *Lancet* 2015; 385:899–909.
Rabe KF, Wedzicha JA. Controversies in the treatment of chronic obstructive pulmonary disease. *Lancet* 2011; 378:1038–1047.
Vestbo J, Edwards LD, Scanlon PD et al. (ECLIPSE). Changes in forced expiratory volume in 1 second over time in COPD. *N Engl J Med* 2011; 365:1184–1192.

ASTHMA

Asthma is a common chronic condition whose cause is incompletely understood. Symptoms include wheeze, chest tightness, cough and shortness of breath, often worse at night. Asthma commonly starts in childhood between the ages of 3 and 5 years and may either worsen or improve during adolescence. Classically, asthma has three characteristics:

- ***airflow limitation***, which is usually reversible spontaneously or with treatment
- ***airway hyper-responsiveness*** to a wide range of stimuli (see below)
- ***bronchial inflammation*** with T lymphocytes, mast cells, eosinophils with associated plasma exudation, oedema, smooth muscle hypertrophy, matrix deposition, mucus plugging and epithelial damage.

In chronic asthma, inflammation may be accompanied by irreversible airflow limitation as a result of airway wall remodelling that may involve large and small airways and mucus impaction.

Prevalence

In many countries, the prevalence of asthma has increased over the past 30 years. This increase is particularly marked in children and young adults, with up to 15% of the population being affected. Asthma is more common in more developed countries, with some of the highest rates in the UK, New Zealand and Australia, and much lower rates in Far Eastern countries such as China and Malaysia, Africa, and Central and Eastern Europe. Long-term follow-up in developing countries suggests that asthma may become more frequent as individuals adopt a more 'Westernized' lifestyle, but the environmental factors accounting for this remain unknown. Studies of occupational asthma suggest that a large proportion of the workforce (15–20%) may become asthmatic if exposed to potent sensitizers. Worldwide, approximately 300 million people have asthma and this is expected to rise to 400 million by 2025.

Classification

Asthma is a complex disorder. Current thinking is that the symptoms can be caused by several different processes. Asthma can be classified according to its trigger factors, by age of onset, by inflammatory subtypes or by response to therapy. There is considerable overlap between populations separated along these different dimensions, and it is now fashionable to describe clinical subtypes (or endotypes).

Many childhood-onset asthmatics have wheezing illness with inhalant allergic triggers. Some 90% of children and 70% of adults with persistent asthma have positive skin-prick tests to common inhalant allergens such as dust mite, animal danders, pollens and fungi. Childhood-onset asthma is often accompanied by eczema (atopic dermatitis; see pp. 1349–1351). Sensitization to chemicals or biological products in the workplace is a frequently overlooked cause of late-onset asthma in adults.

In some people with asthma, inhaled allergens are not relevant. This illness often starts in middle age and attacks are usually triggered by respiratory infections. Nevertheless, many patients with adult-onset asthma show positive allergen skin tests and, on close questioning, some of these will give a history of childhood respiratory symptoms suggesting they have extrinsic asthma.

Non-atopic individuals may develop asthma in middle age from extrinsic causes such as sensitization to occupational agents like toluene diisocyanate, intolerance to NSAIDs such as aspirin, or prescription of β-adrenoceptor-blocking agents that block the protective effect of endogenous catecholamines. Extrinsic causes must be considered in all cases of asthma and, where possible, avoided.

Other clinical phenotypes

Based on the clinical picture, several subtypes or endotypes of asthma are recognized, including 'brittle asthma' and steroid-resistant asthma. While eosinophilic airway inflammation is often present in asthma, there are also patients with eosinophilic bronchitis, who have sputum eosinophilia without wheeze. It remains unclear whether this is a pre-asthmatic state or whether anti-eosinophil treatment is helpful.

Aetiology

The major factors involved in the development of asthma and stimuli that can precipitate attacks are shown in ***Figure 24.29***.

Atopy and allergy

The term 'atopy' was coined in the early 1900s to describe a group of disorders, including asthma and hayfever, which appeared to:

- run in families
- have characteristic wealing skin reactions to common allergens in the environment
- have circulating allergen-specific antibodies (later shown to be IgE).

Allergen-specific IgE is present in 30–40% of the UK population, and elevated serum IgE levels are linked to airway hyper-responsiveness and the prevalence of asthma. Serum total IgE levels are affected by several genetic and environmental factors.

Genetic factors

There is no single gene for asthma, but several genes, in combination with environmental factors, appear to influence the development of asthma.

- Genes controlling the production of the cytokines IL-3, IL-4, IL-5, IL-9, IL-13 and granulocyte–macrophage colony stimulating factor (GM-CSF) are present in a cluster on chromosome 5q31-33 (the IL-4 gene cluster). These cytokines affect the development and survival of mast cells and eosinophils, as well as IgE production.
- Polymorphic variation in proteins along the IL-4/13 signalling pathway is strongly associated with allergy and asthma.
- Novel asthma genes identified by positional cloning from whole-genome scans are the PHF11 locus on chromosome 2 (which includes genes *SETDB2* and *RCBTB1*) and transcription factors, which are implicated in IgE synthesis and associated more with atopy than asthma.
- *ADAM33* (a disintegrin and metalloproteinase) on chromosome 20p13 is associated with airway hyper-responsiveness and tissue remodelling.
- Other genes associated with asthma are those that encode neuropeptide S receptor (*GPRA* or *GPR154*) on chromosome 7p15, *HLA-G* on chromosome 6p21, dipeptidyl peptidase 10 on chromosome 2q14 and *ORMDL3*, a member of a gene family that encodes transmembrane proteins anchored in the endoplasmic reticulum, on chromosome 17q21.

Recent evidence from genome-wide association studies has shown that the epithelial–ILC2 cell axis is involved in the pathogenesis of asthma. ILC2 cells are also known as natural type 2 helper cells or nuocytes. IL33 and its receptor, IL1RL1(ST2), thymic stromal lymphopoietin (*TSLP*), the transcription factor *RORalpha* and *IL13* have been identified as the major asthma susceptibility genes.

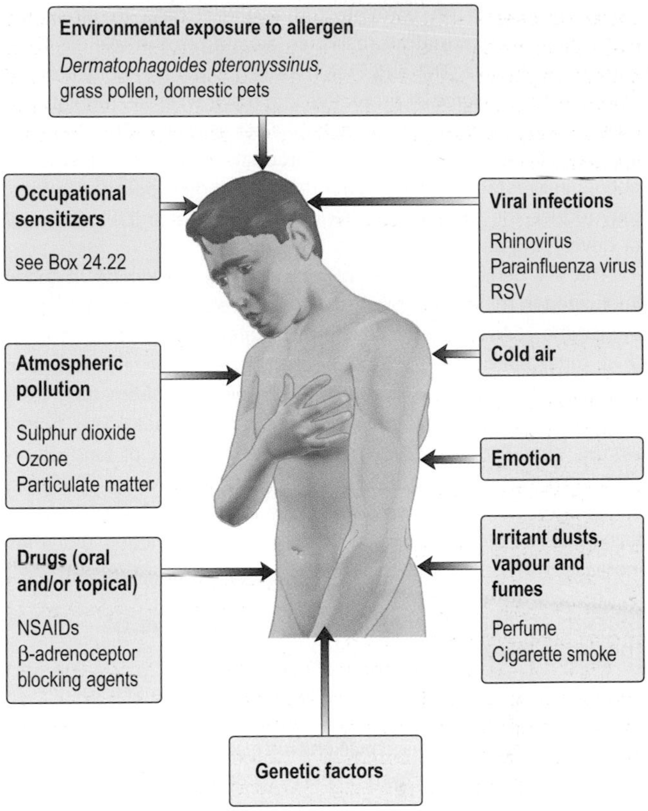

Figure 24.29 Causes and triggers of asthma. NSAIDs, non-steroidal anti-inflammatory drugs; RSV, respiratory syncytial virus.

Environmental factors

Early childhood exposure to allergens and maternal smoking has a major influence on IgE production. Much interest focuses on the role of intestinal bacteria and childhood infections in shaping the immune system in early life. It has been suggested that growing up in a relatively 'clean' environment may predispose towards an IgE response to allergens (the 'hygiene hypothesis'). Conversely, growing up in a 'dirtier' environment may allow the immune system to avoid developing allergic responses. Components of bacteria (e.g. lipopolysaccharide endotoxin, immunostimulatory CpG DNA sequences, flagellin), viruses (e.g. SS- and DS-RNA) and fungi (e.g. chiton, a cell-wall component) stimulate various toll-like receptors

(TLRs) expressed on immune and epithelial cells to direct the immune and inflammatory response away from the allergic (Th2) towards protective (Th1 and Treg) pathways. Th1 immunity is associated with antimicrobial protective immunity, whereas regulatory T cells are strongly implicated in tolerance to allergens. Thus early life exposure to inhaled and ingested products of microorganisms, as occurs in livestock farming communities and developing countries, may reduce the subsequent risk of a child becoming allergic and/or developing asthma.

The allergens involved in allergic asthma are similar to those implicated in rhinitis, although pollens are relatively less implicated in asthma. Most allergic asthmatics are sensitized to house-dust mite allergens. Cockroach allergy has been implicated in asthma in US inner-city children, while allergens from furry pets (especially cats) are increasingly common causes. The fungal spores from *Aspergillus fumigatus* cause a range of lung disorders, including asthma (see pp. 1122–1123). Many allergens, including those from *Aspergillus*, have intrinsic biological properties: for example, enzymes with a proteolytic function that may increase their sensitizing capacity.

Box 24.22 Occupational asthma

Cause	Source/occupation
Low-molecular-weight (non-IgE-related)	
Isocyanates	Polyurethane varnishes Industrial coatings Spray painting
Colophony fumes	Soldering/welders Electronics industry
Wood dust	
Drugs	
Bleaches and dyes	
Complex metal salts, e.g. nickel, platinum, chromium	
High-molecular-weight (IgE-related)	
Allergens from animals and insects	Farmers, workers in poultry and seafood processing industry; laboratory workers
Antibiotics	Nurses, health industry
Latex	Health workers
Proteolytic enzymes	Manufacture (but not use) of 'biological' washing powders
Complex salts of platinum	Metal refining
Acid anhydrides and polyamine hardening agents	Industrial coatings

Increased responsiveness of the airways of the lung (airway hyper-responsiveness)

Airway hyper-responsiveness (AHR) is a characteristic feature of asthma and can be demonstrated by asking patients to inhale gradually increasing concentrations of histamine or methacholine (***bronchial provocation tests***). This induces transient airflow limitation in susceptible individuals (approximately 20% of the population); the severity of AHR can be graded according to the provocation dose (PD) or concentration (PC) of the agonist that produces a 20% fall in FEV_1 (PD_{20} FEV_1 or PC_{20} FEV_1). Patients with clinical symptoms of asthma respond to very low doses of methacholine: that is, they have a low PD_{20} FEV_1. AHR can also be assessed by exercise testing or inhalation of cold, dry air, mannitol or hypertonic saline. These are indirect tests that release endogenous mediators such as histamine, prostaglandins and leukotrienes, which then cause bronchoconstriction. Indirect measures of AHR correlate more closely with symptoms and diurnal PEFR variation than PC_{20} histamine or methacholine; both are useful in diagnosing asthma if there is doubt, and in guiding treatment.

Some patients also react to methacholine but at *higher doses*, including those with:

- attacks of asthma only on extreme exertion
- wheezing or prolonged periods of coughing following a viral infection
- seasonal wheeze during the pollen season
- allergic rhinitis, but not complaining of lower respiratory symptoms until specifically questioned
- some subjects with no respiratory symptoms.

Although the degree of AHR can be influenced by allergic mechanisms (see p. 1094 and ***Fig. 24.32***), its pathogenesis and mode of inheritance involve a combination of airway inflammation and tissue remodelling.

Precipitating factors

Occupational sensitizers

Over 250 materials encountered at the workplace can cause occupational asthma, which accounts for up to 15% of all asthma cases ***(Box 24.22)***. These are recognized occupational diseases in the UK, and patients in insurable employment are eligible for statutory compensation, provided they apply within 10 years of leaving the occupation in which the asthma developed.

Asthma can be due to:

- low-molecular-weight compounds, e.g. reactive chemicals such as isocyanates and acid anhydrides that bond chemically to epithelial cells to activate them, as well as provide haptens recognized by T cells
- high-molecular-weight compounds, e.g. flour, organic dusts and other large protein molecules involving specific IgE antibodies.

Smoking increases the risk of developing some forms of occupational asthma. The proportion of employees developing occupational asthma depends primarily upon the level of exposure. Proper enclosure of industrial processes or appropriate ventilation greatly reduces the risk. Atopic individuals develop occupational asthma more rapidly when exposed to agents causing the development of specific IgE antibody. Non-atopic individuals can also develop asthma when exposed to such agents, but after a longer period of exposure.

Non-specific factors

Due to their AHR, patients with asthma will respond to a wide variety of non-specific direct and indirect stimuli, as well as reacting to specific allergens.

Cold air and exercise

Most asthmatics wheeze after prolonged exercise or inhalation of cold, dry air. Typically, the attack does not occur while exercising but afterwards. Exercise-induced wheeze is driven by release of histamine, prostaglandins (PGs) and leukotrienes (LTs) from mast cells, as well as stimulation of neural reflexes when the epithelial lining fluid of the bronchi becomes hyperosmolar owing to drying and cooling during exercise. The phenomenon can be shown by exercise, cold air and hypertonic provocation tests with saline or mannitol.

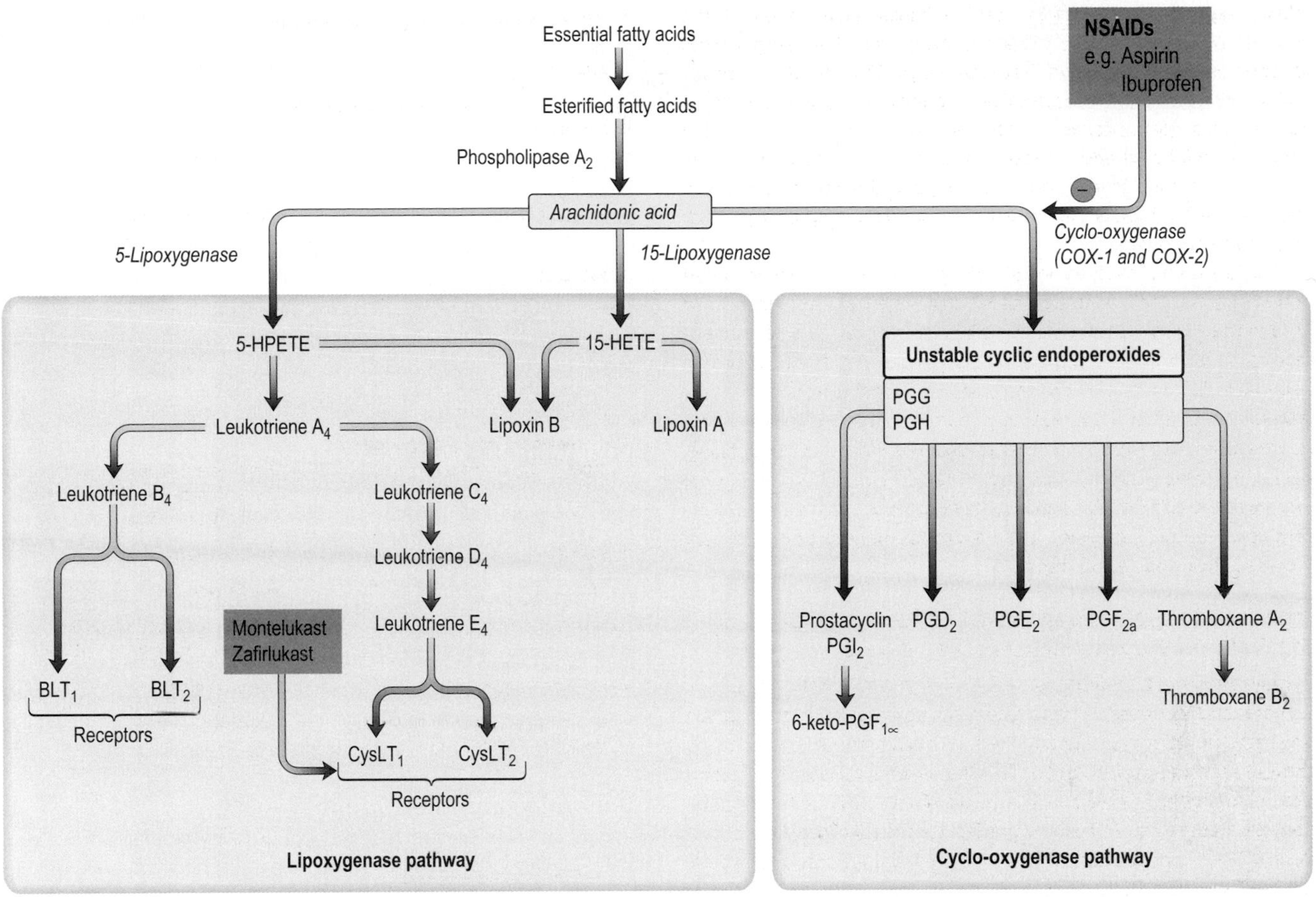

Figure 24.30 Arachidonic acid metabolism and the effect of drugs. The sites of action of non-steroidal anti-inflammatory drugs (NSAIDs, e.g. aspirin, ibuprofen) are shown. The ***enzyme cyclo-oxygenase*** occurs in three isoforms: ***COX-1*** (constitutive), ***COX-2*** (inducible) and ***COX-3*** (in brain). BLT, B leukotriene receptor; CysLT, cysteinyl leukotriene receptor; PG, prostaglandin.

Atmospheric pollution and irritant dusts, vapours and fumes

Many patients with asthma experience worsening of symptoms on exposure to tobacco smoke, car exhaust fumes, solvents, strong perfumes or high concentrations of airborne dust. Major epidemics have been recorded when large amounts of allergens are released into the air: for example, soybean dust in Barcelona. Asthma exacerbations increase during summer and winter air pollution episodes associated with climatic temperature inversions. Epidemics of asthma have occurred in the presence of high concentrations of ozone, particulates and NO_2 in the summer and particulates, NO_2 and SO_2 in the winter.

Diet

Increased intake of fresh fruit and vegetables has been shown to be protective, possibly owing to the increased intake of antioxidants or other protective molecules such as flavonoids. Genetic variation in antioxidant enzymes is associated with more severe asthma.

Emotion

Emotional factors influence asthma both acutely and chronically, but there is no evidence that patients with the disease are any more psychologically disturbed than their non-asthmatic peers. An asthma attack is a frightening experience, especially when its onset is sudden or unexpected. Patients at high risk of life-threatening attacks are understandably anxious.

Drugs

NSAIDs. NSAIDs, particularly aspirin and propionic acid derivatives, such as indometacin and ibuprofen, are implicated in triggering asthma in approximately 5% of patients. NSAID intolerance is especially prevalent in those with both nasal polyps and asthma, and is often associated with rhinitis and flushing on drug exposure. NSAIDs inhibit arachidonic acid metabolism via the cyclo-oxygenase (COX) pathway, preventing the synthesis of certain prostaglandins. In aspirin-intolerant asthma, there is reduced production of PGE_2, which, in a sub-proportion of genetically susceptible subjects, induces the overproduction of cysteinyl leukotrienes by eosinophils, mast cells and macrophages. Genetic polymorphisms involving the enzymes and receptors of the leukotriene-generating pathway are seen ***(Fig. 24.30)***. COX-2 inhibitors do not trigger attacks, indicating that blockade of the COX-1 isoenzyme is the underlying trigger.

Beta-blockers. The airways have a direct parasympathetic innervation that tends to produce bronchoconstriction. There is no direct sympathetic innervation of bronchial smooth muscle, so antagonism of parasympathetically induced bronchoconstriction is critically dependent upon circulating adrenaline (epinephrine) acting through β_2-receptors on the surface of smooth muscle cells. Inhibition of this effect by β-adrenoceptor-blocking drugs, such as propranolol, leads to bronchoconstriction and airflow limitation, but only in asthmatic subjects. Selective β_1-adrenergic-blocking drugs, such as atenolol, may also induce attacks of asthma.

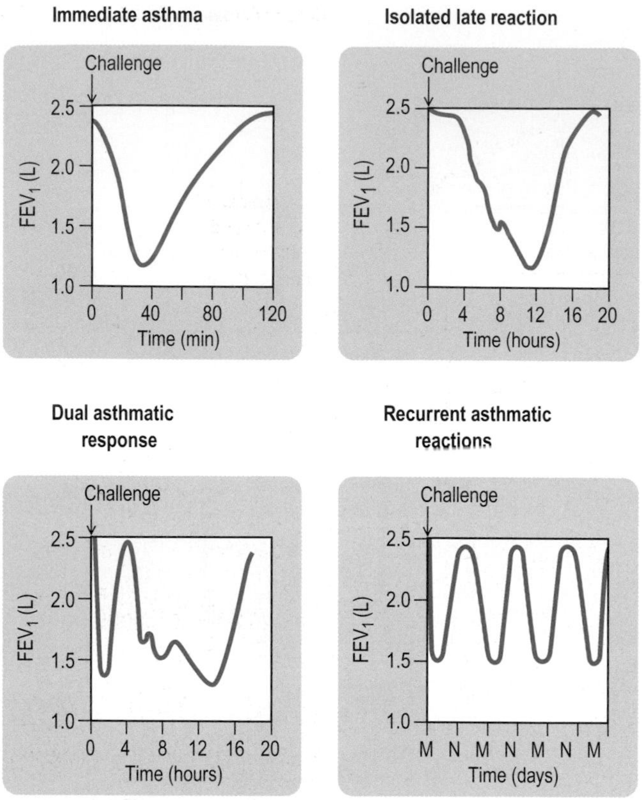

Figure 24.31 Different types of asthmatic reaction following challenge with allergen. M, midnight; N, noon.

Allergen-induced asthma

The experimental inhalation of allergen by atopic asthmatic individuals leads to the development of different types of reaction, as illustrated in ***Figure 24.31***.

Immediate asthmatic reaction. Airflow limitation begins within minutes of contact with the allergen, reaches its maximum in 15–20 minutes and subsides by 1 hour.

Dual and late-phase reactions. Following an immediate reaction, many asthmatics develop a more prolonged and sustained attack of airflow limitation that responds less well to inhalation of bronchodilator drugs such as salbutamol. Isolated late-phase reactions with no preceding immediate response can occur after the inhalation of some occupational sensitizers such as isocyanates. AHR increases during and for several weeks after late-phase reactions, which may explain why symptoms persist after allergen exposure.

Pathogenesis

The pathogenesis of asthma is complex and not fully understood. The role of different cells has been extensively studied to try to find new targets for therapy. Allergen-driven models have dominated this field but some caution is needed in extrapolating to the real disease. Schematically, asthma involves several cells and mediators that can be activated by various different mechanisms, including exposure to allergens ***(Fig. 24.32)***. The varying clinical severity and chronicity of asthma are dependent on an interplay between airway inflammation and airway wall remodelling. The inflammatory component is driven by Th2-type T lymphocytes ***(Fig. 24.32)***. However, as the disease becomes more severe and chronic, and loses its sensitivity to corticosteroids, there is greater evidence of a Th1 response with release of mediators such as TNF-α and associated tissue damage, mucous metaplasia and aberrant epithelial and mesenchymal repair.

Inflammation

Mast cells

Mast cells (see also pp. 125–126) are increased in the epithelium, smooth muscle and mucous glands in asthma, and release mediators, such as histamine, tryptase, PGD_2 and cysteinyl leukotrienes, which act on smooth muscle, small blood vessels, mucus-secreting cells and sensory nerves, causing the immediate asthmatic reaction. Mast cells also release an array of cytokines, chemokines and growth factors that contribute to the late asthmatic response and more chronic aspects of asthma.

Eosinophils

These are found in large numbers in the bronchial wall and secretions of asthmatics. They are attracted to the airways by the cytokines IL-3, IL-5 and GM-CSF, as well as by chemokines that act on type 3 C-C chemokine receptors (CCR-3) (i.e. eotaxin, RANTES, MCP-1, MCP-3 and MCP-4). These mediators also prime eosinophils for enhanced mediator secretion. When activated, eosinophils release LTC_4, and basic proteins that are toxic to epithelial cells. Both the number and activation of eosinophils are rapidly decreased by corticosteroids. Sputum eosinophilia is diagnostically useful and provides a biomarker of response to therapy.

Dendritic cells and lymphocytes

Asthmatic airways show a Th2 pattern of cytokine expression. T-helper lymphocytes ($CD4^+$) in the airways show evidence of activation ***(Fig. 24.32)***; their cytokines aid the migration and activation of mast cells (IL-3, IL-4, IL-9 and IL-13) and eosinophils (IL-3, IL-5, GM-CSF). In mild/moderate asthma, there is selective upregulation of Th2 T cells with reduced evidence of the Th1 phenotype (producing interferon-gamma (IFN-γ), TNF-α and IL-2), although Th1 cells are more prominent in more severe disease. The activity of macrophages and lymphocytes is influenced by corticosteroids but not by β_2-adrenoceptor agonists.

Remodelling

A characteristic feature of chronic asthma is alteration of the structure and functions of the formed elements of the airways. Together, these structural changes interact with inflammatory cells and mediators to alter airways physiology and hence trigger symptoms. Deposition of matrix proteins, swelling and cellular infiltration expand the submucosa beneath the epithelium so that, for a given degree of smooth muscle shortening, there is excess airway narrowing. Swelling outside the smooth muscle layer reduces the retractile forces exerted by the surrounding alveoli so that the airways close more easily. Several factors contribute to these changes.

The epithelium

In asthma, the epithelium of the conducting airways is stressed and damaged with loss of ciliated columnar cells. The epithelium is a major source of mediators, cytokines and growth factors that enhance inflammation and promote tissue remodelling ***(Fig. 24.32)***. Damage and activation of the epithelium make it more vulnerable to infection by common respiratory viruses (e.g. rhinovirus, coronavirus) and to the effects of air pollutants. Increased production of nitric oxide (NO), due to the increased expression of inducible NO synthase, is a feature of epithelial damage and activation.

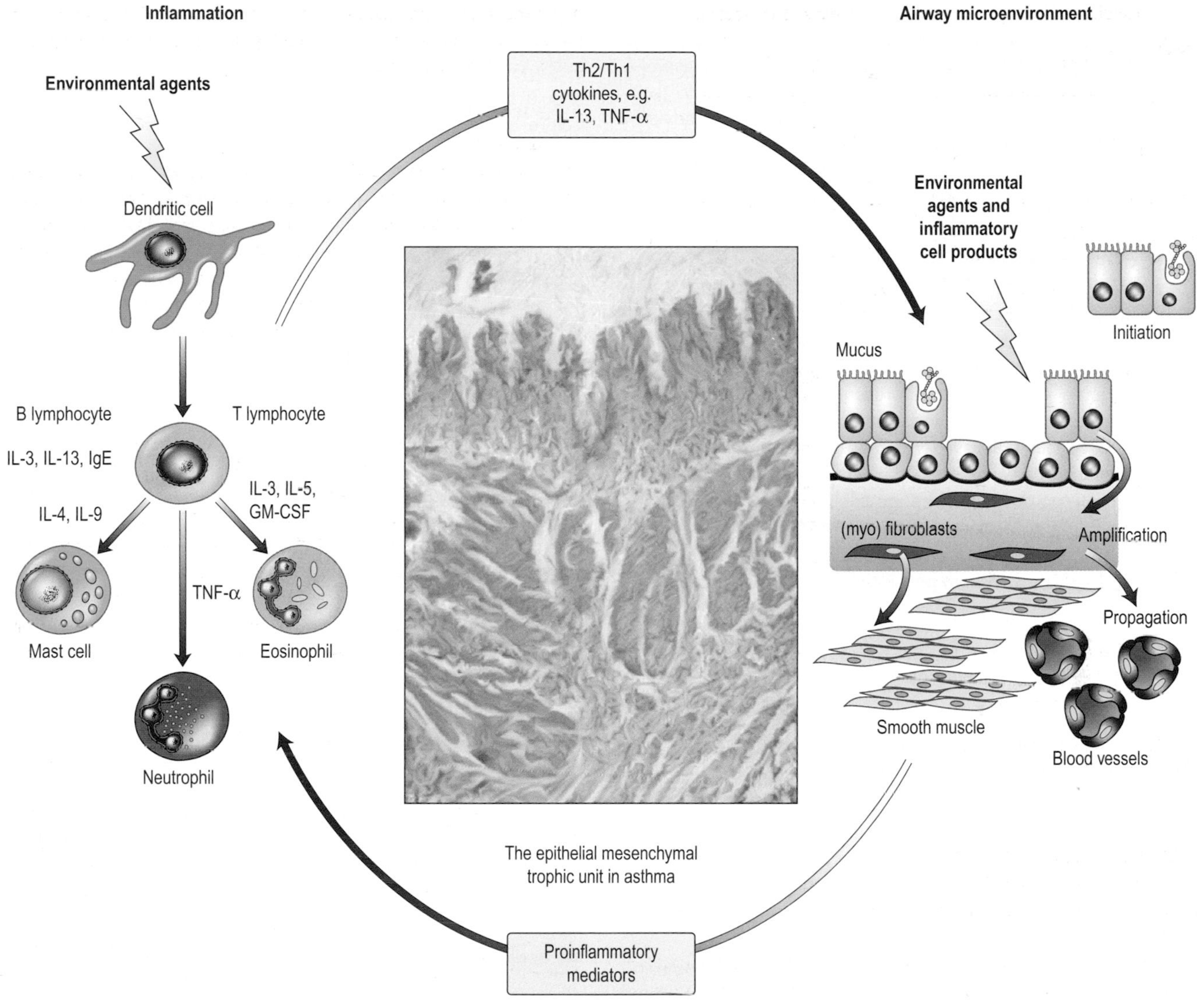

Figure 24.32 **Inflammatory and remodelling responses in asthma with activation of the epithelial mesenchymal trophic unit.** Epithelial damage alters the set point for communication between bronchial epithelium and underlying mesenchymal cells, leading to myofibroblast activation, an increase in mesenchymal volume, and induction of structural changes throughout the airway wall. GM-CSF, granulocyte–macrophage colony stimulating factor; Ig, immunoglobulin; IL, interleukin; TNF-α, tumour necrosis factor alpha. *(Adapted from Holgate ST, Polosa R. The mechanisms, diagnosis, and management of severe asthma in adults.* Lancet *2006; 368:780–793, with permission from Elsevier.)*

Measurement of exhaled NO is a useful non-invasive test of continuing inflammation (see p. 1096).

The epithelial basement membrane

A pathognomonic feature of asthma is the deposition of repair collagens (types I, III and V) and proteoglycans in the lamina reticularis beneath the basement membrane. This, along with the deposition of other matrix proteins such as laminin, tenascin and fibronectin, causes the appearance of a thickened basement membrane observed by light microscopy in asthma. This collagen deposition reflects activation of an underlying sheath of fibroblasts that transform into contractile myofibroblasts, which also have an increased capacity to secrete matrix. Aberrant signalling between the epithelium and underlying myofibroblasts is thought to be the principal cause of airway wall remodelling, since the cells are prolific producers of a range of tissue growth factors such as epidermal growth factor (EGF), transforming growth factor (TGF)-α and β, connective tissue-derived growth factor (CTGF), platelet-derived growth factor (PDGF), endothelin (ET), insulin-like growth factors (IGF), nerve growth factors and vascular endothelial growth factors ***(Fig. 24.32)***.

Smooth muscle

Another prominent feature of asthma is hyperplasia of the helical bands of airway smooth muscle. In addition to increasing in amount, the smooth muscle alters in function so it contracts more easily and stays contracted because of a change in actin–myosin cross-link cycling. These changes allow asthmatic airways to contract too much and too easily at the least provocation. Asthmatic smooth muscle also secretes a wide range of cytokines, chemokines and growth factors that help sustain the chronic inflammatory response.

Nerves

Central and peripheral neural reflexes contribute to the irritability of asthmatic airways. Central reflexes involve stimulation of nerve endings in the epithelium and submucosa with transmission of impulses via the spinal cord and brain back down to the airways, where release of acetylcholine from nerve endings stimulates M_3 receptors on smooth muscle, causing contraction. Local neural reflexes involve antidromic neurotransmission and the release of a variety of neuropeptides, which constrict smooth muscle (substance P, neurokinin A), and affect small blood vessels. Bradykinin generated by tissue and serum proteolytic enzymes (including mast cell tryptase and tissue kallikrein) is also a potent stimulus of local neural reflexes involving (non-myelinated) nerve fibres.

Clinical features

The principal symptoms of asthma are wheezing attacks and episodic shortness of breath. Symptoms are usually worst during the night, especially in uncontrolled disease. Cough is a frequent symptom that sometimes predominates, especially in children, in whom nocturnal cough can be a presenting feature. Attacks vary greatly in frequency and duration. Some patients only have one or two attacks a year that last for a few hours, while others have attacks lasting for weeks. Some patients have chronic persistent symptoms, on top of which there are fluctuations. Attacks may be precipitated by a wide range of triggers (see ***Fig. 24.29***). Asthma is a major cause of impaired quality of life and has an impact on work and recreation, affecting both physical activities and emotions.

Investigations

There is no single satisfactory diagnostic test for all patients with asthma.

Lung function tests

Peak expiratory flow rate* (*PEFR*)** measurements on waking, prior to taking a bronchodilator, and before bed, after a bronchodilator, are particularly useful in demonstrating the variable airflow limitation that characterizes the disease (see ***Fig. 24.14). The diurnal variation in PEFR is a good measure of asthma activity and is of help in the longer-term assessment of the patient's disease and its response to treatment.

Spirometry is useful, especially in assessing reversibility. Asthma can be diagnosed by demonstrating a greater than 15% improvement in FEV_1 or PEFR following the inhalation of a bronchodilator. However, there may be less reversibility when asthma is in remission or in severe chronic asthma, when little reversibility can be demonstrated, or if the patient is already being treated with long-acting bronchodilators.

The carbon monoxide (CO) transfer test is normal in asthma.

Exercise tests

These have been widely used in the diagnosis of asthma in children. Ideally, the child should run for 6 minutes on a treadmill at a workload sufficient to increase the heart rate above 160 b.p.m. Alternative methods use cold air challenge, isocapnic hyperventilation (forced overbreathing with artificially maintained P_ACO_2) or aerosol challenge with hypertonic solutions. A negative test does not automatically rule out asthma.

Histamine or methacholine bronchial provocation test

This test (see p. 1092) indicates the presence of AHR, a feature found in most asthmatics, and can be particularly useful in investigating those patients whose main symptom is cough. The test should not be performed on individuals who have poor lung function (FEV_1 <1.5 L) or a history of 'brittle' asthma. In children, it is often easier to carry out controlled exercise testing as a measure of bronchial hyper-responsiveness.

Trial of corticosteroids

All patients who present with severe airflow limitation should undergo a formal trial of corticosteroids. Prednisolone 30 mg orally should be given daily for 2 weeks, with lung function measured before and immediately after the course. A substantial improvement in FEV_1 (>15%) confirms the presence of a reversible element and indicates that the administration of inhaled steroids will prove beneficial to the patient. If the trial is for ≤2 weeks, the oral corticosteroid can be withdrawn without tailing off the dose, and should be replaced by inhaled corticosteroids in those who have responded.

Exhaled nitric oxide

This test is a measure of airway inflammation and an index of corticosteroid response; it used to assess the efficacy of corticosteroids.

Blood and sputum tests

Patients with asthma sometimes have increased numbers of eosinophils in peripheral blood ($>0.4\times10^9$/L) but sputum eosinophilia is a more specific diagnostic finding.

Chest X-ray

There are no diagnostic features of asthma on the chest X-ray, although overinflation is characteristic during an acute episode or in chronic severe disease. A chest X-ray may be helpful in excluding a pneumothorax, which can occur as a complication, or in detecting the pulmonary infiltrates associated with allergic bronchopulmonary aspergillosis.

Skin tests

Skin-prick tests should be performed in all cases of asthma to help identify allergic trigger factors. Allergen-specific IgE can be measured in serum if skin-prick test facilities are not available, if the patient is taking antihistamines, or if no suitable allergen extracts are available.

Allergen provocation tests

Allergen inhalation challenge is a useful research tool, and is required when investigating patients with suspected occupational asthma, but not in ordinary asthma.

Management

The ***aims of treatment*** are to:

- abolish symptoms
- restore normal or best possible lung function
- reduce the risk of severe attacks
- enable normal growth to occur in children
- minimize absence from school or employment.

This involves:

- patient and family education about asthma
- patient and family participation in treatment
- avoidance of identified causes where possible
- use of the lowest effective doses of convenient medications to minimize short-term and long-term side-effects.

Many asthmatics join self-help groups in order to improve their understanding of the disease and to foster self-confidence and fitness.

Control of extrinsic factors

Where specific allergen triggers are identified, these should be avoided if possible. Unfortunately, there is little evidence that bedding covers or changes to living accommodation improve asthma outcomes. Sublingual allergen immunotherapy (SLIT) with house dust mites has shown a reduction in the number of asthma attacks in early studies. Active and passive smoking should be avoided, as should beta-blockers in either tablet or eye drop form. Individuals intolerant to aspirin should avoid NSAIDs, although they may tolerate COX-2 inhibitors. About one-third of individuals sensitized to occupational agents may be cured if they are kept permanently away from exposure. The remaining two-thirds will continue to have symptoms, and in half of these the symptoms may be as severe as when exposed to materials at work, especially if they were symptomatic for a long time before the diagnosis was made.

This emphasizes that:

- The rapid identification of extrinsic causes of asthma and their removal are necessary wherever possible (e.g. occupational agents, family pets).
- Once extrinsic asthma is initiated, it may become self-perpetuating, possibly by non-immune mechanisms.

Drug treatment

The mainstay of asthma therapy is the use of therapeutic agents delivered as aerosols or powders directly into the lungs ***(Box 24.23)***. The advantages of this method of administration are that drugs are delivered direct to the airways and first-pass metabolism in the liver is avoided; thus lower doses are necessary and systemic unwanted effects are minimized.

Several national and international guidelines have been published on the stepwise treatment of asthma ***(Box 24.24)***, based on three principles:

- Asthma self-management with regular asthma monitoring using PEF meters and individual treatment plans that are discussed with each patient and written down.
- The appreciation that asthma is an inflammatory disease and that anti-inflammatory (controller) therapy should be started, even in mild cases.
- Use of short-acting inhaled bronchodilators (e.g. salbutamol and terbutaline) only to relieve breakthrough symptoms. Increased use of bronchodilator treatment to relieve increasing symptoms is an indication of deteriorating disease.

A list of drugs used in asthma is shown in ***Box 24.25***. These are given in a stepwise fashion, as indicated in ***Box 24.24***.

Once asthma is brought under control, for at least 2–3 months, the drug regimen should be reassessed in order to reduce the dosage of inhaled steroids.

Beta$_2$-adrenoceptor agonists

Beta$_2$-adrenoceptor agonists are selective for the respiratory tract and do not stimulate the β_1 adrenoceptors of the myocardium. These drugs relax the bronchial smooth muscle and are very

Box 24.23 Inhaled therapy for asthma

Patients should be taught how to use inhalers and their technique should be checked regularly.

Use of a metered-dose inhaler

1. The canister is shaken.
2. The patient exhales to functional residual capacity (not residual volume), i.e. normal expiration.
3. The aerosol nozzle is placed to the open mouth.
4. The patient simultaneously inhales rapidly and activates the aerosol.
5. Inhalation is completed.
6. The breath is held for 10 seconds if possible. Even with good technique, only 15% of the contents is inhaled and 85% is deposited on the wall of the pharynx and ultimately swallowed.

Spacers

These are plastic cones or spheres inserted between the patient's mouth and the inhaler. Some inhalers have a built-in spacer extension. These are designed to reduce particle velocity so that less drug is deposited in the mouth. Spacers also diminish the need for coordination between aerosol activation and inhalation. They are useful in children and in the elderly, and reduce the risk of candidiasis.

Box 24.24 The stepwise management of asthma

Step	PEFR	Treatment
1. **Occasional symptoms**; less frequent than daily	100% predicted	***As-required short-acting β_2 agonists*** If used more than once daily, move to step 2
2. **Daily symptoms**	<80% predicted	***Regular inhaled preventer therapy*** Anti-inflammatory drugs: inhaled low-dose corticosteroids up to 800 µg daily Leukotriene receptor antagonists (LTRA), theophylline and sodium cromoglicate are less effective If not controlled, move to step 3
3. **Severe symptoms**	50–80% predicted	***Inhaled corticosteroids and long-acting inhaled β_2 agonist*** Continue inhaled corticosteroid Add regular inhaled long-acting β_2 agonist (LABA) If still not controlled, add either LTRA, modified-release oral theophylline or β_2 agonist If not controlled, move to step 4
4. **Severe symptoms uncontrolled with high dose inhaled corticosteroids**	50–80% predicted	***High-dose inhaled corticosteroid and regular bronchodilators*** Increase high-dose inhaled corticosteroids up to 2000 µg daily Plus regular long-acting β_2 agonists Plus either LTRA or modified-release theophylline or β_2 agonist
5. **Severe symptoms deteriorating**	≤50% predicted	***Regular oral corticosteroids*** Add prednisolone 40 mg daily to step 4
6. **Severe symptoms deteriorating in spite of prednisolone**	≤30% predicted	Hospital admission

Short-acting bronchodilator treatment taken at any step on an as-required basis.

Box 24.25 Drugs used in asthma

Short-acting relievers
- Inhaled β_2 agonists (e.g. salbutamol (albuterol in USA), terbutaline)

Long-acting relievers/disease controllers
- Inhaled long-acting β_2 agonists (e.g. salmeterol, formoterol)
- Inhaled corticosteroids (e.g. beclometasone, budesonide, fluticasone)
- Compound inhaled salmeterol and fluticasone
- Sodium cromoglicate
- Leukotriene modifiers (e.g. montelukast, zafirlukast, zileuton)

Other agents with bronchodilator activity
- Inhaled antimuscarinic agents (e.g. ipratropium, oxitropium, aclidinium)
- Theophylline preparations
- Oral corticosteroids (e.g. prednisolone 40 mg daily)

Steroid-sparing agents
- Methotrexate
- Ciclosporin
- Intravenous immunoglobulin
- Anti-IgE monoclonal antibody – omalizumab
- Etanercept (see p. 680), infliximab, lebrikizumab

effective in relieving symptoms, but do not affect underlying airways inflammation.

- ***Short-acting β agonists* (*SABAs*),** such as salbutamol 100 µg (called albuterol in the USA) or terbutaline 250 µg, can be taken at any step, as and when required, from step 1 to step 5 (see above), and should be prescribed as 'two puffs as required'.
- ***Mildest asthmatics with intermittent attacks***. Only these people should rely on bronchodilator treatment alone. Any patients using β_2-adrenoceptor agonists on a daily basis should be started on inhaled corticosteroids. Excessive use of SABAs was linked to two epidemics of asthma mortality in the 1960s and 1980s.
- ***Poorly controlled asthmatics*** on standard doses of inhaled steroids. These patients require long-acting β_2-adrenoceptor agonists (LABAs) such as salmeterol or formoterol, which are highly selective and potent. LABAs are effective by inhalation for up to 12 hours, and given once or twice daily. LABAs improve symptoms and lung function, and reduce exacerbation rates in patients. They should never be used alone but always in combination with an inhaled corticosteroid. Nowadays, LABAs are usually administered as fixed-dose combinations with corticosteroids (e.g. salmeterol/fluticasone and formoterol/budesonide) in the same inhaler.

To help those who cannot coordinate activation of the aerosol and inhalation, several breath-activated or dry powder devices have been developed. Devices like the Accuhaler and Turbuhaler require a slower steady inhalation to deliver the drug (compared to pressurized metered-dose inhalers). Patients vary in their ability to use such devices; care should be taken to select an appropriate device and train the individual to use it properly.

Antimuscarinic bronchodilators

Muscarinic receptors are found in the respiratory tract; large airways contain mainly M_3 receptors, whereas the peripheral lung tissue contains M_3 and M_1 receptors (see pp. 1060–1061). Non-selective muscarinic antagonists – ipratropium bromide (20–40 µg three or four times daily) or oxitropium bromide (200 µg twice daily) – by aerosol inhalation can be useful during asthma exacerbations, but they are less helpful in stable asthma. Longer-acting antimuscarinics (tiotropium, aclidinium) can be tried in more severe cases.

Anti-inflammatory drugs

Sodium cromoglicate and nedocromil sodium prevent activation of many inflammatory cells, particularly mast cells, eosinophils and epithelial cells, but not lymphocytes, by blocking a specific chloride channel, which in turn prevents calcium *influx*. These drugs are effective in patients with ***milder asthma*** (***step 2***) but are used much less often than in the past.

Inhaled corticosteroids

All patients who have regular persistent symptoms (even mild symptoms) need regular treatment with inhaled corticosteroids delivered in a stepwise fashion (***from step 2 upwards***) or as a high dose followed by a reduction to maintenance levels. Beclometasone dipropionate (BDP) is the most widely used inhaled steroid and is available in doses of 50, 100, 200 and 250 µg per puff. Other inhaled steroids include budesonide, fluticasone propionate, fluticasone furoate, mometasone furoate and triamcinolone.

Much of the inhaled dose does not reach the lung but is either swallowed or exhaled. Deposition in the lung varies between 10% and 25%, depending on inhaler technique and the technical characteristics of the aerosol device. Drug that is deposited in the airways reaches the systemic circulation directly, through the bronchial circulation, while any drug that is swallowed has to pass through the liver before it can reach the systemic circulation. Gram for gram, fluticasone and mometasone are more potent than beclometasone with considerably less systemic bioavailability, owing to their greater sensitivity to hepatic metabolism. Absorption of beclometasone and budesonide does not seem to present a risk at doses up to 800 µg/day, but fluticasone or mometasone may be preferred because of their lower bioavailability when high-dose inhaled steroids are needed. The dose–response curve for inhaled corticosteroids is flat beyond 800 µg beclometasone or equivalent, and in patients with moderate asthma who are taking this daily, addition of a LABA is more effective than doubling the dose of inhaled corticosteroid.

Unwanted effects of inhaled corticosteroids include oral candidiasis (5% of patients) and hoarseness. Sub-capsular cataract formation is rare but can occur in the elderly. Osteoporosis is less likely than with oral steroids but can occur with high-dose inhaled corticosteroids (beclometasone or budesonide >800 µg daily). In children, inhaled corticosteroids at doses >400 µg daily have been shown to retard short-term growth, but final heights are not affected. Inhaled corticosteroid use should be stepped down once asthma comes under control (see p. 1097). Candidiasis and gastrointestinal absorption can be reduced by using spacers, mouth washing and teeth cleaning after use. Systemic effects may also be reduced by choosing corticosteroids that are esterified in the lung (e.g. ciclesonide 80 µg daily).

Asthmatic patients who smoke are less responsive to inhaled corticosteroids due to induction of a range of genes and proteins in their respiratory epithelium. Assistance with smoking cessation should be offered, and additional therapy – for example, with leukotriene receptor antagonists or theophylline – is required.

Patients with anything more than mild/moderate asthma often benefit from combination LABA/corticosteroid therapy and there is some evidence that the two drugs interact therapeutically.

Oral corticosteroids and steroid-sparing agents

Oral corticosteroids are needed for individuals not controlled on inhaled corticosteroids (***step 5***). The dose should be kept as low as possible to minimize side-effects. The effect of short-term treatment with prednisolone 30 mg daily is shown in ***Figure 24.14***. Some patients require continuing treatment with oral corticosteroids. Several studies suggest that treatment with low doses of methotrexate (15 mg weekly) can significantly reduce the dose of prednisolone needed to control the disease in some patients, and ciclosporin also improves lung function in some steroid-dependent asthmatics. Several other steroid-sparing strategies have also been tried, with varying success.

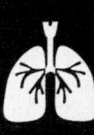

Leukotriene receptor antagonists

This class of anti-asthma therapy targets the cysteinyl LT_1 receptor. A second receptor ($cystLT_2$) has been identified on inflammatory cells. Montelukast, pranlukast (only available in South-east Asia) and zafirlukast are given orally and are effective in a sub-population of asthma patients. However, it is not possible to predict which individuals will benefit; a 4-week trial of leukotriene receptor antagonist (LTRA) therapy is recommended before a decision is made to continue or stop. LTRAs should be tried in any patient who is not controlled on low to medium doses of inhaled steroids (***step 2***; see ***Box 24.24***). Their action is additive to that of LABAs. LTRAs are particularly useful in patients with aspirin-intolerant asthma, in those patients requiring high-dose inhaled or oral corticosteroids, and in asthmatic smokers. Because these drugs are orally active they are helpful in asthma combined with rhinitis and in young children with asthma and/or virus-associated wheezing.

Monoclonal antibodies

Omalizumab, a recombinant humanized monoclonal antibody directed against IgE, chelates free IgE and downregulates the number and activity of mast cells and basophils. It is given subcutaneously every 2–4 weeks, depending on total serum IgE level and body weight. Although expensive, it is cost-effective in patients with frequent exacerbations requiring hospital admission. Proof-of-concept trials have shown that anti-TNF therapy (infliximab or etanercept) may be helpful in severe corticosteroid-refractory asthma. There is still a need to examine other biological agents as potential new controller therapies for the 5–10% of patients with severe disease, who account for a high proportion of the health costs of asthma.

Lebrikizumab, a monoclonal antibody to IL-13, showed improvement in lung function in one study. Mepolizumab and reslizumab, monoclonal antibodies to IL-5, are being introduced in steroid-refractory asthma.

Antibiotics

Although wheezing frequently occurs in infective exacerbations of COPD, there is little evidence that antibiotics are helpful in managing patients with asthma. During acute exacerbations, yellow or green sputum containing eosinophils and bronchial epithelial cells may be coughed up. This is usually due to viral rather than bacterial infection and antibiotics are not required. Occasionally, *Mycoplasma* and *Chlamydia* infections can cause chronic relapsing asthma, and macrolide antimicrobials may be helpful if a bacterial diagnosis has been established by culture or serology.

Bronchial thermoplasty

Bronchial thermoplasty is a novel approach for moderate to severe persistent asthma. This bronchoscopic procedure reduces the mass of airway smooth muscle, decreasing bronchoconstriction, and is currently being evaluated.

Asthma attacks

Although these may occur spontaneously, asthma exacerbations are most commonly caused by lack of treatment adherence, respiratory virus infections associated with the common cold, and exposure to allergen or triggering drug, e.g. an NSAID. Whenever possible, patients should have a written personalized plan that they can implement in anticipation of or at the start of an exacerbation that includes the early use of a short course of oral corticosteroids. If the PEFR is >150 L/min, patients may improve dramatically on nebulized therapy and may not require hospital admission. Their regular treatment should be increased, to include treatment for 2 weeks with 30–60 mg of prednisolone, followed by substitution by an inhaled corticosteroid preparation. Short courses of oral prednisolone can be stopped abruptly without tailing down the dose.

Acute severe asthma

The term acute severe asthma is used to mean an exacerbation of asthma that has not been controlled by the use of standard medication.

Patients with acute severe asthma typically have:

- ***inability to complete a sentence*** in one breath
- a ***respiratory rate*** of ≥25 breaths/min
- ***tachycardia*** of ≥110 b.p.m. (pulsus paradoxus is not useful, as it is only present in 45% of cases)
- ***PEFR <50%*** of predicted normal or best.

Features of life-threatening attacks are:

- a ***silent chest***, cyanosis or feeble respiratory effort
- ***exhaustion***, confusion or coma
- ***bradycardia*** or ***hypotension***
- ***PEFR <30%*** of predicted normal or best (approximately 150 L/min in adults).

Arterial blood gases should always be measured in asthmatic patients requiring admission to hospital, with particular attention paid to the P_aCO_2. ***Pulse oximetry*** is useful in monitoring oxygen saturation during the admission and can reduce the need for repeated arterial puncture.

Features suggesting very severe life-threatening attacks are:

- a high P_aCO_2 >6 kPa
- severe hypoxaemia P_aO_2 <8 kPa despite treatment with oxygen
- a low and/or falling arterial pH.

Management (Box 24.26) consists of nebulized short-acting bronchodilators; nebulized antimuscarinics (e.g. ipratropium bromide) are also helpful. A chest X-ray is helpful to exclude pneumothorax and other causes of dyspnoea. Intravenous hydrocortisone is useful, and in very severe cases, β_2 adrenoceptor agonists and/or magnesium sulphate are also given intravenously. Prednisolone (40–60 mg daily) should be given orally. Ventilation is required for patients who deteriorate despite this initial regimen.

Depending on progress, patients may go home after receiving nebulized therapy. More severe cases should be kept in hospital for 2–5 days with regular monitoring of oxygen saturation and peak flow rates. Downstream assessment of patients admitted with asthma should address trigger factors and aim to reduce the risk of re-admission.

Management of catastrophic sudden severe asthma (brittle asthma)

A small minority of patients with asthma suffer sudden life-threatening attacks despite being well controlled between episodes. These attacks may occur within hours or even minutes, and can cause sudden death. Such patients require a carefully worked-out management plan agreed by patient, primary care physician, hospital emergency services and the respiratory physician, which may include:

- ***optimization of standard therapy***
- ***emergency supplies of medications*** at home, in the car and at work
- ***oxygen and resuscitation equipment*** at home and at work
- ***nebulized β_2-adrenoceptor agonists*** at home and at work
- ***self-injectable adrenaline (epinephrine):*** two autoinjectors of 0.3 mg adrenaline at home, at work and to be carried by the patient at all times
- ***prednisolone tablets 60 mg***
- ***MedicAlert bracelet.***

On developing wheeze, the patient should attend the nearest hospital immediately. Direct admission to intensive care may be required.

Prognosis of asthma

Although asthma often improves in children as they reach their teens, the disease frequently returns in the second, third and fourth decades. In the past, the data indicating a natural decrease in asthma through the teenage years have led to childhood asthma being treated as an episodic disorder. However, airway inflammation is present continuously from an early age and usually persists, even if the symptoms resolve. Moreover, airways remodelling accelerates the process of decline in lung function over time. This has led to a reappraisal of the treatment strategy for asthma, mandating the early use of controller drugs and environmental measures from the time that asthma is first diagnosed.

Box 24.26 Treatment of acute severe asthma

At home

1. The patient is assessed. Tachycardia, a high respiratory rate and inability to speak in sentences indicate a severe attack.
2. If the PEFR is <150 L/min (in adults), an ambulance should be called. (All doctors should carry peak flow meters.)
3. Nebulized salbutamol 5 mg or terbutaline 10 mg is administered.
4. Hydrocortisone sodium succinate 200 mg i.v. is given.
5. Oxygen 40–60% is given if available.
6. Prednisolone 60 mg is given orally.

At the hospital

1. The patient is reassessed.
2. Oxygen 40–60% is given.
3. The PEFR is measured using a low-reading peak flow meter, as an ordinary meter measures only from 60 L/min upwards. O_2 saturation is measured with a pulse oximeter.
4. Nebulized salbutamol 5 mg or terbutaline 10 mg is repeated and administered 4-hourly.
5. Add nebulized ipratropium bromide 0.5 mg to nebulized salbutamol/terbutaline.
6. Hydrocortisone 200 mg i.v. is given 4-hourly for 24 h.
7. Prednisolone is continued at 60 mg orally daily for 2 weeks.
8. Arterial blood gases are measured; if the P_aCO_2 is >7 kPa, ventilation may be required.
9. A chest X-ray is performed to exclude pneumothorax.
10. One of the following intravenous infusions is given if no improvement is seen:
    - Salbutamol 3–20 μg/min, *or*
    - Terbutaline 1.5–5.0 μg/min, *or*
    - Magnesium sulphate 1.2–2 g over 20 min.
11. If there is still no improvement, urgent transfer to the intensive treatment unit is arranged.

Further reading

Beasley R, Semprini A, Mitchell EA. Risk factors for asthma: is prevention possible? *Lancet* 2015; 386:1075–1085.
Holgate ST, Roberts G, Arshad HS et al. The role of the airway epithelium and its interaction with environmental factors in asthma pathogenesis. *Proc Am Thor Soc* 2009; 6:655–659.
Tschumperlin DJ. Physical forces and airway remodelling in asthma. *N Engl J Med* 2011; 364:2057–2058.
https://www.brit-thoracic.org.uk/ *British guideline on the management of asthma 2014, British Thoracic Society/Scottish Intercollegiate Guideline Network.*

PNEUMONIA

Pneumonia is defined as inflammation of the substance of the lungs. It is usually caused by bacteria but can also be caused by viruses and fungi. Clinically, it usually presents as an acute illness with cough, purulent sputum, breathlessness and fever, together with physical signs or radiological changes compatible with consolidation of the lung ***(Fig. 24.33)***. However, it can present with more subtle symptoms, particularly in the elderly.

Pneumonia is usually ***classified*** by the setting in which the person has contracted their infection, for example:

- ***in the community setting*** – community-acquired pneumonia in a person with no underlying immunosuppression or malignancy
- ***in a hospital*** or other institution such as a nursing home – hospital-acquired pneumonia
- in a patient whose ***immune system is compromised***, through either a genetic defect, immunosuppressive medication or acquired immunodeficiency such as human immunodeficiency virus (HIV) infection.

Community-acquired pneumonia

Community-acquired pneumonia (CAP) occurs across all ages but is more common at the extremes of age. There has been an increase in rates of hospital admission due to CAP over the last 10 years, reflecting changes in clinical practice and an ageing population, rather than a true increase in incidence.

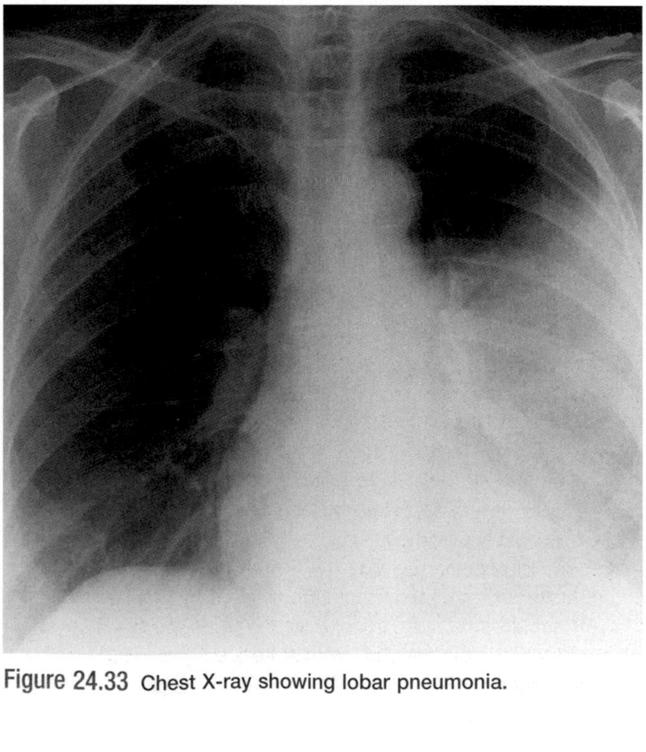

Figure 24.33 Chest X-ray showing lobar pneumonia.

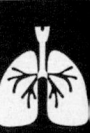

Box 24.27 Risk factors for community-acquired pneumonia

- ***Age***: <16 or >65 years
- ***Co-morbidities***: HIV infection, diabetes mellitus, chronic kidney disease, malnutrition, recent viral respiratory infection
- ***Other respiratory conditions***: cystic fibrosis, bronchiectasis, chronic obstructive pulmonary disease, obstructing lesion (endoluminal cancer, inhaled foreign body)
- ***Lifestyle***: cigarette smoking, excess alcohol, intravenous drug use
- ***Iatrogenic***: immunosuppressant therapy (including prolonged corticosteroids)

Pneumonia can be classified either according to the organism responsible for infection or according to the site of disease. *Pneumococcus* is the most common cause overall; however, in 30–50% of cases, no organism is identifiable, while in about 20% of cases more than one organism is present. Infection can be localized, when the whole of one or more lobes is affected ('lobar pneumonia'), or diffuse, when the lobules of the lung are mainly affected, often due to infection centred on the bronchi and bronchioles ('bronchopneumonia').

Pathophysiology

Several different microorganisms commonly cause CAP. Infection is spread by respiratory droplets. Both the clinical presentation and the range of causative organisms vary with age and with the effectiveness of the host's immune response and innate defence mechanisms. Factors that increase the risk of developing CAP are shown in ***Box 24.27***.

Other causes of pneumonitis are:

- ***chemical insult***, such as in the aspiration of vomit (see p. 1106)
- ***radiotherapy*** (see p. 1124)
- ***allergic mechanisms*** (see pp. 1115–1117).

Clinical features

The clinical presentation varies according to the immune state of the patient and the infecting agent.

- ***Cough***: this may be dry or productive; haemoptysis can occur. In pneumococcal pneumonia, sputum is characteristically rust-coloured.
- ***Breathlessness***: the alveoli become filled with pus and debris, impairing gas exchange. Coarse crackles are often heard on auscultation, due to consolidation of the lung parenchyma. Bronchial breath sounds may be heard over areas of consolidated lung.
- ***Fever***: this can be as high as 39.5–40°C. If swinging fevers are present, this often indicates empyema (see p. 1104).
- ***Chest pain***: this is commonly pleuritic in nature and is due to inflammation of the pleura. A pleural rub may be heard early on in the illness.
- ***Extrapulmonary features (Box 24.28)***: these are more common in certain infections and are not universal. Sometimes the presence of these symptoms gives a clinical clue as to the aetiology
  - Haemolysis due to cold agglutinins occurs in approximately 50% cases of *Mycoplasma* pneumonia. Thrombocytopenia is relatively common.
- ***Other features***: in the elderly, CAP can present with confusion or non-specific symptoms such as recurrent falls. CAP should always be considered in the differential diagnosis of sick elderly patients, given their frequently atypical presentation.

Box 24.28 Extrapulmonary features of community-acquired pneumonia

- ***Myalgia, arthralgia and malaise*** are common, particularly in infections caused by *Legionella* and *Mycoplasma*
- ***Myocarditis and pericarditis*** are cardiac manifestations of infection, most commonly in *Mycoplasma* pneumonia
- ***Headache*** is common in *Legionella* pneumonia. Meningoencephalitis and other neurological abnormalities also occur but are much less common
- ***Abdominal pain, diarrhoea and vomiting*** are common. Hepatitis can be a feature of *Legionella* pneumonia
- ***Labial herpes simplex*** reactivation is relatively common in pneumococcal pneumonia
- ***Other skin rashes***, such as erythema multiforme and erythema nodosum, are found in *Mycoplasma* pneumonia. Stevens–Johnson syndrome (see pp. 1383–1384) is a rare and potentially life-threatening complication of pneumonia

Box 24.29 CURB-65 score

C: ***confusion*** present (abbreviated mental test score <8/10)
U: (plasma) ***urea*** level >7 mmol/L
R: ***respiratory rate*** >30 breaths/min
B: systolic ***blood pressure*** <90 mmHg; diastolic <60 mmHg
65: ***age >65***

1 point for each of the above:

- ***Score 0–1:*** Treat as outpatient
- ***Score 2:*** Admit to hospital
- ***Score 3+:*** Often require care in the intensive treatment unit

Mortality rates increase with increasing score.

Where symptoms have been present for several weeks or have failed to respond to standard antibiotics, ***tuberculosis*** should be excluded.

Investigations and management

The clinical presentation varies between different causative organisms, but there is considerable overlap. *Streptococcus pneumoniae* (pneumococcus) is the most common single cause, and all treatment and investigation strategies need to cover this. The most likely causative pathogens must be treated while considering alternative, less common infectious causes (such as tuberculosis) or an alternative pathology (such as lung cancer). The treatment plan can always be refined and focused later. Pneumonia caused by endobronchial obstruction due to lung cancer is the main concern.

Initial assessment

The type and extent of investigation depend on the severity of the illness, which also guides where the patient should be managed and predicts their outcome. Diagnostic microbiological tests are not needed in mild infection, which should be treated at home with standard antibiotics (amoxicillin, or clarithromycin for those with a history of penicillin allergy). Where patients have mild disease, chest X-ray is not routinely recommended unless they fail to improve after 48–72 hours. Antibiotics can be administered orally.

Severity is commonly assessed by the ***CURB-65 or the CRB-65 score (Box 24.29)***. These give a guide to the likely risk of fatal outcome but antibiotic choice must always be tempered by clinical assessment and judgement, taking into account other factors associated with increased rates of mortality ***(Box 24.30)***. The CRB-65 score is used in the community where the serum urea level is not usually available *(Fig. 24.34)*. Other severity scores are available to predict mortality and where a patient should be cared for, such as the Pneumonia Severity Index (PSI), which is used more widely in the USA. ***Figure 24.34*** shows a diagnostic and treatment algorithm for CAP, which incorporates treatment recommendations from the British Thoracic Society guidance for the management of CAP (2009) and the Infectious Diseases Society of America/American Thoracic Society guidance (2007).

Box 24.30 Other markers of severe community-acquired pneumonia

- ***Chest X-ray*** – more than one lobe involved
- P_aO_2 – <8 kPa
- ***Low albumin*** – <35 g/L
- ***White cell count*** – $<4\times10^9$/L or $>20\times10^9$/L
- ***Blood culture*** – positive
- Other ***co-morbidities***
- ***Absence of fever in the elderly***

Investigations

All patients admitted to hospital with suspected CAP should have a chest X-ray, blood tests and microbiological tests.

Chest X-ray

Radiological abnormalities can lag behind clinical signs. A normal chest X-ray on presentation should be repeated after 2–3 days if CAP is suspected clinically. The chest X-ray must be repeated 6 weeks later to rule out an underlying bronchial malignancy causing pneumonia due to bronchial obstruction. Chest X-ray appearances are not diagnostic of any organism, but in *Mycoplasma* and

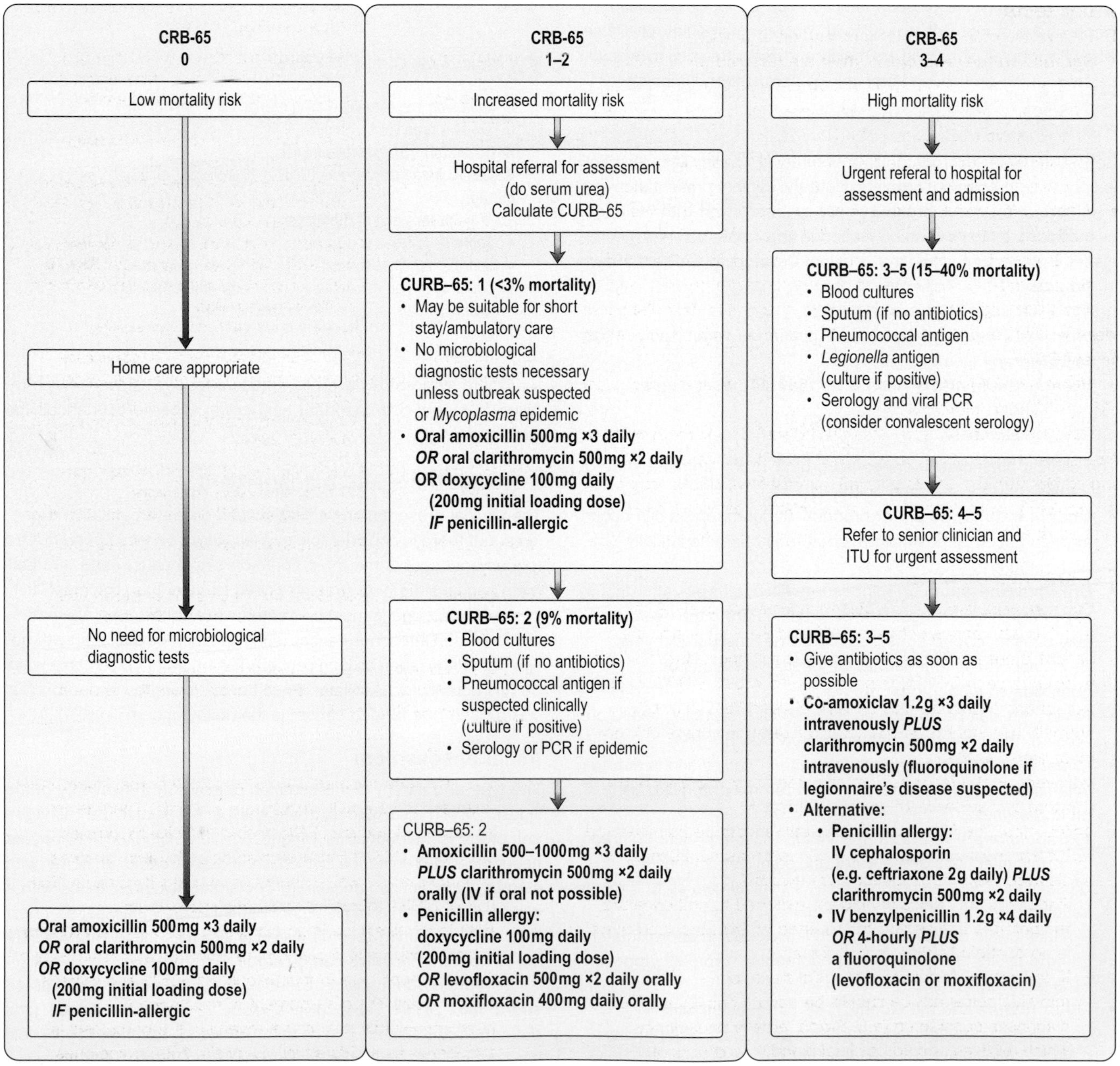

Figure 24.34 Algorithm for the assessment and treatment of community-acquired pneumonia. CRB, confusion, respiratory rate, blood pressure; CURB, includes urea; PCR, polymerase chain reaction.

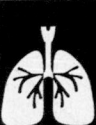

Chlamydophila infection the shadowing is often more extensive than would be expected from the clinical picture.

Blood tests

Full blood count, urea and electrolytes, biochemistry and C-reactive protein (CRP) are helpful.

- ***Strep. pneumoniae***. White cell count is usually $>15\times10^9$/L (90% polymorphonuclear leucocytosis); inflammatory markers are significantly elevated: erythrocyte sedimentation rate (ESR) >100 mm/h; CRP >100 mg/L.
- ***Mycoplasma***. White cell count is usually normal. In the presence of anaemia, haemolysis should be ruled out (direct Coombs' test and measurement of cold agglutinins).
- ***Legionella***. There is lymphopenia without marked leucocytosis, hyponatraemia, hypoalbuminaemia and high serum levels of liver aminotransferases.

Other tests

The causative organism must be identified if possible:

- ***Sputum culture and Gram stain*** are required for all patients:
  - *Strep. pneumoniae*: there are Gram-positive diplococci.
  - *Staph. aureus*: Gram-positive organisms commonly appear in clusters like a bunch of grapes
  - Also diagnostic in infections caused by *Staph. aureus*, *H. influenzae*, *M. catarrhalis* and Gram-negative organisms.
- ***Blood culture*** should be done for all patients who have moderate to severe CAP, ideally before antibiotics are administered. In *Strep. pneumoniae* infection, positive blood cultures indicate more severe disease with greater mortality.

Box 24.31 highlights more specific diagnostic tests used to identify the causative organism in patients with moderate to severe CAP.

Pulse oximetry and ***arterial blood gas analysis*** are necessary if oxygen saturation is <94%.

Since pneumonia is a common initial presenting illness in patients with previously undiagnosed HIV infection, an ***HIV test*** should be offered to all patients with pneumonia, unless the patient is unable to give consent or comfort measures alone are implemented due to poor prognosis.

Box 24.31 Specific diagnostic tests in patients with moderate to severe community-acquired pneumonia

Organism	Diagnostic confirmatory test
Streptococcus pneumoniae	CIE of sputum, urine and serum is 3–4 times more sensitive than sputum or blood cultures Urinary antigen test detects C-polysaccharide. This is rapid and unaffected by antibiotics; sensitivity is 65–80% and specificity about 80% Pneumococcal PCR (not routinely recommended, as inferior to blood cultures and low sensitivity)
Mycoplasma pneumoniae	PCR of respiratory tract samples (throat swab/sputum/BAL fluid) – higher detection rates than serological assays PCR on serum under assessment and likely to become more available CFT (though sensitivity and specificity low) – measure paired samples 10–14 days apart and look for rising titres or single level approximately 7 days after onset of illness
***Legionella* spp.** (also termed legionnaire's disease)	Urinary antigen test detects only serogroup 1, which accounts for most of these infections. Sensitivity (~80%) and specificity are high (almost 99%) DIF staining of organism in the pleural fluid, sputum or bronchial washings Serum antibodies are less reliable. Paired serum antibody titres 10–14 days apart (or single level 7 days after onset of illness) Culture on special media is possible but takes up to 3 weeks. This gives valuable information on antibiotic sensitivity and should be performed if urinary antigen positive *Legionella* is not visible on Gram staining
Chlamydophila pneumoniae	Paired serum antibody titres 10–14 days apart Antigen detection (DIF) on throat swabs/respiratory samples CFT usually only weakly positive and less reliable than in *C. psittaci*
Chlamydophila psittaci	Paired serum antibody titres 10–14 days apart CFT relatively sensitive and specific Antigen detection (DIF) not available for *C. psittaci*
Coxiella burnetti (Q fever)	Paired serum antibody titres 10–14 days apart
All respiratory viruses including influenza A and B	PCR of respiratory tract samples (throat swab/sputum, bronchial aspirate, BAL fluid)

BAL, bronchoalveolar lavage; CFT, complement fixation test; CIE, counter-immunoelectrophoresis; DIF, direct immunofluorescence; PCR, polymerase chain reaction.

General management

- ***Oxygen***. Supplemental oxygen should be administered to maintain saturations between 94% and 98% (provided the patient is not at risk of carbon dioxide retention, due to loss of hypoxic drive in COPD). In patients with known COPD, oxygen saturations should be maintained between 88% and 92%, normally with controlled oxygen via fixed-percentage delivery mask (see ***Fig. 24.25***).
- ***Intravenous fluids***. These are required in hypotensive patients showing any evidence of volume depletion.
- ***Antibiotics***. The first dose of antibiotic should be administered *within 4 h of presentation in hospital* and treatment should not be delayed while investigations are awaited.
  - Parenteral antibiotics should be switched to oral once the temperature has settled for a period of 24 h, provided there is no contraindication to oral therapy.
  - If patients fail to respond to initial treatment, microbiological advice should be sought and alternative diagnoses considered (e.g. *Staph. aureus* pneumonia, which requires addition of flucloxacillin, and possibly cover for MRSA infection). Causes of failure are shown in ***Box 24.32***.
  - The antibiotic regimen should be adjusted specifically once culture and sensitivity results are available. There is an increased incidence of *Clostridium difficile*-associated diarrhoea (CDAD) linked with some antibiotics, such as cephalosporins, which should be avoided if possible. The risk of MRSA increases with antibiotic overuse.
  - Antibiotic resistance is an increasing international problem. In some countries, including the USA, rates of resistance of *Strep. pneumoniae* to macrolides are >25% and there is concern over the development of resistance to fluoroquinolones due to their overuse. If tuberculosis is suspected as a differential diagnosis, fluoroquinolones should never be used as a single agent due to the risk of potentiating monoresistance.

Box 24.32 Causes of slow-resolving pneumonia

Incorrect or incomplete antimicrobial treatment
- Underlying antibiotic resistance
- Inadequate dose/duration
- Non-adherence
- Malabsorption

Complication of community-acquired pneumonia
- Parapneumonic pleural effusion (exudative)
- Empyema
- Lung abscess

Underlying neoplastic lesion or other lung disease
- Obstructing lesion
- Bronchoalveolar cell carcinoma
- Bronchiectasis
- Tuberculosis

Alternative diagnosis
- Pulmonary thromboembolic disease
- Cryptogenic organizing pneumonia
- Eosinophilic pneumonia
- Pulmonary haemorrhage

  - In patients with significant co-morbidities, such as COPD, or those who have received recent antibiotics in the last 90 days, there is an increased risk of drug-resistant pathogens. Antibiotic resistance is a cause of patients failing to improve.
- ***Thromboprophylaxis***. If admitted for >12 h, subcutaneous low-molecular-weight heparin should be prescribed, unless contraindications exist, and thromboembolus deterrent (TED) stockings should be fitted.
- ***Physiotherapy***. Chest physiotherapy is not needed unless sputum retention is an issue.
- ***Nutritional supplementation***. Need is assessed by a dietician, particularly in severe disease.
- ***Analgesia***. Simple analgesia, such as paracetamol or NSAID, helps treat pleuritic pain, thereby reducing the risk of further complications due to restricted breathing because of pain (e.g. sputum retention, atelectasis or secondary infection).

Complications

Complications of pneumonia must be excluded, especially if the patient does not respond quickly to initial treatment (see ***Box 24.34***).

Prevention

Cigarette smoking is an independent risk factor for CAP; if the patient still smokes, cessation advice and support should be given.

Vaccination against influenza is recommended for at-risk groups. All patients over the age of 65 who have not previously been vaccinated and are admitted with CAP should have the pneumococcal vaccine before discharge from hospital.

Types of pneumonia

The clinical presentation of pneumonia varies according to the causative organism but there is considerable overlap ***(Box 24.33)***. Pneumococcal disease is typically acute in onset, with prominent respiratory symptoms and a high fever. Pneumonia due to the so-called atypical pathogens (*Mycoplasma pneumoniae*, *Chlamydophila pneumoniae*, *Legionella pneumophila*) tends to have a slower onset, often with more prominent extrapulmonary symptoms and complications. The radiographic appearances are indistinguishable from those of CAP caused by pneumococcal pneumonia. The other atypical feature is that these organisms do not respond to penicillin because they lack a cell wall. Macrolides (e.g. clarithromycin) and doxycycline are usually effective.

Complications of pneumonia

See ***Box 24.34***.

Parapneumonic effusion and empyema

Pleural effusions are common with pneumonia and complicate around one-third to one-half of cases of CAP. The majority of these are simple exudative effusions but empyema may also develop (purulent fluid in the pleural space). Early indications of empyema are ongoing fever, and rising or persistently elevated inflammatory markers, despite appropriate antibiotic therapy.

Thoracocentesis should be performed to make a diagnosis. Fluid should be aspirated under ultrasound guidance and sent for Gram stain, culture, fluid protein, glucose and lactate dehydrogenase (LDH) (with comparison to serum levels). Light's criteria (see p. 1134) can be applied to assess whether an effusion is transudative or exudative. An exudative effusion with pleural fluid pH <7.2 is strongly suggestive of empyema. Pathogens are often detectable; sensitivity analysis will help guide antimicrobial therapy.

If an empyema develops, the fluid should be urgently drained to prevent further complications, such as development of a thick pleural rind or prolonged hospital admission. The presence of empyema further increases mortality risk. The duration of antibiotic administration will usually need to be extended. Whenever possible, the choice of antimicrobial should be guided by the results of cultures. Thoracic surgical intervention is necessary in severe cases.

Lung abscess

This term is used to describe severe localized suppuration within the lung associated with cavity formation visible on the chest X-ray or CT scan, often with a fluid level (which always indicates an air–liquid interface).

There are several causes of lung abscess ***(Box 24.35)***:
- ***Aspiration pneumonia***: rarely, abscesses develop as a complication of aspiration pneumonia. A history of excessive alcohol consumption or impaired swallowing in a patient with pneumonia suggests aspiration.
- ***Tuberculosis***: see pages 1106–1113.
- ***Pneumonia caused by certain species***, particularly *Staph. aureus* or *Klebsiella pneumoniae*, may lead to abscess development.
- ***Septic emboli usually containing staphylococci***: these can cause multiple lung abscesses. The presence of multiple lung abscesses in an injecting drug user should prompt investigation for infective endocarditis of the tricuspid (or rarely, pulmonary) valves. Infarcted areas of lung (due to pulmonary emboli) occasionally cavitate and become infected.
- ***Inadequately treated CAP.***
- ***Spread from an amoebic liver abscess***: amoebic lung abscesses occasionally develop in the right lower lobe following transdiaphragmatic spread.
- ***Bronchial obstruction by an endoluminal cancer.***
- ***Foreign body inhalation.***

CT scanning is essential and bronchoscopy is often used to obtain samples or remove foreign bodies.

Clinical features

The clinical features are usually persisting or worsening pneumonia associated with the production of large quantities of sputum, which is often foul-smelling owing to the growth of anaerobic organisms. There is usually a swinging fever; malaise and weight loss frequently

Box 24.33 Types of pneumonia and their clinical features

Organism	Features
Streptococcus pneumoniae	Acute onset, often preceded by influenza-like symptoms. Cough with rust-coloured sputum High fevers and pleuritic chest pain common Bacteraemia more common in females, excess alcohol, dry cough and COPD, diabetes or HIV infection
Mycoplasma pneumoniae	Usually mild disease in young patient; occurs in cycles every 3–4 years Usually prominent extrapulmonary symptoms (headache, malaise, myalgia); complications common: haemolytic anaemia, erythema multiforme, hepatitis, meningoencephalitis
***Legionella* spp.** (legionnaire's disease)	Usually *Legionella pneumophila* but other species implicated in around 10% of cases Causes more severe disease with need for early intensive care Usually acquired by inhaling water mist containing bacteria Neurological symptoms frequently seen, along with gastrointestinal involvement and deranged liver enzymes, elevated creatine kinase More common in smokers, in males and in young people with no co-morbidities
Staphylococcus aureus	Evidence of recent influenza found in up to around 40–50% of patients (increasing frequency with greater-severity disease) Usually MSSA but increasing incidence of MRSA, which can produce PVL (see pp. 269–270) and result in necrotizing cavitating pneumonia and bilateral infiltrates
Chlamydophila pneumoniae	Unclear whether this is a causative or associated organism Generally causes mild disease but with prolonged prodrome
Haemophilus influenza, Moraxella catarrhalis	More common in pre-existing structural lung disease (cystic fibrosis, bronchiectasis, COPD) and in the elderly
Chlamydophila psittaci	Acquired from birds (only 20% have positive history) Can be person-to-person spread; usually mild illness
Coxiella burnotti (Q fever)	Tends to occur more commonly in young men. History of dry cough and high fever Recognized cause of endocarditis
Gram-negative organisms	
Klebsiella pneumoniae	More common in men and those with history of excess alcohol (bacteraemia more likely), poor dental hygiene, diabetes and other co-morbidities; often presents with low platelet and white cell count. Systemic upset is usual; high mortality
Pseudomonas aeruginosa	Cavitation and abscess formation seen Infection is associated with underlying lung disease (cystic fibrosis, bronchiectasis, COPD) or immune suppression
All respiratory viruses	Infection more likely in elderly with subsequent staphylococcal pneumonia Usually causes mild disease; not admitted to hospital
Varicella zoster	Causes pneumonitis, which heals, leaving characteristic small, calcified or non-calcified nodules
Influenza A and B	Approximately 10% of adults with confirmed influenza infection have coincident *Staph. aureus* disease Fever, malaise and myalgia common
Other	
Influenza A (H5N1)	Does not usually affect humans Can be transmitted from poultry (causes avian influenza) Fever, breathlessness, cough, diarrhoea Lymphopenia and thrombocytopenia High mortality

COPD, chronic obstructive pulmonary disease; HIV, human immunodeficiency virus; MRSA, meticillin-resistant *Staphylococcus aureus*; MSSA, meticillin-sensitive *Staphylococcus aureus*; PVL, Panton Valentine leucocidin.

Box 24.34 Complications of pneumonia

General
- Respiratory failure
- Sepsis – multisystem failure

Local
- Pleural effusion
- Empyema
- Lung abscess
- Organizing pneumonia

occur. On examination, there may be little to find in the chest. Clubbing occurs in chronic suppuration. Patients have a normocytic anaemia and/or raised inflammatory markers (ESR/CRP).

Management

Treatment should be guided by available culture results or clinical judgement and is often prolonged (4–6 weeks). Surgical drainage is sometimes necessary.

Box 24.35 Common causative organisms in lung abscess

- *Klebsiella pneumoniae*
- *Staphylococcus aureus*
- Gram-negative enteric bacilli
- *Mycobacterium tuberculosis*
- *Streptococcus milleri*
- Anaerobic bacteria (post aspiration)
- *Haemophilus influenzae*

Pneumonia in other settings

Hospital-acquired pneumonia

Hospital-acquired pneumonia (HAP) is defined as new onset of cough with purulent sputum, along with a compatible X-ray demonstrating consolidation, in patients who are beyond 2 days of their

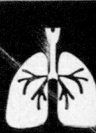

Box 24.36 Organisms implicated in hospital-acquired pneumonia

- Gram-negative bacteria (*Pseudomonas* spp., *Escherichia* spp., *Klebsiella* spp.)
- Anaerobic bacteria (*Enterobacter* spp.)
- *Staphylococcus aureus* (including meticillin-resistant *Staphylococcus aureus*)
- *Acinetobacter* spp.

initial admission to hospital or who have been in a healthcare setting within the last 3 months (including nursing/residential homes, as well as acute care facilities such as hospitals). HAP is the second most common form of hospital-acquired infection after urinary tract infections and carries a significant mortality risk, particularly in the elderly or those with co-morbidities such as stroke, respiratory disease or diabetes. In HAP, the causative organisms differ from those causing CAP ***(Box 24.36)***. Viral or fungal pathogens only affect immunocompromised hosts. Aerobic Gram-negative bacilli are commonly involved (e.g. *P. aeruginosa*, *Escherichia coli*, *K. pneumoniae* and *Acinetobacter* species). *Staph. aureus* is increasingly recognized in HAP, particularly MRSA, in both Europe and the USA. HAP due to *Staph. aureus* is more common in patients with diabetes mellitus or head trauma, and in those on intensive care units. Empirical antimicrobial therapy should be tailored accordingly. Other conditions should be excluded, including aspiration of gastric contents due to impaired swallowing or bulbar weakness.

Elderly residents of long-term care facilities who develop pneumonia have a similar range of pathogens to those found in HAP. In the USA, *Staph. aureus*, Gram-negative rods, pneumococcus and *Pseudomonas* species are the most common causes of pneumonia acquired in nursing homes. Pneumonia associated with ventilation has the same range of organisms as other forms of HAP (see p. 1165). Piperacillin–tazobactam is commonly used in severe HAP.

Aspiration pneumonia

Acute aspiration of gastric contents into the lungs can produce an extremely severe and sometimes fatal illness owing to the intense destructiveness of gastric acid. This can complicate anaesthesia, particularly during pregnancy (Mendelson syndrome). Because of the bronchial anatomy, the most usual sites for aspirated material to end up are the right middle lobe and apical or posterior segments of the right lower lobe. The persistent pneumonia is often due to anaerobes and progresses to lung abscess or even bronchiectasis if protracted. It is vital to identify any underlying problem, since without appropriate corrective measures aspiration will recur.

Treatment should be directed specifically against positive cultures if available. If not, then co-amoxiclav is used for mild to moderate disease, and covers Gram-negative and anaerobic bacteria. Treatment needs to be escalated where there is a lack of response or in severe cases.

Rare causes of pneumonia

Pneumonia can occur as a minor feature during infection by *Bordetella pertussis*, typhoid and paratyphoid bacillus, brucellosis, leptospirosis and a number of viral infections including measles, chickenpox and glandular fever. Details of these infections are provided in Chapter 11.

Pneumonia in immunocompromised patients

Patients who are immunosuppressed (either iatrogenically or due to a defect in host defences) are at risk not only from all the usual organisms that can cause pneumonia but also from opportunistic pathogens that would not be expected to cause disease. These opportunistic pathogens can be commonly occurring microorganisms (i.e. ubiquitous in the environment) or bacteria, viruses and fungi that are found less often (see ***Box 12.21***). The symptom pattern may resemble CAP or be more non-specific. A high degree of clinical suspicion is therefore necessary when assessing an ill patient who is immunocompromised.

Pneumocystis jiroveci pneumonia

Pneumocystis pneumonia is one of the most common opportunistic infections encountered in clinical practice. It affects patients on immunosuppressant therapy, such as long-term corticosteroids, monoclonal antibody therapy or methotrexate for autoimmune disease; those on anti-rejection medication post solid organ transplantation or stem cell transplantation; and those infected with HIV. Individuals with CD4 counts of $<200/mm^3$ are at particular risk. *Pneumocystis jiroveci* is found in the air, and pneumonia arises from re-infection rather than reactivation of persisting organisms acquired in childhood.

Clinically, the pneumonia is associated with a high fever, breathlessness and dry cough. A characteristic feature on examination is rapid desaturation on exercise or exertion. The typical radiographic appearance is one of diffuse bilateral alveolar and interstitial shadowing beginning in the perihilar regions and spreading out in a butterfly pattern. Other chest X-ray appearances include localized infiltration, nodules, cavitation or a pneumothorax. Empirical treatment is justified in very sick high-risk patients; wherever possible, however, the diagnosis should be confirmed by indirect immunofluorescence on induced sputum or bronchoalveolar lavage fluid. First-line treatment of *Pneumocystis* pneumonia is with high-dose co-trimoxazole (see p. 349).

Further reading

Jain S, Self WH, Wunderink S et al. Community-acquired pneumonia requiring hospitalization among US adults. *N Engl J Med* 2015; 373:415–427.
Lim WS, Baudouin SV, George RC et al. British Thoracic Society Guidelines for the management of community-acquired pneumonia in adults: update 2009. *Thorax* 2009; 64(Suppl III):iii1–iii55.
Loke YK, Kwok CS, Niruban A et al. Value of severity scales in predicting mortality from community-acquired pneumonia: systematic review and meta-analysis. *Thorax* 2010; 65(10):884–890.
Musher DM, Thorner AR. Community acquired pneumonia. *N Engl J Med* 2014: 371:1619–1628.

TUBERCULOSIS

Epidemiology

It is estimated that one-third of the world's population are infected with tuberculosis (TB; see also p. 290). The World Health Organization (WHO) declared TB a world emergency in 1993. There were almost 9 million new and relapsed cases of TB worldwide in 2010. Its incidence had been increasing by around 1% per year to a peak in 2005, but since then the global incidence *per capita* has started to decline slowly. The majority of cases (around 65%) are seen in Africa and Asia (India and China). Co-infection with HIV remains a problem, not only because this is a huge health burden on resource-poor nations, but also because of the growing incidence of multi- and extremely drug-resistant strains and the high mortality of the two coexistent diseases. TB was responsible for 1.4 million deaths

Box 24.37 Factors affecting prevalence and risk of developing tuberculosis in the developed world

- Contact with high-risk groups:
  - Origination from a high-incidence country (defined as >40/100 000)
  - Frequent travel to high-incidence areas
- Immune deficiency:
  - HIV infection
  - Corticosteroids or immunosuppressant therapy
  - Chemotherapeutic drugs
  - Nutritional deficiency (vitamin D)
  - Diabetes mellitus
  - Chronic kidney disease
  - Malnutrition/body weight >10% below ideal body weight
- Lifestyle factors:
  - Drug/alcohol misuse
  - Homelessness/hostels/overcrowding
  - Prison inmates
- Genetic susceptibility (twin studies of gene polymorphisms)

in 2010 and a quarter of these were in HIV co-infected individuals. There are a number of factors affecting the prevalence and risk of developing TB ***(Box 24.37)***.

Pathophysiology

TB is caused by four main mycobacterial species, collectively termed *Mycobacterium tuberculosis complex* (MTb):

- *Mycobacterium tuberculosis*
- *Mycobacterium bovis*
- *Mycobacterium africanum*
- *Mycobacterium microti.*

These are obligate aerobes and facultative intracellular pathogens, usually infecting mononuclear phagocytes. They are slow-growing with a generation time of 12–18 hours. Due to their high lipid content in the cell wall, they are relatively impermeable and stain only weakly with Gram stain. When stained with dye combined with phenol and washed with acidic organic solvents, they resist decolorization and therefore are termed 'acid-fast bacilli'.

Pathogenesis

TB is an airborne infection spread via respiratory droplets. Only a small number of bacteria need to be inhaled for infection to develop but not all those who are infected develop active disease. The outcome of exposure is dictated by a number of factors, including the host's immune response ***(Fig. 24.35)***.

Primary tuberculosis

'Primary TB' describes the first infection with MTb. Once inhaled into the lung, alveolar macrophages ingest the bacteria; the bacilli then proliferate inside the macrophages and cause the release of neutrophil chemoattractants and cytokines, resulting in an inflammatory cell infiltrate reaching the lung and draining hilar lymph nodes. Macrophages present the antigen to the T lymphocytes with the development of a cellular immune response. A delayed hypersensitivity-type reaction occurs, resulting in tissue necrosis and formation of a granuloma.

Granulomatous lesions consist of a central area of necrotic material called caseation, surrounded by epithelioid cells and Langhans giant cells with multiple nuclei, both cells being derived from the macrophage. Lymphocytes are present and there is a varying degree of fibrosis. Subsequently, the caseated areas heal

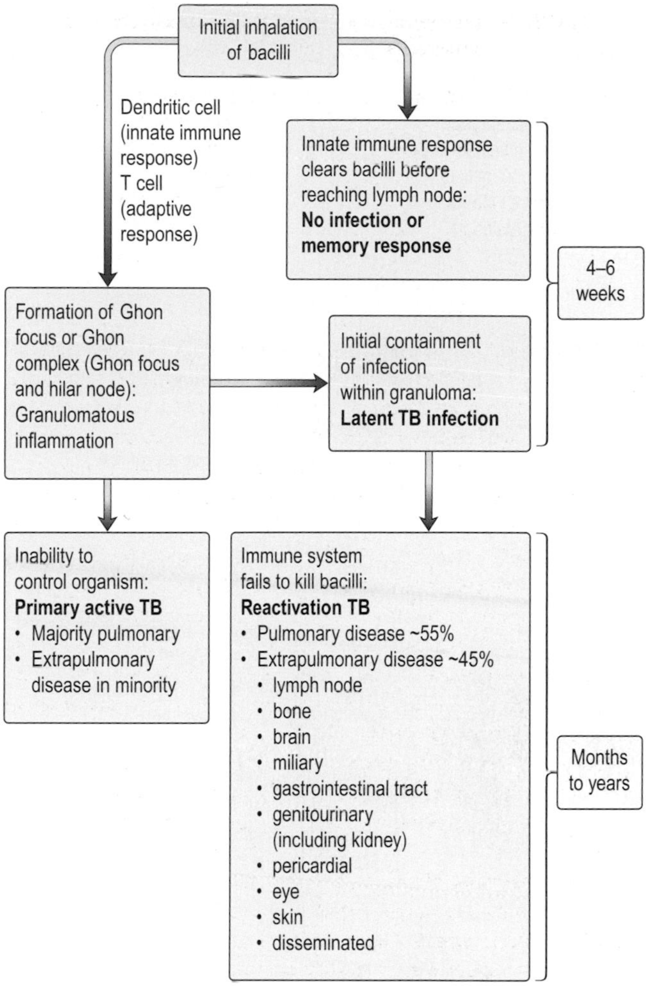

Figure 24.35 The consequences of exposure to tuberculosis.

completely and many become calcified. Some of these calcified nodules contain bacteria, which are contained by the immune system (and the hypoxic acidic environment created within the granuloma) and are capable of lying dormant for many years. The initial focus of disease is termed the 'Ghon focus'.

On a chest X-ray, the Ghon focus is evident as a small, calcified nodule, often within the upper parts of the lower lobes or the lower parts of the upper lobes, seen in the mid-zone. A focus can also develop within the regional draining lymph node (primary complex of Ranke).

Upon initial contact with infection, <5% of patients develop active disease. This percentage increases to 10% within the first year of exposure.

Latent tuberculosis

In the majority of people who are infected by *Mycobacterium* spp., the immune system contains the infection and the patient develops cell-mediated immune memory to the bacteria. This is termed 'latent TB'.

Reactivation tuberculosis

The majority of TB cases are due to reactivation of latent infection. The initial contact usually occurred many years or decades earlier. In patients with HIV infection, newly acquired TB infection is also common. There are several factors implicated in the development

Box 24.38 Factors implicated in the reactivation of latent tuberculosis

- HIV co-infection
- Immunosuppressant therapy (chemotherapy/monoclonal antibody treatment), including corticosteroids
- Diabetes mellitus
- End-stage chronic kidney disease
- Malnutrition
- Ageing

Box 24.39 Some features contrasting latent infection with active tuberculous disease

Latent infection	Active disease
Bacilli present in Ghon focus	Bacilli present in tissues or secretions
Sputum smear- and culture-negative	Sputum commonly smear- and culture-positive in pulmonary disease MTb can usually be cultured from infected tissue
Tuberculin skin test usually positive	Tuberculin skin test usually positive (and can ulcerate)
Chest X-ray normal (small calcified Ghon focus frequently visible)	Chest X-ray shows signs of consolidation/cavitation/effusion in pulmonary disease
Asymptomatic	Symptomatic – night sweats, fevers, weight loss and cough common
Not infectious to others	Infectious to others if bacilli detectable in sputum

MTb, *Mycobacterium tuberculosis complex.*

of active disease ***(Box 24.38)***. The clinical features of latent and reactivation TB are contrasted in ***Box 24.39***.

Clinical features and diagnosis

Any of the manifestations of disease shown in ***Box 24.40*** can occur in primary or reactivation disease, but extrapulmonary involvement is far less common in primary disease and is usually seen only in regions of high endemicity.

In all cases of suspected TB, strong efforts should be made to obtain tissue or fluid for microscopy, smear and culture to obtain information on sensitivities. Tissue samples should also be sent for histopathological examination. Where pulmonary TB is suspected, serial sputum samples should be collected on at least three occasions (ideally, immediately upon waking); where the patient is unable to produce sputum, it is necessary to obtain induced sputum or perform bronchoscopy and lavage to obtain respiratory secretions, not only to make the diagnosis but also to ascertain infectivity of the index case.

Pulmonary TB

Patients are frequently symptomatic with a productive cough and, occasionally, haemoptysis, along with systemic symptoms of weight loss, fevers and sweats (commonly at the end of the day and through the night). Where there is laryngeal involvement, a hoarse voice and a severe cough are found. If disease involves the pleura, then pleuritic pain is a frequent presenting complaint.

The chest X-ray ***(Fig. 24.36)*** demonstrates several findings: consolidation with or without cavitation, pleural effusion or thickening or widening of the mediastinum caused by hilar or paratracheal adenopathy.

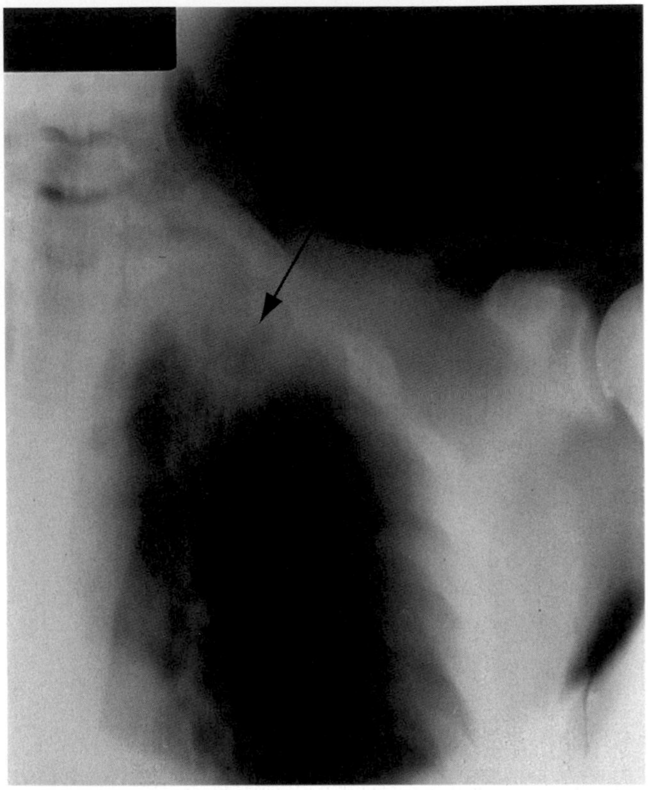

Figure 24.36 **Chest X-ray showing tuberculosis of the left upper lobe with cavitation (arrowed).**

Lymph node TB

The next most common site for infection is lymph node TB. Extrathoracic nodes are more commonly involved than intrathoracic or mediastinal. Usually, this presents as a firm, non-tender enlargement of a cervical or supraclavicular node. The node becomes necrotic centrally and can liquefy and be fluctuant if peripheral. The overlying skin is frequently indurated or there can be sinus tract formation with purulent discharge, but characteristically there is no erythema (cold abscess formation). Nodes typically can be enlarged for several months prior to diagnosis. On CT imaging, the central area appears necrotic (see ***Box 24.40***).

Other forms of TB

Gastrointestinal TB

See page 401.

TB of bone and spine

See pages 718 and 691.

Miliary TB

Miliary disease occurs through haematogenous spread of the bacilli to multiple sites, including the CNS in 20% of cases.

Systemic upset is the rule, with respiratory symptoms in the majority. Other findings are liver and splenic microabscesses with deranged liver enzymes or cholestasis and gastrointestinal symptoms.

The chest X-ray demonstrates multiple nodules, which appear like millet seeds: hence the term 'miliary'.

Box 24.40 Common sites of tuberculosis infection with relevant radiological findings and appropriate diagnostic investigations

Pulmonary, pleural and laryngeal TB

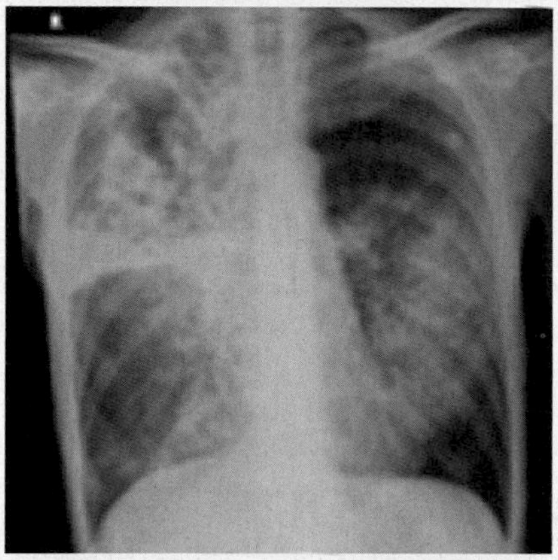

Smear and culture of:
- Sputum (≥2 samples increase diagnostic yield)
- Induced sputum (inhaled hypertonic saline, which induces coughing): diagnostic yield comparable to bronchoscopic samples
- Bronchoalveolar lavage fluid if cough unproductive and induced sputum not possible
- Aspiration of pleural fluid and pleural biopsy
- Gastric aspirates – can be useful in paediatric disease
- Nasoendoscopic or bronchoscopic examination/biopsy of vocal cords with biopsy for smear/culture and histology in laryngeal disease

Miliary TB

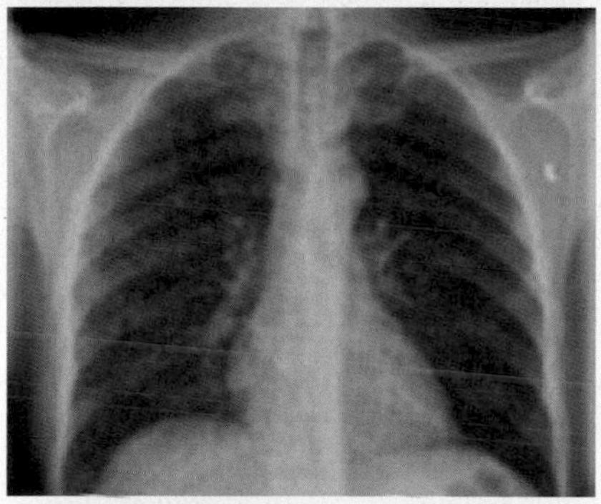

Blood cultures
Bronchoalveolar lavage fluid (usually smear-negative but culture-positive)
Lumbar puncture should be performed in all cases, unless contraindicated, to assess for CNS involvement (affects treatment duration) – see below
Sampling of other involved organs often necessary

Central nervous system TB

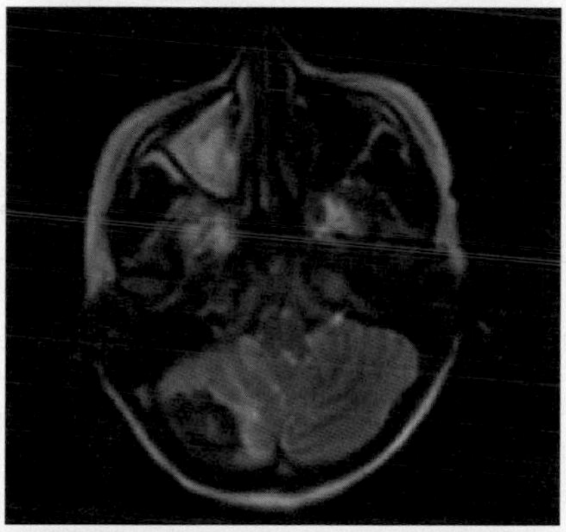

Lumbar puncture if no contraindication. Characteristics of lumbar puncture:
- CSF protein may be very high (usually >2–3 g/L)
- CSF glucose < ½ blood glucose
- CSF lymphocytosis

Lymph node TB

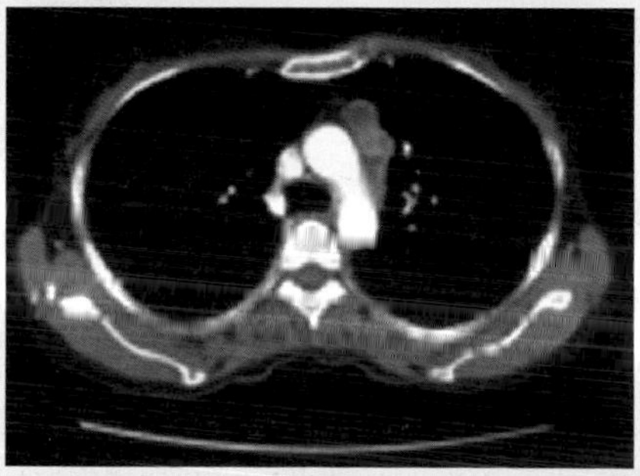

All samples should be sent for histocytopathological examination as well as culture and smear:
- Fine needle aspiration or biopsy of an involved lymph node, usually under radiological guidance
- Mediastinal nodal sampling (endobronchial ultrasound transbronchial needle aspiration, mediastinoscopy/mediastinotomy)

CNS, central nervous system; CSF, cerebrospinal fluid.

Central nervous system TB

See page 865.

Pericardial TB

See page 1043.

Skin

See page 1343.

Microbiological diagnosis

Rapid identification of the presence of bacteria by immediate stains is essential and should be performed within 24 hours; culture of the sample allows determination of the antibiotic sensitivity of the infecting strain.

Stains

Auramine–rhodamine staining is more sensitive (though less specific) than Ziehl–Neelsen; as a result, it is more widely used. It requires fluorescence microscopy and highlights bacilli as yellow-orange on a green background.

Culture

The majority of the developed world uses liquid/broth culture of mycobacteria in addition to solid media (Lowenstein–Jensen slopes or Middlebrook agar), as time to culture is shorter than for solid culture (1–3 weeks compared with 3–8 weeks). Using liquid culture in the presence of anti-mycobacterial drugs (usually first-line therapy initially) establishes the drug sensitivity for that strain and usually takes approximately 3 weeks.

The use of the microscopic-observation drug-sensitivity (MODS) assay allows rapid detection of bacteria and susceptibility by comparing growth in multiple wells with anti-mycobacterial drugs within liquid media. This technique has the advantage of being relatively inexpensive (although is labour-intensive and operator-dependent) and is therefore more widely used in resource-poor areas.

Nucleic acid amplification

Nucleic acid amplification (NAA) is increasingly used for rapid identification of MTb complex and is useful in differentiating between MTb and non-tuberculosis mycobacteria, as well as identifying TB in smear-negative sputum specimens. Culture and staining are still necessary and should not be replaced by PCR. PCR is only useful at the initial stage of diagnosis, as it frequently remains positive despite treatment, due to the detection of dead organisms. This test has a high specificity and moderate sensitivity on cerebrospinal fluid and should be routinely looked for in suspected CNS TB.

The identification of mycobacterial DNA is useful in facilitating rapid commencement of treatment and also rapid identification of drug resistance. Genetic mutations in bacterial DNA conferring rifampicin resistance are highly predictive of multidrug resistance. The development of a highly specific probe designed to detect this mutation thereby allows rapid identification of resistant disease and commencement of appropriate therapy sooner than waiting for cultures to complete (may take up to 8 weeks).

Molecular testing for drug resistance has also become possible using PCR to detect genetic mutations associated with rifampicin resistance. This is performed where resistance is suspected due to specific risk factors in the patient, such as HIV co-infection, previous treatment for TB, location in an area with high rates of resistance or known contact with drug-resistant disease.

Management

Patients with fully sensitive TB require 6 months of treatment; the exception is TB of the CNS, for which the recommended duration is at least 12 months. Shorter-duration courses are being studied, aiming at reducing the duration of treatment and increasing the armamentarium against resistant strains. In CNS and pericardial disease, corticosteroids are used as an adjunct at treatment initiation to reduce long-term complications. ***Box 24.41*** summarizes the standard recommended regimens.

Directly observed therapy (DOT) is widely recommended and employed with an aim to achieve treatment-completion rates of over 85%. DOT is defined as treatment supervised by a healthcare professional or family member, where the person is observed swallowing their medication. WHO advocates universal DOT as one of their strategies to reduce the incidence of TB worldwide, partly because the majority of relapsed disease or treatment failure is due to lack of adherence, interrupted therapy or incorrect treatment ***(Box 24.42)***. Where DOT is used, the dosing frequency may be reduced to three times per week to make treatment more convenient. Success rates for this regimen and standard daily unsupervised therapy are comparable.

Unwanted effects of drug treatment

Rifampicin induces liver enzymes, which may be transiently elevated in the serum of many patients. The drug should be stopped only if the serum bilirubin becomes elevated or if transferases are

Box 24.41 Usual treatment and duration in fully sensitive tuberculosis

Site of disease	Duration of therapy	Drug choice
Pulmonary[a] Extrapulmonary (excluding CNS disease) Miliary (excluding CNS involvement)	6 months (may be extended to 9 months in certain situations): Patient smear-positive 2 months into treatment Some patients with HIV co-infection High burden of disease	Fully sensitive strain: 2HRZE+4HR[b] *Or* 2HRZE+7HR
CNS TB	12 months	2HRZE+10HR *Plus* Prednisolone (20–40 mg o.d.) weaning over 2–4 weeks
Latent TB	3 months *Or* 6 months	3RH *Or* 6H

CNS, central nervous system; E, ethambutol; H, isoniazid; R, rifampicin; Z, pyrazinamide. [a]For pulmonary TB, 2HRZE+4$(HR)_3$, i.e. 3 times weekly for 4HR, is acceptable. [b]2HRZE+4HR, 2 months of HRZE+4 months of HR.

Box 24.42 Criteria for implementation of directly observed therapy (DOT) for tuberculosis

- Patients thought unlikely to comply
  - History of serious mental illness
  - History of non-adherence to TB therapy in past or during current treatment course
- Street- or shelter-dwelling homelessness
- Multidrug-resistant TB

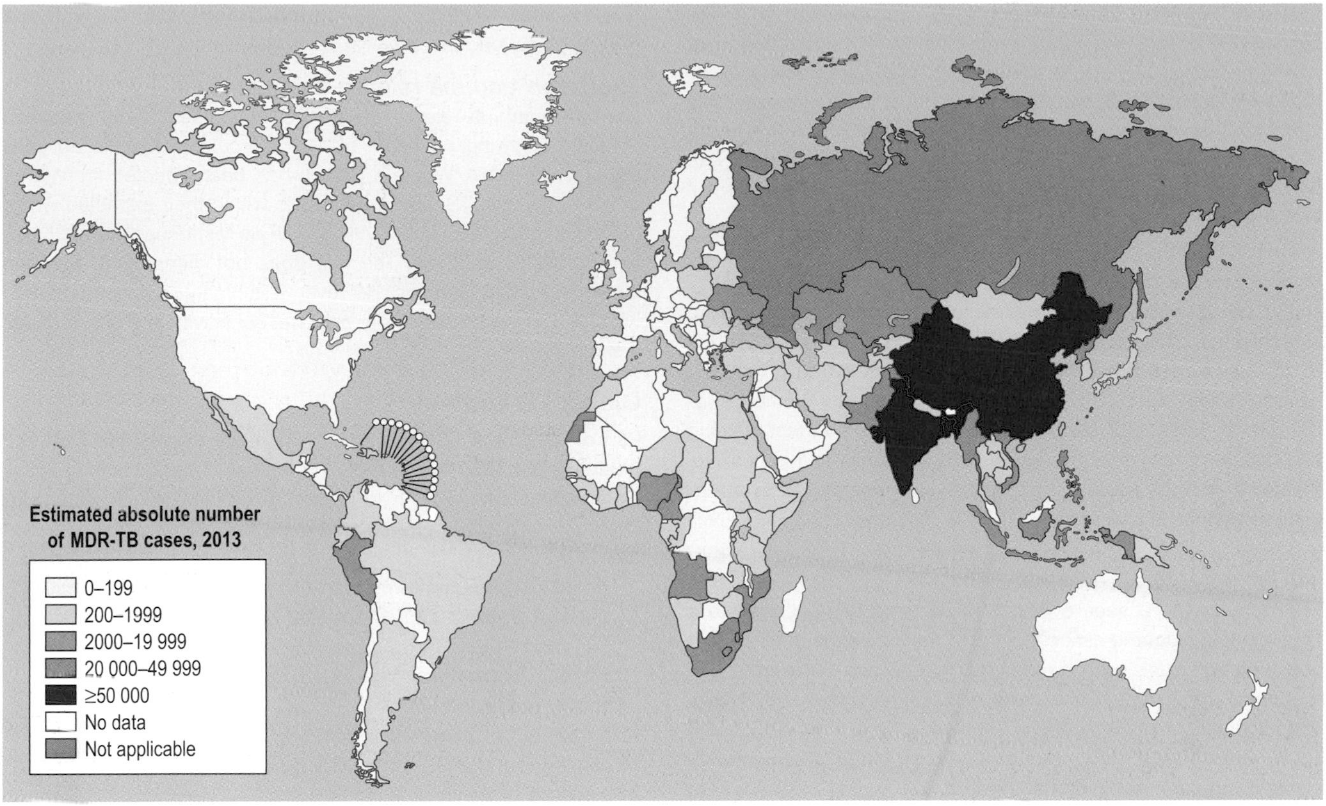

Figure 24.37 Worldwide incidence of multidrug-resistant tuberculosis (MDR-TB), 2013. *(From World Health Organization. Global Tuberculosis Report 2014, with permission from WHO.)*

more than three times elevated, which is uncommon. Induction of liver enzymes means that concomitant drug treatment may be made less effective (see p. 24). Thrombocytopenia has been reported. Rifampicin stains body secretions pink and the patients should be warned of the change in colour of their urine, tears (affects contact lenses) and sweat. Oral contraception will not be effective, so alternative birth-control methods should be used. Rifabutin, a rifamycin, is similar and is used for prophylaxis against *M. avium-intracellulare* complex infection in HIV patients with CD4 counts <200 mm^3.

Isoniazid has very few unwanted effects. At high doses, it may produce a polyneuropathy due to a B_6 deficiency, as isoniazid interacts with pyridoxal phosphate. This is extremely rare when the normal dose of 200–300 mg is given daily. Nevertheless, it is customary to prescribe pyridoxine 10 mg daily to prevent this. Occasionally, isoniazid gives rise to allergic reactions, such as a skin rash and fever. Hepatitis occurs in less than 1% of cases but may be fatal if the drug is continued.

Pyrazinamide may cause hepatic toxicity, though this is much rarer with present dosage schedules. Pyrazinamide reduces the renal excretion of urate and may precipitate hyperuricaemic gout.

Ethambutol can cause a dose-related optic retrobulbar neuritis that presents with colour blindness for green, reduction in visual acuity and a central scotoma (more common at doses of 25 mg/kg). This usually reverses, provided the drug is stopped when symptoms develop; patients should therefore be warned of its effects. All patients prescribed the drug should be seen by an ophthalmologist prior to treatment and doses of 15 mg/kg should be used.

Streptomycin can cause irreversible damage to the vestibular nerve. This is more likely to occur in the elderly and in those with renal impairment. Allergic reactions to streptomycin are more common than those to rifampicin, isoniazid or pyrazinamide. This drug is used only if patients are very ill, have multidrug-resistant TB, or are not responding adequately to therapy.

Box 24.43 Factors associated with an increased risk of drug-resistant tuberculosis

- History of prior drug treatment of TB (particularly if unsupervised, self-administered treatment)
- Co-infection with advanced HIV and previous TB treatment
- Infection acquired in a region with high rates of drug resistance
- Contact with a known case of resistant TB
- Failure to respond to empirical TB therapy despite documented adherence
- Exposure to multiple courses of fluoroquinolone antibiotics for presumed community-acquired pneumonia
- Healthcare workers exposed to cases of resistant TB

Drug resistance

Worldwide, drug resistance is an increasing problem, with an estimated incidence of 444 000 cases in 2008, responsible for around 150 000 deaths (Fig. 24.37 and Box 24.43). It arises due to incomplete or incorrect drug treatment and can be spread from person to person. Mono-resistance is reasonably common: for example, the incidence is approximately 10% in the UK. A risk assessment for drug resistance should be routinely performed. The incidence of multidrug resistance (resistance to both rifampicin and isoniazid, termed MDR-TB) is relatively low in developed countries (around

1%) and only a handful of extensively drug-resistant (XDR-TB) cases have been seen, though most countries have reported at least one case. XDR-TB is defined as high-level resistance to rifampicin, isoniazid, fluoroquinolones and at least one injectable agent such as amikacin, capreomycin or kanamycin. A few cases of total drug resistance (TDR) have been reported from Italy, Iran and Mumbai (India).

TB in special situations

***Mycobacterium bovis* infection** occurs in humans who have consumed unpasteurized milk sometime in their life, in farmers working with infected cows for over 3 years and abattoir workers. TB due to *M. bovis* does not differ from ordinary TB in the chest, but extrapulmonary sites of infection are more common. Immunosuppression is also a risk factor. Diagnosis is with acid fast staining and culture of tissues and sputum. The tuberculin text is positive. Treatment is with isoniazid, rifampicin and ethambutol; pyrazinamide resistance is common.

HIV co-infection

The increase in TB seen over recent decades has occurred to a considerable extent in association with the incidence of HIV infection, with high levels seen in Africa (particularly sub-Saharan Africa), the Indian subcontinent and parts of Eastern Europe and Russia. The incidence of HIV infection in TB worldwide is around 15% and TB is responsible for around one-quarter of acquired immunodeficiency syndrome (AIDS)-related deaths.

Alongside the increased morbidity and mortality of co-infection, there are specific issues relating to the treatment of TB in HIV: namely, the incidence of drug interactions and intolerability, the increased risk of treatment toxicity and the higher incidence of drug resistance. TB/HIV infection should be managed by experts in TB (respiratory or infectious disease physicians) alongside HIV specialists.

Chronic kidney disease

Chronic kidney disease (CKD) is a risk factor for reactivation of latent TB infection (LTBI) due to relative immune paresis. Patients due to undergo renal transplantation may need to be screened for LTBI and given complete chemoprophylaxis if necessary before undergoing their procedure. The presence of CKD also complicates the treatment regimen, as there is an increased risk of toxicity due to altered pharmacokinetics, which necessitates dosage adjustments and therapeutic drug level monitoring. Management should be undertaken by TB specialists in conjunction with renal physicians.

Latent TB infection (LTBI)

LTBI is diagnosed by demonstrating immune memory to mycobacterial proteins. Two tests are available.

Tuberculin skin test

A positive result is indicated by a delayed hypersensitivity reaction evident 48–72 hours after the intradermal injection of purified protein derivative (PPD) resulting in:

- a raised, indurated lesion >6 mm diameter in non-vaccinated adults
- a raised, indurated lesion >15 mm in bacille Calmette–Guérin (BCG)-vaccinated adults.

False-negative (anergic) tuberculin skin tests (TSTs) are common in immunosuppression due to HIV infection ($CD4^+$ <200/mm^3), sarcoidosis, or drugs (chemotherapy, anti-TNF therapy, steroids), at the extremes of age and in active disease. False-positives occur due to cross-reactivity with non-tuberculous mycobacteria and BCG vaccination.

Interferon-gamma release assays

Interferon-gamma release assays (IGRAs) detect T-cell secretion of IFN-γ following exposure to *M. tuberculosis*-specific antigens (ESAT-6, CFP-10). Where a person has been infected (previously or currently) with TB, activated T cells within their extracted whole blood secrete quantifiable levels of IFN-γ in response to re-exposure to TB-specific antigens. The test does not differentiate between active and latent infection. However, it is highly specific compared with the TST and has a similar or better sensitivity and only requires a single visit.

Global TB strategy

Part of the global TB strategy is to increase the identification and treatment of LTBI, thereby reducing the risk of conversion to active disease and transmission to others. In certain groups with LTBI, chemoprophylaxis is offered to reduce the risk of active infection ***(Box 24.44)***.

Active case-finding forms part of a number of programmes:

- ***Contact tracing***: carried out after diagnosis of a new case of TB; involves identifying close contacts who are at risk of infection or who may have active infection and have not yet sought medical attention.
- ***Screening of healthcare workers***: as part of an occupational health programme, with BCG vaccination of those with no evidence of previous TB exposure.
- ***Screening of new entrants***: for those arriving from a country of high incidence of TB, who should be offered screening for latent or active infection and vaccination if not infected and previously unvaccinated.
- ***Street-homeless or hostel dwellers***: at increased risk of active TB and should be offered opportunistic screening for active infection.
- ***Immunocompromised people***:
  - Patients due to commence monoclonal antibody therapy for autoimmune conditions – should be screened for active or latent infection and given appropriate treatment before commencing immunosuppressive therapy, as they are at a particularly high risk for reactivation of LTBI.
  - People with HIV infection (see above).
  - People with underlying haematological malignancies or solid-organ transplants or undergoing chemotherapy – require screening.

BCG vaccination

BCG is a live attenuated vaccine derived from *M. bovis* that has lost its virulence. It has variable efficacy but is still recommended

Box 24.44 People who should be treated for latent tuberculosis infection (after excluding active TB)

- People aged ≤35 years with positive TST or IGRA
- Healthcare workers with positive TST or IGRA
- Patients commencing anti-TNF therapy with positive IGRA
- HIV-positive people with positive IGRA
- People with evidence of previous TB on chest X-ray and inadequate treatment

IGRA, interferon-gamma release assay; TNF, tumour necrosis factor; TST, tuberculin skin test.

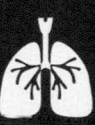

in certain situations in developed countries (but not the USA), though no longer offered routinely to all due to the lack of cost efficacy. It has been shown to reduce the risk of disseminated and CNS TB in babies and children and is therefore used worldwide. There are safety concerns in babies with HIV. Its efficacy in adults is very variable.

Non-tuberculous mycobacterial infection

Non-tuberculous mycobacterial (NTM) infections occur in soil and water and are not usually pathogenic due to their lack of virulence. However, where there is a breach of the normal host defence mechanisms, certain strains have the potential to become pathogenic ***(Box 24.45)***. Factors associated with increased risk of pulmonary NTM infection are shown in ***Box 24.46***. Treatment is suggested if there is a compatible clinical picture and (a) the organism is isolated from an invasive sample or (b) an NTM is isolated from more than one sputum sample obtained at different times.

Box 24.45 Some non-tuberculous mycobacteria strains implicated in disease

Strain	Site of disease
***M. avium intracellulare complex* (MAC)**	Pulmonary (nodular and interstitial infiltrates in middle lobe in women or fibrocavitary disease in smoking middle-aged males) Disseminated (usually in HIV) Hypersensitivity pulmonary disease ('hot-tub lung') Lymphadenitis in children
M. kansasii	Pulmonary (similar presentation to MTb, usually in middle-aged males) Disseminated disease (in HIV)
M. abscessus	Skin, soft tissue and bone disease Pulmonary (usually in bronchiectasis and older, non-smoking females)
M. chelonae	Skin, bone and soft tissue Pulmonary (similar to *M. abscessus*)
M. fortuitum	Pulmonary (similar to *M. abscessus*)
M. gordonae	Only rarely pathogenic (can be significant in immunocompromised host)
M. xenopi	Pulmonary (fibrocavitary disease in COPD) Contaminated surgical instruments causing bone/soft tissue infection
M. malmoense	Pulmonary Lymph node
M. marinum	Soft tissue, skin and bone
M. szulgai	Pulmonary (similar to TB)

COPD, chronic obstructive pulmonary disease; MTb, *Mycobacterium tuberculosis complex*.

Box 24.46 Factors associated with increased risk of pulmonary infection with non-tuberculous mycobacteria

- ***Structural lung disease:***
  - Chronic obstructive pulmonary disease
  - Bronchiectasis: subgroup of women with bronchiectasis, scoliosis, pectus excavatum, mitral valve prolapse and hypermobile joints at particular risk
  - Cystic fibrosis
  - Prior TB
- ***HIV infection*** (CD4 <50/mm^3)
- ***Genetic defects*** of interferon-γ/interleukin-12 pathway

Further reading

Diel R, Goletti D, Ferrara G et al. Interferon-γ release assays for the diagnosis of latent *Mycobacterium tuberculosis* infection: a systematic review and meta-analysis. *Eur Respir J* 2011; 37:88–99.
Kaufmann SH, Hussey G, Lambert PH. New vaccines for tuberculosis. *Lancet* 2010; 375:2110–2119.
Lawn SD, Zumla AI. Tuberculosis. *Lancet* 2011; 378:57–72.
National Institute for Health and Clinical Excellence. *NICE Clinical Guideline CG117: Tuberculosis: Clinical Diagnosis and Management of Tuberculosis, and Measures for its Prevention and Control.* NICE 2011; https://www.nice.org.uk/guidance/cg117.
World Health Organization. *Global Tuberculosis Report 2015*; http://www.who.int/.

DIFFUSE PARENCHYMAL LUNG DISEASES

These are also referred to as **interstitial lung diseases (ILDs)**. They are a heterogeneous group of conditions accounting for about 15% of respiratory clinical practice. They are characterized by varying degrees of inflammation and fibrosis, initially affecting the interstitium of the lung, which typically present with exertional dyspnoea, with or without cough. A classification of ILDs is shown in ***Figure 24.38***.

Idiopathic interstitial pneumonias

The terminology used to describe the idiopathic interstitial pneumonias can be confusing but it is necessary to distinguish between subgroups, as there are significant differences in terms of prognosis and treatment options. Clinical patterns usually link to particular histological subtypes; their classification is shown in ***Box 24.47***.

Idiopathic pulmonary fibrosis

Idiopathic pulmonary fibrosis (IPF) is the most common of the idiopathic interstitial pneumonias. It is a progressive and ultimately fatal disease of unknown cause. There is significant worldwide variation in reported prevalence but the incidence appears to be increasing (6.8–8.8/100 000 in the USA). Mean onset is in the sixties and presentation is very uncommon under the age of 50. Males are twice as likely to be affected.

Pathology

Usual interstitial pneumonia (UIP) is the histological finding in IPF. The key feature is a heterogenous appearance with areas of normal lung punctuated by areas of marked fibrosis, honeycombing mainly in subpleural areas and fibroblastic foci (dense proliferations of fibroblasts and myofibroblasts). The terms IPF and UIP are often used interchangeably but they are *not* synonymous, as UIP is also the primary histological finding in several other diffuse parenchymal lung diseases (e.g. pulmonary autoimmune rheumatic disease).

Pathogenesis

It is thought that repetitive injury to the alveolar epithelium, caused by currently unidentified environmental stimuli, leads to the activation of several pathways responsible for repair of the damaged tissue. However, in IPF, the wound healing mechanisms become uncontrolled, leading to over-production of fibroblasts and deposition of increased extracellular matrix in the interstitium with little inflammation. The structural integrity of the lung parenchyma is therefore disrupted: there is loss of elasticity and the ability to

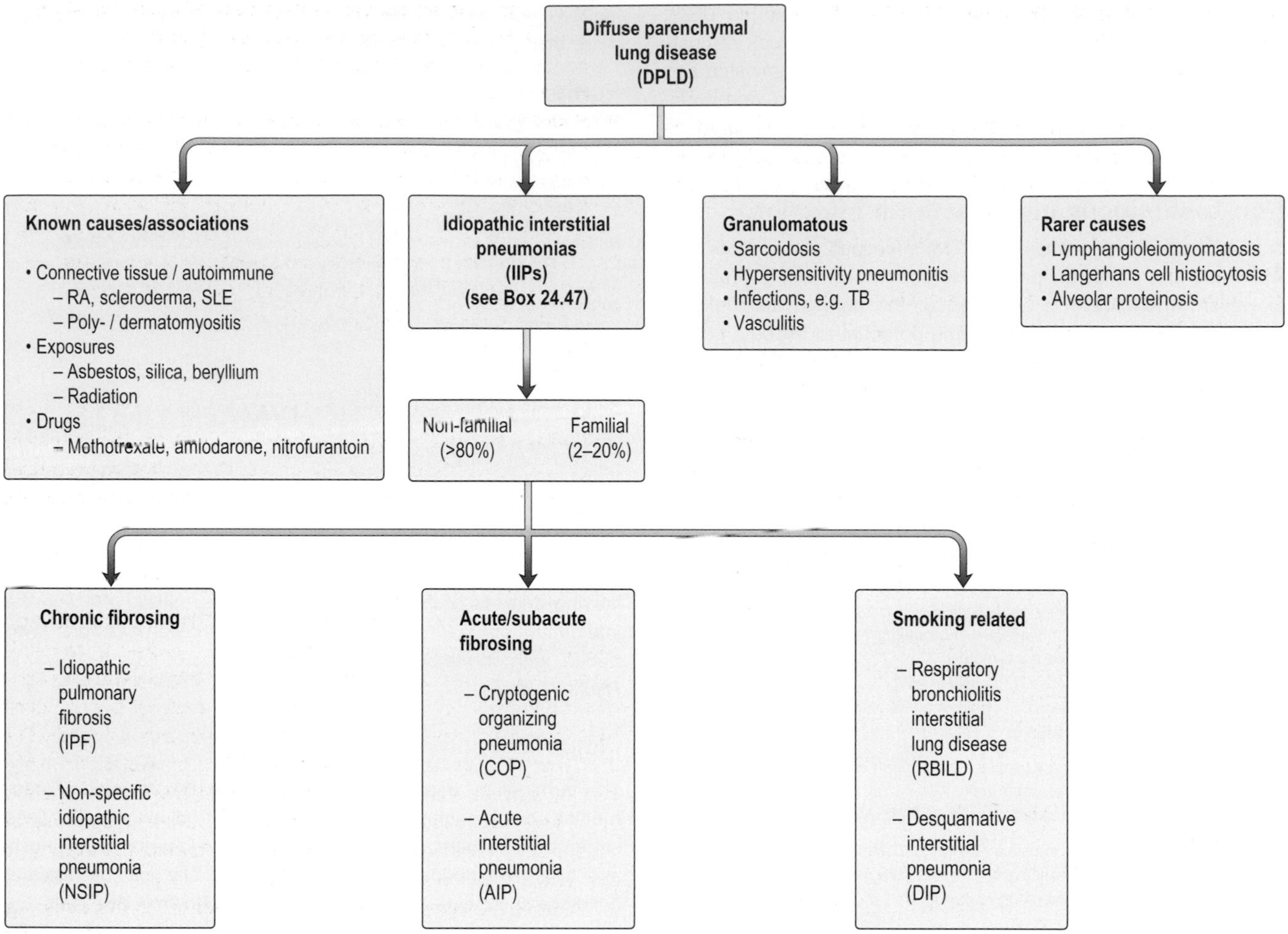

Figure 24.38 Classification of the interstitial lung diseases. RA, rheumatoid arthritis; SLE, systemic lupus erythematosus.

Box 24.47 Classification of idiopathic interstitial pneumonias

Clinical diagnosis	Pathological pattern
Idiopathic pulmonary fibrosis (IPF)	Usual interstitial pneumonia (UIP)
Desquamative interstitial pneumonia (DIP)	Desquamative interstitial pneumonia (DIP)
Respiratory bronchiolitis interstitial lung disease (RBILD)	Respiratory bronchiolitis interstitial lung disease (RBILD)
Acute interstitial pneumonia (AIP)	Diffuse alveolar damage (DAD)
Non-specific interstitial pneumonia (NSIP)	Non-specific interstitial pneumonia (NSIP)
Cryptogenic organizing pneumonia (COP)	Organizing pneumonia (OP)
Lymphoid interstitial pneumonia (LIP)	Lymphoid interstitial pneumonia (LIP)

(From ATS/ERS. American Thoracic Society/European Respiratory Society International Multidisciplinary Consensus Classification of the Idiopathic Interstitial Pneumonias. *American Journal of Respiratory and Critical Care Medicine* 2002; 165:277.)

perform gas exchange is impaired, leading to progressive respiratory failure. Factors implicated in triggering the aberrant wound healing include inhalational insults (cigarette smoke, occupational dust exposure), viruses (e.g. Epstein–Barr), drugs (e.g. methotrexate, nitrofurantoin) and chronic gastro-oesophageal reflux disease (GORD); none of these has been substantiated. There may be a genetic predisposition in a small (2–20%) of patients. Polymorphisms in the MUC5B gene and mutations in genes encoding telomerase and surfactant have been reported.

Clinical features

Patients typically present with insidious onset of progressive dyspnoea that may be accompanied by cough, with or without sputum production. It is not uncommon for patients to be mistakenly treated for heart failure or recurrent chest infections before the diagnosis of IPF is made. The onset is usually in the patient's sixties and is rare below the age of 50. There is a 2 : 1 male : female ratio. Finger clubbing is seen in 25–50% of cases. Examination of the chest shows bi-basal end-inspiratory crackles.

Progressive respiratory failure may be complicated by pulmonary hypertension. Stepwise deterioration can occur due to pneumothorax, pulmonary embolism or intercurrent infection, but acute exacerbations with no identifiable cause are well recognized and are associated with increased mortality. An acute form (also known as Hamman–Rich syndrome) occasionally occurs and has a particularly poor prognosis.

Investigations

The aims of investigation in IPF are to confirm the presence of pulmonary fibrosis and exclude identifiable (and potentially reversible) causes. A combination of typical clinical features and characteristic radiological abnormalities may be sufficient for diagnosis. However, further tests are necessary where the diagnosis is in doubt.

- ***Respiratory function tests*** usually show a restrictive pattern (FEV_1/FVC ratio >70%) with reduced lung volumes and gas transfer. However, spirometry may be normal in early disease and lung volumes can be preserved in the presence of coexisting emphysema.
- ***Blood tests***, including antinuclear antibodies (ANA) and rheumatoid factor (RF), are performed to exclude autoimmune rheumatic disease but there is no specific serological test for IPF.
- ***Chest X-ray*** shows small-volume lungs with increased reticular shadowing at the bases but may be normal in early disease.
- ***HRCT*** is the imaging modality of choice. A confident diagnosis of IPF may be made in patients with typical clinical features and absence of an identifiable cause if the following HRCT abnormalities are present:
  - ***Basal distribution***: abnormalities are more pronounced at the bases.
  - ***Subpleural reticulation***: reticulation is most evident in the lung peripheries.
  - ***Traction bronchiectasis***: the fibrotic process distorts the normal lung architecture, pulling the airways open and causing bronchiectasis.
  - ***Honeycombing***: there are basal layers of small, cystic airspaces with irregularly thickened walls composed of fibrous tissue ***(Fig. 24.39)***.
- ***Bronchoalveolar lavage*** is only necessary if an infective or malignant cause is suspected. A differential cell count may lend support to an alternative diagnosis: a lymphocytosis is suggestive of *hypersensitivity pneumonitis* whereas a neutrophilic pattern (neutrophils >3%) is commonly seen in IPF.
- ***Histological confirmation*** is necessary in some patients. Surgical lung biopsy, usually via video-assisted thoracoscopic surgery (VATS), is the most reliable method for obtaining diagnostic histological samples. Parenchymal tissue can also be obtained bronchoscopically via transbronchial biopsy. This avoids the need for general anaesthetic but the samples obtained are frequently too small for accurate analysis, although may be sufficient to confirm alternative diagnoses such as sarcoidosis.

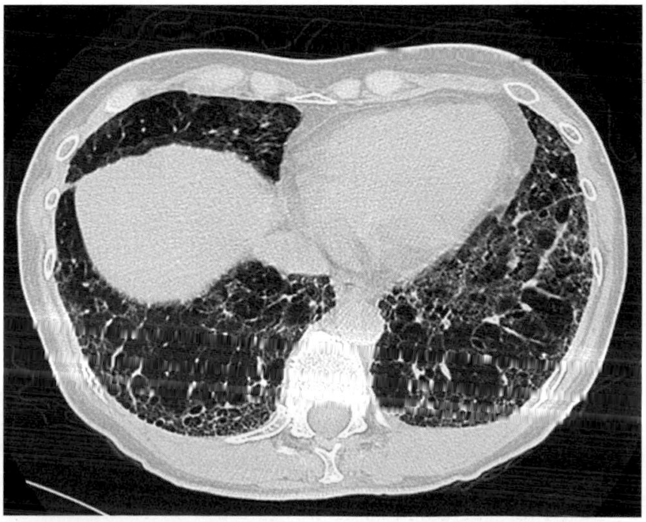

Figure 24.39 CT scan showing idiopathic pulmonary fibrosis. There is reticular shadowing and honeycombing predominantly in the basal and subpleural areas.

Differential diagnosis

The main differential diagnosis for IPF is an alternative interstitial lung disease. Other differentials for the chest X-ray appearances include interstitial pulmonary oedema, infection and lymphangitis carcinomatosa.

Prognosis and management

The median survival time for patients with IPF is 2–5 years, although mortality is higher in the more acute forms. The disease course is highly variable and unpredictable; living with this uncertainty is one of the most difficult aspects of this disease. Serial lung function testing is used to monitor disease progression and a 10% decline in FVC or 15% decline in gas transfer (TLCO) in the first 6–12 months confers a worse prognosis. Periods of stability may be interspersed with periods of more accelerated decline, but failure to recover back to baseline following these episodes is common. Mortality is increased following acute exacerbations.

Previous treatment strategies included a combination of prednisolone, azathioprine and *N*-acetylcysteine. Intravenous methylprednisolone may still be used in acute presentations with life-threatening disease.

Treatment now targets the aberrant fibroblastic proliferation and tissue remodelling implicated in the pathogenesis. ***Pirfenidone***, an antifibrotic agent, has been shown to slow the rate of FVC decline in a number of large randomized controlled trials and has been approved for use in several countries. It is generally well tolerated, with the most common side-effects being a reversible photosensitive rash and gastrointestinal disturbance. Other treatments include ***nintedanib***, an intracellular inhibitor of tyrosine kinases, believed to activate the cell-signalling pathways responsible for the uncontrolled fibroproliferative process.

GORD should be treated, as this is thought to contribute to repetitive alveolar epithelial damage. Even with treatment, IPF is a life-limiting disease and transplant assessment should be undertaken in accordance with local guidelines. All patients should have their need for supportive care assessed with respect to oxygen therapy, pulmonary rehabilitation and palliative care input.

Other idiopathic interstitial pneumonias

These are described in ***Box 24.48***.

Hypersensitivity pneumonitis

Hypersensitivity pneumonitis (HP) is caused by an allergic reaction affecting the small airways and alveoli in response to an inhaled antigen or occasionally following ingestion of a causative drug. Common antigens are illustrated in ***Box 24.49***.

Box 24.48 Other idiopathic interstitial pneumonias (IIPs)

IIP	Presentation	HRCT	Pathology	Treatment
Desquamative interstitial pneumonia (DIP)	Middle-aged smokers Men > women Dyspnoea and cough over weeks to months	Widespread ground glass opacification	Alveolar spaces filled with pigmented macrophages (due to tobacco smoke)	Smoking cessation – may remit spontaneously Corticosteroids in severe or progressive disease ± additional immunosuppressants Response generally good
Respiratory bronchiolitis interstitial lung disease (RBILD)	Current or ex-smokers Similar to DIP	Centrilobular nodules Ground glass opacification	Pigmented macrophages in lumen of respiratory bronchioles	Smoking cessation No clear benefit with corticosteroids Outcome more favourable than in DIP
Acute interstitial pneumonia (AIP) (Hamman–Rich syndrome)	Dyspnoea and progressive respiratory failure over days to weeks Often preceded by viral prodrome	Ground glass opacification Traction bronchiectasis Consolidation Septal thickening	Diffuse alveolar damage (DAD)	Pulsed intravenous methylprednisolone for 3 days followed by maintenance oral corticosteroids Additional immunosuppressants may be required Mortality 50–80%
Non-specific interstitial pneumonia (NSIP)	Similar to IPF but more indolent course May be associated with connective tissue disease	Similar to IPF but increased ground glass opacification, minimal honeycombing	Uniform inflammatory infiltrate with or without fibrosis (fibrotic vs cellular NSIP)	Corticosteroids ± additional immunosuppressants, e.g. azathioprine, cyclophosphamide Prognosis better with cellular form Outcome more favourable than in IPF
Cryptogenic organizing pneumonia (COP)	Influenza-like symptoms, dyspnoea, cough over weeks to months Secondary OP may be related to connective tissue, autoimmune disease or drugs	Bilateral flitting/migratory peripheral consolidation Variable ground glass opacification	Buds of connective tissue (Masson bodies) in alveoli and alveolar ducts	Usually rapidly responsive to corticosteroids but relapses common
Lymphoid interstitial pneumonia (LIP)	Commonly, middle-aged women Insidious dyspnoea, dry cough, systemic upset May be associated with connective tissue disease and HIV	Ground glass opacification Perivascular cysts	Interstitium infiltrated by lymphocytes, macrophages and plasma cells	Corticosteroids Anti-retrovirals in HIV Mortality up to 38%

HRCT, high-resolution computed tomography.

Box 24.49 Some causes of hypersensitivity pneumonitis

Disease	Situation	Antigens
Farmer's lung	Forking mouldy hay or any other mouldy vegetable material	Thermophilic actinomycetes, e.g. *Micropolyspora faeni* Fungi, e.g. *Aspergillus umbrosus*
Bird fancier's lung	Handling pigeons, cleaning lofts or budgerigar cages	Proteins present in the 'bloom' on the feathers and in excreta
Maltworker's lung	Turning germinating barley	*Aspergillus clavatus*
Humidifier fever	Contaminated humidifying systems in air conditioners or humidifiers in factories (especially in printing works)	Possibly a variety of bacterium or amoeba (e.g. *Naegleria gruberi*) Thermophilic actinomycetes
Mushroom worker's lung	Turning mushroom compost	Thermophilic actinomycetes
Cheese washer's lung	Mouldy cheese	*Penicillium casei* *Aspergillus clavatus*
Winemaker's lung	Mould on grapes	Botrytis

One of the most common causes worldwide is farmer's lung, which can affect up to 9% of farmers in humid climates. Interestingly, cigarette smokers have a lower risk of developing HP due to decreased antibody reaction to the antigen, but once established, smoking may lead to a more chronic or severe disease course.

Pathogenesis

Histological features include:

- a chronic inflammatory infiltrate
- poorly defined interstitial granulomas
- interstitial fibrosis and honeycomb change in chronic disease (may be indistinguishable from other causes of pulmonary fibrosis).

The allergic response to the inhaled antigen involves both cellular immunity and the deposition of immune complexes, causing foci of inflammation through the activation of complement via the classical pathway. Some of the inhalant materials may also lead to inflammation by directly activating the alternate complement pathway. These mechanisms attract and activate alveolar and interstitial macrophages so that continued antigenic exposure results in the progressive development of pulmonary fibrosis.

Clinical features

HP can be categorized according to the chronicity of symptoms, as determined by duration and intensity of exposure. Symptoms include malaise, dyspnoea and cough. Weight loss is a prominent feature of subacute and chronic HP. Auscultation reveals inspiratory squeaks due to bronchiolitis, and bilateral fine crackles. Wheeze is uncommon.

- ***Acute***: symptom onset 4–6 h following exposure. Fever is common and patients may be mistakenly diagnosed with a chest infection. Resolution occurs 24–48 h following removal from the inciting antigen.
- ***Subacute***: usually occurs with intermittent or lower-level exposure. Improvement is seen in weeks to months following removal from exposure.
- ***Chronic***: usually no history of preceding acute symptoms. Insidious onset of respiratory and constitutional symptoms is typical. Finger clubbing may be present. Progression to irreversible fibrosis is associated with increased mortality.

Investigations

A diagnosis can often be made by maintaining a high index of suspicion and taking a detailed exposure history. Identification of a culprit antigen in the context of typical clinical and radiological findings often makes lung biopsy unnecessary.

- ***Chest X-ray*** is neither sensitive nor specific for HP and may be normal in acute and subacute disease. When present, abnormalities include diffuse small nodules and increased reticular shadowing.
- ***HRCT*** shows nodules with ground-glass opacity and evidence of air trapping. Increased reticulation and honeycomb change are seen in advanced disease. Abnormalities are most marked in the mid-/upper zones.
- ***Lung function tests*** are used to assess the degree of respiratory impairment but are not diagnostic. A restrictive ventilatory defect with decreased carbon monoxide gas transfer is seen in chronic disease.
- ***Precipitating antibodies*** are present in the serum. One-quarter of pigeon fanciers have precipitating IgG antibodies against pigeon protein and droppings in their serum, but only a small proportion have lung disease. Precipitating antibodies are therefore evidence of exposure, not disease.
- ***Bronchoalveolar lavage*** shows a lymphocytosis. A low CD4:CD8 ratio can help differentiate HP from sarcoidosis.
- ***Lung biopsy*** demonstrates a lymphocyte-rich infiltrate with varying degrees of fibrosis, depending on chronicity of disease.

Differential diagnosis

Although hypersensitivity pneumonitis due to inhalation of the spores of *Micropolyspora faeni* is common among farmers, it is probably more common for these individuals to suffer from asthma related to inhalation of antigens from a variety of mites that infest stored grain and other vegetable material, such as *Lepidoglyphus domesticus, L. destructor* and *Acarus siro*. Symptoms of asthma resulting from inhalation of these allergens are often mistaken for farmer's lung. Alternative differentials include one of the other interstitial lung diseases.

Management

The key to successful treatment is avoidance of exposure to the inciting antigen (if known) and this may be achieved by changes in work practice. Pigeon fancier's lung is more difficult to control since affected individuals remain strongly attached to their hobby. Prednisolone should be initiated in patients whose symptoms persist despite withdrawal from the causative antigen, and in severe disease. Established fibrosis will not resolve and, in some patients, the disease may progress inexorably to respiratory failure despite intensive therapy. Farmer's lung is a recognized occupational disease in the UK and sufferers are entitled to compensation, depending on their degree of disability.

Humidifier fever

Humidifier fever may present with the typical features of hypersensitivity pneumonitis without any radiographic changes, and is caused by humidifiers and air-conditioning units that emit a fine spray of antigenic microorganisms.

Rare interstitial lung diseases

Langerhans cell histiocytosis

This rare disease is characterized histologically by proliferation of Langerhans cells, identified by the presence of Birbeck granules on electron microscopy or the CD1a antigen on the surface of the cells. There is a wide variation in clinical presentation, from isolated lytic bone lesions to multisystem disease involving skin, lymph nodes and major organs (more commonly seen in young children). Pulmonary involvement occurs in 10% of Langerhans cell histiocytosis (LCH) cases and is strongly associated with cigarette smoking. Recurrent spontaneous pneumothorax is seen in up to 25% and is a common mode of presentation. HRCT shows characteristic interstitial thickening, nodules, cysts and honeycombing with mid- and upper zone predominance, which may be sufficient for diagnosis in a young smoker (typical age 20–40 years). Smoking cessation is essential. Various treatment strategies, including corticosteroids, chemotherapy agents and cladribine, have been used with variable success. Lung transplantation may be considered in advanced disease. Outcome varies from spontaneous remission to progressive end-stage fibrosis but overall 5-year survival is 75%.

Pulmonary lymphangioleiomyomatosis

Pulmonary lymphangioleiomyomatosis (LAM) is a rare disorder of premenopausal women, causing hamartomatous smooth muscle infiltration of the lungs. Gene mutations in the hamartin–tuberin complex are present; the gene products regulate the activity of rapamycin complex 1. Extrapulmonary involvement, especially with renal angiomyolipomas (hamartomas), is common. Some 15% of patients with pulmonary LAM have tuberous sclerosis. Presentation is with dyspnoea, chylous pleural effusions and pneumothorax. HRCT shows diffuse thin-walled cysts scattered throughout the lungs. Treatment with hormonal manipulation/oophorectomy has shown a variable response. Sirolimus (rapamycin) can be effective but lung transplantation may be necessary. Prognosis estimates range from 10 to 29 years.

Pulmonary alveolar proteinosis

This is a rare disease in which lipoproteinaceous material accumulates within the alveoli. It can be congenital but most cases are acquired and appear to have an autoimmune basis, with antibodies directed against the cytokine GM-CSF. The disease mostly affects men and presents with progressive exertional dyspnoea and cough. Inspiratory crackles are present in 50%. Diagnosis is made by bronchoalveolar lavage, which reveals a milky appearance and many large, foamy macrophages but few other inflammatory cells. Initial therapy is with whole-lung lavage.

Granulomatous lung disease

A granuloma is a mass or nodule composed of chronically inflamed tissue formed by the response of the mononuclear phagocyte system (macrophages/histiocytes) to an inciting antigen and characterized by the presence of epithelioid multinucleate giant cells. Granuloma formation acts to confine a pathogen and limit the extent of surrounding inflammation and tissue destruction. Granulomas are seen in TB and other infections, including fungal and helminthic ones, in sarcoidosis and in hypersensitivity pneumonitis. Granulomatous lung disease with pulmonary vasculitis is discussed on pages 1120–1121.

Sarcoidosis

Sarcoidosis is a multisystem granulomatous disorder, commonly affecting young adults and typically presenting with bilateral hilar lymphadenopathy, pulmonary infiltration and skin or eye lesions. Beryllium poisoning can produce a clinical and histological picture identical to sarcoidosis, though contact with this element is now strictly controlled.

Epidemiology and aetiology

Sarcoidosis is a common disease of unknown aetiology that is often detected on routine chest X-ray. There is great geographical variation; sarcoidosis is most common in Northern Europe (annual incidence 5–40/100 000) but uncommon in Japan (incidence 1–2/100 000). In the USA, it is 3–4 times more prevalent in blacks than in Caucasians and they are more likely to develop extra-pulmonary or chronic disease. There is a female preponderance with peak incidence in the third and fourth decades. There is no relation with any histocompatibility antigen, but first-degree relatives have an increased risk of developing sarcoidosis (particularly in Caucasians). Other proposed aetiological factors are an atypical mycobacterium or fungus, the Epstein–Barr virus, and occupational, genetic, social or other environmental factors (sarcoidosis is more common in rural than in urban populations and less common in smokers). None of these has been substantiated.

Immunopathology

- Typical sarcoid granulomas consist of focal accumulations of epithelioid cells, macrophages and lymphocytes, mainly T cells.
- There is depressed cell-mediated reactivity to tuberculin; the Mantoux test is usually negative. There is overall lymphopenia; circulating T lymphocytes are low but B cells are slightly increased.
- Bronchoalveolar lavage shows a great increase in the overall number of cells; a lymphocytosis (particularly $CD4^+$ T-helper cells) is common.
- Transbronchial biopsies show infiltration of the alveolar walls and interstitial spaces with leucocytes, mainly T cells, prior to granuloma formation.

It seems likely that the decrease in circulating T lymphocytes and changes in delayed hypersensitivity responses are the result of sequestration of lymphocytes within the lung. There is no evidence to suggest that patients with sarcoidosis suffer from an overall defect in immunity, since the frequency of fungal, viral and bacterial infections is not increased and there is no evidence of any increased risk of developing malignant neoplasms.

Clinical features

Sarcoidosis can affect any organ ***(Box 24.50)*** but has a predilection for the lungs (involvement in up to 90%). Presentation may be with respiratory symptoms but it is not unusual for the diagnosis to be made incidentally on chest X-ray. Common extrathoracic manifestations include eye, skin or lymph node involvement, and constitutional upset with fatigue is a frequent and often refractory symptom. The combination of bilateral hilar lymphadenopathy, erythema nodosum, arthralgia and fever is known as Löfgren syndrome and is a common presentation with a very favourable prognosis. In this

Box 24.50 Clinical presentations of sarcoidosis

Constitutional
- Fever
- Weight loss
- Fatigue

Reticuloendothelial
- Splenomegaly
- Lymphadenopathy

Respiratory
- Stage I–IV pulmonary involvement ***(Box 24.52)***
- Cough
- Dyspnoea
- Wheeze

Hepatic
- Deranged liver function tests
- Hepatomegaly

Ocular
- Anterior uveitis
- Keratoconjunctivitis sicca

Hypercalcaemia/ hypercalciuria
- Hypercalciuria
- Nephrocalcinosis – may cause kidney injury
- Calculi

Cutaneous
- Erythema nodosum
- Lupus pernio

Neurological
- Cognitive dysfunction
- Headache
- Cranial nerve palsies
- Mononeuritis multiplex
- Peripheral neuropathy
- Seizures

Cardiac
- Arrhythmias
- Heart block
- Cardiomyopathy
- Sudden death

case, the constellation of symptoms is usually sufficient to make a clinical diagnosis. In less classic presentations, HRCT may show features highly suggestive of sarcoidosis but the presence of non-caseating granulomas on tissue biopsy of an affected organ is often sought for definitive diagnosis. Skin biopsy is comparatively non-invasive and careful examination for infiltration of scars and tattoos amenable to sampling should be undertaken, even in the absence of overt cutaneous involvement.

Pulmonary manifestations

Although pulmonary involvement may be an incidental finding, cough, exertional breathlessness and vague chest discomfort are common presentations. Even in symptomatic individuals, the chest is often clear to auscultation, although wheeze may be evident if there is significant involvement of the airways with endobronchial disease. There are four radiological stages of lung involvement, which helps inform prognosis ***(Box 24.51)***.

Patients may present with any stage of disease and do not necessarily progress through the stages sequentially. Moreover, the extent of disease on chest X-ray does not correlate with the degree of impairment on pulmonary function testing.

Bilateral hilar lymphadenopathy

Symmetrical bilateral hilar lymphadenopathy (BHL) is a characteristic feature of sarcoidosis; it is usually asymptomatic and only detected on chest X-ray. Occasionally, BHL is associated with a dull ache in the chest, malaise and a mild fever. The differential diagnosis of BHL includes:

- ***Lymphoma:*** this rarely affects the hilar lymph nodes in isolation.
- ***Pulmonary TB:*** hilar lymph nodes are usually asymmetrically enlarged.
- ***Carcinoma of the bronchus*** with malignant spread to the hilar lymph nodes: again, this is rarely symmetrical.

Pulmonary infiltration

Although the lung fields may appear normal on plain chest X-ray, the lung parenchyma is frequently involved, as shown by CT scanning ***(Fig. 24.40)***, transbronchial biopsy and bronchoalveolar lavage. Symptoms may be minimal (or even absent), despite quite marked radiographic abnormalities. Progressive disease may lead to irreversible fibrosis in up to 20% of cases. The principal differential

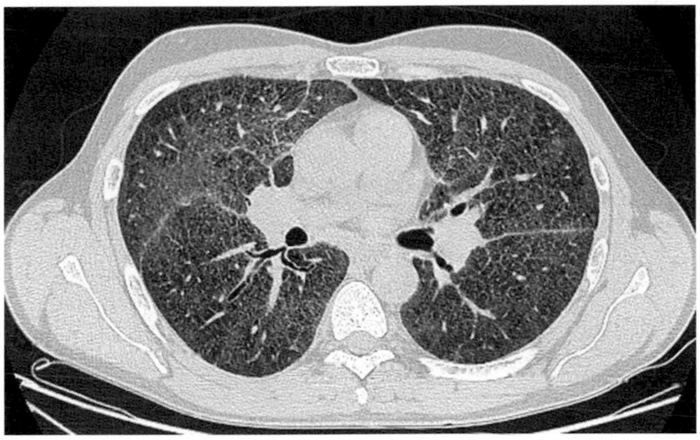

Figure 24.40 High-resolution CT scan in sarcoidosis. Note the bilateral hilar lymphadenopathy and reticular shadowing.

Box 24.51 Radiological stages of pulmonary sarcoidosis

X-ray

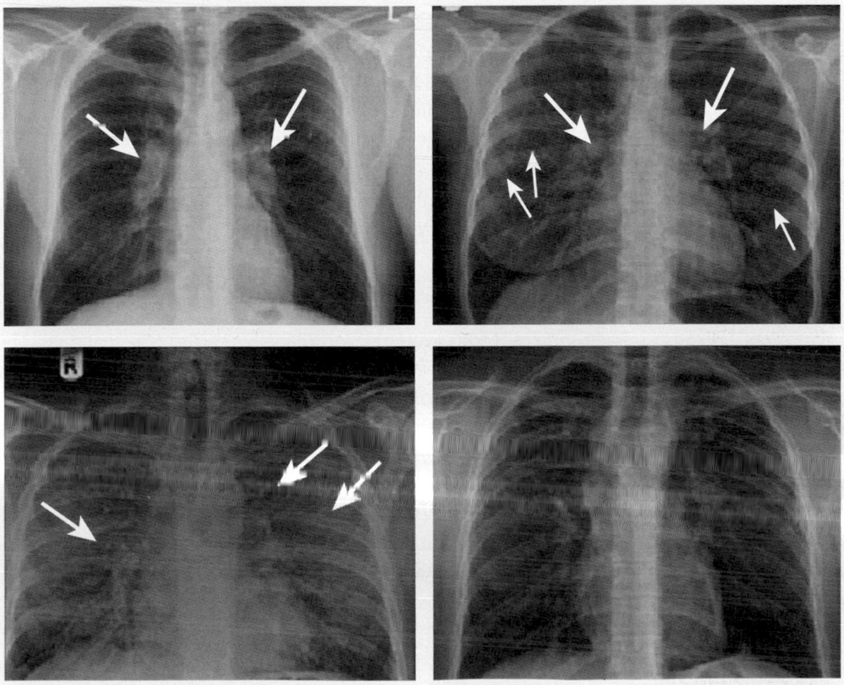

Stage	Chest X-ray appearance	Rate of spontaneous remission
Stage I	Bilateral hilar lymphadenopathy alone (BHL)	55–90%
Stage II	Pulmonary infiltrates with BHL	40–70%
Stage III	Pulmonary infiltrates without BHL	10–20%
Stage IV	Fibrosis	

diagnoses are TB, pneumoconiosis, idiopathic pulmonary fibrosis and hypersensitivity pneumonitis.

Extrapulmonary manifestations

Sarcoidosis can affect any organ. Cutaneous sarcoidosis and ocular sarcoidosis are the most common extrapulmonary presentations but cardiac and CNS involvement are the most important clinically.

Skin lesions. These occur in 10–30% of cases. Sarcoidosis is the most common cause of erythema nodosum (see p. 1363). Lupus pernio, presenting as indurated erythematous or violaceous papules/plaques, may be seen over the nose, cheeks and ears.

Eye lesions. Anterior uveitis is common and presents with misting of vision and a painful, red eye, but posterior uveitis may present simply as progressive loss of vision. Although ocular sarcoidosis accounts for about 5% of uveitis presenting to ophthalmologists, asymptomatic uveitis may be found in up to 25% of patients with sarcoidosis and all patients with a new diagnosis of sarcoidosis should undergo ophthalmological assessment. Keratoconjunctivitis sicca and lacrimal gland enlargement also occur.

Metabolic manifestations. Hypercalcaemia and hypercalciuria can lead to the development of renal calculi, nephrocalcinosis and, ultimately, renal failure.

Central nervous system. CNS involvement is rare (2%) but can lead to severe neurological disease (see p. 862).

Bone and joint involvement. Arthralgia without erythema nodosum is seen in 5% of cases. Bone cysts with associated swelling, particularly affecting the digits, may be seen on X-ray.

Hepatosplenomegaly. Mild derangement of liver function tests is common and granulomas are seen in the majority of biopsy specimens, although these findings are rarely of clinical consequence. Progression to portal hypertension or liver failure is uncommon.

Cardiac involvement. Ventricular dysrhythmias, conduction defects and cardiomyopathy with congestive cardiac failure are rare (3%). Severity ranges from benign rhythm disturbance to sudden cardiac death. All patients with sarcoidosis should have an ECG at presentation.

Investigations

- ***Imaging***. Chest X-ray is the initial modality for staging ***(Box 24.51)***. HRCT is useful for assessment of parenchymal involvement and may show a range of abnormalities, including nodules of 1–10 mm diameter that form a characteristic 'beading' appearance along airways, vessels and fissures; aggregation of nodules into larger nodules or masses (up to 3 cm); increased reticulation due to septal thickening; and honeycombing.
- ***Full blood count***. There may be a mild normochromic, normocytic anaemia with raised ESR.
- ***Biochemistry***. Hypercalcaemia occurs in 10–20% and hypercalciuria in 30–50%. Activated macrophages in lung and lymph nodes are able to hydroxylate vitamin D directly (independent of parathyroid hormone levels), leading to increased intestinal absorption of dietary calcium. Twenty-four-hour urinary calcium excretion should be measured at presentation.
- ***Serum angiotensin-converting enzyme (ACE) level***. This is elevated in over 75% of patients with untreated sarcoidosis. Raised (but lower) levels are also seen in patients with lymphoma, pulmonary TB, asbestosis and silicosis, limiting the diagnostic value of the test. The utility of serum ACE in monitoring disease activity and response to treatment is contentious.
- ***Bronchoalveolar lavage***. This typically shows a lymphocytosis with raised CD4:CD8 ratio.
- ***Transbronchial biopsy***. This is positive in up to 90% of cases of pulmonary sarcoidosis. Pulmonary non-caseating granulomas are found in approximately 50% of patients with extrapulmonary sarcoidosis in whom the chest X-ray is normal.
- ***Endobronchial biopsy***. When performed in addition to transbronchial biopsy, this may significantly increase the yield, even if the macroscopic appearances are normal.
- ***Lung function tests***. These show a restrictive lung defect with reduced gas transfer in patients with parenchymal infiltration or fibrosis. However, an obstructive defect may be seen in endobronchial disease and a mixed pattern is also possible. Lung function is usually normal in patients with isolated hilar adenopathy or extrapulmonary disease.

Prognosis and management

The natural history of sarcoidosis is unpredictable and varies from spontaneous remission to inexorable progression and death in a small number (1–5%). Even once remission has been achieved, relapses are common. Worse outcomes are seen in patients of Afro-Caribbean and Asian descent, and those presenting with extrathoracic disease. By contrast, patients presenting with *Löfgren syndrome* usually experience spontaneous resolution without the need for treatment. Systemic treatment is indicated for hypercalcaemia and extrathoracic major organ involvement, particularly neurological, cardiac or ocular disease resistant to topical therapy. **Treatment** of pulmonary sarcoidosis is less clear-cut, as spontaneous resolution is frequently seen, typically within the first 6 months. Moreover, although corticosteroids improve radiographic appearances, this is not consistently reflected in improved lung function tests. Treatment is therefore reserved for patients with troublesome symptoms, deteriorating lung function or radiological evidence of disease progression. Treatment for symptoms impacting on quality of life but not endangering major organs is a contentious issue and requires individual assessment. First-line treatment is with prednisolone (or equivalent) 0.5 mg/kg for 4–6 weeks, gradually tapering to a maintenance dose for at least 12 months. Alternative immunosuppressants, including methotrexate, azathioprine and hydroxychloroquine, have been used in place of, or in addition to, prednisolone. Relapses are common on withdrawal of therapy. Lung transplantation should be considered for suitable patients with stage IV disease and respiratory failure.

Small-vessel vasculitides

There are several systems for classifying the vasculitides. The nomenclature has moved away from eponymous syndromes in favour of terms describing the underlying disease process. The vasculitides associated with ***anti-neutrophil cytoplasmic antibody*** (***ANCA***) may be differentiated from other systemic small-vessel vasculitides by the lack of immune deposition. ANCA-associated vasculitides include granulomatosis with polyangiitis, microscopic polyangiitis and eosinophilic granulomatosis with polyangiitis. Staining for ANCA shows either a diffuse pattern (c-ANCA) with antibodies directed against proteinase 3 (PR3), or a perinuclear pattern (p-ANCA) with antibodies to myeloperoxidase (MPO) (see also pp. 744–755). The respiratory tract and kidneys are frequently involved and the ESR is often markedly elevated (>100).

Granulomatosis with polyangiitis

Granulomatosis with polyangiitis (GPA) typically affects older adults and is more common in Caucasians. The c-ANCA is usually positive with elevated PR3 antibodies. Constitutional symptoms are prominent and may precede the onset of organ-specific symptoms by many months. The ears and upper respiratory tract are frequently affected with bloody nasal discharge, crusting and destruction, sinusitis and otitis media. Evidence of glomerulonephritis should be sought on urinalysis (see p. 729). Respiratory symptoms include cough, dyspnoea and pleuritic chest pain. Diffuse alveolar haemorrhage occurs in up to 45% and haemoptysis can be life-threatening. Thoracic imaging characteristically shows multiple nodules that often cavitate, areas of consolidation and ground-glass opacification (which may be due to pulmonary haemorrhage). Diagnosis should be confirmed with biopsy of the active site but it is sometimes necessary to initiate empirical treatment in acutely unwell patients. Initial immunosuppressant therapy is with a combination of glucocorticoids and cyclophosphamide, rituximab or methotrexate.

Microscopic polyangiitis

Microscopic polyangiitis (MPA) is primarily associated with p-ANCA positivity. Presentation and treatment are similar to those of granulomatosis with polyangiitis. It is diagnosed on tissue biopsy, where the absence of granuloma formation differentiates it from GPA.

Eosinophilic granulomatosis with polyangiitis

Although ANCA is positive in up to 60% (usually p-ANCA), the presentation and prognosis of eosinophilic granulomatosis with polyangiitis (EGPA) differ from those of the other ANCA-associated vasculitides. The aetiology is uncertain. EGPA classically presents in early adulthood with allergic rhinitis, asthma that is often difficult to control, and peripheral blood eosinophilia (>10%). Systemic vasculitis subsequently develops, sometimes many years later. Involvement of skin (tender subcutaneous nodules, petechiae or purpuric lesions), peripheral nerves (mononeuritis multiplex), heart, kidneys and gastrointestinal tract may occur. The chest X-ray shows migratory patchy opacities that may be accompanied by nodules and pleural effusions. Bronchoalveolar lavage demonstrates an eosinophilia, and biopsy of affected tissues shows eosinophilic infiltration, vasculitis affecting the small arteries, veins and capillaries, and perivascular necrotizing granulomas. EGPA generally responds well to corticosteroids, although additional immunosuppressants are required for severe or refractory disease. Occasionally, EGPA is 'unmasked' when oral steroids are withdrawn in patients being treated for asthma.

Anti-glomerular basement membrane disease (Goodpasture syndrome)

Anti-glomerular basement membrane (anti-GBM) disease is characterized by the triad of pulmonary haemorrhage, glomerulonephritis, and the presence of circulating antibodies directed against an antigen intrinsic to the basement membrane of both kidney and lung. Respiratory symptoms may precede the onset of glomerulonephritis by weeks or months. The chest X-ray shows transient patchy shadows due to intrapulmonary haemorrhage, although haemoptysis can vary from negligible to life-threatening. The carbon monoxide gas transfer is increased due to the presence of haemoglobin in the alveoli. The extent of renal recovery depends on early detection and treatment. Treatment is with plasmapheresis to remove circulating antibodies and immunosuppression (prednisolone and cyclophosphamide) to prevent further antibody production.

Diffuse alveolar haemorrhage

Bleeding into the alveolar spaces occurs in association with certain drugs, infections, autoimmune rheumatic diseases and vasculitis but can also occur without an identifiable precipitating cause. Haemoptysis may be minimal (or even absent), despite significant blood loss into the lungs. It is one of the relatively few causes of raised carbon monoxide gas transfer. Gas exchange is impaired due to the presence of blood in the alveoli and patients may present with severe respiratory failure requiring intensive care support. Treatment is directed at the underlying cause, if known.

Pulmonary manifestations of autoimmune rheumatic diseases

Rheumatoid disease

The lungs can be affected by rheumatoid arthritis (RA) and also by some of the drugs used in its treatment (***Fig. 24.41***; see also pp. 677–678).

- ***Pleural disease*** may take the form of rheumatoid effusions, which are often unilateral and tend to be chronic. Low glucose content is typical but not specific. Several forms of parenchymal disease can occur in patients with RA. These include fibrosis, rheumatoid nodules, cryptogenic organizing pneumonia, lymphoid interstitial pneumonia and bronchiectasis; other pulmonary problems include pulmonary hypertension. Some patients will have modified presentations because they are already on disease-modifying drugs such as prednisolone or methotrexate for their arthritis.
- ***Pulmonary fibrosis*** occurring in RA has similar clinical features to the idiopathic form of the disease but often follows a more chronic course (see p. 1113). In patients taking methotrexate, it is often impossible to determine whether fibrosis is due to the drug or the underlying disease; either way, methotrexate should be substituted for an alternative agent.
- ***Rheumatoid nodules*** appear on the chest X-ray as single or multiple nodules ranging in size from a few millimetres to a

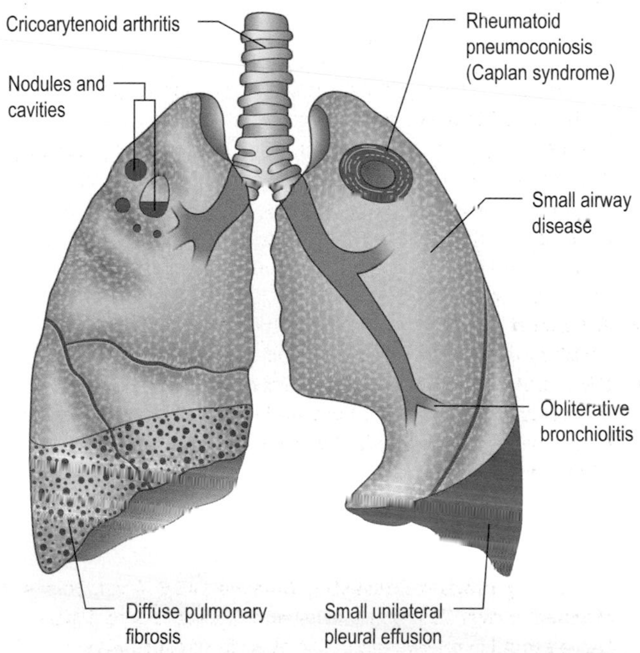

Figure 24.41 Respiratory manifestations of rheumatoid disease. Many drugs affect the lungs; see page 681.

few centimetres. The nodules frequently cavitate. They usually produce no symptoms but can give rise to a pneumothorax or pleural effusion.

- ***Obliterative bronchiolitis*** causing concentric narrowing of the bronchioles is a rare disorder characterized by progressive breathlessness and irreversible airflow limitation. Response to immunosuppressive therapy is generally poor but macrolide antibiotics may have a role.
- ***Cricoarytenoid joint involvement*** in RA gives rise to dyspnoea, stridor and hoarseness. Occasionally, severe obstruction necessitates tracheostomy.
- ***Caplan syndrome*** is due to occupational dust inhalation in the context of the disturbed immunity seen in RA. It occurs particularly in coal worker's pneumoconiosis but can occur in individuals exposed to other dusts, such as silica and asbestos. Typically, the chest X-ray shows rounded nodules 0.5–5.0 cm in diameter but progressive fibrosis can sometimes occur. These lesions may precede the development of arthritis. Rheumatoid factor is positive in the majority of patients.
- ***Drugs*** used in the treatment of RA can cause pulmonary problems, e.g. pneumonitis with methotrexate, gold and NSAIDs; fibrosis with methotrexate; bronchospasm with NSAIDs; infections with corticosteroids and methotrexate; and reactivation of TB with anti-TNF therapy.

Systemic lupus erythematosus

The most common respiratory manifestation of this disease is pleurisy, occurring in up to two-thirds of cases, with or without an effusion (see also p. 693). Effusions are usually small and bilateral. Basal pneumonitis is often present, perhaps as a result of poor movement of the diaphragm, or restriction of chest movements due to pleuritic pain. Pneumonia also occurs because of either infection or the disease process itself. In contrast to RA, diffuse pulmonary fibrosis is uncommon.

Systemic sclerosis

Some degree of lung involvement is present in the majority of cases and pulmonary complications are the leading cause of death (see p. 696). Interstitial fibrosis and pulmonary arterial hypertension are the most common pathologies. Patients should be carefully monitored for their development, as damage may be irreversible by the time symptoms have developed. Serial lung function testing can aid early detection. Other complications include bronchiectasis and aspiration pneumonitis secondary to oesophageal dilatation.

Pulmonary infiltration with eosinophilia

The common types and characteristics of these diseases are shown in **Box 24.52**. They range from simple pulmonary eosinophilia to the often fatal hypereosinophilic syndrome.

Simple and prolonged pulmonary eosinophilia

Simple pulmonary eosinophilia is a relatively mild illness, with a slight fever and cough, and usually lasts for less than 2 weeks. Occasionally, the disease becomes more prolonged, with a high fever lasting for over a month. There is usually an eosinophilia in the blood and the condition is then called prolonged pulmonary eosinophilia. In both conditions, the chest X-ray shows either localized or diffuse opacities. The simple form is probably due to a transient allergic reaction in the alveoli. Many allergens have been implicated, including *Ascaris lumbricoides*, *Ankylostoma*, *Trichuris*, *Trichinella*, *Taenia* and *Strongyloides*. Drugs such as aspirin, penicillin, nitrofurantoin and sulphonamides have also been implicated. However, often no allergen is identified. The disease is self-limiting and no treatment is required, apart from withdrawing culprit drugs and treating identified infective causes. In the more chronic form, all unnecessary treatment should be withdrawn and corticosteroid therapy is indicated, with resolution of the disease over the ensuing weeks.

Asthmatic bronchopulmonary eosinophilia

This is characterized by the presence of asthma, transient fleeting shadows on the chest X-ray, and blood or sputum eosinophilia. By far the most common cause worldwide is allergy to *Aspergillus fumigatus* (see below), although *Candida albicans* and other mycoses may be the inciting allergen in a small number of patients. In many, no allergen can be identified. Whether these cases are intrinsic or driven by an unidentified extrinsic factor is uncertain. Tropical pulmonary eosinophilia is the term reserved for an allergic reaction to microfilaria from *Wuchereria bancrofti*.

Diseases caused by *Aspergillus fumigatus*

The various types of lung disease caused by *A. fumigatus* are illustrated in **Figure 24.42**.

The spores of *A. fumigatus* (diameter 5 mm) are readily inhaled and are present in the atmosphere throughout the year, though they are at their highest concentration in the late autumn. They can be grown from the sputum in up to 15% of patients with chronic lung disease in whom they do not produce disease. They are a cause of extrinsic asthma in atopic individuals.

Allergic bronchopulmonary aspergillosis (asthmatic pulmonary eosinophilia)

This rare disease is caused by a hypersensitivity reaction when the bronchi are colonized by *Aspergillus*. It can complicate asthma and cystic fibrosis. Proximal bronchiectasis occurs.

Clinical features. There are episodes of eosinophilic pneumonia throughout the year, particularly in late autumn and winter. The episodes present with a wheeze, cough, fever and malaise. They are associated with expectoration of firm sputum plugs containing

Box 24.52 Common types and characteristics of pulmonary infiltration with eosinophilia

Disease	Symptoms	Blood eosinophils (%)	Multisystem involvement	Duration	Outcome
Simple pulmonary eosinophilia	Mild	10	None	<1 month	Good
Prolonged pulmonary eosinophilia	Mild/moderate	>20	None	>1 month	Good
Asthmatic bronchopulmonary eosinophilia	Moderate/severe	5–20	None	Years	Fair
Tropical pulmonary eosinophilia	Moderate/severe	>20	None	Years	Fair
Hypereosinophilic syndrome	Severe	>20	Always	Months/years	Poor

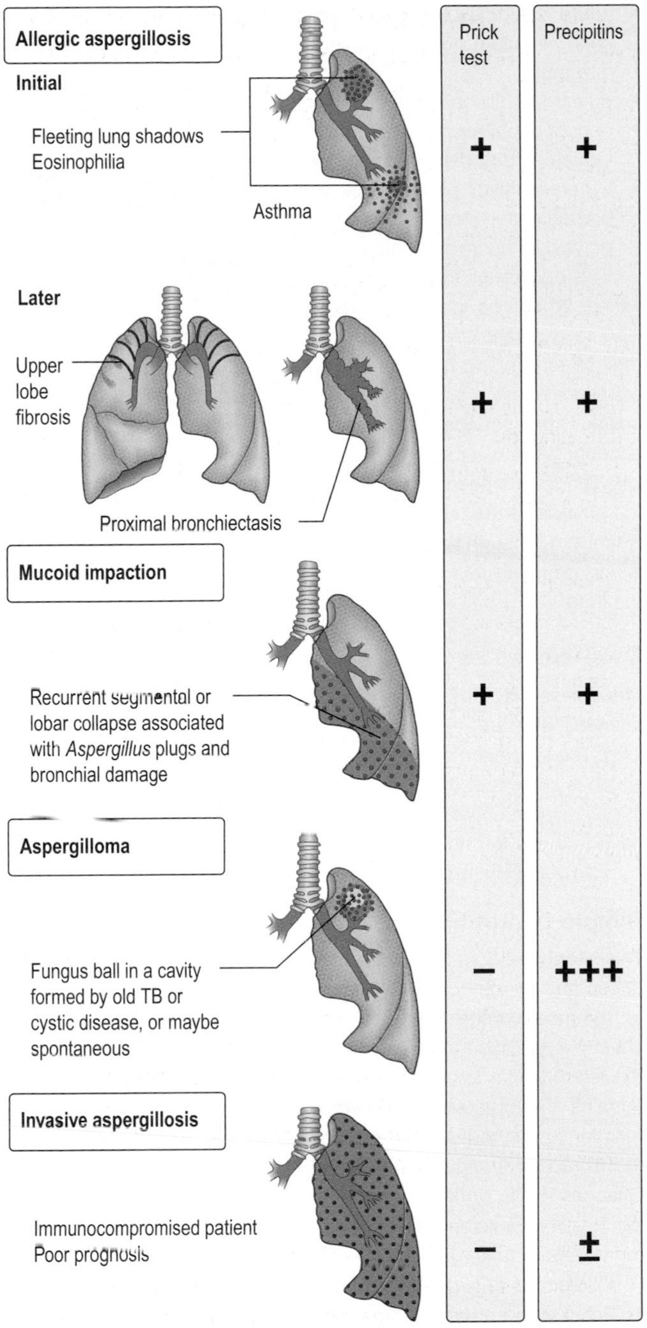

Figure 24.42 Diseases caused by *Aspergillus fumigatus*.

the fungal mycelium, which results in clearing of the pulmonary infiltrates on the chest X-ray. Occasionally, large mucus plugs obliterate the [illegible], causing collapse of the lung.

Left untreated, repeated episodes of eosinophilic pneumonia can result in progressive pulmonary fibrosis that usually affects the upper zones and can give rise to a chest X-ray appearance similar to that produced by TB.

Investigations. The peripheral blood eosinophil count is usually raised, and total levels of IgE are usually extremely high, at >1000 ng/mL (both that specific to *Aspergillus* and nonspecific). Skin-prick testing to protein allergens from *A. fumigatus* gives rise to positive immediate skin tests. Sputum may show eosinophils and mycelia. Precipitating antibodies are usually, but not always, found in the serum.

Lung function tests show a decrease in lung volumes and gas transfer in more chronic cases, but there is evidence of reversible airflow limitation in all cases.

Treatment. Therapy is with prednisolone 30 mg daily, which causes rapid clearing of the pulmonary infiltrates. Frequent episodes of the disease can be prevented by long-term treatment with prednisolone, but doses of 10–15 mg daily are usually required. Antifungal agents (itraconazole, voriconazole) should be used in patients on high doses of steroids; there is evidence that treatment with itraconazole improves pulmonary function. The asthma component responds to inhaled corticosteroids, although these do not influence the occurrence of pulmonary infiltrates. Omalizumab, a humanized monoclonal antibody against IgE, is being trialled.

Aspergilloma and invasive aspergillosis

Aspergilloma is the growth of *A. fumigatus* within previously damaged lung tissue, where it forms a ball of mycelium within lung cavities. Typically, the chest X-ray shows a round lesion with an air 'halo' above it. Continuing antigenic stimulation gives rise to large quantities of precipitating antibody in the serum. The aspergilloma itself causes little trouble, though occasionally massive haemoptysis may occur, requiring resection of the area of damaged lung containing the aspergilloma. The antifungal agent voriconazole is the drug of choice, although isavuconaxole appears to have fewer adverse effects. Amphotericin is used if patients are intolerant of voriconazole. Invasive aspergillosis is a well-recognized complication of immunosuppression and requires aggressive antifungal therapy.

The hypereosinophilic syndrome

This disease is characterized by eosinophilic infiltration in various organs, sometimes associated with an eosinophilic arteritis. The heart muscle is particularly involved, but pulmonary involvement in the form of a pleural effusion or interstitial lung disease occurs in about 40% of cases. Typical features are fever, weight loss, recurrent abdominal pain, persistent non-productive cough and congestive cardiac failure. Corticosteroid treatment may be of value in some cases.

Drug and radiation-induced respiratory reactions

Drugs affecting the respiratory system are shown in ***Box 24.53***, together with the types of reaction they produce. The mechanisms are varied and include direct toxicity (e.g. bleomycin), immune complex formation with arteritis, hypersensitivity (involving both T-cell and IgE mechanisms) and autoimmunity. TB reactivation is seen with immunosuppressive drugs.

Pulmonary infiltrates with fibrosis may result from a number of cytotoxic drugs used in the treatment of cancer. The most common cause of these reactions is bleomycin. The pulmonary damage is dose-related, occurring when the total dosage is >450 mg, but will regress in some cases if the drug is stopped. The most sensitive test is a decrease in carbon monoxide gas transfer, and therefore gas transfer should be measured repeatedly during treatment with the drug. The use of corticosteroids may help resolution. Anaphylaxis with bronchospasm can occur with many drugs. The list is not exhaustive; for example, over 20 different drugs are known to produce a systemic lupus erythematosus-like syndrome, sometimes complicated by pulmonary infiltrates and fibrosis. Paraquat

Box 24.53 Some drug-induced respiratory reactions

Bronchospasm
- Penicillins, cephalosporins
- Sulphonamides
- Aspirin/NSAIDs
- Monoclonal antibodies, e.g. infliximab
- Iodine-containing contrast media
- β-Adrenoceptor-blocking drugs (e.g. propranolol)
- Non-depolarizing muscle relaxants
- Intravenous thiamine
- Adenosine

Interstitial lung disease and/or fibrosis
- Amiodarone
- Anakinra (IL-1 receptor antagonist)
- Nitrofurantoin
- Paraquat
- Continuous oxygen
- Cytotoxic agents (many, particularly busulfan, CCNU, bleomycin, methotrexate)

Pulmonary eosinophilia
- Antibiotics:
  - Penicillin
  - Tetracycline
- Sulphonamides, e.g. sulfasalazine
- NSAIDs
- Cytotoxic agents

Acute lung injury
- (Paraquat – a weedkiller)

Pulmonary hypertension
- Fenfluramine, dexfenfluramine, phentermine

SLE-like syndrome including pulmonary infiltrates, effusions and fibrosis
- Hydralazine
- Procainamide
- Isoniazid
- Phenytoin
- ACE inhibitors
- Monoclonal antibodies

Reactivation of tuberculosis
- Immunosuppressant drugs, e.g. steroids
- Biological agents, e.g. tumour necrosis factor blockers

ACE, angiotensin-converting enzyme; CCNU, chloroethyl-cyclohexyl-nitrosourea (lomustine); IL-1, interleukin 1; NSAIDs, non-steroidal anti-inflammatory drugs; SLE, systemic lupus erythematosus.

ingestion causes severe pulmonary oedema and death, and pulmonary fibrosis develops in many of the few who survive.

Irradiation of the lung during radiotherapy can cause a radiation pneumonitis. Patients complain of breathlessness and a dry cough. Radiation pneumonitis results in a restrictive lung defect. Corticosteroids should be given in the acute stage.

Further reading

Chen M, Kallenberg CG. ANCA-associated vasculitides – advances in pathogenesis and treatment. *Nat Rev Rheumatol* 2010; 6:653–664.
Danoff SK, Terry PB, Horton MR. A clinician's guide to the diagnosis and treatment of interstitial lung disease. *South Med J* 2007; 100:579–587.
Fraser E, Hoyles RK. Therapeutic advances in idiopathic pulmonary fibrosis. *Clin Med (Lond)* 2016; 16:42–51.
King TE. Clinical advances in the diagnosis and therapy of interstitial lung disease. *Am J Respir Crit Care Med* 2005; 172:268–279.
Rockey DC, Darwin Bell P, Hill JA. Fibrosis – a common pathway to organ injury and failure. *N Engl J Med* 2015; 372:1138–1149.
Segal BH. Aspergillosis. *N Engl J Med* 2009; 360:1870.
Tazi A. Adult pulmonary Langerhans' cell histiocytosis. *Eur Respir J* 2006; 27:1272–1285.
Travis WD, Costabel U, Hansell DM et al. An official American Thoracic Society/European Respiratory Society statement: update of the international multidisciplinary classification of the idiopathic interstitial pneumonias. *Am J Respir Crit Care Med* 2013; 188:733–748.

OCCUPATIONAL LUNG DISEASE

Exposure to dusts, gases, vapours and fumes at work can cause several different types of lung disease:

- acute bronchitis and even pulmonary oedema from irritants such as sulphur dioxide, chlorine, ammonia or the oxides of nitrogen
- pulmonary fibrosis due to mineral dust
- occupational asthma (see **Box 24.22**) – now the most common industrial lung disease in the developed world
- hypersensitivity pneumonitis (see **Box 24.49**)
- bronchial carcinoma due to industrial agents (e.g. asbestos, polycyclic hydrocarbons, radon in mines).

The degree of fibrosis that follows inhalation of mineral dust varies. While iron (siderosis), barium (baritosis) and tin (stannosis) lead to dramatic, dense, nodular shadowing on the chest X-ray, their effect on lung function and symptoms is minimal. In contrast, exposure to silica or asbestos leads to extensive fibrosis and disability. Coal dust has an intermediate fibrogenic effect and used to account for 90% of all compensated industrial lung diseases in the UK. The term 'pneumoconiosis' means the accumulation of dust in the lungs and the reaction of the tissue to its presence. The term is not wide enough to encompass all occupational lung disease and is now generally used only in relation to coal dust and its effects on the lung.

Coal-worker's pneumoconiosis

The disease is caused by dust particles approximately 2–5 μm in diameter that are retained in the small airways and alveoli of the lung. The incidence of the disease is related to total dust exposure, which is highest at the coal face, particularly if ventilation and dust suppression are poor. Improved ventilation and working conditions have reduced the risk of this disease.

Two very different syndromes result from the inhalation of coal.

Simple pneumoconiosis

This simply reflects the deposition of coal dust in the lung. It produces fine micronodular shadowing on the chest X-ray and is by far the most common type of pneumoconiosis. It is graded on the chest X-ray appearance according to standard categories set by the International Labour Office (see below). Considerable dispute remains about the effects of simple pneumoconiosis on respiratory function and symptoms. In many cases, the symptoms are due to COPD related to cigarette smoking, but this is not always the case. Changes to UK workers' compensation legislation means that coal miners who develop COPD are compensated for their disability, regardless of their chest X-ray appearance.

Categories of simple pneumoconiosis are as follows:

1. Small round opacities definitely present but few in number.
2. Small round opacities numerous but normal lung markings still visible.
3. Small round opacities very numerous and normal lung markings partly or totally obscured.

Simple pneumoconiosis can progress to the development of progressive massive fibrosis (see below). The latter virtually never occurs on a background of category 1 simple pneumoconiosis but does arise in about 7% of those with category 2 and in 30% of those with category 3 disease. Miners with category 1 pneumoconiosis are unlikely to receive compensation unless they also have evidence of COPD. Those with more extensive radiographic changes are compensated solely on the basis of their X-ray appearances.

Progressive massive fibrosis

In progressive massive fibrosis (PMF), patients develop round fibrotic masses several centimetres in diameter, almost invariably situated in the upper lobes and sometimes having necrotic central cavities. The pathogenesis of PMF is still not understood, though it seems clear that some fibrogenic promoting factor is present in individuals developing the disease, leading to the formation of immune complexes, analogous to the development of large fibrotic nodules in coal miners with rheumatoid arthritis (Caplan syndrome). Rheumatoid factor and anti-nuclear antibodies are both often present in the serum of patients with PMF, and also in those suffering from asbestosis or silicosis. Pathologically, there is apical destruction and disruption of the lung, resulting in emphysema and airway damage. Lung function tests show a mixed restrictive and obstructive ventilatory defect with loss of lung volume, irreversible airflow limitation and reduced gas transfer.

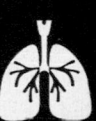

The patient with PMF suffers considerable effort dyspnoea, usually with a cough. The sputum may be black. The disease can progress (or even develop) after exposure to coal dust has ceased and may lead to respiratory failure.

Silicosis

This disease is uncommon, though it may still be encountered in stonemasons, sand-blasters, pottery and ceramic workers, and foundry workers involved in fettling (removing sand from metal castings made in sand-filled moulds). Silicosis is caused by the inhalation of silica (silicon dioxide). This dust is highly fibrogenic. For example, a coal miner can remain healthy with 30 g of coal dust in his lungs but 3 g of silica is sufficient to kill. Silica seems particularly toxic to alveolar macrophages and readily initiates fibrogenesis. The chest X-ray appearances and clinical features of silicosis are similar to those of PMF, but distinctive thin streaks of calcification may be seen around the hilar lymph nodes ('eggshell' calcification).

Diseases caused by asbestos

Asbestos is a mixture of silicates of iron, magnesium, nickel, cadmium and aluminium, and has the unique property of occurring naturally as a fibre. It is remarkably resistant to heat, acid and alkali, and has been widely used for roofing, insulation and fireproofing. Asbestos has been mined in southern Africa, Canada, Australia and Eastern Europe. Several *different types of asbestos* are recognized: about 90% of asbestos is chrysotile, 6% crocidolite and 4% amosite.

Chrysotile (white asbestos) is the softest asbestos fibre. Each fibre is often as long as 2 cm but only a few microns thick. It is less fibrogenic than crocidolite.

Crocidolite (blue asbestos) is particularly resistant to chemical destruction and exists in straight fibres up to 50 mm in length and 1–2 μm in width. Crocidolite is the type of asbestos most likely to produce asbestosis and mesothelioma. This may be due to the fact that it is readily trapped in the lung. Its long, thin shape means that it can be inhaled, but subsequent rotation against the long axis of the smaller airways, particularly in turbulent airflow during expiration, causes the fibres to impact. Crocidolite is also particularly resistant to macrophage and neutrophil enzymatic destruction.

Exposure to asbestos occurred particularly in shipbuilding yards and in power stations, but it was used so widely that low levels of exposure were very common. Up to 50% of city dwellers have asbestos bodies (asbestos fibres covered in protein secretions) in their lungs at postmortem. Regulations in the UK prohibit the use of crocidolite and severely restrict the use of chrysotile. Careful dust control measures are enforced, which should eventually abolish the problem. Workers continue to be exposed to blue asbestos in the course of demolition or in the replacement of insulation, and it should be remembered that there is a considerable time lag between exposure and development of disease, particularly mesothelioma (20–40 years).

The risk of primary lung cancer (usually adenocarcinoma) is increased in people exposed to asbestos, even in non-smokers. This risk is about 5–7-fold greater in those who have parenchymal asbestosis and about 1.5 fold in those with pleural plaques without parenchymal fibrosis. A synergistic relationship exists between asbestosis and cigarette smoking, with the risk of bronchial carcinoma multiplied about 5-fold above the risk attributable to smoking alone.

Diseases caused by asbestos are summarized in ***Box 24.54***. Bilateral diffuse pleural thickening, asbestosis, mesothelioma and asbestos-related carcinoma of the bronchus are all eligible for industrial injuries benefit in the UK.

Box 24.54 The effects of asbestos on the lung

Effect	Exposure	Chest X-ray	Lung function	Symptoms	Outcome
Asbestos bodies	Light	Normal	Normal	None	Evidence of asbestos exposure only
Pleural plaques	Light	Pleural thickening (parietal pleura) and calcification (also in diaphragmatic pleura)	Mild restrictive ventilatory defect	Rare, occasional mild effort dyspnoea	No other sequelae
Effusion	First two decades following exposure	Effusion	Restrictive	Pleuritic pain, dyspnoea	Often recurrent
Bilateral diffuse pleural thickening	Light/moderate	Bilateral diffuse thickening (of both parietal and visceral pleura) >5 mm thick and extending over more than ¼ of the chest wall	Restrictive ventilatory defect	Effort dyspnoea	May progress in absence of further exposure
Mesothelioma	Light (interval of 20–40 years from exposure to disease)	Pleural effusion, usually unilateral	Restrictive ventilatory defect	Pleuritic pain, increasing dyspnoea	Median survival 2 years
Asbestosis	Heavy (interval of 5–10 years from exposure to disease)	Diffuse bilateral streaky shadows, honeycomb lung	Severe restrictive ventilatory defect and reduced gas transfer	Progressive dyspnoea	Poor, progression in some cases after exposure
Asbestos-related carcinoma of the bronchus	The features of asbestosis, bilateral diffuse pleural thickening or bilateral pleural plaques plus those of bronchial carcinoma				Fatal

Asbestosis

Asbestosis is defined as fibrosis of the lungs caused by asbestos dust, which may or may not be associated with fibrosis of the parietal or visceral layers of the pleura. It is a progressive disease characterized by breathlessness and accompanied by finger clubbing and bilateral basal end-inspiratory crackles. Minor degrees of fibrosis that are not seen on chest X-ray are often revealed on HRCT scan. No treatment is known to alter the progress of the disease, though corticosteroids are often prescribed.

Mesothelioma

The number of cases of mesothelioma has increased progressively since the mid-1980s and has now reached 2100 deaths/year in the UK, which has the highest *per capita* death rate from this condition. Rates of mesothelioma in the UK are expected to peak around 2020 at about 2300/year. The most common presentation of mesothelioma is a pleural effusion, typically with persistent chest wall pain, which should raise the index of suspicion even if the initial pleural fluid or biopsy samples are non-diagnostic. Video-assisted thoracoscopic pleural biopsy is often needed to obtain sufficient tissue for diagnosis. Clinical trials of chemotherapy, sometimes combined with surgery, are under way but the outlook for most patients remains very limited.

Byssinosis

This disease occurs worldwide but is declining rapidly in areas where the number of people employed in cotton mills is falling. Typically, symptoms start on the first day back at work after a break (Monday sickness), with improvement as the week progresses. Tightness in the chest, cough and breathlessness occur within the first hour in dusty areas of the mill, particularly in the blowing and carding rooms where raw cotton is cleaned and the fibres are straightened.

The exact nature of the disease and its aetiology remain disputed. Pure cotton does not cause the disease, and cotton dust has some effect on airflow limitation in all those exposed. Individuals with asthma are particularly badly affected by exposure to cotton dust. The most likely aetiology is endotoxins from bacteria present in the raw cotton causing constriction of the airways of the lung. There are no changes on the chest X-ray and there is considerable dispute as to whether the progressive airflow limitation seen in some patients with the disease is due to cotton dust or to other factors such as cigarette smoking or coexistent asthma.

Berylliosis

Beryllium–copper alloy has a high tensile strength and is resistant to metal fatigue, high temperature and corrosion. It is used in the aerospace industry, atomic reactors and many electrical devices.

When beryllium is inhaled, it can cause a systemic illness with a clinical picture similar to sarcoidosis. Clinically, there is progressive dyspnoea with pulmonary fibrosis. However, strict control of levels in the working atmosphere has made this disease a rarity.

Further reading

Lin RT, Takahashi K, Karjalainen A et al. Ecological association between asbestos-related diseases and historical asbestos consumption. *Lancet* 2007; 369:844–849.

LUNG CYSTS

These can be congenital, bronchogenic or the result of a sequestrated pulmonary segment. Hydatid disease causes fluid-filled cysts. Lung abscesses are thin-walled cysts, which are found particularly in staphylococcal pneumonia, tuberculous cavities, septic pulmonary infarction, primary bronchogenic carcinoma, cavitating metastatic neoplasm, or paragonimiasis caused by the lung fluke *Paragonimus westermani*.

TUMOURS OF THE RESPIRATORY TRACT

Malignant tumours

Bronchial carcinoma

Bronchial carcinoma is the most common malignant tumour worldwide, with around 1.4 million deaths annually. It is the third most common cause of death in the UK after ischaemic heart disease and cerebrovascular disease, and is now the most common cause of cancer-related death in both men and women. Rates are declining in men but still increasing overall, reflecting the increasing incidence in women. The ratio in men to women is now 1.2 : 1.

Cigarette smoking (including passive smoke exposure) accounts for >90% of lung cancer. There remains a higher incidence of bronchial carcinoma in urban compared with rural areas, even when allowance is made for cigarette smoking. Other aetiological factors include:

- ***Environmental***: radon exposure, asbestos, polycyclic aromatic hydrocarbons and ionizing radiation; occupational exposure to arsenic, chromium, nickel, petroleum products and oils.
- ***Host factors***: pre-existing lung disease such as pulmonary fibrosis; HIV infection; genetic factors.

Legislative control over smoking in public places in many parts of the world has been introduced to reduce ill health related to cigarette smoke.

Pathophysiology

Historically, lung cancers have been broadly divided into small-cell carcinoma and non-small-cell carcinoma, based on the histological appearances of the cells seen within the tumour. This distinction is necessary with respect to the behaviour of the tumour, providing prognostic information and determining best treatment. Non-small-cell carcinoma is further divided into a number of cell types (adenocarcinoma, squamous cell carcinoma, large-cell carcinoma, large-cell neuroendocrine ***(Box 24.55)***. A number of molecular characteristics have been described more recently (largely affecting adenocarcinoma non-small-cell types), which confer potential prognostic benefit and may result in the ability to deliver a more personalized therapy with targeted agents. The most common of these are activating mutations within epidermal growth factor receptor (EGFR), most commonly encountered in non-smokers, females and those of Asian origin, and the presence of anaplastic lymphoma kinase (*ALK*) fusion oncogene, again more commonly found in non-/ex-smokers and younger patients.

Clinical features

The presentation and clinical course vary between the different cell types ***(Box 24.55)***. Symptoms and signs may be different, depending on the extent and site of disease.

Common presenting features can be divided into those caused by direct/local tumour effects, metastatic spread and non-metastatic extrapulmonary features.

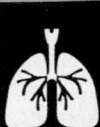

Box 24.55 Lung cancer cell types and clinical features

Cell type	Incidence in UK (%)	Features
Non-small-cell carcinoma		
Squamous cell carcinoma	35	Remain the most common cell type in Europe Arise from epithelial cells, associated with production of keratin Occasionally cavitate with central necrosis Cause obstructing lesions of bronchus with post-obstructive infection Local spread common, metastasize relatively late
Adenocarcinoma	27–30	Likely to become the most common cell type in the UK in the near future (most common cell type in the USA) Increasing incidence over last 10 years possibly linked to low-tar cigarettes Originate from mucus-secreting glandular cells Most common cell type in non-smokers Often cause peripheral lesions on chest X-ray/CT Subtypes include bronchoalveolar cell carcinoma (associated with copious mucus secretion, multifocal disease) Metastases common: pleura, lymph nodes, brain, bones, adrenal glands
Large cell carcinoma	10–15	Often poorly differentiated Metastasize relatively early
Small cell carcinoma	20	Arise from neuroendocrine cells (APUD cells) Often secrete polypeptide hormones Often arise centrally and metastasize early

Local effects

- ***Cough***. This is the most commonly encountered symptom in lung cancer. Because evidence suggests this symptom is neglected by both patients and healthcare professionals, campaigns in the UK have highlighted the '3-week cough' as a symptom that merits a chest X-ray.
- ***Breathlessness***. Central tumours occlude large airways, resulting in lung collapse and breathlessness on exertion. Many patients with lung cancer have coexistent COPD, which is also a cause of breathlessness.
- ***Haemoptysis***. Fresh or old blood is coughed up due to the tumour bleeding into an airway.
- ***Chest pain***. Peripheral tumours invade the chest wall or pleura (both well innervated), resulting in sharp pleuritic pain. Large-volume mediastinal nodal disease often results in a characteristic dull central chest ache.
- ***Wheeze***. This is monophonic when due to partial obstruction of an airway by tumour.
- ***Hoarse voice***. Mediastinal nodal or direct tumour invasion of the mediastinum results in compression of the left recurrent laryngeal nerve.
- ***Nerve compression***. Pancoast tumours in the apex of the lung invade the brachial plexus, causing C8/T1 palsy with small muscle wasting in the hand and weakness, as well as pain, radiating down the arm. An associated Horner syndrome due to compression of the sympathetic chain, with classic features of miosis, ptosis and anhidrosis, also occurs.
- ***Recurrent infections***. Tumour causing partial obstruction of an airway results in post-obstructive pneumonia.
- ***Direct invasion of the phrenic nerve***. Bronchial carcinoma invading the phrenic nerve causes paralysis of the ipsilateral hemidiaphragm. It can involve the oesophagus, producing progressive dysphagia, and the pericardium, resulting in pericardial effusion and malignant dysrhythmias.
- ***Superior vena caval obstruction***. See pages 605–606.
- ***Tracheal tumours***. These present with progressive dyspnoea and stridor. Flow–volume curves show dramatic reductions in inspiratory flow (see ***Fig. 24.7C***).

Metastatic spread

Bronchial carcinoma commonly spreads to mediastinal, cervical and even axillary or intra-abdominal nodes. In addition, the liver, adrenal glands, bones, brain and skin are frequent sites for metastases:

- ***Liver***. Common symptoms are anorexia, nausea and weight loss. Right upper quadrant pain radiating across the abdomen is associated with liver capsular pain.
- ***Bone***. Bony pain and pathological fractures occur as a result of tumour spread. If the spine is involved, there is a risk of spinal cord compression, which requires urgent treatment.
- ***Adrenal glands***. Metastases to the adrenals do not usually result in adrenal insufficiency and are usually asymptomatic.
- ***Brain***. Metastases present as space-occupying lesions with subsequent mass effect and signs of raised intracranial pressure. Less common presentations include carcinomatous meningitis with cranial nerve defects, headache and confusion.
- ***Malignant pleural effusion***. This presents with breathlessness and is commonly associated with pleuritic pain.

Non-metastatic extrapulmonary manifestations of bronchial carcinoma

(***Box 24.56***.) Minor haematological extrapulmonary manifestations of lung cancer, such as normocytic anaemia and thrombocytosis, are reasonably common. Apart from finger clubbing and hypertrophic pulmonary osteoarthropathy (HPOA), most other non-metastatic complications are relatively rare. Approximately 10% of small-cell tumours produce ectopic hormones, giving rise to paraneoplastic syndromes (see ***Box 17.8***).

Investigations

Investigations are necessary to:

- stage the extent of disease
- make a tissue diagnosis (differentiate small-cell from non-small-cell lung cancer (NSCLC), as well as to detail the cell type in NSCLC – increasingly relevant with newer targeted biological agents)
- assess fitness to undergo treatment.

Staging and diagnosis

Chest X-ray

Plain chest radiographs may show obvious evidence of lung cancer or non-specific appearances ***(Box 24.57)***. In some cases, the initial

Box 24.56 Non-metastatic extrapulmonary manifestations of bronchial carcinoma[a]

Metabolic (universal at some stage)
- Loss of weight
- Lassitude
- Anorexia

Endocrine (10%) (usually small-cell carcinoma)
- Ectopic adrenocorticotrophin syndrome
- Syndrome of inappropriate secretion of antidiuretic hormone (SIADH)
- Hypercalcaemia (usually squamous cell carcinoma)
- Rarer: hypoglycaemia, thyrotoxicosis, gynaecomastia

Neurological (2–16%)
- Encephalopathies – including subacute cerebellar degeneration
- Myelopathies – motor neurone disease
- Neuropathies – peripheral sensorimotor neuropathy
- Muscular disorders – polymyopathy, myasthenic syndrome (Eaton–Lambert syndrome)

Vascular and haematological (rare)
- Thrombophlebitis migrans
- Non-bacterial thrombotic endocarditis
- Microcytic and normocytic anaemia
- Disseminated intravascular coagulopathy
- Thrombotic thrombocytopenic purpura
- Haemolytic anaemia

Skeletal
- Clubbing (30%)
- Hypertrophic osteoarthropathy (± gynaecomastia) (3%)

Cutaneous (rare)
- Dermatomyositis
- Acanthosis nigricans
- Herpes zoster

[a]*Percentage of all cases.*

radiograph is normal, either because the lesion is small, or because disease is confined to central structures.

Computed tomography

CT indicates the extent of disease. Imaging should include the liver and adrenal glands, which are common sites for metastases. The International Association for the Study of Lung Cancer (IASLC) has devised the most widely used staging definitions, which are based on CT imaging of tumour size (T), nodal involvement (N) and metastases (M), along with prognostic data. These have been recently updated based on an extensive review of survival in over 80 000 patients ***(Box 24.58)***.

Using CT criteria, lymph nodes that are <1 cm in diameter are not classed as being enlarged, yet they can still contain malignant cells. With increasing size, the positive predictive value of CT in detecting malignant nodes increases; however, it cannot be assumed that enlarged nodes are definitely malignant and further staging tests should be performed if there are no distant metastases and the primary tumour is thought to be eligible for curative treatment. These tests would include direct sampling of affected nodes and PET to assess distant spread of cancer.

Positron emission tomography–computed tomography

This is the investigation of choice for characterizing the extent of mediastinal nodal involvement and highlighting distant metastases either not visualized or indeterminate on CT (see p. 1070). Most commonly, PET images are combined with CT for best correlation. Negative predictive value is high but a positive node on PET–CT should prompt sampling for confirmation of the presence of malignant cells, as the positive predictive value is relatively low.

Other imaging modalities

MRI is not useful for the diagnosis of primary lung tumours other than in Pancoast tumours with nerve invasion or in the assessment of chest wall involvement prior to surgery.

Fibreoptic bronchoscopy

This technique is used to define the bronchial anatomy and to obtain biopsy and cytological specimens ***(Fig. 24.43)***. If the carcinoma involves the first 2 cm of either main bronchus, the tumour is inoperable, as there would be insufficient resection margins for pneumonectomy. Widening and loss of the sharp angle of the carina indicate the presence of enlarged subcarinal lymph nodes, either malignant or reactive. These can be biopsied 'blind' by passage of a needle through the bronchial wall.

Percutaneous aspiration and biopsy

Peripheral lung lesions cannot be seen by fibreoptic bronchoscopy. Samples are obtained by aspiration or biopsy through the chest wall under CT guidance. The most common complication is pneumothorax (around 10% of patients), especially if the mass is deep in the lung, as opposed to lesions next to the parietal pleura. Mild haemoptysis occurs in <5%. Implantation metastases do not occur.

Endobronchial ultrasound

A fibreoptic scope with ultrasound probe is used in the staging of lung cancer, to visualize the majority of mediastinal nodes (not all of which are accessible surgically via mediastinoscopy or mediastinotomy) and then allow fine-needle aspiration.

Endoscopic ultrasound via the oesophagus can also be used with the added advantage of enabling sampling of the left adrenal gland, and posterior and inferior mediastinal lymph node groups. ***Figure 24.44*** shows the lymph node areas that are commonly involved and sampled in the staging investigations.

Ultrasound-guided supraclavicular node sampling

In selected cases, where staging suggests that N3 nodes are involved, even where supraclavicular nodes are not palpable, ultrasound fine-needle aspiration can be diagnostic.

Video-assisted thoracoscopic surgery

Large effusions with evidence of pleural thickening are amenable to biopsy and drainage via minimally invasive surgery. This technique is particularly useful, as pleurodesis to prevent recurrence of effusion can be performed at the same time.

Other investigations

These include a full blood count for the detection of anaemia, and biochemistry for liver involvement, hypercalcaemia and hyponatraemia.

Assessing fitness for treatment

Before radical treatment, an assessment of fitness for treatment should be carried out. This work-up should include full lung function testing with transfer capacity, and if cardiovascular disease is present, cardiopulmonary exercise testing, stress echo or, occasionally, preoperative angiography.

Management

Treatment of lung cancer (see also p. 630) involves several different modalities and should be planned by a multidisciplinary team. Unfortunately, the majority of patients have incurable disease at

Box 24.57 Lung cancer presentations on a chest X-ray

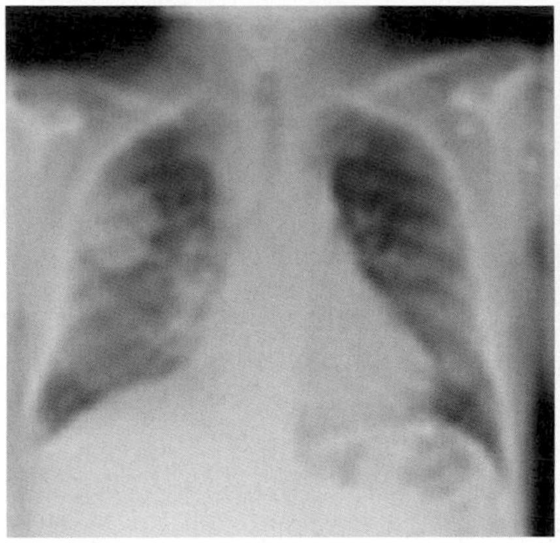

Mass lesion

Lesions visible if >1 cm in diameter. Spiculate, cavitating or smooth-edged. Often an incidental finding, usually asymptomatic if small. By the time symptoms are present, chest X-ray is almost always abnormal

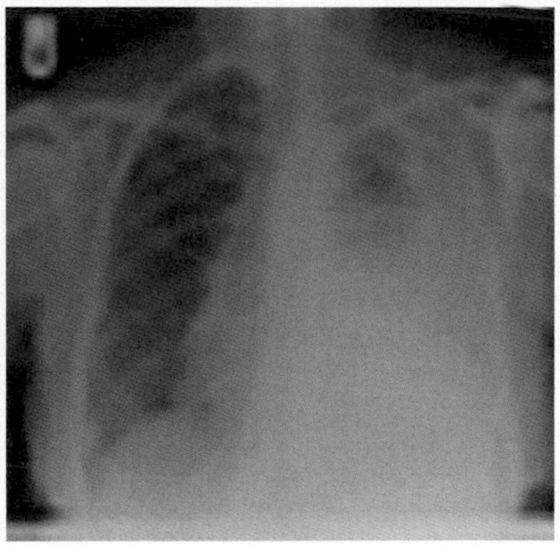

Pleural effusion

Usually unilateral; commonly large, which can obscure an underlying mass or pleural tumour. Mesothelioma is a differential diagnosis

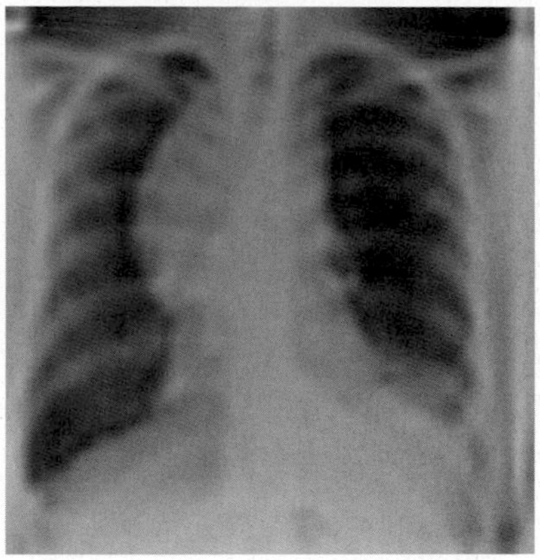

Mediastinal widening or hilar adenopathy

Lymphadenopathy evident on the plain film, manifested by splayed carina, hilar enlargement or paratracheal shadowing

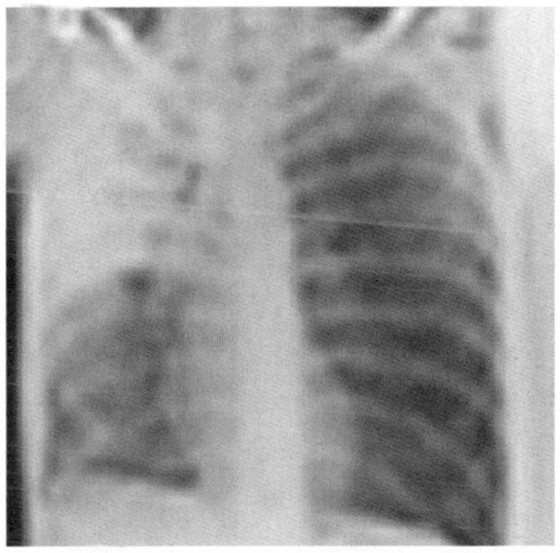

Slow-resolving consolidation

Tumour causes partial obstruction of a bronchus, resulting in retention of secretions, bacterial overgrowth and subsequent infection. (Persistent right upper lobe consolidation due to tumour in right upper lobe)

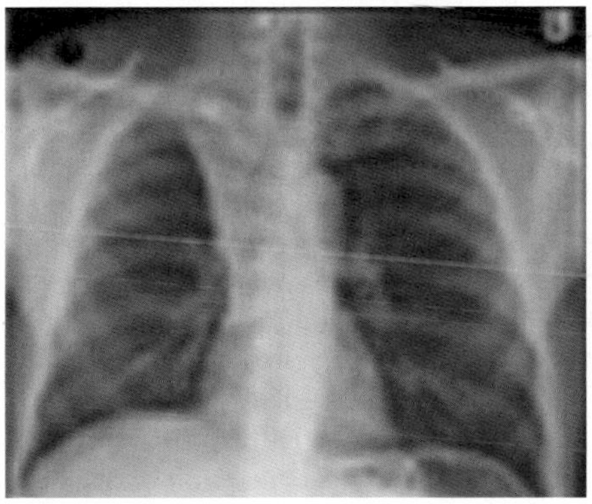

Collapse

Endoluminal tumour causes complete collapse of a lung and associated mediastinal shift, or collapse of a lobe or segment, resulting in volume loss on the affected side with raised hemidiaphragm/deviated trachea

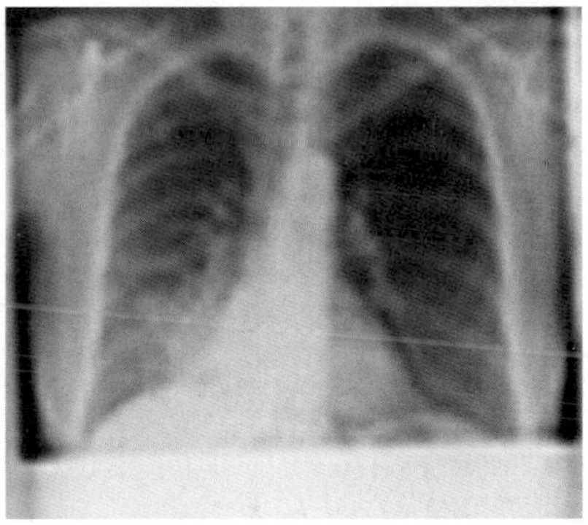

Reticular shadowing

Carcinoma spreads through the lymphatic channels of the lung to give rise to lymphangitis carcinomatosa; in bronchial carcinoma this is usually unilateral and associated with striking dyspnoea. Bilateral lymphangitis should prompt investigation for a primary site other then lung, such as breast, stomach or colon

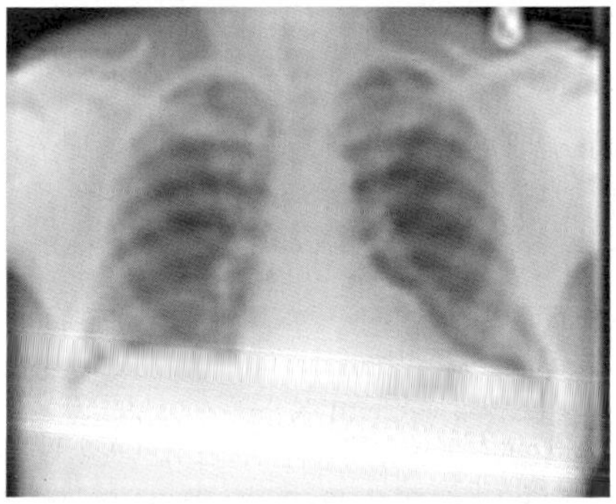

Normal

A normal film does not rule out an underlying tumour. A minority of tumours are confined to the central airways and mediastinum without obvious change on the plain chest X-ray. Although investigation of isolated haemoptysis with a normal chest X-ray is often negative, a normal chest X-ray should not discourage further investigation, especially in smokers over the age of 40 years

Box 24.58 TNM staging system for lung cancer

Notation	Description
T – primary tumour	
TX	Primary tumour cannot be assessed, or tumour proven by the presence of malignant cells in sputum or bronchial washings, but not visualized by imaging or bronchoscopy
T0	No evidence of primary tumour
Tis	Carcinoma *in situ*
T1	Tumour ≤3 cm in greatest dimension, surrounded by lung or visceral pleura, without bronchoscopic evidence of invasion more proximal than the lobar bronchus (i.e. not in the main bronchus)
T1a	Tumour ≤2 cm in greatest dimension
T1b	Tumour >2 cm but not more than 3 cm in greatest dimension
T2	Tumour >3 cm but not more than 7 cm; or tumour with any of the following features: Involves main bronchus, 2 cm or more distal to the carina Invades visceral pleura Associated with atelectasis or obstructive pneumonitis that extends to the hilar region but does not involve the entire lung
T2a	Tumour >3 cm but not more than 5 cm in greatest dimension
T2b	Tumour >5 cm but not more than 7 cm in greatest dimension
T3	Tumour >7 cm or one that directly invades any of the following: chest wall (including superior sulcus tumours), diaphragm, phrenic nerve, mediastinal pleura, parietal pericardium; or tumour in the main bronchus <2 cm distal to the carina but without involvement of the carina; or associated atelectasis or obstructive pneumonitis of the entire lung or separate tumour nodule(s) in the same lobe as the primary
T4	Tumour of any size that invades any of the following: mediastinum, heart, great vessels, trachea, recurrent laryngeal nerve, oesophagus, vertebral body, carina; separate tumour nodule(s) in a different ipsilateral lobe to that of the primary
N – regional lymph nodes	
NX	Regional lymph nodes cannot be assessed
N0	No regional lymph node metastasis
N1	Metastasis in ipsilateral peribronchial and/or ipsilateral hilar lymph nodes and intrapulmonary nodes, including involvement by direct extension
N2	Metastasis in ipsilateral mediastinal and/or subcarinal lymph node(s)
N3	Metastasis in contralateral mediastinal, contralateral hilar, ipsilateral or contralateral scalene, or supraclavicular lymph node(s)
M – distant metastasis	
M0	No distant metastasis
M1	Distant metastasis
M1a	Separate tumour nodule(s) in a contralateral lobe; tumour with pleural nodules or malignant pleural or pericardial effusion
M1b	Distant metastasis
The resultant stage groupings	
Occult carcinoma	TX, N0, M0
Stage 0	TisN0M0
Stage IA	T1a,bN0M0
Stage IB	T2aN0M0
Stage IIA	T2bN0M0; T1a,bN1M0; T2aN1M0
Stage IIB	T2bN1M0; T3N0M0
Stage IIIA	T1a,b, T2a,b, N2M0; T3N1, N2M0; T4N0, N1M0
Stage IIIB	T4N2M0; any T N3M0
Stage IV	Any T any NM1

(Adapted from Goldstraw P, Crowley J, Chansky K et al.; International Association for the Study of Lung Cancer International Staging Committee; Participating Institutions. The IASLC Lung Cancer Staging Project: proposals for the revision of the TNM stage groupings in the forthcoming (7th) edition of the TNM classification of malignant tumours. *Journal of Thoracic Oncology* 2007; 2(8):706–714. Erratum in: *Journal of Thoracic Oncology* 2007; 2(10):985.)

presentation, or have significant co-morbidities that preclude radical treatment. ***Box 24.59*** shows the mean survival based on tumour stage for NSCLC and squamous cell carcinoma: only 25–30% patients are still alive 1 year after diagnosis and only 6–8% after 5 years.

Surgery

Surgery is performed in early-stage NSCLC (stages I, II and selected IIIA) with curative intent. Many patients with stage III disease are treated with chemoradiation with a view to 'downstaging' disease and rendering it amenable to surgical resection. Where surgical

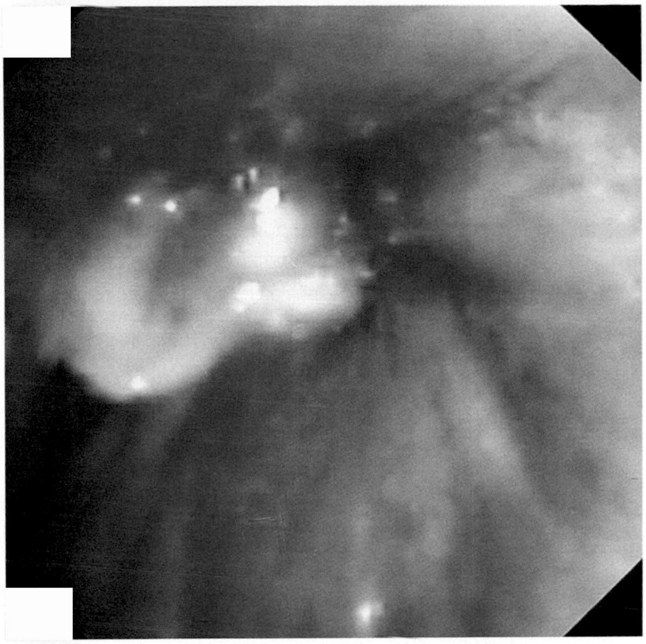

Figure 24.43 Bronchoscopic view of a bronchial carcinoma obstructing a large bronchus.

Box 24.59 Survival in small-cell and non-small-cell cancer based on clinical stage

Stage of disease	Mean 5-year survival (%)	Mean survival time (months)
Non-small-cell lung cancer		
IA	50	60
IB	43	43
IIA	36	34
IIB	25	18
IIIA	19	14
IIIB	7	10
IV	2	6
Small-cell lung cancer		
Limited	10–13	15–20
Extensive	1–2	8–13

(Data from Goldstraw P, Crowley J, Chansky K et al.; International Association for the Study of Lung Cancer International Staging Committee; Participating Institutions. The IASLC Lung Cancer Staging Project: proposals for the revision of the TNM stage groupings in the forthcoming (7th) edition of the TNM classification of malignant tumours. *Journal of Thoracic Oncology* 2007; 2(8):706–714. Erratum in: *Journal of Thoracic Oncology* 2007; 2(10):985.)

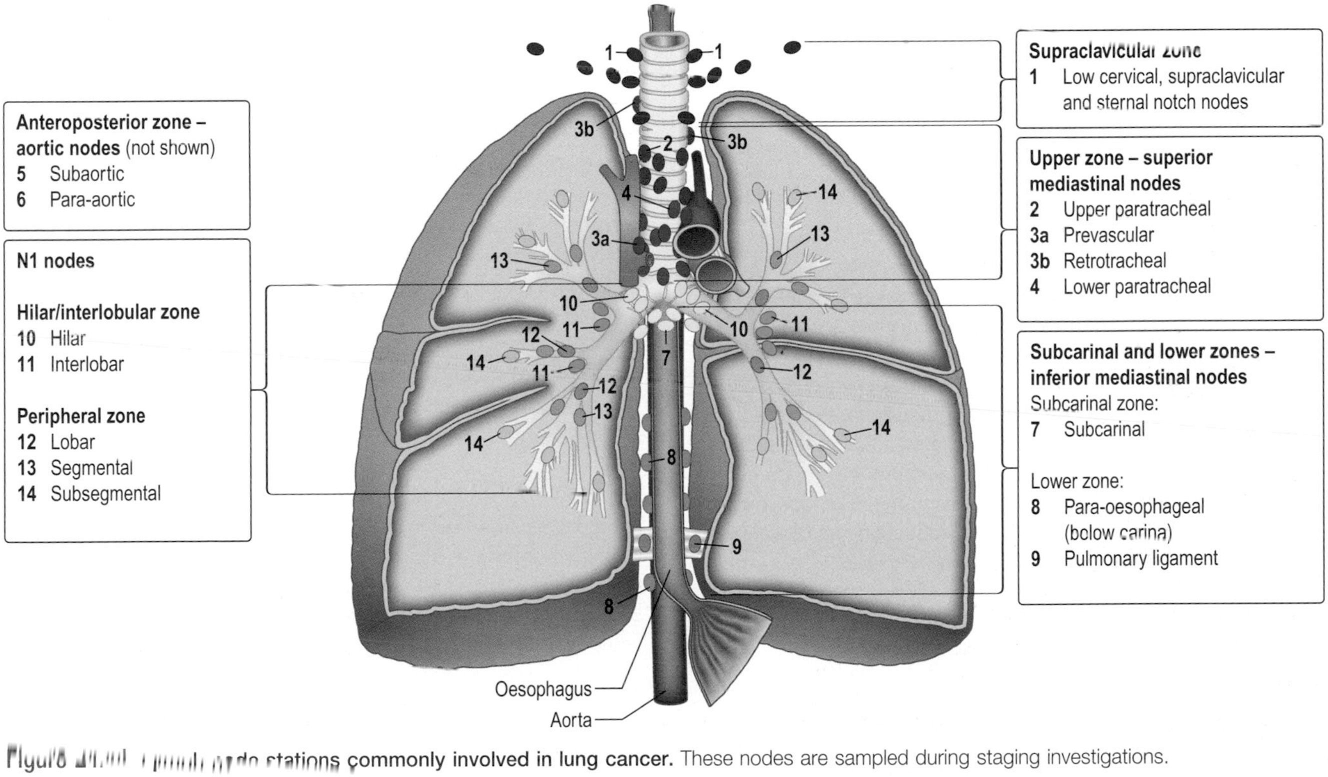

Figure 24.44 Lymph node stations commonly involved in lung cancer. These nodes are sampled during staging investigations.

staging of resected lung cancer demonstrates nodal involvement, patients require adjuvant chemotherapy.

Radiation therapy for cure

In selected patients with adequate lung function and early-stage NSCLC, high-dose radiotherapy or continuous hyperfractionated accelerated regimens (CHART) provide a good alternative to surgical resection with almost comparable outcomes. It is the treatment of choice if surgery is not possible due to co-morbidities. Radiation pneumonitis (defined as an acute infiltrate precisely confined to the radiation area and occurring within 3 months of radiotherapy) develops in 10–15% of cases. Radiation fibrosis, a fibrotic change occurring within a year or so of radiotherapy and not precisely confined to the radiation area, occurs to some degree in all cases. These complications usually cause no problems.

In patients with significant cardiovascular or respiratory co-morbidities and early stage I disease, stereotactic radiotherapy can be used. In the same patient group, radiofrequency ablation is used – an image-guided technique using heat to destroy small peripheral tumours.

Radiation treatment for symptoms

Radiation therapy has a role in palliation of symptoms from lung cancer. Bone and chest wall pain from metastases or direct invasion, haemoptysis, occluded bronchi and superior vena cava obstruction respond favourably to irradiation in the short term. Radiotherapy is also given at the end of chemotherapy to consolidate treatment in small-cell lung cancer.

Chemotherapy and targeted therapy

This is discussed on page 630. Adjuvant chemotherapy with radiotherapy improves response rate and extends median survival in non-small-cell cancer.

Newer targeted agents (p. 630) against epidermal growth factor receptors, tyrosine kinases and anaplastic lymphoma kinase (ALK) in NSCLC (in particular, adenocarcinoma) offer better outcomes in selected patients and can also be used where intravenous chemotherapy offers unacceptable toxicity or as second-line chemotherapy.

Laser therapy, endobronchial irradiation and tracheobronchial stents

These techniques are used in the palliation of inoperable lung cancer in selected patients with tracheobronchial narrowing from intraluminal tumour or extrinsic compression causing disabling breathlessness, intractable cough and complications, including infection, haemoptysis and respiratory failure.

A ***neodymium-Yag (Nd-Yag) laser*** passed through a fibreoptic bronchoscope can be used to vaporize inoperable fungating intraluminal carcinoma involving short segments of trachea or main bronchus. Benign tumours, strictures and vascular lesions can also be treated effectively with immediate relief of symptoms.

Endobronchial irradiation (brachytherapy) is useful for the treatment of both intraluminal tumour and malignant extrinsic compression. A radioactive source is afterloaded into a catheter placed adjacent to the carcinoma under fibreoptic bronchoscope control. Radiation dose falls rapidly with distance from the source, minimizing damage to adjacent normal tissue. Reduction in endoscopically assessed tumour size occurs in 70–95% of cases.

Tracheobronchial stents made of silicone or in the form of expandable metal springs are available for insertion into strictures caused by tumour, external compression, or weakening and collapse of the tracheobronchial wall.

Palliative care

Patients dying of cancer of the lung need attention to their overall wellbeing (see p. 31). Much can be done to make the individual's remaining life symptom-free and as active as possible. Furthermore, compared with patients who have fatal cancers at other sites, patients with lung cancer tend to remain relatively independent and pain-free, but they die more rapidly once they reach the terminal phase. Patient and relatives both require psychological and emotional support, a task that should be shared between the respiratory teams, the primary care team and the nurses, social workers, hospital chaplains and doctors who make up the palliative care team.

Secondary tumours

Metastases in the lung are very common and usually present as round shadows (1.5–3.0 cm in diameter). They are usually detected on chest X-ray in patients already diagnosed as having carcinoma, but can be the first presentation. Typical sites for the primary tumour include the kidney, prostate, breast, bone, gastrointestinal tract, cervix or ovary.

Metastases nearly always develop in the parenchyma and are often relatively asymptomatic, even when the chest X-ray shows extensive pulmonary metastases. Rarely, metastases develop within the bronchi, when they often present with haemoptysis.

Carcinoma, particularly of the stomach, pancreas and breast, can involve mediastinal glands and spread along the lymphatics of both lungs (lymphangitis carcinomatosis), leading to progressive and severe breathlessness. On the chest X-ray, bilateral lymphadenopathy is seen, together with streaky basal shadowing fanning out over both lung fields.

Occasionally, a pulmonary metastasis is detected as a ***solitary round shadow*** on chest X-ray in an asymptomatic patient. The most common primary tumour to do this is a renal cell carcinoma.

The differential diagnosis includes:

- primary bronchial carcinoma
- tuberculoma
- benign tumour of the lung
- hydatid cyst.

Single pulmonary metastases can be removed surgically but, as CT scans usually show the presence of small metastases undetected on chest X-ray, detailed imaging, including PET scanning and assessment, is essential before undertaking surgery.

Investigation of solitary pulmonary nodules

With the increased use of CT scanning for other conditions, there has been greater incidental detection of asymptomatic, small, sub-centimetre nodules. The majority of these are benign; however, radiological follow-up should be arranged at intervals, determined by the size of the nodule in millimetres and the risk of developing malignancy (i.e. high risk associated with either current or previous smoking history, occupational exposure to carcinogens or family history of lung cancer; low risk if the patient never smoked and there was no occupational exposure to potential carcinogens or relevant family history).

Screening for lung cancer

A large trial carried out in the USA has demonstrated a 20% mortality benefit from low-dose helical CT screening for lung cancer in high-risk populations of smokers/ex-smokers between the ages of 55 and 74. A similar trial is under way in Europe. It is likely that CT screening will be employed in the future.

Benign tumours

Pulmonary hamartoma

This is the most common benign tumour of the lung and is usually seen on the X-ray as a very well-defined round lesion 1–2 cm in diameter in the periphery of the lung. Growth is extremely slow but the tumour can reach several centimetres in diameter. Rarely, it arises from a major bronchus and causes obstruction.

Bronchial carcinoid

This rare tumour resembles an intestinal carcinoid tumour and is locally invasive, eventually spreading to mediastinal lymph nodes and finally to distant organs. It is a highly vascular tumour that projects into the lumen of a major bronchus, causing recurrent haemoptysis. It grows slowly and eventually blocks the bronchus, leading to lobar collapse. As foregut derivatives, bronchial carcinoids produce adrenocorticotrophic hormone (ACTH) but do not usually produce the 5-hydroxytryptamine that is seen in midgut or hindgut carcinoid tumours. Staging of carcinoid tumours is the same as for NSCLC.

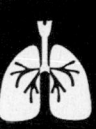

Cylindroma, chondroma and lipoma

These are extremely rare tumours that grow in the bronchus or trachea, causing obstruction.

Tracheal tumours

Benign tumours include squamous papilloma, leiomyoma, haemangiomas and tumours of neurogenic origin.

Further reading

Field JK, Oudkerk M, Pedersen JH, Duffy SW. Prospects for population screening and diagnosis of lung cancer. *Lancet* 2013; 382:732–741.
Goldstraw P, Ball D, Jett JR et al. Non-small cell lung cancer. *Lancet* 2011; 378:1727–1740.
National Institute of Health and Clinical Excellence. *NICE Clinical Guideline 121: Lung Cancer: Diagnosis and Management*. NICE 2011; http://www.nice.org.uk/guidance/cg121.
Rusch VW, Asamura H, Watanabe H et al. Members of IASLC Staging Committee. The IASLC lung cancer staging project: a proposal for a new international lymph node map in the forthcoming seventh edition of the TNM classification for lung cancer. *J Thorac Oncol* 2009; 4:568–577.
Temel JS, Greer JA, Muzikansky A et al. Early palliative care for patients with metastatic non-small-cell lung cancer. *N Engl J Med* 2010; 363:733–742.
Van Meerbeeck JP, Fennell DA, De Ruysscher DK et al. Small cell lung cancer. *Lancet* 2011; 378:1741–1755.
Xie Y, Minna D. A lung cancer molecular prognostic test ready for prime time. *Lancet* 2012; 379:785–787.

DISORDERS OF THE CHEST WALL AND PLEURA

Trauma

Trauma to the thoracic wall can cause penetrating wounds and lead to pneumothorax or haemothorax.

Rib fractures

Rib fractures are caused by trauma or coughing (particularly in the elderly), and can occur in patients with osteoporosis. Pathological rib fractures are due to metastatic spread (most often from carcinoma of the bronchus, breast, kidney, prostate or thyroid). Ribs can also become involved by a mesothelioma. Fractures may not be readily visible on a postero-anterior chest X-ray, so lateral X-rays and oblique views may be necessary.

Pain prevents adequate chest expansion and coughing, and this can lead to pneumonia.

Treatment is with adequate oral analgesia, by local infiltration or an intercostal nerve block.

Two fractures in one rib can lead to a flail segment with paradoxical movement; that is, part of the chest wall moves inwards during inspiration. This can produce inefficient ventilation and may require intermittent positive-pressure ventilation, especially if several ribs are similarly affected.

Rupture of the trachea or a major bronchus

Rupture of the trachea or a major bronchus can occur during deceleration injuries, leading to pneumothorax, surgical emphysema, pneumomediastinum and haemoptysis. Surgical emphysema is caused by air leaking into the subcutaneous connective tissue; this can also occur after the insertion of an intercostal drainage tube. A pneumomediastinum occurs when air leaks from the lung inside the parietal pleura and extends along the bronchial walls.

Rupture of the oesophagus

Rupture of the oesophagus (see p. 374) leads to mediastinitis, usually with mixed bacterial infection. This is a serious complication of external injury, endoscopic procedures, bougienage or necrotic carcinoma, and requires antibacterial chemotherapy.

Lung contusion

This causes widespread fluffy shadows on the chest X-ray owing to intrapulmonary haemorrhage. It may give rise to acute respiratory distress syndrome (see pp. 1167–1169).

Kyphoscoliosis

Kyphoscoliosis may be congenital, due to disease of the vertebrae such as TB or osteomalacia, or due to neuromuscular disease such as Friedreich's ataxia or poliomyelitis. The respiratory effects of severe kyphoscoliosis are often more pronounced than might be expected and respiratory failure and death often occur in the fourth or fifth decade. The abnormality should be corrected at an early stage if possible. Positive airway pressure ventilation delivered through a tightly fitting nasal mask is the treatment of choice for respiratory failure (see pp. 1165–1166).

Ankylosing spondylitis

Limitation of chest wall movement is often well compensated by diaphragmatic movement, and so the respiratory effects of this disease are relatively mild (see also p. 684). It is occasionally associated with upper lobe fibrosis.

Pectus excavatum and carinatum

Pectus excavatum causes few problems other than embarrassment about the deep vertical furrow in the chest, which can be corrected surgically. The heart is seen to lie well to the left on the chest X-ray. Pectus carinatum (pigeon chest) is often the result of rickets but is rarely seen in the West. No treatment is required.

Pleurisy

Pleurisy is pain arising from any disease of the pleura. The localized inflammation produces sharp localized pain, which is worse on deep inspiration, coughing and occasionally on twisting and bending movements. Common causes are pneumonia, pulmonary infarct and carcinoma. Rarer causes include rheumatoid arthritis and systemic lupus erythematosus.

Epidemic myalgia (Bornholm disease) is due to infection by Coxsackie B virus. This illness is common in young adults in the late summer and autumn, and is characterized by an upper respiratory tract illness followed by pleuritic pain in the chest and upper abdomen with tender muscles. The chest X-ray remains normal and the illness clears within a week.

Mesothelioma

Mesothelioma (see also p. 1126) is usually associated with asbestos exposure. It is described with other pleural diseases caused by asbestosis in ***Box 24.54***.

Pleural effusion

A pleural effusion is an excessive accumulation of fluid in the pleural space. It can be detected on X-ray when ≥300 mL of fluid is present,

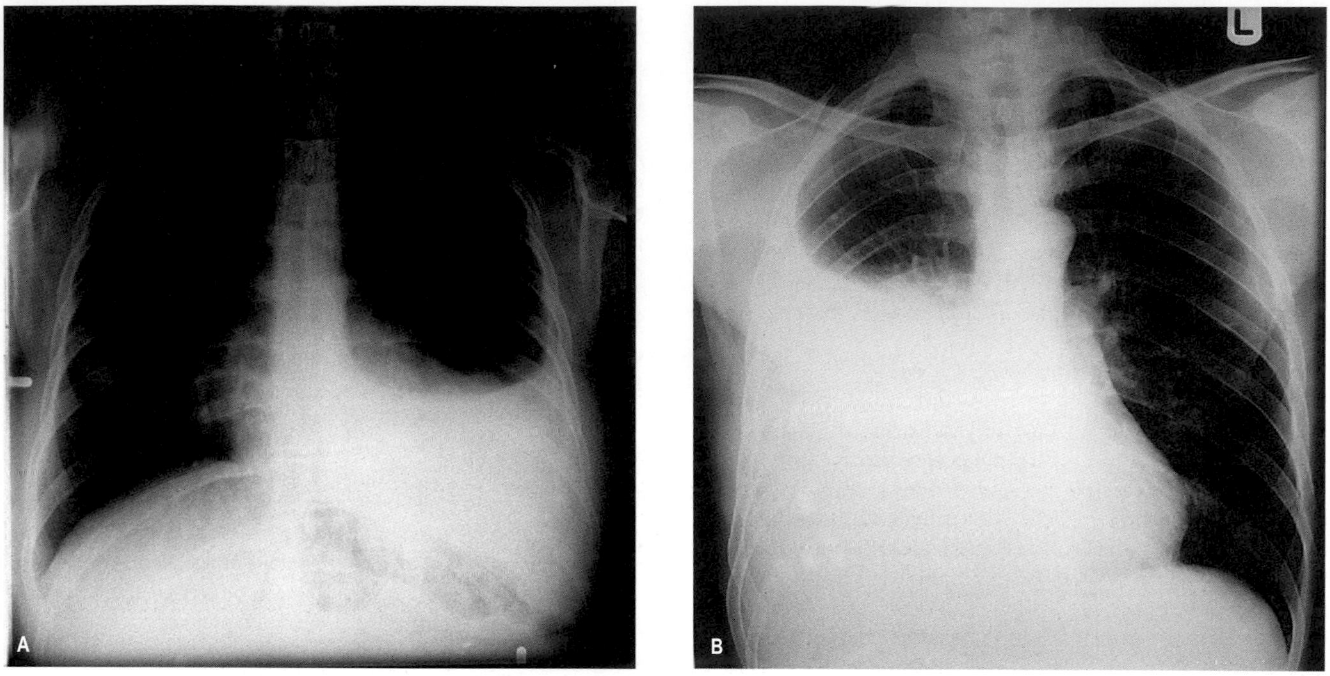

Figure 24.45 Radiographs showing pleural effusions. **A.** Small. **B.** Large.

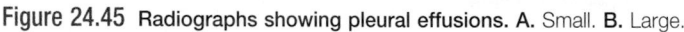

Box 24.60 Light's criteria to diagnose an exudative effusion

- Pleural fluid protein: serum protein >0.5
- Pleural fluid LDH : serum LDH >0.6
- Pleural fluid LDH > ⅔ upper limit of normal for serum (105–333 IU/L)

LDH, lactate dehydrogenase.
(Adapted from Light RW, Macgregor MI, Luchsinger PC et al. Pleural effusions: the diagnostic separation of transudates and exudates. Annals of Internal Medicine *1972; 77(4):507–513.)*

and clinically, when ≥500 mL is present. The chest X-ray appearances ***(Fig. 24.45)*** range from obliteration of the costophrenic angle to dense homogeneous shadows occupying part or all of the hemithorax. Fluid below the lung (a subpulmonary effusion) can simulate a raised hemidiaphragm. Fluid in the fissures may resemble an intrapulmonary mass. The physical signs are shown in ***Box 24.57***.

Diagnosis

This is by pleural aspiration (see p. 1073), usually done with ultrasound guidance. The fluid that accumulates may be a transudate or an exudate ***(Box 24.60)***.

Transudates

Effusions that are transudates can be bilateral but are often larger on the right side. The protein content is <30 g/L, the lactate dehydrogenase (LDH) is <200 IU/L and the fluid to serum LDH ratio is <0.6. Causes include:

- heart failure
- hypoproteinaemia (e.g. nephrotic syndrome)
- constrictive pericarditis
- hypothyroidism
- ovarian tumours producing right-sided pleural effusion – Meigs syndrome.

Exudates

The protein content of exudates is >30 g/L and the LDH is >200 IU/L. Causes include:

- bacterial pneumonia (common)
- carcinoma of the bronchus and pulmonary infarction – fluid may be blood-stained (common)
- TB
- autoimmune rheumatic diseases
- post-myocardial infarction syndrome (rare)
- acute pancreatitis (high amylase content) (rare)
- mesothelioma (rare)
- sarcoidosis (very rare)
- yellow-nail syndrome (effusion due to lymphoedema) (very rare)
- familial Mediterranean fever (rare).

Pleural biopsy (see p. 1073) may be necessary if the diagnosis has not been established by simple aspiration.

Management is of the underlying condition unless the fluid is purulent (empyema), in which case drainage is mandatory.

Management of malignant pleural effusions

Malignant pleural effusions that reaccumulate and are symptomatic can be aspirated to dryness followed by the instillation of a sclerosing agent such as tetracycline or talc. Effusions should be drained slowly since rapid shift of the mediastinum causes severe pain and occasionally shock. This treatment produces only temporary relief.

Chylothorax

This is due to the accumulation of lymph in the pleural space, usually resulting from leakage from the thoracic duct following trauma or infiltration by carcinoma.

Empyema

This is the presence of pus in the pleural space and can be a complication of pneumonia (see p. 1104).

Pneumothorax

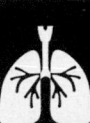

'Pneumothorax' means air in the pleural space. It may be spontaneous or occur as a result of trauma to the chest. Spontaneous pneumothorax is most common in young males, the male-to-female ratio being 6 : 1. It is caused by the rupture of a pleural bleb, usually apical, and is thought to be due to congenital defects in the connective tissue of the alveolar walls. Both lungs are affected with equal frequency. Often these patients are tall and thin. In patients over 40 years of age, the usual cause is underlying COPD. Rarer causes include bronchial asthma, carcinoma, breakdown of a lung abscess leading to bronchopleural fistula, and severe pulmonary fibrosis with cyst formation.

Pneumothorax may be localized if the visceral pleura has previously become adherent to the parietal pleura, or generalized if there are no pleural adhesions. Normally, the pressure in the pleural space is negative but this is lost once a communication is made with atmospheric pressure; the elastic recoil pressure of the lung then causes it to deflate partially. If the communication between the airways and the pleural space remains open, a bronchopleural fistula results. Once the communication between the lung and the pleural space is closed, air will be reabsorbed at a rate of 1.25% of the total radiographic volume of the hemithorax per day. Thus, a 50% collapse of the lung will take about 40 days to reabsorb completely once the air leak is closed.

It has been postulated that a valvular mechanism may develop through which air can be sucked into the pleural space during inspiration but not expelled during expiration. The intrapleural pressure remains positive throughout breathing, the lung deflates further, the mediastinum shifts, and venous return to the heart decreases, with increasing respiratory and cardiac embarrassment. This is called tension pneumothorax and is very rare, except in patients on positive pressure ventilation.

The usual presenting features are sudden onset of unilateral pleuritic pain or progressively increasing breathlessness. If the pneumothorax enlarges, the patient becomes more breathless and may develop pallor and tachycardia. There may be few physical signs if the pneumothorax is small.

The characteristic features and management are shown in ***Figure 24.46***. The main aim is to return the patient to active life as soon as possible. The procedure for simple aspiration is shown in ***Box 24.61***.

Recurrence. One-third of patients will have a recurrence. Chemical pleurodesis with talc is used for patients when surgery is contraindicated. Bleb resection and pleurodesis are achieved using a video-assisted thoracoscopic (VATS) approach or, less often, by open thoracotomy.

Further reading

British Thoracic Society. Investigation of a unilateral pleural effusion in adults: British Thoracic Society pleural disease guideline 2010. *Thorax* 2010; 65:ii4–ii17.

Box 24.61 Simple aspiration of pneumothorax

1. Explain the nature of the procedure and obtain consent.
2. Infiltrate 2% lidocaine down to the pleura in the second intercostal space in the mid-clavicular line.
3. Push a 3–4 cm 16-gauge cannula through the pleura.
4. Connect the cannula to a three-way tap and 50 mL syringe.
5. Aspirate up to 2.5 L of air. Stop if resistance to suction is felt or the patient coughs excessively.
6. Repeat the chest X-ray (in expiration) in the X-ray department.

DISORDERS OF THE DIAPHRAGM

Diaphragmatic fatigue

The diaphragm can become fatigued if the force of contraction during inspiration exceeds 40% of the force it can develop in a maximal static effort. When this occurs acutely, in patients with exacerbations of COPD or cystic fibrosis, or in quadriplegics, positive-pressure ventilation is required. Further rehabilitation requires exercises to increase the strength and endurance of the diaphragm by breathing against resistance for 30 minutes a day.

Unilateral diaphragmatic paralysis

This is common and symptomless. The affected diaphragm is usually elevated and moves paradoxically on inspiration. It can be diagnosed by ultrasound when a sniff causes the paralysed diaphragm to rise, and the unaffected diaphragm to descend. Causes include:

- surgery
- carcinoma of the bronchus with involvement of the phrenic nerve
- neurological disease, including poliomyelitis, herpes zoster
- trauma to cervical spine, birth injury, subclavian vein puncture
- infection, such as TB, syphilis, pneumonia.

Bilateral diaphragmatic weakness or paralysis

This causes breathlessness in the supine position and is a cause of sleep apnoea leading to daytime headaches and somnolence. Tidal volume is decreased and respiratory rate increased. Vital capacity is substantially reduced when lying down, and sniffing causes a paradoxical inward movement of the abdominal wall best seen in the supine position. Causes include viral infections, multiple sclerosis, motor neurone disease, poliomyelitis, Guillain–Barré syndrome, quadriplegia after trauma, and rare muscle diseases. Treatment is either diaphragmatic pacing or night-time assisted ventilation.

Complete eventration of the diaphragm

This is a congenital condition (invariably left-sided) in which muscle is replaced by fibrous tissue. It presents as marked elevation of the left hemidiaphragm, sometimes associated with gastrointestinal symptoms. Partial eventration, usually on the right, causes a hump (often anteriorly) on the diaphragmatic shadow on X-ray.

Diaphragmatic hernias

These are most commonly through the oesophageal hiatus but occasionally occur anteriorly, through the foramen of Morgagni, posterolaterally through the foramen of Bochdalek, or at any site following traumatic tears.

Hiccups

Hiccups are due to involuntary diaphragmatic contractions with closure of the glottis and are extremely common. Occasionally, patients present with persistent hiccups. This can be as a result of diaphragmatic irritation (e.g. subphrenic abscess) or a metabolic cause (e.g. uraemia). Treatment for persistent hiccups is with gabapentin 300 mg or pregabalin 50 mg three times daily. The underlying cause should be treated, if known.

Further reading

McCool ED, Tzelepis GE. Dysfunction of the diaphragm. *N Engl J Med* 2012; 366:932–942.

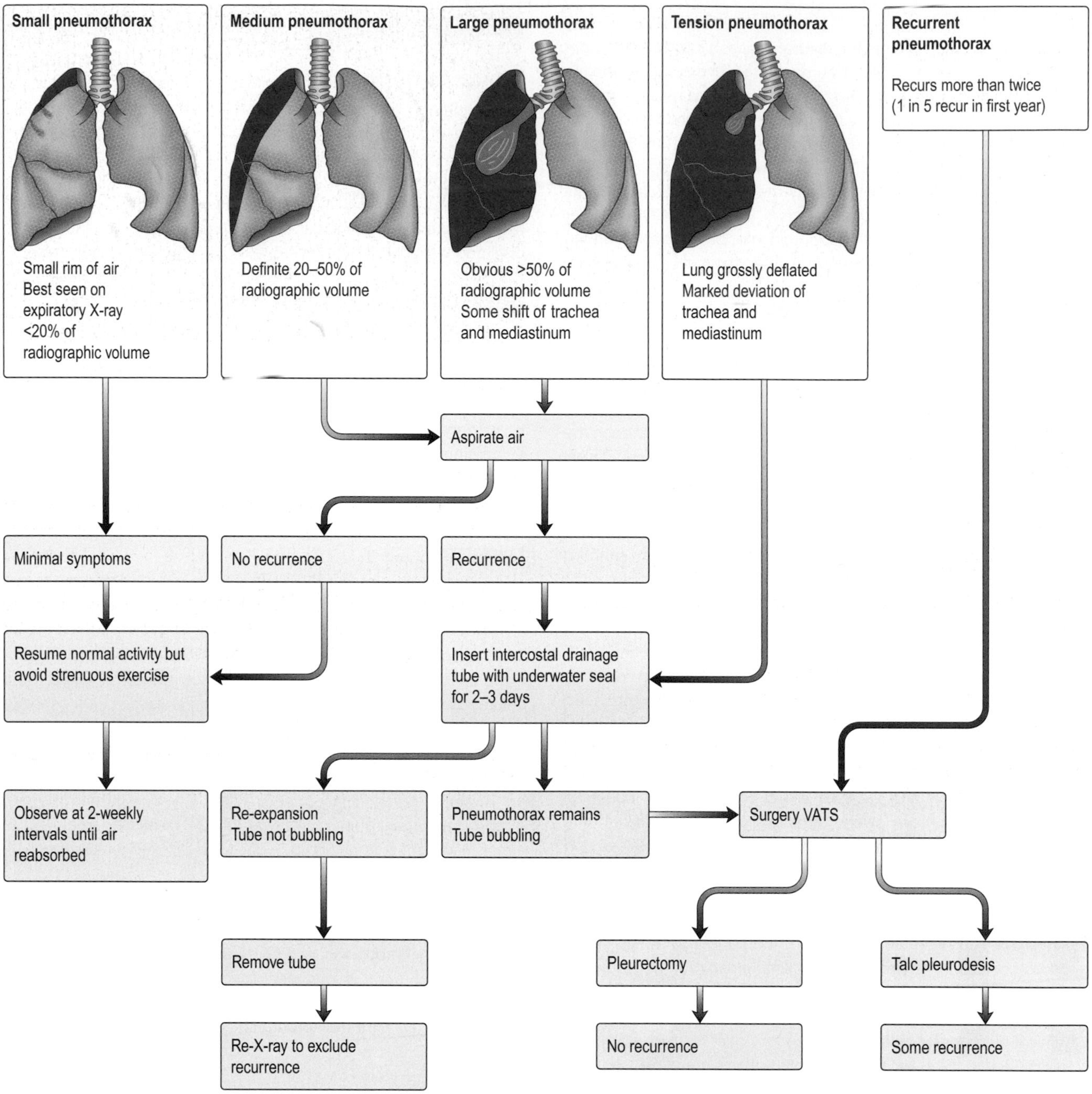

Figure 24.46 Pneumothorax: an algorithm for management. Red: pneumothorax. VATS, video-assisted thoracoscopic surgery.

MEDIASTINAL LESIONS

The mediastinum is defined as the region between the pleural sacs. It is additionally divided as shown in ***Figure 24.47***. Tumours affecting the mediastinum are rare. Masses are detected very accurately on CT, as well as on MRI scan ***(Fig. 24.48)***.

Retrosternal or intrathoracic thyroid

The most common mediastinal tumour is a retrosternal or intrathoracic thyroid, which is nearly always an extension of the thyroid present in the neck. Enlargement of the thyroid by a colloid goitre or malignant disease, or, rarely, in thyrotoxicosis, can cause displacement of the trachea and oesophagus to the opposite side. Symptoms of compression develop insidiously before producing the cardinal feature of dyspnoea. Flow–volume loops are useful to assess the physiological impact. Very occasionally, an intrathoracic thyroid may cause dysphagia or hoarseness and vocal cord paralysis due to stretching of the recurrent laryngeal nerve. The treatment is surgical removal.

Thymic tumours (thymomas)

The thymus is large in childhood and occupies the superior and anterior mediastinum. It involutes with age but may be enlarged by

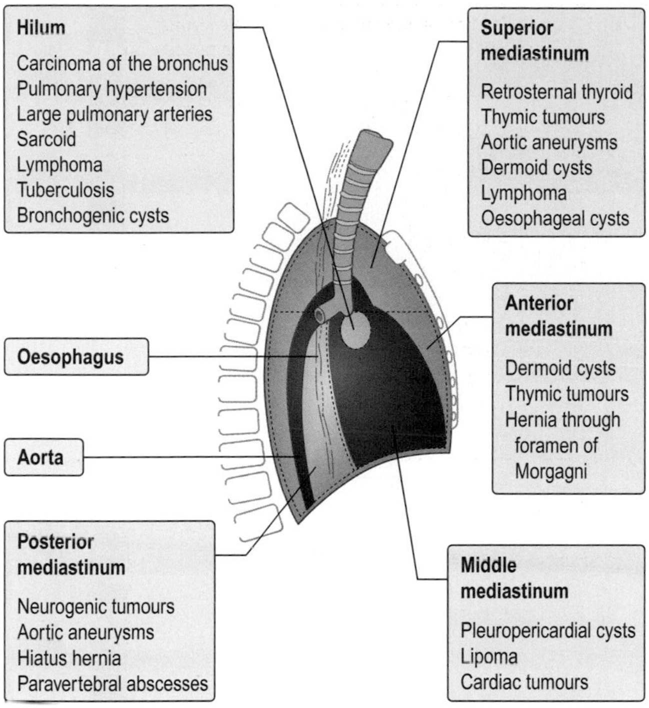

Figure 24.47 Subdivisions of the mediastinum and mass lesions.

cysts, which are rarely symptomatic, or by tumours, which may cause myasthenia gravis or compress the trachea or, rarely, the oesophagus. Surgery is the treatment of choice. Approximately half of the patients presenting with a thymic tumour have myasthenia gravis. Good syndrome, a combined defect in humoral and cellular immunity, is seen in 10% of thymomas.

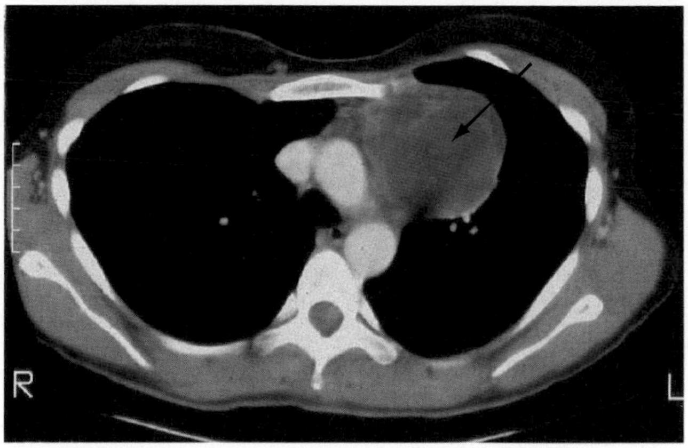

Figure 24.48 CT scan of a dermoid cyst (arrowed) in the mediastinum.

Pleuropericardial cysts

These cysts, which may be up to 10 cm in diameter, are filled with clear fluid. Some 70% of them are situated anteriorly in the cardiophrenic angle on the right side. Infection is rare and malignant change does not occur. The diagnosis is usually made by needle aspiration. No treatment is required, but these patients should be followed up, as an increase in cyst size suggests an alternative pathology; surgical excision is then advisable.

Significant websites

http://www.asthma.org.uk *Asthma UK.*
http://www.brit-thoracic.org.uk *British Thoracic Society.*
http://www.quitsmoking.uk.com *Good site for those wanting to stop smoking or to help patients to stop.*
http://www.thoracic.org *American Thoracic Society.*

25 Critical care medicine

Michael J O'Dwyer, Rupert M Pearse, Charles J Hinds

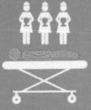

See your e-book for key learning points, clinical tips, drug tips, extra tables, extra images, interactive Figures, audio, videos, learning challenges and MCQs.

INTRODUCTION

Critical care medicine (or 'intensive care medicine') is concerned predominantly with the management of patients with acute life-threatening conditions ('the critically ill') in specialized units. In addition to emergency cases, intensive care units (ICUs) admit high-risk patients electively after major surgery ***(Box 25.1)***. Frequently, ICU staff provide care throughout the hospital in the form of ***medical emergency teams and outreach care***. These teams are trained to recognize and provide resuscitation to patients who become critically ill on the ward and transport them safely to an ICU. Another role for these teams is to identify patients who are deteriorating on the ward and to intervene early, perhaps thereby preventing the need for intensive care admission. Intensive care medicine also encompasses the resuscitation and transport of those who become acutely ill or are injured in the community. Teamwork and a multidisciplinary approach are central to the provision of intensive care and this functions most effectively when directed and coordinated by committed specialists.

ICUs are usually reserved for patients with established or impending organ failure and provide facilities for the diagnosis, prevention and treatment of multiple organ dysfunction. They are fully equipped with monitoring and technical facilities, including an adjacent laboratory and 'near-patient testing' devices for the rapid determination of blood gases and simple biochemical data such as serum potassium, blood glucose and serum lactate levels. Technological advances have led to the development of more compact and complex mechanical ventilators that are adaptable to individual patient demands. Portable ultrasound and echocardiography equipment is commonly available. Patients receive continuous expert nursing care and the constant attention of appropriately trained medical staff.

High-dependency units (***HDUs***) offer a level of care intermediate between that available on the general ward and that provided in an ICU. They provide monitoring and support for patients with acute (or acute-on-chronic) single-organ failure and for those who are at risk of developing organ failure. They can also provide a 'step-down' facility for patients being discharged from intensive care.

The proportion of a hospital's resources dedicated to intensive care varies widely internationally. For example, the UK provides 6.6 ICU and HDU beds per 100 000 population, whereas Germany provides 29.2 such beds per 100 000 population.

CLINICAL APPROACH TO THE CRITICALLY ILL PATIENT

Recognition and diagnosis of critical illness

Early recognition, immediate resuscitation and stabilization are fundamental to the successful management of the critically ill. Previously stable ward patients may deteriorate rapidly. In order to facilitate identification of 'at-risk' patients on the ward and early referral to the critical care team, a number of early warning systems have been devised (e.g. the Modified Early Warning Score, MEWS; ***Box 25.2***). These are based primarily on bedside recognition of deteriorating physiological variables and can be used to supplement clinical intuition. A MEWS score of ≥5 is associated with an increased risk of death and warrants immediate admission to ICU. Another example of a system used to trigger referral to a Medical Emergency Team (MET) is shown in ***Box 25.3*** (see also pp. 1156–1161).

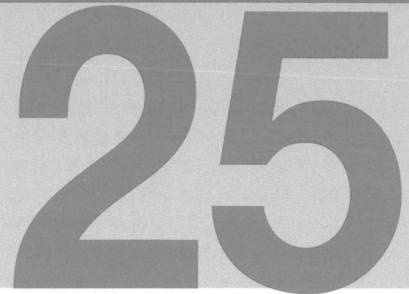

These early warning systems are not infallible and have not been universally implemented. It is therefore imperative that clinicians are trained to recognize critically ill patients at the bedside. The initial assessment may elicit obvious signs. The patient may be unduly agitated or, perhaps more worryingly, unresponsive. Of particular concern is the obtunded patient who is unable to protect their own airway from aspiration of gastric or oral contents. Snoring, grunting or other respiratory sounds may indicate an obstructed airway, which can be caused by posterior displacement of the tongue due to lax oropharyngeal musculature in a comatose patient, or perhaps by secretions pooling in the oropharynx in a patient with a depressed cough reflex. Obvious use of the accessory respiratory muscles and a tracheal tug are sensitive signs of impending respiratory decompensation. Patients in severe respiratory distress frequently sit forwards, grip the sides of the bed and cannot complete sentences in a single breath. Review of the nursing observations may reveal a sudden deterioration in recorded variables, such as a sharp rise in temperature, increasing heart rate, a fall in blood pressure or decreased urine output.

On examination, cool peripheries in conjunction with diaphoresis indicate increased sympathetic drive and may be a sign of cardiogenic shock, hypovolaemia or hypoglycaemia. In contrast, flushed, warm peripheries may be a sign of a hyperdynamic circulation consistent with sepsis. ***Abdominal catastrophes*** are a common cause of an acute deterioration; an abdominal examination should always be performed and may reveal a distended, tender abdomen and often absent or altered bowel sounds consistent with a perforated viscus or ischaemic bowel. ***Blood gas analysis*** is usually readily available and should be performed as soon as possible. Acid–base status, haemoglobin concentration, blood glucose and electrolyte levels obtained from an arterial blood gas sample can all be helpful when assessing the cause and severity of an acute illness. Increased lactate levels usually indicate severe illness. An ***electrocardiogram*** (***ECG***) can allow the rapid diagnosis of treatable conditions, as can a portable chest X-ray.

Frequently, the precise underlying diagnosis is initially unclear but, in all cases, the immediate objective is to preserve life and prevent, reverse or minimize damage to vital organs such as the lungs, brain, kidneys and liver. A systematic approach to the recognition and initial treatment of acute illness should be adopted, as well as performance of investigations to search for the underlying cause. A rapid assessment of the physiological derangement should be carried out, followed by prompt institution of measures to support cardiovascular and respiratory function (following the ABC approach: *A*irway, *B*reathing, *C*irculation; see ***Fig. 25.23***). The patient's condition and response to treatment should be closely monitored throughout. In practice, resuscitation, assessment and diagnosis usually proceed in parallel.

Box 25.1 Some common indications for admission to intensive care

Surgical emergencies
- Acute intra-abdominal catastrophe
  - Perforated viscus, especially with faecal soiling of peritoneum (often complicated by sepsis/septic shock)
  - Ruptured/leaking abdominal aortic aneurysm
- Trauma (often complicated by hypovolaemic and later sepsis/septic shock)
  - Multiple injuries
  - Massive blood loss
  - Severe head injury

Medical emergencies
- Respiratory failure
  - Exacerbation of chronic obstructive pulmonary disease (COPD)
  - Acute severe asthma
  - Severe pneumonia (often complicated by sepsis/septic shock)
- Meningococcal infection
- Status epilepticus
- Severe diabetic ketoacidosis
- Coma

Elective surgical admissions
- Extensive/prolonged procedure (e.g. oesophagogastrectomy)
- Cardiothoracic surgery
- Major head and neck surgery
- Coexisting cardiovascular or respiratory disease

Obstetric emergencies
- Severe pre-eclampsia/eclampsia
- Haemorrhage
- Amniotic fluid embolism

Box 25.3 Calling criteria for the Medical Emergency Team

Parameter	Description
Airway	If threatened
Breathing	All respiratory arrests
	Respiratory rate <5 breaths/min
	Respiratory rate >36 breaths/min
Circulation	All cardiac arrests
	Pulse rate <40 b.p.m.
	Pulse rate >140 b.p.m.
	Systolic blood pressure <90 mmHg
Neurology	Sudden fall in level of consciousness (fall in Glasgow Coma Scale score of >2 points)
	Repeated or prolonged seizures
Other	Any patient who does not fit the criteria above but who seriously worries you

(From Hillman K, Chen J, Cretikos M et al. Introduction of the medical emergency team (MET) system: a cluster-randomized controlled trial. *Lancet* 2005; 365:2091–2097, with permission.)

Box 25.2 Modified Early Warning Score (MEWS) for referral of 'at-risk' patients to the critical care team

Parameter	Score						
	3	*2*	*1*	*0*	*1*	*2*	*3*
Systolic blood pressure (mmHg)	<70	71–80	81–100	101–199		200	
Heart rate (b.p.m.)	<40		41–50	51–100	101–110	111–129	130
Respiratory rate (breaths/min)		<9		9–14	15–20	21–29	30
Temperature (°C)	<34	34–35		35–38.4		38.5	
AVPU score (Alert, Volume, Pain, Unresponsive)				Alert	Reacting to voice	Reacting to pain	Unresponsive

General aspects of managing the critically ill

Critically ill patients require multidisciplinary care with:

- ***Intensive skilled nursing care*** (in the UK, usually with a 1 : 1 nurse/patient ratio in an ICU (level 3 care) or 1 : 2 in a HDU (level 2 care)). Frequent clinical observations are required.
- ***Specialized physiotherapy***. This should include chest physiotherapy, mobilization and rehabilitation.
- ***Management of pain*** and distress. There should be judicious administration of analgesics and sedatives (see p. 1164).
- ***Constant reassurance and support***. Critically ill patients easily become disorientated; delirium (a transient alteration in consciousness, attention, orientation, perception or behaviour) is common. Delirium may be hypoactive, agitated (hyperactive) or a combination of the two. Pain, advanced age, sleep/sensory deprivation, sedative administration (especially benzodiazepines), alcohol/drug withdrawal, neurological injury, severe illness and medical comorbidities all play a role. Patients with delirium are more difficult to wean from ventilation, are at greater risk of self-extubation and require larger doses of sedatives. Delirium has been associated with increased mortality and length of hospital stay. Treatment focuses on effective pain control, minimizing sensory deprivation and early mobilization. Avoid benzodiazepines and limit sedative administration. The use of newer sedative agents, such as the α_2 agonist dexmedetomidine, may reduce the incidence of delirium and time on the ventilator.
- ***H_2-receptor antagonists or proton pump inhibitors***. These agents should be given in selected cases to reduce gastric acidity and prevent stress-induced ulceration. They may, however, encourage bacterial overgrowth in the upper gastrointestinal tract and predispose patients to ventilator-associated pneumonia (VAP) if these bacteria are aspirated.
- ***Compression stockings*** (full-length and graduated), pneumatic compression devices and subcutaneous low-molecular-weight heparin. These help to prevent venous thrombosis.
- ***Mouth care***. Mouth care, particularly the use of chlorhexidine mouth washes, helps to reduce hospital-acquired infections and VAP by reducing the burden of pathogenic oral flora that may be aspirated into the respiratory tree. The recent introduction of chlorhexidine body washes may reduce the total carriage of resistant microorganisms.
- ***Prevention of constipation and pressure ulcers***.
- ***Organ support***. For example, inotropes and vasopressors may be required for cardiovascular support, invasive and non-invasive ventilation for respiratory failure, and dialysis for renal failure. Specialized units may provide extracorporeal membrane oxygenation (ECMO) for severe respiratory failure, mechanical support of the circulation for cardiac failure, and advanced liver support in the form of liver dialysis (e.g. the molecular adsorbent recirculation system, MARS).
- ***Nutritional support*** (see pp. 212–216). Protein energy malnutrition is common in critically ill patients and is associated with muscle wasting, weakness, delayed mobilization, difficulty weaning from ventilation, immune compromise and impaired wound healing. ***Enteral nutrition***, usually delivered via a fine-bore nasogastric tube, is preferred because it is less expensive, preserves gut mucosal integrity, is more physiological and is associated with fewer complications. However, the value of enteral nutrition early in the course of an acute illness remains uncertain, apart from giving small amounts of enteral feed to preserve gut viability.

If enteral feeding is not possible due to the gut dysmotility and malabsorption associated with critical illness, the alternative is ***intravenous (parenteral) nutrition*** (see p. 214). This is more invasive and expensive, and can be complicated by deranged liver function tests, hypertriglyceridaemia, hyperglycaemia and an increased susceptibility to hospital-acquired infections. Usually, hypocaloric enteral nutrition is continued for up to a week in previously well-nourished patients prior to considering parenteral nutrition. Administering parenteral nutrition early in order to maintain caloric input and prevent an energy deficit may be detrimental.

Although all nutrition should contain carbohydrate, protein, lipids and some micronutrients, the precise optimal formulation is unclear. Supplementation with the amino acid glutamine has theoretical advantages and is recommended in some guidelines. The omega-3 fatty acids derived from fish oils also have potentially beneficial antioxidant activity but have not been convincingly shown to improve outcome, as has been the case for micronutrient supplementation with selenium, copper, manganese, zinc, iron and vitamins.

Many critically ill patients are at risk of developing a '***re-feeding syndrome***' (see p. 194) when nutritional support is first initiated.

Critically ill patients commonly require intravenous insulin infusions, often in high doses, to combat insulin resistance and hyperglycaemia (which is associated with hospital-acquired infections, renal impairment and poor wound healing; see p. 1249). Although the use of intensive insulin therapy to achieve 'tight glycaemic control' (blood glucose level between 4.4 and 6.1 mmol/L) was initially shown to improve outcome, subsequent studies found that this approach is associated with an unacceptably high incidence of hypoglycaemia, and possibly increased mortality. Current recommendations suggest that blood glucose levels should be maintained below 8–10 mmol/L.

Discharge from the ICU/HDU

Discharge of patients from intensive care should normally be planned in advance and should ideally take place during normal working hours. Assessment with a quick SOFA is helpful (see p. 1154). Frequently, when the condition of critically ill patients improves, they are initially 'stepped down' to HDU (level 2) care. Premature or unplanned discharge from the ICU or HDU, especially during the night, has been associated with higher hospital mortality rates and should be avoided where possible. A summary including 'points to review' should be included in the clinical notes and there should be a detailed handover to the receiving team (medical and nursing). The intensive care team should continue to review the patient (who might deteriorate following discharge) on the ward and should be available at all times for advice on further management (e.g. tracheostomy care, nutritional support). In this way, deterioration and re-admission to intensive care (which is associated with a particularly poor outcome), or even cardiorespiratory arrest, might be avoided.

This chapter concentrates on cardiovascular, respiratory, renal and neurological problems. Many patients also have failure of other organs, such as the liver; treatment of these is dealt with in more detail in the relevant chapters.

Further reading

Adhikari NKJ, Fowler RA, Bhagwanjee S et al. Critical care and the global burden of critical illness. *Lancet* 2010; 376:1339–1341.

Arabi YM, Aldawood AS, Haddad SH et al. Permissive underfeeding or standard enteral feeding in critically ill adults. *N Engl J Med* 2015; 372:2398–2408.

Casaer MP, Mesotten O, Hermans G et al. Early versus late parenteral nutrition in critically ill adults. *N Engl J Med* 2011; 365:506–517.
Casaer MP, Van den Berghe G. Nutrition in the acute phase of critical illness. *N Engl J Med* **2014; 370:1227–1236.**
Frost PJ, Wise MP. Early management of acutely ill ward patients. *BMJ* 2012; 345:e5677.
Fullerton JN, Perkins GD. Who to admit to intensive care? *Clin Med* 2011; 11:601–604.
NICE-SUGAR Study Investigators. Intensive versus conventional glucose control in critically ill patients. *N Engl J Med* 2009; 360:1293–1297.
Reade MC, Finfer S. Sedation and delirium in the intensive care unit. *N Engl J Med* 2014; 370:444–454.
Vincent JL. Critical care – where have we been and where are we going? *Crit Care* 2013; 17(Suppl 1):S2.

APPLIED CARDIORESPIRATORY PHYSIOLOGY

Oxygen delivery and consumption

Oxygen delivery (DO_2) ***(Fig. 25.1)*** is defined as the total amount of oxygen delivered to the tissues per unit time. It is dependent on the volume of blood flowing through the microcirculation per minute (i.e. the total cardiac output, $\dot{Q}_t$) and the amount of oxygen contained in that blood (i.e. the arterial oxygen content, C_aO_2). Oxygen is transported both in combination with haemoglobin and dissolved in plasma. The amount combined with haemoglobin is determined by the oxygen capacity of haemoglobin (usually taken as 1.34 mL of oxygen per gram of haemoglobin) and its percentage saturation with oxygen (SO_2). The volume dissolved in plasma depends on the partial pressure of oxygen (PO_2). Except when hyperbaric oxygen is administered, the amount of dissolved oxygen in plasma is insignificant.

Clinically, however, the utility of this global concept of oxygen delivery is limited because it fails to account for changes in the relative flow to individual organs and the distribution of flow through the microcirculation (i.e. the efficiency with which oxygen delivery is matched to the metabolic requirements of individual tissues or cells). Furthermore, some organs (such as the heart) have high oxygen requirements relative to their blood flow and may receive insufficient oxygen, even if the overall oxygen delivery is apparently adequate. Lastly, microcirculatory flow can be impaired by an increase in blood viscosity.

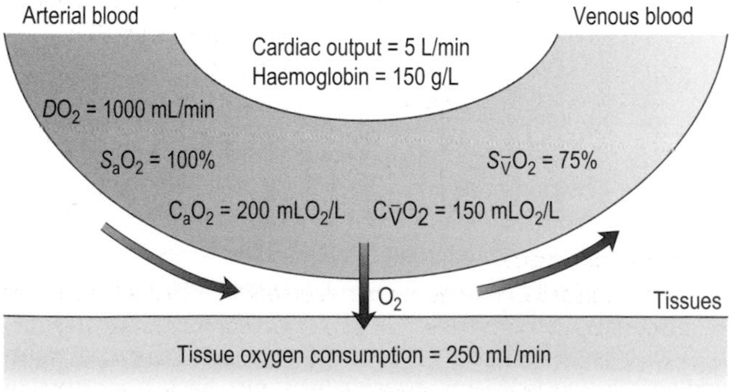

Figure 25.1 Tissue oxygen delivery and consumption in a normal 70 kg person breathing air. Oxygen delivery (DO_2) = cardiac output × (haemoglobin concentration × oxygen saturation (S_aO_2) × 1.34). In normal adults, oxygen delivery is roughly 1000 mL/min, of which 250 mL is taken up by tissues. Mixed venous blood is thus 75% saturated with oxygen. C_aO_2, arterial oxygen content; $C_{\bar{v}}O_2$, mixed venous oxygen content; $S_{\bar{v}}O_2$, mixed venous oxygen saturation.

Oxygenation of the blood

Oxyhaemoglobin dissociation curve

The saturation of haemoglobin with oxygen is determined by the partial pressure of oxygen (PO_2) in the blood, the relationship between the two being described by the oxyhaemoglobin dissociation curve ***(Fig. 25.2)***. The sigmoid shape of this curve is significant for a number of reasons:

- Modest falls in the partial pressure of oxygen in the arterial blood (P_aO_2) may be tolerated (since oxygen content is relatively unaffected), provided that the percentage saturation remains above about 92%.
- Increasing the P_aO_2 to above normal has only a minimal effect on oxygen content unless hyperbaric oxygen is administered (when the amount of oxygen in solution in plasma becomes significant).
- Once on the steep slope of the curve (percentage saturation below about 90%), a small decrease in P_aO_2 can cause large falls in oxygen content, whereas increasing P_aO_2 only slightly, e.g. by administering 28% oxygen to a patient with chronic obstructive pulmonary disease (COPD), can lead to a useful increase in oxygen saturation and content.

If the PCO_2 increases, the oxyhaemoglobin curve moves to the right, facilitating oxygen unloading to the tissues (Bohr effect).

The P_aO_2 is influenced, in turn, by the alveolar oxygen tension (P_AO_2), the efficiency of pulmonary gas exchange, and the partial pressure of oxygen in mixed venous blood ($P_{\bar{v}}O_2$).

Alveolar oxygen tension (P_AO_2)

The partial pressures of inspired gases are shown in ***Figure 25.3***. By the time the inspired gases reach the alveoli, they are fully saturated

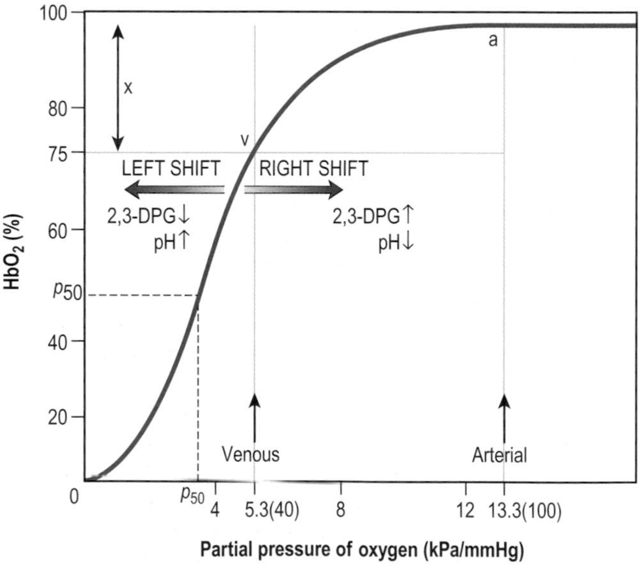

Figure 25.2 The oxyhaemoglobin dissociation curve. HbO_2 (%) is the percentage saturation of haemoglobin with oxygen. The curve will move to the right in the presence of acidosis (metabolic or respiratory), pyrexia or an increased red cell 2,3-diphosphoglycerate (2,3-DPG) concentration. For a given arteriovenous oxygen content difference, the mixed venous PO_2 will then be higher. Furthermore, if the mixed venous PO_2 is unchanged, the arteriovenous oxygen content difference increases and more oxygen is off-loaded to the tissues (see p. 520). P_{50} (the PO_2 at which haemoglobin is half-saturated with O_2) is a useful index of these shifts – the higher the P_{50} (i.e. shift to the right), the lower the affinity of haemoglobin for O_2. a, arterial point; v, venous point; x, arteriovenous oxygen content difference.

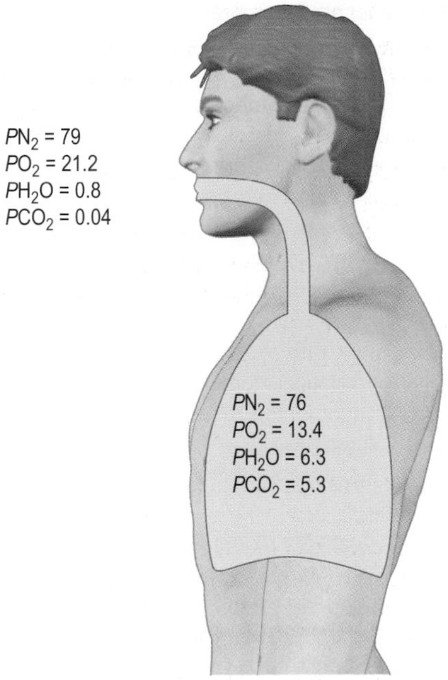

Figure 25.3 The composition of inspired and alveolar gas. (Partial pressures in kPa.)

with water vapour at body temperature (37°C), which has a partial pressure of 6.3 kPa (47 mmHg), and contain CO_2 at a partial pressure of approximately 5.3 kPa (40 mmHg); the P_AO_2 is thereby reduced to approximately 13.4 kPa (100 mmHg).

The clinician can influence P_AO_2 by administering oxygen or by increasing the barometric pressure (hyperbaric therapy).

Pulmonary gas exchange

In *normal* subjects, there is a small alveolar–arterial oxygen difference ($P_{A}–_{a}O_2$). This is due to:

- a small (0.133 kPa, 1 mmHg) pressure gradient across the alveolar membrane
- a small amount of blood (2% of total cardiac output) bypassing the lungs via the bronchial and thebesian veins
- a small degree of ventilation/perfusion mismatch.

Pathologically, there are three possible causes of an increased $P_{A}–_{a}O_2$ difference:

- ***Diffusion defect***. This is not a major cause of hypoxaemia, even in conditions such as lung fibrosis, in which the alveolar–capillary membrane is considerably thickened. Carbon dioxide is also not affected, as it is more soluble than oxygen.
- ***Right-to-left shunts***. In certain congenital cardiac lesions or when a segment of lung is completely collapsed, a proportion of venous blood passes to the left side of the heart without taking part in gas exchange, causing arterial hypoxaemia. This hypoxaemia cannot be corrected by administering oxygen to increase the P_AO_2 because blood leaving normal alveoli is already fully saturated; further increases in PO_2 will not, therefore, significantly affect its oxygen content. On the other hand, because of the shape of the carbon dioxide dissociation curve ***(Fig. 25.4)***, the high PCO_2 of the shunted blood can be compensated for by over-ventilating patent alveoli, thus lowering the CO_2 content of the effluent blood. Indeed, many patients with acute right-to-left shunts hyperventilate in response to the hypoxia and/or to stimulation of mechanoreceptors in the lung, so that their P_aCO_2 is normal or low.

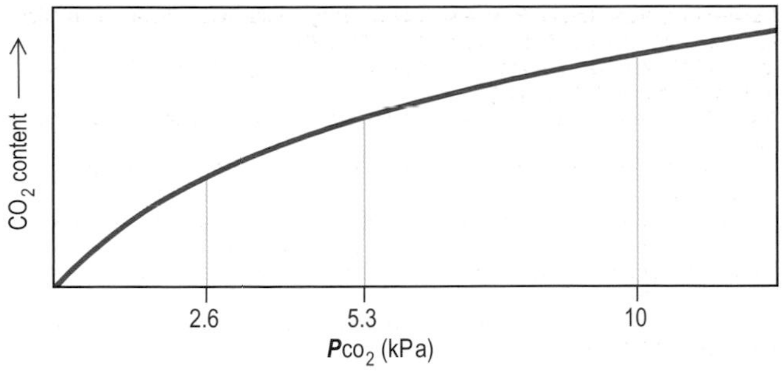

Figure 25.4 The carbon dioxide dissociation curve. Note that, in the physiological range, the curve is essentially linear.

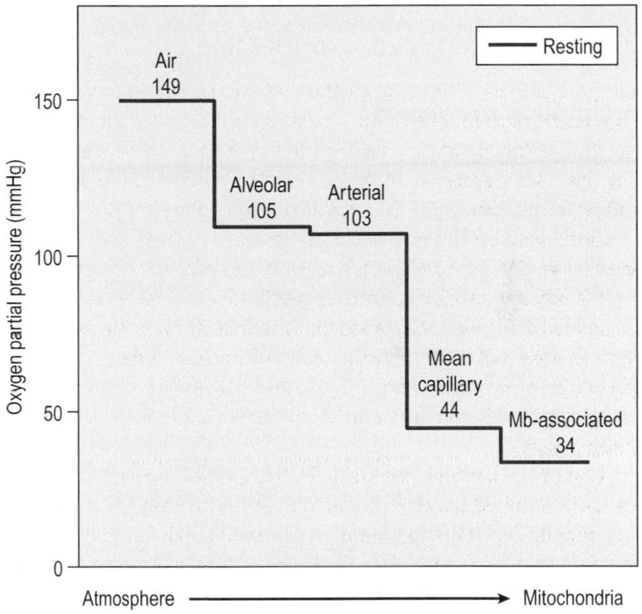

Figure 25.5 The oxygen cascade. Oxygen levels decrease (shown in graph) as oxygen is unloaded into the tissues and diffuses to the mitochondria. Mb, myoglobin.

- ***Ventilation/perfusion ($\dot{V}/\dot{Q}$) mismatch*** (see pp. 1063–1064). Diseases of the lung parenchyma (e.g. pneumonia, pulmonary oedema, acute lung injury) result in $\dot{V}/\dot{Q}$ mismatch, producing an increase in alveolar dead space and hypoxaemia. The increased dead space can be compensated for by increasing overall ventilation. In contrast to the hypoxia resulting from a true right-to-left shunt, that due to areas of low $\dot{V}/\dot{Q}$ can be partially corrected by administering oxygen and thereby increasing the P_AO_2, even in poorly ventilated areas of lung.

Oxygen cascade

Oxygen levels fall further as oxygen is unloaded into the tissues and diffuses to the mitochondria. Tissue oxygen content varies, depending on the distance travelled from the local capillary network. Some mitochondria continue to function at a PO_2 as low as 0.07 kPa (0.5 mmHg) ***(Fig. 25.5)***.

Mixed venous oxygen tension ($P_{\bar{V}}O_2$) and saturation ($S_{\bar{V}}O_2$)

The $P_{\bar{V}}O_2$ is the partial pressure of oxygen in pulmonary arterial blood that has been thoroughly mixed during its passage through the right heart. Assuming P_aO_2 remains constant, $P_{\bar{V}}O_2$ and $S_{\bar{V}}O_2$

will fall if more oxygen has to be extracted from each unit volume of blood arriving at the tissues. A low $P_{\bar{v}}O_2$ therefore indicates either that oxygen delivery has fallen or that tissue oxygen requirements have increased without a compensatory rise in cardiac output. If $P_{\bar{v}}O_2$ falls, the effect of a given degree of pulmonary shunting on arterial oxygenation will be exacerbated. Thus, worsening arterial hypoxaemia does not necessarily indicate a deterioration in pulmonary function but might instead reflect a fall in cardiac output and/or a rise in oxygen consumption.

Conversely, a rise in $P_{\bar{v}}O_2$ and $S_{\bar{v}}O_2$ may reflect impaired tissue oxygen extraction (due to microcirculatory abnormalities) and/or reduced oxygen utilization (e.g. due to mitochondrial dysfunction), as seen in severe sepsis (see below).

Monitoring the oxygen saturation in central venous ($S_{CV}O_2$), rather than pulmonary artery blood is less invasive and may be a useful guide to the resuscitation of some critically ill patients (see p. 1161).

Adaptation to hypoxia

Acute exposure to severe hypoxia may lead to sudden death if the immediate adaptive responses fail to maintain mitochondrial oxygen delivery. Chronic exposure to low oxygen tension, on the other hand, allows time for compensatory mechanisms to develop. Amongst the first is an acute increase in cardiac output, achieved primarily by increasing heart rate. Given the reciprocal relationship between the partial pressures of oxygen and carbon dioxide in the alveoli, as defined by the alveolar gas equation ($P_AO_2 = P_IO_2 - P_ACO_{2/R}$), an increase in respiratory rate serves to decrease alveolar PCO_2 and thereby increase alveolar PO_2 (see also ***Fig. 25.3***). Over time, increased erythropoietin production stimulates haemoglobin synthesis, leading to a marked increase in haematocrit. Over the longer term, capillary bed density in specific tissues adjusts to the physiological demand. In those residing at altitude over generations, the hypoxic ventilatory drive and pulmonary vasoconstrictor response evolve to maximize oxygen uptake. In 2007, a series of arterial blood samples were obtained by a group of critical care doctors on the summit of Mount Everest (see more online). The project included a 4-month acclimatization period at altitude and the samples were eventually obtained at an altitude of 8400 m whilst breathing air. The average PaO_2 was 3.2 kPa (24.6 mmHg). These figures neatly demonstrate features of both acute (hyperventilation) and chronic (increased haematocrit) acclimatization to hypobaric hypoxia.

Further reading

Grocott MPW, Martin DS, Levett DZH et al. Arterial blood gases and oxygen content in climbers on Mount Everest. *N Engl J Med* 2009; 360:140–149.

Cardiac output

Cardiac output is the product of heart rate and stroke volume, and is affected by changes in either of these ***(Fig. 25.6)***.

Heart rate

When heart rate increases, the duration of systole remains essentially unchanged, whereas diastole, and thus the time available for ventricular filling, becomes progressively shorter and the stroke volume eventually falls. In the normal heart, this occurs at rates greater than about 160 beats per minute, but in those with cardiac pathology, especially when ventricular filling is restricted (e.g. mitral stenosis), stroke volume may fall at much lower heart rates. Furthermore, tachycardias cause a marked increase in myocardial oxygen consumption ($\dot{V}_mO_2$) and this may precipitate ischaemia in areas of the myocardium with restricted coronary perfusion. When the heart rate falls, a point is reached at which the increase in stroke volume is insufficient to compensate for bradycardia, and again cardiac output falls.

Alterations in heart rate are often caused by disturbances of rhythm (e.g. atrial fibrillation, complete heart block) in which ventricular filling is not augmented by atrial contraction, exacerbating the fall in stroke volume.

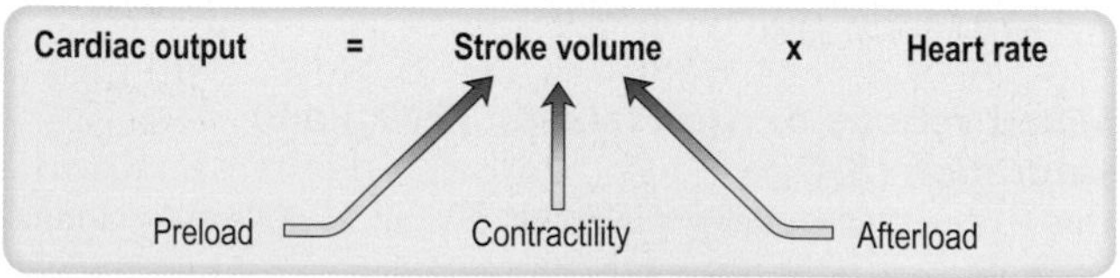

Figure 25.6 The determinants of cardiac output.

Stroke volume

The volume of blood ejected by the ventricle in a single contraction is the difference between the ventricular end-diastolic volume (VEDV) and ventricular end-systolic volume (VESV) (i.e. stroke volume = VEDV−VESV). The ejection fraction describes the stroke volume as a percentage of VEDV (i.e. ejection fraction = (VEDV − VESV)/VEDV × 100%) and is an indicator of myocardial performance.

Three interdependent factors determine the stroke volume (see p. 935).

Preload

This is defined as the tension of the myocardial fibres at the end of diastole, just before the onset of ventricular contraction, and is therefore related to the degree of stretch of the fibres. As the end-diastolic volume of the ventricle increases, tension in the myocardial fibres is increased and stroke volume rises ***(Fig. 25.7)***. Myocardial oxygen consumption ($\dot{V}_mO_2$) increases only slightly with an increase in preload (produced, for example, by a 'fluid challenge', see below) and this is therefore the most efficient way of improving cardiac output.

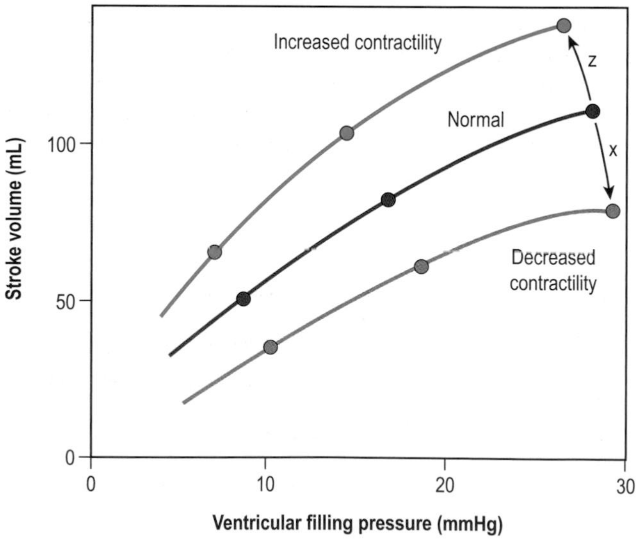

Figure 25.7 The Frank–Starling relationship: as preload is increased, stroke volume rises. If the ventricle is overstretched, stroke volume will fall (x). In myocardial failure, the curve is depressed and flattened. Increasing contractility, such as that due to sympathetic stimulation, shifts the curve upwards and to the left (z).

Myocardial contractility

This refers to the ability of the heart to perform work, independent of changes in preload and afterload. The state of myocardial contractility determines the response of the ventricles to changes in preload and afterload. Contractility is often reduced in critically ill patients, as a result of either pre-existing myocardial damage (e.g. ischaemic heart disease) or the acute disease process itself (e.g. sepsis). Changes in myocardial contractility alter the slope and position of the Starling curve; worsening ventricular performance is manifested as a depressed, flattened curve (***Figs 25.7*** and ***23.5***). Inotropic drugs can be used to increase myocardial contractility (see below).

Afterload

This is defined as the myocardial wall tension developed during systolic ejection. In the case of the left ventricle, the resistance imposed by the aortic valve, the peripheral vascular resistance and the elasticity of the major blood vessels are the major determinants of afterload. Ventricular wall tension will also be increased by ventricular dilatation, an increase in intraventricular pressure or a reduction in ventricular wall thickness.

Decreasing the afterload (through vasodilatation due to exercise, sepsis or vasodilating agents) can increase the stroke volume achieved at a given preload (***Fig. 25.8***), while reducing $\dot{V}_mO_2$. The reduction in wall tension also leads to an increase in coronary blood flow, thereby improving the myocardial oxygen supply/demand ratio. Excessive reductions in afterload will cause hypotension.

Increasing the afterload (vasoconstriction due to increased sympathetic activity, vasoconstrictor agents), on the other hand, can cause a fall in stroke volume and an increase in $\dot{V}_mO_2$.

Right ventricular afterload is normally negligible because the resistance of the pulmonary circulation is very low but is increased in pulmonary hypertension.

Cardiovascular assessment and monitoring of critically ill patients

As well as allowing immediate recognition of changes in the patient's condition, monitoring can also be used to establish or confirm a diagnosis, gauge the severity of the condition, follow the evolution of the illness, guide interventions and assess the response to treatment. Invasive monitoring is generally indicated in the more seriously ill patients and in those who fail to respond to initial treatment. These techniques are, however, associated with a significant risk of complications, as well as additional costs and patient discomfort, and should therefore only be used when the potential benefits outweigh the dangers. Likewise, invasive devices should be removed as soon as possible.

Assessment of tissue perfusion

- ***Pale, cold skin***, delayed capillary refill and the absence of visible veins in the hands and feet indicate poor perfusion. Although peripheral skin temperature measurements can help clinical evaluation, the earliest compensatory response to hypovolaemia or a low cardiac output, and the last to resolve after resuscitation, is vasoconstriction in the splanchnic region.
- ***Metabolic acidosis with raised lactate concentration*** suggests that tissue perfusion is sufficiently compromised to cause cellular hypoxia and anaerobic glycolysis. Persistent, severe lactic acidosis is associated with a very poor prognosis. In addition to being used as a screen for cardiovascular insufficiency and poor tissue perfusion, lactate levels are frequently used to guide resuscitation. Extremely high lactate levels that do not respond to resuscitation are suggestive of reduced splanchnic blood flow and bowel ischaemia. In many critically ill patients, especially those with sepsis, lactic acidosis can also be caused by metabolic disorders unrelated to tissue hypoxia and can be exacerbated by reduced clearance owing to hepatic or renal dysfunction, as well as the administration of adrenaline (epinephrine).
- ***Urinary flow*** is a sensitive indicator of renal perfusion and haemodynamic performance.

Blood pressure

Alterations in blood pressure are often interpreted as reflecting changes in cardiac output. However, if there is vasoconstriction with a high peripheral resistance, the blood pressure may be normal, even when the cardiac output is reduced. Conversely, the vasodilated patient may be hypotensive, despite a very high cardiac output.

Hypotension jeopardizes perfusion of vital organs. The adequacy of blood pressure in an individual patient must always be assessed in relation to the premorbid value. Blood pressure is traditionally measured using a sphygmomanometer, but if rapid alterations are anticipated, continuous monitoring using an intra-arterial cannula is indicated (***Box 25.4*** and ***Fig. 25.9***).

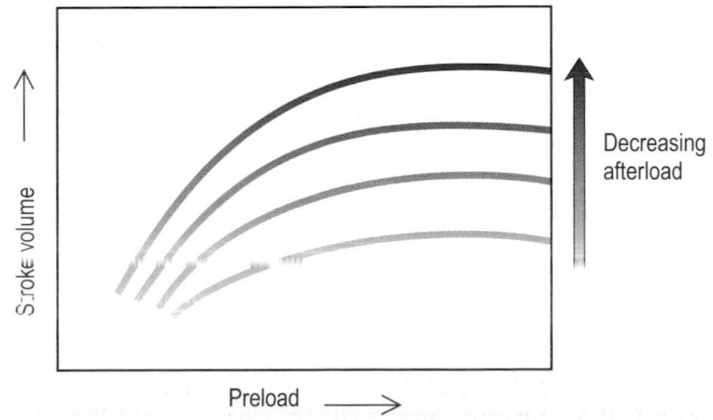

Figure 25.8 The effect of changes in afterload on the ventricular function curve. At any given preload, decreasing afterload increases the stroke volume.

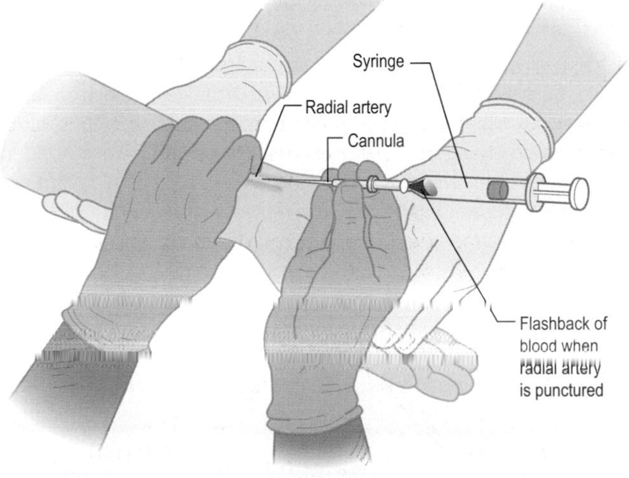

Figure 25.9 Percutaneous cannulation of the radial artery.

Box 25.4 Radial artery cannulation

Technique

1. Explain the procedure to the patient and, if possible, obtain consent.
2. Ask an assistant to support the patient's arm, with the wrist extended. (Gloves should be worn.)
3. Clean the skin with chlorhexidine. Take sterile precautions throughout the procedure.
4. Palpate the radial artery where it arches over the head of the radius.
5. In conscious patients, inject local anaesthetic to raise a weal over the artery, taking care not to puncture the vessel or obscure its pulsation.
6. Make a small skin incision over the proposed puncture site.
7. Use a small, parallel-sided cannula (20 gauge for adults, 22 gauge for children) in order to allow blood flow to continue past the cannula.
8. Insert the cannula over the point of maximal pulsation and advance it in line with the direction of the vessel at an angle of approximately 30°.
9. Look for 'flashback' of blood into the cannula, which indicates that the radial artery has been punctured.
10. To ensure that the shoulder of the cannula enters the vessel, lower the needle and cannula and advance them a few millimetres into the vessel.
11. Thread the cannula off the needle into the vessel and withdraw the needle.
12. Connect the cannula to a non-compliant manometer line filled with saline. Then connect this via a transducer and continuous flush device to a monitor, which records the arterial pressure.

Complications

- Thrombosis
- Loss of arterial pulsation
- Distal ischaemia, e.g. digital necrosis (rare)
- Infection
- Accidental injection of drugs – can produce vascular occlusion
- Disconnection – rapid blood loss

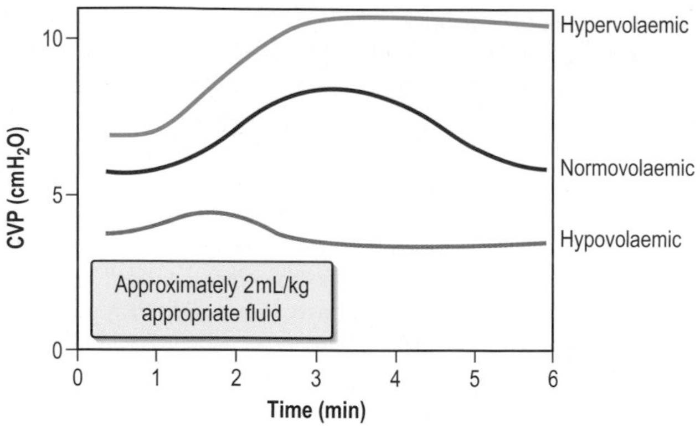

Figure 25.10 The effects on the central venous pressure (CVP) of rapid administration of a 'fluid challenge' to patients with a CVP within the normal range.

Central venous pressure

Assessment of central venous pressure (CVP) provides a fairly simple, but approximate, method of gauging the adequacy of a patient's circulating volume and may reflect the contractile state of the myocardium. The absolute value of the CVP is not as informative as its response to a fluid challenge (the infusion of 100–200 mL of fluid over a few minutes; ***Fig. 25.10***). The hypovolaemic patient will initially respond to transfusion with little or no change in CVP, together with some improvement in cardiovascular function (falling heart rate, rising blood pressure, increased peripheral temperature and urine output). As the normovolaemic state is approached, the CVP may rise slightly and reach a plateau, while other cardiovascular values begin to stabilize. At this stage, volume replacement should be slowed, or even stopped, in order to avoid excessive transfusion (indicated by an abrupt and sustained rise in CVP, often accompanied by some deterioration in the patient's condition). In cardiac failure, the venous pressure is usually high; the patient will not improve in response to volume replacement, which will cause a further, sometimes dramatic, rise in CVP.

The use of CVP to assess cardiovascular function, and the relationship between the response of the CVP to fluid challenge and the intravascular volume, are controversial. Many studies have failed to confirm this relationship and the use of CVP for this purpose is beginning to be supplanted by newer methods, particularly pulse contour analysis and oesophageal Doppler techniques (see below).

Central venous catheters are usually inserted via a percutaneous puncture of the subclavian or internal jugular vein using a guidewire technique (***Box 25.5*** and ***Figs 25.11*** and ***25.12***). The objective is to place the tip of the catheter approximately at the junction of the superior vena cava and the right atrium. Usually, these catheters consist of more than one lumen, some of which may be used for drug or fluid administration. Central venous cannulae may also be inserted via the femoral vein; when this route is used, the tip of the cannula will lie in the inferior vena cava and pressure measurements will not be a reliable guide to the circulating volume. Guidewire techniques can also be used for inserting double-lumen cannulae for haemofiltration or pulmonary artery catheter introducers. The

Box 25.5 Internal jugular vein cannulation

Technique

1. Explain the procedure to the patient and, if possible, obtain consent.
2. Place the patient head down to distend the central veins (this facilitates cannulation and minimizes the risk of air embolism but may exacerbate respiratory distress and is dangerous in those with raised intracranial pressure).
3. Clean the skin with an antiseptic solution such as chlorhexidine. Take sterile precautions throughout the procedure.
4. Inject local anaesthetic (1% plain lidocaine) intradermally to raise a weal at the apex of a triangle formed by the two heads of sternomastoid with the clavicle at its base.
5. Make a small incision through the weal.
6. Insert the cannula or needle through the incision and direct it laterally, downwards and backwards, in the direction of the nipple until the vein is punctured just beneath the skin and deep to the lateral head of sternomastoid.

Ultrasound-guided puncture is recommended to reduce the incidence of complications.

7. Check that venous blood is easily aspirated.
8. Thread the cannula off the needle into the vein or pass the guidewire through the needle (see ***Fig. 25.12***).
9. Connect the central venous pressure manometer line to a manometer/transducer.
10. Take a chest X-ray to verify that the tip of the catheter is in the superior vena cava and to exclude pneumothorax.

Possible complications

- Haemorrhage
- Accidental arterial puncture (carotid or subclavian)
- Pneumothorax
- Damage to thoracic duct on left
- Air embolism
- Thrombosis
- Catheter-related sepsis

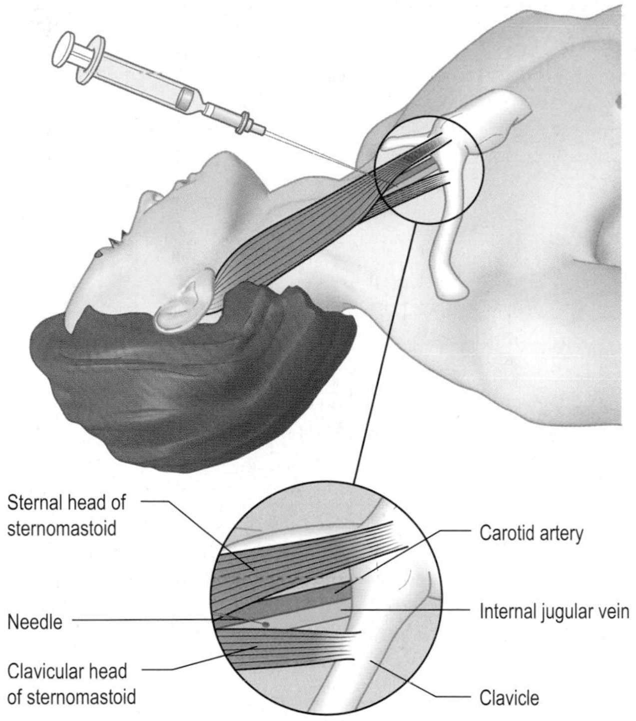

Figure 25.11 Cannulation of the right internal jugular vein.

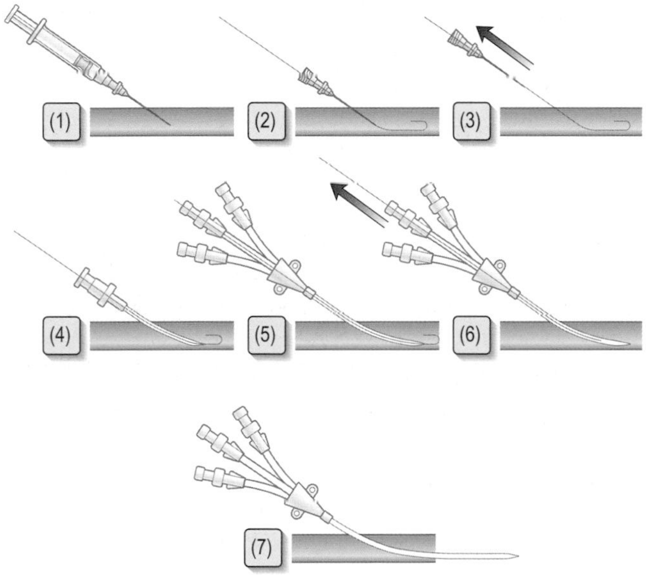

Figure 25.12 Seldinger technique – insertion of a catheter over guidewire. (1) Puncture vessel. (2) Advance guidewire. (3) Remove needle. (4) Dilate vessel. (5) Advance catheter over guidewire. (6) Remove guidewire; (7) Catheter *in situ*.

routine use of ultrasound to guide central venous cannulation reduces complication rates.

The CVP is usually displayed continuously using a transducer and bedside monitor but, in the absence of such equipment, can be recorded intermittently using a manometer system. It is essential for the recorded pressure always to be related to the level of the right atrium. Various landmarks are advocated (e.g. sternal notch with the patient supine; sternal angle or mid-axilla when the patient is at 45°), but the choice is largely immaterial, provided the landmark is used consistently in an individual patient.

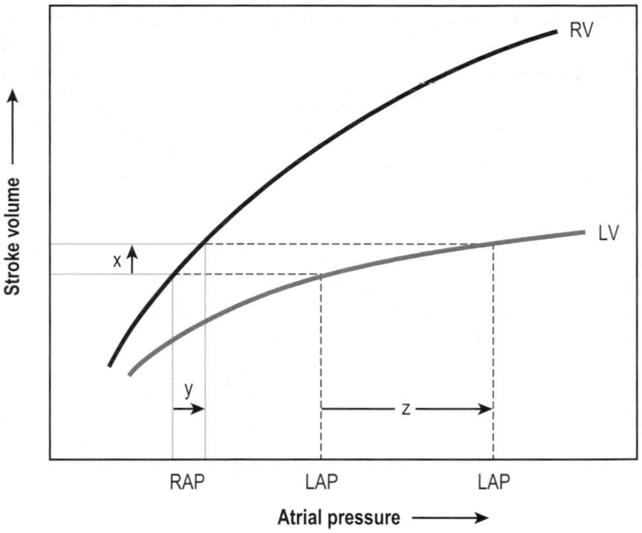

Figure 25.13 Left ventricular (LV) and right ventricular (RV) function curves in a patient with left ventricular dysfunction. Since the stroke volume of the two ventricles must be the same (except, perhaps, for a few beats during a period of circulatory adjustment), left atrial pressure (LAP) must be higher than right atrial pressure (RAP). Moreover, an increase in stroke volume (x) produced by expanding the circulatory volume may be associated with a small rise in RAP (y) but a marked increase in LAP (z)

Left atrial pressure

In uncomplicated cases, careful interpretation of the CVP may provide a reasonable guide to the filling pressures of both sides of the heart. In many critically ill patients, however, there is a disparity in function between the two ventricles. Most commonly, left ventricular performance is worse, so that the left ventricular function curve is displaced downwards and to the right ***(Fig. 25.13)***. High right ventricular filling pressures, with normal or low left atrial pressures, are less common but occur with right ventricular dysfunction and with raised pulmonary vascular resistance (i.e. right ventricular afterload), such as in acute respiratory failure and pulmonary embolism.

Pulmonary artery pressures

A 'balloon flotation catheter' enables reliable catheterization of the pulmonary artery. These 'Swan–Ganz' catheters can be inserted centrally (see ***Fig. 25.11***) or through the femoral vein, or via a vein in the antecubital fossa. Passage of the catheter from the major veins, through the chambers of the heart into the pulmonary artery and into the wedged position, is monitored and guided by the pressure waveforms recorded from the distal lumen (***Box 25.6*** and ***Fig. 25.14***). A chest X-ray should always be obtained to check the final position of the catheter ***(Fig. 25.15)***.

Once in place, the balloon is deflated and the pulmonary artery mean, systolic and end-diastolic pressures (PAEDP) can be recorded. The pulmonary artery occlusion pressure (PAOP; previously referred to as the pulmonary artery or capillary 'wedge' pressure) is measured by re-inflating the balloon, thereby propelling the catheter distally until it impacts in a medium-sized pulmonary artery. In this position, there is a continuous column of fluid between the distal lumen of the catheter and the left atrium, so that the PAOP is usually a reasonable reflection of left atrial pressure.

The technique is generally safe; the majority of complications, such as 'knotting', valve trauma and pulmonary artery rupture (which can be fatal), are related to user inexperience.

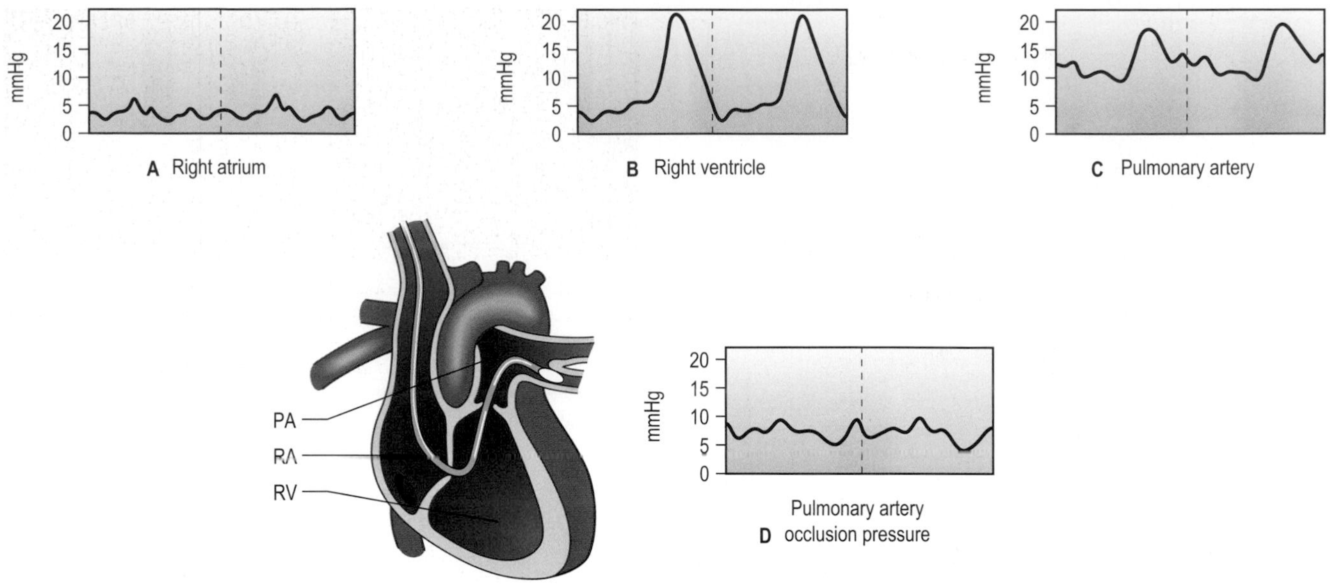

Figure 25.14 Passage of pulmonary artery balloon flotation catheter through the chambers of the heart. The catheter is passed into the 'wedged' position to measure the pulmonary artery occlusion pressure (see ***Box 25.6***). PA, pulmonary artery; RA, right artery; RV, right ventricle.

Box 25.6 Passage of a pulmonary artery balloon flotation catheter

The catheter is passed through the chambers of the heart into the 'wedged' position.

1. Explain the procedure to the patient and, if possible, obtain consent.
2. Insert a balloon flotation catheter through a large vein (see text).
3. Look for respiratory oscillations once the catheter is in the thorax. Advance it further towards the lower superior vena cava/right atrium (see ***Fig. 25.14A***), where pressure oscillations become more pronounced. Then inflate the balloon and advance the catheter.
4. When the catheter is in the right ventricle (see ***Fig. 25.14B***), there is no dicrotic notch and the diastolic pressure is close to 0. Return the patient to the horizontal, or slightly head-up, position before advancing the catheter further.
5. When the catheter reaches the pulmonary artery (see ***Fig. 25.14C***), a dicrotic notch appears and there is elevation of the diastolic pressure. Advance the catheter further with the balloon inflated.
6. Reappearance of a venous waveform indicates that the catheter is 'wedged'. Deflate the balloon to obtain the pulmonary artery pressure. Inflate the balloon intermittently to obtain the pulmonary artery occlusion pressure (also known as pulmonary artery or capillary 'wedge' pressure; see ***Fig. 25.14D***).

Cardiac output

Cardiac output can be continuously monitored using a modified pulmonary artery catheter that transmits low-energy heat from a heating element in the catheter into the surrounding blood. A 'thermodilution curve' is constructed by measuring dissipation of the heat using a thermistor located distal to the heating coil. The dissipation of heat is directly proportional to the cardiac output. These catheters also optically measure and continuously display $S_{\bar{v}}O_2$.

In general, pulmonary artery catheters may help the clinician to optimize cardiac output and oxygen delivery, while minimizing the risk of volume overload. They can also be used to guide the rational use of inotropes and vasoactive agents, and are particularly helpful in patients with pulmonary hypertension. The unselective use of this monitoring device in the absence of evidence-based haemodynamic goals does not, however, lead to improved outcomes and less invasive techniques are preferred, except in the most complex cases (e.g. high-risk cardiac surgery).

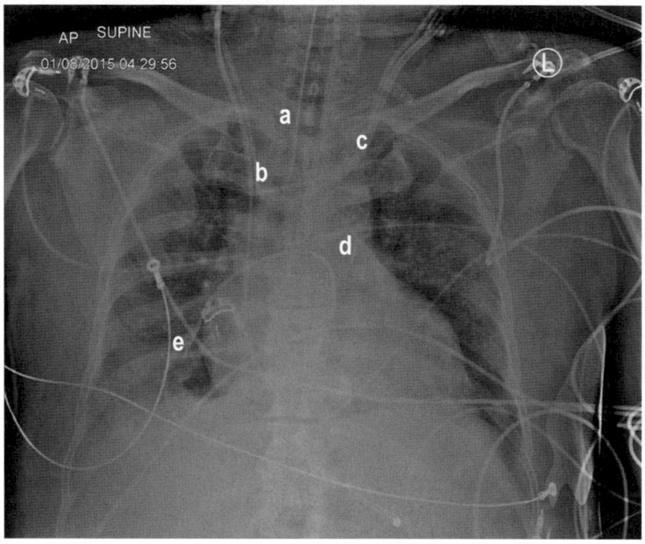

Figure 25.15 Chest X-ray of a critically ill, mechanically ventilated patient. The X-ray shows **(a)** endotracheal tube; **(b)** end of central venous line seen here medial to the proximal end of the pulmonary artery catheter; **(c)** double-lumen catheter for continuous renal replacement therapy placed via the left internal jugular vein; **(d)** tip of the intra-aortic balloon pump travelling superiorly from a femoral artery; and **(e)** pulmonary artery catheter. Note that the tip of the catheter is too distal; it was therefore subsequently withdrawn by a few centimetres.

Less invasive techniques for assessing cardiac function and guiding volume replacement

Arterial pressure variation as a guide to hypovolaemia

Systolic arterial pressure decreases during the inspiratory phase of intermittent positive pressure ventilation (see p. 1163). The

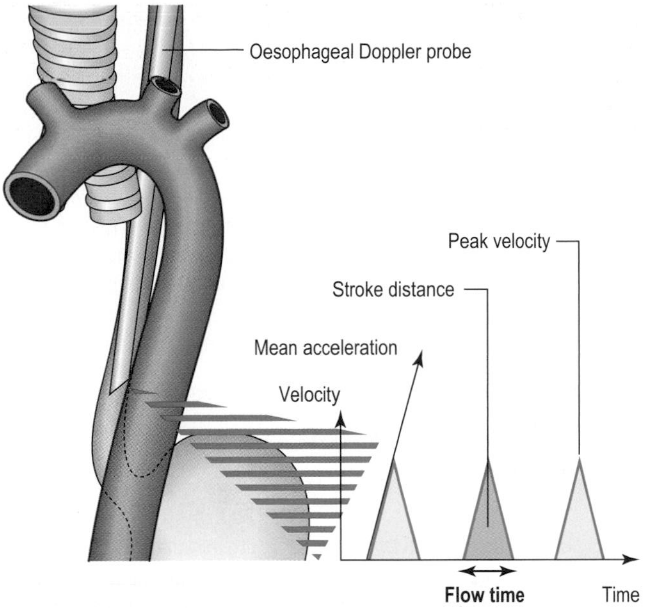

Figure 25.16 Doppler ultrasonography. Velocity waveform traces are obtained using oesophageal Doppler ultrasonography. *(Reproduced from Singer et al (1991), with permission. © 1991 The Williams & Wilkins Co., Baltimore.)*

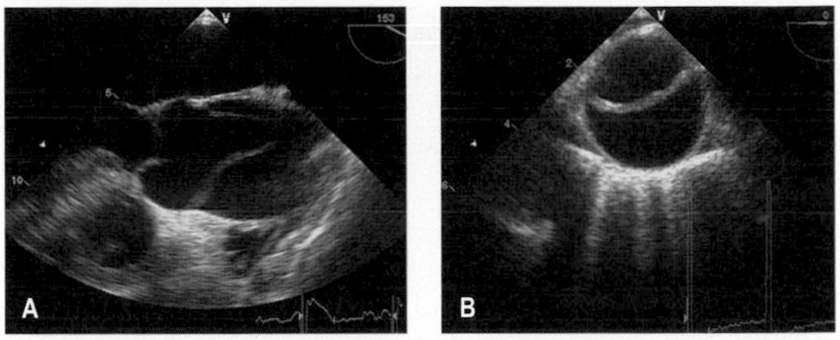

Figure 25.17 Aortic dissection (transoesophageal echocardiography, TOE). A. Mid-oesophageal, long-axis view showing type A aortic dissection. **B.** Short-axis view of descending aorta showing intimal flap with false and true lumen. *(From Hinds CJ, Watson JD.* Intensive Care: A Concise Textbook, *3rd edn. Edinburgh: Saunders; 2008. Courtesy of Dr C. Rathwell.)*

Box 25.7 Key points in monitoring cardiac function

- If there is disagreement between clinical signs and a monitored variable, it should be assumed that the monitor is incorrect until all sources of potential error have been checked and eliminated
- Changes and trends in monitored variables are more informative than a single reading
- Use non-invasive monitoring where possible
- Remove invasive devices as soon as possible

magnitude of this cyclical variability has been shown to correlate more closely with hypovolaemia than other monitored variables, including CVP. Systolic pressure (or pulse pressure) variation during mechanical ventilation can therefore be used as a simple and reliable guide to the adequacy of the circulatory volume. The response to fluid loading can also be predicted simply by observing the changes in pulse pressure during passive leg-raising.

Oesophageal Doppler

Stroke volume, cardiac output and myocardial function can be assessed non-invasively using Doppler ultrasonography. A probe is passed into the oesophagus to monitor velocity waveforms from the descending aorta continuously ***(Fig. 25.16)***. Although reasonable estimates of stroke volume, and hence cardiac output, can be obtained, the technique is best used for trend analysis rather than for making absolute measurements. Oesophageal Doppler probes can be inserted quickly and easily, and are particularly valuable for perioperative optimization of the circulating volume and cardiac performance in the unconscious patient. They are contraindicated in patients with oropharyngeal/oesophageal pathology.

Arterial waveform analysis

Lithium dilution/pulse contour analysis does not require pulmonary artery catheterization or instrumentation of the oesophagus and is suitable for use in conscious patients. A bolus of lithium chloride is administered via a central venous catheter and the change in arterial plasma lithium concentration is detected by a lithium-sensitive [illegible] cannula via a three-way tap. A small battery-powered peristaltic pump is used to create a constant blood flow through the sensor and over the electrode tip. The cardiac output determined in this way can be used to calibrate an arterial pressure waveform ('pulse contour') analysis programme that will continuously monitor changes in cardiac output. Devices that use uncalibrated pulse contour analysis to estimate cardiac output are also available.

Other devices utilize a thermodilution technique, where a small volume of cold fluid is injected into a large central vein and a temperature washout curve is detected via a sensor in a modified arterial line. Following this calibration, beat-to-beat cardiac output is generated by computer-based analysis of the arterial pressure waveform.

As with pulse pressure variation, stroke volume variation, determined by oesophageal Doppler or arterial waveform analysis, can be used to guide fluid replacement.

Echocardiography

Echocardiography is being used increasingly often to provide immediate diagnostic information about cardiac structure and function (myocardial contractility, ventricular filling) in the critically ill patient. Although transoesophageal echocardiography (TOE) may be preferred because of its superior image clarity ***(Fig. 25.17)***, transthoracic probes are increasingly used on general ICUs.

Key points in monitoring cardiac function

These are shown in ***Box 25.7***.

Further reading

Lamperti M, Bodenham AR, Pittiruti M et al. International evidence-based recommendations on ultrasound-guided vascular access. *Intensive Care Med* 2012; 38:1105–1117.

Marik PE, Monnet X, Teboul JL. Hemodynamic parameters to guide fluid therapy. *Ann Intensive Care* 2011; 1:1.

DISTURBANCES OF ACID–BASE BALANCE

The physiology of acid–base control is discussed on pages 174–176. Acid–base disturbances can be described in relation to ***Figure 9.14*** (which shows P_aCO_2 plotted against arterial $[H^+]$).

Box 25.8 Arterial blood gas and acid–base values

Analyte	Normal reference range
H^+	35–45 nmol/L (pH 7.35–7.45)
PO_2 (breathing room air)	10.6–13.3 kPa (80–100 mmHg)
PCO_2	4.8–6.1 kPa (36–46 mmHg)
Base deficit	±2.5
Plasma HCO_3^-	22–26 mmol/L
O_2 saturation	95–100%

Both acidosis and alkalosis can occur, each of which is either metabolic (primarily affecting the bicarbonate component of the system) or respiratory (primarily affecting P_aCO_2). Compensatory changes may also be apparent. In clinical practice, arterial $[H^+]$ values outside the range 18–126 nmol/L (pH 6.9–7.7) are rarely encountered.

Blood gas and acid–base values (normal ranges) are shown in ***Box 25.8***. (For blood gas analysis, see pp. 1161–1162.)

Respiratory acidosis

This is caused by retention of carbon dioxide. The P_aCO_2 and $[H^+]$ rise. A chronically raised P_aCO_2 is compensated by renal retention of bicarbonate, and the $[H^+]$ returns towards normal. A constant arterial bicarbonate concentration is then usually established within 2–5 days. This represents a primary respiratory acidosis with a compensatory metabolic alkalosis (see p. 177). Common causes of respiratory acidosis include ventilatory failure and COPD (type II respiratory failure, where there is a high P_aCO_2 and a low P_aO_2; see p. 1161).

Respiratory alkalosis

In this case, the reverse occurs and there is a fall in P_aCO_2 and $[H^+]$, often with a small reduction in bicarbonate concentration. If hypocarbia persists, some degree of renal compensation may occur, producing a metabolic acidosis, although in practice this is unusual. A respiratory alkalosis may be produced, intentionally or unintentionally, when patients are mechanically ventilated; it may also be seen in patients with hypoxaemic (type I) respiratory failure (see p. 1161), those with spontaneous hyperventilation, and those living at high altitudes (see online, 'Adaptation to hypoxia', for an example of a partly compensated respiratory alkalosis secondary to extreme hypoxaemia).

Metabolic acidosis

Metabolic acidosis (see p. 177) may be due to excessive acid production, often lactate and H^+ (lactic acidosis), as a consequence of anaerobic metabolism during an episode of shock or following cardiac arrest. A metabolic acidosis may develop as a consequence of chronic renal failure or in diabetic ketoacidosis. It can also follow the loss of bicarbonate from the gut or from the kidney in renal tubular acidosis. Respiratory compensation for a metabolic acidosis is usually slightly delayed because the blood–brain barrier initially prevents the respiratory centre from sensing the increased blood $[H^+]$. Following this short delay, however, the patient hyperventilates and 'blows off' carbon dioxide to produce a compensatory respiratory alkalosis. There is a limit to this respiratory compensation, since, in practice, values for P_aCO_2 less than about 1.4 kPa (11 mmHg) are rarely achieved. Spontaneous respiratory compensation cannot occur if the patient's ventilation is controlled or if the respiratory centre is depressed: for example, by drugs or head injury.

Metabolic alkalosis

This can be caused by loss of acid – for example, from the stomach with nasogastric suction, or in high intestinal obstruction, or excessive administration of absorbable alkali. Over-zealous treatment with intravenous sodium bicarbonate is sometimes implicated. Respiratory compensation for a metabolic alkalosis is often slight, and it is rare to encounter a P_aCO_2 above 6.5 kPa (50 mmHg), even with severe alkalosis.

SHOCK, SEPSIS AND ACUTE DISTURBANCES OF HAEMODYNAMIC FUNCTION

Shock is the term used to describe acute circulatory failure with inadequate or inappropriately distributed tissue perfusion, resulting in generalized cellular hypoxia and/or an inability of the cells to utilize oxygen.

Aetiology of shock

Abnormalities of tissue perfusion can result from:

- failure of the heart to act as an effective pump
- mechanical impediments to forward flow
- loss of circulatory volume
- abnormalities of the peripheral circulation.

The causes of shock are shown in ***Box 25.9***; see also page 1154 for definitions of sepsis. Often, shock can result from a combination of these factors (e.g. in sepsis, distributive shock is frequently complicated by hypovolaemia and myocardial depression).

Pathophysiology

The sympatho-adrenal response to shock

Hypotension stimulates the baroreceptors, and to a lesser extent the chemoreceptors, causing increased sympathetic nervous activity with 'spill-over' of noradrenaline (norepinephrine) into the circulation. Later, this is augmented by the release of catecholamines (predominantly, adrenaline (epinephrine)) from the adrenal medulla. The resulting vasoconstriction, together with increased myocardial contractility and heart rate, help to restore blood pressure and cardiac output ***(Fig. 25.18)***.

Box 25.9 Causes of shock

Hypovolaemic
- Exogenous losses (e.g. haemorrhage, burns)

Cardiogenic
- 'Myocardial failure' (e.g. ischaemic myocardial injury)

Obstructive
- Obstruction to cardiac outflow (e.g. pulmonary embolus)
- Restricted cardiac filling (e.g. cardiac tamponade, tension pneumothorax)

Distributive
- (e.g. sepsis, anaphylaxis)
- Vascular dilatation
- Sequestration
- Arteriovenous shunting
- Maldistribution of flow
- Myocardial depression

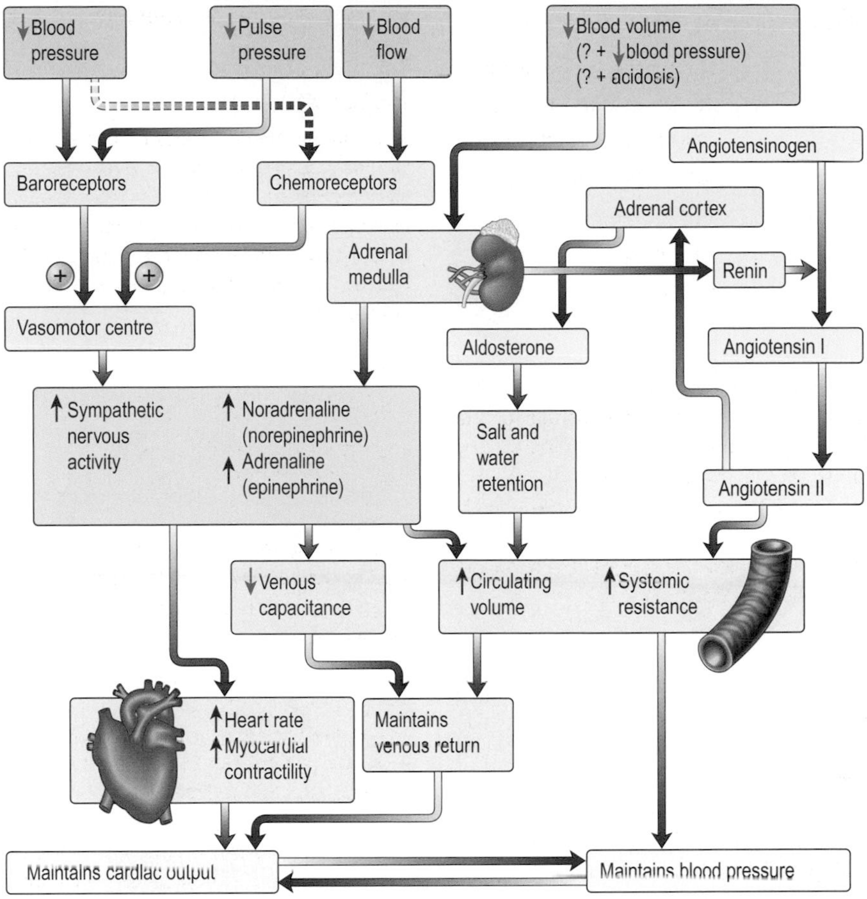

Figure 25.18 The sympatho-adrenal response to shock. The effect of increased catecholamines is shown on the left of the diagram, and the release of angiotensin and aldosterone on the right. Both mechanisms help to maintain the cardiac output and blood pressure in shock.

Reduced perfusion of the renal cortex stimulates the juxtaglomerular apparatus to release renin. This converts angiotensinogen to angiotensin I, which, in turn, is converted in the lungs and by the vascular endothelium to the potent vasoconstrictor angiotensin II. Angiotensin II also stimulates secretion of aldosterone by the adrenal cortex, causing sodium and water retention (see p. 728). This helps to restore the circulating volume (see p. 150).

The neuroendocrine response

- There is ***release of pituitary hormones***, such as adrenocorticotrophic hormone (ACTH), vasopressin (antidiuretic hormone, ADH) and endogenous opioid peptides. (In septic shock, there may be a relative deficiency of vasopressin.)
- There is ***release of cortisol***, which causes fluid retention and antagonizes insulin.
- There is ***release of glucagon***, which raises the blood sugar level.

Although absolute adrenocortical insufficiency (e.g. due to bilateral adrenal haemorrhage or necrosis in meningococcal infection) is rare, there is evidence that patients with septic shock have a blunted response to exogenous ACTH (so-called '***relative***' or '***occult' adrenocortical insufficiency***), and that this could be associated with an impaired vasoconstrictor response to noradrenaline (norepinephrine) and a worse prognosis. The diagnosis, causes and clinical significance of this phenomenon remain unclear.

Release of immune mediators

Severe infection (often with bacteraemia or endotoxaemia), the presence of large areas of damaged tissue (e.g. following trauma or extensive surgery), hypoxia or prolonged/repeated episodes of hypoperfusion can trigger a dysfunctional immune response with alterations in leucocyte activation and release of a variety of potentially damaging 'mediators' (see also pp. 136–138). Although an appropriate immune response is clearly beneficial when targeted against local areas of infection or necrotic tissue, the disseminated, dysregulated response observed in some patients can lead to shock and organ failure. This immune response can be complex, with features of upregulation and downregulation of both the innate and the adaptive immune pathways present at different stages of the illness. Characteristically, the later phase is typified by a period of immune suppression, which, in some cases, may be profound and during which the patient is at increased risk of developing secondary infections.

Microorganisms and their toxic products

In sepsis/septic shock, the innate immune response (*Fig. 25.19*) and inflammatory cascade are triggered by the recognition of pathogen-associated molecular patterns (PAMPs), including bacterial and fungal DNA, cell-wall components (e.g. endotoxin) and/or exotoxins (antigenic proteins produced by bacteria such as staphylococci, streptococci and *Pseudomonas*).

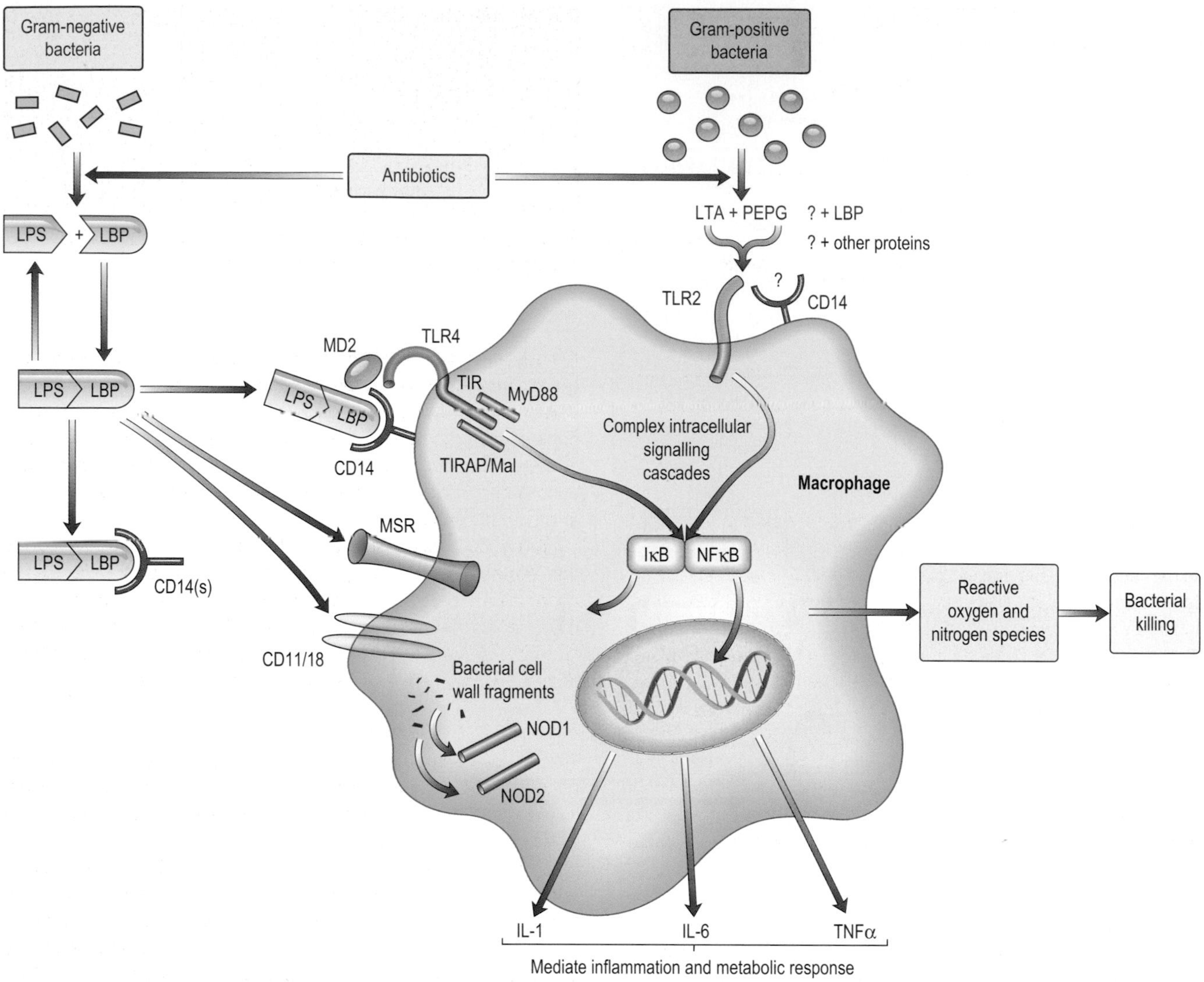

Figure 25.19 **Induction of the innate immune response by the lipopolysaccharide–lipopolysaccharide-binding protein (LPS–LBP) complex.** This simplified figure illustrates the intracellular events initiated by Gram-negative and Gram-positive bacteria, which eventually lead to bacterial killing. IκB, inhibitory factor kappa B; IL, interleukin; LTA, lipoteichoic acid; MD2, a secreted protein involved in binding liposaccharide with TLR4; MSR, macrophage scavenger receptor; MyD88, myeloid differentiation factor 88; NFκB, nuclear factor kappa B; PEPG, peptidoglycan-N; TIR, toll-interleukin receptor; TIRAP, toll-interleukin 1 receptor adaptor protein; TIRAP/Mal, an adaptor protein for TLR2 and TLR4; TLR, toll-like receptors; TNFα, tumour necrosis factor alpha.

Endotoxin is a lipopolysaccharide (LPS) derived from the cell wall of Gram-negative bacteria and is a potent trigger of the innate immune response. The lipid A portion of LPS can be bound by a protein normally present in human serum known as lipopolysaccharide-binding protein (LBP). The LBP–LPS complex attaches to the cell surface marker CD14 and, combined with a secreted protein (MD2), this complex then binds to a member of the toll-like receptor family (TLR4), which transduces the activation signal into the cell. These receptors act through an adaptor molecule, myeloid differentiation factor 88 (MyD88), to regulate the activity of the nuclear transcription factor NFκB, which then passes into the nucleus, where it binds to DNA and promotes the synthesis of a wide variety of immune mediators. Gram-positive bacteria have cell-wall components that are similar in structure to LPS (e.g. lipoteichoic acid), and can also trigger a systemic inflammatory response, probably through similar (TLR2) but not identical pathways ***(Fig. 25.19)***.

Toxic products of tissue injury (surgery and trauma)

Following traumatic or surgical tissue injury, inflammatory pathways may be triggered by damage-associated molecular patterns (DAMPS), such as DNA fragments. Of particular importance is circulating mitochondrial DNA (mtDNA), which retains homology with bacterial DNA in terms of methylation patterns across nucleotides and can be 'mistaken' by the immune system for bacterial DNA. The patient then initiates an immune response apparently almost identical to that observed following bacterial invasion. This is why distributive shock secondary to infection can be difficult to distinguish clinically from that caused by a 'sterile' insult such as severe trauma or surgery.

Cytokines and other immune mediators

An array of cytokines (small proteins released by cells that have specific effects on the interactions between cells, on communications between cells or on the behaviour of cells), chemokines (a

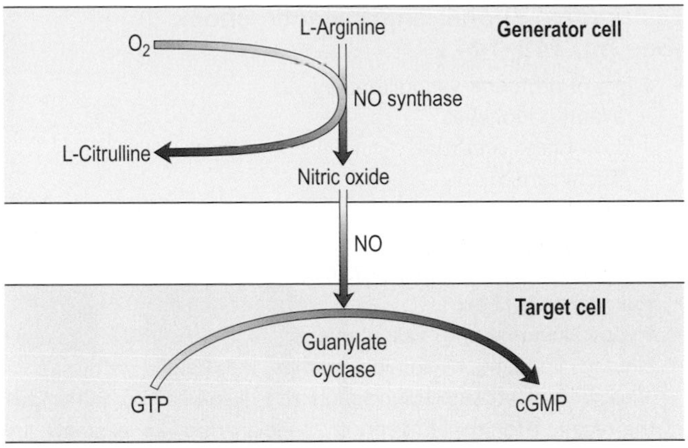

Figure 25.20 Synthesis and biochemical action of nitric oxide (NO). cGMP, cyclic guanosine monophosphate; GTP, guanosine triphosphate.

family of signalling cytokines that induce chemotaxis in nearby cells), prostaglandins, leukotrienes (see ***Fig. 24.30***), heat shock proteins, adhesion molecules and endothelial derived vasoactive factors are induced, particularly during distributive shock. These include pro-inflammatory cytokines (tumour necrosis factor alpha, TNF-α, and interferon gamma, IFN-γ), anti-inflammatory cytokines (interleukin 10, IL-10), mediators promoting extracellular extravasation (intracellular adhesion molecule 1, ICAM-1) (see ***Fig. 8.9***) and vasodilatation (inducible nitric oxide synthase, iNOS; ***Fig. 25.20***). Although there was initial enthusiasm for treatments that dampened the immune response (e.g. high-dose steroids and anti-TNF-α compounds) in cases of distributive shock secondary to infection (septic shock), these strategies failed to improve survival and were sometimes associated with worse outcomes.

Activation of the complement cascade

Fragments of C3 act as opsonins and co-stimulatory molecules that assist lymphocytes with the adaptive immune response, while small peptides derived from C3, C4 and C5 cause leucocyte chemotaxis, release of cytokines and increased vascular permeability (see p. 124).

Influence of genetic variation

Individuals vary considerably in their susceptibility to infection, as well as their ability to recover from apparently similar infections, illnesses or traumatic insults. There is evidence to suggest that inter-individual variations in susceptibility to, and outcome from, sepsis can be partly explained by genetic variation.

Haemodynamic and microcirculatory changes

The dominant haemodynamic feature of severe sepsis/septic shock is peripheral vascular failure with:

- vasodilatation
- maldistribution of regional blood flow
- abnormalities in the microcirculation ***(Fig. 25.21)***:
  - 'stop-flow' capillaries (flow is intermittent)
  - 'no-flow' capillaries (capillaries are obstructed) failure of capillary recruitment
  - increased capillary permeability with interstitial oedema.

Although these ***vascular and microvascular abnormalities*** may partly account for the reduced oxygen extraction often seen, particularly in septic shock, there is also a ***primary defect of cellular oxygen utilization*** caused by mitochondrial dysfunction (see above). Initially, before hypovolaemia supervenes, or when

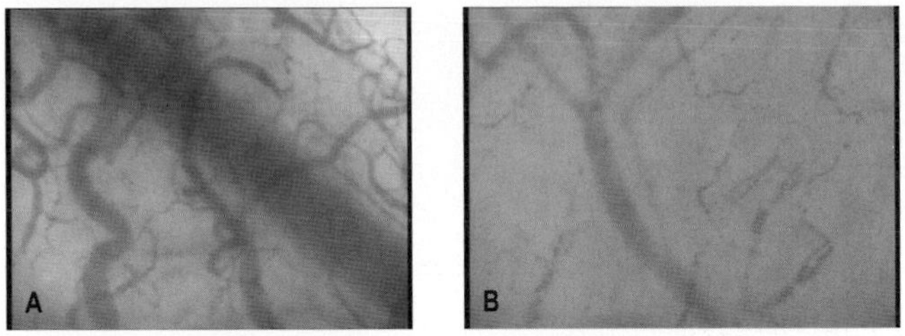

Figure 25.21 Still side-stream dark field (SDF) images of the microcirculation. A. Normal subject. **B.** Septic shock.

therapeutic replacement of the circulating volume has been adequate, ***cardiac output is usually high and peripheral resistance is low***. These changes may be associated with impaired oxygen consumption, a reduced arteriovenous oxygen content difference, an increased $S_{\bar{v}}O_2$ and a lactic acidosis (so-called '***tissue dysoxia***'). Vasodilatation and increased vascular permeability also occur in anaphylactic shock.

The glycocalyx consists of a tight, negatively charged, extremely thin meshwork of proteoglycans on the luminal surface of the endothelium. Oxidative stress, free radicals and endotoxaemia all have specific detrimental effects on the glycocalyx that promote fluid movement into the tissues. Widespread, 'pitting', peripheral oedema is often seen in the most seriously ill patients.

Activation of the coagulation system

The immune response to shock, tissue injury and infection is frequently associated with systemic activation of the clotting cascade, leading to platelet aggregation, widespread microvascular thrombosis and inadequate tissue perfusion.

Initially, the production of prostaglandin I_2 (PGI_2) by the capillary endothelium is impaired. Cell damage (e.g. to the vascular endothelium) leads to exposure to tissue factor (see p. 565), which triggers coagulation. In severe cases, these changes are compounded by elevated levels of plasminogen activation inhibitor type 1, which impairs fibrinolysis, as well as by deficiencies in physiological inhibitors of coagulation (including antithrombin, proteins C and S, and tissue factor-pathway inhibitor). Antithrombin and protein C have a number of anti-inflammatory properties, whereas thrombin is pro-inflammatory. This procoagulant state can lead to end-artery thrombosis and digital and mesenteric ischaemia. Following clot formation, plasminogen is converted to plasmin, which breaks down thrombus, liberating fibrin/fibrinogen degradation products (FDPs). Fibrin formation and fibrinolysis continue unabated and in parallel, leading to a 'consumptive' coagulopathy known as ***disseminated intravascular coagulation*** (***DIC***). Circulating levels of FDPs and D-dimers are therefore increased, the thrombin time, PTT and PT are prolonged, and platelet and fibrinogen levels fall. Clinically, the patient will bleed from trivial venepuncture sites but, paradoxically, may still be at risk of thrombosis. Activation of the coagulation cascade can be confirmed by demonstrating increased plasma levels of D-dimers. The development of DIC often heralds the onset of multiple organ failure. In some cases, a microangiopathic haemolytic anaemia develops. DIC is relatively uncommon but is associated particularly with septic shock, especially when due to meningococcal infection (see p. 281). Management of the ***underlying cause*** is most urgent. Supportive treatment may include infusions of fresh frozen plasma, platelets, cryoprecipitate when fibrinogen levels are low, and occasionally factor VIII concentrates.

Box 25.10 Haemodynamic changes in shock

Hypovolaemic shock
Low central venous pressure (CVP) and pulmonary artery occlusion pressure (PAOP)
- Low cardiac output
- Increased systemic vascular resistance

Cardiogenic shock
Signs of myocardial failure
- Increased systemic vascular resistance
- CVP and PAOP high (except when hypovolaemic)

Cardiac tamponade
Parallel increases in CVP and PAOP
- Low cardiac output
- Increased systemic vascular resistance

Pulmonary embolism
Low cardiac output
- High CVP, high pulmonary artery pressure but low PAOP
- Increased systemic vascular resistance

Anaphylaxis
Low systemic vascular resistance
- Low CVP and PAOP
- High cardiac output

Septic shock
Low systemic vascular resistance
- Low CVP and PAOP
- Cardiac output usually high
- Myocardial depression – low ejection fraction
- Stroke volume maintained by ventricular dilatation
- Cardiac output maintained or increased by tachycardia

Clinical features of shock and sepsis

Although many clinical features are common to all types of shock, the causes may be distinguished by the associated haemodynamic changes ***(Box 25.10)*** and by examination.

Hypovolaemic shock

- ***Inadequate tissue perfusion***:
  - Skin: cold, pale, slate-grey, slow capillary refill, 'clammy'.
  - Kidneys: oliguria, anuria.
  - Brain: drowsiness, confusion and irritability.
- ***Increased sympathetic tone***:
  - Tachycardia, narrowed pulse pressure, 'weak' or 'thready' pulse.
  - Sweating.
  - Blood pressure: may be maintained initially (despite up to a 25% reduction in circulating volume if the patient is young and fit) but hypotension later supervenes.
- ***Lactic acidosis:*** compensatory tachypnoea.

Extreme hypovolaemia may be associated with bradycardia.

Cardiogenic shock

The signs in cardiogenic shock (see p. 989) are the same as for hypovolaemic shock, with the addition of myocardial failure: for example, raised jugular venous pressure (JVP), pulsus alternans, 'gallop' rhythm, basal crackles and pulmonary oedema.

Obstructive shock

Again, the signs are as for hypovolaemic shock with the following additions:

- Elevated JVP.
- Pulsus paradoxus and muffled heart sounds in cardiac tamponade.
- Perhaps signs of pulmonary embolism (see pp. 1031–1035).

Distributive shock: anaphylactic shock (See pp. 143–144.)

- Signs of profound vasodilatation:
  - Warm peripheries.
  - Low blood pressure.
  - Tachycardia.
- Erythema, urticaria, angio-oedema, pallor, cyanosis.
- Bronchospasm, rhinitis.
- Oedema of the face, pharynx and larynx.
- Pulmonary oedema.
- Hypovolaemia due to vascular leak.
- Nausea, vomiting, abdominal cramps, diarrhoea.

Ideally, 10 mL of clotted blood should be taken within 45–60 minutes of the reaction for confirmation of the diagnosis: for example, by measurement of mast cell tryptase. Serum should be separated and stored at −20°C. Follow-up of these patients is essential.

Distributive shock: sepsis and septic shock (see p. 221)

Definition of sepsis (adapted from 3rd International Consensus: Sepsis-3)

- ***Sepsis*** is defined as life-threatening organ dysfunction caused by a dysregulated host response to infection.

  Organ dysfunction can be identified by an acute change in the Sequential Organ Failure Assessment score (SOFA) of >2 points following infection. The baseline SOFA score can be assumed to be zero in patients not known to have pre-existing organ dysfunction. However, a SOFA score ≥2 reflects an overall mortality risk of approximately 10% in a general hospital population with suspected infection. Patients presenting with modest dysfunction can deteriorate further.

  The SOFA severity score (http://clincalc.com/IcuMortality/SOFA.aspx) is derived from:
  - Respiratory system – the ratio of arterial oxygen tension to fraction of inspired oxygen (PaO_2/FiO_2)
  - Cardiovascular system – amount of vasoactive medication necessary to prevent hypotension
  - Hepatic system – bilirubin level
  - Coagulation system – platelet concentration
  - Neurologic system – Glasgow coma score (see p. 825)
  - Renal system – serum creatinine or urine output

    The mean and the highest scores are most predictive of mortality. An increase of 30% is associated with a high mortality of about 50%. (This score has been endorsed by the Society of Critical Care Medicine (SCCM) and the European Society of Intensive Care Medicine (ESICM) as a tool to facilitate the identification of patients at risk of dying from sepsis.)

    A quick SOFA (qSOFA), which is derived from an alteration in mental status (Glasgow coma score), a systolic blood pressure of <100 mmHg or a respiratory rate of >22/min, can be quickly done at the bedside and can identify a patient with suspected infection likely to have a prolonged stay in ICU.
- ***Septic shock*** is a subset of sepsis in which underlying circulatory and cellular/metabolic abnormalities are profound enough to substantially increase mortality.
  - Patients with septic shock can be identified with a clinical construct of sepsis with persisting hypotension requiring vasopressors to maintain MAP (mean arterial pressure) ≥65 mmHg and having a serum lactate level >2 mmol/L (18 mg/dL) despite adequate volume resuscitation. With these criteria, hospital mortality is in excess of 40%.

Symptoms and signs

- Pyrexia and rigors, or hypothermia (unusual, but more common in the elderly and associated with worse prognosis).
- Nausea, vomiting.
- Vasodilatation, warm peripheries.
- Bounding pulse.
- Rapid capillary refill.
- Hypotension, low diastolic pressure, widened pulse pressure.
- Occasionally, signs of cutaneous vasoconstriction.
- Other signs:
  - Jaundice.
  - Coma, stupor.
  - Bleeding due to coagulopathy (e.g. from vascular puncture sites, gastrointestinal tract and surgical wounds).
  - Rash and meningism.
  - Hyperglycaemia; in more severe cases, hypoglycaemia.

The ***diagnosis of sepsis*** is easily missed, particularly in the elderly, when the classical signs may not be present. Some clues to the diagnosis may include mild confusion, tachycardia, tachypnoea, unexplained hypotension, a reduction in urine output, a rising plasma creatinine and glucose intolerance.

The clinical signs of sepsis (triggered by PAMPS) are not always associated with invasive infection and can occur with non-infectious processes such as pancreatitis, cardiopulmonary bypass, severe trauma or major surgery (triggered by DAMPS; see p. 1152). The term ***'systemic inflammatory response syndrome' (SIRS)*** has been superseded in favour of SOFA, which has a better predictive value for in-hospital mortality.

Sepsis and multiple organ failure (multiple organ dysfunction syndrome)

Sepsis is being diagnosed with increasing frequency and is now the most common cause of death in non-coronary adult ICUs. The estimated incidence of severe sepsis has varied from 77 to 300 cases per 100 000 of the population. The most common cause is community-acquired pneumonia ***(Fig. 25.22)***. Mortality rates are high (between 20% and 60%) and are closely related to the severity of illness and the number of organs that fail. Although some early deaths are caused by cardiovascular collapse, advances in ICU care and supportive therapy have reduced early deaths, and now most of those who die are overwhelmed by persistent or recurrent sepsis, with fever, intractable hypotension and failure of several organs.

Sequential failure of vital organs occurs progressively over days or weeks, although the pattern of organ dysfunction is variable. In many cases, the lungs are the first to be affected (acute respiratory distress syndrome, ARDS; see below) in association with cardiovascular instability and deteriorating renal function. Secondary pulmonary infection, complicating ARDS, frequently acts as a further stimulus to the immune response.

Liver dysfunction may develop later. Gastrointestinal failure, with an inability to tolerate enteral feeding and paralytic ileus, is common. Ischaemic colitis, acalculous cholecystitis, pancreatitis and gastrointestinal haemorrhage may also occur. Features of central nervous system dysfunction include impaired consciousness and disorientation, progressing to coma. Characteristically, these patients initially have a hyperdynamic circulation with vasodilatation and a high cardiac output, associated with an increased metabolic rate. Eventually, however, cardiovascular collapse supervenes. It is now often possible to support such patients for weeks or months; most now die following a decision to withdraw or not to escalate treatment (see pp. 1171–1172).

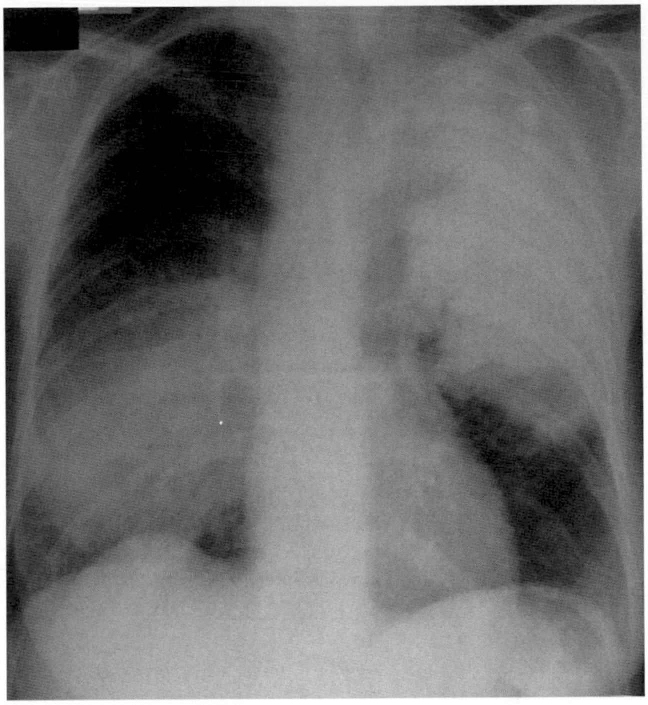

Figure 25.22 Bilateral pneumococcal pneumonia. Community-acquired pneumonia is the most common cause of sepsis requiring admission to intensive care. *(From Hinds CJ, Watson JD.* Intensive Care: A Concise Textbook*, 3rd edn. Edinburgh: Saunders; 2008. Courtesy of Dr SPG Padley.)*

Box 25.11 The metabolic response to trauma, major surgery and severe infection

- ↑ Energy expenditure
- ↑ Gluconeogenesis
- ↑ Mobilization of glucose from glycogen
- Insulin resistance and hyperglycaemia
- ↑ Free fatty acid synthesis
- ↑ Protein breakdown
- ↑ Liver synthesis of acute phase reactants

Metabolic response to trauma, major surgery and severe infection

This response ***(Box 25.11)*** is initiated and controlled by the neuroendocrine system and various cytokines (e.g. IL-6) acting in concert, and is characterized initially by an increase in energy expenditure ('hypermetabolism'; see also p. 212). Gluconeogenesis is stimulated by increased glucagon and catecholamine levels, while hepatic mobilization of glucose from glycogen is increased. Catecholamines inhibit insulin release and reduce peripheral glucose uptake. Combined with elevated circulating levels of other insulin antagonists such as cortisol, and downregulation of insulin receptors, these changes mean that the majority of patients are hyperglycaemic ('insulin resistance'). Later, hypoglycaemia may be precipitated by depletion of hepatic glycogen stores and inhibition of gluconeogenesis. Free fatty acid synthesis is also increased, leading to hypertriglyceridaemia.

Protein breakdown is initiated to provide energy from amino acids, and hepatic protein synthesis is preferentially augmented to produce the 'acute phase reactants'. The amino acid glutamine (which is indispensable in this situation) is mobilized from muscle for use as a metabolic fuel in rapidly dividing cells such as leucocytes and enterocytes. Glutamine is also required for hepatic production of the free radical scavenger glutathione. When severe and prolonged, this catabolic response can lead to considerable weight loss. Protein breakdown is associated with wasting and weakness of skeletal and respiratory muscle, prolonging the need for mechanical ventilation and delaying mobilization. Tissue repair, wound healing and immune function are also compromised.

Management of shock and sepsis

A delay in recognizing a shocked patient and in initiating resuscitation and specific treatments ***(Fig. 25.23)*** (particularly antibiotics when infection is the underlying cause) is associated with substantially increased morbidity and mortality.

A patent airway must be maintained and oxygen given, as is standard for any acutely ill patient. If necessary, an oropharyngeal airway is inserted to alleviate oropharyngeal obstruction. Some patients may require insertion of an endotracheal tube to prevent aspiration of gastric contents, and those with impending respiratory arrest will require immediate mechanical ventilation.

The underlying cause of shock should be sought and corrected where possible; for example, haemorrhage should be controlled or

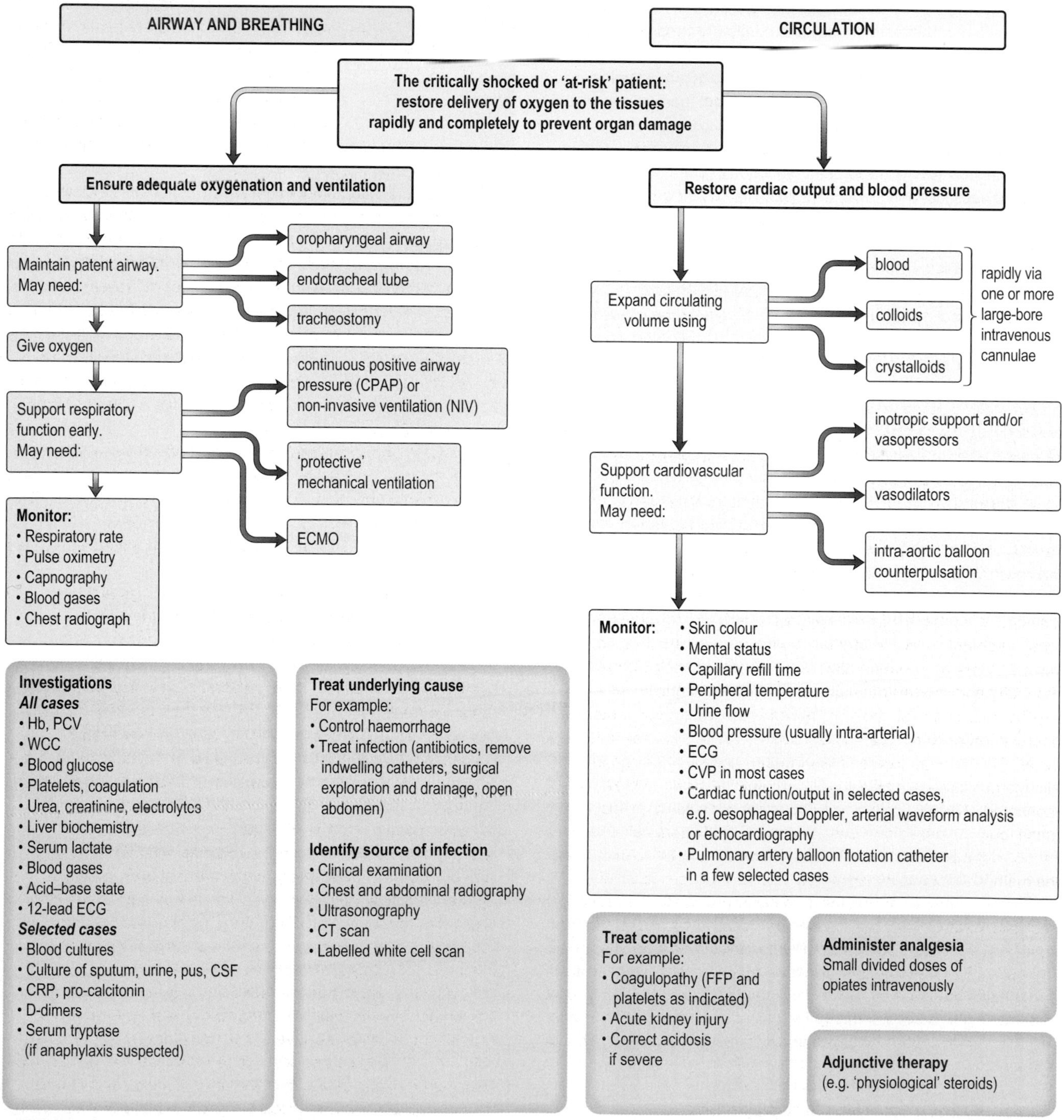

Figure 25.23 **Management of the critically ill, shocked or 'at-risk' patient.** CRP, C-reactive protein; CSF, cerebrospinal fluid; CT, computed tomography; CVP, central venous pressure; ECG, electrocardiogram; ECMO, extracorporeal membrane oxygenation; FFP, fresh frozen plasma; Hb, haemoglobin; PCV, packed cell volume; WCC, white cell count.

infection eradicated. In patients with septic shock, every effort must be made to identify the source of infection and isolate the causative organism. A thorough history, clinical examination and imaging (X-rays, ultrasonography or computed tomography (CT) scanning) should be undertaken. Appropriate samples (urine, sputum, cerebrospinal fluid (CSF), pus drained from abscesses) should be taken for microscopy, culture and sensitivities. Several blood cultures should be performed and empirical, broad-spectrum antibiotic therapy (see pp. 234–245) should be commenced *within the first hour* of recognition of sepsis. If an organism is isolated later, therapy can be adjusted appropriately. The choice of antibiotic depends on the likely source of infection, previous antibiotic therapy and known local resistance patterns, as well as on whether infection was acquired in hospital or in the community. Abscesses must be drained and infected indwelling catheters removed.

Whatever the aetiology of the haemodynamic abnormality:

- ***Tissue blood flow*** must be restored promptly by achieving and maintaining an adequate cardiac output.
- ***Arterial blood pressure*** must be sufficient to maintain perfusion of vital organs.
- ***Published guidelines*** for adult patients suffering septic shock should be followed. These advocate targeting a mean arterial pressure (MAP) of >65 mmHg, CVP of 8–12 mmHg (>12 mmHg if mechanically ventilated), a urine output of >0.5 mL/kg per hour and an $S_{CV}O_2$ of ≥70% (or $S_{\bar{V}}O_2$ of ≥65%) as the initial goals of resuscitation.

Preload and volume replacement

Optimizing preload is the most efficient way of increasing cardiac output. Volume replacement is obviously essential in hypovolaemic shock but is also required in anaphylactic and septic shock because of vasodilatation, sequestration of blood and loss of circulating volume because of vascular leak.

In obstructive shock, high filling pressures may be required to maintain an adequate stroke volume. Even in cardiogenic shock, careful volume expansion may, on occasions, lead to a useful increase in cardiac output. On the other hand, patients with severe cardiac failure, in whom ventricular filling pressures are markedly elevated, often benefit from measures to reduce preload (and afterload), such as the administration of vasodilators and diuretics (see below). Adequate perioperative volume replacement also reduces morbidity and mortality in high-risk surgical patients.

The circulating volume must be replaced quickly (in minutes, not hours) in order to reduce tissue damage and prevent acute kidney injury. Fluid is administered via wide-bore intravenous cannulae to allow large volumes to be given quickly, and the effect is continuously monitored. This involves observing improvements in clinical signs (urine output, consciousness, peripheral perfusion), biochemical variables (falling lactate levels) or increases in stroke volume using the methods discussed earlier (e.g. arterial waveform analysis).

Volume overload, which leads to cardiac dilatation, a reduction in stroke volume, a risk of pulmonary oedema and compromised renal perfusion, must be avoided. Pulmonary and peripheral oedema is more likely in seriously ill patients receiving large-volume fluid resuscitation because of a low colloid osmotic pressure (usually due to a low serum albumin), disruption of the alveolar–capillary membrane, microcirculatory changes and destruction of the endothelial glycocalyx.

Choice of fluid for volume replacement

Blood

This is conventionally given for haemorrhagic shock as soon as it is available. In extreme emergencies, group-specific crossmatch can be performed in minutes (see p. 555). When available and not contraindicated, blood salvage may be employed for those with severe ongoing bleeding. Unmatched blood is frequently administered in trauma patients presenting *in extremis* to the emergency department.

Transfusion of whole blood has largely been replaced by red cell concentrates (see p. 559). The use of leucodepleted blood is considered to be safer in terms of immune-mediated transfusion reactions, disease transmission and immune suppression. Although red cell transfusion can augment oxygen-carrying capacity, and hence global oxygen delivery, transfusion of old stored red blood cells, which become spherical rather than biconcave, and poorly deformable with increased adhesiveness, can compromise microvascular flow. Moreover, the precise objective of blood transfusion will differ depending on the circumstance. In the case of traumatic or intraoperative haemorrhagic shock, many now favour 'hypotensive resuscitation' until surgical control of the bleeding has been achieved. This partial resuscitation has been shown to reduce the rate of bleeding and allows the surgeon a greater chance of achieving definitive haemostasis. Once the patient is stable, higher haemoglobin and blood pressure targets may be pursued.

The absolute haemoglobin target in critically ill patients has changed with increasing awareness of the subtle detrimental immune effects associated with transfusing allogeneic blood. In patients not actively bleeding and without significant cardiovascular risk factors, it is usual to transfuse in order to achieve a target haemoglobin level of ≥70 g/L ('restrictive transfusion strategy'). In patients with significant coronary artery disease or limited respiratory reserve, a target level of 90 g/L ('liberal transfusion strategy') may be more appropriate. Previously healthy individuals can tolerate haemoglobin levels as low as 40 g/L before displaying signs of cardiac ischaemia.

Massive blood transfusion can be defined as a volume of >8–10 units of red cells transfused within a 24-hour period, and ***massive haemorrhage*** as a loss of ≥50% of blood volume within 3 hours or a rate of blood loss exceeding 150 mL/min.

Complications of blood transfusion are discussed on pages 555–559.

Special problems arise as a result of massive transfusion:

- ***Temperature changes***. Bank blood is stored at 4°C; transfusion may result in hypothermia, peripheral venoconstriction (which slows the rate of infusion) and arrhythmias. If possible, blood should be warmed during massive transfusion and in those at risk of hypothermia (e.g. during prolonged major surgery with open body cavity).
- ***Coagulopathy***. Stored blood has virtually no effective platelets or clotting factors. Massive transfusions that frequently include large volumes of colloid/crystalloid can therefore contribute to a coagulopathy that often needs to be treated by replacing clotting factors with fresh frozen plasma and administering platelet concentrates. Many massive transfusion protocols now advocate a balanced ratio of transfusion of units of red cells to units fresh frozen plasma to units platelets (e.g. 1 : 1 : 1), especially in the treatment of severe traumatic haemorrhage. Cryoprecipitate may also play a key role in securing haemostasis. Recombinant factor VIIa may occasionally be indicated in those with uncontrollable bleeding. Prothrombin complex concentrates have some advantages compared with FFP, in that they do not need to be crossmatched or thawed.
- ***Hypocalcaemia***. Citrate in stored blood binds calcium ions. During rapid transfusion, total body ionized calcium levels may be reduced, causing myocardial depression and exacerbating coagulation defects. This is uncommon in practice but can be corrected by administering 10 mL of 10% calcium chloride

intravenously. Routine treatment with calcium is not recommended.

- ***Increased oxygen affinity***. In stored blood, the red cell 2,3-bisphosphoglycerate (2,3-BPG) content is reduced, so that the oxyhaemoglobin dissociation curve is shifted to the left. The oxygen affinity of haemoglobin is therefore increased and oxygen unloading is impaired. Red cell levels of 2,3-BPG are substantially restored within 12 h of transfusion.
- ***Hyperkalaemia***. Plasma potassium levels rise progressively as blood is stored. However, hyperkalaemia is rarely a problem, as rewarming of the blood increases red cell metabolism; the sodium pump becomes active and potassium levels fall.
- ***Microembolism***. Microaggregates in stored blood may obstruct the pulmonary capillaries. This process is thought by some to contribute to acute lung injury.
- ***Immunity***. Blood transfusion has subtle detrimental effects on the host immune system and has been implicated in an increased susceptibility to develop nosocomial infections and an increase in the risk of cancer recurrence.

Crystalloids and colloids

The choice of intravenous fluid for resuscitation and the relative merits of crystalloids or colloids have long been controversial. Crystalloid solutions are cheap and convenient to use. However, they are not completely free of side-effects, as large volumes of solutions with high chloride content, such as 0.9% saline, can cause a hyperchloraemic acidosis and are associated with a greater risk of renal impairment. Balanced solutions, such as compound sodium lactate or plasmalyte, may be preferred (see ***Box 9.8***).

In critically ill patients, resuscitation with equivalent volumes of either 0.9% saline or the colloid 4% albumin has been shown to result in similar outcomes.

Polygelatin solutions have an average molecular weight of 35 000, which is iso-osmotic with plasma. They are cheap and do not interfere with crossmatching. Large volumes can be administered, as clinically significant coagulation defects are unusual and renal function is not significantly impaired. However, because they readily cross the glomerular basement membrane, their half-life in the circulation is only approximately 4 hours and they can promote an osmotic diuresis. These solutions may be useful during the acute phase of resuscitation, especially when volume losses are continuing. Allergic reactions can, however, occur.

Hydroxyethyl starches (***HES***) are available as numerous preparations with differing half-lives. Elimination of HES occurs primarily via the kidneys following hydrolysis by amylase. HES are stored in the reticuloendothelial system, apparently without causing functional impairment, but skin deposits have been associated with persistent pruritus. HES, especially the higher-molecular-weight fractions, have anticoagulant properties, can increase the risk of acute kidney injury and have been associated with an increased mortality. *HES should no longer be used in critically ill patients.*

Human albumin solution (***HAS***) is a natural colloid that has been used for volume replacement in shock and burns, and for the treatment of hypoproteinaemia. HAS is not generally recommended for routine volume replacement because supplies are limited and other cheaper solutions are equally effective. Some use HAS to expand the circulating volume in patients who are hypoalbuminaemic.

Myocardial contractility and inotropic agents

Myocardial contractility can be impaired by many factors, such as hypoxaemia and hypocalcaemia, as well as by some drugs (e.g. beta-blockers, antiarrhythmics and sedatives).

Severe metabolic acidosis conventionally is said to depress myocardial contractility and limit the response to vasopressor agents. Attempted correction of acidosis with intravenous sodium bicarbonate, however, generates additional carbon dioxide, which diffuses across cell membranes, producing or exacerbating intracellular acidosis. Other disadvantages of bicarbonate therapy include sodium overload and a left shift of the oxyhaemoglobin dissociation curve. Ionized calcium levels may be reduced and, combined with the fall in intracellular pH, this may impair myocardial performance. Treatment of lactic acidosis should therefore concentrate on correcting the cause. Bicarbonate should only be administered to correct ***extreme persistent metabolic acidosis*** (see pp. 179–180).

If the signs of shock persist despite adequate volume replacement, and perfusion of vital organs is jeopardized, inotropic/vasopressor agents should be administered to improve cardiac output and blood pressure. Vasopressor therapy may also be required to maintain perfusion in those with life-threatening hypotension, even when volume replacement is incomplete. All inotropes increase myocardial oxygen consumption, particularly if a tachycardia develops, and this can lead to an imbalance between myocardial oxygen supply and demand, with the development or extension of ischaemic areas. Inotropes should therefore be used with especial caution, particularly in cardiogenic shock following myocardial infarction and in known ischaemic heart disease.

Many of the most seriously ill patients become increasingly resistant to the effects of pressor agents, an observation attributed to 'downregulation' of adrenergic receptors and nitric oxide-induced 'vasoplegia' (see p. 1159).

All inotropic agents should be administered via a large central vein and their effects continually monitored ***(Box 25.12)***.

Adrenaline (epinephrine)

Adrenaline stimulates both α- and β-adrenergic receptors but β effects predominate at low doses. Heart rate and cardiac index increase, while peripheral resistance is reduced. If there is an associated increase in perfusion pressure, urine output may improve. Adrenaline at higher doses can cause excessive (α-mediated) vasoconstriction with reductions in splanchnic flow, and cardiac output may fall. Prolonged high-dose administration can cause peripheral gangrene and lactic acidosis. The minimum effective dose of adrenaline should therefore be used for as short a time as possible.

Noradrenaline (norepinephrine)

This is predominantly an α-adrenergic agonist. It is particularly useful in patients with hypotension and a low systemic vascular resistance, such as is seen in septic shock. There is a risk of producing excessive vasoconstriction with impaired organ perfusion and increased afterload, particularly if noradrenaline is administered when fluid resuscitation is inadequate and the circulating volume is reduced.

Dopamine

The haemodynamic effects of dopamine are dose-dependent. At low doses, dopamine is a positive inotrope with vasodilator actions on the renal and splanchnic circulation. Higher doses may be complicated by tachycardia, arrhythmias and vasoconstriction. Dopamine may be used as an alternative to noradrenaline in patients with a low risk of tachyarrhythmia and absolute or relative bradycardia.

Box 25.12 Receptor actions of sympathomimetic and dopaminergic agents

Agent	Receptor β_1	β_2	α_1	α_2	DA_1	DA_2	Dose dependence
Adrenaline (epinephrine)							++++
Low-dose	++	+	+	±	–	–	
Moderate-dose	++	+	++	+	–	–	
High-dose	++(+)	+(+)	++++	+++	–	–	
Noradrenaline (norepinephrine)	++	0	+++	+++	–	–	+++
Isoprenaline	+++	+++	0	0	–	–	
Dopamine							++++
Low-dose	±	0	±	+	++	+	
Moderate-dose	++	+	++	+	++(+)	+	
High-dose	+++	++	+++	+	++(+)	+	
Dopexamine	+	+++	0	0	++	+	++
Dobutamine	++	+	±	?	0	0	++
Action	***Postsynaptic***: positive inotropism and chronotropism; renin release	***Presynaptic***: stimulation of noradrenaline (norepinephrine) release ***Postsynaptic***: positive inotropism and chronotropism; vascular dilatation; relaxation of bronchial smooth muscle	***Postsynaptic***: constriction of peripheral, renal and coronary vascular smooth muscle; positive inotropism; antidiuresis	***Presynaptic***: inhibition of noradrenaline (norepinephrine) release; vasodilatation ***Postsynaptic***: constriction of coronary arteries; promotion of salt and water excretion	***Postsynaptic***: dilatation of renal, mesenteric and coronary vessels; renal tubular effect (natriuresis, diuresis)	***Presynaptic***: inhibition of adrenaline (epinephrine) release	

Dopexamine

Dopexamine is an analogue of dopamine that activates β_2 receptors, as well as DA_1 and DA_2 receptors. Dopexamine is a weak positive inotrope but a powerful splanchnic vasodilator, reducing afterload and improving blood flow to vital organs, including the kidneys. It has been used as an adjunct to the perioperative management of high-risk surgical patients (see below).

Dobutamine

Dobutamine is closely related to dopamine and has predominantly β_1 activity. Dobutamine has no specific effect on the renal vasculature but urine output often increases as cardiac output and blood pressure improve. It reduces systemic vascular resistance, as well as improving cardiac performance, thereby decreasing afterload and ventricular filling pressures. Dobutamine is therefore useful in patients with cardiogenic shock and cardiac failure. In septic shock, it can be used to increase cardiac output and oxygen delivery.

Phosphodiesterase inhibitors (e.g. milrinone, enoximone)

These agents have both inotropic and vasodilator properties. Because the phosphodiesterase type III inhibitors bypass the β-adrenergic receptor they do not cause tachycardia and are less arrhythmogenic than β agonists. They are useful in patients with receptor 'downregulation', those receiving beta-blockers, those being weaned from cardiopulmonary bypass and those with cardiac failure.

Vasopressin

Patients with septic shock have inappropriately low circulating levels of vasopressin. Low-dose vasopressin can increase blood pressure and systemic vascular resistance in patients with vasodilatory septic shock and a high cardiac output unresponsive to other vasopressors ('vasoplegia'). Low-dose vasopressin is sometimes added to conventional vasopressors in patients with septic shock.

Levosimendan

Levosimendan is a myofilament calcium sensitizer. Unlike other inotropes, levosimendan does not exert its action through increases in intracellular Ca^{2+} and, as a result, does not impair diastolic relaxation of the heart. Levosimendan binds to troponin C with high affinity but only during systole when the intracellular calcium concentration is high. Levosimendan has phosphodiesterase inhibitor actions but these are not thought to be clinically significant. The dose is usually infused over 24 hours but, significantly, a long-acting metabolite of levosimendan has similar calcium-sensitizing actions, maintaining the inotropic effect of levosimendan once an infusion is stopped. Adverse cardiovascular effects of levosimendan include tachycardia and hypotension; as a consequence, the addition of a vasopressor may be required.

Summary for use of inotropic and vasopressor agents

A combination of dobutamine and noradrenaline (norepinephrine) is used for the management of patients who are ***shocked with a low systemic vascular resistance*** (e.g. septic shock).

- Dobutamine is given to achieve an optimal cardiac output.
- Noradrenaline, sometimes supplemented by vasopressin, is used to restore an adequate blood pressure by reducing vasodilatation.

Box 25.13 Patients at risk of developing perioperative multiorgan failure

- The elderly
- Patients with co-morbidity, especially limited cardiorespiratory reserve
- Patients with trauma to two body cavities requiring multiple blood transfusions
- Patients undergoing surgery involving extensive tissue dissection, e.g. oesophagectomy, pancreatectomy, aortic aneurysm surgery
- Patients undergoing emergency surgery for intra-abdominal or intrathoracic catastrophic states, e.g. faecal peritonitis, oesophageal perforation

Box 25.14 Some therapeutic strategies for sepsis tested in randomized, controlled, phase II/III trials

- Granulocyte–monocyte colony stimulating factor
- Toll-like receptor/endotoxin antagonists
- Bactericidal permeability-increasing protein
- Tissue necrosis factor (TNF) antibodies
- Soluble TNF receptors
- Interleukin-1 receptor antagonists
- Platelet-activating factor antagonists
- Nitric oxide synthase inhibition
- Antithrombin III
- Activated protein C
- Low-dose steroids

In ***vasodilated septic patients*** with an adequate cardiac output, noradrenaline can be used alone. There is evidence to suggest that adrenaline (epinephrine) may be equally safe and effective as a dobutamine/noradrenaline combination. Because of its potency, adrenaline is particularly useful in patients with ***refractory hypotension***. Phosphodiesterase inhibitors can be used in the management of cardiac failure, especially when associated with pulmonary hypertension, and perioperatively in those undergoing cardiac surgery. Dobutamine is an alternative that is also used in septic patients with fluid overload or myocardial failure. Dopamine is used much less frequently than in the past. The role of levosimendan in the management of shock has yet to be established but it may be useful in resistant cardiogenic shock.

Targeting haemodynamics and oxygen transport

Although resuscitation has conventionally aimed at achieving normal haemodynamics, many of the critically ill patients that survive have raised values for cardiac output, DO_2 and VO_2. However, elevation of DO_2 and VO_2 to these 'supranormal' levels following admission to intensive care produces no benefit and may be harmful. *Early* goal-directed therapy to resuscitate patients in the emergency room, aimed at maintaining a central venous oxygen saturation of more than 70%, does not appear to improve outcome in patients with severe sepsis or septic shock.

High-risk surgical patients

These patients benefit from intensive perioperative monitoring and circulatory support ***(Box 25.13)***. In particular, maintenance of an adequate circulating volume and postoperative admission to a critical care area are advocated. Many believe that volume replacement and administration of inotropes or vasopressors should be guided by monitoring of stroke volume/cardiac output, usually using an oesophageal Doppler or pulse contour analysis. The value of the routine use of inodilators such as dopexamine remains unclear.

Vasodilator therapy

In selected cases, afterload reduction is used to increase stroke volume and decrease myocardial oxygen requirements by reducing the systolic ventricular wall tension. Vasodilatation (see p. 987) also decreases heart size and the diastolic ventricular wall tension, so that coronary blood flow is improved. The relative magnitude of the falls in preload and afterload depends on the pre-existing haemodynamic disturbance, concurrent volume replacement and the agent selected (see below). Vasodilators also improve microcirculatory flow.

Vasodilator therapy can be particularly helpful in patients with cardiac failure in whom the ventricular function curve is flat (see ***Fig. 25.7***), so that falls in preload have only a limited effect on stroke volume. This form of treatment, combined in selected cases with inotropic support, is therefore useful in cardiogenic shock and in the management of patients with cardiogenic pulmonary oedema or mitral regurgitation.

- ***Sodium nitroprusside*** (SNP) dilates arterioles and venous capacitance vessels, as well as the pulmonary vasculature, by donating nitric oxide. SNP therefore reduces the afterload and preload of both ventricles and can improve cardiac output and the myocardial oxygen supply/demand ratio. The effects of SNP are rapid in onset and spontaneously reversible within a few minutes of discontinuing the infusion. Cyanide poisoning is a risk with high-dose, prolonged infusions.
- ***Nitroglycerine*** (*NTG*), at low doses, is predominantly a venodilator, but as the dose is increased, it also causes arterial dilatation, thereby decreasing both preload and afterload. Nitrates are particularly useful in the treatment of cardiac failure with pulmonary oedema and are usually used in combination with intravenous furosemide. NTG reduces pulmonary vascular resistance, an effect that can be exploited in patients with a low cardiac output secondary to pulmonary hypertension.

Mechanical support of the myocardium

Intra-aortic balloon counterpulsation (IABCP) is the technique used most widely for mechanical support of the failing myocardium. It is discussed on pages 961–962. In specialized centres, ventricular assist devices and veno-arterial extra-corporeal membrane oxygenation (ECMO; see below) may be used in the treatment of cardiac failure.

Adjunctive treatment

Initial attempts to combat the high mortality associated with sepsis concentrated on cardiovascular and respiratory support in the hope that surgery, antibiotics and the patient's own defences would eradicate the infection. Despite some success, mortality rates remained unacceptably high. So far, attempts to improve outcome by modulating the immune response (including high-dose steroids) or neutralizing endotoxin ***(Box 25.14)*** have proved disappointing and, in some cases, may even have been harmful.

The administration of relatively low 'stress' doses of hydrocortisone to selected patients with refractory vasopressor-resistant septic shock may assist shock reversal and perhaps improve outcome.

The ***aim of current sepsis guidelines*** (see 'Further reading') is to combine evidence-based interventions with early effective resuscitation (aimed especially at achieving an adequate circulating volume, combined with the rational use of inotropes and/or vasoactive agents to maintain blood pressure, cardiac output and oxygen transport), in order to create 'bundles of care' delivered within specific time limits.

Further reading

Angus DC, Barnato AE, Bell D et al. A systematic review and meta-analysis of early goal-directed therapy for septic shock: the ARISE, ProCESS and ProMISe Investigators. *Intensive Care Med* 2015; 41:1549–1560.
De Backer D, Biston P, Devriendt J et al. Comparison of dopamine and norepinephrine in the treatment of shock. *N Engl J Med* 2010; 362:779–789.
Dellinger RP, Levy MM, Rhodes A et al. Surviving Sepsis Campaign: international guidelines for management of severe sepsis and septic shock: 2012. *Crit Care Med* 2013; 41:580–637.
Haase N, Perner A, Hennings LI et al. Hydroxy ethyl starch 130/0.38-0.45 versus crystalloid or albumin in patients with sepsis: systematic review with meta-analysis and trial sequential analysis. *BMJ* 2013; 346:1839.
Hunt BS. Bleeding and coagulopathies in critical care. *New Engl J Med* 2014: 370:847–859.
Lilly CM. The ProCESS trial – a new era of sepsis management. *New Engl J Med* 2014; 370:18:1750–1751.
Patel A, Laffan MA, Waheed U et al. Randomised trials of human albumin for adults with sepsis: systematic review and meta-analysis with trial sequential analysis of all-cause mortality. *BMJ* 2014; 349:g4561.
Pearse RM, Harrison DA, MacDonald A et al. Effect of a perioperative, cardiac output-guided hemodynamic therapy algorithm on outcomes following major gastrointestinal surgery: a randomized clinical trial and systematic review. *JAMA* 2014; 311:2181–2190.
Rautanen A, Mills TC, Gordon AC et al. Genome-wide association study of survival from sepsis due to pneumonia: an observational cohort study. *Lancet Respir Med* 2015; 3:53–60.
Russell JA. Is there a good MAP for septic shock? *New Engl J Med* 2014; 370:1649–1651.
Singer M, Deutschman CS, Seymour CW et al. The Third International Consensus Definition for Sepsis and Septic Shock (Sepsis-3). *JAMA* 2016; 315:801–810.
Venet F, Lukaszewicz AC, Payen D et al. Monitoring the immune response in sepsis: a rational approach to administration of immunoadjuvant therapies. *Curr Opin Immunol* 2013; 25:477–483.
Zhang D, Raoof M, Chen Y et al. Circulating mitochondrial DAMPs cause inflammatory responses to injury. *Nature* 2010; 464:104–107.
http://www.survivingsepsis.org *Surviving Sepsis Campaign: international guidelines for management of severe sepsis and septic shock: 2012.*

RESPIRATORY FAILURE

(See also Chapter 24.)

Classification and aetiology

The respiratory system consists of a gas-exchanging organ (the lungs) and a ventilatory pump (respiratory muscles/thorax), either or both of which can fail and precipitate respiratory failure. Respiratory failure occurs when pulmonary gas exchange is sufficiently impaired to cause hypoxaemia with or without hypercarbia. In practical terms, respiratory failure is present when the P_aO_2 is <8 kPa (60 mmHg) or the P_aCO_2 is >7 kPa (55 mmHg). It can be divided into:

- type I respiratory failure, in which the P_aO_2 is low and the P_aCO_2 is normal or low
- type II respiratory failure, in which the P_aO_2 is low and the P_aCO_2 is high.

Type I or 'acute hypoxaemic' respiratory failure occurs with diseases that damage lung tissue. Hypoxaemia is due to right-to-left shunts or $\dot{V}/\dot{Q}$ mismatch. Common causes include pneumonia, acute lung injury, cardiogenic pulmonary oedema and lung fibrosis.

Type II or 'ventilatory failure' occurs when alveolar ventilation is insufficient to remove the volume of carbon dioxide being produced by tissue metabolism. Inadequate alveolar ventilation may be due to reduced ventilatory effort, inability to overcome an increased resistance to ventilation, failure to compensate for an increase in dead space and/or carbon dioxide production, or a combination of these factors. The most common cause is COPD. Other causes include chest-wall deformities, respiratory muscle weakness (e.g. Guillain–Barré syndrome) and depression of the respiratory centre (e.g. drug overdose).

Deterioration in the mechanical properties of the lungs and/or chest wall increases the work of breathing and the oxygen consumption/carbon dioxide production of the respiratory muscles. Respiratory muscle fatigue is a factor in the pathogenesis of respiratory failure.

Clinical assessment

The general assessment and recognition of an acutely ill ward patient have been discussed above on pages 1139–1140. A clinical assessment of respiratory distress should be made on the following criteria:

- the use of accessory muscles of respiration
- intercostal recession
- tachypnoea
- tachycardia
- sweating
- pulsus paradoxus (rarely present)
- inability to speak, unwillingness to lie flat
- agitation, restlessness, diminished conscious level
- asynchronous respiration (a discrepancy in the timing of movement of the abdominal and thoracic compartments)
- paradoxical respiration (abdominal and thoracic compartments move in opposite directions)
- respiratory alternans (breath-to-breath alteration in the relative contribution of intercostal/accessory muscles and the diaphragm).

Blood gas analysis should be performed to guide oxygen therapy and to provide an objective assessment of the severity of the respiratory failure. The ***most sensitive clinical indicator*** of increasing respiratory difficulty is a rising respiratory rate. ***Measurement of tidal volume*** is a less sensitive indicator. ***Vital capacity*** is often a better guide to deterioration and is particularly useful in patients with respiratory inadequacy that is due to neuromuscular problems such as the Guillain–Barré syndrome or myasthenia gravis, in which the vital capacity decreases as weakness worsens. Measurement of ***forced expiratory volume in 1 second*** *(FEV_1)* is useful in the assessment of patients suffering acute asthma attacks.

Monitoring

Pulse oximetry

Lightweight oximeters can be applied to an earlobe or finger. They measure the changing amount of light transmitted through the pulsating arterial blood and provide a continuous, non-invasive assessment of arterial oxygen saturation (S_pO_2). These devices are reliable and easy to use, and do not require calibration.

Pulse oximetry is not a sensitive guide to *changes* in oxygenation. An S_pO_2 within normal limits in a patient receiving supplemental oxygen does not exclude the possibility of hypoventilation with carbon dioxide retention. Readings can be inaccurate in those with poor peripheral perfusion.

Blood gas analysis

Normal values of blood gas analysis are shown in ***Box 25.8***. See online for examples of partially compensated respiratory alkalosis.

Errors can result from malfunctioning of the analyser or incorrect sampling of arterial blood. Disposable pre heparinized syringes are available for blood gas analysis.

- The sample should be analysed immediately. Alternatively, the syringe should be immersed in iced water (the end having first been sealed with a cap) to prevent the continuing metabolism of white cells causing a reduction in PO_2 and a rise in PCO_2.
- Air almost inevitably enters the sample. The gas tensions within these air bubbles will equilibrate with those in the blood,

thereby lowering the PCO_2 and usually raising the PO_2 of the sample. However, provided the bubbles are ejected immediately by inverting the syringe and expelling the air that rises to the top of the sample, their effect is insignificant.

Interpretation of the results of blood gas analysis can be considered in two separate parts:

- disturbances of acid–base balance (see pp. 176 and 1149–1150)
- alterations in oxygenation.

Correct interpretation requires a knowledge of the patient's clinical history and age, the inspired oxygen concentration and any other relevant treatment (e.g. the ventilator settings for those on mechanical ventilation or the administration of sodium bicarbonate). The oxygen content of the arterial blood is determined by the percentage saturation of haemoglobin with oxygen. The relationship between the latter and the P_aO_2 is determined by the oxyhaemoglobin dissociation curve (see **Fig. 25.2**).

PaO_2/F_IO_2 ratio

This calculated variable is a simple approximation to the $P_{A-a}O_2$ and can be used to assess the severity of respiratory failure (see p. 1143). It is calculated by taking the arterial PO_2 in mmHg and dividing by the F_IO_2 expressed as a fraction of 1. The 'P/F' ratio has been used to define respiratory impairment in patients with ARDS (see pp. 1167–1168).

Capnography

Continuous breath-by-breath analysis of the expired carbon dioxide concentration can be used to:

- Confirm tracheal intubation.
- Continuously monitor end-tidal PCO_2, which approximates to P_aCO_2 in normal subjects. Continuous capnography is recommended for all mechanically ventilated patients to detect acute airway problems, e.g. tracheal tube/tracheostomy blocked or dislodged (essential when transporting critically ill patients).
- Detect apparatus malfunction.
- Detect acute alterations in cardiorespiratory function (e.g. sudden fall in cardiac output).

Management

Standard management of patients with respiratory failure includes:

- administration of supplemental oxygen through a patent airway
- treatment for distal airways obstruction
- measures to limit pulmonary oedema
- control of secretions
- treatment of pulmonary infection.

The load on the respiratory muscles should be reduced by improving lung mechanics. Correction of abnormalities that may lead to respiratory muscle weakness, such as hypophosphataemia and malnutrition, is also necessary.

Oxygen therapy

Methods of oxygen administration

Oxygen is initially given via a face mask. In the majority of patients (except those with COPD with chronically elevated P_aCO_2), the precise concentration of oxygen given is not vital and oxygen can therefore be given by a 'variable performance' device such as a simple face mask or nasal cannulae **(Fig. 25.24)**.

With these devices, the inspired oxygen concentration varies from about 35% to 55%, with oxygen flow rates of between 6 and 10 L/min. Nasal cannulae are often preferred because they are less claustrophobic and do not interfere with feeding or speaking, but they can cause ulceration of the nasal or pharyngeal mucosa and the inspired oxygen concentration is diluted by mouth breathing. Higher concentrations of oxygen can be administered by using a mask with a reservoir bag attached **(Fig. 25.24C)**. **Figure 25.24** should be compared with the fixed-performance mask shown in **Figure 24.25**; the oxygen concentration can be controlled with the latter and it is used in patients with COPD and chronic type II failure. The hazards of reducing hypoxic drive can be overemphasized and are less dangerous when the patient is in a critical care unit; *remember*, severe hypoxaemia is more dangerous than hypercapnia.

Oxygen toxicity

Experimentally, mammalian lungs have been shown to be damaged by continuous exposure to high concentrations of oxygen, but oxygen toxicity in humans is less well proven. Nevertheless, it is reasonable to assume that high concentrations of oxygen might damage the lungs, and so the lowest inspired oxygen concentration compatible with adequate arterial oxygenation should be used. Although dangerous hypoxia should never be tolerated through a fear of pulmonary oxygen toxicity, oxygen saturations between 90 and 92% are probably adequate for most patients and there is some suggestion that targeting higher oxygen saturations using greater concentrations of inspired oxygen may be detrimental. There has

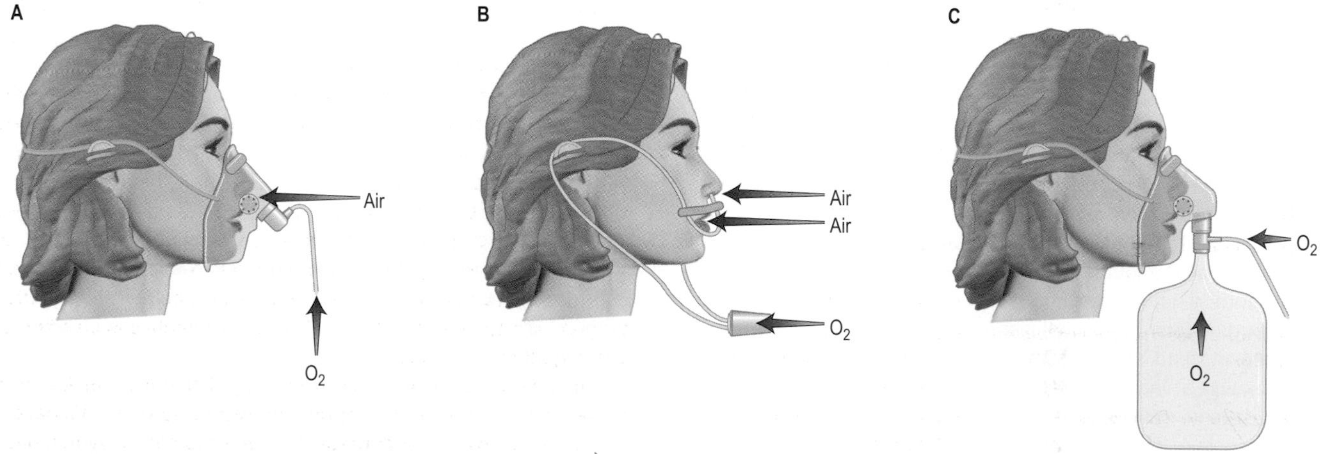

Figure 25.24 Methods of administering supplemental oxygen to the unintubated patient. A. Simple face mask. **B.** Nasal cannulae. **C.** Mask with reservoir bag and non-rebreathing valve.

also been concern that, in some circumstances (e.g. following myocardial infarction), hyperoxia associated with routine administration of supplemental oxygen may be harmful, perhaps because of associated vasoconstriction, and it is now not routinely given.

Respiratory support

If, despite the above measures, the patient continues to deteriorate or fails to improve, the institution of some form of respiratory support is necessary ***(Box 25.15)***. ***Non-invasive ventilation*** via a mask or hood (see p. 1166) can be used, particularly in respiratory failure due to COPD, but in many critically ill patients, ***invasive ventilation*** through an endotracheal tube or tracheostomy is required.

Intermittent positive pressure ventilation (***IPPV***) is achieved by intermittently inflating the lungs with a positive pressure delivered by a mechanical ventilator. There have been a number of refinements and modifications to the manner in which positive pressure is applied to the airway, and to the interplay between the patient's respiratory efforts and mechanical assistance (see pp. 1165–1166).

Controlled mechanical ventilation (***CMV***), with the abolition of spontaneous breathing, rapidly leads to atrophy of respiratory muscles, so that assisted modes that are triggered by the patient's inspiratory efforts (see below) are preferred.

The rational use of mechanical ventilation depends on a clear understanding of its potential beneficial effects, as well as the dangers.

Beneficial effects of mechanical ventilation

- ***Relief from exhaustion***. Mechanical ventilation reduces the work of breathing, 'rests' the respiratory muscles and relieves the extreme exhaustion present in patients with respiratory failure; this exhaustion may culminate in respiratory arrest.
- ***Effects on oxygenation***. Application of positive pressure can prevent or reverse atelectasis. In those with severe pulmonary parenchymal disease, the lungs may be very stiff and the work of breathing is therefore greatly increased. Under these circumstances, the institution of respiratory support significantly reduces total body oxygen consumption; consequently, $P_{\bar{v}}O_2$ and thus P_aO_2 may improve. Because ventilated patients are connected to a leak-free circuit, it is possible to administer high concentrations of oxygen (up to 100%) accurately and to apply a positive end-expiratory pressure (PEEP). In selected cases, the latter may reduce shunting and increase P_aO_2 (see below).
- ***Improved carbon dioxide elimination***. By adjusting the minute volume, the P_aCO_2 can usually be controlled.

Box 25.15 Techniques for respiratory support

Technique		Delivery
Intermittent positive-pressure ventilation (IPPV)		
Controlled mechanical ventilation (CMV) (volume-controlled or pressure-controlled) Synchronized intermittent mandatory ventilation (SIMV)	usually with	Positive end-expiratory pressure (PEEP) *Lung protective ventilation* Pressure-limited or volume-controlled pressure-limited (peak airway pressure <35–40 cmH_2O) Low tidal volume 6–8 mL/kg (± 'permissive hypercarbia') Maintain alveolar volume with PEEP and, in some cases, prolonged inspiratory phase
Pressure support ventilation (PSV)		
Biphasic positive airway pressure (BiPAP)		
Non-invasive ventilation		Nasal mask Face mask Hood
Continuous positive airway pressure (CPAP)		Endotracheal tube, tracheostomy, mask or hood, high-flow nasal prongs
Extracorporeal techniques		Extracorporeal membrane oxygenation (ECMO), extracorporeal CO_2 removal ($ECCO_2$-R)

Indications for mechanical ventilation

- ***Acute respiratory failure***, with signs of severe respiratory distress (e.g. respiratory rate >40 breaths/min, inability to speak, patient exhaustion) persisting despite maximal therapy. Confusion, restlessness, agitation, a decreased conscious level, a rising P_aCO_2 (>8 kPa, >60 mmHg) and extreme hypoxaemia (<8 kPa, <60 mmHg), despite oxygen therapy, are further indications.
- ***Acute ventilatory failure*** due, for example, to myasthenia gravis or Guillain–Barré syndrome. Mechanical ventilation should usually be instituted when the vital capacity has fallen to 10 mL/kg or less. This will avoid complications such as atelectasis and infection, as well as preventing respiratory arrest. The tidal volume and respiratory rate are relatively insensitive indicators of respiratory failure in the above conditions and change late in the course of the disease. A high P_aCO_2 (particularly if rising) is an indication for urgent mechanical ventilation.

Not all patients with respiratory failure and/or a reduced vital capacity require ventilation; clinical assessment of each individual case is essential. The patient's general condition, degree of exhaustion, level of consciousness and ability to protect the airway are often more useful than blood gas values.

Other indications include:

- postoperative ventilation in high-risk patients
- head injury: to avoid hypoxia and hypercarbia, which increase cerebral blood flow and intracranial pressure (see below)
- trauma: chest injury and lung contusion
- severe left ventricular failure with pulmonary oedema
- coma with breathing difficulties, e.g. following drug overdose.

Institution of invasive respiratory support

This requires tracheal intubation. If the patient is conscious, the procedure must be fully explained and written consent obtained before anaesthesia is induced. The complications of tracheal intubation are given in ***Box 25.16***.

Intubating patients in severe respiratory failure is a hazardous undertaking and should be performed only by experienced staff. In extreme emergencies, it may be preferable to ventilate the patient by hand using an oropharyngeal airway and a face mask with added oxygen until experienced help arrives. An alternative is insertion of a laryngeal mask airway.

Intubating a critically ill patient is very different to intubating a patient in the operating theatre prior to elective surgery. The patient is usually hypoxic and hypercarbic, with increased sympathetic activity; the stimulus of laryngoscopy and intubation can precipitate dangerous arrhythmias, bradycardia and even cardiac arrest.

Box 25.16 Complications of tracheal intubation

Complication	Comments
Immediate	
Trauma to the upper airway	Affects lips, teeth, gums, trachea
Tube in oesophagus	Gives rise to hypoxia and abdominal distension Detected by absence of capnography trace Requires immediate removal, bag-mask ventilation with oxygen and re-insertion of the tracheal tube
Tube in one or other (usually the right) main bronchus	Avoid by checking both lungs are being inflated, i.e. both sides of the chest move and air entry is heard bilaterally on auscultation Obtain chest X-ray to check position of tube and to exclude lung collapse
Early	
Migration of the tube out of the trachea Leaks around the tube Obstruction of tube because of kinking or secretions	These are dangerous complications The patient becomes distressed and cyanosed, and has poor chest expansion The following should be performed immediately: Manual inflation with 100% oxygen Tracheal suction Check position of tube Deflation of cuff Check tube for 'kinks' or blockage with secretions or blood (common) If no improvement, remove tube, ventilate with face mask and then insert new endotracheal tube
Late	
Sinusitis	
Mucosal oedema and ulceration	
Laryngeal injury	
Tracheal narrowing and fibrosis	
Tracheomalacia	

Except in an extreme emergency, therefore, the ECG and oxygen saturation should be monitored, and the patient pre-oxygenated with 100% oxygen before intubation. Resuscitation drugs should be immediately available. If time allows, the circulating volume should be optimized and, if necessary, inotropes commenced before attempting intubation. In some cases, it is appropriate to establish intra-arterial and CVP monitoring before instituting mechanical ventilation, although many patients will not tolerate the supine or head-down position. In some deeply comatose patients, no sedation is required, but in the majority, a short-acting intravenous anaesthetic agent, usually with an opiate followed by muscle relaxation, will be necessary. Capnography must be used to confirm tracheal intubation.

Sedation, analgesia and muscle relaxation

Most critically ill patients will require analgesia and many will receive sedatives. The combination of an opiate with a benzodiazepine or propofol is often used to facilitate mechanical ventilation and to obtund the physiological response to stress. Heavy sedation is indicated in those with severe respiratory failure, especially since 'lung-protective' ventilatory strategies (see p. 1166) are inherently uncomfortable. A few may require neuromuscular blockade. It is recognized, however, that minimizing sedation levels using 'sedation scores' and 'daily wakening', or even the avoidance of sedatives altogether, often in combination with spontaneous breathing modes of respiratory support (see pp. 1165–1166), is associated with reductions in the duration of mechanical ventilation and more rapid discharge from the ICU and hospital.

Box 25.17 Complications of tracheostomy

The complications shown for tracheal intubation (see ***Box 26.16***) *plus*:

Early
- Death
- Pneumothorax
- Haemorrhage
- Hypoxia
- Hypotension
- Cardiac arrhythmias
- Tube misplaced in pretracheal subcutaneous tissues
- Subcutaneous emphysema

Intermediate
- Mucosal ulceration
- Erosion of tracheal cartilages (can cause tracheo-oesophageal fistula)
- Erosion of innominate artery (occasionally leads to fatal haemorrhage)
- Stomal infection
- Pneumonia

Late
- Failure of stoma to heal
- Tracheal granuloma
- Tracheal stenosis at level of stoma, cuff or tube tip
- Collapse of tracheal rings at level of stoma
- Cosmetic factors

Tracheostomy

Tracheostomy may be required for the long-term control of excessive bronchial secretions, and in those with a chronically reduced conscious level in order to maintain an airway and protect the lungs if pharyngeal and laryngeal reflexes are impaired. Tracheostomy is also performed when intubation is likely to be prolonged, for patient comfort, reduction of sedation requirements and facilitation of weaning from mechanical ventilation.

Tracheostomy was once performed only in the operating room by a surgeon but it is now usual for this procedure to be carried out by intensive care specialists in the ICU using a percutaneous dilatational approach. This approach is quicker, less resource-intensive, safe and associated with a greatly reduced wound infection rate.

A life-threatening obstruction of the upper respiratory tract that cannot be bypassed with an endotracheal tube can be relieved by a ***cricothyroidotomy***, which is safer, quicker and easier to perform than a formal tracheostomy.

Tracheostomy has a small but significant mortality rate. Complications associated with the technique are shown in ***Box 25.17***.

Complications associated with mechanical ventilation

Airway complications

See ***Boxes 25.16*** and ***25.17***.

Disconnection, failure of gas or power supply, mechanical faults

These are unusual but dangerous. A method of manual ventilation, a face mask and oxygen must always be available by the bedside.

Cardiovascular complications

The application of positive pressure to the lungs and thoracic wall impedes venous return and distends alveoli, thereby 'stretching' the pulmonary capillaries and causing a rise in pulmonary vascular resistance. Both of these mechanisms can produce a fall in cardiac output.

Respiratory complications

Mechanical ventilation can be complicated by a deterioration in gas exchange because of V̇/Q̇ mismatch, fluid retention and collapse of peripheral alveoli. Traditionally, the latter was prevented by using high tidal volumes (10–12 mL/kg) but high inflation pressures, with over-distension of compliant alveoli, perhaps exacerbated by the repeated opening and closure of distal airways, can disrupt the alveolar–capillary membrane. There is an increase in microvascular permeability and release of inflammatory mediators, leading to '***ventilator-associated lung injury***'. Extreme over-distension of the lungs during mechanical ventilation with high tidal volumes and high airway pressures can rupture alveoli and cause air to dissect centrally along the perivascular sheaths. This '***barotrauma***' and '***volutrauma***' may be complicated by pneumomediastinum, subcutaneous emphysema, pneumoperitoneum, pneumothorax and intra-abdominal air. The risk of pneumothorax is increased in those with destructive lung disease (e.g. necrotizing pneumonia, emphysema), asthma or fractured ribs.

A ***tension pneumothorax*** can be rapidly fatal in ventilated patients. Suggestive signs include the development or worsening of hypoxia, hypercarbia, respiratory distress and an unexplained increase in airway pressure, as well as hypotension and tachycardia, sometimes accompanied by a rising CVP. Examination may reveal unequal chest expansion, mediastinal shift away from the side of the pneumothorax (deviated trachea, displaced apex beat) and a hyper resonant hemithorax. Although breath sounds are often diminished over the pneumothorax, this sign can be misleading in ventilated patients. If there is time, the diagnosis can be confirmed by chest X-ray prior to definitive treatment with chest tube drainage.

Ventilator-associated pneumonia

Hospital-acquired pneumonia occurs in as many as one-third of patients receiving mechanical ventilation and is associated with a significant increase in length of stay and mortality. The diagnosis is difficult and controversial because many ventilated patients develop a pyrexia, and infiltrates on the chest X-ray that may not be infective are common. The measurement of serum procalcitonin, a marker of severe bacterial infections, may be helpful. Various organisms may be isolated, such as aerobic Gram-negative bacilli (e.g. *Pseudomonas aeruginosa*, *Klebsiella pneumoniae*, *Escherichia coli*, *Acinetobacter* spp.) and *Staphylococcus aureus*, including meticillin-resistant *Staph. aureus* (MRSA). Deciding whether an organism that has been isolated is causing ventilator-associated pneumonia or is simply colonizing the respiratory tract can also be difficult. Leakage of infected oropharyngeal secretions past the tracheal tube cuff is thought to be largely responsible for ventilator-associated pneumonia. Bacterial colonization of the oropharynx may be promoted by regurgitation of colonized gastric fluid and so the risk of ventilator-associated pneumonia can be reduced by nursing patients in the semi-recumbent, rather than the supine, position and by oropharyngeal decontamination. Treatment is with an appropriate broad-spectrum antibiotic, which can be modified if a causative organism is isolated.

Techniques for respiratory support

(See *Box 25.15*.)

Controlled mechanical ventilation

Controlled mechanical ventilation (CMV) is used when respiratory efforts are absent or have been abolished.

Ventilation involves one of two types:

- ***Volume-controlled ventilation***. The tidal volume and respiratory rate are preset on the ventilator. The airway pressure varies according to both the ventilator setting and the patient's lung mechanics (airways resistance and compliance).
- ***Pressure-controlled ventilation***. Both the inspiratory pressure and the respiratory rate are preset but the tidal volume varies according to the patient's lung mechanics.

Positive end-expiratory pressure

A positive airway pressure can be maintained at a chosen level throughout expiration using a threshold resistor valve in the expiratory limb of the circuit. Positive end-expiratory pressure (PEEP) re-expands under-ventilated lung units, and redistributes lung water from the alveoli to the perivascular interstitial space, thereby reducing shunt and increasing P_aO_2. The inevitable rise in mean intrathoracic pressure associated with the application of PEEP may, however, further impede venous return, increase pulmonary vascular resistance and reduce cardiac output. The fall in cardiac output can be ameliorated by expanding the circulating volume, although, in some cases, inotropic or vasopressor support is required. Thus, although arterial oxygenation is often improved by the application of PEEP, a simultaneous fall in cardiac output can lead to a reduction in total oxygen delivery.

Traditionally, the application of PEEP was considered only if it proved difficult to achieve adequate oxygenation of arterial blood despite raising the inspired oxygen concentration above 50%. Low levels of PEEP (5–7 cmH_2O) are now used in the majority of mechanically ventilated patients in order to maintain lung volume, as well as in those with basal atelectasis and in selected cases with airways obstruction.

Continuous positive airway pressure

The application of continuous positive airway pressure (CPAP) achieves for the spontaneously breathing patient what PEEP does for the ventilated patient. Oxygen and air are delivered under pressure via an endotracheal tube, a tracheostomy, a tightly fitting face mask or a hood (*Fig. 25.25*). Not only can CPAP improve oxygenation, but also the lungs become more compliant and the work of breathing is reduced.

An alternative is to use a very high flow of oxygen and air delivered via large-diameter nasal prongs to create a modest amount of CPAP. This system is often better tolerated, communication is

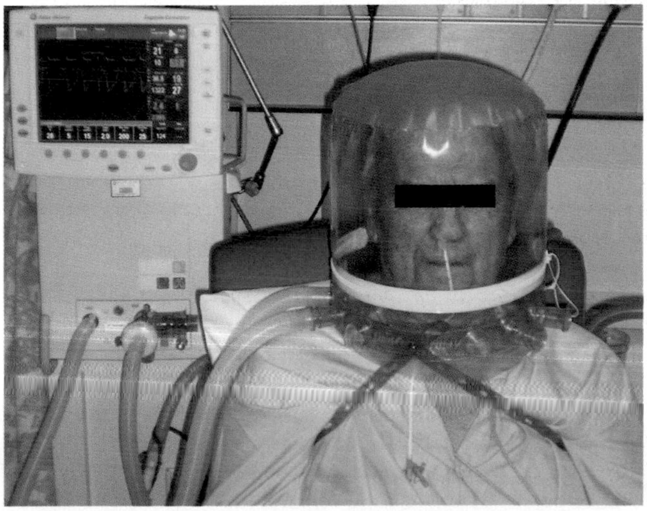

Figure 25.25 Use of a continuous positive airway pressure (CPAP) hood.

easier and the patient can eat. Commencing therapy with high-flow nasal prongs in patients with type I respiratory failure may be equivalent to, or more effective than, non-invasive ventilation in preventing patient deterioration and avoiding subsequent invasive ventilation. However the application of positive airway pressure is compromised if the patient mouth-breathes.

Pressure support ventilation

In pressure support ventilation (PSV), spontaneous breaths are augmented by a preset level of positive pressure (usually between 5 and 20 cmH_2O), triggered by the patient's spontaneous respiratory effort and applied for a given fraction of inspiratory time or until inspiratory flow falls below a certain level. Tidal volume is determined by the set pressure, the patient's effort and pulmonary mechanics. The level of pressure support can be reduced progressively as the patient improves.

Intermittent mandatory ventilation

The intermittent mandatory ventilation (IMV) technique allows the patient to breathe spontaneously between the 'mandatory' tidal volumes delivered by the ventilator. These mandatory breaths are timed to coincide with the patient's own inspiratory effort (synchronized intermittent mandatory ventilation, or SIMV). SIMV can be used with or without CPAP, and spontaneous breaths may be assisted with pressure support ventilation.

'Lung-protective' ventilation

This is designed to avoid exacerbating or perpetuating lung injury by avoiding over-distension of alveoli, minimizing airway pressures, and preventing the repeated opening and closure of distal airways. Alveolar volume is maintained with PEEP, and sometimes by prolonging the inspiratory phase, while tidal volumes are limited to 6–8 mL/kg ideal bodyweight. Peak airway pressures should not exceed 35–40 cmH_2O. An alternative is to deliver a constant preset inspiratory pressure for a prescribed time in order to generate a low tidal volume at reduced airway pressures ('pressure-limited' mechanical ventilation). Respiratory rate can be increased to improve CO_2 removal and avoid severe acidosis (H^+ >63 nmol/L; pH <7.2), but hypercarbia is frequent and should usually be accepted ('permissive hypercarbia'). Both techniques can be used with SIMV. Ventilation with low tidal volumes has been shown to improve outcome in patients with ARDS (see pp. 1168–1169). Lung-protective ventilation should be used in almost all patients undergoing mechanical ventilation.

High-frequency oscillation

High-frequency oscillation (HFO) is administered using a purpose-designed ventilator. With HFO, there is no bulk flow of gas; rather, gas oscillates to and fro at rates of 60–3000 cycles/min with a V_T of 1–3 mL/kg. Both inspiration and expiration are actively controlled with a sine wave pump. The mechanism of gas exchange is not fully understood but lung volume is well maintained and oxygenation may be improved. Whilst this is a well-established and proven treatment in the neonatal ICU, there is some doubt as to its usefulness in adults with acute respiratory failure.

Extracorporeal gas exchange

In patients with severe refractory respiratory failure, pumped, high-flow, veno-venous bypass through a membrane lung is used in specialized centres to achieve adequate oxygenation and increase CO_2 removal (extracorporeal membrane oxygenation, ECMO). Extracorporeal carbon dioxide removal ($ECCO_2$-R) is more easily administered, and uses lower flow rates to provide effective CO_2 removal but less efficient oxygenation. Both techniques have been used to reduce ventilation requirements, thereby minimizing further ventilation-induced lung damage and encouraging resolution of the lung injury.

Non-invasive ventilation

Non-invasive ventilation (NIV) is suitable for patients who are conscious, cooperative and able to protect their airway; they must also be able to expectorate effectively. Positive pressure is applied to the airways using a tight-fitting full-face/nasal mask or a hood. The most popular ventilators for this purpose are those that deliver bi-level positive airway pressure (BiPAP), which are simple to use, cheap and flexible. With the latter technique, inspiratory and expiratory pressure levels and times are set independently and unrestricted spontaneous respiration is possible throughout the respiratory cycle. BiPAP can also be patient-triggered. There is a reduced risk of ventilator-associated pneumonia and improved patient comfort, with preservation of airway defence mechanisms, speech and swallowing (which allows better nutrition). Spontaneous coughing and expectoration are not hampered, permitting effective physiotherapy, and sedation is usually unnecessary. Institution of non-invasive respiratory support can rest the respiratory muscles, reduce respiratory acidosis and breathlessness, improve clearance of secretions and re-expand collapsed lung segments. The intubation rate, length of ICU and hospital stay, and, in some categories of patient, mortality may all be reduced. NIV is particularly useful in acute hypercapnic respiratory failure associated with COPD, provided the patient is not profoundly hypoxic or obtunded. NIV may also be valuable as a means of avoiding tracheal intubation in immunocompromised patients with acute respiratory failure. Evidence suggests that early NIV after extubation of hypercapnic patients with respiratory disorders can reduce the risk of subsequent respiratory failure and mortality. ***Box 25.18*** shows some indications for the use of NIV when standard medical treatment has failed.

Weaning

Weakness and wasting of respiratory muscles are inevitable consequences of the catabolic response to critical illness and are often exacerbated by the reduction in respiratory work during mechanical ventilation ('disuse atrophy'). Often, abnormalities of gas exchange and lung mechanics persist. Not surprisingly, therefore, many patients experience difficulty in resuming unsupported spontaneous ventilation. In a significant proportion of patients who have

Box 25.18 Some indications for, and contraindications to, the use of non-invasive ventilation (NIV)

Indications

- Acute exacerbation of chronic obstructive pulmonary disease (H^+ >44 nmol/L; pH <7.35)
- Cardiogenic pulmonary oedema
- Chest wall deformity/neuromuscular disease (hypercapnic respiratory failure)
- Obstructive sleep apnoea
- Severe pneumonia (see ***Box 24.30***)
- Asthma (occasionally)
- Weaning patients from invasive ventilation

Some contraindications

- Facial or upper airway surgery
- Reduced conscious level
- Inability to protect the airway

(Modified from British Thoracic Society guidelines after 1997, http://www.brit-thoracic.org.uk.)

undergone a prolonged period of respiratory support, the situation is further complicated by the development of a neuropathy, a myopathy or both.

Neuromuscular weakness complicating critical illness

Polyneuromyopathies have most often been described in association with persistent sepsis and multiple organ failure.

Critical illness polyneuropathy is characterized by a primary axonal neuropathy involving both motor and, to a lesser extent, sensory nerves. Clinically, the initial manifestation is often difficulty in weaning the patient from respiratory support. There is muscle wasting, the limbs are weak and flaccid, and deep tendon reflexes are reduced or absent. Cranial nerves are relatively spared. Nerve conduction studies confirm axonal damage. The CSF protein concentration is normal or minimally elevated. These findings differentiate critical illness neuropathy from Guillain–Barré syndrome, in which nerve conduction studies nearly always show evidence of demyelination and CSF protein is usually high.

The cause of critical illness polyneuropathy is not known and there is no specific treatment. Weaning from respiratory support and rehabilitation are likely to be prolonged. With resolution of the underlying critical illness, recovery can be expected after 1–6 months but weakness and fatigue frequently persist.

Critical illness myopathies can also occur, often in association with a neuropathy. A severe quadriplegic myopathy has been associated particularly with the administration of steroids and muscle relaxants to mechanically ventilated patients who have acute, severe asthma.

Criteria for weaning patients from mechanical ventilation

Clinical assessment is the best way of deciding whether a patient can be weaned from the ventilator. The patient's conscious level, mood and cardiovascular performance, as well as the effects of drugs, must all be taken into account. A subjective evaluation by an experienced clinician of the patient's response to a short period of spontaneous breathing (spontaneous breathing trial) is the most reliable predictor of weaning success or failure. Objective criteria are based on an assessment of pulmonary gas exchange (blood gas analysis), lung mechanics and muscular strength.

Techniques for weaning

Patients who have received mechanical ventilation for <24–48 hours, e.g. after elective major surgery, can usually resume spontaneous respiration immediately and no weaning process is required. This procedure can also be adopted for those who have been ventilated for longer periods but who tolerate a spontaneous breathing trial and clearly fulfil objective criteria for weaning. Techniques of weaning include the following:

- The traditional method is to allow the patient to breathe entirely spontaneously for a short time, following which respiratory support is resumed. The periods of spontaneous breathing are gradually increased and the periods of respiratory support are progressively reduced. Initially, it is usually advisable to ventilate the patient throughout the night. This method can be stressful and tiring for both patients and staff, although it is sometimes successful when other methods have failed.
- SIMV (see p. 1166) involves a progressive reduction in the frequency of mandatory breaths. Spontaneous breaths are usually pressure-supported.
- Gradual reduction of the level of pressure support is thought to be the preferred technique.
- CPAP (see p. 1165–1166) can prevent the alveolar collapse, hypoxaemia and fall in compliance that might otherwise occur when patients start to breathe spontaneously. It is therefore used during weaning with SIMV or pressure support, during spontaneous breathing trials and in spontaneously breathing patients prior to extubation.
- Tracheostomy is often used to facilitate weaning from mechanical ventilation.
- Non-invasive respiratory support (BiPAP, CPAP) can be used following extubation to prevent respiratory failure and re-intubation.

Extubation and tracheostomy decannulation

These should not be performed until patients can cough, swallow and protect their own airway, and are sufficiently alert to be cooperative. Patients who fulfil these criteria can be extubated, provided their respiratory function has improved sufficiently to sustain spontaneous ventilation indefinitely. Similar considerations guide the elective removal of tracheostomy tubes.

The ratio of respiratory rate (in breaths/minute) to tidal volume (in litres) can be used to predict which patients will tolerate extubation, provided all other preconditions have been met. This 'rapid shallow breathing index' quantifies the clinical assessment of a patient who breathes slowly and comfortably with adequate tidal volumes. A score of <100 is a relatively good predictor of extubation success.

Further reading

Bouadma L, Luyt CE, Tubach F et al. Use of procalcitonin to reduce patients' exposure to antibiotics in intensive care units. *Lancet* 2010; 375:463–474.
Frat JP, Thille AW, Mercat A et al. High-flow oxygen through nasal cannula in acute hypoxemic respiratory failure. *New Engl J Med* 2015; 372:2185–2196.
Malhotra A, Drazen JM. High-frequency oscillatory ventilation on shaky ground. *N Engl J Med* 2013; 368:863–865.
Nava S, Hill N. Non-invasive ventilation in acute respiratory failure. *Lancet* 2009; 374:250–259.
Peek GJ, Mugford M, Tinwoipati R et al. Efficacy and economic assessment of conventional ventilatory support versus extracorporeal membrane oxygenation for severe adult respiratory failure (CESAR): a multicentre randomised controlled trial. *Lancet* 2009; 374:1351–1363.
Strom T, Martinussen T, Toft P. A protocol of no sedation for critically ill patients receiving mechanical ventilation: a randomized trial. *Lancet* 2010; 375:475–480.
Sud S, Sud M, Friedrich JP. High-frequency oscillation in patients with acute lung injury and acute respiratory distress syndrome (ARDS): systematic review and meta-analysis. *BMJ* 2010; 340:C2327.

ACUTE RESPIRATORY DISTRESS SYNDROME

Definition and aetiology

The acute respiratory distress syndrome (ARDS; ***Box 25.19***) can be defined as follows:

- ***Respiratory distress***.
- ***Stiff lungs*** (reduced pulmonary compliance resulting in high inflation pressures).
- ***Chest X-ray***: new bilateral, diffuse, patchy or homogeneous pulmonary infiltrates.
- ***Cardiac failure***: no apparent cardiogenic cause of pulmonary oedema (pulmonary artery occlusion pressure <18 mmHg if measured or no clinical evidence of left atrial hypertension).
- ***Gas exchange abnormalities***:
  - mild: P_aO_2/F_IO_2 ratio 300–200 mmHg
  - moderate: P_aO_2/F_IO_2 200–100 mmHg
  - severe: P_aO_2/F_IO_2 ratio <100 mmHg

Box 25.19 Disorders associated with acute respiratory distress syndrome

Direct lung injury	Indirect lung injury
Common causes	
Pneumonia	Sepsis
Aspiration of gastric contents	Severe trauma with shock and multiple transfusions
Less common causes	
Pulmonary contusion	Cardiopulmonary bypass
Blast injury	Drug overdose (heroin, barbiturates)
Fat embolism	Acute pancreatitis
Near-drowning	Transfusion-associated lung injury (TRALI)
Inhalational injury (smoke or corrosive gases)	Eclampsia
Reperfusion lung injury after lung transplantation or pulmonary embolectomy	High altitude
	Severe burns
	Pulmonary vasculitis
Amniotic fluid embolism	

all with a PEEP ≥5 cmH_2O (Berlin definition) (in all cases, despite normal arterial carbon dioxide tension).

ARDS can occur as a non-specific reaction of the lungs to a wide variety of direct pulmonary and indirect non-pulmonary insults. By far the most common predisposing factor is sepsis, and 20–40% of patients with severe sepsis will develop ARDS ***(Box 25.19)***.

Pathogenesis and pathophysiology

ARDS can be viewed as an early manifestation of a generalized inflammatory response with endothelial dysfunction and is therefore frequently associated with the development of multiple organ dysfunction syndrome (MODS; see p. 1155).

Non-cardiogenic pulmonary oedema

This is the cardinal feature of ARDS and is the first and clinically most evident sign of a generalized increase in vascular permeability caused by the microcirculatory changes and release of immune mediators described previously (see pp. 1151–1153), with activated neutrophils playing a key role. The pulmonary epithelium is also damaged in the early stages, reducing surfactant production, predisposing to alveolar collapse and lowering the threshold for alveolar flooding.

Pulmonary hypertension

Pulmonary hypertension, sometimes complicated by right ventricular failure (see p. 1030), is a common feature of ARDS. Initially, mechanical obstruction of the pulmonary circulation may occur as a result of vascular compression by interstitial oedema, while local activation of the coagulation cascade leads to thrombosis and obstruction in the pulmonary microvasculature. Later, pulmonary vasoconstriction may develop in response to increased autonomic nervous activity and circulating substances such as catecholamines and thromboxane. Those vessels supplying alveoli with low oxygen tensions constrict (the 'pulmonary hypoxic vasoconstrictor response'), diverting pulmonary blood flow to better-oxygenated areas of lung, thus limiting the degree of shunt.

Haemorrhagic intra-alveolar exudate

This exudate is rich in platelets, fibrin, fibrinogen and clotting factors, and may inactivate surfactant and stimulate inflammation, as well as promoting hyaline membrane formation and the migration of fibroblasts into the air spaces.

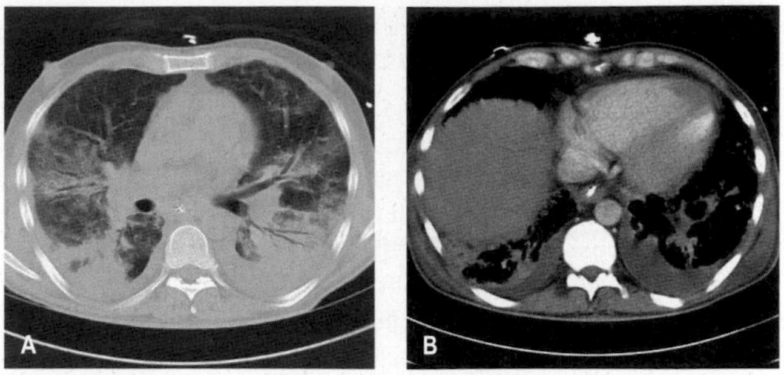

Figure 25.26 Acute respiratory distress syndrome. A. Computed tomography scan of the lung showing ground-glass opacification in non-dependent regions, with atelectasis and consolidation in dependent regions. There are small pleural effusions. **B.** The same patient as shown in **A** using soft-tissue window settings to demonstrate small bilateral effusions layering in the dependent region of both hemithoraces. *(From Hinds CJ, Watson JD.* Intensive Care: A Concise Textbook, *3rd edn. Edinburgh: Saunders; 2008, with permission. Courtesy of Dr SPG Padley.)*

Resolution, fibrosis and repair

Within days of the onset of lung injury, formation of a new epithelial lining is under way and activated fibroblasts accumulate in the interstitial spaces. In some cases, there is progressive interstitial fibrosis. In those who recover, the lungs are substantially remodelled.

Physiological changes

Shunt and dead space increase, compliance falls and there is evidence of airflow limitation. Although the lungs in ARDS are diffusely injured, the pulmonary lesions, when identified as densities on a CT scan, are predominantly located in dependent regions ***(Fig. 25.26)***. This is partly explained by the effects of gravity on the distribution of extravascular lung water and areas of lung collapse. Pleural effusions are common.

Clinical features

The first sign of the development of ARDS is often an unexplained tachypnoea, followed by increasing hypoxaemia with central cyanosis and breathlessness. Fine crackles are heard throughout both lung fields. Later, the chest X-ray shows bilateral diffuse shadowing, interstitial at first, but subsequently with an alveolar pattern and air bronchograms ***(Fig. 25.27)***. The differential diagnosis includes cardiac failure and lung fibrosis.

Management

This is based on treatment of the underlying condition (e.g. eradication of sepsis), supportive measures, and avoidance of complications such as ventilator-induced lung injury and ventilator-associated pneumonia.

Mechanical ventilation

This is the cornerstone of management; strategies designed to minimize ventilator-induced lung injury and encourage lung healing should be used (see p. 1166).

Pulmonary oedema limitation

Pulmonary oedema formation should be limited by fluid restriction, the use of diuretics and, if these measures fail, prevention of fluid overload by haemofiltration. The aim should be to achieve a consistently negative fluid balance.

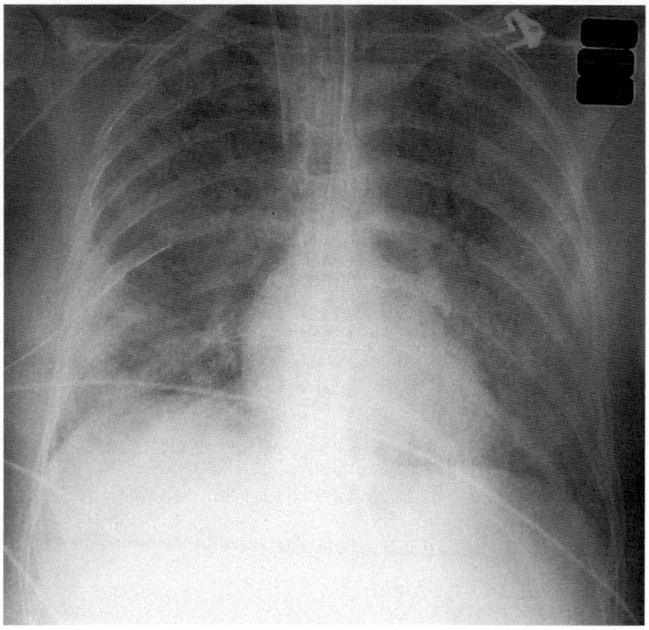

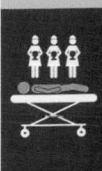

Figure 25.27 Chest radiograph appearances in acute respiratory distress syndrome. Bilateral diffuse alveolar shadowing with air bronchograms and no cardiac enlargement.

Prone position

When the patient is changed from the supine to the prone position, lung densities in the dependent region are redistributed and shunt fraction is reduced. More uniform alveolar ventilation, caudal movement of the diaphragm, redistribution of perfusion and recruitment of collapsed alveoli all contribute to the improvement in gas exchange. Repeated position changes between prone and supine allow reductions in airway pressures and the inspired oxygen fraction. Recent findings suggest that proning early in the course of the disease process and spending longer periods prone than supine are associated with substantial mortality benefits.

Inhaled nitric oxide

This vasodilator, when inhaled, may improve matching by increasing perfusion of ventilated lung units, as well as reducing pulmonary hypertension. It has been shown to improve oxygenation in so-called 'responders' with ARDS but has not been shown to increase survival.

Aerosolized prostacyclin

This appears to have similar effects to inhaled nitric oxide and is easier to deliver. As with inhaled nitric oxide, the response to aerosolized prostacyclin is, however, variable; although it improves oxygenation, its effect on outcome is unclear.

Aerosolized surfactant

Surfactant replacement therapy reduces morbidity and mortality in neonatal respiratory distress syndrome and is beneficial in animal models of ARDS. In adults with ARDS, however, the value of surfactant administration remains uncertain.

Steroids

Administration of steroids to patients with persistent ARDS does not appear to improve outcome.

Prognosis

Mortality from ARDS has fallen over the last decade, from around 60% to between 20% and 40%, perhaps as a consequence of improved general care, lung-protective ventilation strategies, the increasing use of management protocols, and attention to infection control and nutrition. Prognosis is, however, still very dependent on aetiology. When ARDS occurs in association with intra-abdominal sepsis, mortality rates remain very high, whereas much lower mortality rates are to be expected in those with 'primary' ARDS (pneumonia, aspiration, lung contusion). Mortality rises with increasing age and failure of other organs. Most of those dying with ARDS do so as a result of MODS and haemodynamic instability rather than impaired gas exchange.

Further reading

ARDS Definition Task Force. Acute respiratory distress syndrome: the Berlin definition. *JAMA* 2012; 307:2526–2533.
Guérin C, Reignier J, Richard JC et al. Prone positioning in severe acute respiratory distress syndrome. *N Engl J Med* 2013; 368:2159–2168.
Hall JP, Kress JP. The burden of functional recovery from ARDS. *N Engl J Med* 2011; 364:1360–1366.
Herridge MS, Tansey CM, Matté A et al. Functional disability 5 years after acute respiratory distress syndrome. *N Engl J Med* 2011; 364:1293–1304.
Kress JP, Hall JB. ICU-acquired weakness and recovery from critical illness. *N Engl J Med* 2014; 370:1626–1635.

ACUTE KIDNEY INJURY

Acute kidney injury (AKI) is a common and serious complication of critical illness, and is strongly associated with increased morbidity and mortality. The presence and severity of AKI are now formally classified by relative increases in serum creatinine and/or a persistent reduction in urine output (see ***Box 20.27***).

The importance of preventing renal injury by rapid and effective resuscitation, the avoidance of nephrotoxic drugs (especially non-steroidal anti-inflammatory drugs, NSAIDs), and control of infection cannot be overemphasized. While shock and sepsis are the most common causes of AKI in the critically ill, causes requiring specific treatment should be excluded, especially urinary tract obstruction and acute intrinsic renal disease such as rapidly progressive glomerulonephritis (see p. 772).

Acutely, oliguria often accompanies shock and renal hypoperfusion and should prompt attempts to optimize cardiovascular function by expanding the circulating volume and restoring blood pressure, with restoration of urine output a good indicator of successful resuscitation. However, when AKI is established, urine output is often normal or high due to impaired concentrating capacity, so that development of oliguria then implies almost complete loss of renal function; in this case, continued fluid resuscitation will be ineffective and potentially harmful.

There is no evidence to support specific pharmacological interventions to prevent or treat AKI; in particular, low-dose dopamine is ineffective for preventing or reversing renal impairment in sepsis (see p. 772). Thus, treatment of those developing or at risk of AKI should focus on prompt resuscitation with fluid and/or vasopressor therapy, as well treatment of the underlying causes of shock and sepsis. If these measures fail to reverse oliguria, loop diuretics such as furosemide (see p. 156) may be used to treat or prevent fluid overload. However, there is no evidence that diuretics alter the clinical course of AKI, and renal replacement therapy (RRT) should not be delayed if indicated.

In AKI, RRT is indicated for refractory fluid overload, major electrolyte disturbances (especially hyperkalaemia), severe acidosis and, less often, uraemia. There is no evidence to support commencement of RRT for less severe AKI in the absence of these indications. Continuous renal replacement therapy (CRRT; see p. 773) is associated with greater haemodynamic stability and better control of fluid balance than intermittent haemodialysis, while use of peritoneal dialysis is unsatisfactory in critically ill patients (although this may be an option in resource-limited environments). Thus, CRRT is now the preferred method of renal support in the critically ill.

In critical illness complicated by AKI, if the underlying problems resolve, renal function usually recovers over a period of a few days to several weeks. However, there is good evidence to suggest that, after recovery, subtle defects in renal function persist, so that patients requiring RRT in the ICU have a significantly increased risk of developing chronic kidney disease in the months and years after critical illness.

Further reading

Bellomo R, Kellum JA, Ronco C. Acute kidney injury. *Lancet* 2012; 380:756–766.
RENAL Replacement Therapy Study Investigators. Intensity of continuous renal-replacement therapy in critically ill patients. *N Engl J Med* 2009; 361:1627–1638.

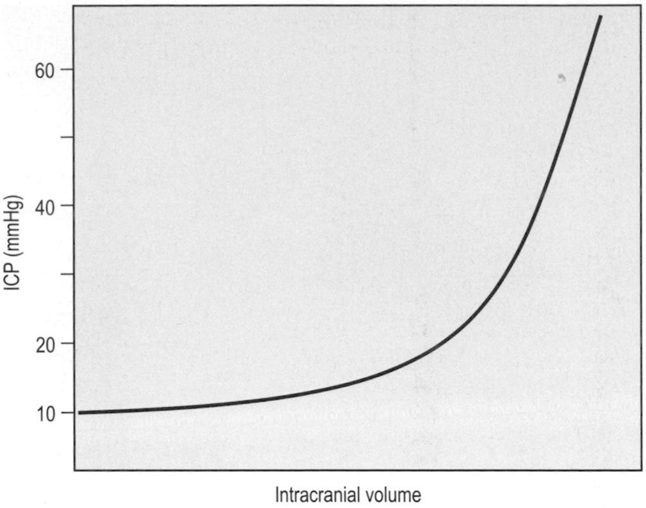

Figure 25.28 Intracranial compliance curve. ICP, intracranial pressure. *(From Hinds CJ, Watson JD.* Intensive Care: A Concise Handbook*, 3rd edn. Edinburgh: Saunders; 2008, with permission).*

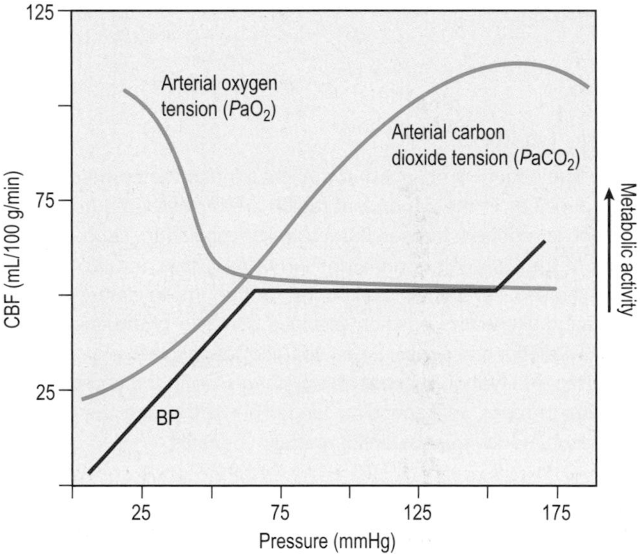

Figure 25.29 Factors influencing cerebral blood flow (CBF). BP, mean arterial blood pressure.

NEUROCRITICAL CARE

Physiology

Neurones are particularly susceptible to acute ischaemic/hypoxic insults, as they have very limited capacity for anaerobic metabolism and are irreversibly lost when blood flow is restricted for as little as 3–8 minutes.

Within the rigid vault of the skull are housed the intracranial contents, which consist of brain parenchyma, blood and CSF. The intracranial pressure (ICP, pressure within the skull) is approximately 7–15 mmHg in a resting, supine adult. Changes in intra-abdominal and intrathoracic pressures, such as occur during coughing or a Valsalva manœuvre, may result in transient increases in ICP that are of no consequence. The ***Monro–Kellie doctrine*** states that, because the cranial compartment is rigid, any increase in the volume of one of the intracranial constituents (blood, CSF, brain tissue) must be compensated by a decrease in the volume of the others. As space-occupying lesions expand or brain tissue swells, the rise in ICP is limited by displacement of CSF and venous blood from the intracranial compartment. Once these compensatory mechanisms are exhausted, further increases in intracranial volume cause exponentially greater increases in ICP ***(Fig. 25.28)***.

In health, ***autoregulation*** maintains constant cerebral blood flow over a range of blood pressures. However, these mechanisms are lost following significant intracranial injury, and cerebral blood flow then becomes directly dependent on cerebral perfusion pressure (CPP). CPP is calculated as the MAP minus the ICP. Occasionally, a very high CVP, greater than the ICP, will also reduce CPP ***(Fig. 25.29)***.

Clinical assessment

The causes of coma are listed in ***Box 21.27***. Conscious level should be documented and any changes noted. The Glasgow Coma Scale (GCS) score ***(Box 21.26)*** is widely used as a semi-quantitative, yet crude, means of gauging the level of consciousness. Assessment of the airway is of particular importance. Patients with airway obstruction due to lax oropharyngeal musculature should be managed as discussed on page 1156. Similarly, patients without a cough or gag reflex may need to be intubated in order to protect the airway. Pupillary signs are crucial. Documentation of pupillary size and reactivity is crucial. A unilaterally dilated pupil that reacts sluggishly or not at all is frequently a sign of increasing ICP. This is caused by compression of the IIIrd cranial nerve by herniating brain; if untreated, it can be rapidly fatal. Immediate treatments to decrease ICP ***(Box 25.20)*** are required whilst a CT scan of the brain is obtained. In some situations, patients may be taken directly to the operating theatre in order to alleviate the raised ICP and to remove expanding space-occupying lesions such as a haematoma. Small or pinpoint pupils may be a sign of mid-brain injury or opioid overdose. New focal neurological signs should be sought, such as cranial nerve palsies, limb weakness or hemiparesis. Seizures should be recognized and treated appropriately (see p. 826).

Box 25.20 Measures to control raised intracranial pressure and prevent secondary brain injury

- Control/restoration of blood pressure
- Control of intracranial pressure:
  - Reduction of intracranial blood volume
  - Mechanical ventilation
  - Sedation
  - Unobstructed venous drainage
  - Control of cerebral oedema
  - Osmotic diuretics (e.g. mannitol)
  - Loop diuretic (e.g. furosemide)
- Other measures:
  - Removal of cerebrospinal fluid via intraventricular catheter
  - Decompressive craniectomy
  - Excision of brain tissue
- Control of seizure activity

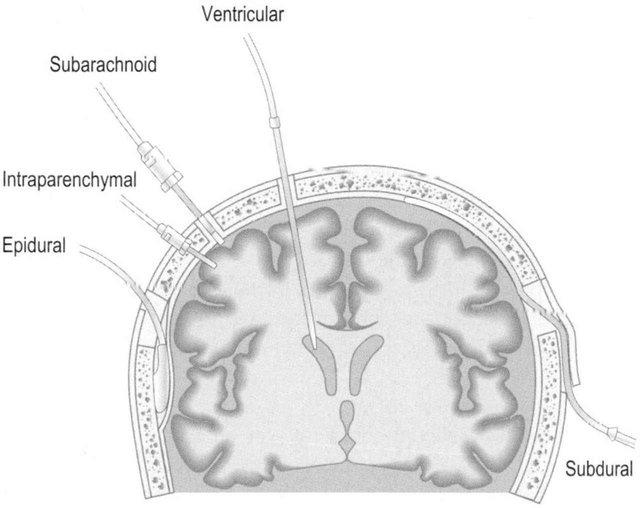

Figure 25.30 Methods for measuring intracranial pressure.

Monitoring

Regular clinical assessments by the bedside nurse are essential, including Glasgow Coma Scale score and pupillary size and reaction to light at least every hour. Neurological assessments are inevitably limited in patients requiring sedation and mechanical ventilation. In these patients, invasive monitoring of ICP may be necessary.

Invasive ICP monitoring devices may be extradural, subdural, subarachnoid, intraparenchymal or intraventricular ***(Fig. 25.30)***. The external ventricular drain (EVD) is the most difficult to insert, particularly when increased ICP causes the ventricles to collapse. EVDs are normally placed through the non-dominant (usually right) hemisphere into the lateral ventricle in the operating theatre. Their main advantage over the other monitoring devices is that they can also be used to treat raised ICP by draining CSF from the ventricular system. They are more prone to infection, however.

Multi-electrode electroencephalography (EEG) monitors give both a waveform and an analogue display that can help in the diagnosis of non-convulsive seizures and are also useful in monitoring the depth of sedation.

Oximeter-tipped catheters can be placed via the internal jugular vein and advanced in a cranial direction to lie in the jugular bulb just external to the skull. These 'jugular bulb oximetry' catheters monitor venous saturation in blood leaving the brain and give an indication of the balance between cerebral oxygen supply and demand. Measurements can be interpreted similarly to the mixed venous oxygen content (see pp. 1143–1144).

Cerebral oximetry uses near-infrared spectroscopy (NIRS) technology to estimate the oxygenation of a small portion of the cerebral cortex. Adhesive pads that both emit and capture near-infrared light waves are placed over the frontal cortex. Cerebral oximetry can provide an early warning of decreased cerebral oxygen delivery.

Management

Because little can be done to reverse the immediate primary brain injury and irreversible loss of neurones that occur as a direct consequence of intracerebral haemorrhage, infarct or traumatic brain injury, ICU care is focused on minimizing secondary brain injury ***(Box 25.20)***. This commonly occurs as a result of increases in ICP and consequent decreases in CPP. Cerebral oedema, expanding mass lesions (e.g. haemorrhage), prolonged seizure activity and hypercarbia (which causes cerebral vasodilatation) are all examples of mechanisms leading to secondary injury. Neurocritical care has therefore focused on monitoring ICP and maintaining CPP. The Brain Trauma Foundation (BTF) guidelines state that an ICP of <20 mmHg and a CPP of between 50 and 70 mmHg should be the aim, with vasopressors and fluid given as required in conjunction with supportive care; the latter should include airway protection, maintenance of normocarbia, reduction of the risk of nosocomial infections and prevention of thromboembolic complications.

Further reading

http://www.braintrauma.org *Brain Trauma Foundation.*

OUTCOMES

Withholding and withdrawing treatment

(See also Ch. 3.)

For many critically ill patients, intensive care is undoubtedly life-saving and resumption of a normal lifestyle is to be expected. It is also widely accepted that the elective admission of high-risk patients into an ICU or HDU, particularly in the immediate post-operative period, can minimize morbidity and mortality and lower costs, as well as reducing the demands on medical and nursing personnel on general wards. In the most seriously ill patients, however, mortality rates are high and a significant number die soon after discharge from the ICU. Mortality rates are particularly high in those who require re-admission to intensive care. Moreover, patients surviving a prolonged ICU admission often do not regain their premorbid functional status, and longer-term mortality rates (for at least 5 years post discharge) remain higher than in a general population matched for age and illness severity. Many centres have established specialist follow-up clinics to address long-term sequelae of critical illness.

Inappropriate use of intensive care facilities has other implications. The patient may experience unnecessary suffering and loss of dignity, while relatives may also have to endure considerable emotional pressures. In some cases, treatment may simply prolong the process of dying or sustain life of dubious quality, and in others the risks of interventions outweigh the potential benefits. Lastly, intensive care is expensive, particularly for those with the worst prognosis, and resources are limited.

To ensure both a humane approach to the management of critically ill patients and the appropriate use of limited resources, it is necessary to:

- avoid admitting patients who cannot benefit from intensive care
- limit further aggressive therapy when the prognosis is clearly hopeless.

Such decisions are extremely difficult; every case must be assessed individually, taking into account previous health and quality of life, primary diagnosis, medium- and long-term prognosis of the underlying condition, and survivability of the acute illness. Age alone should not be the sole consideration. When in doubt, active measures should continue but with regular review in the light of response to treatment and any other changes.

Decisions to limit therapy, not to resuscitate or to withdraw treatment should be made jointly by the ICU medical staff, the primary physician or surgeon, the nurses and, if possible, the patient, normally in consultation with the patient's family. Limitation of active treatment is *not* the cessation of medical or nursing care; rather, a caring approach must be adopted to ensure a dignified death, free of pain and distress, with support for family and friends (see p. 41).

Scoring systems

A variety of scoring systems have been developed that can be used to evaluate the severity of a patient's illness. Some have included an assessment of the patient's previous state of health and the severity of the acute disturbance of physiological function (***acute physiology, age, chronic health evaluation***, or ***APACHE***; and the ***simplified acute physiology score***, or ***SAPS***). Other systems have been designed for particular categories of patient (e.g. the injury severity score for trauma victims).

The APACHE and SAPS scores are widely applicable and have been extensively validated. They can accurately quantify the severity of illness and predict the overall mortality for large groups of critically ill patients, and are therefore useful for defining the 'case mix' of patients when auditing a unit's clinical activity, for comparing results nationally or internationally, and for characterizing groups of patients in clinical studies. Although the APACHE and SAPS methodologies can also be used to estimate risks of mortality, no scoring system has yet been devised that can predict with certainty the outcome in an individual patient. They must not, therefore, be used in isolation as a basis for limiting or discontinuing treatment.

Brain death and organ donation

Brain death means 'the irreversible loss of the capacity for consciousness combined with the irreversible loss of the capacity to breathe'. Both of these are essentially functions of the brainstem. Death, if thought of in this way, can arise either from causes outside the brain (i.e. respiratory and cardiac arrest) or from causes within the cranial cavity. With the advent of mechanical ventilation, it became possible to support such a dead patient temporarily, although, in all cases, cardiovascular failure eventually supervenes and progresses to asystole.

Before deciding on a diagnosis of brainstem death, it is essential for certain preconditions and exclusions to be fulfilled.

Preconditions

- The patient must be in apnoeic coma (i.e. unresponsive and on a ventilator, with no spontaneous respiratory efforts).
- Irremediable structural brain damage due to a disorder that can cause brainstem death must have been diagnosed with certainty (e.g. head injury, intracranial haemorrhage).

Exclusions

- The possibility that unresponsive apnoea is the result of poisoning, sedative drugs or neuromuscular blocking agents must be excluded.
- Hypothermia must be excluded as a cause of coma. The central body temperature should be >35°C.
- There must be no significant metabolic or endocrine disturbance that could produce or contribute to coma or cause it to persist.
- There should be no profound abnormality of the plasma electrolytes, acid–base balance or blood glucose levels.

Diagnostic tests for the confirmation of brainstem death

All brainstem reflexes are absent in brainstem death.

The following tests should not be performed in the presence of seizures or abnormal postures.

- Oculocephalic reflexes should be absent. In a comatose patient whose brainstem is intact, the eyes will rotate relative to the orbit (i.e. doll's eye movements will be present). In a brainstem-dead patient, when the head is rotated from side to side, the eyes move with the head and therefore remain stationary relative to the orbit.
- The pupils are fixed and unresponsive to bright light. Both direct and consensual light reflexes are absent. The size of the pupils is irrelevant, although most often they will be dilated.
- Corneal reflexes are absent.
- There are no vestibulo-ocular reflexes on caloric testing (see p. 810).
- There is no motor response within the cranial nerve territory to painful stimuli applied centrally or peripherally. Spinal reflex movements may be present.
- There is no gag or cough reflex in response to pharyngeal, laryngeal or tracheal stimulation.
- Spontaneous respiration is absent. The patient should be ventilated with 100% O_2 (or 5% CO_2 in 95% O_2) for 10 min and then temporarily disconnected from the ventilator for up to 10 min. Oxygenation is maintained by insufflation with 100% oxygen via a catheter placed in the endotracheal tube. The patient is observed for any signs of spontaneous respiratory efforts. A blood gas sample should be obtained during this period to ensure that the P_aCO_2 is sufficiently high to stimulate spontaneous respiration (>6.7 kPa, 50 mmHg).

The examination should be performed and repeated by two senior doctors.

In the UK, it is not considered necessary to perform confirmatory tests, such as EEG or carotid and vertebral angiography.

The primary purpose of establishing a diagnosis of brainstem death is to demonstrate beyond doubt that it is futile to continue mechanical ventilation and other life-supporting measures.

In suitable cases, and provided the assent of relatives has been obtained (easier if the patient was carrying an organ donor card or is on the organ donor register), the organs of those in whom brainstem death has been established may then be retrieved whilst the heart is still beating and be used for transplantation.

Organ donation may be possible in situations where ongoing life-sustaining treatment in the ICU is deemed futile and a decision is reached in conjunction with the family (and, in rare circumstances, the patient) to withdraw treatments such as invasive ventilation and inotropes that are simply delaying an inevitable death. If the patient and family wish to consider organ donation, then withdrawal of life-sustaining therapies usually occurs in a planned fashion and often in the operating department suite. If the patient does indeed die in a relatively brief period, then organ retrieval may occur immediately following a cardiac death.

Both of these situations require rapport and trust to be established with the family, and many hospitals have a separate team of nurse specialists to help the families through these very difficult situations. In the UK, each region has a transplant coordinator who can help with the process, as well as providing information, training and advice about organ donation. These transplant coordinators should be informed of all patients undergoing brainstem testing and all patients in whom withdrawal of life-sustaining treatment is being considered, so that all families and patients can be offered the opportunity to donate organs if they so wish. The medical teams involved in the ICU care of the patient and those involved in the organ retrieval process must remain completely independent.

Further reading

Curtis JR, Vincent JL. Ethics and end of life care for adults in the intensive care unit. *Lancet* 2010; 376:1347–1353.
Finfer S, Vincent JL. Dying with dignity in the intensive care unit. *N Engl J Med* 2014; 370:2506–2514.

Bibliography

Bersten AD, Soni N. *Oh's Intensive Care Manual*, 7th edn. Oxford: Butterworth–Heinemann; 2014.

Significant websites

http://www.esicm.org *European Society of Intensive Care Medicine*.
http://www.ficm.ac.uk *Faculty of Intensive Care Medicine*.
http://www.icnarc.org *Intensive Care National Audit & Research Centre*.
http://www.ics.ac.uk *UK Intensive Care Society*.
http://www.sccm.org/Research *Society of Critical Care Medicine guidelines*.

26 Endocrine disease

Miles J Levy, Helena Gleeson

See your e-book for key learning points, clinical tips, drug tips, extra tables, interactive Figures, learning challenges and MCQs.

INTRODUCTION

The endocrine system consists of glands that exert their actions at distant parts of the body via the production of biologically active hormones secreted into the bloodstream. Unlike the neurological system, which produces an immediate response, the endocrine system typically has a slower and longer-lasting effect on the body. The main endocrine glands are the pituitary, thyroid, adrenals, gonads, parathyroids and pancreas, and the common endocrine problems seen in clinical practice are shown in ***Figure 26.1*** (see p. 1177). The pituitary gland, a pea-sized structure situated at the base of the brain, plays a key role in the control and feedback mechanisms of the endocrine system and has been termed the 'conductor of the endocrine orchestra'.

CLINICAL APPROACH TO THE PATIENT WITH ENDOCRINE DISEASE

History

Hormones produce widespread effects in the body, and states of hormonal deficiency or excess typically present with symptoms that are generalized, diffuse and non-specific. Symptoms of tiredness, weakness or lack of energy or drive, and changes in appetite or thirst are common presentations. Other typical 'hormonal' symptoms include changes in body size and shape, problems with libido and potency, periods or sexual development, and changes in the skin (dryness, greasiness, acne, bruising, thinning or thickening) and hair (loss or excess). The differential diagnosis is often wide but endocrine disorders should be always considered when assessing a patient with any of these common complaints.

The past, family and social histories are essential for making the diagnosis, planning appropriate management and interpreting results of borderline hormonal blood tests.

- The past history should include previous surgery or radiation involving endocrine glands, menstrual history, pregnancy, and growth and development in childhood.
- A full drug history will identify common iatrogenic endocrine problems ***(Box 26.1)***.
- A family history of autoimmune disease, endocrine disease including tumours, diabetes and cardiovascular disease is frequently relevant, and knowledge of family members' height, weight, body habitus, hair growth and age of sexual development may aid interpretation of the patient's own symptoms.

Examination

A full general examination is essential to endocrine assessment because endocrine disorders affect all organ systems. Weight, height, body mass index (BMI), blood pressure and general habitus should all be documented, together with the presence or absence of specific signs of deficiency or excess of individual hormone axes (signs of hyper- or hypothyroidism, acromegaly, Cushing syndrome or Addison's disease).

In people with suspected pituitary disease, visual fields and adjacent cranial nerves should be assessed clinically. In thyroid disease, the presence of goitre or thyroid eye disease should be documented. Skin changes may give clinical clues, including pigmentation (Addison's and Nelson's), vitiligo (autoimmune endocrinopathies), acanthosis nigricans (polycystic ovary syndrome (PCOS) and diabetes), skin thinning (Cushing's, hypogonadism) or thickening (acromegaly, PCOS), and bruising and striae (Cushing's). Hirsutism is a key sign in women and signs of hair loss from the head (following a change in thyroid function, androgen excess in women or normal virilization in men) or from the body, axillary and pubic areas (hypogonadism) may occur in both sexes.

In children, height and pubertal status are an essential part of the clinical examination.

Specific clinical signs associated with particular endocrine diseases are discussed in detail in the appropriate sections.

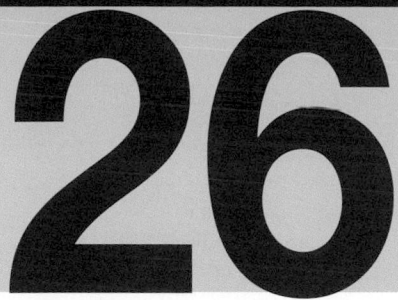

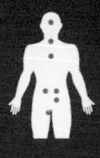

ENDOCRINE DISEASE

Hair
Alopecia
Coarse
Frontal balding

Facial features
Hypothyroid
- coarse
- complexion, peaches and cream
- puffy eyes
- dry skin

Hyperthyroid
- eye problems

Goitre
Nodules

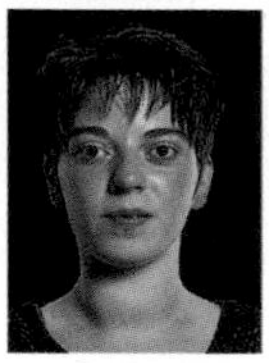

Goitre

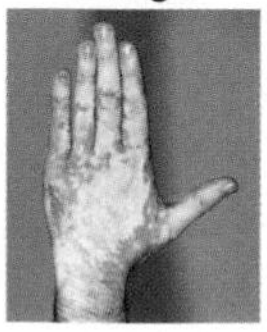

Vitiligo

Skin
Vitiligo (autoimmune disease)
Pigmentation
Hair distribution

Blood pressure
↑ Cushing's
Conn's
Phaeochromocytoma
↓ Adrenal insufficiency

Central
Obesity
Striae (Cushing's)

Genitalia
Testicular volume
Pubertal development
Virilization

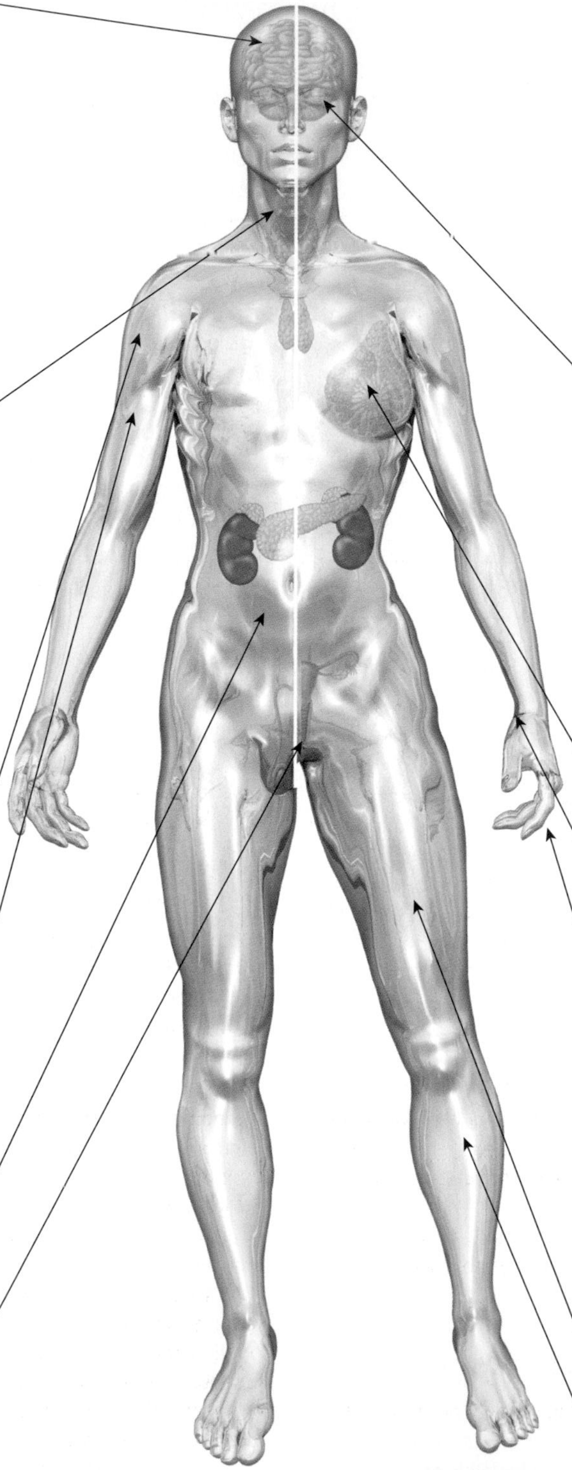

General
Look for features of:
Hypothyroidism
Hyperthyroid
Acromegaly

Mood
- depressed/lethargic
- restlessness
- memory

Voice – hoarse
Weight – loss or gain
Sweating
Hirsutism

Eyes
- Exophthalmos – Graves' disease, stare, lid lag
- Diplopia
- Visual fields defects
- Lid lag
- Ophthalmoscopy
  - Papilloedema
  - Pale optic discs

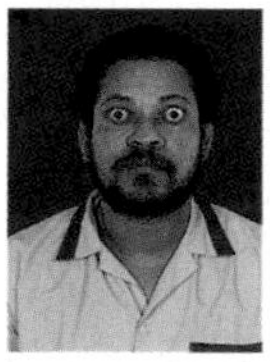

Exophthalmos

Breasts
Gynaecomastia
Galactorrhoea

Pulse
Atrial fibrillation

Hands
Sweating, tremor, palmar erythema
Carpal tunnel
Large, spade-like (acromegaly)
Pigmentation of creases (Addison's)

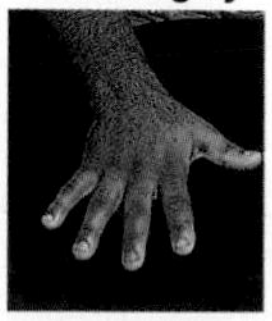

Acromegaly

Proximal myopathy

Pretibial myxedema

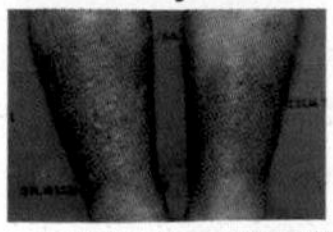

Pretibial myxoedema

(From Rojanametin K, Masaru T. 2015 J Am Coll Dermatol. 73(6): e195-e196, with permission)

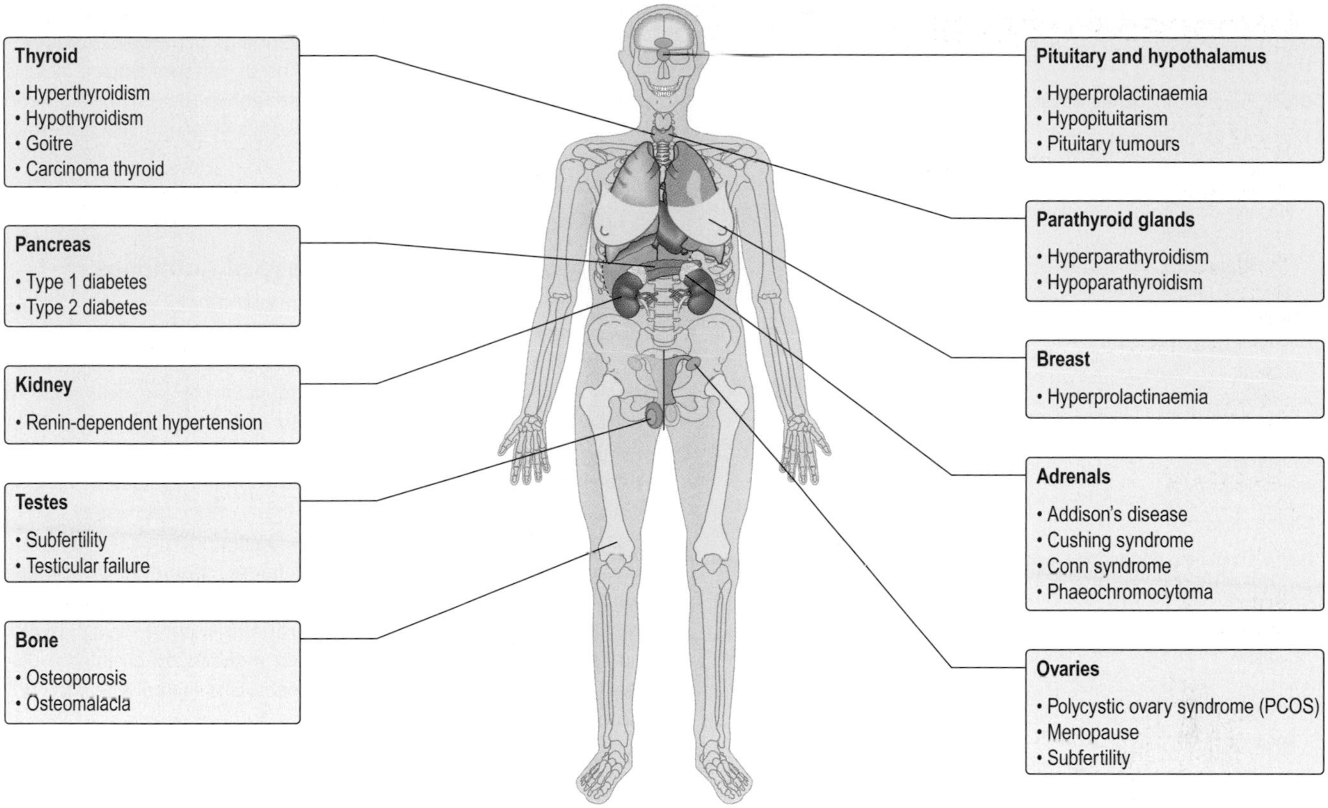

Figure 26.1 The major endocrine organs and common endocrine problems.

Common endocrine conditions

The most common endocrine disorders, excluding obesity (see pp. 206–212) and diabetes mellitus (p. 1241), are:

- thyroid disorders: hypothyroidism, hyperthyroidism, goitre
- menstrual disorders and/or hirsutism, usually due to PCOS
- hypogonadism in association with erectile dysfunction
- osteoporosis and metabolic bone disease
- subfertility
- disorders of growth or puberty.

With the advent of more frequent and detailed head and abdominal scans, another common endocrine referral is for investigation of incidental findings: for example, an empty sella or an incidentaloma, either pituitary or adrenal; all patients require endocrine review and investigation.

While most other endocrine conditions are uncommon, they often affect younger people and are usually curable or completely controllable with appropriate therapy.

Aetiology of endocrine disease

Aetiological mechanisms common to many endocrine disorders are outlined below.

Autoimmune disease

Organ-specific autoimmune diseases can affect every major endocrine organ ***(Box 26.2)***. They are characterized by the presence of specific antibodies in the serum, often present years before clinical symptoms are evident, usually more common in women and have a strong genetic component, often with an identical-twin concordance rate of 50% and with human leucocyte antigen (HLA) associations (see individual diseases). Several of the autoantigens have been identified.

Endocrine tumours

Most endocrine tumours are benign, although a cytological or histological diagnosis may be needed if there is clinical or radiological suspicion of malignancy. Clinical presentation depends on whether the tumour is functional or non-functional, the latter presenting only as a mass clinically or on imaging. Palpable thyroid nodules are common, and mass effects are a frequent presentation of pituitary adenomas, but the increased use of high-resolution ultrasound and detailed cross-sectional imaging has revealed a very high prevalence of asymptomatic, incidentally discovered thyroid, adrenal and pituitary lesions, commonly termed 'incidentalomas' (see p. 1229).

Functional tumours cause their effects via excess secretion of the relevant hormone. While often considered to be 'autonomous' – that is, independent of the physiological control mechanisms – many functional tumours do show evidence of feedback occurring at a higher 'set-point' than normal (e.g. adrenocorticotrophic hormone (ACTH) secretion from a corticotroph adenoma). This is relevant in the dynamic assessment of endocrine diseases, such as in the differential diagnosis of Cushing syndrome.

Endocrine adenomas typically present in a single gland, although rarer multiple endocrine neoplasia (MEN) syndromes exist that are due to very specific mutations of a single gene, such as the mutations of the *RET* proto-oncogene in MEN 2 or the *MEN1* gene mutation in MEN 1 (see p. 1239). The diagnosis of some endocrine tumours, particularly at a young age, or the identification of a family history should prompt discussion about genetic screening.

Box 26.1 Drugs and endocrine disease

Drug[a]	Effect
Drugs inducing endocrine disease	
Traditional antipsychotics (e.g. chlorpromazine, haloperidol, risperidone) Dopamine-antagonist antiemetics (metoclopramide, domperidone, prochlorperazine) Oestrogens	Increase in prolactin, causing galactorrhoea and oligorrhoea/amenorrhoea
Iodine Amiodarone Immune-modulating drugs	Hyperthyroidism
Lithium Amiodarone	Hypothyroidism
Ketoconazole Metyrapone Aminoglutethimide	Hypoadrenalism
Chemotherapy	Ovarian and testicular failure
Drugs simulating endocrine disease	
Sympathomimetics Amfetamines	Mimicking of thyrotoxicosis or phaeochromocytoma
Liquorice	Increase in mineralocorticoid activity; mimicking of aldosteronism
Purgatives	Hypokalaemia
Diuretics	Secondary aldosteronism
ACE inhibitors	Hypoaldosteronism
Drugs affecting hormone-binding proteins	
Oestrogens (e.g. contraceptive pills)	Rise in CBG – increase in total cortisol
Exogenous hormones or stimulating agents	
Use, abuse or misuse, by patient or doctor, of the following:	
Steroids	Cushing syndrome Diabetes
Anabolic steroids (androgens)	Suppression of gonadal axis
Levothyroxine	Thyrotoxicosis factitia
Vitamin D preparations Milk and alkali preparations	Hypercalcaemia
Insulin Sulphonylureas	Hypoglycaemia

[a]Drugs causing gynaecomastia are listed in Box 26.29. Amiodarone may cause both hypo- or hyperthyroidism.
ACE, angiotensin-converting enzyme; CBG, cortisol-binding globulin.

Enzyme defects

The biosynthesis of most hormones involves many stages. Deficient or abnormal enzymes can lead to absent or reduced production of the secreted hormone. In general, severe deficiencies present early in life with obvious signs; partial deficiencies usually present later with mild signs or are only evident under stress. An example of an enzyme deficiency is congenital adrenal hyperplasia (CAH), whose molecular basis has also been identified as mutations or deletions of the gene encoding the relevant enzymes (see p. 1228).

Receptor abnormalities

There are rare conditions in which hormone secretion and control are normal but the receptors are defective; thus, if androgen receptors are defective, normal levels of androgen will not produce masculinization (e.g. androgen insensitivity syndrome). There are also a number of rare syndromes of diabetes and insulin resistance from receptor abnormalities (see p. 1249); other examples include nephrogenic diabetes insipidus, pseudohypoparathyroidism and thyroid hormone resistance, which can cause an unusual pattern of thyroid blood results.

Hormonal activity

Synthesis, storage and release of hormones

Hormones may be of several chemical structures: polypeptide, glycoprotein, steroid or amine. Hormone release is the end-product of a long cascade of intracellular events. In the case of polypeptide hormones, neural or endocrine stimulation of the cell leads to increased transcription from DNA to a specific messenger RNA (mRNA), which is, in turn, translated to the peptide product. This is often in the form of a precursor molecule that may itself be biologically inactive. This 'prohormone' is then further processed before being packaged into granules, in the Golgi apparatus. These granules are then transported to the plasma membrane before release, which is itself regulated by a complex combination of intracellular regulators. Hormone release may be in a brief spurt caused by the sudden stimulation of granules, often induced by an intracellular Ca^{2+}-dependent process, or it is 'constitutive' (immediate and continuous secretion).

Plasma transport

Most classical hormones are secreted into the systemic circulation. In contrast, hypothalamic releasing hormones are released into the pituitary portal system so that much higher concentrations of the releasing hormones reach the pituitary than occur in the systemic circulation.

Many hormones are bound to proteins within the circulation. In most cases, only the free (unbound) hormone is available to the tissues and thus biologically active. This binding serves to buffer against very rapid changes in plasma levels of the hormone, and some binding protein interactions are also involved in the active regulation of hormone action. Many tests of endocrine function measure total rather than free hormone, which can give rise to difficulties in interpretation when binding proteins are altered in disease states or by drugs.

Binding proteins comprise both specific, high-affinity proteins of limited capacity, such as thyroxine-binding globulin (TBG), cortisol-binding globulin (CBG), sex-hormone-binding globulin (SHBG) and insulin-like growth factor (IGF)-binding proteins (e.g. IGF-BP3), and other less specific, low-affinity ones, such as prealbumin and albumin.

Hormone action and receptors

Hormones act by binding to specific receptors in the target cell. Most hormone receptors are proteins with complex tertiary structures. The structure of the hormone-binding domain of the receptor complements the tertiary structure of the hormone, while changes in other parts of the receptor in response to hormone binding are responsible for the effects of the activated receptor within the cell. The structure of common hormones and their receptors is described under individual hormone axes.

Hormone receptors are broadly divided into:

- ***cell surface or membrane receptors***: typically, transmembrane receptors that contain hydrophobic sections spanning the lipid-rich plasma membrane and which trigger internal cellular messengers (see also pp. 88–90)

Box 26.2 Types of autoimmune disease affecting endocrine organs

Organ and frequency, if known[a]	Antibody	Antigen, if known	Clinical syndrome
Stimulating			
Thyroid (1 in 100)	Thyroid-stimulating immunoglobulin (TSI, TSAb)	Thyroid-stimulating hormone (TSH) receptor	Graves' disease, neonatal thyrotoxicosis
Destructive			
Thyroid (1 in 100)	Thyroid microsomal	Thyroid peroxidase enzyme (TPO)	Primary hypothyroidism (myxoedema)
	Thyroglobulin	Thyroglobulin	
	Immunoglobulin (Ig) G4		Riedel's thyroiditis
Adrenal (1 in 20 000)	Adrenal cortex	21-Hydroxylase enzyme	Primary hypoadrenalism (Addison's disease)
Pancreas (1 in 500)	Islet cell	Glutamic acid decarboxylase (GAD; see p. 1248)	Type 1 diabetes
Stomach	Gastric parietal cell	Gastric parietal cell	Pernicious anaemia
	Intrinsic factor	Intrinsic factor	
Skin	Melanocyte	Melanocyte	Vitiligo
Ovary (1 in 500)	Ovary		Primary ovarian failure
Testis	Testis		Primary testicular failure
Parathyroid	Parathyroid chief cell	Parathyroid chief cell	Primary hypoparathyroidism
Pituitary	Pituitary-specific cells		Autoimmune hypophysitis Selective hypopituitarism (e.g. growth hormone (GH) deficiency, diabetes insipidus)

[a]Frequencies are approximate and refer to the population in Northern Europe.
Note: Other related diseases include myasthenia gravis and autoimmune liver diseases.

- ***nuclear receptors***: typically, bind hormones and translocate them to the nucleus, where they bind hormone response elements of nuclear DNA via characteristic amino-acid sequences (e.g. so-called 'zinc fingers'; see p. 98).

Abnormal receptors are an occasional cause of endocrine disease (see pp. 116–117).

Mechanisms of hormone-receptor action

Common structural mechanisms of hormone-receptor action are illustrated in ***Figure 7.12*** (p. 97) and include:

- ***G-protein coupled receptors (7-transmembrane or serpentine receptors)***. These bind hormones on their extracellular domain and activate the membrane G-protein complex with their intracellular domain. The activated complex may then:
  - stimulate cyclic AMP (cAMP) generation by adenylate cyclase – activating further intracellular kinases and leading to phosphorylation
  - activate phospholipase C (PLC), leading to generation of inositol 1,4,5-triphosphate (IP_3) and release of intracellular calcium – in turn, leading to calmodulin-dependent kinase activity and phosphorylation
  - lead to diacylglycerol (DAG) activation of C-kinase and subsequent protein phosphorylation.

  Most peptide hormones act via G-protein coupled receptors.
- ***Dimeric transmembrane receptors***. These receptors, from several receptor superfamilies, bind hormone in their extracellular components (sometimes causing the dimerization of the receptor monomer) and directly phosphorylate intracellular messengers via their intracellular components, leading to a variety of intracellular activation cascades. Growth hormone, prolactin and IGF-1 act via this type of receptor.
- ***Lipid-soluble molecules***. These pass through the cell membrane and typically bind with their ***nuclear receptors*** in the cell cytoplasm before translocation of the activated hormone–receptor complex to the nucleus; here, it binds to nuclear DNA, often in combination with a multi-component complex of promoters, inhibitors and transcription factors. This interaction usually leads to increased transcription of the relevant gene product. Steroid and thyroid hormones act via this type of receptor.

Hormone release and binding to receptors

The activation of intracellular kinases, phosphorylation, release of intracellular calcium and other 'second messenger' pathways, and the direct stimulation of DNA transcription result in some or all of the following:

- stimulation or release of pre-formed hormone from storage granules
- stimulation or synthesis of hormone and other cellular components
- opening or closing of ion or water channels in the cell membrane (e.g. calcium channels or aquaporin water channels)
- activation or deactivation of other DNA binding proteins, leading to stimulation or inhibition of DNA transcription.

In each case, binding of the hormone to its receptor is the first step in a complex cascade of interrelated intracellular events, which eventually lead to the overall effects of that hormone on cellular function.

The sensitivity and/or number of receptors for a hormone are often decreased after prolonged exposure to a high hormone concentration, the receptors thus becoming less sensitive ('downregulation', e.g. angiotensin II receptors, β-adrenoceptors). The reverse is true when stimulation is absent or minimal, the receptors showing increased numbers or sensitivity ('upregulation').

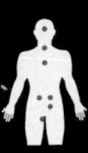

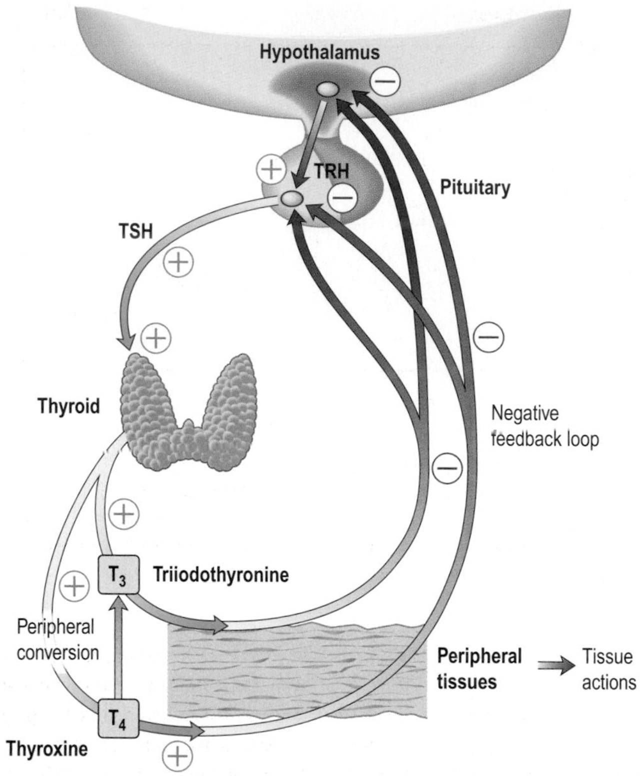

Figure 26.2 The hypothalamic–pituitary–thyroid axis. Pituitary thyroid-stimulating hormone (TSH) is secreted in response to hypothalamic thyrotrophin-releasing hormone (TRH) and stimulates secretion of T_4 and T_3 from the thyroid. T_4 and T_3 have actions in peripheral tissues and exert negative feedback on the pituitary and hypothalamus.

Control and feedback

Most hormone systems are under tight regulatory control (typically by the hypothalamic–pituitary (HP) axis) by a system known as negative feedback. An example of the negative feedback system in the hypothalamic–pituitary–thyroid (HPA) axis is demonstrated in ***Figure 26.2*** and described here:

- Thyrotrophin-releasing hormone (TRH) is secreted in the hypothalamus and travels via the portal system to the pituitary, where it stimulates the thyrotrophs to produce thyroid-stimulating hormone (TSH).
- TSH is secreted into the systemic circulation, where it stimulates increased thyroidal iodine uptake by the thyroid, and the synthesis and release of thyroxine (T_4) and triiodothyronine (T_3).
- Serum levels of T_3 and T_4 are increased by TSH; in addition, the conversion of T_4 to T_3 (the more active hormone) in peripheral tissues is stimulated by TSH.
- T_3 and T_4 then enter cells, where they bind to nuclear receptors and promote increased metabolic and cellular activity.
- Levels of T_3, from the blood and from local conversion of T_4, are sensed by receptors in the pituitary and the hypothalamus. If they rise above normal, TRH and TSH production is suppressed, leading to reduced T_3 and T_4 secretion.
- Peripheral T_3 and T_4 levels fall to normal.
- If, however, T_3 and T_4 levels are low – for example, after thyroidectomy, increased amounts of TRH and TSH are secreted, stimulating the remaining thyroid to produce more T_3 and T_4; blood levels of T_3 and T_4 may be restored to normal, at the expense of increased TSH drive, reflected by a high TSH level: 'compensated euthyroidism'.
- Conversely, in thyrotoxicosis, when factors other than TSH itself are maintaining high T_3 and T_4 levels, the same mechanisms lead to suppression of TSH secretion.

Primary and secondary gland failure

It is useful in clinical endocrinology to distinguish between 'primary' disease of the end-organ gland (e.g. that due to autoimmune destruction, atrophic change, infiltration or surgical removal of the gland) and 'secondary' disorders of the same axis, caused by disease of the pituitary gland. An understanding of the negative feedback system is key to interpreting endocrine blood results and diagnosing the site of the disease process in clinical practice. In general terms:

- ***'Primary' hormone deficiency*** due to a disease process in the endocrine end-organ (thyroid, adrenal or gonad) will lead to a loss of negative feedback and subsequent elevation in the corresponding anterior pituitary hormone.
- In ***'secondary gland failure'***, there are low or 'inappropriately normal' levels of the pituitary trophic hormone in the face of a low end-organ hormone level. For example, if a patient has low circulating free T_3 (fT_3) and T_4 levels in the context of a low TSH, pituitary disease should be suspected.

Hormone excess

Abnormal hormone excess due to a disease process in the primary endocrine gland, or excess amount of exogenous hormone, will lead to increased negative feedback and suppression of the corresponding pituitary hormones. For example, in autoimmune hyperthyroidism, the free fT_3 and T_4 levels are elevated in the context of a suppressed TSH. Equally, the presence of a non-suppressed plasma pituitary hormone in the context of excess primary hormone implies that the pituitary, rather than the primary gland itself, is the cause. For example, in pituitary-driven Cushing's disease, cortisol levels are elevated but ACTH is not suppressed.

Hormone resistance

In certain situations, receptor abnormalities can give rise to abnormal negative feedback due to hormone resistance, which can lead to an unusual pattern of blood results. For example, thyroid hormone resistance, due to mutations in the thyroid hormone receptor, is characterized by an elevation in thyroid hormones with a non-suppressed TSH. With this pattern of thyroid results, the clinician should also consider the rare diagnosis of a TSH-secreting pituitary tumour, in addition to the possibility of assay issues.

Measurement of hormones

Hormones are measured in routine clinical practice by biochemical assays in the laboratory. It is possible to measure pituitary trophic hormones and the hormones produced by the end-organ glands, but hypothalamic hormones are not routinely measured in practice because of their low concentration and local action within the HP axis. Circulating levels of most hormones are very low (10^{-9}–10^{-12} mol/L) and cannot be measured by simple chemical techniques. Hormones are therefore usually measured by immunoassays, which rely on highly specific polyclonal or monoclonal antibodies, which bind to the hormone being measured during the assay incubation. This hormone–antibody interaction is measured by use of labelled hormone after separation of bound and free fractions ***(Fig. 26.3)***.

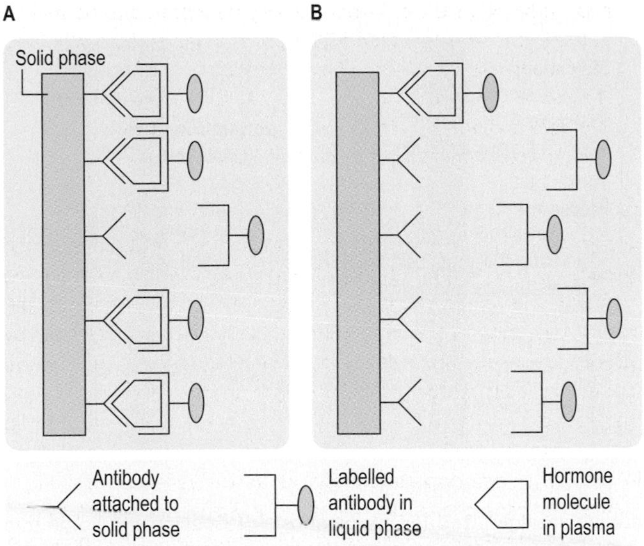

Figure 26.3 Principles of measurement of hormone levels in plasma by immunoassay. (Precise details vary with different assays and manufacturers.) Immunoassays use two antibodies specific to the hormone being measured: one typically attached to a solid phase and one labelled antibody in the liquid phase. **A.** *High hormone levels in plasma*: a large amount of hormone binds to antibody in solid phase, a large amount of labelled antibody is linked to solid phase via molecules of the hormone. **B.** *Low hormone levels in plasma*: less hormone, and therefore less labelled antibody, is linked to the solid phase. Label (radioactive, chemiluminescent, enzymatic or fluorescent) can be measured in either solid or liquid phase after separation of phases; levels of label will be proportional to the amount of hormone in the sample.

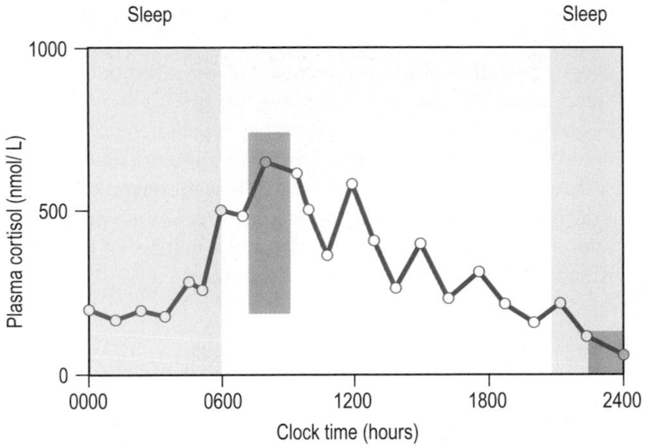

Figure 26.4 Plasma cortisol levels during a 24-hour period. Note both the pulsatility and the shifting baseline. Normal ranges for 09:00 hours (180–700 nmol/L) and 24:00 hours (<100 nmol/L; must be taken when asleep) are shown in the red boxes. Grey shading shows sleep.

Immunoassays are sensitive but have limitations. In particular, the immunological activity of a hormone, as used in developing the antibody, may not necessarily correspond to biological activity and there may be false positive and negative results. The patient's blood may also contain heterophile antibodies, which interact with the animal antibodies used in the assay and produce falsely low or high values. When there is a discrepancy between endocrine blood results and the clinical presentation, the clinician must question the validity of an endocrine result, and a close relationship with the relevant laboratory is essential. It may be necessary for the sample to be measured in a different laboratory using an alternative antibody, or to measure hormones in ways other than by immunoassay. Examples of alternative techniques that quantify and characterize hormone levels accurately include equilibrium dialysis, high-pressure liquid chromatography (HPLC) and, increasingly for the accurate measurement of steroid hormones, mass spectroscopy.

Hormone-binding proteins

Many hormones are transported in the bloodstream from the primary gland to their distant target organ attached to a specific binding protein (see p. 1178). It is more helpful to measure the free hormone rather than total bound hormone level, as this is the part that is biologically active. Some modern assays attempt to measure the free hormone level directly (e.g. free T_4) and are therefore a more accurate reflection of biological activity, although there are often technical problems with this approach and many assays still measure total hormone level.

Cortisol, which is bound to cortisol-binding globulin (CBG), and testosterone, which is bound to sex-hormone-binding globulin (SHBG), are still usually measured in their total form and can be affected by alterations in binding protein levels. In women who are pregnant or on the combined oral contraceptive pill, high oestrogen levels may lead to an elevation in CBG, which can overestimate cortisol and give the false impression of hypercortisolaemia. In people with diabetes mellitus or other insulin-resistant states that may lower SHBG levels, low total testosterone levels may give the false impression of androgen deficiency. Conversely, hyperthyroidism or oestrogen excess can cause an elevation in SHBG, leading to apparently high total testosterone levels. As with all endocrine results, the data need to be interpreted in the clinical context.

Patterns of hormonal secretion

Hormone secretion can be continuous or intermittent, for example:

- ***Continuous secretion*** is shown by the thyroid hormones, with a half-life of 7–10 days for T_4 and 6–10 h for T_3, and with little variation in levels over the day, month and year.
- ***Pulsatile secretion*** is the normal pattern for the gonadotrophins, luteinizing hormone (LH) and follicle-stimulating hormone (FSH), with major pulses released every 1–2 h, depending on the phase of the menstrual cycle. Growth hormone (GH) is also secreted in a pulsatile fashion, with undetectable levels in between pulses. A single measurement is therefore not helpful to diagnose GH deficiency or excess.

Biological rhythms

Circadian means changes over the 24 hours of the day–night cycle and is best shown for the pituitary–adrenal axis. ***Figure 26.4*** shows plasma cortisol levels measured over 24 hours; levels are highest in the early morning and lowest overnight. Additionally, cortisol release is pulsatile, following the pulsatility of pituitary ACTH. Thus, 'normal' cortisol levels vary during the day and great variations can be seen in samples taken only 30 minutes apart.

The menstrual cycle is an example of a longer and more complex (28-day) biological rhythm (see pp. 1213–1214).

Other regulatory factors

- ***Stress***. Physiological 'stress' and acute illness produce rapid increases in ACTH and cortisol, GH, prolactin, adrenaline (epinephrine) and noradrenaline (norepinephrine). These can occur within seconds or minutes.

- ***Sleep***. Secretion of GH and prolactin is increased during sleep, especially the rapid eye movement (REM) phase.
- ***Feeding and fasting***. Many hormones regulate the body's control of energy intake and expenditure, and are therefore profoundly influenced by feeding and fasting. Secretion of insulin is increased, whilst testosterone and GH are decreased after ingestion of food, and secretion of a number of hormones is altered during prolonged food deprivation.

Investigation of endocrine function

Endocrine function is assessed by measurement of hormone levels in blood (or, more precisely, in plasma or serum) and sometimes in other body fluids on samples obtained basally and in response to stimulation and suppression tests.

Basal blood levels

Assays for all clinically relevant pituitary and end-organ hormones are available.

The time, day and conditions of measurement make great differences to hormone levels, and the method and timing of samples therefore depend upon the characteristics of the endocrine system involved. There are also gender, pubertal and age differences.

Basal levels are especially useful for systems with long half-lives (e.g. T_4 and T_3, IGF-1, androstenedione, SHBG). These vary little over the short term and random samples are therefore satisfactory.

Basal samples for many hormones need to be interpreted with respect to normal ranges for the time of day/month, diet or posture concerned. Hormones with a marked circadian rhythm (e.g. testosterone and cortisol) must be measured at an appropriate time of day. Testosterone should be measured before 11:00 hours in the fasting state; cortisol should be checked between 8:00 hours and 10:00 hours to exclude hypoadrenalism, but at midnight to demonstrate normal low levels (to exclude Cushing's). LH/FSH, oestrogen and progesterone vary with time of menstrual cycle, and renin/aldosterone may vary with sodium intake, posture and age. For these hormones, all relevant details must be recorded or the results may prove uninterpretable.

Stress-related hormones

Measurement of stress-related hormones may be problematic either because the patient is stressed by hospital attendance or venepuncture, leading to falsely high levels (e.g. catecholamines, prolactin; sampling via an indwelling needle may be required, some time after initial venepuncture), or because low levels in a non-stressed individual are unable to confirm an adequate reserve required for normal physiological stress (cortisol and GH).

Urine collections

Collections over 24 hours have the advantage of providing an 'integrated mean' of a day's secretion but, in practice, are often incomplete or wrongly timed. They also vary with sex and body size or age. Written instructions should be provided for the patient to ensure accurate collection. Examples of hormones measured in this way are catecholamines and urinary free cortisol levels.

Saliva

Saliva is sometimes used for steroid estimations, especially in children or for samples taken at home. Midnight salivary cortisol levels are increasingly used for the diagnosis of Cushing syndrome due to the practical difficulties in obtaining a midnight blood sample.

Box 26.3 Short ACTH (tetracosactide) stimulation test

Indications
- Diagnosis of Addison's disease
- Screening test for ACTH deficiency

Procedure
- I.v. cannula for sampling
- Any time of day, but best at 09:00 hours; non-fasting
- Tetracosactide 250 µg, i.v. or i.m. at time 0
- Measure serum cortisol at time 0 and time +30 min

Normal response
- 30 min cortisol >600 nmol/L[a]
  - (400–600 nmol/L borderline and may indicate deficiency)

[a]*Precise cortisol normal ranges are variable between laboratories and assays; appropriate local reference ranges must be used.*

Stimulation and suppression tests

These tests are used when basal levels give equivocal information. In general, stimulation tests are used to confirm suspected deficiency of hormone secretion, and suppression tests to confirm suspected excess. These tests are valuable in many instances.

For example, where the secretory capacity of a gland is damaged, maximal stimulation by the trophic hormone will give a diminished output. Thus, in the short ACTH stimulation test for adrenal reserve (***Box 26.3***, ***Fig. 26.5A***), the healthy subject shows a normal response while the subject with primary hypoadrenalism (Addison's disease) demonstrates an impaired cortisol response to tetracosactide (an ACTH analogue).

A patient with a hormone-producing tumour usually fails to show normal negative feedback. A patient with Cushing's disease (excess pituitary ACTH) will thus fail to suppress ACTH and cortisol production when given a dose of synthetic steroid, in contrast to normal subjects. ***Figure 26.5B*** shows the response of a normal subject given dexamethasone 1 mg at midnight; cortisol is suppressed the following morning. The subject with Cushing's disease shows inadequate suppression.

The detailed protocol for each test must be followed exactly, since differences in technique will produce variations in results.

THE PITUITARY GLAND AND HYPOTHALAMUS

Anatomy

Most peripheral hormone systems are controlled by the hypothalamus and pituitary. The hypothalamus is sited at the base of the brain around the third ventricle and above the pituitary stalk, which leads down to the pituitary itself, carrying the hypophyseal–pituitary portal blood supply.

The anatomical relations of the hypothalamus and pituitary ***(Fig. 26.6)*** include the optic chiasm just above the pituitary fossa; any expanding lesion from the pituitary or hypothalamus can thus produce visual field defects by pressure on the chiasm. Such upward expansion of the gland through the diaphragma sellae is termed 'suprasellar extension'. Lateral extension of pituitary lesions may involve the vascular and nervous structures in the cavernous sinus and may rarely reach the temporal lobe of the brain. The

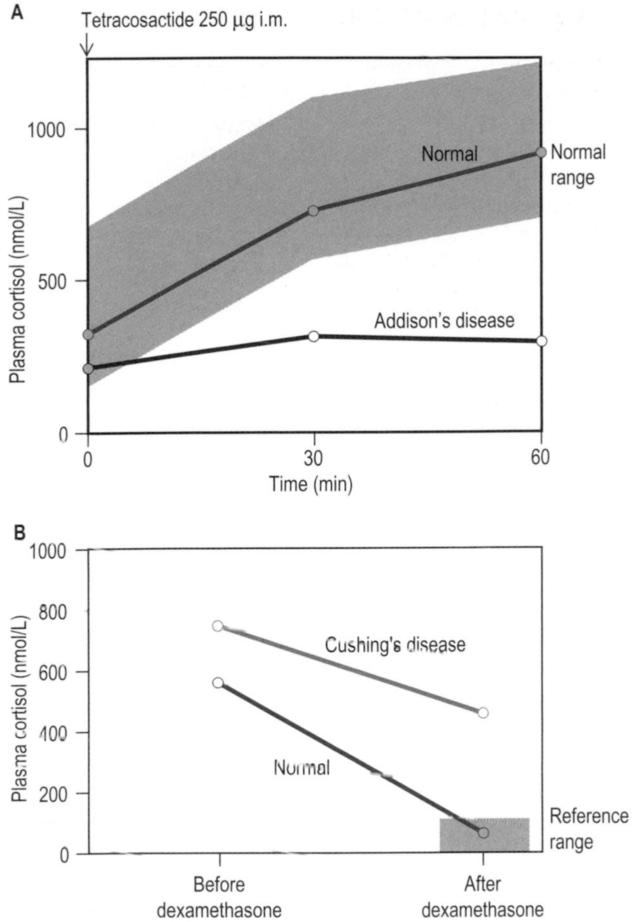

Figure 26.5 Short ACTH stimulation and dexamethasone suppression tests. A. *The short ACTH stimulation test* shows a normal response in a healthy subject and a decreased response in a patient with Addison's disease. **B.** *Dexamethasone suppression tests* in a normal subject and in a patient with Cushing's disease, showing inadequate suppression.

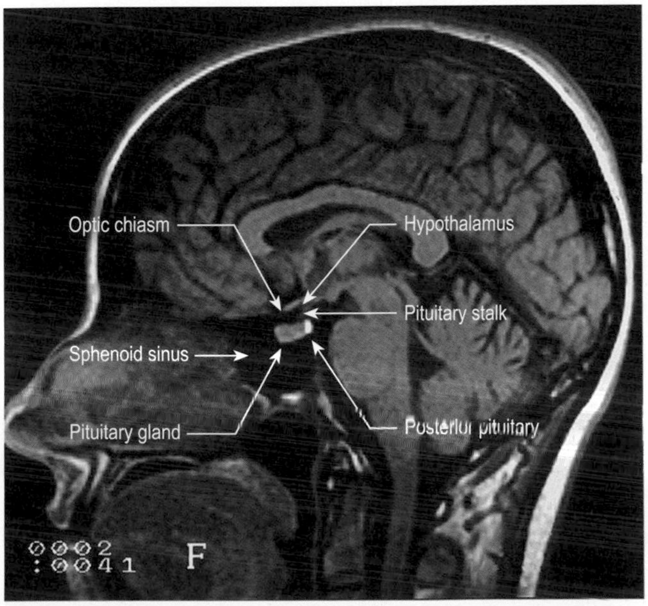

Figure 26.6 Magnetic resonance imaging (MRI) of a sagittal section of the brain, showing the pituitary fossa and adjacent structures. *(By kind permission of Dr Martin Jeffree.)*

pituitary is itself encased in a bony box; therefore, any lateral, anterior or posterior expansion must cause bony erosion.

Embryologically, the anterior pituitary is formed from an upgrowth of Rathke's pouch (ectoderm); this meets an outpouching of the third ventricular floor, which becomes the posterior pituitary. This unique combination of primitive gut and neural tissue provides an essential link between the rapidly responsive central nervous system and the longer-acting endocrine system. Several transcription factors – LHX3, HESX1, PROP1, POU1F1 – are responsible for the differentiation and development of the pituitary cells. Mutation of these produces pituitary disease.

Physiology

Hypothalamus

This contains many vital centres for such functions as appetite, thirst, thermal regulation and sleeping/waking. It acts as an integrator of many neural and endocrine inputs to control the release of pituitary hormone-releasing factors. It plays a role in circadian rhythm, menstrual cyclicity, and responses to stress, exercise and mood.

Hypothalamic neurones secrete pituitary hormone-releasing and inhibiting factors and hormones ***(Box 26.4)*** into the portal system; these run down the stalk to the pituitary. As well as the classical hormones illustrated in ***Figure 26.7***, the hypothalamus also contains large amounts of other neuropeptides and neurotransmitters such as neuropeptide Y, vasoactive intestinal peptide (VIP) and nitric oxide, which can also alter pituitary hormone secretion.

Synthetic hypothalamic hormones and their antagonists are available for the testing of many aspects of endocrine function and for treatment.

Anterior pituitary

The majority of anterior pituitary hormones are under predominantly positive control by the hypothalamic releasing hormones; the exception is prolactin, which is under tonic inhibition by dopamine. Pathological conditions interrupt the flow of hormones between the hypothalamus and pituitary gland, and therefore cause deficiency of most hormones but oversecretion of prolactin. There are five major anterior pituitary axes: the gonadotrophin axis, the growth axis, prolactin, the thyroid axis and the adrenal axis.

Posterior pituitary

The posterior pituitary is neuroanatomically connected to specific hypothalamic nuclei and acts merely as a storage organ. Antidiuretic hormone (ADH, also called vasopressin) and oxytocin, both nonapeptides, are synthesized in the supraoptic and paraventricular nuclei in the anterior hypothalamus. They are then transported along the axon and stored in the posterior pituitary ***(Fig. 26.7)***. This means that damage to the stalk or pituitary alone does not prevent synthesis and release of ADH and oxytocin. ADH is discussed on pages 1232–1235; oxytocin produces milk ejection and uterine myometrial contraction.

Presentations of pituitary and hypothalamic disease

Diseases of the pituitary can cause under- or overactivity of each of the hypothalamic–pituitary–end-organ axes that are under the control of this gland. The clinical features of the syndromes associated with such altered pituitary function, such as Cushing

Box 26.4 Hormones and receptors of the hypothalamic–pituitary axis

Hormone	Source	Site of action	Hormone structure	Receptor	Post-receptor activity
Pituitary growth axis					
Growth hormone-releasing hormone (GHRH)	Hypothalamus	Pituitary	Peptide – 44 AA	Membrane – 7TM	G-proteins cAMP
Somatostatin (inhibitory GHRIH)	Hypothalamus	Pituitary	Cyclic peptide – 14 or 28 AA	Membrane – 7TM SST2 + SST5	G-proteins Inhibit cAMP
Growth hormone	Pituitary	Liver and other tissues	Peptide – 191 AA	Transmembrane Dimerized GHR	JAK2 STAT
Insulin-like growth factor 1 (IGF-1)	Liver and locally elsewhere	Many tissues	Peptide – 70 AA 3 S–S bridges	Transmembrane – IGFR 2α + 2β subunits	Receptor tyrosine kinase
Pituitary–thyroid axis					
Thyrotrophin-releasing hormone (TRH)	Hypothalamus	Pituitary	Peptide – 3 AA	Membrane – 7TM TRHR	G-proteins PLC/IP_3
Thyroid-stimulating hormone (TSH)	Pituitary	Thyroid	Glycoprotein: α and β subunits	Membrane – 7TM TSHR	G-proteins cAMP/PLC/IP_3
Thyroxine and triiodothyronine (T_4 and T_3)	Thyroid	All tissues	Thyronines – 4/3 iodine atoms	Nuclear TR-α and β	Transcription TRE/RXR
Pituitary–gonadal axis					
Gonadotrophin-releasing hormone (GnRH; LHRH)	Hypothalamus	Pituitary	Peptide – 10 AA	Membrane – 7TM GnRH-R1	G-proteins PLC/IP_3
Luteinizing hormone (LH)	Pituitary	Gonad	Glycoprotein: α and β subunits	Membrane – 7TM LHhCGR	G-proteins cAMP
Follicle-stimulating hormone (FSH)	Pituitary	Gonad	Glycoprotein: α and β subunits	Membrane – 7TM FSHR	G-proteins cAMP
Oestradiol	Ovary	Uterus, breast bone, vascular	Steroid ring	Nuclear ER α and β (ESR1/ ESR2)	Homo-/heterodimer ERE Transcription
Testosterone	Testis	Many tissues	Steroid ring	Nuclear AR (NR3C4)	Dimer ARE Transcription
Inhibin and activin	Gonad	Pituitary–hypothalamus	Peptide dimers α and β subunits	Transmembrane dimerized	Phosphorylation by receptor
Prolactin axis					
Dopamine	Hypothalamus	Pituitary	Amine	Membrane – 7TM D2 receptor	G-proteins Inhibit cAMP
Prolactin	Pituitary	Breast Other tissues	Peptide – 199 AA	Transmembrane PRLR Class 1 cytokine	JAK2 and other pathways
Pituitary–adrenal axis					
Corticotrophin-releasing hormone (CRH)	Hypothalamus	Pituitary	Peptide – 41 AA	Membrane – 7TM CRF1	G-proteins cAMP
Adrenocorticotrophic hormone (ACTH)	Pituitary	Adrenal	Peptide – 39 AA	Membrane – 7TM ACTHR (MCR2)	G-proteins cAMP
Cortisol	Adrenal	All tissues	Steroid ring	Nuclear GRα	Transcription GRE
Posterior pituitary axes					
Vasopressin (antidiuretic hormone, ADH)	Hypothalamus → pituitary	Kidney	Peptide – 9 AA	Membrane – 7TM AVPR2	G-proteins cAMP Aquaporin-2
	Hypothalamus → pituitary	Vascular	Peptide – 9 AA	Membrane – 7TM AVPR1A	G-proteins PLC/IP_3
	Hypothalamus → portal veins	Pituitary (ACTH secretion)	Peptide – 9 AA	Membrane – 7TM AVPR1B	G-proteins PLC/IP_3
Oxytocin	Hypothalamus → pituitary	Uterus and breast	Peptide – 9 AA	Membrane – 7TM OXTR	G-proteins

7TM, 7 transmembrane (G-protein coupled receptor); AA, amino acids; ARE, androgen response element; AVPR, arginine vasopressin receptor; cAMP, adenylate cyclase → cyclic adenosine monophosphate; ERE, oestrogen response element; GRE, glucocorticoid response element; GHRIH, growth hormone releasing inhibitory hormone; JAK, Janus kinase; LHhCGR, luteinizing hormone human chorionic gonadotrophin receptor; LHRH, luteinizing hormone-releasing hormone; MCR, melanocortin receptor; OXTR, oxytocin receptor; PLC/IP_3, phospholipase C/inositol triphosphate; STAT, signal transducers and activators of transcriptions; SST, somatostatin receptor subtypes; TRE/RXR, thyroid hormone response element/response silencing region.

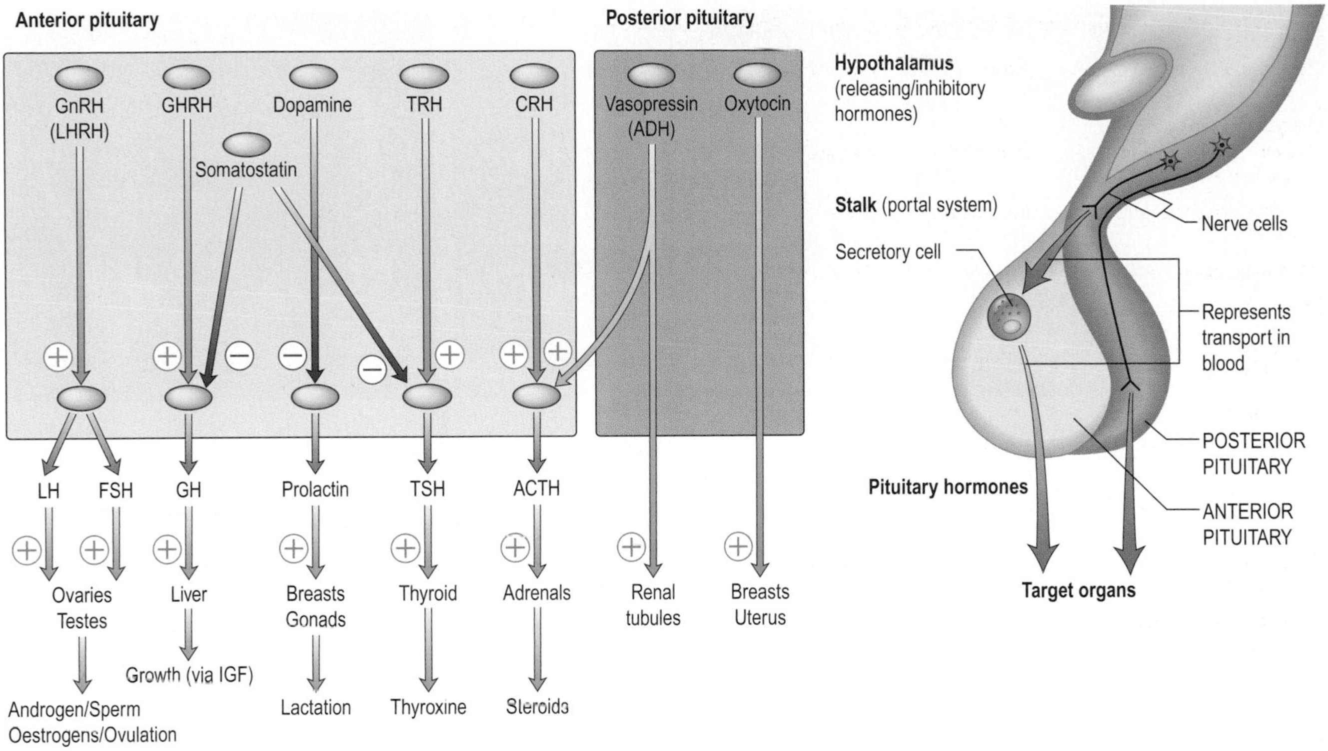

Figure 26.7 **Hypothalamic releasing hormones and the pituitary trophic hormones.** See the text for an explanation and for abbreviations.

Box 26.5 Characteristics of common pituitary and related tumours

Tumour or condition	Usual size	Most common clinical presentation
Prolactinoma	Most <10 mm (microprolactinoma) Some >10 mm (macroprolactinoma)	Galactorrhoea, amenorrhoea, hypogonadism, erectile dysfunction As above plus headaches, visual field defects and hypopituitarism
Acromegaly	Few mm to several cm	Change in appearance, visual field defects and hypopituitarism
Cushing's disease	Most small: few mm (some cases are hyperplasia)	Central obesity, cushingoid appearance (local symptoms rare)
Nelson syndrome	Often large: >10 mm	Post-adrenalectomy, pigmentation, sometimes local symptoms
Non-functioning tumours	Usually large: >10 mm	Visual field defects; hypopituitarism (microadenomas may be incidental finding)
Craniopharyngioma	Often very large and cystic (skull X-ray abnormal in >50%; calcification common)	Headaches, visual field defects, growth failure (50% occur below age 20; about 15% arise from within sella)

syndrome, can be the presenting symptom of pituitary disease or of end-organ disease and are discussed later. First, however, we look at the clinical features of pituitary disease that are common to all hormonal axes.

Pituitary space-occupying lesions and tumours

Pituitary tumours ***(Box 26.5)*** are the most common cause of pituitary disease, and the great majority of these are benign pituitary adenomas, usually monoclonal in origin. Problems are caused by:

- local effects of a tumour
- excess hormone secretion
- the result of inadequate production of hormone by the remaining normal pituitary, i.e. hypopituitarism.

Investigations (for a possible or proven mass)

Is there a tumour?

If there is, how big is it and what ***local anatomical effects*** is it exerting? Pituitary and hypothalamic space-occupying lesions, hormonally active or not, can cause symptoms by pressure on, or infiltration of:

- the visual pathways, with field defects and visual loss (most common)
- the cavernous sinus, with III, IV and VI cranial nerve lesions
- bony structures and the meninges surrounding the fossa, causing headache
- hypothalamic centres: altered appetite, obesity, thirst, somnolence/wakefulness or precocious puberty

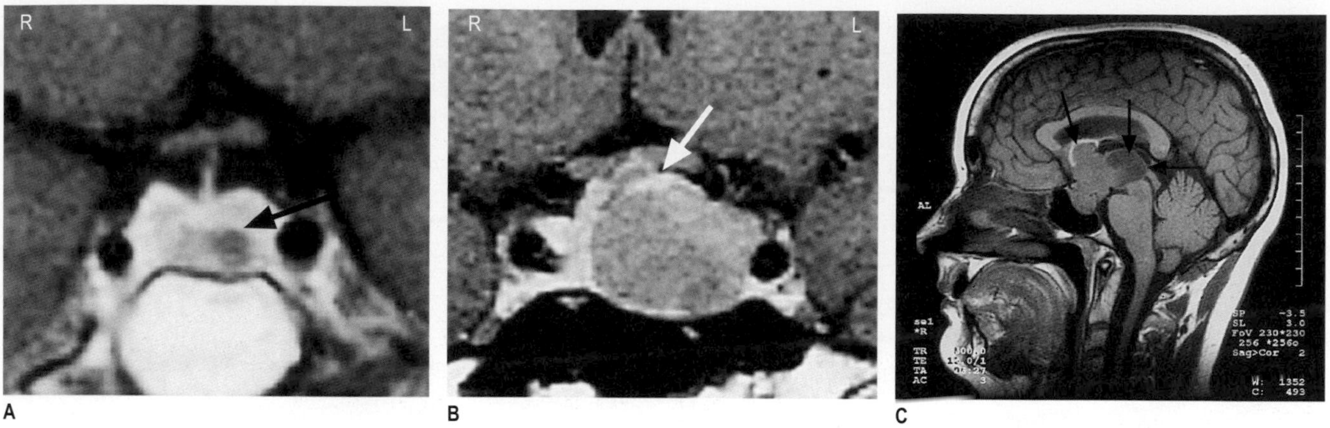

Figure 26.8 Investigation of the pituitary gland. **A** Left-sided *lucent intrasellar microadenoma* (arrowed) (coronal MRI). The pituitary stalk is deviated slightly to the right. **B.** *Macroadenoma with moderate suprasellar extension*, and lateral extension compressing the left cavernous sinus (coronal MRI). The top of the adenoma is compressing the optic chiasm (arrowed). **C.** Pituitary *macroadenoma with massive suprasellar extension* (arrowed) (sagittal MRI).

- the ventricles, causing interruption of cerebrospinal fluid (CSF) flow and leading to hydrocephalus
- the sphenoid sinus with invasion, causing CSF rhinorrhoea.

Investigations

- ***Magnetic resonance imaging (MRI) of the pituitary***. MRI is superior to computed tomography (CT) ***(Fig. 26.8)*** and will readily show any significant pituitary mass. Small lesions within the pituitary fossa, consistent with small pituitary microadenomas, are very common on MRI (10% of normal individuals in some studies). Such small lesions are sometimes detected during MRI of the head for other reasons – so-called 'pituitary incidentalomas'.
- ***Visual fields***. These should be plotted formally by automated computer perimetry or Goldmann perimetry, but clinical assessment by confrontation using a small red pin as the target is also sensitive and valuable. Common defects are upper temporal quadrantanopia and bitemporal hemianopia (see p. 804).

Is there a hormonal excess?

There are three major conditions that are usually caused by excess secretion from pituitary adenomas and which will show positive immunostaining for the relevant hormone:

- prolactin excess (***prolactinoma or hyperprolactinaemia***): histologically, prolactinomas are 'chromophobe' adenomas (a description of their appearance on classical histological staining)
- GH excess (***acromegaly or gigantism***): somatotroph adenomas, usually 'acidophil', and sometimes due to specific G-protein mutations (see p. 1184)
- excess ACTH secretion (***Cushing's disease and Nelson syndrome***): corticotroph adenomas, usually 'basophil'.

Many tumours are able to synthesize several pituitary hormones, and occasionally more than one hormone is secreted in clinically significant excess (e.g. both GH and prolactin).

The clinical features of acromegaly, Cushing's disease or hyperprolactinaemia are usually (but not always) obvious, and are discussed on pages 1193–1194 and 1197–1199. Hyperprolactinaemia may be clinically 'silent'. Tumours producing LH, FSH or TSH are well described but very rare.

Some common pituitary tumours, usually 'chromophobe' adenomas, cause no clinically apparent hormone excess and are referred to as 'non-functioning' tumours. Laboratory studies such as immunocytochemistry or *in situ* hybridization show that these tumours may often produce small amounts of LH and FSH or the α-subunit of LH, FSH and TSH, and occasionally ACTH.

Is there a deficiency of any hormone?

Clinical examination may give clues; thus, short stature in a child with a pituitary tumour is likely to be due to GH deficiency. A slow, lethargic adult with pale skin is likely to be deficient in TSH and/or ACTH. Milder deficiencies may not be obvious and require specific testing (see ***Box 26.8***).

Management

Management depends on the type and size of tumour ***(Box 26.6)***. Decisions about pituitary tumour management are made in a multidisciplinary team (MDT) setting, which typically comprises an endocrinologist, a pituitary surgeon and a radiologist. In general, therapy has three aims: removal/control of the tumour, reduction of excess hormone secretion and replacement of hormone deficiencies.

Removal/control of tumour

This is only required if the tumour is large enough to cause, or is likely to cause, anatomical effects or if the tumour is secreting excess hormones. Small tumours producing no significant symptoms, pressure or endocrine effects may be observed with appropriate clinical, visual field, imaging and endocrine assessments.

- ***Surgery*** via the trans-sphenoidal route is usually the treatment of choice. Very large tumours are occasionally removed via the open transcranial (usually transfrontal) route.
- ***Radiotherapy*** – by conventional linear accelerator or newer stereotactic techniques – is usually employed when surgery is impracticable or incomplete, as it controls but rarely abolishes tumour mass. The conventional regimen involves a dose of 45 Gy, given as 20–25 fractions via three fields. Stereotactic techniques use either a linear accelerator or multiple cobalt sources ('gamma-knife').
- ***Medical therapy*** with somatostatin analogues and/or dopamine agonists sometimes causes shrinkage of specific types of tumour (see p. 1194) and, if successful,

Box 26.6 Comparisons of primary treatments for pituitary tumours

Treatment method	Advantages	Disadvantages
Surgical		
Trans-sphenoidal adenomectomy or hypophysectomy	Relatively minor procedure Potentially curative for microadenomas and smaller macroadenomas	Some extrasellar extensions may not be accessible Risk of CSF leakage and meningitis
Transcranial (usually transfrontal) route	Good access to suprasellar region	Major procedure; danger of frontal lobe damage High chance of subsequent hypopituitarism
Radiotherapy		
External (40–50 Gy)	Non-invasive Reduces recurrence rate after surgery	Slow action, often over many years Not always effective Possible late risk of tumour induction
Stereotactic	Precise administration of high dose to lesion	Long-term follow-up data limited
Medical		
Dopamine agonist therapy (e.g. bromocriptine, cabergoline)	Non-invasive; reversible	Usually not curative; significant side-effects in minority Concerns about fibrotic reactions
Somatostatin analogue therapy (octreotide, lanreotide)	Non-invasive; reversible	Usually not curative; causes gallstones; expensive
Growth hormone receptor antagonist (pegvisomant)	Highly selective	Usually not curative; very expensive

can be used as primary therapy, particularly in the case of prolactinomas.

Reduction of excess hormone secretion

Reduction is usually obtained by surgical removal but sometimes by medical treatment. Useful control can be achieved with dopamine agonists for prolactinomas or somatostatin analogues for acromegaly, but ACTH secretion usually cannot be controlled by medical means. GH antagonists are also available for acromegaly (see p. 1194).

Replacement of hormone deficiencies

Replacement of hormone deficiencies, i.e. hypopituitarism, is discussed below (see ***Box 26.10***).

Differential diagnosis of pituitary or hypothalamic masses

Although pituitary adenomas are the most common mass lesion of the pituitary (90%), a variety of other conditions may also present as a pituitary or hypothalamic mass and form part of the differential diagnosis.

Other tumours

- ***Craniopharyngioma*** (1–2%), a usually cystic hypothalamic tumour that is often calcified and arises from Rathke's pouch, often mimics an intrinsic pituitary lesion. It is the most common pituitary tumour in children but may present at any age ***(Fig. 26.9)***.
- ***Uncommon tumours*** include meningiomas ***(Fig. 26.10)***, gliomas, chondromas, germinomas and pinealomas. Primary pituitary carcinomas are very rare, but occasionally prolactin- and ACTH-secreting tumours can present in an aggressive manner, which may require chemotherapy in addition to conventional treatment. Metastases occasionally present as apparent pituitary tumours, typically accompanied by headache and diabetes insipidus.

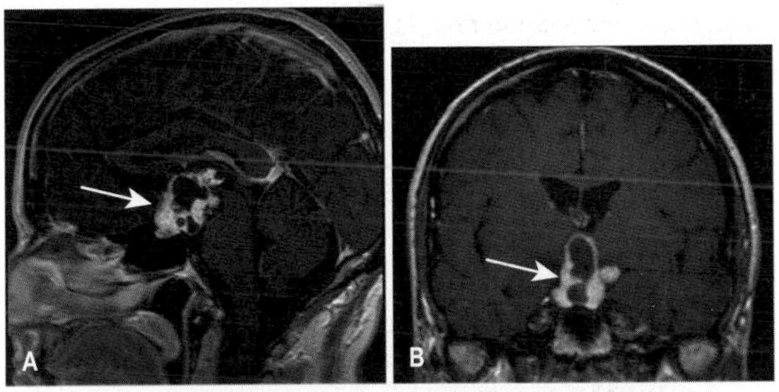

Figure 26.9 Craniopharyngioma (arrowed): a partially cystic pituitary and suprasellar mass. A. Sagittal MRI. **B.** Coronal MRI.

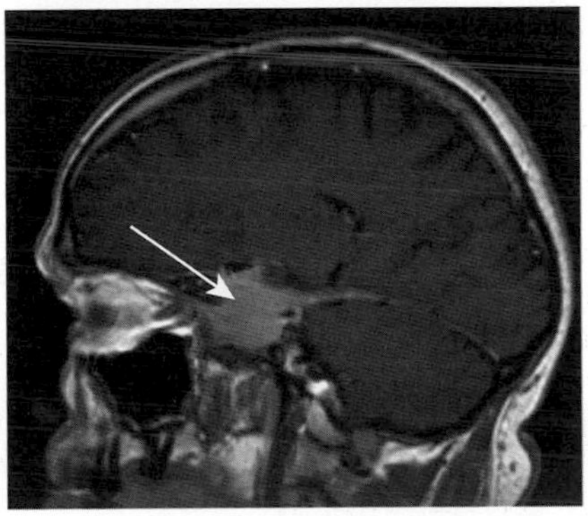

Figure 26.10 Meningioma (arrowed) involving the pituitary fossa. Note the typical 'dural tail'.

Hypophysitis and other inflammatory masses

A variety of inflammatory masses occur in the pituitary or hypothalamus. These include rare pituitary-specific conditions (e.g. autoimmune (lymphocytic) hypophysitis, giant cell hypophysitis, postpartum hypophysitis) or pituitary manifestations of more generalized disease processes (sarcoidosis, Langerhans' cell histiocytosis, granulomatosis with polyangiitis). These lesions may be associated with diabetes insipidus and/or an unusual pattern of hypopituitarism.

Other lesions

Carotid artery aneurysms may masquerade as pituitary tumours and must be diagnosed before surgery. Cystic lesions may also present as a pituitary mass, including arachnoid and Rathke cleft cysts.

Hypopituitarism

Pathophysiology

Deficiency of hypothalamic releasing hormones or of pituitary trophic hormones can be selective or multiple. Thus isolated deficiencies of GH, LH/FSH, ACTH, TSH and vasopressin (ADH) are all seen, some cases of which are genetic and congenital, and others sporadic and autoimmune or idiopathic in nature.

Multiple deficiencies usually result from tumour growth or other destructive lesions. There is generally a progressive loss of anterior pituitary function. GH and gonadotrophins are usually first affected. Hyperprolactinaemia, rather than prolactin deficiency, occurs relatively early because of loss of tonic inhibitory control by dopamine. TSH and ACTH are usually last to be affected.

Panhypopituitarism refers to deficiency of all anterior pituitary hormones; it is most commonly caused by pituitary tumours, surgery or radiotherapy. Vasopressin (ADH) and oxytocin secretion will be significantly affected only if the hypothalamus is involved by a hypothalamic tumour or major suprasellar extension of a pituitary lesion, or if there is an infiltrative/inflammatory process. Posterior pituitary deficiency with diabetes insipidus is rare in an uncomplicated pituitary adenoma.

Genetics

Specific genes are responsible for the development of the anterior pituitary, involving interaction between signalling molecules and transcription factors. For example, mutations in *PROP1* and *POU1F1* (previously PIT-1) prevent the differentiation of anterior pituitary cells (precursors to somatotroph, lactotroph, thyrotroph and gonadotroph cells), leading to deficiencies of GH, prolactin, TSH and gonadotrophin-releasing hormone (GnRH). In addition, novel mutations within GH and growth hormone-releasing hormone (GHRH) receptor genes have been identified, which may explain the pathogenesis of isolated GH deficiency in children. Despite these advances, most cases of hypopituitarism do not have specific identifiable genetic causes.

Aetiology

Disorders that cause hypopituitarism are listed in ***Box 26.7***. Pituitary and hypothalamic tumours, and surgical or radiotherapy treatment, are the most common.

Clinical features

Symptoms and signs depend upon the extent of hypothalamic and/or pituitary deficiencies, and mild deficiencies may not lead to any complaint on the part of the patient. In general, symptoms of deficiency of a pituitary-stimulating hormone are the same as those of primary deficiency of the peripheral endocrine gland (e.g. TSH deficiency and primary hypothyroidism cause similar symptoms due to lack of thyroid hormone secretion).

Box 26.7 Causes of hypopituitarism

Congenital
- Isolated deficiency of pituitary hormones (e.g. Kallmann syndrome)
- *POU1F1* (*Pit-1*), *Prop1*, *HESX1* mutations

Infective
- Basal meningitis (e.g. tuberculosis)
- Encephalitis
- Syphilis

Vascular
- Pituitary apoplexy
- Sheehan syndrome (postpartum necrosis)
- Carotid artery aneurysm

Immunological
- Autoimmune (lymphocytic) hypophysitis
- Pituitary antibodies

Neoplastic
- Pituitary or hypothalamic tumour
- Craniopharyngioma
- Meningioma
- Gliomas
- Pinealoma
- Secondary deposits, especially breast
- Lymphoma

Traumatic
- Skull fracture through base
- Surgery, especially transfrontal
- Perinatal trauma

Infiltrations
- Sarcoidosis
- Langerhans' cell histiocytosis
- Hereditary haemochromatosis
- Hypophysitis:
  - Postpartum
  - Giant cell

Others
- Radiation damage
- Fibrosis
- Chemotherapy
- Empty sella syndrome

'Functional'
- Anorexia nervosa
- Starvation
- Emotional deprivation

- ***Secondary hypothyroidism*** and ***adrenal failure*** both lead to tiredness and general malaise.
- ***Hypothyroidism*** causes weight gain, slowness of thought and action, dry skin and cold intolerance.
- ***Hypoadrenalism*** causes mild hypotension, hyponatraemia and, ultimately, cardiovascular collapse during severe intercurrent stressful illness.
- ***Gonadotrophin*** and thus ***gonadal deficiencies*** lead to loss of libido, loss of secondary sexual hair, amenorrhoea and erectile dysfunction.
- ***Hyperprolactinaemia*** may cause galactorrhoea and hypogonadism, including amenorrhoea.
- ***GH deficiency*** causes growth failure in children and impaired wellbeing in some adults.
- ***Weight may increase*** (due to hypothyroidism; see above) or decrease in severe combined deficiency (pituitary cachexia).
- Longstanding ***panhypopituitarism*** gives the classic picture of pallor with hairlessness ('alabaster skin').

Particular syndromes related to hypopituitarism are described below.

Kallmann syndrome

This syndrome is isolated gonadotrophin (GnRH) deficiency (see p. 1217). It arises due to mutations in the *KAL1* gene, which is located on the short (p) arm of the X chromosome. Kallmann's is classically characterized by anosmia because the *KAL1* gene provides instructions to make anosmin, which has a role both in development of the olfactory system and in migration of GnRH-secreting neurones.

Septo-optic dysplasia

This is a rare congenital syndrome (associated with mutations in the *HESX1* gene), presenting in childhood with a clinical triad of midline forebrain abnormalities, optic nerve hypoplasia and hypopituitarism.

Sheehan syndrome

This is due to pituitary infarction following postpartum haemorrhage and is rare in developed countries.

Pituitary apoplexy

A pituitary tumour occasionally enlarges rapidly owing to infarction or haemorrhage. This may produce severe headache, double vision and sudden severe visual loss, sometimes followed by acute life-threatening hypopituitarism. Often, pituitary apoplexy can be managed conservatively with replacement of hormones and close monitoring of vision, although if there is a rapid deterioration in visual acuity and fields, surgical decompression of the optic chiasm may be necessary ***(Fig. 26.11)***.

'Empty sella' syndrome

An 'empty sella' is sometimes reported on pituitary imaging. This is sometimes due to a defect in the diaphragma and extension of the subarachnoid space (cisternal herniation), or may follow spontaneous infarction or regression of a pituitary tumour. All or most of the sella turcica is devoid of apparent pituitary tissue but, despite this, pituitary function is usually normal, the pituitary being eccentrically placed and flattened against the floor or roof of the fossa.

Investigations

Each axis of the hypothalamic–pituitary system requires separate investigation. However, the presence of normal gonadal function (ovulation/menstruation or normal libido/erections) suggests that multiple defects of anterior pituitary function are unlikely.

Investigations range from measurement of simple basal levels (e.g. free T_4 for the thyroid axis) to stimulatory tests for the pituitary and tests of feedback for the hypothalamus ***(Box 26.8)***. Assessment of the HPA axis is complex: basal 09:00 hours cortisol levels above 400 nmol/L usually indicate an adequate reserve, while levels below 100 nmol/L predict an inadequate stress response. In many cases, basal levels are equivocal and a dynamic test is essential. The insulin tolerance test ***(Box 26.9)*** is widely regarded as the 'gold standard' but the short ACTH stimulation test (see ***Box 26.3***), though an indirect measure, is used by many as a routine test of HPA status. Occasionally, the difference between ACTH deficiency and normal HPA axis can be subtle, and the assessment of adrenal reserve is best left to an experienced endocrinologist.

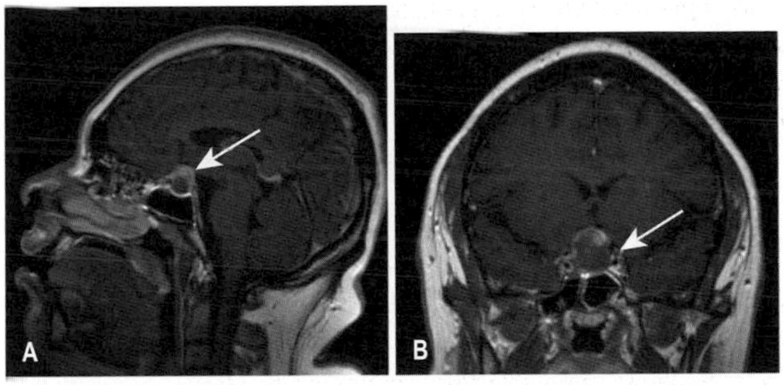

Figure 26.11 Pituitary apoplexy. A bright area of haemorrhage at the top of a pituitary adenoma (arrowed) is shown. **A.** Sagittal MRI. **B.** Coronal MRI.

Box 26.8 Tests of hypothalamic–pituitary (HP) function

All hormone levels are measured in plasma unless otherwise stated.
Tests **shown in bold** are those normally measured on a single basal 09:00 hours sample in the initial assessment of pituitary function.

Axis	Basal investigations: *Pituitary hormone*	Basal investigations: *End-organ product/function*	Common dynamic tests	Other tests
Anterior pituitary				
HP–ovarian	**LH** **FSH**	**Oestradiol** Progesterone (day 21 of cycle)		Ovarian ultrasound LHRH test[a]
HP–testicular	**LH** **FSH**	**Testosterone**		Sperm count LHRH test[a]
Growth	GH	**IGF-1** IGF-BP3	Insulin tolerance test Glucagon test	GH response to sleep, exercise or arginine infusion GHRH test[a]
Prolactin	**Prolactin**	**Prolactin**	–	–
HP–thyroid	**TSH**	**Free T_4, T_3**		TRH test[a]
HP–adrenal	ACTH	**Cortisol**	Insulin tolerance test Short ACTH (tetracosactide) stimulation test	Glucagon test CRH test[a] Metyrapone test
Posterior pituitary				
Thirst and osmoregulation		**Plasma/urine osmolality**	Water deprivation test	Hypertonic saline infusion

[a]Releasing hormone tests were a traditional part of pituitary function testing but have been largely replaced by the advent of more reliable assays for basal hormones. They test only the 'readily releasable pool' of pituitary hormones, and normal responses may be seen in hypopituitarism.
ACTH, adrenocorticotrophic hormone; CRH, corticotrophin releasing hormone; FSH, follicle-stimulating hormone; GH, growth hormone; GHRH, growth hormone-releasing hormone; IGF, insulin-like growth factor; LH, luteinizing hormone; LHRH, luteinizing hormone-releasing hormone; TRH, thyroid-releasing hormone; TSH, thyroid-stimulating hormone.

Box 26.9 Insulin tolerance test

Indications

- Diagnosis or exclusion of ACTH and GH deficiency

Procedure

- Test explained to patient and consent obtained
- Should only be performed in experienced, specialist units
- Exclude cardiovascular disease (ECG), epilepsy or unexplained blackouts; exclude severe untreated hypopituitarism (basal cortisol must be >100 nmol/L; normal free T_4)
- I.v. hydrocortisone and glucose available for emergency
- Overnight fast, begin at 08:00–09:00 hours
- Soluble insulin, 0.15 U/kg, i.v. at time 0
- Glucose, cortisol and GH levels at 0, 30, 45, 60, 90, 120 min

Normal response

- Cortisol rises above 550 nmol/L[a]
- GH rises above 7 ng/L (severe deficiency=<3 ng/L (<9 mU/L))
- Glucose must be <2.2 mmol/L to achieve adequate stress response

[a]Precise cortisol normal ranges are variable between laboratories and assays; appropriate local reference ranges must be used.

ACTH, adrenocorticotrophic hormone; ECG, electrocardiogram; GH, growth hormone.

Box 26.10 Replacement therapy for hypopituitarism

Axis	Usual replacement therapies
Adrenal	Hydrocortisone 15–40 mg daily (starting dose 10 mg on rising/5 mg lunchtime/5 mg evening) (Normally no need for mineralocorticoid replacement)
Thyroid	Levothyroxine 100–150 μg daily
Gonadal	
Male	Testosterone intramuscularly, orally, transdermally or implant
Female	Cyclical oestrogen/progestogen orally or as patch
Fertility	HCG plus FSH (purified or recombinant) or pulsatile GnRH to produce testicular development, spermatogenesis or ovulation
Growth	Recombinant human GH used routinely to achieve normal growth in children
	Also advocated for replacement therapy in adults, where GH has effects on muscle mass and wellbeing
Thirst	Desmopressin 10–20 μg 1–3 times daily by nasal spray or orally 100–200 μg 3 times daily Carbamazepine, thiazides and chlorpropamide are very occasionally used in mild diabetes insipidus
Breast (prolactin inhibition)	Dopamine agonist (e.g. cabergoline 500 μg weekly)

FSH, follicle-stimulating hormone; GH, growth hormone; HCG, human chorionic gonadotrophin.

Management

- Steroid and thyroid hormones are essential for life. Both are given as oral replacement drugs, as in primary thyroid and adrenal deficiency, with the aim of restoring the patient to clinical and biochemical normality ***(Box 26.10)***; levels are monitored by routine hormone assays. ***Note:*** Thyroid replacement should not commence until normal glucocorticoid function has been demonstrated or replacement steroid therapy initiated, as an adrenal 'crisis' may otherwise be precipitated.
- Sex hormones are replaced with androgens and oestrogens, both for symptomatic control and for prevention of long-term problems related to deficiency (e.g. osteoporosis).
- When fertility is desired, gonadal function is stimulated directly by human chorionic gonadotrophin (HCG, mainly acting as LH) or by purified or biosynthetic gonadotrophins, or indirectly by pulsatile gonadotrophin-releasing hormone (GnRH – also known as luteinizing hormone-releasing hormone, LHRH); all are expensive and time-consuming, and their use should be restricted to specialist units.
- GH therapy is given in the growing child, under the care of a paediatric endocrinologist. If the adolescent remains deficient at the achievement of adult height, GH therapy can be offered until patients reach their mid-twenties to support somatic development (increase in muscle and bone mass). In adult GH deficiency, GH therapy also produces improvements in body composition, work capacity and psychological wellbeing, together with reversal of lipid abnormalities associated with a high cardiovascular risk, and often results in significant symptomatic benefit. The National Institute for Health and Care Excellence (NICE) recommends GH replacement for children and adolescents with GH deficiency, and in adults with severe GH deficiency and significant quality of life impairment. It is expensive and in the UK costs £2500–6000 per annum.
- Glucocorticoid deficiency may mask impaired urine concentrating ability, diabetes insipidus only becoming apparent after steroid replacement because steroids are required for excretion of free water.

Further reading

Dattani MT. Growth hormone deficiency and combined pituitary deficiency: does the genotype matter? *Clin Endocrinol* 2005; 63:121–130.

National Institute for Health and Clinical Excellence. *NICE Technology Appraisal 64: Human Growth Hormone (Somatotropin) in Adults with Growth Hormone Deficiency*. NICE 2003; http://www.nice.org.uk/guidance/ta64.

Rajasekaran S, Vanderpump M, Baldeweg S et al. UK guidelines for the management of pituitary apoplexy. *Clin Endocrinol* 2011; 74:9–20.

Schneider HJ, Aimaretti G, Kreitschmann-Andermahr I et al. Hypopituitarism. *Lancet* 2007; 369:1151–1470.

Growth and abnormal stature

Physiology

Growth factor (GH) is the pituitary factor responsible for stimulation of body growth in humans. Its secretion is stimulated by GHRH, released into the portal system from the hypothalamus; it is also under inhibitory control exerted by somatostatin ***(Fig. 26.12)***. A separate GH-stimulating system involves a distinct receptor (GH secretogogue receptor), which interacts with ghrelin (see p. 390). It is not known how these two systems interact but, because ghrelin is synthesized in the stomach, a nutritional role is suggested for GH.

- ***GH*** acts by binding to a specific (single transmembrane) receptor located mainly in the liver (see ***Box 26.4***). This induces an intracellular phosphorylation cascade involving the Janus kinase/signal transducing activators of transcription (JAK/STAT) pathway (see pp. 96–97). STAT proteins are translocated from the cytoplasm into the cell nucleus and cause GH-specific effects by binding to nuclear DNA.
- ***Insulin-like growth factor-1 (IGF-1)***, a somatomedin, stimulates growth. Its hepatic secretion is stimulated by a tissue-specific effect of GH on the liver. There are multiple IGF-binding proteins (IGF-BP) in plasma; IGF-BP3 can be measured clinically to improve assessment of GH status, particularly in children.

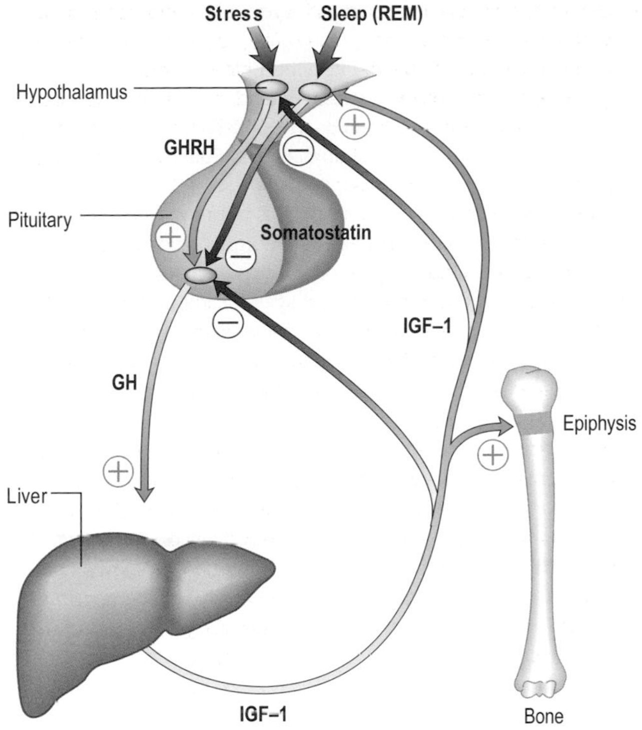

Figure 26.12 The control of growth hormone (GH) and insulin-like growth factor-1 (IGF-1). Pituitary GH is secreted under dual control of growth hormone-releasing hormone (GHRH) and somatostatin, and stimulates release of IGF-1 in the liver and elsewhere. IGF-1 has peripheral actions, including bone growth, and exerts negative feedback to the hypothalamus and pituitary. REM, rapid eye movement.

The metabolic actions of the system are:

- increasing collagen and protein synthesis
- promoting retention of calcium, phosphorus and nitrogen, necessary substrates for anabolism
- opposing the action of insulin (a 'counter-regulatory' hormone effect).

GH release is intermittent and mainly nocturnal, especially during REM sleep. The frequency and size of GH pulses increase during the growth spurt of adolescence and decline thereafter. Acute stress and exercise both stimulate GH release, while, in the normal subject, hyperglycaemia suppresses it.

IGF-1 may, in addition, play a major role in maintaining neoplastic growth. A relationship has been shown between circulating IGF-1 concentrations and breast cancer in premenopausal women and prostate cancer in men.

Normal growth

There are factors other than GH that are involved in linear growth in the human:

- ***Genetic factors***. Children of two short parents will probably be short and vice versa.
- ***Nutritional factors***. Adequate nutrients must be available. Impaired growth can result from inadequate dietary intake or small bowel disease (e.g. coeliac disease).
- ***General health***. Any serious systemic disease in childhood is likely to reduce growth (e.g. chronic kidney disease or chronic infection).
- ***Intrauterine growth retardation***. These infants often grow poorly in the long term, while infants with simple prematurity

Box 26.11 Assessment of problems of growth and development

History

- Pregnancy records
- Rate of growth (home/school records, e.g. heights on kitchen door)
- Comparison with peers at school and siblings
- Change in appearance (old photographs)
- Change in shoe/glove/hat size or frequency of 'growing out' of these
- Age of appearance of pubic hair, breasts, menarche

Physical signs

- Evidence of systemic disease
- Body habitus, size, relative weight, proportions (span versus height)
- Skin thickness, interdental separation
- Facial features
- Spade hands/feet
- Grading of secondary sexual characteristics

usually catch up. There is some evidence that low birth weight may predispose to hypertension, diabetes and other health problems in later adult life (see p. 205).

- ***Emotional deprivation and psychological factors***. These can impair growth by complex, poorly understood mechanisms, probably involving temporarily decreased GH secretion.

In general, there are three overlapping phases of growth: infantile (0–2 years), which appears to be largely dependent on substrates (food); childhood (age 2 years to puberty), which is largely GH-dependent; and the adolescent 'growth spurt', dependent on GH and sex hormones.

The relevant aspects of history and examination in the assessment of problems are shown in ***Box 26.11***.

Assessment of growth

Charts showing normal centiles of height and weight are essential to monitor growth; they are available for normal British children ***(Fig. 26.13)*** and many other national and ethnic groups. Height must be measured, ideally at the same time of day on the same instrument by the same trained observer.

Height velocity is more helpful than current height. It requires at least two measurements some months apart and, ideally, multiple serial measurements. Height velocity is the rate of current growth (centimetres per year), while the current attained height is largely dependent upon previous growth. Standard deviation scores (SDS) based on the degree of deviation from age–sex norms are widely used. Computer programs also allow calculation of many of these indices.

The approximate future height of a child ('mid-parental height') can be simply predicted from the parental heights. For a boy, this is:

$$(\text{Maternal height} + 14\text{ cm }(5.5\text{ inches}) + \text{Paternal height})/2$$

and for a girl:

$$(\text{Paternal height} - 14\text{ cm }(5.5\text{ inches}) + \text{Maternal height})/2$$

Thus, with a father of 180 cm and mother of 154 cm, the predicted heights are 174 cm for a son and 160 cm for a daughter.

Growth failure: short stature

When children or their parents complain of short stature, particular attention should focus on:

- intrauterine growth retardation, and weight and gestation at birth

- possible systemic disorders – any system but especially small bowel disease
- evidence of skeletal, chromosomal or other congenital abnormalities
- endocrine status – particularly thyroid

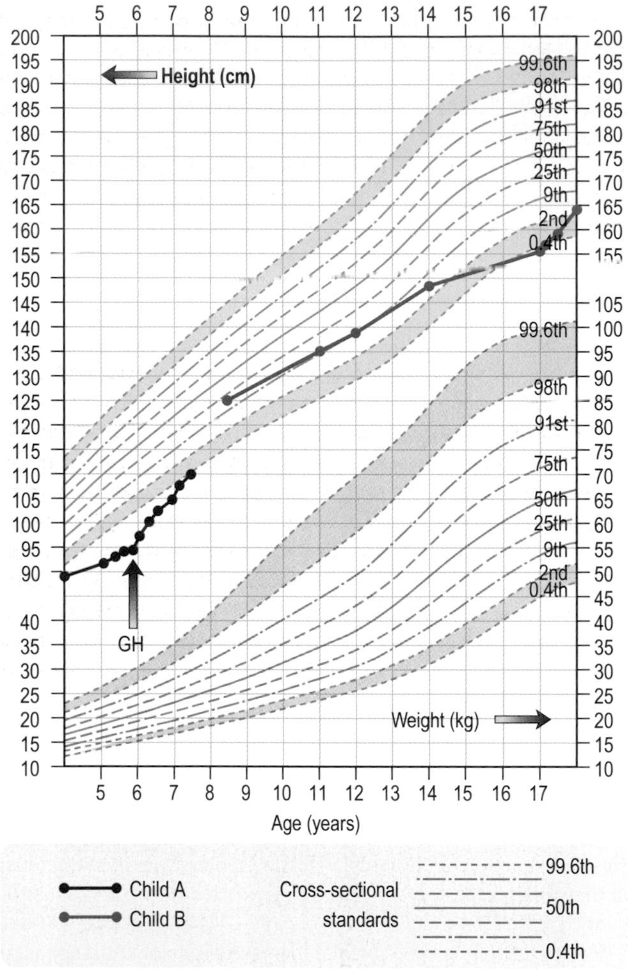

Figure 26.13 A height chart for boys. *Child A* illustrates the course of a child with hypopituitarism, initially treated with cortisol and thyroxine, but showing growth only after growth hormone (GH) treatment. *Child B* shows the course of a child with constitutional growth delay without treatment.

- dietary intake and use of drugs, especially steroids for asthma
- emotional, psychological, family and school problems.

School, general practitioner, clinic and home records of height and weight should be obtained, if possible, to allow growth-velocity calculation. If unavailable, such data must be obtained prospectively.

A child with normal growth velocity is unlikely to have significant endocrine disease and the most common cause of short stature in this situation is pubertal or 'constitutional' delay. However, low growth velocity without an apparent systemic cause requires further investigation. Sudden cessation of growth suggests major physical disease; if no gastrointestinal, respiratory, renal or skeletal abnormality is apparent, then a cerebral tumour or hypothyroidism is most likely.

Consistently slow-growing children require full endocrine assessment. Features of the more common causes of growth failure are given in ***Box 26.12***.

Around the time of puberty, if constitutional delay is clearly shown and symptoms require intervention, then very-low-dose sex steroids in 3- to 6-month courses will usually induce acceleration of growth.

Investigations

Once systemic disease has been excluded, the following tests should be performed:

- ***Thyroid function tests***. Serum TSH and free T_4 should be measured to exclude hypothyroidism.
- ***GH status***. Basal levels are of little value. Validated dynamic tests include the GH response to insulin (the 'gold standard'; see ***Box 26.9***), arginine+GHRH and glucagon. Tests should only be performed in centres experienced in their use and interpretation. Normal responses depend on test and GH assay used.
- ***Blood levels of IGF-1 and IGF-BP3***. These may provide evidence of GH undersecretion.
- ***Assessment of bone age***. Non-dominant hand and wrist X-rays allow assessment of bone age by comparison with standard charts.
- ***Karyotyping in females***. Turner syndrome (see p. 1220) is associated with short stature. It is thought that this is due to a defect in the short stature homeobox (*SHOX*) gene, which has a role in non-GH-mediated growth.

Box 26.12 Clinical features of common causes of short stature

Cause	Family history	Growth pattern, clinical features and puberty	Bone age	Remarks
Constitutional delay	Often present	Slow from birth, immature but appropriate with late but spontaneous puberty	Moderate delay	Often difficult to differentiate from GH deficiency Growth velocity measurement vital
Familial short stature	Positive	Slow from birth, clinically normal with normal puberty	Normal	Need heights of family members Growth velocity normal
GH insufficiency	Rare	Slow growth, immature, often overweight, delayed puberty	Moderate delay, increasing with time	Early investigation and treatment vital Increased suspicion if child is plump
Primary hypothyroidism	Rare	Slow growth, immature and delayed puberty	Marked delay	Measure TSH, T_4 in all cases of short stature Clear clinical signs not obvious
Small bowel disease	Sometimes	Slow, immature, usually thin for height, delayed puberty	Delayed	Diarrhoea and/or macrocytosis/anaemia Occasionally no gastrointestinal symptoms

GH, growth hormone; TSH, thyroid-stimulating hormone.

Management

Systemic illness should be treated and primary hypothyroidism managed with levothyroxine.

For GH insufficiency, recombinant GH (somatropin) is given as nightly injections in doses of 0.17–0.35 mg/kg per week, with dose adjustments made according to clinical response and IGF-1 levels. Treatment is expensive and should be supervised in expert centres.

GH treatment in so-called 'short normal' children has not been shown to produce any worthwhile increase in final height. In Turner syndrome (see p. 1220), large doses of GH are effective in increasing final height, especially in combination with appropriate very-low-dose oestrogen replacement. Familial cases of resistance to GH that is caused by an abnormal GH receptor (Laron-type dwarfism) are well described. They are very rare but may respond to therapy with synthetic IGF-1 (mecasermin).

Tall stature

The most common causes are hereditary (two tall parents), idiopathic (constitutional) or early developmental factors (eventually resulting in short stature). Tall stature can occasionally be due to hyperthyroidism. Other causes include chromosomal abnormalities (e.g. Klinefelter syndrome, Marfan syndrome) or metabolic abnormalities. GH excess is a very rare cause and is usually clinically obvious.

Further reading

Allen DB, Cuttler L. Clinical practice. Short stature in childhood – challenges and choices. *N Engl J Med* 2013; 368:1220–1228.

Savage MO, Burren CP, Rosenfeld RG. The continuum of growth hormone–IGF-I axis defects causing short stature: diagnostic and therapeutic challenges. *Clin Endocrinol* 2010; 72:721–728.

Pituitary hypersecretion syndromes

Acromegaly and gigantism

Growth hormone stimulates skeletal and soft tissue growth. GH excess therefore produces gigantism in children (if acquired before epiphyseal fusion) and acromegaly in adults. Both are due to a GH-secreting pituitary tumour (somatotroph adenoma) in almost all cases. Hyperplasia due to ectopic GHRH excess is very rare. Overall incidence is approximately 3–4/million per year and the prevalence is 50–80/million worldwide. Acromegaly usually occurs sporadically, although gene mutations can rarely give rise to familial acromegaly: typically, the *AIP* gene in familial isolated pituitary adenoma. In familial acromegaly, there is an increased onset before puberty compared to sporadic cases, leading to a higher prevalence of gigantism.

Clinical features

Symptoms and signs of acromegaly are shown in ***Figure 26.14***. One-third of patients present with changes in appearance, and one-quarter with visual field defects or headaches; in the remainder, the diagnosis is made by an alert observer in another clinic: for example, in general practice, or in the diabetes, hypertension, dental, dermatology departments. Sleep apnoea is common and requires investigation and treatment if there are suggestive symptoms (see pp. 1085–1086). Sweating, headaches and soft tissue swelling are particularly useful symptoms of persistent GH secretion. Headache is very common in acromegaly and may be severe, even with small tumours; it is often improved after surgical cure or with somatostatin analogues.

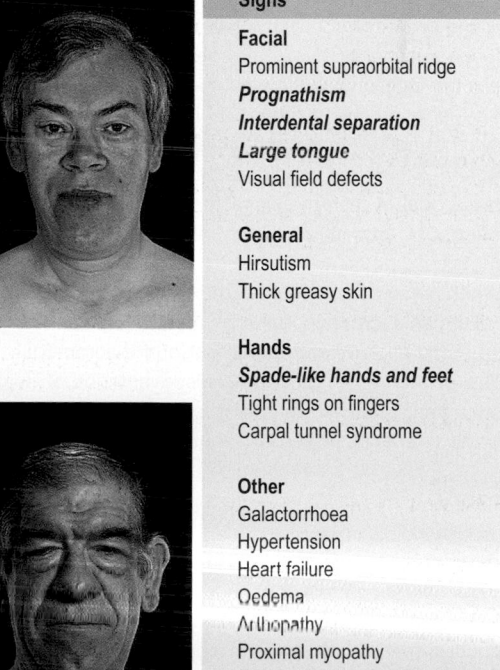

Symptoms

Head and neck
Change in facial appearance
Headaches
Visual deterioration
Deep voice
Goitre

General
Tiredness
Weight gain
Breathlessness
Excessive sweating
Muscular weakness
Joint pain

Hormonal
Amenorrhoea or oligomenorrhoea in women
Galactorrhoea
Impotence or poor libido

Increased glove or hat size

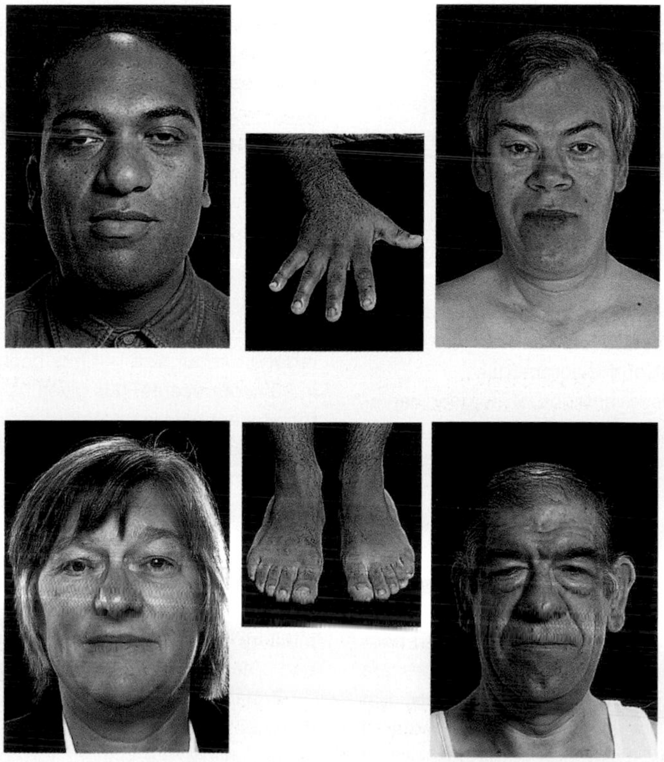

Signs

Facial
Prominent supraorbital ridge
Prognathism
Interdental separation
Large tongue
Visual field defects

General
Hirsutism
Thick greasy skin

Hands
Spade-like hands and feet
Tight rings on fingers
Carpal tunnel syndrome

Other
Galactorrhoea
Hypertension
Heart failure
Oedema
Arthropathy
Proximal myopathy
Glycosuria (plus possible signs of hypopituitarism)

Figure 26.14 **Acromegaly: symptoms and signs.** ***Bold italic*** type indicates signs of greater discriminant value.

Investigations

- ***GH levels*** may exclude acromegaly if they are undetectable, but a detectable value is non-diagnostic taken alone. Normal adult levels are <0.5 µg/L for most of the day, except during stress or a 'GH pulse'.
- ***A glucose tolerance test*** is diagnostic if there is no suppression of GH. Acromegalics fail to suppress GH below 0.3 µg/L and some show a paradoxical rise; about 25% of acromegalics have a positive diabetic glucose tolerance test.
- ***IGF-1 levels*** are almost always raised in acromegaly; a single plasma level of IGF-1 reflects mean 24-h GH levels and is useful in diagnosis. A normal IGF-1, together with random GH of <1 µg/L, may be taken to exclude acromegaly if the diagnosis is clinically unlikely.
- ***Visual field examination*** commonly reveals defects, such as bitemporal hemianopia.
- ***MRI scan*** of the pituitary is carried out if the above tests are abnormal. This will almost always reveal the pituitary adenoma. In cases where no clear lesion is present, or in postoperative cases where residual disease is being sought, there is increasing interest in the use of functional imaging such as positron emission tomography (PET).
- ***Pituitary function*** commonly demonstrates partial or complete anterior hypopituitarism.
- ***Prolactin*** levels show mild to moderate hyperprolactinaemia in 30% of patients (see ***Fig. 26.16***). In some, the adenoma secretes both GH and prolactin.

Management

Untreated acromegaly results in markedly reduced survival. Most deaths occur from heart failure, coronary artery disease and hypertension-related causes. In addition, there is an increase in deaths due to neoplasia, particularly large bowel tumours; guidance advocates regular colonoscopy to detect and remove colonic polyps in order to reduce the risk of colonic cancer, although the evidence is inconclusive. Treatment is therefore indicated in all except the elderly or those with minimal abnormalities. The aim of therapy is to achieve a mean GH level below 2.5 µg/L; this is not always 'normal' but has been shown to reduce mortality to normal levels and is therefore considered a 'safe' GH level. A normal IGF-1 is also a goal of therapy. Occasionally, there can be discordance between GH and IGF-1 levels, which can create management dilemmas.

When present, hypopituitarism should be corrected and concurrent diabetes and/or hypertension should be treated conventionally; both usually improve with treatment of the acromegaly.

The general advantages and disadvantages of surgery, radiotherapy and medical treatment are discussed on page 1190. Progress can be assessed by monitoring GH and IGF-1 levels.

Surgery

Trans-sphenoidal surgery is the appropriate first-line therapy. It will result in clinical remission in a majority of cases (60–90%) with pituitary microadenoma, but in only 50% of those with macroadenoma. Very high preoperative GH and IGF-1 levels are also poor prognostic markers of surgical cure. Surgical success rates are variable and highly dependent upon experience, and a specialist pituitary surgeon is essential. Transfrontal surgery is rarely required except for massive macroadenomas. There is a recurrence rate of approximately 10%.

Pituitary radiotherapy

External radiotherapy is normally used after pituitary surgery fails to normalize GH levels rather than as primary therapy. It is often combined with medium-term treatment using a somatostatin analogue, dopamine agonist or GH antagonist because of the slow biochemical response to radiotherapy, which may take 10 years or more; it is also often associated with hypopituitarism, which makes it unattractive in patients of reproductive age. Stereotactic (gamma-knife) radiotherapy is used in some centres, as it delivers a more concentrated field of radiation.

Medical therapy

There are three receptor targets for the treatment of acromegaly: pituitary somatostatin receptors and dopamine (D_2) receptors, and GH receptors in the periphery.

Somatostatin receptor agonists

Octreotide and ***lanreotide*** are synthetic analogues of somatostatin (see pp. 1190–1191), which act selectively on somatostatin receptor subtypes (SSTR2 and SSTR5) and are highly expressed in GH-secreting tumours. These drugs were used as a short-term treatment whilst other modalities become effective, but now are sometimes used as primary therapy. They reduce GH and IGF levels in most patients but not all achieve treatment targets. Both drugs are typically administered as monthly depot injections and are generally well tolerated; they are, however, associated with an increased incidence of gallstones and are expensive. Pasireotide (acting on SSTR 1, 2, 3 and 5) is a newer agent but its role in acromegaly is still being evaluated.

Dopamine agonists

Dopamine agonists act on D_2 receptors (see p. 1158) and can be given to shrink tumours prior to definitive therapy or to control symptoms and persisting GH secretion; they are probably most effective in mixed GH-producing (somatotroph) and prolactin-producing (mammotroph) tumours. Typical doses are bromocriptine 10–60 mg daily or cabergoline 0.5 mg daily (higher than for prolactinomas). Given alone, they reduce GH to 'safe' levels in only a minority of cases, but are useful for mild residual disease or in combination with somatostatin analogues. Drugs with combined somatostatin and dopamine receptor activity are under development.

Growth hormone antagonists

Pegvisomant (a genetically modified analogue of GH) is a GH receptor antagonist that exerts its effect by binding to and preventing dimerization of the GH receptor. It does not lower GH levels or reduce tumour size but has been shown to normalize IGF-1 levels in 90% of patients. It is given by daily injection and its main role at the present time is treatment of patients in whom GH and IGF levels cannot be reduced to safe levels with somatostatin analogues alone, or by surgery or radiotherapy.

Hyperprolactinaemia

The hypothalamic–pituitary control of prolactin secretion is illustrated in ***Figure 26.15***. Prolactin is a large peptide secreted in the pituitary and acts via a transmembrane receptor stimulating JAK2 and other pathways (see ***Box 26.4***).

Prolactin is under tonic dopamine inhibition; factors known to increase prolactin secretion (e.g. TRH) are probably of less relevance unless the patient has primary hypothyroidism. Prolactin stimulates milk secretion (but not breast tissue development) but

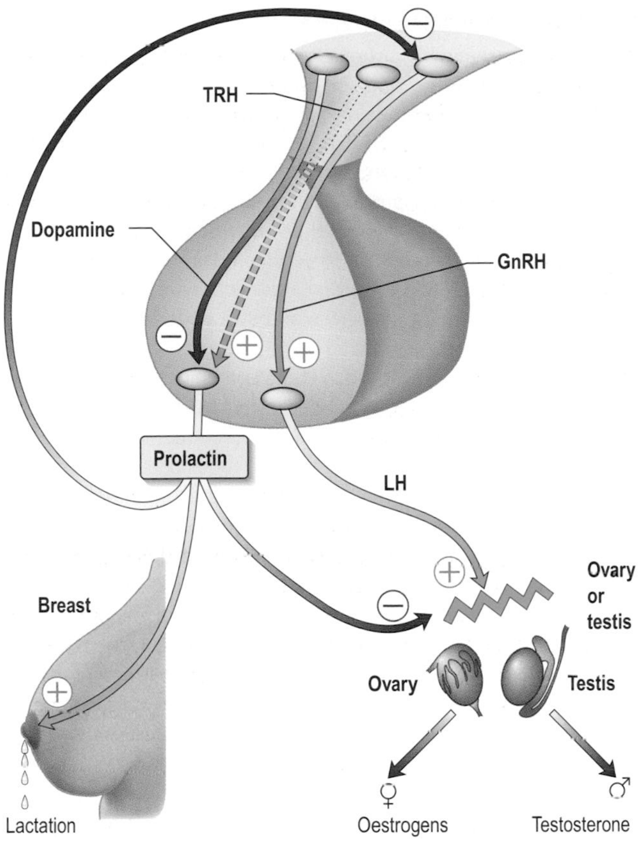

Figure 26.15 The control and actions of prolactin. Prolactin is mainly controlled by tonic inhibition by hypothalamic dopamine. Prolactin stimulates lactation but also inhibits both hypothalamic gonadotrophin-releasing hormone (GnRH) secretion and the gonadal actions of luteinizing hormone (LH). TRH, thyrotrophin-releasing hormone.

also inhibits gonadal activity. It decreases GnRH pulsatility at the hypothalamic level and, to a lesser extent, blocks the action of LH on the ovary or testis, producing hypogonadism even when the pituitary gonadal axis itself is intact.

The role of prolactin outside pregnancy and lactation is not well defined, although there is some epidemiological evidence of a link between high prolactin levels and breast cancer, which has led to an interest in the development of prolactin receptor antagonists.

Physiological hyperprolactinaemia occurs in pregnancy, lactation and severe stress, as well as during sleep and coitus. The range of serum prolactin seen in common causes of hyperprolactinaemia is illustrated in ***Figure 26.16***. Mildly increased prolactin levels (400–600 mU/L) may be physiological and asymptomatic but higher levels require a diagnosis. Levels above 5000 mU/L always imply a prolactin-secreting pituitary tumour.

Aetiology

Hyperprolactinaemia has many causes:

- ***Physiological***. These include pregnancy, lactation, stress, sleep, exercise and coitus.
- ***Pathological***. These include prolactinoma, co-secretion of prolactin in tumours causing acromegaly, stalk compression due to pituitary adenomas and other pituitary masses, polycystic ovarian syndrome, primary hypothyroidism and idiopathic hyperprolactinaemia. Rarer causes include renal failure, liver failure, post-ictal state and chest wall injury (e.g. following herpes zoster).
- ***Drug-induced***. Drug causes include ***oestrogens*** (e.g. contraceptive pill), ***dopamine antagonists*** (e.g. antipsychotics such as phenothiazines), ***antidepressants*** (e.g. tricyclics, selective serotonin reuptake inhibitors (SSRIs)), and ***others*** (e.g. verapamil, cimetidine, methyldopa).

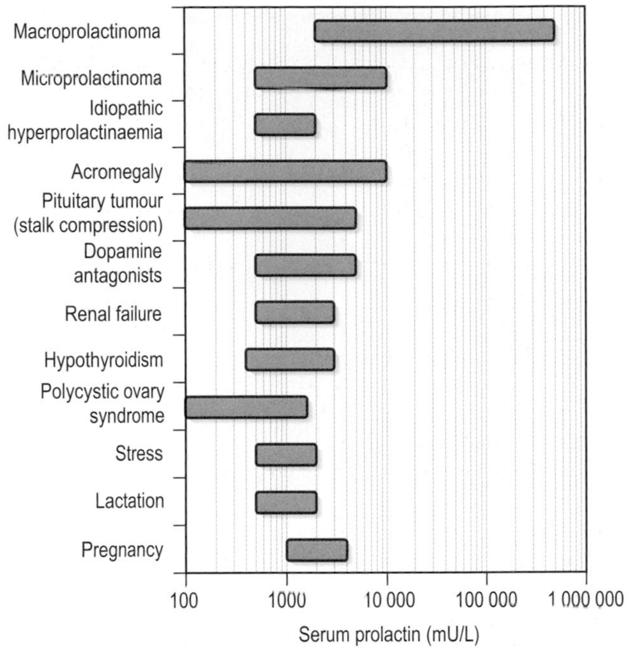

Figure 26.16 Range of serum prolactin seen in common causes of hyperprolactinaemia.

Clinical features

Patients may present with features of hyperprolactinaemia or structural symptoms from a pituitary tumour with headaches and visual loss. This latter presentation is more common in males.

Hyperprolactinaemia stimulates milk production in the breast and inhibits GnRH and gonadotrophin secretion *per se*. It usually presents with:

- galactorrhoea, spontaneous or expressible (60% of cases)
- oligomenorrhoea or amenorrhoea
- decreased libido in both sexes
- decreased potency in men
- subfertility
- symptoms or signs of oestrogen or androgen deficiency – in the long term osteoporosis may result, especially in women
- delayed or arrested puberty in the peripubertal patient
- mild gynaecomastia – often seen in men due to the associated hypogonadism rather than being a direct effect of prolactin.

Additionally, headaches and/or visual field defects occur if there is a pituitary tumour (more common in men). Note that many people with galactorrhoea do not have hyperprolactinaemia – 'normoprolactinaemic galactorrhoea' – and the causes are poorly understood.

Investigations

Hyperprolactinaemia should be confirmed by repeat measurement. If there are no clinical features of hyperprolactinaemia, the possibility of ***macroprolactinaemia*** should be considered. This is a higher-molecular-weight complex of prolactin bound to IgG, which is physiologically inactive but occurs in a small proportion of normal people and can therefore lead to unnecessary treatment. Macroprolactinaemia can be diagnosed in the laboratory by precipitation of immunoglobulin G (IgG) with polyethylene glycol, after which prolactin levels will be normal on testing; most laboratories will do this routinely. Hyperprolactinaemia should be excluded in all patients presenting with a pituitary mass.

Further tests are appropriate after physiological and drug causes have been excluded:

- ***Visual fields*** should be checked.
- ***Primary hypothyroidism*** must be excluded since this is a cause of hyperprolactinaemia.
- ***Anterior pituitary function*** should be assessed if there is any clinical evidence of hypopituitarism or radiological evidence of a pituitary tumour (see ***Boxes 26.3, 26.8 and 26.9***).
- ***MRI of the pituitary*** is necessary if there are any clinical features suggestive of a pituitary tumour, and desirable in all cases when prolactin is significantly elevated (>1000 mU/L).

In the presence of a pituitary mass on MRI, the level of prolactin helps determine whether the mass is a prolactinoma or a non-functioning pituitary tumour causing stalk-disconnection hyperprolactinaemia: levels of above 5000 mU/L in the presence of a macroadenoma, or above 2000 mU/L in the presence of a microadenoma (or with no radiological abnormality), strongly suggest a prolactinoma (see p. 1186). Macroprolactinoma refers to tumours above 10 mm in diameter, microprolactinoma to smaller ones. Tumours that are approximately 10 mm are termed mesoadenomas.

Occasionally, very large prolactinomas can be associated with such high serum prolactin levels that some assays give an artefactual falsely low result (known as the 'hook effect'). If suspected, this can be excluded by serial dilutions of the serum sample.

Management

Hyperprolactinaemia is usually treated to avoid the long-term effects of oestrogen deficiency (even if the patient would otherwise welcome the lack of periods!) or testosterone deficiency in the male. Exceptions include patients with minor elevations (400–1000 mU/L) and preservation of normal regular menstruation (or normal male testosterone levels), and postmenopausal women with microprolactinomas who are not taking oestrogen replacement.

Medical treatment

Hyperprolactinaemia is controlled with a dopamine agonist.

- ***Cabergoline*** (500 µg once or twice a week, judged on clinical response and prolactin levels) is the best-tolerated and longest-acting drug, and is the drug of choice.
- ***Bromocriptine*** is the longest-established therapy and is therefore preferred if pregnancy is planned; initial doses should be small (e.g. 1 mg), taken with food and gradually increased to 2.5 mg two or three times daily. Side-effects, which prevent effective therapy in a minority of cases, include nausea and vomiting, dizziness and syncope, constipation and cold peripheries.
- ***Quinagolide*** (75–150 µg once daily) is an alternative.

Complications, seen when cabergoline is used in higher doses in Parkinson's disease, include pulmonary, retroperitoneal and pericardial fibrotic reactions, and cardiac valve lesions. Patients need monitoring, although studies suggest that adverse effects appear to be very rare in those on lower, 'endocrine', doses.

In most cases, a dopamine agonist will be the first and only therapy, and can be used in the long term, although a trial of discontinuation can be considered in microprolactinomas after 2–3 years, as a significant percentage may not recur, or in females at the onset of the menopause who are not on oestrogen replacement therapy. Prolactinomas usually shrink in size on a dopamine agonist, and in macroadenomas any pituitary mass effects commonly resolve ***(Fig. 26.17)***. Microprolactinomas may not recur after several years of dopamine agonist therapy in a minority of cases, but in the majority hyperprolactinaemia will return if treatment is stopped.

In patients planning ***pregnancy***, it is useful to know the size of the pituitary lesion before starting dopamine agonist therapy. Rarely, tumours enlarge during pregnancy to produce headaches and visual field defects. Dopamine agonists, which are traditionally stopped after conception, particularly when used in the treatment of microprolactinomas, can be restarted if there are any signs of tumour growth during pregnancy.

Trans-sphenoidal surgery

Surgery may rarely be needed in patients who are intolerant of or unresponsive to dopamine agonists. Surgery may restore normoprolactinaemia in people with microadenoma, but is rarely completely successful in those with macroadenomas and risks damage

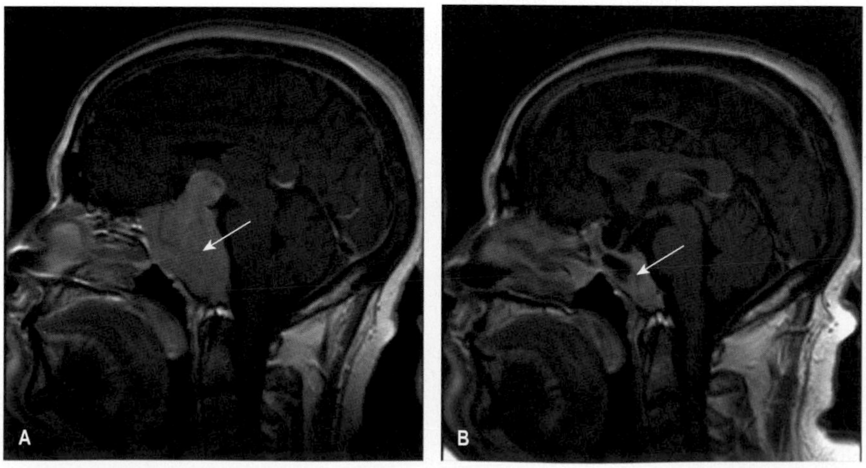

Figure 26.17 **Macroprolactinoma (arrowed). A.** *Before treatment.* **B.** *After 2 years' treatment* with the dopamine agonist cabergoline, showing marked adenoma shrinkage.

to normal pituitary function. Therefore, most patients and physicians elect to continue medical therapy rather than proceed to surgery. Prolactin should therefore always be measured before surgery on any mass in the pituitary region. Some surgeons believe that long-term bromocriptine increases the hardness of the adenoma and makes resection more difficult, but others dissent from this view.

Radiotherapy

Also rarely needed, radiotherapy usually controls adenoma growth and is slowly effective in lowering prolactin, but causes progressive hypopituitarism. It may be advocated after medical tumour shrinkage or after surgery in larger tumours, especially where families are complete or if the drug treatment is poorly tolerated, but most workers simply advocate continuation of dopamine agonist therapy in responsive cases.

Cushing syndrome

Cushing syndrome is the term used to describe the clinical state of increased free circulating glucocorticoid. It occurs most often following the therapeutic administration of synthetic steroids or excess endogenous secretion of ACTH (see below).

Pathophysiology and aetiology

Spontaneous Cushing syndrome is rare, with an incidence of <5/million per year.

Causes of Cushing syndrome are usually subdivided into two groups ***(Box 26.13)***:

1. Increased circulating ACTH from the pituitary (65% of cases), known as Cushing's disease, or from an 'ectopic', non-pituitary, ACTH-producing tumour elsewhere in the body (10%) with consequent glucocorticoid excess ('ACTH-dependent' Cushing's).
2. A primary excess of endogenous cortisol secretion (25%) by an adrenal tumour or, more rarely, by bilateral primary pigmented nodular hyperplasia (PPNH) with subsequent (physiological) suppression of ACTH ('non-ACTH-dependent' Cushing's). Rare cases are due to aberrant expression of receptors for other hormones (e.g. glucose-dependent insulinotrophic peptide (GIP), LH or catecholamines) in adrenal cortical cells. Germline changes in protein kinase A (PKA) can also result in adrenal hyperplasia and adenomas.

Clinical features

The clinical features of Cushing syndrome are those of glucocorticoid excess and are illustrated in ***Figure 26.18***.

- ***Pigmentation*** occurs only with ACTH-dependent causes (most frequently in ectopic ACTH syndrome).
- ***A cushingoid appearance*** can also be caused by excess alcohol consumption (pseudo-Cushing syndrome); the pathophysiology is poorly understood.

Box 26.13 Causes of Cushing syndrome

ACTH-dependent disease	Non-ACTH-dependent disease
• Pituitary-dependent (Cushing's disease)	• Adrenal adenomas
• Ectopic ACTH-producing tumours	• Adrenal carcinomas
	• Exogenous steroids

ACTH, adrenocorticotrophic hormone.

Symptoms

General
Change of appearance
Weight gain (central)
Hair growth/acne
Thin skin/easy bruising

Mental changes
Depression
Psychosis
Insomnia

Muscular weakness
Back pain

Amenorrhoea/oligomenorrhoea

Poor libido

Growth arrest in children

Polyuria/polydipsia

Old photographs may be useful

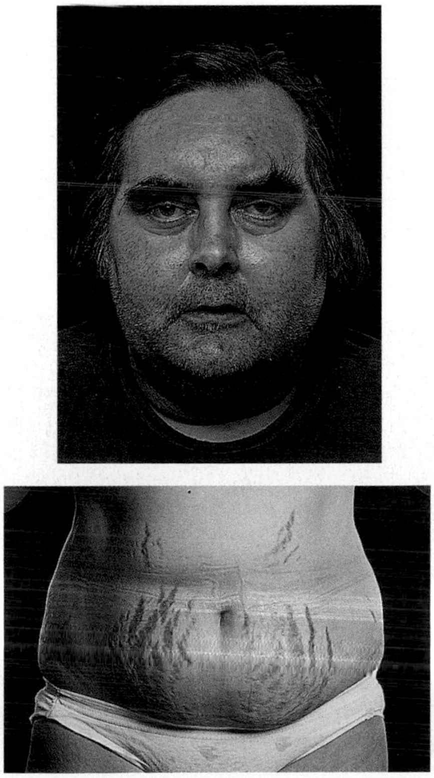

Signs

General
Plethora
Moon face
Hypertension
'Buffalo hump'
Central obesity
Depression/psychosis
Glycosuria
Oedema

Skin
Thin skin
Hirsutism
Acne
Bruising
Poor wound healing
Skin infections
Striae (purple or red)
Pigmentation

Musculoskeletal
Osteoporosis
Pathological fractures (esp. vertebrae and ribs)
Kyphosis
Rib fractures

Proximal myopathy
Proximal muscle wasting

Figure 26.18 Cushing syndrome: symptoms and signs. ***Bold italic*** type indicates signs of most value in discriminating Cushing syndrome from simple obesity and hirsutism.

Box 26.14 Dexamethasone suppression test in the diagnosis of Cushing syndrome

Test and protocol	Measurement[a]	Normal test result or positive suppression	Use and explanation
Dexamethasone (for Cushing's): overnight			
Take 1 mg on going to bed at 23:00 hours	Plasma cortisol at 09:00 hours next morning	Plasma cortisol <100 nmol/L	Outpatient screening test Some 'false-positives'
'Low-dose'			
0.5 mg 6-hourly Eight doses from 09:00 hours on day 0	Plasma cortisol at 09:00 hours on days 0 and +2	Plasma cortisol <50 nmol/L on second sample	For diagnosis of Cushing syndrome
'High-dose' used in differential diagnosis			
2 mg 6-hourly Eight doses from 09:00 hours on day 0	Plasma cortisol at 09:00 hours on days 0 and +2	Plasma cortisol on day +2 <50% of that on day 0 suggests pituitary-dependent disease	Differential diagnosis of Cushing syndrome Pituitary-dependent disease suppresses in about 90% of cases

[a]Plasma cortisol values are very dependent upon the assay used; local reference ranges must be consulted.

- ***Impaired glucose tolerance*** or frank diabetes is common, especially in the ectopic ACTH syndrome.
- ***Hypokalaemia*** due to the mineralocorticoid activity of cortisol is common with ectopic ACTH secretion.
- ***Hypertension*** is common in all causes of Cushing syndrome.

Diagnosis

There are two phases to investigation.

Confirmation

Most obese, hirsute, hypertensive patients do not have Cushing syndrome, and some cases of genuine Cushing's have relatively subtle clinical signs. Confirmation rests on demonstrating inappropriate cortisol secretion, not suppressed by exogenous glucocorticoids; difficulties occur with obesity and depression, where cortisol dynamics are often abnormal. Random cortisol measurements are of no value. Occasional patients are seen with so-called 'cyclical Cushing's', in which the abnormalities come and go.

Investigations to confirm the diagnosis include:

- ***48-h low-dose dexamethasone test (Box 26.14)***. Normal individuals suppress plasma cortisol to <50 nmol/L. People with Cushing syndrome fail to show complete suppression of plasma cortisol levels (although levels may fall substantially in a few cases). This test is highly sensitive (>97%). The overnight dexamethasone test is slightly simpler but has a higher false-positive rate.
- ***24-h urinary free cortisol measurements***. This is simple but less reliable; repeatedly normal values render the diagnosis most unlikely, but some people with Cushing syndrome have normal values on some collections (approximately 10%).
- ***Circadian rhythm***. After 48 h in hospital, cortisol samples are taken at 09:00 hours and 24:00 hours (without warning the patient and ideally when they are asleep). Normal subjects show a pronounced circadian variation (see ***Fig. 26.4***); those with Cushing syndrome have high midnight cortisol levels (>100 nmol/L), though the 09:00 hours value may be normal.
- Midnight or late-night ***salivary cortisol*** collected at home can be used for the diagnosis and surveillance of Cushing's.
- ***Other tests***. There are frequent exceptions to the classic responses to diagnostic tests in Cushing syndrome. If any clinical suspicion of Cushing's remains after preliminary tests, then specialist investigations are still indicated. These may include the insulin stress test, desmopressin stimulation test (see p. 1234) and corticotrophin-releasing hormone (CRH) tests.

Differential diagnosis of the cause

This can be extremely difficult since all causes can result in clinically identical Cushing syndrome. The classical ectopic ACTH syndrome is distinguished by a short history, pigmentation, weight loss, unprovoked hypokalaemia, clinical or chemical diabetes, and plasma ACTH levels above 200 ng/L, but many ectopic tumours are benign and mimic pituitary disease closely, both clinically and biochemically. Severe hirsutism/virilization suggests an adrenal tumour.

Biochemical and radiological procedures for diagnosis include:

- ***Plasma ACTH levels***. Low or undetectable ACTH levels (<10 ng/L) on two or more occasions are a reliable indicator of non-ACTH-dependent disease.
- ***Adrenal CT or MRI scan***. Adrenal adenomas and carcinomas causing Cushing syndrome are relatively large and always detectable by CT scan. Carcinomas are distinguished by their large size and irregular outline, and signs of infiltration or metastases. Bilateral adrenal hyperplasia may be seen in ACTH-dependent causes or in ACTH-independent nodular hyperplasia.
- ***Pituitary MRI***. A pituitary adenoma may be seen but the adenoma is often small and not visible in a significant proportion of cases.
- ***Plasma potassium levels***. Hypokalaemia is common with ectopic ACTH secretion. (All diuretics must be stopped.)
- ***High-dose dexamethasone suppression test (Box 26.14)***. Failure of significant plasma cortisol suppression suggests an ectopic source of ACTH or an adrenal tumour.
- ***CRH test***. An exaggerated ACTH and cortisol response to exogenous CRH suggests pituitary-dependent Cushing's disease, as ectopic sources rarely respond.
- ***Chest X-ray***. A carcinoma of the bronchus or a bronchial carcinoid is sought. Carcinoid lesions may be very small; if ectopic ACTH is suspected, whole-lung, mediastinal and abdominal ***CT scanning*** should be performed.

Further investigations may involve:

- ***Selective catheterization*** of the inferior petrosal sinus to measure ACTH for pituitary lesions, or blood samples taken throughout the body in a search for ectopic sources.

- ***Radiolabelled octreotide*** (^{111}In octreotide) is occasionally helpful in locating ectopic ACTH sites.

Management

Cushing syndrome

Successful treatment with a normal biochemical profile should lead to reversal of the presenting clinical features. However, untreated Cushing syndrome has a very poor prognosis, with death from hypertension, myocardial infarction, infection and heart failure. Whatever the underlying cause, cortisol hypersecretion should be controlled prior to surgery or radiotherapy. Considerable morbidity and mortality are otherwise associated with operating on unprepared patients, especially when abdominal surgery is required.

The usual drug is ***metyrapone***, an 11β-hydroxylase blocker, which is given in doses of 750 mg to 4 g daily in 3–4 divided doses. ***Ketoconazole*** (200 mg three times daily) is also used and is synergistic with metyrapone. Plasma cortisol should be monitored, aiming to reduce the mean level during the day to 150–300 nmol/L, equivalent to normal production rates. ***Aminoglutethimide***, ***trilostane*** (which reversibly inhibits 3-hydroxysteroid dehydrogenase/5–5,4 isomers) and ***etomidate*** infusion (in severe cases) are occasionally used.

Choice of further treatment depends upon the cause.

Cushing's disease (pituitary-dependent hyperadrenalism)

- ***Trans-sphenoidal removal of the tumour*** is the treatment of choice. Selective adenomectomy nearly always leaves the patient ACTH-deficient immediately postoperatively, and this is a good prognostic sign. Overall, pituitary surgery results in remission in 75–80% of cases, but results vary considerably and an experienced surgeon is essential.
- ***External pituitary irradiation*** alone is slow-acting, only effective in 50–60% even after prolonged follow-up, and mainly used after failed pituitary surgery. Children respond much better to radiotherapy, however, 80% being cured. Stereotactic radiotherapy can be useful in selected cases.
- ***Medical therapy*** to reduce ACTH (e.g. bromocriptine, cabergoline and cyproheptadine) is rarely effective. The somatostatin analogue pasireotide may provide medical control of Cushing's in some patients, but is associated with hyperglycaemia as a common side-effect. There is some evidence that aggressive corticotroph adenomas may respond to temozolomide chemotherapy.
- ***Bilateral adrenalectomy*** is an effective last resort if other measures fail to control the disease (see 'Nelson syndrome' below). This can be performed laparoscopically.

Cushing syndrome due to other causes

Adrenal adenomas should be resected laparoscopically after achievement of clinical remission with metyrapone or ketoconazole. Contralateral adrenal suppression may last for a year or more.

Adrenal carcinomas are highly aggressive and the prognosis is poor. In general, if there are no widespread metastases, tumour bulk should be reduced surgically. The adrenolytic drug mitotane may inhibit growth of the tumour and prolong survival, though it can cause nausea and ataxia. Some would also give radiotherapy to the tumour bed after surgery.

Tumours secreting ACTH ectopically should be removed if possible. Otherwise chemotherapy/radiotherapy may be used, depending on the tumour. Control of the Cushing syndrome with metyrapone or ketoconazole is beneficial for symptoms, and bilateral adrenalectomy may be appropriate to give complete control of Cushing syndrome if prognosis from the tumour itself is reasonable.

If the source of ACTH is not clear, cortisol hypersecretion should be controlled with medical therapy until a diagnosis can be made.

Nelson syndrome

Nelson syndrome occurs in about 20% of cases after bilateral adrenalectomy for Cushing's disease and is characterized by increased pigmentation (because of high levels of ACTH), associated with an enlarging pituitary tumour. The syndrome is rare now that adrenalectomy is an uncommon primary treatment, and its incidence may be reduced by pituitary radiotherapy soon after adrenalectomy. The Nelson's adenoma may be treated by pituitary surgery and/or radiotherapy (unless given previously).

Hypersecretion of other pituitary hormones

Pituitary tumours may rarely secrete TSH (and cause thyrotoxicosis). Such 'TSHomas' lead to the unusual biochemical pattern of elevated fT_4 levels with normal or high circulating TSH levels. High fT_4 with non-elevated TSH should also make the physician think of thyroid hormone resistance or a laboratory assay problem (see p. 1181). FSH- and LH-secreting pituitary tumours may cause elevated sex steroids but are usually biologically inactive and seen incidentally on immunostaining after removal of apparent non-functioning pituitary adenomas.

Further reading

Colao A, Petersenn S, Newell-Price J et al. A 12-month phase 3 study of pasireotide in Cushing's disease. *N Engl J Med* 2012; 366:914–924.
Drake WM, Stiles CE, Howlett TA et al. A cross-sectional study of the prevalence of cardiac valvular abnormalities in hyperprolactinemic patients treated with ergot-derived dopamine agonists. *J Clin Endocrinol Metab* 2014; 99:90–6.
Feelders RA, Hofland LJ. Medical treatment of Cushing's disease. *J Clin Endocrinol Metab* 2013; 98:425–438.
Howlett TA, Willis D, Walker G et al. Control of growth hormone and IGF1 in patients with acromegaly in the UK: responses to medical treatment with somatostatin analogues and dopamine agonists. *Clin Endocrinol* 2013; 79:689–699.
Klibanski A. Prolactinomas. *N Engl J Med* 2010; 362:1219–1226.

THE THYROID AXIS

The metabolism of virtually all nucleated cells of many tissues is controlled by the thyroid hormones. Overactivity or underactivity of the gland is the most common of all endocrine problems.

Anatomy

The thyroid gland consists of two lateral lobes connected by an isthmus. It is closely attached to the thyroid cartilage and to the upper end of the trachea, and thus moves on swallowing. It is often palpable in normal women.

Embryologically, it originates from the base of the tongue and descends to the middle of the neck. Remnants of thyroid tissue can sometimes be found at the base of the tongue (lingual thyroid) and along the line of descent. The gland has a rich blood supply from superior and inferior thyroid arteries.

The thyroid gland consists of follicles lined by cuboidal epithelioid cells. Inside is the colloid (the iodinated glycoprotein thyroglobulin), which is synthesized by the follicular cells. Each follicle is surrounded by basement membrane, and between them are parafollicular cells containing calcitonin-secreting C cells.

Physiology

Synthesis

The thyroid synthesizes two hormones:

- triiodothyronine (T_3), which acts at the cellular level
- L-thyroxine (T_4), which is the prohormone.

Inorganic iodide is trapped by the gland via an enzyme-dependent system, oxidized and incorporated into the glycoprotein thyroglobulin to form mono- and diiodotyrosine, and then T_4 and T_3 ***(Fig. 26.19)***.

More T_4 than T_3 is produced, but T_4 is converted in some peripheral tissues (liver, kidney and muscle) to the more active T_3 by 5′-monodeiodination; an alternative 3′-monodeiodination yields the inactive reverse T_3 (rT_3). The latter step occurs particularly in severe non-thyroidal illness (see below).

In plasma, more than 99% of all T_4 and T_3 is bound to hormone-binding proteins (thyroxine-binding globulin, TBG; thyroid-binding prealbumin, TBPA; and albumin). Only free hormone is available for action in the target tissues, where T_3 binds to specific nuclear receptors within target cells. Many drugs and other factors affect TBG; all may result in confusing total T_4 levels in blood, and most laboratories therefore now measure free T_4 levels.

Control of the hypothalamic–pituitary–thyroid axis

Thyrotrophin-releasing hormone (TRH), a peptide produced in the hypothalamus, stimulates the pituitary to secrete thyroid-stimulating hormone (TSH) (see ***Fig. 26.2***). TSH, in turn, stimulates growth and activity of the thyroid follicular cells via the G-protein-coupled TSH membrane receptor (see ***Box 26.4***). The T_3 and T_4 subsequently secreted into the circulation by follicular cells exert negative feedback on the hypothalamus, as described on page 1180.

Circulating T_4 is peripherally deiodinated to T_3, which binds to the thyroid hormone nuclear receptor (TR) on target organ cells to cause modified gene transcription. There are two TR receptors (TR-α and TR-β) and the tissue-specific effects of T_3 are dependent upon the local expression of these TR receptors. TR-α knockout mice show poor growth, bradycardia and hypothermia, whilst TR-β knockout mice show thyroid hyperplasia and high T_4 levels in the presence of inappropriately normal circulating TSH, suggesting a role for the latter receptors in thyroid hormone resistance (see p. 1208).

Physiological effects of thyroid hormones

The physiological effects of thyroid hormones are summarized in ***Box 26.15***.

Dietary iodine requirement

Globally, dietary iodine deficiency is a major cause of thyroid disease, as iodine is an essential requirement for thyroid hormone

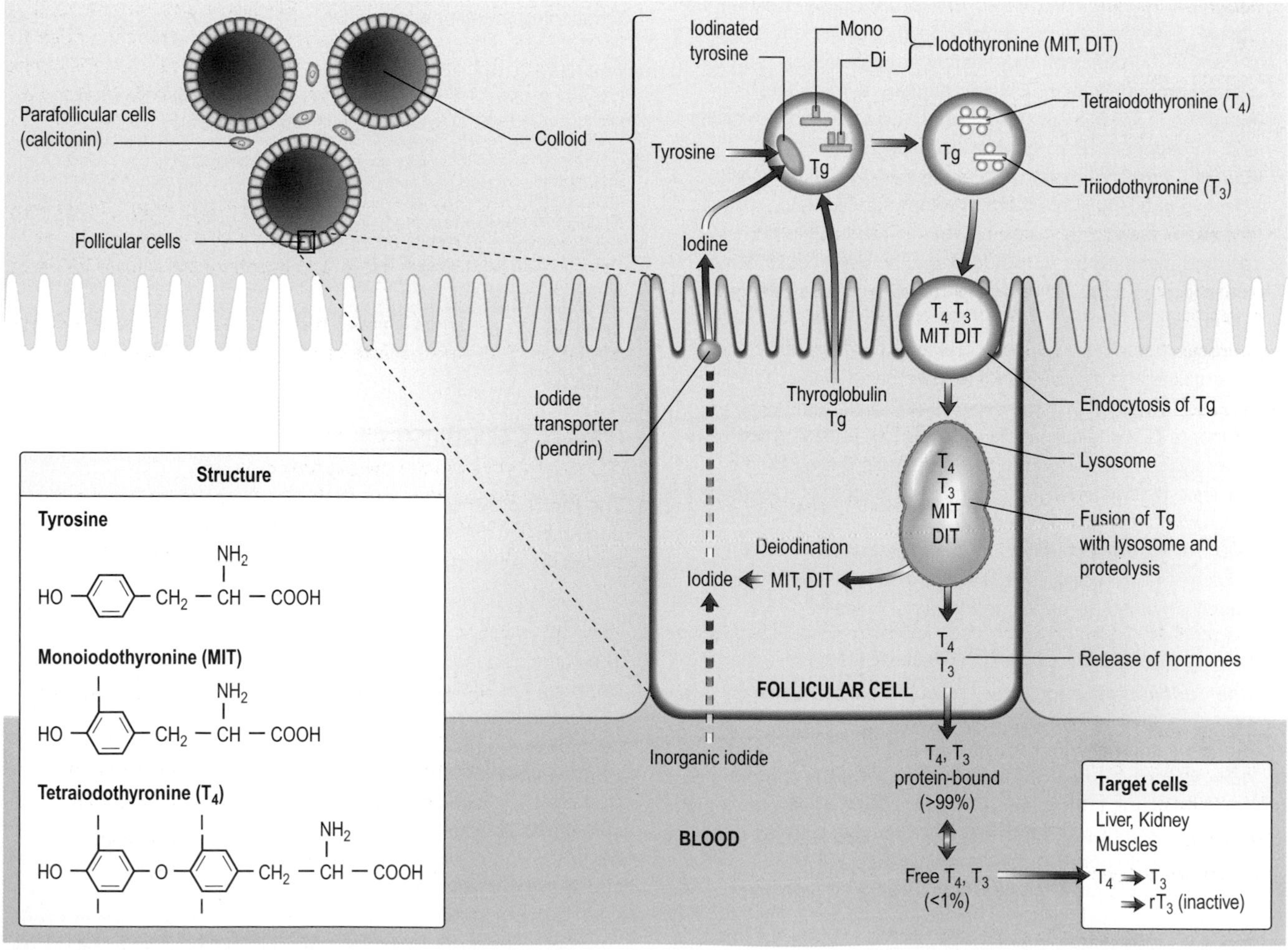

Figure 26.19 Synthesis and metabolism of the thyroid hormones. Tg, thyroglobulin.

synthesis. The recommended daily intake of iodine should be at least 140 µg, and dietary supplementation of salt and bread has reduced the number of areas where 'endemic goitre' still occurs (see below).

Investigations: thyroid function tests

Immunoassays for free T_4, free T_3 and TSH are widely available. There are only minor circadian rhythms and measurements may be made at any time. Particular uses of the tests are summarized in ***Box 26.16***, with typical findings in common disorders.

TSH measurement

In most circumstances, TSH levels can discriminate between hyperthyroidism, hypothyroidism and euthyroidism (normal thyroid gland function). Exceptions are hypopituitarism, and the 'sick euthyroid' syndrome where low levels (which normally imply hyperthyroidism) occur in the presence of low or normal T_4 and T_3 levels. As a single test of thyroid function, TSH measurement is the most sensitive in most circumstances, but accurate diagnosis requires at least two tests: for example, TSH plus free T_4 or free T_3 where hyperthyroidism is suspected; TSH plus serum free T_4 where hypothyroidism is likely.

Box 26.15 Physiological effects of thyroid hormone

Target	Effect
Cardiovascular system	Increases heart rate and cardiac output
Bone	Increases bone turnover and resorption
Respiratory system	Maintains normal hypoxic and hypercapnic drive in respiratory centre
Gastrointestinal system	Increases gut motility
Blood	Increases red blood cell 2,3 BPG[a], facilitating oxygen release to tissues
Neuromuscular function	Increases speed of muscle contraction/relaxation and muscle protein turnover
Carbohydrate metabolism	Increases hepatic gluconeogenesis/glycolysis and intestinal glucose absorption
Lipid metabolism	Increases lipolysis and cholesterol synthesis and degradation
Sympathetic nervous system	Increases catecholamine sensitivity and β-adrenergic receptor numbers in heart, skeletal muscle, adipose cells and lymphocytes Decreases cardiac α-adrenergic receptors

[a]2,3-BPG, 2,3-bisphosphoglyceric acid.

TRH test

This has been rendered almost obsolete by modern sensitive TSH assays, except for investigation of hypothalamic–pituitary dysfunction. TRH (protirelin) is occasionally used to differentiate between thyroid hormone resistance and TSHoma in the context of raised fT_4 and TSH levels. Typically, after TRH administration, there is a rise in TSH in thyroid hormone resistance, whilst in TSHoma there is a flat response due to continued autonomous TSH secretion, which does not respond to TRH.

Problems in interpretation of thyroid function tests

There are three major areas of difficulty: serious acute or chronic illness, pregnancy and use of oral contraceptives, and certain drugs.

Serious acute or chronic illness

Thyroid function is affected in several ways:

- reduced concentration and affinity of binding proteins
- decreased peripheral conversion of T_4 to T_3 with more rT_3
- reduced hypothalamic–pituitary TSH production.

Systemically ill patients can therefore have an apparently low total and free T_4 and T_3 with a normal or low basal TSH (the 'sick euthyroid' syndrome). Levels are usually only mildly below normal and are thought to be mediated by interleukins IL-1 and IL-6; the tests should be repeated after resolution of the underlying illness.

Pregnancy and oral contraceptives

These lead to greatly increased TBG levels and thus to high or high-normal total T_4. Free T_4 is usually normal. Normal ranges for free T_4 and TSH alter with the normal physiological changes during pregnancy and TSH is often slightly suppressed in the first trimester, but this rarely causes clinical problems.

Drugs

Amiodarone decreases T_4 to T_3 conversion and free T_4 levels may therefore be above normal in a euthyroid patient; conversely, amiodarone may induce both hyper- and hypothyroidism – the TSH level is usually reliable.

Many drugs affect thyroid function tests by interfering with protein binding but this now rarely causes a problem with free T_4 assays.

Antithyroid antibodies

Serum antibodies to the thyroid are common.

- ***Destructive antibodies*** are directed against the microsomes or against thyroglobulin; the antigen for thyroid microsomal antibodies is the thyroid peroxidase (TPO) enzyme. TPO

Box 26.16 Characteristics of blood thyroid function tests in common thyroid disorders[a]

	TSH (0.3–3.5 mU/L)	Free T_4 (10–25 pmol/L)	Free T_3 (3.5–7.5 pmol/L)
Thyrotoxicosis	**Suppressed (<0.05 mU/L)**	**Increased**	**Increased**
Primary hypothyroidism	**Increased (>10 mU/L)**	Low/low-normal	Normal or low
TSH deficiency	Low normal or subnormal	**Low/low-normal**	Normal or low
T_3 toxicosis	Suppressed (<0.05 mU/L)	Normal	**Increased**
Compensated euthyroidism	**Slightly increased (5–10 mU/L)**	**Normal**	Normal

[a]The clinically most informative tests in each situation are shown in bold.
TSH, thyroid-stimulating hormone.

Box 26.17 Causes of hypothyroidism

Primary disease of thyroid

Congenital
- Agenesis
- Ectopic thyroid remnants

Defects of hormone synthesis
- Iodine deficiency
- Dyshormonogenesis
- Antithyroid drugs
- Other drugs (e.g. lithium, amiodarone, interferon)

Autoimmune
- Atrophic thyroiditis
- Hashimoto's thyroiditis
- Postpartum thyroiditis

Infective
- Post-subacute thyroiditis

Post-surgery

Post-irradiation
- Radioactive iodine therapy
- External neck irradiation

Infiltration
- Tumour

Secondary (to hypothalamic–pituitary disease)

Hypopituitarism
- Isolated TSH deficiency

Peripheral resistance to thyroid hormone

TSH, thyroid-stimulating hormone.

antibodies are found in up to 20% of the normal population, especially older women, but only 10–20% of these develop overt hypothyroidism.
- ***TSH receptor IgG antibodies*** (***TRAb***) typically stimulate, but occasionally block, the receptor. They are specific for Graves' disease (see p. 1204).

Hypothyroidism

Pathophysiology

Underactivity of the thyroid is usually primary, caused by disease of the thyroid, but may be secondary to hypothalamic–pituitary disease (reduced TSH drive) ***(Box 26.17)***. Primary hypothyroidism is one of the most common endocrine conditions, with an overall UK prevalence of over 2% in women but under 0.1% in men; lifetime prevalence for an individual is higher – perhaps as high as 9% for women and 1% for men, with mean age at diagnosis around 60 years. The worldwide prevalence of subclinical hypothyroidism varies from 1% to 10%.

Aetiology of primary hypothyroidism

See ***Box 26.17***.

Autoimmune

Atrophic (autoimmune) hypothyroidism

This is the most common cause of hypothyroidism and is associated with antithyroid autoantibodies, leading to lymphoid infiltration of the gland and eventual atrophy and fibrosis. It is six times more common in females and the incidence increases with age. The condition is associated with other autoimmune disease, such as pernicious anaemia, vitiligo and other endocrine deficiencies (see p. 1177). Occasionally, intermittent hypothyroidism occurs with subsequent recovery; antibodies that block the TSH receptor may sometimes be involved in the aetiology.

Hashimoto's thyroiditis

This form of autoimmune thyroiditis, again more common in women and most common in late middle age, produces atrophic changes with regeneration, leading to goitre formation. The gland is usually firm and rubbery but may range from soft to hard. TPO antibodies are present, often in very high titres (>1000 IU/L). Patients may be hypothyroid or euthyroid, though they may go through an initial toxic phase, 'Hashi-toxicity'. Levothyroxine therapy may shrink the goitre, even when the patient is not hypothyroid.

Postpartum thyroiditis

This is usually a transient phenomenon observed following pregnancy. It may cause hyperthyroidism, hypothyroidism or the two sequentially. It is believed to result from the modifications to the immune system necessary in pregnancy, and histologically is a lymphocytic thyroiditis. The process is normally self-limiting, but when conventional antibodies are found there is a high chance of this proceeding to permanent hypothyroidism. Postpartum thyroiditis may be misdiagnosed as postnatal depression, emphasizing the need for thyroid function tests in this situation.

Defects of hormone synthesis

Iodine deficiency

Dietary iodine deficiency still exists (see p. 203) as 'endemic goitre' in some areas where goitre, occasionally massive, is common. The patients may be euthyroid or hypothyroid, depending on the severity of iodine deficiency. The mechanism is thought to be borderline hypothyroidism leading to TSH stimulation and thyroid enlargement in the face of continuing iodine deficiency. Iodine deficiency is still a problem in the Netherlands, Western Pacific, India, South-east Asia, Russia and parts of Africa. Efforts to prevent deficiency by providing iodine in salt continue worldwide but often with incomplete success. Even in the late 20th century, of the 500 million with iodine deficiency in India, about 2 million had cretinism (see below).

Dyshormonogenesis

This rare condition is due to genetic defects in the synthesis of thyroid hormones; patients develop hypothyroidism with goitre. One particular familial form is associated with sensorineural deafness due to a deletion mutation in chromosome 7, causing a defect of the transporter pendrin (Pendred syndrome) (see ***Fig. 26.19***).

Clinical features

Hypothyroidism produces many symptoms ***(Fig. 26.20)***. The alternative term 'myxoedema' refers to the accumulation of mucopolysaccharide in subcutaneous tissues. The classic picture of the slow, dry-haired, thick-skinned, deep-voiced patient with weight gain, cold intolerance, bradycardia and constipation makes the diagnosis easy. Milder symptoms are, however, more common and hard to distinguish from other causes of non-specific tiredness. Many cases are detected on biochemical screening.

Special difficulties in diagnosis may arise in certain circumstances:
- ***Children with hypothyroidism*** may not show classic features but often have a slow growth velocity, poor school performance and sometimes arrest of pubertal development.
- ***Young women with hypothyroidism*** may not show obvious signs. Hypothyroidism should be excluded in all people with oligomenorrhoea/amenorrhoea, menorrhagia, infertility or hyperprolactinaemia.
- ***The elderly*** show many clinical features that are difficult to differentiate from normal ageing. Hypothyroidism should be excluded in elderly patients with cognitive impairment.

Investigation of primary hypothyroidism

Serum TSH is the investigation of choice; a high TSH level confirms primary hypothyroidism. A low free T_4 level confirms the

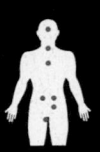

Symptoms

General
Tiredness/malaise
Weight gain
Cold intolerance
Change in appearance
Goitre

Depression
Psychosis
Coma
Poor memory

Hair – dry, brittle, unmanageable
Skin – dry, coarse

Arthralgia
Myalgia
Muscle weakness/stiffness
Poor libido
Puffy eyes
Deafness
Constipation
Anorexia

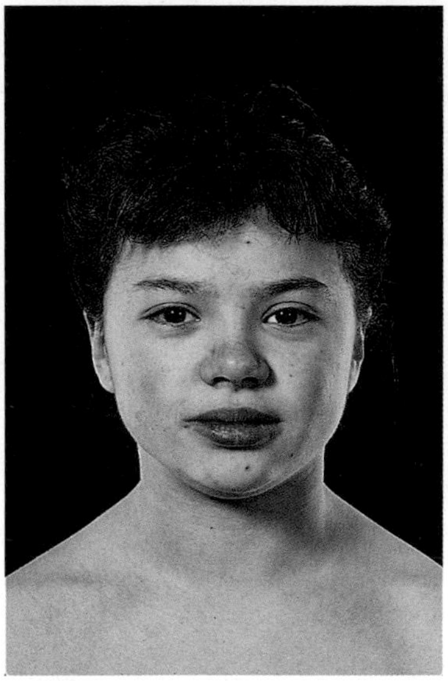

Signs

Mental slowness	
Psychosis/dementia	Periorbital oedema
Ataxia	Deep voice
Poverty of movement	(Goitre)
Deafness	
'Peaches and cream' complexion	***Dry skin***
Dry thin hair	Mild obesity
Loss of eyebrows	
Hypertension	Myotonia
Hypothermia	Muscular hypertrophy
Heart failure	Proximal myopathy
Bradycardia	***Slow-relaxing reflexes***
Pericardial effusion	
Cold peripheries	Anaemia
Carpal tunnel syndrome	
Oedema	

Figure 26.20 Hypothyroidism: symptoms and signs. ***Bold italic*** type indicates symptoms or signs of greater discriminant value. A history from a relative is often revealing. Symptoms of other autoimmune disease may be present.

hypothyroid state (and is also essential to exclude TSH deficiency if clinical hypothyroidism is strongly suspected and TSH is normal or low).

Thyroid and other organ-specific antibodies may be present. Other abnormalities include the following:

- ***anaemia***, which is usually normochromic and normocytic in type but may be macrocytic (sometimes this is due to associated pernicious anaemia) or microcytic (in women, due to menorrhagia or undiagnosed coeliac disease)
- ***increased serum aspartate transferase levels***, from muscle and/or liver
- ***increased serum creatine kinase levels***, with associated myopathy
- ***hypercholesterolaemia*** and hypertriglyceridaemia
- ***hyponatraemia*** due to an increase in ADH and impaired free water clearance.

Management

Replacement therapy

Replacement therapy with levothyroxine (thyroxine, i.e. T_4) is given for life. The starting dose will depend upon the severity of the deficiency and on the age and fitness of the patient, especially their cardiac performance: 100 µg daily for the young and fit, 50 µg (increasing to 100 µg after 2–4 weeks) for the small, old or frail. People with ischaemic heart disease require even lower initial doses, especially if the hypothyroidism is severe and longstanding. Most physicians would then begin with 25 µg daily and perform serial electrocardiograms (ECGs), increasing the dose at 3- to 4-week intervals if angina does not occur or worsen, and the ECG does not deteriorate. Occasional patients develop 'thyrotoxic' (hyperthyroid) symptoms despite normal fT4 levels if the dose is increased too rapidly.

Monitoring

The aim is to restore T_4 and TSH to well within the normal range. Adequacy of replacement is assessed clinically and by thyroid function tests after at least 6 weeks on a steady dose. If serum TSH remains high, the dose of T_4 should be increased in increments of 25–50 µg, and the tests repeated at 6–8-week intervals until TSH becomes normal, ideally in the lower third of the normal range. Complete suppression of TSH should be avoided because of the risk of atrial fibrillation and osteoporosis. The usual maintenance dose is 100–150 µg given as a single daily dose. An annual thyroid function test is recommended – this is usually performed in the primary care setting, often assisted and prompted by district 'thyroid registers'.

Clinical improvement on T_4 may not begin for 2 weeks or more, and full resolution of symptoms may take 6 months. The necessity for lifelong therapy must be emphasized and the possibility of other autoimmune endocrine disease developing, especially Addison's disease or pernicious anaemia, should be considered. During pregnancy, an increase in T_4 dosage of about 25–50 µg is often needed to maintain normal TSH levels, and the necessity for optimal replacement during pregnancy is emphasized by the finding of reductions in cognitive function in children of mothers with elevated TSH during pregnancy.

In cases where there is difficulty normalizing the TSH, compliance issues, concurrent medication that can interfere with thyroxine absorption (such as iron, calcium compounds and proton pump inhibitors), and undiagnosed coeliac disease should be considered.

A few people with primary hypothyroidism complain of incomplete symptomatic response to T_4 replacement. Combination T_4 and T_3 replacement has been advocated in this context, but randomized clinical trials show no consistent benefit in quality-of-life symptoms.

Borderline hypothyroidism or 'compensated euthyroidism'

Patients are frequently seen with low-normal serum T_4 levels and slightly raised TSH levels. Sometimes this follows surgery or radioactive iodine therapy, when it can reasonably be seen as 'compensatory'. Treatment with levothyroxine is normally recommended where the TSH is consistently above 10 mU/L, or when possible symptoms, high-titre thyroid antibodies, or lipid abnormalities are present. Where the TSH is only marginally raised, the tests should be repeated 3–6 months later, as a significant proportion will be normal on repeat testing. Conversion to overt hypothyroidism is more common in men or when TPO antibodies are present. In practice, vague symptoms in people with marginally elevated TSH (below 10 mU/L) rarely respond to treatment, but a 'therapeutic trial' of replacement may be needed to confirm that symptoms are unrelated to the thyroid. It is also considered best to normalize TSH during (and ideally before) pregnancy to avoid potential fetal adverse effects.

Box 26.18 Causes of hyperthyroidism

Common
- Graves' disease (autoimmune)
- Toxic multinodular goitre
- Solitary toxic nodule/adenoma

Uncommon
- Acute thyroiditis
  - Viral (e.g. de Quervain's)
  - Autoimmune
  - Post-irradiation
  - Postpartum
- Gestational thyrotoxicosis (HCG-stimulated)
- Neonatal thyrotoxicosis (maternal thyroid antibodies)
- Exogenous iodine
- Drugs – amiodarone
- Thyrotoxicosis factitia (secret T_4 consumption)

Rare
- TSH-secreting pituitary tumours
- Metastatic differentiated thyroid carcinoma
- HCG-producing tumours
- Hyperfunctioning ovarian teratoma (struma ovarii)

HCG, human chorionic gonadotrophin; TSH, thyroid-stimulating hormone.

Myxoedema coma

Severe hypothyroidism, especially in the elderly, may present with confusion or even coma. Myxoedema coma is very rare; hypothermia is often present and the patient may have severe cardiac failure, pericardial effusions, hypoventilation, hypoglycaemia and hyponatraemia. The mortality was previously at least 50% and patients require full intensive care. Optimal treatment is controversial and data are lacking; most physicians would advise T_3 orally or intravenously in doses of 2.5–5 µg every 8 h, then increasing as above. Large intravenous doses should not be used. Additional measures, though unproven, should include:

- oxygen (by ventilation if necessary)
- monitoring of cardiac output and pressures
- gradual rewarming
- hydrocortisone 100 mg i.v. 8-hourly
- glucose infusion to prevent hypoglycaemia.

Myxoedema madness

Depression is common in hypothyroidism. Rarely, with severe hypothyroidism in the elderly, the patient may become frankly demented or psychotic, sometimes with striking delusions. This may occur shortly after starting T_4 replacement.

Screening for hypothyroidism

The incidence of ***congenital*** hypothyroidism is approximately 1 in 3500 births. Untreated, severe hypothyroidism produces permanent neurological and intellectual damage ('cretinism'). Routine screening of the newborn using a blood spot, as in the Guthrie test, to detect a high TSH level as an indicator of primary hypothyroidism is efficient and cost-effective; cretinism is prevented if T_4 is started within the first few months of life.

Screening of ***elderly*** patients for thyroid dysfunction has a low pick-up rate and is controversial and not currently recommended. However, patients who have undergone thyroid surgery or received radioiodine should have regular thyroid function tests, as should those receiving lithium or amiodarone therapy.

Hyperthyroidism

Hyperthyroidism (thyroid overactivity, thyrotoxicosis) is common, affecting perhaps 2–5% of all females at some time and having a sex ratio of 5 : 1; it most often occurs between the ages of 20 and 40 years. Nearly all cases (>99%) are caused by intrinsic thyroid disease; a pituitary cause is extremely rare ***(Box 26.18)***.

Graves' disease

This is the most common cause of hyperthyroidism and is due to an autoimmune process. Serum IgG antibodies bind to TSH receptors in the thyroid, stimulating thyroid hormone production; that is, they behave like TSH. These TSH receptor antibodies (TSHR-Ab) are specific for Graves' disease. Persistent high levels predict a relapse when drug treatment is stopped. There is an association with HLA-B8, DR3 and DR2; the concordance rate amongst monozygotic twins is 50% and that in dizygotic twins is 5%. There is an association with cytotoxic T lymphocyte-associated antigen 4 (CTLA-4), HLA-DRBP*08 and DRB3*0202 on chromosome 6. The mechanism of immune damage is illustrated in ***Figure 8.15***.

Yersinia enterocolitica, *Escherichia coli* and other Gram-negative organisms contain TSH-binding sites. This raises the possibility that the initiating event in the pathogenesis may be an infection with possible 'molecular mimicry' in a genetically susceptible individual, but the precise initiating mechanisms remain unproven in most cases.

Thyroid eye disease is a feature of Graves' disease. It may accompany the hyperthyroidism in many cases but patients may also be euthyroid or hypothyroid. Other components of Graves' disease, such as Graves' dermopathy, are very uncommon. Rarely, lymphadenopathy and splenomegaly may occur. Graves' disease is also associated with other autoimmune disorders such as pernicious anaemia, vitiligo and myasthenia gravis.

The natural history is one of fluctuation, many patients showing a pattern of alternating relapse and remission; perhaps only 40% of subjects have a single episode. Many patients eventually become hypothyroid.

Other causes of hyperthyroidism/thyrotoxicosis

Solitary toxic adenoma/nodule

This is the cause of about 5% of cases of hyperthyroidism. While the hyperthyroidism will be controlled by the antithyroid drugs, it does not usually remit after a course of antithyroid drugs.

Symptoms

General
Weight loss
Irritability/behaviour change
Restlessness
Malaise
Itching
Sweating
Tall stature (in children)
Breathlessness
Palpitations
Heat intolerance
Stiffness
Muscle weakness

Tremor
Choreoathetosis

Thirst
Vomiting
Diarrhoea

Eye complaints*

Oligomenorrhoea
Loss of libido
Gynaecomastia

Onycholysis
Goitre

*Only in Graves' disease

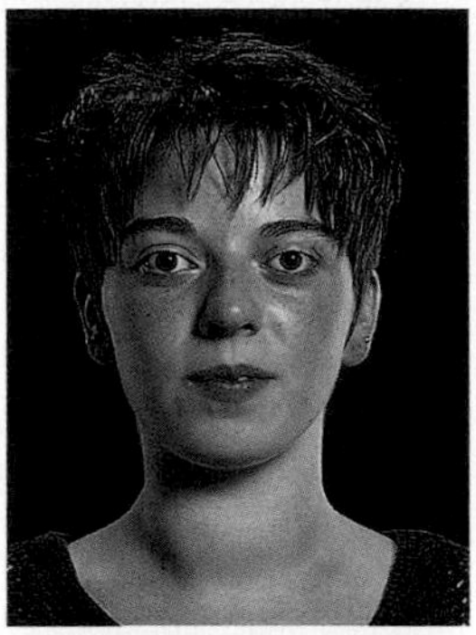

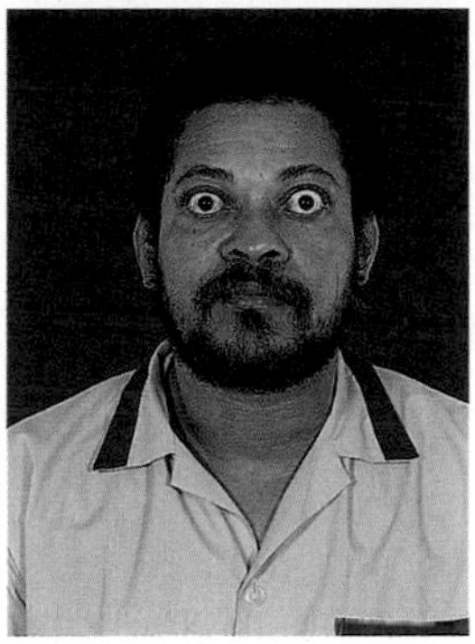

Signs

Tremor
Hyperkinesis
Psychosis

Tachycardia or atrial fibrillation
Full pulse
Warm vasodilated peripheries
Systolic hypertension
Cardiac failure

Exophthalmos*
Lid lag and 'stare'
Conjunctival oedema
Ophthalmoplegia*
Periorbital oedema
Goitre, bruit
Weight loss

Proximal myopathy
Proximal muscle wasting
Onycholysis
Palmar erythema

Graves' dermopathy*
Thyroid acropachy
Pretibial myxoedema

*Only in Graves' disease

Figure 26.21 **Hyperthyroidism: symptoms and signs.** ***Bold italic*** type indicates symptoms or signs of greater discriminant value.

Toxic multinodular goitre

This commonly occurs in older women. Again, antithyroid drugs are rarely successful in inducing a remission, although they can control the hyperthyroidism.

De quervain's thyroiditis

This is transient hyperthyroidism from an acute inflammatory process, probably viral in origin. Apart from the toxicosis, there is usually fever, malaise and pain in the neck with tachycardia and local thyroid tenderness. Thyroid function tests show initial hyperthyroidism, the erythrocyte sedimentation rate (ESR) and plasma viscosity are raised, and thyroid uptake scans show suppression of uptake in the acute phase. Hypothyroidism, usually transient, may then follow after a few weeks. Treatment of the acute phase is with aspirin, using short-term prednisolone in severely symptomatic cases.

Postpartum thyroiditis

[illegible] 1307

Amiodarone-induced thyrotoxicosis

Amiodarone, a class III antiarrhythmic drug (see pp. 978–979), causes two types of hyperthyroidism.

- ***Type I amiodarone-induced thyrotoxicosis (AIT)*** is associated with pre-existing Graves' disease or multinodular goitre. In this situation, hyperthyroidism is probably triggered by the high iodine content of amiodarone.
- ***Type II AIT*** is not associated with previous thyroid disease and is thought to be due to a direct effect of the drug on thyroid follicular cells, leading to a destructive thyroiditis with release of T_4 and T_3. Type II AIT may be associated with a hypothyroid phase several months after presentation. Because amiodarone inhibits the deiodination of T_4 to T_3, biochemical presentation of both types of AIT may be associated with higher T_4:T_3 ratios than usual.

Clinical features of hyperthyroidism

The symptoms and signs of hyperthyroidism affect many systems ***(Fig. 26.21)***.

Symptomatology and signs vary with age and with the underlying aetiology.

- ***The eye signs – lid lag and 'stare'*** – may occur with hyperthyroidism of any cause but other features of thyroid eye disease (see below) occur only in Graves' disease.
- ***Graves' dermopathy*** is rare and can occur on any extensor [illegible] myxoedema is the most commonly described and is an infiltration of the skin on the shin. *Thyroid acropachy* is very rare and consists of clubbing, swollen fingers and periosteal new bone formation.
- ***In the elderly***, a frequent presentation is with atrial fibrillation, other tachycardias and/or heart failure, often with few other signs. Thyroid function tests are mandatory in any patient with atrial fibrillation.

- ***Children*** frequently present with excessive height or excessive growth rate, or with behavioural problems such as hyperactivity. They may also show weight gain rather than loss.
- ***So-called 'apathetic thyrotoxicosis'*** in some elderly patients presents with a clinical picture more like that of hypothyroidism. There may be very few signs and a high degree of clinical suspicion is essential.

Differential diagnosis

Hyperthyroidism is often clinically obvious but treatment should never be instituted without biochemical confirmation.

Differentiation of the mild case from anxiety states may be difficult; useful positive clinical markers are eye signs, a diffuse goitre, proximal myopathy and wasting. Weight loss, despite a normal or increased appetite, is a very useful clinical symptom of hyperthyroidism. The hyperdynamic circulation with warm peripheries seen with hyperthyroidism can be contrasted with the clammy hands of anxiety.

Investigations

- ***Serum TSH*** is suppressed in hyperthyroidism (<0.05 mU/L), except for the very rare instances of TSH hypersecretion.
- ***A raised free T_4 or T_3*** confirms the diagnosis; T_4 is almost always raised but T_3 is more sensitive, as there are occasional cases of isolated 'T_3 toxicosis'.
- ***TSH receptor stimulating antibodies (TSHR-Ab)*** are now measured routinely and the third-generation tests are 97–99% specific for Graves' disease.
- ***Thyroid peroxidase* (*TPO*)** and thyroglobulin antibodies are present in 80% of cases of Graves' disease, but are also found in normals.
- ***Scintiscan ^{99}Tm*** is used when there is doubt as to the nature of the goitre.

Management

Three possibilities are available: antithyroid drugs, radioiodine and surgery. Practices and beliefs differ widely within and between countries.

Antithyroid drugs

Carbimazole is most often used in the UK, and propylthiouracil (PTU) is also an option. ***Thiamazole*** (methimazole), the active metabolite of carbimazole, is used in the USA. These drugs inhibit the formation of thyroid hormones and also have other minor actions; carbimazole/thiamazole is also an immunosuppressive agent. Initial doses and side-effects are detailed in ***Box 26.19***.

Although thyroid hormone synthesis is reduced very quickly, the long half-life of T_4 (7 days) means that clinical benefit is not apparent for 10–20 days. As many of the manifestations of hyperthyroidism are mediated via the sympathetic system, beta-blockers are used to provide rapid partial symptomatic control; they also decrease peripheral conversion of T_4 to T_3. Preferred drugs are those without intrinsic sympathomimetic activity, e.g. propranolol ***(Box 26.19)***. They should not be used alone for hyperthyroidism except when the condition is self-limiting, as in subacute thyroiditis.

Subsequent management is either by gradual dose titration or by a 'block and replace' regimen. Neither regimen has been shown to be unequivocally superior. TSH often remains suppressed for many months after clinical improvement and normalization of T_4 and T_3.

Dosage regimen

Gradual dose titration

1. Start carbimazole 20–40 mg daily.
2. Review after 4–6 weeks and reduce the dose of carbimazole, depending on clinical state and fT_4/fT_3 levels. TSH levels may remain suppressed for several months and are unhelpful at this stage.
3. When the patient is clinically and biochemically euthyroid, stop beta-blockers.
4. Review thyroid function regularly during the planned course of treatment (typically 18 months – but some use courses between 6 and 24 months).
5. Reduce carbimazole if fT_4 falls below or TSH rises above normal, and when approaching the end of the planned course.
6. Increase carbimazole if fT_4 or fT_3 is above normal (and consider if TSH remains suppressed after several months with a normal fT_4).
7. Stop treatment at the end of the course if the patient is euthyroid on 5 mg daily carbimazole.

PTU is used in similar fashion ***(Box 26.19)***.

'Block and replace' regimen

With this policy, full doses of antithyroid drugs, usually carbimazole 40 mg daily, are given to suppress the thyroid completely while replacing thyroid activity with 100 μg of levothyroxine daily once euthyroidism has been achieved. This is continued usually for 18 months, the claimed advantages being the avoidance of over- or undertreatment and the better use of the immunosuppressive action of carbimazole. This regimen is contraindicated in pregnancy, as T_4 crosses the placenta less well than carbimazole.

Relapse

About 50% of patients will relapse after a course of carbimazole or PTU, mostly within the following 2 years but occasionally much

Box 26.19 Drugs used in the treatment of hyperthyroidism

Drug	Usual starting dose	Side-effects	Remarks
Antithyroid drugs			
Carbimazole	20–40 mg daily, 8-hourly or in single dose	Rash, nausea, vomiting, arthralgia, agranulocytosis (0.1%), jaundice	Active metabolite is thiamazole (methimazole) Mild immunosuppressive activity
Propylthiouracil (PTU)	100–200 mg 8-hourly	Rash, nausea, vomiting, agranulocytosis, hepatotoxicity	Additionally blocks conversion of T_4 to T_3
Beta-blocker for symptomatic control May need higher doses than normal			
Propranolol	40–80 mg every 6–8 h		Avoid in asthma Use agents without intrinsic sympathomimetic activity as receptors are highly sensitive

later. Long-term antithyroid therapy is then used, or surgery or radiotherapy is considered (see below). Most patients (90%) with hyperthyroidism have a diffuse goitre but those with large single or multinodular goitres are unlikely to remit after a course of antithyroid drugs and will usually require definitive treatment. Severe biochemical hyperthyroidism is also less likely to remain in remission.

Toxicity

The major side-effect of drug therapy is agranulocytosis, which occurs in approximately 1 in 1000 patients, usually within 3 months of treatment. All patients must be warned to seek immediate medical attention for a white blood cell count if they develop unexplained fever or sore throat; written information is essential. Rashes are more frequent and usually require a change of drug. If toxicity occurs on carbimazole, PTU may be used, and vice versa; side-effects are only occasionally repeated on the other drug.

Radioactive iodine

Radioactive iodine (RAI) is given to patients of all ages, although it is contraindicated in pregnancy and while breast-feeding. RAI is the most common treatment modality in the USA, whereas antithyroid drugs tend to be favoured in Europe.

^{131}***Iodine*** is given in an empirical dose (usually 400–550 MBq) because of variable uptake and radiosensitivity of the gland. It accumulates in the thyroid and destroys the gland by local radiation, although it takes several months to be fully effective.

Patients must be rendered euthyroid before treatment. They should stop antithyroid drugs at least 4 days before radioiodine, and not recommence until 3 days after radioiodine. Patients on PTU should stop antithyroid medication before RAI earlier than those on carbimazole because it has a radioprotective action. Many patients do not need to restart antithyroid medication after treatment.

Early discomfort in the neck and immediate worsening of hyperthyroidism are sometimes seen. If worsening occurs, the patient should receive propranolol ***(Box 26.19)***; if necessary, carbimazole can be restarted. Euthyroidism normally returns in 2–3 months. People with dysthyroid eye disease are more likely to show worsening of eye problems after radioiodine than after antithyroid drugs; this represents a partial contraindication to RAI, although worsening can usually be prevented by steroid administration.

Long-term surveillance

Hypothyroidism affects the majority of subjects over the following 20 years. Some 75% of patients are rendered euthyroid in the short term, but a small proportion remain hyperthyroid and may require a second dose of radioiodine. Long-term surveillance of thyroid function is necessary, with frequent tests in the first year after therapy and at least annually thereafter.

There is no increased risk of malignancy after RAI.

Surgery

Thyroidectomy should be performed only in patients who have previously been rendered euthyroid. Conventional practice is to stop the antithyroid drug 10–14 days before operation and to give potassium iodide (60 mg three times daily), which reduces the vascularity of the gland.

The operation should be performed only by experienced surgeons to reduce the chance of complications:

- Early postoperative bleeding causing tracheal compression and asphyxia is a rare emergency that mandates immediate removal of all clips/sutures to allow escape of the blood/haematoma.
- Laryngeal nerve palsy occurs in 1%. Vocal cord movement should be checked preoperatively. Mild hoarseness is more common and thyroidectomy is best avoided in professional singers!
- Transient hypocalcaemia occurs in up to 10% but with permanent hypoparathyroidism in fewer than 1%.
- Ongoing thyroid function depends on the operation performed. With a single toxic nodule, excision of the lesion is curative. With Graves' disease or multinodular goitre, the traditional 'subtotal' thyroidectomy, aiming for euthyroidism on no treatment, results in recurrent hyperthyroidism in 1–3% within 1 year, then 1% per year and hypothyroidism in about 10% of patients within 1 year, and then increasing with time. 'Near-total' thyroidectomy is therefore now preferred, with inevitable hypothyroidism but a much reduced risk of recurrence.

Indications for either surgery or radioiodine are given in ***Box 26.20***.

Box 26.20 Choice of surgery or radioiodine therapy for hyperthyroidism

Indications for surgery or radioiodine	Indications for surgery
• Patient choice • Persistent drug side-effects • Poor compliance with drug therapy • Recurrent hyperthyroidism after drugs	• A large goitre, which is unlikely to remit after antithyroid medication

Special situations in hyperthyroidism

Thyroid crisis or 'thyroid storm'

This rare condition, with a mortality of 10%, is a rapid deterioration of hyperthyroidism with hyperpyrexia, severe tachycardia, extreme restlessness, cardiac failure and liver dysfunction. It is usually precipitated by stress, infection or surgery in an unprepared patient, or by radioiodine therapy. With careful management, it should no longer occur and most cases referred to as a 'crisis' are simply severe but uncomplicated thyrotoxicosis.

Treatment is urgent. Propranolol in full doses is started immediately together with potassium iodide, antithyroid drugs, corticosteroids (which suppress many of the manifestations of hyperthyroidism) and full supportive measures. Control of cardiac failure and tachycardia is also necessary.

Occasionally, hyperthyroidism can lead to a thyrotoxic cardiomyopathy, which causes ischaemic changes on a 12-lead ECG; these reverse after euthyroidism is achieved ***(Fig. 26.22)***.

Hyperthyroidism in pregnancy and neonatal life

Since hyperthyroidism typically affects young women, pregnancies, both planned and unplanned, inevitably occur during antithyroid treatment. PTU is usually the preferred antithyroid drug at conception and in the first trimester of pregnancy or in any woman planning pregnancy, due to rare reports of congenital abnormalities with carbimazole, which have not been described with PTU (p. 1307). However, carbimazole is recommended in the second and third trimesters, as liver problems are more frequently described on PTU.

The high level of HCG found in normal pregnancy is a weak stimulator of the TSH receptor, commonly causing suppressed TSH with slightly elevated fT_4/fT_3 in the first trimester, which may be

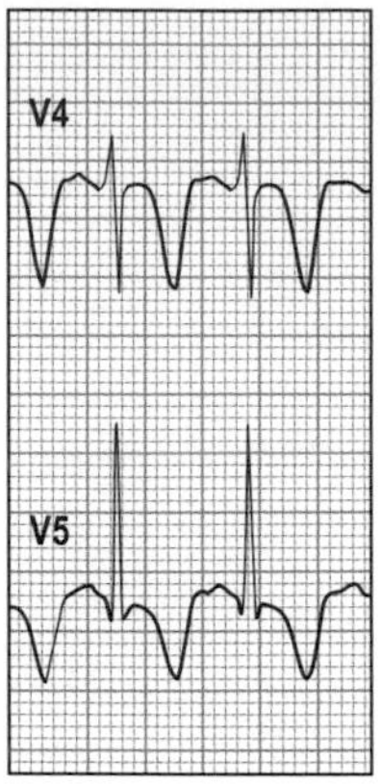

Figure 26.22 Thyrotoxic cardiomyopathies. ECG showing marked lateral T-wave inversion.

associated with hyperemesis gravidarum. True maternal hyperthyroidism occurring *de novo* during pregnancy is, however, uncommon and usually mild. Diagnosis can be difficult because of the overlap with symptoms of normal pregnancy and misleading thyroid function tests, although TSH is largely reliable. The pathogenesis is almost always Graves' disease.

Thyroid-stimulating immunoglobulin (TSI) crosses the placenta to stimulate the fetal thyroid. Carbimazole and PTU (see below) also cross the placenta but T_4 does so poorly, so a 'block and replace' regimen is contraindicated. The smallest dose necessary of PTU or carbimazole (see above) is used and the fetus must be monitored. If necessary (when high doses are needed, or there is poor patient compliance or drug side-effects), surgery can be performed, preferably in the second trimester. RAI is absolutely contraindicated.

The fetus and maternal Graves' disease

Any mother with a history of Graves' disease may have circulating TSI. Even if she is euthyroid after surgery or RAI, the immunoglobulin may still be present to stimulate the fetal thyroid, and the fetus can thus become hyperthyroid.

Any such patient should therefore be monitored during pregnancy. Fetal heart rate provides a direct biological assay of fetal thyroid status, and monitoring should be performed at least monthly. Rates above 160/minute are strongly suggestive of fetal hyperthyroidism, and maternal treatment with PTU and/or propranolol is used. Direct measurement of TSHR-Ab may be helpful to predict neonatal thyrotoxicosis in this situation. To prevent a euthyroid mother becoming hypothyroid, T_4 may be given, as this does not easily cross the placenta. Sympathomimetics, used to prevent premature labour, are contraindicated, as they may provoke fatal tachycardia in the fetus. The paediatrician should be informed and the infant checked immediately after birth, as overtreatment with PTU or carbimazole can cause fetal goitre. Breastfeeding while on the usual doses of carbimazole or PTU appears to be safe.

Hyperthyroidism may also develop in the neonatal period, as TSI has a half-life of approximately 3 weeks. Manifestations in the newborn include irritability, failure to thrive and persisting weight loss, diarrhoea and eye signs. Thyroid function tests are difficult to interpret, as neonatal normal ranges vary with age.

Untreated neonatal hyperthyroidism is probably associated with hyperactivity in later childhood.

Thyroid hormone resistance

Thyroid hormone resistance is an inherited condition, caused by an abnormality of the thyroid hormone receptor. Mutations to the receptor (TR β) result in the need for higher levels of thyroid hormones to achieve the same intracellular effect. As a result, the normal feedback control mechanisms (see ***Fig. 26.2***) result in high blood levels of T_4 with a normal TSH in order to maintain a euthyroid state. This has two consequences:

1. Thyroid function tests appear abnormal, even when the patient is euthyroid and requires no treatment. Specialist review is needed to differentiate this condition from hyperthyroidism due to inappropriate TSH secretion.
2. Different tissues contain different thyroid hormone receptors and, in some families, receptors in certain tissues may have normal activity. In this case, the level of thyroid hormones to maintain euthyroidism at pituitary and hypothalamic levels (which controls secretion of TSH) may be higher than that required in other tissues such as heart and bone, so that these tissues may exhibit 'thyrotoxic' effects in spite of a normal serum TSH. This 'partial thyroid hormone resistance' can be very difficult to manage effectively.

Thyroid hormone resistance is diagnosed on the basis of a raised T_4/T_3 in the context of a non-elevated TSH. The differential diagnosis of this pattern of blood results includes TSHoma and laboratory assay interference.

Long-term consequences of hyperthyroidism

Long-term follow-up studies of hyperthyroidism show a slight increase in overall mortality, which affects all age groups, is not fully explained and tends to occur in the first year after diagnosis. Thereafter, the only long-term risk of adequately treated hyperthyroidism appears to be an increased risk of osteoporosis. People with persistently suppressed TSH levels have an increased likelihood of developing atrial fibrillation, which may predispose to thromboembolic disease.

Graves' orbitopathy (ophthalmopathy)

Pathophysiology

Graves' orbitopathy is due to a specific immune response that causes retro-orbital inflammation ***(Fig. 26.23)***. Swelling and oedema of the extraocular muscles lead to limitation of movement and to proptosis, which is usually bilateral but can sometimes be unilateral. Ultimately, increased pressure on the optic nerve may cause optic atrophy. Histology of the extraocular muscles shows focal oedema and glycosaminoglycan deposition followed by fibrosis. The precise autoantigen that leads to the immune response remains to be identified, but it appears to be an antigen in retro-orbital tissue with similar immunoreactivity to the TSH receptor.

Eye disease is a manifestation of Graves' disease and can occur in patients who may be hyperthyroid, euthyroid or hypothyroid. Thyroid dysfunction and orbitopathy usually occur within 2 years of each other, although sometimes a gap of many years is seen. TSH receptor antibodies are almost invariably found in the serum but their role in the pathogenesis is becoming clearer ***(Fig. 26.23)***. Orbitopathy is more common and more severe in smokers.

Clinical features

The clinical appearances are characteristic (see ***Fig. 26.21***) but thyroid eye disease demonstrates a wide range of severity. A high

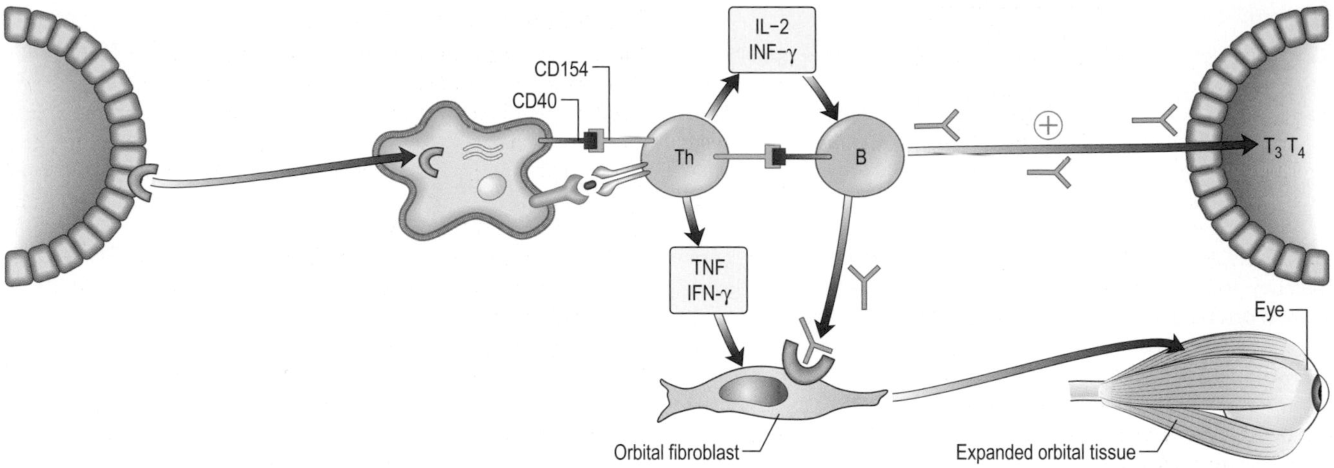

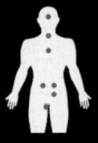

Figure 26.23 Model of the initiation of thyrotrophin-receptor autoimmunity in Graves' ophthalmopathy and its consequences. Thyrotrophin receptor is internalized and degraded by antigen-presenting cells that present thyrotrophin-receptor peptides, in association with major histocompatibility complex (MHC) class II antigens, to helper T (Th) cells. These cells become activated, interact with autoreactive B cells through CD154–CD40 bridges, and secrete interleukin 2 (IL-2) and interferon-gamma (IFN-γ). These cytokines induce the differentiation of B cells into plasma cells that secrete anti-thyrotrophin-receptor antibodies. Anti-thyrotrophin-receptor antibodies (green) recognize the thyrotrophin receptor on orbital fibroblasts and, in conjunction with the secreted type 1 helper T cytokines, IFN-γ and tumour necrosis factor (TNF), initiate the tissue changes characteristic of Graves' ophthalmopathy. These antibodies stimulate the thyrotrophin receptor on thyroid follicular epithelial cells, leading to hyperplasia and increased production of the thyroid hormones triiodothyronine (T_3) and thyroxine (T_4). *(Adapted from Bahn RS. Graves' ophthalmology.* N Engl J Med *2010; 362:726–738.)*

proportion of people with Graves' disease notice some soreness, painful watering or prominence of the eyes, and the 'stare' of lid retraction is relatively common. More severe proptosis occurs in a minority of cases, and limitation and discomfort of eye movement and visual impairment due to optic nerve compression are relatively uncommon. Proptosis and lid retraction may limit the ability to close the eyes completely so that corneal damage may occur. There is periorbital oedema, and conjunctival oedema and inflammation.

Eye manifestations do not parallel the degree of biochemical thyrotoxicosis or the need for antithyroid therapy, but exacerbation of eye disease is more common after radioiodine treatment (15% versus 3% on antithyroid drugs). Sight is threatened in only 5–10% of cases, but the discomfort and cosmetic problems cause great patient anxiety.

Investigations

If the appearance is characteristic, consideration is needed as to whether the patient requires review by an ophthalmologist. Investigation would include:

- TSH, fT_3 and fT_4 measurement.
- MRI or CT of the orbits to exclude retro-orbital, space-occupying lesions. In Graves' orbitopathy, there may be enlarged muscles and oedema, with a taut optic nerve due to raised intra-orbital pressure.
- Assessment of vision, particularly optic nerve function.

Management

If the patient is thyrotoxic, this should be treated, but treatment will not directly result in an improvement of the ophthalmopathy; hypothyroidism must be avoided, as it may exacerbate the eye problem. Smoking should be stopped. Treatment of the eyes may be either local or systemic, and always requires close liaison between specialist endocrinologist and ophthalmologist:

- ***Methylcellulose or hypromellose eyedrops*** or ointment are given to aid lubrication and improve comfort.
- ***Sleeping upright*** affords some patients relief.
- ***Taping the eyelids*** ensures closure at night.
- ***Systemic steroids*** (prednisolone 30–120 mg daily) usually reduce inflammation if more severe symptoms are present. Pulse intravenous methylprednisolone may be used initially and is more rapidly effective in severe cases.
- ***Surgical decompression of the orbit(s)*** may be required, particularly if pressure of orbital contents on the optic nerve threatens vision (often called a 'hot' decompression), and at a later, stable stage for cosmetic reasons ('cold' decompression).
- ***Lid surgery*** will protect the cornea if lids cannot be closed, and can be useful later for cosmetic reasons.
- ***Corrective eye muscle surgery*** may improve diplopia due to muscle changes; it should be deferred until the situation has been stable for 6 months and should follow any orbital decompression.
- ***Irradiation of the orbits*** (20 Gy in divided doses) is used in some centres. This improves inflammation and ocular motility but has little effect on proptosis; its precise role is debated.
- ***Immunomodulatory agents*** may produce a response in some patients when conventional treatments fail, although clinical trial evidence is inconsistent.
- ***Selenium*** may have a beneficial effect on inflammatory thyroid ophthalmopathy in some patients.

Goitre (thyroid enlargement)

Goitre is more common in women than in men and may be either physiological or pathological.

Clinical features

Goitres are present on examination in up to 9% of the population. Most commonly, a goitre is noticed as a cosmetic defect by the patient or by friends or relatives. The majority are painless, but pain or discomfort can occur in acute varieties. Large goitres can produce dysphagia and difficulty in breathing, implying oesophageal or tracheal compression.

A small goitre may be more easily visible (on swallowing) than palpable. Clinical examination should record the size, shape, consistency and mobility of the gland, as well as whether its lower margin can be demarcated (thus implying the absence of retrosternal extension). A bruit may be present. Associated lymph nodes should be sought and the tracheal position determined if possible. Examination should never omit an assessment of the patient's clinical thyroid status.

Specific enquiry should be made about any medication, especially iodine-containing preparations, and possible exposure to radiation.

Particular points of note are as follows:

- Puberty and pregnancy may produce a diffuse increase in size of the thyroid.
- Pain in a goitre may be caused by thyroiditis, bleeding into a cyst or (rarely) a thyroid tumour.
- Excessive doses of carbimazole or PTU will induce goitre.
- Iodine deficiency and dyshormonogenesis (see above) can also cause goitre.

Diagnosis

There are four major aspects to any goitre: its pathological nature, whether it is causing any compressive symptoms, the patient's thyroid status and whether it is of cosmetic concern. The nature can often be judged clinically. Goitres ***(Box 26.21)*** are usually separable into diffuse and nodular types, the causes of which differ.

Diffuse goitre

Simple goitre

In this instance, no clear cause is found for enlargement of the thyroid, which is usually smooth and soft. It may be associated with thyroid growth-stimulating antibodies.

Autoimmune thyroid disease

Hashimoto's thyroiditis and thyrotoxicosis are both associated with firm diffuse goitre of variable size. A bruit is often present in thyrotoxicosis.

? Box 26.21 Goitre: causes and types

Diffuse

- Simple:
  - Physiological (puberty, pregnancy)
- Autoimmune:
  - Graves' disease
  - Hashimoto's disease
- Thyroiditis:
  - Acute (de Quervain's thyroiditis)
- Iodine deficiency (endemic goitre)
- Dyshormonogenesis
- Goitrogens (e.g. sulphonylureas)

Nodular

- Multinodular goitre
- Solitary nodular
- Fibrotic (Riedel's thyroiditis)
- Cysts

Tumours

- Adenomas
- Carcinoma
- Lymphomas

Miscellaneous

- Sarcoidosis
- Tuberculosis

Thyroiditis

Acute tenderness in a diffuse swelling, sometimes with severe pain, is suggestive of an acute viral thyroiditis (de Quervain's). It may produce transient clinical hyperthyroidism with an increase in serum T_4 (see p. 1205).

Nodular goitres

Multinodular goitre

Most common is the multinodular goitre, especially in older patients. The patient is usually euthyroid but may be hyperthyroid or borderline with suppressed TSH levels but normal free T_4 and T_3. Multinodular goitre is the most common cause of tracheal and/or oesophageal compression and can lead to laryngeal nerve palsy. It may also extend retrosternally ***(Fig. 26.24)***.

The classical 'multinodular goitre' is usually readily apparent clinically, but it should be noted that modern, high-resolution ultrasound frequently reports multiple small nodules in glands, which are clinically diffusely enlarged and associated with autoimmune thyroid disease. These nodules are also found in up to 40% of the normal population.

Solitary nodular goitre

Such a goitre presents a difficult problem of diagnosis. Malignancy should be of concern in any solitary nodule; however, the majority of such nodules are cystic or benign and, indeed, may simply be the largest nodule of a multinodular goitre. The diagnostic challenge is to differentiate the small minority of malignant nodules, which require surgery, from the majority of benign nodules, which do not.

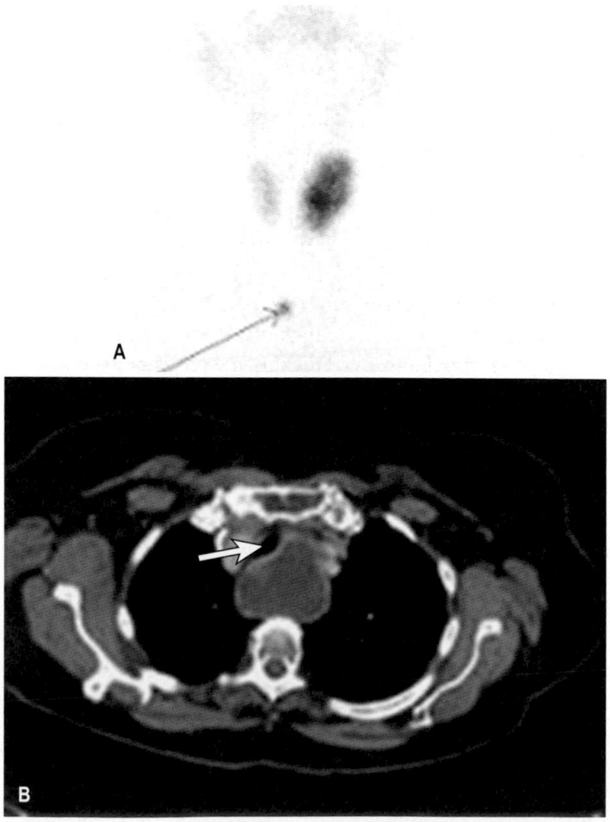

Figure 26.24 Imaging of goitre. A. *Tc scan showing a multinodular goitre*, with predominant involvement of the left lobe of the thyroid (anterior view *with arrowed anatomical marker* at the sternal notch). **B.** *Retrosternal goitre* showing deviation and compression of the trachea (arrowed) on CT.

Sometimes a history of rapid enlargement, associated lymph nodes or pain may suggest an aggressive malignancy, but most thyroid cancers are painless and slow-growing so that investigations are paramount. Risk factors for malignancy include previous irradiation, longstanding iodine deficiency and occasional familial cases.

Solitary toxic nodules are quite uncommon and may be associated with T_3 toxicosis.

Fibrotic goitre (Riedel's thyroiditis)

Fibrotic goitre is a rare condition, usually producing a 'woody' gland. It is associated with other midline fibrosis and is often difficult to distinguish from carcinoma, being irregular and hard. Clinical clues include systemic symptoms of inflammation and elevation in inflammatory markers; it has been shown to be an IgG_4-related disease.

Malignancy

In addition to thyroid carcinomas (see below), the thyroid is rarely the site of a metastatic deposit or the site of origin of a lymphoma.

Investigations

Clinical findings will dictate the appropriate initial tests:

- ***Thyroid function tests*** should include measurement of TSH plus free T_4 or T_3 (see ***Box 26.8***).
- ***Thyroid antibodies*** are assessed to exclude an autoimmune aetiology.
- ***Ultrasound*** with high resolution is a sensitive method for delineating nodules and can demonstrate whether they are cystic or solid. In addition, a multinodular goitre may be demonstrated when only a single nodule is palpable. Unfortunately, even cystic lesions can be malignant and thyroid tumours may arise within a multinodular goitre; therefore fine-needle aspiration (see below) is often required and is performed under ultrasound control at the same time as the scan.
- ***Chest and thoracic inlet X-rays or CT scan*** may detect tracheal compression and large retrosternal extensions in people with a very large goitre or clinical symptoms.
- ***Fine-needle aspiration (FNA)*** should be performed in the outpatient clinic or during ultrasound if the appearance is suggestive of potential malignancy, based on defined ultrasound criteria, as in people with a solitary nodule or a dominant nodule in a multinodular goitre, there is a 5% chance of malignancy. Cytology in expert hands can usually differentiate the suspicious or definitely malignant nodule. FNA reduces the necessity for surgery but there is a 5% false-negative rate, which must be borne in mind (and the patient appropriately counselled). Continued observation is required when an isolated thyroid nodule is assumed to be benign without excision.
- ***Thyroid scan*** (^{99m}Tc) can be useful to distinguish between functioning (hot) or non-functioning (cold) nodules. A hot nodule is only rarely malignant; however, a cold nodule is malignant in only 10% of cases and FNA has largely replaced isotope scans in the diagnosis of thyroid nodules.

Management

Euthyroid goitre

Many goitres are small, cause no symptoms and can be observed (including self-monitoring by the patient in the long term). In particular, during puberty and pregnancy, a goitre associated with euthyroidism rarely requires intervention and the patient can be reassured that spontaneous resolution is likely. Indications for surgical intervention are:

- ***The possibility of malignancy***. A positive or suspicious FNA makes surgery mandatory, and surgery may be necessary if doubt persists, even in the presence of a negative FNA (especially if the patient is concerned by the false-negative rate).
- ***Pressure symptoms on the trachea or, more rarely, oesophagus***. The possibility of retrosternal extension should be excluded.
- ***Cosmetic reasons***. A large goitre often causes considerable anxiety to the patient, even though it is functionally and anatomically benign.

RAI has also been advocated for the treatment of euthyroid goitre, particularly when surgery is an unattractive option.

Toxic nodule

This is initially treated with antithyroid drugs but surgery or radioiodine is often required.

Thyroid carcinoma

Types of thyroid carcinoma, with their characteristics and treatment, are listed in ***Box 26.22***. While not common, these tumours are responsible for 400 deaths annually in the UK and there is an annual incidence of 30 000 cases in the USA. Over 75% occur in women. They present in 90% of cases as thyroid nodules (see above), but occasionally with cervical lymphadenopathy (about 5%), or with lung, cerebral, hepatic or bone metastases.

Carcinomas derived from thyroid epithelium may be papillary or follicular (differentiated), or anaplastic (undifferentiated). Medullary carcinomas (about 5% of all thyroid cancers) arise from the calcitonin-producing C cells. The pathogenesis of thyroid epithelial carcinomas is not understood, except for occasional familial papillary carcinoma, and those cases related to previous head and neck irradiation or ingestion of RAI (e.g. post-Chernobyl). These tumours are minimally active hormonally and are extremely rarely associated with hyperthyroidism; over 90%, however, secrete thyroglobulin, which can therefore act as a tumour marker after thyroid ablation.

Box 26.22 Types of thyroid malignancy

Cell type	Frequency	Behaviour	Spread	Prognosis
Papillary	70%	Occurs in young people	Local, sometimes lung/bone secondaries	Good, especially in young
Follicular	20%	More common in females	Metastases to lung/bone	Good if resectable
Medullary cell	5%	Often familial	Local and metastases	Poor, but indolent course
Anaplastic	<5%	Aggressive	Locally invasive	Very poor
Lymphoma	2%	Variable		Sometimes responsive to radiotherapy

Papillary and follicular carcinomas

The primary treatment is surgical: normally total or near-total thyroidectomy for local disease. Regional or more extensive neck dissection is needed where there is local nodal spread or involvement of local structures.

Most tumours will take up iodine, and UK and other guidelines currently recommend RAI ablation of residual thyroid tissue post-operatively for most people with differentiated thyroid cancer. After ablation of normal thyroid in this way, RAI may be used to localize residual disease (scanning using low doses) or to treat it (using high doses: 5.5–7.5 GBq). When disease does recur, local invasion and lymph node involvement is most common, and lungs and bone are the most common sites of distant metastases.

To minimize risk of recurrence patients are treated with suppressive doses of levothyroxine (sufficient to suppress TSH levels below the normal range). Patient progress is monitored, both clinically and biochemically, using serum thyroglobulin levels as a tumour marker. The measurement of thyroglobulin is most sensitive when TSH is high but this requires the withdrawal of levothyroxine therapy. Recombinant TSH (thyrotropin alpha, rhTSH) 900 μg (2 doses over 48 h) is used to stimulate thyroglobulin without stopping thyroxine therapy. Detectable thyroglobulin suggests recurrence, in which case whole-body ^{131}I scanning is required. Unfortunately, the presence of anti-thyroglobulin antibodies can make the assay unreliable.

The ***prognosis*** is extremely good when differentiated thyroid cancer is excised while confined to the thyroid gland, and the specific therapies available lead to a relatively good prognosis even in the presence of metastases at diagnosis. Accepted markers of high risk include greater age (>40 years), larger primary tumour size (>4 cm) and macroscopic invasion of capsule and surrounding tissues. Recently, oral sorafenib has shown a good short-term response in locally advanced and metastatic differentiated thyroid cancers that were refractory to RAI.

Medullary carcinoma

Medullary thyroid carcinoma (MTC) is a neuroendocrine tumour of the calcitonin-producing C cells of the thyroid. This condition is often associated with MEN 2 (see pp. 1239–1240). Approximately 25% of patients diagnosed with MTC have a mutation of the *RET* proto-oncogene, although the other manifestations of MEN 2 may be absent; hence the importance of genetic counselling and family screening. People with MEN 2 mutations are advised to have a prophylactic thyroidectomy as early as 5 years of age to prevent the development of MTC.

Total thyroidectomy and wide lymph node clearance are usually indicated in MTC. Local invasion or metastasis is frequent, and the tumour responds poorly to treatment, although progression is often slow. Recent biological therapy with vandetanib and cabozantinib have shown benefit in advanced medullary thyroid carcinoma.

Anaplastic carcinomas and lymphoma

These do not respond to RAI, and external radiotherapy produces only a brief respite.

Further reading

Bahn RS. Graves ophthalmopathy. *N Engl J Med* 2010; 362:726–738.
Bartalena L, Baldeschi L, Dickinson A et al. Consensus statement of the European Group on Graves' orbitopathy (EUGOGO) on the management of GO. *Eur J Endocrinol* 2008; 158:273–285.
Brent GA. Thyroid function and screening in pregnancy. *N Engl J Med* 2012; 366:562–568.
Burman KD, Wartofsky L. Thyroid nodules. *N Engl J Med* 2015; 373:2347-2356.
Franklyn JA, Boelaert K. Subclinical thyroid disease: where is the evidence? *Lancet Diabetes Endocrinol* 2013; 1:172–173.
Franklyn JA, Boelaert K. Thyrotoxicosis. *Lancet* 2012; 379:1155–1166.
Perros P, Boelaert K, Colley S et al and the British Thyroid Association. Guidelines for the management of thyroid cancer. *Clin Endocrinol* 2014; 81(S1):1–22.
Ross DS. Radioiodine therapy for hyperthyroidism. *N Engl J Med* 2011; 364:542–550.
Royal College of Physicians. *Report of a Working Party: Radioiodine in the Management of Benign Thyroid Disease – Clinical Guidelines.* London: Royal College of Physicians; 2007; http://www.bnms.org.uk/rcp-guidelines/.
Wartofsky L. Highlights of the American Thyroid Association Guidelines for patients with thyroid nodules or differentiated thyroid carcinoma: the 2009 revision. *Thyroid* 2009; 19:1139–43.
Zimmermann MB, Jooste PL, Pandar CS. Iodine deficiency disorders. *Lancet* 2008; 372:1251–1262.
http://www.ign.org/ *Iodine Global Network*

REPRODUCTION AND SEX

Terminology in reproductive medicine is shown in ***Box 26.23***.

Embryology

Up to 8 weeks of gestation, the sexes share a common development, with a primitive genital tract including the Wolffian and Müllerian ducts. Additionally, there are a primitive perineum and primitive gonads.

- In the presence of a Y chromosome, the potential testis develops while the ovary regresses.
- In the absence of a Y chromosome, the potential ovary develops and related ducts form a uterus and the upper vagina.

Production of Müllerian inhibitory factor from the early 'testis' produces atrophy of the Müllerian duct, while, under the influence of testosterone and dihydrotestosterone, the Wolffian duct differentiates into an epididymis, vas deferens, seminal vesicles and prostate. Androgens induce transformation of the perineum to include a penis, penile urethra and scrotum containing the testes,

Box 26.23 Definitions in reproductive medicine

Term	Definition
Erectile dysfunction	Inability of the male to achieve or sustain an erection adequate for satisfactory intercourse
Azoospermia	Absence of sperm in the ejaculate
Oligospermia	Reduced numbers of sperm in the ejaculate
Libido	Sexual interest or desire; often difficult to assess and greatly affected by stress, tiredness and psychological factors
Menarche	Age at first period
Primary amenorrhoea	Failure to begin spontaneous menstruation by age 16
Secondary amenorrhoea	Absence of menstruation for 3 months in a woman who has previously had cycles
Oligomenorrhoea	Irregular long cycles; often used for any length of cycle above 32 days
Dyspareunia	Pain or discomfort in the female during intercourse
Menstruation	Onset of spontaneous (usually regular) uterine bleeding in the female
Virilization	Occurrence of male secondary sexual characteristics in the female

which descend in response to androgenic stimulation. At birth, testicular volume is 0.5–1 mL. The number of oocytes in the ovaries of a female fetus has reached a maximum by the end of the second trimester of *in utero* development. At birth, the ovaries contain about 3 million oocytes, of which only 400 000 will remain by the time puberty occurs. With the onset of menarche, these oocytes will activate and grow, leading to ovulation and then menstruation.

Physiology

The male

An outline of the hypothalamic–pituitary–gonadal axis is shown in ***Figure 26.25***.

1. Pulses of gonadotrophin-releasing hormone (GnRH) are released from the hypothalamus and stimulate luteinizing hormone (LH) and follicle-stimulating hormone (FSH) release from the pituitary. LH and FSH are composed of two glycoprotein chains (α and β subunits). The α subunits are identical and are shared with TSH, whilst the β subunit confers specific biological activity.
2. LH stimulates testosterone production from Leydig cells of the testis.
3. Testosterone acts via nuclear androgen receptors, which interact with co-regulatory proteins to produce the appropriate tissue responses: male secondary sexual characteristics, anabolism and the maintenance of libido. It also acts locally within the testis to aid spermatogenesis. Testosterone circulates largely bound to sex hormone-binding globulin (SHBG) (see p. 1178). Testosterone feeds back on the hypothalamus/pituitary to inhibit GnRH secretion.
4. FSH stimulates the Sertoli cells in the seminiferous tubules to produce mature sperm and the inhibins A and B.
5. Inhibin feeds back to the pituitary to decrease FSH secretion. Activin, a related peptide, counteracts inhibin.

Secondary sexual characteristics

The secondary sexual characteristics of the male, for which testosterone is necessary, are the growth of pubic, axillary and facial hair, enlargement of the external genitalia, deepening of the voice, sebum secretion, muscle growth and frontal balding.

The female

Female physiology is more complex (***Figs 26.25*** and ***26.26***).

1. In the adult female, higher brain centres impose a menstrual cycle of 28 days upon the activity of hypothalamic GnRH.
2. Pulses of GnRH, at about 2-h intervals, stimulate release of pituitary LH and FSH.
3. LH stimulates ovarian androgen production by the ovarian theca cells.
4. FSH stimulates follicular development and activity of aromatase (an enzyme required to convert ovarian androgens to oestrogens) in the ovarian granulosa cells. FSH also stimulates release of inhibin from ovarian stromal cells, which inhibits FSH release. Activin counteracts inhibin ***(Fig. 26.25)***.
5. Although many follicles are 'recruited' for development in early folliculogenesis, by day 8–10 a 'leading' (or 'dominant') follicle is selected for development into a mature Graafian follicle.
6. Oestrogens have a double feedback action on the pituitary (Fig. 26.25). Initially, they inhibit gonadotrophin secretion (negative feedback) but, later, high-level exposure results in increased GnRH secretion and increased LH sensitivity to

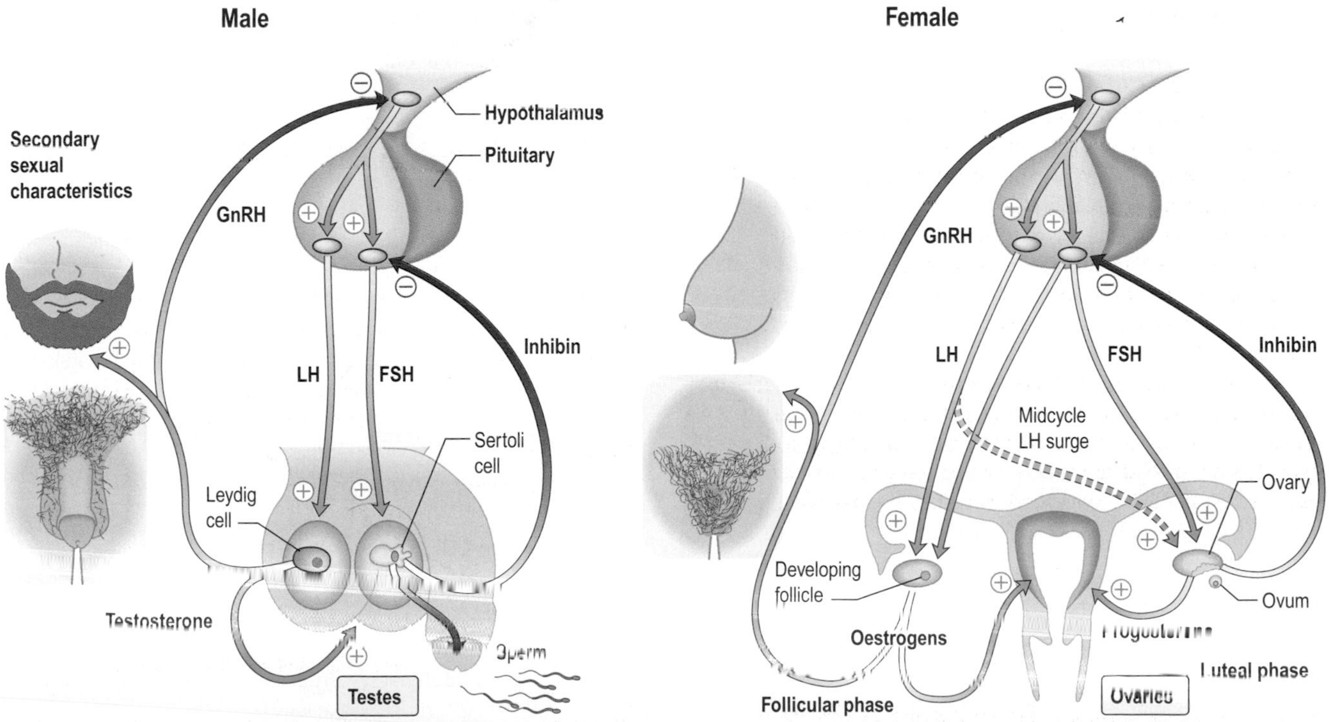

Figure 26.25 Male and female hypothalamic–pituitary–gonadal axes. Luteinizing hormone (LH) and follicle-stimulating hormone (FSH) are secreted in pulses in response to hypothalamic gonadotrophin-releasing hormone (GnRH) and have differential effects on the gonads (see text). Testosterone and oestrogens have multiple peripheral effects and exert negative feedback on LH secretion. Inhibin exerts negative feedback on FSH secretion.

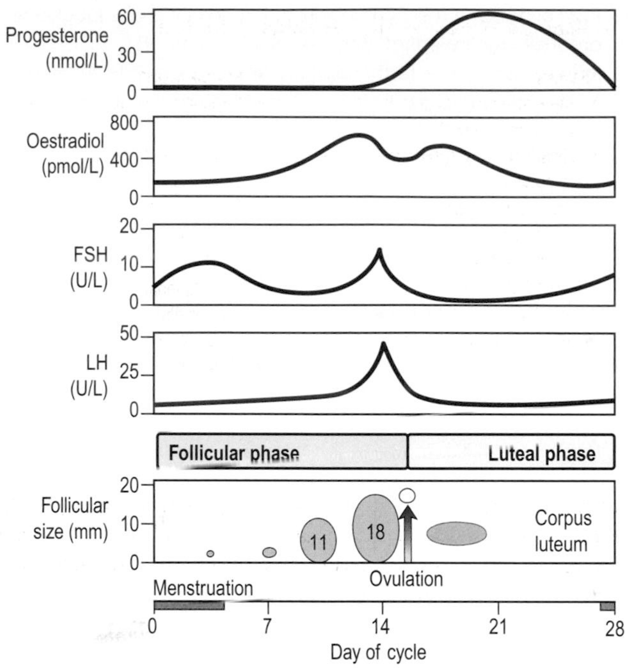

Figure 26.26 Hormonal and follicular changes during the normal menstrual cycle. LH, luteinizing hormone; FSH, follicle-stimulating hormone.

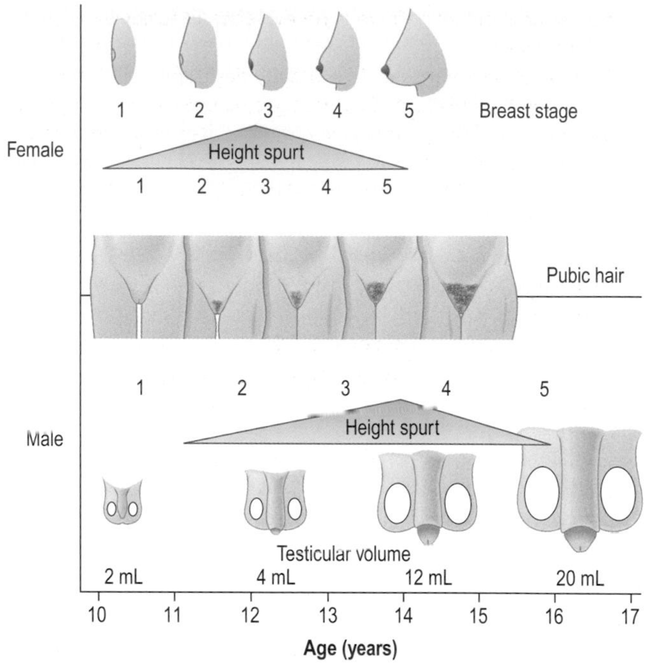

Figure 26.27 The age of development of features of puberty. Stages and testicular size show mean ages, and all vary considerably between individuals. The same is true of the height spurt, shown here in relation to other data. Numbers 2–5 indicate stages of development.

GnRH (positive feedback), which leads to the mid-cycle LH surge, inducing ovulation from the leading follicle ***(Fig. 26.26)***.

7. The follicle then differentiates into a corpus luteum, which secretes both progesterone and oestradiol during the second half of the cycle (luteal phase).
8. Oestrogen initially and then progesterone cause uterine endometrial proliferation in preparation for possible implantation; if implantation does not occur, the corpus luteum regresses and progesterone secretion and inhibin levels fall so that the endometrium is shed (menstruation), allowing increased GnRH and FSH secretion.
9. If implantation and pregnancy follow, human chorionic gonadotrophin (HCG) production from the trophoblast maintains corpus luteum function until 10–12 weeks of gestation, by which time the placenta will be making sufficient oestrogen and progesterone to support itself.

Secondary sexual characteristics

The secondary sexual characteristics of the female are induced by oestrogens, especially development of the breast and nipples, vaginal and vulval growth, and pubic hair development. Oestrogens also induce growth and maturation of the uterus and fallopian tubes. They circulate largely bound to SHBG.

Puberty

The mechanisms initiating puberty are thought to result from withdrawal of central inhibition of GnRH release and involve a complex interplay between hypothalamic peptides, as well as external factors. Environmental and physical factors (including body fat changes and physical exercise) are involved in the timing of puberty, as well as the genetic factors required for pubertal maturation. Kisspeptin is the endogenous ligand for kisspeptin receptor *KISS1R*, formerly known as *GPR54* (a G protein-coupled receptor gene), and this peptide is believed to play a crucial role in the regulation of GnRH production and the timing of puberty.

LH and FSH are both low in the prepubertal child. In early puberty, FSH begins to rise first, initially in nocturnal pulses; this is followed by a rise in LH with a subsequent increase in testosterone/oestrogen levels. The milestones of puberty in the two sexes are shown in ***Figure 26.27***.

In boys, pubertal changes begin with testes enlargement (>4 mL) at 10–14 years and are complete by 15–17 years. The testes enlarge, the genitalia develop and the area of pubic hair increases. Peak height velocity is reached between ages 12 and 17 years during stage 4 of testicular development. Full spermatogenesis occurs comparatively late.

In girls, events start a year earlier. Breast bud enlargement begins at age 9–13 years and continues to 12–18 years. Pubic hair growth commences at ages 9–14 years and is completed at 12–16 years. Menarche occurs relatively late (age 11–15 years) but peak height velocity is reached earlier (at age 10–13 years), and growth is completed much earlier than in boys.

Precocious puberty

Development of secondary sexual characteristics, or menarche in girls before the age of 8 and in boys before the age of 9 years, is premature. True precocious puberty can be divided into gonadotrophin-dependent and gonadotrophin-independent (secondary to exposure to either endogenous or sometimes exogenous sex steroids) types. Gonadotrophin-independent causes can also initiate gonadotrophin-dependent precocious puberty, as is the case in congenital adrenal hyperplasia. All cases require assessment by a paediatric endocrinologist.

True precocious puberty must be distinguished from normal variants:

- ***Premature thelarche***. This is early breast development alone and is usually transient, at age 2–4 years. It may regress or persist until puberty. There is no evidence of follicular development.

- ***Premature adrenarche***. This is early development of pubic hair without significant other changes, usually after the age of 5 years and more commonly in girls. It is also more common in obese children due to reduced SHBG levels, leading to higher free circulating androgens.

Gonadotrophin-dependent precocious puberty

- ***Idiopathic precocity*** is most common in girls and very rare in boys. This is a diagnosis of exclusion. With no apparent cause for premature breast or pubic hair development, and an early growth spurt, it may be normal and may run in families.
- ***Cerebral precocity*** is the mode of presentation of many causes of hypothalamic disease, especially tumours. In boys, these must be rigorously excluded. MRI scan is almost always indicated to exclude this diagnosis.

Gonadotrophin-independent precocious puberty

Causes include testicular or ovarian disorders, such as McCune–Albright syndrome (MAS; see also p. 1240). MAS usually occurs in girls, with precocity, polyostotic fibrous dysplasia and skin pigmentation (café-au-lait patches). HCG-secreting tumours, androgen- and oestrogen-secreting tumours, including teratomas, and congenital adrenal hyperplasia are also important causes of gonadotrophin-independent precocious puberty.

Management

Treatment depends on whether the cause is gonadotrophin-dependent or independent. If the cause is gonadotrophin-dependent, treatment with long-acting GnRH analogues (given by nasal spray, by subcutaneous injection or by implant) causes suppression of gonadotrophin release via downregulation of the receptor – and therefore reduced sex hormone production – and is moderately effective. If the cause is gonadotrophin-independent, inhibitors of steroidogenesis, antiandrogens, and aromatase inhibitors are also used.

Delayed puberty

Over 95% of children show signs of pubertal development by the age of 14 years. In its absence, investigation should begin by the age of 15 years. Causes of hypogonadism (see below) are clearly relevant but most cases represent constitutional delay.

In constitutional delay, pubertal development, bone age and stature are in parallel. A family history may confirm that other family members experienced the same delayed development, which is common in boys but very rare in girls.

In boys, a testicular volume >4 mL indicates the onset of puberty. A rising serum testosterone is an earlier clue.

In girls, the breast bud is the first sign. Ultrasound allows accurate assessment of ovarian and uterine development.

Elevated LH/FSH levels will identify a primary gonadal defect; in other cases, GnRH (LHRH) tests can indicate the stage of early puberty.

If any progression into puberty is evident clinically, investigations are not required. When delay is great and problems are serious (e.g. severe teasing at school), low-dose, short-term sex hormone therapy is used to induce puberty.

Box 26.24 Sexual and menstrual disorders

History

- Menstruation – timing of bleeding and cycle
- Relationship of symptoms to cycle
- Breasts (tenderness/galactorrhoea)
- Hirsutism and acne
- Libido and potency
- Problems with intercourse
- Past fertility and future plans

Physical signs

- Evidence of systemic disease
- Secondary sexual characteristics
- Extent/distribution of hair
- Genital size (testes, ovaries, uterus)
- Clitoromegaly
- Breast development, gynaecomastia
- Galactorrhoea

Clinical features of disorders of sex and reproduction

A detailed history and examination of all systems are required ***(Box 26.24)***. A man having regular satisfactory intercourse or a woman with regular ovulatory periods is most unlikely to have significant endocrine disease, assuming the history is accurate.

Investigation of gonadal function

Much can be deduced from basal measurements of the gonadotrophins, oestrogens/testosterone and prolactin:

- Low testosterone or oestradiol with high gonadotrophins indicates primary gonadal disease.
- Low levels of testosterone/oestradiol with low or normal LH/FSH imply hypothalamic–pituitary disease.
- Demonstration of ovulation (by measurement of luteal phase serum progesterone and/or by serial ovarian ultrasound in the follicular phase) or a healthy sperm count (20–200 million/mL, >60% grade I motility and <20% abnormal forms) provides absolute confirmation of normal female or male reproductive endocrinology, but these tests are not always essential.
- Pregnancy provides complete demonstration of normal male and female function.
- Hyperprolactinaemia can be confirmed or excluded by direct measurement. Levels may increase with stress; if this is suspected, a cannula should be inserted and samples taken through it 30 min later.

More detailed tests are indicated in ***Box 26.25***.

Disorders in the male

Hypogonadism

Clinical features

Male hypogonadism may be a presenting complaint or an incidental finding, such as one that emerges during investigation for subfertility. The testes may be small and soft, and there may be gynaecomastia. Except with subfertility, the symptoms are usually those of androgen deficiency: primarily, poor libido, erectile dysfunction and loss of secondary sexual hair ***(Box 26.26)*** rather than deficiency of semen production. Sperm makes up only a very small proportion of seminal fluid volume; most is prostatic fluid.

Causes of male hypogonadism are shown in ***Box 26.27***.

Investigations

Testicular disease may be immediately apparent but basal levels of testosterone, LH and FSH should be measured. These will allow

Box 26.25 Tests of gonadal function

Test	Uses/comments
Male	
Basal testosterone	Normal levels exclude hypogonadism
Sperm count	Normal count excludes deficiency Motility and abnormal sperm forms should be noted
Female	
Basal oestradiol	Normal levels exclude hypogonadism
Luteal phase progesterone (days 18–24 of cycle)	If >30 nmol/L, suggests ovulation
Ultrasound of ovaries	To confirm ovulation
Both sexes	
Basal LH/FSH	Demonstrates state of feedback system for hormone production (LH) and germ cell production (FSH)
HCG test (testosterone or oestradiol measured)	Response shows potential of ovary or testis; failure demonstrates primary gonadal problem
Clomifene test (LH and FSH measured)	Tests hypothalamic negative feedback system; clomifene is oestrogen antagonist and causes LH/FSH to rise
LHRH test (rarely used)	Shows adequacy (or otherwise) of LH and FSH stores in pituitary

FSH, follicle-stimulating hormone; HCG, human chorionic gonadotrophin; LH, luteinizing hormone; LHRH, luteinizing hormone-releasing hormone.

Box 26.26 Effects of androgens and consequences of androgen deficiency in the male

Physiological effect	Consequences of deficiency
General	
Maintenance of libido	Loss of libido
Deepening of voice	High-pitched voice (if prepubertal)
Frontotemporal balding	No temporal recession
Facial, axillary and limb hair	Decreased hair
Maintenance of erectile and ejaculatory function	Loss of erections/ejaculation
Pubic hair	
Maintenance of male pattern	Thinning and loss of pubic hair
Testes and scrotum	
Maintenance of testicular size/ consistency (needs gonadotrophins as well)	Small, soft testes
Rugosity of scrotum	Poorly developed penis/scrotum
Stimulation of spermatogenesis	Subfertility
Musculoskeletal	
Epiphyseal fusion	Eunuchoidism (if prepubertal)
Maintenance of muscle bulk and power	Decreased muscle bulk
Maintenance of bone mass	Osteoporosis

the distinction to be made between primary gonadal (testicular) failure and hypothalamic–pituitary disease. Depending on the causes, semen analysis, chromosomal analysis (e.g. to exclude Klinefelter syndrome) and bone age estimation are required.

In clear-cut gonadotrophin deficiency, pituitary MRI scan, prolactin levels and other pituitary function tests are needed. However, equivocal lowering of serum testosterone (7–10 nmol/L) without elevation of gonadotrophins is a relatively common biochemical finding, and is a frequent cause of referral in men with poor libido or erectile dysfunction. Such test results are compatible with mild gonadotrophin deficiency, but may also be seen in acute illness of any cause and often simply represent the lower end of the normal range or the normal circadian rhythm of testosterone when bloods are checked in afternoon or evening surgeries, and in the non-fasting state. Regular use of opiate analgesia may lead to gonadotrophin deficiency and should be considered. 'Anabolic' steroid (i.e. androgen) abuse causes similar biochemical findings and is likely if the patient appears well virilized. People with obesity and diabetes mellitus commonly have low circulating SHBG levels associated with insulin resistance and therefore low total testosterone levels.

Box 26.27 Causes of male hypogonadism

- Reduced gonadotrophins (hypothalamic–pituitary disease):
  - Hypopituitarism
  - Selective gonadotrophic deficiency, Kallmann syndrome, normosmic idiopathic hypogonadotropic hypogonadism
  - Severe systemic illness
  - Severe underweight
- Hyperprolactinaemia:
- Primary gonadal disease (congenital):
  - Anorchia/Leydig cell agenesis
  - Cryptorchidism (testicular maldescent)
  - Chromosome abnormality (e.g. Klinefelter syndrome)
  - Enzyme defects: 5α-reductase deficiency
- Primary gonadal disease (acquired):
  - Testicular torsion
  - Orchidectomy
  - Local testicular disease
  - Chemotherapy/radiation toxicity
  - Orchitis (e.g. mumps)
  - Chronic kidney disease
  - Cirrhosis/alcohol
  - Sickle cell disease
- Androgen receptor deficiency/abnormality

A therapeutic trial of testosterone replacement is often justified and forms part of the investigation in some patients; full pituitary evaluation may be required in such cases to exclude other pituitary disease.

Management

The cause of hypogonadism can rarely be reversed and testosterone replacement therapy should be commenced to control current symptoms and prevent osteoporosis in the long term. Replacement is usually given by transdermal gel or by intramuscular injection ***(Box 26.28)***. In gonadotrophin deficiency, LH and FSH (purified or synthetic) or pulsatile GnRH may be used when fertility is required.

Special instances of hypogonadism

Cryptorchidism

Cryptorchidism (or undescended testes) is usually treated by surgical exploration and orchidopexy in early childhood. After that age, the germinal epithelium is increasingly at risk, and lack of descent by puberty is associated with subfertility. A short trial of HCG occasionally induces descent; an HCG test with a testosterone response 72 h later excludes anorchia. Intra-abdominal testes have an increased risk of developing malignancy; if presentation is after puberty, orchidectomy is advised. Patients may present in adulthood with primary testicular failure (due to the testicular damage before or during surgery) or gonadotrophin deficiency (presumably the initial cause of maldescent).

Box 26.28 Androgen replacement therapy

Route	Preparation	Dose	Remarks
Dermal	Testosterone gel Testosterone patch	50–100 mg 300 μg/24 h	Rubs on shoulders Self-adhesive
Intramuscular	Testosterone enanthate Testosterone undecanoate Testosterone propionate	250 mg every 3 weeks 1 g every 3 months 50–100 mg every 2–3 weeks	Frequent injections Painful Large-volume injection Very frequent injections Short half-life
Oral	Testosterone undecanoate	120–160 mg daily, in divided doses	Variable dose, irregular absorption
Implant	Testosterone implant	600 mg every 4–5 months	Requires implant procedure Scarring, infection

Klinefelter syndrome

Klinefelter syndrome is a common congenital abnormality, affecting 1 in 1000 males. It is a chromosomal disorder (47XXY and variants, e.g. 46XY/47XXY mosaicism, i.e. a male with an extra X chromosome). There is both a loss of Leydig cells and seminiferous tubular dysgenesis. Patients usually present in adolescence with poor sexual development, small or undescended testes, gynaecomastia or infertility. In 47XXY, there is long leg length with tall stature, as the androgen deficiency leads to lack of epiphyseal closure in puberty. Patients occasionally have behavioural problems and learning difficulties. There is also a predisposition to diabetes mellitus, breast cancer, emphysema and bronchiectasis; these are all unrelated to the testosterone deficiency.

Clinical examination shows a wide spectrum of features with small, pea-sized but firm testes, usually gynaecomastia and other signs of ***androgen deficiency***. Some patients have a normal puberty and may present later with infertility. Confirmation is by chromosomal analysis.

Treatment is androgen replacement therapy unless testosterone levels are normal. No treatment is possible for the abnormal seminiferous tubules and infertility.

Kallmann syndrome

This is isolated GnRH deficiency. It is associated with decreased or absent sense of smell (anosmia), and sometimes with other bony (cleft palate), renal and cerebral abnormalities (e.g. colour blindness). It is often familial and is usually X-linked, resulting from a mutation in the *KAL1* gene, which encodes anosmin-1 (producing loss of smell); one sex-linked form is due to an abnormality of a cell adhesion molecule. Management is that of secondary hypogonadism (see pp. 1216–1217). Fertility is possible.

Normosmic idiopathic hypogonadotropic hypogonadism

This refers to isolated GnRH deficiency in the absence of anosmia. Known mutations account for less than 15% of normosmic idiopathic hypogonadotropic hypogonadism (nIHH). Mutations include the *KISS1* gene, which codes for kisspeptin, the protein that acts on the GPR54 receptor, and the *FGFR1* gene.

Oligospermia and azoospermia

These may be secondary to gonadotrophin deficiency and can be corrected by gonadotrophin therapy. More often, they result from primary testicular diseases, in which case they are rarely treatable.

Azoospermia with normal testicular size and low FSH levels suggests a vas deferens block, which is sometimes reversible by surgical intervention.

Lack of libido and erectile dysfunction

Lack of libido is a loss of sexual desire; erectile dysfunction (ED) is inability to achieve or maintain erection; they may occur together or separately, and each can precipitate the other. Both are common symptoms in hypogonadism, but most people with either symptom have normal hormones and many have no definable organic cause. ED may be psychological, neurogenic, vascular, endocrine or related to drugs, and often includes contributions from several causes. Vascular disease is a common aetiology, especially in smokers, and is often associated with vascular problems elsewhere. Autonomic neuropathy, most commonly from diabetes mellitus, is a common contributory cause (see pp. 1271–1272) and many drugs produce ED. The endocrine causes are those of hypogonadism (see above) and can be excluded by normal testosterone, gonadotrophin and prolactin levels. The presence of nocturnal emissions and frequent satisfactory morning erections make endocrine disease unlikely.

Psychogenic erectile dysfunction is frequently a diagnosis of exclusion, though complex tests of penile vasculature and function are available in some centres.

Management

Offending drugs should be stopped. Phosphodiesterase type-5 inhibitors (sildenafil, tadalafil, vardenafil), which increase penile blood flow (see pp. 1271–1272), are first choice for therapy. Other treatments include apomorphine, intracavernosal injections of alprostadil, papaverine or phentolamine, vacuum expanders and penile implants.

If no organic disease is found or if there is clear evidence of psychological problems, the couple should receive psychosexual counselling.

Further reading

Shamloul R, Ghanem H. Erectile dysfunction. *Lancet* 2013; 381:153–165.

Gynaecomastia

Gynaecomastia is development of breast tissue in the male. Causes are shown in Box 26.29. It is due to an imbalance between free oestrogen and free androgen effects on breast tissue.

Pubertal gynaecomastia

This occurs in perhaps 50% of normal boys, often asymmetrically. It usually resolves spontaneously within 6–18 months, but after this duration may require surgical removal, as fibrous tissue will have been laid down. The cause is thought to be relative oestrogen

Box 26.29 Causes of gynaecomastia

- Physiological
  - Neonatal
  - Pubertal
  - Old age
- Hyperthyroidism
- Hyperprolactinaemia
- Renal disease
- Liver disease
- Hypogonadism (see Box 26.27)
- Oestrogen-producing tumours (testis, adrenal)
- HCG-producing tumours (testis, lung)
- Starvation/refeeding
- Carcinoma of breast
- Drugs
  - Oestrogenic: oestrogens, digoxin, cannabis, diamorphine
  - Antiandrogens: spironolactone, cimetidine, cyproterone
  - Others: gonadotrophins, cytotoxics

HCG, human chorionic gonadotrophin.

excess, and the oestrogen antagonist tamoxifen is occasionally helpful.

Gynaecomastia in the older male

This requires a full assessment to exclude potentially serious underlying disease, such as bronchial carcinoma and testicular tumours (e.g. Leydig cell tumour). However, aromatase activity (see p. 1213) increases with age and may be the cause of gynaecomastia in this group. Aromatase is an enzyme of the cytochrome P450 family and converts androgens to produce oestrogens. Drug effects are common (especially digoxin and spironolactone), and once these and significant liver disease are excluded, most cases have no definable cause. Painful gynaecomastia may be treated with a 3–6-month trial of tamoxifen, and surgery is occasionally necessary if the symptoms or cosmetic appearance are unacceptable.

The ageing male

In the male, there is no sudden 'change of life'. However, there is a progressive loss of sexual function with reduction in morning erections and frequency of intercourse.

The age of onset varies widely. Typically, overall testicular volume diminishes and SHBG and gonadotrophin levels gradually rise, but other men present with low or borderline testosterone without elevation of LH/FSH. Low testosterone certainly increases the risk of osteoporosis and, in some studies, is associated with increased cardiovascular risk. It remains unclear to what extent general symptoms of lack of energy, drive, muscle strength and general wellbeing may relate to these hormonal changes, but a recent trial of testosterone replacement showed no benefit in general symptoms although there was an improvement in sexual function. Loss of libido and erectile dysfunction are, however, common symptoms, even when hormones are normal, and long-term outcome studies of testosterone replacement are still awaited. Therefore, the decision to offer testosterone replacement to an ageing male is currently based on full clinical and biochemical assessment and full discussion of potential risks (including prostate disease) as well as benefits. If testosterone is unequivocally low (<7 pmol/L) and there are symptoms specific to androgen deficiency (low libido, erectile dysfunction and loss of early morning erections), most authorities would recommend replacement. However, few would treat if testosterone is >12 pmol/L with normal LH/FSH. Clinically, a large proportion of cases are in the borderline range (7–12 pmol/L), which can lead to difficulties in reaching a firm diagnosis. There is an increasing move towards measuring fasting testosterone levels, as food intake may decrease testosterone, leading to an incorrect diagnosis of androgen deficiency.

Disorders in the female

Hypogonadism

Impaired ovarian function, whether primary or secondary, will lead to both oestrogen deficiency and abnormalities of the menstrual cycle. The latter is very sensitive to disruption, cycles becoming anovulatory and irregular before disappearing altogether. Symptoms will depend on the age at which failure develops. Thus, before puberty, primary amenorrhoea will occur, possibly with delayed puberty; after puberty, secondary amenorrhoea and hypogonadism will result.

Oestrogen deficiency

The physiological effects of oestrogens and symptoms/signs of deficiency are shown in ***Box 26.30***.

Amenorrhoea

Absence of periods or markedly irregular infrequent periods (oligomenorrhoea) is the most common presentation of female gonadal disease. The clinical assessment of such patients is shown in ***Box 26.31***, and common causes are listed in ***Box 26.32***. Causes can be divided into whether amenorrhoea is associated with oestrogen deficiency or not, whether it is associated with another condition, whether oestrogen deficiency is due to gonadotrophin deficiency or ovarian damage, and whether amenorrhoea is due to structural problems.

Polycystic ovary syndrome

Polycystic ovary syndrome is an example of amenorrhoea that is not associated with oestrogen deficiency. It is the most common cause of oligomenorrhoea and amenorrhoea (see below).

Box 26.30 Effects of oestrogens and consequences of oestrogen deficiency

Physiological effect	Consequences of deficiency
Breast	
Development of connective and duct tissue	Small, atrophic breast
Nipple enlargement and areolar pigmentation	
Pubic hair	
Maintenance of female pattern	Thinning and loss of pubic hair
Vulva and vagina	
Vulval growth	Atrophic vulva
Vaginal glandular and epithelial proliferation	Atrophic vagina
Vaginal lubrication	Dry vagina and dyspareunia
Uterus and tubes	
Myometrial and tubal hypertrophy	Small, atrophic uterus and tubes
Endometrial proliferation	Amenorrhoea
Skeletal	
Epiphyseal fusion	Eunuchoidism (if prepubertal)
Maintenance of bone mass	Osteoporosis

Box 26.31 Clinical assessment of amenorrhoea

History
- ? Pregnant
- Date of onset
- Age of menarche, if any
- Sudden or gradual onset
- General health
- Weight – absolute and changes in recent past
- Stress (job, lifestyle, examinations, relationships)
- Excessive exercise
- Drugs
- Hirsutism, acne, virilization
- Headaches/visual symptoms
- Sense of smell
- Past history of pregnancies
- Past history of gynaecological surgery

Examination
- General health
- Body shape and skeletal abnormalities
- Weight and height
- Hirsutism and acne
- Evidence of virilization
- Maturity of secondary sexual characteristics
- Galactorrhoea
- Normality of vagina, cervix and uterus

Hypothalamic and weight-related amenorrhoea

Amenorrhoea with low oestrogen and gonadotrophins in the absence of organic pituitary disease is described as hypothalamic amenorrhoea. This may be related to 'stress'; low body weight, excessive exercise or previous weight loss; stopping the contraceptive pill; or severe illness. However, some patients appear to have defective cycling mechanisms without apparent explanation.

A minimum body weight is necessary for regular menstruation. While anorexia nervosa is the extreme form of weight loss (see pp. 927–928), amenorrhoea is common and may be seen at weights within the 'normal' range. It is possible that alterations in leptin levels are responsible for the hypothalamic dysfunction seen in this situation. Restoration of body weight to above the 50th centile for height is usually effective in restoring menstruation, but in the many cases where this cannot be achieved then oestrogen replacement is necessary.

Box 26.32 Differential diagnosis and investigation of amenorrhoea

Hormone results					Possible diagnoses	Secondary tests
LH	*FSH*	*E2*	*PRL*	*T*		
↑	↑	↓	N	N	**Ovarian failure** Ovarian dysgenesis[a] Premature ovarian failure[a] Steroid biosynthetic defect[a] (Oophorectomy) (Chemotherapy) Resistant ovary syndrome	Karyotype Ultrasound of ovary/uterus Laparoscopy/biopsy of ovary HCG stimulation
↓	↓	↓	N	N	**Gonadotrophin failure** Hypothalamic–pituitary disease[a] Kallmann syndrome/nIHH[a] Possible hypothalamic causes: Hypothalamic amenorrhoea[a] Weight-related amenorrhoea[a] Exercise-induced amenorrhoea and anorexia[a] Post-pill amenorrhoea General illness[a]	Pituitary MRI if diagnosis unclear Possibly LHRH test Serum free T_4 Possibly full assessment of pituitary function
↓	↓	↓	↑/↑↑	N	**Hyperprolactinaemia** Prolactinoma[a] Idiopathic hyperprolactinaemia[a] Hypothyroidism[a] Polycystic ovarian disease[a] Physiological in lactation Dopamine antagonist drugs	See pages 1194–1197 (hyperprolactinaemia) Serum free T_4/TSH Pituitary MRI Other tests for PCOS
↑/N	N	N	N/↑	N/↑	**Polycystic ovary syndrome[a]** Rarely, Cushing syndrome	Androstenedione, DHEAS SHBG Ultrasound of ovary Progesterone challenge See pages 1197–1199 (Cushing syndrome)
N/↓	N/↓	N/↓	N	↑↑	**Androgen excess** Gonadal or adrenal tumour Congenital adrenal hyperplasia[a]	Imaging ovary/adrenal 17a-OH-progesterone
N	N	↑	↑	N	**Pregnancy**	Pregnancy test
N	N	N	N	N	**Uterine/vaginal abnormality** Imperforate hymen[a] Absent uterus[a] Lack of endometrium	Examination findings (?EUA) Ultrasound of pelvis Progesterone challenge Hysteroscopy

[a]These conditions may present as primary amenorrhoea.
DHEAS, dehydroepiandrosterone sulphate; E2, oestradiol; EUA, examination under anaesthesia; FSH, follicle-stimulating hormone; HCG, human chorionic gonadotrophin; LH, luteinizing hormone; LHRH, luteinizing hormone-releasing hormone; nIHH, normosmic idiopathic hypogonadotropic hypogonadism; PCOS, polycystic ovary syndrome; PRL, prolactin; SHBG, sex hormone-binding globulin; T, testosterone.

Premature menopause and ovarian failure

The most common cause of premature menopause and, with it, amenorrhoea in women (before age 40) is ovarian failure. This may be autoimmune, and is rarely caused by identifiable genetic causes such as the fragile X pre-mutation or Turner syndrome; most commonly, however, it is of unknown aetiology, although often familial. Repeat measurements of LH/FSH levels are necessary before a diagnosis of premature menopause is given because of the psychological impact of this diagnosis and the possibility that a single elevation of LH/FSH might simply be the mid-cycle ovulatory surge. Bilateral oophorectomy and some chemotherapy regimens cause the same oestrogen deficiency state. In some scenarios, ovarian function can fluctuate; therefore, in younger women, consideration needs to be given as to whether contraception is required, and the combined oral contraceptive pill is the best option for hormone replacement therapy (HRT).

Turner syndrome (see p. 1224) is a cause of primary amenorrhoea. The phenotype is female with female external genitalia. There is gonadal dysgenesis with streak ovaries. Features include short stature, webbing of the neck (up to 40%), a wide carrying angle of the elbows, high-arched palate and low-set ears. These patients also have an increased incidence of autoimmune disease (2%), bicuspid aortic valves, aortic coarctation and dissection, coronary artery disease, hypertension, type 2 diabetes, horseshoe kidneys, lymphoedema, reduced bone density, hearing problems and inflammatory bowel disease (0.3%).

Investigation of oligo-amenorrhoea

Basal levels of FSH, LH, oestrogen and prolactin allow initial distinction between primary gonadal and hypothalamic–pituitary causes ***(Box 26.32)***. Elevation of LH and FSH to menopausal levels usually confirms the diagnosis. Subsequent investigations are also shown in ***Box 26.32***.

Management

Treatment is that of the cause wherever possible (e.g. hypothyroidism, low weight, stress, excessive exercise). Hyperprolactinaemia should be corrected (see below). Polycystic ovary syndrome is discussed in detail below.

When oestrogen deficiency is not reversed, HRT should almost always be given, as the risk of osteoporosis and other conditions related to oestrogen deficiency almost always outweighs the risks of HRT at this younger age. HRT may still also be actively recommended when normal menopause occurs relatively early (e.g. before the age of 50). In some women, in whom ovarian function may recover or fluctuate, consideration should be given to using the combined oral contraceptive pill if fertility is not desired.

In cases of gonadotrophin deficiency, gonadotrophins can be given to achieve ovulation. Primary ovarian disease is rarely treatable except in the rare condition of 'resistant' ovary, where high-dose gonadotrophin therapy can occasionally lead to folliculogenesis.

Hirsutism

Normal hair versus hirsutism

The extent of normal hair growth varies between individuals, families and races, being more extensive in the Mediterranean and some Asian subcontinent populations. These normal variations in body hair, and the more extensive hair growth seen in patients complaining of hirsutism, represent a continuum from no visible hair to extensive cover with thick, dark hair. It is therefore impossible to draw an absolute dividing line between 'normal' and 'abnormal' degrees of facial and body hair in the female. Soft vellus hair is normally present all over the body; this type of hair on the face and elsewhere is 'normal' and is not sex hormone-dependent. Hair in the beard, moustache, breast, chest, axilla, abdominal midline, pubic and thigh areas is sex hormone-dependent. Any excess in the latter regions is thus a marker of increased ovarian or adrenal androgen production: most commonly, polycystic ovary syndrome (PCOS) but occasionally other rarer causes.

Aetiology

- ***Idiopathic hirsutism***. People with hirsutism, no elevation of serum androgen levels and no other clinical features are sometimes labelled as having 'idiopathic hirsutism'. However, studies suggest that most people with 'idiopathic hirsutism' have some radiological or biochemical evidence of PCOS on more detailed investigation, and several studies have demonstrated evidence of mild PCOS in up to 20% of the normal female population. Familial or idiopathic hirsutism does occur, but usually involves a distribution of hair growth that is not typically androgenic.
- ***Ovarian hyperthecosis***. This is a non-malignant ovarian disorder characterized by luteinized thecal cells in the ovarian stroma, which secrete testosterone. The clinical features are similar to those of PCOS but tend to present in perimenopausal women, and serum testosterone levels are higher than typically seen in PCOS.
- ***Iatrogenic hirsutism***. This occurs after treatment with androgens, or more weakly androgenic drugs such as progestogens or danazol.
- ***Non-androgen-dependent hair growth (hypertrichosis)***. This occurs with drugs such as phenytoin, diazoxide, minoxidil and ciclosporin.
- ***Other causes***. Rarer and more serious endocrine causes of hirsutism and virilization include congenital adrenal hyperplasia (CAH; see pp. 1228–1229), Cushing syndrome (pp. 1197–1199), and androgen-secreting (virilizing) tumours of the ovary and adrenal.

Management

See page 1222.

Polycystic ovary syndrome

Polycystic ovary syndrome (PCOS) is the most common cause of hirsutism in clinical practice, affecting about 1 in 5 women worldwide. It is characterized by multiple small cysts within the ovary ***(Fig. 26.28)*** (which represent arrested follicular development) and by excess androgen production from the ovaries (and to a lesser extent from the adrenals).

Measured levels of androgens in blood vary widely from patient to patient and may remain within the normal range, but SHBG levels are often low (due to high insulin levels), leading to high free androgen levels. In PCOS, there is thought to be an increased frequency of the GnRH pulse generator, causing an increase in LH pulses and androgen secretion. The response of the hair follicle to circulating androgens also seems to vary between individuals with otherwise identical clinical and biochemical features, and the reason for this variation in end-organ response remains poorly understood.

PCOS is frequently associated with:

- ***hyperinsulinaemia and insulin resistance***, the prevalence of type 2 diabetes being 10 times higher than in normal women

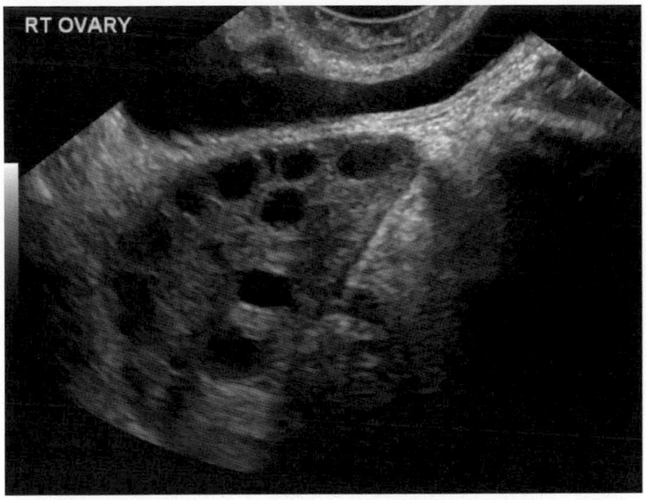

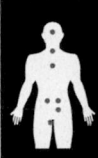

Figure 26.28 **Polycystic ovary syndrome.** Ultrasound of the ovary, revealing multiple cysts with central ovarian stroma showing increased echo texture.

- ***hypertension, hyperlipidaemia and increased cardiovascular risk*** (the metabolic syndrome; see p. 209), which is 2–3 times higher in PCOS, and studies suggest that PCOS *per se* confers an absolute increase in cardiovascular end-points.

Obesity with PCOS is an additional risk factor for insulin resistance. The precise mechanisms that link the aetiology of polycystic ovaries, hyperandrogenism, anovulation and insulin resistance are still to be elucidated, and whether the basic defect is in the ovary, adrenal or pituitary, or is a more generalized metabolic defect, remains unknown. Frequently, there is a family history of either PCOS or type 2 diabetes, suggesting a genetic component.

In routine clinical practice, the majority of people with objective signs of androgen-dependent hirsutism will have PCOS, and investigation is mainly required to exclude rarer and more serious causes of virilization.

Clinical features

Most patients with PCOS present with amenorrhoea/oligomenorrhoea and/or hirsutism and acne, shortly after menarche. Frequently, patients are also obese with evidence of insulin resistance. Clinical, biochemical and radiological features of PCOS merge imperceptibly into those of the normal populations.

- ***Hirsutism***. This should be recorded objectively, ideally using a scoring system, both to document the problem and to monitor treatment. The method and frequency of physical removal (e.g. shaving, plucking) should also be recorded. The development of hirsutism commonly provokes severe distress in young women and may lead to avoidance of normal social activities. Most patients who complain of hirsutism will have an objective excess of hair on examination, but occasionally very little will be found (and appropriate counselling is then indicated).
- ***Age and speed of onset***. Hirsutism related to PCOS usually begins around the time of the menarche and increases slowly and steadily in the teens and twenties. Rapid progression and prepubertal or late onset suggest a more serious cause.
- ***Accompanying virilization***. Hirsutism due to PCOS may be severe and affect all androgen-dependent areas on the face and body. However, more severe virilization (clitoromegaly, recent-onset frontal balding, male phenotype) implies substantial androgen excess, and usually indicates a rarer cause rather than PCOS. Thinning of head hair in a male pattern – androgenic alopecia – occurs in a proportion of women with uncomplicated PCOS, typically with a familial tendency for premature androgen-related hair loss in both sexes.
- ***Menstruation***. Most people with PCOS will have some disturbance of menstruation, typically oligo-/amenorrhoea, although more frequent erratic bleeding can also occur. However, PCOS can present as hirsutism with regular periods or as irregular periods, with no evidence of hirsutism or acne.
- ***Weight***. Many people with PCOS are also overweight or obese. The obesity worsens the underlying androgen excess and insulin resistance, and inhibits the response to treatment; it is an indication for appropriate advice on diet and exercise. In severe cases, the insulin resistance may have a visible manifestation as acanthosis nigricans on the neck and in the axillae. In addition to worsening the symptoms of PCOS, central obesity in PCOS significantly increases the likelihood of developing diabetes and cardiovascular disease.

Investigations and differential diagnosis

- ***Serum total testosterone***. This is often elevated in PCOS and is invariably substantially raised in virilizing tumours (usually >5 nmol/L). People with hirsutism and normal testosterone levels frequently have low levels of SHBG, leading to high free androgen levels. The ***free androgen index*** ([testosterone/SHBG] *100) is often used and is high; free testosterone is difficult to measure directly.
- ***Other androgens***. Androstenedione and dehydroepiandrosterone sulphate are frequently elevated in PCOS, and even higher in congenital adrenal hyperplasia (CAH) and virilizing tumours.
- ***17α-Hydroxyprogesterone***. This is elevated in classical CAH, but may be apparent in late-onset CAH only after stimulation tests.
- ***Gonadotrophin levels***. LH hypersecretion is a frequent feature of PCOS, but the pulsatile nature of secretion of this hormone means that a 'classic' increased LH/FSH ratio is not always observed on a random sample.
- ***Oestrogen levels***. Oestradiol is usually normal in PCOS, but oestrone levels (which are rarely measured) are elevated because of peripheral conversion. Levels are variable in other causes.
- ***Ovarian ultrasound***. This is a useful investigation ***(Fig. 26.28)***. Typical features are those of a thickened capsule, multiple 3–5 mm cysts and a hyperechogenic stroma. Prolonged hyperandrogenization from any cause may lead to polycystic changes in the ovary. Ultrasound may also reveal virilizing ovarian tumours, although these are often small.
- ***Serum prolactin***. Mild hyperprolactinaemia is common in PCOS but rarely exceeds 1500 mU/L.

If an androgen-secreting tumour is suspected clinically or after investigation, then more complex investigations include dexamethasone suppression tests, CT or MRI of adrenals, and selective venous sampling.

Diagnosis

Most patients presenting with a combination of hirsutism and menstrual disturbance will be shown to have PCOS, but the rarer alternative diagnoses should be excluded; the latter include late-onset CAH (early onset, raised serum 17α-hydroxyprogesterone), Cushing syndrome (look for other clinical features), and virilizing tumours of the ovary or adrenals (severe virilization, markedly elevated serum testosterone).

The consensus (***Rotterdam***) ***criteria 2003*** for diagnosis of PCOS are at least two of the following:

- clinical and/or biochemical evidence of hyperandrogenism
- oligo-ovulation and/or anovulation
- polycystic ovaries on ultrasound.

Management

Local therapy for hirsutism

Regular plucking, bleaching, use of depilatory cream, waxing or shaving is used. Such removal neither worsens nor improves the underlying severity of hirsutism. More 'permanent' solutions include electrolysis and a variety of 'laser' hair removal systems; all appear effective but have not been evaluated in long-term studies, are expensive, and still often require repeated long-term treatment. ***Eflornithine cream*** (an antiprotozoal) inhibits hair growth by inhibiting ornithine decarboxylase, but is effective in only a minority of cases and should be discontinued if there is no improvement after 4 months.

Systemic therapy for hirsutism

This always requires a year or more of treatment for maximal benefit, and long-term therapy is frequently required as the problem tends to recur when treatment is stopped. The patient must therefore always be an active participant in the decision to use systemic therapy and must understand the rare risks as well as the benefits. Weight loss should also be encouraged, as many patients have improvement in symptoms.

- ***Oestrogens*** (e.g. oral contraceptives) suppress ovarian androgen production and reduce free androgens by increasing SHBG levels. Combined hormone pills, which contain ethinylestradiol and a non-androgenic progestogen – e.g. desogestrel drospirenone, or cyproterone acetate plus ethinylestradiol (co-cyprindiol) – will produce a slow improvement in hirsutism in a majority of cases and should normally be used first unless there is a contraindication, such as a history of thrombosis. The risk of venous thrombosis appears to be 2–4-fold higher than with other low-dose oral contraceptive pills. After the menopause, HRT preparations that contain medroxyprogesterone (rather than more androgenic progestogens) may be helpful.
- ***Cyproterone acetate*** (50–100 mg daily) is an antiandrogen but is also a progestogen, teratogen and a weak glucocorticoid. Given continuously, it produces amenorrhoea, and so is normally given for days 1–14 of each cycle. In women of childbearing age, contraception is essential.
- ***Spironolactone*** (200 mg daily) also has antiandrogen activity and can cause useful improvements in hirsutism. In women of childbearing age, contraception is essential.
- ***Finasteride*** (5 mg daily), a 5α-reductase inhibitor that prevents the formation of dihydrotestosterone in the skin, has also been shown to be effective but long-term experience is limited. In women of childbearing age, contraception is essential.
- ***Flutamide***, another antiandrogen, is less commonly used owing to the high incidence of hepatic side-effects. In women of childbearing age, contraception is essential.

Treatment of menstrual disturbance

- ***Cyclical oestrogen/progestogen*** administration will regulate the menstrual cycle and remove the symptom of oligo- or amenorrhoea. This is most frequently an additional benefit of the treatment of hirsutism, but may also be used when menstrual disturbance is the only symptom.
- ***Metformin*** (500 mg three times daily) is commonly used in this condition because of the recognised association between PCOS and insulin resistance. It may improve menstrual cyclicity and ovulation; some patients also report improvement in hirsutism and ease of weight loss, but gastrointestinal upset may limit use.

Treatment for fertility in PCOS

- ***Clomifene*** 50–100 mg is given daily on days 2–6 of the cycle and is effective in 75% of women in achieving ovulation. It can occasionally cause the ***ovarian hyperstimulation syndrome***, an iatrogenic complication of ovulation induction therapy, consisting of ovarian enlargement, oedema, hypovolaemia, acute kidney injury and possibly shock; specialist supervision is essential. It is recommended that clomifene should not normally be used for more than six cycles (owing to a possible increased risk of ovarian cancer in patients treated for longer than recommended).
- ***Low-dose FSH*** is used for non-responders to clomifene.
- ***Metformin*** alone may improve ovulation and achieve conception.

Wedge resection of the ovary was a traditional therapy but is now rarely required, although laparoscopic ovarian electrodiathermy may be helpful.

Subfertility

Subfertility, or 'infertility', is defined as the inability of a couple to conceive after 1 year of unprotected intercourse. Investigation requires the combined skills of gynaecologist, endocrinologist and, ideally, andrologist. Both partners must be involved and every aspect of the physiology critically examined.

Aetiology

A significant proportion of couples have both male and female contributing factors ***(Fig. 26.29)***.

Inadequate intercourse, hostile cervical mucus and vaginal factors are uncommon (5%). Some 15% of cases appear to be idiopathic, and natural fertility decreases with increasing age. Conception over 40 years of age for both males and females is reduced to below 30%.

Male factors

About 30–40% of couples have a major identifiable male factor. There is some evidence that male sperm counts are declining in many populations. Untreated male hypogonadism of any cause (see ***Box 26.27***) is likely to be associated with subfertility.

Female factors

Female tubal problems due to pathologies such as pelvic inflammatory disease and endometriosis account for perhaps 20%; a similar proportion have ovulatory disorders. Any cause of

Female factors				Joint factors	Male factors		
Ovulation	Tubal problems	Uterine problems	Cervix Vaginal problems	Adequate intercourse	Normal sperm count		
PCOS	Patency PID, chlamydia, GC Function	Anatomy e.g. fibroids Implantation	Infection e.g. gonorrhoea Cervical hostility	Frequency Timing Technique	Potency, e.g. hypogonadism	Vas blockage e.g. previous STI	Testicular disease e.g. tumour

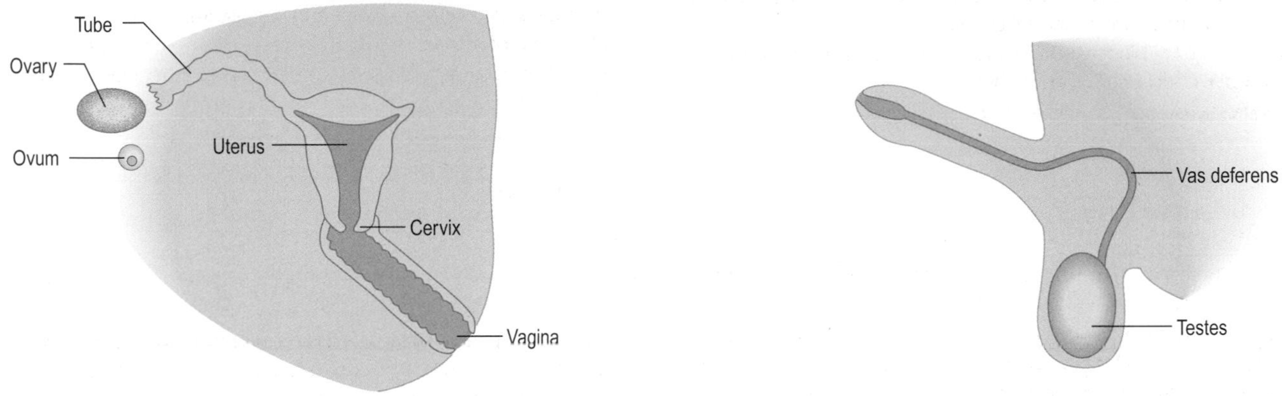

Investigation:				
Pelvic ultrasound; Hysterosalpingogram; Hysteroscopy; Serum progesterone; Laparoscopy / Egg collection	Swabs	History	Semen analysis	Serum LH, FSH Testosterone; Testicular biopsy

Figure 26.29 Major factors involved in subfertility and their investigation. FSH, follicle-stimulating hormone; LH, luteinizing hormone; PCOS, polycystic ovary syndrome; PID, pelvic inflammatory disease; STI, sexually transmitted infection.

oligomenorrhoea or amenorrhoea (see ***Box 26.32***) is likely to be associated with suboptimal ovulation or anovulation.

Clinical features

Both partners should be seen and the following factors checked:

- ***The man***. Look for previous testicular damage (orchitis, trauma), undescended testes, urethral symptoms and evidence of sexually transmitted infection, local surgery, and use of alcohol and drugs. A semen analysis early in the investigations is essential.
- ***The woman***. Look for previous pelvic infection, regularity of periods, previous surgery, alcohol intake, smoking and body weight (see p. 1219).
- ***Together***. Check the frequency and adequacy of intercourse, and the use of lubricants, which may damage sperm and affect their ability to travel to the uterus.

Investigations

See ***Figure 26.29***.

Management

Counselling of both partners is essential. Any defect(s) found should be treated if possible. Ovulation can usually be induced by exogenous hormones if simpler measures fail, while *in vitro* fertilization (IVF) and similar techniques are widely used, especially where there is tubal blockage, oligospermia or 'idiopathic subfertility'. Intracytoplasmic sperm injection (ICSI) appears particularly effective for severe oligospermia and poor sperm function.

Disorders of sexual differentiation

Disorders of sexual differentiation are rare but may affect chromosomal, gonadal, endocrine and phenotypic development ***(Box 26.33)***. Such cases always require extensive, multidisciplinary clinical management. An individual's sex can be defined in several ways:

- ***Chromosomal sex***. The normal female is 46XX, the normal male 46XY. The Y chromosome confers male sex; if it is not present, development follows female lines.
- ***Gonadal sex***. This is determined predominantly by chromosomal sex but requires normal embryological development.
- ***Phenotypic sex***. This describes the normal physical appearance and characteristics of male and female body shape. This, in turn, is a manifestation of gonadal sex and subsequent sex hormone production.
- ***Social sex (gender)***. This is heavily dependent on phenotypic sex and normally assigned on appearance of the external genitalia at birth.
- ***Sexual orientation*** – heterosexual, homosexual or bisexual.

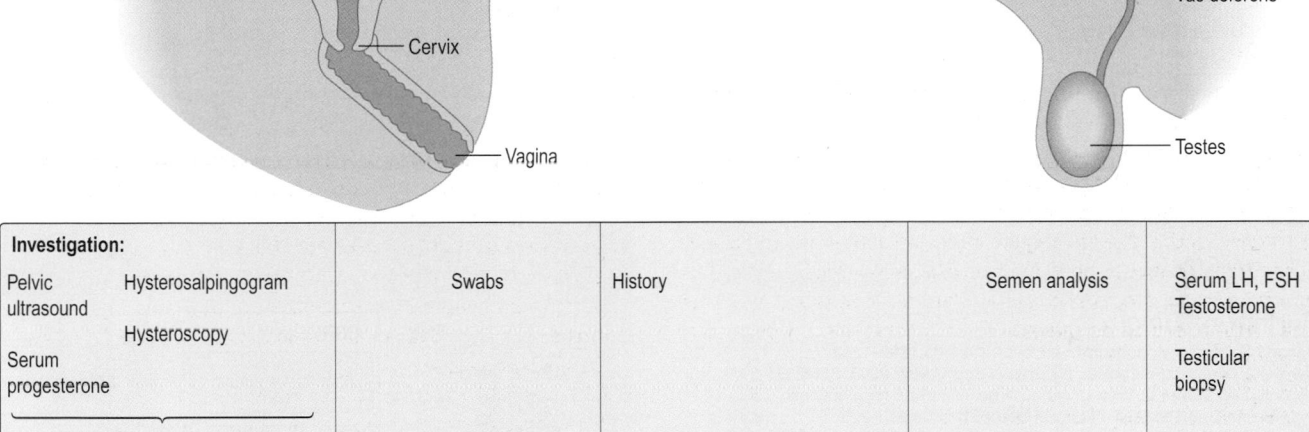

Box 26.33 Disorders of sexual differentiation

Condition	Chromosomes	Gonads	Phenotype	Remarks
Turner syndrome	45X (50%) 46,X,i (Xq) (5–10%) 45,X, mosaicism (remainder)	Streak	Female	Often morphological features (e.g. short stature, web neck, coarctation of aorta)
Gonadal dysgenesis	46XY	Streak or minimal testes[a]	Immature female	
Congenital adrenal hyperplasia	46XX	Ovary	Female with variable virilization	Obvious androgen excess
Virilizing tumour	46XX	Ovary	Female with variable virilization	Obvious androgen excess
True hermaphroditism	46XX/XY or mosaic	Testis and ovary	Male or ambiguous	
Klinefelter syndrome	47XXY	Small testes	Male, often with gynaecomastia	Many are hypogonadal
Testicular feminization	46XY	Testes[a]	Ambiguous or infantile female	Androgen receptor defective
Testicular synthetic defects	46XY	Testes[a]	Cryptorchid, ambiguous	
5α-Reductase deficiency	46XY	Testes	Cryptorchid, ambiguous	Impaired conversion of testosterone to dihydrotestosterone
Anorchia	46XY	Absent	Immature female	

[a]Gonadectomy advised because of high risk of malignancy.
i, isochromosome.

Further reading

Basaria S. Male hypogonadism. *Lancet* 2014; 383:1250–1263.
Carel JC, Léger J. Precocious puberty. *N Engl J Med* 2008; 358:2366–2377.
Caronia LM, Martin C, Welt CK et al. A genetic basis for functional hypothalamic amenorrhea. *N Engl J Med* 2011; 364:215–225.
Gordon CM. Functional hypothalamic amenorrhea. *N Engl J Med* 2010; 363:365–371.
Mani H, Levy MJ, Davies MJ et al. Diabetes and cardiovascular events in women with polycystic ovary syndrome: a 20-year retrospective cohort study. *Clin Endocrinol* 2013; 78:926–934.
Rotterdam ESHRE/ASRM-Sponsored PCOS Consensus Workshop Group. Revised 2003 consensus on diagnostic criteria and long-term health risks related to polycystic ovary syndrome. *Fertil Steril* 2004; 81:19–25.
Snyder PJ, Bhasin S, Cunningham AM et al. Effects of testosterone treatment in older men. *N Engl J Med* 2016; 374:611–624.

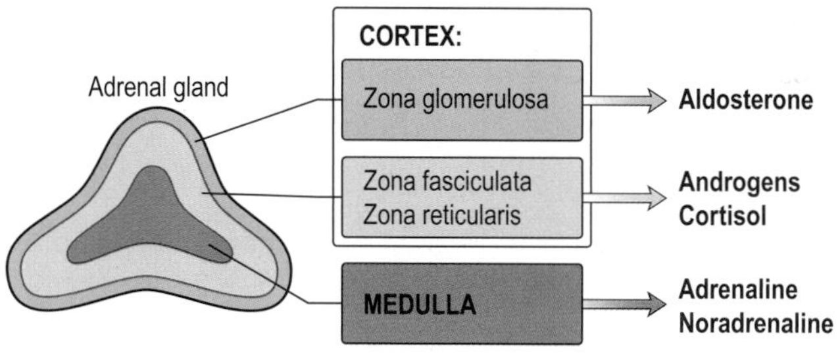

Figure 26.30 The adrenal gland and its hormones.

THE ADRENAL AXIS

Anatomy and function of the adrenal gland

The human adrenals (see ***Box 26.4***) together weigh 8–10 g and comprise an outer cortex and inner medulla. The cortex has three zones: the zona glomerulosa, which secretes aldosterone under the control of the renin–angiotensin system, and the zona reticularis and zona fasciculata, which produce cortisol and androgens under feedback control of the hypothalamic–pituitary–adrenal (HPA) axis. The inner medulla synthesizes, stores and secretes catecholamines (see below and ***Fig. 26.30***).

Box 26.34 The major actions of glucocorticoids

Increased or stimulated	Decreased or inhibited
Gluconeogenesis	Protein synthesis
Glycogen deposition	Host response to infection
Protein catabolism	Lymphocyte transformation
Fat deposition	Delayed hypersensitivity
Sodium retention	Circulating lymphocytes
Potassium loss	Circulating eosinophils
Free water clearance	
Uric acid production	
Circulating neutrophils	

The adrenal cortex

The steroids produced by the adrenal cortex are grouped into three classes, based on their predominant physiological effects: glucocorticoids, mineralocorticoids and androgens.

Glucocorticoids

These are so named after their effects on carbohydrate metabolism. Major actions are listed in ***Box 26.34***. They act on intracellular corticosteroid receptors and combine with coactivating proteins to bind the 'glucocorticoid response element' (GRE) in specific regions of DNA to cause gene transcription. Glucocorticoid action is modified locally by the action of 11β-hydroxysteroid dehydrogenase (11βHSD). 11βHSD type 1 converts inactive cortisone into active cortisol, hence amplifying the hormone signal, whilst 11βHSD type 2 does the opposite.

The relative potency of common steroids is shown in ***Box 26.35***.

Mineralocorticoids

The predominant effect of mineralocorticoids is on the extracellular balance of sodium and potassium in the distal tubule of the kidney. Aldosterone, produced solely in the zona glomerulosa, is the predominant mineralocorticoid in humans (about 50%); corticosterone makes a small contribution to overall mineralocorticoid activity. Mineralocorticoids act on type 1 corticosteroid receptors, whilst glucocorticoids act on type 2 receptors, both having a very similar structure. The mineralocorticoid activity of cortisol is weak but cortisol is present in considerable excess. The mineralocorticoid receptor in the kidney is largely protected from this excess by the intrarenal conversion ('shuttle') of cortisol to cortisone by 11βHSD type 2.

Androgens

Although secreted in considerable quantities, most androgens have only relatively weak intrinsic androgenic activity until metabolized peripherally to testosterone or dihydrotestosterone. Dihydrotestosterone is metabolized from testosterone by 5α-reductase and is a potent androgen receptor agonist. The androgen receptor has been well characterized and mutations within this gene may cause androgen insensitivity syndromes.

Box 26.35 The relative potency of equal amounts of common natural and synthetic steroids

Steroid	Glucocorticoid effect	Mineralocorticoid effect
Cortisol (hydrocortisone)[a]	1	1
Prednisolone	4	0.7
Dexamethasone	40	2
Aldosterone	0.1	400
Fludrocortisone	10	400

[a]Cortisol is arbitrarily defined as 1.

Biochemistry

All steroids have the same basic skeleton ***(Fig. 26.31B)*** and the chemical differences between them are slight. The major biosynthetic pathways are shown in ***Figure 26.31A***.

Physiology

Glucocorticoid production by the adrenal is under hypothalamic–pituitary control ***(Fig. 26.32)***.

Corticotrophin-releasing hormone **(*CRH*)** is secreted in the hypothalamus in response to circadian rhythm, stress and other stimuli. CRH travels down the portal system to stimulate ***adrenocorticotrophin*** **(*ACTH*)** release from the anterior pituitary. Hypothalamic vasopressin (antidiuretic hormone, ADH) also stimulates ACTH secretion and acts synergistically. ACTH is derived from the prohormone pro-opiomelanocortin (POMC), which undergoes complex processing within the pituitary to produce ACTH and a number of other peptides, including beta-lipotrophin and beta-endorphin. Many of these peptides, including ACTH, contain melanocyte-stimulating hormone (MSH)-like sequences, which cause pigmentation when levels of ACTH are markedly raised.

Circulating ACTH stimulates cortisol production in the adrenal. The secreted cortisol (or any other synthetic corticosteroid administered to the patient) causes negative feedback on the hypothalamus and pituitary to inhibit further CRH/ACTH release. The set-point

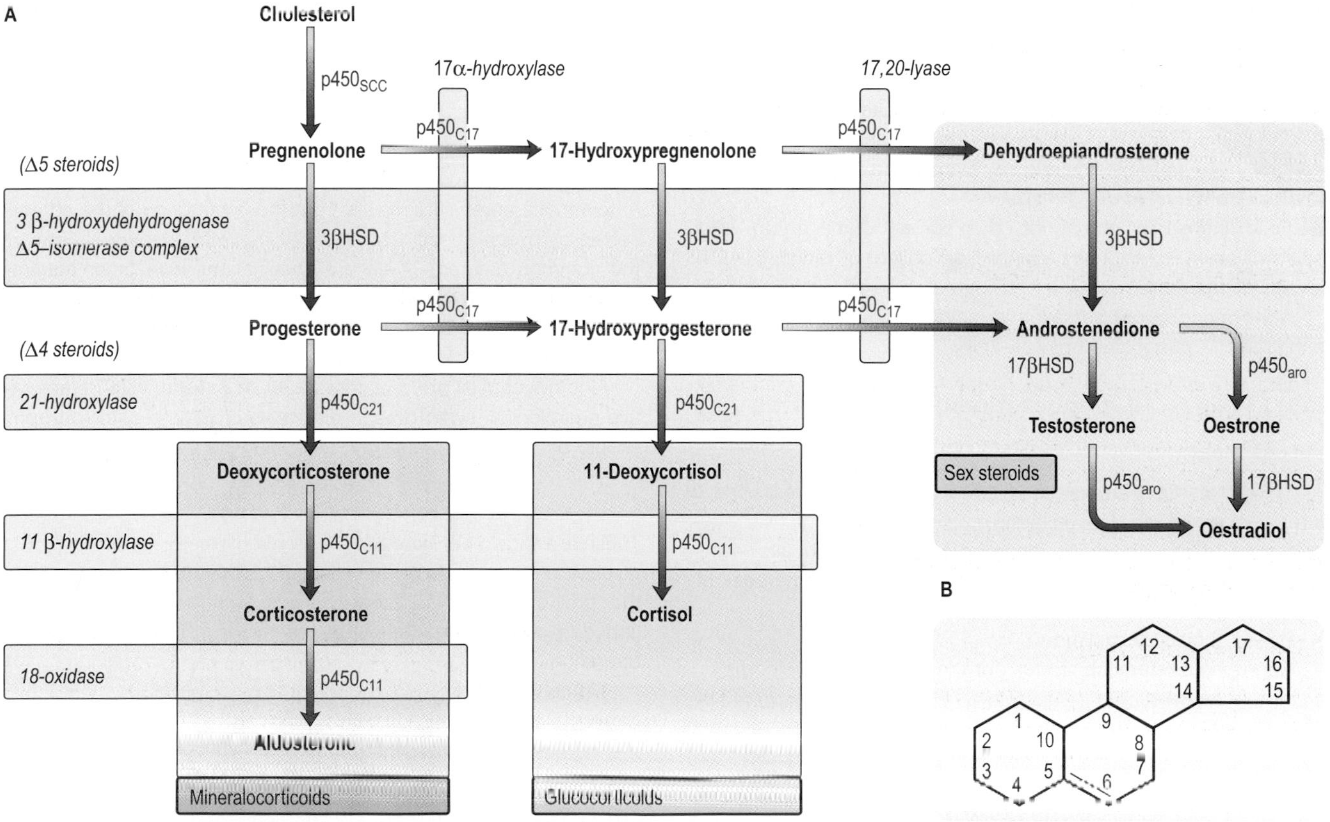

Figure 26.31 Steroid pathways and molecule. A. *The major steroid biosynthetic pathways.* Steroid hormones are synthesized in adrenal and gonads from the initial substrate via a series of interconnected enzymatic steps. The reactions catalysed are shown by shaded boxes with italic labels. The molecular identity of the enzymes is shown in red; some catalyse more than one reaction. The p450 enzymes are in mitochondria, 3β-hydroxysteroid dehydrogenase (3βHSD) in cytoplasm; 17βHSD and $p450_{aro}$ (aromatase) are found mainly in gonads. **B.** *The steroid molecule.*

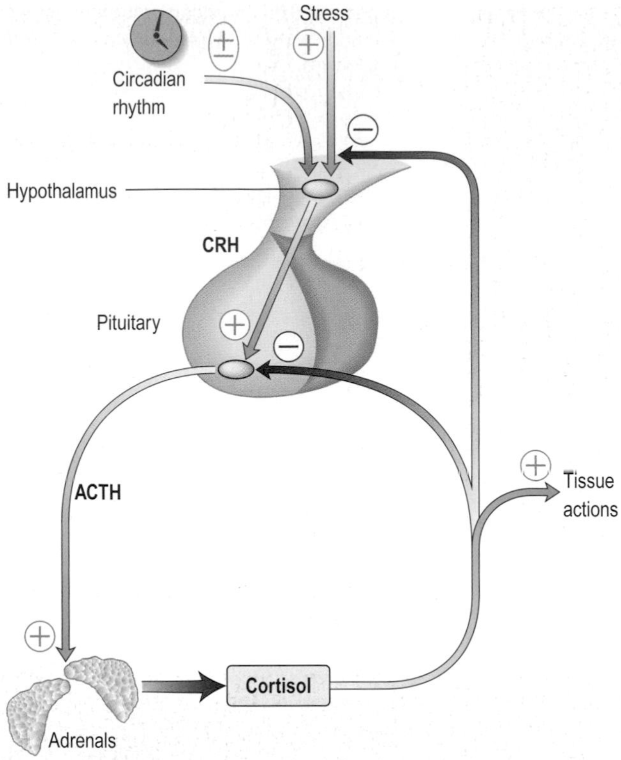

Figure 26.32 Control of the hypothalamic–pituitary–adrenal axis. Pituitary adrenocorticotrophic hormone (ACTH) is secreted in response to hypothalamic corticotrophin-releasing hormone (CRH), triggered by circadian rhythm, stress and other factors, and stimulates secretion of cortisol from the adrenal. Cortisol has multiple actions in peripheral tissues and exerts negative feedback on the pituitary and hypothalamus.

of this system clearly varies through the day according to the circadian rhythm, and is usually overridden by severe stress. Unlike cortisol, mineralocorticoids and sex steroids do not cause negative feedback on the CRH/ACTH axis.

Following adrenalectomy or other adrenal damage (e.g. Addison's disease), cortisol secretion will be absent or reduced; ACTH levels will therefore rise.

Mineralocorticoid secretion is mainly controlled by the renin–angiotensin system (see pp. 727–728).

Investigation of glucocorticoid abnormalities

Basal levels

ACTH and cortisol are released episodically and in response to stress. When taking a blood sample, remember:

- Sampling time should be recorded. Basal levels should be taken between 08:00 hours and 09:00 hours, near the peak of the circadian variation.
- Stress should be minimized.
- Appropriate reference ranges (for time and assay method) should be used.

Suppression tests are used if excess cortisol is suspected, and stimulation tests are used if cortisol deficiency is suspected.

Dexamethasone suppression tests

Administration of a synthetic glucocorticoid (dexamethasone) to a normal subject produces prompt feedback suppression of CRH and ACTH levels, and thus of endogenous cortisol secretion (dexamethasone is not measured by most cortisol assays). Three forms of the test, used in the diagnosis and differential diagnosis of Cushing syndrome, are available (see ***Box 26.14***).

Box 26.36 Causes of primary hypoadrenalism

- Autoimmune disease
- Tuberculosis (<10% in UK)
- Surgical removal
- Haemorrhage/infarction:
  - Meningococcal septicaemia
  - Venography
- Infiltration:
  - Malignant destruction
  - Amyloid
- Schilder's disease (adrenal leukodystrophy)

ACTH stimulation tests

Synthetic ACTH (tetracosactide, which consists of the first 24 amino acids of human ACTH) is given to stimulate adrenal cortisol production. Details are given in ***Box 26.3*** and ***Figure 26.5*** (see p. 1183).

Addison's disease: primary hypoadrenalism

Pathophysiology and aetiology

In this condition, there is destruction of the entire adrenal cortex. Glucocorticoid, mineralocorticoid and sex steroid production are therefore all reduced. (This differs from hypothalamic–pituitary disease, in which mineralocorticoid secretion remains largely intact, being predominantly stimulated by angiotensin II. Adrenal sex steroid production is also largely independent of pituitary action.) In Addison's disease, reduced cortisol levels lead, through feedback, to increased CRH and ACTH production, the latter being directly responsible for the hyperpigmentation.

Addison's disease is rare, with an incidence of 3–4/million per year and prevalence of 40–60/million. Primary hypoadrenalism shows a marked female preponderance and is most often caused by autoimmune disease (>90% in the UK), but in countries with a high prevalence of HIV/AIDS, tuberculosis is an increasing cause. Autoimmune adrenalitis results from the destruction of the adrenal cortex by organ-specific autoantibodies, with 21-hydroxylase as the common antigen. There are associations with other autoimmune conditions in the polyglandular autoimmune syndromes types I and II (e.g. type 1 diabetes mellitus, pernicious anaemia, thyroiditis, hypoparathyroidism, premature ovarian failure; see p. 1239).

All other causes are rare ***(Box 26.36)***. In patients with degenerative neurological symptoms, a diagnosis of adrenoleukodystrophy should be excluded.

Clinical features

These are shown in ***Figure 26.33***. The symptomatology of Addison's disease is often vague and non-specific. These symptoms may be the prelude to an addisonian crisis with severe hypotension and dehydration precipitated by intercurrent illness, accident or operation.

Pigmentation (dull, slaty, grey–brown) is the predominant sign in over 90% of cases.

Postural systolic hypotension, due to hypovolaemia and sodium loss, is present in 80–90% of cases, even if supine blood pressure is normal. Mineralocorticoid deficiency is the cause of the hypotension.

Investigations

Once Addison's disease is suspected, investigation is urgent. If the patient is seriously ill or hypotensive, hydrocortisone 100 mg should

Symptoms

Weight loss
Malaise
Weakness
Fever

Anorexia
Nausea/vomiting
Diarrhoea
Abdominal pain
Constipation
Depression
Confusion
Myalgia
Joint or back pain

Impotence/amenorrhoea

Syncope from postural hypotension

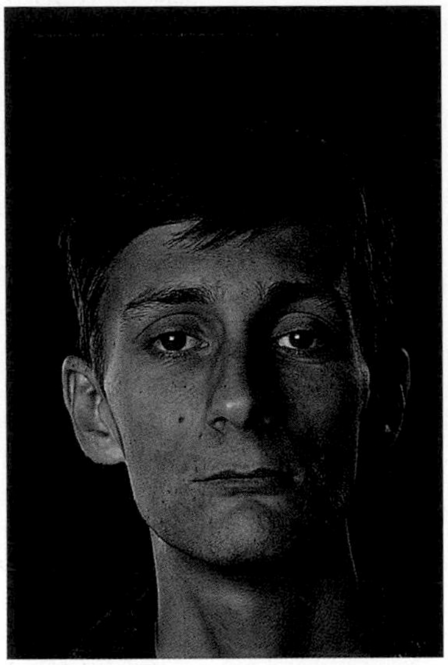

Signs

General
Loss of weight
General wasting
Pigmentation, especially of new scars and palmar creases
Buccal pigmentation
Postural hypotension
Loss of body hair (vitiligo)
Dehydration

Figure 26.33 **Primary hypoadrenalism (Addison's disease): symptoms and signs.** ***Bold italic*** type indicates signs of greater discriminant value.

be given intravenously or intramuscularly, together with intravenous 0.9% saline. Ideally, this should be done immediately after a blood sample is taken for later measurement of plasma cortisol. Alternatively, an ACTH stimulation test can be performed immediately. Full investigation should be delayed until emergency treatment (see below) has improved the patient's condition. Otherwise, tests are as follows:

- ***Single cortisol measurements*** are of little value, although a random cortisol below 100 nmol/L during the day is highly suggestive, and a random cortisol >550 nmol/L makes the diagnosis unlikely.
- ***The short ACTH stimulation test*** should be performed (see ***Box 26.3*** and ***Fig. 26.5***). Note that an absent or impaired cortisol response confirms the presence of hypoadrenalism but does not differentiate Addison's disease from ACTH deficiency or iatrogenic suppression by steroid medication. The long ACTH test is no longer used because of the availability of accurate ACTH assays.
- ***A 09:00 hours plasma ACTH level*** is measured, a high level (>80 ng/L) with low or low-normal cortisol confirming primary hypoadrenalism.
- ***Electrolytes and urea*** classically show hyponatraemia, hyperkalaemia and a high urea, but they can be normal.
- ***Blood glucose*** may be low, with hypoglycaemia.
- ***Adrenal antibodies*** are present in approximately 90% of cases of autoimmune adrenalitis.
- ***Chest and abdominal X-rays*** or cross-sectional imaging of the abdomen (CT or MRI) may show evidence of tuberculosis and/or calcified adrenals ***(Fig. 26.34)***.
- ***Plasma renin activity*** is high due to low ***serum aldosterone***.
- ***Hypercalcaemia and anaemia*** (after rehydration) are sometimes seen.

Management

Acute hypoadrenalism needs urgent treatment ***(Box 26.37)***.

Long-term treatment is with replacement glucocorticoid and mineralocorticoid; tuberculosis must be treated if present or suspected. Replacement dosage details are shown in ***Box 26.38***. A recent dual-release, oral, once-daily hydrocortisone preparation is now on the market. Dehydroepiandrosterone (DHEA) replacement has also been advocated; some studies suggest that this may cause symptomatic improvements, although others show no clear benefit and acne and hirsutism occur.

Adequacy of glucocorticoid dose is judged by:

- clinical wellbeing and restoration of normal, but not excessive, weight
- normal cortisol levels during the day while on replacement hydrocortisone (cortisol levels cannot be used for synthetic steroids).

Adequacy of fludrocortisone replacement is assessed by:

- restoration of serum electrolytes to normal
- blood pressure response to posture (it should not fall >10 mmHg systolic after 2 minutes standing)
- suppression of plasma renin activity to normal.

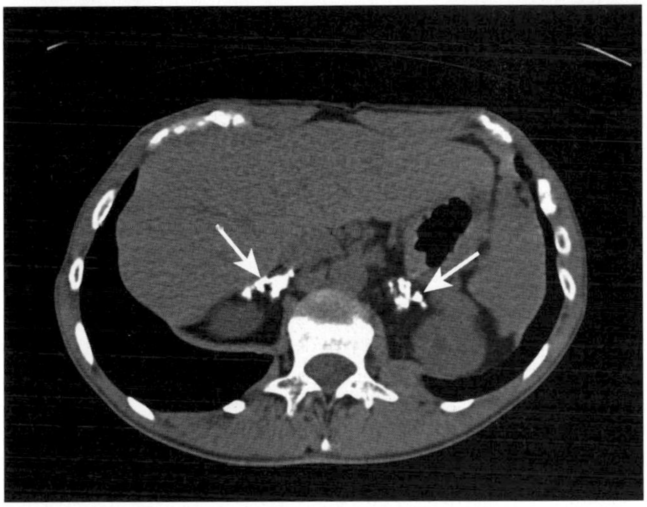

Figure 26.34 **CT scan showing bilateral adrenal calcification.**

Patient advice

All patients requiring replacement steroids should:

- know how to increase steroid replacement by doubling the dose for intercurrent illness

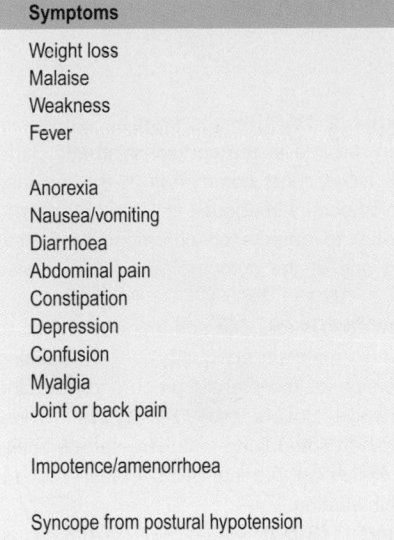

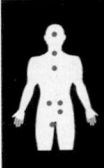

Box 26.37 Management of acute hypoadrenalism

Clinical context

Hypotension, hyponatraemia, hyperkalaemia, hypoglycaemia, dehydration, pigmentation often with precipitating infection, infarction, trauma or operation. The major deficiencies are of salt, steroid and glucose.

Requirements

Assuming normal cardiovascular function, the following are required:

- 1 L of 0.9% saline should be given over 30–60 min with 100 mg of i.v. bolus hydrocortisone
- Subsequent requirements are several litres of saline within 24 h (assessing with central venous pressure line if necessary) plus hydrocortisone, 100 mg i.m., 6-hourly, until the patient is clinically stable
- Glucose should be infused if there is hypoglycaemia
- Oral replacement medication is then started, unless the patient is unable to take oral medication: initially, hydrocortisone 20 mg, 8-hourly, reducing to 20–30 mg in divided doses over a few days (see **Box 26.38**)
- Fludrocortisone is unnecessary acutely, as the high cortisol doses provide sufficient mineralocorticoid activity – it should be introduced later

Box 26.38 Average replacement steroid dosages for adults with primary hypoadrenalism

Drug	Dose
Glucocorticoid	
Hydrocortisone	20–30 mg daily (e.g. 10 mg on waking, 5 mg at 12:00 hours, 5 mg at 18:00 hours)
or	
Prednisolone	7.5 mg daily (5 mg on waking, 2.5 mg at 18:00 hours)
rarely	
Dexamethasone	0.75 mg daily (0.5 mg on waking, 0.25 mg at 18:00 hours)
Mineralocorticoid	
Fludrocortisone	50–300 μg daily

- carry a 'steroid card'
- wear a Medic-Alert bracelet (or similar), which gives details of their condition so that emergency replacement therapy can be given if found unconscious
- keep an (up-to-date) ampoule of hydrocortisone at home in case oral therapy is impossible, for administration by self, family or doctor.

Secondary hypoadrenalism

This may arise from:

- hypothalamic–pituitary disease (inadequate ACTH production) *or*
- long-term steroid therapy leading to hypothalamic–pituitary–adrenal suppression.

Most people with hypothalamic–pituitary disease have panhypopituitarism (see p. 1188) and need T_4 replacement, as well as cortisol; in this case, hydrocortisone must be started before T_4.

Long-term corticosteroid medication for non-endocrine disease is the most common cause of secondary hypoadrenalism. The hypothalamic–pituitary axis and the adrenal may both be suppressed and the patient may have vague symptoms of feeling unwell. ACTH levels are low in secondary hypoadrenalism. Weaning off steroids is often a long and difficult process.

Congenital adrenal hyperplasia

Pathophysiology

Congenital adrenal hyperplasia (CAH) results from an autosomal recessive deficiency of an enzyme in the cortisol synthetic pathways. There are six major types; most common is 21-hydroxylase deficiency (CYP21A2), which occurs in about 1 in 15 000 births and has been shown to be due to defects on chromosome 6 near the HLA region, affecting one of the cytochrome p450 enzymes (p450C21).

As a result, cortisol secretion is reduced and feedback leads to increased ACTH secretion to maintain adequate cortisol, causing adrenal hyperplasia. Diversion of the steroid precursors into the androgenic steroid pathways occurs (see ***Fig. 26.31A***). Thus, 17-hydroxyprogesterone, androstenedione and testosterone levels are increased, leading to virilization. Aldosterone synthesis may be impaired with resultant salt wasting.

The other forms affect 11β-hydroxylase, 17α-hydroxylase, 3β-hydroxysteroid dehydrogenase and a cholesterol side-chain cleavage enzyme (p450scc) (see ***Fig. 26.31A***).

Clinical features

Classical CAH presents at birth with:

- Sexual ambiguity (in the female, clitoral hypertrophy, urogenital abnormalities and labioscrotal fusion are common) *or*
- Adrenal failure (collapse, hypotension, hypoglycaemia), sometimes with a salt-losing state (hypotension, hyponatraemia). The syndrome may be unrecognized in the male until a salt-losing crisis occurs, usually within 10 days of birth.
- Non-classified disease presents later as precocious puberty with hirsutism; rare, milder cases only present in adult life, usually accompanied by primary amenorrhoea. Hirsutism developing before puberty is suggestive of CAH.

Investigations

Expert advice is essential in the confirmation and differential diagnosis of 21-hydroxylase deficiency; with ambiguous genitalia, such advice must be sought urgently before any assignment of gender is made.

A profile of adrenocortical hormones is drawn up before and 1 hour after ACTH administration.

- 17-Hydroxyprogesterone levels are increased.
- Urinary pregnanetriol excretion is increased.
- Androstenedione levels are raised.
- Basal ACTH levels are raised.

Management

Glucocorticoid activity must be replaced, as must mineralocorticoid activity if deficient. The practice in CAH of giving the larger dose of glucocorticoid at night to suppress the morning ACTH peak, with a smaller dose in the morning, is largely outdated. Correct dosage is often difficult to establish in the ***child*** but should ensure normal androstenedione and 17-hydroxyprogesterone levels while allowing normal growth; excessive replacement leads to stunting of growth. In ***adults***, clinical features and biochemistry (plasma renin, androstenedione and 17-hydroxyprogesterone) are used to modify treatment. The use of modified-release hydrocortisone may have a role in the management of CAH.

Prenatal diagnosis

Genetic counselling and antenatal diagnosis is useful (see pp. 116–117). There is a 1:4 chance of recurrence in a family. Dexamethasone given to the mother of a female fetus with a 21-hydroxylase deficiency can prevent virilization by suppressing ACTH levels. There are, however, concerns about the potential adverse consequences of this practice.

Problems of therapeutic steroid therapy

Apart from their use as therapeutic replacement for endocrine deficiency states, synthetic glucocorticoids are widely used for many non-endocrine conditions. Short-term use (e.g. for acute asthma) carries only small risks of significant side-effects, except for the simultaneous suppression of immune responses. The danger lies in their continuance, often through medical oversight or patient default. In general, therapy for 3 weeks or less, or a dose of prednisolone of less than 5 mg per day, will not result in significant long-term suppression of the normal adrenal axis.

Long-term therapy with synthetic or natural steroids will, in most respects, mimic endogenous Cushing syndrome. Exceptions are the relative absence of hirsutism, acne, hypertension and severe sodium retention, as the common synthetic steroids have low androgenic and mineralocorticoid activity.

Excessive doses of steroids may also be absorbed from skin when strong dermatological preparations are used but inhaled steroids rarely cause Cushing syndrome; they commonly cause adrenal suppression, however.

The major hazards are detailed in ***Box 26.39***. In the long term, many are of such severity that the clinical need for high-dose steroids should be continually and critically assessed. Steroid-sparing agents should always be considered, and screening and prophylactic therapy for osteoporosis introduced (see pp. 712–713). New targeted biological therapies for inflammatory conditions may reduce the incidence of steroid-induced adrenal suppression.

Box 26.39 Major adverse effects of corticosteroid therapy

Physiological
- Adrenal and/or pituitary suppression

Pathological

Cardiovascular
- Increased blood pressure

Gastrointestinal
- Pancreatitis

Renal
- Polyuria
- Nocturia

Central nervous
- Depression
- Euphoria
- Psychosis
- Insomnia

Endocrine
- Weight gain
- Glycosuria/hyperglycaemia/diabetes
- Impaired growth
- Amenorrhoea

Bone and muscle
- Osteoporosis
- Proximal myopathy and wasting
- Aseptic necrosis of the hip
- Pathological fractures

Skin
- Thinning
- Easy bruising

Eyes
- Cataracts (including inhaled drug)

Increased susceptibility to infection

(Signs and fever are frequently masked)
- Septicaemia
- Fungal infections
- Reactivation of tuberculosis
- Skin (e.g. fungi)

Supervision of steroid therapy

All patients receiving steroids should carry a 'steroid card'. They should be made aware of the following points:

- Long-term steroid therapy must never be stopped suddenly.
- Doses should be reduced very gradually, with most being given in the morning at the time of withdrawal; this minimizes adrenal suppression. Many authorities believe that 'alternate-day therapy' produces less suppression.
- Doses need to be increased at times of serious intercurrent illness (defined as presence of a fever), accident and stress. Double doses should be taken during these periods.
- Other physicians, anaesthetists and dentists must be told about steroid therapy.

Patients should also be informed of potential side-effects, and all this information should be documented in the clinical record. If prophylactic use of bisphosphonate therapy is required to prevent the development of osteoporosis (National Institute for Health and Care Excellence (NICE) guidance), patients should be informed of the rationale.

Steroids and surgery

Any patient receiving steroids, or who has recently received them (within the last 12 months) and may still have adrenal suppression, requires special control of steroid medication around the time of surgery. Details are shown in ***Box 26.40***.

Incidental adrenal tumours ('incidentalomas')

With the advent of abdominal CT, MRI and high-resolution ultrasound scanning, unsuspected adrenal masses have been discovered in 3–10% of scans (increasing with age). The two issues of concern with an incidental adrenal mass are:

- whether the lesion is functional or non-functional
- whether it is benign or malignant.

Most incidentalomas are asymptomatic and benign, but direct questioning may reveal symptoms of endocrine hypersecretion such as cushingoid features, catecholamine excess, virilization in women, or evidence of endocrine hypertension (see ***Box 23.56***). Even in the absence of symptoms, functional tests to exclude secretory activity should be performed, as adrenal adenomas often secrete cortisol at a low level – 'subclinical Cushing syndrome', which may confer increased cardiovascular risk. If no endocrine activity is found, then most authorities recommend removal only of large adrenal tumours (>4–5 cm) because of the risk of malignancy. Smaller, hormonally inactive lesions are usually observed, as long as there are no worrying radiological features.

Phaeochromocytoma must be excluded before surgery due to the risk of perioperative hypertensive or hypotensive crises (see p. 1231).

Primary hyperaldosteronism

Increased mineralocorticoid secretion from the adrenal cortex, termed primary hyperaldosteronism, is thought to account for 5–10% of all hypertension. Other endocrine causes of hypertension should also be considered if there is clinical suspicion ***(Box 26.41)***. It is impracticable and unnecessary to screen all hypertensive patients for secondary endocrine causes. The highest chances of detecting such causes are in patients:

- under 35 years, especially those without a family history of hypertension
- with accelerated (malignant) hypertension
- with hypokalaemia before diuretic therapy

Box 26.40 Steroid cover for operative procedures[a]

Procedure	Premedication	Intra- and postoperative	Resumption of normal maintenance
Simple procedures (e.g. gastroscopy, simple dental extractions)	Hydrocortisone 100 mg i.m.	–	Immediately if no complications and eating normally
Minor surgery (e.g. laparoscopic surgery, veins, hernias)	Hydrocortisone 100 mg i.m.	Hydrocortisone 20 mg orally 6-hourly or 50 mg i.m. 6-hourly for 24 h if not eating	After 24 h if no complications
Major surgery (e.g. hip replacement, vascular surgery)	Hydrocortisone 100 mg i.m.	Hydrocortisone 50–100 mg i.m. 6-hourly for 72 h	After 72 h if normal progress and no complications Perhaps double normal dose for next 2–3 days
GI tract surgery or major thoracic surgery (not eating or ventilated)	Hydrocortisone 100 mg i.m.	Hydrocortisone 100 mg i.m. 6-hourly for 72 h or longer if still unwell	When patient eating normally again Until then, higher doses (to 50 mg 6-hourly) may be needed

[a]A useful summary of surgical steroid guidelines can be found at: http://www.addisons.org.uk/

Box 26.41 Endocrine causes of hypertension

Excessive renin, and thus angiotensin II, production
- Renal artery stenosis
- Other local renal disease
- Renin-secreting tumours

Excessive production of catecholamines
- Phaeochromocytoma

Excessive growth hormone (GH) production
- Acromegaly

Excessive aldosterone production
- Adrenal adenoma (Conn syndrome)
- Idiopathic adrenal hyperplasia
- Dexamethasone-suppressible hyperaldosteronism

Excessive production of other mineralocorticoids
- Cushing syndrome (massive excess of cortisol, a weak mineralocorticoid)
- Congenital adrenal hyperplasia (in rare cases)
- Tumours producing other mineralocorticoids, e.g. corticosterone

Exogenous 'mineralocorticoids' or enzyme inhibitors
- Liquorice ingestion (inhibits 11β-hydroxylase)
- Misuse of mineralocorticoid preparations

- resistant to conventional antihypertensive therapy (e.g. more than three drugs) *or*
- with unusual symptoms (e.g. sweating attacks or weakness).

Pathophysiology

Primary hyperaldosteronism is a disorder of the adrenal cortex characterized by excess aldosterone production leading to sodium retention, potassium loss and the combination of hypokalaemia and hypertension. This must be distinguished from secondary hyperaldosteronism, which arises when there is excess renin (and hence angiotensin II) stimulation of the zona glomerulosa. Common causes of secondary hyperaldosteronism are accelerated hypertension and renal artery stenosis, when the patient will also be hypertensive. Causes associated with normotension include congestive cardiac failure and cirrhosis, where excess aldosterone production contributes to sodium retention.

Aetiology

Adrenal adenomas (Conn syndrome; see ***Box 26.41***) originally accounted for 60% of cases of primary hyperaldosteronism but represented a rare cause of hypertension. The use of the aldosterone:renin ratio in the routine investigation of hypertension now suggests that hyperaldosteronism due to bilateral adrenal hyperplasia (idiopathic hyperaldosteronism) is much more common than the classical Conn's adenoma. Some claim that idiopathic hyperaldosteronism is the cause of up to 10% of cases of 'essential' hypertension.

Clinical features

The usual presentation is simply hypertension; hypokalaemia (<3.5 mmol/L) is frequently not present. The few symptoms are non-specific; rarely, muscle weakness, nocturia and tetany are seen. The hypertension may be severe and associated with renal, cardiac and retinal damage.

Adenomas, often very small, are more common in young females, while bilateral hyperplasia rarely occurs before the age of 40 years and is more common in males.

Investigations

Beta-blockers and other drugs may interfere with renin activity, and spironolactone, angiotensin-converting enzyme (ACE) inhibitors and angiotensin II receptor antagonists will all affect results; all should be discontinued, if possible. The characteristic features of investigation are as follows:

- ***Plasma aldosterone:renin ratio (ARR)*** is now most frequently used as a screening test for the condition, but raised ARR alone does not confirm the diagnosis (if the renin is low enough, ARR will always be high). Note that normal ranges are highly assay-dependent.
- ***Elevated plasma aldosterone levels*** are not suppressed with 0.9% saline infusion (2 L over 4 h) or fludrocortisone administration. Between 30% and 50% of people with a raised ARR on screening will suppress normally, excluding the diagnosis.
- ***Suppressed plasma renin activity*** or immunoreactivity is seen.
- ***Hypokalaemia*** is often present but a normal serum potassium does not exclude the diagnosis.
- ***Urinary potassium loss*** *of* >30 mmol daily during hypokalaemia is inappropriate.

Once a diagnosis of hyperaldosteronism is established, differentiation of adenoma from hyperplasia involves adrenal CT or MRI, but small adenomas may be missed and non-functioning incidentalomas also occur. Further information is obtained from diurnal/postural changes in plasma aldosterone levels (which tend to rise with adenomas between 09:00 hours supine and 13:00 hours erect samples; in contrast, they fall with hyperplasia), measurement of 18-OH cortisol levels (raised in adenoma), and venous catheterization for aldosterone levels. All of these tests have their pitfalls and exceptions.

Management

An adenoma can be removed surgically, usually laparoscopically; blood pressure falls in 70% of patients. Those with hyperplasia should be treated with the aldosterone antagonist, spironolactone (100–400 mg daily); frequent side-effects include nausea, rashes and gynaecomastia. The pure aldosterone receptor antagonist, eplerenone, can be a useful alternative if side-effects preclude the use of spironolactone (see p. 158) Spironolactone metabolites have been linked with tumour development in animals but this has not been described in humans. Amiloride and calcium-channel blockers are moderately effective in controlling the hypertension but do not correct the hyperaldosteronism.

Glucocorticoid (or dexamethasone)-suppressible hyperaldosteronism

This rare condition is caused by a chimeric gene on chromosome 8. A fusion gene resulting from an unusual crossover at meiosis between the genes encoding aldosterone synthase and adrenal 11β-hydroxylase produces aldosterone, which is under ACTH control. Treatment with glucocorticoid resolves the problem.

Syndrome of apparent mineralocorticoid excess

This causes the clinical syndrome of primary hyperaldosteronism but with low renin and aldosterone levels. Reduced activity of the enzyme 11β-hydroxysteroid dehydrogenase type 2 (11βHSD2) prevents the normal conversion in the kidney of cortisol (which is active at the mineralocorticoid receptor) to cortisone (which is not), and therefore 'exposes' the mineralocorticoid receptor in the kidney to the usual molar excess of cortisol over aldosterone in the blood. While the inherited syndrome is rare, the same clinical syndrome can occur with excessive ingestion of liquorice, which inhibits the 11βHSD2 enzyme.

The adrenal medulla

The adrenal medulla is the innermost part of the adrenal gland, consisting of cells that secrete the major catecholamines, noradrenaline (norepinephrine) and adrenaline (epinephrine), which produce the sympathetic nervous response. The catecholamines are interconverted in the adrenal medulla, and an increase in levels of their metabolites in the urine is a marker of abnormal hypersecretion ***(Fig. 26.35)***.

Phaeochromocytoma and paraganglioma

These are very rare tumours of the sympathetic nervous system (less than 1 in 1000 cases of hypertension) that secrete catecholamines, noradrenaline (norepinephrine), adrenaline (epinephrine) and their metabolites ***(Fig. 26.35)***:

- 90% arise in the adrenal medulla (***phaeochromocytomas***)
- 10% occur elsewhere in the sympathetic chain (***paragangliomas***).

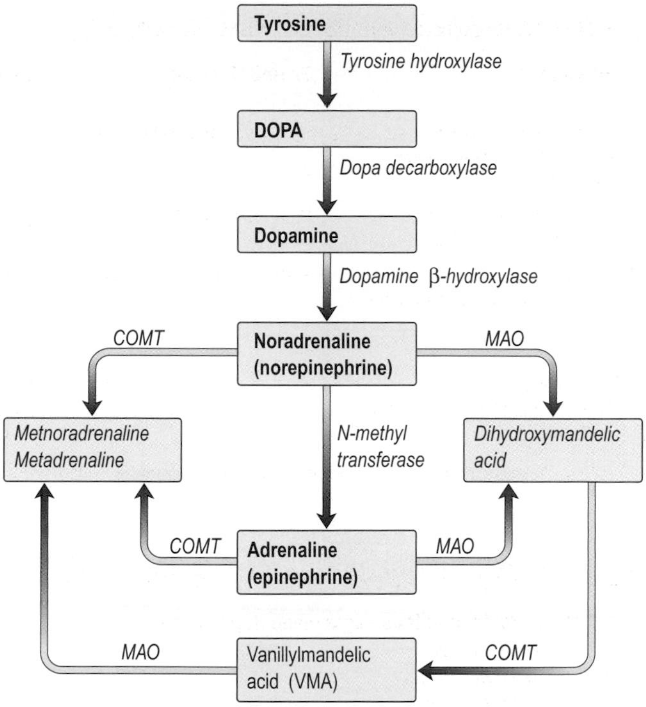

Figure 26.35 The synthesis and metabolism of catecholamines. COMT, catechol-O-methyl transferase; MAO, monoamine oxidase.

Some are associated with MEN 2 syndromes (see below) and the von Hippel–Lindau (VHL) syndrome (see p. 881). Most tumours release both noradrenaline (norepinephrine) and adrenaline (epinephrine), but large tumours and extra-adrenal tumours produce almost entirely noradrenaline.

Paragangliomas typically occur in the head and neck but are also found in the thorax, pelvis and bladder. They are more closely associated with other genetic associations than is phaeochromocytoma. The association of paraganglioma, bilateral adrenal phaeochromocytomas, positive family history or young age at presentation is seen in multiple endocrine neoplasms (see pp. 1239–1240). Mutations in the succinate dehydrogenase (*SDHD*) gene have been shown to be strongly associated with the development of paraganglioma.

Pathology

Oval groups of cells occur in clusters and stain for chromogranin A. Some 25% are multiple and 10% malignant, the latter being more frequent in the extra-adrenal tumours. Malignancy cannot be determined on simple histological examination alone.

Clinical features

The clinical features are those of catecholamine excess and are frequently, but not necessarily, intermittent ***(Box 26.42)***. All people with suspected phaeochromocytomas must be investigated because phaeochromocytomas may cause acute cardiovascular compromise during routine medical procedures, and can also present with sudden death if the diagnosis is missed.

Investigations

Specific tests are:

- ***Measurement of urinary catecholamines and metabolites*** (metanephrines are most sensitive and specific; ***Fig. 26.35***) is a useful screening test; normal levels on three 24-h collections

Box 26.42 Symptoms and signs of phaeochromocytoma

Symptoms
- Anxiety or panic attacks
- Palpitations
- Tremor
- Sweating
- Headache
- Flushing
- Nausea and/or vomiting
- Weight loss
- Constipation or diarrhoea
- Raynaud's phenomenon
- Chest pain
- Polyuria/nocturia

Signs
- Hypertension
- Tachycardia/arrhythmias
- Bradycardia
- Orthostatic hypotension
- Pallor or flushing
- Glycosuria
- Fever
- (Signs of hypertensive damage)

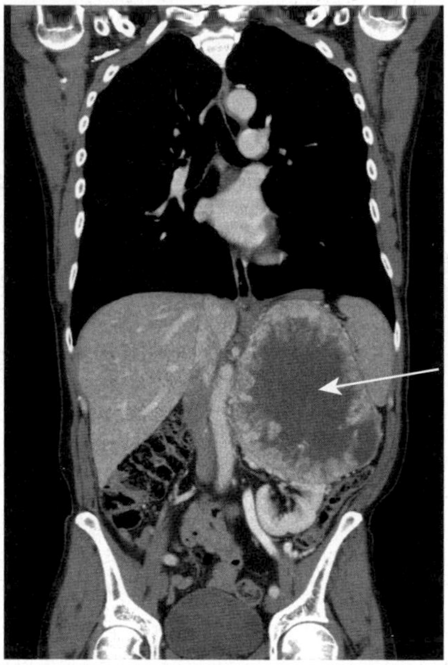

Figure 26.36 MRI scan showing a massive left-sided phaeochromocytoma.

of metanephrines virtually exclude the diagnosis. Many drugs, e.g. tricyclics, and dietary vanilla interfere with these tests.
- ***Resting plasma metanephrines*** are raised.
- ***Plasma chromogranin A*** (a storage vesicle protein) is raised.
- ***Clonidine suppression test*** may be appropriate but should only be performed in specialist centres.
- ***CT/MRI scans***, initially of the abdomen, are helpful to localize the tumours, which are often large ***(Fig. 26.36)***.
- ***Scanning with [^{131}I]meta-iodobenzylguanidine (MIBG)*** produces specific uptake in sites of sympathetic activity with about 90% success. It is particularly useful with extra-adrenal tumours. ^{18}F-deoxyglucose positron emission tomography (PET) is also used by some centres in the localization of phaeochromocytomas ***(Fig. 26.37)***.
- ***Genetic testing*** for *MEN2*, *VHL*, *SDHB* and *SDHD* mutations should be performed in all people with confirmed phaeochromocytoma or paraganglioma.

Management

Tumours should be removed if this is possible; 5-year survival is about 95% for non-malignant tumours. Medical preoperative and

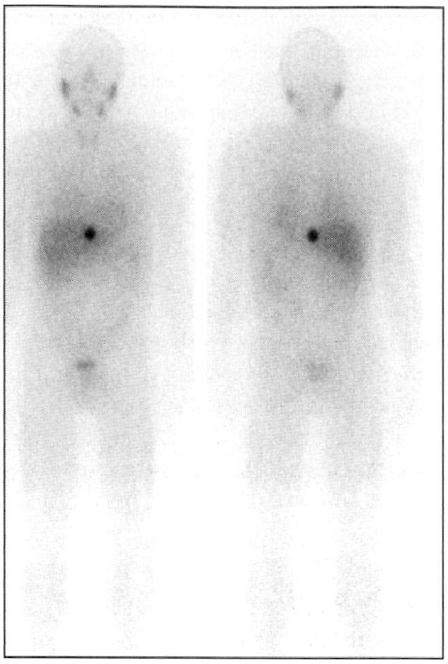

Figure 26.37 MIBG scan showing a solitary area of increased uptake in the liver consistent with metastasis from a phaeochromocytoma.

perioperative treatment is vital and includes complete alpha- and beta-blockade with phenoxybenzamine (20–80 mg daily initially in divided doses), then propranolol (120–240 mg daily), plus intravenous hydration to re-expand the contracted plasma volume. The alpha-blockade must precede the beta-blockade, as worsened hypertension may otherwise result. Labetalol is not recommended. Surgery in the unprepared patient is fraught with dangers of both hypertension and hypotension; expert anaesthesia and an experienced surgeon are both vital, and sodium nitroprusside and phentolamine (a rapid-acting α-blocker) should be available in case sudden severe hypertension develops.

When operation is not possible, combined alpha- and beta-blockade can be used long-term. Radionucleotide treatment with MIBG has been employed but has had limited success in malignant phaeochromocytoma.

Patients should be kept under clinical and biochemical review after tumour resection, as over 10% of tumours recur or a further tumour develops. Catecholamine excretion measurements should be performed at least annually.

Further reading

Auchus RJ, Arlt W. Approach to the patient: the adult with congenital adrenal hyperplasia. *J Clin Endocrinol Metab* 2013; 98:2645–2655.
Lenders JW, Duh QY, Eisenhofer G et al and the Endocrine Society. Pheochromocytoma and paraganglioma: an Endocrine Society clinical practice guideline. *J Clin Endocrinol Metab* 2014; 99:1915–1942.
Merke DP, Bornstein SR. Congenital adrenal hyperplasia. *Lancet* 2005; 365:2125–2136.
Van Nederveen FH, Korpershoek E, Lenders JW et al. Somatic SDHB mutation in an extraadrenal phaeochromocytoma. *N Engl J Med* 2007; 357:306–308.
Young WF. The incidentally discovered adrenal mass. *N Engl J Med* 2007; 356:601–610.

THE THIRST AXIS

Thirst and water regulation are largely controlled by vasopressin, also known as antidiuretic hormone (ADH), which is synthesized in

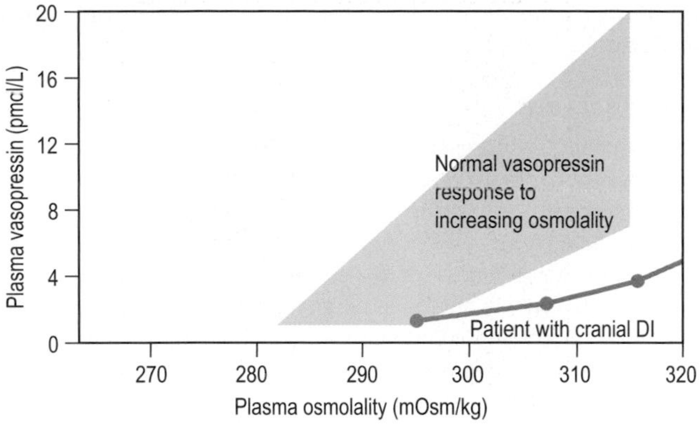

Figure 26.38 Plasma vasopressin response to increasing osmolality in normal subjects and in a patient with diabetes insipidus (DI).

the hypothalamus (see p. 1183) and then migrates in neurosecretory granules along axonal pathways to the posterior pituitary. Pituitary disease alone without hypothalamic involvement therefore does not lead to ADH deficiency, as the hormone can still 'leak' from the damaged end of the intact axon.

At normal concentrations, the kidney is the predominant site of action of vasopressin. Vasopressin stimulation of the V_2 receptors (see ***Box 26.4***) allows the collecting ducts to become permeable to water via the migration of aquaporin-2 water channels, thus permitting reabsorption of hypotonic luminal fluid (see pp. 153–154). Vasopressin therefore reduces diuresis and results in overall retention of water. At high concentrations, vasopressin also causes vasoconstriction via the V_1 receptors in vascular tissue.

Changes in plasma osmolality are sensed by osmoreceptors in the anterior hypothalamus. Vasopressin secretion is suppressed at levels below 280 mOsm/kg, thus allowing maximal water diuresis. Above this level, plasma vasopressin increases in direct proportion to plasma osmolality. At the upper limit of normal (295 mOsm/kg), maximum antidiuresis is achieved and thirst is experienced at about 298 mOsm/kg ***(Fig. 26.38)***.

Other factors affecting vasopressin release are shown in ***Box 26.43***.

Disorders of vasopressin secretion or activity include:

- cranial diabetes insipidus with deficiency as a result of hypothalamic disease
- 'nephrogenic' diabetes insipidus – a rare condition in which the renal tubules are insensitive to vasopressin, and an example of a receptor abnormality
- inappropriate excess of the hormone.

While all these are uncommon, they need to be distinguished from the occasional patient with 'primary polydipsia' and those whose renal tubular function has been impaired by electrolyte abnormalities, such as hypokalaemia or hypercalcaemia.

Diabetes insipidus

Clinical features

Deficiency of vasopressin (ADH) or insensitivity to its action leads to excess excretion of dilute urine with a compensatory increase in thirst (polydipsia). Daily urine output may reach as much as 10–15 L, leading to dehydration that may be very severe if the thirst mechanism or consciousness is impaired or the patient is denied fluid.

Box 26.43 Factors affecting vasopressin (ADH) release

Increased by
- Increased osmolality
- Hypovolaemia
- Hypotension
- Nausea
- Hypothyroidism
- Angiotensin II
- Adrenaline (epinephrine)
- Cortisol
- Nicotine
- Antidepressants

Decreased by
- Decreased osmolality
- Hypervolaemia
- Hypertension
- Ethanol
- α-Adrenergic stimulation

Box 26.44 Causes of diabetes insipidus

Cranial diabetes insipidus
- Familial (e.g. DIDMOAD)
- Idiopathic (often autoimmune)
- Tumours:
  - Craniopharyngioma
  - Hypothalamic tumour, e.g. glioma, germinoma
  - Metastases, especially breast
  - Lymphoma/leukaemia
  - Pituitary with suprasellar extension (rare)
- Infections:
  - Tuberculosis
  - Meningitis
  - Cerebral abscess
- Infiltrations:
  - Sarcoidosis
  - Langerhans' cell histiocytosis
- Inflammatory:
  - Hypophysitis
- Post-surgical:
  - Transfrontal
  - Trans sphenoidal
- Post-radiotherapy (cranial)
- Vascular:
  - Haemorrhage/thrombosis
  - Sheehan syndrome
  - Aneurysm
- Trauma (e.g. head injury)

Nephrogenic diabetes insipidus
- Familial (e.g. vasopressin receptor gene, aquaporin-2 gene defect)
- Idiopathic
- Renal disease (e.g. renal tubular acidosis)
- Hypokalaemia
- Hypercalcaemia
- Drugs (e.g. lithium, demeclocycline, glibenclamide)
- Sickle cell disease
- Prolonged polyuria due to any cause, including cranial DI and primary polydipsia – can cause mild temporary nephrogenic DI

DIDMOAD, diabetes insipidus, diabetes mellitus, optic atrophy and deafness.

Diabetes insipidus (DI) may be masked by simultaneous cortisol deficiency; cortisol replacement allows a water diuresis and DI then becomes apparent.

Aetiology

Causes of DI are listed in ***Box 26.44***. The most common is hypothalamic–pituitary surgery, following which transient DI is common, frequently remitting after a few days or weeks. Typically, inflammatory lesions of the pituitary stalk are associated with DI ***(Fig. 26.39)***.

Familial isolated vasopressin deficiency causes DI from early childhood and is dominantly inherited, caused by a mutation in the *AVP-NPII* gene. ***DIDMOAD (Wolfram) syndrome*** is a rare autosomal recessive disorder comprising diabetes insipidus, diabetes mellitus, optic atrophy and deafness, and is caused by mutations in the *WFS1* gene on chromosome 4. MRI may show an absent or poorly developed posterior pituitary.

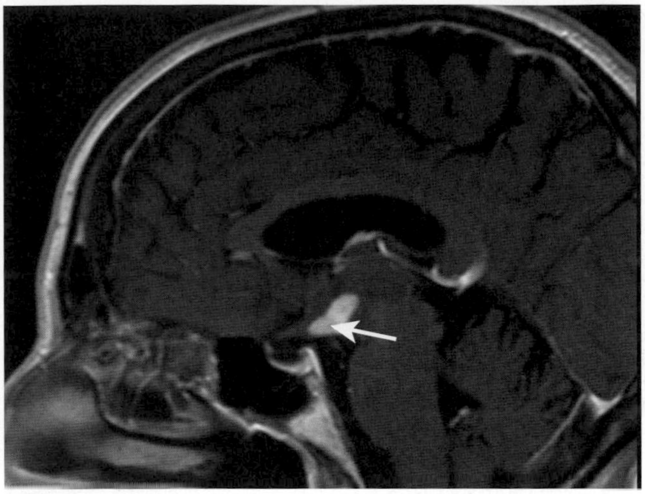

Figure 26.39 MRI showing a thickened pituitary stalk in hypophysitis.

Box 26.45 Water deprivation test

Indications
- Diagnosis or exclusion of diabetes insipidus.

Procedure
- Fasting and no fluids from 07:30 h (or overnight if only mild DI is expected and polyuria is only modest).
- Monitor serum and urine osmolality, urine volume and weight hourly for up to 8 h.
- Abandon fluid deprivation if weight loss >3% occurs.
- If serum osmolality is >300 mOsm/kg and/or urine osmolality <600 mOsm/kg, give desmopressin 2 µg i.m. at end of test. Allow free fluid but measure urine osmolality for 2–4 h.

Interpretation
- ***Normal response*** – serum osmolality remains within normal range (275–295 mOsm/kg). Urine osmolality rises to >600 mOsm/kg.
- ***Diabetes insipidus (DI)*** – serum osmolality rises above normal without adequate concentration of urine osmolality (i.e. serum osmolality >300 mOsm/kg; urine osmolality <600 mOsm/kg).
- ***Nephrogenic DI*** – if desmopressin does not concentrate urine.
- ***Cranial DI*** – if urine osmolality rises by >50% after desmopressin.

Biochemistry

- High or high-normal plasma osmolality with low urine osmolality (in primary polydipsia, plasma osmolality tends to be low).
- Resultant high or high-normal plasma sodium (hypernatraemia).
- High 24-h urine volumes (<2 L excludes the need for further investigation).
- Failure of urinary concentration with fluid deprivation.
- Restoration of urinary concentration with vasopressin or an analogue.

The latter two points are studied with a formal water deprivation test ***(Box 26.45)***. In normal subjects, plasma osmolality remains normal while urine osmolality rises above 600 mOsm/kg. In DI, plasma osmolality rises while the urine remains dilute, only concentrating after exogenous vasopressin is given (in 'cranial' DI), or not concentrating after vasopressin if nephrogenic DI is present. An alternative is measurement of plasma vasopressin during hypertonic saline infusion, but these measurements are not widely available.

Management

The synthetic vasopressin (ADH) analogue, desmopressin, is the treatment of choice in cranial DI. It has a longer duration of action than vasopressin and has no vasoconstrictive effects. It can be given intranasally as a spray 10–40 µg once or twice daily, and orally as 100–200 µg three times daily, or intramuscularly 2–4 µg daily. Response is variable and must be monitored carefully with enquiry about fluid input/output and plasma osmolality measurements. The main problem is avoiding water overload and consequent hyponatraemia (see p. 163). Where there is a reversible underlying cause (e.g. a hypothalamic tumour), this should be investigated and treated.

Alternative agents in mild DI, probably working by sensitizing the renal tubules to endogenous vasopressin, include thiazide diuretics, carbamazepine (200–400 mg daily) or chlorpropamide (200–350 mg daily) but these are rarely used.

Nephrogenic diabetes insipidus

In this condition, renal tubules are resistant to normal or high levels of plasma vasopressin (ADH). Nephrogenic diabetes insipidus may be inherited as a rare sex-linked recessive, with an abnormality in the vasopressin-2 receptor, or as an autosomal post-receptor defect in an ADH-sensitive water channel, aquaporin-2. More commonly, it can be acquired as a result of renal disease, sickle cell disease, drug ingestion (e.g. lithium), hypercalcaemia or hypokalaemia. Wherever possible, the cause should be reversed (see ***Box 26.44***). Polyuria is helped by thiazide diuretics.

Other causes of polyuria and polydipsia

Diabetes mellitus, hypokalaemia and hypercalcaemia should be excluded. In the case of diabetes mellitus, the cause is an osmotic diuresis secondary to glycosuria, which leads to dehydration and an increased perception of thirst owing to hypertonicity of the extracellular fluid.

Primary polydipsia

This is a relatively common cause of thirst and polyuria. It is a psychiatric disturbance characterized by the excessive intake of water. Plasma sodium and osmolality fall as a result and the urine produced is appropriately dilute. Vasopressin levels become virtually undetectable. Prolonged primary polydipsia may lead to the phenomenon of 'renal medullary washout', with a fall in the concentrating ability of the kidney.

Characteristically, the diagnosis is made by a water deprivation test. A low plasma osmolality is usual at the start of the test, and since vasopressin secretion and action can be stimulated, the patient's urine becomes concentrated (although 'maximum' concentrating ability may be impaired); the initially low urine osmolality gradually increases with the duration of the water deprivation.

Syndrome of inappropriate antidiuretic hormone secretion

Clinical features

Inappropriate secretion of antidiuretic hormone (ADH, also called vasopressin) leads to retention of water and hyponatraemia. The presentation of the syndrome of inappropriate antidiuretic hormone secretion (SIADH) is usually vague, with confusion, nausea, irritability

Box 26.46 Common causes of the syndrome of inappropriate antidiuretic hormone secretion (SIADH)

Tumours
- Small-cell carcinoma of lung
- Prostate
- Thymus
- Pancreas
- Lymphomas

Pulmonary lesions
- Pneumonia
- Tuberculosis
- Lung abscess

Central nervous system causes
- Meningitis
- Tumours
- Head injury
- Subdural haematoma
- Cerebral abscess
- Systemic lupus erythematosus
- Vasculitis

Metabolic causes
- Alcohol withdrawal
- Porphyria

Drugs
- Chlorpropamide
- Carbamazepine
- Cyclophosphamide
- Vincristine
- Phenothiazines

and, later, fits and coma. There is no oedema. Mild symptoms usually occur with plasma sodium levels below 125 mmol/L and serious manifestations are likely below 115 mmol/L. The elderly may show symptoms with milder abnormalities.

The syndrome must be distinguished from dilutional hyponatraemia due to excess infusion of glucose/water solutions or diuretic administration (thiazides or amiloride; see p. 164).

Diagnosis

The usual features are:

- dilutional hyponatraemia due to excessive water retention
- euvolaemia (in contrast to hypovolaemia of sodium and water depletion states)
- low plasma osmolality with 'inappropriate' urine osmolality >100 mOsm/kg (and typically higher than plasma osmolality)
- continued urinary sodium excretion >30 mmol/l (lower levels suggest sodium depletion and should respond to 0.9% saline infusion)
- absence of hypokalaemia (or hypotension)
- normal renal and adrenal and thyroid function.

The causes are listed in ***Box 26.46***.

Hyponatraemia is very common during illness in frail elderly patients and it may sometimes be clinically difficult to distinguish SIADH from salt and water depletion, particularly when mixed clinical features are present. Under these circumstances, a trial infusion of 1–2 L 0.9% saline is given. SIADH will not respond (but will excrete the sodium and water load effectively); sodium depletion will respond. ACTH deficiency can give a very similar biochemical picture to SIADH; therefore it is necessary to ensure that the hypothalamic–pituitary–adrenal axis is intact, particularly in neurosurgical patients, in whom ACTH deficiency may be relatively common.

Management

The underlying cause should be corrected where possible. Symptomatic relief can be obtained by the following measures:

- ***Fluid intake*** should be restricted to 500–1000 mL daily. If tolerated and complied with, this will correct the biochemical abnormalities in almost every case.
- ***Frequent measurement*** of plasma osmolality, serum sodium and body weight is needed.
- ***Demeclocycline*** (600–1200 mg daily) is given if water restriction is poorly tolerated or ineffective; this inhibits the action of vasopressin on the kidney, causing a reversible form of nephrogenic diabetes insipidus. It often causes photosensitive rashes, however.
- ***Hypertonic saline*** may be indicated when the syndrome is very severe (i.e. acute and symptomatic), but this is potentially dangerous and should only be used with extreme caution (see pp. 162–163).
- ***Vasopressin V_2 antagonists***, e.g. tolvaptan 15 mg daily, are being used with good results.

Further reading

Spasovski G, Vanholder R et al. Clinical practice guideline on diagnosis and treatment of hyponatraemia. *Eur J Endocrinol* 2014; 170:G1–G47.

DISORDERS OF CALCIUM METABOLISM

Serum calcium levels are mainly controlled by parathyroid hormone (PTH) and vitamin D. Hypercalcaemia is much more common than hypocalcaemia and is frequently detected incidentally with multi-channel biochemical analysers. Mild asymptomatic hypercalcaemia occurs in about 1 in 1000 of the population, with an incidence of 25–30 per 100 000 population. It occurs mainly in elderly females and is usually due to primary hyperparathyroidism.

Parathyroid hormone

There are normally four parathyroid glands, which are situated posterior to the thyroid; occasionally, additional glands exist or they may be found elsewhere in the neck or mediastinum. PTH, an 84-amino-acid hormone derived from a 115-residue pre-prohormone, is secreted from the chief cells of the parathyroid glands. PTH levels rise as serum ionized calcium falls. The latter is detected by specific G-protein-coupled, calcium-sensing receptors on the plasma membrane of the parathyroid cells. PTH has several major actions, all serving to increase plasma calcium by:

- increasing osteoclastic resorption of bone (occurring rapidly)
- increasing intestinal absorption of calcium (a slow response)
- increasing synthesis of 1,25-dihydroxyvitamin D_3
- increasing renal tubular reabsorption of calcium
- increasing excretion of phosphate.

PTH effects are mediated at specific membrane receptors on the target cells, resulting in an increase of adenyl cyclase messenger activity.

Vitamin D metabolism is discussed on page 708.

PTH measurements use two-site immunometric assays that measure only the intact PTH molecule; interpretation requires a simultaneous calcium measurement in order to differentiate most causes of hyper- and hypocalcaemia.

Hypercalcaemia

Pathophysiology and aetiology

The major causes of hypercalcaemia are listed in ***Box 26.47***; primary hyperparathyroidism and malignancies are by far the most common (>90% of cases). Hyperparathyroidism itself may be primary, secondary or tertiary. Primary hyperparathyroidism is caused by single (>80%) parathyroid adenomas or by diffuse hyperplasia of all

Box 26.47 Causes of hypercalcaemia

Excessive parathyroid hormone (PTH) secretion
- Primary hyperparathyroidism (most common by far), adenoma (common), hyperplasia or carcinoma (rare)
- Tertiary hyperparathyroidism
- Ectopic PTH secretion (very rare indeed)

Malignant disease – low PTH levels (second most common cause)
- Myeloma
- Secondary deposits in bone
- Production of osteoclastic factors by tumours
- PTH-related protein secretion

Excess action of vitamin d
- Iatrogenic or self-administered excess
- Granulomatous diseases, e.g. sarcoidosis, tuberculosis
- Lymphoma

Excessive calcium intake
- 'Milk-alkali' syndrome

Other endocrine disease (mild hypercalcaemia only)
- Thyrotoxicosis
- Addison's disease

Drugs
- Thiazide diuretics
- Vitamin D analogues
- Lithium administration (chronic)
- Vitamin A

Miscellaneous
- Long term immobility
- Familial hypocalciuric hypercalcaemia

the glands (15–20%); multiple parathyroid adenomas are rare. Involvement of multiple parathyroid glands may be part of a familial syndrome (e.g. MEN type 1 or 2a). Parathyroid carcinoma is rare (<1%), though it usually produces severe and intractable hypercalcaemia. Hyperparathyroidism–jaw tumour syndrome is a rare familial cause of hyperparathyroidism that may be associated with parathyroid carcinoma and maxillary or mandibular tumours.

Primary hyperparathyroidism

Primary hyperparathyroidism is of unknown cause, though it appears that adenomas are monoclonal. Hyperplasia may also be monoclonal. Chromosomal rearrangements in the 5′ regulatory region of the parathyroid hormone gene have been identified, and inactivation of some tumour suppressor genes at a variety of sites may also be involved.

Secondary hyperparathyroidism

Secondary hyperparathyroidism (see p. 779) is physiological compensatory hypertrophy of all parathyroids because of hypocalcaemia, such as occurs in chronic kidney disease or vitamin D deficiency. PTH levels are raised but calcium levels are low or normal, and PTH falls to normal after correction of the cause of hypocalcaemia where this is possible.

Tertiary hyperparathyroidism

Tertiary hyperparathyroidism is the development of apparently autonomous parathyroid hyperplasia after longstanding secondary hyperparathyroidism, most often in renal failure. Plasma calcium and phosphate are both raised, the latter often grossly so. Parathyroidectomy is necessary at this stage.

Clinical features

Mild hypercalcaemia

Mild hypercalcaemia (e.g. adjusted calcium <3 mmol/L) is frequently asymptomatic, but more severe hypercalcaemia can produce a number of symptoms:

- ***General***. There may be tiredness, malaise, dehydration and depression.
- ***Renal***. Renal colic occurs from stones, polyuria or nocturia, haematuria and hypertension. The polyuria results from the effect of hypercalcaemia on renal tubules, reducing their concentrating ability – a form of mild nephrogenic diabetes insipidus. Primary hyperparathyroidism is present in about 5% of patients who present with renal calculi.
- ***Bones***. There may be bone pain. Hyperparathyroidism mainly affects cortical bone, and bone cysts and locally destructive 'brown tumours' occur but only in advanced disease. Only 5–10% of all cases have definite bony lesions even when sought. Bone disease may be more apparent when there is coexisting vitamin D deficiency.
- ***Abdomen***. There may be abdominal pain.
- ***Chondrocalcinosis*** and ectopic calcification. These are occasional features.
- ***Corneal calcification***. This is a marker of longstanding hypercalcaemia but causes no symptoms.

There may also be symptoms from the underlying cause. Malignant disease is usually advanced by the time hypercalcaemia occurs, typically with bony metastases. The common primary tumours are bronchus, breast, myeloma, oesophagus, thyroid, prostate, lymphoma and renal cell carcinoma. True 'ectopic PTH secretion' by the tumour is very rare, and most cases are associated with raised levels of PTH-related protein. This is a 144-amino-acid polypeptide, the initial sequence of which shows an approximate homology with the biologically active part of PTH, which is necessary in fetal development but does not have a clearly defined role in the adult. Bone-resorbing cytokines and prostaglandins may be involved locally where there are metastatic skeletal lesions, leading to local mobilization of calcium by osteolysis with subsequent hypercalcaemia.

Severe hypercalcaemia

Severe hypercalcaemia (>3 mmol/L) is usually associated with malignant disease, hyperparathyroidism, chronic kidney disease or vitamin D therapy.

Investigations and differential diagnosis

Biochemistry

Several fasting serum calcium and phosphate samples should be taken.

- ***Serum PTH***. The hallmark of primary hyperparathyroidism is hypercalcaemia and hypophosphataemia with detectable or elevated intact PTH levels during hypercalcaemia. When this combination is present in an asymptomatic patient, then further investigation is usually unnecessary. However, an undetectable PTH level in the context of hypercalcaemia always requires further investigation to exclude malignancy or other pathology ***(Box 26.47)***.
- ***Hyperchloraemic acidosis***. This is often mild.
- ***Renal function***. This is usually normal but should be measured as a baseline.

- ***24-h urinary calcium*** or single calcium creatinine ratio. This should be measured in a young patient with modest elevation in calcium and PTH to exclude familial hypocalciuric hypercalcaemia (see p. 1238).
- ***Elevated serum alkaline phosphatase***. This is found in severe parathyroid bone disease, but otherwise it suggests an alternative cause for hypercalcaemia.

Where PTH is undetectable or equivocal, a number of other tests may lead to the diagnosis:

- Protein electrophoresis/immunofixation: to exclude myeloma.
- Serum TSH: to exclude hyperthyroidism.
- 09:00 hours cortisol and/or ACTH test: to exclude Addison's disease.
- Serum ACE: helpful in the diagnosis of sarcoidosis.
- Hydrocortisone suppression test: hydrocortisone 40 mg three times daily for 10 days leads to suppression of plasma calcium in sarcoidosis, vitamin D-mediated hypercalcaemia and some malignancies.

Imaging

The success of parathyroid imaging is highly operator-dependent and choice therefore depends on local skills and experience. Imaging is frequently far less accurate than parathyroid exploration by an expert surgeon, where the success rate is at least 90%. Methods include:

- Radioisotope scanning using ^{99m}Tc-sestamibi, which is approximately 90% sensitive in detecting adenomas; it is enhanced with single-photon emission computed tomography (SPECT).
- Ultrasound, which is simple and safe, although insensitive for small tumours.
- High-resolution CT scan or MRI (more sensitive).

Dual energy X-ray absorptiometry (DXA) bone density scanning is useful to detect bone effects in asymptomatic people with hyperparathyroidism in whom conservative management is planned.

Abdominal X-rays may show renal calculi or nephrocalcinosis. High-definition hand X-rays can show subperiosteal erosions in the middle or terminal phalanges. Neither is required as part of diagnosis unless symptoms of renal calculi are present or there is evidence of renal failure.

Management of hypercalcaemia

Details of emergency treatment for severe hypercalcaemia are given in ***Box 26.48***. This should be followed by oral therapy unless the underlying disease can be treated.

Management of primary hyperparathyroidism

Medical management

There are no effective medical therapies at present for primary hyperparathyroidism, but a high fluid intake should be maintained and replacement of vitamin D in those that are deficient appears to have no detrimental effect on calcium levels. New therapeutic agents that target the calcium-sensing receptors (e.g. cinacalcet) are of proven value in parathyroid carcinoma and in dialysis patients (see p. 780), and are used in primary hyperparathyroidism where surgical intervention is contraindicated.

Surgery

There is agreement that surgery is indicated in primary hyperparathyroidism for:

- people with renal stones or impaired renal function
- bone involvement or marked reduction in cortical bone density
- unequivocal marked hypercalcaemia (UK guidelines advocate consideration of surgery if calcium is >2.85 mmol/L, although many endocrinologists will use a figure of >3.0 mmol/L; USA guidelines state >1 mg/dL above the reference range)
- the uncommon younger patient, below the age of 50 years
- a previous episode of severe acute hypercalcaemia.

The situation where plasma calcium is mildly raised (2.65–3.00 mmol/L) is more controversial. Most authorities feel that young patients should be operated on, as should those who have reduced cortical bone density or significant hypercalciuria, as this is associated with stone formation.

In older patients without these problems, or in those unfit for or unwilling to have surgery, conservative management is indicated. Regular measurement of serum calcium and of renal function is necessary. Bone density of cortical bone should be monitored if conservative management is used. Hyperparathyroidism can cause non-specific symptoms of weakness, fatigue and depression, and it can be difficult to determine whether these symptoms are related to hypercalcaemia or coincidental.

Box 26.48 Management of acute severe hypercalcaemia

Acute hypercalcaemia often presents with dehydration, nausea and vomiting, nocturia and polyuria, drowsiness and altered consciousness. The serum Ca^{2+} is >3 mmol/L and sometimes as high as 5 mmol/L. While investigation of the cause is under way, immediate treatment is mandatory if the patient is seriously ill or if the Ca^{2+} is >3.5 mmol/L.

- ***Rehydrate*** using at least 4–6 L of 0.9% saline on day 1, and 3–4 L for several days thereafter. Central venous pressure (CVP) may need to be monitored to control the hydration rate.
- ***Intravenous bisphosphonates*** are the treatment of choice for the hypercalcaemia of malignancy or of undiagnosed cause. Pamidronate is preferred (60–90 mg as an intravenous infusion in 0.9% saline or glucose over 2–4 h or, if less urgent, over 2–4 days). Levels fall after 24–72 h, lasting for approximately 2 weeks. Zoledronate is an alternative.
- ***Prednisolone*** (30–60 mg daily) is effective in some instances (e.g. in myeloma, sarcoidosis and vitamin D excess) but in most cases is ineffective.
- ***Calcitonin*** (200 units i.v. 6-hourly) has a short-lived action and is little used.
- ***Oral phosphate*** (sodium cellulose phosphate 5 g three times daily) produces diarrhoea.

Surgical technique and complications

Parathyroid surgery should be performed only by experienced surgeons, as the minute glands may be very difficult to define, and it is difficult to distinguish between an adenoma and normal parathyroid. In expert centres, over 90% of operations are successful, involving removal of the adenoma or removal of all four hyperplastic parathyroids. Minimal access surgery is used, and some centres measure PTH levels intraoperatively to ensure that the adenoma has been removed.

Other than postoperative hypocalcaemia (see below), the other rare complications are those of thyroid surgery: bleeding and recurrent laryngeal nerve palsies (<1%). Vocal cord function should be checked preoperatively.

If initial exploration is unsuccessful, a full work-up, including venous catheterization and scanning, is essential, remembering that parathyroid tissue can be ectopic.

Postoperative care

The major danger after operation is hypocalcaemia, which is more common in patients who have significant bone disease and/or vitamin D deficiency – the 'hungry bone' syndrome. Some authorities pre-treat such patients with alfacalcidol 2 µg daily from 2 days preoperatively for 10–14 days, and routine vitamin D replacement (preferably without calcium) is always indicated if deficiency is diagnosed. Chvostek's and Trousseau's signs (see below) are monitored, as well as biochemistry. Plasma calcium measurements are performed at least daily until stable, with or without replacement; a mild transient hypoparathyroidism often continues for 1–2 weeks. Depending on its severity, oral or intravenous calcium should be given temporarily, as only a few patients (<1%) will develop long-standing surgical hypoparathyroidism.

Familial hypocalciuric hypercalcaemia

This uncommon autosomal dominant, and usually asymptomatic, condition demonstrates increased renal reabsorption of calcium despite hypercalcaemia. PTH levels are normal or slightly raised and urinary calcium is low. Familial hypocalciuric hypercalcaemia is caused by loss-of-function mutations in the gene on the long arm of chromosome 3 encoding for the calcium-ion-sensing G-protein-coupled receptor in the kidney and parathyroid gland. Family members are often affected and this is detected by genetic analysis. Parathyroid surgery is not indicated, as the course appears benign. This diagnosis can be differentiated from hyperparathyroidism in an isolated case by the calcium:creatinine ratio in blood and urine.

Hypocalcaemia and hypoparathyroidism

Pathophysiology

Hypocalcaemia may be due to deficiencies of calcium homeostatic mechanisms, or secondary to high phosphate levels or other causes of hypocalcaemia ***(Box 26.49)***. All forms of hypoparathyroidism, except transient surgical effects, are uncommon.

Box 26.49 Causes of hypocalcaemia

Increased phosphate levels
- Chronic kidney disease (common)
- Phosphate therapy

Hypoparathyroidism
- Surgical – after neck exploration (thyroidectomy, parathyroidectomy – common)
- Congenital deficiency (DiGeorge syndrome)
- Idiopathic hypoparathyroidism (rare)
- Severe hypomagnesaemia

Vitamin D deficiency
- Osteomalacia/rickets
- Vitamin D resistance

Resistance to PTH
- Pseudohypoparathyroidism

Drugs
- Calcitonin
- Bisphosphonates

Other
- Acute pancreatitis (quite common)
- Citrated blood in massive transfusion (not uncommon)
- Low plasma albumin, e.g. malnutrition, chronic liver disease
- Malabsorption, e.g. coeliac disease

PTH, parathyroid hormone.

Aetiology

- ***Chronic kidney disease*** is the most common cause of hypocalcaemia.
- ***Severe vitamin D deficiency*** may cause mild, and occasionally severe, hypocalcaemia.
- ***Hypocalcaemia after thyroid or parathyroid surgery*** is common but usually transient; fewer than 1% of thyroidectomies leave permanent damage (see above).
- ***Idiopathic hypoparathyroidism*** is one of the rarer autoimmune disorders, and is often accompanied by vitiligo, cutaneous candidiasis and other autoimmune disease.

DiGeorge syndrome (see p. 140) is a familial condition in which the hypoparathyroidism is associated with intellectual impairment, cataracts and calcified basal ganglia, and occasionally with specific autoimmune disease.

Pseudohypoparathyroidism is a syndrome of end-organ resistance to PTH owing to a mutation in the $G_S\alpha$-protein (GNAS1), which is coupled to the PTH receptor. It is associated with short stature, short metacarpals, subcutaneous calcification and sometimes intellectual impairment. Variable degrees of resistance involving other G protein-linked hormone receptors may also be seen (TSH, LH, FSH).

Pseudo-pseudohypoparathyroidism describes the phenotypic defects but without any abnormalities of calcium metabolism. Individuals with this condition may share the same gene defect as those with pseudohypoparathyroidism and be members of the same families.

Clinical features

Hypoparathyroidism presents as neuromuscular irritability and neuropsychiatric manifestations. Paraesthesiae, circumoral numbness, cramps, anxiety and tetany ***(Box 26.50)*** are followed by convulsions, laryngeal stridor, dystonia and psychosis. Two signs of hypocalcaemia are Chvostek's sign (gentle tapping over the facial nerve causes twitching of the ipsilateral facial muscles) and Trousseau's sign (inflation of the sphygmomanometer cuff above systolic pressure for 3 min induces tetanic spasm of the fingers and wrist). Severe hypocalcaemia may cause papilloedema and, frequently, a prolonged QT interval on the ECG.

Investigations

The clinical history and picture is usually diagnostic and is confirmed by a low serum calcium (after correction for any albumin abnormality). Additional tests include:

- ***Serum and urine creatinine***. These test for renal disease.
- ***PTH levels*** in the serum. These are absent or inappropriately low in hypoparathyroidism, high in other causes of hypocalcaemia.
- ***Parathyroid antibodies***. These are present in idiopathic hypoparathyroidism.

Box 26.50 Causes of tetany

In the presence of alkalosis
- Hyperventilation
- Excess antacid therapy
- Persistent vomiting
- Hypochloraemic alkalosis, e.g. primary hyperaldosteronism

In the presence of hypocalcaemia
- See Box 26.49

- ***25-hydroxyvitamin D serum level***. This is low in vitamin D deficiency.
- ***Magnesium level***. Severe hypomagnesaemia results in functional hypoparathyroidism, which is reversed by magnesium replacement.
- ***X-rays of metacarpals***. Short fourth metacarpals occur in pseudohypoparathyroidism.

Management

In vitamin D deficiency, colecalciferol is the most appropriate treatment (see p. 717). In other cases, alpha-hydroxylated derivatives of vitamin D are preferred for their shorter half-life, and especially in renal disease, as the others require renal hydroxylation. Usual daily maintenance doses are 0.25–2 μg for alfacalcidol (1α-OH-D_3). During treatment, plasma calcium must be monitored frequently to detect hypercalcaemia. Oral calcium supplements may be used in the early stages of treatment, and severe hypocalcaemia presenting as an emergency may occasionally require replacement with intravenous calcium gluconate. In hypoparathyroidism, PTH therapy is being used.

Further reading

Bilezikian JP, Silverberg SJ. Asymptomatic primary hyperparathyroidism. *N Engl J Med* 2004; 350:1746–1751.
Fraser WD. Hyperparathyroidism. *Lancet* 2009; 374:145–158.
Marcocci C, Cetani F. Primary hyperparathyroidism. *N Engl J Med* 2011; 365:2389–2397.
Shoback D. Hypoparathyroidism. *N Engl J Med* 2008; 359:391–403.
Society for Endocrinology. *Emergency Endocrine Guidance: Acute Hypercalcaemia*; Society for Endocrinology 2013; http://www.endocrinology.org/policy.
Society for Endocrinology. *Emergency Endocrine Guidance: Acute Hypocalcaemia*; Society for Endocrinology 2013; http://www.endocrinology.org/policy.

Box 26.51 Multiple endocrine neoplasia (MEN) syndromes

Organ	Frequency	Tumours/manifestations
Type 1		
Parathyroid	95%	Adenomas/hyperplasia
Pituitary	70%	Adenomas – prolactinoma, ACTH- or GH-secreting (acromegaly)
Pancreas	50%	Islet cell tumours (secreting insulin, glucagon, somatostatin, VIP, pancreatic polypeptide, GH-releasing factor) Zollinger–Ellison syndrome (gastrinoma) Non-functional tumour
Adrenal	40%	Non-functional adenoma
Thyroid	20%	Adenomas – multiple or single
Type 2a		
Adrenal	Most	Phaeochromocytoma (70% bilateral) Cushing syndrome
Thyroid	Most	Medullary carcinoma (calcitonin-producing)
Parathyroid	60%	Hyperplasia
Type 2b		
Type 2a with marfanoid phenotype and intestinal and visceral ganglioneuromas but not hyperparathyroidism. Neuromas also present around lips and tongue		

ACTH, adrenocorticotrophic hormone; GH, growth hormone; VIP, vasoactive intestinal peptide.

OTHER ENDOCRINE DISORDERS

Diseases of many glands

Polyglandular autoimmune syndromes

Primary endocrine gland failure is commonly caused by autoantibodies (see ***Box 26.2***) and there may be multiple gland deficiencies. Most common are the associations of primary hypothyroidism and type 1 diabetes, and either of these with Addison's disease or pernicious anaemia.

Autoimmune polyendocrinopathy type 1

Autoimmune polyendocrinopathy type 1 (APS-1) is an autosomal recessive disorder and is caused by *AIRE* gene mutations. This condition is also associated with non-endocrine manifestations. The *AIRE* gene is present in the epithelium of the thymus and is involved in the presentation of self-antigens to thymocytes. Mutations will allow persistence of thymic lymphocytes, which react against self antigens and cause development of autoimmune disorders. Mucocutaneous candidiasis often develops before the onset of endocrine deficiencies, such as hypothyroidism, Addison's disease, type 1 diabetes, hypoparathyroidism, primary hypogonadism, nail dystrophy, vitiligo and dental enamel hypoplasia.

Autoimmune polyendocrinopathy type 2

Autoimmune polyendocrinopathy type 2 (APS-2) is not associated with candidiasis and is also known as Schmidt syndrome, typically when hypothyroidism, Addison's disease, type 1 diabetes, myasthenia gravis and primary hypogonadism are present in combination; coeliac disease is also an association.

Multiple endocrine neoplasias

Multiple endocrine neoplasia (MEN) is the name given to the simultaneous or metachronous occurrence of tumours involving a number of endocrine glands ***(Box 26.51)***. The condition is inherited in an autosomal dominant manner and arises from the expression of recessive oncogenic mutations, most of which have been isolated. Affected persons may pass on the mutation to their offspring in the germ cell, but for the disease to become evident, a somatic mutation must also occur, such as deletion or loss of a normal homologous chromosome.

MEN 1

The defect in MEN 1 is in a novel gene (*menin*) on the long arm of chromosome 11, which encodes for a 610-amino-acid protein. *Menin* represses a transcription factor (*JunD*), and lack of *JunD* suppression leads to decreased apoptosis and oncogenesis. People with the *MEN1* gene carry one mutant gene and a wild-type gene (i.e. are heterozygous). When the wild-type gene undergoes a random somatic mutation during life, this leads to loss of heterozygosity and explains the late onset of tumours at any stage (the 'two hit' hypothesis). MEN 1 is classically associated with pancreatic, parathyroid and pituitary tumours, although other glands may be affected (***Box 26.51, Fig. 26.40***).

MEN 2a and 2b

MEN 2a and 2b are caused by mutations of the *RET* proto-oncogene on chromosome 10 (see medullary thyroid cancer, p. 1212). This gene encodes for a transmembrane glycoprotein receptor. For MEN 2a, the mutation is in the extracellular domain; for 2b, it is in the intracellular domain. MEN 2 is classically associated with

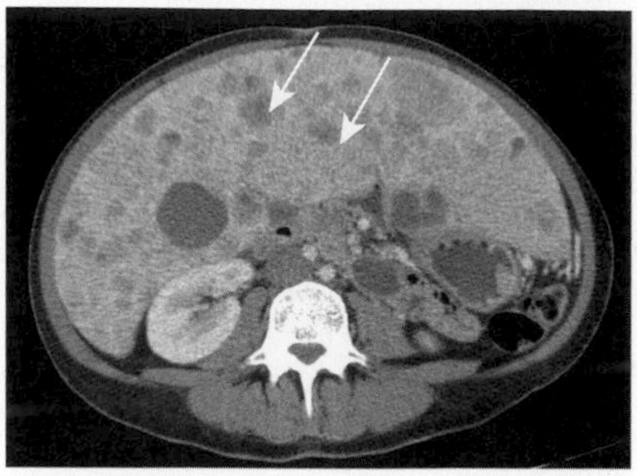

Figure 26.40 Multiple liver metastases (arrowed) from a pancreatic endocrine tumour in multiple endocrine neoplasia type 1.

parathyroid tumours, phaeochromocytoma and medullary thyroid carcinoma ***(Box 26.51)***. Unlike MEN 2a, MEN 2b is associated with a marfanoid phenotype and intestinal and visceral ganglioneuromas, as well as neuromas around the lips and tongue.

Management

Management of established tumours in MEN is largely the same as treatment for similar tumours occurring sporadically. In MEN 1, four-gland parathyroidectomy is usually recommended when surgery is needed since all glands are typically involved. However, the essence of management in MEN is annual screening to detect tumours at an early, treatable stage.

Screening

A careful family history is essential. If the precise gene mutation has been identified in a particular family, then family members at risk can be offered genetic screening for the presence of the mutation, ideally in childhood. In affected individuals, biochemical screening and periodic imaging are then required.

Screening for MEN 1

Hyperparathyroidism is usually the first manifestation, and serum calcium is the simplest screening test in families with no identified mutation. In an established case (or gene-positive family member), other screening bloods include prolactin, GH/IGF-1 and 'gut hormones' (see p. 377). Periodic imaging of pancreas, adrenals and pituitary is usually performed. People with MEN 1 can develop metastases to the liver from non-functional pancreatic tumours that are clinically silent; this emphasizes the need for regular screening imaging.

Screening for MEN 2

Serum calcium levels will easily detect hyperparathyroidism.

- ***Medullary carcinoma of thyroid (MCT)***. With the known presence of the gene defect, total thyroidectomy is recommended in early childhood or as soon as the gene defect is identified. Calcitonin is a useful tumour marker.
- ***Phaeochromocytoma***. Metanephrine or catecholamine estimations are required.

McCune–Albright syndrome

This condition is associated with autonomous hypersecretion of a number of endocrine glands at a young age. Gonadotrophin-independent puberty occurs, with Leydig cell hyperplasia in males and ovarian oestrogen production in girls. Pituitary hypersecretion may lead to hyperprolactinaemia, acromegaly or gigantism. Cushing syndrome due to nodular hyperplasia of the adrenal cortex is observed, as well as autonomous functioning thyroid nodules. Non-endocrine manifestations include café-au-lait patches and increased bone deformity and fractures due to polyostotic fibrous dysplasia. The pathological basis is a point mutation of the *GNAS1* gene that inhibits GTPase activity, leading to persistent activation of cAMP-mediated endocrine secretion.

Ectopic hormone secretion

This term refers to hormone synthesis, and normally secretion, from a neoplastic non-endocrine cell, most usually seen in tumours that have some degree of embryological resemblance to specialist endocrine cells. The clinical effects are those of the hormone produced, with or without manifestations of systemic malignancy. The most common situations seen are the following:

- ***Hypercalcaemia of malignant disease***, often from squamous cell tumours of lung and breast, often with bone metastases. Where metastases are not present, most cases are mediated by secretion of PTH-related protein (PTHrP), which has considerable sequence homology to PTH; a variety of other factors may sometimes be involved but very rarely PTH itself (see p. 1236). Treatment is discussed on page 1237.
- ***SIADH*** (see pp. 1234–1235). Again, this is most commonly caused by a primary lung tumour.
- ***Ectopic ACTH syndrome*** (see p. 1198). Small-cell carcinoma of the lung, carcinoid tumours and medullary thyroid carcinomas are the most common causes, though many other tumours rarely cause it.
- ***Production of insulin-like activity***. This may result in hypoglycaemia (see p. 1276).

Endocrine treatment of other malignancies

See Chapter 17.

Bibliography

Jameson JL, DeGroot L. *Endocrinology*, 6th edn. Philadelphia: WB Saunders; 2010.

Wass JA, Stewart P (eds). *Oxford Textbook of Endocrinology and Diabetes*, 2nd edn. Oxford: Oxford University Press; 2011.

Significant websites

http://www.addisons.org.uk/ *Addison's Self Help Group (UK): information and guidelines on Addison's and steroid replacement*
http://www.endocrine.niddk.nih.gov/ *US National Institutes of Health, National Institute of Diabetes and Digestive and Kidney Diseases*
http://www.endocrineweb.com *Endocrine web resources*
http://www.endocrinology.org *UK Society for Endocrinology*
http://www.endo-society.org *Endocrine Society*
http://www.endotext.org/ *Online endocrinology textbook*
http://www.medicalert.org.uk *Emergency identification system for people with hidden medical conditions*
http://www.pituitary.org.uk *Pituitary Foundation (UK charity): comprehensive information for patients and GPs*
http://www.thyroidmanager.org/ *Online thyroid disease textbook*
http://www.tss.org.uk *UK Turner Syndrome Support Society*

27 Diabetes mellitus

Edwin AM Gale, John V Anderson

See your e-book for key learning points, clinical tips, drug tips, extra tables, learning challenges, case studies, MCQs and Special Topics from the International Advisory Board.

INTRODUCTION

Diabetes mellitus (DM) is a syndrome of chronic hyperglycaemia due to relative insulin deficiency, resistance or both. The International Diabetes Federation (IDF) estimated that 382 million people (8.3% of the global population) had diabetes in 2013, and estimates an increase to 592 million (10.1%) in 2035. Diabetes is generally irreversible and, although patients can lead a reasonably normal lifestyle, its late complications result in reduced life expectancy and major health costs. These include macrovascular disease, leading to an increased prevalence of coronary artery disease, peripheral vascular disease and stroke, and microvascular damage causing diabetic retinopathy and nephropathy. Neuropathy is another major complication.

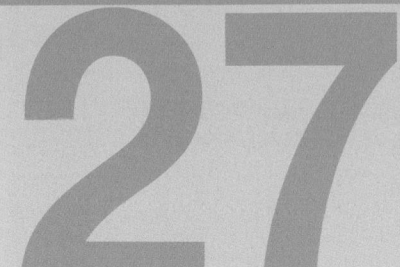

DIABETES MELLITUS

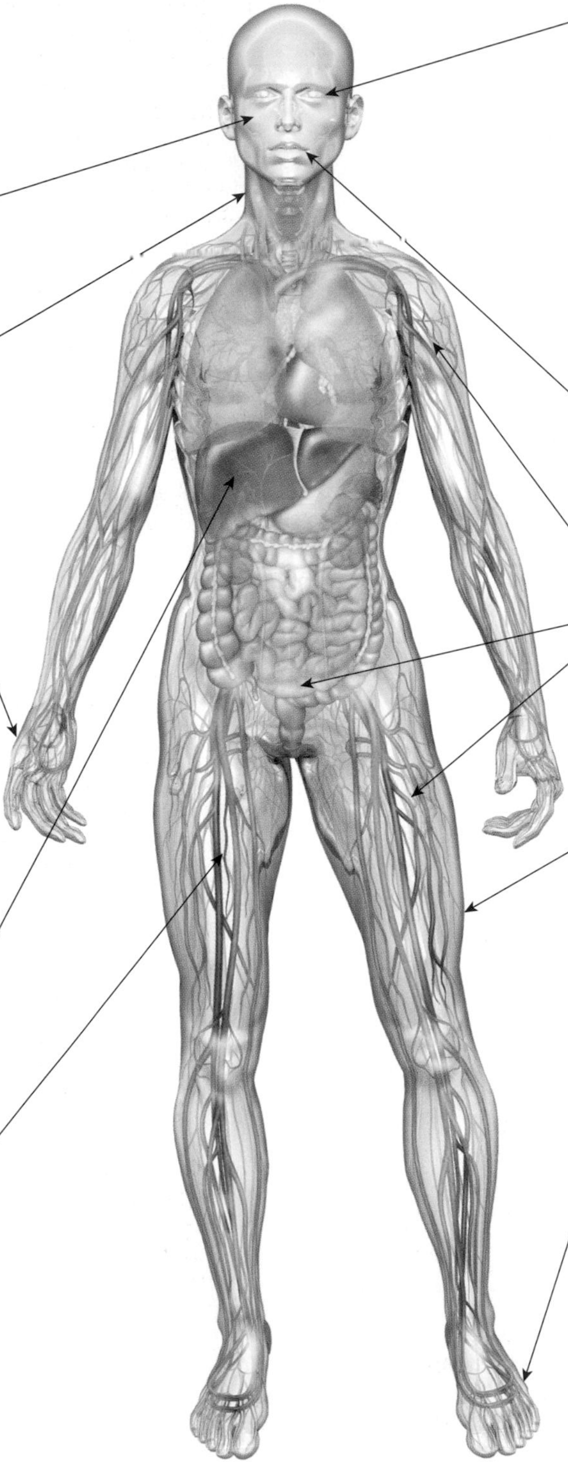

General observation
Does patient look well/ unwell?
Weight loss (DM1)
Weight gain (DM2)
Dehydrated?
Breathing (air hunger, Kussmaul breathing)

Face
Cranial nerve palsy, particularly CN3
Eye movements
Ptosis

Neck
Carotid pulses/bruits
Check thyroid gland for goitre (autoimmune)

Hands
Carpal tunnel
Dupuytren's contracture
Muscle wasting
Limited joint movement

Dupuytren's contracture

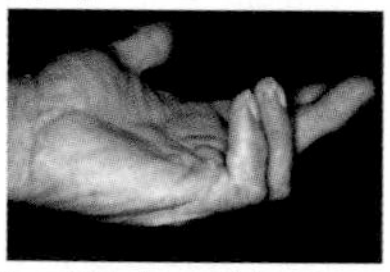

(From Palastanga N Anatomy and Human Movement, 6th Edn, with permission.)

Abdomen
Hepatomegaly (fatty liver)

Skin
Vitiligo (autoimmune)
Pigmentation (e.g. axillary acanthosis nigricans in insulin resistance)
Granuloma annulare
Bullosis

Vitiligo

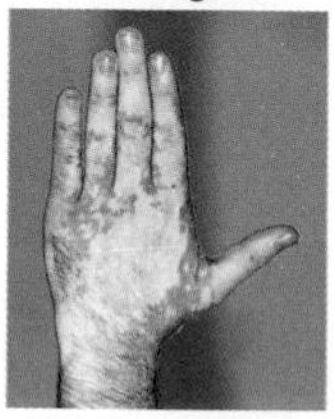

Eyes
Fundoscopy
- Cataracts, against red reflex
- Retinopathy (p. 1266)
- Visual acuity

Eyelids – xanthelasma

Cataracts

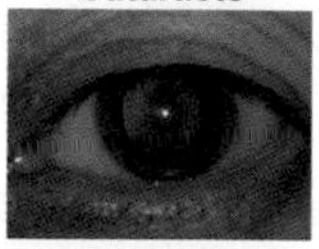

Retinopathy

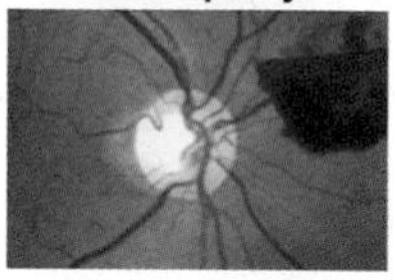

Mouth
Candidiasis

Insulin injection sites
Bruising
Lipohypertrophy
Lipoatrophy (rare)

Legs
Muscle wasting
Hair loss
Sensory neuropathy (glove and stocking)
Reflexes (lost in sensorimotor neuropathy)
Necrobiosis lipoidica

Feet
- Feel for peripheral pulses
- Skin – colour, ulcers, gangrene
- Look between toes for infection
- Sensory loss
  - Neuropathic foot ulcer
  - Charcot neuroarthropathy

Neuropathic ulcer

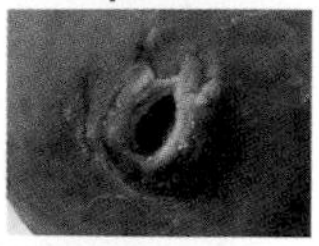

Charcot joints

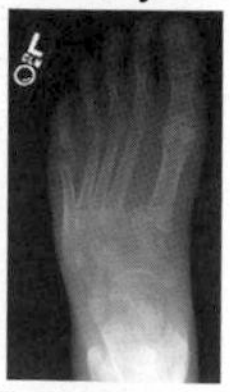

(From Miller MD 2011 Presentation, Imaging and Treatment of Common Musculoskeletal Conditions, Saunders, with permission.)

DIABETES MELLITUS

Practical guide to regular checks (see also *Box 27.12*)

- **Measure**
  - Body weight/BMI
  - Blood pressure
- **Blood tests**
  - FBC
  - Glycated Hb (metabolic control)
  - Fasting plasma lipids (except extreme old age)
- **Renal function**
  - Urea electrolytes
  - Creatinine
  - Estimated glomerular filtration rate (eGFR)
- **Eyes**
  - Acuity
    - Snellen chart at 6 m
    - Near vision – reading chart
    - Normal in most patients with retinopathy
  - Fundoscopy
    - Examine in darkened room. Dilute pupils (i.e. with tropicamide)
    - Note retinopathy ***(Fig 27.14)***
    - Note scars from photocoagulation from laser therapy

Examination of feet (pp. 1272–1273)

Inspection
- Discolouration (ischaemia)
- Loss of plantar arch
- Clawing of toes due to neuropathy
- Check weight bearing areas for callus
- Neuropathic ulcers
- Deformity of joints (Charcot's neuroarthropathy) – lack of sensation
- Between toes for infection

Sensation
- ↓ in glove and stocking distribution (peripheral sensorimotor neuropathy)
- Risk assessment – check with light touch using monofilaments
- Neuropathy – vibration, proprioception, pain

Circulation – check:
- Temperature of foot/toes
- Pulses
- Capillary refill

Reflexes
- Ankle jerks – ↓ in sensorimotor neuropathy
- Plantar reflex

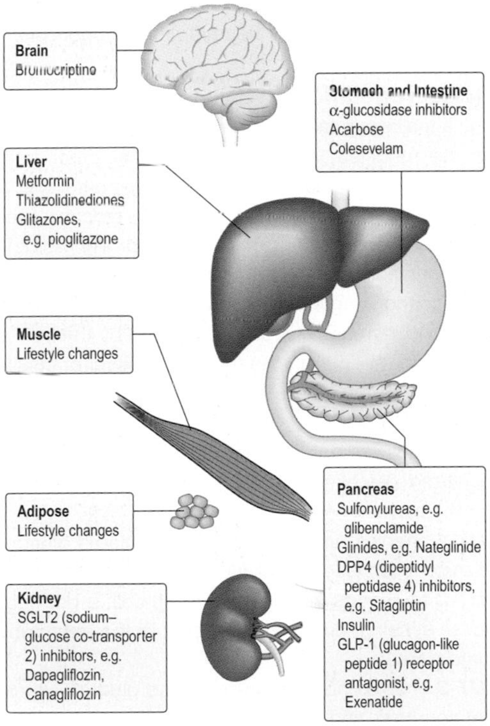

Drugs for treating type 2 diabetes mellitus
SGLT2 sodium–glucose co-transporter 2 inhibitors
DPP4 dipeptidyl peptidase 4 inhibitors
GLP-1 glucagon-like peptide 1 receptor antagonists

Examination of hands

- Joint mobility (cheiroarthopathy), painless stiffness
- Dupuytren's contracture (p. 655)
- Carpal tunnel syndrome (p. 655)
  – Pain radiating from wrist to hands
- Muscle wasting – due to sensorimotor neuropathy
- Trigger finger (flexor tenosynovitis)

Injection sites (see p. 1257)

- **Anterior abdominal wall**
- **Upper thighs/buttocks**
- **Upper outer arms**

Check sites for:
- Bruising
- Lipohypertrophy (subcutaneous fat deposition)
- Lipoatrophy (rare) (subcutaneous fat loss)
- Erythema
- Infection (rare)

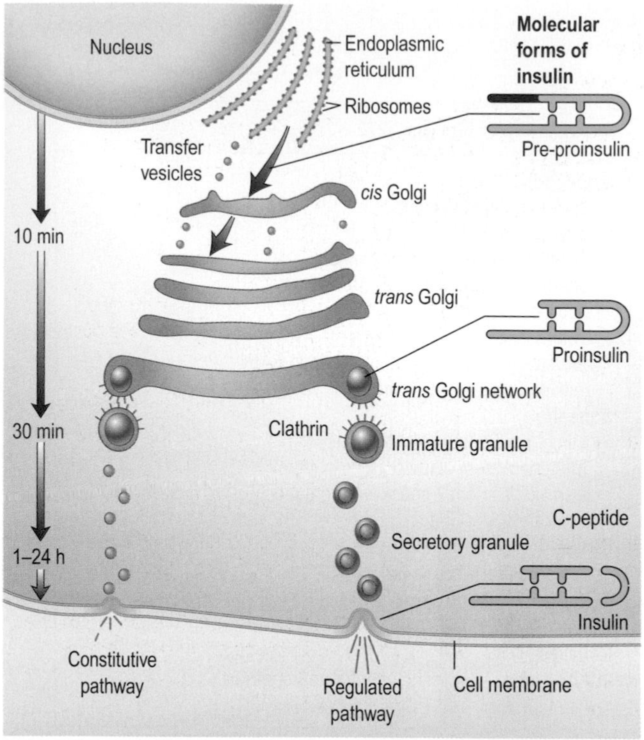

Figure 27.1 **Part of a β cell.** The ribosomes manufacture *pre-proinsulin* from insulin messenger RNA (mRNA). The hydrophobic 'pre' portion of pre-proinsulin allows it to transfer to the Golgi apparatus, and is subsequently enzymatically cleaved off.
Proinsulin is parcelled into secretory granules in the Golgi apparatus. These mature and pass towards the cell membrane, where they are stored before release. The proinsulin molecule folds back on itself and is stabilized by disulphide bonds.
The biochemically inert peptide fragment known as *connecting (C-) peptide* splits off from proinsulin in the secretory process, leaving insulin as a complex of two linked peptide chains. Equimolar quantities of insulin and C-peptide are released into the circulation via the '*regulated pathway*'. A small amount of insulin is secreted by the β cell directly via the '*constitutive pathway*', which bypasses the secretory granules.

Hyperglycaemia, insulin and insulin action

Insulin structure and secretion

Insulin is the key hormone involved in the storage and controlled release within the body of the chemical energy available from food. It is coded for on chromosome 11 and synthesized in the β cells of the pancreatic islets ***(Fig. 27.1)***. The synthesis, intracellular processing and secretion of insulin by the β cell is typical of the way that the body produces and manipulates many peptide hormones. ***Figure 27.2*** illustrates the cellular events triggering the release of insulin-containing granules. After secretion, insulin enters the portal circulation and is carried to the liver, its prime target organ. About 50% of secreted insulin is extracted and degraded in the liver; the residue is broken down by the kidneys. C-peptide is only partially extracted by the liver (and hence provides a useful index of the rate of insulin secretion) but is mainly degraded by the kidneys.

An outline of glucose metabolism

Blood glucose levels are closely regulated in health and rarely stray outside the range of 3.5–8.0 mmol/L (63–144 mg/dL), despite the varying demands of food, fasting and exercise. The principal organ of glucose homeostasis is the liver, which absorbs and stores glucose (as glycogen) in the post-absorptive state and releases it into the circulation between meals to match the rate of glucose utilization by peripheral tissues. The liver also combines three-carbon molecules derived from breakdown of fat (glycerol), muscle glycogen (lactate) and protein (e.g. alanine) into the six-carbon glucose molecule by the process of gluconeogenesis.

Glucose production

About 200 g of glucose is produced and utilized each day. More than 90% is derived from liver glycogen and hepatic gluconeogenesis, and the remainder from renal gluconeogenesis.

Glucose utilization

The brain is the major consumer of glucose and its function depends on an uninterrupted supply of this substrate. Its requirement is 1 mg/kg body weight per minute, or 100 g daily in a 70 kg person. Glucose uptake by the brain is obligatory and is not dependent on insulin, and the glucose used is oxidized to carbon dioxide and water. Tissues such as muscle and fat have insulin-responsive glucose transporters and absorb glucose in response to postprandial peaks in glucose and insulin. At other times, energy requirements are largely met by fatty-acid oxidation. Glucose taken up by muscle is stored as glycogen or metabolized to lactate or carbon dioxide and water. Fat uses glucose as a substrate for triglyceride synthesis; lipolysis releases fatty acids from triglyceride together with glycerol, a substrate for hepatic gluconeogenesis.

Hormonal regulation

Insulin is a major regulator of intermediary metabolism, although its actions are modified in many respects by other hormones. Its actions in the fasting and postprandial states differ ***(Fig. 27.3)***. In the fasting state, its main action is to regulate glucose release by the liver, and in the postprandial state it additionally promotes glucose uptake by fat and muscle. The effect of counter-regulatory hormones (glucagon, adrenaline (epinephrine), cortisol and growth hormone) is to increase glucose production by the liver and reduce its utilization in fat and muscle for a given level of insulin.

Glucose transport

Cell membranes are not inherently permeable to glucose. A family of specialized glucose-transporter (GLUT) proteins carry glucose through the membrane into cells.

- ***GLUT-1*** enables basal non-insulin-stimulated glucose uptake into many cells (see ***Fig. 13.30***).
- ***GLUT-2*** transports glucose into the β cell, a prerequisite for glucose sensing, and is also present in the renal tubules and hepatocytes.
- ***GLUT-3*** enables non-insulin-mediated glucose uptake into brain neurones and placenta.
- ***GLUT-4*** mediates much of the peripheral action of insulin. It is the channel through which glucose is taken up into muscle and adipose tissue cells following stimulation of the insulin receptor ***(Fig. 27.4)***.

The insulin receptor

This is a glycoprotein (400 kDa), coded for on the short arm of chromosome 19, which straddles the cell membrane of many cells ***(Fig. 27.4)***. It consists of a dimer with two α-subunits, which include the binding sites for insulin, and two β-subunits, which traverse the cell membrane. When insulin binds to the α-subunits, it induces a

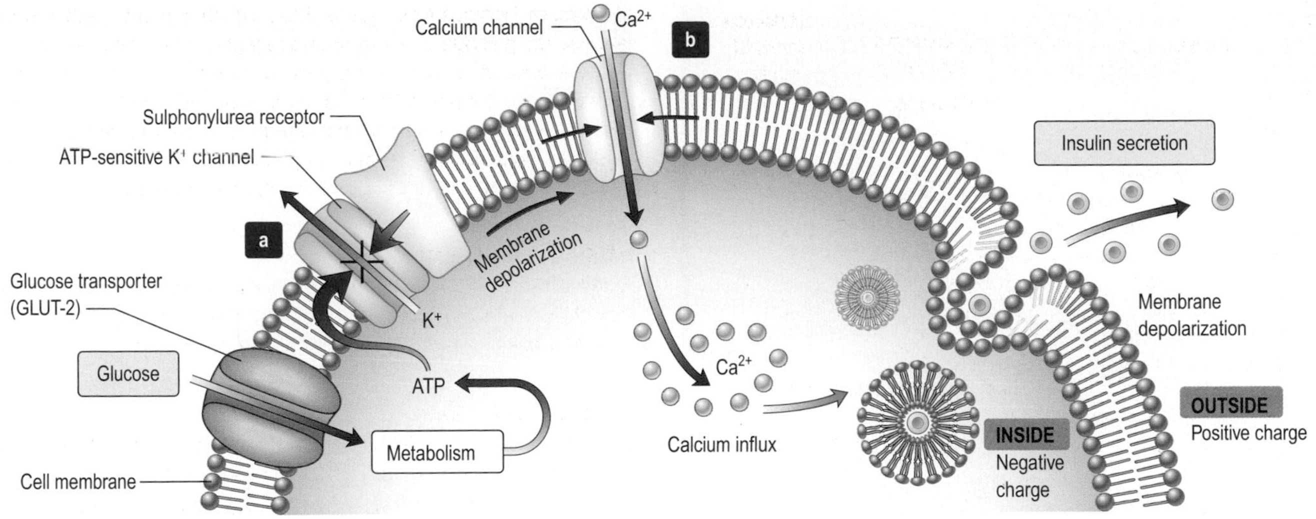

Figure 27.2 Local forces regulating insulin secretion from β cells. Glucose (on the left) enters the β cell via the GLUT-2 transporter protein, which is closely associated with the glycolytic enzyme glucokinase. Metabolism of glucose within the β cell generates adenosine triphosphate (ATP). ATP closes potassium channels in the cell membrane **(a)**. If a sulphonylurea binds to its receptor, this also closes potassium channels. Closure of potassium channels predisposes to cell membrane depolarization, allowing calcium ions to enter the cell via calcium channels in the cell membrane **(b)**. The rise in intracellular calcium triggers activation of calcium-dependent phospholipid protein kinase which, via intermediary phosphorylation steps, leads to fusion of the insulin-containing granules with the cell membrane and exocytosis of the insulin-rich granule contents. Similar mechanisms produce hormone-granule secretion in many other endocrine cells.

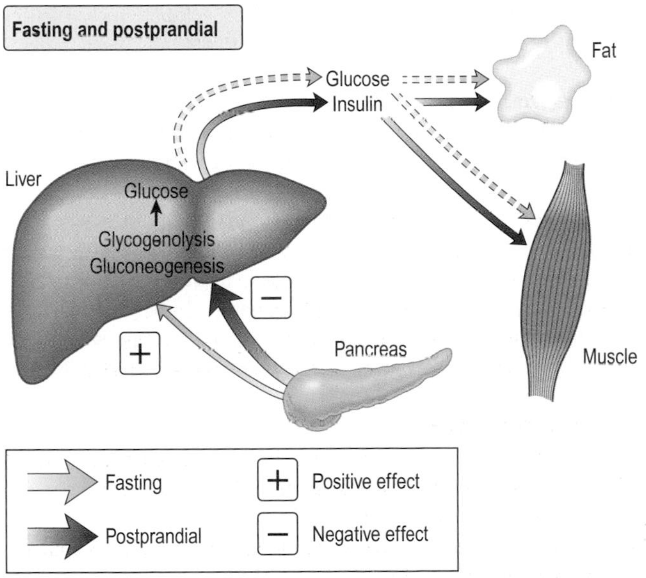

Figure 27.3 Fasting and postprandial effects of insulin. In the ***fasting state***, insulin concentrations are low and it acts mainly as a hepatic hormone, modulating glucose production (via glycogenolysis and gluconeogenesis) from the liver. Hepatic glucose production rises as insulin levels fall. In the ***postprandial state***, insulin concentrations are high and it then suppresses glucose production from the liver and promotes the entry of glucose into peripheral tissues (increased glucose utilization).

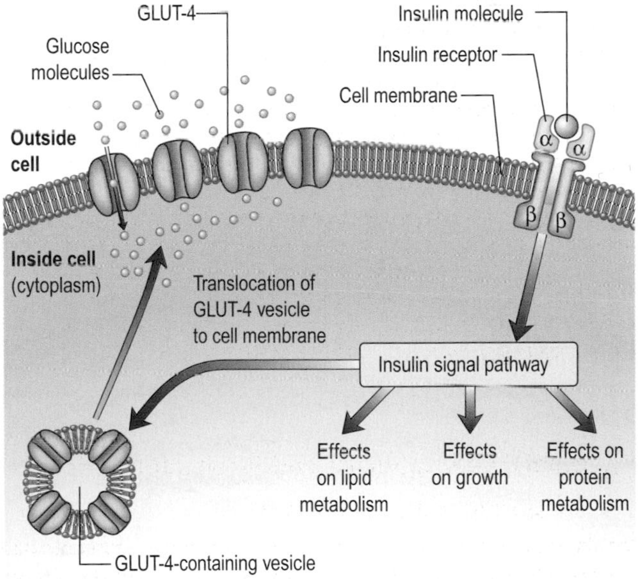

Figure 27.4 Insulin signalling in peripheral cells (e.g. muscle and adipose tissue). The insulin receptor consists of α- and β-subunits linked by disulphide bridges (top right). The β-subunits straddle the cell membrane. The transporter protein GLUT-4 (bottom left) is stored in intracellular vesicles. The binding of insulin to its receptor initiates many intracellular actions, including translocation of these vesicles to the cell membrane, carrying GLUT-4 with them; this allows glucose transport into the cell.

conformational change in the β-subunits, resulting in activation of tyrosine kinase and initiation of a cascade response involving a host of other intracellular substrates. One consequence of this is migration of the GLUT-4 glucose transporter to the cell surface and increased transport of glucose into the cell. The insulin-receptor complex is then internalized by the cell, insulin is degraded, and the receptor is recycled to the cell surface.

CLASSIFICATION OF DIABETES

Diabetes may be primary (idiopathic) or secondary ***(Box 27.1)***. Primary diabetes is classified into:

- ***type 1 diabetes***, which has an immune pathogenesis and is characterized by severe insulin deficiency

Box 27.1 Aetiological classification of diabetes mellitus, based on classification by the American Diabetes Association[a]

Type 1 diabetes
- Beta-cell destruction, usually leading to absolute insulin deficiency:
  - Immune-mediated
  - Idiopathic

Type 2 diabetes
- May range from predominantly insulin resistance with relative insulin deficiency to a predominantly secretory defect with insulin resistance

Other specific types
- Genetic defects of β-cell function
- Genetic defects in insulin action (mainly receptor mutations)
- Diseases of the exocrine pancreas:
  - Pancreatitis
  - Trauma/pancreatectomy
  - Neoplasia
  - Cystic fibrosis
  - Haemochromatosis
  - Fibrocalculous pancreatopathy
  - Other
- Endocrinopathies:
  - Acromegaly
  - Cushing syndrome
  - Glucagonoma
  - Phaeochromocytoma
  - Hyperthyroidism
  - Somatostatinoma
  - Aldosteronoma
  - Others
- Drug- or chemical-induced:
  - Vacor (pyrinuron)
  - Pentamidine
  - Nicotinic acid (niacin)
  - Beta-blockers
  - Thyroid hormone
  - Diazoxide
  - Beta-adrenergic agonists
  - Thiazides
  - Phenytoin
  - Interferon-alfa
  - Protease inhibitors
  - Immunosuppressive agents: glucocorticoids, ciclosporin, tacrolimus, sirolimus
  - Anti-psychotic agents: clozapine, olanzapine, others
- Infections
  - Congenital rubella
  - Cytomegalovirus
  - Others

Uncommon forms of immune-mediated diabetes
- 'Stiff person' syndrome
- Anti-insulin receptor antibodies

Other genetic syndromes sometimes associated with diabetes
- Down syndrome
- Friedreich's ataxia
- Huntington's chorea
- Klinefelter syndrome
- Laurence–Moon–Biedl syndrome
- Myotonic dystrophy
- Porphyria
- Prader–Willi syndrome
- Turner syndrome
- Wolfram syndrome
- Other

Gestational diabetes mellitus

[a]*Patients with any form of diabetes may require insulin treatment at some stage of their disease. Such use of insulin does not, of itself, classify the patient.*
(Adapted from American Diabetes Association. Diagnosis and classification of diabetes mellitus. Diabetes Care *2008; 31(Suppl 1):S55–S60.)*

Box 27.2 The spectrum of diabetes: a comparison of type 1 and type 2 diabetes mellitus

Features	Type 1	Type 2
Age	Younger (usually <30)	Older (usually >30)
Weight	Lean	Overweight
Symptom duration	Weeks	Months/years
Higher-risk ethnicity	Northern European	Asian, African, Polynesian and Native American
Seasonal onset	Yes	No
Heredity	HLA-DR3 or DR4 in >90%	No HLA links
Pathogenesis	Autoimmune disease	No immune disturbance
Ketonuria	Yes	No
Clinical	Insulin deficiency ± ketoacidosis Always need insulin	Partial insulin deficiency initially ± hyperosmolar state Need insulin when β cells fail over time
Biochemical	C-peptide disappears	C-peptide persists

HLA, human leucocyte antigen.

- ***type 2 diabetes***, which results from a combination of insulin resistance and less severe insulin deficiency.

The key clinical features of the two main forms of diabetes are listed in ***Box 27.2***. Type 1 and type 2 diabetes represent two distinct diseases from the epidemiological point of view, but from a clinical point of view the two conditions should be seen as a spectrum, distinct at the two ends but overlapping in the middle. Hybrid forms are increasingly recognized, and patients with immune-mediated diabetes (type 1) may, for example, also be overweight and insulin-resistant. This is sometimes referred to as 'double diabetes'. It is more relevant to give patients the right treatment on clinical grounds than to worry about how to label their diabetes. The classification of primary diabetes continues to evolve. Monogenic forms have been identified (see pp. 1249–1250), in some cases with significant therapeutic implications. Although secondary diabetes accounts for barely 1–2% of all new cases at presentation, it should not be missed because the cause can sometimes be treated. All forms of diabetes derive from inadequate insulin secretion relative to the needs of the body, and progressive insulin secretory failure is characteristic of both common forms of diabetes. Thus, some patients with immune-mediated diabetes type 1 may not at first require insulin, whereas many with type 2 diabetes will eventually do so.

Type 1 diabetes mellitus

Epidemiology

Type 1 diabetes is a disease of insulin deficiency and is subdivided into type 1A (immune-mediated) and type 1B (non-immune-mediated). The great majority of those affected, especially in Western countries, have type 1A disease. This typically manifests in childhood, reaching a peak incidence around the time of puberty, but can present at any age. A 'slow-burning' variant with slower progression to insulin deficiency occurs in later life and is sometimes called ***latent autoimmune diabetes in adults*** (***LADA***). LADA may be difficult to distinguish from type 2 diabetes. Clinical clues are leaner build, rapid progression to insulin therapy following an initial response to other therapies, and the presence of circulating islet autoantibodies. Finland and other Northern European countries have the highest rates of type 1 diabetes ***(Fig. 27.5)***. The incidence of type 1 diabetes appears to be increasing in most populations. In Europe, the annual increase is of the order of 2–3%, and is most marked in children under the age of 5 years. The IDF estimated in 2013 that 0.5 million children aged 0–14 years are currently affected by diabetes, and the figure is increasing by 3% annually.

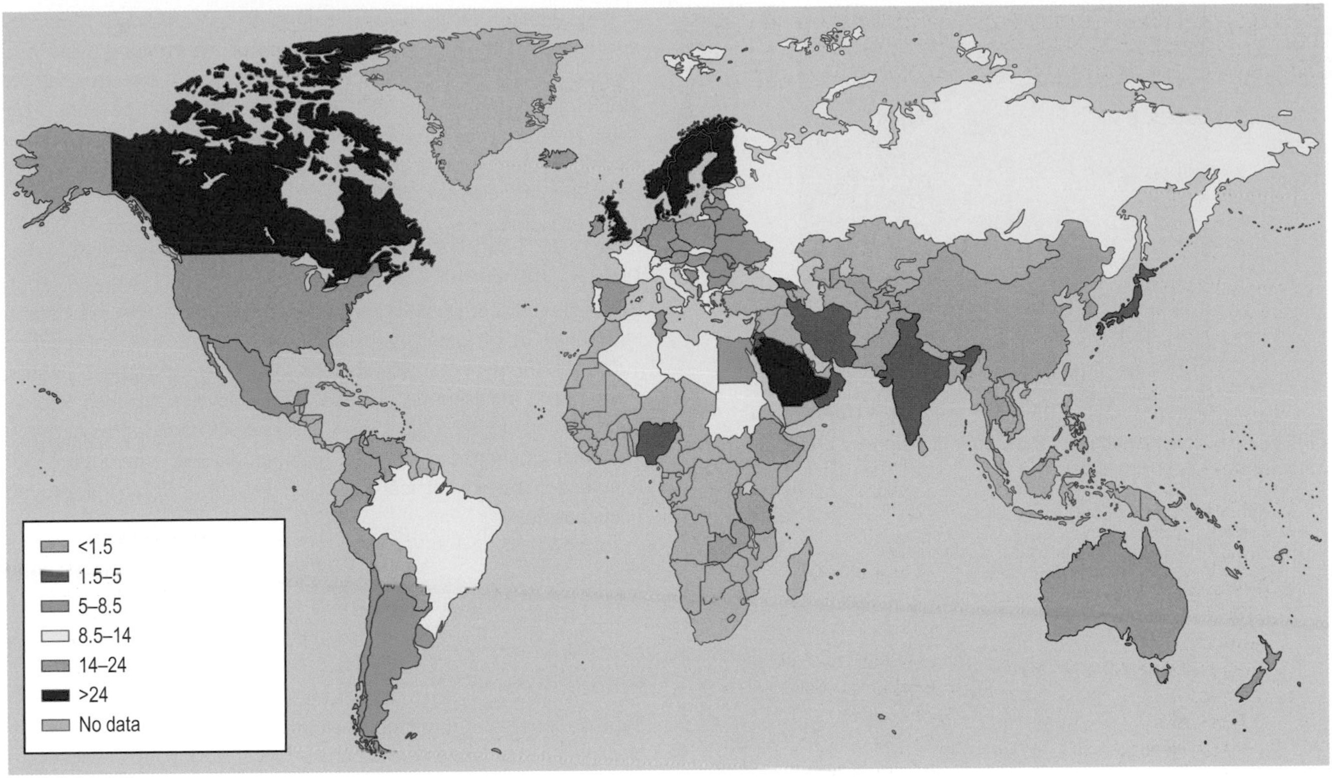

Figure 27.5 **New cases of type 1 diabetes (0–14 years per 100 000/year, 2013).** *(From International Diabetes Federation.* IDF Diabetes Atlas, *6th edn. Brussels: International Diabetes Federation; 2013, with permission.)*

Aetiology

Type 1 diabetes belongs to a family of human leucocyte antigen (HLA)-associated immune-mediated organ-specific diseases. Genetic susceptibility is polygenic, with the greatest contribution from the HLA region. Autoantibodies directed against pancreatic islet constituents appear in the circulation within the first few years of life, and often predate clinical onset by many years. Autoantibodies are also found in older patients with LADA and carry an increased risk of progression to insulin therapy.

Genetic susceptibility and inheritance

Increased susceptibility to type 1 diabetes is inherited but the disease is not genetically predetermined. The identical twin of a patient with type 1 diabetes has a 30–50% chance of developing the disease, which implies that non-genetic factors must also be involved. The risk of developing diabetes by age 20, curiously, is greater with a diabetic father (3–7%) than with a diabetic mother (2–3%). Earlier onset in the parent is associated with increased risk in the child. If one child in a family has type 1 diabetes, each sibling has a approximately 6% risk of developing diabetes by age 20. This risk rises to about 20% in HLA-identical siblings who have the same HLA type as the proband. Since type 1 diabetes can present at any age, the lifetime risk for a sibling or child is at least double the risk by age 20.

HLA system

The HLA genes on chromosome 6 are highly polymorphic and modulate the immune defence system of the body. More than 90% of patients with type 1 diabetes carry HLA-DR3-DQ2, HLA-DR4-DQ8 or both, as compared with some 35% of the background population. All DQB1 alleles with an aspartic acid at residue 57 confer neutral to protective effects, with the strongest effect from DQB1*0602 (DQ6), while DQB1 alleles with an alanine at the same position (i.e. DQ2 and DQ8) confer strong susceptibility. Genotypic combinations have a major influence on risk of disease. For example, HLA-DR3-DQ2/HLA-DR4-DQ8 heterozygotes have a considerably increased risk of disease, and some HLA class I alleles also modify the risk conferred by class II susceptibility genes.

Other genes or gene regions

Genome-wide association studies have greatly broadened our understanding of the genetic background to type 1 diabetes and more than 50 non-HLA genes or gene regions that influence risk have been identified to date. The greatest genetic contribution still comes from the HLA region but this is modulated by a large number of genes with small effects. These include the gene encoding insulin (*INS*) on chromosome 11 and a number of genes involved in immune responses, including the cytotoxic T-lymphocyte-associated protein-4 (*CTLA4*) gene, the lymphoid-specific protein tyrosine phosphatase (*PTPN22*) gene and the interleukin (IL)-2R α-subunit of the IL-2 receptor complex locus (*IL2RA*), all of which are implicated in a variety of HLA-associated autoimmune conditions.

Autoimmunity and type 1 diabetes

Type 1 diabetes is associated with other organ-specific autoimmune diseases, including autoimmune thyroid disease, coeliac disease, Addison's disease and pernicious anaemia. Autopsies of patients who died following a diagnosis of type 1 diabetes show infiltration of the pancreatic islets by mononuclear cells. This appearance, known as insulitis, resembles that in other autoimmune diseases such as thyroiditis ***(Fig. 27.6)***. Several islet antigens have been characterized and these include insulin itself, the enzyme

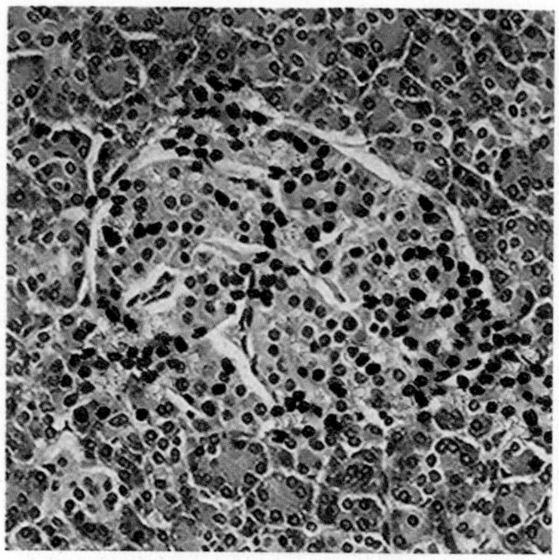

Figure 27.6 **Pancreatic islet showing infiltration by chronic inflammatory cells (insulitis).**

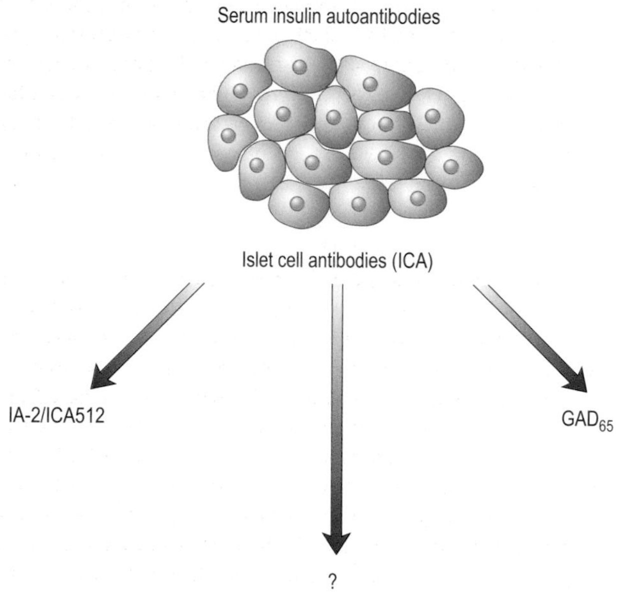

Figure 27.7 **Islet autoantibodies.** Islet cell antibodies (ICA) are detected by a fluorescent antibody technique that detects binding of autoantibodies to islet cells. Much of this staining reaction is due to antibodies specific for *glutamic acid decarboxylase* (GAD) and *protein tyrosine phosphatase* (IA-2, also known as ICA512). Not all the staining seen with ICA is due to these two autoantibodies, so it is assumed that other islet autoantibodies are also involved. Insulin autoantibodies also appear in the circulation but do not contribute to the ICA reaction.

glutamic acid decarboxylase (GAD), protein tyrosine phosphatase (IA-2) ***(Fig. 27.7)*** and the cation transporter ZnT8. The observation that treatment with immunosuppressive agents such as ciclosporin prolongs β-cell survival in newly diagnosed patients has confirmed that the disease is immune-mediated.

Environmental factors

The incidence of childhood type 1 diabetes is rising across Europe at the rate of 2–3% each year, suggesting that environmental factor(s) are involved in its pathogenesis. Islet autoantibodies (see above) appear in the first few years of life, indicating prenatal or early postnatal interactions with the environment. Exposures to dietary constituents, enteroviruses such as Coxsackie B4 and relative deficiency of vitamin D are possible candidates but their role in the causation of the disease has yet to be confirmed. A cleaner environment with less early stimulation of the immune system in childhood may increase susceptibility for type 1 diabetes, as for atopic/allergic conditions (the 'hygiene hypothesis'; see pp. 142–143), and more rapid weight gain in childhood and adolescence leading to increased insulin resistance might accelerate clinical onset (the 'accelerator hypothesis').

Pre-type 1 diabetes and prevention of type 1 diabetes

Children who test positive for two or more autoantibodies have a >80% risk of progression to diabetes, and the risk approaches 100% in those who additionally lose their first-phase insulin response to intravenous glucose and/or develop glucose intolerance. The ability to predict type 1 diabetes with this degree of precision has opened the way to trials of disease prevention, but intervention before clinical onset of diabetes has so far proved unsuccessful.

Type 2 diabetes mellitus

Epidemiology

Type 2 diabetes is common in all populations enjoying an affluent lifestyle, and has increased in parallel with the adoption of a Western lifestyle and increasing obesity. The four major determinants are increasing age, obesity, ethnicity and family history. In poor countries, diabetes is a disease of the rich, but in rich countries, it is a disease of the poor; obesity is the common factor. Glucose intolerance or frank diabetes may be present in a subclinical or undiagnosed form for years before diagnosis, and 25–50% of patients already have some evidence of vascular complications at the time of diagnosis. Onset may be accelerated by the stress of pregnancy, drug treatment or intercurrent illness. The IDF estimates the global lifetime risk of diabetes at 20%, with the highest rates and most rapid increase in the Middle East, South-east Asia and the Western Pacific. There are sometimes 2–3-fold differences in prevalence between populations from different ethnic backgrounds who share the same environment.

Obesity increases the risk of type 2 diabetes 80–100-fold, and this is reflected by the increasing prevalence of diabetes in different populations. On average, the inhabitants of affluent countries gain weight at the rate of 1 g/day or more between the ages of 25 and 55 years. This gain, due to a tiny excess in energy intake over expenditure (90 kcal or one chocolate-coated digestive biscuit per day), is often due to reduced exercise rather than increased food intake. The proportion of obese young adults with type 2 diabetes is rising rapidly, and epidemic obesity will create a huge public health problem for the future.

Type 2 diabetes is associated with central obesity, hypertension, hypertriglyceridaemia, a decreased high-density lipoprotein (HDL) cholesterol, disturbed haemostatic variables and modest increases in a number of pro-inflammatory markers. Insulin resistance is strongly associated with many of these variables, as is increased cardiovascular risk. This group of conditions is referred to as the ***metabolic syndrome*** (see p. 209). The IDF has proposed criteria based on increased waist circumference (or body mass index >30) plus two of the following: diabetes (or fasting glucose >6.0 mmol/L), hypertension, raised triglycerides or low HDL cholesterol. On this definition, about one-third of the adult population has features of the syndrome, not necessarily associated with diabetes. Critics argue that the metabolic syndrome is not a distinct entity, but one end of a continuum in the relationship between lifestyle and body weight on the one hand, and genetic make-up on the other, and that diagnosis adds little to standard clinical practice in terms of diagnosis, prognosis or therapy.

Aetiology

Genetic susceptibility and inheritance

Identical twins of patients with type 2 diabetes have more than a 50% chance of developing diabetes; the risk to non-identical twins or siblings is of the order of 25%, confirming a strong inherited component to the disease. Type 2 diabetes is a polygenic disorder and, as with type 1 diabetes, genome-wide studies of associations between common DNA variants and disease have allowed identification of numerous susceptibility loci. Several of these loci subserve β-cell development or function, and there is no overlap with the immune function genes identified for type 1 diabetes. There is no major gene susceptibility, involving the HLA region. However, transcription factor-7-like 2 (TCF7-L2) is the most common variant observed in type 2 diabetes in Europeans, and KCNQ1 (a potassium voltage-gated channel) in Asians. TCF7-L2 carries an increased risk of around 35%, while other common variants account for no more than 10–20%. TCF7-L2 modulates pancreatic islet cell function. Paradoxically, the genes for type 2 diabetes account for a relatively small fraction of its observed heritability. They do not allow subtypes of the condition to be identified with any confidence; nor do they provide useful disease prediction.

Environmental factors

An association has been noted between low weight at birth and at 12 months of age and glucose intolerance later in life, particularly in those who gain excess weight as adults. The concept is that poor nutrition early in life impairs β-cell development and function, predisposing to diabetes in later life. Low birth weight has also been shown to predispose to heart disease and hypertension.

Inflammation

Subclinical inflammatory changes are characteristic of both type 2 diabetes and obesity; in diabetes, high-sensitivity C-reactive protein (CRP) levels are modestly elevated in association with raised fibrinogen and increased plasminogen activator inhibitor-1 (PAI-1), contributing to cardiovascular risk. Circulating levels of the pro-inflammatory cytokines tumour necrosis factor alpha (TNF-α) and IL-6 are elevated in both diabetes and obesity.

Abnormalities of insulin secretion and action

The relative role of secretory failure versus insulin resistance in the pathogenesis of type 2 diabetes has been much debated, but even massively obese individuals with a fully functioning β-cell mass do not necessarily develop diabetes, which implies that some degree of β-cell dysfunction is necessary. Insulin binds normally to its receptor on the surface of cells in type 2 diabetes, and the mechanisms of 'insulin resistance' are still poorly understood. Insulin resistance is, however, associated with central obesity and accumulation of intracellular triglyceride in muscle and liver in type 2 diabetes, and a high proportion of patients have non-alcoholic fatty liver disease (NAFLD; see p. 465). It has long been stated that patients with type 2 diabetes retain up to 50% of their β-cell mass at the time of diagnosis, as compared with healthy controls, but the shortfall is greater than this when they are matched with healthy individuals who are equally obese. In addition, patients with type 2 diabetes almost all show islet amyloid deposition at autopsy, derived from a peptide known as amylin or islet amyloid polypeptide (IAPP), which is co-secreted with insulin. It is not known if this is a cause or consequence of β-cell secretory failure.

Abnormalities of insulin secretion manifest early in the course of type 2 diabetes. An early sign is loss of the first phase of the normal biphasic response to intravenous insulin. Established diabetes is associated with hypersecretion of insulin by a depleted β-cell mass. Circulating insulin levels are therefore higher than in healthy controls, although still inadequate to restore glucose homeostasis. Relative insulin lack is associated with increased glucose production from the liver (owing to inadequate suppression of gluconeogenesis) and reduced glucose uptake by peripheral tissues. Hyperglycaemia and lipid excess are toxic to β cells, at least *in vitro*, a phenomenon known as glucotoxicity, and this is thought to result in further β-cell loss and further deterioration of glucose homeostasis. Circulating insulin levels are typically higher than in non-diabetics following diagnosis and tend to rise further, only to decline again after months or years due to secretory failure, an observation sometimes referred to as the 'Starling curve' of the pancreas. Type 2 diabetes is thus a condition in which insulin deficiency relative to increased demand leads to hypersecretion of insulin by a depleted β-cell mass and progression towards absolute insulin deficiency, requiring insulin therapy. Its time course varies widely between individuals.

Overview and prevention

Genetic predisposition determines whether an individual is susceptible to type 2 diabetes; if and when diabetes develops largely depends on lifestyle. A dramatic reduction in the incidence of new cases of adult-onset diabetes was documented in the Second World War when food was scarce, and clinical trials in individuals with impaired glucose tolerance have shown that diet, exercise or agents such as metformin have a marked effect in deferring the onset of type 2 diabetes. Established diabetes can be reversed, even if temporarily, by successful dietary changes and weight loss, or by bariatric surgery. Diabetes is therefore largely preventable, although the most effective measures would be directed at the whole population and implemented early in life. Prevention is well worthwhile, for diabetes diagnosed in a man between the ages of 40 and 59 reduces life expectancy by 5–10 years. By contrast, type 2 diabetes diagnosed after the age of 70 has a limited effect on life expectancy.

Monogenic diabetes mellitus

The genetic causes of some rarer forms of diabetes are shown in **Box 27.3**. Considerable progress has been made in understanding these uncommon variants of diabetes. Genetic defects of β-cell function (previously called 'maturity-onset diabetes of the young', MODY) are dominantly inherited, and several variants have been described, each associated with different clinical phenotypes ***(Box 27.4)***. These should be considered in people presenting with early-onset diabetes in association with an affected parent and early-onset diabetes in approximately 50% of relatives.

Infants who develop diabetes before 6 months of age are likely to have a monogenic defect and not true type 1 diabetes. Transient neonatal diabetes mellitus (TNDM) occurs soon after birth and resolves at a median of 12 weeks; some 50% of cases ultimately relapse later in life. Most have an abnormality of imprinting of the *ZAC* and *HYMAI* genes on chromosome 6q. The most common cause of permanent neonatal diabetes mellitus (PNDM) is mutations in the *KCNJ11* gene encoding the Kir6.2 subunit of the β-cell potassium–adenosine triphosphate (ATP) channel.

Neurological features are seen in 20% of patients. Diabetes is due to defective insulin release rather than β-cell destruction, and patients can be treated successfully with sulphonylureas, even after many years of insulin therapy.

Further reading

Atkinson MA, Elsenbarth GS. Type 1 diabetes. *Lancet* 2014; 383:69–82.
Kahn SE, Cooper ME, Del Prato S. Pathophysiology and treatment of type 2 diabetes: perspectives on the past, present and future. *Lancet* 2014; 383:1068–1083.
McCarthy MI. Genomics, type 2 diabetes, and obesity. *N Engl J Med* 2010; 363:2339–2350.
Nathan DM. Navigating the choices for diabetes prevention. *N Engl J Med* 2010; 362:1533–1535.
Nolan CJ, Damm P, Prentki M. Type 2 diabetes across generations: from pathophysiology to prevention and management. *Lancet* 2011; 378:169–181.
Tirosh A, Shai I, Afek A et al. Adolescent BMI trajectory and risk of diabetes versus coronary disease. *N Engl J Med* 2011; 364:1315–1325.
Tuoml T, Santoro N, Caprio S et al. The many faces of diabetes, a disease with increasing heterogenicity. *Lancet* 2014; 383:1081–1097.
Yang W, Lu J, Weng J. Prevalence of diabetes among men and women in China. *N Engl J Med* 2010; 362:1090–1101.

? Box 27.3 Rare genetic causes of type 2 diabetes

Disorder	Features
Insulin receptor mutations	Obesity, marked insulin resistance, hyperandrogenism in women, acanthosis nigricans (areas of hyperpigmented skin)
Maternally inherited diabetes and deafness (MIDD)	Mutation in mitochondrial DNA. Diabetes onset before age 40. Variable deafness, neuromuscular and cardiac problems, pigmented retinopathy
Wolfram syndrome (diabetes insipidus, diabetes mellitus, optic atrophy and deafness, DIDMOAD)	Recessively inherited. Mutation in the transmembrane gene, *WFS1*. Insulin-requiring diabetes and optic atrophy in the first decade. Diabetes insipidus and sensorineural deafness in the second decade, progressing to multiple neurological problems. Few live beyond middle age
Severe obesity and diabetes	Alström, Bardet–Biedl and Prader–Willi syndromes. Retinitis pigmentosa, mental insufficiency and neurological disorders
Disorders of intracellular insulin signalling (all with severe insulin resistance)	Leprechaunism, Rabson–Mendenhall syndrome, pseudoacromegaly, partial lipodystrophy: lamin A/C gene mutation
Genetic defects of β-cell function	See ***Box 27.4***

CLINICAL APPROACH TO THE PATIENT WITH DIABETES

Presentation

Presentation may be acute, subacute or asymptomatic, or a patient may present with one of the complications of diabetes.

Acute presentation

Young people often present with a 2–6-week history and report the classic triad of symptoms:

- ***polyuria*** due to the osmotic diuresis that results when blood glucose levels exceed the renal threshold
- ***thirst*** due to the resulting loss of fluid and electrolytes
- ***weight loss*** due to fluid depletion and the accelerated breakdown of fat and muscle secondary to insulin deficiency.

Ketonuria is often present in young people and may progress to ketoacidosis if these early symptoms are not recognized and treated.

Subacute presentation

The clinical onset may be over several months or years, particularly in older patients. Thirst, polyuria and weight loss are typically present but patients may complain of such symptoms as lack of energy, visual blurring (owing to glucose-induced changes in refraction), or pruritus vulvae or balanitis that is due to *Candida* infection.

Complications as the presenting feature

These include:

- staphylococcal skin infections
- retinopathy noted during a visit to the optician
- a polyneuropathy causing tingling and numbness in the feet

i Box 27.4 Genetic defects of β-cell function[a]

Features	*HNF-4a*	Glucokinase	*HNF-1a*	*IPF-1*	*HNF-1b*
Chromosomal location	20q	7p	12q	13q	17q
Proportion of all cases	5%	15%	70%	<1%	2%
Onset	Teens/thirties	Present from birth	Teens/twenties	Teens/thirties	Teens/twenties
Progression	Progressive hyperglycaemia	Little deterioration with age	Progressive hyperglycaemia	Progression unclear	Progression unclear
Microvascular complications	Frequent	Rare	Frequent	Few data	Frequent
Other features	None	Reduced birth weight	Sensitivity to sulphonylureas	Pancreatic agenesis in homozygotes	Renal cysts, proteinuria, chronic kidney disease

[a]The glucokinase gene is intimately involved in the glucose-sensing mechanism within the pancreatic β cell. The hepatic nuclear factor (*HNF*) genes and the insulin promoter factor-1 (*IPF-1*) gene control nuclear transcription in the β cell, where they regulate its development and function. Abnormal nuclear transcription genes may cause pancreatic agenesis or more subtle progressive pancreatic damage. A handful of families with autosomal dominant diabetes have been described with mutations in neurogenic differentiation factor-1 (NeuroD1).

- erectile dysfunction
- arterial disease, resulting in myocardial infarction or peripheral gangrene.

Asymptomatic diabetes

Glycosuria or a raised blood glucose may be detected on routine examination (e.g. for insurance purposes) in individuals who have no symptoms of ill-health. This is more common in older people, who have a raised renal threshold for glucose. When present, glycosuria is not diagnostic of diabetes but indicates the need for further investigations. Familial renal glycosuria is a monogenic disorder affecting function of the sodium–glucose co-transporter (*SGLT2*) and found in about 1:400 of the population.

Physical examination at diagnosis

Evidence of weight loss and dehydration may be present, and the breath may smell of ketones. Older patients may present with established complications, and the presence of the characteristic retinopathy is diagnostic of diabetes. In occasional patients, there will be physical signs of an illness causing secondary diabetes (see ***Box 27.1***). Patients with severe insulin resistance may have acanthosis nigricans, which is characterized by blackish pigmentation at the nape of the neck and in the axillae (see p. 1364).

Diagnosis and investigations

Diabetes is easy to diagnose when overt symptoms are present and a random blood glucose measurement of >11 mmol/L confirms the diagnosis. In the absence of clear symptoms, diabetes can be diagnosed by any of three measures of glucose metabolism: the oral glucose tolerance test (OGTT), fasting plasma glucose and haemoglobin A_{1c} (HbA_{1c}) (***Boxes 27.5*** and ***27.6***). Unfortunately there is limited overlap between these measures, especially in the 'grey zone' between diabetes and normality.

Box 27.5 World Health Organization diagnostic criteria for diabetes[a]

- Fasting plasma glucose >7.0 mmol/L (126 mg/dL)
- Random plasma glucose >11.1 mmol/L (200 mg/dL)

  One abnormal laboratory value is diagnostic in symptomatic individuals; two values are needed in asymptomatic people. The glucose tolerance test (see ***Box 27.6***) is only required for borderline cases and for diagnosis of gestational diabetes
- HbA_{1c} >6.5 (48 mmol/mol)

[a]*There is no such thing as mild diabetes. All patients who meet the criteria for diabetes are liable to develop disabling long-term complications.*

Box 27.6 The glucose tolerance test: World Health Organization criteria[a]

Timing of test	Normal	Impaired glucose tolerance	Diabetes mellitus
Fasting	<6.0 mmol/L	<7.0 mmol/L	>7.0 mmol/L
2 h after glucose[b]	<7.8 mmol/L	7.8–11.0 mmol/L	>11.1 mmol/L

[a]Only a fasting and a 120-min sample are needed. Results are for venous plasma; whole-blood values are lower. [b]Adult 75 g glucose in 300 mL water; child 1.75 g glucose/kg body weight.

Pre-diabetes

Since any marker of abnormal glucose metabolism is associated with an increased risk of progression to diabetes and/or cardiovascular disease, it can be argued that a single abnormality is sufficient for admission into a risk category, which the American Diabetes Association (ADA) has labelled 'pre-diabetes'. On this basis, 86 million Americans suffer from pre-diabetes, in addition to the 25 million with known or undiagnosed diabetes. The World Health Organization (WHO) and other professional organizations avoid use of the term 'pre-diabetes', on the grounds that the majority will never, in fact, develop diabetes, and that the evidence to support screening and intervention is lacking.

Impaired glucose tolerance

Impaired glucose tolerance (IGT) is not a clinical entity but a risk factor for future diabetes and cardiovascular disease. The diagnosis can only be made with a glucose tolerance test, and is complicated by poor reproducibility of the key 2-hour value in this test. The group is heterogeneous; some patients are obese, some have liver disease and others are on medication that impairs glucose tolerance. Individuals with IGT have the same risk of cardiovascular disease as those with frank diabetes, but do not develop the specific microvascular complications.

Impaired fasting glucose

This diagnostic category (fasting plasma glucose between 6.1 and 6.9 mmol/L) has the practical advantage that it avoids the need for a glucose tolerance test. It is not a clinical entity but indicates future risk of frank diabetes and cardiovascular disease. Impaired fasting glucose (IFG) only overlaps with IGT to a limited extent, and the associated risks of cardiovascular disease and future diabetes are not directly comparable. A lower cut-off of 5.6 mmol/L (rather than 6.1 mmol/L) has been recommended by the ADA and would, if implemented, greatly increase the number of those in this category.

Haemoglobin A_{1c}

Haemoglobin A_{1c} (HbA_{1c}; also referred to as A_{1c} in the USA) is an integrated measure of an individual's prevailing blood glucose concentration over several weeks (see below). Standardization of this measure has enabled it to be proposed as an alternative diagnostic test for diabetes by the ADA. As currently proposed, an HbA_{1c} of >6.5% (48 mmol/mol) would be considered diagnostic of diabetes, whereas a level of 5.7–6.4% (39–46 mmol/mol) would denote increased risk of diabetes. A WHO consultation also concluded that HbA_{1c} 'can be used as a diagnostic test for diabetes'. The ADA has recommended that HbA_{1c} should be used together with IGT and IFG as a marker of 'pre-diabetes', with a range of 5.6–6.4% (38–46 mmol/mol).

Other investigations

No further tests are needed to diagnose diabetes. Other routine investigations include urine testing for protein, a full blood count, urea and electrolytes, liver biochemistry and random lipids. The latter test is useful to exclude associated hyperlipidaemia and, if elevated, should be repeated as a fasting measurement after diabetes has been brought under control. Diabetes may be secondary to other conditions (see ***Box 27.1***), precipitated by underlying illness, and associated with autoimmune disease or hyperlipidaemia. Hypertension is present in 50% of patients with type 2 diabetes and a higher proportion of African and Caribbean patients.

Further reading

American Diabetes Association. Diagnosis and classification of diabetes mellitus. *Diabetes Care* 2014; 37(Suppl 1):S81–S90.

http://www.who.int/diabetes/publications/ *WHO report: Use of Glycated Haemoglobin (HbA1c) in the Diagnosis of Diabetes Mellitus*.

MANAGEMENT OF DIABETES

The role of patient education and community care

The care of diabetes is based on self-management by the patient, who is helped and advised by those with specialized knowledge. The quest for improved glycaemic control has made it clear that whatever the technical expertise applied, the outcome depends on willing cooperation by the patient. This, in turn, depends on an understanding of the risks of diabetes and the potential benefits of glycaemic control and other measures such as maintaining a lean weight, stopping smoking and taking care of the feet. If accurate information is not supplied, misinformation from friends and other patients will take its place. For this reason, the best time to educate the patient is soon after diagnosis. Organized education programmes involve all healthcare workers, including nurse specialists, dieticians and podiatrists, and should include ongoing support and updates wherever possible.

Diet

The diet for people with diabetes is no different from that considered healthy for everyone. ***Box 27.7*** lists recommendations on the ideal composition of this diet. To achieve this, food for people with diabetes should be:

- low in sugar (though not sugar-free)
- high in starchy carbohydrate (especially foods with a low glycaemic index), i.e. slower absorption
- high in fibre
- low in fat (especially saturated fat).

The overweight or obese should be encouraged to lose weight by a combination of changes in food intake and physical activity.

Carbohydrates

The glucose peak seen in the blood after eating pasta is much flatter than that seen after eating the same amount of carbohydrate as white potato. Pasta has a lower 'glycaemic index'. Foods with a low glycaemic index prevent rapid swings in circulating glucose, and are thus preferred to those with a higher glycaemic index.

Prescribing a diet

Most people find it extremely difficult to modify their eating habits, and repeated advice and encouragement are needed if this is to be achieved. A diet history is taken, and the diet prescribed should involve the least possible interference with the person's lifestyle. Advice from dieticians is more likely to affect medium-term outcome than advice from doctors. People taking insulin or oral agents have traditionally been advised to eat roughly the same amount of food (particularly carbohydrate) at roughly the same time each day, so that treatment can be balanced against food intake and exercise. Knowledgeable and motivated patients with type 1 diabetes, who have feedback from regular blood glucose monitoring, can vary the amount of carbohydrate consumed, or mealtimes, by learning to adjust their exercise pattern and treatment. This is the basis of the Dose Adjustment for Normal Eating (DAFNE) regimen.

Box 27.7 Recommended composition of the diet for people with diabetes

Component of diet	How the recommended diet may be achieved
Protein	~1 g/kg ideal body weight
Total fat	<35% of energy intake. Limit: fat/oil in cooking, fried foods, processed meats (burgers, salami, sausages), high-fat snacks (crisps, cake, nuts, chocolate, biscuits, pastry). Encourage: lower-fat dairy products (skimmed milk, reduced-fat cheese, low-fat yoghurt), lean meat
Saturated and *trans*-unsaturated fat	<10% of total energy intake
n-6 polyunsaturated fat	<10% of total energy intake
n-3 polyunsaturated fat	No absolute quantity recommended. Encourage: fish, especially oily fish, once or twice weekly. Not recommended: fish oil supplements
Cis-monounsaturated fat	10–20% of total energy intake (olive oil, avocado)
Total carbohydrate	40–60% of total energy intake Encourage: artificial (intense) sweeteners instead of sugar (sugar-free fizzy drinks, squashes and cordials). Limit: fruit juices, confectionery, cake, biscuits
Sucrose	Up to 10% of total energy intake, provided this is eaten in the context of a healthy diet (e.g. fibre-rich breakfast cereals, baked beans)
Fibre	No absolute quantity recommended. Soluble fibre has beneficial effects on glycaemic and lipid metabolism. Insoluble fibre has no direct effects on glycaemic metabolism, but benefits satiety and gastrointestinal health
Vitamins and antioxidants	Best taken as fruit and vegetables (five portions per day) in a mixed diet. There is no evidence for the use of supplements
Alcohol	Not forbidden. Its energy content should be taken into account, as should its tendency to cause delayed hypoglycaemia in those treated with insulin
Salt	<6 g/day (lower in hypertension)

Exercise

No treatment for diabetes is complete without exercise. Any increase in activity levels is to be encouraged but participation in more formal exercise programmes is best. Where facilities for this exist, exercise should be prescribed for everyone with diabetes. Several trials have shown that regular exercise reduces the risk of progression to type 2 diabetes by 30–60%, and the lowest long-term morbidity and mortality rates are seen in those with established disease who have the highest levels of cardiorespiratory fitness. Both aerobic and resistance training improve insulin sensitivity and metabolic control in type 1 and type 2 diabetes, although reported effects on metabolic control are inconsistent. Patients on insulin or sulphonylureas should be warned that there is an increased risk of hypoglycaemia for up to 6–12 hours following heavy exertion.

Tablet treatment for type 2 diabetes

Diet and lifestyle changes are the key to successful treatment of type 2 diabetes, and no amount of medication will succeed where these have failed. Controlling diabetes is not just a matter of swallowing tablets, and these should never, in general, be prescribed until lifestyle changes have been implemented. Tablets will, however, be needed if satisfactory metabolic control (see pp. 1259–1260) is not established within 4–6 weeks. A consensus treatment pathway is shown in ***Figure 27.9*** (see p. 1255).

Biguanide (metformin)

Metformin is the only biguanide currently in use and remains the best validated primary treatment for type 2 diabetes. It activates the enzyme adenosine monophosphate (AMP) kinase, which is involved in regulation of cellular energy metabolism, but its precise mechanism of action remains unclear. Its effect is to reduce the rate of gluconeogenesis, and hence hepatic glucose output, and to increase insulin sensitivity. It does not affect insulin secretion, does not induce hypoglycaemia and does not predispose to weight gain. It is thus particularly helpful in the overweight, although normal-weight individuals also benefit, and may be given in combination with sulphonylureas, thiazolidinediones, dipeptidyl peptidase-4 (DPP4) inhibitors or insulin. Metformin was as effective as sulphonylurea or insulin in glucose control and reduction of microvascular risk in the UK Prospective Diabetic Study (UKPDS), but proved unexpectedly beneficial in reducing cardiovascular risk, an effect that could not be fully explained by its glucose-lowering actions. This effect has recently been questioned. ***Unwanted effects*** include anorexia, epigastric discomfort and diarrhoea, and these prohibit its use in 5–10% of patients. Diarrhoea should never be investigated in a diabetic patient without testing the effect of stopping metformin or changing to a slow-release preparation. Lactic acidosis has occurred in patients with severe hepatic or renal disease, and metformin is contraindicated when these are present. A Cochrane review showed little risk of lactic acidosis with standard clinical use, but most clinicians withdraw the drug when serum creatinine exceeds 150 μmol/L.

Metformin must be stopped prior to intravascular administration of iodinated contrast agent because of the risk of renal failure and subsequent lactic acidosis. Restart no earlier than 48 h after test of renal function has shown no deterioration.

Sulphonylureas

Sulphonylureas ***(Box 27.8)*** act on the β cell to promote insulin secretion in response to glucose and other secretagogues. They are ineffective in patients without a functional β-cell mass, and are usually avoided in pregnancy. Their action is to bind to the sulphonylurea receptor on the cell membrane, which closes ATP-sensitive potassium channels and blocks potassium efflux. The resulting depolarization promotes influx of calcium, a signal for insulin release (see ***Fig. 27.2***). Sulphonylureas are cheap and more effective than many other oral agents in achieving short-term (1–3 years) glucose control but their effect wears off as the β-cell mass declines. Some studies have associated use of sulphonylureas with the ***unwanted effects*** of increased cardiovascular morbidity and mortality, but the evidence is inconsistent. They promote weight gain and are best avoided in the overweight. They can also cause hypoglycaemia and, although the episodes are generally mild, fatal hypoglycaemia may occur, especially in the elderly. Severe cases should always be admitted to hospital, monitored carefully, and treated with a continuous glucose infusion since some sulphonylureas have long half-lives. They should be used with care in patients with liver disease, and patients with renal impairment should use sulphonylureas primarily excreted by the liver. Tolbutamide is the safest drug in the very elderly because of its short duration of action.

Box 27.8 Properties of the most commonly used sulphonylureas

Drug	Features
Tolbutamide	Lower maximal efficacy than other sulphonylureas Short half-life – preferable in the elderly Largely metabolized by liver – use is possible in renal impairment
Glibenclamide	Long biological half-life Severe hypoglycaemia Not suitable for use in the elderly
Glipizide and glimepiride	Active metabolites Renal excretion – should be avoided in renal impairment
Gliclazide	Intermediate biological half-life Largely metabolized by liver – use is possible in renal impairment More costly
Chlorpropamide	Very long biological half-life Renal excretion – should be avoided in renal impairment 1–2% develop inappropriate antidiuretic hormone (ADH)-like syndrome Facial flush with alcohol Very inexpensive – major issue for developing countries Can produce fatal hypoglycaemia Not recommended in the elderly

Meglitinides

Meglitinides, e.g. repaglinide and nateglinide, are insulin secretagogues. Meglitinides are the non-sulphonylurea moiety of glibenclamide. As with the sulphonylureas, they act via closure of the K^+-ATP channel in the β cells (see ***Fig. 27.2***). They are short-acting agents that promote insulin secretion in response to meals. Their effects are similar to those of the short-acting sulphonylurea tolbutamide but they are much more costly.

Thiazolidinediones

The thiazolidinediones (more conveniently known as the 'glitazones') reduce insulin resistance by interaction with peroxisome proliferator-activated receptor-gamma (PPAR-γ), a nuclear receptor that regulates large numbers of genes, including those involved in lipid metabolism and insulin action. The paradox that glucose metabolism should respond to a drug that binds to nuclear receptors mainly found in fat cells is still not fully understood. One suggestion is that these drugs act indirectly via the glucose–fatty acid cycle, lowering free fatty acid levels and thus promoting glucose consumption by muscle. They reduce hepatic glucose production, an effect that is synergistic with that of metformin, and also enhance peripheral glucose uptake. Like metformin, the glitazones potentiate the effect of endogenous or injected insulin. The glitazones have yet to demonstrate unique advantages in the treatment of diabetes, and their place in routine diabetes care remains uncertain. Troglitazone and rosiglitazone have been withdrawn because of safety concerns (liver failure and increased cardiovascular risk, respectively), and pioglitazone is the only remaining agent in this class. ***Unwanted effects*** of pioglitazone include weight gain of 5–6 kg, together with fluid retention, heart failure and a modestly increased risk of bladder cancer. Mild anaemia and osteoporosis resulting in peripheral bone fractures have also been reported.

Box 27.9 The incretin effect

The insulin response to *oral* glucose is greater than the response to *intravenous* glucose.

Cause

- Two intestinal peptide hormones, glucose-dependent insulinotropic peptide (GIP) and glucagon-like peptide-1 (GLP-1), have a potentiating effect on pancreatic secretion of insulin
- GIP causes 30%, and GLP-1 70%, of the incretin effect
- Both hormones have very short half-lives in the circulation, being degraded predominantly by the enzyme dipeptidyl peptidase-4 (DPP4)
- GIP is secreted from the K cells in the duodenum and GLP-1 from the L cells of the ileum in response to food

Magnitude

- The incretin effect is diminished in type 2 diabetes

Dipeptidyl peptidase-4 inhibitors

These enhance the incretin effect ***(Box 27.9)***. The enzyme dipeptidyl peptidase-4 (DPP4) rapidly inactivates glucagon-like peptide-1 (GLP-1) as this is released into the circulation. Dipeptidyl peptidase-4 inhibitors increase insulin secretion and lower glucagon secretions, and inhibition of this enzyme thus potentiates the effect of endogenous GLP-1 secretion. Five agents are currently available (alogliptin, linagliptin, saxagliptin, sitagliptin and vildagliptin). They have a moderate effect in lowering blood glucose and are weight-neutral. They are most effective in the early stages of type 2 diabetes, when insulin secretion is relatively preserved, and are currently recommended for second-line use in combination with metformin or a sulphonylurea. ***Unwanted effects*** are uncommon: the main side-effect is nausea, and there have been occasional reports of acute pancreatitis. Their place in the management of type 2 diabetes has yet to be fully established and cost remains a constraint. Although the short-term safety record is good, DPP4 is widely distributed in the body, and the long-term consequences of inhibition of this enzyme in other tissues are unknown.

Sodium/glucose transporter 2 inhibitors (inhibition of renal glucose transfer)

The sodium/glucose transporter 2 (SGLT2) is a sodium-dependent glucose transport protein located in the proximal renal tubules, whose function is to reabsorb glucose from the renal filtrate and restore it to the circulation. Its activity thus determines the renal threshold for glucose, which normally averages around 10 mmol/L. Specific inhibitors for this transporter have the effect of lowering this threshold, and consequently of increasing excretion of glucose in the urine. This has the effect of removing both glucose and calories from the circulation, thus lowering blood glucose and facilitating weight loss. Small reductions in systolic blood pressure have also been reported. Canagliflozin, dapagliflozin and empagliflozin are available. ***Unwanted effects*** include an increase in genital candidiasis and a small increase in urinary tract infections. This approach to therapy has the potential advantage of lowering glucose by a mechanism not mediated by insulin. One recent study showed a decrease in cardiovascular mortality when empagliflozin was added to standard care.

Injection therapies for type 2 diabetes

GLP-1 agonists

Exenatide, liraglutide and lixisenatide are injectable, long-acting analogues of glucagon-like peptide-1 (GLP-1), a gut hormone involved in the incretin effect ***(Box 27.9)***. They increase insulin secretion, inhibit glucagon secretion, delay gastric emptying and have central effects on appetite, thus blunting the postprandial rise in plasma glucose and promoting weight loss. Their main clinical disadvantage is the need for subcutaneous injection, and their major advantage is improving glucose control whilst inducing useful weight reduction. They work well in 70% but have limited benefit in 30% of those treated. ***Unwanted effects*** include nausea, acute pancreatitis and acute kidney injury. At present, they are used as an alternative to insulin, particularly in the overweight. A once-weekly version of exenatide has been developed.

GLP-1 promotes β-cell replication in immature rodents, but there is no evidence to suggest that it can do so in adult humans. GLP-1 receptors are also present in the exocrine pancreas and have potential growth-promoting effects, but the long-term clinical implications of this observation remain unclear.

Other therapies

- ***Intestinal enzyme inhibitors*** include acarbose, a sham sugar that competitively inhibits α-glucosidase enzymes situated in the brush border of the intestine, reducing absorption of dietary carbohydrate. Undigested starch may then enter the large intestine, where it will be broken down by fermentation. Abdominal discomfort, flatulence and diarrhoea can result, and dosage needs careful adjustment to avoid these side-effects.
- ***Orlistat*** is a lipase inhibitor that reduces the absorption of fat from the diet. It benefits diabetes indirectly by promoting weight loss in patients under careful dietary supervision on a low-fat diet. This is necessary to avoid unpleasant steatorrhoea.
- ***Colesevelam***, a bile acid-binding resin that lowers cholesterol, can reduce blood glucose concentrations by reducing release of gastrointestinal peptides.
- ***Gastric banding and gastric bypass surgery*** (see pp. 210–211) have been used in those with marked obesity unresponsive to 6 months' intensive attempts at dieting and graded exercise. The National Institute for Health and Care Excellence (NICE) recommends consideration of surgery in those with a body mass index (BMI) of >40, or in those with a BMI of >35 and co-morbidities such as diabetes or hypertension likely to be alleviated by weight loss. In the USA, the Food and Drug Administration (FDA)-recommended BMI thresholds are lower. The risks of surgery are not insignificant, and long-term specialist care and follow-up are needed, including psychological support and nutritional supplements for those with bowel resection, but these concerns should be balanced against the risk of patients staying as they are. Gastric banding is safer than gastric bypass (which involves permanent loss of gastric and duodenal tissue) but is also somewhat less effective. Evidence from randomized controlled clinical trials (RCTs) shows that about one-third of patients become non-diabetic after gastric bypass, but the procedure has life-long implications and diabetes may recur.

Insulin treatment

Insulin is found in every vertebrate and the key parts of the molecule show few species differences. Small differences in the amino acid sequence may alter the antigenicity of the molecule. The glucose and insulin profiles in normal subjects are shown in ***Figure 27.8***.

Short-acting insulins

Insulins were historically derived from beef or pig pancreas but these have now been almost entirely replaced by biosynthetic human insulin. This is produced by adding a DNA sequence coding for insulin or proinsulin into cultured yeast or bacterial cells. Short-acting insulins are used for pre-meal injection in multiple-dose regimens, for continuous intravenous infusion in labour or during medical emergencies, and for use in patients using insulin pumps. Human insulin is absorbed slowly, reaching a peak 60–90 minutes after subcutaneous injection, and its action tends to persist after meals, predisposing to hypoglycaemia. Absorption is delayed because soluble insulin is in the form of stable hexamers (six insulin molecules around a zinc core) and needs to dissociate to monomers or dimers before it can enter the circulation. ***Short-acting insulin analogues*** have been engineered to dissociate more rapidly following injection without altering the biological effect. ***Insulin analogues (Fig. 27.9)*** such as the ***rapid-acting insulins*** (***insulin lispro, insulin aspart*** and ***insulin glulisine***) enter the circulation more rapidly than human soluble insulin, and also disappear more rapidly. Although widely used, the short-acting analogues have little effect on overall glucose control in most patients, mainly because improved postprandial glucose is balanced by higher levels before the next meal. A Cochrane review has concluded that there is little evidence of their benefit in type 2 diabetes.

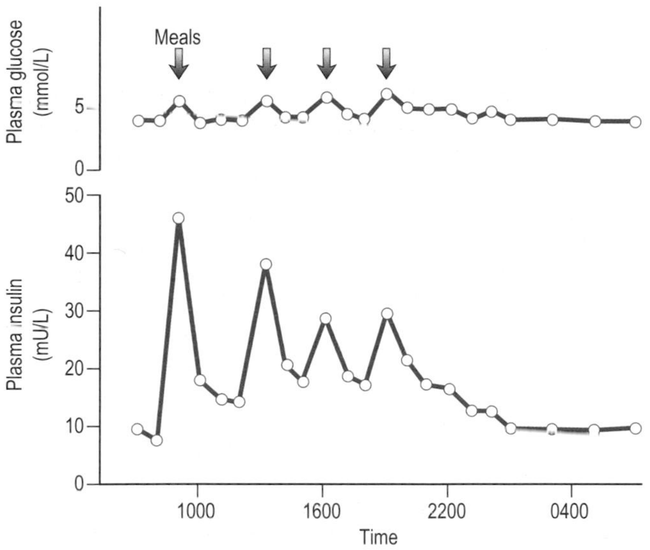

Figure 27.8 Glucose and insulin profiles in normal subjects.

Intermediate and longer-acting insulins

The action of human insulin can be prolonged by the addition of zinc or protamine derived from fish sperm. The most widely used form is NPH (isophane insulin), which has the advantage that it can be premixed with soluble insulin to form stable mixtures (biphasic insulins); the combination of 30% soluble with 70% NPH is most widely used. Long-acting analogues have their structure modified to delay absorption or to prolong their duration of action. ***Insulin glargine*** is soluble in the vial as a slightly acidic (pH 4) solution but precipitates at subcutaneous pH, thus prolonging its duration of action. ***Insulin detemir*** has a fatty acid 'tail' that allows it to bind to serum albumin, and its slow dissociation from the bound state prolongs its duration of action. ***Insulin degludec*** is a newer, long-term insulin that has proved non-inferior to insulin glargine, with a small reduction in nocturnal hypoglycaemia. Although popular and widely used, these insulins are much more expensive than, and have little demonstrated advantage over, human NPH, especially in the management of type 2 diabetes, although they are useful in those on intensified therapy or with troublesome hypoglycaemia. NICE advises that insulin analogues should be reserved for those who fail to respond well to human NPH insulin.

Inhaled insulin

The first inhaled insulin was withdrawn from the market in 2007 on the grounds of limited clinical demand, although lung cancer was

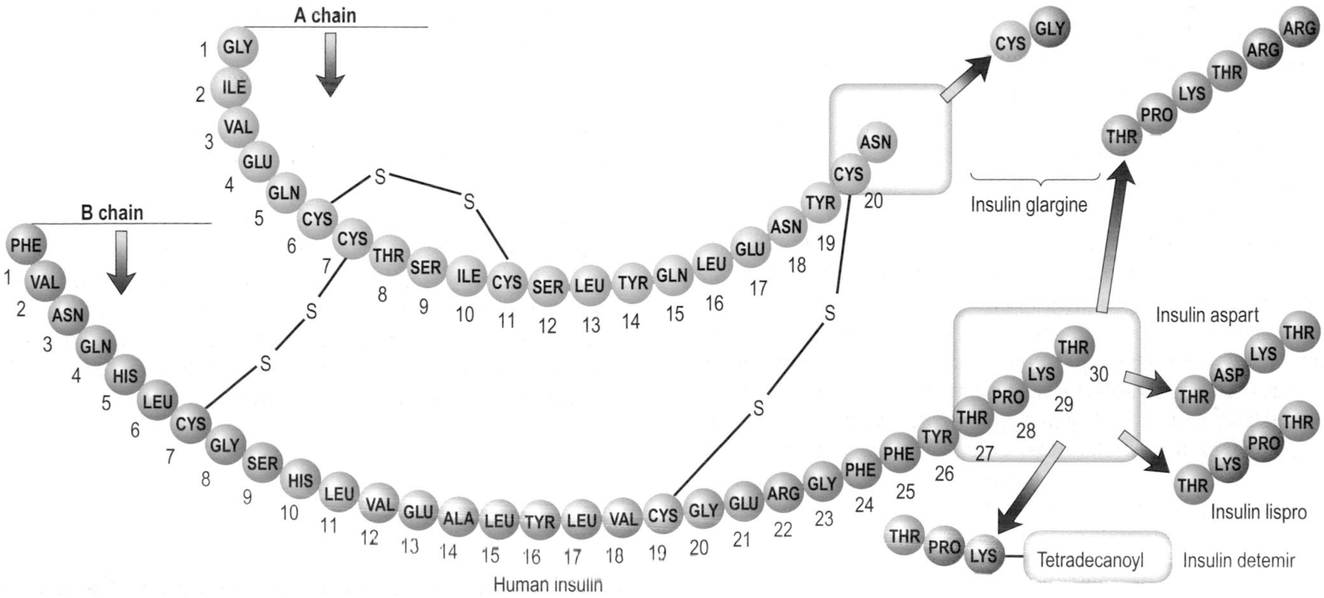

Figure 27.9 Amino acid structure of human insulin. Modification of human insulin produces rapid-acting insulins, of which two examples (lispro and aspart) are shown, and long-acting insulins (glargine and detemir). *Lispro* is created by reversing the order of the amino acids proline and lysine in positions 28 and 29 of the B chain. *Aspart* is a similar analogue created by replacing proline at position 28 of the B chain with an aspartic acid residue. *Insulin glargine* is created by replacing asparagine in position 21 of the A chain with a glycine residue and adding two arginines to the end of the B chain. *Detemir* discards threonine in position 30 of the B chain and adds a fatty acyl chain to lysine in position B29.

also observed. A new formulation (Afrezza®) received FDA approval in July 2014.

Practical management of diabetes

All patients with diabetes require advice about diet and lifestyle. Lifestyle changes – that is, controlling weight, stopping smoking and taking regular exercise – can prevent or delay the onset of type 2 diabetes in people with glucose intolerance. Good glycaemic control is unlikely to be achieved with insulin or oral therapy when diet is neglected, especially when the patient is also overweight. Regular exercise helps to control weight and reduces cardiovascular risk. Blood pressure control is vital using an angiotensin-converting enzyme (ACE) inhibitor or angiotensin II receptor antagonist (see pp. 985–987). Most patients will also benefit from a statin and low-dose aspirin (see p. 1265).

Type 2 diabetes

The great majority of patients presenting over the age of 40 will have type 2 diabetes but clinicians should be alert for the occasional type 1 patient presenting late. An approach to their management is illustrated in ***Figure 27.10***. Goals of treatment are described on page 1260. Type 2 diabetes is characterized by progressive β-cell failure, and glucose control deteriorates over time, requiring a progressive and pre-emptive escalation of diabetes therapy. Regular review is essential for this to be achieved. Most patients on tablets will eventually require insulin and it is helpful to explain this from the outset. The most widespread error in management at this stage is procrastination; the patient whose control is inadequate on oral therapy should start insulin without undue delay. Targets for glucose control are discussed later (see p. 1260).

NICE recommends NPH as the initial insulin to use in type 2 diabetes, and metformin is a useful adjunct in those able to tolerate it. NPH insulin at night, together with metformin during the day, is initially as effective as multidose insulin regimens in controlling glucose levels and is less likely to promote weight gain. Addition of a morning dose of insulin may become necessary to control post-prandial hyperglycaemia. Twice-daily injections of pre-mixed soluble and NPH (biphasic isophane) insulin are widely used and effective (***Fig. 27.11***, top panel). More aggressive treatment, with multiple injections or continuous infusion pumps, is increasingly used in younger patients with type 2 diabetes.

Type 1 diabetes

Insulin is always indicated in a patient who has been in ketoacidosis, and is usually required in lean patients who present under the age of 40 years.

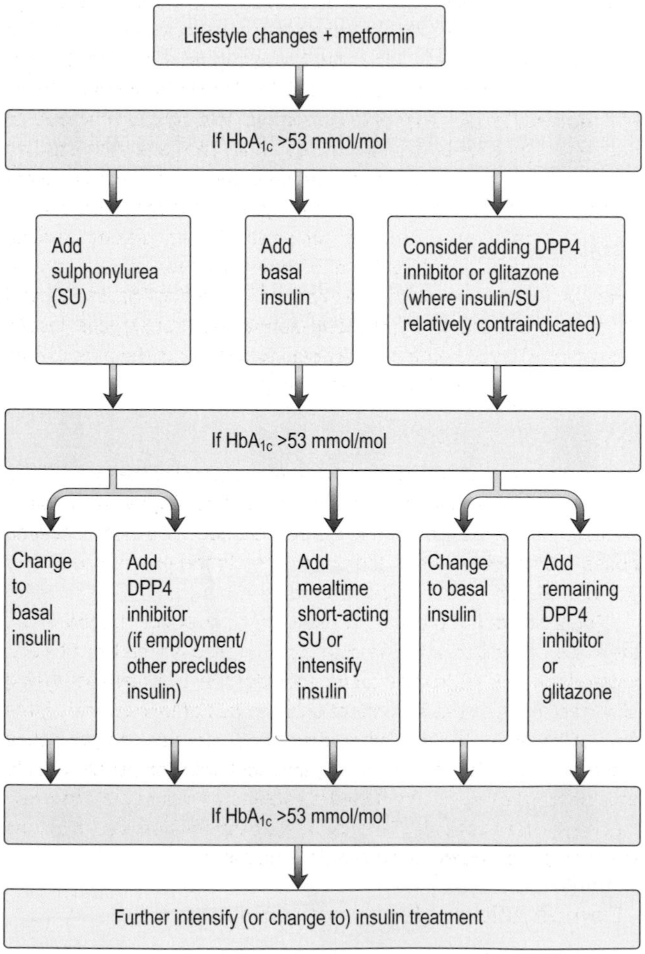

Figure 27.10 A treatment pathway for type 2 diabetes mellitus. Discussion of lifestyle changes and compliance should be undertaken at every stage. All patients require blood pressure control, statin therapy and low-dose aspirin. GLP-1 agonists and sodium glucose co-transporter 2 inhibitors are also used in many countries. DPP4, dipeptidyl peptidase-4.

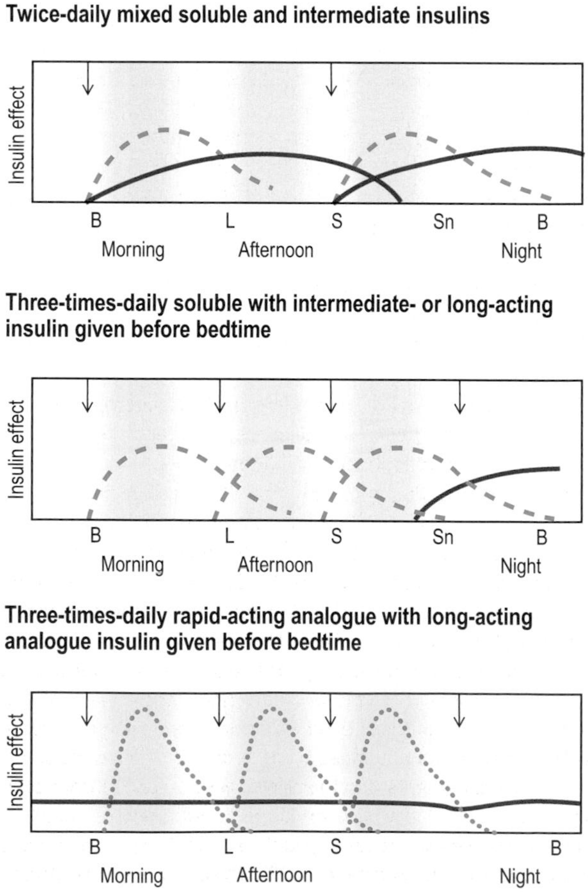

Figure 27.11 Insulin regimens. Profiles of soluble insulins are shown as dashed lines; intermediate- or long-acting insulin as solid lines (purple); and rapid-acting insulin as dotted lines (blue). The arrows indicate when the injections are given. B, breakfast; L, lunch; S, supper; Sn, snack (bedtime).

Principles of insulin treatment

Injections

The needles used to inject insulin are very fine and sharp. Even though most injections are virtually painless, patients are understandably apprehensive and treatment begins with a lesson in injection technique. Insulin is usually administered by a pen injection device but can be drawn up from a vial into special plastic insulin syringes marked in units (100 U in 1 mL). Injections are given into the fat below the skin on the abdomen, thighs or upper arm, and the needle is usually inserted to its full length. Slim adults and children usually use a 31-gauge 6-mm needle and fatter adults a 30-gauge 8-mm needle. Both reusable and disposable pen devices are available, together with a range of devices to aid injection. The injection site should be changed regularly to prevent areas of lipohypertrophy (fatty lumps). The rate of insulin absorption depends on local subcutaneous blood flow and is accelerated by exercise, local massage or a warm environment. Absorption is more rapid from the abdomen than from the arm, and is slowest from the thigh. All these factors can influence the shape of the insulin profile.

Insulin administration

In healthy individuals, a sharp increase in insulin occurs after meals; this is superimposed on a constant background of secretion (see ***Fig. 27.8***). Insulin therapy attempts to reproduce this pattern but ideal control is difficult to achieve for four reasons:

- In normal subjects, insulin is secreted directly into the portal circulation and reaches the liver in high concentration; about 50% of the insulin produced by the pancreas is cleared on first passage through the liver. By contrast, insulin injected subcutaneously passes into the systemic circulation before reaching the liver. Insulin-treated patients therefore have lower portal levels of insulin and higher systemic levels relative to the physiological situation.
- Subcutaneous soluble insulin takes 60–90 min to achieve peak plasma levels, so it is slower to reach its peak, and slower to leave the circulation.
- The absorption of subcutaneous insulin into the circulation is variable.
- Basal insulin levels are constant in healthy people but injected insulin invariably peaks and declines, with resulting swings in metabolic control in those with diabetes.

A multiple-injection regimen with short-acting insulin and a longer-acting insulin at night is appropriate for most younger patients (***Fig. 27.11***, middle panel). The advantages of multiple-injection regimens are that the insulin and the food go together, so that meal times and sizes can vary without greatly disturbing metabolic control. The flexibility of multiple-injection regimens is of great value to patients who have busy jobs, work shifts and travel regularly. Some recovery of endogenous insulin secretion may occur over the first few months (the 'honeymoon period') in type 1 patients and the insulin dose may need to be reduced or even stopped for a period. Requirements rise thereafter. Strict glucose control from diagnosis in type 1 diabetes prolongs β-cell function, resulting in better glucose levels and less hypoglycaemia. Target blood glucose values should normally be 4–7 mmol/L before meals and 4–10 mmol/L after meals, assuming that this can be achieved without troublesome hypoglycaemia.

All patients need careful training for a life with insulin. This is best achieved outside hospital, provided that adequate facilities exist for outpatient diabetes education. A scheme for adjusting insulin regimens is given in ***Box 27.10***. DAFNE is described on page 1252.

Box 27.10 Guide to adjusting insulin dosage according to blood glucose test results

Time	Blood glucose persistently too high	Blood glucose persistently too low
Before breakfast	Increase evening long-acting insulin	Reduce evening long-acting insulin
Before lunch	Increase morning short-acting insulin	Reduce morning short-acting insulin or increase mid-morning snack
Before evening meal	Increase morning long-acting insulin or lunch short-acting insulin	Reduce morning long-acting insulin or lunch short-acting insulin or increase mid-afternoon snack
Before bed	Increase evening short-acting insulin	Reduce evening short-acting insulin

When to use insulin analogues

Hypoglycaemia between meals and particularly at night is the limiting factor for many patients on multiple-injection regimens. The more expensive rapid acting insulin analogues (***Fig. 27.11***, bottom panel) are a useful substitute for soluble insulin in some patients, and reduce the frequency of nocturnal hypoglycaemia due to reduced carry-over effect from the daytime. They are often used on grounds of convenience, since patients can inject shortly before meals, but overall control is unchanged if standard insulins are injected at the same time. High or erratic fasting plasma glucose can prove a problem for patients on conventional multiple-injection regimens because the bedtime intermediate-acting insulin falls and the absorption is variable. The long-acting insulin analogues, insulin glargine and insulin detemir, may help to overcome these problems and reduce the risk of nocturnal hypoglycaemia.

Infusion devices

Continuous subcutaneous insulin infusion (CSII) is delivered by a small pump strapped around the waist that infuses a constant trickle of insulin via a needle in the subcutaneous tissues. Mealtime doses are delivered when the user instructs the pump to deliver a bolus of insulin at the start of a meal.

This approach is particularly useful in the overnight period, since the basal overnight infusion rate can be programmed to fit each patient's needs. Disadvantages include the nuisance of being attached to a gadget, skin infections, the risk of ketoacidosis if the flow of insulin is broken (since these patients have no protective reservoir of injected depot insulin), and cost. Infusion pumps should only be used by specialized centres able to offer a round-the-clock service to their patients. This form of treatment has revolutionized the lives of some people with type 1 diabetes.

Complications of insulin therapy

Injection site

Shallow injections result in intradermal insulin delivery and painful reddened lesions or even scarring. Injection site abscesses occur but are extremely rare. Fatty lumps, known as lipohypertrophy, may occur as the result of overuse of a single injection site with any type of insulin. Local allergic responses sometimes occur early in therapy but usually resolve spontaneously. Generalized allergic responses are exceptionally rare.

Insulin resistance

The most common cause of mild insulin resistance is obesity. Occasional unstable patients require massive insulin doses, sometimes with a fluctuating requirement. Some patients benefit from use of U500-strength insulin, which allows them to inject the same dose of insulin in one-fifth of the usual volume. Rare syndromes of insulin resistance may be present but most cases are unexplained. Insulin resistance associated with antibodies directed against the insulin receptor has been reported in patients with acanthosis nigricans (see ***Box 27.3***).

Weight gain

Many patients show weight gain on insulin treatment, especially if the insulin dose is increased inappropriately, but this can, to some extent, be overcome by an emphasis on the need for diet and exercise, with the addition of metformin. Patients who are in poor control when insulin is started are more likely to gain weight.

Hypoglycaemia during insulin treatment

This is the most common complication of insulin therapy and limits what can be achieved with insulin treatment. It is a major cause of anxiety for patients and relatives. It results from an imbalance between injected insulin and a patient's normal diet, activity and basal insulin requirement. The times of greatest risk are before meals, during the night and during exercise. Irregular eating habits, unusual exertion and alcohol excess may precipitate episodes; other cases appear to be due simply to variation in insulin absorption.

Symptoms

Symptoms develop when the blood glucose level falls below 3 mmol/L and typically develop over a few minutes, with most patients experiencing 'adrenergic' features of sweating, tremor and a pounding heartbeat. Virtually all patients with type 1 diabetes experience intermittent hypoglycaemia and 1 in 3 will go into a coma at some stage in their lives. A small minority suffer attacks that are so frequent and severe as to be virtually disabling.

Physical signs

These include pallor and a cold sweat. Many patients with long-standing diabetes report loss of these warning symptoms (***hypoglycaemic unawareness***) and are at a greater risk of central nervous dysfunction (neuroglycopenia), resulting in altered behaviour or conscious level. Such patients appear pale, drowsy or detached, signs that their relatives quickly learn to recognize. Behaviour is clumsy or inappropriate, and some individuals become irritable or even aggressive. Others slip rapidly into a hypoglycaemic coma. Occasionally, patients develop convulsions during a hypoglycaemic coma, especially at night. This must not be confused with idiopathic epilepsy. Another presentation is with a hemiparesis that resolves when glucose is administered.

People with diabetes have an impaired ability to counter-regulate glucose levels after hypoglycaemia. The glucagon response is invariably deficient, even though the α cells are preserved and respond normally to other stimuli. The adrenaline (epinephrine) response may also fail in patients with a long duration of diabetes, and this is associated with hypoglycaemia unawareness. Recurrent hypoglycaemia may itself induce a state of hypoglycaemia unawareness, and the ability to recognize the condition may sometimes be restored by relaxing control for a few weeks.

Nocturnal hypoglycaemia

Basal insulin requirements fall during the night but increase again from about 4 a.m. onwards, at a time when levels of injected insulin are falling. As a result, many patients wake with high blood glucose levels, but find that injecting more insulin at night increases the risk of hypoglycaemia in the early hours of the morning. The problem may be helped by the following measures:

- checking that a bedtime snack is taken regularly
- advising patients taking twice-daily mixed insulin that they can separate their evening dose and take the intermediate insulin at bedtime rather than before supper
- reducing the dose of soluble insulin before supper, since the effects of this persist well into the night
- changing to a rapid-acting insulin analogue, with a long-lasting insulin analogue at night
- changing to an insulin infusion pump that can be programmed to deliver lower doses of insulin at the time of night when a patient has been experiencing hypoglycaemia.

Mild hypoglycaemia

Any form of rapidly absorbed carbohydrate will relieve the early symptoms, and glucose or sweets should always be carried. Drowsy individuals will be able to take carbohydrate in liquid form (e.g. Lucozade®). All patients and their close relatives need training about the risks of hypoglycaemia. More carbohydrate than necessary should not be taken during the recovery period, since this causes a rebound to hyperglycaemia. Alcohol excess increases the risk of hypoglycaemia and this requires careful explanation, together with a warning about the need to guard against hypoglycaemia while driving.

Severe hypoglycaemia

The diagnosis of severe hypoglycaemia resulting in confusion or coma is simple and can usually be made on clinical grounds, backed by a bedside blood test. If real doubt exists, blood should be taken for glucose estimation before treatment is given. Patients should carry a card or wear a bracelet or necklace to say that they have diabetes, and these should be looked for in unconscious patients.

Unconscious patients should be given either intramuscular glucagon (1 mg) or intravenous glucose (25–50 mL of 50% glucose solution) followed by a flush of 0.9% saline to preserve the vein (since 50% glucose scleroses veins). Glucagon acts by mobilizing hepatic glycogen, and works almost as rapidly as glucose. It is simple to administer and can be given at home by relatives. It does not work when liver glycogen levels are low, as after a prolonged fast. Oral glucose is given to replenish glycogen reserves once the patient revives.

Whole-pancreas and pancreatic islet transplantation

Whole-pancreas transplantation has been performed for some 30 years, usually in diabetic patients who require immunosuppression for a kidney transplant. Surgical advances have greatly improved the outcome of this procedure. In experienced hands, graft function lasts longer with considerable improvement in quality of life. Patient survival is better in those who receive simultaneous pancreas and kidney grafts, mainly because of the delay involved in waiting for a pancreas to become available following renal transplantation. There is some evidence of protection against or reversal of some complications of diabetes, but this comes at the cost of long-term immunosuppression.

Islet transplantation is performed by harvesting pancreatic islets from cadavers (two or three pancreata are usually needed); these are then injected into the portal vein and seed themselves into the liver. This form of treatment had limited success for many years but improved treatment protocols have now achieved more promising results. The main indication for islet transplantation is disabling hypoglycaemia, and the main disadvantage is the need for powerful immunosuppressive therapy, with its associated costs and complications.

Measuring the metabolic control of diabetes

Urine tests

Urine dipstick tests, although less informative than blood tests, offer some feedback on metabolic control. Patients with consistently negative tests and no symptoms of hypoglycaemia are generally well controlled. Nevertheless, the correlation between urine tests and simultaneous blood glucose is poor for three reasons:

- Changes in urine glucose lag behind changes in blood glucose.
- The mean renal threshold is around 10 mmol/L but the range is wide (7–13 mmol/L). The threshold also rises with age.
- Urine tests can give no guidance concerning blood glucose levels below the renal threshold

Home blood glucose testing

Blood tests offer invaluable feedback to everyone affected by diabetes but their routine use varies according to need. Patients soon learn to provide their own profiles using finger-prick blood samples and reagent strips, which can be read with the aid of a meter. Blood is taken from the side of a finger-tip (not from the top, which is densely innervated) using a special lancet that is usually fitted to a spring-loaded device; a range of these is available. The fasting blood glucose concentration is reproducible in diet- or tablet-treated type 2 diabetes and is therefore a useful guide to therapy, supplemented by occasional tests after meals. Those on insulin treatment require more frequent testing in order to adjust their therapy and avoid hypoglycaemia. Regular profiles (e.g. 4 daily samples on at least 2 days each week) are needed in those on intensified therapy, and should be recorded electronically or in a record book. Patients on insulin are encouraged to adjust their insulin dose as appropriate ***(Box 27.10)*** and should be able to obtain advice over the telephone when needed. Blood glucose monitoring does not, in itself, result in better control but is essential to those wishing to achieve it.

Glycosylated haemoglobin (HbA_1 or HbA_{1c}) and fructosamine

Glycosylation of haemoglobin occurs as a two-step reaction resulting in the formation of a covalent bond between the glucose molecule and the terminal valine of the β chain of the haemoglobin molecule. The rate at which this reaction occurs is related to the prevailing glucose concentration. Glycosylated haemoglobin is expressed as a percentage of the normal haemoglobin (standardized range 4–6.1%; 20–44 mmol/mol). This test provides an index of the average blood glucose concentration over the life of the haemoglobin molecule (approximately 6 weeks). The figure will be misleading if the lifespan of the red cell is reduced or if an abnormal haemoglobin or thalassaemia is present. There is considerable inter-individual variation in HbA_{1c} levels, even in health. Although the glycosylated haemoglobin test provides a rapid assessment of glycaemic control in a given patient, blood glucose testing is needed before the clinician can know what to do about it.

Glycosylated plasma proteins ('***fructosamine***') may also be measured as an index of control. Glycosylated albumin is the major component, and fructosamine measurement relates to glycaemic control over the preceding 2–3 weeks. It is useful in patients with anaemia or haemoglobinopathy, and in pregnancy (when haemoglobin turnover is changeable) and other situations where a swift means of assessing progress is needed for changes of treatment.

Does good glucose control matter?

Diabetes affects not only carbohydrate metabolism, but also the metabolism of lipids and proteins. The microvascular complications of diabetes are, however, glucose-specific (i.e. they occur only in the presence of hyperglycaemia), whereas hyperglycaemia is merely one of a number of risk factors for arterial disease, which is not specific to diabetes. Furthermore, microvascular complications generally occur above a threshold level of glycaemia, which forms the basis for our definition of diabetes, whereas the association of glucose with large-vessel disease extends well into the glucose range of the general population, with no clear cut-off for risk. In light of these observations, it is not surprising that the impact of improved glucose control on small-vessel complications such as retinopathy and nephropathy has been compellingly demonstrated, whereas the benefit of improved glucose control has not been unequivocally demonstrated in large-vessel disease. This distinction has been demonstrated in a series of major outcome trials.

The Diabetes Control and Complications Trial (DCCT) in the USA compared standard and intensive insulin therapy in a large prospective controlled trial of young patients with type 1 diabetes. Two groups were recruited: those with no evidence of retinopathy or microalbuminuria (primary prevention group), and those with evidence of retinopathy or microalbuminuria (secondary prevention group). Despite intensive therapy, mean blood glucose levels were still 40% above the non-diabetic range, but even at this level of control, the risk of primary progression to retinopathy was reduced by 60%, nephropathy by 30% and neuropathy by 20% over the 7 years of the study. The effect on progression of established microvascular disease was less evident. Coronary disease is uncommon in this age group but long-term follow-up after the end of the study indicated a benefit for tight control.

Near-normoglycaemia should therefore be the goal for all young patients with type 1 diabetes. The unwanted effects of this policy include weight gain and a two- to threefold increase in the risk of severe hypoglycaemia.

The UK Prospective Diabetes Study (UKPDS) compared standard and intensive treatment in a large prospective controlled trial in recently diagnosed type 2 diabetes patients. Intensive treatment was associated with a 25% overall reduction in microvascular disease end-points, a 33% reduction in albuminuria and a 30% reduction in the need for laser treatment for retinopathy in the more intensively treated patients. These benefits persisted for many years after conclusion of the trial (the 'legacy effect'). This study also showed blood pressure control to be equally necessary in the prevention of retinopathy, but there is no legacy effect and good blood pressure control needs to be maintained. There appeared to be little difference in outcome between the agents used to achieve good metabolic control (metformin, sulphonylurea or insulin).

Cardiovascular risk was not reduced by intensive therapy during the trial but did improve in post-trial follow-up, markedly so in those on metformin.

Three large outcome studies have confirmed the benefits of good glucose control on microvascular complications in type 2 diabetes, although these benefits diminish with increasing age. Once again, no short-term cardiovascular benefit or reduction in overall mortality was observed.

Glucose targets for diabetes management

It follows that glucose control is a high priority for the prevention of microvascular complications, although blood pressure control is also essential to prevent progression of established disease. Glucose control appears of less value in prevention of arterial disease, and the current trend is to aim for more relaxed glucose control in older patients (e.g. HbA_{1c} <8% (<64 mmol/mol)), while attention to blood pressure and lipids should take priority. In the ACCORD study, the use of intensive therapy to target a glycated haemoglobin level <6% in people with type 2 diabetes increased 5-year mortality. Such an intensive strategy thus cannot be recommended, particularly for high-risk patients with advanced complications of type 2 diabetes.

Ideally, all patients should therefore aim to run their glycosylated haemoglobin readings <7.0% (53 mmol/mol) in order to reduce the risk of long-term microvascular complications ***(Box 27.11)***. Hypoglycaemia, patterns of eating and lifestyle, weight problems, and difficulties accepting and coping with diabetes limit what can be achieved. Some will be able to reach these target values but most will not, particularly as their duration of diabetes increases. Realistic goals should be set for each patient, taking into account what is likely to be achievable, and this applies in particular to elderly patients and those with a limited prognosis.

Regular checks for patients with diabetes

Box 27.12 is modified from the guidelines set out in *The European Patients' Charter*, published by the St Vincent Declaration Steering Committee of the WHO. The charter sets out goals for both the healthcare team and the patient.

Psychosocial implications of diabetes

Patients starting tablet or insulin treatment should live as normal a life as possible but this is not always easy. Tact, empathy, encouragement and practical support are needed from all members of the clinical team. Diabetes, like any chronic disease, has psychological sequelae. Most patients will experience periods of not coping, of helplessness, of denial and of acceptance, often fluctuating over time. Other problems include the following:

- ***You cannot take a 'holiday' from diabetes*** – yet the human psyche is poorly developed to cope with unremitting adversity.
- ***Concessions or sympathy are often denied*** to the person with diabetes, since its presence is invisible.
- ***The treatment is complex and demanding***, and the person with diabetes must make trade-offs between short-term and long-term wellbeing.
- ***Embarrassing loss of control over personal behaviour*** or consciousness can occur in insulin-treated patients when minor miscalculation leads to hypoglycaemia.
- ***Risk-taking behaviour*** is indulged in by all humans when emotion is in conflict with logical thought but its effects can be much greater for the person with diabetes (particularly the risks of unplanned pregnancy, alcohol and tobacco).
- ***Poor self-image*** is a very common problem.
- ***Eating disorders*** are more common in people with diabetes – 30–40% of young women will report disordered eating at some stage of their diabetes.
- ***Omission of tablets or insulin*** is common since non-adherence to treatment regimens is universal in all illness. Between 1 in 4 and 1 in 5 tablets prescribed for diabetes is not consumed within the designated treatment period. Insulin omission is not uncommon in young women, in whom the motivation to stay slim may overcome concerns about long-term complications.

Adolescence

Lapses into poor metabolic control, or dropping out of medical care for a time and re-emerging with complications, are very common in adolescence. Diabetic summer camps (e.g. those run by Diabetes UK) help prevent a feeling of isolation and not knowing anyone else with the same problem. Separate adolescent clinics allow:

- ***treatment without marginalization*** in a larger group of older people
- ***meeting peers with similar problems*** in the waiting room

Box 27.11 Target goals of risk factors for diabetic patients

Parameter	Ideal	Reasonable but not ideal
HbA_{1c}	<7% (53 mmol/mol)	<8% (64 mmol/mol)
Blood pressure (mmHg)	<130/80	<140/80
Total cholesterol (mmol/L)	<4.0	<5.0
Low-density lipoprotein	<2.0	<3.0
High-density lipoprotein[a]	>1.1	>0.8
Triglycerides	<1.7	<2.0

[a]In women, >1.3 mmol/L. Standards from American Diabetes Association (2016).

Box 27.12 Regular checks for patients with diabetes

Checked each visit

- Review self-monitoring results and HbA_{1C} results
- Review balance between food, exercise and treatment
- Talk about targets and change where necessary
- Talk about any general or specific problems
- Review diabetes educational needs

Checked at least annually

- Carry out biochemical assessment of metabolic control (e.g. glycosylated Hb test)
- Measure body weight and body mass index
- Measure blood pressure
- Measure plasma lipids (except in extreme old age)
- Measure visual acuity
- Examine state of retina (ophthalmoscope or retinal photo)
- Test urine for proteinuria/microalbuminuria (albumin:creatinine ratio)
- Test blood for renal function (creatinine, estimated glomerular filtration rate)
- Check condition of feet, pulses and neurology
- Review cardiovascular risk factors
- Review self-monitoring and injection techniques
- Review eating habits

- ***gradual separation from parents*** and assumption of personal responsibility for the illness
- ***age-appropriate literature*** to be made available.

Practical aspects

Patients need to inform the driving and vehicle licensing authority and their insurance companies after diagnosis. They would also be wise to inform their family, friends and employers, in case unexpected hypoglycaemia occurs. Insulin treatment can be undertaken by people in most walks of life. A few jobs are unsuitable; these include driving heavy goods or public service vehicles, working at heights, piloting aircraft, or working close to dangerous machinery in motion. Certain professions, such as the police and the armed forces, are barred to all diabetic patients. There are few other limitations, although a considerable amount of ill-informed prejudice exists. Doctors can sometimes help support patients in the face of misinformed work practices.

Further reading

Ajala O, English P, Pinkney J. Systematic review of diet in type 2 diabetes mellitus. *Am J Clin Nutr* 2013; 97:505–516.

Boussageon R, Gueyffier F, Cornu C. Metforming as firstline treatment for type 2 diabetes: are we sure? *BMJ* 2016; 352:h6748.

DCCT/Epidemiology of Diabetes Interventions and Complications Research Group. Retinopathy and nephropathy in patients with type 1 diabetes four years after a trial of intensive insulin therapy. *N Engl J Med* 2000; 342:381–389.

Gloy VL, Briel M, Bhatt DL et al. Bariatric surgery versus non-surgical treatment for obesity: a systematic review and meta-analysis of randomized controlled trials. *BMJ* 2013; 347:f5934.

Holman RR, Paul SK, Bethel MA et al. Long-term follow-up after tight control of blood pressure in type 2 diabetes. *N Engl J Med* 2008; 359:1565–1576.

Holman RR, Paul SK, Bethel MA et al. 10 year follow-up of intensive glucose control in type 2 diabetes. *N Engl J Med* 2008; 359:1577–1589.

Ingelfinger JR, Rosen CJ. Cardiovascular risk and sodium-glucose cotransporter 2 inhibition in type 2 diabetes. *N Engl J Med* 2015; 373:2178–2179.

Inzucchi SE, Bergenstal RM, Buse JB et al. Management of hyperglycemia in type 2 diabetes: a patient-centered approach. Position statement of the American Diabetes Association (ADA) and the European Association for the Study of Diabetes (EASD). *Diabetes Care* 2012; 35:1346–1379.

Pickup JC. Insulin-pump therapy for type 1 diabetes mellitus. *N Engl J Med* 2012; 366:1616–1624.

Rejeski W, Ip EH, Bertoni AG et al. Lifestyle change and mobility in obese adults with type 2 diabetes. *N Engl J Med* 2012; 366:1209–1217.

Schellenberg ES, Dryden DM, Vandermeer B et al. Lifestyle for type 2 diabetes mellitus. *Ann Intern Med* 2013; 159:543–551.

DIABETIC METABOLIC EMERGENCIES

The main terms used are defined in ***Box 27.13***.

Diabetic ketoacidosis

Diabetic ketoacidosis (DKA) is the hallmark of type 1 diabetes. It is usually seen in the following circumstances:

- previously undiagnosed diabetes
- interruption of insulin therapy
- the stress of intercurrent illness.

The majority of cases reaching hospital could have been prevented by earlier diagnosis, better communication between patient and doctor, and better patient education. The most common error of management is for patients to reduce or omit insulin because they feel unable to eat, owing to nausea or vomiting. This is a factor in at least 25% of all hospital admissions. ***Insulin may need adjusting up or down but should never be stopped***.

Pathogenesis

Ketoacidosis is a state of uncontrolled catabolism associated with insulin deficiency. Insulin deficiency is a necessary precondition since only a modest elevation in insulin levels is sufficient to inhibit hepatic ketogenesis, and stable patients do not readily develop ketoacidosis when insulin is withdrawn. Other factors include counter-regulatory hormone excess and fluid depletion. The combination of insulin deficiency with excess of its hormonal antagonists leads to the parallel processes shown in ***Figure 27.12***. In the

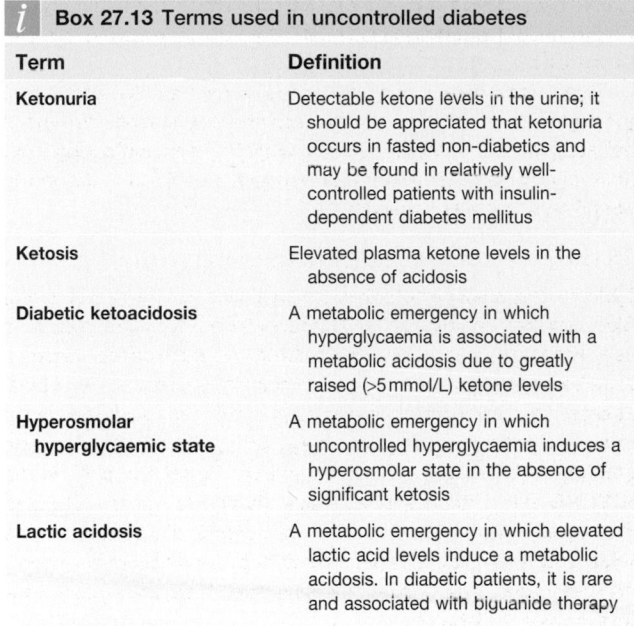

Box 27.13 Terms used in uncontrolled diabetes

Term	Definition
Ketonuria	Detectable ketone levels in the urine; it should be appreciated that ketonuria occurs in fasted non-diabetics and may be found in relatively well-controlled patients with insulin-dependent diabetes mellitus
Ketosis	Elevated plasma ketone levels in the absence of acidosis
Diabetic ketoacidosis	A metabolic emergency in which hyperglycaemia is associated with a metabolic acidosis due to greatly raised (>5 mmol/L) ketone levels
Hyperosmolar hyperglycaemic state	A metabolic emergency in which uncontrolled hyperglycaemia induces a hyperosmolar state in the absence of significant ketosis
Lactic acidosis	A metabolic emergency in which elevated lactic acid levels induce a metabolic acidosis. In diabetic patients, it is rare and associated with biguanide therapy

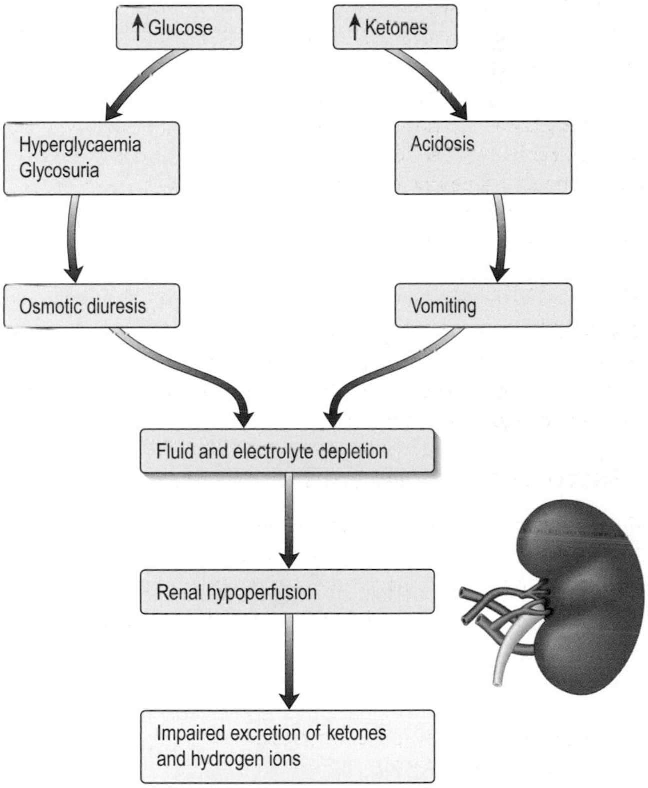

Figure 27.12 Dehydration occurs during ketoacidosis as a consequence of two parallel processes. Hyperglycaemia results in osmotic diuresis, and hyperketonaemia results in acidosis and vomiting. Renal hypoperfusion then occurs and a vicious circle is established as the kidney becomes less able to compensate for the acidosis.

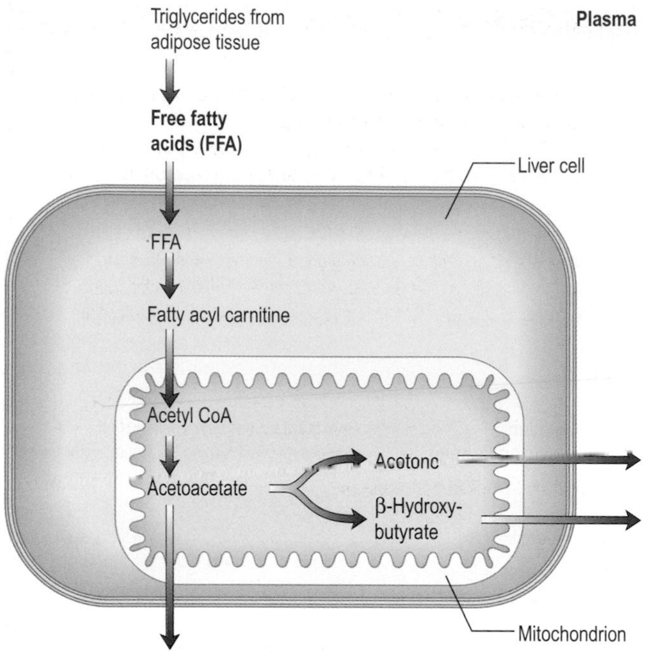

Figure 27.13 Ketogenesis. During insulin deficiency, lipolysis accelerates and free fatty acids taken up by liver cells form the substrate for ketone formation (acetoacetate, acetone and β-hydroxybutyrate) within the mitochondrion. These ketones pass into the blood, producing acidosis. CoA, coenzyme A.

absence of insulin, hepatic glucose production accelerates and peripheral uptake by tissues such as muscle is reduced. Rising glucose levels lead to an osmotic diuresis, loss of fluid and electrolytes, and dehydration. Plasma osmolality rises and renal perfusion falls. In parallel, rapid lipolysis occurs, leading to elevated circulating free fatty-acid levels. The free fatty acids are broken down to acetyl-coenzyme A (CoA) within the liver cells, and this, in turn, is converted to ketone bodies within the mitochondria ***(Fig. 27.13)***. Accumulation of ketone bodies produces a metabolic acidosis. Vomiting leads to further loss of fluid and electrolytes. The excess ketones are excreted in the urine but also appear in the breath, producing a distinctive smell similar to that of acetone. Respiratory compensation for the acidosis leads to hyperventilation, graphically described as 'air hunger'. Progressive dehydration impairs renal excretion of hydrogen ions and ketones, aggravating the acidosis. As the pH falls below 7.0 ($[H^+]$ >100 nmol/L), pH-dependent enzyme systems in many cells function less effectively. Untreated, severe ketoacidosis is invariably fatal.

Clinical features

The features of ketoacidosis are those of uncontrolled diabetes with acidosis, and include prostration, hyperventilation (Kussmaul respiration), nausea, vomiting and, occasionally, abdominal pain. The latter is sometimes so severe that it can be confused with a surgical acute abdomen.

Some patients are mentally alert at presentation but confusion and stupor are present in more severe cases. Up to 5% present in coma. Evidence of marked dehydration is present and the eyeball is lax to pressure in severe cases. Hyperventilation is present but becomes less marked in very severe acidosis, owing to respiratory depression. The smell of ketones on the breath allows an instant diagnosis to be made by those able to detect the odour. The skin is dry and the body temperature is often subnormal, even in the presence of infection; in such cases, pyrexia may develop later.

Diagnosis

This is confirmed by demonstrating hyperglycaemia with ketonaemia or heavy ketonuria, and acidosis. No time should be lost and treatment is started as soon as the first blood sample has been taken. Hyperglycaemia is demonstrated by dipstick, while a venous blood sample is sent to the laboratory for confirmation. Ketonaemia is confirmed by centrifuging a blood sample and testing the plasma with a dipstick that measures ketones. Hand-held sensors measuring β-hydroxybutyrate in 30 s are available. An arterial blood sample is taken for blood gas analysis.

The severity of DKA can be assessed as follows. One or more of these features suggests severe DKA.

Clinical observations

- Pulse >100 b.p.m. or <60 b.p.m.
- Systolic blood pressure <90 mmHg.
- Glasgow Coma Scale score of <12 (see ***Box 21.26***) or abnormal 'Alert, Voice, Pain, Unresponsive' (AVPU) scale.
- O_2 saturation <92% on air (if normal respiratory function).

Blood tests

- Blood ketones >6 mmol/L.
- Bicarbonate <12 mmol/L.
- Venous/arterial pH <7.1 ([H+] >80 nmol/L).
- Hypokalaemia on admission <3.5 mmol/L.

Management (and pathophysiology)

The principles of management are as follows and as shown in ***Box 27.14***; these measures should be carried out in a high-dependency area.

- ***Replace the fluid losses*** with 0.9% saline. Average loss of water is 5–7 L with a sodium loss of 500 mmol.
- ***Replace the electrolyte losses***. Patients have a total body potassium deficit of 350 mmol, although initial plasma levels may not be low. Insulin therapy leads to uptake of potassium by the cells with a consequent fall in plasma K^+ levels. Potassium is therefore given as soon as insulin is started.
- ***Restore the acid–base balance***. A patient with healthy kidneys will rapidly compensate for the metabolic acidosis once the circulating volume is restored. Bicarbonate is seldom necessary and is used only if the pH is <7.0 ($[H^+]$ >100 nmol/L); it is best given as an isotonic (1.26%) solution.
- ***Replace the deficient insulin***. Relatively modest doses of insulin lower blood glucose by suppressing hepatic glucose output rather than by stimulating peripheral uptake, and are therefore much less likely to produce hypoglycaemia. Insulin and glucose together both inhibit gluconeogenesis, and thus ketone production, and are needed to metabolize ketones into less harmful substances. Short-acting insulin is given as an intravenous infusion where facilities for adequate supervision exist or as hourly intramuscular injections. The subcutaneous route is avoided because subcutaneous blood flow is reduced in shocked patients.
- ***Monitor blood glucose closely (Box 27.14)***.
- ***Seek the underlying cause***. Physical examination may reveal a source of infection (e.g. a perianal abscess). Two common markers of infection are misleading: fever is unusual, even

Box 27.14 Guidelines for the diagnosis and management of diabetic ketoacidosis

Diagnosis

- Hyperglycaemia: measure blood glucose
- Ketonaemia: test plasma with Ketostix. Finger-prick sample for β-hydroxybutyrate
- Ketonuria: measure urine ketone levels where plasma ketone measurements are not available
- Acidosis: measure:
  - pH in arterial blood
  - Bicarbonate in venous blood.

Immediate measures

1. Assess
2. Send blood samples to laboratory
3. Set up intravenous infusion
   - Blood glucose:
     - Measure baseline and hourly initially
     - Aim for fall of 3–6 mmol/L (55–110 mg/dL) per hour
   - Urea and electrolytes – measure at baseline and hourly until 6 h, then at 12 h and 24 h:
     - Potassium: add when K^+ <3.5 mmol/L. Give 20 mmol with each litre infusion; give 10 mmol/h when K^+ = 3.5–5 mmol
   - Full blood count
   - Blood gases: at 0, 2, 6 h
   - Creatinine: at 0, 6, 12, 24 h
   - Bicarbonate: at 0, 1, 2, 3, 6, 12, 24 h.

Phase 1

- Admit to an area where staffing and facilities allow more detailed clinical observation and more frequent medical and nursing assessment than may be found on a general ward
- ***Insulin***: soluble insulin i.v. 0.1 U/kg/h by infusion, or 20 U i.m. stat. followed by 6 U i.m. hourly
- ***Fluid and electrolyte replacement***: i.v. 0.9% sodium chloride with 20 mmol KCl/L[a]
  - 1 L in 30 min, then
  - 1 L in 1 h
  - 1 L in 2 h
  - 1 L in 4 h
  - 1 L in 8 h
- Adjust KCl concentration depending on results of regular blood K^+ measurement

IF:

- Blood pressure <80 mmHg, give 500 mL 0.9% sodium chloride over 15 min; if no response, give plasma expander
- pH <7.0 ($[H^+]$ >100 nmol/L) give 500 mL of sodium bicarbonate 1.26% plus 10 mmol KCl. Repeat if necessary to bring pH up to 7.0

Phase 2

- ***Insulin and glucose***: when blood glucose falls to 10–12 mmol/L, change infusion fluid to 1 L 5% glucose plus 20 mmol KCl 6-hourly. Continue insulin with dose adjusted according to hourly blood glucose test results (e.g. i.v. 3 U/h glucose 15 mmol/L; 2 U/h when glucose 10 mmol/L).

Phase 3

- Once stable and able to eat and drink normally, transfer patient to 4-times-daily s.c. insulin regimen (based on previous 24 hours' insulin consumption and trend in consumption)

Other semi-urgent procedures

- Blood and urine culture
- Cardiac enzymes
- Chest X-ray
- Electrocardiogram (monitor if electrolyte problems or severe diabetic ketoacidosis)
- Catheterization if no urine passed after 3 h of hydration

Special measures

- Broad-spectrum antibiotic if infection likely
- Nasogastric tube if drowsy
- Central venous pressure monitoring if shocked or if previous cardiac or renal impairment
- Give s.c. prophylactic low-molecular-weight heparin

Subsequent management

- Monitor glucose hourly for 8 hours
- Monitor electrolytes 2-hourly for 8 hours
- Adjust potassium replacement according to blood results

[a]The regimen of fluid replacement set out above is a guide for patients with severe ketoacidosis. Excessive fluid can precipitate pulmonary and cerebral oedema; inadequate replacement may cause renal failure. Fluid replacement must therefore be tailored to the individual and monitored carefully throughout treatment.

when infection is present; and polymorpholeucocytosis is present, even in the absence of infection. Relevant investigations include a chest X-ray, urine and blood cultures, and an electrocardiogram (to exclude myocardial infarction). The serum amylase may be elevated in the absence of pancreatitis. If infection is suspected, broad-spectrum antibiotics are started once the appropriate cultures have been taken.

Problems of management

- ***Hypotension***. This may lead to renal shutdown. Sodium chloride 0.9% is the fluid of choice to increase circulating volume and thus blood pressure and renal perfusion. A central venous pressure line is useful in this situation. A bladder catheter is inserted if no urine is produced within 2 h but routine catheterization is not necessary.
- ***Coma***. The usual principles apply (see pp. 825–829). It is essential to pass a nasogastric tube to prevent aspiration, since gastric stasis is common and carries the risk of aspiration pneumonia if a drowsy patient vomits.
- ***Cerebral oedema***. This is a rare but serious complication and has mostly been reported in children or young adults. Excessive rehydration and use of hypertonic fluids such as 8.4% bicarbonate may sometimes be responsible. The mortality is high.
- ***Hypothermia***. Severe hypothermia with a core temperature <33°C may occur and can be overlooked unless a rectal temperature is taken with a low-reading thermometer.
- ***Late complications***. These include pneumonia and deep-vein thrombosis (DVT; prophylaxis is essential – see p. 580) and occur especially in the comatose or elderly patient.
- ***Complications of therapy***. These include hypoglycaemia and hypokalaemia, due to loss of K^+ in the urine from osmotic diuresis. Over-enthusiastic fluid replacement may precipitate pulmonary oedema in the very young or the very old. Hyperchloraemic acidosis may develop in the course of treatment since patients have lost a large variety of negatively charged electrolytes, which are replaced with chloride. The kidneys usually correct this spontaneously within a few days.

Subsequent management

Intravenous glucose and insulin are continued until the patient feels able to eat and keep food down. The drip is then taken down and a similar amount of insulin is given as four injections of soluble insulin subcutaneously at mealtimes and a dose of intermediate-acting insulin at night.

Sliding-scale regimens are unnecessary and may even delay the establishment of stable blood glucose levels.

The mortality of DKA is around 5% and is increased in older patients. Its treatment is incomplete without a careful enquiry into the causes of the episode and advice as to how to avoid its recurrence.

Hyperosmolar hyperglycaemic state

This condition, in which severe hyperglycaemia develops without significant ketosis, is the characteristic metabolic emergency of uncontrolled type 2 diabetes. Patients present in middle or later life, often with previously undiagnosed diabetes. Common precipitating factors include consumption of glucose-rich fluids, concurrent medication such as thiazide diuretics or steroids, and intercurrent illness. The hyperosmolar hyperglycaemic state and ketoacidosis represent two ends of a spectrum rather than two distinct disorders ***(Box 27.15)***. The biochemical differences may partly be explained as follows:

- ***Age***. The extreme dehydration characteristic of the hyperosmolar hyperglycaemic state may be related to age. Old people experience thirst less acutely and become dehydrated more readily. In addition, the mild renal impairment associated with age results in increased urinary losses of fluid and electrolytes.
- ***The degree of insulin deficiency***. This is less severe in the hyperosmolar hyperglycaemic state. Endogenous insulin levels are sufficient to inhibit hepatic ketogenesis but insufficient to inhibit hepatic glucose production.

Box 27.15 Electrolyte changes in diabetic ketoacidosis and the hyperosmolar hyperglycaemic state

Examples of blood values	Severe ketoacidosis	Hyperosmolar hyperglycaemic state
Na^+ (mmol/L)	140	155
K^+ (mmol/L)	5	5
Cl^- (mmol/L)	100	110
HCO_3^- (mmol/L)	5	25
Urea (mmol/L)	8	15
Glucose (mmol/L)	30	50
Arterial pH	7.0[a]	7.35

The normal range of osmolality is 285–300 mOsm/kg. It can be measured directly, or can be calculated approximately from the formula:

$$\text{Osmolality} = 2(Na^+ + K^+) + \text{glucose} + \text{urea}.$$

For instance, in the example of severe ketoacidosis given above:

$$\text{Osmolality} = 2(140+5)+30+8 = 328\ \text{mOsm/kg}$$

and in the example of the hyperosmolar hyperglycaemic state:

$$\text{Osmolality} = 2(155+5)+50+15 = 385\ \text{mOsm/kg}$$

The normal anion gap is <17. It is calculated as $(Na^+ + K^+) - (Cl^- + HCO_3^-)$. In the example of ketoacidosis, the anion gap is 40, and in the example of the hyperosmolar hyperglycaemic state, the anion gap is 25. Mild hyperchloraemic acidosis may develop in the course of therapy. This will be shown by a rising plasma chloride and persistence of a low bicarbonate, even though the anion gap has returned to normal.

[a] $[H^+]$ >100 nmol/L.

Clinical features

The characteristic clinical features on presentation are dehydration and stupor or coma. Impairment of consciousness is directly related to the degree of hyperosmolality. Evidence of underlying illness, such as pneumonia or pyelonephritis, may be present, and the hyperosmolar state may predispose to stroke, myocardial infarction or arterial insufficiency in the lower limbs.

Investigations and management

These are (with some exceptions) according to the guidelines for ketoacidosis. The plasma osmolality is usually extremely high. It can be measured directly or calculated as $(2(Na^+ + K^+) + \text{glucose} + \text{urea})$, all in mmol/L. Many patients are extremely sensitive to insulin and the glucose concentration may plummet. The resultant change in osmolality may cause cerebral damage. It is sometimes useful to infuse insulin at a rate of 3 U/h for the first 2–3 h, increasing to 6 U/h if glucose is falling too slowly. The standard fluid for replacement is 0.9% saline. Avoid 0.45% saline, since rapid dilution of the blood may cause more cerebral damage than a few hours of exposure to hypernatraemia. Prophylactic low-molecular-weight heparin should be given.

Prognosis

The reported mortality ranges as high as 20–30%, mainly because of the more advanced age of the patients and the frequency of intercurrent illness. Unlike ketoacidosis, the hyperosmolar hyperglycaemia state is not an absolute indication for subsequent insulin therapy, and survivors may do well on diet and oral agents.

Lactic acidosis

The risk of lactic acidosis in patients taking metformin is extremely low, provided that the therapeutic dose is not exceeded and the drug is withheld in patients with advanced hepatic or renal dysfunction.

Patients present in severe metabolic acidosis with a large anion gap (normally <17 mmol/L), usually without significant hyperglycaemia or ketosis. Treatment is by rehydration and infusion of isotonic 1.26% bicarbonate. The mortality is in excess of 50%.

Further reading

Joint British Diabetes Societies Inpatient Care Group. *The Management of Diabetic Ketoacidosis in Adults*, 2nd edn. London: Diabetes Care UK; 2013.

Kamel KS, Halperin ML. Acid–base problems in diabetic ketoacidosis. *N Engl J Med* 2015; 372:546–554.

COMPLICATIONS OF DIABETES

People with diabetes still have a reduced life expectancy, although the prognosis has improved considerably over recent decades. The major cause of death in treated patients is cardiovascular problems (60–70%) followed by renal failure (10%) and infections (6%). There is no doubt that the duration and degree of hyperglycaemia play a major role in the production of complications. Improved glucose control can reduce the rate of progression of both nephropathy and retinopathy, and the DCCT trial (see p. 1259) showed a 60%

reduction in developing complications over 9 years when the HbA_{1c} was kept at around 7% in type 1 diabetes.

Pathophysiology

The mechanisms leading to damage are ill defined. The following are consequences of hyperglycaemia and may play a role:

- ***Non-enzymatic glycosylation*** of a wide variety of proteins, such as haemoglobin, collagen, low-density lipoprotein (LDL) and tubulin in peripheral nerves. This leads to an accumulation of advanced glycosylated end-products, causing injury and inflammation via stimulation of pro-inflammatory factors, such as complement and cytokines.
- ***Polyol pathway***. The metabolism of glucose by increased intracellular aldose reductase leads to accumulation of sorbitol and fructose. This causes changes in vascular permeability, cell proliferation and capillary structure via stimulation of protein kinase C and transforming growth factor beta (TGF-β).
- ***Abnormal microvascular blood flow***. This impairs the supply of nutrients and oxygen. Microvascular occlusion is due to vasoconstrictors, such as endothelins and thrombogenesis, and leads to endothelial damage.
- ***Other factors***. These include the formation of reactive oxygen species and stimulation of growth factors TGF-β and vascular endothelial growth factor (VEGF). These growth factors are released by ischaemic tissues and cause endothelial cells to proliferate.
- ***Haemodynamic changes***. These take place, for example, in the kidney (see pp. 1269–1270).

It has been proposed that all of the above mechanisms stem from a single hyperglycaemia-induced process of overproduction of superoxide by the mitochondrial electron chain. This paradigm offers an integrated explanation of how complications of diabetes develop.

Macrovascular complications

(See ***Box 27.16***.) Diabetes is a risk factor for the development of atherosclerosis. This risk is related to that of the background population. For example, people with diabetes in Japan are less likely than European patients to develop atherosclerosis, but more likely to develop it than non-diabetic Japanese.

- Stroke is twice as likely.
- Myocardial infarction is 2–4 times as likely, and women with diabetes lose their premenopausal protection from coronary artery disease.
- Amputation of a foot for gangrene is 50 times as likely.

Several large trials have shown that intensive glucose-lowering treatment of diabetes has a relatively minor effect on cardiovascular risk; it is vital to tackle all cardiovascular risk factors together in diabetes, and not just to focus on glucose levels.

- ***Hypertension***. The UKPDS demonstrated that aggressive treatment of hypertension produces a marked reduction in adverse cardiovascular outcomes, both microvascular and macrovascular. To achieve the target for blood pressure (see ***Box 27.11***), the UKPDS found that one-third of patients needed three or more antihypertensive drugs in combination, and two-thirds of treated patients needed two or more.
- ***Smoking***: This is the avoidable risk factor (see pp. 1074–1075). Efforts to help patients stop smoking should never be given up.
- ***Lipid abnormalities***. Clinical trials suggest that there is no 'safe' cut-off for serum cholesterol. It seems best to aim for the lowest achievable level, and in practice this means that almost all people with type 2 diabetes will be treated with a statin (see p. 1284).
- ***Low-dose aspirin*** can reduce macrovascular risk but is associated with a morbidity and mortality from bleeding. The benefits of aspirin outweigh the bleeding risk when the risk of a cardiovascular end-point is >30% in the next 10 years. This risk is reached in patients aged under 45 with three strong additional cardiovascular risk factors, those aged 45–54 with three additional risk factors, those aged 54–65 with two additional risk factors, or those aged over 65 with just one additional risk factor.
- ***ACE inhibitors/angiotensin II receptor antagonists.*** Treating people with diabetes and at least one other major cardiovascular risk factor with an ACE inhibitor produces a 25–35% lowering of the risk of heart attack, stroke, overt nephropathy or cardiovascular death. Angiotensin II receptor antagonists are sometimes preferred initially and are also used for those intolerant to ACE inhibitors. The two agents are not used together.

Box 27.16 Diabetic risk factors for macrovascular complications

- Duration
- Increasing age
- Systolic hypertension
- Hyperinsulinaemia due to insulin resistance associated with obesity and the metabolic syndrome
- Hyperlipidaemia, particularly hypertriglyceridaemia/low high-density lipoprotein (HDL)
- Proteinuria (including microalbuminuria)
- Other factors as for the general population

Microvascular complications

In contrast to macrovascular disease, which is prevalent in the West as a whole, microvascular disease is specific to diabetes. Small blood vessels throughout the body are affected but the disease process is of particular danger in three sites:

- retina
- renal glomerulus
- nerve sheaths.

Diabetic retinopathy, nephropathy and neuropathy tend to manifest 10–20 years after diagnosis in young patients but may present earlier in older patients, probably because these individuals have had unrecognized diabetes for months or even years prior to diagnosis. Genetic factors appear to contribute to the susceptibility to microvascular disease. Diabetic siblings of diabetic patients with renal and eye disease have a three- to fivefold increased risk of the same complication in both type 1 and type 2 patients. There are racial differences in the overall prevalence of nephropathy. In the USA, prevalence is: Pima American Indian > Hispanic/Mexican > US black > US white patients.

Diabetic eye disease

At least 90% of young patients with type 1 diabetes will develop retinal changes but these only progress to sight-threatening retinopathy in a minority. Some 30–50% will require laser photocoagulation to prevent or limit progression to proliferative retinopathy, and good control of blood pressure is essential. Diabetes is still the most common cause of blindness in under-65-year-olds. It affects the eye in a variety of ways:

- ***Cataract*** is denaturation of the protein and other components of the lens of the eye, which renders it opaque.
- ***Diabetic retinopathy*** is damage to the retina and iris caused by diabetes, which can lead to blindness.
- ***External ocular palsies*** (see p. 806) most commonly affect the sixth and the third nerves. Third nerve palsy is not associated with pain. These nerve palsies usually recover spontaneously within a period of 3–6 months.

Natural history

Cataracts

Cataract develops earlier in people with diabetes than in the general population. Sustained very poor diabetes control with a degree of ketosis can cause an acute cataract (snowflake cataract), which comes on rapidly. Fluctuations in blood glucose concentration can cause refractive variability, as a result of osmotic changes within the lens (the absorption of water into the lens causes temporary hypermetropia). This presents as fluctuating difficulty in reading. It resolves with better metabolic control of the diabetes.

Diabetic retinopathy

Diabetic retinopathy ***(Fig. 27.14)*** is the most commonly diagnosed diabetes-related complication. Its prevalence increases with the duration of diabetes ***(Fig. 27.15)***. Some 20% of people with type 1 diabetes will have retinal changes after 10 years, rising to >95% after 20 years ***(Box 27.17)***; 20–30% of people with type 2 diabetes have retinopathy at diagnosis. The metabolic consequences of poorly controlled diabetes cause intramural pericyte death, and thickening of the basement membrane in the small blood vessels of the retina. This leads initially to increased permeability of the vascular walls, and later to occlusion of the vessels (capillary closure). This process has somewhat different consequences in the peripheral retina and in the macular area.

Box 27.17 Grading and management of pathological changes in diabetic retinopathy

Retinopathy grade	Retinal abnormality (cause)	Action needed
Peripheral retina		
Background (R1)	Dot haemorrhages (capillary microaneurysms) (usually appear first) Blot haemorrhages (leakage of blood into deeper retinal layers) Hard exudates (exudation of plasma rich in lipids and protein)[a] Cotton wool spots/cytoid bodies[b]	Annual screening only
Pre-proliferative (R2)	Venous beading/loops Intraretinal microvascular abnormalities (IRMAs) Multiple deep, round haemorrhages	Non-urgent referral to an ophthalmologist
Proliferative (R3)	New blood-vessel formation/ neovascularization Preretinal or subhyaloid haemorrhage Vitreous haemorrhage	Urgent referral to an ophthalmologist
Advanced retinopathy	Retinal fibrosis Traction retinal detachment	Urgent referral to an ophthalmologist – but much vision already lost
Central retina		
Maculopathy (M1)	Hard exudates within 1 disc-width of macula Lines or circles of hard exudates within 2 disc-widths of macula Microaneurysms or retinal haemorrhages within 1 disc-width of macula if associated with an unexplained visual acuity 6/12 or worse	Prompt referral to an ophthalmologist

[a]Hard exudates have a bright yellowish-white colour and are often irregular in outline with a sharply defined margin. [b]Cotton-wool spots are greyish-white and have indistinct margins and a dull matt surface, unlike the glossy appearance of hard exudates.

Peripheral retina

Damage to the wall of small vessels causes ***microaneurysms*** (small red dots) within the retina. When vessel walls are breached, ***superficial (blot) haemorrhages*** occur in the ganglion cell and outer plexiform layers. Damaged blood vessels leak fluid into the retina. The fluid is cleared into the retinal veins, leaving behind protein and lipid deposits and causing ***hard exudates***. These are eventually cleared by macrophages.

Micro-infarcts within the retina due to occluded vessels cause ***cotton wool spots***. The spot itself is due to the accumulation of axoplasmic debris. This debris is removed by macrophages. As this occurs, there may be white dots at the site of the previous cotton wool spot (***cytoid bodies***). Damage to the walls of veins causes their calibre to vary (***venous beading***) and elongation to occur, causing ***venous loops***. Blockage of blood vessels leads to areas of capillary non-perfusion. Ischaemia in these areas causes the release of vascular growth factors such as VEGF. These factors cause new blood vessels to grow in the retina (***neovascularization***). Some of these new blood vessels are inside the retina and are helpful. These new intraretinal vessels, and other vessels whose walls are damaged and dilated, give the appearance of ***intraretinal microvascular abnormalities*** (***IRMAs***).

Other new vessels emerge through the retina and lie on its surface, usually at the margin of an area of capillary closure. The normal shearing stresses that occur within the eye can cause these poorly supported new vessels to bleed. Small haemorrhages give rise to ***pre-retinal haemorrhages*** (boat-shaped haemorrhages). With further bleeding, ***vitreous haemorrhage*** occurs with consequent sudden loss of vision. Later, collagen tissue grows along the margins of the new vessels and gives rise to ***fibrotic bands***. These bands may contract and pull on the retina, causing further haemorrhage and ***retinal detachment***. Sometimes, vessels may be induced to grow on the pupil margin (***rubeosis***) and in the angle of the anterior chamber of the eye, giving rise to a rapid increase in intraocular pressure (***rubeotic glaucoma***). These features of retinopathy in the peripheral retina are grouped, according to the risk of visual loss, into three stages ***(Box 27.17)***.

Macular area

Fluid from leaking vessels is cleared poorly in the macular area because its anatomy differs from that of the rest of the retina. Above a certain rate of formation, clearance fails and ***macular oedema***

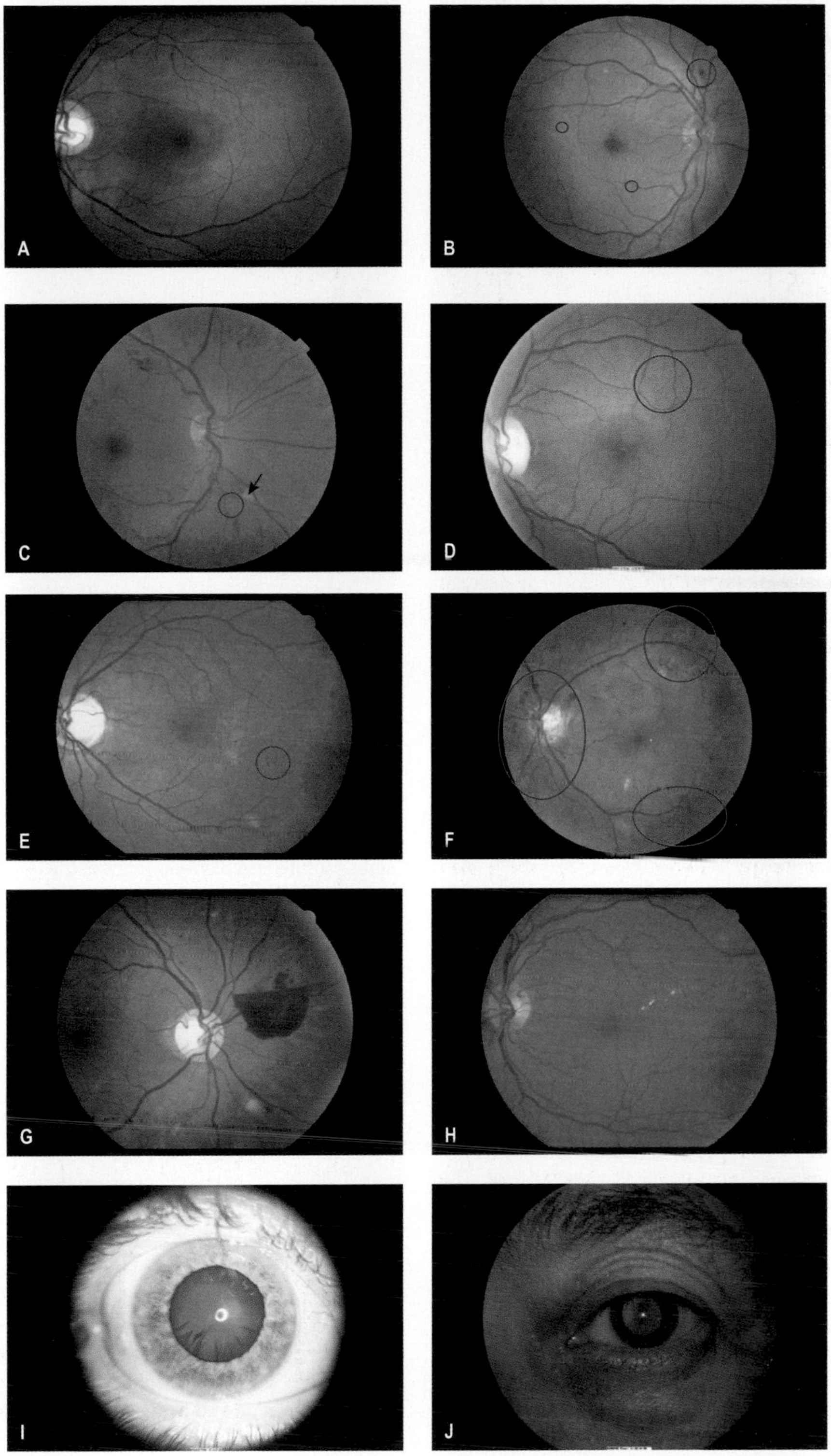

Figure 27.14 Features of diabetic eye disease. A. The normal macula (centre) and optic disc (to left). **B.** Microaneurysms (small circles) and blot haemorrhage (larger circle) – early background retinopathy. **C.** Hard exudates (circled) and single cotton wool spot (arrowed) in addition to multiple blot haemorrhages in background retinopathy. **D.** Intra-retinal microvascular abnormalities (IRMA) – pre-proliferative retinopathy (circled). **E.** Venous loop (circled) also indicates pre-proliferative change. **F.** Fronds of new vessels on the disc and elsewhere (proliferative; circled). **G.** Pre-retinal haemorrhage in proliferative disease. **H.** Hard exudates within a disc-width of the macula (maculopathy). **I.** Cortical cataracts and **J.** central cataracts can be seen against the red reflex with the ophthalmoscope.

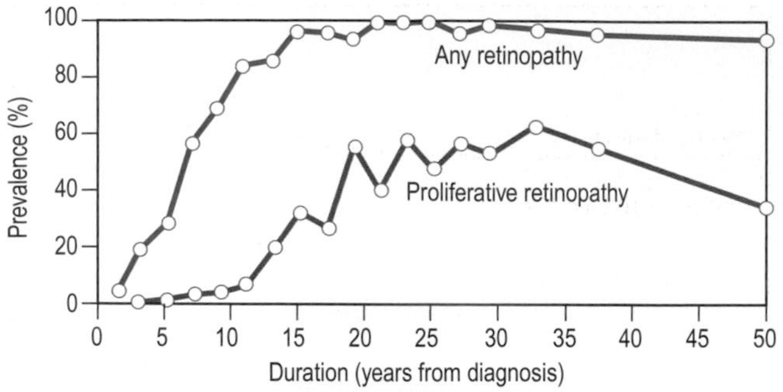

Figure 27.15 Prevalence of retinopathy. Prevalence is shown in relation to duration of the disease in patients with type 1 diabetes mellitus diagnosed under the age of 33 years. Almost all eventually develop background change and 60% progress to proliferative retinopathy. *(Data from* Archives of Ophthalmology *1984; 102:520.)*

occurs. This distorts and thickens the retina at the macula. If sustained, this distortion causes loss of central vision. Macular oedema is not visible with the ophthalmoscope or with retinal photography. For this reason, surrogate markers for the presence of macular oedema are used ***(Box 27.17)***. Capillary occlusion in the macular area will also cause loss of central vision.

Examination

Bedside examination of the eye

Visual acuity should be checked using both a pinhole and the patient's distance spectacles. The ***ocular movements*** are assessed to detect any ocular motor palsies. The ***iris*** is examined for rubeosis and then the pupils dilated with 1% tropicamide. About 20 minutes later, the eye is examined for the presence of a cataract by looking at the lens with a +10.00 lens in the ophthalmoscope and viewing the lens against the red reflex. The ***retina*** is then examined systematically looking at the disc, then all four quadrants, and finally the macula. The macula is examined last because this induces the greatest discomfort, and pupillary constriction.

Eye screening

Screening for sight-threatening eye disease with universal access is seen as offering the best hope of displacing diabetes as the most common cause of blindness in those under 65 years of age. The National Screening Committee in the UK has helped establish digital photography-based screening across the country, based on a national set of standards. All people with diabetes who are over the age of 12 are offered annual measurement of their acuity and photographs of their retina. ***Box 27.18*** shows standardized criteria for screening schemes; these are regularly inspected.

Box 27.18 Criteria for a successful local screening scheme for sight-threatening diabetic retinopathy

- Clearly defined geographical area for the screening programme
- Adequate number of people with diabetes for viability (>12 000)
- Identified screening programme manager
- Identified clinical screening lead
- Identified hospital eye service for diagnosis and laser treatment
- Computer software capable of supporting call/recall of patients and image grading
- Centralized appointment administration
- Single collated list of all people with diabetes in the area over the age of 12
- Equipment to obtain adequate disc- and macula-centred images of each eye
- Single image grading centre
- Process to manage people with poor-quality images
- Clear route of referral for treatment, and for feedback from treatment centre to screening unit
- Accreditation of screening staff
- Annual reporting of service performance

Management of diabetic eye disease

(See ***Box 27.17***.)

Cataract

Extraction and intraocular lens implantation is indicated if the cataract is causing visual disability or an inability to view the retina adequately. Cataract extraction is straightforward if there is no retinopathy present. Pre-existing retinopathy may worsen after cataract extraction.

Retinopathy

The DCCT and UKPDS trials (see pp. 1259–1260) show that the risk of developing diabetic eye disease and the risk of established retinopathy progressing can be reduced by tight metabolic control of both diabetes and blood pressure. Development or progression of retinopathy may be accelerated by rapid improvement in glycaemic control, by pregnancy and by nephropathy, and these groups need frequent monitoring. Fluorescein angiography (a fluorescent dye is injected into an arm vein and photographed in transit through the retinal vessels) is used to define the extent of the potentially sight-threatening diabetic retinopathy. Ocular coherence tomography (OCT) is used to image the content of the layers of the retina at the macula, and in particular to measure retinal thickness. It can detect macular oedema and other macular abnormalities.

Proliferative retinopathy

New vessels are an indication for laser photocoagulation therapy. New vessels on the disc carry the worst prognosis and warrant urgent laser therapy. The laser should be directed at the new vessels and, in addition, at the associated areas of capillary non-perfusion (ischaemia). If the proliferative retinopathy has progressed to development of new vessels on the optic disc, then a technique known as ***panretinal photocoagulation*** (***PRP***) is carried out. This involves multiple laser burns to the peripheral retina, especially in the areas of capillary non-perfusion. Rubeosis is also treated with panretinal photocoagulation. If some bleeding has occurred but there is a good view, then laser treatment should be applied. Vitreoretinal surgery is used if bleeding is recurrent and preventing laser therapy. It is also employed to try to salvage some vision after vitreous haemorrhage and to treat fibrotic traction retinal detachment in advanced retinopathy.

Maculopathy

Extrafoveal exudates can be watched. However, if they are beginning to encroach on the fovea, then the centre of any rings of exudates can be treated by laser photocoagulation. This treatment has largely been replaced by new therapies (see below).

New therapies

Anti-VEGF drugs, such as bevacizumab, aflibercept and ranibizumab (see p. 1334), are being used to control diabetic retinopathy and diabetic maculopathy, particularly that which involves the centre of the macula and is causing sight loss. Studies have shown benefit over laser for this type of maculopathy.

The diabetic kidney

The kidney may be damaged by diabetes in three main ways:

- glomerular damage
- ischaemia resulting from hypertrophy of afferent and efferent arterioles
- ascending infection.

Diabetic nephropathy

Epidemiology

Clinical nephropathy secondary to glomerular disease usually manifests 15–25 years after diagnosis of diabetes and affects 25–35% of patients diagnosed under the age of 30 years. It is the leading cause of premature death in young diabetic patients. Older patients also develop nephropathy but the proportion affected is smaller. The incidence of end-stage kidney disease has fallen in recent decades, probably due to better control of blood glucose and blood pressure, but this benefit has been cancelled out by the rising incidence of both types of diabetes.

Pathophysiology

The earliest functional abnormality in the diabetic kidney is renal hypertrophy associated with a raised glomerular filtration rate. This appears soon after diagnosis and is related to poor glycaemic control. As the kidney becomes damaged by diabetes, the afferent arteriole (leading to the glomerulus) becomes vasodilated to a greater extent than the efferent glomerular arteriole. This increases the intraglomerular filtration pressure, further damaging the glomerular capillaries. This raised intraglomerular pressure also leads to increased local shearing forces, which are thought to contribute to mesangial cell hypertrophy and increased secretion of extracellular mesangial matrix material. This process eventually leads to glomerular sclerosis. The initial structural lesion in the glomerulus is thickening of the basement membrane. Associated changes result in disruption of the protein cross-linkages that normally make the membrane an effective filter. In consequence, there is a progressive leak of large molecules (particularly protein) into the urine.

Albuminuria

The earliest evidence of this is 'microalbuminuria' – amounts of urinary albumin so small as to be undetectable by standard dipsticks (see p. 730). Microalbuminuria may be tested for with radioimmunoassay or special dipsticks. It is a predictive marker of progression to nephropathy in type 1 diabetes, and of increased cardiovascular risk in type 2 diabetes. Microalbuminuria may, after some years, progress to intermittent albuminuria followed by persistent proteinuria. Light-microscopic changes of glomerulosclerosis become manifest, both diffuse and nodular glomerulosclerosis can occur. The latter is sometimes known as the Kimmelstiel–Wilson lesion. At the later stage of glomerulosclerosis, the glomerulus is replaced by hyaline material.

At the stage of persistent proteinuria, the plasma creatinine is normal but the average patient is only some 5–10 years from end-stage kidney disease. The proteinuria may become so heavy as to induce a transient nephrotic syndrome, with peripheral oedema and hypoalbuminaemia.

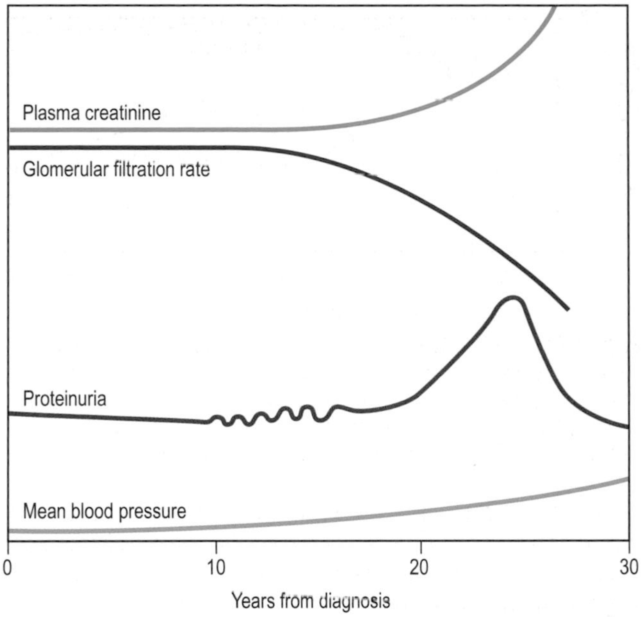

Figure 27.16 Schematic representation of the natural history of nephropathy. The typical onset is 15 years after diagnosis. Intermittent proteinuria leads to persistent proteinuria. In time, the plasma creatinine rises as the glomerular filtration rate falls.

Patients with nephropathy typically show a normochromic normocytic anaemia and a raised erythrocyte sedimentation rate (ESR). Hypertension is a common development and may itself damage the kidney still further. A rise in plasma creatinine is a late feature that progresses inevitably to renal failure, although the rate of progression may vary widely between individuals.

The natural history of this process is shown in ***Figure 27.16***.

Ischaemic lesions

Arteriolar lesions, with hypertrophy and hyalinization of the vessels, can occur in patients with diabetes. The appearances are similar to those of hypertensive disease and lead to ischaemic damage to the kidneys.

Infective lesions

Urinary tract infections are relatively more common in women with diabetes, but not in men. Ascending infection may occur because of bladder stasis resulting from autonomic neuropathy, and infections more easily become established in damaged renal tissue. Autopsy material frequently reveals interstitial changes suggestive of infection, but ischaemia may produce similar changes and the true frequency of pyelonephritis in diabetes is uncertain. Untreated infections in diabetics can result in renal papillary necrosis, in which renal papillae are shed in the urine, but this complication is now very rare.

Diagnosis

The urine of all diabetic patients should be checked regularly (at least annually) for the presence of protein. Many centres also screen younger patients for microalbuminuria since there is evidence that meticulous glycaemic control and early antihypertensive treatment, particularly with ACE inhibitors and angiotensin II blockers, may delay the onset of frank proteinuria. The albumin:creatinine ratio (ACR, tested on a mid-stream first morning urine sample) is <2.5 in healthy men and <3.5 mg/mmol in healthy women. Once proteinuria

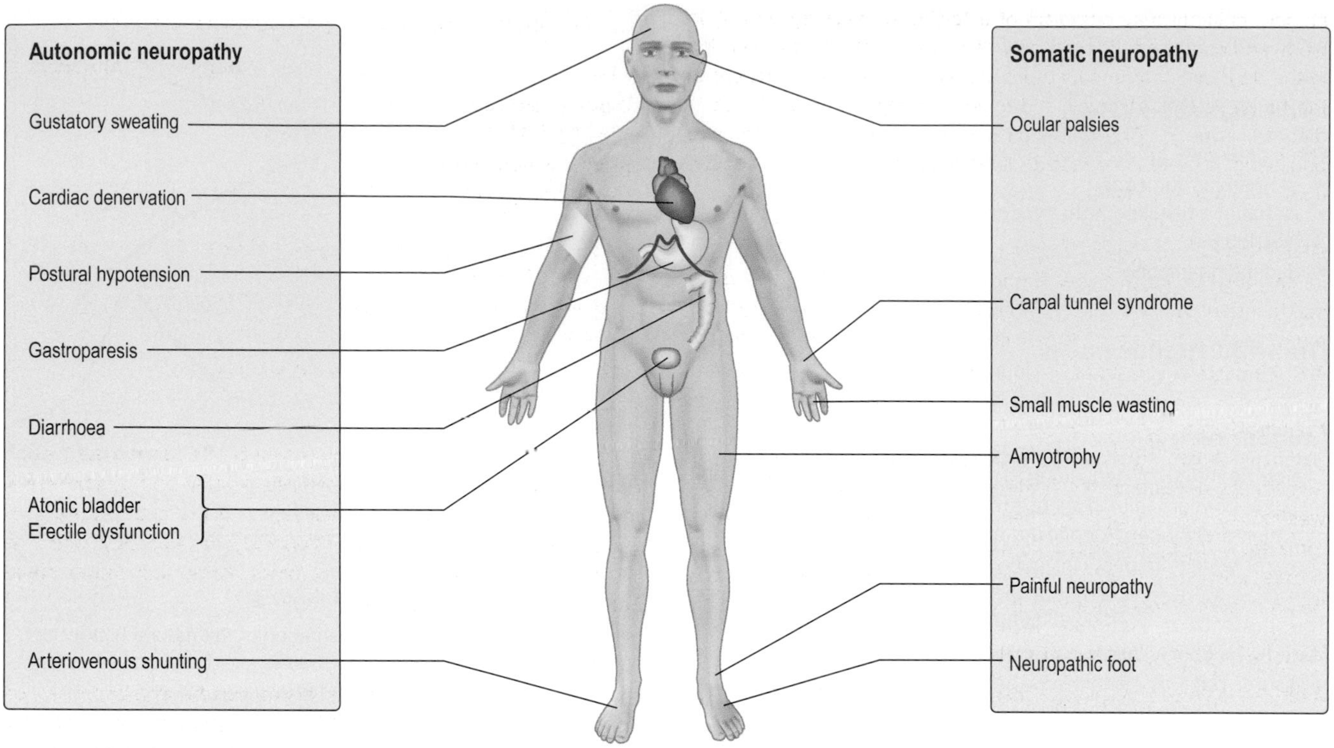

Figure 27.17 The neuropathic man.

is present, other possible causes should be considered (see below), but once these are excluded, a presumptive diagnosis of diabetic nephropathy can be made. For practical purposes, this implies inevitable progression to end-stage kidney disease, although the time course can be markedly slowed by early aggressive antihypertensive therapy. Clinical suspicion of a non-diabetic cause of nephropathy may be provoked by an atypical history, the absence of diabetic retinopathy (usually, but not invariably, present with diabetic nephropathy) and the presence of red-cell casts in the urine. Renal biopsy should be considered in such cases but is rarely necessary or helpful. Regular measurement is made of the plasma creatinine level with estimated glomerular filtration rate (eGFR).

Management

The management of diabetic nephropathy is similar to that of other causes of chronic kidney disease, with the following provisos:

- Aggressive treatment of blood pressure with a target <130/80 mmHg has been shown to slow the rate of deterioration of renal failure considerably. An ACE inhibitor or angiotensin II receptor antagonist is the drug of choice (see p. 1047). These drugs should also be used in normotensive patients with persistent microalbuminuria. Reduction in albuminuria occurs with this treatment.
- Oral hypoglycaemic agents partially excreted via the kidney (e.g. glibenclamide and metformin) should be avoided.
- Insulin sensitivity increases and drastic reductions in insulin dosage may be needed.
- Associated diabetic retinopathy tends to progress rapidly, and frequent ophthalmic supervision is essential.

Management of end-stage disease is made more difficult by the fact that patients often have other complications of diabetes, such as blindness, autonomic neuropathy or peripheral vascular disease. Vascular shunts tend to calcify rapidly and hence chronic ambulatory peritoneal dialysis may be preferable to haemodialysis.

The failure rate of renal transplants is somewhat higher than in non-diabetic patients. A segmental pancreatic or islet graft is sometimes performed under cover of the immunosuppression needed for the renal graft, and this has been shown to improve survival, as well as offering freedom from insulin injections.

Diabetic neuropathy

Diabetes can damage peripheral nervous tissue in a number of ways. The vascular hypothesis postulates occlusion of the vasa nervorum as the prime cause. This seems likely in isolated mononeuropathies but the diffuse symmetrical nature of the common forms of neuropathy implies a metabolic cause. Since hyperglycaemia leads to increased formation of sorbitol and fructose in Schwann cells, accumulation of these sugars may disrupt function and structure.

The earliest functional change in diabetic nerves is delayed nerve conduction velocity; the earliest histological change is segmental demyelination, caused by damage to Schwann cells. In the early stages, axons are preserved, implying prospects of recovery; at a later stage, irreversible axonal degeneration develops.

The following varieties of neuropathy occur ***(Fig. 27.17)***:

- symmetrical, mainly sensory polyneuropathy (distal)
- acute painful neuropathy
- mononeuropathy and mononeuritis multiplex
  - cranial nerve lesions
  - isolated peripheral nerve lesions
- diabetic amyotrophy (asymmetrical motor diabetic neuropathy)
- autonomic neuropathy.

Symmetrical, mainly sensory polyneuropathy

This is often unrecognized by the patient in its early stages. Early clinical signs are loss of vibration sense, pain sensation (deep before superficial) and temperature sensation in the feet. At later stages, patients may complain of a feeling of 'walking on cotton wool' and can lose their balance when washing the face or walking in the dark owing to impaired proprioception. Early involvement of the hands is less common and should prompt a search for non-diabetic causes. Complications include unrecognized trauma, beginning as blistering due to an ill-fitting shoe or a hot-water bottle, and leading to ulceration.

Sequelae of neuropathy

Involvement of motor nerves to the small muscles of the feet gives rise to interosseous wasting. Unbalanced traction by the long flexor muscles leads to a characteristic shape of the foot, with a high arch and clawing of the toes, which in turn causes abnormal distribution of pressure on walking, resulting in callus formation under the first metatarsal head or on the tips of the toes and perforating neuropathic ulceration. ***Neuropathic arthropathy*** (***Charcot's joints***) may sometimes develop in the ankle. The hands show small-muscle wasting, as well as sensory changes, but these signs and symptoms must be differentiated from those of the carpal tunnel syndrome, which occurs with increased frequency in diabetes and may be amenable to treatment (see p. 655).

Acute painful neuropathy

A diffuse, painful neuropathy is less common. The patient describes burning or crawling pains in the feet, shins and anterior thighs. These symptoms are typically worse at night and pressure from bedclothes may be intolerable. The condition may present at diagnosis or after sudden improvement in glycaemic control (e.g. when insulin is started). It usually remits spontaneously after 3–12 months if good control is maintained. A more chronic form, developing later in the course of the disease, is sometimes resistant to almost all forms of therapy. Neurological assessment is difficult because of the hyperaesthesia experienced by the patient, but muscle wasting is not a feature and objective signs can be minimal.

Management is firstly to explore for non-diabetic causes (see pp. 884–885). Explanation and reassurance about the likelihood of remission within months may be all that is needed. Duloxetine (NICE recommends this as first-line therapy), tricyclics, gabapentin or pregabalin, mexiletine, valproate and carbamazepine all reduce the perception of neuritic pain somewhat, but usually not as much as patients hope for. Transepidermal nerve stimulation (TENS) benefits some patients. Topical capsaicin-containing creams help occasionally. A few report that acupuncture has been of value.

Mononeuritis and mononeuritis multiplex (multiple mononeuropathy)

Any nerve in the body can be involved in diabetic mononeuritis; the onset is typically abrupt and sometimes painful. Radiculopathy (i.e. involvement of a spinal root) may also occur.

Isolated palsies of nerves to the external eye muscles, especially the third and sixth nerves, are more common in diabetes. A characteristic feature of diabetic third nerve lesions is that pupillary reflexes are retained owing to sparing of pupillomotor fibres. Full spontaneous recovery is the rule for most episodes of mononeuritis over 3–6 months. Lesions are more likely to occur at common sites for external pressure palsies or nerve entrapment (e.g. the median nerve in the carpal tunnel; see p. 882).

Diabetic amyotrophy

This condition is usually seen in older men with diabetes. Presentation is with painful wasting, usually asymmetrical, of the quadriceps muscles. The wasting may be very marked and knee reflexes are diminished or absent. The affected area is often extremely tender. Extensor plantar responses sometimes develop and cerebrospinal fluid (CSF) protein content is elevated. Diabetic amyotrophy is usually associated with periods of poor glycaemic control and may be present at diagnosis. It often resolves in time with careful metabolic control of the diabetes.

Box 27.19 Bedside testing of autonomic function

Test	Normal	Abnormal
Supine to erect blood pressure		
Systolic BP fall (mmHg)	10	≥30
Heart rate responses to:		
Deep breathing (6 breaths over 1 min) max. to min. HR	≥15	≤10
Valsalva manœuvre (15 s): ratio of longest to shortest R–R interval	≥1.21	≤1.20
Lying to standing ratio of R–R interval of 30th to 15th beats	≥1.04	≤1.00

HR, heart rate; R–R, time between R and next R on ECG.

Autonomic neuropathy

Asymptomatic autonomic disturbances can be demonstrated on testing in many patients ***(Box 27.19)*** but symptomatic autonomic neuropathy is rare. It affects both the sympathetic and parasympathetic nervous systems and can cause disabling postural hypotension.

The cardiovascular system

Vagal neuropathy results in tachycardia at rest and loss of sinus arrhythmia. At a later stage, the heart may become denervated (resembling a transplanted heart). Cardiovascular reflexes, such as the Valsalva manœuvre (see p. 970), are impaired. Postural hypotension occurs owing to loss of sympathetic tone to peripheral arterioles. A warm foot with a bounding pulse is often seen in a polyneuropathy as a result of peripheral vasodilatation.

The gastrointestinal tract

Vagal damage can lead to gastroparesis, often asymptomatic but sometimes leading to intractable vomiting. Implantable devices that stimulate gastric emptying, and injections of botulinum toxin into the pylorus (to paralyse the sphincter partly), have each shown benefit in cases of this previously intractable problem. Autonomic diarrhoea characteristically occurs at night, accompanied by urgency and incontinence. Diarrhoea and steatorrhoea may be present, owing to small bowel bacterial overgrowth; treatment is with antibiotics such as tetracycline.

Bladder involvement

Loss of tone, incomplete emptying and stasis (predisposing to infection) can occur and may ultimately result in an atonic, painless, distended bladder. Treatment is with intermittent self-catheterization, permanent catheterization if that fails, and prophylactic antibiotic therapy for those prone to recurrent infection.

Male erectile dysfunction

This is common. The first manifestation is incomplete erection, which may, in time, progress to total failure; retrograde ejaculation also occurs in patients with autonomic neuropathy. Erectile dysfunction in diabetes has many causes, including anxiety, depression, alcohol excess, drugs (e.g. thiazides and beta-blockers),

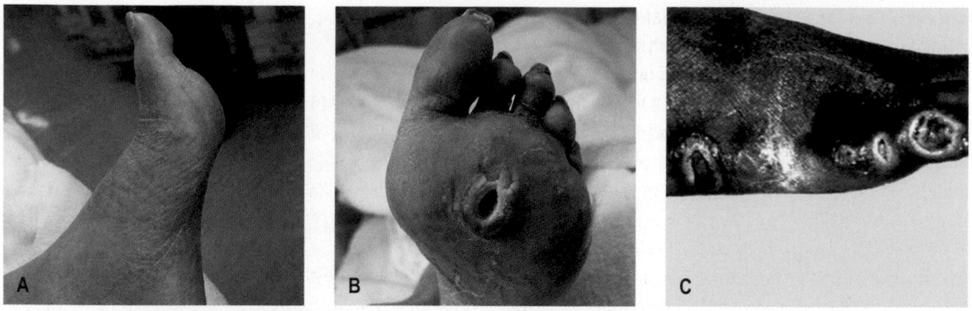

Figure 27.18 **Diabetic foot. A.** High arch and clawing of toes. **B.** Typical neuropathic plantar ulceration. **C.** Vascular pattern of ulceration.

primary or secondary gonadal failure, hypothyroidism and inadequate vascular supply owing to atheroma in pudendal arteries. The history and examination should focus on these possible causes. Blood is taken for luteinizing hormone, follicle stimulating hormone, testosterone, prolactin and thyroid function. Treatment should ideally include sympathetic counselling of both partners.

Phosphodiesterase type 5 inhibitors (sildenafil, tadalafil, vardenafil, avanafil), which enhance the effects of nitric oxide on smooth muscle and increase penile blood flow, are used in those who do not take nitrates for angina. Some 60% of patients can be expected to benefit from this therapy.

Alternatives for those who fail to improve with a phosphodiesterase inhibitor or who dislike the side-effects (headache and a green tinge to vision the next day), and for those in whom it is contraindicated, are:

- Apomorphine 2 or 3 mg sublingually 20 min before sexual activity.
- Alprostadil (prostaglandin E1 preparation), given as a small pellet inserted with a device into the urethra (125 μg initially to a maximum of 500 μg). If the partner is pregnant, barrier contraception must be used to keep prostaglandin away from the fetus.
- Intracavernosal injection or insertion of a pellet of alprostadil into the urethra (2.5 μg initially to a maximum of 40 μg). Side-effects include priapism, which needs urgent treatment should erection last >3 h.
- Vacuum devices.

Box 27.20 Distinguishing features between ischaemia and neuropathy in the diabetic foot

Feature	Ischaemia	Neuropathy
Symptoms	Claudication Rest pain	Usually painless Sometimes painful neuropathy
Inspection	Dependent rubor Trophic changes	High arch Clawing of toes No trophic changes
Palpation	Cold Pulseless	Warm Bounding pulses
Ulceration	Painful Heels and toes	Painless Plantar

Box 27.21 Principles of diabetic foot care

- Inspect feet daily
- Moisturize dry skin
- Seek early advice for any damage
- Check shoes inside and out for sharp bodies/areas before wearing
- Use lace-up shoes with plenty of room for the toes
- Keep feet away from sources of heat (hot sand, hot-water bottles, radiators, fires)
- Check the bath temperature before stepping in
- Attend a podiatrist regularly

The diabetic foot

A total of 10–15% of diabetic patients develop foot ulcers at some stage in their lives. Diabetic foot problems ***(Fig. 27.18)*** are responsible for nearly 50% of all diabetes-related hospital admissions. Many diabetic limb amputations could be delayed or prevented by more effective patient education and medical supervision. Ischaemia, infection and neuropathy combine to produce tissue necrosis. Although all these factors may coexist, the ischaemic and the neuropathic foot ***(Box 27.20)*** can be distinguished. In rural India, foot ulcers are commonly due to neuropathic and infective causes rather than vascular causes.

Management

Many diabetic foot problems are avoidable, so patients need to learn the principles of foot care ***(Box 27.21)***. Older patients should visit a chiropodist/podiatrist regularly and should not cut their own toenails. Once tissue damage has occurred in the form of ulceration or gangrene, the aim is preservation of viable tissue. The four main threats to the skin and subcutaneous tissues are:

- ***Infection***. This can take hold rapidly in a diabetic foot. Early antibiotic treatment is essential, with antibiotic therapy adjusted in the light of culture results. The organism grown from the skin surface may not be the organism causing deeper infection. Collections of pus are drained and excision of infected bone is needed if osteomyelitis develops and does not respond to appropriate antibiotic therapy. Regular X-rays of the foot are needed to check on progress.
- ***Ischaemia***. The blood flow to the feet is assessed clinically and with Doppler ultrasound. Femoral angiography is used to localize areas of occlusion amenable to bypass surgery or angioplasty. Relatively few patients fall into this category.
- ***Abnormal pressure***. An ulcerated site must be kept non-weight-bearing. Resting the affected leg may need to be supplemented with special deep shoes and insoles to move pressure away from critical sites, or by removable or non-removable casts of the leg. After healing, special shoes and insoles are likely to continue to be needed to protect the feet and prevent abnormal pressure repeating damage to a healed area. In neuropathic feet, particularly, sharp surgical debridement by a chiropodist is necessary to prevent callus

distorting the local wound architecture and causing damage through abnormal pressure on normal skin nearby.
- ***Wound environment***. Dressings are used to absorb or remove exudate, maintain moisture, and protect the wound from contaminating agents; they should be easily removable. The role of expensive new dressings containing growth factors and other biologically active agents is being assessed.

Good liaison between physician, chiropodist/podiatrist and surgeon is essential if periods in hospital are to be used efficiently. When irreversible arterial insufficiency is present, it is often quicker and kinder to opt for an early major amputation rather than subject the patient to a debilitating sequence of conservative procedures.

Infections

There is no evidence that diabetic patients with good glycaemic control are more prone to infection than normal subjects. However, poorly controlled diabetes entails increased susceptibility to the following infections:

- ***Skin***
  - staphylococcal infections (boils, abscesses, carbuncles)
  - mucocutaneous candidiasis
- ***Gastrointestinal tract***
  - periodontal disease
  - rectal and ischiorectal abscess formation (when control is very poor)
- ***Urinary tract***
  - urinary tract infections (in women)
  - pyelonephritis
  - perinephric abscess
- ***Lungs***
  - staphylococcal and pneumococcal pneumonia
  - Gram-negative bacterial pneumonia
  - tuberculosis
- ***Bone***
  - spontaneous staphylococcal spinal osteomyelitis.

One reason why poor control leads to infection is that chemotaxis and phagocytosis by polymorphonuclear leucocytes are impaired because, at high blood glucose concentrations, neutrophil superoxide generation is impaired.

Conversely, infections may lead to loss of glycaemic control and precipitate hyperglycaemic emergencies. Insulin-treated patients need to increase their dose by up to 25% in the face of infection, and non-insulin-treated patients may need insulin cover while the infection lasts. Patients should be told never to omit their insulin dose, even if they are nauseated and unable to eat; instead, they should test their blood glucose frequently and seek urgent medical advice. Patients should receive pneumococcal vaccine and yearly influenza vaccine.

Diabetes and cancer

Certain types of cancer are more common in type 2 diabetes. The risk of carcinoma of the uterus and of the pancreas is approximately doubled, and there is a 20–50% increase in the risk of colorectal and breast cancer. These associations appear to be mediated by obesity, which confers similar levels of risk in the absence of hyperglycaemia, although there is also an element of reverse causation with carcinoma of the pancreas, which can precipitate or cause diabetes. Metformin-treated patients have been reported to have a lower cancer risk than those on other therapies, and this agent is under investigation for possible anti-tumour properties.

Skin and joints

Joint contractures in the hands are a common consequence of childhood diabetes. The sign may be demonstrated by asking the patient to join the hands as if in prayer; the metacarpophalangeal and interphalangeal joints cannot be opposed. Thickened, waxy skin can be noted on the backs of the fingers. These features may be due to glycosylation of collagen and are not progressive (see also p. 1364). The condition is sometimes referred to as diabetic cheiroarthropathy.

Osteopenia in the extremities is also described in type 1 diabetes but rarely has clinical consequences.

Further reading

Antonetti DA, Klein R, Gardner TW. Diabetic retinopathy. *N Engl J Med* 2012; 366:1227–1239.
DCCT/EDIC Research Group, de Boer IH, Sun W et al. Intensive diabetes therapy and glomerular filtration rate in type 1 diabetes mellitus. *N Engl J Med* 2011; 365:2366–2376.
Jude EB, Eleftheriadou I, Tentolouris N. Peripheral arterial disease in diabetes – a review. *Diabetes Med* 2010; 27:4–14.
Martin DF, Maguire MG. Treatment choice for diabetic macular edema. *N Engl J Med* 2015; 372:1260–1261.
Pernicova I, Korbonits M. Metformin – mode of action and clinical implications for diabetes and cancer. *Nat Rev Endocrinol* 2014; 10:143–156.
White NH, Sun W, Cleary PA. Prolonged effect of intensive therapy on the risk of retinopathy complications in patients with type 1 diabetes mellitus: 10 years after the Diabetes Control and Complications Trial. *Arch Ophthalmol* 2008; 126:1707–1715.

SPECIAL SITUATIONS IN DIABETES

Surgery in diabetes

Smooth control of diabetes minimizes the risk of infection and balances the catabolic response to anaesthesia and surgery. The procedure for insulin-treated patients is simple:

- Long-acting and/or intermediate insulin should be stopped the day before surgery, and soluble insulin substituted.
- Whenever possible, diabetic patients should be first on the morning theatre list.
- An infusion of glucose, insulin and potassium is given during surgery. The insulin can be mixed into the glucose solution or administered separately by syringe pump. A standard combination is 16 U of soluble insulin with 10 mmol of KCl in 500 mL of 10% glucose, infused at 100 mL/h.
- Postoperatively, the infusion is maintained until the patient is able to eat. Other fluids needed in the perioperative period must be given through a separate intravenous line and must not interrupt the glucose/insulin/potassium infusion. Glucose levels are checked every 2–4 h and potassium levels are monitored. The amount of insulin and potassium in each infusion bag is adjusted either upwards or downwards, according to the results of regular monitoring of the blood glucose and serum potassium concentrations.

The same approach is used in the emergency situation, with the exception that a separate variable-rate insulin infusion may be needed to bring blood glucose under control before surgery.

Non-insulin-treated patients should stop medication 2 days before the operation. Patients with mild hyperglycaemia (fasting blood glucose <8 mmol/L) can be treated as non-diabetic. Those with higher levels are treated with soluble insulin prior to surgery, and with glucose, insulin and potassium during and after the procedure, as for insulin-treated patients.

Pregnancy in established diabetes

Pregnancy in diabetes was, in the past, associated with high fetal mortality, which has been dramatically reduced by meticulous metabolic control of the diabetes and careful obstetric management. Despite this, the rates of congenital malformation and perinatal mortality remain several times higher than in the non-diabetic population. Type 2 diabetes is now much more prevalent in the maternal population as a result of the changing natural history of this condition.

Metabolic control of diabetes in pregnancy

Congenital malformations are associated with poor glucose control in the early weeks of pregnancy, and good control should therefore be in place before conception, wherever possible. The mother should perform daily home blood glucose profiles, recording blood tests before and 2 hours after meals. The renal threshold for glucose falls in pregnancy and urine tests are therefore of little value. Insulin requirements rise progressively and intensified insulin regimens are generally used. The aim is to maintain blood glucose and fructosamine (or HbA_{1c}) levels as close to the normal range as can be tolerated. Oral antidiabetic therapy should be avoided, except for metformin, which is recognized to be safe in pregnancy.

General management

The patient is seen at intervals of 2 weeks or less at a clinic managed jointly by physician and obstetrician. Circumstances permitting, the aim should be outpatient management with a spontaneous vaginal delivery at term. Retinopathy and nephropathy may deteriorate during pregnancy. Digital photographic eye screening and urine testing for protein should be undertaken at booking, at 28 weeks and before delivery.

Obstetric problems associated with diabetes

Congenital malformations associated with maternal diabetes affect cardiac and skeletal development, of which the caudal regression syndrome is an example. Poorly controlled diabetes later in gestation is associated with stillbirth, shoulder dystocia owing to fetal macrosomia, polyhydramnios and pre-eclampsia. Ketoacidosis in pregnancy carries a 50% fetal mortality, but maternal hypoglycaemia, although highly undesirable, is relatively well tolerated by the fetus.

Neonatal problems

Maternal diabetes, especially when poorly controlled, is associated with fetal macrosomia. The infant of a diabetic mother is more susceptible to hyaline membrane disease than non-diabetic infants of similar maturity. In addition, neonatal hypoglycaemia may occur. The mechanism is as follows: maternal glucose crosses the placenta but insulin does not; the fetal islets hypersecrete to combat maternal hyperglycaemia, and a rebound to hypoglycaemic levels occurs when the umbilical cord is cut. These complications are due to hyperglycaemia in the third trimester.

Gestational diabetes

This term refers to glucose intolerance that develops or is first recognized in the course of pregnancy; it is typically asymptomatic and usually remits following delivery. Gestational diabetes has been estimated to complicate about 7% of all pregnancies, with wide variation due to differences between populations and diagnostic criteria. Women with a previous history of gestational diabetes, older or overweight women, those with a history of large-for-gestational-age babies, and women from certain ethnic groups are at particular risk, but many affected women are not in any of these categories. For this reason, some advocate screening of all pregnant women on the basis of random plasma glucose testing in each trimester and by oral glucose tolerance testing if the glucose concentration is, for example, 7 mmol/L or more. The Hyperglycemia and Adverse Pregnancy Outcomes (HAPO) study found that the risk of adverse outcomes increased as a function of maternal glucose levels at 24–28 weeks of pregnancy, even when these were within the normal reference range. This has added to the controversy concerning the appropriate cut-off levels for screening and intervention, since the benefits of intervention are marginal at lower glucose levels, while labelling a mother as diabetic may have unwanted consequences, such as a higher rate of caesarean section.

Treatment is with diet in the first instance, followed by metformin if blood glucose targets (fasting 5.3 mmol/L; 2 h after meals 6.4 mmol/L) are not met using changes in diet and exercise within 1–2 weeks. Initial treatment with insulin is used in those with a fasting plasma glucose level >7.0 mmol/L at diagnosis, or between 6.0 and 6.9 mmol/L if macrosomia or hydramnios is present, although many patients come to require insulin as their pregnancy advances. Insulin does not cross the placenta. Many oral agents cross the placenta and are usually avoided because of the potential risk to the fetus, although glibenclamide has been used in gestational diabetes presenting later in pregnancy.

Gestational diabetes has been associated with all the obstetric and neonatal problems described above for pre-existing diabetes, except that there is no increase in the rate of congenital abnormalities. Gestational diabetes typically remits after delivery but signals an increased risk of type 2 diabetes in later life; maintaining a low body weight and keeping physically active reduce this risk.

Not all diabetes presenting in pregnancy is gestational. True type 1 diabetes may develop and swift diagnosis is essential to prevent the development of ketoacidosis. Hospital admission is required if the patient is symptomatic, or has ketonuria or a markedly elevated blood glucose level.

Unstable diabetes

This term is used to describe the condition of patients with recurrent ketoacidosis and/or recurrent hypoglycaemic coma. Of these, the largest group is made up of those who experience recurrent severe hypoglycaemia.

Recurrent severe hypoglycaemia

This affects 1–3% of insulin-dependent patients. Most are adults who have had diabetes for >10 years. By this stage, endogenous insulin secretion is negligible in the great majority of patients. Pancreatic α cells are still present in undiminished numbers but the glucagon response to hypoglycaemia is virtually absent. Long-term patients are thus subject to fluctuating hyperinsulinaemia owing to erratic absorption of insulin from injection sites, and lack a major component of the hormonal defence against hypoglycaemia. In this situation, adrenaline (epinephrine) secretion becomes vital, but this too may become impaired in the course of diabetes. Loss of adrenaline (epinephrine) secretion has been attributed to autonomic neuropathy but this is unlikely to be the sole cause; central adaptation to recurrent hypoglycaemia may also be a factor.

The following factors may also predispose to recurrent hypoglycaemia:

- ***Over-treatment with insulin***. Frequent biochemical hypoglycaemia lowers the glucose level at which symptoms develop. Symptoms often reappear when overall glucose control is relaxed.
- ***An unrecognized low renal threshold for glucose***. Attempts to render the urine sugar-free will inevitably produce hypoglycaemia.
- ***Excessive insulin doses***. A common error is to increase the dose when a patient needs more frequent injections to overcome a problem of timing.
- ***Endocrine causes***. These include pituitary insufficiency, adrenal insufficiency and premenstrual insulin sensitivity.
- ***Alimentary causes***. These include exocrine pancreatic failure and diabetic gastroparesis.
- ***Chronic kidney disease***. Clearance of insulin is diminished.
- ***Patient causes***. Patients may struggle to understand the principles of diabetes management, may be uncooperative or may manipulate their therapy.

Recurrent ketoacidosis

This usually occurs in adolescents or young adults, particularly girls. Metabolic decompensation may develop very rapidly. A combination of chaotic food intake and insulin omission, whether conscious or unconscious, is the primary cause of this problem. It almost always occurs in the context of considerable psychosocial problems, particularly eating disorders. This area needs careful and sympathetic exploration in any patient with recurrent ketoacidosis. It is perhaps not surprising that in an illness where much of one's life is spent thinking of and controlling food intake, 30% of women with diabetes have had some features of an eating disorder at some time. Other causes include:

- ***Iatrogenic factors***. Inappropriate insulin combinations may be a cause of swinging glycaemic control. For example, a once-daily regimen may cause hypoglycaemia during the afternoon or evening and pre-breakfast hyperglycaemia due to insulin deficiency.
- ***Intercurrent illness***. Unsuspected infections, including urinary tract infections and tuberculosis, may be present. Thyrotoxicosis can also manifest as unstable glycaemic control.

Further reading

International Association of Diabetes in Pregnancy Study Groups Consensus Panel. International Association of Diabetes in Pregnancy Study Groups recommendations on the diagnosis and classification of hyperglycemia in pregnancy. *Diabetes Care* 2010; 33:676–682.

HYPOGLYCAEMIA IN THE NON-DIABETIC PATIENT

Hypoglycaemia develops when hepatic glucose output falls below the rate of glucose uptake by peripheral tissues. Hepatic glucose output may be reduced by:

- inhibition of hepatic glycogenolysis and gluconeogenesis by insulin
- depletion of hepatic glycogen reserves by malnutrition, fasting, exercise or advanced liver disease
- impaired gluconeogenesis (e.g. following alcohol ingestion).

In the first of these categories, insulin levels are raised, the liver contains adequate glycogen stores and the hypoglycaemia can be reversed by injection of glucagon. In the other two situations, insulin levels are low and glucagon is ineffective. Peripheral glucose uptake is accelerated by high insulin levels and by exercise, but these conditions are normally balanced by increased hepatic glucose output.

The most common symptoms and signs of hypoglycaemia are neurological. The brain consumes about 50% of the total glucose produced by the liver. This high energy requirement is needed to generate ATP, used to maintain the potential difference across axonal membranes.

Box 27.22 Presenting features of insulinoma

- Diplopia
- Sweating, palpitations, weakness
- Confusion or abnormal behaviour
- Loss of consciousness
- Grand mal seizures

Insulinomas

Insulinomas are pancreatic islet cell tumours that secrete insulin. Most are sporadic but some patients have multiple tumours arising from neural crest tissue (multiple endocrine neoplasia). Some 95% of these tumours are benign. The classic presentation is with fasting hypoglycaemia, but early symptoms may also develop in the late morning or afternoon. Recurrent hypoglycaemia is often present for months or years before the diagnosis is made, and the symptoms may be atypical or even bizarre; the presenting features in one series are given in ***Box 27.22***. Common misdiagnoses include psychiatric disorders, particularly pseudodementia in elderly people, epilepsy and cerebrovascular disease. Whipple's triad remains the basis of clinical diagnosis. This is satisfied when:

- symptoms are associated with fasting or exercise
- hypoglycaemia is confirmed during these episodes
- glucose relieves the symptoms.

A fourth criterion – demonstration of inappropriately high insulin levels during hypoglycaemia – may usefully be added.

The diagnosis is confirmed by the demonstration of hypoglycaemia in association with inappropriate and excessive insulin secretion. Hypoglycaemia is demonstrated by:

- Measurement of overnight fasting (16 h) glucose and insulin levels on three occasions. About 90% of patients with insulinomas will have low glucose and non-suppressed (normal or elevated) insulin levels.
- A prolonged 72-h supervised fast if overnight testing is inconclusive and symptoms persist.

Autonomous insulin secretion is demonstrated by lack of the normal feedback suppression during hypoglycaemia. This may be shown by measuring insulin, C-peptide or proinsulin during a spontaneous episode of hypoglycaemia.

Management

The most effective therapy is surgical excision of the tumour but insulinomas are often very small and difficult to localize. Many techniques can be used to attempt to localize insulinomas. Sensitivity and specificity vary between centres and between operators. These include highly selective angiography, contrast-enhanced high-resolution computed tomography scanning, scanning with radiolabelled somatostatin (some insulinomas express somatostatin receptors), and endoscopic and intraoperative ultrasound scanning. Venous sampling for the detection of 'hot spots' of high insulin concentration in the various intra-abdominal veins is still used occasionally.

Medical treatment with diazoxide is useful when the insulinoma is malignant, when a tumour cannot be located and when elderly patients have mild symptoms. Symptoms may also remit on treatment with a somatostatin analogue (octreotide or lanreotide).

Hypoglycaemia with other tumours

Hypoglycaemia may develop in the course of advanced neoplasia and cachexia, and has been described in association with many tumour types. Certain massive tumours, especially sarcomas, may produce hypoglycaemia owing to the secretion of insulin-like growth factor-1. True ectopic insulin secretion is extremely rare.

Postprandial hypoglycaemia

If frequent venous blood glucose samples are taken following a prolonged glucose tolerance test, about 1 in 4 subjects will have at least one value below 3 mmol/L. The arteriovenous glucose difference is quite marked during this phase, so that very few are truly hypoglycaemic in terms of arterial (or capillary) blood glucose content. Failure to appreciate this simple fact led some authorities to believe that postprandial (or reactive) hypoglycaemia was a potential 'organic' explanation for a variety of complaints that might otherwise have been considered psychosomatic. An epidemic of false 'hypoglycaemia' followed, particularly in the USA. Later work showed a poor correlation between symptoms and biochemical hypoglycaemia. Even so, a number of otherwise normal people occasionally become pale, weak and sweaty at times when meals are due, and report benefit from advice to take regular snacks between meals.

True postprandial hypoglycaemia may develop in the presence of alcohol, which 'primes' the cells to produce an exaggerated insulin response to carbohydrate. The person who substitutes alcoholic beverages for lunch is particularly at risk. Postprandial hypoglycaemia sometimes occurs after gastric surgery, owing to rapid gastric emptying and mismatching of nutrient absorption and insulin secretion. This is referred to as 'dumping' but it is now rarely encountered (see p. 381).

Hepatic and renal causes of hypoglycaemia

The liver can maintain a normal glucose output despite extensive damage, and hepatic hypoglycaemia is uncommon. It is, however, a particular problem with acute hepatic failure.

The kidney has a subsidiary role in glucose production (via gluconeogenesis in the renal cortex), and hypoglycaemia is sometimes a problem in terminal renal failure.

Hereditary fructose intolerance occurs in 1 in 20 000 live births and can cause hypoglycaemia (see p. 1285).

Endocrine causes of hypoglycaemia

Deficiencies of hormones antagonistic to insulin are rare but well-recognized causes of hypoglycaemia. These include hypopituitarism, isolated adrenocorticotrophic hormone (ACTH) deficiency and Addison's disease.

Drug-induced hypoglycaemia

Many drugs have been reported to produce isolated cases of hypoglycaemia, but usually only when other predisposing factors are present:

- Sulphonylureas may be used in the treatment of diabetes or may be taken by non-diabetics in suicide attempts.
- Quinine may produce severe hypoglycaemia in the course of treatment for *falciparum* malaria.
- Salicylates may cause hypoglycaemia, usually after accidental ingestion by children.
- Propranolol can induce hypoglycaemia in the presence of strenuous exercise or starvation.
- Pentamidine, used in the treatment of resistant *Pneumocystis* pneumonia, may produce hypoglycaemia (see p. 349).

Alcohol-induced hypoglycaemia

Alcohol inhibits gluconeogenesis. Alcohol-induced hypoglycaemia occurs in poorly nourished chronic alcohol users, binge drinkers, and children who have taken relatively small amounts of alcohol, since they have a diminished hepatic glycogen reserve. They present with coma and hypothermia (hypothermia is a feature of hypoglycaemia, due to the suppression of central thermoregulation, particularly the shivering response; children manifest hypothermia more frequently due to their high ratio of surface area to body mass).

Factitious hypoglycaemia

This is a relatively common variant of self-induced disease and is more common than an insulinoma. Hypoglycaemia is produced by surreptitious self-administration of insulin or sulphonylureas. Many patients in this category have been extensively investigated for an insulinoma. Measurement of C-peptide levels during hypoglycaemia should identify patients who are injecting insulin; sulphonylurea abuse can be detected by chromatography of plasma or urine.

Significant websites

http://www.diabetes.ca *Canadian Diabetes Association site – well-designed, practical site with many links to other diabetes-related sites; a good starting point.*

http://www.diabetes.org *American Diabetes Association – heavyweight and authoritative, with an American flavour.*

http://www.diabetes.org.uk *Diabetes UK charity – information for patients, researchers and health professionals.*

http://www.diapedia.org *The Living Textbook of Diabetes, sponsored by the European Association for the Study of Diabetes (EASD).*

http://www.dtu.ox.ac.uk *Diabetes Trials Unit (University of Oxford) – research information, particularly the UK Prospective Diabetes Study results.*

http://www.eatlas.idf.org *International Diabetes Federation.*

http://www.sign.ac.uk *Scottish Intercollegiate Guidelines Network – guidelines on a range of subjects including diabetes.*

28 Lipid and metabolic disorders

Edwin AM Gale, John V Anderson

See your e-book for clinical tips, drug tips, extra tables, interactive Figures and MCQs.

DISORDERS OF LIPID METABOLISM

Physiology

Lipids are insoluble in water and are transported in the bloodstream as macromolecular complexes. In these complexes, lipids (principally triglyceride, cholesterol and cholesterol esters) are surrounded by a stabilizing coat of phospholipid. Proteins (called apoproteins) embedded into the surface of these 'lipoprotein' particles exert a stabilizing function and allow the particles to be recognized by receptors in the liver and the peripheral tissues. The structure of a chylomicron (one type of lipoprotein particle) is illustrated in ***Figure 28.1***.

Five principal types of lipoprotein particles are found in the blood ***(Fig. 28.2)***. They are structurally different and can be separated in the laboratory by their density and electrophoretic mobility. The larger particles give postprandial plasma its cloudy appearance. More than half of all patients under 60 years of age who have angiographically confirmed coronary artery disease have a lipoprotein disorder.

The genes for all the major apoproteins and that for the low-density lipoprotein (LDL) receptor have been isolated and sequenced, and their chromosomal sites have been mapped. Production of abnormal apoproteins is known to give rise, or predispose, to several types of lipid disorder, and it is likely that others will be discovered.

Chylomicrons

Chylomicrons (see ***Fig. 28.1***) are synthesized in the small intestine postprandially, passing initially into the intestinal lymphatic drainage, then along the thoracic duct into the bloodstream. They contain triglyceride and a small amount of cholesterol and its ester, and provide the main mechanism for transporting the digestion products of dietary fat to the liver and peripheral tissues. Each newly formed chylomicron contains several different apoproteins (B48, AI, AII), and acquires apoproteins CII and E by transfer from high-density lipoprotein (HDL) particles in the bloodstream. Apoprotein CII binds to specific receptors in adipose tissue, skeletal muscle and the liver, where the endothelial enzyme, lipoprotein lipase, hydrolyses most of the triglyceride into fatty acids, which are used as an energy source or stored. The remaining chylomicron remnant particle, which contains the bulk of the original cholesterol, is taken up by the liver. Apoprotein E on the particle's surface binds with liver clearance receptors.

Very-low-density lipoprotein particles

Very-low-density lipoprotein (VLDL) particles are synthesized continuously in the liver; they contain most of the body's endogenously synthesized triglyceride and a smaller quantity of cholesterol. They are the body's main source of energy during prolonged fasting. Apoprotein B100 is an essential component of VLDL. Apoproteins CII and E are incorporated later into VLDL by transfer from HDL particles. As they pass round the circulation, VLDL particles bind through apoprotein CII, allowing triglyceride to be progressively removed by lipoprotein lipase in the capillary endothelium. This leaves a particle, now depleted of triglyceride and apoprotein CII, called an intermediate-density lipoprotein particle.

Intermediate-density lipoprotein particles

Intermediate-density lipoprotein (IDL) particles have apoprotein B100 and apoprotein E molecules on the particle surface. Most IDL particles bind to liver LDL receptors through the apoprotein E molecule and are then catabolized. Some IDL particles have further triglyceride removed (by the enzyme hepatic lipase), producing LDL particles.

Low-density lipoprotein particles

Low-density lipoprotein (LDL) particles are the main carrier of cholesterol, and deliver it both to the liver and to peripheral cells. The surface of the LDL particle contains apoprotein B100 and also apoprotein E. Apoprotein B100 is the principal ligand for the LDL clearance receptor. This receptor lies within coated pits on the surface of the hepatocyte. Once bound to the receptor, the coated pit invaginates and fuses with liposomes, which destroy the LDL particle ***(Fig. 28.3)***.

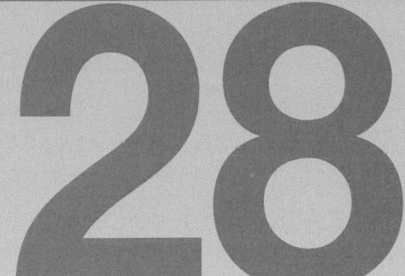

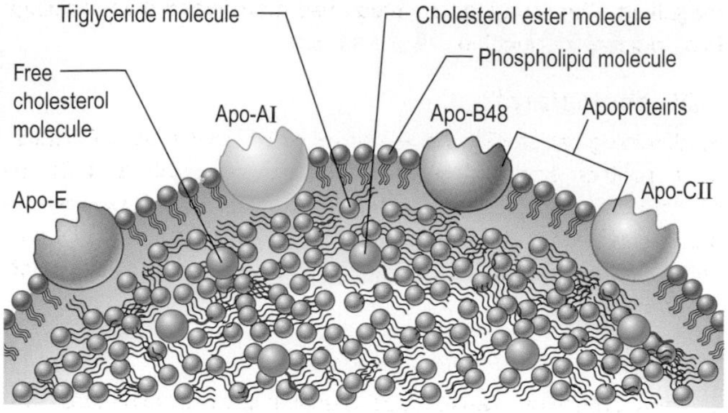

Figure 28.1 **A chylomicron particle (75–1200 nm) showing apoproteins lying in the surface membrane.**

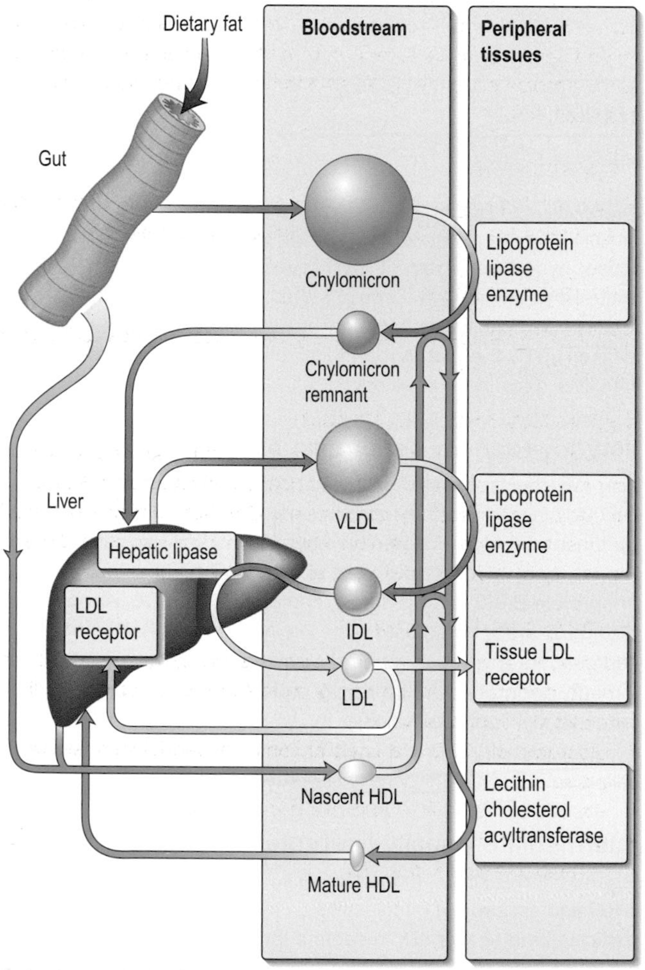

Figure 28.2 **The sites of origin of the major lipoprotein particles, showing their interaction and fate.** HDL, high-density lipoprotein; IDL, intermediate-density lipoprotein; LDL, low-density lipoprotein; VLDL, very-low-density lipoprotein

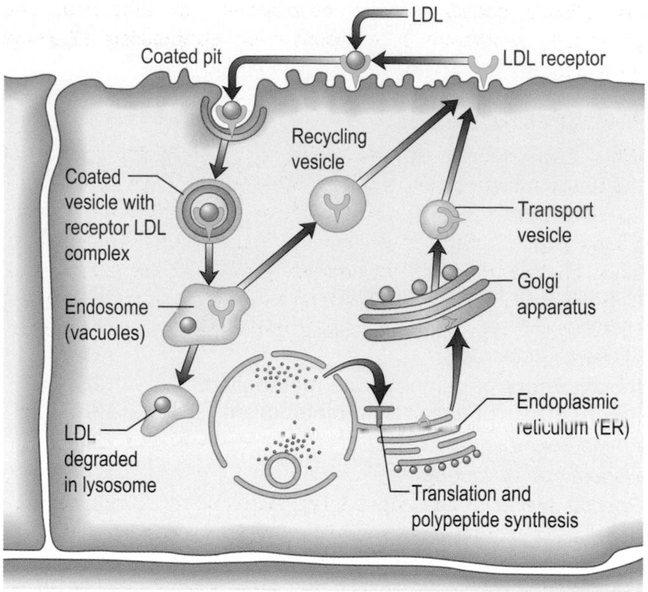

Figure 28.3 **Receptor-mediated endocytosis.** Low-density lipoprotein (LDL) receptors are formed in the endoplasmic reticulum and transported via the Golgi apparatus to the surface of a hepatocyte. LDLs bind to these receptors, and are internalized and taken up by the endosome. The receptor is recycled back to the surface, while the LDL is broken down by the lysosomes, freeing the cholesterol needed for membrane synthesis.

This process is, in part, regulated by a serine protease, proprotein convertase subtilisin/kexin type 9 (PCSK9). When PCSK9 binds to an LDL–LDL clearance receptor complex, the receptor is destroyed along with the LDL particle. If PCSK9 does not bind, the receptor returns to the surface of the cell and removes more cholesterol. The number of hepatic LDL clearance receptors regulates the circulating LDL concentration. This is also influenced by the activity of the rate-limiting enzyme in the cholesterol synthetic pathway, hydroxymethylglutaryl coenzyme A (HMG-CoA) reductase.

LDL particles can deposit lipid into the walls of the peripheral vasculature. Not all the cholesterol synthesized by the liver is packaged immediately into lipoprotein particles. Some is oxidized into bile salts. Both bile salts and cholesterol are excreted in the bile; both are then reabsorbed through the terminal ileum and recirculated (enterohepatic circulation; see p. 443).

LDL particles become Lp(a) lipoproteins as a result of the linkage of apoprotein (a) to apoprotein B100 with a single disulphide bond. Raised levels of Lp(a) lipoprotein are a risk factor for cardiovascular disease.

High-density lipoprotein particles

Nascent high-density lipoprotein (HDL) particles are produced in both the liver and the intestine. They are disc-shaped and seemingly inert, and contain apoprotein AI. They are transmuted into mature particles by the acquisition of phospholipids, and the E and C apoproteins from chylomicrons and VLDL particles in the circulation. The more mature HDL particles take up cholesterol from cells in the peripheral tissues, aided by cholesterol-efflux regulatory protein – a product of the ATP-binding cassette transporter 1 gene (*ABC1* gene). As it is taken up, the enzyme lecithin cholesterol acyltransferase (LCAT), activated by the apoprotein A on the particle's surface, esterifies the sequestered cholesterol. The HDL particle transports cholesterol away from the periphery and may transfer it indirectly to other particles, such as VLDL, in the circulation, or deliver its cholesterol directly to the liver (reverse cholesterol transport) and steroid-synthetic tissues (ovaries, testes, adrenal cortex).

This direct delivery takes place through scavenger-receptor B1. In experimental animals, the absence of scavenger-receptor B1 dramatically accelerates the development of atheroma, and genetically programmed over-production suppresses atheroma formation.

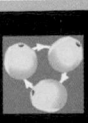

Measurement

When a laboratory measures fasting serum lipids, the majority of the total cholesterol concentration consists of LDL particles with a 20–30% contribution from HDL particles. The triglyceride concentration largely reflects the circulating number of VLDL particles, since chylomicrons are not normally present in the fasted state. If the patient is not fasted, the total triglyceride concentration will be raised, owing to the additional presence of triglyceride-rich chylomicrons.

Epidemiology

LDL and total cholesterol

Population studies have repeatedly demonstrated a strong association between both total and LDL cholesterol concentration and coronary heart risk. There is a strong link between mean fat consumption, mean serum cholesterol concentration and the prevalence of coronary heart disease between countries. The exception is France, where the cardiovascular risk is only moderate – perhaps owing to high alcohol consumption. Studies of migrants, particularly of Japanese men migrating to Hawaii, have shown that, as diet changes and cholesterol concentrations rise, so does the cardiovascular risk. Such studies demonstrate the role of the environment rather than the genetic make-up of a population.

The Multiple Risk Factor Intervention Trial (MRFIT) screened one-third of a million American men for various cardiovascular risk factors and then followed them for 6 years. Data from this study have shown that, although cardiovascular risk rises progressively as total cholesterol concentration increases ***(Fig. 28.4)***, the increase in risk is modest for individuals with no other cardiovascular risk factors. With each additional risk factor, the effect produced by the same difference in cholesterol concentration becomes greatly magnified. The Framingham Study has reproduced these findings in a separate population.

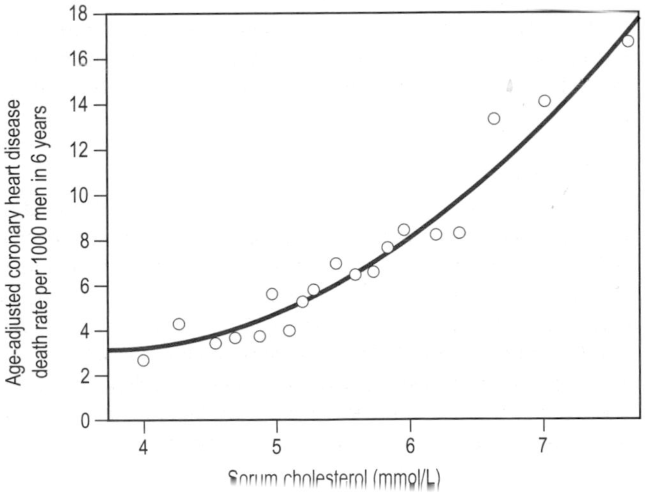

Figure 28.4 The Multiple Risk Factor Intervention Trial. Relationship between levels of serum cholesterol and risks of fatal coronary artery disease in a longitudinal study of more than 361 000 men screened for entry into the trial. *(Data from Stamler J, Wentworth D, Neaton JD. Is relationship between serum cholesterol and risk of death from coronary heart disease continuous and graded? Findings in 356 222 primary screenees of the Multiple Risk Factor Intervention Trial (MRFIT).* JAMA *1986; 256:2823.)*

HDL cholesterol

Epidemiological studies have shown that higher HDL concentrations protect against cardiovascular disease. Raising HDL by pharmacological means does not, however, necessarily reduce cardiovascular risk. HDL also has effects on the function of platelets and of the haemostatic cascade. These properties may favourably influence thrombogenesis.

VLDL particles (triglycerides)

There is a relatively weak independent link between raised concentrations of (triglyceride-rich) VLDL particles and cardiovascular risk. Very raised triglyceride concentrations (>6 mmol/L) cause a greatly increased risk of acute pancreatitis and retinal vein thrombosis. Hypertriglyceridaemia tends to occur in association with a reduced HDL concentration. Much of the cardiovascular risk associated with 'hypertriglyceridaemia' turns out, on multivariate analysis, to be due to the associated low HDL levels and not to the hypertriglyceridaemia itself.

Chylomicrons

Excess chylomicrons do not confer an excess cardiovascular risk but do raise the total plasma triglyceride concentration.

Hyperlipidaemia

Hyperlipidaemia results from genetic predisposition interacting with an individual's diet.

Secondary hyperlipidaemia

If a lipid disorder has been detected, it is vital to carry out a clinical history, examination and simple special investigations to detect the causes of secondary hyperlipidaemia ***(Box 28.1)***, which may need treatment in their own right. Hypothyroidism, diabetes, renal disease and abnormal liver function can all raise plasma lipid levels.

Primary hyperlipidaemia

The functional/genetic classification has the advantage that the genetic disorders may be grouped on the results of simple lipid biochemistry into causes of:

- disorders of VLDL and chylomicrons – hypertriglyceridaemia alone
- disorders of LDL – hypercholesterolaemia alone
- disorders of HDL
- combined hyperlipidaemia.

? Box 28.1 Causes of secondary hyperlipidaemia

- Hypothyroidism
- Diabetes mellitus (when poorly controlled)
- Obesity
- Chronic kidney disease
- Nephrotic syndrome
- Dysglobulinaemia
- Hepatic dysfunction and cholestasis
- Alcohol in susceptible individuals
- Anorexia nervosa
- Drugs:
  - Oral contraceptives in susceptible individuals
  - Retinoids, thiazide diuretics, corticosteroids, beta-blockers, sirolimus (and other immunosuppressive agents), anti-retrovirals

Box 28.2 Genetic defects underlying some lipoprotein disorders

Disorder	Affected gene	Chromosome	Frequency
Common disorders			
Heterozygous familial hypercholesterolaemia	LDL receptor	19	1:500
Familial defective apoprotein B	*Apo-B100*	2	1:700
Hypobetalipoproteinaemia	*Apo-B100*	2	1:1000
Familial combined hyperlipidaemia	As yet unknown	As yet unknown	1:200
Familial hypertriglyceridaemia	As yet unknown	As yet unknown	1:200
Some rarer disorders			
Homozygous familial hypercholesterolaemia	LDL receptor	19	1:1000000
Lipoprotein lipase deficiency	As yet unknown	8	1:1000000 (homozygous)
Apoprotein CII deficiency	*Apo-CII*	19	40 cases
Tangier disease	ATP binding cassette (*ABC1*)	9	Very rare
Lecithin cholesterol acyltransferase deficiency	*LCAT*	16	Very rare
Apoprotein A1 deficiency	*Apo-A1*	1	Very rare

Disorders of VLDL and chylomicrons – hypertriglyceridaemia alone

The majority of cases appear to be due to multiple genes acting together to produce a modest excess of circulating concentration of VLDL particles, such cases being termed polygenic hypertriglyceridaemia.

In a proportion of cases, there will be a family history of a lipid disorder or its effects (e.g. pancreatitis). Such cases are often classified as familial hypertriglyceridaemia. The defect underlying the majority of such cases is not understood. Apoprotein A5 deficiency underlies some cases. The main clinical feature is a history of attacks of pancreatitis or retinal vein thrombosis in some individuals.

Lipoprotein lipase deficiency and apoprotein CII deficiency

These are rare diseases that produce greatly elevated triglyceride concentrations owing to the persistence of chylomicrons (and not VLDL particles) in the circulation. The chylomicrons persist because the triglyceride within cannot be metabolized if the enzyme lipoprotein lipase is defective, or because the triglycerides cannot gain access to the normal enzyme owing to deficiency of the apoprotein CII on their surface. Patients present in childhood with eruptive xanthomas, lipaemia retinalis and retinal vein thrombosis, pancreatitis and hepatosplenomegaly. If disease is not identified in childhood, it can present in adults with gross hypertriglyceridaemia resistant to simple measures. The presence of chylomicrons floating like cream on top of fasting plasma suggests this diagnosis. It is confirmed by plasma electrophoresis or ultracentrifugation. An abnormality of apoprotein C can be deduced if the hypertriglyceridaemia improves temporarily after infusing fresh frozen plasma, and lipoprotein lipase deficiency is likely if it does not.

Disorders of LDL – hypercholesterolaemia alone

Heterozygous familial hypercholesterolaemia

This is an autosomal dominant monogenic disorder present in 1 in 500 of the normal population. The average primary care physician would therefore be expected to have four such patients, but because of clustering within families the prevalence varies. There is an increased prevalence in some racial groups (e.g. French Canadians, Finns, South Africans). Surprisingly, most individuals with this disorder remain undetected. Patients may have no physical signs, in which case the diagnosis is made on the presence of very high plasma cholesterol concentrations that are unresponsive to dietary modification and are associated with a typical family history of early cardiovascular disease. Diagnosis can more easily be made if typical clinical features are present. These include xanthomatous thickening of the Achilles tendons and xanthomas over the extensor tendons of the fingers. Xanthelasma may be present but is not diagnostic of familial hypercholesterolaemia.

The most common genetic defect is under-production or mal-production of the LDL cholesterol clearance receptor in the liver **(Box 28.2)**. Over 150 different mutations in the LDL receptor have been described to date. Mutations affecting the serine protease activity of PCSK9 (see p. 1278) are rarer and also cause familial hypercholesterolemia. Fifty per cent of men with the disease will die by the age of 60, most from coronary artery disease, if untreated.

Homozygous familial hypercholesterolaemia

This condition is very rare indeed. Affected children have no LDL receptors in the liver. They have a hugely elevated LDL cholesterol concentration, and massive deposition of lipid in arterial walls, aorta and skin. The natural history is for death from ischaemic heart disease in late childhood or adolescence. Repeated plasmapheresis has been used to remove LDL cholesterol with some success. Liver transplantation is a 'cure'. Plasma lipids normalize and xanthomas regress after transplantation, but the number of patients having undergone this procedure is small. Two orphan drugs are licensed for use **(Box 28.3)**.

Mutations in the apoprotein B100 gene

These cause another relatively common single-gene disorder. Since LDL particles bind to their clearance receptor in the liver through apoprotein B100, this defect also results in high LDL concentrations in the blood, and a clinical picture that closely resembles classical heterozygous familial hypercholesterolaemia. The two disorders can be distinguished clearly only by genetic tests. The approach to treatment is the same.

Polygenic hypercholesterolaemia

This is a term used to lump together patients with raised serum cholesterol concentrations, but without one of the monogenic disorders above. They exist in the right-hand tail of the normal

Box 28.3 Drugs used in the treatment of hyperlipidaemia

Drug/examples	Mechanism of action	Contraindications	Adverse effects	Expected therapeutic effect	Safety
Statins					
Simvastatin Pravastatin Fluvastatin Atorvastatin Rosuvastatin	Inhibit the rate-limiting step in cholesterol synthesis (HMG-CoA reductase)	Active liver disease, pregnancy, lactation	Constant aches/muscle stiffness, derangement of liver biochemistry, diarrhoea, myopathy Raised ciclosporin level in blood	Reduce LDL cholesterol by 30–60% Have modest lowering effect on triglycerides Have tiny effect on HDL cholesterol Atorvastatin and particularly rosuvastatin have the most potent cholesterol-lowering effects	Simvastatin, atorvastatin and pravastatin have good long-term safety in large-scale trials and in clinical practice Avoid if possible in women of childbearing age
Cholesterol absorption inhibitors					
Ezetimibe	Inhibits gut absorption of cholesterol from food and also from bile; inhibits activity of VPCILI, a lipid transporter found in liver and intestine	Lactation	Occasional diarrhoea, abdominal discomfort	Reduce LDL cholesterol by an additional 10–15% if given with a statin Reduce triglyceride concentrations by 10% Increase HDL cholesterol by 5%	Mostly act in gut and little is absorbed. Short/medium-term safety good; long-term safety seems good
Bile acid sequestrants					
Colestyramine Colestipol Colesevelam	Bind bile acids in the gut, preventing enterohepatic circulation; liver makes more bile acids from cholesterol, depleting the cholesterol pool	Biliary obstruction	Gastrointestinal side-effects predominantly (constipation, diarrhoea, bloating, flatulence); sometimes reduce vitamin absorption Palatability is a problem Other drugs bind to resins and should be taken 1 h before or 4 h afterwards	Reduce LDL cholesterol by 8–15% Have little or no effect on HDL cholesterol Increase triglyceride concentration by 5–15%	Not systemically absorbed. Safety profile is good Appear safe in women of childbearing age Fat-soluble vitamin supplements may be required in children, and pregnant and breastfeeding women
Fibric acid derivatives					
Gemfibrozil Bezafibrate Ciprofibrate Fenofibrate	Activate peroxisome proliferator-activated nuclear receptors (esp. PPAR-α), producing protean effects on lipid metabolism	Severe hepatic or renal impairment, gall bladder disease, pregnancy	Reversible myositis, nausea, predisposition to gallstones, non-specific malaise, impotence	Reduce LDL cholesterol by 10–15% and triglycerides by 25–35% Increase HDL cholesterol concentrations by 10–50% (newer agents often have greater beneficial effect on HDL)	No knowledge of effect on developing fetus. Avoid in women of childbearing age Long-term safety appears good
Nicotinic acid (NA) derivatives					
Modified-release NA (also used with laropiprant, which stops flushing) Acipimox	Unclear: probably inhibit lipid synthesis in the liver by reducing free fatty acid concentrations through an inhibitory effect on lipolysis in fat tissue	Pregnancy, breast-feeding	Value limited by frequent side-effects: headache, flushing, dizziness, nausea, malaise, itching, abnormal liver biochemistry Glucose intolerance, hyperuricaemia, dyspepsia, hyperpigmentation may occur	Reduce LDL cholesterol by 5–10% Reduce triglycerides by 15–20% Increase HDL cholesterol by 10–20%	Medium-term safety good but marred by the adverse effects listed Modified-release preparation or combination with laropiprant reduces side-effect incidence
Fatty acid compounds					
Omega-3 acid ethyl esters Omega-3 marine triglycerides	Reduce hepatic VLDL secretion	Avoid with anticoagulants since bleeding time is prolonged	Occasional nausea and belching	Reduce triglycerides in severe hypertriglyceridaemia Effect no favourable change in other lipids May aggravate hypercholesterolaemia in a few patients	Long-term safety is not yet known but seems unlikely to be poor
Microsomal triglyceride transfer protein (MTP) inhibitors					
Lomitapide	Inhibits MTP, which is necessary for VLDL assembly and secretion in the liver	Unclear		Lowers LDL cholesterol Orphan drug licensed only for homozygous familial hypercholesterolaemia	Long-term safety is not yet known
Antisense therapeutic drugs					
Mipomersen	Targets the messenger RNA for apolipoprotein B	Liver toxicity possible – monitor		Lowers LDL cholesterol Orphan drug licensed only for homozygous familial hypercholesterolaemia	Long-term safety is not yet known

HMG-CoA, hydroxymethylglutaryl coenzyme A; LDL, low-density lipoprotein; VLDL, very-low-density lipoprotein.

distribution of cholesterol concentration. The precise nature of the polygenic variation in plasma cholesterol concentration remains unknown. Variations in the apoprotein E gene (chromosome 19) and in the sterol-regulatory element-binding protein (*SREBP*)-2 gene are involved in some individuals in this heterogeneous group.

Disorders of HDL (very low HDL, low total cholesterol)

Tangier disease

This is an autosomal recessive disorder characterized by a low HDL cholesterol concentration. Cholesterol accumulates in reticulo-endothelial tissue and arteries, causing enlarged, orange-coloured tonsils and hepatosplenomegaly. Cardiovascular disease, corneal opacities and a polyneuropathy also occur. It is due to a gene mutation (*ABC1* gene; see **Box 28.2**), which normally promotes cholesterol uptake from cells by HDL particles.

Other mutations in this gene have been found in a few families with autosomal dominant HDL deficiency. It is as yet unknown whether abnormalities of this gene contribute to the low HDL cholesterol concentrations commonly seen in cardiovascular disease patients.

Combined hyperlipidaemia (hypercholesterolaemia and hypertriglyceridaemia)

The most common patient group is characterized by a polygenic combined hyperlipidaemia. Patients have an increased cardiovascular risk due to both high LDL concentrations and suppression of HDL by the hypertriglyceridaemia.

Familial combined hyperlipidaemia

This is relatively common, affecting 1 in 200 of the general population. The genetic basis for the disorder has not yet been characterized. It is diagnosed by finding raised cholesterol and triglyceride concentrations in association with a typical family history. There are no typical physical signs.

Remnant hyperlipidaemia

This is a rare (1 in 5000) cause of combined hyperlipidaemia. It is due to accumulation of LDL remnant particles and is associated with an extremely high risk of cardiovascular disease. It may be suspected in a patient with raised total cholesterol and triglyceride concentrations by finding xanthomas in the palmar creases (diagnostic) and the presence of tuberous xanthomas, typically over the knees and elbows ***(Fig. 28.5)***. Remnant hyperlipidaemia is almost always due to the inheritance of a variant of the apoprotein E allele (apoprotein E2), together with an aggravating factor such as another primary hyperlipidaemia. When suspected clinically, the diagnosis can be confirmed using ultracentrifugation of plasma or by phenotyping apoprotein E.

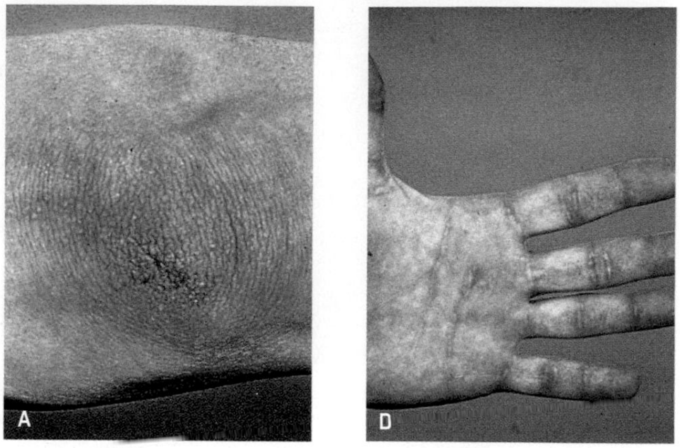

Figure 28.5 Remnant hyperlipidaemia. A. Tuberous xanthomas behind the elbow. **B.** Lipid deposits in the hand creases.

Management of hyperlipidaemia

The lipid-lowering diet

Studies have shown that dieticians helping patients to adjust their own diet to meet the nutritional targets set out below produce a better lipid-lowering effect than does the issuing of standard diet sheets and advice from a doctor. The main elements of a lipid-lowering diet are similar to those for people with diabetes (see ***Box 27.7***). Additional specific measures are to:

- reduce consumption of liver, offal and fish roes to lower dietary cholesterol
- reduce alcohol consumption, since this may worsen primary lipid disorders at doses that would not affect normal individuals
- include foods containing plant stanols in the diet.

Plant stanols reduce the absorption of cholesterol from the intestine by competing for space in the micelles that deliver lipid to the mucosal cells of the gut. They are largely unabsorbed and are excreted in the stool. Increasing the amount of plant stanol in the diet tenfold by using a margarine (e.g. Benecol) containing added stanol esters lowers LDL cholesterol by approximately 0.35–0.5 mmol/L. A reduction in the risk of heart disease of about 25% would be expected if this reduction in LDL cholesterol were applied to a population.

Exercise, weight loss and smoking

Taking regular physical exercise, losing weight and stopping smoking all reduce the level of cardiovascular risk, irrespective of lipid levels.

Drugs

The classes of drugs used to treat hyperlipidaemia are described in ***Box 28.3*** and principles of use in ***Box 28.4***. Statins are the most widely used lipid-lowering agents. Generalized muscular aches are the most common adverse effect, occasionally leading to a frank myopathy. These adverse events occur more frequently in people with a single nucleotide polymorphism (SNP) in a gene region coding for a liver specific organic anion transporter protein (*so*lute carrier organic anion transporter *IBI* – SLCOIBI), which leads to a decreased hepatic uptake of the statin and higher statin levels in the serum. New classes of lipid-lowering drugs in development are listed in ***Box 28.5***.

Screening

Most patients with hyperlipidaemia are asymptomatic and have no clinical signs. Many are discovered during the screening of high-risk individuals. Whose lipids should be measured? There are great doubts as to whether blanket screening of plasma lipids is warranted. Selective screening of people at high risk of cardiovascular disease should be undertaken in these circumstances:

- a family history of coronary heart disease (especially below 50 years of age)
- a family history of lipid disorders
- the presence of a xanthoma

Box 28.4 Drug therapy for hyperlipidaemia

Hypertriglyceridaemia (predominantly)	Combined hyperlipidaemia	Hypercholesterolaemia (predominantly)
First-line agents		
Fibric acid derivative	Fibric acid derivative	Statin: simvastatin 40 mg initially; atorvastatin 80 mg for greater cholesterol lowering (Cholesterol-binding resin instead if pregnancy possible)
Additional/alternative agents		
Fish oil capsules Nicotinic acid derivatives	Statin may be required in addition to lower cholesterol adequately (monitor carefully for muscle aches, creatine kinase rise or worsening liver function) Ezetimibe (to lower cholesterol further) Nicotinic acid derivative (to lower cholesterol and triglycerides further)	Ezetimibe if statin not tolerated or greater cholesterol lowering needed Cholesterol-binding resin Nicotinic acid derivative

Box 28.5 Classes of drugs in clinical trials for the potential treatment of hyperlipidaemia

Drug class	Mechanism of action
Cholesteryl ester transfer protein (CETP) inhibitors e.g. anacetrapib, evacetrapib	Monoclonal antibodies that inhibit the action of CETP. Increase LDL cholesterol and raise HDL cholesterol. The ACCELERATE and ACCENTUATE phase III trials may report on cardiovascular outcome in 2016, but outcome is currently not known
Proprotein convertase subtilisin/kexin type 9 (PCSK9) inhibitors e.g. alirocumab, evolocumab, bococizumab	Drugs that block PCSK9 and thus lower LDL with significant reduction in risk of coronary artery disease. Phase III clinical trials are in progress, but their effect on cardiovascular outcome is currently unknown
Squalene synthase inhibitors	Squalene synthase catalyses the branching point between sterol and non-sterol biosynthesis, and moves farnesyl pyrophosphate towards production of sterols, especially cholesterol. Inhibitors decrease cholesterol synthesis and lower triglyceride levels, but their effect on cardiovascular outcome is currently unknown

HDL, high-density lipoprotein; LDL, low-density lipoprotein.

- the presence of xanthelasma or corneal arcus before the age of 40 years
- obesity
- diabetes mellitus
- hypertension
- acute pancreatitis
- patients undergoing renal replacement therapy.

Where one family member is known to have a monogenic disorder, such as familial hypercholesterolaemia (1 in 500 of the population), siblings and children must have their plasma lipid concentrations measured. It is also worth screening the prospective partners of any patients with this heterozygous monogenic lipid disorder because of the [illegible] of producing children who are homozygous for the condition.

Acute severe illnesses, such as myocardial infarction, can derange plasma lipid concentrations for up to 3 months. Plasma lipid concentrations should be measured either within 48 hours of an acute myocardial infarction (before derangement has had time to occur) or 3 months later.

Serum cholesterol concentration does not change significantly after a meal and as a screening test a random blood sample is sufficient. If the total cholesterol concentration is raised, HDL cholesterol, triglyceride and LDL cholesterol concentrations should be quantitated on a fasting sample. If a test for hypertriglyceridaemia is needed, a fasting blood sample is mandatory.

Management of hypertriglyceridaemia

A serum triglyceride concentration below 2.0 mmol/L is normal. In the range 2.0–6.0 mmol/L, no specific intervention will be needed unless there are coincident cardiovascular risk factors, and in particular a strong family history of early cardiovascular death. In general, patients should be alerted to the fact that they have a minor lipid problem; they should be offered advice on weight reduction if obese, and on correction of other cardiovascular risk factors.

If the triglyceride concentration is above 6.0 mmol/L, there is a risk of pancreatitis and retinal vein thrombosis. Patients should be advised to reduce their weight if overweight and start a formal lipid-lowering diet (see above). A proportion of individuals with hypertriglyceridaemia have livers that respond to even moderate degrees of alcohol intake by allowing accumulation or excess production of VLDL particles. If hypertriglyceridaemia persists, lipid measurements should be repeated before and after a 3-week interval of complete abstinence from alcohol. If a considerable improvement results, life-long abstinence may prove necessary. Other drugs, including thiazides, oestrogens and glucocorticoids, can have a similar effect to alcohol in susceptible patients.

If the triglyceride concentration remains above 6.0 mmol/L, despite the above measures, drug therapy is warranted (see ***Boxes 28.3*** and ***28.4***). The severe hypertriglyceridaemia associated with the rare disorders of lipoprotein lipase deficiency and apoprotein CII deficiency may require restriction of dietary fat to 10–20% of total energy intake and the use of special preparations of medium-chain triglycerides in cooking in place of oil or fat. Medium-chain triglycerides are not absorbed via chylomicrons (see p. 1277).

Management of hypercholesterolaemia (without hypertriglyceridaemia)

Familial hypercholesterolaemia

Individuals often require treatment with dietary measures and more than one cholesterol-lowering drug. The cholesterol absorption inhibitor ezetimibe is a logical addition to a statin and has a low side-effect profile (see ***Boxes 28.3*** and ***28.4***). Bile acid sequestrants are an alternative to ezetimibe but there are problems with tolerability. Concurrent therapy with statins and fibrates, particularly fenofibrate, can be used in severe cases. Checking for muscle symptoms and measuring creatine kinase are necessary.

Primary prevention for people with risk factors

Lipid-lowering therapy with a statin, or alternatives as above, is used in asymptomatic individuals with type 2 diabetes alone, unless there are no other risk factors and the LDL cholesterol is particularly low (<1.8 mmol/L). It is also used in people with two or more of the following factors: positive family history of cardiovascular disease, albuminuria, hypertension and smoking.

Primary prevention for people without risk factors

In the absence of risk factors, lipid-lowering therapy can be used in asymptomatic men with LDL cholesterol levels persistently above 5.0 mmol/L despite dietary change. The situation for women is less clear.

Secondary prevention

As a generality, statin treatment is warranted for any patient with known macrovascular disease (coronary artery disease, transient ischaemic attack or stroke, peripheral vascular disease), irrespective of the total or LDL cholesterol level (treatment target is total cholesterol <4.0 mmol/L and LDL <2 mmol/L; alternatively, the maximum tolerated statin dose can be used). If a statin is not tolerated, combinations of other agents are tried (see ***Box 28.4***).

Risk prediction tables

An array of risk prediction tables (see p. 993) is available to allow quantification of the risk of a patient having a cardiovascular event within the next 10 years. The authors side with those who have reservations over their use. Such risk analyses are a useful approach in helping to decide whether to use treatments such as aspirin. Aspirin probably has no effect until the day an atherosclerotic plaque ruptures, when it may then prevent thrombosis leading to a heart attack or stroke. Furthermore, it has a significant associated morbidity and mortality (from bleeding). At a 10-year cardiovascular risk level of 15%, the benefit : risk ratio for aspirin becomes favourable. At the 30% level, the benefits are clear.

By contrast, the use of lipid-lowering agents, if initially tolerated, has a low associated morbidity and mortality. These agents probably reduce the rate of atheroma accumulation over decades. When a patient is young, the chance that atheroma will be bad enough to cause a heart attack or stroke within the next 10 years will be small, even if atheroma is accumulating at a swift rate. The level of cardiovascular risk will only rise when the patient gets older. It seems bizarre, however, not to treat the gradual accumulation of atheroma when the patient is young with a low 10-year risk, and then to start treatment when age causes the 10-year risk levels to rise to a particular threshold, if all other factors are the same. In choosing whether or not to prescribe, the authors prefer to consider whether the patients will live long enough to collect some pension and see their grandchildren, rather than asking whether they will have a heart attack or stroke within the next 10 years. The answers to these two questions are very different. The American Heart Association risk calculator predicts both 10-year risk and lifetime risk, and aids discussion of treatment with patients.

Management of combined hyperlipidaemia

Treatment is the same for all varieties of combined hyperlipidaemia (hypercholesterolaemia and hypertriglyceridaemia). For any given cholesterol concentration, the hypertriglyceridaemia found in the combined hyperlipidaemias increases the cardiovascular risk considerably. Treatment is aimed at reducing serum cholesterol below 4.0 mmol/L and triglycerides below 2.0 mmol/L. Therapy is with diet in the first instance and then with drugs if an adequate response has not occurred. Fibrates are the treatment of choice since these reduce both cholesterol and triglyceride concentrations, and also have the benefit of raising cardioprotective HDL concentrations. Combination with other agents is often needed (see ***Box 28.4***).

Other lipid disorders

Hypolipidaemia

Low lipid levels can be found in severe protein–energy malnutrition. They are also seen occasionally with severe malabsorption and in intestinal lymphangiectasia.

Hypobetalipoproteinaemia (see ***Box 28.2***) is a benign familial condition that is increasingly recognized. The cholesterol levels are in the range 1–3.5 mmol/L.

Abetalipoproteinaemia

This is described on page 402.

Further reading

Link E, Parish S, Armitage J et al. and SEARCH Collaborative Group. SLCO 1B1 variants and statin-induced myopathy – a genomewide study. *N Engl J Med* 2008; 359:789–799.

Mammen AL. Statin-associated autoimmune myopathy. *N Engl J Med* 2016; 374:664–669.

Robinson JG, Farnier M, Krempf M et al. Efficiency and safety of alirocumab in reducing lipids and cardiovascular events. *N Engl J Med* 2015; 72:1489–1499.

http://www.cvriskcalculator.com *American College of Cardiology/American Heart Association cardiovascular risk calculator.*

INBORN ERRORS OF CARBOHYDRATE METABOLISM

Glycogen storage disease

All mammalian cells can manufacture glycogen, but the main sites of production are the liver and muscle. Glycogen is a high-molecular-weight glucose polymer made up of 1–4 linked glucose units, with a 1–6 branch point every 4–10 residues. In glycogen storage disease (GSD), there is either an abnormality in the molecular structure or an increase in glycogen concentration owing to a specific enzyme defect. Almost all of these conditions are autosomal recessive in inheritance and present in infancy, except for McArdle's disease, which presents in adults.

Box 28.6 shows the classification and clinical features of some of these diseases. Five types – GSDI, GSDIII, GSDVI and GSD VIII involving liver, and GSDII involving skeletal muscle – make up the majority of cases.

Galactosaemia

Galactose is normally converted to glucose. However, a deficiency of the enzyme ***galactose-1-phosphate uridyl-transferase*** or, less commonly, ***uridine diphosphate galactase-4-epimerase***, results in accumulation of galactose-1-phosphate in the blood. The transferase deficiency, inherited as an autosomal recessive condition, is due in 70% of patients to a glutamine-to-arginine missense mutation in *Q188R*. Galactose ingestion (i.e. milk) leads to inanition, failure to thrive, vomiting, hepatomegaly and jaundice, diabetes, cataracts and developmental delay. A lactose-free diet stops

Box 28.6 The most common glycogen storage diseases

Type	Affected tissue	Enzyme deficiency	Clinical features	Diagnosis (DNA abnormality and tissue[a], if necessary)	Comments
Liver glycogenoses					
Ia (Von Gierke) (25%)	Liver, intestine, kidney	Glucose-6-phosphatase	Hepatomegaly, ketotic hypoglycaemia, short stature, obesity, hypotonia	Liver R83C, Q347X (Caucasian) 130X, R83C (Hispanic) R83A (Chinese) R83C (Ashkenazi Jew)	If patients survive initial hypoglycaemia, prognosis is good; allopurinol for hyperuricaemia (a late complication); corn starch
Ib	Liver	Glucose-6-phosphatase transporter	Hepatomegaly, ketotic hypoglycaemia, short stature, obesity, hypotonia	DNA testing	Granulocyte colony-stimulating factor (G-CSF)
III (Forbes–Cori) (24%)	Liver, muscle (abnormal glycogen structure)	Glycogen debranching enzyme	Like type I In adults, muscle weakness predominates	Fibroblasts, liver, muscle biopsies Amyloglucosidase (*AGL*) gene or 1p21	Good prognosis but progressive neuropathy and cardiomyopathy
VI (Hers)	Liver	Liver phosphorylase (PGYL)	Hepatomegaly with hypoglycaemia in childhood	Liver biopsy *PGYL* or 14q21	Good prognosis
VIII	Liver	Phosphorylase kinase (PBK)	Hepatomegaly, hypoglycaemic hyperlipidaemia, fatiguability, growth retardation	Liver, muscle PBK at β-subunit gene (*PHBK*) at 16q12 and Xq13, X-linked	No treatment
Muscle glycogenoses					
II (Pompe) (15%)	Liver, muscle, heart	Lysosomal acid, maltase	Respiratory muscle hypotonia, heart failure, hepatomegaly cardiomyopathy	Fibroblasts, muscles Lysosomal α-1,4 glucosidase at 17q 25.2–q25.3 200+ mutations DNA testing	α-glucosidase treatment every 2 weeks; high-protein, low-carbohydrate diet

[a]Tissue obtained is used for the biochemical assay of the enzyme. % = percentage of total number of cases in USA and Europe.

the acute toxicity, but poor growth and problems with speech and mental development still occur with the transferase deficiency. A newborn screening programme to detect galactosaemia is in place in parts of the USA and other countries.

Prenatal diagnosis and diagnosis of the carrier state are possible by measurement of red cell galactose-1-phosphate activity. DNA analysis is available for common mutations.

Galactokinase deficiency also results in galactosaemia and early cataract formation.

Defects of fructose metabolism

Absorbed fructose is chiefly metabolized in the liver to lactic acid or glucose. Three defects of metabolism in the liver and intestine occur, all of which are inherited as autosomal recessive traits:

- ***Fructosuria*** is due to fructokinase deficiency. It is a benign asymptomatic condition.
- ***Hereditary fructose intolerance*** is due to fructose-1-phosphate aldolase deficiency. Fructose-1-phosphate accumulates after fructose ingestion, inhibiting both glycogenolysis and gluconeogenesis, resulting in symptoms of severe hypoglycaemia. Hepatomegaly and renal tubular defects occur but are reversible on a fructose- and sucrose-free diet. Intelligence is normal and there is an absence of dental caries.
- ***Hereditary fructose-1,6-diphosphatase deficiency*** leads to a failure of gluconeogenesis. Infants present with hypoglycaemia, ketosis and lactic acidosis. Dietary control can lead to normal growth.

INBORN ERRORS OF AMINO ACID METABOLISM

Inborn errors of amino acid metabolism are chiefly inherited as autosomal recessive conditions. The major ones are shown in ***Box 28.7***.

Amino acid transport defects

Amino acids are filtered by the glomerulus, but 95% of the filtered load is reabsorbed in the proximal convoluted tubule by an active transport mechanism. Aminoaciduria results from:

- abnormally high plasma amino acid levels (e.g. phenylketonuria)
- any inherited disorder that damages the tubules secondarily (e.g. galactosaemia)
- tubular reabsorptive defects, either generalized (e.g. Fanconi syndrome) or specific (e.g. cystinuria).

Amino acid transport defects can be congenital or acquired.

Box 28.7 The major inborn errors of amino acid metabolism[a]

Disease	Enzyme defect	Incidence	Biochemical and clinical features	Management	Prognosis
Albinism	Tyrosinase	1 in 13 000	Amelanosis: whitish hair, pink–white skin, grey–blue eyes Nystagmus, photophobia, strabismus	Symptomatic	Good
Alkaptonuria	Homogentisic acid oxidase	1 in 100 000	Homogentisic acid polymerizes to produce a brown–black product that is deposited in cartilage and other tissues (ochronosis)	None	Good
Homocystinuria Type I	Cystathionine synthase	1 in 65 000	Homocystine is excreted in urine Learning difficulties Marfan-like syndrome Thrombotic episodes Survivors have learning difficulties	Pyridoxine supplement Diet low in methionine Folic acid supplement Trimethylglycine (betaine) supplement Cystine supplement	Before age 30, a quarter of patients die from thrombotic complications, e.g. heart attack. Treatment improves life expectancy towards normal
Type II	Methylene tetrahydrofolate reductase				
Phenylketonuria	Phenylalanine hydroxylase	1 in 20 000	Phenylpyruvate and its derivatives excreted in urine Brain damage with learning difficulties and epilepsy	Diet low in phenylalanine in first few months of life prevents damage	Good but some intellectual impairment
Histidinaemia	Histidase	Very rare	Learning difficulties	–	–
'Maple syrup' disease	Branched-chain ketoacid dehydrogenase	Very rare	Failure to thrive Fits, neonatal acidosis and severe cerebral degeneration Valine, isoleucine and their derivatives excreted in urine A milder form is seen	–	Early death
Oxalosis (hyperoxaluria)	Type 1: alanine: glyoxylate aminotransferase Type 2: glyoxylate reductase–hydroxypyruvate reductase Type 3: 4-hydroxy-2-oxoglutarate aldolase	Rare	Nephrocalcinosis, renal stones, chronic kidney disease due to deposition of calcium oxalate Prenatal and early diagnosis possible	–	Liver transplantation ?Gene therapy

[a]There are many other enzyme defects producing, for example, alaninaemia, ammonaemia, argininaemia, citrullinaemia, isovaleric acidaemia, lysinaemia, ornithinaemia or tyrosinaemia.

Generalized aminoacidurias

Fanconi syndrome

This occurs in a juvenile form (De Toni–Fanconi–Debré syndrome); in adult life, it is often acquired through, for example, heavy metal poisoning, drugs or some renal diseases. There is a generalized defective proximal tubular reabsorption of most amino acids, glucose, urate and phosphate, resulting in hypophosphataemic rickets and bicarbonate, with failure to transport hydrogen ions, causing a renal tubular acidosis that then produces a hyperchloraemic acidosis (see pp. 177–178).

Other abnormalities include potassium depletion, primary or secondary to the acidosis, polyuria, and increased excretion of immunoglobulins and other low-molecular-weight proteins.

Various combinations of the above abnormalities have been described.

The juvenile form begins at the age of 6–9 months, with failure to thrive, vomiting and thirst. The clinical features are as a result of fluid and electrolyte loss and the characteristic vitamin D-resistant rickets.

In the adult, the disease is similar to the juvenile form but osteomalacia is a major feature.

Treatment of the bone disease is with large doses of vitamin D (e.g. 1–2 mg of 1-α-hydroxycholecalciferol with regular blood calcium monitoring). Fluid and electrolyte loss needs to be corrected.

Specific aminoacidurias

Cystinuria

There is a defective tubular reabsorption and jejunal absorption of cystine and the dibasic amino acids, lysine, ornithine and arginine. Cystinuria is either a completely or an incompletely autosomal recessive disorder with mutations in two genes, *SLC3A1* and *SLC7A9*. Cystine absorption from the jejunum is impaired but, nevertheless, cystine in peptide form can be absorbed. Cystinuria leads to urinary stones and is responsible for approximately 1–2% of all urinary calculi. The disease often starts in childhood, although most cases present in adult life.

Treatment is described on pages 756–757.

The condition cystinosis must not be confused with cystinuria. Cystinosis is characterized by the accumulation of cystine in different organs, leading to organ dysfunction, e.g. photophobia and ocular problems, and chronic kidney disease. Management is with cysteamine.

Hartnup's disease

There is defective tubular reabsorption and jejunal absorption of most neutral amino acids but not their peptides. The resulting tryptophan malabsorption produces nicotinamide deficiency (see p. 199). Patients can be asymptomatic but others develop evidence of pellagra (see pp. 199–200).

Management is with nicotinamide.

Other aminoacidurias

Tryptophan malabsorption syndrome (blue diaper syndrome), familial iminoglycinuria and methionine malabsorption syndrome have all been described.

Further reading

Blau N, van Spronsen FJ, Levy HL. Phenylketonuria. *Lancet* 2010; 376:1417–1427.

Inglefinger JR. Primary hyperoxaluria. *New Engl J Med* 2013; 369:649–658.

www.hgmd.cf.ac.uk *Human gene mutation database.*

LYSOSOMAL STORAGE DISEASES

Lysosomal storage diseases are due to inborn errors of metabolism, which are mainly inherited in an autosomal recessive manner.

Glucosylceramide lipidoses: Gaucher's disease

This is the most prevalent lysosomal storage disease and is caused by a deficiency in glucocerebrosidase, a specialized lysosomal acid β-glucosidase. This results in accumulation of glucosylceramide in the lysosomes of the reticuloendothelial system, particularly the liver, bone marrow and spleen. Over 200 mutations have been characterized in the glucocerebrosidase gene (*1g21*), the most common being a single base change (N370S) that causes the substitution of arginine for serine; this is seen in 70% of Jewish patients. The typical Gaucher cell, a glucocerebroside-containing reticulo-endothelial histiocyte, is found in the bone marrow, producing many cytokines such as CD14.

There are three clinical types, the most common presenting in childhood or adult life with an insidious onset of hepatosplenomegaly (***type 1***). There is a high incidence in Ashkenazi Jews (1 in 3000 births), and patients have characteristic pigmentation on exposed parts, particularly the forehead and hands. The clinical spectrum is variable, with patients developing anaemia, evidence of hypersplenism and pathological fractures that are due to bone involvement. Nevertheless, many have a normal lifespan. The diagnosis is made on finding reduced glucocerebrosidase in leucocytes. Mutational analysis will confirm the diagnosis. Plasma chitotriosidase (an enzyme secreted by activated macrophages) is grossly elevated in Gaucher's disease and other lysosomal disorders; it is used to monitor enzyme replacement therapy.

Acute Gaucher's disease (***type 2***) presents in infancy with rapid onset of hepatosplenomegaly, and neurological involvement owing to the presence of Gaucher cells in the brain. The outlook is very poor.

Type 3 presents in childhood or adolescence with a variable progression of hepatosplenomegaly, neurodegeneration and bone disease. Again, the outlook is poor.

Management

There are currently four glucocerebrosidases available (eliglustat, imiglucerase, taliglucerase alfa and velaglucerase). These are produced by recombinant DNA technology and are given intravenously; they are typical 'orphan drugs'. They are used in people with type 1 disease, and in most with type 3 disease. This enzyme replacement treatment decreases liver and splenic size and reverses other manifestations. Glucocerebrosidase treatment costs the price of a small house per patient per year. Oral miglustat (an inhibitor of glucosylceramide synthase) prevents the production of glucocerebroside and is used for mild to moderate type 1 Gaucher's disease.

Sphingolipidoses: Niemann–Pick disease

This condition is due to a deficiency of lysosomal sphingomyelinase, which results in the accumulation of sphingomyelin cholesterol and glycosphingolipids in the reticuloendothelial macrophages of many organs, particularly the liver, spleen, bone marrow and lymph nodes. The disease usually presents within the first 6 months of life with mental retardation and hepatosplenomegaly; a particular type (11c) presents in adults with dementia. The gene frequency is 1:100 in Ashkenazi Jews, the diagnosis being made in the group by targeted mutation analysis. Typical foam cells are found in the marrow, lymph nodes, liver and spleen.

Mucolipidosis

The mucolipidoses are a group of disorders caused by the deficiency of lysosomal enzymes (e.g. α-L-iduronidase) required for the catabolism of glycosaminoglycans (mucopolysaccharides).

The catabolism of dermatan sulphate, heparan sulphate, keratin sulphate or chondroitin sulphate may be affected either singularly or together.

Accumulation of glycosaminoglycans in the lysosomes of various tissues results in the disease. Ten forms of mucopolysaccharidosis (MPS) have been described; all are chronic but progressive, and a wide spectrum of clinical severity can be seen within a single enzyme defect. The MPS types show many clinical features, though in variable amounts, with dysostosis, abnormal facies, poor vision and hearing, and joint dysmobility (either stiff or hypermobile) frequently seen. Mental retardation is present in, for example, Hurler (MPS IH) and San Filippo A (MPS IIIA) types, but normal intelligence and lifespan are seen in Scheie syndrome (MPS IS). L-aronidase infusion reduces lysosomal storage, resulting in clinical improvement.

The GM2 gangliosidoses

In these conditions, there is accumulation of GM2 gangliosides in the central nervous system and peripheral nerves. It is particularly common (1 in 2000) in Ashkenazi Jews. Tay–Sachs disease is the severest form, where there is a progressive degeneration of all cerebral function, with fits, epilepsy, dementia and blindness, and death usually occurs before 2 years of age. The macula has a characteristic cherry spot appearance.

Fabry's disease

This X-linked recessive condition involves the glycosphingolipid pathway. There is a deficiency of lysosomal hydrolase (α-galactosidase A). This enzyme is encoded by the gene on the Xq22.1 region of the X chromosome. Many mutations have been described and genetic analysis is used in the diagnosis, causing an accumulation of globotriaosylceramide with terminal α-galactosyl moieties in the lysosomes of various tissues, including the liver, kidney, blood vessels and the ganglion cells of the nervous system. The patients present with peripheral nerve involvement, gastrointestinal symptoms/abdominal pain, diarrhoea and early satiety, but eventually most have a cardiomyopathy, strokes and kidney disease in adult life. An absent or very low level of α-galactosidase A in leucocytes confirms the diagnosis. Genetic testing is available. Treatment is with agalsidase α-β infusions.

Diagnosis

Many of the sphingolipidoses can be diagnosed by demonstrating the enzyme deficiency, usually in peripheral blood leucocytes.

Prenatal diagnosis is possible in a number of the conditions by obtaining specimens of amniotic cells. Carrier states can also be identified, so that sensible genetic counselling can be given.

Further reading

Fletcher J, Wilcken B. Neonatal screening for lysosomal storage disorders. *Lancet* 2012; 379:294–295.
www.genetests.org *Information on genetic testing.*

AMYLOIDOSIS

Amyloidosis is a disorder of protein metabolism, in which there is extracellular deposition of pathological insoluble fibrillar proteins in organs and tissues. Characteristically, the amyloid protein consists of β-pleated sheets that are responsible for its insolubility and resistance to proteolysis.

Amyloidosis can be acquired or inherited. Classification is based on the nature of the precursor plasma proteins (at least 20) that form the fibrillar deposits. The process for the production of these fibrils appears to be multifactorial and differs amongst the various types of amyloid.

AL amyloidosis (immunoglobulin light chain-associated)

This is a plasma cell dyscrasia, related to multiple myeloma, in which clonal plasma cells in the bone marrow produce immunoglobulins that are amyloidogenic. This may be the outcome of destabilization of light chains owing to substitution of particular amino acids into the light chain variable region. There is a clonal dominance of amyloid light (AL) chains – either the dominant κ or γ isotype – which are excreted in the urine (Bence Jones proteins). This type of amyloid is often associated with lymphoproliferative disorders, such as myeloma, Waldenström's macroglobulinaemia or non-Hodgkin's lymphoma. It rarely occurs before the age of 40 years.

The clinical features are related to the organs involved. These include the kidneys (presenting with proteinuria and the nephrotic syndrome) and the heart (presenting with heart failure). Autonomic and sensory neuropathies are relatively common, and carpal tunnel syndrome with weakness and paraesthesia of the hands may be an early feature. Sensory neuropathy is common. There is an absence of central nervous system involvement.

On examination, hepatomegaly and, rarely, splenomegaly, cardiomyopathy, polyneuropathy and bruising may be seen. Macroglossia occurs in about 10% of cases and periorbital purpura in 15%.

Familial amyloidoses (transthyretin-associated, ATTR)

These are autosomally dominant transmitted diseases where the mutant protein forms amyloid fibrils, starting usually in middle age. The most common form is due to a mutant – transthyretin – which is a tetrameric protein with four identical subunits. It is a transport protein for thyroxine and retinol-binding protein, and is mainly synthesized in the liver. Over 80 amino acid substitutions have been described; for example, a common substitution is that of methionine for valine at position 30 (Met 30) in all racial groups, and alanine for threonine (Ala 60) in the English and Irish. These substitutions destabilize the protein, which precipitates following stimulation, and can cause disorders such as familial amyloidotic polyneuropathy (FAP), cardiomyopathy or the nephrotic syndrome. Major foci of FAP occur in Portugal, Japan and Sweden.

Other less common variants include mutations of apoprotein AI, gelsolin, fibrinogen Aα and lysozyme.

Clinically, peripheral sensorimotor and autonomic neuropathy is common, with symptoms of autonomic dysfunction, diarrhoea and weight loss. Renal disease is less prevalent than with AL amyloidosis. Macroglossia does not occur. Cardiac problems are usually those of conduction. There may be a family history of unidentified neurological disease.

Other hereditary systemic amyloidoses include various familial amyloid polyneuropathies (e.g. Portuguese, Icelandic, Dutch). There is a familial Creutzfeldt–Jakob disease. In familial Mediterranean fever, renal amyloidosis is a common serious complication.

Reactive systemic (secondary AA) amyloidoses

These are due to amyloid formed from serum amyloid A (SAA), which is an acute phase protein. It is, therefore, related to chronic inflammatory disorders and chronic infection.

Clinical features depend on the nature of the underlying disorder. Chronic inflammatory disorders include rheumatoid arthritis, inflammatory bowel disease and untreated familial Mediterranean fever. In developing countries, it is still associated with infectious diseases such as tuberculosis, bronchiectasis and osteomyelitis. AA amyloidosis often presents with chronic kidney disease, with hepatomegaly and splenomegaly. Macroglossia is not a feature and cardiac involvement is rare. The degree of renal failure correlates with the SAA level in a more favourable outcome in patients with low normal levels.

Other amyloids

Cerebral amyloidosis, Alzheimer's disease and transmissible spongiform encephalopathy

The brain is a common site of amyloid deposition, although it is not directly affected in any form of acquired systemic amyloidosis. Intracerebral and cerebrovascular amyloid deposits are seen in Alzheimer's disease. Most cases are sporadic, but hereditary forms caused by mutations have been reported. In hereditary spongiform encephalopathies, several amyloid plaques have been seen.

Amyloid deposits are frequently found in the elderly, particularly cerebral deposits of A4 protein. This is also seen in Down syndrome. Apoprotein E (involved in LDL transport; see pp. 1277–1278) interacts directly with β-A4 protein in senile plaques and neurofibrillary tangles in the brain. The gene for apoprotein E is on chromosome 19 and may be a susceptibility factor in the aetiology of Alzheimer's disease.

Local amyloidosis

Deposits of amyloid fibrils of various types can be localized to various organs or tissues (e.g. skin, heart and brain).

Dialysis-related amyloidosis

This is due to the β_2-microglobulin-producing amyloid fibrils in chronic dialysis patients (see p. 784). It frequently presents with the carpal tunnel syndrome.

Diagnosis

This is based on clinical suspicion and, if possible, on tissue histology. Amyloid in tissues appears as an amorphous, homogeneous substance that stains pink with haematoxylin and eosin, and stains red with Congo red. It also has a green fluorescence in polarized light. Tissue can be obtained from the rectum, gums or fat pad. The bone marrow may show plasma cells in amyloidosis or a lymphoproliferative disorder. A paraproteinaemia and proteinuria with light chains in the urine may also be seen in AL amyloidosis. In secondary or reactive amyloidosis, there will be an underlying disorder. Scintigraphy using ^{123}I-labelled serum amyloid P component is useful for the assessment of AL, ATTR and AA amyloidosis, but it is not widely available and is expensive.

Management

This is symptomatic or relates to the associated disorder. The nephrotic syndrome and congestive cardiac failure require the relevant therapies. Treatment of any inflammatory source or infection should be instituted. Colchicine may help familial Mediterranean fever. Eprodisate, which interferes with interactions between amyloid proteins and glycosaminoglycans, inhibits polymerization of amyloid fibroids; it slows the fall in renal function in AA amyloidosis. Chemotherapy is with melphalan plus dexamethasone in AL amyloidosis. Stem cell therapy is also used. In ATTR amyloidosis, where transthyretin is predominantly synthesized in the liver, liver transplantation (when there would be a disappearance of the mutant protein from the blood) is considered as the definitive therapy.

Further reading

Lachmann HJ. A new era in the treatment of amyloidosis? *N Engl J Med* 2013; 369:866–868.

THE PORPHYRIAS

This heterogeneous group of rare inborn errors of metabolism is caused by abnormalities of enzymes involved in the biosynthesis of haem, resulting in overproduction of the intermediate compounds called 'porphyrins' ***(Fig. 28.6)***. The porphyrias show extreme genetic heterogeneity. For example, in acute intermittent porphyria, more than 90 mutations have been identified in the porphobilinogen deaminase gene. One mutation has a high prevalence in patients in northern Sweden, suggesting a common ancestor.

Structurally, porphyrins consist of four pyrrole rings. These pyrrole rings are formed from the precursors glycine and succinyl-CoA, which are converted to δ-aminolaevulinic acid (δ-ALA) in a reaction catalysed by the enzyme δ-ALA synthase. Two molecules of δ-ALA condense to form a pyrrole ring.

Porphyrins can be divided into uroporphyrins, coproporphyrins or protoporphyrins, depending on the structure of the side-chain. They are termed type I if the structure is symmetrical, and type III

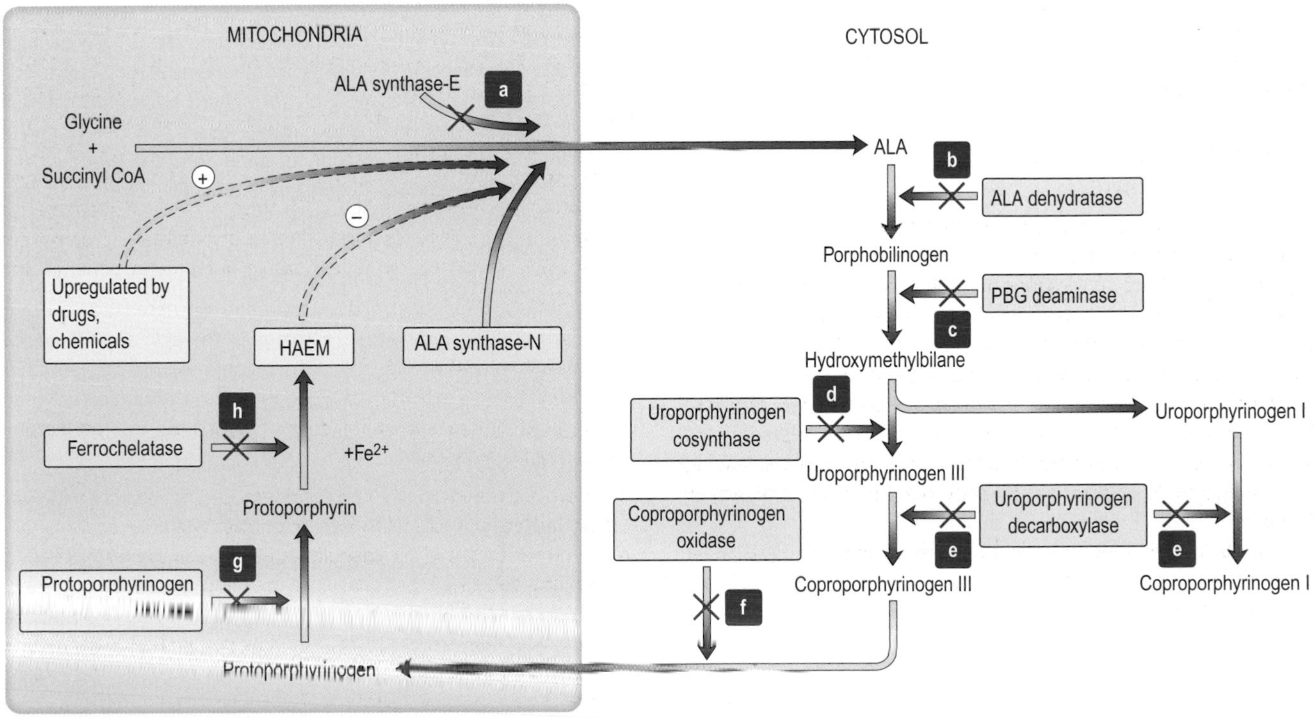

Figure 28.6 Porphyrin metabolism showing the various porphyrias. ALA synthase is the rate-limiting enzyme. Deficiencies of the other seven enzymes (crosses) cause the different porphyrias: **(a)** X-linked sideroblastic anaemia; **(b)** ALA dehydratase porphyria (ADP); **(c)** acute intermittent porphyria (AIP); **(d)** congenital erythropoietic porphyria (CEP); **(e)** porphyria cutanea tarda (PCT) and hepatoerythropoietic porphyria (HEP); **(f)** hereditary coproporphyria (HCP); **(g)** variegate porphyria (VP); **(h)** erythropoietic protoporphyria (EPP). ALA, aminolaevulinic acid; PBG, porphobilinogen.

Box 28.8 Porphyria: neurovisceral symptoms

Neuropsychiatric	Visceral
• Neuropathy	• Abdominal pain (up to 90%)
– Motor (70%)	• Vomiting (up to 90%)
– Sensory	• Constipation (up to 90%)
• Epilepsy (15%)	• Diarrhoea (occasional)
• Psychiatric disorders (50%)	• Fever (~30%)
– Depression	• Hypertension (up to 50%)
– Anxiety	• Tachycardia (up to 80%)
– Psychosis	• Muscular pain (~50%)

if it is asymmetrical. Both uroporphyrins and coproporphyrins can be excreted in the urine.

The sequence of enzymatic changes in the production of haem is shown in ***Figure 28.6***. The chief rate-limiting step is the enzyme δ-ALA synthase. This has two isoforms, ALA-N (non-erythroid) and ALA-E (erythroid). ALA-N is under negative feedback by haem but is upregulated by drugs and chemicals; there is no known inherited deficiency and the gene is on 3p21. Conversely ALA-E, encoded by Xp11.21, is unaffected by drugs or haem, and an inherited deficiency causes X-linked sideroblastic anaemia ***(Fig. 28.6)***. Consequently:

- Haem (endogenous or exogenous) produces remission of hepatic porphyria.
- Chemicals and drugs can produce disease.
- Erythropoietic porphyria gives constant symptoms and is affected by sunlight.

Clinical features

All of the haem intermediates shown in ***Figure 28.6*** are potentially toxic. Three patterns of symptoms occur in the various types of porphyria:

- neurovisceral ***(Box 28.8)***
- photosensitive
- haemolytic anaemia.

The most common types of porphyria are acute intermittent porphyria (AIP), porphyria cutanea tarda (PCT) and erythropoietic porphyria (EPP).

Neurovisceral pattern

Acute intermittent porphyria

Acute intermittent porphyria (AIP) is an autosomal dominant disorder ***(Fig. 28.6)***. Presentation is in early adult life, usually around the age of 30 years, and women are affected more than men. It may be precipitated by alcohol and by drugs such as barbiturates and oral contraceptives; these are mostly cytochrome P450-inducers but a wide range of lipid-soluble drugs has also been incriminated. Acute attacks present with neurovisceral symptoms ***(Box 28.8)***. Symptoms of the rare, autosomal recessive aminolaevulinic acid dehydrogenase porphyria (ADP) are similar.

Investigations

A rapid semi-quantitative spot urine test for porphobilinogen (PBG) is often available. The urine turns red–brown or red on standing.

- ***Blood count*** is usually normal, with occasional neutrophil leucocytosis.
- ***Liver biochemical tests*** demonstrate elevated bilirubin and aminotransferases.
- ***Serum urea*** is often raised.
- ***Urinary ALA and PBG*** are raised (24-h collection).
- ***Erythrocyte PBG deaminase*** is decreased.

Screening

Family members should be screened to detect latent cases. Urinalysis is not adequate but measurement of erythrocyte PBG deaminase and ALA synthase is extremely sensitive.

Mixed neurovisceral and photocutaneous pattern

Variegate porphyria

Variegate porphyria (VP) combines neurovisceral symptoms with those of a cutaneous photosensitive porphyria ***(Fig. 28.6)***. A bullous eruption develops on exposure to sunlight owing to the activation of porphyrins deposited in the skin.

Investigation shows an elevated urinary ALA and PBG. Fluorescence emission spectroscopy of plasma differentiates this from other cutaneous porphyrias.

Hereditary coproporphyria

Hereditary coproporphyria (HCP) is extremely rare but is broadly similar in presentation to variegate porphyria.

Photocutaneous pattern

Porphyria cutanea tarda (cutaneous hepatic porphyria)

Porphyria cutanea tarda (PCT), which has a genetic predisposition, presents with a bullous blistering eruption on exposure to sunlight; the eruption heals with scarring. Alcohol is the most common aetiological agent but smoking, oestrogens, hepatitis C, iron overload/haemochromatosis or human immunodeficiency virus (HIV) can also precipitate the disease. Evidence of biochemical or clinical liver disease may also be present. Polychlorinated hydrocarbons have been implicated and porphyria cutanea tarda has been seen in association with benign or malignant tumours of the liver.

Hepatoerythropoietic porphyria (HEP; ***Fig. 28.6***) is a rare disease that is clinically very similar to congenital erythropoietic porphyria and presents in childhood; haemolytic anaemia occurs. The defect in HEP is similar to that in PCT.

Diagnosis depends on demonstration of increased levels of plasma or urinary porphyrins. Histology of the skin shows subepidermal blisters with perivascular deposition of periodic acid–Schiff-staining material. The serum iron and transferrin saturation are often raised. Liver biopsy shows mild iron overload, as well as features of alcoholic liver disease.

Congenital erythropoietic porphyria

Congenital erythropoietic porphyria (CEP) is extremely rare and is transmitted as an autosomal recessive trait. Patients show extreme sensitivity to sunlight and develop disfiguring scars. Dystrophy of the nails, blindness due to lenticular scarring, and brownish discoloration of the teeth also occur.

Erythropoietic protoporphyria

Erythropoietic protoporphyria (EPP) is more common than congenital erythropoietic porphyria and is inherited as an autosomal dominant trait. It presents with irritation and a burning pain in the skin, non-blistering, on exposure to sunlight. The liver is usually normal but protoporphyrin deposition can occur. ***Diagnosis*** is made by fluorescence of the peripheral red blood cells and by detection of increased protoporphyrin (total and free) in the red cells and stools.

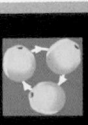

Management of porphyrias

Neurovisceral pattern

Acute episodes

The management of acute episodes is largely supportive. Precipitating factors, such as drugs, should be stopped. Analgesics should be given (avoiding drugs that may aggravate an attack). Intravenous carbohydrates, such as glucose, inhibit ALA synthase activity. Intravenous haem arginate (human haemin) infusion reduces ALA and PBG excretion by exerting a negative effect on ALA synthase-N activity ***(Fig. 28.6)*** and shortens the duration of an attack; this is useful in a severe attack. Calorie and fluid intake should be maintained.

Prevention in remission period

This is by avoidance of possible precipitating factors, such as drugs and alcohol. Smoking cessation, treatment of infections and stress avoidance are helpful. Surgery can precipitate attacks. A high-carbohydrate diet should be maintained and haemin infusions may also help.

Photocutaneous episodes

Acute episodes

Acute attacks following exposure to ultraviolet light can only be treated symptomatically. However, venesection, which reduces urinary porphyria, can be used for PCT in both acute and remission phases. Chloroquine can also aid excretion by forming a water-soluble complex with uroporphyrins. Liver transplantation is used for severe cases.

Prevention

This is with avoidance of sunlight, and use of zinc-containing sunscreens and protective clothing. Oral β-carotene, which quenches free radicals, provides effective protection against solar sensitivity in EPP.

Further reading

Puy H, Gouya L, Deybach JC. Porphyrias. *Lancet* 2010; 375:924–937.

Bibliography

Scriver CR, Beaudet AL, Sly WS et al. *The Metabolic Basis of Inherited Disease*, 9th edn. New York: McGraw-Hill; 2008.

Significant websites

http://www.porphyriafoundation.com *American Porphyria Foundation.*

http://www.sign.ac.uk *Scottish Intercollegiate Guidelines Network – guidelines on a range of subjects, including diabetes and lipid disorders.*

29 Women's health

Catherine Nelson-Piercy, Edward WS Mullins, Lesley Regan

See your e-book for clinical tips, drug tips, extra tables and MCQs.

INTRODUCTION

Women are affected by both general and gender-specific medical problems. They have predictable long-term reproductive healthcare needs and more frequent interactions with health services than men. Some 70% of women will have one or more pregnancies during their lives. In addition to complications relating to pregnancy and childbirth, and genital tract and breast cancers (see pp. 631–635), they also experience more severe forms of anaemia and osteoporosis (see pp. 711–715).

Women are also adversely affected by domestic violence and rape to a far greater extent than men. These determinants of ill-health and morbidity remain largely unrecognized alongside more general socioeconomic factors and mental health; women are more likely than men to report symptoms of common mental disorders.

THE LIFE COURSE APPROACH

A life course approach ***(Fig. 29.1)*** addresses the long-term effects of biological, social and behavioural [illegible] during gestation, childhood, adolescence and young adulthood upon health, wellbeing and disease in later life and across generations. This perspective recognizes that early life events can have an impact on long-term outcomes, and that early interventions may reduce the risk and severity of disease.

Women's reproductive and sexual health needs are largely predictable across their lifespan. The vast majority of women want to enjoy healthy sexual relationships and control their own fertility.

Sexual health education

Early sexual health education for girls provides information on:

- optimal methods of contraception to avoid unplanned pregnancy
- risks of sexually transmitted diseases
- vaccination and screening programmes to prevent adult disease.

For example, human papillomavirus (HPV) vaccination for girls aged 11–13 years and *Chlamydia trachomatis* screening for those under 25 are linked to the prevention of cervical cancer, ectopic pregnancy and tubal infertility. These encounters provide early opportunities to discuss the long-term benefits of adopting a healthier lifestyle before embarking on a first pregnancy.

Early sex education has been shown to reduce the teenage pregnancy rate. Teenage mothers have some of the worst obstetric outcomes; 90% drop out of school and 20% become pregnant again. Forty per cent of pregnancies in the UK are unplanned and opportunities to provide general preconceptual advice on diet, weight, exercise, smoking, alcohol use and folic acid intake are often missed until the young woman presents pregnant.

- The provision of contraceptive, preconception and antenatal services is poorly integrated.
- Pre-pregnancy counselling allows a review of recent medication and [illegible] management plan for the pregnancy is in place.

The UK Confidential Enquiry into maternal mortality and morbidity reported in December 2014 that three-quarters of all the women who died had coexisting medical or mental health problems identified before they became pregnant and should have been offered pre-pregnancy advice and joint specialist and maternity care (see pp. 1302–1309).

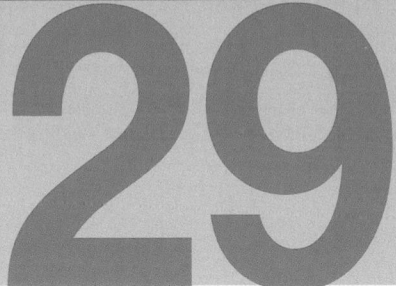

CHANGES IN PREGNANCY

Haematology
↑ Plasma volume (by 50%)
↓ Haemoglobin
↓ Platelets
↑ Fibrinogen (by 50%)
↑ Clotting factors VIII, IX, X
Venous stasis (L >R)

Respiratory
↑ Oxygen consumption (by 20%)
↑ Minute ventilation (by 40–50%)
↑ pO_2
↓ pCO_2
↓ FVC (3rd trimester)

Cardiac
↑ Cardiac output (by 40%)
↑ Stroke volume
↑ Heart rate (by 10–20 bpm)
↓ Blood pressure (↓ in 1st and 2nd trimesters)
↓ Systemic vascular resistance (by 25–30%)
↓ Serum colloid osmotic pressure (by 10–15%)

Renal
↑ Renal plasma flow (by 60–80%)
↑ Glomerular filtration rate (by 55%)
↑ Protein excretion (up to 300 mg / 24 hours)
↓ Serum creatinine (max = 75 μmol/l)
Glycosuria
Physiological hydronephrosis (R>L)

Gastroenterology
↓ Motility
↑ Alkaline phosphatase
↓ Albumin (by 20–40%)

Endocrine
Impaired glucose tolerance
Insulin resistance
↑ Prolactin (10 fold)
↑ Cortisol
↑ Renin, angiotensin, aldosterone

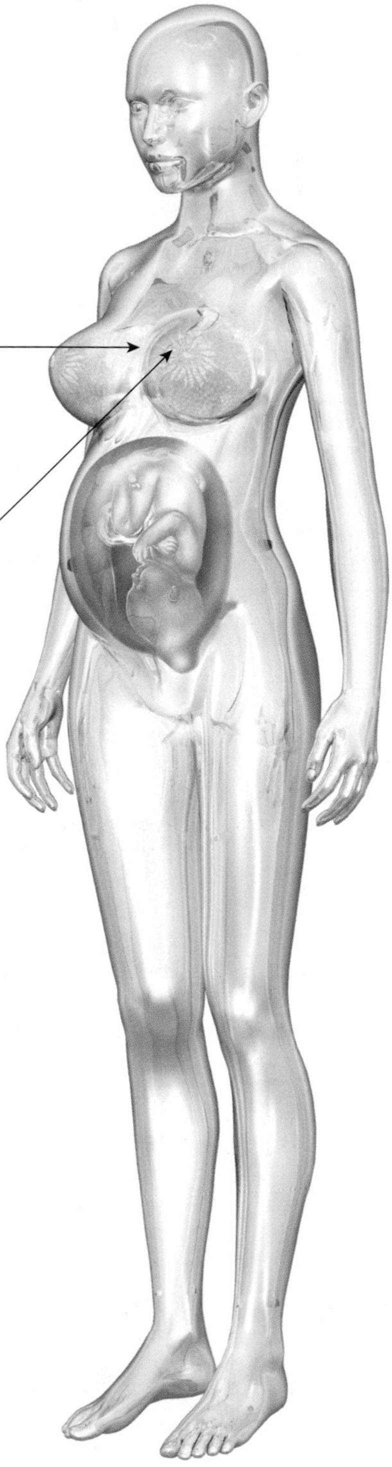

General
Fatigue
Weight gain
Nausea/Vomiting
Constipation
Breathlessness
Palpitations
Ankle oedema

Skin
Palmar erythema
Dry skin
Telangiectasia
Pruritus (in 20%)

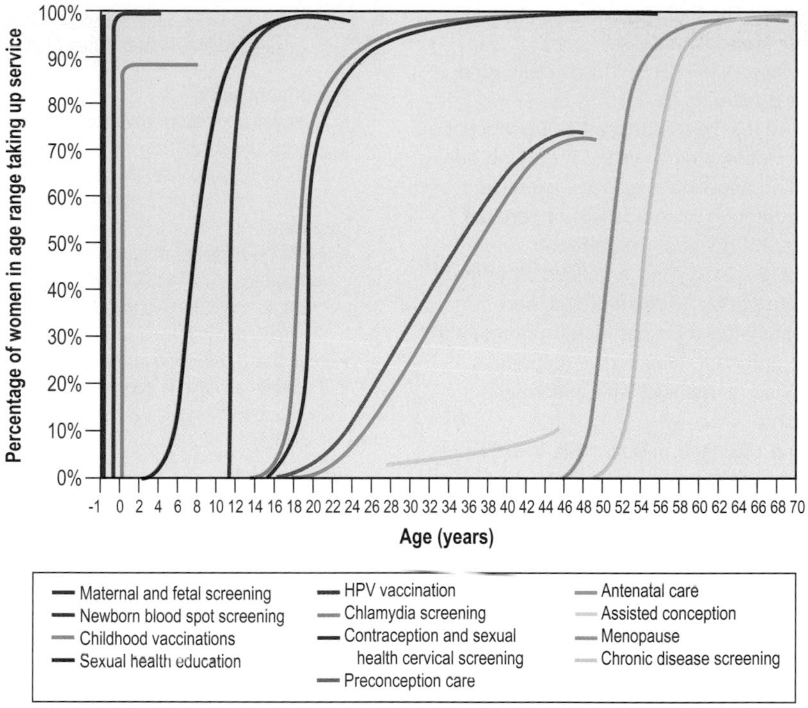

Figure 29.1 The life course approach: major health issues specifically affecting women as they age. HPV, human papillomavirus. *(After Royal College of Obstetricians and Gynaecologists.* SEC Opinion Paper 27; *August 2011.)*

The physiological response to pregnancy

The mother's physiological response to her pregnancy reveals information about risks of disease in later life. For example:

- Pre-eclampsia and gestational diabetes resolve after delivery but are associated with higher cardiovascular mortality in later life.
- Roughly 50% of women with gestational diabetes will develop type 2 diabetes within 10 years and children born of diabetic pregnancies are more likely to develop diabetes.
- Teenage pregnancies and premature deliveries repeat across generations.
- Mental health problems during pregnancy and the puerperium are associated with low birth weight and impaired intellectual development, as measured by lower IQ at age 3 years.

Pregnancy should be viewed as the Health Care Opportunity of Two Lifetimes (HOOTL, ***Fig. 29.2***), which offers major potential for population health gain and is the first step on the way to tackling and interrupting the cross-generational transmission of ill-health.

The postnatal visit

The postnatal visit is an ideal time to plan future healthcare needs for mother and baby, and can have a positive impact on lifestyle issues such as obesity, exercise, dental health, contraception, smoking and drug misuse. Review of the recent pregnancy will provide valuable predictions about future problems and their long-term prevention.

Nearly 20% of women in the UK now choose to remain childless. A smaller, but growing, number of women are pursuing assisted conception to overcome their age-related decline in fertility. These are at increased risk of serious complications during pregnancy due to medical co-morbidities.

The normal menstrual cycle

Definitions, including some disorders

- ***Puberty*** (see p. 1214). The mean age of menarche is 12.8 years but it may take several years for the menstrual cycle

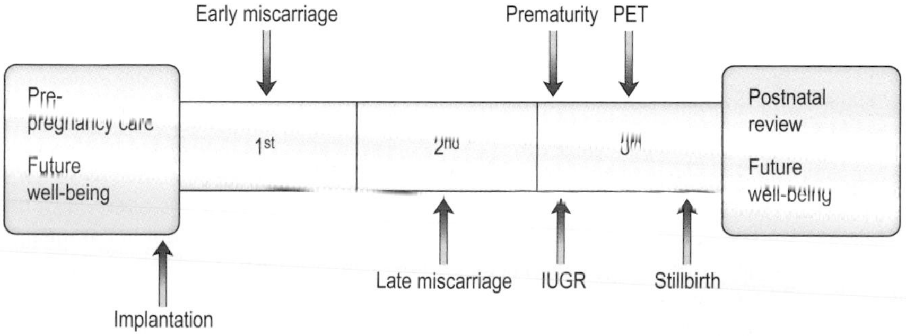

Figure 29.2 The Healthcare Opportunity of Two Lifetimes – HOOTL. IUGR, intrauterine growth retardation; PET, pre-eclampsia.

to establish a regular pattern. The initial cycles are usually anovulatory and frequently unpredictable.

- ***Precocious puberty*** (see pp. 1214–1215). This is defined as menses before the age of 8 years.
- ***Delayed puberty*** (see p. 1215). This is defined as the absence of secondary sex characteristics after 14 years. It may be due to a central defect (including anorexia, excessive exercise, chronic illness or pituitary tumour) or to a failure of gonadal function (Turner syndrome, XX gonadal dysgenesis).
- ***Amenorrhoea*** (see pp. 1218–1219). This is defined as primary in a girl who fails to menstruate by 16 years of age, and secondary when the menses stop for more than 6 months in a normal female who is not pregnant, lactating or menopausal.
- ***Menorrhagia***. This is defined as menses with abnormally heavy or prolonged bleeding.
- ***Premenstrual syndrome*** (PMS) (see p. 002). This is extremely common. In 5–15%, the severity of the progesterone-induced bloating, weight gain, mastalgia, headaches, depression and irritability in the luteal phase are so debilitating that lifestyle and personal relationships are adversely affected. Treatment success, using lifestyle modifications, hormonal preparations, cognitive behavioural therapy, selective serotonin reuptake inhibitors (SSRIs) and surgery, is highly variable.
- ***Premature ovarian insufficiency*** (POI) (see p. 1220). This is defined as cessation of periods before 40 years of age and occurs in 1% of women.
- ***Menopause***. The average age of menopause among Western women is 51–52 years (see below).
- ***Postmenopausal bleeding*** (PMB). The majority of cases of PMB are due to benign atrophic vaginitis and respond to topical oestrogens. Approximately 10% of cases of PMB will have atypical hyperplasia or cancer requiring staging and surgical clearance of the uterus and ovaries, with or without adjuvant therapy. Investigate by ultrasound to assess endometrial thickness, proceeding to tissue sampling when it exceeds 3–5 mm. Women on tamoxifen medication for breast disease may have irregular, thickened and cystic endometrium, and require hysteroscopy and directed tissue biopsy.

Menopause

The menopause, or cessation of periods, naturally occurs at about the age of 45–55 years. Female life expectancy has increased significantly over the last century, with many women now living into their eighties or nineties. During the late forties, follicle stimulating hormone (FSH) concentrations initially and then luteinizing hormone (LH) concentrations begin to rise, probably as follicle supply diminishes. Oestrogen levels fall and the cycle becomes disrupted. Most women notice irregular, scanty periods coming on over a variable period, though, in some, sudden amenorrhoea or menorrhagia occurs. Eventually, the menopausal pattern of low oestradiol levels with grossly elevated LH and FSH levels (usually >50 and >25 U/L, respectively) is established. Premature menopause may also occur surgically, with radiotherapy to the ovaries and with ovarian disease.

Clinical features

Features of oestrogen deficiency are hot flushes (which occur in most women and can be disabling), vaginal dryness and atrophy of the breasts. There may also be symptoms of loss of libido, loss of self-esteem, non-specific aches and pains, sleep disturbance, irritability, depression, loss of concentration and weight gain.

Box 29.1 Risks and benefits of hormone replacement therapy[a]

Potential benefits

- ***Symptomatic improvement in most menopausal symptoms*** for the majority of women. Oestrogen-deficient symptoms respond well to oestrogen replacement; the vaguer general symptoms may or may not improve. Vaginal symptoms also respond to local oestrogen preparations.
- ***Protection against fractures of wrist, spine and hip, secondary to osteoporosis*** (~24–33%) (see pp. 711–715), owing to protection of predominantly trabecular bone (see p. 707). However, this is not a recommended indication to prevent osteoporosis.
- ***Significant reduction in the risk of large bowel cancer*** (~33%).
- ***Possible increase in general wellbeing***, although hopes for a reduction in the incidence of Alzheimer's disease have not been confirmed.

Potential risks

- ***Significant increase in the risk of breast cancer*** (+26%) but no change in breast cancer mortality. This is primarily a risk of combined oestrogen–progesterone HRT. Some studies suggest that breast cancers diagnosed on HRT are easier to treat effectively.
- ***Significant increase in the risk of endometrial cancer*** when unopposed oestrogens are given to women with a uterus.
- ***Significant increase in the risk of ischaemic heart disease*** (+29%) and stroke (+41%).
- ***Inconvenience of withdrawal bleeds***, unless a hysterectomy has been performed or regimens used that include continuous oestrogen and progesterone.

[a]Percentages are from the Women's Health Initiative (WHI) study of 16 600 women.

Women show a rapid loss of bone density in the 10 years following the menopause (osteoporosis; see pp. 711–715) and the premenopausal protection from ischaemic heart disease disappears.

Management

Hormone replacement therapy

Symptomatic patients should usually be treated but the previous widespread use of hormone replacement therapy (HRT) has been thrown into doubt by a number of large prospective studies that have reported in recent years. Although scientific debate continues, the overall benefits and risks are summarized in ***Box 29.1***. Absolute risks and benefits for individual women clearly depend on their background risk of a specific disease, and there is as yet no evidence on the relative risks of different hormone preparations or routes of administration (oral, transdermal or implant). Overall, the Women's Health Initiative (WHI) study estimated that, over 5 years of treatment, one extra woman in every 100 would develop an illness that would not have occurred had she not been taking HRT. However, the decision about whether or not a woman takes HRT is now very much an individual one and is based on:

- the severity of the woman's menopausal symptoms
- her personal risk of conditions that may be prevented or made more likely by HRT
- individual patient choice.

HRT is not recommended purely for prevention of postmenopausal osteoporosis in the absence of menopausal symptoms.

Symptomatic treatment is the main indication, with the lowest effective dose being given for short-term rather than long-term treatment.

Selective oestrogen receptor modulators (SERMs; e.g. raloxifene) offer a potentially attractive combination of positive oestrogen effects on bone and cardiovascular system with no effects on oestrogen receptors of uterus and breast, and a possible reduction in breast cancer incidence; long-term outcome studies, however, are still awaited.

The Women's Health Initiative and Million Women Study suggested an association between longer-term usage of HRT and an increased risk of breast cancer, stroke and venous thromboembolism, but this has recently been challenged. The incidence of ischaemic heart disease increases after the menopause but this is 10 years later than in men. There is increasing evidence of the value of HRT in menopausal women to prevent cardiovascular morbidity.

Further reading

Beral V. Million Women Study Collaborators. Breast cancer and hormone-replacement therapy in the Million Women Study. *Lancet* 2003; 362:419–427.

Chlebowski RT, Schwartz AG, Wakelee H et al. Oestrogen plus progestin and lung cancer in postmenopausal women (Women's Health Initiative trial): a post-hoc analysis of a randomised controlled trial. *Lancet* 2009; 374:1243–1251.

Manson JE, Chlebowski RT, Stefanick ML et al. Menopausal hormone therapy and health outcomes during the intervention and extended poststopping phases of the Women's Health Initiative randomized trials. *JAMA* 2013; 310:1353–1368.

National Institute for Health and Care Excellence. *NICE Clinical Guideline NG23: Menopause: diagnosis and treatment*. NICE 2015; https://www.nice.org.uk/guidance/ng23.

Palmert MR, Dunkel L. Delayed puberty. *N Engl J Med* 2012; 336:443–453.

Royal College of Obstetricians and Gynaecologists. *Why Should we Consider a Life Course Approach to Women's Health Care?* Scientific Impact Paper No. 27. London: RCOG; 2011.

Contraception

Control of fertility has positive effects on a woman's health and wellbeing. Those who lack access to contraceptive methods are at increased risk of mortality and morbidity, due to obstetric complications and the consequences of illegal abortion. More than 30% of maternal deaths and 10% of child mortality can be prevented by ensuring a 2-year interval between each pregnancy.

Women require expert advice about the safest and most suitable methods of contraception available to them at different ages. In general, contraception is extremely safe, although some methods do have rare but serious side-effects. The combined oestrogen–progestogen pill also protects against both ovarian and endometrial cancer, and many hormonal methods help control heavy or painful periods. Barrier methods prevent sexually transmitted infections and protect against cervical cancer.

The efficacy of any contraceptive method depends on how it works and how easy it is to use. There is a wide choice of contraception options now available. They include barrier methods (condoms, diaphragms), the combined oestrogen–progestogen or progestogen-only pill, long-acting progestogen injection or implant, and intrauterine systems. Each has its advantages and disadvantages.

Oral contraception

The combined oestrogen–progestogen pill is widely used for contraception and has a low failure rate (<1 per 100 woman-years). 'Pills' contain 20–40 μg of oestrogen, usually ethinylestradiol, together with a variable amount of one of several progestogens. The mechanism of action is twofold:

- suppression by oestrogen of gonadotrophins, thus preventing follicular development, ovulation and luteinization
- progestogen effects on cervical mucus, making it hostile to sperm, and on tubal motility and the endometrium.

Side-effects of these preparations are shown in ***Box 29.2***. Most of the serious ones are rare and are less common with typical modern 20–30 μg oestrogen pills, although evidence suggests that

Box 29.2 Adverse effects and drug interactions of oral contraceptives (mixed oestrogen–progesterone combinations)

General
- Weight gain
- Loss of libido
- Pigmentation (chloasma)
- Breast tenderness
- Increased growth rate of some malignancies

Cardiovascular
- Increased blood pressure[a]
- Deep vein thrombosis[a]
- Myocardial infarction
- Stroke (migraine is a risk factor)

Gastrointestinal
- Nausea and vomiting
- Abnormal liver biochemistry
- Gallstones increased
- Hepatic tumours

Nervous system
- Headache
- Migraine[a]
- Depression[a]

Malignancy
- Increase in cancer of the breast (but reduced risk of ovarian and endometrial cancer)

Gynaecological
- Amenorrhoea
- 'Spotting'
- Cervical erosion

Haematological
- Increased clotting tendency

Endocrine/metabolic
- Mild impairment of glucose tolerance
- Worsened lipid profile, though variable

Drug interactions[b]
- Antibiotics
- Barbiturates
- Phenytoin
- Carbamazepine
- Rifampicin
- St John's wort

[a]Common reasons for stopping oral contraceptives. [b]Reduced contraceptive effect owing to enzyme induction.

thromboembolism may be slightly more common with 'third-generation pills' containing desogestrel and gestodene (approximately 30/100 000 woman-years compared with 15/100 000 on older pills and 5/100 000 on no treatment). While some problems require immediate cessation of the pill, other milder side-effects must be judged against the hazards of pregnancy occurring with inadequate contraception, especially if other effective methods are not practicable or acceptable.

Hazards of the combined pill are increased in smokers, in obesity and in those with other risk factors for cardiovascular disease (e.g. hypertension, hyperlipidaemia, diabetes), especially in women aged over 35 years (avoid if over 50 years). The 'mini-pill' (progestogen-only, usually norethisterone) is less effective but is often suitable where oestrogens are contraindicated (***Box 29.2***).

Long-acting reversible contraceptives

Long-acting reversible contraceptive (LARC) methods, such as implants, injectables and intrauterine devices, all have lower failure rates than user-dependent contraception and tend to have better continuation rates since they cannot be easily abandoned. They have also been shown to be more cost-effective than oral contraceptives.

Barrier methods

Condoms, diaphragms, spermicides and sponges, which require users to remember to employ them correctly every time they have sexual intercourse, have the highest failure rates but offer protection against sexually transmitted infections.

Combined oral contraceptive pills, patches and vaginal rings

These prevent ovulation, make the endometrium hostile to implantation and alter the cervical mucous. They are highly effective but only if used correctly and consistently. Minor side-effects may lead to discontinuation and include headaches, mood swings, bloating, weight gain and breast tenderness. The more significant risks relate to cardiovascular disease, including venous thromboembolism (three- to fivefold increase), myocardial infarction and stroke (rare). Progestogen-only preparations avoid the side-effects of oestrogen and are available as a pill, subdermal implant (Implanon), injectables (Depoprovera) and intrauterine system (Mirena). They all act on cervical mucous and the endometrium, but the higher-dose preparations also inhibit ovulation. Common side-effects include irregular bleeding, simple ovarian cysts, breast tenderness and acne.

- ***Pills*** are taken every day and have a higher failure rate but are suitable for women who are breast-feeding, are older, are smokers and have cardiovascular risks (hypertension, diabetes).
- ***Injectables*** are given intramuscularly and are effective for 12 weeks. Side-effects include weight gain, irregular periods or amenorrhoea, and delays in return of fertility of up to 6 months.
- ***Subdermal implants*** are inserted in the upper arm with local anaesthetic and last for 3 years. They are a highly effective long-term method of contraception and offer a rapid return of fertility after removal. Irregular bleeding is common.

Intrauterine contraceptive devices

Intrauterine contraceptive devices (IUDs) are a highly effective and increasingly popular method of contraception that is independent of intercourse and user compliance. The device is inserted into the uterine cavity by trained healthcare personnel and a thread is left protruding from the cervix into the vagina, which allows the IUD to be removed by traction.

Copper IUDs are cheap, licensed for 10 years of use, and cause much less menstrual disruption than the older plastic models. They have a toxic effect on both egg and sperm before fertilization occurs.

Mirena is a levonorgestrel hormone-releasing intrauterine system and is licensed for contraception, the treatment of heavy menstrual bleeding and use as part of HRT regimens. The duration of use is 5 years, during which time many women become amenorrhoeic. Irregular vaginal spotting is common initially but may resolve. Some women complain of greasier skin, breast tenderness and mood swings but these symptoms often settle with time.

Emergency contraception

Emergency contraception can be used following unprotected intercourse. Levonorgestrol is available over the counter and needs to be taken within 72 hours. Ulipristal acetate can be used up to 120 hours after intercourse but is available on prescription only. Insertion of a copper IUD within 5 days is highly effective. Permanent contraception may be achieved by male or female sterilization, but both carry a late failure rate quoted as 1:2000 and 1:200, respectively.

MISCARRIAGE

Miscarriage is a pregnancy that ends spontaneously before the fetus reaches a viable gestational age. The term includes all pregnancy losses between the time of conception and 24 weeks of gestation. Sporadic miscarriage is the most common complication of pregnancy and the majority are due to random genetic abnormalities in the embryo or fetus. The incidence of clinically recognized miscarriage is generally quoted as 15–20%, but the total number of very early conceptions that are lost is in the region of 50%. The miscarriage rate decreases with advancing gestation, reaching 10% by 8 weeks and 3% after a heartbeat is seen on ultrasound scan. By 13 weeks (the start of the second trimester), no more than 1% of viable pregnancies are lost.

Box 29.3 Practical classification of miscarriage

Type of miscarriage	Ultrasound findings	Clinical presentation
Biochemical pregnancy	Uterine cavity empty	PV bleeding 'late period' after positive pregnancy test
Threatened miscarriage	Intrauterine pregnancy	PV bleeding and pain Speculum: cervical os closed
Inevitable miscarriage	Intrauterine pregnancy	PV bleeding and pain Speculum: cervical os open
Incomplete miscarriage	Retained products of conception in cavity	PV bleeding and pain Speculum: cervical os open ± products in cervical os
Complete miscarriage	Uterine cavity empty, no retained products	Pain and PV bleeding resolved Speculum: cervical os closed
Missed miscarriage	Fetal pole present, no heartbeat present	± PV bleeding and pain
Blighted ovum 'anembryonic' pregnancy	Empty gestation sac (>20 mm) no fetal pole	± PV bleeding and pain

PV, *per vaginam*.

Maternal age at conception and previous reproductive history are strong and independent risk factors for miscarriage. The risk of fetal loss rises steeply after the age of 35 years, reaching 75% by 45 years, as the increase in poor-quality oocytes leads to chromosomally abnormal conceptions. Delayed childbearing has resulted in increased rates of miscarriage, ectopic pregnancy, stillbirth and other later complications of pregnancy. Less common factors contributing to early pregnancy loss are uterine abnormalities, infections, medical/endocrine disorders and exposure to drugs and chemicals.

The different types of miscarriage can be classified by the clinical presentation and the results of investigations ***(Box 29.3)***. Vaginal bleeding in early pregnancy is common and the differential diagnosis includes a threatened, inevitable or incomplete miscarriage, bleeding from a viable pregnancy, ectopic pregnancy, lower genital tract pathology or trophoblastic disease. Sensitive home pregnancy testing kits have identified many biochemical pregnancies that fail to implant successfully and resolve spontaneously as a delayed and/or heavy menstrual period.

Women presenting with vaginal bleeding in pregnancy need to have a detailed clinical history and examination performed.

- Speculum examination assesses the state of the cervix and excludes lower genital tract pathology such as cervical polyps or ectropion.
- Transvaginal ultrasound determines the location, gestation, nature and viability of the pregnancy. It also offers the woman valuable reassurance if fetal heart activity can be shown.

Bleeding and pain associated with products of conception distending the cervical canal can be very severe and prompt removal with sponge forceps should be performed. Serial measurements of serum beta-human chorionic gonadotrophin (β-HCG) levels may be necessary when the site of pregnancy is unknown.

Severe pain localized to either iliac fossa and peritonism are suggestive of ectopic pregnancy and may warrant urgent laparoscopic assessment and treatment. However, many ectopic gestations resolve spontaneously by being resorbed or miscarried from the tube into the peritoneal cavity.

Management

This depends on clinical presentation and patient choice. Most miscarriages can be managed expectantly, although urgent surgical evacuation may be required if the bleeding becomes heavy.

- ***Follow-up urinary pregnancy test or pelvic scan*** confirms whether the miscarriage is complete.
- ***Prostaglandins*** (oral or vaginal misoprostol) to induce uterine contractions and expulsion are cheap and effective.
- ***Subsequent surgical evacuation of the uterus*** is required by a small number of women.

The success rate of medical management is increased by using a progesterone antagonist (mifepristone) prior to administering the misoprostol. Surgical evacuation of the retained products of conception (ERPC) can be performed by suction under general anaesthesia or by manual vacuum aspiration (MVA) under local anaesthesia. It is associated with a small but finite morbidity, including uterine perforation, cervical trauma, intrauterine adhesion formation and postoperative pelvic infection.

Recurrent miscarriage

Recurrent miscarriage (RM), the loss of three or more consecutive pregnancies, affects 1–2% of women trying to conceive and is associated with significant psychological morbidity. Investigation includes a search for parental translocations and for anatomical, infective, endocrine, immune and thrombophilic causes. Most cases remain unexplained, which is a good prognosis for future pregnancy outcome.

Currently, the most treatable cause of RM is the antiphospholipid syndrome (see p. 695), which is present in 15–20% of all women with RM. When it is managed with low-dose aspirin and heparin, a live birth rate of more than 75% can be achieved.

Women with a history of recurrent miscarriage are at greater risk of pre-eclampsia, fetal growth restriction and prematurity when they achieve a successful pregnancy because all of these problems are determined by the quality and depth of early implantation. They are also more likely to suffer strokes at an earlier age than women with no miscarriage history.

Miscarriages can cause acute anxiety, depression, denial, anger, blame, severed relationships and a sense of loss and inadequacy. Compassionate counselling services and access to support groups for women who have experienced pregnancy loss are needed.

Stillbirths

Miscarriage and stillbirth are pregnancy losses defined on when the loss occurs. This varies from 20 to 28 weeks. WHO bases this on fetal weight of 1000 g or more, an assumed equivalent of 28 weeks' gestation. Worldwide, there were 2.6 million [illegible] stillbirths in 2015. Although there was a reduction in maternal and child mortality, both targeted in the Millennium Development Goals (MDGs), the number of stillbirths annually remains high with sadly little reduction in the past decade. Intrapartum losses are extremely high, at 1.3 million, and are preventable.

Further reading

Lancet Series 1, 2, 3. Ending preventable stillbirths. *Lancet* 2016; 387:374, 387 and 604.

HEAVY MENSTRUAL BLEEDING

Heavy menstrual bleeding (HMB) accounts for 1 in 5 gynaecology clinic consultations and is the most common cause of iron deficiency anaemia. Objective methods to quantify menstrual blood loss are inaccurate and therefore clinical assessment based on the woman's perception of blood loss and how it impacts on her quality of life is needed. Periods characterized by the passage of large blood clots, severe pain or flooding that prevents the woman leaving home require investigation and management.

Take a detailed menstrual and general medical history. On examination, search for signs of anaemia. Abdominal and pelvic examination is carried out to exclude pelvic masses, visualize the cervix, perform a smear if needed, and take swabs if infection is suspected. Investigations are as follows:

- ***full blood count*** – to assess the need for iron replacement and, in extreme cases, blood transfusion
- ***history*** consistent with a coagulation disorder – refer for a haematological opinion
- ***ultrasound scan*** – if a pelvic mass is palpated or the bleeding pattern suggests endometrial pathology
- ***endometrial biopsy*** (at the outpatient clinic or at hysteroscopy in women aged > 45 years) – for irregular or intermenstrual bleeding and where drug therapy fails
- ***ultrasound and haematological investigation*** – young women presenting with menorrhagia from their first period.

Selecting the most appropriate treatment for HMB involves patient preference, risk/benefit analysis of available options, the woman's fertility and contraceptive requirements, and any contraindications to medical or surgical therapies. A summary of the National Institute for Health and Care Excellence (NICE) guidelines for HMB is shown in ***Figure 29.3***.

Management

First-line medical therapies

These include:

- ***Tranexamic acid***. This antifibrinolytic agent is associated with a 50% reduction in HMB *and/or*
- ***Mefenamic acid***. This non-steroidal anti-inflammatory drug (NSAID) is associated with a 25% reduction in bleeding and is taken during the menses.
- ***The combined oral contraceptive pill***. This has the added advantage of providing effective contraception but may be contraindicated in women with risk factors for thromboembolism or breast cancer, smokers over the age of 35 and obese women.
- ***Oral progestogens***. Taken on days 6–26 of the menstrual cycle, these may regulate the bleeding pattern, but are not contraceptive and can cause breakthrough bleeding.
- ***Levonorgestrel intrauterine system*** (LNG-IUS or Mirena coil). This has revolutionized the treatment of HMB. It results in a 95% reduction in blood loss (30% of women are amenorrhoeic within 1 year of insertion), is an effective contraceptive, [illegible] dysmenorrhoea and has few side-effects. It should be considered in the majority of women with HMB [illegible] alternative to surgical treatment. Some women are troubled by irregular bleeding and persistent spotting for the first 3–9 months after insertion.

Gonadotrophin-releasing hormone (GnRH) agonist drugs act on the pituitary and result in amenorrhoea. They are only suitable for short-term use because they produce a hypo-oestrogenic state that predisposes to osteoporosis.

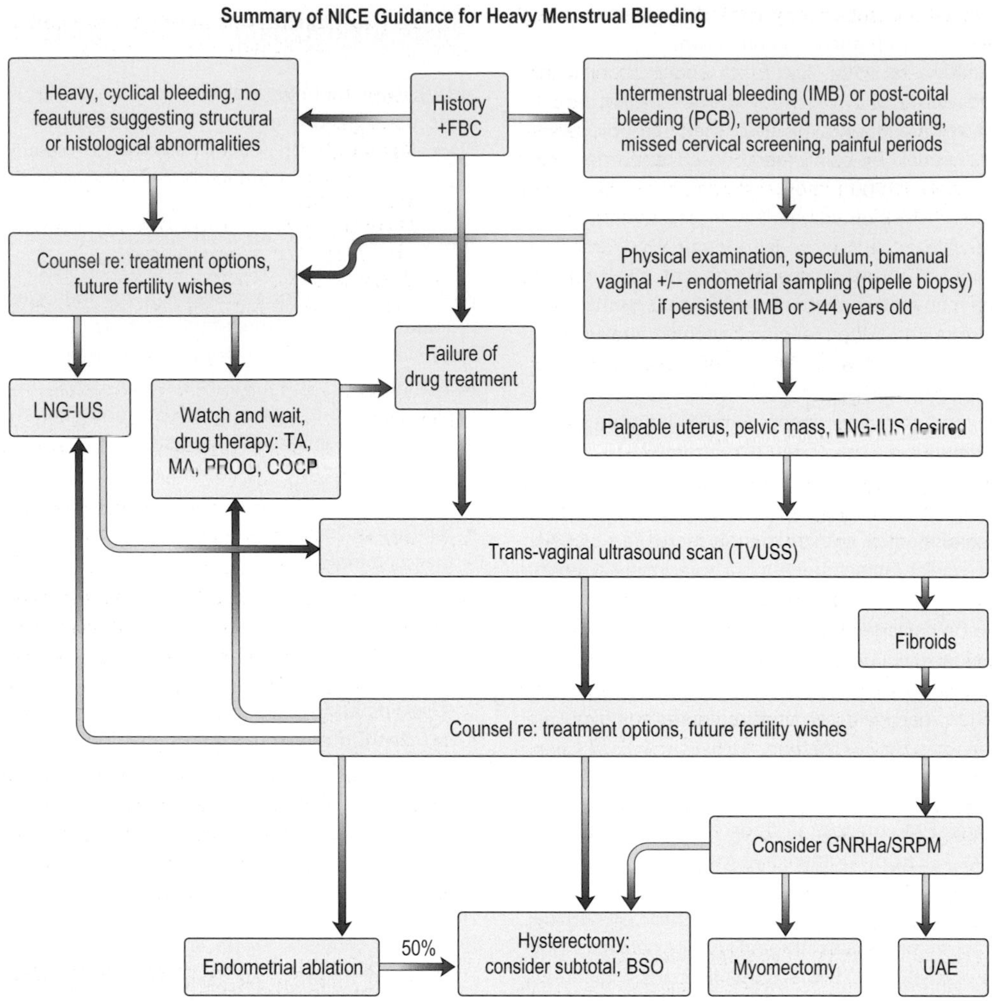

Figure 29.3 **A summary of NICE 2007 guidance for heavy menstrual bleeding.** BSO, bilateral salpingo-oophorectomy; COCP, combined oral contraceptive pill or patch; FBC, full blood count; GNRHa, gonadotrophin releasing hormone analogue; LNG-IUS, levonorgestrel intrauterine system; MA, mefenamic acid; PROG, progesterone-only pill or injection; SPRM, selective progesterone receptor modulator; TA, tranexamic acid; UAE, uterine artery embolization.

Surgical treatments

Surgical treatments for HMB should be restricted to women for whom medical treatments have failed and who have completed their family.

- ***Endometrial ablation techniques***. These destroy the endometrial lining to a depth that prevents cyclical regeneration. The second-generation microwave and thermal ablation techniques are highly successful in treating HMB and are undertaken as day-case procedures.
- ***Hysterectomy***. Removal of the uterus may be abdominal, vaginal or laparoscopic, depending on the size of the uterine body, the degree of laxity of the pelvic muscular floor and the skill set of the surgeon. Histology of the uterus is normal in about 40% of cases. The vaginal and laparoscopic surgical procedures usually mean shorter hospital stays and a faster return to normal activities.

Uterine fibroids (leiomyomata)

These are the most common solid pelvic tumours in women of reproductive age. The prevalence increases with age and is higher in Afro-Caribbean women. Heavy and/or prolonged periods, pressure symptoms due to the pelvic mass, and reproductive dysfunction are common presenting symptoms. The mechanism(s) by which fibroids cause HMB are poorly understood but submucosal lesions within the uterine cavity are particularly troublesome.

Management

Treatment is surgical excision or uterine artery embolization, both of which may adversely affect fertility. GnRH agonists or selective progesterone receptor modulators (SPRM) can be used to alleviate HMB as a short-term measure or to shrink the overall size and vascularity of the fibroids prior to surgery.

ABORTION/TERMINATION OF PREGNANCY

Unintended pregnancy is common and abortion is one of the most frequently performed gynaecological procedures. One in three women will have an abortion in their lifetime. However, abortion remains a controversial subject, mostly related to cultural, moral and religious beliefs.

Every year, an estimated 210 million pregnancies occur worldwide: 80 million are unplanned and 50 million are terminated by abortion, 20 million of them illegally. Where abortion for unintended pregnancy is illegal, it is invariably unsafe and frequently has tragic sequelae. Approximately 70 000 maternal deaths occur each year due to unsafe abortion, 99% of them in developing countries.

In developed countries that have legalized abortion, the procedure is extremely safe. The risk of death from an early surgical termination of pregnancy is less than 1 per 100 000, which is far lower than the maternal mortality associated with a full-term pregnancy. Abortion was legalized in the UK in 1967 and 95% of the 190 000 procedures performed yearly are for Clause C of the Abortion Act. This states that the pregnancy has not exceeded its 24th week and that continuance of the pregnancy would involve risk, greater than if the pregnancy were terminated, of injury to the physical or mental health of the pregnant woman. Only 1% of abortions are done because of a risk that the child would be born handicapped.

Induced abortion can be undertaken surgically under local or general anaesthesia or using drug regimens that induce miscarriage. The type of procedure is generally dictated by the gestation of the pregnancy, availability of methods and the wishes of the woman concerned. The earlier an abortion is performed, the safer it is. Currently, 91% of abortions in the UK are carried out before 13 weeks' gestation.

Early medical abortion (before 9 weeks' gestation) using the antiprogestogen drug mifepristone, followed 36–48 hours later by vaginal misoprostol to expel the products, achieves a complete abortion in over 95% of cases. Asthma and cardiac disease are contraindications to medical abortion. Most women remain in the clinical facility for 4–6 hours after the misoprostol insertion to abort the pregnancy, but some units support women to remain at home during an early medical abortion.

Surgical abortions before 14 weeks are usually performed as suction terminations under general anaesthesia. Preoperative priming of the cervix with oral or vaginal misoprostol reduces the risk of cervical trauma and haemorrhage. Early abortions before 7 weeks can be performed with a manual vacuation aspiration (MVA) syringe under local anaesthesia.

With modern early abortion techniques and routine screening for pelvic infection in high-risk women, the risk of future subfertility is extremely low. Later medical and surgical abortions are associated with more complications: in particular, incomplete procedures, pelvic infection and trauma to the genital tract. Contraception should be discussed before the abortion and started immediately after the procedure to avoid a further unplanned pregnancy.

Many women are emotionally vulnerable following an abortion. Feelings of guilt and regret are frequently mixed with relief that the ordeal is over. There is no evidence of an increase in serious psychiatric disease after abortion. Psychological problems can be minimized with careful counselling before the procedure and access to post-abortion support services.

URINARY INCONTINENCE

Urinary incontinence (UI; see also p. 793) is common and has a negative impact on a woman's quality of life. One in three women over the age of 60 years suffers from some urinary leakage and the majority are too embarrassed to seek help for their problem, despite

Box 29.4 Classification of urinary incontinence (UI) in women

- ***Stress UI*** is involuntary urine leakage on effort or exertion or on sneezing or coughing
- ***Urgency UI*** is involuntary urine leakage accompanied or immediately preceded by urgency (a sudden compelling desire to urinate that is difficult to delay)
- ***Mixed UI*** is involuntary urine leakage associated with both urgency and exertion, effort, sneezing or coughing
- ***Overactive bladder*** (***OAB***) is defined as urgency that occurs with or without urgency UI, and usually with frequency and nocturia

the fact that the symptoms can often be alleviated by simple, non-pharmacological interventions. As our ageing population continues to expand, UI will become an even more prevalent problem, placing an increasingly large demand on our healthcare resources.

The NICE guidelines offer a simple classification of female UI (summarized in ***Box 29.4***; see also p. 793).

Lifestyle interventions, including weight loss, smoking cessation, caffeine reduction and timed fluid restriction, can alleviate the symptoms of UI significantly. Physiotherapy and bladder retraining may be helpful in cases of stress and urgency, respectively, and also for mixed UI. In postmenopausal women, oestrogen deficiency exaggerates many urinary symptoms and topical vaginal or systemic HRT is a treatment option.

Referral for specialist management may include detailed assessment of the pelvic floor and any prolapse, urinary tract imaging and urodynamic evaluation where appropriate. Discussion of further management is based on the type of incontinence, the woman's preferences and future fertility wishes.

DOMESTIC ABUSE AND VIOLENCE

Domestic violence is the cause of considerable hidden morbidity and mortality. One in four women in England and Wales experience some form of domestic abuse or violence – whether it be psychological, physical, sexual, financial or emotional – during their lifetime. One in ten women experience rape. Domestic violence accounts for one-third of violent crimes, and the cost of domestic violence in human and economic terms is enormous – an estimated £23 billion per annum in the UK alone.

There are several groups of people who are more vulnerable to becoming victims. Around 30% of domestic abuse begins or escalates during pregnancy. After road accidents, domestic abuse is the second leading cause of trauma during pregnancy, and pregnant women are more likely to have multiple sites of injury. The prevalence among women requesting a termination of pregnancy is six times higher than among women attending antenatal clinics. The disabled are also at greater risk of abuse: the odds of being a victim of violence are twofold higher in people with a physical disability and threefold higher for those with a mental illness. Sex workers, trafficked women and certain ethnic groups also have a higher prevalence of domestic violence.

Victims of domestic abuse are significantly more likely to commit suicide. Domestic violence and abuse are serious health concerns and healthcare professionals are particularly well placed to identify abuse and intervene, as the victims frequently present to departments of Emergency Medicine, Psychiatry, and Obstetrics and Gynaecology. Healthcare professionals have an important role to play in tackling the problem and are often the first and only point

Protection – delivering an effective criminal justice system:
Investigation; prosecution; victim support and protection; perpetrator programmes

Provision – helping women and girls to continue with their lives:
Effective provision of services, advice and support; emergency and acute services; refuges and safe accommodation

Prevention – changing attitudes and preventing violence:
Awareness-raising campaigns; safeguarding and educating children and young people; early identification/intervention and training

Figure 29.4 **Key actions to reduce violence against women and girls.** *(After NICE 2014.)*

of contact to whom the isolated and vulnerable victim reaches out. All healthcare workers need to be trained to recognize the signs of violence and abuse, use targeted questioning, and know how to act and refer to ensure the women's safety. The key actions to reduce violence against women and girls are shown in ***Figure 29.4***.

Further reading

Faculty of Sexual and Reproductive Healthcare, Royal College of Obstetricians and Gynaecologists. *The UK Medical Eligibility Criteria for Contraceptive Use.* London: RCOG; 2009; http://www.fsrh.org.

Knight M, Kenyon S, Brocklehurst P et al (eds). Maternal, Newborn and Infant Clinical Outcome Review Programme 2014. *Saving Lives, Improving Mothers' Care: Lessons Learned to Inform Future Maternity Care from the UK and Ireland Confidential Enquiries into Maternal Deaths and Morbidity 2009–2012.* Oxford: MBRRACE-UK/ National Perinatal Epidemiology Unit; 2014.

National Institute for Health and Care Excellence. *NICE Clinical Guideline 171: Urinary Incontinence: The Management of Urinary Incontinence in Women.* NICE 2013; http://www.nice.org.uk/guidance/cg171.

National Institute for Health and Care Excellence. *NICE Public Health Guidance 50: Domestic Violence and Abuse: How Health Services, Social Care and the Organisations they Work with can Respond Effectively.* NICE 2014; http://www.nice.org.uk/guidance/ph50.

National Institute for Health and Care Excellence and British Medical Association Board of Science. *Domestic Abuse – Updated BMA Policy Report.* London: BMA; 2014.

Royal College of Obstetricians and Gynaecologists. *The Care of Women Requesting Induced Abortion.* Evidence-based Clinical Guideline no. 7. London: RCOG; 2011.

Royal College of Obstetricians and Gynaecologists. *The Investigation and Treatment of Couples with Recurrent First-trimester and Second-trimester Miscarriage.* Green-top guideline no. 17. London: RCOG; 2011.

Royal College of Obstetricians and Gynaecologists. *National Heavy Menstrual Bleeding Audit: Final Report.* London: RCOG; 2014.

MEDICAL PROBLEMS IN PREGNANCY

The prevalence of medical conditions complicating pregnancy is increasing, partly because:

- Women in Western countries are delaying childbearing until they are older.
- Fifty per cent of pregnant women are now overweight or obese, resulting in more women with diabetes, hypertension and associated co-morbidities.
- Women with chronic medical diseases, such as congenital heart disease, diabetes, chronic kidney disease (CKD) and cystic fibrosis, now survive into their child-bearing years because of better medical care.
- Widening access to assisted conception services, including the use of donor eggs, mean that age is no longer a barrier to pregnancy.
- Maternal death (during or soon after pregnancy) in the UK is now more often due to medical than obstetric complications. Confidential enquiries show that inadequate knowledge and care are implicated in one-quarter of deaths from medical conditions in pregnancy.

The anatomical and physiological changes that occur as an adaptation to normal pregnancy can result in a number of symptoms and signs. These overlap with those associated with diseases outside pregnancy. Most of the symptoms and signs are benign, but clinicians need to be aware of those that warrant further investigation and may be associated with disease.

Women with pre-existing disease should be made aware of the normal adaptation to pregnancy, as symptoms may worsen or improve, depending on the body system involved. The stress of pregnancy may also result in previously subclinical disease presenting for the first time.

Infectious diseases are a major problem in pregnancy, particularly in low- and middle-income countries. There is an increased mortality in both the mother and the fetus. See individual diseases in Chapter 11.

Hypertensive disorders

During normal pregnancy, there is a reduction in blood pressure due to a fall in systemic vascular resistance that is maximal by weeks 22–24.

Chronic/pre-existing hypertension

This is present at the initial booking visit or before 20 weeks, or the patient is already taking medication for hypertension.

Management

- ***Angiotensin-converting enzyme (ACE) inhibitors, angiotensin II receptor blockers (ARBs) and chlorothiazide agents*** that are associated with congenital abnormalities should be **discontinued**.
- ***Dietary salt intake*** should be kept low (2 g or 100 mmol daily).
- ***Aspirin 75 mg*** should be given from 12 weeks until birth to women at moderate or high risk of pre-eclampsia.
- ***Oral labetalol*** is first-line therapy during pregnancy. Second-line agents are ***methyldopa*** and ***nifedipine***. Treatment may be required for several weeks postpartum.
- ***Target blood pressure*** is <150 mmHg systolic and 80–85 mmHg diastolic. If blood pressure is <160/110 mmHg, birth should not be offered before 37 weeks.

In **breast-feeding**, ACE inhibitors, beta-blockers and nifedipine are safe. Methyldopa should be avoided because of the risk of depression.

Gestational hypertension

This is defined as blood pressure of >140/90 mmHg after 20 weeks' gestation in a previously normotensive woman.

Investigations and management

- ***Blood tests*** should include full blood count, urea and electrolytes with serum creatinine, calcium, liver biochemistry and liver function tests. Estimated glomerular filtration rate (eGFR) is not validated for use in pregnancy.
- ***Blood pressure measurements*** once a week.
- ***Urine tests*** for protein, as there is an increased risk of pre-eclampsia developing.

- ***Treatment of moderate hypertension*** (159–150/109–100 mmHg) with oral labetalol.
- ***Admission to hospital*** if blood pressure is ≥160/110 mmHg. Treatment may be required for several weeks post-partum.

Pre-eclampsia

Pre-eclampsia is a common direct (obstetric) cause of maternal and perinatal death, and a significant cause of maternal and neonatal morbidity. The risk factors are shown in ***Box 29.5***. It is a heterogeneous multisystem endothelial disorder that has widespread effects.

There is some evidence that low dose aspirin is beneficial in patients with mid to high risk of developing pre-eclampsia; it is safe in pregnancy and is stopped 10 days before delivery.

Clinical features

Pre-eclampsia varies in severity, timing, progression and order of onset of different clinical features. Symptoms include severe headache, visual blurring or flashing, nausea and vomiting, severe epigastric or right upper quadrant pain, and rapidly progressive oedema of the hands, feet and face. Signs include new hypertension >20 weeks, oedema and proteinuria (>0.3 g/24 h or urinary protein : creatinine ratio >30 mg/mmol on a 'spot' sample); these are the most common manifestations of pre-eclampsia. Hyper-reflexia may be seen. Pre-eclampsia (including eclampsia) may present ante-, intra- or postpartum. Postpartum disease is more likely to be associated with symptoms. Complications and crises are shown in ***Box 29.6***.

Investigations

- ***Full blood count*** – thrombocytopenia.
- ***Urea, electrolytes, creatinine*** – to monitor for acute kidney injury.
- ***Liver biochemistry*** – raised transferases.
- ***Urine protein : creatinine ratio.***
- ***Ultrasound fetus*** – for fetal growth.
- sFlt-1/PlGF ratio is a novel immunoassay recommended by NICE to rule out pre-eclampsia, following clinical assessment.

Box 29.5 Risk factors for pre-eclampsia

- Age >40 years
- Obesity: body mass index (BMI) >30
- Family history
- Primiparity
- Multiple pregnancy
- Previous pre-eclampsia
- Long birth interval
- Hydrops with a large placenta
- Hydatidiform mole
- Triploidy (particular association with pre-eclampsia of very early onset (before 24 weeks' gestation))
- Medical disorders:
  - Pre-existing hypertension
  - Renal disease (even without renal impairment)
  - Diabetes mellitus (pre-existing or gestational)
  - Antiphospholipid syndrome
  - Autoimmune rheumatic diseases
  - Sickle cell disease

Box 29.6 Complications and crises seen in pre-eclampsia

- Eclampsia
- HELLP syndrome (haemolysis, elevated liver enzymes, low platelets)
- Pulmonary oedema
- Placental abruption
- Cerebral haemorrhage
- Cortical blindness
- Disseminated intravascular coagulation
- Acute kidney injury
- Hepatic rupture
- Transient left ventricular systolic or diastolic dysfunction

Management

Patients should be admitted and treated for hypertension with regular blood pressure measurements (4 times/day) and blood tests (2–3/week).

Close fetal monitoring is required because of the risks of placental insufficiency and intrauterine growth restriction.

Delivery is the only cure for pre-eclampsia and this may be indicated for fetal or maternal reasons. The recurrence risk of pre-eclampsia is increased with early-onset disease.

Women whose pregnancy has been complicated by pre-eclampsia are significantly more likely to develop hypertension, ischaemic heart disease, cerebrovascular disease and CKD in later life.

If a patient develops eclampsia (convulsions or coma) and/or HELLP syndrome, she should be admitted to a critical care or high-dependency unit and may require intravenous hydralazine, labetalol and magnesium sulphate 4 g over 5 minutes then maintenance 1 g/h (for convulsions), and prompt delivery. Patients should be given steroids (betamethasone 12 mg i.m. for fetal lung maturation, repeated at 24 h if delivery is likely within 7 days). **HELLP** is a syndrome describing ***h***aemolysis, ***e***levated ***l***iver enzymes and ***l***ow ***p***latelets ($<100 \times 10^9$/L) in a pregnant woman. It is a form of severe pre-eclampsia, more common in multiparous women, and can occur in the second and third trimesters or postpartum. The haemolysis is due to a microangiopathic haemolytic anaemia (see p. 548). Hypertension and proteinuria may be absent or mild. Clinically, patients complain of epigastric/right upper quadrant pain, nausea, vomiting and jaundice (5%). If symptoms are severe, prompt delivery is necessary and is advised in all patients who are beyond 34 weeks' gestation.

Further reading

Bartsch E, Medcalf KE, Park AL et al. Clinical risk factors for pre-eclampsia determined in early pregnancy: systemic review and meta analysis of large cohort studies. *BMJ* 2016; 353:i1753.

National Institute for Health and Care Excellence. *NICE Clinical Guideline 107: Hypertension in Pregnancy: The Management of Hypertensive Disorders During Pregnancy*. NICE 2010; http://www.nice.org.uk/guidance/CG107.

Liver disease

Liver function is not impaired in pregnancy. Any liver disease (see p. 437), from whatever cause, can occur incidentally and coincide with pregnancy. For example, viral hepatitis accounts for 40% of all cases of jaundice during pregnancy. Pregnancy does not necessarily exacerbate established liver disease, but it is uncommon for women with advanced liver disease to conceive.

The following effects are seen:

- Plasma and blood volumes increase during pregnancy but the hepatic blood flow remains constant.
- The proportion of cardiac output delivered to the liver therefore falls from 35% to 29% in late pregnancy; drug metabolism can thus be affected.
- The size of the liver remains constant.
- Liver biochemistry remains unchanged, apart from a rise in serum alkaline phosphatase from the placenta (up to three to four times increased) and a decrease in total protein owing to increased plasma volume.
- Triglycerides and cholesterol levels rise, and caeruloplasmin, transferrin, α_1-antitrypsin and fibrinogen levels are elevated owing to increased hepatic synthesis.

- During pregnancy and particularly postpartum, there is a tendency to hypercoagulability, and acute Budd–Chiari syndrome (see p. 482) can occur.

There are a number of liver diseases that complicate pregnancy.

Hyperemesis gravidarum

Pathological vomiting during pregnancy can be associated with liver dysfunction and jaundice. Liver dysfunction resolves when vomiting subsides.

Intrahepatic cholestasis of pregnancy

This condition of unknown aetiology usually presents with pruritus alone in the third trimester. It has a familial tendency and there is a higher prevalence in Scandinavia, Chile and Bolivia.

Investigations

Liver biochemistry shows raised aminotransferases, which occasionally can be very high. The hallmark is raised bile acids but serum bilirubin and gamma-glutamyl transferase (γ-GT) may be slightly raised. Jaundice is rare. Liver biopsy is not indicated but would show centrilobular cholestasis.

Management

Treatment is symptomatic with ursodeoxycholic acid 1–2 g daily in divided doses. **Prognosis** is usually excellent for the mother but there is increased fetal loss. The condition resolves after delivery. Recurrent cholestasis may occur during subsequent pregnancies or with the ingestion of oestrogen-containing oral contraceptive pills.

Acute fatty liver of pregnancy

Acute fatty liver of pregnancy (AFLP) is a rare but serious condition occurring in the third trimester and affecting 1 in 6000–20 000 pregnancies. It is more common in women with multiple gestations. Patients present with abdominal pain, vomiting and jaundice. Polyuria and thirst due to diabetes insipidus may occur because of reduced breakdown of placentally derived vasopressinase. In fulminant AFLP patients, haematemesis, encephalopathy, coagulopathy, hypoglycaemia, lactic acidosis and acute kidney injury can occur. It may be associated with features of pre-eclampsia.

Investigations

- Full blood count
- Urea, electroytes, serum creatinine
- Serum glucose ↓
- Serum uric acid ↑
- Liver biochemistry shows hepatocellular damage (raised serum aminotransferase and raised bilirubin).
- Thrombocytopenia and rarely disseminated intravascular coagulation (DIC)
- ***Liver biopsy*** is rarely performed; it shows fine droplets of fat (microvesicular) in the hepatocytes with a little necrosis but is not necessary for diagnosis.

Management

Treatment is as for acute liver failure (see p. 463). Immediate delivery may save both the baby and the mother. Early diagnosis and treatment have reduced the mortality to less than 20%.

Cardiac disease

Cardiac disease, both congenital and acquired, is commonly encountered in pregnancy and is mostly benign. Many women experience palpitations and breathlessness due to awareness of physiological sinus tachycardia, ventricular premature/ectopic beats and increased minute ventilation.

Cardiac disease, predominantly acquired, is the most common cause of maternal death in the UK. The main conditions causing severe morbidity and mortality are myocardial infarction, aortic dissection, and peripartum cardiomyopathy.

- ***Myocardial infarction*** in pregnancy is more often due to coronary artery dissection or thrombus than in non-pregnant women. Intervention with primary angioplasty and coronary artery stenting is appropriate.
- ***Peripartum cardiomyopathy*** is defined as the development of heart failure with left ventricular ejection fraction <45% at the end of pregnancy or in the months following delivery, where no other cause of heart failure is found. It is a dilated cardiomyopathy (see p. 1040) and is more common in obese and multiparous women. It should be treated with conventional heart failure therapy (including thromboprophylaxis), except that ACE inhibitors and ARBs are withheld until after delivery. Nearly half of these patients will recover to normal within 6 months.
- ***Pulmonary hypertension*** (see pp. 1029–1030) and fixed pulmonary vascular resistance are dangerous and often (10–20%) fatal in pregnancy.

Box 29.7 Counselling against pregnancy where risk to the mother from cardiac conditions is high

- Pulmonary arterial hypertension
- Systemic ventricular dysfunction – left ventricular ejection fraction <30% (New York Heart Association (NYHA) class III/IV; see p. 984)
- Previous peripartum cardiomyopathy (PPCM) with any residual left ventricular impairment
- Severe mitral stenosis
- Severe symptomatic aortic stenosis
- Aortic root >4.5 cm in Marfan syndrome
- Ascending aorta >5 cm with bicuspid aortic valve
- Severe aortic coarctation

Other contraindications to pregnancy are shown in ***Box 29.7*** and include a dilated aortic root >4.5 cm, severe left heart obstruction from critical mitral or aortic stenosis, and severe impairment of left ventricular function.

Women with significant heart disease need multidisciplinary care in a specialist centre by obstetricians, cardiologists and anaesthetists who have expertise in the care of heart disease in pregnancy. Agreed management plans should be documented.

If **pregnancy is contraindicated**, then appropriate contraceptive advice is essential. The levels of risk associated with pregnancy for individual conditions are summarized in ***Box 29.8***, based on the European Society of Cardiology Guidelines.

Pregnancy and prosthetic heart valves

See page 1017.

Any strategy for anticoagulation for a pregnant woman with a mechanical heart valve is associated with risks to the mother and/or fetus. ***Pre-pregnancy counselling***, explaining that warfarin is the safest option for the mother but associated with a 5% risk of warfarin embryopathy and increased risks of miscarriage, stillbirth and fetal intracranial haemorrhage, is essential. The alternative is full anticoagulant doses of low-molecular-weight heparin, given twice daily and titrated upwards in pregnancy based on ***regular monitoring of anti-factor Xa*** levels.

Box 29.8 Pregnancy-associated risks of different cardiac diseases

Low risk

- Uncomplicated small or mild PS, PDA, MVP
- Successfully repaired ASD, VSD, PDA
- Atrial and ventricular ectopic beats

Small increased risk of mortality/moderate increased risk of morbidity

- Unrepaired ASD, VSD
- Repaired tetralogy of Fallot
- Most arrythmias

Moderate increased risk of mortality or severe morbidity

- Mild LV dysfunction, HCM
- Repaired coarctation
- Most native or tissue valve disease (except those in extremely high risk)

Significant increased risk of mortality or severe morbidity

- Mechanical valves
- Systemic RV
- Fontan circulation
- Unrepaired cyanotic congenital heart disease

Extremely high risk of mortality or severe morbidity

- Pulmonary arterial hypertension
- Severe LV impairment (<30%), NYHA III/IV
- Previous PPCM with any residual LV impairment
- Severe MS/symptomatic AS
- Severe aortic coarctation

AS, aortic stenosis; ASD, atrial septal defect; HCM, hypertrophic cardiomyopathy; LV, left ventricular; MS, mitral stenosis; MVP, mitral valve prolapse; NYHA, New York Heart Association; PDA, patent ductus arteriosus; PPCM, peripartum cardiomyopathy; PS, pulmonary stenosis; RV, right ventricle; VSD, ventricular septal defect.

Further reading

Regitz-Zagrosek V, Blomstrom Lundqvist C, Borghi C et al. ESC guidelines on the management of cardiovascular diseases during pregnancy: the Task Force on the Management of Cardiovascular Diseases during Pregnancy of the European Society of Cardiology (ESC). *Eur Heart J* 2011; 32:3147–3197.

Thromboembolic disease

Pulmonary embolism is the most common direct cause of death in pregnancy and the puerperium. Pregnancy and especially the puerperium are associated with a sixfold increased risk of thrombosis. Although the risks are highest after emergency caesarean section, women with risk factors ***(Box 29.9)*** are at risk antenatally, especially if admitted to hospital, and after vaginal delivery.

Diagnosis

Objective diagnosis of deep vein thrombosis (DVT) and pulmonary embolism (PE) must be made in those with a suggestive history and risk factors. ***D-dimers*** are not useful in pregnancy, as the levels are often raised. DVT is much more common in the left leg (ratio 9:1) than the right in pregnancy because the gravid uterus compresses the left common iliac vein, which lies under the right common iliac artery. ***Ventilation/perfusion ($\dot{V}/\dot{Q}$) scans*** and computed tomography ***pulmonary angiograms*** (***CTPAs***) are associated with negligible radiation to the fetus and are safe, but $\dot{V}/\dot{Q}$ scans are preferred, as they do not irradiate the maternal breast and increase the risk of breast cancer.

Management

Treatment of venous thromboembolism (VTE) in pregnancy involves the following:

- Larger doses of low-molecular-weight heparins (LMWHs), e.g. enoxaparin, are given.
- Warfarin and new oral anticoagulants are avoided.

Box 29.9 Risk factors for venous thromboembolism in pregnancy

- Previous VTE
- Thrombophilia
- Active medical disease, e.g. inflammatory bowel disease, systemic lupus erythematosus, pyelonephritis, nephrotic syndrome
- Age >35 years
- Obesity (body mass index (BMI) >30 kg/m^2) either pre-pregnancy or in early pregnancy
- Parity ≥3 (a woman becomes 'para 3' after her third delivery)
- Smoking
- Gross varicose veins (symptomatic or above the knee or with associated phlebitis, oedema/skin changes)
- Dehydration, hyperemesis gravidarum, ovarian hyperstimulation syndrome
- Paraplegia, immobility
- Multiple pregnancy
- Current pre-eclampsia
- Caesarean section
- Prolonged labour (>24 h)
- Mid-cavity rotational operative delivery
- Stillbirth
- Preterm birth
- Postpartum haemorrhage (>1 L)/requiring transfusion
- Surgery in pregnancy or the puerperium

- LMWH must be continued for the rest of the pregnancy and the puerperium.

Decisions regarding thromboprophylaxis in pregnancy relate to past history of VTE, the presence of thrombophilia and other risk factors ***(Box 29.9)***.

Women with previous VTE should receive antenatal and postnatal thromboprophylaxis with LMWH. This should begin as early in pregnancy as possible. LMWH and warfarin are safe to use in lactating mothers.

Further reading

Royal College of Obstetricians and Gynaecologists. *Green-top Guideline No. 37a: Thrombosis and Embolism during Pregnancy and the Puerperium, Reducing the Risk*. RCOG 2015; http://www.rcog.org.uk/.

Royal College of Obstetricians and Gynaecologists. *Green-top Guideline No. 37b: Thrombosis and Embolism during Pregnancy and the Puerperium, the Acute Management of*. RCOG 2015; http://www.rcog.org.uk/.

Respiratory disease

Asthma

The treatment of asthma (see pp. 1096–1110) in pregnancy does not differ from management in the non-pregnant patient. Pregnancy itself does not usually influence the severity of asthma. For the majority of women, asthma has no adverse effect on pregnancy outcome.

- Poorly controlled severe asthma presents more of a risk to the fetus than the medication used to prevent or treat it. This small risk is minimized with good control.
- Education and reassurance, ideally prior to pregnancy, concerning the safety of asthma medications during pregnancy are integral parts of management.
- Decreasing or stopping inhaled anti-inflammatory therapy during pregnancy causes deterioration in disease control.
- Inhaled, oral and intravenous steroids, inhaled, nebulized and intravenous short- and long-acting β_2-agonists, and the leukotriene receptor antagonist montelukast are safe to use in pregnancy and while breast-feeding.

- Effective control of the disease process and its accompanying symptoms is a priority. An increase in the dose or frequency of inhaled steroids should be the first step if symptoms are not optimally controlled on the current dose of inhaled steroids and the inhaler technique is good.

Pneumonia

The bacteria that cause pneumonia (see p. 1105) are no different in pregnancy. Chest X-rays are safe in pregnancy. Most antibiotics are safe to use in pregnancy and during lactation. Aminoglycosides should not be used unless essential and tetracycline/doxycycline should not be given. A high dose (500 mg x 3 daily) of amoxicillin is required in pregnancy. Varicella and influenza A pneumonia may be fatal in pregnancy and active steps must be taken to prevent chickenpox infection. Non-immune pregnant women exposed to varicella or prescribed steroids in pregnancy should be given varicella zoster immunoglobulin (VZIG). If a pregnant woman does contract chickenpox, she should be treated with aciclovir as soon as possible.

All pregnant women should receive immunization against seasonal influenza and influenza A H1N1.

Tuberculosis

Tuberculosis (TB) is particularly common in Asia and Africa. Perform a chest X-ray if TB is suspected and seek the advice of a respiratory physician. Extrapulmonary TB is as common as pulmonary TB in pregnancy. Diagnosis must be confirmed bacteriologically, which may necessitate bronchoscopy or biopsy, and is often delayed because of inappropriate reluctance to perform invasive investigations in pregnancy. The neonate should be given bacille Calmette–Guérin (BCG) vaccination.

Sarcoidosis

The course of sarcoidosis is unaltered by pregnancy. Flare-up of the disease is more likely postpartum. Erythema nodosum may occur in a normal pregnancy. Serum ACE is not reliable for the diagnosis of sarcoidosis in pregnancy. Systemic steroids should be used if indicated (see p. 1120).

Cystic fibrosis

Women with cystic fibrosis often reach child-bearing age with adequate lung function or will have received a lung transplant to be able to consider pregnancy. Pre-pregnancy counselling, with consideraton of lung function and concomitant diabetes, is required. Joint care with a cystic fibrosis centre should be maintained throughout pregnancy. Pregnancy outcome is related to pre-pregnancy lung function. Perinatal outcome is usually good but preterm delivery rates are high. Maternal outcome is variable, and worse in the presence of pulmonary hypertension. Specialist dietary advice with additional energy supplements should be given. Chest physiotherapy can and should be continued in pregnancy and infective exacerbations should be treated aggressively. There is a risk of gestational diabetes.

Severe restrictive lung disease

Women with severe lung disease are better able to tolerate pregnancy than women with severe cardiac insufficiency. If the forced vital capacity (FVC) is over 1 litre, a successful pregnancy is usually possible but individual assessment is necessary. Immunosuppression for diffuse parenchymal lung disease should be continued in pregnancy. Respiratory diseases complicated by pulmonary hypertension have a poor prognosis in pregnancy.

Neurological disease

Epilepsy

Birth defects

The overall risk of birth defects in babies of mothers who take one antiepileptic drug (AED) is around 7%, as compared with 3% in women without epilepsy. In most women, the frequency of seizures is not altered in pregnancy, provided there is compliance to the AEDs. Free drug levels tend to fall in pregnancy and increased doses of AEDs, particularly lamotrigine, may be required. The risk to the fetus of uncontrolled seizures is greater than the risks of continuing AED treatment; poorly controlled epilepsy and recurrent seizures are associated with adverse outcomes for the fetus, such as an increased risk of sudden unexplained death in epilepsy (SUDEP). If drugs cannot be safely stopped, monotherapy is preferable at the minimum effective dose. Sodium valproate is associated with a higher rate of serious malformations (e.g. neural tube defects) and long-term neurodevelopmental defects (e.g. a reduced IQ, increased risk of autism spectrum disorder and attention deficit disorder (ADHD)), and should be stopped or substituted if necessary.

Management

Counselling before conception is essential. Folic acid (5 mg/day) supplements should be taken before conception and throughout the first trimester. Vitamin K (10–20 mg orally) should also be taken by women receiving enzyme-inducing AEDs in the last 4 weeks before delivery to prevent neonatal haemorrhage. Antenatal screening for congenital abnormalities is necessary.

Breast-feeding

Mothers taking AEDs need not, in general, be discouraged from breast-feeding, though manufacturers are often hesitant in assuring that there is no risk to the baby.

Contraception

AEDs inducing hepatic enzymes (e.g. carbamazepine, phenytoin and phenobarbital) reduce the efficacy of oral contraceptives. A combined contraceptive pill containing a higher dose of oestrogen or the progesterone-only pill provides greater contraceptive security. An IUD or barrier method of contraception is often used in preference to oral contraceptives.

Migraine

Migraine can occur as a pregnancy-related phenomenon in women without a prior history of migraine. Those with pre-existing migraine often improve in pregnancy. Hemiplegic migraine, particularly aura without headache, can mimic transient ischaemic attacks (TIAs). Ergotamine should be avoided in pregnancy. Sumatriptan may be used to treat migraine. Low-dose aspirin, beta-blockers, tricyclic antidepressants and pizotifen are used for prophylaxis.

Multiple sclerosis

Pregnancy has no effect on the long-term prognosis of multiple sclerosis. Relapses are less likely during pregnancy but more likely in the postpartum period. Prophylactic treatments, such as interferon beta, glatiramer and natalizumab, are usually avoided in pregnancy and breast-feeding but benefit may outweigh risk for some women. Those with disability may require extra help during pregnancy and while caring for the infant following delivery. There is no contraindication to epidural anaesthesia, except that documentation of pre-existing neurological deficit in the legs is necessary to avoid any postpartum exacerbation of multiple sclerosis being inappropriately attributed to the regional block.

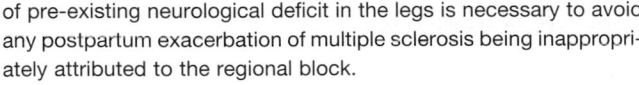

Myasthenia gravis

The course of myasthenia gravis (MG) in pregnancy is unpredictable, but in women with stable disease pregnancy outcome is usually normal. Postpartum exacerbations occur in 30% of women. Usual immunosuppressant therapy with steroids, azathioprine and calcineurin inhibitors should be continued. Increased doses of long-acting anticholinesterases may be required. Many drugs should be avoided in MG and consultation with an experienced obstetric anaesthetist should be obtained. Transient neonatal MG may develop in 10–20% of neonates born to myasthenic mothers due to transplacental passage of immunoglobulin G acetylcholine receptor antibodies.

Stroke

The risks of arterial ischaemic stroke, cerebral venous thrombosis and intracranial haemorrhage are increased, particularly in the puerperium. In pregnancy, the prevalence of haemorrhagic stroke equals that of ischaemic stroke, in contrast to non-pregnant women, where ischaemic stroke is more common (>75% of strokes).

Ischaemic causes of stroke in pregnancy include:

- cardiac causes, e.g. arterial emboli or arrhythmias
- peripartum cardiomyopathy (see p. 1042)
- paradoxical embolus (in situations causing increased right compared with left atrial pressure) through an atrial septal defect or patent foramen ovale
- aortic/carotid artery dissection
- antiphospholipid syndrome
- sickle-cell disease

Haemorrhagic causes include:

- pre-eclampsia/eclampsia.

Depression

This is discussed on pages 907 and 914.

Endocrine disease

Diabetes mellitus

This is discussed on page 1274.

Thyroid and parathyroid disease

Thyrotoxicosis

Untreated thyrotoxicosis (see pp. 1207–1208) is dangerous for both the mother and her fetus, increasing the risk of miscarriage, fetal growth restriction and preterm delivery. Graves' disease affects about 0.2% of pregnancies and often improves during pregnancy, but there is a risk of flare postpartum. Both carbimazole and propylthiouracil (PTU) cross the placenta, and in high doses may cause fetal hypothyroidism and goitre. The lowest possible maintenance dose of antithyroid drug should be used. Despite the advice in guidelines to avoid carbimazole in the first trimester, the risk of teratogenesis is very low. It is therefore also not logical to avoid PTU because of the risk of liver failure in the general population, but use it specifically in women planning pregnancy or in the first trimester. Women do not need to be swapped from one antithyroid drug to another before or during pregnancy; they should remain on whichever drug is controlling their disease. For those with good control of thyrotoxicosis on doses of carbimazole <15 mg/day or PTU <150 mg/day, the maternal and fetal outcome is usually good and unaffected by the thyrotoxicosis. Women may safely breast-feed on these doses of antithyroid drugs. Beta-blockers are safe to use in the short term, if required for control of thyrotoxic symptoms. Neonatal or fetal thyrotoxicosis due to transplacental passage of thyroid-stimulating antibodies is rare, but occurs most commonly in women with active disease in pregnancy and those with high levels of thyroid-stimulating antibodies.

Hypothyroidism

Hypothyroidism (see pp. 1202–1204) affects about 1% of pregnancies. Untreated hypothyroidism is associated with infertility, an increased rate of miscarriage, and fetal loss. For those on adequate replacement therapy, maternal and fetal outcome is usually good and is unaffected by the hypothyroidism. Very little thyroxine crosses the placenta and the fetus is not at risk of thyrotoxicosis from maternal thyroxine replacement therapy. Provided they are euthyroid at the beginning of pregnancy, most women do not usually require any adjustment to thyroxine dose during pregnancy or in the puerperium. Any dose increase should be based on thyroid function tests, interpreted using reference ranges for pregnancy (see p. 1203). There is no evidence to support the widespread recommendation for a target thyroid-stimulating hormone (TSH) of <2.5 mU/L.

Subclinical hypothyroidism affects 5% of the general population and is more common in women, particularly those who have anti-thyroid antibodies. Studies fail to demonstrate a consistent association between any adverse pregnancy outcome and subclinical hypothyroidism in pregnancy, and there is insufficient evidence that thyroxine replacement in subclinical hypothyroidism affects pregnancy outcome.

Postpartum thyroiditis is more common in women with a family history of hypothyroidism, thyroid peroxidase antibodies and type 1 diabetes. Presentation is usually between 3 and 4 months postpartum. Disease may present with symptoms of hyper- or hypothyroidism but a high index of suspicion is needed. The condition is caused by a destructive autoimmune lymphocytic thyroiditis. Most patients recover spontaneously and treatment is not always required. Postpartum thyroiditis often recurs and is a significant predictor of future hypothyroidism.

Hyperparathyroidism

Hypercalcaemia may be improved by pregnancy and the fetal demand for calcium. The risks to the mother are from acute pancreatitis and hypercalcaemic crisis, especially postpartum, when maternal transfer of calcium to the fetus stops abruptly. There is an increased risk of miscarriage, intrauterine death and preterm labour. Fetal mortality rates are up to 40% when the maternal hypercalcaemia is severe (>3.5 mmol/L). Up to 25% of women with hyperparathyroidism develop hypertension or pre-eclampsia. The risk to the neonate is from tetany and hypocalcaemic convulsions, caused by suppression of fetal parathyroid hormone (PTH) by high maternal calcium levels. Acute neonatal hypocalcaemia usually presents at 5–14 days after birth but may be delayed by up to 1 month if the infant is breast-fed. The ideal treatment is surgery and this may be safely performed in pregnancy. Surgery is usually delayed until the second trimester.

Pituitary disease (pp. 1183–1190)

Prolactinomas

Prolactinomas are the most common pituitary tumours encountered in pregnancy but rarely cause problems. The prolactin level should not be measured during pregnancy, as it is invariably raised. Those with microprolactinomas usually have no problems in pregnancy. The risk of tumour enlargement during pregnancy is increased with macroprolactinomas. Dopamine-receptor agonists are safe for use in pregnancy and are usually continued in women with macroprolactinomas. Visual fields should be measured in each trimester in those with macroprolactinomas. If tumour enlargement is suspected, magnetic resonance imaging (MRI) of the pituitary is indicated. If women with macroprolactinomas wish to breast-feed, their dopamine-receptor agonists may be discontinued in the last few weeks of pregnancy and during breast-feeding, but serial visual field examinations and pituitary MRIs are required, and cabergoline or bromocriptine should be reintroduced if there is concern regarding tumour expansion.

Diabetes insipidus (pp. 1233–1234)

Established or subclinical diabetes insipidus (DI) may worsen in pregnancy due to increased vasopressinase production by the placenta, or decreased vasopressinase breakdown by the liver. Extended fluid-deprivation tests should be avoided in pregnancy and close observation with paired urine and plasma osmolality measurements may be sufficient to exclude DI. Desmopressin is safe for use in pregnancy for diagnosis or treatment of DI. Transient DI may occur in pregnancy and is often associated with acute fatty liver of pregnancy and, more rarely, with pre-eclampsia and HELLP syndrome (see p. 1303).

Hypopituitarism

Hypopituitarism (see pp. 1188–1190) is rare in pregnancy but may be caused by the following:

- pituitary surgery
- radiotherapy
- pituitary or hypothalamic tumours
- pituitary haemorrhage
- postpartum pituitary infarction (Sheehan syndrome)
- lymphocytic hypophysitis.

Sheehan syndrome usually presents after delivery following postpartum haemorrhage and may lead to partial or complete pituitary failure. There may be a delay in diagnosis, as the symptoms may be attributed to the postpartum state. ***Lymphocytic hypophysitis*** is an uncommon autoimmune disorder due to extensive infiltration of the anterior pituitary by chronic inflammatory cells, predominantly lymphocytes, causing pituitary expansion. Antipituitary antibodies have been described and this condition is associated with autoimmune thyroiditis or adrenalitis in 20% of cases. It is most common in late pregnancy and the postpartum period. It presents with features suggestive of an expanding pituitary tumour and 85% of cases have endocrine hypofunction.

Adrenal disease

See also page 1224.

Conn syndrome and hyperaldosteronism

This is rare in pregnancy but hypertension, particularly in the absence of a positive family history, and hypokalaemia are indications for screening. High levels of progesterone in pregnancy may antagonize aldosterone and ameliorate the hypokalaemia. Renin and aldosterone levels are increased in pregnancy, and diagnosis requires the use of pregnancy-specific normal ranges. Hypertension is controlled in the usual way with labetalol, methyldopa or nifedipine, and hypokalaemia is treated with potassium supplementation or potassium-sparing diuretics. Amiloride is safe to use in pregnancy and high doses (e.g. 20 mg) may be needed. Spironolactone, which is used as a potassium-sparing diuretic in Conn syndrome outside pregnancy, should be avoided, as it may cause feminization of a male fetus because it is an antiandrogen. Surgery for adrenal adenomas can usually be safely deferred until after delivery.

Phaeochromocytoma and paraganglioma

Phaeochromocytoma and paraganglioma (see pp. 1231–1232) are a rare but dangerous cause of hypertension in pregnancy. Women with hypertension associated with unusual features of palpitations, anxiety, sweating or headache should be screened. Management involves adequate α-blockade with phenoxybenzamine to control hypertension, followed by β-blockade, if required, to control tachycardia. Alpha-blockade is imperative prior to delivery. Surgical removal is the only cure, and optimal timing of tumour resection depends on the point of gestation at which the diagnosis is made. There is an increasing vogue to delay tumour resection until the puerperium.

Renal disease

Urinary tract infection

See pages 762–767.

Bacteriuria in pregnancy

The urine of all pregnant women must be cultured, as 2–6% have asymptomatic bacteriuria. While asymptomatic bacteriuria in the non-pregnant female seldom leads to acute pyelonephritis and often does not require treatment, acute pyelonephritis frequently occurs in pregnancy under these circumstances. Failure to treat may thus result in severe symptomatic pyelonephritis later in pregnancy, with the possibility of preterm labour. *Therefore, bacteriuria must always be treated and be shown to be eradicated.* Re-infection may require prophylactic therapy. Tetracycline, sulphonamides and 4-quinolones must be avoided in pregnancy. Trimethoprim should be avoided in the first trimester. Amoxicillin, nitrofurantoin and cephalosporins may safely be used in pregnancy.

Chronic kidney disease

Women with chronic kidney disease (CKD) are at increased risk of pre-eclampsia, fetal growth restriction (FGR), preterm delivery and caesarean section; the perinatal mortality rate is increased. These obstetric complications and the risk of permanent deterioration in renal function are increased by the presence and severity of any renal impairment or hypertension.

In women with ***moderate or severe renal impairment*** (CKD stage 3–5), GFR 45 to 15 mL/min/1.73 m^2), 60–90% of infants are born preterm and there is a risk of accelerated decline in renal function of 20–50% in the mother.

An increase in the degree of proteinuria is very common in pregnancy and does not necessarily imply pre-eclampsia or worsening renal disease.

Management

Management should include regular monitoring of blood pressure, renal function and fetal wellbeing. In view of the increased risk of pre-eclampsia, treatment with low-dose aspirin (75 mg daily from week 12 to delivery) is used, especially in those with hypertension and renal impairment or a previous poor obstetric history.

Renal transplantation

If graft function is normal, pregnancy outcome is excellent and there is no adverse long-term effect on renal allograft function or survival.

The chance of successful pregnancy outcome is reduced and the risk of long-term deterioration in graft function increased with poor baseline graft function. Pregnancy outcome is optimal in those without hypertension, proteinuria or recent episodes of graft rejection.

The doses of immunosuppressive drugs are maintained at prepregnancy levels. Prednisolone, azathioprine, ciclosporin and tacrolimus are safe for use in pregnancy without any reported increase in the risk of congenital malformations. Mycophenolate mofetil and sirolimus are contraindicated. Prophylactic antibiotics should be given for recurrent UTIs and to cover any surgical procedure. The risks of pre-eclampsia, graft rejection, fetal growth restriction (FGR), preterm delivery and infection are increased. Caesarean section is only required for obstetric indications but the rate is increased.

Acute kidney injury

Because serum creatinine falls in pregnancy, acute kidney injury (AKI) is defined as an abrupt deterioration in renal function with a serum creatinine >90 µmol/L. Mild degrees of AKI are not uncommon, particularly immediately postpartum. The most common underlying causes are:

- ***Infection***: septic abortion, puerperal sepsis, acute pyelonephritis.
- ***Blood loss***: postpartum haemorrhage, placenta abruption.
- ***Volume contraction***: pre-eclampsia, eclampsia, hyperemesis gravidarum, diarrhoea.
- ***Post-renal failure***: ureteric damage or obstruction.
- ***Drugs***: NSAIDs, antibiotics (e.g. aminoglycosides).

Women with pre-eclampsia are particularly prone to pulmonary oedema and therefore management protocols include fluid restriction, even in the presence of oliguria. If these patients develop AKI, this is usually rapidly reversible upon recovery and less dangerous than pulmonary oedema, which may result if the AKI is treated with repeated fluid challenges. In this respect, therefore, the management of AKI differs from that outside pregnancy.

Skin disorders in pregnancy

Common skin changes that occur in pregnancy include striae (see p. 1378), spider naevi, melasma (pigmentation on the face) and linea nigra (midline pigmentation on the abdomen). A shift in maternal immune profile from predominantly Th1 to Th2 may underlie the tendency for atopic dermatitis to develop or worsen during pregnancy. Psoriasis usually improves.

The specific dermatoses of pregnancy have recently been reclassified as follows:

- ***Atopic eruption of pregnancy***:
  - ***Atopic eczema*** (see pp. 1349–1351).
  - ***Prurigo of pregnancy*** usually starts on the abdomen in the third trimester but may persist for some months after delivery. Clustered excoriated papules (prurigo-like lesions) occur on the abdomen and extensor surfaces of the limbs. The cause is unknown but pregnancy-related itch (pruritus gravidarum) may be due to cholestasis (see p. 1304). Rarely, liver biochemical tests are abnormal and urinary HCG levels may be elevated. Prurigo can recur in subsequent pregnancies. Treatment is with topical steroids and oral antihistamines.
  - ***Pruritic folliculitis of pregnancy*** is characterized by an itchy folliculitis, which looks similar to steroid-induced 'acne'. It is not associated with any increased maternal or fetal risk. Treatment is with topical benzoyl peroxide, and hydrocortisone cream helps to relieve symptoms.

Box 29.10 Drug use during pregnancy in treatment of rheumatoid arthritis

- ***Paracetamol***: the oral analgesic of choice
- ***Oral NSAIDs and selective COX-2 inhibitors***: can be used after implantation up until the last trimester if symptoms justify their use
- ***Corticosteroids***: may be used to control disease flares (main maternal risks are hypertension, glucose intolerance and osteoporosis)
- ***DMARDs***:
  - ***May be used***: sulfasalazine, hydroxychloroquine, azathioprine or ciclosporin if required to control inflammation
  - ***Must be avoided***: methotrexate, leflunomide and cyclophosphamide; women should not conceive while taking methotrexate or leflunomide
  - ***Biological agents***: safety during pregnancy is currently unclear
- ***Contraindicated in breast-feeding***: methotrexate, leflunomide, cyclophosphamide

COX-2, cyclo-oxygenase 2; DMARDs, disease-modifying anti-rheumatic drugs; NSAIDs, non-steroidal anti-inflammatory drugs.

- ***Polymorphic eruption of pregnancy*** (pruritic urticated papules of pregnancy) is a relatively common, intensely itchy rash that starts on the abdomen, often within striae, in the last trimester; it is associated with multiple births. It is uncomfortable but harmless. Symptomatic topical therapy and antihistamines are helpful until after delivery, when the rash resolves.
- ***Pemphigoid gestationis*** is a rare disease that is analogous to bullous pemphigoid (see pp. 1369–1370). It is associated with prematurity and stillbirth, and transplacental passage of pathogenic immunoglobulin G (IgG) antibodies can lead to transient blistering in the neonate. It often starts around the umbilicus with itchy, inflamed papules; then blistering appears and the eruption may become generalized. Onset may be in the first or second trimester, and it typically flares postpartum. The diagnosis is confirmed with direct immunofluorescence (see p. 1368). Systemic steroid therapy is required. Recurrences may occur with subsequent pregnancies and with the oral contraceptive pill, which should be avoided.

Further reading

Vaughan Jones S, Ambros-Rudolph C, Nelson-Piercy C. Skin diseases in pregnancy. *BMJ* 2014; 348:g3489.

Rheumatoid arthritis in pregnancy

50–80% of women with rheumatoid arthritis usually go into remission in pregnancy. However, about 90% will flare during the postpartum period. Disease-modifying anti-rheumatic drugs (DMARDs) are contraindicated in pregnancy. Women should take advice from their rheumatologist and obstetrician ***prior*** to conception. ***Box 29.10*** shows the use of drugs in pregnancy.

PRESCRIBING IN PREGNANCY

Many clinicians are understandably reluctant to prescribe drugs for pregnant women. This relates mainly to concern regarding teratogenic risk. The following general principles should be remembered:

- ***Older generic drugs***. Use older generic drugs within each class, since there are likely to be more data on use in pregnancy.

- ***Dosages***. Resist the temptation to prescribe lower doses. Pregnant women usually need *higher* doses because of increased renal and liver clearance.
- ***Disease control***. Control of underlying diseases, such as arthritis, inflammatory bowel disease, epilepsy, asthma and thyrotoxicosis, with appropriate drug therapy is likely to reduce adverse fetal and neonatal outcomes such as preterm birth and growth restriction.
- ***Treatment for unfamiliar diseases***. When considering treatment for these, always ask the specialist physician, 'What would you do if this woman was not pregnant?' Then assess the risks of this strategy in pregnancy.
- ***Risks to the fetus***. These must be balanced against potential benefits to the mother (and therefore indirectly the fetus).

The ***teratogenic potential*** of some drugs classified as '***absolutely contraindicated***' (see ***Box 2.6***, p. 22) is sufficiently high to justify termination of a pregnancy following inadvertent exposure, e.g. methotrexate (see p. 680) or thalidomide. For others, there are theoretical reasons to avoid their use in pregnancy, but they carry a low risk of teratogenesis and therefore there is no justification for termination (e.g. rubella vaccine, simvastatin, ACE inhibitors).

For drugs that are '***relatively contraindicated***', there are situations in which use is appropriate and where no safer alternative exists: for example, warfarin in women with prosthetic heart valves or AEDs in women with epilepsy.

- Beta-blockers should not be used as first-line treatment of hypertension, but may be indicated to control tachyarrhythmias, for migraine prophylaxis, thyrotoxicosis and mitral stenosis, and in those at risk of aortic dissection.
- Diuretics should be avoided in the treatment of hypertension but are appropriate in the treatment of pulmonary oedema.

Further reading

Huybrechlsk, Palmsten K, Avorn J et al. Anti-depressant use in pregnancy and the rise of cardiac defects. *N Engl J Med* 2014; 370:2397–2407.

30 Ear, nose and throat and eye disease

Francis Vaz, Nishchay Mehta, Robin D Hamilton

See your e-book for key learning points, summaries, clinical tips, drug tips, extra tables, extra images, interactive Figures, learning challenges and MCQs.

EAR, NOSE AND THROAT AND EYE DISEASE

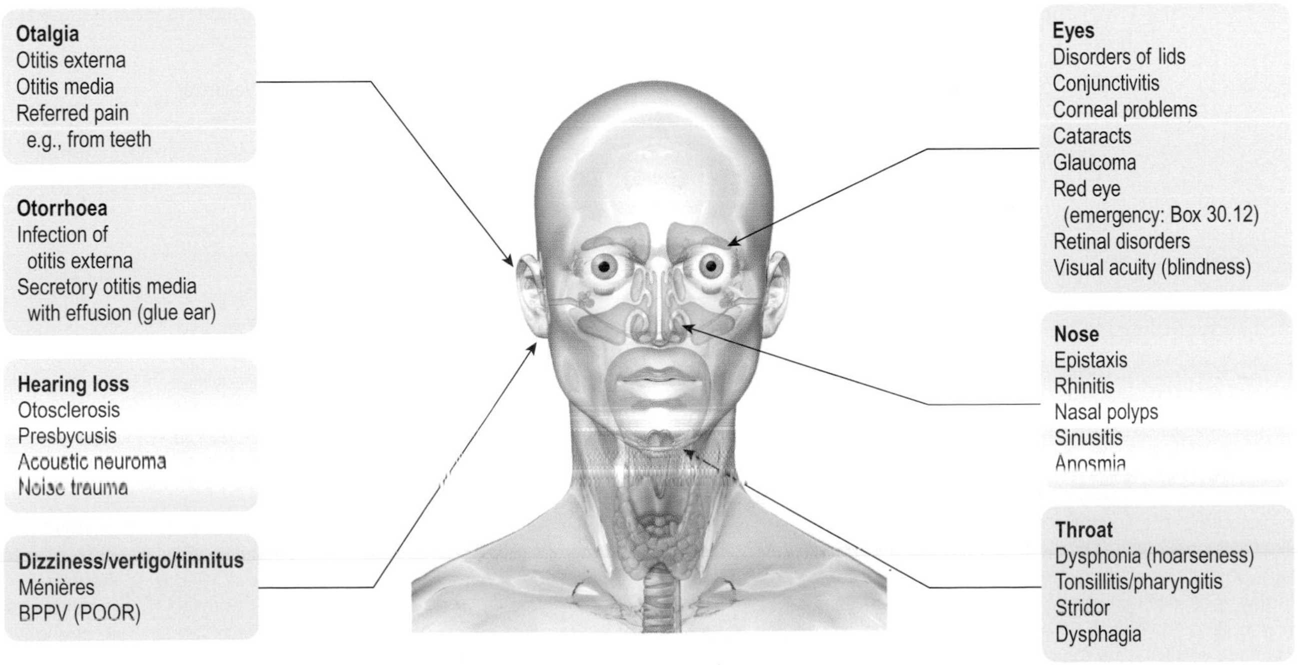

DISORDERS OF THE EAR

ANATOMY AND PHYSIOLOGY

The ear can be divided into three parts: outer, middle and inner ***(Fig. 30.1)***.

The ***outer ear*** has a skin-lined tube 2.5 cm long leading down to the tympanic membrane (the ear drum). Its outer third is cartilaginous and contains hair and sebaceous and ceruminous glands, but the walls of the inner two-thirds are bony. The outer ear is self-cleaning, as the skin is migratory so there are no indications to use cotton wool buds. Wax should only be seen in the outer third.

The ***middle ear*** is an air-containing cavity derived from the branchial clefts. It communicates with the mastoid air cells superiorly, and the Eustachian tube connects it to the nasopharynx medially. The Eustachian tube ventilates the middle ear and maintains equal air pressure across the tympanic membrane. It is normally closed but opens via the action of the palatal muscles to allow air entry when swallowing or yawning. A defect in this mechanism, such as with a cleft palate, will prevent air entering the middle ear cleft, which may then fill with fluid. Lying within the middle ear cavity are the three ossicles (malleus, incus and stapes), which transmit sound from the tympanic membrane ***(Fig. 30.2)*** to the inner ear. On the medial wall of the cavity is the horizontal segment of the facial nerve, which can be damaged during surgery or by direct extension of infection in the middle ear.

The ***inner ear*** contains the cochlea for hearing and the vestibule and semicircular canals for balance. There is a semicircular canal arranged in each body plane and these canals are stimulated by rotatory movement. The facial, cochlear and vestibular nerves emerge from the inner ear and run through the internal acoustic meatus to the brainstem (see ***Fig. 21.8***).

Physiology of hearing

The ossicles, in the middle ear, transmit sound waves from the tympanic membrane to the cochlea. They amplify the waves by

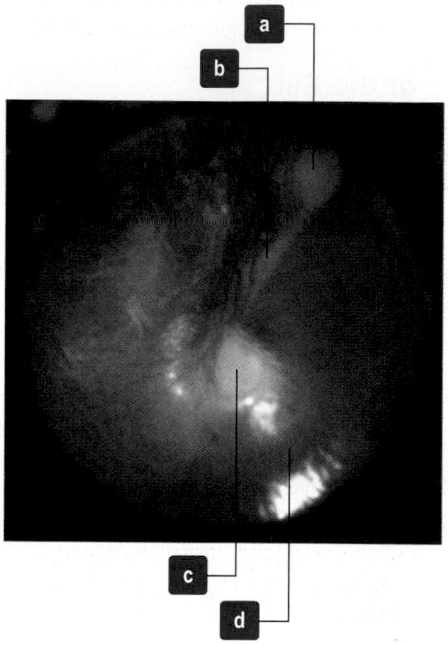

Figure 30.2 Normal tympanic membrane. (a) Lateral process of malleus. **(b)** Handle of malleus. **(c)** Umbo. **(d)** Light reflex.

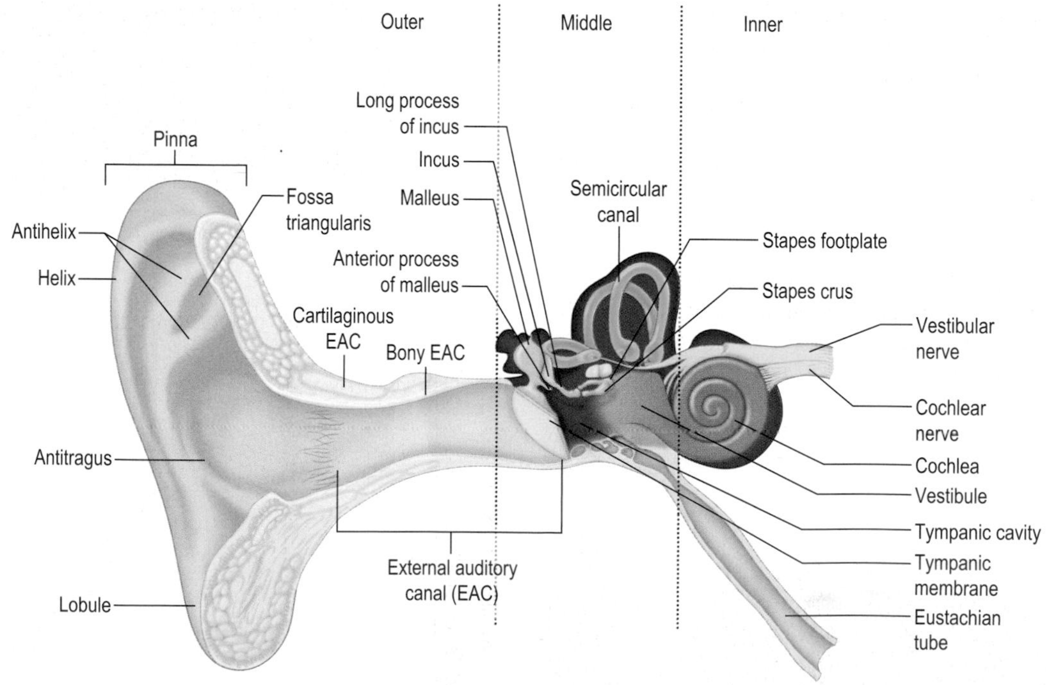

Figure 30.1 The anatomy of the ear. The ear is anatomically divided into outer, middle and inner ear, as indicated at the top. The ***outer ear*** consists of the pinna and external auditory meatus, and funnels sound energy to the middle ear, selectively amplifying sounds in the 2–4 kHz range by 15 decibels (dB, speech sounds). When sound energy passes from air in the outer ear to fluid in the inner ear, it loses 30 dB due to energy that is reflected at the interface of the two mediums. The ***middle ear*** acts as a transformer, increasing the pressure of the acoustic wave to account for the energy lost at this air–fluid interface. As the acoustic wave moves across the tunnel of the ***inner ear***, passing from the oval window to the round window, it causes maximal vibration of the basilar membrane in a location that is specific to its resonant frequency. This vibration causes the hair cell to open its ion gates and an action potential to be propagated along a fibre of the cochlear nerve. The location of the nerve fibre and the strength of its action potential allow the central nervous system to construct meaning from the sound we hear.

about 18-fold to compensate for the loss of sound waves moving from the air-filled middle ear to the fluid-filled cochlea. Hair cells in the basilar membrane of the cochlea detect the vibrations and transduce these into nerve impulses, which pass to the cochlear nucleus and then eventually to the superior olivary nuclei of both sides; thus lesions central to the cochlear nucleus do not cause unilateral hearing loss.

If the ossicles are diseased, sound can also reach the cochlea by vibration of the temporal bone (bone conduction).

CLINICAL APPROACH TO THE PATIENT WITH A DISORDER OF THE EAR

Examination

The pinna and post-auricular region should first be examined for erythema, scars or swellings. An auroscope is used to examine the external ear canal whilst the pinna is retracted backwards and upwards to straighten the canal. Look for wax, discharge or foreign bodies. The tympanic membrane should always be seen with a light reflex anteroinferiorly. Previous repeated infections may cause a thickened, whitish drum but fluid in the middle ear may show as dullness of the drum. Perforations can be described as marginal if they involve the annulus, subtotal if the pars tensa is absent, and total if both pars tensa and the annulus are absent.

Rinne test

(***Fig. 30.3.***)

- Normally, a tuning fork, 512 Hz, will be heard as louder if held next to the ear (i.e. air conduction) than it will if placed on the mastoid bone (***Rinne-positive***).
- If the tuning fork is perceived louder when placed on the mastoid (i.e. via bone conduction), then a defect in the conducting mechanism of the external or middle ear is present (true ***Rinne-negative***).

Weber test

(***Fig. 30.4.***) A tuning fork placed on the forehead or vertex of a patient with normal hearing (or with symmetrical hearing loss) should be perceived centrally by the patient. A patient with unilateral conductive hearing loss will hear the sound loudest in the affected ear, whereas a patient with unilateral sensorineural hearing loss will report the sound to be loudest in the unaffected ear.

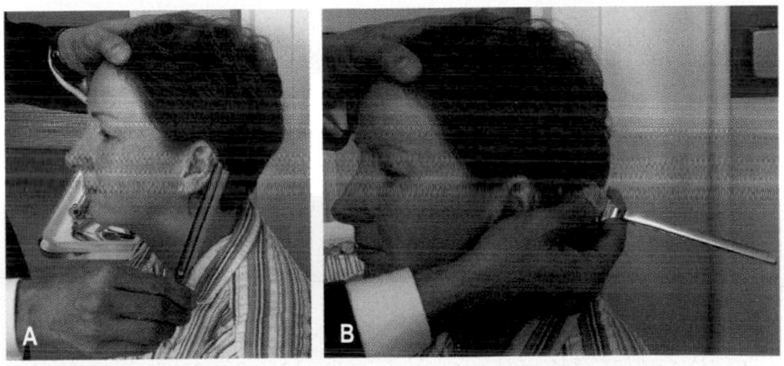

Figure 30.3 **Rinne test.** Comparing conduction of sound. **A.** Air conduction. **B.** Bone conduction.

Pure-tone audiometry

The patient is asked to respond when they hear sounds presented as pure tones at varying sound intensities and frequencies. Sounds are presented to each ear (representing air conduction) and then to each mastoid in turn (representing bone conduction). An audiogram is produced by the lowest sound intensity that is reliably perceptible at each frequency tested at both ears and mastoids ***(Fig. 30.5)***.

COMMON DISORDERS OF THE EAR

There are four main symptoms related to ear pathology: pain (otalgia), discharge (otorrhoea), hearing loss and dizziness (vertigo). The sequence and combination of symptoms can differentiate between most conditions and therefore history is often the most useful diagnostic tool.

The painful ear (otalgia)

A painful ear is a common complaint but, due to the complex innervation, may be referred from distant sites and can thus on occasion have an obscure aetiology.

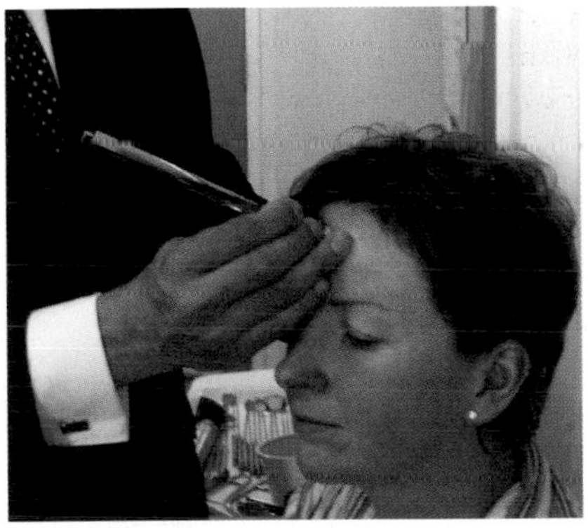

Figure 30.4 **Weber test.**

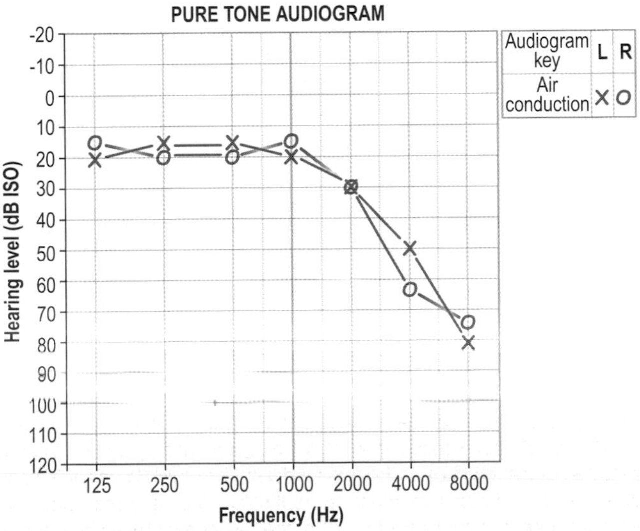

Figure 30.5 **Audiogram showing presbycusis (high-frequency loss).**

Otitis externa

When the natural barriers to infection are overcome, the skin of the ear canal can become infected. Discharge and itch are the initial presenting symptoms, followed by pain and then reduction in hearing as the ear canal closes off. Infection can spread to the pinna, causing cellulitis. Although the causative organism is most commonly bacterial (pseudomonal species, followed by staphylococcal species), it can also be fungal. There may be swelling of the pre-auricular or post-auricular lymph nodes that can be mistaken for mastoiditis.

Examination often reveals debris in the canal, which needs to be removed either by gentle mopping or preferably by suction, viewed directly under a microscope. The tympanic membrane is normal, when visible. In severe cases, the canal may be swollen and a view of the tympanic membrane impossible. Any foreign body seen should be removed with great care by trained personnel.

Treatment is with topical antibiotics in the first instance: drops such as dexamethasone 0.05%, framycetin sulphate 0.5%, gramicidin 0.005% drops, hydrocortisone acetate 1% or gentamicin 0.3%, or a spray such as dexamethasone 0.1%, neomycin sulphate 3250 units. If it does not resolve in 3–4 days, then microsuction in an Ear, Nose and Throat (ENT) department is necessary.

Finafloxacin ear drops are used if there is a perforation, to reduce ototoxicity.

Otitis media

Otitis media is an infection of the middle ear seeded from the upper respiratory tract through the Eustachian tube. Therefore most commonly encountered pathogens are similar to those that cause upper respiratory tract infections: respiratory syncytial virus (RSV), *Streptococcus pneumoniae*, *Haemophilus influenzae* and *Moraxella catarrhalis*. Otitis media most commonly affects children under the age of 10. Infection causes inflammation of the middle ear mucosa and inflammatory exudate in the middle ear space. Due to the middle ear fluid, otitis media presents with otalgia and hearing disturbance. If it does not resolve, it can lead to tympanic membrane perforation and discharge. There are no mucous glands in the external ear canal. If the discharge is serous, then middle ear pathology is unlikely. Otitis media classically presents with otalgia followed by discharge, whereas otitis externa presents with discharge followed by otalgia. Rare complications of otitis media include mastoiditis as the middle ear inflammatory fluid escapes from the middle ear into the mastoid, or meningitis as the infection spreads through the tegmen into the intracranial cavity. Examination shows a healthy ear canal with an erythematous and occasionally bulging tympanic membrane.

Treatment of the acute case is initially with non-steroidal anti-inflammatory drugs. Otitis media is often viral in origin – for example, following a cold – and will settle within 72 hours without antibacterial treatment. In people with systemic features or after 72 hours, a systemic antibiotic, such as amoxicillin, should be given, particularly in children under 2 years old. Topical therapy is of no value. If there is tenderness and swelling over the mastoid, then an urgent ENT opinion should be obtained.

Referred otalgia

Pain may be referred from:

- the teeth and temporomandibular joint from the auriculotemporal nerve (a branch of the mandibular (Vth cranial) nerve)
- cervical spinal problems from C1 to C3
- tonsil and tongue base problems from the glossopharyngeal (Jacobson's) nerve
- the larynx and pharynx from the vagus (Arnold's) nerve
- Ramsay Hunt syndrome, causing vesicles along the distribution of the VIIth cranial nerve.

The innervation of the pinna is from the auriculotemporal branch of the trigeminal and the first two cervical nerves ***(Fig. 30.6)***. Therefore, dental pain, temporomandibular joint dysfunction and upper cervical osteoarthritis can all present as otalgia. The ear canal is innervated by the above-mentioned nerves, and also by the facial and vagus nerves ***(Fig. 30.6)***. Hence Ramsay Hunt syndrome (varicella reactivation along the sensory division of the facial nerve) causes otalgia with ear canal vesicles, whereas cancer of the larynx and pharynx can occasionally present as otalgia due to referred pain along the vagus nerve. The middle ear is innervated by the glossopharyngeal nerve and therefore infections of the pharynx are associated with otalgia.

The discharging ear (otorrhoea)

Discharge from the ear is usually due to infection of the outer or middle ear. The most common cause is otitis externa, followed by otitis media with a perforated tympanic membrane (see above).

Cholesteatoma

Although cholesteatoma is a rarer cause of the otorrhoea, it has severe implications if missed and should be considered in any non-resolving or recurrent case of otorrhoea. Cholesteatoma is defined as keratinizing squamous epithelium within the middle ear cleft and can present with foul-smelling otorrhoea. Examination shows a defect in the tympanic membrane full of white, cheesy material. Mastoid surgery is required to remove this sac of squamous debris, as it can erode local structures such as the ossicles or facial nerve, or even extend intracranially to cause meningitis or an intracranial abscess.

Hearing loss

Deafness can be conductive or sensorineural and these can be differentiated at the bedside by the Rinne and the Weber tests ***(Box 30.1)*** or with pure-tone audiometry. ***Conductive hearing loss*** has many causes ***(Box 30.2)*** but wax is the most common.

Perforated tympanic membrane

This arises from trauma or chronic middle ear disease when recurrent infection results in a permanent defect. Surgical repair is indicated only if the patient is symptomatic with recurrent discharge. The larger the perforation, the greater the impact on hearing.

Box 30.1 Testing hearing loss

Type	Defect	Rinne test	Weber test
Conductive	Outer or middle ear	Negative	Sound heard louder on the affected side
Sensorineural	Inner ear or more centrally	Positive	Sound heard louder in the normal ear

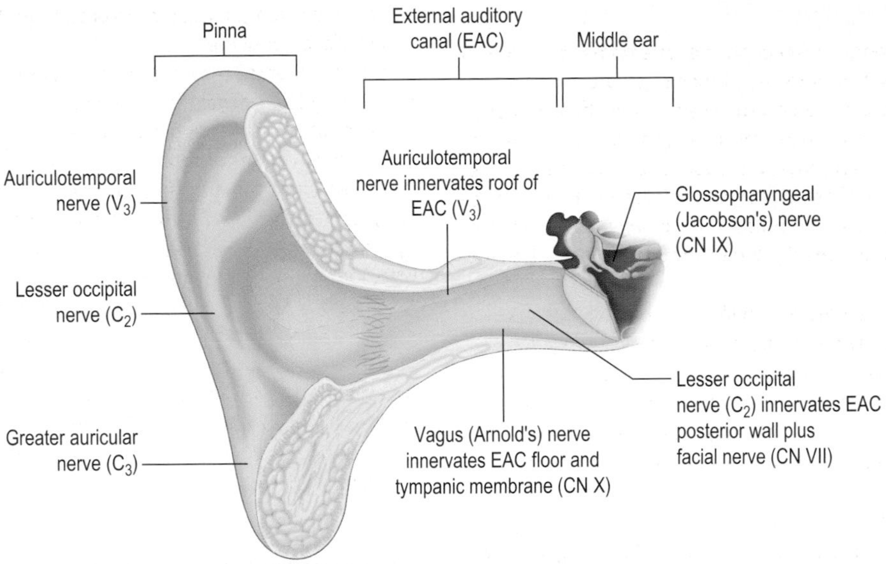

Figure 30.6 Sensory innervation of the ear. Due to the sophisticated embryology of ear structures, the sensory innervation is complicated. Therefore otalgia can be referred from many sites, and knowledge of aural sensory innervation is a good guide for a comprehensive examination in idiopathic ear pain. The ***auriculotemporal nerve*** (a branch of the mandibular division of the trigeminal nerve) supplies innervation to the superolateral pinna and roof of the external auditory canal (EAC). Pathology related to the upper teeth, temporomandibular joint and parotid gland can cause referred otalgia through this nerve. The ***lesser occipital nerve*** (a branch from the second cervical nerve) supplies most of the medial surface of the pinna and the posterior wall of the EAC. Cervical osteoarthritis can cause referred otalgia through this nerve. The ***greater auricular nerve*** (a branch from the third cervical nerve) supplies the inferior portion of the pinna, including the lobule. Cervical osteoarthritis can cause referred otalgia through this nerve. ***Arnold's nerve (a branch of the vagus cranial nerve)*** supplies the EAC floor and lateral surface of the tympanic membrane. Tumours of the larynx and pharynx can cause referred otalgia through this nerve. ***Jacobson's nerve (a branch of the glossopharyngeal nerve)*** supplies innervation to the mucosa of the middle ear, including the medial surface of the tympanic membrane. Tonsillitis and pharyngitis can cause referred otalgia through this nerve. CN, cranial nerve.

Box 30.2 Causes of deafness

Conductive

External meatus
- Wax
- Foreign body
- Otitis externa
- Chronic suppuration

Drum
- Perforation/trauma

Middle ear
- Otosclerosis
- Ossicular bone problems
- Suppuration (otitis media)

Sensorineural

Congenital
- Pendred syndrome (see p. 1202)
- Long QT syndrome
- Björnstad syndrome (pili torti)

End-organ
- Advancing age
- Occupational acoustic trauma
- Ménière's disease
- Drugs (e.g. gentamicin, furosemide)

VIIIth nerve lesions
- Acoustic neuroma
- Cranial trauma
- Inflammatory lesions:
  - Tuberculous meningitis
  - Sarcoidosis
  - Neurosyphilis
  - Carcinomatous meningitis

Brainstem lesions (rare)
- Multiple sclerosis
- Infarction

Otitis media and otitis externa

As discussed above, both of these infections lead to hearing loss but the sequence of events will help differentiate the conditions: hearing loss is common and early in otitis media, but rare and late in otitis externa.

Secretory otitis media with effusion ('serous otitis media' or 'glue ear')

This is common in children because Eustachian tube dysfunction may lead to poorly ventilated middle ears. The vacuum created by poor ventilation leads to a non-inflammatory effusion. The effusion resolves naturally in the majority of cases but can persist or recur, causing a hearing loss that impacts on speech and language skills and on educational progress. The presenting complaint is hearing loss or speech delay but little association with otalgia.

Examination shows a dull tympanic membrane with loss of light reflex ***(Fig. 30.7)*** and occasionally fluid with air bubbles visible in the middle ear. Children with glue ear frequently have adenoidal hypertrophy and nasal blockage.

Management involves insertion of a grommet (tympanostomy tube) into the tympanic membrane, which ventilates the middle ear cavity, if the symptoms are persistent and troublesome. Antibiotic–glucocorticoid ear drops are more effective than oral antibiotics. Adenoidectomy can be added to the procedure if there is a strong history of complete nasal blockage or recurrent upper respiratory tract infections. Grommets are extruded from the tympanic

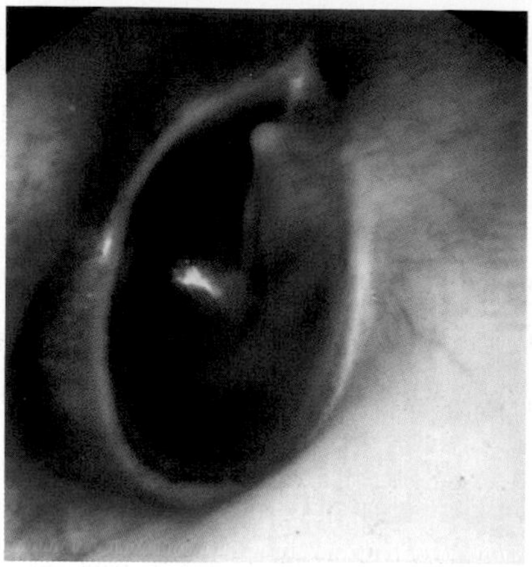

Figure 30.7 Secretory otitis media (glue ear). Auroscopic view of the tympanic membrane, which is dull with loss of light reflex.

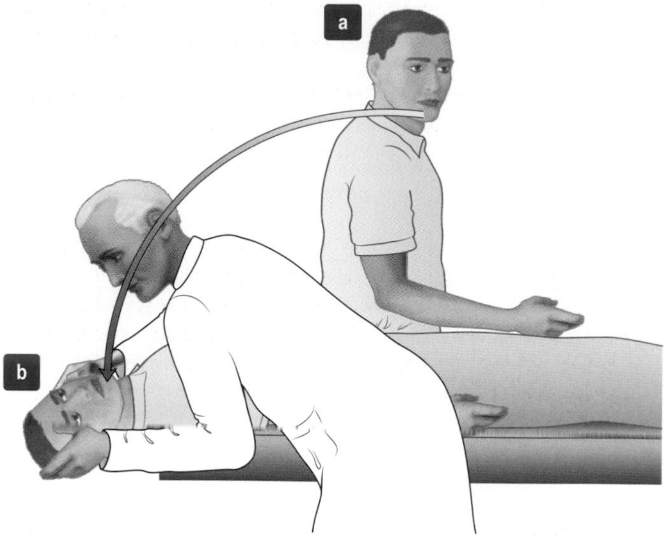

Figure 30.8 Hallpike manœuvre for diagnosis of benign paroxysmal positional vertigo. This can be done in the outpatient department. **(a)** The patient sits on a couch, his head turned towards one ear. **(b)** The head is supported by the examiner while the patient lies down so that his head is just below the horizontal. Nystagmus (following a latent interval of a few seconds) is commonly noted when the head has been turned towards the affected ear. This can be repeated with the patient's head turned towards the other ear.

membrane as it heals (over 6 months to 2 years). Developmental outcomes are not improved by grommet insertions. In most children, the middle third of the face grows around the age of 7–14 years and Eustachian tube dysfunction is rare after this.

Otosclerosis

This is usually a hereditary disorder, in which new bony deposits occur within the stapes footplate and the cochlea. Characteristically seen in the second and third decades, it is more common in females and can become worse during pregnancy. The hearing loss may be mixed, and management includes a hearing aid or replacement of the fixed stapes with a prosthesis (stapedectomy). The choice of treatment is dependent on the patient. Surgery is an excellent option, with very good success rates in regular stapedectomists' hands, but it always carries a small risk of a complete hearing loss. Hearing aids, whilst safe, require the patient's compliance if they are to afford benefit.

Presbycusis

This is the most common cause of deafness. It is a degenerative disorder of the cochlea and is typically seen in old age. It can be due to the loss of outer hair cells (sensory), loss of the ganglion cells (neural) or strial atrophy (metabolic), or there can be a mixed picture. Ageing itself does not cause outer hair cell loss but environmental noise toxicity over the years is a major factor. The onset is gradual and the higher frequencies are affected most (see ***Fig. 30.5***). Speech has two components: low frequencies (vowels) and high frequencies (consonants). When the consonants are lost, speech loses its intelligibility. Increasing the volume merely increases the low frequencies and the characteristic response of 'Don't shout. I'm not deaf!'

A high-frequency-specific hearing aid will do much to ease the frustrations of both the patients and their close contacts.

Noise trauma

Cochlear damage can occur, for example, from shooting without ear protectors or from industrial noise (see p. 59), and characteristically has a loss at 4 kHz.

Acoustic neuroma

This is a slow-growing benign schwannoma of the vestibular nerve (see p. 868), which can present with progressive sensorineural hearing loss. Any patient with an asymmetric sensorineural hearing loss or sudden sensorineural hearing loss should be investigated: for example, with a magnetic resonance imaging (MRI) scan.

Dizziness/vertigo

Vertigo is usually rotatory when it arises from the ear. The presence of otalgia, otorrhoea, tinnitus or hearing loss suggests an otologic aetiology. Vestibular causes can be classified according to the duration of the vertigo. Common causes are summarized below.

- seconds (<1 minute) – benign paroxysmal positional vertigo
- minutes to hours – Ménière's disease
- hours to days – labyrinthine or central pathology.

Benign paroxysmal positional vertigo

Benign paroxysmal positional vertigo (BPPV) is thought to occur when otoconia (tiny crystals of calcium carbonate) are dislodged from the utricle into the semicircular canals, commonly the posterior canal. Positional vertigo is precipitated by head movements, usually to a particular position, and often occurs when turning in bed or on sitting up. The onset is typically sudden and distressing. The vertigo lasts seconds (<1 minute) and the phenomenon becomes less severe on repeated movements (fatigue). There is no serious underlying cause but it sometimes follows vestibular neuronitis (see p. 810), head injury or ear infection. It occurs in 50% of older people and is the most common cause of head injury in those under 50 years of age.

Diagnosis

Diagnosis is made on the basis of the history and by the ***Hallpike manœuvre (Fig. 30.8)***. A positive Hallpike test confirms BPPV, which can be cured in over 90% of cases by the Epley manœuvre. This involves gentle but specific manipulation and rotation of the patient's head to shift the loose otoliths from the semicircular canals.

The differential diagnosis includes a cerebellar mass, but in that case positional nystagmus (and vertigo) is immediately apparent (no latent interval) and does not fatigue.

Ménière's disease

This is a rare condition characterized by recurring, episodic, rotatory vertigo lasting 30 minutes to a few hours; attacks are recurrent over months or years. Classically, it is associated with a low-frequency sensorineural hearing loss, a feeling of fullness in the affected ear, loss of balance, tinnitus and vomiting. There is a build-up of endolymphatic fluid in the inner ear, although its precise aetiology is still unclear.

Management

Vestibular sedatives, such as cinnarizine, are used in the acute phase. Preventative measures, such as a low-salt diet, betahistine and avoidance of caffeine, are useful. If the disease cannot be controlled, then a chemical labyrinthectomy, perfusing the round window orifice with ototoxic drugs such as gentamicin, is used. Gentamicin destroys the vestibular epithelium; therefore the patient has severe vertigo for around 2 weeks until the body compensates for the lack of vestibular input on that side. The patient will happily trade occasional mild vertigo when the balance system is challenged against the unpredictable, severe and disabling attacks of vertigo involved in Ménière's disease. There is a risk of sensorineural hearing loss and complete vestibular failure if Ménière's starts in the previously unaffected side. The final option is surgical decompression of the endolymphatic compartment of the inner ear to relieve the endolymphatic hydrops.

Labyrinthine or central causes of vertigo

(See **Box 21.13**.) These are managed with vestibular sedatives in the acute phase. Most patients will settle over a few days but continuous true vertigo with nystagmus suggests a central lesion. A patient with a deficit of vestibular function due to viral labyrinthitis or neuronitis should be able to cease vestibular sedatives within 2 weeks; long-term use can give parkinsonian side-effects, delay central compensation and thus prolong the vertigo. Vestibular rehabilitation by a physiotherapist or audiological scientist can speed up the compensation process, although most patients will be able to do this themselves with time.

Tinnitus

This is a sensation of a sound when there is no auditory stimulus. It can occur without hearing loss and results from heightened awareness of neural activity in the auditory pathways. Patients describe a hissing or ringing in their ears and this can cause much distress. It usually does not have a serious cause but vascular malformation, such as aneurysms or vascular tumours can be associated. In these cases, the tinnitus is pulsatile and most commonly unilateral.

Management

This is difficult. A tinnitus masker (a mechanically produced, continuous soft sound) can help. Cognitive behavioural therapy through audiological services are of use and rehabilitate patients well.

Further reading

Kim J, Zee DS. Benign paroxysmal positional vertigo. *N Engl J Med* 2014; 370:1138–1147.

Kral A. Profound deafness in children. *N Engl J Med* 2010; 363:1438–1450.

Schreiber BE, Agrup C, Haskard DO et al. Sudden sensorineural hearing loss. *Lancet* 2010; 375:1203–1211.

DISORDERS OF THE NOSE

ANATOMY AND PHYSIOLOGY

(**Fig. 30.9**.) The function of the nose is to facilitate smell and respiration:

- Smell is a sensation conveyed by the olfactory epithelium in the roof of the nose. The olfactory epithelium is supplied by the Ist cranial nerve (see p. 802).
- The nose also filters, moistens and warms inspired air and, in doing so, assists the normal process of respiration.

The external portion of the nose consists of two nasal bones attached to the rest of the facial skeleton and to the upper and lower lateral cartilages. The internal nose is divided by a midline septum that comprises both cartilage and bone. This divides the internal nose in two, from the external nostril to the posterior choanae. The posterior choanae are in continuity with the nasopharynx posteriorly. The paranasal sinuses open into the lateral wall of the nose and form a system of aerated chambers within the facial skeleton.

The blood supply of the nose is derived from branches of both the internal and external carotid arteries. The internal carotid artery supplies the upper nose via the anterior and posterior ethmoidal arteries. The external carotid artery supplies the posterior and inferior portion of the nose via the superior labial artery, greater palatine artery and sphenopalatine artery. On the anterior nasal septum there is an area of confluence of these vessels (Little's area; **Fig. 30.10A**).

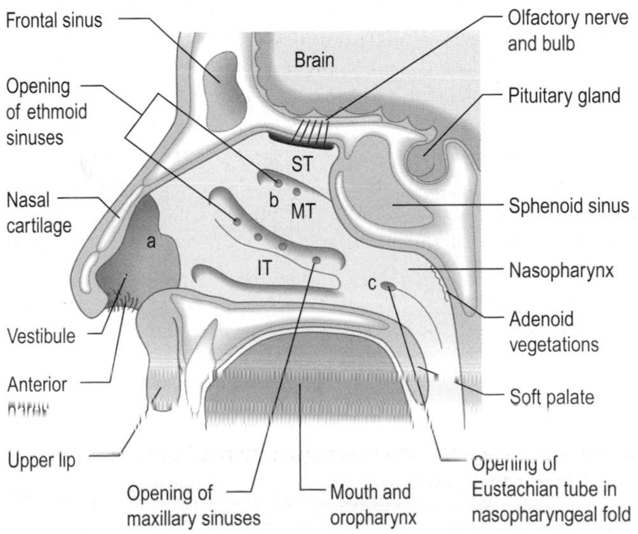

Figure 30.9 The anatomy of the nose in longitudinal section. IT, inferior turbinate; MT, middle turbinate; ST, superior turbinate; a, internal ostium; b, respiratory region; c, choanae.

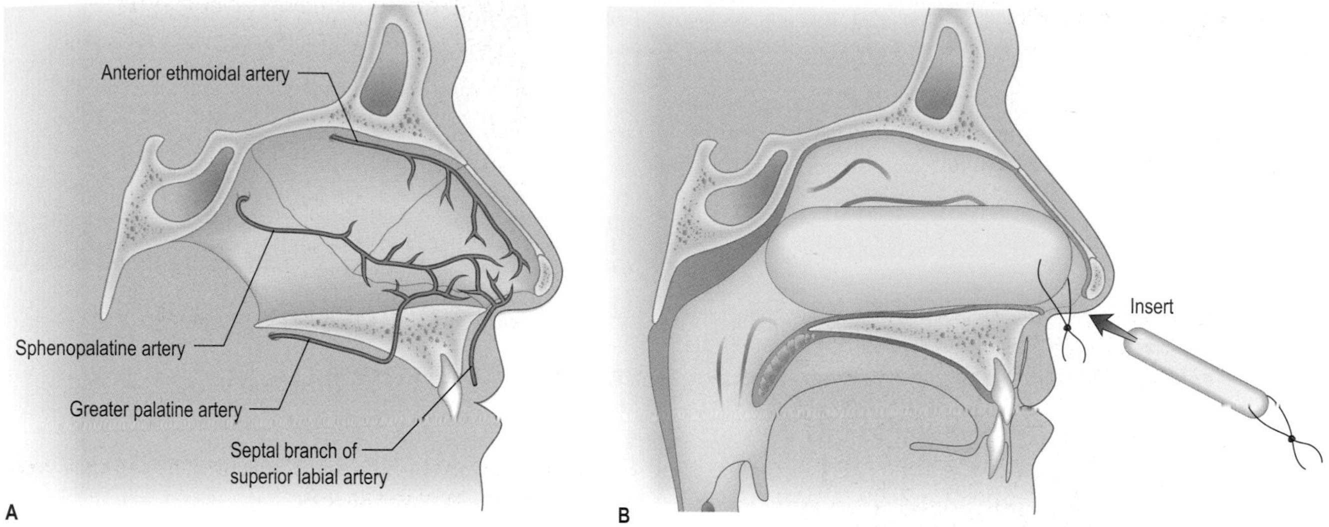

Figure 30.10 **Little's area and nasal packing. A.** Blood supply of Little's area on the septum of the nose. **B.** Nasal pack.

CLINICAL APPROACH TO THE PATIENT WITH A DISORDER OF THE NOSE

Examination

The anterior part of the nose can be examined using a nasal speculum and light source. Endoscopes are required to examine the nasal cavity and postnasal space.

COMMON DISORDERS OF THE NOSE

Epistaxis

Nose bleeds vary in severity from minor to life-threatening. Little's area ***(Fig. 30.10A)*** is a frequent site of nasal haemorrhage. First aid measures should be administered immediately, including external digital compression of the anterior lower portion of the external nose, ice packs and leaning forward. The patient should be asked to avoid swallowing any blood running posteriorly, as this causes nausea.

Not infrequently, small, recurrent epistaxes occur and these may require a visit to the emergency clinic for an examination and simple local anaesthetic cautery with a silver nitrate stick. If the bleeding continues profusely, then resuscitation in the form of intravenous access, fluid replacement or blood, and oxygen can be administered. If further intervention is necessary, consideration should be given to intranasal cautery of the bleeding vessel, or intranasal packing using a variety of commercially available nasal packs ***(Fig. 30.10B)***. In addition to direct treatment of the epistaxis, a cause should be sought and treated appropriately ***(Box 30.3)***. If the above treatments fail, surgical ligation of the sphenopalatine artery can be undertaken endoscopically or an interventional arterial embolization can be performed for the problematic vessel.

Rhinitis

See pages 1076–1077.

Box 30.3 Aetiology of epistaxis

Local
- Idiopathic
- Trauma – foreign bodies, nose-picking and nasal fractures
- Iatrogenic – surgery, intranasal steroids
- Neoplasm – nasal, paranasal sinus and nasopharyngeal tumours

General
- Anticoagulants/antiplatelet agents
- Coagulation disorders
- Severe hypertension
- Osler–Weber–Rendu syndrome (familial haemorrhagic telangiectasia)

Nasal obstruction

Nasal obstruction is a symptom and not a diagnosis. It can significantly affect a patient's quality of life. Causes include:
- ***Rhinitis*** (see pp. 1076–1077). The most common aetiology is allergy-based. Rhinitis results in erythema of the nasal mucosa and hypertrophy of inferior turbinates. If an allergen is identified, then allergen avoidance is the mainstay of treatment. Topical steroids and/or antihistamines can be tried. If rhinitis is severe, then referral to an allergy clinic for immunotherapy is warranted. Short-term benefit can be gained in severe nasal blockage by surgically reducing the inferior turbinate.
- ***Septal deviation***. Correction can be undertaken surgically.
- ***Nasal polyps***. This condition occurs with inflammation and oedema of the sinus nasal mucosa. This oedematous mucosa prolapses into the nasal cavity and can cause significant nasal obstruction. In allergic rhinitis (see p. 1075), the mucosa lining the nasal septum and inferior turbinates are swollen and a dark-red or plum colour. Nasal polyps can be identified as glistening swellings, which are insensate. Treatment with intranasal steroids helps, but if polyps are large or unresponsive to medical treatment, then surgery is necessary.
- ***Foreign bodies***. These are usually seen in children who present with unilateral nasal discharge. Clinical examination of the nose with a light source often reveals the foreign body, which requires removal, either in clinic or in theatre, with a general anaesthetic.

Box 30.4 Types of sinusitis

Type	Duration of symptoms
Acute	1 week to 1 month
Recurrent acute	>4 episodes of acute sinusitis per year
Subacute	1–3 months
Chronic	>3 months

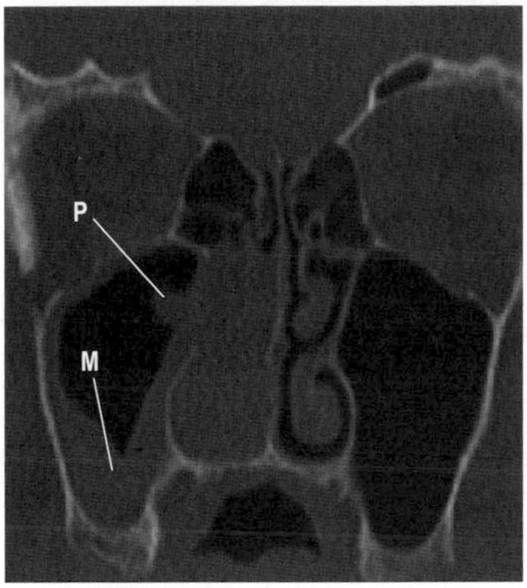

Figure 30.11 **CT of the sinuses.** An inverting papilloma (P) can be seen obstructing the right nostril, and there is mucosal thickening (M) of the right maxillary sinus.

- ***Sinonasal malignancy***. This is extremely rare. The diagnosis must be considered if unusual unilateral symptoms are seen, including nasal obstruction, epistaxis, pain, epiphora (watery eye), cheek swelling, paraesthesia of the cheek, unilateral serous otitis media and proptosis of the orbit.

Sinusitis

Sinusitis is an infection of the paranasal sinuses that is bacterial (mainly *Streptococcus pneumoniae* and *Haemophilus influenzae*) or occasionally fungal. It is most commonly associated with an upper respiratory tract infection and can occur with asthma. Symptoms include frontal headache, purulent rhinorrhoea, facial pain with tenderness, and fever. Sinusitis can be confused with a variety of other conditions, such as migraine, trigeminal neuralgia and cranial arteritis.

Management

Treatment for a bacterial sinusitis includes nasal decongestants, such as xylometazoline; broad-spectrum antibiotics, such as co-amoxiclav because *H. influenzae* can be resistant to amoxicillin; anti-inflammatory therapy with topical corticosteroids, such as fluticasone propionate (nasal spray) to reduce mucosal swelling; and steam inhalations.

If the symptoms of sinusitis are recurrent ***(Box 30.4)*** or complications such as orbital cellulitis arise, then an ENT opinion is appropriate and a computed tomography (CT) scan of the paranasal sinuses is undertaken. Plain sinus X-rays are now rarely used to image the sinuses.

CT scan of the sinuses ***(Fig. 30.11)*** or an MRI scan can demonstrate bony landmarks and soft tissue planes.

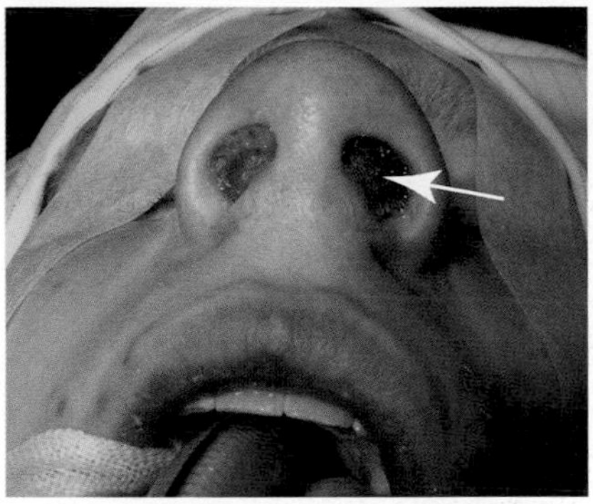

Figure 30.12 **Septal haematoma.**

Functional endoscopic sinus surgery (***FESS***) is used for ventilation and drainage of the sinuses.

Anosmia

Olfaction is mainly under the control of cranial nerve I, although irritant, unpleasant nasal sensations are carried by cranial nerves V, IX and X. Anosmia is a complete loss of the sense of smell and ***hyposmia*** is a decreased sense of smell:

- A ***conductive deficit*** of smell occurs if odorant molecules do not reach the olfactory epithelium high in the nose.
- A ***sensorineural loss*** of smell is incurred if the neural transmission of smell is affected.
- Some conditions predispose to a mixed (conductive and sensorineural) loss of smell.

The main cause of a loss of smell is nasal obstruction due to upper respiratory infection or nasal polyps. Other causes include sinonasal disease, old age, drug therapy and head injury/trauma. It is difficult to predict the speed and extent of recovery in the latter causes. In many, anosmia is idiopathic, but before this diagnosis is accepted, an assessment of the patient for the possibility of an intranasal tumour or intracranial mass should be undertaken.

Fractured nose

People with a fractured nose present with epistaxis, bruising of the eyes and nasal bridge swelling. Initially, it is often difficult to assess whether the bones are deviated, particularly if there is significant swelling. Reduction of the fracture should be undertaken in the first 2 weeks after injury and can be achieved by manipulation. However, if the fracture sets, a more formal rhinoplasty may have to be undertaken at a later stage. The patient should be examined for a head injury and the nose should also be checked for a septal haematoma ***(Fig. 30.12)***. This is painful, can cause nasal obstruction, is fluctuant to touch on the nasal septum, and requires immediate drainage to prevent destruction of the septal cartilage.

DISORDERS OF THE THROAT

ANATOMY AND PHYSIOLOGY

The throat can be considered as the oral cavity, the pharynx and the larynx ***(Fig. 30.13)***. The oral cavity extends from the lips to the tonsils. The pharynx can be divided into three areas:

- ***The nasopharynx*** extends from the posterior nasal openings to the soft palate

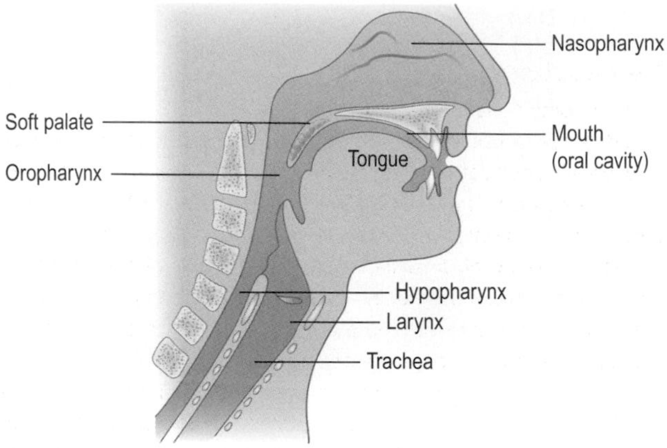

Figure 30.13 Normal anatomy of the throat.

- ***The oropharynx*** extends from the soft palate to the tip of the epiglottis
- ***The hypopharynx*** extends from the tip of the epiglottis to just below the level of the cricoid cartilage, where it is continuous with the oesophagus.

Lying within the hypopharynx is the larynx. This consists of cartilaginous, ligamentous and muscular tissue that has the primary function of protecting the distal airway. The pharynx is innervated from the pharyngeal plexus.

In the larynx, there are two vocal cords that abduct (open) during inspiration and adduct (close) to protect the airway and for voice production (phonation). The main nerve supply of the vocal cords comes from the recurrent laryngeal nerves (branches of the vagus nerve), which arise in the neck, but on the left side pass down around the aortic arch and then ascend in the tracheo-oesophageal groove to the larynx.

Normal vocal cords in phonation vibrate between 90 (male) and 180 (female) times per second, giving the voice its pitch or frequency. A healthy voice requires full closure of the vocal cords with a smooth, regular pattern of vibration, and any pathology that prevents full closure will result in air escaping between the vocal cords during phonation and a 'breathy' voice.

CLINICAL APPROACH TO THE PATIENT WITH A DISORDER OF THE THROAT

Examination

Good illumination is essential. Look at the teeth, gums, tongue, floor of mouth and oral cavity. The tonsils, soft palate and uvula are easily seen, and a gag reflex (see p. 810) is present. The remainder of the pharynx and larynx can be inspected with a laryngeal mirror or flexible nasendoscope.

Examination of the neck for lymph nodes and other masses is also performed.

COMMON DISORDERS OF THE THROAT

Hoarseness (dysphonia)

There are three essential components for voice production: an air source (the lungs); a vibratory source (the vocal cords); and a resonating chamber (the pharynx and nasal and oral cavities). Although chest and nasal disorders can affect the voice, the majority of hoarseness is due to laryngeal pathology.

Inflammation that increases the 'mass' of the vocal cords will cause the vocal cord frequency to fall, giving a much deeper voice. Thus listening to a patient's voice can often give a diagnosis before the vocal cords are examined.

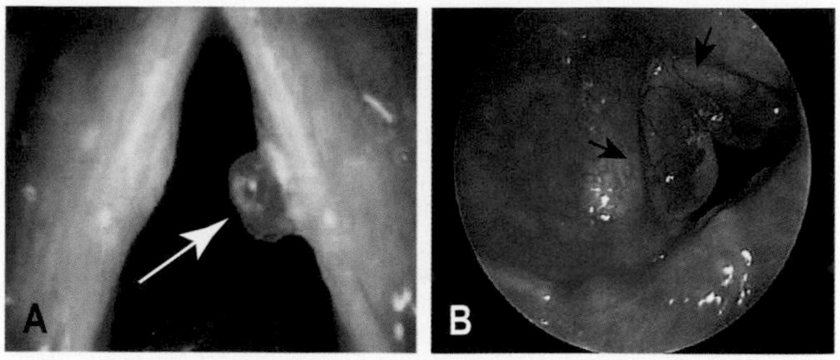

Figure 30.14 Disorders of the vocal cords. A. Vocal cord polyp. B. Reinke's oedema of the vocal cords.

Box 30.5 Red flags for hoarseness requiring urgent laryngoscopy

- Heavy smoking
- High alcohol intake
- Haemoptysis
- Dysphagia
- Pain, including otalgia
- Increasing dyspnoea

Nodules

Nodules (always bilateral and more common in females) and polyps ***(Fig. 30.14A)*** are found on the free edge of the vocal cord, preventing full closure and giving a 'breathy, harsh' voice. They are commonly found in professionals who rely on their voice for their livelihood, such as teachers, singers and lawyers. They are usually related to poor technique of voice production and can usually be cured with speech therapy. If surgery is needed, great care must be taken to remain in the superficial layers of the vocal cord in order to prevent deep scarring, which leaves the voice permanently hoarse.

Reinke's oedema

This is due to a collection of tissue fluid in the subepithelial layer of the vocal cord ***(Fig. 30.14B)***. The vocal cord has poor lymphatic drainage, predisposing it to oedema. Reinke's oedema is associated with irritation of the vocal cords by smoking, voice abuse, acid reflux and, very rarely, hypothyroidism. Treatment is to remove the irritation in most cases, but surgery to incise the cords and reduce the oedema will also allow the voice to return to its normal pitch.

Acute-onset hoarseness

Hoarseness, in a smoker, is a danger sign. Any patient with a hoarse voice for over 6 weeks should be seen by an ENT surgeon. Other red flag symptoms will require urgent laryngoscopy ***(Box 30.5)***. The voice may be deep, harsh and breathy, indicating a mass on the vocal cord ***(Fig. 30.15)***, or it can be weak, suggesting a paralysed left vocal cord secondary to mediastinal disease, such as bronchial carcinoma.

Early squamous cell carcinoma of the larynx has a good prognosis. Treatment is with carbon dioxide laser resection or radiotherapy. Spread and growth of the tumour can lead to referred otalgia, and, if the tumour is significant in its size, requires a laryngectomy (removal of the voicebox), with a neck dissection to remove the affected glands in the neck. A patient with a paralysed left vocal cord must have a CT of the neck and chest. Medialization of the paralysed cord to allow contact with the opposite cord can return the voice and give a competent larynx. This can be done under local or general anaesthesia, producing an immediate result whatever the long-term prognosis of the chest pathology.

Stridor

Stridor, or noisy breathing, can be divided into the following types:

- ***Inspiratory***: obstruction is at the level of the vocal cords or above.
- ***Mixed*** (both inspiratory and expiratory): obstruction is in the subglottis or extrathoracic trachea.
- ***Expiratory***: obstruction is in the intrathoracic trachea or distal airways.

All people with stridor, both paediatric and adult, are potentially at risk of asphyxiation and should be investigated fully. Severe stridor may be an indication for either intubation or a tracheostomy ***(Box 30.6)***.

Box 30.6 Indications for tracheostomy

- Upper airway obstruction (real or anticipated)
- Long-term ventilation
- Bronchial lavage
- Incompetent larynx with aspiration

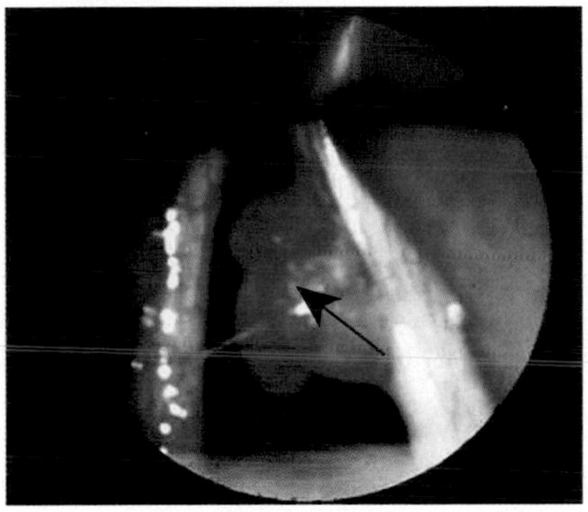

Figure 30.15 **Carcinoma of the right cord.**

Management

Tracheostomy

Tracheostomy tubes ***(Fig. 30.16)*** are:

- ***Cuffed or uncuffed***. A high-volume, low-pressure cuff is used to prevent aspiration and to allow positive-pressure ventilation.
- ***Fenestrated or unfenestrated***. A fenestrated cuff has a small hole on the greater curvature of the tube (both outer and inner), allowing air to escape upwards to the vocal cords; the patient can therefore speak. This tube often has a valve that allows air to enter from the stoma but closes on expiration, directing the air through the fenestration.

Most long-term tracheostomy tubes have an inner and an outer tube. The inner tube fits inside the outer tube and projects beyond its lower end. A major problem with a tracheostomy tube is crusting of its distal end with dried secretions, and this arrangement allows the inner tube to be removed, cleaned and replaced as frequently as required, without disrupting the outer tube.

When to decannulate a patient is often a difficult issue if laryngeal competence is unclear. Movement of the vocal cords requires an ENT examination and a speech therapist's involvement. The tracheostomy tube itself can also produce problems due to compression of the oesophagus with a cuffed tube and prevention of the larynx from rising during normal swallowing.

Tonsillitis and pharyngitis

Viral infections of the throat are common and, although many practitioners may be under pressure from the patient to give antibiotics, they should not be used. The vast majority of infections are usually self-limiting, settling with bed rest, analgesia and encouragement of fluid intake. Fungal infections, usually candidiasis, are uncommon and may indicate an immunocompromised patient or undiagnosed diabetes.

Tonsillitis

Tonsillitis, with a good history of pyrexia, dysphagia, lymphadenopathy and severe malaise, is usually bacterial; β-haemolytic streptococcus is the most common organism, which responds to penicillin V.

Glandular fever

Glandular fever (see p. 258) can also present with tonsillitis. Although, clinically, the tonsils have a confluent white exudate, there is often a petechial rash on the soft palate and an accompanying lymphadenopathy.

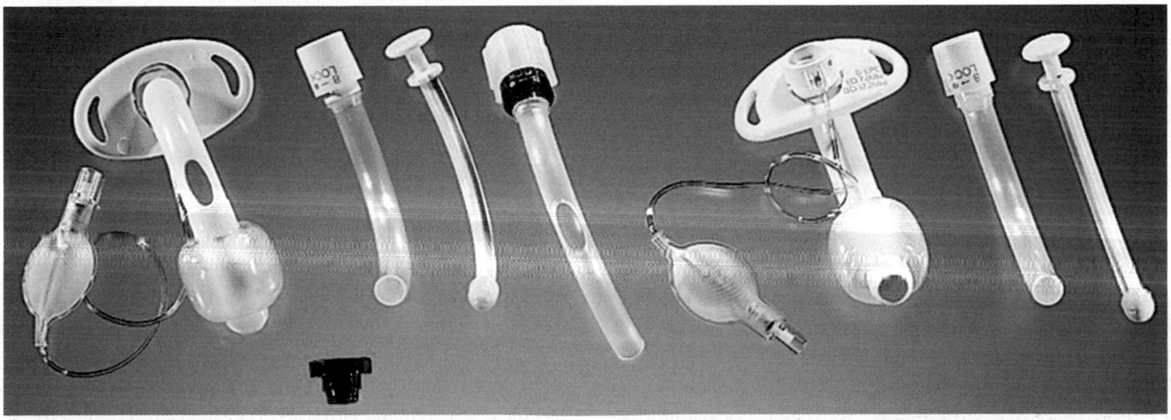

Figure 30.16 **Tracheostomy tubes and their accompanying components.**

Box 30.7 Indications for tonsillectomy

- Suspected malignancy
- Obstructive sleep apnoea due to tonsillar hypertrophy
- Recurrent tonsillitis: 5 attacks a year for at least 2 years
- Quinsy in a patient with a history of recurrent tonsillitis

Quinsy (peritonsillar abscess)

Quinsy is a collection of pus outside the capsule of the tonsil, usually located adjacent to its superior pole. The patient often has trismus, making examination difficult, but the pus pushes the uvula across the midline to the opposite side. The area is usually hyperaemic and smooth but unilateral tonsil ulceration is more likely to be a malignancy. In either case, urgent referral to an ENT specialist is essential.

Indications for a ***tonsillectomy*** are shown in ***Box 30.7***. This is carried out under a general anaesthetic and current surgical techniques include diathermy dissection, laser excision and coblation (using an ultrasonic dissecting probe). There are strong advocates for each technique and much will depend on the individual surgeon's preference. Some departments carry out tonsillectomy as a day-case procedure, as most reactionary bleeding will occur within the first 8 hours postoperatively.

Snoring

Snoring is caused by high-pressure airflow, resulting in vibration of soft tissue above the level of the larynx. It is a common symptom (50% of 50-year-old males will snore to some extent) and can be considered to be related to obstruction of three potential areas: the nose, the palate or/and the hypopharynx (see ***Fig. 24.26***). There is a strong association between snoring and sleep-disordered breathing, such as in obstructive sleep apnoea (see pp. 1085–1086).

The Epworth questionnaire (see ***Box 24.17***) can assist in identification of sleep apnoea. People with a history of habitual, non-positional, heroic snoring (can be heard through a wall) require a full ENT examination and can be investigated by sleep nasendoscopy, in which a sedated, snoring patient has a flexible nasendoscope inserted to identify the source of vibration.

Nasal pathology, such as polyps, can be removed surgically with good results and most patients will benefit from lifestyle changes, such as weight loss. Stiffening or shortening the soft palate via surgery, often using a laser, can help for palatal snorers but hypopharyngeal snorers require either a dental prosthesis at night to hold the mandible forwards or continuous positive airway pressure (CPAP) via a mask (see p. 1086).

Dysphagia

Dysphagia (see pp. 365–366) occurs because of any lesion between the throat and stomach. The two conditions described here are the ones usually dealt with by ENT departments. Gastroenterology departments see causes further down the gullet.

Pharyngeal pouch

A pharyngeal pouch is a herniation of mucosa through the fibres of the inferior pharyngeal constrictor muscle (cricopharyngeus) ***(Fig. 30.17A)***. An area of weakness known as Killian's dehiscence allows a pulsion diverticulum to form. Patients present with a neck swelling following a failed swallow attempt. They can occasionally compress the swelling to allow food particles to be pushed back into the oesophagus. They may also complain that a gurgling sound is heard in the neck following a swallow as liquid and food collect in the pouch. Occasionally, patients present with recurrent pneumonia following aspiration of food into the trachea. Diagnosis is made with a barium swallow ***(Fig. 30.18)*** and treatment is surgical, either via an external approach through the neck where the pouch is excised or, more commonly, via endoscopy with stapling of the party wall ***(Fig. 30.17B)***.

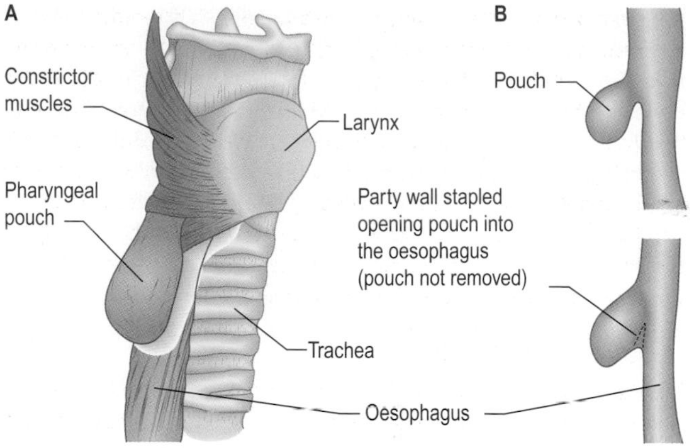

Figure 30.17 Pharyngeal pouch. A. Position of pharyngeal pouch. **B.** Stapling of the party wall between oesophagus and pouch.

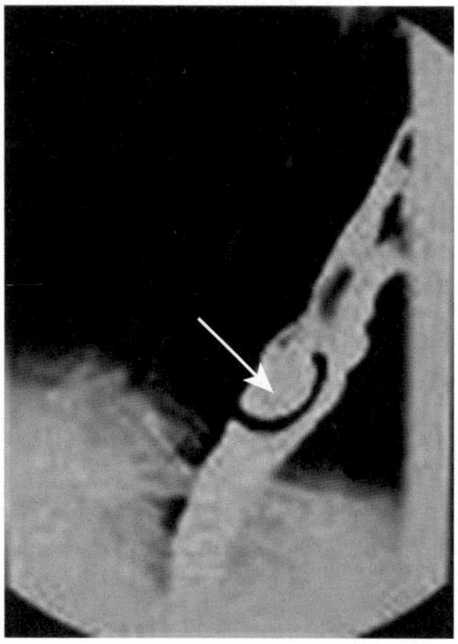

Figure 30.18 Pharyngeal pouch shown on barium swallow.

Foreign bodies

Foreign bodies in the pharynx can be divided into three general categories: soft food bolus, coins (smooth) and bones (sharp). Soft food bolus can be initially treated conservatively with muscle relaxants for 24 hours. Impacted coins should be removed at the earliest opportunity but sharp objects require emergency removal to avoid perforation of the muscle wall.

If the patient perceives the foreign body to be to one side, then it should be above the cricopharyngeus and an ENT examination will locate it; common areas are the tonsillar fossae, base of tongue, posterior pharyngeal wall and valleculae. Radiology will identify coins, and a clinical decision can be made to see whether a coin will pass down to the stomach; in this case no further treatment, is required as it will exit naturally. Some departments advocate the use of a metal detector to monitor the position of the coin in the patient, who is usually a child or has a mental disorder. Fish can be divided into those with a bony skeleton (teleosts) and those with a cartilaginous skeleton (elasmobranchs), and therefore radiology is useful only in some cases. Radiology can also identify air in the cervical oesophagus, indicating a radiolucent foreign body lying distally. A soft tissue lateral neck radiograph is the investigation of choice to delineate some of the features above.

Globus pharyngeus

This is a functional disorder and is not a true dysphagia. It is a condition with classic symptoms of an intermittent sensation of a lump in the throat. This is perceived to be in the midline at the level of the cricoid cartilage and is worse when swallowing saliva; indeed, it often disappears when ingesting food or liquids. ENT examination is clear and normal laryngeal mobility can be felt when gently rocking the larynx across the postcricoid tissues. A contrast swallow will not only show the structures below the pharynx but also assess the swallowing dynamically. Treatment is with explanation and reassurance. Antidepressants may be tried. Any suspicious area will require an endoscopy with biopsy.

Further reading

Dhillon RS, East CA. *Ear, Nose and Throat and Head and Neck Surgery*, 4th edn. Edinburgh: Churchill Livingstone; 2013.
Warner G, Burgess A, Patel S et al. *Otolaryngology and Head and Neck Surgery*. Oxford: Oxford University Press; 2009.
http://www.britishsnoring.co.uk *Interactive version of the Epworth Sleepiness Scale*.

DISORDERS OF THE EYE

Most of the major and common types of eye disease are covered below. However, diabetic eye disease (pp. 1265–1269) and hypertensive eye disease (p. 1046) are discussed elsewhere.

APPLIED ANATOMY AND PHYSIOLOGY

The average length of the human eye is 24 mm. It is essentially made up of two segments:

- The smaller anterior segment is transparent and coated by the cornea; its radius is approximately 8 mm.
- The larger posterior segment is coated by the opaque sclera; its radius is approximately 12 mm.

It is the cornea and the sclera that give the mechanical strength and shape to the exposed surface of the eye.

The cornea occupies the central aspect of the globe and is one of the most richly innervated tissues in the body. This clear, transparent, avascular structure, measuring 12 mm horizontally and 11 mm vertically, provides 78% of the focusing power of the eye. The eyelids prevent the cornea from drying and becoming an irregular surface by distributing the tear film over the surface of the globe with each blink.

Anatomically, the cornea is made up of five layers:

- epithelium
- Bowman's layer (membrane)
- stroma
- Descemet's membrane
- endothelium.

The endothelial cells lining the inner surface of the cornea are responsible for maintaining the clarity of the cornea by continuously pumping fluid out of the tissue. Any factor that alters the function of these cells will result in corneal oedema and cause blurred vision.

The sclera is an opaque white structure covering four-fifths of the globe and is continuous with the cornea at the limbus. The six extraocular muscles responsible for eye movements are attached to the sclera, and the optic nerve perforates it posteriorly.

The conjunctiva covers the anterior surface of the sclera. This richly vascularized and innervated mucous membrane stretches from the limbus over the anterior sclera (where it is called the bulbar conjunctiva) and is then reflected on to the undersurface of the upper and lower lids (the tarsal conjunctiva). The area of conjunctival reflection under the lids makes up the upper and lower fornix.

The anterior chamber is the space between the cornea and the iris, and is filled with aqueous humour ***(Fig. 30.19)***. This fluid is produced by the ciliary body (2 μL/min) and provides nutrients and oxygen to the avascular cornea. The outflow of aqueous humour is through the trabecular meshwork and canal of Schlemm adjacent to the limbus. Any factor that impedes its outflow will increase the intraocular pressure. The upper range of normal for intraocular pressure is 21 mmHg.

The uveal tract is made up of the iris anteriorly, the ciliary body and the choroid. The ***iris*** is the coloured part of the eye under the transparent cornea. The muscles of the iris diaphragm regulate the size of the pupil, thereby controlling the amount of light entering the eye. The muscles of the ***ciliary body*** control the accommodation of the lens, and the secretory epithelium produces the aqueous humour (see above). The highly vascular ***choroid*** lines the inner aspect of the sclera and upon this lies the retina.

The lens lies immediately posterior to the pupil and anterior to the vitreous humour. It is a transparent biconvex structure and is responsible for 22% of the refractive power of the eye. By changing its shape, it can alter its refractive power and help to focus objects at different distances from the eye. By the fourth decade of life, this ability to change shape starts to decline and, with time, the lens starts to become less transparent and cataracts begin to develop.

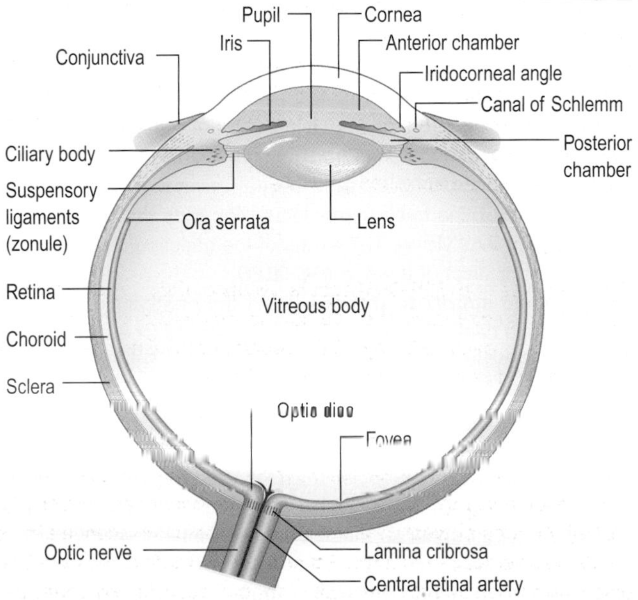

Figure 30.19 Cross-section of the eyeball.

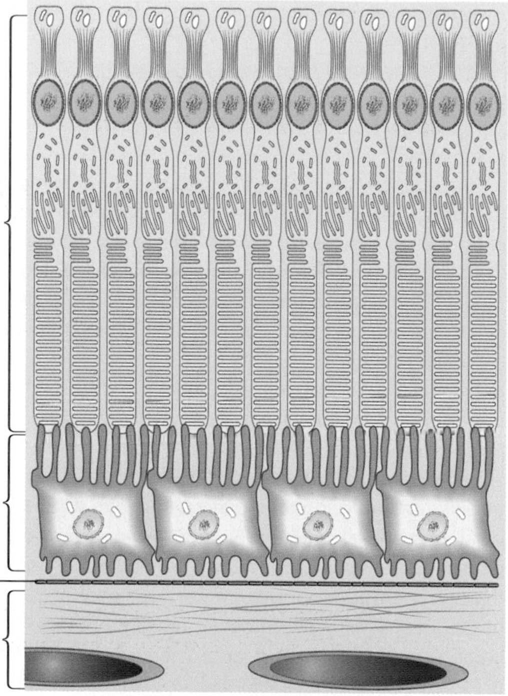

Figure 30.20 Schematic diagram of the retina.

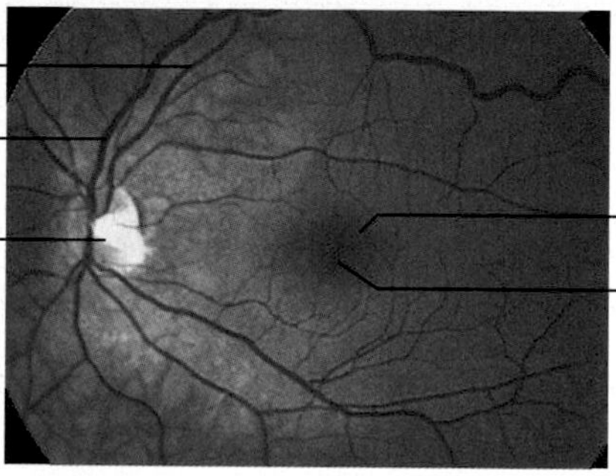

Figure 30.21 Fundus photograph of the left eye.

The vitreous humour fills the cavity between the retina and the lens.

The retina is a multilayered structure. The metabolically active region of the retina is represented in ***Figure 30.20***. There are two types of photoreceptors in the retina: rods and cones. There are approximately 6 million cones, mainly confined to the ***macula***, and these are responsible for detailed central vision and colour vision. The peripheral retina has around 125 million rods that are responsible for peripheral vision. The axons of the ganglion cells form the optic nerve (or disc) of the eye ***(Fig. 30.21)***.

The blood supply to the eye is via the ophthalmic artery; in particular, the central retinal artery is responsible for supplying the inner retinal layers. Venous return is through the central retinal and ophthalmic veins. Local lymphatic drainage is to the pre-auricular and submental nodes.

The sensory innervation of the eye is through the trigeminal (Vth) nerve. The six extraocular muscles are supplied by different nerves (see pp. 805–806):

- oculomotor (IIIrd) nerve: medial, superior, inferior rectus and inferior oblique
- trochlear (IVth) nerve: superior oblique
- abducens (VIth) nerve: lateral rectus.

The oculomotor (IIIrd) nerve also supplies the upper lid and, indirectly, the pupil (parasympathetic fibres are attached to it). The facial (VIIth) nerve supplies the orbicularis and other muscles of facial expression.

CLINICAL APPROACH TO THE PATIENT WITH A DISORDER OF THE EYE

History and examination

A detailed history gives most of the facts needed to make a working diagnosis. The eye has limited mechanisms by which it can convey a diseased state. Common symptoms include alteration in visual acuity, redness, pain, discharge and photophobia.

It is essential to adopt a systematic approach to the examination of the eye. Different approaches and instruments (including direct ophthalmoscope, slit lamp with or without Goldman or Volk lens) are necessary for examination of the lids and anterior and posterior segments, as well as extraocular movements.

Visual acuity

It is vital for an accurate assessment of visual acuity to be recorded in all people with an eye problem. The visual acuity of each eye is recorded in two ways: distance visual acuity and near visual acuity. Distance vision is measured in Snellen letters or, ever more commonly, in LogMAR letters or figures of different sizes (see below). The recording is given as an expression of the line of letters that can be discerned at a particular distance, usually 6 metres (20 feet): for example 6/60, where 6 equals the distance of the chart from the eye in metres and 60 equals the distance at which the letter subtends 5′ at the nodal point.

The Snellen visual acuity chart ***(Fig. 30.22)*** is most commonly employed, but use of the LogMAR chart (*log*arithm of the *M*inimum *A*ngle of *R*esolution; ***Fig. 30.23***) is increasing, largely due to its necessity in studies or research, since it allows better statistical analysis of results. Unlike the Snellen and other visual acuity charts, the LogMAR chart has equal graduation between the letters on a line, as well as the space between lines. There is also a fixed number of letters – five – on each line. Research conducted using a logarithmic progression in size of letters on a test chart provides the most accurate visual acuity measurement. Snellen equivalents can be calculated from the LogMAR charts if necessary ***(Fig. 30.24)***.

COMMON DISORDERS OF THE EYE

Refractive errors

The eye projects a sharp and focused image on to the retina. Refractive errors refer to any abnormality in the focusing mechanism of the eye and not to any opacity in the system, such as a corneal or retinal scar.

The refraction of light in emmetropic (normal), myopic (short-sighted; negative lenses will correct) and hypermetropic (long-sighted; positive lenses will correct) eyes is shown in ***Figure 30.25***.

Astigmatism is a refractive error of the eye in which there is a different degree of refraction in the different meridians of curvature. It may be myopic in one plane and hypermetropic or emmetropic in the other plane. In this situation, the front surface of the eye is shaped more like a rugby ball than a football.

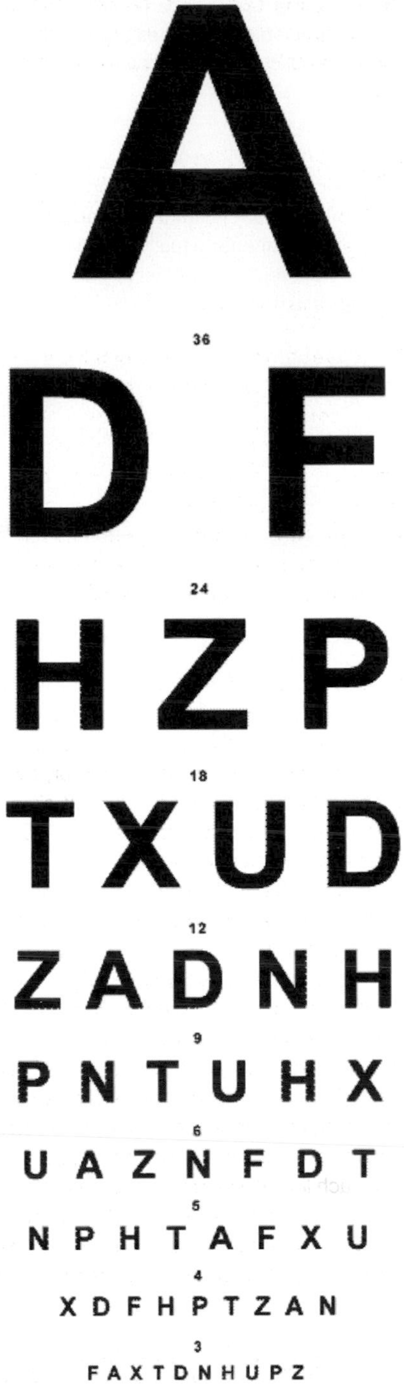

Figure 30.22 Snellen chart.

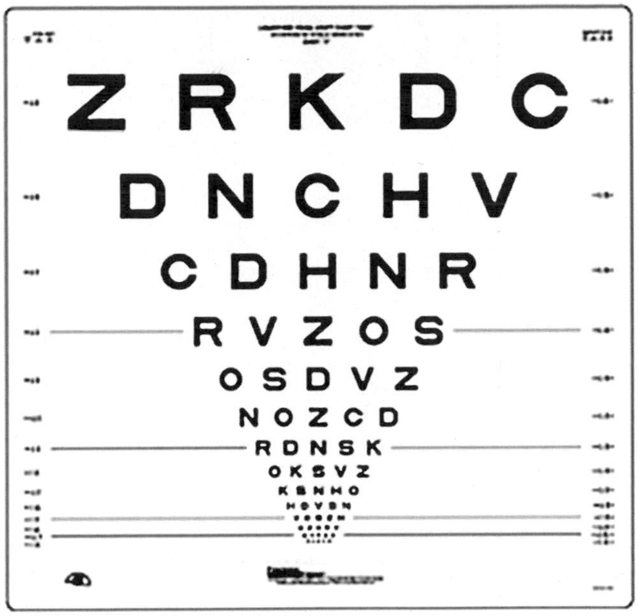

Figure 30.23 LogMAR chart (*log*arithm of the *M*inimum *A*ngle of *R*esolution).

20 feet (Snellen)	6 metres (Snellen)	Decimal	4 metres	logMAR
20/200	6/60	0.1	4/40	+1.0
20/160	6/48	0.125	4/32	+0.9
20/125	6/38	0.16	4/25	+0.8
20/100	6/30	0.2	4/20	+0.7
20/80	6/24	0.25	4/16	+0.6
20/63	6/19	0.32	4/12.5	+0.5
20/50	6/15	0.4	4/10	+0.4
20/40	6/12	0.5	4/8	+0.3
20/32	6/9.5	0.63	4/6.3	+0.2
20/25	6/7.5	0.8	4/5	+0.1
20/20	6/6	1.0	4/4	+0.0
20/16	6/4.8	1.25	4/3.2	-0.1
20/12.5	6/3.8	1.60	4/2.5	-0.2
20/10	6/3	2.0	4/2	-0.3

Figure 30.24 Snellen equivalents can be calculated from the LogMAR charts if necessary. Vision is often recorded at 4 metres in studies, and logMAR equivalents or decimals are used in statistics.

Presbyopia is the term used to describe the normal ageing of the lens, which leads to a change in the refractive state of the eye. As the lens ages, it becomes less able to alter its curvature and this causes difficulty with near vision, especially reading.

Management

Errors of refraction can be corrected by using spectacles or contact lenses. The latter often result in better-quality vision but carry the risk of infection. They may be the only option in some refractive states such as keratoconus, a degenerative disorder of the eye in which structural changes within the cornea cause it to thin and to take on a more conical shape than its normal gradual curve. A number of surgical techniques can correct these errors of refraction, with varying degrees of accuracy. Phakic intraocular lenses may be used to treat high degrees of myopia but the most popular method remains the excimer laser to re-profile the corneal curvature (using PRK, LASIK and LASEK techniques). The laser either removes corneal tissue centrally to flatten the cornea in myopia or it removes tissue from the peripheral cornea to steepen it in hypermetropia.

Disorders of the lids

The lids afford protection to the eyes and help to distribute the tear film over the front surface of the globe. Excess tears are drained via the puncta and lacrimal system to the nose ***(Fig. 30.26)***. Malposition of the lids, factors that affect blinking and lacrimal drainage can all cause problems.

Entropion

The lid margin rolls inwards so that the lashes are against the globe ***(Fig. 30.27A)***. The lashes act as a foreign body and cause

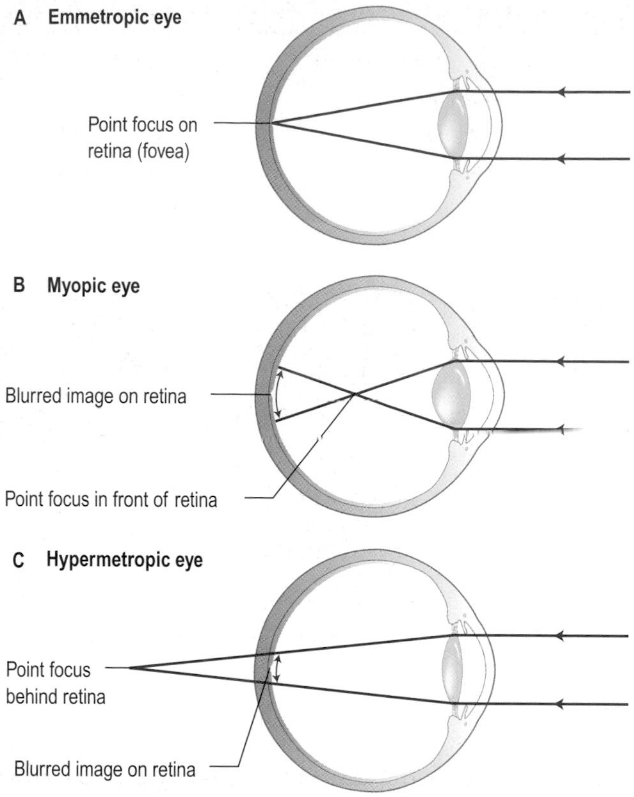

Figure 30.25 **Refraction. A.** Emmetropic (normal). **B.** Myopic (short-sighted). **C.** Hypermetropic (long-sighted).

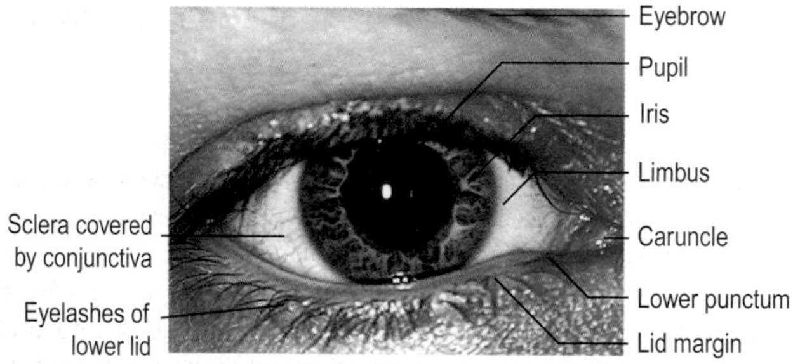

Figure 30.26 **The right eye.**

irritation, leading to a red eye that can mimic conjunctivitis. Occasionally, the constant rubbing of lashes against the cornea causes an abrasion. The most common cause is ageing and surgery is usually required.

Ectropion

The lid margin rolls outwards and is not apposed to the globe. As a result, the lacrimal punctum is not in the correct anatomical position to drain tears and patients usually complain of a watery eye. Underlying factors include age, VIIth nerve palsy and cicatricial skin conditions. Surgery is usually required.

Dacryocystitis

Patients who have inflammation of the lacrimal sac usually present with a painful lump at the side of the nose adjacent to the lower lid ***(Fig. 30.27B)***. This should be treated with oral broad-spectrum antibiotics such as a cephalosporin, and patients should be watched carefully for signs of cellulitis. All patients should be referred to the ophthalmologist, as some have an underlying mucocele or dilated sac, and will require surgery.

Blepharitis

This is an extremely common condition in which inflammation of the lid margins may involve the lashes and lash follicles ***(Fig. 30.28A)***, resulting in styes, or inflammation and blockage of meibomian glands ***(Fig. 30.28B)*** leading to chalazion ***(Fig. 30.28C)***. Common underlying causes of blepharitis include meibomian gland dysfunction, seborrhoea and *Staphylococcus aureus* infection. Patients can be asymptomatic or complain of itchy, burning eyes because of tear film instability resulting from meibomian gland dysfunction. *Staph. aureus* is frequently responsible for chronic blepharoconjunctivitis and some patients may develop keratitis in the cornea ***(Fig. 30.29)***.

Management

Lid hygiene is the mainstay of treatment for blepharitis, as it helps to reduce the bacterial load and unblock meibomian glands. A short course of topical chloramphenicol or fusidic acid is useful in chronic cases, but in severe cases or cases where acne rosacea is suspected, oral doxycycline is used. Some patients are left with a lump once the acute inflammatory phase has subsided. Most of these patients find the lump, or chalazion, cosmetically unacceptable and require incision and curettage. People with keratitis should be referred to the ophthalmologist for topical steroids.

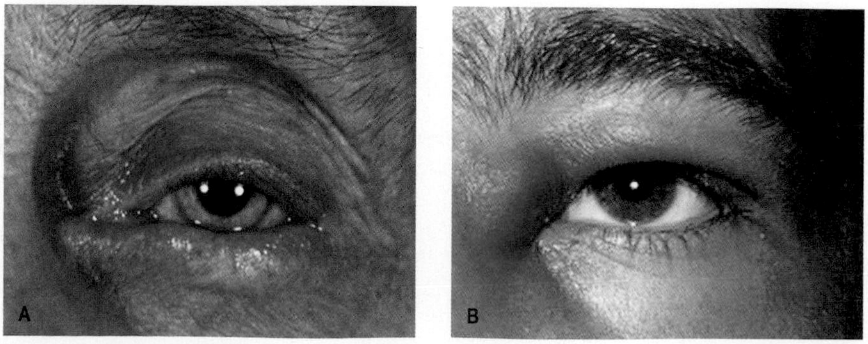

Figure 30.27 **Disorders of the eyelid. A.** Lid entropion. The lower lid appears inverted. **B.** Acute dacryocystitis, showing a lump on the side of the nose.

Box 30.8 Conjunctivitis

Type	Discharge	Pre-auricular node	Corneal involvement	Comment
Bacterial	Mucopurulent	–ve (except gonococci)	+ve Gonococcus	Rapid onset
Viral	Watery	+ve	+ve Adenovirus	Cold and/or sore throat
Chlamydial	Watery	+ve	+ve	Genitourinary discharge
Allergic	Stringy	–ve	+ve	Itchiness

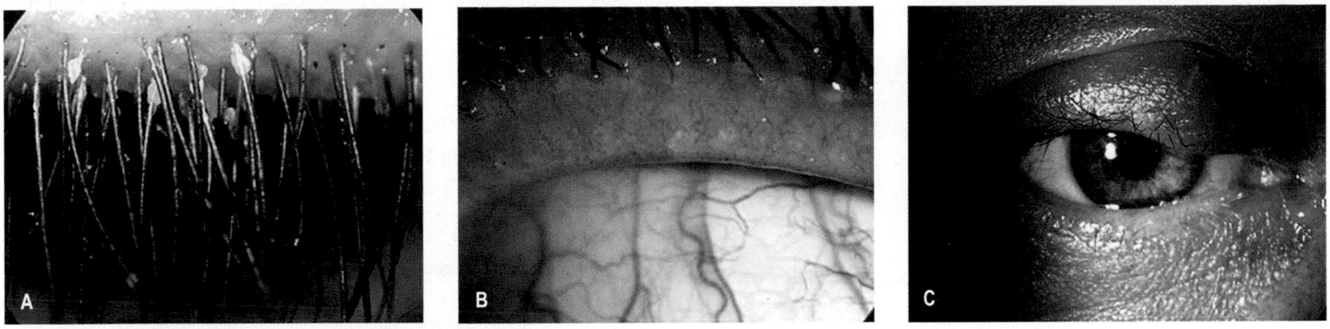

Figure 30.28 Blepharitis. A. Crusty and scaly deposits on the lashes and lash bases. **B.** Upper lid showing meibomian glands plugged with oily secretions. **C.** Blockage of the meibomian glands leads to swelling of the lid (chalazion).

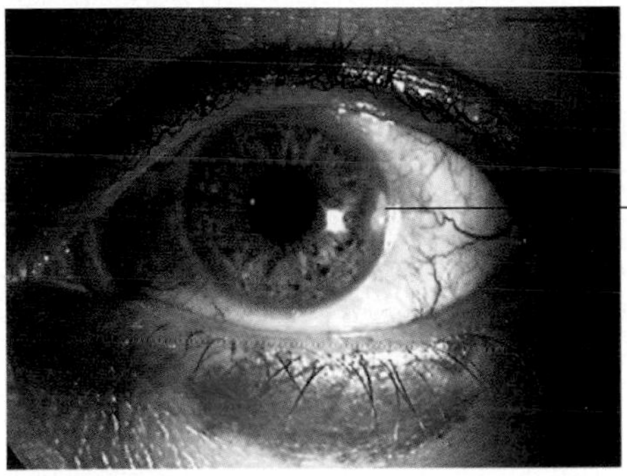

Figure 30.29 Marginal keratitis.

Conjunctivitis

The most common cause of a red eye, inflammation of the conjunctiva can arise from a number of causes, viral, bacterial and allergic being the most frequently encountered. Common features in all types include soreness, redness and discharge; in general, the visual acuity is good. History should include the speed of onset of the inflammation, the colour and consistency of the discharge, whether the eye is itchy, and if there has been a recent history of a cold or sore throat. In the neonate, it is vital to exclude gonococcal or chlamydial conjunctivitis associated with maternal sexually transmitted infection. The differential diagnosis of conjunctivitis is shown in ***Box 30.8***.

Bacterial conjunctivitis

Bacterial conjunctivitis is uncommon, making up 5% of all cases of conjunctivitis. In the vast majority of patients, it causes a sore or gritty eye in the presence of good vision. Bacterial conjunctivitis is invariably bilateral and should be suspected when conjunctival inflammation is associated with a purulent discharge.

Clinical features

Gonococcal conjunctivitis should be suspected when the onset of symptoms is rapid, the discharge is copious, and ocular inflammation includes chemosis (conjunctival oedema) and lid oedema. Gonococci are a cause of conjunctivitis, giving rise to a palpable pre-auricular node. Less acute or subacute purulent conjunctivitis with moderate discharge can be attributed to organisms such as *Haemophilus influenzae* and *Streptococcus pneumoniae*. Chronic conjunctivitis is usually associated with mild conjunctival injection and scant purulent discharge. Common organisms include *Staphylococcus aureus* and *Moraxella lacunata*.

Management

Prompt treatment with oral and topical penicillin is given in gonococcal conjunctivitis to ensure a reduced rate of corneal perforation. A Gram stain of the conjunctival swab can quickly confirm the presence of diplococci. Gonococcal conjunctivitis is a notifiable disease in the UK. Empirical treatment for both subacute and chronic conjunctivitis involves a topical broad-spectrum antibiotic, such as chloramphenicol. Swabs should be taken if these cases do not respond to this initial treatment. Antibiotic resistance is increasing.

Chlamydial conjunctivitis

Chlamydia trachomatis (see pp. 321–322) in developed countries causes a sexually transmitted infection that is most prevalent in sexually active adolescents and young adults. Direct or indirect contact with genital secretions is the usual route of infections but shared eye cosmetics can also be involved. Neonatal chlamydial conjunctivitis is a notifiable disease in the UK and should be suspected in newborns with a red eye. Mothers should be asked about sexually transmitted infections.

Clinical features

The onset of symptoms is slow, and patients may complain of mild discomfort for weeks. In these cases, the red eye is associated with

Box 30.9 Trachoma

- A very common cause of blindness worldwide (see p. 288)
- Found mainly in the tropics and the Middle East
- Caused by *Chlamydia trachomatis* but not usually sexually transmitted
- Chronic conjunctival inflammation causes progressive scarring, trichiasis, entropion and subsequent corneal scarring
- The result may be severe visual impairment or blindness from corneal opacification or ulceration

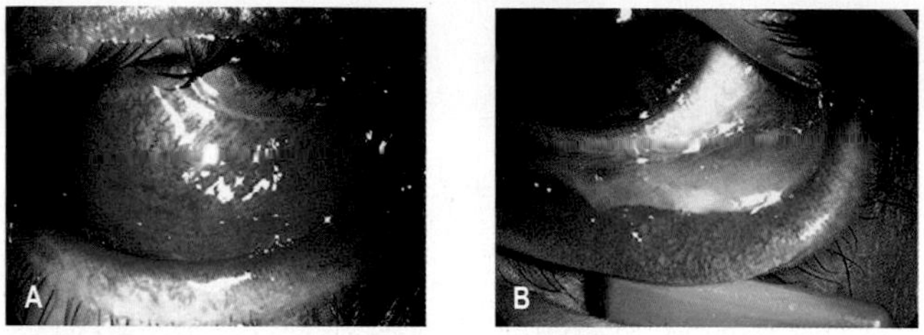

Figure 30.30 Viral conjunctivitis. A. Conjunctival chemosis. **B.** Pseudomembrane on lower lid.

a scanty mucopurulent discharge and a palpable pre-auricular lymph node. In chronic cases, it is not unusual to see superior corneal vascularization. In neonates, the onset of the red eye is typically around 2 weeks after birth, whereas gonococcal conjunctivitis occurs within days of birth. Conjunctival swabs should be taken and a nucleic acid amplification test (NAAT; see p. 321) performed prior to commencement of treatment.

Management

Topical erythromycin twice daily is commenced and patients referred to the genitourinary physician. Neonates should be started on topical erythromycin and referred to the paediatrician, as there may be associated otitis media or pneumonitis.

Trachoma

See ***Box 30.9***.

Viral conjunctivitis

Adenoviral conjunctivitis

This is highly contagious and can cause epidemics in communities. Transmission is through direct or indirect contact with infected individuals. The onset of symptoms may be preceded by a cold or influenza-like symptoms. Inflammation is commonly associated with chemosis, lid oedema and a palpable pre-auricular lymph node. Some patients develop a membrane on the tarsal conjunctiva ***(Fig. 30.30)*** and haemorrhage on the bulbar conjunctiva. Viral conjunctivitis can cause deterioration in visual acuity owing to corneal involvement (focal areas of inflammation). In 50% of these patients, the conjunctivitis is unilateral.

The condition is largely self-limiting in the majority of cases. Lubricants, together with a cold compress, can be a soothing element of ***management*** for patients. Adhering to strict hygiene and keeping towels separate from those of the rest of the household go a long way towards reducing the spread of the infection. In people with corneal involvement or intense conjunctival inflammation, topical steroids are indicated.

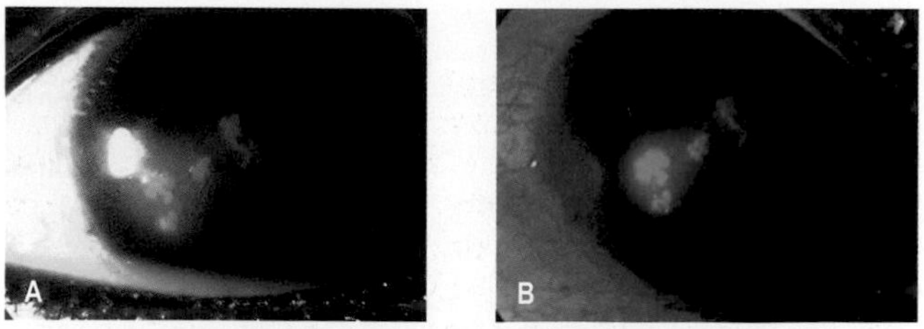

Figure 30.31 Dendritic ulcers on the cornea. A. Stained with fluorescein. **B.** Stained with fluorescein and viewed with blue light.

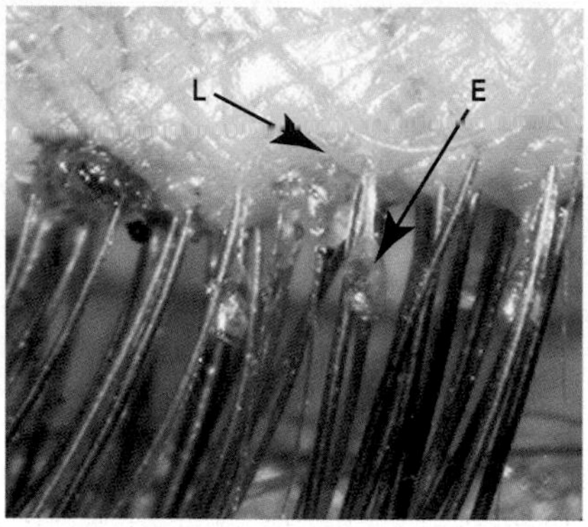

Figure 30.32 Phthiriasis palpebrarum. The lice (L) and the nits (eggs) can be seen on the lid margins. E, empty egg.

Herpes simplex conjunctivitis

Primary ocular herpes simplex conjunctivitis is typically unilateral. It usually causes a palpable pre-auricular lymph node, and cutaneous vesicles develop on the eyelids and the skin around the eyes in the majority. Over 50% of these patients develop a dendritic corneal ulcer ***(Fig. 30.31)***. The organism responsible for this condition is the herpes simplex virus (HSV), usually HSV-1, although HSV-2 can give rise to ocular infection.

Primary ocular HSV infection is self-limiting but most clinicians choose ***treatment*** with topical aciclovir in order to limit the risk of corneal epithelial involvement.

Molluscum contagiosum conjunctivitis

This is typically unilateral; it produces a red eye that generally goes unrecognized and comes to the forefront because patients fail to improve and the cornea starts to become involved. On close inspection, pearly, umbilicated nodules, filled with the DNA poxvirus, can be seen on the lid margin.

Management includes curetting the central portion of the lesion, freezing the centre or completely excising the lesion. If the corneal involvement is severe or the eye is very inflamed, a short course of topical steroids, such as prednisolone 0.5% or dexamethasone 0.1%, is helpful.

Phthiriasis palpebrarum

Phthiriasis palpebrarum ***(Fig. 30.32)*** is an eyelid infestation caused by *Phthirus pubis*, or the crab louse. Infestation of the cilia and eyelid is rare. It leads to blepharitis with marked conjunctival inflammation, pre-auricular lymphadenopathy and, rarely, secondary infection at the site of louse bite.

Management

Mechanical removal of the lice with fine forceps, physostigmine 1.25% and pilocarpine gel 4% are all effective treatments.

Allergic conjunctivitis

There are five main types of allergic conjunctivitis: seasonal, perennial, vernal, atopic and giant papillary. Both seasonal and perennial allergic conjunctivitis are acute allergic conjunctival disorders. Symptoms include itching and pink to reddish eyes. These two eye conditions are mediated by mast cells and can be treated easily with cold compresses, eye washes with tear substitutes, and avoidance of allergens. The last three are difficult to treat; they are chronic and can be sight-threatening, so should be referred to an ophthalmologist.

Seasonal/perennial conjunctivitis

Seasonal allergic conjunctivitis and perennial conjunctivitis, affecting 20% of the general population in the UK, are allergic reactions to grass and tree pollen and fungal spores. Seasonal allergic conjunctivitis occurs mainly in spring and summer. Perennial allergic conjunctivitis occurs all year round but peaks in the autumn; causes include allergens, such as house-dust mites.

The main symptoms include itching, redness, soreness, watering and a stringy discharge. Occasionally, the conjunctiva may become so hyperaemic that chemosis results. This is usually associated with swollen lids.

Lowering the allergen load (reducing dust; see p. 1077) is helpful. Medical ***treatment*** includes the use of antihistamine drops such as azelastine and emedastine, together with topical mast-cell-stabilizing agents such as sodium cromoglicate and nedocromil. Olopatadine (twice daily) has dual action and is very effective. Corticosteroid drops should be avoided. Oral antihistamines help the itching.

Corneal disorders

Trauma

Corneal abrasions

Trauma resulting in the removal of a focal area of epithelium on the cornea is very common. Abrasions usually occur when the eye is accidentally poked with a finger, a foreign body flies into the eye or something brushes against the eye.

Symptoms include severe pain, due to exposure of the corneal nerve endings, lacrimation and inability to open the eye (blepharospasm). Blinking and eye movement can aggravate the pain and foreign body sensation. The visual acuity is usually reduced. Most cases will need topical anaesthetic drops such as oxybuprocaine or tetracaine to be administered before it is possible to examine the eye. The cornea should be inspected with a blue light after instillation of fluorescein drops. The orange dye will stain the area of the abrasion. Under blue light, the abrasion lights up as green. Occasionally, foreign bodies can lodge on the undersurface of the upper lid and give rise to linear vertical abrasions. Eversion of the upper lid is necessary in all cases of abrasions ***(Fig. 30.33)***.

Treatment consists of a broad-spectrum topical antibiotic, such as chloramphenicol drops or ointment four times a day for 5 days. The role of padding is controversial but common practice is to pad the affected eye for 24 hours once chloramphenicol ointment has been applied to the eye.

Corneal foreign body

Occasionally, when something flies into the eye, it sticks on the cornea ***(Fig. 30.34A)***. It may be associated with lacrimation and photophobia. Examination is best attempted following instillation of a topical anaesthetic and should include eversion of the upper lid ***(Fig. 30.34B)***. Corneal foreign bodies can usually be seen directly with a white light.

The corneal foreign body should be removed. ***Treatment*** involves a topical antibiotic, such as chloramphenicol four times a day for 5 days, or fusidic acid twice a day for 5 days.

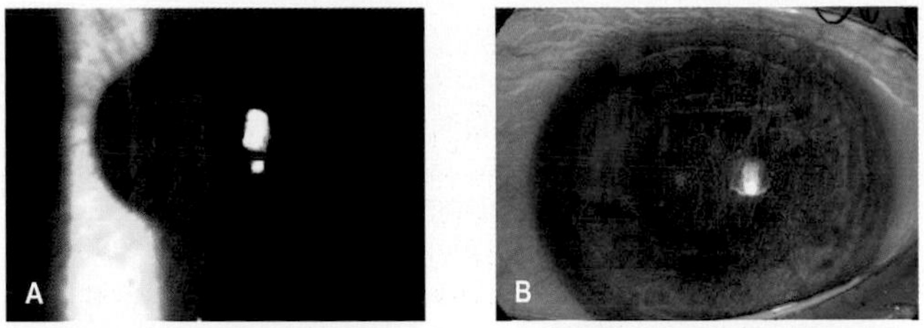

Figure 30.33 Linear corneal abrasion. A. Stained with fluorescein. **B.** Stained with fluorescein and viewed with blue light.

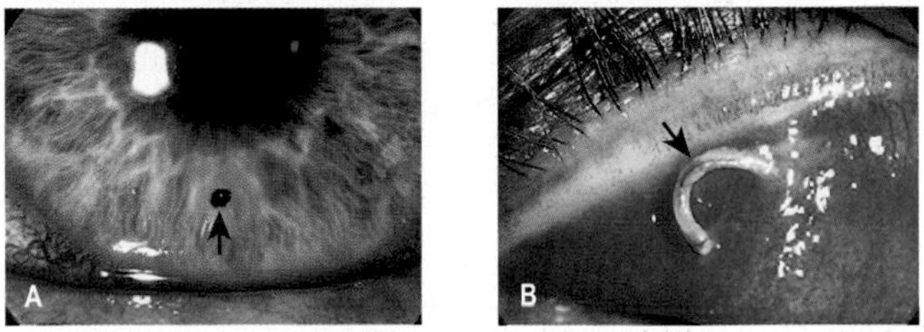

Figure 30.34 Foreign bodies (arrowed). A. Corneal. **B.** Subtarsal.

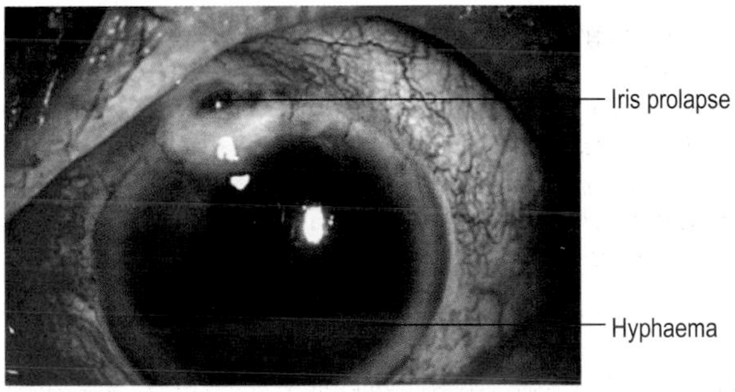

Figure 30.35 Blunt trauma. Hyphaema and globe rupture with iris prolapse.

High-velocity trauma

In cases of high-velocity trauma, corneal perforation or an intraocular foreign body should be suspected. Examination may show a corneal laceration and a foreign body may also be embedded in the cornea. The foreign body may be present on the iris or in the lens or vitreous. Other clues pointing towards a penetrating injury include a large subconjunctival haemorrhage, a flat anterior chamber with low intraocular pressure, and the presence of blood in the anterior chamber (hyphaema). Urgent referral to the ophthalmologist is mandatory, ensuring that no drops are instilled into the eye and that a plastic shield is placed over the eye to minimize further risk of trauma.

Blunt trauma usually results in periorbital bruising and gross lid oedema, which can make examination to exclude perforating injury difficult. These patients should be referred to the ophthalmologist for a detailed ocular examination to exclude a perforation, retinal detachment or a traumatic hyphaema ***(Fig. 30.35)***.

Keratitis

This is a general term used to describe corneal inflammation. Common causes include herpes simplex virus, contact lens-associated infection and blepharitis. Symptoms include the sensation of a foreign body or pain (depending on the size and depth of the ulcer), photophobia and lacrimation. Vision is reduced if the ulcer affects the visual axis.

Herpes simplex keratitis

Corneal epithelial cells infected with the virus eventually undergo lysis and form an ulcer, which is typically dendritic in shape (see Fig. 30.31). The ulcer stains with fluorescein and can be observed easily with a blue light. Topical immunosuppression, such as with steroid drops, or systemic immunosuppression, such as in AIDS, can lead to the centrifugal spread of the virus, such that the ulcer increases in area and is referred to as a geographic ulcer. Recurrent attacks of HSV keratitis can be triggered by ultraviolet light, stress and menstruation. All these factors are responsible for activating the virus, which normally lies dormant in the ganglion of the Vth nerve.

Treatment consists of aciclovir ointment five times a day for 2 weeks; this is usually very effective.

Contact lens-related keratitis

A small number of contact lens wearers develop infective corneal ulcers, which are potentially sight-threatening ***(Fig. 30.36)***. The organisms usually responsible include Gram-positive and Gram-negative bacteria. Patients should be referred to an ophthalmologist for scraping of the ulcer and commencement of antibiotic treatment.

Keratoconus

Keratoconus is an eye condition in which the normally round, dome-shaped cornea progressively thins and causes a cone-shaped bulge to develop. Aetiology is uncertain but genetic factors play a role, and the condition is more common in people with allergic diseases such as asthma, in Down syndrome and in some disorders of collagen such as Marfan's disease. Keratoconus affects up to 1 in 1000 people and is more common in individuals of Asian heritage. It is usually diagnosed in teenagers and young people.

Management

In the early stages, spectacles or soft contact lenses may be used to correct vision. As the cornea becomes thinner and steeper, rigid gas-permeable contact lenses may be necessary.

Corneal cross-linking is a new treatment that can stop keratoconus becoming worse. It is effective in more than 9 out of 10 patients, with a single 30-minute day-case procedure, but is only suitable when the corneal shape is continuing to deteriorate. In very advanced cases, where contact lenses fail to improve vision, a corneal transplant may be needed.

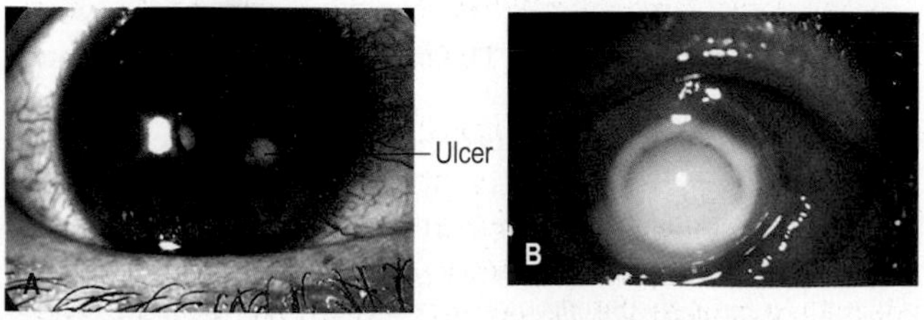

Figure 30.36 **Contact lens-related keratitis. A.** Corneal ulcer. **B.** Severe keratitis with a corneal abscess and a hypopyon.

Corneal dystrophy

Corneal dystrophies may be classified anatomically as consisting of:

- epithelial and subepithelial dystrophies
- epithelial–stromal *TGFBI* corneal dystrophies
- stromal dystrophies
- endothelial dystrophies.

The most common endothelial dystrophy, Fuchs' corneal dystrophy, is a genetically associated degenerative disorder leading to corneal oedema and vision loss. The gene involved is *TCF4*. The condition affects both eyes; it is more common in females and is of gradual onset, leading to blindness in the 40–60 age group. There is an accumulation of deposits (guttae) in the cornea with thickening of Descemet's membrane. Treatment is by corneal transplantation.

Cataracts

Cataract ***(Fig. 30.37)*** is by far the most common cause of preventable blindness in the world, having an effective surgical treatment. In the UK, approximately 250 000 cataract operations are performed each year, making it the most common surgical procedure.

Aetiology

Age-related opacification of the lens (cataract) is the commonest cause of visual impairment, with 30% of people over 65 years having visual acuities below that required for driving (Snellen acuity less than 6/12). The common causes of cataracts are summarized in ***Box 30.10***.

In young patients, familial or congenital causes should be excluded. Any history of ocular inflammation is noted. Cataracts diagnosed in infants demand urgent referral to the ophthalmologist in order to minimize the subsequent development of amblyopia.

Clinical features

Gradual painless deterioration of vision is the most common symptom. Other symptoms are dependent on the type of cataract:

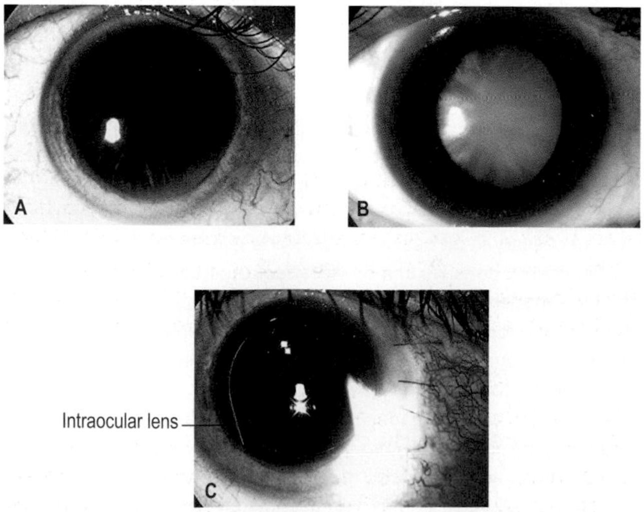

Figure 30.37 **Cataracts. A.** Early cataract. **B.** White mature cataract. **C.** Artificial intraocular lens following phacoemulsification.

Box 30.10 Cataracts: aetiology

Congenital
- Maternal infection
- Familial

Age
- Elderly

Metabolic
- Diabetes
- Galactosaemia
- Hypocalcaemia
- Wilson's disease

Drug-induced
- Corticosteroids
- Phenothiazines
- Miotics
- Amiodarone

Traumatic
- Post-intraocular surgery

Inflammatory
- Uveitis

Disorder-associated
- Down syndrome
- Dystrophia myotonica
- Lowe syndrome

for example, a posterior capsular type would lead to glare and problems with night driving. Early changes in the lens are correctable by spectacles but eventually the opacification needs surgical intervention.

Investigations

Blood glucose, serum calcium and liver biochemistry should be measured to diagnose metabolic disorders.

Management

Small-incision extracapsular or phacoemulsification cataract extraction with the insertion of an intraocular lens is the treatment of choice ***(Fig. 30.37C)***. Recent advances have enabled surgeons to perform multiple steps in the surgical process with the Excimer laser to enhance visual outcomes. Lens technology has also improved and Toric lenses are available to treat astigmatism, and multifocal or accommodative lenses to overcome intraocular lens-induced presbyopia.

Glaucoma

Glaucoma is due to increased pressure inside the eye, which is sufficiently elevated to cause optic nerve damage and result in visual field defects, with loss of sight ***(Fig. 30.38)***. Normal intraocular pressure (IOP) is 10–21 mmHg. Some types of glaucoma can result in an IOP exceeding 70 mmHg. Glaucoma is the second most common cause of blindness worldwide and the third most common cause of blind registration in the UK.

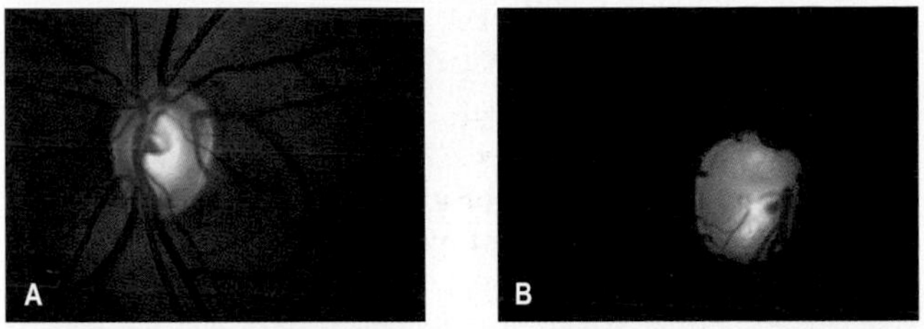

Figure 30.38 **The optic disc. A.** Normal optic disc. **B.** Glaucomatous optic disc. The central cup is enlarged and deepened.

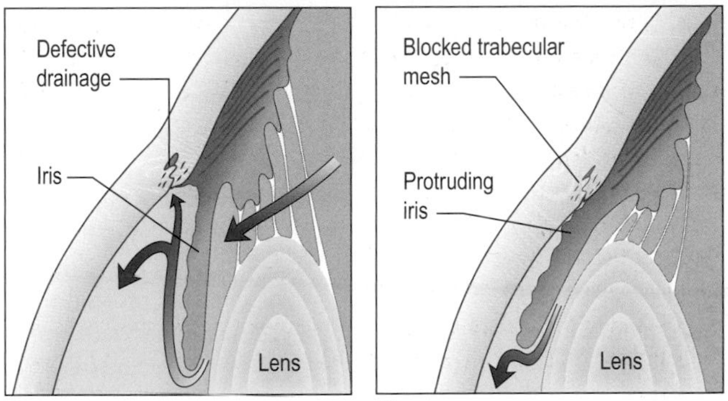

A B

Figure 30.39 **Glaucoma. A.** Primary open-angle glaucoma. **B.** Angle-closure glaucoma.

Primary open-angle glaucoma

Primary open-angle glaucoma (POAG) is the most common form of glaucoma. High intraocular pressures result from reduced outflow of aqueous humour through the trabecular meshwork ***(Fig. 30.39A)***. Common risk factors include age (0.02% of 40-year-olds versus 10% of 80-year-olds), race (black Africans are at five times greater risk than whites), positive family history and myopia.

Clinical features

POAG causes a gradual, insidious, painless loss of peripheral visual field, causing loss of vision. It is initially asymptomatic and the central vision remains good until the end-stage of the disease. Usually, glaucoma is identified during a routine ophthalmic examination. Diagnosis is only made if the IOP is measured. The optic disc is inspected and shows an enlarged cup with a thin neuroretinal rim. Visual fields are assessed and show a normal blind spot with scotomas.

Management

Treatment aims to reduce the IOP, either by reducing aqueous production or by increasing aqueous drainage:
- ***Beta-blockers***, such as timolol, carteolol and levobunolol, reduce aqueous production and are the most commonly prescribed topical agents. These drugs are contraindicated in people with chronic obstructive pulmonary disease, asthma or heart block.
- ***Prostaglandin analogues***, such as latanoprost, bimatoprost and travoprost, increase aqueous outflow and are also used (alone or in combination with beta-blockers) for POAG, as they can reduce IOP by 30%.
- ***Carbonic anhydrase inhibitors***, such as dorzolamide and acetazolamide, reduce aqueous production and are available in topical preparations. Acetazolamide is also available orally and, in this form, is the most potent drug for reducing IOP. It should not be used in patients who have a sulphonamide allergy.
- ***Selective laser trabeculoplasty*** (***SLT***) is a form of laser surgery that can lower the IOP by about 30% when used as initial therapy. It is useful when eye-drop medications are not lowering the eye pressure enough or are causing significant side-effects. It may sometimes be used as initial treatment in glaucoma, although effects commonly last 1–5 years only.

Acute angle-closure glaucoma

Acute angle-closure glaucoma (AACG) is an ophthalmic emergency. There is a sudden rise in intraocular pressure to levels over 50 mmHg. This occurs due to reduced aqueous drainage when the ageing lens pushes the iris forwards against the trabecular meshwork ***(Fig. 30.39B)***. People most at risk of developing AACG are those with shallow anterior chambers, such as hypermetropes and women. The attack is more likely to occur under reduced light conditions when the pupil is dilated.

Clinical features

AACG causes ***sudden onset of a red, painful eye*** and ***blurred vision***. Patients become unwell, with nausea and vomiting, and complain of headache and severe ocular pain. The eye is injected and tender, and feels hard. The cornea is hazy and the pupil is semi-dilated ***(Fig. 30.40)***. ***Box 30.11*** shows the differential diagnosis of the acute red eye. ***Box 30.12*** shows features that require ***urgent referral*** to an ophthalmologist.

Management

Prompt treatment is required to preserve sight and includes:

- i.v. acetazolamide 500 mg (provided there are no contraindications) to reduce IOP, *and*
- instillation of pilocarpine 4% drops to constrict the pupil to improve aqueous outflow and prevent iris adhesion to the trabecular meshwork.

Other topical drops, such as beta-blockers and prostaglandin analogues, can also be instilled if available, provided there are no contraindications. Analgesia and antiemetics are given as required.

Patients must be referred to an ophthalmologist immediately so that reduction in IOP can be monitored and other agents, such as oral glycerol or i.v. mannitol, can be administered to non-responding patients. Definitive treatment involves making a hole in the periphery of the iris of both eyes either by laser or by surgical means.

Uveitis

Uveitis is inflammation of the uveal tract, which includes the iris, ciliary body and choroid. It is classified according to the part of the uveal tract that the inflammation affects:

- ***Anterior uveitis*** is inflammation that affects the anterior part of the uveal tract. This can include the iris (iritis), or both the iris and the ciliary body (iridocyclitis). It is the most common type of uveitis.
- ***Intermediate uveitis*** is inflammation that affects the middle part of the uveal tract or eye, mainly the vitreous. It can also affect the underlying retina.
- ***Posterior uveitis*** is inflammation that affects the posterior part of the eye. It can affect the choroid, optic nerve head and the retina (or any combination of these structures). It includes chorioretinitis, retinitis and neuroretinitis.
- ***Panuveitis*** is inflammation affecting the whole of the uveal tract.

The most common symptoms of uveitis are blurred vision, pain, redness, photophobia and floaters. Each symptom is determined by the location of the inflammation, such that photophobia and pain are common features of iritis whilst floaters are commonly seen with posterior uveitis.

Anterior uveitis (iritis)

The classic presentation entails a triad of eye symptoms: redness, pain and photophobia. Vision can be normal or blurred, depending on the degree of inflammation. The eye can be generally red or the injection can be localized to the limbus. The anterior chamber shows features consistent with inflammation, including cells, keratic precipitates on the corneal endothelium, fibrin or hypopyon (pus), and the pupil may have adhered to the lens (posterior synechiae) ***(Fig. 30.41)***. The IOP may be normal or raised, either due to cells clogging up the trabecular meshwork, or due to posterior synechiae causing aqueous humour to build up behind the iris and force the iris against the trabecular meshwork and so reduce aqueous drainage.

Management

This consists of reducing inflammation with the use of topical steroids such as dexamethasone 0.1% and dilating the pupil with cyclopentolate 1% to prevent formation of posterior synechiae.

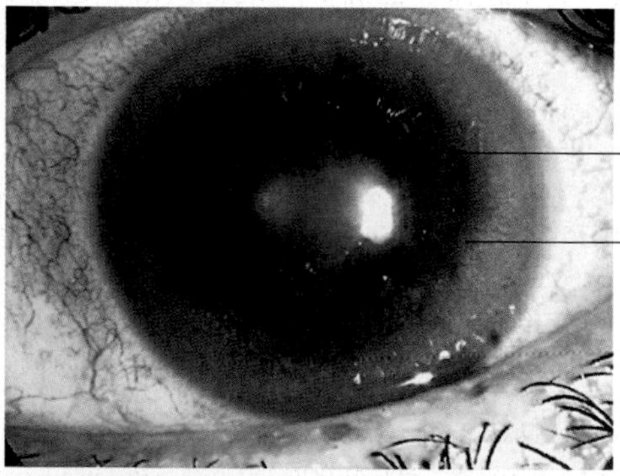

Figure 30.40 Acute angle-closure glaucoma.

Box 30.12 Red flags for a red eye

The following symptoms require **urgent** referral:

- Severe pain
- Photophobia
- Reduced vision, particularly if sudden
- Coloured halos around point of light in a patient's vision
- Proptosis
- Smaller pupil in affected eye

Plus on medical assessment:

- High intraocular pressure
- Corneal epithelial disruption
- Shallow anterior chamber depth
- Ciliary flush

Box 30.11 Differential diagnosis of the acute red eye

Cause	Conjunctival injection	Unilateral or bilateral	Pain	Photophobia	Vision	Pupil	Intraocular pressure
Conjunctivitis	Diffuse	Bilateral (often unilateral initially)	Gritty	Occasionally with adenovirus	Normal	Normal	Normal
Keratitis	Diffuse	Unilateral	Gritty	Yes	Reduced	Normal	Normal
Anterior uveitis	Circumcorneal	Unilateral	Painful	Yes	Reduced	Constricted	Normal or raised
Acute glaucoma	Diffuse	Unilateral	Severe pain	Mild	Reduced	Mid-dilated	Raised

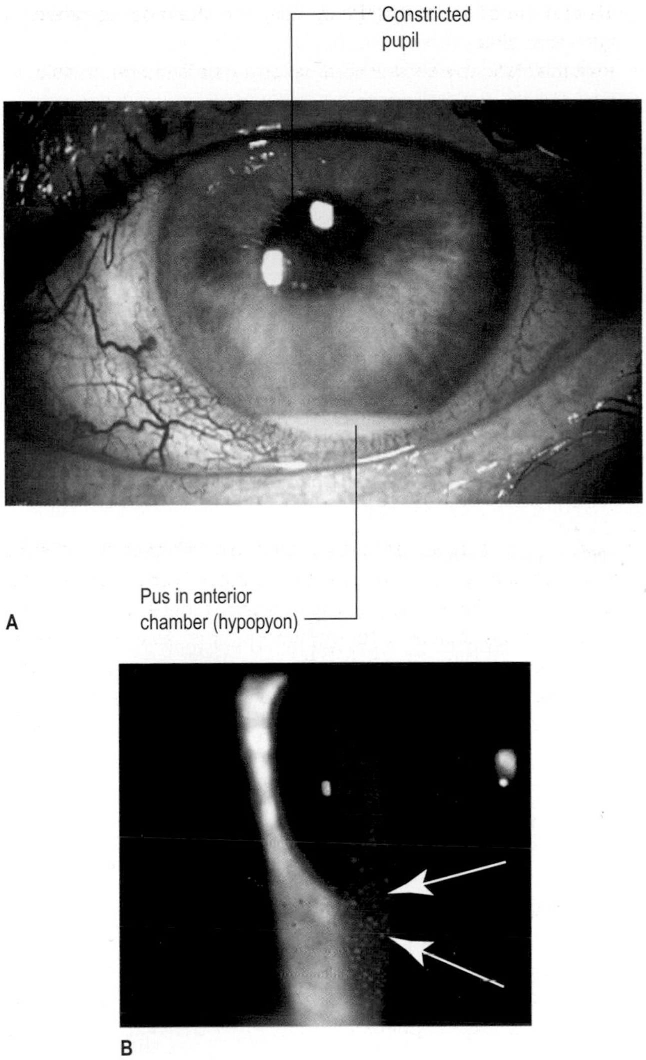

Figure 30.41 **Anterior uveitis. A.** Acute uveitis with hypopyon. **B.** Keratic precipitates (arrowed) on the corneal endothelium.

Dilatation also allows fundoscopy to exclude posterior segment involvement. If the IOP is raised, this is treated with topical beta-blockers, prostaglandin analogues, or oral or i.v. acetazolamide. Referral should be made to the ophthalmologist.

Intermediate uveitis

This usually causes painless blurred vision, most commonly associated with floaters. It is unusual to experience photophobia and redness. Both eyes are commonly affected in intermediate uveitis.

Management

This consists of a combination of treatment for anterior and posterior uveitis depending on the degree of anterior and posterior involvement.

Posterior uveitis

This commonly causes painless, blurred vision and can progress to severe visual loss. It is commonly associated with floaters and scotomata, or blind spots in the visual field.

Posterior uveitis is often found with systemic autoimmune diseases or infections; appropriate investigations should be performed and treatment given that is aimed at the cause.

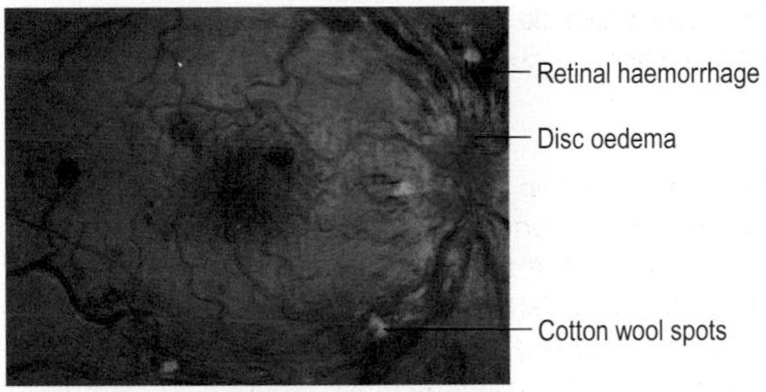

Figure 30.42 **Central retinal vein occlusion.**

Autoimmune diseases associated with uveitis include rheumatoid arthritis and Behçet's disease, ankylosing spondylitis and positive HLA-B27 (see p. 683), reactive arthritis, sarcoidosis, psoriasis and inflammatory bowel disease (Crohn's disease and ulcerative colitis; see p. 407). Infections, a rare cause of uveitis, include herpes simplex, herpes zoster, toxoplasmosis, cytomegalovirus, syphilis, tuberculosis, HIV infection and Lyme disease. In a number of patients, no cause is found (idiopathic uveitis).

Management

Steroids are commonly given orally, or more locally by injection into or around the eye. If steroid treatment is needed to treat uveitis in the longer term, second-line immunosuppressive drugs, such as mycophenolate mofetil, ciclosporin or azathioprine, are used. Biological agents, such as rituximab or adalimumab, are showing increasing promise in more severe cases.

Disorders of the retina

Central retinal vein occlusion

Central retinal vein occlusion (CRVO) usually leads to profound, sudden, painless loss of vision with thrombosis of the central retinal vein at or posterior to the lamina cribrosa, where the optic nerve exits the globe. The thrombus causes obstruction to the outflow of blood, leading to a rise in intravascular pressure. This results in dilated veins, retinal haemorrhage, cotton wool spots and abnormal leakage of fluid from vessels, causing retinal oedema ***(Fig. 30.42)***. In severe cases, an afferent papillary defect (p. 804) is present and this suggests the ischaemic variant.

Predisposing factors include increasing age, hypertension and cardiovascular disease, diabetes, glaucoma and, in the younger age group, blood dyscrasias and vasculitis.

Management

Treatment of any underlying medical condition is mandatory. Referral to an ophthalmologist is essential to monitor the eye, as some patients can develop retinal ischaemia with resulting neovascularization of the retina and iris. Panretinal photocoagulation should be commenced if there is neovascularization, and intravitreal steroid or anti-vascular endothelial growth factor (anti-VEGF) therapy is also used if there is macular oedema. Patients who develop iris neovascularization – rubeosis – where these new blood vessels block the drainage angle are at risk of developing rubeotic glaucoma.

Central retinal artery occlusion

Central retinal artery occlusion (CRAO) results in sudden, painless severe loss of vision. Retinal arterial occlusion results in infarction of the inner two-thirds of the retina. The arteries become narrow and the retina becomes opaque and oedematous. A cherry-red spot

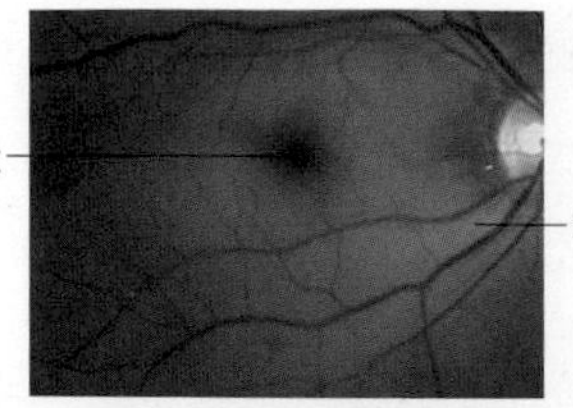

Figure 30.43 Central retinal artery occlusion.

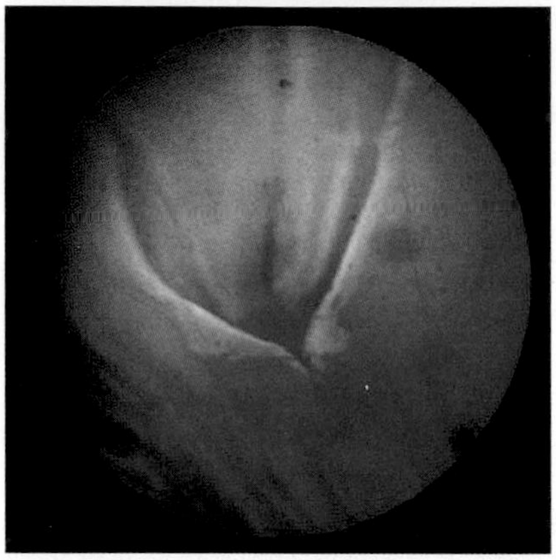

Figure 30.44 Retinal tear leading to detachment.

is seen at the fovea because the choroidal vasculature shows up through the thinnest part of the retina ***(Fig. 30.43)***. An afferent papillary defect is usually present.

Arteriosclerosis-related thrombosis is the most common cause of CRAO. Emboli from atheromas and diseased heart valves are other causes. Giant cell arteritis (see pp. 700–701) must be excluded.

Management

CRAO is an ophthalmic emergency since studies have shown that irreversible retinal damage occurs *within 90 minutes of onset*. Ocular massage and 500 mg i.v. acetazolamide help to reduce ocular pressure and may assist in dislodging the emboli. Breathing into a paper bag allows a build-up of carbon dioxide, which acts as a vasodilator and so helps dislodge the emboli. Other options include making a corneal paracentesis to drain off some aqueous humour, thereby reducing the IOP.

People with CRAO should have a thorough medical evaluation to determine the aetiology of the emboli or thrombus. Some patients may present with transient loss of vision or amaurosis fugax (see p. 832). All people with CRAO and amaurosis fugax should be started on oral aspirin if it is not medically contraindicated.

Retinal detachment

This causes a painless, progressive visual field loss. The shadow corresponds to the area of detached retina. If the detachment affects the macula, central vision will be lost. Following a tear in the retina, fluid collects in the potential space between the sensory retina and the pigment epithelium ***(Fig. 30.44)***. Patients usually report a sudden onset of floaters, often associated with flashes of light (photopsia) prior to the detachment. These individuals should be referred to an ophthalmologist for a detailed fundal examination.

Retinitis pigmentosa

This is a common chronic, inherited, degenerative disease of the retina, which can be primary or part of a syndrome, and leads to blindness. There is constriction of the peripheral vision, leading to tunnel vision and progressive loss of night vision.

Ophthalmoscopy shows bone spicule deposits and attenuated retinal vessels. Several genes are implicated.

There is no treatment but high-dose vitamin A supplementation may slow progression. Gene therapy is being investigated.

Age-related macular degeneration

Age-related macular degeneration (AMD) is the most common cause of visual impairment in patients over 50 years in the Western world, and the most common cause of blind registration in this age group. It affects 10% of people over 65 years and 30% over 80 years. Mutations in various genes have been reported: fibulin 5, complement factor H, and the Arg 80 Gly variant of oom plement C3.

The cause is unknown but suggested risk factors include increasing age, smoking, hypertension, hypercholesterolaemia and ultraviolet exposure.

There are two types:

- ***Non-exudative (dry) macular degeneration*** describes a painless and progressive loss of central vision. With age, lipofuscin deposits (drusen) are found between the retinal pigment epithelium (RPE) and Bruch's membrane (Fig. 30.45A; see Fig. 30.20). Drusen may be hard or soft, and there may be focal RPE detachment. Not all people with these changes will be affected visually but some develop distortion and blurring of their central vision. Extensive atrophy of RPE can occur (geographic atrophy).
- ***Exudative (wet) AMD*** (10% of cases) occurs with the development of abnormal subfoveal choroidal neovascularization in the region of the macula and causes severe central visual loss ***(Fig. 30.45B)***.

Management

The Age-Related Eye Disease Study (AREDS) has shown that vitamins C and E, β-carotene, zinc and copper slow progression of the disease. The subsequent study, AREDS 2, suggests that adding lutein, zeaxanthin and omega 3 does not improve the original AREDS formula overall, unless subjects had little of the supplements in their diets.

People with central distortion or with frank macular pathology should be referred *urgently* to the ophthalmologist for assessment of treatment. Anti-VEGF, such as ranibizumab, aflibercept and bevacizumab, are given by intravitreal injections with great success; the last of these is unlicensed yet less expensive. The treatment course should be commenced *as a matter of urgency*, as vision is maintained in up to 95% of patients and improves in approximately one-third. Initial monthly monitoring with optical coherence tomography (OCT) is recommended ***(Fig. 30.46)***. Laser treatment and photodynamic therapy with verteporfin constituted the treatment of choice in the past for wet AMD but now have limited roles.

Severe visual loss is possible and low-vision aids, such as magnifying glasses, may help to improve a patient's independence.

Visual loss

Every patient with unexplained sudden visual loss requires ophthalmic referral. The initial history and examination are summarized in ***Box 30.13***.

The common causes of blindness are similar across the world ***(Box 30.14)***. In developing countries, trachoma due to *Chlamydia*

Box 30.13 The initial history and examination in the patient presenting with sudden loss of vision

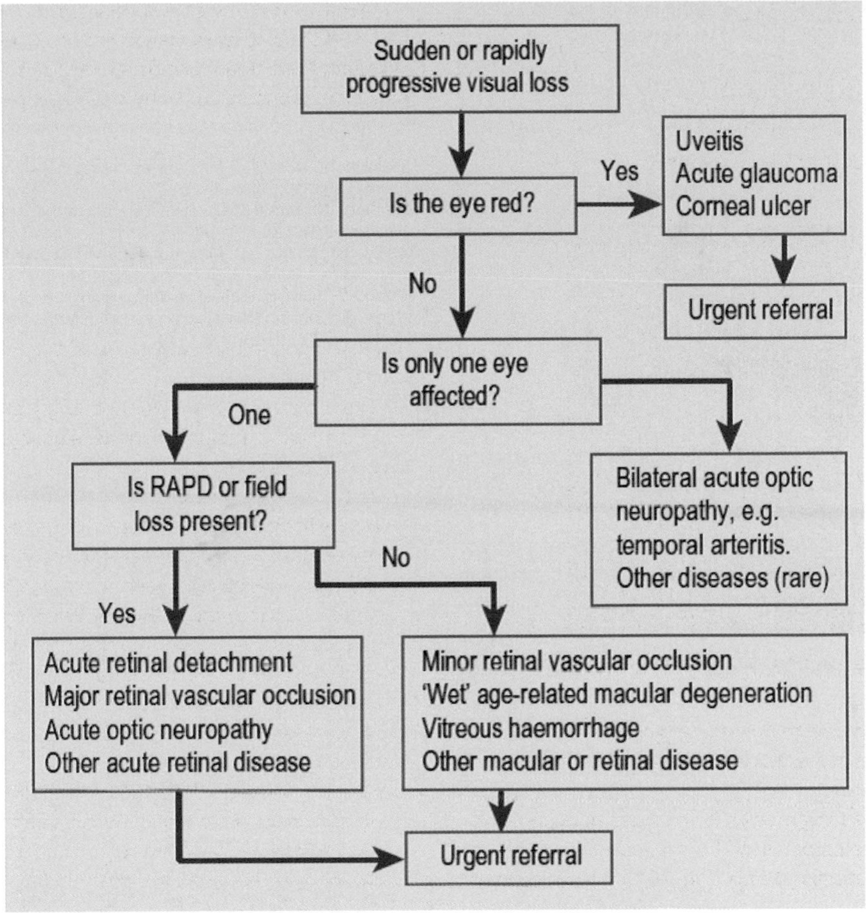

RAPD, relative afferent papillary defect.
(After Pane A, Simcock P. Practical Ophthalmology. *Edinburgh: Churchill Livingstone; 2005.)*

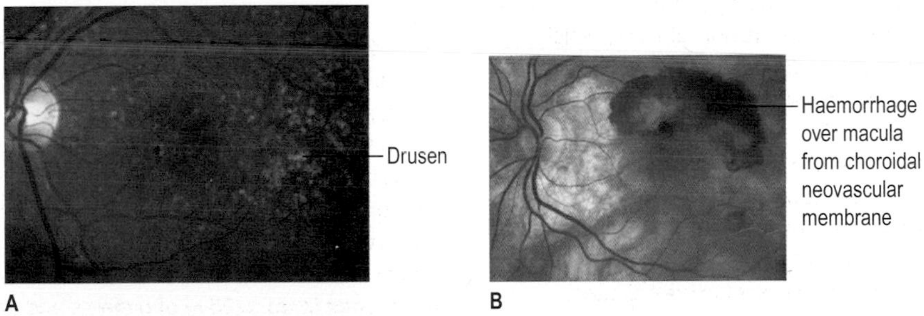

Figure 30.45 Age-related macular degeneration. A. With deposition of material (drusen) over the macula. **B.** With choroidal neovascularization.

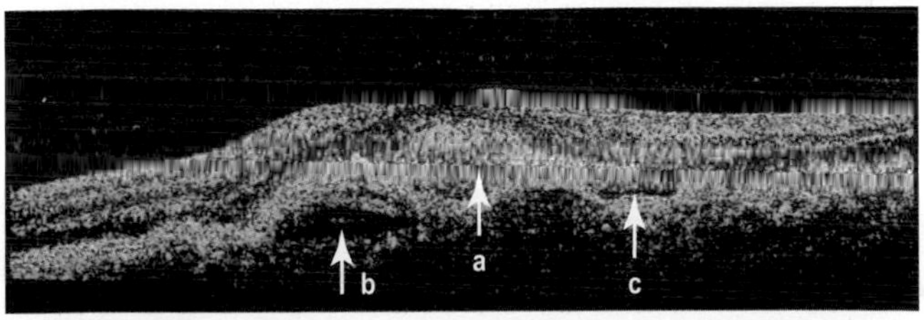

Figure 30.46 Age-related macular degeneration seen by optical coherence tomography. (a) Area of thickened retina. **(b)** Pigment epithelial detachment. **(c)** Subretinal fluid.

trachomatis (see p. 288) is also a major cause, accounting for 10% of global blindness; onchocerciasis (river blindness, due to *Onchocerca volvulus*; see p. 309) accounts for blindness in about 1 million people, although this figure is decreasing with treatment. In leprosy, 70% of patients have ocular involvement, and blindness occurs in 5–10% of these. Ocular involvement is common in cerebral malaria (see p. 299), although loss of vision is rare.

HIV infection can produce uveitis but the major problem is severe opportunistic infection of the eye when the CD4 count falls (see pp. 338–339) and anti-retroviral therapy is not available.

Box 30.14 Causes of loss of vision

Painless loss of vision
- Cataract
- Open-angle glaucoma
- Retinal detachment
- Central retinal vein occlusion
- Central retinal artery occlusion
- Diabetic retinopathy
- Vitreous haemorrhage
- Posterior uveitis
- Age-related macular degeneration
- Optic nerve compression
- Cerebral vascular disease

Painful loss of vision
- Acute angle-closure glaucoma
- Giant cell arteritis
- Optic neuritis
- Uveitis
- Scleritis
- Keratitis
- Shingles
- Orbital cellulitis
- Trauma

Vitamin A deficiency and xerophthalmia affect millions each year; the World Health Organization (WHO) classification of xerophthalmia by ocular signs is shown in ***Box 10.15***.

The WHO lists the most common causes of blindness across the world as cataract, glaucoma, acute macular degeneration, corneal opacity, diabetic retinopathy, and infections from bacteria or parasites.

Further reading

Lynn WA, Lightman S. The eye in systemic infection. *Lancet* 2004; 364:1439–1450.
Quigley MA. Glaucoma. *Lancet* 2011; 377:1367–1377.
Rosenfeld PJ. Bevacizumab versus ranibizumab for AMD. *N Engl J Med* 2011; 364:1966–1967.
Sakimoto E, Roseblatt MI, Azar DT. Laser eye surgery for refractive errors. *Lancet* 2006; 367:1432–1447.
Sheffield VC, Stone EM. Genomics and the eye. *N Engl J Med* 2011; 364:1932–1942.
Weiss JS1, Møller HU, Aldave AJ et al. IC3D classification of corneal dystrophies – edition 2. *Cornea* 2015; 34:117–159.
Wong TY, Scott IV. Retinal vein occlusion. *N Engl J Med* 2010; 363:2135–3144.
Wright AF, Dhillon B. Major progress in Fuchs's corneal dystrophy. *N Engl J Med* 2010; 363:1072–1075.

31 Skin disease

David G Paige, Sarah H Wakelin

See your e-book for key learning points, clinical tips, drug tips, extra images, extra tables and MCQs.

INTRODUCTION

Skin diseases are common throughout the world. In the UK, they account for about 1 in 10 consultations in primary care. In tropical and often poorer areas, infections such as leprosy and onchocerciasis predominate, while in more affluent temperate countries, chronic inflammatory disorders such as atopic eczema occur most commonly. Skin disorders can be an isolated complaint, part of an inherited disorder such as Ehlers–Danlos syndrome, or a feature of systemic disease such as systemic lupus erythematosus (SLE).

The common presenting symptoms of a rash or lesion(s) are itch, pain, disturbed sleep and anxiety/psychological upset. Because of their visibility, skin diseases can affect self-esteem and quality of life. They may also impair the ability to work: for example, hand eczema in a chef. Skin disease is rarely life-threatening, although, for example, malignant melanoma, toxic epidermal necrolysis and pemphigus can be fatal.

STRUCTURE AND FUNCTION OF THE SKIN

With an average surface area of 2 m^2 in the adult, the skin is the largest organ in the human body. It consists of three main layers:

1. the epidermis
2. the dermis
3. the subcutis ***(Fig. 31.1)***.

The functions of the skin are summarized in ***Box 31.1***.

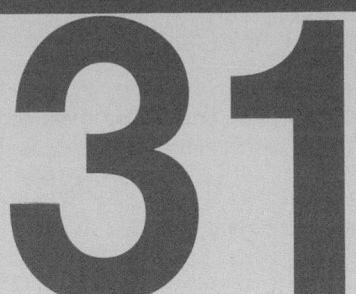

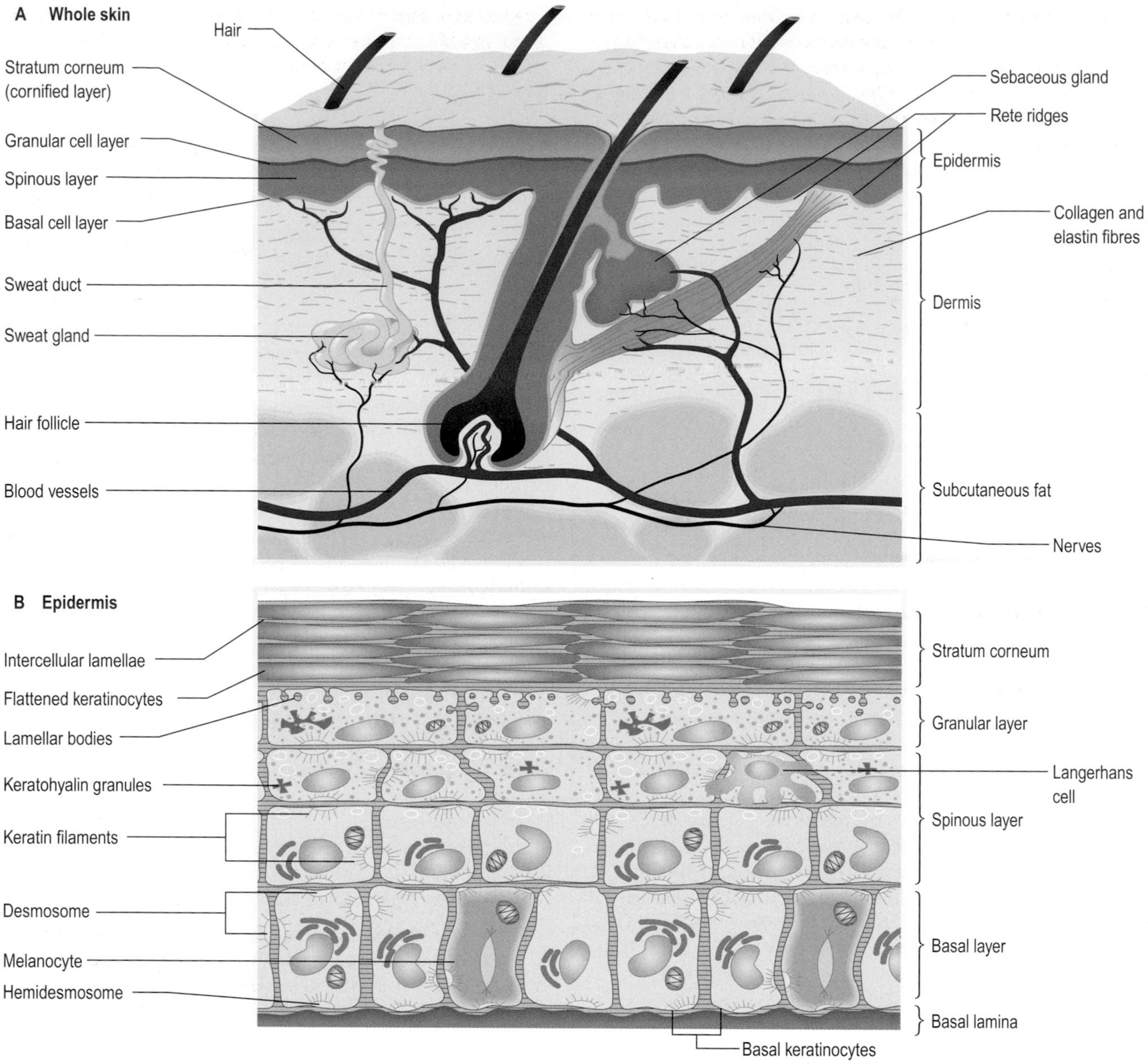

Figure 31.1 **The structure of the skin.** (See also ***Fig. 31.34***.)

Box 31.1 Functions of the skin

- Physical barrier against friction and shearing forces
- Protection against infection (immune and innate), chemicals, ultraviolet irradiation
- Prevention of excessive water loss or absorption
- Ultraviolet-induced synthesis of vitamin D
- Temperature regulation
- Sensation (pain, touch and temperature)
- Antigen presentation/immunological reactions/wound healing
- Hormonal, e.g. testosterone synthesis

The epidermis

The epidermis is a ***stratified squamous epithelium*** of ectodermal origin. It varies in thickness according to body site (from 0.05 to 1.5 mm) and provides an essential barrier against the environment and pathogens. Downward projections of the epidermis into the dermis are called the rete ridges. The epidermis is mainly composed of keratinocytes, which originate from a proliferating ***basal layer*** and differentiate as they migrate outwards to the surface, where they are shed. This process involves a carefully autoregulated sequence of protein and lipid synthesis. In the basal layer, keratinocytes synthesize a variety of keratin filaments and desmosomal proteins (desmoglein and desmoplakin), which make up the 'cytoskeleton' and give cells their strength and cohesion. Higher up in the ***granular layer***, lipid and lipid hydrolases are synthesized, then secreted by lamellar bodies to form a water-tight intercellular lipid bilayer. These lamellar bodies also produce abundant quantities of pro-filaggrin, which is converted to filaggrin in the outer layer of cells or ***stratum corneum***. Filaggrin has a dual role, holding moisture within cells – so-called 'natural moisturizing factor' – and as a component of the tough protein cell envelope. As the cells migrate outwards, they die, lose their nuclei and flatten into squames. The ***outer stratum corneum*** is tissue-paper thin but provides most of the barrier function of the epidermis. Filaggrin deficiency leads to a 'leaky' skin that loses water and allows entry of allergens that trigger an immunological response. Loss-of-function mutations in the filaggrin gene cause the dry, scaly skin complaint, ichthyosis vulgaris, and are a major risk factor for atopic eczema and associated allergies. Changes in lipid metabolism and protease activity in the outermost layers cause skin shedding (desquamation). It takes approximately 30 days for keratinocytes to migrate from the basal layer to the skin surface in normal skin, but is considerably faster in, for example, psoriasis.

Keratinocytes secrete a variety of cytokines (e.g. interleukins, interferon-gamma (IFN-γ), tumour necrosis factor-alpha (TNF-α)) in response to tissue injury, which stimulate wound healing and protect the body against microbial invasion. They also produce antimicrobial peptides (β-defensins and cathelicidins) that are part of the innate immune system. A deficiency of these peptides may underline the increased susceptibility to certain infections in people with atopic eczema.

Other cells in the epidermis

Melanocytes originate from the neural crest and reside in the basal layer in a ratio of approximately 1 per 10 keratinocytes. They synthesize the pigment melanin, which is transferred into surrounding keratinocytes to give protection against ultraviolet (UV) radiation. Racial differences in skin colour are due to variation in melanin production, not melanocyte numbers.

Merkel cells are also found in the basal layer. They are numerous on fingertips and in the oral cavity, and play a role in sensation.

Langerhans cells are dendritic cells derived from the bone marrow. They form a network across the supra-basal layer and play a role in antigen presentation and in immunoregulation.

The epidermis is anchored to the dermis by a complex meshwork of proteins that link the keratin intermediate filaments of basal keratinocytes to collagen fibres in the superficial dermis. This area is called the ***basement membrane zone*** (see ***Fig. 31.34***). Inherited or autoimmune-induced deficiencies of these proteins can cause skin fragility and a variety of blistering diseases (see pp. 1368–1371).

The dermis

The dermis is of mesodermal origin and is a matrix of collagen and elastin fibres, surrounded by an extracellular gel-like substance (ground substance). These fibres give skin its strength and elasticity. The dermis contains a range of cells: fibroblasts, mast cells, lymphocytes and dermal dendritic cells. It also contains blood and lymphatic vessels, nerves, muscle and appendages (sweat glands, sebaceous glands and hair follicles). In the upper ***papillary dermis***, there are finger-like projections that contain terminal capillary networks. The lower ***reticular dermis*** is thicker and denser.

Eccrine sweat glands are found throughout the skin, except at the mucosal surfaces, and are responsible for most thermoregulatory sweating. ***Apocrine sweat glands*** are found in the axillae and anogenital area, and do not function until puberty. ***Sebaceous glands*** are also inactive until puberty, when they excrete an oily substance called sebum under the influence of androgens. Sebum passes on to the skin surface via the pilosebaceous duct (hair follicle). Its lipids contribute to the skin barrier and have antimicrobial actions. Sebaceous glands are found in the highest density on the face, scalp and upper torso.

The skin is richly innervated. Sensory ***nerve fibres*** transmit stimuli of touch, pain, itch, vibration, pressure and temperature. Innervation of dermal autonomic structures, including sweat glands, blood vessels and arrectores pilorum muscles, control the skin's thermoregulatory mechanisms.

Hair

The skin surface is covered with hair, except for the mucous membranes and the glabrous skin of the palms and soles. Hairs arise from modified downgrowth of epidermal keratinocytes into the dermis. The hair shaft has an inner and outer root sheath, a cortex and sometimes a medulla. The lower portion of the hair follicle consists of an expanded bulb (which also contains melanocytes) surrounding a richly innervated and vascularized dermal papilla. The hair regrows from the bulb after shedding. All hair follicles go through a cycle of anagen (growth), catagen (involution) and telogen (shedding). At any one time, most hairs (>90%) will be in the anagen phase, which is usually 3–5 years for scalp hair. Grey hair is due to decreased tyrosinase activity in the hair bulb melanocytes. White hair is due to a total loss of these melanocytes. There are three types of hair:

- ***terminal***: medullated coarse hair, e.g. scalp, beard, pubic
- ***vellus***: non-medullated fine, downy hairs seen on the face of women and in pre-pubertal children
- ***lanugo***: non-medullated fetal hair, seen in premature babies and occasionally in malnourished people, e.g. those with anorexia nervosa.

Nails

Nails are tough plates of hardened keratin, which arise from the nail matrix (just visible as the moon-shaped lunula) under the nail fold. It takes 6 months to grow a fingernail and 1 year to grow a toenail.

The subcutis

The subcutaneous layer consists predominantly of adipose tissue arranged into lobules and separated by fibrous septa. It also contains blood vessels and nerves. This layer provides insulation and cushioning against trauma; in non-obese subjects, it contains about 80% of all body fat.

CLINICAL APPROACH TO THE PATIENT WITH SKIN DISEASE

Dermatological history and examination

The ***history*** should include the following:

- time course and distribution of rash/lesion(s)
- symptoms (e.g. itch or pain)
- family history (e.g. atopy and psoriasis)
- drug/allergy history (oral and topical medication)
- general medical history
- provoking factors (e.g. sunlight or medication)
- occupational, recreational and travel history.

Examination entails careful inspection of the whole skin – looking *and* feeling (for terminology, see ***Box 31.2***) – and should include nails, hair and mucosal surfaces. The following terms are used to describe distribution: flexural, extensor, acral (hands and feet), symmetrical, localized, widespread, facial, unilateral, linear, centripetal (trunk more than limbs), annular and reticulate (lacy network or mesh-like).

Box 31.2 Morphological description of skin lesions

Term	Description		Term	Description	
Atrophy	Thinning of the skin		**Papule**	Small, palpable, circumscribed lesion (<0.5 cm)	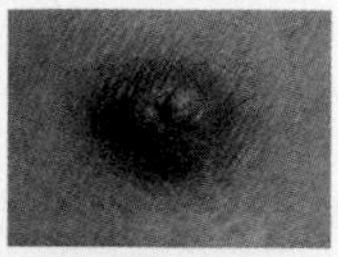
Bulla	A large, fluid-filled blister (>1 cm diameter)	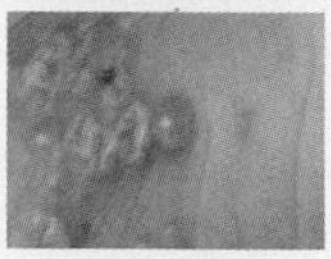	**Petechia**	Pinhead-sized, non-blanching area of haemorrhage	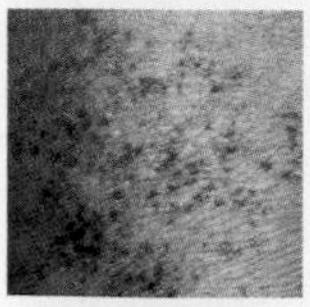
Crusted	Dried serum or exudate on the skin surface	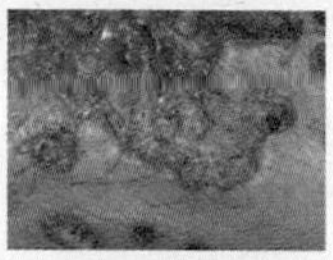	**Plaque**	Large, flat-topped, elevated, palpable lesion	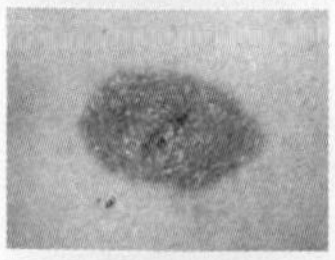
Ecchymosis	Large, confluent area of purpura ('bruise')	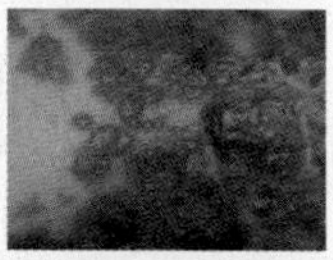	**Purpura**	Larger macule or papule of blood in the skin that does not blanch on pressure	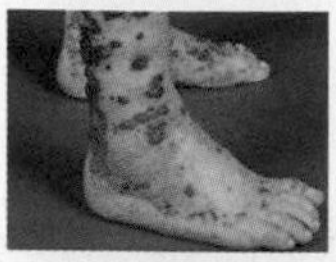
Erosion	Denuded area of skin (partial epidermal loss)	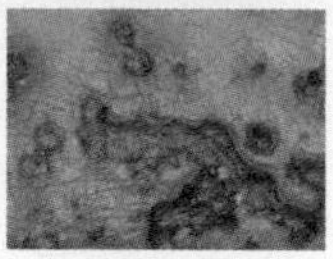	**Pustule**	Yellow–white pus-filled lesion	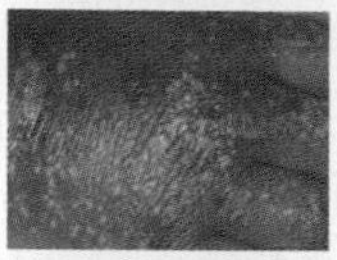
Excoriation	Scratch mark	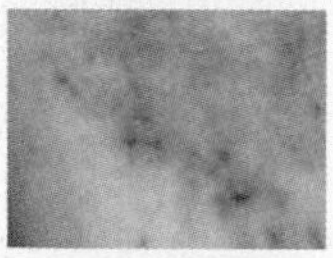	**Scaly**	Visible flaking and shedding of surface skin	
Fissure	Deep linear crack or crevice (often in thickened skin)	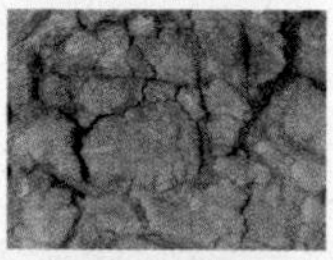	**Telangiectasia**	Abnormal visible dilatation of blood vessels	
Lichenified	Thickened epidermis with prominent normal skin markings	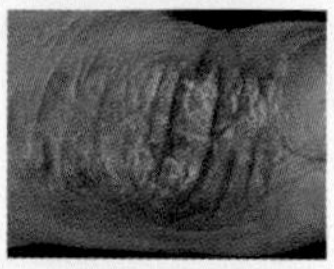	**Ulcer**	Deeper denuded area of skin (full-thickness epidermal loss and dermal loss)	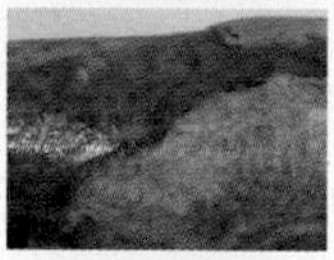
Macule	Flat, circumscribed, non-palpable lesion	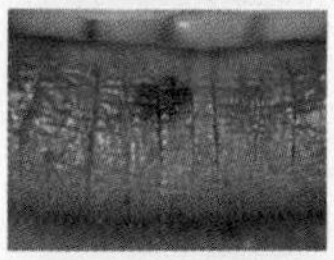	**Vesicle**	A small, fluid-filled blister	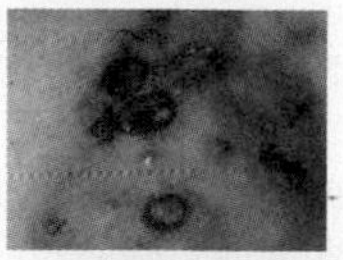
Nodule	Large papule (>0.5 cm)	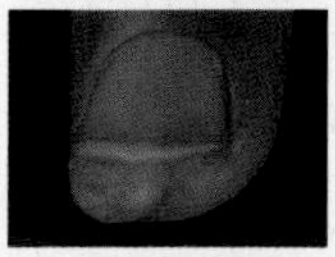	**Weal**	Smooth, itchy, raised swelling like 'nettle rash' ('hive') caused by dermal oedema	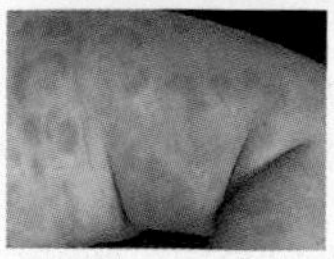

(Petechia image reproduced with permission from W Piette. Purpura and coagulation. In: Bolognia JL, Jorizzo JL (eds). *Dermatology*, 2nd edn. London: Elsevier; 2003.)

Box 31.3 Investigations used in skin disorders

Test	Use	Clinical examples
Skin swabs	Microscopy and culture of bacteria and yeast	Impetigo, candidiasis
Blister fluid	Electron microscopy, viral culture and PCR	Herpes simplex
Skin scrapes	Microscopy and fungal culture	Tinea pedis
	Microscopy of KOH preparation	Scabies
Nail sampling	Microscopy and fungal culture	Onychomycosis
Wood's light (ultraviolet A)	Microbial fluorescence	Scalp ringworm Erythrasma
Blood tests	Serology Autoantibodies	Streptococcal cellulitis Systemic lupus erythematosus
	HLA typing DNA analysis	Dermatitis herpetiformis Epidermolysis bullosa
Skin biopsy	Histology Immunohistochemistry Immunofluorescence Culture	General diagnosis Cutaneous lymphoma Immunobullous disease Mycobacteria/fungi
Patch tests	Allergic contact eczema	Hand eczema
Urine	Dipstick (glucose) Cytology (red cells)	Diabetes mellitus Vasculitis
Dermoscopy (direct microscopy of skin)	Assessment of pigmented lesions	Malignant melanoma

HLA, human leucocyte antigen; KOH, potassium hydroxide; PCR, polymerase chain reaction.

Investigations

Many rashes and lesions can be diagnosed by their appearance. Laboratory tests are useful if the diagnosis is uncertain, to reach a prognosis and to identify pathogens ***(Box 31.3)***.

INFECTIONS

The skin's surface is covered with an array of microbes that protect against pathogens. This natural flora or 'microbiome' may be disturbed by a range of factors, including altered host immunity, impaired skin barrier function or trauma, and this can lead to infection. Nasal carriage of bacteria can also be a source of infection.

Bacterial infections

(See also pp. 268–271.)

Impetigo

Impetigo is a highly infectious skin disease that usually affects children ***(Fig. 31.2)*** and is spread by direct contact. Infected areas appear as inflamed plaques with a golden, crusted surface, typically around the mouth and nose. It is caused by *Staphylococcus aureus* or *Streptococcus pyogenes*. Toxin-producing strains of staphylococcus can also cause blisters (bullous impetigo; see below). Skin

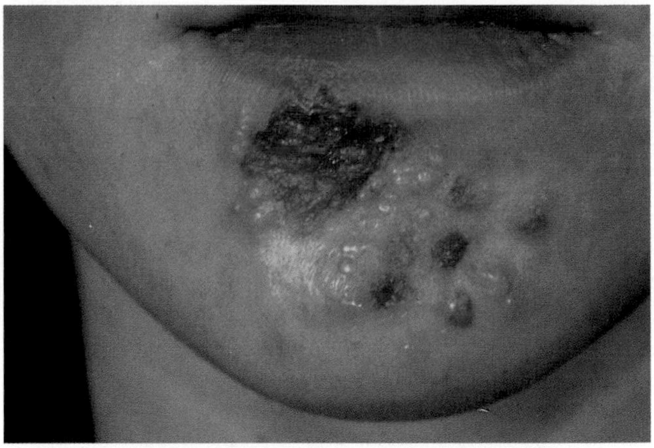

Figure 31.2 **Impetigo.** Crusted, blistering lesions on the chin.

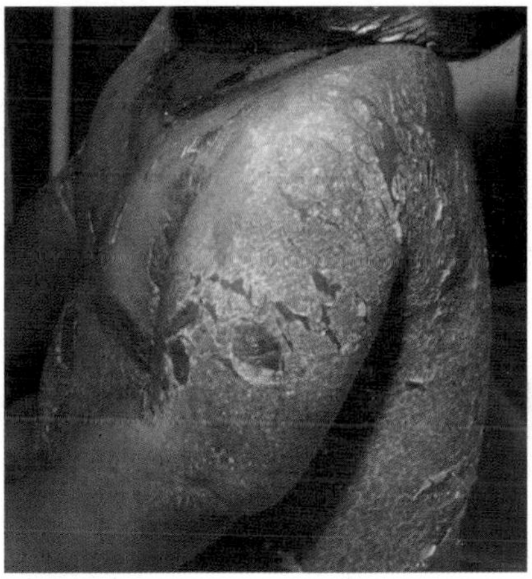

Figure 31.3 Staphylococcal scalded skin syndrome.

and nasal swabs should be taken if the complaint is extensive or recurrent, or constitutes a suspected outbreak.

Management

Localized impetigo may be treated with topical fusidic acid. Mupirocin should be reserved for cases caused by meticillin-resistant *Staphylococcus aureus* (MRSA). The new topical antibiotic retapamulin is also effective but is considered a second-line treatment due to its expense. Widespread infection or bullous impetigo should be treated with oral antibiotics for 7 days (flucloxacillin 500 mg four times daily, or erythromycin or clarithromycin if the patient is penicillin-allergic). Five days' treatment with once-daily co-trimoxazole is also an option. Affected individuals should avoid school or work until the lesions are dry or for 48 hours after starting antibiotics.

Staphylococcal scalded skin syndrome

Certain strains of staphylococci secrete exfoliative toxins (ETs) that can cause widespread areas of desquamation – staphylococcal scalded skin syndrome (SSSS; ***Fig. 31.3***) – or the localized blistering of bullous impetigo (see ***Fig. 31.2***). ETs are serine proteases that hydrolyse desmosomal proteins in the granular layer, leading to detachment of the superficial epidermis. In SSSS, ETs spread haematogenously from a source of infection and can cause septic shock and pneumonia. SSSS is more common in newborns than adults. However, in adults, it is often associated with underlying illness such as renal disease or immunosuppression, and has a higher mortality rate of up to 50%.

SSSS can resemble toxic epidermal necrolysis (TEN; see pp. 1383–1384) but the mucous membranes are not involved in SSSS and the level of epidermal detachment is higher. Histology therefore shows a more superficial split in SSSS (intra-epidermal) than in TEN (sub-epidermal). Frozen section processing can expedite the diagnosis. SSSS requires systemic treatment with anti-staphylococcal antibiotics (e.g. flucloxacillin) and full supportive care.

Cellulitis and erysipelas

Cellulitis and erysipelas are caused by superficial and deeper infection of the dermis and subcutaneous tissues, respectively. It is not always possible to make a clear distinction. Both complaints present with tender confluent areas of inflamed skin and are often associated with fever and malaise. Cellulitis typically affects the lower leg or arm and may spread proximally. Other sites that may be affected include the abdomen and perianal and periorbital areas. Erysipelas is more common on the face and is more sharply demarcated. Localized blistering (clear or blood-stained), necrosis, abscess formation, lymphangitis and lymphadenopathy may occur. The most common infective organisms are β-haemolytic streptococcus and *Staph. aureus*. Gram-negative or anaerobic bacteria may cause infection in those with diabetes or the immunocompromised.

Lymphoedema, leg ulcer, toe-web intertrigo and traumatic wounds are risk factors for cellulitis and erysipelas, and the skin should be carefully examined to look for any broken areas that act as an entry point for infection. Skin swabs are usually negative unless taken from broken skin. Serological tests can be used to confirm a streptococcal infection (antistreptolysin O titre, ASOT) and anti-DNAse B titre.

Management

Systemic antibiotics (flucloxacillin or erythromycin, both 500 mg four times daily) are usually the drugs of choice; depending on the patient's age, disease severity and co-morbidities; options range from high-dose oral therapy at home to urgent hospital admission for intravenous therapy. Toe-web fungal infection should be treated, as this may reduce the risk of recurrent infection.

About 25% of patients suffer from recurrent episodes of cellulitis and it is not clear whether prophylactic treatment with low-dose antibiotics (e.g. phenoxymethylpenicillin 500 mg twice daily) is beneficial.

Necrotizing fasciitis

This is a rapidly spreading, deeper bacterial infection of the subcutaneous tissues that may complicate surgical or traumatic wounds. It is characterized by severe pain that is out of proportion to the degree of skin inflammation and systemic upset. Urgent medical and surgical intervention is required for this severe, life-threatening infection (see pp. 270–271).

Folliculitis

Folliculitis is an inflammatory disorder of the hair follicle, which presents as itchy or tender small papules and pustules. It may be caused by a range of microbes, most commonly *Staph. aureus*. Predisposing factors include humid climates, occlusive clothing, obesity and diabetes. A localized variant affecting the beard area ('sycosis barbae') is more common in black African men and is caused by ingrowth of curly hairs. Extensive, itchy folliculitis of the upper trunk and limbs may be a manifestation of human immunodeficiency virus (HIV) infection. The Gram-negative bacterium, *Pseudomonas aeruginosa*, may cause outbreaks of folliculitis from inadequately disinfected hot tubs and pools.

Treatment is with topical antiseptics, topical antibiotics or oral antibiotics, and management of underlying predisposing factors.

Boils (furuncles)

Boils or furuncles are deeper infections of hair follicles and are painful, red, pus-filled swellings. They are usually caused by *Staph. aureus*. Boils are most common in young men and may spread from person to person due to poor hygiene or overcrowding. They may also be a manifestation of diabetes or malnutrition. Multiple coalescing boils are sometimes called 'carbuncles'. The rapid emergence of highly pathogenic strains of *Staph. aureus* that secrete a toxin called ***Panton–Valentine leukocidin*** (***PVL***) (pp. 269–270) is causing concern. It is associated with outbreaks of severe recurrent boils and skin abscesses in healthy adults. MRSA is also involved in an increasing number of cases of furunculosis in some parts of the world, such as the USA. Skin swabs should be taken from all patients with severe or recurrent folliculitis to determine antibiotic sensitivities and screen for PVL toxin-producing strains of staphylococci.

Management

Isolated boils can be treated with hot bathing alone. Antistaphylococcal oral antibiotics (flucloxacillin, erythromycin 500 mg four times daily or clarithromycin 250 mg twice daily) for 10–14 days are required for widespread infection or facial involvement. PVL-positive strains require more prolonged therapy with a combination of antibiotics such as rifampicin and clindamycin. Larger boils and abscesses may need incision and drainage. Screening of family contacts, nasal decolonization and use of antiseptic washes (e.g. chlorhexidine) are recommended.

Ecthyma

Ecthyma is also caused by streptococci (group A β-haemolytic), *Staph. aureus*, or occasionally both. It presents as chronic, well-demarcated, deep ulcers with a necrotic crust and exudate. It is associated with malnutrition and poor hygiene: for example, in intravenous drug users.

Management is with systemic antibiotics, phenoxymethylpenicillin 500 mg four times daily and flucloxacillin 500 mg four times daily for 10–14 days, and improved nutrition.

Erythrasma and pitted keratolysis

Erythrasma is an orange–beige rash that affects the large flexures (axillae and groin) and is caused by *Corynebacterium minutissimum* ***(Fig. 31.4)***. It is often misdiagnosed as a fungal infection. Corynebacteria are part of the normal skin microbiome but can also act as pathogens. They can be identified by their characteristic coral-pink fluorescence when examined with Wood's light (UVA). Corynebacteria are also implicated in pitted keratolysis.

Management is with topical or oral erythromycin 500 mg four times daily. Antiperspirants may also be helpful.

Pitted keratolysis is a superficial infection of the horny layer of the skin. It frequently involves the soles of the forefoot and appears as numerous small, punched-out, circular lesions of rather macerated skin (e.g. as seen after prolonged immersion). There may be associated hyperhidrosis of the feet and a prominent odour.

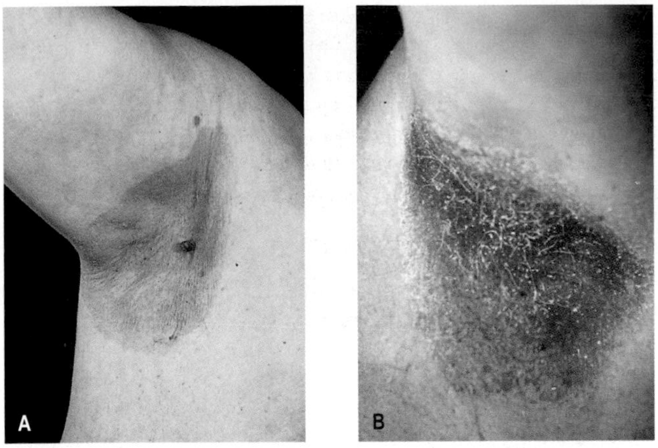

Figure 31.4 **Erythrasma. A.** Erythrasma of the axilla. **B.** Showing pink fluorescence under a Wood's lamp.

Management is with topical antibiotics (e.g. sodium fusidate or clindamycin, applied three times daily for 2–4 weeks) and topical antiperspirants, which are effective therapies.

Further reading

Grice EA, Segre JA. The skin microbiome. *Nat Rev Microbiol* 2011; 9:244–253.
Handler NZ, Schwartz RA. Staphylococcal scalded skin syndrome: diagnosis and management in children and adults. *J Eur Acad Dermatol Venereol* 2014; 28:1418–1423.
Irvine AD, McLean WHI, Leung DYM. Filaggrin mutations: associations with allergic, dermatologic and other epidermal diseases. *N Engl J Med* 2011; 365:1315–1327.
National Institute for Health and Care Excellence. *Impetigo – Summary*. NICE 2015; http://cks.nice.org.uk/impetigo#!topicsummary
Thomas KS, Crooke AM, Nunn AJ et al. Penicillin to prevent recurrent leg cellulitis. *N Engl J Med* 2013; 368:1695–1703.

Mycobacterial infections

Leprosy (Hansen's disease)

Leprosy (see pp. 285–286) usually involves the skin and nerves, and the clinical features depend on the host's immune response to the infecting organism, *Mycobacterium leprae*.

Indeterminate leprosy is the most common clinical type, especially in children. It presents as small, hypopigmented or erythematous, circular, scaly macules with reduced sensation. It may resolve spontaneously or progress to one of the other types. Biopsy reveals a perineural granulomatous infiltrate and scant acid-fast bacilli.

Tuberculoid leprosy presents with a few larger, hypopigmented (see ***Fig. 11.32***) or erythematous plaques with an inflamed border. Sensation is absent within lesions, which are dry and hairless, due to nerve damage. Nerves may be enlarged and palpable. Biopsy shows a granulomatous infiltrate around nerves but no organisms.

Lepromatous leprosy presents with multiple inflammatory papules, plaques and nodules. Loss of the eyebrows ('madarosis') and nasal stuffiness are common. Skin thickening and severe disfigurement may follow. Anaesthesia is much less prominent. Biopsy shows numerous acid-fast bacilli.

Diagnosis and management are discussed on page 286.

Skin manifestations of tuberculosis

Tuberculosis can occasionally cause skin manifestations:

- ***Lupus vulgaris*** usually arises as a post-primary infection. It commonly presents on the head or neck with red–brown nodules that look like apple jelly when pressed with a glass slide ('diascopy'). They heal with scarring, and new lesions slowly spread out to form a chronic solitary, erythematous plaque. Chronic lesions are at high risk of developing into squamous cell carcinoma.
- ***Tuberculosis verrucosa cutis*** arises in people who are partially immune to tuberculosis but who suffer a further direct inoculation in the skin. It presents as warty lesions on a 'cold' erythematous base.
- ***Scrofuloderma*** arises when an infected lymph node discharges on to the skin with ulceration and scarring.
- ***The tuberculides*** are a group of rashes caused by hypersensitivity reactions within the skin to underlying *Mycobacterium tuberculosis* infection. Erythema nodosum is the most common and is discussed on page 1363. Erythema induratum ('Bazin's disease') is a similar rash with deep red nodules on the calves rather than the shins; lesions can ulcerate.

Mycobacterium marinum infection ('fish tank/swimming pool granuloma')

This atypical/non-tuberculous mycobacterial infection presents with one or more painless granulomatous nodules on a hand or upper limb, which usually follow mild trauma. Local lymphadenopathy may also be present. Infection is usually acquired by coming into contact with non-chlorinated water or by cleaning out a fish tank without gloves. The diagnosis is usually made from the occupational or recreational history and clinical features. A skin biopsy shows granulomatous inflammation in the dermis and *Mycobacterium marinum* may be isolated from prolonged culture at low temperature. Polymerase chain reaction (PCR) of tissue can also confirm the diagnosis but this is not widely available.

Treatment is with combination oral antibiotics (e.g. clarithromycin and ciprofloxacin) for 4–8 weeks. Other antibiotics, such as tetracyclines, trimethoprim–sulfamethoxazole and anti-tuberculous drugs, can be used. Occasionally, mild infections will clear themselves without treatment.

Viral infections

Viral exanthem

An exanthem is the most common cutaneous manifestation of viral infection and is an erythematous maculopapular rash that predominantly affects the torso and proximal limbs. It is probably caused by deposits of immune complexes of antibody and viral antigen within dermal blood vessels. Many different viruses can cause exanthems, e.g. echovirus (see p. 260), erythrovirus (see p. 252), human herpesvirus 6 (see pp. 252–253), Epstein–Barr virus (see p. 258). The rash resolves spontaneously in 7–10 days.

Slapped cheek syndrome (erythema infectiosum, fifth disease)

See page 252.

Herpes simplex virus

Herpes simplex virus (HSV, see also pp. 247–249) occurs as two genomic subtypes. Most people are affected in early childhood with HSV type 1 but the infection is usually subclinical. Occasionally, it can present with either clusters of painful blisters on the face ***(Fig. 31.5)*** or a painful gingivostomatitis. In some individuals, cell-mediated immunity is poor and they experience recurrent attacks of HSV, often manifest as cold sores. Immunosuppression can also cause a

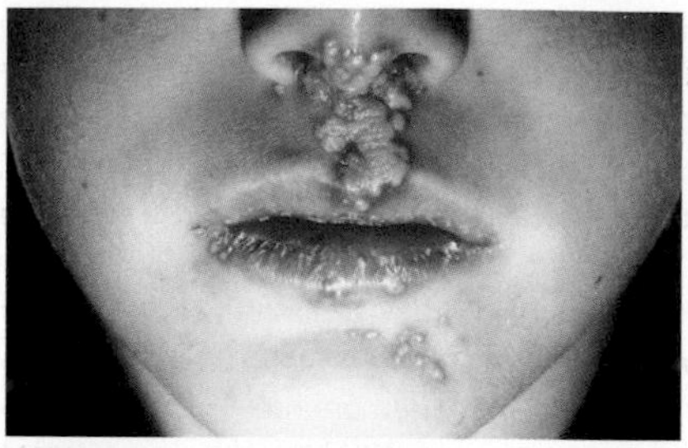

Figure 31.5 Primary herpes simplex infection.

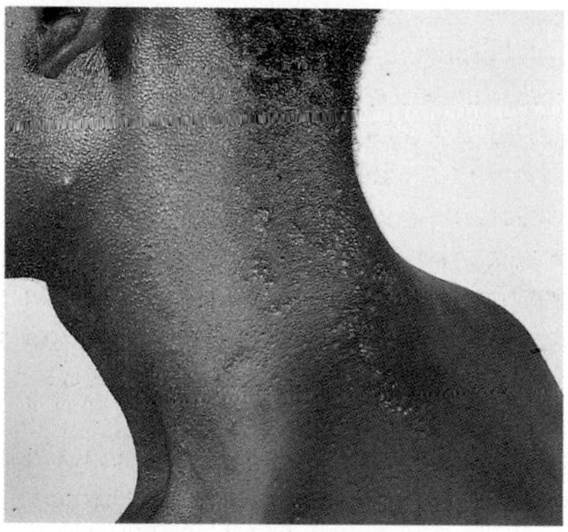

Figure 31.6 Herpes zoster in an African male. *(Courtesy of Dr P Matondo, Lusaka, Zambia.)*

recrudescence of HSV. HSV can also autoinoculate into sites of trauma and present as painful blisters or pustules that may be seen, for example, on the fingers of healthcare workers ('herpetic whitlow').

HSV type 2 infections are discussed on page 249. Other rare complications of HSV infection include corneal ulceration, eczema herpeticum, chronic perianal ulceration in acquired immunodeficiency syndrome (AIDS) patients, and erythema multiforme.

Management

Oral valaciclovir (500 mg twice daily for 5 days) is used for primary HSV and painful genital HSV. Cold sores are treated with aciclovir cream but this must be used early to shorten an attack; frequent recurrences can be treated with prophylactic oral therapy. Attacks of herpes become less frequent with time. Intravenous aciclovir must be used in immunosuppressed patients.

Varicella zoster virus

Varicella zoster virus (VZV) causes the common childhood infection, chickenpox. It is discussed on pages 249–250. It also causes herpes zoster.

Herpes zoster (shingles)

'Shingles' results from reactivation of latent VZV infection. It may be preceded by a prodromal phase of tingling or pain, which is followed by a painful, unilateral, blistering eruption in a dermatomal distribution (***Fig. 31.6***; see also ***Fig. 11.16***). The blisters occur in crops and may become purulent before crusting. The rash lasts 2–4 weeks and is usually more severe in the elderly. Occasionally, more than one dermatome is involved.

Complications of shingles include severe, persistent pain (postherpetic neuralgia), ocular disease (if the ophthalmic nerve is involved) and, rarely, a motor neuropathy.

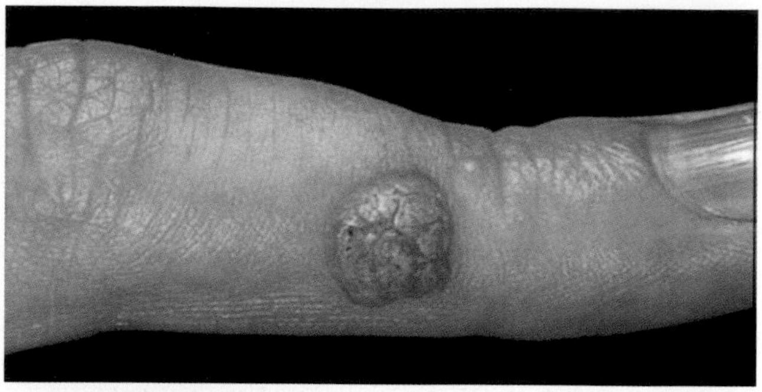

Figure 31.7 Viral wart.

Management

Herpes zoster requires adequate analgesia and antibiotics (if secondary bacterial infection is present). Valaciclovir 1 g or famciclovir 250 mg three times daily for 7 days is used; alternatively, oral aciclovir 800 mg five times daily for 7 days helps shorten the attack if given early in the illness.

High-dose intravenous aciclovir is used in immunosuppressed patients. A live-attenuated varicella zoster virus vaccine is available to boost immunity against VZV in the elderly and reduce the risk of developing herpes zoster.

Human papillomavirus

Human papillomavirus (HPV) is responsible for the common cutaneous infection of 'viral warts' (see also p. 265).

Common warts are papules with a coarse, roughened surface, often seen on the hands and feet but also on other sites. Small black dots (thrombosed vessels) are often seen within the lesion ***(Fig. 31.7)***. Warts on the face may become elongated ('filiform'). Children and adolescents are usually affected. Spread is by direct contact and can be facilitated by trauma.

Plantar warts (***verrucae***) affect the soles of the feet. They are flattened due to pressure but still have a characteristic warty (papillomatous) surface. Black dots can be seen if the skin is pared down (unlike callosities). Warts may be tender if they affect pressure points or are sited around nail folds.

Plane warts are much less common and are caused by certain HPV subtypes. They are clinically different and appear as very small, flesh-coloured or pigmented, flat-topped lesions (best seen with side-on lighting) with little surface change and no black dots. They are usually multiple and are frequently found on the face or the backs of the hands.

Anogenital warts (see p. 326).

Management

There is no definitive cure and warts may persist for months or years before spontaneously clearing. They are often recalcitrant in those with impaired immunity (e.g. transplant recipients).

Regular use of a topical keratolytic agent (e.g. 10–26% salicylic acid) after removal of hyperkeratotic skin may hasten resolution and is the mainstay of treatment. Liquid nitrogen cryotherapy can also be effective. Other destructive treatments include cantharadin, curettage and cautery, and laser therapy, but these may cause considerable pain and scarring.

Molluscum contagiosum

Molluscum contagiosum is a common cutaneous infection of childhood and is caused by a pox virus. Lesions are multiple small

(1–3 mm) translucent, firm papules, which may look as though they contain fluid – '***water blisters***' – but in fact contain soft, white matter that can be extruded through a central (umbilicated) depression and on squeezing. Mollusca may exhibit the Köbner phenomenon (see p. 1353). They can affect any body site, including the genitalia, and are transmitted by contact. Occasionally, lesions may be up to 1 cm in diameter ('giant molluscum').

Lesions usually recur in crops over 6–12 months before resolving spontaneously. Treatment is not required, but localized trauma, such as cryotherapy or curettage, may be helpful in older children. Hydrogen peroxide 1% cream or 5% imiquimod cream can be used in younger children. Mollusca are usually sexually transmitted in adults, and giant lesions or widespread involvement should raise the possibility of immunosuppression, especially HIV infection.

Orf

Orf is a pox virus infection of sheep and goats that causes a vesicular and pustular rash around the mouths of young offspring. People who handle the infected animal may become infected. Orf has long been recognized in farm workers but has recently been reported in children who catch the infection at 'petting stations' in city farms. Lesions appear as 1–2 cm red papules on the hands with an inflamed border that blisters; alternatively, they turn into pustules and resolve spontaneously after 4–6 weeks, conferring life-long immunity. Occasionally, orf is complicated by erythema multiforme (see p. 1363).

Further reading

Chen N, Li Q, Yang J et al. Antiviral treatment for preventing postherpetic neuralgia. *Cochrane Database Syst Rev* 2014; 2:CD006866.
Cohen JJ. Clinical practice: herpes zoster. *N Engl J Med* 2013; 369:255–263 (1765–1767 for comment).
Johnson RW, Rice AS. Clinical practice: post herpetic neuralgia. *N Engl J Med* 2014; 371:1526–1533.
Sterling JC, Gibbs S, Haque Hussain SS. British Association of Dermatologists' guidelines for the management of cutaneous warts 2014. *Br J Dermatol* 2014; 171:696–712.

Fungal infections

Fungal skin diseases have a high prevalence in humans, 'thrush' and 'athlete's foot' being two extremely common examples. In most cases, infection is confined to the stratum corneum (superficial mycoses), which elicits no inflammation, or the deeper layers of the epidermis, including hair and nails (cutaneous mycoses), where inflammation may be triggered by the fungus or its products. Subcutaneous mycoses include a range of infections of the subcutaneous tissues, usually following traumatic inoculation. The inflammatory response may extend upwards to the epidermis.

There are three groups of pathogenic fungi that commonly affect the outer layer of skin or keratinizing epithelium: dermatophytes, *Candida albicans* and *Malassezia* (formerly pityrosporum).

Dermatophyte infection

Dermatophyte (tinea) fungi invade and grow in dead keratin. The three main genera that affect humans are *Trichophyton*, *Microsporum* and *Epidermophyton*. They tend to form an expanding annular lesion due to lateral growth: hence the name 'ringworm'. Tinea may be transmitted to humans by other people (anthropophilic), from animals (zoophilic) or from soil (geophilic). The clinical appearance depends on the infecting organism, the site affected and the host reaction.

Tinea of the body usually presents with asymmetrical, scaly, inflamed patches with clearer centres and a scaly, raised border. Occasionally, vesicles or pustules may be seen. Treatment with topical steroids will modify the appearance, reducing scaling and erythema due to the anti-inflammatory effect and thereby masking some of the clinical signs – '***tinea incognito***'. However, the rash typically flares when steroids are stopped. Tinea infections are classified according to body site: tinea corporis (body), tinea facei (face), tinea barbae (beard), tinea cruris (groin), tinea manuum (hand), tinea pedis (foot), tinea capitis (scalp) and tinea unguium (nails). Multiple sites may be affected, and skin, hair and nails should be examined.

Asymmetrical scaly rashes should be investigated for fungal infection by mycology of skin scrapings.

Tinea cruris is more common in men than women and presents with an intensely itchy rash in the groin, with a scaly border that extends on to the thighs ***(Fig. 31.8)***.

Tinea pedis (athlete's foot) is extremely common in adults and is often confined to the toe webs, where the skin looks white, macerated and fissured. It may extend more widely on to the soles and sides of the feet, causing dryness, scaling and erythema, and the toenails are also often affected. Tinea pedis frequently flares in hot weather, causing pustules or blisters, and this can be misdiagnosed as eczema. Infection may also spread to the palm (***tinea manuum***), especially in manual workers. Annular lesions are rarely seen on palmoplantar skin.

Tinea capitis is the most common dermatophyte infection in young children, especially those of black African origin, whose hair and scalp seem more susceptible to fungal invasion. Adults and the elderly are rarely affected. Fungus may confine itself to within the hair shaft (endothrix) or spread out over the hair surface (ectothrix). The latter may fluoresce under a Wood's lamp (UV light). Scalp ringworm is spread by close contact (especially in schools and households) and by sharing of brushes or clippers. Immigration has led to changing patterns of fungal infections in Europe (e.g. *Trichophyton tonsurans* from Central America, *Trichophyton violaceum* from India and Pakistan). The majority of UK cases are due to *T. tonsurans* (which does not fluoresce).

The clinical appearance of scalp ringworm varies from mild diffuse scaling with no hair loss (similar to dandruff) to the more typical appearance of bald, scaly patches with broken hairs. An increased host response causes pustules and an inflammatory exudate, and certain types of tinea can trigger a severe inflammatory reaction with a swollen purulent mass or 'kerion'. This may be mistaken for a bacterial infection and inappropriately treated with an antibiotic. Extensive infection is occasionally accompanied by a widespread papulopustular rash on the trunk. This is a so-called 'id

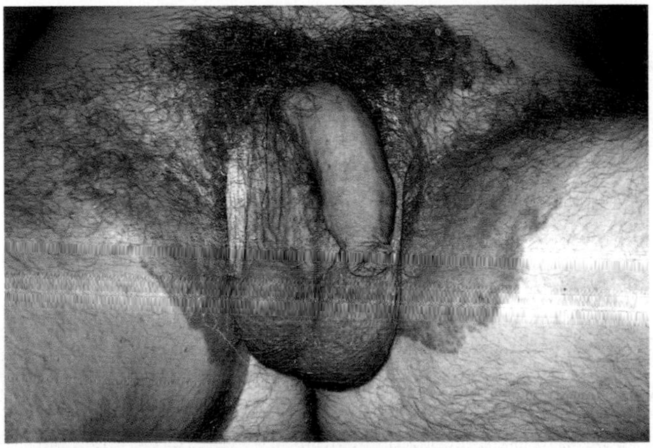

Figure 31.8 Tinea cruris. Ringworm of the groin.

reaction' and probably relates to the host immune response to the fungus. It resolves when the infection is treated.

Tinea unguium and onychomycosis

Onychomycosis is a broad term for fungal nail infection. Tinea unguium refers to a dermatophyte infection of the fingernails or toenails ***(Fig. 31.9)***. Tinea toenail infection is a common finding in the elderly and is usually asymptomatic. Fingernail infection is less common. Affected nails are dystrophic, thick (subungual hyperkeratosis) and discoloured (white–yellow–beige). Infection usually starts at the distal or lateral nail edges, then spreads proximally. The whole nail plate may be destroyed with advanced disease. The ***differential diagnoses*** include nail psoriasis and traumatic nail dystrophy (which may coexist with fungal infection). Diseased nails should be clipped back and the crumbly white nails analysed by microscopy and mycological culture to confirm the diagnosis and identify the organism. *Trichophyton rubrum* is the most common pathogen.

Management

Localized tinea of the body or flexures is treated with an antifungal cream (clotrimazole, miconazole or terbinafine applied three times daily for 1–2 weeks). Nystatin is ineffective. More widespread infection, tinea pedis, tinea manuum and tinea capitis require oral antifungal therapy with itraconazole (100 mg daily) or terbinafine (250 mg per day) for 1–2 months. Griseofulvin is a less effective drug, but is still used for childhood tinea capitis.

Tinea unguium of the toenails requires prolonged oral antifungal therapy. Itraconazole (as a continuous or pulsed regimen) or terbinafine for 3–6 months can clear up to 80% of cases but relapses are common.

Candida albicans

Candida albicans (see also p. 295) is a commensal yeast within the gastrointestinal tract. It can overgrow on occluded moist skin, causing nappy rash, intertrigo of the large flexures in obese people ***(Fig. 31.10)***, and vulvovaginal candidiasis or 'thrush'. The glans penis may be affected in uncircumcised males (candidal balanitis).

Candidal intertrigo causes irritation and soreness; affected areas are glazed and inflamed, with a ragged peeling edge that may contain a few small pustules. Spotty erythema may extend beyond the affected border (satellite lesions).

Candida may also affect the moist interdigital clefts of the toes and mimic tinea pedis. In people who frequently immerse their hands in water (e.g. cleaners, caterers), *Candida* may cause chronic infection of the nail folds ('paronychia') and nail infection (candidal onychomycosis). *Candida* can also infect the oral mucosa, especially in those who have taken broad-spectrum antibiotics and in the immunosuppressed and elderly. Affected mucosal surfaces are inflamed with superficial white or creamy pseudomembranous plaques, which can easily be scraped away.

Management

Predisposing factors should be treated. Diabetes should be excluded. Topical therapy (azoles or nystatin) is usually adequate, except for nail infection, and may take the form of creams, pessaries, lozenges or powder, depending on body site. Recurrent vulvovaginal candidiasis (see p. 325) is a common complaint in women and may require oral azole antifungal therapy.

Malassezia

This lipophilic yeast family (formerly called pityrosporum; see p. 297) form part of the normal skin microbiome. Colonization is prominent in the scalp, flexures and upper trunk. At least 10 different species have been identified and there is increasing evidence of their causal role in three common dermatoses:

- pityriasis versicolor
- seborrhoeic eczema (see pp. 1351–1352)
- *Pityrosporum* folliculitis.

Pityriasis versicolor is a common complaint in young adults and *Malassezia globosa* appears to be the causative agent; in fair-skinned people, it typically causes pink–beige scaly macules on the torso. Pale areas may be prominent after suntanning and in darker-skinned individuals as the yeast impairs melanin synthesis.

The ***diagnosis*** is usually made clinically but can be confirmed by microscopy of skin scrapings, which shows the characteristic 'meatballs and spaghetti' appearance of spherical yeast and short pseudohyphae.

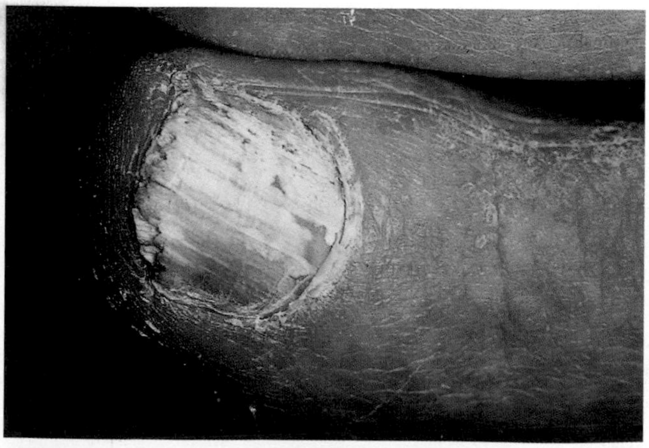

Figure 31.9 Dermatophyte infection of the nail. White, crumbling dystrophy is shown.

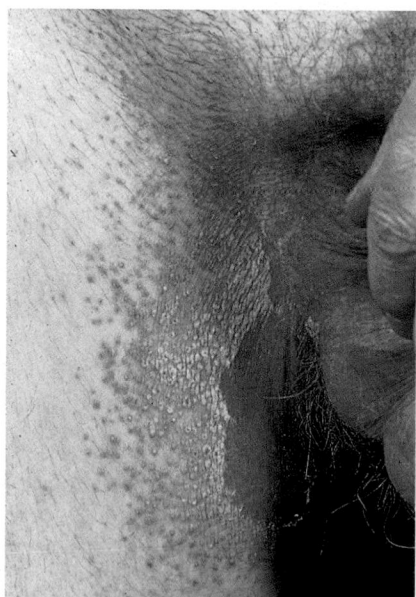

Figure 31.10 Intertrigo with the satellite lesions typical of candidiasis.

Management is with topical azoles or oral itraconazole for resistant cases. Antifungal shampoos containing selenium sulphide or ketoconazole may also be used as a body wash. The pigment changes can take months to resolve and recurrences are common.

Pityrosporum folliculitis is also common in young men and causes small, itchy, monomorphic papules and pustules on the upper back, shoulders and face. It may be confused with acne. Topical and oral azole antifungals can be effective but the complaint often relapses quickly.

Subcutaneous mycoses

Subcutaneous mycoses (see p. 297) are a rare group of localized infections of the skin and subcutaneous tissues that follow traumatic implantation of the fungal agent, a soil saprophyte. The causative organisms vary geographically and disease examples include sporotrichosis (worldwide), chromoblastomycosis and mycotic mycetoma (tropical and subtropical). Sporotrichosis or 'rose gardener's disease' usually causes a slowly growing, inflamed nodule at the site of skin inoculation, with new lesions developing along lymphatics and blood vessels – 'sporotrichoid spread'. Treatment is with oral itraconazole.

Further reading

Ahmeen M, Lear JT, Madan V et al. British Association of Dermatologists' guidelines for the management of onychomycosis 2014. *Br J Dermatol* 2014; 171:937–958.

Infestations

Scabies

Scabies is an ectoparasite infestation with the mite *Sarcoptes scabiei*. It can affect all races and people of any social class. It is most common in children and young adults but can affect any age group. There are 300 million cases of scabies in the world each year. It is more common in poorer countries with social overcrowding, especially sub-Saharan Africa. At any time there are approximately 130 million untreated cases. Although scabies is a trivial complaint, the infectious complications include neonatal septicaemia, post-streptococcal nephritis and rheumatic fever, and cause considerable morbidity. Scabies is spread by close or prolonged contact, such as within households or institutions, and by sexual contact. It presents with an intensely itchy, excoriated rash that resembles eczema. Pruritus is usually worse at night and disturbs sleep. Small, red papules, vesicles and occasionally pustules occur anywhere on the body but rarely on the face, except in neonates. The distribution of lesions is helpful in making a diagnosis ***(Fig. 31.11)***. Sites of predilection are the finger webs, palms, soles, wrists, axillae, the male genitalia, and around the nipples and umbilicus.

The diagnostic sign is fine linear or curved burrows but these are not always visible. Dermoscopy may help. The rash may be complicated by secondary bacterial infection. Scabies can be confirmed by microscopy of potassium hydroxide-treated skin scrapings from the tip of a burrow, which reveal the mite and/or its eggs.

Management

A topical scabicide (e.g. 5% permethrin) is applied overnight. For the treatment to be successful, the following should be noted:

- Treat all skin below the neck, including the genitalia, palms and soles, and under the nails. Treat the head and neck regions in infants (up to age 2 years).
- All close contacts should be treated at the same time, even if asymptomatic.

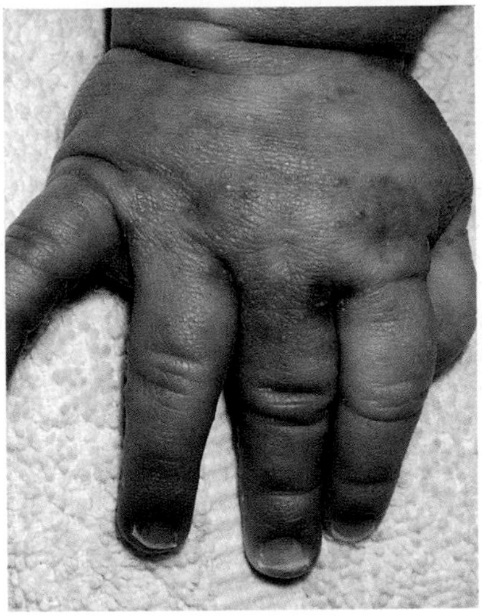

Figure 31.11 Scabies. Itchy papules and pustules centred on the web spaces of the hand.

- Reapply scabicide to the hands if they are washed during the treatment period.
- Wash or clean recently worn clothes (preferably at 60°C) to avoid re-infection.
- Advise that pruritus may persist for up to 4 weeks after successful treatment.
- The application should be repeated after 1 week.

Malathion can be used if permethrin is unavailable; benzyl benzoate is employed occasionally but is very irritant and should not be used in children. Lindane is a cheap therapy but there are concerns about resistance to this drug and neurotoxicity. Oral ivermectin 200 µg/kg, as 2 doses 2 weeks apart, is effective, especially for use in institutions, but remains unlicensed for this indication.

Crusted scabies (Norwegian scabies)

Crusted scabies is a variant that occurs in immunosuppressed individuals when huge numbers of mites are carried in the skin ***(Fig. 31.12)***. Pruritus may be mild or absent. Individuals are highly infectious and may be the source of outbreaks if the diagnosis is delayed. Hyperkeratotic crusted lesions characteristically affect the hands and feet. This may progress to a widespread erythema with irregular crusted plaques, mimicking infected eczema or psoriasis.

Management is with careful barrier nursing, repeated applications of a scabicide and oral ivermectin (200 µg/kg – at least 2 doses 1 week apart).

Lice infection

Lice are blood-sucking ectoparasites that cause three patterns of infection in humans.

Head lice (pediculosis capitis)

Head lice infestation is an extremely common problem in schoolchildren, especially young girls. Lice spread by close contact and cause pruritus, leading to excoriations and papules around the hairline of the neck and ears.

Diagnosis can be confirmed by identifying the eggs ('nits'), which are firmly stuck to the hair shaft, or the adult lice, which can be caught between the teeth of a fine comb.

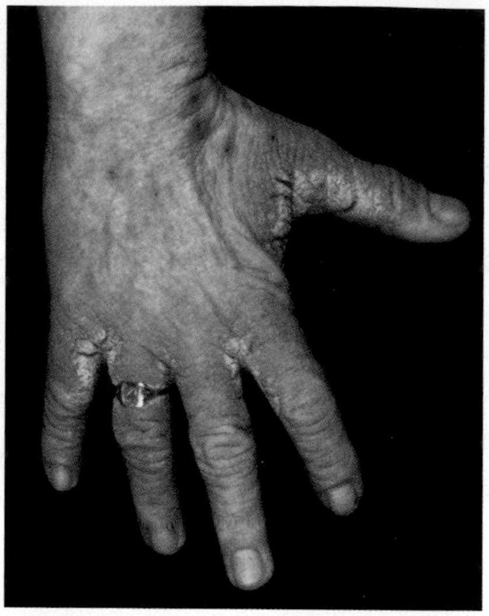

Figure 31.12 Crusted scabies in a patient with chronic myeloid leukaemia.

Management aims at eradication but this is difficult because of the time-consuming nature of treatment and frequent re-infestations. Lotions containing traditional topical insecticides, such as malathion, carbaryl and phenothrin, are used less widely because of resistance and are being replaced with physical treatment (wet combing). This involves use of a fine-toothed comb to remove young lice before they mature and needs to be repeated meticulously until all eggs have hatched. Oral ivermectin is an option in recalcitrant infestations but is unlicensed in the UK.

Body lice (pediculosis corporis)

Infestation with body lice is a disease of poverty and neglect. It is rarely seen in developed countries except in homeless individuals and vagrants. It is spread by direct contact or by sharing of infested clothing. The lice and eggs are rarely seen on the patient but are commonly found on the clothing. Infestation with body lice presents with itch, excoriations and, sometimes, post-inflammatory hyperpigmentation of the skin.

Management consists of malathion or permethrin for the patient and high-temperature washing and drying of clothing.

Pubic lice (crabs, *Phthiriasis pubis*)

Pubic lice are transmitted by direct contact, usually sexual (see p. 331). Infestation presents with itching, especially at night. Lice can be seen near the base of the hair with eggs somewhat further up the shaft. Occasionally, eyebrows, eyelashes and the beard area are affected.

Management is as for head lice but all sexual contacts should be treated and the patient screened for other sexually transmitted diseases. Eyelash infestation is treated with white soft paraffin three times daily for 1–2 weeks.

Arthropod-borne diseases ('insect bites' or papular urticaria)

These depend on contact with an animal (e.g. dog, cat, bird) that is infested with fleas (*Cheyletiella*) or on bites from flying insects (e.g. midges, mosquitoes). In the case of flea bites, the animal itself may be itchy with scaly and thickened skin. Flea eggs can lie dormant in soft furnishings (e.g. carpets) for many months. Bites present as itchy, urticated lesions, which are often grouped in clusters or lines. The legs are most commonly affected and lesions can blister in hot weather. It is not unusual for an individual to react badly to bites when other family members seem unaffected. Anti-flea treatment of the animal and furnishings is required. Insect repellents and appropriate clothing help lessen bites from flying insects.

Infestations with bed bugs have increased enormously in the past decade in the developed world. Bed bugs are small, brown/black, lentil-sized insects, which emerge from the seams of bedding at night-time when attracted to the warmth of sleeping humans and the carbon dioxide they produce. Their bites cause clustered, itchy papules on exposed areas, including the eyelids, face and neck. Infestations require professional insecticide treatment of properties. Advice can be obtained from the National Pest Technicians Association in the UK (see 'Further reading').

Further reading

Chosidow O, Giraudeau B, Cottrell J et al. Oral ivermectin versus malathion lotion for difficult to treat headlice. *N Engl J Med* 2010; 362:896–905.
Currie BJ, McCarthy JS. Permethrin and ivermectin for scabies. *N Engl J Med* 2010; 362:717–725.
Quach KA, Zaenglein AL. The eyelid sign: a clue to bed bugs. *Paediatr Dermatol* 2014; 31:353–355.
http://www.npta.org.uk *UK National Pest Technicians Association*.

Tropical dermatoses

Skin diseases feature among a group of 'neglected tropical diseases' defined by the World Health Organization WHO): leprosy, leishmaniasis, dracunculiasis (guinea worm), lymphatic filariasis and onchocerciasis. These are endemic in poor countries and constitute a huge physical and financial burden. Travellers returning to the West from tropical or subtropical countries may also be affected by skin diseases, especially cutaneous leishmaniasis, cutaneous larva migrans and myiasis. In addition, rashes may be a feature of systemic infections such as dengue, schistosomiasis and rickettsial diseases.

Leishmaniasis (see pp. 303–305) is an infection with the protozoon *Leishmania*, and is acquired from the bite of a sandfly vector. Cutaneous, mucocutaneous and visceral disease (kala azar) may occur, depending on the infecting organism and host response. ***Cutaneous leishmaniasis*** (see p. 304) is the most common form and presents as a chronic ulcer (oriental sac), which heals slowly over many months with scarring.

Cutaneous larva migrans is caused by direct contact with the larvae of hookworm from animal faeces – usually acquired by walking or lying on sandy beaches. Larvae penetrate the skin and cause an intensely itchy serpiginous lesion, which migrates as the larva burrows within the epidermis.

Myiasis is an infestation of the skin with developing fly larvae (maggots). Species that can penetrate intact skin to cause boil-like lesions include botfly and tumbu fly.

PAPULO-SQUAMOUS/ INFLAMMATORY RASHES

Eczema

The terms eczema and dermatitis are used interchangeably to describe a common group of inflammatory skin diseases. In the developed world, eczema may affect about 10% of the population at any one time, with up to 40% experiencing an episode of eczema

Box 31.4 Classification of eczema

Endogenous
- Atopic eczema
- Seborrhoeic eczema
- Discoid eczema
- Chronic hand/food eczema
- Venous ('gravitational') eczema
- Asteatotic eczema
- Lichen simplex/nodular prurigo

Exogenous
- Irritant contact eczema
- Allergic contact eczema

during their lifetime. Eczema is classified as constitutional or endogenous, and contact or exogenous ***(Box 31.4)***. It can also be classified according to duration (acute, subacute or chronic).

The inflammation common to all forms of eczema causes erythema and surface change (dryness, scaling), as well as itch, which ranges from mild to intolerable. In acute eczema, tiny vesicles or larger bullae may be seen within oedematous, inflamed skin. Scratching leads to sero-sanguinous exudate and crusts. In subacute eczema, there is less oedema and some flaking and scaling. Chronic eczema is thickened and dry with prominent skin creases (lichenification). Secondary bacterial infection may occur and cause crusts, papules and pustules. The histology of eczema correlates with the clinical signs: in acute eczema the keratinocytes are swollen with increased intercellular fluid ('spongiosis'), while in chronic disease there is little oedema but prominent thickening of the epidermis (acanthosis) and scaling (hyperkeratosis). Inflammatory cells are present around the upper dermal vessels in all patterns.

Atopic eczema

This type of constitutional eczema is extremely common affecting up to 20% of children. It usually starts under the age of 2 years and is often associated with other atopic diseases, which present in a sequence described as the 'atopic march'.

Aetiology

Atopic eczema is a genetically complex, familial disease with a strong maternal influence. A positive family history of atopic disease is often present: there is a 90% concordance in monozygotic twins but only 20% in dizygotic twins. If one parent has atopic disease, the risk of a child developing eczema is about 20–30%. If both parents have atopic eczema, the risk is greater than 50%.

The exact pathophysiology is not fully understood but abnormalities in skin barrier function, combined with abnormalities in both adaptive and innate immunity, seem to be crucial. In at least 80% of cases, there is a raised serum total immunoglobulin E (IgE) level, but it is not clear whether this is of primary importance or a secondary effect.

Genetic studies have shown a primary problem of skin barrier function. Loss-of-function mutations in the epidermal barrier protein filaggrin cause ichthyosis vulgaris but also strongly predispose to atopic eczema. This work has been reproduced in different ethnic groups around the world. Filaggrin is coded by the *FLG* gene in the epidermal differentiation complex on chromosome 1q21.

Filaggrin deficiency leads to poor barrier function and dry skin, and allows antigen penetration into the epidermis. There is an initial selective activation of Th2-type CD4 lymphocytes in the skin, which drives the inflammatory process (adaptive immunity). This causes an increase in the cytokines interleukin (IL)-4, IL-5 and IL-13, as well as high IgE levels. During the chronic phase of the disease, both Th1 and Th2 cells are involved.

There are also defects in the innate immune system in atopic eczema. There is a decrease in epidermal antimicrobial peptides, Toll-like receptor 2 expression and epidermal tight junctions, and this, in turn, may explain why cutaneous infection (*Staphylococcus* and herpes simplex) is common in eczema (but rare in psoriasis).

Recent research shows the IL-4/IL-13 pathway is critical in Th2 activation. Blockade of this pathway is now being used as a new treatment for both eczema and asthma. IL-31 (which is induced by IL-4) may be a key player in 'itch'.

Exacerbating factors

Infection, either in the skin or systemically, can lead to an exacerbation, possibly by a super-antigen effect. Paradoxically, lack of infection (in infancy) may cause the immune system to follow a Th2 pathway and allow eczema to develop (the so-called 'hygiene hypothesis'). Soap, bubble bath and woollen fabric can irritate and aggravate eczema. Teething is another factor in young children. Severe anxiety or stress appears to exacerbate eczema in some individuals. Cat and dog dander can aggravate eczema. The role of house dust mites and diet is less clear-cut. Immediate/type 1 hypersensitivity to food allergens (cow's milk, egg, soya, wheat, fish and nuts) are common in young children with severe eczema. It causes urticaria (hives) and gastrointestinal symptoms (reflux, vomiting and diarrhoea) but not eczema. Rarely, there may be a delayed reaction to foods such as cow's milk that cause an eczema flare after 12–24 hours. Delayed food hypersensitivity cannot be investigated with prick tests or blood tests and the mechanism is unknown. The diagnosis is made by taking a careful dietary history, followed by oral food challenge tests. There is some evidence that food allergens may play a role in triggering atopic eczema and that dairy products or eggs cause exacerbation of eczema in a minority of infants under 12 months of age.

Clinical features

Atopic eczema has a variable clinical presentation. The most common involves itchy, erythematous, scaly patches, especially in the flexures of the elbows, knees, ankles and wrists ***(Fig. 31.13)***, and around the neck. In infants, eczema often starts on the cheeks before spreading to the body. Very acute lesions may weep or exude and can show small vesicles. Scratching can produce excoriations, and repeated rubbing produces skin thickening (lichenification) with exaggerated skin markings.

In people with pigmented skin, eczema may be more prominent on the extensor surfaces of the sites mentioned above, and the follicles can be prominent. Lichenification is common. Pigmentary changes – hyper- and hypopigmentation – may follow the inflammatory phase of eczema and are often slow to resolve.

Associated features

In some atopic individuals, the skin of the upper arms and thighs may feel roughened due to follicular hyperkeratosis ('keratosis pilaris'). The palms may show very prominent skin creases ('hyperlinear palms'). There may be an associated dry, 'fish-like' scaling of the skin, which is non-inflammatory and often prominent on the lower legs ('ichthyosis vulgaris').

Complications

Broken skin can become secondarily infected by bacteria, usually *Staph. aureus*, although streptococci may be involved, especially in macerated flexural areas such as the neck and groin. Pustules, crusted papules with exudate and impetigo-like lesions suggest secondary infection. Cutaneous viral infections (e.g. viral warts and

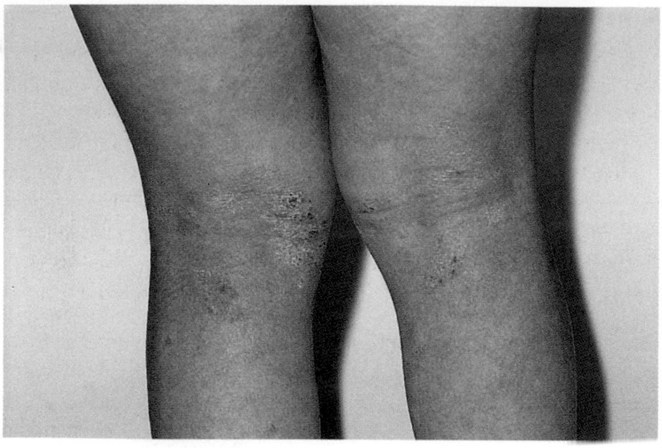

Figure 31.13 Atopic eczema behind the knees.

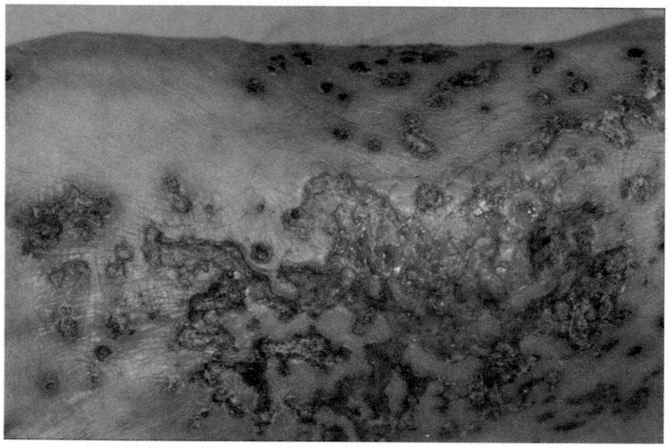

Figure 31.14 **Eczema herpeticum.** Multiple punched-out crusted erosions are shown.

molluscum) may be more widespread in atopic eczema. HSV can cause a widespread infection of the skin, ***eczema herpeticum*** (***Kaposi's varicelliform eruption***). It appears as multiple small blisters or monomorphic, painful, punched-out crusted papules ***(Fig. 31.14)*** associated with malaise and pyrexia. Very rarely, infection may become disseminated and life-threatening. Eczema herpeticum needs urgent treatment with systemic aciclovir. An unusually extensive form of hand, foot and mouth disease has been recently described in children with eczema, in which blistering, crusted lesions may extend to involve large areas of the limbs and face ('eczema coxsackium'). This resolves spontaneously but secondary bacterial infection may require antibiotics.

Ocular complications of atopic eczema include conjunctival irritation and, less commonly, keratoconjunctivitis and cataract.

Investigations

Atopic eczema is diagnosed by the history and clinical features. About 80% of patients also have laboratory features of atopy (raised total serum IgE and allergen-specific IgE and mild eosinophilia).

Prognosis

The majority (80–90%) of children with early-onset atopic eczema will spontaneously improve and 'clear' before the teenage years, 50% being clear by the age of 6. A few will experience a recurrence as adults, even if just in the form of hand eczema. However, if the onset of eczema is late in childhood or in adulthood, the disorder follows a more chronic remitting/relapsing course.

Box 31.5 Management of atopic eczema

- Education and explanation
- Avoidance of irritants/allergens
- Emollients
- Bath oils/soap substitutes
- Topical therapies:
  - Steroids
  - Immunomodulators
- Adjunct therapies:
  - Oral antibiotics
  - Sedating antihistamines
  - Bandaging
- Phototherapy
- Systemic therapy, e.g. oral prednisolone, ciclosporin

Management

(See ***Box 31.5***.)

General measures

These include avoiding irritants (especially soaps or furry animals), wearing cotton clothes and not getting too hot. Manipulating the diet (e.g. following a dairy-free or egg-free diet) may be helpful in a minority of infants with moderate to severe eczema. However, dietary modification should only be made with expert supervision, to ensure adequate intake of nutrients such as calcium.

Topical therapies

Topical therapies (see pp. 1385–1386) are sufficient to control atopic eczema in most people. The three components are usually a topical steroid, bland moisturizer and soap substitute/bath oil. Moisturizers should be used liberally on all dry skin areas and reapplied as often as needed (see ***Box 31.26***). Dermatology nurse-led education of eczema sufferers and their families can help provide psychological support and improve adherence to treatment.

Topical steroids

Topical corticosteroids remain the mainstay of eczema treatment. Selecting an appropriate dose and potency of steroid according to the body site, surface area and age of the patient is necessary to minimize the risk of adverse effects and allow safe, long-term intermittent treatment. Unfortunately, 'steroid phobia' is common among patients or their carers and leads to under-use of an otherwise effective treatment. Steroids should only be used on inflamed skin. Potent steroids should only be used for short periods. Regular use of emollients may lessen steroid usage. Topical steroids are classified into four main groups according to potency ***(Box 31.6)***. They are usually applied once or twice a day to inflamed areas.

While mild steroids rarely cause atrophy, this is a significant risk with potent and superpotent steroids, especially if used under occlusion or with keratolytics such as salicylic acid. Milder steroids should be used on the face and flexures, especially in the periocular area and in young children. The palmoplantar skin usually requires potent steroid therapy due to the thicker stratum corneum. The 'fingertip unit' can be used to guide topical steroid dosage. The ***adverse effects of topical steroids*** include:

- cutaneous atrophy and telangiectasia
- striae
- steroid-induced rosacea, perioral dermatitis and folliculitis
- tinea incognito (a tinea infection modified by a topical steroid applied inappropriately)
- ocular adverse effects – cataract, glaucoma.

Box 31.6 Classification of topical steroids by potency

Very potent
- 0.05% clobetasol propionate
- 0.3% diflucortolone valerate

Potent
- 0.1% betamethasone valerate
- 0.025% fluocinolone acetonide

Moderately potent
- 0.05% clobetasone butyrate
- 0.05% alclometasone dipropionate

Mild
- 2.5% hydrocortisone
- 1% hydrocortisone

Topical calcineurin inhibitors

Tacrolimus ointment (0.1% and 0.03%) and the less potent 1% pimecrolimus cream, applied twice daily, are licensed for the treatment of atopic eczema in children over 2 and adults. They do not cause skin atrophy and are a good option for treating eczema on delicate areas such as the face and eyelids. They are less effective on thicker, lichenified skin due to poorer penetration. The main adverse effect is a burning or prickling sensation when first used, which improves with continued treatment. Alcohol-induced flushing can affect a minority. Initial concerns that the immunosuppressant effects of topical calcineurin inhibitors (TCIs) would increase the risk of skin cancer have not materialized, but patients using these preparations are advised to avoid sun exposure and vaccinations. Tacrolimus ointment is also used twice weekly to prevent eczema flares.

Antibiotics

These are needed for bacterial infection and are usually given orally for 7–10 days. Flucloxacillin (500 mg four times daily) is effective against *Staphylococcus*, and phenoxymethylpenicillin (500 mg four times daily) acts against *Streptococcus*. Erythromycin (500 mg four times daily) is useful if there is allergy to penicillin. Topical antiseptics are used in cases of recurrent infection but they can be irritant. They are usually added to the bath water rather than applied directly to the skin.

Sedating antihistamines

These (e.g. oral hydroxyzine hydrochloride 10–25 mg) are useful at night-time.

Bandaging

Paste bandaging can be useful for resistant or lichenified eczema of the limbs. It helps absorption of treatment and acts as a barrier to prevent scratching. Wet tubular gauze bandages are used for inpatient therapy but are difficult and time-consuming to apply at home.

Second-line agents

These are used in severe, unresponsive eczema, especially if it is significantly interfering with an individual's life (e.g. growth, sleeping, school work or job). Ultraviolet phototherapy (see p. 1362), ciclosporin (3–5 mg/kg daily), azathioprine (1–3 mg/kg daily) and methotrexate can be helpful. Short, tapering courses of oral prednisolone usually give rapid disease control but relapse is common on withdrawal. The risks and benefits of long-term systemic therapy require careful evaluation and should be discussed with the patient.

New drugs

The new anti-IL-4/IL-13 monoclonal antibody dupilumab has been shown to have great efficacy and speed of action in atopic eczema. A new anti-IL-31 drug is in phase 3 trials in adults with eczema.

Omalizumab (anti-IgE monoclonal antibody) is already licensed for use in resistant asthma and chronic urticaria. There are conflicting reports as to whether it helps eczema, especially in those with very high IgE levels, but it may act via a non-anti-IgE mechanism. It is currently under trial in the UK in children with eczema. Apremilast (a phosphodiesterase-4 inhibitor) is also being studied in both eczema and psoriasis.

Seborrhoeic eczema

Clinical features

Seborrhoeic eczema is extremely common in adults of all ages and in its mildest form is often overlooked. As the name implies, it occurs in greasy body areas. On the face, it presents with scaling and erythema around the nose ***(Fig. 31.15)***, medial eyebrows, hairline and ear canals. Itch is variable. Dandruff is thought to be the mildest manifestation of scalp seborrhoeic dermatitis. More severe scalp involvement can look like psoriasis. The pre-sternal area may be affected in men and other sites include the large flexures and anogenital area. A generalized form of seborrhoeic eczema presents as erythroderma in the elderly (see pp. 1362–1363). Children are not affected until puberty, but a self-limiting infantile form is recognized, with scalp scaling/cradle cap and a non-itchy napkin dermatitis.

Aetiology

There is increasing evidence that the lipophilic commensal yeast, *Malassezia* (see p. 297), plays a role in triggering the inflammatory skin changes of seborrhoeic dermatitis in susceptible individuals. Host immunity is also involved, and seborrhoeic dermatitis is one of the earliest skin manifestations of HIV infection (see p. 337). Its prevalence is also increased in Parkinson's disease.

Management

Seborrhoeic dermatitis usually runs a chronic course with relapses, and treatment is suppressive rather than curative. Topical azole antifungal creams, with short-term use of mild- to moderate-potency steroids according to body site, are usually helpful. Topical

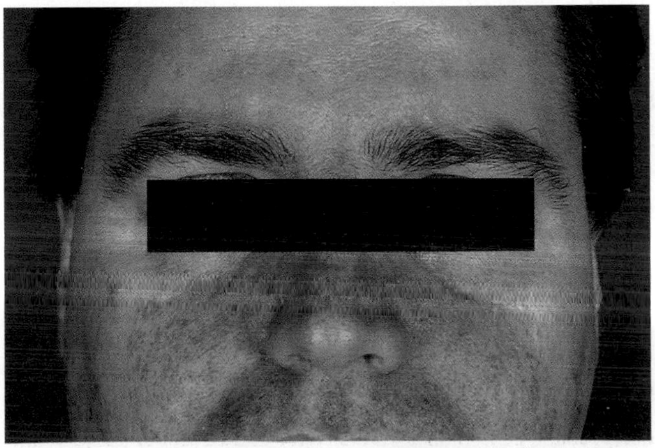

Figure 31.15 Seborrhoeic eczema affecting the sides of the nose.

calcineurin inhibitors (TCIs) are an effective option but are unlicensed in the UK for this form of dermatitis. A ketoconazole shampoo is useful to treat scalp involvement and as maintenance therapy.

Venous eczema (varicose eczema, stasis, gravitational eczema)

Venous eczema usually affects the elderly and those with varicose veins or a history of venous thrombosis. The inner calf is involved and there are usually coexistent signs of venous hypertension (see pp. 1375–1376), including haemosiderin deposition, lipodermatosclerosis and varicose ulceration. The eczematous changes range from mild erythema and scaling to an acute exudative inflammatory rash. It may be complicated by allergic contact dermatitis to medicated creams or bandages, and patch tests should be used if there is an inadequate response to treatment.

Management

This should include bland emollients, such as a liquid paraffin and white soft paraffin mix, and short-term use of a moderately potent topical steroid. Underlying venous hypertension may also benefit from compression hosiery or surgical intervention (see p. 1376).

Discoid eczema (nummular eczema)

Discoid eczema is characterized by well-demarcated, inflamed scaly patches, sometimes with tiny vesicles. It usually affects the limbs and torso, and is intensely itchy, which helps differentiate it from psoriasis. Lesions may be secondarily infected with *Staph. aureus*. The cause is unknown. Potent topical steroids are usually required to clear individual lesions.

Asteatotic eczema (winter eczema, eczema craquelé)

This form of eczema often affects the elderly in wintertime and can be intensely pruritic. It involves the lower legs, lower back and other areas that have few sebaceous glands. These areas are particularly vulnerable to the drying effects of soap and water. The skin resembles crazy paving with dry scales and inflamed cracks. Frequent use of a bland moisturizer and soap substitute is usually all that is needed.

Hand eczema

Hand eczema is a common problem in adults ***(Fig. 31.16)*** and has different patterns and causes. The causes are broadly classified as:

- ***Contact dermatitis/eczema*** – due to an external harsh substance (irritant) or allergy-provoking substance (allergen).
- ***Endogenous dermatitis/eczema*** – where no external factors can be identified. There may also be involvement of the feet.

In reality, it is often a mixed complaint with an underlying endogenous eczema tendency and an additional irritant and/or allergic component.

Mild ***irritant hand eczema*** in the finger webs and backs of the hands, with dry, sore, chapped skin, is extremely common in cold, dry weather and in those who wash their hands frequently, either at home (especially those who care for young children) or in occupations such as catering, healthcare and hairdressing. Hand eczema can also occur as part of ***atopic eczema*** and it is sometimes the only site in which this complaint persists beyond the teens. A ***hyperkeratotic*** form of eczema is characterized by dry, scaly plaques and cracks on the palms and soles, and shares similarities with psoriasis at these sites. In other cases, the features are non-specific and the complaint lasts for months – chronic hand eczema. Localized eczema of the finger pads is called 'pulpitis'. Even mild and localized hand eczema can be debilitating, as it affects the ability to do manual tasks.

Patch testing should be used in anyone with chronic hand eczema to investigate contact allergies, as it is not possible to identify which patients have an allergic contact dermatitis by clinical features alone. A careful history of occupation and hobbies may indicate the need to test with extra allergens: for example, plants in a gardener or garlic in a chef.

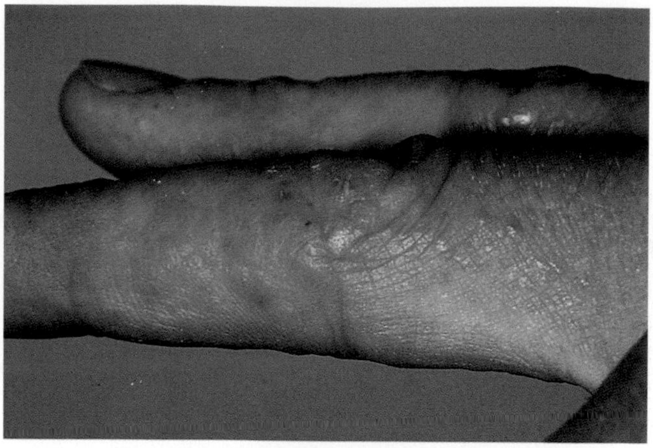

Figure 31.16 **Pompholyx eczema.** *(Courtesy of Dr A Bewley, London.)*

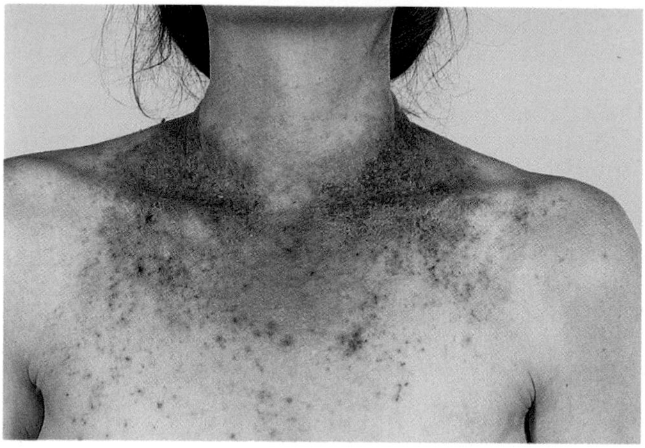

Figure 31.17 **Contact eczema secondary to perfume allergy.**

Allergic contact and irritant contact eczema

The most common causes of allergic contact dermatitis are as follows:

- fragrance – e.g. perfume ***(Fig. 31.17)***, toiletries, soap and moisturizers
- rubber chemicals – in household and examination gloves and footwear
- metals – in jewellery, buckles and gadgets, including mobile phones
- chemical hair dye – in permanent and semi-permanent colorants
- preservative chemicals – in cosmetics, toiletries, and household and occupational products
- other ingredients in medicated creams, such as lanolin, hydrocortisone and topical antibiotics.

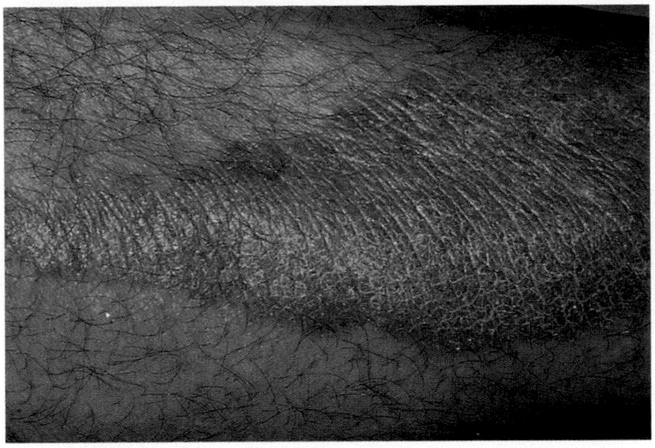

Figure 31.18 Lichen simplex from chronic rubbing.

Allergic contact dermatitis is an example of a delayed-type hypersensitivity reaction and the rash does not usually appear until at least 12–24 hours after skin contact. Other areas of the body that are prone to allergic contact dermatitis include the face (due to cosmetics and toiletries) and the lower leg, outer ear and anogenital area (due to medicaments).

Management involves managing eczema actively (as for atopic eczema; see pp. 1350–1351), minimizing contact with irritants and avoiding exposure to allergens. This may include wearing protective clothing such as gloves or, in extreme cases, even changing occupation or hobbies. The oral retinoid, alitretinoin, is an effective treatment for severe chronic hand eczema and can clear or significantly improve eczema in over half of all patients over a 6-month course. Like all oral retinoids, it is a teratogen, and a pregnancy prevention programme (see p. 897) must be followed.

Lichen simplex

This is a chronic form of eczema in which the skin is thickened and lined (lichenified) in response to repeated rubbing and scratching ***(Fig. 31.18)***. Common sites are the nape of the neck, outer calves and anogenital area. Topical antipruritics, short-term treatment with a potent topical steroid, and advice about habit reversal are usually helpful. There may be underlying emotional stress: hence the alternative name 'neurodermatitis'.

Nodular prurigo

This is a very persistent and itchy nodular eruption that is also perpetuated by picking and scratching. It may develop on a background of atopic eczema. Scattered eroded and hyperkeratotic nodules are typically found on the upper trunk and the extensor surfaces of the limbs. Unfortunately, topical corticosteroids, sedating antihistamines and antipruritics usually give temporary relief at best, and the complaint runs a chronic course.

The diagnosis is made by exclusion of other pathologies and may require a skin biopsy. General medical causes of pruritus should be excluded, including HIV infection (see p. 995).

Further reading

Banks TA, Gada SM. Filaggrin mutations as an archetype for understanding the pathophysiology of atopic dermatitis. *J Am Acad Dermatol* 2014; 71:592–593.
Beck LA, Thaçi D, Hamilton JD et al. Dupilumab treatment in adults with moderate-to-severe atopic dermatitis. *N Engl J Med* 2014; 371:130–139.
Paulden M, Rodgers M, Griffin S et al. Alitretinoin for the treatment of severe chronic hand eczema. *Health Technol Assessments* 2010; 14(Suppl 1):39–46.
Tsianakas A. Dupilumab: a milestone in the treatment of atopic dermatitis. *Lancet* 2016; 386:4–5.

Psoriasis

Psoriasis is a common papulo-squamous disorder affecting 2% of the population and is characterized by well-demarcated, red, scaly plaques. The skin becomes inflamed and hyperproliferates at about ten times the normal rate. It affects males and females equally and can involve all races. The age of onset occurs in two peaks. Early onset (age 16–22) is more common and is often associated with a positive family history. Late-onset disease peaks at age 55–60 years.

Aetiology

The condition appears to be polygenic but is also dependent on certain environmental triggers. Twin studies show 73% concordance in monozygotic twins compared with 20% in dizygotic pairs. Nine genetic psoriasis susceptibility loci have been identified (PSORS 1–9). Some loci seem shared with other diseases: atopic eczema (1q21, 3q21, 17q25, 20p), rheumatoid arthritis (3q21, 17q24–25) and Crohn's disease (16). The most studied locus, PSORS1 (which accounts for 35–50% of the heritable component), lies in the major histocompatibility (MHC) region of chromosome 6 (human leucocyte antigen (HLA) Cw6).

The exact aetiology is unknown but evidence suggests that psoriasis is a T-lymphocyte driven disorder that is a response to an unidentified antigen(s). ***Figure 31.19*** shows the trigger factors that activate the antigen-presenting cell (dendritic/Langerhans). This activation results in upregulation of Th1-type T-cell cytokines, such as IFN-γ, IL-1, 2 and 8, growth factors (tumour growth factor alpha (TGF-α) and TNF-α) and adhesion molecules (ICAM-1). The pro-inflammatory cytokine TNF-α is also produced by keratinocytes and this may be involved in both initiation and maintenance of psoriatic lesions. TNF-α-blocking drugs have proved highly effective in treatment ***(Fig. 31.19)***. IL-17 and IL-22 are thought to work together to produce clinical psoriasis (see p. 1356).

Pathology

Skin biopsy shows epidermal acanthosis and parakeratosis, reflecting the increase in skin turnover, and the granular layer is often absent. Polymorphonuclear abscesses may be seen in the upper epidermis. The epidermal rete ridges appear elongated and clubbed as they fold down into the dermis. Dermal changes include capillary dilatation surrounded by a mixed neutrophilic and lymphohistiocytic perivascular infiltrate.

Clinical features

Different patterns of psoriasis are recognized and can occur together. Certain drugs can make psoriasis worse: notably, lithium, antimalarials and beta-blockers.

Chronic plaque psoriasis

This is the most common type of psoriasis. It is characterized by pink-red, well-demarcated plaques, with a silver scale seen especially on extensor surfaces of the knees ***(Fig. 31.20A)*** and elbows ***(Fig. 31.20B)***. The lower back, ears and scalp are also commonly involved. New plaques of psoriasis occur at sites of skin trauma: the so-called 'Köbner phenomenon'. The lesions can become itchy or sore.

Flexural psoriasis

This tends to occur in later life. It is characterized by well-demarcated, red, glazed plaques with little, if any, scaling affecting

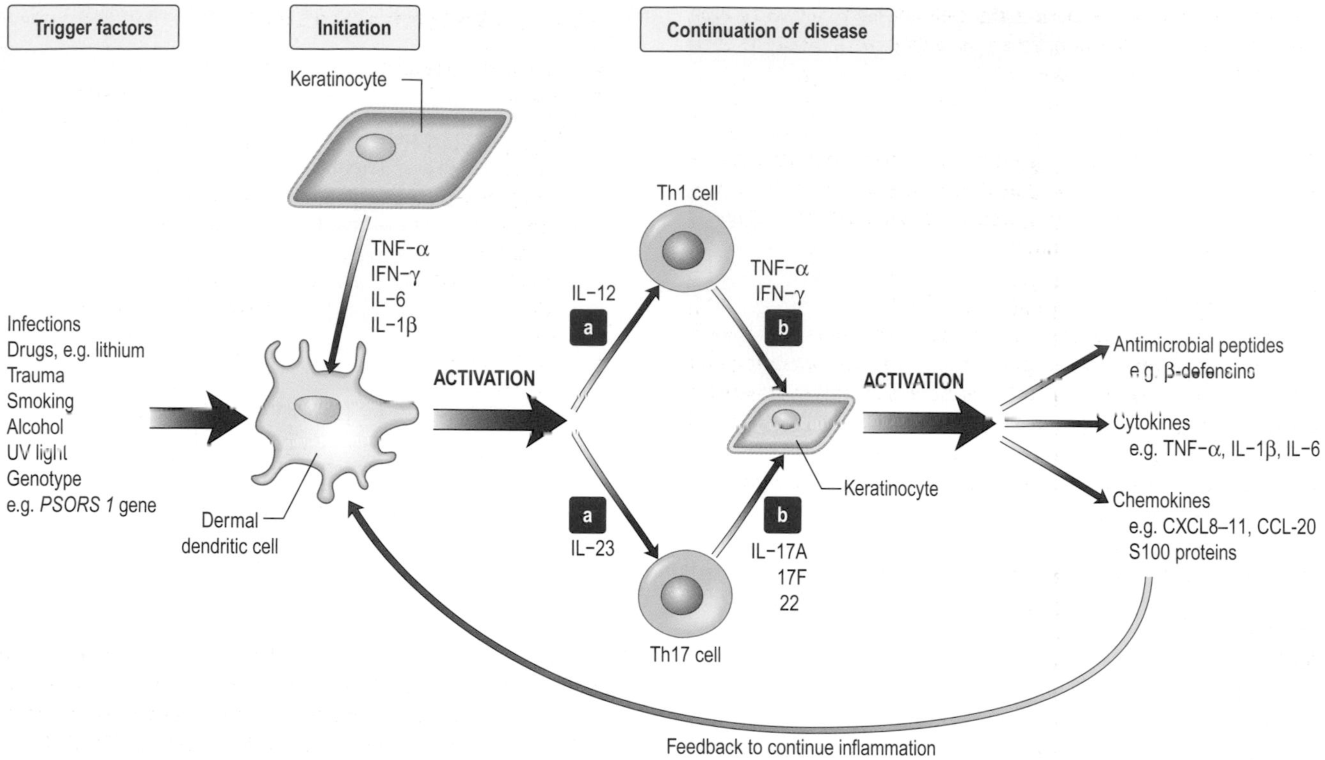

Figure 31.19 Pathogenesis of psoriasis. Trigger factors activate the dendritic cell and, in turn, Th1 and Th17 via IL-12 and IL-23. These T cells secrete mediators to activate keratinocytes to produce antimicrobial peptides, cytokines and chemokines. These maintain the inflammation and feedback to activate the dendritic cell. **(a)** Site of action of ustekinumab and briakinumab. **(b)** Site of action of infliximab, etanercept and adalimumab. IFN-γ, interferon-gamma; IL, interleukin; TNF-α, tumour necrosis factor-alpha; UV, ultraviolet.

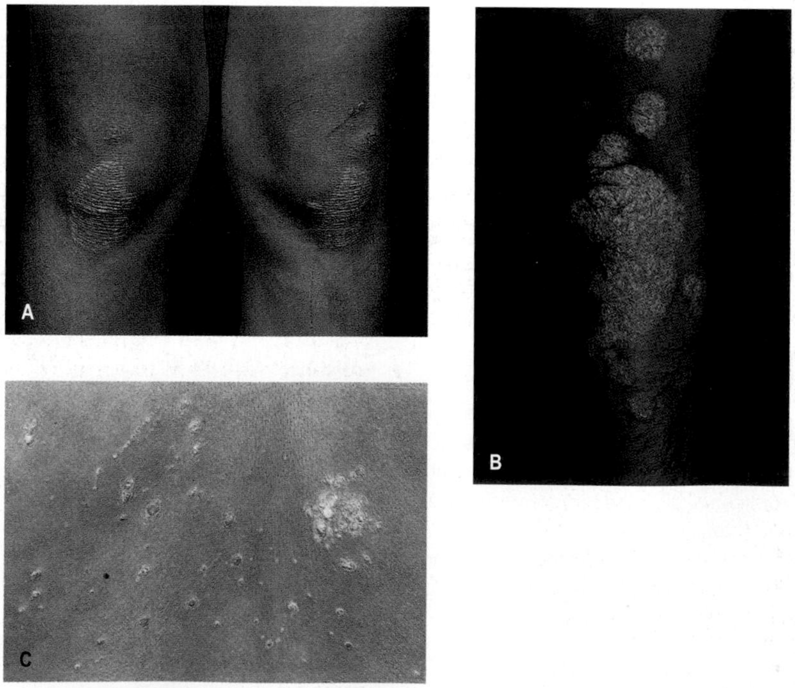

Figure 31.20 Psoriasis. A. Chronic plaque psoriasis of the knees. **B.** Chronic plaque psoriasis on the elbows in an Indian patient. **C.** Guttate psoriasis in an African patient. *(Courtesy of Dr P Matondo, Lusaka, Zambia.)*

the large flexures of the groin, natal cleft and sub-mammary area. The rash is often misdiagnosed as candida intertrigo but the latter usually shows satellite lesions.

Guttate psoriasis

'Raindrop-like' psoriasis is a variant most commonly seen in children and young adults ***(Fig. 31.20C)***. An explosive eruption of very small circular or oval plaques appears over the trunk about 2 weeks after a streptococcal sore throat.

Erythrodermic and pustular psoriasis

These are the most severe types of psoriasis, reflecting a widespread, intense inflammation of the skin. They can occur together ('Von Zumbusch' psoriasis) and may be associated with malaise, pyrexia and circulatory disturbance. This form can be life-threatening. The pustules are not infected but are sterile collections of inflammatory cells. There is also a more localized variant of pustular psoriasis that confines itself to the hands and feet (palmoplantar psoriasis) and is not associated with severe systemic symptoms. This latter type is more common in heavy cigarette smokers.

Associated features

Nails

Up to 50% of individuals with psoriasis develop nail changes ***(Fig. 31.21)*** and, rarely, these can precede the onset of skin disease. There are five types of nail change:

- pitting of the nail plate
- distal separation of the nail plate (onycholysis)
- yellow–brown discoloration
- subungual hyperkeratosis
- rarely, a damaged nail matrix and lost nail plate.

Topical therapy is usually ineffective, but systemic medication and biologics can improve nail dystrophy.

Arthritis and enthesitis

Some 5–10% of individuals develop psoriatic arthritis and most of these will have nail changes (see pp. 685–686). Asymptomatic enthesitis may be an early manifestation.

Metabolic syndrome

(See p. 209.) Psoriasis patients have a higher prevalence of cardiometabolic diseases and these may reflect a common underlying chronic, systemic inflammatory state.

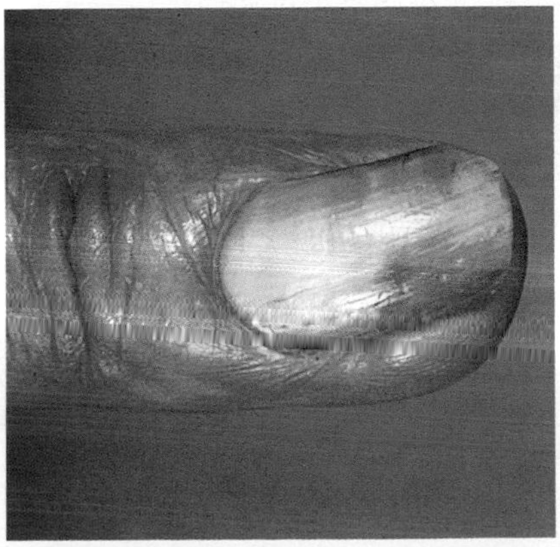

Figure 31.21 Psoriasis of the nail. Yellowish brown discoloration and distal nail plate separation (onycholysis).

Box 31.7 Management of psoriasis

- Education and explanation
- Emollients
- Topical therapies:
  - Mild to moderate steroids
  - Vitamin D analogues
  - Tazarotene
  - Tacrolimus
  - Purified coal tar
  - Salicylic acid
  - Dithranol
- Topical therapy in combination with UVB or PUVA
- Systemic therapy if conventional treatments have failed (monitoring for toxicity is required):
  - Methotrexate
  - Ciclosporin
  - Mycophenolate
  - Hydroxycarbamide
  - Acitretin
- Cytokine modulators if systemic therapy has failed:
  - Etanercept
  - Adalimumab
  - Infliximab
  - Ustekinumab

PUVA, psoralens + ultraviolet A; UVB, ultraviolet B.

Management

There is no curative treatment and the choice of therapy will be determined on an individual basis, according to the site and severity of disease, its psychological impact, co-morbidities such as cardiovascular or liver disease, and the individual's wishes ***(Box 31.7)***.

Chronic plaque psoriasis

Localized disease is usually managed with a vitamin D analogue (calcipotriol, calcitriol, tacalcitol) and an emollient to reduce scaling. Moderate to potent corticosteroids may also be used. Other topical therapy includes tazarotene (a retinoid), purified coal tar and dithranol, though these are less popular due to irritancy. Salicylic acid can be a useful adjunct for removing scales. Topical therapy is applied once or twice daily to palpable lesions. Once lesions have flattened, therapy can be discontinued. Vitamin D analogues used in extensive psoriasis may lead to hypercalcaemia if more than 100 g is given per week.

Dithranol stains the skin and clothes and has become less popular, as treatment is messy and time-consuming. Short-contact dithranol therapy is applied in increasing concentrations for 10–30 minutes and then washed off. Topical therapies are sometimes used in combination with UVB or psoralens + ultraviolet A (PUVA; see p. 1362) phototherapy. The 'Goeckerman regimen' consists of tar and UVB; the 'Ingram regimen' consists of dithranol and UVB. The latter has similar results to oral PUVA in terms of clearance rates and lengths of remission: approximately 75% in 6 weeks.

Flexural psoriasis

This is usually treated with mild steroid and/or tar topical creams. Calcitriol and 0.1% tacrolimus ointment are also useful for treating flexural (facial and genital) psoriasis, where irritation can be a problem.

Guttate psoriasis

This is usually treated with topical therapies and/or UVB phototherapy.

Palmoplantar psoriasis

Treatment is with very potent topical steroids, coal tar paste or local hand and foot PUVA.

Systemic therapy

Agents such as methotrexate, acitretin, mycophenolate, ciclosporin or hydroxycarbamide (hydroxyurea) are used for moderate to severe psoriasis. ***Erythrodermic psoriasis*** usually requires systemic therapy (but not phototherapy), as well as general supportive measures (see p. 1363).

All systemic treatments must be monitored for toxicity.

Methotrexate

Low-dose methotrexate is given once a week for severe psoriasis and psoriatic arthritis. Additional treatment with folic acid may improve gastrointestinal tolerance. Both men and women should avoid conception during, and for 3 months after, therapy. Regular blood tests need to be carried out to monitor for bone marrow suppression and liver damage. Alcohol should be avoided, as this can increase the risk of hepatotoxicity. Non-steroidal anti-inflammatory drugs (NSAIDs) should also be avoided, as these impair renal excretion of methotrexate. Lower doses of methotrexate should be used in the elderly. Long-term use can cause hepatic fibrosis, and serial monitoring of serum pro-collagen III peptide level or elastography (see p. 446) is increasingly being used as a non-invasive alternative to liver biopsy.

Ciclosporin

Ciclosporin is a selective immunosuppressant that inhibits IL-2 production by T lymphocytes. It is used for the long-term treatment of severe psoriasis. The main adverse effects are renal damage and hypertension, and so close monitoring of blood pressure and renal function (estimated glomerular filtration rate) is required throughout treatment. Ciclosporin interacts with many drugs (e.g. erythromycin, NSAIDs), which should be avoided.

Cytokine modulators

In the UK, the use of cytokine modulators ('biologics'; see ***Fig. 31.19***) is restricted to patients who have severe disease (Psoriasis Area Severity Index (PASI) >10, Dermatology Life Quality Index (DLQI) >10) and in whom phototherapy and conventional systemic treatment (ciclosporin, methotrexate, acitretin) have failed or cannot be tolerated due to toxicity.

- ***Etanercept, infliximab and adalimumab*** (TNF-α blockers). These are highly effective and tend to be used as first-line treatments in the UK, as they have the longest safety data. There is about 7% attrition per year ('tachyphylaxis').
- ***Ustekinumab*** (a human IL-12/23 monoclonal antibody). This is also highly effective but its safety data are limited so it is most commonly used in those patients in whom a TNF-α blocker has failed. There appears to be less tachyphylaxis than with TNF-α blockers and it has a favourable dosage schedule (four injections a year for maintenance therapy). Secukinumab, an IL-17A blocker, is also effective.

Both TNF-α blockers and anti-IL-12/23 drugs are also effective in treating psoriatic arthritis. Apremilast, an oral PDE4 inhibitor, has been shown to be effective in psoriatic arthritis.

New drugs

A number of anti-IL-17 monoclonal antibody drugs have been developed. Brodalumab (an anti-IL-17 receptor), ixekizumab (anti-IL-17) and secukinumab (anti-IL-17A) are all highly effective in psoriasis. Other anti IL-23 drugs are also in development.

All these new injectable biologic drugs are very expensive. Long-term side-effects of these new agents are unknown. The side-effects of TNF-α blockers are discussed on pages 680–682. One biologic drug (efalizumab) has been withdrawn due to the risk of prion brain disease.

Two new but somewhat less effective oral drugs are on the horizon. The small-molecule kinase inhibitors apremilast (a phosphodiesterase-4 blocker) and tofacitinib (a Janus kinase inhibitor) have also shown effectiveness in psoriasis.

Prognosis

Most individuals who develop chronic plaque psoriasis will have the condition for life but 80% will experience remission at times. Disease fluctuates in severity and there are no available tests to predict outcome. Guttate psoriasis resolves spontaneously and in up to one-third of individuals does not recur. However, two-thirds will go on to have recurrent guttate attacks or will progress to chronic plaque psoriasis.

Other papulo-squamous/inflammatory rashes

Urticaria and angio-oedema

Urticaria (hives, 'nettle rash') is a common skin condition characterized by short-lived, itchy swellings –'weals' – which usually clear within minutes to hours without residual dryness of the skin ***(Fig. 31.22)***. ***Angio-oedema*** is a similar disorder involving deeper tissues and usually affecting the lips, tongue and eyelids. Urticaria and angioedema may occur together or separately, and have a range of causes.

Aetiology and clinical features

Both conditions are caused by degranulation of dermal mast cells, which leads to the release of a range of inflammatory mediators (including histamine and/or bradykinin) that cause vasodilatation and increased capillary permeability. Mast cell degranulation may be triggered by various different stimuli, including ***drugs*** (opiates, aspirin), ***physical triggers*** (friction, pressure, sweating), allergens and ***autoantibodies***. Urticaria is classified as acute or chronic (>6 weeks' duration); the latter is divided into spontaneous (or idiopathic) and inducible types ***(Fig. 31.23)***.

Acute urticaria may be triggered by infections or can be a manifestation of immediate (type 1) allergy, especially in young children with atopic eczema. Common causes include food (nuts, egg, milk), drugs (penicillin) and natural rubber latex. It may be localized, as in contact urticaria, or part of a more widespread allergic reaction that can progress to anaphylaxis (see pp. 143–144).

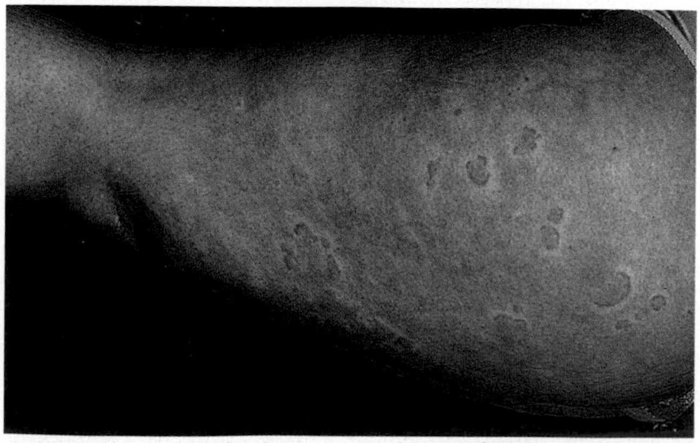

Figure 31.22 Urticaria.

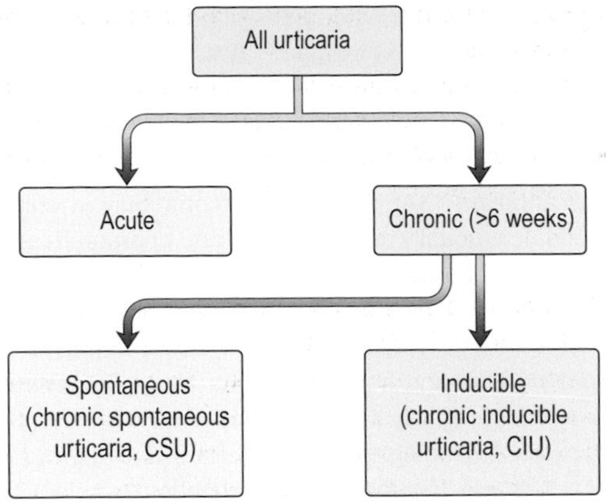

Figure 31.23 Classification of urticaria.

Box 31.8 Hereditary angio-oedema

Subtype	Gene (inheritance)	Biochemistry
Type I	*SERPING1* (AD)	C1-INH low C1-INH function low C4 low C1q normal
Type II	*SERPING1* (AD)	C1-INH normal/raised C1-INH function low C4 low C1q normal
Type III	*FacXII* (XLD)	C1-INH normal C1-INH function normal C4 normal
Acquired	Secondary to lymphoma/SLE	C1-INH low C4 low C1q low

AD, autosomal dominant; C1-INH, C1 esterase inhibitor; SLE, systemic lupus erythematosus; XLD, X-linked dominant.

Measurement of allergen-specific IgE and/or skin prick tests and allergen challenge tests are used to confirm an allergic cause.

Chronic inducible urticaria has a range of causes, including friction (symptomatic dermographism), pressure (delayed pressure urticaria), cold (cold urticaria), sunshine (solar urticaria) and sweating (cholinergic urticaria). Physical tests, such as lightly scratching the skin for dermographism or an ice cube test for cold urticaria, are helpful in demonstrating the nature of the problem.

Chronic spontaneous urticaria (***CSU***). The underlying cause may be autoimmune; in some individuals, functional autoantibodies against the high-affinity IgE receptor on mast cells and basophils or against IgE antibodies can be identified. There is also an association with autoimmune thyroid disease. Chronic urticaria is seldom caused by food allergy, and so food allergy testing is not routinely indicated.

Angio-oedema without urticaria is classified into hereditary and acquired varieties. ***Hereditary angioedema*** (***HAE***) (***Box 31.8***) is a rare autosomal dominant condition that can cause recurrent severe swellings of the skin, upper airways and intestinal tract. Laryngeal involvement may be life-threatening. Attacks usually start in childhood and can be spontaneous or triggered by minor trauma. Skin swellings are not itchy and usually last for several days. They may be preceded by a non-specific erythema (erythema marginatum). HAE types I and II are caused by mutations in the *SERPING1* gene that result in decreased plasma levels of functional C1 esterase inhibitor (C1INH). This allows unchecked activation of the complement cascade. Measurement of serum complement C4 can be used as a screening test. HAE type III is the rarest type and is caused by increased kininogenase activity. All lead to increased levels of bradykinin. HAE usually presents in childhood; severity is highly variable and is influenced by factors such as hormones, trauma, stress and infection.

Acquired angioedema may be idiopathic or associated with lymphoproliferative or autoimmune disorders. Drugs can also cause angioedema, especially angiotensin-converting enzyme (ACE) inhibitors, and black people are more commonly affected. The onset can be delayed by months or years after starting therapy and so a careful drug history is necessary.

Management

Acute urticaria is usually self-resolving. Acute allergic urticaria and angioedema may require emergency treatment with intramuscular adrenaline (epinephrine) and intravenous steroids (see ***Box 8.24***). ***Chronic urticaria*** is managed with non-sedating antihistamines such as loratadine 10 mg daily, which may be 'up-dosed' to four times the usual daily dose if needed for symptom control. Montelukast may also be helpful in those with aspirin sensitivity. NSAIDs and opiate analgesics should be avoided, as they can aggravate urticaria. Some physicians advocate low-salicylate, low-histamine and pseudoallergen-free diets for CSU, but these are difficult to follow in the long term. IgE therapy with omalizumab is used for treatment of severe CSU in addition to allergic asthma.

Management of ***HAE*** used to be limited to prophylaxis with attenuated androgens (stanozolol, danazol), which were poorly tolerated, and treatment of acute attacks was with fresh frozen plasma. Newer selective therapies include C1-inhibitor – both human plasma-derived and recombinant – a kallikrein inhibitor (ecallantide) and a specific antagonist of bradykinin B2 receptors (icatibant). These newer products can be used for treatment of acute attacks of HAE, and C1-inhibitors can also be used for prophylaxis.

Urticarial vasculitis

If urticarial weals are painful and persist for more than 12–24 hours with residual bruising or skin staining, this may indicate an underlying cutaneous or systemic vasculitis. It requires thorough assessment with a vasculitis screen of blood tests, skin biopsy and urinalysis.

Pityriasis rosea

Pityriasis rosea is an acute, self-limiting exanthem, which is thought to be caused by a viral infection, possibly human herpesvirus (HHV)-6 and HHV-7. It usually affects older children or young adults and there is an increased incidence in spring and autumn.

The rash is most prominent on the torso and proximal limbs, and consists of circular or oval pink macules with a collarette of fine scale. It is usually preceded by a larger solitary patch – the 'herald patch'. Lesions tend to run along dermatomal lines of the back, giving a 'Christmas tree' pattern. The rash is usually asymptomatic or mildly itchy and resolves within 4–8 weeks. Treatment is not usually required but emollients and a mild steroid cream may be used for pruritus.

Lichen planus

Lichen planus (LP) is a chronic inflammatory rash of unknown cause. It is speculated that a viral infection triggers an autoimmune

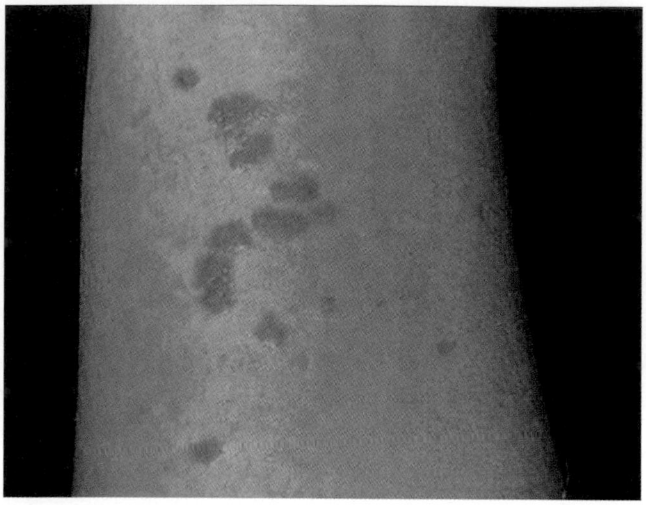

Figure 31.24 Lichen planus.

attack on keratinocytes by cytotoxic T cells. Conflicting results have been reported for an association with hepatitis viruses (HBV and HCV). Mucosal involvement may be seen in about 50% of patients with cutaneous LP and the oral mucosa may also be affected in isolation. Less commonly, LP may involve the scalp or nails, causing scarring. LP-like (lichenoid) rashes may be triggered by drugs (e.g. beta-blockers, gold, levamisole, ACE inhibitors and antimalarials) and are rarely due to sunlight. A widespread lichenoid eruption is also a feature of chronic graft-versus-host disease.

The rash of LP usually consists of clusters of intensely pruritic, purple–pink, polygonal papules ***(Fig. 31.24)***. It is most common on the flexors of the wrists and the lower legs but can be widespread. Close inspection of the papules shows fine, lacy white streaks (Wickham's striae). Lesions can fuse into plaques, especially on the lower legs, where they can become hyperkeratotic. After resolution, post-inflammatory hyperpigmentation may be prominent, especially in people with darker skin. Atrophic, hypertrophic and annular variants can occur. LP may köbnerize: that is, localize to areas of superficial trauma. Involvement of the scalp causes scarring alopecia, and nail involvement can cause permanent dystrophy with wing-like scars (pterygion) and loss of the nail plate.

Mucosal involvement is common. Changes range from asymptomatic, reticulate, white streaks on the buccal mucosa and lateral tongue to a severe, painful, erosive gingivitis and glossitis. Delayed-type hypersensitivity to metals in amalgam fillings may cause localized LP-like changes on the oral mucosa, which resolve on removal of the filling. The anogenital mucosa may be affected by LP and lesions on the penis are often annular. A rare chronic, severe, erosive form with vulval, vaginal and oral involvement is recognized in women.

Histology of LP usually shows diagnostic features of a dense infiltrate of T lymphocytes along the dermo-epidermal junction, which becomes damaged and 'saw-toothed', and degenerate basal keratinocytes (liquefaction degeneration). Apoptotic keratinocytes may also be identified as densely eosinophilic colloid bodies.

Cutaneous LP usually resolves within 1–2 years, though it may relapse at intervals. Hypertrophic and mucosal disease may be more persistent. Malignant change and development of squamous cell carcinoma may rarely complicate chronic ulcerated LP. Skin and mucosal lesions usually show some response to potent or superpotent topical corticosteroids. Topical calcineurin inhibitors (TCIs) may also be of benefit. Widespread skin disease or scalp disease may require tapering courses of oral steroids. Other therapies for recalcitrant disease include PUVA, methotrexate, oral retinoids, azathioprine and thalidomide.

Granuloma annulare

Granuloma annulare (GA) is seen most commonly in children and young adults. It is usually asymptomatic and characterized by clusters of small flesh-coloured or slightly erythematous papules (with no surface change), which tend to form rings or part of a ring with a dusky centre. They typically affect the dorsal hands and/or feet. Generalized papular and annular variants also exist. The cause of GA is unknown; several systemic associations have been proposed but not proven, including diabetes mellitus and thyroid disease. Histological features include a granulomatous dermal infiltrate and focal degeneration of collagen (necrobiosis). Localized GA is often self-limiting, resolving within 2 years. Papules may respond to intralesional corticosteroids or cryotherapy. Generalized disease can be persistent and many interventions have been proposed, but there is no clearly effective therapy.

Lichen sclerosus

Lichen sclerosus (LS) is a common inflammatory dermatosis that usually affects the genital area. The cause is unknown but may be autoimmune, and preceding infection or trauma and an occluded, moist environment may act as triggers. In females, the usual age of onset is before puberty or after the menopause. Males may develop LS at any age. Lesions are intensely pruritic or sore, and appear as shiny, ivory–white, fissured patches on the vulva, or on the glans penis (ballanitis xerotica obliterans) and distal foreskin or penile shaft. Perianal involvement is common in females, giving a 'figure-of-eight' distribution. Telangiectasia may be evident. Early lesions in girls may present with haemorrhagic blisters and these are occasionally mistaken for signs of sexual abuse.

The scarring and atrophy that accompany longstanding LS cause change in the vulval architecture, with loss and fusion of the labia minora and scarring of the clitoral hood. Involvement of the foreskin can cause phimosis, and urethral disease may cause strictures and impaired micturition. Profound sexual dysfunction can result from LS in both men and women. Perianal lesions may fissure and cause constipation. Rarely, LS may involve non-anogenital sites, especially in women, and lesions are typically more hyperkeratotic with plugged follicles. The diagnosis is usually made by the clinical appearance. The dominant feature on histology is condensation 'hyalinization' of the dermal collagen.

Management

Short-term courses of potent or superpotent topical corticosteroids improve the signs and symptoms of LS. TCIs may also be helpful. The condition may remit spontaneously after several years, especially in children. Male patients may require circumcision if phimosis does not respond to topical therapy. Longstanding anogenital LS is associated with an increased risk of squamous cell carcinoma of the penis and vulva.

Hidradenitis suppurativa (acne inversa)

This chronic inflammatory disorder affects the apocrine pilosebaceous follicles of the axillae, the inguinal area and around the breasts. It is characterized by recurrent abscesses, draining sinuses and scarring, and is associated with the metabolic syndrome, obesity and smoking. Patients often struggle with debilitating pain, odour and discharging lesions; there is no definitive treatment.

Bacterial biofilms within the occluded follicles may explain the disappointing results of treatment with acne antibiotics. Other options include acitretin, combined rifampicin and clindamycin, TNF-α and IL-1 inhibitors and laser therapy. Surgery may be required to drain abscesses and to excise the affected areas of skin.

Further reading

Boehncke W-H, Schön MP. Psoriasis. *Lancet* 2015; 386:983–994.
Irvine AD, McLean WH, Leung DY. Filaggrin mutations associated with skin and allergic diseases. *N Engl J Med* 2011; 365:1315–1327.
Jemec GBE. Hidradenitis suppurativa. *N Engl J Med* 2012; 366:158–164.
Langley RG, Elewski BE, Lebwohl M et al. Secukinumab in plaque psoriasis–results of two phase 3 trials. ERASURE Study Group; FIXTURE Study Group. *N Engl J Med* 2014; 371:326–338.
Le Cleach L, Chosidow O. Lichen planus. *N Engl J Med* 2012; 366:723–732.
Longhurst H, Cicardi M. Hereditary angio-oedema. *Lancet* 2012; 379:474–481.
Neill SM, Lewis FM, Tatnall FM et al. British Association of Dermatologists' guidelines for the management of lichen sclerosus 2010. *Br J Dermatol* 2010; 163:672–682.
National Institute for Health and Care Excellence. *NICE Clinical Guideline 153: Psoriasis: Assessment and Management.* NICE 2012; http://www.nice.org.uk/guidance/cg153.
Papp K, Cather JC, Rosoph L et al. Efficacy of apremilast in the treatment of moderate to severe psoriasis: a randomised controlled trial. *Lancet* 2012; 380:738–746.
Samarasekera EJ, Smith CH. Psoriasis: guidance on assessment and referral. *Clin Med* 2014; 14:178–182.
Tausend W, Downing C, Tyring S. Systematic review of interleukin-12, interleukin-17, and interleukin-23 pathway inhibitors for the treatment of moderate-to-severe chronic plaque psoriasis: ustekinumab, briakinumab, tildrakizumab, guselkumab, secukinumab, ixokizumab, and brodalumab. *J Cutan Med Surg* 2014; 18:156–169.
Waisma A. To be 17 again – anti-leukin-17 treatment for psoriasis. *N Engl J Med* 2012; 366:1251–1252.

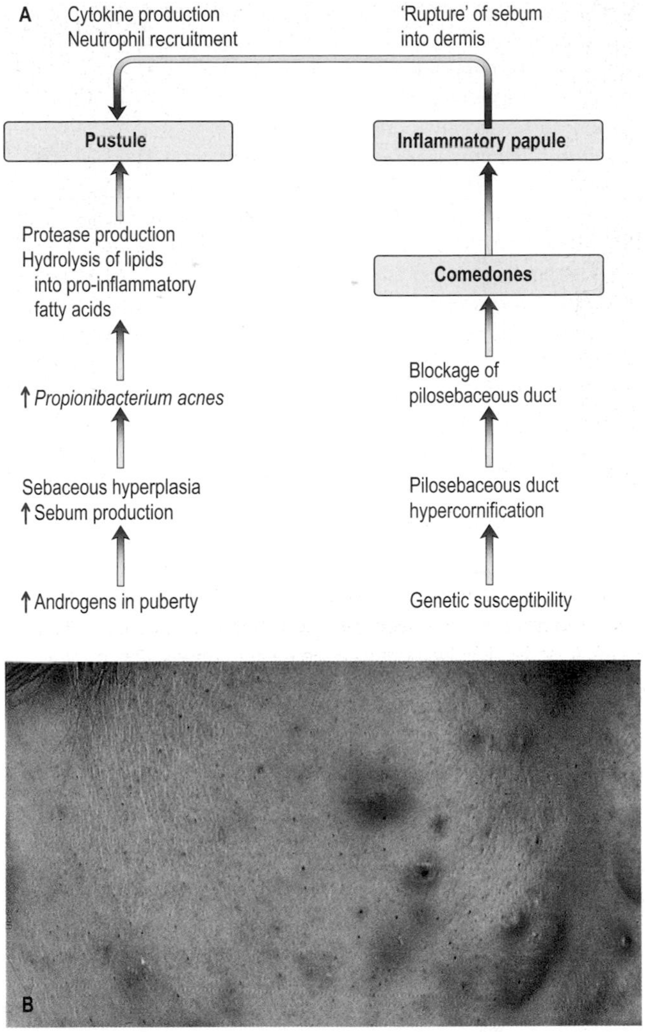

Figure 31.25 Acne vulgaris. **A.** Pathophysiology. **B.** Skin lesions.

FACIAL RASHES

Facial rashes often cause diagnostic confusion but a close examination of the clinical signs should help differentiate the underlying cause ***(Box 31.9)***. All facial rashes, by virtue of their visibility, can cause significant distress to the patient.

Acne vulgaris

Acne is one of the most common skin complaints and affects over 85% of adolescents. It may persist into adulthood and, in women, a late-onset chronic variant starting in the twenties is increasingly recognized. Acne can have a significant effect on self-esteem and mood, leading to anxiety, depression and an increased risk of suicide. Lesions arise in the pilosebaceous follicle, which becomes blocked due to abnormal keratinization and increased production of sebum. This leads to overgrowth of *Propionibacterium acnes*, which triggers an inflammatory response by activation of Toll-like receptors and induction of pro-inflammatory cytokines ***(Fig. 31.25A)***. The hallmark of acne is the comedo or blocked pore. Early microscopic comedones – microcomedones – can be seen in acne-prone skin. Comedones may be obscured in moderate to severe acne where inflammatory lesions predominate. Release of elastase by activated neutrophils causes connective tissue damage and scarring, which has long-lasting psychological sequelae. Post-inflammatory hyperpigmentation is common in dark-skinned patients.

Clinical features

Acne occurs on the face and upper torso, where the sebaceous glands are very dense and affected areas are usually greasy (seborrhoea). Lesions are classified as:

- ***non-inflammatory*** – open comedones (blackheads) or closed comedones (whiteheads)
- ***inflammatory*** – papules, pustules ***(Fig. 31.25B)***, nodules and cysts
- ***scars*** – raised (hypertrophic) or depressed/pitted (box, rolling and ice-pick).

A number of clinical variants exist.

- ***Infantile acne*** is occasionally seen in infants and is sometimes cystic. It is thought to be triggered by maternal androgens and resolves spontaneously.
- ***Acneiform eruptions*** may be caused by systemic steroid therapy, which cause a pustular folliculitis without comedones, and by epidermal growth factor receptor (EGFR) inhibitors.

Box 31.9 Causes of facial rashes

- Acne vulgaris
- Rosacea
- Perioral dermatitis
- Seborrhoeic eczema
- Atopic eczema
- Allergic and irritant contact eczema
- Impetigo
- Erysipelas
- Dermatomyositis
- Lupus erythematosus
- Photosensitivity
- Sarcoidosis (lupus pernio)
- Tuberculosis (lupus vulgaris)
- Sweet syndrome

- ***Oil acne*** is an occupational skin complaint caused by prolonged contact with oils or other hydrocarbons, and is common on the legs.
- '***Acne conglobata***' is a severe form of cystic acne with abscesses and interconnecting sinuses.
- ***Acne fulminans*** is a rare form of severe acne with systemic upset, seen mostly in male adolescents. Deeply inflamed, ulcerated nodules occur in association with fever, weight loss and musculoskeletal pain. Systemic steroids and oral isotretinoin are required.
- ***SAPHO syndrome*** (synovitis, acne, pustulosis, hyperostosis, osteitis) also features acne, but skin and osteoarticular changes do not often occur simultaneously and it may affect older individuals.
- '***Acne excoriée***' is a chronic form of acne typically affecting women, in which minor lesions are repeatedly picked/excoriated and there is underlying psychological upset.
- '***Follicular occlusion triad***' is a rare disorder most commonly seen in black Africans. It is characterized by the presence of severe nodulocystic acne, dissecting cellulitis of the scalp (see p. 1381) and hidradenitis suppurativa (pp. 1358–1359). This may be caused by a problem of follicular occlusion.

Management

Acne treatment should include therapy to target the primary pathogenic lesion: the ***microcomedo***. The choice of agents broadly depends on the predominant acne lesions, severity and response to earlier treatment ***(Box 31.10)***.

Patients should be told that topical retinoids, azelaic acid, salicylic acid and benzoyl peroxide (BPO) cause dryness and flaking of the skin due to their keratolytic effects. Tetracyclines and erythromycin are licensed for oral use in acne. Treatment may need to be continued for up to 6 months for maximum benefit. They should not be prescribed for non-inflammatory acne and should be used in conjunction with a non-antibiotic topical agent, as this improves effectiveness and reduces bacterial resistance. In females, the ***combined oral contraceptive pill*** and a formulation containing additional ***cyproterone acetate*** (a mild antiandrogen) may be of benefit, primarily due to a reduction in sebum excretion. ***Oral isotretinoin*** is a highly effective treatment for inflammatory acne; it is indicated for severe or unresponsive acne and where there is scarring or psychological upset. It is a potent teratogen, and females of child-bearing potential must use effective contraception and be carefully monitored with monthly pregnancy tests if at risk of pregnancy. All patients should be monitored for mood change but this usually improves as the acne clears. Several forms of high-energy light therapy have recently been advocated for treatment of acne, including blue light, intense pulsed light and photodynamic therapy. Ablative laser therapy and physical treatment, such as dermabrasion, may improve the appearance of scars.

Box 31.10 Treatment of acne

Severity	Treatment
Mild acne	
Comedonal	Topical retinoid, azelaic acid or salicylic acid
Inflammatory	Topical retinoid + topical antimicrobial or azelaic acid + topical antimicrobial
Moderate acne	Oral antibiotic + topical retinoid ± BPO
(Alternative for females)	Oral antiandrogen + topical retinoid/azelaic acid ± topical antimicrobial
Severe acne	Oral isotretinoin High-dose oral antibiotic + topical retinoid + BPO
(Alternative for females)	Oral antiandrogen + topical retinoid ± topical antimicrobial BPO (topical)

BPO, benzoyl peroxide.
(Adapted from Cunliffe WJ, Gollnick H. *J Am Acad Dermatol* 2003; 49:S1–S37.)

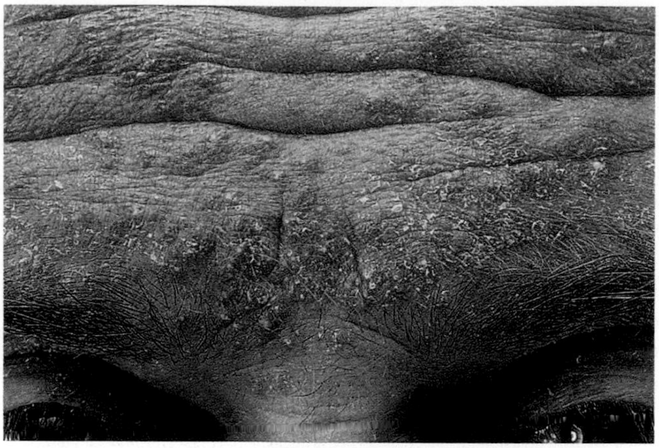

Figure 31.26 Rosacea. Papules and pustules on background erythema. There are no comedones.

Rosacea

Rosacea ***(Fig. 31.26)*** is a common inflammatory facial rash. The onset is usually in mid-adult life and it is more common in women.

The cause is unknown. Recent attention has turned to abnormalities in the innate immune system, including cathelicidin antimicrobial peptides and the proteases that convert them into pro-angiogenic and pro-inflammatory mediators. The commensal mite *Demodex folliculorum* is speculated to be one of the primary triggers of this abnormal immune response.

Clinical features

The main features are diffuse erythema and inflammatory papules and pustules affecting the convexities of the central face: that is, nose, forehead and cheeks. Flushing and blushing are often the earliest sign and can be triggered by hot drinks, alcohol, sunlight and changes in temperature. As the disease progresses, fixed erythema occurs due to dilated blood vessels (telangiectatic rosacea). This is followed by papules and pustules (papulopustular rosacea) but, unlike in acne, there are no comedones. Ocular involvement can lead to blepharitis, keratitis and conjunctivitis. Later complications include sebaceous gland and soft tissue overgrowth, especially of the nose in men, causing rhinophyma and facial lymphoedema. Prolonged use of topical steroids can exacerbate or trigger rosacea.

Management

Treatment is suppressive rather than curative. Metronidazole or azelaic acid cream or gel may be used for long-term control, with intermittent courses of oral tetracyclines for more resistant inflammatory disease. Sub-antimicrobial doses of doxycycline are effective due to their anti-inflammatory effects. The flushing and erythema do not respond to antibacterial drugs; treatment options include cosmetic concealers, topical brimonidine and vascular laser therapy. Rhinophyma can be debulked surgically or with the CO_2 laser.

Perioral dermatitis

Perioral dermatitis is a distinctive rosacea-like rash that typically affects the area around the mouth in young women. It is characterized by small inflammatory papules and pustules with overlying scaling and often runs along the nasolabial folds. Topical steroids may trigger the complaint in susceptible individuals and are often continued inadvertently as they appear to help temporarily. Treatment is with an oral tetracycline as for rosacea and weaning off topical steroids.

Flushing

Facial flushing in response to emotional stimuli (blushing) is a normal physiological response that can cause embarrassment and may be associated with social phobia. Non-emotional causes should be excluded, such as menopause, drugs, carcinoid syndrome and mastocytosis. ***Management*** includes cognitive behavioural therapy, cosmetic camouflage, beta-blockers and clonidine. Selective serotonin reuptake inhibitors may help associated depression and anxiety.

Other rarer causes of facial rashes include autoimmune rheumatic diseases and granulomatous infiltrates (see ***Box 31.9***).

Further reading

Bhate K, Williams HC. What's new in acne? An analysis of systematic reviews published in 2011–2012. *Clin Exp Dermatol* 2014; 39:273–277.
Dorschner RA, Williams MR, Gallo RL. Rosacea, the face of innate immunity. *Br J Dermatol* 2014; 171:1282–1284.
Lipozencic J, Ljubojevic MD. Perioral dermatitis. *Clin Dermatol* 2011; 29:157–161.
Van Zuuren EJ, Kramer S, Carter B et al. Interventions for rosacea. *Cochrane Database Syst Rev* 2011; 3:CD003262.
Williams HC, Dellavalle RP, Garner RS et al. Acne vulgaris. *Lancet* 2012; 379:361–372.

PHOTODERMATOLOGY

The solar spectrum includes visible light and UV radiation, which is divided into short, medium and long wavelengths (UVC, UVB and UVA, respectively; ***Box 31.11***). UVB and UVA penetrate the Earth's atmosphere and reach the skin, where they are potentially mutagenic and carcinogenic. They cause premature ageing (photodamage) and skin cancer, but can also suppress cutaneous inflammation.

Box 31.11 Visible and ultraviolet radiation

Visible radiation	Light	400–700 nm	Visible light
Ultraviolet A	UVA	400–315 nm	Long wave, black light, not absorbed by the ozone layer
Ultraviolet B	UVB	315–280 nm	Medium wave, mostly absorbed by the ozone layer
Ultraviolet C	UVC	280–100 nm	Short wave, germicidal, completely absorbed by the ozone layer and atmosphere

Box 31.12 Differential diagnosis of photosensitive rashes

Photoexacerbated/provoked rashes

Systemic disease
- Systemic lupus erythematosus (see pp. 692–695)
- Chronic discoid lupus erythematosus (see p. 1366)
- Subacute cutaneous lupus erythematosus (see p. 1367)

Metabolic disease
- Porphyrias (see pp. 1289–1291)
- Pellagra (see pp. 199–200)

Drugs
- Thiazides
- Phenothiazines
- Tetracyclines
- Amiodarone

Plant phototoxins
- Phytophotodermatitis (photosensitivity induced by contact of the skin with certain plants, e.g. celery, hogweed, rue, lime, fig tree)

Skin disease
- Rosacea
- Rarely, atopic eczema, psoriasis, lichen planus (these usually improve in sunlight)

Idiopathic photodermatoses
- Polymorphic light eruption
- Chronic actinic dermatitis
- Solar urticaria

Sunburn is caused by UVB and photosensitive drug rashes are predominantly caused by UVA (***Box 31.11***).

Photosensitive rashes arise on sun-exposed sites, such as the face, the 'V' of the chest, the ears and the dorsa of the hands and forearms. Shaded areas, such as under the chin, the upper eyelid and between the fingers, are characteristically spared. Porphyria, drug sensitivity and lupus erythematosus should be excluded in all photosensitive patients.

Photosensitive rashes may be divided into photo-exacerbated/provoked rashes and the idiopathic photodermatoses (***Box 31.12***). Examples of this include systemic lupus erythematosus (see pp. 692–695), pellagra (pp. 199–200) and porphyria (pp. 1289–1291). The only common photodermatosis is polymorphic light eruption. Very rarely, eczema and urticaria can be light-induced.

Polymorphic light eruption

Polymorphic light eruption (PLE) is a very common photosensitive rash that affects up to 10–20% of the population in temperate regions. It is most common in young women. In many cases, it is mild and undiagnosed, and simply a nuisance on tropical holidays. Typically, an itchy papular rash develops several hours after sun exposure and is confined to the exposed sites. Vesicles or plaques may occur: hence 'polymorphic'. These last for several days. A minority of patients are also affected in temperate zones; the rash appears in spring, but may improve during the summer because of acquired UV tolerance ('skin hardening'). PLE is thought to be an immunologically mediated condition where there is a failure of UV-induced immunosuppression, which allows a delayed-type hypersensitivity response to an as yet unidentified endogenous photoantigen.

Management

Mild cases can be managed by avoiding sun exposure with clothing and sunscreens. Topical steroids are of limited effectiveness, and individuals who are troubled by more severe PLE after intense sun exposure can be given prophylaxis or treatment with a short course of oral prednisolone (e.g. 30 mg daily for 7 days). Resistant cases can be managed with a short course of phototherapy (narrow-band UVB or PUVA) in early spring to induce photo-tolerance. Regular natural sunlight exposure is needed to maintain this effect over the summer season.

Phototherapy and photoprotection

Phototherapy

UVB and UVA have localized immunosuppressive effects in the skin and there is increasing evidence that they can also suppress systemic immunoreactivity: hence their use in the treatment of several inflammatory dermatoses. However, they also cause skin ageing and predispose to skin malignancy especially in fair-skinned individuals. UVB is less carcinogenic than UVA and is the preferred treatment for most dermatoses. Sunbeds are used for tanning and predominantly deliver UVA; they are of limited effectiveness in treating skin disease. If used frequently, there is an increased risk of skin cancer and premature ageing. The following types of phototherapy are used therapeutically:

- broad-band UVB
- narrow-band UVB (311 nm or TL01)
- psoralen and UVA (PUVA)
- high-intensity long wave UVA (UVA-1).

Narrow-band UVB therapy is widely employed in the treatment of eczema and psoriasis, and is usually given three times a week for 6–10 weeks. It has superseded broad-band UVB, as it is more effective. UVA is relatively ineffective alone, and so is used with a psoralen photosensitizer, which may be applied topically or taken orally (PUVA therapy). PUVA is usually given twice a week, and if the psoralen is taken orally, UV-protective glasses must be worn for the day of treatment to protect the retina. The use of PUVA is limited because long-term treatment increases the risk of skin cancer development, especially squamous cell carcinoma.

The maximum recommended lifetime dose is 1000 joules (approximately 200 treatments).

Unaffected regions of skin or high-risk areas like the scrotum can be screened during phototherapy. High-intensity UVA-1 penetrates more deeply into the dermis and can be of benefit in autoimmune rheumatic diseases such as morphea, but it is not widely available.

Photoprotection

Sunscreens protect against UVA and UVB irradiation but they are no substitute for covering the skin and restricting exposure, especially in young children. They work by absorbing/filtering UV radiation (e.g. benzophenones, cinnamates, salicylates) or reflecting it (zinc/titanium dioxide). New sunscreen chemicals have been developed to give better protection, and the particle size of reflective sunscreens can be reduced (micronized) to improve their cosmetic acceptability. Modern creams are formulated to give broad-spectrum protection against UVA and UVB. The sun protection factor (SPF) is a measure of UVB protection and the degree to which exposure can be prolonged before burning. However, in many cases, sunscreens are not applied in adequate amounts so do not provide the SPF as labelled. UV-absorbing chemicals may occasionally cause allergic contact dermatitis and, in rare instances, photoallergic contact dermatitis (where the sunscreen becomes allergenic with UV exposure).

Sunlight is the main source of vitamin D and individuals who do not have photosensitivity benefit from short-term sun exposure (without burning) to maintain levels, particularly in those with darker skins living in temperate climates; advice about sun protection therefore needs to take into account the individual's skin type.

Further reading

Gruber-Wackernagel A, Byrne SN, Wolf P. Polymorphous light eruption: clinic aspects and pathogenesis. *Dermatol Clin* 2014; 32:315–334.

Lehmann P. Sun exposed skin disease. *Clin Dermatol* 2011; 29:180–188.

http://www.bad.org.uk/for-the-public/skin-cancer/ *British Association of Dermatologists Sunscreen Fact Sheet.*

http://www.sunsmart.org.uk/ *Information from Cancer Research UK on sun, UV and cancer.*

ERYTHRODERMA

Erythroderma (literally, 'red skin') is a term applied to inflammatory complaints that cause redness of 90% or more of the body surface.

Aetiology and clinical features

There are a number of causes ***(Box 31.13)***, of which underlying skin disease and drugs are the most common. It is more frequently found in males and older people. The skin may feel 'tight' and itchy. Systemic symptoms are common and include malaise, fever or chills; there may be generalized lymphadenopathy. Because the normal functions of the skin are disturbed (see below) – that is, there is skin failure – erythroderma may be life-threatening and is regarded as a medical emergency. Longstanding erythroderma may be associated with hair loss, ectropion of the eyelids and nail shedding.

Examination should look for features of an underlying dermatosis, such as pustules and nail changes suggestive of psoriasis. A skin biopsy may help with diagnosis, especially in cutaneous lymphoma. Lymph node biopsy and T-cell receptor gene rearrangement studies (seeking evidence of clonal T cell expansion in the skin and blood) are also useful in the diagnosis of lymphoma. In non-malignant disease, enlarged lymph nodes usually show non-specific, reactive (dermatopathic) changes.

Complications

The skin is the largest organ of the body and, given its essential role in regulating body temperature and water loss, it is no surprise that extensive inflammation causes metabolic and haemodynamic problems. These may include:

- high-output cardiac failure from increased blood flow
- hypothermia from heat loss
- pre-acute kidney injury from fluid depletion
- hypoalbuminaemia
- catabolism and increased basal metabolic rate
- 'capillary leak syndrome'.

Capillary leak syndrome is the most severe complication and has been responsible for a fatal outcome in some cases of psoriasis, although this is extremely rare. It is thought that the inflamed skin releases large quantities of cytokines that cause generalized

Box 31.13 Causes of erythroderma

Common
- Atopic eczema
- Psoriasis
- Drugs (e.g. sulphonamides, gold, sulphonylureas, penicillin, allopurinol, captopril)
- Seborrhoeic eczema
- Idiopathic

Rare
- Chronic actinic dermatitis
- Cutaneous T-cell lymphoma (Sézary syndrome)
- Malignancy (especially leukaemias)
- Pemphigus foliaceus
- Pityriasis rubra pilaris (a hereditary disorder of keratinization)
- HIV infection
- Toxic shock syndrome

vascular leakage. This can lead to cutaneous oedema, hypovolaemic shock and acute respiratory distress syndrome (ARDS) (see pp. 1167–1169).

Management

Supportive treatment includes maintaining body temperature (with space blankets and heaters) and close monitoring of vital signs and of fluid and electrolyte balance. Skin swabs should be taken if secondary infection is suspected. All non-essential medication should be stopped. Topical therapy with a bland emollient or mild topical steroid can be initiated until the underlying cause is established, when systemic therapy may be indicated: for example, ciclosporin for psoriasis.

CUTANEOUS SIGNS OF SYSTEMIC DISEASE

Some dermatoses are associated with a variety of underlying systemic diseases. Furthermore, some medical conditions may present with cutaneous features.

Erythema nodosum

Erythema nodosum (see also p. 705) has a number of underlying causes ***(Box 31.14)***. It presents as painful or tender dusky blue–red nodules, commonly over the shins or lower limbs, which fade over 2–3 weeks, leaving a bruised appearance (see ***Fig. 31.52***). It is most common in young adults, especially females. It may be associated with arthralgia, malaise and fever. Inflammation occurs in the dermis and the subcutaneous layer (panniculitis).

Management consists of treatment of the symptoms with NSAIDs (avoid in pregnancy), light compression bandaging and bed rest, as the condition resolves spontaneously. The underlying cause should be treated. In very persistent cases, dapsone (100 mg daily), colchicine (500 µg twice daily) or prednisolone (up to 30 mg daily) can be useful.

Box 31.14 Causes of erythema nodosum

- Streptococcal infection[a]
- Drugs (e.g. sulphonamides, oral contraceptive)
- Sarcoidosis[a]
- Idiopathic[a]
- Bacterial gastroenteritides, e.g. *Salmonella*, *Shigella*, *Yersinia*
- Fungal infection (histoplasmosis, blastomycosis)
- Tuberculosis
- Leprosy
- Inflammatory bowel disease
- *Chlamydia* infection

[a]*Common causes.*

Erythema multiforme

Erythema multiforme is a self-limiting, symmetrical rash characterized by target lesions on the distal limbs, palms and soles. These are concentric rings of erythema with a dusky centre, which may occasionally blister. The mucous membranes may be involved, with oro-genital ulceration, erosions and conjunctivitis – so-called 'erythema multiforme major' ***(Fig. 31.27)***. The most common trigger is herpes simplex virus. Erythema multiforme may occasionally be a recurrent problem, in which case prophylactic aciclovir can be used. Other causes include orf (see p. 1345), *Mycoplasma* and drugs (sulphonamides, anticonvulsants). In 50% of cases, there is no identifiable cause.

Management is supportive, with analgesia and short-term parenteral fluids if there is dysphagia. The role of systemic steroids in erythema multiforme major remains controversial.

The clinical features of 'erythema multiforme major' – Stevens–Johnson syndrome – are show in ***Box 31.15***.

Pyoderma gangrenosum

Pyoderma gangrenosum is a condition of unknown aetiology. It presents with painful erythematous nodules or pustules that rapidly evolve into large ulcers ***(Fig. 31.28)***. The ulcer often has a purple margin, undermined edge and a purulent surface ('pyoderma'). Lesions may occasionally be triggered by trauma or surgery, and debridement is contraindicated, as it worsens the condition. Biopsy

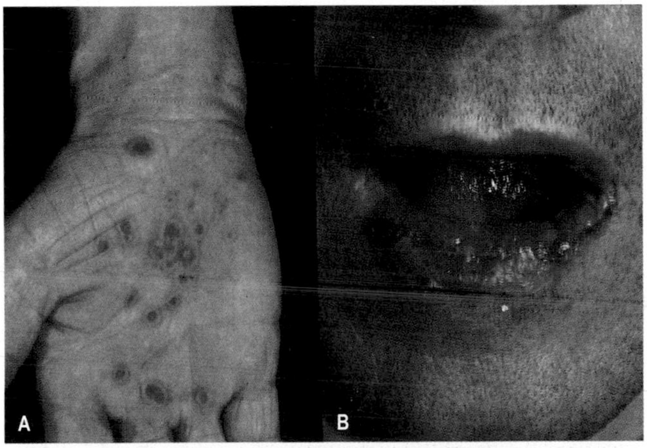

Figure 31.27 **Erythema multiforme major. A.** Target lesions of the palm. **B.** Mucosal involvement around the mouth.

Box 31.15 Clinical spectra of erythema multiforme, Stevens–Johnson syndrome and toxic epidermal necrolysis

Diagnosis	Skin lesions	Mucosal lesions	Other signs/symptoms
Erythema multiforme (EM)	Three-ring target lesions, often hands and feet	EM major only	Recent infection (herpes simplex virus, *Mycoplasma*)
Stevens–Johnson syndrome (SJS)	Scattered macules/blisters scattered over face, trunk proximal limbs (<10% body surface area) Occasional two-ring target lesion	Always	Fever Skin tenderness Recent drug exposure
Toxic epidermal necrolysis (TEN)	As for SJS but >30% body surface area involved	Always	As for SJS Respiratory and gastrointestinal lesions Hypotension Decreased consciousness
SJS/TEN overlap	As for SJS (10–30% body surface area involved)	Always	

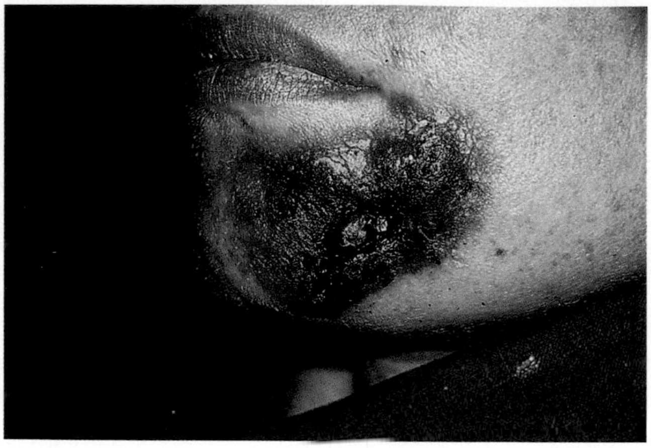

Figure 31.28 Pyoderma gangrenosum.

of the ulcer edge shows an intense neutrophilic infiltrate but the diagnosis is based largely on clinical appearance. Most cases occur in association with:

- inflammatory bowel disease
- rheumatoid arthritis
- haematological malignancy – myeloma, monoclonal gammopathy, leukaemia, lymphoma
- liver disease (e.g. primary biliary cholangitis).

Very potent topical steroids or tacrolimus ointment may help mild disease, but high-dose oral steroids are usually needed to halt rapidly progressive ulceration. Systemic immunosuppressants or dapsone may be required for long-term control, and any underlying disease should be treated.

Endocrine disease

Acanthosis nigricans

Acanthosis nigricans presents as thickened, hyperpigmented, velvet-textured skin around the large flexures ***(Fig. 31.29)***. It can appear warty when advanced. The commonest and mildest form is associated with obesity and insulin resistance ('pseudo-acanthosis nigricans', ***Fig. 31.29***). Late onset and severe disease is usually a paraneoplastic phenomenon caused by underlying malignancy (especially gastrointestinal tumours). Rarely it is associated with hyperandrogenism in females.

Diabetes mellitus

Diabetes mellitus (see also p. 1241) can have a number of cutaneous manifestations and complications, including:

- fungal infection (e.g. *Candidiasis*; see p. 295)
- bacterial infections (e.g. recurrent boils; see p. 1342)
- xanthomas
- arterial disease (ulcers, gangrene)
- neuropathic ulcers.

Specific dermatoses of diabetes include:

- necrobiosis lipoidica (a patch of spreading erythema over the shin, which becomes yellowish and atrophic in the centre and may ulcerate; ***Fig. 31.30***)
- diffuse granuloma annulare (see p. 1358)
- diabetic dermopathy (red–brown, flat-topped papules)
- diabetic stiff skin (tight, waxy skin over the fingers with limitation of joint movement owing to thickened collagen; also called cheiroarthropathy).

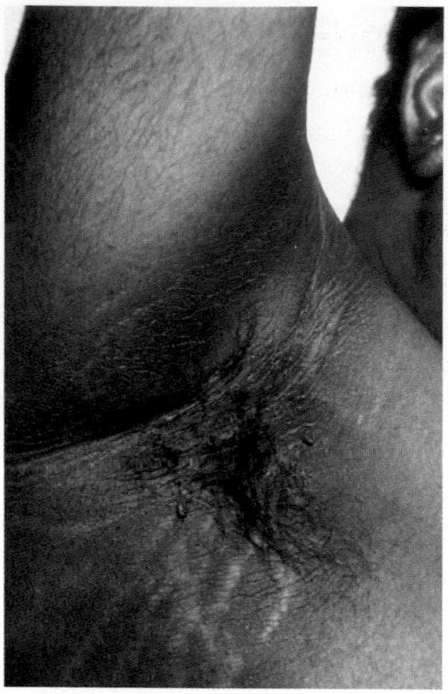

Figure 31.29 Acanthosis nigricans in axilla of an obese individual.

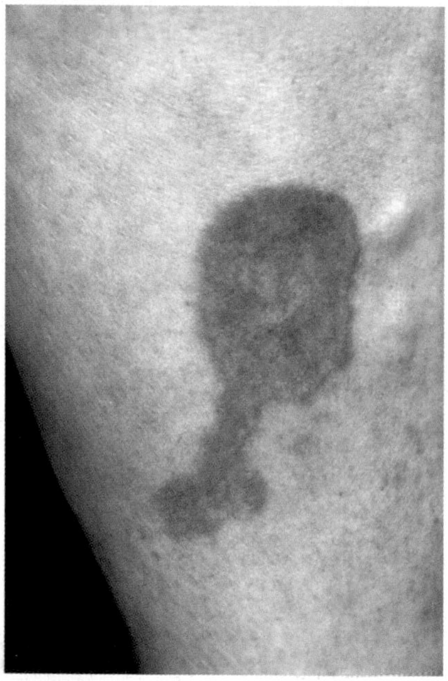

Figure 31.30 Necrobiosis lipoidica on the shin in type 1 diabetes mellitus.

Thyroid disease

(See also pp. 1199–1212.) Hypothyroidism may cause dry, firm, gelatinous (myxoedematous) skin with diffuse hair thinning and loss of the outer third of the eyebrows. Hyperthyroidism may be associated with warm, sweaty skin and a diffuse alopecia. Graves' disease is rarely associated with thyroid acropachy ('clubbing' with underlying bone changes) and pretibial myxoedema (a red–brown mucinous infiltration of the shins, which can become lumpy and tender).

Cushing syndrome

(See also pp. 1197–1199.) Skin manifestations include hirsutism, a moon face, a buffalo hump, striae, telangiectasia and folliculitis (often called steroid acne; see p. 1342).

Metabolic disease

Hyperlipidaemias

Hyperlipidaemias (see also pp. 1279–1284) can present with xanthomas, which are abnormal collections of lipid in the skin. All people with xanthomas should be investigated for hyperlipidaemia, although the most common type, called xanthelasmas (yellow plaques around the eyes), are usually associated with normal lipids. There are a number of other clinical variants of ***xanthomas***, such as:

- ***tuberous xanthoma*** (firm orange–yellow nodules and plaques on extensor surfaces)
- ***tendon xanthoma*** (firm subcutaneous swellings attached to tendons)
- ***plane xanthoma*** (orange–yellow macules often affecting palmar creases)
- ***eruptive xanthoma*** (numerous small, yellowish papules commonly on the buttocks).

Amyloidosis

Macular amyloid is a common, purely cutaneous variant seen in Asians. It is characterized by itchy brown, rippled macules on the upper back.

Systemic amyloid may be associated with reddish-brown papules, nodules or plaques, especially around the eyes, the flexural areas and mucosal surfaces. Distinctive periorbital bruising and macroglossia may also be present.

Porphyria cutanea tarda

Porphyria cutanea tarda (PCT; see p. 1290) is a rare metabolic disorder associated with liver disease; it is usually precipitated by alcohol excess or hepatitis C virus (HCV) infection and 20% of cases have underlying haemochromatosis (see pp. 477–479). Approximately 75% of cases are sporadic and 25% familial. PCT presents with sun-induced blisters, skin fragility, scarring, milia, especially on the dorsal hands, and hypertrichosis.

Management is with repeated venesection to reduce iron load, alcohol avoidance and low-dose chloroquine. Antiviral therapy for HCV may also help the skin, presumably by improving liver function. All people with PCT are at risk of hepatic carcinoma.

Pruritus

The pathophysiology of pruritus (itch) is complex and incompletely understood. It may be caused by peripheral mechanisms (as in skin disease), central or neuropathic mechanisms (as in multiple sclerosis), neurogenic mechanisms (as in cholestasis/μ-opioid receptor stimulation) or psychogenic mechanisms (e.g. parasitophobia). Evidence suggests that low stimulation of unmyelinated C-fibres in the skin is associated with the sensation of itch (high stimulation produces pain). Histamine, tachykinins (e.g. substance P) and cytokines (e.g. IL-31) may also play a role peripherally in the skin. The major nerve pathways for itch and the influence of the central nervous system are not well characterized but processes that are dependent on μ-opioid receptors can regulate the perception and intensity of itch.

Asteatotic eczema and cholinergic urticaria are common causes of pruritus in which the rash is often missed. The term idiopathic pruritus or 'senile' pruritus is often due to skin dryness (xerosis) and is common in the elderly.

Pruritus in the absence of a demonstrable rash can be caused by a number of different medical problems ***(Box 31.16)***.

Box 31.16 Medical conditions associated with pruritus

- Iron deficiency anaemia
- Internal malignancy (especially lymphoma)
- Diabetes mellitus
- Chronic kidney disease
- Chronic liver disease (especially primary biliary cholangitis)
- Thyroid disease
- HIV infection
- Polycythaemia vera

Management involves avoidance of soaps and symptomatic measures (as for asteatotic eczema). Phototherapy, low-dose amitriptyline or gabapentin may help intractable cases. Any underlying medical problem should be treated.

Haematological disease

Both anaemia (especially iron deficiency) and polycythaemia can cause pruritus. It can also be a feature of lymphoproliferative disease, such as lymphoma.

Liver disease

Chronic liver disease

Chronic liver disease may present with jaundice, palmar erythema, spider naevi, white nails, hyperpigmentation and pruritus.

Renal disease

Chronic kidney disease

Chronic kidney disease (CKD; see also pp. 774–789) is commonly associated with intractable pruritus. Pallor, hyperpigmentation and ecchymoses are commonly seen. Rarely, it is associated with non-inflammatory blisters, pseudo-porphyria cutanea tarda and cutaneous calcification. Longstanding renal transplant recipients often suffer with recurrent viral warts and squamous cell carcinomas due to the immunosuppression.

'***Nephrogenic fibrosing dermopathy***' (also known as '***nephrogenic systemic fibrosis***') is a severe scleroderma-like skin disease found in a subset of patients who have CKD (usually those on dialysis). The disease is rapid in onset (days to weeks) with skin discoloration and thickening, joint contractures, muscle weakness and generalized pain. Widespread tissue fibrosis may ensue, causing severely restricted mobility. The condition is strongly associated with the contrast medium, gadolinium, used in magnetic resonance imaging (MRI) scans, and such contrast agents are best avoided in people with low glomerular filtration rates. There is no accepted treatment but some advocate PUVA and extracorporeal photophoresis. No spontaneous remissions have been recorded. Rapid correction of renal function generally stops the condition progressing.

Calciphylaxis is discussed on page 780.

Autoimmune rheumatic diseases

Dermatomyositis

The rash of dermatomyositis (see also pp. 697–698) is distinctive and often photosensitive. There is facial erythema and a magenta rash with oedema around the eyes. There may be areas of poikiloderma (reticulate pigmentation, atrophy and telangiectasia). Bluish-red nodules or plaques may be present over the knuckles (Gottron's papules; see ***Fig. 18.37***) and extensor surfaces. The nail folds are frequently ragged with dilated capillaries. The diagnosis is made from the clinical appearance, muscle biopsy, electromyography and a serum creatine phosphokinase. Skin biopsy is not diagnostic. MRI scanning is useful to assess myositis. Newer antibody tests are of use in diagnosis and prediction of complications; they include anti-Mi-2 antibodies (highly specific for dermatomyositis), anti-MDA-5 antibody (interstitial lung disease) and anti-TIF1-gamma antibodies (associated malignancy) (see p. 698).

Juvenile dermatomyositis usually starts before the age of 10 and eventually resolves. This variant is associated with cutaneous calcinosis and muscle contractures. The adult form usually occurs after the age of 40. Some cases are associated with malignancy, especially gynaecological, and this requires thorough investigation. Other cases are linked with autoimmune rheumatic diseases and may share overlapping features with scleroderma and lupus erythematosus.

Management

Skin disease may respond to sunscreens and hydroxychloroquine (200 mg twice daily). Myositis usually requires high-dose corticosteroids and immunosuppressant drugs, such as azathioprine or ciclosporin.

Scleroderma

The term scleroderma refers to a thickening or hardening of the skin owing to abnormal dermal collagen. It is not a diagnostic entity in itself. Systemic sclerosis and morphea both show sclerodermatous changes but are separate conditions.

Systemic sclerosis (often called scleroderma) has cutaneous and systemic features, and is discussed fully on pages 695–697.

Morphea (localized cutaneous scleroderma) is confined to the skin and usually presents in children or young adults. It is more common in females and the cause is unknown. Lesions are usually on the trunk and appear as bluish-red plaques, which progress to induration and then central white atrophy ***(Fig. 31.31)***. A linear variant exists in childhood, which is more severe as it can cause atrophy of underlying deep tissues and thus lead to unequal limb growth or scarring alopecia.

Rarely, sclerodermatous skin changes may be seen in Lyme disease (acrodermatitis chronica atrophicans), chronic graft-versus-host disease, polyvinyl chloride disease, eosinophilic myalgia syndrome (due to tryptophan therapy) and bleomycin therapy.

Management

Potent topical steroids, oral (or pulsed intravenous) steroids and phototherapy can be used. Treatment needs to be more aggressive if there is deep cutaneous involvement, as scarring is irreversible once it has occurred. Methotrexate and mycophenolate have also been used.

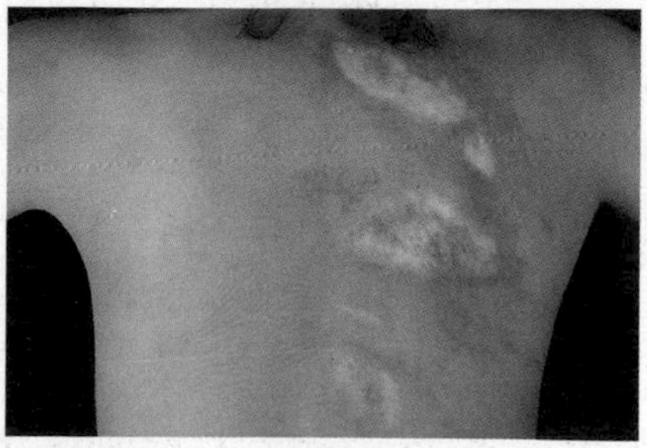

Figure 31.31 Morphea. Hyperpigmentation and scarring on the trunk.

Lupus erythematosus

Lupus is a chronic autoimmune disease characterized by acute and chronic inflammation in various body tissues (see pp. 692–695). Skin involvement falls into three broad categories:

- chronic discoid lupus erythematosus (CDLE)
- subacute cutaneous lupus erythematosus (SCLE)
- systemic lupus erythematosus (SLE).

The cause is unknown but inherited factors, drugs and UV exposure may be relevant. All forms of lupus erythematosus are more common in women.

Chronic discoid lupus erythematosus

Chronic discoid lupus erythematosus (CDLE) is characterized by erythematous, scaly, atrophic plaques with telangiectasia, especially on the face or other sun-exposed sites ***(Fig. 31.32)***. Hypopigmentation is common and follicular plugging may be apparent. Scalp involvement may lead to a scarring alopecia. Oral involvement (erythematous patches or ulceration) occurs in 25% of cases. A minority of patients also suffer with Raynaud's phenomenon or chilblain-like lesions (chilblain lupus). Disease is usually localized to the skin and fewer than 5% of cases will go on to develop systemic disease, but this is more common in children. Serum anti-nuclear factor (ANF) is positive in 30% of cases.

Skin biopsy shows a dense patchy, lymphocytic infiltrate around the dermal appendages. Epidermal basal layer damage, follicular plugging and hyperkeratosis may be present. Direct immunofluorescence of lesional skin may show IgM and C3 deposition in a granular band at the dermo-epidermal junction ('lupus band').

First-line ***treatment*** is with sunscreens and potent topical steroids. Unresponsive disease may require antimalarial therapy (hydroxychloroquine 100–200 mg twice daily and mepacrine 100 mg daily). Smoking reduces their effectiveness. Systemic steroids and immunosuppressants may be required for resistant disease or associated arthritis. Thalidomide has been used for recalcitrant CDLE.

The disease is usually chronic, with fluctuations in severity, and eventually undergoes remission in up to 50% of cases after many years.

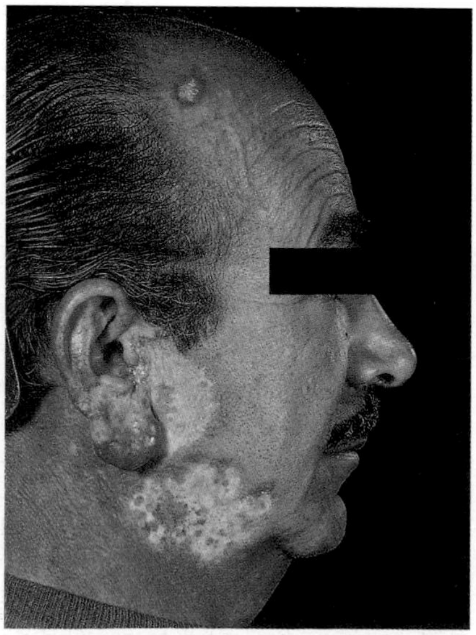

Figure 31.32 Chronic discoid lupus erythematosus. Scaling, atrophy and hypopigmentation.

Subacute cutaneous lupus erythematosus

Subacute cutaneous lupus erythematosus (SCLE) is a rare variant that presents with widespread annular, papulosquamous lesions and plaques on the upper torso and upper limbs. Photosensitivity is often a prominent feature. Complications, such as arthralgia and mouth ulceration, are seen but significant organ involvement is rare. ANF and extractable nuclear antibodies (anti-Ro and anti-La) are usually positive (see p. 694).

Treatment is with oral dapsone, antimalarials or systemic immunosuppression (prednisolone and ciclosporin).

Systemic lupus erythematosus

The cutaneous manifestations of systemic lupus erythematosus (SLE; see also p. 693) are not usually the presenting complaint, as other organ involvement such as joints or kidneys predominates. The classical 'butterfly' rash affects the cheeks, nose and forehead ***(Fig. 31.33)***. Palmar erythema, dilated nail-fold capillaries, splinter haemorrhages and digital infarcts of the fingertips may also be seen; livedo reticularis and purpura are occasionally present. Rarely, SLE can be complicated by an atypical erythema multiforme-like rash ('Rowell syndrome').

Treatment is described on pages 694–695.

Livedo reticularis

This is also seen in non-autoimmune rheumatic disorders. It is a disorder of blood vessels. Livedo reticularis is the term used to describe a bluish-red discoloration of the skin in a network or lacy pattern. It occurs on the limbs (especially the legs) and sometimes the trunk. It looks worse in the cold but does not disappear on rewarming (unlike cutis marmorata in babies). The colour change is due to dilatation of capillaries and small venules in the affected areas. When biopsying livedo reticularis, the sample should be taken from the middle of the 'mesh' and not through the visibly apparent vessels or the pathology is often missed. If the network/mesh pattern is broken, it is more likely that there will be an underlying secondary cause.

There are many causes of livedo reticularis:

- idiopathic livedo reticularis (young adults and middle-aged females, rarely with leg ulceration)

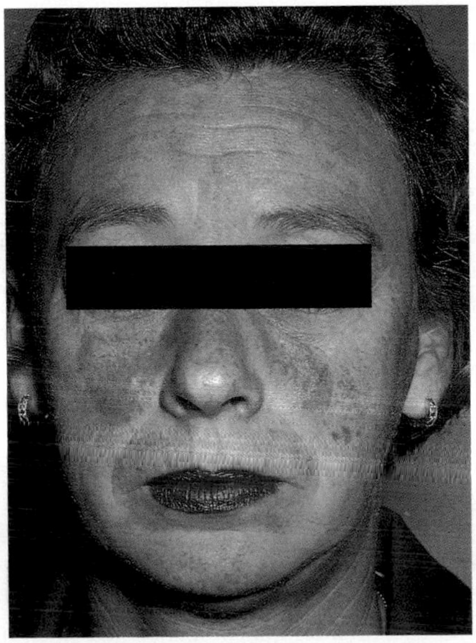

Figure 31.33 **Systemic lupus erythematosus.** Macular erythema on the cheeks ('butterfly rash').

- systemic disease (rheumatoid arteritis, lupus erythematosus, antiphospholipid syndrome, dermatomyositis, cryoglobulinaemia)
- livedoid vasculopathy (associated with painful leg ulcers, atrophie blanche and venous insufficiency)
- polyarteritis nodosa (cutaneous or systemic; see p. 701)
- Sneddon syndrome (associated with widespread evidence of arterial disease involving cerebral, ocular, coronary and peripheral arteries)
- calciphylaxis (chronic kidney disease)
- cutis marmorata telangiectatica (fixed livedo reticularis in neonates – may associate with abnormal limb growth or skin ulceration)
- post-cosmetic 'filler' (hyaluronic acid) injections.

There is no specific treatment for livedo reticularis but any underlying cause that is identified should be treated.

Miscellaneous systemic disorders

Behçet's disease

Behçet's disease (see p. 702) is a syndrome characterized by oral ulcers combined with two of the following: eye lesions, genital ulcers or skin lesions.

Cutaneous features include erythema nodosum/panniculitis, acneiform papulopustular lesions, thrombophlebitis or skin pathergy (blistering at the site of needleprick or other skin injuries). The syndrome is probably a vasculitis and many organs can be involved. Whilst systemic disease is usually treated with immunosuppression, skin disease may respond well to oral colchicine or dapsone.

Sarcoidosis

Sarcoidosis (see also pp. 1118–1120) is a multisystem granulomatous disorder of unknown aetiology. Cutaneous infiltrates usually present with reddish-brown dermal papules and nodules, especially around the eyelid margins and the rim of the nostrils. Extensive infiltration around the nose is called lupus pernio. Lesions on the body may be polymorphic (papules, nodules and plaques) and accompanied by hypo- or hyperpigmentation, especially in dark skin. Swollen fingers from a dactylitis may also be present. Erythema nodosum (see p. 1363) is sometimes seen in acute sarcoidosis. Although sarcoidosis may be confined to the skin, all patients should be investigated for evidence of systemic disease (see p. 1120).

Treatment of cutaneous lesions includes very potent topical steroids (0.05% clobetasol propionate), intralesional steroids or oral steroids; methotrexate or an antimalarial is also used.

Neurofibromatosis type 1 (von Recklinghausen's disease)

Type 1 neurofibromatosis is an autosomal dominant condition with high levels of penetrance. It often presents in childhood with a variety of cutaneous features. Many cases are new mutations in the *NF1* gene. Early signs include café-au-lait spots (brown macules, >5 mm in diameter, and more than five lesions) and axillary freckling. Lisch nodules (hyperpigmented iris hamartomas) may be seen in the eyes by slit-lamp examination. Learning difficulties and skeletal dysplasia occur. Later on, fleshy skin tags and deeper soft tumours (neurofibromas) appear and they can progress to cover the skin completely, causing significant cosmetic disability. A number of endocrine disorders are rarely associated, including phaeochromocytoma, acromegaly and Addison's disease.

Tuberous sclerosis

The tuberous sclerosis complex (TSC) is an autosomal dominant condition of variable severity, which may not present until later childhood. It is characterized by a variety of hamartomatous growths. The three cardinal features are:

- mental retardation
- epilepsy
- cutaneous abnormalities

but not all have to be present. In most cases, it is due to a mutation in either the *TSC1* gene (encodes hamartin) or the *TSC2* gene (encodes tuberin). Genetic testing is available but the diagnosis still remains clinical, requiring two major features or one major and two minor features. The ***skin signs*** include:

- adenoma sebaceum (reddish papules/fibromas around the nose)
- periungual fibroma (nodules arising from the nail bed)
- shagreen patches (firm, flesh-coloured plaques on the trunk)
- ash-leaf hypopigmentation (pale macules best seen with Wood's UV lamp)
- forehead plaque (indurated, flesh-coloured patch)
- café-au-lait patches
- pitting of dental enamel.

Internal hamartomas can arise in the heart, lung, kidney, retina and central nervous system. Parents of a suspected case should be examined (under UV light), as they may have a 'forme fruste' of the condition, which can manifest just as hypopigmented patches. This and gonadal mosaicism can have genetic implications for future offspring. A large contiguous gene defect may involve *TSC2* and *PKD1* genes, causing tuberous sclerosis and polycystic kidney disease together in the same patient. A recent major advance in treatment has been the use of mTOR inhibitor drugs, such as rapamycin. This has useful effects against various hamartomas, including skin angiofibromas, cardiac rhabdomyomas and renal angiomyolipomas.

Systemic malignant disease

Certain rashes may be a non-metastatic manifestation of an underlying malignancy: paraneoplastic dermatoses ***(Box 31.17)***. Rarely, internal malignancies can metastasize to the skin, where they usually present as papules or nodules that may ulcerate.

Box 31.17 Non-metastatic cutaneous manifestations of underlying malignancy

Dermatosis	Tumour
Dermatomyositis	Lung, gastrointestinal tract, genitourinary tract
Acanthosis nigricans	Gastrointestinal tract, lung, liver
Paget's disease (localized patch of eczema around the nipple)	Ductal breast carcinoma
Erythroderma	Lymphoma/leukaemia
Tylosis (thickened palms/soles)	Oesophageal carcinoma
Tripe palms (velvet palms)	Pulmonary, gastric
Ichthyosis (dry flaking of skin)	Lymphoma
Erythema gyratum repens (concentric rings of erythema, which change rapidly)	Lung, breast
Necrolytic migratory erythema (burning, geographic and spreading annular areas of erythema)	Glucagonoma
Paraneoplastic pemphigus	Lymphoproliferative

Further reading

Abreu Velez AM, Howard MS. Diagnosis and treatment of cutaneous paraneoplastic disorders. *Dermatol Ther* 2010; 23:662–675.
Aguilera P, Laguno M, To-Figueras J. Treatment of chronic hepatitis C with boceprevir leads to remission of porphyria cutanea tarda. *Br J Dermatol* 2014; 171:1595–1596.
Balestri R, Neri I, Patrizi A et al. Analysis of current data on the use of topical rapamycin in the treatment of facial angiofibromas in tuberous sclerosis complex. *J Eur Acad Dermatol Venereol* 2015; 29:14–20.
Bohelay G, Bouaziz JD, Nunes H et al. Striking leflunomide efficacy against refractory cutaneous sarcoidosis. *J Am Acad Dermatol* 2014; 70:e111–113.
Fett N. Scleroderma: nomenclature, etiology, pathogenesis, prognosis, and treatments: facts and controversies. *Clin Dermatol* 2013; 31:432–437.
Ko MJ, Peng YS, Chen HY et al. Interleukin-31 is associated with uremic pruritus in patients receiving hemodialysis. *J Am Acad Dermatol* 2014; 71:1151–1159.
Kuhn A, Landmann A. The classification and diagnosis of cutaneous lupus erythematosus. *J Autoimmun* 2014; 48–49:14–19.
Obermoser G, Sontheimer RD, Zelger B. Overview of common, rare and atypical manifestations of cutaneous lupus erythematosus and histopathological correlates. *Lupus* 2010; 19:1050–1070.
Stone JH, Zen Y, Deshpande V. IgG_4-related disease. *N Engl J Med* 2012; 366:539–551.

BULLOUS DISEASE

There are many causes of skin blisters; the most common are infection (herpes simplex virus, chickenpox, impetigo, tinea pedis, cellulitis), insect bites – especially on the lower legs – and trauma (burns and friction). Blistering may also be a feature of eczema, especially on the hands and feet ('pompholyx').

More rarely, blistering is due to skin fragility secondary to a genetically determined abnormality in the structural proteins of the skin (mechanobullous diseases) or an autoimmune disease targeting antigens in keratinocytes or the basement membrane zone of the dermo-epidermal junction (immunobullous). The level of the skin where fragility and blistering occur varies according to disease and will influence the clinical presentation and prognosis. The level can be identified by light and electron microscopy and by immunofluorescence (IMF) studies ***(Fig. 31.34)***. Direct immunofluorescence investigates the presence of antibody (with or without complement) deposition in affected (perilesional) skin; indirect immunofluorescence identifies the presence of circulating skin autoantibodies.

Immunobullous disease

Pemphigus vulgaris and pemphigus foliaceus

Pemphigus vulgaris is a rare and potentially life-threatening blistering disease. It is more common in Ashkenazi Jews and people from the Indian subcontinent. It may affect all ages but usually starts in mid-adult life. Pathogenic IgG4 antibodies against desmosomal proteins (desmoglein 1 and 3) cause loss of keratinocyte adhesion in the skin and mucous membranes, leading to superficial blisters (intraepidermal), erosions and oral ulceration. The cause of pemphigus is unknown but viral triggers have been speculated.

Pemphigus foliaceus is a rarer variant of pemphigus, in which the target antigen is desmoglein 1. This antigen is not expressed in the oral mucosa, which is therefore unaffected. Histology of pemphigus vulgaris shows intraepidermal cleavage above the basal cell layer with separation of individual keratinocytes (acantholysis). The split occurs higher in the epidermis in pemphigus foliaceus where there is greater target antigen expression.

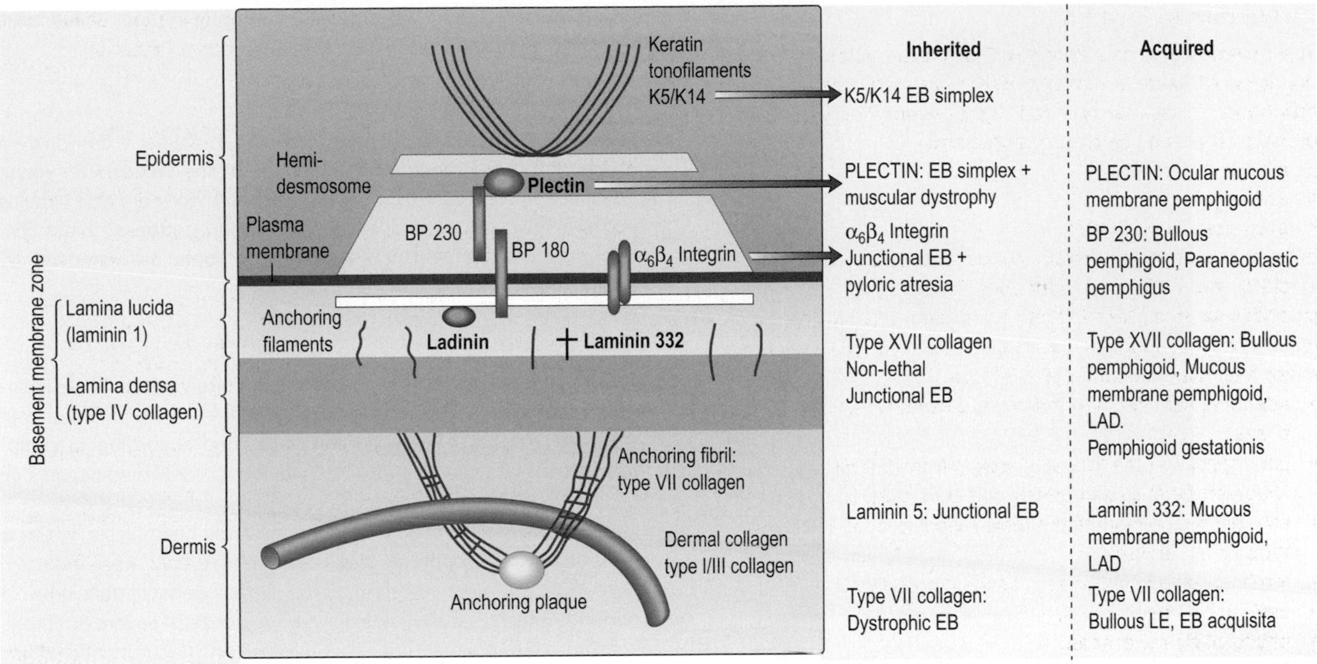

Figure 31.34 **Section of the basement membrane zone.** The structural sites of damage in bullous disorders. EB, epidermolysis bullosa; K, keratin; LAD, linear IgA disease; LE, lupus erythematosus.

An endemic form of pemphigus foliaceus occurs in the Limão Verde area of Brazil and is thought to be triggered by an infectious agent carried by the black fly and other biting insects. A pemphigus foliaceus-like rash can also be induced by drugs (e.g. captopril, penicillamine).

Direct immunofluorescence of perilesional skin in pemphigus demonstrates intercellular IgG deposition. Circulating anti-epidermal antibodies can also be detected and their titre correlates with disease activity.

Clinical features

Mucosal involvement (especially oral ulceration) is common and is the presenting sign in up to 50% of patients with pemphigus vulgaris. Development of non-itchy, flaccid blisters may follow, especially on the torso. Large areas may be involved, but as blisters are fragile (intraepidermal), they rupture easily, leaving erythematous, weeping erosions. Blisters can be extended with gentle lateral pressure (Nikolsky's sign). Flexural lesions often have a vegetative appearance. In pemphigus foliaceus, blisters are rarely seen and the rash has a crusted appearance, often affecting the seborrhoeic areas (scalp, face and upper chest) before becoming more widespread.

Management

High-dose systemic corticosteroids are usually effective in controlling pemphigus, but due to their long-term adverse effects, immunosuppressive drugs are usually introduced for a steroid-sparing effect. These include azathioprine, cyclophosphamide, methotrexate, ciclosporin, mycophenolate mofetil, dapsone and, more recently, rituximab (an anti-CD20 monoclonal antibody). High-dose intravenous immunoglobulin may also be of benefit in severe, unresponsive pemphigus vulgaris.

Paraneoplastic pemphigus

This is a rare pemphigus-like disorder that occurs in association with neoplasms, especially lymphoproliferative malignancy. Features include severe oral erosions and the rash may show additional changes resembling pemphigoid, erythema multiforme and lichen planus. Autoantibodies can be demonstrated against a range of desmosomal proteins and a broad-range protease inhibitor. Therapy includes immunosuppressants and treatment of the underlying malignancy.

Bullous pemphigoid

Bullous pemphigoid is more common than pemphigus and usually affects those over the age of 60 years. Autoantibodies against a 230 kDa or 180 kDa hemidesmosomal protein ('bullous pemphigoid antigen 1' and 'type XVII collagen') play a pathogenic role and cause a split through the basement membrane zone. This can be demonstrated on routine histology as a sub-epidermal split, and direct IMF shows deposition of IgG and complement at the dermo-epidermal junction.

Clinical features

Large, tense, serous or haemorrhagic blisters (bullae) appear anywhere on the body, especially the limbs and torso *(Fig. 31.35)*. The underlying skin is usually inflamed; early lesions may resemble urticaria but persist for days or weeks. Pemphigoid can be very itchy. Mucosal ulceration is uncommon except in a rare variant of pemphigoid – mucous membrane pemphigoid (formerly called cicatricial pemphigoid) – in which erosions and ulceration of the mucosal surfaces lead to scarring. Ocular involvement in mucous membrane pemphigoid can cause fusion of the eyelids, corneal damage and visual loss. Pemphigoid gestationis is rarely seen in pregnancy (p. 1309).

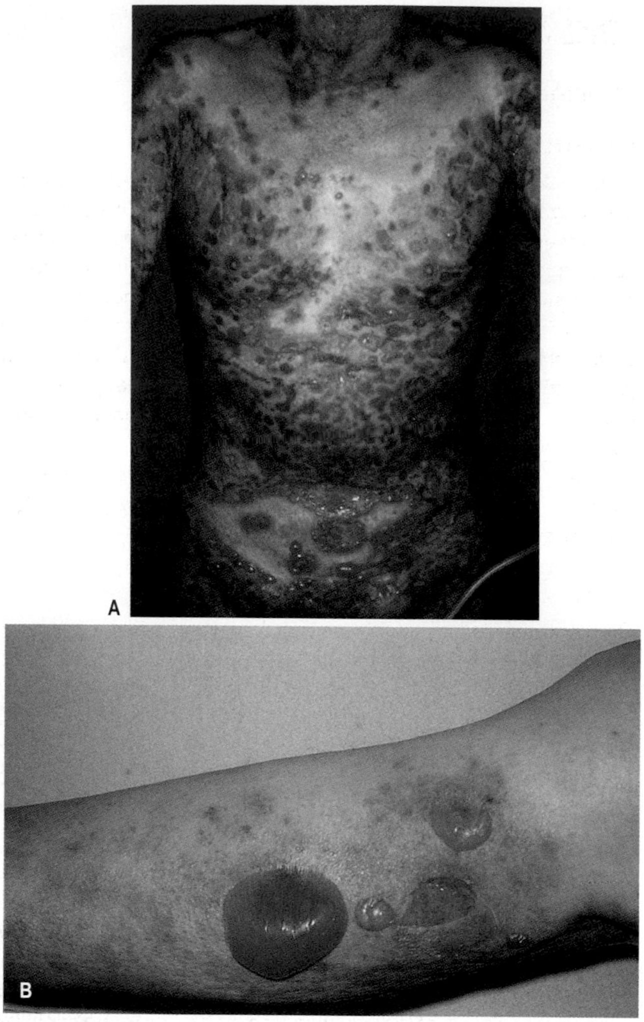

Figure 31.35 **Bullous pemphigoid. A.** Widespread blistering. **B.** Large, tense bullae.

Management

Oral corticosteroids in moderate to high dose are used initially for disease control, with introduction of a steroid-sparing agent such as azathioprine or mycophenolate mofetil for long-term disease control. This requires monitoring, as the elderly are at increased risk of the adverse effects of steroids and immunosuppressant agents, and these drugs contribute to the increased mortality associated with pemphigoid. In mild, localized pemphigoid, use of a very potent topical steroid and minocycline may provide adequate disease control. Treatment can sometimes be withdrawn within a few years but relapses occur.

Dermatitis herpetiformis

Dermatitis herpetiformis is a rare blistering disorder associated with gluten-sensitive enteropathy (coeliac disease; see p. 398). Dermatitis herpetiformis and coeliac disease are associated with other organ-specific autoimmune disorders.

Skin biopsy shows a sub-epidermal blister with neutrophil microabscesses in the dermal papillae. Direct immunofluorescent studies of uninvolved skin show IgA deposits in the dermal papillae and patchy granular IgA along the basement membrane. The small bowel mucosa shows a partial villous atrophy in most cases but a total villous atrophy in a small percentage.

Clinical features

Dermatitis herpetiformis is more common in males; it can present at any age but is most likely to appear for the first time in young adult life. It presents with small, intensely itchy blisters and papules on the elbows, extensor forearms, scalp and buttocks. Intact blisters may not be evident because their roofs are removed by scratching, leaving crusted erosions.

Management

Patients should avoid all dietary forms of gluten (see p. 397). Treatment with dapsone or sulphonamides usually gives rapid relief from itch and blistering. The dose can be titrated according to symptoms. If a strict gluten-free diet is followed, oral medication can usually be withdrawn after 2 years.

Dapsone usually causes mild dose-related haemolysis, which is well tolerated except in those with cardiorespiratory disease. Screening for glucose-6-phosphate dihydrogenase deficiency is performed to identify individuals who are at risk of severe haemolysis. Other rare adverse effects of dapsone include hepatitis, which may be associated with a hypersensitivity syndrome including rash and fever (see p. 1384), and peripheral neuropathy. Treatment requires regular monitoring of the full blood count and liver function tests.

Linear IgA disease (chronic bullous dermatosis of childhood)

Linear IgA disease is a rare sub-epidermal blistering disorder of adults and children. Pathogenic IgA autoantibodies bind to several basement membrane proteins, including type XVII collagen and laminin-332 (see ***Fig. 31.34***). The cause is unknown but disease may be induced by drugs, especially vancomycin.

Clinical features

Linear IgA disease characteristically presents with circular clusters of blisters, described as a 'string of jewels' ***(Fig. 31.36)***. The oral, vulval and ocular mucosa may be involved and can be scarred. Direct IMF of skin shows linear IgA deposition along the dermo-epidermal junction.

Management

There is usually a good response to dapsone or sulphonamides, with disease resolution after several years.

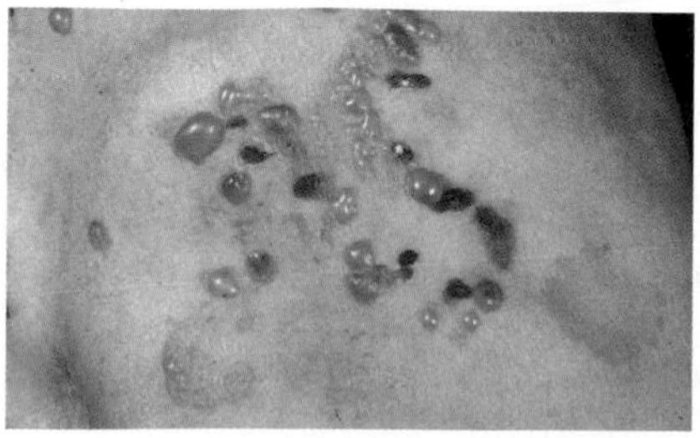

Figure 31.36 **Linear IgA disease.** Typical circular clustering of blisters.

Mechanobullous disease (epidermolysis bullosa)

This rare group of genodermatoses are disorders caused by defective or absent structural skin proteins, leading to 'skin fragility'. This causes trauma-induced blisters and erosions that often appear at or shortly after birth. The degree of blistering varies considerably between diseases, ranging from mild friction blisters to severe extensive skin loss, with life-threatening complications. There are three broad groups of disorders:

- ***Epidermolysis bullosa simplex*** is characterized by 'superficial' localized blistering of the hands and feet, especially in hot weather. Scarring is absent and the nails and teeth are normal. It is inherited as an autosomal dominant trait and caused by abnormal synthesis of cytoskeleton proteins within the basal layer of the epidermis, e.g. keratins 5 and 14.
- ***Epidermolysis bullosa dystrophica*** is characterized by deeper blistering within the basement membrane and scarring. The underlying abnormalities are mutations in the *COL-7A1* gene, which cause a reduction or absence of collagen VII in the anchoring fibrils. Nails and mucosae, including the larynx, may be involved. The autosomal dominant form usually manifests as mild disease, but the autosomal recessive form usually causes widespread, painful erosions that heal with scarring, leading to fusion of digits, joint contractures and dysphagia. Life expectancy is significantly reduced and this is usually due to an associated high risk of developing multiple aggressive squamous cell carcinomas within areas of chronically inflamed skin. There is no curative therapy at present and management is supportive.
- ***Junctional epidermolysis bullosa*** is the most severe form of epidermolysis bullosa and is s characterized by a split in the lamina lucida of the basement membranes due to mutations in various proteins (laminin-332, $\alpha_6\beta_4$ integrin, type XVII collagen). It presents at birth with widespread blistering and areas of absent skin. Erosions of the central face and hoarseness from laryngeal involvement are common. Nail and teeth abnormalities are also frequently present. Both a lethal and a rarer non-lethal form of junctional epidermolysis bullosa exist and they show an autosomal recessive inheritance. The lethal form causes death in infancy or early childhood.

Investigations and management

Investigation and treatment of epidermolysis bullosa should be carried out in a specialist centre. The precise diagnosis depends on ultrastructural analysis of the skin and immunohistochemistry, which can be further confirmed with genetic testing. This enables a more accurate prognosis and genetic counselling of parents. Prenatal diagnosis and pre-implantation diagnosis are available for the more severe forms of epidermolysis bullosa. Gene therapy and bone marrow transplantation are two new approaches that are currently undergoing clinical trials.

Further reading

Aoki V, Rivitti EA, Diaz LA; Cooperative Group on Fogo Selvagem Research. Update on fogo selvagem, an endemic form of pemphigus foliaceus. *J Dermatol* 2015; 42:18–26.

Atzmony L, Hodak E, Gdalevich M et al. Treatment of pemphigus vulgaris and pemphigus foliaceus: a systematic review and meta-analysis. *Am J Clin Dermatol* 2014; 15:503–515.

Uitto J, McGrath JA, Rodeck U et al. Progress in epidermolysis bullosa research: toward treatment and cure. *J Invest Dermatol* 2010; 130:1778–1784.

Wagner JE, Yamamoto AI, McGrath JA et al. Bone marrow transplantation for recessive dystrophic epidermolysis bullosa. *N Engl J Med* 2010; 363:629–639, 680–682.

SKIN TUMOURS

Benign cutaneous tumours

Melanocytic naevi (moles)

Moles are benign proliferations of overgrowth of melanocytes and are common in fair-skinned people. Congenital melanocytic naevi are present at birth. Acquired naevi appear in childhood, adolescence and early adult life, increasing in size and number. Benign naevi usually have even pigmentation and regular borders. They start as flat brown macules with proliferation of melanocytes at the dermo-epidermal junction (junctional naevi). With later downward growth of melanocytes into the dermis (compound naevi), the mole becomes raised and palpable, eventually maturing into an intradermal naevus with loss of pigment.

Blue naevus is an acquired asymptomatic blue–grey mole caused by a deeper proliferation of melanocytes in the mid-dermis.

Basal cell papilloma (seborrhoeic keratosis/wart)

This is an extremely common, harmless growth that affects older adults and is caused by overgrowth of the basal keratinocytes. Lesions range from flesh-coloured to very dark brown, and have a greasy 'stuck-on' appearance ***(Fig. 31.37)***. The surface is rough and warty and may contain tiny keratin cysts. They can be removed under local anaesthetic with curettage or treated with cryotherapy or electrodesiccation.

Dermatofibroma (histiocytoma)

Dermatofibromas are pink–beige, firm dermal nodules, which may be surrounded by a peripheral ring of hyperpigmentation. They are often found on the leg and are more common in females. There is sometimes a history of trauma or an insect bite. The lesion consists of histiocytes, blood vessels and varying degrees of fibrosis. Excision is not needed unless lesions are symptomatic or there is diagnostic uncertainty.

Epidermoid cyst ('sebaceous cyst')

Epidermoid cysts are cystic swellings derived from an occluded follicle. They have a central punctum and contain 'cheesy' keratinous matter. Cysts may enlarge and can become secondarily infected and inflamed.

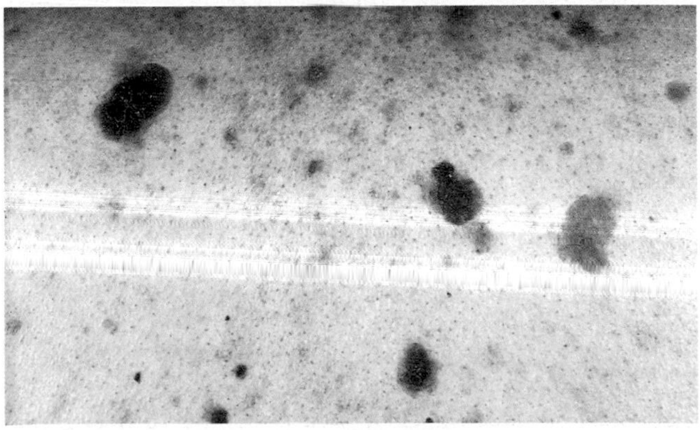

Figure 31.37 Seborrhoeic warts (basal cell papillomas).

Pilar cyst (trichilemmal cyst)

Pilar cysts are smooth cysts without a punctum, usually found on the scalp. They may be multiple and familial.

Pyogenic granuloma (granuloma telangiectaticum)

Pyogenic granulomas are benign vascular proliferations that present as rapidly growing, friable red nodules. They may follow minor trauma and often occur on the face or fingers. Excision is advisable and lesions should be sent for histology to exclude amelanotic malignant melanoma.

Cherry angioma (Campbell de Morgan spots)

Cherry angiomas are benign angiokeratomas that appear as tiny, pinpoint, red papules, especially on the trunk, and increase with age. No treatment is required.

Dysplastic/pre-malignant cutaneous lesions

Solar keratoses (actinic keratoses)

These are common on the sun-exposed areas of fair-skinned individuals in later life, especially bald scalps. They appear as rough, scaly, erythematous papules or patches and the surrounding skin usually shows signs of chronic sun damage ***(Fig. 31.38)***, with wrinkles and solar lentigines. A small minority (<1%) of lesions may undergo malignant transformation into squamous cell carcinoma after many years. Lesion-based treatments include cryotherapy and curettage. Field treatments, aimed at removing early and subclinical lesions in a larger area, include topical 5-fluorouracil cream, imiquimod cream, diclofenac gel and ingenol mebutate gel. Topical photodynamic therapy (PDT) using aminolaevulinic acid or its methyl ester is another option, but is painful and requires special expertise.

Bowen's disease

This is an indolent form of intraepidermal carcinoma-in-situ, which rarely progresses to invasive squamous cell carcinoma. It typically affects the lower legs in fair-skinned women or the torso in men, and is thought to be caused by chronic UV exposure. Lesions appear as a slowly enlarging, well-demarcated, scaly red patch or plaque resembling psoriasis but lacking thick silvery scale. A variant of Bowen's disease can affect the mucosal sites of the genital area and is referred to as vulval-, penile- or anal-intraepithelial neoplasia ***(Fig. 31.39)***. This presents with non-specific erythematous patches ('erythroplasia') or warty areas. There is a strong link with oncogenic infection, and genital Bowen's disease probably has a greater malignant potential than non-mucosal disease. It is more common in immunosuppressed individuals, including those with HIV. The anal form is increasingly reported in HIV-positive patients (as, indeed, is anal carcinoma) and extension into the rectum may occur. Treatment is with topical 5-fluorouracil, 5% imiquimod cream, cryotherapy, curettage, topical photodynamic therapy or a tissue-destructive laser.

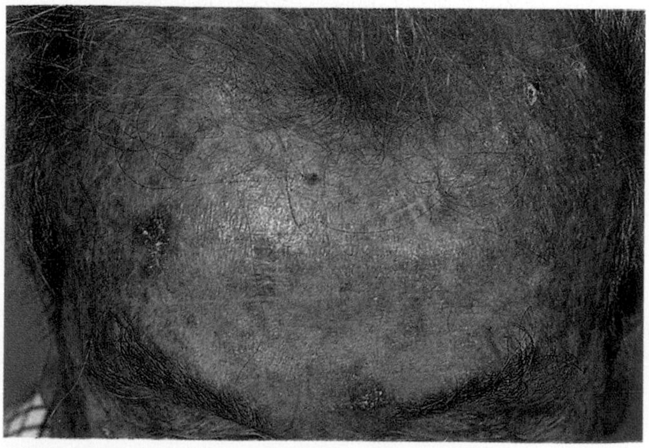

Figure 31.38 Solar keratoses with background actinic damage.

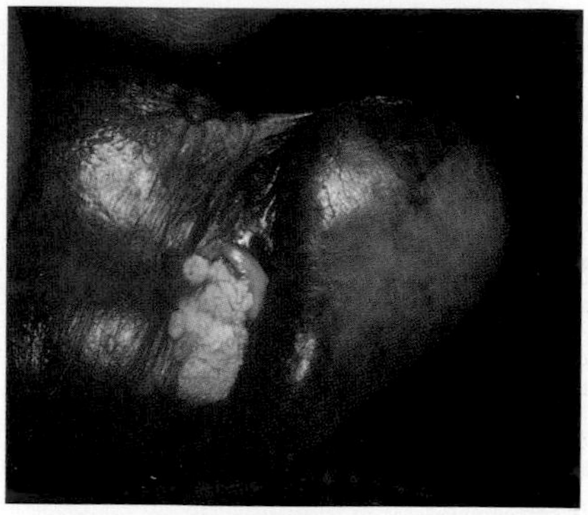

Figure 31.39 Erythroplasia of glans penis (penile intraephithelial neoplasia).

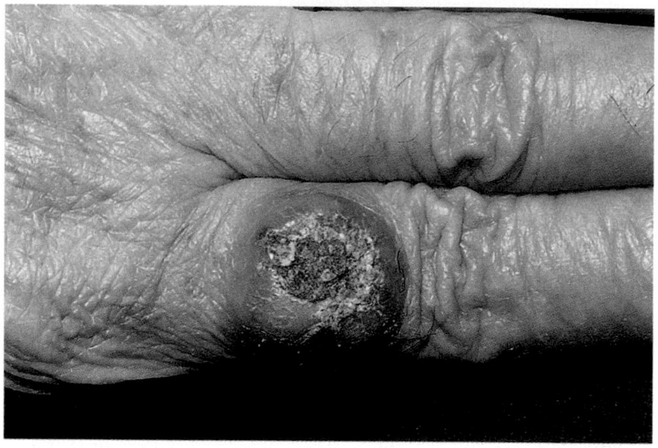

Figure 31.40 Keratoacanthoma.

Keratoacanthoma

Keratoacanthomas are rapidly growing epidermal tumours that develop central necrosis and ulceration ***(Fig. 31.40)***. They occur on sun-exposed skin in later life and often reach 2–3 cm in diameter. Although they resolve spontaneously after several months, they are usually excised to exclude a squamous cell carcinoma (which they can closely resemble.)

Familial atypical multiple mole melanoma (FAMMM)

This is often familial. A large number of melanocytic naevi begin to appear in childhood, even on unexposed sites. Individual lesions may be large with irregular pigmentation and border; histologically, they may show cytological and architectural atypia but no frank malignant change. Individuals with this condition have an increased risk of developing malignant melanoma, pancreatic and other malignancies. They should have their moles photographed and be regularly reviewed. Suspicious lesions should be excised.

Giant congenital melanocytic naevi

These are very large moles present at birth. Very large lesions (>20 cm across) show an increased risk of developing malignant melanoma (up to 5%). Excision may be considered but is rarely possible without multiple operations and marked disfigurement, so regular monitoring is advised. There have been a number of reports showing that a few of these lesions improve spontaneously and partially resolve during childhood.

Lentigo maligna

This is a slow-growing macular area of pigmentation seen in elderly people, commonly on the face. The border and pigmentation are often irregular. Some people regard this lesion as a melanoma-in-situ. There is an increased risk of developing invasive malignant melanoma. Treatment is by excision if possible but 5% imiquimod cream is currently being tried in the very large lesions where surgery would be disfiguring.

Malignant cutaneous tumours

Basal cell carcinoma ('rodent ulcer')

Basal cell carcinomas (BCCs) are the most common malignant skin tumour and are increasingly prevalent in ageing populations. The exact aetiology of BCCs is unknown, but it is thought that they arise from pluripotential cells in the basal epidermis or follicular structures. Mutations in *PTCH1*, the human homolog of the 'Patched' gene that regulates the Hedgehog intracellular signalling pathway (see p. 98), have been detected in sporadic BCCs and Gorlin syndrome (hereditary BCC syndrome). BCCs typically appear as a slowly enlarging, shiny nodule on the head and neck area, which bleeds following minor trauma and does not heal (nodulocystic BCC). The border of ulcerated lesions is raised with a pearly appearance ***(Fig. 31.41)*** and overlying telangiectasia. Pigmented, superficial and morpheic (scar-like) variants exist. BCCs can cause significant morbidity by eroding into adjacent tissues but have minimal metastatic potential.

Management

In most cases, the treatment of choice is a wide excision with histology to ensure clear and adequate tumour margins. Mohs micrographic surgery is preferred for morpheic BCCs and lesions involving the nasal creases, as these are more likely to recur. Superficial BCCs can be managed with non-surgical treatment, including cryotherapy, photodynamic therapy and topical imiquimod. Radiotherapy remains an option in those who are unable to tolerate surgery. Vismodegib is a new oral therapy for advanced/inoperable BCC that inhibits the Hedgehog signalling pathway by binding to Smoothened transmembrane protein, thereby normalizing basal keratinocyte proliferation. The majority of tumours respond (60%) and a small number may actually clear.

Squamous cell carcinoma

Squamous cell carcinoma (SCC) is a more aggressive tumour than BCC and has a higher metastatic potential. There is a clearer correlation with chronic UV damage than for BCC and sun protection measures reduces its incidence. SCC can arise in pre-existing solar keratoses or Bowen's disease and can also complicate areas of chronic inflammation, as in lupus vulgaris. Rarely, multiple tumours may arise due to arsenic ingestion in early life. Multiple tumours also occur in people who have had prolonged periods of immunosuppression, such as renal transplant patients, where certain HPV subtypes may be involved in malignant transformation.

Clinically, the lesions are often keratotic, rather ill-defined nodules that may ulcerate ***(Fig. 31.42)***. They can grow very rapidly. They are most common on sun-exposed sites in later life. Ulcerated lesions on the lower lip or ear are often more aggressive. Examination of regional lymph nodes is essential.

Management

Treatment is complete surgical excision with a minimal margin of 5 mm. Radiotherapy is also used.

Malignant melanoma

Malignant melanoma is the most serious form of skin cancer, as metastasis can occur early; it causes a number of deaths, even in

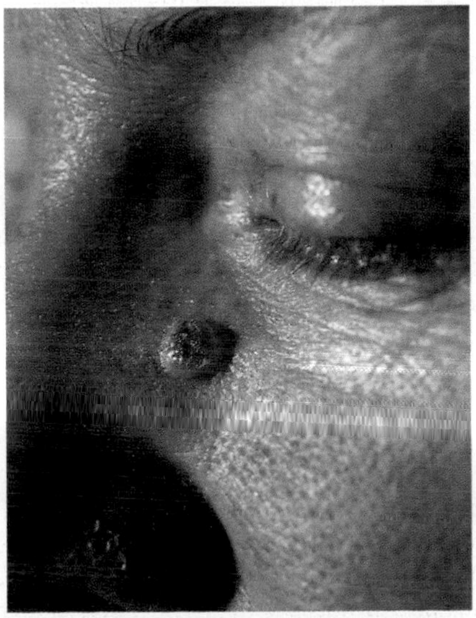

Figure 31.41 Ulcerating basal cell carcinoma.

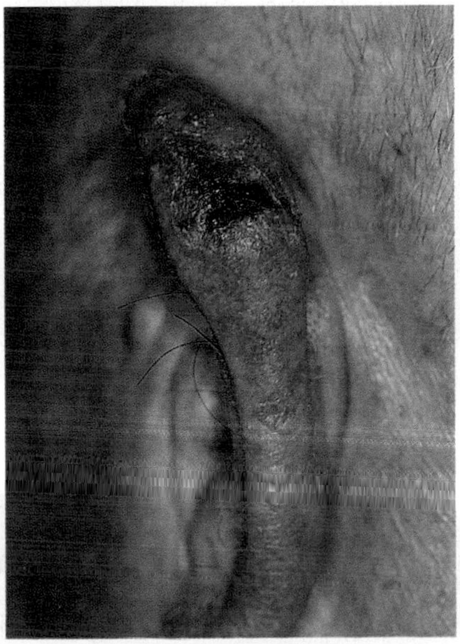

Figure 31.42 Squamous cell carcinoma.

young people. The increasing incidence in recent years is thought to be due to excessive exposure to sunlight, especially intermittent intense exposure and sunburn in childhood. Other risk factors include pale skin, multiple melanocytic naevi (>50), sun sensitivity, immunosuppression, atypical mole syndrome, giant congenital melanocytic naevi, lentigo maligna and a positive family history of malignant melanoma. Malignant melanoma is more common in later life but many young adults are also affected. A number of oncogenes and tumour suppressor proteins have been implicated in the pathogenesis of melanoma. Some 60% of human melanomas have an activating mutation (V600E) in the serine protein kinase B-RAF, which has now become a target for 'personalized' therapy (see p. 1374).

Diagnosis of melanoma is not always easy but the clinical signs listed in ***Box 31.18*** help distinguish malignant from benign moles. Examination with a dermatoscope (a hand-held polarized light source with magnification) can aid clinical diagnosis.

Four clinical types exist:

- ***Lentigo maligna melanoma*** is a patch of lentigo maligna that develops a papule or nodule, signalling invasive tumour.
- ***Superficial spreading malignant melanoma*** is a large, flat, irregularly pigmented lesion that grows laterally before vertical invasion develops.
- ***Nodular malignant melanoma (Fig. 31.43)*** is the most aggressive type. It presents as a rapidly growing pigmented nodule, which bleeds or ulcerates. Rarely, it is amelanotic (non-pigmented) and can mimic pyogenic granuloma.

Box 31.18 Clinical criteria for the diagnosis of malignant melanoma

ABCDE criteria (USA)
- Asymmetry of mole
- Border irregularity
- Colour variegation
- Diameter >6 mm
- Elevation

The Glasgow seven-point checklist

Major criteria
- Change in size
- Change in shape
- Change in colour

Minor criteria
- Diameter >6 mm
- Inflammation
- Oozing or bleeding
- Mild itch or altered sensation

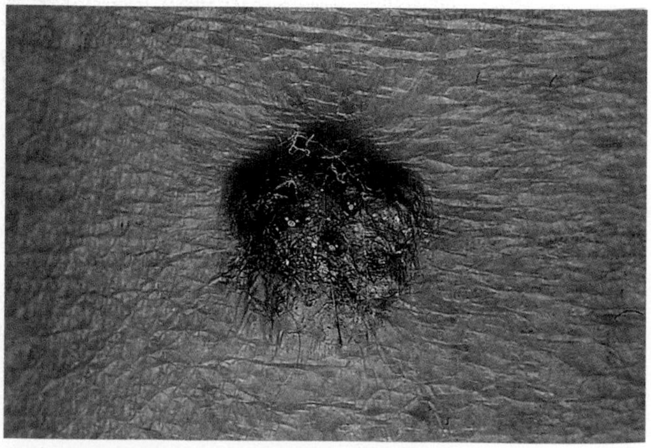

Figure 31.43 Nodular malignant melanoma.

- ***Acral lentiginous malignant melanomas*** arise as pigmented lesions on the palm or sole or under the nail, and usually present late. They may not be related to sun exposure.

Management

In the UK, all people with melanoma >1 mm thick should be referred to their regional multidisciplinary team for expert management. Surgery is the only curative treatment: urgent wide excision with a 1 cm margin for thin melanomas (<1 mm), increasing to a 3 cm margin for thicker melanomas (>2 mm). Histological analysis will determine the depth of invasion ('Clark's level') and the thickness of the tumour ('Breslow thickness'). People with thick melanomas are staged according to the ***American Joint Committee on Cancer (AJCC) 2009 criteria*** (tumour, nodes, metastases – TNM), which help predict prognosis and 5-year survival rates. Sentinel node biopsy for people with thicker lesions remains under assessment as a tool for predicting prognosis, determining therapy (e.g. lymph node dissection) and improving survival.

Treatment for metastatic disease includes removal of regional lymph nodes, isolated limb perfusion, radiotherapy, immunotherapy and chemotherapy. Until recently, none of these altered the disease outcome. However, a variety of new treatments have been developed over the last 5 years, which are now beginning to improve survival. The first was the selective mitogen-activated protein (MAP) kinase inhibitor, BRAF inhibitors (vemurafenib) and MEK inhibitors (trametinib). These drugs proved better than conventional chemotherapy, but early resistance and toxicity were limitations. The second major advance is the development of immune checkpoint-blocking agents, including CTLA4 antibody (ipilimumab) and programmed death 1 protein antibody (PD-1 antibody – pembrolizumab, nivolumab).

Results from combination treatments with ipilimumab and nivolumab have shown good results with acceptable toxicity.

Primary cutaneous T-cell lymphoma (mycosis fungoides)

Mycosis fungoides is a rare lymphoproliferative disease that usually follows an indolent course. It presents with pruritic, scaly patches, which typically start on the buttocks and can resemble eczema or psoriasis; asymmetry and atrophy are useful clues ***(Fig. 31.44)***. Skin biopsy shows invasion of the epidermis by atypical T lymphocytes (exocytosis), and T-cell receptor gene rearrangement studies show that the infiltrate is clonal.

Occasionally, patches evolve into nodules or tumours, which may metastasize to lymph nodes and internal organs. ***Sézary syndrome*** (see p. 625) is a rare erythrodermic variant of cutaneous T-cell lymphoma with peripheral lymphadenopathy and peripheral blood involvement; it is seen mostly in elderly men. Mycosis fungoides and Sézary syndrome usually run chronic relapsing courses. Treatment choices depend on disease stage and extent. Patch and plaque-stage mycosis fungoides usually responds to potent topical corticosteroids, topical nitrogen mustard or low-dose PUVA. Radiotherapy and systemic therapy are used for aggressive/recalcitrant early-stage disease and advanced-stage disease; options include IFN-α, oral retinoids (acitretin) and bexarotine (an agonist of the retinoid x receptor), histone deacetylase inhibitors and chemotherapy drugs. However, evidence of their effectiveness is lacking.

Kaposi's sarcoma

This is a tumour of vascular and lymphatic endothelium that presents as purplish nodules and plaques. There are three types:

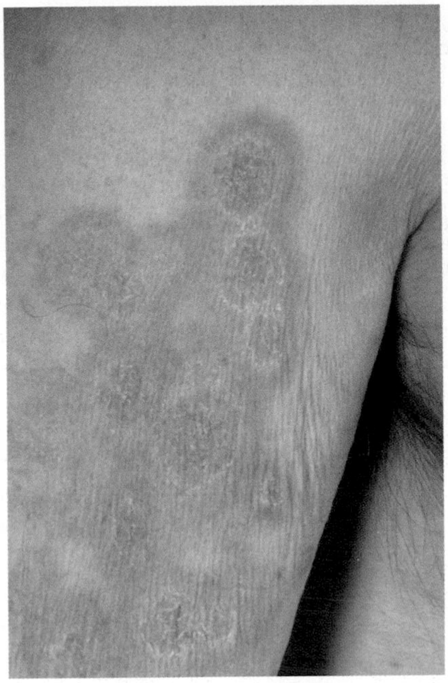

Figure 31.44 Patch-stage mycosis fungoides.

- ***The 'classic' or 'sporadic' form*** (as described by Kaposi) occurs in elderly males, especially Jewish people from Eastern Europe. It presents as slow-growing, purple tumours in the foot and lower leg, which rarely cause any significant problem.
- ***The 'endemic' form*** occurs in males from Central Africa and shows more widespread cutaneous involvement, as well as lymph node (or occasionally systemic) involvement. Oedema is a prominent feature.
- ***The immunosuppression-related form*** is more severe and is most common in HIV-positive men who have sex with men. Lesions are widespread and often affect the skin, bowel, oral cavity and lungs.

All three types have a strong association with human herpesvirus-8 (HHV-8) but other factors must be involved, as HHV-8 seroprevalence is up to 10% in the USA and 50% in some African countries. Anti-retroviral therapy (ART; see pp. 341–346) has significantly reduced the incidence of Kaposi's sarcoma in HIV infection, although the prevalence has started to increase again over the last few years for as yet unexplained reasons.

Management

Treatment of advanced Kaposi's sarcoma is with radiotherapy, immunotherapy or chemotherapy.

Further reading

Balch CM, Gershenwald JE, Soong SJ et al. Final version of 2009 AJCC melanoma staging and classification. *J Clin Oncol* 2009; 27:6199–6206.
Editorial. Melanoma research gathers momentum. *Lancet* 2015; 385:2323.
Eggermont AM, Spatz A, Robert C. Cutaneous melanoma. *Lancet* 2014; 383:816–827.
Gbabe OF, Okwundu CI, Dedicoat M et al. Treatment of severe or progressive Kaposi's sarcoma in HIV-infected adults. *Cochrane Database Syst Rev* 2014; 8:CD003256.
Hughes CF, Khot A, McCormack C et al. Lack of durable disease control with chemotherapy for mycosis fungoides and Sézary syndrome: a comparative study of systemic therapy. *Blood* 2015; 125:71–81.
Madan V, Lear JT, Szeimies RM. Non-melanoma skin cancer. *Lancet* 2010; 375:673–685.
Menzies AM, Long GV. Systemic treatment for BRAF-mutant melanoma: where do we go next? *Lancet Oncol* 2014; 15:e371–381.
Morton DL, Thompson JF, Cochran AJ. Final trial report of sentinel-node biopsy versus nodal observation in melanoma. *N Engl J Med* 2014; 370:599–609.
Postow MA, Chesney J, Pavlick AC et al. Nivolumab versus ipilimumab in untreated melanoma. *N Engl J Med* 2015; 372:2006–2017.
Sekulic A, Migden MR, Oro AE et al. Efficacy and safety of vismodegib in advanced basal-cell carcinoma. *N Engl J Med* 2012; 366:2171–2179.

DISORDERS OF BLOOD VESSELS AND LYMPHATICS

Leg ulcers

Leg ulcers are common and can have many causes ***(Box 31.19)***. Venous ulcers are the most common type in developed countries.

Venous ulcers

Venous ulcers are the result of sustained venous hypertension in the superficial veins, owing to incompetent valves in the deep or perforating veins or to previous deep vein thrombosis. The increased pressure causes extravasation of fibrinogen through the capillary walls, giving rise to perivascular fibrin deposition, which leads to poor oxygenation of the surrounding skin.

Venous ulcers are common in later life and constitute a significant drain on healthcare budgets, as they are often chronic and recurrent; they affect 1% of the population over the age of 70 years. They are most commonly found on the lower leg in a triangle above the ankles ***(Fig. 31.45)***, and may be associated with:

- oedema of the lower legs
- venous eczema (see p. 1352)
- brown pigmentation from haemosiderin
- varicose veins

Box 31.19 Causes of leg ulceration

- Venous hypertension
- Arterial disease (e.g. atherosclerosis)
- Neuropathic (e.g. diabetes, leprosy)
- Neoplastic (e.g. squamous or basal cell carcinoma)
- Vasculitis (e.g. rheumatoid arthritis, systemic lupus erythematosus, pyoderma gangrenosum)
- Infection (e.g. ecthyma, tuberculosis, deep mycoses, Buruli ulcer, syphilis, yaws)
- Haematological (e.g. sickle cell disease, spherocytosis)
- Drug (e.g. hydroxycarbamide (hydroxyurea))
- Other (e.g. necrobiosis lipoidica, trauma, artefact)

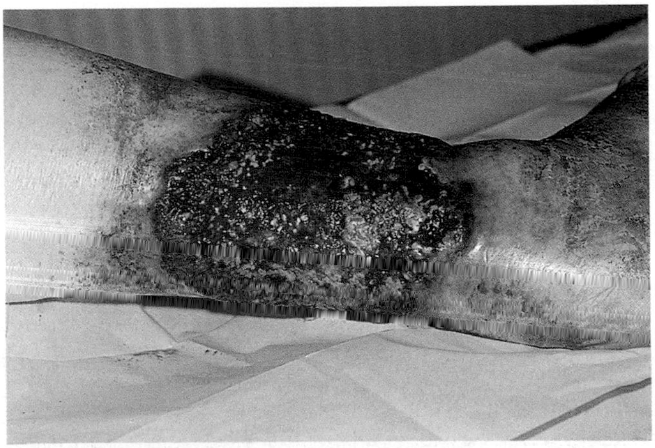

Figure 31.45 Venous leg ulcer.

- lipodermatosclerosis (the combination of induration, reddish-brown pigmentation and inflammation) – a fibrosing panniculitis of the subcutaneous tissue
- scarring white atrophy with telangiectasia (atrophie blanche).

Management is with high-compression bandaging (e.g. four-layer bandaging) and leg elevation to reduce venous hypertension. Similar healing results can be obtained with a two-layer support hosiery technique, although more dressing changes are needed. Doppler studies should be done before compression to exclude significant arterial disease. This treatment can be delivered effectively in the community by appropriately trained nurses. Ulcer dressings are used to keep the ulcer moist and free of slough and exudates. Up to 80% of ulcers can be healed within 6 months. Slower healing rates occur in patients who have decreased mobility and in those with ulcers that are very large, present for longer than 6 months or bilateral. Diuretics are sometimes helpful to reduce the oedema. Antibiotics are necessary only for overt bacterial infection.

Venous leg ulcers can be painful so adequate analgesia should be given, including opiates if required. Split-thickness skin grafting is used in resistant cases. Support stockings (individually fitted) should be worn for life after healing, as this lessens recurrence.

Underlying venous disease is best investigated with duplex ultrasound or plethysmography. Therapeutic ultrasound is now proven not to help ulcer healing. Surgery for purely superficial venous disease does not assist ulcer healing but it is proven to help prevent ulcer recurrence (ESCHAR study).

Arterial ulcers

Arterial ulcers present as punched-out, painful ulcers higher up the leg or on the feet. There may be a history of claudication, hypertension, angina or smoking. Clinically, the leg is cold and pale. Absent peripheral pulses, arterial bruits and loss of hair may be present. Doppler ultrasound studies will confirm arterial disease.

Management depends on keeping the ulcer clean and covered, adequate analgesia and vascular reconstruction if appropriate. Compression bandaging must not be used.

Neuropathic ulcers

Neuropathic ulcers tend to be seen over pressure areas of the feet, such as the metatarsal heads, owing to repeated trauma. They are most commonly found in diabetics due to peripheral neuropathy. In some developing countries, leprosy is a common cause.

Management depends on keeping the ulcer clean and removing pressure or trauma from the affected area. Diabetics should pay particular attention to foot care and correctly fitting shoes with the help of a specialist podiatrist (see pp. 1272–1273).

Pressure ulcers (decubitus ulcers, bedsores)

These occur in elderly, immobile, unconscious or paralysed patients. They are due to skin ischaemia from sustained pressure over a bony prominence: most commonly, the heel and sacrum. Normal individuals feel the pain of continued pressure, and even during sleep movement takes place to change position continually. Pressure ulcers may be graded:

- Stage I: non-blanchable erythema of intact skin.
- Stage II: partial-thickness skin loss of epidermis/dermis (blister or shallow ulcer).
- Stage III: full-thickness skin loss involving subcutaneous tissue but not fascia.
- Stage IV: full-thickness skin loss with involvement of muscle/bone/tendon/joint capsule.

Box 31.20 Risk factors for the development of pressure ulcers

Prolonged immobility
- Paraplegia
- Arthritis
- Severe physical disease
- Apathy
- Operation and postoperative states
- Plaster casts
- Intensive care

Decreased sensation
- Coma, neurological disease, diabetes mellitus
- Drug-induced sleep

Vascular disease
- Atherosclerosis, diabetes mellitus, scleroderma, vasculitis

Poor nutrition
- Anaemia
- Hypoalbuminaemia
- Vitamin C or zinc deficiency

There are numerous risk factors for the development of pressure ulcers ***(Box 31.20)***.

The majority of pressure ulcers occur in hospital. Some 70% appear in the first 2 weeks of hospitalization; 70% are in orthopaedic patients, especially those on traction. Between 20% and 30% of pressure ulcers occur in the community. Some 80% of patients who have deep ulcers involving the subcutaneous tissue die in the first 4 months.

The early sign of red/blue discoloration of the skin can lead rapidly to ulcers in 1–2 hours. Leaving patients on hard emergency room trolleys or sitting them in chairs for prolonged periods must be avoided.

Management

- Bed rest with pillows and fleeces to keep pressure off bony areas (e.g. sacrum and heels) and prevent friction.
- Air-filled cushions for patients in wheelchairs.
- Special pressure-relieving mattresses and beds.
- Regular turning but avoidance of pressure on hips.
- Adequate nutrition.
- Non-irritant occlusive moist dressings (e.g. hydrocolloid).
- Adequate analgesia (may need opiates).
- Plastic surgery (debridement and grafting in selected cases).
- Treatment of underlying condition.

Prevention

Prevention is better than cure. Specialist 'tissue-viability nurses' help identify at-risk patients and train other clinical staff. Several risk assessment tools have been devised for the immobile patient, based on the known risk factors. The 'Norton scale' and Waterlow Pressure Ulcer Risk Assessment ***(Box 31.21)*** are two such validated systems; they produce a numerical score, enabling staff to identify those at most risk. Braden, Walsall and Maelor scales are also used.

Vasculitis

Vasculitis (see also pp. 699–702) is an inflammatory disorder of blood vessels that causes endothelial damage. Cutaneous vasculitis (confirmed by skin biopsy) may be an isolated problem or part of a systemic disease with involvement of other organs. The most commonly used classification is based on the size of blood vessel involved (see ***Boxes 18.37*** and ***18.38***).

Box 31.21 Pressure ulcer risk assessment tools

NORTON SCALE FOR PRESSURE ULCERS

Physical		Neurology		Activity		Mobility		Incontinence	
4	Good	4	Alert	4	Ambulant	4	Full	4	None
3	Fair	3	Apathetic	3	Walks with help	3	Slightly	3	Occasionally incontinent
2	Poor	2	Confused	2	Not bound	2	Limited[a]	2	Usually incontinent
1	Very poor	1	Stupor	1	Bedfast	1	Very limited; immobile	1	Doubly incontinent

[a]Low scores carry a high risk.

WATERLOW PRESSURE ULCER RISK ASSESSMENT

Build/weight for height		Visual skin type		Continence		Mobility		Sex/Age		Appetite	
Average	0	Healthy	0	Complete	0	Fully mobile	0	Male	1	Average	0
Above average	2	Tissue paper	1	Occasionally incontinent	1	Restricted/difficult	1	Female	2	Poor	1
Below average	3	Dry	1	Catheter/incontinent of faeces	2	Restless/fidgety	2	14–18	1	Anorectic	2
		Oedematous	1	Doubly incontinent	3	Apathetic	3	50–64	2		
		Clammy	1			Inert/traction	4	65–75	3		
		Discoloured	2					75–80	4		
		Broken/spot	3					81+	5		

Special risk factors		Assessment value	
1. Poor nutrition, e.g. terminal cachexia	8	At risk	10
2. Sensory deprivation, e.g. diabetes, paraplegia, cerebrovascular disease	6	High risk	15
3. High-dose anti-inflammatory or steroid in use	3	Very high risk	20
4. Smoking 10+ per day	1		
5. Orthopaedic surgery/fracture below waist	3		

The cutaneous features are haemorrhagic papules, pustules, nodules or plaques, which may erode and ulcerate. These purpuric lesions do not blanch with pressure from a glass slide ('diascopy'). Occasionally, a fixed livedo reticularis pattern may appear, which does not disappear on warming. Pyrexia and arthralgia are common associations, even in the absence of significant systemic involvement. Other clinical features depend on the underlying cause.

Leucocytoclastic vasculitis (LCV) or angiitis is the most common cutaneous vasculitis affecting small vessels. This usually appears on the lower legs as a symmetrical palpable purpura. It is rarely associated with systemic involvement. It can be caused by drugs (15%), infection (15%), inflammatory disease (10%) or malignant disease (<5%) but often no cause is found (55–60%). Investigations are only necessary with persistent lesions or associated signs and symptoms. Whilst LCV often settles spontaneously, treatment with analgesia, support stockings, dapsone or prednisolone may be needed to control the pain and to heal any ulceration. ***Urticarial vasculitis*** is discussed on page 1357.

Calciphylaxis (***calcific uraemic arteriopathy***) is described on page 780.

Lymphatics

Lymphoedema

Lymphoedema refers to a chronic, non-pitting oedema caused by lymphatic insufficiency. It most commonly affects the legs and tends to progress with age. The legs can become enormous and prevent normal shoes being worn. Chronic disease may cause a secondary 'cobblestone' thickening of the skin. Lymphoedema can be primary (and present early in life) due to an inherited deficiency of lymphatic vessels (e.g. Milroy's disease) or can be secondary due to obstruction of lymphatic vessels (e.g. filarial infection or malignant disease).

Management is with compression stockings and physical massage. If there is recurrent cellulitis, long-term antibiotics are advisable, as each episode of cellulitis will further damage the lymph vessels. Surgery should be avoided.

Lymphangioma circumscriptum

This is a rare hamartoma of lymphatic tissue. It usually presents in childhood with multiple small vesicles in the skin, which weep lymphatic fluid and sometimes blood. They reflect deeper vessel involvement and so surgery should be avoided. Cryotherapy or CO_2 laser treatment may help the superficial lesions.

Further reading

Ashby RL, Gabe R, Ali S et al. Clinical and cost-effectiveness of compression hosiery versus compression bandages in treatment of venous leg ulcers (Venous leg Ulcer Study IV, VenUS IV): a randomised controlled trial. *Lancet* 2014; 383:871–879.

Chen C, Hou W, Chan ESY et al. Phototherapy for treating pressure ulcers. *Cochrane Database Syst Rev (Online)* 2014; 7:CD009224.

Kirsner RS, Marston WA, Snyder RJ et al. Spray-applied cell therapy with human allogeneic fibroblasts and keratinocytes for the treatment of chronic venous leg ulcers: a phase 2, multicentre, double-blind, randomised, placebo-controlled trial. *Lancet* 2012; 380:977–985.

Langer G, Fink A. Nutritional interventions for preventing and treating pressure ulcers. *Cochrane Database Syst Rev (Online)* 2014; 6:CD003216.

Moore ZEH, Webster J. Dressings and topical agents for preventing pressure ulcers. *Cochrane Database Syst Rev (Online)* 2013; 8:CD009362.

National Institute for Health and Care Excellence. *NICE Clinical Guideline 179: Pressure Ulcers: Prevention and Management*. NICE 2014; https://www.nice.org.uk/guidance/CG179.

Nelson EA, Bell-Syer SE. Compression for preventing recurrence of venous leg ulcers. *Cochrane Database Syst Rev (Online)* 2014; 9:CD002303.
O'Meara S, Cullum N, Nelson EA et al. Compression for venous leg ulcers. *Cochrane Database Syst Rev (Online)* 2012; 11:CD000265.

DISORDERS OF COLLAGEN AND ELASTIC TISSUE

Ehlers–Danlos syndrome

Ehlers–Danlos syndrome (see also pp. 666–667) is a term that refers to a group of inherited autoimmune rheumatic diseases that manifest with abnormalities in the skin, ligament, joints, blood vessels and internal organs. The underlying defects are varied and involve abnormalities of synthesis of collagen fibrils and extracellular matrix molecules (see p. 04). Cutaneous features include hyper-extensible skin, tissue paper scarring and pseudo-tumours at the sites of scars. Skin biopsy with electron microscopy can be helpful in guiding the need for genetic testing. The beta-blocker celiprolol significantly decreases the severe arterial complications of the vascular form of type IV Ehlers–Danlos syndrome.

Pseudoxanthoma elasticum

Pseudoxanthoma elasticum is a rare disease involving abnormal mineralization of connective tissue, characterized by changes in the skin, eye and blood vessels. It is caused by mutations in the cell transporter gene *ABCC6*. The skin may be slack and wrinkled with a yellow, papular, 'plucked chicken' appearance. These changes are best seen in the flexures, especially the sides of the neck. Non-cutaneous features include recurrent gastrointestinal bleeding, early myocardial infarction, claudication and angioid streaks on the retina.

Striae distensae (stretch marks)

Striae are linear scars caused by dermal collagen damage and fragmentation of elastic tissue. They occur commonly over the abdomen and breasts in pregnancy, and on the thighs and trunk in adolescents and obese individuals. Striae are usually red–blue then fade to white atrophic lines. The cause is unknown but excessive skin tension, high levels of cortisol (as in Cushing syndrome) and genetics may play a role. Striae are also seen in Marfan syndrome.

Keloids and hypertrophic scars

Abnormal wound healing with excessive dermal fibrosis leads to hypertrophic scars and keloid formation. Hypertrophic scars remain confined to the borders of the original wound and usually regress spontaneously. Keloids ***(Fig. 31.46)*** can arise spontaneously or after trauma and continue to proliferate and enlarge beyond the wound margins. They are often itchy and tend to affect young, dark-skinned adults. Sites of predilection include the shoulders, upper back and chest, earlobes and chin. Treatment options include silicone gel or dressings, cryotherapy and intralesional triamcinolone. Newer agents include intralesional chemotherapeutic agents (5-fluorouracil or bleomycin) and laser therapy (pulsed dye laser, non-ablative fractional lasers).

Further reading

Arno AI, Gauglitz GG, Barret JP et al. Up-to-date approach to manage keloids and hypertrophic scars: a useful guide. *Burns* 2014; 40:1255–1266.
Sobey G. Ehlers–Danlos syndrome: how to diagnose and when to perform genetic tests. *Arch Dis Child* 2015; 100:57–61.

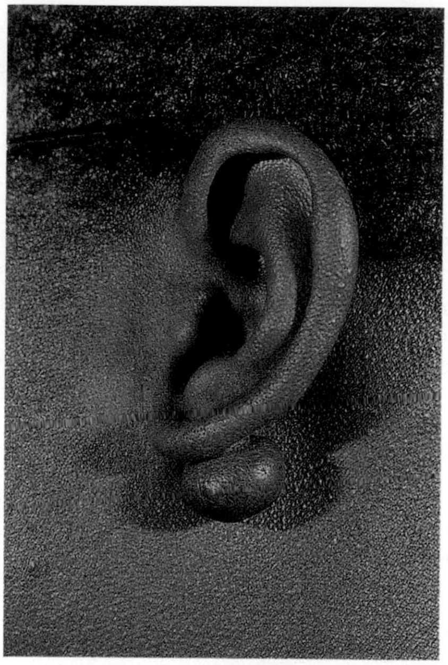

Figure 31.46 Keloid scar of the lobe of the ear.

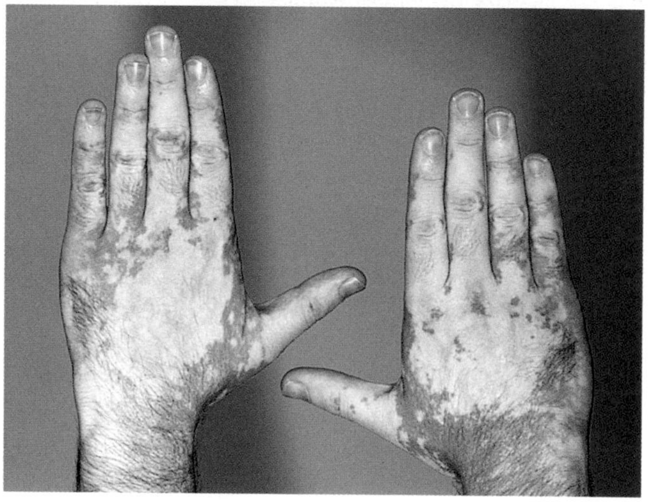

Figure 31.47 Vitiligo of the hands. Areas of depigmentation.

DISORDERS OF PIGMENTATION

Hypopigmentation

Vitiligo

Vitiligo is chronic depigmenting skin disorder that affects 1–2% of the world population; about a third of all cases start in childhood. Vitiligo has features of an autoimmune disorder with an aberrant T-cell response against melanocytes, and is associated with other organ-specific autoimmune diseases. It presents with asymptomatic, symmetrical, well-demarcated macules of complete pigment loss and typically affects the face, genitalia and bony prominences ***(Fig. 31.47)***. Pigment may be lost from overlying hair. There is no history of preceding inflammation. Treatment is often unsatisfactory and has no impact on the long-term outcome. Potent topical corticosteroids, topical tacrolimus and phototherapy (UVB, PUVA or excimer laser) may stimulate repigmentation, and this usually starts around hair follicles, giving a speckled appearance. Repigmentation is less likely in established lesions and acral sites. Sunblocks should be used to prevent burning. Patients may benefit from psychological support and skin camouflage advice. If vitiligo is extensive and fixed, the remaining pigment can be removed with monobenzone.

Post-inflammatory hypopigmentation

This phenomenon is sometimes noticeable in dark-skinned individuals when inflammatory rashes such as eczema and psoriasis clear. It may be mistaken for vitiligo, but lesions are usually hypopigmented rather than depigmented, and recover spontaneously over several months, as long as the underlying disease is controlled.

Oculocutaneous albinism

This group of rare autosomal recessive disorders are caused by reduced or absent pigment synthesis in the skin, hair and eyes. It can affect all races. Affected individuals have pale skin, white or yellow hair, and a pink iris. Ocular manifestations include photophobia, nystagmus and a squint. Meticulous UV protection is required to prevent sunburn and reduce the risk of skin cancer.

Idiopathic guttate hypomelanosis

This occurs most commonly in black African people and is of unknown aetiology. It presents with small (2–4 mm), asymptomatic, porcelain-white macules, often on skin exposed to sunlight. The borders are frequently sharply defined and angular. There is no effective treatment.

Leprosy

Both tuberculoid leprosy and indeterminate leprosy (see also pp. 285–286) can present with anaesthetic hypopigmented patches and should always be considered in people from endemic regions. Lesions may also show hair loss and decreased sweating.

Hyperpigmentation

Freckles (ephelides)

These appear in childhood as small brown macules after sun exposure. They fade in the winter.

Lentigines

These are persistent pigmented macules that look similar to freckles. They may rarely be associated with systemic syndromes (e.g. Peutz–Jeghers (see p. 403), LEOPARD/Noonan (*L*entigines, *E*CG abnormalities, *O*cular hypertension, *P*ulmonary stenosis, *A*bnormalities of genitalia, *R*etardation of growth and *D*eafness). Solar lentigines ('age spots', 'liver spots') are common on the dorsal hands and face and on bald scalps in older, fair-skinned people.

Café-au-lait macules

These may occur as an isolated abnormality. Multiple lesions are also a feature of neurofibromatosis types 1 and 2, tuberous sclerosis, ataxia telangiectasia, Fanconi's anaemia, multiple endocrine neoplasia type 1 and McCune–Albright syndrome.

Chloasma (melasma)

This is a common complaint in pregnancy and women taking hormonal contraception. Asymptomatic beige–brown patches develop on the forehead, temples and cheeks. Topical treatment with azelaic acid or retinoic acid (which should be avoided in pregnancy) and 2–5% hydroquinone may help. High-factor sunscreens are needed to prevent relapse.

Post-inflammatory hyperpigmentation

This phenomenon occurs in dark-skinned individuals at the sites of skin trauma or inflammatory rashes, such as acne, lichen planus and eczema. It improves slowly over many months.

Metabolic/endocrine effects

Generalized skin darkening can occur with chronic liver disease, especially haemochromatosis. It is also seen sometimes in Cushing syndrome, Addison's disease (more marked in palmar creases and buccal mucosa) and Nelson syndrome.

Urticaria pigmentosa (cutaneous mastocytosis)

This disorder is caused by a benign proliferation of cutaneous mast cells. It presents most commonly in childhood as multiple pigmented macules that become red, itchy and urticated if they are rubbed (Darier's sign). Occasionally, lesions may blister. Extensive mast cell degranulation can lead to systemic symptoms, such as wheeze, flushing, syncope or diarrhoea and, very rarely, anaphylaxis. This may be triggered by drugs, including aspirin and opiates. Childhood urticaria pigmentosa usually resolves spontaneously but adult-onset disease is often persistent. Histology of skin lesions shows increased numbers of mast cells. Most cases are due to somatically acquired activating mutations of the *KIT* receptor that controls mast cell proliferation and apoptosis. Rarely, in adult and neonatal disease, urticaria pigmentosa may progress with mast cell infiltration of internal organs (bone, gastrointestinal tract, liver, spleen – ***systemic mastocytosis***). There is a small risk of developing leukaemia if the bone marrow is heavily infiltrated. Therapy of cutaneous mastocytosis is aimed at controlling the symptoms of mast cell mediator release with antihistamines and cromoglicate, and minimizing the risk of anaphylaxis.

Further reading

Ezzedine K, Eleftheriadou V, Whitton M et al. Vitiligo. *Lancet* 2015; 386:74–84.
Nicolaidou E, Katsambas AD. Pigmentation disorders: hyperpigmentation and hypopigmentation. *Clin Dermatol* 2014; 32:66–72.

DISORDERS OF THE NAILS

- ***Psoriasis*** (see pp. 1353–1356), ***fungal infection*** (pp. 1345–1347) and ***trauma*** are the most common causes of abnormal nail growth (dystrophy).
- ***Pitting*** can be caused by psoriasis, alopecia areata, atopic eczema and trauma.
- ***Onycholysis*** (distal nail plate separation) is caused by psoriasis, thyrotoxicosis, trauma and, rarely, a phototoxic drug reaction (e.g. with tetracyclines).
- ***Koilonychia*** (thin, spoon-shaped nails) can be caused by iron deficiency anaemia.
- ***Leuconychia*** (white nails) is seen in hypoalbuminaemia.
- ***Beau's lines*** (transverse lines) are horizontal grooves that grow distally with the nail over several months. They are associated with an acute severe illness that causes a temporary arrest in nail growth.
- ***Yellow-nail syndrome*** is a rare disorder of lymphatic drainage. It presents with thickened, slow-growing, yellow

nails, which may be associated with pleural effusions, bronchiectasis and lymphoedema of the legs.

- ***Sub-ungual hyperkeratosis*** is thickening of the nail plate – usually due to tinea infection (see p. 1346), psoriasis, trauma or a combination of these.
- ***Onychogryphosis*** is severe nail thickening and curvature (ram's horn), which is common in the elderly, especially in the big toe-nail, where trauma from ill-fitting footwear may be relevant.
- ***Longitudinal melanonychia*** (brown streaks) of multiple nails is a common finding in dark-skinned people. An acquired solitary pigmented streak may be caused by a melanocytic naevus and needs to be differentiated from subungual melanoma (see pp. 1373–1374), especially if the pigmentation spreads on to the adjacent nail fold ('Hutchinson's sign').
- ***Sub-ungual haemorrhage*** is common in the great toe-nails after trauma (football, running downhill). The red–brown pigmentation grows out with the nail over several months with clear proximal growth.
- ***Clubbing*** is discussed on page 1067.

Nail dystrophy is also a feature of various genodermatoses including ***nail patellar syndrome*** (triangular lunulae, dystrophic nails and absent or hypoplastic patellae; ***ectodermal dysplasias*** (abnormal hair, teeth and nail) and ***pachyonychia congenita*** ('hoof' nails and keratoderma).

Further reading

Iorizzo M. Tips to treat the 5 most common nail disorders: brittle nails, onycholysis, paronychia, psoriasis, onychomycosis. *Dermatol Clin* 2015; 33:175–307.

Khan S, Basit S, Habib R et al. Genetics of human isolated hereditary nail disorders. *Br J Dermatol* 2015; 173:922–929.

DISORDERS OF HAIR

Hair loss

Hair loss can be due to either a disorder of the hair follicle in which the scalp skin looks normal (non-scarring alopecia), or a disorder within the scalp skin that causes permanent loss of the follicle (scarring or cicatricial alopecia). This latter form causes shiny, atrophic bald areas in the scalp, which are devoid of follicular openings. There are many causes of alopecia ***(Box 31.22)***.

Androgenic alopecia

Androgenic alopecia (male-pattern baldness) is the most common type of non-scarring hair loss and depends on genetic factors and an abnormal sensitivity to androgens. It presents in young men with frontal receding followed by thinning of the crown, and there is often a positive family history. It also occurs in females but tends to occur at a later age, be milder and show little in the way of frontal recession. If acne and menstrual disturbance are also present, the cause may be polycystic ovary syndrome or another endocrine disorder of androgens.

Treatment may not be required. Topical 5% minoxidil lotion or oral 5-alpha-reductase inhibitors (finasteride or dutasteride) can help arrest progression and may induce modest regrowth, providing they are used early in disease, but the treatment needs to be continued indefinitely. Approximately one-third of patients will not respond to either therapy. Finasteride is well tolerated but causes sexual adverse effects, such as loss of libido in about 1% of men. It should not be used in females, as it can affect the sexual development of a male fetus. However, antiandrogen therapy (e.g. cyproterone acetate or spironolactone) may help some women.

Box 31.22 Causes of alopecia

Scarring alopecia	Non-scarring alopecia
• Discoid lupus erythematosus	• Androgenic alopecia
• Kerion (tinea capitis)	• Telogen effluvium
• Lichen planus	• Alopecia areata
• Dissecting cellulitis	• Trichotillomania (self-induced hair-pulling)
• X-irradiation	• Tinea capitis
• Idiopathic ('pseudopelade')	• Traction alopecia
	• Metabolic (iron deficiency, hypothyroidism)
	• Drugs (e.g. heparin, isotretinoin, chemotherapy)

Alopecia areata

Alopecia areata is thought to be an autoimmune disease, as it is often associated with other organ-specific autoimmune diseases. Recent genome-wide association studies have implicated ligands for the NKG2D receptor (the product of the *KLRK1* gene) in disease pathogenesis.

Alopecia areata presents in children or young adults with patches of baldness ***(Fig. 31.48)***. These may regrow, to be followed by new patches of hair loss. The presence of broken exclamation mark hairs (narrow at the scalp and wider and more pigmented at the tip) at the edge of a bald area is diagnostic. Regrowth may initially be with white hairs and often occurs slowly over months. Occasionally, all of the scalp hair is lost (alopecia totalis) and, rarely, all body hair is lost (alopecia universalis). The nails may be pitted or roughened.

Management has no effect on the long-term progression. Potent topical or injected steroids may trigger regrowth of localized patchy hair loss. Topical immunotherapy with diphencyprone can be helpful in more extensive disease. There is insufficient evidence to justify using PUVA, topical minoxidil or tacrolimus ointment. Oral ruxolitinib (a JAK1 and 2 inhibitor) has recently been shown to be highly effective in a mouse model of alopecia, as well as in three patients with alopecia areata. Larger studies are currently under way. Wigs can be provided for severe cases and patient support groups are often beneficial.

Traction alopecia

This refers to the 'mechanical damage' type of hair loss that arises from pulling the hair back into a bun or tight plaits. It is more common in black Africans.

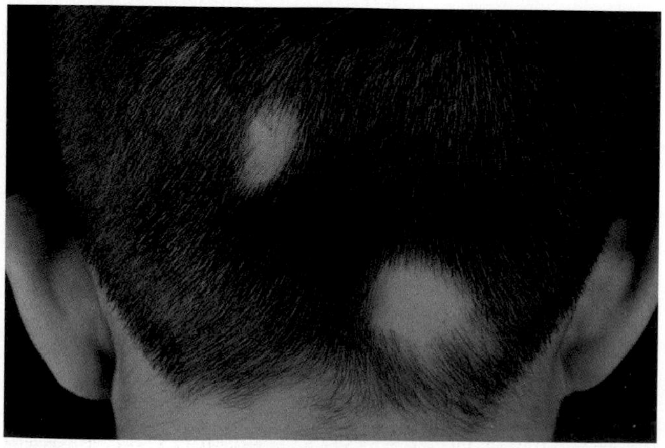

Figure 31.48 Alopecia areata.

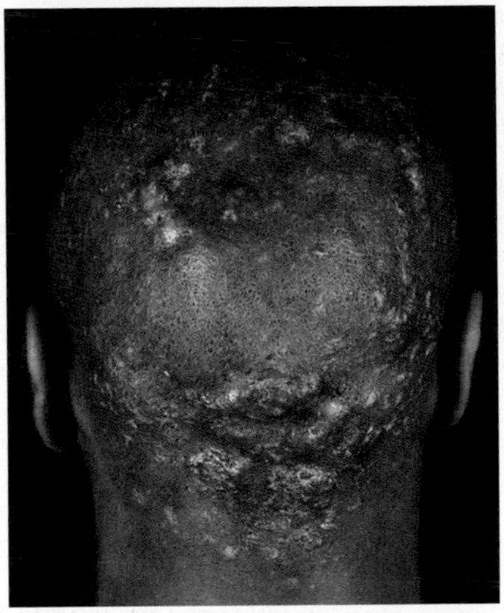

Figure 31.49 Dissecting cellulitis of the scalp in an African–Caribbean male.

Telogen effluvium

Telogen effluvium refers to the pattern of diffuse hair loss that occurs some 3 months after pregnancy or a severe illness. It occurs because 'stress' puts all the hairs into the telogen phase of hair shedding at the same time. The hair fully recovers and the normal staggered hair growth/hair shedding cycle resumes within a few months.

Dissecting cellulitis

This is a chronic folliculitis of the scalp that predominantly affects young black men. Papules and pustules occur over the back of the scalp with scarring hair loss, and the skin may become chronically swollen and purulent with a boggy texture ***(Fig. 31.49)***. Prolonged courses of oral antibiotics, including a combination of rifampicin and clindamycin, may be helpful.

Increased hair growth

Hirsutism

Hirsutism (see p. 1220) refers to the male pattern of hair growth seen in females. The racial variation in hair growth must be considered. Certain races (e.g. Mediterranean and Asian) have more male-pattern hair growth than Northern European females. This is not due to excess androgens but may reflect a genetically determined altered sensitivity to them. If virilizing features (deep voice, clitoromegaly, dysmenorrhoea, acne) are present, a full endocrine assessment is necessary. Hirsutism can cause severe psychological distress in some individuals.

Management involves physical methods, such as bleaching, waxing, electrolysis, intense pulsed light (IPL) and laser therapy. Oral anti-androgen therapy is occasionally helpful.

Hypertrichosis

Hypertrichosis refers to the state of excessive hair growth at any site and occurs in both sexes. It can be seen in anorexia nervosa, porphyria cutanea tarda and underlying malignancy, and is caused by certain drugs (e.g. ciclosporin, minoxidil).

Further reading

Mella JM, Perret MC, Manzotti M et al. Efficacy and safety of finasteride therapy for androgenetic alopecia: a systematic review. *Arch Dermatol* 2010; 146:1141–1150.

Xing L, Dai Z, Jabbari A et al. Alopecia areata is driven by cytotoxic T lymphocytes and is reversed by JAK inhibition. *Nat Med* 2014; 20:1043–1049.

BIRTH MARKS/NEONATAL RASHES

Infantile haemangioma (strawberry naevus, cavernous haemangioma)

Infantile haemangioma affects up to 1% of infants ***(Fig. 31.50)***. It presents at, or shortly after, birth as a single red, lumpy nodule that grows rapidly for the first few months. Multiple lesions can be present. They will spontaneously resolve with good cosmesis but complete resolution may take up to 7 years. Occasionally, plastic surgery is needed after resolution to remove residual slack skin. Reassurance of parents is usually all that is required.

Urgent treatment is indicated if the lesion:

- interferes with feeding or vision
- ulcerates or bleeds frequently
- is associated with high-output cardiac failure from shunting of large volumes of blood
- consumes platelets and/or clotting factors, causing potentially life-threatening haemorrhage ('Kasabach–Merritt syndrome').

The last two complications are very rare and tend to occur only in large lesions with significant deep-vessel involvement.

Treatment has been revolutionized by the discovery that oral propranolol (3 mg/kg per day in 3 divided doses) rapidly shrinks infantile haemangiomas, even the deep or sub-glottic lesions. The mechanism of action is unclear. Treatment may need to be continued for up to a year. Side-effects (acrocyanosis, disturbed sleep, hypotension) are usually mild. In life-threatening cases, high-dose systemic steroids, vincristine or embolization may be used.

Port-wine stain (naevus flammeus)

Port-wine stain is also called a capillary haemangioma but, strictly speaking, it is not a haemangioma, just an abnormal dilatation of dermal capillaries. It presents at birth as a flat, red, macular area and is commonly found on the face. It does not improve spontaneously and may become thickened with time. If the lesion is found in the distribution of the first division of the trigeminal nerve, it may be associated with ipsilateral meningeal vascular anomalies that can cause epilepsy and even hemiplegia (Sturge–Weber syndrome). Periocular lesions may be associated with glaucoma and so ophthalmological follow-up is required.

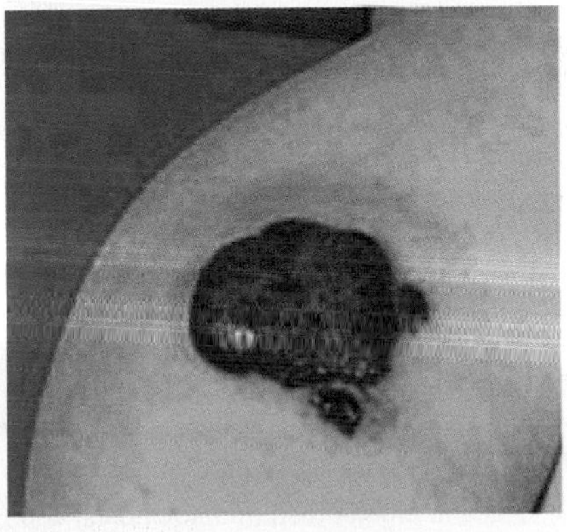

Figure 31.50 Strawberry naevus (cavernous haemangioma).

Management of port-wine stains is ideally with a vascular selective laser, such as the tunable dye (pulsed dye) laser. Facial lesions respond best but lesions can darken after several years and require retreatment.

Milia

'Milk spots' are small follicular epidermal cysts. These small, pinhead, white papules are commonly found on the face of infants. They resolve spontaneously, unlike in adults.

Congenital melanocytic naevi

Some children are born with small melanocytic naevi (<2 cm in diameter). In later life, they are usually larger than acquired naevi and often have coarse hair. They may display some irregularity in colour and border but malignant change is extremely rare, so prophylactic excision is not necessary. It is only the giant congenital melanocytic naevus (>20 cm) that has a high risk for malignant transformation (see p. 1373).

Mongolian blue spot

This appears in infants as a deep blue–grey, bruise-like area, usually over the sacrum or back ***(Fig. 31.51)***; it is occasionally mistaken for a sign of child abuse. Mongolian blue spot is due to presence of melanocytes in the deeper dermis. It is very common in Oriental children, less common in black Africans and rare in Caucasians. It usually disappears by the age of 7 years.

Toxic erythema of the newborn (erythema neonatorum)

Toxic erythema of the newborn is a term used to describe a common transient, blotchy, maculopapular rash in newborns. The rash is occasionally pustular but the child is not toxic or unwell. It disappears spontaneously within a few days.

Nappy rash ('diaper dermatitis')

This is a form of irritant contact dermatitis caused by prolonged skin contact with faeces and urine. It is much less common nowadays due to the high absorbency of disposable nappies. The flexures are usually spared, which is a useful differentiating feature from atopic eczema. Satellite lesions around the edge may indicate a superimposed candidal infection. A recalcitrant purpuric nappy rash in the groins and axillae should be biopsied to exclude rarer pathology such as Langerhans cell histiocytosis.

Management involves frequent changing of the nappy and regular application of a barrier cream.

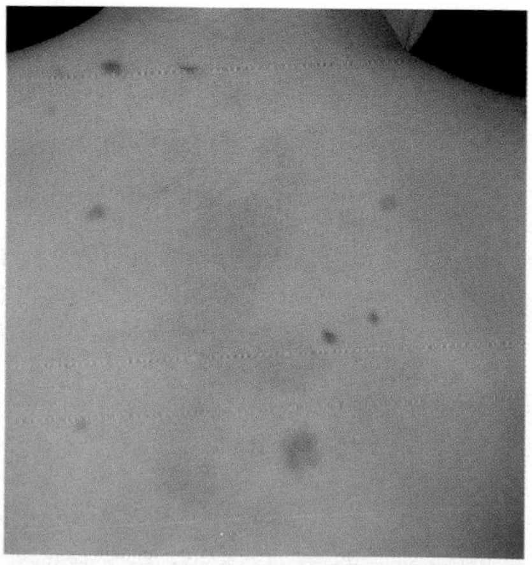

Figure 31.51 Urticaria pigmentosa (mastocytosis) and Mongolian blue spots in a baby.

Acrodermatitis enteropathica

This rare but distinctive rash (see p. 203) is a manifestation of zinc deficiency, which can occur in three settings:

- an inherited defect in zinc transporter protein in the gastrointestinal tract (presents after breast-feeding finishes)
- low levels in breast milk in breast-fed infants (presents during breast-feeding)
- patients on total parenteral nutrition without adequate zinc replacement.

There is an erythematous, sometimes blistering, rash around the perineum, mouth, hands and feet. It may be associated with photophobia, diarrhoea and alopecia.

In the inherited form the rash presents when breast-feeding finishes, as breast milk usually has high levels of zinc that override the poor absorption. These cases will need life-long oral zinc replacement therapy, not just to improve the skin but also to ensure normal neurological development. The second type needs replacement only until breast-feeding finishes. The response to zinc is rapid and dramatic.

Further reading

Ji Y, Chen S, Xu C et al. The use of propranolol in the treatment of infantile haemangiomas: an update on potential mechanisms of action. *Br J Dermatol* 2015; 172:24–32.

Léauté-Labrèze C, Hoeger P, Mazereeuw-Hautier J et al. A randomised control trial of oral propranolol in infantile hemangiomas. *N Engl J Med* 2015; 372:735–746.

Schmitt S, Küry S, Giraud M et al. An update on mutations of the SLC39A4 gene in acrodermatitis enteropathica. *Hum Mutat* 2009; 30:926–933.

Shirley MD, Tang H, Gallione CJ et al. Sturge-Weber syndrome and port-wine stains caused by somatic mutation in GNAQ. *N Engl J Med* 2013; 368:1971–1979.

DRUG ERUPTIONS

Drugs can cause predictable, dose-related adverse effects in the skin, such as phototoxicity from doxycycline or mucocutaneous dryness from oral isotretinoin. They may also cause hypersensitivity rashes ranging from mild exanthems to severe, life-threatening eruptions (severe cutaneous adverse drug reactions). These are idiopathic and can be difficult to diagnose because individual drugs can lead to different rashes, and these sometimes mimic constitutional dermatoses such as dermatitis or viral rashes. A high index of suspicion and a detailed drug history are essential. Underlying viral infection, especially HIV, and systemic disease, such as systemic lupus and leukaemia, may also increase the risk of drug rashes ***(Fig. 31.52)***. Allergy tests (prick tests and patch tests) have a limited role, especially in the acute setting, and drug challenge tests are time-consuming and potentially risky.

Maculopapular (morbilliform) exanthems

These are the most common type of hypersensitivity rash ***(Fig 31.53)***. They start on the torso and spread to the face and limbs, but spare the mucosae. They are self-limiting and usually clear within 1–2 weeks.

Fixed drug eruptions

These are inflamed patches that recur at the same site each time a drug is taken. They may blister, and often resolve with hyperpigmentation.

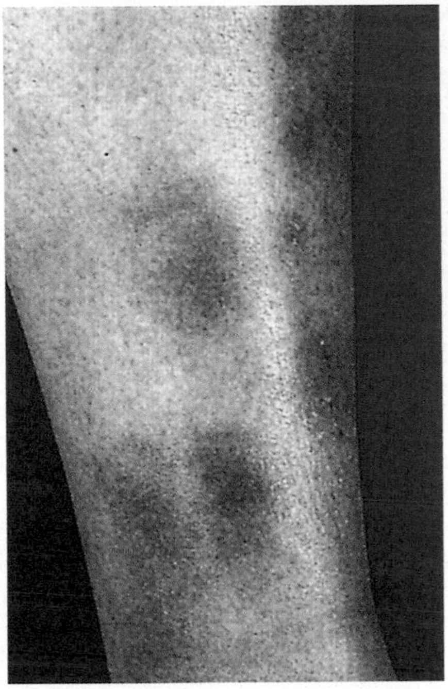

Figure 31.52 Erythema nodosum in a patient with HIV on co-trimoxazole.

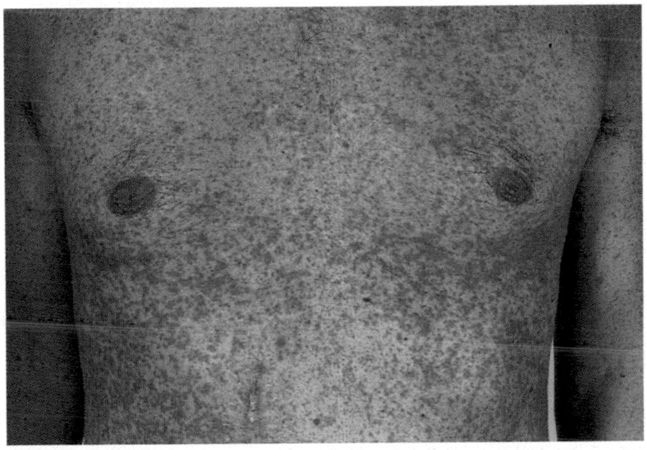

Figure 31.53 Morbilliform drug rash due to penicillin allergy.

Drug-induced and drug-exacerbated dermatoses

Drugs may exacerbate pre-existing skin disease and can also trigger/induce skin disease that resembles a constitutional dermatosis. Examples are shown in ***Box 31.23***.

Severe cutaneous adverse drug reactions

Severe drug rashes are listed below ***(Box 31.24)***. Common causes include antibiotics, NSAIDs, anticonvulsants, allopurinol, Dapsone and nevirapine. Early recognition and drug withdrawal can minimize morbidity and mortality. Recent advances in pharmacogenetics have identified HLA associations, and cytochrome P450 polymorphisms which are associated with an increased risk of reaction to certain drugs.

Box 31.23 Dermatoses induced or aggravated by drugs

Dermatosis	Drugs
Acne	Androgens (danazol)
Acneiform	Corticosteroids, EGFR inhibitors
Angioedema	ACE inhibitors
Urticaria	Penicillin, aspirin, NSAIDs, iodine contrast media
Vasculitis	Gold, hydralazine, NSAIDs, proton pump inhibitors
Fixed drug eruption	Phenolphthalein in laxatives, tetracyclines, paracetamol
Pigmentation	Minocycline (black), amiodarone (slate-grey)
Lupus erythematosus	Minocycline, anti-TNF biologics, isoniazid, interferons
Photosensitivity	Thiazides, quinolones, tetracyclines, diuretics, amiodarone
Pseudoporphyria	Naproxen, diuretics
Leg ulcers	Hydroxyurea
Anogenital ulcers	Nicorandil
Erythema nodosum	Sulphonamides, oral contraceptive
Erythema multiforme	Barbiturates, etravirine
Lichen planus-like (lichenoid)	Antimalarials, thiazides, statins, diuretics
Psoriasiform	Methyldopa, gold, lithium, beta-blockers
Toxic epidermal necrolysis	Penicillin, co-trimoxazole, carbamazepine, NSAIDs, nevirapine, efavirenz
Pemphigus	Penicillamine, ACE inhibitors
Erythroderma	Gold, sulphonylureas, allopurinol, nevirapine, efavirenz

ACE, angiotensin-converting enzyme; EGFR, epidermal growth factor receptor; NSAIDs, non-steroidal anti-inflammatory drugs; TNF, tumour necrosis factor.

Box 31.24 Severe cutaneous adverse drug reactions

- Stevens–Johnson syndrome (SJS) and toxic epidermal necrolysis (TEN)
- Drug reaction with eosinophilia and systemic symptoms (DRESS)
- Acute generalized exanthematous pustulosis (AGEP)
- Erythroderma/exfoliative dermatitis
- Serum sickness-like reactions

Stevens–Johnson syndrome and toxic epidermal necrolysis

Stevens–Johnson syndrome (SJS) and toxic epidermal necrolysis (TEN) are severe mucocutaneous disorders, which are considered variants of a disease spectrum. They are characterized by varying extents of blistering/epidermal detachment and mucosal ulceration:

- ***SJS***: <10% skin detachment; one or two mucosal sites involved (oral, genital, ocular)
- ***SJS–TEN*** overlap: 10–30% skin detachment
- ***TEN***: >30% skin detachment: all mucosal sites involved in most cases.

The onset is usually 1–2 weeks after drug exposure. Initial symptoms are non-specific (malaise, myalgia, fever and cough). These are followed by very tender areas of maculopapular erythema on the torso with inflammation of mucosal surfaces. Target lesions may

Box 31.25 SCORTEN prognostic score in toxic epidermal necrolysis

Risk factor	0	1
Age	<40 years	>40 years
Associated malignancy	No	Yes
Heart rate (b.p.m.)	<120	>120
Serum urea (mmol/L)	<9.6	>9.6
Detached or compromised body surface	<10%	>10%
Serum bicarbonate (mmol/L)	>20	<20
Serum glucose (mmol/L)	<13.9	>13.9

The more risk factors present, the higher the SCORTEN score, and the higher the mortality rate:
0–1 risk factors: 3.2% mortality
2: 12.1%
3: 35.3%
4: 58.3%
≥5: >90%

(From Bastuji-Garin S, Fouchard N, Bertocchi M et al. SCORTEN: a severity-of-illness score for toxic epidermal necrolysis. *J Invest Dermatol* 2000; 115: 149–153.)

occur on the hands and feet in SJS. In TEN there is widespread flaccid blistering with skin that wrinkles like wet wallpaper on gentle pressure (Nikolsky's sign). Features of 'skin failure' can ensue, with defective fluid and temperature regulation leading to hypotension and renal impairment. Respiratory mucosal and pulmonary involvement may require ventilation, and upper gastrointestinal involvement can cause haemorrhage. Patients are at high risk of sepsis and require expert intensive supportive care, as for extensive burns. Multiorgan failure may occur and the mortality for TEN ranges from 30% to 50%. 'SCORTEN' is a clinical severity score that can help assess prognosis ***(Box 31.25)***. All potential drug causes should be stopped.

Treatment with high-dose steroids, ciclosporin and intravenous immunoglobulin therapy remains controversial, as high-quality clinical trials are lacking.

Drug reaction with eosinophilia and systemic symptoms/drug hypersensitivity syndrome

Drug reaction with eosinophilia and systemic symptoms (DRESS)/drug hypersensitivity syndrome usually starts 2–6 weeks after initial exposure and is characterized by widespread erythema, facial oedema, fever, lymphadenopathy and hepatosplenomegaly. Blood eosinophilia is usual with elevated hepatic transferases. Pneumonia and nephritis can develop and a mortality rate of 10% has been reported. Treatment is with oral steroids tapered over at least 3 months. Aromatic anticonvulsants are one of the most common causes of DRESS and, as they cross-react, all drugs of this group must be avoided in the future. Sodium valproate is a suitable alternative.

Acute generalized exanthematous pustulosis/toxic pustuloderma

Acute generalized exanthematous pustulosis (AGEP)/toxic pustuloderma is an exanthem with numerous small, non-follicular, sterile pustules that usually develop around the neck, axillae and groin. It usually starts a few days after drug exposure and resolves with peeling. There may be mild systemic upset but internal organs are not involved. Topical steroids and emollients can be used to relieve symptoms.

Further reading

Dodiuk-Gad RP, Laws PM, Shear NH. Epidemiology of severe drug hypersensitivity. *Semin Cutan Med Surg* 2014; 33:2–9.
Farquharson NR, Coulson IH. Drug eruptions. *Medicine* 2013; 41:360–364.
Litt JZ. *Litt's Drug Eruption Reference Manual*, 22nd edn (Boca Raton: CRC Press; 2016).
Schwartz RA, McDonough PH, Lee BW. Toxic epidermal necrolysis: Part II. Prognosis, sequelae, diagnosis, differential diagnosis, prevention, and treatment. *J Am Acad Dermatol* 2013; 69:187.e1–187.e16.

HUMAN IMMUNODEFICIENCY VIRUS AND THE SKIN

HIV infection (see pp. 331–355) commonly causes significant dermatological problems and a rash may even be the presenting feature of HIV infection. Rashes may be severe or atypical and difficult to diagnose; histology or culture of skin biopsies is sometimes required for diagnosis. Prior to anti-retroviral therapy (ART; see pp. 341–346), many dermatoses associated with advanced HIV infection were recalcitrant, but this treatment has considerably reduced their prevalence.

Seroconversion rash

This is a non-specific maculopapular exanthem that occurs in up to 75% of individuals a few weeks after contracting the virus as they start to make an anti-HIV antibody response. There may be an associated fever, malaise, myalgia, lymphadenopathy and mouth ulceration (or oral candidiasis). Symptoms usually resolve within a few weeks. This episode is often dismissed as influenza and the diagnosis missed. Patients are extremely infectious at this time due to very high viral loads.

Cutaneous infection and opportunistic infection

These are increased due to HIV-induced immune deficiency. ***Molluscum contagiosum*** is particularly common, especially on the face. Lesions are often multiple and of a 'giant' size, measuring over 1 cm across. Molluscum is rarely seen in immunocompetent adults but can be the presenting feature of HIV. Other viral infections, such as extensive ulcerative herpes or widespread viral warts, are seen. Bacterial infections (e.g. staphylococcal boils) and fungal infections (e.g. ringworm and *Candida*) are also common. Recalcitrant and recurrent oropharyngeal candidiasis is a particular problem.

Opportunistic infections, such as cutaneous cytomegalovirus (pustules or necrotic ulcers), sporotrichosis (linear nodules) or *Cryptococcus* (red papules, psoriasiform or molluscum-like lesions), can pose diagnostic difficulties, stressing the need for skin biopsy and culture.

Inflammatory dermatoses

These show an increased incidence with HIV infection, probably due to an immune dysfunction or imbalance. Severe, extensive seborrhoeic eczema is very common and is often a presenting sign of HIV. Ichthyosis (dry, scaly skin), nodular prurigo, pruritus and psoriasis are all more common in HIV infection and can be very severe. The treatment of these conditions can be difficult in patients who have low CD4 counts (<200/mm^3), as oral immunosuppressive therapies (e.g. prednisolone, ciclosporin) are best avoided. Topical therapies and phototherapy seem relatively safe and oral retinoids are a safe option for psoriasis.

'Autoimmune dermatoses'

Dermatoses such as bullous pemphigoid, thrombocytopenic purpura and vitiligo seem to increase in incidence. The aetiology is related to polyclonal stimulation of B lymphocytes by HIV with a resulting abnormal antibody production. Erythroderma is sometimes seen in HIV disease where skin biopsy suggests a 'graft-versus-host disease' mechanism. This presumably reflects a severe underlying immune dysfunction of T-lymphocyte control.

Drug rashes

These are much more common in HIV patients. Reactions (maculopapular rash) to co-trimoxazole, dapsone (used in *Pneumocystis* prophylaxis) and anti-retroviral drugs appear particularly common. Drug rashes may be severe (especially with nevirapine and efavirenz), resulting in erythroderma or toxic epidermal necrolysis. Other unusual rashes include a striking nail/mucosal pigmentation from zidovudine, paronychia from indinavir and lipodystrophy (of the face and abdomen/buttocks) from protease inhibitors. As protease inhibitors and zidovudine are now used much less often in first-line drug combinations, the latter side-effects are rare today.

Cutaneous tumours

Benign tumours, such as extensive persistent viral warts and melanocytic naevi, are more common with HIV infection. Premalignant conditions, such as the intraepithelial dysplasias (cervix – CIN, penis – PIN, anal – AIN), are all much increased, possibly due to persistent human papillomavirus infection. The risk of malignant transformation in all these three sites is high and should be assessed by screening.

Kaposi's sarcoma (see pp. 1374–1375) is much more common in men who have sex with men with HIV than other groups. Basal and squamous cell carcinomas are also increased in incidence, presumably reflecting a loss of immune surveillance.

Interestingly, ART has had little impact on reducing rates of anal, penile or cervical cancer, and although Kaposi's sarcoma seemed almost to disappear early on when CD4 counts rose, it has recently shown a resurgence, even in those with high CD4 counts and fully suppressed virus.

'Specific' HIV dermatoses

'Itchy folliculitis' of HIV

Itchy folliculitis (also called papular pruritic eruption) is common in HIV as CD4 counts decline. Its aetiology is unknown. The previously described staphylococcal folliculitis, eosinophilic folliculitis, pityrosporum folliculitis and *Demodex* mite folliculitis are probably all part of a spectrum and the term 'itchy folliculitis' is useful to encompass these. It presents with intensely itchy papules centred on hair follicles and occurs most commonly over the upper trunk and upper arms ***(Fig. 31.54)***. The face is more commonly involved in black patients. Individual lesions frequently have the top scratched off, leaving a crateriform appearance.

Management with oral minocycline, potent topical steroids and emollients helps. Phototherapy or oral isotretinoin is useful in resistant cases.

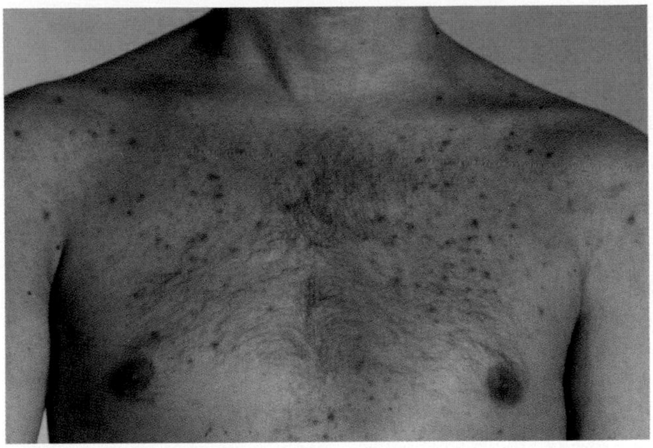

Figure 31.54 **Itchy folliculitis of HIV infection on upper trunk and proximal limbs.**

Oral hairy leucoplakia

This is characterized by white plaques with vertical ridging on the sides of the tongue. Unlike in oral candidiasis, the lesions cannot be peeled off. It was first recognized in HIV disease but can rarely occur in other forms of immunosuppression. It is thought to be due to co-infection with Epstein–Barr virus.

Treatment is with aciclovir, ganciclovir or foscarnet.

Immune reconstitution inflammatory syndrome

Many infections can manifest 2–4 months after commencing ART as the CD4 lymphocyte count recovers – so-called Immune reconstitution inflammatory syndrome (IRIS). Most commonly described are ano-genital herpes simplex virus infection, viral warts, tinea folliculitis, molluscum and genital warts. IRIS affects up to 25% of patients on ART and may simply reflect the fact that the recovering immune system can now react against pathogens that were already present. IRIS may also be responsible for an increase in inflammatory rashes, such as folliculitis and subacute lupus erythematosus. It can affect internal organs, such as with an exacerbation of pulmonary tuberculosis or cytomegalovirus retinitis.

Further reading

Chang CC, Sheikh V, Sereti I et al. Immune reconstitution disorders in patients with HIV infection: from pathogenesis to prevention and treatment. *Curr HIV/AIDS Rep* 2014; 11:223–232.

Rodgers S, Leslie KS. Skin infections in HIV-infected individuals in the era of HAART. *Curr Opin Infect Dis* 2011; 24:124–129.

PRINCIPLES OF TOPICAL THERAPY

The easy accessibility of the skin means that many dermatoses can be treated effectively with topical therapy. This reduces the likelihood of systemic adverse effects compared with oral therapy. Topical formulation consists of an ***active ingredient***, in an appropriate ***vehicle*** or ***base***, and ***excipients*** such as ***preservatives*** or ***emulsifiers*** to maintain the product's shelf-life. Cosmetic acceptability and clear instructions are important in achieving good adherence and efficacy – creams do not work if they stay in the pot! Patients should be advised of common adverse effects, such as irritancy with topical retinoids, and risks, such as atrophy with potent corticosteroids. Clear information, such as the 'fingertip unit' for topical corticosteroids, helps guide correct dosage.

- ***Creams are oil-in-water emulsions***, which are light and easily absorbed. They usually contain preservatives, such as parabens (hydroxybenzoates), which can cause sensitization. Aqueous cream is a popular and inexpensive soap substitute.

Box 31.26 Emollients commonly used in the UK

Greasy emollients	Lighter creams
• Epaderm ointment[a]	• E45 cream[a]
• Oily cream	• Diprobase cream[a]
• Unguentum Merck[a]	• Aveeno cream[a]
• 50 : 50 white soft paraffin/ liquid paraffin	• Aqueous cream

[a]*Trade names.*

- ***Ointments are greasy preparations based in vehicles*** such as polyethylene glycol (water-soluble) or petrolatum (insoluble). They feel sticky and are used to treat dry, flaky skin disorders ***(Box 31.26)***.
- ***Lotions*** have a liquid vehicle, such as water or alcohol, which evaporates on contact with the skin, giving a cooling effect. They are useful for weeping skin conditions and hairy skin (e.g. the scalp), but alcohol based-lotions should be avoided on broken skin, as they sting.
- ***Gels*** are semi-solid preparations of high-molecular-weight polymers. They are non-greasy and liquefy on contact with the skin. They are used to treat oily or hairy areas (e.g. scalp).
- ***Pastes*** are thick, adherent preparations containing a high percentage (>40%) of powder in an ointment base: e.g. dithranol in Lassar's paste, used for plaque psoriasis. They are seldom used now due to poor cosmetic acceptability.

Adverse effects of topical therapies

- ***Systemic absorption*** may occur but is significant only if large areas of inflamed skin are treated topically, especially with occlusive bandages or dressings. Neonates are particularly susceptible due to their relatively high body surface area and immature stratum corneum.
- ***Contact allergy*** may develop to the active drug (e.g. hydrocortisone, neomycin) vehicle (e.g. lanolin, cetearyl alcohol) or excipient (e.g. chlorocresol, parabens). It should be suspected in patients with an unresponsive dermatitis or new dermatitis following application of topical treatment. Ointments contain fewer excipients and are therefore less likely to cause contact allergy.
- ***Folliculitis*** can occur due to blockage of hair follicles especially with use of ointments in hot weather and on occluded skin (bandages, tight clothing).

Corticosteroids can cause a range of adverse effects (see p. 1350). However, they have a very good safety profile when used correctly under supervision.

Bibliography

Burns T, Breathnach S, Cox N et al. (eds). *Rook's Textbook of Dermatology*, 8th edn. Oxford: Blackwell Scientific; 2010.

Patterson J. *Weedon's Skin Pathology*, 4th edn. Edinburgh: Churchill Livingstone; 2015.

Significant Websites

http://dermnetnz.org/ *Dermatology information and images.*
http://hardinmd.lib.uiowa.edu/dermpictures.html *Dermatology images (atlas).*
http://www.aad.org *American Academy of Dermatology.*
http://www.bad.org.uk *British Association of Dermatologists.*
http://www.debra.org.uk *Dystrophic Epidermolysis Bullosa Association.*
http://www.eczema.org *National Eczema Society.*
http://www.evidence.nhs.uk/ *Clinical guidelines, systematic reviews, evidence-based synopses, image database.*
http://www.guidance.nice.org.uk/ *Dermatology treatment guidelines in the UK.*
http://www.psoriasis-association.org.uk *Psoriasis Association.*
http://www.skin-camouflage.net *British Association of Skin Camouflage.*
http://www.thecochranelibrary.com *Cochrane Database systematic reviews of treatment.*
http://www.vitiligosociety.org.uk *Vitiligo Society.*

Index

Page numbers followed by '*f*' indicate figures, '*b*' indicate boxes, and '*e*' indicate online content.

E

F

H

M

O

Q

R

S

T